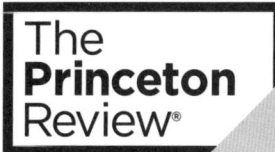

MCAT®

Organic Chemistry Review

4th Edition

The Staff of The Princeton Review

Penguin
Random
House

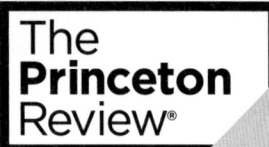

The Princeton Review
110 E. 42nd Street, 7th Floor
New York, NY 10017

Published in the United States by Penguin Random House
LLC, New York, and in Canada by Random House of Canada,
a division of Penguin Random House Ltd., Toronto.

Terms of Service: The Princeton Review Online Companion
Tools ("Student Tools") for retail books are available for
only the two most recent editions of that book. Student
Tools may be activated only once per eligible book purchased for a total of 24 months of access. Activation of
Student Tools more than once per book is in direct violation of these Terms of Service and may result in discontinuation of access to Student Tools Services.

ISBN: 978-0-593-51626-3
ISSN: 2150-8887

MCAT is a registered trademark of the Association of
American Medical Colleges.

The Princeton Review is not affiliated with Princeton
University.

The material in this book is up-to-date at the time of publication. However, changes may have been instituted by the
testing body in the test after this book was published.

If there are any important late-breaking developments,
changes, or corrections to the materials in this book, we
will post that information online in the Student Tools.
Register your book and check your Student Tools to see if
there are any updates posted there.

Every attempt has been made to obtain permission to
reproduce material protected by copyright. Where
omissions may have occurred the editors will be happy
to acknowledge this in future printings.

Editor: Laura Rose
Production Editor: Becky Radway, Kathy Carter
Production Artist: Jason Ullmeyer

Manufactured in China.

10 9 8 7 6 5 4 3 2 1

4th Edition

The Princeton Review Publishing Team
Editorial Rob Franek, Editor-in-Chief
David Soto, Senior Director, Data Operations
Stephen Koch, Senior Manager, Data Operations
Deborah Weber, Director of Production
Jason Ullmeyer, Production Design Manager
Jennifer Chapman, Senior Production Artist
Selena Coppock, Director of Editorial
Aaron Riccio, Senior Editor
Meave Shelton, Senior Editor
Chris Chimera, Editor
Orion McBean, Editor
Patricia Murphy, Editor
Laura Rose, Editor
Alexa Schmitt Bugler, Editorial Assistant

Random House Publishing Team
Tom Russell, VP, Publisher
Alison Stoltzfus, Senior Director, Publishing
Brett Wright, Senior Editor
Emily Hoffman, Assistant Managing Editor
Ellen Reed, Production Manager
Suzanne Lee, Designer
Eugenia Lo, Publishing Assistant

For customer service, please contact
editorialsupport@review.com,
and be sure to include:

- full title of the book

- ISBN

- page number

CONTRIBUTORS

Peter J. Alaimo, Ph.D.
Senior Author

TPR MCAT O-Chem Development Team:

Alan M. Marchand, Ph.D.

Jason Osman, Ph.D., Senior Editor, Lead Developer

Edited for Production by:

Judene Wright, M.S., M.A.Ed.
National Content Director, MCAT Program, The Princeton Review

The TPR MCAT O-Chem Team and Judene would like to thank the following people for their contributions to this book:

Farhad Aziz, B.S., Bethany Blackwell, M.S., Kristen Brunson, Ph.D., Brian Butts, B.S., B.A., Douglas S. Daniels, Ph.D., Amanda Edward, H.BSc, H.BEd, William Ewing, Ph.D., Carlos Guzman, Adam Johnson, Brandon Kelley, Ph.D., Omair Adil Khan, Stefan Loren, Ph.D., Joey Mancuso, D.O., M.S., Janet Marshall, Ph.D., Douglas K. McLemore, B.S., Katherine Miller, B.A., Tenaya Newkirk, Ph.D., Daniel J. Pallin, M.D., Tyler Peikes, Chris Rabbat, Ph.D., Steven Rines, Ph.D., Jayson Sack, M.D., M.S., Karen Salazar, Ph.D., Sina Shahbaz, B.S., Christopher Volpe, Ph.D.

PERIODIC TABLE OF THE ELEMENTS

1																	18
1 **H** 1.0	2											13	14	15	16	17	2 **He** 4.0
3 **Li** 6.9	4 **Be** 9.0											5 **B** 10.8	6 **C** 12.0	7 **N** 14.0	8 **O** 16.0	9 **F** 19.0	10 **Ne** 20.2
11 **Na** 23.0	12 **Mg** 24.3	3	4	5	6	7	8	9	10	11	12	13 **Al** 27.0	14 **Si** 28.1	15 **P** 31.0	16 **S** 32.1	17 **Cl** 35.5	18 **Ar** 39.9
19 **K** 39.1	20 **Ca** 40.1	21 **Sc** 45.0	22 **Ti** 47.9	23 **V** 50.9	24 **Cr** 52.0	25 **Mn** 54.9	26 **Fe** 55.8	27 **Co** 58.9	28 **Ni** 58.7	29 **Cu** 63.5	30 **Zn** 65.4	31 **Ga** 69.7	32 **Ge** 72.6	33 **As** 74.9	34 **Se** 79.0	35 **Br** 79.9	36 **Kr** 83.8
37 **Rb** 85.5	38 **Sr** 87.6	39 **Y** 88.9	40 **Zr** 91.2	41 **Nb** 92.9	42 **Mo** 95.9	43 **Tc** (98)	44 **Ru** 101.1	45 **Rh** 102.9	46 **Pd** 106.4	47 **Ag** 107.9	48 **Cd** 112.4	49 **In** 114.8	50 **Sn** 118.7	51 **Sb** 121.8	52 **Te** 127.6	53 **I** 126.9	54 **Xe** 131.3
55 **Cs** 132.9	56 **Ba** 137.3	57 ***La** 138.9	72 **Hf** 178.5	73 **Ta** 180.9	74 **W** 183.9	75 **Re** 186.2	76 **Os** 190.2	77 **Ir** 192.2	78 **Pt** 195.1	79 **Au** 197.0	80 **Hg** 200.6	81 **Tl** 204.4	82 **Pb** 207.2	83 **Bi** 209.0	84 **Po** (209)	85 **At** (210)	86 **Rn** (222)
87 **Fr** (223)	88 **Ra** (226)	89 **†Ac** (227)	104 **Rf** (267)	105 **Db** (268)	106 **Sg** (271)	107 **Bh** (270)	108 **Hs** (269)	109 **Mt** (278)	110 **Ds** (281)	111 **Rg** (282)	112 **Cn** (285)	113 **Nh** (286)	114 **Fl** (289)	115 **Mc** (289)	116 **Lv** (293)	117 **Ts** (294)	118 **Og** (294)

	58 **Ce** 140.1	59 **Pr** 140.9	60 **Nd** 144.2	61 **Pm** (145)	62 **Sm** 150.4	63 **Eu** 152.0	64 **Gd** 157.3	65 **Tb** 158.9	66 **Dy** 162.5	67 **Ho** 164.9	68 **Er** 167.3	69 **Tm** 168.9	70 **Yb** 173.0	71 **Lu** 175.0
*Lanthanoids														
†Actinoids	90 **Th** 232.0	91 **Pa** (231)	92 **U** 238.0	93 **Np** (237)	94 **Pu** (244)	95 **Am** (243)	96 **Cm** (247)	97 **Bk** (247)	98 **Cf** (251)	99 **Es** (252)	100 **Fm** (257)	101 **Md** (258)	102 **No** (259)	103 **Lr** (266)

MCAT ORGANIC CHEMISTRY REVIEW CONTENTS

Get More (Free) Content
at PrincetonReview.com/prep

As easy as 1·2·3

1 Go to PrincetonReview.com/prep or scan the **QR code** and enter the following ISBN for your book: **9780593516263**

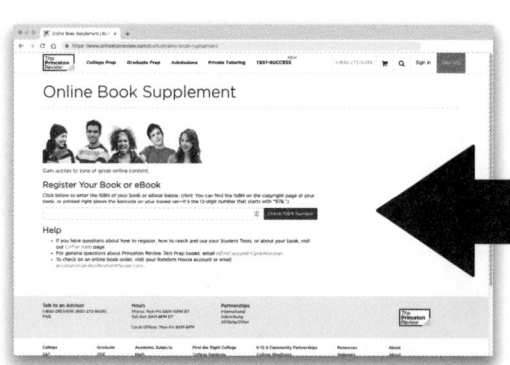

2 Answer a few simple questions to set up an exclusive Princeton Review account. *(If you already have one, you can just log in.)*

3 Enjoy access to your **FREE** content!

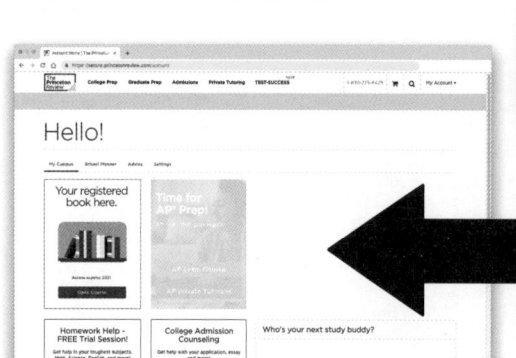

Once you've registered, you can...

- Take **3** full-length practice MCAT exams

- Find useful information about taking the MCAT and applying to medical school

- Check to see if there have been any corrections or updates to this edition

- Get our take on any recent or pending updates to the MCAT

Need to report a potential **content** issue?

Contact **EditorialSupport@review.com** and include:

- full title of the book
- ISBN
- page number

Need to report a **technical** issue?

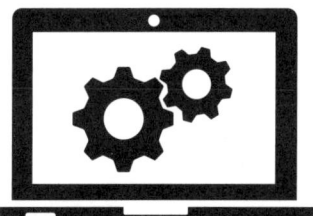

Contact **TPRStudentTech@review.com** and provide:

- your full name
- email address used to register the book
- full book title and ISBN
- Operating system (Mac/PC) and browser (Chrome, Firefox, Safari, etc.)

Chapter 1
MCAT Basics

SO YOU WANT TO BE A DOCTOR

So...you want to be a doctor. If you're like most premeds, you've wanted to be a doctor since you were pretty young. When people asked you what you wanted to be when you grew up, you always answered "a doctor." You had toy medical kits, bandaged up your dog or cat, and played "hospital." You probably read your parents' home medical guides for fun.

When you got to high school, you took the honors and AP classes. You studied hard, got straight As (or, at least, really good grades!), and participated in extracurricular activities so you could get into a good college. And you succeeded!

At college you knew exactly what to do. You took your classes seriously, studied hard, and earned a great GPA. You talked to your professors and hung out at office hours to get good letters of recommendation. You were a member of the premed society on campus, volunteered at hospitals, and shadowed doctors. All that's left to do now is to achieve a good MCAT score.

Just the MCAT.

Just the most confidence-shattering, most demoralizing, longest, most brutal entrance exam for any graduate program. At about 7.5 hours (including breaks), the MCAT tops the list; even the closest runners up, the LSAT and GMAT, are only about 4 hours long. The MCAT tests significant science content knowledge along with the ability to think quickly, reason logically, and read comprehensively, all under the pressure of a timed exam.

The path to a good MCAT score is not as easy to see as the path to a good GPA or the path to a good letter of recommendation. The MCAT is less about what you know and more about how to apply what you know—and how to apply it quickly to new situations. Because the path might not be so clear, you might be worried. That's why you picked up this book.

We promise to demystify the MCAT for you, with clear descriptions of the different sections, how the test is scored, and what the test experience is like. We will help you understand general test-taking techniques as well as provide you with specific techniques for each section. We will review the science content you need to know as well as give you strategies for the Organic Chemistry section. We'll show you the path to a good MCAT score and help you walk the path.

After all, you want to be a doctor. And we want you to succeed.

WHAT IS THE MCAT...REALLY?

Most test-takers approach the MCAT as though it were a typical college science test, one in which facts and knowledge simply need to be regurgitated in order to do well. They study for the MCAT the same way they did for their college tests, by memorizing facts and details, formulas and equations. And when they get to the MCAT they are surprised...and disappointed.

It's a myth that the MCAT is purely a content-knowledge test. If medical school admission committees want to see what you know, all they have to do is look at your transcripts. What they really want to see is how you think, especially under pressure. That's what your MCAT score will tell them.

The MCAT is really a test of your ability to apply basic knowledge to different, possibly new, situations. It's a test of your ability to reason out and evaluate arguments. Do you still need to know your science content? Absolutely. But not at the level that most test-takers think they need to know it. Furthermore, your science knowledge won't help you on the Critical Analysis and Reasoning Skills (CARS) section. So how do you study for a test like this?

You study for the science sections by reviewing the basics and then applying them to MCAT practice questions. You study for the CARS section by learning how to adapt your existing reading and analytical skills to the nature of the test (more information about the CARS section can be found in *MCAT Critical Analysis and Reasoning Skills Review*).

The book you are holding will review all the relevant MCAT Organic Chemistry content you will need for the test, and a little bit more. It includes hundreds of questions (printed and online) designed to make you think about the material in a deeper way, along with full explanations to clarify the logical thought process needed to get to the answer. It also comes with access to three full-length online practice exams to further hone your skills. For more information on accessing those online exams, please refer to the "Get More (Free) Content" spread on page viii.

A Note About Flashcards

For most of the exams you've taken previously, flashcards were likely very helpful. This was because those exams mostly required you to regurgitate information, and flashcards are pretty good at helping you memorize facts. However, the most challenging aspect of the MCAT is not that it requires you to memorize the fine details of content knowledge, but that it requires you to apply your basic scientific knowledge to unfamiliar situations: flashcards alone may not help you there.

Flashcards can be beneficial if your basic content knowledge is deficient in some area. For example, if you don't know the definitions of all the possible types of isomers or if you are unsure of some of the functional groups you need to know, flashcards can certainly help you memorize these facts. Or, you may need to learn and recognize polar, nonpolar, acidic, and basic amino acids and their 1-letter abbreviations. You might find that flashcards can help you memorize these. But unless you are trying to memorize basic facts in your personal weak areas, you are better off doing and analyzing practice passages than carrying around a stack of flashcards.

MCAT NUTS AND BOLTS

Overview

The MCAT is a computer-based test (CBT) that is *not* adaptive. Adaptive tests base your next question on whether or not you've answered the current question correctly. The MCAT is linear, or fixed-form, meaning that the questions are in a predetermined order and do not change based on your answers. However, there are many versions of the test so that on a given test day, different people will see different versions. The following table highlights the features of the MCAT exam.

Registration	Online via www.aamc.org. Begins as early as six months prior to test date; available up until week of test (subject to seat availability).
Testing Centers	Administered at small, secure, climate-controlled computer testing rooms.
Security	Photo ID with signature, electronic fingerprint, electronic signature verification, assigned seat.
Proctoring	None. Test administrator checks examinee in and assigns seat at computer. All testing instructions are given on the computer.
Frequency of Test	Many times per year distributed over January, April, May, June, July, August, and September.
Format	Exclusively computer-based. NOT an adaptive test.
Length of Test Day	7.5 hours
Breaks	Optional 10-minute breaks between sections, with a 30-minute break for lunch.
Section Names	1. Chemical and Physical Foundations of Biological Systems (Chem/Phys) 2. Critical Analysis and Reasoning Skills (CARS) 3. Biological and Biochemical Foundations of Living Systems (Bio/Biochem) 4. Psychological, Social, and Biological Foundations of Behavior (Psych/Soc)
Number of Questions and Timing	59 Chem/Phys questions, 95 minutes 53 CARS questions, 90 minutes 59 Bio/Biochem questions, 95 minutes 59 Psych/Soc questions, 95 minutes
Scoring	Test is scaled. Several forms per administration.
Allowed/ Not Allowed	No timers/watches. Noise reduction headphones available. Noteboard and wet-erase marker given at start of test and taken at end of test. Locker or secure area provided for personal items.
Results: Timing and Delivery	Approximately 30 days. Electronic scores only, available online through AAMC login. Examinees can print official score reports.
Maximum Number of Retakes	The test can be taken a maximum of three times in one year, four times over two years, and seven times over the lifetime of the examinee. An examinee can be registered for only one date at a time.

Registration

Registration for the exam is completed online at www.aamc.org/students/applying/mcat/reserving. The AAMC opens registration for a given test date at least two months in advance of the date, often earlier. It's a good idea to register well in advance of your desired test date to make sure that you get a seat.

Sections

There are four sections on the MCAT, all of which consist of multiple-choice questions:

Section	Concepts Tested	Number of Questions and Timing
Chemical and Physical Foundations of Biological Systems (Chem/Phys)	Basic concepts in chemistry and physics, including biochemistry, scientific inquiry, reasoning, research and statistics skills.	59 questions in 95 minutes
Critical Analysis and Reasoning Skills (CARS)	Critical analysis of information drawn from a wide range of social science and humanities disciplines.	53 questions in 90 minutes
Biological and Biochemical Foundations of Living Systems (Bio/Biochem)	Basic concepts in biology and biochemistry, scientific inquiry, reasoning, research and statistics skills.	59 questions in 95 minutes
Psychological, Social, and Biological Foundations of Behavior (Psych/Soc)	Basic concepts in psychology, sociology, and biology, research methods and statistics.	59 questions in 95 minutes

Most questions on the MCAT (44 in the science sections, all 53 in the CARS section) are passage-based; the science sections have 10 passages each and the CARS section has 9. A passage consists of a few paragraphs of information on which several following questions are based. In the science sections, passages often include equations or reactions, tables, graphs, figures, and experiments to analyze. CARS passages come from literature in the social sciences, humanities, ethics, philosophy, cultural studies, and population health, and do not test content knowledge in any way.

Some questions in the science sections are freestanding questions (FSQs). These questions are independent of any passage information and appear in four groups of about three to four questions, interspersed throughout the passages. Fifteen of the questions in the science sections are freestanding, and the remainder are passage-based.

Each section on the MCAT is separated by either a 10-minute break or a 30-minute lunch break. We recommend that you take these breaks.

Section	Time
Test Center Check-In	Variable, can take up to 40 minutes if center is busy
Tutorial	10 minutes
Chemical and Physical Foundations of Biological Systems	95 minutes
Break (optional)	10 minutes
Critical Analysis and Reasoning Skills	90 minutes
Lunch Break (optional)	30 minutes
Biological and Biochemical Foundations of Living Systems	95 minutes
Break (optional)	10 minutes
Psychological, Social, and Biological Foundations of Behavior	95 minutes
Void Option	5 minutes
Survey (optional)	5 minutes

The survey includes questions about your satisfaction with the overall MCAT experience, including registration, check-in, etc., as well as questions about how you prepared for the test.

Scoring

The MCAT is a scaled exam, meaning that your raw score will be converted into a scaled score that takes into account the difficulty of the questions. There is no guessing penalty. All sections are scored from 118–132, with a total scaled score range of 472–528. Because different versions of the test have varying levels of difficulty, the scale will be different from one exam to the next. Thus, there is no "magic number" of questions to get right in order to get a particular score. Plus, some of the questions on the test are considered "experimental" and do not count toward your score; they are just there to be evaluated for possible future inclusion in a test.

At the end of the test (after you complete the Psychological, Social, and Biological Foundations of Behavior section), you will be asked to choose one of the following two options: "I wish to have my MCAT exam scored" or "I wish to VOID my MCAT exam." You have five minutes to make a decision, and if you do not select one of the options in that time, the test will automatically be scored. If you choose the VOID option, your test will not be scored (you will not now, or ever, get a numerical score for this test), medical schools will not know you took the test, and no refunds will be granted. You cannot "unvoid" your scores at a later time.

So, what's a good score? The AAMC is centering the scale at 500 (i.e., 500 will be the 50th percentile), and recommends that application committees consider applicants near the center of the range. To be on the safe side, aim for a total score of around 510. Remember that if your GPA is on the low side, you'll need higher MCAT scores to compensate, and if you have a strong GPA, you can get away with lower MCAT scores. But the reality is that your chances of acceptance depend on a lot more than just your MCAT scores. It's a combination of your GPA, your MCAT scores, your undergraduate coursework, letters of recommendation, experience related to the medical field (such as volunteer work or research), extracurricular activities, your personal statement, etc. Medical schools are looking for a complete package, not just good scores and a good GPA.

GENERAL LAYOUT AND TEST-TAKING STRATEGIES

Layout of the Test

In each section of the test, the computer screen is divided vertically, with the passage on the left and the range of questions for that passage indicated above (e.g., "Passage 1 Questions 1–5"). The scroll bar for the passage text appears in the middle of the screen. Each question appears on the right, and you must click "Next" to move to each subsequent question.

In the science sections, the freestanding questions are found in groups of 3–4, interspersed with the passages. The screen is still divided vertically; on the left is the statement "Questions [X–XX] do not refer to a passage and are independent of each other," and each question appears on the right as described above.

CBT Tools

There are a number of tools available on the test, including highlighting, strike-outs, the Flag for Review button, the Navigation and Review Screen buttons, the Periodic Table button, and of course, the noteboard booklet. All tools are available with both mouse control (buttons to click) or keyboard commands (Alt+ a letter). As everyone has different preferences, you should practice with both types of tools (mouse and keyboard) to see which is more comfortable for you personally.

The following is a brief description of each tool.

1) **Highlighting:** This is done in the passage text (including table entries and some equations, but excluding figures and molecular structures), in the question stems, and in the answer choices (including Roman numerals). Select the words you wish to highlight (left-click and drag the cursor across the words), and in the upper left corner click the "Highlight" button to highlight the selected text yellow. Alternatively, press "Alt+H" to highlight the words. Highlighting can be removed by selecting the words again and in the upper left corner clicking the down arrow next to "Highlight." This will expand to show the "Remove Highlight" option; clicking this will remove the highlighting. Removing highlighting via the keyboard is cumbersome and is not recommended.

2) **Strike-outs:** This can be done on the answer choices, including Roman numeral statements, by selecting the text you want to strike out (left-click and drag the cursor across the text), then clicking the "Strikethrough" button in the upper left corner. Alternatively, press "Alt+S" to strike out the words. The strike-out can be removed by repeating these actions. Figures or molecular structures cannot be struck out; however, the letter answer choice of those structures can.

3) **Flag for Review button:** This is available for each question and is found in the upper right corner. This allows you to flag the question as one you would like to review later if time permits. When clicked, the flag icon turns yellow. Click again to remove the flag. Alternatively, press "Alt+F."

4) **Navigation button:** This is found near the bottom of the screen and is only available on your first pass through the section. Clicking this button brings up a navigation table listing all questions and their statuses (unseen, incomplete, complete, flagged for review). You can also press "Alt+N" to bring up the screen. The questions can be sorted by their statuses, and clicking a question number takes you immediately to that question. Once you have reached the end of the section and viewed the Review screen (described below), the Navigation screen is no longer available.

5) **Review Screen button:** This button is found near the bottom of the screen after your first pass through the section, and when clicked, brings up a new screen showing all questions and their statuses (either incomplete, unseen, or flagged for review). Questions that are complete are assigned no additional status. You can then choose one of three options by clicking with the mouse or with keyboard shortcuts: Review All (Alt+A), Review Incomplete (Alt+I), or Review Flagged (Alt+R); alternatively, you can click a question number to go directly back to that question. You can also end the section from this screen.

6) **Periodic Table button:** Clicking this button will open a periodic table (or press "Alt+T"). Note that the periodic table is large, covering most of the screen. However, this window can be resized to see the questions and a portion of the periodic table at the same time. The table text will not decrease, but scroll bars will appear on the window so you can center the section of the table of interest in the window.

7) **Noteboard Booklet (Scratch Paper):** At the start of the test, you will be given a spiral-bound set of four laminated 8.5″ × 14″ sheets of paper and a wet-erase marker to use as scratch paper. You can request a clean noteboard booklet at any time during the test; your original booklet will be collected. The noteboard is only useful if it is kept organized; do not give in to the tendency to write on the first available open space! Good organization will be very helpful when/if you wish to review a question. Indicate the passage number, the range of questions for that passage, and a topic in a box near the top of your scratch work, and indicate the question you are working on in a circle to the left of the notes for that question. Draw a line under your scratch work when you change passages to keep the work separate. Do not erase or scribble over any previous work. If you do not think it is correct, draw one line through the work and start again. You may have already done some useful work without realizing it.

General Strategy for the Science Sections

Passages vs. FSQs in the Science Sections: What to Start With

Since the questions are displayed on separate screens, it is awkward and time consuming to click through all of the questions up front to find the FSQs. Therefore, go through the section on a first pass and decide whether to do the passage now or to save it for later, basing your decision on the passage text and the first question. Tackle the FSQs as you come upon them. More details are below.

Here is an outline of the procedure:

1) For each passage, write a heading on your noteboard with the passage number, the general topic, and its range of questions (e.g., "Passage 1, thermodynamics, Q 1–5" or "Passage 2, enzymes, Q 6–9). The passage numbers do not currently appear in the Navigation or Review screens, thus having the question numbers on your noteboard will allow you to move through the section more efficiently.

2) Skim the text and rank the passage. If a passage is a "Now," complete it before moving on to the next passage (also see "Attacking the Questions" below). If it is a "Later" passage, first write "SKIPPED" in block letters under the passage heading on your noteboard and leave room for your work when you come back to complete that passage. (Note that the specific passages you skip will be unique to you; in the Bio/Biochem section, you might choose to do all Biology passages first, then come back for Biochemistry. Or in Chem/Phys you might choose to skip experiment-based or analytical passages. Know ahead of time what type of passage you are going to skip and follow your plan.)

3) Next, click on the "Navigation" button at the bottom to get to the Navigation screen. Click on the first question of the next passage; you'll be able to identify it because you know the range of questions from the passage you just skipped. This will take you to the next passage, where you will repeat steps 1–3.

4) Once you have completed the "Now" passages, go to the Review screen and click the first question for the first passage you skipped. Answer the questions, and continue going back to the Review screen and repeating this procedure for other passages you have skipped.

Attacking the Questions

As you work through the questions, if you encounter a particularly lengthy question, or a question that requires a lot of analysis, you may choose to skip it. This is a wise strategy because it ensures you will tackle all the easier questions first, the ones you are more likely to get right. If you choose to skip the question (or if you attempt it but get stuck), write down the question number on your noteboard, click the Flag for Review button to flag the question in the Review screen and move on to the next question. At the end of the passage, click back through the set of questions to complete any that you skipped over the first time through, and make sure that you have filled in an answer for every question.

General Strategy for the CARS Section

Ranking and Ordering the Passages: What to Start With

Ranking: Since the questions are displayed on separate screens, it is awkward and time consuming to click through all of the questions before ranking each passage as "Now" (an easier passage), "Later" (a harder passage), or "Killer" (a passage that you will randomly guess on). Therefore, rank the passage and decide whether or not to do it on the first pass through the section based on the passage text, skimming the first 2–3 sentences.

Ordering: Because of the additional clicking through screens (or use of the Review screen) that is required to navigate through the section, the "Two-Pass" system (completing the "Now" passages as you find them) is likely to be your most efficient approach. However, if you find that you are continuously making a lot of bad ranking decisions, it is still valid to experiment with the "Three-Pass" approach (ranking all nine passages up front before attempting your first "Now" passage).

Here is an outline of the basic Ranking and Ordering procedure to follow:

1) For each passage, write a heading on your noteboard with the passage number and its range of questions (e.g., "Passage 1 Q 1–7). The passage numbers do not currently appear in the Navigation or Review screens, thus having the question numbers on your noteboard will allow you to move through the section more efficiently.

2) Skim the first 2–3 sentences and rank the passage. If the passage is a "Now," complete it before moving on to the next. If it is a "Later" or "Killer," first write either "Later" or "Killer" and "SKIPPED" in block letters under the passage heading on your noteboard and leave room for your work if you decide to come back and complete that passage. Then click through each question, flagging each one and filling in random guesses, until you get to the next passage.

3) Once you have completed the "Now" passages, come back for your second pass and complete the "Later" passages, leaving your random guesses in place for any "Killer" passages that you choose not to complete. Go to the Review screen and use your noteboard notes on the question numbers; click on the number of the first question for that passage to go back to that question, and proceed from there. Alternatively, if you have consistently flagged all the questions for passages you skipped in your first pass, you can use "Review Flagged" from the Review screen to find and complete your "Later" passages.

4) Regardless of how you choose to find your second pass passages, unflag each question after you complete it, so that you can continue to rely on the Review screen (and the "Review Flagged" function) to identify questions that you have not yet attempted.

Previewing the Questions

The formatting and functioning of the tools facilitates effective previewing. Having each question on a separate screen will encourage you to really focus on that question. Even more importantly, you can highlight in the question stem and in the answer choices.

Here is the basic procedure for previewing the questions:

1) Start with the first question, and if it has lead words referencing passage content, highlight them. You may also choose to jot them down on your noteboard. Once you reach and preview the last question for the set on that passage, THEN stay on that screen and work the passage (your highlighting appears and stays on every passage screen, and persists through the whole 90 minutes).

2) Once you have worked the passage and defined the Bottom Line—the main idea and tone of the entire passage—work **backward** from the last question to the first. If you skip over any questions as you go (see "Attacking the Questions" below), write down the question number on your noteboard. Then click **forward** through the set of questions, completing any that you skipped over the first time through. Once you reach and complete the last question for that passage, clicking "Next" will send you to the first question of the next passage. Working the questions from last to first the first time through the set will eliminate the need to click back through multiple screens to get to the first question immediately after previewing, and will also make it easier and more efficient to do the hardest questions last (see "Attacking the Questions" on the next page).

3) Remember that previewing questions is a CARS-only technique. It is not efficient to preview questions in the science sections.

Attacking the Questions

The question types and the procedure for actually attacking each type will be discussed later. However, it is still important **not** to attempt the hardest questions first (potentially getting stuck, wasting time, and discouraging yourself).

So, as you work the questions from last to first (see "Previewing the Questions" above), if you encounter a particularly difficult and/or lengthy question (or if you attempt a question but get stuck), write down the question number on your noteboard (you may also choose to flag it) and move on backward to the next question. Then click **forward** through the set and complete any that you skipped over the first time through the set, unflagging any questions that you flagged that first time through and making sure that you have filled in an answer for every question.

Pacing Strategy for the MCAT

Since the MCAT is a timed test, you must keep an eye on the timer and adjust your pacing as necessary. It would be terrible to run out of time at the end only to discover that the last few questions could have been easily answered in just a few seconds each.

In the science sections you will have about one minute and thirty-five seconds (1:35) per question, and in the CARS section you will have about one minute and forty seconds (1:40) per question (not taking into account time reading the passage before answering the questions).

Section	# of Questions in passage	Approximate time (including reading the passage)
Chem/Phys, Bio/Biochem, and Psych/Soc	4	6.5 minutes
	5	8 minutes
	6	9.5 minutes
CARS	5	8.5 minutes
	6	10 minutes
	7	11.5 minutes

When starting a passage in the science sections, make note of how much time you will allot for it, and the starting time on the timer. Jot down on your noteboard what the timer should say at the end of the passage. Then just keep an eye on it as you work through the questions. If you are near the end of the time for that passage, guess on any remaining questions, make some notes on your noteboard, flag the questions, and move on. Come back to those questions if you have time.

For the CARS section, keep in mind that many people will maximize their score by *not* trying to complete every question or every passage in the section. A good strategy for test-takers who cannot achieve a high level of accuracy on all nine passages is to randomly guess on at least one passage in the section, and spend your time getting a high percentage of the other questions right. To complete all nine CARS passages, you have about ten minutes per passage. To complete eight of the nine, you have about 11 minutes per passage.

To help maximize your number of correct answer choices in any section, do the questions and passages within that section in the order *you* want to do them in. See "General Strategy" above.

Process of Elimination

Process of elimination (POE) is probably the most useful technique you have to tackle MCAT questions. Since there is no guessing penalty, POE allows you to increase your probability of choosing the correct answer by eliminating those you are sure are wrong.

1) Strike out any choices that you are sure are incorrect or that do not address the issue raised in the question.

2) Jot down some notes to help clarify your thoughts if you return to the question.

3) Use the "Flag for Review" button to flag the question for review. (Note, however, that in the CARS section, you generally should not be returning to rethink questions once you have moved on to a new passage.)

4) Do not leave it blank! For the sciences, if you are not sure and you have already spent more than 60 seconds on that question, just pick one of the remaining choices. If you have time to review it at the end, you can always debate the remaining choices based on your previous notes. For CARS, if you have been through the choices two or three times, have reread the question stem and gone back to the passage, and you are still stuck, move on. Do the remaining questions for that passage, take one more look at the question you were stuck on, then pick an answer and move on for good.

5) Special Note: If three of the four answer choices have been eliminated, the remaining choice must be the correct answer. Don't waste time pondering *why* it is correct; just click it and move on. The MCAT doesn't care if you truly understand why it's the right answer, only that you have the right answer selected.

6) More subject-specific information on techniques will be presented in the next chapter.

Guessing

Remember, there is NO guessing penalty on the MCAT. NEVER leave a question blank!

QUESTION TYPES

In the science sections of the MCAT, the questions fall into one of three main categories:

1) Memory questions: These questions can be answered directly from prior knowledge and represent about 25 percent of the total number of questions.

2) Explicit questions: These questions are those for which the answer is explicitly stated in the passage. To answer them correctly, for example, may just require finding a definition, reading a graph, or making a simple connection. Explicit questions represent about 35 percent of the total number of questions.

3) Implicit questions: These questions require you to apply knowledge to a new situation; the answer is typically implied by the information in the passage. These questions often start "if... then..." (for example, "if we modify the experiment in the passage like this, then what result would we expect?"). Implicit style questions make up about 40 percent of the total number of questions.

In the CARS section, the questions fall into four main categories:

1) Specific questions: These either ask you for facts from the passage (Retrieval questions) or require you to deduce what is most likely to be true based on the passage (Inference questions).

2) General questions: These ask you to summarize themes (Main Idea and Primary Purpose questions) or evaluate an author's opinion (Tone/Attitude questions).

3) Reasoning questions: These ask you to describe the purpose of, or the support provided for, a statement made in the passage (Structure questions) or to judge how well the author supports his or her argument (Evaluate questions).

4) Application questions: These ask you to apply new information from either the question stem itself (New Information questions) or from the answer choices (Strengthen, Weaken, and Analogy questions) to the passage.

More detail on question types and strategies can be found in Chapter 2.

TESTING TIPS

Before Test Day

- Take a trip to the test center at least a day or two before your actual test date so that you can easily find the building and room on test day. This will also allow you to gauge traffic and see if you need money for parking or anything like that. Knowing this type of information ahead of time will greatly reduce your stress on the day of your test.
- During the week before the test, adjust your sleeping schedule so that you are going to bed and getting up in the morning at the same times as on the day before and morning of the MCAT. Prioritize getting a reasonable amount of sleep during the last few nights before the test.
- Don't do any heavy studying the day before the test. This is not a test you can cram for! Your goal at this point is to rest and relax so that you can go into test day in a good physical and mental condition.
- Eat well. Try to avoid excessive caffeine and sugar. Ideally, in the weeks leading up to the actual test you should experiment a little bit with foods and practice tests to see which foods give you the most endurance. Aim for steady blood sugar levels during the test: sports drinks, peanut-butter crackers, trail mix, etc., make good snacks for your breaks and lunch.

General Test Day Info and Tips

- On the day of the test, arrive at the test center at least a half hour prior to the start time of your test.
- Examinees will be checked in to the center in the order in which they arrive.
- You will be assigned a locker or secure area in which to put your personal items. Textbooks and study notes are not allowed, so there is no need to bring them with you to the test center.
- Your ID will be checked, a scan of your palm will be taken, and you will be asked to sign in.
- You will be given a noteboard booklet and a wet-erase marker, and the test center administrator will take you to the computer on which you will complete the test. You may not choose a computer; you must use the computer assigned to you.
- Nothing is allowed at the computer station except your photo ID, your locker key (if provided), and a factory sealed packet of ear plugs; not even your watch.
- If you choose to leave the testing room at the breaks, you will have your palm scanned again, and you will have to sign in and out.
- You are allowed to access the items in your locker, except for notes and cell phones. (Check your test center's policy on cell phones ahead of time; some centers do not even allow them to be kept in your locker.)
- Don't forget to bring the snack foods and lunch you experimented with in your practice tests.
- At the end of the test, the test administrator will collect your noteboard and clean off your notes.
- Definitely take the breaks! Get up and walk around. It's a good way to clear your head between sections and get the blood (and oxygen!) flowing to your brain.
- Ask for a clean noteboard at the breaks if you want a fresh one for the next section.

Chapter 2
Organic Chemistry
Strategy for the MCAT

2.1 GENERAL SCIENCE SECTIONS OVERVIEW

There are three science sections on the MCAT:

- Chemical and Physical Foundations of Biological Systems
- Biological and Biochemical Foundations of Living Systems
- Psychological, Social, and Biological Foundations of Behavior

The Chemical and Physical Foundations of Biological Systems section (Chem/Phys) is the first section on the test. It includes questions from General Chemistry (about 35%), Physics (about 25%), Organic Chemistry (about 15%), and Biochemistry (about 25%). Further, the questions often test chemical and physical concepts within a biological setting, for example, pressure and fluid flow in blood vessels. A solid grasp of math fundamentals is required (arithmetic, algebra, graphs, trigonometry, vectors, proportions, and logarithms) however, there are no calculus-based questions.

The Biological and Biochemical Foundations of Living Systems section (Bio/Biochem) is the third section on the test. Approximately 65% of the questions in this section come from Biology, approximately 25% come from Biochemistry, and approximately 10% come from Organic and General Chemistry. Math calculations are generally not required on this section of the test; however, a basic understanding of statistics as used in biological research is helpful.

The Psychological, Social, and Biological Foundations of Behavior section (Psych/Soc) is the fourth and final section on the test. About 65% of the questions will be drawn from Psychology (and about 5% of these will be Biological Psychology), about 30% from Sociology, and about 5% from Biology. As with the Bio/Biochem section, calculations are generally not required; however, a basic understanding of statistics as used in research is helpful.

Most of the questions in the science sections (44 of the 59) are passage-based, and each section has ten passages. Passages consist of a few paragraphs of information and include equations, reactions, graphs, figures, tables, experiments, and data. Four to six questions will be associated with each passage.

The remaining 25% of the questions (15 of 59) in each science section are freestanding questions (FSQs). These questions appear in approximately four groups interspersed between the passages. Each group contains three to four questions.

You are allowed 95 minutes to complete each of the science sections. This breaks down to approximately one minute and 35 seconds per question.

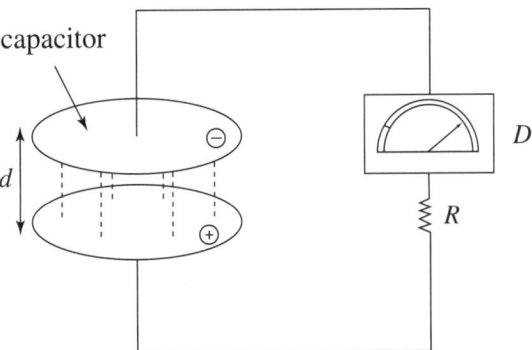

2.2 GENERAL SCIENCE PASSAGE TYPES

The passages in the science sections fall into one of three main categories: Information and/or Situation Presentation, Experiment/Research Presentation, or Persuasive Reasoning.

Information and/or Situation Presentation

These passages either present straightforward scientific information or they describe a particular event or occurrence. Generally, questions associated with these passages test basic science facts or ask you to predict outcomes given new variables or new information. Here is an example of an Information/Situation Presentation passage:

Figure 1 shows a portion of the inner mechanism of a typical home smoke detector. It consists of a pair of capacitor plates, which are charged by a 9-volt battery (not shown). The capacitor plates (electrodes) are connected to a sensor device, D; the resistor R denotes the internal resistance of the sensor. Normally, air acts as an insulator and no current would flow in the circuit shown. However, inside the smoke detector is a small sample of an artificially produced radioactive element, americium-241, which decays primarily by emitting alpha particles, with a half-life of approximately 430 years. The daughter nucleus of the decay has a half-life in excess of two million years and therefore poses virtually no biohazard.

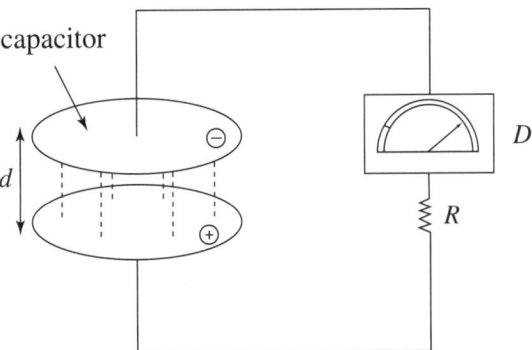

Figure 1 Smoke detector mechanism

The decay products (alpha particles and gamma rays) from the ^{241}Am sample ionize air molecules between the plates and thus provide a conducting pathway, which allows current to flow in the circuit shown in Figure 1. A steady-state current is quickly established and remains as long as the battery continues to maintain a 9-volt potential difference between its terminals. However, if smoke particles enter the space between the capacitor plates and thereby interrupt the flow, the current is reduced, and the sensor responds to this change by triggering

the alarm. (Furthermore, as the battery starts to "die out," the resulting drop in current is also detected to alert the homeowner to replace the battery.)

$$C = \varepsilon_0 \frac{A}{d}$$

Equation 1

where ε_0 is the universal permittivity constant, equal to 8.85 $\times$ 10^{-12} $C^2/(N \cdot m^2)$. Since the area A of each capacitor plate in the smoke detector is 20 cm^2 and the plates are separated by a distance d of 5 mm, the capacitance is 3.5×10^{-12} F = 3.5 pF.

Experiment/Research Presentation

These passages present the details of experiments and research procedures. They often include data tables and graphs. Generally, questions associated with these passages ask you to interpret data, draw conclusions, and make inferences. Here is an example of an Experiment/Research Presentation passage:

The development of sexual characteristics depends upon various factors, the most important of which are hormonal control, environmental stimuli, and the genetic makeup of the individual. The hormones that contribute to the development include the steroid hormones estrogen, progesterone, and testosterone, as well as the pituitary hormones FSH (follicle-stimulating hormone) and LH (luteinizing hormone).

To study the mechanism by which estrogen exerts its effects, a researcher performed the following experiments using cell culture assays.

Experiment 1:

Human embryonic placental mesenchyme (HEPM) cells were grown for 48 hours in Dulbecco's Modified Eagle Medium (DMEM), with media change every 12 hours. Upon confluent growth, cells were exposed to a 10 mg per mL solution of green fluorescent-labeled estrogen for 1 hour. Cells were rinsed with DMEM and observed under confocal fluorescent microscopy.

Experiment 2:

HEPM cells were grown to confluence as in Experiment 1. Cells were exposed to Pesticide A for 1 hour, followed by the 10 mg/mL solution of labeled estrogen, rinsed as in Experiment 1, and observed under confocal fluorescent microscopy.

Experiment 3:

Experiment 1 was repeated with Chinese Hamster Ovary (CHO) cells instead of HEPM cells.

Experiment 4:

CHO cells injected with cytoplasmic extracts of HEPM cells were grown to confluence, exposed to the 10 mg/mL solution of labeled estrogen for 1 hour, and observed under confocal fluorescent microscopy.

The results of these experiments are given in Table 1.

Table 1 Detection of Estrogen (+ indicates presence of Estrogen)

Experiment	Media	Cytoplasm	Nucleus
1	+	+	+
2	+	+	+
3	+	+	+
4	+	+	+

After observing the cells in each experiment, the researcher bathed the cells in a solution containing 10 mg per mL of a red fluorescent probe that binds specifically to the estrogen receptor only when its active site is occupied. After 1 hour, the cells were rinsed with DMEM and observed under confocal fluorescent microscopy. The results are presented in Table 2.

The researcher also repeated Experiment 2 using Pesticide B, an estrogen analog, instead of Pesticide A. Results from other researchers had shown that Pesticide B binds to the active site of the cytosolic estrogen receptor (with an affinity 10,000 times greater than that of estrogen) and causes increased transcription of mRNA.

Table 2 Observed Fluorescence and Estrogen Effects (G = green, R = red)

Experiment	Media	Cytoplasm	Nucleus	Estrogen effects observed?
1	G only	G and R	G and R	Yes
2	G only	G only	G only	No
3	G only	G only	G only	No
4	G only	G and R	G and R	Yes

Based on these results, the researcher determined that estrogen had no effect when not bound to a cytosolic, estrogen-specific receptor.

Persuasive Reasoning

These passages typically present a scientific phenomenon along with a hypothesis that explains the phenomenon, and may include counter-arguments as well. Questions associated with these passages ask you to evaluate the hypothesis or arguments. Persuasive Reasoning passages in the science sections of the MCAT tend to be less common than Information Presentation or Experiment/Research Presentation passages. Here is an example of a Persuasive Reasoning passage:

Two theoretical chemists attempted to explain the observed trends of acidity by applying two interpretations of molecular orbital theory. Consider the pK_a values of some common acids listed along with the conjugate base:

acid	pK_a	conjugate base
H_2SO_4	< 0	HSO_4^-
H_2CrO_4	5.0	$HCrO_4^-$
H_2PO_4	2.1	$H_2PO_4^-$
HF	3.9	F^-
HOCl	7.8	ClO^-
HCN	9.5	CN^-
HIO_3	1.2	IO_3^-

Recall that acids with a $pK_a < 0$ are called strong acids, and those with a $pK_a > 0$ are called weak acids. The arguments of the chemists are given below.

Chemist #1:

"The acidity of a compound is proportional to the polarization of the H—X bond, where X is some nonmetal element. Complex acids, such as H_2SO_4, $HClO_4$, and HNO_3 are strong acids because the H—O bonding electrons are strongly drawn towards the oxygen. It is generally true that a covalent bond weakens as its polarization increases. Therefore, one can conclude that the strength of an acid is proportional to the number of electronegative atoms in that acid."

Chemist #2:

"The acidity of a compound is proportional to the number of stable resonance structures of that acid's conjugate base. H_2SO_4, $HClO_4$, and HNO_3 are all strong acids because their respective conjugate bases exhibit a high degree of resonance stabilization."

MAPPING A PASSAGE

"Mapping a passage" refers to the combination of on-screen highlighting and noteboard notes that you take while working through a passage. Typically, good things to highlight include the overall topic of a paragraph, unfamiliar terms, unusual terms, italicized terms, numerical values, hypotheses, and experimental results. Noteboard notes can be used to summarize the paragraphs and to jot down important facts and connections that are made when reading the passage. More details on passage mapping will be presented in Section 2.5.

2.3 GENERAL SCIENCE QUESTION TYPES

Questions in the science sections are generally one of three main types: Memory, Explicit, or Implicit.

Memory Questions

These questions can be answered directly from prior knowledge, with no need to reference the passage or question text. Memory questions represent approximately 25 percent of the science questions on the MCAT. Usually, Memory questions are found as FSQs, but they can also be tucked into a passage. Here's an example of a Memory question:

> Which of the following acetylating conditions will convert diethylamine into an amide at the fastest rate?
>
> A)   Acetic acid/HCl
> B)   Acetic anhydride
> C)   Acetyl chloride
> D)   Ethyl acetate

Explicit Questions

Explicit questions can be answered primarily with information from the passage, along with prior knowledge. They may require data retrieval, graph analysis, or making a simple connection. Explicit questions make up approximately 35–40 percent of the science questions on the MCAT; here's an example (taken from the sample Information/Situation Presentation passage):

> The sensor device D shown in Figure 1 performs its function by acting as:
>
> A)   an ohmmeter.
> B)   a voltmeter.
> C)   a potentiometer.
> D)   an ammeter.

Implicit Questions

These questions require you to take information from the passage, combine it with your prior knowledge, apply it to a new situation, and come to some logical conclusion. They typically require more complex connections than do Explicit questions, and may also require data retrieval, graph analysis, etc. Implicit questions usually require a solid understanding of the passage information. They make up approximately 35–40 percent of the science questions on the MCAT; here's an example (taken from the sample Experiment/Research Presentation passage):

If Experiment 2 were repeated, but this time exposing the cells first to Pesticide A and then to Pesticide B before exposing them to the green fluorescent-labeled estrogen and the red fluorescent probe, which of the following statements will most likely be true?

A) Pesticide A and Pesticide B bind to the same site on the estrogen receptor.
B) Estrogen effects would be observed.
C) Only green fluorescence would be observed.
D) Both green and red fluorescence would be observed.

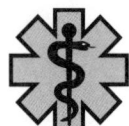

The Rod of Asclepius

You may notice this Rod of Asclepius icon as you read through the book. In Greek mythology, the Rod of Asclepius is associated with healing and medicine; the symbol continues to be used today to represent medicine and healthcare. You won't see this on the actual MCAT, but we've used it here to call attention to medically related examples and questions.

2.4   ORGANIC CHEMISTRY ON THE MCAT

The science sections of the MCAT have 10 passages and 15 freestanding questions (FSQs). Organic chemistry is the least prevalent subject tested on the MCAT, and will make up roughly 15% of the Chemical and Physical Foundations of Biological Systems section and only about 5% of the questions on the Biological and Biochemical Foundations of Living Systems section. In the Chemical and Physical Foundations section of the test, the questions will be distributed between two to four freestanding questions and either one longer passage (with five or six questions) or two very short passages (usually with four questions each). In the Biological and Biochemical Foundations section, the three or four O-Chem questions are likely to be either FSQs, or mixed in with either a biology or biochemistry passage. The O-Chem topics covered span roughly two college semesters' worth of material but focus most on carbonyl chemistry and laboratory techniques. For now, let's talk about what you can expect from O-Chem passages more generally, and we'll get to specific content in the coming chapters.

2.5 TACKLING AN ORGANIC CHEMISTRY PASSAGE

In general, some sort of biologically important compound or reaction provides the context for O-Chem passages. The text of the passage might contain biologically related concepts or facts, but a sure sign that you're reading an O-Chem passage and not a Biology passage will be chemical structures, usually lots of them.

Your approach to reading and mapping an O-Chem passage should be a bit different than your approach for all other subjects. The reason? There is hardly ever information within the text of an O-Chem passage that will be useful or needed to answer passage-based questions. The most important information in these passages will be in the form of chemical structures from synthetic or mechanistic schemes, or experimental data from a table, graph, or figure. Often, complicated syntheses and mechanisms can be intimidating because of all the detail presented, and they can slow you down considerably if you pay too much attention to this information during your first run through the passage. Be sure to read the titles of figures or schemes to get a sense of the big picture being presented, then jump into answering the questions quickly.

Passage Types as They Apply to Organic Chemistry

The main science passage types mentioned previously, when considered in the context of O-Chem, look something like this:

Information and/or Situation Presentation

These are the most common types of O-Chem passages, and generally present:

- A multistep synthetic scheme, a novel reaction, or atypical outcomes of reactions you might already be familiar with. Questions associated with these passages might ask you to analyze or classify the steps of the process described, or use common laboratory techniques to analyze intermediate compounds in the synthesis. You might need to justify the exceptions to the rules as described.

- A class of biologically important molecules. Questions associated with these passages could ask you to analyze the molecules with a common laboratory technique, or simply ask about their structure or their relationship to each other. You might also need to predict the reactivity of the molecules if treated with a given reagent.

- A biochemical process or mechanism. Questions here often test your understanding of the stability of intermediates and ask you to explain why the reaction occurs in the manner described. Given a new reactant, you might need to use the mechanistic steps to predict the product of a reaction.

Experiment/Research Presentation

This type of passage presents the details of an experiment or a mechanistic study, and often includes spectroscopy data (IR or NMR) in the form of lists or tables. Questions ask you to interpret data and identify the likely pathway of reaction. You might also need to identify compounds, or simply choose the appropriate technique to achieve the desired purification or product identification.

Persuasive Reasoning

This is the least common type of O-Chem passage, but can appear as a comparison of two mechanisms that attempt to explain the outcome of a reaction. Questions ask you to evaluate the arguments presented and will likely relate to the stability of intermediates.

Reading an O-Chem Passage

You should never really *read* much of the text of an O-Chem passage, but rather, just skim through the text. Remember that most of the important information you'll use from an O-Chem passage will be in the form of the structures and data presented. O-Chem passage-based questions are often essentially freestanding questions. They require only reference to a structure given in the passage in order to answer. However, as you're skimming the passage, you won't know which structures, reaction steps, or data will be the useful bits, AND you won't be able to mark or highlight structures in any way using your on-screen tools. That means that when skimming, you should get a general sense of the importance of each figure or table by reading titles and headings, but not get bogged down in the details of the figures in any way. You want to know where to go to examine the details when a question refers you to a particular synthetic step or structure along the pathway, something the MCAT is amazingly kind enough to do in most cases.

While you're reading, be on the lookout for new *italicized* terms in the text to highlight, or unexpected outcomes of experiments and exceptions to rules. The MCAT will ask you to apply the science fundamentals you've studied to novel situations, so look for and highlight anything that might be out of the ordinary.

Mapping an O-Chem Passage

It will often be the case that the text of a passage will reproduce information presented in a more visually useful manner, such as a flowchart, reaction scheme, or mechanism. Try to focus on the structures, and resist the urge to make a lot of yellow marks in the text.

Since you cannot highlight any structures in the passage (this is unfortunate, since structures are the place you'll get most of your necessary information), remember to use your noteboard to make note of anything related to a reaction scheme or mechanism, especially if it's taken you some time to come to your conclusion. Keep your noteboard organized so it will be a useful tool if you need to refer to it while checking back over your answers toward the end of the section. Label each new passage with a number and the range of questions attached to that passage, and give it an identifying title that summarizes the main point of the passage.

If you reach an important conclusion while answering questions, be sure to make note of it on your note-board as well. Other questions may require this information in order to proceed, and a brief note beats wasted time reconfirming your conclusion while trying to answer a subsequent question. Your O-Chem passage map will begin to develop as you answer your questions, but before jumping into answering them, you will likely have very little to jot down.

The passage below is an example of an Information Presentation passage (of the second type described previously). Note the minimal highlighting. The highlighted text was seemingly important upon a first pass to identify what the passage was about and to predict the types of questions with which it might be associated. You'll find upon review of the questions, however, that nothing but structures was necessary to answer any of the passage-based questions.

2.5

The small milkweed bug, *Lygaeus kalmii*, produces and emits a number of C_5-C_8 alkenals. Some of these small, fragrant, organic molecules are used to attract conspecific males or females for mating; thus, they act as sex pheromones. Others of the molecules are strongly malodorous and are used for defense.

Collaborating scientists in Brazil, the Netherlands, and Maryland have recently developed a method of noninvasive sampling and identification of these small organic molecules from live insects. This method involves the use of gas chromatography and mass spectrometry for the separation and identification of the components of the mixture of molecules involved in the sex- and defense-pheromone response in *L. kalmii*. Several of the molecules identified in this manner are shown in Figure 1.

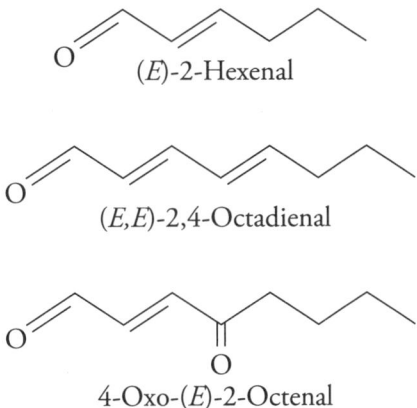

(*E*)-2-Hexenal

(*E,E*)-2,4-Octadienal

4-Oxo-(*E*)-2-Octenal

Figure 1   Molecules Identified Using Gas Chromatography and Mass Spectrometry

In addition to its mass spectrum, Molecule A, shown below, was also identified by its ^{1}H NMR spectrum:

Molecule A

Remember not to get bogged down in spectroscopic data before a question specifically asks you to analyze it. Here is an example of a passage map for the passage above. This is what you might jot down on your noteboard:

P1 – alkenals
P2 – separation and identification of alkenals
P3 – NMR data

The passage below is another example of an Information Presentation passage (of the third type described previously). While the passage has much more text to wade through, only one small piece of it proves to be important in an Explicit question (addressed in detail later). Highlighted items are related to the main point of each paragraph, include new definitions, or provide examples of phenomena. The figures presented are more complex than those in the first passage, and the questions related to them are likely to be more involved as well.

Dyes are ionizable, aromatic compounds that absorb visible light due to the presence of a highly conjugated system of *p* orbitals. The observed color is one that is complementary to the wavelength of light absorbed by the molecule (complementary color pairs are red/green, orange/blue, and yellow/violet). Dyes bind to the materials to be colored, such as fabrics or paper, through inter- and intramolecular interactions, including hydrogen bonds, ionic interactions, covalent bonds, and coordinate covalent bonds. The stronger the interaction between dye molecule and fiber, the more permanent the color will be. When a dye covalently bonds to a fiber, it becomes a part of the fabric itself and cannot be washed away.

Two of the most common dye types are mordant dyes and direct dyes. A mordant is a polyvalent metal ion (usually Al^{3+} or Fe^{3+}) that forms a coordination complex with certain dyes. Mordants chelate to the fabric as well as the dye molecule, thereby improving their colorfastness. Mordant dyes are primarily used on protein-based fibers such as wool, silk, angora, and cashmere since the mordant can bind to the constituent amino acids of these fibers. Direct dyes are typically charged molecules, and interact with the material to be dyed through ionic forces or hydrogen bonding. As such they tend to bleed more than mordant dyes. Direct dyes are more commonly used on cellulose fibers such as cotton, linen, or hemp.

Azo dyes, a subclass of direct dyes, may be used in a dyeing technique in which an insoluble azo compound is produced directly onto or within a fiber. This is achieved by treating the fiber first with a diazonium component, followed by a coupling component. With suitable adjustment of dye bath conditions the two components react to produce the required insoluble azo dye. The coupling reagent used in the final step is typically a molecule containing either a phenolic hydroxyl group or an arylamine. The synthesis of methyl orange, an azo dye, is shown in Figure 1.

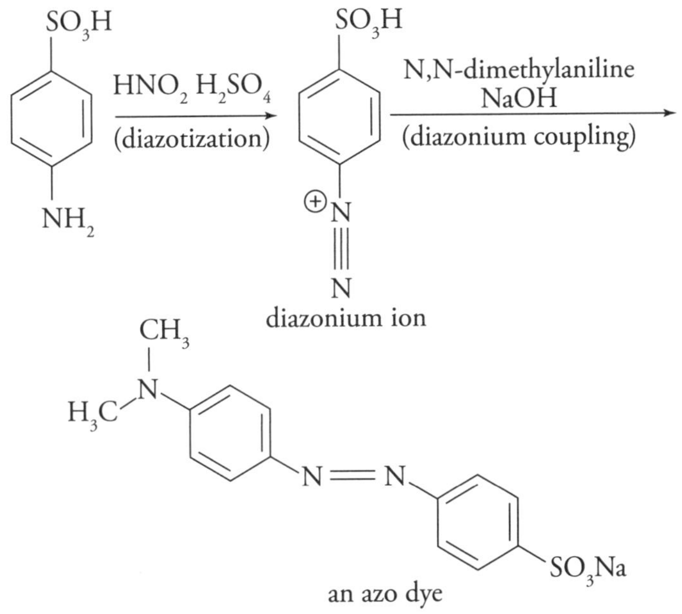

Figure 1 Synthesis of methyl orange

Figure 2 below represents the mechanism of the diazonium coupling reaction in the synthesis of methyl orange.

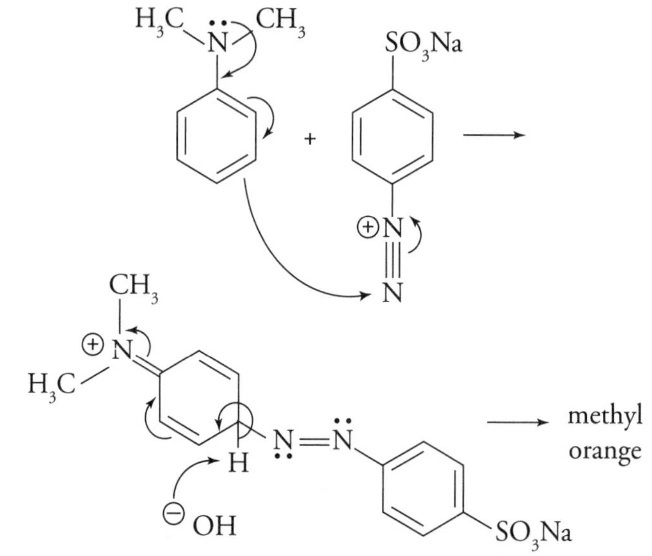

Figure 2 Mechanism of diazonium coupling

This is what you might jot down on your noteboard for the passage above:

P1 – what dyes are and how they work
P2 – Definitions: mordant dye vs. direct dyes, fiber types dyed
P3 – Structure requirements for diazocoupling

2.6 TACKLING THE QUESTIONS

The Organic Chemistry passage-based questions are some of the most straightforward ones on the entire exam and, as a result, some of the quickest ones to answer. It may be a wise strategy to consider doing the O-Chem passages before the Biology, Physics, or General Chemistry ones to help bank up some extra time to spend on the wordier, more involved Biology passages.

However, you should also consider starting with whichever subject you feel the most comfortable with, saving your more difficult subject for last. Whatever subject you choose, do all of the passages in one subject first before switching. In addition, do the passages within a subject in the order with which you feel most comfortable, leaving the topic you struggle with most, or the passage that appears to be the most difficult, for last. Within the passages themselves, tackle the easier questions first, leaving the most time-consuming ones for last. See Chapter 1, "MCAT Basics," for more information on efficiently moving around in the test.

O-Chem Memory Questions

These questions can be answered directly from prior knowledge. You can often recognize this question type by the length of the answer choices; one- or two-word answer choices are a good indication that you have the answer to these questions in your head already. Freestanding questions are commonly Memory questions since there is no passage to refer to. In addition, O-Chem passages often have "hidden" FSQs associated with them. This is another good reason to get to the questions quickly, rather than getting stuck reading details within the passage text.

Here is a true freestanding question that is also a Memory question:

Which of the following acetylating conditions will convert diethylamine into an amide at the fastest rate?

A) Acetic acid/HCl
B) Acetic anhydride
C) Acetyl chloride
D) Ethyl acetate

2.6

Your first step to attacking this question should be to consider what type of reaction is described. The conversion of an amine to an amide is a nucleophilic addition-elimination, where the amine acts as the nucleophile. Therefore, you're looking for the answer choice with the best electrophile, thereby increasing the reaction rate. Knowing the relative reactivities of carboxylic acids derivatives (amide < ester < anhydride < acid halide) allows you to eliminate choices B and D. In order to choose between the remaining answers that include a carboxylic acid and an acid derivative, rely on your fundamentals. Ask yourself: How would an amine be expected to behave under each set of conditions? When you consider that amines are not only nucleophilic but also basic, you can deduce that they will be protonated by both the HCl and the acetic acid to yield a non-nucleophilic conjugate acid under the conditions of answer choice A. The nucleophilic addition reaction is therefore faster with the acid chloride derivative, making answer choice C correct.

O-Chem Explicit Questions

These questions have answers that are explicitly stated in the passage. To answer them correctly, for example, may just require finding a definition, reading a graph, or making a simple connection. Explicit questions are much more common in passages of the test that rely more on reading comprehension. Since chemical structures are the most common source of referenced information in an O-Chem passage, Explicit questions in this section might ask you to identify the number of chiral centers in a given molecule, or to identify whether a particular functional group is present or not.

Here's an example of an Explicit question from the azo dye passage:

Mordant dyes are used in biological assays in addition to the textile industry. Which of the following biologically important molecules is most likely to be labeled by a mordant dye?

A) Glycogen
B) Chromatin
C) Cholesterol
D) Starch

You should recognize the term "mordant" as a new term you highlighted while reading the passage, so go back to the text to retrieve the important information. The passage states that mordants generally bind to protein-based fibers. Without this information, you might be able to eliminate choices A and D (glycogen and starch) since they are both carbohydrates, and as such, are not likely to be the answer. With the passage information at your disposal, however, this becomes a bit of a Memory question, and you need only determine which of your answer choices contain proteins. Cholesterol, a lipid, can be eliminated in addition to the two carbohydrates, leaving choice B as the correct answer (note that chromatin contains both proteins and DNA).

O-Chem Implicit Questions

These questions require you to apply knowledge to a new situation or make a more complex connection; the answer is typically implied by the information in the passage. Answer choices are generally longer, and may come in two parts, where the second half provides an explanation for the first. As mentioned before, the relevant information in the passage is often a molecular structure, but the analysis required to answer the question is more involved than for Explicit questions that rely on structures. Implicit style questions are the most common types of O-Chem questions.

Here's an example of an Implicit question from the azo dye passage:

The diazonium coupling reaction in Figure 2 is faster than most electrophilic substitutions of benzene. Which of the following statements best explains this fact?

A) The diazonium ion is an electron withdrawing substituent, making its benzene ring a better electrophile than benzene.
B) The diazonium ion is a good nucleophile.
C) The dimethylamino group is an electron donating substituent, making its benzene ring a better electrophile than benzene.
D) The dimethylamino group is an electron donating substituent, making its benzene ring a better nucleophile than benzene.

Since these answer choices are relatively long (and most have a second clause), try to use POE to eliminate choices based on obvious false statements in the first part of the answer. Remember, if any part of an answer choice is false, the entire statement can be eliminated. The first half of all the choices makes a statement about the inductive effects of substituents, or, in the case of answer choice B, the nucleophilicity of a compound. Refer to the structures in Figure 2. You should note that the diazonium ion is positively charged and therefore electron deficient. Since nucleophiles are by definition electron rich, choice B can be eliminated. The first halves of the remaining answer choices are all valid statements, since a positively charged substituent will pull electron density toward it, while an amine with a lone pair of electrons on the nitrogen will push electron density toward the ring. This question requires a more critical approach to distinguish between answer choices.

You should identify this as an Implicit question since it asks you to compare a new reagent to one you might already be familiar with. Consider, then, what you already know about benzene. Since benzene has six π electrons and is electron rich, it should behave as a nucleophile. This fundamental piece of information about the reactivity of benzene allows you to eliminate choices A and C. It does not matter whether the indicated substituents in Figure 2 make benzene a better or worse electrophile, since in the context of this reaction benzene behaves as a nucleophile. The remaining answer (choice D) is not only internally consistent but also answers the question.

Content Categories

O-Chem questions can be further classified from a content perspective into four main categories. Instead of trying to memorize a lot of detailed information, try to generalize as much as possible, and focus on the fundamentals of structure and stability when approaching questions. Remember that the MCAT is more likely to ask you to apply fundamental concepts to novel situations rather than ask you to recall an exception to a rule and regurgitate trivia. Just about every O-Chem question can be put into one of the following four categories:

Structure

Questions are generally about functional groups, stereochemistry, isomers, electron density (nucleophiles vs. electrophiles), and nomenclature.

Stability

This generally refers to stability of products or reaction intermediates. These questions often ask about inductive effects, resonance, steric strain, torsional strain, ring strain, etc.

Laboratory Practices

These questions may ask you to identify an appropriate separation technique (extraction, chromatography, distillation, etc.) for a given mixture of compounds, or ask you to interpret/predict the results of a separation procedure. You might also be asked to choose an appropriate spectroscopic technique (IR, NMR, mass spec, UV-vis, etc.) to identify a compound, or interpret spectroscopic data.

Predict the Product

Given a starting material and reaction conditions, choose the major product of the reaction. This will only be a one-step synthesis; no multistep processes will be presented. These questions will generally be associated with a passage in which a reaction type is explained in detail rather than as a freestanding question.

Finally, let's take a look at some sound advice about how to manage your time effectively while answering individual questions, as well as good strategies or rules of thumb you can apply to attack some of the most common formats of questions you'll see on the MCAT.

ORGANIC CHEMISTRY QUESTION STRATEGIES

1. Remember that Process of Elimination is paramount! The strikeout tool allows you to eliminate answer choices; this will improve your chances of guessing the correct answer if you are unable to narrow it down to one choice.

2. Answer the straightforward questions first. Leave questions that require analysis of experiments and graphs for later.

3. Make sure that the answer you choose actually answers the question, and isn't just a true statement.

4. Roman numeral questions: Whenever possible, start by evaluating the Roman numeral item that shows up in exactly two answer choices. This allows you to quickly eliminate two wrong answer choices regardless of whether the item is true or false. Typically then, you will only have to assess one of the other Roman numeral items to determine the correct answer. Always work between the I-II-III items and the answer choices. Once an item is found to be true (or false), strike out answer choices which do not contain (or do contain) that item number. Make sure to strike out the actual Roman numeral item as well, and highlight those items that are true.

5. Ranking questions: Look for an extreme in whatever is being ranked, then look at the answer choices. Use the strikeout feature to eliminate choices as you go. In some cases, you may immediately get the answer as only one choice lists the appropriate option as "least" or "greatest." Usually you will, at minimum, be able to strikeout two answer choices. Then just examine the remaining possibilities to determine which of the items at the other end of the ranking can be correct.

6. 2 x 2 style questions: These questions require you to know two pieces of information to get the correct answer, and are easily identified by their answer choices, which commonly take the form A because X, B because X, A because Y, B because Y. Tackle one piece of information at a time, which should allow you to quickly eliminate two answer choices.

7. LEAST/EXCEPT/NOT questions: Don't get tricked by these questions that ask you to pick the answer that doesn't fit (the incorrect or false statement). It's often good to use your noteboard and write "A B C D" with a T or F next to each answer choice. The one that stands out as different is the correct answer!

8. If you read a question and do not know how to answer it, look to the passage for help. It is likely that the passage contains information pertinent to answering the question, either within the text or in the form of experimental data.

9. Math: Any questions that involve calculations should be left for last (there aren't many in O-Chem, but they happen). You should always round numbers and estimate while working out calculations on your scratch paper.

10. Don't ever leave a question blank since there is no penalty for guessing.

Chapter 3
Organic Chemistry
Fundamentals

3.1   BACKGROUND AND INTRODUCTION

This section covers the fundamentals of nomenclature in organic chemistry. Although this section will require memorization as your primary study technique, it is in your best interest to be comfortable reading, hearing, and using this terminology. Although most of the terminology that appears on the MCAT is IUPAC (International Union of Pure and Applied Chemistry), some common nomenclature is also used.

Basic Nomenclature

Carbon Chain Prefixes and Alkane Names			
Number of carbon atoms in a row	Prefix	Alkane	Name
1	meth-	CH_4	methane
2	eth-	CH_3CH_3	ethane
3	prop-	$CH_3CH_2CH_3$	propane
4	but-	$CH_3CH_2CH_2CH_3$	butane
5	pent-	$CH_3(CH_2)_3CH_3$	pentane
6	hex-	$CH_3(CH_2)_4CH_3$	hexane
7	hept-	$CH_3(CH_2)_5CH_3$	heptane
8	oct-	$CH_3(CH_2)_6CH_3$	octane
9	non-	$CH_3(CH_2)_7CH_3$	nonane
10	dec-	$CH_3(CH_2)_8CH_3$	decane

In the case of an all-carbon containing ring, these are preceded by the prefix **cyclo-**. Hence, a six-membered ring containing all $-CH_2-$ units is called *cyclohexane*.

Nomenclature for Substituents	
Substituent	Name
$-CH_3$	methyl
$-CH_2CH_3$	ethyl
$-CH_2CH_2CH_3$	propyl
$H_3C-\overset{H}{\underset{\vert}{C}}-CH_3$	isopropyl
$-CH_2CH_2CH_2CH_3$	butyl (or *n*-butyl)
$CH_3\underset{\vert}{C}HCH_2CH_3$	*sec*-butyl
$-\overset{CH_3}{\underset{CH_3}{\overset{\vert}{\underset{\vert}{C}}}}-CH_3$	*tert*-butyl (or *t*-butyl)

Common Functional Groups

R = alkyl group   X = halogen (F, Cl, Br, I)

R_3C—CR_3 R_2C=CR_2 RC≡CR R—X R—$\ddot{O}H$

alkane   alkene or olefin   alkyne   alkyl halide   alcohol

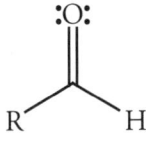   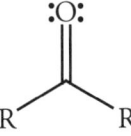   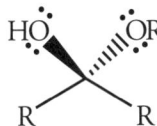   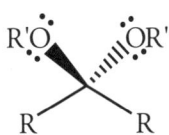

R—$\ddot{S}H$ R—$\ddot{O}$—R

thiol   ether   epoxide or oxirane   phenol

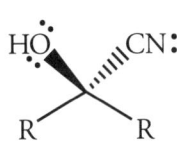   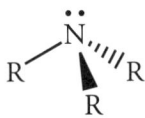   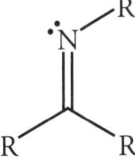   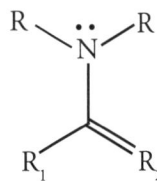

aldehyde   ketone   hemiacetal   acetal

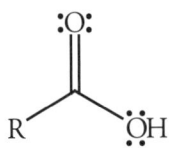   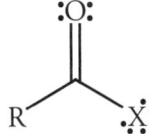

cyanohydrin   amine   imine   enamine

carboxylic acid   acid halide   acid anhydride

ester   lactone   amide   lactam

3.2 ABBREVIATED LINE STRUCTURES

The prevalence of carbon-hydrogen (C—H) bonds in organic chemistry has led chemists to use an abbreviated drawing system, merely for convenience. Just imagine having to draw every C—H bond for a large molecule like a steroid or polymer! Abbreviated line structures use only a few simple rules:

1. Carbons are represented simply as vertices.
2. C—H bonds are not drawn.
3. Hydrogens bonded to any atom *other* than carbon must be shown.

To illustrate rules 1 and 2, pentane can be represented using the full Lewis structure:

or using the abbreviated line structure:

Although C—H bonds are not drawn, the number of hydrogens required to complete carbon's valency are assumed. To clarify this, let's look more closely at the abbreviated line structure of pentane:

These three carbon atoms are each bonded to two other carbon atoms. In order to complete carbon's valency, we assume there are two hydrogens bonded to each of these carbons.

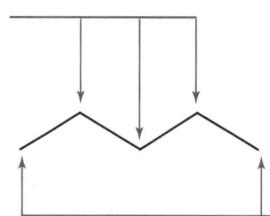

These two carbon atoms are each bonded to one other carbon atom. In order to complete carbon's valency, we assume there are three hydrogens bonded to each of these carbons.

This must be correct, because if we draw out all of the hydrogens in pentane, we get the full Lewis structure shown above.

To illustrate rule 3, consider dimethyl amine:

full Lewis structure

abbreviated line structure

Remember that hydrogens bonded to carbon can be assumed (the methyl groups in dimethyl amine, for example), but hydrogens bonded to any other atom must be shown. Lone pairs of electrons are often omitted.

Example 3-1: Translate each of the following Lewis structures into an abbreviated line structure:

(a)

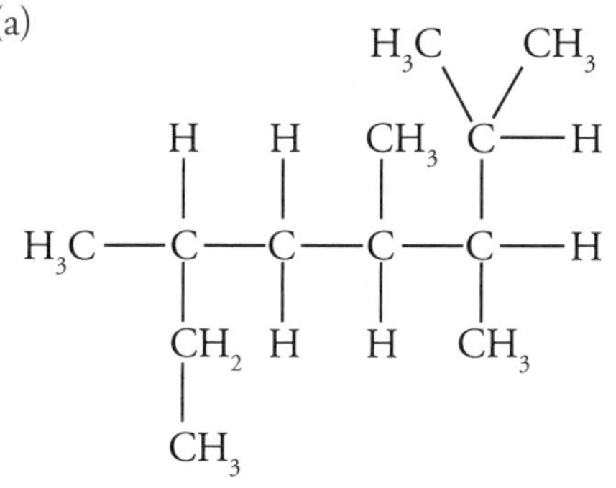

(b)

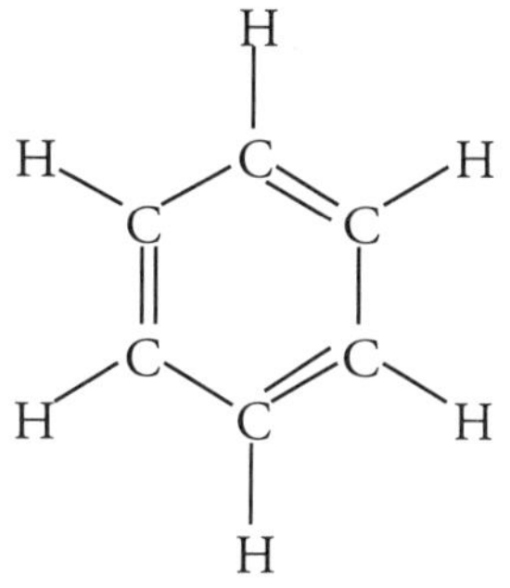

(c)

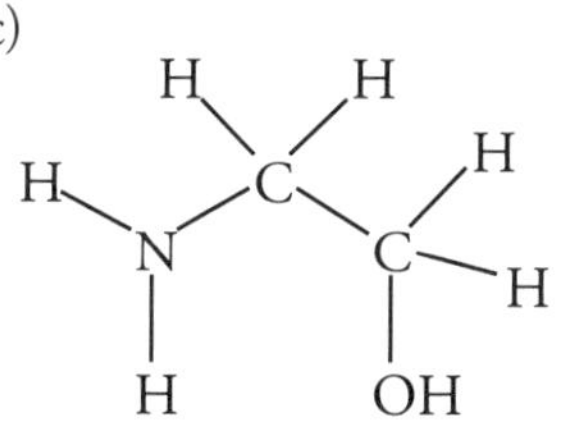

(d)

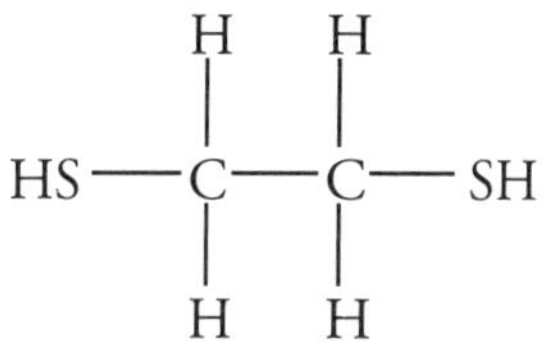

Solution:

(a)

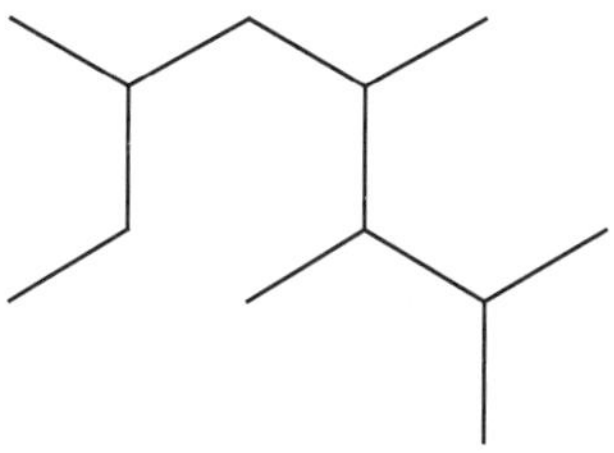

(b)

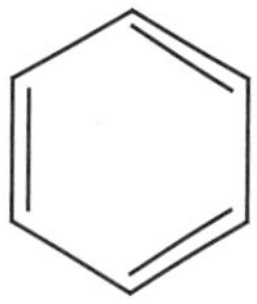

(c)

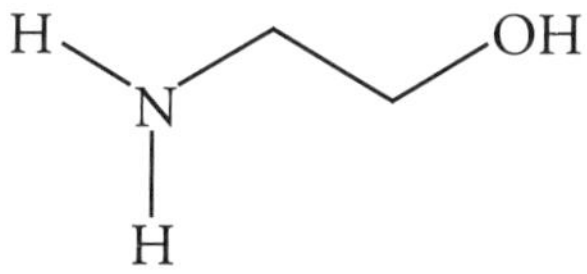

(d)

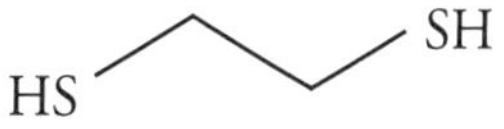

Example 3-2: Translate each of the following abbreviated line structures into a Lewis structure:

(a)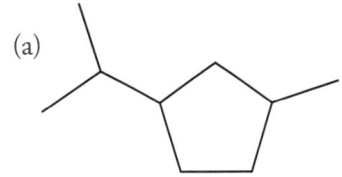

(b)

(c)

(d)

Solution:

(a)

(b)

(c)

(d)

3.3 NOMENCLATURE OF ALKANES

Alkanes are named by a set of simple rules. One particular alkane (shown below) will be used to illustrate this process:

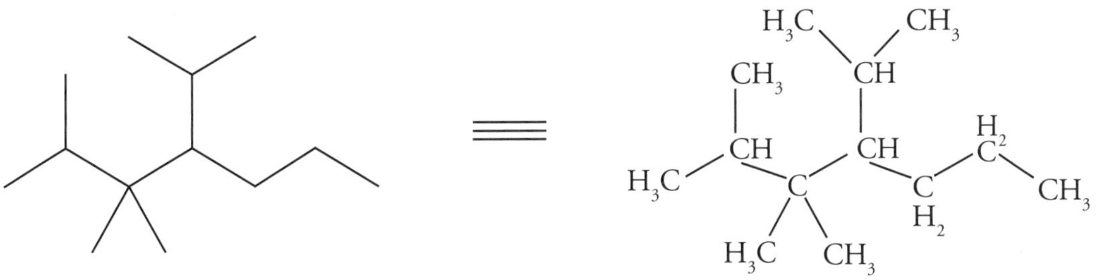

1. Identify the longest continuous carbon chain. The names of these chains are given in the first table in this chapter ("Carbon Chain Prefixes and Alkane Names").

    The longest chain in the compound above is a 7-carbon chain, which is called *heptane*. (This chain is shown below, outlined by dashed lines.)

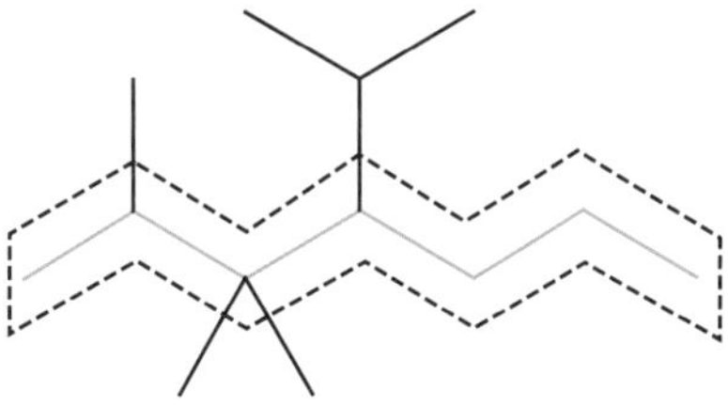

2. Identify any substituents on this chain. The names of some common hydrocarbon substituents are given in the second table in this chapter ("Nomenclature for Substituents").

    There are four substituents in this example: three methyl groups and one isopropyl group.

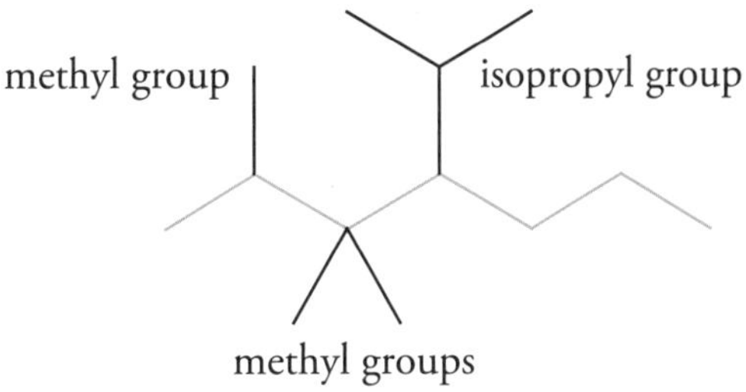

3. Number the carbons of the main chain such that the substituents are on the carbons with lower numbers.

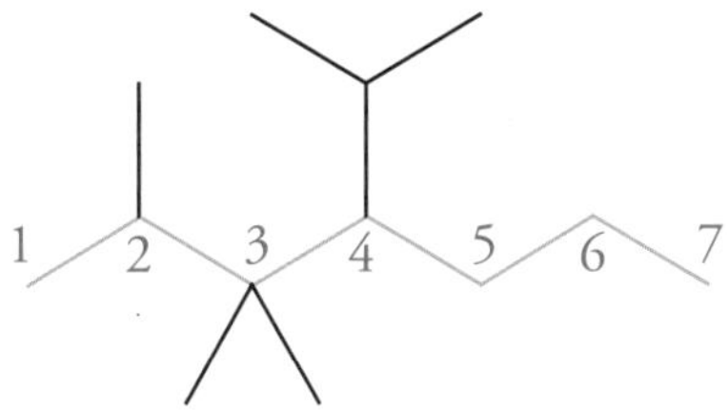

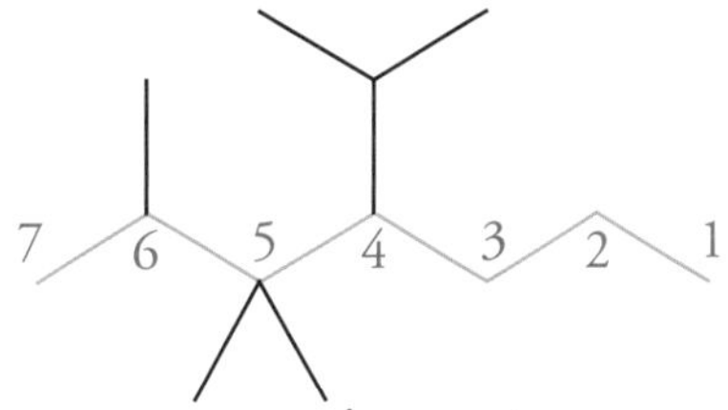

3.3

Now each substituent can be associated with the carbon atom to which it's attached:

2 – methyl
3 – methyl
3 – methyl
4 – isopropyl

4. Identical substituents are grouped together; the prefixes **di-**, **tri-**, **tetra-**, and **penta-** are used to denote how many there are, and their carbon numbers are separated by a comma.

In this case we have:

$$\left.\begin{array}{l} 2-\text{methyl} \\ 3-\text{methyl} \\ 3-\text{methyl} \end{array}\right\} \longrightarrow \text{2,3,3-trimethyl}$$

5. Alphabetize the substituents, ignoring the prefixes di-, tri-, etc., and *n-*, *sec-*, *tert-*, and separate numbers from words by a hyphen and numbers from numbers by a comma. Note that "iso" is not a prefix but is part of the name of the substituent, so it is NOT ignored when alphabetizing.

The complete name for our molecule is therefore **4-isopropyl-2,3,3-trimethylheptane.**

Let's do another example and find the name of this molecule:

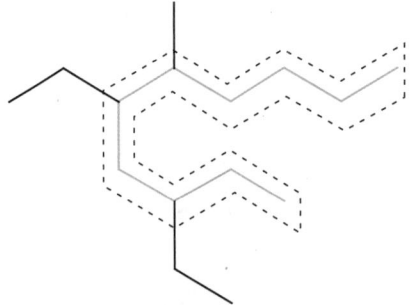

1. The longest continuous carbon chain is a 10-carbon chain, called **decane**.

2. There are three substituents on this chain: two ethyl groups and a methyl group.

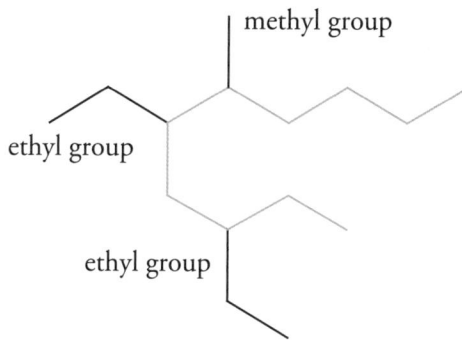

3. The correct numbering of the carbons in the main chain is as follows:

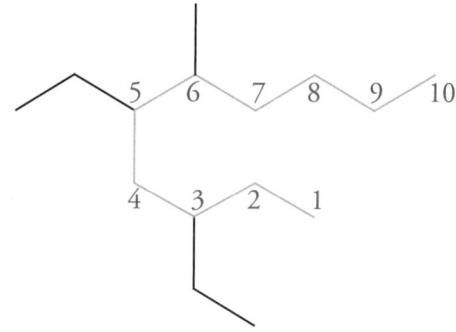

4. The substituents are now identified as:
    3,5-diethyl
    6-methyl

5. The complete name of the molecule is therefore **3,5-diethyl-6-methyldecane**.

Example 3-3: Name each of the following alkanes:

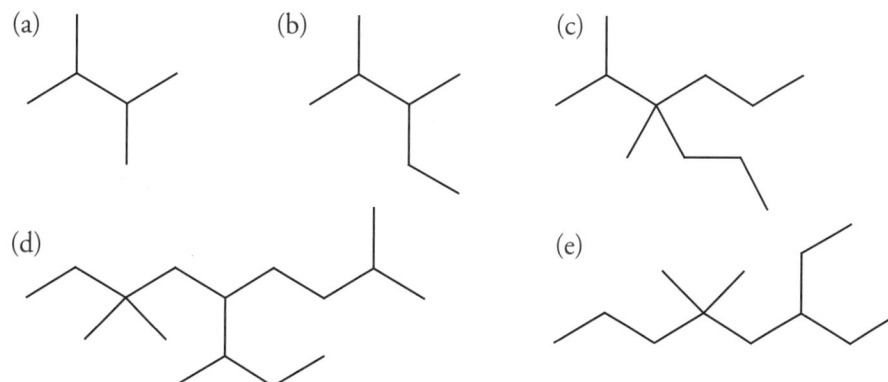

Solution:

(a) 2,3-dimethylbutane
(b) 2,3-dimethylpentane
(c) 4-isopropyl-4-methylheptane
(d) 5-*sec*-butyl-2,7,7-trimethylnonane
(e) 3-ethyl-5,5-dimethyloctane

3.4   NOMENCLATURE OF HALOALKANES

Alkanes with halogen (F, Cl, Br, I) substituents follow the same set of rules as simple alkanes. Halogens are named using these prefixes:

Halogen	Prefix
fluorine	fluoro-
chlorine	chloro-
bromine	bromo-
iodine	iodo-

By applying the same rules as for naming simple alkanes, verify the following names:

Structure   Name

2-chlorobutane

2-chloro-1-fluoro-4-methylpentane

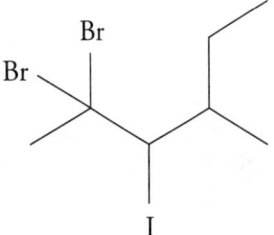

2,2-dibromo-3-iodo-4-methylhexane

Example 3-4: Name each of the following haloalkanes:

(a)
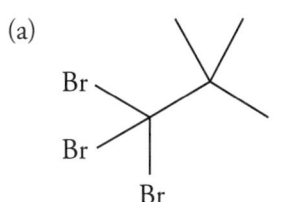

(b)
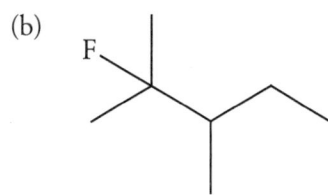

(c)
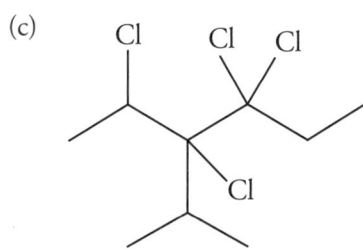

(d)
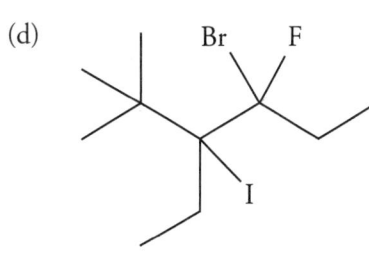

Solution:

(a) 1,1,1-tribromo-2,2-dimethylpropane
(b) 2-fluoro-2,3-dimethylpentane
(c) 2,3,4,4-tetrachloro-3-isopropylhexane
(d) 4-bromo-3-ethyl-4-fluoro-3-iodo-2,2-dimethylhexane

Example 3-5: For each name, draw the structure:

(a) 3-chloro-2,2-dimethylbutane
(b) 3-bromo-4-chloro-5,5-diethylnonane
(c) 2,3-dibromo-1,1-diiodopropane
(d) 3,4-difluoro-2,2,3-trimethylpentane

Solution:

(a)
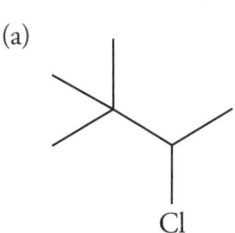

(b)
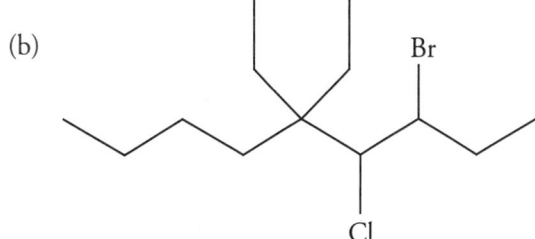

(c)
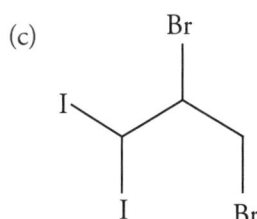

(d)
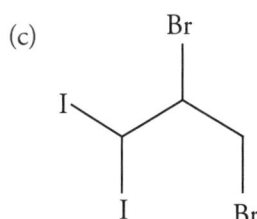

3.5 NOMENCLATURE OF ALCOHOLS

Alcohols also follow many of the same nomenclature rules as alkanes. Hydroxyl groups (–OH), however, are typically denoted by a suffix to the main alkyl chain. The table of straight-chain alcohols given below shows that to denote a hydroxyl group, the suffix **–ol** replaces the last **–e** in the name of the alkane.

Alkanes		Alcohols	
Structure	**Name**	**Structure**	**Name**
CH_4	methane	CH_3OH	methanol
CH_3CH_3	ethane	CH_3CH_2OH	ethanol
$CH_3CH_2CH_3$	propane	$CH_3CH_2CH_2OH$	propanol
$CH_3CH_2CH_2CH_3$	butane	$CH_3CH_2CH_2CH_2OH$	butanol

When the position of the hydroxyl group needs to be specified, the number is placed after the name of the longest carbon chain and before the –ol suffix, separated by hyphens. For example:

OH

butan-2-ol
(or 2-butanol)
or *sec*-butanol

OH

pentan-2-ol
(or 2-pentanol)

Priorities are assigned (the way the main carbon chain is numbered) to give the lowest number to the hydroxyl group. For example:

OH

3-methylbutan-2-ol
not
2-methylbutan-3-ol

Cl

OH

6-chloro-5-methylhexan-3-ol

Example 3-6: Name each of the following molecules:

(a)

(b)

(c)

(d)

Solution:

(a)   4,4-dichloro-2-methylpentanol (the "-1-" is assumed if no number is given)
(b)   propane-1,2-diol (or 1,2-propandiol)
(c)   2-chloro-2-fluoro-3-methylbutane-1,1-diol
(d)   6-chloro-4-ethylhexan-2-ol

Other organic functional groups have small nuances to their nomenclature, but this introduction to nomenclature should allow you to interpret chemical names on the MCAT.

Chapter 4
Structure and Stability

4.1 THE ORGANIC CHEMIST'S TOOLBOX

In the following chapters, we will frequently discuss several fundamental principles necessary to understand the reactivity of organic molecules. These "tools" are collected here.

Structural Formulas

By definition, an organic molecule is said to be **saturated** if it contains no π bonds and no rings; it is **unsaturated** if it has at least one π bond or a ring. A saturated compound with n carbon atoms has exactly $2n + 2$ hydrogen atoms, while an unsaturated compound with n carbon atoms has fewer than $2n + 2$ hydrogens.

The formula below is used to determine the **degree of unsaturation** (d) of simple organic molecules:

n = number of carbons

x = number of hydrogens*

$$\text{degree of unsaturation} = \frac{(2n + 2) - x}{2}$$

* x represents the number of hydrogens and any monovalent atoms (such as the halogens: F, Cl, Br, or I).
Since the number of oxygens has no effect, it is ignored.
For nitrogen-containing compounds, replace each N by 1 C and 1 H when using this formula.

One degree of unsaturation indicates the presence of one π bond or one ring; two degrees of unsaturation means there are two π bonds (two separate double bonds or one triple bond), or one π bond and one ring, or two rings, and so on. The presence of heteroatoms can also affect the degree of unsaturation in a molecule. This is best illustrated through a series of related molecules that all have one degree of unsaturation.

Butene (C_4H_8) has one degree of unsaturation, since $d = [(2 \times 4 + 2) - 8]/2 = 1$, in the form of a double bond:

4-Chlorobutene (C_4H_7Cl) also has one degree of unsaturation, but the number of hydrogens is different. Each halogen atom (fluorine, chlorine, bromine, iodine) or other monovalent atom "replaces" one hydrogen atom, so $d = [(2 \times 4 + 2)-(7 + 1)]/2 = 1$:

Methoxyethene (C_3H_6O) also has one degree of unsaturation. Since a divalent atom can take the place of a methylene group, it doesn't affect the degree of unsaturation, and can be ignored. The calculation for this formula, then, should look like this: $[(2 \times 3 + 2) - 6]/2 = 1$

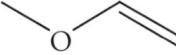

Methyl vinyl amine (C_3H_7N) has one degree of unsaturation as well. Each nitrogen (or other trivalent atom) "replaces" one carbon and one hydrogen atom. Therefore, adjust the formula to be C_4H_8, then do the calculation. The new formula thus gives $d = [(2 \times 4 + 2) - 8]/2 = 1$:

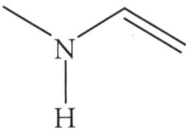

Example 4-1: Determine the degree of unsaturation of each of these molecules. Which, if any, are saturated?

(a) C_6H_8
(b) C_4H_6O
(c) $C_{20}H_{30}O$
(d) C_3H_8O
(e) C_3H_5Br

Solution:

(a) $d = [(2 \times 6 + 2) - 8]/2 = 3$.
(b)   Just ignore the O, and find that $d = [(2 \times 4 + 2) - 6]/2 = 2$.
(c)   Ignoring the O, we get $d = [(2 \times 20 + 2) - 30]/2 = 6$.
(d)   Ignore the O, and find that $d = [(2 \times 3 + 2) - 8]/2 = 0$. *This molecule is saturated.*
(e)   Since Br is a halogen, we treat it like a hydrogen, so $d = [(2 \times 3 + 2) - (5 + 1)]/2 = 1$.

Hybridization

Although hybridization theory is covered in more detail in the *MCAT General Chemistry Review*, it's useful here to briefly outline how to determine an atom's hybridization.

Every pair of electrons must be housed in an electronic orbital (either an *s, p, d,* or *f*). For example, the carbon atom in methane, CH_4, has *four* pairs of electrons surrounding it (four single covalent bonds and no lone pairs), so it must provide *four* orbitals to house these electrons.

Orbitals always get "used" in the following order:

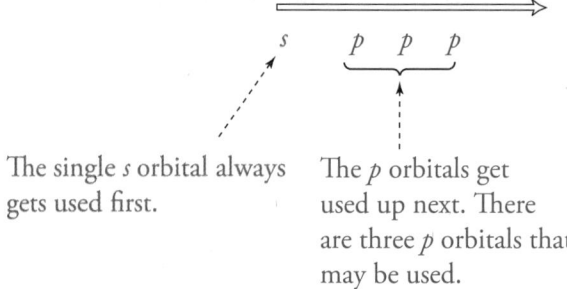

The single *s* orbital always gets used first.

The *p* orbitals get used up next. There are three *p* orbitals that may be used.

So, since the carbon atom in methane must provide *four* orbitals, we just count: 1...2...3...4:

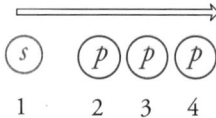

Therefore, the hybridization of the carbon atom in methane is $s + p + p + p$, which is written as sp^3. The sum of the exponents in the hybridization nomenclature tells us how many orbitals of this type are used. So, in methane, there are $1 + 3 = 4$ hybrid orbitals. The following table gives the hybridization of the central atom for each of the orbital geometries:

Number of Electron Groups	Orbital Geometry	Hybridization of Central Atom
2	Linear	sp
3	Trigonal Planar	sp^2
4	Tetrahedral	sp^3

Reaction Intermediates

Some organic reactions proceed through carbocations (carbonium ions), while others make use of carbanions.

Carbocations, or **carbonium ions**, are positively charged species with a full positive charge on carbon. The reactivity of these species is determined by what type of carbon bears the positive charge. On the MCAT, carbocations will always be sp^2 hybridized with an empty *p* orbital.

Carbanions are negatively charged species with a full negative charge localized on carbon. The reactivity of these species is determined by what type of carbon bears the negative charge.

Stability Continuum				
Carbocations	3°	2°	1°	methyl
Carbanions	methyl	1°	2°	3°
	more stable	→		less stable
	less reactive	→		more reactive
	lower energy	→		higher energy

It's essential to understand the stabilities of reaction intermediates, because generally the reactivity of a molecule is inversely related to its stability. This means the molecules that are more stable are less reactive, while higher energy species will be more reactive. This theme will resurface over and over again in organic chemistry, and is a useful rule of thumb to keep in mind when you need to predict how a reaction might proceed.

Organic intermediates are stabilized in two major ways: **inductive effects** stabilize charge through σ bonds, while **resonance effects** stabilize charge by delocalization through π bonds.

Inductive Effects

All substituent groups surrounding a reaction intermediate can be thought of as electron-withdrawing groups or electron-donating groups. **Electron-withdrawing** groups pull electrons toward themselves through σ bonds. **Electron-donating** groups donate (push) electron density away from themselves through σ bonds. Groups *more* electronegative than carbon tend to withdraw, while groups *less* electronegative than carbon tend to donate. On the MCAT, alkyl substituents are always electron-donating groups.

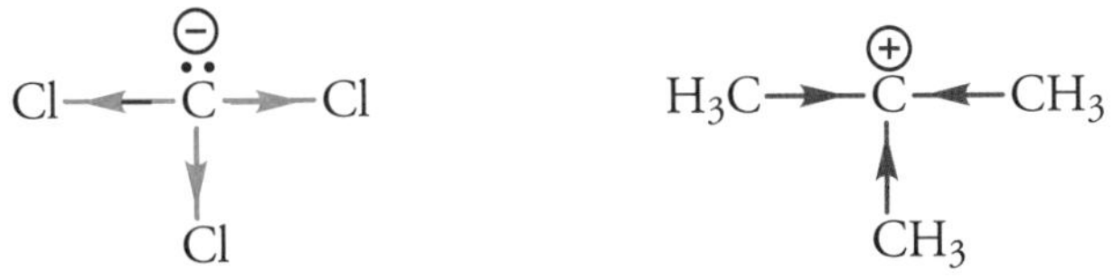

Electron
Withdrawal

Electron
Donation

Electron-donating groups tend to stabilize electron-deficient intermediates (carbocations), while electron-withdrawing groups tend to stabilize electron-rich intermediates (carbanions). The stabilization of reaction intermediates by the sharing of electrons through σ bonds is called the **inductive effect**.

Example 4-2: Inductive effects frequently alter the reactivity of molecules. Justify the fact that trichloroacetic acid (pK_a = 0.6) is a better acid than acetic acid (pK_a = 4.8).

Solution: The chlorine atoms in trichloroacetic acid are electron withdrawing. This decreases the amount of electron density elsewhere in the molecule, especially in the O–H bond. With less electron density, the O–H bond is weaker, making it more acidic than the O–H bond in acetic acid.

An alternative explanation would be to consider the stability of the conjugate bases of these acids.

The chlorine atoms in the trichloroacetate anion distribute the negative charge better, making it more stable than the acetate anion. Therefore, because trichloroacetate anion is a weaker base (is more stable) than acetate anion, trichloroacetic acid is a stronger acid than acetic acid. Acidity will be reviewed in more detail a bit later in the Toolbox.

Resonance Stabilization

While induction works through σ bonds, resonance stabilization occurs in conjugated π systems. A **conjugated system** is one containing three or more atoms that each bear a p orbital. These orbitals are aligned so they are all parallel, creating the possibility of delocalized electrons.

Electrons that are confined to one orbital, either a bonding orbital between two atoms or a lone-pair orbital, are said to be **localized**. When electrons are allowed to interact with orbitals on adjacent atoms, they are no longer confined to their original "space," and so are termed **delocalized**. Consider the allyl cation:

The electrons in the π bond can interact with the empty *p* orbital on the carbon bearing the positive charge. This is illustrated by the following resonance structures:

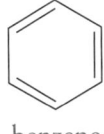

delocalized picture, or resonance hybrid

The electron density is spread out—delocalized—over the entire 3-carbon framework in order to stabilize the carbocation. So, we might say of the allyl cation that both the electrons and the positive charge are delocalized.

As the allyl cation demonstrates, it often happens that a single Lewis structure for a molecule is not sufficient to most accurately represent the molecule's true structure. It is important to remember that resonance structures are just multiple representations of the actual structure. The molecule does not become one resonance structure or another; it exists as a combination of all resonance structures, although all may not contribute equally. All resonance structures must be drawn to give an accurate picture of the real nature of the molecule. In the case of the allyl cation, the two structures are equivalent and will have equivalent energy. They will also contribute equally to the delocalized picture of what the molecule really looks like. This average of all resonance contributors is called the **resonance hybrid**.

Benzene (C_6H_6) is another common molecule that exhibits resonance. Looking at a Lewis representation of benzene might lead one to believe that there are two distinct types of carbon-carbon bonds: single σ bonds (this structure of benzene has three such bonds) and double bonds (of which there are also three):

benzene

Thus one might expect two distinct carbon-carbon bond lengths: one for the single bonds, and one for the double bonds. Yet experimental data clearly demonstrates that all the C—C bond lengths are identical in benzene. All the carbons of benzene are sp^2 hybridized, so they each have an unhybridized *p* orbital. Two structures can be drawn for benzene, which differ only in the location of the π bonds. The true structure of benzene is best pictured as a resonance hybrid of these structures. Perhaps a better representation of benzene shows both resonance contributors, like this:

Notice that these resonance structures differ only in the arrangement of their π electrons, not in the locations of the atoms. All six unhybridized *p* orbitals are aligned parallel with one another. This alignment of adjacent unhybridized *p* orbitals allows for delocalization of π electrons over the entire ring. Whenever we have a delocalized π system (aligned *p* orbitals), resonance structures can be drawn.

Delocalization of electrons is also observed in thiophene:

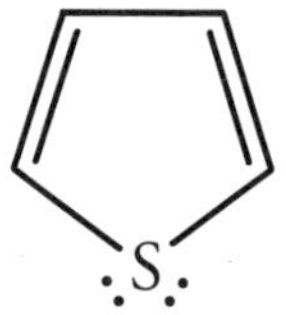

Here the sulfur atom has two pairs of non-bonding electrons. Notice that these electrons are one atom away from two π bonds. One pair of these electrons is actually in an unhybridized *p* orbital, such that it can be delocalized into the cyclic π system. Here are the representative resonance structures:

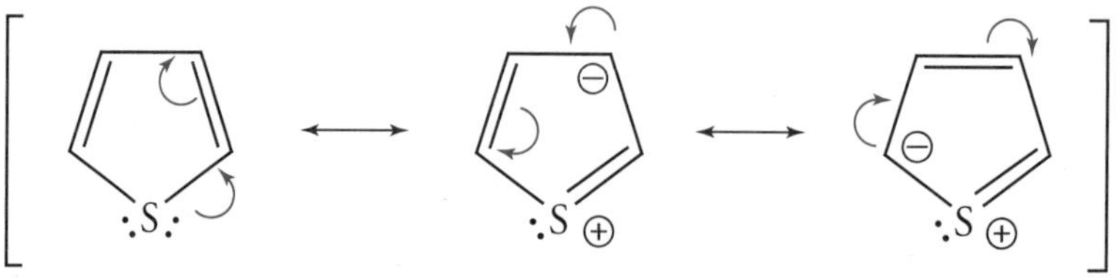

The other pair of electrons, however, is in a hybrid orbital and cannot delocalize into the π system. Here the delocalization of sulfur's electrons imparts aromatic stability to the molecule. The hybridization of the sulfur is therefore most correctly represented as *sp*².

Let's consider one more example:

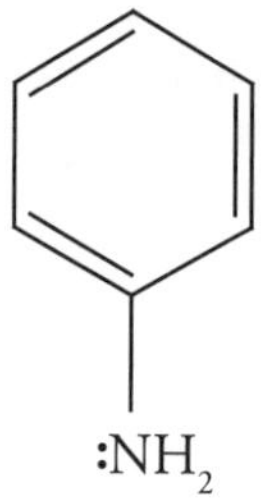

The nitrogen in aniline has an unshared electron pair that is one atom removed from a cyclic π system. Again these electrons can be delocalized by overlap of the lone pair-containing orbital with the *p* orbitals of the benzene ring. This can be demonstrated by the following resonance structures:

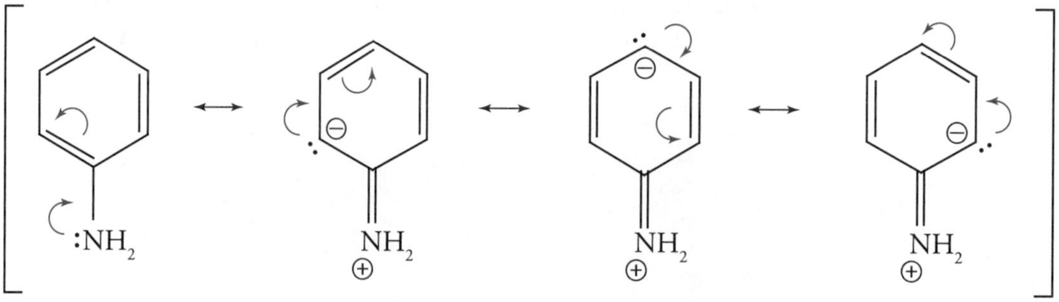

In this case, the delocalization of the nitrogen's electrons disrupts the aromaticity of the benzene ring and is therefore less favorable. Experimental determination of the nitrogen's bond angles reveals that they are actually intermediate between 120° and 109°, so the hybridization of the nitrogen can best be described not as sp^2 or sp^3, but as something intermediate between them. The important point, however, is that the electrons are at least somewhat delocalized into the π system. Therefore, the nitrogen's hybridization is not strictly sp^3.

Example 4-3: For the following molecules, indicate the hybridization and idealized bond angles for the indicated atoms.

(a)

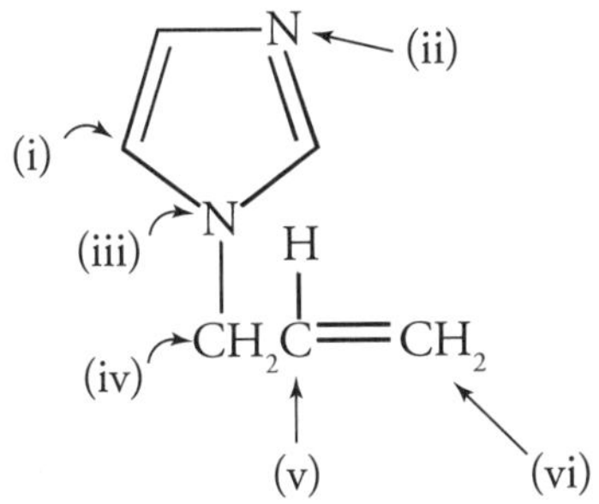

(b)

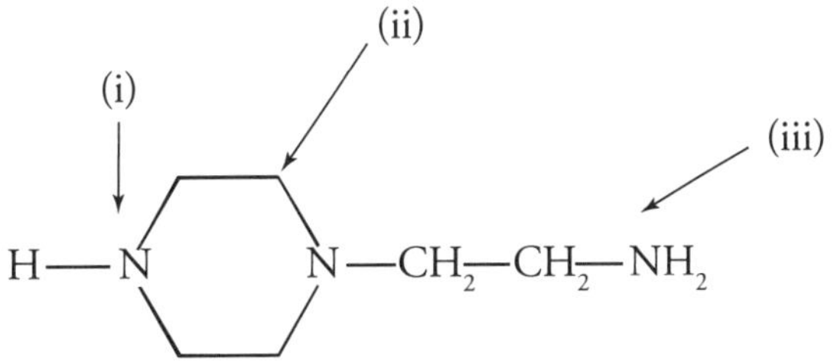

(c)

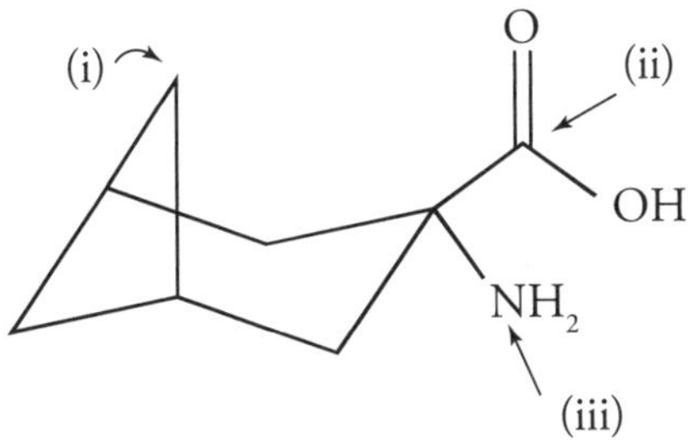

(d)

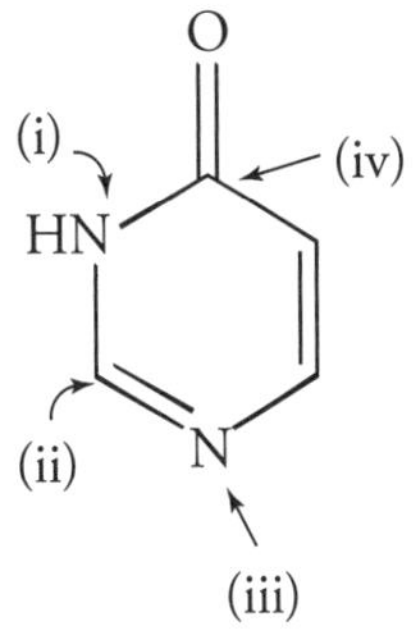

(e)

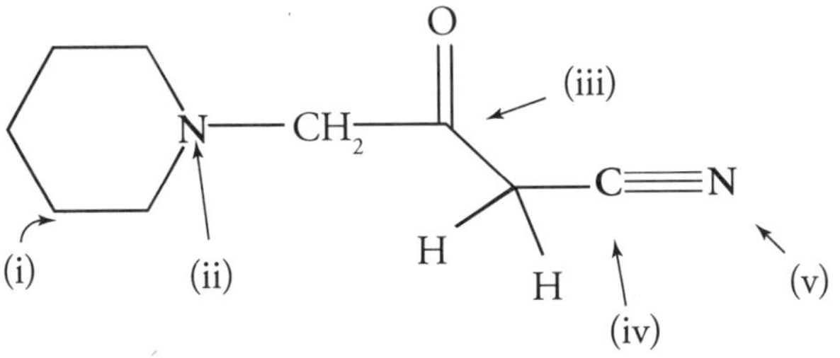

(f)

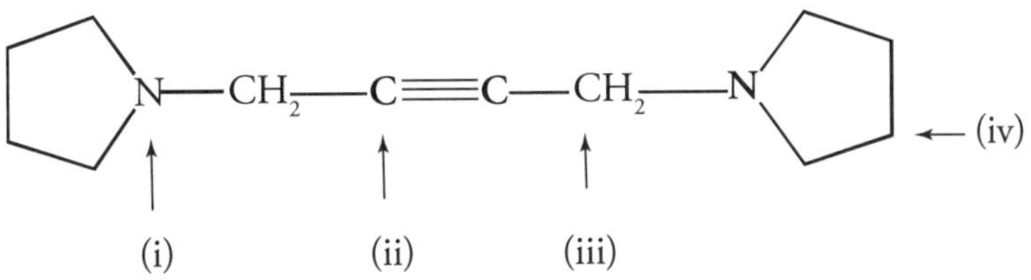

Solution: Remember to always draw the electrons on nitrogen if they are not drawn in the structure.

(a) i) sp^2, 120°   ii) sp^2, 120°   iii) sp^2, 120° (The lone pair is delocalized, so it's not counted.)
     iv) sp^3, 109°   v) sp^2, 120°   vi) sp^2, 120°
(b) i) sp^3, 109°   ii) sp^3, 109°   iii) sp^3, 109°
(c) i) sp^3, 109°   ii) sp^2, 120°   iii) sp^3, 109°
(d) i) sp^2, 120°   ii) sp^2, 120°   iii) sp^2, 120°   iv) sp^2, 120°
(e) i) sp^3, 109°   ii) sp^3, 109°   iii) sp^2, 120°   iv) sp, 180°   v) sp, 180°
(f) i) sp^3, 109°   ii) sp, 180°   iii) sp^3, 109°   iv) sp^3, 109°

So why all this focus on resonance? In general, the more stable a molecule is, the less reactive it will be. Since the delocalization of charge tends to stabilize molecules, resonance has a big impact on the reactivity of molecules.

Since it's important to recognize molecules that are stabilized by resonance, we'll next review the three basic principles of resonance delocalization.

1. Resonance structures can never be drawn through atoms that are truly sp^3 hybridized. Remember that an sp^3-hybridized atom is one with a total of four σ bonds and/or lone electron pairs.

No resonance
structures possible!

No resonance structures are
possible with these electrons.

No resonance structures are
possible with these electrons.

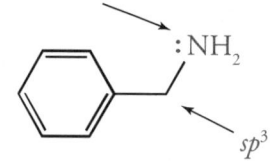

2. Resonance structures usually involve electrons that are adjacent to (one atom away from) a π bond or an unhybridized *p* orbital. Here are some examples of molecules that are resonance stabilized:

3. Resonance structures of lowest energy are the most important. Remember that the evaluation of resonance structure stability involves three main criteria:
   a. Resonance contributors in which the octet rule is satisfied for all atoms are more important than ones in which it is not. This is the most important of the three criteria listed here and takes priority over items b and c below.
   b. Resonance contributors that minimize separation of charge (formal charge) are better than those with a large separation of charge.
   c. In structures with formal charge(s), the more important resonance contributor has negative charges on the more electronegative atom(s), and positive charge(s) on the less electronegative atom(s).

Now that we can identify valid resonance structures of any given molecule and rank those resonance structures based on their relative energies, let's use this information to demonstrate the close relationship between stability and reactivity by examining acidity.

Acidity

While acids and bases are covered in detail in Chapter 11 of the *MCAT General Chemistry Review,* we will now examine how the organic chemistry principles we've just discussed can help explain the acidity of a compound, as well as help us understand the relative acidity of several functional groups.

Firstly, let's review the definition of a Brønsted-Lowry acid. Simply put, it's a molecule that can donate a proton (H^+), and once the molecule has done so, it most commonly takes on a negative charge. This deprotonated structure is referred to as the conjugate base of the acid.

$$HCl \longrightarrow H^+ \quad + \quad Cl^-$$

acid   conjugate
                                              base

The strength of an acid refers to the degree to which it dissociates (or donates its proton) in solution. The more the acid dissociates, the stronger the acid is said to be. Acids that dissociate completely are said to be strong. Most organic acids, and all organic acids you're likely to see on the MCAT, are said to be weak acids because they do NOT dissociate completely in solution.

The strength of the acid is determined by the extent to which the negative charge on the conjugate base is stabilized. This means all you need to rank the relative acidity of organic compounds on the MCAT is your background in ranking the stability of reactive intermediates.

Electronegativity Effects

For example, let's compare the acidity of an alcohol like propanol and an alkane like propane. If we compare the stability of each conjugate base, we find that the alkoxide ion is a relatively stable species compared to the carbanion since the negative charge is located on the very electronegative oxygen atom rather than on a carbon atom.

CH$_3$CH$_2$CH$_2$——Ö——H   CH$_3$CH$_2$CH$_2$——Ö:$^{\ominus}$

an alcohol   *an alkoxide ion*

CH$_3$CH$_2$CH$_2$——H   CH$_3$CH$_2$CH$_2$$^{\ominus}$

an alkane   *a carbanion*

Therefore, alcohols are considerably more acidic than hydrocarbons.

Resonance Effects

Let's next compare the relative acidities of propanol and propanoic acid.

a carboxylic acid

a carboxylate ion

In the carboxylate ion, the electrons on the negatively charged oxygen are adjacent to a π bond and can therefore be delocalized. This leads to greater stability of the carboxylate anion and thus to higher acidity of the conjugate acid.

sp² hybridized carbon

These electrons are one atom away from a π bond and therefore can be delocalized.

a carboxylate ion

Note that the two resonance structures of the carboxylate ion are equivalent, and are therefore of equal energy.

resonance structures for carboxylate ion

In contrast, the electrons on the oxygen of the propoxide ion below have no adjacent empty *p* orbital or π system. Therefore, they are localized and highly reactive, making an alkoxide ion a very strong base (much like OH⁻) and the alcohol a weak acid.

an alkoxide ion

sp³ hybridized carbon

This carbon has no unhybridized *p* orbital. Therefore no resonance delocalization of the adjacent lone pairs is possible.

n-propoxide

This makes carboxylic acids, as their name suggests, much more acidic than alcohols.

Example 4-4: Rank the following acids in order of increasing acidity:

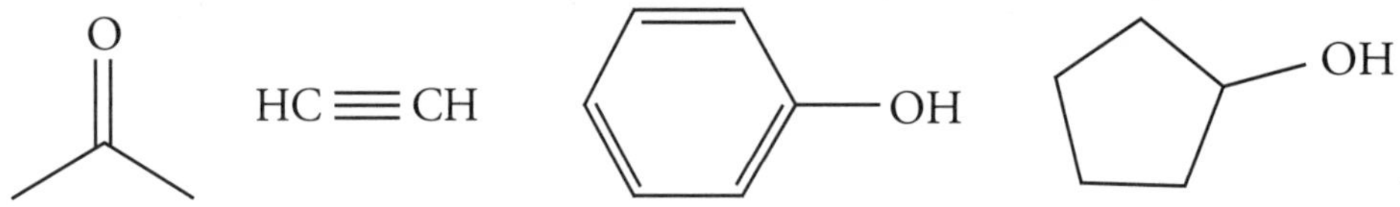

Solution: We examine the conjugate base of each acid in order to determine which one will have the more stabilized anion.

For the acetylene, there are no possible resonance structures for its conjugate base, and the negative charge is localized on carbon, an element with low electronegativity; **rank 1st** as the weakest acid.

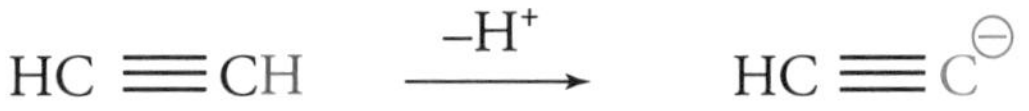

In acetone, the hydrogens next to the carbonyl are acidic because there are two resonance structures for the conjugate base of a ketone. One is stable with the negative charge on oxygen, and one is higher in energy with the negative charge on carbon. Even though it has resonance, it is less acidic than cyclopentanol (see below) because some of the charge resides on the carbon; **rank 2nd.**

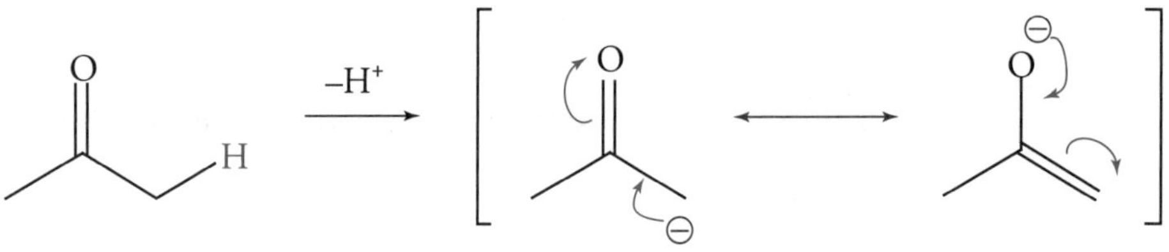

There are no possible resonance structures for this molecule, but the negative charge resides on an electronegative oxygen; **rank 3rd.**

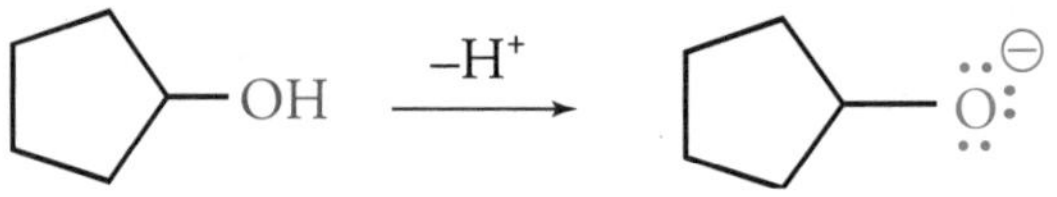

Four resonance structures are possible for the phenoxide ion because the negative charge on the oxygen is adjacent to a benzene ring. However, they are not all of equivalent energy because the negative charge resides on the less electronegative C in three of the four structures. The delocalization of charge means that a phenol (–OH group attached to a benzene ring) is more acidic than an alkyl alcohol; **rank 4th** as the strongest acid.

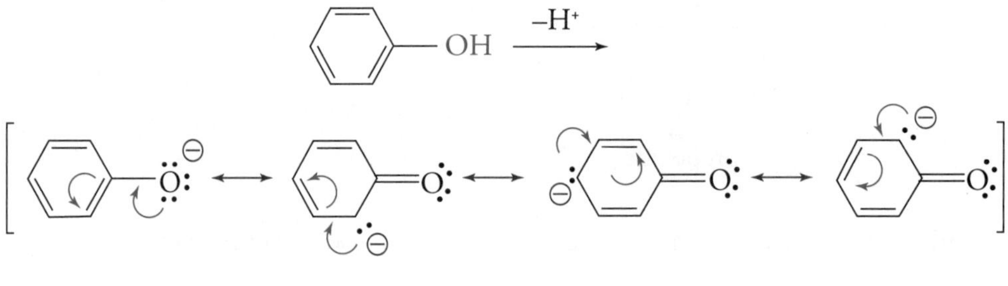

Note that the phenol on the previous page would still be less acidic than a carboxylic acid since both resonance structures of a carboxylate ion have the negative charge on oxygen, rather than the less electro-negative carbon in the phenoxide ion.

To summarize, here is a general ranking of the relative acidities of the most important organic functional groups you are likely to see on the MCAT:

General Rule of Thumb for Organic Compound Acidity

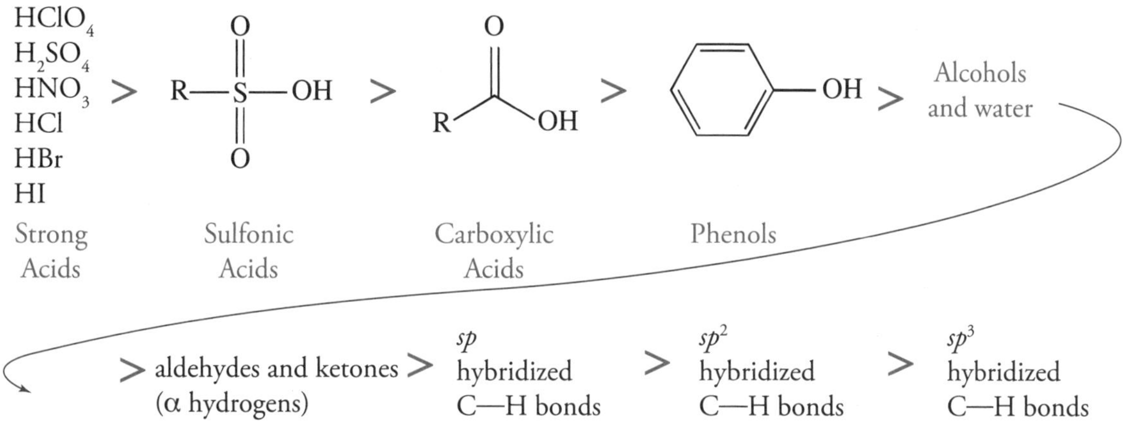

$HClO_4$
H_2SO_4
HNO_3 > R—S—OH > (carboxylic) > (phenol)—OH > Alcohols and water >
HCl
HBr
HI

Strong Acids   Sulfonic Acids   Carboxylic Acids   Phenols

> aldehydes and ketones > sp hybridized C—H bonds > sp^2 hybridized C—H bonds > sp^3 hybridized C—H bonds
(α hydrogens)

Inductive Effects

As we've just learned, the acidity of carboxylic acids compared to alcohols results from the resonance stability of the carboxylate anion. In addition, Example 4-2 briefly illustrated how electron-withdrawing substituents next to the carboxylic acid group can increase the acidity of this (or any) functional group by increasing the stability of the negative charge on the anion. To expand upon this idea, inductive effects decrease with increasing distance; the closer the electron-withdrawing group is to the acidic proton (or the negative charge on the conjugate base), the greater the stabilizing effect. The following order of acidity for the isomers of fluorobutanoic acid should help clarify this point.

Order of Acidity

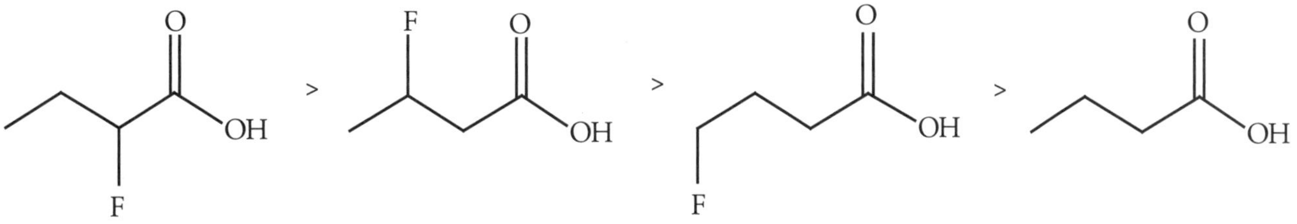

most acidic   least acidic

The magnitude of the effect is also dependent on the strength of the electron withdrawing substituent. In general, the more electronegative a substituent is, the greater its inductive effect will be. As shown below, while trifluoro-, trichloro-, and tribromoacetic acid all have substantially lower pK_a values than standard acetic acid (pK_a = 4.76), the trend in their acidities mirrors the electronegativity of their respective inductive group.

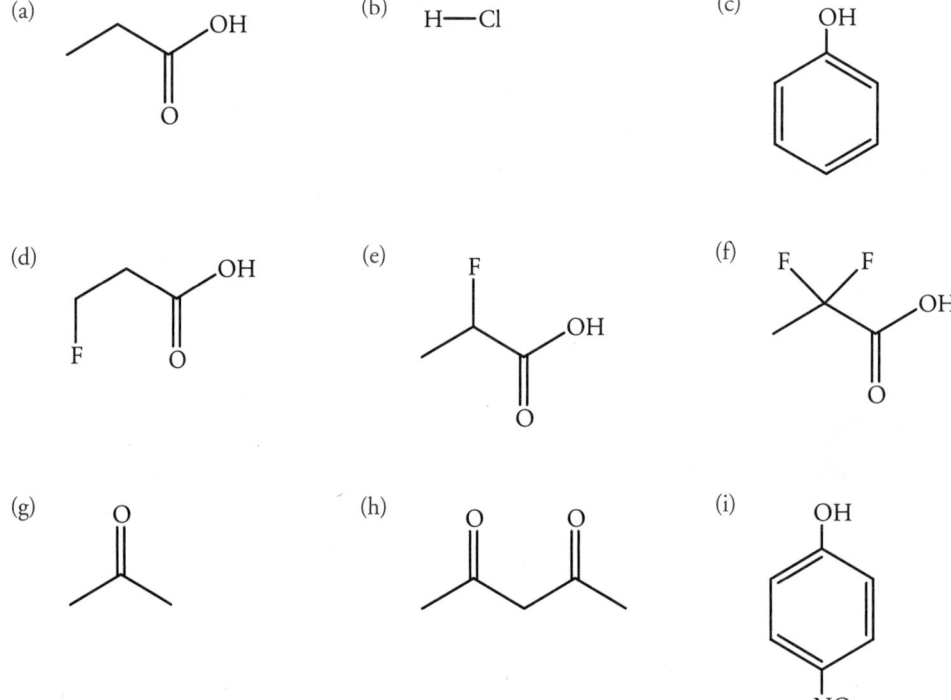

Example 4-5: Rank the following nine compounds in order of decreasing acidity.

Solution:

(b)	>	(f)	>	(e)	>	(d)	>	(a)
strong acid		difluorinated carboxylic acid		monofluorinated carboxylic acid in α position		monofluorinated carboxylic acid in β position		carboxylic acid

	>	(i)	>	(c)	~	(h)	>	(g)
		phenol with electron withdrawing nitro group		phenol		diketone with 2 α protons adjacent to 2 carbonyls		ketone

Effects of Substituents on Acidity

Electron-withdrawing substituents on phenols increase their acidity. As an example, consider *para*-nitrophenol. The nitro group is strongly electron-withdrawing and greatly stabilizes the phenoxide ion through resonance. Once the *para*-nitrophenol is deprotonated, it's easy to see how the nitro group can withdraw electrons through the delocalized π system such that the negative charge on the phenoxide oxygen can be delocalized all the way to an oxygen atom of the nitro group. This electron-withdrawing resonance stabilization of the nitro group increases the acidity of *para*-nitrophenol as compared to a phenol that does not have electron-withdrawing substituents.

On the other hand, consider a substituted phenol that has an electron-*donating* group rather than an electron-*withdrawing* group. A good example of this is *para*-methoxyphenol. Here, it is easy to see how once *para*-methoxyphenol is deprotonated, the negative charge on the oxygen can be destabilized by the donation of a lone pair of electrons from the methoxy oxygen so a negative charge is placed on a carbon that's adjacent to the negatively charged phenoxide oxygen. Electron-donating groups tend to destabilize a phenoxide ion and decrease the acidity of substituted phenols.

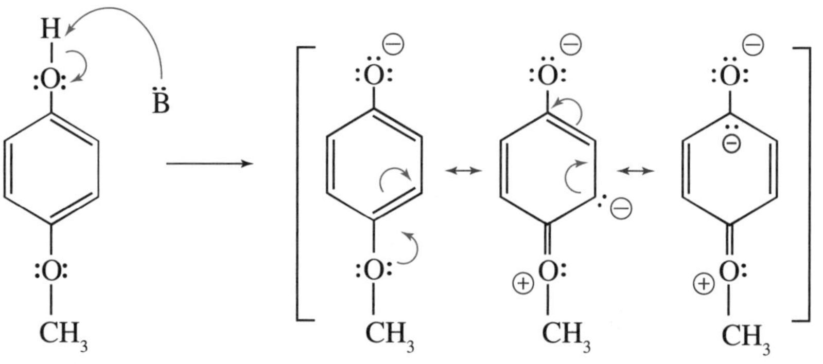

Example 4-6: For each of the following groups of three phenols, rank them in order of decreasing acidity.

(i)

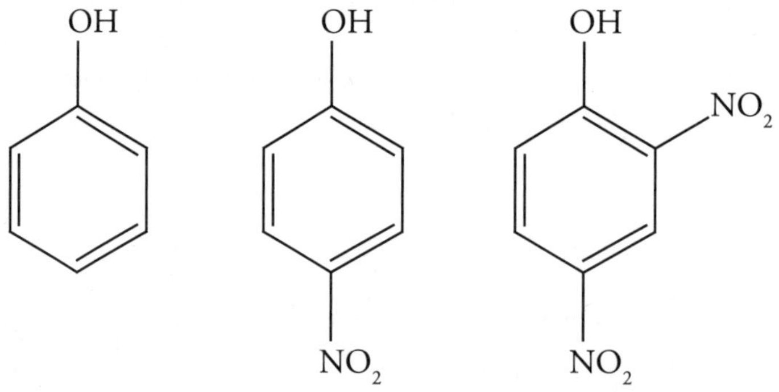

A   B   C

(ii)

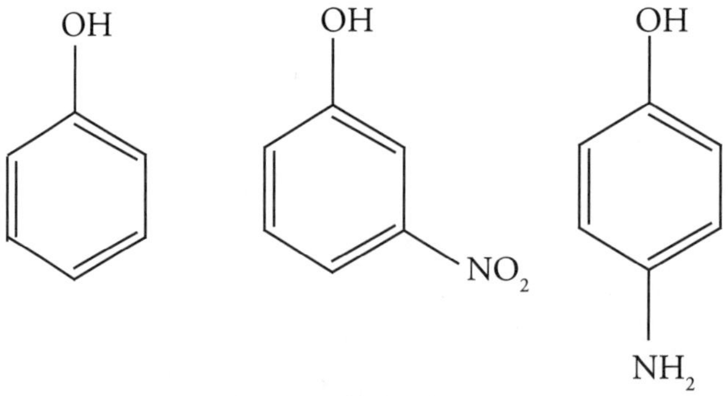

A   B   C

Solution:

(i)   C > B > A. Compound C is the most acidic because of the two electron-withdrawing nitro groups. They delocalize the charge of the conjugate base, making C a stronger acid. The *para*-nitro group in B can also delocalize the charge by resonance, though not as well as the two nitro groups in choice C. Finally, A is the least acidic, since it has no electron-withdrawing groups to stabilize the charge.

(ii)   B > A > C. Since the amino group in choice C is similar to the OCH_3 group discussed above due to the lone pair of electrons on the N, it is also an electron-donating group. As such, it will decrease the acidity of the phenol, making it the least acidic of the three compounds.

Nucleophiles and Electrophiles

Most organic reactions occur between nucleophiles and electrophiles. **Nucleophiles** are species that have unshared pairs of electrons or π bonds and, frequently, a negative (or partial negative, δ^-) charge. As the name *nucleophile* implies, they are "nucleus-seeking" or "nucleus-loving" molecules. Since nucleophiles are electron pair donors, they are also known as **Lewis bases**. Here are some common examples of nucleophiles:

Nucleophilicity is a measure of how "strong" a nucleophile is. There are general trends for relative nucleophilicities:

1. **Nucleophilicity increases as negative charge increases.** For example, NH_2^- is more nucleophilic than NH_3.
2. **Nucleophilicity increases going down the periodic table within a particular group.** For example, $F^- < Cl^- < Br^- < I^-$.
3. **Nucleophilicity increases going left in the periodic table across a particular period.** For example, NH_2^- is more nucleophilic than OH^-.

Trend #2 is directly related to a periodic trend introduced in general chemistry: **polarizability**. Polarizability is the measure of how easy it is for the electrons surrounding an atom to be distorted. As you go down any group in the periodic table, atoms become larger and generally more polarizable and more nucleophilic.

Trend #3 is related to the electronegativity of the nucleophilic atom. The more electronegative the atom is, the better it is able to support its negative charge. Therefore, the less electronegative an atom is, the higher its nucleophilicity.

You should note that Trend #2 should only be applied for atoms within a column of the periodic table, while Trend #3 should be applied for atoms across a row of the periodic table.

Example 4-7: In each of the following pairs of molecules, identify the one that is more nucleophilic.

(a)   H—$\ddot{\ddot{O}}$:$^\ominus$ or   H—$\ddot{\ddot{S}}$:$^\ominus$

(b)   H—$\ddot{\ddot{O}}$:$^\ominus$ or $\ddot{O}$ with H and H

(c) $\overset{\ominus}{\ddot{N}}$ with H and H   or   :$\ddot{\ddot{F}}$:$^\ominus$

(d) $\overset{\ominus}{\ddot{N}}$ with H and H   or   H—$\overset{\ominus}{C}$—H with H below

Solution:

(a)   SH⁻, since by Trend #2 on the previous page, S is more nucleophilic than O.
(b)   OH⁻, because OH⁻ carries a negative charge, while H_2O does not (Trend #1, previous page).
(c) NH_2^-, since F is more electronegative than N.
(d) CH_3^-, because N is more electronegative than C.

Electrophiles are electron-deficient species. They have a full or partial positive (δ^+) charge and "love electrons." Frequently, they have an incomplete octet. **Electrophilicity** is a measure of how strong an electrophile is. Since electrophiles are electron pair acceptors, they are also known as **Lewis acids**. Here are some common examples of electrophiles:

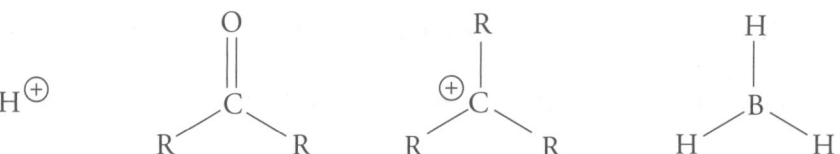

In all organic reactions (except free-radical and pericyclic reactions), nucleophiles are attracted—and donate a pair of electrons—to electrophiles. When the electrophile accepts the electron pair (a Lewis acid/Lewis base reaction), a new covalent bond forms between the two species, which we can represent symbolically like this:

E$^\oplus$ + :Nu$^\ominus$ ⟶ E—Nu

Leaving Groups

While students of organic chemistry often associate the discussion of leaving groups with substitution and elimination reactions, these reaction types are beyond the scope of the MCAT. However, a good understanding of leaving group ability will be useful for several reactions we'll review in Chapter 6.

Generally speaking, the biggest take-home message about leaving groups is that they are more likely to dissociate from their substrate (i.e., do their "leaving") if they are more stable in solution. Sound familiar? Our understanding of stability and reactivity is all we need to explain relative leaving group ability. For example, leaving groups that are resonance-stabilized (like tosylate, mesylate, and acetate) are some of the best ones out there. We'll discuss these groups in more detail in Chapter 6.

Resonance Structures of the Mesylate Leaving Group

In addition, weak bases (I⁻, Br⁻, Cl⁻, etc.) are good leaving groups because their negative charge is stabilized due to their large size. In fact, it's because basicity decreases down a family in the periodic table that leaving group ability increases. This periodic trend will be true for any family, though the halogens are the most common leaving groups you'll likely come across.

Strong bases (HO⁻, RO⁻, NH₂⁻, etc.), on the other hand, are great electron donors because they cannot stabilize their negative charge very well, making them very reactive. As a result, these groups are more likely to stay bound to their substrate rather than dissociate in solution. As you might expect, strong bases are therefore bad leaving groups.

Now just because you're a bad leaving group one minute doesn't mean you can't be made better. For example, while the –OH group of an alcohol is unlikely to dissociate as OH⁻, treating the compound with acid protonates a lone pair of electrons on the oxygen, thereby making the –OH into –OH₂⁺. The altered group can dissociate as a neutral water molecule, and *voila*!—no negative charge to stabilize. This trick will work for any of the strong bases listed above, and is the reason why many organic reactions are acid-catalyzed.

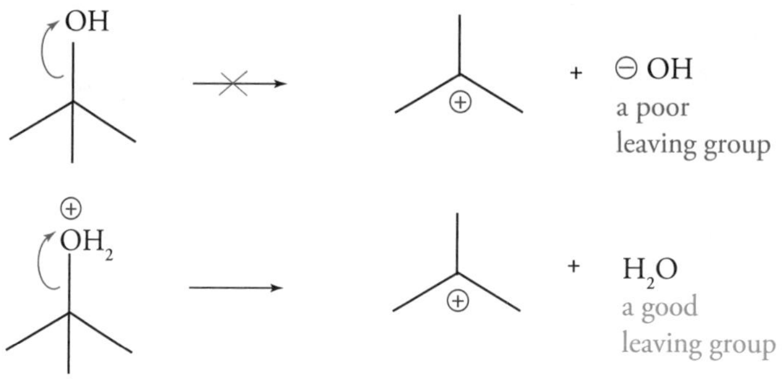

+ $\ominus$ OH
a poor
leaving group

+ H_2O
a good
leaving group

Ring Strain

The last item in our toolbox is a feature of organic molecules that, unlike inductive and resonance effects, contributes to instability in a molecule: **ring strain**. Ring strain arises when bond angles between ring atoms deviate from the ideal angle predicted by the hybridization of the atoms. Let's examine several cycloalkanes in turn.

Cyclopropane (C_3H_6) is very strained because the carbon-carbon bond angles approach 60° rather than the idealized 109° for sp^3 hybridized carbons.

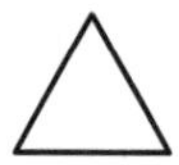

Cyclopropane

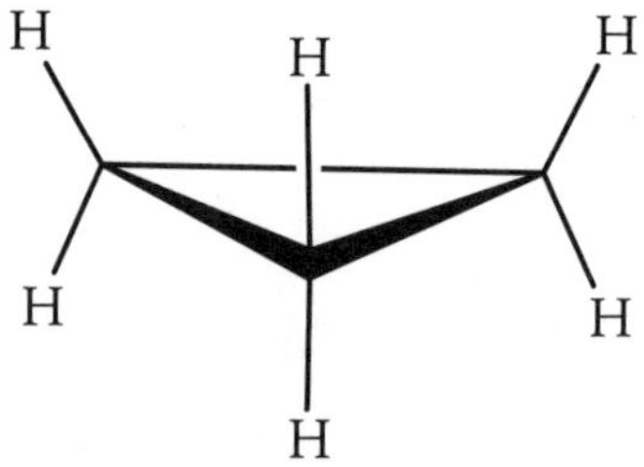

Cyclobutane (C_4H_8) might be expected to have 90° bond angles. However, one of the carbons is bent out of the plane, such that all of the bond angles are 88°. The distortion of the cyclobutane ring minimizes the eclipsing of carbon-hydrogen σ bonds on adjacent carbon atoms.

Cyclobutane

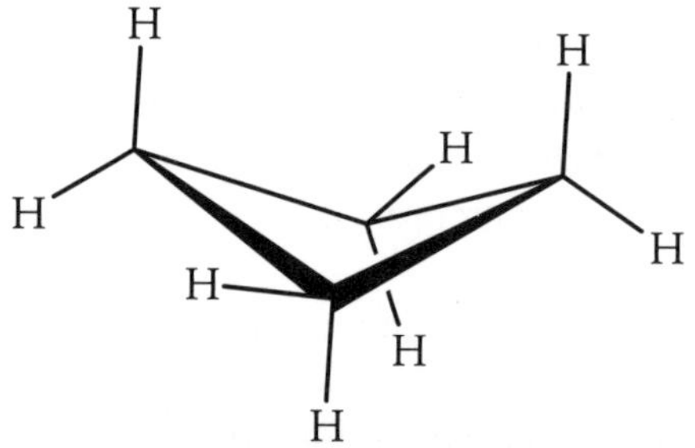

The deviation of the bond angles from the normal tetrahedral 109° causes cyclopropane and cyclobutane to be high energy compounds. The strain weakens the carbon-carbon bonds and increases reactivity of these cycloalkanes in comparison to other alkanes. For example, while it is essentially impossible to cleave the average alkane C—C single bond via hydrogenation, C—C bonds in these highly strained cyclic molecules are significantly more reactive. However, they are still much less reactive than C=C double (π) bonds.

Hydrogenation Reactions of Cyclopropane and Cyclobutane

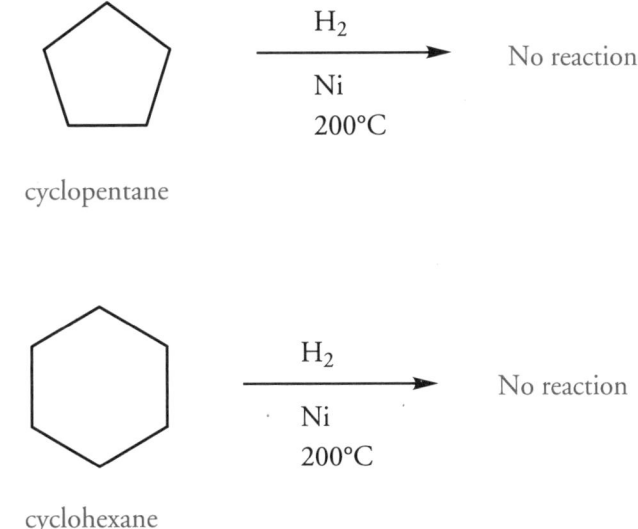

Unlike cyclopropane and cyclobutane, cyclopentane has a low degree of ring strain, and cyclohexane is strain free. Both molecules have near-tetrahedral bond angles (109°) due to the conformations they adopt. Consequently, these cycloalkanes do not undergo hydrogenation reactions under normal conditions, and react similarly to straight chain alkanes.

4.2 ISOMERISM

Constitutional Isomerism

Constitutional (or, less precisely, *structural*) **isomers** are compounds that have the same molecular formula but have their atoms connected together differently. Take pentane (C_5H_{12}), for example. *n*-Pentane is a fully saturated hydrocarbon that has two additional constitutional isomers:

n-pentane   isopentane   neopentane

Example 4-8: Draw (and name) all the constitutional isomers of hexane, C_6H_{14}. (*Hint*: There are five of them altogether.)

Solution:

n-hexane   2-methylpentane   3-methylpentane

2,3-dimethylbutane   2,2-dimethylbutane

Conformational Isomerism

Conformational isomers are compounds that have the same molecular formula and the same atomic connectivity, but differ from one another by rotation about a σ bond. In truth, they are the exact same molecule. For saturated hydrocarbons, there are two orientations of σ bonds attached to adjacent sp^3 hybridized carbons on which we will concentrate. These are the **staggered** conformation and the **eclipsed** conformation. In staggered conformations, a σ bond on one carbon bisects the angle formed by two σ bonds on the adjacent carbon. In an eclipsed conformation, a σ bond on one carbon directly lines up with a σ bond on an adjacent carbon. Both conformations can be visualized using either the flagged bond notation, or the Newman projection, as shown with ethane (C_2H_6) on the next page.

This vertex represents
the closer (front)
carbon atom.

If we were to look
down the C–C bond,
we would see:

A staggered conformation

A staggered conformation

This circle represents
the back carbon atom.

An eclipsed conformation

An eclipsed conformation

Example 4-9: For (a) and (b), represent the flagged bond notation conformation as a Newman projection. For (c) and (d), represent the Newman projection using flagged bond notation, and be sure to label which bond you are looking down when translating from the Newman projection.

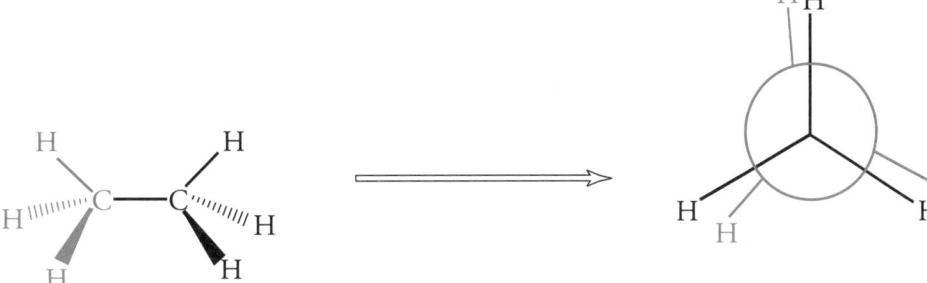

(a)

(b)

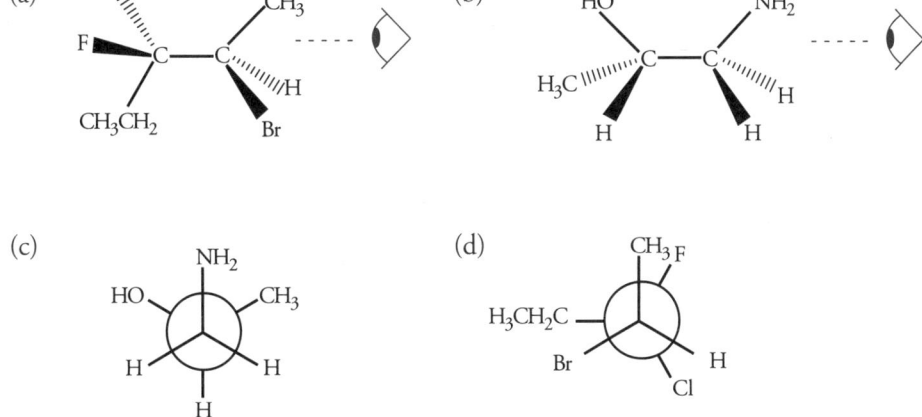

(c)

(d)

Solution:

(a)

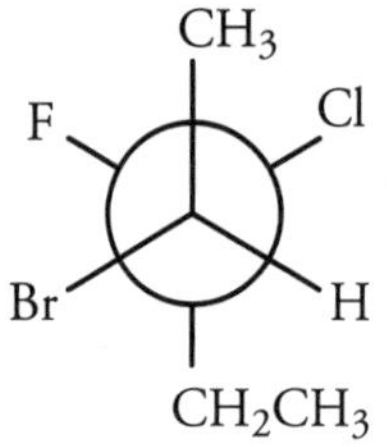

(b)

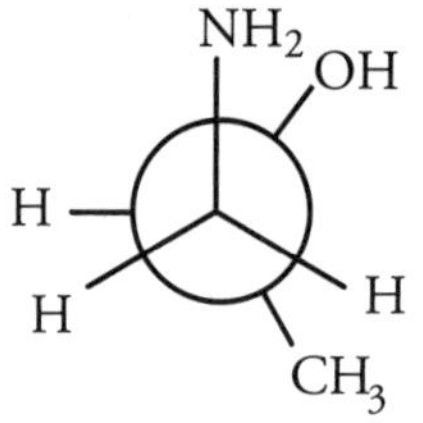

(c)

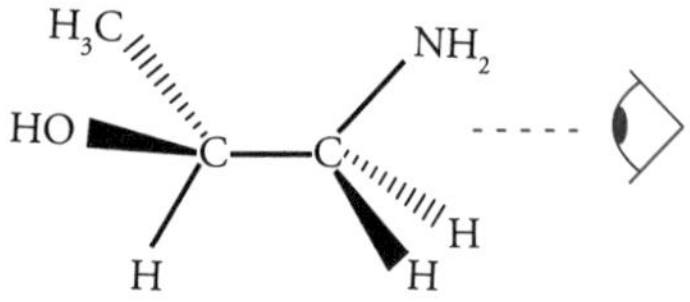

(d)

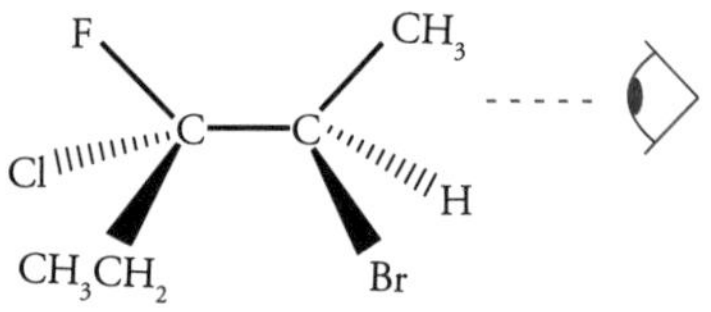

Using these notations, we turn our attention to the conformational analysis of hydrocarbons as demonstrated for *n*-butane.

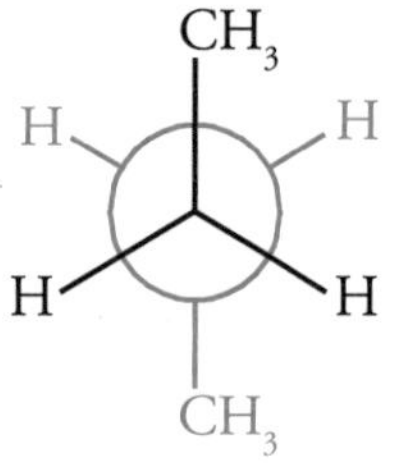

staggered conformation

less crowded
more stable

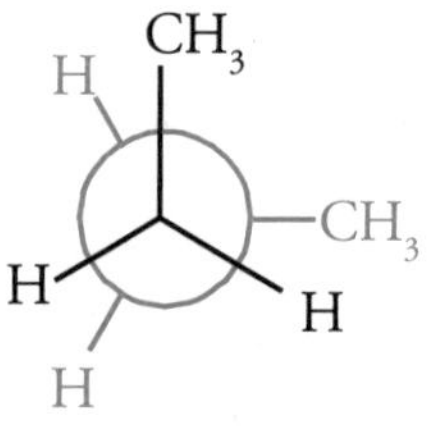

eclipsed conformation

more crowded
electronic repulsion
less stable

The σ bonds should
actually directly
line up with each other.
For clarity here,
they are not
directly aligned.

It's important to note, however, that there are an infinite number of conformations for a molecule that has free rotation around a C—C bond, and that all of these other conformations are energetically related to the staggered and eclipsed conformations on which we will concentrate. For example, relative to the carbon atom in the rear of a Newman projection, the front carbon atom could be rotated *any number of degrees*. Any change in the rotation of one carbon, relative to its adjacent neighbor, is a change in molecular conformation.

What are the relative stabilities of the staggered conformations, the eclipsed conformations, and the infinite number of conformations that are in between them? A staggered conformation is more stable than an eclipsed conformation for two reasons. First, the staggered conformation is more stable than the eclipsed conformation because of electronic repulsion. Covalent bonds repel one another simply because they are composed of (negatively charged) electrons. That being the case, the staggered conformation is more stable than the eclipsed, since in the staggered conformation, the σ bonds are as far apart as possible, while in the eclipsed conformation they are directly aligned with one another. The other major reason the staggered conformation is more stable than the eclipsed conformation is steric hindrance. It is more favorable to have atoms attached to the σ bonds in the roomier staggered conformation where they are 60° apart, rather than the eclipsed conformation where they are directly aligned with one another. There are further aspects to consider in conformational analysis. Not all staggered conformations are of equal energy. Likewise, not all eclipsed conformations are of equal energy. There are particularly stable staggered conformations and particularly unstable eclipsed conformations. The following demonstrates this by examining all staggered and eclipsed conformations for *n*-butane.

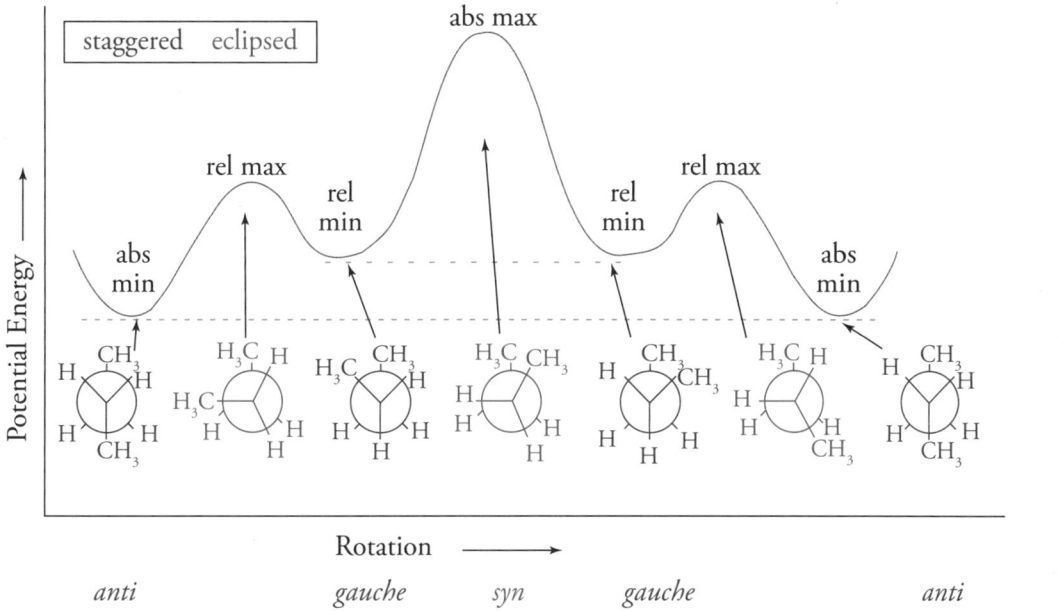

We begin our discussion with the most stable conformation of *n*-butane. This staggered conformation is referred to as the ***anti* conformation** and arises when the two largest groups attached to adjacent carbons are 180° apart. This produces the most sterically favorable, and hence the most energetically favorable (lowest energy) conformation. Now we proceed through a series of 60° rotations around the C2—C3 σ bond until we return to the initial conformation (360°). In our first rotation, we go from the *anti* staggered to an eclipsed conformation and observe the relative energy maximum that results from the alignment of the methyls and hydrogens. Next as we rotate another 60°, we fall again into a staggered conformation that resides in a relative energy minimum. Notice that this energy minimum is not as low as the *anti* conformation. In this structure, the methyl substituents are closer together than in the *anti* conformation. They are now 60° apart; this is referred to as a ***gauche* conformation**. A *gauche* conformation arises when the two largest groups on adjacent carbon atoms are in a staggered conformation 60° apart. In our next 60° rotation, we travel to the absolute maximum on our potential energy diagram. In this eclipsed conformation, the two methyl groups are directly aligned behind one another and are therefore in the most crowded and unfavorable environment. This conformation is referred to as the ***syn* conformation**. As we continue our rotation, we fall from the absolute energy maximum and go through the corresponding staggered and eclipsed conformations encountered before.

Example 4-10: Draw a Newman projection for the most stable conformation of each of these compounds:

(a) 2,2,5,5-tetramethylhexane (about the C3—C4 bond)
(b) 2,2-dimethylpentane (about the C2—C3 bond)
(c) 1,2-ethandiol

Solution:

(a) (b)

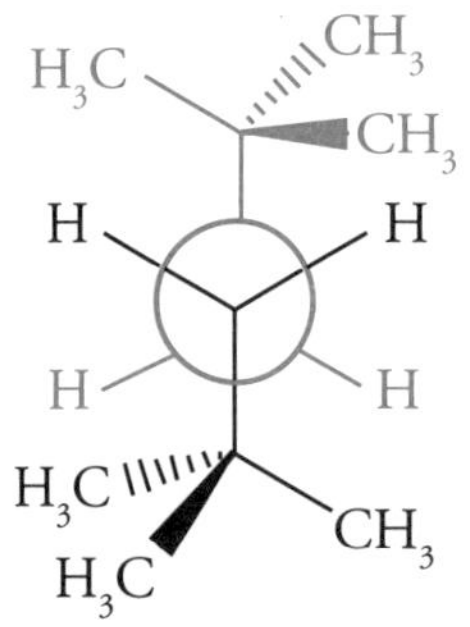

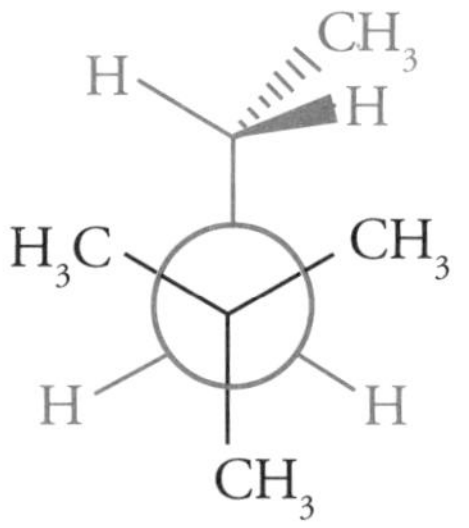

(c) In this molecule, the *gauche* conformation is more stable than the *anti* conformation, because an intramolecular hydrogen bond can be formed in the *gauche* but not in the *anti* conformation.

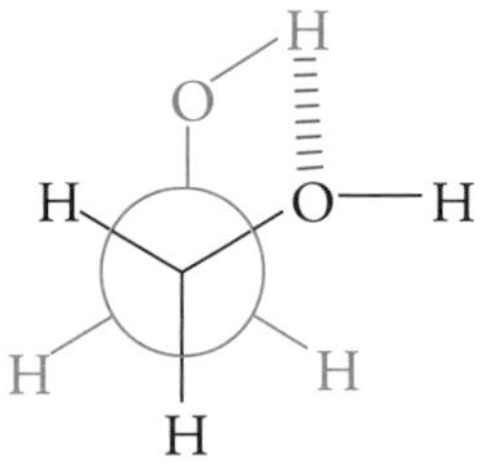

Remember that it's usually the case that the *anti* conformation is the more stable. In general, the two largest groups on adjacent carbon atoms would like to be *anti* to one another since this will minimize steric interactions. However, if the two groups are not too large and can form intramolecular hydrogen bonds with one another, then the *gauche* conformation can be more stable.

Thus far we've limited our discussion of conformational isomers to molecules with unrestricted rotation around σ bonds. Let's now consider the conformational analysis of two very common cycloalkanes, cyclopentane (C_5H_{10}) and cyclohexane (C_6H_{12}).

In cyclopentane, the pentagonal bond angle is 108° (close to normal tetrahedral of 109°), so we might expect cyclopentane to be a planar structure. If all of the carbons of cyclopentane were in a plane, however, all of the carbon-hydrogen σ bonds on adjacent carbons would eclipse each other. In order to compensate for the eclipsed C—H σ bonds, cyclopentane has one carbon out of the plane of the other carbons and so adopts a puckered conformation. This puckering allows the carbon-hydrogen σ bonds on adjacent carbons to be somewhat staggered, and thus reduces the energy of the compound. This puckered form of cyclopentane is referred to as the "envelope" form.

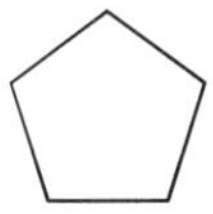

Cyclopentane

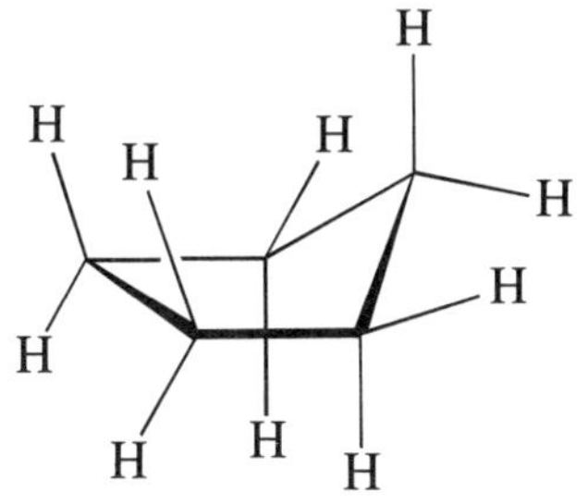

If cyclohexane were planar, it would have bond angles of 120°. This would produce considerable strain on sp^3 hybridized carbons as the ideal bond angle should be around 109°. Instead, the most stable conformation of cyclohexane is a very puckered molecule referred to as the chair form. In the **chair conformation**, four of the carbons of the ring are in a plane with one carbon above the plane and one carbon below the plane. There are two chair conformations for cyclohexane, and they easily interconvert at room temperature:

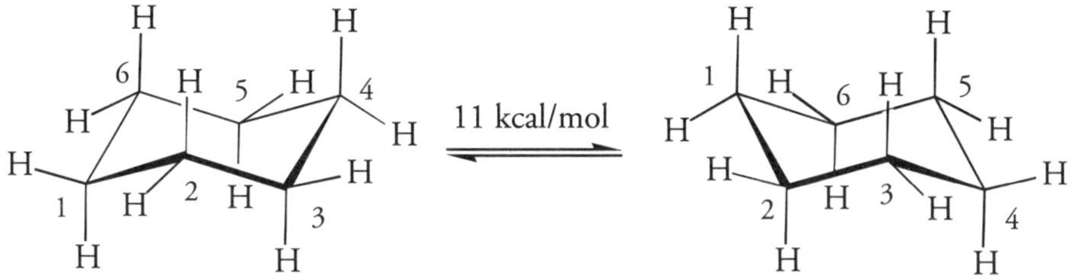

Chair representations of cyclohexane

As one chair conformation flips to the other chair conformation, it must pass through several other less stable conformations including some (referred to as *half-chair* **conformations**) that reside at energy maxima and one (the ***twist boat* conformation**) at a local energy minimum (but still of much higher energy than the chair conformations). The boat conformation represents a transition state between twist boat conformations. It is important to remember, however, that all of these conformations are much more unstable than the chair conformations and thus do not play an important role in cyclohexane chemistry.

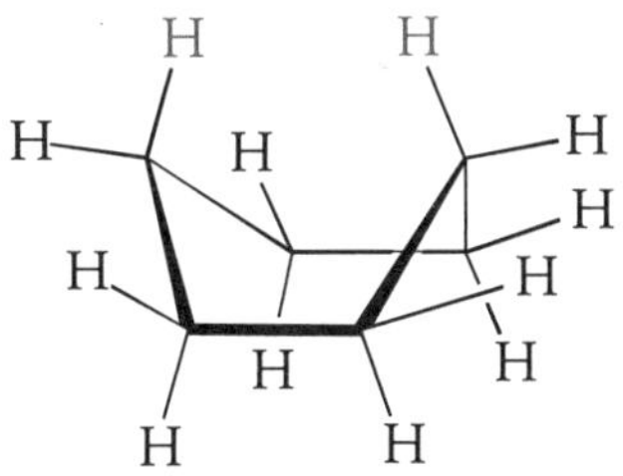

Boat conformation

4.2

Notice that there are two distinct types of hydrogens in the chair forms of cyclohexane. Six of the hydrogens lie on the equator of the ring of carbons. These hydrogens are referred to as **equatorial hydrogens**. The other six hydrogens lie above or below the ring of carbons, three above and three below; these are called **axial hydrogens**.

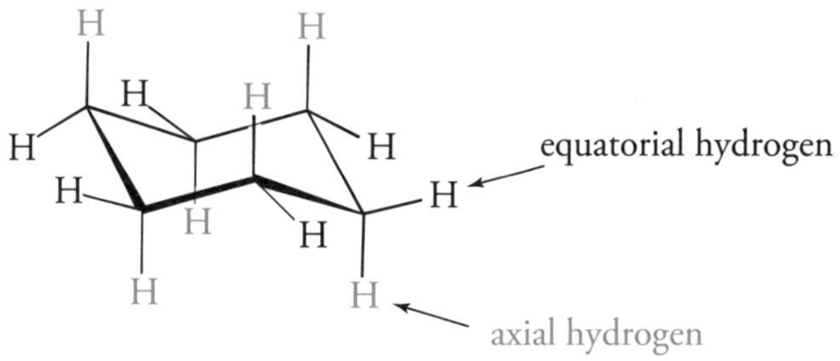

There is an energy barrier of about 11 kcal/mol between the two equivalent chair conformations of cyclohexane. At room temperature there is sufficient thermal energy to interconvert the two chair conformations about 10,000 times per second. Note that when a hydrogen (or any substituent group) is axial in one chair conformation, it becomes equatorial when cyclohexane flips to the other chair conformation. The same is also true for an equatorial hydrogen that flips to an axial position when the chair forms interconvert. This property is demonstrated for deuterocyclohexane:

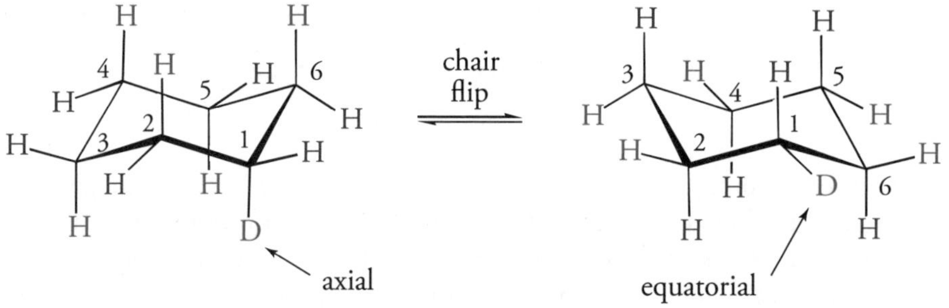

These factors become important when examining substituted cyclohexanes. Let's first consider methylcyclohexane. The methyl group can occupy either an equatorial or axial position:

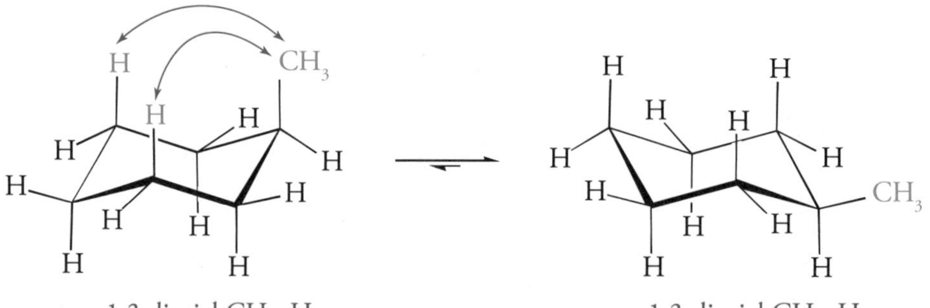

two 1,3-diaxial CH₃–H interactions

no 1,3-diaxial CH₃–H interactions

Is one conformation more stable than the other? *Yes*. It is more favorable for large groups to occupy the equatorial position rather than a crowded axial position. For a methyl group, the equatorial position is more stable by about 1.7 kcal/mol over the axial position. This is because in the axial position, the methyl group is crowded by the other two hydrogens that are also occupying axial positions on the same side of the ring. This is referred to as a **1,3-diaxial interaction**. It is more favorable for methyl to be in an equatorial position where it is pointing out, away from other atoms.

Example 4-11: In each of the following pairs of substituted cyclohexanes, identify the more stable isomer:

4.2

Solution: Draw chair conformations of each isomer and compare them to see which is more stable. As a good rule of thumb, it's best to first put the bulkier (i.e., the larger) substituent in a roomier equatorial position and decide if it's the more stable of the two chair conformations; it usually is. (See figures below.)

(a)

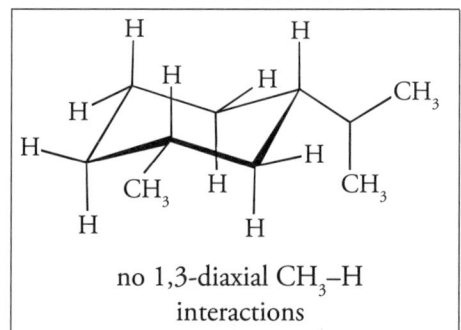

This is the more stable isomer.

two 1,3-diaxial CH₃–H
interactions

vs.

no 1,3-diaxial CH₃–H
interactions

(b)

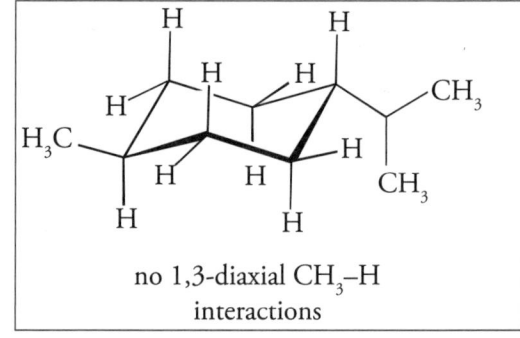

This is the more stable isomer.

two 1,3-diaxial CH₃–H
interactions

vs.

no 1,3-diaxial CH₃–H
interactions

(c)

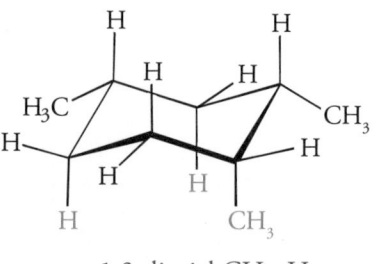

This is the more stable isomer.

two 1,3-diaxial CH₃–H
interactions

vs.

no 1,3-diaxial CH₃–H
interactions

(d)

This is the more stable isomer.

no 1,3-diaxial CH₃–H
interactions

vs.

two 1,3-diaxial CH₃–H
interactions

Stereoisomerism

Stereoisomerism is of major importance in organic chemistry, especially when looking at biological molecules, so several questions relating to stereochemistry routinely appear on the MCAT. **Stereoisomers** are molecules that have the same molecular formula and connectivity but differ from one another only in the spatial arrangement of the atoms. They cannot be interconverted by rotation of σ bonds. For example, consider the following two molecules:

Molecule I   Molecule II

Both molecules have the same molecular formula, C_2H_5ClO, with the same atoms bonded to each other. However, if one superimposes II onto I without any rotation, the result is:

Note that while the –CH_3 and –OH groups superimpose, the –Cl and –H do not. Likewise, if we rotate Molecule II so that the –OH is pointing directly up (12 o'clock) and the –CH_3 is pointing at about 7 o'clock, and then attempt to superimpose II on I, the result is:

While the –Cl and the –H groups are now superimposed, the –CH_3 and the –OH are not. No matter how one rotates Molecules I and II, two of the substituent groups will be superimposed, while the other two will not. Hence they are indeed different molecules; they are stereoisomers.

4.2

Chirality

Any molecule that cannot be superimposed on its mirror image is said to be **chiral**, while a molecule that *can* be superimposed on its mirror image has a plane of symmetry and is said to be **achiral**. It's important that you be able to identify **chiral centers**. For carbon, a chiral center will have four different groups bonded to it. Note that since a carbon atom has four different groups attached to it, it must be sp^3 hybridized with (approximately) 109° bond angles and tetrahedral geometry. Such a carbon atom is also sometimes referred to as a **stereocenter**, a **stereogenic center**, or an **asymmetric center**.

Example 4-12: Identify all the chiral centers in the following molecules and determine how many possible stereoisomers each compound has by placing a star next to each chiral center. (Note: The number of possible stereoisomers equals 2^n, where n is the number of chiral centers.)

(a)

(b)

(c)

(d)

(e)

(f)

(g)

(h)

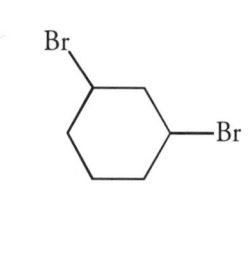

(i)

Solution:

(a) This molecule has no chiral centers.

(b) This molecule has 1 chiral center and, therefore, 2 possible stereoisomers:

*
H

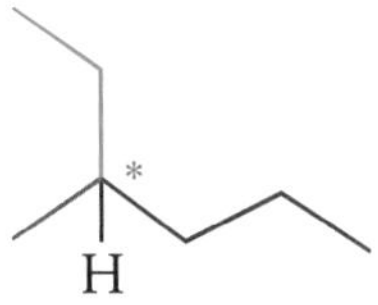

(c) There is 1 chiral center and, therefore, 2 possible stereoisomers:

CH3 H H
H3C C C* C CH3
H CH3 H

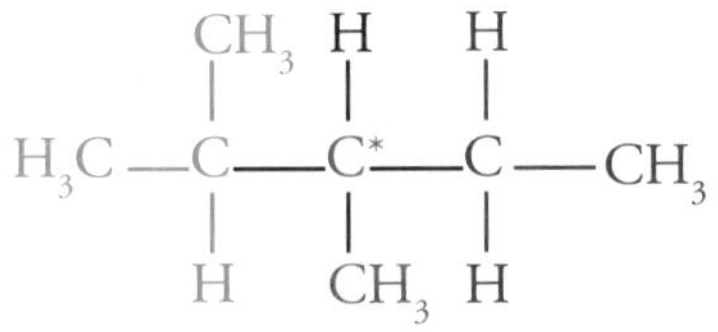

(d) This molecule has 1 chiral center and, therefore, 2 possible stereoisomers:

Br
the back carbon
*
H3C
CH3
H3C
H
OH

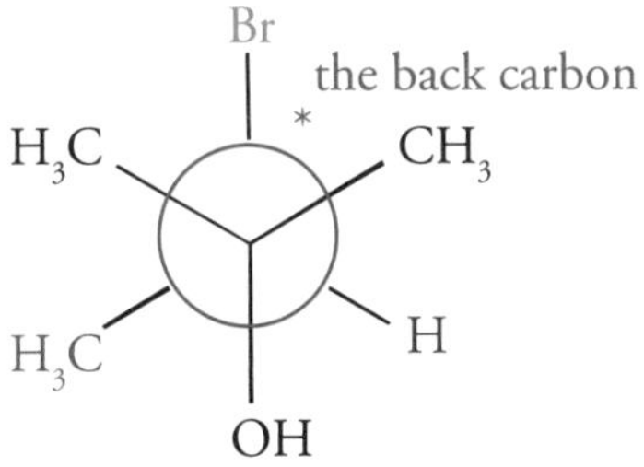

(e) There are 2 chiral centers and, therefore, 4 possible stereoisomers:

CH3
*
H3C
Br
*
HO
D
OH

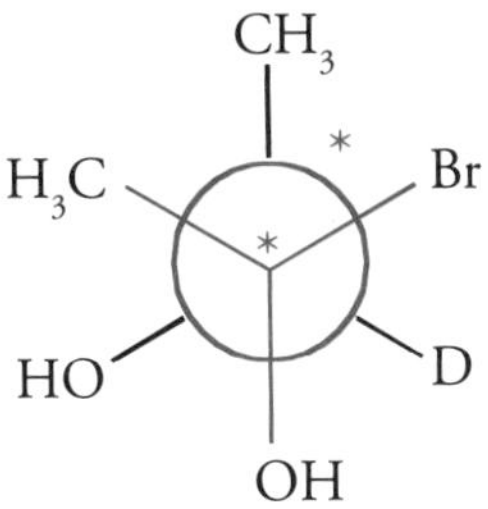

(f)   There are 2 chiral centers, which would seem to indicate 4 possible stereoisomers:

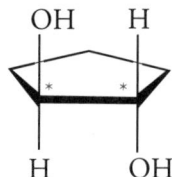

However, there are only 3, because the following "two" molecules are actually the same:

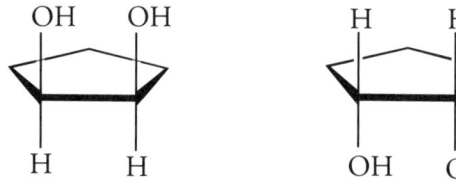

(g)   This molecule has no chiral centers.

(h)   This molecule has 9 chiral centers but because the two leftmost epoxide carbon atoms have two possible configurations (not four), the possible number of stereosiomers is $2^8 = 256$:

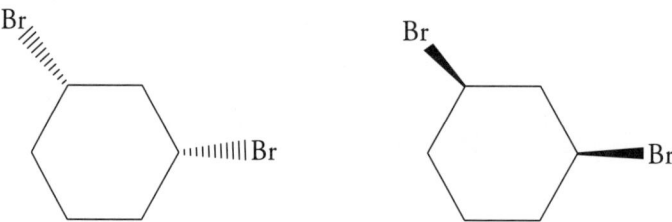

(i)   Although there are two chiral centers,

there are 3, not 4 stereoisomers, because—see (f) above—the following "two" molecules are actually the same:

Absolute Configuration

Chiral centers (carbon atoms bearing four different substituents) can be assigned an **absolute configuration**. There is an arbitrary set of rules for assigning absolute configuration to a stereocenter (known as the **Cahn-Ingold-Prelog rules**), which can be illustrated using Molecule A:

Molecule A

1. Priority is assigned to the four different substituents on the chiral center according to increasing atomic number of the atoms directly attached to the chiral center. Going one atom out from the chiral center, bromine has the highest atomic number and is given highest priority, #1; oxygen is next and is therefore #2; carbon is #3, and the hydrogen is the lowest priority group, #4:

   If isotopes are present, then priority among these are assigned on the basis of atomic weight with the higher priority being assigned to the heavier isotope (since they are all of the same atomic number). For example, the isotopes of hydrogen are ^1H, ^2H = D (deuterium), and ^3H = T (tritium), and for the following molecule, we'd assign priorities as shown:

If two identical atoms are attached to a stereocenter, then the next atoms in both chains are examined until a difference is found. Once again this is done by atomic number. Note the following example:

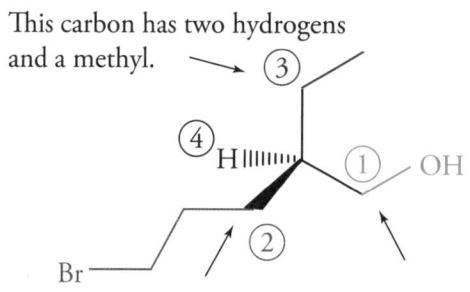

This carbon has two hydrogens and a methyl.

This carbon has two hydrogens followed by a –CH₂CH₂Br.

This carbon has two hydrogens and an –OH.

2. A multiple bond is counted as two single bonds for both of the atoms involved. For example:

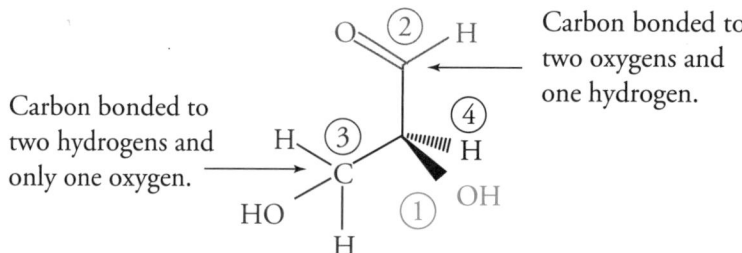

Carbon bonded to two hydrogens and only one oxygen.

Carbon bonded to two oxygens and one hydrogen.

3. Once priorities have been assigned, the molecule is rotated so that the lowest priority group points directly away from the viewer. Then simply trace a path from the highest priority group to the lowest remaining priority group. If the path traveled is *clockwise*, then the absolute configuration is **R** (from the Latin *rectus*, right). Conversely, if the path traveled is *counterclockwise*, then the absolute configuration is **S** (from the Latin *sinister*, left).

Note: The two-dimensional representation (on the left) of the following hypothetical molecule is known as the "Fischer projection," named after famous organic chemist Emil Fischer.

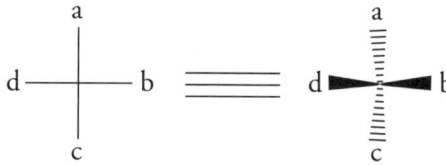

The Fischer projection is a simplification of the actual three-dimensional structure. In the Fischer projection, as shown on the right, vertical lines are assumed to go back into the page, and horizontal lines are assumed to come out of the page.

The Fischer projection will be very important in our discussion of carbohydrates and will be covered extensively in future chapters.

Example 4-13: Assign absolute configurations to the following molecules.

(a)

(b) CH₃
H‖‖‖‖ D
HO

(c) OH
H₂N——C——CH₃
H

(d) H
HO⟍ ‖‖‖‖D
CH₃

(e) ‖‖‖‖ Br
H

(f) O ⟍OH
H NH₂
CH₃

(g)
H ⟍OH

Solution:

(a) *R*. Either rotate the molecule so the lowest priority group is in the back,

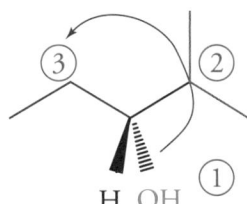

or simply trace it as it stands and invert the configuration (since the lowest priority group is coming toward you):

(b)   *R*. The lowest priority group is already pointing away from you and the trace is clockwise.

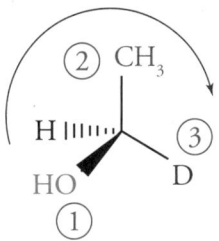

(c)   *S*. Recall Fischer notation for molecules, note that the lowest priority group is pointing away from you, and the trace is counterclockwise.

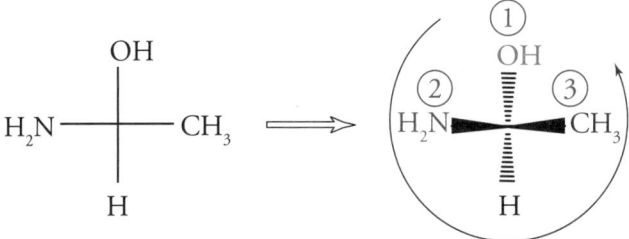

(d)   *R*. The lowest priority group is neither going into nor coming out of the plane of the page. One method is to rotate the molecule so the lowest priority group is in the back and redraw the molecule. Since the path is traveled clockwise, the configuration is *R*.

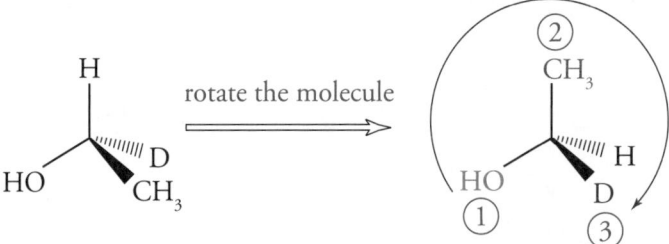

Here's a trick to help in the rotation of molecules. Exchanging two groups on a chiral center necessarily changes the absolute configuration. So in this case, it is perhaps most convenient to exchange any two groups such that the lowest priority group is going into the page:

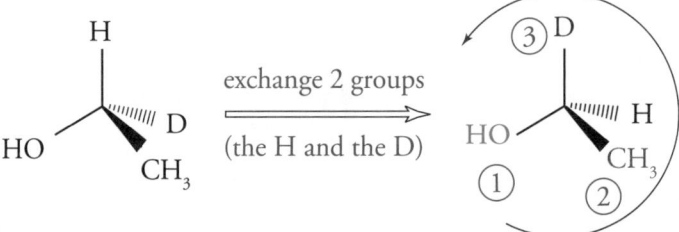

Note that this trace is going counterclockwise. Remember, however, that we exchanged two groups (the hydrogen and the deuterium), which necessarily changes the absolute configuration. Since the counterclockwise trace in the altered molecule means an *S* configuration, the true configuration is *R*.

(e)   Because this molecule is not chiral, we cannot assign it an absolute configuration.

(f)   *S*. Rotate so the lowest priority group is in back,

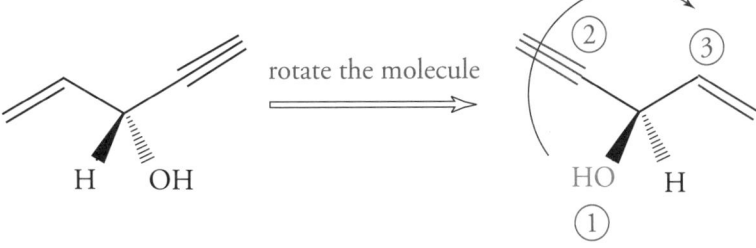

or exchange two groups, –H and –NH₂:

Clockwise trace.
But remember that two groups
on the chiral center were exchanged,
so the absolute configuration of the
given molecule is the opposite;
therefore, *S*.

(g)   *R*. Rotate so the lowest priority group is in the back:

Enantiomers

It is important to be able to identify chiral centers because, as we have seen, when there are four different groups attached to a centralized carbon, there are two distinct arrangements or configurations possible for these groups in space. Consider the following two molecules:

Molecule A   Molecule B

mirror plane

Molecule A has one chiral center with four different groups attached. Notice that Molecule B also has a chiral center and that the four groups attached to it are the same as those in Molecule A. Observe the mirror plane that has been drawn between Molecules A and B. Molecules A and B are mirror images of each other, but they are not superimposable; therefore, they are chiral.

or

These molecules are **enantiomers**: non-superimposable mirror images.

Enantiomers can occur when chiral centers are present. Note that two molecules that are enantiomers will always have opposite absolute configurations; for example:

S   *R*

What are the properties of enantiomers? That is, how do they differ from one another? Most chemical properties such as melting point, boiling point, polarity, and solubility are the same for both pure enantiomers of an enantiomeric pair. That is, the pure enantiomers shown above will have many identical physical properties.

Optical Activity

One important property that differs between enantiomers is the manner in which they interact with plane-polarized light. A compound that rotates the plane of polarized light is said to be **optically active**. A compound that rotates plane-polarized light clockwise is said to be **dextrorotatory** (*d*), also denoted by (+), while a compound that rotates plane-polarized light in the counterclockwise direction is said to be **levorotatory** (*l*), also denoted by (−). The magnitude of rotation of plane-polarized light for any compound is called its **specific rotation**. This property is dependent on the structure of the molecule, the concentration of the sample, and the path length through which the light must travel.

A pair of enantiomers will rotate plane-polarized light with equal magnitude, but in opposite directions. For example, pure (+)-2-bromobutanoic acid has a specific rotation of +39.5°, while (−)-2-bromobutanoic acid has a specific rotation of −39.5°.

(+) and (−)-2-bromobutanoic acid

What do you think the specific rotation of an equimolar mixture of the two enantiomers above will be? Since one enantiomer will rotate plane-polarized light in one direction, while the other enantiomer will rotate light by the same magnitude in the opposite direction, the specific rotation of a 50/50 mixture of enantiomers —a **racemic mixture**—is 0°. Therefore, a racemic mixture of enantiomers, also known as a *racemate*, is not optically active.

Example 4-14: What is the specific rotation of the *R* enantiomer of 2-bromobutanoic acid? Of the *S* enantiomer?

Solution:

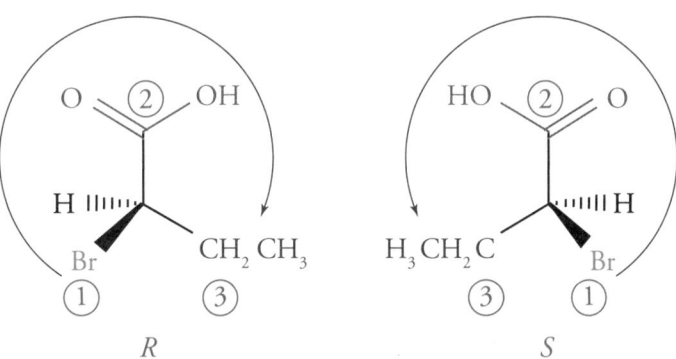

The magnitude of rotation cannot be predicted; it must be experimentally determined. It just so happens in this case that the *R* enantiomer has the (+) rotation [while the *S* enantiomer has the (−) rotation.] But be careful: ***This is only coincidental. (+) and (−) say nothing about whether the absolute configuration is R or S.*** There is no correlation between the sign of rotation and the absolute configuration.

Diasteromers

Diastereomers

In the preceding discussions on stereoisomerism, we have focused on molecules that have only one chiral center. What about molecules with multiple stereocenters? Remember that the number of possible stereoisomers is 2^n, where n is the number of chiral centers. If there is one chiral center, then there are two possible stereoisomers: the enantiomeric pair R and S. Two chiral centers means there are four possible stereoisomers. Consider the following molecule (3-bromobutan-2-ol), for example:

Each of the two chiral centers in 3-bromobutan-2-ol can have either R or S absolute configuration. This leads to four possible combinations of absolute configurations at the chiral centers. Both carbons could be of the S configuration or both could be of the R configuration; or, the left carbon could be R and the right carbon S, or vice versa. Here are the four possible combinations:

What's the relationship between Molecules I and II? Each of the two chiral centers in Molecule I is of the opposite configuration of Molecule II: S,S vs. R,R. Note that they are non-superimposable mirror images:

4.2

Therefore, these molecules are enantiomers. What about Molecules III and IV? Once again, each of the two chiral centers in Molecule III is of the opposite configuration of those in Molecule IV. This makes Molecules III and IV an enantiomer pair, just as we noted for Molecules I and II on the previous page. Is there a relationship between Molecules I and III?

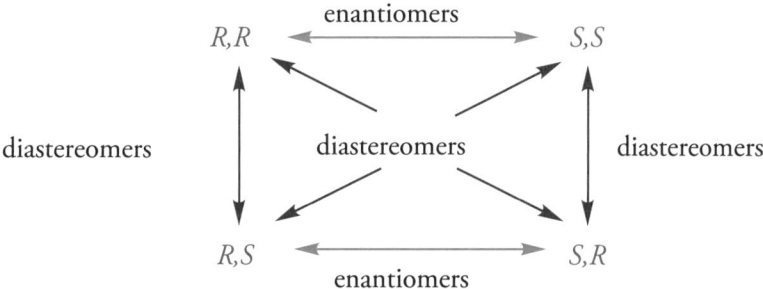

By mentally moving Molecule III to the left and aligning it over Molecule I, we see that the right chiral centers of both molecules are directly superimposable (*S* superimposes onto *S*). Also note that no matter what we do, we cannot get the left chiral centers of Molecules I and III to superimpose (*S* does not superimpose onto *R*).

Molecules I and III are diastereomers. **Diastereomers** are stereoisomers that are not enantiomers. That is, diastereomers are stereoisomers that are non-superimposable, non-mirror images. The same is true for Molecules I and IV. One of the chiral centers is of the same absolute configuration, while the other chiral center is of the opposite configuration:

The figure below summarizes all possible stereochemical relationships between isomers containing two stereocenters. Inverting at least one, but not all, of the chiral centers within a molecule will form a diastereomer of that molecule. Enantiomers can be formed by inverting every stereocenter within the molecule.

Example 4-15: For each pair of molecules below, state the relationship between them.

(a)

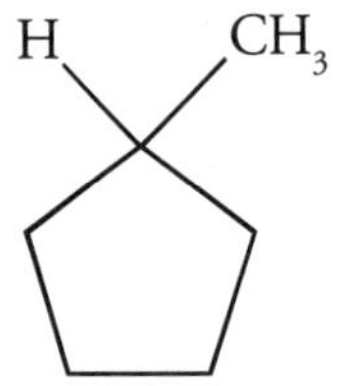

and

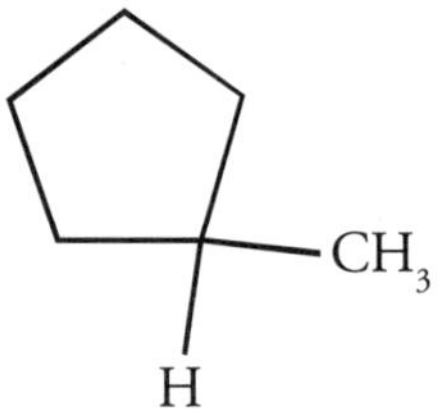

(b)

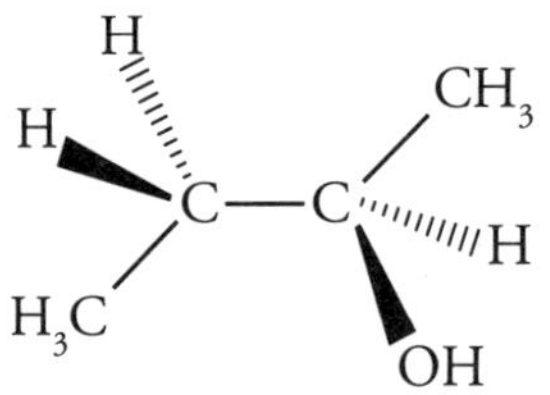

and

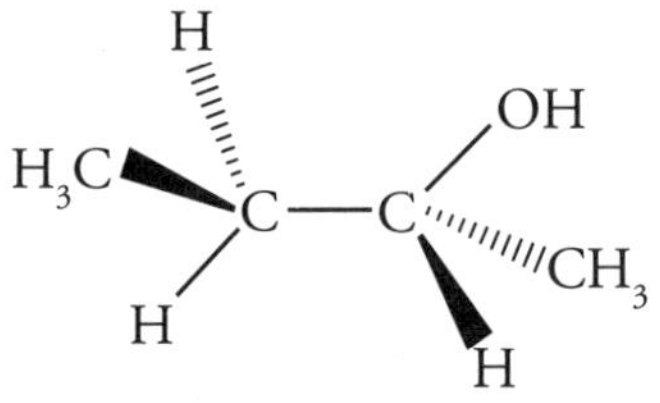

(c)

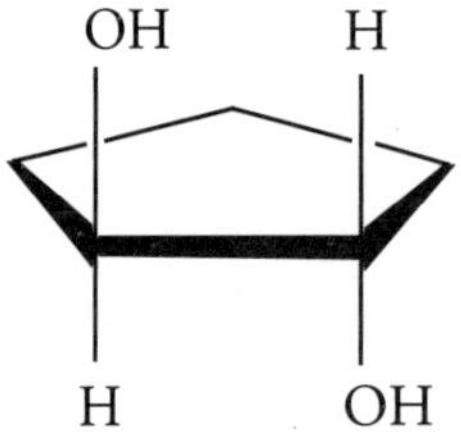

and

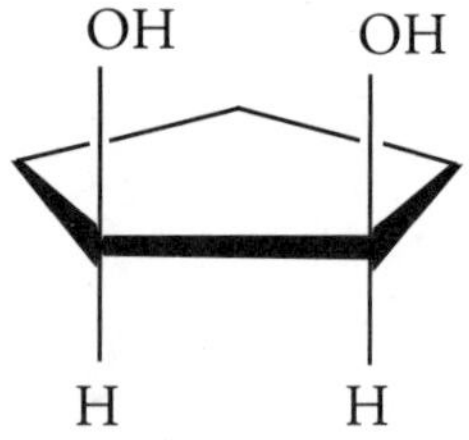

(d)

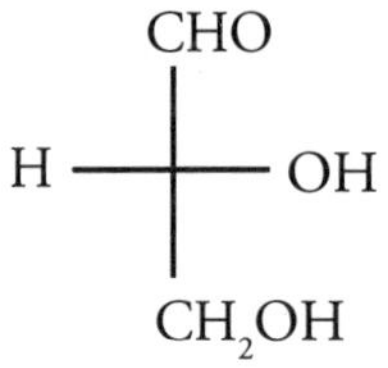

and

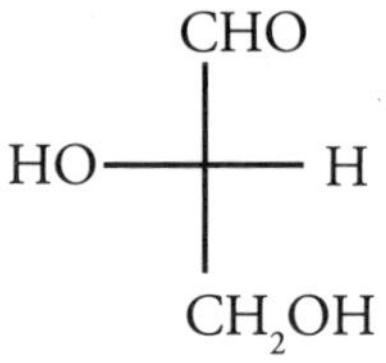

(e)

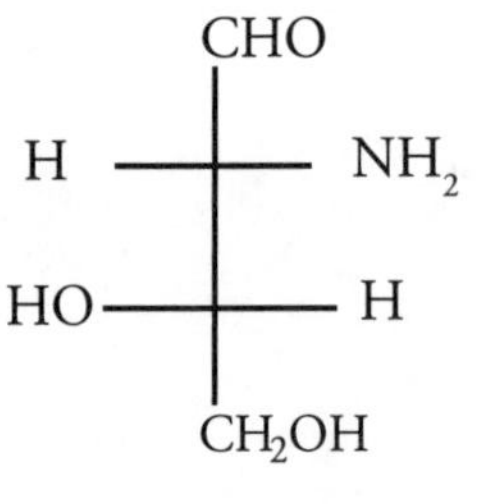

and

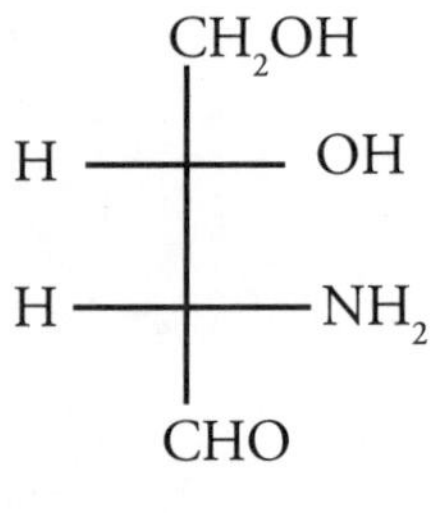

Solution:

(a)   The molecules are superimposable and therefore *identical*.

(b)   The molecules are *identical*. (The left carbon is not a chiral center.)

(c)   *Diastereomers.*

(d)   *Enantiomers.*

(e)   *Diastereomers.*

While the structures of diastereomers are similar, their physical and chemical properties can vary dramatically. They can have different melting points, boiling points, solubilities, dipole moments, specific rotations, etc. Most importantly for the MCAT, the specific rotation of diastereomers is also different, but *there is no relationship between the specific rotations of diastereomers as there is for enantiomers.* There is no way to predict the specific rotation of one diastereomer if you know the degree of rotation of another.

Resolution of Enantiomers

Nature has evolved intricate mechanisms for the biosynthesis of enantiomerically pure, optically active compounds. For example, L-(+)-tartaric acid, D-(+)-fructose, and L-(+)-valine are all isolated as a single enantiomer from their respective biological sources.

L-(+)-tartaric acid
(2R,3R)-tartaric acid

D-(+)-fructose

L-(+)-valine

Unfortunately, the laboratory syntheses of enantiomerically pure compounds is often laborious and expensive. It is generally more time- and cost-effective to synthesize chiral targets as racemic mixtures. For example, the reduction of 2-butanone (achiral) to 2-butanol (chiral) yields both enantiomers.

2-butanone   (S)-2-butanol   (R)-2-butanol

If only one enantiomer of 2-butanol is needed, the two alcohols must be separated. Since enantiomers have identical chemical and physical properties, separating a racemic mixture is a nontrivial process called **resolution**.

The traditional method for resolving a racemic mixture is through the use of an enantiomerically pure chiral probe, or resolving agent, that associates with the components of the mixture through either covalent bonds or intermolecular forces (like hydrogen bonds or salt interactions). The resulting products will be diastereomers, capable of separation due to their different physical properties.

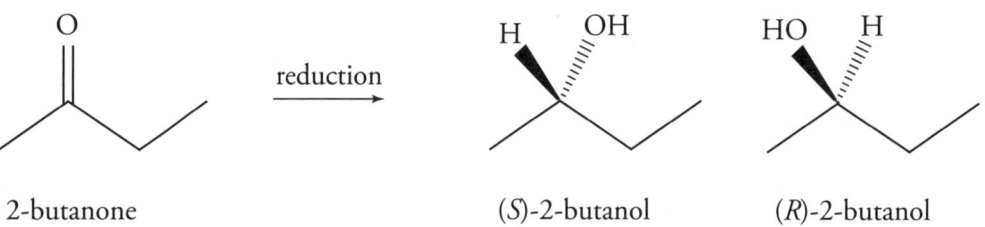

$(R) + (S)$ +   chiral probe $\rightleftharpoons$ (R)-----chiral probe
(racemic mixture) (S)-----chiral probe
                                                         diastereomeric association complexes

For example, racemic (±)-2-amino-2-phenylacetic acid can be resolved with enantiomerically pure (1R,4R)-(+)-10-camphorsulfonic acid, as shown in the figure below.

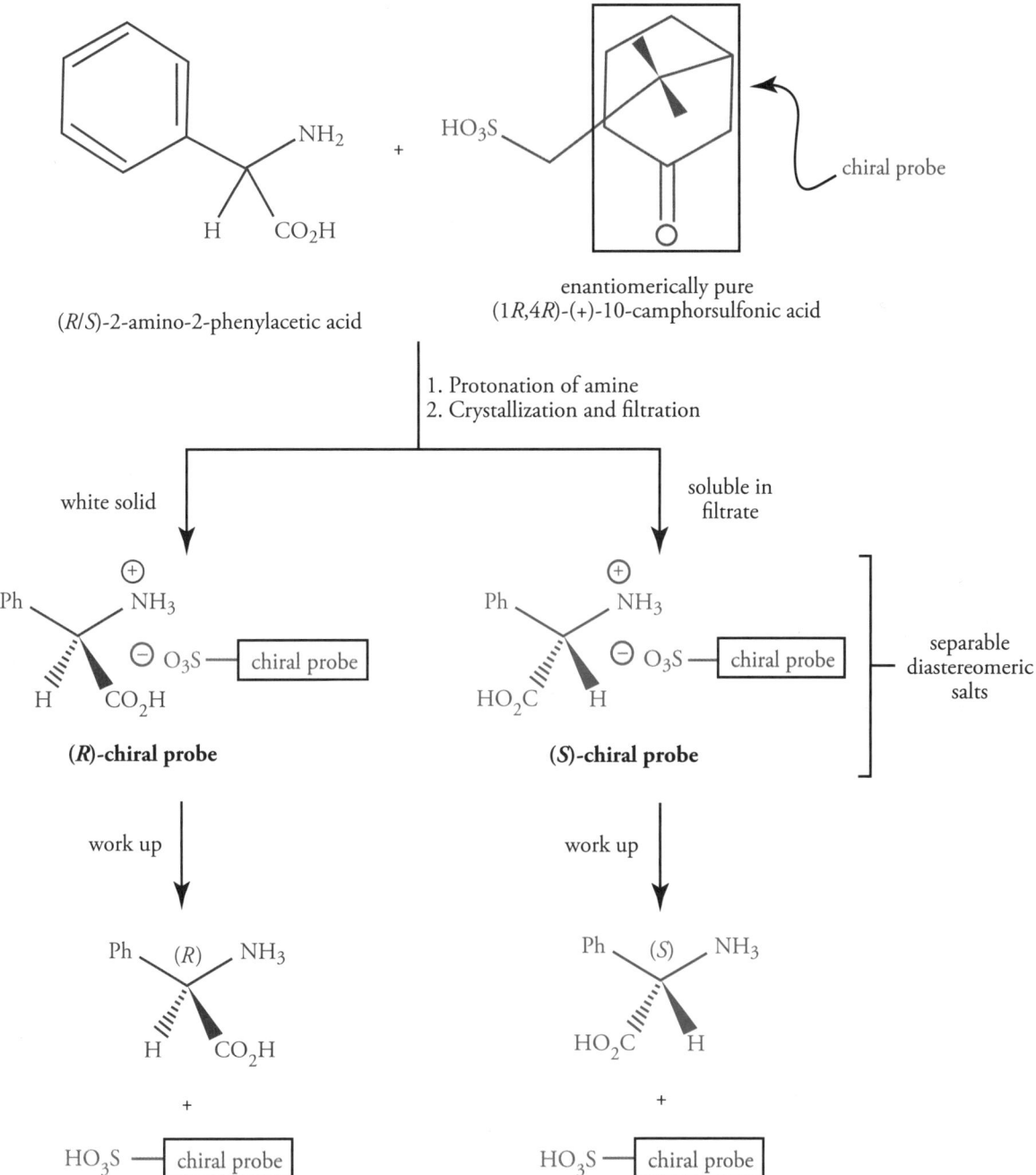

Protonation of the amine by the sulfonic acid produces two diastereomeric salts with different chemical and physical properties. In this particular instance, these salts have different solubilities; the R salt precipitates as a crystalline solid while the S salt remains dissolved in the filtrate. A simple filtration process is used to separate the two, which can be released from the probe and isolated as enantiomerically pure material in a subsequent work-up step.

4.2

Epimers

Epimers are a subclass of diastereomers that differ in their absolute configuration at a single chiral center (only *one* stereocenter is inverted). To illustrate epimeric relationships, let's look at the Fischer projections of some sugars (see Chapter 7):

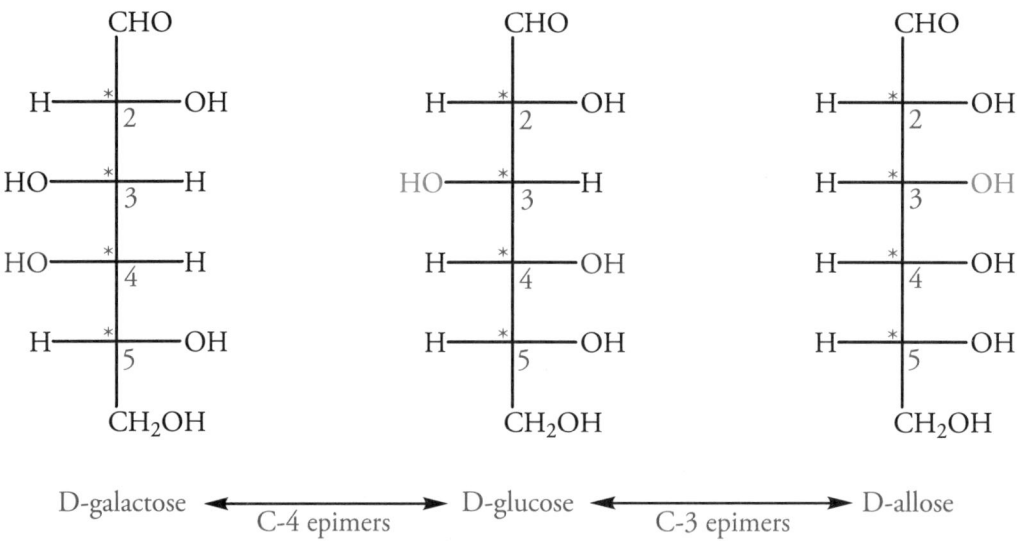

The prefix D on the name of these molecules refers to the orientation of the hydroxyl group (–OH) on the highest-numbered chiral center in a Fischer projection (C-5 in these cases). When the hydroxyl group is on the *right* of this carbon in the Fischer projection, the molecule is a D sugar. (When the hydroxyl group is on the *left*, the molecule is an L sugar.)

You must understand that D and L, like *R* and *S*, are entirely unrelated to optical activity, (+) or (–). Distinctions between D and L (or between *R* and *S*) can be made just by looking at a drawing of the molecule, but distinctions between (+) and (–) can be made only by running experiments in a polarimeter.

- *R* or *S* = absolute configuration (structure)
- D or L = relative configuration (structure)
- (+) or (–) = observed optical rotation (property)

Concerning the three sugars above, we see that D-glucose and D-galactose differ in stereochemistry at only one chiral center (C-4). Thus, D-glucose and D-galactose are said to be C-4 epimers, and C-4 is called the **epimeric carbon**. Likewise, D-glucose and D-allose differ in structure at a single chiral center (C-3). D-Glucose and D-allose are C-3 epimers, with C-3 being the epimeric carbon.

What about D-galactose and D-allose? What is the relationship between these two molecules? We can see that these two sugars differ at two chiral centers (C-3 and C-4). At least one, but not all, of the stereocenters have been inverted. Therefore they are diastereomers, but *NOT* epimers. Note that all epimers are diastereomers, but not all diastereomers are epimers.

Anomers

Epimers that form as a result of ring closure are known as **anomers**. For the MCAT, anomers will be encountered only with regard to sugar chemistry. To illustrate anomerism, consider D-glucose. Open-chain glucose exists in equilibrium with cyclic glucose, known as *glucopyranose*. Cyclization occurs when the C-5 hydroxyl group attacks the carbonyl (C=O) carbon, C-1. This converts a carbon with three substituents to a carbon with four different substituents. Thus, a new stereocenter is formed (C-1), and it can assume one of two possible forms: with the hydroxyl group *down*, it is α; with the hydroxyl group *up*, it is β. It is the orientation at C-1 that distinguishes the two anomers, and C-1 is known as the **anomeric center** (or **anomeric carbon**).

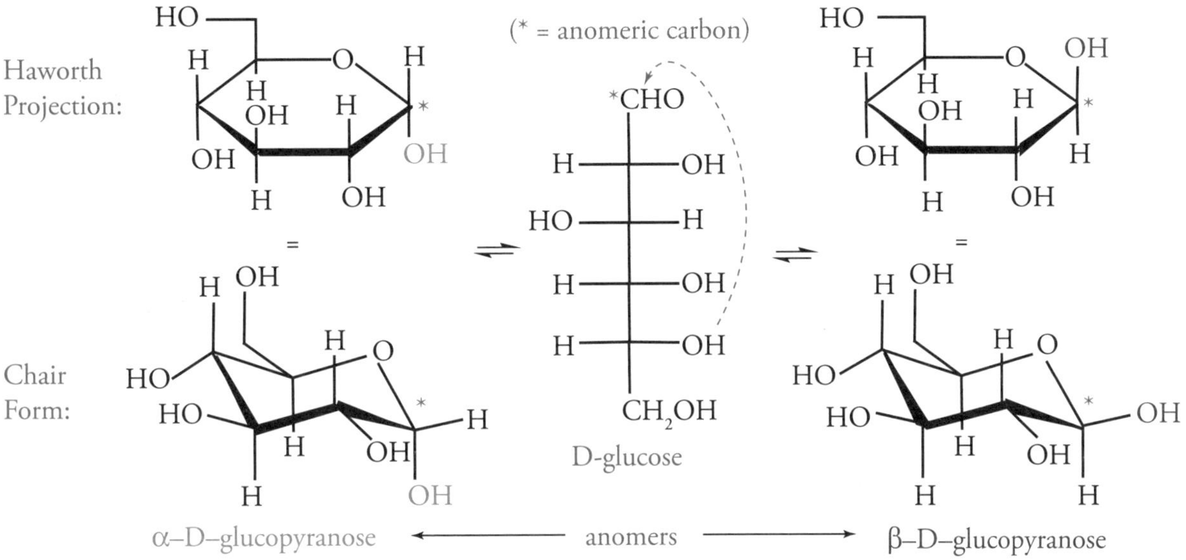

Meso Compounds

Let's look at another molecule with more than one stereocenter. Consider 2,3-butanediol:

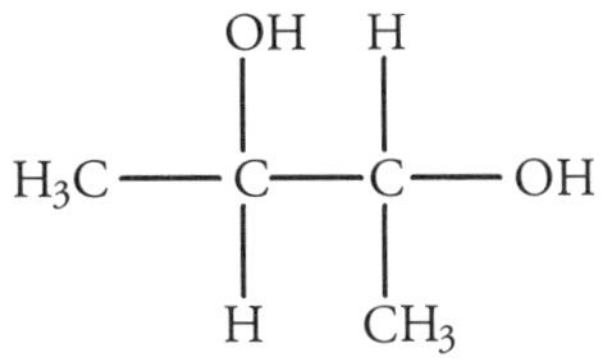

Upon inspection, we determine that there are two chiral centers and therefore four possible stereoisomers. Notice that both chiral centers have the same groups attached to them: –H, –CH$_3$, –OH, and –CH(OH)CH$_3$. When the same four groups are attached to two chiral centers, the molecule can have an internal plane of symmetry. Let's examine this a little more closely.

4.2

We first consider the *R,R* stereoisomer and the *S,S* stereoisomer of 2,3-butanediol:

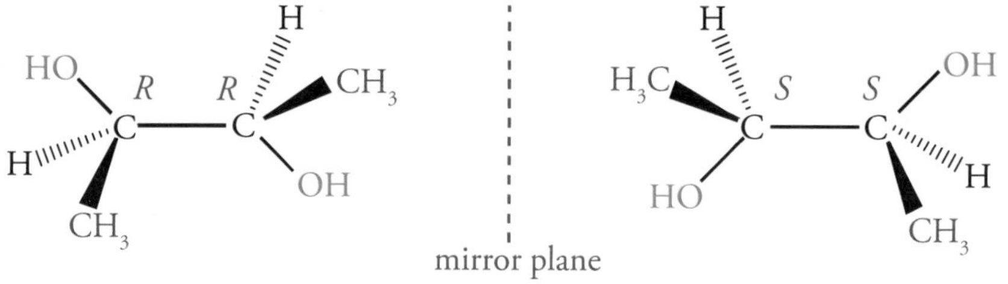

mirror plane

I   II

There are two things to notice here. First, I and II are non-superimposable mirror images and therefore enantiomers. Second, in both I and II there is no internal plane of symmetry. This is demonstrated for Molecule II:

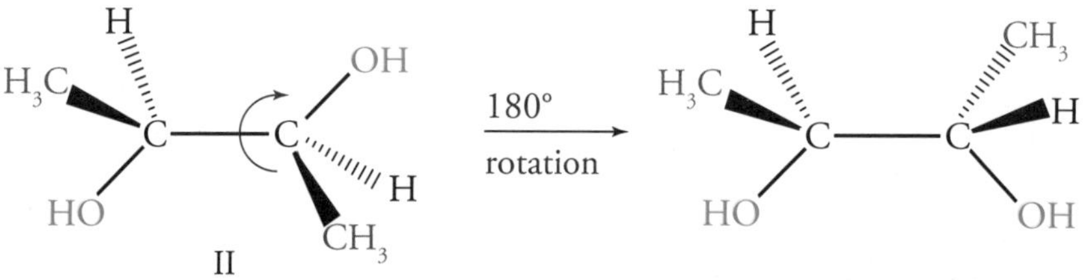

$$\xrightarrow[\text{rotation}]{180°}$$

II

The –OH groups line up on the two chiral centers, but the –CH$_3$ groups and –H atoms do not. The optical rotation of a 50/50 mixture of Molecules I and II would measure zero because this is a racemic mixture.

Now look at the *R,S* stereoisomer and its mirror image:

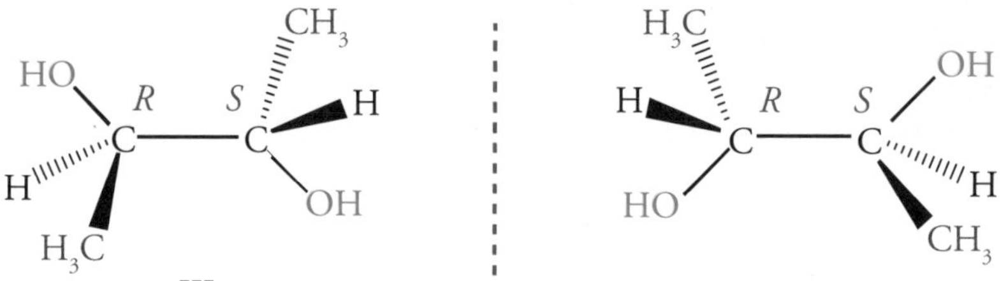

III

III and IV are actually the same molecule.

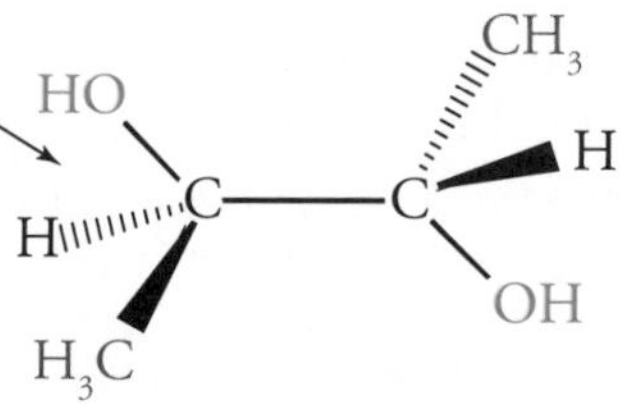

Rotate the entire molecule so that the two –OH groups are as in III.

IV

It turns out that Molecules III and IV are directly superimposable and therefore identical. This is because there is an internal plane of symmetry within the molecule.

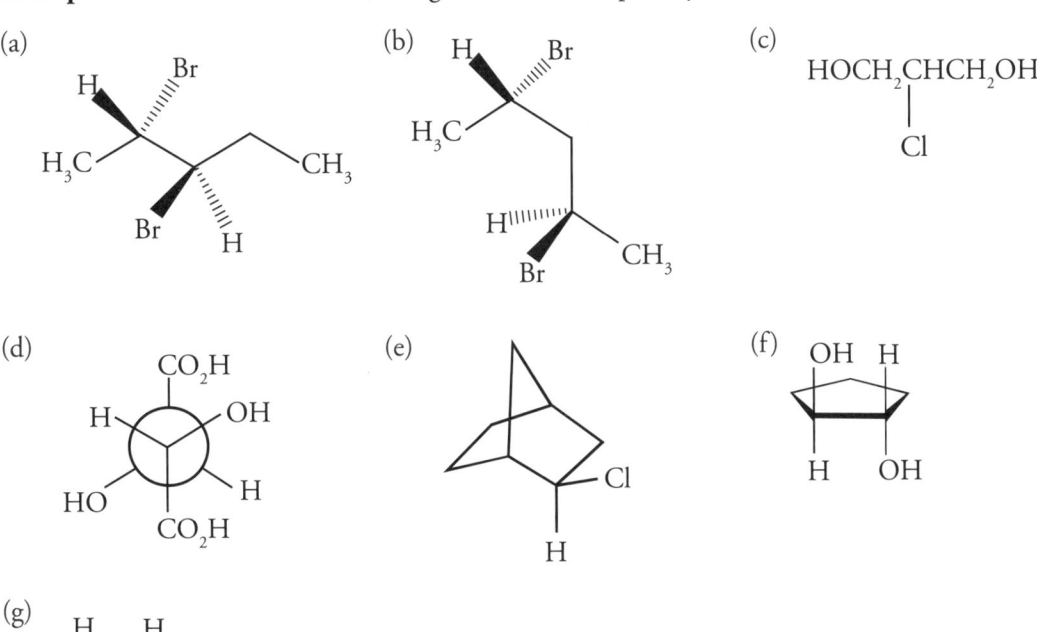

III

Rotate 180° about the
C_2–C_3 σ bond

One side of the molecule is the mirror image of the other side. This is a *meso* compound.

When there's an internal plane of symmetry in a molecule that contains chiral centers, the compound is called a **meso** compound. Actually then, 2,3-butanediol has only *three* stereoisomers, not four. Molecules I and II are enantiomers, while III and IV are the same molecule. Molecule III (or IV) is an example of a meso compound. Meso compounds have chiral centers but are not optically active (so they are achiral) because one side of the molecule is a mirror image of the other. In a sense, the optical activity imparted by one side of the molecule is canceled by its other side.

Example 4-16: Which of the following molecules are optically active?

(a)

(b)

(c) $HOCH_2CHCH_2OH$
      |
      Cl

(d)

(e)

(f)

(g)

4.2

Solution:

(a) This molecule is optically active. It has two chiral centers, but no internal mirror plane. Therefore it is not a meso compound and will rotate plane-polarized light.

(b) This molecule is a meso compound due to its two chiral centers and internal mirror plane. It will be optically inactive. Be sure to look for rotations around σ bonds in order to find the mirror planes of some molecules.

(c) This molecule has no chiral centers, so it will have no optical activity.

(d) By rotating around the C-2 to C-3 bond to put the molecule into an eclipsed conformation, you can see that there is an internal mirror plane in the molecule. Since C-2 and C-3 are also chiral centers with four different substituents, this is a meso compound, and will be optically inactive.

(e) This molecule has three chiral centers (the two bridgehead carbons are chiral), but no plane of symmetry. It is therefore chiral and optically active.

(f) There is no mirror image in this molecule even though it has two chiral centers (they have the same absolute configuration). It will therefore be optically active.

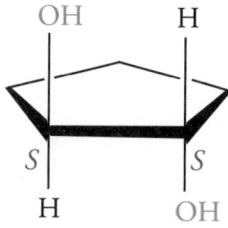

(g)   This molecule does have an internal mirror plane, and its two chiral centers have opposite absolute configurations. It is therefore meso, and not optically active.

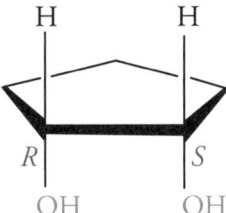

Geometric Isomers

Geometric isomers are diastereomers that differ in orientation of substituents around a ring or a double bond. Cyclic hydrocarbons and double bonds (alkenes) are constrained by their geometry, meaning they do not rotate freely about all bonds. So, there's a difference between having substituents on the same side of the ring (or double bond) and having substituents on opposite sides. For example, the following are geometric isomers of 1,2-dimethylcyclohexane:

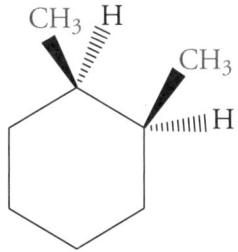
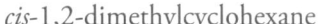
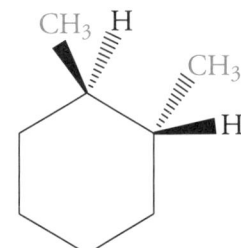

cis-1,2-dimethylcyclohexane   trans-1,2-dimethylcyclohexane

Priority of substituent groups is assigned the same way as for absolute configuration. On C-1, the methyl group is given higher priority than the H, and the same is true on C-2. The molecule in which the two higher-priority groups are on the same side is termed **cis**, and the molecule in which the two higher-priority groups are on opposite sides of the ring is termed **trans**.

4.2

The same-side/opposite-side substituent relativity also occurs with double bonds, but in this case the stereochemistry is officially designated by *Z* or *E*. The *Z/E* notation is a completely unambiguous way to specify the appropriate stereochemistry at the double bond. In this system, a high and low priority group are assigned at each carbon of the double bond based on atomic number, just as with absolute configuration. If the two high priority groups are on the *same* side, the configuration at the double bond is *Z* (from the German *zusammen*, meaning *together*). On the other hand, if the two high priority groups are on opposite sides of the double bond, the configuration is referred to as *E* (from the German *entgegen*, meaning *opposite*). Be aware that the MCAT may also use the terms *cis* and *trans* when referring to double bonds. However, this is usually reserved for the case when there is one H attached to each carbon of the double bond, as shown below. The geometric isomers of 2-bromo-1-chloropropene and of 1,2-dibromoethene are shown below:

Highest priority groups (Br and Cl) on same side, so *Z*.

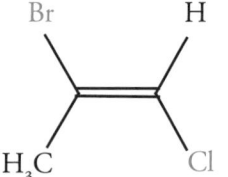

Highest priority groups (Br and Cl) on opposite side, so *E*.

(*Z*)-2-bromo-1-chloropropene   (*E*)-2-bromo-1-chloropropene

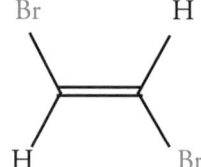

cis-1,2-dibromoethene   *trans*-1,2-dibromoethene

SUMMARY OF ISOMERS

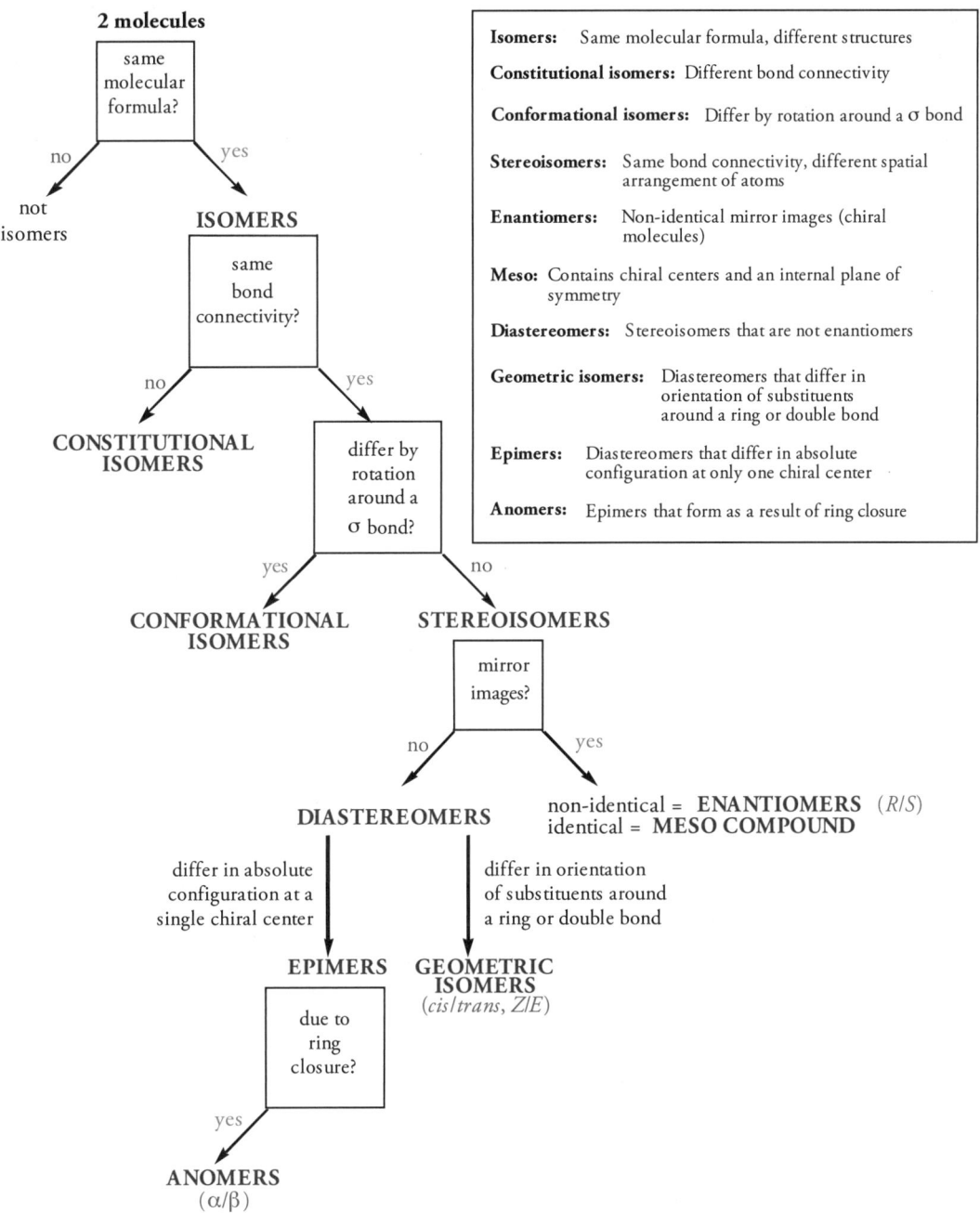

Isomers: Same molecular formula, different structures

Constitutional isomers: Different bond connectivity

Conformational isomers: Differ by rotation around a σ bond

Stereoisomers: Same bond connectivity, different spatial arrangement of atoms

Enantiomers: Non-identical mirror images (chiral molecules)

Meso: Contains chiral centers and an internal plane of symmetry

Diastereomers: Stereoisomers that are not enantiomers

Geometric isomers: Diastereomers that differ in orientation of substituents around a ring or double bond

Epimers: Diastereomers that differ in absolute configuration at only one chiral center

Anomers: Epimers that form as a result of ring closure

Chapter 4 Summary

- Saturated compounds have the general formula C_nH_{2n+2}; unsaturated molecules contain rings or π bonds.

- As the substitution of carbocations increases, so does their stability due to the inductive effect; carbanions are more stable when they are less substituted.

- Resonance stabilization results from the ability of π electrons or charge to move and delocalize through a system of conjugated π bonds or unhybridized p orbitals.

- Brønsted-Lowry acids are proton donors, and are stronger (dissociate more) when their conjugate bases are most stable in solution.

- Acidity of carboxylic acids results from the resonance stability of the carboxylate anion.

- Electron-withdrawing groups increase the acidity of carboxylic acids by stabilizing the negative charge of the carboxylate anion via the inductive effect.

- Nucleophiles are Lewis bases and are electron rich, while electrophiles are Lewis acids and are electron deficient.

- Nucleophiles are stronger when negatively charged, less electronegative, or larger in size.

- Leaving groups are more likely to leave as their stability in solution increases (uncharged and/or larger groups are usually better LGs).

- Compounds with the same molecular formula are known as *isomers*; structural or constitutional isomers differ by the connectivity of atoms in the molecule.

- Conformational isomers differ by rotation around a σ bond.

- Stereoisomers have the same atom connectivity, but different spatial orientation of atoms.

- Chiral molecules have chiral centers (carbon with four different substituents), are not superimposable on their mirror image, and rotate plane-polarized light.

- Enantiomers are non-superimposable mirror images and have opposite absolute configuration at all chiral centers.

- Enantiomers rotate plane-polarized light an equal magnitude, but in opposite direction, therefore a 50:50 mixture of enantiomers, or a racemic mixture, is not optically active.

- The process of separating a mixture of enantiomers is called resolution, and entails conversion of the racemic mixture into a pair of separable diastereomers temporarily before converting back to the pure, chiral enantiomers.

- Diastereomers are stereoisomers that are not mirror images; they differ in absolute configuration for at least one, but not all carbons.

- Epimers are diastereomers that differ in absolute configuration at only one stereocenter.

- Geometric isomers are diastereomers that are *cis/trans* (or *Z/E*) pairs on a ring or double bond. When highest priority groups are on the same side of a ring or bond the molecule is *cis* (or *Z*); when they're on opposite sides, the compound is *trans* (or *E*).

- Meso compounds are achiral molecules with chiral centers and an internal mirror plane.

CHAPTER 4 FREESTANDING PRACTICE QUESTIONS

1. In the molecule below, what are the hybridizations of C_1, C_2, C_3, and C_4 respectively?

A) sp, sp, sp^2, sp^2
B) sp, sp, sp, sp^2
C) sp^2, sp^2, sp, sp
D) sp^2, sp, sp, sp

2. Which of the following structures represents the most stable possible resonance structure for acetic acid (CH_3CO_2H)?

3. Rank the conformations of 2-aminoethanol by increasing stability.

A) *anti* < *gauche* < eclipsed
B) eclipsed < *anti* < *gauche*
C) *gauche* < *anti* < eclipsed
D) eclipsed < *gauche* < *anti*

4. The most stable conformation of the following substituted cyclohexane has the methyl groups in which of the following positions?

A) 2 equatorial and 1 axial
B) All axial
C) All equatorial
D) 2 axial and 1 equatorial

5. How many stereoisomers are possible for cortisone acetate (shown below)?

A) 32
B) 64
C) 128
D) 256

6. What is the correct IUPAC name for the following molecule?

A) (*E*)-3-heptenoic acid
B) (*E*)-4-heptenoic acid
C) (*Z*)-3-heptenoic acid
D) (*Z*)-4-heptenoic acid

7. Which of the following is the strongest nucleophile?

A) CN^-
B) OH^-
C) CH_3OH
D) NH_3

8. Which of the following lists two pairs of diastereomers?

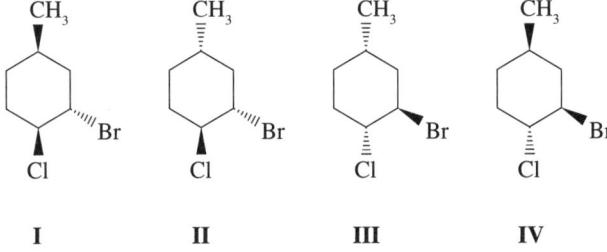

I   II   III   IV

A) I, III and II, IV
B) I, II and II, III
C) I, III and I, IV
D) II, IV and III, IV

9. How many chiral centers are contained in the compound below?

A) 4
B) 5
C) 6
D) 7

CHAPTER 4 PRACTICE PASSAGE

In mammalian systems, aromatic hydrocarbons are enzymatically metabolized by cytochrome P_{450} into arene oxides when ingested or inhaled. Arene oxides are compounds in which one of the double bonds of an aromatic ring has been converted into an epoxide. These molecules can rearrange to form phenols, which are harmlessly excreted. As shown in Figure 1, arene oxide rearrangement requires the formation of an intermediate carbocation and subsequent hydride shift.

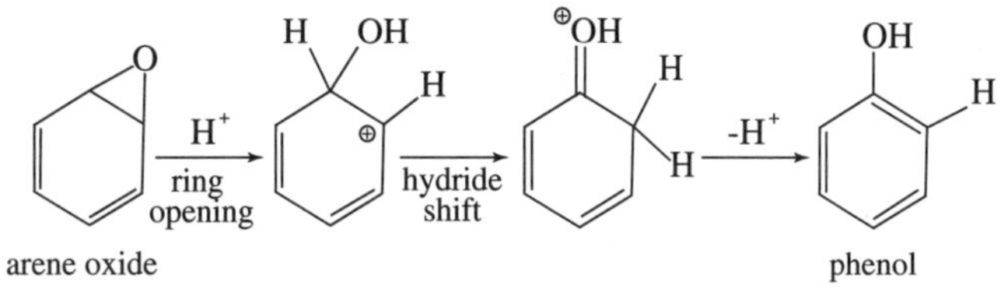

Figure 1 Arene oxide rearrangement

Benzo[a]pyrene, found in tobacco smoke and automobile exhaust, is one of the most troublesome natural arene oxides because it is a procarcinogen due to its bioconversion to a number of harmful molecules such as the 7,8-diol epoxide shown in Figure 2. The danger of the 7,8-diol epoxide lies in the unwillingness of the epoxide ring to rearrange and form a phenol. Instead, the diol epoxide intercalates in DNA and is covalently bound by 2′-deoxyguanosine nucleosides, leading to point mutations in the course of DNA replication.

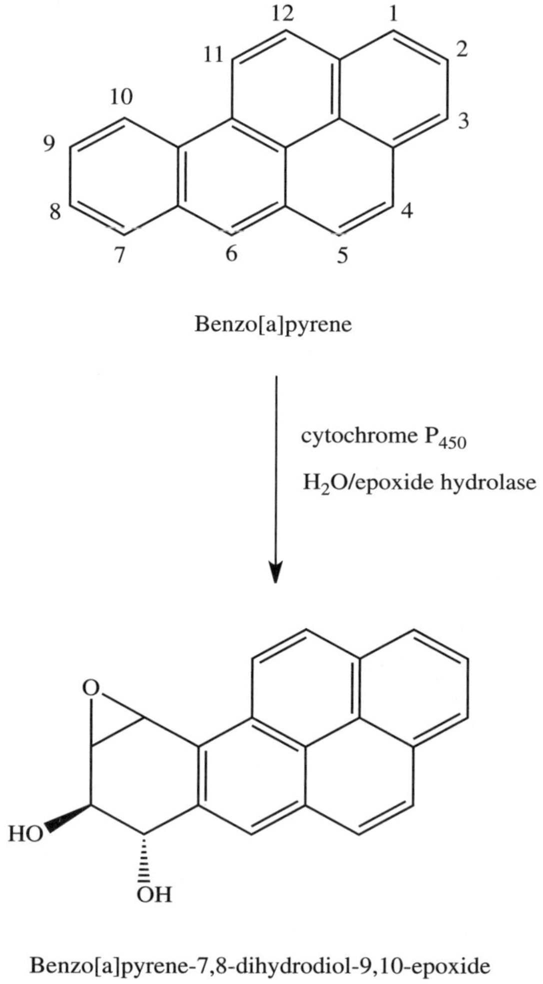

Benzo[a]pyrene

cytochrome P_{450}

H_2O/epoxide hydrolase

Benzo[a]pyrene-7,8-dihydrodiol-9,10-epoxide

Figure 2 Oxidation of Benzo[a]pyrene

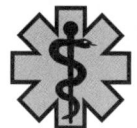

1. Determine the absolute configurations of Carbons 7 and 8 of the diol epoxide shown in Figure 2.

A) 7*R*, 8*R*
B) 7*R*, 8*S*
C) 7*S*, 8*S*
D) 7*S*, 8*R*

2. All of the following statements about the diol epoxide shown in Figure 2 are correct EXCEPT:

A) the epoxide bears the same type of leaving group as an ether.
B) ring strain and torsional strain increase the free energy of the epoxide.
C) the epoxide may react under strongly acidic conditions.
D) the epoxide oxygen atom is capable of donating a hydrogen bond.

3. Rank the following four substances in order of increasing reactivity with an arene oxide.

   I.   Hydroxide
   II. Ammonia
   III. Methide
   IV. Water

A) III < I < II < IV
B) IV < II < I < III
C) IV < II < III < I
D) II < IV < I < III

4. Which labeled atom of the nucleoside shown below is responsible for intercalation of the diol epoxide?

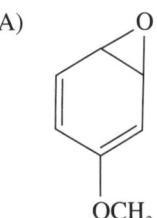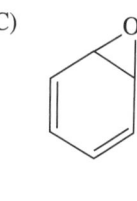

A) 1
B) 2
C) 3
D) 4

5. Which of the following arene oxides will react as in Figure 1 to form the most stable carbocation intermediate?

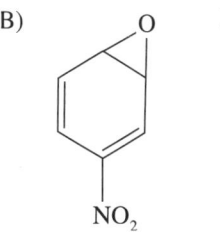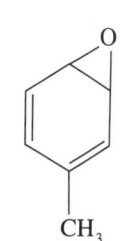

SOLUTIONS TO CHAPTER 4 FREESTANDING PRACTICE QUESTIONS

1. **B** Both C_1 and C_2 make up the triple bond. They are both *sp* hybridized so you can eliminate choices C and D. C_3 is part of an allene. The bonds that it forms with its neighbors are linear (180°), so it is also *sp*. You can eliminate choice A, which leaves choice B as the correct choice. C_4 has a double bond and two single bonds so it is *sp²*.

2. **B** Good resonance structures must do the following: obey the octet rule, accrue the fewest charges possible, and place negative charges on electronegative atoms and positive charges on electropositive atoms (listed in priority). Further, resonance structures don't represent oxidation or reduction of molecules, and as such the total charge of each structure must be the charge of the molecule. This eliminates choices C and D. Choices A and B are both valid resonance structures, but only choice B places a full octet on all non-H atoms.

3. **B** Since this is a ranking question, look for obvious extremes and eliminate answers. Choices A and C should be eliminated because the eclipsed conformation is always the least stable due to sterics and electron repulsions in aligned bonds. Choice D is the more enticing answer of the remaining two because the general rule of thumb is that the *anti* conformation is the most stable because the bulky groups are farthest apart, while they are 60° apart in a *gauche* conformation. This question is tricky, however, because in this case there is intramolecular hydrogen bonding which can occur in the *gauche* conformation, making it the most stable one (eliminate choice D).

4. **A** Choice B can be eliminated before analyzing the structure since if all three substituents could be axial, then by a ring flip, all three could also be equatorial. The more stable chair conformation puts substituents in an equatorial position since they are less sterically crowded than those in axial positions. Similarly, if choice A is true of the molecule, then by ring flip, choice D must be also. Therefore, choice D should be eliminated since it has more axial substituents. Between choices A and C, only choice A fits the compound shown because the relationship between the methyl groups on Carbons 1 and 2 is *trans* and the relationship between the methyl groups on Carbons 1 and 4 is *cis*. In this conformation, the methyl groups on Carbons 1 and 2 would be found in the equatorial position and the methyl group on Carbon 4 would be axial, making A the better choice.

5. **B** The maximum number of stereoisomers is given by the formula 2^n, where *n* equals the number of stereocenters. Cortisone acetate has six stereocenters and $2^6 = 64$. Five of the six ring junctures are chiral centers (all *sp³* carbons), as is the carbon with the OH substituent. Choice A would correspond to five stereocenters, choice C would require seven stereocenters, and choice D would correspond to a compound with eight stereocenters.

6.   **A**   When naming a compound, number the carbons starting at the end nearest a functional group (the carboxylic acid in this case). Based on the position of the double bond in the molecule, you can eliminate choices B and D. Since the two largest substituents on each carbon of the double bond are on opposite sides of the bond, the double bond has *E* stereochemistry; therefore, eliminate choice C.

7.   **A**   Nucleophiles are electron rich. While neutral compounds that have lone pairs can be nucleophilic, negatively charged nucleophiles tend to be stronger (eliminate choices C and D). The stronger nucleophile is the more reactive nucleophile; more reactive corresponds to less stable. Therefore, the nucleophile that is less able to stabilize a negative charge will be the stronger nucleophile. For choices A and B, the negative charge resides on the C and O, respectively. Since carbon is less electronegative than oxygen, it is therefore less able to stabilize a negative charge, making cyanide the best nucleophile (eliminate choice B).

8.   **B**   Stereoisomers in which all stereocenters are inverted are enantiomers, while stereoisomers with at least one, but not all, inverted chiral centers are diastereomers. Molecules I and III are an enantiomeric pair (eliminate choices A and C); Molecules II and IV are enantiomers as well (eliminate choice D). All other pairs of molecules are diastereomers.

9.   **D**   The molecular structure given in the question contains seven chiral centers, which are located at C(1), C(2), C(6), C(7) C(9), C(10), and C(11). Each of these centers is marked by an asterisk in the structure shown below.

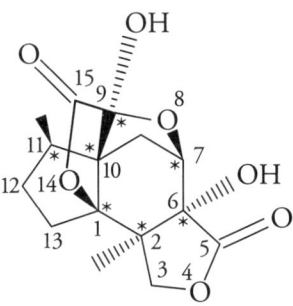

SOLUTIONS TO CHAPTER 4 PRACTICE PASSAGE

1. **D**

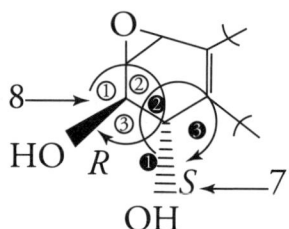

Note that the configuration for Carbon 7 reads as *R*, but because the hydroxyl group occupies an into-plane position, this assignment is incorrect. One way to get around this is to exchange the hydroxyl group's position with the hydrogen also on this carbon. Doing so will place the hydroxyl group in a correct position, which results in a clockwise trace. This reads as *R* but because two groups have been exchanged, the true configuration is *S*. Once the configuration of Carbon 7 is determined to be *S*, choices A and B can be eliminated.

2. **D** Make sure to highlight the word "except" and write "A B C D" on your noteboard. Then evaluate each answer choice, writing "T" if it is true or "F" if it is not. Then choose the answer that stands out. Epoxides and ethers all bear an OR leaving group (write "T" next to "A" on the noteboard). Epoxides, due to their 3-point ring structure, possess ring strain and torsional strain, which imparts a relatively high free energy (write "T" next to "B" on the noteboard). Under acidic conditions, the epoxide oxygen atom will be protonated, which permits a nucleophile to perform an S_N2 reaction (write "T" next to "C" on the noteboard). However, epoxides are only capable of accepting hydrogen bonds, not donating them (write "F" next to "D" on the noteboard). Since choice D stands out with an "F" instead of a "T", it is the correct answer choice.

3. **B** Each of the four substances listed will act as nucleophiles with an arene oxide. The strongest nucleophile has a negative charge on the least electronegative atom, which is carbon. Choices B and D both list methide as the strongest nucleophile (eliminate choices A and C). The weakest nucleophile is going to be listed first. The choice is between water and ammonia. Since nitrogen is less electronegative than oxygen, NH_3 is a stronger nucleophile than water (eliminate choice D).

4. **C** As stated in the passage, intercalation of the 2′-deoxyguanosine nucleoside occurs via a covalent bond with the diol epoxide. As all labeled atoms in the molecule shown contain a lone pair of electrons, this suggests that the 2′-deoxyguanosine nucleoside can act as a nucleophile. The site that is most nucleophilic will therefore be the site most likely to react. O-1 is unlikely to react, as oxygen is not as electron-donating as the three remaining nitrogen-based choices (eliminate choice A). N-2 is an amide nitrogen engaged in resonance with the adjacent carbonyl, decreasing its ability to donate electrons (eliminate choice B). The lone pairs available on N-3 and N-4 are localized and not engaged in resonance, making both of these options the most nucleophilic. However, the N-4 nitrogen, being a secondary nitrogen, is more sterically hindered and therefore less nucleophilic than the primary N-3 nitrogen (eliminate choice D).

5.   **A**   The nature of the substituents on each ring acts to stabilize or destabilize the carbocation that forms. The methoxy substituent in choice A is an electron-donating group, which will stabilize the carbocation through resonance due to the lone electron pairs on the oxygen.

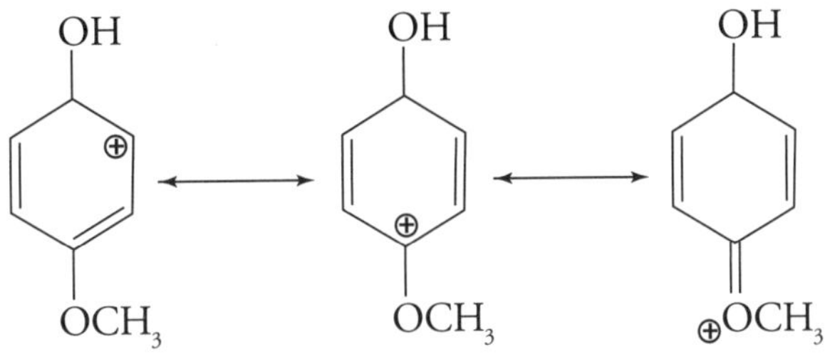

On the other hand, the nitro group in choice B will destabilize the intermediate since one resonance structure, shown below, puts two atoms with a positive charge next to each other (eliminate choice B). Choice C affords no increase or decrease in stability. Choice D will show mild stabilization due to the inductive donation offered by its methyl group (also shown below).

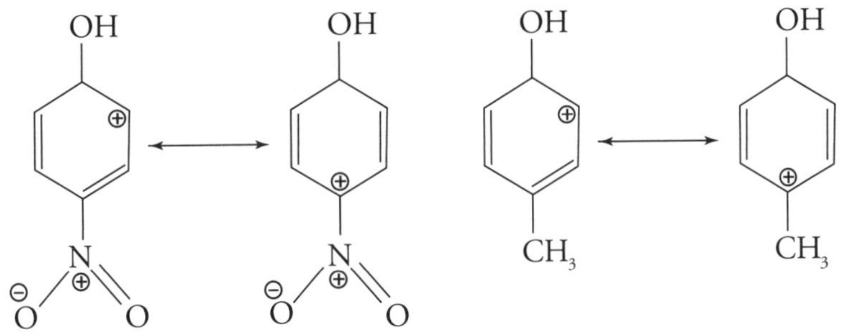

Overall, choice A shows the strongest carbocation stabilization since resonance effects are generally stronger than inductive ones.

DIRECT CATALYTIC *N*-ALKYLATION OF α-AMINO ACID ESTERS AND AMIDES USING ALCOHOLS WITH HIGH RETENTION OF STEREOCHEMISTRY

Tao Yan, Ben L. Fering, and Katalin Barta

N-alkyl amino acid esters and amides are frequently encountered chiral moieties in bioactive compounds (Figure 1). For example, Cilazapril and Enalapril are enzyme inhibitors, while Ximelagatran is an anticoagulant that has been investigated as an alternative for warfarin therapy. Furthermore, Lidocaine and Bupivacaine are well-known and widely used drug molecules that are included in the World Health Organization (WHO) list of essential medicines. Traditional pathways to obtain *N*-alkyl amino acid esters commonly include reductive amination of aldehydes or nucleophilic substitution with alkyl halides (Scheme 1A). While the former pathway may be limited by the availability and stability of the aldehyde substrates as well as the formation of side products, the latter pathway generally suffers from poor selectivity and atom economy due to the formation of stoichiometric amount of undesired halogen-containing salts.

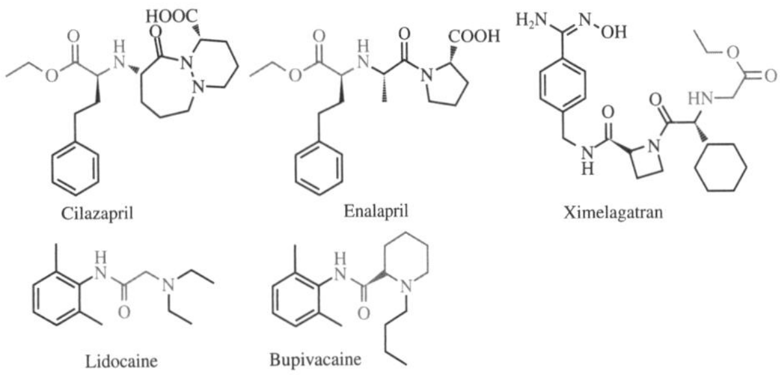

Alcohols are vastly abundant substrates and would be optimal alkylation agents and excellent alternatives to the commonly used alkyl-halogenides or aldehydes. Despite tremendous developments in catalytic borrowing hydrogen strategies the direct *N*-alkylation of natural amino acid esters via this methodology has remained largely unaddressed and there is lack of general methods that would allow for preserving the valuable chiral information in the amino acid backbone. While there are a number of examples that involve the use of chiral substrates, to the best of our knowledge, only one example for the *N*-alkylation of an unnatural amino acid ester has been reported employing an Ir-based homogeneous catalytic system and 1,5-pentane-diol, which was limited to using NaHCO$_3$ as base and a substrate that comprised a quaternary stereocenter (Scheme 1B). Indeed, most of the borrowing hydrogen methodologies rely on the use of a base for activation of the catalyst or substrates. Considering the use of natural amino acid esters as substrates, the chiral α-carbon would be sensitive to racemization due to its acidic proton in the presence of a base, as previously described.

In order to accomplish the challenging *N*-alkylation of natural or synthetic amino acid esters with alcohols without racemization on α-carbon, a robust, base-free

Figure 1. Important pharmaceutically active compounds containing a chiral *N*-alkyl amino acid ester or amide moiety.

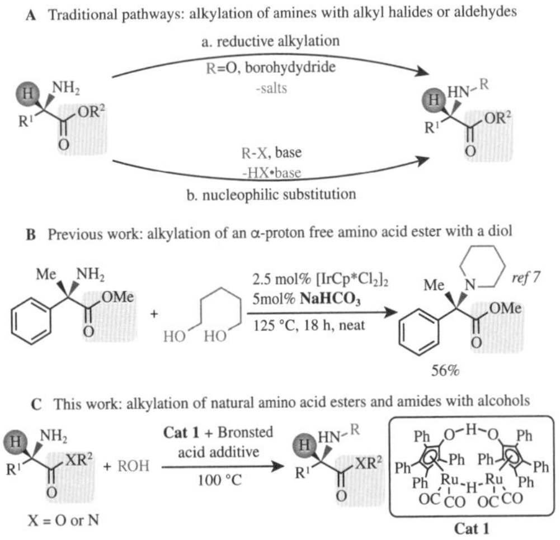

Scheme 1. Synthesis of functionalized *N*-alkyl amino esters and amides via *N*-alkylation of amino acids and/or esters.

catalyst system is needed. Importantly such catalyst should be tolerant to strong chelating coordination of the highly functionalized amino acid ester or amide substrates or derived reaction intermediates (Scheme 1C) that may block important coordination sites and thus might slow or shut down catalysis.

We have previously introduced the first homogeneous Fe-catalyzed direct *N*-alkylation of amines with alcohols (with Knölker's complex) without any addition of base. Next, we have also developed a powerful, base-free method

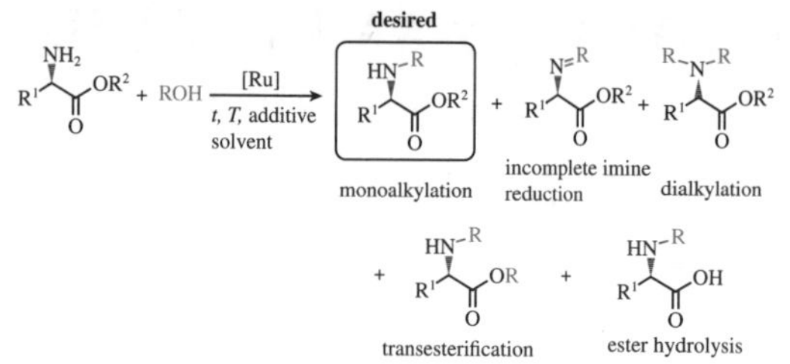

Scheme 2. Reaction scheme of mono *N*-alkylation of amino acid esters: desired product and possible side reactions.

for the direct coupling of unprotected amino acids with alcohols as well as the direct amination of β-hydroxyl acid esters and the decarboxylative *N*-alkylation of cyclic amino acids with alcohols using the Ru-based Shvo's catalyst (**Cat 1**). These findings serve as excellent starting point for establishing a novel catalytic methodology for the direct coupling of amino acid amides and esters with alcohols (Scheme 1). Initial study revealed that amino acid esters behave differently from unprotected amino acids, since the lack of free carboxylic acid moiety may influence the imine formation or reduction rates and transesterification may also occur at higher temperatures. The method requires unique reaction conditions (temperature, catalyst loading, potential additives) to allow for sufficiently facile imine formation and reduction without competing side reactions (i.e., transesterification, dialkylation) and avoiding racemization (Scheme 2).

To establish suitable conditions for the selective *N*-alkylation of amino acid esters, we have selected phenylalanine pentyl ester (**1 a**) and 4-methylbenzyl alcohol (**2 a**) as substrates and toluene as the solvent. The use of 0.5 mol% **Cat 1**, at 120°C for 18 h, gave full conversion of **1 a**, but only 55% selectivity of the desired mono-alkylation product **3 a** (Table 1, entry 1) due to the formation of 35% alkylated transesterification side product, as expected. With the benzyl ester of phenylalanine (**1 b**) the reaction was more sluggish, displaying only 69% conversion (Table 1, entry 2). Lowering the reaction temperature to 90°C with phenylalanine pentyl ester (**1 a**) gave minimal (< 5%) conversion (Table 1, entry 3), but no transesterification was seen.

Realizing that at lower temperatures the competing transesterification step is much less pronounced, we have searched for alternative ways to enhance reactivity at 90°C, by employing an appropriate Brønsted acid co-catalyst. Previous studies have described cooperative catalysis in ruthenium-catalyzed imine hydrogenation using chiral or achiral Brønsted acids, and we have earlier reported the enhancement of both the imine formation as well as the imine reduction step involved in the hydrogen borrowing sequence during the amination of β- hydroxy acids employing the same Ru catalyst. Indeed, both the conversion of **1 a** (23%) and **3 a** selectivity (22%) improved upon addition of 4 mol% of diphenyl phosphate (**A1**) (Table 1, entry 4). The

Table 1. Direct *N*-alkylation of L-phenylalanine ester with 4-methylbenzyl alcohol.[a]

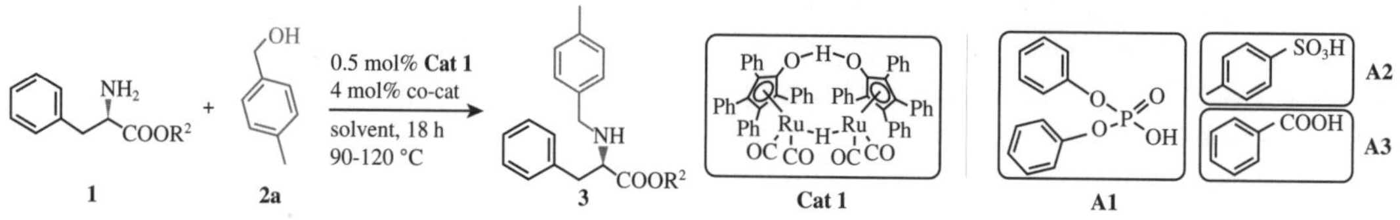

Entry	R2/1	2 a [equiv.]	solvent	co-cat.	T [°C]	Conv. 1 [%]	Sel. 3 [%]	
1	*n*-pentyl/**1a**	1.5	toluene	–	120	>99	**3a**	55[b]
2	Bn/**1b**	1.5	toluene	–	120	69	**3b**	60
3[c]	*n*-pentyl/**1 a**	2	toluene	–	90	<5	**3a**	–
4[c]	*n*-pentyl/**1 a**	2	toluene	**A1**	90	23	**3a**	22
5[c]	*n*-pentyl/**1 a**	2	toluene	**A2**	90	14	**3a**	13
6[c,d]	*n*-pentyl/**1 a**	2	toluene	**A3**	90	–	**3a**	–
7	*n*-pentyl/**1 a**	2	CPME	**A1**	100	26	**3a**	23
8	*n*-pentyl/**1 a**	2	THF	**A1**	100	18	**3a**	10
9	*n*-pentyl/**1 a**	2	heptane	**A1**	100	34	**3a**	32
10	*n*-pentyl/**1 a**	2	toluene	**A1**	100	63	**3a**	62
11	*n*-pentyl/**1 a**	4	toluene	**A1**	100	>99	**3a**	93 (86), 96% *ee*

[a] General reaction conditions: general procedure, 0.5 mmol **1**, 1.5–4 equiv. **2 a**, 0.5 mol% **Cat 1**, 2 mL solvent, 18 h, 90–120°C, isolated yield in parentheses, unless otherwise specified. Conversion and selectivity were determined by GC-FID based on the integration ratio among amino acid contained moieties. [b] 35% Alkylated transesterification side-product was observed. [c] 24 h. [d] Decomposition of ester **1 a** was observed.

use of other Brønsted acids [*p*-toluenesulfonic acid (**A2**) and benzoic acid (**A3**)] resulted only in moderate improvement (Table 1, entries 5 and 6) and screening a range of solvents at 100°C with **A1** also showed poor results (Table 1, entries 7–9). Therefore, further optimization of reaction temperature and **2 a** amount in toluene was carried out, while keeping **A1** as the co-catalyst in toluene (Table 1, entries 10 and 11). The best result was obtained at 100°C, leading to full conversion of **1 a**, and 93% selectivity (86% isolated yield) of the desired product **3a** with and 96% retention of enantiomeric excess (*ee;* Table 1, entry 11). The positive results with diphenyl phosphate (**A1**) are likely due to the enhancement of imine formation as well as imine reduction steps involved in the hydrogen borrowing cycle.

Next, the reaction scope was explored with selected examples of methyl-, ethyl-, isopropyl-, and pentyl esters of diverse amino acids including phenylalanine (**Phe**), alanine (**Ala**), valine (**Val**), leucine (**Leu**), proline (**Pro**) and glutamic acid (**Glu**) (Scheme 3). Various esters of phenylalanine (**Ph**) were efficiently *N*-alkylated with substituted benzyl alcohols (**2 a**, **2 b**, **2 d**) or pentanol (**2 c**) with excellent selectivity, high isolated yields, and high retention of *ee* in the corresponding products **3 c–3 f**. The functionalization of the alanine (**Ala**) backbone was evaluated using isopropyl and pentyl esters.

Gratifyingly, the pentyl esters resulted in the formation of the corresponding mono-alkylated products (**3 i–3 k**) in 66–79% isolated yields and 92–97% *ee* retention. Interestingly, slight racemization was observed for the isopropyl ester **3 h** (83% *ee*). Next, the pentyl ester of valine (**Val**) was subjected to this optimized *N*-alkylation protocol with benzyl alcohols (**2 a**, **2 b**, **2 e**) affording the corresponding *N*-alkyl analogues (**3 m–3 o**) with 82–87% isolated yield and outstanding *ee* (99%), while also the pentyl analogue **3 l** was obtained in 86% isolated yield. Similarly, the ethyl ester of leucine (**Leu**) provided the desired products **3 p** and **3 q** with 96 and 94% *ee*, respectively.

Interestingly, the reaction of 4-methyl-benzyl alcohol (**2 a**) with glutamic acid (**Glu**) diethyl ester (**1 i**) lead to the formation of the cyclic 2-pyrrolidinone derivative **3 r** with excellent stereoselectivity (99% *ee*) albeit moderate isolated yield (35%), due to an intramolecular amide formation. Finally, when the pentyl ester of proline (**Pro**) was selected to react with alcohol **2 a**, the corresponding product **3 t** was obtained with 42% isolated yield and 70% retention of *ee*.

We also performed a specific comparison between our Ru- based catalytic system with the previously described Ir-based system shown on Scheme 1B, in the direct alkylation of phenylalanine ethyl ester (**1 d**) with 1,5-pentanediol (**2 f**).

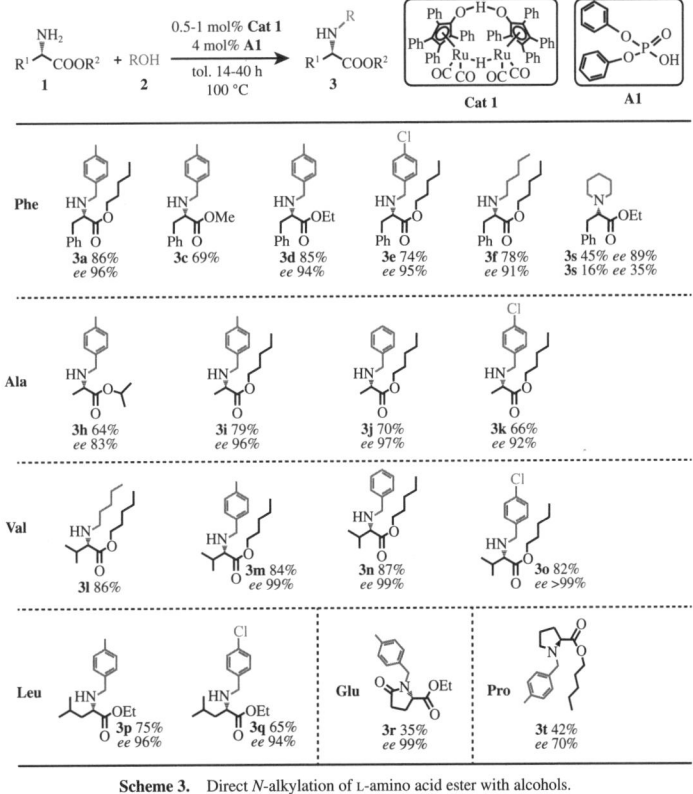

Scheme 3. Direct *N*-alkylation of L-amino acid ester with alcohols.

While our base-free system (comprising **Cat 1** and **A1**) resulted in **3 s** in 48% yield and 89% *ee*, the base-containing Ir system displayed lower conversion and significant racemization (16% **3 s** yield, 35% *ee).*

Next, we addressed challenging examples of direct alkylation of amino acid amides with alcohols (Scheme 4). Gratifyingly, when prolinamide (**1 k**) and 4-methylbenzyl alcohol (**2 a**) were selected as substrates (Scheme 4A), 83% isolated yield of the desired *N*-alkylation product *N*-(4-methyl)-benzyl prolinamide (**3 u**) was obtained, with as low as 0.5 mol% **Cat 1** and 4 mol% **A1**. Unfortunately, only 59% *ee* was obtained in this case, which indicates easier racemization of amino amides than esters in the working condition. Interestingly, when the Fe-based **Cat 2** (Knölker's complex), previously applied in *N*-alkylation by our group, was used in the same reaction, the cyclic product 4-imidazonone **3 w** was obtained instead, via intramolecular nucleophilic attack of the iminium intermediate by the amide group (Scheme 4A), likely due to the sluggish iminium reduction step. This underscores the efficiency of our Ru-based, base free method and the advantages of using the acid co-catalyst **A1** expected to facilitate the important reduction step.

Finally, to demonstrate the versatility of our methodology, we turned our attention to the straightforward synthesis of the pharmaceutical compound Ropivacaine (**3 v**). Previously, Leonard et al. attempted the direct Ru-catalyzed *N*-alkylation of the specific amino amide **1 l** with *n*-propanol to access Ropivacaine (**3 v**); however, the imidazolidinone derivative (**3 x**) was obtained instead, similarly to what we observed with **Cat 2** in the case of **3 w** (Scheme 4A). Gratifyingly, with our catalytic system, quantitative yield of Ropivacaine (**3 v**) was obtained with 90% *ee* when the *N*-alkylation of aminoamide **1 l** was performed in neat *n*-propanol at 90°C, using 1 mol% **Cat 1** and 4 mol% **A1** (Scheme 4C). This demonstrates the superior performance of our newly developed Ru-catalyzed method for preparing pharmaceutically relevant *N*-alkyl amino amides.

In summary, this study demonstrates an efficient method (0.5–1 mol% Ru loading) for the direct selective mono-*N*-alkylation of natural amino acid esters and amides with alcohols, with good to excellent yields and retention of the stereochemical integrity. This provides an excellent opportunity for the direct coupling of naturally abundant amino acid derivatives with widely accessible and potentially bio-based alcohols. Moreover, this method allowed for the challenging direct *N*-alkylation of amino-acid amides, while taking advantage of the facile iminium reduction step, thus overcoming a common cyclization side reaction. The successful synthesis of Ropivacaine, which was prepared in quantitative yield and excellent *ee* retention, underscores the power of this methodology.

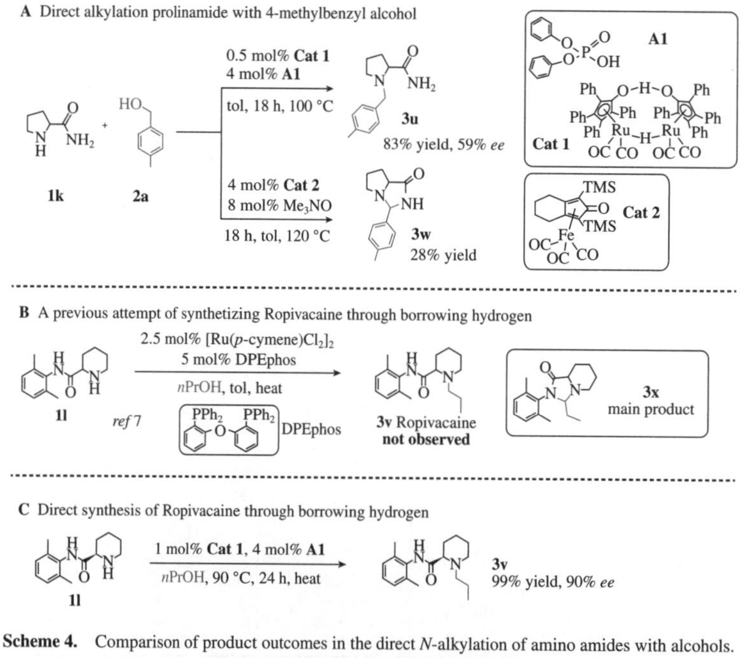

Scheme 4. Comparison of product outcomes in the direct *N*-alkylation of amino amides with alcohols.

JOURNAL ARTICLE EXERCISE 1

The science sections on the MCAT include a significant number of passages with experiments. Questions for these passages often ask you to analyze data, read charts and graphs, and come to some reasonable conclusion based on the information they give you. If you don't know how to extract information efficiently and analyze data effectively, you will be at a distinct disadvantage. Therefore, it's important to be comfortable with skimming and locating information in both text and nontext sources.

There are three "Journal Article Exercises" in this book that will show you how to start locating and considering this type of information in organic chemistry-oriented journal publications. In this first exercise, we'll show you the type of information you should be able to extract from the article and the sorts of things to pay attention to in the data. In a subsequent exercise, you'll do more of that on your own, and in the final exercise we'll show you how that article might get turned into an MCAT-style passage.

This first exercise demonstrates what to pay attention to in a journal article discussing organic synthesis by asking some generalized questions, then showing you what responses are appropriate and where the information for that response can be found within the article.

The questions we will be addressing are:

1. What is the purpose of this study?
2. What problem is this study trying to address or solve?
3. What functional groups appear in the molecules being studied?
4. Do any familiar reactions appear in this study?
5. How are the results presented? Tables/graphs/figures?
6. What approaches are presented in this study?
7. What unique terms are provided in the experimental data?
8. What results are found from the experimental data?
9. Are there any unexpected/unexplained results?
10. What final summary of the study and results can you conclude?

Remember, the goal of these exercises is NOT to learn content from the articles, just to get a little more comfortable reading and extracting information from them. As you read, you should avoid getting bogged down by details. Instead, focus on the bottom line and pay attention to where information is located, then read through the response to each question to help clarify your understanding of the meaningful aspects gleaned from the article. On the following pages, let's answer the above questions for Journal Article 1.

SOLUTIONS TO JOURNAL ARTICLE EXERCISE 1

1. **What is the purpose of this study?**

   The study examines a nontraditional method of selective N-alkylation of α-amino acid esters and/or amides using alcohols by employing a base-free, ruthenium-based catalyst. By designing a series of N-alkylation reactions, the study seeks to identify a selective method of mono-N-alkylation with high yield and retention in stereochemistry.

2. **What problem is this study trying to address or solve?**

   The introduction to this study states that a base is required for most methods that provide direct N-alkylation of amino acid derivatives. Since the α-carbon in amino acids is sensitive to base and may undergo racemization in its presence, this study seeks to provide a method to deliver direct N-alkylation of amino acid esters while retaining α-carbon chirality.

3. **What functional groups appear in the molecules being studied?**

   N-alkyl amino acid esters and/or amides are featured throughout the study. From the figures, you should note that these structures contain a combination of individual functional groups. For example, an amino acid ester is a molecule based on an amino acid structure but where instead of a COOH (carboxylic acid) group a COOR (ester) group appears.

   Mono-N-alkylation means that the amino nitrogen atom has been modified with a single alkyl (R) group. The process of N-alkylation of an amino acid ester can be viewed in a generalized way in Scheme 1A in the article. As a further example of this, the structure for Enalapril shown in Figure 1 can be identified as an N-alkylated amino acid ester whereas Lidocaine would be an example of an N-alkylated amino acid amide.

4. **Do any familiar reactions appear in this study?**

   By and large the reactions being used in this study should not be recognizable and are not testable on the MCAT, but the reaction shown in Scheme 1A (lower pathway, b) follows a nucleophilic substitution, which is a common MCAT reaction. You should thus be able to identify the amino group nitrogen atom as a nucleophile, the carbon atom of the R group in R–X as the electrophile, with X being a leaving group for this reaction.

   Scheme 2 notes multiple (desired and undesired) products from the mono-N-alkylation of amino acid esters. Notable among these are the transesterification and hydrolysis products which result from nucleophilic addition-elimination processes.

5. **How are the results presented? Tables/graphs/figures?**

   The results are presented in tables and figures. Table 1, Scheme 3, and Scheme 4 show results. The remaining figures throughout the article outline schemes for the reactions being discussed but do not contain data.

6. **What approaches are presented in this study?**
Scheme 1C shows the general *N*-alkylation process being followed in this study, which includes a ruthenium-based catalyst, called Shvo's catalyst (Cat 1). This method of *N*-alkylation was then tested with five separate approaches.

This first approach is outlined in paragraphs 5 and 6 with results given in Table 1. This approach includes:

- Phenylalanine pentyl ester and 4-methylbenzyl alcohol as substrates.
- Toluene as solvent.
- Heat and a co-catalyst (diphenyl phosphate), a Brønstead-Lowry acid. Both conditions are needed to overcome the competing transesterification reaction shown in Scheme 2.
- Other Brønstead-Lowry co-catalysts (*p*-toluenesulfonic acid and benzoic acid).

The second approach involves a wide range of substrates consisting of methyl-, ethyl-, isopropyl-, and pentyl- esters of Phe, Ala, Val, Leu, Pro, and Glu along with the same conditions employed in the first approach (namely, toluene as solvent with Cat 1 and diphenyl phosphate as co-catalyst under heating conditions). The results from these reactions are displayed in Scheme 3.

The third approach compares *N*-alkylation reactions from a Ru-based catalyst to that of an Ir-based system (outlined in Scheme 1B).

The fourth approach addresses direct *N*-alkylation of the amino acid amide, prolinamide. The results from this reaction are displayed in Scheme 4A.

The final approach addresses the direct synthesis of the pharmaceutically relevant amino acid amide, Ropivacaine, by comparing an earlier method with the Ru-based method from this study. The results from these reactions are displayed in Schemes 4B and 4C.

7. **What unique terms are provided in the experimental data?**
Table 1, and Schemes 3 and 4 address **conversion** and **selectivity**. These terms can be better understood by reading paragraph 5 which describes the first entry in Table 1 giving "full conversion of 1A but only 55% selectivity of the desired" product. This indicates the reactant is fully consumed but does not produce a high yield of the desired product. Ideally, full conversion with high selectivity (as close to 100% as possible for both numbers) would reflect an optimized reaction. Reading the data provided from Table 1 and Schemes 3 and 4 in this way is how one should process the results.

The term *ee* also appears in each location indicating enantiomeric excess, or yield of the specific enantiomer formed. An *ee* value that is high indicates that predominantly one enantiomer is produced which means there is high stereoselectivity in the process of forming that product (i.e., good purity).

8. **What results are found from the experimental data?**

Based on the details given in Table 1 for the reaction shown, you should notice that there are several variables to consider, including:

a. the R^2 group in **1**: *n*-pentyl or benzyl.
b. the equivalents of **2**: 1.5, 2, or 4 eq.
c. the solvent: toluene, CPME, or TMF (all nonpolar solvents).
d. the co-catalyst used: no co-catalyst, A1, A2, or A3.
e. the temperature: 90, 100, or 120°C.

Good practice is to observe the results and work backward to the corresponding conditions to establish useful connections. For example, entry 11 in Table 1 shows the optimal trial with the following combination of variables from those above: *n*-pentyl on **1**, 4 eq. of **2**, toluene as solvent, A1 co-catalyst, and 100°C. From this, one might then notice that entry 10 features one difference in variable: half the eq. of **2** is used. This produces a decrease in conversion and selectivity by roughly one-third, which suggests an excess of alcohol is important for optimizing the reaction. When more variables are changed, the conclusions weaken, so focus on single variable changes like this to draw out possible meaning in data sets.

For Scheme 3, a reaction is shown at the top, where only the substrates are manipulated, and products formed are represented with molecular structures below. The most important details to note here are the substrate combinations and patterns in the resulting products for specific % yields and % *ee*. For instance, it appears that pentyl esters of the various amino acids yield good results (3a, 3e, 3f, 3h–o) with the pentyl ester of Pro being a notable exception.

For Scheme 4, one might note that attempts at direct *N*-alkylation of amino acid amides shown using Cat 1 gives more successful results than with previous methodologies. This is revealed by the product **3u**, which is the desired *N*-alkylated product in Scheme 4A. Cat 2, a previously tested catalyst, does not produce the desired product at all. The fact that a low % *ee* is observed for **3u** further allows the researchers to conclude that it is more difficult to *N*-alkylate amino acid amides compared to amino acid esters. This finding is also supplemented by the attempt to synthesize Ropivacaine, which a previous attempt (Scheme 4B) did not successfully produce, but here Cat 1 reports in high success (Scheme 4C).

9. **Are there any unexpected/unexplained results?**

Many unexplained nuances can emerge when examining data, so for the purpose of this question, we will look at one such example in Table 1, entry 6. Decomposition of phenylalanine pentyl ester was observed in the reaction using benzoic acid acting as co-catalyst. It is unclear what the substrate decomposes to or why this occurs.

10. **What final summary of the study and results can you conclude?**

The methodology proposed in this study shows that direct mono-*N*-alkylation of amino acid esters and amides using alcohols is possible by employing a base-free, Ru-based system. The results show good yield and a high degree of retention of stereochemistry of the α-carbon in a range of substrates. These substrates include esters of Phe, Ala, Val, Leu, Pro, and Glu, and the amino acid amide, prolinamide. Results with prolinamide, and amino acid amides in general, indicated greater difficulty in employing the proposed methodology using those substrates. This study also shows the successful direct synthesis of a pharmaceutically active molecule, Ropivacaine.

Chapter 5
Lab Techniques: Separations and Spectroscopy

5.1 SEPARATIONS

Extractions

One of the more useful techniques in experimental organic chemistry is solvent extraction. Isolation of natural products from marine organisms, plants, and other natural sources is facilitated by exploiting the particular solubilities of organic compounds in various solvents. Complex mixtures of organic compounds can be separated using a careful choice of solvents based on the differential solubilities of the various components of the mixture. We'll see that the acid/base properties of organic molecules play an important role in the extraction process.

Extraction allows the chemist to separate one substance from a mixture of substances by adding a solvent in which the compound of interest is highly soluble. If the solution containing the compound of interest is shaken with a second solvent (completely immiscible with the first) and allowed to separate into two distinct phases, the compound of interest will distribute itself between the two phases based upon its solubility in each of the individual solvents. This is called a **liquid-liquid extraction**. The ratio of the substance's solubilities in the two solvents is called the **distribution** (or **partition**) **coefficient**.

Solubility largely depends on two things: the polarity of the solute and the polarity of the solvent. When it comes to solubility, *like dissolves like*. Polar molecules are soluble in polar solvents, and nonpolar molecules are soluble in nonpolar solvents. For example, water is a polar solvent and hydrocarbons are nonpolar molecules. Hydrocarbons will therefore have very low solubility in water.

The simplest liquid-liquid extraction is accomplished when an organic compound is extracted with water. A simple water extraction can remove substances that are highly polar or charged, including inorganic salts, strong acids and bases, and polar, low molecular weight compounds (less than five carbons) such as alcohols, amines, and carboxylic acids.

A second class of organic extraction involves the use of acidic or basic water solutions. Organic compounds that are basic (e.g., amines) can be extracted from mixtures of organic compounds upon treatment with dilute acid (usually 5–10% HCl). This treatment will protonate the basic functional group, forming a positively charged ion. The resulting cationic salts of these basic compounds are usually freely soluble in aqueous solution and can be removed from the organic compounds that remain dissolved in the organic phase.

Extraction of Organic Amines

$$R-\overset{\displaystyle ..}{N}H_2 \xrightarrow{\text{10\% HCl}} R-\overset{\displaystyle \overset{H}{|}}{\underset{\displaystyle \underset{H}{|}}{N}}\!\!\overset{\oplus}{}-H \;\; + \;\; Cl^-$$

On the other hand, extraction with a dilute weak base—typically 5 percent sodium bicarbonate ($NaHCO_3$) —results in converting carboxylic acids into their corresponding anionic salts.

Extraction of Carboxylic Acids

$$R-COOH \xrightarrow{\text{5\% NaHCO}_3} R-COO^-Na^+ \;\; + \;\; H_2O \;\; + \;\; CO_2$$

These anionic salts are generally soluble in aqueous solution and can be removed from the organic compounds that remain dissolved in the organic phase. Dilute sodium hydroxide could also be used for this kind of extraction, but it is basic enough to also convert phenols into their corresponding anionic salts. When phenols are present in a mixture of organic compounds and need to be removed, a dilute sodium hydroxide solution (usually about 10%) will succeed in converting phenols into their corresponding anionic salts. The anionic salts of the phenols are generally soluble in the aqueous phase and can therefore be removed from the organic phase.

Extraction of Phenols

(*Note:* NaOH will also extract carboxylic acids.)

The apparatus in which these extractions are typically carried out is called a **separatory funnel**. To perform a solvent-solvent extraction, the solution containing the mixture of organic compounds and the extraction solvent of choice are poured into the separatory funnel, and the apparatus is fitted with a stopper. After mixing, the two layers may be separated from one another by removing the stopper at the top and slowly collecting each phase into separate receiving flasks by opening the stopcock at the bottom of the funnel.

As an example, let us step through an extraction that will separate four organic compounds from one another. The original mixture consists of *para*-cresol, benzoic acid, aniline, and naphthalene, all of which are dissolved in diethyl ether. This mixture is first extracted with an equal volume of aqueous sodium bicarbonate. The weakly basic bicarbonate is sufficiently basic to deprotonate benzoic acid and convert it to an anionic salt, but not strong enough to deprotonate *para*-cresol (a phenol). Likewise, a bicarbonate extraction will not affect aniline (a base itself) or naphthalene (a hydrocarbon). Thus, *para*-cresol, aniline, and naphthalene will remain dissolved in the ether phase, while the benzoic acid, now in its anionic salt form, will be extracted into the aqueous layer.

The ether layer, which now contains three components, is extracted with a sodium hydroxide solution. The strongly basic hydroxide ion is strong enough to deprotonate *para*-cresol and convert it to its anionic salt form. The basic conditions will not affect aniline or naphthalene, so *para*-cresol is the only compound that is extracted into the aqueous phase. The aniline and naphthalene will remain dissolved in the ether layer.

Finally, the remaining two components can be separated from one another by an acidic extraction with a 10% HCl solution. The solution is acidic enough to protonate the lone pair of electrons of aniline and to convert aniline to its cationic salt. Naphthalene will not be affected and will remain dissolved in the ether layer. The final extraction of aniline into the aqueous phase completes the separation. Naphthalene can be isolated by evaporating off the diethyl ether.

These steps are summarized on the following page.

All four components dissolved in diethyl ether

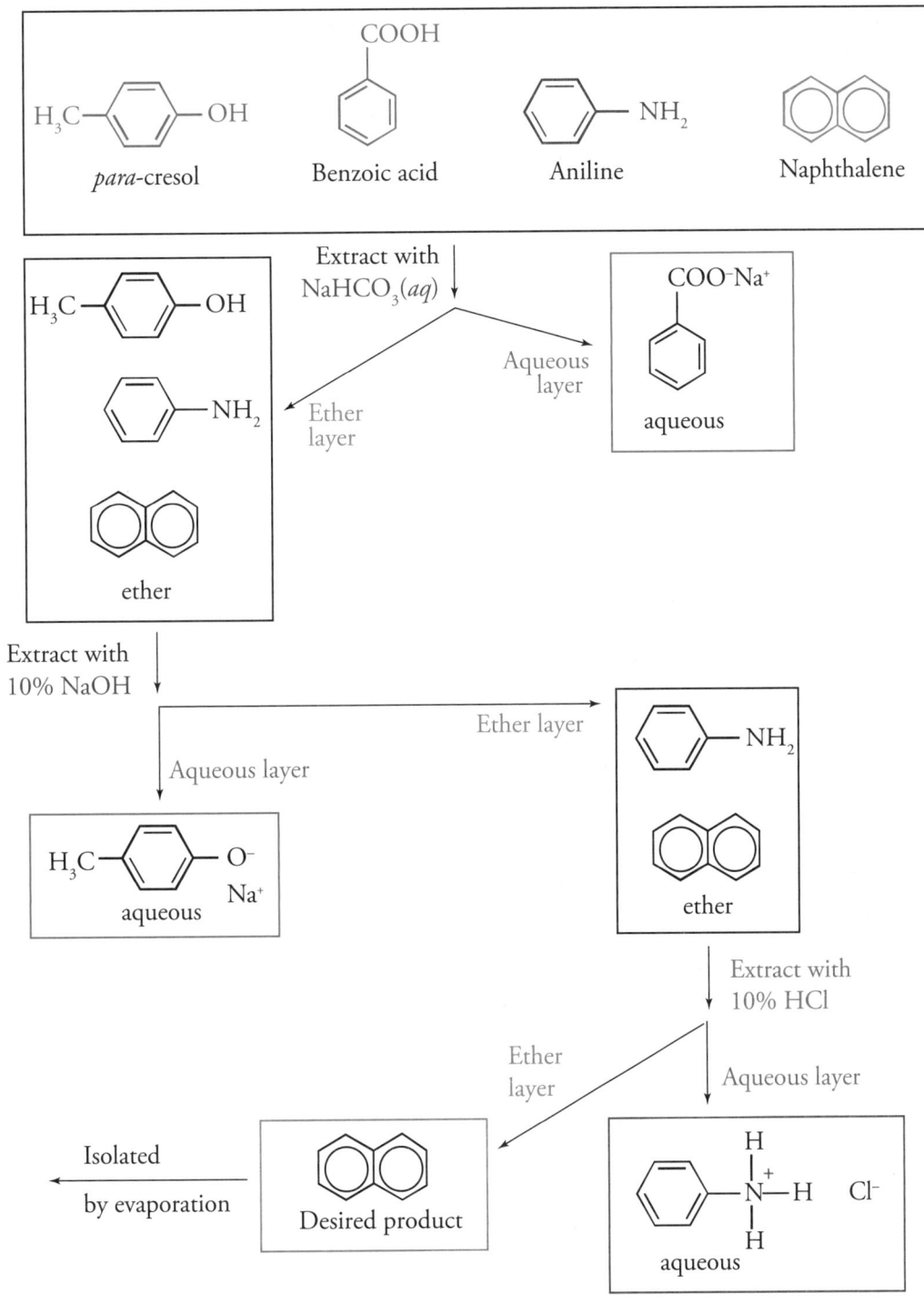

Chromatography

While there are many types of chromatography, they all have a number of basic features in common. All types of chromatography are used to separate mixtures of compounds, though some are used mostly for identification purposes, while others are generally used as purification methods. First, we will consider thin-layer chromatography to outline the basic features. Then we will describe several other types, high-lighting for each how the separation process works and the types of compounds that are most commonly separated by that method.

Thin-Layer Chromatography (TLC)

In TLC, compounds are separated based on differing polarities. Because of the speed of separation and the small sample amounts that can be successfully analyzed, this technique is frequently used in organic chemistry laboratories. **Thin-layer chromatography** is a solid-liquid partitioning technique in which the **mobile liquid phase** ascends a thin layer of absorbent (generally silica, SiO_2) that is coated onto a supporting material such as a glass plate. This thin layer of absorbent acts as a **polar stationary phase** for the sample to interact with. To perform TLC, a very small amount (about 1 microliter) of sample is spotted near the base of the plate (about 1 cm from the bottom) before placing the plate upright in a sealed container with a shallow layer of solvent.

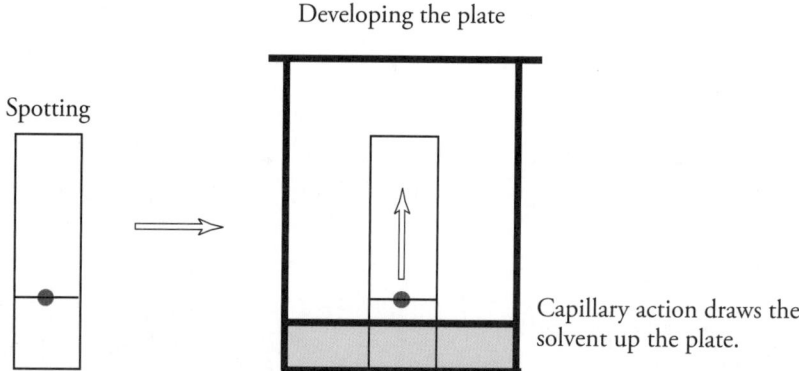

Developing the plate

Spotting

Capillary action draws the solvent up the plate.

As the solvent slowly ascends the plate via capillary action, the components of the spotted sample are partitioned between the mobile phase and the stationary phase. This process is referred to as **developing**, or **running**, a thin layer plate. Each component of the sample experiences many equilibrations between the mobile and the stationary phases as the development proceeds.

Separation of the compounds occurs because different components travel along the plate at different rates. The more polar components of the mixture interact more with the polar stationary phase and travel at a slower rate. The less polar components have a greater affinity for the solvent than the stationary phase and travel with the mobile solvent at a faster rate than the more polar components. Once the solvent nearly reaches the top of the plate, the plate is removed and allowed to dry. If the compounds in the mixture are colored, we would see a vertical series of spots on the plate; however, it is more likely that the components are not colored and need to be detected by some other means. Visualization methods include shining ultraviolet light on the plate, placing the thin layer plate in the presence of iodine vapor, and a host of other chemical staining techniques.

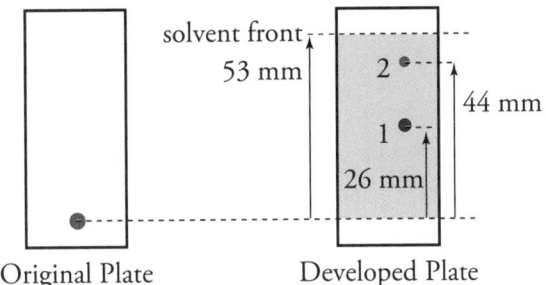

Original Plate   Developed Plate

Once the separated components have been visualized, R_f values can be computed. This "ratio to front" value (R_f) is simply the distance traveled by an individual component divided by the distance traveled by the solvent front. For example, from the illustration above, we would find

$$R_f \text{ (Compound 1)} = \frac{26 \text{ mm}}{53 \text{ mm}} = 0.49 \qquad R_f \text{ (Compound 2)} = \frac{44 \text{ mm}}{53 \text{ mm}} = 0.83$$

(Note that R_f is always positive and never greater than 1.)

Column (Flash) Chromatography

While TLC is a good technique for separating very small amounts of material in order to assess how many compounds make up a mixture, it's not a good technique for isolating bulk compounds. A common technique known as column or flash chromatography employs the same principles behind TLC toward just such a goal. Shown on the next page is a chromatography column. This column is filled with silica gel (predominantly SiO_2, as in the TLC plate). The silica gel is saturated with a chosen organic solvent, and the mixture of compounds to be separated is then added to the top and allowed to travel down through the silica-packed column. Excess solvent is periodically added to the top of the column, and the flow of solvent (along with the separated compounds) is collected from the bottom. Just as is the case in TLC, polar compounds will spend more time adsorbed on the polar solid phase, and as such travel more slowly down the column than nonpolar compounds. Therefore, compounds can be expected to leave the column, and be collected, in order of polarity (least polar to most polar).

Column Chromatography

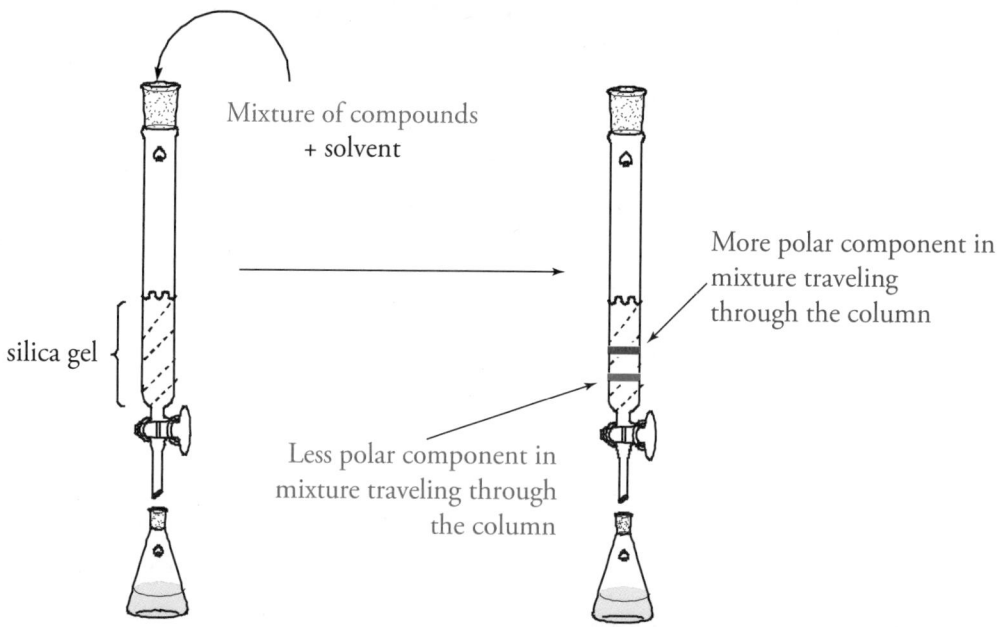

silica gel

Mixture of compounds + solvent

More polar component in mixture traveling through the column

Less polar component in mixture traveling through the column

Ion Exchange Chromatography

In applications where the materials to be separated have varying charge states, ion exchange chromatography may be employed. This method, again involving passing a mobile liquid phase containing the analyte through a column packed with a solid stationary phase, utilizes a polymeric resin functionalized with either positively or negatively charged moieties on the polymer surface.

The schematic on the next page depicts the passage of an analyte containing both positively and negatively charged ionic species, as well neutral molecules, through a pore of an ion exchange resin. The particular stationary phase resin depicted on the following page is functionalized with anionic sulfonate groups, initially coordinated to sodium cations.

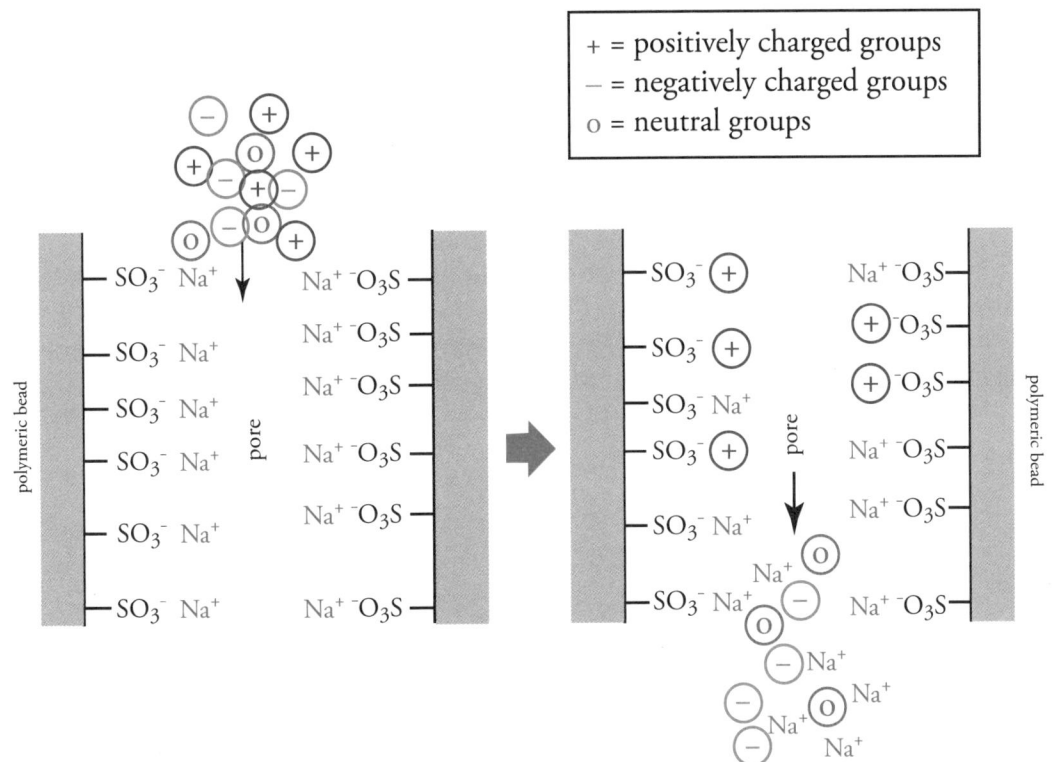

+ = positively charged groups
− = negatively charged groups
o = neutral groups

As the analyte passes through the resin, positively charged groups displace sodium ions and coordinate to the anionic functionalities tethered to the polymer surface. While these groups are retained, and their progress through the column retarded, the negatively charged groups and neutral species quickly pass through the material and are eluted first. Once all the negatively charged and neutral species have been eluted, the column can be treated with a concentrated sodium-containing solution to displace all adsorbed positively charged species.

Ion exchange chromatography is frequently used in the separation of mixtures of proteins. At any given pH, proteins within a mixture may exist in a variety of charge states (more on this in Chapter 7). If such a mixture is passed through a cation exchange resin (one functionalized with negatively charged groups and cationic counterions as shown in the figure above), those proteins with pI values greater than the pH of the mobile phase will be positively charged and elute slowly compared to those with pI values below the solution pH. If the same mixture at the same pH were passed through an anion exchange resin, the opposite would be true, and proteins with pI values above the pH of the solution will elute first. If the pI values of the proteins to be separated are known, the pH of the mobile phase may be buffered to a specific pH, thereby ensuring different charge states and hence good separation.

High Performance Liquid Chromatography (HPLC)

HPLC uses the same principles as all chromatographic separation techniques, and takes advantage of the differing affinities of various compounds for either a stationary phase or a mobile phase. However, because the mobile phase is forced through the stationary phase at very high pressures, both the speed and efficiency of the separation is increased, making this technique an improvement over column chromatography.

The basic configuration of an HPLC system is shown in the figure below. The pumping unit is where pressurization of the mobile phase first occurs. The sample to be separated is solubilized and injected by syringe, then the mobile phase carries the sample to the column. The sample is separated into its constituent components, which are detected and analyzed as they exit the column. The eluent is collected after detection, and the components can be isolated after evaporation of the solvent, if desired.

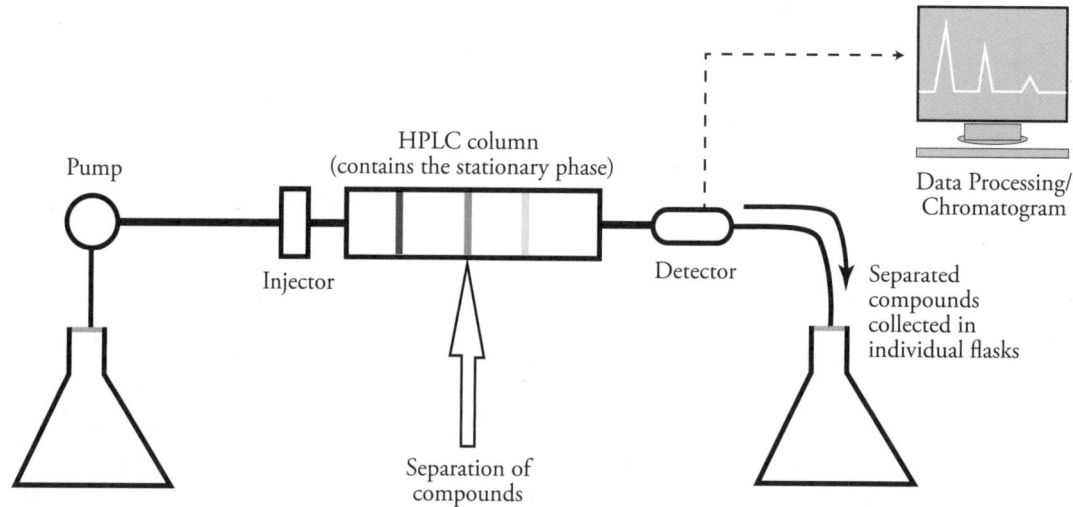

The elution time of any compound is dependent upon the mobile and stationary phases used. For most HPLC separations of organic compounds, the stationary phase is a silica gel that has been bonded to a nonpolar group (e.g., octadecylsilane), creating a relatively *nonpolar* stationary phase. This is called reverse phase HPLC. The mobile phase used is generally *more polar* than the stationary phase. This means the order of elution will be the reverse of what occurs on a TLC plate or in simple column chromatography. More polar compounds elute first in HPLC as they have a high affinity for the mobile phase. The less polar compounds are slowed by their interactions with the nonpolar stationary phase, and therefore elute last.

For the analysis of charged compounds, such as amino acids, the stationary phase is often an ion exchange column, usually cation exchange. The mobile phase is a polar, protic (e.g, CH_3OH or H_2O) or acidic solvent that ensures solubility and suppresses the dissociation of the COOH group on the amino acid. The difference in affinity to the column is attributed to the effects of the various R groups of the amino acids. Elution order can be predicted based on an analysis of the intermolecular forces of these side chains.

Size Exclusion Chromatography

Size exclusion chromatography is a technique used to separate bulk materials based on molecular size. Much like flash chromatography, the materials to be separated are dissolved in solvent, loaded onto a column packed with a stationary phase, and allowed to travel to the bottom of the column where they are collected.

In contrast to flash chromatography, which uses a polar silicate stationary phase, the stationary phase employed in size exclusion chromatography most often consists of chemically inert, porous polymer beads. The sizes of the pores in the bead are carefully controlled to allow permeation of small molecules in the eluent, while excluding larger ones. A schematic for the beads and the paths taken by large and small molecules is depicted below.

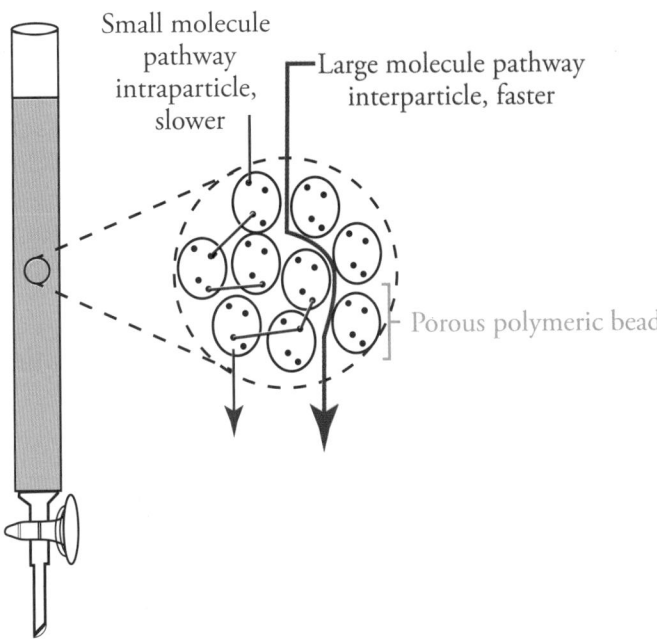

The exclusion of large molecules from the pore volume creates a more direct path down the column for large species than the more complicated intraparticle pathway taken by compounds small enough to permeate the beads. The overall result is the quick elution of large molecules and longer retention of smaller species.

Size exclusion chromatography is frequently used for the separation of large polymers from small oligomeric fragments, or the separation of full proteins from smaller peptide chains. The lack of chemical interaction between the mobile and stationary phases results in relatively speedy elution (compared to chromatography on silica) and minimal loss of material on the column. However, though materials of very different sizes are easily separated, the technique is not particularly effective at separating different compounds of similar sizes.

Affinity Chromatography

Affinity chromatography is most commonly used to purify proteins or nucleic acids from complex biochemical mixtures like cell lysates, growth media, or blood, rather than a reaction mixture. It is based on highly specific interactions between macromolecules. As a result of this specific binding, the target molecule is trapped on the stationary phase, which is then washed to remove the unwanted components of the mixture. The target protein is then released (or eluted) off the solid phase in a highly purified state.

In large-scale work, the stationary phase is a column packed with a solid resin, and the sample is poured through the column. In smaller scale experiments, the solid phase can be mixed in a small tube with the sample to allow interaction with the components of the mixture. The sample is then centrifuged (spun at high speeds) so the heavy solid resin settles to the bottom of the tube. Since the protein of interest is bound to the solid resin, the liquid (or supernatant) is simply decanted, leaving the desired compound behind.

In order to isolate a protein of interest, the highly specific interactions of antibodies can be used, as shown in the figure below. A commercially available antibody specific for the protein is added to the lysate sample. To isolate the antigen-antibody complex, one of three common microbe-derived proteins (Protein A, Protein G, or Protein L) is covalently linked to a solid support. These proteins are useful because they bind mammalian antibodies, so upon mixing, complexes made of *Protein of Interest – Antibody – Protein A/G/L – Solid Support Bead* form in solution. The target is then isolated after centrifuging the sample and decanting the supernatant.

Purifying a Protein of Interest using an Antibody and Protein A-linked Beads

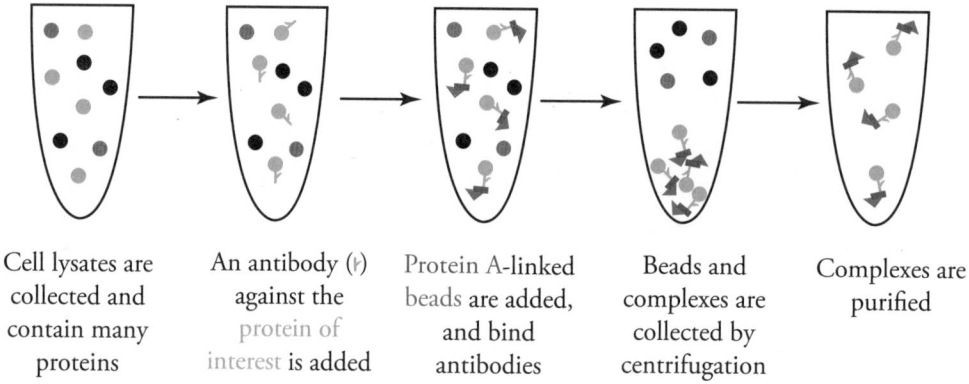

| Cell lysates are collected and contain many proteins | An antibody (⊦) against the protein of interest is added | Protein A-linked beads are added, and bind antibodies | Beads and complexes are collected by centrifugation | Complexes are purified |

Instead of centrifugation, magnetic beads can be used as the solid phase, as shown on the next page. The beads are isolated from the solution by using a magnet to hold them (bound to the protein of interest) against the sides of the tube, while the solution containing any undesired compounds is decanted. Then the desired compound can be released from the beads in a pure state.

Using Magnetic Beads as the Solid Phase in Affinity Chromatography

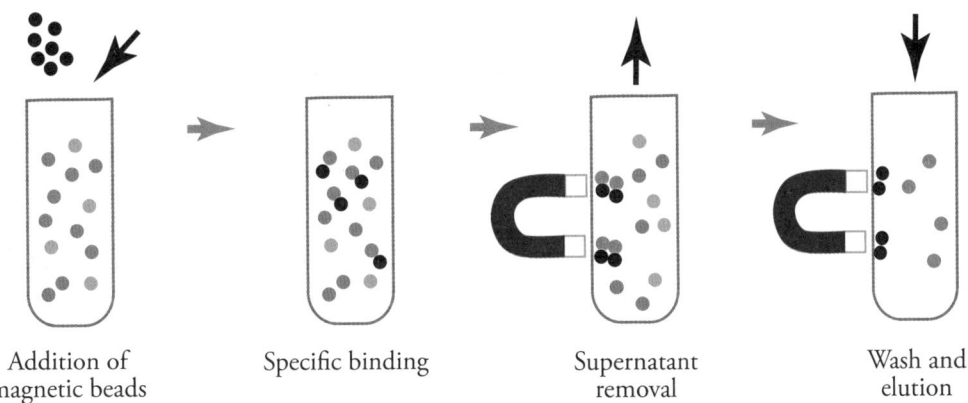

Addition of magnetic beads   Specific binding   Supernatant removal   Wash and elution

Not all proteins of interest have a commercial antibody available. In this case, researchers can use an **affinity tag.** Using recombinant technology (described in Appendix 1 of the *MCAT Biology Review*), a small molecular tag is added to the N-terminus or the C-terminus of the protein. DNA sequences coding for affinity tags are well known, and these can be subcloned into a plasmid with the gene of interest. Affinity-tagged proteins can be produced in large amounts in laboratory bacteria, and the cell lysate collected is rich in tagged protein.

There are many types of affinity tags, and they are generally small enough that they don't interfere with protein folding or function. One class of commonly used affinity tags includes the His tags (made of 6–10 histidine amino acids), which bind ions such as nickel. When a cell lysate is applied to a column packed with nickel-based resin, the His-tagged proteins bind to the resin. This is done under high pH conditions, and the His-tagged protein can be eluted off the solid phase using lower pH conditions.

Gas Chromatography

Gas chromatography (GC) is a form of column chromatography in which the partitioning of the components to be separated takes place between a **mobile gas phase** and a **stationary liquid phase**. This partitioning, or separation, between mixtures of compounds occurs based on their *different volatilities*. In a typical gas chromatograph, a sample is loaded into a syringe and injected into the device through a rubber septum. The sample is then vaporized by a heater in the injection port and carried along by a stream of inert gas (typically helium). The vaporized sample is quickly moved by the inert gas stream into a column composed of particles that are coated with a liquid absorbent. As the components of the sample pass through the column, they interact differently with the absorbent based on their relative volatilities. Each component of the sample is subjected to many gas-liquid partitioning processes which separates the individual components.

As each component exits the column, it is burned, and the resulting ions are detected by an electrical detector that generates a signal that is recorded by a chart recorder. The chart recorder printout enables us to determine the number of components and their relative amounts.

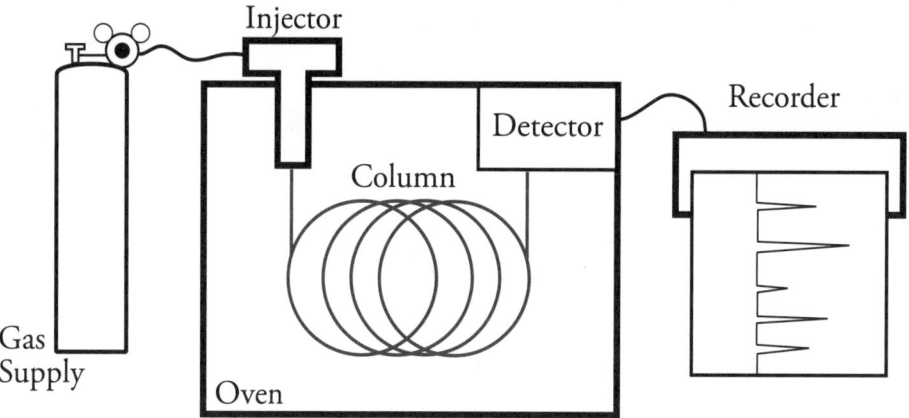

Let's now take a closer look at the separation process by examining a typical GC column. To do so, we will consider a mixture of two individual components. As the mixture enters the column, it begins to interact with the stationary phase, which is composed of support material coated with a liquid absorbent. The liquid absorbents can range from hydrocarbon mixtures that are very nonpolar to polyesters that are polar. As the mixture passes through the column, the components equilibrate between the carrier gas and the liquid phase. The less volatile components will spend more time dissolved in the liquid stationary phase than the more volatile component that will be carried along by the carrier gas at a faster rate. It is this equilibrium between the component (the absorbed liquid phase and the carrier gas mobile phase) that results in the separation of the mixture. If the interactions of the substrates with the column are similar (this is usually the case with most GC columns), the more volatile components emerge from the column first, while the less volatile components emerge from the column later.

Physical Properties of Organic Compounds

As we just discussed, it's the volatility, or boiling point, of a compound that is most important to consider when conducting a gas chromatography experiment. Generally speaking, this technique separates only small amounts of material, whereas the next technique, distillation, does the same thing, just for larger amounts of material.

In order to best understand the principles behind distillations, as well as predict when it's appropriate to use, we should first discuss some fundamentals about the physical properties of compounds, namely melting points and boiling points, and how they are related to the intermolecular forces of molecules.

Melting and Boiling Points

Melting point (mp) and **boiling point (bp)** are indicators of how well identical molecules interact with (attract) each other. Nonpolar molecules, like hydrocarbons, interact principally because of an attractive force known as the London dispersion force, one of the intermolecular (van der Waals) forces. This force exists between temporary dipoles formed in nonpolar molecules as a result of a temporary asymmetric electron distribution. Such intermolecular forces must be overcome to melt a nonpolar compound (solid → liquid) or to boil a nonpolar compound (liquid → gas). The greater the attractive forces between molecules, the more energy will be required to get the compound to melt or boil. The weaker these forces, the lower the melting or boiling point.

Many factors determine the degree to which molecules of a given compound will interact. For hydrocarbons, the most significant of these factors is *branching*. Branching tends to inhibit van der Waals forces by reducing the surface area available for intermolecular interaction. Thus, branching tends to reduce attractive forces between molecules and to lower both melting point and boiling point. Consider the following two constitutional isomers:

Molecule I
n-octane

Molecule II
2,4-dimethylhexane

Molecule I, *n*-octane, is unbranched. Molecule II, 2,4-dimethylhexane, is a branched isomer of *n*-octane. Although each compound has the same molecular formula, C_8H_{18}, these two constitutional isomers have dramatically different melting points and boiling points. *n*-octane requires much more energy to melt or boil, because unbranched, it experiences greater van der Waals forces than does the branched isomer 2,4-dimethylhexane. Therefore, *n*-octane has both a higher melting point and a higher boiling point than does 2,4-dimethylhexane.

The second factor influencing melting point and boiling point for hydrocarbons is molecular weight. The greater the molecular weight of a compound, the more surface area there is to interact, the greater the number of van der Waals interactions, and the higher the melting point and boiling point. Therefore, hexane—a six-carbon alkane—has a higher mp and bp than propane, a three-carbon alkane.

The influence of molecular weight on melting point and boiling point is readily seen when considering the following trends for hydrocarbons:

- Small hydrocarbons (1 to 4 carbons) tend to be gases at room temperature.
- Intermediate hydrocarbons (5 to 16 carbons) tend to be liquids at room temperature.
- Large hydrocarbons (more than 16 carbons) tend to be (waxy) solids at room temperature.

Example 5-1: Rank the following six hydrocarbons in order of increasing boiling point:

Solution: Since branching lowers the boiling point, each of the branched hydrocarbons has a lower boiling point than the unbranched hydrocarbon of the same molecular formula. Also, the larger the molecule, the greater the surface area over which van der Waals forces can act, so heavier molecules have higher boiling points. We can now put the whole sequence in order of increasing bp:

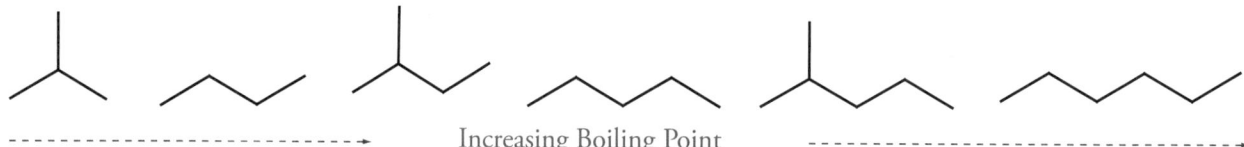

Increasing Boiling Point

Hydrogen Bonding

Another important type of intermolecular force that has a large effect on the physical properties of organic molecules is the hydrogen bond. In order to examine the effect of hydrogen bonding on melting or boiling points, let's examine two molecules that are isomers of one another, *n*-butanol and diethyl ether. Both have the same molecular formula ($C_4H_{10}O$), yet there is a dramatic difference in their boiling points (117°C for *n*-butanol vs. 34.6°C for diethyl ether). This difference arises from the ability of *n*-butanol to form intermolecular hydrogen bonds, while diethyl ether *cannot*.

Recall from General Chemistry that hydrogen bonding occurs between a hydrogen-bond donor—a hydrogen covalently bonded to a nitrogen, oxygen, or fluorine atom, and a hydrogen-bond acceptor—a lone pair of electrons on a nitrogen, oxygen, or fluorine in another molecule, or part of the first molecule. Alcohols form intermolecular hydrogen bonds because they have hydroxyl (–OH) groups. This results from a strong dipole in which the hydroxyl group's hydrogen acquires a substantial partial positive charge (δ^+) and the oxygen acquires a substantial partial negative charge (δ^-). The partial positive hydrogen can interact electrostatically with a non-bonding pair of electrons on a nearby oxygen, resulting in a hydrogen bond.

On the other hand, diethyl ether has an oxygen atom with non-bonding electrons but all hydrogen atoms are bound to carbons. Since carbon and hydrogen have similar electronegativity values, the bond is not very polarized, and these hydrogens cannot participate in hydrogen bonding. It's important to remember that a hydrogen bond is *not* a covalent bond; in this case it's an intermolecular interaction.

Intermolecular hydrogen bonding between molecules of *n*-butanol.

molecular weight = 74
bp = 117°C

$$H_3CH_2CH_2CH_2C \overset{\delta^-}{\underset{}{O}} \cdots \overset{\delta^+}{H} \cdots \overset{\delta^-}{O} \cdots CH_2CH_2CH_2CH_3$$

Intermolecular hydrogen bonding is not possible between molecules of diethyl ether

molecular weight = 74
bp = 34.6°C

The hydrogen bonding pattern in phenols provides insight into *inter*molecular vs. *intra*molecular hydrogen bonding. Let's consider the two isomers, 4-nitrophenol and 2-nitrophenol. First, examine the hydrogen bonding pattern in 4-nitrophenol. Notice that hydrogen bonding can occur with both the nitro and the hydroxyl groups in this molecule and that the bonding is exclusively intermolecular. That is, all hydrogen bonding takes place between individual molecules of 4-nitrophenol. These hydrogen bonding interactions hold molecules of 4-nitrophenol together and increase their boiling and melting points.

Now, examine the hydrogen bonding pattern in 2-nitrophenol. Notice that for this molecule, the nitro group and the hydroxyl group are in close proximity so that intramolecular hydrogen bonding can occur between the hydrogen of the hydroxyl group and a lone pair of electrons on the nitro group *on the same molecule*. These intramolecular hydrogen bonding interactions decrease the amount of intermolecular hydrogen bonding interactions that can occur between molecules thereby decreasing the melting and boiling points of 2-nitrophenol (46°C) relative to 4-nitrophenol (114°C).

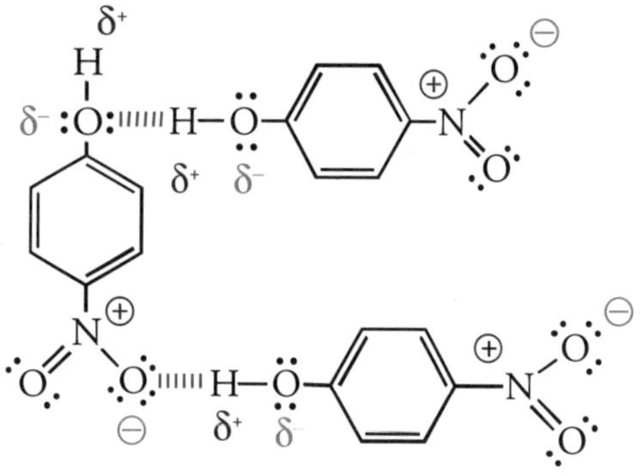

4-nitrophenol
Intermolecular hydrogen bonding

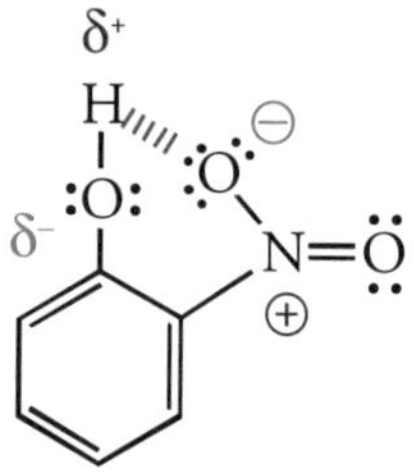

2-nitrophenol
Intramolecular hydrogen bonding

Example 5-2: Rank the following three compounds in order of increasing boiling point:

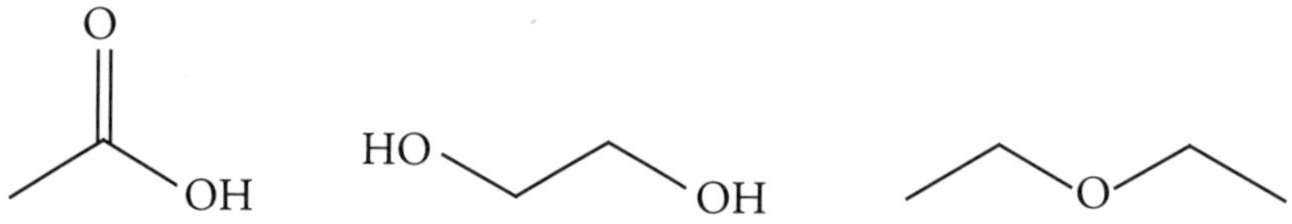

Solution: The more hydrogen-bond donors and hydrogen-bond acceptors there are in a molecule, the higher the boiling and melting points will be. This is because the hydrogen bonds, like dispersion forces, act to *hold* the molecules together, resisting the change to becoming either a liquid or a gas. The first molecule, acetic acid ($C_2H_4O_2$), has one hydrogen-bond donor and four hydrogen-bond acceptors. The second molecule, 1,2-ethanediol ($C_2H_6O_2$), has two hydrogen-bond donors and four hydrogen-bond acceptors. The third molecule, diethyl ether ($C_4H_{10}O$), has two hydrogen-bond acceptors, but no hydrogen bond donors. From this we can now correctly assign the order of their boiling points:

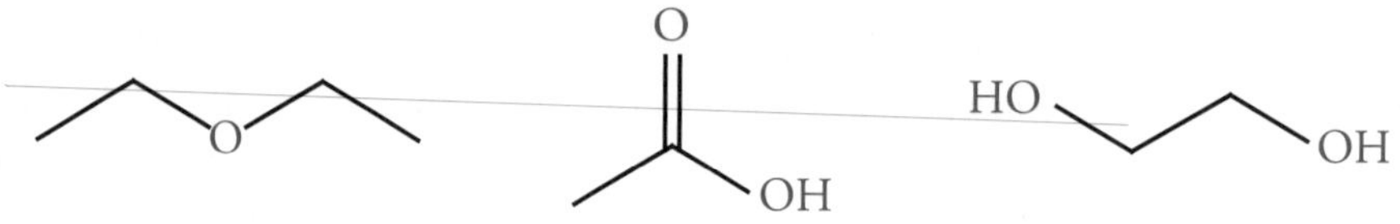

- - - - - - - - - - - - - →   Increasing Boiling Point   - - - - - - - - - - - - →

Example 5-3: For each of the following pairs of compounds, predict which molecule will have the higher boiling point.

(i)

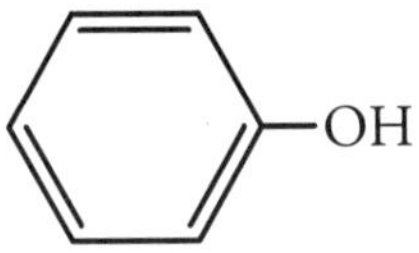

OH   or   Br

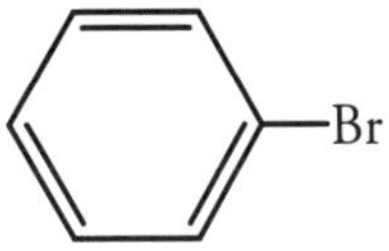

(ii)

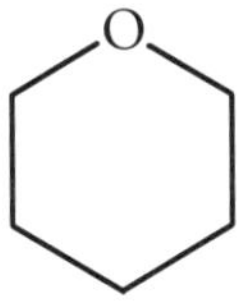

or

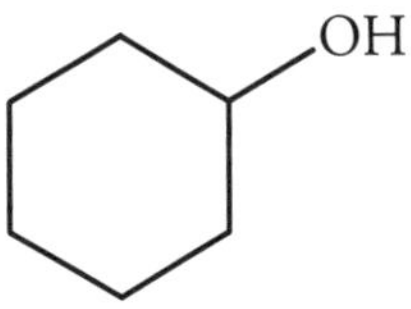

(iii)

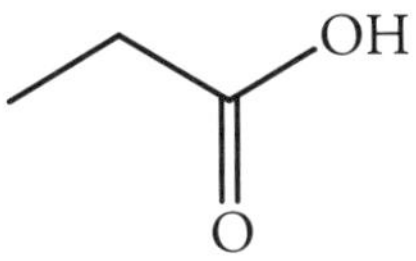

or

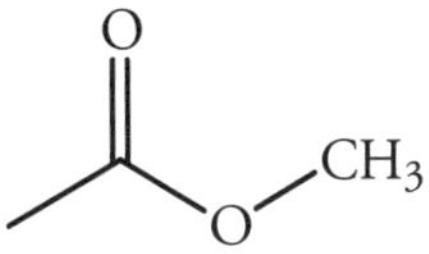

(iv)

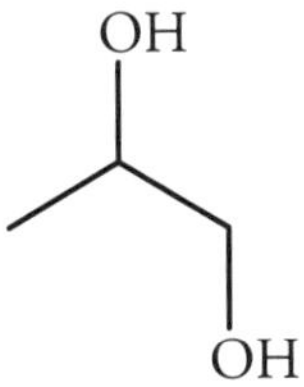

or

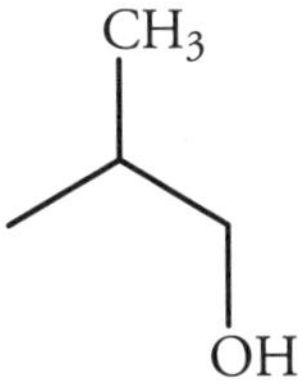

(v)

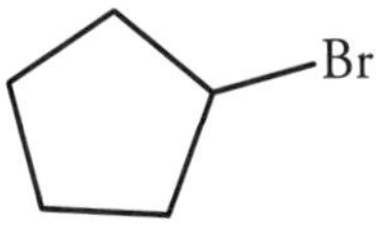

Br   or   CH₃

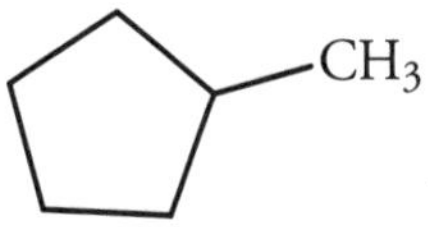

Solution:

(i)

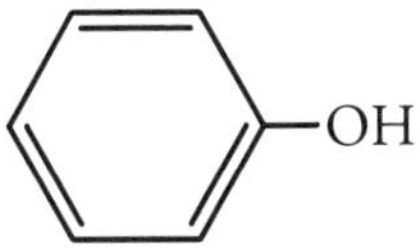

(ii)

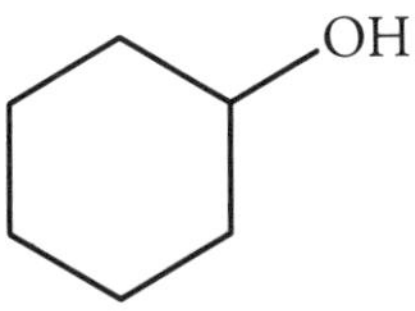

(iii)

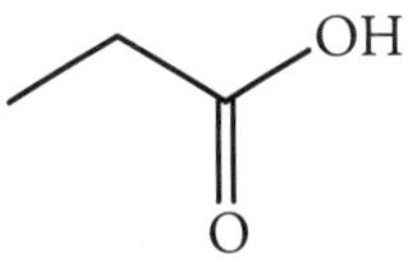

(iv)

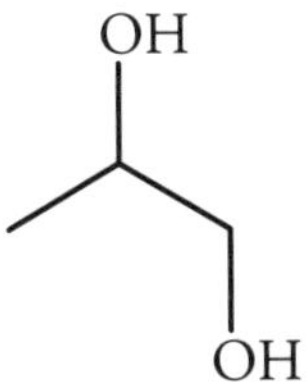

(v)

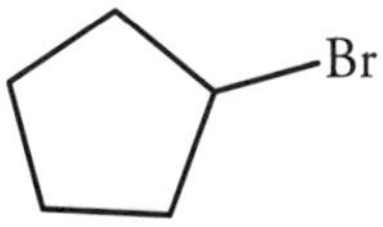

(primarily because of its greater mass)

With a better understanding of what helps to determine the boiling point of an organic molecule, let's now discuss the next important separation technique for the MCAT—distillations.

Distillations

Distillation is the process of raising the temperature of a liquid until it can overcome the intermolecular forces that hold it together in the liquid phase. The vapor is then condensed back to the liquid phase and subsequently collected in another container.

Simple Distillation

A simple distillation is performed when trace impurities need to be removed from a relatively pure compound, or when a mixture of compounds with significantly different boiling points needs to be separated. For example, an appropriate use of a simple distillation would be to purify fresh drinking water away from a salt water solution. The more volatile water can be boiled away, then condensed and collected, leaving behind the nonvolatile salts.

Fractional Distillation

Fractional distillation is a different type of distillation process that is used when the difference in boiling points of the components in the liquid mixture is not large. A fractional distillation column is packed with an appropriate material, such as glass beads or a stainless steel sponge. The packing of the column results in the liquid mixture being subjected to many vaporization-condensation cycles as it moves up the column toward the condenser. As the cycles progress, the composition of the vapor gradually becomes enriched in the lower boiling component. Near the top of the column, nearly pure vapor reaches the condenser and condenses back to the liquid phase where it is subsequently collected in a receiving flask.

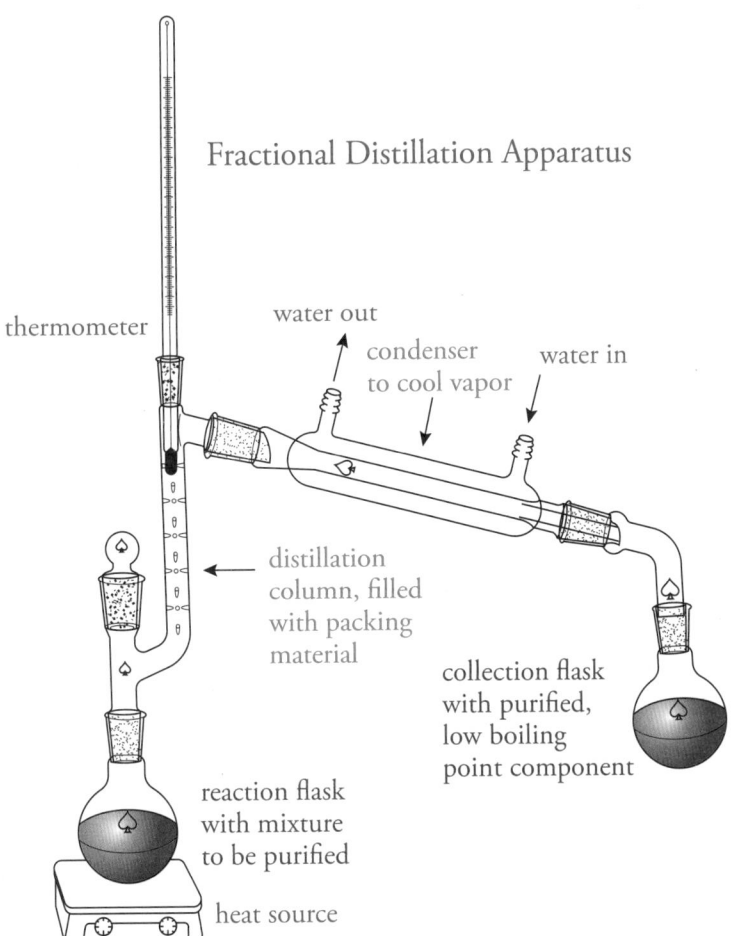

Fractional Distillation Apparatus

thermometer

water out

condenser to cool vapor

water in

distillation column, filled with packing material

collection flask with purified, low boiling point component

reaction flask with mixture to be purified

heat source

Example 5-4: A chemist wishes to separate a mixture of Compounds A and B. He decides to distill the mixture; however, he is unsure of their respective boiling points. After several minutes of heating, he collects the distillate, takes a small sample, and injects it into a gas chromatograph. The output is:

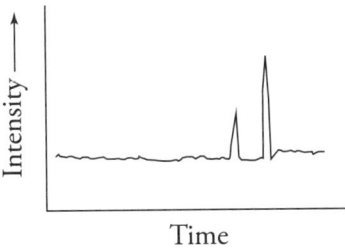

What can this chemist conclude about the separation, and how could it be improved?

Solution: Based on the data from the GC, his separation was only partial (because two different peaks are recorded). Because the second peak is larger than the first, the distillate consists primarily of one of the two compounds, but their boiling points may have been similar enough such that a complete separation was not possible. Perhaps the chemist should try fractional distillation.

5.2 SPECTROSCOPY

A basic understanding of the general principles of spectroscopy will enable you to answer important questions regarding the structure of organic molecules. In this section, we'll examine the general principles of spectroscopy with the goal of interpreting the spectra of simple organic molecules.

Most types of spectroscopy that we will discuss are examples of absorption spectroscopy. A short explanation of the molecular events involved in absorption spectroscopy will help you remember the details of IR and NMR spectroscopy. Molecules normally exist in their lowest energy form, called their **ground state**. When a molecule is exposed to light it *may* absorb a photon, provided the energy of this photon matches the energy between two of the fixed electronic energy levels of the molecule. When this happens, the molecule is said to be in an **excited state**. Molecules tend to prefer their ground state to an excited state, but in order for them to return to their ground state, they must lose the energy they have gained. This loss of energy can occur by the emission of heat, or less commonly, light. In absorption spectroscopy, scientists induce the absorption of energy by a sample of molecules by exposing the sample to various forms of light, thereby exciting molecules to a higher energy state. They then measure the energy released as the molecules relax back to their ground state. This measured energy can reveal structural features of the molecules in the sample.

There are many different forms of light, as displayed in the electromagnetic spectrum. In principle, any of these forms of light could be used to do absorption spectroscopy on molecules, and, in fact, many are! The different forms of light induce different transitions in ground state molecules to different excited states of the molecules and allow for the acquisition of different structural information about the molecules.

Mass Spectrometry

Mass spectrometry is a very useful technique that allows researchers to determine the mass of compounds in a sample. Within the mass spectrometer, molecules are ionized in a high vacuum, usually by bombarding them with high energy electrons. Once ionized, compounds enter a region of the spectrometer where they are acted on by a magnetic field. This field causes the flight path of the charged species to alter, and the degree to which the path is changed is determined by the mass of the ion. This difference is detected and translated into a mass readout in the detector.

On the following page is a schematic of a portion of the mass spectrum for *n*-nonane (MW = 128 g/mol).

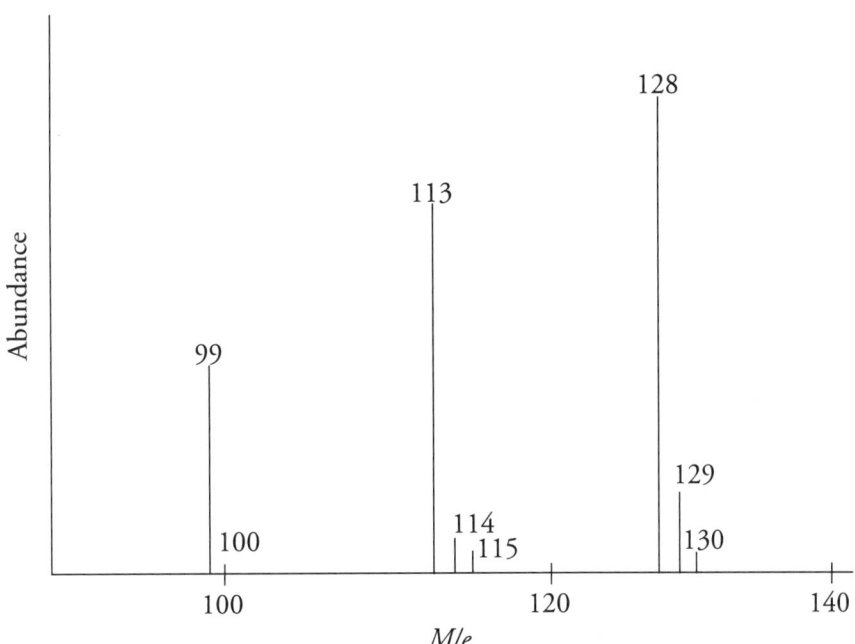

The *M/e* label on the *x*-axis represents the ratio of mass (*M*) to charge (*e*). In most cases *e* = +1, so peaks can simply be viewed as molecular mass. The *y*-axis represents the relative abundance of each species of a particular mass detected in the sample. Masses, though generally not labeled as such, are measured in amu.

Two aspects of the above spectrum may be puzzling: 1) If the molecular weight of nonane is 128 g/mol, why are there peaks greater than this value, and 2) why are there significant peaks in the sample with masses lower than 128?

Remember, atoms can come in a number of different isotopes. For example, the most prevalent mass of hydrogen in nature is 1, but deuterium has an extra neutron and weighs 2 (natural abundance = .015%). Likewise, the most abundant isotope of carbon is ^{12}C, but ^{13}C exists as 1.1% of all carbon atoms. So, the small peaks with masses larger than the main peak represent molecules that have one or more of these less abundant isotopes.

The masses lower than 128 in the above scan represent the masses of molecular fragments. The high energy beam of electrons used to ionize molecules in the mass spectrometer can cause the molecule to break into smaller parts. The figure below shows where *n*-nonane might have been broken to produce peaks with the masses found above. The outer, curved brackets represent a fragment which has lost the terminal CH_3 group and hence is 15 less than the peak at 128. The inner, square brackets show a fragment weighing 99, having lost CH_2CH_3.

Particular atoms present in a molecule may give characteristic peaks in their mass spectra thanks to isotopic ratios. The two most important are Br and Cl. Bromine naturally occurs in two isotopes (79 and 81) of nearly identical natural abundance. This means that any mass spectrum involving a brominated compound will have two major peaks, nearly equal in height, 2 amu apart. Chlorine also occurs as two main isotopes: 35 (75% natural abundance) and 37 (25% natural abundance). Mass spectra for chlorinated molecules will have a peak 2 amu heavier than the main peak, and about one-third its height.

Ultraviolet/Visible (UV/Vis) Spectroscopy

UV/Vis spectroscopy is a type of absorption spectroscopy used in organic chemistry. It is very similar to IR (which we'll discuss next), but instead focuses on the slightly shorter, more energetic wavelengths of radiation in the ultraviolet and visible area of the spectrum. The wavelengths in the UV and visible ranges of the electromagnetic spectrum are strong enough to induce electronic excitation, promoting ground state valence electrons into excited states.

In general, UV/Vis spectroscopy is used with two kinds of molecules. It is very useful in monitoring complexes of transition metals. The easy promotion of electrons from ground to excited states in the closely spaced d-orbitals of many transition metals gives them their bright color (by absorbing wavelengths in the visible region), and since many of these promotions involve energies in the UV range, these promotions allow study of these species.

More importantly in organic chemistry, UV/Vis spectroscopy is used to study highly conjugated organic systems. Molecular orbital theory tells us that when molecules have conjugated π-systems, orbitals form many bonding, non-bonding, and anti-bonding orbitals. These orbitals can be reasonably close together in energy, and in fact, close enough to allow promotion of electrons between electronic states through absorption of ultraviolet, or even visible photons. The wavelength of maximum absorption for any compound is directly related to the extent of conjugation in the molecule. The more extensive the conjugated system is, the longer the wavelength of maximum absorption will be. To illustrate this relationship, let's look at a series of polycyclic aromatic hydrocarbons in Table 5.1 below.

Table 5.1 UV/Vis Spectroscopic Data for Select Polycyclic Aromatic Hydrocarbons

		λ_{max}	absorbs	appears
Anthracene		363 nm	UV	white
Tetracene		475 nm	blue	orange
Pentacene		595 nm	yellow/ orange	blue/ violet

With the addition of each aromatic ring, the conjugated system grows longer and the wavelength of maximum absorption increases. Since each λ_{max} corresponds to a particular color of light, a simple color wheel can be used to predict the color the compound will appear. As a general rule, the color a compound maximally absorbs is complementary to the color it will appear to our eyes. For a compound that absorbs only ultraviolet radiation, ALL of the visible wavelengths will be reflected and thus the compound will appear white or colorless. However, a compound that absorbs blue light will appear to us as orange, since blue and orange are complementary colors on opposites sides of the color wheel (Figure 5.1).

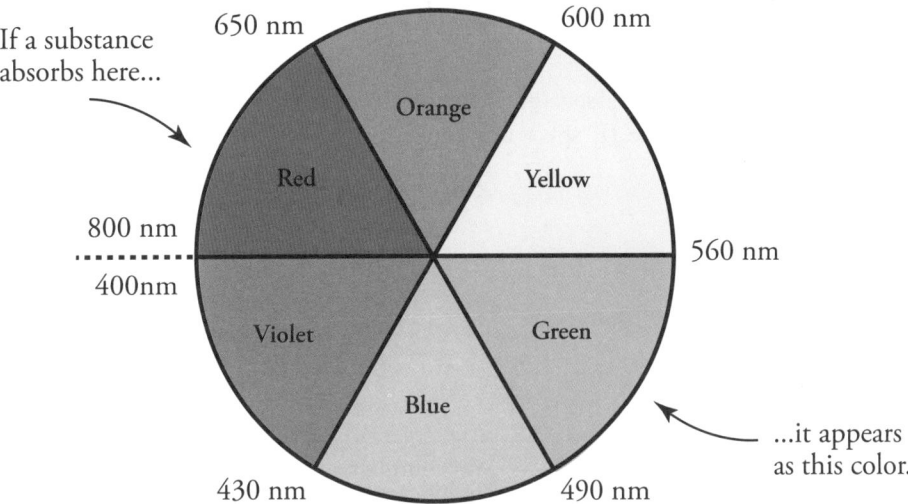

Figure 5.1 Color wheel showing complementary colors

Infrared (IR) Spectroscopy

Electromagnetic radiation in the infrared (IR) range λ = 2.5 to 20 μm has the proper energy to cause bonds in organic molecules to become vibrationally excited. When a sample of an organic compound is irradiated with infrared radiation in the region between 2.5 and 20 μm, its covalent bonds will begin to *vibrate at distinct energy levels* (wavelengths, frequencies) within this region. These wavelengths correspond to frequencies in the range of 1.5×10^{13} Hz to 1.2×10^{14} Hz. In IR spectroscopy, vibrational frequencies are more commonly given in terms of the **wavenumber**. Wavenumber ($\overline{\nu}$) is simply the reciprocal of wavelength:

$$\overline{\nu} = \frac{1}{\lambda} = \frac{1}{c}\nu$$

and is therefore directly proportional to both the frequency (since $\lambda\nu = c = 3 \times 10^{10}$ cm/sec) and the energy of the radiation (since $E = h\nu$). That is, the higher the wavenumber, the higher the frequency and

the greater the energy. Wavenumbers are usually expressed in *reciprocal centimeters*   AT IR
spectra will typically cover the range from 4000 to 1000 cm^{-1}.

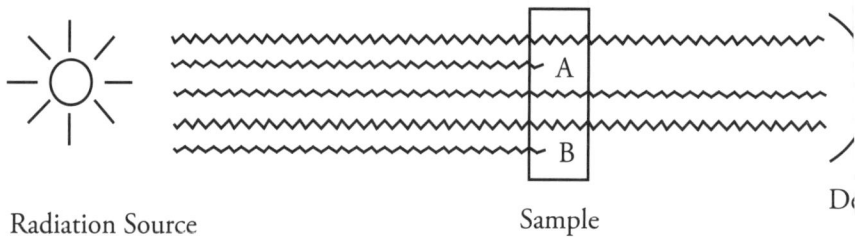

Radiation Source   Sample   D

When a bond absorbs IR radiation of a specific frequency, that frequency is not recorded by the detector and is thus seen as a peak in the IR spectrum (since low transmittance corresponds, naturally, to
absorbance):

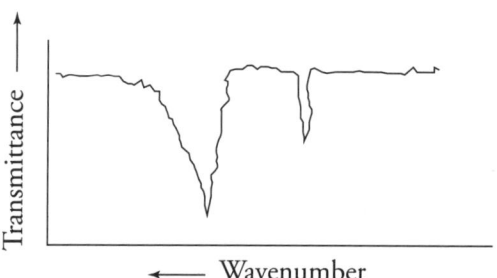

Important Stretching Frequencies

In order to do well on the MCAT, it is important that you know the stretching frequencies of the common functional groups. The most important ones are listed below.

The Double Bond Stretches

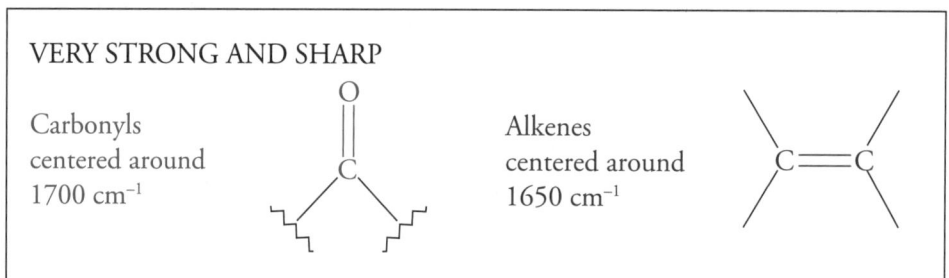

VERY STRONG AND SHARP

Carbonyls
centered around
1700 cm^{-1}

Alkenes
centered around
1650 cm^{-1}

We'll begin by examining the carbonyl, or C=O, stretch. The carbonyl stretch is centered around 1700 cm^{-1}
and is very **strong** and very **intense**. *Strength* is reflected in the percent absorbance (or transmittance). *Intensity* is reflected in the sharpness or distinctiveness ("V" shape) of the spike appearing on the spectrum.
The carbonyl stretch is one of the most important absorptions, and you should commit its location to
memory. In any spectrum, always look for this stretch first. If it is *not* present, you can eliminate a wide
range of compounds that contain a carbonyl group, including aldehydes, ketones, carboxylic acids, acid

chlorides, esters, amides, and anhydrides. On the other hand, if the carbonyl stretch *is* present, you know that one of the carbonyl-containing functional groups is indeed present.

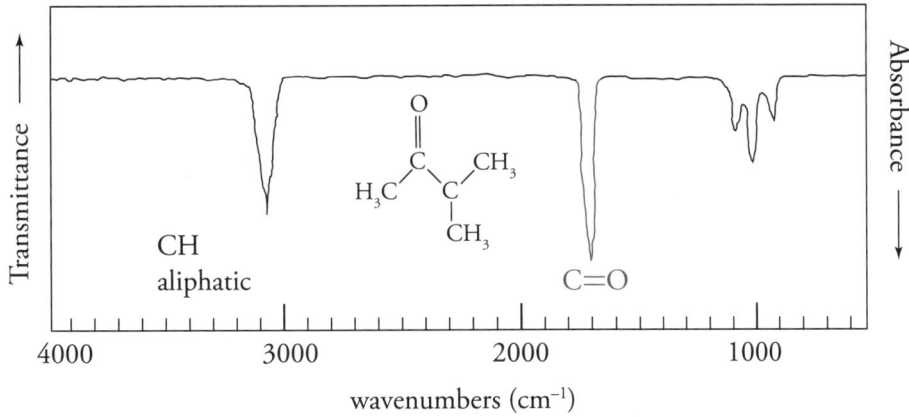

The C=C double bond stretch will appear slightly lower in the spectrum, near 1650 cm^{-1}.

The Triple Bond Stretch

The next stretch to consider is the triple bond. This is an easy one because few molecules possess these functional groups. If they are present, however, the following characteristic stretches will be seen:

C≡C or C≡N
2260–2100 cm^{-1}

The O—H Stretch

Next we come to the hydroxyl stretch. *The O—H stretch is strong and very broad.* **Strength** is reflected as the degree of absorption a peak displays in the spectrum. **Broadness** is reflected as a wide "U"-shaped appearance on the absorption spectrum, as opposed to a "V," or spiked, shape. The broadness is due to hydrogen bonding. Like the carbonyl stretch that occurs at 1700 cm^{-1}, one should always look for the O—H stretch at 3600–3200 cm^{-1}. Amines also have stretches in this region although they vary in intensity.

O—H
3600–3200 cm^{-1}

Alcohols

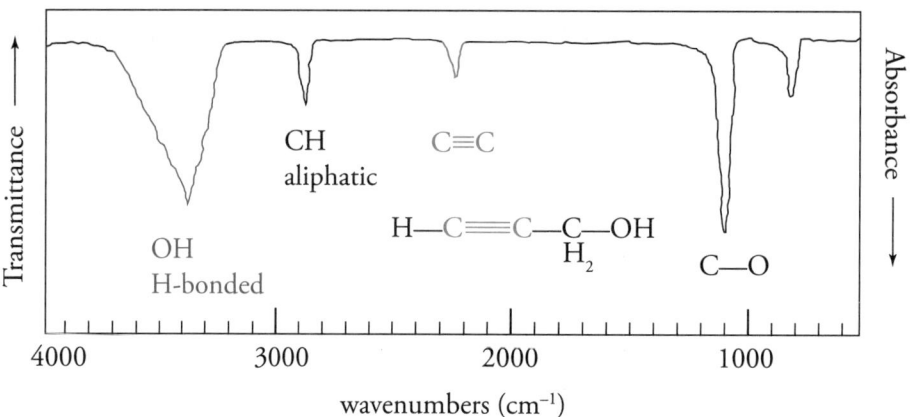

The C—H Stretches

Finally we come to the C—H stretching region (3300–2850 cm^{-1}). Since the vast majority of organic compounds contain C—H bonds, you will almost always see absorbances in this region. Note that aliphatic C—H bonds stretch at wavenumbers a little less than 3000 cm^{-1}, and aromatic C—H bonds stretch at wavenumbers slightly greater than 3000 cm^{-1}.

C—H	for sp^3 carbon: 3000–2850 cm^{-1}
C—H	for sp^2 carbon: 3150–3000 cm^{-1}
C—H	for sp carbon: 3300 cm^{-1}

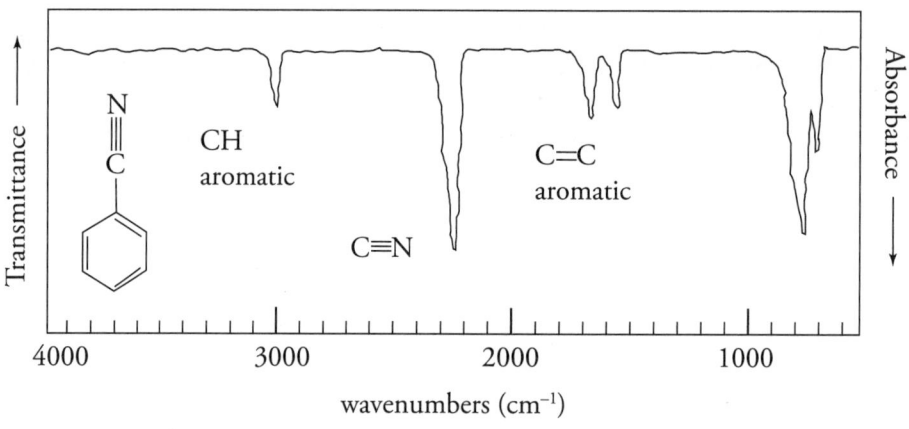

Summary of Relevant Infrared (IR) Stretching Frequencies

Bond	Frequency (Wavenumber) Range (cm^{-1})	Intensity
C=O	1735–1680	strong
C=C	1680–1620	variable
C≡C	2260–2100	variable
C≡N	2260–2220	variable
C—H	3300–2700	variable
N—H	3150–2500	moderate
O—H	3650–3200	broad

^{1}H Nuclear Magnetic Resonance (NMR) Spectroscopy

^{1}H NMR spectroscopy, commonly called proton NMR, is the third type of absorption spectroscopy that we will consider. In all types of NMR spectroscopy, light from the radio frequency range of the electromagnetic spectrum is used to induce energy absorptions. The interpretation of ^{1}H NMR spectral data is important for the MCAT, but the theory underlying NMR spectroscopy is beyond the scope of the exam. Here, we'll only cover the interpretation of ^{1}H NMR spectra.

Four essential features of a molecule can be deduced from its ^{1}H NMR spectrum, and while we'll review all four, it is most important for the MCAT to focus on the first two. First, the number of sets of peaks in the spectrum tells one the number of chemically nonequivalent sets of protons in the molecule. Second, the splitting pattern of each set of peaks tells how many protons are interacting with the protons in that set. Third, the mathematical integration of the sets of peaks indicates the relative numbers of protons in each set. Fourth, the chemical shift values of those sets of peaks give information about the environment of the protons in that set. These four key features of ^{1}H NMR spectroscopy are explained in the next four sections.

Chemically Equivalent Hydrogens

Determining which hydrogens, or protons, are **equivalent** in an organic molecule is the first important skill to master with respect to NMR spectroscopy. Equivalent hydrogens in a molecule are those that have *identical electronic environments*. Such hydrogens have identical locations in the ^{1}H NMR spectrum, and are therefore represented by the same signal, or resonance. Nonequivalent hydrogens will have different locations in the ^{1}H NMR spectrum and be represented by different signals. You must be able to determine which hydrogens (or, usually, groups of hydrogens) are equivalent to which other groups, so that you can predict how many distinct NMR signals there will be in any ^{1}H NMR spectrum. Hydrogens are considered equivalent if they can be interchanged by a free rotation or a symmetry operation (mirror plane or rotational axis). Check yourself on the following examples:

Example 5-5: A hydrocarbon C_5H_{12} shows only one peak on its ^1H NMR spectrum. Identify its structure.

Solution: Compute the degrees of unsaturation: $d = [2(\#C) + 2 - (\#H)]/2$. In this case, $d = 0$, so there are no double bonds or rings. Because there is only one peak in the ^1H NMR spectrum, all protons are equivalent, and thus our molecule must be:

Example 5-6: C_5H_{10} also has an ^1H NMR spectrum showing only one peak. Identify its structure.

Solution: Here, $d = [2(\#C) + 2 - (\#H)]/2 = 1$, so the molecule has a double bond or ring. All C_5H_{10} variations with a double bond have more than one type of proton. But in cyclopentane, all hydrogens are equivalent due to the presence of a five-fold axis of symmetry:

Splitting

The second aspect of NMR spectroscopy that you should be familiar with is the **spin-spin splitting phenomenon**. This occurs when nonequivalent hydrogens interact with each other. This interaction exists because the magnetic field felt by a proton is influenced by surrounding protons. This effect tends to fall off with distance, but it can often extend over two adjacent carbons. Nearby protons that are nonequivalent to the proton in question will cause a splitting in the observed ^{1}H NMR signal. The degree of splitting depends on the number of adjacent hydrogens, and a signal will be split into $n + 1$ lines, where n is the number of nonequivalent, neighboring (interacting) protons. The important information one must determine is how a proton or a group of chemically equivalent protons will be split by their hydrogen neighbors.

This is best demonstrated by an example:

Three distinct types of hydrogens:
3 H_a hydrogens
2 H_b hydrogens
2 H_c hydrogens

H_a signal split into **three** peaks due to the two neighboring, but different, H_b atoms.

H_b signal split into **six** peaks due to the five neighboring, but different, H_a and H_c atoms.

H_c signal split into **three** peaks due to the two neighboring, but different, H_b atoms.

Note that, for MCAT purposes, the H_a and H_c protons neighboring H_b do not have to be equivalent in order to add them together to get $n = 5$.

$n + 1$ RULE

n = Number of neighboring nonequivalent hydrogens	Splitting ($n + 1$)
0	1—Singlet
1	2—Doublet
2	3—Triplet
3	4—Quartet
4	5—Quintet (or multiplet)
5	6—Sextet (or multiplet)

Consider the NMR spectrum of CH_3CH_2I:

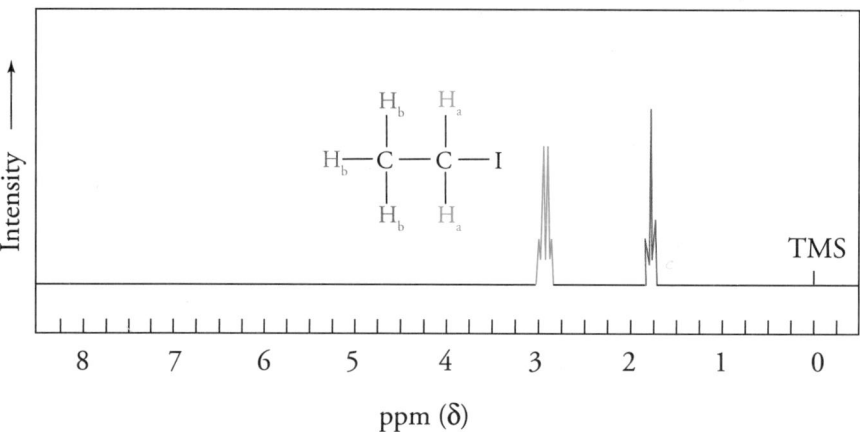

The α-hydrogens have three neighboring hydrogens and are therefore split into a quartet, according to the $n + 1$ rule. The β-hydrogens are split into a triplet because they have two neighboring hydrogens.

Example 5-7: How many ^1H NMR signals would you expect to find for the following molecules? What is the splitting pattern of each signal?

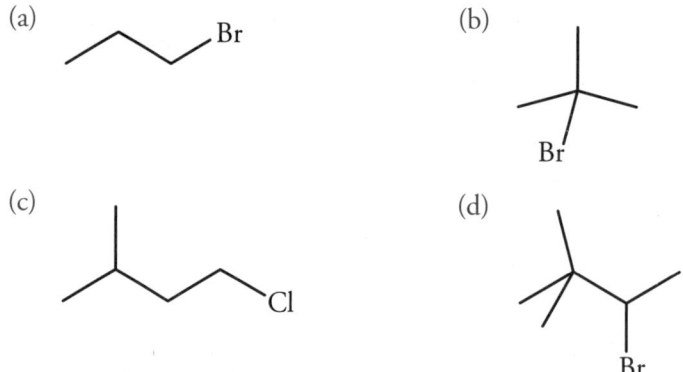

(a)

(b)

(c)

(d)

Solution:

(a) Three signals. C1's equivalent protons are split by two Hs on C2 to make a triplet. C2's protons are split by a total of five Hs on C1 and C3 to make a sextet, or multiplet. C3's protons are split by two Hs on C2 to make a triplet.

(b) One signal; all are equivalent, therefore no splitting.

(c) Four signals. C1's equivalent protons are split by two Hs on C2 to make a triplet. C2's protons are split by a total of three Hs on C1 and C3 to make a quartet. C3's proton is split by eight neighboring protons to make a multiplet. C4 and C5 have equivalent protons, split by C3's proton and forming a doublet.

(d) Three signals. The first proton signal is from the H on C3 (the one bearing the Br). It is split by three Hs on C4 to make a quartet. The Hs on C4 are split by the one H on C3 to yield a doublet. The remaining Hs on the *tert*-butyl group are equivalent (nine total), have no neighbors, and appear as a singlet.

Integration

The third important piece of information obtained from the ^{1}H NMR spectrum of a molecule is the mathematical integration. As the NMR instrument obtains a spectrum of the sample, it performs a mathematical calculation, called an **integration**, thereby measuring the area under each absorption peak (resonance). The calculated area under each peak is proportional to the relative number of protons giving rise to each peak. Thus, the integration indicates the relative number of protons in each set in the molecule.

The Chemical Shift

The fourth and final aspect of an NMR spectrum is the **chemical shift**, which indicates the location of the resonance (set of peaks) in the ^{1}H NMR spectrum. Differences in the chemical shift values for different sets of protons in a molecule are the result of the differing electronic environments that different sets of protons experience. The magnetic field created by electrons near a proton will **shield** the nucleus from the applied magnetic field created by the instrument, shifting the resonance **upfield**. The more a proton is **deshielded** (i.e., the more distorted away from the atom the electron cloud is), the further **downfield** (to the left) in an NMR spectrum it will appear. For example, a set of protons *near* an electronegative group is said to be deshielded and will appear downfield (to the left) in the ^{1}H NMR spectrum, relative to a set of protons that are farther away from the electronegative group, which is more shielded and appears more upfield (to the right) in the ^{1}H NMR spectrum.

We now briefly examine the factors involved in proton deshielding. These include:

1. the electronegativity of the neighboring atoms
2. hybridization
3. acidity and hydrogen bonding

Electronegativity Effects on Chemical Shift Values

If an electronegative atom is in close proximity to a proton, it will decrease the electron density near the proton and thereby deshield it. This will result in a *down*field shift in the chemical shift value. Examples:

$\delta = 0.26$ ppm $\delta = 3.06$ ppm $\delta = 3.25$ ppm

The spectrum of methyl acetate on the next page shows how the two electronegative groups in the molecule (the O of the ester and the carbonyl) contribute to shifting both methyl signals downfield.

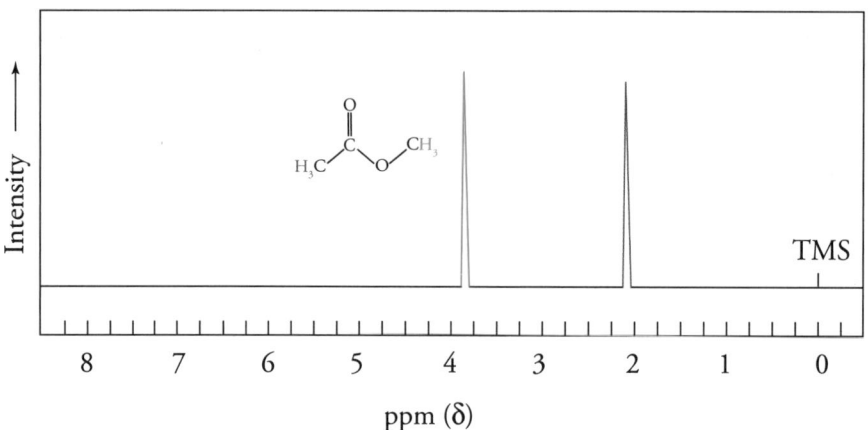

Hybridization Effects on Chemical Shift Values

The **hybridization effect** occurs as a result of the varying bond characteristics of carbon atoms *connected* to the hydrogens. The greater the *s*-orbital character of a C—H bond, the less electron density on the hydrogen. Thus, when considering the hybridization effect alone, the greater the *s*-orbital character, the more deshielded the set of protons is, which will result in a downfield shift for the peak corresponding to that set of protons. Here is an example:

$$\delta = 1 \text{ ppm} \qquad\qquad H_3C\!-\!C\!\equiv\!C\!-\!H \qquad \delta = 2 \text{ ppm}$$

Hybridization effects alone would indicate the alkyne proton to be more deshielded than the alkene proton. However, due to a more complicated physical phenomenon, which is beyond the scope of the MCAT, this turns out not to be the case. To simplify for the MCAT, two other very characteristic chemical shifts you should be familiar with are that of the aromatic protons (δ = 6.5–8 ppm) and alkene protons (δ = 5–6 ppm).

$$\delta = 6.5\text{–}8 \text{ ppm} \qquad\qquad \delta = 6 \text{ ppm}$$

Acidity and Hydrogen Bonding Effects on Chemical Shift Values

Protons that are attached to **heteroatoms** (oxygen and nitrogen, for example) are quite deshielded. Acidic protons on a carboxylic acid are an extreme example of a very large downfield shift. In addition, hydrogen bonding can cause a wide variation of **chemical shift**. For example, the resonance of the alcohol proton in methanol varies with both solvent and temperature (different degrees of H bonding).

You should also be aware that the chemical shifts of alcohol protons are quite variable depending upon the particular compound, but are in the range of δ = 2–5 ppm.

H_3C—OH

δ = 2–5 ppm

δ = 10–13 ppm

As with IR stretching frequencies, memorizing some commonly encountered ^1H NMR chemical shift values will be helpful. Below is a correlation chart for some common chemical shifts, the most important of which are in red:

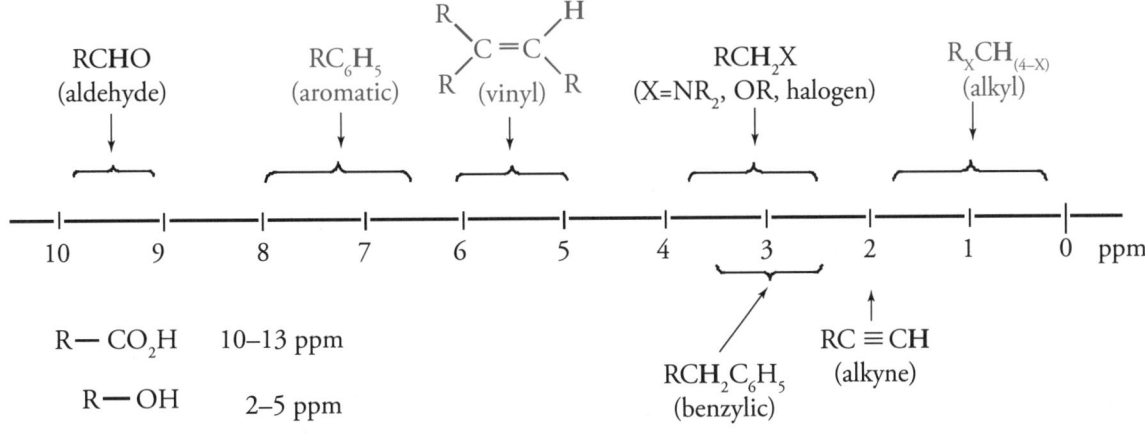

R—CO_2H	10–13 ppm
R—OH	2–5 ppm

Chapter 5 Summary

- Organic compounds are separated via extraction based on their differing solubility in aqueous or organic solvents.

- Organic acids (COOHs and PhOHs) and bases (amines) can undergo acid-base reactions to generate ions, which preferentially dissolve in the aqueous layer during an extraction.

- Thin layer chromatography (TLC) separates molecules based on polarity; the more polar compound travels the least distance up the plate and has the lowest R_f value.

- Ion exchange, HPLC, size exclusion, and affinity chromatography are similar in nature to column chromatography and generally use a mobile and stationary phase for separating compounds. They are generally used to separate biomolecules like amino acids, proteins, or nucleic acids.

- Distillation and gas chromatography separate compounds based on boiling point.

- UV/Vis spectroscopy indicates the presence of a conjugated π system in a molecule, whereas IR spectroscopy identifies the functional groups present in molecules.

- The most common IR resonances tested on the MCAT are the C=O bond ($\approx 1700 \text{ cm}^{-1}$), the C=C bond ($\approx 1650 \text{ cm}^{-1}$) and the O—H bond ($\approx 3600 \text{ cm}^{-1}$).

- The number of resonances in a ^{1}H NMR spectrum indicates the number of nonequivalent hydrogens present in a molecule.

- Splitting in a ^{1}H NMR spectrum occurs when one H has nonequivalent protons located on an adjacent atom (signal will be split into $n + 1$ lines; n = # of nonequivalent adjacent hydrogens).

- The number of Hs each signal represents is determined by the integration of the peak.

- Protons that are more deshielded (near electronegative groups) will be further downfield (at higher ppm), and protons that are more shielded (near electron donating groups) will be more upfield (at lower ppm).

CHAPTER 5 FREESTANDING PRACTICE QUESTIONS

1. The ^{1}H NMR spectrum for Compound X shows one peak at 7.4 ppm. If elemental analysis shows that the compound has an empirical formula of CH, how many possible stereoisomers could Compound X have?

A) 0
B) 1
C) 2
D) 4

2. How many resonances would appear in a ^{1}H NMR spectrum of the following compound?

A) 3
B) 5
C) 7
D) 13

3. Consider the following reaction:

Which of the following observations about the infrared spectrum of the reaction mixture would indicate that the reaction above went to completion yielding the expected product?

A) The appearance of a stretch at 1700 cm^{-1}
B) The disappearance of a stretch at 3300 cm^{-1}
C) The disappearance of a stretch at 3300 cm^{-1} and the appearance of a stretch at 1700 cm^{-1}
D) The disappearance of a stretch at 1700 cm^{-1} and the appearance of a stretch at 3300 cm^{-1}

4. For the following reaction, how would the R_f value of the product compare to that of the starting material if monitored by TLC on a normal silica gel plate?

A) The R_f value of the product would be greater than that of the reactant because the product is more polar.
B) The R_f value of the product would be greater than that of the reactant because the product is less polar.
C) The R_f value of the product would be smaller than that of the reactant because the product is more polar.
D) The R_f value of the product would be smaller than that of the reactant because the product is less polar.

5. The ^{1}H NMR spectrum of Compound X consists of a singlet, a triplet, and a quartet. The ^{1}H NMR spectrum of Compound Y contains only singlets. The IR spectra of both Compounds displays a signal near 1730 cm^{-1}. Which of the following choices is most likely to correspond to the structures of Compounds X and Y, respectively?

A)

B)

C)

D)

6. Which of the following fatty acids has the highest melting point?

A) (3E, 5E)-octa-3,5-dienoic acid
B) (3E, 5E)-deca-3,5-dienoic acid
C) (3Z, 5Z)-octa-3,5-dienoic acid
D) (3Z, 5Z)-deca-3,5-dienoic acid

7. Infrared spectroscopy could be used to discern which two molecules from each other?

   I.   An amine and an imine
   II. An alcohol and a carboxylic acid
   III. Glucose and fructose

A) II only
B) I and II only
C) I and III only
D) I, II, and III

8. DEAE-C (shown below) is a type of resin employed in ion-exchange chromatography. Which one of the following statements correctly describes a property of DEAE-C resin?

Diethylaminoethyl Cellulose

A) DEAE-C resin is employed as a stationary phase in cation-exchange chromatography.
B) DEAE-C resin is best used to separate and purify proteins when the pH of mobile phase is buffered above the pK_a of the diethylamino groups.
C) Proteins that bear smaller charges are eluted from a column packed with DEAE-C resin more rapidly than those bearing larger charges.
D) Binding of proteins on a column packed with DEAE-C resin is best performed by using a buffer with a high concentration of buffer anions.

9. A solvent extraction scheme employs diethyl ether as the organic phase and 5% dilute aqueous acid or base as the aqueous phase. Which of the following procedures could best be employed to separate an ether solution containing a mixture of benzoic acid, phenol, and aniline?

A) Extract the ether solution with HCl, then separate the layers; extract the remaining ether layer with NaOH, then separate the layers.
B) Extract the ether solution with NaOH, then separate the layers; extract the remaining ether layer with HCl, then separate the layers.
C) Extract the ether solution with NaOH, then separate the layers; extract the remaining ether layer with $NaHCO_3$, then separate the layers.
D) Extract the ether solution with $NaHCO_3$, then separate the layers; extract the remaining ether layer with HCl, then separate the layers.

10. A mixture containing five amino acids was separated via reverse-phase HPLC by elution with 10% aqueous methanol. What is the expected order of increasing retention time of the amino acids in the mixture?

A) M < Y < D < W < F
B) Y < F < D < M < W
C) D < Y < M < F < W
D) W < F < M < Y < D

CHAPTER 5 PRACTICE PASSAGE

13-Deoxytetrodecamycin (**1**) was isolated from WAC04657, a wild-isolate *Streptomyces* that has antibiotic activities against drug resistant Gram-negative and Gram-positive pathogens. 13-Deoxytetrodecamycin is a congener of the tetrodecamycin family (Figure 1), lacking the *trans* hydroxyl on C-13 on the decalin type ring. 13-Deoxytetrodecamycin was isolated as a white residue and is soluble in DMSO and CHCl$_3$. It has a molecular formula of C$_{18}$H$_{22}$O$_5$, and its exact mass was found via high-resolution mass spectrometry as the sodium complex.

13-deoxytetrodecamycin (**1**)

tetrodecamycin (**2**)

dihydrotetrodecamycin (**3**)

Figure 1 Tetrodecamycin family of molecules

In order to isolate the compounds associated with the bioactivity, solid agar cultures of WAC04657 were grown and extracted with ethyl acetate. The ethyl acetate was concentrated, and the crude extract was dissolved in chloroform. The extracts were separated by TLC, and the plates were overlaid with the bacterium *Bacillus subtilis*. In order to analyze the plate, the cells were stained with a yellow dye, MTT, after which, the appropriate band of silica was extracted with chloroform and subjected to reverse-phase HPLC analysis. The chromatogram revealed that the band of silica consisted of one primary peak (Figure 2). This peak was determined to be **1**. The semi-pure product was used to develop an HPLC purification of the compound from large-scale crude extracts (Figure 3).

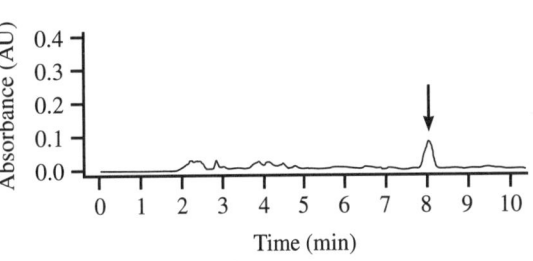

Figure 2 HPLC trace of TLC purified compound

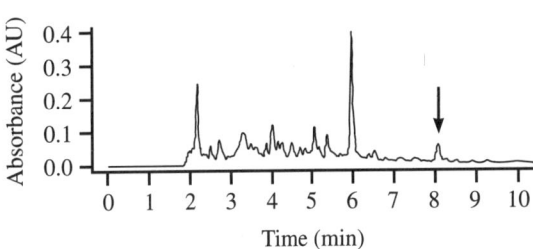

Figure 3 HPLC trace of crude extract

In order to sufficiently study the bioactivity of **1**, a large-scale isolation and purification procedure was developed. The solid MYM agar (12.8 L) was macerated and extracted with an equal volume of ethyl acetate. The ethyl acetate was filtered and concentrated under vacuum giving a brown extract. The extract was suspended in 50% H$_2$O/acetonitrile and loaded onto a Sep-Pak C18 column. The column was washed with 10 mL each of H$_2$O and 30% aqueous acetonitrile, then the desired compound was eluted with 70% aqueous acetonitrile. The solvent was evaporated and redissolved in 50% aqueous acetonitrile. After two HPLC purifications, 1.1 mg of pure **1** was isolated as a white residue.

(Adapted from Gverzdys, T.; Hart. M. K.; Pimentel-Elardo, S.; Tranmer, G.; Nodwell, J. R. J. *Antibiot. (Tokyo)*, 2010, *63*, 1.)

1. Mitochondrial dehydrogenase in living cells converts the yellow dye MTT, commonly used in cell proliferation assays, into MTT-formazan, which is purple in color. What feature(s) of the TLC plate would allow for the isolation of the appropriate compound from the silica gel?

   A) The TLC plate would be white and the appropriate band would be purple.
   B) The TLC plate would be yellow and the appropriate band would be purple.
   C) The TLC plate would be purple and the appropriate band would be white.
   D) The TLC plate would be purple and the appropriate band would be yellow.

2. What m/z value was experimentally determined in the isolation of 13-deoxytetrodecamycin?

   A) 317
   B) 341
   C) 340
   D) 319

3. Both 13-deoxytetrodecamycin and the C-14 epimer of tetrodecamycin were independently reacted with p-toluenesulfonyl chloride (TsCl) in the presence of base, and each gave distinct products. Which of the following steps is LEAST likely to occur in either mechanism of the reactions?

   A) TsCl will react with the alcohol of 13-deoxytetrodecamycin to generate a good leaving group, which will eliminate at C-13 to yield an alkene.
   B) TsCl will react with the secondary alcohol of the C-14 epimer of tetrodecamycin to generate a good leaving group, which the C-13 hydroxyl will displace to yield an epoxide.
   C) TsCl will react with the tertiary alcohol of the C-14 epimer of tetrodecamycin to generate a good leaving group, which the C-14 hydroxyl will displace to yield an epoxide.
   D) TsCl will react with the alcohol of 13-deoxytetrodecamycin to generate a good leaving group, which can leave to yield a carbocation intermediate.

4. Supercritical fluid chromatography (SFC) uses supercritical fluid CO_2 in the mobile phase, and like HPLC, both normal and reverse phase methods can be used. If the crude extract in the passage was purified by reverse phase SFC, how would the analysis chromatogram for the separation of the indicated product compare to Figure 3?

   A) The desired product would have a longer retention time because CO_2 is a nonpolar solvent.
   B) The desired product would have a similar retention time because both purifications use a reverse phase column.
   C) The desired product would have a similar retention time because retention time is independent of the type of column used.
   D) The desired product would have a shorter retention time because CO_2 is a polar solvent.

5. Which of the following describes the absolute configuration at the carbon atom containing the OH group in 13-deoxytetrodecamycin and the position of its OH group?

   A) R, axial
   B) R, equatorial
   C) S, axial
   D) S, equatorial

SOLUTIONS TO CHAPTER 5 FREESTANDING PRACTICE QUESTIONS

1. **A** One signal on the ^{1}H NMR spectrum tells us that the molecule has only one type of hydrogen. Since the empirical formula of Compound X is CH and the molecule contains no electronegative elements to shift the signal downfield, the single peak, located in the region common for aromatic hydrogens (7–8 ppm), must represent an aromatic H. Any compound with only aromatic Hs must have carbons that are all sp^2 hybridized, and as such will have no stereoisomers. In this case, the compound is benzene (C_6H_6).

2. **B** By showing the hydrogens, one would expect the molecule to have five resonances in a ^{1}H NMR spectrum. Note the plane of symmetry through the molecule (as shown with the dotted line). Both sets of CH_2 hydrogens on the carbons adjacent to the bromo and methyl substituents are chemically equivalent to each other.

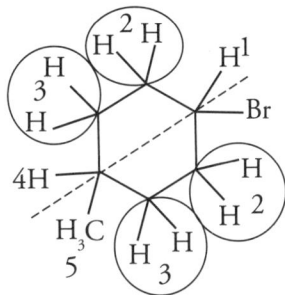

3. **C** The reaction is a transformation from an alcohol to a ketone. In an infrared spectrum, this can be noticed by the disappearance of the broad O—H stretch around 3300 cm^{-1}, and the appearance of the C=O stretch at 1700 cm^{-1}. Choices A and B are incorrect because the appearance of the C=O stretch does not automatically translate that the oxidation reaction went to completion and the disappearance of the O—H stretch doesn't mean that the desired product is formed. In order for the reaction to be complete, one must disappear as the other appears. Choice D is incorrect as the stretches that would appear and disappear are incorrect for the corresponding functional group transformation.

4. **C** TLC separates compounds based on their polarities. The more polar a compound is, the more it adheres to the silica gel plate, giving it a smaller R_f value. Choices A and D are inconsistent with this type of interaction. The product for this reaction is bromocyclohexane, which is more polar than the reactant due to the presence of the halogen.

5. **C** The stem indicates that both compounds produce an IR spectroscopy signal at 1730 cm^{-1}, which indicates both must contain a carbonyl functional group (eliminate choices A and B). Next consider the simpler ^{1}H NMR spectrum result of Compound Y, which contains only singlets (signals indicating the presence of no neighboring hydrogen atoms). In the Compound Y structure for choice C, only singlets are expected, but in choice D one singlet, two doublets, and one multiplet are expected (eliminate choice D; choice C is correct). While unnecessary to consider, the singlet, triplet, and quartet signals for Compound X are confirmed by the structure given in choice C, but they are not found in choice D. The corresponding structure for Compound X in choice D produces a singlet, a doublet, and a multiplet.

6. **B** In general, larger molecules have higher melting points due to increased London dispersion forces. Eliminate choices A and C since they have eight carbons (octa), while the molecules in choices B and D have ten carbons (deca). The remaining difference between B and D is the presence of *E* or *Z* double bonds. *Z* double bonds introduce kinks in the fatty acid chain, making it more difficult for the molecules to pack together, therefore reducing their melting point. This eliminates choice D.

7. **B** Since this is a Roman numeral question, start by evaluating the item that appears in exactly two answer choices; in this case Item III. Whether it is true or false you can eliminate half the answers. Item III is false: even though glucose is an aldose (contains an aldehyde), these functional groups both have the C=O bond and their possible regions in the IR spectrum overlap. Thus these molecules would be difficult to distinguish using infrared spectroscopy (choices C and D can be eliminated). Since both remaining choices include Item II it must be true, and you can evaluate Item I. Item I is true: this refers to a molecule with a C—N bond (amine) and a molecule with a C=N bond (imine) which will generate different resonances (choice A can be eliminated and choice B is correct). Note that Item II is in fact true: this compares an alcohol with an –OH group to a carboxyl group (–COOH). While this compound will have an –OH signal in its spectrum, it will also have a peak for the carbonyl making it distinguishable from the alcohol.

8. **C** When protonated, the diethylamino group on DEAE-C bears a positive charge to which negatively charged proteins will become bound via electrostatic interactions. Therefore, DEAC-C resin is employed as a stationary phase in anion-exchange chromatography (choice A is wrong).

In order to maintain protonation, and positive charge, on the side-chain diethylamino group on DEAE-C, the pH of the mobile phase must be significantly below the p*K*a of the dimethylamino group (eliminate choice B). Negatively charged proteins become adsorbed onto the surface of DEAE-C resin by an electrostatic interaction with the positively charged diethylammonium group in protonated DEAE-C. Since the primary interaction is electrostatic in nature, it follows that proteins bearing larger charges will be more strongly adsorbed and proteins bearing smaller charges will be eluted more rapidly (choice C is correct). Increasing the concentration of buffer anion creates competition for binding between negatively charged proteins and buffer anions for the stationary phase; this will tend to favor this ion and disfavor binding of proteins to protonated DEAE-C (eliminate choice D).

9. **D** To approach this question efficiently, consider choices B and C first, where NaOH is repeated as the first aqueous solvent. Extraction of an ether solution containing benzoic acid, phenol, and aniline with 5% NaOH is expected to convert both acids, benzoic and phenol, into their corresponding salts. These salts will be transported into the aqueous layer and cannot be separated further by using the procedures described in either choice (eliminate choices B and C). Extraction of an ether solution of the original mixture with 5% HCl permits separation

of the amine-containing aniline as a salt, which is transported into the aqueous layer. However, extraction of the remaining ether layer containing benzoic acid and phenol with 5% NaOH is not effective and thus will not be separated (eliminate choice A). The procedure described in choice D takes advantage of the fact that phenol, a weaker acid than benzoic acid, is soluble in 5% NaOH but insoluble in 5% $NaHCO_3$. Thus, $NaHCO_3$ is first expected to extract benzoic acid as a salt and, following separation, extraction of the remaining ether layer with HCl will result in aniline being extracted as a salt, leaving phenol in the final ether layer (choice D is correct).

10. **C** This ranking question should be approached by evaluating the extremes. Recall that reverse-phase HPLC utilizes a nonpolar stationary phase and a moderately polar aqueous solvent (mobile phase). Amino acids with nonpolar, hydrophobic side chains adhere to the stationary phase most strongly and thus experience the longest retention times (i.e., these species are eluted last). W (Trp) and F (Phe) contain nonpolar side chains, are expected to display the longest retention times, and would elute last (choice D can be eliminated). D (Asp) and Y (Tyr) contain polar side chains, are expected to display the shortest retention times, and elute first (choice A can be eliminated). While the subtle polarity differences between D/Y or W/F can be exploited, a more overt detail can be found in choice B, which shows F eluting quickly. This will not occur under reverse-phase conditions (choice B can be eliminated and choice C is correct).

SOLUTIONS TO CHAPTER 5 PRACTICE PASSAGE

1. **D** The TLC plate in the passage is overlaid with *Bacillus subtilis*, which possess the cellular activity to convert the yellow MTT to purple MTT-formazan. Thus the plate will have a purple color (eliminate choices A and B). Since the TLC plate is separating the molecules that are active against *Bacillus subtilis*, the bands of silica at the R_f values for those molecules will not have microbial growth. With no cellular activity, those bands will remain yellow, the color of MTT (choice D is correct).

2. **B** A *m/z* value represents the mass of a substance. The passage states that 13-deoxytetrodecamycin has a molecular formula of $C_{18}H_{22}O_5$ and that the exact mass was experimentally found as the sodium complex. The molar mass of 13-deoxytetrodecamycin is 318 g/mol, and sodium has a molar mass of ~23 g/mol, giving 318 + 23 = 341 (choice B is correct).

3. **C** In the presence of TsCl and base, 13-deoxytetrodecamycin should generate an alkene between C-13 and C-14 via a carbocation intermediate (eliminate choices A and D), while the C-14 epimer of tetrodecamycin should produce an epoxide between carbons C-13 and C-14 (via an S_N2-like reaction) as the answer choices suggest. However, in both reactions the secondary alcohol will be activated with the tosyl group, as it's the least sterically hindered alcohol. Therefore, choice C is the correct answer, as the tertiary alcohol will NOT get activated as the leaving group.

4. **B** SFC uses supercritical fluid CO_2 as a nonpolar solvent for the separation of compounds (eliminate choice D). As the question states, it can use both normal and reverse phase, and regardless of that, the column is critical for separating polar and nonpolar compounds (eliminate choice C). Finally since the purification is occurring by a reverse phase process similar to that in Figure 3, the retention time of the indicated product purified by SFC would be similar to that of Figure 3 (eliminate choice A). Therefore, choice B is the correct answer.

5. **D** The figure below shows the appropriate prioritization of the four groups that must be considered when determining the absolute configuration of the carbon atom in question:

The OH group has the highest priority because oxygen has the highest atomic number of the four groups, and hydrogen is the lowest priority as it has the lowest atomic number. The remaining priority assignments are between two carbon substituents, so we must find the first point of difference. Since the oxygen has the higher atomic number, the carbon on the right gets the higher priority than the carbon on the left. When the arc from 1 → 2 → 3 is traced in a counterclockwise direction with the lowest priority group oriented in back of the molecule, the configuration is *S* (eliminate choices A and B).

13-Deoxytetrodecamycin has a *trans*-fused decalin ring system, making the hydrogens on the fused carbons axial. This is the case for all *trans*-fused decalins, since if the hydrogens were equatorial, the fused ring would have to adopt an impossible geometry (see figure below) in order to make a six-membered ring.

Since the hydrogen is axial, the OH group is equatorial. Thus, choice D is the correct answer.

Chapter 6
Carbonyl Chemistry

In this chapter we will discuss the major reaction types: nucleophilic substitution and addition. Each reaction type is defined by the bonding changes that occur over the course of the reaction.

In a substitution reaction, one σ bond in the starting material is converted into a new σ bond in the product. We will briefly explore the two most common substitution reactions.

In an addition reaction, one π bond in the starting material is converted into 2 new σ bonds in the product. Addition will be the principal focus of this chapter as it relates to the carbonyl functional group, a group that appears in all major biomolecules. In addition to this reactivity, carbonyl-containing compounds will undergo deprotonation of the α-carbon atom. We will learn in this chapter how these two reactivities interrelate.

6.1 NUCLEOPHILIC SUBSTITUTIONS

Nucleophilic substitution reactions replace a leaving group in an electrophilic substrate with a nucleophile. In this context, the bonds that break during the substitution will do so via a heterolytic cleavage in which the leaving group takes both electrons from the bond that connected it to the electrophile. This also means you can recognize a substitution reaction by the fact that one σ bond is broken to the leaving group while another is formed to the incoming nucleophile. Therefore, there is no net change in the number of σ bonds or π bonds over the course of the reaction.

Before you read on about the two main nucleophilic substitution mechanisms—S_N1 and S_N2—go back to the Organic Chemist's Toolbox in Section 4.1 to review the three main players involved in all nucleophilic substitution reactions: nucleophiles, electrophiles, and leaving groups.

The S_N2 Mechanism

The first nucleophilic mechanism we'll examine is the S_N2 mechanism. Typical electrophiles (also known as the substrates) for this type of reaction are alkyl halides. Alkyl halides are alkanes that contain at least one halogen (fluorine, chlorine, bromine, or iodine). Since halogen atoms are electronegative, are large in size, and are the conjugate bases of strong acids (except for F^-), most halides (Cl^-, Br^-, I^-) make good leaving groups.

For example, when 1-iodobutane is treated with a Br^- nucleophile, an S_N2 reaction occurs in which bromide replaces the I^- group (known as the leaving group) to yield 1-bromobutane.

1-iodobutane   1-bromobutane

In the first (and only) step of this reaction (see the mechanism on the next page), because the nucleophilic bromide anion attacks the electrophilic carbon at the *same time* that the leaving group leaves, the attack must occur *from the backside* of the substrate. The bromine-carbon bond forms as the iodine-carbon bond is broken, *in a single step*, to yield bromobutane.

The Mechanism

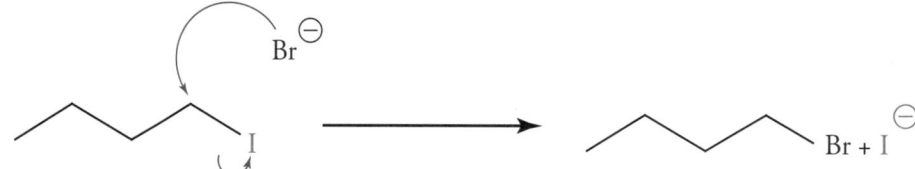

Let's look at a chiral substrate in order to see the stereochemical implications of this concerted mechanism. When (*R*)-1-deutero-1-chloroethane is treated with iodide, the typical backside attack occurs. As the new C—I bond begins to form while the C—Cl bond breaks, the reaction proceeds through a *pentavalent transition state.* As you can see in the product below, there is complete *inversion of configuration* at the carbon being attacked by the nucleophile. This is always the case in an S_N2 reaction on a chiral substrate.

backside attack   pentavalent   inverted product
                        transition state

Furthermore, the rate of the reaction is a function of two variables—that is, **bimolecular**. The rate of the reaction depends on the concentrations of both the nucleophile and the electrophile, and is equal to the product of the rate constant (*k*), the concentration of the nucleophile ([I⁻]), and the concentration of the electrophile ([R-Cl]).

reaction rate = *k*[nucleophile][electrophile]

We can now explain what we mean when we say that this reaction proceeds by an "S_N2" mechanism. The "S" indicates that it is a <u>s</u>ubstitution reaction mechanism, the subscript "N" indicates that it is <u>n</u>u-cleophilic, and the "2" indicates that it is <u>b</u>imolecular (see *General Chemistry Review* Section 9.4 for more details on rate laws).

The rate of the reaction depends not only on the concentration of the electrophile, but also on the degree of substitution of the electrophilic carbon. Since the transition state is sterically crowded with five groups attached, the more bulky those groups are, the harder it is for the nucleophile to gain access to the reactive site. Therefore, less substituted substrates react faster than more substituted ones via the S_N2 mechanism.

The last factor to consider in substitution reactions is the solvent. To favor an S_N2 mechanism, protic solvents such as water and alcohols should be avoided. Since these hydrogen bonding solvents are able to strongly solvate the nucleophile, they hinder the backside attack necessary for the concerted reaction. To prevent this interference, polar, *aprotic* solvents such as acetone, DMF (dimethylformamide), or DMSO (dimethylsulfoxide) should be used. Their polar nature allows the charged nucleophiles and leaving groups to remain dissolved, but they are not as efficient at completely solvating the nucleophile.

Key Features of an S_N2 Reaction

Reactivity of substrate:	$CH_3 > 1° > 2° >> 3°$ (Because of steric hindrance)
Stereochemistry:	Complete stereochemical inversion of the carbon that is attacked by the nucleophile.
Kinetics:	reaction rate = k[nucleophile][electrophile]
Solvent:	S_N2 reactions are favored by polar, aprotic (non-hydrogen bonding) solvents.
Rearrangements:	Not possible due to concerted mechanism. No carbocations are present in solution.
Favoring Conditions:	Strong, non-bulky nucleophile will favor S_N2 reactions over S_N1 (see next section).

The S_N1 Mechanism

In contrast to the concerted S_N2 mechanism, the course of S_N1 substitution reactions, a carbocation (carbonium ion) forms. Let's take a moment to review the relative stability of carbocations. Remember that the formation of charged species from neutral ones is generally an energetically disfavorable process; that is, it is energetically *uphill*. But some ions are more stable than others. For alkyl cations, the relative stabilities due to the inductive effect (Section 4.1) are given below.

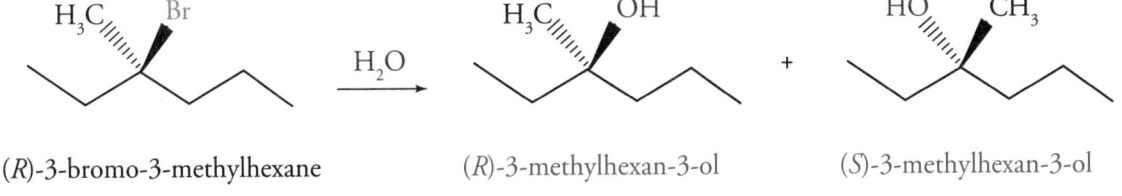

Now that we have reviewed the basics of carbocation stability, let's consider an example in which a chiral halide undergoes an S_N1 substitution reaction. When (*R*)-3-bromo-3-methylhexane is treated with H_2O, a racemic mixture of 3-methylhexan-3-ol is formed:

S_N1 substitution occurs in *two distinct steps*, unlike S_N2 reactions that occur in one step. In the first step of the S_N1 reaction, a *planar carbocation* with 120° bond angles forms (see mechanism below). This occurs when the leaving group falls off (dissociates). This is the slow step of the mechanism, or the rate limiting step. In the final step of this reaction, *racemization* occurs as the nucleophile attacks equally *on either side* of the carbocation. The result is a racemic mixture.

The Mechanism

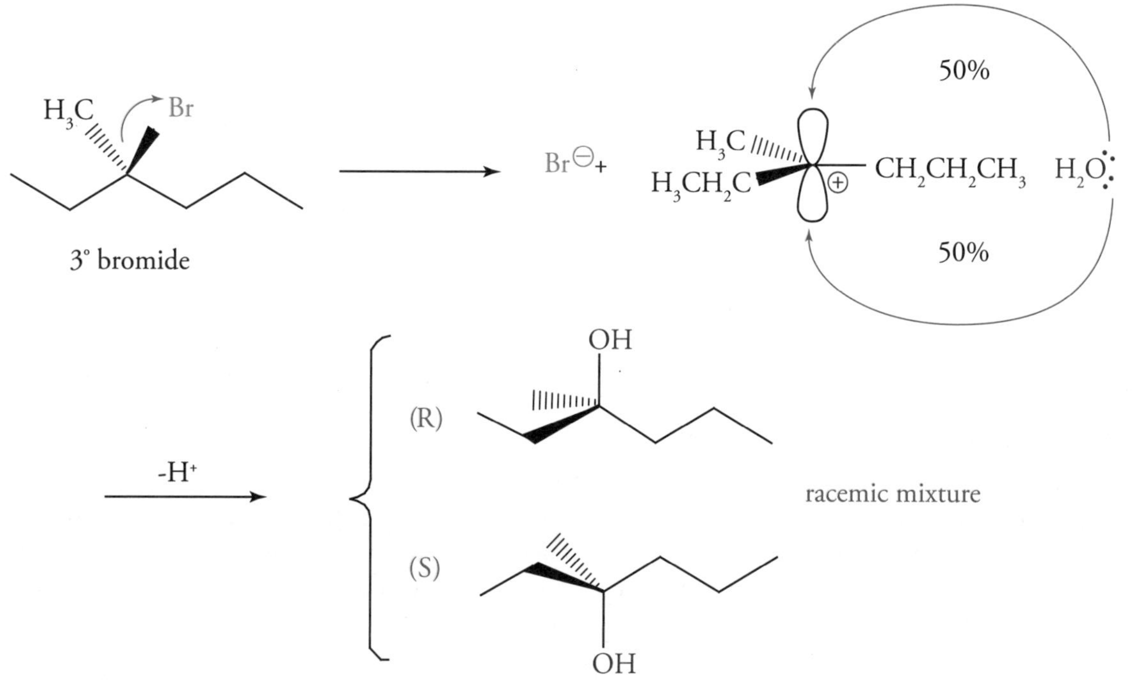

3° bromide

50%

Br⁻ +

50%

-H⁺

(R)

racemic mixture

(S)

Unlike the S_N2 reaction explained above in which the rate of the reaction was a function of two variables, the S_N1 reaction rate is a function of only one variable, that is, **unimolecular**. The rate of the S_N1 reaction depends only upon the concentration of the electrophile (the species that loses the leaving group over the course of the reaction). The rate of the reaction is equal to the product of the rate constant (k), and the electrophile concentration ([R-Br]):

$$\text{reaction rate} = k[\text{electrophile}]$$

As before, we can now explain what we mean when we say that this reaction proceeds by an "S_N1" mechanism. The "S" indicates that it is a <u>s</u>ubstitution reaction mechanism, the subscript "N" indicates that it is <u>n</u>ucleophic, and the "1" indicates that it is <u>uni</u>molecular.

The rate of the reaction depends not only on the concentration of the electrophile, but also on the degree of substitution of the electrophilic carbon. Since the dissociation of the leaving group is the slow step of the mechanism, anything that makes that step more favorable will speed up the reaction. As was just discussed, the more substituted the carbocation intermediate, the more stable it is. Therefore, more substituted substrates will dissociate to make more stable intermediates faster, speeding up the rate of the entire reaction.

To favor an S_N1 mechanism, protic solvents such as water and alcohols should be used. The role of the solvent is twofold. The protic solvent helps to stabilize the forming carbocation and solvate the leaving group, thereby facilitating the first, or slow step of the mechanism. Secondly, the solvent then behaves as the nucleophile in a **solvolysis** reaction, attacking the carbocation intermediate. This produces an alcohol product if water is used as the solvent and an ether if the reaction is run in an alcoholic solvent.

Key Features of an S_N1 Reaction

Reactivity of substrate: 3° > 2° >> 1° (Due to stabilization of the carbocation)

Stereochemistry: Almost complete racemization due to nucleophilic attack on either side of p orbital.

Kinetics: reaction rate = k[electrophile]

Solvent: S_N1 reactions are favored by protic (hydrogen bonding) solvents. (This stabilizes the carbocation.)

Rearrangements: Carbocation rearrangement is possible; if the carbocation can rearrange to one that is more stable, it will.

Favoring conditions: Non-basic, weaker nucleophiles favor unimolecular substitutions. Often the solvent acts as the nucleophile (solvolysis).

Alcohols undergo substitution reactions just as alkyl halides do. They can undergo either S_N1 or S_N2 substitution reactions depending upon the degree of substitution of the alcohol. Alcohols are treated with strong mineral acids to make their bad –OH leaving group into a good one (H_2O). In S_N2 reactions, the conjugate base of the mineral acid will attack while the leaving group leaves. In S_N1 reactions, the water will first dissociate, followed by nucleophilic attack of the halide ion on the carbocation intermediate.

Example 6-1: Predict whether the following substitution reactions will proceed via an S_N1 or an S_N2 mechanism.

(a)

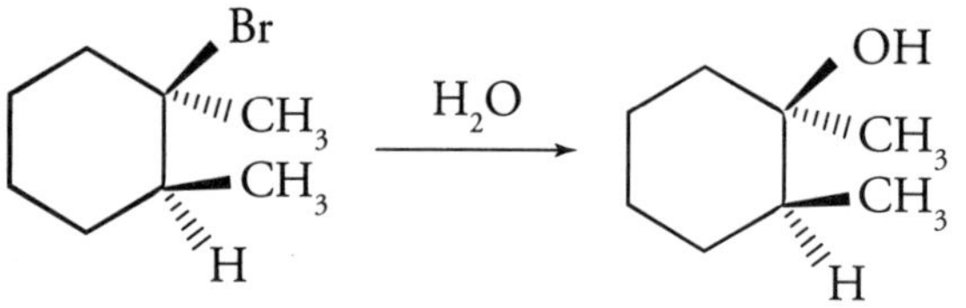

(b)

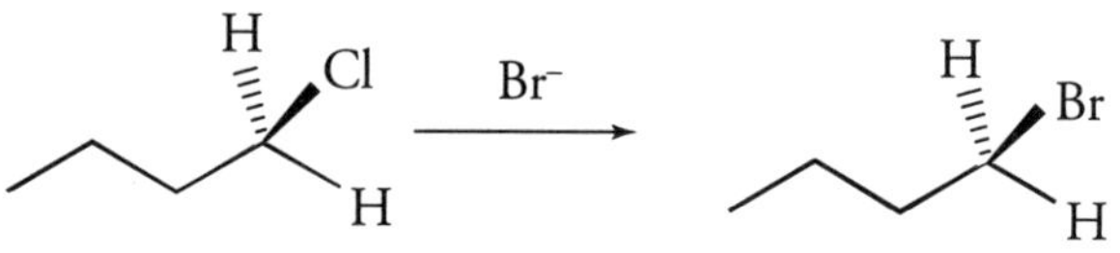

(c)

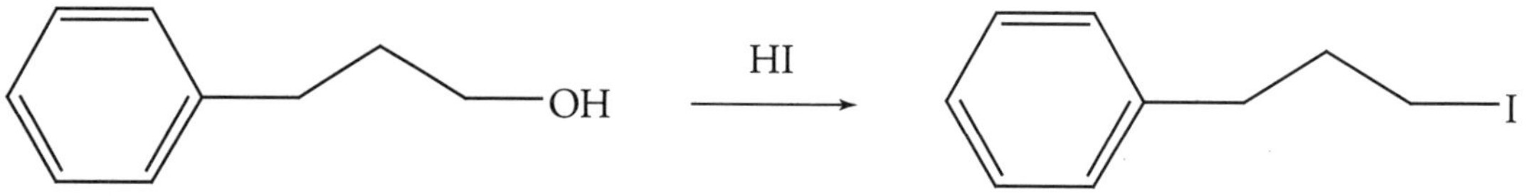

(d)

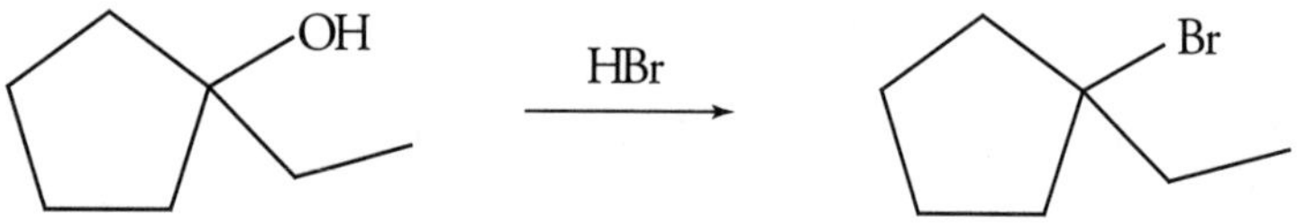

Solution:

(a) 3° bromide, S_N1
(b) 1° chloride, S_N2
(c) 1° alcohol, S_N2
(d) 3° alcohol, S_N1

6.2 ALDEHYDES AND KETONES

Two very important classes of oxygen-containing organic compounds are **aldehydes** and **ketones**. We begin the discussion of these functional groups by looking at a common way carbonyls are formed—the oxidation of an alcohol:

Note: Since the oxidizing agent removes a hydrogen from the carbon, tertiary alcohols are not able to react to form carbonyls since they have no hydrogen at the reactive site.

Oxidizing agents are able to absorb electrons (and be reduced). Below are some common oxidizing agents that appear on the MCAT. Note that only the anhydrous oxidant (PCC) will NOT overoxidize the primary alcohol to the carboxylic acid (we'll talk more about this functional group later). All oxidizing agents shown can be used to form ketones from secondary alcohols.

Aqueous Oxidants	Anhydrous Oxidant
Chromic Acid (H_2CrO_4)	
Chromate Salts (CrO_4^{2-})	
Dichromate Salts ($Cr_2O_7^{2-}$)	Pyridinium Chlorochromate (PCC)
Permanganate (MnO_4^-)	
Chromium Trioxide (CrO_3)	

Now that we understand how aldehydes and ketones are formed, let's look at their reactivities. The key to understanding the chemistry of aldehydes and ketones is to understand the electronic structure and properties of the carbonyl group. The C=O double bond is very polarized because oxygen is much more electronegative than carbon, and so it is able to pull the π electrons of the C=O double bond toward itself and away from carbon. This is illustrated by the following resonance structures:

So overall, carbonyls react like

This bond polarization renders the carbon atom electrophilic (δ^+) and accounts for two kinds of reactions of aldehydes and ketones. First, these molecules have *acidic protons* α *to (i.e., next to) the carbonyl group.*

An α-proton is acidic because the electrons left behind upon deprotonation can delocalize into the π system of the carbonyl. Second, the electrophilic carbon of the carbonyl group makes aldehydes and ketones *susceptible to nucleophilic attack.* In the aldol condensation, which we will study in some detail, both of these types of reactivity are involved in a single reaction.

Acidity and Enolization

The first type of reaction that is commonly observed with aldehydes and ketones is the result of the relative acidity of protons that are α to the carbonyl group. These α-protons are sufficiently acidic that they can be removed by a strong base [such as hydroxide ion (OH⁻) or an alkoxide ion (OR⁻)] to yield a carbanion. This carbanion can be easily formed because the electrons that are left behind on the carbon can be delocalized into the carbonyl π system. In this way, the negative charge can be delocalized onto the electronegative oxygen atom. A resonance-stabilized carbanion of this type is referred to as an **enolate ion**. *An enolate ion* *is negatively charged and nucleophilic.* The nucleophilic character of an enolate ion lies predominantly at the carbon at which the proton was abstracted, *not* the oxygen atom of the carbonyl. This is why the α-carbon of enolates is the nucleophile in most common enolate reactions.

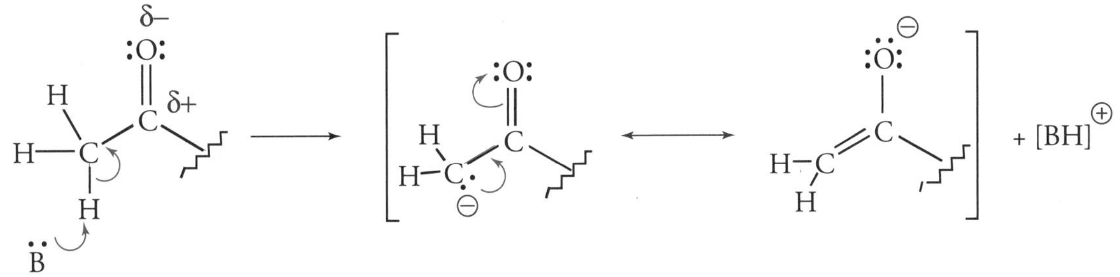

resonance forms of enolate anion

An example that demonstrates the acidity of α-protons is the exchange reaction that occurs between the α-proton of Compound I (below) and deuterium from D_2O. Compound I has a single α-proton that is α to *two* carbonyl groups in comparison to the six other α-protons in the molecule that are α to only *one* carbonyl group. It is this lone α-proton that exchanges with a deuterium of D_2O over the course of a couple of days, even in the absence of base. Being next to two carbonyl groups greatly enhances the acidity of this α-proton and allows it to exchange (although slowly) with a deuterium from D_2O. The mechanism of this exchange, which essentially consists of protonation of the intermediate enolate ion, is shown in the following figure:

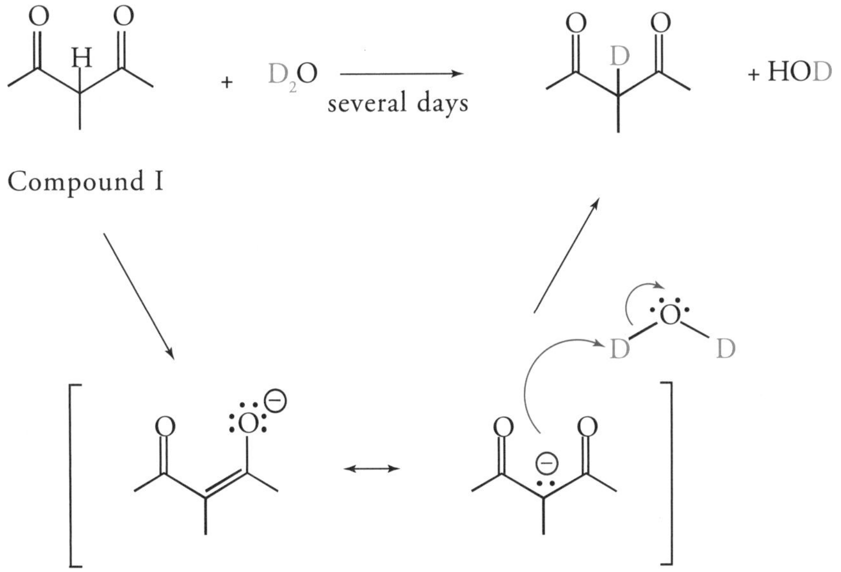

Example 6-2: As a review of acidity, for each of the following pairs of compounds, identify the one with the more acidic proton.

(a) 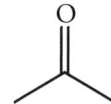 vs.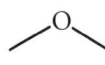

(b) 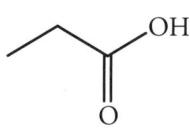 vs.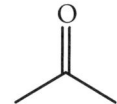

(c) 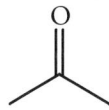 vs.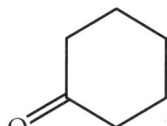

(d) 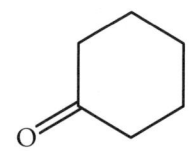 vs.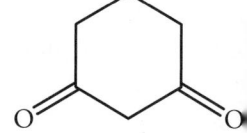

(e) 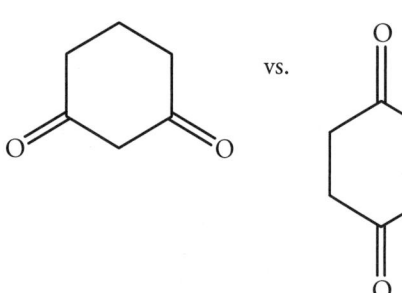 vs.

(f) vs.

(g) vs.

Solution:

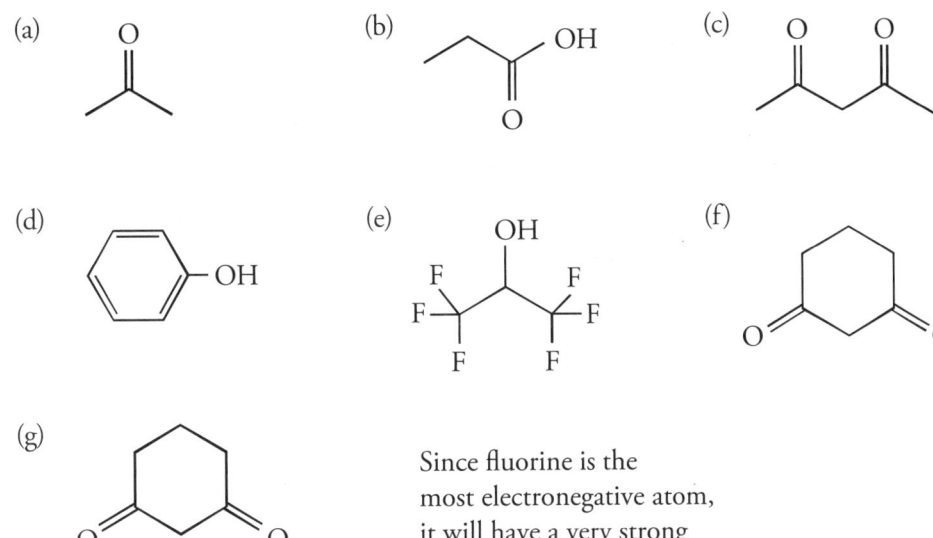

(a)

(b)

(c)

(d)

(e)

(f)

(g)

Since fluorine is the most electronegative atom, it will have a very strong inductive effect.

Keto-Enol Tautomerism

A ketone is converted into an enol by deprotonation of an α-carbon atom and subsequent protonation of the carbonyl oxygen. These two forms of the molecule are very similar to one another and differ only by the position of a proton and a double bond. This is referred to as **keto-enol tautomerism**. Two molecules are **tautomers** if they are readily interconvertible constitutional isomers in equilibrium with one another.

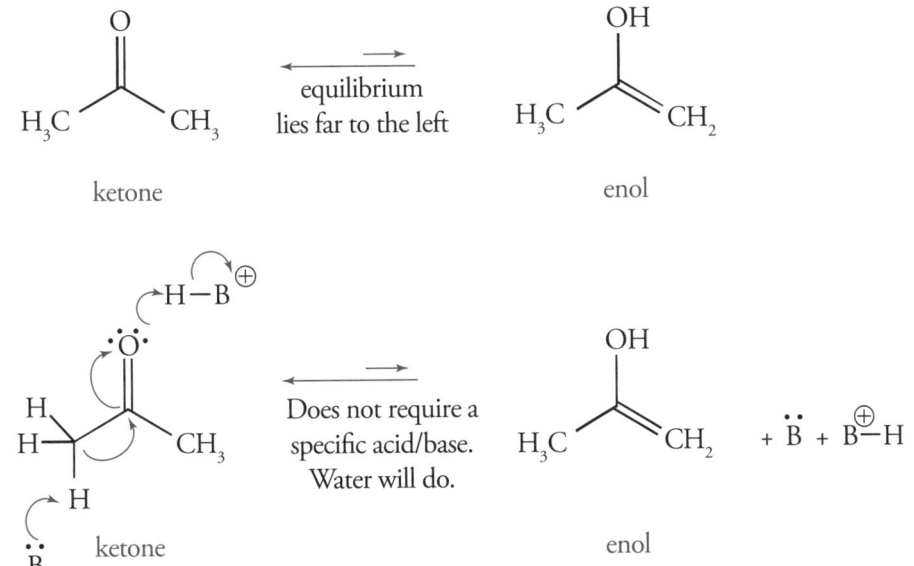

Tautomerization has consequences for molecules with chiral α-carbons. Imagine an alcohol with a chiral center adjacent to the hydroxyl group (as shown below). If this stereochemically defined alcohol were oxidized, the corresponding ketone would have racemic stereochemistry.

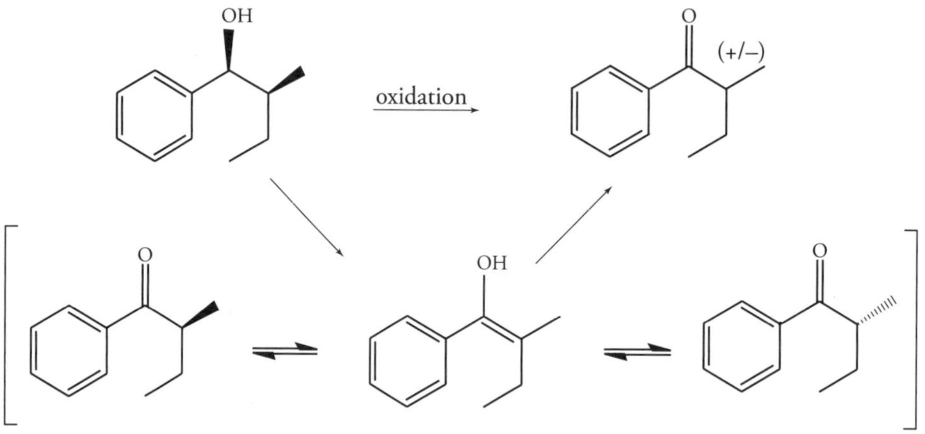

Because the α-carbon of the compound is sp^2 hybridized and planar in the enol tautomer, protonation to form the keto tautomer can occur from both the top and bottom faces of the double bond. This loss of defined stereochemistry, which results in a mixture of R and S configurations at the once chiral α-carbon, is termed **racemization**.

Nucleophilic Addition Reactions to Aldehydes and Ketones

Because of the polarized nature of the C=O double bond in aldehydes and ketones, the carbon of the carbonyl group is very electrophilic. This means that it will attract nucleophiles and can readily be reduced. The attack of a nucleophile upon the carbon of a carbonyl group, called a nucleophilic addition reaction, is shown below with a generic nucleophile (Nu:).

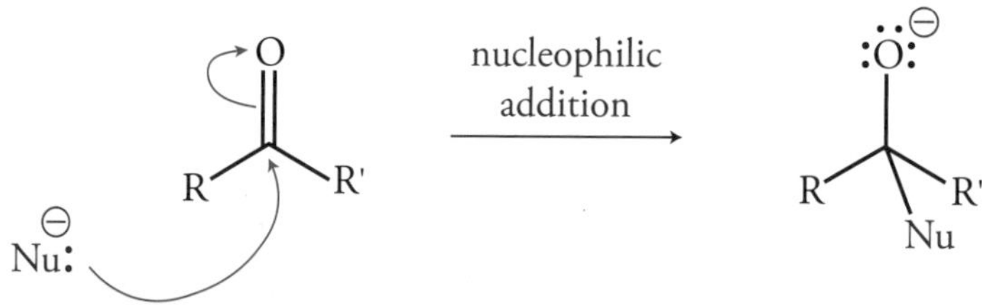

Nucleophilic addition reactions are defined by the bonding changes that occur over the course of the reaction. In these reactions, a π bond in the starting material is broken, and two σ bonds in the product result. This very general reaction allows for the conversion of aldehydes or ketones into a variety of other functional groups, such as alcohols, via hydride reduction: (top of next page)

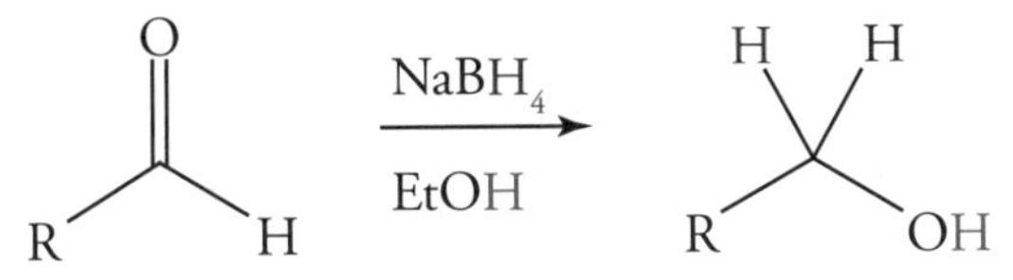

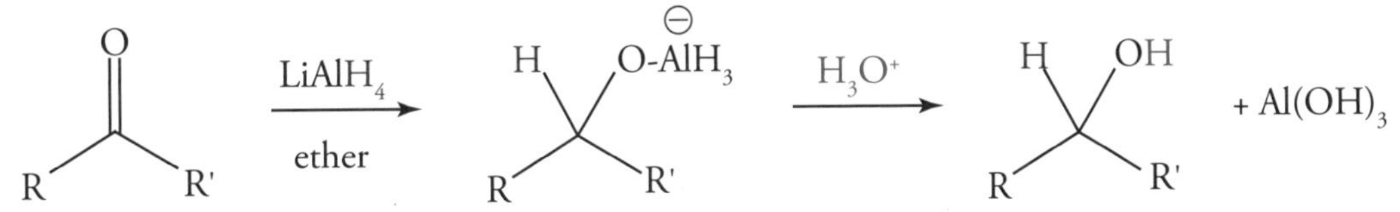

Note: Sodium borohydride (NaBH₄) and lithium aluminum hydride (LiAlH₄) are common reducing agents seen on the MCAT. In general, strong reducing agents easily lose electrons by adding hydride (a hydrogen atom and a pair of electrons) to the carbonyl. Reducing agents often have many hydrogens attached to other elements with low electronegativity.

Organometallic Reagents

Organometallic reagents are commonly used to perform nucleophilic addition to a carbonyl carbon. The basic structure of an organometallic reagent is R^-M^+. They act as electron rich, or anionic, carbon atoms and therefore function as either strong bases or nucleophiles. Grignard and lithium reagents are the most common organometallic reagents.

Grignard reagents are generally made via the action of an alkyl or acyl halide on magnesium metal, as depicted below.

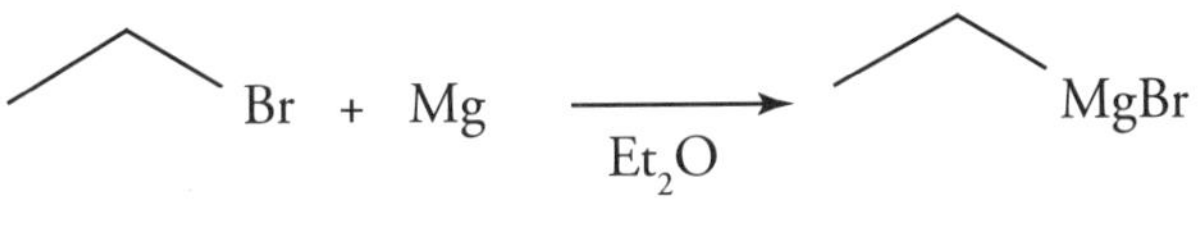

To avoid unwanted protonation of the very basic Grignard reagent, the reaction is carried out in an aprotic solvent such as diethyl ether.

The carbonyl containing compounds are then added to the Grignard reagents to yield alcohol products. In the reaction below, the ethyl magnesium bromide acts as a nucleophile and adds to the electrophilic carbonyl carbon. An intermediate alkoxide ion is formed that is rapidly protonated to produce the alcohol during an aqueous acidic workup step.

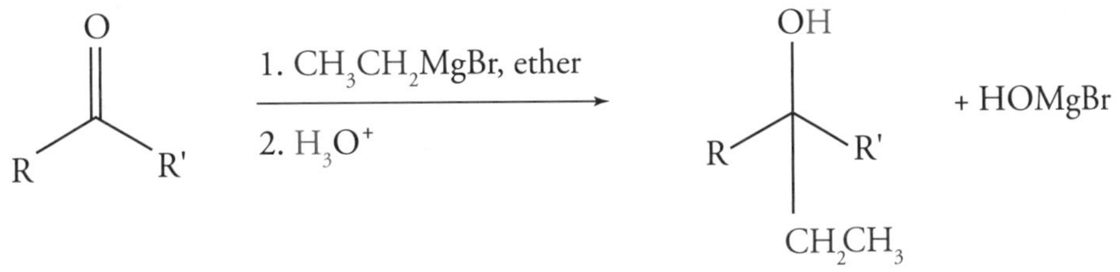

In addition to using an aprotic solvent, care must also be taken to avoid the presence of any other acidic hydrogens in the substrate molecule bearing the carbonyl. This means that alcohol groups or carboxylic acid groups must be absent, or else first be protected, before the Grignard reagent can be added to the carbonyl compound.

Mesylates and Tosylates

Two commonly used strategies for the protection of alcohols are their transformation into mesylates and tosylates. By adding a mesyl (methanesulfonyl, $CH_3-SO_3^-$) or tosyl group (toluenesulfonyl, $CH_3C_6H_4-SO_3^-$) in the place of hydroxyl, the reactive nature of the protic, and potentially nucleophilic, −OH group is removed, allowing the molecule to participate in reactions the presence of the hydroxyl may have prevented.

The formation of mesylates and tosylates from alcohols is shown below. Reaction of a sulfonyl chloride, either mesyl chloride or tosyl chloride, with an alcohol in the presence of a base (generally triethylamine or pyridine) leads to nucleophilic attack at the sulfur, followed by expulsion of the chloride.

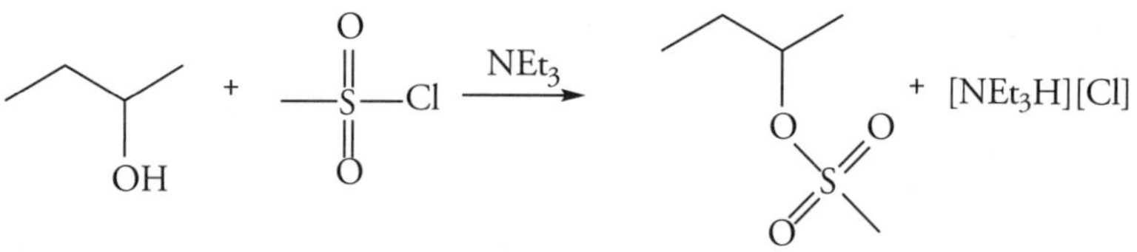

sec-butyl alcohol   mesyl chloride   sec-butyl mesylate

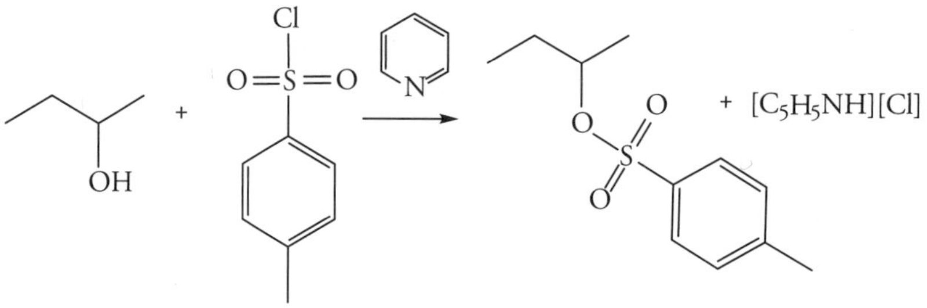

sec-butyl alcohol   tosyl chloride   sec-butyl tosylate

The base in each reaction is required to neutralize the HCl (consisting of the hydroxyl proton and the chloride from the sulfonyl group) and pull it out of the solution as an ammonium or pyridinium chloride salt.

These groups, particularly the tosyl group, may be similarly utilized in the protection of amino (−NH$_2$) groups. In either case, hydroxyl or amino, the protected functionality is rendered sufficiently inert for the purposes of the subsequent reaction steps. Once the protection is no longer required, the protecting group may be removed and the hydroxyl or amine functionality regenerated, generally under reductive conditions.

In addition to their use as protecting groups, both mesylates and tosylates are good leaving groups in reactions featuring nucleophilic attack. Whereas hydroxyl is a poor leaving group requiring a very strong nucleophile for displacement, conversion of a hydroxyl into a mesylate or tosylate makes attack and displacement facile.

Acetals and Hemiacetals

Acetals and hemiacetals, which are of fundamental importance in biochemical reactions that occur in living organisms, can be synthesized from nucleophilic addition reactions to aldehydes or ketones. There are many examples of these molecules in common biochemical pathways. Before we learn the chemistry of these groups, we must be able to identify acetals and hemiacetals.

Note: The terms *ketal* and *hemiketal* refer to acetals and hemiacetals made from *ketones*, but this nomenclature appears infrequently.

General Formulas

acetals   hemiacetals

Some Specific Examples

an acetal   a hemiacetal

Example 6-3: For each of the following compounds, identify whether it's an acetal, hemiacetal, or neither:

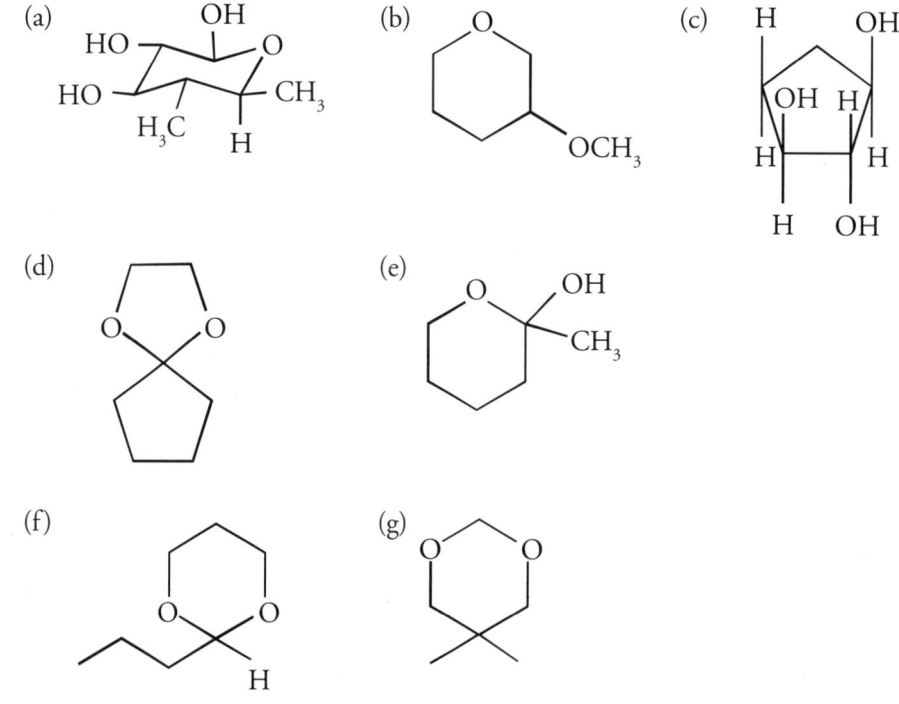

Solution:

(a) hemiacetal
(b) neither
(c) neither
(d) acetal
(e) hemiacetal
(f) acetal
(g) acetal

Acetals are formed when aldehydes or ketones react with alcohols in the presence of acid. This occurs by a nucleophilic addition mechanism. It is easy to predict the product of an acetal formation reaction. Notice that *hydrogens or carbons attached to the carbonyl carbon* of the aldehyde or ketone *remain attached* in the acetal product with the subsequent addition of two –OR groups from the alcohol. Also, note that an intermediate hemiacetal results from the addition of one –OR group to an aldehyde or ketone with subsequent protonation of the carbonyl oxygen. The aldehyde or ketone, the hemiacetal, and the acetal are all in equilibrium with one another. In order for the hemiacetal to form the acetal, a molecule of water must be lost.

Acetal Formation

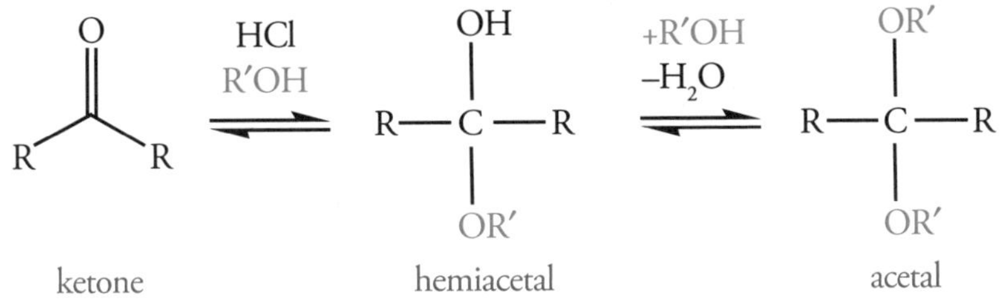

The mechanism of this important reaction is shown below. In the first step, the carbonyl oxygen is protonated, making the carbonyl carbon even more susceptible to nucleophilic attack by the oxygen of the attacking alcohol molecule. Following nucleophilic attack, the oxygen of the alcohol nucleophile is positively charged. This positive charge is unfavorable, and neutrality is achieved by loss of a proton, which yields the intermediate hemiacetal. Remember that the reaction mixture is acidic so that a lone pair of electrons on the hemiacetal –OH can be protonated, thereby converting a poor leaving group into a good leaving group. Once again, this increases the electrophilicity of the carbon and makes it more susceptible to a second nucleophilic attack by an alcohol molecule. All that remains is for the positively charged oxygen from the attacking alcohol to lose a proton to yield the acetal product.

The Mechanism

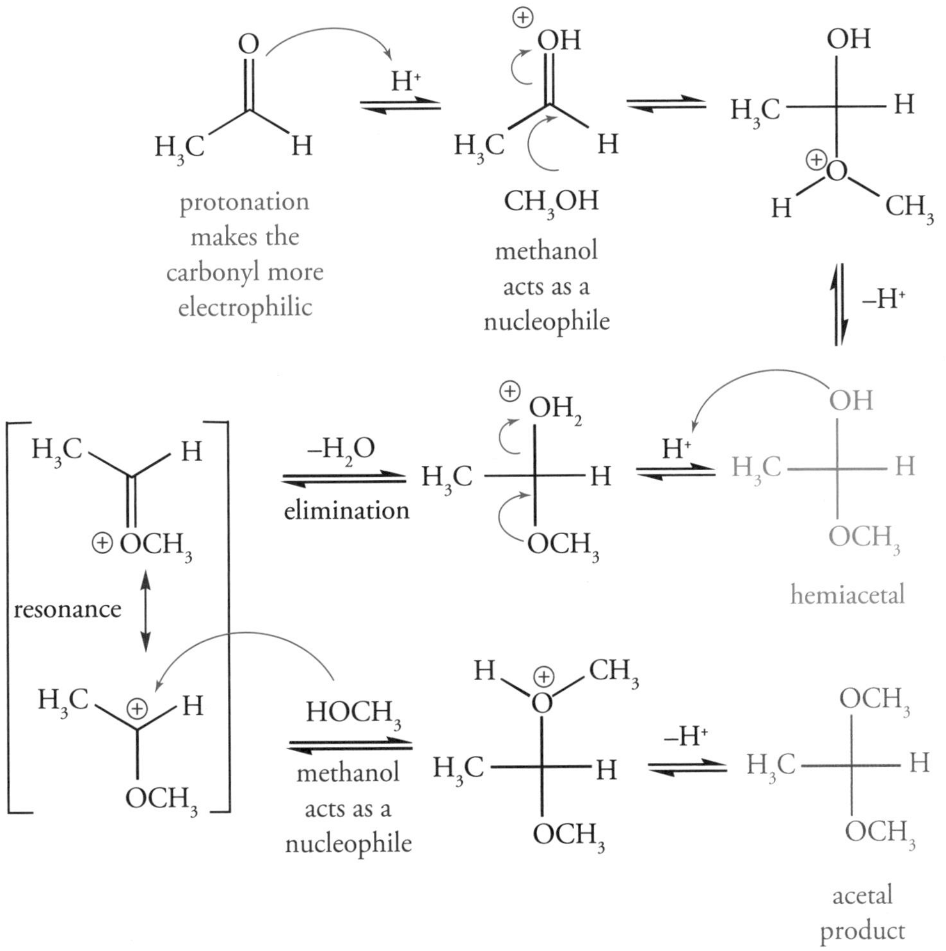

The Overall Reaction

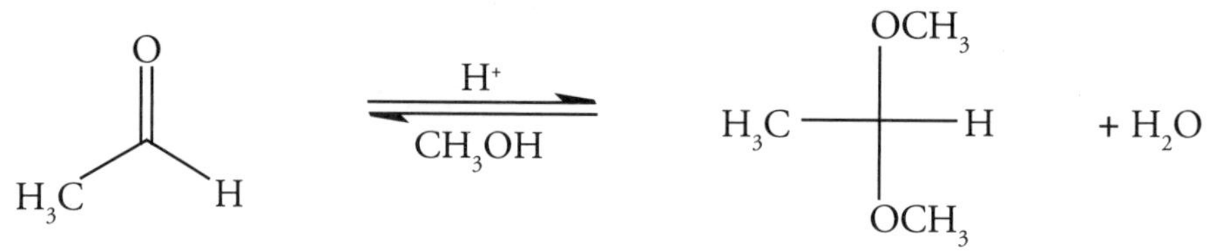

Example 6-4: Predict the acetal product from the following reactions:

(a)

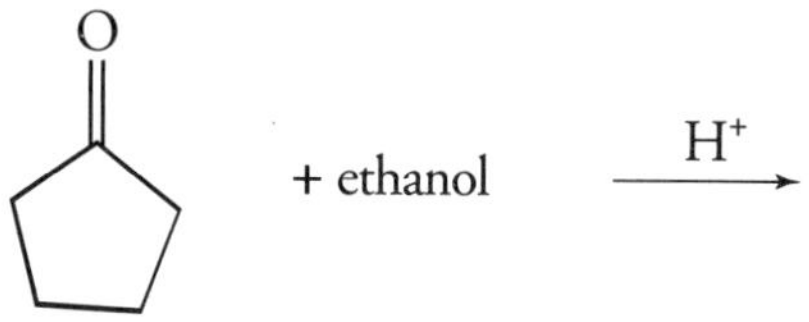

(b)

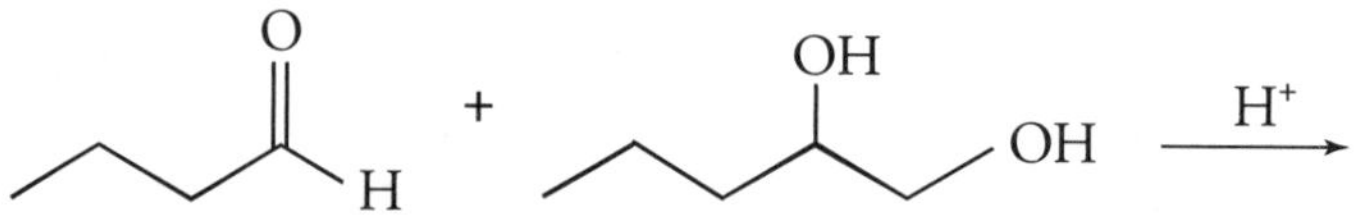

(c)

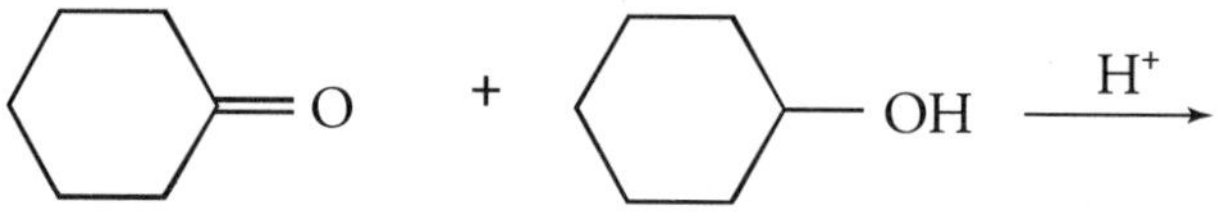

(d)

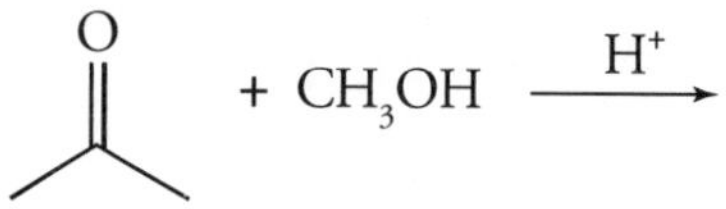

Solution:

(a)

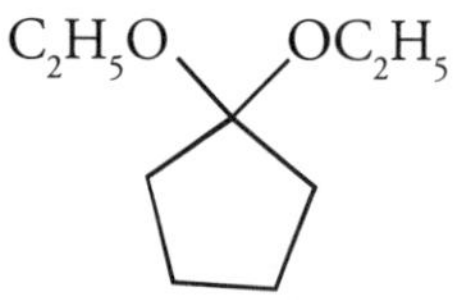

(b)

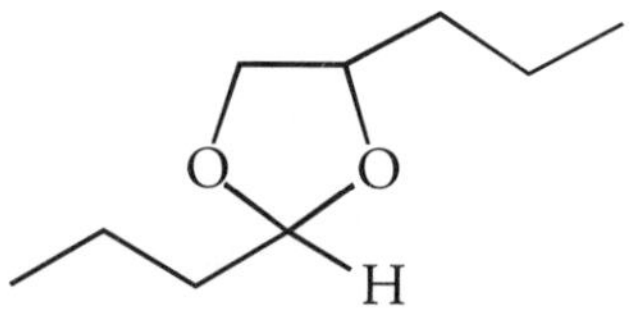

(c)

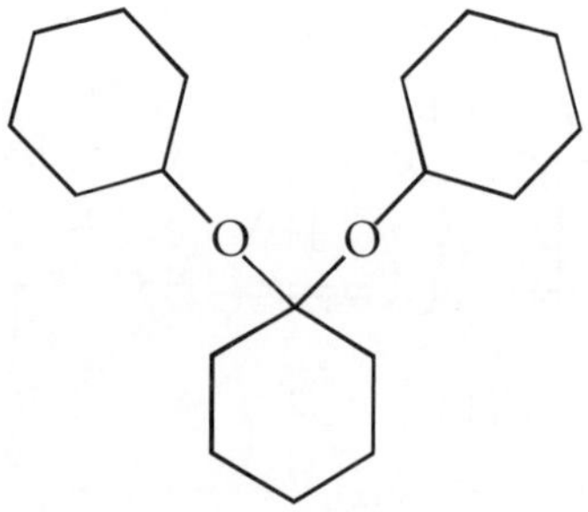

(d)

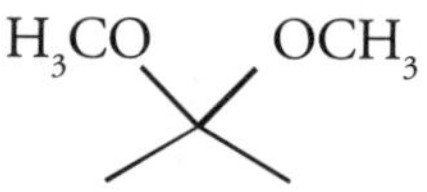

Cyanohydrin Formation

Whereas the nucleophilic attack of an alcohol or alkoxide on a ketone or aldehyde leads to the formation of a tetrahedral hemiacetal, attack by cyanide ($^{-}C{\equiv}N$) results in the formation of a cyanohydrin. The mechanism, shown below, is very similar to the one at work in the formation of hemiacetals. While cyanohydrin formation can be technically envisioned as an equilibrium process, much like the formation of hemiacetals, the equilibrium heavily favors the products and can practically be envisioned as a one-way reaction.

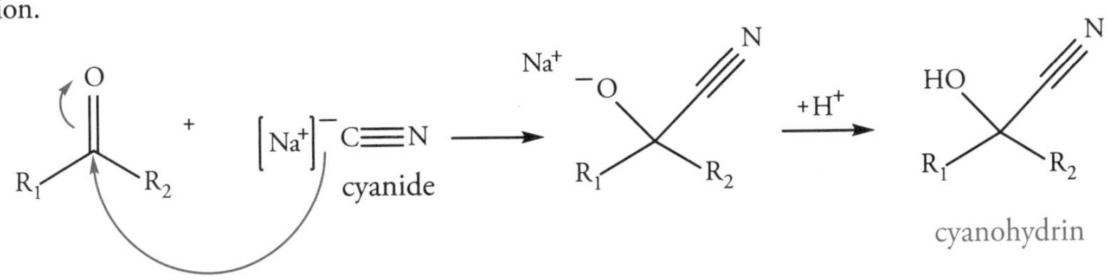

Amines

Before looking at the next few examples of nucleophilic addition reactions, we should first briefly discuss the nucleophile used in the reactions—namely amines. Organic compounds that contain nitrogen are of fundamental importance in biological systems. The most common nitrogen-containing compounds are the **amines**, which have the general structure of $R{-}NH_2$. Amines can be further classified as either **alkyl amines** or **aryl amines**. *Alkyl* amines are compounds in which nitrogen is bound to an *sp*^{3}-hybridized carbon, while *aryl* amines are compounds in which nitrogen is bonded to an *sp*^{2}-hybridized carbon of an aromatic ring.

Below are a few examples of common amines.

$CH_3CH_2\ddot{N}H_2$

ethylamine

(–)-nicotine

epinephrine

benzyltrimethyl-ammonium chloride

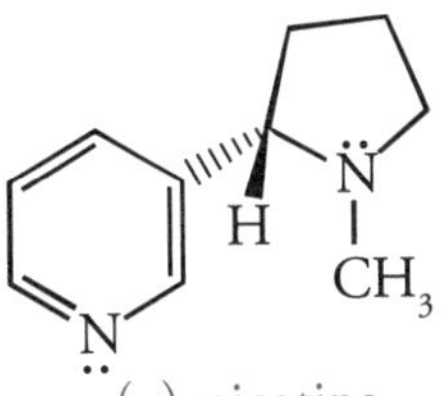

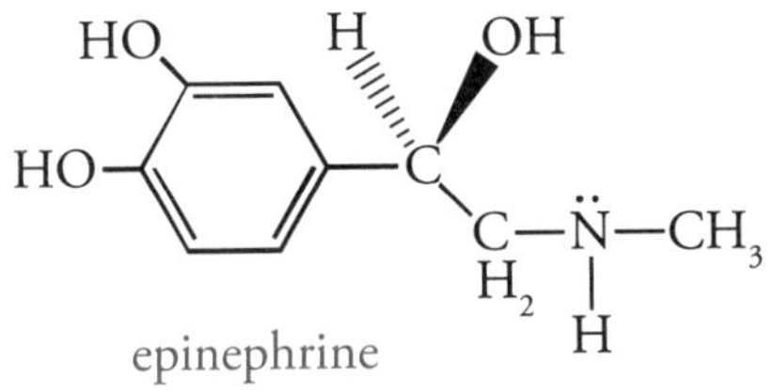

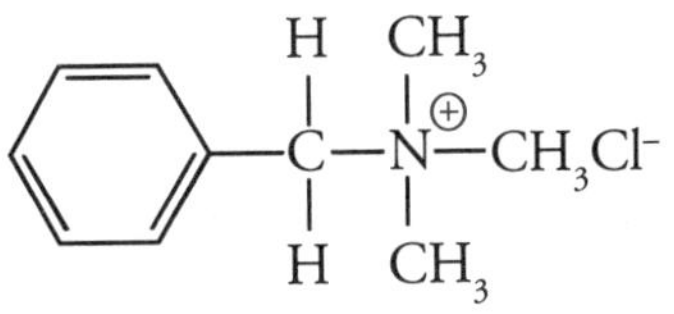

Amines can be further categorized as primary amines, secondary amines, tertiary amines, and quaternary ammonium ions.

A primary amine   A secondary amine   A tertiary amine   A quaternary ammonium ion

In the simple methyl amine, CH_3NH_2, notice that the nitrogen has three σ bonds and one lone electron pair. Its hybridization is therefore sp^3 with approximately 109° bond angles. The molecular geometry of an alkyl amine is pyramidal.

Methyl amine

Nitrogen Hybridization	sp^3
Bond Angles	109°
Molecular Geometry	pyramidal

Most importantly, because of the lone pair of electrons on the N, amines behave as either Brønsted-Lowry bases or as nucleophiles. Let's now look at a few reactions in which the nucleophile is an amine.

Imine Formation

A class of reactions that closely resembles acetal formation are the reactions of aldehydes or ketones with amines. These reactions are often catalyzed under weakly acidic conditions (pH about 4–5). When an aldehyde or ketone reacts with a primary amine (RNH_2), an imine will form.

an aldehyde or ketone   an imine

As in the acetal formation reaction, whatever R groups are originally attached to the carbonyl carbon stay attached in the product, and a molecule of water is liberated as a byproduct. A brief examination of the reaction mechanism will help illustrate these common features.

Mechanism

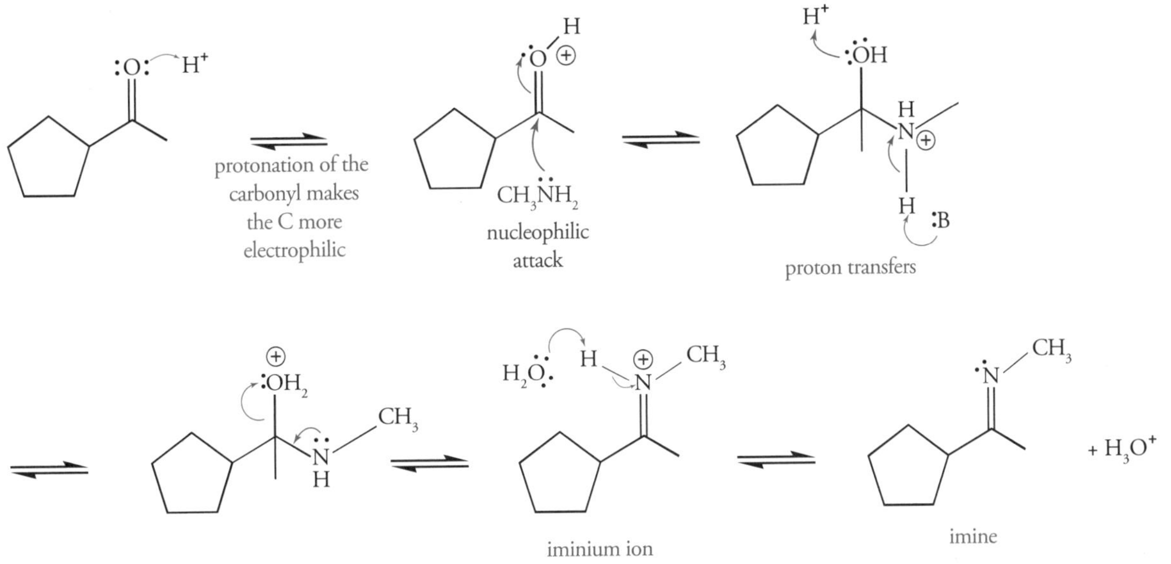

In the first step of this reaction, a lone pair of electrons on the carbonyl oxygen is protonated by the acidic medium. As in acetal formation, protonation of the carbonyl oxygen makes the carbonyl carbon more electrophilic and therefore more susceptible to nucleophilic attack. This time, the nucleophile is a primary amine, but attack by the nucleophilic nitrogen on the electrophilic carbon results in a similar tetrahedral intermediate. This intermediate is then deprotonated at the nitrogen and protonated at the oxygen, thereby converting a poor leaving group (–OH) into a good one ($-OH_2^+$). Next, the oxygen departs as a neutral water molecule, leaving behind a carbocation that is resonance-stabilized by the lone pair of electrons on nitrogen, reminiscent of the stabilization by the incoming oxygen during acetal formation. (*Note*: Only the more stable resonance form is shown in the mechanism above.) The similarities to acetal formation end here, as the final step of imine production is the deprotonation of the iminium ion to regenerate the acid catalyst.

Enamine Formation

While imines are derived from primary amines, if a secondary amine (R_2NH) is used under similar reaction conditions, the result is a functional group called an enamine. The overall reaction of a typical enamine synthesis is shown below. Note that this is another reversible reaction, and that enamines can be hydrolyzed to the carbonyl compound under aqueous acidic conditions.

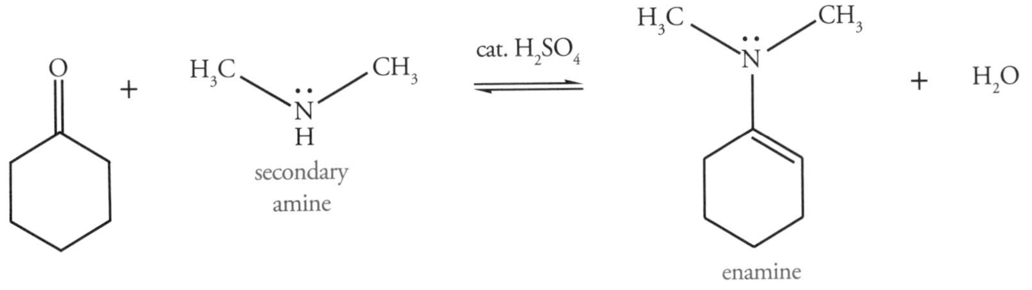

The mechanism of enamine formation is identical to imine formation until the final step. Since the incoming amine is secondary rather than primary, the iminium ion cannot be deprotonated as in the imine mechanism. Instead, deprotonation of a hydrogen α to the double bond, now substantially more acidic on account of the positive charge on nitrogen, yields the enamine.

iminium ion   enamine

Enamines are a class of organic molecules resembling enols, in which the enol-oxygen of the aldehyde or ketone is replaced by a secondary amine. The chemistry of enamines is similar to enol chemistry in that it is largely governed by the resonance between the enamine and iminium structures. The partial double-bond character in the C—N bond, implied by the iminium resonance structure, results in the sp^2–hybridization of the enamine nitrogen and hindered rotation around the C—N bond (and the C—C_α bond in acyclic compounds).

enamine form   iminium form

As the iminium resonance form above suggests, the α-carbon of the enamine is nucleophilic and will readily react with electrophiles. The increased donor ability of nitrogen, as compared to oxygen, results in enamines being more nucleophilic than neutral enols, but less nucleophilic than charged enolates (as we'll see shortly). As shown on the next page, attack by the nucleophilic α-carbon on the polarized carbon of an alkyl halide results in the expulsion of the halide leaving group. This generates an iminium ion, which, as mentioned above, will reform the carbonyl under acidic, aqueous workup conditions.

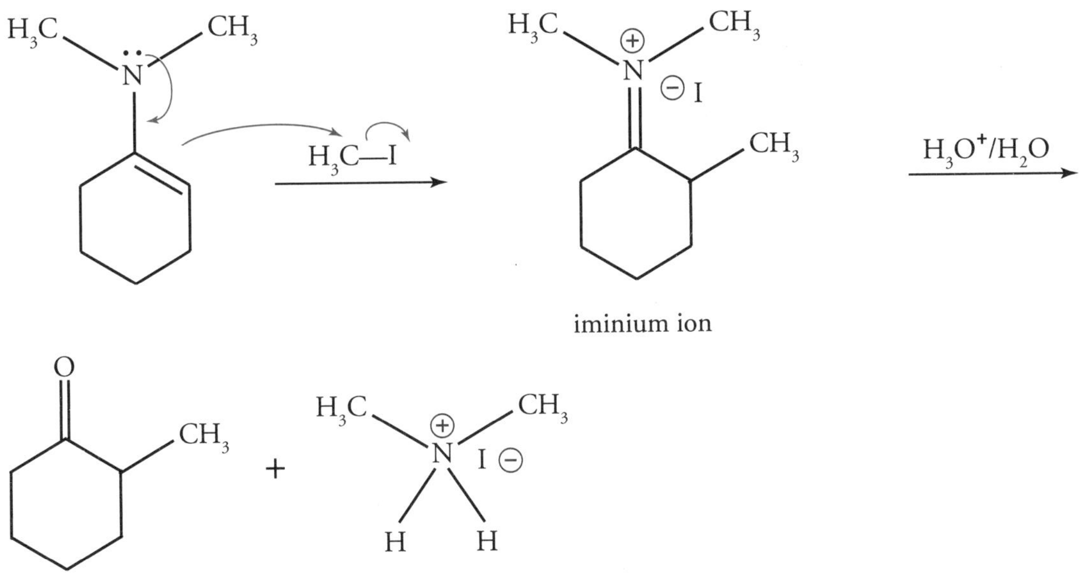

H3C
CH3
N
H3C—I
H3C
CH3
N
I
CH3
H3O+/H2O
iminium ion
O
CH3
+
H3C
CH3
N
I
H
H

Example 6-5: Predict the major organic product of each of the following reactions:

(a)

O
H
+
NH2CH(CH3)2
mildly acidic
pH 5

(b)

O
+
NH
mildly acidic
pH 5

(c)

O
H
+
H
N
mildly acidic
pH 5

(d)

CH3
O
+
O
H2N
N
H
NH2
mildly acidic
pH 5

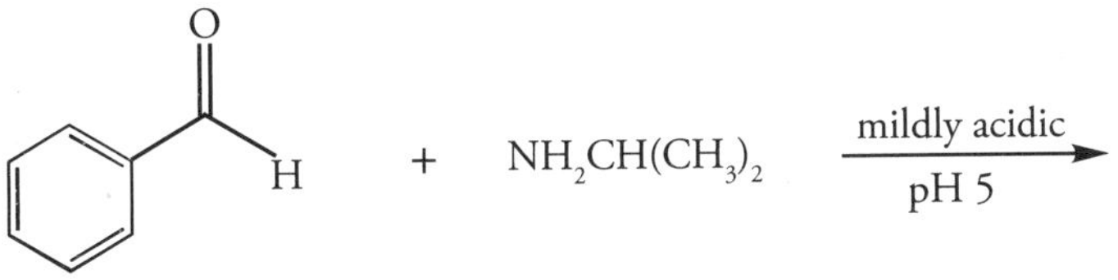

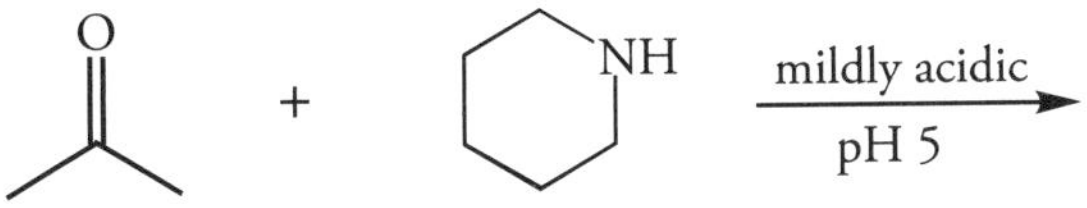

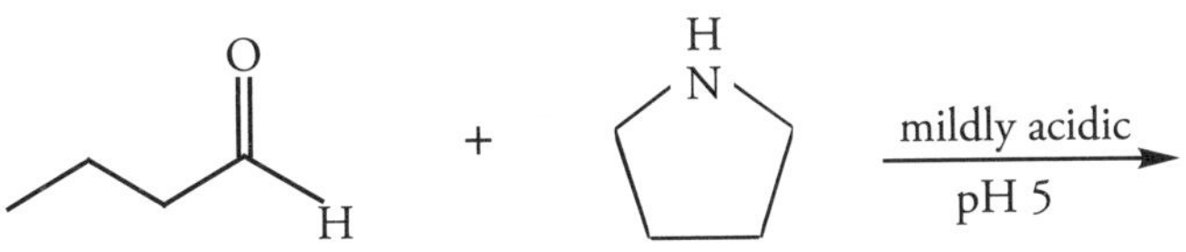

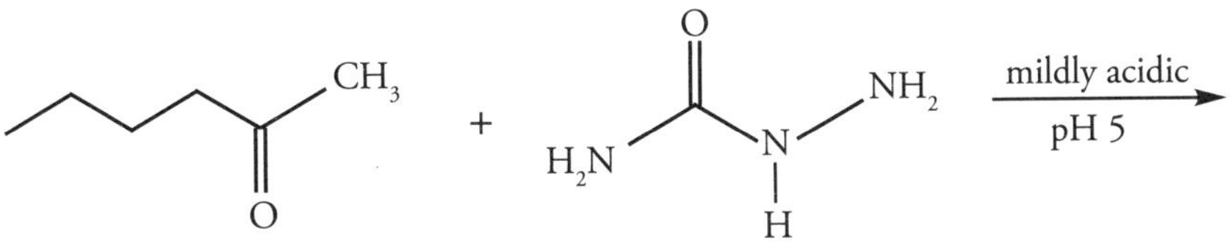

Solution:

(a)

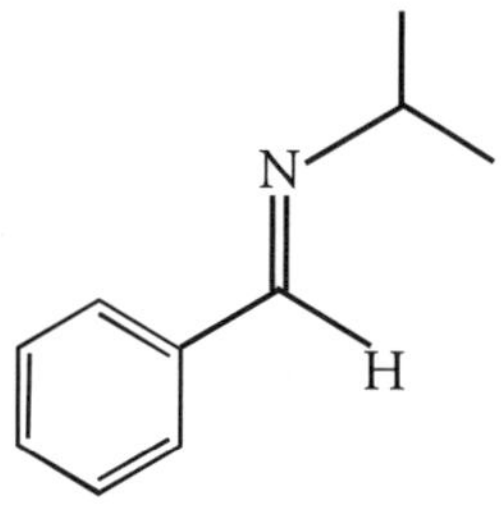

(b)

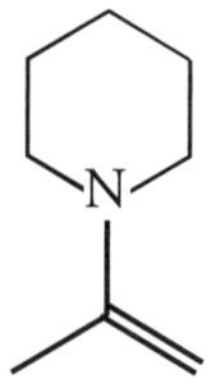

(c)

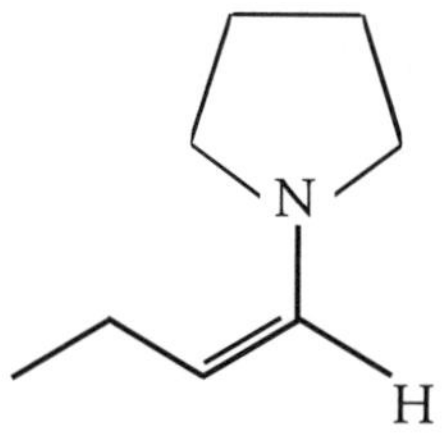

(d)

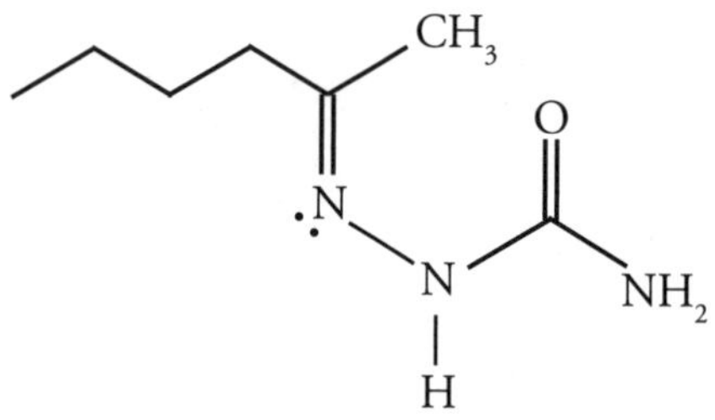

Aldol Condensation

A classic reaction in which the enolate anion of one carbonyl compound reacts with the carbonyl group of another carbonyl compound is called the **aldol condensation**. This reaction combines the two types of aldehyde/ketone reactivities: the acidity of the α-proton and the electrophilicity of the carbonyl carbon, and forms a β-hydroxycarbonyl compound as the product.

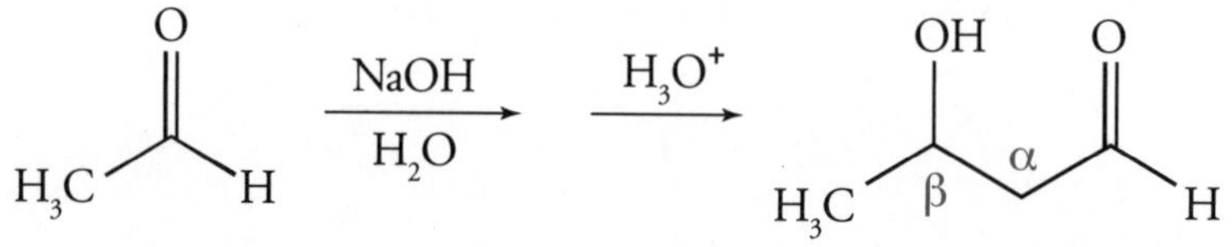

β–hydroxyaldehyde

As the mechanism below shows, in the first step of this reaction, a strong base removes an α-proton from the aldehyde or ketone, resulting in the formation of a resonance-stabilized enolate anion. (Remember, the enolate anion is nucleophilic and usually reacts at the carbon atom that was deprotonated.) Next, the α-carbon of the enolate anion attacks the carbonyl carbon of another aldehyde molecule, thereby generating an alkoxide ion that is subsequently protonated by a molecule of water. This results in the formation of a general class of molecules referred to as β-hydroxy carbonyl compounds.

The Mechanism

β–hydroxy aldehyde

There are three important points to note about this reaction. First, it requires a strong base (typically hydroxide, OH⁻, or an alkoxide ion RO⁻) to remove an α-proton adjacent to the carbonyl group. Second, one of the aldehydes or ketones must act as a source for the enolate ions while the other aldehyde or ketone will come under nucleophilic attack by the enolate carbanion. Third, the aldol condensation does not require the two carbonyl groups that participate in the reaction to be the same. When they are different, it is called a **crossed aldol condensation** reaction. In order to avoid obtaining a complex mixture of products in a crossed aldol condensation, it is often the case that one of the carbonyl compounds is chosen such that it does not have any acidic α-protons, and therefore *cannot* act as the nucleophile (enolate ion); it *must* be the electrophile.

6.2

Kinetic vs. Thermodynamic Control of the Aldol Reaction

When asymmetric ketones with more than one set of α-protons are treated with base, two different enolates are possible. When these ketones are used to perform aldol reactions, different products are formed depending on which enolate is used. Regiochemical control of such a reaction can be achieved through the choice of base and the reaction conditions, as depicted below.

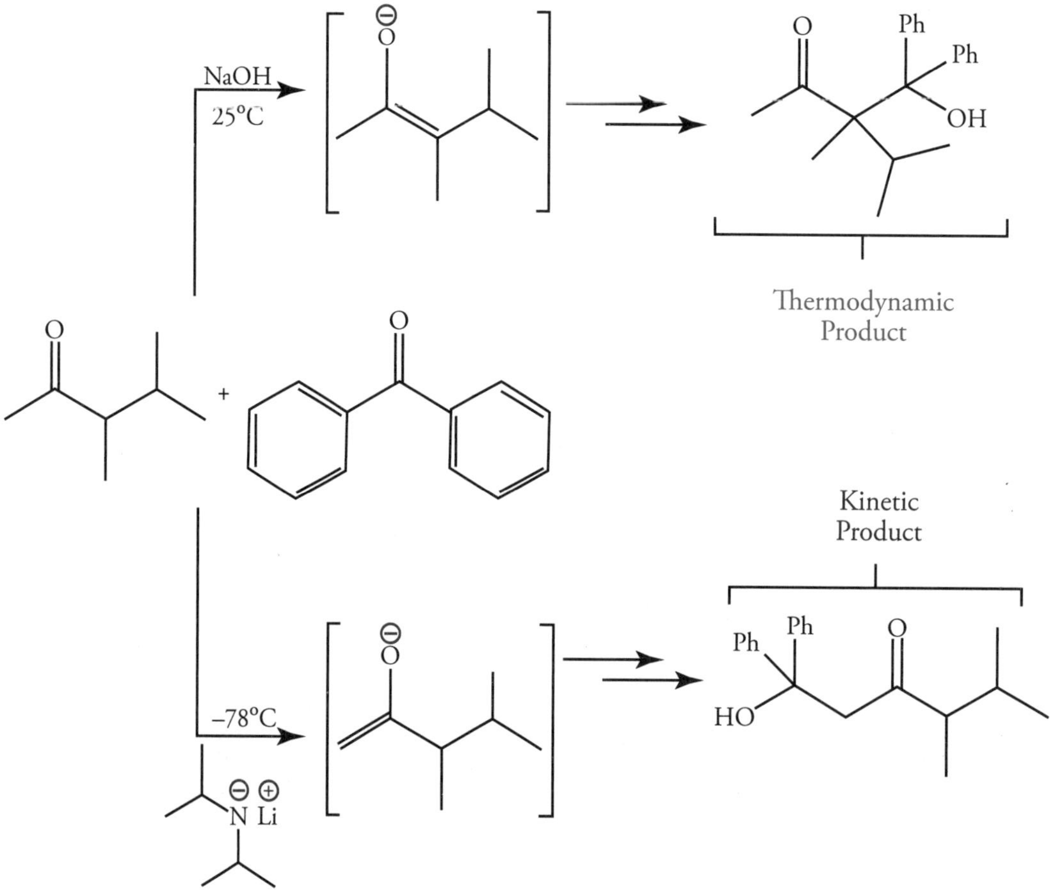

The upper pathway, run at room temperature with an unencumbered base, is said to be under *thermodynamic* control. In general, double bonds with more carbon-substituents (fewer vinyl-hydrogens) are more thermodynamically stable than less-substituted alkenes. In the absence of other constraints, the enolate formed by removing protons from the more sterically crowded α-carbon will be favored.

Formation of the less-substituted enolate (the lower pathway) may be achieved by denying the base access to the more sterically hindered α-carbon. Two ways to do this include using a bulky base that cannot fit into the area required to remove the sterically shielded proton (in this case, lithium diisopropyl amide, or LDA), or by doing the reaction at very low temperature. At a reduced temperature, there is not enough energy to overcome the activation barrier associated with the base approaching the more crowded α-carbon. Through use of these constraints, the base will deprotonate the less hindered, more kinetically accessible α-carbon. These reactions are said to be under **kinetic control**.

Retro-Aldol Reaction and Dehydration

Though stabilized by an intramolecular hydrogen bond between the hydroxyl and carbonyl groups, and hence generally thermodynamically stable at moderate temperatures and pH levels, β-hydroxy aldehydes and ketones are not immune to further transformations. When treated with strong bases, deprotonation of the free hydroxyl group may induce the reverse of the initial aldol condensation in a reaction known as a retro-aldol reaction. It is useful to note that the constitutive pieces of any β-hydroxy aldehyde or ketone synthesized via an aldol reaction may be determined by working through the mechanism of the retro-aldol.

If the β-hydroxyaldehyde or ketone products are heated, they will undergo an elimination reaction (dehydration) to form an α,β-**unsaturated carbonyl compound**. Notice that the newly formed carbon-carbon π bond is in conjugation with the carbonyl group; this stabilizes the molecule.

β-hydroxy carbonyl

α,β-unsaturated carbonyl compound
(some *Z* compound will also form)

Example 6-6: Predict the condensation products of each of the following reactions. Show both the β-hydroxy carbonyl product and the elimination product.

(a)

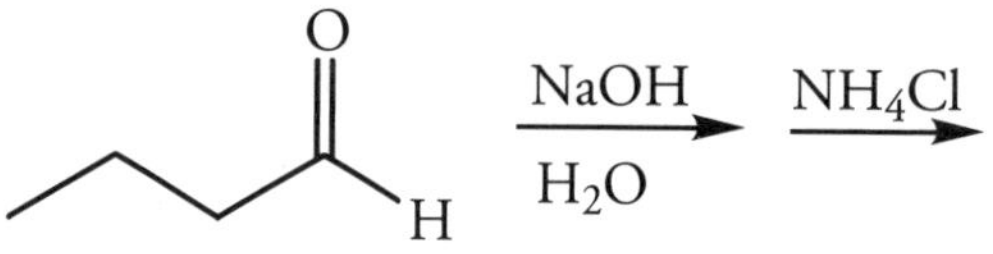

(b)

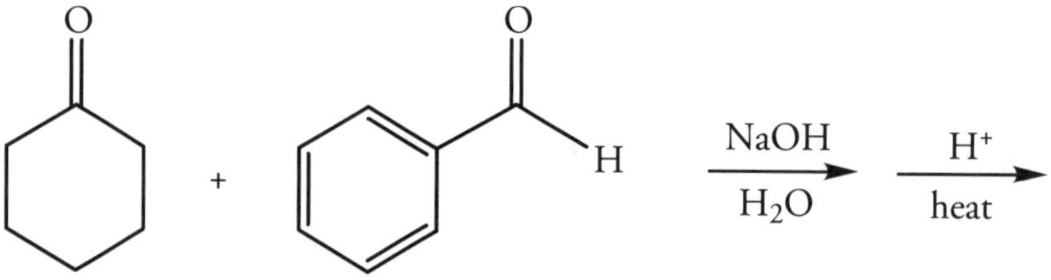

(c)

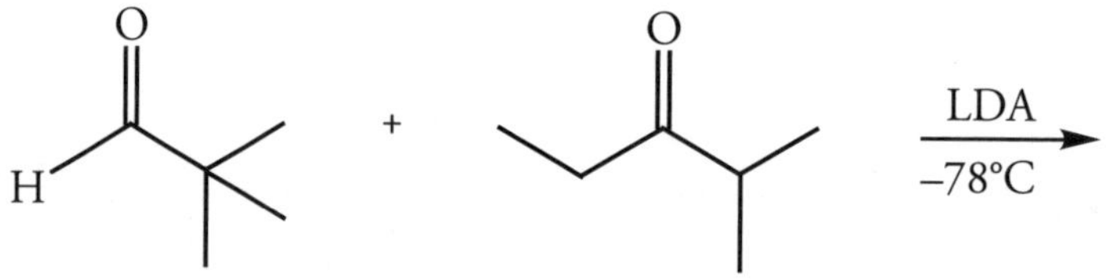

(d)

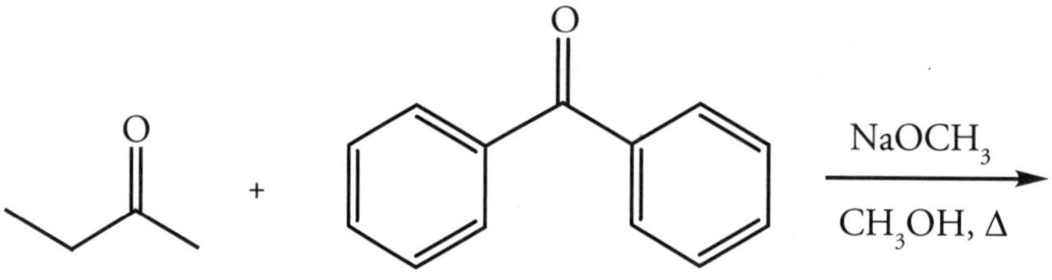

Solution:

(a)

(b)

(c)

(d)

6.3 CARBOXYLIC ACIDS

Carboxylic acids are of fundamental importance in many biological systems. Fatty acids, for example, are long chain carboxylic acids that play important roles in both cellular structure and metabolism (as we'll see in Section 7.4). In the following sections, we'll explore the basic physical properties and common chemical reactions of carboxylic acids and their derivatives.

Hydrogen Bonding

Carboxylic acids form strong hydrogen bonds because the carboxylate group contains both a hydrogen bond donor and a hydrogen bond acceptor. This can be seen in the intermolecular hydrogen bonding of acetic acid. Notice that the acidic proton is the hydrogen bond donor and a lone pair of electrons on the carbonyl oxygen is the hydrogen bond acceptor. For this reason, carboxylic acids can form stable hydrogen bonded dimers, giving them high melting and boiling points.

Reduction of Carboxylic Acids

Earlier in the chapter we discussed the use of boron and aluminum hydrides in the reduction of ketones and aldehydes to their respective alcohols. Carboxylic acids can similarly be reduced to primary alcohols, with one important difference: $LiAlH_4$ is effective, but $NaBH_4$ is not.

As aluminum is slightly more electropositive than boron, the Al—H bond is more highly polarized, more reductive, and ultimately capable of performing these more challenging reductions.

Decarboxylation Reactions of β-Keto Acids

Carboxylic acids that have carbonyl groups β to the carboxylate are unstable because they are subject to decarboxylation. The reaction proceeds through a cyclic transition state and results in the loss of carbon dioxide from the β-keto acid.

6.4 CARBOXYLIC ACID DERIVATIVES

Carboxylic acid derivatives include acid chlorides, acid anhydrides, esters, and amides. The general chemical structures for these acid derivatives are:

(eN = electronegative group)

As you might expect, the derivatives of carboxylic acids react similarly to aldehydes because they are also electrophilic at the carbonyl carbon atom. However, unlike reactions with aldehydes and ketones, nucleophilic additions to carboxylic acid derivatives are usually followed by elimination. (Note that additions and eliminations are opposites—while you can recognize an addition reaction because a π bond is broken and replaced by two new σ bonds, eliminations are the reverse. A new π bond is formed while two σ bonds break.) This is because the tetrahedral intermediate formed upon attack of the nucleophile on the carbonyl carbon has both a negatively charged oxygen atom (the former carbonyl oxygen) and a good leaving group (the eN-group of the carboxylic acid derivative). This elimination by the electrons on the oxygen atom regenerates the carbonyl, thereby displacing the leaving group (eN⁻). This is called a **nucleophilic addition-elimination reaction,** and is sometimes referred to as an acyl substitution.

| Acid derivative | Tetrahedral intermediate | New acid derivative |

Esterification Reactions

An **esterification reaction** occurs when a carboxylic acid reacts with an alcohol in the presence of a catalytic amount of acid.

Esterification

a carboxylic acid   an alcohol   an ester

The following mechanism shows that protonation of the carbonyl oxygen makes the carbonyl carbon more electrophilic, and nucleophilic attack by the oxygen of the alcohol results in a tetrahedral intermediate that is neutralized by deprotonation. An –OH group of the tetrahedral intermediate is then protonated, converting a poor leaving group (–OH) into a good one ($-OH_2^+$). As a result, a water molecule departs, leaving behind the protonated form of the ester. Deprotonation of the carbonyl oxygen yields the ester product and regenerates the acid catalyst.

The Acid-Catalyzed Mechanism

Acidic and Basic Hydrolysis of Esters

Let's now examine both the acidic and basic hydrolysis of the ester *methyl benzoate* to form the carboxylic acid and alcohol. First, we look at the acid-catalyzed reaction:

| methyl benzoate | benzoic acid | methanol |

In the first step of this reaction, the carbonyl oxygen is protonated. As before, the protonation of the carbonyl oxygen makes the carbon more electrophilic. Nucleophilic attack by a water molecule, followed by deprotonation, leads to the formation of a tetrahedral intermediate. *In any nucleophilic addition-elimination reaction of an acid derivative, there will always be a tetrahedral intermediate.*

Acid-Catalyzed Ester Hydrolysis Mechanism

tetrahedral intermediate

Next, the leaving group of the tetrahedral intermediate is protonated under the acidic reaction conditions. Notice that protonation of the hydroxyl oxygens can also occur. This leads to the reverse reaction. Protonation of the leaving group converts a poor leaving group (RO^-, an alkoxide ion) into a good one (ROH, a neutral alcohol molecule). The alcohol leaves and yields a protonated acid that only has to undergo a deprotonation to give the carboxylic acid product.

Acid-Catalyzed Mechanism, Continued

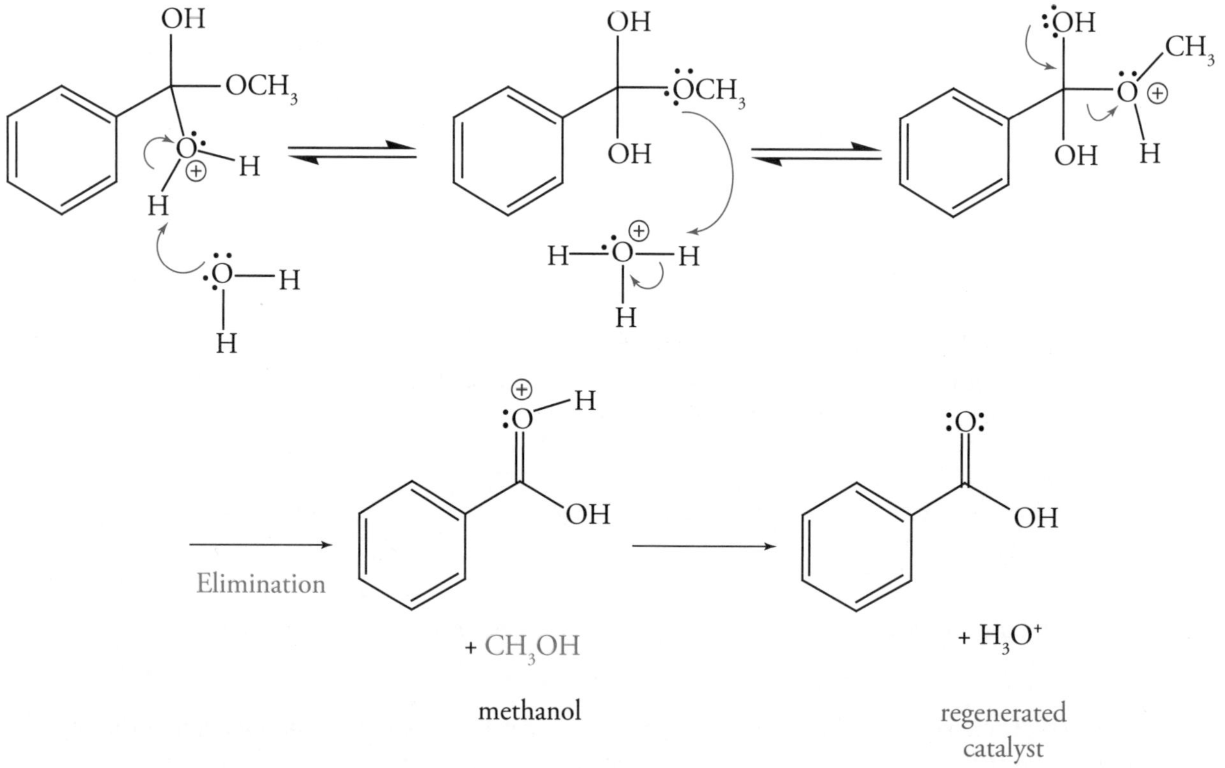

Elimination

+ CH_3OH

methanol

+ H_3O^+

regenerated catalyst

Transesterification

Not only can esters be hydrolyzed to carboxylic acids, but treatment of esters with alcohols, generally with acid catalysis, results in a process known as transesterification. Following an equivalent mechanism as shown above for hydrolysis, the nucleophilic attack by an alcohol on the electrophilic carbonyl-carbon of the ester results in the replacement of the original –OR (below depicted as EtO–) with the incoming alcohol (depicted below as isobutanol).

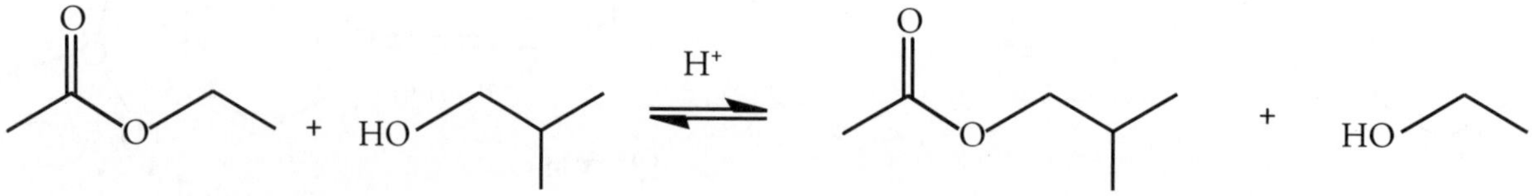

Like the esterification/hydrolysis reactions, the two esters exist in equilibrium, but there are a number of ways to favor the formation of the desired ester. One way is to employ conditions that remove by-products of the reaction from the solution. For example, since ethanol is more volatile than isobutanol, mildly heating the reaction on the previous page will drive ethanol into the vapor phase and push the reaction to the right via Le Châtelier's principle. Similarly, using a large excess of the alcohol constituting the desired –OR in the product serves to shift the equilibrium in the desired direction. Such conditions are indicated as in the equation below.

Placing isobutanol above or below the arrow denotes that it is used as the solvent, and is therefore in great excess. As a result, the equilibrium is essentially halted and the reaction is driven completely to the right. The reverse reaction is, of course, still possible if the isobutanol solvent is removed and replaced with ethanol.

Base-Mediated Ester Hydrolysis Mechanism

We now consider the corresponding *base*-mediated hydrolysis of methyl benzoate. In the first step of the reaction, the strongly nucleophilic hydroxide ion directly attacks the electrophilic carbonyl carbon. The nucleophilic attack results in the formation of a tetrahedral intermediate.

6.4

The tetrahedral intermediate then undergoes an elimination reaction, reforming the carbonyl when a pair of electrons on the negatively charged oxygen regenerates the carbon-oxygen π bond. This eliminates the alkoxide ion as a leaving group. However, since the reaction is carried out under basic conditions and the alkoxide ion is a strong enough base to deprotonate the newly formed carboxylic acid, the final step of the mechanism is the acid-base reaction shown on the previous page. In order to recover the carboxylic acid from this process, the reaction must have a final aqueous acidic workup.

In summary, these two reactions, the acid-catalyzed hydrolysis of an ester and the base-mediated hydrolysis of an ester, display the most common reactivities of all of the carboxylic acid derivatives. Both of these reactions give the same products, but by different mechanisms. Most importantly, both of the mechanisms proceed through nucleophilic addition and elimination steps. A good understanding of these two reaction mechanisms leads to a solid understanding of all of the reactions of carboxylic acids and their derivatives.

Saponification: An Example of a Base-Mediated Ester Hydrolysis Reaction

The hydrolysis of fats and glycerides is a chemical reaction that has been practiced for many centuries in the process of making soap. Typically, large vats of animal fat are treated with lye (NaOH or KOH) and stirred over a roaring fire. This bubbling cauldron liberates free fatty acids from the animal fat, which then can be utilized as soap.

Upon inspection, it is clear that this ancient method is simply the basic hydrolysis of a triacylglyceride to yield a molecule of glycerol and three fatty acids. This is the reaction mechanism we just reviewed.

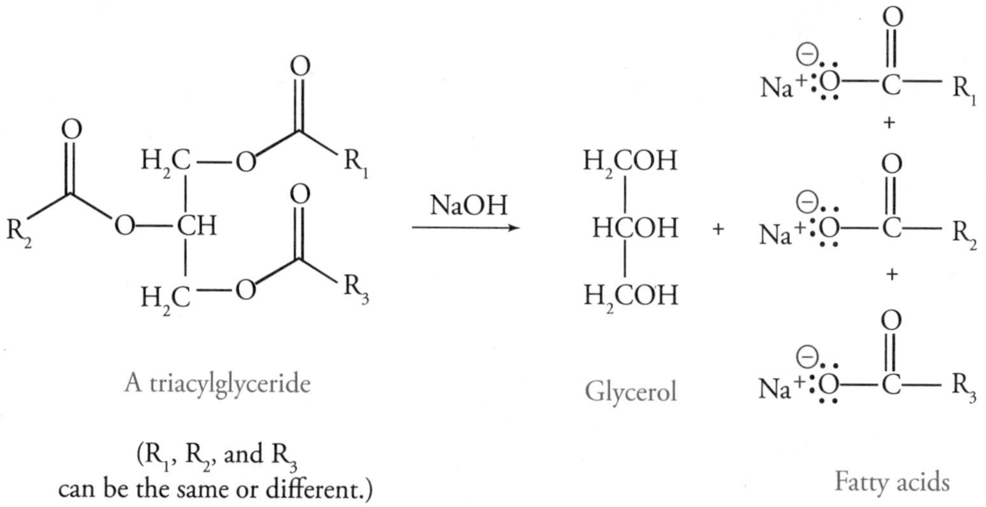

A triacylglyceride

Glycerol

Fatty acids

(R_1, R_2, and R_3 can be the same or different.)

The three electrophilic carbonyl carbons of the triacylglyceride sequentially undergo nucleophilic attack by hydroxide ions to produce an oxyanion tetrahedral intermediate. Then the tetrahedral intermediate eliminates the –OR portion of the ester as an alkoxide ion which is then protonated to form the alcohol. This happens three times to ultimately yield glycerol and three molecules of fatty acid.

Fatty acids are **amphipathic** molecules because they contain a negatively charged carboxylate group that is hydrophilic and a long hydrocarbon tail that's hydrophobic. As a result, these amphipathic fatty acid molecules form micelles in water in which the hydrophobic tails associate with one another to exclude water, while the charged carboxylate groups are localized on the exterior of the micelles. Greases and fats are adsorbed by the fatty portion of these micelles and the whole micelle is "washed" away by water. This is the physical basis of soap. We will discuss this further in Chapter 7.

Synthesis of the Carboxylic Acid Derivatives

Now that we understand how the electronic structure of the carboxylic acid derivatives relates to their reactivity, the synthesis of carboxylic acid derivatives should be straightforward. For the most part, we shall only be concerned with the interconversion of one derivative to another.

Acid Halides

Carboxylic acid halides are made from the corresponding carboxylic acid and either $SOCl_2$ or PX_3 (X = Cl, Br).

Acid Anhydrides

As their name implies, anhydrides (meaning "without water") can be prepared by the condensation of two carboxylic acids with the loss of water.

Acid anhydrides are also prepared from addition of the corresponding carboxylic acid (or carboxylate ion) to the corresponding acid halide.

Esters

Esters are most easily synthesized from the corresponding carboxylic acid and an alcohol, as we saw earlier. This reaction is referred to as **esterification**. Esters can also be prepared from an acid halide, an anhydride, or another ester and a corresponding alcohol.

Amides

Amides can be prepared from the corresponding acid halide, anhydride, or ester with the desired amine. They *cannot* be prepared from the carboxylic acid directly. This is because amines are very basic and carboxylic acids are very acidic; an acid-base reaction occurs much faster than the desired addition-elimination reaction.

Carboxylic acids can be prepared from *any* of the derivatives merely by heating the derivative in acidic aqueous solutions.

Relative Reactivity of Carboxylic Acid Derivatives

Now that we are familiar with the general reactivity of carboxylic acid derivatives, we will examine how chemical *structure* affects the *relative* chemical reactivity of common acid derivatives. The order of reactivity in nucleophilic addition-elimination reactions for acid derivatives is:

| Acid chlorides | Acid anhydrides | Esters | Amides |

If we examine the leaving groups of these acid derivatives, it is clear that the reactivity of acid derivatives in nucleophilic addition-elimination reactions decreases with increasing basicity of the leaving group.

Acid Derivative Reactivity

Acid Derivative	*Leaving Group*	

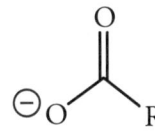

acid chloride

Chloride anion is a very good leaving group. It is a very weak base since it is the conjugate base of the strong acid HCl ($pK_a = -7$).

acid anhydride

This is a fairly good leaving group. It is the conjugate base of the weakly acidic carboxylic acid ($pK_a = 4$–5).

ester

An alkoxide ion is a rather poor leaving group. It is moderately basic since it is the conjugate base of alcohol, which is a fairly weak acid ($pK_a = 15$–19).

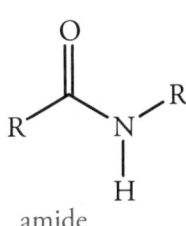

amide

This is a horrible leaving group. It is strongly basic since it is the conjugate base of an amine, which is a terrible acid ($pK_a = 35$–40).

While acid chlorides and anhydrides are readily hydrolyzed in water, esters and amides are much more stable. Esters require either acidic or basic conditions and elevated temperatures in order to effect hydrolysis, and amides are generally only hydrolyzed under acidic conditions, high temperatures, and long reaction times.

Chapter 6 Summary

- The C=O bond is very polarized due to the high electronegativity of oxygen, resulting in the carbon of the carbonyl group being electrophilic.

- Protons α to a carbonyl are acidic and can be removed by a strong base to yield a nucleophilic carbanion, or enolate.

- Keto-enol tautomerism is the rapid equilibration of the more stable keto form of a carbonyl and the less stable enol form where the α-proton shifts to the carbonyl oxygen.

- Nucleophilic additions involve the attack of a nucleophile on the carbon of an aldehyde or ketone; these reactions break one π bond to form two σ bonds.

- Hydride reduction, a type of nucleophilic addition, can convert ketones or aldehydes into alcohols; alcohols can be converted back to carbonyl compounds using oxidizing agents.

- An aldol condensation is a C—C bond forming reaction where the carbonyl carbon of one molecule is the electrophile, while the α-carbon of another carbonyl compound is the nucleophile.

- The formation of a specific enolate from an asymmetrical ketone can be controlled by carefully manipulating reaction conditions. The less substituted (kinetic) enolate is formed at low temperatures with bulky bases, while the more substituted (thermodynamic) enolate is formed at higher temperatures with small bases.

- The reactivity of carboxylic acid derivatives decreases as follows: acid halide > acid anhydride > ester > amide.

- Nucleophilic addition to the carbonyl carbon in a carboxylic acid derivative is usually followed by elimination due to the presence of a good electronegative leaving group.

CHAPTER 6 FREESTANDING PRACTICE QUESTIONS

1. Rank the protons from least acidic to most acidic.

A) $H^a < H^b = H^d < H^c$
B) $H^c < H^d < H^b < H^a$
C) $H^c < H^b = H^d < H^a$
D) $H^c < H^b < H^d < H^a$

2. Predict a possible product of the following reaction:

A) C)

B) D)

3. The enol and keto tautomers of 3-pentanone (shown below) are best described as:

A) resonance structures.
B) geometric isomers.
C) constitutional isomers.
D) diastereomers.

4. Which of the following carbonyl compounds cannot undergo a self aldol condensation?

A) 2,2,4,4-tetramethylpentan-3-one
B) 1,2,2-triphenylethanone
C) *3,3-dimethylbutan-2-one*
D) pentan-2-one

5. Which of the following would increase the rate of the reaction shown below?

I. Addition of acid
II. Addition of base
III. Increased concentration of EtOH

A) I only
B) I and II only
C) II and III only
D) I, II, and III

6. A reaction is performed at 20°C to form a mixture of two products, L (20%) and M (80%). When heated to 60°C and allowed to stand overnight, the composition of the mixture slowly changes to 80% L/20% M and does not change at longer reaction times. Which one of the following statements is most consistent with these observations?

A) An equilibrium mixture of L and M is formed at 60°C.
B) The activation energy for formation of L is lower than that for M.
C) M is more stable than L.
D) L is formed faster than M.

7. Which of the following reactions presents the fastest reaction?

A) C)

B) D)

CHAPTER 6 PRACTICE PASSAGE

The *Robinson annulation* reaction is a widely used, multistep process for generating cyclic α,β-unsaturated ketones. The first step (known as a *Michael reaction*) involves conjugate addition of an enol or enolate to an α,β-unsaturated carbonyl (Molecule 1). The reaction then proceeds with ring closure and loss of water (cyclodehydration) to give a cyclic α,β-unsaturated ketone (Molecule 8).

Scientists have found a way to catalyze the Robinson annulation by using artificial enzymes made from antibodies (Zhong, *et. al., J. Am. Chem. Soc.* 1997, *119*, 8131). As shown in Figure 1, these catalytic antibodies speed up the reaction by using a lysine side chain to form an imine with Molecule 3. The imine more readily undergoes tautomerization and cyclodehydration to give Molecule 7, which is easily hydrolyzed to Molecule 8. An important result is that Molecule 8 is produced as a single enantiomer.

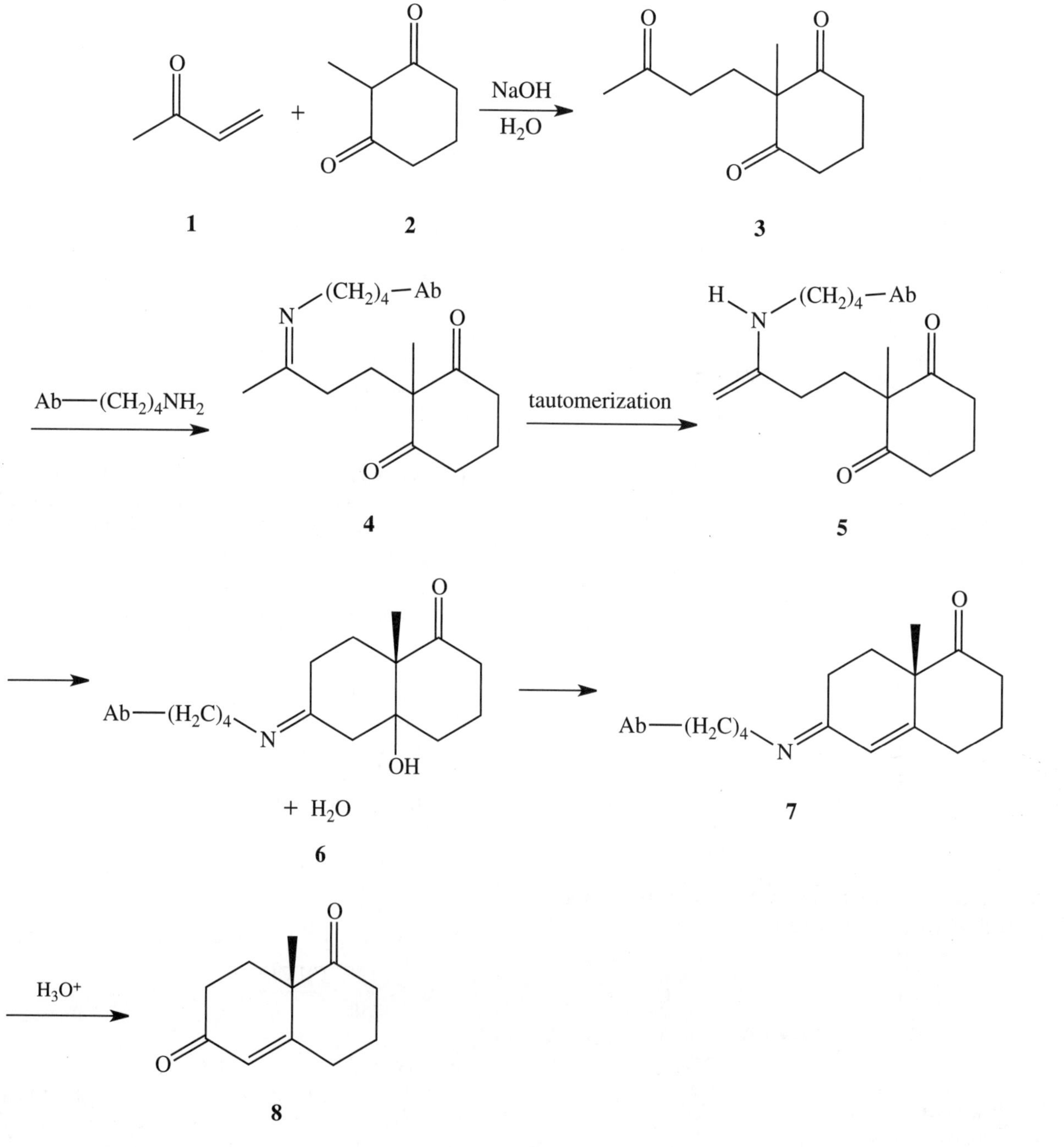

Figure 1 Enzymatic catalysis of Robinson annulation

1. In the first step shown in Figure 1, which of the following acts as the nucleophile?

A) Enol of Molecule 1
B) Enolate of Molecule 1
C) Enol of Molecule 2
D) Enolate of Molecule 2

2. The antibody described in the passage catalyzes an enantioselective Robinson annulation reaction. What is the stereochemistry of the single enantiomer that is produced?

A) (E)-(R)
B) (E)-(S)
C) (Z)-(R)
D) (Z)-(S)

3. The reaction of Molecule 3 with the lysine side chain of the catalytic antibody can best be described as what type of reaction?

A) Hydrolysis
B) Alkylation
C) Addition–elimination
D) Esterification

4. If the first step in Figure 1 was carried out in NaOD/D$_2$O, which of the following molecules would NOT be produced?

A)

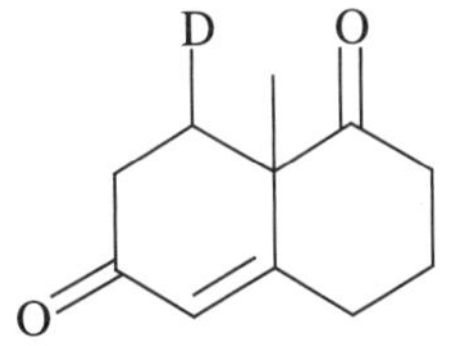

B)

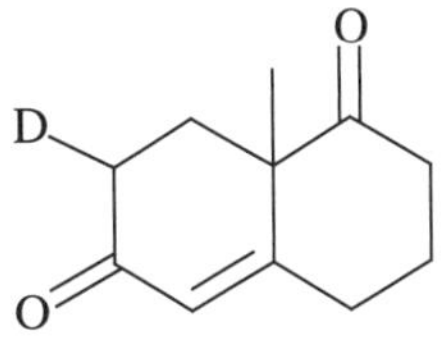

C)

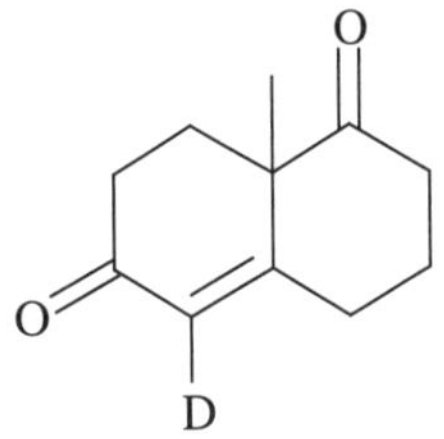

D)

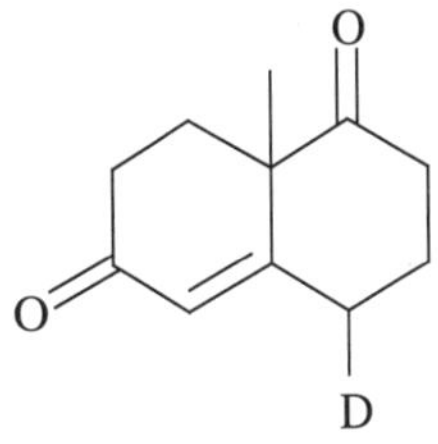

5. An aldol condensation between which two compounds could be used to generate Molecule 1?

A)

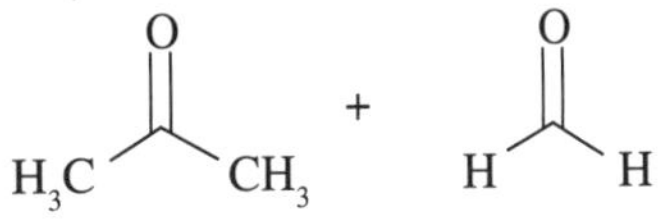

B)

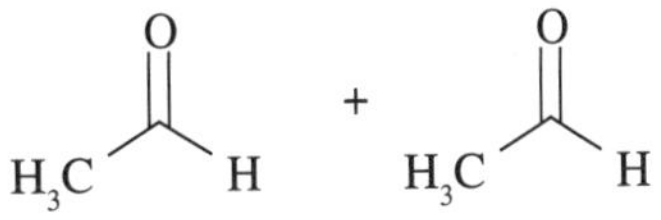

C)

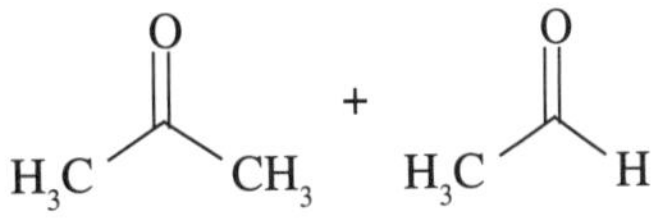

D)

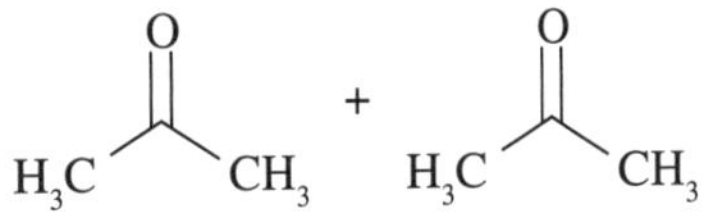

SOLUTIONS TO CHAPTER 6 FREESTANDING PRACTICE QUESTIONS

1. **C** Because H^a is bound to a carbon that is adjacent to two carbonyl groups, it is the easiest proton for a base to abstract since the conjugate base has the most resonance structures. Therefore, you can eliminate choice A. Because this molecule has a mirror plane, H^b and H^d are equivalent, so you can eliminate choices B and D, which leaves choice C as the correct choice. H^c is on a carbon that is not adjacent to any electron withdrawing groups or pi electrons, so it is the least acidic.

2. **B** This is an addition reaction involving a ketone and a Grignard reagent (RMgX). The R group in the Grignard reagent, in this case the phenyl, adds on to the carbonyl carbon, and the acid workup step is used to protonate the carbonyl oxygen into an alcohol. This gives the product shown in choice B. Choice A can be eliminated as ketones cannot undergo substitution reactions with Grignard reagents due to lack of an appropriate leaving group. Choices C and D can be eliminated since the halogen is not the nucleophilic atom in a Grignard reagent.

3. **C** Tautomers do not have the same connectivity of atoms; they are constitutional isomers which are in equilibrium with one another. Choices A, B, and D all have the same connectivity of atoms.

4. **A** A self aldol condensation occurs between two molecules of the same compound. In order for an aldol condensation to occur, at least one of the carbonyl compounds must be able to form an enolate through deprotonation of an α-carbon. Since 2,2,4,4-tetramethylpentan-3-one contains no α-hydrogens, it cannot form an enolate, and therefore cannot undergo a self-condensation reaction. All of the other molecules listed have at least one α-hydrogen, and therefore can undergo self-condensation reactions.

5. **A** Since this is a Roman numeral question, start by evaluating the item that appears in exactly two answer choices, in this case Item III. Item III is false: although hemiacetal formation occurs through nucleophilic addition (a bimolecular mechanism that involves both the carbonyl compound and the nucleophile, in this case, EtOH), the rate-limiting step of this reaction is the conversion of the hemiacetal to the acetal. This conversion requires formation of a high-energy carbocation intermediate. Therefore, the kinetics of the rate-limiting step are independent of the concentration of EtOH, and increasing its concentration would not increase the rate of the reaction (choices C and D can be eliminated). Since both remaining answer choices include Item I, it must be true and you can evaluate Item II. Item II is false: although hemiacetal formation is catalyzed by both acid and base, conversion of the hemiacetal to the acetal requires a catalytic amount of acid to protonate the hemiacetal OH group so it can leave as water. The presence of base would prevent this from occurring, and slow acetal formation (choice B can be eliminated and choice A is correct).

6. **A** The observation that the composition of the reaction mixture remains constant at 80% L/20% M when the reaction mixture is maintained at 60°C over a long period of time indicates that this product ratio represents the equilibrium product composition at that temperature (choice A), thereby demonstrating that L is more stable than M (eliminate choice C). The fact that M is the major product when the reaction is performed at 20°C

suggests that the activation energy for formation of M is lower than that for L (eliminate choice B) and, hence, that M is formed faster than L (eliminate choice D). Choice A is the correct answer.

7. **A** All choices present a range of carboxylic acid derivatives (acid halide, ester, amide) reacting with an alcohol. A faster reaction will be based on a more reactive carboxylic acid derivative, or one containing a better leaving group. Eliminate choices C and D which contain poor leaving groups ($^-$OR and $^-$NR$_2$, respectively). Between choices A and B, the best halide leaving group will be the larger one, Br$^-$, making choice A correct.

SOLUTIONS TO CHAPTER 6 PRACTICE PASSAGE

1. **D** As the passage states, the first step of the reaction involves the conjugate addition of an enol or enolate to an α,β-unsaturated carbonyl. Since Molecule 1 is the α,β-unsaturated carbonyl (the electrophile), Molecule 2 must act as the nucleophilic enol or enolate. Given the basic conditions, the enolate of Molecule 2 will be formed.

2. **D** The alkene product (Molecule 8) has both highest-priority groups on the same side of the double bond, giving it (Z) stereochemistry, so eliminate answer choices A and B. To assign (R) or (S) configuration to the single stereocenter, we must first assign priority to its substituents according to the Cahn-Ingold-Prelog Rules for assigning stereochemistry (see below).

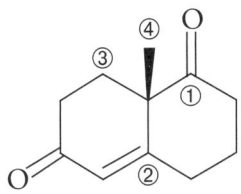

Now, looking down the bond from the stereocenter to the lowest-priority group (from below the plane of the page), the substituents progress from highest to lowest priority in a counterclockwise direction, giving this stereocenter the (S) configuration.

3. **C**   Formation of the imine from Molecule 3 begins with addition of the nucleophilic lysine nitrogen atom to the electrophilic carbonyl group. Water is then eliminated to complete formation of the imine.

4. **A**   In the presence of a base, enolates can be reversibly formed, resulting in deuterium labeling at the α-carbons in the first step of the reaction. Thus, the α-carbons labeled a (choice C), b (choice B), c, d (choice D), and e, shown below, may all be deuterated:

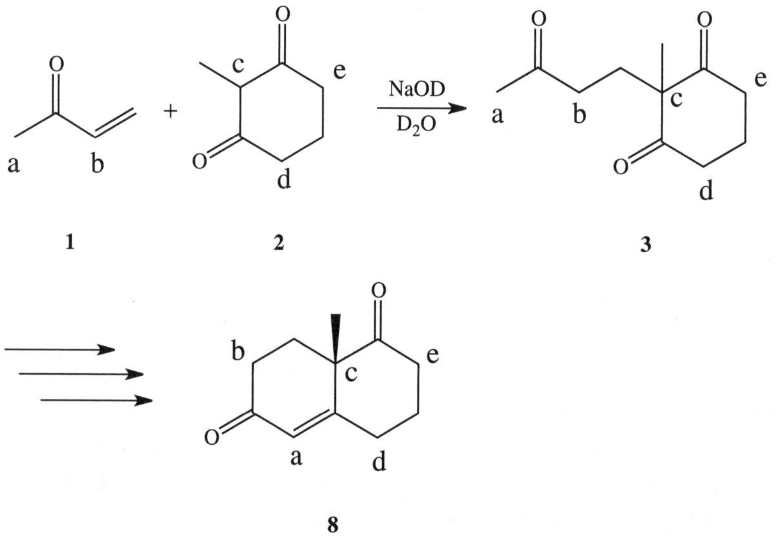

Since the position labeled in choice A is not an α-carbon and cannot be deprotonated, it will not be deuterated.

5. **A**   An aldol condensation between an enol and ketone or aldehyde yields an α,β-unsaturated carbonyl compound. The alkene marks the newly formed bond between the two molecules. Therefore, using retrosynthetic analysis of Molecule 1, we see that it may be formed from acetone and formaldehyde (choice A).

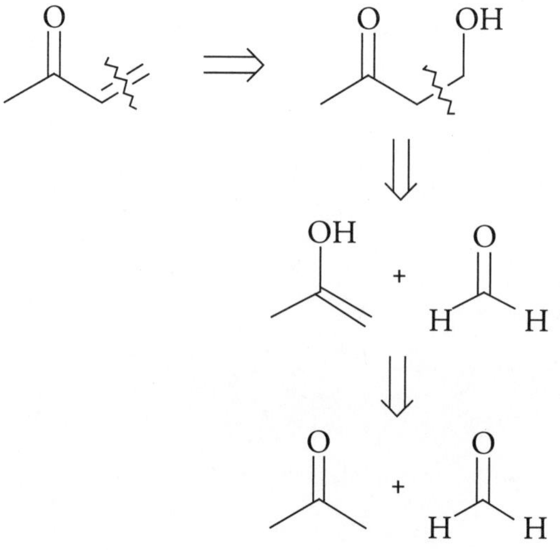

TETRAMETHYL ORTHOSILICATE (TMOS) AS A REAGENT FOR DIRECT AMIDATION OF CARBOXYLIC ACIDS

D. Christopher Braddock, Paul D. Lickiss, Ben C. Rowley, David Pugh, Teresa Purnomo, Gajan Santhakumar, and Steven J. Fussell

Methodologies that facilitate direct amidation of a carboxylic acid with an amine avoiding poor atom economy are of much current interest. Significant progress has been made with thermal amidations, boron based catalysts and reagents, oxophilic transition metal catalysts, and other systems. However, limitations remain, including multistep synthesis of catalysts, the use of nonstoichiometric acid-to-amine quantities, extended reflux with azeotropic removal of water in refluxing aromatic solvents, the need for chromatographic purification of the amide product, and/or the inability to mediate the more challenging amidation types. In the mid-2000s, a series of seminal papers by Mukaiyama describe the use of imidazoylsilanes, tetrakis(pyridine-2- yloxy) silane, and tetrakis(1,1,1,3,3,3-hexafluoro-2-propoxy)- silane as reagents for direct amidation reactions at room temperature in ethereal solvents. These silicon-based reagents perform excellently for all the major classes of acidamine combinations, but require prior synthesis from tetrachlorosilane, and with the exception of the latter silane, they do not afford pure amide upon workup: further purification is required to remove the ancillary ligand. In addition, other silicon-based reagents and silicas have also been found to be useful in amide synthesis. A recent perspective from industry on amidation technologies states, "The ideal reagent is inexpensive, widely available, nontoxic, safe, simple to handle, easy to purge from reaction mixtures, and contributes only minimally to waste streams." This desire for convenient and inexpensive reagents, coupled with the literature precedent for silicas as reagents for amidation, prompted us to investigate the widely available and inexpensive tetraalkyl orthosilicates [$Si(OR)_4$; R= Me (TMOS, **1**), Et (TEOS, **2**)] as potential direct amidation reagents.

We now report that TMOS **1** is an excellent reagent for effecting direct amidations, where preliminary comparisons with TEOS **2** showed the former to be more effective. Thus, at 200–250 mol % TMOS **1** loading in refluxing toluene, direct amidation of phenylacetic acid as a representative aliphatic acid with a primary amine, cyclic secondary amines, an acyclic secondary amine, and an aniline amidations of increasing difficulty gave amides **3–7** in excellent to quantitative yield (Figure 1, top). Notable features of this amidation protocol include the use of the ideal 1:1 stoichiometry of acid and amine, the toleration of nondried toluene, and *the isolation of the pure amide product directly after a simple workup procedure*. The workup procedure acts to destroy any excess TMOS **1** or any other residual silicon-containing components, by rapid basic hydrolysis in a homogeneous THF–aqueous potassium carbonate solution to produce silica, followed by addition of solid sodium chloride to effect phase separation. Any residual amidation components are also removed in the workup procedure allowing for the isolation of the amide product in pure form without the need for chromatography.

This protocol also successfully transfers to the inherently more difficult amidations of benzoic acid as a representative aromatic carboxylic acid with primary amines and cyclic secondary amines giving amides **8–10** (Figure 1, bottom) making this method highly competitive with other methods reported for these direct amidation classes. To effect the still more challenging amidations of benzoic acid with acyclic secondary amines and anilines to give amides **11** and **12**, higher reaction concentrations, an excess of carboxylic acid (for **12**), and the use of 4 Å MS sieves suspended in the reaction headspace were necessary. There is only limited literature precedent for high yielding reactions of the former and latter amidation reaction types, and to the best of our knowledge, no quantitative yields have been reported. The quantitative yield obtained for amide **12** is therefore notable. In all cases the amide products were obtained in pure form directly after workup.

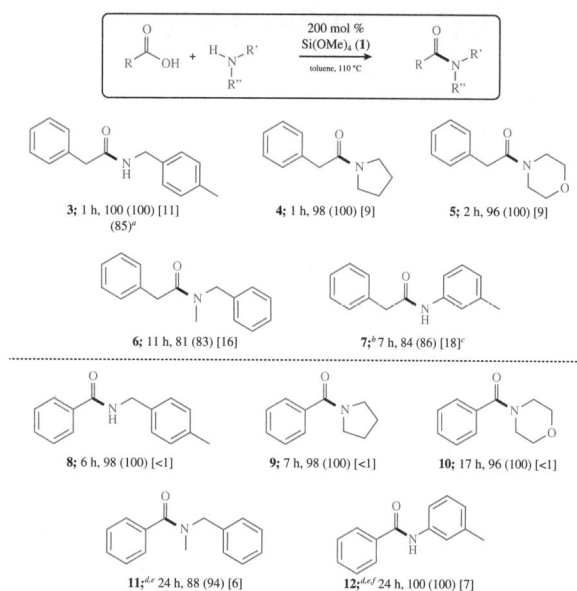

Figure 1. Direct amidations of phenylacetic acid (top) and benzoic acid (bottom) as representative aliphatic and aromatic carboxylic acids with [acid] = 0.2 M, [amine] = 0.2 M. Isolated percentage yields after workup are shown, where the value in parentheses is the percentage conversion. The value in square brackets is the percentage background conversion without added TMOS **1** under the stated conditions. All reactions were performed in triplicate; the variation in observed percentage conversions are ±1%. [a] 200 mol % TEOS **2**. [b] [acid] = 0.5 M, [aniline] = 0.5 M; 250 mol % TMOS. [c] Background conversion after 16 h. [d] 250 mol % TMOS, N₂; [acid] = 2.0 M, [amine] = 2.0 M. [e] With 4 Å MS suspended in the head space. [f] 2 equiv of BzOH (the conversion to amide **12** using 1.1 equiv of BzOH was 84%).

Figure 2. Direct amidations with TMOS **1** from the corresponding carboxylic acid (shown in blue postamidation) and amine/aniline (shown in red postamidation). Reaction conditions: toluene, reflux, N₂, 200 mol % TMOS **1**, [acid] = 0.2 M, [amine] = 0.2 M. [a] toluene, reflux, N₂, 250 mol % TMOS, N₂, [acid] = 4.0 M, [amine] = 2.0 M. [b] Toluene, reflux, N₂, 250 mol % TMOS, N₂, [acid] = 1.0 M, [amine] = 0.5 M. [c] Conversion.

Mechanistically, we consider that silyl esters are the likely *de facto* acylating agents in these direct amidation reactions by formation as per the equilibrium shown in Scheme 1. In accord with this hypothesis, silyl ester **13** was observed by ¹H, ¹³C, and ²⁹Si NMR as the only other species as a minor component when benzoic acid was heated with TMOS in toluene for 1 h. Furthermore, when aliquots were taken from a TMOS mediated direct amidation of benzoic acid with benzylamine (1 M in both components), the characteristic ¹H NMR resonances for silyl ester **13** (ca. 4%, 5 h) could also be observed.

Scheme 1. Silyl Esters as Postulated *de Facto* Intermediates

Further exemplification of the method using branched aliphatic carboxylic acids, and *ortho*-substituted benzoic acids as amidations of increased difficulty gave amides **14–18** in good to quantitative yields (Figure 2). The method was further utilized to obtain Moclobemide **19** (an antidepressant), nitrobenzenamide **20** (a viable precursor to the antiarrhythmic agent procainamide), and amides **21** and **22** containing basic heterocyclic rings from their corresponding acids and amines. These examples, and the amidation of the heteroaromatic indomethacin to give amide **23**, reveals the functional group tolerance of the method. Free hydroxyl groups are tolerated either in the acid or amine component as evidenced by amidation using lithocholic acid or ethanolamine to give amides **24** and **25**. In these reactions, the hydroxyl groups presumably undergo silylation, but the resulting silyl ethers are cleaved in the workup procedure. We were delighted to observe that a *N*-Cbz protected amino acid underwent direct amidation providing amide **26** without detectable racemization. In all cases, the amides were obtained pure directly after a suitable workup.

Having demonstrated that TMOS is an effective reagent for a range of direct amidations, we sought to exemplify the method on scale. Preliminary investigations on a 1 mol scale at 2 M concentration using benzoic acid and benzylamine as a representative acid–amine combination were unanticipatedly slow. Here, we conjectured that *on this scale* quantities of methanol may be deleteriously retained in the reaction mixture. Accordingly, a 1 mol scale reaction of benzoic acid with pyrrolidine (Scheme 2) with fractional distillation of methanol gave a 91% conversion to product after 12 h at reflux and, after suitable workup, gave pure amide 9 in 90% isolated yield (158 g), with a process mass intensity (PMI) of 43. A comparison of green chemistry metrics for amide-forming reactions has recently been reported: the PMI of this method compares favorably with representative conditions for those reported therein via acid chloride (PMI: 292) versus HATU (PMI: 178) versus boric acid catalysis (PMI: 89).

Scheme 2. 1 mol Scale Amidation To Give Amide 9

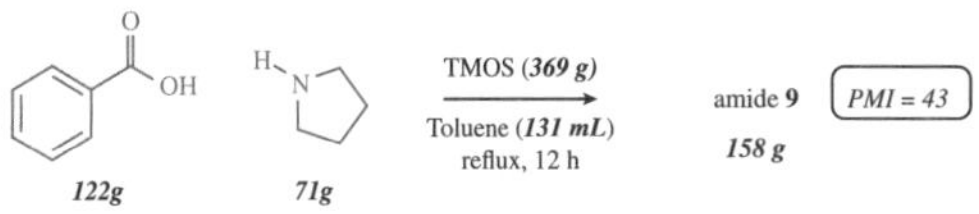

In conclusion, we have reported the use of TMOS **1** as a readily available and inexpensive commodity for the high yielding direct amidation of representative aliphatic and aromatic carboxylic acids with primary, cyclic, and acyclic secondary amines and anilines (i.e., increasingly difficult amidations) including the first quantitative direct amidation of an aromatic carboxylic acid with an aniline. The one-pot protocol, which does not require dried toluene nor necessitates preactivation of the carboxylic acid, is operationally simple, and the workup annihilating any excess reagent and other silicon species by its conversion to silica gel provides the pure amide products directly in excellent to quantitative yield without the need for chromatographic purification. A range of other biologically/medicinally relevant and/or challenging direct amidations are demonstrated. The method is amenable to scale-up with competitive process mass intensities compared to other procedures.

JOURNAL ARTICLE EXERCISE 2

Remember that the science sections on the MCAT include a significant number of passages with experiments. You'll need to be able to extract information efficiently and analyze data effectively in order to do well on these passages.

This is the second of three "Journal Article Exercises" in this book. In the first exercise, we showed you the type of information you should be able to extract from the article and the sorts of things to pay attention to. In this second journal review exercise, it's now your turn to extract information and respond to the same generalized questions you encountered before. You can compare your responses to the questions below to the correct responses at the end of the exercise to see how close you are.

As you read the article on pages 213–215, focus on the introduction to first get an understanding of the premise of the study, then investigate where results are given and what approaches are used to obtain the results as you get a deeper idea of the details. Lastly, read the conclusion for a final takeaway.

Write brief responses to the questions below:

1. What is the purpose of this study?

_____

_____

_____

2. What problem is this study trying to address or solve?

_____

_____

_____

3   What functional groups appear in the molecules being studied?

_____

_____

_____

4. Do any familiar reactions appear in this study?

_____

_____

_____

5. How are the results presented? Tables/graphs/figures?

_____

_____

_____

6. What approaches are presented in this study?

_____

_____

_____

7. What unique terms are provided in the experimental data?

_____

_____

_____

8. What results are found from the experimental data?

_____

_____

_____

9. Are there any unexpected/unexplained results?

_____

_____

_____

10. What final summary of the study and results can you conclude?

_____

_____

_____

Completed responses can be found on the following page.

SOLUTIONS TO JOURNAL ARTICLE EXERCISE 2

1. **What is the purpose of this study?**

   The study examines a method of direct conversion of carboxylic acids to amides (amidation). A series of reactions are reported with different aliphatic and aromatic carboxylic acids and a range of amines and aniline using tetramethylorthosilicate (TMOS) as a reagent.

2. **What problem is this study trying to address or solve?**

   The introduction to this study states that direct amidation of a carboxylic acid is problematic for a variety of reasons, including:

   - poor atom economy (low percentage of reactants that convert to products)
   - multistep synthesis of catalysts
   - disproportionate carboxylic acid-to-amine stoichiometries
   - extended reflux time in aromatic solvents while removing water from the reaction
   - the need for purification
   - the inability to perform more challenging amidation reactions

   To overcome these challenges, this study seeks to investigate tetraalkyl orthosilicates as convenient and inexpensive reagents for the potential direct amidation of carboxylic acids.

3. **What functional groups appear in the molecules being studied?**

   A range of carboxylic acids and amines are used in the numerous reactions investigated in this study to produce amides. A range of amines are used, including a primary amine, cyclic secondary amine, an acyclic secondary amine, and aniline. You should be familiar with the structure proposed by each amine name and aniline, which describes benzene substituted with an NH_2 group.

   Also note that silyl esters appear as intermediates in this study representing a variation on an ester structure, as shown in Scheme 1. You are not expected to recognize a silyl ester but you should note its similarity to a traditional ester and therefore expect it to react as an ester would.

4. **Do any familiar reactions appear in this study?**

   Carboxylic acids and derivatives (esters and amides, in particular) react by an addition-elimination reaction. You should note that direct amidation of carboxylic acids is not possible due to an acid-base reaction between a carboxylic acid and an amine so no addition-elimination reaction occurs under equimolar conditions. Normally this can be overcome by using an excess of amine, but this study seeks to provide a more efficient solution to this typical problem.

   The pathway for amidation this study proposes uses a silyl ester as an intermediate, shown in Scheme 1. The overall process this study accomplishes thus occurs in two steps:

   1. carboxylic acid + TMOS → silyl ester
   2. silyl ester + amine → amide

   To better understand what might occur in the first step, recognize that MeOH is identified as a leaving group in Scheme 1. This suggests the hydroxyl oxygen atom in a carboxylic acid acts as a nucleophile to attack Si in TMOS to displace MeOH in a substitution reaction.

   In the second step, an addition-elimination reaction occurs with the amine nitrogen acting as a nucleophile to attack the carbonyl C atom in the carboxylic acid. This results in the TMOS component being released as a leaving group.

The passage discusses in paragraph 1 how basic hydrolysis degrades the silicate components left over, including the leaving group and any unreacted TMOS reagent, leaving only the amide behind.

5. **How are the results presented? Tables/graphs/figures?**
The results are reported in figures. Notably, Figures 1, 2, and Scheme 2 provide results.

6. **What approaches are presented in this study?**
The boxed reaction given at the top of Figure 1 presents the scheme being followed in this study. The approach in Figure 1 includes:

- phenylacetic acid and benzoic acid plus a range of different amines as substrates
- equimolar amounts of substrate
- TMOS 1 reagent
- toluene as solvent
- refluxing conditions (heating)

Figure 2 presents the same approach as in Figure 1, but with variations in the carboxylic acid used to create challenging or biologically/medicinally relevant amides. In some cases a 2:1 ratio of acid to amine is used, as indicated by the Figure 2 description, but the remaining conditions are otherwise identical to those indicated in Figure 1.

Scheme 2 examines a "1 mol scale" approach to amidation using TMOS **1**. A "1 mol scale" means that the molecular weight of each substance is used in the reaction. For instance, the molecular weight of benzoic acid is 122 g/mol, therefore 122 g are reacted in a "1 mol scale" study.

7. **What unique terms are provided in the experimental data?**
As indicated in Figures 1 and 2, isolated percentage yields, percentage conversion, and background conversion are being measured for most of the products obtained. Isolated percentage yield is a measure of reaction success. It compares the amount of product obtained to the amount of product that was expected. Percentage conversion is the amount of starting materials converted to product. Background conversion is the amount of starting materials converted to product without TMOS 1.

In the discussion, PMI is identified as process mass intensity. This term reflects how "green" or efficient a method is by comparing the mass of all substances used against the mass of product obtained. In this way, a PMI value that is low is desirable.

8. **What results are found from the experimental data?**
Based on the details presented for the reaction being studied in Figure 1, there are two major results to note: isolated percentage yields and percentage conversion. Background conversion is also indicated as low for all reactions, which is to be expected. As higher values for the first two terms indicate an optimal reaction, a good starting question to ask is *which products reflect the most optimized reactions in Figure 1?*

Amides **3** and **12** do with 100% for both values. However, note that amides **3** and **12** employ different conditions than most other trials which makes them difficult to compare to the other results. Amide **3** is formed with TEOS **2**, a different reagent than all other reactions. Amide **12** is formed using an excess of BzOH (benzoic acid).

If we next examine the reactions that follow standard conditions, the reactions leading to amides **4**, **8**, and **9** stand out. These amides are formed from either phenylacetic acid or benzoic acid and a primary amine or pyrrolidine (a cyclic secondary amine) with TMOS **1**. These results suggest that amidation reactions with primary or cyclic secondary amines proceed more easily.

What can be said about the reactions that do not perform as well? Amides **6**, **7**, **11**, and **12** all have lower percentage yields and percentage conversions in the 80% range (amide **12** formed under standard conditions results in an 84% yield, as indicated in the Table 1 caption). All of these amides are formed from an acyclic secondary amine or aniline as the amine substrate, suggesting that these amines present a greater challenge to direct amidation.

Are these results consistent with the broader range of amidation reactions given in Figure 2? For the most part, yes. The best percentage yield values (which are the only percentages shown for most results) are associated with amines that provide primary amine or cyclic secondary amines as substrates, as in amides **14–16**, **19–21**, and **23–26**. Amides **17**, **18**, and **22** again stand out with lower percentages due to the use of acyclic secondary amines and aniline serving as amine substrates.

Scheme 2 is the last area that presents results from a 1 mol scale process that reacts benzoic acid with pyrrolidine and TMOS **1**. The results show a PMI of 43, which is a favorable value indicating an efficient reaction. Note that the amine substrate, pyrrolidine, is a cyclic secondary amine which previous results identified as a good choice for an optimized reaction.

9. **Are there any unexpected/unexplained results?**
Several results may be considered unexpected/unexplained, including:

The time taken to form certain amides (e.g., amide **18**) can be much longer than others. The study suggests branched substituted carboxylic acids and *ortho*-substituted benzoic acids are more challenging to work with without providing reasoning.

Amides **12** and **17** are both formed using benzoic acid and aniline compounds. They both employ a 2:1 ratio of acid to amine so why are the amide yields so different?

Amide **26** is reported to have formed without racemization but no reasoning for this observation is given.

For the reaction in Scheme 2, the study indicates that distillation was employed to remove methanol from the reaction. It is speculated that methanol accumulation caused the "unanticipatedly slow" 1 mol scale reaction with benzoic acid and benzylamine at 2 M concentration. Why wasn't distillation performed, as in Scheme 2, to overcome this problem?

10. **What final summary of the study and results can you conclude?**
The methodology proposed in this study shows that TMOS is an effective reagent for the high-yielding direct amidation of aliphatic and aromatic carboxylic acids with primary amines, cyclic, and acyclic secondary amines, and anilines. Amidation yields were reported to be lower using the latter two substrates. This method provides several distinct advantages, including a direct reaction, no need for excess reagents, no need for purification, and it provides excellent yield. A successful large-scale result was obtained with this method with good efficiency.

Chapter 7
Biologically Important Molecules

INTRODUCTION

As you begin reading and working through this chapter of the text, you will notice that it is a little different than the other chapters. Up to now, this book has presented you with lots of information, then offered you practice questions and passages to help you test yourself. But this book's real purpose is not to just stuff you with detail—it is to make you think. Thus, this chapter is written in a style intended to do just that.

This chapter offers you *grillage*; that is, it puts you "on the grill" by asking you questions on the material you're reading and studying. In other words, the approach is Socratic. The grillage takes the form of questions between paragraphs, but also rears its head as queries that interrupt the flow of text. Some of the questions test factual knowledge that has already been presented. Others ask you to speculate, based on new information. Others force you to integrate factual knowledge and speculation. The idea is to wake you up and remind you that you're not supposed to be memorizing, but rather thinking about the information flowing past your eyes, speculating about it, integrating it with what you know, what you'd like to know, and what you'd like to do with all that knowledge (help sick people).

It is crucial that you take advantage of the grillage. How? When the book asks you a question, you'll usually find the answer in a footnote on the same page. DON'T READ THE FOOTNOTE UNTIL YOU'VE ANSWERED THE QUESTION! Some of the answers are as simple as "C" or "No," and others are complex conceptual explanations. In any case, take the time to formulate a thorough answer before you go to the footnote. If you think you're too rushed to "waste" time doing this, we've got news for you: you are studying the wrong way. The real waste of time is doing nothing but memorizing details. The profitable time is spent pondering concepts, as you'll do on the day of the MCAT. Though you shouldn't read the footnotes too soon, do be sure to read them, as sometimes they contain important information or vocabulary not given in the main body of the text.

7.1   AMINO ACIDS

Proteins are biological macromolecules that act as enzymes, hormones, receptors, antibodies, and support structures inside and outside cells. Proteins are composed of twenty different amino acids linked together in polymers. The composition and sequence of amino acids in the polypeptide chain is what makes each protein unique and enables it to fulfill its special role in the cell. In this section of Chapter 7, we will start with amino acids, the building blocks of proteins, and work our way up to three-dimensional protein structure and function.

Amino Acid Structure and Nomenclature

Understanding the structure of amino acids is key to understanding both their chemistry and the chemistry of proteins. The generic formula for all twenty amino acids is shown below.

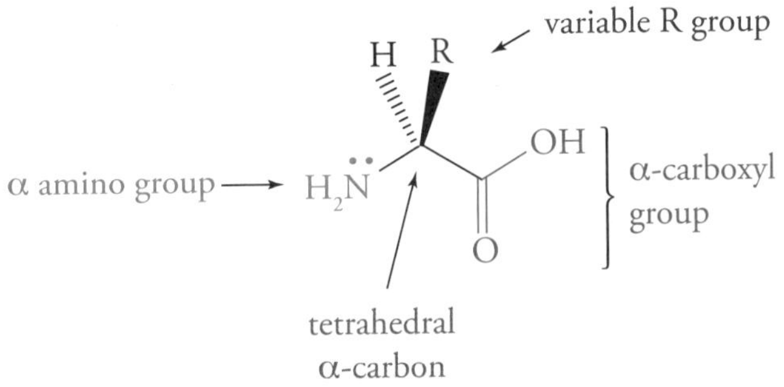

Generic Amino Acid Structure

All twenty amino acids share the same nitrogen-carbon-carbon backbone. The unique feature of each amino acid is its **side chain** (variable R group), which gives it the physical and chemical properties that distinguish it from the other nineteen. Note that the α-carbon of each of the twenty amino acids is a stereocenter (has four different groups), except in the case of glycine, whose α-carbon is bonded to two hydrogen atoms. This means that all of the amino acids are chiral except for glycine.

L- and D-Amino Acids

Chemists often draw chiral molecules in their **Fischer projection** to illustrate stereochemistry. Let's review how Fischer projections denote the absolute stereochemistry of molecules. The conformation of a molecule that is shown in a Fischer projection happens to be the least stable, fully eclipsed form of the molecule. In Fischer projections the most oxidized carbon is at the top, and the structure is extended vertically until the final carbon atom is reached. This leaves the substituents on each carbon atom to occupy the horizontal positions of each carbon atom in the chain. This is illustrated on the next page.

L-amino acid   D-amino acid

In the Fischer projection, it's understood that all horizontal lines are projecting from the plane of the page toward the viewer, and all vertical lines are projecting into the plane of the page, away from the viewer.

*All animal amino acids are of the **L** configuration, with the amino group drawn on the left in Fischer notation.* Some **D**-amino acids, with the amino group on the right, occur in a few specialized structures, such as bacterial cell walls. The L and D classification system can be a source of great confusion. For the MCAT, it is most important to remember that *all animal amino acids have the L configuration and that all naturally occurring carbohydrates have the D configuration.* (Carbohydrates are discussed in a later section of this chapter.) For completeness, though, we'll take the time to discuss the meaning of D and L now.

Assigning the Configuration to a Chiral Center

L- and D-amino acids and L- and D-carbohydrates are **enantiomeric stereoisomers**. The simplest (smallest) carbohydrate has only three carbons and only one chiral center. It is called **glyceraldehyde**. Since it has one chiral center, this molecule can exist in one of two enantiomeric forms, (+)-glyceraldehyde and (–)-glyceraldehyde. In reactions occurring in living organisms, CHOH groups are added to carbon #1 of glyceraldehyde to form larger carbohydrate molecules with more than one chiral center. In this synthetic process the configuration at the original glyceraldehyde chiral carbon (#2) is not changed. So, if you start with (–)-glyceraldehyde and build a longer carbohydrate chain, that carbohydrate chain will have a penultimate (second-to-last) carbon atom with the same configuration as (–)-glyceraldehyde. So why not just call the new, larger carbohydrate "(–)"? You cannot refer to the new carbohydrate as (–) because you have added several new chiral centers, and now if you put the new molecule in solution and measure its optical rotation with a polarimeter, the optical activity may in fact be (+). What is needed is a way to name a carbohydrate that would specify that it had been built up from (–)- or (+)-glyceraldehyde without worrying about its actual optical activity.

L-(–)-Glyceraldehyde   D-(+)-Glyceraldehyde

The solution is to nickname (–)-glyceraldehyde as "L-glyceraldehyde," and to likewise refer to (+)-glyceraldehyde as "D-glyceraldehyde." Now we can refer to all carbohydrates built up from (–)-glyceraldehyde as "L" carbohydrates, without specifying whether they rotate plane-polarized light to the left (–) or to the right (+). All we have to do is look at the last chiral carbon in the chain and decide whether it looks like C2 from L- or D-glyceraldehyde.

Once again, the important thing to remember is that *all animal amino acids are derived from L-glyceraldehyde* (because they share the same basic structure at the penultimate carbon). Hence, they all have the L configuration. *Animal carbohydrates are chemically derived from D-glyceraldehyde*, and are thus all D.

As we discussed in Chapter 4, there is another classification system, in which chiral centers are denoted either *R* or *S*. This system describes the *absolute configuration* of the chiral center; it refers to the actual three-dimensional arrangement of groups, as in a model or drawing; it says nothing about what the molecule will do to plane-polarized light.

In summary, you can see that three classification systems are used to organize amino acids and carbohydrates:

1. (+) and (–) describe optical activity, and mean the same thing as D and L, respectively;
2. *R* and *S* describe actual structure or absolute configuration; and
3. D and L tell us the basic precursor of a molecule (D- or L-glyceraldehyde).

You can also see that the three different classification systems don't describe each other in any way. A molecule that has the *R* configuration of its only stereocenter might rotate plane-polarized light *either* clockwise *or* counterclockwise, and hence be *either* (+) *or* (–). And a molecule that is experimentally determined to be (+) might be either D or L. However, two of the three classification systems go together for certain molecules. All D-sugars have the *R* configuration at the penultimate carbon atom because they are all derived from D-glyceraldehyde. Similarly, all L-sugars have the *S* configuration at the penultimate carbon atom. This is true only because carbohydrates are named according to the configuration of the last chiral center in the chain (which, remember, is synthetically derived from glyceraldehyde). By the same rationale, all L-amino acids are *S*, and all D-amino acids are *R*. (Note that the only exception is for cysteine, because the R group (CH_2SH) of this amino acid has a higher priority than the COOH group.)

1) You crash-land on Mars without any food but notice that Mars is loaded with edible-looking plants. Martian life has evolved with all L-carbohydrates. Can you metabolize carbohydrates from Mars?[1]

---

[1] No. Enzyme activity depends on three-dimensional shape, and all animal digestive enzymes have active sites specific for substrate carbohydrates with the D configuration.

Classification of Amino Acids

Each of the 20 amino acids is unique because of its side chain, but many of t   in their chemical properties. You should be familiar with the side chains, and it is impc   and the chemical properties that characterize them, such as their varying *shape, ability to   and ability to act as acids or bases (which determines their charge at physiological pH).*

As you study the 20 amino acids, do so by organizing them into four broad categ   . BASIC, NONPOLAR, and POLAR amino acids. Each amino acid has a three-letter abbr   ne-letter abbreviation, which are both important to know for the MCAT. This may seem l   to keep track of, but if you prioritize memorizing the codes of the acidic and basic amin   likely to be able to answer the vast majority of amino acid-related MCAT questions.

Acidic Amino Acids

Aspartic acid and glutamic acid are the only amino acids with carboxylic acid functional groups ($pK_a \approx$ 4) in their side chains, thereby making the side chains acidic. Thus, there are three functional groups in these amino acids that may act as acids—the two backbone groups and the R group. You may hear the terms aspart*ate* and glutam*ate*—these simply refer to the anionic (deprotonated) form of each molecule, which is how these amino acids are observed at physiological pH.

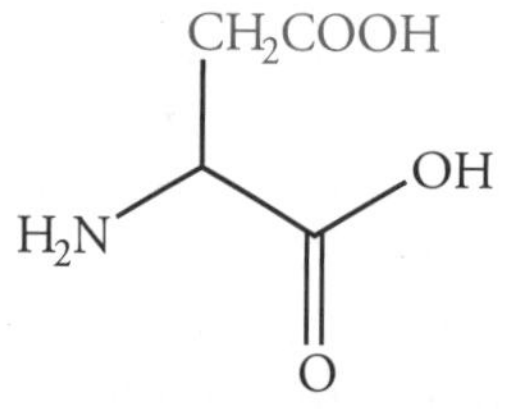

ASPARTIC ACID   D
Asp

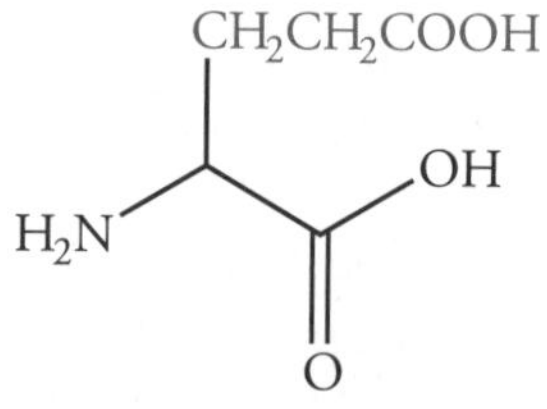

GLUTAMIC ACID   E
Glu

Basic Amino Acids

Lysine, arginine, and histidine have basic R group side chains. The pK_a values for the side chains in these amino acids are 10 for Lys, 12 for Arg, and 6.5 for His. Both Lys and Arg are cationic (protonated) at physiological pH, but histidine is unique in having a side chain with a pK_a close to physiological pH. At pH 7.4, histidine may be either protonated or deprotonated—we put it in the basic category, but it often acts as an acid, too. This makes it a readily available proton acceptor or donor, explaining its prevalence at protein active sites. A mnemonic is "His goes both ways." This contrasts with amino acids containing COOH or NH_2 side chains, which are *always* anionic ($RCOO^-$) or cationic (RNH_3^+) at physiological pH. [By the way, *histamine* is a small molecule that has to do with allergic responses, itching, inflammation, and other processes. (You've heard of antihistamine drugs.) It is not an amino acid; don't confuse it with *histidine*.]

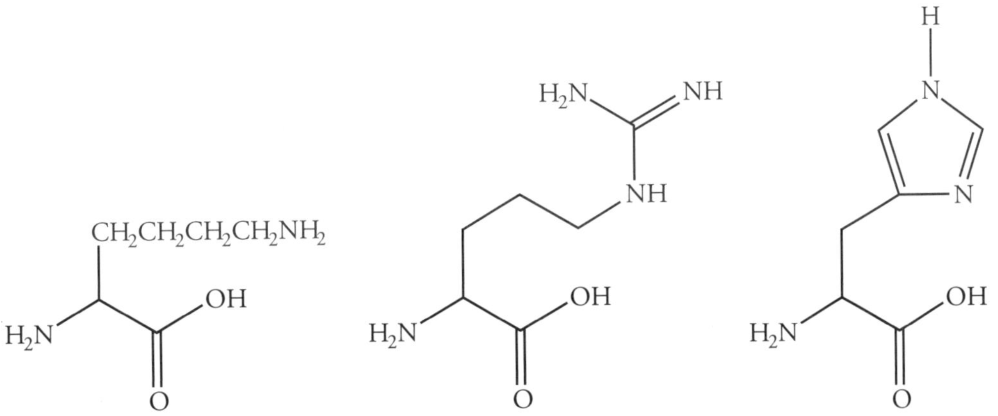

LYSINE
Lys
K

ARGININE
Arg
R

HISTIDINE
His
H

Hydrophobic (Nonpolar) Amino Acids

Hydrophobic amino acids have either aliphatic (alkyl) or aromatic side chains. Amino acids with aliphatic side chains include glycine, alanine, valine, leucine, and isoleucine. Amino acids with aromatic side chains include phenylalanine, tryptophan, and tyrosine (though the latter is a polar amino acid). Hydrophobic residues tend to associate with each other rather than with water, and therefore are found on the interior of folded globular proteins, away from water. The larger the hydrophobic group, the greater the hydrophobic force repelling it from water.

GLYCINE Gly G

ALANINE Ala A

VALINE Val V

LEUCINE Leu L

ISOLEUCINE Ile I

PHENYLALANINE Phe F

TRYPTOPHAN Trp W

Polar Amino Acids

These amino acids are characterized by an R group that is polar enough to form hydrogen bonds with water but which does not act as an acid or base. This means they are hydrophilic and will interact with water whenever possible. The hydroxyl groups of serine, threonine, and tyrosine residues are often modified by the attachment of a phosphate group by a regulatory enzyme called a kinase. The result is a change in structure due to the very hydrophilic phosphate group. This modification is an important means of regulating protein activity. This category also includes the amide derivatives of aspartic acid and glutamic acid, which are named asparagine and glutamine, respectively.

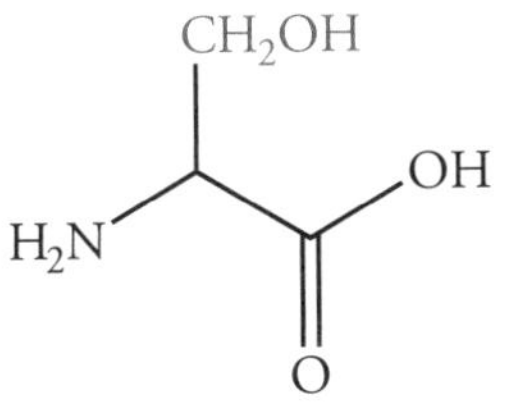

SERINE
Ser
S

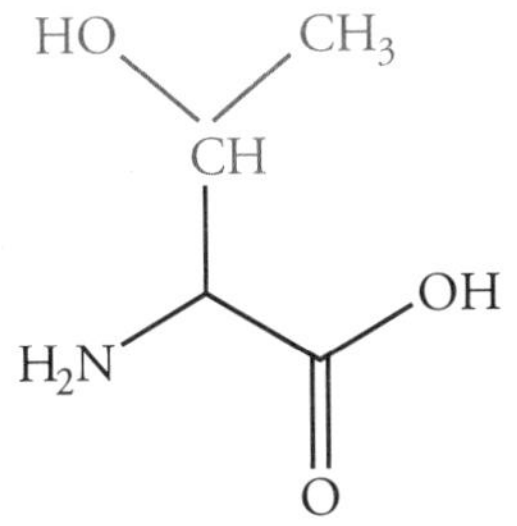

THREONINE
Thr
T

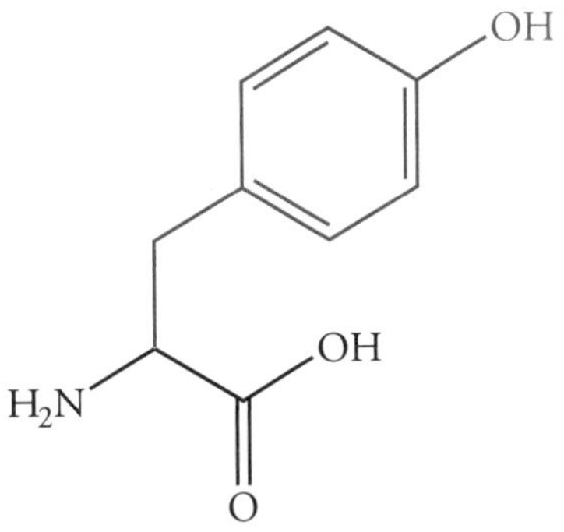

TYROSINE
Tyr
Y

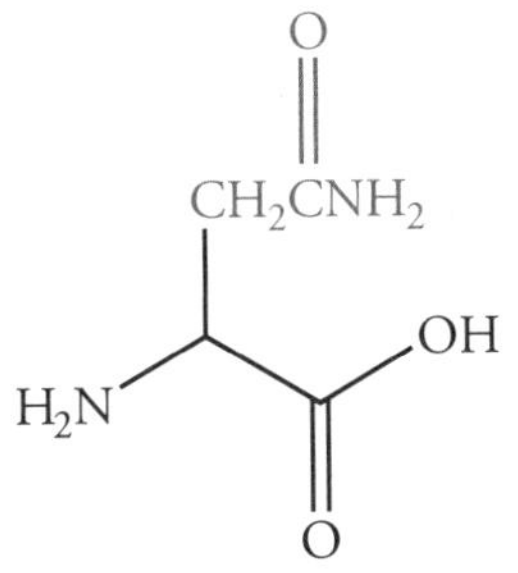

ASPARAGINE
Asn
N

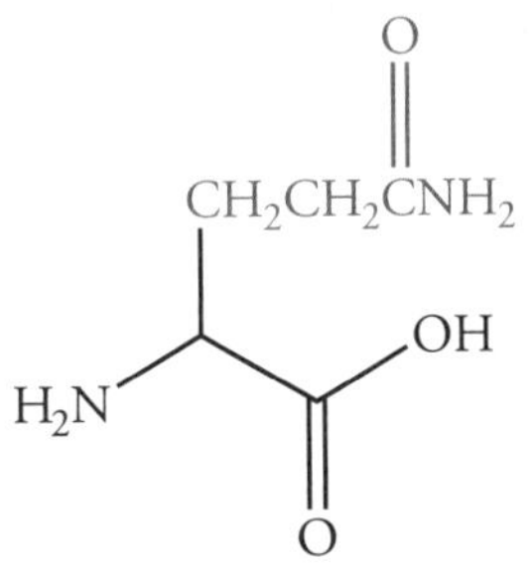

GLUTAMINE
Gln
Q

Sulfur-Containing Amino Acids

Amino acids with sulfur-containing side chains include cysteine and methionine. Cysteine, which contains a thiol (also called a sulfhydryl—like an alcohol that has an S atom instead of an O atom), is fairly polar, and methionine, which contains a thioether (like an ether that has an S atom instead of an O atom) is fairly nonpolar.

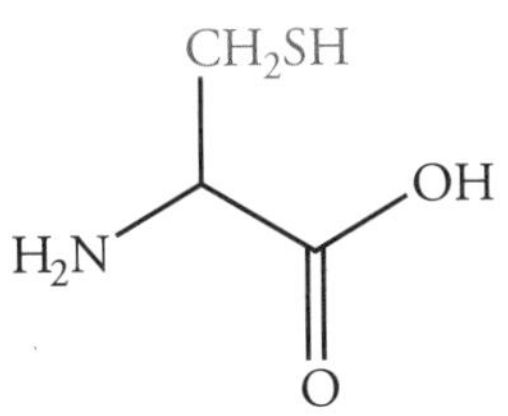

CYSTEINE
Cys
C

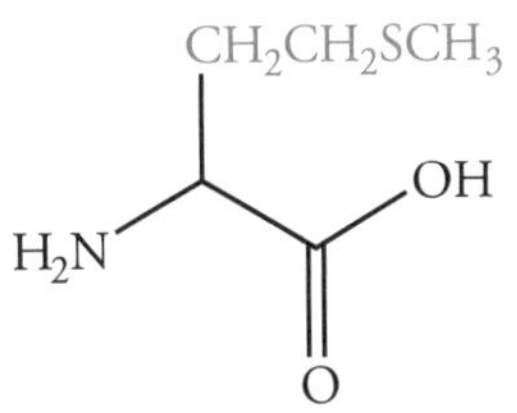

METHIONINE
Met
M

Proline

Proline is unique among the amino acids in that its amino group is covalently bound to its nonpolar side chain, creating a secondary α-amino group and a distinctive ring structure. This unique feature of proline has important consequences for protein folding (see Section 7.2).

PROLINE
Pro

Hydrophilic			Hydrophobic
ACIDIC	BASIC	POLAR	NONPOLAR
Aspartic acid Glutamic acid	Lysine* Arginine Histidine*	Serine Cysteine Tyrosine Threonine* Asparagine Glutamine	Glycine Alanine Valine* Leucine* Isoleucine* Phenylalanine* Tryptophan* Methionine* Proline

*Denotes one of the **nine essential** amino acids, those that cannot be synthesized by adult humans and must be obtained from the diet.

Summary Table of Amino Acids

Synthesis of Amino Acids

Nature has developed complicated mechanisms for the syntheses of the amino acids it uses to build proteins. In the laboratory, synthetic chemists have developed their own set of tools with which to make these essential building blocks available. Two important synthetic methods for the production of amino acids are the Strecker and Gabriel syntheses.

Strecker Synthesis

The Strecker synthesis utilizes ammonium and cyanide salts to transform aldehydes into α-amino acids. While naturally occurring amino acids are stereochemically pure (L-enantiomers), those produced via this process are racemic. Despite this drawback, a variety of both naturally occurring and non-natural amino acids may be easily synthesized, depending on the substitution of the aldehyde. An example of the Strecker synthesis applied to the production of (D,L)-valine is shown on the next page:

2-methylpropanal   (D,L)-valine

The combination of an ammonium halide and alkali cyanide results in the formation of alkali halide salts and the *in situ* production of the active species, NH_3 and HCN. In the first step of the reaction, the aldehyde reacts with ammonia to yield an imine as described previously in Section 6.2.

When protonated by HCN, the imine becomes more electrophilic, enabling attack by the remaining cyanide ion on the imine-carbon and concomitant formation of an α-amino nitrile. This attack by cyanide on an unsaturated carbon electrophile resembles the mechanism previously described for the formation of cyanohydrins. The difference is that the Strecker synthesis utilizes an imine (rather than a carbonyl) as substrate for the attack.

imine   α-amino nitrile

In a subsequent step, acid catalyzed hydrolysis of the α-amino nitrile gives the α-amino acid.

α-amino nitrile   α-amino acid

Gabriel-Malonic Ester Synthesis

The Gabriel-malonic ester synthesis is another useful method for the production of α-amino acids. Over the course of the reaction, the nitrogen in a molecule of phthalimide is converted into a primary amine. To begin, phthalimide is deprotonated with potassium hydroxide (KOH) to give the resonance-stabilized phthalimide anion, as shown below:

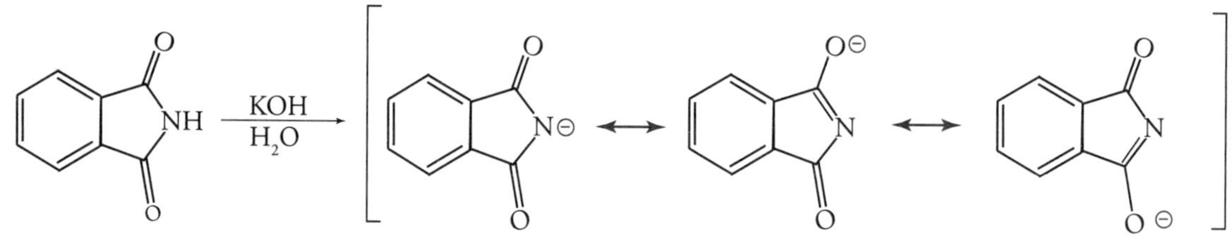

phthalimide   resonance-stabilized phthalimide anion

The phthalimide anion is a strong nucleophile, and when treated with α-bromomalonic ester, it displaces bromide from the central carbon, yielding an N-phthalimidomalonic ester.

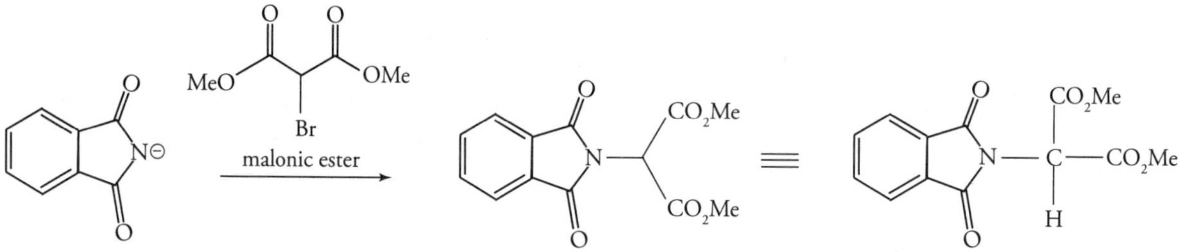

N-phthalimidomalonic ester

Enolization of the α-carbon with a strong base creates a nucleophilic carbon, which can be functionalized with the desired amino acid side chain. The example below shows the reaction of the enolate with methyl-(2-bromoethyl)-sulfide to give a precursor of methionine. The phthalimido group and both esters are then subjected to acid hydrolysis, and after heat-induced decarboxylation, the racemic amino acid may be isolated.

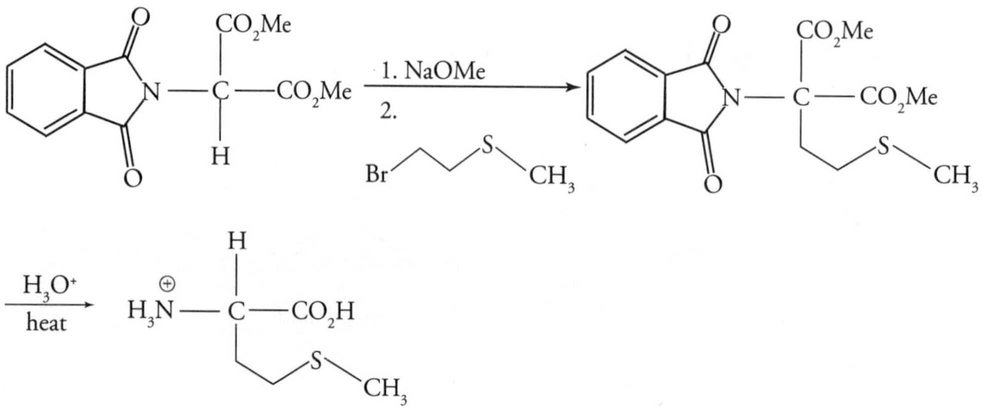

racemic methionine

Amino Acid Reactivity

Since amino acids are composed of an acidic group (the carboxylic acid) and a basic group (the amine), we must be sure to understand the acid/base chemistry of amino acids. Later, we will review amide bond formation by examining formation of the peptide bond in protein synthesis.

Reviewing the Fundamentals of Acid/Base Chemistry

Before we can discuss amino acids, we must be sure to understand the fundamentals of acid/base chemistry because each amino acid is **amphoteric**, which means it has both acidic and basic activity. This should make sense since an amino acid contains the acidic carboxylic acid group and the basic amino group.

Remember from general chemistry that acids can be defined as proton (H^+) donors, and bases can be defined as proton acceptors. Thus, in the case of the equation below, H_2A^+ is a proton donor (acid), and A^- is a proton acceptor (base); HA may act as either acid or base. The equations below also show how to calculate the equilibrium constant (K) for an acid dissociation reaction. The equilibrium constant for an acid dissociation reaction is given a special name: **acid dissociation constant**, abbreviated "K_a." The equilibrium reactions for the first and second proton dissociation reactions are described by the equations for the acid dissociation constants K_{a1} and K_{a2}.

$$H_2A^+ \underset{}{\overset{(K_{a1})}{\rightleftharpoons}} HA + H^+ \underset{}{\overset{(K_{a2})}{\rightleftharpoons}} A^- + 2H^+$$

$$K_a = \frac{[\text{products}]}{[\text{reactants}]} \implies \boxed{K_{a1} = \frac{[HA]\,[H^+]}{[H_2A^+]}} \quad \boxed{K_{a2} = \frac{[A^-]\,[H^+]}{[HA]}}$$

The Acid Dissociation Reaction

2) In the equilibrium between H_2A^+, HA, and A^- above, which statement is true?[2]
   A. HA will act as a base by donating a proton.
   B. HA will act as an acid by accepting a proton.
   C. HA can act as either an acid or a base, depending on whether it accepts or donates a proton.
   D. HA is in chemical equilibrium with H_2A^+ and A^- and in that capacity cannot act as either an acid or a base.

Whether a molecule (or a functional group) is protonated depends on its affinity for protons and the concentration of protons in solution that are available to it. Let's discuss both and do a few practice problems.

The concentration of available protons is simply $[H^+]$ (moles/liter), but it is usually expressed as **pH**, defined as $-\log [H^+]$. If you're wondering why pH is used instead of $[H^+]$, it has to do with the fact that $[H^+]$ values tend to be clumsy numbers, so a logarithmic scale reduces the amount of writing we have to do; we use the *negative* logarithm simply to avoid writing an extra minus sign. For example, instead of writing "$[H^+] = 10^{-3.46}$," we can write "pH = 3.46." The pH inside cells is 7.4. This is often referred to as **physiological pH**, and is carefully regulated by buffers in the blood because extremes of pH disrupt protein structure.

---

[2] Choice **C** is correct: In the equilibrium shown, HA can either act as an acid by donating a proton (choice B is wrong) or as a base by accepting a proton (choice A is wrong). Remember also that equilibrium is not a fixed state; in other words, HA is not doomed to stay HA forever, it can move forward and back between the states shown (choice D is wrong).

The affinity of a functional group (such as an amino or carboxyl group) for protons is given by the acid dissociation constant K_a for that functional group, which is simply the equilibrium constant for the dissociation of the acid form (HA) into a proton (H^+) plus the conjugate base (A^-). The equilibrium constant describes a reaction's tendency to move right or left as it moves toward equilibrium from some starting point. This affinity can also be expressed as pK_a, defined as $-\log K_a$. Carboxyl groups of amino acids generally have a pK_a of about 2 (stronger acid), while the ammonium groups generally have a pK_a of 9 or 10 (weaker acid).

The mathematical formula that describes the relationship between pH, pK_a, and the position of equilibrium in an acid-base reaction is known as the **Henderson–Hasselbalch** equation:

$$pH = pK_a + \log \frac{[A^-]}{[HA]} = pK_a + \log \frac{[\text{base form}]}{[\text{acid form}]}$$

Given the pH and the pK_a, we can calculate the ratio of the base and acid forms of a compound at equilibrium. Just remember these rules:

- Low pH means high $[H^+]$.
- Lower pK_a (same as higher K_a) describes a stronger acid that can donate a proton even when there are already excess protons (high $[H^+]$, low pH).

3) The text above states that physiological pH is 7.4. Is this more or less acidic—and are there more or fewer extra protons—than in pure water?[3]
4) Pure water at 25°C has a balance of 10^{-7} M H^+ and 10^{-7} M OH^- resulting from the spontaneous breakdown of water itself. What pH does pure water have?[4]
5) What is the pH of a solution of 0.1 M HCl (assuming the HCl dissociates fully)?[5]
6) Acetic acid (CH_3COOH) has pK_a = 4.7. Calculate the equilibrium ratio of $[CH_3COO^-]$ to $[CH_3COOH]$ at pH 4.7.[6]
7) Which functional group of amino acids has a stronger tendency to donate protons: carboxyl groups (pK_a = 2.0) or ammonium groups (pK_a = 9)? Which group will donate protons at the lowest pH?[7]

---

[3] Remember that a larger pH implies *fewer* extra protons, since pH = $-\log[H^+]$. A pH of 7.4 describes a solution with slightly fewer extra free protons, i.e., a slightly less acidic (more basic) solution, relative to a pH 7.0 solution.

[4] Simply use the formula for pH. Pure water has a pH of $-\log(10^{-7})$ = 7.

[5] The solution will have a proton concentration equal to 0.1 or 10^{-1} M. The pH of a solution with $[H^+]$ = 10^{-1} M is determined by the formula for pH: pH = $-\log(10^{-1}$ $M)$ = 1.

[6] First, substitute into the equation: 4.7 = 4.7 + log $[CH_3COO^-]/[CH_3COOH]$. Then, solve:
0 = log $[CH_3COO^-]/[CH_3COOH]$.
What has a log of 0? In other words, 10 to the power of 0 is equal to what?
10^0 = $[CH_3COO^-]/[CH_3COOH]$ = 1.0
So when the pH = pK_a, the ratio of base to acid is 1 to 1. That's a fact worth memorizing.

[7] A higher pK_a means that a higher proportion of the protonated form is present relative to the unprotonated form, according to the H-H equation. High pK_a indicates a weak acid. Acids with low pK_as, tend to deprotonate more easily. Therefore, ammonium groups have a stronger tendency to keep their protons and carboxyl groups will donate protons at the lowest pH (highest $[H^+]$).

Application of Fundamental Acid/Base Chemistry to Amino Acids

With that review of acids and bases, we are now prepared to discuss amino acid reactivity. The review is important because all amino acids contain an amino group that acts as a base and a carboxyl group ($pK_a \approx 2$) that acts as an acid. In its protonated, or acidic form, the amine is called an **ammonium group**, and has a pK_a between 9–10. For example:

$$-NH_3^+ \rightleftharpoons -NH_2 + H^+ \qquad pK_a \approx 9$$

$$-COOH \rightleftharpoons -COO^- + H^+ \qquad pK_a \approx 2$$

8) Assuming a pK_a of 2, will a carboxylate group be protonated or deprotonated at pH 1.0?[8]
9) Will the amino group be protonated or deprotonated at pH 1.0?[9]
10) Glycine is the simplest amino acid, with only hydrogen as its R group. Its only functional groups are the backbone groups discussed above (amino and carboxyl). What will be the net charge on a glycine molecule at pH 12?[10]
11) At pH 6.0, between the pK_as of the ammonium and carboxyl groups, what will be the net charge on a molecule of glycine?[11]

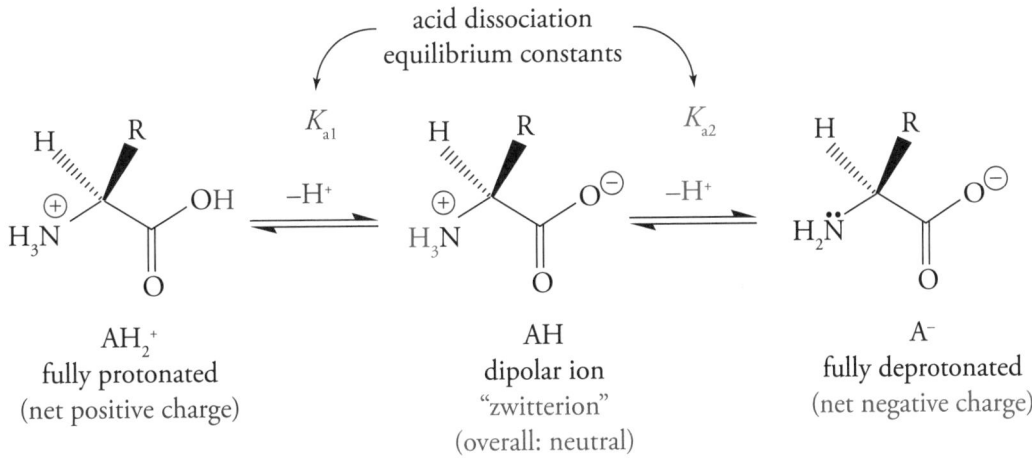

Important Amino Acid Conjugate Acid/Base Pairs

The Isoelectric Point of Amino Acids

There is a pH for every amino acid at which it has no overall net charge (the positive and negative charges cancel). A molecule with positive and negative charges that balance is referred to as a dipolar ion or **zwitterion**. The pH at which a molecule is uncharged (zwitterionic) is referred to as its **isoelectric point** (pI). "Zwitter" is German for "hybrid," implying that an amino acid at its pI has both (+) and (–) charges.

---

[8] The pH is less than the pK_a here, so protonation wins over dissociation, and the group will be protonated. The correct answer is –COOH.

[9] The pH is much lower than the pK_a for the ammonium group, so the amino group is protonated: NH_3^+.

[10] Since pH 12 represents a very low [H^+], both groups will become deprotonated (COO^- and NH_2), creating a net charge of –1 per glycine molecule.

[11] The carboxyl group will be deprotonated (COO^-) with a charge of –1 and the amino group will be protonated (NH_3^+) with a charge of +1, creating a net charge of 0 per glycine molecule.

It is possible to calculate the pI of an amino acid—in other words, to figure out the pH value at which (+) and (–) charges balance (that's the definition of pI). For a molecule with two functional groups, such as glycine, the calculation is simple: just *average the pK$_a$s of the two functional groups*. The pI of an amino acid with three functional groups can be calculated by averaging the two numerically closer pK^a values of the three. Another important thing to know for the MCAT is how to compare the pH of a solution to the pK_a of a functional group of an amino acid and determine if a site is mostly protonated or deprotonated. If the pH is higher than the pK_a, the site is mostly deprotonated; if the pH is lower than the pK_a, the site is mostly protonated. This can be illustrated in the titration curve for glycine:

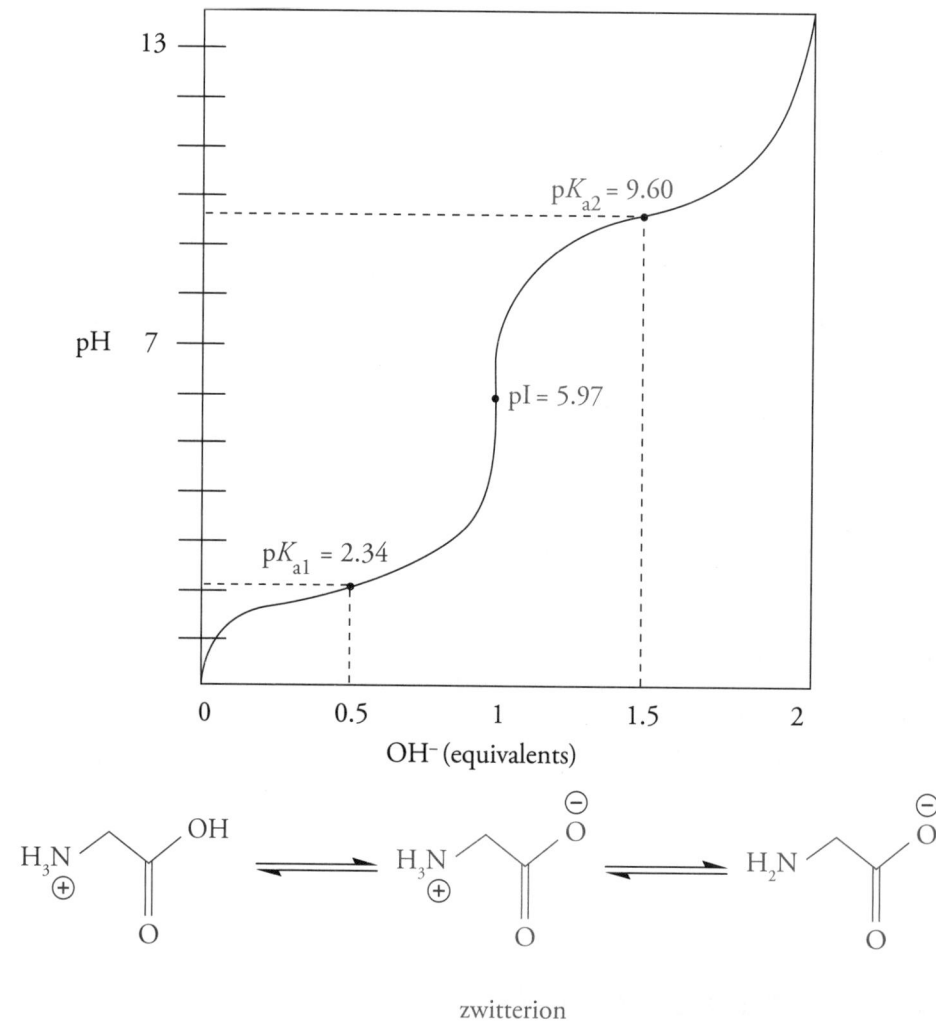

zwitterion

12) What is the pI of glycine?[12]
13) What is the pI of aspartic acid?[13]

---

[12] To calculate the pI, just average the pK_as of the two functional groups: $(9.60 + 2.34)/2 = 5.97$, or roughly 6.

[13] To calculate the pI of an amino acid with three functional groups like aspartic acid, average the two closer together pK_a values: $(1.88 + 3.65) = 2.77$, or roughly 3.

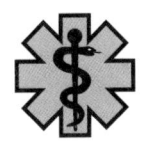

Amino Acid Separation—Gel Electrophoresis

Gel electrophoresis is a general separation technique that can be used to separate amino acids based on their charge. In general, when employing this technique, amino acids are loaded onto a gel that is held at a constant pH, then exposed to an electric field. When the pH of the gel is different than the pI of the amino acids, each amino acid will bear an overall charge because pI is specific to the unique structure of the side chain of each amino acid. The amino acids will therefore migrate through the gel based on their charge and the external electric field. The MCAT tends to ask about how specific amino acids will migrate relative to each other in these separation conditions. In order to answer these questions, an understanding of the relationship between pH, pK_a, and pI (as discussed previously) is required. See the table below, which summarizes how pH will determine the direction of amino acid migration during an electrophoresis separation:

pH	Charge on Amino Acid	Direction of Migration
greater than pI	negative	toward positive electrode
lower than pI	positive	toward negative electrode
equal to pI	neutral (zwitterion)	no migration

14) A sample of glycine is loaded on a gel in a pH = 6.0 solution with a (+) electrode at one end and a (–) electrode at the other end. Will the majority of the glycine migrate toward the negative terminal, migrate toward the positive terminal, or not migrate in either direction?[14]

15) The pK_as for the three functional groups in aspartic acid are 9.8 for the amino group, 2.1 for the α–carboxyl, and 3.9 for the side chain carboxyl. What pole (– or +) will aspartic acid migrate toward in an electric field at physiological pH (7.4)?[15]

16) What pole (– or +) would aspartic acid migrate toward in an electric field in a pH 1.0 solution?[16]

17) Which of these amino acids is most likely to be found on the interior of a protein at pH 7.0?[17]
    A. Alanine
    B. Glutamic acid
    C. Phenylalanine
    D. Glycine

18) Which of the following amino acids is most likely to be found on the exterior of a protein at pH 7.0?[18]
    A. Leucine
    B. Alanine
    C. Serine
    D. Isoleucine

---

[14] At this pH level, glycine has a net charge of zero. Hence, it will not move in an electric field.

[15] The amino group will be protonated ($-NH_3^+$), and both carboxyl groups deprotonated ($-COO^-$), producing an average charge per aspartic acid molecule of –1. Thus, aspartic acid will migrate toward the oppositely charged (+) pole at pH 7.4.

[16] Both carboxyl groups would be protonated and uncharged (–COOH), and the amino group would be protonated and charged ($-NH_3^+$). The net charge is +1, so aspartic acid would migrate toward the (–) pole.

[17] Glu is incorrect, since this amino acid is charged at a pH of 7. Of the three remaining, phenylalanine has the largest hydrophobic group, and is therefore the most likely to be found on the interior of a protein. The answer is **C**.

[18] Leucine, alanine, and isoleucine are all hydrophobic residues more likely to be found on the interior than the exterior of proteins. Serine (choice **C**), which has a hydroxyl group that can hydrogen bond with water, is the correct answer.

7.2 PROTEINS

There are two common types of covalent bonds between amino acids in proteins: the **peptide bonds** that link amino acids together into polypeptide chains and **disulfide bridges** between cysteine R groups.

The Peptide Bond

Polypeptides are formed by linking amino acids together in peptide bonds. A peptide bond is formed between the carboxyl group of one amino acid and the α-amino group of another amino acid with the loss of water. This occurs by the same nucleophilic addition-elimination mechanism shown in Section 6.4 for formation of any one of the carboxylic acid derivatives from any other carboxylic acid derivative. Remember that a peptide bond is just an amide bond between two amino acids. The figure below shows the formation of a dipeptide from the amino acids glycine and alanine.

Peptide Bond (Amide Bond) Formation

Note: The above diagram showing formation of a peptide bond via a simple condensation reaction is not entirely accurate. As seen in the following graph, the formation of a peptide bond with two amino acids is not thermodynamically favorable and requires energy. This naturally occurring reaction, which takes place during translation in cells, involves enzyme catalysis, is RNA directed, and co-factor mediated.

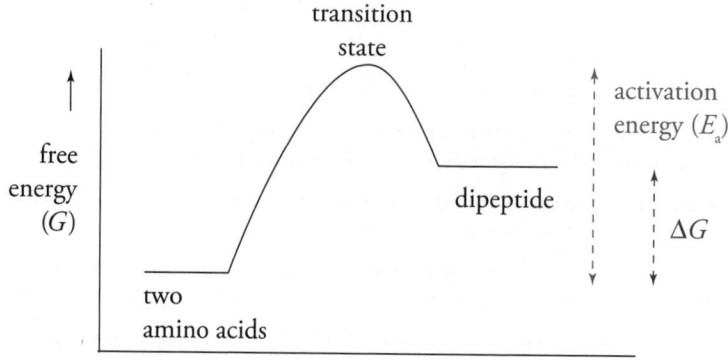

DCC Coupling

In order to synthesize peptides artificially in the laboratory, **DCC coupling** is used. In the first step of the coupling process, DCC, or dicyclohexyl carbodiimide, converts the OH of the caboxylate group in an amino acid into a good leaving group. In the next step, the amino group of a second amino acid attacks the carbonyl carbon of the "activated" amino acid. Finally, the DCC leaves with the oxygen to which it is bonded. To assure that amino acids are added in a unidirectional manner and in the proper order for the desired peptide, the reaction is run using protecting groups so that only one of the carboxyl groups and one of the amino groups are available to react. See the example reaction that follows.

In a polypeptide chain, the N–C–C–N–C–C pattern formed from the amino acids is known as the **backbone** of the polypeptide. An individual amino acid is termed a **residue** when it is part of a polypeptide chain. The amino terminus is the first end made during polypeptide synthesis, and the carboxy terminus is made last. Hence, by convention, the amino-terminal residue is also always written first.

19) In the oligopeptide Phe-Glu-Gly-Ser-Ala, state the number of acid and base functional groups, which residue has a free α-amino group, and which residue has a free α-carboxyl group. (Refer to the beginning of the chapter for structures.)[19]

20) Thermodynamics states that free energy must decrease for a reaction to proceed spontaneously and that such a reaction will spontaneously move toward equilibrium. The reaction coordinate diagram above shows the free energy changes during peptide bond formation. At equilibrium, which is thermodynamically favored: the dipeptide or the individual amino acids?[20]

---

[19] As stated above, the amino end is always written first. Hence, the oligopeptide begins with an exposed Phe amino group and ends with an exposed Ala carboxyl; all the other backbone groups are hitched together in peptide bonds. Out of all the R groups, there is only one acidic or basic functional group, the acidic glutamate R group. This R group plus the two terminal backbone groups gives a total of three acid/base functional groups.

[20] The dipeptide has a higher free energy, so its existence is less favorable. In other words, existence of the chain is less favorable than existence of the isolated amino acids.

21) In that case, how are peptide bonds formed and maintained inside cells?[21]

Planarity of the Peptide Bond

The peptide bond is planar and rigid because the resonance delocalization of the nitrogen's electrons to the carbonyl oxygen gives substantial double bond character to the bond between the carbonyl carbon and the nitrogen, as shown below. Hence there can be no rotation around the peptide bond.

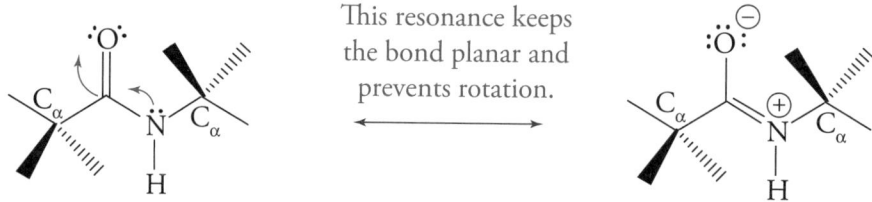

This resonance keeps the bond planar and prevents rotation.

Resonance Structure of the Planar, Rigid Peptide Bond

22) If the peptide bond is rigid and planar, then is the entire polypeptide rigid and incapable of rotation?[22]

Hydrolysis of the Peptide Bond

Hydrolysis refers to any reaction in which water is inserted in a bond to cleave it. We have already discussed the details of hydrolysis reactions in Chapter 6, which covered the hydrolysis of an ester under both acidic and basic reaction conditions (see Section 6.4). Hydrolysis of the peptide bond (amide bond) to form a free amine and a carboxylic acid is thermodynamically favored (products have lower free energy), but kinetically slow. There are two common means of accelerating the rate of peptide bond hydrolysis (i.e., two common ways to destroy proteins): strong acids and proteolytic enzymes.

Acid hydrolysis is the cleaving of a protein into its constituent amino acids with strong acid and heat. This is a non-specific means of cleaving peptide bonds. The amount of each amino acid present after hydrolysis can then be quantified to determine the overall amino acid content of the protein.

23) If a tripeptide of Gly-Phe-Ala is subjected to acid hydrolysis, can the order of the residues in the tripeptide be determined afterward?[23]

---

[21] During protein synthesis, stored energy is used to force peptide bonds to form. Once the bond is formed, even though its destruction is thermodynamically favorable, it remains stable because the activation energy for the hydrolysis reaction is so high. In other words, hydrolysis is thermodynamically favorable but kinetically slow.

[22] No, only the peptide bond (between amino acids) is rigid due to resonance. The bonds to the α-carbon (within each amino acid) are free to rotate.

[23] No. After hydrolysis, all amino acids are separate and have free amino and carboxyl groups.

Hydrolysis of a protein by another protein is called **proteolysis** or **proteolytic cleavage**, and the protein that does the cutting is known as a **proteolytic enzyme** or **protease**. Proteolytic cleavage is a specific means of cleaving peptide bonds. Many enzymes only cleave the peptide bond adjacent to a specific amino acid. For example, the protease trypsin cleaves on the carboxyl side of the positively charged (basic) residues arginine and lysine, while chymotrypsin cleaves on the carboxyl side of residues containing an aromatic side chain such as phenylalanine. (Do *not* memorize these examples.)

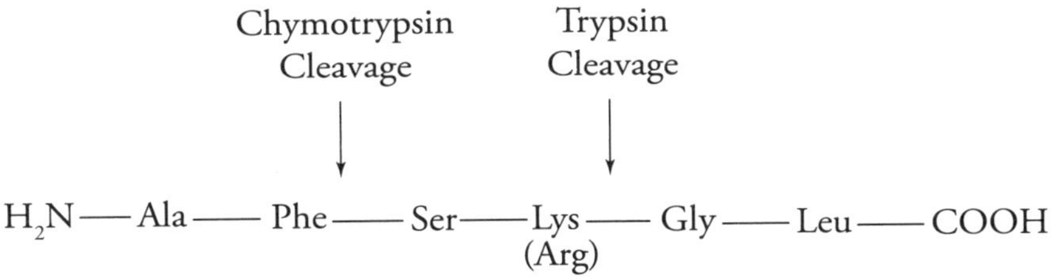

Chymotrypsin
Cleavage

Trypsin
Cleavage

H₂N—Ala——Phe——Ser——Lys——Gly——Leu——COOH
(Arg)

Specificity of Protease Cleavage

24) Based on the above, if the following peptide is cleaved by trypsin, what amino acid will be on the new N-terminus and how many fragments will result: Ala-Gly-Glu-Lys-Phe-Phe-Lys?[24]

The Disulfide Bond

Cysteine is an amino acid with a reactive thiol (sulfhydryl, SH) in its side chain. The thiol of one cysteine can react with the thiol of another cysteine in an oxidation reaction to produce a covalent sulfur-sulfur bond known as a **disulfide bond**, as illustrated below. The cysteines forming a disulfide bond may be located in the same or different polypeptide chain(s). The disulfide bridge plays an important role in stabilizing tertiary protein structure; this will be discussed in the section on protein folding. Once a cysteine residue becomes disulfide-bonded to another cysteine residue, it is called *cystine* instead of cysteine.

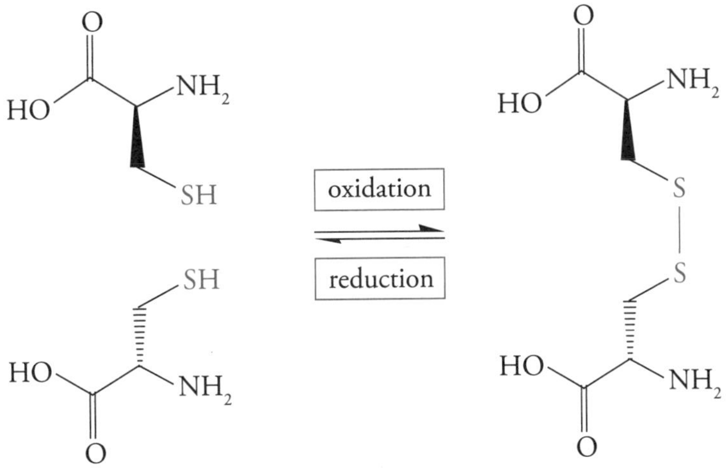

Formation of the Disulfide Bond

---

[24] Trypsin will cleave on the carboxyl side of the Lys residue, with Phe on the N-terminus of the new Phe-Phe-Lys fragment. There will be two fragments after trypsin cleavage: Phe-Phe-Lys and Ala-Gly-Glu-Lys.

25) Which is more oxidized, the sulfur in *cysteine* or the sulfur in *cystine*?[25]
26) The inside of cells is known as a reducing environment because cells possess antioxidants (chemicals that prevent oxidation reactions). Where would disulfide bridges be more likely to be found, in extracellular proteins, under oxidizing conditions, or in the interior of cells, in a reducing environment?[26]

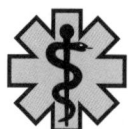

Protein Structure in Three Dimensions

Each protein folds into a unique three-dimensional structure that is required for that protein to function properly. Improperly folded, or **denatured**, proteins are nonfunctional. There are four levels of protein folding that contribute to their final three-dimensional structure. Each level of structure is dependent upon a particular type of bond, as discussed in the following sections.

Denaturation is an important concept. It refers to the **disruption of a protein's shape without breaking peptide bonds**. Proteins are denatured by *urea* (which disrupts hydrogen bonding interactions), by *extremes of pH*, by extremes of *temperature*, and by *changes in salt concentration (tonicity)*.

Primary (1°) Structure: The Amino Acid Sequence

The simplest level of protein structure is the order of amino acids bonded to each other in the polypeptide chain. This linear ordering of amino acid residues is known as primary structure. Primary structure is the same as **sequence**. The bond which determines 1° structure is the peptide bond, simply because this is the bond that links one amino acid to the next in a polypeptide.

Secondary (2°) Structure: Hydrogen Bonds Between Backbone Groups

Secondary structure refers to the initial folding of a polypeptide chain into shapes stabilized by hydrogen bonds between backbone NH and CO groups. Certain motifs of secondary structure are found in most proteins. The two most common are the α-**helix** and the β-**pleated sheet**.

All α-helices have the same well-defined dimensions that are depicted below with the R groups omitted for clarity. The α-helices of proteins are always right handed, 5 angstroms in width, with each subsequent amino acid rising 1.5 angstroms. There are 3.6 amino acid residues per turn with the α-carboxyl oxygen of one amino acid residue hydrogen-bonded to the α-amino proton of an amino acid three residues away. (*Don't* memorize these numbers, but *do* try to visualize what they mean.)

---

[25] The sulfur in cysteine is bonded to a hydrogen and a carbon; the sulfur in cystine is bonded to a sulfur and a carbon. Hence, the sulfur in cystine is more oxidized.

[26] In a reducing environment, the S-S group is reduced to two SH groups. Disulfide bridges are found only in extracellular polypeptides, where they will not be reduced. Examples of protein complexes held together by disulfide bridges include antibodies and the hormone insulin.

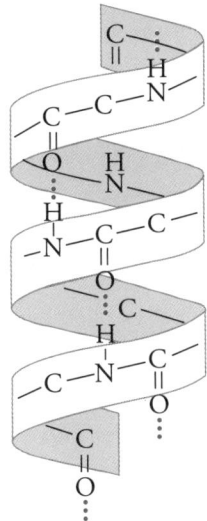

An α Helix

The unique structure of **proline** forces it to kink the polypeptide chain; hence, proline residues never appear within the α-helix.

Proteins such as hormone receptors and ion channels are often found with α-helical transmembrane regions integrated into the hydrophobic membranes of cells. The α-helix is a favorable structure for a hydrophobic transmembrane region because all polar NH and CO groups in the backbone are hydrogen bonded to each other on the inside of the helix, and thus don't interact with the hydrophobic membrane interior. α-Helical regions that span membranes also have hydrophobic R groups, which radiate out from the helix, interacting with the hydrophobic interior of the membrane.

β-Pleated sheets are also stabilized by hydrogen bonding between NH and CO groups in the polypeptide backbone. In β-sheets, however, hydrogen bonding occurs between residues distant from each other in the chain or even on separate polypeptide chains. Also, the backbone of a β-sheet is extended, rather than coiled, with side groups directed above and below the plane of the β-sheet. There are two types of β-sheets, one with adjacent polypeptide strands running in the *same* direction (**parallel** β-pleated sheet) and another in which the polypeptide strands run in *opposite* directions (**antiparallel** β-pleated sheet).

A β-Pleated Sheet

27) If a single polypeptide folds once and forms a β-pleated sheet with itself, would this be a parallel or antiparallel β-pleated sheet?[27]

28) What effect would a molecule that disrupts hydrogen bonding, e.g., urea, have on protein structure?[28]

Tertiary (3°) Structure: Hydrophobic/Hydrophilic Interactions

The next level of protein folding, tertiary structure, concerns interactions between amino acid residues located more distantly from each other in the polypeptide chain. The folding of secondary structures such as α-helices into higher order tertiary structures is driven by interactions of R groups with each other and with the solvent (water). Hydrophobic R groups tend to fold into the interior of the protein, away from the solvent, and hydrophilic R groups tend to be exposed to water on the surface of the protein (shown for the generic globular protein).

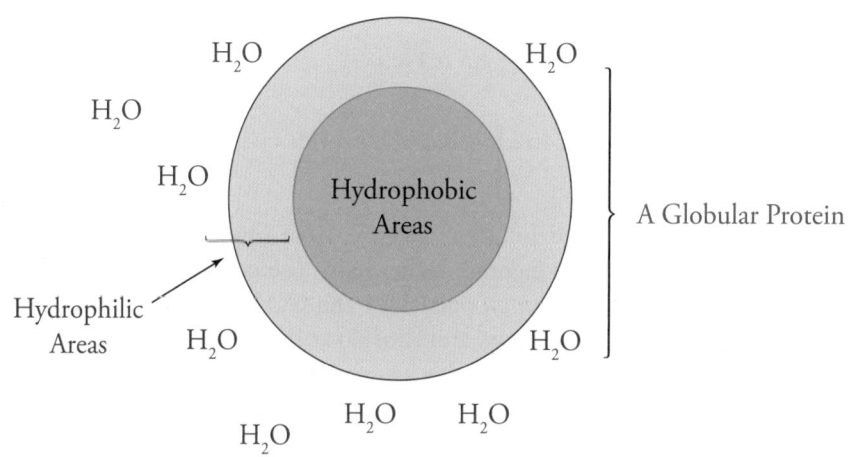

Folding of a Globular Protein in Aqueous Solution

Under the right conditions, the forces driving hydrophobic avoidance of water and hydrogen bonding will fold a polypeptide spontaneously into the correct conformation, the lowest energy conformation. In a classic experiment by Christian Anfinsen and coworkers, the effect of a denaturing agent (urea) and a reducing agent (β-mercaptoethanol) on the folding of a protein called ribonuclease were examined. In the following questions, you will reenact their thought processes. Figure out the answers before reading the footnotes.

29) Ribonuclease has eight cysteines that form four disulfide bonds. What effect would a reducing agent have on its tertiary structure?[29]

30) If the disulfides serve only to lock into place a tertiary protein structure that forms first on its own, then what effect would the reducing agent have on correct protein folding?[30]

---

[27] It would be antiparallel because one participant in the β-pleated sheet would have a C to N direction, while the other would be running N to C.

[28] Putting a protein in a urea solution will disrupt H-bonding, thus disrupting secondary structure by unfolding α-helices and β-sheets. It would not affect primary structure, which depends on the much more stable peptide bond. Disruption of 2°, 3°, or 4° structure without breaking peptide bonds is *denaturation*.

[29] The disulfide bridges would be broken. Tertiary structure would be less stable.

[30] The shape should not be disrupted if breaking disulfides is the only disturbance. It's just that the shape would be less sturdy—like a concrete wall without the rebar.

31) Would a protein end up folded normally if you (1) first put it in a reducing environment, (2) then denatured it by adding urea, (3) next removed the reducing agent, allowing disulfide bridges to reform, and (4) finally removed the denaturing agent?[31]

32) What if you did the same experiment but in this order: 1, 2, 4, 3?[32]

The disulfide bridge is perhaps not a good example of 3° structure because it is a covalent bond, not a hydrophobic interaction. However, because the disulfide is formed after 2° structure and before 4° structure, it is usually considered part of 3° folding.

33) Which of the following may be considered an example of tertiary protein structure?[33]
   I.   van der Waals interactions between two Phe R groups located far apart on a polypeptide
   II. Hydrogen bonds between backbone amino and carboxyl groups
   III. Covalent disulfide bonds between cysteine residues located far apart on a polypeptide

34) What effect would dissolving a globular protein in a hydrophobic organic solvent such as hexane have on tertiary protein structure?[34]

Quaternary (4°) Structure: Various Bonds Between Separate Chains

The highest level of protein structure, quaternary structure, describes interactions between polypeptide subunits. A **subunit** is a single polypeptide chain that is part of a large complex containing many subunits (a **multisubunit complex**). The arrangement of subunits in a multisubunit complex is what we mean by quaternary structure. For example, mammalian RNA polymerase II contains 12 different subunits. The interactions between subunits are instrumental in protein function, as in the cooperative binding of oxygen by each of the four subunits of hemoglobin.

The forces stabilizing quaternary structure are generally the same as those involved in secondary and tertiary structure—non-covalent interactions (the hydrogen bond and the van der Waals interaction). However, covalent bonds may also be involved in quaternary structure. For example, antibodies (immune system molecules) are large protein complexes with disulfide bonds holding the subunits together. It is key to understand, however, that there is one covalent bond that may not be involved in quaternary structure—the peptide bond—because this bond defines sequence (1° structure).

35) What is the difference between a disulfide bridge involved in quaternary structure and one involved in tertiary structure?[35]

---

[31] No. If you allow disulfide bridges to form while the protein is still denatured, it will become locked into an abnormal shape.

[32] You should end up with the correct structure. In step one, you break the reinforcing disulfide bridges. In step two, you denature the protein completely by disrupting H-bonds. In step four, you allow the H-bonds to reform; as stated in the text, normally the correct tertiary structure will form spontaneously if you leave the polypeptide alone. In step three, you reform the disulfide bridges, thus locking the structure into its correct form.

[33] This is a simple question provided to clarify the classification of the disulfide bridge. Item I is a good example of 3° structure. Item II describes 2°, not 3°, structure. Item III describes the disulfide, which is considered to be tertiary because of when it is formed, despite the fact that it is a covalent bond.

[34] The protein would be turned inside out.

[35] Quaternary disulfides are bonds that form between polypeptide chains that aren't linked by peptide bonds. Tertiary disulfides are bonds that form between residues in the same polypeptide.

7.3   CARBOHYDRATES

Carbohydrates are chains of hydrated carbon atoms with the molecular formula $C_nH_{2n}O_n$. The chain usually begins with an aldehyde or ketone and continues as a polyalcohol in which each carbon has a hydroxyl substituent. Carbohydrates are produced by photosynthesis in plants and by biochemical synthesis in animals. Carbohydrates can be broken down to CO_2 in a process called **oxidation**, which is also known as burning or combustion. Because this process releases large amounts of energy, carbohydrates serve as the principle energy source for cellular metabolism. Glucose in the form of the polymer cellulose is also the building block of wood and cotton. Understanding the nomenclature, structure, and chemistry of carbohydrates is essential to understanding cellular metabolism. This chapter will also help you understand key facts such as why we can eat potatoes and cotton candy but not wood and cotton T-shirts, and why milk makes some adults flatulent.

Structure and Nomenclature of Monosaccharides

A single carbohydrate molecule is a **monosaccharide** (meaning "single sweet unit"), also known as a **simple sugar**. Two monosaccharides bonded together form a **disaccharide**; several bonded together make an **oligosaccharide**, and many make a **polysaccharide**. If these polymers are subjected to strong acid, they are hydrolyzed to monosaccharides, which are not further hydrolyzed.

Classes of monosaccharides are given a two-part name. The first part is either "aldo" or "keto," depending on whether an aldehyde or a ketone is present. The second part reveals the number of carbon atoms in the chain: trioses are the smallest and have three carbons; tetroses have four, pentoses five, hexoses six, and heptoses seven. For example, the *polyhydroxy aldehyde glucose* is an *aldohexose* because it is a six-carbon chain beginning in an aldehyde. "Glucose" and "fructose" are examples of **common names**. IUPAC nomenclature is not usually used with individual carbohydrates because the systematic names are so long.

The carbons in monosaccharides are numbered beginning with carbon #1 at the *most oxidized end* of the carbon chain, which is the end with the aldehyde or ketone.

Some Metabolically Important Simple Sugars and Common Sugars on the MCAT

36)   Which of the sugars in the figure above is a ketohexose?[36]
37)   Which carbon (#?) is the most oxidized in fructose?[37]

[36] Fructose. It has six carbons, making it a hexose, and the carbonyl group is located on carbon #2, making it a ketose. Fructose is a polyhydroxy ketone, or a ketohexose.

[37] Carbon #2.

Absolute Configuration of Monosaccharides

Because carbohydrates contain chiral carbons, it is also necessary to classify them according to stereochemistry. Like amino acids, carbohydrates are assigned one of two configurations, either D or L, based on the configuration of the last chiral carbon in the chain (farthest from the aldehyde or ketone). By convention, this configuration is determined by comparison with glyceraldehyde. If a monosaccharide's last chiral carbon matches the chiral carbon of D-glyceraldehyde, it will be assigned the "D" label. The sugars in our bodies have the D configuration. When you are drawing a Fischer projection of a monosaccharide, put the aldehyde or ketone on top and the CH_2OH group (last carbon) on the bottom. The last chiral carbon will have its OH on the **Left** for **L** monosaccharides. However, we have only D-sugars in our bodies. Remember that we have only L-amino acids and only D-sugars.

The Fischer Notation for Carbohydrates

For a given class of monosaccharide (like any other chiral molecule), there are 2^n different stereoisomers, where n is the number of chiral carbons.

Four Monosaccharide Stereoisomers

7.3

38) Consider the four monosaccharides on the previous page. Which one of the following is correct?[38]

    A. Carbohydrate #2 is a D sugar and an enantiomer of #4.

    B. Carbohydrate #2 is an enantiomer of #3.

    C. Carbohydrates #1 and #3 are epimers and enantiomers.

    D. Carbohydrates #1 and #3 are enantiomers.

39) There are __ aldohexoses and __ D-aldohexoses (tough question but you *do* have all the information you need to figure it out).[39]

40) Is it possible to produce a diastereomer of D-glyceraldehyde? How about an epimer?[40]

Since we already discussed the relationships between the terms *isomer, stereoisomer, enantiomer, diastereomer,* and *epimer* in Chapter 4, we will not discuss them again here. The following Venn diagram represents a concise way of categorizing these terms. It shows which groups are subsets of which. *Isomers* have the same atoms but different bonds, unless they are also stereoisomers. Stereoisomers have the same atoms and the same bonds, but different bond geometries. All stereoisomers are either enantiomers or diastereomers. Some diastereomers are epimers.

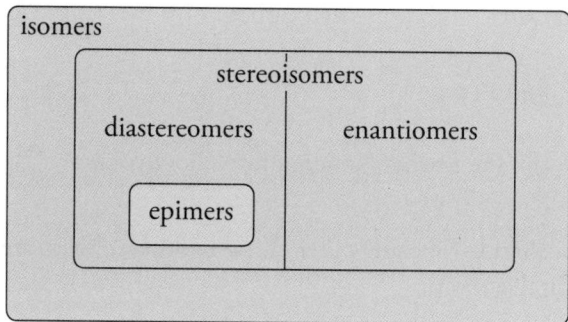

A Venn Diagram for Stereoisomers

Cyclic Structures of Monosaccharides

So far, we have represented the monosaccharides as straight chain structures. In solution, however, hexoses and pentoses spontaneously form five- and six-membered rings. In fact, the cyclic structures are thermodynamically favored, so that only a small percentage usually exist in the open chain form. The six-membered ring structures are termed **pyranoses** due to their resemblance to pyran, and five-membered sugar rings are termed **furanoses** due to their resemblance to furan.

---

[38] Sugar #2 is an L sugar, since the last chiral OH is on the left (choice A is false and can be eliminated). Sugars #2 and #3 are not mirror images, so they cannot be enantiomers (choice B is false and can be eliminated). Since sugars #1 and #3 are non-superimposable images, the are enantiomers (choice D is the correct statement), and remember that epimers are never enantiomers (choice C is false and can be eliminated).

[39] There are 2^4 aldohexoses, because there are 4 chiral carbons (#2, 3, 4, and 5). There are only 2^3 D-aldohexoses, because when you specify the "D" configuration, you leave only 3 variable chiral centers.

[40] No, it is not possible to make a glyceraldehyde diastereomer, because the molecule has only one chiral carbon. The only stereoisomer of D-glyceraldehyde is L-glyceraldehyde, an enantiomer. You can't make an epimer because the word *epimer* is reserved for sugars with more than one chiral center.

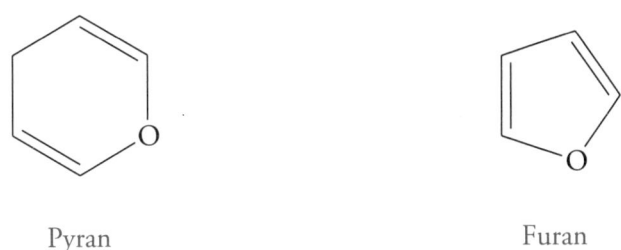

Pyran   Furan

Let's take glucose as an example. The ring forms when the OH on C5 nucleophilically attacks the carbonyl carbon (C1), forming a **hemiacetal**. The reactions involved, in which an alcohol reacts with an aldehyde to produce a hemiacetal (one –OR group and one –OH group) and subsequently an acetal (two –OR groups), are shown below (see also Section 6.2). The difference between an acetal and a hemiacetal is that the hemiacetal is in constant equilibrium with the carbonyl form. The acetal form, in contrast, is quite stable, requiring an enzyme to react.

Aldehyde   Hemiacetal   Acetal
                            (labile)   (stable)

Formation of a Hemiacetal and an Acetal

The figure below shows the reaction for glucose. This manner of drawing ring structures is a modified form of Fischer notation, useful for indicating which carbons are involved in forming the cyclical structure, but unrealistic in terms of bond lengths and angles.

α-D-glucose   β-D-glucose

Glucopyranose Formation: A Nucleophilic Addition Reaction

The more realistic "chair" representations of these structures are shown on the next page. Note that two different ring structures are shown, α and β. The α or β ring is formed depending upon from which face of the carbonyl the C5-hydroxyl group attacks. If the attack comes from one face, the carbonyl oxygen will become an equatorial hydroxyl group; if the attack comes from the other face, the carbonyl oxygen will become an axial hydroxyl group. [To distinguish the forms, remember, "It's always better to βE up (happy)!" This will help you remember that in β-D-Glucose, the anomeric hydroxyl group is up.] The two forms are called **anomers**, and C1 (designated with an asterisk in the figures) is called the **anomeric carbon**. The anomeric carbon is always the carbonyl carbon, so in aldoses it is C1, but in ketoses it is C2. The interconversion between the two anomers is called **mutarotation**.

The groups on the *left* in Fischer notation are *above* the ring in chair notation. Also, remember that *axial* substituents on six-membered chair rings are those that point *straight up or down*. The *equatorial* substituents point *out* from the ring. Equatorial substituents have less steric hindrance with the ring and are thus thermodynamically more favorable.

Chair Representation of Glucopyranose Formation

41) Why doesn't glucose cyclize into three- or four-membered rings?[41]
42) Are the OHs in β-D-glucopyranose axial or equatorial?[42]
43) A solution of glucose may contain both furanose and pyranose rings. How can the same sugar exist in both forms?[43]

Another way to represent cyclic sugars is called Haworth notation. The groups on the *left* in Fischer notation are *above* the ring in Haworth notation (as in the chair form). A summary of how to convert Fischer Projections of sugars to Haworth Projections is as follows:

1. Draw the basic structure of the sugar.
2. If the sugar is a D-sugar, place a –CH$_2$OH above the ring on the carbon to the left of the oxygen. For an L-sugar, place it below the ring.
3. For an α-sugar, place an –OH below the ring on the carbon to the right of the ring oxygen. For a β-sugar, place the –OH above the ring.
4. Finally, –OH groups on the right go below the ring and those on the left above, using the –CH$_2$OH group as the reference point for both projections.

---

[41] Smaller rings necessitate bond angles that are much narrower than the normal tetrahedral angle. Strained bonds are unfavorable because they are high energy.

[42] They are all equatorial. This makes it a very stable molecule, and may explain why it is the most prevalent sugar in nature. It stores a lot of energy, and yet is very stable. (Key fact.)

[43] The structure that forms depends on which OH attacks the carbonyl carbon (C#1). If OH4 attacks the carbonyl, the result will be a five-membered ring. If OH5 attacks, the result will be a six-membered ring. If you actually counted the structures in solution, you'd find more six-membered rings, since these are inherently more stable due to bond angles.

α-D-glucose   β-D-glucose

Haworth Representation of Glucopyranose

44) A monosaccharide is represented below in Haworth notation. What number is the carbon that the arrow is pointing toward? Is this a furanose or a pyranose? Is it the α- or β-anomer?[44]

45) Is this a D- or L-sugar? How many chiral carbons does it have?[45]

Structure and Nomenclature of Disaccharides

Recall that two monosaccharides bonded together form a disaccharide, a few form an oligosaccharide, and many form a polysaccharide. The bond between two sugar molecules is called a **glycosidic linkage**. This is a covalent bond, formed in a dehydration reaction that requires enzymatic catalysis.

Typically, the glycosidic bond joins C1 of one pyranose or furanose to C4 (sometimes C2 or C6) of another pyranose or furanose through an oxygen atom. Is the anomeric carbon in a hemiacetal form, or is it in an acetal form once it is part of a glycosidic bond? It has two –OR constituents, so it forms an acetal group. The significance of this is that the glycosidic linkage stays in the α or β configuration until an enzyme breaks the bond, because the acetal is a stable functional group. In other words, once a monosaccharide has attacked another sugar to form a glycosidic linkage, it is no longer free to mutarotate. This is an important concept, and we will discuss it further in the section on reducing sugars.

---

[44] It is the one farthest from the anomeric carbon, so it is #6. It is in a five-membered ring, so it is a furanose. The anomeric OH (former carbonyl O) is up, so it's β.

[45] It is D-fructose, with three chiral carbons (four when cyclic). One way to determine that it's a D sugar is to identify the penultimate chiral carbon, mentally open the chain, and visualize it as a Fischer structure. Another is to assign absolute configuration. D sugars have *R* configurations at the penultimate carbon.

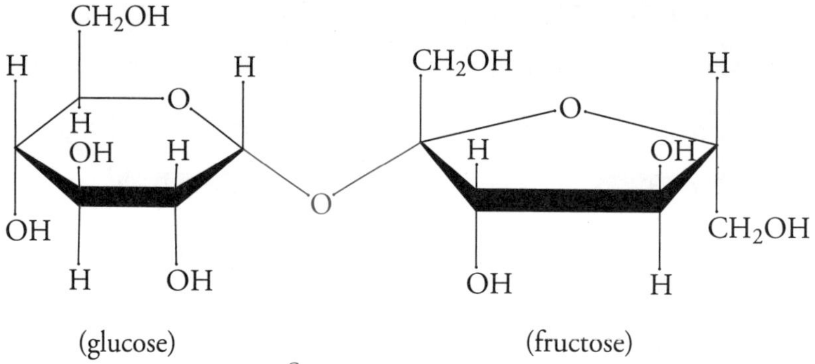

(glucose)   (fructose)

Sucrose

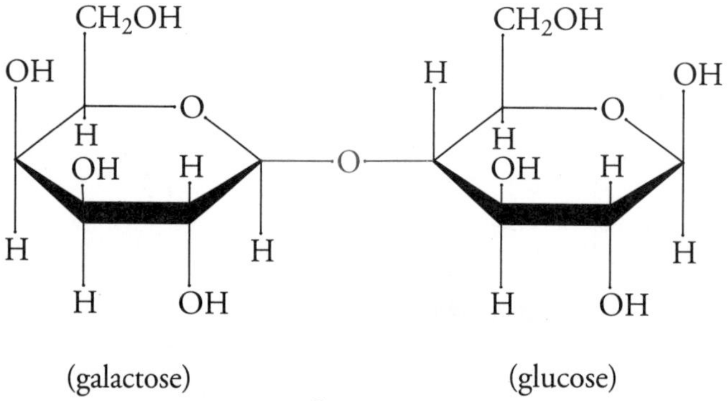

(galactose)   (glucose)

Lactose

Disaccharides and the α- or β-Glycosidic Bond

Glycosidic linkages are named according to which carbon in each sugar comprises the linkage. The configuration (α or β) of the linkage is also specified. For example, lactose (milk sugar) is a disaccharide joined in a galactose-β-1,4-glucose linkage (above). Sucrose (table sugar) is also shown above, with a glucose unit and a fructose unit.

46)   Does sucrose contain an α- or β-glycosidic linkage?[46]

Some common disaccharides you might see on the MCAT are sucrose (Glc-α-1,2-Fru), lactose (Gal-β-1,4-Glc), maltose (Glc-α-1,4-Glc), and cellobiose (Glc-β-1,4-Glc). However, you should NOT try to memorize these linkages.

Polymers made from these disaccharides form important biological macromolecules. Glycogen serves as an energy storage carbohydrate in animals and is composed of thousands of glucose units joined in α-1,4 linkages; α-1,6 branches are also present. Starch is the same as glycogen (except that the branches are a little different), and serves the same purpose in plants. Cellulose is a polymer of cellobiose; the β-glycosidic bonds allow the polymer to assume a long, straight, fibrous shape. Wood and cotton are made of cellulose.

---

[46] The anomeric carbon of glucose is pointing down, which means the linkage is α-1,2. So, sucrose is Glc-α-1,2-Fru.

The hydrolysis of polysaccharides into monosaccharides is essential for monosaccharides to enter metabolic pathways (e.g., glycolysis) and be used for energy by the cell. Different enzymes catalyze the hydrolysis of different linkages. The enzyme is named for the sugar it hydrolyzes. For example, the enzyme that catalyzes the hydrolysis of maltose into two glucose monosaccharides is called **maltase**. Each enzyme is highly specific for its linkage.

This specificity is a great example of the significance of stereochemistry. Consider cellulose. A cotton T-shirt is pure sugar. The only reason we can't digest it is that mammalian enzymes can't deal with the β-glycosidic linkages that make cellobiose from glucose. Cellulose is actually the energy source in grass and hay. Cows are mammals, and all mammals lack the enzymes necessary for cellobiose breakdown. To live on grass, cows depend on bacteria that live in an extra stomach called a rumen to digest cellulose for them. If you're really on the ball, you're next question is: Humans are mammals, so how can we digest lactose, which has a β linkage? The answer is that we have a specific enzyme, **lactase**, which can digest lactose. This is an exception to the rule that mammalian enzymes cannot hydrolyze β-glycosidic linkages. People without lactase are **lactose malabsorbers**, and any lactose they eat ends up in the colon. There it may cause gas and diarrhea, if certain bacteria are present; people with this problem are said to be **lactose intolerant**. People produce lactase as children so that they can digest mother's milk, but most adults naturally stop making this enzyme, and thus become lactose malabsorbers and sometimes intolerant.

The Polysaccharide Glycogen

Hydrolysis of Glycosidic Linkages

Disaccharides and polysaccharides are broken down into their component monosaccharides by enzymatic hydrolysis. This just means water is the nucleophile, and one of the sugars is the leaving group (the one that was the attacker during bond formation). In other words, the cleavage reaction is precisely the reverse of the formation reaction.

Hydrolysis of polysaccharides into monosaccharides is favored thermodynamically. This means the hydrolysis of polysaccharides releases energy in the cell. However, it does not occur at a significant rate without enzymatic catalysis. As catalysts, enzymes increase reaction rates by lowering the activation energy but do not change final concentrations of reactants and products.

47) Which requires net energy input: polysaccharide synthesis or hydrolysis?[47]
48) If the activation energy of polysaccharide hydrolysis were so low that no enzyme was required for the reaction to occur, would this make polysaccharides better for energy storage?[48]

Reducing Sugars

This is a simple concept that often confuses students. **Benedict's test** is a chemical assay that detects the carbonyl units of sugars. It is useful because it distinguishes hemiacetals from acetals [only hemiacetals are in equilibrium with the carbonyl (open-chain) form]. For example, if you had a white powder that you knew to be composed of glucose, you would be able to say whether the glucose existed in the free monosaccharide form or was in the form of glycogen. How? Well, if it's in the monosaccharide form, there will be many hemiacetals, and Benedict's test will be strongly positive. However, if the powder consists of only relatively few glycogen molecules, Benedict's will be only weakly positive. This is because all the glucose units in a glycogen polymer are tied up in acetal linkages, except for the very first one in the chain (the one which was first attacked during polymerization).

Benedict's Test for Reducing Sugars

Benedict's test is performed as follows: Benedict's reagent, an oxidized form of copper, is used to oxidize a sugar's aldehyde or ketone to the corresponding carboxylic acid, yielding a reddish precipitate. Any carbohydrate that can be oxidized by Benedict's reagent is referred to as a **reducing sugar** because it *reduces the Cu^{2+} to Cu^+ while itself being oxidized. All monosaccharides are reducing sugars. More generally, all aldehydes, ketones, and hemiacetals give a positive result in Benedict's test for reducing sugars; acetals give a negative result because they do not react with Cu^{2+}, and they are not in equilibrium with the open-chain (carbonyl) form.*

49) Which carbon of glucose can be oxidized by Benedict's reagent? What about fructose?[49]

---

[47] Because hydrolysis of polysaccharides is thermodynamically favored, energy input is required to drive the reaction toward polysaccharide synthesis.

[48] No, because then polysaccharides would hydrolyze spontaneously (they'd be unstable). The high activation energy of polysaccharide hydrolysis allows us to use enzymes as gatekeepers—when we need energy from glucose, we open the gate of glycogen hydrolysis.

[49] The anomeric carbon, which is #1 for aldoses like glucose and #2 for ketoses like fructose.

Recall that we've said once a monosaccharide has attacked another sugar to form a glycosidic linkage, it is no longer free to mutarotate. Now we can expand this statement as follows: once a monosaccharide has attacked another sugar to form a glycosidic linkage, its anomeric carbon is in an acetal configuration and is thus no longer free to mutarotate *nor to reduce Benedict's reagent*.

50) If 98% of a monosaccharide is present as the ring form at equilibrium in solution, then how much of the sugar can be oxidized in Benedict's reaction?[50]

51) Is lactose a reducing sugar? What about sucrose? (You may refer back to the text and figures previously.)[51]

7.4 LIPIDS

Lipids are oily or fatty substances that play three physiological roles, summarized here and discussed below.

- In cellular membranes, phospholipids constitute a barrier between intracellular and extracellular environments.
- In adipose cells, triglycerides (fats) store energy.
- Finally, cholesterol is a special lipid that serves as the building block for the hydrophobic steroid hormones.

The cardinal characteristic of the lipid is its **hydrophobicity**. Hydrophobic means *water-fearing*. It is important to understand the significance of this. Since water is very polar, polar substances dissolve well in water; these are known as *water-loving*, or **hydrophilic** substances. Carbon-carbon bonds and carbon-hydrogen bonds are nonpolar. Hence, substances that contain only carbon and hydrogen will not dissolve well in water. Here are some examples. Table sugar dissolves well in water, but cooking oil floats in a layer above water or forms many tiny oil droplets when mixed with water. Cotton T-shirts become wet when exposed to water because they are made of glucose polymerized into cellulose, but a nylon jacket does not become wet because it is composed of atoms covalently bound together in a nonpolar fashion. A synonym for hydrophobic is **lipophilic** (which means lipid-loving); a synonym for hydrophilic is **lipophobic**. We return to these concepts below.

Fatty Acid Structure

Fatty acids are composed of long unsubstituted alkanes that end in a carboxylic acid. The chain is typically 14 to 18 carbons long, and because they are synthesized two carbons at a time from acetate, only *even-numbered* fatty acids are made in human cells. A fatty acid with no carbon-carbon double bonds is said to be **saturated** with hydrogen because every carbon atom in the chain is covalently bound to the

---

[50] 100% will be oxidized. In a monosaccharide, the ring form is in equilibrium with the open chain form. So when the open chain form is used up in the oxidation reaction, it will be replenished by other rings opening up (Le Châtelier's principle).

[51] Lactose (Gal-β-1-,4-Glc) is a reducing sugar. Although the attacking anomeric carbon becomes locked in an acetal, the anomeric carbon of the *attacked* monosaccharide is still free to mutarotate or react with Benedict's reagent. Sucrose (Glc-α-1-,2-Fru) is not a reducing sugar, because it is made of glucose and fructose, which are both joined at their anomeric carbons. Carbon #1 of glucose is the anomeric carbon, since glucose is an aldose; carbon #2 of fructose is the anomeric carbon, since fructose is a ketose.

7.4

maximum number of hydrogens. **Unsaturated** fatty acids have one or more double bonds in the tail. These double bonds are almost always (Z) (or *cis*). The position of a double bond in the alkyl chain of a fatty acid is denoted by the symbol Δ and the number of the first carbon involved in the double bond. Carbons are numbered starting with the carboxylic acid carbon. For example, a (Z) double bond between carbons 3 and 4 in a fatty acid would be referred to as (Z)-Δ^3 (or *cis*-Δ^3).

Saturated fatty acid

Unsaturated fatty acid

52) What is the correct nomenclature for the double bond in the unsaturated fatty acid above?[52]
53) How does the shape of an unsaturated fatty acid differ from that of a saturated fatty acid?[53]
54) If fatty acids are mixed into water, how are they likely to associate with each other?[54]

The drawing on the next page illustrates how free fatty acids interact in an aqueous solution; they form a structure called a **micelle**. The force that drives the tails into the center of the micelle is called the **hydrophobic interaction**. The hydrophobic interaction is a complex phenomenon. In general, it results from the fact that water molecules must form an orderly **solvation shell** around each hydrophobic substance. The reason is that H_2O has a dipole that "likes" to be able to share its charges with other polar molecules. A solvation shell allows for the most water-water interaction and the least water-lipid interaction. The problem is that forming a solvation shell is an increase in order and thus a decrease in entropy ($\Delta S < 0$), which is unfavorable according to the second law of thermodynamics. In the case of the fatty acid micelle, water forms a shell around the spherical micelle with the result being that water interacts with polar carboxylic acid head groups while hydrophobic lipid tails hide inside the sphere.

Soaps are the sodium salts of fatty acids ($RCOO^-Na^+$). They are **amphipathic**, which means both hydrophilic and hydrophobic.

---

[52] This double bond extends between carbons 7 and 8, and is *cis*. The bond therefore is *cis*-Δ^7.

[53] An unsaturated fatty acid is bent, or "kinked," at the *cis* double bond.

[54] The long hydrophobic chains will interact with each other to minimize contact with water, exposing the charged carboxyl group to the aqueous environment.

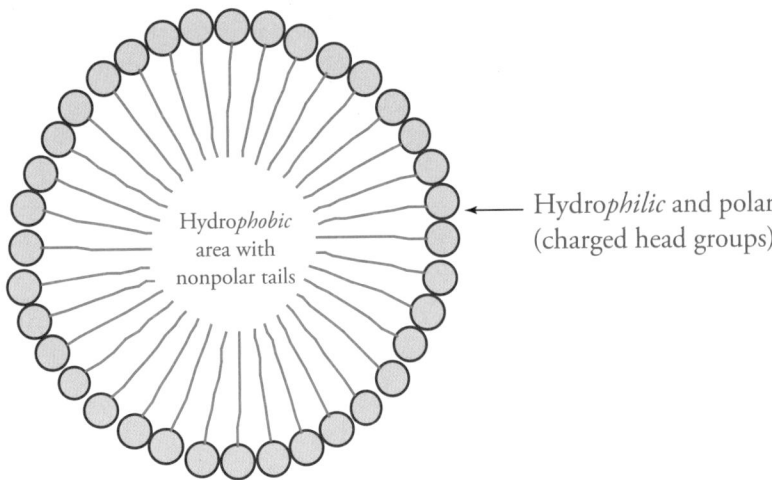

Hydro*philic* and polar
(charged head groups)

Hydro*phobic* area with nonpolar tails

A Fatty Acid Micelle

55) How does soap help to remove grease from your hands?[55]

Triacylglycerols (TG)

The storage form of the fatty acid is fat. The technical name for fat is **triacylglycerol** or **triglyceride** (shown below). The triglyceride is composed of three fatty acids esterified to a glycerol molecule. Glycerol is a three-carbon triol with the formula $HOCH_2$–$CHOH$–CH_2OH. As you can see, it has three hydroxyl groups that can be esterified to fatty acids. It is necessary to store fatty acids in the relatively inert form of fat because free fatty acids are reactive chemicals.

$$
\begin{array}{c}
\text{H}_2\text{C} - \text{O} - \overset{\displaystyle \text{O}}{\overset{\displaystyle \|}{\text{C}}} - \text{R}_1 \\
\text{HC} - \text{O} - \overset{\displaystyle \text{O}}{\overset{\displaystyle \|}{\text{C}}} - \text{R}_2 \\
\text{H}_2\text{C} - \text{O} - \overset{\displaystyle \text{O}}{\overset{\displaystyle \|}{\text{C}}} - \text{R}_3
\end{array}
$$

R groups may be the same or different.

A Triglyceride (Fat)

—

[55] Grease is hydrophobic. It does not wash off easily in water because it is not soluble in water. Scrubbing your hands with soap causes micelles to form around the grease particles.

The triacylglycerol undergoes reactions typical of esters, such as base-catalyzed hydrolysis. Soap is economically produced by base-catalyzed hydrolysis of triglycerides from animal fat into fatty acid salts (soaps). This reaction is called **saponification** and is illustrated below.

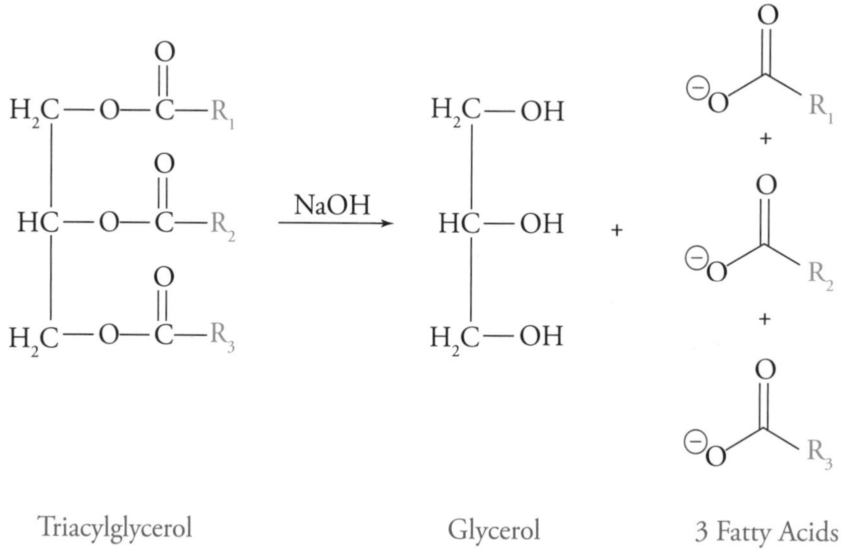

Triacylglycerol   Glycerol   3 Fatty Acids

Saponification

Lipases are enzymes that hydrolyze fats. Triacylglycerols are stored in fat cells as an energy source. Fats are more efficient energy storage molecules than carbohydrates for two reasons: packing and energy content.

<u>Packing:</u> Their hydrophobicity allows fats to pack together much more closely than carbohydrates. Carbohydrates carry a great amount of water-of-solvation (water molecules hydrogen bonded to their hydroxyl groups). In other words, the amount of carbon per unit area or unit weight is much greater in a fat droplet than in dissolved sugar. If we could store sugars in a dry powdery form in our bodies, this problem would be obviated.

<u>Energy content:</u> All packing considerations aside, fat molecules store much more energy than carbohydrates. In other words, regardless of what you dissolve it in, a fat has more energy carbon-for-carbon than a carbohydrate. The reason is that fats are much more *reduced*. Remember that energy metabolism begins with the *oxidation* of foodstuffs to release energy. Since carbohydrates are more oxidized to start with, oxidizing them releases less energy. Animals use fat to store most of their energy, storing only a small amount as carbohydrates (glycogen). Plants such as potatoes commonly store a large percentage of their energy as carbohydrates (starch).

Introduction to Lipid Bilayer Membranes

Membrane lipids are **phospholipids** derived from diacylglycerol phosphate or DG-P. For example, phosphatidyl choline is a phospholipid formed by the esterification of a choline molecule $[HO(CH_2)_2N^+(CH_3)_3]$ to the phosphate group of DG-P. Phospholipids are **detergents**, substances that efficiently solubilize oils while remaining highly water-soluble. Detergents are like soaps, but stronger.

$$\text{H}_2\text{C}-\text{O}-\overset{\displaystyle \overset{O}{\|}}{\text{C}}-\text{R}_1$$
$$\text{HC}-\text{O}-\overset{\displaystyle \overset{O}{\|}}{\text{C}}-\text{R}_2$$
$$\text{H}_2\text{C}-\text{O}-\overset{\displaystyle \overset{O}{\|}}{\text{P}}-\text{O}^{\ominus}$$
$$\overset{|}{\text{O}}_{\ominus}$$

A Phosphoglyceride (Diacylglycerol Phosphate, or DGP)

We saw previously how fatty acids spontaneously form micelles. Phospholipids also minimize their interactions with water by forming an orderly structure—in this case, it is a **lipid bilayer** (below). Hydrophobic interactions drive the formation of the bilayer, and once formed, it is stabilized by van der Waals forces between the long tails.

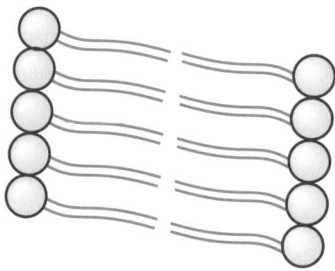

A Small Section of a Lipid Bilayer Membrane

56) Would a saturated or an unsaturated fatty acid residue have more van der Waals interactions with neighboring alkyl chains in a bilayer membrane?[56]

A more precise way to give the answer to the question above is to say that double bonds (unsaturation) in phospholipid fatty acids *tend to increase membrane fluidity*. Unsaturation prevents the membrane from solidifying by disrupting the orderly packing of the hydrophobic lipid tails. This decreases the melting point. The right amount of fluidity is essential for function. Decreasing the *length* of fatty acid tails also increases fluidity. The steroid **cholesterol** (discussed a bit later) is a third important modulator of membrane fluidity. At low temperatures, it increases fluidity in the same way as kinks in fatty acid tails; hence, it is known as membrane antifreeze. At high temperatures, however, cholesterol attenuates (reduces) membrane fluidity. Don't ponder this paradox too long; just remember that cholesterol keeps fluidity at an *optimum level*. Remember, the structural determinants of membrane fluidity are degree of saturation, tail length, and amount of cholesterol.

---

[56] The bent shape of the unsaturated fatty acid means that it doesn't fit in as well and has less contact with neighboring groups to form van der Waals interactions. Unsaturation makes the membrane less stable, less solid.

The lipid bilayer acts like a plastic bag surrounding the cell in the sense that it seals the interior of the cell from the exterior. However, the cell membrane is much more complex than a plastic bag. Since the plasma bilayer membrane surrounding cells is impermeable to charged particles such as Na^+, protein gateways such as ion channels are required for ions to enter or exit cells. Proteins that are integrated into membranes also transmit signals from the outside of the cell into the interior. For example, certain hormones (peptides) cannot pass through the cell membrane due to their charged nature; instead, protein **receptors** in the cell membrane bind these hormones and transmit a signal into the cell in a **second messenger cascade.**

Terpenes

A terpene is a member of a broad class of compounds built from isoprene units (C_5H_8) with a general formula $(C_5H_8)_n$.

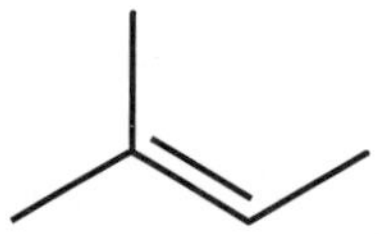

isoprene

Terpenes may be linear or cyclic, and are classified by the number of isoprene units they contain. For example, monoterpenes consist of two isoprene units, sesquiterpenes consist of three, and diterpenes contain four.

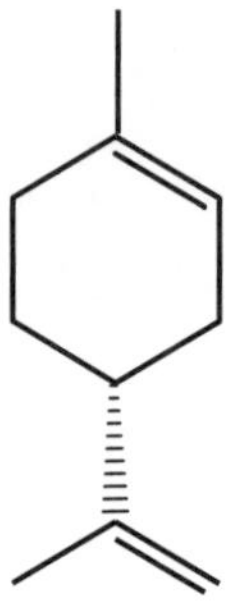

limonene
$C_{10}H_{16}$
(a monoterpene)

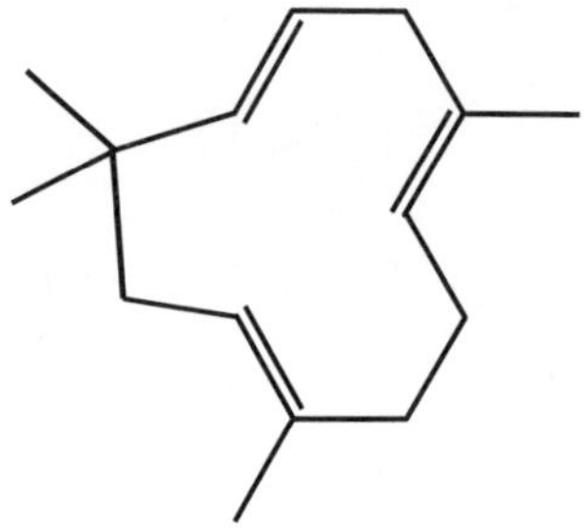

humulene
$C_{15}H_{24}$
(a sesquiterpene)

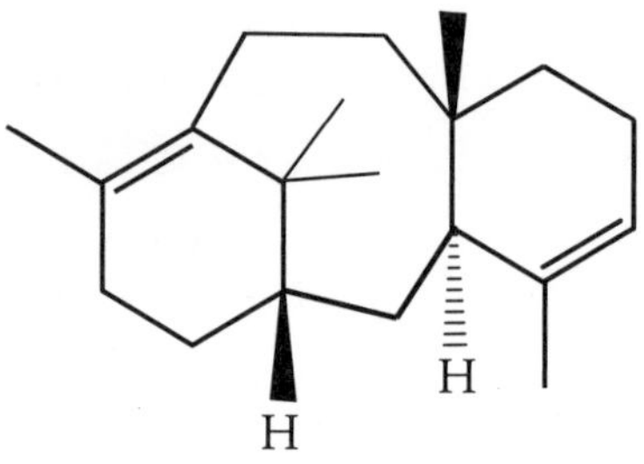

taxadiene
$C_{20}H_{32}$
(a diterpene)

Squalene is a triterpene (made of six isoprene units), and is a particularly important compound as it is biosynthetically utilized in the manufacture of steroids.

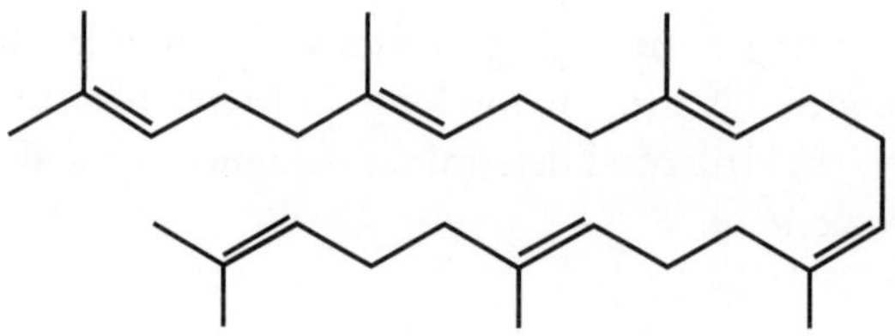

Whereas a terpene is formally a simple hydrocarbon, there are a number of natural and synthetically derived species that are built from an isoprene skeleton and functionalized with other elements (O, N, S, etc.). These functionalized-terpenes are known as *terpenoids*. Vitamin A ($C_{20}H_{30}O$) is an example of a terpenoid.

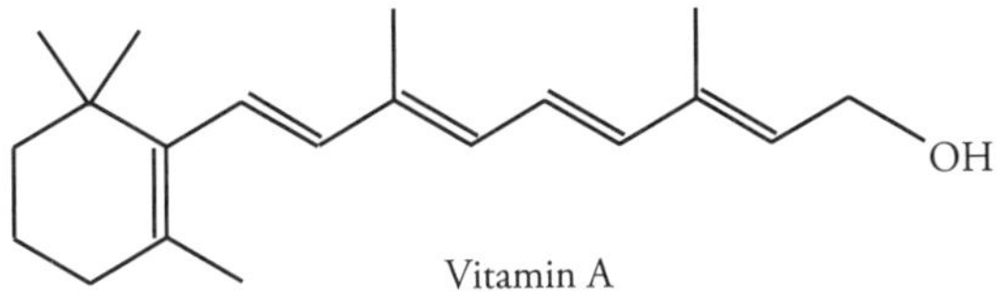

Vitamin A

Steroids

Steroids are included here because of their hydrophobicity, and, hence, similarity to fats. Their structure is otherwise unique. All steroids have the basic tetracyclic ring system (see below), based on the structure of **cholesterol**, a polycyclic amphipath. (Polycyclic means several rings, and amphipathic means displaying both hydrophilic and hydrophobic characteristics.)

As discussed above, the steroid cholesterol is an important component of the lipid bilayer. It is obtained from the diet and synthesized in the liver. It is carried in the blood packaged with fats and proteins into **lipoproteins**. One type of lipoprotein has been implicated as the cause of atherosclerotic vascular disease, which refers to the build-up of cholesterol "plaques" on the inside of blood vessels.

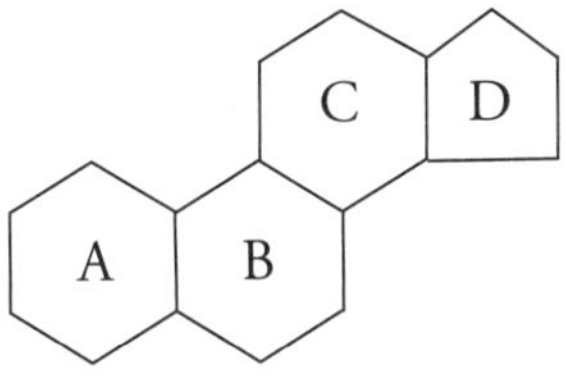

tetracyclic ring system

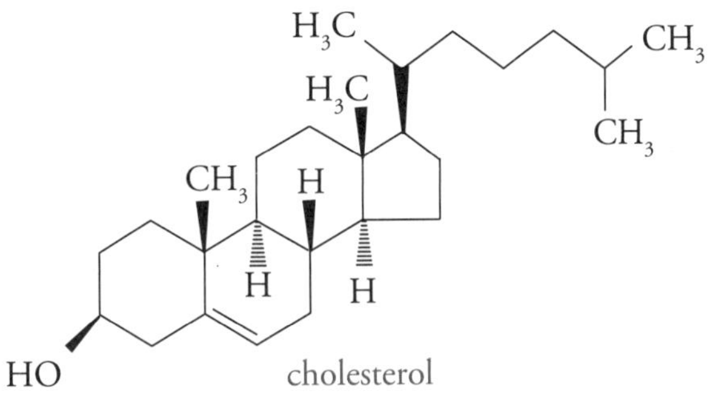

cholesterol

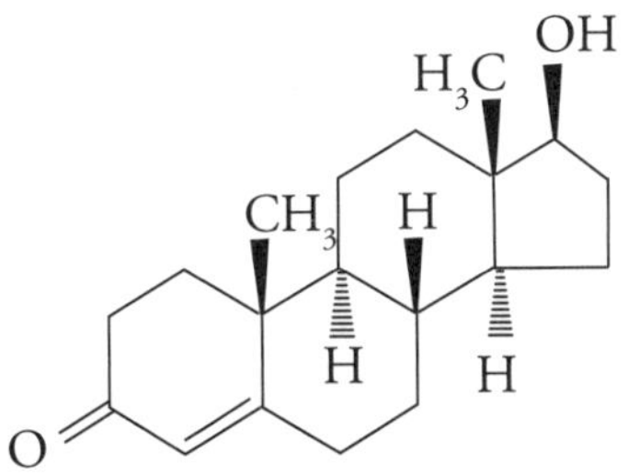

testosterone

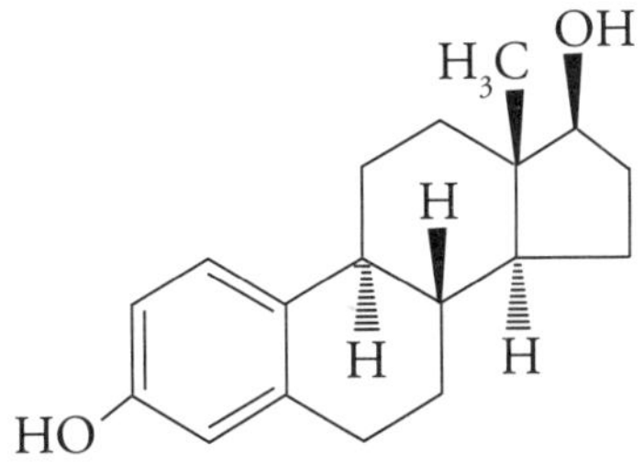

estrogen

Cholesterol-Derived Hormones

Steroid hormones are made from cholesterol. Two examples are **testosterone** (an androgen or male sex hormone) and **estradiol** (an estrogen or female sex hormone). There are no receptors for steroid hormones on the surface of cells. If this is true, how can they exert an influence on the cell? Because steroids are highly hydrophobic, they can diffuse right through the lipid bilayer membrane into the cytoplasm. The receptors for steroid hormones are located within cells rather than on the cell surface. This is an important point! You must be aware of the contrast between *peptide* hormones, such as insulin, which exert their effects by binding to receptors at the cell-surface, and *steroid* hormones, such as estrogen, which diffuse into cells to find their receptors.

7.5 NUCLEIC ACIDS

Before we can talk about nucleic acids, we must first briefly review some background.

Phosphorus-Containing Compounds

Phosphoric acid is an *inorganic* acid (it does not contain carbon) with the potential to donate three protons. The pK_as for the three acid dissociation equilibria are 2.1, 7.2, and 12.4. Therefore, at physiological pH, phosphoric acid is significantly dissociated, existing largely in anionic form.

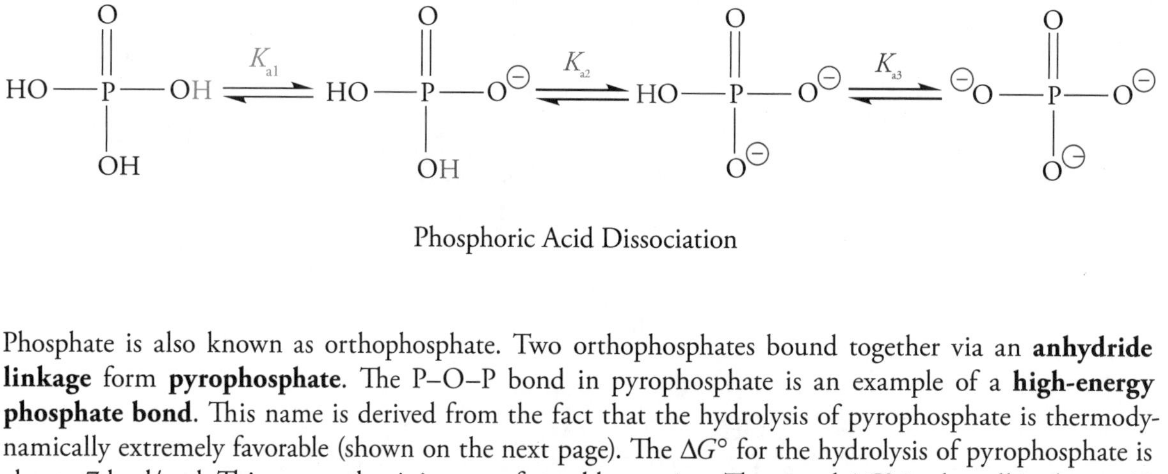

Phosphoric Acid Dissociation

Phosphate is also known as orthophosphate. Two orthophosphates bound together via an **anhydride linkage** form **pyrophosphate**. The P–O–P bond in pyrophosphate is an example of a **high-energy phosphate bond**. This name is derived from the fact that the hydrolysis of pyrophosphate is thermodynamically extremely favorable (shown on the next page). The $\Delta G°$ for the hydrolysis of pyrophosphate is about –7 kcal/mol. This means that it is a very favorable reaction. The actual $\Delta G°$ in the cell is about –12 kcal/mol, which is even more favorable.

There are three reasons that phosphate anhydride bonds store so much energy:

1. When phosphates are linked together, their negative charges repel each other strongly.
2. Orthophosphate has more resonance forms and thus a lower free energy than linked phosphates.
3. Orthophosphate has a more favorable interaction with the biological solvent (water) than linked phosphates.

The details are not crucial. What is essential is that you fix the image in your mind of linked phosphates acting like compressed springs, just waiting to fly open and provide energy for an enzyme to catalyze a reaction.

The Hydrolysis of Pyrophosphate

Nucleotides

Nucleotides are the building blocks of nucleic acids (RNA and DNA). Each nucleotide contains a **ribose** (or **deoxyribose**) **sugar** group; a **purine** or **pyrimidine base** joined to carbon number one of the ribose ring; and one, two, or three phosphate units joined to carbon five of the ribose ring. The nucleotide **a**denosine **tri**phosphate (ATP) plays a central role in cellular metabolism in addition to being an RNA precursor.

ATP is the universal short-term energy storage molecule. Energy extracted from the oxidation of foodstuffs is immediately stored in the phosphoanhydride bonds of ATP. This energy will later be used to power cellular processes; it may also be used to synthesize glucose or fats, which are longer-term energy storage molecules. This applies to *all* living organisms, from bacteria to humans. Even some viruses carry ATP with them outside the host cell, though viruses cannot make their own ATP.

Adenosine Triphosphate (ATP)

Chapter 7 Summary

- Amino acids (AAs) consist of a tetrahedral α-carbon connected to an amino group, a carboxyl group, and a variable R group, which determines the AA's properties.

- The isoelectric point of an AA is the pH at which the net charge on the molecule is zero; this structure is referred to as the *zwitterion*.

- Electrophoresis separates mixtures of AAs and is conducted at buffered pH. Positively charged AAs move to the "–" end of the gel, and negative AAs move to the "+" end. Zwitterions will not move.

- Proteins consist of amino acids linked by peptide bonds, or amide bonds, which have partial double bond characteristics, lack rotation, and are very stable.

- The secondary structure of proteins (α-helices and β-sheets) is formed through hydrogen bonding interactions between atoms in the backbone of the molecule.

- The most stable tertiary protein structure generally places polar AAs on the exterior and nonpolar AAs on the interior of the protein. This minimizes interactions between nonpolar AAs and water, while optimizing interactions between side chains inside the protein.

- All animal amino acids are L-configuration and all animal sugars are D-configuration.

- Carbohydrates are chains of hydrated carbon atoms with the molecular formula $C_nH_{2n}O_n$.

- Sugars in solution exist in equilibrium between the straight chain form and either the furanose (five-atom) or pyranose (six-atom) cyclic forms.

- The anomeric forms of a sugar differ by the position of the OH group on the anomeric carbon; OH down = α, OH up = β.

- All monosaccharides will give a positive result in a Benedict's test because they contain an aldehyde, ketone or hemiacetal, and are therefore reducing sugars.

- The glycosidic linkage in a disaccharide is named based on which anomer is present for the sugar containing the acetal and the numbers of the carbons linked to the bridging O.

- Saponification (base-mediated hydrolysis) of a triglyceride produces three equivalents of fatty acid carboxylates. These amphipathic molecules form micelles in solution.

- Lipids are found in several forms in the body, including triglycerides, phospholipids, cholesterol, and steroids.

- The building blocks of nucleic acids (DNA and RNA) are nucleotides, which are comprised of a pentose sugar, a purine or pyrimidine base, and 2–3 phosphate units.

CHAPTER 7 FREESTANDING PRACTICE QUESTIONS

1. Which of the following best explains the strength of the peptide bond in a protein?

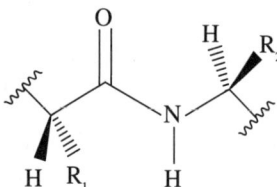

A) The steric bulk of the R groups prevents nucleophilic attack at the carbonyl carbon.
B) The electron pair on the nitrogen atom is delocalized by orbital overlap with the carbonyl group.
C) Peptide bonds are never exposed to the exterior of a protein.
D) The peptide bond is resistant to hydrolysis by many biological molecules.

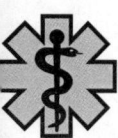

2. Why is ATP known as a "high energy" structure at neutral pH?

A) It exhibits a large decrease in free energy when it undergoes hydrolytic reactions.
B) The phosphate ion released from ATP hydrolysis is very reactive.
C) It causes cellular processes to proceed at faster rates.
D) Adenine is the best energy storage molecule of all the nitrogenous bases.

3. Which of the following best describes the secondary structure of a protein?

A) Various folded polypeptide chains joining together to form a larger unit
B) The amino acid sequence of the chain
C) The polypeptide chain folding upon itself due to hydrophobic/hydrophilic interactions
D) Peptide bonds hydrogen-bonding to one another to create a sheet-like structure

4. Which of the following fatty acids has the highest melting point?

A) 4,5-Dimethylhexanoic acid
B) Octanoic acid
C) 2,3-Dimethylbutanoic acid
D) Hexanoic acid

5. Which of the following terms best describes the interconversion between α-D-glucose and β-D-glucose?

A) Tautomerism
B) Nucleophilic addition
C) Mutarotation
D) Elimination

6. A dipeptide is synthesized with the sequence Asp-Glu. The aspartic acid residue has an observed pK_a of 2.10 for its side chain. In free glutamic acid, the side chain has an expected pK_a of 2.15. However, in this dipeptide, it is likely that the observed pK_a of the glutamic acid side chain will be:

A) higher due to a favorable ionic interaction between the deprotonated side chains.
B) lower due to a favorable ionic interaction between the deprotonated side chains.
C) higher due to an unfavorable ionic interaction between the deprotonated side chains.
D) lower due to an unfavorable ionic interaction between the deprotonated side chains.

7. In the dipeptide shown below, all of the labeled dihedral angles may freely rotate EXCEPT:

A) ω
B) ψ
C) χ
D) φ

8. Gel electrophoresis is used to separate a mixture of arginine, tryptophan, and aspartic acid. Relevant pK_a information is given below:

Amino Acid	pK_{a1}	pK_{a2}	pK_{a3}
Arginine	2.17	9.04	12.48
Tryptophan	2.83	9.39	—
Aspartic acid	1.88	9.60	3.65

Which of the following matrix pH values could best be used to separate the mixture of three amino acids into pure components by using gel electrophoresis?

A) pH 2.1
B) pH 3.2
C) pH 6.0
D) pH 12.1

9. How many fragments are expected to result via acid-catalyzed hydrolysis of the compound below?

A) 3
B) 4
C) 5
D) 6

CHAPTER 7 PRACTICE PASSAGE

In the body, proteins are constantly being synthesized and degraded in order to maintain and modulate protein concentration and enzyme activity levels. In eukaryotic cells, a 76-residue protein called *ubiquitin* is used as a tag to label proteins destined for degradation.

Ubiquitin forms an amide bond between its glycine residue at position 76 and the side chain of a lysine residue of the target protein. Three enzymes are required in the attachment of ubiquitin to the target protein. The steps of ubiquitination at pH 7 are shown in Figure 1. The first step is coupled to ATP hydrolysis.

First, a single ubiquitin is attached to the target protein via the reaction shown in Figure 1. Subsequently, a second ubiquitin is attached to a lysine residue of the first ubiquitin, a third ubiquitin is attached to a lysine residue of the second ubiquitin, and so on, until a chain consisting of four ubiquitin monomers is attached to the target protein (Figure 1). The ubiquitinated protein is then sent to the proteosome where it is degraded into single amino acids. In the proteosome, threonine proteases cleave solvent-exposed peptide bonds using a threonine active site residue. A representative cleavage of a diglycine peptide at pH 7 is shown in Figure 2.

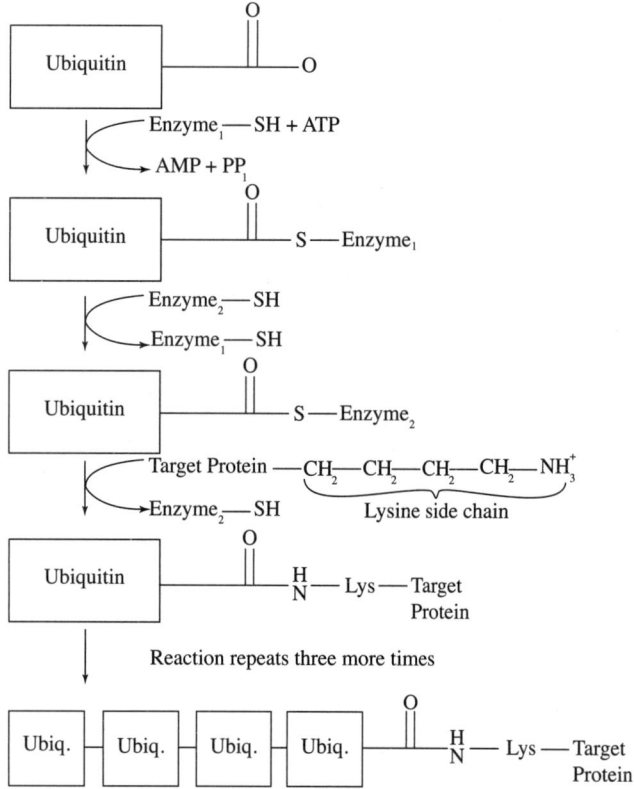

Figure 1   Ubiquitination

(Adapted from Stryer, *Biochemistry,* 3rd edition)

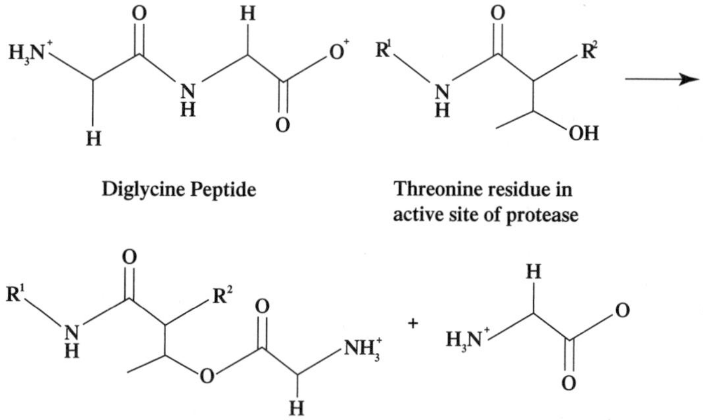

Figure 2   Threonine-dependent peptide hydrolysis

1. The amide bond between ubiquitin and its target protein is formed between the side chain of a lysine residue and the:

A) C-terminus of glycine 76.
B) N-terminus of glycine 76.
C) side chain of glycine 76.
D) α–carbon of glycine 76.

2. In Step 2 of ubiquitination, the ubiquitin is transferred from Enzyme$_1$ to Enzyme$_2$. This reaction is most accurately described as:

A) nucleophilic substitution.
B) transesterification.
C) trans(thio)esterification.
D) nucleophilic addition.

3. In the absence of ATP, the ubiquitination reaction would:

A) occur more slowly than in the presence of ATP.
B) occur more quickly than in the presence of ATP.
C) not be affected.
D) not occur.

4. In the threonine-dependent hydrolysis of proteins, the primary function of the threonine residue is to act as a(n):

A) acid.
B) base.
C) nucleophile.
D) electrophile.

5. Which of the following techniques would be most effective in separating lysine from a mixture of lysine, glycine, and threonine in aqueous buffer at pH 7?

A) Extraction
B) Gel electrophoresis
C) Silica-gel column chromatography
D) Distillation

SOLUTIONS TO CHAPTER 7 FREESTANDING PRACTICE QUESTIONS

1. **B** Because the peptide bond is delocalized, the C—N bond has double-bond character and is difficult to break. Choice A can be eliminated because steric hindrance describes the electron density surrounding an atom, not the density associated with bonds. Choice C can be eliminated because the folding of a peptide within a protein does not affect bond strength. Choice D can be eliminated because proteins are susceptible to hydrolysis from enzymes.

2. **A** Choice A is the best because it directly addresses the energetics of ATP hydrolysis. Choice B discusses the reactivity of the released phosphate ion and not the structure of ATP itself, so it can be eliminated. Choice C can be eliminated because it describes the rate of cellular processes not the energy of ATP. Choice D can be eliminated because the structure of adenine is not related to why ATP is a good energy storage molecule.

3. **D** The secondary structure of proteins is the initial folding of the polypeptide chain into α-helices or β-pleated sheets. Choice A describes the formation of a quaternary protein, choice B can be eliminated because it describes the primary protein structure, and choice C can be eliminated because it describes the tertiary protein structure.

4. **B** Two points to consider in the melting point of fatty acids are 1) molecular weight, and 2) branching. Choices A and B both consist of eight carbons, while choices C and D each have six. Thus, it is likely that choice A or B will be the better choice based on molecular weight. Since choice A is branched and choice B is not, choice A has the lower melting point. Although all four structures may be drawn to answer this question, it is not necessary. The carbons can be counted based on the names (2 *methyl* = 2 carbons + *hexan* = 6 carbons or *but* = 4 carbons), and the methyl substituents are indicative of branching in choices A and C.

5. **C** The interconversion between α and β anomers of the same sugar is known as mutarotation. Although the mechanism of mutarotation involves both elimination, then nucleophilic addition, individually each of these two answers is incomplete (eliminate choices B and D). Tautomerism describes the equilibration between structural isomers (eliminate choice A), not anomers, which are stereoisomers.

6. **C** This problem can be approached as a 2x2. First, consider that when aspartic acid and glutamic acid are deprotonated, they go from having neutral side chains to having a negative charge. Repulsion between these two negative charges creates an unfavorable ionic interaction (eliminate choices A and B). If the side chain of glutamic acid has a higher observed pK_a, the repulsion can be avoided somewhat since the group will be deprotonated only at higher pH, and therefore a narrower range of conditions (eliminate choice D).

7. **A** Since the peptide bond has partial double bond character, it cannot freely rotate. The peptide bond is labeled as ω, making choice A the correct answer. The rest of the labeled dihedral angles are all single bonds, and therefore can freely rotate.

8. **C** Overall charges can be predicted by comparing pH to pI (the isoelectric point). When pH = pI, an amino acid exists as a (neutral) zwitterion, which does not migrate when an electric field is applied. However, when pH < pI, the amino acid will be positively charged; when pH > pI, the amino acid will be negatively charged. pI values for the three amino acids of interest can be estimated as indicated below by using pK_a information contained in the stem.

pI (arginine) = (9.04 + 12.48) / 2 = 11 (rounded)
pI (tryptophan) = (2.83 + 9.39) / 2 = 6 (rounded)
pI (aspartic acid) = (1.88 + 3.65) / 2 = 3 (rounded)

The widest separation among the three amino acids under an electric field is made possible when the net charges differ on all three amino acids. At pH 2.1 (choice A), the pH < pI condition applies for all amino acids and all will be positively charged, resulting in poor separation (eliminate choice A). The same applies at pH 12.1 (choice D), where pH > pI for all amino acids and all are thus negatively charged (eliminate choice D). At pH 3.2 (choice B), two amino acids, Arg and Trp, will be in a pH < pI condition and are thus positively charged, again resulting in poor separation (eliminate choice B). Lastly, at pH 6.0 (choice C), all three amino acids fall into different conditions. Asp will be negatively charged as pH > pI and Arg will be positively charged because pH < pI. Trp will not migrate as pH = pI. At this matrix pH, arginine and aspartic acid migrate to opposite electrodes while tryptophan remains at the origin (choice C is correct).

9. **B** Inspection of the structure provided reveals that it contains carbohydrate and steroid moieties joined by glycosidic linkages. Acid-catalyzed hydrolysis will break glycosidic linkages (acetals) in a carbohydrate polymer to give hemiacetal components. Three acetal carbons [indicated by dark circles ("●") in the structure shown below] participate in the formation of glycosidic linkages, and each of these is expected to be hydrolyzed. This acid-catalyzed hydrolysis process is summarized below.

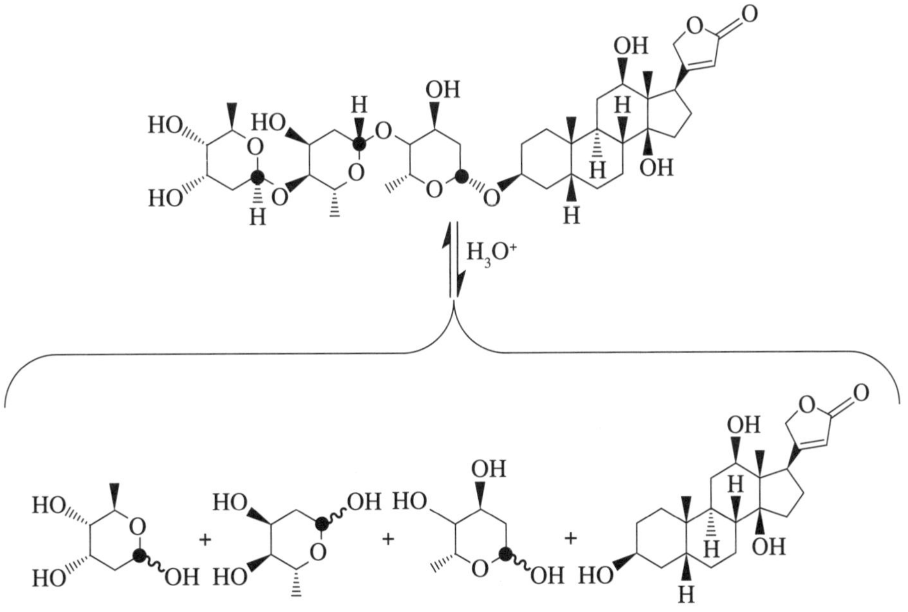

Hydrolyzing all glycosidic linkages reveals that four fragments are expected, making choice B the correct answer.

SOLUTIONS TO CHAPTER 7 PRACTICE PASSAGE

1. **A**   Since proteins are written from N-terminus to C-terminus, glycine 76 is the C-terminal residue with the free carbonyl shown (eliminate choice B). Glycine does not have a side chain (its R group attached to the α-carbon is a single H) so choice C can be eliminated. The α-carbon of an amino acid is next to the carbonyl, not the carbonyl carbon itself, so choice D can be eliminated.

2. **C**   At the beginning of Step 2, the ubiquitin is linked to Enzyme$_1$ through a thioester bond, not a simple ester, due to the presence of sulfur in the molecule. At the end of the reaction it emerges linked to Enzyme$_2$ through a new thioester bond. Transesterification and trans(thio)esterification involve the exchange of one alcohol or thiol group, respectively, on one ester compound for another. Therefore, this reaction is best described as a trans(thio)-esterification (eliminate choice B). Substitution is a tempting answer since one enzyme has been replaced by another, maintaining the same number of sigma bonds from reactant to product. However, since the interconversion of carboxylic acid derivatives occurs through an addition-elimination mechanism, choice C is a more specific answer, and choice A can be eliminated. Choice D can be eliminated since it only describes part of the mechanism.

3. **D**   ATP coupling is used to drive thermodynamically unfavorable reactions that would otherwise be nonspontaneous. Therefore, in the absence of ATP this reaction would not occur. Choices A and B imply that the kinetics of the reaction would change, not the thermodynamics, and can therefore be eliminated.

4. **C**   The hydroxyl group on the threonine side chain carries two lone pairs and can act as a nucleophile. Reaction 2 shows that this hydroxyl group attacks the electrophilic carbonyl carbon of the peptide bond, further implicating threonine as a nucleophile. While there is some proton transfer in this reaction, the main function of threonine is not to act as an acid or base (eliminate choices A and B), but to cause the cleavage of the peptide bond via nucleophilic addition-elimination.

5. **B**   The major physical difference between lysine and the other two amino acids at pH 7 is that lysine carries an overall positive charge, as shown in Figures 1 (lysine side chain) and 2 (threonine and glycine). Gel electrophoresis separates molecules with different charges, and therefore would be the best choice for the separation. Extraction would not be effective since all of the species are charged and soluble in aqueous solution at pH 7 (eliminate choice A). Silica gel is a polar substance that would strongly attract all of the amino acids, therefore it would be very difficult to separate them using silica-gel column chromatography (eliminate choice C). The high molecular weight of the amino acids and ionic interactions between them will cause them to have a high vaporization point, making them nearly impossible to distill (eliminate choice D).

CONTROL OF ALDOL REACTION PATHWAYS OF ENOLIZABLE ALDEHYDES IN AN AQUEOUS ENVIRONMENT WITH A HYPERBRANCHED POLYMERIC CATALYST

Yonggui Chi, Steven T. Scroggins, Emine Boz, and Jean M. J. Fréchet

A central challenge of organic chemistry resides in the control of reaction pathways to avoid undesired reactions and develop new or more efficient syntheses. Nature uses precise control to amplify kinetically or thermodynamically unfavorable transformations with the assistance of enzymes, catalytic biopolymers that fold into sophisticated tertiary structures in water. A number of important advances have been made in approximating enzymes with synthetic materials. These include for example Miller's synthetic peptide catalysts, Breslow's polymer/pyridoxamine enzyme mimics, Reymond's peptide dendrimer catalysts, Moore's catalytic phenylene ethynylene foldamer, the metal complex self-assemblies of Bergman and Raymond, and the unimolecular free energy pump reactor of Fréchet and Hawker. However, it is still extremely difficult to mimic the complex and precise functional makeup of an enzyme. In this study we attempted to replicate an enzyme's ability to control competing reaction pathways by using synthetic polymers that promote reactions in an aqueous environment. We anticipated that such macromolecule catalysts might be used to direct the reaction pathways in a way not readily achievable with typical small molecule catalysts.

A class of reactions that attracted our attention are aldehyde transformations, such as cross ketone/aldehyde aldol condensations. These reactions are of fundamental importance in organic chemistry and have broad applications from the manufacture of basic chemicals to the preparation of fine pharmaceuticals. Indeed, aldehydes are the most common substrates in the recent explosive development of enamine, iminium, and SOMO catalysis. However, since enolizable aldehydes are often very reactive as both nucleophiles and electrophiles, controlling the competing pathways to avoid self-aldol reactions is an intrinsically unsolved chemoselectivity challenge. Usually, a large excess of one reagent is used to ensure high yielding reactions. For example, cross ketone/aldehyde reactions are typically carried out using the ketone substrates as solvent in the presence of either inorganic bases such as NaOH or amines such as proline as the catalyst. Here we report a soluble polymer catalyst that can eliminate the self-aldol reactions in an aqueous environment by suppressing an irreversible aldol pathway, thereby allowing for the amplification of otherwise unfavorable reactions without the need for excess reactants.

Our investigation began with a careful re-examination of the widely studied proline-catalyzed aldol reaction with enolizable aldehydes as the substrates. A typical model self-aldol of butanal (**1**) shows two major competing pathways at room temperature (rt) (Scheme 1). One is the *irreversible* formation of α,β-unsaturated aldehyde **2**, presumably through a Mannich-type pathway involving an iminium intermediate formed between aldehyde **1** and proline; the other is the *reversible* formation of β-hydroxy-aldehyde **3** via an enamine intermediate. These results were consistent with observations and postulations in the literature. Our aim was to eliminate the irreversible pathway leading to the formation of **2**. Thus the reversible formation of **3** can be turned into dynamic catalysis in developing new or more efficient syntheses. We speculated that the undesired pathway might be disrupted by controlling the charged iminium species involved in the Mannich-type reaction leading to **2**. Initial studies indicated that the use of typical small molecule amine catalysts (e.g., proline, pyrrolidine), changes in solvent polarity, or the use of water as solvent or cosolvent failed to suppress the formation of **2**. Here we are interested in the development of soluble synthetic polymers to address this chemoselectivity problem.

Scheme 1. Competing Pathways of Enolizable Aldehyde Self-Aldol Reactions

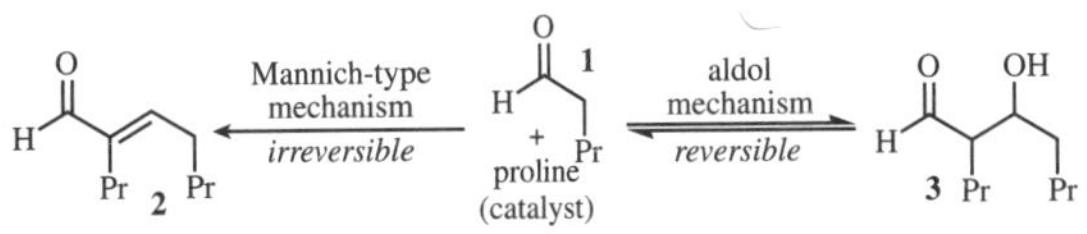

We chose a commercial hyperbranched polyethyleneimine (PEI) as the scaffold to develop our polymer catalyst. In contrast to the use of PEI and related amine polymers and dendrimers as catalyst supports (e.g., for metal nanoparticles), we aimed to use this type of water-soluble highly branched polymer to facilitate catalytic reactions in an aqueous environment. Pristine commercial

PEI contains primary and secondary amine groups and is thus not suitable for our purpose because these amino groups catalyze the aldol reaction without any control over the competing pathways shown in Scheme 1. However, simple chemical modification of PEI readily affords polymers of tunable structures and properties; for example, reaction of PEI with propylene oxide gave a water-soluble polymer (a possible structure is illustrated by **4**) that met our requirements (Scheme 2). Instead of introducing catalytically active sites via covalent linkages, we took advantage of the tertiary amino groups in **4** as noncovalent handles to attract proline catalysts via electrostatic interactions, affording the desired polymer catalyst (**5**). This polymer catalyst **5** provided nearly complete control over the two reaction pathways when the aldol reaction was carried out in water (Scheme 2).

The formation of β-hydroxy aldehyde **3** is facile and reversible. Very little (typically less than 1%) unsaturated aldehyde **2** was detected even at long reaction times (2 days or longer). Very interestingly, **5** did not provide any control over the two competing pathways when the reaction is carried out in *organic solvents* such as DMF, dimethyl sulfoxide, or CH$_2$Cl$_2$. For example, a typical self-aldol reaction of **1** with 10 mol% catalyst **5** in water reached equilibrium with reversible formation of 50–70% β-hydroxy aldehyde **3**. The remainder was starting aldehyde **1** while essentially no unsaturated aldehyde **2** was observed after 24 h (chemoselectivity, the ratio between **3** and **2** is greater than 60; Table 1, entry 3). The same reaction (with **5** as the catalyst) carried out in organic solvents such as DMF under otherwise identical conditions led to poor chemoselectivity with the irreversible formation of **2** as the major product (Table 1, entry 4). In initial studies, triethylamine (TEA) tested as the small molecule analogue of polymer **4** under otherwise identical conditions showed poor reaction control (Table 1, entry 5). Further experiments using tertiary amines containing alcohol groups (*N*-methyl-diethanolamine, triethanol-amine) in an aqueous medium gave results better than that with TEA (Table 1, entry 6−9). The pH values of the reaction medium were measured. It appears that pH has an effect on the reaction selectivity, and reactions in aqueous media with pH ∼9.0 gave optimal results. The catalytic conditions provided by the polymer can be approximated but are difficult to duplicate; therefore significant formation of the undesired self-aldol product **2** was still observed with the small molecule tertiary amines tested under various conditions, including different pH's. The use of alcohols, such as methanol, 2-propanol, and 2,2,2-trifluoro-ethanol as additives or cosolvents, does not improve reaction selectivity. In all cases, polymer catalyst **5** performs best in controlling the aldol reaction pathways (Scheme 2).

Scheme 2. Control of Aldol Reaction Pathways with a Hyperbranched Polymer Catalyst in Aqueous Environment

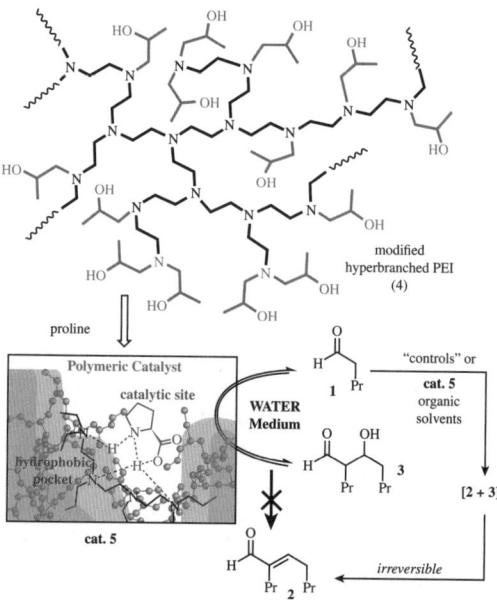

Table 1.   Self-Aldol Reaction of Enolizable Aldehyde

entry	cocatalyst	solvent	conv. (2+3)%^{a}	selectivity (3:2)	pH^b
1	–	DMF	82	1.4	–
2	–	H$_2$O	<1	–	–
3	polymer **4**	**H$_2$O**	**56**	**63**	**9.2**
4	polymer **4**	DMF	86	0.6	–
5	Et$_3$N	H$_2$O	80	1.0	11.1
7	CH$_3$N(EtOH)$_2$^{c}	H$_2$O	82	5.3	10.1
8	CH$_3$N(EtOH)$_2$^{d}	H$_2$O	77	3.3	–
9	N(EtOH)$_3$	H$_2$O	86	15	9.5

^{a} Measured by ^{1}H NMR of the crude reaction mixture; diastereoselectivity of aldol product **3** is ∼1.2:1; enanti-oselectivity was not determined. ^{b} pH of the catalyst solution in water (before the addition of aldehyde substrate). ^{c} *N*-Methyldiethanolamine. ^{d} Sodium dodecyl sulfate (a surfactant) was added.

Scheme 3. Dynamic Catalytic Cross Ketone/Aldehyde Reaction

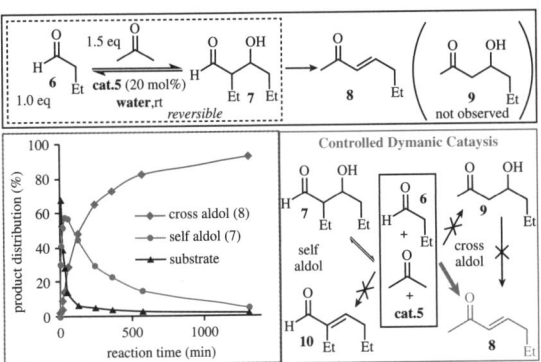

In view of the numerous chemical transformations involving enolizable aldehydes as substrates, the catalyst system with polymer complexes such as **5** might prove useful in the development of more efficient syntheses. In particular, a dynamic catalytic process might be developed for the amplification of desired products by reactions involving either the aldehyde substrate or the reversibly formed β-hydroxy aldehyde adduct. Initially, we chose to study the cross-aldol condensation between butanal and acetone to demonstrate this concept and highlight the potential of this catalytic system. The product of this condensation, an α,β-unsaturated ketone, is a key intermediate in the commercial production of methyl amyl ketone, an FDA listed food additive. In general, α,β-unsaturated ketones are both important commercial chemicals and common functional groups found in complex molecules such as natural products. Previous methods used to prepare these compounds typically require the use of a large excess of ketone to compete with the generally more rapid aldehyde self-condensation.

In a model cross aldol reaction between acetone and butanal using catalytic complex **5** in water (Scheme 3), the self-aldol reaction of **6** to form β-hydroxy aldehyde **7** proceeded much faster than the cross-aldol reaction, reaching maximum conversion in ~30 min. However, the facile reversibility of the self-aldol reaction in our catalytic system led to the eventual formation of the kinetically disfavored cross-aldol product **8** in more than 90% yield in 22 h. In this instance, a slight excess of ketone was used to facilitate monitoring of reaction progress, but it is not necessary in preparative scale syntheses. Surprisingly, little β-hydroxy ketone **9** was detected in the reaction. A sample of **9** prepared using a literature procedure did not yield any dehydration product (the unsaturated ketone) when subjected to the same catalytic condition, suggesting

that the cross condensation proceeds exclusively via a Mannich-type mechanism. The Mannich-type pathway is proposed to involve the reaction of an enamine intermediate formed between acetone and proline as well as an iminium ion derived from aldehyde and a second molecule of proline. It remains unclear exactly why the same iminium intermediate does not react with the enamine derived from aldehyde and proline to yield the aldehyde self-condensation product under the aqueous catalytic conditions with polymer complex **5**.

To probe the substrate scope, we first examined cross acetone/aldehyde condensations with unhindered straight-chain aliphatic aldehydes of different size and hydrophobicity. Increasing aldehyde hydrophobicity leads to a large decrease in reaction efficiency due to the polar nature of the aqueous polymer catalytic phase. This selectivity determined by substrate hydrophobicity may be used to design polymer-assisted polarity gradient-directed chemoselective reactions, such as aldehyde/aldehyde cross-aldol reactions. The mild catalytic conditions that prevail with **5** should enable the use of this catalyst with substrates containing

Scheme 4. Catalytic Cross Ketone/Aldehyde Condensation

11a
conversion: > 90%
(11a:12a = 25:1)

11f
67% (> 95:1)

11l
88% (> 95:1)

11g
67% (25:1)

11m
74% (5:1)

11b
>90% (> 95:1)

11h
>95% (95:1)

11n
56% (13:1)

11c
>90% (> 95:1)

11i
86% (> 95:1)

11o
90% (25:1)

11d
79% (83:1)

11j
67% (> 95:1)

11p
67% (8:1)

11e
77% (> 95:1)

11k
65% (> 95:1)

11q
50% (20:1)

functional groups such as esters, which are not compatible with the use of strong bases (e.g., NaOH) as catalysts. A small set of cross-aldol condensation products, including variations in ketone substrates, is illustrated in Scheme 4. Our method provides access to α,β-unsaturated ketones in an efficient manner without the need for excess reagents. While our polymer catalyst was solely designed to control reaction pathways, a side benefit of such polymer catalyst systems is the relative ease of catalyst recycling without further proline addition. In summary, we have developed an aqueous polymer catalyst system that controls the challenging aldol reaction pathways of enolizable aldehydes, a problem that had remained intrinsically unsolved previously. Such control of reaction pathways allows dynamic catalytic processes for the amplification of otherwise unfavorable reactions. Although we have primarily focused on addressing the chemoselectivity problems at this point, studies in progress indicate that stereoselective reactions are achievable using this catalyst system. Ongoing work also suggest that very challenging reactions, such as those involving hindered and unreactive substrates with the generation of quaternary carbon centers, can be developed. Given the large number of transformations that involve enolizable aldehydes as substrates, we anticipate that this catalyst and its polymer or small molecule analogues may be useful in a broad range of new or more efficient syntheses. Overall, the design of macromolecule catalysts that can address fundamental challenges is of both conceptual and practical importance in chemistry.

JOURNAL ARTICLE EXERCISE 3

The science sections on the MCAT include a significant number of passages with experiments. Questions for these passages often ask you to analyze data, read charts and graphs, and come to some reasonable conclusion based on the information they give you. If you don't know how to extract information efficiently and analyze data effectively, you will be at a distinct disadvantage.

There are three "Journal Article Exercises" in this book. In this third and final exercise, you will again be asked to extract information from a journal article and respond to the same generalized questions you encountered before, then complete an MCAT passage based on this article. After that, we'll show you the "correct" information to pull out and the answers to the passage.

And, as before, the goal of these exercises is NOT to learn content from the articles, just to get a little more comfortable reading and extracting information from them.

As a reminder, when reading the article on pages 273–276, you should focus on the introduction to first get an understanding of the premise of the study, then investigate where results are given and what approaches are used to obtain the results as you get a deeper idea of the details. Lastly, read the conclusion for a final takeaway.

Write brief responses to the questions below:

1. What is the purpose of this study?

   _____

   _____

   _____

2. What problem is this study trying to address or solve?

   _____

   _____

   _____

3. What functional groups appear in the molecules being studied?

   _____

   _____

   _____

4. Do any familiar reactions appear in this study?

   _____

   _____

   _____

5. How are the results presented? Tables/graphs/figures?

_____

_____

_____

6. What approaches are presented in this study?

_____

_____

_____

7. What unique terms are provided in the experimental data?

_____

_____

_____

8. What results are found from the experimental data?

_____

_____

_____

9. Are there any unexpected/unexplained results?

_____

_____

_____

10. What final summary of the study and results can you conclude?

_____

_____

_____

Completed responses can be found on pages 282–283.

JOURNAL ARTICLE 3 PASSAGE

The Hajos-Parrish-Eder-Sauer-Wiechert reaction employs proline to catalyze aldol reactions. The results of a recent study to control reaction pathways available via proline-catalyzed aldol reaction of enolizable aldehydes and ketones have been reported. As part of this study the investigators developed a new polymeric catalyst, shown in Figure 1, which employs proline combined with a water-soluble hyperbranched polyethyleneimine (PEI) cocatalyst (cocatalyst 1).

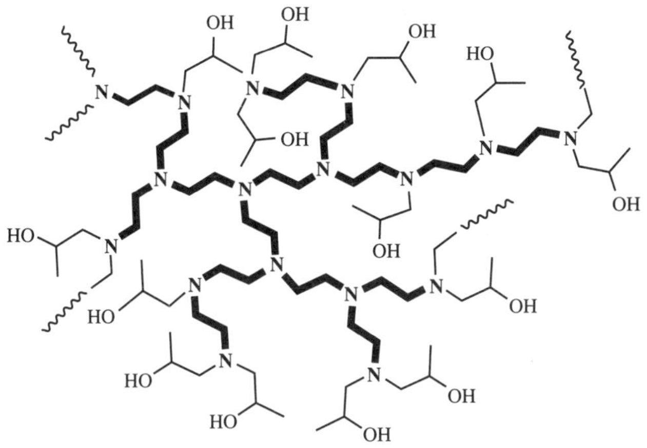

Figure 1   Structure of hyperbranched PEI cocatalyst **1**

Cross-aldol reaction between acetone and *n*-butanal performed in the presence of a complex catalyst composed of proline and cocatalyst **1** at 25°C afforded the products shown in Figure 2.

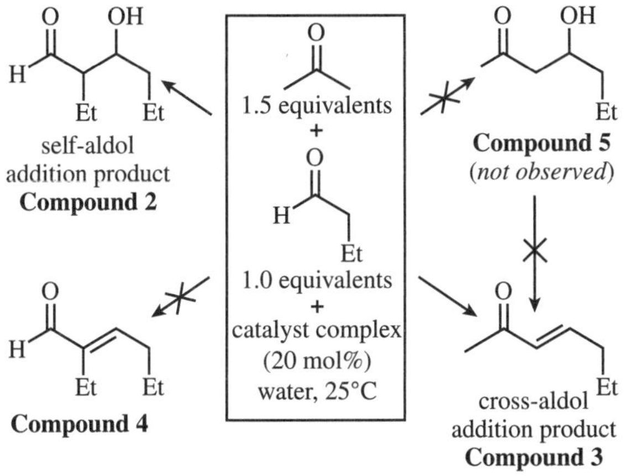

Figure 2   Catalytic aldehyde/cross-ketone aldol reaction

The self-aldol addition product (Compound **2**, Figure 2) was formed as a mixture of diastereomers along with a corresponding cross-aldol condensation product (Compound **3**). The product distribution arising from the reaction shown in Figure 2 as a function of time appears in Figure 3.

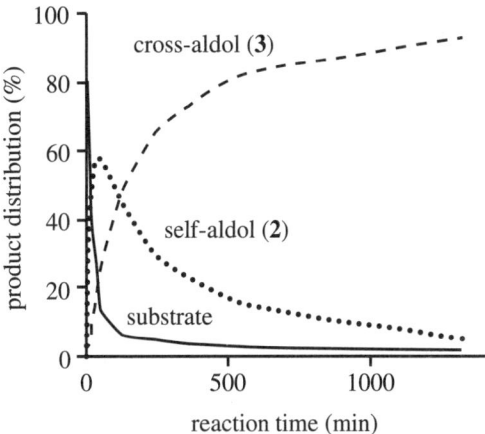

Figure 3   Product distribution in the (proline + **1**) catalyzed *n*-butanal/acetone aldol reaction

Interestingly, two other potential reaction products from the reaction in Figure 2, Compounds **4** and **5**, were not found. In the absence of the hyperbranched PEI cocatalyst, the cross-aldol reaction shown in Figure 2 performed by using only conventional organocatalysts afforded all four products (Compounds **2–5**). To better understand the absence of Compounds **4** and **5** from the aldol reaction depicted in Figure 2, two control experiments were conducted with the following results:

1. When prepared separately by using a literature procedure and then subjected to the catalytic conditions shown in Figure 2, Compound **5** failed to produce the corresponding α,β-unsaturated ketone (**3**).

2. The potential reversibility of formation of the cross-aldol addition reaction shown in Figure 2 was clarified by subjecting pure **3** to the indicated catalytic conditions. The results show that formation of **3** proceeds irreversibly.

1. D-and L-Proline catalyzed aldol condensations have been used to perform a stereocontrolled synthesis of monosaccharides beginning with propanal. The first two steps leading to formation of a key intermediate in this process are summarized below.

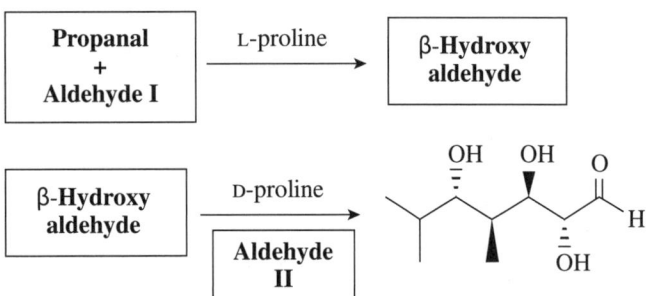

Which of the following offers the most useful combination of aldehydes I and II, respectively, to prepare this key intermediate?

A) 2-Hydroxyacetaldehyde and 2-methylpropanal
B) 2-Hydroxyacetaldehyde and propanal
C) 2-Methylpropanal and 2-hydroxyacetaldehyde
D) Propanal and 2-hydroxyacetaldehyde

2. One model proposed to account for the interaction between proline and the hyperbranched PEI cocatalyst is shown in scheme **A**. Consider a hypothetical enzyme shown in scheme **B** that approximates the shape and hydrophobic properties of the catalytic complex shown in scheme **A**.

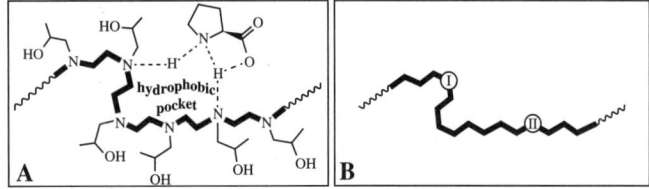

Which pair of amino acid residues (I and II) in the enzyme are most likely to favor formation of a catalytic complex with proline in an aqueous environment?

A) Lys and Met
B) Asp and Leu
C) Phe and Trp
D) Arg and His

3. The self-aldol reaction of *n*-butanal affords Compound **2** as a mixture of diastereomers. Which one of the structures shown below corresponds to the 2*R*,3*S* diastereomer of Compound **2**?

A)

B)

C)

D)

4. Four cross-aldol addition products (W–Z, structures shown below) were isolated from the gross mixture of compounds obtained after workup of a solution of acetone and 2-butanone in 10% aqueous NaOH that had been stirred at ambient temperature during several hours.

Compound W   **Compound X**

Compound Y   **Compound Z**

The proton NMR spectrum of which one of these compounds is expected to display a doublet in the spectral region δ 1.1–1.3?

A) Compound W
B) Compound X
C) Compound Y
D) Compound Z

5. Which one of the following conclusions is most consistent with the results shown in Figure 3?

A) Compound **3** is formed via (proline + **1**) catalyzed aldol reaction between an electron-rich species derived from *n*-butanal and an electron-poor species derived from acetone.
B) Formation of Compound **2** under the reaction conditions shown in Figure 2 occurs irreversibly.
C) The catalytic environment induced by the catalyst complex (proline + **1**) alters the reaction kinetics by disfavoring pathways that lead to formation of the kinetically favored product **2**.
D) The catalytic environment induced by the catalyst complex (proline + **1**) alters the relative stabilities of **2** and **3**, thereby favoring formation of **3**.

SOLUTIONS TO JOURNAL ARTICLE EXERCISE 3

1. **What is the purpose of this study?**
   This study examines a mechanistic approach to controlling the aldol reaction to favor cross-aldol products by employing a modified hyperbranched PEI catalyst.

2. **What problem is this study trying to address or solve?**
   Aldol reactions result in mixtures of self- and cross-aldol products, which is often undesirable. The introduction states that in cross aldehyde/ketone aldol reactions, an excess of ketone and NaOH or proline as a catalyst is required to produce high yields of the cross-aldol product in aqueous solution. This study reports the use of a soluble polymeric catalyst to suppress the self-aldol pathway and encourage cross-aldol products.

3. **What functional groups appear in the molecules being studied?**
   Aldehydes and ketones are substrates used in each Scheme in the article. The β-hydroxy aldehyde/ketone and α,β-unsaturated aldehyde/ketone products formed in aldol reactions are recognizable structures.

   As described in paragraph four, the catalyst used in the aldol reactions performed in this study employ proline, an amino acid. The hyperbranched PEI catalyst is a co-catalyst that complexes with proline to perform the catalytic function observed in this study.

4. **Do any familiar reactions appear in this study?**
   The aldol reaction is the central reaction examined in the article.

   The aldol reaction is an organic reaction important for the MCAT, which uses a base to catalyze the enolization of an aldehyde or ketone, which then nucleophilically attacks the carbonyl carbon of a second aldehyde or ketone molecule. The aldol reaction can follow a self-aldol or a cross-aldol pathway. Self-aldol describes a process whereby two of the same aldehyde/ketone molecules react together. Cross-aldol describes two different aldehydes/ketones reacting together.

   The article states in the third paragraph and shows in Scheme 1 that self-aldol reactions of an enolizable aldehyde can produce a reversible product (a β-hydroxyaldehyde) or an irreversible product (an α,β-unsaturated aldehyde).

   Proline's role as a catalyst is clarified in the second paragraph. Proline serves to form an iminium intermediate in the reversible self-aldol pathway and an enamine intermediate in the irreversible self-aldol condensation pathway. An enamine formation process is therefore important, which considers proline's nitrogen atom as a nucleophile to attack the electrophilic carbonyl carbon atom in the aldehyde reactant.

5. **How are the results presented? Tables/graphs/figures?**
   Tables and graphs. Table 1, Schemes 3 and 4 contain the results obtained in this study.

6. **What approaches are presented in this study?**
   Scheme 2 displays the PEI catalyst that was produced for this study. This water-soluble polymer was designed to "attract proline catalysts via electrostatic interactions," as described in paragraph four.

   Scheme 2 further details how this catalyst complex was then applied to a self-aldol reaction of pentanal in water and in organic solvents, notably DMF. In most aqueous trials, a basic pH of 9 or greater is used for optimal results.

   Scheme 3 outlines a cross-aldol reaction between 1.5 equivalents of acetone and 1 equivalent of butanal with the same catalyst complex.

Scheme 4 outlines a cross-aldol reaction that employs different aldehyde and ketone substrates with variable equivalents used in a range of 1.0–1.5 for the ketone and 1.0 for the aldehyde.

7. **What unique terms are provided in the experimental data?**

Conversion percentage and product selectivity are discussed for products 2 and 3 in the Table 1 results from the self-aldol reaction of pentanal. Conversion percentage is the percentage of reactant molecules converted to products. The passage clarifies in paragraph five that product selectivity reflects the ratio of the two products forming in a ratio of product 3:product 2. Product distribution is presented in the Scheme 3 graph. This graph shows the production of each product as a percentage from the reaction reported in Scheme 3 over time.

Note that the Table 1 caption mentions diastereoselectivity and enantioselectivity. These terms arise for product **3** because it contains two chiral centers and can produce 4 total stereoisomers (meaning any product will have one enantiomer and two diastereomers to consider against it). Enantioselectivity describes the preferential formation of one enantiomer over the other in a reaction and diastereoselectivity is the preferential formation of one diastereomer over another.

8. **What results are found from the experimental data?**

Entries 3 and 4 in Table 1 provide directly comparable results for the reaction in Scheme 2 (self-aldol reaction of pentanal) because they both employ the catalyst complex. Entry 3 indicates that in aqueous solution the self-aldol reaction with pentanal yields the reversible β-hydroxy aldehyde as the major product. Entry 4 indicates that in an organic solvent the same reaction favors the irreversible α,β-unsaturated aldehyde as the major product.

The results from Scheme 3 (cross-aldol reaction of acetone and butanal) indicate a rapid self-aldol reaction of butanal to produce the reversible β-hydroxy aldehyde. However, concomitant decline of this product and production of the irreversible crossed aldol α,β-unsaturated carbonyl product ensues, leading to the irreversible product "in more than 90% yield in 22 hours" as given in paragraph seven.

Leading up to the results shown in Scheme 4, paragraph eight remarks that cross acetone/aldehyde aldol reactions show that as aldehyde hydrophobicity increases a significant decrease in reaction efficiency is observed. This feature can be viewed in the range of products displayed in Scheme 4, with the most hydrophobic (carbon-heavy) structures being those listed with the lower percentage conversion values, such as 11 (g, j, k, p, q).

9. **Are there any unexpected/unexplained results?**

Several results may be considered unexpected/unexplained, including:

- the need for a high pH to encourage reaction selectivity.
- better selectivity in the absence of the catalyst complex, as shown for the results obtained in trials with an organic solvent (Table 1, entries 1 and 4).
- the variation in selectivity indicated for the products shown in Scheme 4, even for those products that show high conversion rates.

10. **What final summary of the study and results can you conclude?**

The methodology reported in this study shows that the use of an aqueous polymeric catalyst in conjunction with proline can allow for control over the aldol reaction. Results indicate that self-aldol reactions with aldehydes can be catalyzed by this method to favor β-hydroxy aldehyde products while cross-aldol condensation reactions can be catalyzed to favor α,β-unsaturated carbonyl compounds.

SOLUTIONS TO JOURNAL ARTICLE EXERCISE 3 PASSAGE

1. **C**   Note that the key intermediate produced from the scheme in this question is a nine-carbon aldehyde; hence, propanal + aldehyde I + aldehyde II must sum to nine carbon atoms. However, answer choices B and D offer reactants that when combined with propanal total only eight carbons (eliminate choices B and D). It is apparent that two successive aldol reactions are required to account for the formation of the key intermediate from the materials offered in each of the four choices. When approaching an organic synthesis problem, it often is helpful to employ a retrosynthetic approach by working backward from the target molecule. In this case, consider the retro-aldol process which requires identification of the α,β C–C sigma bond formed from each aldol addition:

Identifying the σ-bond between C(2) and C(3) in the key intermediate (leftmost structure in the scheme above) and cleaving there, indicates a 7-carbon and a 2-carbon component. Thus, aldehyde II must be a two-carbon aldehyde (i.e., 2-hydroxyacetaldehyde, eliminate choice A). By having identified aldehyde II and by noting that the β-hydroxyaldehyde formed via the first aldol addition must contain seven carbons, it follows that the first aldol reaction must incorporate a four-carbon aldehyde with propanal; thus 2-methylpropanal is aldehyde I (choice C is correct).

2. **D**   Note that the two nitrogen atoms in the PEI backbone (scheme **A**), which participate in electrostatic interactions with proline, are tertiary amines and thus function as hydrogen bond acceptors. It follows that groups in the corresponding positions in the enzyme should provide a similar function to form a catalytic complex with proline. In choice A, Lys contains a primary amine side chain while Met contains a side chain sulfur atom that cannot function effectively as a hydrogen bond acceptor (eliminate choice A). In choice B, Asp contains a carboxyl group in its side chain, which either in its protonated form or as the corresponding carboxylate anion contains oxygen atoms that are effective hydrogen bond acceptors. However, Leu offers only a hydrophobic hydrocarbon side chain, which cannot participate in hydrogen bonding. Similarly in choice C, both Phe and Trp contain hydrophobic side chains (eliminate choices B and C). Recall that Arg and His each contain a basic side chain that can function as a hydrogen bond acceptor, making choice D the best response.

3. **B**   Note that Compound **2** in the passage contains two adjacent chiral centers, which are displayed in the four choices as Newman projections. The choices offered thus constitute the four possible diastereomers of this compound. To manage time efficiently in this question, it is advised to solve it as a 2x2 question. For example, notice that the C(2) atom, the background

carbon in each Newman projection, is drawn the same in choices A and C, while choices B and D are also drawn the same as each other. By applying Cahn-Ingold-Prelog (CIP) rules first to one diastereomer and then to other choices, the choices can be narrowed down quickly. Starting with the C(2) atom (the background carbon) in choice A, CIP priorities follow the order O=CH > C(3) > Et > H (see diagram below). By looking down the bond of lowest priority (i.e., the C—H bond), the order of priorities is seen to produce a counterclockwise trace. Thus, C(2) in choice A possesses the 2S configuration, as does the corresponding carbon atom in choice C (eliminate choices A and C).

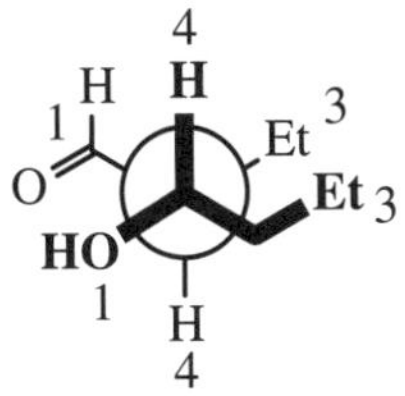

Choice A

Similar analysis of C(3) in choice A, the carbon in the foreground of the Newman projection, leads to the conclusion that this carbon atom possesses the S configuration. Eliminate choice D, which must possess the 3R configuration. This leaves only choice B, which corresponds to the 2R,3S form of Compound **2**.

4. **B** The proton NMR spectral region of interest is associated with a proton located upfield and thus is well-removed from electron-withdrawing groups, e.g., C=O or OH, present elsewhere in the molecule. All four compounds contain CH_3 and/or CH_2 functionalities that meet this criterion. However, only Compound X contains a methyl group adjacent to a C—H proton, which can account for the appearance of a doublet splitting pattern.

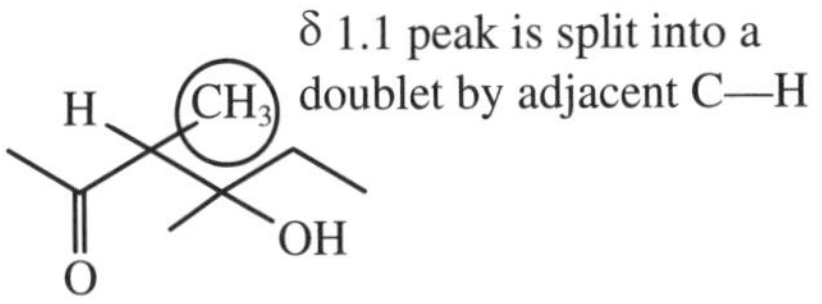

Compound X

5. **C** As this question requires interpretation of various details given in the passage, it is best to proceed by process of elimination. First, in choice A it is instructive to apply a retro-aldol approach to identifying the new C—C σ-bond formed via the cross-aldol addition reaction that results in **3** (see below). Therein it can be seen that acetone provides the electron-rich enolate component whereas *n*-butanal serves as the electron-poor component of the (forward) cross-aldol addition reaction. This demonstrates the exact opposite of the statement appearing in choice A (eliminate choice A).

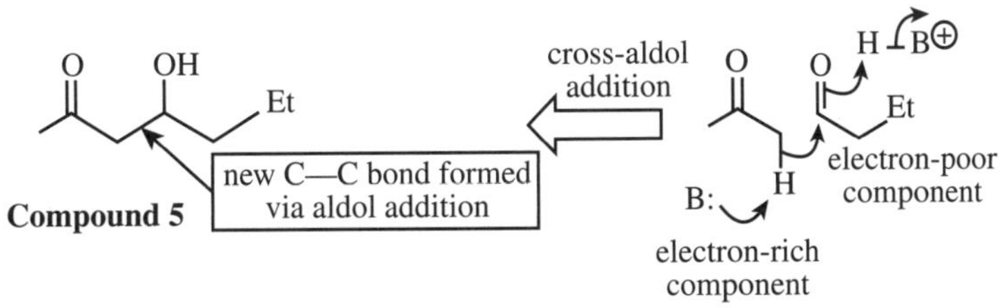

When considering choice B, examination of the product distribution vs. time plot in Figure 3 reveals that the self-aldol reaction leading to the formation of Compound **2** occurs much faster than the corresponding cross-aldol reaction that affords **3**. However, Compound **2** slowly disappears over time as production of Compound **3** increases.

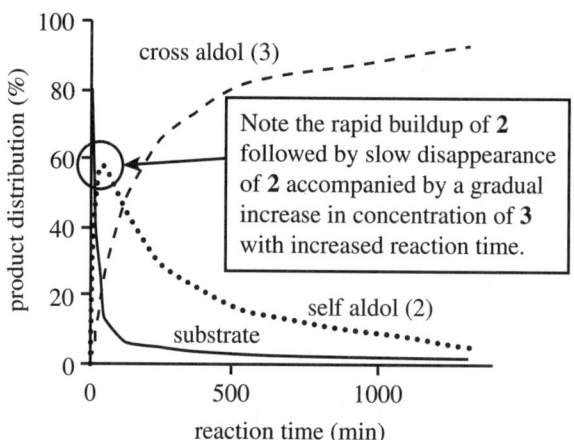

The time-dependent behavior shown in the plot suggests that initial formation of **2** proceeds both rapidly and reversibly. Recall the results of a control experiment described in the passage, which concluded that formation of **3** proceeds irreversibly. As the reaction progresses, irreversible conversion of **2** to **3** occurs, resulting in a shift of the initial equilibrium to the right in accordance with Le Châtelier's principle. It follows that the conclusion stated in choice B, i.e., that **2** is formed irreversibly, is incorrect (eliminate choice B).

When considering choice C, note that the plot shown in Figure 3 indicates that the catalytic environment induced by the catalyst complex (proline + **1**) alters the reaction kinetics by disfavoring pathways that lead to formation of **2**. It should be noted that inclusion of the polymeric catalyst permits preferential formation of the *kinetically disfavored* cross-aldol product (**3**) thereby attesting to the ability of this methodology to exert dynamic control over competing aldol reaction pathways in an aqueous environment (choice C is correct).

Lastly, applying knowledge of the differences between kinetic and thermodynamic processes is useful in considering choice D. Catalysis is a kinetic phenomenon, which affects the rate of a given reaction and/or the relative rates of competing reactions. The stabilities of reactants and products are not affected by the presence of a catalyst (eliminate choice D).

Organic Chemistry Glossary

After each entry, the section number in *MCAT Organic Chemistry Review* where the term is discussed is given.

1,3-diaxial interaction
A destabilizing interaction between substituents that occupy axial positions on the same side of a cyclohexane ring. **[Section 4.2]**

achiral
A molecule that is superimposable on its mirror image. **[Section 4.2]**

aldehyde
A functional group where a carbonyl is attached to one carbon group and one hydrogen. **[Section 6.2]**

aldol condensation
A reaction in which the enolate anion of one carbonyl reacts with the carbonyl of another compound. **[Section 6.2]**

alkanes
Saturated hydrocarbons of the form C_nH_{2n+2}. **[Section 3.3]**

amphipathic
A molecule that is both hydrophilic and hydrophobic. **[Section 6.3]**

anomers
Epimers formed by ring closure. **[Section 4.2]**

***anti* conformation**
A conformation in which the two largest groups are 180° apart. **[Section 4.2]**

axial
A substituent orientation on rings where the group is pointed up or down, perpendicular to the plane of the ring. **[Section 4.2]**

Benedict's test
A test to detect aldehydes, ketones, and hemiacetals in sugars. **[Section 7.3]**

boiling point
The temperature at which a compound changes from a liquid into a gas. **[Section 5.1]**

Cahn-Ingold-Prelog rules
A set of rules for assigning absolute configuration to a stereocenter. **[Section 4.2]**

carbanions
Negatively charged species with a negative formal charge on carbon. **[Section 4.1]**

carbocations or carbonium ions
Positively charged species with a positive formal charge on carbon. **[Section 4.1]**

carbohydrate
A chain of hydrated carbon atoms with the molecular formula $C_nH_{2n}O_n$. **[Section 7.3]**

chair conformation
The most stable conformation of cyclohexane. **[Section 4.2]**

chemical shift
The location of a resonance in an NMR spectrum. **[Section 5.2]**

chiral
A molecule that cannot be superimposed on its mirror image is chiral. Most frequently this refers to an sp^3 hybridized carbon with four different groups attached to it. **[Section 4.2]**

cis
Substituents on the same side of a double bond or ring. **[Section 4.2]**

conformational isomers
Any compounds that have the same molecular formula and the same connectivity but that differ from one another by rotation about a σ bond. **[Section 4.2]**

constitutional isomers
Any compounds with the same molecular formula but whose atoms have different connectivity. **[Section 4.2]**

degree of unsaturation
A degree of unsaturation is either one ring or one π bond in a molecule. [**Section 4.1**]

delocalized
Electron density that is spread over multiple atoms is said to be delocalized. [**Section 4.1**]

diastereomers
Stereoisomers that are not enantiomers. [**Section 4.2**]

disaccharide
Two monosaccharides bonded together. [**Section 7.3**]

distillation
A purification method based on a difference in boiling points. [**Section 5.1**]

disulfide bonds
A sulfur-sulfur bond between two cysteines that stabilizes protein structure. [**Section 7.2**]

(E)-alkenes
Alkenes where the two higher priority groups are on the opposite side of the double bond. [**Section 4.2**]

electron-donating groups
Groups that push (donate) electron density toward another functional group through σ or π bonds. [**Section 4.1**]

electron-withdrawing groups
Groups that pull (withdraw) electron density toward themselves through σ or π bonds. [**Section 4.1**]

electrophiles
Electrophiles ("electron loving") are electron-deficient and typically react with nucleophiles by accepting electrons. [**Section 4.1**]

enantiomers
Molecules that are mirror images and non-superimposable. [**Section 4.2**]

enolate ion
A resonance-stabilized anion resulting from the deprotonation of a carbon atom adjacent to a carbonyl functional group. [**Section 6.2**]

epimers
Diastereomers that differ in configuration at only one of many chiral centers. [**Section 4.2**]

equatorial
A substituent orientation on rings where the group is pointed away from the center of the ring. [**Section 4.2**]

extraction
A separation technique that relies on relative solubilities of the two solvents used. [**Section 5.1**]

gas chromatography
A method that separates compounds based on their volatilities. [**Section 5.1**]

gauche conformation
A conformation in which the two largest groups are 60° apart when viewed in a Newman projection. [**Section 4.2**]

geometric isomers
Diastereomers that differ in orientation of substituents around a ring or double bond. [**Section 4.2**]

glycosidic linkage
The bond between two saccharides. [**Section 7.3**]

half-chair conformation
The high-energy intermediate conformation of cyclohexane as it converts from one chair conformation into the other. [**Section 4.2**]

hybrid orbitals
Hybrid orbitals are a mathematical combination of atomic orbitals centered on the same atom. The total number of orbitals is conserved in their formation (i.e., the number of atomic orbitals equals the number of hybrid orbitals). [**Section 4.1**]

hydrophilic
Literally "water loving." [Section 7.4]

hydrophobic
Literally "water fearing." [Section 7.4]

imine formation
A reaction between an aldehyde or ketone and a primary amine to form an imine. [Section 6.2]

inductive effect
The sharing of electrons through σ bonds. [Section 4.1]

infrared spectroscopy
A method that detects the vibrations of covalent bonds and can differentiate their frequencies, which is related to the type of bond. [Section 5.2]

isomers
Any compounds that have the same molecular formula. [Section 4.2]

ketone
A functional group in which a carbonyl is attached to two carbon groups. [Section 6.2]

lipase
Enzymes that hydrolyze fats. [Section 7.4]

lipid bilayer
A double layer of lipids in which the polar groups line the outside and the non-polar tails compose the inside. [Section 7.4]

lipids
Oily or fatty substances that are part of cellular membranes (phospholipids), can store energy as triglycerides (in adipose cells), and can serve as the building block for steroid hormones (cholesterol). [Section 7.4]

localized
Electrons that are confined to one orbital, either a bonding orbital or a lone-pair orbital. [Section 4.1]

melting point
The temperature at which a compound changes from a solid into a liquid. [Section 5.1]

meso
A molecule that contains chiral centers and an internal plane of symmetry. [Section 4.2]

monosaccharide
Literally a "single sweet unit," also known as a simple sugar (e.g., fructose, glucose, etc.). [Section 7.3]

mutarotation
Interconversion between anomers. [Section 7.3]

nucleophile
Nucleophiles ("nucleus loving") have an unshared pair of electrons or a π bond and react with electrophiles by donating these electrons. [Section 4.1]

nucleotides
The building blocks of nucleic acids. [Section 7.5]

oligosaccharide
Several monosaccharides bonded together. [Section 7.3]

optically active
Compounds that rotate the plane of polarized light are optically active. A pair of enantiomers will rotate the plane of polarized light in equal, but opposite directions. [Section 4.2]

peptide bond
The bond that links amino acids together formed between the carboxyl group of one amino acid and the amino group of another. [Section 7.2]

pi (π) bonds
A π bond consists of two electrons localized above and below a nodal plane; π bonds are formed from overlap of two unhybridized p orbitals on adjacent atoms. [Section 4.1]

polysaccharide
Many monosaccharides bonded together.
[Section 7.3]

protease
A protein enzyme that performs proteolysis.
[Section 7.2]

proteolysis
Hydrolysis of a protein by another protein.
[Section 7.2]

racemic mixture
An equal mixture of two enantiomers is said to be racemic; racemic mixtures do not rotate the plane of polarized light because one enantiomer cancels out the rotation of the other. **[Section 4.2]**

resonance
The sharing of electrons through π bonds.
[Section 4.1]

ring strain
Instability due to deviation of bond angles from optimal geometry. **[Section 4.1]**

saponification
The hydrolysis of esters by treatment with a basic solution. **[Section 7.4]**

saturated
A molecule is saturated if it contains no π bonds and no rings. **[Section 4.1]**

sigma (σ) bonds
A σ bond consists of two electrons localized between two nuclei; σ bonds are formed by overlap of two hybridized orbitals. **[Section 4.1]**

stereoisomers
Any compounds with the same molecular formula and connectivity, that differ only in the spatial arrangement of atoms, are known as stereoisomers. Note that if the compounds only differ by rotation around a sigma bond, they are not stereoisomers but *conformational* isomers.
[Section 4.2]

tautomers
Readily interconvertible constitutional isomers.
[Section 6.2]

thin-layer chromatography (TLC)
A rapid technique used to separate compounds based on their polarity. **[Section 5.1]**

trans
Substituents on opposite sides of a double bond or ring. **[Section 4.2]**

twist boat conformation
The local energy minimum for cyclohexane as it converts from one chair conformation to the other. **[Section 4.2]**

unsaturated
A molecule is unsaturated if it contains at least one π bond or ring. **[Section 4.1]**

van der Waals forces
A general term for intermolecular forces, often used to describe London dispersion forces: forces between temporary dipoles formed in nonpolar molecules formed because of a temporary asymmetric electron distribution. **[Section 5.1]**

wavenumber
The reciprocal of wavelength, expressed in reciprocal centimeters (cm^{-1}). **[Section 5.2]**

(Z)-alkenes
Alkenes in which the two high priority groups are on the same side of the double bond.
[Section 4.2]

zwitterion
A molecule with both positive and negative formal charges. **[Section 7.1]**

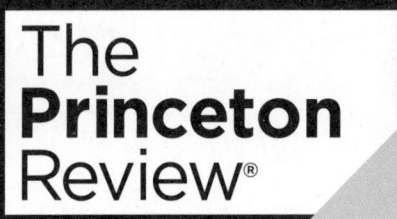
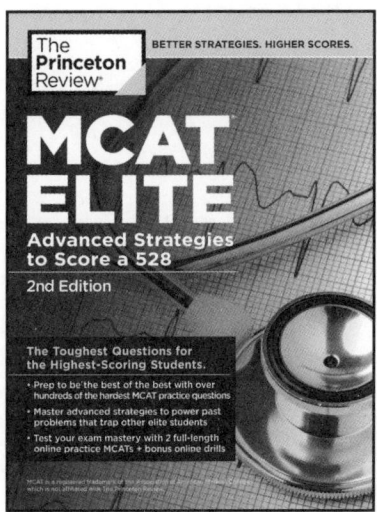
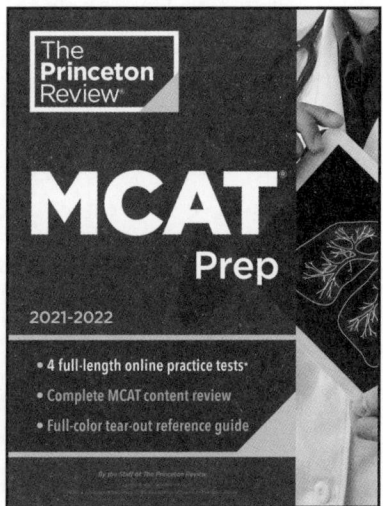
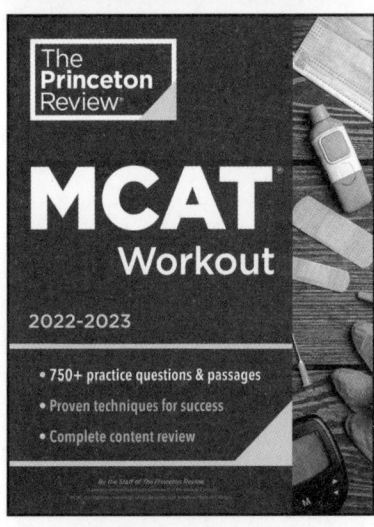
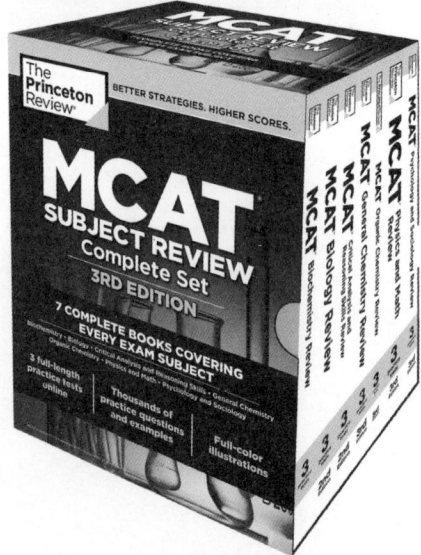

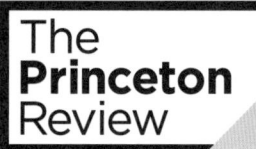

MCAT®

Psychology and Sociology Review

4th Edition

The Staff of The Princeton Review

Penguin
Random
House

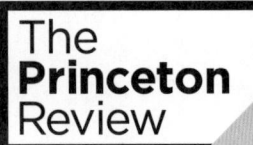

The Princeton Review
110 E. 42nd Street
New York, NY 10017

Published in the United States by Penguin Random
House LLC, New York, and in Canada by Random House
of Canada, a division of Penguin Random House Ltd.,
Toronto.

The material in this book is up-to-date at the time of
publication. However, changes may have been instituted by the testing body in the test after this book was
published.

If there are any important late-breaking developments,
changes, or corrections to the materials in this book, we
will post that information online in the Student Tools.
Register your book and check your Student Tools to see
if there are any updates posted there.

ISBN: 978-0-593-51622-5
ISSN: 2332-8495

MCAT is a registered trademark of the Association of
American Medical Colleges.

The Princeton Review is not affiliated with Princeton
University.

Editor: Patricia Murphy
Production Artist: Jennifer Chapman
Production Editor: Sarah Litt and Liz Dacey

Manufactured in China.

10 9 8 7 6 5 4 3 2 1

4th Edition

The Princeton Review Publishing Team
Rob Franek, Editor-in-Chief
David Soto, Senior Director, Data Operations
Stephen Koch, Senior Manager, Data Operations
Deborah Weber, Director of Production
Jason Ullmeyer, Production Design Manager
Jennifer Chapman, Senior Production Artist
Selena Coppock, Director of Editorial
Aaron Riccio, Senior Editor
Meave Shelton, Senior Editor
Chris Chimera, Editor
Orion McBean, Editor
Patricia Murphy, Editor
Laura Rose, Editor
Alexa Schmitt Bugler, Editorial Assistant

Random House Publishing Team
Tom Russell, VP, Publisher
Alison Stoltzfus, Senior Director, Publishing
Brett Wright, Senior Editor
Emily Hoffman, Assistant Managing Editor
Ellen Reed, Production Manager
Suzanne Lee, Designer
Eugenia Lo, Publishing Assistant

For customer service, please contact
editorialsupport@review.com,
and be sure to include:

- full title of the book

- ISBN

- page number

CONTRIBUTORS

Nadia L. Johnson, M.A., M.S.
        Senior Author
Rizwan Ahmad, M.A.
        Senior Author
Tomislav Kurtović, M.A.
        Senior Author

TPR MCAT Psychology and Sociology Team:

Matthew Dempsey, Ph.D., Lead Developer and Senior Editor
Christine Lindwall, M.A., J.D.

Edited for Production by:

Judene Wright, M.S., M.A.Ed.
        National Content Director, MCAT Program, The Princeton Review

The TPR MCAT Psychology and Sociology Team and Judene would like to thank the following people for their contributions to this book :

Erika C. Castro, B.A., Maria S. Chushak, M.S., Guenevieve O. del Mundo, B.A., B.S., C.C.S., Jon Fowler, M.A., Michelle E. Fox, B.S., Kevin Keogh, Anthony Krupp, Ph.D., Christine Lindwall, M.A., J.D., Ali Landreau, B.A., Toni Lupro, Mike Matera, Jennifer A. McDevitt, Paola A. Munoz , M.A., B.A., Jonathan Nasrallah, Bikem Ayse Polat, Shalom Shapiro, Andrew D. Snyder, M.S., M.A., Gordy Steil, M.A., M.F.T., David Stoll, Chelsea K. Wise, M.S., Alexandra Vinson, Betsy Walli, M.S., Ph.D.

JOURNAL ARTICLE PERMISSIONS

PERIODIC TABLE OF THE ELEMENTS

1	2	3	4	5	6	7	8	9	10	11	12	13	14	15	16	17	18
1 **H** 1.0																	2 **He** 4.0
3 **Li** 6.9	4 **Be** 9.0											5 **B** 10.8	6 **C** 12.0	7 **N** 14.0	8 **O** 16.0	9 **F** 19.0	10 **Ne** 20.2
11 **Na** 23.0	12 **Mg** 24.3											13 **Al** 27.0	14 **Si** 28.1	15 **P** 31.0	16 **S** 32.1	17 **Cl** 35.5	18 **Ar** 39.9
19 **K** 39.1	20 **Ca** 40.1	21 **Sc** 45.0	22 **Ti** 47.9	23 **V** 50.9	24 **Cr** 52.0	25 **Mn** 54.9	26 **Fe** 55.8	27 **Co** 58.9	28 **Ni** 58.7	29 **Cu** 63.5	30 **Zn** 65.4	31 **Ga** 69.7	32 **Ge** 72.6	33 **As** 74.9	34 **Se** 79.0	35 **Br** 79.9	36 **Kr** 83.8
37 **Rb** 85.5	38 **Sr** 87.6	39 **Y** 88.9	40 **Zr** 91.2	41 **Nb** 92.9	42 **Mo** 95.9	43 **Tc** (98)	44 **Ru** 101.1	45 **Rh** 102.9	46 **Pd** 106.4	47 **Ag** 107.9	48 **Cd** 112.4	49 **In** 114.8	50 **Sn** 118.7	51 **Sb** 121.8	52 **Te** 127.6	53 **I** 126.9	54 **Xe** 131.3
55 **Cs** 132.9	56 **Ba** 137.3	57 ***La** 138.9	72 **Hf** 178.5	73 **Ta** 180.9	74 **W** 183.9	75 **Re** 186.2	76 **Os** 190.2	77 **Ir** 192.2	78 **Pt** 195.1	79 **Au** 197.0	80 **Hg** 200.6	81 **Tl** 204.4	82 **Pb** 207.2	83 **Bi** 209.0	84 **Po** (209)	85 **At** (210)	86 **Rn** (222)
87 **Fr** (223)	88 **Ra** (226)	89 **†Ac** (227)	104 **Rf** (267)	105 **Db** (268)	106 **Sg** (271)	107 **Bh** (270)	108 **Hs** (269)	109 **Mt** (278)	110 **Ds** (281)	111 **Rg** (282)	112 **Cn** (285)	113 **Nh** (286)	114 **Fl** (289)	115 **Mc** (289)	116 **Lv** (293)	117 **Ts** (294)	118 **Og** (294)

*Lanthanoids

58 **Ce** 140.1	59 **Pr** 140.9	60 **Nd** 144.2	61 **Pm** (145)	62 **Sm** 150.4	63 **Eu** 152.0	64 **Gd** 157.3	65 **Tb** 158.9	66 **Dy** 162.5	67 **Ho** 164.9	68 **Er** 167.3	69 **Tm** 168.9	70 **Yb** 173.0	71 **Lu** 175.0

†Actinoids

90 **Th** 232.0	91 **Pa** (231)	92 **U** 238.0	93 **Np** (237)	94 **Pu** (244)	95 **Am** (243)	96 **Cm** (247)	97 **Bk** (247)	98 **Cf** (251)	99 **Es** (252)	100 **Fm** (257)	101 **Md** (258)	102 **No** (259)	103 **Lr** (266)

CONTENTS

CONTENTS

Get More (**Free**) Content
at **PrincetonReview.com/prep**

As easy as **1·2·3**

1 Go to PrincetonReview.com/prep or scan the **QR code** and enter the following ISBN for your book: **9780593516225**

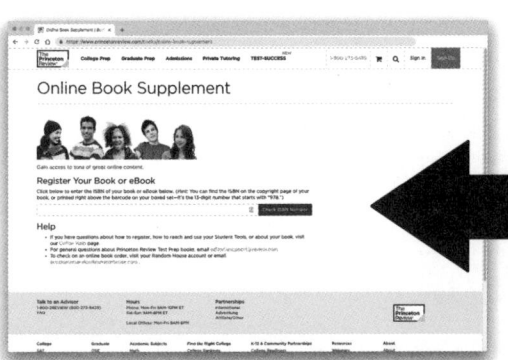

2 Answer a few simple questions to set up an exclusive Princeton Review account. *(If you already have one, you can just log in.)*

3 Enjoy access to your **FREE** content!

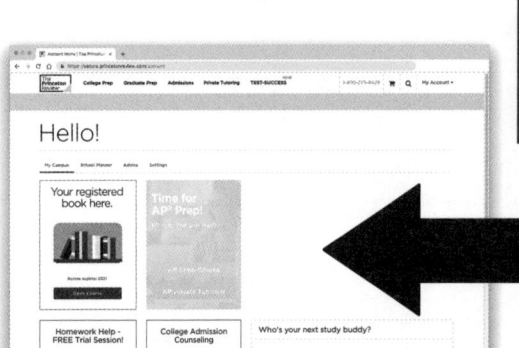

Once you've registered, you can...

- Take **3** full-length practice MCAT exams

- Find useful information about taking the MCAT and applying to medical school

- Check to see if there have been any corrections or updates to this edition

- Get our take on any recent or pending updates to the MCAT

Need to report a potential **content** issue?

Contact **EditorialSupport@review.com** and include:

- full title of the book
- ISBN
- page number

Need to report a **technical** issue?

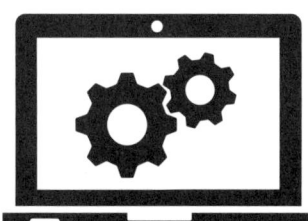

Contact **TPRStudentTech@review.com** and provide:

- your full name
- email address used to register the book
- full book title and ISBN
- Operating system (Mac/PC) and browser (Firefox, Safari, etc.)

Chapter 1
MCAT Basics

SO YOU WANT TO BE A DOCTOR.

So...you want to be a doctor. If you're like most premeds, you've wanted to be a doctor since you were pretty young. When people asked you what you wanted to be when you grew up, you always answered "a doctor." You had toy medical kits, you bandaged up your dog or cat, and you played "hospital." You probably read your parents' home medical guides for fun.

When you got to high school you took the honors and AP classes. You studied hard, got straight As (or at least really good grades!), and participated in extracurricular activities so you could get into a good college. And you succeeded!

At college you knew exactly what to do. You took your classes seriously, studied hard, and got a great GPA. You talked to your professors and hung out at office hours to get good letters of recommendation. You were a member of the premed society on campus, volunteered at hospitals, and shadowed doctors. All that's left to do now is get a good MCAT score.

Just the MCAT.

Just the most confidence-shattering, most demoralizing, longest and most brutal entrance exam for any graduate program. At about 7.5 hours (including breaks), the MCAT tops the list...even the closest runners-up, the LSAT and GMAT, are only about 4 hours long. The MCAT tests significant science content knowledge along with the ability to think quickly, reason logically, and read comprehensively, all under the pressure of a timed exam.

The path to a good MCAT score is not as easy to see as the path to a good GPA or the path to a good letter of recommendation. The MCAT is less about what you know, and more about how to apply what you know...and how to apply it quickly to new situations. Because the path might not be so clear, you might be worried. That's why you picked up this book.

We promise to demystify the MCAT for you, with clear descriptions of the different sections, how the test is scored, and what the test experience is like. We will help you understand general test-taking techniques as well as provide you with specific techniques for each section. We will review the science content you need to know as well as give you an overview of the Psychology/Sociology section of the MCAT. We'll show you the path to a good MCAT score and help you walk the path.

After all...you want to be a doctor. And we want you to succeed.

WHAT IS THE MCAT...REALLY?

Most test-takers approach the MCAT as though it were a typical college science test, one in which facts and knowledge simply need to be regurgitated in order to do well. They study for the MCAT the same way they did for their college tests, by memorizing facts and details, formulas and equations. And when they get to the MCAT, they are surprised...and disappointed.

It's a myth that the MCAT is purely a content-knowledge test. If medical school admission committees want to see what you know, all they have to do is look at your transcripts. What they really want to see, is how you *think*, especially how you think under pressure. That's what your MCAT score will tell them.

The MCAT is really a test of your ability to apply basic knowledge to different, possibly new, situations. It's a test of your ability to reason out and evaluate arguments. Do you still need to know your science content? Absolutely. But not at the level that most test-takers think they need to know it. Furthermore, your science knowledge won't help you on the Critical Analysis and Reasoning Skills (CARS) section. So how do you study for a test like this?

You study for the science sections by reviewing the basics and then applying them to MCAT practice questions. You study for the Psychology and Sociology section of the MCAT by reading this book, and by studying the people, and world, around you.

The book you are holding will review all the relevant MCAT Psychology and Sociology content you will need for the test, and a little bit more. Plus, it includes questions designed to make you think about the material in a deeper way, along with full explanations to clarify the logical thought process needed to get to the answer. It also comes with access to three full-length online practice exams to further hone your skills. For more information on accessing those online exams, please refer to the "Get More (Free) Content" spread on page viii.

MCAT NUTS AND BOLTS

Overview

The MCAT is a computer-based test (CBT) that is *not* adaptive. Adaptive tests base your next question on whether or not you've answered the current question correctly. The MCAT is *linear*, or *fixed-form*, meaning that the questions are in a predetermined order and do not change based on your answers. However, there are many versions of the test, so that on a given test day, different people will see different versions. The following table highlights the features of the MCAT exam.

Registration	Online via www.aamc.org. Begins as early as six months prior to test date; available up until week of test (subject to seat availability).
Testing Centers	Administered at small, secure, climate-controlled computer testing rooms.
Security	Photo ID with signature, electronic fingerprint, electronic signature verification, assigned seat.
Proctoring	None. Test administrator checks examinee in and assigns seat at computer. All testing instructions are given on the computer.
Frequency of Test	Many times per year distributed over January, April, May, June, July, August, and September.
Format	Exclusively computer-based. NOT an adaptive test.
Length of Test Day	7.5 hours
Breaks	Optional 10-minute breaks between sections, with a 30-minute break for lunch.
Section Names	1. Chemical and Physical Foundations of Biological Systems (Chem/Phys) 2. Critical Analysis and Reasoning Skills (CARS) 3. Biological and Biochemical Foundations of Living Systems (Bio/Biochem) 4. Psychological, Social, and Biological Foundations of Behavior (Psych/Soc)
Number of Questions and Timing	59 Chem/Phys questions, 95 minutes 53 CARS questions, 90 minutes 59 Bio/Biochem questions, 95 minutes 59 Psych/Soc questions, 95 minutes
Scoring	Test is scaled. Several forms per administration.
Allowed/ Not allowed	No timers/watches. Noise reduction headphones available. Noteboard booklet and wet-erase marker given at start of test and taken at end of test. Locker or secure area provided for personal items.
Results: Timing and Delivery	Approximately 30 days. Electronic scores only, available online through AAMC login. Examinees can print official score reports.
Maximum Number of Retakes	The MCAT can be taken a maximum of three times in one year, four times over two years, and seven times over the lifetime of the examinee. An examinee can be registered for only one date at a time.

Registration

Registration for the exam is completed online at www.aamc.org/students/applying/mcat/reserving. The AAMC opens registration for a given test date at least two months in advance of the date, often earlier. It's a good idea to register well in advance of your desired test date to make sure that you get a seat.

Sections

There are four sections on the MCAT, all of which consist of multiple-choice questions:

Section	Concepts Tested	Number of Questions and Timing
Chemical and Physical Foundations of Biological Systems (Chem/Phys)	Basic concepts in chemistry and physics, including biochemistry, scientific inquiry, reasoning, research and statistics skills.	59 questions in 95 minutes
Critical Analysis and Reasoning Skills (CARS)	Critical analysis of information drawn from a wide range of social science and humanities disciplines.	53 questions in 90 minutes
Biological and Biochemical Foundations of Living Systems (Bio/Biochem)	Basic concepts in biology and biochemistry, scientific inquiry, reasoning, research and statistics skills.	59 questions in 95 minutes
Psychological, Social, and Biological Foundations of Behavior (Psych/Soc)	Basic concepts in psychology, sociology, and biology, research methods and statistics.	59 questions in 95 minutes

Most questions on the MCAT (44 in the science sections, all 53 in the CARS section) are passage-based; the science sections have 10 passages each and the CARS section has 9. A passage consists of a few paragraphs of information on which several following questions are based. In the science sections, passages often include graphs, figures, and experiments to analyze. CARS passages come from literature in the social sciences, humanities, ethics, philosophy, cultural studies, and population health, and they do not test content knowledge in any way.

Some questions in the science sections are freestanding questions (FSQs). These questions are independent of any passage information and appear in four groups of about four to five questions interspersed throughout the passages. About 15 of the questions in the sciences sections are freestanding, and the remainder are passage-based.

Each section on the MCAT is separated by either a 10-minute break or a 30-minute lunch break:

Section	Time
Test Center Check-In	Variable, can take up to 40 minutes if center is busy.
Tutorial	10 minutes
Chemical and Physical Foundations of Biological Systems	95 minutes
Break (optional)	10 minutes
Critical Analysis and Reasoning Skills	90 minutes
Lunch Break (optional)	30 minutes
Biological and Biochemical Foundations of Living Systems	95 minutes
Break (optional)	10 minutes
Psychological, Social, and Biological Foundations of Behavior	95 minutes
Void Option	5 minutes
Survey (optional)	5 minutes

The survey includes questions about your satisfaction with the overall MCAT experience, including registration, check-in, etc., as well as questions about how you prepared for the test.

Scoring

The MCAT is a scaled exam, meaning that your raw score will be converted into a scaled score that takes into account the difficulty of the questions. There is no guessing penalty. All sections are scored from 118–132, with a total scaled score range of 472–528. Because different versions of the test have varying levels of difficulty, the scale will be different from one exam to the next. Thus, there is no "magic number" of questions to get right in order to get a particular score. Plus, some of the questions on the test are considered "experimental" and do not count toward your score; they are just there to be evaluated for possible future inclusion in a test.

At the end of the test (after you complete the Psychological, Social, and Biological Foundations of Behavior section), you will be asked to choose one of the following two options, "I wish to have my MCAT exam scored" or "I wish to VOID my MCAT exam." You have five minutes to make a decision, and if you do not select one of the options in that time, the test will automatically be scored. If you choose the VOID option, your test will not be scored (you will not now, or ever, get a numerical score for this test), medical schools will not know you took the test, and no refunds will be granted. You cannot "unvoid" your scores at a later time.

So, what's a good score? The AAMC is centering the scale at 500 (i.e., 500 will be the 50th percentile), and recommends that application committees consider applicants near the center of the range. To be on the safe side, aim for a total score of around 510. Remember that if your GPA is on the low side, you'll need higher MCAT scores to compensate, and if you have a strong GPA, you can get away with lower MCAT scores. But the reality is that your chances of acceptance depend on a lot more than just your MCAT scores. It's a combination of your GPA, MCAT scores, undergraduate coursework, letters of recommendation, experience related to the medical field (such as volunteer work or research), extracurricular activities, your personal statement, and so on. Medical schools are looking for a complete package, not just good scores and a good GPA.

GENERAL LAYOUT AND TEST-TAKING STRATEGIES

Layout of the Test

In each section of the test, the computer screen is divided vertically, with the passage on the left and the range of questions for that passage indicated above (e.g., "Passage 1 Questions 1–5"). The scroll bar for the passage text appears in the middle of the screen. Each question appears on the right, and you need to click "Next" to move to each subsequent question.

In the science sections, the freestanding questions are found in groups of 4–5, interspersed with the passages. The screen is still divided vertically; on the left is the statement "Questions [X–XX] do not refer to a passage and are independent of each other," and each question appears on the right as described above.

CBT Tools

There are a number of tools available on the test, including highlighting, strike-outs, the Flag for Review button, the Navigation and Review Screen buttons, the Periodic Table button, and of course, the noteboard booklet. All tools are available with both mouse control (buttons to click) or keyboard commands (Alt+ a letter). As everyone has different preferences, you should practice with both types of tools (mouse and keyboard) to see which is more comfortable for you personally. The following is a brief description of each tool.

1) **Highlighting:** This is done in the passage text (including table entries and some equations, but excluding figures and molecular structures), in the question stems, and in the answer choices (including Roman numerals). Select the words you wish to highlight (left-click and drag the cursor across the words), and in the upper left corner click the "Highlight" button to highlight the selected text yellow. Alternatively, press "Alt+H" to highlight the words. Highlighting can be removed by selecting the words again and in the upper left corner clicking the down arrow next to "Highlight." This will expand to show the "Remove Highlight" option; clicking this will remove the highlighting. Removing highlighting via the keyboard is cumbersome and is not recommended.

2) **Strike-outs:** This can be done on the answer choices, including Roman numeral statements, by selecting the text you want to strike out (left-click and drag the cursor across the text), then clicking the "Strikethrough" button in the upper left corner. Alternatively, press "Alt+S" to strikeout the words. The strike-out can be removed by repeating these actions. Figures or molecular structures cannot be struck out, however, the letter answer choice of those structures can.

3) **Flag for Review button:** This is available for each question and is found in the upper right corner. This allows you to flag the question as one you would like to review later if time permits. When clicked, the flag icon turns yellow. Click again to remove the flag. Alternatively, press "Alt+F."

4) **Navigation button:** This is found near the bottom of the screen and is only available on your first pass through the section. Clicking this button brings up a navigation table listing all questions and their statuses (unseen, incomplete, complete, flagged for review). You can also press "Alt+V" to bring up the screen. The questions can be sorted by their statuses, and clicking a question number takes you immediately to that question. Once you have reached the end of the section and viewed the Review screen (described below), the Navigation screen is no longer available.

5) **Review Screen button:** This button is found near the bottom of the screen after your first pass through the section and, when clicked, brings up a new screen showing all questions and their statuses (either incomplete, unseen, or flagged for review). Questions that are complete are assigned no additional status. You can then choose one of three options by clicking with the mouse or with keyboard shortcuts: Review All (Alt+A), Review Incomplete (Alt+I), or Review Flagged (Alt+R); alternatively, you can click a question number to go directly back to that question. You can also end the section from this screen.

6) **Periodic Table button:** Clicking this button will open the periodic table (or press "Alt+T"). Note that the periodic table is large, covering most of the screen. However, this window can be resized to see the questions and a portion of the periodic table at the same time. The table text will not decrease, but scroll bars will appear on the window so you can center the section of the table of interest in the window.

7) **Noteboard Booklet (Scratch Paper):** At the start of the test, you will be given a spiral-bound set of four laminated 8.5"×14" sheets of paper and a wet-erase black marker to use as scratch paper. You can request a clean noteboard booklet at any time during the test; your original booklet will be collected. The noteboard is only useful if it is kept organized; do not give in to the tendency to write on the first available open space! Good organization will be very helpful when/if you wish to review a question. Indicate the passage number, the range of questions for that passage, and a topic in a box near the top of your scratch work, and indicate the question you are working on in a circle to the left of the notes for that question. Draw a line under your scratch work when you change passages to keep the work separate. Do not erase or scribble over any previous work. If you do not think it is correct, draw one line through the work and start again. You may have already done some useful work without realizing it.

General Strategy for the Science Sections

Passages vs. FSQs in the Science Sections: What to Start With

Since the questions are displayed on separate screens, it is awkward and time consuming to click through all of the questions up front to find the FSQs. Therefore, go through the section on a first pass and decide whether to do the passage now or to save it for later, basing your decision on the passage text and the first question. Tackle the FSQs as you come upon them. More details are below.

Here is an outline of the procedure:

1) For each passage, write a heading on your noteboard with the passage number, the general topic, and its range of questions (e.g., "Passage 1, thermodynamics, Q 1–5" or "Passage 2, enzymes, Q 6–9"). The passage numbers do not currently appear in the Navigation or Review screens, thus having the question numbers on your noteboard will allow you to move through the section more efficiently.

2) Skim the text and rank the passage. If a passage is a "Now," complete it before moving on to the next passage (also see "Attacking the Questions" below). If it is a "Later" passage, first write "SKIPPED" in block letters under the passage heading on your noteboard and leave room for your work when you come back to complete that passage. (Note that the specific passages you skip will be unique to you; in the Bio/Biochem section, you might choose to do all Biology passages first, then come back for Biochemistry. Or in Chem/Phys you might choose to skip experiment-based or analytical passages. Know ahead of time what type of passages you are going to skip and follow your plan.)

3) Next, click on the "Navigation" button at the bottom to get to the Navigation screen. Click on the first question of the next passage; you'll be able to identify it because you know the range of questions from the passage you just skipped. This will take you to the next passage, where you will repeat steps 1–3.

4) Once you have completed your first pass through the section, go to the Review screen and click the first question for the first passage you skipped. Answer the questions, and continue going back to the Review screen and repeating this procedure for other passages you have skipped.

Attacking the Questions

As you work through the questions, if you encounter a particularly lengthy question, or a question that requires a lot of analysis, you may choose to skip it. This is a wise strategy because it ensures you will tackle all the easier questions first, the ones you are more likely to get right. If you choose to skip the question (or if you attempt it but get stuck), write down the question number on your noteboard, click the Flag for Review button and move on to the next question. At the end of the passage, click "Previous" to move back through the set of questions and complete any that you skipped over the first time through. Make sure that you have filled in an answer for every question.

General Strategy for the CARS Section

Ranking and Ordering the Passages: What to Start With

Ranking: Since the questions are displayed on separate screens, it is awkward and time consuming to click through all of the questions before ranking each passage as Now (an easier passage), Later (a harder passage), or Killer (a passage that you will randomly guess on). Therefore, rank the passage and decide whether or not to do it on the first pass through the section based on the passage text, skimming the first 2–3 sentences.

Ordering: Because of the additional clicking through screens (or, use of the Review screen) that is required to navigate through the section, the "Two-Pass" system (completing the "Now" passages as you find them) is likely to be your most efficient approach. However, if you find that you are continuously making a lot of bad ranking decisions, it is still valid to experiment with the "Three-Pass" approach (ranking all nine passages up front before attempting your first "Now" passage).

Here is an outline of the basic Ranking and Ordering procedure to follow.

1) For each passage, write a heading on your noteboard with the passage number and its range of questions (e.g., "Passage 1 Q 1–7"). The passage numbers do not currently appear in the Navigation or Review screens, thus having the question numbers on your noteboard will allow you to move through the section more efficiently.

2) Skim the first 2–3 sentences and rank the passage. If the passage is a "Now," complete it before moving on to the next. If it is a "Later" or "Killer," first write either "Later" or "Killer" and "SKIPPED" in block letters under the passage heading on your noteboard and leave room for your work if you decide to come back and complete that passage. Then click through each question, flagging each one for review and filling in random guesses, until you get to the next passage.

3) Once you have completed the "Now" passages, come back for your second pass and complete the "Later" passages, leaving your random guesses in place for any "Killer" passages that you choose not to complete. Go to the Review screen and use your noteboard notes on the question numbers. Click on the number of the first question for that passage to go back to that question, and proceed from there. Alternatively, if you have consistently flagged all the questions for passages you skipped in your first pass, you can use "Review Flagged" from the Review screen to find and complete your "Later" passages.

4) Regardless of how you choose to find your second pass passages, unflag each question after you complete it, so that you can continue to rely on the Review screen (and the "Review Flagged" function) to identify questions that you have not yet attempted.

Previewing the Questions

The formatting and functioning of the tools facilitates effective previewing. Having each question on a separate screen will encourage you to really focus on that question. Even more importantly, you can now highlight in the question stem and the answer choices.

Here is the basic procedure for previewing the questions:

1) Start with the first question, and if it has lead words referencing passage content, highlight them. You may also choose to jot them down on your noteboard. Once you reach and preview the last question for the set on that passage, THEN stay on that screen and work the passage (your highlighting appears and stays on every passage screen, and persists through the whole 90 minutes).

2) Once you have worked the passage and defined the Bottom Line—the main idea and tone of the entire passage—work **backward** from the last question to the first. If you skip over any questions as you go (see "Attacking the Questions" below), write down the question number on your noteboard. Then click **forward** through the set of questions, completing any that you skipped over the first time through. Once you reach and complete the last question for that passage, clicking "Next" will send you to the first question of the next passage. Working the questions from last to first the first time through the set will eliminate the need to click back through multiple screens to get to the first question immediately after previewing, and will also make it easier and more efficient to do the hardest questions last (see "Attacking the Questions" below).

3) Remember that previewing questions is a CARS-only technique. It is not efficient to preview questions in the science sections.

Attacking the Questions

The question types and the procedure for actually attacking each type is discussed in much greater detail in the *MCAT CARS Review*. However, it is still important **not** to attempt the hardest questions first (potentially getting stuck, wasting time, and discouraging yourself).

So, as you work the questions from last to first (see "Previewing the Questions" above), if you encounter a particularly difficult and/or lengthy question (or if you attempt a question but get stuck), write down the question number on your noteboard (you may also choose to Flag for Review) and move on backward to the next question. Then click **forward** through the set and complete any that you skipped over the first time through the set, unflagging any questions that you flagged that first time through and making sure that you have filled in an answer for every question.

Pacing Strategy for the MCAT

Since the MCAT is a timed test, you must keep an eye on the timer and adjust your pacing as necessary. It would be terrible to run out of time at the end only to discover that the last few questions could have been easily answered in just a few seconds each.

If you complete every question, in the science section you will have about one minute and thirty-five seconds (1:35) per question, and in the CARS section you will have about one minute and forty seconds (1:40) per question (not taking into account time spent reading the passage before answering the questions).

Section	# of Questions in passage	Approximate time (including reading the passage)
Chem/Phys, Bio/Biochem, and Psych/Soc	4	6.5 minutes
	5	8 minutes
	6	9.5 minutes
CARS	5	8.5 minutes
	6	10 minutes
	7	11.5 minutes

When starting a passage in the science sections, make note of how much time you will allot for it, and the starting time on the timer. Jot down on your noteboard what the timer should say at the end of the passage. Then just keep an eye on it as you work through the questions. If you are near the end of the time for that passage, guess on any remaining questions, make some notes on your noteboard, flag the questions for review, and move on. Come back to those questions later if you have time.

For the CARS section, keep in mind that many people will maximize their score by *not* trying to complete every question or every passage in the section. A good strategy for test-takers who cannot achieve a high level of accuracy on all nine passages is to randomly guess on at least one passage in the section, so that you can spend your time getting a high percentage of the other questions right. To complete all nine CARS passages, you have about ten minutes per passage. To complete eight of the nine, you have about 11 minutes per passage.

To help maximize your number of correct answer choices in any section, do the questions and passages within that section in the order *you* want to do them in. See "General Strategy" above.

Process of Elimination

Process of Elimination (POE) is probably the most useful technique you have to tackle MCAT questions. Since there is no guessing penalty, POE allows you to increase your probability of choosing the correct answer by eliminating those you are sure are wrong.

1) Strike out any choices that you are sure are incorrect or that do not address the issue raised in the question.
2) Jot down some notes to help clarify your thoughts if you return to the question.
3) Use the "Flag for Review" button to identify questions you may want to return to. (Note, however, that in the CARS section, you generally should not be returning to rethink questions once you have moved on to a new passage.)

4) Do not leave it blank! For the sciences, if you are not sure and you have already spent more than 60 seconds on that question, just pick one of the remaining choices. If you have time to review it at the end, you can always debate the remaining choices based on your previous notes. For CARS, if you have been through the choices two or three times, have re-read the question stem and gone back to the passage and you are still stuck, move on. Do the remaining questions for that passage, take one more look at the question you were stuck on, then pick an answer and move on for good.

5) Special Note: if three of the four answer choices have been eliminated, the remaining choice must be the correct answer. Don't waste time pondering *why* it is correct; just click it and move on. The MCAT doesn't care if you truly understand why it's the right answer, only that you have the right answer selected.

6) More subject-specific information on techniques is presented in the next chapter.

Guessing

Remember, there is NO guessing penalty on the MCAT. NEVER leave a question blank!

QUESTION TYPES

In the science sections of the MCAT, the questions fall into one of three main categories:

1) Memory questions: These questions can be answered directly from prior knowledge and represent about 25 percent of the total number of questions.
2) Explicit questions: These questions are those for which the answer is explicitly stated in the passage. To answer them correctly, for example, may just require finding a definition, or reading a graph, or making a simple connection. Explicit questions represent about 35 percent of the total number of questions.
3) Implicit questions: These questions require you to apply knowledge to a new situation; the answer is typically implied by the information in the passage. These questions often start "If…. Then…." (for example, "if we modify the experiment in the passage like this, then what result would we expect?"). Implicit style questions make up about 40 percent of the total number of questions.

In the CARS section, the questions fall into four main categories:

1) Specific questions: These either ask you for facts from the passage (Retrieval questions) or require you to deduce what is most likely to be true based on the passage (Inference questions).
2) General questions: These ask you to summarize themes (Main Idea and Primary Purpose questions) or evaluate an author's opinion (Tone/Attitude questions).
3) Reasoning questions: These ask you to describe the purpose of, or the support provided for, a statement made in the passage (Structure questions) or to judge how well the author supports his or her argument (Evaluate questions).
4) Application questions: These ask you to apply new information from either the question stem itself (New Information questions) or from the answer choices (Strengthen, Weaken, and Analogy questions) to the passage.

More detail on question types and strategies can be found in Chapter 2.

TESTING TIPS

Before Test Day

- Take a trip to the test center at least a day or two before your actual test date so that you can easily find the building and room on test day. This will also allow you to gauge traffic and see if you need money for parking or any other unexpected expenses. Knowing this type of information ahead of time will greatly reduce your stress on the day of your test.
- During the week before the test, adjust your sleeping schedule so that you are going to bed and getting up in the morning at the same times as on the day before and morning of the MCAT. Prioritize getting a reasonable amount of sleep during the last few nights before the test.
- Don't do any heavy studying the day before the test. This is not a test you can cram for! Your goal at this point is to rest and relax so that you can go into test day in a good physical and mental condition.
- Eat well. Try to avoid excessive caffeine and sugar. Ideally, in the weeks leading up to the actual test you should experiment a little bit with foods and practice tests to see which foods give you the most endurance. Aim for steady blood sugar levels during the test: sports drinks, peanut-butter crackers, trail mix, etc. make good snacks for your breaks and lunch.

General Test Day Info and Tips

- On the day of the test, arrive at the test center at least a half hour prior to the start time of your test.
- Examinees will be checked in to the center in the order in which they arrive.
- You will be assigned a locker or secure area in which to put your personal items. Textbooks and study notes are not allowed, so there is no need to bring them with you to the test center.
- Your ID will be checked, your palm vein will be scanned, and you will be asked to sign in.
- You will be given a noteboard booklet and a wet-erase pen, and the test center administrator will take you to the computer on which you will complete the test. You may not choose a computer; you must use the computer assigned to you.
- Nothing is allowed at the computer station except your photo ID, your locker key (if provided), and a factory sealed packet of ear plugs; not even your watch.
- If you choose to leave the testing room at the breaks, you will have your palm vein scanned again, and you will have to sign in and out.
- You are allowed to access the items in your locker, except for notes and cell phones. (Check your test center's policy on cell phones ahead of time; some centers do not even allow them to be kept in your locker.)
- Don't forget to bring the snack foods and lunch you experimented with in your practice tests.
- At the end of the test, the test administrator will collect your noteboard and pen.
- Definitely take the breaks! Get up and walk around. It's a good way to clear your head between sections and get the blood (and oxygen!) flowing to your brain.
- Ask for a clean noteboard at the breaks if you want a fresh one.

Chapter 2
Psychology
and Sociology
Strategy for the MCAT

2.1 SCIENCE SECTIONS OVERVIEW

There are three science sections on the MCAT:

- Chemical and Physical Foundations of Biological Systems
- Biological and Biochemical Foundations of Living Systems
- Psychological, Social, and Biological Foundations of Behavior

The Chemical and Physical Foundations of Biological Systems section (Chem/Phys) is the first section on the test. It includes questions from General Chemistry (about 30%), Physics (about 25%), Organic Chemistry (about 15%), Biochemistry (about 25%), and Biology (about 5%). Further, the questions often test chemical and physical concepts within a biological setting, for example, pressure and fluid flow in blood vessels. A solid grasp of math fundamentals is required (arithmetic, algebra, graphs, trigonometry, vectors, proportions, and logarithms), however, there are no calculus-based questions.

The Biological and Biochemical Foundations of Living Systems section (Bio/Biochem) is the third section on the test. Approximately 65% of the questions in this section come from biology, approximately 25% come from biochemistry, and approximately 10% come from Organic and General Chemistry. Math calculations are generally not required on this section of the test, however, a basic understanding of statistics as used in biological research is helpful.

The Psychological, Social, and Biological Foundations of Behavior section (Psych/Soc) is the fourth and final section on the test. About 65% of the questions will be drawn from Psychology (with about 5% of these having biological relevance), about 30% from Sociology, and about 5% from Biology. As with the Bio/Biochem section, calculations are generally not required, however, a basic understanding of statistics as used in research is helpful.

Most of the questions in the science sections (44 of the 59) are passage-based, and each section has ten passages. Passages consist of a few paragraphs of information and include equations, reactions, graphs, figures, tables, experiments, and data. Four to six questions will be associated with each passage.

The remaining 25% of the questions (15 of 59) in each science section are freestanding questions (FSQs). These questions appear in approximately four groups interspersed between the passages. Each group contains four to five questions.

95 minutes are allotted to each of the science sections. This breaks down to approximately one minute and 35 seconds per question.

2.2   SCIENCE PASSAGE TYPES

The passages in the science sections fall into one of three main categories: Information and/or Situation-Presentation, Experiment/Research Presentation, or Persuasive Reasoning.

Information and/or Situation Presentation

These passages either present straightforward scientific information or they describe a particular event or occurrence. Generally, questions associated with these passages test basic science facts or ask you to predict outcomes given new variables or new information. Here is an example of an Information/Situation Presentation passage:

Figure 1 shows a portion of the inner mechanism of a typical home smoke detector. It consists of a pair of capacitor plates which are charged by a 9-volt battery (not shown). The capacitor plates (electrodes) are connected to a sensor device, D; the resistor R denotes the internal resistance of the sensor. Normally, air acts as an insulator and no current would flow in the circuit shown. However, inside the smoke detector is a small sample of an artificially produced radioactive element, americium-241, which decays primarily by emitting alpha particles, with a half-life of approximately 430 years. The daughter nucleus of the decay has a half-life in excess of two million years and therefore poses virtually no biohazard.

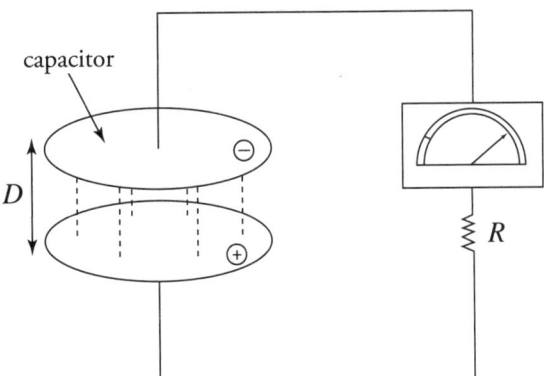

Figure 1   Smoke detector mechanism

The decay products (alpha particles and gamma rays) from the ^{241}Am sample ionize air molecules between the plates and thus provide a conducting pathway which allows current to flow in the circuit shown in Figure 1. A steady-state current is quickly established and remains as long as the battery continues to maintain a 9-volt potential difference between its terminals.

However, if smoke particles enter the space between the capacitor plates and thereby interrupt the flow, the current is reduced, and the sensor responds to this change by triggering the alarm. (Furthermore, as the battery starts to "die out," the resulting drop in current is also detected to alert the homeowner to replace the battery.)

$$C = \varepsilon_0 \frac{A}{d}$$

Equation 1

Where ε_0 is the universal permittivity constant, equal to 8.85 $\times 10^{-32}$ $C^2/(N \cdot m^2)$. Since the area A of each capacitor plate in the smoke detector is 20 cm^2 and the plates are separated by a distance d of 5 mm, the capacitance is 3.5×10^{-12} F = 3.5 pF.

Experiment/Research Presentation

These passages present the details of experiments and research procedures. They often include data tables and graphs. Generally, questions associated with these passages ask you to interpret data, draw conclusions, and make inferences. Here is an example of an Experiment/Research Presentation passage:

The development of sexual characteristics depends upon various factors, the most important of which are hormonal control, environmental stimuli, and the genetic makeup of the individual. The hormones that contribute to the development include the steroid hormones estrogen, progesterone, and testosterone, as well as the pituitary hormones FSH (follicle-stimulating hormone) and LH (luteinizing hormone).

To study the mechanism by which estrogen exerts its effects, a researcher performed the following experiments using cell culture assays.

Experiment 1:

Human embryonic placental mesenchyme (HEPM) cells were grown for 48 hours in Dulbecco's Modified Eagle's Medium (DMEM), with media change every 12 hours. Upon confluent growth, cells were exposed to a 10 mg per mL solution of green fluorescent-labeled estrogen for 1 hour. Cells were rinsed with DMEM and observed under confocal fluorescent microscopy.

Experiment 2:

HEPM cells were grown to confluence as in Experiment 1. Cells were exposed to Pesticide A for 1 hour, followed by the 10 mg/mL solution of labeled estrogen, rinsed as in Experiment 1, and observed under confocal fluorescent microscopy.

Experiment 3:

Experiment 1 was repeated with Chinese Hamster Ovary (CHO) cells instead of HEPM cells.

Experiment 4:

CHO cells injected with cytoplasmic extracts of HEPM cells were grown to confluence, exposed to the 10 mg/mL solution of labeled estrogen for 1 hour, and observed under confocal fluorescent microscopy.

The results of these experiments are given in Table 1.

Table 1 Detection of Estrogen (+ indicates presence of Estrogen)

Experiment	Media	Cytoplasm	Nucleus
1	+	+	+
2	+	+	+
3	+	+	+
4	+	+	+

After observing the cells in each experiment, the researcher bathed the cells in a solution containing 10 mg per mL of a red fluorescent probe that binds specifically to the estrogen receptor only when its active site is occupied. After 1 hour, the cells were rinsed with DMEM and observed under confocal fluorescent microscopy. The results are presented in Table 2.

The researcher also repeated Experiment 2 using Pesticide B, an estrogen analog, instead of Pesticide A. Results from other researchers had shown that Pesticide B binds to the active site of the cytosolic estrogen receptor (with an affinity 10,000 times greater than that of estrogen) and causes increased transcription of mRNA.

Table 2 Observed Fluorescence and Estrogen Effects (G = green, R = red)

Experiment	Media	Cytoplasm	Nucleus	Estrogen effects observed?
1	G only	G and R	G and R	Yes
2	G only	G only	G only	No
3	G only	G only	G only	No
4	G only	G and R	G and R	Yes

Based on these results, the researcher determined that estrogen had no effect when not bound to a cytosolic, estrogen-specific receptor.

Persuasive Reasoning

These passages typically present a scientific phenomenon along with a hypothesis that explains the phenomenon, and may include counter-arguments as well. Questions associated with these passages ask you to evaluate the hypothesis or arguments. Persuasive Reasoning passages in the science sections of the MCAT tend to be less common than Information Presentation or Experiment-based passages. Here is an example of a Persuasive Reasoning passage:

Two theoretical chemists attempted to explain the observed trends of acidity by applying two interpretations of molecular orbital theory. Consider the pK_a values of some common acids listed along with the conjugate base:

acid	pK_a	conjugate base
H_2SO_4	< 0	HSO_4-
H_2CrO_4	5.0	$HCrO_4-$
H_2PO_4	2.1	H_2CrO_4-
HF	3.9	F–
HOCI	7.8	CIO–
HCN	9.5	CN–
HIO_3	1.2	IO_3-

Recall that acids with a $pK_a < 0$ are called strong acids, and those with a $pKa > 0$ are called weak acids. The arguments of the chemists are given below.

Chemist #1:

"The acidity of a compound is proportional to the polarization of the H—X bond, where X is some nonmetal element.

Complex acids, such as H_2SO_4, $HClO_4$, and HNO_3 are strong acids because the H—O bonding electrons are strongly drawn toward the oxygen. It is generally true that a covalent bond weakens as its polarization increases. Therefore, one can conclude that the strength of an acid is proportional to the number of electronegative atoms in that acid."

Chemist #2:

"The acidity of a compound is proportional to the number of stable resonance structures of that acid's conjugate base. H_2SO_4, $HClO_4$, and HNO_3 are all strong acids because their respective conjugate bases exhibit a high degree of resonance stabilization."

Mapping a Passage

"Mapping a passage" refers to the combination of on-screen highlighting and noteboard notes that you take while working through a passage. Typically, good things to highlight include the overall topic of a paragraph, familiar terms, unusual terms, italicized terms, numerical values, hypothesis, and experimental results. Noteboard notes can be used to summarize the paragraphs and to jot down important facts and connections that are made when reading the passage. More details on passage mapping will be presented in section 2.5.

2.3 SCIENCE QUESTION TYPES

Questions in the science sections are generally one of three main types: Memory, Explicit, or Implicit.

Memory Questions

These questions can be answered directly from prior knowledge, with no need to reference the passage or question text. Memory questions represent approximately 25 percent of the science questions on the MCAT. Usually, Memory questions are found as FSQs, but they can also be tucked into a passage. Here's an example of a Memory question:

> Which of the following acetylating conditions will convert diethylamine into an amide at the fastest rate?
>
> A) Acetic acid / HCl
> B) Acetic anhydride
> C) Acetyl chloride
> D) Ethyl acetate

Explicit Questions

Explicit questions can be answered primarily with information from the passage, along with prior knowledge. They may require data retrieval, graph analysis, or making a simple connection. Explicit questions make up approximately 35–40 percent of the science questions on the MCAT; here's an example (taken from the Information/Situation Presentation passage above):

> The sensor device D shown in Figure 1 performs its function by acting as:
>
> A) an ohmmeter.
> B) a voltmeter.
> C) a potentiometer.
> D) an ammeter.

Implicit Questions

These questions require you to take information from the passage, combine it with your prior knowledge, apply it to a new situation, and come to some logical conclusion. They typically require more complex connections than do Explicit questions, and may also require data retrieval, graph analysis, etc. Implicit questions usually require a solid understanding of the passage information. They make up approximately 35–40 percent of the science questions on the MCAT; here's an example (taken from the Experiment/Research Presentation passage above):

> If Experiment 2 were repeated, but this time exposing the cells first to Pesticide A and then to Pesticide B before exposing them to the green fluorescent-labeled estrogen and the red fluorescent probe, which of the following statements will most likely be true?

A) Pesticide A and Pesticide B bind to the same site on the estrogen receptor.
B) Estrogen effects would be observed.
C) Only green fluorescence would be observed.
D) Both green and red fluorescence would be observed.

2.4 PSYCHOLOGY AND SOCIOLOGY ON THE MCAT

This section will test your content knowledge of psychological, biological, and sociological factors that shape human thought, perception, behavior, attitude, and learning. Furthermore, you will be expected to have a basic understanding of mental illness, social structure, and global disparities in health, health care, and social class. The MCAT will test your knowledge and application of these subjects at approximately the level that you would be expected to understand them in an introductory psychology class (one semester), introductory sociology class (one semester), and an introductory biology class (two semesters, though you should be prepared for more advanced physiology concepts, like you would see on the MCAT Biological and Biochemical Foundations of Living Systems section). The application of this material is potentially vast; passages can discuss anything from the specifics about a psychological research study to the complexities of studying population dynamics to the nuances of an unusual neurological disease. Additionally, questions on the Psych/Soc section will require you to demonstrate your scientific inquiry, reasoning, and understanding of basic research and statistical methods as applied to concepts in the psychological, sociological, and biological sciences. Overall, this section is designed to test your knowledge and application of the behavioral, biological, and social determinants of health and wellness.

The science sections of the MCAT have 10 passages and 15 freestanding questions (FSQs). On the Psych/Soc section, introductory biology will comprise approximately 5% of the questions, introductory sociology concepts will comprise roughly 30% of the questions, and introductory psychology concepts will comprise about 65% of the questions, with 5% having biological relevance.

2.4

2.5 TACKLING A PSYCH/SOC PASSAGE

In order to complete all of the passages and freestanding questions on the Psych/Soc section, it will be important to tackle this section strategically. An understanding about the types of passages you will encounter should help you accomplish this.

Experiment/Research Presentation

This type of passage on the Psych/Soc section will typically present some information about a relevant topic, and also present the details behind an experiment relating to that topic. Data will be presented in the tables, graphs, figures, and within the passage. These passages are challenging because they require an understanding of the reasoning and logic behind the experiment and research, the ability to analyze the results and form conclusions, and a basic understanding of statistics.

Information/Situation Presentation

This type of passage will generally present a basic concept with additional detail (that goes well beyond an introductory-level understanding) or a novel concept (like a rare neurological disease) that extrapolates information from more basic information. In order to tackle these passages, first, do not panic if you see information that you've never heard about! Rather, look for concepts that parallel what you *do* know about. For example, if you see a question about a rare neurological disorder, look for information that applies to your basic knowledge of the nervous system.

However, in order to answer passage questions and freestanding questions effectively and efficiently, you *will* need to know your basics. Don't waste time staring at a passage or question wondering, "Should I know this?" Instead, with a solid foundation in the basic core knowledge, you will be confident that you are *not* expected to know about this random, rare disease, and rather will find information in the passage and/or apply core concepts.

READING A PSYCH/SOC PASSAGE

Although tempting, try not to get too bogged down in reading all of the little details in a passage. While it is easy to get lost in the science or the glut of background information in a passage, it isn't necessary to read every nuance. Almost every psychology/sociology passage—including information/situation passages —will, in some way, describe research that was conducted. When skimming the passage, look for the key elements of any study: the methods, participants, hypotheses, and results. Your goal is to skim, and as quickly as possible get a gist for what the study was about and what the results suggested.

For Experiment/Research Presentation passages, you will need to read more closely and carefully. You will likely have questions concerning the experimental design and/or the data and results. Therefore, invest a little more time reading so you understand the experiment and the outcomes, but don't worry about completely absorbing the results until you see what types of questions are asked.

Information/Situation Presentation passages can be skimmed to get a general sense of where the information is located within the passage. The research that is described in these passages tends to be more of a general overview of findings and less detail about the methodology of the study is generally provided. Furthermore, these passages may contain a fair amount of detailed information that you may not need, so save your time—don't bother reading all of the details until you come to a question that asks about them; then go back and read more closely.

Advanced Reading Skills

To improve your ability to read and glean information from a passage, you need to practice. Be critical when you read the content; watch for vague areas or holes in the passage that aren't explained clearly. Remember that information about new topics will be woven throughout the passage; you may need to piece together information from several paragraphs and a figure to get the whole picture.

After you've read, highlighted, and mapped a passage (more on this in a bit), stop and ask yourself the following questions:

- What was this passage about? What was the conclusion or main point?
- Was there a paragraph that was mostly background?
- What question were the researchers trying to explore?
- Who were the participants?
- What groups did researchers divide the participants into, or what groups were present in the research that was described?
- What were the hypotheses?
- What were the results?
- Were there any unexpected results, or did they confirm the hypotheses?

This takes a while at first, but eventually becomes second nature and you will start doing it as you are reading the passage. With practice, you will begin to notice patterns in the way that passages are presented: they usually begin with background information (of varying complexity and utility), then frame a specific area of researchers that social scientists have been interested in. Once this frame is established, a research question is explored either through a study or information that has been gathered. Then, in some order, there are groups, hypotheses, results, and conclusions. This is more of a general guideline than a hard and fast rule, but identifying these patterns (and noticing exceptions and deviations when they arise) during abundant practice will greatly increase the efficiency and effectiveness with which you are able to skim the passage. If you have a study group you are working with, consider doing this as an exercise with your study partners. Take turns asking and answering the questions above. Having to explain something to someone else not only solidifies your own knowledge, but helps you see where you might be weak.

MAPPING A PSYCH/SOC PASSAGE

Mapping a Psych/Soc passage is a combination of highlighting and noteboard notes that can help you organize and understand the passage information.

Resist the temptation to highlight everything (everyone has done this: you're reading a psychology textbook with a highlighter, and then look back and realize that the whole page is yellow!). Restrict your highlighting to a few things:

2.5

- the main theme of a paragraph (does it describe background, methods, results, etc.?)
- an unusual or unfamiliar term that is defined specifically for that passage (e.g., something that is italicized)
- each of the important details of the study that we described earlier: methods, participants, groups, hypotheses, results, and conclusions

Your noteboard notes should be organized. Make sure the passage number, the range of questions for that passage, and a topic appear at the top of your notes. For each paragraph, note "P1," "P2," etc., on the noteboard, and jot down a few notes about that paragraph. Try to translate science-y jargon into your own words using everyday language (this is particularly useful for experiments). Also, make sure to jot down simple relationships (e.g., the relationship between two variables).

Pay attention to figures and tables to see what type of information they contain. Don't spend a lot of time analyzing at this point, but do jot down on your noteboard "Fig 1" and a brief summary of the data. Also, if you've discovered a list in the passage, note its topic and location down on your noteboard.

Let's take a look at how we might highlight and map a practice passage:

Psychotic disorders—most notably schizophrenia and bipolar disorder with psychotic features—affect approximately 2% of Americans. These disorders are extremely manageable with psychotropic medications—to relieve symptoms such as hallucinations and delusions—and behavioral therapy, such as social skills training and hygiene maintenance.

However, individuals with psychotic disorders have the lowest level of medication compliance, as compared to individuals with mood or anxiety disorders. Antipsychotic medications can have extremely negative side effects, including uncontrollable twitching of the face or limbs, blurred vision, and weight gain, among others. They also must be taken frequently, and at high doses, in order to be effective. While relatively little is known about the reasons for noncompliance, studies do suggest that in schizophrenia, age of schizophrenia diagnosis and medication compliance is positively correlated. Evidence also suggests that medication noncompliance is disproportionally prevalent in individuals of a low socioeconomic status (SES) due to issues such as homelessness, lack of insurance benefits, and lack of familial or social support.

Researchers were interested to see how drug education might affect compliance or noncompliance with psychotropic medications based on patient socioeconomic status. In a study of 1200 mentally ill individuals in the Los Angeles metro area, researchers measured baseline psychotropic medication compliance, then provided patients with a free educational seminar on drug therapy, and then measured psychotropic medication compliance six months later. The one-day, 8-hour seminar included information on positive effects of psychotropic medication, side effects of psychotropic medication, psychotropic medication interactions with other substances such as alcohol and non-prescribed drugs, and information on accessing Medicare benefits. Compliance was measured by the number of doses of prescribed psychotropic medication that the patients took in a week, over the course of 12 weeks, as compared to the number of doctor-recommended doses per week. Compliance was measured using a self-report questionnaire.

Results indicated that post-seminar, mentally ill patients from middle or upper class backgrounds (Upper and Middle SES) were significantly more compliant with their psychotropic medication regimens than prior to the seminar. However, no significant differences were found in patients at or below the poverty level (Lower SES). Table 1 displays psychotropic medication compliance by SES and disorder.

Table 1 Psychotropic Medication Compliance by Socioeconomic Status (SES) and Disorder

Disorder	SES	Pre-Seminar Compliance	Post-Seminar Compliance
Bipolar I	Upper	60%	73%
	Middle	57%	61%
	Lower	25%	27%
Schizophrenia	Upper	53%	65%
	Middle	51%	62%
	Lower	22%	26%

Analysis and Passage Map

This Experiment/Research Presentation passage follows a very common pattern for psychology/sociology passages. It starts off with an introduction of a topic and background information, provides a frame for the research, describes methodology, and presents results. The way this is presented varies, but in this example each point is given its own paragraph. The first paragraph starts with an introduction to the topic, psychotic disorders (specifically schizophrenia and bipolar disorder). This is primarily a background information paragraph and can be skimmed quickly, with a few specific words/phrases highlighted.

The second paragraph starts with "however," indicating a change in direction. This change in direction establishes the frame for the research. The first paragraph said that schizophrenia is easily managed with drugs and therapy, but the second paragraph indicates that that isn't the whole story; in fact, the main topic of the passage is presented—medication noncompliance, particularly in low socioeconomic (SES) individuals.

The third paragraph presents relevant information about the study conducted to determine the impact of drug education on medication noncompliance in various SES groups. This is essentially the methodology section. It is important to highlight the key features of the study here—what is it looking at, and how is data collected. You do not necessarily need to highlight every single detail, but understand the basic premise of the study.

The final paragraph describes the results of the study, and presents the data in Table 1. The paragraph provides you with the significant finding that is demonstrated by the data in the table—while upper and middle SES individuals demonstrated an increased medication compliance after the drug education seminar, low SES individuals did not.

Here is what your noteboard should look like:

> (Your heading would go above this list)
> *P1—psychotic disorders are manageable with medication and therapy*
> *P2—but medication compliance is a big problem, especially for low SES*
> *P3—STUDY: medication compliance by SES before and after a drug education seminar*
> *P4—RESULTS: medication compliance increases for upper and middle SES, no improvement for low SES*

One more thing about passages on the MCAT: you can do the passages in any order you want to. There are no bonus points for taking the test in order. Therefore, tackle the passages that you are most comfortable with first, and save the harder ones for last (see "General Strategy" in Chapter 1 for more information on how to move around efficiently in the test).

2.6 TACKLING THE QUESTIONS

Questions on the Psych/Soc section mimic the three typical science question types: Memory, Explicit, and Implicit.

Memory Questions in the Psych/Soc Section

Memory questions are exactly what they sound like: they test your knowledge of some specific fact or concept. While Memory questions are typically found as freestanding questions, they can also be tucked into a passage. The questions, aside from requiring memorization, do not generally cause problems for students because they are similar to the types of questions that would appear on a typical college psychology or sociology exam. Below are two examples of Memory questions, taken from the passage above:

1. What is one "positive" symptom of schizophrenia?

    A) Catatonia
    B) Weight gain
    C) Flattened affect
    D) Auditory or visual hallucinations

2. Bipolar disorder involves periods of mania and depression, and for some, episodes of hypomania. Hypomania, a state that is less severe than mania, is characterized by "feeling good/high" and increased well-being and productiveness. Which of the mechanisms is most likely involved with the hypomanic episodes experienced by individuals diagnosed with bipolar disorder?

    A) Increased dopamine in the brain
    B) Decreased stimulation of the enteric plexus
    C) Increased activation of the posterior pituitary
    D) Decreased serotonin in the central nervous system

These are Memory questions because, even though they are associated with the passage, you could have answered them (and should be able to answer them) without reading the passage. It is important that you recognize them as Memory questions so you don't go back to the passage and waste time looking for answers that are not there! There is no specific "trick" to answering Memory questions; either you know the correct answer or you don't.

If you find that you are missing a fair number of Memory questions, it is a sure sign that you do not know the content well enough. Go back and review.

Here are the answers for the questions above.

1. **D**   A "positive" symptom of schizophrenia is an addition to, excess of, or distortion of normal functions; auditory or visual hallucinations are positive symptoms of the illness (choice D is correct). A "negative" symptom of schizophrenia is a diminishment or absence of normal function; catatonia (lack or responsiveness to stimuli) and flattened affect (lack of emotion) are both negative symptoms (choices A and C are wrong). Weight gain is often a side effect of psychotropic medications, not a symptom of schizophrenia (choice B is wrong).

2. **A**   Dopamine is the primary neurotransmitter involved with the "reward centers" of the brain; since hypomania is characterized by "feeling good/high," it can reasonably be concluded that an increase of dopamine in the brain could produce this effect (choice A is correct). The enteric plexus or enteric nervous system is a portion of the autonomic nervous system that controls the gastrointestinal tract; decreased stimulation of the enteric nervous system would not produce any of the characteristics of hypomania described (choice B is wrong). The posterior pituitary is responsible for producing oxytocin, a hormone that controls lactation and uterine contractions, and vasopressin, a hormone that controls how much water the kidneys resorb; therefore, increased activation of the posterior pituitary would not produce any of the characteristics of hypomania described (choice C is wrong). Serotonin is a neurotransmitter with widespread effects in the brain; a decrease of serotonin in the brain has been shown to produce symptoms of depression, not hypomania (choice D is wrong).

2.6

Explicit Questions in the Psych/Soc section

True, pure Explicit questions are rare in the Psych/Soc section. A purely Explicit question can be answered with only information in the passage. Below is an example of a pure Explicit question from the passage above:

3. What is the incidence of psychotic disorders in the American population?

A) 1%
B) 2%
C) 4%
D) Unknown

Referring back to the first paragraph of the passage, it clearly states that "Psychotic disorders—most notably schizophrenia and bipolar disorder with psychotic features—affect approximately 2% of Americans;" therefore, choice **B** is correct.

However, more often on the Psych/Soc section, Explicit questions are more of a blend of Explicit and Memory; they require not only retrieval of passage information, but also recall of some relevant information. They usually do not require in-depth analysis or connections. Here is an example of a common type of Explicit question:

4. Based on the design of the study described in the passage, what limits the researchers' abilities to draw conclusions about the causal relationship between socioeconomic status and psychotropic medication compliance?

A) Age at first diagnosis was not measured.
B) Participants were not randomly assigned to socioeconomic status.
C) The sample contained only Los Angeles metro area residents.
D) Severity of symptoms were not measured.

2.6

To answer this question, you first need to retrieve information from the passage about the study's experimental design (from paragraph 3). You also need to recall some information about experimental design, and what sort of factors limit a researcher's ability to infer a causal relationship.

Here is the solution to the question above:

4. **B** Causation is extremely difficult to determine when experimenting with humans, particularly because all of the variables in a given experiment must by controlled by the researcher, and subjects must be randomly assigned to experimental and control groups. Therefore, random assignment of subjects to a group (in this case, a socioeconomic status group) is one of the many variables that should have been controlled for in order to determine a causal relationship between socioeconomic status and psychotropic medication compliance (choice B is correct). While age at first diagnosis and symptom severity are important variables that could have been measured, neither specifically limits the researchers' ability to draw conclusions about the causal relationship between socioeconomic status and psychotropic medication compliance (choices A and D are wrong). The fact that the sample only contained participants from the Los Angeles metro area limits the researchers' ability to draw conclusions about how their results might apply to the general population, not about causality (choice C is wrong).

A final subgroup in the Explicit question category is graph or data interpretation questions. These questions will either ask you to take graphical information from the passage and convert it into a text answer, or they will ask you to take text from the passage and convert it into a graph. Below is an example from the passage above:

2.6

5. Which of the following graphs would best illustrate the relationship between age of schizophrenia diagnosis and medication compliance described in the passage?

A)
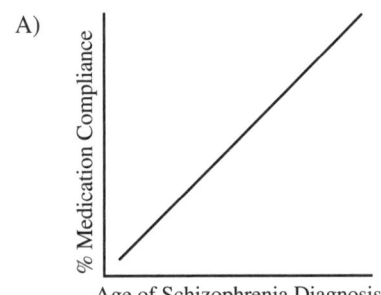

B)
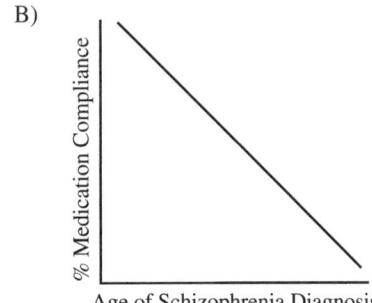

C)
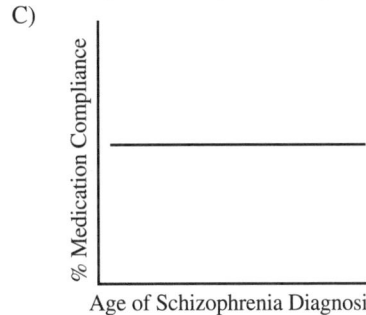

D)
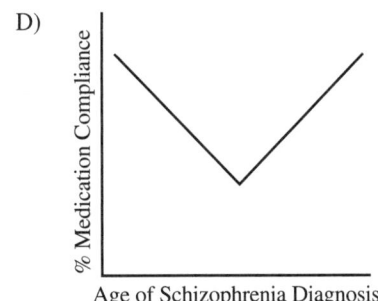

The passage states, in the second paragraph, that "…studies do suggest that in schizophrenia, age of schizophrenia diagnosis and medication compliance is positively correlated." Therefore, as age of diagnosis increases, so does compliance. So, a graphical representation should look like the figure in choice **A**.

If you find you are missing Explicit questions, practice your passage mapping. Make sure you aren't missing the critical items in the passage that lead you to the right answer. Slow down a little; take an extra 15 to 30 seconds per passage to read or think about it more carefully.

Implicit Questions

Implicit questions require the most thought. These require recall not only of Psych/Soc content information but also information gleaned from the passage, and a more in-depth analysis of how the two relate. Implicit questions require more analysis and connections to be made than Explicit questions. Often they take the form "If…then…." Below is an example of a classic Implicit question, based on the passage above:

6. The experiment described in the passage was repeated, but instead of testing how drug education affects compliance, researchers measured how incentives affect compliance in low SES schizophrenics. The low SES schizophrenia group was broken into two groups. Group A received an incentive every time they took their medication for seven consecutive days, while Group B received an incentive every two weeks, regardless of compliance level. Based on operant conditioning principles, what results should the researchers see?

A) There should be no difference in compliance levels from the first study.
B) Group A's compliance should be higher than Group B's compliance.
C) Group B's compliance should be higher than Group A's compliance.
D) Both groups should demonstrate increased compliance from the first study but it is impossible to tell which group's compliance is expected to be higher.

To answer this question, conclusions have to be drawn about the experiment described in the passage, and the new experiment described in the question stem, and then applied to your content knowledge about reward schedules in operant conditioning. Many, many more connections need to be made than when answering an Explicit question. A detailed explanation for this question is below.

6. **B** According to the question, Group A is receiving an incentive on a fixed-ratio schedule (after every seven consecutive days of medication compliance) and Group B is receiving an incentive on a fixed-interval schedule (every two weeks, regardless of compliance). According to operant conditioning principles, a fixed-ratio schedule should produce a high rate of desired behavior (in this case, medication compliance), while a fixed-interval schedule produces

a steady rate of response that tends to increase closer to the reward, but is not nearly as frequent as what is expected from a fixed-ratio reward schedule (choice B is correct; choice C is wrong). Based on operant conditioning principles, rewarding desired behavior should increase behavior (choice A is wrong), and applying a fixed-ratio and fixed-interval reward schedule should increase behavior in predictable ways (choice D is wrong).

If you find that you are missing a lot of Implicit questions, first of all, make sure that you are using POE aggressively. Second, go back and review the explanations for the correct answers, and figure out where your logic went awry. Did you miss an important fact in the passage? Did you forget the relevant Psych/Soc content? Did you follow the logical train of thought to the right answer? Once you figure out where you made your mistake, you will know how to correct it.

2.7 SUMMARY OF THE APPROACH TO PSYCHOLOGY AND SOCIOLOGY

How to Map the Passage and Use Your Noteboard

1) The passage should be skimmed, NOT be read like textbook material. Do not try to learn something from every sentence (science majors especially will be tempted to read this way). Passages should be read to get a feel for the type of questions that will follow, and to get a general idea of the location of information within the passage.

2) Highlighting—Use this tool sparingly, or you will end up with a passage that is completely covered in yellow highlighter! Highlighting in a Psych/Soc passage should be used to draw attention to a few words that demonstrate one of the following:
   - the main theme of a paragraph
   - an unusual or unfamiliar term that is defined specifically for that passage (e.g., something that is italicized)
   - main points of the research: methods, participants, groups, hypotheses, results, conclusions

3) Pay brief attention to figures and experiments, noting only what information they deal with. Do not spend a lot of time analyzing at this point.

4) For each passage, start by noting the passage number, the general topic, and the range of questions on your noteboard. You can then work between your noteboard and the Review screen to easily get to the questions you want (see Chapter 1).

5) For each paragraph, note "P1," "P2," etc. on the noteboard and jot down a few notes about that paragraph. Try to translate psych/soc jargon into your own words using everyday language. Especially note down simple relationships (e.g., the relationship between two variables). Be brief here. Use annotations and symbols to represent main ideas and results.

6) The noteboard is only useful if it is kept organized! Make sure that your notes for each passage are clearly delineated and marked with the passage number and question range. This will allow you to easily read your notes when you come back to a review a flagged question. Resist the temptation to write in the first available blank space, as this makes it much more difficult to refer back to your work.

Psych/Soc Question Strategies

1) Remember that the content in Psychology and Sociology is broad, but not necessarily super deep, so don't panic if something seems completely unfamiliar. Understand the basic content well, find the basics in the unfamiliar topic, and apply them to the question.

2) Process of Elimination is paramount! The strikeout tool allows you to eliminate answer choices; this will improve your chances of guessing the correct answer if you are unable to narrow it down to one choice.

3) Answer the straightforward questions first (typically the memory questions). Leave questions that require analysis of experiments and graphs for later. Take the test in the order YOU want. Make sure to use your noteboard to indicate questions you skipped.

4) Make sure that the answer you choose actually answers the question, and isn't just a true statement.

5) Try to avoid answer choices with extreme words such as "always," "never," etc. In psych/soc, there is almost always an exception and answers are rarely black-and-white.

6) I-II-III questions: Whenever possible, start by evaluating the Roman numeral item that shows up in exactly two answer choices. This will allow you to quickly eliminate two wrong answer choices regardless of whether the item is true or false. Typically then, you will only have to assess one of the other Roman numeral items to determine the correct answer. Always work between the I-II-III statements and the answer choices. Once an item is found to be true (or false), strike out answer choices which do not contain (or do contain) that item number. Make sure to strike out the actual Roman numeral item as well, and highlight those items that are true.

7) LEAST/EXCEPT/NOT questions: Don't get tricked by these questions that ask you to pick the answer that doesn't fit (the incorrect or false statement). It's often good to use your note-board and write a T or F next to answer choices A–D. The one that stands out as different is the correct answer!

8) Again, don't leave any question blank.

A Note About Flashcards

For most of the exams you've taken previously, flashcards were likely very helpful. This was because those exams mostly required you to regurgitate information, and flashcards are pretty good at helping you memorize facts. However, the most challenging aspect of the MCAT is not that it requires you to memorize the fine details of content knowledge, but that it requires you to apply your basic scientific knowledge to unfamiliar situations: flashcards alone may not help you there.

Flashcards can be beneficial if your basic content knowledge is deficient in some area. For example, if you don't know the stages of Erikson's psychosocial model of development, flashcards can certainly help you memorize these facts. Or, maybe you are unsure of the functions of the different brain regions. You might find that flashcards can help you memorize these. But unless you are trying to memorize basic facts in your personal weak areas, you are better off doing and analyzing practice passages than carrying around a stack of flashcards.

Chapter 3
Research Methods and Study Design

To understand human behavior and the complex interplay of human societies, researchers in the social sciences use a variety of methodologies to test hypotheses regarding behavior. Conducting social science research presents ethical and logistical complications that are unique from those faced by scientists in the physical and biological sciences. As a result, social scientists must be creative about how they combine methodologies, design research, and especially how they draw conclusions from the research they conduct. Determining causal relationships between variables is especially difficult when complex human behavior is considered. This chapter explores the types of problems researchers face, and the different tools at their disposal to assess human behavior and draw conclusions on why we do the things we do and what makes us who we are.

In addition to psychology and sociology content at the first-year undergraduate level, the MCAT Psychology and Sociology section will also feature many questions that incorporate research methods and study design (about 20-25% of the section). These questions will require knowledge of the elementary aspects of social research, such as types of study design, especially the experimental method, and what types of conclusions can be drawn from each. Almost all Psychology/Sociology passages will contain a study, and the majority of these passages will contain at least one question in which you are asked to evaluate the study or make a prediction about the implications of the research. Fortunately, the amount of content associated with these questions is manageable and is not heavy in statistics. What *is* required is knowledge of the common types of research conducted by social scientists, the strengths and weaknesses of each method, and the types of conclusions that can reasonably be drawn from each.

3.1 EXPERIMENTAL DESIGN

Because the word "experiment" is often used interchangeably with "research," it is easy to forget that "experimental design" is a technical term for a *specific type* of research. To emphasize this difference, let's examine an area of research in which social scientists might be interested. Many different types of studies have shown that a Mediterranean diet (one rich in seafood, legumes, nuts, olive oil, fruits, and vegetables) is associated with cardiovascular health and longevity. However, to show that consuming a Mediterranean diet helps *cause*, or helps *lead* to cardiovascular health and longevity, an experimental design is needed.

To see why this is the case, imagine a study in which a team of social scientists creates a scale to measure the extent to which an individual follows the Mediterranean diet: the subject would answer questions about how frequently she eats foods associated with that diet. Based on the responses on this food-frequency questionnaire, researchers assign a score for each individual from 1 (diet least resembles a traditional Mediterranean diet) to 12 (diet most resembles a traditional Mediterranean diet). Let's call this scale the Mediterranean Diet Index (MDI). Suppose researchers find that as individual MDI scores increase, so do measures of cardiovascular health. This finding does not show that adherence to the Mediterranean diet causes cardiovascular health to improve.

What the team has found is a positive correlation (discussed below) between the MDI and cardiovascular fitness, but correlation is not causation. For example, it is possible that people with a genetic predisposition toward good cardiovascular health produce a profile of digestive enzymes that leads to a natural preference for a Mediterranean-style diet. This implies that a predisposition to good cardiovascular health causes high MDI scores. This actually flips the causal direction! Another possible explanation is that some third factor, such as exercise or social support, leads to both greater cardiovascular health *and* a preference for Mediterranean foods (see Figure 1). A fourth possibility is that some third factor causes an increase in cardiovascular health, but does not actually lead to consuming a Mediterranean diet. This causal factor is merely positively correlated with Mediterranean-diet consumption. To rule out these other possible explanations and determine that a Mediterranean diet actually does cause improved cardiovascular health, the team must conduct a follow-up study with an experimental design.

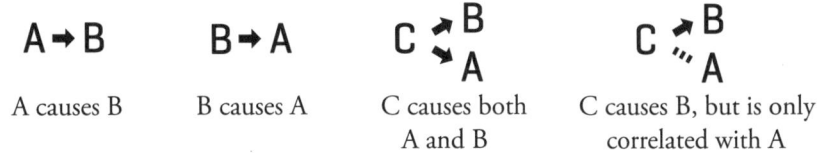

A → B	B → A	C ⤲ B A	C ⤲ B A
A causes B	B causes A	C causes both A and B	C causes B, but is only correlated with A

Figure 1 Possible causal relationships that could explain a correlation that is found between two variables, A and B.

There are several steps to good experimental design. In this case, the researchers hope to show that adherence to a Mediterranean diet actually *causes* greater cardiovascular health.

1) <u>Select the population.</u> The first thing the researchers must agree on is the population of interest. Whom do they want to study? It may seem obvious that they would be interested in "all humans;" however, for various reasons, this may not be the best group to select. For example, many experiments in the social sciences are done by scholars at universities. Suppose our team of researchers were all tenured at a university—let's call it Healthy Living U. Then the easiest way for the researchers to get a large group of participants at low cost would be to use students at Healthy Living U as participants in the experiment.

Of course, our researchers would ideally like their findings to apply to everyone, but if they select the greater population as the population of interest, the researchers would have to find older (and younger) participants. Researchers would have to come up with ways to incentivize them to participate in the research and follow through to make sure they follow the experimental protocol correctly. Because this would be very taxing in terms of resources and logistics, the researchers are likely to decide that their population of interest will be healthy young adults in their early twenties. The research team now has access to thousands of willing participants that they can recruit by offering course credit or a small cash payment, and follow up on more easily since they are all located at the university.

Think about what this (very reasonable) decision about what population to study implies for later findings. If they *do* find that Mediterranean diet adherence leads to cardiovascular health, can they say that this result is also true for individuals in their 50s or 60s? It very well might, but this conclusion now lies outside the scope of the Healthy Living U experiment. Follow-up studies would be needed to say for sure whether the effect also applies to older adults. The researchers have compromised the reach and scope of their experiment, but they now have the advantage of a large pool of willing participants that they can sample for their experiment. In practice, social science researchers often make the (very dubious) assumption that the findings they made while studying a group of young adults in college apply to all adults in a society.

2) Operationalize the independent and dependent variables. The **independent variable** is the variable manipulated by the research team. The **dependent variable** is the variable that is measured. In the correlational study described earlier, researchers found that high MDI scores were associated with better cardiovascular health. In this follow-up experimental study, the *causal* relationship that researchers want to test experimentally is whether eating a Mediterranean diet *leads* to greater cardiovascular health. The researchers must specify exactly what they mean by this.

The independent variable in this experiment is adherence to a Mediterranean diet; to qualify as an experimental design, this variable must be *directly manipulated* by the researchers. Researchers want to have maximum control over the experimental environment so that they can be sure that differences between the groups actually led to the effect, assuming one is measured. Good experimental design requires experiments that can be reproduced by other researchers, an important quality of research design known as **reproducibility**. These other researchers may want to verify the results or adapt some aspect of the experiment. For this reason, precise definitions are key. A related concept to reproducibility, **replicability**, refers to obtaining consistent results across various studies attempting to answer the same scientific question but using different data and/or new statistical methods.

The researchers at Healthy Living U decide that they will work with the cafeteria on campus to serve a special diet to participants. They team up with a group of nutritionists to create a six-month-long diet plan of twenty-one meals per week that participants will be required to consume. Participants can also consume a set of preselected snacks and beverages for their dorm rooms, but outside foods are not allowed. The diet the team constructs is such that it would score a perfect 12 on the MDI scale.

The dependent variable in the experiment is cardiovascular health. This is the variable that the researchers will measure to see if their diet has an effect. To obtain rigorous results, the researchers must create an **operational definition**, a specification of precisely what they mean by each variable. The independent variable was operationalized as a very specific set of foods consumed over a 6-month period. The dependent variable must be equally well-defined and must also meet the criterion of being **quantitative**, or numerical, as opposed to **qualitative**, or descriptive. Quantitative data will be necessary later to conduct statistical analyses that will test the research hypothesis. The researchers decide that the dependent variables they will measure are heart rate, blood pressure, peak oxygen uptake, aerobic recovery rate, blood glucose levels, and ejection fraction. Each of these will produce a numerical value that they will measure before and after the 6-month period. The difference in these values will test the effect of the dietary regimen on health.

These are strong operational definitions. Both the independent and dependent variable definitions are specific and replicable, and the dependent variable is sufficiently quantitative to allow for statistical analyses. However, notice that the researchers have introduced new limitations to the experiment. Look first at the independent variable. What if the Mediterranean diet only starts to be effective after many years? Perhaps there is an adjustment period to the new dietary protocol and we only start to see benefits over time spans much longer than 6 months. If that were the case, the present experiment would not detect a result, and the research team might wrongly conclude that the diet is ineffective.

The operationalization of the dependent variable also introduced limitations. The variable is quantitative and rigorous; however, it only indirectly measures what we are really interested in: cardiovascular health (and ultimately increased longevity). The variables the researchers selected can only *indirectly* suggest that the quality-of-life variables we really care about are improving. Again, good experimental design often involves making compromises to meet conditions or to make conducting a study realistic.

It would be great if we could verify experimentally that eating a specific diet decreases the risk of heart attack and leads to increased longevity. However, let's reflect for a moment on how difficult that would be in practice. The Healthy Living U experiment we are developing is already shaping up to be *very* restrictive for participants, even though we have created a rather optimal scenario by defining variables so that many able participants who live in the research environment could be used. Imagine if we extended the dietary regimen for a lifetime, then measured average life expectancy and morbidity due to cardiovascular disease over the course of decades. This would be nearly impossible to accomplish in practice, but that is what we would need to do to conclusively show that the diet led to health benefits! To conduct experiments that are realistically feasible, the Healthy Living U researchers must compromise by narrowing the scope of their study and selecting measurable dependent variables like heart rate and blood pressure that *imply* cardiovascular health, rather than trying to measure cardiovascular morbidity and life expectancy directly.

3) Carefully select control and experimental groups. The group of participants that receives treatment is the **experimental** group. To draw conclusions about the effect of the treatment, researchers also need a **control** group, which acts as a point of reference and comparison.

Suppose the high-MDI six-month-long diet leads to improvements for participants with respect to each of the cardiovascular variables measured. This would seem to be a great success for the experiment, but it could not confirm the experimental hypothesis without a control group. For example, it is probable that being given *any* dietary regimen would offer some health benefits. The researchers need a point of comparison to rule this possibility out and conclude that it was actually the Mediterranean diet, and not following a dietary regimen that offered benefits, if any are found.

Having a control group is critical to this experimental design; otherwise the study would not qualify as experimental and no causal conclusions could be drawn. Researchers want to show that eating a Mediterranean diet causes cardiovascular health. To show this, they need a control group that is **homogenous**, the same throughout, and as similar as possible to the experimental group except for the variable of interest —the treatment.

The objective of having a similar control group is to rule out **extraneous (or confounding) variables**, variables other than the treatment that could potentially explain an experimental result. What sorts of variables could affect the current experiment? Gender, age, and socioeconomic status might play a role. Certainly exercise, BMI, and stress levels could play a role as well. If researchers agreed on this list of potential extraneous variables, they would carefully select experimental and control groups that were as similar as possible in age, gender, status, serum cortisol levels, and BMI. To control for exercise, they might create a regulated regimen for both groups to follow.

Remember that to optimize study design, the experimental and control groups must be *as similar as possible*. When evaluating research methodology in published articles, you might think the care that researchers take to maintain this quality can seem extreme. However, many studies have shown that unexpected and seemingly unrelated variables can lead to an effect. One of the many phenomena that complicate social research and can lead to erroneous results is the **placebo effect**, the well-known fact that just *believing* that treatment is being administered can lead to a measurable result.

It works like this. Tell a group of depressed subjects that they are getting a cutting-edge neurological treatment for depression, confirmed through years of double-blind clinical trials. Bring them into a state-of-the-art medical research center and test them through EEG, fMRI, and stress hormone exams to "establish a baseline measure of cortical activity." Then, give them each a sugar pill to take twice a day for six weeks. It is likely, if the environment and protocol seemed authentic, that depression would actually decrease. This would be especially likely if the doctors and medical aides administering the tests and giving the prescriptions also believed the pill was the real thing. That's right, if researchers know that they are administering a treatment, that can also lead to a placebo effect! To help counter the placebo effect, studies must be **double blind**: neither the person administering treatment nor the participants truly know if they are assigned to the treatment or control groups.

If we apply these considerations to the Healthy Living U experiment, then the control group subjects need their own special diet, with physiologists taking their readings, and special chefs to cook the meals in the cafeteria. Neither the physiologists taking the readings nor the chefs should be privy to the hypotheses of the experiment, and both the experimental and control groups should be operating under the belief that they will potentially receive health benefits from participating in the study. Now, finally, we are almost ready to recruit participants and begin the procedure.

But before we start recruiting participants and conduct the study, we must take one more thing into account. The study is designed to test for the *Mediterranean* diet, specifically. To appropriately isolate this variable (also for ethical reasons, see below), researchers had better give a healthy alternative diet to the control group. The researchers might select a diet that scores a 6 on the MDI so it is relatively average in "Mediterranean-ness," but is known to also be composed of fresh, healthy foods. Then later, if a difference were to be measured, researchers could be relatively sure that this result was due to the Mediterranean diet specifically, and not just the effect of eating a healthy diet designed by a team of professional nutritionists.

Researchers can never account for *every* potential extraneous variable. Firstly, *any* variable could theoretically be a potential confound, so researchers must focus on the most likely candidates. Beyond that, it may not be possible to control for a variable even if researchers would like to.

4) <u>Randomly sample from the population.</u> Finally, researchers can start recruiting participants for the study. The sampling should be random: it should be equally likely for any member of the population to be a participant in the study. This is an ideal that is almost never accomplished in practice. For the Healthy Living U study, any healthy young adult in their early 20s should have an equal chance of participating in the study. However, since the study is done at a specific university, only students at that school can be used. One of the most common flaws in social research is the fact that most studies are done on undergraduate students, and results are then applied to the greater population. This is often a dubious and highly precarious leap in logic. If it is not equally likely for all members of a population to be sampled, this is known as **sampling bias**.

Selection bias is a more general category of systemic flaws in a design that can compromise results. Aside from sampling bias, another type of selection bias is purposefully selecting which studies to evaluate in a **meta-analysis**, a big-picture analysis of many studies to look for trends in the data. Attrition, discussed below, is also a type of selection bias.

Usually, participants in a study are incentivized in some way, which could range from monetary compensation to access to new treatments and medication. The team at Healthy Living U might use extra points on an exam or nominal tuition rebates as an incentive for students to participate. This introduces another potential problem into the study—**attrition**, participants dropping out of the study. If the reason that participants are dropping out is non-random, this might introduce an extraneous variable.

5) <u>Randomly assign individuals to groups.</u> Once the individuals who will participate in the study have been incentivized and rounded up, it is time to assign them to the experimental and control groups. In a well-designed experiment, it should be equally likely that they are assigned to either group. In contrast to the previous step, this one is relatively easy to pull off. In this study, there are many extraneous variables that the researchers decided to account for, so they might use a **randomized block technique.** In this technique, researchers evaluate where participants fall along the variables they wish to equalize across experimental and control groups. Then they randomly assign individuals from these groups so that the treatment and control groups are similar along the variables of interest.

6) <u>Measure the results.</u> For this experiment, the dependent variable is a set of well-known physiological measurements with standardized collection procedures and error measures. In more general situations, they must check to make sure that their measurements are valid. The most important aspects of measurement for an experiment are that the dependent variable is quantitative (and therefore measurable) and that instruments used are **reliable** and **valid**. Reliability means that an instrument produces stable and consistent results; validity means that it actually measures what it's supposed to measure. For example, if every morning when you step on

your bathroom scale it indicates that you weigh three pounds, that scale is reliable but not valid. Replicability means that the experiment would produce similar findings if conducted by another researcher on different subjects. This requires clarity and precision in terms of the experimental procedure and measurements that are used. This is often a point of consideration for psychological studies that test dependent variables like mood, memory, and attitude. **Psychometrics** is the study of how to measure psychological variables through testing. Another concern with surveys is **response bias**, the tendency for respondents to not have perfect insight into their state and provide inaccurate responses.

There are many ways that researchers could choose to compare groups and measure results. In the Healthy Living U study, researchers are comparing two different groups: one experimental group that receives a high-MDI diet, and a control group with an alternative dietary regimen. This is known as a **between-subjects** design; the comparisons are made between subjects, from one group to another. An alternative approach is to use a **within-subjects** design and compare the same group at different time points. For example, the research team could also choose to measure cardiovascular fitness before and after the dietary regimen, thereby making the comparisons within subjects. If researchers were to use both techniques, and make both within-subjects and between-subjects comparisons, this would be a type of **mixed methods** research. Mixed methods are any combination of different research techniques, such as within-subjects and between subjects, or qualitative and quantitative.

7) Test the Hypothesis. Scientists and philosophers of science over the years have generally agreed that it is better to incorrectly conclude that there is no effect (**type 2 error**, or false negative) than to falsely suppose the veracity of a result that does not actually exist (**type 1 error**, or false positive). In fact, a way to remember this distinction is to think of type 1 error as predominant, because it is a graver problem in hypothesis-testing. Much like the legal concept of "innocent until proven guilty," it is better to reason from a point of skepticism. For this reason, scientists generally start with the **null hypothesis**: they assume that there is no causal relationship between the variables and any effect that they measure, if there is one, is due to chance. Then, they see whether evidence from the experiment suggests that the null hypothesis is true or false. Taking this position and reasoning in this way places the "burden of proof" on the **experimental hypothesis,** the proposition that variations in the independent variable cause changes in the dependent variables.

To reject the null hypothesis, it is not satisfactory simply to observe a difference between two groups. After all, the observed difference may simply be due to chance. Even two identical groups or identical measures are subject to randomness and can therefore produce different measures even if there is no fundamental difference. To see why, and to get an idea of how social scientists and statisticians conduct hypothesis-testing, consider the following example.

Imagine you and a friend roll two dice (each a cube with six faces labeled from "1" to "6"). Suppose you roll a 3, and your friend rolls a 5. Should you conclude that your friend cheated, and is using an unfair die? Of course not. Chances are, the difference in that individual roll is simply due to chance. If the dice are in fact fair, after many rolls, you will find that both your averages start to converge to the natural average, 3.5[1]. If, for example, you each roll 1,000 times, and your average score is 3.497 while your friend's average score is 3.501, you will conclude that the dice were fair and the slight difference measured is simply due to chance.

[1] The sum of the possible scores divided by the number of possibilities (1 + 2 + 3 + 4 + 5 + 6).

Likewise, if the Healthy Living U researchers find slight differences between the experimental and control groups in cardiovascular fitness, they will not rush to conclude that the difference was *significant*. In statistics and hypothesis-testing, a **significant difference** is a measured difference between two groups that is large enough that it is probably not due to chance. The vagueness of this definition is intentional. It is up to the researchers to determine when the difference is big enough.

To see how this works in practice, let's return to the example of rolling dice. Suppose that this time around, when you and your friend roll 1,000 times, your average is 3.506 and your friend's average is 3.813. Did your friend cheat? It is not immediately obvious what you should conclude. Maybe they just got lucky. Although you can never be absolutely sure, using statistics it is possible to calculate the probability that your friend obtained this value using a fair die. The mathematics used to compute this probability are briefly covered in the statistics chapter and generally are beyond the scope of Psychology/Sociology questions on the MCAT.

Now, suppose that you ran the necessary statistical tests and they show that the chance of the measured difference in dice scores was 17%. What would you conclude? Using the legal analogy from above, you would not want to wrongfully incriminate your friend. But what if the probability you found was 6%? 3%? 0.04%? At what point would you accuse your friend of cheating? It is not an easy decision to make, since whatever value you choose as the threshold point will inherently be arbitrary.

Scientists evaluating data from experiments have the same problem. They can never be certain that a difference measured in an experiment actually reflects a fundamental difference between the groups. They must arbitrarily pick a cutoff point at which it is reasonable to conclude "beyond reasonable doubt" that there was a difference. Conventionally, social scientists have decided that if the probability of an observed difference is found to be 5% (or 0.05) or less, this constitutes a significant difference. A **p-value** is a number from 0 to 1 that represents the probability that a difference observed in an experiment is due to chance. By convention, if (and only if) $p < 0.05$, scientists reject the null hypothesis. Other p-values such as 0.01 or 0.001 are also used as the threshold for significance in some cases. To make sure that the experiment picks up an effect, it is necessary to have a large enough **sample size**, or number of participants. Usually 30 or more participants are necessary to meet the mathematical criteria needed to conduct statistical tests. A larger sample size is usually preferred. This increases the **power** of the experiment, or the ability to pick up an effect if one is actually present.

Whatever researchers decide to do, they must select the significance threshold in advance, or they might be extremely tempted to change the number so that their data reach significance. For the MCAT, make sure you know what p-values represent, and that a lower value suggests a stronger relationship.

Table 1 Summary of Good Experimental Design

Step:	Objective:	Common Flaws in Design:
1. Select the population	• Determine the population of interest • Consider what group will be pragmatic to sample	• Population is too restrictive • Sampling all individuals of interest is not practical
2. Operationalize variables	• Determine the independent and dependent variables • Specify exactly what is meant by each • Make sure the dependent variable can be measured quantitatively within the parameters of the study	• Insufficient rigor in description • Manipulation of the independent variable presents practical problems
3. Divide into groups	• Carefully select experimental and control groups • Homogenize the two groups • Isolate the treatment by controlling for potential extraneous variables	• Control group does not resemble treatment group along important variables • Experiment is not double-blind • Participants can guess the hypothesis, purpose of the study, and ways in which they're expected to behave
4. Random sampling	• Make sure all subsets of the population are represented • Ideally each member has an equal chance of being selected • Meeting these criteria is often not possible for practical reasons	• Sampling is not truly random • Sample does not represent the population of interest
5. Random assignment	• Individuals who have been sampled are equally likely to be assigned to treatment or control groups • Consider matching along potential extraneous variables which have been pre-selected	• Groups are not properly matched • Assignment is not perfectly random
6. Measurement	• Make sure measurements are standardized • Make sure instruments are reliable and valid	• Tools are not precise enough to detect a result • Instruments used for measurement are not reliable and valid
7. Test the hypothesis	• Use statistics to check for a significant difference • Assign a pre-established threshold at which the null hypothesis will be rejected	• Small sample size leads to insufficient power • Researchers do not set thresholds in advance and make after-the-fact conclusions that are suspect

3.2 EXPERIMENTAL DESIGN CONSIDERATIONS

Validity

As we took a step-by-step look at experimental design, we looked at some of the potential flaws that come up in experiments, and how they might compromise our ability to draw conclusions about the real world from our study. These flaws can be placed into two categories. In one case, the flaw or limitation might make it difficult to apply our conclusion to the real world. This is known as a flaw in **external validity**. For example, the fact that only students of Healthy Living U can participate in the study is a threat to external validity. We cannot be absolutely sure that a result that rejects the null hypothesis applies to all healthy young adults in their twenties.

Another threat to external validity is that the subjects in this experiment ate a special diet, constructed by professional researchers, cooked by culinary professionals at a university, and monitored by a team of scientists. Can we really expect an average person trying to eat an experimental diet to match this rigor? An affirmative finding that a high-MDI diet leads to healthier outcomes might not apply to conditions outside the conditions of the study.

On the other hand, a limitation of the study might be such that the experiment is not "well done," leaving doubts about the conclusion because of some inherent flaw in the design. This is known as **internal validity**. Internal validity is high if confounding variables have been considered and minimized, and the causal relationship between the independent and dependent variable can be established by the way the experiment was set up. Another important component of a well-done study is construct validity, or the extend to which a psychometric instrument measure what it purports to. If the researchers forgot to control for sex differences, used a diet that was not actually Mediterranean, or gave the control group unhealthy foods, for example, internal validity could be threatened. **Demand characteristics**, or subtle cues (usually subconscious or inadvertent) that let subjects know how they are expected to behave, can also threaten internal validity.

Another consideration, especially when psychometric evaluations are used, is **predictive validity**. For example, consider the MCAT. Does the test predict performance after the exam-taker enters school (or becomes a doctor)? This is a question about predictive validity: does the test tell us about the variable of interest? Below is a summary of the frequently-tested common threats to validity in social science experiments.

Table 2 Threats to Internal Validity

Impression Management	Participants adapt their responses based on social norms or perceived researcher expectations; self-fulfilling prophecy; methodology is not double-blind; Hawthorne Effect
Confounding Variables	Extraneous variables not accounted for in the study; another variable offers an alternative explanation for results; lack of a useful control
Lack of Validity/Reliability	Measurement tools do not measure what they purport to, lack consistency
Sampling Bias	Selection criteria are not random; population used for sample does not meet conditions for statistical test (e.g., population is not normally distributed)
Attrition Effects	Participant fatigue; participants drop out of study
Demand Characteristics	Researchers inadvertently give subtle cues about the hypothesis and how subjects are expected to behave

Table 3 Threats to External Validity

Experiment doesn't reflect real world	Laboratory setups that don't translate to the real world; lack of generalizability
Selection Criteria	Too restrictive of inclusion/exclusion criteria for participants (i.e., sample is not representative)
Situational Effects	Presence of laboratory conditions changes outcome (e.g., pre-test and post-test, presence of experimenter, claustrophobia in an MRI machine)
Lack of Statistical Power	Sample groups have high variability; sample size is too small

Ethical Considerations

Finally, all researchers should consider the ethical implications of the procedures they employ. Ethical problems tend to arise more frequently in experimental designs because researchers are directly manipulating variables, not just observing what they see in nature. Ethical controversies arose regarding many social science experiments of the early 20th century as researchers, institutions, and society gradually came to an agreement as to the correct protocol for running experiments. Some studies became infamous for their egregious breach of ethical protocols. One such experiment was the Tuskegee syphilis experiment. In this study, African-American males in Alabama who had contracted syphilis were not told they had the disease after they tested positive, and were not treated for the disease, even though treatments were available. The participants were recruited under false pretexts and treated with an inhumane disregard for their health and well-being. This experiment and others have become classic examples of ethical breaches that researchers must avoid. Any procedures that could lead to detrimental health consequences must be ruled out. If researchers become aware that patients have a condition or disease they must be immediately notified and given treatment options. Over time, ethical standards for human experiments have strengthened to include the emotional health of participants and potentially traumatic experimental procedures must include protocols for dealing with the harm they might cause, such as counseling or other clinical treatment.

To be sure that these ethical standards are met, modern experiments must be cleared by an independent internal commission. They must also contain some type of **disclosure**, an outline given to participants before the experiment begins that clarifies incentives and expectations while reminding them of their right to terminate the experiment at any time. Finally, experimental protocol should include **debriefing**, in which participants are told after the experiment exactly what was done and why the experiment was conducted. In some cases, particularly if the experiment may have triggered psychological vulnerability, participants may be offered access to treatment or counseling services as part of debriefing.

3.3 NON-EXPERIMENTAL DESIGNS

We have seen that experiments are difficult to conduct, sometimes prohibitively, and introduce many possible problems concerning validity and ethics. However, they are often worth the trouble. Experimental design offers the only way to confidently establish a causal relationship between two variables. When, however, experiments are not feasible for practical or ethical reasons, researchers in the social sciences have many other types of design at their disposal. Each offers its own benefits and potential drawbacks. In general, non-experimental designs tend to offer the benefit of observing phenomena in a more naturalistic setting, often improving external validity. The trade-off is reduced control of the variables of interest, which tends to reduce the internal validity. Below are the most frequently tested non-experimental research designs that appear on the MCAT.

1) **Correlational studies** explore the relationship between two quantitative variables. The most commonly used type of correlation is the **Pearson correlation**. A Pearson correlation assigns a number from −1 to +1 to a pair of variables. If the value is negative, the two variables are negatively correlated. This means that if one increases, the other will decrease, and vice versa. On the other hand, a positive value represents a positive correlation, which means that as one variable increases, the other also increases, and if one variable decreases the other will also decrease. A value of zero indicates no correlation, that there is no *linear* relationship between the two variables, although a nonlinear relationship is still plausible. Significance testing can be combined with Pearson correlations to see if the computed correlation is likely to have occurred by chance or not.

   For example, many studies have shown that size and mass of the amygdala, a brain area associated with fear and primal emotions, is positively correlated with subjective reports of anxiety. We expect that as reported anxiety increases, so too will measures of amygdala size. Note that this does not imply that one variable *causes* the other. As we mentioned earlier, the causal relationship could go in either direction, or some third variable (say, childhood abandonment) could be responsible for both.

   An example of a negative correlation is the relationship between social support and introversion. Some studies have shown that as social support increases, measures of introversion tend to decrease, and vice versa. Correlational studies offer the advantage of showing a numerical relationship between two variables, and are usually easier to conduct than experiments. Researchers can take the measurements of a population as it exists and do not need to directly manipulate the variables. The main disadvantage, as we've discussed, is that causality cannot be inferred.

2) **Ethnographic studies** are a qualitative method in which researchers immerse themselves completely in the lives, culture, or way of life of the people they are studying. These studies tend to be lengthy and thorough and involve as little interference or intervention by the researchers as possible. The culture studied is often unique or remote in some way, or offers a special insight into a scientific question. A researcher interested in the effects of the Mediterranean diet on health might go to a remote Sicilian village and study the lives of the participants, scrutinizing their everyday lives and recording everything they possibly can over the span of several years.

   Many of the early ethnographic studies were anthropological in nature: they often explored the lives and habits of remote cultures with little outside contact. Over time, ethnographic methods came to be used throughout the social sciences.

Nowadays, a lot of ethnographic research is conducted through online tools and technology. By utilizing social media, researchers can explore the habits, lifestyles, and social interactions of millions of individuals, then use data analytics to analyze the research and draw conclusions. There are many web tools that now make this type of research relatively easy to conduct, and it can be less resource intensive and time consuming than traditional forms of ethnographic research.

In general, perhaps the greatest strength of the ethnographic method is depth of analysis. Researchers can get a thorough understanding of a culture and the factors that influence it over many years. There are also many potential weaknesses. The researcher in an ethnographic study is often working alone, so there is no one to critique the methodology. Also, the mere presence of the researcher can affect the findings. It is likely that the members of the group will probably want to present themselves and their group/culture in a good light. This also makes replication of the study difficult, and deep immersion in a culture can result in feelings of association and attachment with the culture by the researchers, which threatens objectivity.

3) **Twin studies** are often run to test the relationship between nature and nurture. They are the best way to measure **heritability**, the extent to which an observed trait is due to genetics versus the environment. For example, twin studies interested in the heritability of intelligence might look at correlations in IQ scores between monozygotic (identical) twins and dizygotic (fraternal) twins. It is reasonable to conclude that any differences between these two correlations are due to genetics, since both types of twins share an environment. Similarly, an intelligence study might look at the difference in correlations between IQs of identical twins reared together versus reared apart. These differences would likely be due to the environment, since both sets of twins would share the same percentage of genes, namely 100.

4) **Longitudinal studies** can be run when researchers may be interested in how individuals develop over time along some research variable. While some longitudinal research is experimental, most longitudinal studies do not involve independent-variable manipulation. The New York longitudinal study is a classic example of the **longitudinal method**, which involves intervallic measurements of a dependent variable over long time frames. The New York longitudinal study asked a simple research question: what effect does our disposition at birth have on the life we lead? Researchers categorized newborns according to their dispositions: agreeable or irritable, healthy or sickly, regular or irregular in biological functions. Then they checked in on subjects over periodic intervals to see if temperament at birth was consistent throughout life. These types of research are costly, difficult to execute, time-and-resource intensive, and likely to have high attrition rates. The benefit is the ability to detail how an effect or factor can develop over time. This allows researchers to have high accuracy when observing for change. A related (but slightly different) methodology is known as a **cross-sectional study**, data collection or survey of a population or sample at a specific time.

5) **Case studies** involve in-depth exploration of individual, small group, entity, event, or phenomenon. Suppose that a researcher from Healthy Living U met a native Sicilian in her late 90s with extraordinary health and fitness. The researcher might want to know everything possible about this person's diet and lifestyle to understand how she was able to obtain such a high level of fitness, including dietary habits over time, exercise frequency, interaction with family, and sleep patterns. They would then compile this data and offer a report for critique by the scientific community. This would offer an excellent way to thoroughly explore the potential causes that

lead to a phenomenon, but of course the limitation is that there is no isolation of variables or control over the conditions. It is also difficult to determine how the different variables involved in a phenomenon interact.

6) **Phenomenological studies** are interested in describing phenomena, using the introspective method to explore research questions. All the studies we have discussed so far have involved researchers studying another individual or group of individuals. Another type of study could involve researchers studying themselves, or researchers recording what individuals report about their own personal experiences. Hermann Ebbinghaus made many groundbreaking discoveries in learning and forgetting by taking detailed data and notes on his own learning and memory performance. These investigations were phenomenological; Ebbinghaus attempted to understand his own perceptions and understandings, rather than make a comparison between variables or draw a causal conclusion.

Not all phenomenological studies are confined to self-observation. A phenomenological study attempts to understand people's perceptions, perspectives, and understandings of a situation (or phenomenon). Although the sample size may be greater than one, it is almost always small. Phenomenological studies offer the advantage of detail and in-depth understanding, but the data is subjective, potentially affecting validity. It is also difficult to generalize data, and the small sample sizes reduce external validity.

7) The **survey** is a method for collecting information or data as reported by individuals. Participants answer a series of questions and self-report the information. Surveys are used to ascertain the beliefs and attitudes of a particular group about issues such as politics and religion, as well as their opinions about, for example, the quality of new businesses, academic classes, consumer products, etc. Additionally, surveys can be a way for people to measure how often or how little people engage in different behaviors, such as smoking or drinking alcohol. The benefits of surveys are that they are easy to administer and tend to be cost effective. Nowadays, they can be administered online, which further boosts the reach and facility of conducting survey studies. Potential flaws are that respondents may not feel encouraged to provide honest and accurate answers and that validity can be adversely affected by an unrepresentative sample or poor survey questions. Surveys must be assessed for reliability and validity to make sure they are consistently measuring what they're supposed to measure.

8) A few other types of studies are worth mentioning briefly since they may appear on the MCAT Psychology/Sociology section. **Archival studies** analyze already collected data from historical records and authentic original documents. **Biographical studies** are exhaustive accounts of an individual's life experience. Finally, many of the study types we've looked at fall under the category of **Observational Studies**. An observational study is any study in which individuals are observed and outcomes measured with no attempt to control the outcome. Table 4 provides a summary of the non-experimental designs that are likely to show up on the MCAT.

Table 4 Summary of Non-Experimental Designs

Type of Study:	Description	Strengths	Weaknesses
Correlational	• Measures the quantitative relationship between two variables	• Great preliminary technique • Usually easy to conduct	• Does not establish causality • May not pick up nonlinear relationship
Ethnographic	• Deep, lengthy qualitative analysis of a culture and its characteristics	• Provides detailed analysis and comprehensive evaluation	• Researcher's presence may affect individuals' behavior • Heavily dependent on the researcher conducting the study, difficult to replicate, and objectivity may be compromised
Twin	• Analysis of heritability through measuring characteristics of twins	• Offers insight into how nature and nurture might interact to lead to various characteristics	• Difficult to find participants who meet criteria • Difficult to analyze the complex variables involved and how they interact
Longitudinal	• Long-term analysis that intermittently measures the evolution of some behavior or characteristic; usually nonexperimental	• Scientists can understand how trait of interest changes over time	• Logistically demanding, expensive and difficult to implement • High attrition rate
Case	• Deep analysis of a single case or example	• Offers comprehensive details about the single case	• Results may not be generalizable • Does not offer points of reference or comparison
Phenomenological	• Self-observation of a phenomenon by researcher or small group of participants	• Introspection can provide insight into behaviors and occurrences that are difficult to measure	• Lacks objectivity due to results coming from self-analysis • Difficult to generalize results to other circumstances or individuals
Survey	• Use of a series of questions to allow participants to self-report behaviors or tendencies	• Easy to administer • Can provide quantitative data that can be compared to large participant pools	• Self reporting creates limitations in objectivity

Archival	• Analysis of historical records for insight into a phenomenon	• Provide insight into events from the past that are different from everyday behavior	• Quality of analysis subject to the quality and integrity of records • Difficult to conduct follow-ups • Data are unlikely to be comprehensive, leaving ambiguity and unanswered questions
Biographical	• Exploration of all the events and circumstances of an individual's life	• Comprehensive knowledge of all the details of an individual's life	• Limitations in objectivity • Difficult to generalize observations
Observational	• Broad category that includes any research in which experimenters do not manipulate the situation or results	• Naturalistic observation of circumstances as they are	• Difficult to tease out the complex interplay of many variables

Chapter 3 Summary

- The experimental method is the primary method used by researchers to establish causality.

- Several steps must be scrupulously followed in order to meet the rigorous requirements of experimental research: selecting the population, operationalizing variables, creating the different groups and the protocols for each, randomly sampling from the population, and randomly assigning subjects to groups.

- The independent variable is the variable manipulated by the researcher.

- The dependent variable, or measurement variable, is the variable that is measured to test for an effect.

- An operational definition is a precise and concrete definition of a research variable.

- Quantitative indicates numerical, whereas qualitative indicates descriptive or categorical.

- A control group is the group researchers use as a point of comparison; it does not receive the treatment.

- An experimental group is the group that does receive the treatment in a study.

- Extraneous (or confounding) variables are variables other than the research variable that could potentially explain a result in an experiment.

- A research sample should reflect the population from which it is drawn.

- Individuals who are sampled from the population should be randomly assigned to the control and experimental groups.

- In hypothesis testing, researchers assign the null hypothesis: the hypothesis that any effects are due to chance and there is no experimental result.

- Type 1 error is known as a false positive, rejecting the null hypothesis: any observed effects are not systematic and are simply due to chance.

- Internal validity is how well done a study is, or how well it allows researchers to draw conclusions from measured effects. External validity is how well a research result applies to the population at large and real-life scenarios.

- Non-experimental methodologies, which do not allow researchers to draw conclusions about causality, include the correlational method, the observational method, the longitudinal method, ethnographic studies, and case studies.

CHAPTER 3 FREESTANDING PRACTICE QUESTIONS

1. A team of researchers measures a negative correlation between income and length of labor time in a group of pregnant women. It is expected that as income increases, labor time:

   A) decreases.
   B) increases.
   C) stays the same.
   D) The change in labor time cannot be determined.

2. Due to scheduling and logistical limitations, researchers conducting a study could only conduct the study on Tuesdays and Thursdays between 7 P.M. and 9 P.M. They were therefore limited to individuals who were available at this time to participate in the study. This set up would have created issues in:

   A) external validity, due to the selection criteria.
   B) internal validity, due to a potential Hawthorne effect.
   C) external validity, due to the lack of a control group.
   D. internal validity, due to impression management.

3. Researchers want to explore the experience of subjects as they engage in the Stroop task, a task in selective attention that measures the ability to distinguish between discordant stimuli. The researchers are not merely interested in response time but want to know qualitative details about the subjects' internal experiences. Which of the following methodologies should the researchers implement?

   A) Correlational method
   B) Observational method
   C) Survey method
   D) Phenomenological method

4. Which of the following is a limitation of the ethnographic method?

   A) Cultural validity is low, since the observer is not a member of the society of interest
   B) External validity is low, because the conditions under which the research is conducted do not match the real world
   C) External validity is low, because only one culture is sampled
   D) Construct validity is low, since the instruments have not been checked for reliability

5. A team of researchers finds that there is a complex relationship between IQ and sociability. Measures of sociability were found to be high for individuals within one standard deviation of the mean for intelligence, and gradually decreased for individuals with both very high and very low IQ scores. Which of the following correlations would be measured in this instance?

   A) A strong positive correlation
   B) A weak negative correlation
   C) No correlation
   D) A moderate negative correlation

6. In a study of the impact of personality type on the interpretation of a social symbol, which of the following is a possible operational definition of the independent variable?

   A) Personality type is the independent variable, so it can be defined as results on a questionnaire designed to measure five-factor model personality traits.
   B) Personality type is the independent variable, so it can be defined as degree of sympathetic arousal and amygdala activation when seeing a symbol.
   C) Symbol interpretation is the independent variable, so it can be defined as average ranking, from positive to negative, of a series of neutral symbols.
   D) Symbol interpretation is the independent variable, so it can be defined as degree of sympathetic arousal and amygdala activation when seeing a symbol.

7. Attrition, or subjects dropping out of a study before its completion, is a threat to:

   A) internal validity, because it introduces a potential confounding variable.
   B) internal validity, because the group may no longer be representative.
   C) external validity, because it introduces a potential confounding variable.
   D) external validity, because the group may no longer be representative.

8. Which of the following research methodologies would best explore the development of human memory over time?

   A) Case study
   B) Longitudinal study
   C) Observational study
   D) Archival study

CHAPTER 3 PRACTICE PASSAGE

Recent adaptations in technology, such as smartphones and the Internet, have been found to have potentially negative effects on physical and psychological well-being. Sociologists refer to the time it takes to catch up to technology as cultural lag. Researchers have been interested in studying the effects of cultural lag on attention, cognition, and psychopathology.

A study was conducted by recruiting 347 students from first year introductory psychology courses at a four-year state university in the Midwest, where a large majority of students were in-state residents. They were incentivized with extra credit in their course, and of the 347 that were invited, 62 participants that chose to participate were first asked to respond on a Likert scale from 1 to 5 on how often they used their cell phones, social media, and the Internet. Based on the results, participants were divided into 2 groups of 31 students each. Both groups contained more females, 21 and 23 in the low usage and high usage groups, respectively. Researchers also considered GPA, and found that the cumulative GPAs for both groups were similar, 3.16 and 3.32, respectively, a difference that was not found to be significant. It was hypothesized that the group that used various types of digital media more would manifest detrimental effects along a range of variables, measured by a battery of exams on reaction time, working memory, and ability to conduct tasks while ignoring a distractor. Participants were given a questionnaire designed to measure depression and a second questionnaire designed to measure anxiety.

Results supported the research hypotheses. Based on the results, researchers determined that the stress response may have been the link between technology use and the measurement variables, since various studies showed that stress was known to have detrimental effects on each of these areas. The group suggested to campus health experts that they should recommend students limit their use of digital media to mitigate the effects of cultural lag.

1. If the researchers are correct in their conclusion, what is likely to happen in a second study of elderly adults who are known to be more sensitive in their response to stress?

A) They will have difficulty attending to stimuli.
B) They will score higher on depression.
C) The low digital usage group will have slower reaction times.
D) The high digital usage group will demonstrate increased anxiety.

2. Which of the following conclusions can be most reasonably drawn from the study in passage?

A) Stress plays a critical role in the relationship between technology and cognitive effects, because it provides the most plausible mediating variable.
B) There was a relationship between technology use and psychopathology because the research utilized various psychometrics.
C) Cultural lag regarding digital media is an ongoing problem on college campuses because the research conducted used random assignment and random sampling to test the hypotheses.
D) Use of social media caused detrimental effects on cognition because of the strain placed on the attentional mechanism, as demonstrated by comparison with the control group.

3. A likely confounding variable created by the experimental design was:

A) school performance.
B) gender.
C) extraversion.
D) academic major.

4. The methodology described in the passage created threats to external validity due to each of the following considerations EXCEPT:

A) geographic location.
B) lack of a control group.
C) student availability.
D) age.

5. Which of the following pairs represents a qualitative and quantitative variable, respectively?

A) Reaction time and coping ability
B) Reaction time and depression score
C) Type of coping response and level of depression
D) Attending fluidity ability and reaction time

6. Each of the following could be an operational definition of the dependent variable EXCEPT:

A) depression inventory score.
B) sympathetic nervous system arousal.
C) size of social media network.
D) time attending to distracting variables.

SOLUTIONS TO CHAPTER 3 FREESTANDING PRACTICE QUESTIONS

1. **A** A negative correlation suggests that as the value measured for one variable increases, the other decreases, and vice versa. Therefore, as income increases, labor time is expected to decrease (choice A is correct). Labor time would increase if the correlation were positive (choice B is wrong). There was a result measured, so the measurement would not stay the same (choice C is wrong), and the direction of change is known because the type of correlation is given in the question stem (choice D is wrong).

2. **A** This question can be attacked more quickly with the observation that the second part of the answer choices cuts the set of choices in half. The first step is to determine if the situation described in the question stem is a threat to internal or external validity. The recruitment method is problematic because the experiment will not sample individuals who have different schedules and are not available at that time. A sample that is not representative of the population is a threat to external validity (choices B and D are wrong). Selection criteria are the processes used to select participants for an experiment. This describes the scheduling issue presented in the question stem (choice A is correct). A lack of control group is a threat to internal (not external) validity, as this factor is related to how well-designed the study is and to what extent researchers can draw conclusions based on findings (choice C is wrong).

3. **D** The phenomenological method is a technique used to evaluate the experience of some phenomenon and often obtains more introspective details about an event than is possible with other methods. This method is also usually qualitative, or descriptive, as the question stem suggests (choice D is correct). The correlational method is a quantitative measure of the relationship between two variables (choice A is wrong). The observational method involves observation and minimal interference by the researcher. It would be very difficult to know about subjects' internal experiences by simply observing them (choice B is wrong). The survey method tends to reveal only general aspects of an event or experience, since it contains general questions that are tested on numerous individuals. This characteristic would make it difficult to know about subjects' unique internal experiences. The survey method is also quantitative in most cases, since subjects often provide a numerical assessment of their self-reported beliefs or feelings (choice C is wrong).

4. **C** External validity is an issue in ethnographic studies, mainly because the methodology involves deep exploration of a single culture or subculture, so it provides limited information on how the results might apply to other cultures (choice C is correct). Cultural validity is not a type of validity checked for by researchers (choice A is wrong). Conditions in ethnographic research are usually very close to the real world, since the researcher makes every attempt to not disrupt the environment. The goal of ethnographic research is to observe the culture in a naturalistic setting (choice B is wrong). Ethnographic researchers do not usually use surveys, but deep analysis, in their evaluations of the cultures they study, so construct validity is very unlikely to be a consideration. Construct validity usually applies to psychometric instruments such as surveys (choice D is wrong).

5. **C** The results described in the question are curvilinear in nature. They do not represent a linear relationship and would show up as a bell on a graph. Correlational research does not pick up nonlinear trends (choice C is correct; choices A, B, and D are wrong).

6. **A** This question can be resolved more quickly by noticing that the first part of the answer choices is divided in half. The first step is to determine whether personality type or symbolic interpretation is the independent variable. The study described is designed to measure how personality affects symbolic interpretation. Therefore, the independent variable—the variable manipulated by the researcher—is personality type (choices C and D are wrong). The five-factor model is a common measure of personality (choice A is correct). Sympathetic arousal and amygdala activation do not define personality type (choice B is wrong).

7. **A** Attrition is primarily a threat to internal validity, because there may be some non-trivial reason that subjects are dropping out. This would present a confounding variable, because if the reason for attrition were related to the hypothesis, it could provide an alternative explanation for the results (choice A is correct). Non-representative samples are a threat to external, not internal, validity (choice B is wrong). Confounding variables are a threat to internal, not external, validity (choice C is wrong). It is less likely that enough subjects drop out to threaten the external validity of the study. Also, if participants began to drop out, internal validity would be threatened first, such that it would be difficult to draw a conclusion that would then be applied to the external population (choice D is wrong).

8. **B** Longitudinal studies are best for exploring how variables develop over time. They involve conducting periodic measurements of the same individuals over many years to see how certain variables change. This is the ideal methodology for exploring the question presented in the stem (choice B is correct). Case studies are best for understanding individuals in a comprehensive way. This would be an ideal methodology for understanding one person's memory development, but would not allow for generalization to human memory (choice A is wrong). An observational study could meet the criteria, but observational studies do not specifically deal with the development of variables over a long period of time. This study methodology usually involves observing events in a naturalistic setting, and although this could be done over time intervals, this is not usually a feature of observational research (choice C is wrong). Archival studies would be best for exploring how a phenomenon was different many years ago, to use as a comparison with other epochs. However, archival research would not be ideal for understanding how memory evolved for groups of individuals, since it is impossible to control for variables with data taken many years ago, and there are often gaps in the data available (choice D is wrong).

SOLUTIONS TO CHAPTER 3 PRACTICE PASSAGE

1. **D** The researchers concluded that stress was a potential mediating result because of its known relationship with the cognitive variables. Stress and anxiety are known to be related to each other, so high digital usage would be associated with increased anxiety (choice D is correct). The research described showed a relationship between digital usage and attention, not stress response and attention. Note that stress response does not necessarily mean that the group will actually experience more stress, but that they will respond with greater sensitivity if stress occurs. Therefore, the known relationships between stress and attention and stress and depression do not necessarily apply (choices A and B are wrong). Slower reaction time was associated with the high digital use group, not the low digital use group (choice C is wrong).

2. **B** Psychopathology refers to mental disorders or abnormal behavior. The research described found a relationship between time spent using various forms of technology and slowed cognitive function. The psychometrics used were the battery of exams on cognitive functions (reaction time, working memory, and multitasking) as well as the Likert scale that was used to assess technology use (choice B is correct). The researchers proposed stress as a possible mediator in paragraph 3, however, the actual research to establish this relationship was not actually conducted. A mediating variable is a variable that provides a link in a causal relationship and helps to show why that relationship exists. The researchers did not conduct any tests on stress and how stress relates to technology use (choice A is wrong). The research did suggest that cultural lag was a point of concern since new technologies seemed to be related to cognitive problems. However, the study did not contain random sampling from the population described in the answer choice, namely college campuses. The study only sampled from one university, and without follow-up research, we cannot be sure that the results apply to students on other campuses (choice C is wrong). The researchers cannot be sure that social media caused the detrimental effects because the independent variable is not manipulated directly by the researchers in this case. Instead, it is measured and the subjects are placed into groups. Also, there was no control group. There was only a high technology and low technology group (choice D is wrong).

3. **C** Extraversion is a characteristic related to how energizing individuals find social interactions which others. Individuals who are high in extraversion tend to be more sociable, garrulous, and spend more time interacting with others. It may therefore be more likely that they engage more with social media and technology, spending more time on their phones. This could make high extraversion individuals more susceptible to the effects of the study (choice C is correct). School performance and gender were both measured in the study, and the researchers did not find large differences between the two groups in either variable (choices A and B are wrong). Academic major is unlikely to be a confounding variable since there is not a clear link between major and digital media usage. Also, there are many academic majors, and variables with many groups are less likely to confound, since any effect will be distributed across a spectrum (choice D is wrong).

4. **B** For except/not/least questions, evaluate each answer choice and eliminate the answer choices that are true. Only using subjects from one geographic location (a Midwestern university) is a threat to external validity because these individuals may not be representative of the larger population (choice A is true and can be eliminated). The study did lack a control group, but this is a threat to internal validity, not external validity, because it is a flaw in the way the research is designed that affects the ability to draw conclusions from the variables (choice B is false and the correct answer choice). Student availability is a threat to external validity, because only some students participated in the study, so the research results may not apply as well to the entire student population, which includes students who may be too busy to participate in the research (choice C is true and can be eliminated). Age is a threat to external validity since most students will be in their early 20s. This means the results may not apply to older adults (choice D is true and can be eliminated).

5. **C** The correct answer choice will pair a qualitative variable with a quantitative variable. Type of coping response suggests that coping responses will be broken into categories, a sign that it is a qualitative variable, since it would not involve a numerical continuum but rather placement into one of several different coping styles. Depression level can be measured quantitatively, since "level" suggests a score along a scale (choice C is correct). Reaction time is a quantitative variable (choices A and B are wrong). Attending fluidity ability suggests a measure along a continuum. Most variables along a continuum tend to be quantitative in nature, whereas most categorical variables tend to be qualitative. Since attending fluidity ability suggests a range of abilities along a single variable, attending fluidity, this suggests a quantitative variable (choice D is wrong).

6. **C** For except/not/least questions, evaluate each answer choice and eliminate the answer choices that are "true" or work for this question (i.e., could be an operational definition of the dependent variable). A dependent variable is an outcome variable measured by the researchers to test the extent of effect of the manipulation in the study. Depression is one of the dependent, or measurement, variables (choice A works for this question and can be eliminated). Sympathetic nervous arousal is related to anxiety, one of the dependent variables (choice B works for this question and can be eliminated). Size of social media network is related to how much time an individual spends using digital media, which is an independent, not dependent, variable in the study (choice C does not work for this question and is therefore the correct answer choice). Attention and ability to tune out distracting variables is a dependent variable in the study (choice D works for this question and can be eliminated).

Chapter 4
Sociological Theories and Social Institutions

Sociologists employ various theoretical lenses to provide a framework for how individuals and social structures interact with each other. Each theory provides a perspective for understanding social phenomena and guides the type of research conducted by social scientists. Theories can focus on society as a whole and other big-picture issues, or individual interactions, or both. One of the primary large scale issues sociologists explore is the nature of social institutions: how they organize, evolve, and impact the lives of individuals within the society.

4.1 SOCIOLOGY: THEORETICAL APPROACHES

A **society** can be defined as a group of people who share a culture and live/interact with each other within a definable area. **Sociology** is the study of how individuals interact with, shape, and are subsequently shaped by the society in which they live. Because culture influences individuals and individuals influence their culture, sociologists consider both individual actions and the patterns of behavior of groups.

There are four major sociological theories that explain society: functionalism, conflict theory, symbolic interactionism, and social constructionism. The first two, functionalism and conflict theory, are macro-level theories which focus on the effects of large scale social structures. Macro-level theories try to answer fundamental questions such as why societies form, why societies change, and why their social structures function in the manner that they function.

The third major perspective is **symbolic interactionism**, which analyzes society on a **micro-level**. Micro-sociologists are interested in small-scale individual considerations, most prominently one-on-one and small group interactions. From the micro-sociological perspective, societies are best understood as emergent properties of individual human social interactions and best understood by analyzing very specific relationships among individuals and small groups. The fourth theory, **social constructionism**, can be either macro or micro, depending on the context.

Presented in this section are these four major theories along with the **feminist**, and **rational choice/ social exchange theories**.

Functionalism (also known as Structural Functionalism)

The oldest of the three major theories of sociology, **functionalism** is a paradigm that conceptualizes society as a living organism with many different interrelated and interdependent parts, each of which has a distinct and necessary purpose. Functionalism can trace its genesis to the philosopher **Herbert Spencer** (1820–1903). Spencer postulated that just as the various organs and systems in a human body work together to keep the body functioning and regulated, the various structures and institutions of a society work together to keep that entire society functioning and regulated. Spencer also contended that societies were subject to evolutionary pressures and could evolve in response to these pressures just as organisms do.

The functionalist perspective focuses on the social functions of different social structures by asking what these structures contribute to society at large. For example, the contribution of our lungs to the body is to orchestrate the exchange of air. Similarly, we can think about the function of schools, churches, hospitals, and other social structures. Just as organs function interdependently to help the organism survive, social structures work together to sustain society. According to the functionalist perspective, societies can thrive and grow or become disease-addled and die, like living organisms.

Émile Durkheim (1858–1917) was a pioneer in modern social research and a major proponent of functionalism. Durkheim established sociology as an academic field of study separate and distinct from psychology and political philosophy. Through the influential scientific journal he edited and his groundbreaking scientific work, Durkheim is considered by many to be the founder of sociology. Durkheim extended Spencer's analogy to explain how societies form, grow, persist, and function. To Durkheim, a society's capacity to maintain social order and stability is paramount to its functional success.

Durkheim believed that modern societies were more complex than primitive societies. In primitive societies, people are held together because they are all quite similar, sharing a common language as well as common tasks, values, and symbols. In modern societies, Durkheim argued, people rely upon each other to make the society function as a whole. According to functionalist theory, all the interrelated parts of modern societies, including all major social structures such as the government, the police force, the educational system, and the medical system have interdependent roles to play. For society to thrive, all of these complex, interdependent parts must work together to keep society ordered, balanced, and stable. When a healthy society faces an imbalance or crisis, functionalist theory proposes that the major structures of society will work together to return to a state of **dynamic equilibrium**. Healthy societies can successfully achieve and maintain this dynamic equilibrium; unhealthy ones cannot.

Durkheim further believed that society should always be viewed holistically—as a collective of social facts, rather than individuals. **Social facts** are the elements that serve some function in society, such as the laws, morals, values, religions, customs, rituals, and rules that make up a society. Durkheim felt that such cultural links create societal "solidarity." He proposed the existence of a "collective conscience," his name for how people of a shared culture come to think in the same manner due to their shared beliefs, ideas, and moral attitudes, all which operate to unify society.

There is an important distinction in the functionalist framework made between manifest and latent functions. **Manifest functions** are the official, intended, and anticipated consequences of a structure. Manifest functions are at least arguably beneficial. For example, the manifest functions of a police department include enforcing laws against violent crime and property crime. In contrast, **latent functions** are consequences of a structure that are not officially sought or sanctioned. Latent functions can be beneficial, neutral, or harmful. For example, the latent functions of a police department can include providing employment to community residents, raising government revenue by issuing traffic tickets, or even promoting social inequality through selective law enforcement.

Functionalism recognizes that not all of the effects of social structures are beneficial. A **social dysfunction** is a process that has undesirable consequences and may actually reduce the stability of society. For example, a dysfunctional police department could routinely commit police brutality. However, functionalist theory predicts that in a healthy society other social structures such as a free press and a responsive government will, over time, work together to mitigate such dysfunctions.

While functionalism was the prevailing theory in sociology in the 1950s, many sociologists began to argue that functionalism's focus on the structures of healthy society working together to maintain societal order, balance, and stability could not accurately account for the many rapid sociological advances taking place in the 1960s and 1970s. Though functionalism is still considered useful in many respects, other sociological theories have become more popular in recent decades.

Conflict Theory

Like functionalism, **conflict theory** is also a macro-level theory that focuses primarily on large-scale social structures and their effects on individuals. However, conflict theory views society as a never-ending competition for limited resources, and at least in some respects, conflict theory is diametrically opposed to the functionalist perspective. According to conflict theory, all past and current societies have had unequally distributed resources; therefore, individual members of these societies must compete for social, political, and material resources such as money, land, power, and leisure. Furthermore, social structures and institutions will reflect this competition in their degree of inherent inequality. Those with the most resources, power, and influence will use their relative advantages to amass more resources, power, and influence by suppressing the advancement of others.

Karl Marx (1818–1883), who is closely identified with conflict theory, looked at the economic conflict between different social classes. According to Marx, every society is divided into two major classes based upon the ownership of the means of production (such as tools, factories, and land). In the economic system of **capitalism**, which encourages competition and private ownership, the bourgeoisie, or ruling class, owns the means of production, while the proletariat, or working class, provides labor. The working class is oppressed and exploited by the capitalist bourgeois class that pays the members of the working class only a fraction of the production value of their labor. These differences result in an inherent conflict of interests between the two groups. Those who already have want to use their advantages to maintain their position at the top of society, while the interests of the have-nots is to overthrow the haves in order to create an egalitarian society.

According to conflict theorists, this unequal social order is maintained through ideological coercion that creates societal consensus, or **hegemony**—a coerced acceptance of the values, expectations, and conditions as determined by the capitalist class. Conflict theorists maintain that societal "consensus" is imposed by the "superstructure" of society, comprised of social institutions, political structures, and culture. This coerced consensus justifies the social, political, and economic status quo as natural, inevitable, and perpetual, as well as beneficial for everyone in society rather than only for the capitalist class that engenders this cultural hegemony.

Marx believed that revolution was inevitable in any capitalist society because of the inherent instability of the extreme class inequality that capitalism promotes. To maximize profits, members of the capitalist class pay the lowest possible wages while providing the worst possible working conditions. Such exploitation will eventually result in the development of **class consciousness**, which Marx defined as exploited workers' awareness of the reasons for their oppression. This in turn would inevitably lead the more numerous workers to revolt against less numerous capitalists, overthrow their oppressors, and replace capitalism with an extreme form of **socialism**, that Marx called **communism** in which all means of production are owned by all workers equally.

Max Weber (1864–1920), who is best known for refining and critiquing many of Marx's tenets of conflict theory, agreed with Marx that inequalities in a capitalist system would lead to conflict, but Weber did not believe that the collapse of capitalism was inevitable. Instead, Weber believed that Marx's focus on economic inequality alone was too narrow and extreme. Weber also believed that Marx did not pay enough attention to the power of values and beliefs to influence, transform, and stabilize societies. Weber theorized that the **Protestant/Puritan work ethic**, a widely held religious belief that lauded the morality of hard work for the sake of godliness, was a critical factor in the success of the capitalist system in replacing the feudalist system that preceded it in Western Europe. Weber contended that the fundamental trend of modern society was the increasing **rationalization of society**, which he defined as our increasing concern with efficiency (achieving the maximum result with the minimum amount of effort). Weber also argued that several factors moderate people's reaction to inequality, such agreement with authority figures, high rates of social mobility, and low rates of class difference.

Like functionalism, conflict theory strongly emphasizes the effects of large-scale structures of society over individuals, making it a macro-sociological theory. Although the perspectives of Karl Marx and Max Weber fundamentally differ from the perspective of Émile Durkheim, these three men are generally considered the founders of sociology.

The major criticism of conflict theory is that it focuses too much on competition and does not recognize the role of stability within society. Critics of conflict theory contend that conflict theorists focus too myopically on economic factors, view society only from the perspective of those who lack power, and ignore the cooperative ways in which people and groups can reach pragmatic agreements for the good of society as a whole.

Symbolic Interactionism

While the first two sociological perspectives look at society from a macro (top-down and zoomed-out) perspective, **symbolic interactionism** starts at the micro (bottom-up and zoomed-in) level and views society as built up from typical everyday interactions. Rather than considering individuals as entities who are acted upon by the large-scale structures of their society, symbolic interactionism emphasizes the ways by which individuals actively shape their world through their understanding and subsequent behavioral responses to the meanings they attribute to the societal symbols through which individuals define their reality.

While symbolic interactionism's focus was presaged by Max Weber's assertion that individuals act according to their respective interpretations of the meaning of their world, the term "symbolic interactionism" was not officially coined until 1969 (by Herbert Blumer, a proponent of the theory). However, the works of **George Herbert Mead** (1863–1931) are considered most important in the initial development of the paradigm.

Symbolic interactionism examines the relationships between individuals and society by focusing on the exchange of information through language and symbols in one-on-one and small-group communication. According to symbolic interactionism, individuals can make sense of the world around them by ascribing meaning to the symbols and language of their shared culture, and these meanings depend on both individual interpretations and social context.

Symbolic interactionism analyzes society by addressing the subjective meanings that people impose upon objects, events, and behaviors. Subjective meaning is important because people behave based on what they believe to be true, whether or not their beliefs are actually true. Therefore, society is constructed through human interpretation; people must continually interpret their own behaviors as well as those of others around them, and these interpretations form a social bond.

Symbolic interactionism holds the principle of meaning to be the central aspect of human behavior: (1) humans ascribe meaning to things and act toward those things based on their ascribed meaning; (2) language allows humans to generate meaning through social interaction with each other and society; (3) humans modify meanings through an interpretive thought process that observes and considers the reactions of others as well as the social context of these interactions.

Mead and other interactionists have also been interested in identity and the development of the self. For interactionists, the self is developed through three important activities: language, games, and play. Language is probably the most prominent system of symbols in all human interactions and incorporates not only what we say and hear, but all modes of communication including body language and interpretation of meaning. The distinction between play and games is also worth noting. These are words that often suggest interactions among children and are sometimes used interchangeably. However, Mead meant for them to apply to all humans and established a clear distinction between them. Social play is characterized by spontaneity and freedom, with minimal social rules and limited stakes. Two children playing in a sandbox and building castles with the sand would be an example of play, as would two adults meeting for coffee. Social games, on the other hand, have a much stricter set of rules and have greater stakes. Classic board games like monopoly are clearly a type of social game, but so is taking the MCAT: the rules are clearly defined and there are spoils that go to the winner. Language, play, and games are the primary ways that we interact with each other and interpret the role of the self, and each plays a critical role in the formation of identity.

Another important distinction Mead proposed was the difference between the "I" and the "me." Mead thought there were two important components to identity: the individualistic self, which sought to establish its own unique identity through social interactions in the face of social pressures and expectations, and the social self, which internalized the characteristics of the social environment. The "I" represents the individualistic self. There is a connection with grammar and linguistics. I, as a subject pronoun, represents the part of the self that is the active agent, the part that acts on other people and things and has its own autonomy and will. On the other hand, the object pronoun "me" is used to represent the social self. This governs when others are acting and interpreting our behavior and we are the object of their actions and interpretations. Both the "I" and "me" are in constant dialogue with each other, sometimes agreeing, sometimes in conflict; and thinking itself, Mead believed, represents the internal dialogue between the individualistic and social self.

People interpret one another's behavior, and it is these interpretations that form our social bonds. These interpretations are called the "definition of the situation." An example of this phenomenon is called the **Thomas theorem**, the theory that interpretation of a situation affects the response to that situation.

A specific type of interactionist philosophy is called the **dramaturgical approach**, which was developed by **Erving Goffman** (1922–1982), a prominent proponent of symbolic interactionism. As the name suggests, this paradigm views people as theatrical performers and everyday life as a stage. Just as actors project a certain on-screen image, people in society choose what kind of image they want to communicate to those they interact with. For example, a college student who lands a coveted internship downtown will project a different image while at her internship than she will in class, and an even different image still when hanging out with her friends at a bar, or visiting her family in her childhood home.

Critics of symbolic interactionism contend that the theory neglects the macro-level of social interpretation and may miss the larger issues of society by focusing too closely on individual interactions.

Social Constructionism

Like symbolic interactionism, **social constructionism** asserts that people actively shape their reality through social interactions; reality is therefore something that is socially constructed rather than inherent. Both social constructionism and symbolic interactionism share the **belief** that society is subject to cultural "meaning-making" and collective definition-building and that the primary way that societies evolve is through changes in collective meaning-making. This similarity is not coincidental and derives from the fact that most social constructionists have been greatly influenced by the tenets of symbolic interactionism. Both of these theories challenge the scientific viewpoint that there is one objective reality shared by all humans.

Social constructionists focus on **social constructs** (mechanisms or practices created and sustained by society) that change across cultures and within a single culture over time. Social constructionism claims that social attributes such as race, gender, sexuality, and class are constructs of society, and that the same is true of our concepts of occupational status, power, and mental health/illness. Even concepts we typically think of as completely measurable physical characteristics, such as money, wealth, age and even time itself, are only social constructs. Whether the phenomenon in question is depression or higher education, social constructionists argue that the "reality" people see when they consider such phenomena is actually socially constructed, or an "artifice of society."

A major difference between symbolic interactionism and social constructionism is that while symbolic interactionists focus almost exclusively on one-on-one and small group interactions, social constructionists examine the constructs of society from both macro- and micro-sociological perspectives.

Other interests of social constructionists include our individual **stocks of knowledge** that allow us to classify objects and actions we observe quickly and to routinely structure our own actions in immediate response through a process called **typification**. Frequently repeated actions evolve into patterns that we learn to reproduce without much effort. As these actions become routines, they form a general store of knowledge that can be institutionalized by society. Once knowledge becomes institutionalized, we experience it as objective, unquestionable reality, the truth of which is continuously affirmed by others around us as well as concretized by the language we use to describe as "real" what was previously only a routine.

Social constructionism also analyzes the effects of mass media and contends that mass media corporations have become the main mechanisms by which our social institutions transmit culture to preserve power and authority. Echoing conflict theorists, these social constructionists feel that disempowering societal constructs are derived from, or at least bound up with, larger social structures and institutional practices.

Feminist Theory

Feminist theory is concerned with the social experiences of both men and women and the differences between these experiences (for example, manhood versus womanhood and masculine versus feminine). Feminist sociologists strive to understand both the social structures that contribute to gender differences (macro-level questions) and the effects of gender differences on individual interactions (micro-level questions). Feminist theory is related to the concept of feminism, but feminism is better described as a collection of social movements with the purpose of establishing men and women as equals in terms of social rights, roles, statuses, etc.

The feminist perspective sometimes extends to the idea of active oppression in which both individuals and structures maintain inequalities. Micro-level oppression can occur as the result of authoritative principles that allow men to restrict women. Domestic violence is an example of this. Macro-level oppression can occur when economic, political, and other social structures permit the domination of women. The driving ban for women in Saudi Arabia is a high-profile modern example of this.

Feminist theory can also extend to questions of **intersectionality**. Intersectionality posits that various human aspects subject to societal oppression (such as class, race, sexual orientation, and gender) do not exist isolated and separated from each other, but instead have complex, influential, and interwoven relationships.

Rational Choice and Social Exchange Theories

Economic considerations also have a place in the sociological tradition. Economics is a social science concerned with resources, whether goods or services, and their production, distribution, and consumption by both individuals and groups (for example, corporations). Capitalist societies, in particular, are built on competition, and thus economics influences social behavior. Under the broad heading of **rational choice theory** can be included **social exchange theory**, **game theory**, and **rational actor theory**. No matter what name is used, the rational choice paradigm brings a decidedly economic approach to the analysis of why, when, and how people interact.

In all rational choice theories, individuals seek to maximize the benefits they gain and minimize the disadvantages they sustain in all of their social interactions. If an individual decides that the benefits of an interaction outweigh its disadvantages, this individual will initiate the interaction (or continue it if it has already begun). If an individual instead decides that an interaction's disadvantages outweigh its benefits, this individual will decline interacting (or stop the interaction if it has already started). Social order is possible because individuals realize that their best interests are often served through cooperation and compromises with others.

All rational choice paradigms share the fundamental premise that human behaviors are utilitarian. **Utilitarianism** is based on two assumptions: (1) that individual humans are rational in their actions, and (2) that in every human interaction, individuals will seek to maximize their own self-interest. Since utilitarianism focuses on the individual social choices that individuals make, rational choice theory and all of its related theories, such as social exchange theory, are often **micro-sociological theories**. However, because they can also look at the tendencies and behaviors of large groups of people, they are also capable of being **macro-sociological theories**.

Rational choice theorists tend to treat society as a kind of market or game in which each person is constantly making choices among available options, based on a cost-benefit or risk-reward analysis and according to his or her own set of value preferences. The players in the game may not have perfect information about exactly what their options are or about the rewards, costs, and risks of each option. Rational choice theorists examine the relative power of interacting individuals and analyze how differing parameters of an exchange relationship can shape an individual's ability to get favorable returns from that exchange.

Rational choice theory is widely criticized for assuming the inherent rationality of human actions and minimizing the role of culture and subjective meaning in individual and group behavior. Advocates claim that rational choice theory provides an integrated theoretical analysis of human behavior that has the potential to unify many branches of social science.

4.2 SOCIAL INSTITUTIONS

Social institutions are complexes of roles, norms, and values organized into a relatively stable form that contribute to social order by governing the behavior of people. Social institutions provide predictability and organization for individuals within a society and mediate social behavior between people. Social institutions provide harmony and allow for specialization and differentiation of skills. Examples of social institutions in the United States include our educational systems, family, religions, government, and health care systems.

Family

The family, in all of its many different forms, is part of all human cultures. A family may be defined as a set of people related by blood, marriage, adoption, or some other agreed-upon relationship that signifies some responsibility to one another. Throughout history families have tended to serve five functions:

1) Reproduction and the monitoring of sexual behavior
2) Protection
3) Socialization—passing down norms and values of society
4) Affection and companionship
5) Social status—social position is often based on family background and reputation

One way of conceptualizing family is to distinguish **nuclear family**, consisting of direct blood relations, and **extended** family, in which grandparents, aunts, uncles, and others are included. Across cultures and even within a culture, the members of the family that typically live together may vary.

The extension of a family through marriage can occur in many different ways. **Monogamy** refers to a form of marriage in which two individuals are married only to each other. **Polygamy** allows an individual to have multiple wives or husbands simultaneously. Throughout world history, polygamy has actually been more common than the monogamous relationships currently considered the norm in the United States. There are two subtypes of polygamy. **Polygyny** refers to a man married to more than one woman, while **polyandry** refers to a woman married to more than one man. In choosing a mate, **endogamy** refers to the practice of marrying within a particular group. **Exogamy** refers to a requirement to marry outside a particular group, with it being the norm in almost all cultures to prohibit sexual relationships between certain relatives.

How we think about who we are related to is referred to as **kinship**. Kin do not have to live together, and kin is considered a cultural group rather than a biological one. Kinship groups may include extended family and members of the community or friends (like godparents and close family friends that are referred to as "aunts" and "uncles"). If kin groups involve both the maternal and paternal relations, this is called **bilateral descent**. Preference for paternal and maternal relations is called **patrilineal** and **matrilineal** descent, respectively.

Families may differ in terms of who has the power and authority to make decisions. In some families, each individual is given power over certain tasks, such as cooking, shopping, working, cleaning, and finances. There are three types of authority patterns based on gender. In a **patriarchy**, men have more authority than women, and in a **matriarchy**, women have more authority than men. In an **egalitarian family**, spouses are treated as equals and may be involved in more negotiation when making decisions.

There are many alternatives to the traditional family. A few of the differences seen in the United States are described as follows:

1) *Cultural differences:* many cultures emphasize the importance of extended family, often living with grandparents, cousins, and the like. In some cases, "kin" who are non-blood related members of the community may be considered part of the family.
2) *Divorce:* The divorce rate has generally risen in the United States due to several factors. First, there is a growing social and religious acceptance of divorce. Second, more and more opportunities are becoming available for women to succeed autonomously, making divorce a realistic possibility. Third, the financial and legal barriers to divorce have lessened over time as it has become more common.
3) *Cohabitation:* there has been a large increase, especially among couples in their 20s and 30s in living together without getting married. Sometimes these couples will have children and do many of the same things "traditionally" married couples do (like buy property and have a joint checking account) but remain legally unmarried.
4) *Lesbian and gay marriage/relationships:* Lesbian and gay couples often engage in all of the same behaviors that a "traditionally" married couple might, including property ownership and raising children.

Both individual and group experiences can threaten the strength of families. **Family violence** is a dramatic example in which one member of the family is directly responsible for the threat through their mistreatment of another person, often in an attempt to gain power, leaving the target fearful and powerless. **Child abuse** involves abusive behavior directed toward a child target. There are four categories of child abuse: physical abuse, emotional abuse, sexual abuse, and neglect. **Domestic abuse**, also referred to as dating abuse or spousal abuse, involves abuse directed toward one partner of an intimate relationship, where the abuser is the second partner. **Elder abuse** involves abuse directed toward an older target. The added element in elder abuse is that there is an expectation of trust from the older person, which is violated in the course of violence or other mistreatment. Abuse has been linked to alcohol consumption, mental illness, and certain social conditions.

Education

Educational institutions have both manifest and latent functions. Their manifest functions are to systematically pass down knowledge and to give status to those who have been educated. For example, patients trust doctors mainly because of the conferral of an awarded degree and subsequent licensure. This degree and licensure represents an agreed-upon amount of information, skills, and training acquired in order to practice medicine. Latent functions include socialization, serving as agents of change, and maintaining social control.

As a social institution, schools transmit aspects of the dominant culture. School plays a role in teaching the dominant language and literature, holidays and traditions, historical figures and events, and exposes people to existing beliefs. This involves a significant degree of interpretation. Schooling also helps maintain social norms by disciplining students and otherwise teaching them socially acceptable behavior.

While many forms of student socialization are intentional (manners, learning to talk only when called on, learning to work independently), there are other lessons learned in school known as the **hidden curriculum**. The hidden curriculum often conflicts with the manifest curriculum. For example, medical educators know that medical students experience a conflict between the stated values of their curriculum and the lived reality of hospital work they encounter during their third and fourth years. While students may have learned about the sanctity of patient care during their lectures, they often encounter hospital staff whose actions inadvertently teach them that patients are nuisances.

Within schools, benefits such as small class size, excellent teachers, and the availability of the latest technology and resources, are based on the socioeconomic status of the school district for public schools. The option of private school is only really an option for those in the higher income brackets. Access to higher education, a key factor in getting a good job, is also highly dependent on family income, as well as other factors. Level of education then continues to be influential in terms of power, respect, and social standing. Therefore, the education system has often been criticized as one that serves to maintain or widen socioeconomic and privilege gaps. This is accomplished through the processes of educational segregation and stratification.

These processes lead to an informal type of **educational segregation**, the widening disparity between children from high-income neighborhoods and those from low-income neighborhoods. In wealthier neighborhoods, parents have the time and resources to be more involved, and would potentially intervene in the event of poor teacher performance. On the other hand, children in poorer neighborhoods have public schools that are poorly funded, and teachers that may not get enough resources to do their job well. Consequently, research has found that poorer schools may be more likely to have higher teacher turnover, lower quality instruction, and provide a lower quality of education to students.

- tend to attend poorer schools and receive poorer educations
- are far less likely than children from wealthier neighborhoods to pursue a four-year college degree, and even more unlikely to pursue education beyond college, like a graduate or medical degree
- are more likely to end up with lower-paying jobs, and perpetuate the cycle of poverty for themselves

Additionally, teachers can greatly affect students' achievement. Research has shown that teachers tend to quickly form expectations of individual students, and once they have formed these expectations, they tend to act toward the student with these expectations in mind. If the student accepts the teacher's expectations as reasonable, the student will begin to perform in accordance with them as well. This is known as **teacher expectancy theory**.

While education has long been touted as the path to upward mobility in the United States, it can also reinforce and perpetuate social inequalities. This is known as **educational stratification**.

Religion

Organized religion is a social institution involving beliefs and practices. These practices are based on objects and ideas that are recognized as sacred and worthy of reverence. The MCAT may include information regarding the forms of religious organizations, common information on the five major world religions, and the social functions of religion. The forms of religious organizations include the following:

1) **Ecclesia:** a dominant religious organization that includes most members of society, is recognized as the national or official religion, and tolerates no other religions. It is often integrated into political institutions, and people do not choose to participate but are born into the social institution. Examples of countries with this social structure are Sweden (Lutheranism is the official state religion) and Iran (Islam is the official state religion).

2) **Church:** a type of religious organization that is well-integrated into the larger society. Church membership tends to occur by birth, but most churches allow people to join. Congregations are typically concerned both with the sacred and ordinary aspects of life and have well-stipulated rules and regulations. An example in the United States is the Catholic Church.

3) **Sect:** a religious organization that is distinct from that of the larger society. Sects are often formed from breaking away from larger religious institutions. Over time, some sects may develop into churches. Membership may be by birth or through conversion. Examples of sects in the United States include the Mormon community and the Amish community.

4) **Cult/New religious movement:** a religious organization that is far outside society's norms and often involves a very different lifestyle. Examples of cults in the United States include the Branch Davidians and Heaven's Gate.

From a functionalist standpoint, religion can create social cohesion (as well as dissent), social change (as well as control), and provide believers with meaning and purpose. Social cohesion is often experienced by members of religious groups due to the system of shared beliefs and values that they provide. Religious communities can be a source of emotional, spiritual, and material support in difficult times. However, religion can also be a source of social dissent, as a history of violence between religious factions indicates. Religion can be a vehicle for social change. Teachings such as the Protestant work ethic can have a profound impact on how members live their lives. Liberation theology refers to the use of the church in a political effort against various social issues, such as poverty and injustice.

Religion can prompt social change as mentioned above, but there are also cases wherein it must respond to social change. The classical sociologists predicted that as societies became more modern, there would be a decline in religious practice in favor of more rational thought. **Secularization** is the process through which religion loses its social significance in modern societies. However, evidence of secularization is contested, and even in the United States, religious factors continue to influence economics and politics. **Fundamentalism** is a second response to modernist societies in which there is strong attachment to traditional religious beliefs and practices and a strict adherence to basic religious doctrines resulting from a literalist interpretation of these texts.

A very brief overview of the five major world religions is as follows:

1) **Christianity** is the largest single faith in the world, with about 30% of the population across the globe identifying as Christian, though there are multiple denominations. About two-thirds of people in the United States identify as Christian, and although church and state are legally separate, many social and political matters reference God. Christianity is monotheistic (one God), and its followers also believe in prophets (Jesus as the Son of God), an afterlife, and a judgment day.

2) **Islam** is the second largest religion in the world. Its followers are known as Muslims, and it is estimated that between 20–25% of the world's population is Muslim. It is also monotheistic (Allah), and its followers believe in prophets (with the final one being Mohammad), an after-life, and a judgment day. Muslim governments often do not separate religion and state, and religion frequently dictates law in Muslim countries. Muslim cultures vary in their norms, with issues such as the hijab worn by women being cultural rather than religious.

3) **Hinduism** developed in India and is a polytheistic religion (many gods) practiced by about 14% of the world's population, although there are major deities such as Shiva and Vishnu. Hinduism also includes a belief in reincarnation, or rebirth after death.

4) **Buddhism**, a religion that recognizes no deity, also originated in India. Based on the teach-ings of Siddhartha Gautama (the Buddha), Buddhism centers on the goal of achieving enlightenment. Buddhism teaches overcoming cravings for physical or material pleasures primarily through meditative practices.

5) **Judaism** is monotheistic and formed the historical basis for Christianity and Islam. Jews believe that God formed a covenant with Abraham and Sarah, and that if certain rules were followed (the Ten Commandments), God would bring paradise to Earth. Jews make up about 0.2% of the world's population.

There are many individual differences among people who consider themselves members of a particular reli-gion. **Religiosity** refers to the extent that religion influences a person's life. Some may be very devout, with the extreme form being **fundamentalists**, who adhere strictly to religious beliefs. Others may adhere more to the beliefs of the religion without the rituals or to the rituals without the beliefs. Still others may define them-selves by some sort of religion but do not practice their religion actively or attend any formal religious events.

Government and Economy

Our political and economic structures both influence and are influenced by social structure. Power structures are a fundamental part of both politics and economics. Governments across the world derive their power from different places. The United States government is one based on **rational-legal authority**, legal rules and regulations are stipulated in a document like the Constitution. Many corporations, including health care organizations, work within this structure and are often organized in a similar way. Other governments around the world may derive power from **traditional authority**, from custom, tradition, or accepted practice. Still other leaders may be powerful due to **charismatic authority**, the power of their persuasion.

Political sociologists are interested in the relationship between the government and the people; these scholars are concerned with the organization of governments in terms of the distribution of power and the effects of this distribution on social control. **Aristarchic governments** are controlled by a small group of people, selected based on specific qualifications, with decision-making power; the public is not involved in most political decisions. Aristarchies include **aristocracies** (those ruled by elite citizens, like those of noble birth) and **meritocracies** (those ruled by the meritorious, like those with a record of meaningful social contributions). **Autocratic governments** are controlled by a single person, or a selective small group, with absolute decision-making power. Autocracies include **dictatorships** (those ruled by one person) and **fascist governments** (those ruled by a small group of leaders). **Monarchic governments** are controlled by a single person, or by a select small group who inherited the leadership role, like kings and queens. In addition to absolute monarchies, there are constitutional monarchies, in which leaders are limited through formal constitutions.

There are also concerns of how the leadership is elected. **Authoritarian governments** consist of unelected leaders; the public might have some individual freedoms but have no control over representation. Authoritarianisms include **totalitarianism** (those in which unelected leaders regulate both public and private life through coercive means of control). **Democratic governments** consist of elected leaders; the public has some degree of political decision-making power through either direct decisions or representation. Democracies include **direct democracies** (governments in which there is direct public participation) and **representative democracies** (governments in which there is indirect public participation through the election of representatives). Democratic structures are common in the Western world, such as in the United States, where most of the population is granted the right to vote through public elections, although there might not be an equal distribution of this decision-making power (for example, minorities have been denied the right to vote in the past). This often results in the formation of **political parties**, formal groups of people that share the same principal political beliefs and organize with a common purpose of ensuring governance that supports these principles through appropriate policies. **Oligarchic governments** are less clear as leaders can be elected or unelected; the public might have the power to elect representation, but people have little influence in directing decisions and social change. Oligarchies are controlled by a small group of people with shared interests; for example, theocracies are governments ruled by the religious elite.

Finally, the structure of governments can be studied. **Republican governments** consider their countries to be public concerns and are thus democratic in nature, meaning that the people have the supreme power in these societies. **Federalist governments** include a governing representative head that shares power with constituent groups. There is the division between the central government, or the federal government, and the constituent governments, or the state, provincial, and local governments. **Parliamentary governments** include both executive and legislative branches that are interconnected; members of the executive branch (ministers) are accountable to members of the legislature. **Presidential governments** also include organizing branches, as well as a head of state. Other political concepts include **anarchy**, which refers to societies without a public government; here, there is a common implication of "lawlessness."

Economics is concerned with the production, distribution, and consumption of resources, both goods and services. Most economic structures fit into one of four categories: command, market, mixed, or traditional. In **command economies**, also known as **planned economies**, economic decisions are based on a plan of production and the means of production are often public (state-owned); these include socialism and communism. In **market economies**, economic decisions are based on the market ("supply and demand") and the means of production are often private; these include laissez-faire and free market economies. **Mixed economies** blend elements of command and market economies with both public and private ownership. There are various forms of mixed economics; for example, in some societies, there is public oversight, and even funding, of private production, such as in the United States. **Traditional**

economies consider social customs in economic decisions; this practice is most common in rural areas and often involves bartering and trading.

In addition to deriving power from rational-legal authority (i.e., governmental power is legitimized by laws and rules), our political and economic system is influenced greatly by capitalist ideals, although the United States is not purely capitalist. **Capitalism** is an economic system in which resources and production are mainly privately owned, and goods/services are produced for a profit. The driving force in capitalist societies is the pursuit of personal profit. It is thought that the advantages of capitalism are that it benefits the consumer by allowing for competition, which theoretically promotes higher quality and lower price of goods and services. Capitalism is also thought to emphasize personal freedom, by limiting government restrictions and regulations.

On the other hand, **socialism** is an economic system where resources and production are collectively owned. Socialism includes a system of production and distribution designed to satisfy human needs (good/services are produced for direct use instead of for profit). Private property is limited and government intervenes to share property amongst all. The driving force in socialist societies is collective goals; everyone is given a job and everyone is provided with what they need to survive. In socialist societies, the economy is usually centrally controlled and run by the government. **Communism** is a specific socialist structure in which there is common ownership of the means of production, as well as the absence of currencies, classes, and states, based on shared economic, political, and social ideologies.

Most nations incorporate both capitalist and socialist ideas. **Welfare capitalism** is a system in which most of the economy is private with the exception of extensive social welfare programs to serve certain needs within society. Most countries in Western Europe demonstrate welfare capitalism because most of their economies are based on capitalist principles, but universal health care is provided by the state. **State capitalism** is a system in which companies are privately run, but work closely with the government in forming laws and regulations. In the United States, most businesses are privately owned, but the government runs many operations, such as schools, the postal service, and the military. However, most hospitals and other health care providers, as well as insurance companies, remain privately run in the United States.

Numerous trends have led to the economic system that currently exists. Notably, the Information Revolution has been followed by a deindustrialization. Instead of focusing on tangible products, the emphasis has shifted to intangible products, such as information technology and services. This has changed the focus from factory work to work that can be done almost anywhere, and emphasizes literacy over mechanical skills. This shift has led to a focus on **professions**, highly esteemed white-collar occupations that require a great deal of education.

The **division of labor** occurs as societies become so complex that it is not possible for an individual to meet all of his or her needs alone, such as happened with the rise of capitalism. Different occupations emerge as a response; these occupations are specialized to serve a specific social need (for example, doctors can treat medical problems and mechanics can address our automobile issues). Because individuals no longer participate in all of the activities required for survival, there is an increase in interdependence. The division of labor has had both positive and negative consequences for social order; for example, it has increased the rate of production but it has also decreased the similarities in social experience among individuals, contributing to class differences. Thus, the division of labor is about more than economic interests.

Durkheim contributed to our current understanding of the division of labor and differentiated between two forms of social solidarity in relation to economic approaches. **Mechanical solidarity** allows society to remain integrated because individuals have common beliefs that lead to each person having the same fundamental experience. **Organic solidarity** allows society to integrate through a division of labor, which leads to each person having a different personal experience; thus, each movement is distinguishable and separate.

Health and Medicine

Medicine is the social institution that governs health and illness, particularly with respect to diagnosis, treatment, and prevention of illness. The **delivery of health care** in the United States is accomplished by teams of health-care providers with different training backgrounds and specialty areas, such as physicians and nurses of all specialties, physical and occupational therapists, dentists, hospitalists, social workers, community health workers, caregivers, pharmacists, alternative medicine providers, and rehabilitative therapists—to name only a few! The delivery of health care is organized into different levels: primary, secondary, and tertiary care. Primary care describes the care provider responsible for ongoing preventative care or disease management, or community-based care (such as an urgent care center). Secondary care includes acute care (emergency department), as well as specialty care, which is often received following a referral from a primary care provider. Tertiary care is a very specialized form of health care. It is based on consultations with specialist care providers and often occurs in hospitals or care facilities designed just for the purpose of caring for patients with a limited set of conditions. Examples of tertiary care include cancer hospitals, burn centers, and palliative care (end-of-life care) facilities. It is also important to remember that community centers and agencies can provide para-medical care, such as patient education, in-home care work, and public health outreach.

Society plays a large role in defining health/illness and acceptable health care practices. For example, societies differ in the degree of emphasis that they put on physical health versus mental health. In many nations, ADHD and depression are not considered illnesses and are not treated. The United States has experienced the spread of the **medical model of disease**, which emphasizes physical or medical factors as being the cause of all illness. Because the medical model characterizes all illness as having a physiological or pathological basis, the medical profession has been able to reframe many conditions as disease states based on the success of empirical treatment or the hope that scientific research will eventually expose the underlying cause of disease. The process by which a condition comes to be reconceptualized as a disease with a medical diagnosis and a medical treatment is known as **medicalization**. When medicalization results in medical explanations for social problems, the physician can act as the expert on a variety of issues including child development, criminality, drug addiction, and depression. However, the medical model is only one way of understanding illness, and it does not always describe illness from the patient's point of view.

An alternate way of understanding illness is known as the **social model of disease**. The social model of disease emphasizes the effect one's social class, employment status, neighborhood, exposure to environmental toxins, diet, and many other factors can have on a person's health. While someone working from the perspective of the medical model might look for the *ultimate* cause of a person's illness, someone working from the social model would be attuned to a more *proximate* cause—something about the patient's life circumstances that put him/her at greater risk of exposure.

The social model of disease, as discussed above, postulates that social pressures create the conditions for health and illness. The field that studies how social organization contributes to the prevalence, incidence, and distribution of disease across and within populations is known as **social epidemiology**. Being low-income can predispose individuals to conditions that limit individuals' ability to eat healthy food, exercise, get enough sleep, and avoid the long-term effects of severe stressors. Low-income individuals often work multiple jobs, which may cause sleep deprivation and leave little time for the exercise needed to maintain a healthy weight. Very low-income neighborhoods are often food deserts. A **food desert** is an area where healthy, fresh food is difficult to find because there are no proper grocery stores, making people more likely to eat high-calorie foods that have low nutritional value. Also, living paycheck-to-paycheck is extremely stressful. The effects of chronic stress on the body take their toll as poor health: low infant birth weight, high blood pressure, obesity, and cognitive deficits, to name only a few.

Being ill impacts not only the patient, but also the patient's social networks. Two main sociological concepts describe what illness can be like for a patient. One concept, the sick role, describes society's response to illness. The second concept, illness experience, explains the patient's subjective experience of illness.

The **sick role** is a concept developed by American sociologist Talcott Parsons. According to this concept, when a person is ill, he or she is not able to be a contributing member of society. Being ill, from Parsons' point of view, is a type of deviance. For others to take up the extra work in this person's absence they must consider the person's illness to be legitimate—they must sanction this person's deviance by exempting him/her from normal social roles and by not blaming the person for his or her illness. In return, the person must fulfill the role obligations of an ill person: the person should seek medical care and the person should make a sincere attempt to get well.

However, the sick role concept does not always hold up empirically. Other sociologists have pointed out the limitations of this role for those with chronic disease, stigmatized diseases, and "lifestyle" diseases. For example, if a person is suffering from a condition about which little is known, such as fibromyalgia, others may not accept that the person is actually ill and not confer the legitimation of the sick role. Second, the sick role concept was developed to describe acute illness and cannot explain chronic illness, where a person has good days and bad days, and often must carry on with normal life despite poor health.

Other research has examined the type of doctor-patient relationship the concept of the sick role implies. The sick role implies a passive patient and an authoritative physician. Research on **illness experience** takes the patient's subjective experience of illness as its main concern. When studying illness experience, sociologists are not just interested in the meanings people give to their illness, but also how the experience of being ill affects patients' daily lives—their ability to work, spend time with friends and family, and cultivate their identities. With a chronic disease a patient can have no reasonable expectation of getting better; thus, she or he must adjust normal daily life to fit the constraints of the illness.

Chapter 4 Summary

- A society is defined as the group of people who share a culture and live/interact with each other within a definable area.

- Functionalism is a sociological theory that conceptualizes society as a living organism with many different parts and organs, each of which has a distinct purpose; Émile Durkheim was a major proponent of functionalism.

- Manifest functions are the intended and obvious consequences of a structure; latent functions are unintended or less recognizable consequences of a structure.

- Conflict theory views society as a place where there will be inequality in resources, therefore individuals will compete for social, political, and material resources like money, land, power, and leisure; Karl Marx, a proponent of conflict theory, advocated for socialism.

- Symbolic interactionism examines the relationship between individuals and society by focusing on communication, the exchange of information through language and symbols.

- The dramaturgical approach suggests that people in society choose what kind of image they want to communicate verbally and nonverbally to others.

- Social constructionism argues that people actively shape their reality through social interactions; it is therefore something that is constructed, not inherent.

- Social institutions are a complex of roles, norms, and values organized into a relatively stable form that contributes to social order by governing the behavior of people. They provide predictability and organization for individuals within a society and mediate social behavior between people.

- Social institutions include family, education, organized religion, government and economy, and medicine.

CHAPTER 4 FREESTANDING PRACTICE QUESTIONS

1. Social institutions include all of the following, EXCEPT:

A) social networks.
B) families.
C) schools.
D) churches.

2. Joy lives in a neighborhood where 40% of the population is obese. Almost half of the adults in her neighborhood are unemployed and rely on food stamps. There are no grocery stores within a ten block radius of where Joy lives, but there are many fast-food chains. The economic and social situation in Joy's neighborhood could be described as:

   I. a food desert.
   II. absolute poverty.
   III. relative poverty.

A) I only
B) II only
C) I and II
D) I and III

3. A country where the economy is profit-driven and privately-owned, but public services like health care and education are state-funded, would be considered:

A) socialist.
B) capitalist.
C) collectivist.
D) welfare capitalist.

4. A study finds that lower-income Hispanic women from a specific urban community located near a factory are more than twice as likely to develop a rare form of cancer than women in the general population. This finding could be potentially attributed to all of the following, EXCEPT:

A) class-dependent health care disparities.
B) environmental injustice.
C) gender-dependent health care disparities.
D) ethnicity-dependent health care disparities.

5. Which of the following is NOT a macro theory of sociology?

A) Functionalism
B) Conflict theory
C) Feminist theory
D) Symbolic interactionism

6. Which of the following is NOT true regarding the sociology theory structural functionalism?

A) Functionalism is less concerned about the interactions of small groups.
B) Functionalism involves the idea that society is like an organism.
C) Functionalism encourages people to actively change the status quo of society for their own benefit.
D) Functionalism believes that once one part of an institution changes, it will always affect the other parts of the institution.

7. An adolescent gets into a fight with her parents over curfew rules. Her parents tell her that she is often irresponsible and gets distracted from her school work when her friends invite her out, so she must respect their rules. The girl responds that she knows how to manage her time and when she can spend more time with her friends without sacrificing her grades. When the girl returns to her room she is likely to experience a conflict between:

A) the "I" and "me."
B) the "I" and the individualistic self.
C) the "me" and the social self.
D) her real self and her ideal self.

8. Religion has been famously described as "the opiate of the masses" since it keeps poorer members of societies from attaining class consciousness. This concept is most consistent with:

A) exchange-rational theory.
B) structural functionalism.
C) conflict theory.
D) symbolic interactionism.

CHAPTER 4 PRACTICE PASSAGE

The term *arbovirus* is used to describe the hundreds of predominantly RNA viruses that are transmitted by mosquitoes and other arthropods. One of these, Zika virus, was first discovered in Uganda in 1947. For many years, the virus was found predominantly in primates and was restricted to a thin, equatorial belt running from Africa through Asia. Only in the second decade of the 21st century did a Zika pandemic spread to the West.

The symptoms of Zika, which is related to dengue but displays milder symptoms, include eye pain, fever, maculopapular rash, muscle aches, and prostration. Zika is also believed to sometimes carry complications. In Brazil, the incidence of microcephaly increased about 20-fold from 2014 to 2015; many public health officials believe the condition is linked to a significantly increased incidence of Zika among pregnant mothers in the region. Although a causal relationship between Zika in pregnant women and microcephaly was not definitively established, pregnant women and women planning to become pregnant were advised to refrain from traveling to areas in which the virus is apparent.

Some of the best preventive measures include applying insect repellent as well as wearing long pants and shirts. Other precautions that may be taken are using screens, mosquito nets, and air-conditioning as well as eliminating debris and still water that provide conditions for mosquito-breeding. Access to these items can be limited in developing regions, and this partially explains the prevalence of the disease in countries with less robust economies. Also, Zika is classified as a disease of poverty, meaning it is a disease that is endemic to poor regions with underdeveloped public health systems that can allow diseases to spread unchecked. Confronting these diseases in regions where the capacity of public health officials to respond in a systematic and orchestrated way is limited is an ongoing challenge for health policy officials and governments, due to limited availability and accessibility of preventative measures in lower income regions. Historically, studies have found that the most effective preventative measures are much more available and accessible in higher income regions.

Adapted from A.S. Fauci & D.M. Morens. "Zika virus in the Americas—Yet another arbovirus threat." The New England Journal of Medicine. © 2016 Massachusetts Medical Society.

1. Ana lives in a small village in Latin America. Her parents, like many other parents in the area, have always struggled to provide food and clean water for their five children. When Anna becomes sick with Zika, she does not have access to healthcare and must suffer the symptoms with no reprieve or definitive diagnosis. This situation demonstrates:

A) absolute poverty.
B) cyclical poverty.
C) relative poverty.
D) situational poverty.

2. Which type of research design would be most appropriate to determine the hypothesized relationship between Zika and pregnant women mentioned in paragraph 2?

A) A correlational study
B) An experimental design
C) A phenomenological study
D) A case study design

3. A team of researchers is testing an intravenous vaccine to prevent the spread of Zika. One hundred participants are divided into two groups. Members of the first group are given glucose fluid intravenously, while members of the second group are given the vaccine. Which of the following is true in this study?

A) The independent variable is vaccine efficacy, and the dependent variable is health outcomes.
B) The independent variable is type of fluid, and the dependent variable is health outcomes.
C) The independent variable is the type of fluid, and the dependent variable is the vaccine.
D) The independent variable is the vaccine, and the dependent variable is vaccine efficacy.

4. Which sociological theory would be most consistent with the findings regarding the availability and accessibility of Zika virus preventative measures mentioned in the final paragraph?

A) Structural functionalism
B) Symbolic interactionism
C) Social constructionism
D) Conflict theory

SOLUTIONS TO CHAPTER 4 FREESTANDING PRACTICE QUESTIONS

1. **A** Social institutions are complexes of roles, norms, and values organized into a relatively stable form that contribute to social order by governing the behavior of people. Families, schools, and churches are all examples of social institutions (choices B, C, and D can be eliminated), while social networks are not (choice A is not a social institution and is the correct answer choice).

2. **D** Item I is true: a food desert refers to an area, typically in a highly populated lower-income urban environment, where healthy, fresh food is difficult to find. Joy's neighborhood does not have a nearby grocery store but does have a plethora of fast-food restaurants, therefore, it would arguably qualify as a food desert (choice B can be eliminated). Item II is false: absolute poverty is the inability to meet a bare minimum of basic necessities, including clean drinking water, food, safe housing, and reliable access to health care; the scenario described is not absolute poverty (choice C can be eliminated). Item III is true: relative poverty is defined as an inability to meet the average standard of living within a society. The fact that so many people in Joy's neighborhood are unemployed suggests that she is living in relative poverty (choice A can be eliminated, and choice D is correct).

3. **D** Welfare capitalism refers to a system of government where most of the economy is private with the exception of extensive social welfare programs to serve certain social needs within society (such as health care and education; choice D is correct). Socialism is an economic system where resources and production are collectively owned. Socialism includes a system of production and distribution designed to satisfy human needs; good/services are produced for direct use instead of for profit (choice A is wrong). Capitalism is an economic system in which resources and production are mainly privately owned, and goods/services are produced for a profit; strict capitalism does not include state-funded public services (choice B is wrong). Collectivism is an economic or social outlook that emphasizes interdependence between people; a profit-driven economy would not be a part of a collectivist country (choice C is wrong).

4. **C** Gender-dependent health care disparities highlight differences in the treatment and outcomes between men and women; because this question relates lower-income Hispanic women to women in the general population, there is no evidence that the disparity is based on gender because no comparison is made to men (this finding is not attributable to choice C, so it is the correct answer choice). Class-dependent health care disparities are based on socioeconomic differences between classes and ethnicity-dependent health care disparities are based on ethnic differences between groups; because this question relates lower-income Hispanic women to women in the general population, it is possible that this disparity exists due to either class and/or ethnicity (the finding could be attributable to either choices A or D, so both choices can be eliminated). Environmental injustice refers to the fact that people in poorer communities are more likely to be subjected to negative environmental impacts on their health and well-being; because these women live near a factory, this health care disparity could be the result of environmental injustice (the finding could be attributable to choice B, so it can be eliminated).

5.   **D**   Macro theories are concerned with interactions between groups of people, while micro-level theories are concerned with interactions between individuals. Symbolic interactionism, which is concerned with the way individuals use symbols to communicate in society, is the only micro-level theory listed (choice D is not a macro-level theory and is the correct answer choice). Functionalism explains how social processes work on a broad scale. It considers the function and purpose of large groups within society, e.g., churches, schools, hospitals, and the like, and is considered a macro-level theory (choice A can be eliminated). Conflict theory explains society based on constant competition between groups for limited resources and is considered a macro-level theory (choice B can be eliminated). Feminist theory is concerned with inequality between the genders (whole groups of people) rather than inequalities between particular individuals (choice C is a macro-level theory and can be eliminated).

6.   **C**   Functionalism discourages people from changing the norm because it emphasizes the idea of stability through the universal agreement to abide by the norms of society (choice C is false and therefore the correct answer). Functionalism focuses on society as a whole rather than the individual aspects of society (choice A is true and can be eliminated). Organic solidarity is an idea within functionalism that compares society to an organism (choice B is true and can be eliminated). Functionalists believe that if one part of the system changes, then the rest of the system will have to adjust to the dysfunction until social stability can be restored (choice D is true and can be eliminated).

7.   **A**   The adolescent in the question stem has just received an interpretation of her identity from her parents that she is at odds with. Her individualistic belief of her own character is different from the feedback she is getting from her social environment. This is exactly the difference between the "I" and the "me," the individualistic self and the social self (choice A is correct). The I and the individualistic self are one and the same, so would not cause a conflict (choice B is wrong). This is also true for the me and the social self (choice C is wrong). Real versus ideal self is a gap between who one is in the real world and who one wishes to be. This is a concept in Humanistic psychology and client-centered therapy that does not apply to the situation (choice D is wrong).

8.   **C**   Karl Marx, one of the founders of modern sociology, said that religion was "the opiate of the masses." This statement is most consistent with conflict theory, as he saw the state's use of religion to ensure the continued inequality of the system (choice C is correct). Exchange-rational theory asserts that people use cost-benefit analyses to choose which action will be most beneficial to them (choice A can be eliminated). Structural functionalism says that there are individual structures in society that all work together for the good of the whole—for dynamic equilibrium. Religion is one of these structures (choice B can be eliminated). Symbolic interactionism is a micro-level theory that says that people use language express what objects mean individually to them. While Marx might be expressing his own symbolic understanding of religion, the quote itself refers not to an individual interpretation on the micro-level, but rather to how the larger society uses religion as a tool (choice D can be eliminated).

SOLUTIONS TO CHAPTER 4 PRACTICE PASSAGE

1. **A**   Absolute poverty is when individuals do not have access to basic necessities such as clean water, food, and healthcare (choice A is correct). Cyclical poverty usually lasts for a transient period and is related to the overall state of the economy (choice B is wrong). Relative poverty refers to the idea that some persons may not be able to attain the average standard of living within a given society, but it does not indicate absence of the basic necessities (choice C is wrong). Situational poverty arises because of a change in circumstances, which may be related to health, environmental, or personal issues, among others. The question stem does not indicate a change in circumstances, and it emphasizes that the family has always struggled to make ends meet (choice D is wrong).

2. **B**   Paragraph 2 mentions that "a causal relationship between Zika in pregnant women and microcephaly was not definitively established...". To determine causality, an experimental design must be used (choice B is correct). Choices A, C, and D may give insight to a relationship between two variables but would not allow researchers to infer any cause-and-effect relationship (choices A, C, and D are incorrect).

3. **B**   In this scenario, the independent variable (the one that can be manipulated or controlled) is whether or not the subject receives the vaccine. Thus, there are two conditions for the independent variable: vaccine and placebo (glucose fluid), and the independent variable is best described as the type of fluid given, not one of the two conditions (choices A and D can be eliminated). The dependent variable is the type of health outcome observed (choice C can be eliminated, and choice B is correct). Note that vaccine and vaccine efficacy are both conditions, not variables.

4. **D**   The final paragraph discusses both limited access and availability of the Zika virus preventative measures, as well as economic disparities in terms of the availability and accessibility. The sociological theory that would be most concerned with limited resources and economic discrepancies would be conflict theory (choice D is correct). Structural functionalism is more concerned with the institutions and groups of society functioning together to maintain social stability, which does not clearly apply (choice A is incorrect). Symbolic interactionism is a micro-level theory, and the final paragraph is discussing macro-level trends (choice B is incorrect). Social constructionism is concerned with socialization and the construction of social realities, neither of which clearly apply to this scenario (choice C is incorrect).

Chapter 5
Culture, Demographics, and Social Inequality

Human beings live within societies, so in order to best understand human behavior, we must consider both the impact of the individual on the collective and that of the collective on the individual. By understanding social structures we can better understand the individual. Moreover, these social structures, along with cultural and demographic factors, play a key role in determining a person's health. Social stratification and inequality affect all societies across the globe, and afford power and privilege to some while denying it to others.

5.1 CULTURE AND DEMOGRAPHICS

Culture

Culture simply refers to a shared way of life, including the beliefs and practices that a social group shares. Although cultures can vary a great deal, they are composed of some common elements. **Symbolic culture** consists of symbols that are recognized by people of the same culture. Symbols convey agreed-upon meaning, can communicate the values and norms of the culture, and include rituals, gestures, signs, and words that help people within a society communicate and understand each other.

Symbols and rituals can differ between cultures, for example, some cultures celebrate the life of a deceased relative with a party, while others mourn at a more somber funeral. While symbolic elements of culture involve values and norms, **material culture** involves physical objects or artifacts. This includes clothing, hairstyles, food, and the design of homes. The importance placed on material objects can reflect the culture's values; for example, the American dream often includes a car, a symbol of mobility and independence. In contrast, **non-material culture** is specific to social thoughts and ideas, such as values.

Popular culture is a phrase used to describe features of culture that appeal to the masses, often those communicated through mass media such as radio and television. This is distinguished from **high culture**, which describes those features often limited to the elite, like the ballet or opera.

While comparing different cultures is useful for noticing differences, some anthropologists assert that there are also some **cultural universals**—patterns or traits that are common to all people. Cultural universals tend to pertain to basic human survival and needs, such as securing food and shelter, and also pertain to events that every human experiences, including birth, death, and illness. Despite these very important similarities that unite us all, cultural differences are far more common than cultural universals.

Two of the most crucial elements of culture are its values and beliefs, which people within a given culture tend to share. **Values** can be defined as a culture's standard for evaluating what is good or bad, while **beliefs** are the convictions or principles that people hold. Values often define how people in a society should behave, but they may not actually reflect how people do behave. For example, in the United States, open-mindedness and tolerance are considered to be values, yet examples of racism and homophobia abound. In order to promote societal values, laws, sanctions, or rewards may be in place to encourage behavior in line with social values and discourage behavior counter to social values. For example, it is against the law to discriminate based on race, color, religion, gender, or national origin when making employment decisions. **Norms** are the visible and invisible rules of social conduct within a society.

Culture and Social Groups

Sociobiology is a study of how biology and evolution have affected human social behavior. Primarily, it applies Darwin's principle of natural selection to social behavior, suggesting there is a biological basis for many behaviors. That is, particular social behaviors persist over generations because they are adaptive for survival. Sociobiologists would argue that biological predisposition is influenced by social factors; an aggressive individual may learn to channel these tendencies away from socially unacceptable acts (for example, assault) and toward socially accepted activities (for example, cage-fighting).

Scientists also believe that the origins of culture lie in human evolution. Through time, humans in various societies evolved the ability to categorize and communicate human experience through the use of symbols (as discussed above). As these codified systems for communication were learned and taught to future generations, they began to develop independently of human evolution. While people living in different areas will likely develop their own unique cultures, culture can still be taught and learned. Therefore, anthropologists consider culture to be not just a product of human evolution, but a complement to it; it is a means of social adaptation to the natural world.

Cultural Construction and Transformation

Cultural diffusion is the transfer of elements of culture from one social group to another. This contributes to cultural similarities between different societies. Diffusion can be direct or indirect, or sometimes even forced, as with cultural imperialism. The rate of diffusion has increased as a result of cross-cultural communication, like modern media and transportation. This is important for **cultural competence** or effective interactions between people from different cultures. For example, in medicine, the diffusion of cultural understanding—which leads to effective communication—is an important element in reducing disparities in health and health care. **Cultural transmission** is the process through which this information is passed down to successive generations.

Elements of culture are not static. In some cases, **social change** occurs, in which societies experience a change in state. This can be subtle, like with the development of new linguistic phrases, or radical, like with **revolutions**. Transformative social changes, such as technological innovations, often challenge our understanding of the world because there is no social consensus about the new innovation; the creation of new social rules "lags" behind. This is described as **cultural lag**. The foundational work on cultural lag explains that material culture changes much faster than non-material culture, which often resists change.

When individuals experience changes that necessitate a period of adjustment, there is often **transition shock**. When this disorientation is the result of an individual being subjected to alternative cultures and foreign environments, such as through leisure travel or permanent relocation, it is called **culture shock**. This is a real experience that involves deeper emotions than homesickness; it challenges an individual's assumptions about their social surroundings. Different cultures have different cuisines, fashions, languages, gestures, etc., and individuals must grow accustomed to all of these changes. For example, the transition to medical school causes a definite reaction for most students; there is a feeling of "information overload" as the result of exposure to unfamiliar content and the disruption of established schedules. **Reverse culture shock** involves the same experiences but upon an individual's return to their initial environment.

Sociocultural evolution is a set of theories describing the processes through which societies and cultures have progressed over time. Both individuals and social structures experience continuous transformation in response to their complex needs. Sociologists argue that these changes are the result of social factors, such as social interactions, rather than biological factors. Thus, sociocultural evolution is less concerned with the evolution of human bodies, but instead questions how human minds have evolved for us to succeed as beings with natural social tendencies. While myriad societies have existed throughout the centuries, as revealed by historical research, most of these have declined naturally and only a couple hundred remain today. Two modern theories of sociocultural evolution, *modernization* and *sociobiology*, are discussed previously.

POPULATION STUDIES

Human **population** is the collection of people in a defined geographical area, and also refers to the number of people in the area. Population studies are interested in demographic shifts and can be quite complex. There is periodic population growth and population decline as a result of birth rates, death rates, and migration rates. The world as a whole is experiencing a period of population growth that is predicted to continue for many decades. Much of this growth is attributed to advances in agricultural production and innovations in medicine that have contributed to changes in birth and death rates. In contrast, studies of population decline are often concerned with great reductions in population as a result of catastrophes, such as epidemics and massacres, or widespread social changes (such as rural flight). Population growth and decline are measured using the **population growth rate**: the rate of population change in a specified time period, reported as a percent of the initial population.

In societies experiencing population growth, there is concern of reaching **overpopulation**, at which point there are more people than can be sustained; in societies experiencing decline, there are concerns about maintaining economic success. The total possible population that can be supported with needed resources and without significant negative effects in a given area is referred to as the **carrying capacity**. Populations tend to increase and decrease until **population equilibrium** is met at this maximum load.

Population projections are estimates of future populations made from mathematical extrapolations of previous data. Traditional projections are based on birth rates, death rates, and migration rates, and thus do not consider unpredicted effects on population, like the chance of catastrophes. The global population reached 7.9 billion in 2021. Experts project an increase in this population until at least 2050 with upper estimates ranging from 9 to 11 billion despite decreases in worldwide fertility rates. The projections suggest that the greatest contributions will be made in less-developed regions. In fact, nine countries are expected to contribute to more than half of the world's population; these countries are underdeveloped regions, including China and India, with the exception of the United States where international migration rates are an important consideration. In contrast, in some developed regions the death rate exceeds the birth rate which, coupled with increasing life expectancies, suggests population decline. In the United States, national population growth rates have been in decline since the turn of the century.

Population distributions—in particular, age and sex distributions—are sometimes represented through graphical illustrations called **population pyramids** (Figure 1). These representations create age- and sex-specific groups (cohorts) using either total population or percentages. The *x*-axis represents the population and the *y*-axis separates men and women with the tradition positioning males on the left and females on the right. This creates a clear and distinct shape that describes the social structure. For example, an expansive population pyramid is wide at the base, representing a high birth rate and a high death rate. Thus, population pyramids can help predict population trends and determine the social needs for dependents, such as children and people of retirement age.

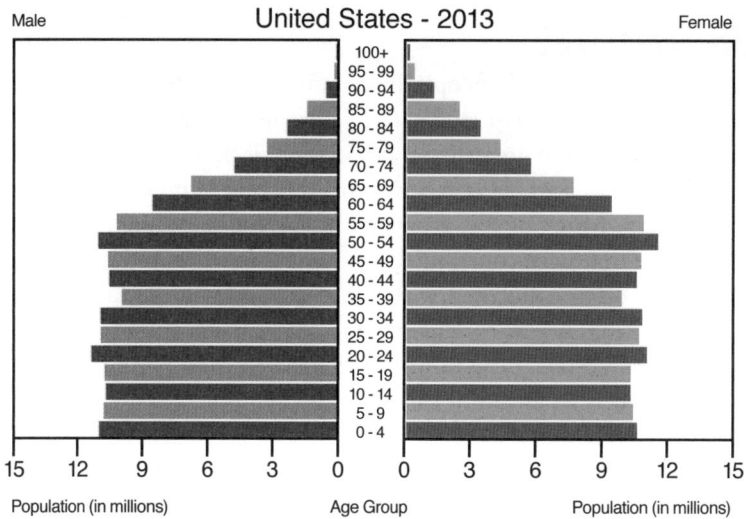

Figure 1   Population pyramid: birth rates, death rates, and migration rates
are the main determinants of changes in population

Fertility and Mortality

Birth rates and death rates are often reported through statistical measures. The **crude birth rate** (CBR) is the annual number of births per 1,000 people in a population. Experts consider crude birth rates of 10–20 to be low and those of 40–50 to be high. The **crude death rate** (CDR) is the annual number of deaths per 1,000 people in a population. Experts consider crude death rates below 10 to be low and those above 20 to be high. The **rate of population change** is the difference between the crude birth rate and crude death rate. There are also **age-specific birth rates** and **age-specific death rates**, which are the annual number of births or deaths per 1,000 persons in an age group.

In broad terms, **fertility** is the ability of a woman to reproduce. The **general fertility rate** is the annual number of births per 1,000 women in a population. The more complicated measure of **total fertility rate** predicts the total number births per single woman in a population with the assumption that the woman experiences the current recorded age-specific fertility rates and reaches the end of her reproductive life. Most women are capable of reproduction between the ages of 15 and 45 ("childbearing years"). The **replacement fertility rate** is the fertility rate at which the population will remain balanced, and **sub-replacement fertility** indicates that the birth rate is less than the death rate, thus the population size will not be sustained. The **population-lag effect** refers to the fact that changes in total fertility rates are often not reflected in the birth rate for several generations. This is the result of **population momentum**, in which the children produced during periods of higher fertility rates reproduce; there are more women of reproductive age and thus more births overall, regardless of the number of births per woman. Because crude birth rates do not consider age or sex differences, fertility rates offer a clearer idea of demographic trends.

Regarding decreases in population, **mortality** refers to the death rate in a population, and this also includes both general and specific measures. This is distinguished from **morbidity**, which refers to the nature and extent of disease in a population; the **prevalence rate** measures the number of individuals experiencing a disease and the **incidence rate** measures the number of new cases of a disease. Reference to death rates in medicine often concern the **case fatality rate**, which measures deaths as the result of a set diagnosis or procedure, sometimes specific to the beginning or late stages. The current leading cause of death worldwide is ischemic heart disease, but there are also variations in causes of death by location; for example, age-related issues are a major cause of death in developed countries, while malnutrition is a major cause of death in developing countries. There is an inverse correlation between a nation's crude death rate and its gross domestic product (GDP). There are two additional common and reliable indicators of important qualities of life: the infant mortality rate and life expectancy. The **infant mortality rate** is the annual number of deaths per 1,000 infants under one year of age. This rate is lowest in European countries, such as Iceland, at a low of 5 and highest in the sub-Saharan regions of Africa, such as Sierra Leone, at a high of 170. **Life expectancy** is the number of years that individual can expect to live based on year of birth and other demographic factors. Estimates of global life expectancies range from 36 to 79 years.

Developed regions tend to have lower birth rates and death rates. Factors contributing to decreasing crude birth rates include access to contraception, costs associated with raising a child, and other social changes. For example, teenage births are at a historic low in the United States and an increasing number of older couples are choosing to postpone reproduction, or to not reproduce at all. Factors contributing to decreasing crude death rates include improvements in agriculture, medicine, and sanitation.

Migration

In addition to birth rates and death rates, population is also determined through rates of **migration**, the geographical movement of individuals, families, or other small or large groups of people. Migration is distinct from non-permanent movement. For example, non-permanent travel for leisure, pilgrimage, or seasonal reasons and **nomadism**, which is a traditional method of continuous travel in search of natural resources as a method of sustenance ("hunting and gathering"), are not considered migration because there is no intention to settle. **External migration**, also referred to as cross-border or international migration, involves migration to another nation. Motivations for external migration are often economic or political in nature. **Internal migration** involves migration to another region of the same nation. Motivations for internal migration are often more economic in nature as individuals pursue better opportunities, such as education. **Voluntary migration** is the result of internal factors (a personal decision). **Involuntary migration**, or forced migration, is the result of external factors that pose a threat to the individual in their initial environment and are often a form of social control, such as ethnic cleansing. Those who migrate to unsettled areas are **settlers** and those who migrate to settled areas as a result of displacement are **refugees**. More complicated is **colonization**, which involves migration to settled areas in which dominance is exerted over the foreign state. **Immigration** involves entering a new area and these people are called immigrants (and can be either legal or illegal residents); **emigration** involves leaving an area and those who do so are called emigrants. For example, there is a high rate of emigration from Mexico and a high rate of immigration to the United States. There is also a high rate of illegal immigration, which has disadvantages for both the migrant individual and their new home. **Reverse migration**, or return migration, is the return of individuals to their former homes.

There are numerous historical theories describing the reasons for migration and its effects. Everett Lee, a popular theorist, differentiated between push and pull factors in migration. **Push factors** are those features that are unattractive about an area and "push" people to leave. Push factors are often economic, political, or religious (e.g., housing **discrimination** or insufficient access to social resources). There are also more extreme examples, such as destructive violence or natural disasters, and **genocide**, or mass execution with the intention of eliminating a specific social group. **Pull factors** are those features that are attractive about an area and "pull" people there. These often include opportunities for economic, political, or religious freedom and success. The interaction between push and pull factors contributes to the rates of migration.

Urban Growth, Decline, and Renewal

Internal migration includes the movement between rural and urban areas. The spatial distribution of individuals and social groups is an interest of **social geography**. **Urbanization** refers to the growth of urban areas (as people move from rural to urban areas) as the result of global change. Urbanization is tied to **industrialization**, the process through which societies transform from agrarian to industrial, and industrialized countries have more people living in urban areas than non-industrialized countries do. The global urbanization rate is roughly 55%, and approximately 80% of the U.S. population lives in urban areas (including cities and suburbs). People move to urban areas predominantly for the economic advancement that cities provide. Furthermore, people can access more social services in cities. This is related to **rural flight**, the migration from rural areas to urban areas. Emigration from rural areas is often related to a decreasing emphasis on agricultural processes.

In contrast to urban growth, suburbanization leads to urban decline. **Suburbanization** refers to population growth on the fringes of urban areas (as people move from urban areas to suburban areas). The **suburbs** are residential satellite communities located in the peripheral regions of major urban centers that are often connected to the cities in some fashion. In the United States more people live in the suburbs (which are considered "urban" for statistical purposes) than in the cities themselves. **White flight** is a historical example of suburbanization that involved the migration of whites from cities to more racially homogenous suburbs. Migration to such areas that are adjacent to the cities is an example of **urban sprawl**, or the migration of people from urban areas to otherwise remote areas. The negative effects of urban sprawl include **urban blight**, which occurs when less functioning areas of large cities degrade as a result of urban decline. These forms of migration can thus lead to desolate properties, such as condemned houses, and the resulting dangerous conditions can contribute to an increase in crime levels in blighted areas. Those who remain in the blighted areas are often poor and have less access to social amenities and opportunities.

Gentrification refers to the renovation of urban areas in a process of urban renewal. Gentrification is often specific to the introduction of wealthier residents to the cities who then help to restore the existing infrastructure, which alters the region's demographics and economics. Gentrification is a form of **urban renewal**, or the redevelopment of urban areas. This causes much social change with both positive and negative effects; for example, it can increase the tax base, but it can also lead to the displacement of the original local people. Urban renewal can be a mechanism for reform or a mechanism for control (for example, eminent domain).

Theories of Population Change

There are multiple theories of population change. **Demographic transition** (DT) is the transition from overall higher to overall lower birth and death rates as a result of a country's development from a pre-industrial to industrial framework due to both economic and social changes; thus, both fertility and mortality rates decrease as in the transition from an agricultural to a manufacturing society. This has long-term effects, such as a stable population. The model includes specific stages of transition and, in general, developed countries are further along in this transition than developing countries but most countries have started to experience changes in crude birth rate and crude death rate. However, the model is limited; for example, it does not consider additional social factors that affect birth rates, like religious influences.

Thomas Robert Malthus argued that population is the result of available resources for sustenance, such as productive farmland. Humans are inclined to reproduce and thus population growth is often exponential, especially during times of excess. However, **Malthusianism** states that the possible rate of population increase exceeds the possible rate of resource increase. Malthus described two forms of checks on population growth: **positive checks** that raise the death rate, like disease, disasters, hunger, and wars, and **preventative checks** that lower the birth rate, like abstinence, birth control, late marriage, and same-sex relationships. A **Malthusian Catastrophe** occurs when the means of sustenance are not enough to support the population, resulting in population reduction through famine or predicted famine (i.e., people have fewer children because they fear serious food shortages in the future). **Neo-Malthusianism** is a movement based on these principles that advocates for population control in order to reduce the negative effects of population strain.

Demographics in U.S. Society

Demography is the study of human population dynamics, including the size, structure, and distribution of a population, and changes in the population over time due to birth, death, and migration. An analysis of the demographics of a given society can provide powerful information about many sociological phenomena. Demographic data are largely derived from censuses.

As of 2020, the population of the United States was approximately 331,449,000, roughly 50.8% of whom were female. Approximately 22.3% of the population were eighteen years old or younger, while approximately 16.5% were sixty-five or older.

In 2020, approximately 13.6% of the population was foreign-born, including approximately 11 million noncitizens. Latin America accounts for just over half of all of the people who are foreign-born in the United States, so is thus the largest source of both legal and illegal immigration to the United States.

In regards to population studies, there has been a rapid decline in the total global fertility rate; this is of particular concern in the United States where the average woman has fewer than two children, which is below the population replacement level. The infant mortality rate has decreased in recent years and is now approximately 6 deaths per 1,000 live births. The current life expectancy at birth is approximately 79 years (76 for males and 81 for females). The current migration rates (external migration) have caused increases in population despite low birth rates and death rates (although population growth is nonetheless near a historical low). There are also examples of internal migration. There have been historic migrations from the eastern states to the western states (expansion), as well as the migration of African Americans from the rural south to the urban north after abolition of slavery, called the Great Migration. The **New Great Migration** is an example of a domestic reverse migration. During this period, there was an increase in Black migration to the now urban South as racial relations improved.

Researchers often use aggregate statistics to provide a demographic profile of a specific population (based on region or time). **Minorities** are those demographic groups that receive differential treatment through processes of prejudice and discrimination due to their shared characteristics. These groups have lower statuses than other groups, and may be viewed as inferior. It is important to note that despite the title, these groups are termed minorities not for their size but instead for their disparate social experiences and the description holds regardless of population size. Thus, despite the gender and sex distributions being near equal in most societies, women are sometimes considered minorities because of their perceived status as inferior and subordinate to men. The **dominant groups** are those with the social power to assign these labels.

Demographic measures discussed on the next pages include age, gender, race and ethnicity, sexual orientation, and immigration status.

Age

People's temporal position between birth and death is measured through **age**. In Western societies, the most common use is numerical age, a chronological measurement that begins at birth (thus babies are age 0 at birth). This is distinguished from measures of prenatal development, such as gestational age, although some societies do consider this period (thus babies are age 9 months at birth if full-term). Years are the most common units of measurement for age, but months or even weeks are also used in certain situations, such as with infants.

Age cohorts are an example of statistical cohorts in which a group of subjects share the characteristic of age. Generational cohorts, or **generations**, are groups of people born in the same period. Demographic age profiles describe populations in terms of age groups. Populations with a proportionate distribution are the most stable. **Population aging** occurs when there is a disproportionate percentage of older people in a population. This raises concerns such as health-care demands and provider shortages. **Ageism** is prejudice or discrimination against a person based on age, often against older people.

The concept of aging has both biological and social components. *Social aging* reflects the biological changes in a multidimensional process in which individuals experience complex emotional and social changes. There are serious social implications of an aging population. Economic consequences of a rising median age include increased requirements for pension liabilities, retirement packages, and worker's compensation. In contrast, an increase in children leads to greater demands for social resources such as education. Furthermore, younger people are more likely to contribute to social changes, such as the creation of new technologies or the push for political changes.

There are theories that explain the social construction of age. These perspectives assert that perceptions of age are not inherent but instead social creations based on cultural customs, traditions, and values. Eastern cultures tend to respect older people for their experience and wisdom. Western cultures, however, tend to see aging as undesirable. It is thus common to take measures to control appearances and impressions, such as cosmetic surgeries. The response to aging parents exemplifies these cultural differences. Retirement homes are more popular in developed societies and public perceptions of these resources are accepting; in less modern societies, it is expected that children will care for their parents and assisted living options might be seen as disrespectful.

Gender

Sex is a biological characteristic that is assigned at birth and permanent in most cases; it is based on chromosomes, external genitalia, gonads, and hormones. Thus, categories of sex are male (XY) and female (XX). The third sex, albeit rare, is intersex. This classification is applicable when a single sex cannot be identified. **Gender** is a social characteristic that is based on behavioral role expectations. Thus, categories of gender are masculine and feminine. Developed societies often discuss gender in dichotomous terms, where masculine and feminine are opposites, but in some societies, there are third genders, such as the Native American two-spirit: individuals who are neither male nor female, and are held in high regard in some traditional Native American tribes.

Gender is thought to be influenced by both nature and nurture. In terms of nature, biological measures can have behavioral effects (for examples, hormones influence emotions). The natural sciences are interested in the consequences of biological differences between men and women on gender. In some cases, genetic abnormalities (such as the XXY chromosomal abnormality in Klinefelter's syndrome) might cause unexpected presentations in light of one's biological sex. In terms of nurture, our social surroundings have a profound effect on the development of our gender identities. Gender identification occurs through multiple agents of socialization and **gender roles** (the socialization of gender roles is also known as **gender conditioning**) describe the social and behavioral expectations for men and women. These expectations are internalized and become connected to our self-identities (how we think about ourselves) and thus influence our behaviors. **Gender expression** is the external manifestation of these roles. **Gender schema theory** is the study of how gender beliefs become socialized in society. A similar theory states that individuals learn sexual behavior through gender scripts, a series of predictable patterns that are internalized through socialization.

Sexism is prejudice or discrimination against a person based on gender or sex, often against women. Despite revolutionary social changes, there continues to be a flawed perception in which men are viewed as dominant and women are viewed as subordinate; men are the reference group and women are the "other" group in continuous reference to men. Men and women are different and unequal in the social resources afforded to them; women are marginalized and given less power at birth and fewer opportunities throughout their lifetime to gain power. A classic example of gender inequality concerns the institution of marriage. Upon entering into a marriage, women often gain many more responsibilities. The division of labor further limits the representation of women in the public sphere, which also limits the opportunities women have to develop the intellectual reasoning skills that society values. These disparate experiences are an interest of the previously discussed Feminist Theory.

Gender roles are those behaviors that are considered appropriate or proper for men and women. Gendered behaviors that follow social conventions are approved while those that do not are disapproved; thus, deviation from gender roles tends to create social disorder. **Transgender** individuals have gender identities that are inconsistent with their biological sex. Some transgender individuals decide to make permanent changes to their bodies through hormone therapy, surgery, or some other means. There is much prejudice and discrimination against transgender communities.

Race and Ethnicity

Race and ethnicity are related concepts that are of much interest to sociologists because of their importance in human interactions. **Race** is a description of a distinct social group based on certain shared characteristics. These shared characteristics are often inherited biological traits or genetic differences (and thus manifest in physical appearances). According to the U.S. Census Bureau, the currently accepted race categories include Black/African American, white, Asian, American Indian/Alaska Native, Native Hawaiian/Other Pacific Islander, and "Other." **Ethnicity** is cultural and ethnicities are distinct from nationalities. For example, Arab populations originate in the Arabian Peninsula, which includes several modern nations including (1) Egypt, (2) Algeria, (3) Iraq, (4) Sudan, and (5) Morocco. In addition to Arab populations, Egypt also includes ethnic minorities, such as the Beja, Berber, Dom, and Nubian peoples. **Ethnogenesis** is a social process that results in the creation of separate ethnicities. Historical examples of this include the development of small sub-ethnic groups, **tribes**, into independent ethnic groups.

Members of the same racial or ethnic group do not develop a common identity based on shared characteristics alone; such identities are also formed on the basis of shared historical and social experiences. It is not the common origin that forms the group but the shared consciousness of the common origin, and the meanings ascribed to that specific origin. Prejudices and actions that discriminate based on race, or hold that one race is inferior to another, are called **racism**. While the exact definitions of "race," "ethnicity," and "racism" have been subject to much debate over the years, racism tends to be seen when the dominant or majority group holds a prejudice or engages in discrimination, whether intentional or not, against non-dominant or minority groups. Sometimes racism is used to describe discrimination on an ethnic or cultural basis, independent of whether these differences are described as racial. The ambiguity largely stems from confusion about the definitions of the terms "race" and "ethnicity." Ethnocentrism is a related concept that describes biases that result when people look at issues from the perspective of a particular cultural background. It is often whites who are said to be ethnocentric in sociological studies, but this is not absolute.

Michael Omi and Howard Winat's **racial formation perspective** was created with the purpose of deconstructing race in its modern form. Race is seen as a complex and fluid social construct, enforced through both micro- and macro-level social processes. In contrast to other theories that do not present race exclusively as a social construct, the racial formation perspective asserts that without these processes, the differences in biological features are meaningless.

Racialization, or **ethnicization**, is the social process by which the dominant group ascribes racial or ethnic identities, perceived or real, to groups that do not otherwise relate to the labels. These processes are used as forms of social control, often as a part of imperialism or nationalism. Historical examples of racialization and ethnicization have resulted in the eventual self-identification of these groups with the ascribed race or ethnicity.

Sexual Orientation

Sexual orientation concerns the target of a person's romantic or sexual attraction or behavior. There are three main sexual orientations:

- **Heterosexual**: the orientation toward the opposite gender or sex
- **Homosexual**: the orientation toward the same gender or sex
- **Bisexual**: the orientation toward both genders or sexes

Bisexual identities do not necessitate an equal attraction toward both genders or sexes; in some cases, there is a distinct, but not exclusive, sexual preference toward one gender or sex. Bisexual communities include those who are **pansexual** and attracted to people irrespective of gender or sex. **Asexuality** involves the lack of sexual attraction. This is different from the decision to be abstinent or celibate for personal reasons, such as religious beliefs. In fact, those with little or no sexual attraction sometimes participate in sexual behavior nonetheless for reasons like reproduction. Sexual orientation exists along a continuum, with the extremes being exclusive attraction to the opposite gender or sex (heterosexual) and exclusive attraction to the same gender or sex (homosexual). The Kinsey Scale, also called the Heterosexual-Homosexual Rating Scale assigns a number from 0 (exclusively heterosexual) to 6 (exclusively homosexual) that places each individual along this continuum.

Heterosexism is prejudice or discrimination against a person based on their sexual orientation toward the same sex (for example, homophobic attitudes). **Heteronormative beliefs** often enforce strict gender roles and involve prejudice and discrimination against non-heterosexual individuals. There are sometimes public sanctions, such as formal policies, reinforcing these beliefs. This has led to modern social movements for the recognition of legal rights, such as adoption rights, marriage rights, and health-care rights for same-sex couples.

There is much debate about the causes of sexual orientation, including both biological theories that consider factors like genetics and hormones and environmental theories that consider factors like parenting. Some argue that non-heterosexual behavior is unnatural for certain reasons (for example, it does not permit reproduction). However, research suggests that sexual orientation is a human characteristic that is generally resistant to change, leading to the argument that non-heterosexual behavior can be natural. Furthermore, there is no substantive scientific evidence to support the argument that sexual orientation can be changed through interventions.

Immigration Status

Immigration was introduced above as the migration of people to a new area. Immigration status is another common demographic measure. In the past, the United Nations estimated the international migrant population to be near 3 percent of the total world population. Most of these migrants moved to developed countries. European countries host the most immigrants worldwide (around 70 million); North American countries host the second most (around 45 million). Recent research recorded that the highest percentage of respondents (23%) in a study who identified as being interested in migration named the United States as their preferred destination. This can be attributed in part to the **American Dream**, an ideological construct that offers individuals the opportunities for happiness and success with the proper amount of determination. This central promise has contributed to the rise in migration to the United States in the search of a better life with enhanced personal freedoms.

The United States has had four main periods of immigration, based on the social context, as well as the distinct demographics (ethnicities, nationalities, and races) of the migrants.

1) **The seventeenth and eighteenth centuries**: During this period, English colonists migrated to the United States (the colonial period). Indentured servants also migrated through this process, accounting for more than half of all immigrants from Europe during the period.

2) **The mid-nineteenth century**: During this period, the most migrants came from northern Europe.

3) **The early twentieth century**: During this period, the most migrants came from southern and Eastern Europe. The peak of European migration was 1907, after which the social context of the United States made conditions less suitable for immigration. The Great Depression, for example, led to a period of higher national emigration rates than immigration rates (this occurred in the early 1930s).

4) **The late twentieth century (post-1965) to the present**: During this period, the majority of migrants have been from Asia and Latin America. The rates of immigration during this period have been unprecedented. For example, the decade with the historically highest rate of immigration was from 1990 to 2000; between 10 and 11 million legal and illegal immigrants entered the United States during this phase. There are now more than 44 million immigrants living in the United States; approximately 10.5 million of those are undocumented, according to 2017 estimates.

The United States has restrictive legal limits on immigration. There are current quotas based on origin, and these limits do not consider populations (thus, the maximum number of visas offered is the same for all countries). **Immigration controls** are formal policies that define and regulate who has the right to settle in an area. Today, most legal immigration is granted on the basis of family reunification (this accounts for two-thirds of all cases), employment skills, and humanitarian reasons. Historically, immigration decisions have been made for other reasons, such as ethnic selection. In some cases, the U.S. government has granted amnesties for undocumented immigrants. The presence of illegal immigrants presents definite challenges in describing the complex demographics of the United States.

The shared experiences of immigrants are of concern to sociologists. These individuals are often mistreated, and in some cases their rights are violated, in the immigration process. Immigrants are also a common target of prejudice and discrimination. Public attitudes, in general, are more positive toward established migrants (such as the Polish and Italian communities) and more negative toward recent migrants (such as Hispanic communities). For these reasons, there are often intersections between immigration status and race and ethnicity, as well as social class. There is also a distinction in the public opinion of legal and illegal immigrants, often fueled by media coverage of migration. Furthermore, immigrant status can have implications for social functioning due to the differences in the social conventions of developing and developed countries. For example, arranged marriages are more common in the East than in the West, which requires immigrants to reconcile these practices with the accepted traditions of their new homes.

DEMOGRAPHIC SHIFTS AND SOCIAL CHANGE

Globalization

Modern advancements in telecommunications and transportation have contributed to the rates of **globalization**, the process of increasing interdependence of societies and connections between people across the world. **Telecommunications**, in particular, use modern technologies to ease the challenges of communication across distances, and like most information and communication technologies, contribute to the integration of economic, political, and social processes worldwide. In response to an increase in global competition, multinational corporations and transnational companies have formed in order to gain the benefits of cooperation and pursue new investment opportunities. This is made possible through new technologies that ease the challenges of international communication, such as videoconferences for business, as well as the possibilities for international exchange of resources through automatic electronic transactions. **Economic interdependence** can be thought of as the division of labor on a global scale; countries might have the demand for products without the internal means of production. For example, the United States is dependent on other countries for some natural resources, like oil. These new markets can pose concerns. The example of **outsourcing** involves the contracting of third parties for specific operations. This can be domestic or foreign, but the financial savings associated with foreign outsourcing have led to its increase and made it a focus of much opposition.

Politics are also an important component of globalization. The increased opportunities for international communication contribute to an increased awareness of relevant global issues through the diffusion of knowledge. This has led to the development of international organizations, like the popular intergovernmental organization known as the United Nations. **Non-governmental organizations** (NGOs) are those organizations without an official government affiliation with the intention of contributing to the lessening of global issues. Médecins Sans Frontières (MSF), or Doctors Without Borders, is a good example of an international humanitarian NGO; MSF is committed to lessening global inequalities in health. Thus, globalization eases borders and allows international cooperation in the fight for human rights.

There are also cultural consequences of globalization as the sharing of cultures leads to more foreign choices, such as cuisines and media options. In some cases, this interchange can lead to the disintegration of local culture as new ideas are welcomed. Furthermore, globalization contributes to rates of migration, thus changing the demographics of an area. This can also create environmental challenges, such as air pollution resulting from increased transportation. Two dramatic examples of resulting social changes in globalization are civil unrest and terrorism. Periods of **civil unrest**, or civil disorder, involve forms of collective behavior in which there is public expression of the group's concern, often in response to major social problems, like with political demonstrations and protests. This can have serious consequences for societies, such as the destruction of public properties and the interruption of important services. **Terrorism** involves the use of violence with the intention to create fear in the target communities. There is no single form of terrorism: it can be committed for ideological, nationalistic, political, religious, or other reasons. The defining characteristic of terrorist acts is indiscriminate violence; thus, terrorism involves violence directed toward non-combatants. The United States experienced a series of terrorist attacks on September 11, 2001, and this is one of the most-discussed examples of terrorism in the world. The result of the extremist organization known as Al Qaeda, this is the deadliest terrorist attack recorded. The aftermath of these attacks, including the Global War on Terrorism, have had serious domestic and international consequences, such as an increase in hate crimes committed against American Muslims.

Perspectives on globalization are varied, and some of the positives and negatives of three main aspects of globalization (economic, political, and sociocultural globalization) are discussed above. One can expand upon these contrasting perspectives using the example of the political consequences. Proponents consider the positive consequences of globalization. As mentioned above, processes of globalization offer greater democratic representation of less-developed countries as a result of new political institutions. These international bodies are often concerned with human issues, such as environmental issues, like chlorofluorocarbon (CFC) emissions and nuclear proliferation, and promote international cooperation in addressing these issues, such as researching alternative energies and conservation. There are some in favor of organized world governments to address the needs of world citizens. Opponents consider the negative consequences of globalization. In contrast to the arguments of democratic globalization, critics believe it contributes to the disintegration of democratic values. The economic issues inherent in globalization, such as the concentration of economic power in developed countries, contribute to oppressive politics; thus, globalization is not seen as a contributor to social cohesion but to social control.

Social Movements

The section on collective behavior introduces social movements as a method of achieving social change. In this sense, social movements are a reflection of public dissatisfaction and a collective response to economic, political, or social issues. This necessitates the existence of two opposing groups: those who support the current social structure and those who support change. For example, the social issue of abortion has created two distinct social movements: pro-choice and pro-life. It is common that social movements arise when the formal means of participation, like voting, do not address the concerns of the public. For this reason, much social movement is seen as the people's opposition to those in power, and in particular those who have vested interests so strong that there is resulting corruption at the expense of the public. The processes involved in social movements might contribute to an intermediate disruption of social order, but the purpose is to protect the core values of modern societies: civil rights, freedom, justice, protection, etc. Thus, the most successful social movements are the result of critical social problems that violate these central values. This makes the concern relevant to the general population and necessitates that the issue be resolved through progressive social change.

There has been an unprecedented increase in the use of public participation to challenge existing social structures and facilitate positive changes in modern times (consider the increased freedoms for minorities, for example). This is often seen as a function of the founding principles of democracies, such as the freedom of speech, as well as a result of the related processes of industrialization and urbanization. **Relative**

deprivation has also been suggested as a contributing factor. Relative deprivation refers to the conscious experience of individuals or groups that do not have the resources needed for the social experiences and services that are seen as appropriate to their social position. In essence, there is a feeling of being entitled to more than what one has in their current situation, based on relative, not absolute, standards. This perceived deprivation can be economic, political, or social. Relative deprivation can also contribute to social deviance.

The organization of social movements varies, but the most successful movements tend to have strong leadership. These often charismatic leaders help create allied communities of consensus, and later have coordinating roles. The overall organization might be loose, but there is nonetheless a divide between those who support the cause (insiders) and those who do not (outsiders). Popular social movements are often supported through the efforts of multiple social movement organizations. For example, People for the Ethical Treatment of Animals (PETA) is a single organization that participates in the broader social movement for animal rights and its members are part of an even larger group of advocates.

The use of telecommunications is one of the most important strategies used in modern social movements. The Internet, and social networking in particular, has made it easier to accomplish the successful formation of groups, and provides an effective means of directing efforts once these groups are formed. The rapid dissemination of information through the Internet contributes to the success of activist groups in educating the masses. For example, the Internet group known as Anonymous describes itself as an "Internet gathering" and its followers, called Anons, have taken collective action against injustices, often recognized through their use of identifiable Guys Fawkes masks. The power of Internet communication as a means of activism is so strong that it is considered a contributing factor in the increase of government censorship online.

Furthermore, peaceful, rather than violent, social movements are often more successful in gaining the public's support. This is more in line with the principal concept of social movements: protecting central beliefs (such as peace), which is here used to its advantage. It is also less threatening, which allows more people to participate because it is more difficult for the movement to be discredited; for example, peaceful action has a lower chance of leading to arrest. Movements that are violent in nature ("rebellions") are often self-destructive.

5.2 STRATIFICATION, HEALTH, AND HEALTH CARE DISPARITIES

Stratification and Inequality

Social stratification refers to the way that people are categorized in society; people can be categorized by race, education, wealth, and income (among other factors). People with the most resources comprise the top tiers of the stratification, while people with the least resources comprise the bottom tiers. Social stratification is a system that not only serves to define differences (or inequalities) but also serves to reinforce and perpetuate them. The **caste system** describes a closed stratification where people can do nothing to change the category that they are born into. On the other hand, the **class system** considers both social variables and individual initiative; the class system groups together people of similar wealth, income, education, etc. but the classes are open, meaning that people can strive to reach a higher class (or fall to a lower one). However, a person's upward social mobility is constrained; a person's class position affords them only a certain amount of resources. A **meritocracy** is another stratification system that uses merit (or personal effort) to establish social standing; this is an idealized system—no society solely stratifies based on effort. Most sociologists define stratification in terms of socioeconomic status. **Socioeconomic status** (SES) can be defined in terms of power (the ability to get other people to do something), property (sum of possessions and income), and prestige (reputation in society), because these three concepts tend to (but not always) be related in U.S. society.

Social mobility refers to the ability to move up or down within the social stratification system. **Upward mobility** refers to an elevation in social class; in America, we applaud examples of upward mobility because everyone wants to believe that it is possible to achieve the American Dream. **Downward mobility** refers to a decline in social class. **Intergenerational mobility** occurs when there is an elevation or decline in social class between parents and children within a family, and **intragenerational mobility** describes the differences in social class between different members of the same generation.

Social reproduction refers to the structures and activities in place in a society that serve to transmit and reinforce social inequality from one generation to the next. Cultural capital and social capital are two mechanisms by which social reproduction occurs. **Cultural capital** refers to the non-financial social assets that promote social mobility. Education is an excellent example of cultural capital; an education gives someone the potential to be upwardly mobile (though there are a lot of reasons why inequalities in U.S. educational system might actually serve to prevent someone from becoming upwardly mobile as well). **Social capital** refers to the potential for social networks to allow for upward social mobility. Social capital is a powerful way to tap into vast networks of resources, but it can also serve to reinforce inequalities already present in society.

Power (the ability to get other people to do something) and **prestige** (reputation in society) are two related components of socioeconomic status in U.S. society. Both power and prestige rely on privilege, a less often discussed aspect of social life. **Privilege** is a set of advantages available exclusively to a person or group.

When social scientists study privilege, they conceptualize different privileged identities as intersecting with each other and affording individuals advantage in a non-additive way. This analytical approach, which seeks to highlight the ways different identities intersect within individuals and social groups to produce unique social positions, is called **intersectionality**. Sociologists conducting intersectional analyses assert that, for example, the social position of a Black lesbian cannot be understood by considering her Blackness and then her homosexuality; rather, the unique social position of Black lesbian must be considered in its own right. Identities, whether privileged or disadvantaged, do not combine additively and should not be considered in isolation.

Health care is a very significant institution in U.S. society, and there are notable disparities between groups who can access the health care they need and those who cannot. One of the major factors that affects access is one's ability to pay for health care. Because health care must be bought just like other goods, the same socioeconomic gradient that affects individuals' ability to buy goods affects their ability to pay for health care. For this reason, we can consider the effect of a **socioeconomic gradient in health**. The socioeconomic gradient applies within countries (higher SES individuals tend to have better outcomes, across many variables) and between countries (countries with higher gross domestic product, for example, tend to have better outcomes). However, this socioeconomic gradient transcends the ability to pay for medical care and extends to the conditions in which people live. One's socioeconomic status also affects where one can live and corresponds to the type of work one does. Lower paid work, such as manual labor, is often dirty, dangerous, and difficult (the 3 Ds). This type of work may predispose laborers to injury or ill health, all while affecting their ability to pay for their health care. The socioeconomic gradient is a global effect, influencing individuals across a variety of nations, even, to varying degrees, those with socialized healthcare. Environmental injustice (sometimes referred to as environmental justice) refers to the location of and exposure to health risks. For example, smog producing factories, landfills, and other pollutants are more likely to be located in and around lower income communities than higher income communities, potentially exposing residents of lower income neighborhoods to more pollutants than residents of higher income neighborhoods.

Global stratification refers to the unequal distribution of resources among the world's nations that produces a hierarchical framework. A comparison across the globe highlights the worldwide patterns of **global inequality:**

- certain countries hold a majority of the resources
- access to resources among countries seriously impacts other social factors, such a mortality
- the burden of inequality is placed on certain segments of the population

For example, the poorest people in the wealthiest countries (such as the United States) are far better off than the poorest people in the poorest countries. Likewise, women and racial and ethnic minorities often bear the brunt of unequal distributions of resources. High-income countries include the United States, Canada, and many Western European countries. Low-income countries include India, Nigeria, and China, among several others. In these countries, women are disproportionately affected by poverty. Poverty can be defined as being either relative or absolute. **Relative poverty** is the inability to meet the average standard of living within a society whereas **absolute poverty** is the inability to meet a bare minimum of basic necessities, including clean drinking water, food, safe housing, and reliable access to health care. Another important distinction is between **marginal poverty** and **structural poverty**. Marginal poverty is due to a lack of stable employment, whereas structural poverty is due to underlying and pervasive effects of the society's institutions.

Health and Health Care Disparities

On a broader scale, **social epidemiology** is the study of the distribution of health and disease across a population, with the focus on using social concepts to explain patterns of health and illness in a population. Many factors influence the accessibility and availability of health care across various social groups. **Health care disparities** include the population-specific differences in the presence of disease, health outcomes, and quality of health care across various social groups. Social epidemiology can help to explain some of the health care disparities that exist across multiple social constructs, including gender, race, and class.

Gender

Historically, medical research, treatment, and pharmacological studies have been conducted on men. Some studies suggest that over 90% of medical research was conducted on male subjects only, and that the findings were extrapolated to women. Women were traditionally excluded from medical research for a number of reasons; medical research was conducted predominantly on men, and the results were then assumed to be similar for women. We are now seeing that this is not a responsible or ethical way to conduct research. For example, women and men experience heart attack symptoms differently; men tend to experience "crushing" chest pain, but women are more likely to experience abdominal pain, indigestion, difficulty breathing, or fatigue. The fact that most early heart attack studies were conducted almost entirely on men led to a general misperception that women would experience the same symptoms as men, which is in fact not the case. Furthermore, there exists a disparity between how women and men are treated for heart disease, likely due to a

gender bias (when women and men receive different treatment for the same disease or illness) and a lack of information. For example, women tend to be treated less aggressively than men for heart disease, primarily because studies on men have set the standard for detection and treatment.

Drug dosing provides another example of the potentially deleterious effects of conducting medical research on men and extrapolating to women. Recently, the Food and Drug Administration (FDA) pulled a popular prescription sleep aid from the market because women were experiencing drowsiness and impairment the morning following prescribed usage that was leading to an increase in car accidents. Further testing demonstrated that the recommended dosage was too high for women: a costly mistake that could have been prevented had drug-dosage studies been conducted on both women and men before the drug was approved.

Race and Social Class

While race and social class (or socioeconomic status) are two very different social constructs, when discussing health and health care disparities, it makes sense to look at these two factors together, partially because in the United States a large proportion of minority groups are also socioeconomically disadvantaged. Large health-care disparities exist between minorities and whites in the United States. For example, infant mortality rates are almost twice as high for African Americans as they are for white people, the risks for cancer, heart disease, and diabetes are higher for African Americans than for white people, and studies suggest that Hispanics receive 60% inferior health care than non-Hispanics. Access to health care and accurate health information is a large part of the problem. Lower-income areas (with larger proportions of minorities) have fewer health care facilities, and a lack of health insurance prevents many lower-income people from seeking regular or preventative health care. Typically, once an uninsured person makes it into the health care system, a problem that was potentially treatable has developed into a much larger (and much more expensive) problem, thus perpetuating the cycle of avoiding the doctor until it is, or is almost, too late.

Chapter 5 Summary

- Symbolic culture consists of symbols that carry a particular meaning and are recognized by people of the same culture.

- Material culture involves the physical objects that are particular to that culture.

- Values can be defined as a culture's standard for evaluating what is good or bad, while beliefs are the convictions or principles that people hold.

- Demography is the study of human population dynamics.

- Social stratification refers to the way that people are categorized in society; people can be categorized by race, education, wealth, and income (among other factors).

- Social mobility refers to the ability to move up or down within the social stratification system.

- Global stratification involves the relative wealth, economic stability, and power of various countries and the hierarchy that results.

- Relative poverty is defined as an inability to meet the average standard of living within a society, while absolute poverty is the inability to acquire a bare minimum of basic necessities.

CHAPTER 5 FREESTANDING PRACTICE QUESTIONS

1. The Louisiana Basin in many ways represents a subculture of American society where French language and culture has had a significant impact on norms and rituals. The famous Mardi Gras festival is an example of an imported cultural ritual which has, over the years, come to dominate much of what the world associates with the New Orleans area and its culture, at the expense of many other traditions and norms. Which term most closely describes this scenario?

A) Cultural lag
B) Cultural transmission
C) Cultural diffusion
D) Culture shock

2. Life expectancy in most developed countries is currently increasing while fertility rates are decreasing. In Japan, for example, recent data showed life expectancy in the mid-80s and average fertility at approximately 1.5 births per female. Both these trends are expected to stabilize in the coming years. We would expect Japan to experience:

A) population growth due to reduced mortality rates.
B) population decline due to sub-replacement-level birth rates.
C) population growth due to replacement-level birth rates.
D) population decline due to mortality rate stabilization.

3. Each of the following is consistent with the socioeconomic gradient in health EXCEPT:

A) a state university makes a push to accept more students from its immediate vicinity and this leads to improved health measures in the neighborhood.
B) teachers are found to have higher life expectancy than a collection of blue collar workers, despite similar median incomes and income distributions.
C) an African American male living in a wealthy community is more likely to have better health outcomes despite a low income.
D) a wealthy business owner in a poor neighborhood is shielded against detrimental effects despite low health care outcomes in her community.

4. One employee quits a job to take a similar position at another firm. Her subordinate is promoted to replace her in the position. Which of the following has occurred?

A) An employee exercising vertical mobility to replace another employee who has exercised vertical mobility
B) An employee exercising horizontal mobility to replace another employee who has exercised horizontal mobility
C) An employee exercising vertical mobility to replace another employee who has exercised horizontal mobility
D) An employee exercising horizontal mobility to replace another employee who has exercised vertical mobility

5. Recent demographic information shows that for the first time in many generations, American children are not expected to earn more real (inflation-adjusted) income than their parents, and there seems to be a decrease in meritocracy. This is evidence that:

A) intergenerational mobility is stagnant, and stratification may be on the rise.
B) generational stagnation is leading to social reproduction.
C) social reproduction is leading to stagnant intergenerational mobility.
D) intergenerational mobility is stagnant, and stratification is relatively stable.

Use the following table to answer questions 6–8.

	Ethnicity: White	Ethnicity: Black	Ethnicity: Latino	Income: <$20,000	Income: $20,000-40,000	Income: $40,000+
2016	8.6	11.7	16.9	18.6	15.9	8.3

Figure 1 Uninsured rates among various demographics of nonelderly adults.

6. The trends in ethnicity and uninsured rates are most indicative of:

A) latent functions negatively affecting the dominant culture.
B) intersectionalism exacerbating the effects of the socioeconomic gradient.
C) demographic variables impacting a social institution.
D) manifest functions of health insurance interacting with subcultures.

7. The trend in income and uninsured rates demonstrated in Figure 1 is most indicative of:

A) issues of accessibility consistent with the socioeconomic gradient in health.
B) issues of availability consistent with the socioeconomic gradient in health.
C) issues of accessibility at odds with the socioeconomic gradient in health.
D) issues of availability at odds with the socioeconomic gradient in health.

8. Suppose that the data in Figure 1 were assessed in light of comparable data from 2015 and 2014, and the comparison strongly suggested that coverage rates are converging among ethnic groups. This would suggest increasing:

A) assimilation.
B) multiculturalism.
C) ethnocentrism.
D) cultural relativity.

CHAPTER 5 PRACTICE PASSAGE

Historical data on life expectancies for the wealthy show that, since the Sanitary Act in the nineteenth century, mortality rates have decreased. The human life span has continued to increase over time, as countries have modernized. Among all of the age groups, decreases in infant mortality rates are the most dramatic because infant exposure to environmental pathogens is a huge factor affecting their mortality. In recent years, the elderly age group has begun to demonstrate an increase in life expectancy compared to the infant age group, which is beginning to demonstrate little or no change over time. Figure 1 displays the rise of modern life expectancy for the different age groups in the United States from 1900 to 2000.

Life Expectancy in the United States, 1900 to 2000							
Gender	**Age**	**1900**	**1920**	**1940**	**1960**	**1980**	**2000**
Male	0	43.9	62.4	65.3	75.9	77.3	77.5
	15	32.4	34.0	40.5	55.8	68.9	71.3
	35	28.3	27.3	23.5	28.4	38.4	41.4
	55	19.9	23.5	28.2	33.9	34.2	35.9
	75	5.2	5.7	3.3	3.8	4.5	4.9
Female	0	40.3	42.9	50.2	69.8	75.8	75.9
	15	34.5	39.1	40.3	58.3	60.3	69.3
	35	30.9	27.4	35.9	46.7	43.4	49.7
	55	23.4	24.2	29.6	32.3	36.8	34.3
	75	5.8	3.2	4.3	5.9	6.1	6.4

Figure 1 Life expectancy in years for various age groups between 1900–2000

Generally, females have higher life expectancy rates than males in modern societies. There is biological evidence that shows that women are more impervious to pathogens compared to men. For example, some theorize that the X-chromosome and hormonal mechanisms influence the efficiency of the immune system. There is also psychosocial evidence that supports this finding. Women in pre-modern societies have a higher mortality rate due to sexist practices, which can lead to neglect or even infanticide of female infants. Figure 2 displays the gender mortality ratio of men and women in the United States from 1900 to 2000. Gender mortality ratio is the male-to-female proportion in death rates.

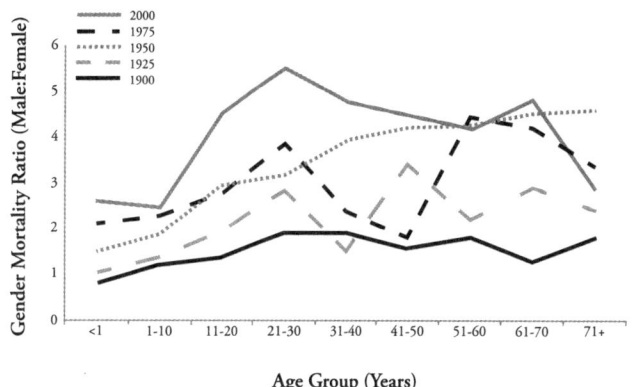

Figure 2 Gender mortality ratio in the united states between 1900–2000

In pre-modern societies, there are high mortality rates due to poverty and governmental persecution. Most people in pre-modern societies believe that daily oppression is beyond their control, and that they have no choice but to accept their fate. On the other hand, people in modern societies believe that they can proactively strive for change when facing a difficult situation. Alex Inkeles was a sociologist who administered interviews to over 6,000 men from Argentina, Chile, India, Israel, Nigeria, and Pakistan to prove that modernization changes the personality structure of people. Inkeles discovered that during the course of modernization, individuals became more involved with the steps necessary to improve their society.

Source: Adapted from Leonard A. Sagan, *The Health of Nations: True Causes of Sickness and Well-Being*. ©1987 by Basic Books, Inc.

1. According to Figure 1, what is true about life expectancy in the United States?

A) In recent years, the life expectancy for infants has plateaued for both sexes.
B) Age 35 is the ideal age to accurately determine the expectancy of life for both sexes.
C) In 1980, males at age 55 had a higher life expectancy compared females at age 55.
D) At the age of 75, life expectancy consistently increased over time for both sexes.

2. Suppose that in a pre-modernist society, a lower-class woman tries to join a conversation among a group of upper-class men. As a result, the men ridicule the woman. This scenario most accurately portrays:

A) prejudice against the in-group.
B) prejudice against the out-group.
C) discrimination against the in-group.
D) discrimination against the out-group.

3. Suppose that a pre-modernist moves up from the lower class to the upper class because the government recognized his skills as a craftsman. Which of the following is true about this pattern of social mobility?

   I.   The pre-modernist experienced intergenerational mobility.
   II. The pre-modernist experienced intragenerational mobility.
   III. This pre-modern society practiced meritocracy.

A) I only
B) II only
C) I and III only
D) II and III only

4. According to Figure 2, at what age do the mortality rates of males widely differ from the mortality rates of females in 1925?

A) 21–30
B) 31–40
C) 41–50
D) 51–60

5. Poor people in pre-modern societies are forced to live in a place where they lack food, water, and shelter needed for them to survive. Which of the following most closely defines the struggles that lower class pre-modernists face?

A) Absolute poverty
B) Social change
C) Relative poverty
D) Global inequality

6. Which ideology best describes Alex Inkeles's findings?

A) Traditional theory, in which society is observed at its current state in order to learn and understand its systems
B) Critical theory, in which people continually evaluate and change society in order to attain progress
C) Functionalism, in which the interdependence of institutions strives to maintain stability in a society
D) Conflict theory, in which the inequality among classes ultimately forces change on a society

SOLUTIONS TO CHAPTER 5 FREESTANDING PRACTICE QUESTIONS

1. **C** Cultural diffusion describes the spread of cultural beliefs, values, and norms from one culture to another. In this scenario, culture is imported from another country (France) to the United States. The Mardi Gras festival is an example of a cultural ritual passed on to New Orleans through cultural diffusion (choice C is correct). Cultural lag refers to the time it takes for society to catch up to technological innovations and come up with solutions for the issues created. The question stem does not introduce any new technology or how the society deals with it (choice A is wrong). Cultural transmission occurs when cultural values are passed along within the same culture. In this case, the culture is brought in from another culture (choice B is wrong). Culture shock refers to the disorientation experienced by an individual, not a society, when that individual comes into contact with a new culture significantly different from their own (choice D is wrong).

2. **B** This question can be done more quickly by noticing the two different parts of the answer choices. Low fertility and stable life expectancy would lead to population decline, not growth (choices A and C are wrong). Replacement level fertility is 2.1 births per female. This is the number of births per female necessary to maintain a stable population. The number given for Japan in the question stem, 1.5, is significantly less than replacement level, and therefore likely to lead to population decline (choice B is correct). A stable mortality rate would lead to stable population size in the absence of other factors, so this is not enough by itself to cause the population to decline (choice D is wrong).

3. **D** The socioeconomic gradient in health implies that incremental increases in socioeconomic status lead to a corresponding increase in health and health outcomes. Context and situation are also important, so that an individual's surroundings also matter. On except/not/least questions, use Process of Elimination and eliminate answer choices that make true statements. Education is an important aspect of socioeconomic status, so more students accepted to a university in a neighborhood would lead to improved health measures according to the socioeconomic gradient (choice A is true and can be eliminated). Socioeconomic status encompasses more than just income. Prestige associated with an occupation is also an important part. Teaching has a higher status associated with it than typical blue collar work, so the socioeconomic gradient would predict that teachers would have better health outcomes than blue collar workers despite similar salaries (choice B is true and can be eliminated). Context is also a critical part of the socioeconomic gradient, so the individual living in a wealthy community is expected to see a benefit despite low income (choice C is true and can be eliminated). Because of contextual influences, a wealthy business owner is likely to see negative consequences from a poor environment (choice D is false and is the correct answer choice).

4. **C** This is a two-by-two type question, which divides the answer choices in half along two dimensions. For the first part of the answer choice, the employee who is promoted is exercising vertical mobility, because she is moving up to a higher position within the firm and likely a higher salary (choices B and D are wrong). The employee who left, on the other hand, is leaving for a similar position, so she is exercising horizontal mobility, shifting to a new position, but not making a significant change in salary or status (choice C is correct, and choice A is wrong).

5. **A** Intergenerational mobility is the ability of one generation to improve socioeconomic status relative to earlier generations. In the question stem, later generations are described as not making improvements relative to prior generations. Also, the question stem states that meritocracy is decreasing, which is likely to lead to an increase in stratification, as individuals are reduced in their ability to work their way into a higher social class (choice A is correct). Generational stagnation is not a term in demographics and socioeconomic status (choice B is wrong). Social reproduction is the passing on from generation to generation of the same social position. This is suggested by the decrease in meritocracy mentioned in the question stem. However, there is no way to gauge, from the question stem, that either of these two variables causes the other (choice C is wrong). Stratification seems to be on the rise based on the fact that meritocracy is decreasing (choice D is wrong).

6. **C** Ethnicity is an example of a demographic variable, and healthcare is a social institution. The differences in insurance rates among ethnic groups suggest that the demographic variable is influencing the social institution (choice C is correct). The dominant culture in this case would be represented by individuals in the white ethnicity category, and they are showing positive, not negative, effects (choice A is wrong). Intersectionalism refers to multiple levels of oppression and how they interact. Here, only one type of oppression, racial or ethnic, is shown (choice B is wrong). Manifest functions of a social instruction are the professed or stated functions. For healthcare, the primary manifest function is to provide medical treatment for individuals who are sick. Possible racial disparities would be a type of latent function (choice D is wrong).

7. **A** This is a two-by-two question, and in this case it is easier to determine the second half of the answer choices. In the figure, as income increases, so does health coverage, so this is consistent with the socioeconomic gradient in health, not at odds (choices C and D are wrong). Insurance rates are related to accessibility, since they represent an individual's ability to receive healthcare treatment given that services are actually available (choice A is correct). Availability, on the other hand, refers to the actual presence of healthcare resources. No information related to availability is presented in the figure (choice B is wrong).

8. **B** Convergent coverage rates among ethnicities suggest that society is becoming more equitable in the distribution of healthcare access. This is closest to multiculturalism, the phenomenon of different cultures living in the same society cohesively (choice B is correct). Assimilation refers to an individual or group taking on the attributes of a dominant culture. In this scenario it is not clear that any group is assimilating, or changing, in response to the dominant culture (choice A is wrong). Ethnocentrism is the belief in the superiority of one ethnicity or cultural perspective. There is no value judgement indicated in the figure of the relative merits of any ethnicity (choice C is wrong). Cultural relativity is understanding an individual's culture through the perspective of his or her own experiences or background. The data in the figure do not relate to cultural understanding or perspective-taking (choice D is wrong).

SOLUTIONS TO CHAPTER 5 PRACTICE PASSAGE

1. **A** According to Figure 1, for both males and females at the age of 0, life expectancy 1980–2000 has not increased significantly; therefore, this figure illustrates that the life expectancy of infants has plateaued (choice A is correct). There is not enough information given in the passage or the figure to determine the age that is most ideal for accurately calculating life expectancy (choice B is wrong). In 1980, males at the age of 55 had a lower life expectancy rate (34.2) than females (36.8; choice C is wrong). Between the years 1900–2000, life expectancy rates at age 75 decreased for females in 1920 and for males in 1940 (choice D is wrong).

2. **D** Discrimination is the mistreatment of others based on their perceived differences in characteristics and social position. The men view the woman as an out-group member because they do not identify themselves as being in the same group as her based on their status and gender (choice D is correct, and choice C is wrong). Prejudice leads to discrimination. It is the positive or negative attitude that people have about another group of people based on their perceptions of the group. The scenario does not closely relate to the concept of prejudice because the men have already committed the action of discrimination against the woman by mocking her (choices A and B are wrong).

3. **D** Item I is false: intergenerational mobility is the mobility across generations. This usually occurs when the child has a higher or lower social class than their parents (choices A and C can be eliminated). Note that both remaining answer choices include Item II, so it must be true: unlike intergenerational mobility, intragenerational mobility is the mobility within the generation for an individual. The pre-modernist moved up in social class within his lifetime. Item III is true: meritocracy is the system in which power and prestige are given to those who have the skills to be appointed to the upper class. The pre-modernist gained mobility through his craftsmanship skills (choice B can be eliminated, and choice D is correct).

4. **C** By following the gender mortality ratio in 1925, ages 41–50 have a mortality ratio of roughly 3.4, meaning that for every 1 female who dies, 3.4 males die within this age range; therefore, this is the highest mortality ratio between men and women (choice C is correct). Although ages 21–30 have the highest ratio in 2000, the same trend does not apply for the year 1925 (choice A is wrong). Ages 31–40 show gender mortality ratio at its lowest in 1925 (choice B is wrong). Although ages 51–60 have a high gender mortality ratio in 1975, it is not the same case for 1925 (choice D is wrong).

5. **A** Absolute poverty is defined as the inability to obtain basic resources necessary for daily living; poor pre-modernists have no choice but to live in a society in which they struggle to acquire those necessities (choice A is correct). Social change is the adjustment of social systems that can occur over a time; pre-modernists in poverty were less likely to participate in creating social changes because of their fatalistic point of view (choice B is wrong). Relative poverty involves a reference point of the group of people in comparison to another group of people based on socioeconomic status and living conditions; the question stem is closely related to absolute poverty because it focuses more on the physical resources needed for survival (choice C is wrong). Global inequality can be eliminated as an answer because the question does not go into the inequalities from a global perspective (choice D is wrong).

6. **B**   According to the last paragraph, "Inkeles discovered that during the course of modernization, individuals became more involved with the steps necessary to improve their society." Critical theory as defined in the answer choices is most applicable to the scenario described in the passage (choice B is correct). Traditional theory is focused on learning and understanding a given society rather than proactively making change, as Inkeles described in his study (choice A is wrong). Functionalism strives for stability and prompts people to stay with the status quo; furthermore, Inkeles does not make any conclusions about "institutions" (choice C is wrong). Conflict theory involves the power struggle among classes; there is no information in the passage that supports the idea that class struggle was one of Inkeles's discoveries (choice D is wrong).

REBEL WITHOUT A CAUSE EFFECT: BIRTH ORDER AND SOCIAL ATTITUDES

Jeremy Freese; Brian Powell; Lala Carr Steelman
American Sociological Review; Apr 1999; 64, 2; Research Library Core pg. 207

Sociologists of the family have long tried to direct more attention to how individuals are affected by basic components of family structure and early childhood environment. In recent years, these efforts have sparked considerable debate about the effects of family size (Downey 1995; Downey et al. 1999; Guo and VanWey 1999; Phillips 1999) and of being raised in single- versus two-parent homes (Cherlin, Chase-Lansdale, and McRae 1998; Furstenberg 1990; McLanahan and Sandefur 1994). Historically, however, the family structure variable that has perhaps received the most lively scrutiny both within and outside the realm of sociology has been birth order. Indeed, birth order has inspired some of the most striking dialogues among sociologists and between sociologists and other social scientists (Bayer 1967; Hauser and Sewell 1985; Retherford and Sewell 1991; Schachter 1963; Steelman and Mercy 1980; Zajonc and Markus 1975; Zajonc et al. 1991). Sociologists have examined the effects of birth order on achievement, educational performance, and personality, and have critiqued some of the more ambitious claims that have been made about birth order. Until recently, scholars have shown little empirical interest in the relationship between birth order and social attitudes, despite the persistent (and often taken-for-granted) notion that adults who are firstborn children are more conservative than adults who are not. Instead, to comprehend the determinants of social attitudes, sociologists have typically emphasized the role of social structural position, cultural norms, and group identity, and they have relied on a relatively limited set of explanatory variables, most prominently gender, race, age, and social class.

We examine the relationship between birth order and social attitudes using data from a contemporary survey of adults in the United States. We test whether firstborns are more conservative than laterborns.

DATA AND MEASURES

Data

We use data from the 1994 General Social Survey (GSS), conducted by the National Opinion Research Center (Davis and Smith 1994). The GSS is a full probability sample of noninstitutionalized, English-speaking adults in the United States. In 1994, as part of a special module on family mobility, GSS respondents were asked to provide background information on each of their siblings, including their year of birth. To our knowledge, no other data set that contains information on a respondent's birth order combines the GSS's large, nationally representative sample, high-quality data-collection techniques, and variety of questions on social and political attitudes.

A difficulty in testing birth-order theories is that many individuals' early family lives do not lend themselves to easy classification as firstborns or laterborns. We use a subsample of GSS respondents that excludes only children, respondents with any step- or half-siblings, and respondents who report having a sibling born the same year as they were born. Only children differ from firstborns in that they do not compete with younger siblings for parental attention. Step- and half-siblings imply varying relations in a family between children and caregivers that may complicate the allocation of parental resources and may unfairly undermine the expectations of birth-order theories. We assume that most pairs of siblings born in the same year are twins, and twins, unfortunately, have received little consideration in the birth-order literature. In auxiliary analyses, we retain only children and respondents with step- or half-siblings; retaining these individuals in our sample has little effect on the overall patterns we observe (these results are available from the authors on request).

After also excluding respondents who failed to report the birth year of any of their siblings, the sample used in our main analyses contains 1,945 of the original 2,992 respondents. The number of cases used in our analyses is sometimes considerably fewer than 1,945 because the 1994 GSS used a split-ballot design, and most of the questions eliciting social attitudes were administered only to a randomly selected subset (one-third to two-thirds) of all respondents. Preliminary analyses using items administered to the whole sample suggest no systematic differences among respondents receiving different ballots.

Measures of Birth Order

We measure birth order as a dichotomous variable indicating whether the respondent is the firstborn child in his or her family, as indicated by the year-of-birth information provided by respondents. This tactic is the most common way of measuring birth order in previous research. In addition, we also tested other operationalizations of birth order: the number of older siblings (birth rank); the number of older siblings divided by the total number of siblings (relative birth rank); the number of older brothers; the number of older children of the same sex; and a trichotomous variable differentiating firstborns, middleborns, and lastborns. None of these alternative measures yielded patterns substantively different from those presented here.

Measures of Social Attitudes

The GSS contains a large number of questions on social attitudes. We sought to test a respondent's social attitudes in six domains: (1) political identification; (2) opposition to liberal social movements; views on (3) race and (4) gender; (5) support for existing authority; and (6) "tough-mindedness." Initially, we chose 24 items and scales that represented these broad headings.

Other Independent Variables

As noted above, our research seeks not only to examine the effect of birth order on social attitudes, but also to compare the influence of birth order on social attitudes with that of other variables that have received more sustained attention from sociologists. Consequently, after examining the bivariate relationships between birth order and our measures of social attitudes, we look at birth order in the context of multiple regression models that also include sex, age, race (coded as dummy variables), parents' education, and sibship size. Because each of these variables has been posited to affect social attitudes directly and because each may be correlated with birth order, including these variables as controls also permits better estimates of actual birth-order effects.

In addition, subsequent models employ more stringent controls. Because birth-order theories typically place emphasis on childhood environment, our next model adds controls for parents' occupational prestige (using recent recodings by Hauser and Warren [1997]), parents' marital status, the loss of a parent to death before age 16, childhood religion, and the region of the country in which the respondent was raised. To account for the possibility that observed birth-order effects may be caused by birth-order differences in achievement, our final model adds controls for the respondent's education and occupational prestige.

RESULTS

Table 1 presents estimates of the effect of birth order on the different measures of social attitudes. All measures are coded so that positive coefficients are consistent with the hypothesis that firstborns are more conservative, supportive of authority, and "toughminded" than laterborns.

If we look first at the results of the bivariate regression (Model 1), the data do not appear to support the hypothesis. The observed effect of birth order is indistinguishable from chance for 22 out of the 24 measures of social attitudes, and only one of the two significant effects is in the predicted direction: firstborns were more likely than laterborns to have supported Bush in 1992. Meanwhile, contradicting Sulloway's findings about the "tough-mindedness" of laterborns, firstborn respondents are significantly more likely than laterborns to believe that the nation's courts are too harsh with criminals.

CONCLUSION

We find no evidence that birth order affects social attitudes. Instead, our data strongly contradict the assertion that birth order is a better predictor of social attitudes than are gender, class, or race.

Table 1. Coefficients from the OLS and Logistic Regression of Selected Measures of Social Attitudes on Birth Order: U.S. Adults with Full Siblings, GSS, 1994

Social Attitude Measure	Model 1		Model 2		Model 3		Model 4		Model 4 Results in Predicted Direction?
	Coef.	S.E.	Coef.	S.E.	Coef.	S.E.	Coef.	S.E.	
Political Identification									
Identifies self as:									
Conservative	–0.57	(.069)	–.006	(.072)	–.021	(.071)	–.034	(.071)	No
Republican	.092	(.100)	.050	(.100)	.024	(.099)	.003	(.098)	Yes
Bush supporter in 1992 [c]	.220*	(.104)	.193	(.111)	.155	(.113)	.141	(.114)	Yes
Opposition to Liberal Movements									
Opposes:									
Abortion rights	.154	(.155)	.307	(.159)	.289	(.158)	.298	(.157)	Yes
Assisted suicide laws [c]	.039	(.139)	.229	(.150)	.194	(.154)	.206	(.154)	Yes
Legalization of marijuana [c]	–.167	(.142)	–.029	(.151)	–.078	(.155)	–.089	(.155)	No
Animal rights [b]	–.076	(.134)	–.005	(.141)	–.052	(.143)	–.032	(.144)	No
Environmental movement	.059	(.056)	.102	(.058)	.101	(.059)	.103	(.059)	Yes
Free speech	–.038	(.182)	.078	(.179)	.043	(.176)	.014	(.171)	Yes
Social welfare programs	.080	(.043)	.034	(.043)	.023	(.043)	.013	(.043)	Yes
Resistance to Racial Reforms									
Thinks government is too generous to Black Americans [a]	.083	(.059)	.093	(.061)	.076	(.060)	.065	(.060)	Yes
Excluding Black Americans is OK [a]	–.003	(.062)	.048	(.060)	.024	(.060)	.014	(.058)	Yes
Racial inequality due to Black American's lack of ability/will power [a]	–.142	(.076)	–.101	(.078)	–.127	(.076)	–.127	(.075)	No
Against benefits for immigrants [a, b]	–.008	(.149)	–.026	(.155)	–.063	(.157)	–.090	(.158)	No
Supports English-only laws [a]	–.079	(.074)	–.121	(.076)	–.129	(.077)	–.145	(.077)	No
Belief in Traditional General Roles									
Against mothers working	.005	(.081)	–.020	(.079)	–.019	(.079)	–.021	(.079)	No
Supports traditional division of labor between spouses	.008	(.077)	.027	(.071)	.016	(.071)	.003	(.069)	Yes
Against women in politics [b]	–.019	(.152)	.153	(.162)	.150	(.165)	.133	(.166)	Yes
Support for Existing Authority									
Children should obey [b]	–.095	(.110)	.051	(.115)	.001	(.117)	.010	(.117)	Yes
Trusts social institutions	–.005	(.100)	.027	(.104)	.032	(.105)	.024	(.105)	Yes
Patriotism [b]	–.156	(.136)	–.292*	(.145)	–.309*	(.147)	–.332*	(.148)	No
"Tough-Mindedness"									
Tough on crime [c]	–.350*	(.155)	–.401*	(.164)	–.412*	(.165)	–.424*	(.166)	No
Supports:									
Capital punishment [c]	–.172	(.124)	–.269*	(.134)	–.284*	(.135)	–.305*	(.136)	No
Corporal punishment [b]	–.001	(.112)	.114	(.117)	.092	(.119)	.086	(.119)	Yes

Notes: Numbers in parentheses are standard errors. Model 1 is the bivariate regression. Model 2 controls for sibship size, age, sex, race, and parents' education. Model 3 adds controls for parents' marital status and occupational prestige, parental loss, respondents' religion, and region where respondent was raised. Model 4 adds controls for current income and education. Positive coefficients are consistent with the hypothesis that firstborns are more conservative, supportive of authority, and "tough-minded" than laterborns. Number of cases range from 595 to 1,894.

[a] Racial equality items include only white respondents

[b] Ordered logistic regression used for ordinal dependent variables.

[c] Binary logistic regression used for dichotomous dependent variables.

* $p < .05$ ** $p < .01$ *** $p < .001$ (two-tailed tests)

JOURNAL ARTICLE EXERCISE 1

The science sections on the MCAT include a significant number of passages with experiments. Questions for these passages often ask you to analyze data, read charts and graphs, and come to some reasonable conclusion based on the information they give you. If you don't know how to extract information efficiently and analyze data effectively, you will be at a distinct disadvantage.

There are three "Journal Article Exercises" in this book. In this first exercise, we'll show you the type of information you should be able to extract from the article and the sorts of things to pay attention to in the data. In subsequent exercise, you'll do more of that on your own, and in the final exercise we'll show you how that article might get turned into an MCAT-style passage.

When analyzing an experiment, you should be able to:

- identify the control group(s)
- extract information from graphs and data tables
- determine how the experimental group(s) change relative to the control
- determine if the results are statistically significant
- come to a reasonable conclusion about WHY the results were observed
- consider potential weaknesses in the study
- determine how to increase the power of the study
- decide what the next most logical experiment or study should be

The goal of these exercises is NOT to learn content from the articles, just to get a little more comfortable reading and extracting information from them.

For the (abridged) article on pages 111–113, try to summarize the purpose of the experiment and the methods in 4–5 sentences. Consider the following mnemonic: Oh ouR Car Won't Start (ORCWS).

- **O = Organism and Organization**: is the research being conducted on humans or on animals or on bacteria in a petri dish, or something else? What is being done to these organisms? Are there any unique qualities to these organisms? Are there multiple groups? Is the study conducted over a long period of time with multiple data points, or is it a short-term study? Does it have a large or small n?

- **R = Results**: where and how are the results presented? Is it a graph? A data table? Figures and images? What is/are the independent variable(s)? What is/are the dependent variable(s)? What are the results? Do the results show correlation or cause and effect, or both? Describe.

- **C = Control and Comparison**: is there a control group? How does it differ from the experimental group? Is it given a placebo or nothing at all? Is it held under different conditions? If there are multiple experimental groups, how do they differ from one another? Is it a blinded study? If so, double-blind or single-blind?

- **W = Weirdness**: does anything or do any of the results stand out as unexpected?

- **S = Statistics**: was any sort of statistical analysis done? How is it presented? Are there error bars on a graph? Standard errors around a mean? Are there p-values? Is there an asterisk indicating statistical significance? Is there any data that is not statistically significant?

Try interpreting the data on your own before reading the results/discussion section. When you do read the discussion, consider:

- What are the conclusions of the study?
- How are the conclusions supported by the data?
- What potential weaknesses or flaws do you see in the experimental design? Are these addressed in the discussion section?
- How might this study be potentially biased?
- How might this study be improved?
- What would be the next most logical experiment?

Let's answer the above questions for the article on pages 111–113.

SOLUTIONS TO JOURNAL ARTICLE EXERCISE 1

1. **O = Organism and Organization:**
   - Is the research being conducted on humans or on animals or on bacteria in a petri dish, or something else? *Humans*
   - What is being done to these organisms? *Participants responded to a survey/questionnaire (the General Social Survey)*
   - Are there any unique qualities to these organisms? *noninstitutionalized, English-speaking adults in the United States*
   - Are there multiple groups? *No*
   - Is the study conducted over a long period of time with multiple data points, or is it a short-term study? *Short-term*
   - Does it have a large or small *n*? *Large: 1,945 respondents in the sample*

2. **R = Results:**
   - Where and how are the results presented? Is it a graph? A data table? Figures and images? *Data table*
   - What is/are the independent variable(s)? *Birth order*
   - What is/are the dependent variable(s)? *(1) political identification; (2) opposition to liberal social movements; views on (3) race and (4) gender; (5) support for existing authority; and (6) "tough-mindedness"*
   - What are the results of the study? *Authors find no evidence that birth order affects social attitudes.*
   - Do the results show correlation or cause and effect, or both? Describe. *Correlation*

3. **C = Control and Comparison:**
   - Is there a control group? *No*
   - How does it differ from the experimental group? Is it give a placebo or nothing at all? Is it held under different conditions? *N/A*
   - If there are multiple experimental groups, how do they differ from one another? *N/A*
   - Is it a blinded study? If so, double-blind or single-blind? *Not a blinded study*

4. **W = Weirdness:**
   - Does anything or do any of the results stand out as unexpected? *Results were contrary to the hypothesis.*

5. **S = Statistics:**
   - Was any sort of statistical analysis done? *Yes*
   - How is it presented? Are there error bars on a graph? Standard errors around a mean? Are there *p*-values? Is there an asterisk indicating statistical significance? *Regression coefficients with standard error reported; yes, an asterisk is used to indicate statistical significance*
   - Is there any data that is not statistically significant? *Yes, nearly all of the data*

6. **Interpreting the data:**
   - What are the conclusions of the study? *Authors find no evidence that birth order affects social attitudes.*
   - How are the conclusions supported by the data? *Most of the data is not statistically significant.*
   - What potential weaknesses or flaws do you see in the experimental design? Are these addressed in the discussion section? *Only data from 1994 is used. Perhaps that year is an anomaly.*
   - How might this study be potentially biased? *Sample bias: it was only conducted on English- speaking Americans; perhaps birth-order effects would be found in other cultures/ languages?*
   - How might this study be improved? *More diversity in subjects' culture/country/native language*
   - What would be the next most logical experiment? *Repeat the exercise using different participants with different cultures, different languages, and a longer time span.*

7. **Final Summary of Experiment and Results:**
   - *In this journal article, the responses of 1,945 English-speaking respondents to the General Social Survey in the United States were studied. The researchers were attempting to confirm the hypothesis that firstborn children are more conservative than later-born children. The authors' statistical analysis found no support for their hypothesis.*

Chapter 6
Social Psychology

Development of identity can be viewed from a psychological or sociological perspective. In order to fully understand identity, the self, and the collective, it is important to look at these concepts from multiple perspectives. Understanding the individual as part of a group is central to understanding human nature, as we are inherently social creatures who cannot exist in a vacuum.

6.1 SELF-CONCEPT AND IDENTITY FORMATION

Self-concept or **self-identity** is broadly defined as the sum of an individual's knowledge and understanding of his- or herself. Differing from **self-consciousness**, which is awareness of one's self, self-concept includes physical, psychological, and social attributes, which can be influenced by the individual's attitudes, habits, beliefs, and ideas. For example, if you asked yourself the question "Who am I?" your responses would form the basis of your self-concept. Self-concept is how an individual defines him- or herself based on beliefs that person has about him- or herself, known as **self-schemas**. For example, an individual might hold the following self-concepts: female, African American, student, smart, funny, future doctor.

Different Types of Identities

These qualities can be further divided into those that form personal identity and those that form social identity. **Personal identity** consists of one's own sense of personal attributes (in the example above, smart and funny constitute attributes of personal identity). **Social identity** consists of social definitions of who one is; these can include race, religion, gender, occupation, and such (in the example above, female, African American, student, and future doctor constitute attributes of social identity). Thus, the "self" is a personal and social construction of beliefs. Individuals are very sensitive to others' perceptions of their self-identities. The theory of **self-verification** asserts that individuals want to be understood in terms of their deeply held core beliefs.

As a quick way to remember different aspects of one's identity, consider the ADRESSING framework: each letter stands for a different characteristic. These characteristics are age, disability status, religion, ethnicity/race, sexual orientation, socioeconomic status, indigenous background, national origin, and gender. Note that gender is a socially constructed concept while sex is biologically determined. Each of these categories contains a dominant group as well as groups that are less dominant in society. For example, here is the breakdown (generally) in American society:

Table 1 ADRESSING Framework

Cultural Characteristics	Power	Less Power
Age	Adults	Children, adolescents, elders
Disability status	Temporarily able-bodied	Persons with disabilities
Religion	Christians	Jews, Muslims, other non-Christians
Ethnicity/race	Euro-American	People of color
Sexual orientation	Heterosexuals	LGBTQ+
Socioeconomic class	Owning and middle classes (those with access to higher education)	Poor and working classes
Indigenous background	Non-native	Native
National origin	U.S. born	Immigrants and refugees
Gender	Male	Female, transgender, intersex

Old information that is consistent with one's self-concept is easy to remember, and new information coming in that is consistent with one's self-schemas is easily incorporated. This tendency to better remember information relevant to ourselves is known as the **self-reference effect**. Inconsistent information is more difficult. For example, if someone considers herself to be intelligent but receives an extremely low score on an exam, this would oppose her self-concept. Therefore, this person may choose to externalize the new information from her self-concept by attributing it to a lack of sleep or an unfair test. It is often easier to externalize information that opposes a self-concept by attributing it to an outside factor than it is to internalize the information and adjust one's self-concept.

When people have positive self-concepts (I am intelligent), they tend to act positively and have more optimistic perceptions of the world. When people have negative self-concepts (I am stupid), they tend to feel that they have somehow fallen short, and they are usually dissatisfied and unhappy.

Carl Rogers, founder of the **humanistic psychology** perspective, pioneered a unique approach to understanding personality and human relationships (see Chapter 7 for more on Carl Rogers). According to Rogers, personality is composed of the ideal self and the real self. The **ideal self** is constructed out of your life experiences, societal expectations, and the traits you admire about role models. The ideal self is the person *you ought to be*, while the real self is the person *you actually are*. When the ideal self and the real self are similar, the result is a positive self-concept. However, Rogers suggests that the ideal self is usually an impossible standard to meet, and that when the real self falls short of the ideal self, the result is **incongruity**.

The Role of Self-Esteem, Self-Efficacy, and Locus of Control in Self-Concept and Self-Identity

In addition to how the "self" is defined, there are three powerful influences on an individual's development of self-concept. These are self-efficacy, locus of control, and self-esteem.

1) **Self-efficacy** is a belief in one's own competence and effectiveness. It's how capable we believe we are of doing things. It turns out that this is no small factor; studies have shown that simply believing in our own abilities actually improves performance. Self-efficacy can vary from task to task; an individual may have high self-efficacy for a math task and low self-efficacy for juggling.

2) **Locus of control** can be internal or external. Those with an **internal locus of control** believe they are able to influence outcomes through their own efforts and actions. Those with an **external locus of control** perceive outcomes as controlled by outside forces. Someone with an internal locus may attribute a good grade to his or her own intelligence and hard work. The same score may lead someone with an external locus to assume that the test was especially easy or that he or she got lucky. In an extreme situation, in which people are exposed to situations in which they have no control, they may learn not to act because they believe it will not affect the outcome anyway. Even once this situation passes and they find themselves once again in arenas in which they can exert some control, this lack of action may persist. This phenomenon is known as **learned helplessness**. It has been shown that believing more in an internal locus of control can be empowering and lead to proactivity. An external locus of control and learned helplessness are characteristics of many depressed and oppressed people, and they often result in passivity.

3) **Self-esteem** is one's overall evaluation of one's self-worth. This may be based on different factors for different individuals, depending on which parts of a person's identity he or she has determined to be the most important. For some, self-esteem may rest on intelligence. How would you value yourself if you had low versus high intelligence? For others, it may rest on athletic ability, beauty, or moral character. Self-esteem is related to self-efficacy; self-efficacy can improve self-esteem if one has it for an activity that one values. However, if the activity is not one that is valued, it may not help self-esteem. For example, a person may have high self-efficacy as a soldier, but still struggle with low self-esteem if this is not her desired occupation. Low self-esteem increases the risk of anxiety, depression, drug use, and suicide. However, inflated self-esteem is also present in gang members, terrorists, and bullies, and may be used to conceal deep-seated insecurities. Unrealistic self-esteem to either extreme can be painful.

Stages of Identity Development

Identity formation or individuation is the development of a distinct individual personality. Identity changes throughout different life stages, but includes the characteristics an individual considers his or her own, which distinguish the individual from others. Erik Erikson's theory of psychosocial development (see Chapter 7) includes a series of crises and conflicts experienced throughout a person's lifetime that help to define and shape identity. According to Erikson, the particular stage relevant to identity formation takes place during adolescence (roughly ages 12–20): the "Identity versus Role Confusion" stage. In this stage, adolescents try to figure out who they are and form basic identities that they will build on throughout the rest of their lives. Other psychological theories concur with Erikson's that adolescence is an important time for establishing identity. Some theories posit that in order to establish identity, an individual has to explore various possibilities and then make commitments to an occupation, religion, sexual orientation, and political viewpoint. Gender, moral, psychosexual, and social development are all important elements of identity development. For a review of psychosexual development, see the discussion of Freud in Chapter 7. Interactions with individuals, as well as socialization into broader cultural groups, also affect the development of identity.

Influence of Social Factors on Identity Formation

Influence of Individuals

Charles Cooley, an American sociologist, posited the idea of the **looking-glass self**, which is the idea that a person's sense of self develops from interpersonal interactions with others in society and the perceptions of others. According to this idea, people shape their self-concepts based on their understanding of how others perceive them. The looking-glass self begins at an early age and continues throughout life; we never stop modifying it unless all social interactions cease. **George Herbert Mead**, another American sociologist, developed the idea of **social behaviorism**: the mind and self emerge through the process of communicating with others. The idea that the mind and self emerge through the social process of communication or use of symbols was the beginning of the **symbolic interactionism** school of sociology. Mead believed that there is a specific path to development of the self. During the preparatory stage, children merely imitate others, as they have no concept of how others see things. In the play stage, children take on the roles of others through playing (as when playing house and taking on the role of "mom"). During the game stage, children learn to consider multiple roles simultaneously, and can understand the responsibilities of multiple roles. Finally, the child develops an understanding of the **generalized other**, the common behavioral expectations of general society. Mead also characterized the "me" and the "I." The "me" is how the individual believes the generalized other perceives him or her. The "me" could also be defined as the social self. The "I" is the response to the "me;" in other words, the "I" is the response of the individual to the attitudes of others. The "I" is the self as subject; the "me" is the self as object.

Influence of Culture and Socialization on Identity Formation

Socialization is the process through which people learn to be proficient and functional members of society; it is a lifelong sociological process by which people learn the attitudes, values, and beliefs that are reinforced by a particular culture. For older adults, this process often involves teaching the younger generation their way of life; for young children, it predominantly involves incorporating information from their surrounding culture as they form their personalities (the patterns for how they think and feel). It is socialization that allows a culture to pass on its values from one generation to the next.

Clearly, this is a process that occurs through socializing (interacting with others in society). The necessity for social organisms to have early social contact has been demonstrated through deprivation studies. For example, Harlow's monkeys (Chapter 9) were extremely socially deprived from infancy, and were therefore unable to re-integrate successfully with other monkeys. Disturbingly, there are some examples of extreme deprivation in humans as well. Termed **feral children**, these children are individuals who were not raised with human contact or care, and a large part of our understanding about the importance of socialization is derived from what has been learned about their experiences and the terrible consequences of growing up without proper human care and contact.

Norms

Every society has spoken and unspoken rules and expectations for the behavior of its members, called **norms**; social behaviors that follow these expectations and meet the ideal social standard are described as **normative behavior**. Such behavior is strongly encouraged in everyday social interactions by **sanctions**—rewards and punishments for behaviors that are in accord with or against norms. For example, in some nations, it is considered the norm to offer your food to others when eating in a public place. To offer food to a stranger on a bus in the United States, though, would likely result in a sanction such as a disapproving or uncomfortable look.

Norms can be classified in multiple ways, and one way is by formality. **Formal norms** are generally written down; laws are examples of formal norms. They are precisely defined, publicly presented, and often accompanied by strict penalties for those who violate them. **Informal norms** are generally understood but are less precise and often carry no specific punishments. One example is not covering one's nose and mouth when sneezing in a public setting. Not to do so does not carry a fine, but it may affect how others perceive the sneezing individual.

Another way of classifying norms is based on their importance. **Mores** ("more-ays") are norms that are highly important for the benefit of society and so are often strictly enforced. For example, animal abuse and treason are actions that break mores in the United States and carry harsh penalties. **Folkways** are norms that are less important but shape everyday behavior (for example, styles of dress, ways of greeting). Although there is a strong relationship between mores and formal norms, and folkways and informal norms, this division is not absolute. Society may have a formal norm such as walking within a crosswalk when crossing the street; however, the lack of strong enforcement of this formal norm suggests that it is not that important and is more a folkway than a more.

In contrast, those behaviors that customs forbid are described as **taboo**. In the case of a taboo, the endorsement of the norm is so strong that its violation is forbidden and oftentimes punishable through formal or non-formal methods. Taboo behaviors, in general, result in disgust toward the violator. There is often a moral or religious component to the taboo, and violation of the norm poses the threat of divine penalties. For example, in accordance with religious laws, Muslims denounce the consumption of pork; thus, in Muslim countries, eating such products would be considered taboo. More widespread examples of taboo behaviors include cannibalism, incest, and murder. Furthermore, forms of prejudice and discrimination might be viewed as taboo, depending on the perspective. Modern research suggests that taboo behavior is a social construct that varies around the world; the idea of taboo changes in response to changes in social structure and there is no universal taboo.

Anomie

The normative effects of social values contribute to social cohesion and social norms are involved in maintaining order. In some cases, societies lack this cohesion and order. This is referred to as **anomie**, a concept that describes the social condition in which individuals are not provided with firm guidelines in relation to norms and values and there is minimal moral guidance or social ethics. For this reason, anomie is often thought of as a state of *normlessness*. The concept was developed through the work of the famous sociologist Émile Durkheim (section 4.1). In researching patterns of suicide in the context of nineteenth-century Europe, Durkheim used the term anomie as an explanation for the differences in suicide rates between Catholics and Protestants. His research suggested that suicide rates were lower in cultures that valued communal ties, as this provided a form of support during times of emotional distress. Anomie, then, is characteristic of societies in which social cohesion is less pronounced; for example, anomie may be more likely to occur in societies where individualism and autonomous decision-making predominate, even at the expense of the greater social order. Anomie suggests the disintegration of social bonds between individuals and their communities, which causes the fragmentation of social identities in exchange for an emphasis on personal success. Discrepancies between personal and social values are thought to contribute to moral deregulations.

Deviance

Complex social processes regulate social behaviors by positioning social norms as the correct method of action. However, there are cases where individuals do not conform to the expectations implicit in social structures. In contrast to normative behavior, **non-normative behavior** is viewed as incorrect because it challenges shared values and institutions, thus threatening social structure and cohesion. These behaviors are seen as abnormal and thus discouraged. Actions that violate the dominant social norms, whether formal or informal, are described as forms of **deviance**. In some cases, deviant behavior is seen as criminal, in which case it violates public policies; thus, studies of deviance are popular among criminologists.

The construction of deviance has important social functions. For example, the process of creating deviant labels affirms and reinforces social norms and values through the dichotomous presentation of the acceptable (normative) behavior and unacceptable (non-normative) behavior. The distinction between normal and deviant behavior is maintained through the punishment of transgressions through both formal and informal methods, such as means of criminal justice (for example, court hearings) and unofficial social processes (for example, public condemnation causing humiliation and shame).

However, the concept is problematic because deviance, similar to taboo, is a social construct. There are no behaviors in which deviance is inherent; instead, deviance is situational and contextual. For example, in most circumstances, murder is considered an illegal deviant behavior. However, this non-normative behavior is considered acceptable in certain contexts, such as warfare and self-defense when governments permit it. Furthermore, because social norms are subject to change, examples of deviance are also subject to change, both across time and cultures. For example, in the United States it is considered acceptable for interviewers and interviewees to shake hands, regardless of gender differences; in fact, it is considered a form of respect. However, in some Eastern cultures, this non-verbal form of communication would be offensive because of the different perspectives on relationships between men and women. Thus, it is important to consider differences in cross-cultural communication and the cultural meanings of behaviors in determining their appropriateness.

It is common that deviance is studied through the lens of crime; however, there are additional institutions in societies responsible for controlling deviance. In fact, deviance is an important concept in the context of health care. The purpose of the medical institution is to maintain health and control illness, which involves more than biological concerns. For example, according to the functionalist perspective, individuals experiencing illness are considered deviant because their condition violates conforming behavior and threatens social cohesion by limiting the individual's social contributions.

Functionalism, conflict theory, and symbolic interactionism all provide different descriptions of deviant behavior based on their respective premises (section 4.1). In addition to these three perspectives, the following are specific theories often used in the discussion of deviance.

1) Edwin Sutherland's **differential association**: This perspective asserts that deviance is a learned behavior resulting from interactions between individuals and their communities (for example, the communication of ideas). The process of learning deviance involves learning the techniques of deviant behaviors as well as the motives and values that rationalize these behaviors, and it is no different from other learning processes in its mechanism. The principal source of exposure is an individual's closest personal groups, whether formal groups, such as professional business associates, or informal groups, such as urban gangs. These groups determine the specific behaviors learned (for example, corporate, organized crime such as fraud, insider trading, or tax evasion versus gang-related offenses such as vandalism or violence). In either case, when an individual participates in communities that condone deviant behaviors, it becomes easier for the individual to learn these behaviors and thus become deviant themselves. The extent of learning is dependent on certain features, such as the frequency and intensity of the interactions. In social situations, it is inevitable that individuals will encounter others with both favorable and unfavorable views of deviance. Sutherland posits that individuals become deviant when their contacts with favorable attitudes toward deviance outweigh their contacts with unfavorable attitudes.

A criticism of differential association is the idea that individuals are reduced to their environments; instead of considering people as independent, rational actors with personal motivations, this perspective suggests that deviant behavior is learned from one's environment without choice. It fails to consider individual characteristics and experiences and how these considerations affect a person's reaction to deviant influences in their current surroundings.

2) Howard Becker's **labeling theory**: This perspective suggests that deviance is the result of society's response to a person rather than something inherent in the person's actions; behaviors become deviant through social processes (it assumes the act itself is not deviant for intrinsic moral reasons). This approach is one of the most important theories in understanding

deviance from a social perspective. The use of negative labels can have serious consequences, both on our perception of the deviant person and the person's self-perception. For example, individuals might internalize labels and redefine their concept of the self, which can lead to **self-fulfilling prophecies** (section 6.2). Because of the societal preoccupation with labels, the individual might begin to exhibit more deviant behaviors to fulfill the expectations associated with specific ascribed labels (a form of conforming behavior). Furthermore, because deviance is a social construct, there is no absolute set of characteristics that are viewed as deviant; instead, deviance is contextual. In fact, across the same social context, there are often double standards: the same behavior might be viewed as acceptable in one group and unacceptable in another (for example, the virgin woman versus the virgin man).

Because this perspective views deviance as a social construct, it is often used in interactionist arguments. However, the use of social labels also concerns conflict theorists. Those with the most power in societies, such as politicians, are able to impose the most severe labels, while those with the least power in societies, such as criminals, are those whom labels are most often directed toward. In general, it is often the dominant groups (majorities) labeling the subordinate groups (minorities); for example, men labeling women as "less capable" in professional contexts or the upper class labeling the lower class as "less motivated" to achieve economic success. In fact, social structures often contribute to this by allowing the dominant groups the power to enforce the boundaries of normal behavior and thus define the difference between non-deviant and deviant behaviors, perhaps institutionalizing these differences through legal policies. These groups are often referred to as **agents of social control** because of their ability to attach stigmas to certain behaviors (for example, a doctor can define obsessive-compulsive behavior as a mental illness, a form of deviance). The creation of stigmatic roles, in turn, reinforces the power structures and hierarchies inherent in most societies and serves to limit deviant behavior. Furthermore, there is also a functional component to labels, as labeling satisfies the social need to control behaviors and maintain order.

A criticism of the labeling theory is the idea that deviance is assumed to be an automatic process: individuals are seen to be influenced through the use of labels, which ignores their abilities to resist social expectations.

3) Robert Merton's **structural strain theory:** This perspective posits that deviance is the result of experienced strain, either individual or structural. Modern societies have shared perceptions of the ideal life (social goals). These societies also have accepted means of achieving these established goals. In expanding upon Durkheim's research, Merton specified that anomie is the state in which there is a mismatch between the common social goals and the structural or institutionalized means of obtaining these goals. In this state, individuals experience social strain; because existing social structures are inadequate, there is pressure to use deviant methods to prevent failure. When the social goals and means are balanced, deviance is not expected.

For example, economic success is a common goal for most individuals and societies and the legitimate means for obtaining this goal include continued education and professional positions that compensate well. However, in the United States, it is known that there is not equal access to resources among social groups (see section 4.2 for more details on social inequalities). For example, individuals born into lower class families have less financial resources available to obtain an education. Because the means are not serving these individuals in accomplishing the goal of economic success, the result is structural strain, which in turn leads to deviance. Merton's perspective, then, suggests that lower class individuals are more expected to use deviant methods of reaching economic success (for example, stealing, selling drugs).

A criticism of the structural strain theory is the fact that some deviant behaviors, and in particular criminal behaviors, are seemingly excessive and serve no useful purpose. Merton's perspective is applicable to fraud and theft, for example, in the cases where the economic structure is not serving individuals as best as possible (such as the means of earning is not the best option for the goal of obtaining financial assets). However, it is less applicable to deviant behaviors that are malicious and violent in nature, such as forms of sexual assault. Furthermore, this perspective is more applicable to material, rather than social, goals.

Collective Behavior

In addition to normative or conforming behaviors and non-normative or deviant behaviors, there is a third form of social behavior that is described through the separate and distinct concept of **collective behavior**, in which social norms for the situation are absent or unclear. This concept describes the actions of people operating as a collective group; however, it is important to distinguish collective behavior from group behavior. In general, collective behavior is more short-lived and less conventional values influence the group's behavior and guidelines for membership. Examples of collective behavior, as opposed to those of group behavior, do not reflect the existing social structure but are instead spontaneous situations in which individuals engage in actions that are otherwise unacceptable and violate social norms. Research on collective behavior has suggested that there are characteristics of the behavior that cannot be compared to the independent effect of numerous individual actions. Instead, with collective behavior, there is a loss of the individual and independent moral judgment in exchange for a sense of belonging to the group. This can be destructive (for example, mobs and riots) or harmless (for example, fads and popular catchphrases), depending on the diverse episode. It is important to understand collective behavior to limit its negative consequences—in particular, those negative consequences which are the result of human response rather than unpreventable circumstances. For example, an understanding of collective behavior could help establish effective and safe crowd management and design planning to accommodate for potential issues.

The classification of collective behavior is a point of contention. However, **Herbert Blumer**, a sociologist whose ideas were foundational in the understanding of collective behavior, identified four main forms of collective behavior:

1) **Crowds:** The **crowd** is defined as a group that shares a purpose. The crowd is the most agreed-upon example of collective behavior and is the most common in modern life (for example, orchestras, theaters, and other performances). In general, crowds are thought to be emotional; often, in the context of the crowds, there is a non-permanent loss of rational thought and the crowd influences individual behaviors, sometimes referred to as **herd behavior**. However, not all crowd behavior is irrational. For example, although the thought of stampedes suggests chaos, in the face of threats, such as during bombings or fires, it is not irrational for individuals to run, rather than walk, to the nearest exit as a response to fear. Crowds can be classified based on their specific intention: acting crowds gather for a specific cause or goal (for example, protesters or revolutionaries), casual crowds emerge spontaneously and include people who are not really interacting (for example, people waiting in line for something), conventional crowds gather for a planned event (for example, football fans or religious congregants), and expressive crowds aggregate to express an emotion (for example, funeral attenders or rock-concert goers). Crowds can be further classified based on the closeness of the individuals (for example, compact or diffuse crowds) and the emotions caused (for example, fear in the panic, happiness in the craze, and anger in the hostile outburst). The idea of panic is a common theme in examples of collective behavior; **panic** is a situation in which fear escalates to the point that it dominates thinking and thus affects entire groups (for example, during disaster situations). A **mob** is a specific example of a crowd in which emotion is heightened and behavior is directed toward a specific and violent cause. Historical examples of mobs include lynching.

2) **Publics:** A **public** is defined as a group of individuals discussing a single issue, which conflicts with the common usage of the term. This form of collective behavior begins as the discussion begins and ceases as the discussion ceases and there can exist various publics to reflect various discussions. People in publics share ideas.

3) **Masses:** A **mass** is defined as a group whose formation is prompted through the efforts of mass media; masses consist of a relatively large number of people who may not be in close proximity but nevertheless share common interests.

4) **Social movements:** A **social movement** is defined as collective behavior with the intention of promoting change. There are two main categories of social movements: **active movements**, which attempt to foster social change (for example, revolutions), and **expressive movements**, which attempt to foster individual change (for example, support groups). There are numerous forms of social movements identified in sociological tradition: global or local (range), old or new (origin), peaceful or violent (method), etc. In contrast to other forms of collective behavior, social movements can become established and permanent social institutions.

There are additional aspects of collective behavior with which you should be familiar. A **fad**, also known as a **craze**, is an example of a collective behavior in which something (1) experiences a rapid and dramatic boost in reputation, (2) remains popular among a large population for a brief period, and (3) experiences a rapid and dramatic decline in reputation. The enthusiasm for the particular thing is driven through methods such as peer pressure and social media and through actors such as peers and famous celebrities. Examples of fads include clothing, food, language, and other novel ideas that often fade not long after catching on. Internet phenomena are an excellent example of fads; viral videos that have lost momentum include dances such as Gangnam Style and the Harlem Shake. It is important to note that fads are separate from **trends**, which are longer-lived and often lead to permanent social changes; for example, the hippie movement created visible trends, such as peace signs, but also prompted widespread social change.

Another aspect of collective behavior is the concept of **mass hysteria**, which is a diagnostic label that refers to the collective delusion of some threat that spreads through emotion (for example, fear) and escalates until it spirals out of control (for example, panic). Mass hysteria is the result of public reactions to stressful situations; common examples include medical problems and supernatural occurrences, such as periodic interest in crop circles. In these situations, the collective behavior is often irrational as a result of emotional excesses and thus mass hysteria has been described as a form of groupthink (section 6.2). For example, in the context of medical problems, there might be a spontaneous spread of related diseases. Those affected might manifest similar medical symptoms, such as fatigue, headaches, or nausea. It is curious that these popular signs are also connected to high levels of stress. In most cases, the illness cannot be linked to an external source, such as an infectious agent.

It is thus important to distinguish this form of collective behavior from the concepts of **outbreaks**, **epidemics**, and **pandemics**. These cases involve an unexpected increase in the incidence of an infectious disease in a given region, with outbreaks being the most limited and pandemics being the most widespread. For example, the Bubonic plague is a well-known historical epidemic; in modern times, the extent of the dangerous COVID-19 virus reached pandemic proportions, spreading across the world. In contrast, famous examples of mass hysteria include larger movements without clear medical explanation, such as the Salem witch trials. This series of trials and prosecutions began as the result of a group of adolescent girls experiencing "fits" that were thought to exceed the power of the more common epileptic fits. This caused a **moral panic**—a specific form of panic as a result of a perceived threat to social order—which lead to numerous executions.

Riots are a third example of collective behavior. Riots are a form of crowd behavior (see page 128). Most riots occur as the result of general dissatisfaction with social conditions, with examples including food and bread, police, prison, race, religion, sports, student, and urban riots. In general, collective behavior is often thought to be irrational. However, some research suggests that riots are not irrational as there are examples where the source of dissatisfaction is less political and more fundamental; for example, some riots begin as a response to a lack of basic needs (for example, hunger riots). The most famous historical examples include reactions to government oppression, poor living conditions, racial or religious conflicts, and other serious social issues. In these cases, riots can have serious measurable consequences for economics and politics; these effects are often complex. For example, the Arab Spring was a revolution that included riots. It first began in Tunisia but spread across the Arab world, causing civil uprisings that contributed to the eventual fall of governments. The power of riots has led to increased public attention and participation, due in part to mass media coverage, and certain representations, which were once intended to conceal identities and offer protection (such as facemasks and scarves), have become iconic.

In general, riots are chaotic and disorganized due to a sudden onset, often described as states of civil disorder, civil distress, or civil unrest. There is an increase in criminal behaviors, such as vandalism and violence. The target of this destruction can include both private and public properties, depending on the source of the grievance, but often include institutions such as government or religious buildings. Because of the state of distress common in riots, crowd control is an important consideration. Police measures tend to be non-lethal in nature (for example, arrest or tear gas), but police intervention does lead to occasional injuries and deaths.

Agents of Socialization

There are many different social forces that influence our lives and the development of culture over time. Six of these "agents of socialization" are family, school, peers, the workplace, religion/government, and mass media/technology.

1) *Family*

    The lifelong process of socialization begins shortly after birth and is generally driven first by family members. Family members attend to a baby's physical needs but also to social development. First relationships heavily influence how an individual will interact in future relationships. Family members teach children the customs, beliefs, and traditions of their cultures through both instruction and modeling. They also influence the situations to which children are exposed, especially in the early years of life.

2) *School*

    Like family, schools explicitly teach children the norms and values of their culture. Schools can also affect children's self-identities by accentuating those intellectual, physical, and social strengths that society endorses. For example, schools may differ in how they value logic and linear thinking versus creativity, and can influence children toward one or the other. Finally, schools can reinforce divisive aspects of society, because the quality and availability of schooling is influenced by socioeconomic status.

3) *Peer Groups*

    As children grow older, the family typically becomes less important in social development and peer groups become more significant. Fashion, style of speech, gender-role identity, sexual activity, drug/alcohol use, and other behaviors are affected by peers and by the influence of hierarchies such as popularity.

4) *Workplace*

People typically spend a good portion of their time at work. The workplace influences behavior through written codes and rules as well as through informal norms. There is pressure to fit in at the workplace that often alters behavior; occupation can also be a large part of one's identity.

5) *Religion/Government*

Both government and organized religion influence the course of cultural change by creating "rites of passage." In religion, this might include traditional milestones and celebrations such as coming of age and marriage. Government sets legal ages for drinking, voting, joining the military, and so on. Laws both influence and are influenced by the societies to which they apply. For example, in the United States, stricter laws apply to crack than to cocaine, and this affects society's perceptions of these drugs and of drug addicts.

6) *Mass Media/Technology*

Mass media and technology have extended themselves to influence almost everyone on the planet, through television, movies, the Internet, cell phones, and other communications. The impact of television on culture through displays of sex, violence, and impossible-to-achieve ideals has been much debated. It has also affected culture in ways that most people agree are positive, such as educational programming and introductions to other cultures and lifestyles. The Internet can similarly help shrink the world and increase social influences through tools such as online social networking and blogs.

Cultural Assimilation

Assimilation and amalgamation are two possible outcomes of interactions among multiple cultures in the same space. **Assimilation** is the process by which an individual forsakes aspects of his or her own cultural tradition to adopt those of a different culture. Generally, this individual is a member of a minority group who is attempting to conform to the culture of the dominant group.

$$A + B + C \rightarrow A$$

In the diagram above, A is the dominant group that minority groups B and C work to imitate and become absorbed by. In order to assimilate, members of the minority group may make great personal sacrifices, such as changing their spoken languages, their religions, how they dress, and their personal values. In the United States, minority groups attempting to assimilate not only must learn English if it is not their native language, but must adopt the values of a capitalist society with a heavy emphasis on the individual and independence—a tough transition for those from collectivist cultures. In addition, assimilation does not guarantee that one will not be the victim of discrimination.

Amalgamation occurs when majority and minority groups combine to form a new group.

$$A + B + C \rightarrow D$$

In this case, a unique cultural group is formed that is distinct from any of the initial groups.

Multiculturalism

Multiculturalism or **pluralism** is a perspective that endorses equal standing for all cultural traditions. It promotes the idea of cultures coming together in a true melting pot, rather than in a hierarchy. The United States, despite the common description as a melting pot, includes elements of hierarchy. For example, English is the dominant language, and national holidays tend to reflect Eurocentricism.

$$A + B + C \rightarrow A + B + C$$

In true multiculturalism, each culture is able to maintain its practices. It is especially apparent in cities such as New York where there exist pockets of separate cultures (Chinatown, Little Italy, Koreatown). As a practice, multiculturalism is under debate. Supporters say it increases diversity and helps empower minority groups. Opponents say it encourages segregation over unity by maintaining physical and social isolation and hinders cohesiveness within a society.

Subcultures

Bike enthusiasts, bartenders, and medical personnel are examples of groups that can be called subcultures. A **subculture** is a segment of society that shares a distinct pattern of traditions and values that differs from that of the larger society. As the name suggests, a subculture can be thought of as a culture existing within a larger, dominant culture. Members of a subculture do participate in many activities of the larger culture, but also have unique behaviors and activities that are specific to their subculture. This often includes having unique slang, such as that used by medical personnel (for example, *cabbage* for "coronary artery bypass graft"). Sometimes, subcultures are the result of countercultural backlash, an opposition to views widely accepted within a society. Hippies in the late 1960s and early 1970s would be considered a counterculture, because they opposed certain aspects of the dominant culture, such as middle class values and the Vietnam War.

Moral Development

Moral development is an important aspect of socialization and identity formation. Lawrence Kohlberg, an American psychologist, expanded upon Jean Piaget's theory (Chapter 11) of moral development in children. **Kohlberg's stages of moral development** include six identifiable developmental stages of moral reasoning, which form the basis of ethical behavior. Kohlberg's stages are grouped into three levels with two stages each (see Table 2). According to Kohlberg, stages cannot be skipped. Each stage provides a new and necessary moral perspective, and the understanding from each stage is retained and integrated at later stages. Interestingly, most adults attain but do not surpass the fourth stage, in which morality is dictated by outside forces (laws, rules, social obligations). Few people attain a post-conventional level of moral reasoning. In fact, though Kohlberg insisted that stage 6 exists, he found it difficult to identify people who operated at that level.

Table 2   Kohlberg's Stages of Moral Development

Level 1	Pre-conventional level of moral reasoning: morality judged by direct consequences to the self (no internalization of "right" and "wrong") Typical of children	Stage 1: Obedience and punishment orientation	Individuals focus on the direct consequences to themselves of their actions ("How can I avoid punishment?")
		Stage 2: Self-interest orientation	Individuals focus on the behavior that will be in their best interests, with limited interest in the needs of others ("What's in it for me?")
Level 2	Conventional level of moral reasoning: morality judged by comparing actions to society's views and expectations (acceptance of conventional definitions of "right" and "wrong") Typical of adolescents and adults	Stage 3: Interpersonal accord and conformity	Individuals focus on the approval and disapproval of others, and try to be "good" by living up to expectations ("What will make others like me?")
		Stage 4: Authority and social-order maintaining orientation	Beyond a need for individual approval, individuals feel a duty to uphold laws, rules, and social conventions ("What am I supposed to do?")
Level 3	Post-conventional level of moral reasoning: morality judged by internal ethical guidelines; rules viewed as useful but malleable guidelines Many people never reach this abstract level of moral reasoning	Stage 5: Social contract orientation	Individuals see laws as social contracts to be changed when they do not promote general welfare ("The greatest good for the greatest number of people")
		Stage 6: Universal ethical principles	Morality is based on abstract reasoning using universal ethical principles; laws are only valid if they are grounded in justice

6.2   POSITIVE AND NEGATIVE ELEMENTS OF SOCIAL INTERACTION

Attribution

Attribution theory is rooted in social psychology and attempts to explain how individuals view behavior, both our own behavior and the behavior of others. Given a set of circumstances, individuals attribute behavior to internal causes (**dispositional attribution**) or external causes (**situational attribution**). Driving tends to be a situation that generates plenty of salient examples. Imagine you are driving and someone cuts you off. You might think, "Wow, that driver is a real jerk." This would be a dispositional attribution, because the driver's behavior is attributed to an internal cause (he is a jerk). On the other hand, you could alternatively think, "Wow, that driver must be in a hurry because of an emergency; maybe he just found out his mom is in the hospital." This would be a situational attribution (there is an emergency).

How often do you think that someone who cut you off might have had a good reason to do so? People tend to assign dispositional attributions to others (they are just jerks), but give themselves the benefit of situational attributions. For example, the last time you cut someone off while driving, did you feel like you had a good reason to do so? Did you then think to yourself, "Wow, I am a real jerk"?

What determines whether we attribute behavior to internal or external causes? There are three factors that influence this decision: consistency, distinctiveness, and consensus. To consider these, imagine a simple situation: you are walking past your friend, who looks angry and walks past you without saying hello.

1) **Consistency:** is anger consistent with how your friend typically acts? If it is, then you might explain it with internal causes (dispositional). If not, you might think there are external factors that explain it (situational).

2) **Distinctiveness:** is your friend angry toward everyone or just toward you? If your friend is angry toward everyone, the cause likely has to do with your friend (dispositional). If your friend is just angry toward you, it may be situational; perhaps you did something irritating.

3) **Consensus:** is your friend the only one angry or is everyone angry? If your friend is the only one angry, then it is more likely that the anger has something to do with your friend (dispositional). If everyone is angry, then it might be situational (the team lost the playoffs).

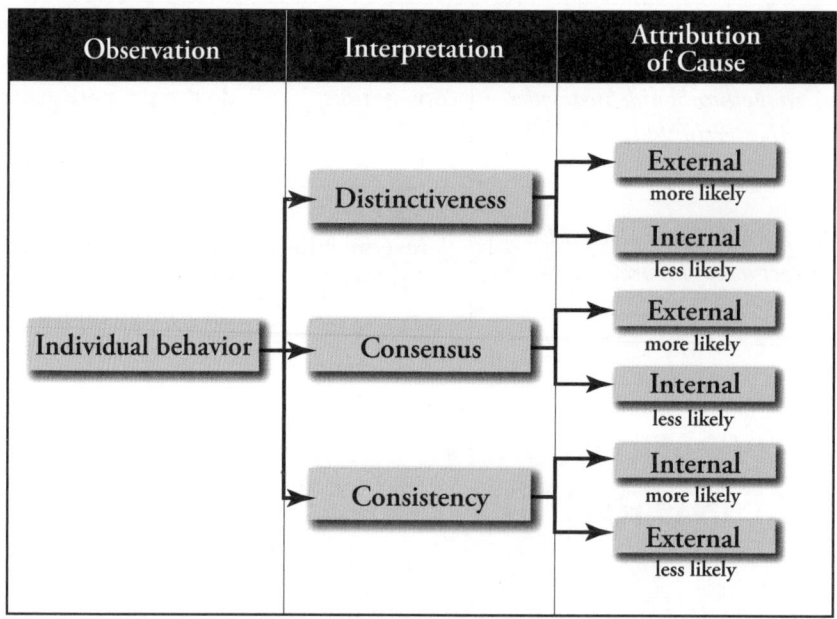

Figure 1   Attributing behavior to external or internal causes

Attributional Biases

Despite the apparent logic in our methods of identifying whether someone's behavior is due to internal or external causes, we are frequently wrong in our analysis of others. We often make the **fundamental attribution error**, which is that we tend to underestimate the impact of the situation and overestimate the impact of a person's character or personality. Another way of saying this is that we tend to assume that people *are* how they act. Thus, we are more likely to think that the driver who cuts us off is a jerk in general, rather than assuming the driver acted that way because he has to rush to the hospital to be with his ailing mother. Remember, when we attribute our own actions to something, we tend to attribute to external rather than internal causes. So if I cut someone off, it is because I had a good reason to. This tendency to blame our actions on the situation and blame the actions of others on their personalities is also called the **actor-observer bias**.

People tend to give themselves much more credit than they give others. We are wired to perceive ourselves favorably. The **self-serving bias** is the tendency to attribute successes to ourselves and our failures to others or the external environment. If we perform well academically, it is because we are smart and worked hard. If we perform poorly academically, it was because the test was unfair or the teacher graded too hard.

Similarly, we have a tendency to be optimistic and want to believe that the world is a good place. We want to believe that life is predictable and that actions influence outcomes. The **optimism bias** is the belief that bad things happen to other people, but not to us. This goes hand-in-hand with the fact that we want to believe that life is fair, which also impacts how we think about others. The **just world phenomenon** is a tendency to believe that the world is fair and people get what they deserve. When bad things happen to others, it is the result of their actions or their failure to act, not because sometimes bad things happen to good people. Similarly, when good things happen to us, it is because we deserved it. **Hindsight bias,** or the knew-it-all-along effect, is the tendency to believe that an event that has already occurred was predictable.

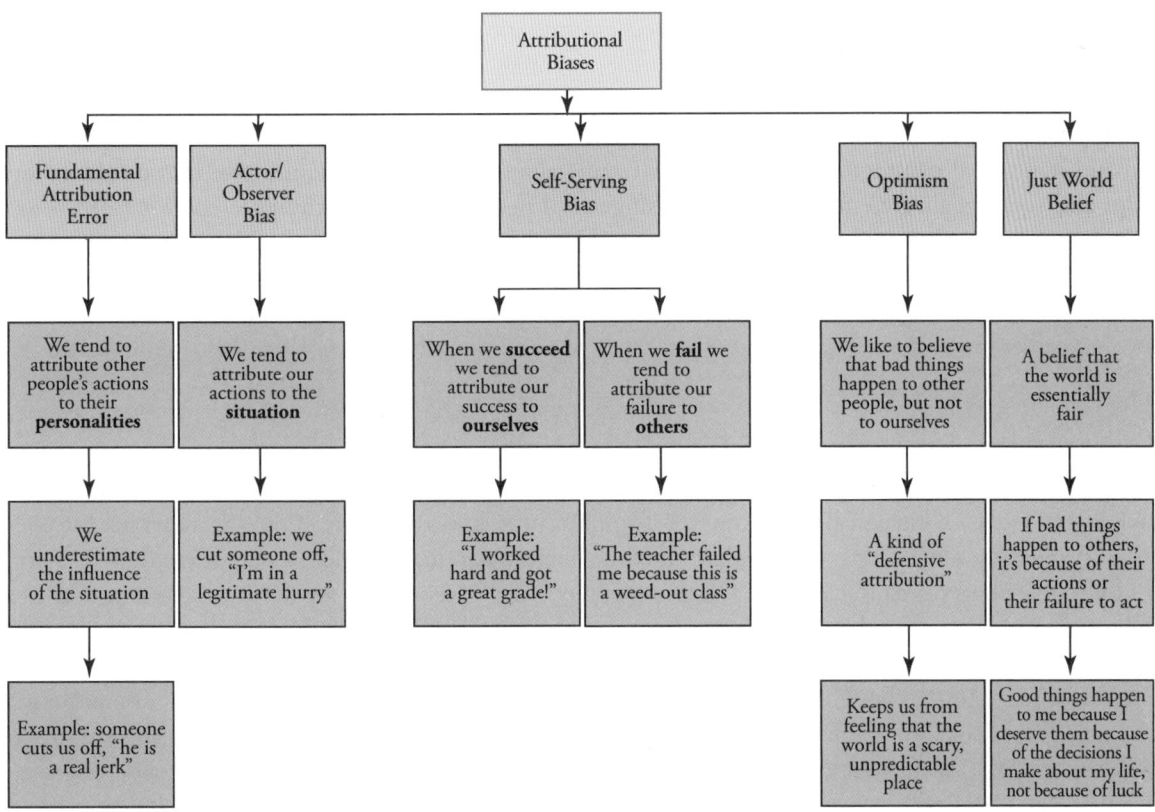

Figure 2   Attributional biases

Another type of error that occurs when we make assumptions about others is the halo effect (or halo error). The **halo effect** is a tendency to believe that people have inherently good or bad natures, rather than looking at individual characteristics. Our overall impression of a person is influenced by how we feel or think about his or her character. For example, your overall impression of your neighbor might be "he is nice," therefore, you make other assumptions about him ("he must be a good dad"). The **physical attractiveness stereotype** is a specific type of halo effect; people tend to rate attractive individuals more favorably on personality traits and characteristics than they do those who are less attractive.

Culture Affects Attributions

There are cultural differences that influence how attributions are made. Western cultures tend to endorse an individualistic attitude: "You can do anything you put your mind to!" This influences people toward more internal attributions for success and failure. Unemployment is sometimes explained as laziness or stupidity. In Eastern Asian cultures, external attribution is more predominant. Thus, the system as a whole is scrutinized more than the individual. If an insider trading scandal occurs, this attitude would emphasize controlling the financial organization, rather than finding and prosecuting the guilty individuals.

Self-Perceptions Shape Our Perceptions of Others

Social perception involves the understanding of others in our social world; it is the initial information we process about other people in order to try to understand their mindsets and intentions. **Social cognition** is the ability of the brain to store and process information regarding social perception. Social perception is the process responsible for our judgments and impressions about other people, and it allows us to recognize how others impact us, and predict how they might behave in given situations. We rely upon our social perception and cognition in order to interpret a range of socially relevant information, such as verbal and non-verbal communication, tone, facial expressions, and an understanding of the social relationships and social goals present in situations. Using social perception, we try to figure out what others are thinking. Sometimes our tendencies lead us to mistakes in social perception. A **false consensus** occurs when we assume that everyone else agrees with what we do (even though they may not). A **projection bias** happens when we assume others have the same beliefs we do. Since people have a tendency to look for similarities between themselves and others, they often assume them even when this is unfounded.

Stereotypes, Prejudice, and Discrimination

Many people may not know the differences between the terms stereotype, prejudice, discrimination, and racism, but from a sociological perspective, it is important to know their meanings. **Stereotypes** are oversimplified ideas about groups of people, based on characteristics (race, gender, sexual orientation, religion, disability). Stereotypes can be positive ("X group is successful because they are hard workers") or negative ("Y group is poor because they are lazy").

Prejudice refers to the thoughts, attitudes, and feelings someone holds about a group that are not based on actual experience. As the name implies, prejudice is a prejudgment or biased thinking about a group and its members. The group that one is biased against can be one defined by race, age, gender, religion, or any other characteristic. Some forms of prejudice are blatant or overt, such as the prejudice used to justify the actions taken by Hitler and his regime against the Jews and other groups during World War II. Other forms are more subtle, such as the finding that employers in a study considered more resumes for employment from candidates with "white-sounding names" than "Black-sounding names." In this situation, an employer may not even be aware of his or her prejudice. In fact, prejudice has been found at a subconscious level when studying individuals' reactions to pleasant and unpleasant words. For example, when primed with a Black face rather than a white face, people are more likely to predict the subject is carrying a gun rather than another object, such as a tool or wallet.

While prejudice involves thinking a certain way, **discrimination** involves acting a certain way toward a group or group member. People can discriminate against any number of characteristics and, unfortunately, American history is rife with examples of discrimination. Moreover, traditions, policies, ideas, practices, and laws that are discriminatory still exist in many institutions. Attempts to limit discrimination, such as **affirmative action** (policies that take factors like race or sex into consideration to benefit underrepresented groups in admissions or job hiring decisions) have been used to benefit those believed to be current or past victims of discrimination. However, these attempts have been controversial, and some have deemed these practices "discrimination against the majority," or **reverse discrimination**.

Prejudices and actions that discriminate based on race, or hold that one race is inferior to another, are called **racism**. While the exact definitions of "race," "ethnicity," and "racism" have been subject to much debate over the years, racism tends to be seen when the dominant or majority group (usually white) holds a prejudice or engages in discrimination, whether intentional or not, against non-dominant or minority groups (usually non-white). Sometimes racism is used to describe discrimination on an ethnic or cultural basis, independent of whether these differences are described as racial. The confusion largely stems from confusion about the definitions of the terms "race" and "ethnicity."

Institutional discrimination refers to unjust and discriminatory practices employed by large organizations that have been codified into operating procedures, processes, or institutional objectives. An example of institutional discrimination was the "don't ask, don't tell" policy of the U.S. military, which frowned upon openly gay men and women serving in the armed forces. In general, members of minority groups are much more likely to encounter institutional discrimination than members of majorities.

A society's prescriptions for which groups attain more power, prestige, and social standing can account for prejudice toward those on the lower rungs of that society. In general, any unequal status sets the stage for prejudice. These symbols of status are all relative, so in order to be of a higher status, one needs other people to be of a lower status. Thus, some people at the "top" are motivated to try to justify and maintain these differences, sometimes using prejudice as a tool. For example, very wealthy individuals may justify their wealth by insinuating that poorer members of society are lazy, and they seek to maintain this gap by voting against welfare programs for this group. Social institutions can also be designed to maintain these differences. For example, in the United States, good, well-funded schools are in wealthier neighborhoods and below-average, poorly-funded schools are in poorer neighborhoods.

In the United States, wealth is an important source of power and class, with the wealthiest shaping the laws and agenda of the society. Prestige is often based on occupation. Doctors get more respect than janitors, not just in their occupations but also as people. Higher prestige positions are usually taken by members of the dominant groups in societies, as can be seen by the disparate number of men compared to women in many of these prestigious roles.

Emotion and Cognition in Prejudice

Prejudice is an attitude. Remember that attitudes have three components (the ABCs): affect (feelings), behavioral inclinations/tendencies, and cognition (beliefs). Therefore, emotion and cognition both play roles in contributing to prejudice. In addition, there are several social sources of prejudice. Let's consider each of these contributing factors.

Emotion can play a role in feeding prejudices. At the core of prejudice is often fear or frustration. When someone is faced with something intimidating or unknown, especially if it is presumed to be blocking that person from some goal (frustration), hostility can be a natural reaction. There is a tendency to want to direct that hostility at someone, and history shows that displaced aggression often falls on marginalized people. **Scapegoats** are the unfortunate people at whom displaced aggression is directed. Many Germans blamed the Jews for the economic struggles that preceded the genocide of World War II. In the United States, fear and hostility were redirected onto women who were accused as "witches" in the 1600s. In subtler forms, scapegoats for an economic collapse can be those who are impoverished and on welfare.

This is not to say that one has to be some kind of "monster" to experience feelings of prejudice. Although in some of the above examples, drastic actions were taken, the underlying emotions can also influence those who do not take action. For example, when seated next to someone who is clearly very different from them on a bus, even people who do not see themselves as prejudiced may be uncomfortable. When a person sees an unfamiliar person of another race, emotion processing centers in the brain become more active automatically. It is only through active self-monitoring and reflection that people are able to inhibit prejudiced responses despite the presence of prejudiced feelings. Some may feel guilty for having the feelings at all, though they are not unusual. These self-inhibition abilities weaken with age, so many older adults find it hard to inhibit the prejudiced thoughts that they may have suppressed during their younger years.

There are also some aspects of normal thinking and information processing that contribute to prejudice. Our brains seek to categorize and organize data based on similarities, as a shortcut. We create conceptual categories such as "white" just as we do categories like "furniture" and "toys." These conceptualizations can lead to stereotypes. Stereotypes, both positive and negative, stem from our mental shortcuts that simplify our conceptualizations of the world.

Our brains also hone in on differences. Even babies are more interested in new objects presented in their field of vision than they are in things they've seen before. Thus, people who are seen as distinctive draw more attention and are often likely to be seen as representative of groups. For example, all Black people may be incorrectly considered good athletes based on examples of distinctive Black athletes like Michael Jordan. There is an **illusory correlation** created between a group of people and a characteristic based on unique cases.

Attributional biases (described above), particularly the optimism bias and just-world belief, also suggest that we are more likely to believe that the world is fair and predictable, things happen for a reason, and people get what they deserve. Thus, the sick or disadvantaged often face prejudice because others believe that they have done something wrong that led them to be in their position. Thus, someone with HIV may face prejudice, including the assumption that he or she contracted the disease through irresponsible behavior, despite how the disease was actually transmitted.

Self-Fulfilling Prophecy and Stereotype Threat

These stereotypes can lead to behaviors that affirm the original stereotypes in what is known as a **self-fulfilling prophecy**. For example, if a college guy believes that the girls in a certain sorority are snobby and prudish, he may avoid engaging in conversations with the girls from that sorority at parties. Because he does not engage them in conversation, his opinion of them as snobby and prudish will probably be reinforced. People may also be affected by stereotypes they know others have of a group to which they belong. **Stereotype threat** refers to a self-fulfilling fear that one will be evaluated based on a negative stereotype. For example, the idea that males are better at math than females is a negative stereotype. In studies where females are asked to complete a math test, if the female is first told that males do better than females on the math test, the female's performance on the test is lower than if she was not first presented with this information. Similarly, if the female is being tested on math concepts with males present, she will perform more poorly than if there are no males present. This phenomenon helps to explain the dearth of women in math and engineering fields.

Ethnocentrism Versus Cultural Relativism

On a broader level, when different cultures interact, there is often a tendency to judge people from another culture by the standards of one's own culture, a phenomenon known as **ethnocentrism**. It is an example of favoritism for one's in-group over out-groups (see Groups below). For example, the tension that exists between those who live in the city and those who live in rural areas is often due to judgments about each other's ways of life. City dwellers may look down on those in rural areas based on their standards of occupation and wealth. Those in the country may look down on city dwellers based on standards of morality, practicality, and quality of life. An alternative to ethnocentrism is **cultural relativism**: judging another culture based on its own standards. This can be very difficult to do, especially when the values of another culture clash with the values of one's own. For example, in India, child labor is common and is often seen as a way in which children can help their families. This may be a difficult viewpoint to accept for someone from a culture in which childhood is equated with a carefree time of play, and child labor is seen as abusive. However, practicing cultural relativism would involve judging this practice in the context of that culture's values.

Groups

A **group** is a collection of any number of people (as few as two) who regularly interact and identify with each other, sharing similar norms, values, and expectations. A team of neurologists may be considered a group, while the entire hospital staff may not be considered a group if there is little interaction between departments. The concept of social groups is complex, and groups come in numerous varieties. There are sociologists who might view societies as large groups in the context of cohesive social identities. Within a social structure, groups are often the setting for social interaction and influence. Groups help clearly define social roles and statuses.

Groups can be further divided into primary groups and secondary groups. **Primary groups** play a more important role in an individual's life; these groups are usually smaller and include those with whom the individual engages with emotionally, in-person on a long-term basis. A **secondary group** is larger and more impersonal, and may interact for specific reasons for shorter periods. Primary groups serve **expressive functions** (meeting emotional needs) and secondary groups serve **instrumental functions** (meeting pragmatic needs). A family would be an example of a primary group (regardless of how family is defined), whereas the MCAT study group would be an example of a secondary group.

In-groups and out-groups are subcategories of primary and secondary groups. An **in-group** is a group that an individual belongs to and believes to be an integral part of who she is. A group that an individual does not belong to is her **out-group**. Social identity theory asserts that when we categorize other people, we identify with some of them, whom we consider our in-groups, and see differences with others, whom we consider our out-groups. We tend to have favorable impressions of our in-groups because they bolster our social identities and self-esteem. People tend to have positive stereotypes about their own in-groups ("we are hard-working"). It feels good to have a sense of belonging, and feel positive about the groups to which you belong. On the other hand, we may have more negative impressions of members of out-groups. Different can be seen as worse (for example, "I feel sorry for those who don't believe the same things I do"). People also tend to have more negative stereotypes about out-groups ("they are lazy"). In-groups and out-groups help to explain some negative human behaviors like exclusion and bullying. When certain groups of people are defined as different, they may also be seen as inferior (when people assume that their in-group is the best, everyone in the out-group is somehow less); therefore, in-groups may engage in sexism, racism, ethnocentrism, heterosexism, and other such behaviors. (These ideas are discussed in more detail below.)

A **reference group** is a standard measure to which people compare themselves. For example, peers who are also studying for the MCAT might be a reference group for you. This is a group to which you might compare yourself. What are the people in this group studying? What classes are they taking? When are they taking the exam? To which medical schools are they applying? An individual can have multiple reference groups, and these different groups may convey different messages. For example, you might view your friends in class who are all taking the MCAT as one reference group, and your older sibling, who is in medical school, and his or her medical school friends as another reference group.

Furthermore, there are descriptions of **group size**. The number of people present within the group has consequences for group relations. The smallest social group, known as the **dyad**, contains two members. Dyadic interaction is often more intimate and intense than that in larger groups because there is no outside competition. However, the small size also requires active cooperation and participation from both members to be stable. In some cases of dyads, such as within marriages, there are laws that enforce the strength of the pair. Dyads can involve equal relationships, such as with monogamous romantic partners, or unequal relationships, such as with master-servant relationships. The next largest group, known as the **triad**, contains three members. In the dyad, there is a single relationship, but in the triad, there are three relationships, one between each pair of members. For this reason, triads can be more or less stable. It is possible for the group to become more stable because there is an additional person to mediate tension; it is possible for the group to become less stable because it is an observed rule that two people will tend to unite, causing conflict with the final group member. Triads can also be equal or unequal, and a common example of hierarchical triads involves groups in which there is a single dominant member, such as in an MCAT tutoring group (one tutor and two students).

People who exist in the same space but do not interact or share a common sense of identity make up an **aggregate**. For example, an MCAT study group that meets after class regularly at a coffee shop to prepare for the exam is a group. All of the people that frequent that coffee shop on a regular basis (but do not interact or share a common identity) are an aggregate. Similarly, people who share similar characteristics but are not otherwise tied together would be considered a **category**. All of the people studying for the MCAT this year make up a category of people.

Bureaucracy is a term used to describe an administrative body and the processes by which this body accomplishes tasks. Bureaucracies arise from an advanced division of labor in which each worker does his or her small task. These tasks are presided over and coordinated by managers. Bureaucracies can be a very efficient way to complete complicated tasks because each member of the organization has a specific role. A major theory of bureaucracy was developed by sociologist Max Weber, who considered bureaucracy to be a necessary aspect of modern society. Weber outlined the following characteristics of an ideal bureaucracy:

1. It covers a fixed area of activity.
2. It is hierarchically organized.
3. Workers have expert training in an area of specialty.
4. Organizational rank is impersonal, and advancement depends on technical qualification, rather than favoritism.
5. Workers follow set procedures to increase predictability and efficiency.

One major concept related to bureaucracy is rationalization. Rationalization describes the process by which tasks are broken down into component parts to be efficiently accomplished by workers within the organization. Because the workers follow set procedures in completing tasks, it is easy to predict the outcome of the process. Manufacturers have taken advantage of these aspects of bureaucracy when designing production processes. One of the first manufacturers to popularize this process was Henry Ford, who implemented assembly lines in his automobile plants. Ford rationalized the process of building a car by breaking it down into component parts and assigning the assembly of each part to a worker. In this way, he was able to have cars efficiently assembled and each car was exactly the same as the ones coming before and after it. Sociologist George Ritzer studied a similar process—the design of McDonald's restaurants to produce food quickly, and to produce uniform products across all franchises. He describes the rationalization of fast food production as **McDonaldization**. This process has four components that reflect the principles of bureaucracy: efficiency, calculability (assessing performance through quantity and/or speed of output), predictability, and control (automating work wherever possible in order to make results more predictable).

While a bureaucracy, in its ideal form, may be the most efficient way to accomplish complicated tasks, this organizational form can have several drawbacks. First, because workers follow set procedures, this can cause the organization to struggle when adapting to challenges that require it to change its way of coordinating tasks. Second, workers may become overly attached to their individual task and lose sight of the organizational mission as a whole. Third, workers may become overly attached to the set procedures and not respond flexibly to new challenges on an interpersonal level.

One paradoxical feature of organizations is that, although they may be founded to tackle new challenges in revolutionary ways, as their organizational structure becomes more complex, it also becomes more conservative and less able to adapt. Thus, revolutionary organizations inevitably become less revolutionary as their organizational structures develop and become entrenched. This pattern is known as the **Iron Law of Oligarchy**. Oligarchy means rule by an elite few, and it comes about through the very organization of the bureaucracy itself. Bureaucracies depend on increased centralization of tasks as one moves up the hierarchy. That is, there are many layers of managers in a bureaucracy, each one responsible for coordinating (centralizing) a set of tasks. The individuals who are responsible for coordinating the coordinators have the most power, and those individuals become an oligarchy at the top of the organizational structure. Furthermore, these oligarchs become specialized at their task (management), just as other members of the organization become specialists in their tasks. As discussed above, one downside to bureaucracy is that workers will fight to maintain control over their task and their established way of carrying it out. Thus, managers defend their position at the top of the organizational structure, thereby entrenching the oligarchy.

Social Facilitation

Social psychology seeks to understand how people influence one another through their interactions. The most basic level of experience between members of society is "mere presence." **Mere presence** means that people are simply in one another's presence, either completing similar activities or apparently minding their own business. For example, the task of grocery shopping usually involves the mere presence of other shoppers, without direct engagement. What's fascinating is that it turns out that the mere presence of others has a measurable effect on an individual's performance.

People tend to perform simple, well-learned tasks better when other people are present. For example, people can do simple math problems more quickly and run slightly faster when in the presence of others. People's color preferences are even stronger when they make judgments in the presence of others (a task that has no competitive influence). This finding has been called the **social facilitation effect**, and it may help explain why some of us study in the library (in the presence of others) or walk faster when in the presence of other pedestrians. However, the social facilitation effect only holds true for simple or practiced tasks. The presence of others can impair performance when completing complex or novel tasks. Thus, people do not complete complex math problems as quickly and may have a harder time navigating in novel environments when others are present.

The prevailing explanation for these phenomena involves arousal. The presence of others stimulates arousal, which serves to activate our dominant responses (the practiced responses that come most easily to us). When completing tasks that are easy and well-practiced, these dominant responses are exactly what is called for; thus, performance improves with arousal stimulated by the presence of others. When completing tasks that are more complex or novel, the dominant responses are likely to be incorrect for the situation; thus, performance declines with arousal, and in the presence of others. A basketball player who is a good, well-practiced shooter will experience an improvement in performance when there is an audience, because making baskets is his or her dominant response. A player who does not often shoot the ball will suffer with an audience, because shooting is not his or her dominant response.

There are other factors that also impact one's performance in the presence of others. Overwhelming fear of evaluation reduces performance even on behaviors that were previously automatic, because self-consciousness and doubt can lead to overanalysis. Athletes struggle if they tend to overthink their body movements at critical times. Distraction is also a factor, with the presence of others sometimes serving to divert our attention from tasks. This can be due to external events, such as others' behavior, or internal events, such as our thoughts of what others might be thinking or doing.

Deindividuation

When situations provide a high degree of arousal and a very low sense of responsibility, people may act in startling ways, surprising both to themselves at a later time and to others who know them closely. In these situations, people may lose their sense of restraint and their individual identity by identifying with a group or mob mentality, a situation called **deindividuation**. Its effects can be seen in examples ranging from atrocious acts during wartime to mosh pits at concerts. Deindividuation involves a lack of self-awareness and is the result of a disconnection of behavior from attitudes.

The confluence of several factors creates the ideal conditions for deindividuation to occur. These factors include:

- Group size: larger groups create a diminished sense of identity and responsibility, and may allow people to achieve anonymity by getting "lost in the crowd"
- Physical anonymity: using face paint, masks, or costumes (or communicating anonymously online) makes one less identifiable
- Arousing activities: rather than beginning with a frenzy, deindividuating circumstances usually start with arousing activities that escalate

The bottom line is that factors that reduce self-awareness increase a sense of deindividuation. This can further include social roles (as evidenced by Zimbardo's prison study) and the use of drugs or alcohol, which serve to disinhibit and reduce self-consciousness.

Bystander Effect

The **Kitty Genovese** case involved the stabbing of a woman in New York City late at night. Research spawned by this event revealed what is known as the **bystander effect**: the finding that a person is less likely to provide help when there are other bystanders. This occurs because the presence of bystanders creates a diffusion of responsibility—the responsibility to help does not clearly reside with one person in the group. When faced with circumstances in which one is the only individual available to assist, one may be more likely to act. Interestingly, the likelihood that someone will stop to help is inversely correlated with the number of people around; therefore, if you ever find yourself in a life-threatening emergency, you would be better off in a small town with a few folks around than in the middle of Times Square with thousands of people around.

Social Loafing

The bystander effect involves a diffusion of responsibility when in the presence of others. Taken further, this effect extends to circumstances in which people are working together toward common goals. In these situations, there is a tendency for people to exert less effort if they are being evaluated as a group than if they are individually accountable, a phenomenon called **social loafing**. It is something that you may have experienced in your everyday life, and it does not necessarily mean that the "loafer" is someone who is lazy or irresponsible. For example, as an audience member in a small group of five, you are likely to clap louder for a presenter than if you were in an audience of 500 people. This is thought to occur because there can be less pressure on individuals as parts of a group on some tasks, leading to a tendency to take a little bit of a free ride, getting the benefit from the group while putting less effort in than one might on one's own.

Social facilitation and social loafing are both responses to the group situation and the task at hand. Which one tends to occur is based in part on evaluation. When being part of a group increases concerns over evaluation, social facilitation occurs. When being part of a group decreases concerns over evaluation, social loafing occurs. In order to fight against the threat of social loafing, companies in which people work in groups often use measures of group performance (for example, a store's total revenue) as well as of individual performance (for example, individual sales).

Group Polarization

We've seen how groups can influence one's performance, either by facilitating or hindering it based on circumstances. But how does group influence affect beliefs and opinions? It turns out that groups tend to intensify the preexisting views of their members—that is, the average view of a member of the group is accentuated. This tendency is called **group polarization**. It does NOT indicate that the group becomes more divided on an issue, but rather, suggests that the entire group tends toward more extreme versions of the average views they initially shared before discussion.

Group polarization occurs at every level in society—in families, schools, political parties, communities, and such. Consider a political debate on whether a wetland area should be converted into a shopping center. Although they likely each initially held a belief in the importance of conserving the wetlands, members of an environmental political party who interact with each other end up adopting a more extreme stance toward conservation than previously held by the average member. Similarly, members of another political party that focuses on the importance of jobs would emphasize this focus even more after discussions within the group. Thus, each group adopts a more extreme stance than its initial position. This creates more divisiveness between the two groups. When you consider the group polarization phenomenon together with the fact that people tend to preferentially interact with like-minded people, you can see why group negotiations are so difficult.

There are two reasons why group polarization occurs. The first is **informational influence**; in group discussion, the most common ideas to emerge are the ones that favor the dominant viewpoint. This serves to persuade others to take a stronger stance toward this viewpoint and provides an opportunity to rehearse and validate these similar opinions, further strengthening them. In fact, just thinking about an opinion for a couple of minutes can strengthen your support of it, because we tend to mostly think of facts that support it. The second reason is **normative influence**, which is based on social desirability, that is, wanting to be accepted or admired by others. If you want to identify with a particular group, then you may take a stronger stance than you initially would have in order to better relate to and internalize the group's belief system. The influence of **social comparison** (evaluating our opinions by comparing them to those of others) extends far beyond high school.

Groupthink

Pressure not to "rock the boat" in a group by providing a dissenting opinion can lead to what is known as groupthink. Although **groupthink** is a state of harmony within a group (because everyone is seemingly in a state of agreement), it can lead to some pretty terrible decisions. Groupthink manifests in a group when certain factors come together. Groups that are at risk tend to be overly friendly and cohesive, isolated from dissenting opinions, and inclined to favor the decisions of a directive leader.

There are certain symptoms that are often clues to the presence of groupthink:

- the group is optimistic about its capabilities and has unquestioned belief in its stances—an overestimation of "might and right"
- the group becomes increasingly extreme by justifying its own decisions while demonizing those of opponents
- some members of the group prevent dissenting opinions from permeating the group by filtering out information and facts that go against the beliefs of the group (a process called **mindguarding**)
- there is pressure to conform, and so individuals censor their own opinions in favor of consensus, which creates an illusion of unanimity

Stigma and Deviance

As discussed earlier in this chapter, **deviance** involves a violation of society's standards of conduct or expectations. Deviant behavior can range from being late to an interview to smuggling drugs. In the United States, there are many groups who are classified as deviants, including drug pushers and gang members. However, more harmless groups can also be labeled deviants, including the obese and the mentally ill. Deviance can even involve positive acts, for example, Rosa Parks and other African Americans who refused to sit in the back of the bus were acting deviantly in an attempt to change norms they saw as unfair.

Society often devalues deviant members by assigning demeaning labels, called **stigma**. Entire groups may be labeled based on physical or behavioral qualities. For example, the term "fob" (for "fresh off the boat") has been used to refer to recent immigrants. Once these identities have been assigned, they can follow individuals and affect their lives based on the reactions other people have when they discover the labels. How might your behavior toward an individual change (for example, how likely would you be to hire the person) if you learned that he or she carried the label "felon"?

Conformity and Obedience

Behavior can often be contagious; for example, have you ever walked past someone on the street who is staring up at something on a tall building or in the sky? If you have never had this experience, try it and see what happens—more than likely other people around you will also start looking up. People, as social creatures, tend to do what others are doing. This can have an interesting impact on behavior. There are two well-known experiments that sought to investigate the influence of conformity and obedience.

Solomon Asch wanted to test the effects of **group pressure** (or **peer pressure**) on individuals' behavior, so he designed a series of simple experiments where subjects would be asked to participate in a study on visual perception. In the experiment, subjects were asked to determine which of three lines was most similar to a comparison line (there was one line that was clearly identical to the comparison line and the other two were clearly longer). When subjects completed this task alone, they erred less than 1% of the time. When subjects were placed in a room with several other people who they thought were also participating in the study, but who were actually **confederates** (meaning that they were part of the experiment), the results were quite different. On the first few tests, all of the confederates responded correctly. However, after a little while, the confederates began all choosing one of the incorrect lines. What's interesting is that Asch found that more than one-third of subjects conformed to the group by answering incorrectly. They chose to avoid the discomfort of being different, rather than trust their own judgment in answering. The phenomenon of adjusting behavior or thinking based on the behavior or thinking of others is called **conformity**.

Another commonly referenced experiment is **Stanley Milgram**'s study of obedience involving fake shocks. The participants in this study believed that they were in control of equipment that delivered shocks to another subject (the "learner") who was attempting to pass a memory test. No shocks were actually used. A researcher was in the room and directed the participant to administer increasing levels of shock to this purported subject, a confederate, by turning a dial whenever he or she answered incorrectly. The only contact the participant had with the learner was to hear the student's voice from the other room. When shocks were given at particular levels, the participants would hear moans, shouts of pain, pounding on the walls, and after that, dead silence. Milgram found that participants in the study were surprisingly obedient to the researcher's demands that they continue to administer the shocks. Out of 40 subjects, few questioned the procedure before reaching 300 volts and 26 of the subjects continued all the way to the maximum 450 volts. Milgram conducted many variations on his original experiment, to see how various independent variables affected obedience. He found that decreased distance of the "learner," increased distance of the authority figure, more casual wardrobe of the authority figure, and a shabbier office location all decreased obedience among subjects. While this series of experiments has long been considered a seminal study in the area of obedience research, many have sharply questioned not only Milgram's ethics (this experiment would never be permitted today) but also his methodology and the importance of his findings. Many note that only one variation of the original experiment yielded the oft-cited high rates of obedience. Moreover, there is evidence that many subjects did not believe they were actually administering shocks to the learner.

There are three ways that behavior may be motivated by social influences:

1) *Compliance*: compliant behavior is motivated by the desire to seek reward or to avoid punishment. There is likely to be a punishment for disobeying authority. Compliance is easily extinguished if rewards or punishments are removed.
2) *Identification*: identification behavior is motivated by the desire to be like another person or group. A participant who conformed in Asch's experiment likely did not want to be disapproved of for choosing a different answer than the rest of the group. Identification endures as long as there is still a good relationship with the person or group being identified with and there are not convincing alternative viewpoints presented.
3) *Internalization*: internalized behavior is motivated by values and beliefs that have been integrated into one's own value system. Someone who has internalized a value not to harm others may have objected to the shocks administered in Milgram's study. This is the most enduring motivation of the three.

When the motivation for compliance is desire for the approval of others and to avoid rejection, this is called **normative social influence**. With normative social influence, people conform because they want to be liked and accepted by others. This often leads to public compliance, but not necessarily private acceptance of social norms. **Informational social influence** is the process of complying because we want to do the right thing and we feel like others "know something I don't know." Informational social influence is more likely to apply to new situations, ambiguous situations, or situations in which an obvious authority figure is present.

There are several factors that influence conformity:

1) *Group Size:* a group doesn't have to be very large, but a group of 3–5 people will elicit more conformity than one with only 1–2 people.
2) *Unanimity:* there is a strong pressure not to dissent when everyone else agrees. However, if just one person disagrees, others are more likely to voice their real opinions.
3) *Cohesion:* an individual will more likely be swayed to agree with opinions that come from someone within a group with which the individual identifies.
4) *Status:* higher-status people have stronger influence on opinions.
5) *Accountability:* People tend to conform more when they must respond in front of others rather than in closed formats in which they cannot be held accountable for their opinions.
6) *No Prior Commitment:* once people have made public commitments, they tend to stick to them. For example, once someone has taken a pledge to become a fraternity brother, he is more likely to follow the norms of that group.

6.3 SOCIAL INTERACTION AND BEHAVIOR

All social interactions take place within social structures, which are composed of five elements: statuses, social roles, groups (previously discussed), social networks, and organizations. These five elements are developed through the process of socialization, discussed earlier. Social interactions include behaviors such as expressing emotion, managing others' impressions, and communicating.

Social Structures

Statuses and Roles

Status is a broad term in sociology that refers to all the socially defined positions within a society. These can include positions such as "president," "parent," "resident of Wisconsin," and "Republican." Needless to say, one person can hold multiple statuses at the same time. Some of these statuses may place someone in a higher social position while others may imply a lower position. One's **master status** is the one that dominates the others and determines that individual's general position in society. For example, an A-list movie star's life is typically completely dominated by the master status of "famous celebrity;" few people ever consider her other statuses, such as "wife," "mother," "American," etc. Sometimes the master status is not one the individual prefers; someone with a disability may be strongly identified by others as holding that status, with less attention paid to her other statuses, which she may find more important and fulfilling.

Statuses may be ascribed or achieved. **Ascribed statuses** are those that are assigned to a person by society regardless of the person's own efforts. For example, gender and race are ascribed statuses. **Achieved statuses** are considered to be due largely to the individual's efforts. These can include statuses such as "doctor," "parent," or "Democrat."

Roles

Social roles are expectations for people of a given social status. It is expected that doctors will possess strong medical knowledge and be intelligent. Role expectations can also come with ascribed statuses. There may be an expectation that a female is more likely to be a babysitter than a male. Roles help contribute to society's stability by making things more predictable.

However, roles can also be sources of tension in multiple ways. **Role conflict** happens when there is a conflict in society's expectations for *multiple statuses* held by the same person (for example, a male nurse or a gay priest). **Role strain** occurs when a *single status* results in conflicting expectations. For example, a homosexual man may feel pressure to avoid being "too gay" and also "not gay enough." **Role exit** is the process of disengaging from a role that has become closely tied to one's self-identity to take on another. Some examples include the transition from high school student to more independent college student living on campus with peers. Another would be transitioning from the workforce to retirement. These transitions are difficult because they involve the process of detaching from something significant, as well as embarking on something new and unknown.

Networks and Organizations

Networks

Think about the people you know. Now think about the people that those people know. As you keep extrapolating to more distant connections, you can get a sense of your **social network**. A social network is a web of social relationships, including those in which a person is directly linked to others as well as those in which people are indirectly connected through others. Facebook is a popular online social network. Social networks are often based on groups to which individuals belong. Network ties may be weak, but they can be powerful resources for meeting people (for example, using a network like LinkedIn to find a job).

Organizations

6.3

Large, more impersonal groups that come together to pursue particular activities and meet goals efficiently are called **organizations**. They tend to be complex and hierarchically structured. Formal organizations can include businesses, governments, and religious groups. Organizations serve the purpose of increasing efficiency, predictability, control, and uniformity in society. They also allow knowledge to be passed down more easily, so that individual people become more replaceable. As an example, consider going to a McDonald's. Because this corporation is an organization, one may expect a particular experience and menu options regardless of who is actually working at that particular restaurant.

There are three types of organizations. **Utilitarian organizations** are those in which members get paid for their efforts, such as businesses. **Normative organizations** motivate membership based on morally relevant goals, for example, Mothers Against Drunk Driving (MADD). **Coercive organizations** are those for which members do not have a choice in joining (for example, prisons). Like groups, organizations are influenced by statuses and roles and also help define statuses and roles.

Social Interactions

Expressing and Detecting Emotion

The physiological basis of emotion will be discussed in Chapter 7. Emotion is also vital in explaining how we react to situations and others. Emotions arise based on our (typically unconscious) appraisals of situations. The ability to quickly appraise situations using emotion has evolutionary significance: if we hear something and feel fearful, we might have the opportunity to escape a threatening situation faster than if we were to wait to see what was causing the noise, and then make a decision about whether it would be a good idea to escape. Some emotional responses, such as likes, dislikes, and fears, involve no conscious thought. More complex emotions, like hatred, love, guilt, and happiness, can have important influences on our memories, expectations, and interpretations. Take a simple example: if you are having an awful day and are in a really crummy mood when your mother calls you, you might have an expectation that she is calling to nag you about something, even when she is actually calling for some other reason.

We detect emotion in others using clues: their body language, tone and pitch in their voices, and expression on their faces, which can display an impressive array of emotions that humans are precisely wired to detect (Chapter 7). For example, through experiments it was determined that if we glimpse a face for a mere tenth of a second, we can accurately judge the emotion it portrays. The eyes and mouth are the two areas of the face that convey the most emotion: we can detect fear and anger in the eyes and happiness in the mouth. Some of our facial muscles can actually betray our emotions if we are trying to conceal our feelings. For example, lifting the inner part of the eyebrow conveys distress or concern. Raising the eyebrows and pulling them together conveys fear. Muscles in the eyes and cheeks convey happiness through smiling. Some people are more sensitive to emotional cues than others, and introverts are better at reading others' emotions, while extroverts are generally easier to read.

Gender Shapes Expression

Some studies suggest that women surpass men at reading emotional cues. Women's greater sensitivity to nonverbal cues perhaps explains their greater emotional literacy, or ability to describe their emotions. Men tend to describe emotions in simpler ways, while women are generally capable of describing more complex emotions. Women also demonstrate greater emotional responsiveness in positive and negative situations, with the one exception being anger. Anger is the one emotion that seems to be considered by most a "masculine" emotion. For example, when shown pictures of a gender-neutral face that was either smiling or angry, people were more likely to assume the face was male if it was angry, and female if it was smiling. **Empathy**, the ability to identify with others' emotions, is relatively equal between the sexes. Both men and women can "put themselves in someone else's shoes" and feel that person's pain or elation. But women are more likely than men to *express* empathy by crying or reporting genuine distress at another's misfortune. In studies, women tend to experience emotional events more deeply, with greater brain activation in the areas that process emotion, and are better able to remember emotional events later.

Culture Shapes Expression

Culture provides an additional filter for interpreting emotion. In other cultures, common emotions like fear and happiness are expressed in ways that Americans may find difficult to interpret. Gestures (movements of the hands and body that are used to express emotion) vary widely among cultures. For example, the use of a thumbs-up sign indicates to an American that things are "okay," but is used as an insult in some other cultures, whereas the extension of just the middle finger expresses anger or discourtesy in America, but is a neutral symbol in several other cultures. Certain facial expressions, however, seem to be universal; babies and blind people make the same universal emotional expressions with their faces. While cultures do share universal facial expressions, the degree to which emotion is expressed is influenced by culture. Cultures that promote individuality (such as Western cultures) also encourage emotional expressiveness. Like many other facets of human interaction, emotion is best understood by considering its biological, psychological, and sociological aspects.

Impression Management

In sociology and psychology, **impression management** or **self-presentation** is the conscious or unconscious process whereby people attempt to manage their own images by influencing the perceptions of others. This is achieved by controlling either the amount or type of information, or the social interaction. People construct images of themselves and want others to see them in certain lights. There are multiple impression management strategies that people employ. Assertive strategies for impression management include the use of active behaviors to shape our self-presentations, such as talking oneself up and showing off flashy status symbols to demonstrate a desired image. Defensive strategies for impression management include avoidance or self-handicapping. **Self-handicapping** is a strategy in which people create obstacles and excuses to avoid self-blame when they do poorly. It is easier to erect external hindrances to explain our poor performances than to risk considering, or having others consider, an internal characteristic to be the cause of a poor performance. A classic example is the student who loudly lets everyone know before an exam that she did not study. Her strategy is such that if she receives a poor grade on the exam, it can't be blamed on her intelligence (an internal characteristic that is likely an important element of her self-esteem), but must rather be blamed on an external factor, the fact that she didn't study.

Front Stage Versus Back Stage Self

The **dramaturgical perspective** in sociology stems from symbolic interactionism and posits that we imagine ourselves as playing certain roles when interacting with others. This perspective uses the theater as a metaphor for the way we present ourselves; we base our presentations on cultural values, norms, and expectations, with the ultimate goal of presenting an acceptable self to others. Dramaturgical theory suggests that our identities are not necessarily stable, but dependent on our interactions with others; in this way, we constantly remake who we are, depending on the situations we are in. Social interaction can be broken into two types: front stage and back stage. On the **front stage**, we play a role and use impression management to craft the way we come across to other people. On the **back stage**, we can "let down our guard" and be ourselves. For example, the way you dress and behave at work (front stage) is potentially very different from your dress and behavior at home (back stage).

Verbal and Nonverbal Communication

Nonverbal communication involves all of the methods for communication that we use that do not include words. Because humans are inherently visual creatures, a majority of these cues are visual, but we employ other cues as well. Nonverbal communication includes gestures, touch, body language, eye contact, facial expressions, and a host of finer subtleties. The act of communicating verbally also employs a lot of nonverbal cues, such as pitch, volume, rate, intonation, and rhythm. In a society in which written communication is exploding in popularity (for example, emails and text messaging), we also employ nonverbal cues in our writing, such as emoticons and emojis, use of capitalization and punctuation, and spacing. Consider the following three text messages. Each uses the same three words, yet they each express slightly different ideas:

OH MY GOSH!!!!!

Oh. My. Gosh.

Oh my… Gosh?

Social Behavior

Social behavior occurs between members of the same species within a given society. Communication occurs between members of the same species, and not usually between different species. Specific social behaviors include attraction, aggression, attachment, and social support.

Attraction

Attraction between members of the same species is a primary component of love, and explains much about friendship, romantic relationships, and other close social relationships. Researchers in social psychology are particularly interested in studying human attraction because it helps to explain how much we like, dislike, or hate others. Research into human attraction has found that the following three characteristics foster attraction: proximity, physical attractiveness, and similarity.

Proximity

Proximity (geographic nearness) is the most powerful predictor of friendship. Think of the people you consider your closest friends. How many of them shared a grade school classroom or a neighborhood with you growing up? How many people from your freshman dorm or living situation do you still consider to be close friends? People are more inclined to like, befriend, and even marry others from the same class, neighborhood, or office. People prefer repeated exposure to the same stimuli; this is known as the **mere exposure effect**. With certain exceptions, familiarity breeds fondness. This partially explains the common affinity for celebrities, and the fact that many people vote based on name recognition alone, regardless of whether or not they know much about a candidate. The tendency to like those in close proximity probably has an evolutionally foundation; for our ancestors, the familiar faces were likely the ones that could be trusted.

Appearance

Appearance also has a powerful impact on attraction. Physical attractiveness is an important predictor of attraction; in fact, studies show that people rate physically attractive people higher on a number of characteristics and traits, indicating that physically attractive people are somehow more likeable. While many aspects of attractiveness vary across cultures, some appear to be culturally universal, such as youthful appearance in women (perhaps reflecting a biological constraint of fertility), and maturity, dominance, and affluence in men. Humans also tend to prefer average, symmetrical faces. Attractiveness is also influenced by personality traits; people believed to have positive personality traits are judged more attractive.

Similarity

Similarity between people also impacts attraction. Friends and partners are likely to share common values, beliefs, interests, and attitudes. The more alike people are, the more their liking for each other endures over time.

Aggression

While attraction is an important unifying force in society, aggression is the opposite: a potentially destructive force to social relations. **Aggression** is broadly defined as behavior that is forceful, hostile, or attacking. In sociology, aggression is considered something that is intended to cause harm or promote social dominance within a group. Aggression can be communicated verbally or by actions or gestures. While aggression is employed for a variety of reasons by humans today (competitive sports, war, getting ahead at work), in non-human animals it is generally employed as a means for protecting resources, such as food, territory, and mates. Indeed, aggression was likely employed for similar reasons by prehistoric humans, and as our society evolved, we began using aggression in additional ways.

Aggression is considered an instinct, but biology and society can influence aggression. There are three types of predictors for aggressive behavior: genetic, neural, and biochemical. Identical twin studies suggest that there is some genetic predisposition toward aggressiveness; if one twin has a temper, the other tends to as well. Humans and other animals are naturally wired both to inhibit and to exhibit aggressive behavior. While no particular locus in the brain controls aggression, certain areas are thought to facilitate aggression, while other areas (in the frontal lobe) inhibit aggression. Many biochemical factors can alter the neural control of aggression. Alcohol, for example, can lower aggression inhibition, making someone more aggressive while drunk. Animals also tend to exhibit less aggression when they are castrated.[1]

Many psychological and social factors are thought to trigger aggression in humans. The **frustration-aggression principle** suggests that when someone is blocked from achieving a goal, this frustration can trigger anger, which can lead to aggression. Other frustrating stimuli, such as physical pain, unpleasant odors, and hot temperatures can also lead to aggression. Aggression is more likely to occur in situations in which prior experience has somehow promoted aggression. For example, if a child acts aggressively toward another child and ends up getting what she wants (lunch money, for example), she is more likely to behave in an aggressive manner in the future. People who are ostracized are also more likely to behave aggressively, which may partially explain some of the mass shootings that have occurred in schools and public spaces. While it would be a mistake to oversimplify the roots of aggression, it seems clear that biology, experience, and society combine to provide the fodder for aggression.

---

[1] Though castration does not *completely* remove aggression, as territorial battles between "fixed" housecats illustrate.

6.3

Social Support

Social support is a major determinant of health and wellbeing for humans and other animals. Family relationships provide comfort, and close relationships are predictive of health outcomes. Happily married people live longer, healthier lives, regardless of age, sex, and race. People who have social support have been shown to engage in healthier behaviors; they are less likely to smoke, more likely to exercise, and report a better capacity to cope with adversity and stress. Interestingly, social support is not confined to human-human interactions. People with dogs or other pets also reap some of the benefits of social support.

Biological Explanations of Social Behavior in Animals

Many animals also exhibit a wide range of social behavior. Some species (such as ants, bees, and wasps) engage in highly organized and hierarchical social behaviors, with each individual playing a specific role within the group. Most mammals also engage in social behavior, and many interesting phenomena have been elucidated by studying how mammals interact with members of their own species.

Foraging Behavior

Foraging behavior describes the search for and exploitation of food resources by animals. Securing food can come at a high energetic cost, which is an important consideration for organisms; the amount of energy it requires a lion to track, chase, and kill an antelope, or the amount of energy it takes an antelope to search for and graze upon enough foliage to sustain itself matters greatly to that organism's patterns of behavior. Ethologists believe that organisms employ learning behavior in the search for food. Since an organism's environment is constantly changing, it is important that foraging behavior be adaptable. Many organisms employ observational learning of older members in the group to learn behaviors such as knowing what is safe to eat.

Mating Behavior and Mate Choice

Mating behavior involves the pairing of opposite-sex organisms for the purposes of reproduction and the propagation of genes. Mating behaviors include courtship rituals, copulation, the building of nests, and the rearing of offspring for specific periods. For animals, mating strategies include random mating, disassortative mating, and assortative mating. In random mating, all members of a species are equally likely to mate with each other, meaning that there are no spatial, genetic, or behavioral limitations on mating. This ensures the largest amount of genetic diversity, and protects against genetic drift and bottlenecking. Assortative mating is a nonrandom mating pattern in which individuals with similar genotypes or phenotypes mate with each other more frequently than would be expected with random mating. In negative assortative mating, also known as disassortative mating, individuals with more disparate traits mate more frequently than would be expected with random mating.

Inclusive Fitness and Altruism

The **inclusive fitness** of an organism is defined by the number of offspring the organism has, how it supports its offspring, and how its offspring support others in a group. The inclusive fitness theory proposes that an organism can improve its overall genetic success through altruistic social behaviors. An **altruistic behavior** is one that helps ensure the success or survival of the rest of a social group, possibly at the expense of the success or survival of the individual. For example, the ground squirrel, a social mammal that lives in dens underground, will sound an alarm call if it sees a predator near the group. The alarm call does two things: first, it alerts the rest of the group to danger, and second, it calls the predator's attention to the particular squirrel that makes the noise. Therefore, in many instances, alerting the group results in the demise of the individual that sounded the alarm. Even though the alerter has not survived to reproduce, it has helped promote the survival of the rest of the clan, many of whom are probably close genetic relatives. In this way, the altruistic behavior of the ground squirrel has increased its own inclusive fitness by ensuring the survival of its siblings and other genetic relatives.

Applying Game Theory

Evolutionary **game theory** is used to try and predict large, complex systems, such as the overall behavior of a population. Evolutionary game theory has been used to explain many complex and challenging aspects of biology, such as how altruistic behaviors work in the context of Darwinian natural selection. While it may seem that large groups of animals and large crowds of people are too complex to accurately predict behavior, game theory suggests that it might be possible to do so. This type of analysis might be useful, for instance, in predicting the behavior of a large crowd of people in an enclosed space during a disaster. While this field is still emerging, it may be quite possible to accurately predict behavior in complex living systems in the future.

6.4   SOCIAL COGNITION AND INTELLIGENCE

Attitudes are an important part of what makes us human and what makes us unique. Our attitudes about people, places, and things are shaped by experience, but can be highly mutable. Attitude and behavior are intimately related, and it is important to understand how both develop and change over time.

Elaboration Likelihood Model

Persuasion is one method of attitude and behavior change. When you change your beliefs about something, there are a few factors that likely come into play. For example, say you are listening to two speeches about the importance of expanding the ban on smoking in public spaces. The first orator is attractive, but his argument is not well-formulated. The second orator's speech has better, more logical arguments, but he is not as attractive. Whose argument will persuade you more? The **elaboration likelihood model** explains when people will be influenced by the content of the speech (or the logic of the arguments), and when people will be influenced by other, more superficial characteristics like the appearance of the orator or the length of the speech.

Since persuasion can be such a powerful means for influencing what people think and do, much research has gone into studying the various elements of a message that is likely to be highly persuasive. The three key elements are message characteristics, source characteristics, and target characteristics.

1) The **message characteristics** are the features of the message itself, such as the logic and number of key points in the argument. Message characteristics also include more superficial factors, such as the length of the speech or article and its grammatical complexity.
2) The **source characteristics** of the person or entity delivering the message, such as expertise, knowledge, and trustworthiness, are also of importance. People are much more likely to be persuaded by a major study described in the *New England Journal of Medicine* than in the pages of the local supermarket tabloid.

6.4

3) Finally, the **target characteristics** of the person receiving the message, such as self-esteem, intelligence, mood, and other such personal characteristics, have an important influence on whether a message will be perceived as persuasive. For instance, some studies have suggested that those with higher intelligence are less easily persuaded by one-sided messages.

The two **cognitive routes** that persuasion follows under this model are the central route and the peripheral route. Under the **central route,** people are persuaded by the *content* of the argument. They ruminate over the key features of the argument and allow those features to influence their decisions to change their points of view. The **peripheral route** functions when people focus on superficial or secondary characteristics of the speech or the orator. Under these circumstances, people are persuaded by the attractiveness of the orator, the length of the speech, whether the orator is considered an expert in his field, or other features. The elaboration likelihood model asserts that people will choose the central route only when they are both motivated to listen to the logic of the argument (they are interested in the topic), and they are not distracted, thus focusing their attention on the argument. If those conditions are not met, individuals will choose the peripheral route, and, if persuaded at all, will be persuaded by more superficial factors. Messages processed via the central route are more likely to have longer-lasting persuasive outcomes than messages processed via the peripheral route.

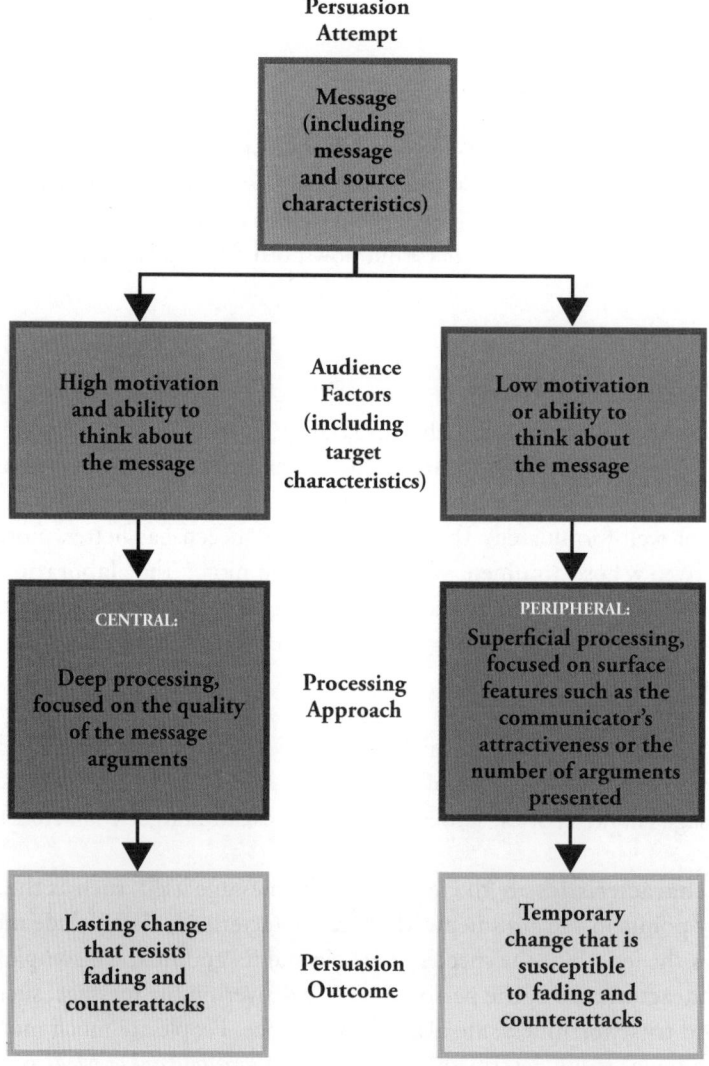

Figure 3   Elaboration likelihood model: central vs. peripheral processing routes

Social Cognitive Theory

The social cognitive perspective incorporates elements of cognition, learning, and social influence. **Social Cognitive Theory** is a theory of behavior change that emphasizes the interactions between people and their environment. However, unlike behaviorism (where the environment controls us), cognition (how we process our environment) is also important in determining our behavior. Social cognitive theory focuses on how we interpret and respond to external events and how our past experiences, memories, and expectations influence our behavior. According to social cognitive theory, **social factors**, observational learning, and environmental factors can also influence a person's attitude change. The opinions and attitudes of your friends, family members, and other peer groups often have a major influence on your beliefs.

Reciprocal determinism is the interaction between a person's behaviors (conscious actions), personal factors (individual motivational forces or cognitions; personality differences that drive a person to act), and environment (situational factors). There are three different ways that individuals and environments interact.

1) People choose their environments which in turn shape them. For example, the college that you chose to attend had some sort of unique impact on you.
2) Personality shapes how people interpret and respond to their environment. For example, people prone to depression are more likely to view their jobs as pointless.
3) A person's personality influences the situation to which she then reacts. Experiments have demonstrated that how you treat someone else influences how they will treat you. For example, if you call customer service because you are furious about something, you are more likely to receive a defensive or aggressive response on the phone.

In these three ways people both shape, and are shaped by, their environments.

Behavioral Genetics

Genetics plays an important role in the behavior of humans and other animals. **Behavioral genetics** attempts to determine the role of inheritance in behavioral traits; the interaction between heredity and experience determines an individual's personality and social behavior.

Almost every cell in the body contains DNA [which cells in humans do not contain DNA?[2]], and this DNA contains genes, some 20,000 or so in humans. Genes encode the information for creating proteins, the building blocks of physical development. To help determine what makes us different (for example, why one person suffers from schizophrenia while his brother does not), it is vital to understand the variations in both our genes and our environments. The **genotype** is the genetic makeup of an organism, while the **phenotype** is the observable characteristics and traits. Behavioral genetics seeks to understand how the genotype and environment affect the phenotype.

Most phenotypes are influenced by several genes and by the environment; for example, tallness in humans is the result of the interaction between several genes, and is also the result of proper nutrition at key developmental stages. If someone is born with genes for tallness, but is malnourished as a child, they will not grow nearly as tall as their genotype might indicate. Therefore, in order to determine the influence of genes versus the environment (the old "nature versus nurture" argument!), behavioral genetics uses two types of studies in humans: twin studies and adoption studies.

---

[2] Mature red blood cells do not contain DNA.

6.4

Twin studies compare traits in monozygotic (identical) and dizygotic (fraternal) twins. Monozygotic (MZ) twins have essentially identical genotypes[3] and an almost identical environment (assuming they are reared together), starting from the womb[4]. Dizygotic (DZ) twins share roughly 50% of their DNA (they are genetically no more similar than ordinary siblings), and an arguably similar environment, starting in the womb. The classic twin study attempts to assess the variance of a phenotype (behavior, psychological disorder) in a large group in order to estimate genetic effects (heritability) and environmental effects (both from shared environment or experiences and unshared/unique environment or experiences). If identical twins share the phenotype more than fraternal twins (which is the case for most traits), genes likely play an important role. For example, if one MZ twin develops Alzheimer's disease, the other MZ twin has a 60% chance of developing it as well. Alternatively, if one DZ twin develops the disease, the other only has a 30% chance of developing it. By comparing hundreds of twin pairs, researchers can understand more about the roles of genetic effects, shared environment, and unique environment in shaping behavior.

Adoption studies present another unique way to study the effects of genetics and environment on phenotype. Adoption creates two groups: genetic relatives and environmental relatives. Adopted individuals can be compared with both groups to determine if they are more similar to their genetic relatives or their environmental relatives. The advantage of adoption studies over twin studies is that they can help to elucidate the impact of both heredity and environment on phenotype. Twin studies can only examine the impact of genetics because the environment is so similar for each twin. Interestingly, hundreds of studies have shown that people who grow up together do not much resemble one another's personalities. Adopted children have personalities more similar to their biological parents than their adopted parents; traits such as agreeableness, extraversion, introversion, etc. tend to pass from parents to biological offspring. However, adopted children are more similar to their adoptive families in terms of attitudes, values, manners, faith, and politics.

There have been some cases of identical twins separated at birth and raised independently by different adopted families. Psychologists have noted that these individuals, despite being raised in completely different environments with no contact with each other while growing up, are remarkably similar in terms of their tastes, physical abilities, personality, interests, attitudes, and fears.

Using twin and adoption studies, behavioral geneticists can mathematically estimate heritability for many phenotypes. Heritability does not pertain to an individual, but rather to how two individuals differ. For example, the estimated heritability of intelligence (the variation of intelligence scores attributable to genetic factors) is roughly 50%. This does not mean that your genes are responsible for 50% of your intelligence, rather, it means that heredity is responsible for 50% of the variation in intelligence between you and someone else. In fact, it means that genetic differences account for 50% of the variation in intelligence *among all people*.

---

[3] Though MZ twins have the same genes, they don't always have the same number of copies of a gene; this may help to explain why one develops a disease, while the other does not. Furthermore, X inactivation in female somatic cells is not identical between MZ female twins; therefore, female MZ twins are actually not *quite* as identical as male MZ twins!

[4] About 70% of MZ twins share a placenta in the womb, and in some instances, one twin will receive more blood flow, resulting in differential nutrition and growth between the two. Additionally, approximately 30% of MZ twins develop separate placentas and therefore may have slightly different prenatal conditions, as well.

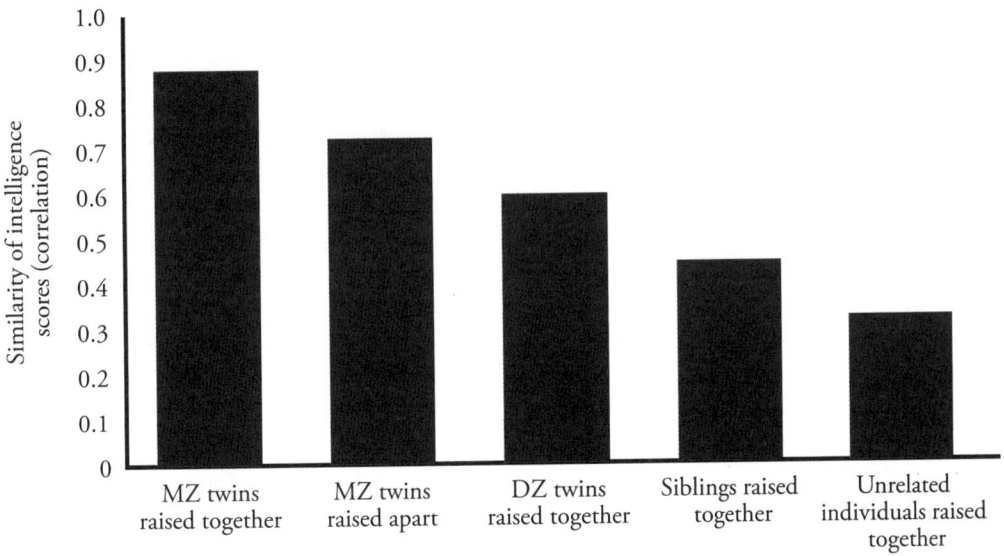

6.4

Figure 4   The heritability of intelligence, estimated using twin studies and adoption studies

In animals, the interaction between genotype and phenotype is easier to study because genes and environment can be more tightly controlled. Researchers can use **transgenesis** (the introduction of an exogenous[5] or outside gene) or knockout genes to alter genotype while controlling for environment. Transgenic animal models are useful for helping researchers understand what happens when a certain gene is present. For example, transgenic mice that have had human cancer genes introduced can help researchers study how and when cancer develops, and how cancer responds to various treatments in the mouse model (before trying the treatments on humans). Knockout animal models are useful for helping researchers understand what happens when a gene is absent. For example, knockout mice that are missing a specific gene known to protect against cancer can also help researchers understand how and why cancer develops, and how it responds to treatment.

One of the most important aspects of all life—from single-celled organisms to human beings—is the capacity for adaptation. Genes and environment work together; not only do genes code for proteins, but they also respond to the environment. Genes might be turned on in one environment and turned off in another. For example, in response to an ongoing stressor, one gene might begin producing more of a neurotransmitter involved in overeating, which then leads to obesity. The gene itself was not hard-wired to produce obesity, but an interaction between the gene and the environment resulted in obesity.

Genes and environment interact. Consider the example of **temperament** (emotional excitability): infants who are considered "difficult" have a temperament that is more irritable and unpredictable, while infants who are considered "easy" have a more placid, quiet, and easygoing temperament. While heredity might predispose infants toward these temperament differences, an easy baby will be treated differently than a difficult baby, and studies have shown that temperament persists through childhood and beyond. Do difficult babies grow up to be aggressive, pugnacious teenagers because their temperament is genetically wired, or because their parents reacted to their irritability and unpredictability in infancy with frustration and unsupportive caregiving? It is difficult to say, but it is important to understand that both heredity and environment play an important role in many complex human traits, such as personality (of which temperament is one aspect), intelligence, and motivation.

---

[5] In Greek, "exo" means "outside" and "gignomi" means "to come to be."

Intellectual Functioning

Multiple Definitions of Intelligence

What is intelligence? We often think of it as something objective that can be measured like height and weight, but the concept of intelligence is a human creation. A common definition is the ability to learn from experience, problem-solve, and use knowledge to adapt to new situations. But there is no neurological trait that defines intelligence. Consider the concept of athleticism. Athleticism can be broadly defined as physical prowess. However, it becomes difficult to define details since athleticism could be defined by one's speed, agility, ability to lift weights, or visual motor skills. Based on the criteria, a golfer or a football player may or may not be considered an athlete.

Theories of Intelligence

Francis Galton first proposed a theory of general intelligence in the mid 1800s. Galton believed intelligence had a strong biological basis and could be quantified by testing certain cognitive tasks. Galton's book, *Hereditary Genius*, argues that intelligence is genetically determined. In the early 1900s, **Alfred Binet** administered intelligence tests to schoolchildren in France, with the goal of developing a measure to determine which children were in need of special education. The intelligence test, better known as an IQ (intelligence quotient) test, created by Binet (and his collaborator, Theodore Simon) was later revised by a psychologist at Stanford University and renamed the Stanford-Binet Intelligence Scale. Also in the early 1900s, **Charles Spearman** first coined the term **general intelligence** (also referred to as "Spearman's g"); Spearman, like Binet, believed that intelligence could be strictly quantified through cognitive tests, and those who possessed high general intelligence would do well on lots of different measures of cognitive ability.

In the mid-twentieth century, psychologist **Raymond Cattell** proposed two types of intelligence: fluid intelligence (Gf), which is the ability to "think on your feet" and solve novel problems, and crystallized intelligence (Gc), which is the ability to recall and apply already-learned information (which is the majority of what you are expected to do in school—learn and memorize information, then apply it on test day). In the 1980s, **Howard Gardner** put forth a theory on multiple intelligences, which breaks intelligence down into eight different modalities: logical, linguistic, spatial, musical, kinesthetic, naturalist, intrapersonal, and interpersonal intelligences. This theory is a nice counter to the idea that intelligence is a single general ability that can be conveniently measured and quantified by an IQ test. While Gardner was not the first to consider the importance of social intelligence (**Edward Thorndike** first proposed the idea of social intelligence in the 1920s, defined as the ability to manage and understand people), the theory of multiple intelligences did renew interest in the concept of social intelligence. This renewed interest led to the idea of emotional intelligence in the 1990s. Emotional intelligence involves being well attuned to one's own emotions, being able to accurately intuit the emotions of others, and using this information as a guide for thinking and acting. Studies suggest that both emotional intelligence and social intelligence are correlated with good leadership skills, good interpersonal skills, positive outcomes in classroom situations, and better functioning in the world.

Influence of Heredity and Environment on Intelligence

Is it natural ability, or is it the environment and experiences that determine one's intellectual abilities? As you might expect, it's a little bit of both. Studies of twins, family members, and adopted children indicate that there is significant heritability of intelligence. Scores on intelligence tests taken by identical twins correlate highly, while those of adopted children more closely resemble scores of their birth parents than of their adoptive parents. However, although genes are a predisposing factor, life experiences affect one's performance on intelligence tests. Malnutrition, sensory deprivation, social isolation, and trauma can affect normal brain development in childhood. On the other hand, early intervention and schooling can increase intelligence scores.

Also remember that intelligence is a social construct. The way it is measured is determined by cultural context. In many Western cultures, intelligence is often thought of as superior performance on academic and cognitive tasks. Some of these tasks emphasize speed, because it is valued in those societies. However, other cultures may emphasize emotional and spiritual knowledge, or social skills.

Variations in Intellectual Ability

Some differences have been found in how various groups perform on intelligence tests. These differences have often been attributed to biases within the tests themselves or related to outside confounding factors. For example, controversial but well-established findings are that racial groups differ in their average scores on intelligence tests, and that high-scoring people are more likely to attain high levels of education and income. However, these differences are potentially due to environmental factors, such as the availability of quality schooling.

Intellectual abilities at the upper and lower extremes have profound social and functional implications. At the lower extreme are individuals whose intelligence scores fall below 70. On intelligence tests, a score of 70 is two standard deviations below the average score of 100. Individuals who not only have a score below 70, but also have difficulty adapting to everyday demands of life are classified as having an **intellectual disability**. Sometimes, intellectual disability is the product of a physical cause, such as Down's syndrome or an acquired brain injury. Students with mild intellectual disabilities are educated in the least restrictive environments in which they can learn, and they are integrated into regular classrooms with accommodations if possible. At the upper extreme, high intelligence scores (130+) often serve as selection criteria for gifted education.

Experience and Behavior

While it is true that our genes play an important role in our behavior, our individual experiences and our social experiences also shape our behavior in important ways. The **life course perspective**, or **life course approach** looks at how key events in a person's life such as marriage, professional milestones, and the birth of children unfold over time and lead to a person's development. As social animals, we learn ways of thinking and behavior from our families and peer groups. An individual's development, then, is determined by a complex interplay of biology, psychology, society, and culture. Biological influences include the inherited genome, prenatal development, sex-related genes, hormones, and physiology. Psychological influences include gene-environment interactions, significant experiences, responses evoked in others by our own traits (such as our temperament or gender), and beliefs, feelings, and expectations. Social and cultural influences include families, peers, friends, cultural ideals, cultural mores, and cultural norms.

Chapter 6 Summary

- Culture refers to the beliefs and practices that a social group shares.

- Socialization is the process by which people learn the norms, values, attitudes, and beliefs necessary to become proficient members of society.

- Norms are spoken or unspoken rules and expectations for the behavior in society.

- Cultural assimilation occurs when an individual forsakes their own culture to completely adopt another culture; amalgamation occurs when majority and minority groups combine to form a new group.

- Multiculturalism or pluralism endorses equal standing for all cultural traditions within a society.

- A subculture is a segment of society that shares a distinct pattern of traditions and values that differs from that of the larger society.

- Self-concept or self-identity is the sum of an individual's understanding of him- or herself, including physical, psychological, and social attributes.

- Personal identity includes personal attributes (such as age, disability status, ethnicity/race), while social identity consists of social definitions (such as religion, gender, occupation).

- Self-efficacy is a belief in one's own competence and effectiveness, while self-esteem is an individual's evaluation of his or her overall worth.

- Those with an internal locus of control believe they are able to influence outcomes through their own effort; those with an external locus of control believe outcomes are controlled by outside forces.

- Multiculturalism or pluralism endorses equal standing for all cultural traditions within a society.

- Kohlberg described six stages of moral development; most adults reach stage 4, but few reach stage 6.

- In order to determine whether behavior should be attributed to internal or external causes, consistency, distinctiveness, and consensus must be considered.

- The fundamental attribution error occurs when people tend to underestimate the impact of the situation and overestimate the impact of a person's character or personality on observed behavior.

- The self-serving bias is the tendency to attribute our successes to ourselves and our failures to others or to the external environment.

- The optimism bias is the belief that bad things happen to other people, but not to us; the just world phenomenon is a tendency to believe that the world is fair and people get what they deserve.

- Stereotypes are oversimplified ideas about groups of people, based on characteristics (race, gender, sexual orientation, religion, disability, etc.).

- A self-fulfilling prophecy occurs when stereotypes lead to behaviors that affirm the original stereotypes; stereotype threat refers to a self-fulfilling fear that one will be evaluated based on a negative stereotype.

- The social facilitation effect occurs when people perform simple, well-learned tasks better when other people are present.

- Deindividuation occurs in situations that provide a high degree of arousal and a very low sense of responsibility, when people lose their sense of restraint and their individual identity by identifying with a group or mob mentality.

- The bystander effect predicts the finding that a person is less likely to provide help when there are other bystanders.

- Social loafing is the tendency for people to exert less effort when they are being evaluated as a group than when they are individually accountable.

- Group polarization occurs when group members adopt more extreme versions of their original viewpoints as the result of group membership.

- Groupthink is a phenomenon that occurs within a group when the desire for harmony or conformity in the group results in a consensual perspective without much thought of alternative viewpoints.

- Deviance is a violation of society's expectations or standards of conduct.

- Behavior is motivated by social influences when there is compliance, identification, and internalization.

- Several factors influence conformity: group size, unanimity, cohesion, status, accountability, and lack of prior commitment.

- The elaboration likelihood model of persuasion is the theory that attitudes are formed by dual processes: the central processing route (which includes high motivation and deep processing of the message) or by the peripheral processing route (which includes low motivation and superficial processing of the messenger).

- Behavioral genetics attempts to determine the role of inheritance in behavioral traits; the interaction between heredity and experience determines an individual's personality and social behavior.

CHAPTER 6 FREESTANDING PRACTICE QUESTIONS

1. Agent(s) of socialization include:

    I. parents.
    II. teachers.
    III. friends.

    A) I only
    B) I and II
    C) II and III
    D) I, II, and III

2. Eli studies really hard for his chemistry class but keeps getting poor scores on quizzes and lab assignments. Eventually, he begins to feel like nothing he does will improve his performance in chemistry. When faced with future chemistry assignments, Eli doesn't even bother trying because he feels destined to fail at chemistry. This can best be described as:

    A) learned helplessness.
    B) an internal locus of control.
    C) incongruity.
    D) the fundamental attribution error.

3. Marcia wears clothing that she thinks are appropriate but that are also sharply criticized by her community. Upon learning of the criticism, Marcia is overcome with guilt and feelings of shame. As a result, she vows never to wear that type of clothing again. According to Kohlberg, Marcia is most likely at which level/stage of moral development?

    A) Preconventional morality
    B) Stage 1: Punishment and obedience orientation
    C) Conventional morality
    D) Stage 6: Universal ethical principles

4. When new members of a society eventually become indistinguishable from the rest of society, adopting the language, norms, and customs, which process has occurred?

    A) Multiculturalism
    B) Amalgamation
    C) Assimilation
    D) Groupthink

5. A researcher randomly surveys people, asking them how they found out about their most recent job: either through an acquaintance or through a close friend. The researcher concluded that the results proved the social network theory, which suggests:

    A) more respondents found their jobs from an acquaintance rather than a close friend.
    B) more respondents found their jobs from a close friend rather than an acquaintance.
    C) half of the respondents found their jobs from an acquaintance, while the other half of the respondents found their jobs from a close friend.
    D) a majority of respondents found their jobs on their own.

6. A doctor does a checkup on a 40-year-old patient and talks to him in a serious and professional manner. A few moments later, the same doctor goes to a different room to do a routine checkup on a 5-year-old patient. The doctor makes funny faces throughout the checkup in order to make the patient laugh. This scenario is most closely related to which concept?

A) Deviance
B) Impression management
C) Conflict theory
D) Symbolic interactionism

7. College students have started an environmental awareness club on their campus. At the first meeting, they gave out a questionnaire, which indicated that the students in attendance strongly favored policies protecting the environment. At the end of the school year, the questionnaire was re-administered to the same students. The results indicated that the membership had become even more strongly in favor of environmental protection policies. This scenario most likely illustrates which of the following phenomenon?

A) Groupthink
B) Group polarization
C) Deindividuation
D) Peer pressure

8. Despite having a stake in an upcoming election, a citizen eligible to vote declines to go to the polls, declaring that her vote is too insignificant to make a difference and she knows her candidate will win anyway. Her behavior is most demonstrative of which of the following?

A) Social loafing theory
B) Opponent-process theory
C) Regression to the mean
D) Group polarization

CHAPTER 6 PRACTICE PASSAGE

When people want to establish a new form of identity, they undergo an exiting process to transition from their ex-role to their new role. The exiting process from their ex-role will be satisfied once society gives acknowledgment to the individual's change in identity. This is a difficult transition because society has already set expectations for the individual based on their ex-role. Through a series of interviews with people who have undergone role exiting, ranging from ex-nuns to ex-convicts, researchers found several issues that individuals encounter in the process of creating new roles.

The first issue that individuals face is the presentation of self. Individuals use external and internal indicators to publicly show others that they would like to be treated differently from their past selves. For example, transgender individuals, who identify with a gender that is the opposite of their biological sex, alter their clothes and mannerisms based on what they believe society considers acceptable for the sex they want to convey in their new role. It is the responsibility of others in society to recognize the individual's new identity through the newly acquired props and mannerisms the individual employs.

Social reaction is another issue for those exiting an old role and assuming a new one. During the exiting process, individuals are affected by reactions they receive from society based on their ex-role. Role exits are either socially desirable (such as being a drug user turning into an ex-drug user) or socially undesirable (such as being a doctor and turning into an ex-doctor). People continue to hold positive or negative expectations about the old role that an individual is trying to break away from as they continue through the exiting process. However, the more society expects certain behaviors from an individual, the more likely the individual will act in a way they are expected to act. For instance, if parents and teachers continue to treat a student like a delinquent, it is likely that the student will continue to misbehave because he is fulfilling the role assigned. The presentation of self and social reaction to the ex-role together determine the difficulty of adapting to the new role for the individual.

Another challenge is the change of friendship networks for the individual. People who shift identities are inclined to distance themselves from their old peers in order to be surrounded with a network that would encourage and facilitate their new role. For example, individuals who are married surround themselves with other married couples. However, if they become "ex-spouses," they are likely to begin associating with single people and fellow divorcées because their interactions with other married couples are different and uncomfortable. Additionally, while in their old role, individuals formed bonds with other people. After role-exiting, individuals have to manage their relationships with people who continue to be a part of their ex-role as well as those who are part of their new role.

Finally, individuals face role residuals, which can also be known as "hangover identity." This concept describes the number of aspects that persist for an individual from an ex-role even after completing the exiting process to their newly formed identity. Overall, the more involved an individual was in his former role, the more likely he is to have a higher role residual compared to someone who was not as committed to his previous role.

Source: Adapted from H.R.F. Ebaugh, *Becoming an Ex: The Process of Role Exit*. ©1988 by The University of Chicago Press

1. Which of the following theories best describes the process of presentation of self in creating an ex-role?

A) Social facilitation
B) Dramaturgy
C) Social support
D) Peer pressure

2. Which of the following scenarios describes the self-serving bias?

A) An employee who receives a bonus believes this reward was well-deserved because of how hard she worked and all of the extra hours she put into her job.
B) A man who is ignored by a salesperson at a high-end suit store believes the salesperson is just a rude jerk.
C) A survey finds that most people think that attractive celebrities are good people.
D) An employee receives a promotion and feels lucky to have been "in the right place at the right time."

3. Based on the passage, which of the following types of social identities do transgender individuals try to express through their self-presentation?

    I. Sexual orientation
    II. Gender
    III. Biological sex

A) I only
B) II only
C) III only
D) II and III

4. A felon fails to find a job because potential employers are aware of his role as a convict. Which of the following concepts best describes this social reaction?

A) Social stigma
B) Social support
C) False consensus
D) Socialization

5. All of the following are ways that an individual's behavior may be motivated by social influences, EXCEPT:

A) compliance.
B) identification.
C) aggregation.
D) internalization.

6. Which of the following individuals would most likely experience "hangover identity?"

A) A biological male who identifies as a female, but has not yet begun the transition to the female gender
B) An alcoholic who was sober for six months and then relapsed
C) Someone who was married for six weeks and then gets a divorce
D) A recent retiree who worked at the same company for 45 years, had a tight group of friends at work, participated in the company Thursday night bowling league, and volunteered with her colleagues every holiday season in a neighborhood soup kitchen

SOLUTIONS TO CHAPTER 6 FREESTANDING PRACTICE QUESTIONS

1. **D** Item I is true: family, including parents, are considered agents of socialization (choice C can be eliminated). Item II is true: educators, like teachers, are agents of socialization (choice A can be eliminated). Item III is true: peers and friends are also agents of socialization (choice B can be eliminated; choice D is correct).

2. **A** Learned helplessness occurs when someone tries hard but fails repeatedly at a task. Eventually, the individual believes that they have no control over the outcome, develops an external locus of control (choice B is wrong), and stops trying (choice A is correct). Incongruity refers to the idea that the real self has fallen short of the ideal self; while this might pertain to the situation described in the question stem, there is not enough evidence to assume that succeeding in chemistry is part of Eli's idealized self (choice C is wrong). The fundamental attribution error occurs when an individual attributes the actions of others (but not their own actions) to dispositional factors (choice D is wrong).

3. **C** The question asks how far Marcia appears to have progressed in terms of Kohlberg's stages of moral development. Marcia views her behavior as bad if other people view it as bad, feeling shame and guilt when others criticize her. Thus, she is in the "conventional" level of morality. More specifically, she is most likely in stage 3 (the "good boy/girl" stage) in which morality is determined by others' approval (choice C is correct). If you didn't remember Kohlberg, you can use POE to eliminate some of the choices. Marcia seems to be past the stage 1: preconventional level of moral development in which good = avoidance of punishment (this is common among very young children). Marcia genuinely feels guilty and ashamed because she believes she did something wrong; she's not simply conforming to escape some punishment (choices A and B can be eliminated). Stage 6: universal ethical principles wouldn't seem to fit here either. Marcia sees an action as "wrong" because others see it that way, not because it violates some higher universal moral code that she's developed (choice D can be eliminated).

4. **C** Assimilation occurs when a new member forgoes her own culture in order to adapt to the dominant culture. When new members of society eventually become indistinguishable from the rest of society, assimilation has occurred (choice C is correct). Multiculturalism asserts that different cultures can live harmoniously without newcomers feeling the need to adjust or adapt to the dominant culture (choice A is wrong). Amalgamation occurs when two cultures combine to form a new culture, different from both of the original cultures (choice B is wrong). Groupthink is the phenomenon whereby a cohesive group establishes a consensual perspective without much thought to alternative viewpoints (choice D is wrong).

5. **A** The social network theory posits that people's networks are important and necessary for the spread of ideas and resources; there is much strength in weak ties because weak ties allow the sharing of new resources to a vast network. It is more likely for participants to find jobs through an acquaintance (weak tie) than a close friend (strong tie; choice A is correct). Although having strong ties has an advantage with respect to people's networks, there is a sense of redundancy with the information and resources provided; generally people's strong ties have information that the person is already aware of since they are a part of the same

cluster (choice B is wrong). Since the researcher concluded that the results "proved the social network theory," it wouldn't make sense for the results to be half and half (choice C is wrong), nor would it make sense that most respondents found their jobs on their own (choice D is wrong).

6. **B**   Impression management involves expressing different aspects of oneself, depending on the person on the receiving end of the interaction. The doctor acts differently toward the 40-year-old patient and the 5-year-old patient (choice B is correct). Deviance occurs when an individual is violating social norms. It is socially acceptable for the doctor to act professionally with the adult and silly with the child (choice A is wrong). Conflict theory is the belief that inequality exists due to an uneven distribution of power and resources in society; this theory is unrelated to the scenario described in the question (choice C is wrong). Symbolic interactionism asserts that the way individuals interpret interactions affects how they choose to interact. In comparison with impression management, symbolic interactionism is not more closely related to the scenario and does not fully explain the doctor's different behavior toward the two patients (choice D is wrong).

7. **B**   The key words are "strongly favored policies protecting the environment" and "even more strongly in favor of environmental protection policies." The correct answer choice will be a concept in social psychology that explains how like-minded people, when they have been meeting over time, tend to become even more intensely aligned with their original points of view. That is choice B, group polarization (choices A, C, and D do not match the scenario and are incorrect).

8. **A**   According to social loafing theory, people working in groups will exert less effort when they are not held individually accountable, downplaying the importance of their own contribution while assuming that someone else will take up the slack. Because the citizen described does have a stake in the election, but decides not to vote because she believes her vote won't make a difference (she assumes that the candidate will win because everyone else will vote for that candidate), her behavior can best be explained by social loafing (choice A is correct). The opponent-process theory has to do with color perception, not group behavior (choice B is wrong) and regression to the mean is a statistical phenomenon, not a social one (choice C is wrong). Group polarization describes the phenomenon whereby a group's views become more extreme; it does not explain the scenario presented in the question stem (choice D is wrong).

SOLUTIONS TO CHAPTER 6 PRACTICE PASSAGE

1. **B**   In the second paragraph, the mention of "props" is a strong indicator that dramaturgy is implicated, which is the concept that individuals' lives are a stage and they use the appropriate props to portray their respective roles (choice B is correct). Social facilitation is the idea that an individual will perform better on simple or familiar tasks because of the presence of other people; this concept does not apply to the process of presentation of self (choice A is incorrect). Social support involves having a strong network to assist the individual in times of need; this does not best explain the process of presentation of self (choice C is incorrect). Peer pressure involves peers influencing one another to conform; the passage implies that the individuals choose to change themselves as opposed to being pressured into doing so (choice D is incorrect).

2. **A**   Self-serving bias occurs when we attribute our successes to ourselves and our failures to external factors; the employee who attributes her promotion to her own hard work is the best example of the self-serving bias (choice A is correct). Self-serving bias does not attribute success to external factors like luck (choice D is wrong). The man who believes a salesperson is a rude jerk after he is ignored by the salesperson is committing a fundamental attribution error, by attributing the salesperson's actions to some internal element of personality (choice B is wrong). The physical attractiveness stereotype explains why people tend to believe that attractive people are also "good" people (choice C is wrong).

3. **B**   Item I is false: sexual orientation describes an individual's sexual attraction and preference; while this is a social identity, transgender individuals are not attempting to convey information about their sexual preferences through presentation of self (choice A can be eliminated). Item II is true: gender is a social identity; transgender individuals express their self-perceived gender through the use of outward indicators. The passage specifies that transgender individuals use clothing and a change in behavior to adjust to gender norms of society (choice C can be eliminated). Item III is false: biological sex is not a social identity; rather, it is based on human biology. The passage example focuses on the act of presenting the individual's self through props and characteristics rather than body parts (choice D can be eliminated, and choice B is correct).

4. **A**   Social stigma involves negative societal attitudes toward an individual or group due to some perceived mark of shame or inferiority; ex-felons have high social stigma since their former role as a convict is greatly disapproved of in society (choice A is correct). Social support describes close relationships people have with each other, typically within a family; the scenario presented in the question stem does not demonstrate social support (choice B is incorrect). A false consensus occurs when an individual believes that everyone else agrees with what they do; like social support, false consensus has no relevance to the scenario (choice C is incorrect). Socialization is the process of creating an individual identity based on what one learns from society's norms, values, and customs; socialization does not explain the social reaction to the ex-felon (choice D is incorrect).

5. **C** There are three ways that an individual's behavior may be motivated by social influences. Compliance is a desire to seek rewards or avoid punishment (choice A is a motivating factor and can be eliminated). Identification is the desire to be like another person or group (choice B is a motivating factor and can be eliminated). Internalization happens when values and beliefs are integrated into a person's own value system and then drives their behavior (choice D is a motivating factor and can be eliminated). However, aggregation is not a term in sociology; an *aggregate* describes people who exist in the same space but do not share a common sense of identity (choice C is not a motivating behavior and is the correct answer choice).

6. **D** A "hangover identity" (also known as a role residual) can occur when several aspects persist for an individual from an ex-role even after completing the exiting process to a newly formed identity. According to the final paragraph, "the more involved an individual was in his former role, the more likely he is to have a higher role residual compared to someone who was not as committed to his previous role." Therefore, a newly retired individual who worked at the same company for a long time and was very involved with her coworkers would be most likely to experience "hangover identity" upon transitioning into her new role as retiree (choice D is correct). A biological male who has not begun the process of transitioning to female has not yet abandoned his former role (choice A is wrong), and neither the alcoholic nor the married person was committed to the role at issue for a significant amount of time (choices B and C are wrong).

Chapter 7
Personality, Motivation, and Emotion

Many different qualities make up an individual; our personalities are a big part of who we are (some might say *all* of who we are!). Each of us has a personality shaped over time by both internal and external factors. We all develop our own unique sets of attitudes and opinions and are driven by different motivating forces: these are also important aspects of who we are as individuals.

7.1 PERSONALITY

Theories of Personality

Personality, while very hard to precisely define, is essentially the individual pattern of thinking, feeling, and behavior associated with each person. Personalities are nuanced and complex. Various theories and perspectives on personality have evolved to help explain this fundamental aspect of individuality, including the psychoanalytic perspective, the humanistic perspective, the behaviorist perspective, the social-cognitive perspective, the trait perspective, and the biological perspective. Therapies to treat personality disorders are based on the first four perspectives (psychoanalytic therapy, humanistic or person-based therapy, behavioral therapy, and cognitive behavioral therapy).

Psychoanalytic Perspective

According to **psychoanalytic theory**, personality (made up of patterns of thoughts, feelings, and behaviors) is shaped by a person's unconscious thoughts, feelings, and memories. These unconscious elements are derived from past experiences, particularly interactions with primary early caregivers. What a person is conscious of is quite limited, like the tip of an iceberg compared with his or her vast unconscious stores of experiences, memories, needs, and motivations below the surface. According to psychoanalytic theory, the existence of the unconscious is inferred from behaviors such as dreams, slips of the tongue, posthypnotic suggestions, and free associations.

Within classical psychoanalytic theory as developed by **Sigmund Freud**, two instinctual drives motivate human behavior. The **libido**, or life drive, generates behaviors focused on survival, growth, creativity, pain avoidance, and pleasure. Note that libido is commonly defined as "sex drive," but libido includes more than just sexual energy. The **death drive** generates aggressive behaviors fueled by an unconscious wish to die or to hurt oneself or others.

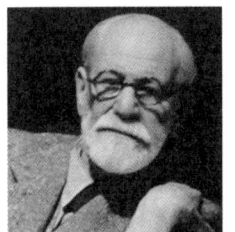

Sigmund Freud

Psychic energy is distributed among three personality components that function together: id, ego, and superego.

1) The largely unconscious **id** is the source of energy and instincts. Ruled by the **pleasure principle**, the id seeks to reduce tension, avoid pain, and gain pleasure. It does not use logical or moral reasoning, and it does not distinguish mental images from external objects. According to Freud, young children function almost entirely from the id.

2) The **ego**, ruled by the **reality principle**, uses logical thinking and planning to control consciousness and the id. The ego tries to find realistic ways to satisfy the id's desire for pleasure.

3) The **superego** inhibits the id and influences the ego to follow moralistic and idealistic goals rather than just realistic goals; the superego strives for a "higher purpose." Based on societal values as learned from one's parents, the superego makes judgments of right and wrong and strives for perfection. The superego seeks to gain psychological rewards such as feelings of pride and self-love, and to avoid psychological punishment such as feelings of guilt and inferiority.

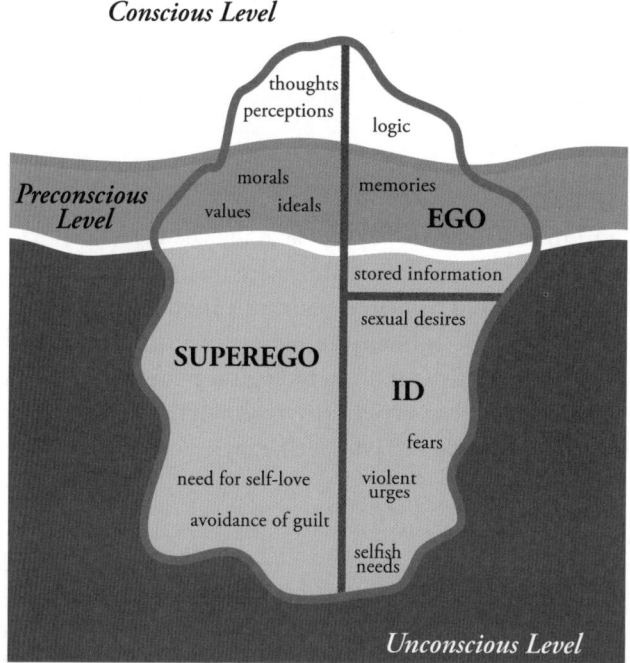

Figure 1 Freud's iceberg analogy to the human mind and personality

According to Freud, anxiety is a feeling of dread or tension, a warning of potential danger, that occurs when a person begins to become aware of repressed feelings, memories, desires, or experiences. To cope with this anxiety and protect the ego, all people develop **ego defense mechanisms** that unconsciously deny or distort reality. Ego defense mechanisms are therefore normal, and become unhealthy only when taken to extremes. The psychoanalyst Anna Freud published a book-length discussion of the ego and its defenses. Several (but not all) common ego defense mechanisms are described in Table 1.

Table 1 Some Common Ego Defense Mechanisms

Defense Mechanism	Description
Repression	Lack of recall of an emotionally painful memory
Denial	Forceful refusal to acknowledge an emotionally painful memory
Reaction Formation	Expressing the opposite of what one really feels, when it would feel too dangerous to express the real feeling (such as acting hateful toward someone to whom one is inappropriately sexually attracted)
Projection	Attributing one's own unacceptable thoughts or feelings to another person ("I'm not angry; you are!")
Displacement	Redirecting aggressive or sexual impulses from a forbidden action or object onto a less dangerous one (as when a person goes home and kicks the dog instead of expressing anger at a boss)
Rationalization	Denying the true motivations for one's behavior while believing false ones that are reassuring or otherwise self-serving (such as believing that embezzling from one's company was an act of politically-motivated "wealth distribution" as opposed to base greed)
Regression	Reverting to an earlier, less sophisticated behavior (as when a child reverts to bedwetting after a trauma)
Sublimation	Channeling aggressive or sexual energy into positive, constructive activities, such as producing art

According to psychoanalytic theory, at each developmental stage throughout the lifespan, certain needs and tasks must be satisfied. When these needs and tasks are not met, a person harbors unresolved unconscious conflicts that lead to psychological dysfunction. There are two different theories of developmental stages that you should be familiar with: Sigmund Freud's psychosexual stages and Erik Erikson's psychosocial stages.

Freud suggested that sexual energy is present from infancy, and that each person matures through **five psychosexual stages** (the oral, anal, phallic, latent, and genital stages), each corresponding to whichever part of the body is the focus of sensual pleasure. In the **oral stage**, the child seeks sensual pleasure through oral activities such as sucking and chewing. In the **anal stage**, the child seeks sensual pleasure through control of elimination. In the **phallic stage**, the child seeks sensual pleasure through the genitals. At this stage, the child is both sexually attracted to the opposite-sex parent and hostile toward the same-sex parent, who is seen as a rival. This is known as the **Oedipus complex** in a boy, and the **Electra complex** in a girl. Girls are also said to experience **penis envy** during the phallic stage (as they discover that they do not have penises). During the **latency stage**, sexual interests subside and are replaced by interests in other areas such as school, friends, and sports. The **genital stage** begins in adolescence, when sexual themes resurface and a person's life/sexual energy is not only directed toward various rewarding activities, but also toward members of the opposite sex outside the family unit.

According to Freud, adult personality is largely determined during the first three psychosexual stages. If parents either frustrate or overindulge the child's expression of sensual pleasure at a certain stage so that the child does not resolve that stage's developmental conflicts, the child becomes **psychologically fixated** at that stage, and will, as an adult, continue to seek sensual pleasure through behaviors related to that stage. For example, if an infant is not fed adequately he or she might become an orally-fixated adult, continually overeating, smoking cigarettes, and abusing alcohol.

Several prominent theorists emerged from the community around Sigmund and Anna Freud and developed their own versions of psychodynamic theory. These include Carl Gustav Jung, Alfred Adler, Karen Horney, and Melanie Klein, among others.

In particular, **Erik Erikson** extended Freud's theory of developmental stages in two ways. Erikson added social and interpersonal factors to supplement Freud's focus on unconscious conflicts within a person. And Erikson delineated eight developmental stages and conflicts in adolescence and adulthood to supplement Freud's focus on early childhood. Also, note that Erikson's stages are much less rigid than Freud's with respect to age range, and he accounted for considerable variability from person to person. The ages given (table, next page) are approximations.

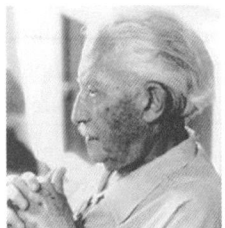

Erik Erikson

1) In Erikson's first stage, the infant's task is to resolve the crisis of **trust versus mistrust**. If an infant's physical and emotional needs are not met, as an adult he or she may mistrust the world and interpersonal relationships.

2) In the second stage, the toddler must resolve the crisis of **autonomy versus shame and doubt**. If a toddler's need to explore, make mistakes, and test limits is not met, as an adult he or she may be dependent rather than autonomous.

3) In the third stage, the preschool-age child must resolve the crisis of **initiative versus guilt**. If a young child's need to make decisions is not met at this stage, as an adult he or she may feel guilty taking initiative and instead allow others to choose.

4) In Erikson's fourth stage, the school-age child must resolve the crisis of **industry versus inferiority**. If a child's need to understand the world, develop a gender-role identity, succeed in school, and set and attain personal goals is not met at this stage, as an adult he or she may feel inadequate.

5) The fifth stage occurs in adolescence and involves resolving the crisis of **identit**
   confusion. If an adolescent does not test limits and clarify his or her identity,
   meaning, he or she may develop role confusion.

6) The young adult faces the sixth stage: resolving the crisis of **intimacy versus isolat**   n
   does not form intimate relationships at this stage, he or she may become alienated

7) In the seventh stage, which occurs in middle age, a person must resolve the cri
   generativity versus stagnation. If a person does not feel productive by helpin;
   generation and resolving differences between actual accomplishments and earli
   or she may become psychologically stagnant.

8) Finally, in later life, a person must resolve the crisis of **integrity versus despaii**
   eighth and final stage. If a person looks back with regrets and a lack of personal worth at this
   stage, he or she may feel hopeless, guilty, resentful, and self-rejecting.

Table 2   Freud's and Erikson's Developmental Stages

Age	Psychosexual Stages (Freud)	Age	Psychosocial Stages (Erikson)
Birth to 1 year	Oral • Sensual pleasure in mouth area	Birth to 1.5 years	Infancy • Trust vs. mistrust • Physical and emotional needs met
1–3 years	Anal • Sensual pleasure in controlling elimination	1.5–3 years	Early childhood • Autonomy vs. shame and doubt • Explore, make mistakes, test limits
3–6 years	Phallic • Sensual pleasure in genital area • Incestuous desire for the opposite-sex parent	3–5 years	Preschool age • Initiative vs. guilt • Make decisions
6–12 years	Latency • Localized sensual pleasures disappear • Pursue school, friends, sports	6–12 years	School age • Industry vs. inferiority • Gender-role identity, school success, attain personal goals, understand the world
12 +	Genital • Sensual pleasure returns to genital area • Life/sexual energy fuels friendships, art, sports, careers, and relationships with the opposite sex	12–18 years	Adolescence • Identity vs. role confusion • Identity, goals, life meaning, limit-testing
		18–40 years	Young adulthood • Intimacy vs. isolation • Form intimate relationships
		40–65 years	Middle age • Generativity vs. stagnation • Help next generation and resolve the difference between dreams and accomplishments
		65+ years	Later life • Integrity vs. despair • Look back with no regrets and feel personal worth

Psychoanalytic therapy uses various methods to help a patient become aware of his or her unconscious motives and to gain insight into the emotional issues and conflicts that are presenting difficulties. Therefore, one of the goals of therapy is to help the patient become more able to choose behaviors consciously. Another goal of therapy is to strengthen the ego, so that choices can be based on reality rather than on instincts (id) or guilt (superego). Psychoanalytic therapy is sometimes referred to as "talk therapy" because therapy sessions usually focus on patients talking about their lives. The therapist will listen for patterns or significant events that may play a role in the client's current difficulties. Psychoanalysts believe that childhood events and unconscious feelings, thoughts, and motivations play a role in mental illness and maladaptive behaviors. Psychoanalytic therapy may also use other techniques such as free association, role-play, and dream interpretation.

Humanistic Perspective

In contrast to classical psychoanalytic theory, which tends to focus on conflicts and psychopathology, the **humanistic theory** focuses on healthy personality development. According to this theory, humans are seen as inherently good and as having free will, rather than having their behavior determined by their early relationships. In humanistic theory, the most basic motive for all people is the **actualizing tendency**, which is an innate drive to maintain and enhance the organism. Like a child learning to walk, a person will grow toward **self-actualization**, or realizing his or her human potential, as long as no obstacle intervenes.

According to humanistic theory, as developed by **Carl Rogers**, when a child receives disapproval from a caregiver for certain behavior, he or she senses that the caregiver's positive regard is conditional. In order to win the caregiver's approval and still see both self and caregiver as good, the child introjects the caregiver's values, taking them on as part of his or her own self-concept. The **self-concept** is made up of the child's conscious, subjective perceptions and beliefs about his or her self. The child's true values remain but are unconscious, as the child pursues experiences consistent with the introjected values rather than the true values. The discrepancy between conscious introjected values and unconscious true values is the root of psychopathology. This discrepancy between the conscious and unconscious leads to tension, not knowing oneself, and a feeling that something is wrong.

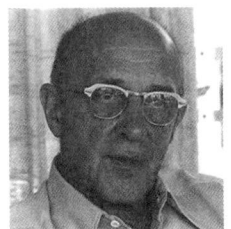

Carl Rogers

People choose behavior consistent with their self-concepts. If they encounter experiences in life that contradict their self-concepts, they feel uncomfortable **incongruence**. By paying attention to his or her emotional reactions to experiences, a person in an incongruent state can learn what his or her true values are, and then become healthy again by modifying the introjected values and self-concept and growing toward fulfillment and completeness of self. However, people usually find it easier to deny or distort such experiences than to modify their self-concepts.

The goal of **humanistic therapy** (also called **person-centered therapy**) is to provide an environment that will help clients trust and accept themselves and their emotional reactions, so they can learn and grow from their experiences. According to Rogers, the essential elements of such an environment are the therapist's trust in the client, and the therapist communicating genuineness (congruence), unconditional positive regard, and empathic understanding to the client. Using the term "client" rather than "patient" is meant to suggest the inherent health of the person and place the person on an equal level with the therapist.

Behaviorist Perspective

According to the **behaviorist perspective**, personality is a result of learned behavior patterns based on a person's environment. Behaviorism is **deterministic**, proposing that people begin as blank slates, and that environmental reinforcement and punishment completely determine an individual's subsequent behavior and personalities. This process begins in childhood and continues throughout the lifespan.

According to behaviorism, learning (and thus the development of personality) occurs through two forms of conditioning: classical conditioning and operant conditioning. In classical conditioning, a person acquires a certain response to a stimulus after that stimulus is repeatedly paired with a second, different stimulus that already produces the desired response. Classical conditioning is also called associational learning (see Chapter 9). In operant conditioning, behaviors are influenced by the consequences that follow them. An operant is a person's action or behavior that operates on the environment and produces consequences. Consequences are either reinforcements (which make it more likely that the operant will be repeated) or punishments (which make it less likely that the operant will be repeated). Both reinforcements and punishments can be positive or negative. In this context, the terms "positive" and "negative" are used to describe whether the consequence involves the presence or the absence of a particular stimulus. A positive reinforcement is the presence of a rewarding stimulus (e.g., money), and a negative reinforcement is the absence of an aversive stimulus (e.g., a respite from daily chores). A positive punishment is the presence of an aversive stimulus (e.g., an electric shock), and a negative punishment is the absence of a rewarding stimulus (e.g., taking away a teenager's car) (see Chapter 9 for more details on conditioning).

Table 3 Positive and Negative Reinforcement and Punishment

	Reinforcement	Punishment
Positive	Presence of rewarding stimulus	Presence of aversive stimulus
Negative	Absence of aversive stimulus	Absence of rewarding stimulus

Behavioral therapy uses conditioning to shape a client's behavior in the desired direction. Using the ABC model, the therapist first performs a functional assessment to determine the antecedents (A) and consequences (C) of the behavior (B). Therapy then proceeds by changing antecedents and consequences, using the least aversive means possible. Common applications of behavioral therapy include relaxation training and systematic desensitization to help clients manage fear and anxiety. In systematic desensitization, the client is helped to relax while repeatedly being exposed to real or imagined anxiety-producing stimuli, the intensity of which increase incrementally. This technique involves creating a hierarchy of fear-inducing versions of the disturbing object or situation (e.g., seeing a picture of a snake, seeing a snake across the room, holding a snake in one's hands, etc.).

Social Cognitive Perspective

According to the **social cognitive perspective**, personality is formed by a reciprocal interaction among behavioral, cognitive, and environmental factors. The behavioral component includes patterns of behavior learned through classical and operant conditioning, as well as **observational learning**. Observational, or **vicarious**, learning occurs when a person watches another person's behavior and its consequences, thereby learning rules, strategies, and expected outcomes in different situations. For example, studies found that children who watched aggressive and violent behavior in a video subsequently behaved with more aggression and violence toward a doll[1]. People are more likely to imitate models whom they like or admire, or who seem similar to themselves.

---

[1] The infamous "Bobo doll" experiments conducted by Albert Bandura in the early 1960s will be covered in more detail in Chapter 9.

The cognitive component of personality includes the mental processes involved in observational or vicarious learning, as well as conscious cognitive processes such as self-efficacy beliefs (beliefs about one's own abilities). The environmental component includes situational influences, such as opportunities, rewards, and punishments.

Behavioral therapy is usually combined with a cognitive approach and called **cognitive behavioral therapy** (CBT). From the cognitive perspective, a person's feelings and behaviors are seen as reactions not to actual events, but to the person's thoughts about those events. Each person thus lives by self-created, subjective beliefs about him- or herself, other people, and the world, and these beliefs color the person's interpretations of events. Many of these beliefs are formed during childhood, and they are often unconscious. From the cognitive perspective, the roots of psychopathology are irrational or dysfunctional thoughts and beliefs. The goal of cognitive psychotherapy is to help the client become aware of these and substitute rational or accurate beliefs and thoughts, which will lead to more functional feelings and behaviors.

Table 4   Comparison of the Major Therapy Types

Therapy	Assumed Problem	Therapy Goals	General Method
Psychoanalytic (also known as psychodynamic or talk therapy)	Unconscious forces and deleterious childhood experiences	Reduction of anxiety through self-insight	Analysis and interpretation
Humanistic (also known as client-centered or person-centered)	Barriers to self-understanding and self-acceptance	Personal growth through self-insight	Active listening and unconditional positive regard
Cognitive Behavioral (CBT)	Maladaptive behavior and/or negative, self-defeating thoughts	Extinction and relearning of undesired thoughts/behaviors and healthier thinking and self-talk	Reconditioning, desensitization, reversal of self-blame

Trait Perspective

A **personality trait** is a generally stable predisposition toward a certain behavior. Trait theories of personality focus on identifying, describing, measuring, and comparing individual differences and similarities with respect to such traits.

Trait theorists distinguish between surface and source traits. **Surface traits** are evident from a person's behavior. For example, a person might be described as talkative or exuberant. There are as many surface traits as there are adjectives for describing human behavior. Conversely, **source traits** are the factors underlying human personality and behavior; source traits are fewer and more abstract (see Table 5). Each trait is not binary but rather a continuum ranging between two or more extremes, such as extroversion and introversion.

The **Five-Factor Model** described by McCrae and Costa is widely accepted. The five factors in their model are extroversion, neuroticism, openness to experience, agreeableness, and conscientiousness.

Table 5   McCrae & Costa Personality Traits

Big Five Personality Traits (McCrae & Costa)	
Source Traits	**Surface Trait Examples**
Extroversion	Reserved / Affectionate Loner / Joiner Quiet / Talkative Internal stimuli / External stimuli
Neuroticism	Calm / Worrying Even-tempered / Emotional Secure / Sensitive Confident / Nervous Emotionally stable / Unstable
Openness to experience	Down-to-earth / Imaginative Uncreative / Original Prefer routine / Prefer variety Cautious / Curious Consistent / Inventive
Agreeableness	Antagonistic / Acquiescent Ruthless / Softhearted Suspicious / Trusting Cold / Friendly Unkind / Compassionate Obstinate / Cooperative Not pleasing / Pleasing others
Conscientiousness	Lazy / Hardworking Aimless / Ambitious Quitting / Persevering Ineffectual / Efficient Careless / Organized

Personality traits are thought to help predict a person's performance and enjoyment in certain careers. Assessments of personality traits are often used for career counseling, and by human resources departments as an aid to hiring and promotion decisions. Trait-based personality assessments are also used to help people understand and accept themselves and others. Each personality type is seen as having its own strengths and weaknesses. No type is identified as pathological, and weaknesses are viewed as characteristics to be aware of and manage, rather than to change. Trait theories are generally not concerned with explaining why a person has particular traits, although some have proposed that certain traits are biologically based.

Biological Perspective

From the biological perspective, much of what we call personality is at least partly due to innate biological differences among people. Support for this view is found in the heritability of basic personality traits, as well as in correlations between personality traits and certain aspects of brain structure and function.

Hans Eysenck proposed that a person's level of extroversion is based on individual differences in the reticular formation (which mediates arousal and consciousness). In this view, introverts are more easily aroused and therefore require and tolerate less external stimulation, whereas extroverts are less easily aroused and are therefore comfortable in more stimulating environments. Eysenck also proposed that a person's level of neuroticism is based on individual differences in the limbic system (which helps mediate emotion and memory). Correlations have been found between extroversion and the volume of brain structures involved with processing rewards, and between neuroticism and the volume of brain regions involved with processing negative emotions and punishment. In addition, twin studies and adoption studies (discussed in Chapter 6) have found strong evidence for the heritability of extroversion and neuroticism.

Jeffrey Alan Gray proposed that personality is governed by interactions among three brain systems that respond to rewarding and punishing stimuli. In this view, fearfulness and avoidance are linked to the "fight-or-flight" sympathetic nervous system, worry and anxiety are linked to the behavioral inhibition system, and optimism and impulsivity are linked to the behavioral approach system. **C. Robert Cloninger** also linked personality to brain systems involved with reward, motivation, and punishment. Cloninger proposed that personality is linked to the level of activity of certain neurotransmitters in three interacting systems. In this view, low dopamine activity correlates with higher impulsivity and novelty-seeking, low norepinephrine activity correlates with higher approval-seeking and reward dependence, and low serotonin activity correlates with risk avoidance. Correlations have been found between novelty-seeking and grey matter volume in the cingulate cortex, between reward dependence and grey matter volume in the caudate nucleus, and between harm avoidance and grey matter volume in the orbitofrontal, occipital, and parietal cortices.

Situational Approach to Explaining Behavior

The **person-situation controversy** (also known as the **trait versus state controversy**) considers the degree to which a person's reaction in a given situation is due to their personality (trait) or is due to the situation itself (state). **Traits** are considered to be internal, stable, and enduring aspects of personality that should be consistent across most situations. **States** are situational; they are unstable, temporary, and variable aspects of personality that are influenced by the external environment. For example, extroversion is a trait, stress is a state. The primary question is whether personality is consistent over time and across situations and contexts. A fair amount of research suggests that while people's personality *traits* are fairly stable, their *behavior* in specific situations can be variable. In other words, people do not act with predictable consistency, even if their personality traits are predictably consistent. In unfamiliar situations, people tend to modify their behavior based on **social cues** (verbal or nonverbal hints that guide social interactions); therefore, specific traits may remain hidden. For example, a person who is normally quite extroverted may seem quiet and reserved in an unfamiliar formal situation. In familiar situations, people may "act more like themselves" (the same extroverted person may be considerably more talkative in a familiar situation with friends). Averaging behavior over many situations is the best way to reveal distinct personality traits.

7.2 MOTIVATION

Out of all the behaviors that are possible, what motivates us (and all animals) to act in particular ways in particular moments? This process can be as simple as being motivated to take a drink of water due to a feeling of thirst or as complex as being motivated to undertake a difficult studying regimen and training program in order to become a physician due to a desire to help others.

Factors that Influence Motivation

Instincts

There are several factors that are understood to influence motivation. The first is **instinct**: behaviors that are unlearned and present in fixed patterns throughout a species. An example is imprinting in chicks, who learn to follow objects or organisms that are present when they hatch. In humans, instincts in babies include sucking behaviors, naturally holding the breath under water, and demonstrating fear when approaching drops in elevation. Instincts represent the contribution of genes, which predispose species to particular behaviors.

Drives / Negative Feedback Systems

Physiological drives can also push organisms to act in certain ways, as is the case when we are thirsty. A **drive** is an urge originating from a physiological discomfort such as hunger, thirst, or sleepiness. Drives can be useful for alerting an organism that it is no longer in a state of homeostasis, an internal state of equilibrium. They suggest that something is lacking: food, water, or sleep, for example. Drives often work through negative feedback systems, which are abundant in human physiology. The process of **negative feedback** works by maintaining stability or homeostasis; a system produces a product or end result, which feeds back to stop the system and maintains the product or end result within tightly controlled boundaries. Biological examples of negative feedback include regulation of blood pressure, blood glucose levels, and body temperature. These biological systems can have an important impact on behavior. For example, if blood glucose drops because you haven't eaten in hours, you will feel hungry and have a strong drive to eat. If your temperature begins to drop, you will feel cold and have a strong drive to seek warmth.

Arousal

However, instincts and drives cannot explain some of the artistic accomplishments of humans or the exploratory behavior of infants and animals. Even a toddler whose needs have all seemingly been met will wander around the room, putting objects in his or her mouth. This suggests that some behaviors are motivated by a desire to achieve an optimum level of arousal. A toddler who is not stimulated enough may seek stimulation by exploring the surroundings. An adult who is feeling bored will do the same. On the other hand, feeling overstimulated can lead to feelings of stress, which may lead one to seek ways to relax or sleep. Different people may have different optimal levels of arousal.

Needs

While including basic biological needs (physiological drives), this category also includes higher-level needs than those previously discussed. Instincts, drives, and arousal do not explain why a student may aspire to become a physician. In addition to drives, one may experience various needs, including a need for safety, a need for belonging and love, and a need for achievement.

Theories that Explain How Motivation Affects Human Behavior

Drive Reduction Theory

Since drives are physiological states of discomfort, it follows that we are motivated to reduce these drives through behaviors such as eating and drinking. Drive-reduction theory suggests that a physiological need creates an aroused state that drives the organism to reduce that need by engaging in some behavior. If your blood glucose drops, you feel hungry (or light-headed), and have a drive to eat. The greater the physiological need, the greater the physiological drive (an aroused and motivated state).

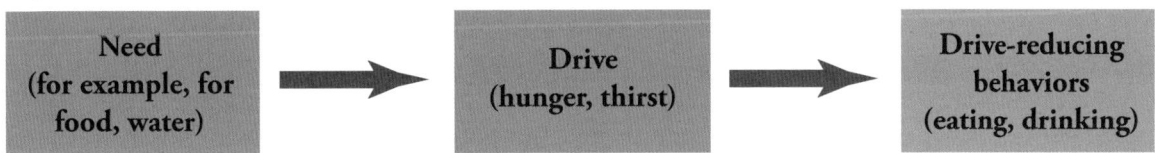

Figure 2   Drive-reduction theory

Incentive Theory

While drives are internal physiological needs, **incentives** are external stimuli in the environment that either encourage or discourage certain behaviors. Incentives can be positive and drive us to do something, or they can be negative and repel us from doing something. For example, if you were offered a new job accompanied by a large increase in salary, the salary might serve as a positive incentive. If the job also involved an increase in work hours, the increased workload might serve as a negative incentive. In general, behaviors are most strongly motivated when there are physiological needs, strong positive incentives, and a lack of negative incentives. For example, if you were walking down the street and were very hungry, smelled delicious pizza, and found out it was being given away for free, you'd have a strong motivation to eat it.

Expectancy-Value Theory

Expectancy-value theory posits that the extent to which human beings are motivated to act in a certain way is a function of 1) **expectancy**: the likelihood that the action under consideration will bring about a desired result; and 2) **value**: the degree to which the individual desires the anticipated result. When either of these two factors is very low, there will be little or no motivation to act. For example, a woman who learns of an essay contest, with the first prize being a free trip to France, might want desperately to win that contest. If she knows she has little or no chance of doing so, however, she is unlikely to put in much effort and may not even submit an entry. Conversely, a professional writer who has an excellent chance of winning, but who has no desire to visit France, would be similarly unmotivated. A gifted writer with a passion for everything French, however, may very well make an arduous effort to win that contest.

Self-Determination Theory

The basic tenet of **self-determination theory** is that human beings are inherently motivated to achieve personal growth and well-being. This ideal state of psychological health is thought to come essentially from **intrinsic** sources (i.e., from inside the person) as opposed to **extrinsic** sources (i.e., from the external world). For example, a social worker who strives to perform well at her job in order to receive a raise in salary will not consequently grow as a person. However, if she does her best simply for the satisfaction of knowing that she is a noble human being who is helping society, she will truly benefit from her hard work. Self-determination theorists believe that three core factors facilitate personal growth: 1) **autonomy**: one must feel in control of one's actions and free to make his or her own choices; 2) **competence**: one must believe that he or she possesses skills and abilities capable of producing results; and 3) **connection**: one must feel a sense of relatedness to the world and to other people such that his or her actions matter. When these three critical needs are met, the process of self-determination can occur.

Maslow's Hierarchy of Needs

Abraham Maslow sought to explain human behavior by creating a hierarchy of needs (Figure 3). At the base of this pyramid are physiological needs, or the basic elements necessary to sustain human life. If these needs are met, we will seek safety; if the need for safety is met, we will seek love, and so on. His pyramid suggests that not all needs are equal; some needs take priority over others. For example, an individual who is struggling every day to work and put food on the table will place a higher value on meeting physiological needs than on fulfilling a cognitive need for belongingness by joining a community organization that hopes to increase awareness of global warming. Maslow's hierarchy is somewhat arbitrary—it comes from a Western emphasis on individuality, and some individuals have shown the ability to reorganize these motives (for example, hunger strikes or eating disorders). Nevertheless, it has been generally accepted that we are only motivated to satisfy higher-level needs once certain lower-level needs have been met. The inclusion of higher-level needs, such as self-actualization and the need for recognition and respect from others, also explains behaviors that the previous theories do not.

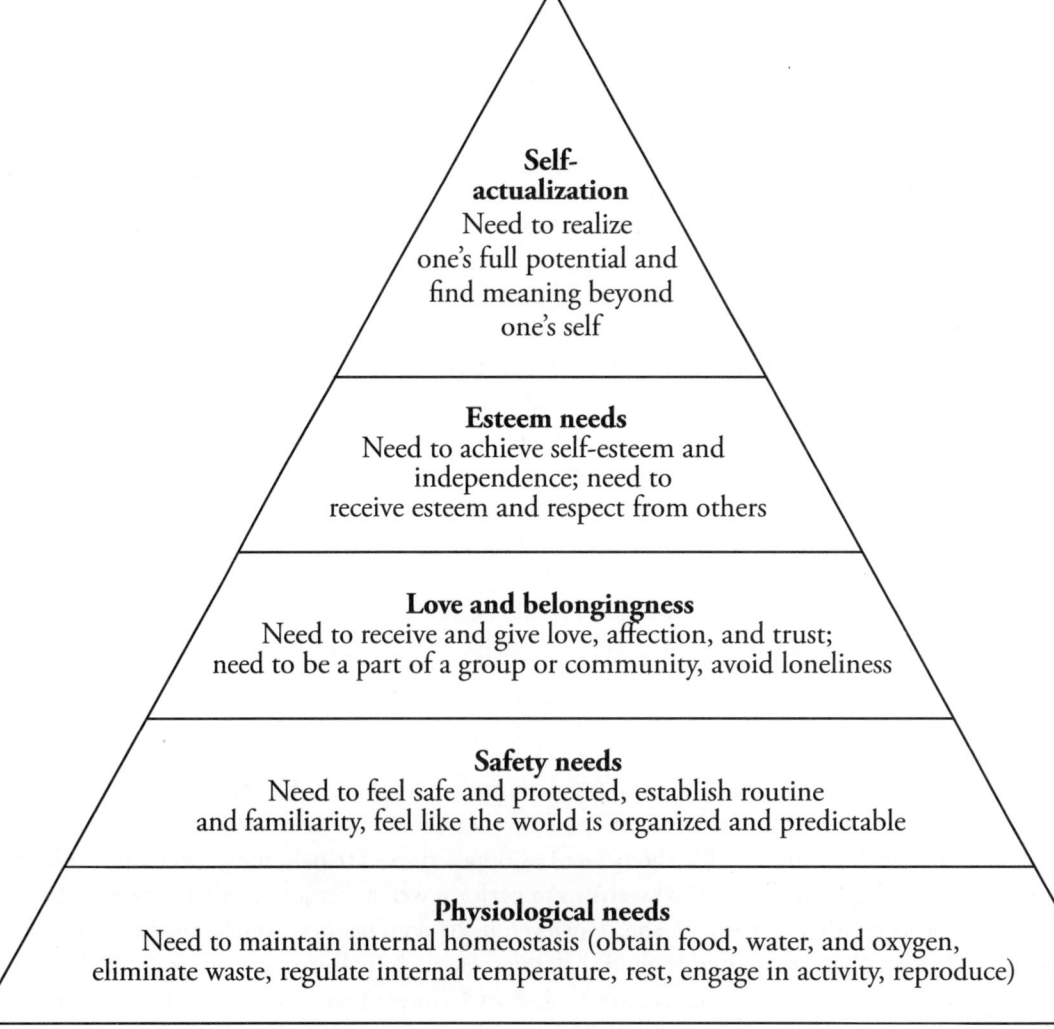

Figure 3 Maslow's hierarchy of needs

Application of Theories of Motivation to Understand Behaviors

Biological Factors that Regulate Motivation

As drive-reduction theory suggests, biological factors can play a large part in motivation. For many physiological processes, it is theorized that our bodies have a "set point" or a "sweet spot" at which things are in homeostasis. Our bodies also have mechanisms for detecting deviations from the set point and stimulating us to react either internally or behaviorally to regain the set point. Responses to body temperature variations, fluid intake, weight variations, and sexual stimulation are regulated to a large extent by biological processes.

Regulating body temperature is important for survival because it affects protein function, cellular membranes, and the like. Even small elevations in blood temperature can result in heat stroke. The hypothalamus is the primary control center for detecting changes in temperature and receives input from skin receptors. When the hypothalamus determines that the body is cold, it causes vasoconstriction and shivering. When the hypothalamus determines that the body is hot, it causes vasodilation and sweating. Behaviorally, we respond to heat by stretching out to maximize surface area and shedding layers of clothing, as on a hot summer day; we respond to cold by curling inward, snuggling up, and adding layers of clothing, as on a cold winter day.

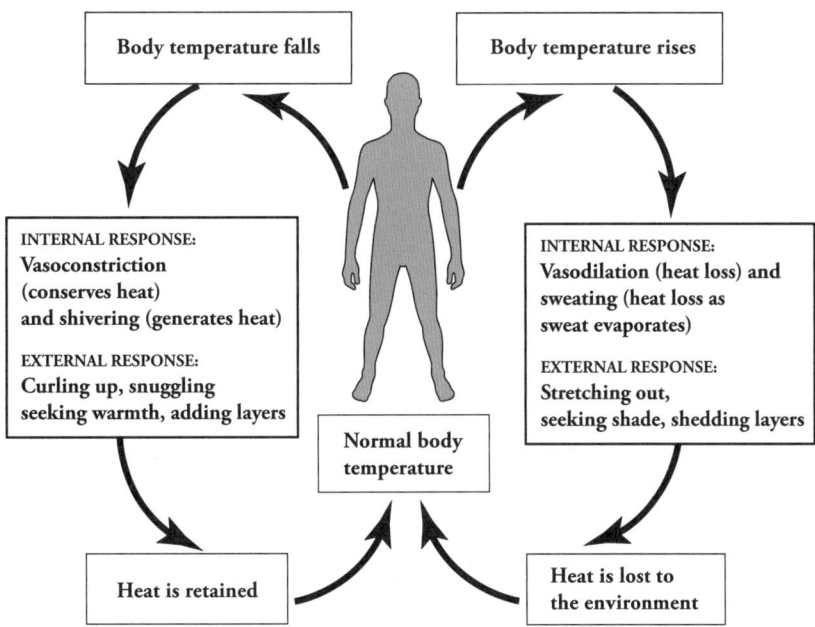

Figure 4 Physiological and behavioral processes regulating body temperature

Monitoring fluid levels includes the intake of fluids as well as excretion. The intake of fluids is stimulated by specialized osmoreceptors in the brain that detect dehydration. These receptors communicate with the pituitary gland to stimulate the release of antidiuretic hormone (ADH), which in turn communicates with the kidneys to reduce urine production by reclaiming water. When blood volume is low, including when one has sustained an injury and is losing a significant amount of blood, the desire for sodium is stimulated to increase the concentration of salt in the blood. Thirst is also stimulated to replace the lost fluid.

7.3 ATTITUDE AND BEHAVIOR

When psychologists refer to a person's **attitude**, they are referring to a person's feelings and beliefs about other people or events around them as well as their tendency to react behaviorally based on those underlying evaluations. Attitudes are useful in that they provide a quick way to size things up and make decisions. However, they can also lead us astray when they lead to inaccurate snap judgments or when they remain fixed beliefs in the face of disconfirming evidence.

Components of Attitudes

Attitudes are considered to have three main components (the ABCs): affect (emotion), behavioral tendencies, and cognition (thought).

The Link Between Attitudes and Behavior

Processes by Which Attitudes Influence Behavior

To what extent do our attitudes affect our behaviors? As is the case with most answers in psychology, it depends. At times, behavior does not accurately reflect attitudes. Consider the following common experiences:

- an individual believes in a healthy lifestyle, but is unable to sustain a healthy diet
- a man believes in not judging others, but finds himself avoiding eye contact and the seat next to a dirty homeless man on the bus
- a juror believes in a guilty verdict but finds himself conforming to the opinions of other jurors to vote "not guilty"

These scenarios suggest that the relationship between who we believe we are and what we do is complex. Social psychologists have found that there are some situations in which attitudes better predict behavior. Those are as follows:

1) *When social influences are reduced*
   Compared to attitudes, which are more internal, external behavior is much more susceptible to social influences. People are much more likely to be honest in a secret ballot process than if they must overtly express their opinions. This is in large part due to fear of criticism and the powerful influence of factors such as conformity and groupthink (discussed in Chapter 6).

2) *When general patterns of behavior, rather than specific behaviors, are observed*
   Our attitudes are better at predicting overall decision-making rather than specific behaviors. For example, one who believes in a healthy lifestyle will tend to make healthier decisions than someone who does not, yet this attitude does not necessarily prevent someone from occasionally reaching for a slice of cheesecake. This is known as the **principle of aggregation**; an attitude affects a person's aggregate or average behavior, but not necessarily each isolated act.

3) *When specific, rather than general, attitudes are considered*
   Belief in a healthy lifestyle can be a poor predictor of a specific behavior, such as eating properly. It would be wiser to compare the specific attitude that the individual has toward eating properly, because it will be a better predictor of this particular behavior. Thus, it is most accurate to consider specific attitudes closely related to the specific behavior of interest.

4) *When attitudes are made more powerful through self-reflection*
People are more likely to behave in accordance with their attitudes if they are given some time to prepare themselves to do so. When people act automatically, they may be impulsive and act in ways that do not match their beliefs. However, when given more time to deliberate over actions, they are more likely to act in ways that match. In addition, when people are made more self-conscious, often through the use of mirrors in experiments, they are more likely to behave morally. Self-awareness reminds us of the beliefs that we have attached to our identities.

Processes by Which Behavior Influences Attitudes

What is perhaps more interesting is the notion that behavior sometimes precedes and affects our attitudes. This comports with the James-Lange theory of emotion (section 7.4), which proposes that behaviors may precede and influence emotions. It has been found that just the act of smiling can somewhat boost mood, and that the act of running away may contribute to a sensation of fear.

There are several situations in which behaviors are likely to influence attitudes.

1) *Role-playing*
The most notable influence of behavior on attitudes is **role-playing**. Like a role in a play, a social role is a script for how to act. The most powerful demonstration of the power of roles is Zimbardo's **prison study** at Stanford. In this experiment, **Philip Zimbardo** randomly divided Stanford students into prisoners and guards in a mock prison. What happened over the course of the study was astonishing. After an initial lighthearted period, the guards and prisoners began really acting out their characters to the point that the guards were actively humiliating and degrading the prisoners. Some prisoners rebelled while others broke down or became apathetic. Participants in the study reported feeling a sense of confusion about reality and fantasy as they became caught up in their roles. The study, which was intended to be two weeks long, had to be discontinued after six days. While some have called Zimbardo's findings and methodology into question in recent years (e.g., only a few "guards" behaved abusively and some of them admit to posturing), the study demonstrates a powerful lesson about the influence that social roles can have.[2] Consider how social roles such as "soldier" and "slave" may have affected how people have acted over the course of history. In wartime, soldiers' beliefs about the enemy become dramatically altered over time, with feelings of ambivalence giving way to perceiving the enemy as "evil." Actions, such as singing the national anthem and saluting the flag, tend to increase patriotic beliefs. How does your own role of "student" affect your behavior? The same influences can stem from positive roles. Zimbardo has also researched positive roles, like that of "hero." Someone who identifies with the role of citizen, parent, or spiritual teacher may be influenced toward wholesome actions in order to better play out that role.

2) *Public Declarations*
In order to please others, people may feel pressure to adapt what they say. What's interesting is that saying something publicly—a **public declaration**—can cause the declarant to believe it in the absence of bribery, coercion, or some other blatant external motive. Since the individual may not be aware of the social pressure that might have influenced the statement, he

---

2 Note that the Stanford Prison experiment, if conducted today, would violate modern ethical rules governing experimentation on human subjects.

or she may justify it by concluding that the statement is a personal belief. As we continue to express ourselves, we become more and more entrenched in believing what we say, a habit that is even stronger for statements made publicly. Consider a politician who voices an opinion on the issue of abortion that mirrors the belief of the majority of her supporters, although she is somewhat ambivalent about the issue herself. As she continues to express their opinion, she will find herself becoming more polarized toward that opinion and her feelings of ambivalence will start to subside. Because her statements were made publicly, think how hard it would be for the politician to shift positions if she had a change of heart through her own development. Thus, she will be more likely to maintain a belief that is consistent with the actions she has taken. An emphasis on "political correctness" has developed from the idea that saying can become believing. The use of a term such as "gay" in a derogatory manner can lead to the development of beliefs that justify use of the term; therefore, many people feel terms of that sort should not be used.

3) *Justification of Effort*

Just as people may modify their attitudes to match their language, they may also modify them to match other behavior. A prominent example of this phenomenon is **justification of effort**. For example, consider a student who works hard to study for the MCAT and earns a fantastic score, only to feel a calling toward becoming an actor rather than going to medical school at the end of the process. In order to justify the effort already put into the process, the student will feel pressure to go to medical school. Another interesting example of justification of effort is the finding that doing favors for someone increases feelings of liking for that person. The internal dialogue is something like: "I must really like this person; otherwise, why would I be doing so many favors for him?"

4) *Foot-in-the-Door*

Salespeople, political activists, and others trying to influence behavior often take advantage of what is known as the **foot-in-the-door** phenomenon. The strategy involves enticing people to take small actions, such as signing a free petition or joining a mailing list, at first. Upon obtaining this level of involvement, the stakes are raised to accepting bumper stickers or lawn signs. Then, further involvement is encouraged when donations or volunteer time is requested. While people may have agreed to the earlier steps because they required minimal commitment, they will find themselves feeling internal pressure to consent to larger requests to justify their acceptance of the smaller requests. Over time, their attitudes will reflect those of someone who has taken a strong stance on the issue, in order to justify all the steps that they have taken.

Cognitive Dissonance Theory

When considering how behaviors can shape attitudes, self-justification plays an important part. In role-playing, public declarations, justification of effort, and foot-in-the-door scenarios, individuals justify their actions (including language) through beliefs. The theory that seeks to explain why self-justification is such a powerful influence on attitude modification is cognitive dissonance theory.

Cognitive dissonance theory explains that we feel tension ("dissonance") whenever we hold two thoughts or beliefs ("cognitions") that are incompatible, or when attitudes and behaviors don't match. When this occurs, we may feel like hypocrites or feel confused as to where we stand. The theory explains that in order to reduce this unpleasant feeling of tension, we make our views of the world match how we feel or what we've done.

Cognitive dissonance theory can explain people's reactions to situations in which there is insufficient justification for actions that were taken. Without sufficient justification for an action, people are likely to experience dissonance, and thus adjust their beliefs to match what they have done. For example, consider two parents trying to motivate their respective children to study and earn good grades. To accomplish this, one parent institutes a reward system in which the child gets $100 for every A. The second parent rewards their child with $5 for every A. In the first situation, the child may feel coerced into earning good grades. Thus, although he or she may study hard for the reward and earn a lot of money, the child will be less likely to have an internal belief that the grades themselves are important. The behavior of studying hard is easily justified by the reward. In the second situation, the child may work to receive As but have insufficient external justification for having done so, because the reward is insufficient. In cases of insufficient justification, cognitive dissonance theory indicates that there will be some tension that needs to be resolved. The child has earned some As (behavior) but does not have a supporting attitude available to explain the behavior. Thus, the child is likely to adopt the attitude that grades are important to him or her. Consider how cognitive dissonance theory can similarly be used to explain why mild punishment of appropriate severity is more effective at creating internal attitude change than unjustifiably harsh punishment.

Cognitive dissonance can also be used to explain the way people react after they make decisions. Imagine that a woman is trying to decide between two men who have expressed their romantic interest in her. One is exciting and passionate, but utterly undependable and irresponsible. The other is somewhat subdued, but very considerate and dependable. After making her decision, no matter which way she decides, she is sure to experience some dissonant thoughts about the man she rejected. If she chooses the exciting man, she may miss the dependability and consideration of the subdued man; if she chooses the subdued man, she may lament the lack of excitement and passion. According to cognitive dissonance theory, she will tend to change her attitudes to accentuate the positive qualities of her choice and the negative qualities of the alternative. Thus, if she chooses the exciting man, she may internalize beliefs that excitement and passion are important to a relationship and that dependability is overrated. If she chooses the subdued man, she may instead espouse the belief that it is consideration and dependability that are the centerpieces of a relationship and that passion and excitement are fleeting. The important point is that her endorsement of either of these beliefs will come after she makes her decision in order to alleviate the tension of losing what she turned down.

7.4 EMOTION

You walk through your front door, set your keys down, and turn on the light just like you always do when, "Surprise!" Balloons fall from the ceiling, friends jump out of their hiding places, and a cake is brought out. Without any conscious effort, you scream, cover your mouth with your hands, and explode into a giant grin. You feel a pang as your heart skips a beat and then feel a warm glow as you look around at the smiling faces. The thought pops into your head, "A surprise party! How exciting!"

Emotion is quite an interesting phenomenon. It blurs the arbitrary boundary between what we consider mental and what we consider physical. What is really going on when an emotional state arises?

Three Components of Emotion

Emotion is complex and consists of three components: a physiological (body) component, a behavioral (action) component, and a cognitive (mind) component. The physical aspect of emotion is one of **physiological arousal**, or an excitation of the body's internal state. For example, when being startled at a surprise party, you may feel your heart pounding, your breathing becoming shallow and rapid, and your palms becoming sweaty. These are the sensations that accompany emotion (in this instance, surprise).

The behavioral aspect of emotion includes some kind of expressive behavior; for example, spontaneously screaming and bringing your hands over your mouth. The cognitive aspect of emotion involves an appraisal or interpretation of the situation. Initially upon being startled, the thought "dangerous situation" or "fear" may arise, only to be reassessed as "surprise" and "excitement" after recognizing the circumstances as a surprise party. This describes how the situation is interpreted or labeled. Interestingly, many emotions share the same or very similar physiological and behavioral responses; it is the mind that interprets one situation that evokes a quickened heart rate and tears as "joyful" and another with the same responses as "fearful."

Universal Emotions

Darwin assumed that emotions had a strong biological basis. If this is true, then emotions should be experienced and expressed in similar ways across cultures, and in fact, this has been found to be the case. There are six major universal emotions: happiness, sadness, surprise, fear, disgust, and anger. Regardless of culture, most people can readily identify these emotions simply by observing facial expressions. Further supporting the idea that emotions have an innate basis is the finding that children's capacities for emotional expression and recognition appear to develop along similar timelines, regardless of their environments. However, environmental factors like culture do play a role in how emotion is expressed.

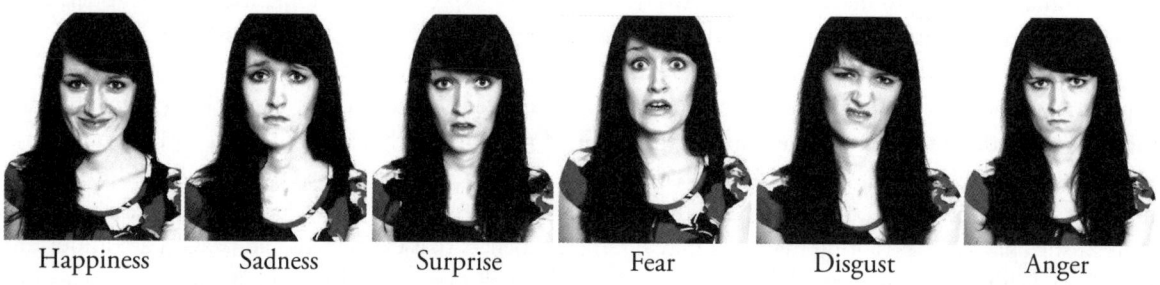

| Happiness | Sadness | Surprise | Fear | Disgust | Anger |

Courtesy Wikimedia Commons

Figure 5   Universal emotions

Adaptive Role of Emotion

The relationship between performance and emotional arousal is a U-shaped correlation: people perform best when they are moderately aroused. This is known as the **Yerkes-Dodson law** (often referred to as Optimal Arousal theory). A student will perform best when neither too complacent nor too overwhelmed, but rather in a "sweet spot" of optimum arousal (though this "sweet spot" can vary greatly from person to person and from task to task). The **optimal-arousal theory**, based on the Yerkes-Dodson law, further predicts that, while moderate arousal is ideal for optimum success, a higher level of arousal is better for easier tasks than for harder ones. For example, the Yerkes-Dodson law has been used to understand the social facilitation effect (see Chapter 6): performing difficult tasks that haven't been practiced sufficiently in front of others makes us overly nervous, beyond the optimal level of arousal for performance, whereas simple, well-practiced tasks move closer to optimal arousal with the presence of others and increased emotional activation.

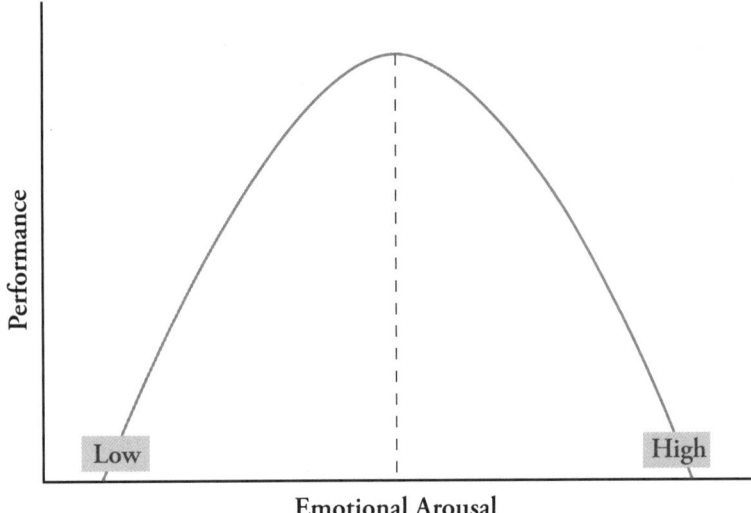

Figure 6   Yerkes-Dodson law regarding the relationship between arousal and performance

In addition to moderating performance, emotion has several other adaptive roles. It enhances survival by serving as a useful guide for quick decisions. A feeling of fear when walking alone down a dark alley while a shadowy figure approaches can be a valuable tool to indicate that the situation may be dangerous. A feeling of anger may enhance survival by encouraging attack on an intruder. The MCAT exam often emphasizes the adaptive benefits of emotional arousal. The most intensely unpleasant negative emotions, such as rage and terror, enhance survival by restricting the individual's attention and focusing it upon whatever is causing the emotional response.

Other emotions may have a role in influencing individual behaviors within a social context. For example, embarrassment may encourage social conformity. Additionally, in social contexts, emotions provide a means for nonverbal communication and empathy, allowing for cooperative interactions.

On a more subtle level, emotions are a large influence on our everyday lives. Our choices often require consideration of our emotions. A person with a brain injury to their prefrontal cortex (which plays a role in processing emotion) has trouble imagining their own emotional responses to the possible outcomes of decisions. This can lead to inappropriate decisions that can cost someone a job, a marriage, or his or her savings. Imagine how difficult it would be to refrain from risky behaviors, such as gambling or spending huge sums of money, without the ability to imagine your emotional response to the possible outcomes.

Theories of Emotion

The most commonsense way to think about emotion is that something happens (a stimulus), then you experience the emotion, and then you have a physiological and behavioral response. For example, you're walking down the street and a scary dog starts chasing you (stimulus), you first experience the emotion (fear), then the physiological response (your heart begins to race) and behavioral response (you run away). Indeed, this commonsense logic was how emotions were assumed to operate until the late 1800s, when scientists began proposing very different theories. There are three predominant theories that attempt to explain how the components of emotion—the physiological, the behavioral, and the cognitive—are interconnected.

James-Lange Theory

The James-Lange theory of emotion was proposed in the late 1800s and basically flips the commonsense notion of how emotion is experienced: instead of first experiencing the emotion and then the physiological reaction, the James-Lange theory proposes that first we experience the physiological response and then we experience the emotion. In other words, if a scary dog begins to chase you, first you experience an increased heart rate and this is followed by the conscious labeling of the experience as "fear." This may seem counterintuitive; it implies you feel afraid because your heart is racing. This theory suggests that the emotional experience (the brain labeling the situation as fear-inducing) is the result of the physiological response.

We frequently experience situations and events (stimuli) that result in various physiological reactions like increased muscle tension, increased heart rate, sweating, and many others, which are caused by the autonomic nervous system. This theory suggests that emotions are a result of these physiological responses, and not their cause. James and Lange suggested that autonomic activity induced by emotional stimuli generate the feeling of emotion, not the other way around.

There is some evidence in support of the James-Lange theory. For example, breathing patterns can also lead to certain emotions; short, shallow breathing creates a feeling of panic, while long, deep breathing creates a feeling of calm. People with cervical spine damage often experience less arousal and reduced emotions, because they no longer perceive physiological arousal from their bodies. However, the theory does not explain all scenarios and makes two assumptions that may be problematic. First, it assumes that each emotion originates from a distinctive physiological state. However, many emotions share very similar if not identical physiological profiles; for example, fear and sexual arousal involve very similar physiological patterns. Second, the theory assumes that we possess the ability to label these physiological states accurately. However, there is some evidence that the same physiological state can be interpreted differently based on context. For example, a physiological state similar to fear can be interpreted as excitement at a surprise party.

Cannon-Bard Theory

Walter Cannon, a critic of the James-Lange theory, suggested (1) that in order for the James-Lange theory to adequately describe the process of emotion, there must be different physiological responses corresponding to each distinct emotion; and (2) that physiological experiences do not appear to differ from one another to the extent that would be essential to discriminate one emotion from another based only on our bodily reactions. Cannon also conducted a series of experiments in the early 1900s on cats whereby he severed the afferent nerves of the sympathetic branch of the autonomic nervous system (thereby preventing the cats from receiving any physiological input from their bodies) and exposed them to emotion-inducing stimuli. Cannon (and his grad student, Philip Bard) found that the cats still experienced emotion, even in the absence of physiological input from their bodies, thus casting significant doubt on the James-Lange theory. Therefore, the Cannon-Bard theory of emotion suggests that after a stimulus, the physiological response and the experience of emotion occur simultaneously and independently of each other. For example, a scary dog comes running after you (stimulus) and you then experience fear (emotion) and an increased heart rate (physiological response) at the same time; the fear does not cause the increased heart rate and the increased heart rate does not cause the fear. The Cannon-Bard theory is able to explain the overlap in physiological states between emotions like fear and sexual arousal, because the cognitive labeling is independent from the physiological reaction, rather than directly caused by it. However, it struggles to explain phenomena in which controlling the physiological response influences the experience of emotion (e.g., deep breathing causes us to feel more calm).

Schachter-Singer Theory

According to the **Schachter-Singer theory** of emotion, once we experience physiological arousal, we make a conscious cognitive interpretation based on our circumstances, which allows us to identify the emotion that we are experiencing. Thus, like the James-Lange theory, this suggests that each emotional experience begins with an assessment of our physiological reactions. Unlike James-Lange, however, it suggests that the cognitive label is given based on the situation, rather than being a one-to-one correlate of the physiological experience. Therefore, as with this Cannon-Bard theory, physiological states can be similar but cognitively labeled differently (for example, fear and sexual arousal). Therefore, the sight of the scary dog would cause the physiological change of an increased heart rate, which would be interpreted as the result of fearing the dog because of the situation. This would then inspire a behavioral response (running away). This theory accounts for several situations, but suffers from the same shortcoming as the Cannon-Bard theory in that it does not explain how physiological responses influence cognitive aspects of emotion.

7.4

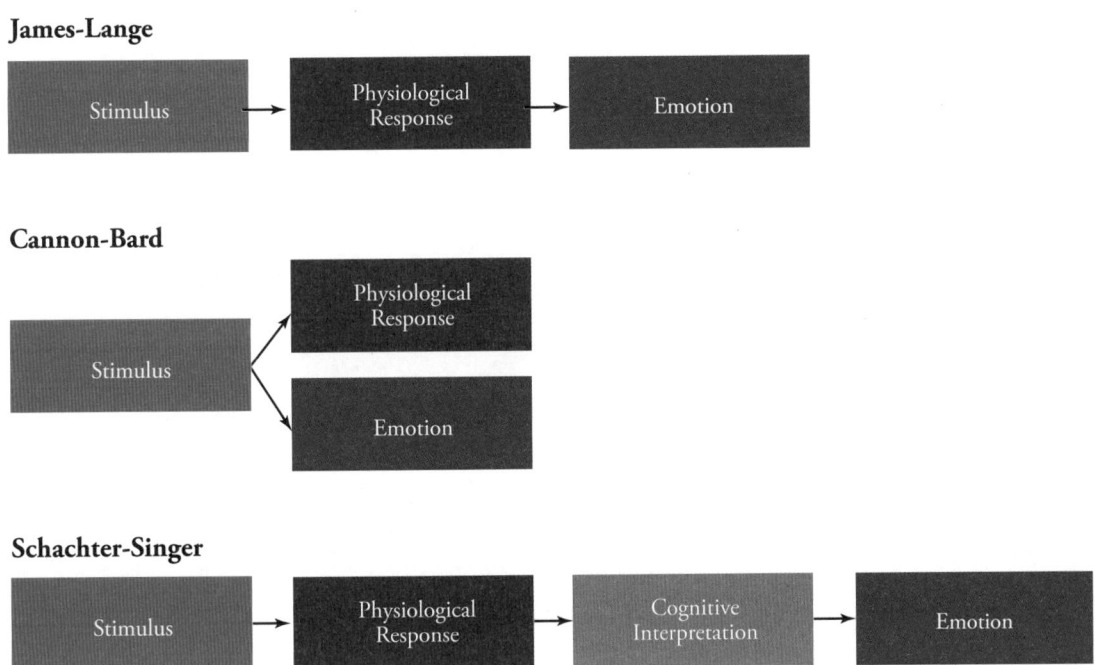

Figure 7   Schematic comparison of the theories of emotion

Chapter 7 Summary

- Personality is defined as the individual pattern of thinking, feeling, and behavior associated with each person.

- Sigmund Freud pioneered psychoanalytic theory, which proposes that personality is the result of an individual's unconscious thoughts, feelings, and memories.

- The id is ruled by the pleasure principle and is unconscious, the ego is ruled by the reality principle and uses logical thinking and planning to control consciousness and the id, and the superego inhibits the id and influences the ego to follow moralistic, rather than realistic, goals.

- According to Freud, people develop through five psychosexual stages: the oral stage, the anal stage, the phallic stage, the latent stage, and the genital stage; failure to resolve developmental conflicts within each stage leads to fixation.

- Erik Erikson added social and interpersonal factors to supplement Freud's theory; Erikson's developmental stages involve the resolution of the following crises: trust vs. mistrust, autonomy vs. shame, initiative vs. guilt, industry vs. inferiority, identity vs. role confusion, intimacy vs. isolation, generativity vs. stagnation, and integrity vs. despair.

- Carl Rogers pioneered the humanistic perspective in psychology and believed that incongruence between behavior and self-concept causes psychopathology.

- Behaviorists believe that personality is determined by conditioning; environmental reinforcements and punishments determine an individual's personality and behaviors.

- The social cognitive perspective suggests that personality is formed by a reciprocal interaction among behavioral, cognitive, and environmental factors.

- The Five-Factor Model describes five major personality traits: extroversion, neuroticism, openness to experience, agreeableness, and conscientiousness.

- Motivation is influenced by drives, instincts, feedback, arousal, and needs.

- The drive-reduction theory suggests that individuals engage in certain behavior in an attempt to alleviate physiological states of discomfort.

CHAPTER 7 FREESTANDING PRACTICE QUESTIONS

1. Which of the following is a universal emotion likely to occur with learned helplessness?

A) Guilt
B) Disgust
C) Sadness
D) Hopelessness

2. Research shows that emotions with salient labels are easier to remember, and when the recall state is similar to the initial state. This is most consistent with the:

A) dual coding hypothesis and the Optimal Arousal theory.
B) depth of processing model and the Optimal Arousal theory.
C) method of loci and the self-reference effect.
D) the self-reference effect and the dual coding hypothesis.

3. Psychoanalytic psychotherapy is a long-term therapeutic approach in which the therapist and client engage in deep analysis of the client's dreams, childhood, and life experiences in an attempt to gain insight into the unconscious. One important process in this type of therapy is known as transference, in which the client associates feelings with the therapist that originated in feelings for another person, in many cases a parent. If this resulted in the client accusing the therapist of angry feelings she herself held, this would be most reminiscent of the ego defense mechanism of:

A) repression.
B) reaction formation.
C) projection.
D) displacement.

4. According to the James-Lange theory:

A) motivation follows action.
B) emotion follows physiologic arousal.
C) physiologic arousal follows emotion.
D) emotions are validated by inner dialogue.

5. Pooja is hungry and buys a sandwich at the nearby sandwich shop. According to drive-reduction theory, she:

A) has returned her body to homeostasis.
B) has raised her glucose levels to an unhealthy level.
C) will have created another imbalance and feel thirsty.
D) will continue to feel hungry.

6. An individual despairs because she senses a lack of purpose in her work. Although she is considered successful within her career and earns enough to support her family, she feels as though her work has lacked purpose and has not benefited society as much as she would like. As her first grandchild is born, she reflects on whether she wants to consider a radical career change to a more fulfilling career that she believes does more social good and allows her to feel a greater sense of purpose. Which Erikson stage is she likely in, paired with the correct Maslow need she is striving to fulfill?

A) Integrity vs. despair seeking self-actualization needs
B) Generativity vs. stagnation seeking esteem needs
C) Integrity vs. despair seeking esteem needs
D) Generativity vs. stagnation seeking self-actualization needs

7. Rafael walks into a dark room, turns on the light, and his friends yell "surprise." Rafael's racing heartbeat is interpreted as surprise and joy instead of fear. Which theory of emotion is supported by his reaction?

A) Optimal arousal
B) Schachter-Singer
C) Cannon-Bard
D) James-Lange

8. A married couple has gone camping with their son and are discussing site protocol with a park ranger when suddenly a bear appears from the woods. Which sympathetic response is most consistent with the Schachter-Singer theory of emotion?

A) The park ranger feels an increased heart rate, then connects the event with several past experiences, and feels a sense of anxious alertness while holding bear spray to use in the event of an emergency.

B) The mother feels intense fear as she tries to catch her breath, which has instantly increased.

C) The father clutches his wife's wrist as he goes into shock, realizing when he is unable to move his hand that he is paralyzed with fear.

D) The son feels a rush of adrenaline and runs immediately into the tent, realizing once he is inside that he is in a state of panic.

9. Which of the following best summarizes Carl Rogers' view of personality?

A) Personality traits such as inhibition, extroversion, and conscientiousness are constant over time.

B) Individual, adult personalities are the result of repressed childhood memories.

C) People's personality traits are overwhelmingly positive and goal-directed.

D) Personality is mainly formed by behavioral expectations.

CHAPTER 7 PRACTICE PASSAGE

Maslow's hierarchy of needs is a well-established model of motivation within the humanistic framework. Maslow asserted that the ultimate goal of the individual is self-actualization, to become the best version of oneself, or who one was meant to be. However, many obstacles stand in the way of this path to self-actualization.

One method researchers have used to model self-actualization is to measure degree of convergence between the real and ideal selves. In humanistic psychology, the gap between these two aspects of self-concept is a predictor of psychopathology, on the one hand, and degree of life satisfaction on the other. Researchers created an instrument to measure this convergence, the Self Perceived Actualization Index (SPAI). The SPAI began as a 103-item questionnaire, but factor analysis showed that certain clusters of questions correlated with one another, and researchers were able to narrow the number of questions down to 34. The final version of the SPAI contained questions such as "In an ideal world, I would love to have more education" and "I sometimes wish I could start over in a new career and get back the time I lost" rated on a Likert Scale from 1 to 7. The SPAI was then checked against similar instruments for reliability and consistency.

A group of researchers in the field of clinical psychology created a study to explore how self-perceived actualization was related to motivation from the perspective of a Maslowian hierarchy. They created a study with three groups: high actualization, low actualization, and control. The researchers then checked for interactions between self-actualization and motivation, and how they affected mood and altruistic behavior. Each group was told not to eat before coming to the research laboratory then given a small meal before participating in the study. Over time, as hunger increased, the researchers wanted to see the extent to which participants were willing to engage in altruistic behaviors, modeled by the extent to which they were willing to share their winnings from a game. The researchers found that as participants became hungrier, they were less likely to share their winnings with other participants. There was also a mediating effect of actualization, such that individuals who scored higher on the SPAI were less susceptible to hunger effects on their altruism and mood.

In a follow-up study, the same team of researchers conducted a personality assessment and found significant correlations with certain personality characteristics and positive affect and altruistic behavior.

1. The checks in the research methodology were to check for

    I. internal validity.
    II. external validity.
    III. construct validity.

    A) I only
    B) I and III only
    C) II and III only
    D) I, II, and III

2. Which of the following conclusions is best supported by the research?

    A) Altruism is a surface trait dependent on context.
    B) Altruism is a source trait that is relatively stable.
    C) Altruism is a surface trait that is relatively stable.
    D) Altruism is a source trait that is dependent on context.

3. Which of the following is the most likely connection the researchers were trying to establish with respect to the Maslowian hierarchy?

    A) Meeting love and belonging needs plays a stabilizing role in the effects of not getting esteem needs met.
    B) Meeting self-actualization needs plays a stabilizing role in the effects of not getting physiological needs met.
    C) Meeting esteem needs plays a stabilizing role in the effects of not getting safety needs met.
    D) Meeting physiological needs plays a stabilizing role in the effects of not getting esteem needs met.

4. A low rating on which of the following items is most likely to be interpreted as having high self-actualization?

    A) Love and belonging needs
    B) Integrity
    C) Conscientiousness
    D) Neuroticism

5. Which of the following pairs of correlations did researchers most likely find in the follow-up study?

A) A positive correlation between neuroticism and positive affect and a positive correlation between conscientiousness and altruistic behavior

B) A positive correlation between neuroticism and positive affect and a negative correlation between conscientiousness and altruistic behavior

C) A negative correlation between neuroticism and positive affect and a positive correlation between conscientiousness and altruistic behavior

D) A negative correlation between neuroticism and positive affect and a negative correlation between conscientiousness and altruistic behavior

6. Which of the following is likely to lead to convergence similar to the type mentioned in the passage between real and ideal self?

A) Unconditional positive regard and successful resolution during the autonomy vs. shame and doubt phase

B) High self-concept and successful resolution during the latency phase

C) Strong emotional regulation due to positive cognitive appraisals of potentially threatening stimuli

D) Unstable source traits that are congruent with an idealized self-concept

SOLUTIONS TO CHAPTER 7 FREESTANDING PRACTICE QUESTIONS

1. **C** Learned helplessness occurs when an organism learns through experience that it has no control over a situation and gives up, despite the fact that the environment has changed in such a way that it now has autonomy. Among the answer choices, this is closest to sadness, which is characterized by low energy and feelings of being unable to change the environment, and often results in decreased activity (choice C is correct). Guilt is not one of the six universal emotions (choice A is wrong). The expression of disgust originates in the reaction often displayed when one consumes disagreeable food, and now includes situations where we observe someone else acting in a way with which we strongly disagree. The phenomenon of learned helplessness is not associated with a negative judgement of another person's actions (choice B is wrong). Hopelessness is not one of the six universal emotions (choice D is wrong).

2. **B** The depth-of-processing model states that experiences which receive a greater depth of neural and cognitive processing are more likely to be remembered. This is consistent with deep emotions with salient labels leading to greater recall. Optimal Arousal theory states that there is an optimal level of emotional arousal, consistent with the emotional arousal implied in the recall state, which the question stem suggests is like the initial state (choice B is correct). The dual-coding hypothesis refers to the fact that it is easier to remember words when they are related to images and is not related to emotions (choice A is wrong). The method of loci is a recall strategy in which an individual imagines that she is moving through a space and connects images with the objects or ideas that she is trying to remember. This is unrelated to emotional arousal (choice C is wrong). The self-reference effect refers to the fact that it is easier to recall events that have personal relevance. This can connect to greater emotional salience, but this is not necessarily so (choice D is wrong).

3. **C** Projection involves an attempt to disown one's own unacceptable feelings or characteristics by falsely attributing them to others. The question stem describes such a situation, in which the patient projects her feelings onto the therapist (choice C is correct). Repression is an attempt to ignore or forget strong emotional memories, often related to childhood. No repression of memories is mentioned in the question stem (choice A is wrong). Reaction formation is characterized by behaving in a manner that is actually the opposite of one's true feelings. The question stem does not indicate that the client acts in a way that is the opposite of her feelings, rather that she attributes her own feelings to the therapist (choice B is wrong). Displacement involves shifting a forbidden desire or impulse onto another object of desire or interest that is more acceptable (choice D is wrong).

4. **B** The James-Lange theory of emotion posits that emotion is experienced after the body's physiological response to a stimulus (choice B is correct; choice C is wrong). Motivation is not part of the James-Lange theory (choice A is wrong), and neither is inner dialogue (choice D is wrong).

5. **A** According to drive-reduction theory, the drive is hunger in this case; to reduce the need, Pooja needs to eat something. Since she does this, theoretically she will return to homeostasis (choice A is correct). The sandwich could conceivably increase glucose levels in the body, but it is not certain that they will be raised to unhealthy levels (choice B is incorrect). Yes,

she may be thirsty as well, but that is not stated in the question, nor will a sandwich necessarily make one thirsty (choice C is incorrect). Lastly, as the sandwich will likely satiate the hunger, there is not enough evidence to support the idea that she might remain hungry (choice D is incorrect).

6. **D** This is a two-by-two question; approach one part of the answer choice at a time and use Process of Elimination. For the Erikson phase, the question stem states that the individual is experiencing doubt about the impact of her career. This is connected with the phase of generativity vs. stagnation. Integrity vs. despair involves reflecting back on one's life and evaluating whether it was a life worth living (choices A and C are wrong). The question stem states that the individual was already successful in her career, so it is unlikely that she is striving for esteem needs (choice B is wrong). The question also states that she would like to feel a greater sense of purpose, which corresponds closely to self-actualization (choice D is correct).

7. **B** Rafael can cognitively appraise the situation to know he is not in danger. Thus, while he is experiencing a physiological response to a stimulus, he is ultimately demonstrating cognitive interpretation of that physiological response, which is consistent with the two-factor theory of Schachter and Singer (choice B is correct). The Optimal Arousal theory (often referred to as the Yerkes-Dodson law) is not a theory of emotion (choice A is incorrect). The Cannon-Bard theory does not connect the cognitive interpretation of the physiological response (choice C is incorrect). The James-Lange theory also does not work here because the physiological response would only lead to one emotional output, most likely fear (choice D is incorrect).

8. **A** The Schachter-Singer theory of emotion is characterized by the role of cognitive evaluation and context. Emotions with identical physiological markers can be experienced differently based on the interpretation of the situation. A park ranger who experiences a sympathetic response but experiences alertness instead of fear because of memories and experiences is an example of the Schacter-Singer theory (choice A is correct). The mother's experience is consistent with Canon-Bard because the emotion and physiological responses occur simultaneously (choice B is wrong). The father's shock does not specify any sympathetic response, as indicated by the answer choice (choice C is wrong). The son realizes his emotion after the physiological response. This is consistent with the James-Lange theory (choice D is wrong).

9. **C** Rogers believed in the intrinsic goodness of the humans, hence why he belongs to the humanistic school of psychology; choice C most mirrors his views (choice C is correct). Choice A is somewhat extreme in claiming personality traits are "constant over time," they are not; nonetheless, this is not Rogers' perspective (choice A is incorrect). Choice B is the psychoanalytic perspective of personality (choice B is incorrect), and choice D is the behavioral explanation of personality (choice D is incorrect).

SOLUTIONS TO CHAPTER 7 PRACTICE PASSAGE

1. **B** The passage states that the researchers checked for reliability and consistency, and these are both attributes related to the validity of psychometric instruments: whether they measure what they purport to, and whether repeated assessments lead to similar results. The validity of a measurement tool is related to internal validity, so Item I is true (choice C is wrong). Neither of the checks made by researchers for reliability and consistency is related to whether the research applies to real world situations in the greater population, so Item II is not true (choice D is wrong). Construct validity is specifically related to how well-designed an instrument is, which is exactly what the researchers checked for. Therefore, Item III is true (choice B is correct, and choice A is wrong).

2. **A** This question can be answered more quickly by dividing it into two parts. First, note that altruism in the passage is dependent on context. Individuals became less altruistic as they got hungrier. Source traits tend to be largely stable across situations, whereas surface traits are largely dependent on context so can vary widely depending on the situation. The fact that altruism tends to change for participants in the study suggests that it is a surface trait (choices B and D are wrong). Surface traits tend to be more dependent on context and are not stable because they can vary widely from situation to situation (choice A is correct, and choice C is wrong).

3. **B** The passage indicates that individuals who scored high on the SPAI, a measure of self-actualization, were more stable and saw less of a decline in altruism when they were hungry. Since hunger is a physiological need, this suggests that self-actualization played a stabilizing role on not getting physiological needs met (choice B is correct). The SPAI measures self-actualization, how much individuals feel that they are leading the life they want, not love and belonging, the extent to which they feel loved and cared for (choice A is wrong). Esteem needs refer to a sense of accomplishment and high self-esteem, not self-actualization, and safety needs refer to the absence of threat, as opposed to not having a physiological need (hunger) met (choice C is wrong). Physiological needs are the needs that were tested in the passage, as individuals became more hungry. Therefore, this is not the need that played a stabilizing role (choice D is wrong).

4. **D** Neuroticism is associated with negative emotions and difficulty dealing with stress. Low levels of neuroticism would indicate a more positive emotional experience and better stress management. This is likely to be associated with self-actualization (choice D is correct). Love and belonging needs would need to be met first, according to Maslow, before achieving self-actualization. Therefore, high levels of love and belonging, not low levels, would be associated with self-actualization (choice A is wrong). Integrity would result in positive resolution of Erikson's last stage of development, integrity vs. despair. This positive resolution would be associated with a sense of a life well-lived, which is a sense of self-actualization. Therefore, high levels, not low levels, of integrity would be associated with self-actualization (choice B is wrong). Conscientiousness is associated with awareness of others' conditions, thoughtfulness, and responsibility. It is not clear that this attribute is directly related to self-actualization, but conscientiousness is generally considered to be socially desirable, so it is more likely that high levels are associated with self-actualization than low levels (choice C is wrong).

5.   **C**   For two-by-two question types, evaluate one part of the answer choice at a time and use POE. Neuroticism is associated with negative emotions, so a negative correlation is expected between neuroticism and positive emotions (choices A and B are wrong). Conscientiousness is related to thoughtfulness and consideration for others' states, so a positive correlation is expected between conscientiousness and altruistic behavior (choice C is correct, and choice D is wrong).

6.   **A**   Unconditional positive regard is a concept in humanistic psychology that, when provided by parents, caregivers, therapists, or other significant figures provides an individual the best chance at reaching self-actualization. Also, successful resolution of the autonomy vs. shame and doubt phase would lead to a sense of independence and autonomy that would make it more likely that an individual could lead a life congruent with his or her ideals (choice A is correct). Self-concept is not conceptualized as being high or low, like perhaps self-esteem would be. It is more likely to be referred to in terms of how integrated or differentiated it is. Also, the latency phase in Freud's stage theory is not associated with psychosexual conflict, so successful resolution here would lead to minimal benefits. Freud considered the first three stages directly before the latency phase to be far more important (choice B is wrong). Resilient response to potentially threatening stimuli is a positive attribute that would probably be associated with greater life satisfaction, but how this would be related to real and ideal selves and their convergence is not clear (choice C is wrong). Source traits are considered the more stable traits, as opposed to surface traits, which vary more from situation to situation (choice D is wrong).

EXPLORING THE RELATIONSHIP BETWEEN FREQUENCY OF INSTAGRAM USE, EXPOSURE TO IDEALIZED IMAGES, AND PSYCHOLOGICAL WELL-BEING IN WOMEN

Sherlock, Mary; Wagstaff, Danielle L.

Psychology of popular media culture Vol. 8, Iss. 4, (Oct 2019): 482-490. DOI:10.1037/ppm0000182

The appealing features of social networking sites (SNSs), such as the ability to communicate with others despite geographical distance, have attracted billions of users worldwide, with many incorporating social networking into their daily routine (Boyd & Ellison, 2007). Between 2014 and 2015, 72% of Australians accessed the Internet for social networking purposes, with younger age groups (<35 years) being the heaviest Internet users (Australian Bureau of Statistics, 2016). Indeed, 80% of university students use their devices (i.e., laptops, tablets, and mobile phones) for social networking purposes.

METHOD

Participants were 129 women, ranging in age from 18 to 35 years (M = 24.60 years, SD = 4.54), who indicated they currently used Instagram. Participants were recruited from the authors' university's undergraduate psychology participant pool, as well as volunteers recruited via SNSs and flyer advertisements on university campuses. The research was approved by the institutional human ethics research committee, and all participants provided their informed consent. The study was hosted on SurveyMonkey and included two parts. Participation took approximately 30 to 40 min, and upon completion, participants were presented with a debriefing statement regarding the nature of the manipulation.

Materials and Procedure

Participants completed a survey containing the following scales presented in random order:

The 20-item Centre for Epidemiologic Studies Depression Scale (Radloff, 1977) was used to measure depressive symptoms. Participants were asked to answer a number of questions relating to how they felt or behaved in the week prior, including "I felt depressed" and "I had crying spells," on a scale from 1 (*rarely or none of the time*) to 4 (*all of the time*). Higher scores indicate higher depressive symptoms.

The Centre for Epidemiologic Studies Depression Scale had high internal reliability (α = .93).

The Heatherton Self-Esteem Scale (Heatherton & Polivy, 1991) measures state self-esteem across three domains: performance, social interaction, and appearance. Participants respond to 20 items such as "I feel self-conscious" and "I feel as smart as others," on a 5-point scale from 1 (*not at all*) to 5 (*extremely*). Higher scores indicate higher self-esteem. The Heatherton Self-Esteem Scale had high internal reliability (α = .96).

The State-Trait Anxiety Inventory (Spielberger, Gorsuch, Lushene, Vagg, & Jacobs, 1983) is a commonly used measure of general anxiety and contains 20 items for assessing state anxiety and 20 for trait anxiety. Items include "I am tense" and "I am a steady person," which participants answer on a 4-point scale from 1 (*almost never*) to 4 (*almost always*). Higher scores indicate greater anxiety. The State-Trait Anxiety Inventory had high internal reliability (α = .96).

The Physical Appearance State and Trait Anxiety Scale (PASTAS; Reed, Thompson, Brannick, & Sacco, 1991) measures an individual's body image anxiety as they generally feel (trait) and as they currently feel (state). The trait scale asks participants to best indicate the extent to which they generally feel anxious, tense, or nervous about specific body parts such as "my hips" and "my buttocks" on a 5-point scale from 1 (*never*) to 5 (*always*). The state scale asks how they feel about the same body parts "right now" on a scale from 1 (*not at all*) to 5 (*exceptionally so*). Higher scores indicate higher physical appearance anxiety. The scale had high internal reliability (α = .91).

Self-rated physical attractiveness was measured by two questions: "Rate what you perceive to be your own physical attractiveness compared to your same sex friends" and "Rate what you perceive to be your own physical attractiveness compared to the general population," on a scale from 1 (*extremely less attractive*) to 9 (*extremely* more attractive). Scores were summed to create a single value for self-rated attractiveness. The items correlated strongly ($r = .72$).

The Body Image Disturbance Questionnaire (BIDQ; Cash, Phillips, Santos, & Hrabosky, 2004) assesses concerns about physical appearance. The Body Image Disturbance Questionnaire consists of seven items such as "Are you concerned about the appearance of some part(s) of your body, which you consider especially unattractive?" which participants answer on a scale from 1 (not at all concerned) to 5 (extremely concerned). Higher scores indicate higher body image disturbance. The scale showed high internal consistency ($\alpha = .93$).

Social comparison was measured using the Iowa-Netherlands Comparison Orientation Scale (INCOM; Gibbons & Buunk, 1999), with 11 items measuring how frequently individuals compare themselves with others. Items include "I always like to know what others in a similar situation would do," measured on a 5-point scale from 1 (disagree strongly) to 5 (agree strongly). Higher scores indicate higher frequency of social comparison. The Iowa-Netherlands Comparison Orientation Scale showed high internal reliability ($\alpha = .83$).

Instagram use was measured using questions derived by the researchers. Items related to frequency of use. That is, "how many followers do you have on Instagram?" from 1 (1–10) to 11 (1,000+), "How many accounts do you follow on Instagram?" from 1 (1–10) to 11 (1,000+), and "In the past week, on average, approximately how much time per day have you spent actively using Instagram," from 1 (less than 10 min) to 6 (more than 3 hr).

Design

Part 1 consisted of a correlational design in which we correlated Instagram use with each of the psychological well-being variables, and with age. Because Lup et al. (2015) found that the relationship between Instagram use and depression was mediated by social comparison, we attempted to replicate these findings, as well as explore the mediation by social comparison of the relationship between Instagram use and other psychological well-being variables.

RESULTS

Instagram Use and Psychological Well-being

As shown in Table 1, the average time spent on Instagram correlated positively with depressive symptoms, trait anxiety, social comparison orientation, physical appearance anxiety, and body image disturbance. The time spent on Instagram also correlated negatively with self-esteem, and thus findings are consistent with the hypothesis. Exploring the other Instagram measures taken, we found that number of followers correlated positively with depression and trait anxiety, and negatively with self-esteem. The number of accounts followed correlated positively with depression and negatively with self-esteem. Additionally, age correlated negatively with Instagram use, $r = -0.36$, $p < .001$, and negatively with social comparison, $r = -0.21$, $p = .019$.

Descriptive Statistics for Each Scale, Plus Correlations Between Scales

Table 1   Descriptive Statistics for Each Scale, Plus Correlations Between Scales

Variable	Descriptive statistics		Pearson's correlation coefficients								
	M	SD	1	2	3	4	5	6	7	8	9
1. Time spent on Instagram	2.65	1.65									
2. Number of accounts followed	7.06	2.69	.58**								
3. Number of followers	6.97	2.43	.53**	.77**							
4. Depressive symptoms	22.65	12.77	.49**	.21*	.22*						
5. Trait anxiety	49.88	11.93	.42**	.30**	.28**	.81**					
6. Physical appearance anxiety	41.55	13.47	.47**	.29**	.16	.48**	.59**				
7. Body image disturbance	16.91	6.62	.33**	.26*	.16	.48**	.63**	.64**			
8. Self-rated attractiveness	8.21	2.91	−.11	−.05	.11	−.26**	−.49**	−.48**	−.56**		
9. Self-esteem	59.91	17.77	−.47**	−.24**	−.18*	−.74**	−.84**	−.75**	−.65**	.55**	
10. Social comparison	40.17	7.22	.42**	.25**	.15	.43**	.59**	.57**	.43**	−.28**	−.62**

* $p < .05$ ** $p < .01$

DISCUSSION

Instagram Use and Psychological Well-being

There is an array of evidence demonstrating excessive Facebook use is related to negative mental health outcomes (Błachnio et al., 2013, 2015; Fardouly et al., 2014; Haferkamp & Krämer, 2011; Labrague, 2014). In this study, we demonstrated that heavier Instagram use (as well as number of followers and number of people followed) correlated with a range of psychological well-being outcomes, including depressive symptoms, general anxiety, physical appearance anxiety, self-esteem, and body image disturbance. Previously, Lup et al. (2015) showed that the relationship between Instagram use and depressive symptoms was mediated by social comparison. Here, we discovered a similar relationship, with social comparison having a significant mediating effect on the relationship between Instagram use and depressive symptoms, as well as general anxiety, physical appearance anxiety, self-esteem, and body image disturbance. These results are also in line with previous research demonstrating that social comparison behavior after exposure to social media has a negative effect on mental health (Feinstein et al., 2013; Labrague, 2014; Vogel et al., 2014). Similarly, Hendrickse et al. (2017) found that appearance-related comparisons on Instagram mediated the relationship between Instagram photo activity and the drive for thinness and body dissatisfaction.

This research is important, as Instagram has some distinguishing features that set it apart from Facebook and relatively fewer studies have focused on Instagram. Importantly, Instagram is associated with a range of social trends, such as "fitspiration," which can lead to negative body image outcomes (Tiggemann & Zaccardo, 2015). Thus, excessive Instagram exposure may have an effect on other aspects of psychological well-being that extend beyond depressive symptoms to self-esteem and body image (e.g., Hendrickse et al., 2017). Although Facebook use is linked to negative outcomes, our assertion that exposure to visual media, specifically, can lead to negative outcomes is complemented by research by Meier and Gray (2014). Meier and Gray showed that Facebook photo activity, rather than total Facebook activity, correlated positively with body dissatisfaction. Therefore, based on our findings, increased use of the image-based platform Instagram, in which users post idealized images, is likely putting users at higher risk of negative outcomes than the users of other forms of social media.

In our sample, younger participants spent more time on Instagram, and engaged in higher levels of social comparison. Although our sample was restricted to a young adult to adult demographic (i.e., age 18–35 years), these findings suggest that Instagram use could pose an even higher risk to psychological well-being in adolescents.

In this study, we showed that the number of followers also correlated with the range of psychological well-being variables. Because Facebook and Instagram users are likely to share positive and idealistic portrayals of themselves, teenagers may feel they are "missing out" or "everyone is doing better" than themselves when making social comparisons online. This seems to relate to the extent to which individuals follow others who are unknown to them, with Chou and Edge (2012) showing that those who used Facebook for longer, and who followed more strangers, agreed more that others had better lives. These negative outcomes may be larger for teenagers who are less popular than their peers (Nesi & Prinstein, 2015).

Finally, although the aim of this research was to explore the effects of Instagram use on female psychological well-being, men are also prone to body dissatisfaction after exposure to idealized images (Galioto & Crowther, 2013; Hargreaves & Tiggemann, 2004), and social comparison can also mediate the link between social media use and depressive symptoms in men (Steers et al., 2014). Hence, it is worthwhile for future research to address the outcomes of excessive Instagram use in both adolescent samples and in men, including long-term impact.

JOURNAL ARTICLE EXERCISE 2

Remember that the science sections on the MCAT include a significant number of passages with experiments. You'll need to be able to extract information efficiently and analyze data effectively in order to do well on these passages.

This is the second of three "Journal Article Exercises" in this book. In the first exercise, we showed you the type of information you should be able to extract from the article and the sorts of things to pay attention to in the data. In this exercise, you'll do more of that on your own, and in the final exercise we'll show you how that article might get turned into an MCAT-style passage.

As a reminder, when analyzing an experiment, you should be able to:

- identify the control group(s)
- extract information from graphs and data tables
- determine how the experimental group(s) change relative to the control
- determine if the results are statistically significant
- come to a reasonable conclusion about WHY the results were observed
- consider potential weaknesses in the study
- determine how to increase the power of the study
- decide what the next most logical experiment or study should be

Again, the goal of these exercises is NOT to learn content from the articles, just to get a little more comfortable reading and extracting information from them.

For the (abridged) article on pages 203–205, try to summarize the purpose of the experiment and the methods in 4–5 sentences. Consider the following mnemonic: Oh ouR Car Won't Start (ORCWS).

- **O = Organism and Organization**: Is the research being conducted on humans or on animals or on bacteria in a petri dish, or something else? What is being done to these organisms? Are there any unique qualities to these organisms? Are there multiple groups? Is the study conducted over a long period of time with multiple data points, or is it a short-term study? Does it have a large or small n?

- **R = Results**: Where and how are the results presented? Is it a graph? A data table? Figures and images? What is/are the independent variable(s)? What is/are the dependent variable(s)? What are the results? Do the results show correlation or cause and effect, or both? Describe.

- **C = Control and Comparison**: Is there a control group? How does it differ from the experimental group? Is it given a placebo or nothing at all? Is it held under different conditions? If there are multiple experimental groups, how do they differ from one another? Is it a blinded study? If so, double-blind or single-blind?

- **W = Weirdness**: Does anything or do any of the results stand out as unexpected?

- **S = Statistics**: Was any sort of statistical analysis done? How is it presented? Are there error bars on a graph? Standard errors around a mean? Are there p-values? Is there an asterisk indicating statistical significance? Is there any data that is not statistically significant?

Try interpreting the data on your own before reading the results/discussion section. When you do read the discussion, consider:

- What are the conclusions of the study?
- How are the conclusions supported by the data?
- What potential weaknesses or flaws do you see in the experimental design? Are these addressed in the discussion section?
- How might this study be potentially biased?
- How might this study be improved?
- What would be the next most logical experiment?

Let's answer the above questions for the article on pages 203–205.

Write brief responses to the questions below:

1. **O = Organism and Organization:**
   - Is the research being conducted on humans or on animals or on bacteria in a petri dish, or something else?

     _____

     _____

   - What is being done to these organisms?

     _____

     _____

   - Are there any unique qualities to these organisms?

     _____

     _____

   - Are there multiple groups?

     _____

     _____

   - Is the study conducted over a long period of time with multiple data points, or is it a short-term study?

     _____

     _____

   - Does it have a large or small n?

     _____

     _____

2. **R = Results:**
   - Where and how are the results presented? Is it a graph? A data table? Figures and images?

     _____

     _____

   - What is/are the independent variable(s)?

     _____

     _____

   - What is/are the dependent variable(s)?

     _____

     _____

   - What are the results of the study?

     _____

     _____

- Do the results show correlation or cause and effect, or both? Describe.

  _____

  _____

3. **C = Control and Comparison:**
   - Is there a control group?

     _____

     _____

   - How does it differ from the experimental group? Is it given a placebo or nothing at all? Is it held under different conditions?

     _____

     _____

   - If there are multiple experimental groups, how do they differ from one another?

     _____

     _____

   - Is it a blinded study? If so, double-blind or single-blind?

     _____

     _____

4. **W = Weirdness:**
   - Does anything or do any of the results stand out as unexpected?

     _____

     _____

5. **S = Statistics:**
   - Was any sort of statistical analysis done?

     _____

     _____

   - How is it presented? Are there error bars on a graph? Standard errors around a mean? Are there p-values? Is there an asterisk indicating statistical significance?

     _____

     _____

   - Is there any data that is not statistically significant?

     _____

     _____

6. **Interpreting the data:**
   - What are the conclusions of the study?

     _____

     _____

- How are the conclusions supported by the data?

  _____

  _____

- What potential weaknesses or flaws do you see in the experimental design? Are these addressed in the discussion section?

  _____

  _____

- How might this study be potentially biased?

  _____

  _____

- How might this study be improved?

  _____

  _____

- What would be the next most logical experiment?

  _____

  _____

7. **Final Summary of Experiment and Results:**

   _____

   _____

   _____

   _____

   _____

   _____

   _____

SOLUTIONS TO JOURNAL ARTICLE EXERCISE 2

1. **O = Organism and Organization:**
   - Is the research being conducted on humans or on animals or on bacteria in a petri dish, or something else? *Humans*
   - What is being done to these organisms? *Participants filled out surveys*
   - Are there any unique qualities to these organisms? *All participants were women, all 18-35*
   - Are there multiple groups? *No*
   - Is the study conducted over a long period of time with multiple data points, or is it a short-term study? *Very short, 30–40 minutes*
   - Does it have a large or small *n*? *Relatively small: 129 participants*

2. **R = Results:**
   - Where and how are the results presented? Is it a graph? A data table? Figures and images? *Data table*
   - What is/are the independent variable(s)? *None, this is a correlational study.*
   - What is/are the dependent variable(s)? *None, this is a correlational study.*
   - What are the results of the study? *The average time spent on Instagram correlated positively with depressive symptoms, trait anxiety, social comparison orientation, physical appearance anxiety, and body image disturbance. The time spent on Instagram also correlated negatively with self-esteem. The number of followers also correlated positively with depression and trait anxiety, and negatively with self-esteem. The number of accounts followed correlated positively with depression and negatively with self-esteem. Additionally, age correlated negatively with Instagram use and negatively with social comparison.*
   - Do the results show correlation or cause and effect, or both? Describe. *The study is correlational and thus does not allow us to infer a cause and effect relationship.*

3. **C = Control and Comparison:**
   - Is there a control group? *No*
   - How does it differ from the experimental group? Is it given a placebo or nothing at all? Is it held under different conditions? *N/A*
   - If there are multiple experimental groups, how do they differ from one another? *N/A*
   - Is it a blinded study? If so, double-blind or single-blind? *Not a blinded study*

4. **W = Weirdness:**
   - Does anything or do any of the results stand out as unexpected? *No.*

5. **S = Statistics:**
   - Was any sort of statistical analysis done? *Yes*
   - How is it presented? Are there error bars on a graph? Standard errors around a mean? Are there *p*-values? Is there an asterisk indicating statistical significance? *R-values, standard deviation around the mean, asterisks*
   - Is there any data that is not statistically significant? *There are a few measures that are not statistically significant (e.g., self-rated attractiveness is not significant for low amount of time spent on Instagram).*

6. **Interpreting the data:**
   - What are the conclusions of the study? *Authors demonstrated that heavier Instagram use (as well as number of followers and number of people followed) correlated with a range of psychological well-being outcomes, including depressive symptoms, general anxiety, physical appearance anxiety, self-esteem, and body image disturbance.*
   - How are the conclusions supported by the data? *R-values are used to indicate both the direction and the strength of a correlation.*
   - What potential weaknesses or flaws do you see in the experimental design? Are these addressed in the discussion section? *Relatively small sample size, largely university students (who might react differently than those not in university), men were not included in the study.*
   - How might this study be potentially biased? *By the limited (mostly university student, all female) sample.*
   - How might this study be improved? *A wider participant pool, including men*
   - What would be the next most logical experiment? *Repeat the study, with a larger n, but also potentially with males, or participants from various countries/cultures.*

7. **Final Summary of Experiment and Results:**
   - *This correlational research implies that excessive exposure to Instagram can be damaging to users, especially when they engage in negative social comparisons. Exposure to content of idealistic beauty and fitness standards could be harmful in the long-term, considering the achievement of many of these ideals is unrealistic. This may be of particular importance in adolescents, who are heavy users of social media and engage in more social comparisons than do older adults.*

Chapter 8
Psychological
Disorders and Stress

Psychological disorders affect personality, motivation, and attitude. The study and treatment of psychological disorders is an important field of psychology. Not only do the disorders help us understand how our minds and bodies function properly (by understanding what happens when something goes awry), but they also constitute a huge area of clinical practice.

8.1 PSYCHOLOGICAL DISORDERS

It is estimated that, in America, roughly one in every four adults (ages 18 and over) meets the diagnostic criteria for a psychological disorder. Psychological disorders are therefore an important part of our culture and comprise a significant component of our health care system. Psychological disorders, particularly when they go untreated, also affect our economy by impacting our social welfare and criminal justice systems.

Understanding Psychological Disorders

Although psychological disorders affect about one-quarter of the population, serious psychological disorders are less common, affecting roughly one in 17 people, or 6% of the U.S. population. A **psychological disorder** is a set of behavioral and/or psychological symptoms that are not in keeping with cultural norms, and that are severe enough to cause significant personal distress and/or significant impairment to social, occupational, or personal functioning. Sometimes cultural norms can be ruled out as a source of behavior; for example, when what appears to be a delusion or even a hallucination can be better understood in terms of religious or spiritual practice, that belief or experience would not count as a symptom of a psychological disorder. When cultural norms cannot explain behavior, the core components of diagnosis for a psychological disorder are *symptom quantity and severity*, and *impact on functioning*. A psychological disorder is *diagnosable* based on specific symptoms and symptom thresholds, and *treatable* (or at least *manageable*) with various types of medication and/or therapy.

Biopsychosocial Approach to Mental Health

As the three parts of the term indicate, the bio-psycho-social approach recognizes the interaction between nature (the biological, such as genetic predispositions) and nurture (the psychological, such as individual environmental forces), as well as the social (including cultural forces). For example, while not exclusive to Western cultures, eating disorders appear to be far more common in wealthier countries that espouse a thin ideal (like the United States) than they are in other parts of the world. It is also possible, for a given psychological disorder, that the underlying genetic and physiological dynamics are similar, but that the manifestation of the disorder for a particular person is influenced by cultural or social factors. Figure 1 presents the separate and overlapping influences that have been shown to correlate with psychological disorders.

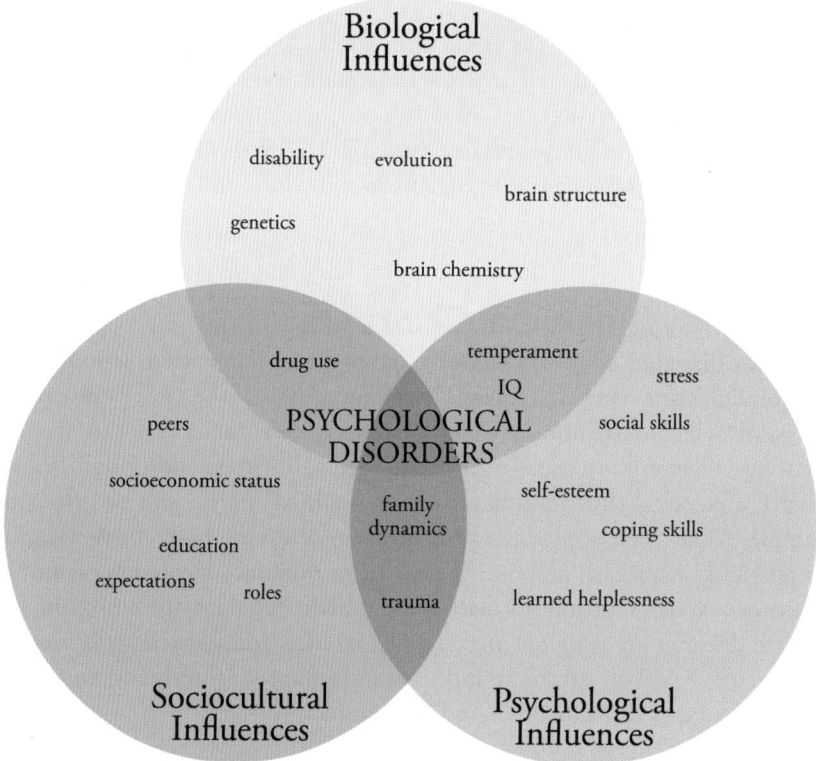

Figure 1   Biopsychosocial model of psychological disorders

Classifying Psychological Disorders

It is important to understand the classification of psychological disorders in order to understand the symptoms and prevalence of each. Without classification, it would be impossible to know what the biological and genetic risk factors are, which treatments work the best, and so on. In the United States and elsewhere in the world, current standards for classification and diagnosis are gathered in the **Diagnostical and Statistical Manual of Mental Disorders, Fifth edition (DSM-5)**, published in May 2013. Each new edition of the DSM reflects changes in research and clinical perspectives. For example, since the publication of the fourth edition in 1994, research findings and clinical experience prompted the publishers of the DSM-5 to combine the four separate autism disorders into one—Autism Spectrum Disorder—and to change the symptom categories from three to two areas. In several areas, in fact, the newest version of the DSM emphasizes the existence of a spectrum of behavior ranging from normal to disordered. Accurate diagnosis is critical; most insurance companies require a diagnosis based on DSM criteria before they will cover the cost of therapy.

For the purposes of the MCAT, familiarize yourself with the categories of disorders presented on the following pages in Table 1. Note that this list is not all-inclusive but instead presents the psychological disorders that are most likely to be tested.

Table 1 Categories of Psychological Disorders

Broad Ca...ory	...iption	Specific Psychological Disorders
Anxiety Disorders	...ty disorders are characterized by ...ive fear (of specific real things or ...generally) and/or anxiety (of real ...agined *future* things or events) ...ooth physiological and psycho-...l symptoms.	• Separation Anxiety Disorder • Specific Phobia(s) • Social Anxiety Disorder • Panic Disorder • Generalized Anxiety Disorder
Obsessive Compulsive and Related Disorders	...ders in this category are distinct from anxiety disorders in that they involve a pattern of obsessive thoughts or urges that are coupled with maladaptive behavioral compulsions; the compulsions are experienced as a necessary/urgent response to the obsessive thoughts/urges, creating rigid, anxiety-filled routines.	• Obsessive-Compulsive Disorder • Body Dysmorphic Disorder • Hoarding Disorder
Trauma- and Stressor-Related Disorders	Traumas and stressors are central to the definition of these disorders, which involve unhealthy or pathological responses to one or more harmful or life-threatening events, including witnessing such an event. Subsequent symptoms include patterns of anxiety, depression, depersonalization, nightmares, insomnia, and/or a heightened startle response.	• Posttraumatic Stress Disorder • Acute Stress Disorder • Adjustment Disorders
Somatic Symptom Disorders	Somatic symptom disorders are characterized by physical symptoms that cannot be explained by a medical condition or substance use, and are not attributable to another psychological disorder, but that nonetheless cause emotional distress.	• Somatic Symptom Disorder • Illness Anxiety Disorder • Conversion Disorder • Factitious Disorder (imposed on self or another)
Bipolar and Related Disorders	Bipolar and related disorders involve mood swings or cycles (called episodes) ranging from manic to depressive, in which manic episodes tend to be followed by depressive episodes, and vice versa.	• Bipolar I Disorder • Bipolar II Disorder • Cyclothymic Disorder
Depressive Disorders	Depressive disorders are characterized by a disturbance in mood or affect. Specific symptoms include difficulties in sleep, concentration, and/or appetite; fatigue; and inability to experience pleasure (anhedonia).	• Major Depressive Disorder • Persistent Depressive Disorder (dysthymia) • Premenstrual Dysphoric Disorder

Broad Category	Description	Specific Psychological Disorders
Schizophrenia Spectrum and Other Psychotic Disorders	Psychotic disorders are characterized by a general "loss of contact with reality" which can include "positive" symptoms, such as delusions and hallucinations, and/or "negative" symptoms, such as flattened affect (e.g., monotone vocal expression).	• Delusional Disorder • Brief Psychotic Disorder • Schizophreniform Disorder • Schizophrenia • Schizoaffective Disorder
Dissociative Disorders	Dissociative disorders are characterized by disruptions in memory, awareness, identity, or perception. Many dissociative disorders are thought to be caused by psychological trauma.	• Dissociative Identity Disorder • Dissociative Amnesia • Depersonalization/Derealization Disorder
Personality Disorders	Personality disorders are characterized by enduring maladaptive patterns of behavior and cognition that depart from social norms, present across a variety of contexts, and cause significant dysfunction and distress. These patterns permeate the broader personality of the person and typically solidify during late adolescence or early adulthood.	Cluster A: • Paranoid • Schizoid • Schizotypal Cluster B: • Antisocial • Borderline • Histrionic • Narcissistic Cluster C: • Avoidant • Dependent • Obsessive-compulsive
Neurodevelopmental Disorders	Neurodevelopmental disorders are characterized by developmental deficits varying from specific learning impairments to global impairments of social skills or intelligence.	• Intellectual Disability • Attention-Deficit/Hyperactivity Disorder (ADHD) • Autism Spectrum Disorder (ASD)
Neurocognitive Disorders	Neurocognitive disorders are characterized by cognitive abnormalities or general decline in memory, problem-solving, and/or perception.	• Major and Mild Neurocognitive Disorders (MMND) • MMND Due to Alzheimer's Disease • MMND Due to Parkinson's Disease • Major or Mild Vascular Neurocognitive Disorder
Feeding and Eating Disorders	Feeding and eating disorders are characterized by abnormal eating behaviors such as severe undereating (anorexia nervosa) and purging to maintain unhealthy weight (bulimia nervosa).	• Anorexia Nervosa • Bulimia Nervosa • Pica • Binge Eating Disorder

Types of Psychological Disorders

The nine categories of psychological disorders discussed in this section correspond to the nine categories of disorders listed by the AAMC that you should be familiar with for the MCAT: Anxiety Disorders, Obsessive-Compulsive and Related Disorders, Trauma- and Stressor-Related Disorders, Somatic Symptom and Related Disorders, Bipolar and Related Disorders, Depressive Disorders, Schizophrenia Spectrum and Other Psychotic Disorders, Dissociative Disorders, and Personality Disorders. The following section discusses neurodevelopmental and neurocognitive disorders.

1. Anxiety Disorders

Anxiety is an emotional state of unpleasant physical and mental arousal—a preparation to fight or flee. For a person with an anxiety disorder, the anxiety is intense, frequent, irrational (out of proportion), and uncontrollable; it causes significant distress or impairment of normal functioning (at-work productivity, success in intimate relationships, and so on). Four types of anxiety disorders are discussed here: panic disorder, generalized anxiety disorder, specific phobia, and social phobia (now called "Social Anxiety Disorder").

Symptoms mimicking an anxiety disorder can also be caused by general medical conditions, alcohol, certain recreational drugs, or medication use or withdrawal. If a person has a medical condition or uses substances that are likely to be causing the symptoms, the diagnosis is "anxiety disorder due to a general medical condition" or "substance-induced anxiety disorder." This approach to specifying non-psychological causes applies to the other sections of the DSM-5 as well.

Panic Disorder A person with **panic disorder** has suffered at least one **panic attack** and is worried about having more of them. The panic attacks can be triggered by certain situations, but they are more often uncued or "spontaneous," occurring unexpectedly and with sometimes unpredictable frequency.

During a **panic attack**, a person commonly experiences intense dread, along with shortness of breath, chest pain, a choking sensation, and cardiac symptoms such as a rapid heartbeat or palpitations. There may also be trembling, sweating, lightheadedness, or chills. Many fear they are dying of a heart attack or stroke during a panic attack. One danger of panic attacks is that they can mask other illnesses, such as heart attacks and **mood disorders**. Although panic attacks are brief (often less than 30 minutes in duration), they can be excruciating, and people with panic disorder live in fear of having more panic attacks. Panic disorder can be debilitating if left untreated, but people with this disorder do respond well to treatment.

Generalized Anxiety Disorder A person with **generalized anxiety disorder** (GAD) feels tense or anxious much of the time about many issues, but does not experience panic attacks. The source of this underlying, chronic nervousness can seem like a moving target, shifting from one situation to another, or there may be no identifiable source. The distress and impairment associated with GAD is not often severe; it may include restlessness, tiring easily, poor concentration, irritability, muscle tension, and insomnia or restless sleep.

Specific Phobia and Social Phobia There are several types of **phobias**. In specific and social phobias, the sufferer feels a strong fear that he or she recognizes as unreasonable. He or she nevertheless almost always experiences either general anxiety or a full panic attack when confronted with the feared object or situation. People with phobias often go to great lengths to avoid the triggers they fear, and this avoidance itself is part of the symptom profile.

Specific phobia is a persistent, strong, and unreasonable fear of a certain object or situation. Specific phobias are classified into four types (plus "other") depending on the types of triggers they involve (see Table 2).

Table 2 Types of Specific Phobias

Type of Specific Phobia	Example of Triggers
Situational	Flying, elevators, bridges, crowds (in agoraphobia)
Natural Environment	Thunderstorms, heights, water, lightning
Blood-Injection-Injury	Injections, blood, surgical procedures
Animal	Spiders, snakes, dogs

Social Anxiety Disorder, or **Social Phobia**, is an unreasonable, paralyzing fear of feeling embarrassed or humiliated while one is seen or watched by others, even while performing routine activities such as eating in public or using a public restroom. Here too a prominent symptom is avoidance, which can lead to social isolation.

2. Obsessive-Compulsive and Related Disorders

Separated now from anxiety disorders, these disorders feature at least one pronounced repetitive behavior that exceeds cultural norms and rituals such as grooming practices or maintaining a healthy body weight. Unsuccessful attempts to decrease or otherwise manage these behaviors are also central to the diagnosis. Without therapeutic intervention, these conditions tend to increase over time in terms of severity or level of self-harm, or both.

Obsessive-Compulsive Disorder A person with **obsessive-compulsive disorder (OCD)** has obsessions, compulsions, or both. **Obsessions** are repeated, intrusive, uncontrollable thoughts or impulses that cause distress or anxiety. The person knows the thoughts are irrational, and despite attempts to disregard or suppress them, typically resorts to responding to them through a compulsive behavior. **Compulsions** are repeated physical or mental behaviors (e.g., counting) that are performed in response to an obsession or in accordance with a set of strict rules, in order to reduce distress or prevent something dreaded from occurring. The person realizes that the compulsive behavior is not rational, being either unrelated to the dreaded event, or related but clearly excessive. Nevertheless, if the person does not perform the behavior, he or she feels intense anxiety and a conviction that the terrible event will happen. Some common obsessions and compulsions are listed in Table 3.

Table 3 Common Obsessions and Compulsions

Obsessions (Thoughts)	Compulsions (Actions)
• Irrational fear of contamination by dirt, germs, or toxins • Pathological doubt that a task was done, or fear of having inadvertently harmed someone or violated a law • Fear of harming someone violently or sexually, or otherwise behaving in an unacceptable way	• Washing self (often hands) or surroundings repeatedly, sometimes with a lengthy ritual • Checking repeatedly that a task was done, sometimes with a lengthy ritual • Counting to a certain number before certain tasks, or performing a behavior a certain number of times (such as folding a shirt) • Arranging objects or performing actions with perfect symmetry or precision

3. Trauma- and Stressor-Related Disorders

Like the disorders in the previous section, these were also separated in the DSM-5 from what used to be a much broader category of anxiety disorders. Although anxiety can accompany a response to a traumatic or stressful event, many people who have been exposed to such an event display primarily symptoms other than anxiety (such as dysphoria, aggression, and/or dissociation).

Posttraumatic Stress Disorder **Posttraumatic stress disorder (PTSD)** can arise when a person feels intense fear, horror, or helplessness after experiencing, witnessing, or otherwise confronting an extremely traumatic event that involves actual or threatened death, serious injury, or sexual violence to the self or others. It is estimated that most people (more than half) will experience at least one traumatic event in their lifetime, but only a small subset of those will develop PTSD. Approximately 8% of men and 20% of women develop PTSD after a trauma. Rates of PTSD are higher in males of Latino heritage and males who have served in active combat, for whom the estimated prevalence reaches 20%.

The traumatic event is often *relived* (not just remembered) through dreams and flashbacks in which the person feels as though the event is currently happening, and which can include multisensory reprocessing, such as the intrusion of smells and sounds from the original event context. Some experience mental or physiological distress (e.g., elevated heart rate or blood pressure) when reminded of the event, however indirectly. A person with PTSD tries to avoid people, places, feelings, thoughts, or conversations that are reminders of the event, or even avoids people and feelings in general. The person may also be chronically physiologically hyperaroused, with symptoms such as an increased startle response, insomnia, angry outbursts, poor concentration, and extreme alertness (called **hypervigilance**). For a diagnosis of PTSD, these symptoms must have been present for more than a month. Symptoms may not begin until months or even years after the trauma.

Acute stress disorder Similar to PTSD, but its symptoms last between 3 days and 1 month. Indeed, some instances of PTSD begin as acute distress disorder.

Adjustment disorders In adjustment disorders, the maladaptive response is to a stressor (a romantic break-up, job issues, marital issues) rather than a trauma. This response may last between 3 and 6 months. The diagnosis also applies in cases where the subsequent distress appears in some way to be disproportionate to the cause.

For all three conditions, it is noteworthy that individuals from low-SES communities, or who are otherwise disadvantaged, encounter more stressors in their everyday lives and are thus at increased risk for a disorder in this category.

4. Somatic Symptom and Related Disorders

A **somatic symptom disorder** is a psychological disorder characterized primarily by distress and decreased functioning due to persistent physical symptoms and concerns, which may mimic physical (somatic) disease but generally are not rooted in any detectable pathophysiology. Further, the somatic symptoms do not improve with medical treatment. This symptom/behavior pattern is commonly referred to as "hypochondriasis," but as the differences between these disorders should make clear, that term lacks precision.

Though they are often treated with skepticism even by physicians (a large majority of these diagnoses occur in the primary care setting), most people with somatic symptom disorders—the exception being factitious disorders—genuinely experience their symptoms and/or believe that there is something physically wrong with them. The DSM-5 accounts for this complexity with streamlined presentation of four subtypes: somatic symptom disorder, illness anxiety disorder, conversion disorder, and factitious disorder.

Somatic Symptom Disorder For someone with **somatic symptom disorder**, the central complaint is one or more somatic symptoms—such as chronic pain or headaches or fatigue—and diagnosis also requires evidence of diminished functioning stemming from excessive preoccupation with and/or anxiety about the symptoms. Whether the symptoms in any way coincide with a related medical problem or illness, the distress and/or disruption of daily life caused by the symptoms warrants at least consideration of the diagnosis.

Illness Anxiety Disorder One reason **"hypochondriasis"** can be considered imprecise is that it refers to concern about both illness and somatic symptoms. **Illness anxiety disorder** differs from somatic symptom disorder insofar as the somatic aspect of the illness is not as central or can even be nonexistent. In illness anxiety disorder, the distress is predominantly psychological, with people experiencing persistent preoccupation with both their health condition and health-related behaviors, including seeking treatment.

Conversion Disorder A person with **conversion disorder** experiences a change in sensory or motor function—such as weakness, tremors, seizures, or difficulty talking or eating—that has no discernible physical or physiological cause and that seems to be significantly affected by psychological factors. The symptoms of conversion disorder typically begin or worsen after an emotional conflict or other stressor. As the terminology suggests, the emotion or anxiety is "converted" into a physical symptom. The change in function is severe enough to warrant medical attention, or to cause significant distress or impairment in work, social, or personal functioning. Diagnosis of conversion disorder is possible, for example, when a person suddenly experiences blindness but his or her blink reflex remains intact.

Factitious Disorder This disorder is colloquially referred to as "Münchhausen Syndrome" (when imposed on oneself) or "Münchhausen by proxy" (when imposed on someone else). In **factitious disorder imposed on self**, a person has not just fabricated an illness but has gone the further step of either falsifying evidence or symptoms of the illness or inflicting harm to him- or herself to induce injury or illness. Though the person presents the illness to others and thus attracts interpersonal and/or medical attention, diagnosis requires evidence that the person behaves this way even without obvious benefit. When someone induces physical or psychological symptoms in someone else, often a child—and then presents the other person as ill or injured—the perpetrator of the deception is diagnosed with **factitious disorder imposed on another**.

5. Bipolar and Related Disorders

Bipolar Disorders Most people with a **bipolar disorder** (formerly called manic depression) experience cyclic mood episodes oscillating between the extremes or 'poles' of depression and mania.

Table 4 Diagnostic Criteria for Bipolar and Related Disorders and Depressive Disorders

	Manic Episode	Hypomanic Episode	Major Depressive Episode
Duration	At least one week, nearly every day	At least four consecutive days	At least two weeks
Mood	Elevated, expansive, or irritable mood	Elevated, expansive, or irritable mood	Depressed; diminished interest or pleasure in almost all activities
Self-image	Inflated, grandiose	Inflated, grandiose	Feelings of worthlessness or excessive guilt
Appetite/weight	May show diminished appetite or interest in food	May show diminished appetite or interest in food	Increase or decrease in body weight by 5% or more in a month
Sleep need	Decreased	Decreased	Insomnia or hypersomnia
Cognition	Flight of ideas or racing thoughts; distractibility	Flight of ideas or racing thoughts; distractibility	Diminished ability to think or concentrate; recurrent thoughts of death or suicide
Speech	Rapid, pressured	Rapid, pressured	May manifest muted or flat affect in speech
Energy/behavior	Increased energy and goal-directed activity and/or psychomotor agitation	Increased energy and goal-directed activity and/or psychomotor agitation	Fatigue or loss of energy; psychomotor agitation or slowness
Judgment	Lack of consequential thinking	Lack of consequential thinking	May include suicide attempt or a specific plan for committing suicide
Impairment in functioning	Severe, marked impairment; may require hospitalization (to prevent harm to self or others); may include psychotic features	Unequivocal, observable change that is not typical of the individual; not severe enough to cause marked impairment or to necessitate hospitalization	Clinically significant distress or marked impairment in one or more areas of functioning

In a **manic episode**, a person has experienced an abnormal euphoric, unrestrained, or irritable mood for at least one week, as well as a marked increase in either goal-directed activity (e.g., increased energy and productivity at work) or in psychomotor agitation, which stems from an urge to be engaged in goal-directed activity but without the focus necessary to do so. (Hence, the "surplus" energy causes agitation and irritability.) For example, someone experiencing a manic episode may feel compelled to spend hours shopping online or looking for an activity to absorb the energy. These symptoms are severe enough to cause psychotic features, hospitalization, or impairment of work, social, or personal function.

Bipolar I disorder is diagnosed only if there has been a spontaneous manic episode not triggered by treatment for depression or caused by another medical condition or medication. The disorder may include a swing to a full depressive episode, or only to partial or moderate depression (dysthymic symptoms), or no depression at all (although this is rare). In a **mixed episode**, a person has met the symptoms for both major depressive and manic episodes nearly every day for at least a week, and the symptoms are severe enough to cause psychotic features, hospitalization, or impaired work, social, or personal functioning. In the simplest terms, the only requirement for a diagnosis of **bipolar I disorder** is that the person has experienced at least one manic or mixed episode.

In a person with **bipolar II disorder**, the manic phases are less extreme. A person with bipolar II disorder has experienced cyclic moods, including at least one major depressive episode and one hypomanic episode, but has not met the criteria for a manic or mixed episode. In a **hypomanic episode**, for at least four days a person has experienced an abnormally euphoric or irritable mood, with at least three of the symptoms for a manic episode, but at a less severe level. With hypomania, the impairment or distress is less serious, and there is no psychosis or hospitalization. In a **major depressive episode**, a person has felt worse than usual for most of the day, nearly every day, for at least two weeks. The individual also has at least five of the following emotional, behavioral, cognitive, and physical symptoms: depressed mood or decreased interest in activities, significant increase or decrease in weight or appetite, excessive or insufficient sleep, agitated or slowed psychomotor activity, fatigue or loss of energy, feelings of low self-worth or excessive guilt, impaired concentration or decision-making, and thoughts of death or suicide. The diagnosis of bipolar II disorder requires both types of episodes.

Cyclothymic Disorder **Cyclothymic disorder** is similar to the bipolar disorders, but the moods are less extreme, with symptoms not meeting the criteria for either a manic or a major depressive episode. A person with cyclothymic disorder has experienced cyclic moods, including multiple hypomanic episodes, as well as episodes of depressed mood that are milder than a major depressive episode, for at least two years. These mood swings have never been absent for more than two months.

6. Depressive Disorders

A **depressive disorder** is more than acute moodiness; it is a persistent pattern of abnormal and often painful mood symptoms severe enough to cause significant personal distress and/or impairment to social, occupational, or personal functioning. While **emotions** or **feelings** are measurable in terms of seconds, minutes, or hours, **mood** describes a baseline of weeks or months; mood is a person's sustained internal emotion that colors his or her view of life. Three depressive disorders are discussed in this section: major depressive disorder, persistent depressive disorder (dysthymia), and premenstrual dysphoric disorder (this last condition is new in DSM-5).

Major Depressive Disorder A person with **major depressive disorder** (MDD) has suffered one or more major depressive episodes (as discussed in the previous section). Ten percent of people with major depressive disorder attempt suicide and many more contemplate it or devise a suicide plan. These symptoms do not indicate major depression if they occur within two months of bereavement, as they may be part of a normal grieving reaction. In seasonal affective disorder (or what DSM-5 refers to as MDD "with seasonal pattern"), episodes of depression occur during certain seasons, usually fall and winter.

Persistent Depressive Disorder (Dysthymia) **Persistent depressive disorder** (PDD), also called **dysthymic disorder** or **dysthymia**, is a less intense, but typically more chronic form of depression. A person with PDD has experienced milder symptoms of depression most days for at least two years, with symptoms never absent for more than two months, but without a major depressive episode. Onset is typically adolescence or early adulthood, and the persistence of the condition often leaves people feeling like they've "always felt this way" or as if they are a "depressed person" to their core.

Premenstrual Dysphoric Disorder In **premenstrual dysphoric disorder**, which is diagnosed only in women, many of the symptoms of a major depressive episode are present, with the caveat that they intensify in the final week before the onset of menses and then improve, and in many cases disappear, in the week after menstruation has ended. There are a few symptoms that distinguish the illness from the other two depressive disorders discussed here: feeling keyed up or on edge, specific food cravings, a sense of being overwhelmed or out of control, as well as the physical symptoms of the body's preparation for menstruation: tenderness or swelling in the breasts, joint or muscle pain, and bloating.

Figure 2 compares the various mood states or episodes for depressive disorders and bipolar and related disorders. Persistent depressive disorder is thus a milder (though often more persistent) form of major depressive disorder, whereas bipolar disorder I, bipolar disorder II, and cyclothymia generally involve cycling through either manic or hypomanic episodes, and dysthymic or depressed episodes.

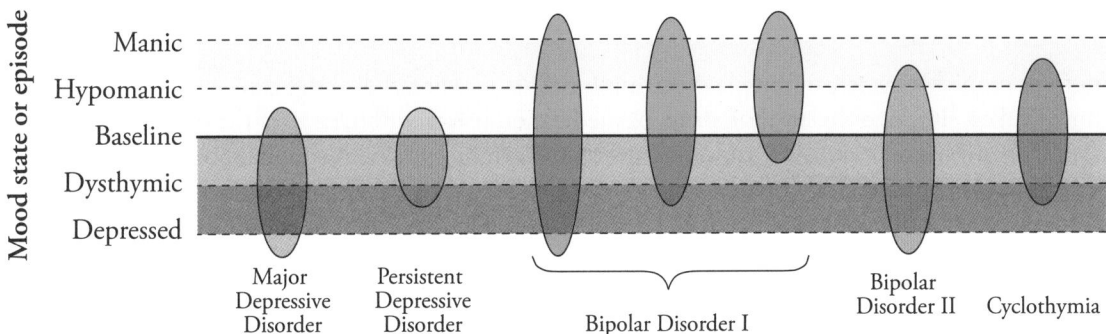

Figure 2   Depressive disorders and bipolar (and related) disorders based on diagnostic criteria for mood state or episode

7. Schizophrenia Spectrum and Other Psychotic Disorders

Schizophrenia spectrum and other psychotic disorders are diagnosed when someone has been experiencing one or more of the following **positive symptoms**: delusions, hallucinations, disorganized thinking (as manifested in disorganized speech), disorganized or abnormal motor behavior, and/or one or more **negative symptoms**, such as decreased emotional expression (presentation of "flat" **affect**), *avolition* (lack of motivation or purpose), and/or *alogia* (decreased or absent speech). Positive symptoms indicate the presence of an atypical behavior or other characteristic. Negative symptoms indicate a decrease in, or lack of, a typical behavior or other characteristic. The general profile of the disorders in this section is that they involve some sort of splitting off or distancing of the person from aspects of his or her everyday reality.

Although schizophrenia literally means "split mind," the term refers to a split in mental functions, or a split from reality; it does not indicate a split in identity. Many people incorrectly use the term schizophrenia to mean "multiple personality disorder" (a condition now called dissociative identity disorder).

A **delusion** is a false belief that is not due to culture, and is not relinquished despite evidence that it is false. For example, a person might believe that he or she is a certain movie star. Delusions are different from strongly held non-psychotic beliefs, both in intensity and plausibility. For someone with **delusional disorder**, one or more delusions have been present for at least a month, and counterevidence is generally denied or distorted to keep the delusion intact. Common delusions include erotomania (the belief that someone is in love with you), grandiosity (the belief that you have a special talent or insight), and persecution (the belief that you are being followed, drugged, harassed, and so on).

A **hallucination** is a false sensory perception that occurs while a person is conscious (not during sleep or delirium). It is important to distinguish between true hallucinations, which occur in the absence of related sensory stimuli, and illusions, which are misperceptions of actual sensory stimuli (which may occur in low light). The most common hallucinations are auditory and visual.

Schizophrenia is diagnosed when someone has been experiencing positive, and sometimes negative, symptoms for longer than six months. Here the impact on functioning is greatest, with impairment in work, relationships, and/or self-care. Though the symptoms may subside at times to a prodromal level (just below the diagnostic threshold), there is no complete remission without medication. On the schizophrenia spectrum, schizophrenia proper thus represents the chronic version of the disorder.

Symptoms mimicking a schizophrenia spectrum (or other psychotic) disorder can also be caused by a general medical condition, or by alcohol, drug, or medication use or withdrawal. If the person has a medical condition or uses substances that could be causing the symptoms, the diagnosis should be psychotic disorder due to a general medical condition or substance-induced psychotic disorder. Symptoms of psychosis can also occur with mood or developmental disorders. All of these disorders must be ruled out before one can make diagnosis of one of the disorders in this section.

8. Dissociative Disorders

During a dissociative experience, some of a person's thoughts, feelings, perceptions, memories, or behaviors are separated from conscious awareness and control, in a way that is not explainable as mere forgetfulness. This separation sometimes occurs as a defense against a traumatic situation that is too overwhelming to hold in awareness. In a **dissociative disorder**, the disruptions in awareness, memory, and identity are extreme and/or frequent, and they cause distress or impair the person's functioning. Dissociative disorders can be triggered by severe stress or psychological conflicts, and they usually begin and end suddenly.

Dissociative Identity Disorder A person with **dissociative identity disorder** alternates among two or more distinct personality states (or identities), only one of which interacts with other people at a given time. The condition may be experienced as a "possession" by another personality or identity, as it involves amnesia—loss of awareness or memory—for one or more of the personality states. These distinct identities may vary widely in age, gender, and personality traits, and they may or may not be aware of one another. This disorder was previously known as multiple personality disorder.

Dissociative Amnesia A person with **dissociative amnesia** has had at least one episode of forgetting some important personal information, creating gaps in memory that are usually related to severe stress or trauma. The person may wander aimlessly during the episode or experience it as a kind of journey, in what is called a **dissociative fugue**. Most often, the amnesia is localized, meaning that everything that happened during a particular time frame is forgotten, but it can also be selective (only some events during a particular time frame are forgotten), generalized (the person's whole lifetime is forgotten), continuous (everything since a certain time is forgotten), or systematized (only particular categories of information are forgotten, such as everything relating to the person's family). The disorder usually begins and ends suddenly, with full recovery of memory, though it may also linger with some information only gradually, if ever, fully coming back to consciousness. Unfortunately, when remission means recovery of disturbing memories, amnesia may give way to suicidal ideation or behavior, or to PTSD or another condition.

Depersonalization/Derealization Disorder A person with **depersonalization disorder** has a recurring or persistent feeling of being cut off or detached from his or her body or mental processes, as if observing themselves from the outside, in something like an out-of-body experience. In a **derealization disorder**, on the other hand, a person experiences a feeling that people or objects in the external world are unreal. In both cases, the person knows that the feeling is not accurate—his or her "reality testing" remains intact—and the depersonalization and/or derealization, plus awareness of this incongruity, causes distress or impairs functioning. The disorder usually first occurs in late adolescence, with almost all cases having a first onset before the person is 25 years old. Onset and remission can be sudden or gradual, with stress or novel situations often playing an exacerbating role.

9. Personality Disorders

Personality traits are stable patterns of thought, feeling, and behavior that influence how a person experiences, thinks about, and interacts with the people and events in his or her life. A **personality disorder** is an enduring, rigid set of personality traits that deviates from cultural norms, impairs functioning, and causes distress either to the person with the disorder or to those in his or her life. The symptom profile therefore involves a list of the prominent traits that characterize each "disordered" personality. Because many personality disorders are **egosyntonic**—generally in harmony with a person's ego or self-image—it is usually the consequences of the personality disorder, such as depression, rather than its symptom structure, that cause a person to seek treatment.

The degree of distress or impairment is important. Because personality traits are not simply binary— "normal" versus "pathological"—but instead represent a continuum (for example, from independent to nonconforming to antisocial), the same constellations of traits that are found in personality disorders can also be present to varying degrees in normal people. A difficult or rigid personality becomes a personality disorder when the pattern causes significant distress or impairment, has been present since adolescence or young adulthood, affects nearly all personal and social situations, and creates dysfunction in two or more of the following areas: affect, cognition, impulse control, and interpersonal functioning.

In the DSM-5, the personality disorders have been organized, or "clustered," into three categories. **Cluster A** includes the paranoid, schizoid, and schizotypal personality disorders associated with irrational, withdrawn, odd, or suspicious behaviors. **Cluster B** includes the antisocial, borderline, histrionic, and narcissistic personality disorders associated with emotional, dramatic, and self-centered behaviors, and intense interpersonal conflict. **Cluster C** includes the avoidant, dependent, and obsessive-compulsive personality disorders, associated with fearful, anxious, over-controlled behaviors.

Table 5 Personality Disorders

Category	Personality Disorder	Traits
Cluster A	Paranoid Schizoid Schizotypal	Irrational, Withdrawn, Odd, Suspicious
Cluster B	Antisocial Borderline Histrionic Narcissistic	Emotional, Dramatic, Self-centered, Intense
Cluster C	Avoidant Dependent Obsessive-Compulsive	Fearful, Anxious, Over-controlled

Cluster A

Paranoid Personality Disorder A person with **paranoid personality disorder** mistrusts and misinterprets others' motives and actions without sufficient cause, suspecting them of deceiving, harming, betraying, or attacking him or her. The person tends to be guarded, tense, and self-sufficient, generally in counterproductive/maladaptive ways.

Schizoid Personality Disorder A person with **schizoid personality disorder** is a loner with little interest or involvement in close relationships, even those with family members. The person seems unaffected emotionally by interactions with other people, appearing instead detached or cold. This disorder is thus characterized by one of the negative symptoms of schizophrenia.

Schizotypal Personality Disorder A person with **schizotypal personality disorder** has several traits that cause problems interpersonally, including limited or inappropriate affect; magical or paranoid thinking; and odd beliefs, speech, behavior, appearance, and perceptions. This disorder is thus characterized by some of the positive symptoms of schizophrenia. The person tends to have no confidantes other than close relatives. Many cases eventually develop into schizophrenia (the disorder is cross-listed in the DSM-5 in the section on Schizophrenia Spectrum and Other Psychotic Disorders).

Cluster B

Antisocial Personality Disorder A person with **antisocial personality disorder** has a history of serious behavior problems beginning as a young teen (often even younger), including significant aggression against people or animals, deliberate property destruction, lying or theft, and serious rule violation. In addition, the person must have a history (since age 15) of repeatedly disregarding the rights of others in various ways without remorse, through illegal activities, dishonesty, impulsiveness, physical fights, disregard for safety, and financial irresponsibility. This disorder is cross-listed in the DSM-5 in the section on Disruptive, Impulse-Control, and Conduct Disorders. It is more frequently encountered in men and specifically in incarcerated men.

Borderline Personality Disorder A person with **borderline personality disorder** suffers from enduring or recurrent instability in his or her impulse control, mood, and image of self and others. Impulsive and reckless behavior, together with extreme mood swings, reactivity, and anger, can lead to unstable relationships and to damage, both to the person with the disorder and to others in his or her life. Feeling empty, with an unstable sense of self, the person is terrified of abandonment by others, whom the person may first idealize and then devalue or demonize. Self-harming and suicidal behaviors may also occur. There is some evidence that this disorder is a generalized and more severe form of a bipolar disorder and/or that it is linked to childhood sexual abuse. It is more frequently encountered in women.

Histrionic Personality Disorder A person with **histrionic personality disorder** strongly desires to be the center of attention, and often seeks to attract attention through personal appearance and seductive behavior. The person's expressions of emotion are dramatic, yet the emotions themselves are often shallow and shifting, and the person may believe that his or her relationships are more intimate than they are. The person may also be suggestible, and vague in his or her speech.

Narcissistic Personality Disorder A person with **narcissistic personality disorder** feels grandiosely self-important, with fantasies of beauty, brilliance, and power. The person feels a desperate need for admiration in a variety of contexts and may be intensely envious. Lacking empathy, he or she may continually exploit others and behave in an arrogant, haughty, and entitled manner.

Cluster C

Avoidant Personality Disorder A person with **avoidant personality disorder** feels inadequate, inferior, and undesirable and is preoccupied with fears of criticism and conflict. The person feels ashamed, and avoids interpersonal contact and new activities, unless he or she is certain of being liked. The person is also restrained and inhibited in relationships.

Dependent Personality Disorder A person with **dependent personality disorder** feels a need to be taken care of by others and an unrealistic fear of being unable to take care of him- or herself. The person also has trouble assuming responsibility and making decisions, preferring to gain approval by making others responsible and seeking others' advice and reassurance regarding decisions. In relationships, he or she is clingy, submissive, and afraid to express disagreement. Others often take advantage of the person because he or she is willing to do or tolerate almost anything, even abuse, in order to gain support and nurturing, and to avoid abandonment. He or she urgently seeks another relationship if one is lost.

Obsessive-Compulsive Personality Disorder A person with **obsessive-compulsive personality disorder** (OCPD) may be perfectionistic, rigid, and stubborn, with a strong need for control. The person resists others' authority, and will not cooperate with or delegate to others unless things are done his or her way. Often workaholic and moralistic beyond the level of the surrounding culture or religion, the person also may be depressed and have trouble expressing affection. A preoccupation with orderliness and list-making across a variety of situations can interfere with effectiveness and efficiency. OCPD is cross-listed in the DSM-5 in the section on Obsessive-Compulsive and Related Disorders.

Biological Bases of Nervous System Disorders

Schizophrenia

Recall that schizophrenia is a disorder characterized by positive symptoms, such as delusions, hallucinations, and disorganized speech, as well as negative ones, such as flat affect, decreased or absent speech, and avolition. Although schizophrenia presents as a thought disorder, it is important to remember that psychological characteristics have a physical or neurological basis; the division between these two is largely a conceptual one (based on an outdated **mind-body dualism** framework). Schizophrenia is a neurological disorder with a strong genetic basis. Studies have found that in identical twins, if one twin has schizophrenia, the other has about a 50% chance of also having it; if the second twin does not have schizophrenia, the first twin is likely to have a lesser form of it (e.g., schizophreniform disorder). The onset of schizophrenia happens around adolescence. The **stress-diathesis theory** suggests that while genetic inheritance provides a biological predisposition for schizophrenia, stressors elicit the onset of the disease.

There are numerous brain changes that have been noted in people with schizophrenia. One idea formed from observations is the **dopamine hypothesis**, which suggests that the pathway for the neurotransmitter dopamine is hyperactive in people with schizophrenia. This is due both to an overabundance of dopamine and to hypersensitive dopamine receptors. This finding, along with evidence of hyperactivation of the temporal lobes in people with this condition, may explain the presence of the positive signs of schizophrenia (like auditory hallucinations). Dopamine antagonist medications have been found to be helpful as antipsychotics.

Additionally, *hypo*activation of the frontal lobes may be responsible for the negative signs of schizophrenia, creating a kind of pseudo-depression, flat affect, and impaired speech. Individuals with schizophrenia have also been found to have smaller brains due to atrophy: schizophrenic individuals display increased ventricles (cavities in the brain), and enlarged sulci and fissures (less folding).

Depression

Depression also appears to have a strong genetic basis—there is increased risk of developing depression when a first-degree family member has it. Depression has been linked to diminished functioning in pathways in the brain that involve the neurotransmitters dopamine, serotonin, and norepinephrine. Antidepressants thus target and try to stimulate these pathways. Depression can often accompany other neurological diseases, such as Parkinson's and traumatic brain injury, due to damage to similar or overlapping areas of the brain.

Neurodevelopmental Disorders

As the name "neurodevelopmental" implies, something abnormal occurred to the brain during early development, whether *in utero* or shortly after birth. While **intellectual disability** can have several causes, a notable one is Down syndrome (trisomy 21) in which a third copy of chromosome 21 is present in the genome. In the case of **attention-deficit/hyperactivity disorder (ADHD)**, PET scans have suggested a general understimulation of the brain, which helps explain why stimulants may alleviate some of the behavioral symptoms. In the case of **autism spectrum disorder (ASD)**, brain structure and chemistry are still being studied; one leading hypothesis involves the underformation of mirror neurons.

Neurocognitive Disorders

Dementia (the general term for what is called a neurocognitive disorder in DSM-5) is a severe loss of cognitive ability beyond what would be expected from normal aging. **Alzheimer's disease** ("major or minor neurocognitive disorder due to Alzheimer's disease") is the most prevalent form of dementia, affecting a large number of people who reach their 80s and especially their 90s (over 50% for this latter group, according to some estimates). It is a disease that is characterized by **anterograde amnesia**, the inability to form new memories, as well as stepwise **retrograde amnesia**, with more recent memories degrading first, such that the last memories to fade are typically the oldest. Alzheimer's patients may thus be able to recall events from decades earlier but forget people and events that were encountered recently. Their visual memory will be impaired as well, such that they may get lost and confused. Needless to say, living with Alzheimer's disease can be very confusing, frustrating, and emotionally painful both for the patient and for family members and friends.

Alzheimer's disease is a cortical disease, meaning that it affects the cortex, the outermost tissue of the brain. It is caused by the formation of **neuritic plaques**, hard formations of beta-amyloid protein and **neurofibrillary tangles** (clumps of tau protein). It is unclear why these plaques and tangles form, though there is some evidence of at least partial genetic susceptibility. Some theories suggest that when these plaques build up, they reach a critical mass and then begin to cause cell death by "gunking up" neuronal connections, preventing nutrients and waste from traveling to and from some neurons. Currently, there is no cure for Alzheimer's, and treatments are directed at slowing the progress of the illness rather than reversing it.

Finally, there is some evidence of abnormalities in the activity of the neurotransmitter acetylcholine in the hippocampus. It should be no surprise that the hippocampus could be involved, because this is the area of the brain that plays a major role in the formation of new memories. As mentioned above, the disease tends to progress in a predictable pattern: as it progresses, the patient loses increasingly older memories, as well as language function and spatial coordination. Eventually, patients are not able to perform daily functions without assistance.

Parkinson's disease ("major or mild neurocognitive disorder due to Parkinson's disease" in the DSM-5) is a movement disorder caused by the death of cells that generate dopamine in the **basal ganglia** and **substantia nigra**, two subcortical structures in the brain. Among the symptoms are a resting tremor (shaking), slowed movement, rigidity of movements and facial expressions, and a shuffling gait. As the disease progresses, language is typically spared. However, depression and visual-spatial problems may arise. It is estimated that 50% to 80% of Parkinson's patients eventually experience dementia as their disease progresses. In order to treat Parkinson's, patients are given L-dopa treatments. L-dopa is a precursor to dopamine and is used because it is able to pass the blood-brain barrier, entering the brain's blood supply (dopamine is not able to cross the blood-brain barrier).

8.2   STRESS

The Nature of Stress

Stress is a great reminder that often what is considered to be psychological is simultaneously physiological. Under acute conditions of stress, such as while giving a formal presentation, it is common to feel physical symptoms such as increased heart rate and sweating. Prolonged periods of stress can have negative consequences, including immunosuppression, infertility, and hypertension. However, stress is not a simple stimulus-response phenomenon. How a stimulus is perceived plays a large role in how much stress is experienced.

Appraisal

Not everyone responds the same way to events that can trigger a stressful reaction. For example, imagine that a couple is at home in bed when suddenly they hear a creaking sound in another room. One person may assume that the sound is due to the age of the house or the steps of a pet, while the other may attribute the sound to a possible burglar sneaking around the house. Obviously, though the stimulus is the same, one person is going to become much more stressed than the other. What is most important for determining the stressful nature of an event is its **appraisal**, or how it is interpreted by the individual. When stressors are appraised as being challenges, as one may perceive the MCAT, they can actually be motivating. On the other hand, when they are perceived as threatening aspects of our identity, well-being, or safety, they may cause severe stress. Additionally, events that are considered negative and uncontrollable produce a greater stress response than those that are perceived as negative but controllable.

Different Types of Stressors

There are three main types of stressors, which differ in terms of their severity: catastrophes, significant life changes, and daily hassles.

1) **Catastrophes** are unpredictable, large-scale events that include natural disasters and war. They are events that almost everyone would appraise as dangerous and stress-inducing. The repercussions of a catastrophic event are often felt for years after the event. In the months following 9/11, many people developed psychological disorders including anxiety, depression, and posttraumatic stress disorder (PTSD). Health consequences can also follow prolonged periods of stress, as may be common in refugee camps or shelters.

2) **Significant life changes** include events such as moving, leaving home, losing a job, marriage, divorce, death of a loved one, and other such changes. The frequency of these events during young adulthood may explain the high degree of stress during this time. These events can be risk factors for disease and death, with several concurrent events creating greater risk than single stressful events would.

3) **Daily hassles** are the everyday irritations of life including bills, traffic jams, misplacing belongings, and scheduling activities. These things are fairly universal events, but some people take them lightly, while others may become overwhelmed. These little stressors can accumulate and lead to health problems such as hypertension and immunosuppression.

Effects of Stress on Psychological Functions

Moderate amounts of stress can actually improve psychological functioning by providing more energy and motivation for cognitive activities (for example, cramming the day before a final exam). However, when stress is not at an optimal level, it can impair psychological functioning by leading to fatigue, decreased ability to concentrate, and irritability. In addition, when stress is accompanied by a perceived lack of control over the stress-inducing events, over time someone may develop **learned helplessness**, which is a sense of exhaustion and lack of belief in one's ability to manage situations. With severe or prolonged stress, some people may develop PTSD. This disorder is characterized by symptoms of re-experiencing the traumatic event through flashbacks or nightmares, hypervigilance to one's surroundings, and avoidance of situations related to the stressful event.

Stress Outcomes/Response to Stressors

Physiological

Our bodies respond to stress by activating two parallel systems. The first is the **sympathetic nervous system**, the "fight or flight" response. This system responds to acute stress situations; it releases the stress hormones epinephrine (adrenaline) and norepinephrine (noradrenaline) into the bloodstream from the adrenal glands. This response causes increased heart and respiratory rates, directs blood flow toward the skeletal muscles rather than the digestive system, releases sugar into the bloodstream, and dulls pain. It is a fast-acting response.

The second is a cognitive system initiated by the hypothalamus, located just above the brainstem. The hypothalamus releases corticotropin-releasing hormone (CRH), a messenger that stimulates the pituitary gland to release **adrenocorticotropic hormone (ACTH)**. ACTH then signals the adrenal glands to release cortisol into the bloodstream. **Cortisol** is a glucocorticoid, a hormone that shifts the body from using sugar (glucose) as an energy source toward using fat as an energy source. This "glucose-sparing" effect keeps blood sugar levels high during stress situations (important because the only energy source the brain can use is glucose), thus ensuring that the brain will have enough fuel to stay active. This chain of events is a slower process than the near-instantaneous fight or flight response, and it is primarily triggered during long-term stress.

While short-term cortisol release can be helpful, prolonged release due to chronic stressors is harmful. Most notably, prolonged cortisol release inhibits the activity of white blood cells and other functions of the immune system. Thus, stress itself does not make us sick but rather increases the vulnerability to illness. It has been shown that stress can exacerbate the course of diseases including AIDS, cancer, and heart disease.

Emotional

Emotional stresses can be correlated with worse medical outcomes. For example, anger can trigger cardiac events such as heart attacks, arrhythmias, and even sudden death in people who already have heart disease. High levels of stress can contribute to the development of anxiety and depressive disorders, which are characterized by negative mood and irritability.

Behavioral

People respond in many different ways to stress, and an individual may respond differently to the same stressor depending on the circumstances. Sometimes we confront stressful situations, while at other times we avoid uncomfortable situations or emotions. Avoidance can be accompanied by habits such as cigarette smoking, consuming alcohol, or eating as a means of temporary physical comfort. In response to high stress situations, some people develop PTSD, which involves three clusters of symptoms: avoidance, hyperarousal, and re-experiencing. Avoidance involves avoiding both circumstances that remind one of the trauma and emotions associated with the trauma. Thus, someone with PTSD may tell a horrific story of personal trauma in a flat tone that is disconnected from the associated emotion. Hyperarousal involves heightened sensitivity (making a person easily startled) and hypervigilance to surroundings due to fear of danger. Re-experiencing symptoms are responses to triggers related to the traumatic event, such as flashbacks and nightmares. Sleep disturbances are common side effects of stress.

Managing Stress

There is an optimal level of stress that is motivating and invigorating. Too little stress can lead to complacency, while too much can be overwhelming and debilitating. However, stress is largely a personal experience based on an appraisal of situations. People vary in their ability to modulate their stress levels to remain close to the optimum.

One effective way of coping with stress is aerobic exercise. Exercise has been shown to be a useful adjunct to antidepressant drugs and psychotherapy, and is about as effective as these treatments in reducing depression. In addition to lowering blood pressure, aerobic exercise may help by increasing the production of neurotransmitters that boost mood, including norepinephrine, serotonin, and endorphins.

A second means for managing stress is through the use of biofeedback and relaxation. **Biofeedback** is a means of recording and feeding back information about subtle autonomic responses in an attempt to train the individual to control those involuntary responses. For example, people can be trained to adjust their muscle tension, heartbeats, and respiratory rates. This has been a particularly effective means of treating tension headaches. Many of the same benefits can occur through relaxation training, including meditation, progressive muscle relaxation, visual imagery, and yoga.

A third means of effectively managing stress is through the utilization of social support. Stronger social support has been associated with lower blood pressure, lower stress hormones, and stronger immune system function. The impact of stressful events can be mediated when individuals can express their emotional reactions and recollection of traumatic events through talking about them, writing in journals, or other means best suited to those individuals.

There is an unclear relationship between spirituality and health. Many studies have established that religious activity is associated with longer life expectancy and healthier immune functioning; however, it is unclear whether this is a causal relationship. Those who are more involved religiously also tend to have healthier diets and are less likely to smoke or drink. They also tend to have stronger social support systems within the religious community of which they are part. Thus, it is unclear whether other variables explain the improvement in health. Regardless, there may be important aspects inherent in or associated with spirituality and religion that can promote health.

Chapter 8 Summary

- Psychological disorders are sets of symptoms at odds with societal norms that are severe enough to cause personal distress or significantly impair functioning.

- The DSM-5 categorizes disorders according to symptoms and offers research-based treatments.

- Anxiety disorders, including panic disorders and phobias, involve an unpleasant and unwanted fight-or-flight-like response in situations where there is no immediate threat or danger and are not related to acute trauma.

- Obsessive-compulsive disorders are characterized by uncontrollable thoughts or behaviors that are often repeated as rituals and interrupt normal functioning.

- Trauma-or-stressor-related disorders include posttraumatic stress disorder, a disorder caused by a stressful life event that leads to a fear response in the presence of triggering stimuli.

- Somatic symptom disorders mimic the symptoms of some physical disorder in the absence of a diagnosable condition.

- Bipolar disorders are characterized by a fluctuation between a depressive state and a manic state.

- Depressive disorders involve a lowered mood and feelings of dejection or worthlessness.

- Schizophrenic disorders often include delusions, disorganized and abnormal behavior, hallucinations, and impaired social functioning.

- Dissociative identity disorder, previously known as multiple personality disorder, involves a disintegrated identity in which individuals can appear to assume different personalities in different states.

- Personality disorders are inflexible patterns of thought and behavior that create problems in day-to-day functioning and well-being.

CHAPTER 8 FREESTANDING PRACTICE QUESTIONS

1. A patient suffering from social anxiety disorder has been referred to two different therapists with different approaches. The first therapist uses the psychoanalytic approach, while the second therapist uses a cognitive-behavioral approach. Which answer choice most accurately reflects the beliefs and goals of these two therapists, respectively?

A) The first therapist will focus his efforts on analyzing and interpreting the patient's behaviors and interactions, with the end goal of helping his patient reach insight into their unconscious desires. The second therapist will focus on identifying and subsequently replacing her patient's learned behaviors with new, healthier behaviors.
B) The first therapist will focus on identifying and subsequently replacing his patient's unhealthy habits and cognitive processes. The second therapist will focus her efforts on analyzing and interpreting the patient's behaviors and interactions, with the end goal of helping her patient reach insight into their unconscious desires.
C) The first therapist will focus his efforts on analyzing and interpreting the patient's behaviors and interactions, with the end goal of helping his patient reach insight into their unconscious desires. The second therapist will focus on identifying and subsequently replacing her patient's unhealthy habits and distorted cognitive processes.
D) The first therapist will focus his efforts on exploring his patient's childhood experiences, to uncover any psychosexual fixation that they may have developed. The second therapist will focus on showing her patients unconditional positive regard and helping them remove barriers toward self-actualization.

2. Conversion disorder is characterized by:

A) a constant fear of being ill.
B) panic attacks and severe anxiety.
C) frequent vague complaints about a physical symptom.
D) functional impairment of a limb or sensory ability with no apparent physical cause.

3. All the following are Cluster B personality disorders EXCEPT:

A) histrionic behavior disorder.
B) schizoid personality disorder.
C) narcissistic personality disorder.
D) borderline personality disorder.

4. A child shows difficulty engaging with other children and needs to follow a very strict routine every day to function properly. If the routine is broken, he cries and has a very difficult time adjusting. These symptoms may satisfy which of the following diagnoses?

A) Attention-deficit hyperactivity disorder
B) Obsessive-compulsive personality disorder
C) Obsessive-compulsive disorder
D) Autism spectrum disorder

5. Parkinson's disease involves:

I.   overstimulation of dopamine-producing neurons in the peripheral nervous system.
II. cell death in the basal ganglia and substantia nigra.
III. neurofibrillary tangles and neuritic plaques in the brain.

A) I only
B) II only
C) I and II
D) II and III

6. Which of the following represents a stressor that would be considered a "catastrophe?"

I.   A terrorist attack that kills hundreds of people
II. Divorce
III. Death of a child

A) I only
B) III only
C) I and III
D) I, II, and III

CHAPTER 8 PRACTICE PASSAGE

In the late 1800s, psychiatrist William Gull described one of his patients as suffering from a "perversion of the will" that resulted in "simple starvation." Today, Gull's patient would likely be diagnosed with *anorexia nervosa* (AN), which is characterized by a dramatic distortion of perceived body image and dangerously low weight achieved through food restriction, excessive exercise, or other extreme means (abuse of diet pills, laxatives, etc.). According to multiple studies, AN has the highest mortality rate of all mental illnesses. This finding is likely due to the severe health consequences associated with AN, including cardiovascular stress, gastrointestinal dysfunction, and malnutrition.

Several theories have been advanced to explain the etiology or risk factors of AN and other eating disorders. Some researchers posit that AN is primarily a sociocultural phenomenon rooted in Western culture's espousal of a thin body ideal. According to these theorists, the disorder initially progresses through three stages: exposure to the thin ideal, internalization of the thin ideal, and perceived discrepancy between oneself and the thin ideal. In an effort to conform to the thin ideal, individuals who have AN employ extreme behaviors to reduce their weight. Other researchers point to personality traits or family dynamics as the primary sources of AN pathology. Finally, some theorists prefer to view AN from an addiction perspective.

In an effort to determine best treatment practices for AN and other eating disorders, some studies have compared treatment results of various clinical interventions. For example, Britain's National Institute for Clinical Excellence (NICE) conducted a comprehensive review of both inpatient and outpatient interventions for all of the AN treatment centers in the United Kingdom, collecting data on psychoanalytic therapy, behavioral therapy (BT), cognitive behavioral therapy (CBT), and family-based treatment (FBT). Published in 2004, the NICE study concluded that no particular treatment approach was significantly superior to any other particular approach in terms of treatment outcome. In another study conducted in 2010, researchers examined treatment outcome differences between FBT and ego-oriented individual therapy (EOIT) with adolescent patients. Selection criteria required a diagnosis of AN between twelve and eighteen months prior to therapy, as well as therapy duration between twelve and twenty sessions.

The FBT group contained fifty-two subjects, while the EOIT group contained fifty subjects. Figure 1 displays the results of this study.

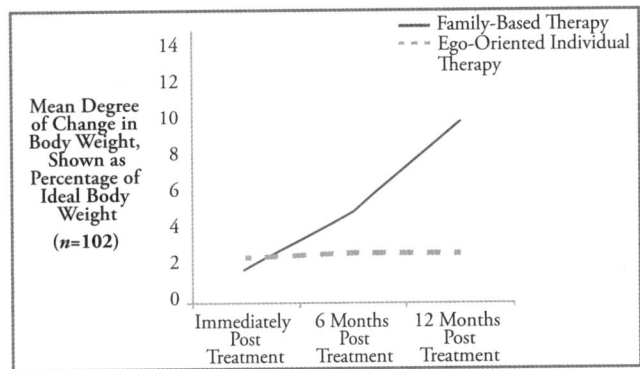

Figure 1   Treatment outcome results for FBT and EOIT

Material used in this passage was adapted from the following sources:

Risk Factors for Eating Disorders, R. H. Striegel-Moore and C.M. Bulik, in *American Psychologist*. © 2007 by the American Psychological Association.

Eating Disorders: Core interventions in the treatment and management of anorexia nervosa, bulimia nervosa, and related eating disorders. © 2004 by the British Psychological Society and the Royal College of Psychiatrists.

Randomized clinical trial comparing family-based treatment with adolescent-focused individual therapy for adolescents with anorexia nervosa. J. Lock, D. Le Grange, W. S. Agras, A. Moye, S. W. Bryson, and B. Jo, in the Archives of General Psychiatry. © 2010 by the American Medical Association.

1. Most AN sufferers demonstrate largely consistent eating patterns marked by some sporadic binging; AN sufferers generally stick to a very specific restrictive diet, eating only "safe foods" a majority of the time, but binging occasionally on other foods. Despite this irregularity in behavior, AN sufferers' attitudes about food remain consistent. What concept best describes this behavior, in terms of AN sufferers maintaining a specific attitude about food, but demonstrating slightly inconsistent eating behavior?

A)   The reality principle
B)   The principle of aggregation
C)   The self-actualizing tendency
D)   Vicarious learning

2. Heather was recently diagnosed with anorexia nervosa, and she has experienced continued weight loss and severe stomach pain. According to learning theory, for Heather, her physical symptoms would be considered:

    I.   positive reinforcement.
    II. extinction.
    III. punishment.

A) I only
B) III only
C) I and III only
D) I, II, and III

3. An empirical basis for the addiction model of AN would most likely come from research that:

A) discovers that a majority of those diagnosed with AN have at least one parent who is alcohol dependent.
B) identifies high comorbidity of AN and tobacco dependence.
C) proves that there is an inverse relationship between dopamine production in the brain and the activity of the satiety center controlled by the hypothalamus in individuals with AN.
D) shows that those with AN have a higher mortality rate than individuals dependent on methamphetamines.

4. Which of the following scenarios best reflects how a psychoanalytic therapist would treat a patient with AN?

A) The therapist would make sure to establish a relationship with the client based on rapport and mutual trust, and would always provide unconditional positive regard to the client.
B) The therapist would help the patient gain awareness of his or her unconscious motives for AN-related behavior, and help the patient to transition from self-loathing and guilt to reality.
C) The therapist would attempt to recondition negative behaviors.
D) The therapist would help the patient pinpoint negative thoughts and feelings, and help the patient learn positive self-talk and healthier behaviors.

5. Noreen, who was diagnosed with AN, now participates in family therapy. Based on the chart in Figure 1, what should the therapist expect?

A) Noreen will gain approximately 10% of her ideal body weight by the end of 12 months.
B) Noreen will gain approximately five pounds by the end of six months.
C) Noreen's weight will double halfway through the treatment.
D) Noreen will gain ten pounds by the end of treatment.

6. Which of the following conclusions can be inferred from the results displayed in Figure 1?

A) Family-based therapy is superior to ego-oriented individual therapy in reducing the negative thought processes associated with AN.
B) The distortions in self-image characteristic of those with AN derive from an underdeveloped ego.
C) Attachment theory is relevant to treating AN.
D) AN typically derives from poor parenting.

SOLUTIONS TO CHAPTER 8 FREESTANDING PRACTICE QUESTIONS

1. **C** In choice C, the first therapist focuses on uncovering unconscious desires, which is consistent with the psychoanalytic method, and the second therapist is concerned with correcting maladaptive patterns, consistent with the cognitive behavioral method. In choice A, the second therapist does not seem to focus on any cognitive influences. Based on the description, the second therapist is taking a behavioral approach, not a cognitive-behavioral approach (choice A is incorrect). In choice B, the approach of the first therapist is consistent with cognitive-behavioral therapy, and the second therapist's approach is consistent with psychoanalytic therapy. This is the opposite of the question stem (choice B is incorrect). In choice D, the first therapist's goals are consistent with psychoanalysis, but the second therapist is using a humanist perspective, rather than cognitive behavioral therapy (choice D is incorrect).

2. **D** Conversion disorder is a somatoform disorder in which a person displays blindness, deafness, or other symptoms of sensory or motor failure without a physical cause (choice D is correct). A constant fear of illness refers to illness anxiety disorder (hypochondriasis), not conversion disorder (choice A is wrong). Panic attacks and severe anxiety are symptoms of anxiety disorders, while conversion disorder is a type of somatoform disorder (choice B is wrong). Frequent vague complaints about physical symptoms are characteristic of somatization disorder, not conversion disorder (choice C is wrong).

3. **B** Schizoid personality disorder is classified under Cluster A personality disorders, not Cluster B (choice B is correct). This person will likely be markedly detached from friends and family members and have a flat affect, whereas Cluster B disorders are more emotional and dramatic (choices A, C, and D are incorrect).

4. **D** Many diagnoses like obsessive-compulsive disorder and personality disorders are diagnosed only in adolescence/adulthood. This is a child, so this must be a neurodevelopmental disorder (choices B and C can be eliminated). The child is not exhibiting impulsivity/hyperactivity nor inattention (choice A can be eliminated), but rather restrictive behavior and difficulty in social situations, since he is having difficulty engaging with peers. This is descriptive of autism spectrum disorder (ASD, choice D is correct).

5. **B** Item I is false: Parkinson's disease is the result of the death of dopamine-producing neurons in the brain; furthermore, while there are *some* dopamine-producing neurons in the peripheral nervous system, the primary neurotransmitter responsible for muscle movement is acetylcholine, not dopamine (choices A and C can be eliminated). Note that both remaining answer choices include Item II, so it must be true: Parkinson's is primarily caused by cellular death of neurons in the basal ganglia and substantia nigra of the brain; these neurons are dopamine-producing and inhibitory, connecting with the motor cortices in the brain and help to smooth out movement and inhibit excessive movement. Death of neurons in these areas results in the characteristic shaking, rigidity, and slowness of movement initiation. Item III is false: neurofibrillary tangles and neuritic plaques in the brain are characteristic of Alzheimer's disease, not Parkinson's disease (choice D can be eliminated, and choice B is correct).

6.   **A**   Item I is true: catastrophes are unpredictable, large-scale events that include natural disasters and wartime devastation. Catastrophes are events that almost everyone would appraise as dangerous and stress-inducing (choice B can be eliminated). Item II is false: divorce is considered a significant life change, not a catastrophe (choice D can be eliminated). Item III is false: while emotionally devastating, the death of a child would be considered a significant life change, not a catastrophe, because it is not a large-scale event affecting many people (choice C can be eliminated, and choice A is correct).

SOLUTIONS TO CHAPTER 8 PRACTICE PASSAGE

1. **B** The principle of aggregation explains how attitudes are better at predicting general patterns of behavior, but cannot always account for specific behaviors. The principle of aggregation best explains the periodically inconsistent behavior of binging, despite the fact that the attitude of AN sufferers toward food remains consistent (choice B is correct). According to Freud, the ego is ruled by the reality principle, which employs logical thinking to control consciousness and the id; while the reality principle may be involved in the choices AN sufferers make about eating, it does not explain the inconsistent behavior in light of a consistent attitude (choice A is wrong). The self-actualizing tendency is an innate drive toward recognizing one's full potential; it does not explain the scenario described in the question stem (choice C is wrong). Vicarious learning involves an individual learning by observing another individual; this does not explain the scenario described in the question stem (choice D is wrong).

2. **C** Item I is true: according to learning theory, positive reinforcement is an operant conditioning term that refers to a favorable consequence that reinforces a particular behavior. In Heather's case, the physical symptom of weight loss is considered a reward for her eating behavior (because she has AN and weight loss is desirable for her) and is thus a positive reinforcement (choice B can be eliminated). Item II is false: extinction is the process by which the behavior in question ceases due to the absence of a favorable consequence; since the question stem makes no mention of Heather ceasing her behavior, extinction does not explain her physical symptoms (choice D can be eliminated). Item III is true: punishment refers to a negative consequence experienced as a result of the behavior; Heather's stomach pain is a punishment for her eating behaviors (choice A can be eliminated, and choice C is correct).

3. **C** The hypothalamus is the brain structure associated with appetite regulation, while dopamine is the neurotransmitter associated with the pleasure pathways of the brain. Many illicit and addictive substances manipulate the dopamine system in some fashion, either by stimulating the release of dopamine or by inhibiting its absorption. If AN is a form of addiction, there would likely be an inverse relationship between the brain region that communicates satiety and the pleasure center of the brain; in other words, when the satiety center is not active (an individual with AN is not sated or full), dopamine is produced. This would indicate that the pleasure center of the brain is triggered when an individual with AN starves him- or herself, thus establishing a biochemical basis for the addiction model (choice C is correct). It is important to recognize that the context in which the passage mentions an addictions model suggests that AN is itself a type of addiction. It does not refer to mere correlations with addiction, such as family members with addictions (choice A is wrong) or comorbidity with other addictions (choice B is wrong). Finally, the possibility that AN is more lethal than substance abuse does not logically yield the conclusion that AN is also an addiction (choice D is wrong).

4. **B** Psychoanalytic therapy focuses on helping the patient gain awareness of his or her unconscious motives, and then make choices that are based on reality rather than on drives (id) or guilt (superego; choice B is correct). Humanistic therapy is more concerned with establishing a relationship between the therapist and the "client" based on mutual trust and unconditional positive regard (choice A is wrong). Behavioral therapy might involve reconditioning of negative behaviors (choice C is wrong) and cognitive-behavioral therapy best describes targeting negative thoughts/feelings and learning positive self-talk and healthier behaviors (choice D is wrong).

5. **A** The vertical axis of the chart in Figure 1 reflects the percentage of ideal body weight. Therefore, Figure 1 demonstrates that those in family-based therapy will gain 10% of their ideal body weight by the end of 12 months (choice A is correct). The vertical axis of Figure 1 does not represent pounds gained (choices B and D are wrong). Additionally, although the percentage of ideal body weight doubles six months post-treatment, weight gained during treatment is not depicted in Figure 1. Further, the six-month marker shows a doubling of *percentage* of ideal body weight rather than a doubling of total baseline weight (choice C is wrong).

6. **C** The chart in Figure 1 suggests that family-based therapy is superior to ego-oriented individual therapy in helping those with AN to gain weight post-treatment; but it does not suggest that family-based therapy is superior to individual therapy at reducing the negative thought processes associated with AN (choice A is wrong). However, it does imply that family relationships play a key role in AN pathology, which is consistent with attachment theory (choice C is correct). Attachment theory maintains that parent-child relationships strongly influence the child's attitudes about the self and the world. Nevertheless, a relevance of attachment and relationships to successful treatment of the disorder does not automatically imply that the disorder was caused by poor parenting. It may simply mean that familial relationships can help the patient to develop more positive self-images or become more aware of unhealthy behavior (choice D is wrong). Although psychodynamic theory may view distorted body image as a function of poor reality-testing, which is the domain of the ego, this focus would not be supported (or contradicted) by the relative superiority of family-based therapy to individual therapy (choice B is wrong).

A RANDOMIZED CONTROLLED TRIAL OF EMOTION REGULATION THERAPY FOR GENERALIZED ANXIETY DISORDER WITH AND WITHOUT CO-OCCURRING DEPRESSION

Mennin, Douglas S; Fresco, David M; O'Toole, Mia Skytte; Heimberg, Richard G.

Journal of Consulting and Clinical Psychology Vol. 86, Iss. 3, (Mar 2018): 268-281. DOI:10.1037/ccp0000289

Generalized anxiety disorder (GAD) is a burdensome condition marked by chronic and excessive worry (American Psychiatric Association, 2013) and considerable suffering. Highly impairing when occurring alone, GAD is especially impacting when it co-occurs with major depressive disorder (MDD; e.g., Whisman, Sheldon, & Goering, 2000; Henning, Turk, Mennin, Fresco, & Heimberg, 2007). Given high rates of comorbidity and overlapping symptoms, GAD and MDD are often regarded as "distress disorders" (e.g., Watson, 2005; also "emotional disorders"; Barlow, Sauer-Zavala, Carl, Bullis, & Ellard, 2014). Despite the availability of efficacious treatments, GAD and MDD frequently exhibit suboptimal long-term treatment response (e.g., Farabaugh et al., 2012; Newman, Przeworski, Fisher, & Borkovec, 2010).

EMOTION REGULATION THERAPY

In an effort to integrate and synthesize theory and findings from traditional cognitive behavior therapy and affect science, Mennin and Fresco (2013, 2014) have advanced an emotion dysregulation model that characterizes distress disorders as marked by heightened emotional experience (i.e., motivational intensity) coupled with NSRP, which functions as a compensatory strategy to manage the experience of strongly felt emotional and somatic experiences. Building on this framework, Emotion Regulation Therapy (ERT; e.g., Fresco, Mennin, Heimberg, & Ritter, 2013; Mennin & Fresco, 2014) represents a mechanism-targeted intervention that integrates findings from affect science with principles from cognitive–behavioral therapy (CBT; see Mennin, Ellard, Fresco, & Gross, 2013). This model posits that dysfunction in distress disorders can best be understood by (a) motivational mechanisms, reflecting the functional and directional properties of an emotional response tendency; (b) regulatory mechanisms, reflecting the alteration of emotional response trajectories utilizing less (i.e., attentional) and more (i.e., metacognitive) cognitively

elaborative systems; and (c) contextual learning consequences, reflecting the promotion of broad and flexible behavioral repertoires (Renna, Quintero, Fresco, & Mennin, 2017). With respect to GAD, dysfunction results from a failure in each of these normative systems of functioning. Specifically, GAD is characterized by heightened emotional experience (i.e., motivational intensity) coupled with negative self-referential processing, which functions as compensatory strategy to manage the experience of strongly felt emotional and somatic experiences. Using a motivational framework (i.e., identifying reward- and risk-based impulses), ERT instructs patients to engage in mindful emotion regulation skills to counteract negative self-referential processing (e.g., worry, rumination, and self-criticism) in service of pursuing intrinsically rewarding and goal-directed actions in their lives.

Building on these encouraging findings, the present study sought to further examine the efficacy of ERT using a controlled research design. Consistent with the stage model of psychosocial intervention development (e.g., Onken, Carroll, Shoham, Cuthbert, & Riddle, 2014), the current study utilized a randomized controlled trial (RCT) design comparing patients randomly allocated to immediate ERT with patients assigned to a modified attention control condition (MAC), wherein patients received periodic contact from study therapists to assess clinical status and offer encouragement while they completed assessments and then awaited their turn to receive open label ERT following their participation in the MAC. We hypothesized that ERT would demonstrate superiority to the MAC in reducing symptoms associated with anxiety, depression, and disability, while increasing quality of life. We further hypothesized that ERT would exceed the MAC in ameliorating deficits in hypothesized mechanisms reflecting mindful attention and metacognitive regulation (i.e., trait mindfulness, decentering, cognitive reappraisal, and trait emotion dysregulation). We also examined long-term outcome (at 3- and 9-month following treatment) of both acutely and post-MAC treated patients to determine the enduring effects of ERT on all study outcomes. Here, we expected the largest change to be found in the acute phase after which trajectories would maintain effects into the follow-up periods.

Importantly, given the deliberate focus in ERT on the development of adaptive regulatory skills and the successful probing and improvement of these regulation-related variables in our prior OT (Mennin et al., 2015), we also hypothesized that improvements in less and more elaborative regulatory abilities (i.e., trait mindfulness, decentering, cognitive reappraisal, and trait emotion dysregulation) would mediate primary outcomes (i.e., GAD severity, worry, depression, disability, and life satisfaction) of those treated with ERT compared with the MAC condition. Finally, we examined indices of clinical significance in GAD- and MDD-related outcomes to show that improvements reflect gains of considerable magnitude beyond mere statistical change (Kazdin, 1999).

METHOD

Participants

One Hundred Thirty-Four individuals sought treatment both as part of routine care or specifically in response to directed recruitment efforts for the study (e.g., fliers). All individuals were assessed for general eligibility for clinical care using diagnostic assessment (see below). Fifty-three adults at two psychology training clinic sites in the Northeastern United States (Site 1 was located in Philadelphia, PA, $n = 28$; Site 2 was located in New Haven, CT, $n = 25$) ultimately expressed interest in the study and consented to be randomized. Institutional Review Boards approved procedures for the study at both sites, and all patients provided informed consent. The targeted sample size was based on a power analysis proposed in the NIMH funded R34 to enroll 34 patients drawing on meta-analytic effect sizes comparing an active treatment to WL control. This proposed sample size also anticipated expected attrition during the RCT of 4 patients leaving 30 completers. As such we would be powered to detect group by time interaction effect sizes ranging from Cohen's $d = .44$ (no attrition) to 48 (with expected attrition). Seeing as we successfully enrolled 53 patients with 44 completers, our study was actually powered to detect group by time interaction effect sizes ranging from $d = .36$ (full sample) to .38 (completers).

Interviewers at both sites were clinical psychologists or doctoral students in clinical psychology trained according to the guidelines of the ADIS or SCID. Patients were required to have a primary or coprimary diagnosis (based on clinical severity) of GAD to be admitted into the study. In addition, an independent assessor also administered the GAD module at pre-, mid-, posttreatment, and at the follow-up assessments. Further, modules with positive diagnoses at pretreatment were readministered at posttreatment and into the follow-up periods. Diagnostic agreement (in diagnosis and CSR within 1 point; ADIS CSR was used at both sites) for GAD between the intake clinician and the independent assessor at pretreatment was necessary for study inclusion. Agreement rate was 100% across both sites.

Additional inclusion criteria consisted of fluency in spoken and written English; and willing and able to give informed written consent.

The sample was mostly women (75%), with a mean age of 39 ($SD = 14.5$), primarily White (87%; Asian American/Pacific Islander 2%; African American 6%; other 6%), non-Hispanic (91%), and well-educated (64% had at least a college education). Twenty-five patients were employed full time followed by working part-time ($n = 7$), being full-time students ($n = 5$), unemployed ($n = 10$), a homemaker ($n = 4$), or retired ($n = 2$). Median annual family income for the sample was $48,819 (Range = $0 to $176,000). Twenty-three patients had a concurrent MDD diagnosis. Thirty-one patients had at least one additional current diagnosis (Range: 1–5) including obsessive–compulsive disorder ($n = 7$), panic disorder ($n = 10$), posttraumatic stress disorder ($n = 4$), social phobia ($n = 17$), specific phobia ($n = 7$), dysthymic disorder ($n = 5$), and eating disorder ($n = 1$). Thirteen patients participated while receiving concurrent antidepressant medication; 7 patients enrolled receiving benzodiazepines. Of the 53 consented patients, 28 were randomized to treatment and 25 were randomized to the MAC condition. Group assignment was determined by a random-number generator at the outset of the trial. Patients and clinicians remained unaware of randomization condition until after the signing of informed consent.

Twenty-five patients in the immediate treatment condition (89%) and 20 in the MAC condition (80%) completed the acute phase of the study. Reasons for attrition from acute ERT included a patient's mother had a major mental health issue that required leaving the area, a patient decided to leave the area to transfer to another university, a patient did not return after reporting an abuse history, a patient began taking psychotropic medication, and divorce proceedings made it difficult for another patient to regularly attend sessions. Twenty MAC completers initiated open-label ERT and 15 completed treatment (75%). Three- and 9-month follow-up assessments were conducted for all patients who completed the treatment. There were no demographic differences across the two sites, and no baseline clinical and demographic differences associated with treatment response (analyses available upon request). Thus, analyses were conducted on the full sample aggregated across sites. RCT analyses compared ERT with MAC patients at pre-, mid-, and postacute treatment. Follow-up analyses were conducted on all patients who received ERT (immediate ERT + MAC patients who received open-label ERT).

Treatment

ERT consisted of 20 weekly sessions of 60-min duration except for Sessions 11–16 which lasted 90 min to accommodate exposure exercises. In the first half, sessions focused on teaching emotion regulation strategies via attention regulation and more verbally elaborate metacognitive regulation. In the second half of ERT, patients were encouraged to deploy regulation skills during in-session and out-of-session exposures that simultaneously invoked both engagement of a context that is both rewarding and threatening. The final sessions focused on consolidating gains and preparing for termination (Fresco et al., 2013; Mennin & Fresco, 2014).

Ten clinical psychology doctoral students trained to administer ERT by the first and second authors served as protocol therapists, and received 2 hours of weekly group supervision to discuss active cases. All therapists reviewed their session video to generate a detailed timestamped and annotated note detailing how each intervention was received and what issues arose in implementation. Every video and accompanying note was reviewed by the first and second authors prior to supervision. Each case was discussed for approximately 20 min with additional time provided when emergent clinical management issues came to light.

Measures

Patients completed clinician-assessed and self-report measures of anxiety, depression, worry, disability, and quality of life as well as hypothesized mechanisms. The assessment schedule for these measures was pretreatment, midtreatment, postacute treatment, and three- and 9-month follow-up. Intake interviewers and independent assessors (all assessment points) were blind to patients' assignment in the RCT.

Clinician and diagnostic assessment

Independent assessors provided clinical assessment of patients at all points utilizing the ADIS CSR and a modified version of the *Clinical Global Impression Rating Scales* (CGI; Guy, 1976). A version with anchor points developed specifically for rating improvement (CGI-I) in symptoms associated with GAD was utilized. Patients received a rating of 1 (very much improved) or 2 (much improved) were classified as responders.

Self-report symptom and severity measures

The *Penn State Worry Questionnaire (*PSWQ; Meyer, Miller, Metzger, & Borkovec, 1990) is a widely used 16-item measure of trait worry ($\alpha = .85$). The 7-item *State–Trait Anxiety Inventory* (STAI; Bieling, Antony, & Swinson, 1998) is an abbreviated version of this frequently used measure, comprised of the seven items that loaded most highly on an anxiety factor (present sample $\alpha = .85$). The *Mood and Anxiety Symptom Questionnaire-Short Form* (MASQ; Watson & Clark, 1991) is a 62-item instrument that comprises four subscales: General Distress Anxious Symptoms (GDA; present sample $\alpha = .79$), General Distress Depressive Symptoms (GDD; present sample $\alpha = .92$), Anxious Arousal (AA; present sample α $\alpha = .89$), and Anhedonic Depression (AD; present sample $\alpha = .66$). The *Beck Depression Inventory-II* (BDI–II; Beck, Steer, & Brown, 1996) is a 21-item self-report measure that assesses the affective, cognitive, behavioral, and somatic symptoms of depression (present sample $\alpha = .90$). The Brooding subscale of *Rumination Scale* (RS; Treynor, Gonzalez, & Nolen-Hoeksema, 2003) is a five-item measure of self-reported rumination uncontaminated by depression symptom content (present sample $\alpha = .77$; only given at Site 2). The Sheehan Disability Scale (SDS; Sheehan, 1983) is a commonly utilized measure assessing impairment at work, in social relationships, and in responsibilities at home and with family (present sample α = .60). The *Quality of Life Inventory* [QOLI; Frisch, Cornell, Villanueva, & Retzlaff, 1992] assesses the degree to which an individual is satisfied with 16 areas of his or her life (e.g., health, standard of living, friendships, relationship with family, community, etc.; present sample α = .81).

Hypothesized mechanism measures

The *Five Facet Mindfulness Questionnaire* (FFMQ; Baer, Smith, Hopkins, Krietemeyer, & Toney, 2006) is a 39-item self-report measure assessing trait mindfulness (present sample α = .90). The 11-item Decentering subscale of the *Experiences Questionnaire* (EQ; Fresco et al., 2007) assessed decentering (i.e., the metacognitive ability to observe items that arise in the mind with distance and perspective; present sample α = 71). The *Difficulties in Emotion Regulation Scale* (DERS; Gratz & Roemer, 2004) is a 36-item measure of the acceptance of emotions, ability to engage in goal-directed behavior when distressed, impulse control, awareness of emotions, access to strategies for regulation, and clarity of emotions (present sample α = .93). The Cognitive Reappraisal subscale of the *Emotion Regulation Questionnaire* (ERQ; Gross & John, 2003) is a 6-item measure of cognitive reappraisal (present sample α = .91).

The following measures were considered "primary outcomes" (given centrality to hypotheses and primary focus of other GAD trials) and only these measures were utilized in mediation analyses: GAD CSR, PSWQ, BDI, SDS, & QOLI. Although MDD CSR and the RSQ are centrally related to hypotheses, there were limitations in data collection of these latter two measures, and, thus, they were not suitable to examine as outcomes in mediation analyses (i.e., MDD CSR was only assessed at pre- and posttreatment; RSQ was only administered at site 2).

RESULTS

Acute Treatment Effects

Means and standard deviations for all outcomes at the three acute time points are reported in Table 1. There were no significant between-groups differences at pretreatment on any of the measures. The Time × Group interaction effects for all three of the diagnostic measures (GAD CSR and MDD CSR, and mean CSR of additional diagnoses) were significant and of moderate to large effect sizes (Hedge's gs ranging from .72 to .83). The Time × Group interaction effects for all self-reported anxiety outcomes (PSWQ, STAI-7, MASQ-AA, MASQ-GDA), self-reported depression outcomes (BDI, RSQ Brooding, MASQ-AD, MASQ-GDD), disability/quality of life outcomes (SDS, QOLI), and the hypothesized mechanism variables (FFMQ, EQ Decentering, ERQ Reappraisal, DERS) were significant in the expected direction, ranging in effect size from .51 to 1.50. All results survived the correction for multiple comparisons according to the Benjamini-Hochberg critical value. Result statistics can be found in Table 1.

Mediation Analyses

Mediation analyses were conducted on the six primary outcomes for the four hypothesized mechanisms utilized as mediators. Result statistics are reported in Table 2. All proposed mediators showed an indirect effect of group on the primary outcomes.

Table 1 Treatment Effects Presented as Means (*M*), Standard Deviations (*SD*), *Z* Statistics, and Hedge's *g* Effect Size

Measure	Emotion regulation therapy (*n* = 28)			Modified attention control (*n* = 25)			Time × Group interaction effect		
	Pre	Mid	Post	Pre	Mid	Post	*z*	*p*	*g*
Diagnostic measure									
GAD CSR[a]	5.6 (.6)	4.1 (1.1)	3.0 (1.3)	5.9 (.6)	5.4 (1.2)	5.5 (.9)	−6.5	<.001	.83
MDD CSR[b]	4.3 (.5)	—	1.4 (2.0)	4.7 (.5)	—	3.5 (1.9)	−2.2	.030	.82
Mean CSR of additional diagnoses other than GAD[b]	4.3 (.4)	—	1.1 (1.3)	4.4 (.6)	—	2.5 (2.0)	−2.9	.004	.72
Self-reported anxiety									
PSWQ[a]	67.5 (7.3)	55.3 (10.2)	44.0 (9.9)	68.1 (11.8)	68.6 (10.3)	67.2 (10.9)	−6.9	<.001	1.50
STAI-7	18.6 (4.2)	15.3 (3.1)	12.3 (2.6)	19.7 (3.9)	19.9 (4.3)	19.7 (4.2)	−5.3	<.001	1.22
MASQ AA	29.1 (10.7)	24.0 (6.4)	21.0 (3.8)	33.0 (10.6)	32.2 (10.5)	31.0 (11.3)	−2.1	.037	.51
MASQ GDA	30.2 (9.6)	25.1 (5.2)	21.3 (4.7)	30.8 (7.8)	29.5 (7.6)	29.0 (7.2)	−4.1	<.001	.87
Self-reported depression									
BDI[a]	19.8 (9.9)	11.3 (7.7)	5.8 (5.8)	21.2 (10.7)	19.9 (10.3)	18.7 (11.3)	−4.2	<.001	.93
RSQ Brooding[a,b]	12.5 (2.4)	12.9 (3.0)	10.3 (2.3)	13.6 (2.9)	15.0 (3.4)	14.0 (3.2)	−3.7	<.001	.74
MASQ AD	69.6 (12.3)	61.0 (812.8)	53.0 (811.4)	74.8 (13.6)	76.5 (10.1)	73.1 (15.6)	−3.0	.002	.62
MASQ GDD	32.6 (8.8)	27.4 (5.2)	20.5 (5.3)	36.5 (10.9)	29.5 (7.6)	34.4 (12.5)	−3.1	.002	.69
Disability/quality of life									
SDS[a]	15.1 (6.2)	10.6 (5.7)	7.3 (5.4)	15.4 (5.8)	16.4 (6.5)	14.7 (7.2)	−3.8	<.001	.87
QOLI[a]	.7 (1.8)	1.2 (1.5)	2.2 (1.2)	−.1 (1.9)	.2 (1.7)	−.1 (1.8)	2.6	.009	.48
Proposed mediators									
FFMQ total	109.8 (15.5)	122.2 (20.7)	131.6 (17.7)	107.9 (23.6)	109.0 (20.9)	112.6 (23.0)	3.6	<.001	.83
ERQ Reappraisal	22.6 (6.2)	26.4 (5.2)	29.7 (4.4)	21.6 (9.2)	21.6 (9.7)	24.0 (9.9)	2.2	.031	.54
EQ Decentering	29.5 (6.7)	33.7 (7.0)	39.2 (5.1)	29.6 (5.2)	29.4 (5.1)	30.4 (6.5)	4.5	<.001	1.00
DERS total	98.2 (23.1)	82.3 (20.3)	74.6 (19.0)	104.8 (22.4)	102.2 (23.2)	96.0 (22.0)	−3.4	.001	.80

Note. *g* = Hedge's *g* Effect size; GAD = Generalized Anxiety disorder; CSR = Clinician's Severity Rating from the Anxiety Disorders Interview Schedule for *DSM-IV,* Lifetime Version; PSWQ = Penn State Worry Questionnaire; STAI = State Trait Anxiety Inventory; MASQ = Mood and Anxiety Symptom Questionnaire; AA = Anxious Arousal; GDA = General Distress Anxiousness; MDD = Major Depressive Disorder; BDI-II = Beck Depression Inventory II; RSQ = Response Style Questionnaire; AD = Anhedonic Depression; GDD = General Distress Depression; SDS = Sheehan Disability Scale; QOLI = Quality of Life Inventory; FFMQ = Five Facet Mindfulness Questionnaire; ERQ = Emotion Regulation Questionnaire; EQ = Experiences Questionnaire; DERS = Difficulties in Emotion Regulation Scale.
[a] Primary outcomes. [b] Clinician assessment not conducted at midtreatment.

Table 2 Indirect Effects of Proposed Mediators on Primary Outcomes

Mediator	B	BSSE	BCLL	BCUL
GAD CSR mediated by:				
FFMQ total Score	−.30	.18	−.73	−.01
DERS total score	−.39	.18	−.81	−.10
ERQ Reappraisal	−.27	.13	−.67	−.07
EQ Decentering	−.41	.19	−.87	−.10
PSWQ mediated by:				
FFMQ total score	−2.76	1.36	−6.33	−.40
DERS total score	−4.32	1.78	−8.51	−1.23
Reappraisal	−2.79	1.57	−7.40	−.62
EQ Decentering	−4.57	1.75	−8.22	−1.36
BDI mediated by:				
FFMQ total Score	−2.71	1.45	−5.89	−.12
DERS total score	−4.02	1.69	−7.65	−.97
ERQ Reappraisal	−2.34	1.18	−5.04	−.34
EQ Decentering	−3.12	1.26	−5.86	−.87
QOLI mediated by:				
FFMQ total Score	.29	.16	.02	.64
DERS total score	.42	.18	.11	.83
ERQ Reappraisal	.24	.13	.04	.54
EQ Decentering	.30	.13	.09	.61
SDS mediated by:				
FFMQ total Score	−1.58	.86	−3.52	−.10
DERS total score	−2.40	1.01	−4.51	−.58
ERQ Reappraisal	−1.48	.74	−3.15	−.21
EQ Decentering	−1.61	.69	−3.17	−.47

Note. BSSE = Bootstrapped standard error; BCLL = Bias-corrected lower level of 95% confidence interval; BCUL = Bias-corrected upper level of 95% confidence interval; GAD = generalized anxiety disorder; Schedule for DSM-IV, Lifetime Version; PSWQ = Penn State Worry Questionnaire; BDI-II = Beck Depression Inventory II; RSQ = Response Style Questionnaire; SDS = Sheehan Disability Scale; QOLI = Quality of Life Iventory; FFMQ = Five Facet Mindfulness Question-naire; ERQ = Emotion Regulation Questionnaire; EQ = Experiences Questionnaire; DERS = Difficulties in Emotion Regulation Scale. Re-sults refer to the indirect effect of the proposed mediators investigated separately. Significant (p < 0.05) indirect effects are in bold.

Follow-Up Effects and Clinical Response

Means and standard deviations from all patients who received ERT of all outcome variables at the five time points are reported in Table 3. All but one of the effect sizes was of a large magnitude, ranging from .70 to 1.77. Result statistics can be found in Table 3.

The proportion of participants meeting the criteria for treatment response is reported in Table 4. Employing both simple criteria and more stringent indices showed that participants continued to improve over the follow-up period on all the GAD-related response measures. Concerning the MDD-related response measures, the same pattern was detected although there was a slight decrease in response over the follow-up period on the two more stringent indices of clinical response (i.e., 30% improvement and high endstate functioning).

Further, although in the acute treatment phase, no patients initiated medication or additional psychotherapy, at the 3-month follow-up, 1 patient initiated antidepressant medication. At the 9-month follow-up, 2 additional patients initiated antidepressant medication and 1 patient initiated anxiolytic medication. With respect to psychotherapy, 1 patient at the 3-month follow-up and 4 patients at the 9-month follow-up initiated new psychological treatment.

DISCUSSION

The current study provides additional evidence for the efficacy of ERT following the promising findings of an earlier open label trial (Mennin et al., 2015). ERT was well tolerated as reflected in the high rate of treatment completion among all patients receiving ERT (83%) as well as among patients with comorbid MDD (83%). In terms of treatment efficacy, patients receiving immediate ERT versus the MAC demonstrated statistically and clinically meaningful improvement on measures of GAD and MDD symptoms, additional anxiety disorder severity, functional impairment, quality of life, worry, rumination, as well as theoretically consistent mechanism factors reflecting mindful attentional, metacognitive, and overall emotion dysregulation. This superiority of immediate ERT over MAC equaled or exceeded conventions for a medium effect size with many outcomes surpassing conventions for a large effect. Importantly, treatment effects attributable to ERT were largely maintained for nine months following the end of acute treatment.

Despite these promising findings, notable limitations must be considered that may also suggest directions for further investigation. First, the sample was relatively small and patients were only followed for nine months. Future studies would ideally treat and follow a larger sample for a longer period of time (~2 years) to better determine durability of treatment gains. Second, the sample was largely White and non-Hispanic. Future investigations with more racially and ethnically heterogeneous samples are needed to ideally show that ERT effects generalize to the full population of those suffering with distress disorders. Third, although the MAC included active attention from a clinician during the waitlist period and is appropriate for this stage of treatment development (e.g., Onken et al., 2014), the control comparison was relatively inert and not optimally equated against active treatment such as ERT.

In conclusion, the current findings provide considerable preliminary efficacy for ERT in treating GAD as well as associated MDD and other anxiety problems. Building on these encouraging findings, an important next step will be to determine the optimal duration and intensity of ERT (e.g., Renna, Quintero, et al., in press). On balance, the present results provide encouraging initial support for the efficacy and potential mechanisms of ERT in a sample of patients with GAD with and without comorbid MDD and suggest fruitful directions for improving our understanding and treatment of complicated clinical conditions such as the distress disorders.

Table 3   Long-Term Treatment Effects Presented as Means (*M*), Standard Deviations (*SD*), *Z* Statistics, and Hedge's *g* Effect Size

Measure	Time point *M* (*SD*)					Effect of time		
	Pre	Mid	Post	3-month follow-up	9-month follow-up	*z*	*p*	*g*
Diagnostic measure								
GAD CSR[a]	5.4 (.9)	4.3 (1.2)	2.9 (1.5)	2.9 (1.4)	2.6 (1.2)	−13.93	<.001	1.77
MDD CSR[b]	4.5 (.5)		2.8 (1.8)	2.8 (1.1)	2.1 (1.2)	−7.80	<.001	1.39
Mean CSR of additional diagnoses other than GAD[b]	4.4 (.6)		2.7 (1.4)	2.6 (1.1)	2.4 (1.1)	−11.81	<.001	1.47
Self-reported anxiety								
PSWQ[a]	67.9 (8.7)	57.3 (10.2)	47.4 (10.6)	48.0 (11.8)	49.9 (10.5)	−9.97	<.001	1.41
STAI-7	19.1 (4.2)	15.9 (3.3)	12.7 (3.3)	13.6 (3.9)	13.7 (3.7)	−8.64	<.001	1.28
MASQ AA	30.0 (6.9)	26.0 (8.4)	22.4 (5.7)	22.3 (5.4)	24.9 (6.1)	−4.53	<.001	.83
MASQ GDA	29.8 (6.9)	25.5 (6.0)	21.9 (4.9)	21.3 (5.1)	21.2 (5.7)	−8.77	<.001	1.34
Self-reported depression								
BDI[a]	19.2 (10.5)	11.7 (8.8)	6.4 (7.1)	8.8 (8.0)	9.4 (9.3)	−8.47	<.001	1.12
RSQ Brooding[a,c]	13.2 (2.9)	13.4 (2.5)	10.8 (2.5)	11.0 (2.8)	11.0 (2.5)	−4.46	<.001	1.04
MASQ AD	71.1 (13.9)	63.7 (13.8)	55.1 (12.0)	61.9 (13.7)	62.1 (13.9)	−5.43	<.001	.70
MASQ GDD	33.2 (10.5)	28.5 (9.6)	22.0 (7.1)	24.3 (7.7)	25.4 (9.4)	−6.71	<.001	.93
Disability/quality of life								
SDS[a]	15.1 (6.6)	12.6 (6.3)	7.5 (5.4)	7.3 (5.3)	7.3 (6.2)	−10.09	<.001	1.23
QOLI[a]	.2 (1.8)	.8 (1.7)	1.9 (1.4)	1.4 (1.4)	1.4 (1.5)	5.56	<.001	.81
Proposed mediators								
FFMQ total	111.2 (19.1)	118.0 (18.9)	130.6 (18.0)	131.4 (20.3)	130.8 (19.1)	9.03	<.001	1.30
ERQ Reappraisal	23.1 (8.1)	26.4 (6.1)	31.0 (5.8)	29.6 (5.3)	27.4 (5.9)	4.49	<.001	.80
EQ Decentering	29.9 (6.6)	32.9 (6.0)	38.5 (5.6)	36.8 (5.4)	36.5 (4.8)	8.62	<.001	1.17
DERS total	97.0 (22.6)	91.2 (20.5)	75.4 (20.8)	79.1 (19.8)	76.5 (18.9)	−9.72	<.001	1.24

Note. *g* = Hedge's *g* Effect size; GAD = Generalized Anxiety disorder; CSR = Clinician's Severity Rating from the Anxiety Disorders Interview Schedule for *DSM-IV*, Lifetime Version; PSWQ = Penn State Worry Questionnaire; STAI = State Trait Anxiety Inventory; MASQ = Mood and Anxiety Symptom Questionnaire; AA = Anxious Arousal; GDA = General Distress Anxiousness; MDD = Major Depressive Disorder; BDI-II = Beck Depression Inventory II; RSQ = Response Style Questionnaire; AD = Anhedonic Depression; GDD = General Distress Depression; SDS = Sheehan Disability Scale; QOLI = Quality of Life Inventory; FFMQ = Five Facet Mindfulness Questionnaire; ERQ = Emotion Regulation Questionnaire; EQ = Experiences Questionnaire; DERS = Difficulties in Emotion Regulation Scale.
[a] Primary outcomes. [b] Clinician assessment not conducted at midtreatment. [c] Only administered at Site 2.

Table 4   Percentages of Patients Receiving ERT Meeting Criteria for Treatment Response

Response	Posttreatment: No. responders (% ITT)	3-month follow-up: No. responders (% ITT)	9-month follow-up: No. responders (% ITT)
GAD clinical response			
ADIS GAD CSR <4	33/48 (69%)	29/40 (73%)	35/40 (88%)
CGI-improvement <3	37/48 (77%)	36/40 (90%)	39/40 (98%)
30% improvement (4+ of 6 criteria met)	36/48 (75%)	35/40 (88%)	36/40 (90%)
High endstate functioning (4+ of 6 criteria met)	32/48 (67%)	30/40 (75%)	32/40 (80%)
MDD clinical response			
ADIS MDD CSR <4	15/23 (65%)	15/19 (79%)	16/19 (84%)
CGI-improvement <3	16/23 (70%)	15/19 (79%)	17/19 (89%)
30% improvement (3+ of 4 criteria met)	13/23 (57%)	14/19 (74%)	12/19 (63%)
High endstate functioning (3+ of 4 criteria met)	14/23 (61%)	14/19 (74%)	12/19 (63%)

Note. ERT = Emotion Regulation Therapy; ITT = Intention to Treat: ITF = Intention to Follow; GAD = generalized anxiety disorder; ADIS = Anxiety Disorders Interview Schedule; CSR = Clinician's Severity Rating from the Anxiety Disorders Interview Schedule for *DSM-IV*, Lifetime Version; CGI = clinical global impression; MDD = major depressive disorder.

JOURNAL ARTICLE EXERCISE 3

The science sections on the MCAT include a significant number of passages with experiments. Questions for these passages often ask you to analyze data, read charts and graphs, and come to some reasonable conclusion based on the information they give you. If you don't know how to extract information efficiently and analyze data effectively, you will be at a distinct disadvantage.

There are three "Journal Article Exercises" in this book. In this final exercise, you'll read and extract information from the article, then complete an MCAT passage based on this article. After that, we'll show you the "correct" information to pull out and the answers to the passage.

As before, when analyzing an experiment, you should be able to:

- identify the control group(s)
- extract information from graphs and data tables
- determine how the experimental group(s) change relative to the control
- determine if the results are statistically significant
- come to a reasonable conclusion about WHY the results were observed
- consider potential weaknesses in the study
- determine how to increase the power of the study
- decide what the next most logical experiment or study should be

And, as before, the goal of these exercises is NOT to learn content from the articles, just to get a little more comfortable reading and extracting information from them.

For the (abridged) article on pages 243–249, try to summarize the purpose of the experiment and the methods in a few sentences. Remember the mnemonic: Oh ouR Car Won't Start (ORCWS).

- O = Organism and Organization
- R = Results
- C = Control and Comparison
- W = Weirdness
- S = Statistics

Try interpreting the data on your own before reading the results/discussion section. When you do read the discussion, consider:

- What are the conclusions of the study?
- How are the conclusions supported by the data?
- What potential weaknesses or flaws do you see in the experimental design? Are these addressed in the discussion section?
- How might this study be potentially biased?
- How might this study be improved?
- What would be the next most logical experiment?

Write brief responses to the questions below for the article on pages 243–249:

1. **O = Organism and Organization:**
   - Is the research being conducted on humans or on animals or on bacteria in a petri dish, or something else?

     _____

     _____

   - What is being done to these organisms?

     _____

     _____

   - Are there any unique qualities to these organisms?

     _____

     _____

   - Are there multiple groups?

     _____

     _____

   - Is the study conducted over a long period of time with multiple data points, or is it a short-term study?

     _____

     _____

   - Does it have a large or small n?

     _____

     _____

2. **R = Results:**
   - Where and how are the results presented? Is it a graph? A data table? Figures and images?

     _____

     _____

   - What is/are the independent variable(s)?

     _____

     _____

   - What is/are the dependent variable(s)?

     _____

     _____

   - What are the results of the study?

     _____

     _____

- Do the results show correlation or cause and effect, or both? Describe.

  _____

  _____

3. **C = Control and Comparison:**
   - Is there a control group?

     _____

     _____

   - How does it differ from the experimental group? Is it given a placebo or nothing at all? Is it held under different conditions?

     _____

     _____

   - If there are multiple experimental groups, how do they differ from one another?

     _____

     _____

   - Is it a blinded study? If so, double-blind or single-blind?

     _____

     _____

4. **W = Weirdness:**
   - Does anything or do any of the results stand out as unexpected?

     _____

     _____

5. **S = Statistics:**
   - Was any sort of statistical analysis done?

     _____

     _____

   - How is it presented? Are there error bars on a graph? Standard errors around a mean? Are there *p*-values? Is there an asterisk indicating statistical significance?

     _____

     _____

   - Is there any data that is not statistically significant?

     _____

     _____

6. **Interpreting the data:**
   - What are the conclusions of the study?

     _____

     _____

- How are the conclusions supported by the data?

  _____

  _____

- What potential weaknesses or flaws do you see in the experimental design? Are these addressed in the discussion section?

  _____

  _____

- How might this study be potentially biased?

  _____

  _____

- How might this study be improved?

  _____

  _____

- What would be the next most logical experiment?

  _____

  _____

7. **Final Summary of Experiment and Results:**

  _____

  _____

  _____

  _____

  _____

JOURNAL ARTICLE EXERCISE 3 PASSAGE

Generalized anxiety disorder (GAD) is marked by chronic and excessive worry and considerable suffering. Highly impairing when occurring alone, GAD is especially impacting when it co-occurs with major depressive disorder (MDD). Given high rates of comorbidity and overlapping symptoms, GAD and MDD are often regarded as "distress disorders". Despite the availability of efficacious treatments, GAD and MDD frequently exhibit suboptimal long-term treatment response.

A study randomly allocated participants to either an immediate Emotion Regulation Therapy (ERT) condition or to a modified attention control condition (MAC). ERT utilizes principles from cognitive–behavioral therapy, while the MAC condition participants received periodic contact from study therapists to assess clinical status and offer encouragement. Researchers hypothesized that ERT would demonstrate superiority to the MAC in reducing symptoms associated with anxiety, depression, and disability, while increasing quality of life. Participants were also examined in terms of their long-term outcomes (at 3- and 9-month intervals following treatment).

Overall, 53 adults at two psychology training clinic sites in the Northeastern United States expressed interest in the study and consented to be randomized. The participants with a primary diagnosis of GAD (43% with comorbid MDD) were randomly assigned to immediate treatment with ERT ($n = 28$) or a modified attention control condition (MAC, $n = 25$). The sample was mostly women (75%), with a mean age of 39, primarily White (87%), non-Hispanic (91%), and well-educated (64% college educated).

The study found that participants receiving immediate ERT versus the MAC demonstrated statistically and clinically meaningful improvement on measures of GAD and MDD symptoms, additional anxiety disorder severity, functional impairment, quality of life, worry, rumination, as well as theoretically consistent mechanism factors reflecting mindful attentional, metacognitive, and overall emotion dysregulation. Importantly, treatment effects attributable to ERT were largely maintained for nine months following the end of acute treatment. These findings provide encouraging support for the efficacy and hypothesized mechanisms underlying ERT and point to fruitful directions for improving our understanding and treatment of complex clinical conditions such as GAD with co-occurring MDD.

1. The researchers in the study utilized which of the following study designs?

A) Cross-sectional
B) Longitudinal
C) Historical research
D) Case study

2. Emotion Regulation Therapy, as defined in the passage, is based on which of the following psychological perspectives on personality?

A) Humanistic approach
B) Psychoanalytic approach
C) Social cognitive approach
D) Behavioralist approach

3. Which of the following can be concluded from the results of the study?

A) Participants in the Modified Attention Control demonstrated superior improvement on clinician rated and self-reported anxiety and depression, satisfaction with life, worrying and ruminating, and in self-perceived ability to manage emotions with mindfulness and perspective taking, relative to patients receiving immediate treatment.
B) Participants in the Emotion Regulation Therapy condition did not demonstrate long-term benefit from their assigned treatment condition.
C) Participants in the Modified Attention Control condition did not demonstrate long-term benefit from their assigned treatment condition.
D) Emotion Regulation Therapy participants demonstrated superior improvement on clinician rated and self-reported anxiety and depression, satisfaction with life, worrying and ruminating, and in self-perceived ability to manage emotions with mindfulness and perspective taking, relative to patients receiving delayed treatment.

4. Each of the following is a limitation of the study design EXCEPT:

A) the study only compared two types of treatment methods.
B) patients were only followed for nine months.
C) the sample was largely White and non-Hispanic.
D) the sample was largely female.

SOLUTIONS TO JOURNAL ARTICLE EXERCISE 3

1. **O = Organism and Organization:**
   - Is the research being conducted on humans or on animals or on bacteria in a petri dish, or something else? *Humans*
   - What is being done to these organisms? *They are subjected to two different types of treatment for GAD (generalized anxiety disorder) and MDD (major depressive disorder).*
   - Are there any unique qualities to these organisms? *The sample was mostly women (75%) with a mean age of 39 and also primarily white (87%).*
   - Are there multiple groups? *Yes, an ERT (emotion regulation therapy) treatment group, which is compared to the MAC (modified attention control) treatment group*
   - Is the study conducted over a long period of time with multiple data points, or is it a short-term study? *Long. The ERT group consisted of 20 weekly sessions of 60 to 90 minute durations. The MAC group received less contact, consisting of four 15-minute telephone contacts.*
   - Does it have a large or small *n*? *Small n: 28 in the ERT group and 25 in the MAC condition*

2. **R = Results:**
   - Where and how are the results presented? Is it a graph? A data table? Figures and images? *Data tables*
   - What is/are is the independent variable(s)? *Type of treatment received*
   - What is/are is the dependent variable(s)? *Clinical indicators of GAD and MDD (worry, rumination, disorder severity, functional impairment, and quality of life)*
   - What are the results of the study? *ERT patients evidenced statistically meaningful improvement in clinical indicators compared to the MAC group, even after the study concluded.*
   - Do the results show correlation or cause and effect, or both? Describe. *Cause and effect: the treatment group showed more improvement compared to the MAC group.*

3. **C = Control and Comparison:**
   - Is there a control group? *Yes (MAC group)*
   - How does it differ from the experimental group? Is it given a placebo or nothing at all? Is it held under different conditions? *The control group received a different type of treatment.*
   - If there are multiple experimental groups, how do they differ from one another? *Only one experimental group*
   - Is it a blinded study? If so, double-blind or single-blind? *Single-blind; the participants did not know the treatment method of the other group*

4. **W = Weirdness:**
   - Does anything or do any of the results stand out as unexpected? *No*

5. **S = Statistics:**
   - Was any sort of statistical analysis done? *Yes*
   - How is it presented? Are there error bars on a graph? Standard errors around a mean? Are there *p*-values? Is there an asterisk indicating statistical significance? *P values, standard deviations, Z-scores, and Hedge's g*
   - Is there any data that is not statistically significant? *No*

6. **Interpreting the data:**
   - What are the conclusions of the study? *Emotion Regulation Therapy (ERT) demonstrates superior improvement on clinician rated and self-reported anxiety and depression, satisfaction with life, worrying and ruminating, and in self-perceived ability to manage emotions with mindfulness and perspective taking, relative to patients receiving delayed treatment.*
   - How are the conclusions supported by the data? *Data shows significant differences between the ERT and MAC groups.*
   - What potential weaknesses or flaws do you see in the experimental design? Are these addressed in the discussion section? *Biased sample, mostly women and white*
   - How might this study be potentially biased? *Demographics of sample*
   - How might this study be improved? *More varied demographics (racially, sex, age, etc.)*
   - What would be the next most logical experiment? *Repeat the experiment with subjects in varying demographic groups.*

7. **Final Summary of Experiment and Results:**
   - *53 patients with a primary diagnosis of GAD (43% with comorbid MDD) were randomly assigned to immediate treatment with ERT (n = 28) or a modified attention control condition (MAC, n = 25). ERT patients, as compared with MAC patients, evidenced statistically and clinically meaningful improvement on clinical indicators of GAD and MDD. Treatment effects were maintained for nine months following the end of acute treatment. Overall, ERT resulted in high rates endstate functioning for both GAD and MDD that were maintained into the follow-up period.*

SOLUTIONS TO JOURNAL ARTICLE EXERCISE 3 PASSAGE

1. **B**   The passage states that participants were examined in terms of their long-term outcomes (at 3- and 9-months following treatment). A study design that permits comparison of identical measures and groups at two or more points in time is known as a longitudinal study (choice B is correct). Cross-sectional designs measure at one specific point in time (choice A is incorrect), historical research focuses on examining past events, usually through primary or archival sources (choice C is incorrect), and a case study focuses on the examination of a single case (choice D is incorrect).

2. **C**   Paragraph 2 states that ERT is based on the principles of cognitive-behavioral therapy (CBT). CBT, in turn, is based on the social cognitive perspective on personality, pioneered by psychologists such as Albert Bandura (choice C is correct). The humanistic approach lead to the creation of client-centered therapy, pioneered by Carl Rogers (choice A is incorrect). The psychoanalytic approach led to the creation of psychotherapy, pioneered by Sigmund Freud (choice B is incorrect). The behavioralist perspective on personality lead to behavioral therapy, pioneered by B.F. Skinner (choice D is incorrect).

3. **D**   The final paragraph of the passage states that ERT participants had superior improvement, relative to the MAC condition, and displayed the beneficial treatment effects for nine months following the end of treatment (choice D is correct, and choice B is false). Choice A, which reverses the two participants groups, is incorrect. The results do not state that the MAC condition did not improve at all, only that their improvement was not as pronounced as that of the ERT condition (choice C is incorrect).

4. **A**   Since this is an EXCEPT question, highlight the word "EXCEPT" and write "A B C D" on the noteboard. Then evaluate each answer choice, writing "Y" if it is a limitation of the study or "N" if it is not. Comparing two therapeutic approaches is not inherently a limitation in this study's design; while there certainly could be other, potentially more effective, methods of addressing either GAD or MDD in a therapeutic setting, this is not a limitation (write "N" next to "A" on the noteboard). Given that the paragraph 1 states GAD and MDD frequently exhibit suboptimal long-term treatment response, the fact that the patients were only followed for nine months could be a limitation. Future studies would ideally treat and follow a larger sample for a longer period (~2 years) to better determine durability of treatment gains (write "Y" next to "B" on the noteboard). The sample was largely white, non-Hispanic, and female. Future investigations with more racially and ethnically heterogeneous samples, in addition to being more diverse in terms of sex/gender, are needed to ideally show that ERT effects generalize to the full population of those experiencing distress disorders (write "Y" next to both "C" and "D" on the noteboard). Since choice A stands out with an "N" instead of a "Y," it is the correct answer choice.

Chapter 9
Learning, Memory, and Development

Learning is an important way that organisms interact with, are changed by, and change their environment. The basis of learning is that experiences can alter and change behavior, sometimes permanently. While learning occurs in many organisms, humans demonstrate the broadest range of different types of learning.

Human learning is influenced by many factors, including both innate and environmental variables. Learning and memory are intimately related and both play critical roles in human behavior, personality, attitudes, and development over the entire lifetime of an individual.

9.1 TYPES OF LEARNING

We have been learning since the day we were born. At times it comes more formally, like learning how to add and subtract in school, throw a baseball, or studying for the MCAT. Other times, learning occurs more informally, like learning how to walk, how to behave in certain social situations, or how to talk. Any way it happens, learning is an important part of how humans (and other animals) interact with one another and with the world around them.

Nonassociative Learning

Nonassociative learning occurs when an organism is repeatedly exposed to one type of stimulus. Two important types of nonassociative learning are habituation and sensitization. A **habit** is an action that is performed repeatedly until it becomes automatic, and **habituation** follows a very similar process. Essentially, a person learns to "tune out" the stimulus. For example, suppose you live near train tracks and trains pass by your house on a regular basis. When you first moved into the house, the sound of the trains passing by was annoying and loud, and it always made you cover your ears. However, after living in the house for a few months, you become used to the sound and stop covering your ears every time the trains pass. You may even become so accustomed to the sound that it becomes background noise and you don't even notice it anymore.

Dishabituation occurs when the previously habituated stimulus is removed. More specifically, after a person has been habituated to a given stimulus, and the stimulus is removed, this leads to dishabituation; the person is no longer accustomed to the stimulus. If the stimulus is then presented again, the person will react to it as if it were a new stimulus, and is likely to respond even more strongly to it than before. In the train example above, dishabituation could occur when you go away on vacation for a few weeks to a quiet beach resort. The train noise is no longer present, so you become dishabituated to that constant noise. Then, when you return to your home and the noisy train tracks, the first time you hear the train after you return, you notice it again. The noise may cause you to cover your ears again or react even more strongly because you have become dishabituated to the sound of the trains passing.

Sensitization is, in many ways, the opposite of habituation. During sensitization, there is an increase in responsiveness due to either a repeated application of a stimulus or a particularly aversive or noxious stimulus. Instead of being able to "tune out" or ignore the stimulus and avoid reacting at all (as in habituation), the stimulus actually produces a more exaggerated response. For example, suppose that instead of trains passing by outside your house, you attend a rock concert and sit near the stage. The feedback noise from the amplifier may at first be merely irritating, but as the aversive noise continues, instead of getting used to it, it actually becomes much more painful and you have to cover your ears and perhaps even eventually move. Sensitization may also cause you to respond more vigorously to other similar stimuli. For example, suppose that as you leave the rock concert, an ambulance passes. The siren noise, which usually doesn't bother you, seems particularly loud and abrasive after being sensitized to the noise of the rock concert. Sensitization is usually temporary and may not result in any type of long-term behavior change (you may or may not avoid rock concerts in the future and you are unlikely to respond so strongly to an ambulance siren when you hear one next week). Desensitization occurs when a stimulus that previously evoked an exaggerated response (something that we were sensitized to), no longer evokes an exaggerated response. Going back to the example of leaving a rock concert and being more sensitized to noise: at first the sound of the siren is very abrasive, but by the next morning loud noises no longer bother you—you have become desensitized.

Associative Learning

Associative learning describes a process of learning in which one event, object, or action is directly connected with another. There are two general categories of associative learning: classical conditioning and operant conditioning.

Classical Conditioning

Classical (or respondent) **conditioning** is a process in which two stimuli are paired in such a way that the response to one of the stimuli changes. The archetypal example of this is Pavlov's dogs. **Ivan Pavlov**, who first named and described the process of classical conditioning, did so by training his dogs to salivate at the sound of a ringing bell. Dogs naturally salivate at the sight and smell of food; it is a biological response that prepares the dogs for food consumption. The stimulus (food) naturally produces this response (salivating), however, dogs do not intrinsically react to the sound of a bell in any particular way. Pavlov's famous experiment paired the sound of a bell (an auditory stimulus) with the presentation of food to the dogs, and after a while, the dogs began to salivate to the sound of a bell even in the absence of food. The process of pairing the two initially unrelated stimuli changed the dogs' response to the sound of the bell over time; they became conditioned to salivate when they heard it. The dogs effectively learned that the sound of the bell was meant to announce food.

This example demonstrates a few key concepts about classical conditioning. This type of learning relies on specific stimuli and responses.

- A **neutral stimulus** is a stimulus that initially does not elicit any intrinsic response. For Pavlov's dogs, this was the sound of the bell prior to the experiment.
- An **unconditioned stimulus** (US) is a stimulus that elicits an **unconditioned response** (UR). Think of this response like a reflex. It is not a learned reaction, but a biological one: in this case, the presentation of food is the unconditioned stimulus and the salivation is the unconditioned response.
- A **conditioned stimulus** (CS) is an originally neutral stimulus (bell) that is paired with an unconditioned stimulus (food) until it can produce the conditioned response (salivation) without the unconditioned stimulus (food).
- Finally, the **conditioned response** (CR) is the learned response to the conditioned stimulus. It is the same as the unconditioned response, but now it occurs without the unconditioned stimulus. For the dogs, salivating at the sound of the bell is the conditioned response.

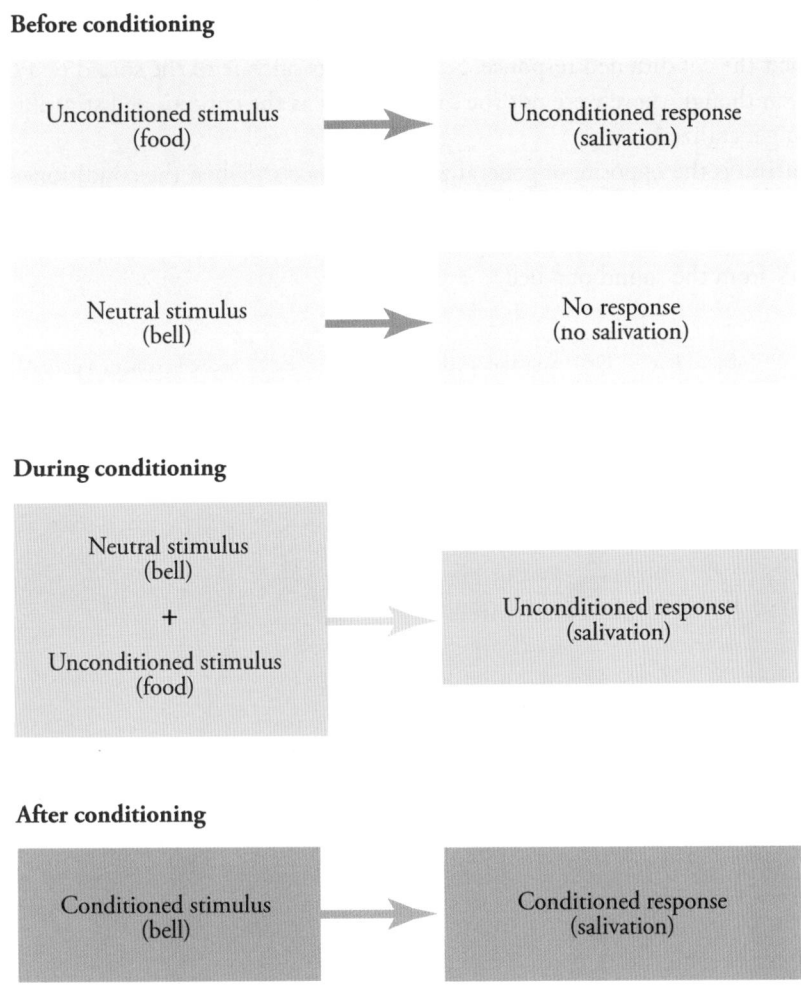

Before conditioning

Unconditioned stimulus
(food) → Unconditioned response
(salivation)

Neutral stimulus
(bell) → No response
(no salivation)

During conditioning

Neutral stimulus
(bell)

+

Unconditioned stimulus
(food) → Unconditioned response
(salivation)

After conditioning

Conditioned stimulus
(bell) → Conditioned response
(salivation)

Figure 1   Conditioning in Pavlov's dogs

Acquisition, extinction, spontaneous recovery, generalization, and discrimination are the processes by which classically-conditioned responses are developed and maintained.

1) **Acquisition** refers to the process of learning the conditioned response. This is the time during the experiment when the bell and food are always paired.

2) **Extinction**, in classical conditioning, occurs when the conditioned and unconditioned stimuli are no longer paired, so the conditioned response eventually stops occurring. After the dogs have been conditioned to salivate at the sound of the bell, if the sound is presented to the dogs over and over without being paired with the food, then after some time the dogs will eventually stop salivating at the sound of the bell.

3) **Spontaneous recovery** happens when an extinct conditioned response occurs again when the conditioned stimulus is presented after some time. For example, if the behavior of salivating to the sound of the bell becomes extinct in a dog, and the paired stimuli are then presented to the dog again after some amount of lapsed time and the dog salivates, the conditioned response was spontaneously recovered.

4) **Generalization** refers to the process by which stimuli other than the original conditioned stimulus elicit the conditioned response. So, if the dogs salivate to the sound of a chime or a doorbell, even though those were not the same sounds as the conditioned stimulus, the behavior has been generalized.

5) **Discrimination** is the opposite of generalization and occurs when the conditioned stimulus is differentiated from other stimuli; thus, the conditioned response only occurs for conditioned stimuli. If the dogs do not salivate at the sound of a buzzer or a horn, they have differentiated those stimuli from the sound of a bell.

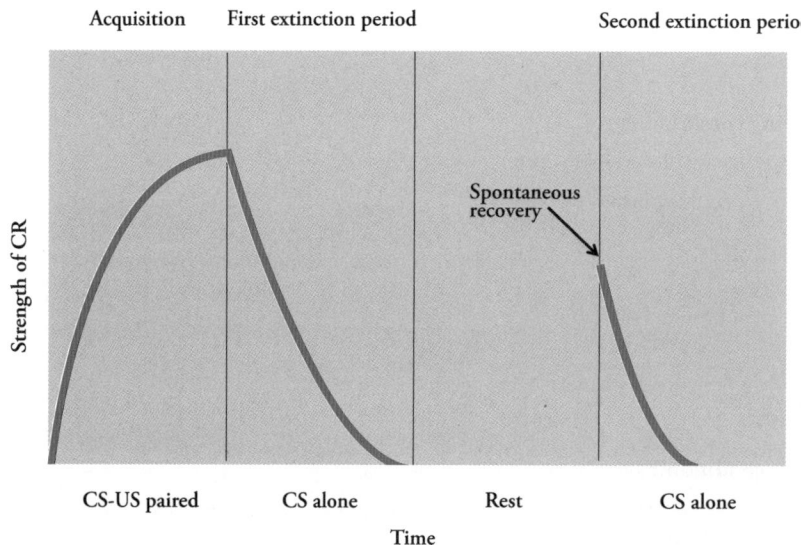

Figure 2   Curve of acquisition, extinction, and spontaneous recovery in classical conditioning

Organisms seem predisposed to learn associations that are adaptive in nature. One powerful and very long-lasting association in most animals (including humans) is **taste-aversion** caused by nausea and/or vomiting. An organism that eats a specific food and becomes ill a few hours later will generally develop a strong aversion to that food. Most organisms develop the aversion specifically to the smell or taste of the food (occurs in most mammals), but it is also possible to develop an aversion to the sight of the food (occurs in birds). The function of this quickly-learned response is to prevent an organism from consuming something that might be toxic or poisonous in the future. This response happens to be one that does not need a long acquisition phase (it is typically acquired after one exposure) and has a very long extinction phase; in fact for most organisms, it never extinguishes.

Operant Conditioning

The other category of associative learning is **operant** (or instrumental) **conditioning.** Whereas classical conditioning connects unconditioned and neutral stimuli to create conditioned responses, operant conditioning uses reinforcement (pleasant consequences) and punishment (unpleasant consequences) to mold behavior. However, just as with classical conditioning, timing is everything. In classical conditioning, it was important for the neutral stimulus to be paired with the unconditioned stimulus (that is, for them to occur together or very close together in time) in order for the neutral stimulus to become conditioned. In operant conditioning, it is just as important for the reinforcement or the punishment to occur around the same time as the behavior in order for learning to occur.

One of the most famous people to conduct research in the area of operant conditioning was **B.F. Skinner**. Skinner worked with animals and designed an operant conditioning chamber (later called a "Skinner box") that he used in a series of experiments to shape animal behavior. For example, in one series of experiments, a hungry rat would be placed inside a Skinner box that contained a lever. If the rat pressed the lever, a food pellet would drop into the box. Often the rat would first touch the lever by mistake, but after discovering that food would appear in response to pushing the lever, the rat would continue to do so until it was sated. In another series of experiments, the Skinner box would be wired to deliver a painful electric shock until a lever was pushed. In this example, the rat would run around trying to avoid the shock at first, until accidentally hitting the lever and causing the shock to stop. On repeated trials, the rat would quickly push the lever to end the painful shock.

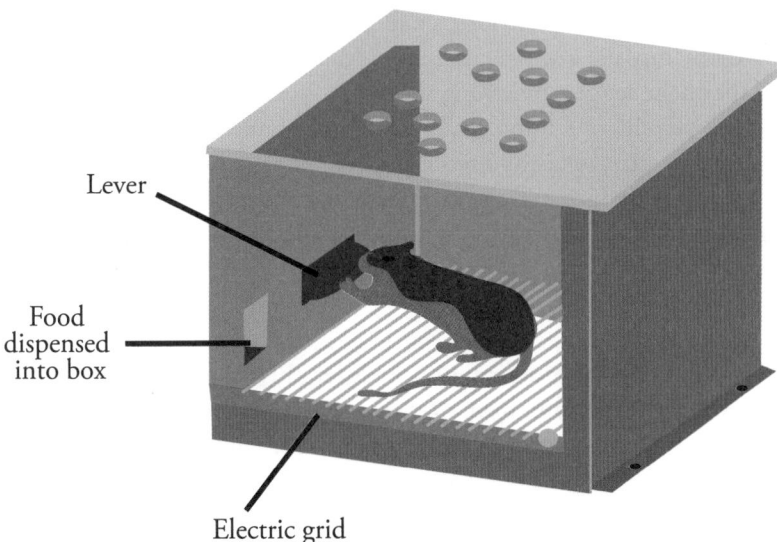

Lever

Food dispensed into box

Electric grid

Figure 3 Example of a "Skinner Box"

These examples demonstrate a few key concepts about operant conditioning.

> **Reinforcement**: A reinforcer is anything that will increase the likelihood that a preceding behavior will be repeated; the behavior is supported by reinforcement. There are two major types of reinforcement: positive and negative.
> - **Positive reinforcement** is the presentation of some sort of desirable stimulus that occurs immediately following a behavior. In the above experiments, the food pellet was a positive reinforcer for the hungry rat because it caused the rat to repeat the desired behavior (push the lever).
> - **Negative reinforcement** is the *removal* of some sort of undesirable stimulus immediately following a behavior. In the above experiments, the removal of the electric shock is negative reinforcement for the rat because it causes the rat to repeat the desired behavior (again, push the lever) to remove the undesirable stimulus (the painful shock).

Anything that *increases* a desired behavior is a reinforcer; both positive and negative reinforcements increase the desired behavior, but the process by which they do so is different. Positive reinforcement does it by adding a positive stimulus (something desirable) and negative reinforcement does it by removing a negative one (something undesirable). Positive reinforcement *adds* and negative reinforcement *subtracts* (this will be important when contrasted with punishment later). While several brain structures are involved in operant conditioning, the amygdala is understood to be particularly important in negative conditioning, while the hippocampus is believed to be particularly important in positive conditioning.

Another key distinction for reinforcement is between primary and secondary (or unconditioned and conditioned) reinforcers.

1) **Primary** (or unconditioned) **reinforcers** are somehow innately satisfying or desirable. These are reinforcers that we do not need to learn to see as reinforcers because they are integral to our survival. Food is a primary positive reinforcer for all organisms because it is required for survival. Avoiding pain and danger are primary negative reinforcers for the same reason; avoidance is important for survival.

2) **Secondary** (or conditioned) **reinforcers** are those that are learned to be reinforcers. These are neutral stimuli that are paired with primary reinforcers to make them conditioned. For example, suppose that every time a child reads a book, she receives a stamp. After accruing ten stamps, she can exchange these for a small pizza. The pizza, being food, is the primary reinforcer, and the stamps are a secondary reinforcer. The child learns to find the stamps desirable because they help her get something she wants—pizza. Secondary reinforcers can also be paired with other secondary reinforcers. For example, suppose that after collecting ten stamps, instead of receiving a pizza, the child receives a coupon that is good for one small pizza. In this example, both the stamps and the coupon are secondary reinforcers. Almost any stimulus can become a secondary reinforcer, but it must be paired with a primary reinforcer in order to produce learned behavior.

Operant conditioning relies on a **reinforcement schedule**. This schedule can be **continuous**, in which every occurrence of the behavior is reinforced, or it can be **intermittent**, in which occurrences are sometimes reinforced and sometimes not. Continuous reinforcement will result in rapid behavior **acquisition** (or rapid learning), but it will also result in rapid **extinction** when the reinforcement ceases. Intermittent reinforcement typically results in slower acquisition but great persistence (or resistance to extinction) of that behavior over time. Therefore, it is possible to initially condition a behavior using a continuous reinforcement schedule, and then **maintain** that behavior using an intermittent reinforcement schedule. For instance, a dog can be trained to sit in response to a hand motion on a continuous reinforcement schedule where a treat is given every time the dog sits; once the dog has sufficiently mastered this behavior, you can switch to an intermittent reinforcement schedule, where the dog receives a treat only occasionally when it sits in response to the hand motion.

There are four important intermittent reinforcement schedules: fixed-ratio, variable-ratio, fixed-interval, and variable-interval. Ratio schedules are based on the number of instances of a desired behavior required for the reward, and interval schedules are based on time.

1) A **fixed-ratio schedule** provides the reinforcement after a set number of instances of the behavior. Returning to the example of a hungry rat in a Skinner box, if the rat receives a food pellet every 10 times it pushes the lever after it has been conditioned, the rat will demonstrate a high rate of response (in other words, it will push the lever rapidly, many times to get the food).

2) A **variable-ratio schedule** provides the reinforcement after an unpredictable number of occurrences. A classic example of reinforcement provided on a variable-ratio schedule is gambling (e.g., a slot machine); the reinforcement may be unpredictable, but the behavior will be repeated with the hope of a reinforcement. Both fixed-ratio schedules and variable-ratio schedules produce high response rates; the chances that a behavior will produce the desired outcome (a treat or a jackpot or some other reinforcement) increases with the number responses (times the behavior is performed).

3) A **fixed-interval schedule** provides the reinforcement after an amount of time that is constant. The behavior will increase as the reinforcement interval comes to an end. For example, if an employee is reinforced by attention from the boss, the employee might work hard all the time, thinking the boss will walk by at any second and notice the hard work (and provide the positive reinforcement, attention). Once the employee learns that the boss only walks by at the top of the hour every hour, the employee may become an ineffective worker throughout the day, but be more effective as the top of the hour approaches.

4) A **variable-interval schedule** provides the reinforcement after an inconsistent amount of time. This schedule produces a slow, steady behavior response rate, because the amount of time it will take to get the reinforcement is unknown. In the employee-boss example, if the boss walks by at unpredictable times each day, the employee does not know when he or she might receive the desired reinforcement (attention). Thus, the employee will work in a steady, efficient manner throughout the day, but not very quickly. The employee knows it doesn't matter how quickly he works at any given time, because the potential reinforcement is tied to an unpredictable schedule.

Figure 4 demonstrates behavior response patterns to each of the four reinforcement schedules.

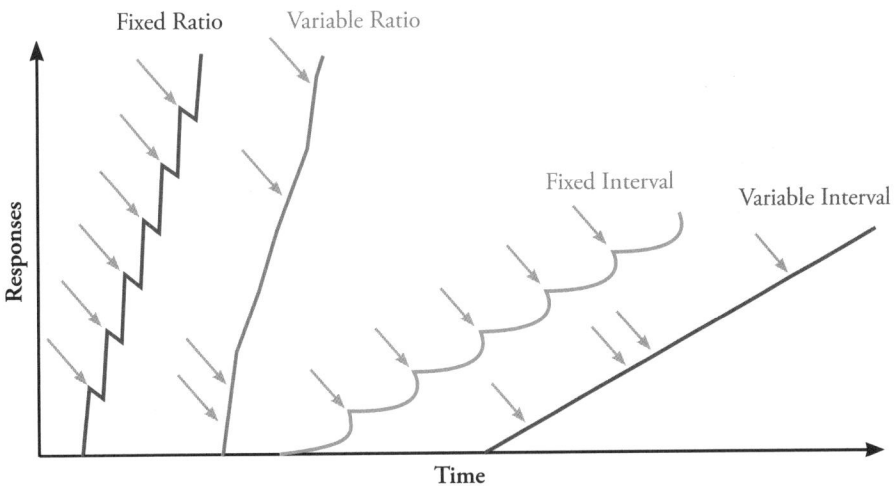

Figure 4   Behavior response patterns to each of the four reinforcement schedules

Table 1   Reinforcement Schedules: Response and Extinction Rates

	Definition	Response Rate	Extinction Rate	Notable Behavior Patterns
Continuous	Reinforcer given after every single response	SLOW	FAST	**Best way to teach new behavior,** but has the fastest rate of extinction
Fixed Ratio	Reinforcer given after set number of responses	FAST	MEDIUM	Post-reinforcement pause may be an analogue to procrastination
Fixed Interval	Reinforcer given after set amount of time	MEDIUM	MEDIUM	Long pause in responding following reinforcement, followed by accelerating rate
Variable Ratio	Reinforcer given after variable number of responses	FAST	SLOW	**Slowest rate of extinction** (behavior persists longest despite lack of reinforcer)
Variable Interval	Reinforcer given after variable amount of time	MEDUIM-FAST	SLOW	Tends to produce a low to moderate steady rate of responding

Note: these same schedules can also be used for punishments.

Reinforcement and reinforcement schedules explain how behaviors can be learned, but not every behavior is learned by simply providing a reinforcement. For example, think about how a baby learns to walk. Do babies spontaneously walk one day and then receive some sort of reinforcement from their parents for doing so? Of course not. Instead, parents **shape** the desired behavior by reinforcing the smaller intermediate behaviors necessary to achieve the final desired behavior, walking. Thus, parents will reinforce their child's attempts to pull herself up, so she will try again. Once she's mastered pulling herself up and standing while holding onto something, they will reinforce the child's attempts to stand while not holding anything. And so on until the child is able to walk on her own. Shaping is a way to learn more complex behaviors by breaking them down and reinforcing the "pieces of the puzzle" until the whole behavior is strung together.

Like reinforcement, punishment is also an important element of operant conditioning, but the effect is the opposite: reinforcement *increases* behavior, while punishment *decreases* it. **Punishment** is the process by which a behavior is followed by a consequence that decreases the likelihood that the behavior will be repeated. Like reinforcement, punishment can be both positive AND negative. **Positive punishment** involves presenting an undesirable stimulus after a behavior that one wishes to decrease. For example, if cadets speak out of turn in military boot camp, the drill sergeant makes them do twenty push-ups. Conversely, **negative punishment** involves the removal of a desirable stimulus after the **behavior has occurred.** For example, if a child breaks a window while throwing a baseball in the house, they lose TV privileges for a week. Positive punishment *adds* and negative punishment *subtracts*. Commonly, reinforcement and punishment are used in conjunction when shaping behaviors; however, it is uncommon for punishment to have as much of a lasting effect as reinforcement. Once the punishment has been removed, then it is no longer effective. Furthermore, punishment only instructs what *not* to do, whereas reinforcement instructs what *to* do. Reinforcement is therefore a better alternative to encourage behavior change and learning. Additionally, the processes described for classical conditioning (acquisition, extinction, spontaneous recovery, generalization, and discrimination) occur in operant conditioning, as well.

Note that the term "negative reinforcement" is often used incorrectly; colloquially, people use the term when they mean punishment.

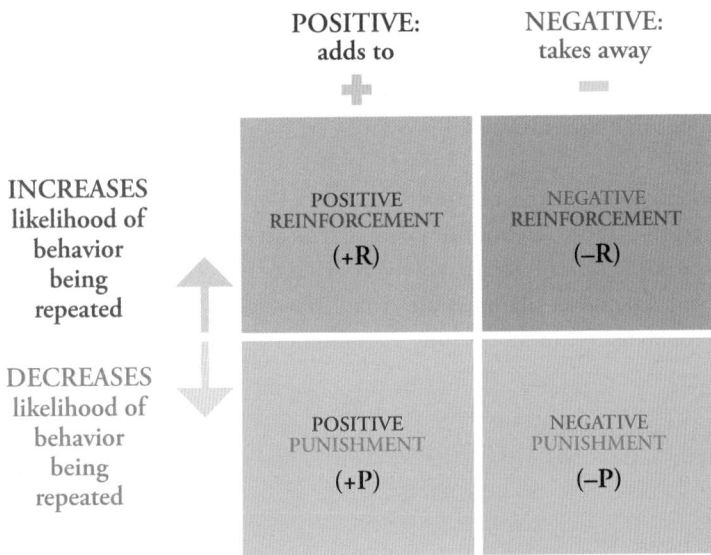

POSITIVE: adds to

NEGATIVE: takes away

INCREASES likelihood of behavior being repeated

POSITIVE REINFORCEMENT (+R)

NEGATIVE REINFORCEMENT (–R)

DECREASES likelihood of behavior being repeated

POSITIVE PUNISHMENT (+P)

NEGATIVE PUNISHMENT (–P)

Figure 5   Schematic of positive and negative reinforcement and punishment

In conclusion, let's examine two specific types of operant learning: escape and avoidance. In **escape learning,** an individual learns how to get away from an aversive stimulus by engaging in a particular behavior. This helps negatively reinforce the behavior so that it is more likely to be repeated. For example, a child does not want to eat her vegetables (aversive stimulus) so she throws a temper tantrum. If the parents respond by not making the child eat the vegetables, then tantrums will be negatively reinforced, as they cause the removal of the aversive stimulus (the vegetables). On the other hand, **avoidance** occurs when a person performs a behavior to ensure an aversive stimulus is not presented. For example, a child notices Mom cooking vegetables for dinner and fakes an illness so Mom will send him to bed with ginger ale and crackers. The child has effectively avoided confronting the aversive stimulus (the offensive vegetables) altogether. As long as either of these techniques work (meaning the parents do not force the child to eat the vegetables), the child is reinforced to perform the escape and/or avoidance behaviors.

Cognitive Processes that Affect Associative Learning

Classical and operant conditioning fall under the behaviorist tradition of psychology, which is most strongly associated with Skinner. In **behaviorism**, all psychological phenomena are explained by describing the observable antecedents of behaviors and their consequences. Behaviorism is not concerned with the unobservable events occurring within the mind. This perspective views the brain as a "black box" which does not need to be incorporated into the discussion. While Skinner and other behaviorists contributed a great deal to science, this extreme form of behaviorism has lost favor. As a reaction to behaviorism, **cognitive psychology** emerged. In cognitive psychology, researchers began to focus on the brain, cognitions (thoughts), and their effects on how people navigate the world. Cognitive psychologists do not see learning as simply due to stimulus-pairing and reinforcement. Although its importance is acknowledged, cognitive psychologists do not believe that all learning can be explained in this way. For example, say a child learns that he can slide on his belly to reach a toy he wants under the bed. Then he learns that a grabbing tool can be used to pick up his toys from the ground. What will the child do when his toy is under the bed out of reach? He may figure out that he can combine the two behaviors: sliding on his belly and using the grabbing tool to get the toy. **Insight learning** is the term used to describe when previously learned behaviors are suddenly combined in unique ways. For the child, the two behaviors (sliding on the belly and using the grabbing tool) were previously reinforced because he got the toy he wanted each time. A new situation was presented (the toy is out of reach under the bed), and he was able to combine previously reinforced behavior in a novel way on his own to attain the desired outcome (retrieval of the toy).

This also works the other way around: previously unseen behavior can manifest quickly when required. In **latent learning**, something is learned but not expressed as an observable behavior until it is required. For instance, if a child in middle school always receives a ride to school from his dad, he may latently learn the route to school, even if he never demonstrates that knowledge. One day, when his dad is on a business trip, the child is able to navigate to school along the same route by bike.

Finally, conditioning is not only behavioral learning. For instance, in operant conditioning, certain behaviors are reinforced and the likelihood of that behavior being repeated increases as a result. Cognitively, the reinforcement establishes an expectation for a future reinforcer, so the process is not exclusively behavioral. There is thinking involved in this kind of learning. Expectations may also present themselves in stimulus generalization. If you were rewarded in one class for raising your hand before speaking, then you would expect that to be reinforced in another class as well.

Table 2 Comparison of Classical Conditioning and Operant Conditioning

	Classical Conditioning	**Operant Conditioning**
Defined	Organisms learn associations between stimuli that they don't control	Organisms learn associations between behaviors and resulting consequences
Response	Involuntary, automatic	Voluntary
Acquisition	Associating two stimuli	Associating response with consequence (reinforcement or punishment)
Extinction	Conditioned response decreases as the conditioned stimulus is continually presented alone	Response decreases without reinforcement
Spontaneous recovery	Reappearance, after a rest period, of a response	Reappearance, after a rest period, of a response
Generalization	Response to a stimulus similar (but not identical) to the conditioned stimulus	Response to a similar stimulus is also reinforced
Discrimination	Ability to distinguish between conditioned stimulus and other stimuli	Learning that certain responses, not others, will be reinforced

Biological Factors that Affect Nonassociative and Associative Learning

Learning is a change in behavior as a result of experience. While many extrinsic factors can influence learning, learning is also limited by biological constraints of organisms. For example, chimpanzees can learn to communicate using basic sign language, but they cannot learn to speak, in part because they are constrained by a lack of specialized vocal chords that would enable them to do so. It was long believed that learning could occur using any two stimuli or any response and any reinforcer. But again, biology serves as an important constraint. Associative learning is most easily achieved using stimuli that are somehow relevant to survival. Furthermore, not all reinforcers are equally effective. As previously discussed, a dramatic example of this is illustrated by food aversions. If an organism consumes something that tastes strongly of vanilla and becomes nauseated a few hours later (even if the nausea was not caused by the vanilla food), that organism will develop a strong aversion to both the taste and the smell of vanilla, even if the nausea occurred hours after consuming the food. This aversion defies many of the principles of associative learning previously discussed because it occurs after one instance, it can occur after a significant delay of hours, and it is often an aversion that can last for a very long time, sometimes indefinitely. In studies, researchers tried to condition organisms to associate the feeling of nausea with other stimuli, such as a sound or a light, but were unable to do so. Therefore, food aversions demonstrate another important facet of learning: learning occurs more quickly if it is biologically relevant.

The process of learning results in physical changes to the central nervous system (see Chapter 10). Different areas of the brain are involved with different types of learning. For example, the cerebellum is involved with learning how to complete motor tasks and the amygdala is involved with learning fear responses (brain lesion studies have helped scientists determine this).

Learning and memory are two processes that work together in shaping behavior, and it is impossible to discuss how learning is processed in the brain without discussing memory. Certain synaptic connections develop in the brain when a memory is formed. **Short-term memory** typically lasts only a matter of seconds, but can potentially be converted into **long-term memory** through a process called **consolidation**. Newly acquired information (such as the knowledge that a reward follows a certain behavior) is temporarily stored in short-term memory and can be transferred into long-term memory under the right conditions.

Long-term Potentiation

When something is learned, the synapses between neurons are strengthened and the process of long-term potentiation begins. **Long-term potentiation** occurs when, following brief periods of stimulation, an increase in the synaptic strength between two neurons leads to stronger electrochemical responses to a given stimulus. When long-term potentiation occurs, the neurons involved in the circuit develop an increased sensitivity (the sending neuron needs less prompting to fire its impulse and release its neurotransmitter, and/or the receiving neurons have more receptors for the neurotransmitter), which results in increased potential for neural firing after a connection has been stimulated. This increased potential can last for hours or even weeks. Synaptic strength is thought to be the process by which memories are consolidated for long-term memory (so learning can occur). At a given synapse, long-term potentiation involves both presynaptic and postsynaptic neurons. For example, dopamine is one of the neurotransmitters involved in pleasurable or rewarding actions. In operant conditioning, reinforcement activates the limbic circuits that involve memory, learning, and emotions. Since reinforcement of a desired behavior is pleasurable, the circuits are strengthened as dopamine floods the system, making it more likely the behavior will be repeated.

After long-term potentiation has occurred, passing an electrical current through the brain doesn't disrupt the memory associations between the neurons involved, although other memories will be wiped out. For example, when a person receives a blow to the head resulting in a concussion, he or she loses memory for events shortly preceding the concussion. This is due to the fact that long-term potentiation has not had a chance to occur (and leave traces of memory connections), while old memories, which were already potentiated, remain.

Long-term memory storage involves more permanent changes to the brain, including structural and functional connections between neurons. For example, long-term memory storage includes new synaptic connections between neurons, permanent changes in pre- and postsynaptic membranes, and a permanent increase or decrease in neurotransmitter synthesis. Furthermore, visual imaging studies suggest that there is greater branching of dendrites in regions of the brain thought to be involved with memory storage. Other studies suggest that protein synthesis somehow influences memory formation; drugs that prevent protein synthesis appear to block long-term memory formation.

Not all behaviors are learned, of course. The neural processes described above occur when animals or people learn new behaviors, or change their behaviors based on experience (that is, environmental feedback). As our learned behaviors change, our synapses change too. On the other hand, some behaviors are **innate**. These are all the actions we know how to do instinctively (or our body just does without us consciously thinking about it), not because someone taught us to do them (for example, breathing or pulling away from a hot stove). Further, innate behaviors are always the same among members of the species, even for the ones performing them for the first time.

Observational Learning

More advanced organisms, particularly humans, do not learn only through direct experience. **Observational learning,** also known as **social learning** or **vicarious learning,** is learning through watching and imitating others.

Modeling

Modeling is one of the most basic mechanisms behind observational learning. In modeling, an observer sees the behavior being performed by another person. Later, with the model in mind, the observer **imitates** the behavior she or he observed. You likely participated in this behavior as a child (or even now). Think back to when you were little and you played with your friends; perhaps you played house or pretended to be a superhero. Typically, you would play your role ("mom" or "Superman") according to the model you have seen: your mother, or Superman (on TV). As an adult, your appearance may be based on models in society; you dress, talk, and walk like your friends. Modeling is not limited to humans either; think about how lions learn to hunt in the wild. A lioness will take her cubs with her to hunt and her cubs watch her during the process and hunt based on what they observe.

Typically, the likelihood of imitating a modeled behavior is based on how successful someone finds that behavior to be, or the type of reinforcement that the model received for his behavior. However, individuals may choose to imitate behaviors even if they do not observe the consequences of the model's behavior. For instance, **Albert Bandura** (considered a pioneer in the field of observational learning) conducted a series of experiments using a Bobo doll (a large inflatable toy with a heavy base that will spring back up after being punched). Bandura showed children videos of adults either behaving aggressively toward the Bobo doll (punching, kicking, and shouting at the doll) or ignoring the doll altogether. Even when children did not see the consequences of the adult's behavior, they tended to imitate the behavior they saw. Later studies conducted by others support that humans are prone to imitation and modeling, and we are particularly likely to imitate those whom we perceive as similar to ourselves, as successful, or as admirable in some way. Therefore, modeling, and social learning in general, is a very powerful influence on individuals' behaviors.

Biological Processes that Affect Observational Learning

Mirror neurons have been identified in various parts of the human brain, including the premotor cortex, supplementary motor area, primary somatosensory cortex, and the inferior parietal cortex. In monkeys, mirror neurons fire when the monkey performs a task, as well as when the monkey observes another monkey performing the task. Humans also possess mirror neurons, and while there is still some debate about the exact function of these neurons, there are several hypotheses. Some believe that mirror neurons are activated by connecting the sight and action of a movement (that is, they are programmed to mirror). Some postulate that mirror neurons help us understand the actions of others and help us learn through imitation. It has also been proposed that mirror neurons in humans are responsible for **vicarious emotions**, such as empathy, and that a problem in the mirror neuron system might underlie disorders such as autism. However, this has yet to be proven, and there is clearly still much research needed to determine the exact function or functions of mirror neurons. Despite that, many believe that they are somehow involved in observational learning in animals, including humans.

Applications of Observational Learning to Explain Individual Behavior

As social organisms, human beings connect through observational learning. We learn from and behave like one another, but this mimicking is not perfect. There are individual differences between people and animals. Personality differences and psychological disorders can affect observational learning. For example, much of the research on observational learning has focused on violence and how observing violence increases violence in society, but not everyone who observes violence is violent. Cognition plays a role in how we use what we learn.

9.2 MEMORY

Encoding

Process of Encoding Information

As you may recall from information-processing models, information first enters a sensory register before encoding occurs. **Encoding** is the process of transferring sensory information into our memory system.

Working memory—where information is maintained temporarily as part of a particular mental activity (learning, solving a problem)—is thought to include a phonological loop, visuospatial sketchpad, central executive, and episodic buffer (Chapter 11). Working memory is quite limited, and this model helps to explain the **serial position effect**. This effect occurs when someone attempts to memorize a series, such as a list of words. In an immediate recall condition (shortly after the information is first presented), the individual is more likely to recall the first and last items on the list. These phenomena are called the

primacy effect and the **recency effect**. It is hypothesized that first items are more easily recalled because they have had the most time to be encoded and transferred to long-term memory. Last items may be more easily recalled because they may still be in the phonological loop, and thus may be readily available. When the individual is asked to recall the list at a later point, the individual tends to remember only the first items well. This may be because that was the only information that was transferred to long-term memory, whereas recent information from the phonological loop would quickly decay and be lost.

Processes That Aid in Encoding Memories

A **mnemonic** is any technique for improving retention and retrieval of information from memory. One simple process that aids memory is use of the phonological loop through **rehearsal**. If someone were to give you a phone number and you didn't have any way to record the information, you might repeat the digits over and over in your head until you were able to write them down. In some cases, such as the recital of the Pledge of Allegiance, repeated rehearsal can lead to encoding into long-term memory.

Chunking is a strategy in which information to be remembered is organized into discrete groups of data. For example, with phone numbers, one might memorize the area code, the first three digits, and the last four digits as discrete chunks. Thus, the number of "things" being remembered is decreased—in the case of a phone number, there are now three "things" to memorize instead of 10 individual digits. This is an important strategy because the limit of working memory is generally understood to be about seven digits. Even the process of remembering that a group of letters makes a particular word involves chunking.

When memorizing information, people make use of **hierarchies** for organization. For example, imagine that a child is learning about the different animals in the zoo. It would be useful to have a category of "birds" to include ostriches, penguins, etc. and a category of "big cats" to remember lions, tigers, and so on. As the child learns more, these hierarchies are reorganized to match incoming information. When words are organized into groups, recall significantly improves. For example, it would be easier to remember the list "chair, table, desk, lamp, recliner, sofa" if you realized that all of these words are pieces of furniture.

There is some evidence that the **depth of processing** is important for encoding memories. Information that is thought about at a deeper level is better remembered. For example, it is easier to remember the general plot of a book than the exact words, meaning that semantic information (meaning) is more easily remembered than grammatical information (form) when the goal is to learn a concept. On the other hand, rhyme can be useful in aiding phonological processing. Another useful mnemonic device is to use short words or phrases that represent longer strings of information. For example, ROYGBIV is an **acronym** that is helpful in memorizing the colors of the rainbow (red, orange, yellow, green, blue, indigo, violet).

The **dual-coding hypothesis** asserts that it is easier to remember words with associated images than either words or images alone. By encoding both a visual mental representation and an associated word, there are more connections made to the memory and an opportunity to process the information at a deeper level. For this reason, imagery is a useful mnemonic device. One aid for memory is to use the **method of loci**. This involves imagining moving through a familiar place, such as your home, and in each place, leaving a visual representation of a topic to be remembered. The images of the places are then called upon to bring into awareness the associated topics. Similarly, **the peg word method** involves assigning images to a sequence of numbers.

It is also easier to remember things that are personally relevant, known as the **self-reference effect**. We have excellent recall for information that we can personally relate to because it interacts with our own views or because it can be linked to existing memories. A useful tool for memory is to try to make new information personally relevant by relating it to existing knowledge.

Memory Storage

Types of Memory Storage

Different stores of memory include sensory memory, short-term memory, and long-term memory. **Sensory memory,** the initial recording of sensory information in the memory system, is a very brief snapshot that quickly decays. Three types of sensory memory are iconic memory, eidetic memory, and echoic memory. **Iconic memory** is brief photographic memory for visual information, which decays in a few tenths of a second. **Eidetic memory** is an ability found in some children to remember an image in vivid detail for several minutes after brief exposure. **Echoic memory** is memory for sound, which lasts for about 3–4 seconds. This is why sometimes in a conversation you might ask what someone said if you had trouble hearing him or her, only to hear and make sense of the words yourself a second later. Information from sensory memory decays rapidly if it is not passed through Broadbent's filter into short-term memory. **Short-term memory** is also limited in duration and in capacity. Recall capacity for an adult is typically around seven items, plus or minus two. This is why phone numbers with seven digits (excluding the area code) are conveniently remembered. As discussed earlier, although chunking increases the amount of information remembered by putting more information into each chunk, it is still subject to this limit of about seven chunks. Information in short-term memory is retained only for about 20 seconds, unless it is actively processed so that it can be transferred into long-term memory. **Long-term memory** is information that is retained sometimes indefinitely; it is believed to have an infinite capacity.

It is important to draw a distinction between short-term memory and working memory. Short-term memory, which is strongly associated with the hippocampus, is where new information sought to be remembered resides temporarily and is then encoded to long-term memory or forgotten. Thus, if you meet a new person, you will store the person's name in short-term memory and, perhaps through rehearsal, encode the name into long-term memory. Working memory, which is strongly associated with the prefrontal cortex, is a storage bin to hold memories (short-term or long-term) that are needed at a particular moment in order to process information or solve a problem. For example, if you need to mentally determine the area of a triangle, you will bring the formula and your knowledge of multiplication into your working memory while you process the result.

Implicit or **procedural memory** refers to conditioned associations and knowledge of how to do something, while **explicit** or **declarative memory** involves being able to "declare" or voice what is known. Explicit memory involves conscious recall of information, while implicit memory does not. For example, one could read a book on how to develop a great shot in basketball from cover to cover and be able to explain in great detail the necessary steps. However, this book knowledge would not likely translate into being able to execute the shot on the court without practice. Explaining the concept involves explicit or declarative memory, while not having practiced it indicates a lack of implicit or procedural memory. Semantic and episodic memory are two subdivisions of explicit memory. **Semantic memory** is memory for factual information, such as the capital of England. **Episodic memory** is autobiographical memory for information of personal importance, such as the situation surrounding a first kiss. Typically, semantic memory deteriorates before episodic memory does.

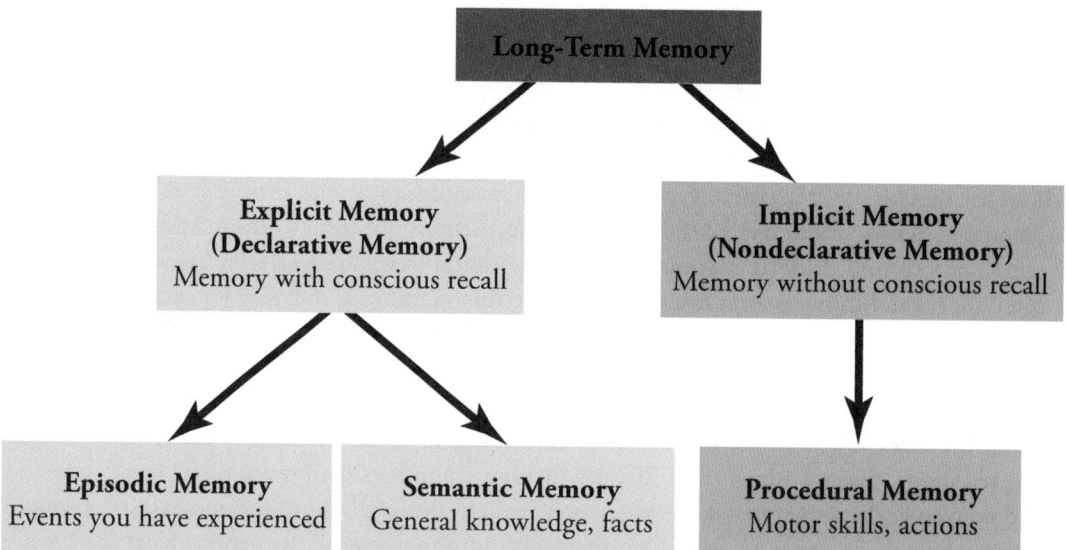

Figure 6 Types of long-term memory

The distinction between explicit and implicit memory is supported by neurological evidence. Brain structures involved in memory include the hippocampus, cerebellum, and amygdala. The hippocampus is necessary for the encoding of new explicit memories. The cerebellum is involved in learning skills and conditioned associations (implicit memory). The amygdala is involved in associating emotion with memories, particularly negative memories; for example, a fear response to a dentist's drill involves fear conditioning. The roles of the hippocampus, cerebellum, and amygdala are shown by studies on patients who have the capacity for either implicit or explicit memory (but not both). For example, amnesic patients with hippocampal damage may not have declarative memory for a skill they have recently learned (due to amnesia), and yet may be able to demonstrate the skill, indicating that implicit memory exists. Interestingly, the implicit memories that infants form are retained indefinitely, but the explicit memories that infants form are largely not retained beyond about age four—a phenomenon known as infantile amnesia. It is only later, after the hippocampus has fully developed, that explicit memories are retained long-term.

Retrieval

Recall, Recognition, and Relearning

Retrieval is the process of finding information stored in memory. When most people think of retrieval, they think of **recall**, the ability to retrieve information. **Free recall** involves retrieving the item "out of thin air," while **cued recall** involves retrieving the information when provided with a cue. For example, a test of free recall would be to ask a student to name all of the capital cities of the world. A test of cued recall would be to provide the student with a list of countries and then ask him or her to name all of the capital cities of the world. Another type of retrieval is **recognition,** which involves identifying specific information from a set of information that is presented. One recognition task would be a multiple-choice question. **Reproductive memory** is storage of the original stimulus input and subsequent recall (i.e., remembering something accurately without significantly altering it). Finally, **relearning** involves the process of learning material that was originally learned. Once we have learned and forgotten something, we are able to relearn it more quickly than when it was originally learned, which suggests that the information was in the memory system to be retrieved.

Retrieval Cues

Retrieval cues provide reminders of information. Within the network model of memory, we have already discussed how hints may activate a closely related node, making it easier to retrieve the node being searched for. Prior activation of these nodes and associations is called **priming**. Often, this process occurs without our awareness. For example, if you are shown several red items and then asked to name a fruit, you will be more likely to name a red fruit. The best retrieval cues are often contextual cues that had associations formed at the time that the memory was encoding, such as tastes, smells, and sights. Almost everyone has had the experience of not recognizing someone familiar because of seeing the person in another context. For example, running into your coffee shop barista at a concert might make it harder to recognize her or him. Or a man may associate happiness with beagles because he had one as a child. When looking in a shelter to adopt a dog decades later, he may find himself emotionally drawn to select a beagle. Although he may not consciously be thinking of his childhood dog, his memories predispose him to connect a beagle with feeling happy.

The Role of Emotion in Retrieving Memories

In addition to words, events, and sensory input serving as retrieval cues, emotion can also serve as a retrieval cue. What we learn in one state is most easily recalled when we are once again in that emotional state, a phenomenon known as **mood-dependent memory**. Thus, when someone is depressed, events in the past that were sad are more likely to emerge to the forefront of his or her mind. This plays a role in maintaining the cycle of depression. When we are happy, we tend to remember past times that were also happy. In addition, emotion can bias the recall of memories. If someone is angry at a friend, the person is more likely to feel that the friendship has always been rotten, whereas in a moment when the friendship feels joyful, the person is more likely to perceive the relationship as having always been a joyful one. Emotion has a powerful effect on the experience of memory, often leading to increased recall for emotionally intense experiences. **Flashbulb memories** are intense, vivid "snapshots" of an emotionally intense experience. These intense memories are often experienced by PTSD patients during recollection of the traumatic event.

Forgetting

Remembering information is achieved through the process of paying attention, encoding, retaining information (storage), and finally retrieval. Failure along any step of this process can cause forgetting. A failure to pay attention or encode means that the information never got into the memory system. A failure to store information is decay. A failure in retrieval could result from a lack of retrieval cues or interference.

Aging and Memory

Older adults vary in their memory abilities. Decline in memory is influenced by how active the person is: increased activity (both physical and mental) is a protective factor against neuronal atrophy. Memory loss may parallel the age-related loss of neurons. As we age, memory decline tends to follow some common trends, with certain types of memory being affected earlier. As you might expect, older adults have accumulated many experiences and so have a rich network of nodes and associations. Information that is meaningful and connects well to that existing web of information, and information that is skill-based, shows less decline with age. However, there is greater decline for information that is less meaningful and less richly connected.

Due to having a more extensive memory network, retrieval can also become trickier with time. Older adults show minimal decline in recognition, but greater decline in free recall. One type of recall is **prospective memory**, remembering to do things in the future. Prospective memory is stronger when there are cues in the environment. For example, an older adult may be asked to remember to take a particular medication three times a day. However, unless there is a reminder cue such as a readily visible pillbox or an alarm, it may be difficult to remember that there is a task that needs to be completed. Thus, the person fails to "remember to remember." Difficulty with prospective memory without cues also makes it difficult to complete time-based tasks, since one must remember to look at a clock or keep track of a schedule.

Memory Dysfunctions

Remember that memory has a neurological basis, with the hippocampus playing a role in the encoding of new explicit memories, the cerebellum playing a role in encoding implicit memories, and the amygdala helping to tie emotion to memories. Once information is in long-term memory, it is stored in various areas spread throughout the brain. Damage to parts of the brain by strokes, brain tumors, alcoholism, traumatic brain injuries, and other events can cause memory impairment. Patients with damage to the hippocampus could develop **anterograde amnesia**, an inability to encode new memories, or **retrograde amnesia**, an inability to recall information that was previously encoded (or both types of amnesia). In addition, neurological damage involving neurotransmitters can also cause memory dysfunction. One theory about the cause of Alzheimer's disease, for example, involves an inability to manufacture enough of the neurotransmitter acetylcholine, which results in, among other things, neuronal death in the hippocampus.

Decay

Memory decay results in a failure to retain stored information. Even if information is successfully encoded into memory, it can decay from our memory storage and be forgotten. However, decay does not happen in a linear fashion. Rather, the "forgetting curve" indicates that the longer the **retention interval**, or the time since the information was learned, the more information will be forgotten, with the most forgetting occurring rapidly in the first few days before leveling off. It is unclear why memories fade or erode with the passage of time. It is possible that the brain cells involved in the memory may die off, or perhaps that the associations among memories need to be refreshed in order not to weaken.

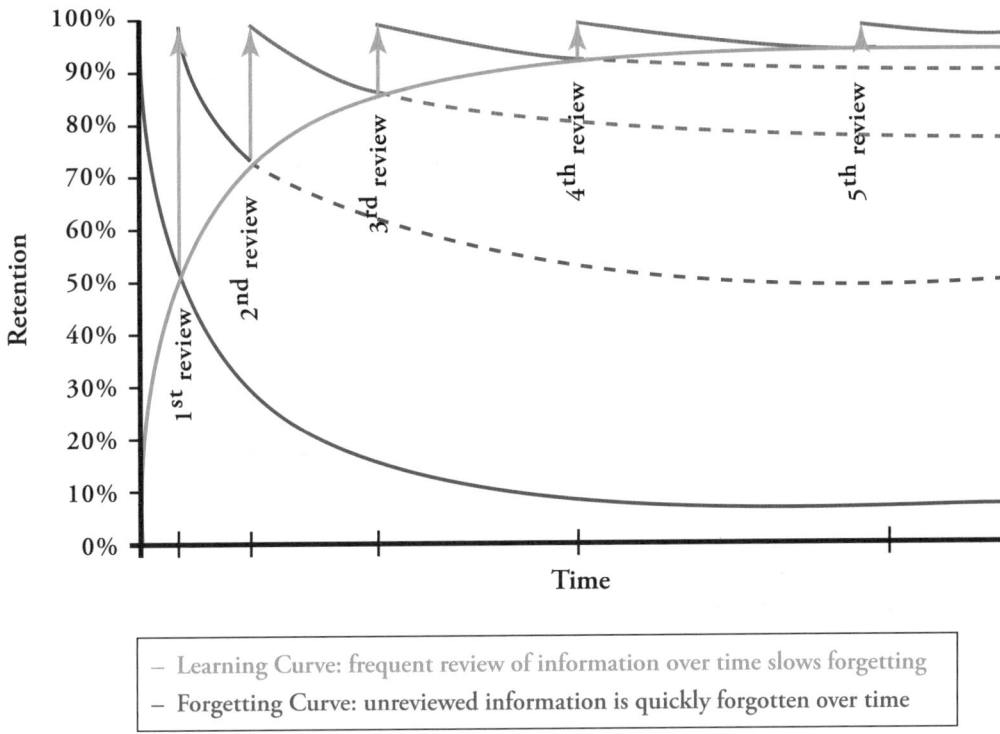

Retention

Time

- Learning Curve: frequent review of information over time slows forgetting
- Forgetting Curve: unreviewed information is quickly forgotten over time

Figure 7 Forgetting curve

Interference

Interference can result in a failure to retrieve information that is in storage. The passage of time may create more opportunity for newer learning to interfere with older learning, which is especially common if the learned information is similar. **Proactive interference** happens when information previously learned interferes with the ability to recall information learned later. For example, remembering where you had parked your car in a parking garage will be more difficult once you have parked in that parking garage for months in different locations. **Retroactive interference** happens when newly learned information interferes with the recall of information learned previously. For example, someone who has moved frequently may find that learning new addresses and directions interferes with his or her ability to remember old addresses and directions. Of course, old and new information do not always interfere. Sometimes, old information facilitates the learning of new information through **positive transfer**. For example, knowing how to play American football may make it easier for someone to learn how to play rugby.

Memory Construction and Source Monitoring

Our memories are far from being snapshots of actual experience. We already know that when memories are encoded, they pass through a "lens;" the mood and selective attention of the observer influence how they are encoded. Memory is once again altered when passing through the "lens" of retrieval. When we remember something, we do not pull from a mental photo album, but rather, we draw a picture, *constructing* the recalled memory from information that is stored. This process is not foolproof.

Sometimes the information that we retrieve is based more on a **schema** than on reality. A schema is a mental blueprint containing common aspects of some part of the world. For example, if asked to describe what your fourth-grade classroom looked like, you might "remember" a chalkboard, chalk, desks, posters encouraging reading, and books, based on your schema for such a classroom, even though the actual room may not have had posters. In this way, when we construct a memory, we tend to "fill in the blanks" by adding details that may not have been present at the time. We may also unknowingly alter details. For example, in eyewitness testimony, leading questions often cause witnesses to misestimate or misremember. When participants in an experiment were asked how fast cars were going when they *smashed* into each other, instead of just *hit* each other, they indicated higher speeds. Individuals in the first group also reported seeing broken glass and car parts, when there actually were none. After people are exposed to subtle misinformation, they are usually susceptible to the **misinformation effect**, a tendency to misremember.

Individuals may also misremember when asked to repeatedly imagine nonexistent actions and events. Simply repeatedly imagining that one did something can create **false memories** for an event. False memories are inaccurate recollections of an event and may be the result of the implanting of ideas. For example, if one repeatedly imagined being lost as a child in a shopping mall, this imagined occurrence would begin to feel familiar, and as it felt more familiar, it would take on the flavor of a real memory. In fact, it can be very difficult for people to distinguish between real memories and false memories by feeling, because both can be accompanied by emotional reactions and the sense of familiarity. The theory of **reconstructive memory** posits that rather than an episodic recall of events that took place, memory is a constructive process that involves building a memory from similar experiences, social expectations, perceptions, cues, and feelings, all of which are combined with recollection of the event itself to form a memory experience. For this reason, an individual's confidence in the validity of a memory has not been found to be a good indication of how valid it actually is.

When recalling information, people are also susceptible to forgetting one particular fact—the information's source. This is an error in **source monitoring**. For example, you may find yourself angry with an individual in your life for doing something hurtful, only to later realize that the action occurred in a dream. Or you may recognize someone, but have no idea where you have seen the person before.

Changes in Synaptic Connections Underlie Memory and Learning

Neuroscientists have had a difficult time in their search for a physical basis for memory. There has been no central location found for memories, and there seem to be no such thing as special memory neurons. The process of forming memories involves electrical impulses sent through brain circuits. Somehow, these impulses leave permanent neural traces that are physical representations of information. More and more evidence indicates that what is important for memory and for learning is the synapses—those sites where nerve cells communicate with one another through neurotransmitters.

9.3 HUMAN DEVELOPMENT

Developmental psychology is the study of how humans develop physically, cognitively, and socially, throughout their lifetime. As previously discussed, genetics and environment play an important role in human development.

Early Brain Development

During prenatal development, the brain actually produces more neurons than needed. At birth, humans have the highest number of neurons at any point in their life, and these are pruned throughout the ensuing lifetime. However, the immature brain does not have many **neural networks**, or codified routes for information processing (the types that are generated in response to learning and experience throughout a lifetime). During infancy and early childhood development, these neurons form neural networks, and networks are reinforced by learning and behavior. From ages 3 to 6, the most rapid growth occurs in the frontal lobes, corresponding to an increase in rational planning and attention. The association areas, linked with thinking, memory, and language, are the last cortical areas to develop. (For more information on cognitive development, see Jean Piaget in Chapter 11.)

Maturation is the sequence of biological growth processes in human development. Maturation, while largely genetic, is still influenced by environment. For example, while humans are programmed to learn how to speak, first using one-word utterances, then developing progressively more complex speech, severe deprivation can significantly delay this process, while an incredibly nurturing environment might speed it up. The developing brain allows for motor development; as the nervous system and muscles mature, more and more complex physical skills develop. The sequence of motor development is almost entirely universal. Babies learn to roll over, then sit, then crawl, then stand, then walk. The development of the cerebellum is a necessary precursor to walking, and most humans learn to walk around age one.

The average age of earliest conscious memory is roughly 3.5 years. Before this age, we are unable to remember much, if anything; this is referred to as **infantile amnesia**. Even though humans are unable to recall memories from this period, babies and young children are still capable of learning and memory. In one famous experiment, a researcher tied a string to an infant's foot and attached the other end of the string to a mobile. When the baby kicked its foot, the mobile moved. Babies demonstrated learning—they associated kicking with mobile movement—because they kicked more when attached to the mobile, both on the day of the experiment and the day after. Interestingly, if the babies were attached to a different mobile, they did not kick more; however, when attached to the same mobile a month later, they remembered the association and began kicking again.

Social Development and Attachment

Humans are social organisms. From approximately 8–12 months of age, young children display **stranger anxiety** (crying and clinging to caregiver). Around this time, infants have developed schemas for familiar faces, and when new faces do not fit an already developed schema, the infant becomes distressed. Infant-parent attachment bonds are an important survival impulse. Stranger anxiety seems to peek around 13 months for children and then gradually declines. For many years it was assumed that infants attached to their parents because they provided nourishment, but an accidental experiment actually countered this assumption.

In the 1950s, two psychologists (**Harry Harlow** and **Margaret Harlow**) bred monkeys for experiments. To control for environment and to reduce the incidence of disease, infant monkeys were separated from their mothers at birth (maternal deprivation) and provided with a baby blanket. When the blankets were removed for laundering the baby monkeys became very distressed because they had formed an intense attachment to the object. This physical attachment seemed to contradict the idea that attachment was formed based on nourishment, so the Harlows designed a series of experiments to further investigate. In one experiment, the Harlows fashioned two artificial mothers—one nourishing (a wire frame with a wooden head and a bottle) and the other cloth (wire frame with a wooden head and a cloth blanket wrapped around it). They found that the baby monkeys preferred the cloth mother, clinging to her and spending the majority of their time with her, and visiting the other mother only to feed. Harlow concluded that "contact comfort" was an essential element of infant/mother bonding, as well as to psychological development. Keep in mind, however, that even though these baby monkeys were provided with a surrogate wire mother, this mother was still largely inadequate. Therefore, when the monkeys from these experiments matured, they demonstrated social deficits when reintroduced to other monkeys. Harlow's monkeys demonstrated aggressive behavior as adults, were unable to socially integrate with other monkeys, and did not mate. If female monkeys were artificially inseminated, they would neglect, abuse, or even kill their offspring.[1]

Mary Ainsworth conducted a series of experiments called the "strange situation experiments," wherein mothers would leave their infants in an unfamiliar environment (usually a laboratory playroom) to see how the infants would react. These studies suggested that attachment styles vary among infants. **Securely attached** infants in the presence of their mothers (or primary caregivers) will play and explore; when the mother leaves the room, the infant is distressed, and when the mother returns, the infant will seek contact with her and is easily consoled. **Insecurely attached** infants in the presence of their mothers (or primary caregivers) are less likely to explore their surroundings and may even cling to their mothers; when the mother leaves, they will either cry loudly and remain upset or will demonstrate indifference to her departure and return. Observations indicate that securely attached infants have sensitive and responsive mothers (or primary caregivers) who are quick to attend to their child's needs in a consistent fashion. Insecurely attached infants have mothers (or primary caregivers) who are insensitive and unresponsive, attending to their child's needs inconsistently or sometimes even ignoring their children. In the Harlow monkey experiments described above, the cloth mother would be considered rather insensitive and unresponsive; when these monkeys were put into situations without their artificial mothers, they became terrified.

Psychologists believe that early interactions with parents and caregivers lay the foundation for future adult relationships. Securely attached infants grow up to demonstrate better social skills, a greater capacity for effective intimate relationships, and a superior ability to promote secure attachments in their children. Alternatively, children who are neglected or abused are *more likely* to neglect or abuse their own children. Note that more likely does not imply a destiny; most abused children do not grow up to abuse their own children. Humans display a large degree of resiliency, and most insecurely attached or abused children grow into normal adults.

Parenting styles vary but tend to fall largely into three categories: authoritarian, permissive, and authoritative:

- **Authoritarian** parenting involves attempting to control children with strict rules that are expected to be followed unconditionally. Authoritarian parents will often utilize punishment instead of discipline, and will not explain the reasoning behind their rules. Typically, authoritarian parents are very demanding, but not very responsive to their children, and do

---

[1] Note: this type of extreme deprivation experiment would no longer be considered ethical or humane today; research animals in captivity are treated much better.

not provide much warmth or nurturing. Children raised by authoritarian parents may display more aggressive behavior toward others, or may act shy and fearful around others, have lower self-esteem, and have difficulty in social situations.

- **Permissive** parents, on the other hand, allow their children to lead the show. With few rules and demands, these parents rarely discipline their children. Permissive parents are very responsive and loving toward their children, but are rather lenient; if rules exist, they are enforced inconsistently. Children raised by permissive parents tend to lack self-discipline, may be self-involved and demanding, and may demonstrate poor social skills.

- **Authoritative** parents listen to their children, encourage independence, place limits on behavior and consistently follow through with consequences when behavior is not met, express warmth and nurturing, and allow children to express their opinions and to discuss options. Authoritative parents have expectations for their children, and when children break the rules they are disciplined in a fair and consistent manner. Authoritative parenting is the "best" parenting style, as it tends to produce children that are happier, have good emotional control and regulation, develop good social skills, and are confident in their abilities.

Please remember that parenting style and children's dispositions are merely correlated; while it is possible that parenting style causes these outcomes in children, there are other possible explanations, as well [what are some potential alternative explanations for these results?[2]].

Adolescence

Despite the fact that infancy is crucial for development, development continues throughout our lifetime. **Adolescence**[3] is the transitional stage between childhood and adulthood; this period roughly begins at puberty and ends with achievement of independent adult status. Therefore, adolescence generally encompasses the teenage years. Adolescence involves many important physical, psychological, and social changes. The onset of puberty (typically around age 10 or 11 in girls, and age 11 or 12 in boys) involves surging estrogens and androgens (sex hormones) that cause a cascade of physical changes. In girls, increased estrogen causes the development of secondary sex characteristics (increased body and pubic hair, increased fat distribution, breast development) as well as the initiation of the menstrual cycle. In boys, increased testosterone (the primary androgen) also causes the development of secondary sex characteristics (increased body and pubic hair, increased muscle mass, voice deepening, enlargement of the penis and testes), and the onset of ejaculation. While the sequence of events in puberty is fairly predictable, the onset of these events is less so, which can be distressing. For example, early puberty for a girl means that she will begin developing breasts and menstruating before her peers do, which can be psychologically upsetting.

During adolescence, the brain undergoes three major changes: cell proliferation (in certain areas, particularly the prefrontal lobes and limbic system), synaptic pruning (of unused or unnecessary connections), and myelination (which strengthens connections among various regions). The prefrontal cortex—responsible for abstract thought, planning, anticipating consequences, and personality—continues to develop

---

[2] It is possible that certain children have a genetic disposition to be easygoing, confident, and socially adjusted, so the authoritative parent has an "easy time" raising this easy child, and their resultant behavior is attributed to the parent when, in actuality, there was something innate about the child that caused the parent to respond to him in that way.

[3] From the Latin word *adolescere*, which means "to grow up."

during this period.[4] The limbic system—involved in emotion—develops more rapidly than the prefrontal cortex during adolescence, which may explain behavior that appears to be emotionally, rather than rationally, driven. Though it may seem contradictory, adolescents are actually improving their self-control, judgment, and long-term planning abilities during this time.

Adulthood and Later Life

While the transition to "adulthood" is not marked by any definitive biological event (indeed, the term is essentially defined by society), attainment of adulthood is marked by a feeling of comfortable independence. Interestingly, while childhood and adolescence are marked by clear developmental milestones and attainment of physical abilities, adulthood is less clearly defined. For example, if you met a 4-year old and a 14-year old, you would probably be able to reasonably guess at some of the actions they were and were not capable of, and the differences between them would be drastic. If, on the other hand, you met a 40-year old and 50-year old, it may be much harder to pinpoint the difference, if there was much of one at all.

---

[4] In fact the frontal lobes are not completely developed until roughly age 26!

Chapter 9 Summary

- Nonassociative learning occurs when an organism is repeatedly exposed to a stimulus and includes habituation and sensitization.

- Associative learning occurs when an organism learns that an event, object, or action is connected with another; the two major types are classical conditioning and operant conditioning.

- Classical conditioning pairs a neutral stimulus with an unconditioned stimulus to generate a conditioned stimulus and conditioned response (for example, Pavlov's dogs). In acquisition the response is learned, in extinction the response is "lost," and in spontaneous recovery, an extinct response occurs again when the stimulus is presented after some length of time.

- Taste aversion is a very strong and long-lasting association between a specific taste or smell and illness; taste aversion challenges some of the tenets of classical conditioning because it is learned quickly (after one time) and is very slow to extinguish.

- Operant conditioning uses reinforcement and punishment to mold behavior and eventually cause associative learning; B. F. Skinner and his work with rats and pigeons in a "Skinner box" is a famous example of operant conditioning.

- Reinforcement increases the likelihood that a preceding behavior will be repeated; positive reinforcement is a desirable stimulus that occurs immediately following a behavior, whereas negative reinforcement is an undesirable stimulus that is removed immediately following a behavior.

- A fixed-ratio schedule provides the reinforcement after a set number of instances of the behavior while a variable-ratio schedule provides the reinforcement after an unpredictable number of occurrences.

- A fixed-interval schedule provides the reinforcement after a set amount of time, while a variable-interval schedule provides the reinforcement after an inconsistent amount of time.

- Punishment is a consequence that follows a behavior and decreases the likelihood that the behavior will be repeated; positive punishment presents an undesirable stimulus after an instance of the target behavior, while negative punishment removes a desirable stimulus after an instance of the target behavior.

- Insight learning occurs when previously learned behaviors are suddenly combined in unique ways.

- Latent learning occurs when previously unseen behavior can manifest quickly when required.

- Long-term potentiation occurs when, following brief periods of stimulation, a persistent increase in the synaptic strength between two neurons leads to stronger electrochemical responses to a given stimulus.

- Observational learning is a social process; in modeling, an observer sees behavior and later imitates it; Albert Bandura's Bobo doll experiment is a famous example of modeling.

- Mirror neurons have been identified in various parts of the human brain and are believed to fire when we observe another person performing a task.

- Short-term memory is limited in duration and in capacity; recall capacity for an adult is typically around seven items, plus or minus two.

- Long-term memory is information that is retained sometimes indefinitely; it is believed to have an infinite capacity. Long-term memory consists of implicit (procedural) memory and explicit (declarative) memory; explicit memory includes episodic and semantic memory.

- The spreading activation theory of memory posits that during recall, nodes (concepts) are activated, which are connected to other nodes, and so on.

- Anterograde amnesia is an inability to encode new memories, while retrograde amnesia is an inability to recall information that was previously encoded.

- Important information about attachment was discovered through studies conducted by Mary Ainsworth; the impact of deprivation was discovered through studies conducted by Harry and Margaret Harlow.

CHAPTER 9 FREESTANDING PRACTICE QUESTIONS

1. Retroactive interference occurs when:

   A) old information interferes with learning new material.
   B) new material interferes with recalling old material.
   C) new information decays over time.
   D) old information decays over time.

2. Which of the following types of memory does not affect behavior consciously and can be measured only indirectly?

   A) Nondeclarative memory
   B) Declarative memory
   C) Episodic memory
   D) Explicit memory

3. A five-year-old boy has formed a habit of writing on his parents' living room walls. Based on operant conditioning principles, which of the following types of punishment would be least effective in stopping this behavior?

   A) Giving the child a time out immediately after he writes on the wall, every time the child writes on the wall.
   B) Providing the child with a cookie at the end of each day that he abstains from writing on the walls.
   C) Harshly scolding the child (an intense punishment) every time that the child writes on the wall.
   D) Punishing the child occasionally, when the parents happen to notice writing on the wall.

4. Jay joins a social media website to lose weight, and he receives points based on the intensity of his daily exercise and praise from fellow website users for each workout he logs on the website. This increases his exercise frequency and intensity. Eventually he stops logging onto the website, but continues to exercise with increased frequency. This is an example of:

   A) vicarious reinforcement.
   B) operant conditioning.
   C) innate behavior.
   D) classical conditioning.

5. A student cramming for finals memorizes the steps in solving a physics problem early in the afternoon and then studies for his other subjects for several hours before his physics exam. When he arrives at the exam, he can no longer remember how to solve the physics equation. This is an example of:

   A) retroactive interference.
   B) proactive interference.
   C) retrieval cues.
   D) long-term potentiation.

6. A researcher studying several patients gives each of them the same maze to solve. Although each works independently on it for 30 minutes—with varying degrees of success—none of them recalls seeing the maze when presented with it the next day. Nonetheless, their overall speed and success in solving it has improved significantly. These patients are likely experiencing impairment in:

   I. procedural memory.
   II. episodic memory.
   III. echoic memory.

   A) I only
   B) II only
   C) I and II
   D) II and III

7. Knowing how to ride a bike is a type of:

   A) procedural, long-term, implicit memory.
   B) explicit, short-term, procedural memory.
   C) prospective, long-term, implicit memory.
   D) procedural, mood-dependent, source memory.

8. An individual attempting to memorize a series of complex steps for the first time is most likely to have the most success if he uses:

   A) priming that incorporates proactive interference.
   B) chunking and serial position.
   C) source-monitoring and rehearsal.
   D) a mnemonic that incorporates spaced repetition of the steps.

CHAPTER 9 PRACTICE PASSAGE

Elizabeth Loftus is widely known as one of the leading experts in the field of false memories, especially regarding childhood sexual abuse. However, this particular topic is deeply controversial, with many experts divided over whether these memories are truly false, or if they are instead repressed to protect the individual from reliving further trauma. Loftus is most famous for her theory of the *misinformation effect*, which refers to the phenomenon in which exposure to incorrect information between the encoding of a memory and its later recall causes impairment to the memory. That is to say, if you witnessed a hit-and-run car accident, and heard a radio commercial for Ford before giving your testimony to the police, you might incorrectly recall that the offending vehicle was a Ford, even if it was not. Loftus' research has been used in many cases of eyewitness testimony in high-profile court cases to demonstrate the malleability of the human memory.

To test this theory, researchers in New York City set up a "crime" for participants to "witness" (unbeknownst to them). 175 local female college students were recruited to participate in a study about memory, and were directed to complete some computer tasks involving word and picture recall in a room overlooking an alley. While completing the computer tasks, participants witnessed a young woman being "mugged" by a young man in the alley outside the lab—both individuals were confederates of the researchers. After reporting the "crime" to the researchers, participants were escorted out of the lab and told that this crime would be reported to the local police, and that they might be called back in to give a testimony. For half of the participants, a research confederate acting as a custodial worker was present as they were being escorted out. For the other half, no decoys were present. Participants were randomly assigned to either the decoy or non-decoy groups. Participants who did not report the "crime" to the researchers were excluded from the study (25 women were excluded).

One week later, participants were called back to the lab to give their testimony to a police officer—another confederate. Participants were told that the police had several leads on who the mugger might be, and were asked to pick out the suspect from five different photo options. Included in the photo set were photos of the mugger, the custodial worker, and three neutral faces chosen to be similar to the two experimental faces. After recalling the event to the police officer and choosing a face, participants were debriefed (they were told that the mugging was fake) and awarded course credit for their participation. The results of this study are summarized in Table 1.

Table 1 Number of Positive Identifications in Photo Line-up

	Photo				
	"Mugger"	"Custodial Worker"	Neutral Photo #1	Neutral Photo #2	Neutral Photo #3
Decoy Group (n = 75)	18	37	7	5	8
Non-Decoy Group (n = 75)	23	13	12	14	13

1. What conclusions can be drawn from the data presented in Table 1?

A) The misinformation effect is present in the decoy group.
B) The non-decoy group had better memory than the decoy group.
C) There are no significant differences between the decoy and non-decoy groups.
D) No conclusions can be drawn from these data.

2. The inability to form new memories is called:

A) retrograde amnesia.
B) anterograde amnesia.
C) source amnesia
D) infantile amnesia.

3. Suppose that after selecting someone from the photo line-up, all of the subjects in the non-decoy group watched a ten-minute film presentation in which a "police officer" provided additional evidence about why the custodial worker was suspected to be the culprit responsible for the mugging. Half of the subjects had a "very handsome" police officer presenting the information, and the other half had an "unattractive" police officer presenting the same information. 85% of the subjects who watched the video with the handsome police officer either changed their answer to the custodial worker or confirmed that selection. 35% of the subjects who watched the video with the unattractive police officer changed their answer to the custodial worker. The elaboration likelihood model suggests that the discrepancy in the two groups is based on:

A) the peripheral route of information processing.
B) target characteristics.
C) message characteristics.
D) the central route of information processing.

4. What type of memory is used in a multiple-choice test, such as this one?

A) Recall
B) Recognition
C) Repressed
D) Déjà vu

5. What are the three main stages of memory, according to the information-processing perspective?

A) Encoding, storage, and retrieval
B) Recognition, detection, and regurgitation
C) Consolidation, reconsolidation, and recovery
D) Identification, encrypting, and reclamation

SOLUTIONS TO CHAPTER 9 FREESTANDING PRACTICE QUESTIONS

1. **B** Retroactive interference is a type of memory interference in which new information interferes with our ability to recall older material (choice B is correct). Proactive interference occurs when old information interferes with learning new material (choice A is wrong). Choices C and D refer to memory decay which occurs regardless of interference (choices C and D are wrong).

2. **A** Nondeclarative memory, or implicit memory, is a form of memory that is not conscious. It is the autopilot of memory (so it does not affect behavior consciously) and may be difficult to verbalize, making it measurable only indirectly (choice A is correct). Declarative memory, also referred to as explicit memory, involves long-term memories that can be consciously or intentionally called upon (choices B and D are wrong). Episodic memory is a type of declarative memory that is responsible for the recall of autobiographical events (choice C is wrong).

3. **D** Operant conditioning employs consequences to modify behavior. Reinforcement is more effective at modifying behavior than punishment is, but for both, the timing/schedule and intensity of the reinforcement or punishment is important. In general, delivering punishment consistently for every occurrence of the behavior produces more effective suppression of the behavior than does delivering punishment intermittently or inconsistently. Punishing the child only when the negative behavior happens to be noticed would not qualify as consistent and would thus not be very effective (choice D is correct). Immediacy, or delivering the punishment immediately after the act, will increase the effectiveness of the punishment, as will consistency (choice A would be more effective than D, and is therefore wrong). Positive reinforcement is generally more effective than punishment for increasing the frequency of a desired behavior (not writing on the walls) and diminishes the child's motivation to engage in the undesired response (choice B is more effective than D, and is therefore wrong). Finally, while severe punishment can have undesirable side effects, in general, the more intense the punishment, the more effective the punishment is in producing major, rapid, and long-lasting suppression (choice C is more effective than D, and is therefore wrong).

4. **B** Positive reinforcement (one type of operant conditioning) is accomplished when someone receives a reward after performing a task; after the person has performed the task and received the reward enough times, they will perform the task without the reward (choice B is correct). Vicarious reinforcement involves watching another person receive a reward for his or her behavior; there is no mention of Jay being motived by other people getting rewarded (choice A is wrong). An innate behavior is one that does not need to be conditioned, and therefore not what is being described in the question stem (choice C is wrong). Classical conditioning is accomplished by pairing two stimuli, one that is neutral with another that is unconditioned. Over time, the neutral stimulus becomes the conditioned stimulus. Since the question is not describing the pairing of two stimuli, nor is a stimulus presented before the behavior, classical conditioning does not explain the behavior described in the question stem (choice D is wrong).

5. **A** Retroactive interference occurs when new information interferes with the storage of information learned beforehand (choice A is correct). Proactive interference occurs when information that is learned first interferes with the ability to recall information learned subsequently; the opposite is described in this question (choice B is wrong). Retrieval cues are used to retrieve stored memories; there is no mention of retrieval cues in this question (choice C is wrong). Long-term potentiation is part of long-term memory storage; while a failure to remember information is partially a result of a failure to convert information

via long-term potentiation, it does not explain the interference of information learned after memorizing the steps to a physics problem (choice D is wrong).

6. **B**   Item I is false: the subjects have no recall of the maze, meaning that their *declarative* memory (long-term, concerning specific facts, details, situations, and context) is not functioning properly; *procedural* memory, which concerns development of specific skills for how to do something, is biologically distinct from declarative memory, and must be functioning if they display improvement on the maze (choices A and C can be eliminated). Note that both remaining answer choices include Item II, so Item II must be true: episodic memory (part of declarative memory) includes memory of events that have been experienced personally. Amnesic patients with hippocampal damage may not have declarative memory for a skill they have recently learned (due to amnesia), and yet may be able to demonstrate the skill, indicating that implicit (procedural) memory exists, much like the patients described in the question stem. Item III is false: echoic memory, part of the short-term sensory memory system, is brief memory for sound. The question stem does not provide any information about the patients' ability to process or remember sound information (choice D can be eliminated, and choice B is correct).

7. **A**   Procedural memory is related to actions, implicit memory is unconscious memory without conscious recall, and long-term memory is memory stored indefinitely. Each of these attributes applies to riding a bike (choice A is correct). Explicit memory is memory that involves conscious recall, which does not apply to riding a bike. Riding a bike is also part of long-term, not short-term or working memory (choice B is wrong). Prospective memory refers to remembering to perform planned actions (choice C is wrong). Mood-dependent memory refers to memories that are more easily accessed during the experience of similar moods and emotions. Source memory does not refer to a type of memory, but is a trap answer taken from "source monitoring error" (choice D is wrong).

8. **D**   A mnemonic is a memory retention tool, and spaced repetition is known to reduce forgetting and allow for long-term retention (choice D is correct). Priming would be a memory aid, but would not help to memorize the steps independently of the presence of the aid. Proactive interference refers to forgetting and would reduce memory retention (choice A is wrong). Chunking would be a helpful tool, but serial position refers to the location of a word in a list and does not to refer to a memorization technique (choice B is wrong). Source-monitoring refers to knowing the source from which a memory came from and is not likely to help memorization of a series of complex steps. That is, knowing where one originally learned the steps does not address the problem of trying to memorize them (choice C is wrong).

SOLUTIONS TO CHAPTER 9 PRACTICE PASSAGE

1. **A**   Based on the data presented in Table 1, one can reasonably conclude that the misinformation effect is present in the decoy group. The overwhelming majority of participants in that group positively identified the custodial worker as the mugger, most likely because his face was presented to them before the memory of the mugging could be fully encoded (choice A is correct). Although the non-decoy group chose the mugger at a higher rate than did the decoy group, this is not enough information to reasonably conclude that the non-decoy group has better memory (choice B is wrong). Forty-nine percent (37) of the subjects in the decoy group identified the custodial worker as the mugger, whereas only 17% (13) of the non-decoy subjects did so (choice C is wrong). Based on these findings, some conclusions can indeed be drawn from these data (choice D is wrong).

2. **B**   Anterograde amnesia is defined as the inability to form new memories (choice B is correct). Retrograde amnesia is defined as the inability to retrieve information from one's past (choice A is wrong). Source amnesia is defined as the attribution of an event one has experienced, heard about, or imagined to the wrong source (choice C is wrong). Infantile amnesia is used to explain why individuals are typically unable to remember anything from before the age of 3; the human brain pathways are not yet fully developed enough to form memories at this age (choice D is wrong).

3. **A**   The elaboration likelihood model theorizes that attitudes are formed by dual processes, via the central processing route or by the peripheral processing route. Since the subjects with the handsome police officer were far more likely to be persuaded that the photo of the custodial worker was the mugger, this suggests that both groups were focusing on characteristics of the person delivering the message (attractiveness). In the peripheral processing route, people are more likely to be persuaded by attractive messengers (choice A is correct). The central processing route involves focusing on the information of the message; in this scenario, the message was the same for both groups, so the central processing route does not explain the difference in outcome (choice D is wrong). Target characteristics describe the characteristics of the person receiving the message (motivation, interest); there is no information provided in the stem that would indicate that any characteristics of the two groups were responsible for the different outcome (choice B is wrong). Similarly, the message characteristics include specific features of the message itself (like length, logic, and evidence). Since the message was the same for the two groups, message characteristics do not explain the difference in outcomes (choice C is wrong).

4. **B**   Multiple-choice tests rely most heavily on recognition memory; that is, test-takers do not have to generate the correct response, but rather have to recognize the correct response from several options (choice B is correct). On the flip side, a test that involved short-answer or essay questions would rely on recall memory, which requires individuals to retrieve previously learned information and repeat it in some context (choice A is wrong). Repressed memories are a phenomenon that is hotly debated in the legal and psychological fields, and would likely not come into play during a multiple-choice test (choice C is wrong). Déjà vu is the phenomenon in which cues from the current situation subconsciously trigger retrieval of an earlier experience, creating that "I've been here before" feeling. This phenomenon is not typically associated with testing (choice D is wrong).

5. **A**   The three main stages of memory are encoding (receiving, processing, and combining information), storage (the creation of a permanent record of the encoded information), and retrieval (the recovery of the stored information in response to a particular cue or activity; choice A is correct). The other terms, while sometimes associated with the study of memory, are not part of the formal stages of memory (choices B, C, and D are wrong).

Chapter 10
Behavioral
Neuroscience

We now mostly take for granted that the brain is the primary seat of behavior, where our thoughts, feelings, reflections, and perceptions take place. However, it took many years for scientists and philosophers to arrive at this conclusion. Gradually, through work with patients who had suffered traumatic brain injury and strokes, it became clear to neurologists and psychologists that our brains contain regions that are largely responsible for specific functions. This lead to an effort to "map the brain" by compiling clinical data from lesions, using molecular techniques to study neural activity, and using brain imaging to determine functionality. These various methods show that the brain is more integrated and complex than anyone could previously have imagined, and different regions and networks play crucial roles in learning, memory, emotion, stress, and indeed, all behavior.

10.1 MEASUREMENT TOOLS FOR STUDYING THE BRAIN

Behavioral neuroscience is the area of psychology that looks for the neurophysiological correlates of behavior. This search can be broken down to two questions: "What parts of the brain are active during specific behaviors?" and "How do neurotransmitters and other chemicals affect behavior?" These two questions will remain central as we explore the way that the brain gives life to experiences we are all familiar with like fear, stress, happiness, confusion—in fact, there is probably no area of psychology that today does not fall within the purview of neuroscience and exploration of brain-behavior correlates. First, it is important to understand what tools researchers have at their disposal for exploring the brain. There are three general categories: molecular methods, brain lesions, and neuroimaging. Molecular methods are beyond the scope of the MCAT Psychology/Sociology section and some of these methods will be covered in Biology and Organic Chemistry. Let's take a closer look at the other two methods: the clinical study of brain lesions and neuroimaging.

Brain Lesions

A landmark case in the history of neuroscience was the case of Phineas Gage. In the 1800s, Phineas Gage, a 25-year-old railroad worker, suffered an accident in which a railroad tie blasted through his head, entering under his cheekbone and exiting through the top of his skull. Gage survived, but after the accident, he was described by friends and associates as "no longer himself," prone to impulsivity, unable to stick to plans, and seemingly unable to demonstrate empathy. People who knew him said he was like a completely different person. The accident had severely damaged his **prefrontal cortex,** an area of the brain that is now known to be involved in reflection, planning, emotional regulation, and **theory of mind**—the ability to understand the perspectives of others.

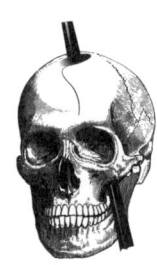

Phineas Gage Injury

The case of Phineas Gage was groundbreaking as it was a first step toward the discovery of the role of the prefrontal cortex in personality. Psychologists had also stumbled on an important methodology for mapping the brain: by observing the clinical changes in behavior that occurred after a lesion or accident, they could infer the role that the damaged area played in behavior and personality. The case study method (described in Chapter 3) has been critical to the study of behavioral neuroscience and discovering brain-behavior correlates. Throughout the 20th century, psychologists continued to study and document traumatic brain injuries such as Phineas Gage's as well as the effects of acute strokes. The rationale was simple: if damage to an area of the brain resulted in a change in behavior, then that area must be directly involved in, or part of a network of regions that is involved in, the functioning of that behavior.

Of course, this method had limitations because scientists could not conduct double-blind, randomized experimental studies (sign us up for the control group, please!) and researchers had to wait for a stroke or accident to occur, which could then only be studied one incident at a time. Later in the 20th century and continuing into the present, technological innovations have allowed neuroscientists to use various imaging techniques to study the brain in a more controlled fashion, and design studies—many of them experimental—to address specific hypotheses, rather than waiting for the data to come to them.

Neuroimaging Techniques

Neuroimaging techniques are either structural or functional. **Structural imaging** techniques provide a picture of the brain; they show anatomical regions and where they are located with respect to one another. They do not, however, offer any insight into which regions are active at any given time. For this, neuroscientists use **functional imaging** techniques, which demonstrate which parts of the brain are active, and to what extent, as experimental participants manifest a behavior. Let's look first at the two important types of structural techniques; Computerized Tomography (CT) and Magnetic Resonance Imaging (MRI).

Computerized Tomography (CT) scans, also known as CAT (computerized axial tomography) scans, use a computer to combine many cross-sectional (tomographic) images generated from the differential absorption of X-rays of an anatomical part, in this case the human brain, or a subsection of it. These differential absorptions are used to create a three-dimensional structural "snapshot" that appears as a series of cross-sectional images.

Magnetic Resonance Imaging (MRI) uses strong magnets which cause protons to align, spin, and generate a detectable radio-frequency signal that is measured by antennas close to the anatomy being examined. Regular MRI (in contrast to "functional" MRI, see below) provides only structural data, high quality "snapshots" that provide three-dimensional views of the target tissue. Structural MRI cannot be used to analyze the function of the brain across time.

When comparing CT scans and MRIs, advantages of CT scans include a very rapid acquisition of images of a large portion of the body, generally lower cost, more open and less noisy machinery, no requirement that subjects remain completely motionless, and no prohibition on implanted medical devices. For brain imaging, CT scans are preferred when speed is important, such as during a suspected stroke. Advantages of MRIs include higher resolution and therefore a more detailed image. MRI provides much more detail about soft tissues. Also, MRIs do not use X-rays, and do not include significant exposure to ionizing radiation, which make MRIs safer in most instances.

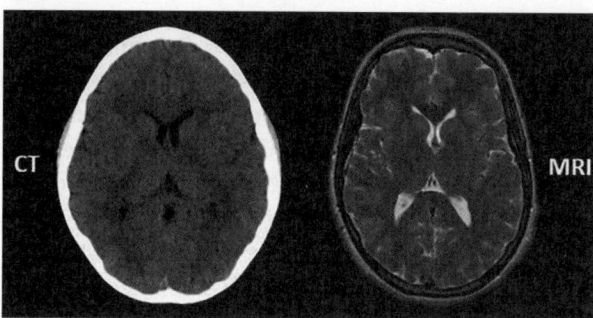

Figure 1   CT scan vs. MRI

The other important types of imaging techniques are functional: they provide insight into which brain regions are active during any given time. We'll look at four types of functional imaging: EEG, MEG, fMRI, and PET.

Electroencephalography (EEG) is a relatively noninvasive method of gathering functional information about brain activity. Electrodes are placed on the scalp to measure voltage fluctuations in the ionic currents of brain neurons. The resulting traces are known as electroencephalograms (EEGs), and each trace represents the net electrical signal of a large number of neurons. EEGs provide functional data about the brain's electrical neural oscillations (often referred to as "brain waves") that have extremely precise temporal resolution.

To prepare a subject for an EEG, a number of electrodes are placed on the subject's face and scalp, which allows the electrical potential of each electrode to be measured. Depending on a person's state of consciousness (awake, REM sleep, N1 sleep, N2 sleep, N3 sleep, etc.), the frequency, amplitude, and waveforms of the measured EEG traces differ. EEGs are useful in the diagnosis of seizures, sleep disorders, and other conditions that involve activity imbalances in certain parts of the brain.

Advantages of EEG compared to fMRI and PET (below) include less hardware bulk, lower hardware costs, relative tolerance of movement, much higher temporal resolution, non-aggravation of claustrophobia, and silence. However, disadvantages of EEG include far lower spatial resolution, poor measurement of neural activity that occurs below the cortex, poor signal-to-noise ratio, and significant additional preparation time.

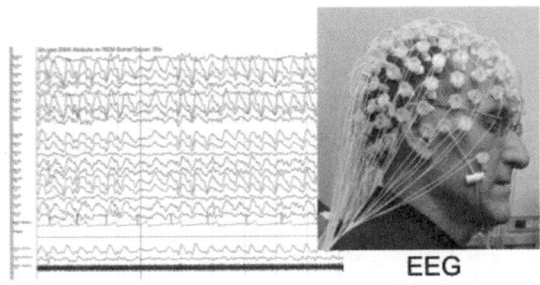

Figure 2   EEG and results

Magnetoencephalography (MEG) is a functional neuroimaging technique for mapping brain activity that records the magnetic fields produced by the brain's electrical currents. MEG uses very sensitive magnetometers, typically using an array of SQUIDs (superconducting quantum interference devices).

MEG has more or less the same advantages and disadvantages as EEG compared to fMRI and PET. Compared to EEG, MEG has better spatial resolution of the brain activity it can detect, while EEG can detect activity in more areas of the brain. In addition, MEG requires expensive bulky machinery as well as a magnetically shielded room.

Functional magnetic resonance imaging (fMRI) uses a computer to combine a series of magnetic resonance images (see MRI, above) taken less than a second apart to provide a functional picture of how brain activity changes over time. fMRI can display changes in oxygen levels (which indicate blood flow) in various regions of the brain in real time and can be used to produce activation maps that indicate the areas of the brain involved in particular mental processes.

fMRI technology has several advantages over other methods of measuring brain structure (regular MRI) by providing evidence of real-time activity in the brain. fMRI is also considered safer than PET (below) because PET requires subjects to be injected with radioactive substances. The locational precision of fMRI data is more precise than PET and far more precise than EEG. fMRI is also generally more cost effective than PET. The major disadvantage of fMRI (as with MRI, above) is that the subject has to remain completely still in a noisy, cramped space while the imaging is performed. For example, it is not possible to query a subject to answer simple questions during the fMRI of the brain.

Positron emission tomography (PET) is a nuclear medicine imaging technique that produces a three-dimensional image of functional metabolic processes across time. PET scans require the subject to be injected with a positron-emitting radionuclide tracer, which is introduced into the body on a biologically active molecule, such as glucose. Three-dimensional images of the tracer concentration within the body are then constructed by computer analysis that allows the movement of, and changes in, the tracer concentration to be displayed in real time.

In modern PET-CT scanners, three-dimensional PET imaging is often augmented with a CT X-ray scan performed on the patient during the same session, in the same machine. This combination (as well as the less common PET/MRI combination) can provide a detailed structural image of the brain together with functional data. PET is a valuable technique for some diseases and disorders because it is possible to image specific radio-chemicals used for particular bodily functions. For example, if a patient is injected with a radioactive glucose analog, a PET scan can be used to image and then analyze the uptake of this specific glucose analog in the brain.

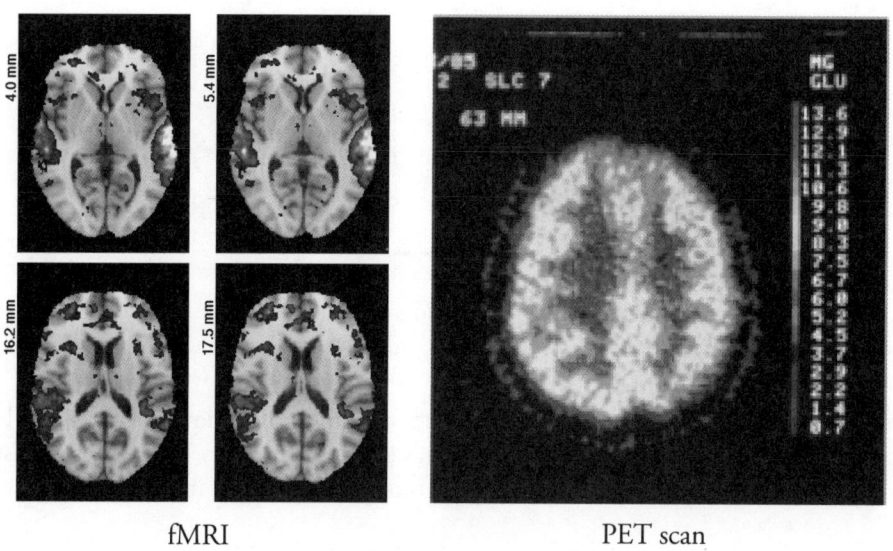

fMRI   PET scan

Figure 3   fMRI vs. PET

These are the primary methods of observing the brain itself. However, researchers are often also interested in understanding how the rest of the body is responding by measuring physiological markers that are associated with personality or behavior. For example, if a researcher were investigating the stress response, they would likely take data on electrical skin conductance, cortisol levels, heart rate, blood pressure, pupil dilation, etc. These indicators are also frequently used in behavioral neuroscience studies, especially research into stress and stress management, which we cover below.

10.2 BRAIN STRUCTURE AND NEUROTRANSMITTERS

Now that we have looked at some of the techniques neuroscientists use to study functionality in the brain, let's take a deeper look at what their work has revealed about the brain and behavior. We hope to understand not only what the anatomical parts of the brain are, but how those parts interact with one another to give rise to behavior. Then, we'll look more closely at the neurotransmitters in the brain and their functions as understood by neuroscientists.

Anatomical Organization of the Nervous System

The main anatomical division of the nervous system is between the **central nervous system (CNS)** and the **peripheral nervous system (PNS)**. The central nervous system is the brain and spinal cord. The peripheral nervous system includes all other axons, dendrites, and cell bodies. The great majority of neuronal cell bodies are found within the central nervous system. Sometimes they are bunched together to form structures called **nuclei** (not to be confused with the nucleic-acid-containing nuclei of cells). Somas located outside the central nervous system are found in bunches known as **ganglia**. In this section, we'll look at the anatomy of the central nervous system. The peripheral nervous system is covered in Chapter 12.

CNS Anatomical Organization

The CNS includes the **spinal cord** and the brain. The brain has three subdivisions: the **hindbrain,** the **midbrain**, and the **forebrain**. These four regions of the CNS (which will be discussed individually below) perform increasingly complex functions, with the forebrain considered the seat of complex behavior and planning. The entire CNS (brain and spinal cord) floats in **cerebrospinal fluid (CSF),** a clear liquid that serves various functions such as shock absorption and exchange of nutrients and waste with the CNS.

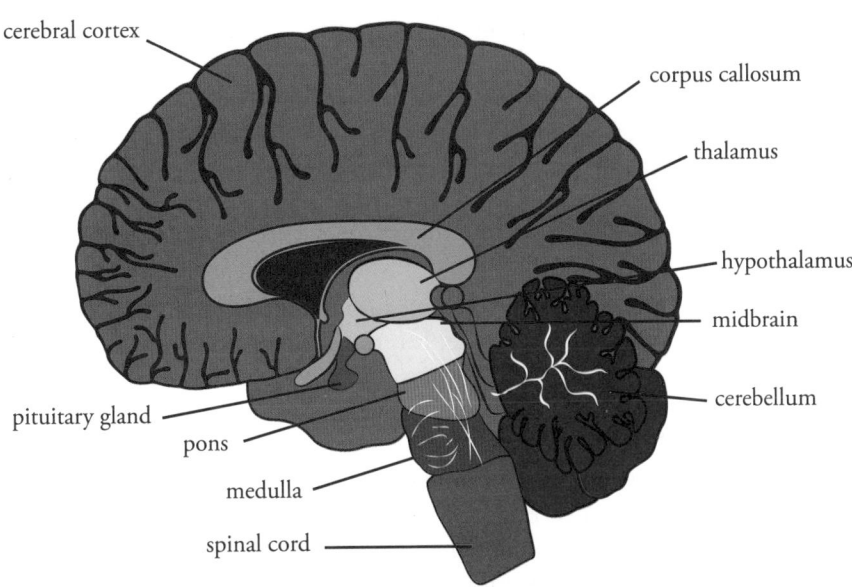

Figure 4   Medial cross-section of the brain

1) The spinal cord is connected to the brain and is protected by the CSF and the vertebral column. It is a pathway for information to and from the brain. Most sensory data is relayed to the brain for integration, but the spinal cord is also a site for information integration and processing. The spinal cord is responsible for simple spinal reflexes (like the muscle stretch reflex) and is also involved in primitive processes such as walking, urination, and sex organ function.

2) The hindbrain includes the medulla, the pons, and the cerebellum.
   - The **medulla** (or medulla oblongata) is located below the pons and is the area of the brain that connects to the spinal cord. It functions in relaying information between other areas of the brain, and regulates vital autonomic functions such as blood pressure and digestive functions (including vomiting). Also, the respiratory rhythmicity centers are found here.
   - The **pons** is located below the midbrain and above the medulla oblongata. It is the connection point between the brain stem and the cerebellum (see below). The pons controls some autonomic functions and coordinates movement; it plays a role in balance and antigravity posture.
   - The **cerebellum** (or "little brain") is located behind the pons and below the cerebral hemispheres. It is an integrating center where complex movements are coordinated. An instruction for movement from the forebrain must be sent to the cerebellum, where the billions of decisions necessary for smooth execution of the movement are made. Damage to the cerebellum results in poor hand-eye coordination and balance. Both the cerebellum and the pons receive information from the vestibular apparatus in the inner ear, which monitors acceleration and position relative to gravity.

3) The midbrain is a relay for visual and auditory information and contains much of the **reticular activating system** (RAS), which is responsible for arousal or wakefulness. Another term you should be familiar with is **brainstem**. Together, the medulla, pons, and midbrain constitute the brainstem, which contains important processing centers and relays information to and from the cerebellum and cerebrum.

4) The forebrain includes the **diencephalon** and the **telencephalon**.
   a) The diencephalon includes the thalamus and hypothalamus:
      - The thalamus is located near the middle of the brain below the cerebral hemispheres and above the midbrain. It contains relay and processing centers for sensory information.
      - The hypothalamus interacts directly with many parts of the brain. It contains centers for controlling emotions and autonomic functions, and has a major role in hormone production and release. It is the primary link between the nervous and the endocrine systems, and, by controlling the pituitary gland, it is the fundamental control center for the endocrine system (discussed later in this chapter).

   b) All parts of the CNS up to and including the diencephalon form a single symmetrical stalk, but the telencephalon consists of two separate cerebral hemispheres. Generally speaking, the areas of the left and right hemispheres have similar functions, with some exceptions. However, the left hemisphere primarily controls the motor functions of the right side of the body, and the right hemisphere controls those of the left side. Also, in most people, the left side of the brain is said to be dominant; it is generally responsible for speech. The right hemisphere is more involved in visual-spatial reasoning and music.

- The **cerebral hemispheres** are connected by a thick bundle of axons called the **corpus callosum**. A person with a cut corpus callosum has two independent cerebral cortices and to a certain extent two independent minds!
- The **cerebrum** is the largest region of the human brain and consists of the large, paired cerebral hemispheres. The hemispheres of the cerebrum consist of the **cerebral cortex** (an outer layer of gray matter) plus an inner core of white matter connecting the cortex to the diencephalon. The gray matter is composed of trillions of somas; the **white matter** is composed of myelinated axons (see Chapter 12 for information on somas, axons, and myelination). The cerebral hemispheres are responsible for conscious thought processes and intellectual functions. They also play a role in processing somatic sensory and motor information. The cerebral cortex is divided into four lobes, each of which is subdivided according to specific functions:
    - i) The **frontal lobes** initiate all voluntary movement and are involved in complex reasoning skills and problem-solving.
    - ii) The **parietal lobes** are involved in general sensations (such as touch, temperature, pressure, vibration, etc.) and in gustation (taste). The parietal lobes receive input from mechanoreceptors and proprioceptors.
    - iii) The **temporal lobes** process auditory and olfactory sensation and are involved in short-term memory, language comprehension, and emotion.
    - iv) The **occipital lobes** process visual sensation.

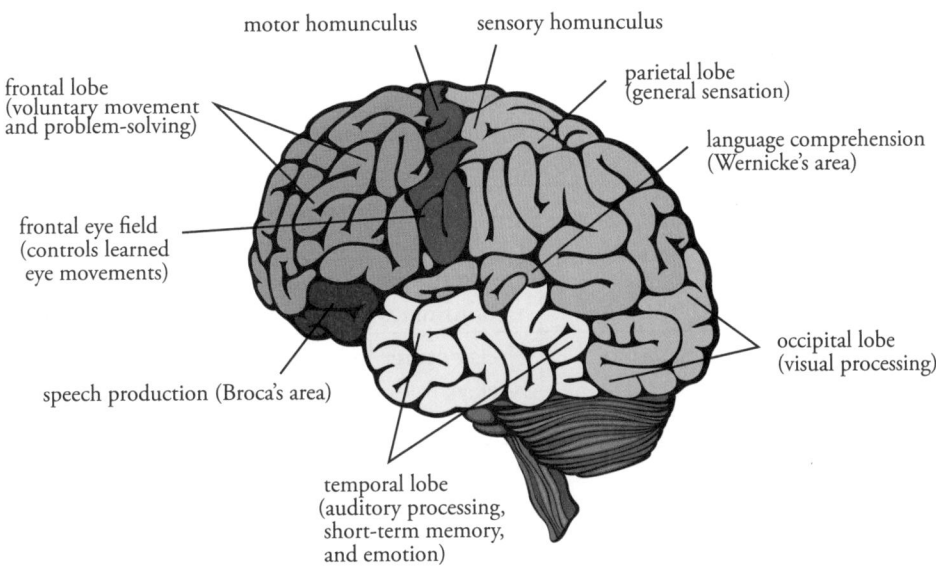

Figure 5 Principal areas of the cerebral cortex

Two other regions of the brain deserve mention:

- The **basal nuclei** (also called the "cerebral nuclei," and also sometimes referred to as the basal ganglia) are composed of gray matter and are located deep within the cerebral hemispheres. They include several functional subdivisions, but broadly function in voluntary motor control and procedural learning related to habits. The basal nuclei and cerebellum work together to process and coordinate movement initiated by the primary motor cortex; the basal nuclei are inhibitory (preventing excess movement), while the cerebellum is excitatory.

- The **limbic system** is located between the cerebrum and the diencephalon. It includes several substructures (such as the amygdala, the cingulate gyrus, and the hippocampus) and works closely with parts of the cerebrum, diencephalon, and midbrain. The limbic system is important for emotion and memory.

The information above describes the general functions of each region of the brain. Table 1, below, summarizes the brain functions and provides a little more specific detail for each region.

Table 1   Parts of the Brain

Structure	General Function	Specific Functions
Spinal cord	Simple reflexes	• controls simple stretch and tendon reflexes • controls primitive processes such as walking, urination, and sex organ function
Medulla	Involuntary functions	• controls autonomic processes such as blood pressure, blood flow, heart rate, respiratory rate, swallowing, vomiting • controls reflex reactions such as coughing or sneezing • relays sensory information to the cerebellum and the thalamus
Pons	Relay station and balance	• controls antigravity posture and balance • connects the spinal cord and medulla with upper regions of the brain • relays information to the cerebellum and thalamus
Cerebellum	Movement coordination	• integrating center • coordination of complex movement, balance and posture, muscle tone, spatial equilibrium
Midbrain	Eye movement	• integration of visual and auditory information • visual and auditory reflexes • wakefulness and consciousness • coordinates information on posture and muscle tone
Thalamus	Integrating center and relay station	• relay center for somatic (conscious) sensation • relays information between the spinal cord and the cerebral cortex
Hypothalamus	Homeostasis and behavior	• controls homeostatic functions (such as temperature regulation, fluid balance, appetite) through both neural and hormonal regulation • controls primitive emotions such as anger, rage, and sex drive • controls the pituitary gland
Basal nuclei	Movement	• regulate body movement and muscle tone • coordination of learned movement patterns • general pattern of rhythm movements (such as controlling the cycle of arm and leg movements when walking) • subconscious adjustments of conscious movements
Limbic system	Emotion, memory, and learning	• controls emotional states • links conscious and unconscious portions of the brain • helps with memory storage and retrieval

Structure	General Function	Specific Functions
Cerebrum	Perception, skeletal muscle movement, memory, attention, thought, language, and consciousness	• divided into four lobes (frontal, parietal, temporal, and occipital) with specialized subfunctions • conscious thought processes and planning, awareness, and sensation • perception and processing of the special senses (vision, hearing, smell, taste, touch) • intellectual function (intelligence, learning, reading, communication) • abstract thought and reasoning • memory storage and retrieval • initiation and coordination of voluntary movement • complex motor patterns • language (speech production and understanding) • personality
Corpus callosum	Connection	• connects the left and right cerebral hemispheres

The motor and sensory regions of the cortex are organized such that a very specific, small area of cortex controls a specific body part. A larger area is devoted to body parts which require more motor control or more sensation, such as facial muscles and fingers (Figure 6). For example, more cortex is devoted to the lips than to the entire leg. The body parts represented on the cortex can be sketched according to the body part controlled by each part of the cortex. When sketched out, this drawing looks like a distorted person, known as a **homunculus** (little man).

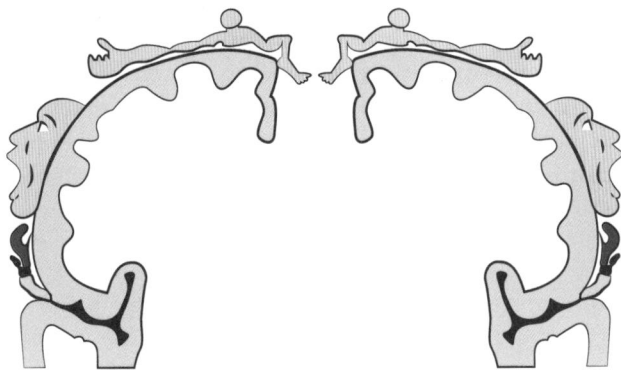

Figure 6   The sensory homunculus

Neurotransmitters

Neurotransmitters are chemicals released by neurons into synapses that affect the next neuron (or organ). They can generally can generally be divided into excitatory neurotransmitters, which increase the likelihood of the postsynaptic neuron firing, and inhibitory neurotransmitters, which decrease the likelihood of firing (for more detail on synaptic transmission, see Chapter 12). Although, be careful! The actual function of each neurotransmitter varies widely based on the part of the nervous system or part of the brain where it is active, and how it interacts with other neurotransmitters.

Table 2 Summary of Neurotransmitters

Neurotransmitter	Primary Functions
Dopamine	• Reward, mood, pleasure, smooth motor movements, focus and attention • Shortages can lead to depression, lethargy, and difficulty coordinating motion
Serotonin	• Mood, digestion, sleep, memory, sexual desire • Shortages can lead to aggression, compulsive behavior, overeating, and depression
Melatonin	• Circadian rhythm, sleepiness, sleep initiation (melatonin is technically a "neurotransmitter-like substance") • Shortages can lead to insomnia
Gamma Aminobutyric Acid (GABA)	• Primary inhibitory neurotransmitter in the brain • Shortages can lead to stress and anxiety, depression, ADHD, panic disorders, and a host of other disorders
Acetylcholine	• Excitation at neuromuscular junction, parasympathetic nervous system activity • Shortages can lead to dysfunction of the GI tract and paralysis
Epinephrine (adrenaline) and norepinephrine (noradrenaline)	• Two similar molecules both involved in fight-or-flight response, sympathetic nervous system activation (both are hormones and neurotransmitters) • Shortages can lead to fatigue, lack of focus, apathy
Glutamate	• Primary excitatory neurotransmitter the brain; learning, memory, long-term potentiation • Shortages can lead to fatigue, low concentration and energy

Dopamine and serotonin are two of the most important, and thoroughly studied, neurotransmitters in the brain. A summary of their circuits, and the effects they have on behavior, can be found in Figure 7 on the next page. Serotonin pathways project from the raphe nucleus, whereas there are three dopaminergic pathways: the **mesolimbic circuit** is known as a natural pathway for feelings of reward and pleasure (covered in more detail in addiction below), the **nigrostriatal circuit** is heavily involved in movement and coordination, and the **mesocortical circuit** is involved in higher cortical functions, thought, planning, and emotional regulation.

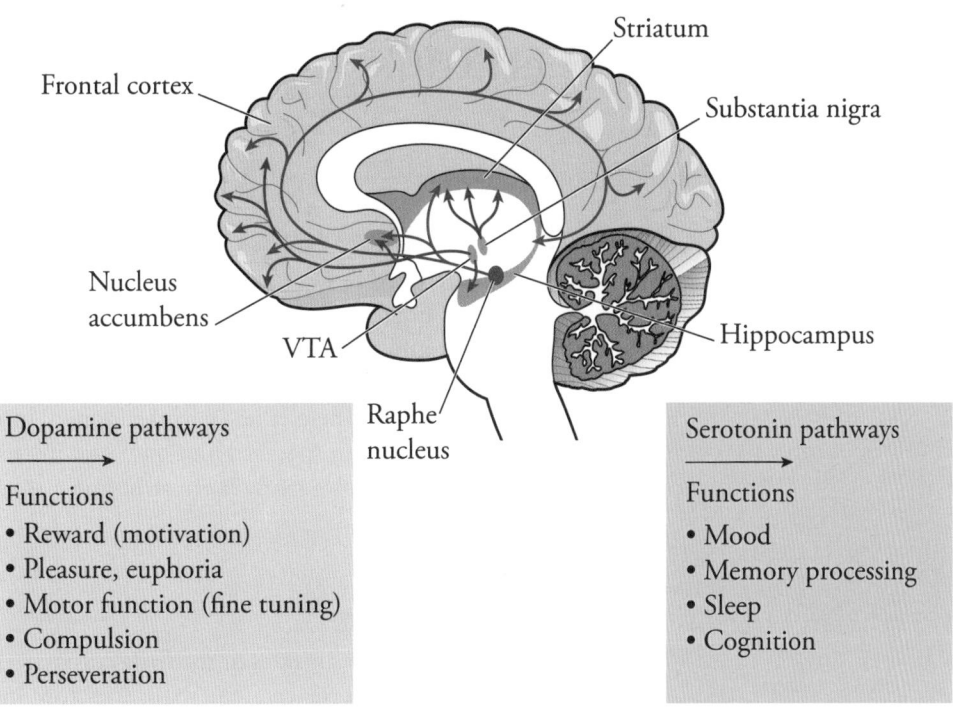

Figure 7   Dopamine and serotonin pathways in the brain

In addition to neurotransmitters, there are various hormones that impact behavior and produce psychological effects. Note that the primary difference between the two is that neurotransmitters are considered the signaling chemicals of the *nervous* system, and hormones are considered the signaling chemicals of the *endocrine* system, although there can be considerable overlap.

Table 3   Summary of Hormones

Hormone	Primary Functions
Cortisol	Stress, sympathetic nervous system response
Oxytocin	Trust, formation of social bonds, sexual reproduction, mother-infant bonding
Endorphins	Pleasure, arousal, pain suppression
Leptin	Regulation of energy, inhibition of hunger

Other differences between neurotransmitters and hormones can be seen in the table below:

Table 4   Neurotransmitters vs. Hormones

	Neurotransmitters	Hormones
Area of Operation	Synaptic cleft between neurons	Bloodstream
Produced by	Neurons	Endocrine glands
Activation Period	Extremely fast (a few milliseconds)	Can be longer (a few seconds to a few days)
Target Cells	Neighboring neurons or cells	Can be more distant cells throughout the body

10.3   NEUROSCIENCE OF EMOTION, MEMORY, STRESS, AND LANGUAGE

The Role of Biological Processes in Perceiving Emotion

Someone who openly expresses emotions is sometimes referred to as "wearing his heart on his sleeve." But while romantics tend to believe that emotion is purely a matter of the heart, it turns out that the brain is very much involved in emotional states. The generation and experience of emotions involve many brain regions. Mapping emotions to brain regions is difficult because thinking of different emotions as based in different parts of the brain has proven to be too simplistic. There is no "surprise center" in the brain. Rather, widespread areas of the brain appear to be associated with specific emotions. And instead of emotional "centers," there appear to be emotional "circuits" that involve many brain structures.

The Role of the Limbic System in Emotion

The limbic system is a collection of brain structures that lies on both sides of the thalamus; together, these structures appear to be primarily responsible for emotional experiences. The main structure involved in emotion in the limbic system is the **amygdala**, an almond-shaped structure deep within the brain. The amygdala serves as the conductor of the orchestra of our emotional experiences. It can communicate with the **hypothalamus**, a brain structure that controls the physiological aspects of emotion, such as sweating and a racing heart. It also communicates with the **prefrontal cortex**, located at the front of the brain, which controls approach and avoidance behaviors—the behavioral aspects of emotion (the prefrontal cortex is not, however, part of the limbic system). The amygdala plays a key role in the identification and expression of fear and aggression.

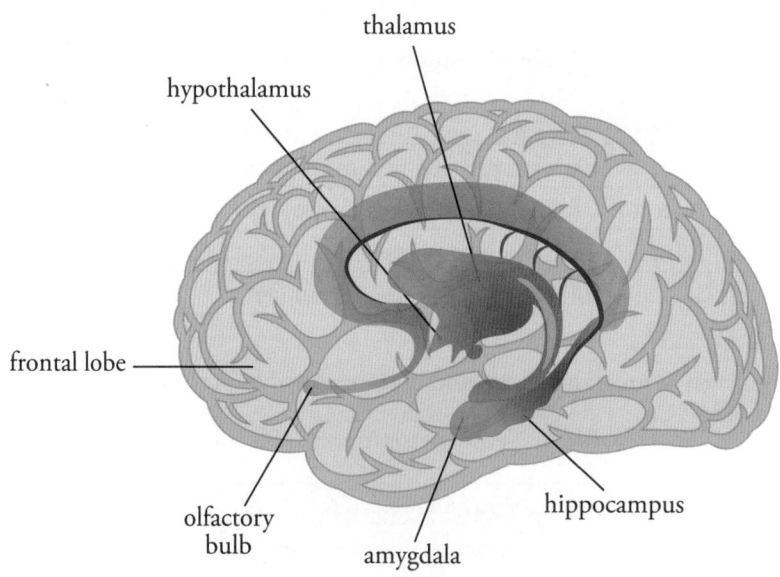

Figure 8   The limbic system

Emotion and the Autonomic Nervous System (ANS)

The **autonomic nervous system** is responsible for controlling the activities of most of the organs and glands, and controls arousal. It answers primarily to the hypothalamus. The sympathetic nervous system (SNS) provides the body with brief, intense, vigorous responses. It is often referred to as the "fight or flight" system because it prepares an individual for action. It increases heart rate, blood pressure, and blood sugar levels in preparation for action. It also directs the adrenal glands to release the stress hormones epinephrine and norepinephrine. The parasympathetic nervous system (PNS) provides signals to the internal organs during a calm resting state when no crisis is present. When activated, it leads to changes that allow for recovery and the conservation of energy, including an increase in digestion and the repair of body tissues.

Physiological Markers of Emotion (Signatures of Emotion)

Many physiological states associated with emotion have been discussed. These include heart rate, blood pressure, respiratory rate, sweating, and the release of stress hormones. An increase in these physiological functions is associated with the sympathetic (fight-or-flight) response. In order to measure autonomic function, clinicians can measure heart rate, finger temperature, skin conductance (sweating), and muscle activity. Keep in mind that different patterns tend to exist during different emotional states, but states such as fear and sexual arousal may display very similar patterns.

Emotions, Temperament, and Decision-Making

As mentioned earlier, the prefrontal cortex is critical for emotional experience, and is also important in temperament and decision-making. Increased activity in the prefrontal cortex is associated with a reduction in emotional feelings, especially fear and anxiety. It is the soft voice that calms down the amygdala when it is overly aroused. Methods of emotion regulation and stress relief often activate the prefrontal cortex. The prefrontal cortex also plays a role in **executive functions**—higher order thinking processes such as planning, organizing, inhibiting behavior, and decision-making. Damage to this area may lead to inappropriateness, impulsivity, and trouble with initiation. This area is not fully developed in humans until they reach their mid-twenties, explaining the sometimes erratic and emotionally-charged behavior of teenagers.

Another behavior that is connected to self-control and impulse regulation is addiction. **Addiction** has a strong biological basis. Many addictive drugs, as well as other pleasurable behaviors and primary reinforcers such as food or sex, share the characteristic of stimulating the release of dopamine in the nucleus accumbens. As such, the **nucleus accumbens** is often described as the primary center for reward in the brain, and dopamine is often thought of as the primary neurotransmitter in reward, although many other brain areas and chemicals also play a lesser role.

Other important cortical structures that have also been implicated in the experience of reward include the amygdala, a part of the limbic system that is involved in many different types of emotion, the insula, or insular cortex, which is closely connected to the striatum, and the lateral hypothalamus, which releases hormones such as endorphins that induce the physiological changes we often associate with pleasure and reward.

Emotion and Memory

Emotional experiences can be stored as memories that can be recalled by similar circumstances. The limbic system also includes the **hippocampus**, a brain structure that plays a key role in forming memories. When memories are formed, often the emotions that are associated with these memories are also encoded. Emotion can therefore aid and enhance memory and thus provides adaptive benefits. Take a second to close your eyes and imagine someone whom you love very much. Notice the emotional state that arises with your memory of that person. Recalling an event can bring about the emotions associated with it. Note that this isn't always a pleasant experience. It has an important role in the suffering of patients who have experienced traumatic events. Similar circumstances to a traumatic event can lead to recall of the memory of the experience, referred to as "flashback." Sometimes this recall isn't even conscious; for example, for someone who was involved in a traumatic car accident, driving past the intersection where the incident occurred might cause increased muscle tension, heart rate, and respiratory rate.

However, memory also involves changes directly to the neural structures in the brain. Let's transition from our discussion of emotion to look more closely at memory and how it is stored within the brain by neurons and neural networks.

The Neuroscience of Memory

When something is learned, the synapses between neurons are strengthened and the process of **long-term potentiation** begins. Following brief periods of stimulation, neurons reorient themselves to increase the likelihood of firing within the connection, leading to an increase in the synaptic strength between two neurons and stronger electrochemical responses to a given stimulus. When long-term potentiation occurs, the neurons involved in the circuit develop an increased sensitivity, which results in increased potential for neural firing after a connection has been stimulated. This increased potential can last for hours or even weeks. Synaptic strength is thought to be the process by which memories are consolidated for long-term memory (so learning can occur). At a given synapse, long-term potentiation involves both presynaptic and postsynaptic neurons. For example, dopamine is one of the neurotransmitters involved in pleasurable or rewarding actions. In operant conditioning, reinforcement activates the limbic circuits that involve memory, learning, and emotions. Since reinforcement of a desired behavior is pleasurable, the circuits are strengthened as dopamine floods the system, making it more likely the behavior will be repeated.

After long-term potentiation has occurred, passing an electrical current through the brain doesn't disrupt the memory associations between the neurons involved, although other memories will be wiped out. For example, when a person receives a blow to the head resulting in a concussion, he or she loses memory for events shortly preceding the concussion. This is due to the fact that long-term potentiation has not had a chance to occur (and leave traces of memory connections), while old memories, which were already potentiated, remain.

Long-term memory storage involves more permanent changes to the brain, including structural and functional connections between neurons. For example, long-term memory storage includes new synaptic connections between neurons, permanent changes in pre- and postsynaptic membranes, and a permanent increase or decrease in neurotransmitter synthesis. Furthermore, visual imaging studies suggest that there is greater branching of dendrites in regions of the brain thought to be involved with memory storage. Other studies suggest that protein synthesis somehow influences memory formation; drugs that prevent protein synthesis appear to block long-term memory formation.

If our long-term memories contained isolated pockets of information without any organization, they might be more difficult to access. A person might have numerous memories for directions, people's faces, the definitions of tens of thousands of words, and other such content; with that much information, it could be nearly impossible to find anything. Just as hierarchies are a useful tool for processing information during the encoding process, it is believed that information is stored in long-term memory as an organized network. In this network exists individual ideas called **nodes**, which can be thought of like cities on a map. Connecting these nodes are **associations**, which are like roads connecting the cities. Not all roads are created equal; some are superhighways and some are dirt roads. For example, for a person living in a city, there may be a stronger association between the nodes "bird" and "pigeon" than between "bird" and "penguin." According to this model, the strength of an association in the network is related to how frequently and how deeply the connection is made. Processing material in different ways leads to the establishment of multiple connections. In this model, searching through memory is the process of starting at one node and traveling the connected roads until one arrives at the idea one is looking for. Retrieval of information improves if there are more and stronger connections to an idea. Because all memories are, in essence, neural connections, the road analogy provides a useful visual aid in understanding access to memories; strong neural connections are like better roads.

Like any neural connection, a node does not become activated until it receives input signals from its neighbors that are strong enough to reach a **response threshold**. The effect of input signals is cumulative: the response threshold is reached by the **summation** of input signals from multiple nodes. Stronger memories involve more neural connections in the form of more numerous dendrites, the stimulation of which can summate more quickly and powerfully to threshold. Once the response threshold is reached, the node "fires" and sends a stimulus to all of its neighbors, contributing to their activation. In this way, the activation of a few nodes can lead to a pattern of activation within the network that spreads onward. This process is known as **spreading activation**. It suggests that when trying to retrieve information, we start the search from one node. Then, we do not "choose" where to go next, but rather that activated node spreads its activation to other nodes around it to an extent related to the strength of association between that node and the others. This pattern continues, with well-established links carrying activation more efficiently than more obscure ones. The network approach helps explain why hints may be helpful. They serve to activate nodes that are closely connected to the node being sought after, which may therefore contribute to that node's activation. It also explains the relevance of contextual cues. If you are reading this book while jumping up and down on a trampoline, you are more likely to later recall this information if you are once again on the trampoline. This is because you would have developed some associations between the learned information and the cues in the environment when learning the information.

Not all behaviors are learned, of course. The neural processes described above occur when animals or people learn new behaviors, or change their behaviors based on experience (that is, environmental feedback). As our learned behaviors change, our synapses change too. On the other hand, some behaviors are **innate**. These are the things we know how to do instinctively (or our body just does without us consciously thinking about it), not because someone taught us to do them (for example, breathing or pulling away from a hot stove). Further, innate behaviors are always the same between members of the species, even for the ones performing them for the first time.

Neuroscientists have had a difficult time in their search for a physical basis for memory. There has been no central location found for memories, and there seem to be no such thing as special memory neurons. The process of forming memories involves electrical impulses sent through brain circuits. Somehow, these impulses leave permanent neural traces that are physical representations of information. More and more evidence indicates that what is important for memory and for learning is the synapses—those sites where nerve cells communicate with each other through neurotransmitters.

Neural Plasticity

It was once believed that after the brain develops in childhood, it remains fixed. However, scientists are finding that the brain is not a static organ. **Neural plasticity** refers to the malleability of the brain's pathways and synapses based on behavior, the environment, and neural processes. In fact, the brain undergoes changes throughout life. As you will see, changes in memory and learning are reflected physiologically by changes in the associations between neurons. Connections in the brain are constantly being removed and recreated. In fact, if someone sustains a brain injury, neurons will reorganize in an attempt to compensate for or work around the impaired connections. As an example, shortly after someone becomes blind, neurons that were devoted to vision take on different roles, potentially improving other sensory perception. Furthermore, while it was previously thought that neurons of the central nervous system were irreplaceable, **neurogenesis**, the birth of new neurons, has been found to occur to a small extent in the hippocampus and cerebellum. NMDA receptors (targets of the neurotransmitter glutamate) within the hippocampus are thought to play an important role in long-term potentiation and neural plasticity by inducing new connections, cell growth, and consolidation of new memories.

Memory and Learning

"What fires together, wires together." In other words, nearby neurons that fire impulses simultaneously form associations with one another. These associations can create neural nets, or patterns of activation, that represent information that is learned or stored in memory. Therefore, if any part of the neural net is activated, a memory may be recalled. This provides a neurological basis for the usefulness of retrieval cues discussed earlier. The process of learning and memory throughout the lifetime does not involve the enlarging of the brain or the gaining of neurons, but rather involves increased interconnectivity of the brain by increasing the synapses between existing neurons. As neurons fire together, more associations are formed. The strength of these associations is further based on the frequency with which simultaneous firing occurs, and other aspects such as the presence of emotion (which strengthens associations).

Neuroscience of Stress

In addition to the sympathetic fight-or-flight response, the hypothalamus, located just above the brain stem, releases corticotropin-releasing hormone (CRH), a messenger that stimulates the pituitary gland to release adrenocorticotropic hormone (ACTH). ACTH then signals the adrenal glands to release cortisol into the bloodstream. **Cortisol** is a glucocorticoid, a hormone that shifts the body from using sugar (glucose) as an energy source toward using fat as an energy source. This "glucose-sparing" effect keeps blood sugar levels high during stress situations (important because the only energy source the brain can use is glucose), thus ensuring that the brain will have enough fuel to stay active. This chain of events is a slower process than the near-instantaneous fight or flight response, and it is primarily triggered during long-term stress.

While short-term cortisol release can be helpful, prolonged release due to chronic stressors is harmful. Most notably, prolonged cortisol release inhibits the activity of white blood cells and other functions of the immune system. Thus, stress itself does not make us sick but rather increases the vulnerability for illness. It has been shown that stress can exacerbate the course of diseases including AIDS, cancer, and heart disease.

10.4 NEUROBIOLOGY OF NERVOUS SYSTEM DISORDERS

Schizophrenia

Recall that schizophrenia is a disorder characterized by positive symptoms, such as delusions and hallucinations, as well as negative ones, such as flat affect, disorganized speech, and avolition. Although schizophrenia presents as a thought disorder, it is important to remember that psychological characteristics have a physical or neurological basis; the division between these two is largely a conceptual one (based on an outdated **mind-body dualism** framework).

Additionally, *hypo*activation of the frontal lobes may be responsible for the negative signs of schizophrenia, creating a kind of pseudo-depression, flat affect, and impaired speech. Decreased working memory is also thought to be associated with decreased volume of the hippocampus. Individuals with schizophrenia have also been found to have smaller brains due to atrophy: schizophrenic individuals display increased ventricles (cavities in the brain), and enlarged sulci and fissures (less folding).

Further, the biochemical factor most associated with schizophrenia is excess levels of dopamine in the brain. The first drugs used for psychopathology, antipsychotics, were used to treat the positive symptoms of schizophrenia, such as hallucinations and delusions, by blocking the dopamine receptors, thus inhibiting the production of dopamine in the brain.

In addition to abnormal brain chemistry, abnormalities in brain structure may also play a role in schizophrenia. Enlarged brain ventricles are seen in some schizophrenics, indicating a deficit in the volume of brain tissue. There is also evidence of abnormally low activity in the frontal lobe, the area of the brain responsible for planning, reasoning, and decision-making. Some studies also suggest that abnormalities in the temporal lobes, hippocampus, and amygdala are connected to schizophrenia's positive symptoms. But despite the evidence of brain abnormalities, it is highly unlikely that schizophrenia is the result of any one problem in any one region of the brain.

Depression

Depression also appears to have a strong genetic basis—there is increased risk of developing depression when a first-degree family member has it. Depression has been linked to diminished functioning in pathways in the brain that involve the neurotransmitters dopamine, serotonin, and norepinephrine. Antidepressants thus target and try to stimulate these pathways. Depression can often accompany other neurological diseases, such as Parkinson's and traumatic brain injury, due to damage to similar or overlapping areas of the brain.

Stem Cell-based Therapy to Regenerate Neurons in the CNS

Cell death is a characteristic of most CNS disorders and neurodegenerative diseases. It has been theorized that neural stem cells, which have the capacity to differentiate into any of the cell types in the nervous system, hold the key to curing damage to the central nervous system caused by trauma or illness. Experiments have demonstrated that neural stem cells can migrate and replace dying neurons in the CNS. These studies hold promise for an eventual cure for diseases such as Parkinson's disease, Alzheimer's disease, multiple sclerosis, and Huntington's disease.

Chapter 10 Summary

- Neuroscientists use many different methods to understand how the brain is related to behavior and which brain regions are responsible for which functions.

- Structural imaging techniques give cross-sectional images of anatomical regions, whereas functional imaging provides insight into which brain regions are active during certain behaviors.

- Drug use causes increased dopamine activity in the nucleus accumbens, which can lead to drug addiction.

- The nervous system is divided into two parts: the central nervous system and the peripheral nervous system.

- The central nervous system is composed of the brain and spinal cord.

- Different brain regions, such as the thalamus, hippocampus, and amygdala, are responsible for specific functions.

- The central nervous system contains neurotransmitter systems that are important for modulating behavior.

- Important neurotransmitters are dopamine, serotonin, acetylcholine and others.

- The limbic system, made up of the amygdala, hippocampus, hypothalamus, thalamus, olfactory bulb, and frontal lobe, is known to play a critical role in emotion.

- The prefrontal cortex plays a critical role in executive functions such as long-term planning and emotional regulation.

- The hippocampus is critical in forming new memories.

- Physiological changes in neuron structure and neural network activation are associated with the formation of new memories.

- Spreading activation theory suggests that connections are made in memory with similar or related concepts.

- Stress has many important neurochemical implications, such as sympathetic nervous system activation and the release of cortisol, resulting in a fight-or-flight response.

- Nervous system disorders such as Alzheimer's, Parkinson's, depression, and schizophrenia are also correlated with neurophysiological changes.

CHAPTER 10 FREESTANDING PRACTICE QUESTIONS

1. Which imaging technique is best suited for measuring changes in brain activity that require the highest possible spatial resolution?

A) Computerized tomography (CT)
B. Positron emission tomography (PET)
C) Electroencephalography (EEG)
D) Functional magnetic resonance imaging (fMRI)

2. In an experiment, primates are injected with a newly synthesized chemical compound. Which of the following observed effects would provide the best evidence that this drug is a stimulant that is pharmacologically active in these primates?

A) Increased alpha waves in the primates' brain
B) Significant constriction of the primates' pupils
C) Increased glucose metabolism in the primates' brains
D) Increased absorption of norepinephrine agents inside neurons in the primates' brains

3. Which of the following structures of the human brain is LEAST likely to show increased activity when an extremely thirsty experimental participant drinks a glass of water?

A) Reticular activating system
B) Amygdala
C) Hypothalamus
D) Nucleus accumbens

4. A lesion in which of these areas is most likely to adversely affect an individual's vision?

A) Occipital lobe
B) Frontal lobe
C) Hypothalamus
D) Pons

5. Of the following, which neurotransmitter and hormone pair is most reliably associated with aggression?

A) Serotonin and testosterone
B) Glutamate and dopamine
C) Melatonin and norepinephrine
D) GABA and endorphins

6. Group A consists of socially anxious individuals sitting down to meet their peers on the first day of a new job. Group B consists of non-anxious individuals listening to white noise. In which of the following areas of the brain would we expect to see the largest difference in activity between these two groups?

A) Cerebellum
B) Thalamus
C) Amygdala
D) Basal ganglia

7. Each of the following has been demonstrated in the brains of schizophrenics EXCEPT:

A) enlarged ventricles.
B) smaller hippocampus.
C) abnormal levels of acetylcholine.
D) abnormal levels of dopamine.

8. Which part of the brain initiates signals to the endocrine system?

A) Hippocampus
B) Thalamus
C) Prefrontal cortex
D) Hypothalamus

CHAPTER 10 PRACTICE PASSAGE

Recent research has explored the neurophysiological correlates of various therapies to assess their efficacy. Reduced cortical mass in areas associated with negative emotions are interpreted as indications of effective therapeutic intervention. Also, researchers looked at the mass of various regions associated with emotional regulation, such that increased mass in these regions also suggested that the therapies had helped patients improve their ability to modulate emotional experience.

Study 1: Cognitive Behavioral Therapy

A team of researchers conducted an fMRI study that looked at activation levels in a cohort of 20 patients who were given a 10-week treatment protocol, meeting with a psychologist for 45 minutes in each session. During sessions, participants explored maladaptive thought patterns, and created a plan for more effective coping mechanisms that was encouraged by positive secondary reinforcement by the therapist at the next session. To track thoughts while subjects were alone during the week, participants were told to keep a journal. Pretest and posttest measures of cortical activity were measured and compared.

Study 2: Psychoanalytic Psychotherapy

Increase in cortical mass in areas associated with self-awareness and the top-down regulation of emotion was measured through the use of positron emission tomography (PET). At the end of the 3-month program, researchers saw changes in the mass of regions of the prefrontal cortex, amygdala, and hippocampal projections to the sensory cortices. Researchers conducted the study on 10 male and female participants who had grown up in single-parent homes, based on the premise that the absence of a parent made them good candidates for psychoanalytic therapy. Researchers hypothesized that awareness and analysis of repressed thoughts, and not emotional regulation, would mediate effectiveness of therapy and improved clinical outcomes.

Study 3: Behavioral Therapy

A reinforcement schedule was paired with aversion therapy, which was used to rewire the reward circuit in individuals with various types of addiction. 18 male and female undergraduate students who had been diagnosed with alcohol and drug addiction were given treatment. The treatment involved exposure to alcohol or the drug and nasal inhalation of an aversive agent meant to induce mild nausea. Application of the aversive treatment was potentially dangerous, so it was done in a supervised clinical environment twice a week according to a schedule. Researchers also checked in once a week at random times to see if patients had successfully avoided drug or alcohol use, and gave points that could be used towards various prizes if they had. Afterwards, dopaminergic circuits and density of regions associated with impulse control were assessed.

1. Based on the information in the passage, and assuming validity of the research hypotheses, reductions in mass to which of the following regions would be evidence of the efficacy of a therapeutic intervention?

   A) Superior posterior frontal lobe
   B) Lateral hypothalamus
   C) Superior anterior parietal lobe
   D) Prefrontal cortex

2. Which of the following would be the most adequate substitute as a neuroimaging technique in the study on cognitive behavioral therapy?

   A) Magnetic resonance imaging (MRI)
   B) Positron emission tomography (PET)
   C) Electroencephalography (EEG)
   D) Magnetoencephalography (MEG)

3. Which of the following correctly describes the reinforcement schedule used in Study 3?

   A) Fixed interval
   B) Variable ratio
   C) Fixed ratio
   D) Variable interval

4. Data analysis revealed that of the three therapies, the psychoanalytic method was the least associated with growth of the prefrontal cortex. Which of the following is a potential problem with the conclusion that psychoanalysis was the least effective of the three therapies?

   A) The length of time of treatment
   B) Growth in the prefrontal cortex is evidence of reduced efficacy
   C) The neurophysiological exams used
   D) Study 2 did not include information on the reward circuit

5. If the hypothesis in Study 2 turned out to be correct, which of the following would most likely be the reason that the psychoanalytic psychotherapy had been effective?

A) Increased neural integration in the amygdala
B) Increased integration between the prefrontal cortex and limbic circuits
C) Increased rates of firing between hippocampal and primary sensory cortices
D) Increased volume of the prefrontal cortex

6. Suppose the subjects in Study 3 were presented with the addictive substances for which they received treatment. If the treatment was effective, one would expect measurements to show LESS cortical mass in each of the following, EXCEPT:

A) dopaminergic neurons in the basal ganglia.
B) dopaminergic neurons in the nucleus accumbens.
C) dopaminergic neurons in the ventral tegmental area.
D) serotonergic neurons in the amygdala.

SOLUTIONS TO CHAPTER 10 FREESTANDING PRACTICE QUESTIONS

1. **D** Imaging techniques that measure changes in brain activity require functional techniques, and CT scan is a structural technique (choice A is wrong). Although EEG has higher temporal resolution than the other imaging techniques, EEG has a very low spatial resolution compared to other functional techniques (choice C is wrong). Between fMRI and PET, fMRI is known to have the highest spatial resolution (choice D is correct). Although PET offers the advantage of measuring neuronal activity directly, the question stem is only concerned with spatial resolution (choice B is wrong).

2. **C** Pharmacological activity is best measured by the effect on neurotransmitters, which bind to receptors on the outside. Stimulants are known to increase blood metabolism; therefore, increased glucose metabolism would likely be measured (choice C is correct). Alpha waves are associated with a more relaxed state, which is unlikely to be induced by a stimulant (choice A is wrong). Also, stimulants are associated with pupil dilation, a sympathetic nervous system response, not pupil constriction, which is a parasympathetic response associated with depressants (choice B is wrong). Since pharmacological agents bind to receptors on the outside, internalization of the neurotransmitter is highly unlikely to occur. Rather, ions will be absorbed into the postsynaptic cell, not the neurotransmitter itself (choice D is wrong).

3. **A** Water is a primary reinforcer, and will therefore lead to activation of the reward circuit, especially in a participant who is extremely thirsty. Using the except/not/least technique, go through each answer choice one at a time. The reticular activating system is responsible for conscious awareness, not reward. Therefore, this structure is least likely to show increased activity and is the correct answer (choice A is correct). The amygdala, hypothalamus, and nucleus accumbens are all part of the brain's reward circuit (choices B, C, and D are wrong).

4. **A** The occipital lobe contains the primary visual cortex, and is the primary region for higher-order visual processing in the brain (choice A is correct). The frontal lobe is implicated in higher-level cortical functioning such as planning, attention, and emotional regulation. A lesion here would not be likely to affect vision (choice B is wrong). The hypothalamus' primary function is control of the endocrine system and hormone release, not visual processing or relay (choice C is wrong). The pons is associated with neurotransmitter synthesis and connectivity between the midbrain and hindbrain (choice D is wrong).

5. **A** Serotonin is a mood stabilizer, and depleted levels are known to be involved in aggressive behaviors. Testosterone is a hormone associated with aggressive behavior and fight-or-flight response (choice A is correct). Glutamate is an abundant neurotransmitter implicated in many behaviors, and some research shows associations with aggressive behavior, however, a relationship between dopamine and aggression has not been firmly established. In addition, glutamate and dopamine are neurotransmitters, so the answer choice does not include a hormone as indicated by the question stem (choice B is wrong). Norepinephrine is also known to be associated with sympathetic nervous system responses, such as fight or flight, however, melatonin release is associated with sleepiness and drowsiness, and decreases in melatonin would primarily result in sleeplessness and insomnia, not necessarily aggression (choice C is wrong). Increases in both GABA (usually inhibitory) and endorphins (pleasure and satisfaction) would have anti-aggressive effects, and low levels of neither is thought to be associated with aggression but primarily anxiety (GABA) and depression (endorphins) (choice D is wrong).

6. **C** The amygdala is associated primarily with negative emotions such as anxiety, so there would be a large difference in amygdala activity between anxious and relaxed groups of participants (choice C is correct). The cerebellum is primarily associated with movement (choice A is wrong), the thalamus is the brain's sensory relay station (choice B is wrong), and the basal ganglia are also associated with movement (choice D is wrong).

7. **C** Notice that this is an except/not/least question. Schizophrenia has not been associated with abnormal levels of acetylcholine (choice C is correct). It has, however, been associated with enlarged ventricles, a smaller hippocampus, and abnormal levels of dopamine (choices A, B, and D are wrong).

8. **D** The hypothalamus is the brain region most associated with control of the endocrine system (choice D is correct). The hippocampus is primarily associated with memory (choice A is wrong). The thalamus is primarily associated with sensory relay (choice B is wrong). The prefrontal cortex is primarily associated with executive control and emotional regulation (choice C is wrong).

SOLUTIONS TO CHAPTER 10 PRACTICE PASSAGE

1. **B** The passage states that reduction in mass in areas associated with negative emotionality would suggest that the therapy was effective. The lateral hypothalamus is part of the stress-release mechanism, leading to release of cortisol and other stress hormones, and is therefore known to be involved in negative primitive emotions such as anger and rage. Reduced mass in this area would make stressful or angry responses less likely (choice B is correct). The superior posterior frontal lobe is the location of the motor cortex and motor homunculus, responsible for motor control in the contralateral hemisphere (choice A is wrong). The superior anterior parietal lobe is the location of the sensory cortex and sensory homunculus, responsible for feeling and tactile awareness in the contralateral hemisphere (choice C is wrong). Increased activity in the prefrontal cortex is associated with improved emotional control and positive emotionality. Therefore, reduction in mass in this area would suggest that a given therapeutic intervention was not effective (choice D is wrong).

2. **B** The study on cognitive behavioral therapy used fMRI, and the description suggests that a functional technique with high resolution is needed to evaluate the hypotheses of the study. Of the answer choices, only PET is a functional imaging technique with high resolution (choice B is correct). MRI is a structural, not a functional technique, so it does not make a good substitute for fMRI as it would not produce functional data (choice A is wrong). EEG is a functional technique, but with low spatial resolution that would not let researchers draw conclusions about specific brain regions or areas deep in the cortex such as the limbic system (choice C is wrong). MEG is also a functional technique, but shares most of the benefits and limitations of EEG (choice D is wrong).

3. **D** For the reinforcement schedule of Study 3, the passage states that participants were contacted randomly and reinforced with tokens for successfully abstaining from drug or alcohol use. Because intervals of time are used, and not number of occurrences, this is an interval schedule (choices B and C are wrong). Because researchers contacted participants at random, and not fixed intervals, the reinforcement schedule is variable interval (choice D is correct, and choice A is wrong).

4. **A** Psychoanalytic psychotherapy is typically a long therapeutic intervention, requiring many months to many years to start to show results. Patients and therapists become part of a transference relationship in which patients will eventually transfer emotions associated with parents onto the therapist, and the therapist then works to bring these repressed feelings and behaviors further and further into conscious awareness. With such a lengthy process, three months may not have been enough time for patients to start to see results, so this would undermine the conclusion that psychoanalysis was not effective (choice A is correct). Growth in the prefrontal cortex is associated with increased emotional regulation, and therefore increased therapeutic effectiveness (choice B is wrong). The neurophysiological exams used are fMRI and PET, both functional exams with high spatial resolution. Although using the same type of exam would be preferable for points of comparison, both provide similar data about brain activity and would allow for valid comparisons and valid conclusions (choice C is wrong). The passage suggests that areas associated with negative emotionality and emotional regulation would be used to draw conclusions about therapeutic efficacy, and the reward circuit is associated with positive emotionality. Including it in Study 2, therefore, would not have provided much insight into the efficacy of therapy according to the research hypotheses (choice D is wrong).

5. **C** The study hypothesis states that awareness and analysis of repressed memories would be the determining factor of whether the therapy was effective. This suggests that integration of memory regions is the cause of improved outcomes. The hippocampus is involved in memory formation and transference into long-term memory, as well as memory recall processes in which long-term memory and short-term memory interact. Long-term memories are also believed to be stored in the area in which they are formed, so that the visual part of a long-term memory is stored in the occipital lobe, the auditory aspect is stored in the temporal lobe, etc. This indicates that integration between the hippocampus and these regions would lead to increased awareness of repressed memories, which the study hypothesizes improves therapeutic outcomes (choice C is correct). The amygdala is primarily associated with negative emotions, so increased integration there would suggest therapy was not effective (choice A is wrong). Increased integration between the prefrontal cortex and limbic circuits suggests improved emotional regulation, which the study hypothesizes is not the primary reason for improved outcomes (choice B is wrong). Increased volume of the prefrontal cortex would also suggest improved emotional regulation (choice D is wrong).

6. **A** This question constitutes an except/not/least question, so each answer choice should be evaluated one by one. If patients received treatment for addiction, you would expect less activation in the reward circuit in response to the addictive substance. Dopaminergic neurons in the basal ganglia are known to be primarily associated with movement, not reward. Therefore, it is not expected that there would be less cortical mass in this area. Therefore, choice A is a false statement and, in this case, the correct answer (choice A is correct). Dopaminergic neurons in the nucleus accumbens and ventral tegmental area are known to be associated with reward (choices B and C are wrong). The amygdala is also a part of the reward circuit, so although serotonin is not considered the primary neurotransmitter associated with reward and addiction, a decrease in cortical mass here would suggest that the substance was having less rewarding and addictive effects within the brain.

Chapter 11
Sensation, Perception, and Cognition

Organisms interact with their environments by taking in information (sensation) and deciding what information is important while filtering out the rest (attention), making complex decisions about that information (cognition), sometimes in a split-second, and reacting (behavior). Reacting includes a number of complex events, some conscious and some subconscious, some physical and some emotional. Humans are complex creatures, and emotion and stress play important roles in our interactions with the environment. Also, language is an important means for communicating with the environment for humans, and indeed, language is so important to what it means to be human, that it is difficult to imagine what "thinking" even means without language.

11.1   SENSATION

Types of Sensory Receptors

Sensory receptors are designed to detect one type of stimulus from either the interior of the body or the external environment. Each sensory receptor receives only one kind of information and transmits that information to sensory neurons, which can in turn convey it to the central nervous system. Sensory receptors that detect stimuli from the outside world are **exteroceptors** and receptors that respond to internal stimuli are **interoceptors**. A more important distinction between sensory receptors is based on the type of stimulus they detect. The types of sensory receptors are listed below.

1) **Mechanoreceptors** respond to mechanical disturbances. For example, **Pacinian corpuscles** are pressure sensors located deep in the skin. The Pacinian corpuscle is shaped like an onion. It is composed of concentric layers of specialized membranes. When the corpuscular membranes are distorted by firm pressure on the skin, the nerve ending becomes depolarized and the signal travels up the dendrite (note that these are graded potential changes—not action potentials). Another important mechanoreceptor is the **auditory hair cell**. This is a specialized cell found in the cochlea of the inner ear. It detects vibrations caused by sound waves. **Vestibular hair cells** are located within special organs called semicircular canals, also found in the inner ear. Their role is to detect acceleration and position relative to gravity. **Baroreceptors** are mechanoreceptors that respond to changes in pressure; these are commonly found in the walls of arteries.

2) **Chemoreceptors** respond to particular chemicals. For example, **olfactory receptors** detect airborne chemicals and allow us to smell things. Taste buds are **gustatory receptors**. Autonomic chemoreceptors in the walls of the carotid and aortic arteries respond to changes in arterial pH, PCO_2, and PO_2 levels.

3) **Nociceptors** are pain receptors. They are stimulated by tissue injury. Nociceptors are the simplest type of sensory receptor, generally consisting of a free nerve ending that detects chemical signs of tissue damage. (In that sense the nociceptor is a simple chemoreceptor.) Nociceptors may be somatic or autonomic. Autonomic pain receptors do not provide the conscious mind with clear pain information, but they frequently give a sensation of dull, aching pain. They may also create the illusion of pain on the skin when their nerves cross paths with somatic afferents from the skin. This phenomenon is known as **referred pain**.

4) **Thermoreceptors** are stimulated by changes in temperature. There are autonomic and somatic examples. Peripheral thermoreceptors fall into three categories: cold-sensitive, warm-sensitive, and thermal nociceptors, which detect painfully hot stimuli.

5) **Electromagnetic receptors** are stimulated by electromagnetic waves. In humans, the only examples are the rod and cone cells of the retina of the eye (also termed **photoreceptors**). In other animals, electroreceptors and magnetoreceptors are separate. For example, some fish can detect electric fields with electroreceptors, and magnetoreceptors allow animals to sense Earth's magnetic field, which can help them navigate during migration.

Encoding of Sensory Stimuli

All sensory receptors need to encode relevant information regarding the nature of the stimulus being detected. There are four properties that need to be communicated to the CNS:

1) Stimulus **modality** is the type of stimulus. As mentioned above, the CNS determines the stimulus modality based on which type of receptor is firing.

2) Stimulus **location** is communicated by the receptive field of the sensory receptor sending the signal. Localization of a stimulus can be improved by overlapping receptive fields of neighboring receptors. This works like a Venn diagram, and allows the brain to localize a stimulus activating neighboring receptors to the area in which their receptive fields overlap. Discrimination between two separate stimuli can be improved by lateral inhibition of neighboring receptors.

3) Stimulus **intensity** is coded by the frequency of action potentials. The dynamic range, or range of intensities that can be detected by sensory receptors, can be expanded by range fractionation—including multiple groups of receptors with limited ranges to detect a wider range overall. One example of this phenomenon is human cone cells responding to different but overlapping ranges of wavelengths to detect the full visual spectrum of light.

4) Stimulus **duration** may or may not be coded explicitly. *Tonic receptors* fire action potentials as long as the stimulus continues. However, these receptors are subject to adaptation, and the frequency of action potentials decreases as the stimulus continues at the same level (see below). *Phasic receptors* only fire action potentials when the stimulus begins and do not explicitly communicate the duration of the stimulus. These receptors are important for communicating changes in stimuli and essentially adapt immediately if a stimulus continues at the same level.

The ability to adapt to a stimulus is an important property of sensory receptors. This allows the brain to tune out unimportant information from the environment. **Adaptation** is a decrease in firing frequency when the intensity of a stimulus remains constant. For example, if you walk into a kitchen where someone is baking bread, the bread odor molecules stimulate your olfactory receptors to a great degree and you smell the bread baking. But if you remain in the kitchen for a few minutes, you stop smelling the bread; the continuous input to the olfactory receptors causes them to stop firing even though the odor molecules are still present. This is what allows us to "get used to" certain environments and situations, for example, cold pool water, loud background noise, etc. The receptors don't stop being able to respond; they can be retriggered if the stimulus intensity increases. For example, if you open up the oven door, you will smell the bread again. Likewise, if you are used to the background noise in a restaurant, but someone drops a plate, you'll hear it. In other words: the nervous system is programmed to respond to changing stimuli and not so much to constant stimuli, because for the most part, constant stimuli are not a threat, whereas changing stimuli might need to be addressed. (Note that nociceptors do not adapt under any circumstance. We can learn to ignore them, but pain is something that the nervous system wants us to do something about since it is an indication that something is wrong.)

Proprioceptors

This is a broad category including many different types of receptors. **Proprioception**[1] refers to awareness of self (that is, awareness of body position) and is closely related to your **kinesthetic sense** (your awareness of your body movement or "muscle memory," which is critical to learning and performing complex physical routines). An important example of a proprioceptor is the **muscle spindle**, a mechanoreceptor. This is a sensory organ specialized to detect muscle stretch. You are already familiar with it because it is the receptor that senses muscle stretch in the muscle stretch reflex. Other proprioceptors include **Golgi tendon organs**, which monitor tension in the tendons, and **joint capsule receptors**, which detect pressure, tension, and movement in the joints. By monitoring the activity of the musculoskeletal system, the proprioceptive component of the somatic sensory system allows us to know the positions of our body parts. This is most important during activity, when precise feedback is essential for coordinated motion. [What portion of the CNS would you expect to require input from proprioceptors?[2]]

Gustation and Olfaction

Taste and smell are senses that rely on chemoreceptors in the mouth and nasal passages. **Gustation** is taste, and **olfaction** is smell. Much of what is assumed to be taste is actually smell. (Try eating with a bad head cold.) In fact, taste receptors (known as **taste buds**) can only distinguish five flavors: sweet (glucose), salty (Na^+), bitter (basic), sour (acidic), and umami (amino acids and nucleotides). Each taste bud responds most strongly to one of these five stimuli. The taste bud is composed of a bunch of specialized epithelial cells, shaped roughly like an onion. In its center is a **taste pore**, with **taste hairs** that detect food chemicals. Information about taste is transmitted by cranial nerves to an area of the brain in the temporal lobe not far from where the brain receives olfactory information.

Olfaction is accomplished by olfactory receptors in the roof of the **nasopharynx** (nasal cavity). The receptors detect airborne chemicals that dissolve in the mucus covering the nasal membrane. Humans can distinguish thousands of different smells. Olfactory nerves project directly to the **olfactory bulbs** of the brain. The olfactory bulbs are located in the temporal lobe of the brain near the limbic system, an area important for memory and emotion (which may explain why certain smells can bring back vivid memories and feelings).

Interestingly, the perception of a smell as "good" or "bad" is entirely learned, based on experiences with those smells. There is no smell that is universally noxious to people (though the military has tried to find one in order to develop a "stink" bomb), because different smells can be associated with good or bad experiences based on culture and upbringing.

Pheromones are chemical signals that cause a social response in members of the same species. Though not well understood in humans, pheromones have been studied extensively in insects, particularly those species with complex social structures (such as bees and ants). Pheromones are an important means of communicating information; for example, alarm pheromones will alert the rest of the beehive of danger, food-trail pheromones allow ants to follow a trail to a promising food source, and sex pheromones play an important role in mating for most species. In humans, pheromones are much harder to study.

---

[1] *Proprio-* means *of or pertaining to the self,* as in "proprietary."

[2] The cerebellum, which is responsible for motor coordination.

Hearing and the Vestibular System

Structure of the Ear

The **auricle,** or **pinna,** and the external **auditory canal** comprise the **outer ear.** The **middle ear** is divided from the outer ear by the **tympanic membrane** or eardrum. The middle ear consists of the **ossicles,** three small bones called the **malleus** (hammer), the **incus** (anvil), and the **stapes** (stirrup). The stapes attaches to the **oval window,** a membrane that divides the middle and **inner ear.** Structures of the inner ear include the **cochlea,** the **semicircular canals,** the **utricle,** and the **saccule.** The semicircular canals together with the utricle and saccule are important to the sense of balance. The **round window** is a membrane-covered hole in the cochlea near the oval window. It releases excess pressure. The **Eustachian tube** (also known as the **auditory tube**) is a passageway from the back of the throat to the middle ear. It functions to equalize the pressure on both sides of the eardrum and is the cause of the "ear popping" one experiences at high altitudes or under water.

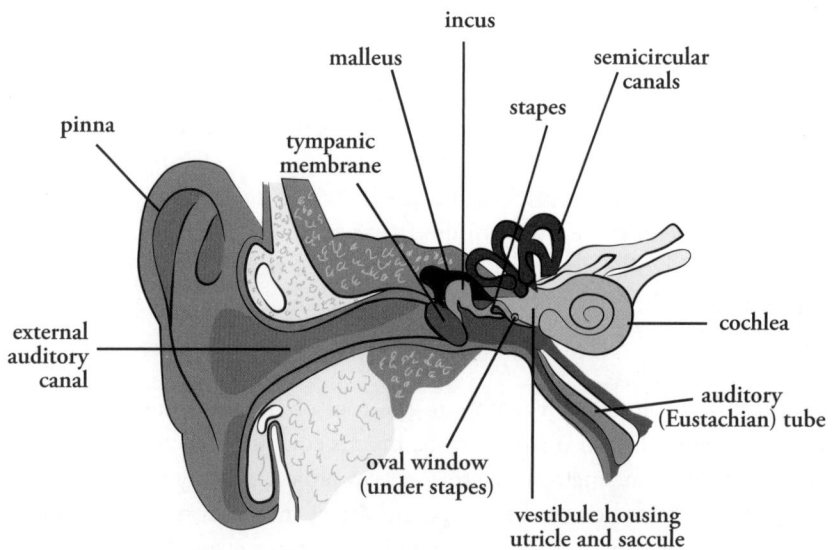

Figure 1   The ear

Mechanism of Hearing

Sound waves enter the external ear to pass into the auditory canal, causing the eardrum to vibrate. The malleus attached to the eardrum receives the vibrations, which are passed on to the incus and then to the stapes. The bones of the middle ear are arranged in such a way that they amplify sound vibrations passing through the middle ear. The stapes is the innermost of the three middle-ear bones, contacting the oval window. Vibration of the oval window creates pressure waves in the **perilymph** and **endolymph,** the fluids in the cochlea. Note that sound vibrations are first conveyed through air, next through bone, and then through liquid before being sensed. The pressure waves in the endolymph cause vibration of the **basilar membrane,** a thin membrane extending throughout the coiled length of the cochlea. The basilar membrane is covered with the auditory receptor cells known as **hair cells.** These cells have **cilia** (hairs) projecting from their apical (top) surfaces (opposite the basilar membrane). The hairs contact the **tectorial membrane** (tectorial means "roof"), and when the basilar membrane moves, the hairs are dragged across the tectorial membrane and they bend. This displacement opens ion channels in the hair cells, which results in neurotransmitter release. Dendrites from bipolar auditory afferent neurons are stimulated by hair cells, and tectorial membrane together are known as the **organ of Corti**. The outer ear and middle ear convey sound waves to the cochlea, and the organ of Corti in the cochlea is the primary site at which auditory stimuli are detected.

Summary: From Sound to Hearing sound waves → auricle → external auditory canal → tympanic membrane → malleus → incus → stapes → oval window → perilymph → endolymph → basilar membrane → auditory hair cells → tectorial membrane → neurotransmitters stimulate bipolar auditory neurons → brain → perception

Pitch (frequency) of sound is distinguished by which *regions* of the basilar membrane vibrate, stimulating different auditory neurons. The basilar membrane is thick and sturdy near the oval window and gradually becomes thin and floppy near the apex of the cochlea. Low frequency (long wavelength) sounds stimulate hair cells at the apex of the cochlear duct, farthest away from the oval window, while high-pitched sounds stimulate hair cells at the base of the cochlea, near the oval window. **Loudness** of sound is distinguished by the *amplitude* of vibration. Larger vibrations cause more frequent action potentials in auditory neurons.

Locating the source of sound is also an important adaptive function. Having two ears allows for stereophonic (or three-dimensional) hearing. The auditory system can determine the source of a sound based on the difference detected between the two ears. For example, if a horn blasts to your right, your right ear will receive the sound waves slightly sooner and slightly more intensely than your left ear. Sound stimuli are processed in the **auditory cortex**, located in the temporal lobe of the brain.

In humans, audition is highly adaptive. While we are able to hear a wide range of sounds, those sounds with frequencies within the range corresponding to the human voice are heard best, and we are able to differentiate variations among human voices. For example, when answering the phone, you will recognize your mom's voice within a fraction of a second.

- If a sensory neuron leading from the ear to the brain fires an action potential more rapidly, how will the brain perceive this change?
- In some cases of deafness, sound can still be detected by conduction of vibration through the skull to the cochlea. If the auditory nerve is severed, can sound still be detected by conductance through bone?
- If the bones of the middle ear are unable to move, would this impair the detection of sound by conductance through bone?

Equilibrium and Balance

The vestibular complex is made up of the **three semicircular canals**: the **utricle**, the **saccule**, and the **ampullae**. All are essentially tubes filled with endolymph; like the cochlea, they contain hair cells that detect motion. However, their function is not to detect sound, but rather rotational acceleration of the head. They are innervated by afferent neurons which send balance information to the pons, cerebellum, and other areas. The vestibular complex monitors both static equilibrium and linear acceleration, which contribute to your sense of balance.

Vision: Structure and Function

The eye is the structure designed to detect visual stimuli. The structures of the eye first form an image on the retina, which detects light and converts the stimuli into action potentials to send to the brain. Light enters the eye by passing through the **cornea**, the clear portion at the front of the eye. Light is bent or **refracted** as it passes through the cornea (which is highly curved and thus acts as a lens), since the refractive index of the cornea is higher than that of air. The cornea is continuous at its borders with the white of the eye, the **sclera**. Beneath the sclera is a layer called the **choroid**. It contains darkly-pigmented cells; this pigmentation absorbs excess light within the eye. Beneath the choroid is the **retina**, the surface upon which light is focused.

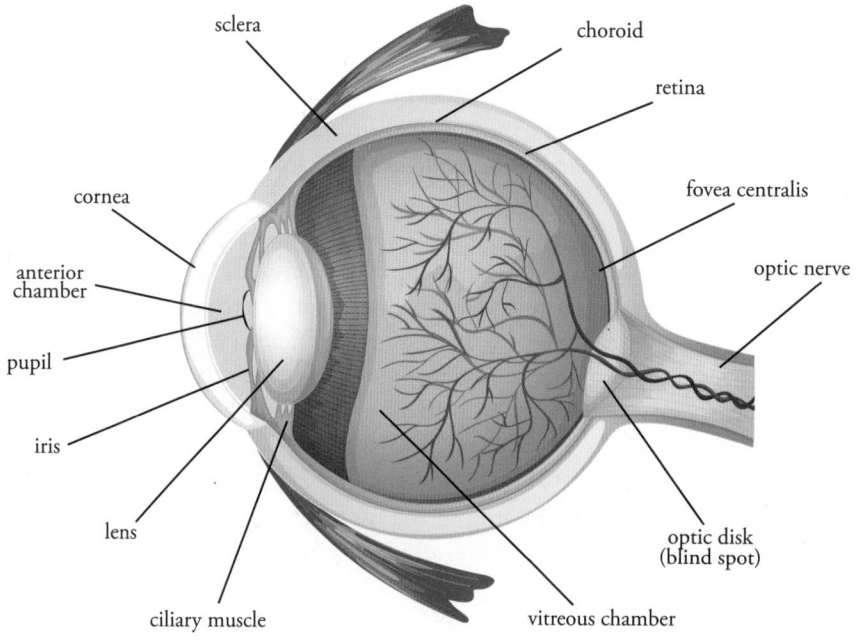

Figure 2   The eye

Just inside the cornea is the **anterior chamber** (front chamber), which contains a fluid termed **aqueous humor**. At the back of the anterior chamber is a membrane called the **iris** with an opening called the **pupil**. The iris is the colored part of the eye, and muscles in the iris regulate the diameter of the pupil. Just behind the iris is the **posterior chamber**, also containing aqueous humor. In the back part of the posterior chamber is the **lens**. Its role is to fine-tune the angle of incoming light, so that the beams are perfectly focused upon the retina. The curvature of the lens (and thus its refractive power) is varied by the **ciliary muscle**.

Light passes through the **vitreous chamber** en route from the lens to the retina. This chamber contains a thick, jelly-like fluid called **vitreous humor**. The retina is located at the back of the eye. It contains electromagnetic receptor cells (photoreceptors) known as **rods** and **cones** and which are responsible for detecting light. The rods and cones synapse with nerve cells called **bipolar cells**. In accordance with the name "bipolar," these cells have only one axon and one dendrite. The bipolar cells in turn synapse with **ganglion cells**, whose axons comprise the **optic nerve**, which travels from each eye toward the occipital lobe of the brain where complex analysis of a visual image occurs. In Figure 3, you may notice that light has to pass through two layers of neurons before it can reach the rods and cones. The neurons are fine enough to not significantly obstruct incoming rays.

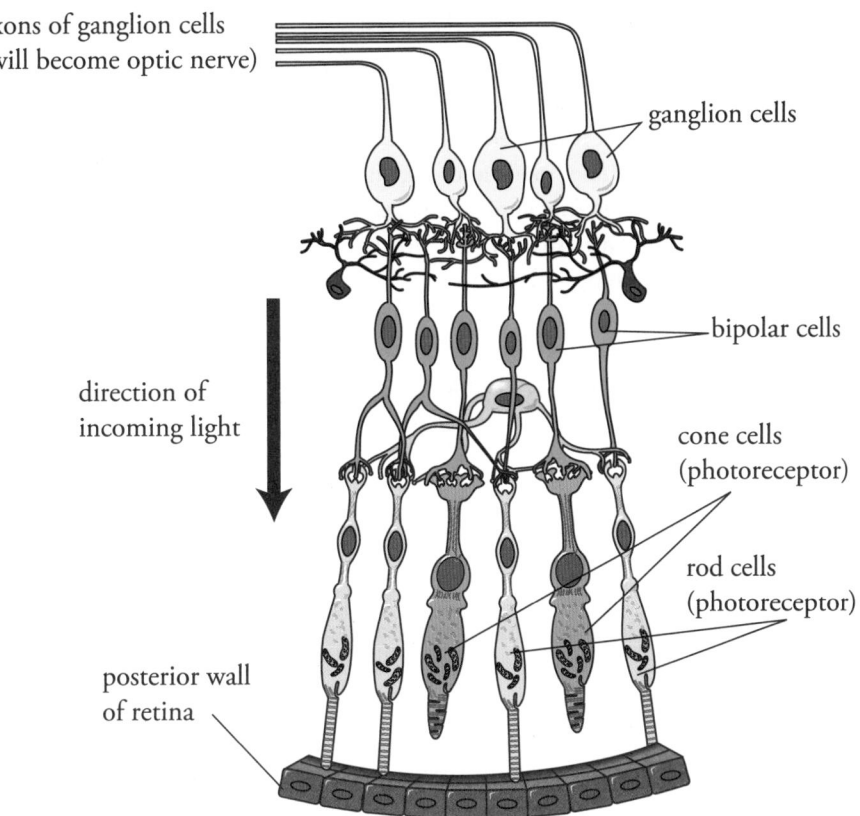

axons of ganglion cells
(will become optic nerve)

ganglion cells

bipolar cells

direction of
incoming light

cone cells
(photoreceptor)

rod cells
(photoreceptor)

posterior wall
of retina

Figure 3   Organization of the retina

The point on the retina where many axons from ganglion cells converge to form the optic nerve is the **optic disk**. It is also known as the **blind spot** (Figure 4) because it contains no photoreceptors. Another special region of the retina is the **macula**. In the center of the macula is the **fovea centralis** (focal point), which contains only cones and is responsible for extreme visual acuity. When you stare directly at something, you focus its image on the fovea.

A   ●   ●   B

Cover your left eye and focus your right eye on dot A while holding the page about 5 inches away from your face. Move the page forward and back. You will find that at a certain distance, dot B becomes invisible. You are placing dot A on the fovea by focusing on it, and at the correct distance, dot B becomes focused on the blind spot.

Figure 4   Demonstrating the blind spot

The Photoreceptors: Rods and Cones

Rods and cones, named because of their shapes, contain special pigment proteins that change their tertiary structure upon absorbing light. Each protein, called an opsin, is bound to one molecule and contains one molecule of **retinal**, which is derived from vitamin A. In the dark, when the rods and cones are resting, retinal has several *trans* double bonds and one cis double bond. In this conformation, retinal and its associated opsin keep a sodium channel open. The cell remains depolarized. Upon absorbing a photon of light, retinal is converted to the **all-trans form**. This triggers a series of reactions that ultimately closes the sodium channel, and the cell hyperpolarizes.

Rods and cones synapse on bipolar cells. Because of their depolarization in the dark, both types of photoreceptors release the neurotransmitter **glutamate** onto the bipolar cells, inhibiting them from firing. Upon the absorption of a photon of light and subsequent hyperpolarization, the photoreceptor stops releasing glutamate. Because glutamate has an inhibitory effect on the bipolar cells, when glutamate is no longer present, the bipolar cell can depolarize (removal of inhibition causes excitation in this system). This then causes depolarization of the ganglion cells and an action potential along the axon of the ganglion cell. All of the axons of the ganglion cells together make up the optic nerve to the brain.

Night vision is accomplished by the rods, which are more sensitive to dim light and motion, and are more concentrated in the periphery of the retina. Cones require abundant light and are responsible for color vision and high-acuity vision, and hence are more concentrated in the fovea. Color vision depends on the presence of three different types of cones. One is specialized to absorb blue light, one absorbs green, and one absorbs red. The brain perceives hues by integrating the relative input of these three basic stimuli.

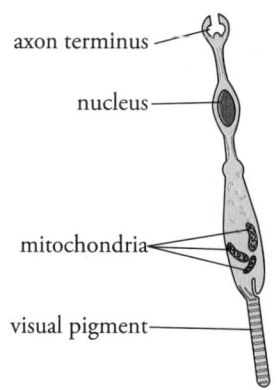

axon terminus

nucleus

mitochondria

visual pigment

Figure 5   Rod cell structure

Defects in Visual Acuity

Normal vision is termed **emmetropia**. Too much or too little curvature of the cornea or lens results in visual defects. Too much curvature causes light to be bent too much and to be focused in front of the retina. The result is **myopia**, or nearsightedness. Myopia can be corrected by a concave (diverging) lens, which will cause the light rays to diverge slightly before they reach the cornea. **Hyperopia**, farsightedness, results from the focusing of light behind the retina. Hyperopia can be corrected by a convex (converging) lens, which causes light rays to converge before reaching the cornea. **Presbyopia** is an inability to **accommodate** (focus). It results from loss of flexibility of the lens, which occurs with aging.

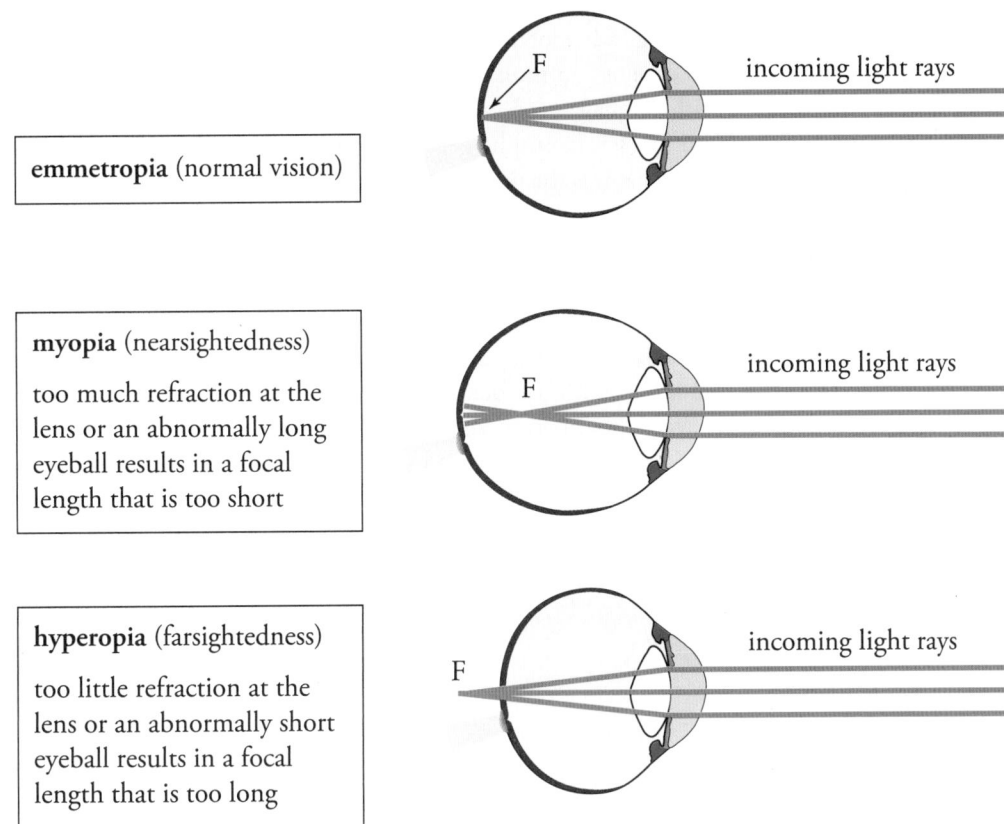

Figure 6   Deficits in visual acuity ("F" denotes the focal point)

Primary Visual Pathways

The photoreceptors and other neuronal cells of the retina send varied types of information to the brain including the light intensity, colors, and spatial distribution of the information received. The neural signals initially processed by the retina travel via the axons of the ganglion cells and leave the posterior poles of the eyes as the optic nerves. The area where the axons exit the eye is called the optic disc. Since no receptors exist in this region, it is technically a blind spot. However, when both eyes are open, each eye's blind spot is filled in with neuronal information provided by the other eye.

At the point where the optic nerves unite, the optic chiasm is found. At the optic chiasm, fibers carrying information from the nasal half of each retina (the half of each retina nearer to the nose) cross over to the opposite side of the brain. Information from the nasal half of the retina of the left eye (the left eye's information about the left visual field) crosses over to the right side of the brain. Information from the nasal half of the retina of the right eye (the right eye's information about the right visual field) crosses over to the left side of the brain. Information from the temporal part of each eye (the half of each retina further from the nose) does not cross over at the optic chiasm. Thus, the left side of the brain receives all information about the right visual field of each eye, and the right side of the brain receives all information about the left visual field of each eye.

This results in an interesting effect among individuals whose corpus callosums are severed to the point that their left and right brain hemispheres cannot communicate (sometimes termed "split-brain"). Since areas of the brain most strongly associated with language processing (Wernicke's area and Broca's area) are located in the dominant hemisphere of the brain (the left hemisphere for about 97% of people), many individuals with severed corpus callosums cannot vocally express the names of objects displayed only in their left visual field.

After the optical chiasm, the optical axons are called the optic tract. The optic tract wraps around the midbrain to get to the lateral geniculate nucleus (LGN) of the thalamus. The majority of visual information flows through the LGN into optic radiations terminating in an occipital lobe, which contains the primary visual cortex. Each side of the brain has its own neural visual pathway consisting of the optic tract, LGN body, optic radiations, and occipital lobe. Each of these pathways contain neural information from both eyes. If the right optic tract were destroyed, a person would lose partial vision in both eyes, the right temporal and the left nasal fields of vision. In such a case, neither eye would be able to perceive the left field of vision.

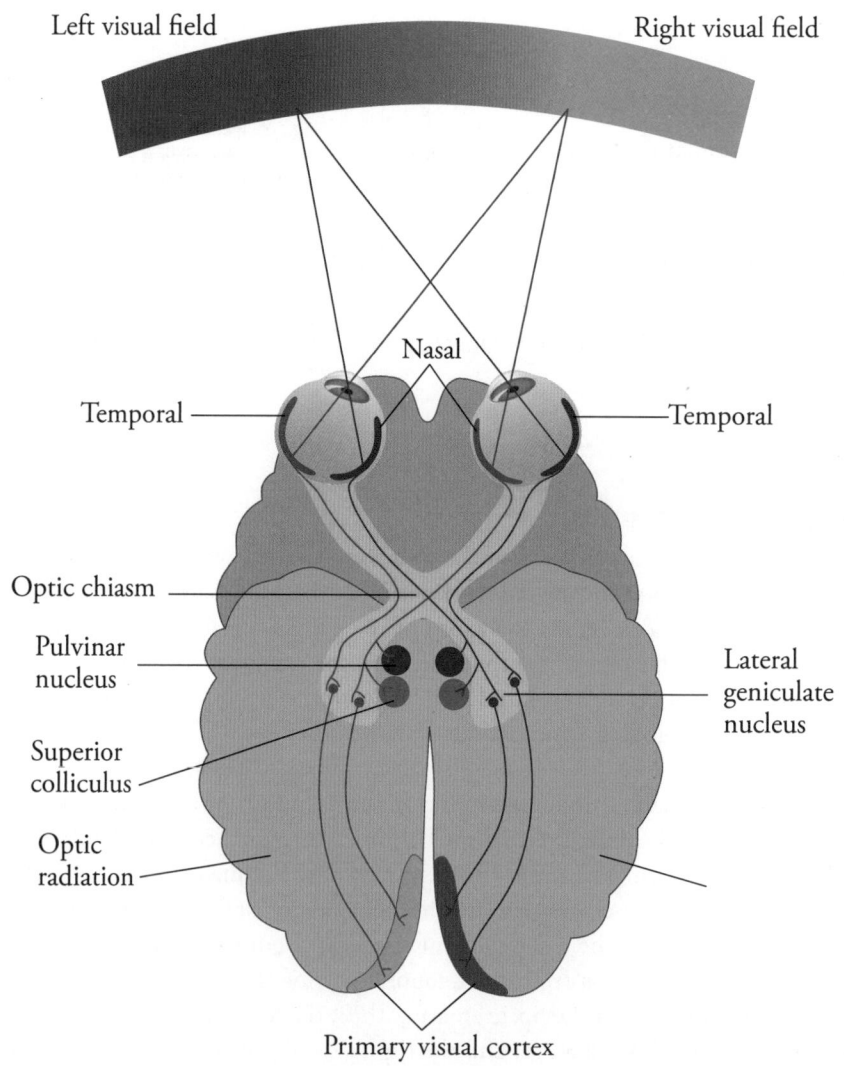

Figure 7   Visual pathways in the brain

Table 1 Summary of Sensory Modalities

Modality	Receptor	Receptor type	Organ	Stimulus
Vision	• rods and cones	• electromagnetic	• retina	• light
Hearing	• auditory hair cells	• mechanoreceptor	• organ of Corti	• vibration
Olfaction	• olfactory nerve endings	• chemoreceptor	• individual neurons	• airborne chemicals
Taste	• taste cells	• chemoreceptor	• taste bud	• food chemicals
Touch (a few examples)	• Pacinian corpuscules • free nerve endings • temperature receptors	• mechanoreceptor • nociceptor • thermoreceptor	• skin	• pressure • pain • temperature
Interoception (two examples)	• aortic arch baroreceptors • pH receptors	• baroreceptor • chemoreceptor	• aortic arch • aortic arch / medulla oblongata	• blood pressure • pH

11.2   PERCEPTION

Vision: Information Processing and Perception

For humans, vision is the primary sense; even if other information (such as sound or smell) counters visual information, we are more likely to "believe our eyes." The processing of visual information is extremely complex, and highly reliant on expectations and past experience. Neurons in the **visual cortex** fire in response to very specific information; feature-detecting neurons are specific neurons in the brain that fire in response to particular visual features, such as lines, edges, angles, and movement. This information is then passed along to other neurons that begin to assimilate these distinct features into more complex objects, and so on. Therefore, **feature-detection theory** explains why a certain area of the brain is activated when looking at a face, a different area is activated when looking at the letters on this page, etc. In order to process vast amounts of visual information quickly and effectively, our brain employs **parallel processing**, whereby many aspects of a visual stimulus (such as form, motion, color, and depth) are processed simultaneously instead of in a step-by-step or serial fashion. [Note: parallel processing is also employed for other stimuli as well.] The occipital lobe constructs a holistic image by integrating all of the separate elements of an object, in addition to accessing stored information. For example, the brain is simultaneously processing the individual features of an image, while also accessing stored information, to rapidly come to the conclusion that you are not only viewing a face, but you are specifically viewing your mom's face. All of this requires a tremendous amount of resources; in fact, the human brain dedicates approximately 30% of the cortex to processing visual information, while only 8% is devoted to processing touch information, and a mere 3% processes auditory information!

Depth perception is the ability to see objects in three dimensions despite the fact that images are imposed on the retina in only two dimensions. Depth perception allows us to judge distance, oftentimes with amazing accuracy. Experiments conducted on babies using something called a visual cliff demonstrate that depth perception appears to be largely innate. For these visual cliff experiments, babies were placed on a clear glass surface above a steep drop-off (Figure 8). The glass surface would allow the babies to safely crawl over the steep drop to their mothers, but most babies would not venture out over the visual cliff, indicating that their depth perception was developed enough to understand that the drop was dangerous.

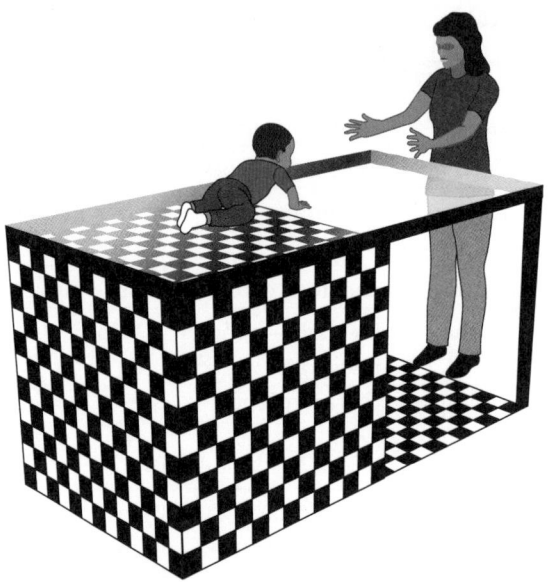

Figure 8   Visual cliff experiments show depth perception in infants

Binocular cues and monocular cues are responsible for our ability to perceive depth and distance. **Binocular cues** are depth cues that depend on information received from both eyes and are most important for perceiving depth when objects are close to us in our visual field.

Retinal disparity is a binocular cue whereby the brain compares the images projected onto the two retinas in order to perceive distance. The greater the difference or disparity between the images on the two retinas, the shorter the distance to the observer. For example, suppose you are looking at a tree far in the distance, and hold your thumb about 18 inches in front of your face (feel free to try this!). When you focus on the tree far in the distance (or any object farther away than your thumb), your thumb appears to "double" (you see two sort of see-through versions of your thumb while you focus on the object farther from you). These two versions of your thumb are the two different images from the two retinas. If you move your thumb farther from your face (while still focusing past it), the two images of your thumb get closer together. If you move your thumb closer to your face, the two images get farther apart. Now focus on your thumb. Your brain is still receiving two disparate representations of your thumb, but now it converges these two representations into one, and also provides information about how far your thumb is from your face. This is how retinal disparity works. Farther images have less disparity (the images from the two retinas are more similar, indicating to your brain that the object is farther away), while closer images have more disparity, indicating to your brain that they are closer to your face.

Convergence is another binocular cue that describes the extent to which the eyes turn inward when looking at an object; the greater the angle of convergence or inward strain, the closer the object. In other words, if you hold your thumb right in front of your nose, your eyes have to turn inward a great deal to focus on your thumb (this is known as going "cross-eyed"), which signals to your brain that the object you are focusing on is quite close.

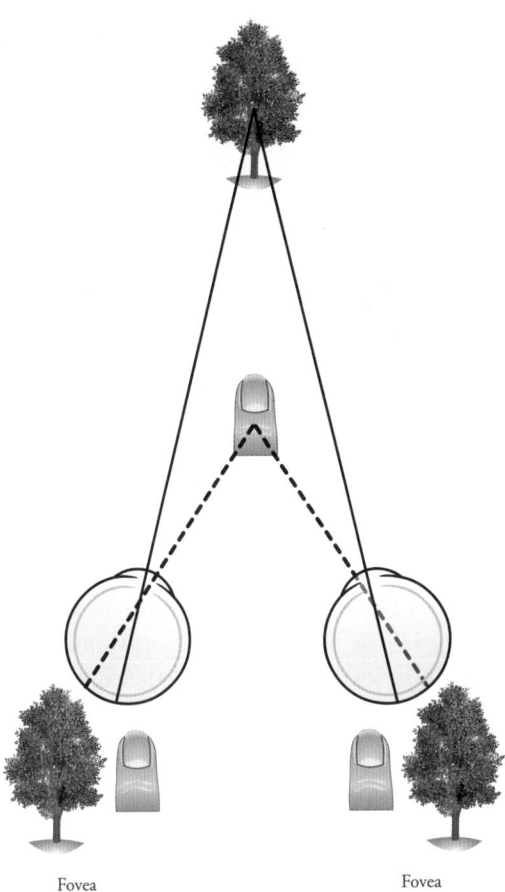

Figure 9 Retinal disparity helps us to determine distance

Monocular cues are depth cues that depend on information that is available to either eye alone and are important for judging distances of objects that are far from us, since the retinal disparity is only slight. Since we cannot rely on binocular cues for objects at farther distances, we rely on any combination of the following monocular cues:

- **Relative Size**: If objects are assumed to be the same size, the one that casts the smaller image on the retina appears more distant. For example, in Figure 10, our brains assume the elk in the foreground are roughly the same size as those in the background; therefore, since some of the elk are perceived by our retinas as smaller, those that are smaller are perceived as farther away than those elk that are perceived by our retinas as larger.
- **Interposition**: If one object blocks the view of another, we perceive it as closer. In Figure 10, the horns of the elk in the foreground partially obscure the elk in the immediate background (and the elk in the immediate background is partially obscuring elk in the more distant background and so on); therefore, the elk that are partially blocking the view of other elk are perceived by our brains as closer.
- **Relative Clarity**: We perceive hazy objects as being more distant than sharp, clear objects. In Figure 10, the elk in the far background are fuzzier and less sharp than the elk in the foreground; therefore, we perceive the sharper elk as closer and the fuzzier elk as farther away.

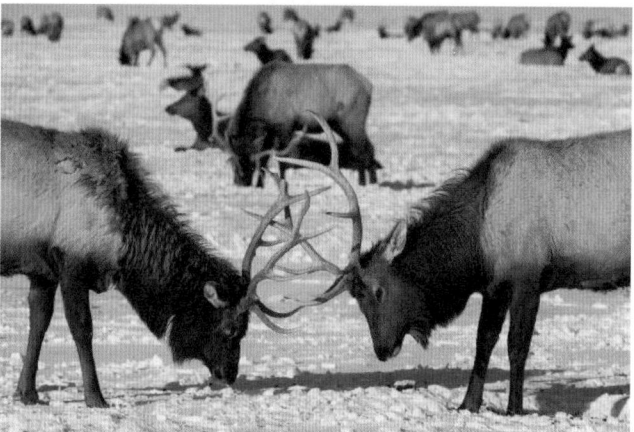

Figure 10

- **Texture Gradient**: Change from a coarse, distinct texture to a fine, indistinct texture indicates increasing distance. In Figure 11, the poppies in the foreground appear as distinct flowers, but those in the background begin to sort of blend in together until it looks like a continuous stretch of red. The distinct poppies are perceived as closer and the indistinct poppies that all blend into a stretch of red are perceived as farther away.
- **Relative Height**: We perceive objects that are higher in the visual field as farther away. In Figure 11, the red area of poppies higher in the visual field (and on the hill) are perceived as farther away than the poppies at the bottom of the visual field.

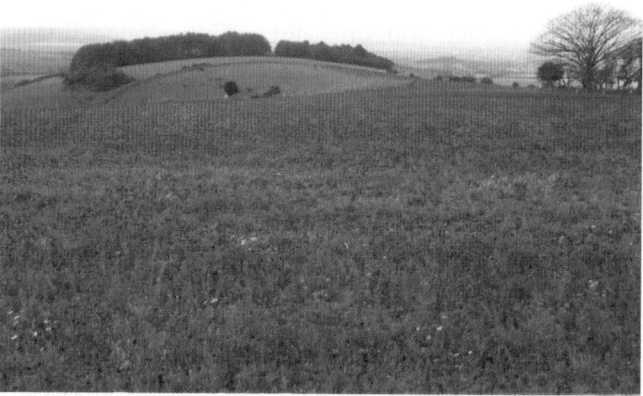

Figure 11

- **Relative Motion**: As we move, stable objects appear to move as well. Objects that are near to us appear to move faster than objects that are farther away. This is easily demonstrated whenever you are in a car or train—the farther away something is on the horizon, the slower it moves past you, while nearby objects fly past. This difference in motion cues our brains that the objects moving quickly by are close, while those moving by more slowly are farther away.
- **Linear Perspective**: Parallel lines appear to converge as distance increases. The greater the convergence, the greater the perceived distance. This is seen in Figure 12, where the parallel lines of the rail tracks appear to get closer together, which signals our brains that as the lines converge, the distance increases.

- **Light and Shadow**: Closer objects reflect more light than do distant objects. The dimmer of two identical objects will seem farther away. In Figure 12, the closer rail tracks are brighter than the more distant tracks, signaling our brains that the brighter tracks are closer, while the dimmer tracks are farther away.

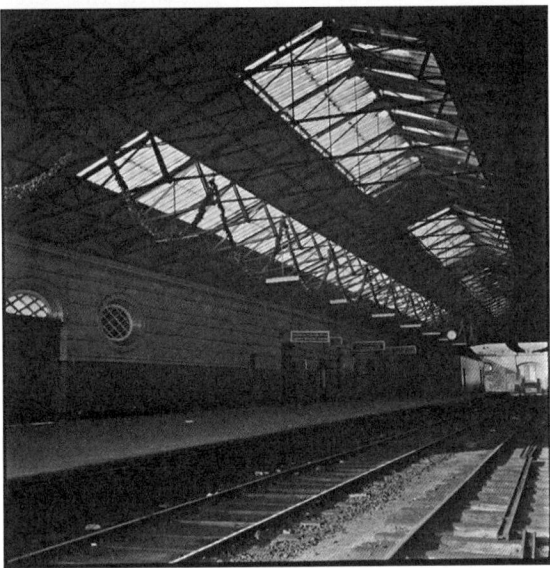

Figure 12

Absolute Thresholds

We are very sensitive to certain types of stimuli. The minimum stimulus intensity required to activate a sensory receptor 50% of the time (and thus detect the sensation) is called the **absolute threshold**. In other words, for each special sense, the 50% recognition point defines the absolute threshold. (Note that this threshold can vary among individuals and different organisms—the absolute smell threshold for a human and a dog differs greatly.) Absolute thresholds also vary with age. For example, as we age, we gradually lose our ability to detect higher-pitched sounds. [What is the anatomical reason for this?[3]]

---

[3] Loud sounds can mechanically harm the hair cells, causing them to die. When this occurs, the hair cell can no longer send sound signals to the brain. In people, once a hair cell dies, it will never regrow. The hair cells that detect higher frequency sounds are the smallest and the most easily damaged; therefore, as people age and more hair cells are damaged and lost, hearing loss occurs. Since the smallest hair cells are the ones most likely lost, loss of sensitivity to high-pitched sounds is common in older people.

Difference Thresholds

Absolute thresholds are important for detecting the presence or absence of stimuli, but the ability to determine the change or difference in stimuli is also vital. The **difference threshold** (also called the *just noticeable difference*, or JND) is the minimum noticeable difference between any two sensory stimuli, 50% of the time. The magnitude of the initial stimulus influences the difference threshold; for example, if you lift a one-pound weight and a two-pound weight, the difference will be obvious, but if you lift a 100-pound weight and 101-pound weight, you probably won't be able to tell the difference. Indeed, **Weber's law** dictates that two stimuli must differ by a constant *proportion* in order for their difference to be perceptible. Interestingly, the exact proportion varies by stimulus; but for humans, two objects must differ in weight by 2% [in the weight example above, what is the minimum weight needed to detect a difference between it and the 100-pound weight?[4]], two lights must differ in intensity by 8%, and two tones must differ in frequency by 0.3%.

Signal Detection Theory

Detecting sensory stimuli not only depends on the information itself, but also on our psychological state, including alertness, expectation, motivation, and prior experience. **Signal detection theory** attempts to predict how and when someone will detect the presence of a given sensory stimulus (the "signal") amidst all of the other sensory stimuli in the background (considered the "noise"). There are four possible outcomes: a hit (the signal is present and was detected), a miss (the signal was present but not detected), a false alarm (the signal was not present but the person thought it was), and a correct rejection (the signal was not present and the person did not think it was). Signal detection can have important life-or-death consequences—imagine how crucial it is for doctors to be able to detect the signal (perhaps a tumor on a CT scan) from the noise.

Gestalt Psychology

Gestalt is the German word for "form" or "shape," and has come to mean, in English, an organized whole perceived as more than the sum of its individual parts. Therefore, in psychology, gestalt refers to the idea that the whole exceeds the sum of its parts; in other words, when humans perceive an object, rather than seeing lines, angles, colors, and shadows, they perceive the whole—a face or a table or a dog. Importantly, gestalt does not explain *how* the brain is able to perceive in such a way, merely that it does. There are many different gestalt principles to explain perceptual organization; below the most common are covered. (Note that gestalt principles can be applied to any sensory modality, but they are most often described using visual perception examples, as we have here).

Emergence. Look at the image in Figure 13. This is essentially a series of black irregular shapes on a white background. Those are the individual *parts* of the image. However, the whole that our brain perceives is a dog. You did not recognize the dog by first identifying its parts and constructing the whole ("there is the nose, there is the collar, there is a leg, this must be a dog!"), rather, the dog appears as a whole, all at once—it sort of pops out at you. This is an example of the gestalt principle of emergence. According to this gestalt principle, when attempting to identify an object, we first identify its outline, which then allows us to figure out what the object is. Only after the whole emerges do we start to identify the parts that make up the whole, such as the dog's face, legs, or the chain attached to his collar in Figure 13.

---

[4] 102 pounds, which is 2% heavier than 100 pounds.

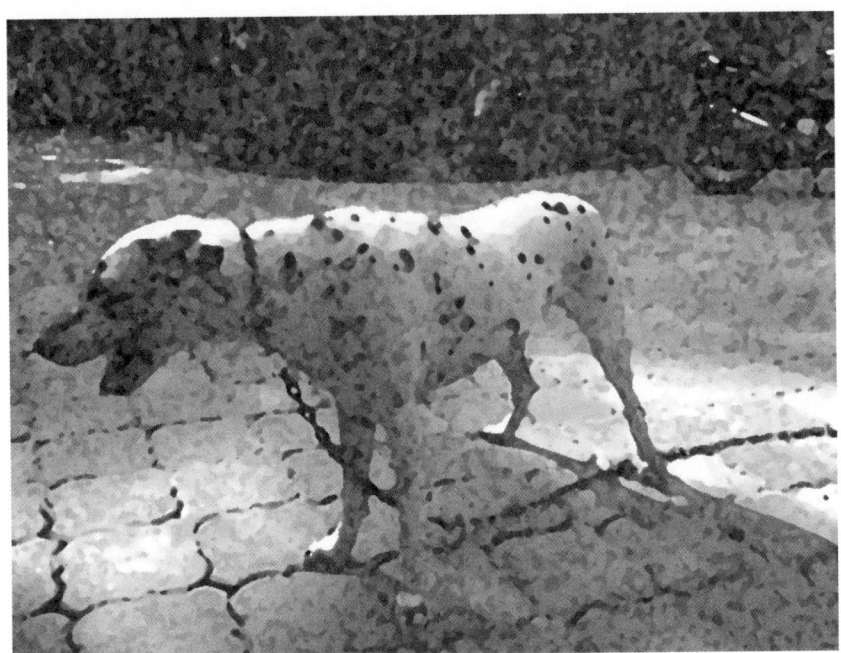

Figure 13

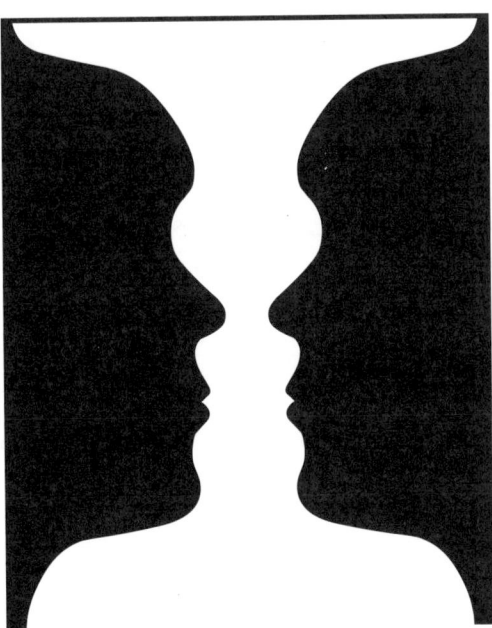

Figure 14

Multistability. The image in Figure 14 is also a great example of the gestalt principle of multistability or multistable perception, which is the tendency for ambiguous images to pop back and forth unstably between alternative interpretations in our brains. Other examples include the images of two impossible objects in Figure 15. Again, gestalt does not explain *how* images appear multistable, only that they *do*.

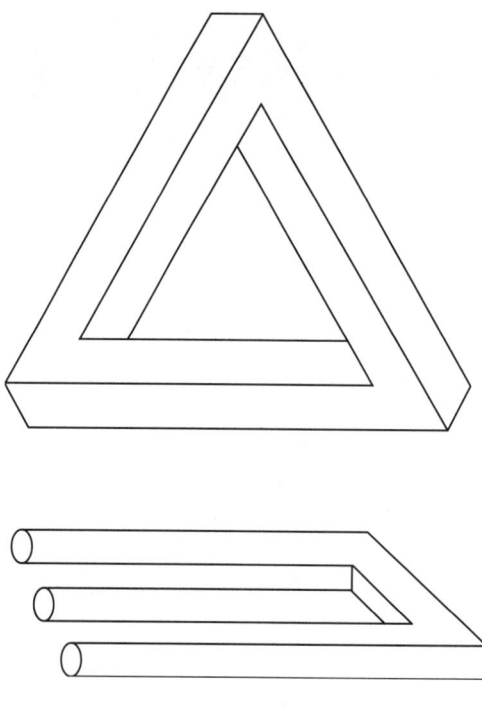

Figure 15

Gestalt Laws of Grouping. There are also several gestalt grouping laws meant to help explain how we tend to perceive things. While there are more than five laws, the five most common are discussed here. The **law of proximity** suggests that things that are near one another seem to be grouped together. Nearby objects tend to be perceived as a unit or group (see A in Figure 16: do you perceive 25 individual dots, or a square composed of dots? The law of proximity predicts that you perceive a square composed of dots). The law of similarity suggests that things that are similar tend to appear grouped together. In other words, we tend to perceive similar items as a unit or group (see B in Figure 16 below: what do you see? According to the law of similarity, you are likely to perceive the columns as important, and will perceive columns composed of circles and squares). The **law of continuity** (also known as the law of good continuation) suggests that we perceive smooth, continuous lines and forms, rather than disjointed ones. For example, in Figure 16, the law of continuity predicts that we will perceive the image in C as two overlapping circles, rather than two black semicircular lines and a red football shape in the middle. Even though the lines are different colors, we still tend to perceive the lines as continuous, forming two circles. The gestalt **law of closure** predicts that we will perceive things as complete logical entities, because our brains will fill in the gaps in the information. For example, what do you see in D in Figure 16? The law of closure predicts that you will perceive a triangle! The **gestalt law of common fate** predicts that objects moving in the same direction, or moving in synchrony, are perceived as a group or unit. This applies to things like a group of dancers moving in unison or a flock of birds all moving together (like E in Figure 16). The gestalt **law of connectedness** predicts that things that are joined or linked or grouped are perceived as connected. In Figure 16, F shows the same set of circles in the shape of a square as in A, but the box around some of those circles connects them in our brains. The law of connectedness predicts that we are likely to perceive those nine circles as connected and differentiated from the rest.

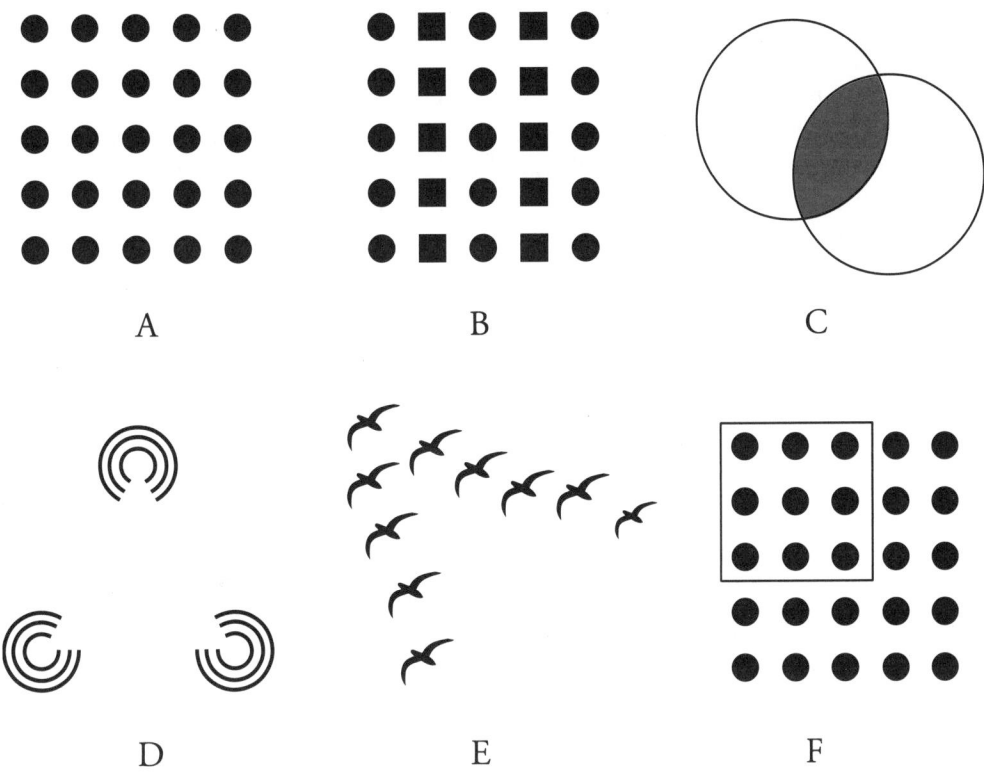

Figure 16

If a lot of these gestalt principles and laws seem similar to you, it is because there is a fair amount of overlap (it doesn't help that they are described as either principles or laws by different sources, called by multiple different names, and exemplified by many of the same images.). Therefore, familiarize yourself with the basic principles here and try not to get too wrapped up in differentiating between each individual law or principle—our visual perception is the result of many of these principles or laws working simultaneously!

Perceptual Processing

Bottom-up processing begins with the sensory receptors and works up to the complex integration of information occurring in the brain. Bottom-up processing is also known as data-driven processing; information enters the eyes in one direction (this sensory input is the "bottom"), and is then turned into an identifiable image by the brain (this final image is the "top"). We tend to use more of a bottom-up approach when we have no or little prior experience with a stimulus. **Top-down processing** occurs when the brain applies experience and expectations to interpret sensory information. Instead of focusing on the sensory input (the "bottom"), we can use our prior experience and knowledge to impose our expectations on the stimulus, which tends to occur with stimuli with which we are more familiar. Note that the brain in fact uses a combination of the two: information is received in a bottom-up fashion from sensory receptors, while the brain is superimposing assumptions in a top-down manner.

11.3 ATTENTION

Imagine the attention to detail necessary to perform a complicated procedure such as a heart transplant. These details may include the tools being utilized, the various monitors, the incision site, the support staff, the status of the patient, etc. There might also be countless other things that the surgeon could pay attention to…the trim on the walls, the numbers on the clock, the glasses on the face of the nurse…in fact, if the surgeon *did* pay attention to these things, he or she would find it more difficult to complete the surgery successfully. How is it that the surgeon is able to avoid distractions, choosing instead to pay attention to only particular inputs out of the many available in the environment? What limits people in general from paying attention to all objects and entities at once? Further, imagine that the surgeon was chewing gum while performing the surgery (not recommended!). This would likely not have an impact on the surgeon's performance; however, if the surgeon were giving a speech while performing the surgery (definitely not recommended!), the surgeon's performance would likely be impaired. All of the above are examples of different aspects of attention. Let's look at two unique components of attention—selective attention and divided attention—and the models that have been used to explain each.

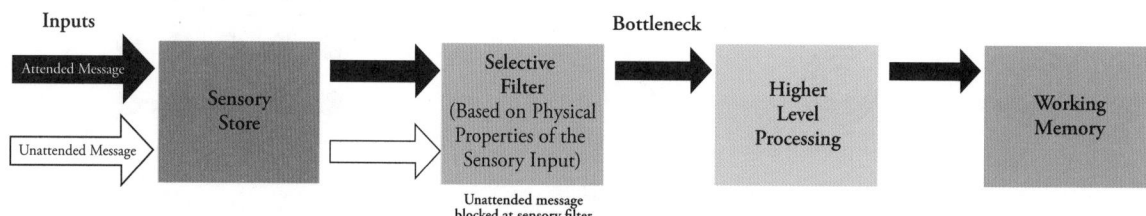

Figure 17   Broadbent Filter Model of Selective Attention

Selective Attention

Selective attention is the process by which one input is attended to and the rest are tuned out. This is necessary because we do not have the capacity to pay attention to everything in our environments. A resource model suggests that we only have a limited capacity to pay attention and so must devote our resources carefully.

One way that selective attention has been studied is using a dichotic listening setup. A person wears headphones and each ear hears a different dialogue. The individual is instructed to listen to information coming into one ear, called the **attended channel**, and to ignore input to the other ear, the **unattended channel**. When people do this, they are able to remember some of the message from the attended ear but lose almost everything from the unattended ear. The same observation has been made with visual stimuli; when people are told to focus on one visual aspect, they may miss other visual details.

Donald Broadbent thought of the brain as a processing system with a limited capacity and sought to map out the steps that went into creating memories from raw sensory data. He developed the **Broadbent Filter Model of Selective Attention** (Figure 17). In this model, inputs from the environment first enter a sensory buffer. One of these inputs is then selected and filtered based on physical characteristics of the input (e.g., sensory modality). This theoretical filter is designed to keep us from becoming overloaded and overwhelmed with information. Other sensory information stays in the sensory buffer briefly, but then quickly decays. At this point in the process, the information is still raw data that has just been filtered—it has not yet been transformed. It is in the next step, when the information enters short-term memory storage, where semantic (meaning-making) processes occur.

In the dichotic listening task described above, only information from the attended ear is allowed to pass through the filter. If an input in the sensory buffer does not go through the filter, the theory proposes that it remains briefly but then quickly decays and disappears.

To make matters more complicated, it seems that some unattended inputs are still detected. Imagine you are in a conversation with someone at a party in a room full of people. You are not aware of the content of any of the other conversations until suddenly you hear the name of your best friend mentioned in a conversation behind you. This phenomenon is known as the **cocktail party effect**. It happens when information of personal importance from previously unattended channels catches our attention. This observation cannot be well accounted for by the filter model of attention. Later adaptations of the original model have thus suggested that information from the unattended ear is not completely filtered out, but rather dampened, like turning the volume down on a television. Information from the unattended ear can still be processed at some level.

Anne Treisman's Attenuation Model tried to account for the cocktail party effect. Treisman believed that rather than a filter, the mind has an attenuator, which works like a volume knob—it "turns down" the unattended sensory input, rather than eliminating it.

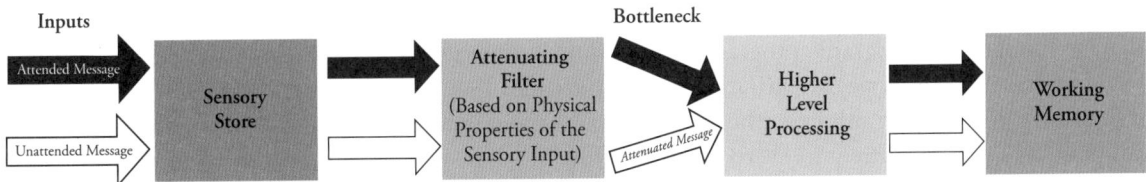

Figure 18   Treisman Attenuation Model of Selective Attention

The cocktail party effect has also been explained through the concept of **selective priming**. This idea suggests that people can be selectively primed to observe something, either by encountering it frequently or by having an expectation. If one is primed to observe something, one is more likely to notice it when it occurs. Over the course of our lifetimes, we have frequently encountered our own names and the names of our friends and are thus primed to hear them. The more something is primed, the more it will be picked up despite distractions. Researchers have also studied priming by providing people with stimuli, sometimes subliminally, and testing whether these stimuli have an impact on later performance.

For example, if asked to read a list of words including the word "lettuce" before embarking on a word completion task, subjects are more likely to complete "LET____" with T-U-C-E to make the word "lettuce" than people who were not initially primed with the list of words. Even if people are not conscious of remembering the stimuli, it can still have an impact on later performance.

Visual attention has often been explained via a **spotlight model**. In this model, the spotlight is a beam that can shine anywhere within an individual's visual field. It is important to note that this beam describes the movement of attention, not the movement of the eyes. Shifts in attention actually precede the

11.3

corresponding eye movements. The shifting of attention requires us to unlock the beam from its current target, move the focus, and lock onto a new target.

Information from visual perception is processed in the brain by feature detectors that examine the different aspects of an object, such as color, shape, orientation, etc. One problem with visual processing is called the **binding problem**—the problem of how all these different aspects are assembled together and related to a single object, rather than something else in the visual field. Visual attention is the solution to this problem. If our visual attention is on a particular object such as a cup, then the feature detectors' input of shape, color, etc. will all be related to the object being attended to—the cup. It has been found that when people are distracted while viewing two items, they may have issues with binding; for example, the color of one item may be attributed to the other.

Divided Attention

Divided attention concerns when and if we are able to perform multiple tasks simultaneously. It turns out that this depends on the characteristics of the activities one is trying to multitask. The **resource model of attention** says that we have a limited pool of resources on which to draw when performing tasks, both modality-specific resources and general resources. In general, if the resources required to perform multiple tasks simultaneously exceed the available resources to do so, then the tasks cannot be accomplished at the same time. Three factors are associated with performance on multi-tasking: task similarity, task difficulty, and task practice.

Imagine listening to a talk radio program while trying to write a paper. It is likely that these two activities would be very difficult to pay attention to at the same time. They would interfere with each other because of their task similarity, in this case, the use of the same modality for processing. One activity requires verbal input, while the other requires verbal output. However, if instead you were listening to classical music, you might be able to write a paper at the same time because you would be doing two dissimilar tasks; one requires auditory input resources, while the other requires verbal output.

Task difficulty also plays a role. If a task is more difficult, it requires more resources in general and would be hard to do simultaneously with another task without passing resource capacity. Imagine driving a car while conversing with your passengers. When driving through familiar neighborhoods in a single lane (an easy task), you may have no trouble carrying on a conversation. However, if you are about to enter a complicated intersection involving a lane change and a quick turn, attention to the conversation may have to stop or you may become silent or miss what was said during that time. Alternatively, while deep in conversation, it is easy to miss a turn!

11.4 COGNITION

Information-Processing Models

With the advent of computers, psychologists were influenced to think about the human mind as if it were a computer processor. Contrary to behaviorism, which is concerned mostly with the link between stimulus and response, **information-processing models** focus on what happens between the ears. These models have a few basic assumptions. They assume that information is taken in from the environment and processed through a series of steps including **attention**, **perception**, and **storage into memory**. Along the way, information is systematically transformed. Thus, our minds are like mental computer programs or assembly lines that change, store, use, and retrieve information.

Two theories of attention and perception were described above (Broadbent filter model of selective attention and the Treisman attenuation model of selective attention). **Alan Baddeley's model** sought to better define short-term memory, which he renamed **working memory**. In his model, working memory consists of four components—a phonological loop, a visuospatial sketchpad, an episodic buffer, and a central executive. The **phonological loop** allows us to repeat verbal information to help us remember it. This may be what you use to remember a phone number that someone tells you when you have nothing with which to write it down. The **visuospatial sketchpad** serves a similar purpose for visuospatial information through the use of mental images. The **episodic buffer** is theorized to integrate information from the phonological loop and visuospatial sketchpad with a sense of time, and to interface with long-term memory stores. In other words, the episodic buffer is responsible for combining information from a variety of sources into coherent episodes (hence the name, episodic buffer). For example, if a man sees a station wagon much like the one his father used to drive, he is able to make this connection through the interaction between his memory of his father's car and his current visual experience in the episodic buffer. The **central executive** is the overseer of the entire process and orchestrates it by shifting and dividing attention.

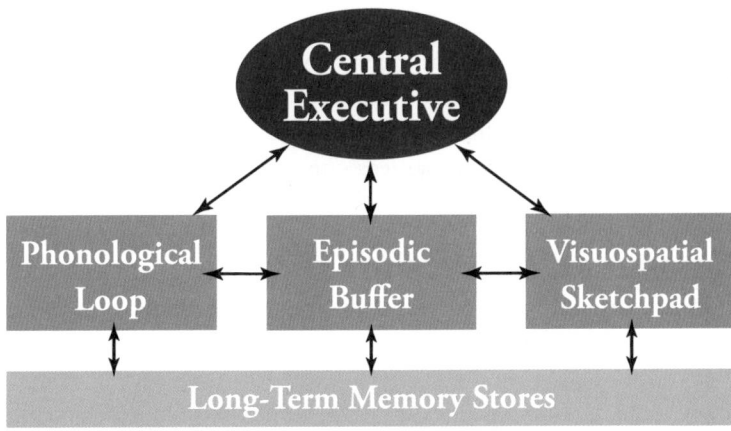

Figure 19   Baddeley Model of Working Memory

Cognitive Development

Piaget's Stages of Cognitive Development

Jean Piaget was one of the first developmental psychologists who studied cognitive development in children; he argued against the prevailing belief that children were much like miniature adults in their thought processes and abilities. He thought that the process of cognitive development involved forming **schemas**, or mental frameworks that shape and are shaped by our experience. As we encounter new experiences, Piaget believed that we either **assimilate** those experiences by fitting them into our existing schemas or we **accommodate** by adjusting our schemas to take into account the new experiences. For example, if a young girl believes that there is a monster under the bed but her parent turns on the light to reveal that there is nothing there, the girl can take two paths. She can assimilate this experience by believing that the monster still exists but runs away from light, or accommodate her schema by agreeing that there must be no monster.

Piaget's theory included four developmental stages. They are as follows:

1) **Sensorimotor Stage:** from birth to roughly age 2. Babies and young infants experience the world through their senses and movement, such as looking, touching, mouthing, and grasping. During this time, they learn about **object permanence**—the understanding that things continue to exist when they are out of sight. They also demonstrate stranger anxiety: distress when confronted with an unfamiliar person.

2) **Preoperational Stage:** roughly from ages 2 to 7. During this time, children learn that things can be represented through symbols such as words and images. This accompanies their learning during pretend play and development of language, but they still lack logical reasoning. They also are egocentric, meaning they do not understand that others have different perspectives.

3) **Concrete Operational Stage:** roughly from ages 7 to 11. Children learn to think logically about concrete events. This helps them learn the principle of **conservation**: the idea that quantity remains the same despite changes in shape. For example, if water from a wide bowl is poured into a thin cylinder, it still has the same volume despite the difference in height. They also grasp mathematical concepts during this time.

4) **Formal Operational Stage:** roughly from age 12 through adulthood. People learn abstract reasoning (e.g., hypothesizing) and moral reasoning.

Cognitive Changes in Late Adulthood

During early and middle adulthood, most cognitive abilities remain stable or increase. Beyond the age of 60, the following cognitive declines have been noted:

1) The elderly show some memory declines in recall, while their recognition abilities remain relatively intact. **Recall** involves retrieving information from memory without any clues, while **recognition** involves retrieving information from memory with clues. Asking an eyewitness to describe the face of a suspect is a test of recall; asking an eyewitness to identify a suspect out of a lineup is a test of recognition.

2) Time-based tasks can also be challenging for older adults, such as a regimen involving medication taken three times a day.

3) Older adults also have slower information-processing abilities, as evidenced by slower reaction times and speech.

Role of Culture in Cognitive Development

The process of learning is in many ways the process of internalizing information provided by a given culture. Higher mental processes may have their roots in broader social processes. Thus, instead of the individual developing and learning how to utilize developed skills in a social context, consider the possibility that the individual learns social relationships and converts these into mental capabilities. The developing individual and the environment are in a reciprocal relationship in which the social context can shape thinking and behavior. For example: the expression of thoughts is limited by the thinker's language. Furthermore, internalized speech is only developed after a child speaks out loud and receives feedback from others in the environment. As you can imagine, different languages result in different ways of thinking. Multilingual people have even been shown to perform differently on personality tests depending on the language in which the test is given.

Influence of Heredity and Environment on Cognitive Development

Heredity and the environment interact during the course of an individual's life to create a developmental trajectory. One way of thinking about this is that genetics provides the biological predispositions, or raw material that an individual has. Sociocultural influences then help mold and channel this potential into the development of particular capabilities. The amount and quality of schooling and the richness of the child's environment can heavily influence performance on tests of cognitive functioning. Thus, neither "nature" (genetics) nor "nurture" (environment) may be sufficient to explain the developmental path of an individual—it may instead be explained by a complex interaction. For an example, consider the case of language. Noam Chomsky convincingly argued that children could not learn the wealth of vocabulary that they quickly acquire simply through environmental influence; genetics and heredity are also involved. At the same time, the quality of reading education in school influences a child's ability to acquire this skill.

Biological Factors that Affect Cognition

Many aspects of cognitive functioning can be traced back to structures in the brain. Sensory information provides the raw material for cognitive processes and is transmitted to the parietal, occipital, and temporal lobes of the brain (discussed in Chapter 10). In fact, the inability to recognize objects through sensory mechanisms (a vital aspect of perception and cognition) despite intact function of the underlying sense itself is called **agnosia**; it is often due to damage at the occipitoparietal border. The frontal lobes play a role in executive functions, including planning, organizing, inhibiting impulses, and thinking flexibly. The hippocampus has been shown to be involved in the formation of new memories. Furthermore, emotional arousal is necessary to provide the motivation and alertness necessary to complete tasks and is managed by the amygdala and the rest of the limbic system. The interconnectivity of these various regions underlies our cognitive skills.

Problem-Solving and Decision-Making

Types of Problem-Solving and Problem-Solving Approaches

What detours can I take to get out of this traffic jam? How do I change a flat tire? Should I hitchhike with this stranger? A strange morning commute may require us to use various strategies for solving problems. For some problems, we may use a strategy of **trial and error**. For others, we may rely on following an **algorithm**, a step-by-step procedure. For others, we may use mental shortcuts, called **heuristics**. At times, we may use a combination of these strategies. For example, when changing a tire, an algorithm may be followed until it is discovered that a needed wrench is missing. At this point, other tools may be pulled out and experimented with through trial and error until an appropriate one for the bolts is found. Sometimes we use problem-solving strategies consciously, while at other times this is an unconscious process. For example, we may not be actively thinking about a problem, but may be struck later in the shower with a sudden flash of inspiration called **insight**.

Barriers to Effective Problem-Solving

Think about a time when you struggled with solving a problem to no avail. There are two cognitive tendencies that can lead us astray when looking for solutions: confirmation bias and fixation.

Confirmation bias is a tendency to search only for information that confirms our preconceived thinking, rather than information that might not support it. This can prevent you from approaching a problem from multiple perspectives, because you are more likely to view it from one way—your way. As a result, this bias can lead to faulty decision-making; one-sided information may leave you without a complete picture of the situation. For example, suppose you are in charge of staffing the nurses at the hospital ER where you work, and you believe that during college football game nights there are more admissions than on other days. You will tend to take notice of admissions during college football game nights, but be inattentive to admissions during other nights of the month. A tendency to do this over time unjustifiably strengthens your belief, and it could lead to poor staffing decisions.

A second obstacle to problem-solving is **fixation**, an inability to see the problem from a fresh perspective. At times, fixation results from the existence of a **mental set**, a tendency to fixate on solutions that worked in the past though they may not apply to the current situation. For example, a parent trying to control their child's behavior may not realize that time-outs at age 15 are just not as effective as they were at age 5. Another type of fixation is **functional fixedness**, a tendency to perceive the functions of objects as fixed and unchanging. Thus, one may search high and low to find a box-cutter to open a package, when a readily available key would work just as well.

Heuristics, Biases, Intuition, and Emotion

It may not surprise you to know that humans are not always logical in their decision-making. Often we don't put a great deal of time and effort into a decision because the decision may be trivial, or because it must be made quickly, or because no clear logical path for problem-solving is available.

Mental shortcuts, or heuristics, can increase efficiency in decision-making and although they are helpful most of the time, they can also lead to errors in judgment. Who was a more prolific composer, Joseph Haydn or Ludwig van Beethoven? Most of us would assume Beethoven, because his name and possibly even examples of his work come more readily to mind. Haydn was actually Beethoven's teacher, and he composed nearly three times more music than did Beethoven! When you make a decision about something based on the examples that are most available in your mind, this is known as the **availability heuristic**. While the availability heuristic relies more on our memory of specific instances, the **representativeness heuristic** has more to do with our generalizations about people and events. For example, let's say you go to the post office three different times and each time a different employee is rude to you. You might conclude, "people who work at the post office are rude!" This would be an example of the representativeness heuristic—you have developed a generalization about postal workers. Another example: what does a taxicab look like? Most Americans would use the adjective "yellow" when describing a taxicab, because a yellow car fits our prototype of what a taxicab looks like. Again, this generalization is the result of the representativeness heuristic. The representativeness and availability heuristics may seem quite similar, but the representativeness heuristic is based more on generalizations (rather than specific examples), whereas the availability heuristic is based on how readily particular examples come to mind.

Another susceptibility is **belief bias**, which is the tendency to judge arguments based on what one believes about their conclusions rather than on whether they use sound logic. In other words, we tend to accept conclusions that fit with our beliefs and tend to reject conclusions that do not fit with our beliefs. For example, you probably believe that doctors are good people; therefore, if you read a story about a doctor who allegedly murdered his wife, no matter the strength of the evidence, you might be more inclined to believe that the death was an accident. On the other hand, you might easily believe that a drug-dealer killed his wife, despite the lack of any compelling evidence. Once these preexisting beliefs are formed, they become resistant to change through a phenomenon known as **belief perseverance**, a tendency to cling to beliefs despite the presence of contrary evidence.

Overconfidence and Belief Perseverance

The use of intuitive heuristics and a tendency to confirm preconceived beliefs combine to lead to **overconfidence**, an overestimation of the accuracy of knowledge and judgments. For example, after hearing that a classmate completed an assignment quickly, along with their belief that a particular class is easy, students can be overconfident in how much time it would take to complete assignments or write papers, estimating that they would take less time than they actually do. People can also be influenced by how information is **framed**. For example, one study found that consumers are more likely to buy meat advertised as 75% lean than that labeled 25% fat. Similarly, rather than informing customers that they will be charged a "fee" for using a credit card, a company may choose to offer those who use cash a "discount" to make the same situation more palatable.

11.5 CONSCIOUSNESS

Consciousness is something that science has not yet been able to pin down and with which religion has wrestled. It has been explained through concepts such as the soul by some and thought of as inseparable from the body by others. **Consciousness** is defined as the awareness that we have of ourselves, our internal states, and the environment. It is also important for reflection and exerts control by directing our attention. Thus, consciousness is always needed to complete novel and complex tasks, although we may complete practiced and simple tasks, such as driving a familiar path, with little conscious awareness. We may also be influenced by subconscious cues without them entering our consciousness. These subconscious cues can be a basis for first impressions of others and even for prejudice.

States of Consciousness

Alertness

Alertness and arousal involve the ability to remain attentive to what is going on. It is something that we often take for granted, however, many patients who arrive in an emergency room are not alert for various reasons. These can include head injuries and toxins. The ability to be alert is also impaired in a variety of disorders, including narcolepsy, attention deficit disorder, depression, and chronic fatigue syndrome. Even without these disorders, it is not possible to maintain a heightened state of alertness indefinitely, and alertness varies over a 24-hour cycle. Alertness and arousal are controlled by structures within the brainstem. These structures are known as the **reticular formation** (also known as the reticular activating system, or RAS).

Sleep

Stages of Sleep

Although the purpose of sleep and exact definition of sleep are unclear, the stages of sleep have been empirically determined. The best way to explain the stages of sleep is to put them in context of how they are measured and distinguished. **Polysomnography** (PSG) is a multimodal technique to measure physiological processes during sleep. PSG includes electroencephalogram (EEG—measures of electrical impulses in the brain), **electromyogram** (EMG—measures of skeletal muscle movements), **electrooculogram** (EOG— measures of eye movement), and other physiological indicators of sleep. Through experiments using PSG, research has shown there are several distinct stages of sleep.

When a person is awake, but sleepy and relaxed, the individual's EEG changes from when they are alert. In this relaxed state, the EEG shows **alpha waves**, which have low amplitudes and high frequencies (8–12 Hz; Figure 20). These waves are the first indicator that a person is ready to drift off to sleep: the body relaxes; the person feels drowsy and closes his or her eyes. Compare these waves to **beta waves**, the waves demonstrated during alert, focused, and active consciousness. These waves have even higher frequencies (between 12.5 Hz and 30 Hz) than alpha waves and also lower amplitudes.

When sleep begins, the first stage of non-REM (**rapid eye movement**) sleep is entered. This is called **Stage 1 sleep**. During this stage, the EEG is dominated by **theta waves**: waves of low to moderate intensity and intermediate frequency (3–7 Hz; Figure 20). Further, EOG measures slow-rolling eye movements and EMG measures moderate activity. The person becomes less responsive to stimuli and has fleeting thoughts.

Stage 2 sleep is denoted by a change to two distinct wave patterns on the EEG. Although a person still experiences theta waves, these waves are intermixed with these two patterns: K-complexes and sleep spindles. A **K-complex** typically has a duration of a half second and is large and slow. These each occur as a single wave amongst the theta waves. **Sleep spindles** are bursts of waves. They have a frequency of 12–14 Hz and are moderately intense. Like K-complexes, these spindles do not last long: only a half to one and a half seconds. During Stage 2, there is no eye movement and EMG measures moderate activity. This stage brings increased relaxation to in the body that is characteristic of sleep, such as decreased heart rate, respiration, and temperature.

During **Stage 3 and Stage 4 sleep**, a person transitions into slow wave sleep. Stage 3 and Stage 4 are characterized by **delta waves**, which are high amplitude, low frequency waves (0.5–3 Hz) and signify the deepest level of sleep. Initially, delta waves are mixed with higher-frequency waves, but as Stage 3 progresses to Stage 4, delta waves come to dominate. During slow wave sleep, a person continues to show no eye movement and moderate muscle movement. The heart rate and digestion slow, and growth hormones are secreted.

The final stage of sleep is **REM sleep**, which is characterized by bursts of quick eye movements. Also unique to REM sleep, the EEG measures waves that most resemble the beta waves seen in individuals when awake. However, the waves in REM sleep are sawtooth waves with low intensity and variable frequency. These waves are more jagged in appearance than beta waves, which are also low intensity, but high frequency (16–25 Hz). Unlike the conscious state, REM sleep is characterized by low (almost no) skeletal muscle movement: hence the name "**paradoxical sleep**." Although the person physiologically appears to be awake, their muscle movement does not corroborate, as the individual is nearly paralyzed except for sudden bursts or twitches. REM sleep is generally when dreams occur.

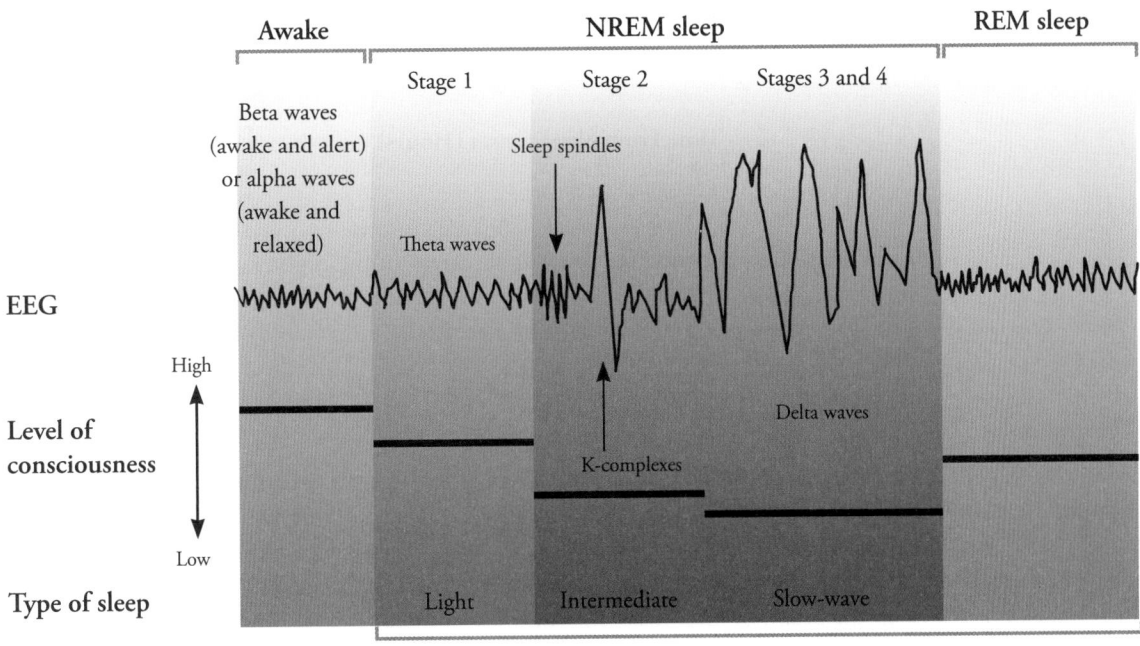

Figure 20   EEG wave forms during wakefulness and sleep

11.5

11.5

During normal sleep, an individual passes through the non-REM sleep stages, then enters into REM sleep, then passes back through the non-REM sleep stages. This may happen in sequence (Stages 1, 2, 3, 4, then REM), but it is also possible to jump between various stages while sleeping. Regardless, the average sleep cycle is about 90 minutes (for a typical adult), and includes periods of non-REM and REM sleep. We complete multiple sleep cycles per night. Periods of REM sleep are shortest early in the night, and get longer as the night progresses. Deep sleep (Stages 3 and 4) periods are longest early in the night and less frequent as the night progresses (Figure 21). The amount of sleep needed for optimal functioning changes throughout one's lifespan. Infants spend a much larger fraction of their sleep in REM than adults do (and need much more sleep—young babies spend about 16 out of every 24 hours sleeping!). Teens need, on average, about 9–10 hours a night of uninterrupted sleep. As we age, we require less and less sleep—it is not uncommon for individuals in their 60s and 70s to sleep about 6 hours a night. Without an adequate amount of sleep, the body is not able to complete all of the restorative phases needed for muscle repair, memory consolidation, and the release of various hormones, including those that regulate growth and appetite. When we do not get enough sleep, we wake up less prepared to concentrate, focus, and engage in decision-making.

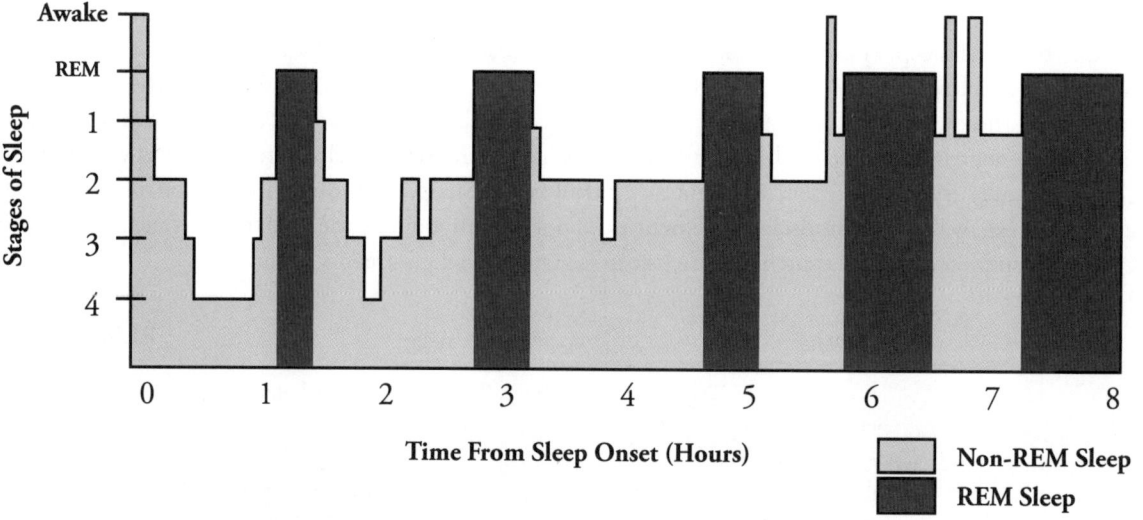

Figure 21   Normal sleep stages throughout the night

Sleep and Circadian Rhythms

There are several possible explanations for why organisms sleep. Since humans (and most other non-nocturnal animals) are better suited to survival in the daytime when we can best use our vision to navigate and stay out of harm's way, sleep may have served as a survival mechanism to reduce nighttime activity (when our ancestors were more likely to become prey). A second theory is that sleep helps heal the body by restoring tissues, including those in the brain. While we are asleep, the brain is still active, and could be reorganizing connections and consolidating memories into long-term memory storage. A third idea is that sleep plays a role in growth. During sleep, the pituitary gland releases growth hormone, with lower levels of the hormone released as an individual ages. **Circadian rhythms** (sometimes referred to as the biological clock) are the biological waxing and waning of alertness over the 24-hour day. Most people feel their most alert during the mid-morning, experience an energy dip in early afternoon (when some people take siestas or grab a second cup of coffee!), and then feel alert again in the early evening; later in the evening, as alertness wanes, sleep becomes more and more enticing. Although this is a general description of the ebb and flow of alertness throughout the day, it varies by individual, and circadian rhythms also vary with age. Newborns can spend two-thirds of a day asleep. Older adults tend to peak in the morning and decline as the day progresses, while adolescents and young adults tend to be more energetic in the mid-to-late evening.

A key factor in how sleep is regulated involves exposure to light, which stimulates a nerve pathway from the retina to the suprachiasmatic nucleus (SCN) in the hypothalamus. The SCN signals other parts of the brain, which regulate body temperature and control the production and release of hormones. The SCN is essentially our internal clock; it helps regulate the pattern of neurophysiological activities that affect the entire body. When exposed to light at the beginning of the day, our body temperature begins to rise and hormones (like cortisol) are released; these signals indicate that it is time to wake up.

Melatonin is a hormone made by the **pineal gland** in the brain. Darkness causes the SCN to signal the pineal gland to start producing and releasing melatonin. As melatonin levels rise, you begin to feel tired. Melatonin levels stay elevated throughout the night; the light of a new day causes melatonin levels to fall. Bright light both regulates the function of the SCN and directly inhibits the release of melatonin. Artificial indoor lighting can also sometimes be bright enough to prevent the release of melatonin (which is why some studies suggest that turning off mobile devices an hour before bedtime can improve your sleep!).

Core body temperature fluctuates between about 96.8° and 100.4°F over a 24-hour period, and this is also regulated by the hypothalamus. For most of us with normal circadian rhythms, sleep tends to occur when the core temperature is dropping at the end of the day. The average adult experiences their lowest core body temperature about two hours before waking time in the morning.

Dreaming

As mentioned earlier, the REM stage of sleep is when dreams typically occur. This stage is absolutely necessary. Missing REM sleep for one night results in an increase in REM sleep later to make up for it, called **REM rebound**. Some of the dreams during the REM stage can be exciting, including lucid dreams (in which one might be aware that one is dreaming and have some conscious control of the dreams). Most dreams are about daily events, like missing an exam, playing a sport, or talking to a friend. But why is it that we dream? Freud believed that the plotlines of dreams, or **manifest content**, were symbolic versions of underlying **latent content**, unconscious drives and wishes that are difficult to express. Thus, he believed that dreams are a way of understanding our inner conflicts. Other theories for why dreams exist have emerged since Freud. Some studies have found that dreaming can improve learning and problem-solving. It was found that brain regions used by rats to navigate a maze while they were awake were also active while the rats slept, as if the rats were running the maze in their dreams. When they woke, the rats demonstrated improved performance compared to both their previous performances and the performances of other rats that did not get REM sleep. The same is true for human performance on tasks. You may find that a night of consolidating information you've learned while studying for the MCAT is beneficial to retaining that information. The **activation-synthesis theory** suggests that dreams are byproducts of brain activation during REM sleep. This theory allows for the possibility that dreams are far from purposeful. Finally, some proponents have suggested that the purpose of dreams is to provide a template of consciousness on which the mind can practice consciousness-development.

Sleep Disorders

While there may be some debate as to the purpose of sleep, it cannot be disputed that sleep is necessary when we consider how debilitating sleep disorders can be. Sleep disorders can be subdivided into dyssomnias and parasomnias.

Dyssomnias are abnormalities in the amount, quality, or timing of sleep, and include insomnia, narcolepsy, and sleep apnea. **Insomnia** is the most common sleep disorder and is characterized by difficulty falling or staying asleep. Insomnia is not the occasional inability to fall asleep due to anxiety or excitement, but rather a persistent problem that can stem from chronic stress. Common quick treatments are sedatives such as sleeping pills, but these have a risk of dependency and overdose, and become less effective with time. They also create abnormal sleep cycles that include less time in REM and slow-wave stages, which can lead to drowsy carry-over effects. Natural alternatives include relaxation before bedtime, avoiding stimulants and exercise in the evening, and sleeping on a regular schedule. Those with **narcolepsy** experience periodic, overwhelming sleepiness during waking periods that usually last less than 5 minutes. They can occur without warning at dangerous times, such as while driving or walking down stairs. Recent research suggests that the cause of narcolepsy is a dysfunction in the region of the hypothalamus that produces the neurotransmitter hypocretin (also called orexin). Narcolepsy has been treated with stimulants with modest success. **Sleep apnea** is a disorder that causes people to intermittently stop breathing during sleep, which results in waking after a minute or so without air. This process can repeat hundreds of times a night, and can deprive sufferers of deep sleep. Those with sleep apnea may not even be aware that they have it, although their partners may be, as it can be accompanied by heavy snoring. The incidence of sleep apnea is associated with obesity.

Parasomnias are abnormal behaviors that occur during sleep and include somnambulism and night terrors. **Somnambulism** (or sleepwalking) tends to occur during slow-wave sleep (Stage 3), usually during the first third of the night. There may be genetic predispositions for sleepwalking and sleeptalking. **Night terrors** also usually occur during Stage 3 (unlike nightmares, which occur during REM sleep toward morning). A person experiencing a night terror may sit up or walk around, babble, and appear terrified, although none of this is recalled the next morning. Both of these disorders are more likely to appear in children.

Hypnosis and Meditation

Hypnotism has been portrayed in so many different ways in movies and other media that it is important to separate fact from fiction. **Hypnotism** is an interpersonal interaction in which a hypnotist has a subject focus attention on what is being said, relax and feel tired, "let go," and accept suggestions easily through the use of vivid imagination. Nearly everyone is hypnotizable to some extent, although some have a stronger capacity. Hypnotized people do NOT acquire superhuman physical abilities—this is a myth. Hypnotism can promote recall of some long-term memories by putting someone in a relaxed state, but a patient is also susceptible to constructing **false memories**—that is, using imagination to create inaccurate memories. It cannot help a patient remember events from infancy. Finally, hypnotism cannot force people to commit extreme acts against their will or moral code, such as commit murder. Studies show that the presence of the authoritative hypnotist equally influences hypnotized and non-hypnotized people to commit acts that are of similar danger levels.

This does not imply that hypnotized people are "faking it." In fact, posthypnotic suggestions have been utilized to help alleviate headaches, asthma, and stress-related skin disorders. In addition, 50% of people can gain some pain relief from hypnosis. Hypnosis works not by preventing sensory input, but by blocking attention to those sensory inputs. People may experience physiological states such as pain or a pounding heart, but are not consciously aware of these sensations. Some studies indicate that hypnotism results in changes in brain activity, insinuating that it is an actual altered state of consciousness (although this idea is controversial). There are two theories for how it works. The **dissociation theory** suggests that hypnotism is an extreme form of divided consciousness. In hypnosis, just as in everyday life, many behaviors occur on autopilot. Have you ever driven somewhere and not recalled anything about the actual drive? Thus, hypnotism may be an extended form of this normal dissociation in which the individual is on autopilot and the hypnotist takes over the executive control, which directs action. The **social influence theory** suggests that people do, and report, what's expected of them. They are not consciously faking it, but are like actors who get caught up in their roles and thus behave in ways that fit them.

Meditation refers to a variety of techniques, many of which have been practiced for thousands of years, and which usually involve the training of attention. Meditators may focus intensely on one object of attention, such as their breathing, or they may broaden their attention and be aware of multiple stimuli, such as anything in their auditory field. Meditation has been utilized successfully to manage pain, stress, and anxiety disorders. **Mindfulness-based stress reduction** (MBSR) is a protocol commonly used in the medical setting to help alleviate stress. Meditators have increased alpha and theta waves while they are meditating (and to some extent an increase above baseline after they stop), with more experienced meditators showing greater improvements.

Consciousness-Altering Drugs

There are three main categories of psychoactive drugs: depressants, stimulants, and hallucinogenics. All of these drugs work by altering actions at the neuronal synapses, either enhancing, dampening, or mimicking the activity of the brain's natural neurotransmitters.

Depressants include alcohol, barbiturates (tranquilizers), and opiates. They work by depressing, or slowing down, neural activity. When drinking alcohol, people are more likely to be impulsive and may appear hyperactive, but this is due to the slowing of brain activity related to judgment and inhibition in the frontal lobe. In larger doses, alcohol can lead to deterioration in skilled motor performance, decreased reaction time, and slurring of speech [which brain area is impacted when this occurs?[5]]. Excessive drinking can lead to memory blackouts for recent memories (those that have not been consolidated into long-term memory). Alcohol also suppresses REM sleep, which may contribute to the loss of short-term memory and less restful sleep the night of drinking. Thus, a heavy drinker may not remember what happened the night before when they wake up the next morning. While impaired motor control after drinking has caused countless vehicular deaths, an "overdose" of alcohol can also cause death by depressing the respiratory control centers in the medulla to the point that breathing ceases. Alcohol works by stimulating GABA and dopamine systems. GABA is an inhibitory neurotransmitter and is associated with reduced anxiety, while dopamine leads to the feeling of minor euphoria. Prolonged and excessive alcohol use can actually shrink the brain.

---

[5] The cerebellum, which is responsible for smoothing out motor commands from the primary motor cortex of the frontal lobe. The cerebellum controls precision, timing, coordination, and plays a role in muscle memory. The altered speech demonstrated with inebriation might lead you to believe that Broca's area is impaired; actually, slurred speech is the result of loss of motor control of the lips.

11.5

Both alcohol and **barbiturates** depress the sympathetic nervous system ("fight or flight") activity. Barbiturates are often prescribed as sleep aids. They are dangerous in combination with alcohol and prone to overdose—too much of a depressive effect can actually shut down life-sustaining organs. **Opiates**, which are derivatives of opium (including morphine and heroin), also depress neural functioning. They temporarily reduce pain by mimicking the brain's own pain relievers, neurotransmitters known as endorphins; pain is replaced with a blissful feeling. With prolonged use, the brain may stop producing endorphins, leading to a painful withdrawal from the drug.

Stimulants include caffeine, nicotine, cocaine, and amphetamines ("speed"). They typically work by either increasing the release of neurotransmitter, reducing the reuptake of neurotransmitter, or both. Their overall effect is to speed up body functions, resulting in increased energy, respiratory rate, heart rate, and pupil dilation. People use stimulants to stay awake, enhance physical performance, and boost mood. Cocaine works by causing a "rush," a release of the brain's supply of neurotransmitters including dopamine, serotonin, and norepinephrine. While this creates a brief period of intense pleasure, it is followed by a depressive crash. MDMA, also known as ecstasy, is a stimulant and a mild hallucinogen. It works by triggering the release of dopamine and serotonin, as well as by blocking the reabsorption of serotonin so that it stays in the synapse longer. It causes emotional elevation, but long-term effects include damage to serotonin-producing neurons. The resulting reduction in serotonin levels can cause a depressed mood.

Hallucinogens, also known as psychedelics, distort perceptions in the absence of any sensory input, creating hallucinations. These include LSD (lysergic acid diethylamide), mescaline, and, to a much lesser extent, marijuana. After taking LSD, a user may see vivid images and colors. The experience may peak with a feeling of being separated from one's body or experiencing imagined scenes as if they were reality. Emotions related to LSD can vary from euphoria to panic, depending on the person's mood and the context. Marijuana's active ingredient is THC, which affects functioning by stimulating cannabinoid receptors in the brain. It relaxes and disinhibits like alcohol, but it also acts as a hallucinogen by amplifying sensory perceptions including colors, sounds, tastes, and smells. Marijuana can also impair motor skills, reaction time, and judgment. Marijuana has been used medically to help with nausea and pain. Hallucinogens are thought to be the least addictive of the psychoactive drug classes.

Drug Addiction, Dependence, and Tolerance

The defining feature of drug addiction is a compulsion to use a drug repeatedly. Users can have psychological and/or physical dependence on drugs. A **psychological dependence** is often associated with the use of a drug in response to painful emotions related to depression, anxiety, or trauma. For example, an individual with social anxiety may feel compelled to drink alcohol excessively in order to lower anxiety at parties. Sometimes this dependence can be stopped by removing the individual from a painful situation. **Physical dependence** is evidenced by withdrawal. **Withdrawal** involves an uncomfortable and often physically painful experience without the use of a drug. This discomfort is alleviated when the user takes the drug, thus reinforcing further drug use. Alcohol withdrawal is especially dangerous—excessive users must be slowly detoxified, as stopping suddenly is life-threatening. Even caffeine addiction can cause withdrawal, with the user experiencing headache, fogginess, and irritability that end when more caffeine is taken.

Tolerance effects of drugs can vary. For example, alcohol abuse is associated with increased baseline blood pressure, potentially to dangerous levels. Alcohol is known to act as a stimulant for a brief period (up to two or three drinks) before depressant effects begin. Long-term abuse can lead an individual's intrinsic stress-reduction mechanisms to be debilitated. Caffeine, to take another example, is known to have acute effects, but does not change baseline measures such as blood pressure except at extreme doses above 600 mg.

Tolerance to caffeine will actually return an individual to baseline blood pressure after a period during which the individual demonstrates elevated levels. The effects of caffeine are therefore transient and reversible. Different drugs have different effects on baseline measures after tolerance.

11.6 LANGUAGE

One of the most characteristically *human* ways of interacting with the environment is to communicate using language. Indeed, our ability to learn and use language is often cited as the most defining human characteristic, that which distinguishes us from all the other animals. Even today, questions about what exactly language *is*, how it develops, and the role it plays in cognition remain important topics of debate and research.

Debates about these questions echo larger divisions in psychology. Behaviorists who argue that language is just another example of conditioned behavior are *empiricist* in their approach; they believe that the study of psychology should focus on directly observable environmental factors as opposed to abstract mental states. In contrast, nativists, who argue that language is a human ability prewired into the brain, are *rationalist* in their approach; they hold that certain ideas and capabilities cannot come from experience, and so must be innate. Still other researchers take a *materialist* approach to language and cognition, grounding their work in the belief that all discussion of "ideas," linguistic "expression," and the like is a set of convenient metaphors for real physical changes in the brain and actions of the body. Materialists believe that "only grey matter matters," and study thoughts and words by looking at what happens in the brain when people think, speak, write, and listen. In this section, we will define the ways these different schools of thought have explained how people learn language and how language relates to mental processes.

Theories of Language Development

Language acquisition is the term used by psychologists to refer to the way infants learn to understand and speak their native language (usually the language used by their parents). Language acquisition is the process of language learning in school or that of learning a foreign language. These other forms of language acquisition seem to work much differently.

B.F. Skinner's **behaviorist** model of language acquisition holds that infants are trained in language by operant conditioning (see Chapters 7 and 9 for more on behaviorism). Skinner argued that language use, though complex, is a form of behavior like any other, and so it is as subject to conditioning as a rat pulling a lever to receive a food pellet. Describing a beautiful sunset or persuading a friend to help you move obviously result in more complicated outcomes than receiving a food pellet after pulling a lever, but all three can be described as physical actions intended to produce effects (e.g., the production of sound using your vocal chords or the movement of your arm). How can learning to speak be analogous to learning other behaviors? Consider an infant babbling nonsense as its father repeats "bottle" while holding a bottle. By random chance, the baby will eventually make some noise like "bu-ba," at which point daddy will say "very good!" and smile delightedly before calling in mommy to praise their little genius. This positive reinforcement accomplishes two things: first, it conditions the infant to make the sound in association with the stimulus (the sight of the bottle), and second and more important, it encourages imitative behavior, so that the baby begins more regularly to copy the sounds made by the parent. This imitation is how the second, third, and five-hundredth words and phrases are learned progressively faster, as each subsequent "correct" utterance produces some reinforcing behavior like a hug or a piece of candy, whereas nonsense utterances achieve no reinforcement and are abandoned.

11.6

Linguist **Noam Chomsky** pointed out several major flaws with the application of behaviorism to language acquisition, and proposed an alternative to Skinner's model. Chomsky suggested that we all possess an innate feature unique to the human mind **(the language acquisition device)** that allows people to gain mastery of language from limited exposure during the sensitive developmental years in early childhood. This idea was later named "**universal grammar**" (UG). Chomsky's device was theoretical in that he provided no anatomical evidence for the exact location or structure of this device in the brain. However, research into the function of the device is empirical; linguists study UG by studying actual languages and actual cases of language acquisition. Their goal is to find the basic rules that apply to all or almost all languages and that are presumably innate in the brain, allowing the child to, for example, distinguish nouns, verbs, and adjectives without ever being taught these terms. It is important to note the distinction between language rules being prewired in the brain and language itself being hardwired: many songbirds, for example, are hatched knowing how to sing the territorial songs of their species, but no human is ever born knowing English or Mandarin. Rather, the theory states that humans have an innate ability to make grammatical distinctions and do so naturally when exposed to (not actively taught) language at a young age.

Influence of Language on Cognition

The relationship between language and cognition is still under debate. Some experts argue that language is first and foremost a social phenomenon, and that speech is not developmentally equivalent with thought. In other words, children first learn how to think and how to speak as separate enterprises, and only later is there overlap between the two. The first stage of acquiring language is immersion in "social speech," which is analogous to other social phenomena. This moves gradually into "egocentric speech" or "private speech," wherein children begin talking to themselves, experimenting with language as kind of thinking out loud. The final stage of language acquisition is "inner speech," the point at which a child's understanding of grammar and the relationship between words and objects is sufficiently advanced to allow him to think in words without mouthing them. This is a critical stage in the development of the relationship between language and thought. Prior to this point, speech and thought are separate activities, but at this point, some thought becomes "verbal," able to be expressed in words and clauses.

The **"linguistic relativity hypothesis"** asserts that not only do language and thought overlap, but cognition and perception are *determined* by the language one speaks. Unlike Chomsky's universal grammar, which emphasizes the commonality among all human languages, this hypothesis focuses on important distinctions among families of languages, such as Western European versus East Asian languages. Because of these distinctions, the argument goes, native speakers in these language groups conceptualize the world differently. The famous example is that Inuit peoples conceive of snow differently from English speakers, as evidenced by the fact that they have so many more words for snow. Subsequent research has called this "fact" into question, pointing out, for example, that Inuits do not have a very large number of words for snow compared to speakers of other languages and that skiers who speak different languages also have many different words in each to describe conditions of snow.

Different Brain Areas Control Language and Speech

Broca's area, located in the dominant hemisphere (usually left) of the frontal lobe of the brain, is involved in the complicated process of speech production. Broca's area was discovered when several people who had an injury to this area lost the ability to speak—a disorder now termed **Broca's aphasia**[6]. People with Broca's aphasia (also known as *expressive aphasia*) know what they want to say, but are unable to communicate it. They are typically able to comprehend words and simple sentences but are unable to generate fluent speech. Sometimes they can produce very simple, telegraphic speech ("Take. Car. Store."), or are limited to one or two words that they repeat over and over.

Wernicke's area, located in the posterior section of the temporal lobe in the dominant hemisphere of the brain (the left for most people), is involved in the comprehension of speech and written language. Wernicke's area was also discovered with the help of people with injuries to this area; in these individuals, speech production retains a natural sounding rhythm and syntax, but is completely meaningless. In other words, people with **Wernicke's aphasia** (also known as *receptive aphasia*) do not have a problem producing speech, but are incapable of producing intelligible, meaningful language. For example, someone with Wernicke's aphasia might say something like: "You know how go what moodle winkered and what you can't toodle doodle do so show him little litty round and cake you make more want to." A sentence such as this would be uttered with fluidity, with normal-sounding inflections. So, it would sound as though the person were merely speaking in an unknown language. As you might imagine, it is often difficult to decipher what the person is trying to communicate. People with Wernicke's aphasia usually have great difficulty understanding speech, and they are often unaware of their mistakes. Furthermore, these individuals usually have no body weakness or movement issues because their injury is not near the parts of the brain that control movement. Another type of aphasia, **conduction aphasia**, involves poor speech repetition despite intact comprehension and fluent speech.

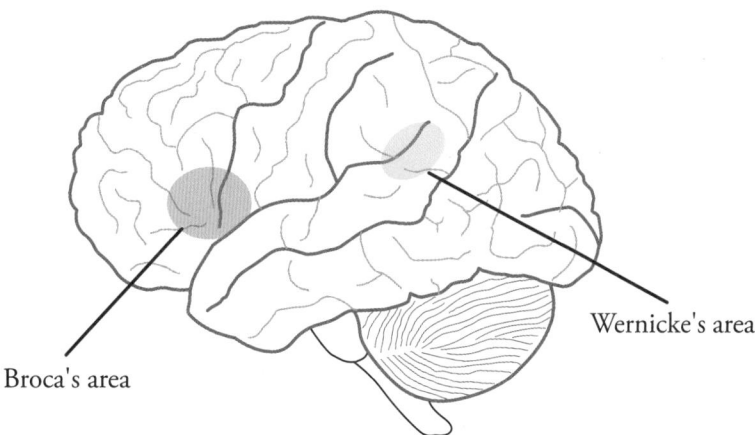

Figure 22   Approximate locations of Broca's area and Wernicke's area in the brain

---

[6]   From the Greek word aphatos meaning "speechlessness."

11.6

Chapter 11 Summary

- Humans have several types of receptors (mechanoreceptors, chemoreceptors, nociceptors, thermoceptors, electromagnetic receptors, and proprioceptors) that allow us to detect a variety of stimuli.

- Weber's law dictates that two stimuli must differ by a constant proportion in order for their difference to be perceptible.

- Gestalt psychology asserts that when humans perceive an object, rather than seeing lines, objects, colors, and shadows, they perceive the whole, not just the individual parts.

- The Broadbent filter model of selective attention proposes that all sensory input first enters a buffer, then is selectively filtered so that only some of the information is sent on for higher processing.

- Treisman's attenuation model proposed that rather than being filtered, sensory input is attenuated—turned up or turned down—before moving on to working memory.

- The resource model of attention asserts that there are limited resources for tasks in general.

- Baddeley's model of working memory considered working memory to have four components: a phonological loop, a visuospatial sketchpad, an episodic buffer, and a central executive (which oversees the process).

- Jean Piaget proposed a four-stage theory of cognitive development, which included: the sensorimotor stage, preoperational stage, concrete operations stage, and formal operations stage.

- Sleep progresses through four stages, each characterized by specific physiological differences.

- Broca's area is involved with speech production, while Wernicke's area is involved with speech comprehension.

CHAPTER 11 FREESTANDING PRACTICE QUESTIONS

1. Suppose that a researcher subliminally flashed words for negative and positive emotions (e.g., sad, happy) for a millisecond before showing subjects a neutral picture of people in a room. The words flashed so quickly that they were only perceived as a flash of light, but subjects were more likely to describe the scene in negative or positive terms (corresponding to the word that was flashed before the image), than subjects who did not see a subliminal word beforehand. What phenomenon does this describe?

   A) Primacy effect
   B) Priming
   C) Divided attention
   D) Episodic memory

2. If a two-year-old child repeatedly asks his mother for his favorite toy after it has been lost, what understanding has the child obtained, according to Piaget's theory of cognitive development?

   A) Schemas
   B) Conservation
   C) Object permanence
   D) Formal operations

3. The "candle problem" is a famous experiment whereby the subject is given a wax candle, a small cardboard box containing several thumbtacks, and a book of matches. The subject is asked to affix the candle to a corkboard so that wax will not drip onto the floor below. The only correct way to solve the task is to empty the box of thumbtacks, tack the box onto the corkboard, and light the candle and place it inside the box. Most subjects are unable to figure out the solution to this task, but if the thumbtacks are presented next to the box, not inside of it, they can solve the task easily. Why can't the subjects solve the task in the first scenario?

   A) They are bound by a mental set that does not comprehend how to light a candle in this way.
   B) They are unable to employ trial and error quickly enough to solve the task.
   C) They are overconfident about their own strategies for solving the task.
   D) They are unable to see alternative uses for the box containing the thumbtacks due to functional fixedness.

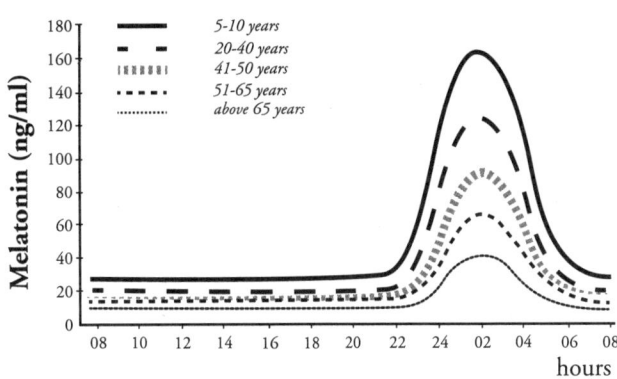

Figure 1 Average melatonin production (in ng/mL) over a 24-hour period by age group

4. A normal 15-year-old is participating in a sleep study and falls asleep at 10:30. This subject enters her first REM cycle at midnight. According to Figure 1 above, which of the following measures would most likely be recorded at midnight?

   I. Melatonin levels of 90 ng/mL
   II. Moderate to high EMG activity
   III. EEG measures that include theta waves and K-complexes

   A) I only
   B) III only
   C) I and III only
   D) I, II, and III

5. Alcohol withdrawal syndrome occurs when an individual with a dependence on alcohol suddenly limits or stops alcohol consumption. Symptoms of withdrawal can be very dangerous, including seizures, uncontrollable shaking of the extremities, and other nervous system issues. What is the most plausible mechanism of action for these physical symptoms?

   A) Chronic alcohol consumption causes down-regulation of GABA receptors, leading to a reduction in CNS inhibition, and excito-neurotoxicity.
   B) Long-term alcohol abuse stimulates the autonomic nervous system, causing tremors.
   C) Cessation of alcohol consumption leads to a reduction in dopamine production in the nucleus accumbens.
   D) Alcohol is a hallucinogenic, and withdrawal acts by relaxing, disinhibiting, and amplifying sensory information.

6. A patient recently admitted to the ER is reported to have had a stroke. At present, he is having some trouble communicating with hospital staff. When he addresses the doctor, he seems to have great difficulty forming sentences. His speech is rather monotone and lacks many function words. This patient is most likely experiencing:

A) somnambulism.
B) Wernicke's aphasia.
C) Broca's aphasia.
D) receptive aphasia.

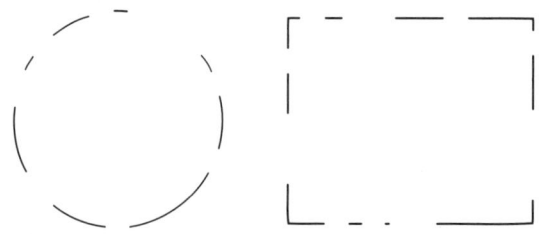

7. Instead of perceiving a series of lines in the figure above, humans perceive two shapes: a circle and a rectangle. What best accounts for this phenomenon?

A) The principles of Gestalt psychology
B) Bottom-up processing
C) Parallel processing
D) Weber's law

8. What structure in the middle ear generates vibrations that match the sound waves striking it?

A) Basilar membrane
B) Tympanic membrane
C) Cochlea
D) Malleus

9. In the human visual pathway, what cell type comprises the bundle of fibers called the optic nerve?

A) Photoreceptors
B) Bipolar cells
C) Ganglion cells
D) Fovea cells

10. After hearing a telephone number, one only has a few seconds to write it down before the information is lost. What aspect of Baddeley's information processing model accounts for this ability?

A) Phonological loop
B) Visuospatial sketchpad
C) Episodic buffer
D) Central executive

CHAPTER 11 PRACTICE PASSAGE

Guided meditation and deep-breathing exercises have long been used as effective techniques for stress reduction. The mechanism of action for this non-pharmacologic intervention is not entirely known, but scientists believe that the act of focusing ones thoughts and deep belly-breathing both serve to somehow inhibit the stress response activated by the hypothalamic-pituitary-adrenal axis. Practitioners of meditation are capable of reducing their heart and respiration rates seemingly on command.

Irritable Bowel Syndrome (IBS) is a disorder that causes a range of abdominal discomfort and bowel irregularities, but unlike bowel diseases with similar symptoms, there are no physical abnormalities; rather, the disorder appears to be the physical manifestation of psychological triggers. For example, IBS is often comorbid with anxiety disorders or episodes of extreme stress. Acute anxiety and stress are known triggers for IBS symptoms, which usually include severe abdominal cramping, bloating, gassiness, constipation and/or diarrhea (sometimes sufferers experience one or the other more frequently, and a minority of sufferers experience both in an alternating pattern). IBS symptoms usually begin during late teen or early adult years, and a majority of sufferers are women.

The current standard non-pharmacologic treatment for IBS is cognitive behavior therapy (CBT). CBT treats IBS sufferers by treating the emotional and psychological triggers that cause physical symptoms. A trained therapist uses a structured, goal-oriented plan to identify thought patterns and behaviors that trigger IBS symptoms, and provides patients with very specific tools for recognizing these, and also for implementing techniques to replace these negative thoughts and behaviors with more positive ones. In an attempt to determine if meditation is as beneficial as CBT for treating IBS, a recent six-month study was conducted on female IBS sufferers.

Eligible participants had active IBS symptoms for at least three months during the past year. Participants with and without a diagnosed anxiety disorder were recruited to participate in this study. Subjects were randomly assigned to one of three groups: a CBT group, a guided-meditation group, and a no-treatment group. Approximately 65% of the participants had an anxiety disorder, and these subjects were roughly equally represented in each of the three groups. The results of this study, measured by percent reduction of IBS symptoms after treatment, are summarized in Figure 1.

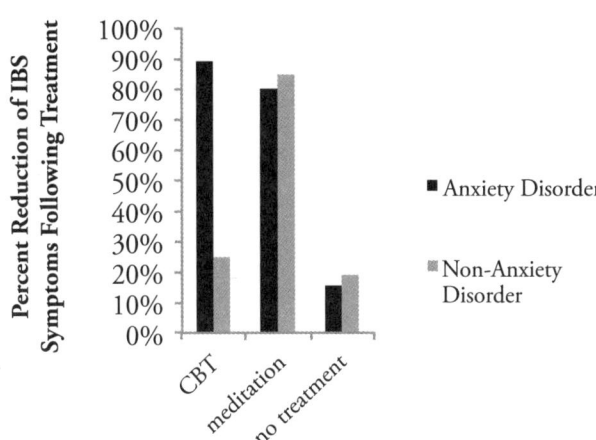

Figure 1   IBS symptom reduction for participants with and without anxiety disorders, by treatment condition

1. Based on the results of this study, what can be most reasonably concluded about the efficacy of CBT for IBS sufferers who do not have an anxiety disorder?

A) CBT is more effective than no treatment and more effective than meditation.
B) CBT and meditation combined provide the most effective treatment possible.
C) CBT is not as effective as meditation.
D) CBT is equally effective for IBS sufferers with and without anxiety disorders.

2. What is the role of the adrenal gland in the stress response?

A) The adrenal gland produces epinephrine and norepinephrine as part of the parasympathetic response to stressful triggers.
B) At the onset of a stressful event, the adrenal gland triggers a cascade of events in the hypothalamus and pituitary, resulting in activation of the sympathetic nervous system's "fight or flight" response.
C) The adrenal medulla produces cortisol, which helps regulate blood pressure and heart rate, in response to stress.
D) The adrenal medulla produces adrenaline in response to acute stressors and the adrenal cortex produces cortisol in response to longer-term, low-grade stressors.

3. The average individual diagnosed with IBS is a 40–50 year old female who is white, educated, married, and middle to upper-middle class. Based on this information, which of the following is most likely to be true about IBS?

A) IBS is underdiagnosed in less-affluent populations.
B) IBS rarely affects younger men and women.
C) There is a causal relationship between educational status and IBS.
D) Getting a divorce could be an effective treatment for married women who develop IBS.

4. Given the description of the study in this passage, which unknown factor might have the most influence on the validity of the results?

A) Sample size
B) Duration of IBS symptoms before entering the study
C) Participants' previous exposure to medication to treat IBS symptoms
D) Length of the treatment protocols

5. Suppose that a recent study, using advanced neuroimaging techniques, found increased activity in the anterior cingulate cortex during meditation. Given the types of physical responses to meditation described in the passage, what functions are likely associated with this area of the brain?

A) Sympathetic functions, including inhibition of the hypothalamus to prevent release of corticotropin releasing hormone (CRH)
B) Somatic functions, including control of the diaphragm
C) Autonomic functions, including heart rate and blood pressure
D) Rational cognitive functions, including decision-making

SOLUTIONS TO CHAPTER 11 FREESTANDING PRACTICE QUESTIONS

1. **B** The scenario in this question stem is describing priming, whereby subjects are provided with some sort of subliminal information (in this instance, the word for a negative or positive emotion) before another stimulus, and their response is impacted by the primed word (choice B is correct). The primacy effect refers to the phenomenon wherein people are more likely to recall the first information they hear or see, and less likely to recall later information (choice A is wrong). Divided attention refers to the ability to complete multiple tasks at once, and the ability to pay attention to one or both of those tasks; because the images were not flashed simultaneously, nor were the subjects even aware of the subliminal image, this scenario is not demonstrating divided attention (choice C is wrong). Episodic memory refers to the type of memory that would be encoded surrounding an event that is of personal significance; this scenario is not demonstrating episodic memory (choice D is wrong).

2. **C** A two-year-old is likely in the earliest stages of preoperational thought and has thus attained object permanence, the ability to understand that something still exists even if they cannot see it (choice C is correct). Schemas are mental frameworks for organizing concepts; while the child likely has a schema for "toy" that he fits his favorite toy into mentally, this does not describe why the child would ask for the toy after it is lost (choice A is wrong). Conservation (the ability to understand that quantity does not change despite a change in size or shape) is attained during the concrete operational stage (ages 7 to 11), and does not explain the described scenario (choice B is wrong). Formal operational thought occurs around age 12 (choice D is wrong).

3. **D** Functional fixedness is the inability to envision various possibilities for an object. In this scenario, when presented with a box of thumbtacks, the subjects do not see the box as a potential tool for solving the task, because they are fixed on the idea that the box is merely a tool for holding the thumbtacks (choice D is correct). A mental set is the tendency to focus on past solutions to a problem, even if they do not apply to the problem at hand; there is no evidence in the question stem that subjects are bound by a mental set (choice A is wrong). Similarly, there is no mention of a time constraint, and trial and error does not best describe what is happening in this scenario (choice B is wrong). There is no indication that overconfidence was a factor here either (choice C is wrong).

4. **A** Item I is true: according to Figure 1, 90 ng/mL of melatonin would be within the normal range for a 15-year-old at approximately midnight (choice B can be eliminated). Item II is false: during REM sleep, the brain stem inhibits movement, therefore EMG activity is very low or absent (choice D can be eliminated). Item III is false: theta waves and K-complexes are present during stage 2 sleep, but absent during REM sleep (choice C can be eliminated, and choice A is correct).

5. **A** Alcohol is a depressant (choice D is wrong) and inhibits neural activity. GABA receptors in the central nervous system respond to GABA, an inhibitory neurotransmitter. Alcohol acts on GABA receptors, inhibiting neuronal signaling. Chronic alcohol consumption causes a down-regulation of GABA receptors; therefore, once the artificial depressant (alcohol) is removed from the system, the CNS no longer has an inhibitory influence, and excito-neurotoxicity occurs, which can result in seizures and tremors (choice A is correct).

Alcohol is a depressant and does not stimulate the autonomic nervous system (choice B is wrong). While alcohol consumption does promote dopamine release in the nucleus accumbens (which stimulates the reward pathway in the brain and helps to explain why alcohol is addictive), and cessation of alcohol consumption would surely lead to a decrease in dopamine, this does not explain the physical symptoms of withdrawal described in the question stem (choice C is wrong).

6. **C**   Broca's aphasia is characterized by difficulty producing speech; moreover, inflection and function words (such as pronouns or prepositions) may disappear (choice C is correct). Somnambulism is sleepwalking, which is not typically a result of stroke and does not explain the patient's impairments described in the question stem (choice A is wrong). In cases of Wernicke's aphasia, speech is preserved; however, some words are substituted for others or used incorrectly. Utterances may seem confusing or nonsensical (choice B is wrong). Receptive aphasia is another term for Wernicke's aphasia (choice D is wrong; note also that there cannot be two correct answers).

7. **A**   Gestalt psychology proposes that humans tend to see objects in their entirety, and our visual processing systems and brain will superimpose larger organization or structure that makes holistic sense. The "shapes" are technically composed of a series of unconnected lines, but according to Gestalt psychologists, humans are more likely to use both top-down and bottom-up processing to perceive them as a complete circle or a complete rectangle (choice A is correct). Bottom-up processing begins with the sensory receptors and works up to the complex integration of information occurring in the brain; while bottom-up processing is a requirement of perceiving the lines in the figure, it does not explain why we see two shapes instead of a bunch of unconnected lines (choice B is wrong). Parallel processing refers to the fact that the brain is capable of processing multiple sensory inputs simultaneously and Weber's law explains how much two stimuli must differ in order for their difference to be perceptible; neither accounts for the phenomenon described in the question stem (choices C and D are wrong).

8. **B**   The tympanic membrane (also known as the eardrum), located in the middle ear, generates vibrations that match the sound waves striking it (choice B is correct). Vibrations generated in the tympanic membrane pass through three small bones—the malleus (the hammer), the incus (anvil), and the stapes (stirrup); these bones magnify the incoming vibrations by focusing them onto a structure known as the oval window (choice D is wrong). Once the vibrations pass through the oval window, they enter the cochlea, a fluid-filled spiral structure in the inner ear (choice C is wrong). The base of the cochlea is lined with a long, fluid-filled duct known as the basilar membrane (choice A is wrong). Sound waves passing along the basilar membrane cause it to move up and down, stimulating hair cells in the organ of Corti. These hair cells, in turn, connect with the acoustic, or auditory nerve.

9. **C**   The axons of ganglion cells in the retina make up the optic nerve, which carries visual information to the brain (choice C is correct). Photoreceptors are specialized cells in the retina that transduce light energy into nerve cell activity; they synapse with bipolar cells (which synapse with ganglion cells), but neither is part of the optic nerve (choices A and B are wrong). The fovea is the area of highest visual acuity and contains a high concentration of cones, which are a type of photoreceptor, and do not comprise the optic nerve (choice D is wrong).

10. **A** According to Alan Baddeley's information processing model, the phonological loop is the component of working memory that allows us to remember auditory information for a very brief amount of time before it is either processed or lost; therefore, this is the best explanation for why, after hearing a telephone number, we only have a few seconds to write it down before forgetting it (choice A is correct). The visuospatial sketchpad works similarly to the phonological loop, but is specific for visual, not auditory, information (choice B is wrong). The episodic buffer does not store auditory information for short periods of time (the phonological loop does), but rather allows information from the phonological loop and visuospatial sketchpad to interact, incorporates a temporal element to information, and communicates with long-term memory (choice C is wrong). The central executive is the overseer of the entire system, responsible for shifting and dividing attention; while the central executive is responsible for the ability to focus on the important information—the telephone number—it is not the part of the system that explains why this information decays so quickly if it isn't written down (choice D is wrong).

SOLUTIONS TO CHAPTER 11 PRACTICE PASSAGE

1. **C** According to Figure 1, CBT appears to be far less effective than meditation at reducing IBS symptoms for participants without an anxiety disorder (choice C is correct, and choice A is wrong). It is also far less effective for participants without an anxiety disorder than it is for participants with an anxiety disorder (choice D is wrong). CBT and meditation were not tested in combination (choice B can be eliminated).

2. **D** The adrenal glands are endocrine glands above the kidneys; in response to stress, they release hormones. The adrenal medulla (inner portion) produces epinephrine and norepinephrine (choice C is wrong) in response to direct input from the sympathetic nervous system (not the parasympathetic, choice A is wrong). This is the body's response to acute stress. The adrenal cortex (outer portion) produces corticosteroids, including cortisol; the amount of cortisol released increases as a result of long-term stress (choice D is correct). The hypothalamus and pituitary gland release hormones that trigger the release of hormones from the adrenal gland, not the other way around (choice B is wrong).

3. **A** Since the passage states at the end of the second paragraph that "IBS symptoms usually begin during late teen or early adult years," choice B is wrong, and we might conclude that these individuals are not being diagnosed because they are less affluent, and have perhaps less access to medical care (choice A is correct). In fact, many psychiatric illnesses and disorders are underdiagnosed in less affluent populations. Based solely on the information provided, you cannot conclude that there is a causal relationship between the listed factors and IBS (choice C is wrong), nor can you assume that any of these factors increase one's risk for developing IBS, such that eliminating one of the factors (marriage) will cause the IBS to go away (choice D is wrong). Correlation does not imply or prove causation.

4. **A** In statistics, validity refers to whether the results of a given study are able to answer the question being posed by that study. In the case of this study, the question is whether meditation is as effective as the current standard therapy (CBT) at reducing IBS symptoms for participants with and without an anxiety disorder. Based on the description provided in the passage, we do not know all of the specifics about this study, though we do know that the

study duration is six months (choice D is wrong). While we do not know the overall duration of IBS symptoms for participants, we do know that participants must have had active IBS for at least three months in the past year (choice B is wrong). Prior exposure to medication to treat IBS symptoms is of unknown importance, but the sample size of this study is definitely not known, and the results cannot prove that meditation is as effective as CBT without an appropriately large sample size (choice A is better than choice C).

5.   **C**   The first paragraph of the passage describes the physical responses to meditation as reduced heart rate and respiration rate. Thus, it is most likely that the anterior cingulate cortex plays a role in autonomic functions (in this case parasympathetic activity, so choice A is wrong, and choice C is correct), including the regulation of heart rate, resting respiratory rate, and blood pressure. While practitioners of meditation can reduce their respiratory rate, and while this might involve the somatic nervous system (the diaphragm is a skeletal muscle), this would not account for the reduction in heart rate (choice B is wrong). The anterior cingulate cortex is involved with rational cognitive functions, however this does not help to explain how activity in this area during meditation might inhibit the stress response (choice D is wrong).

Chapter 12
Biological Processes in the Brain

All human behavior has a biological foundation; psychological, sociological, and biological drivers influence how we perceive and respond to our environment. The ability to receive and process sensory information is dependent on several specialized cells, receptors, and biochemical pathways. The mechanisms of sensation can be understood largely from a biological perspective. The way we perceive, interpret, and respond to sensory information, however, can be infinitely more complex. It is important to keep a psychological, social, and cultural perspective in mind when understanding perception and behavior. This chapter covers the biological foundations of behavior, including the nervous system and endocrine system, as well as some of the genetic and environmental factors that play a role in behavior.

12.1 NEURONAL STRUCTURE AND FUNCTION

Neurons are specialized cells that transmit and process information from one part of the body to another. This information takes the form of electrochemical impulses known as **action potentials**. The action potential is a localized area of depolarization of the plasma membrane that travels in a wave-like manner along an axon. When an action potential reaches the end of an axon at a synapse, the signal is transformed into a chemical signal with the release of neurotransmitter into the synaptic cleft, a process called **synaptic transmission** (Section 12.2). The information of many synapses feeding into a neuron is integrated to determine whether that neuron will in turn fire an action potential. In this way, the action of many individual neurons is integrated to work together in the nervous system as a whole.

Structure of the Neuron

The basic functional and structural unit of the nervous system is the **neuron** (Figure 1). The structure of these cells is highly specialized to transmit and process **action potentials**, the electrochemical signals of the nervous system (Figure 3). Neurons have a central cell body, the **soma**, which contains the nucleus and is where most of the biosynthetic activity of the cell takes place. Slender projections, termed **axons** and **dendrites**, extend from the cell body. Neurons have only one axon (as long as a meter in some cases), but most possess many dendrites. Neurons with one dendrite are **bipolar neuron**; those with many dendrites are **multipolar neuron**. Neurons generally carry action potentials in one direction, with dendrites receiving signals and axons carrying action potentials away from the cell body. Axons can branch multiple times and terminate in **synaptic knobs** that form connections with target cells. When action potentials travel down an axon and reach the synaptic knob, chemical messengers are released and travel across a very small gap called the **synaptic cleft** to the target cell. The nature of the action potential and the transmission of signals across the synaptic cleft are key aspects of nervous system function. [In Figure 1, in what direction does an action potential travel in the axon shown?[1] What's the difference between a neuron and a nerve?[2]]

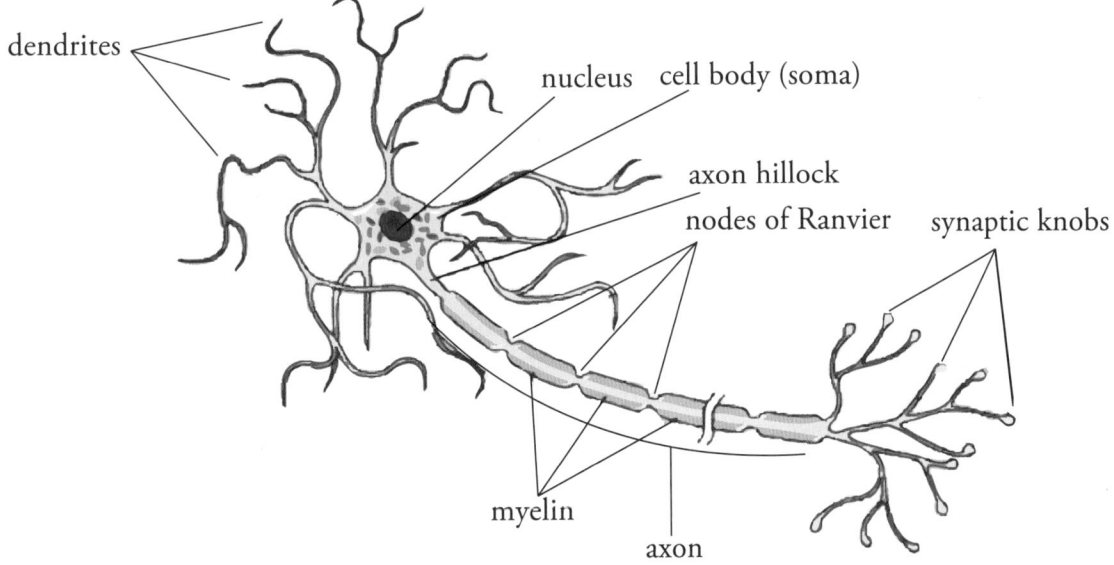

Figure 1 A multipolar neuron

---

[1] Action potentials travel from the cell body down the axon, or from left to right in Figure 1.

[2] A neuron is a single cell. A nerve is a large bundle of many different axons from different neurons.

The Action Potential

The Resting Membrane Potential

The **resting membrane potential** is an electric potential across the plasma membrane of approximately –70 millivolts (mV), with the interior of the cell negatively charged with respect to the exterior of the cell. Two primary membrane proteins are required to establish the resting membrane potential: the Na^+/K^+ ATPase and the potassium leak channels. The **Na^+/K^+ ATPase** pumps three sodium ions out of the cell and two potassium ions into the cell with the hydrolysis of one ATP molecule. The result is a sodium gradient with high sodium outside of the cell and a potassium gradient with high potassium inside the cell. **Leak channels** are channels that are open all the time and that simply allow ions to "leak" across the membrane according to their gradient. Potassium leak channels allow potassium, but no other ions, to flow down their gradient out of the cell. The combined loss of many positive ions through Na^+/K^+ ATPases and the potassium leak channels leaves the interior of the cell with a net negative charge, approximately 70 mV more negative than the exterior of the cell; this difference is the resting membrane potential. Note that there are very few sodium leak channels in the membrane (the ratio of K^+ leak channels to Na^+ leak channels is about 100:1), so the cell membrane is virtually impermeable to sodium.

The resting membrane potential establishes a negative charge along the interior of axons (along with the rest of the neuronal interior). Thus, the cells can be described as **polarized**: negative on the inside and positive on the outside. An action potential is a disturbance in this membrane potential, a wave of **depolarization** of the plasma membrane that travels along an axon. Depolarization is a change in the membrane potential from the resting membrane potential of approximately –70 mV to a less negative, or even positive, potential. After depolarization, **repolarization** returns the membrane potential to normal. The change in membrane potential during passage of an action potential is caused by movement of ions into and out of the neuron through ion channels. The action potential is therefore not strictly an electrical impulse, like electrons moving in a copper telephone wire, but an electro*chemical* impulse.

Depolarization

Key proteins in the propagation of action potentials are the **voltage-gated sodium channels** located in the plasma membrane of the axon. In response to a change in the membrane potential, these ion channels open to allow sodium ions to flow down their gradient into the cell and depolarize that section of membrane. These channels are opened by depolarization of the membrane from the resting potential of –70 mV to a **threshold potential** of approximately –50 mV. Once this threshold is reached, the channels are opened fully, but below the threshold, they are closed and do not allow the passage of any ions through the channel. When the channels open, sodium flows into the cell, down its concentration gradient, depolarizing that section of the membrane to about +35 mV before inactivating. Some of the sodium ions flow down the interior of the axon, slightly depolarizing the neighboring section of membrane. When the depolarization in the next section of membrane reaches threshold, those voltage-gated sodium channels open as well, passing the depolarization down the axon (Figure 2).

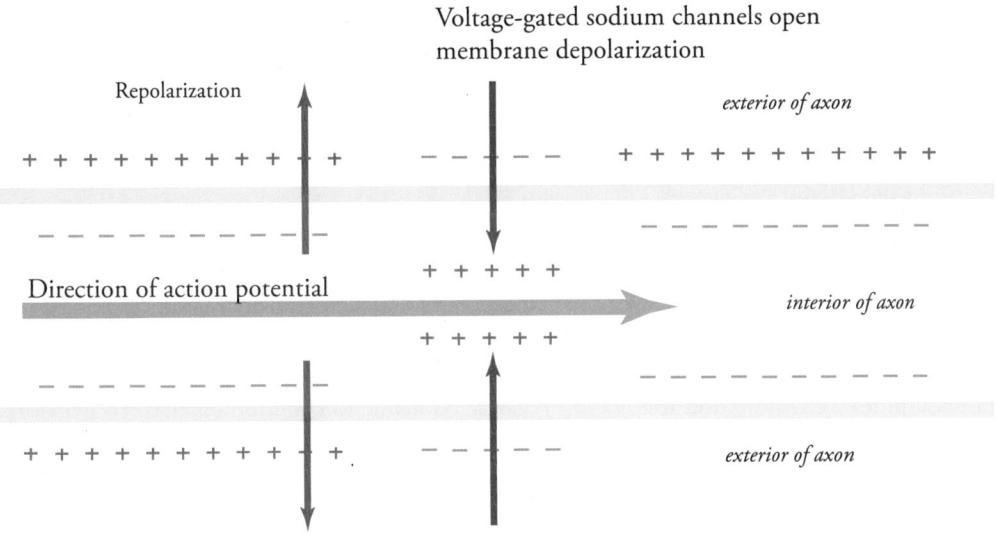

Figure 2   The action potential is a wave of membrane depolarization

Repolarization

With the opening of voltage-gated sodium channels, sodium flows into the cell and depolarizes the membrane to positive values. As the wave of depolarization passes through a region of membrane, the membrane does not remain depolarized (Figure 3).

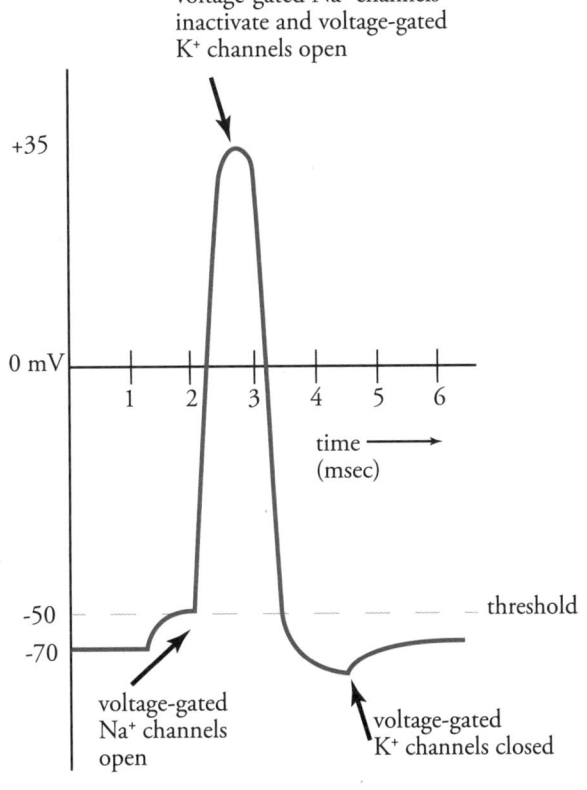

Figure 3   The action potential at a single location

After depolarization, the membrane is **repolarized**, re-establishing the original resting membrane potential. A number of factors combine to produce this effect:

1) Voltage-gated sodium channels inactivate very quickly after they open, shutting off the flow of sodium into the cell. The channels remain **inactivated** until the membrane potential nears resting values again.

2) Voltage-gated potassium channels open more slowly than the voltage-gated sodium channels and stay open longer. Voltage-gated potassium channels open in response to membrane depolarization. As potassium leaves the cell down its concentration gradient, the membrane potential returns to negative values, actually overshooting the resting potential by about 20 mV (to about −90 mV). At this point, the voltage-gated potassium channels close.

3) Potassium leak channels and the Na⁺/K⁺ ATPase continue to function (as they always do) to bring the membrane back to resting potential. These factors alone would repolarize the membrane potential even without the voltage-gated potassium channels, but it would take a lot longer.

Saltatory Conduction

The axons of many neurons are wrapped in an insulating sheath called **myelin** (Figure 4). The myelin sheath is not created by the neuron itself, but by cells called **Schwann cells**, a type of glial cell, that exist in conjunction with neurons, wrapping layers of specialized membrane around the axons. Note that Schwann cells are found in the peripheral nervous system (PNS). In the central nervous system (CNS), myelination of axons is accomplished via similar cells called oligodendrocytes. No ions can enter or exit a neuron where the axonal membrane is covered with myelin. There is no membrane depolarization and no voltage-gated sodium channels in regions of the axonal plasma membrane that are wrapped in myelin. There are periodic gaps in the myelin sheath, however, called **nodes of Ranvier** (Figures 1, 4, and 5). Voltage-gated sodium and potassium channels are concentrated in the nodes of Ranvier in myelinated axons. Rather than impeding action potentials, the myelin sheath dramatically speeds the movement of action potentials by forcing the action potential to jump from node to node. This rapid jumping conduction in myelinated axons is termed **saltatory conduction**.

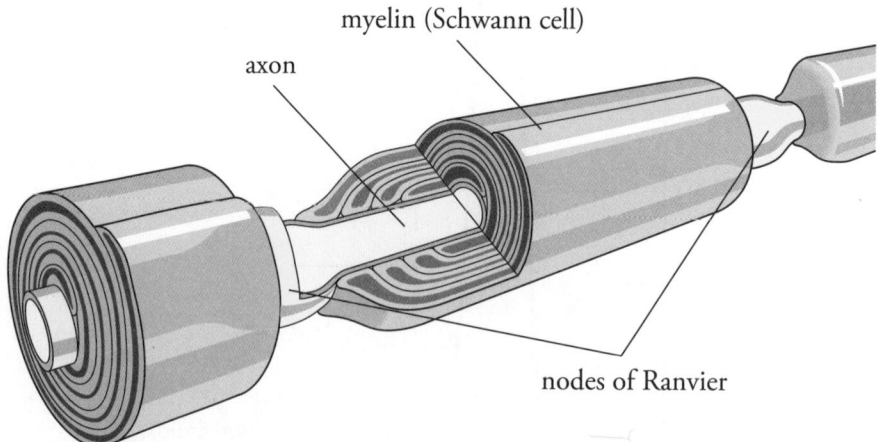

myelin (Schwann cell)

axon

nodes of Ranvier

Figure 4 A Schwann cell wrapping an axon with myelin

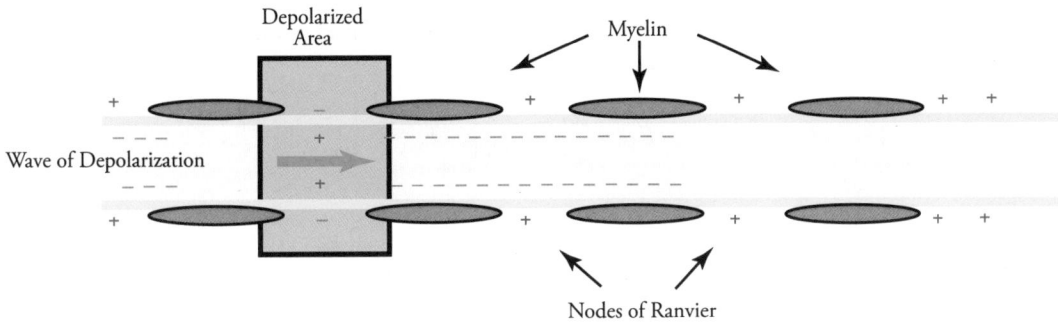

Figure 5 Propagation of the AP in a myelinated axon (cross section)

Glial Cells

As mentioned above, the myelin sheath is formed by a type of glial cell called a Schwann cell. However, Schwann cells are not the only type of glial cell. **Glial cells** are specialized, non-neuronal cells that typically provide structural and metabolic support to neurons (Table 1). Glia maintain a resting membrane potential but do not generate action potentials.

Table 1 Types of Glial Cells and Their Functions

Cell Type	Location	Primary Functions
Schwann cells	PNS	Form myelin—increase speed of conduction of APs along axon
Oligodendrocytes	CNS	Form myelin—increase speed of conduction of APs along axon
Astrocytes	CNS	Guide neuronal development Regulate synaptic communication via regulation of neurotransmitter levels
Microglia	CNS	Remove dead cells and debris
Ependymal cells	CNS	Produce and circulate cerebrospinal fluid

Equilibrium Potentials

During the action potential, the movement of Na^+ and K^+ ions across the membrane through the voltage-gated channels is *passive*; driven by gradients. The **equilibrium potential** is the membrane potential at which this driving force (the gradient) does not exist; in other words, there would be no net movement of ions across the membrane. Note that the equilibrium potential is specific for a particular ion. For example, the Na^+ equilibrium potential is *positive*, approximately +50 mV. Na^+ ions are driven inward by their concentration gradient. However, if the interior of the cell is too positive, the positively-charged ions are repelled; in other words, the *electrical* gradient would drive sodium *out*. These forces, the chemical gradient driving sodium in and the electrical gradient driving sodium out, balance each other at about +50 mV, so this is the equilibrium potential for Na^+.

K^+, however, has a *negative* equilibrium potential. K^+ ions are driven outward by their concentration gradient. However, if the interior of the cell is too negative, the positively-charged ions cannot escape the attraction; the electrical gradient drives potassium *in*. The chemical gradient driving potassium out and the electrical gradient driving potassium in balance each other at about –90 mV, so this is the equilibrium potential for K^+.

The equilibrium potential for any ion is based on the electrochemical gradient for that ion across the membrane, and can be predicted by the **Nernst equation**:

$$E_{ion} = \frac{RT}{zF} \ln \frac{[X]_{outside}}{[X]_{inside}}$$

where E_{ion} is the equilibrium potential for the ion, R is the universal gas constant, T is the temperature (in Kelvin), z is the valence of the ion, F is Faraday's constant, and $[X]$ is the concentration of the ion on each side of the plasma membrane. Note that the relative concentrations of the ion on each side of the membrane create the *chemical* gradient, while the valence (charge of the ion) helps determine the *electrical* gradient.

Note that the fact that the resting membrane potential is –70 mV reflects both the differences in the equilibrium potentials for Na^+ and K^+, and also the relative numbers of leak channels for these two ions. If the cell were completely permeable to K^+, the resting potential would be about –90 mV. The fact that the resting potential is *very close* to the K^+ equilibrium potential indicates that there are a large number of K^+ leak channels in the membrane; the cell at rest is almost completely permeable to potassium. However, the resting potential is slightly more positive than –90 mV, indicating that there are a few Na^+ leak channels allowing Na^+ in. There are not very many Na^+ leak channels, though, otherwise the resting potential would be much more positive—closer to the Na^+ equilibrium potential. (This is in fact what we see when the cell *does* become completely permeable to Na^+ at the beginning of the action potential; the membrane potential shoots upward to +35 mV.)

The Refractory Period

Action potentials can pass through a neuron extremely rapidly, thousands each second, but there is an upper limit to how soon a neuron can conduct an action potential after another has passed. The passage of one action potential makes the neuron nonresponsive to membrane depolarization and unable to transmit another action potential, or **refractory**, for a short period of time. There are two phases of the refractory period, caused by two different factors. During the **absolute refractory period**, a neuron will not fire another action potential no matter how strong a membrane depolarization is induced. During this time, the voltage-gated sodium channels have been *inactivated* (not the same as *closed*) after depolarization. They will not be able to be opened again until the membrane potential reaches the resting potential and the Na^+ channels have returned to their "closed" state. During the **relative refractory period**, a neuron can be induced to transmit an action potential, but the depolarization required is greater than normal because the membrane is **hyperpolarized**. When repolarization occurs, there is a brief period in which the membrane potential is more negative than the resting potential (Figure 3), caused by voltage-gated potassium channels that have not closed yet. Because it is further from threshold, a greater stimulus is required to open the voltage-gated sodium channels to start an action potential.

12.2 SYNAPTIC TRANSMISSION

A **synapse** is a junction between the axon terminus of a neuron and the dendrites, soma, or axon of a second neuron. It can also be a junction between the axon terminus of a neuron and an organ. There are two types of synapses: electrical and chemical. **Electrical synapses** occur when the cytoplasms of two cells are joined by gap junctions. If two cells are joined by an electrical synapse, an action potential will spread directly from one cell to the other. Electrical synapses are not common in the nervous system, although they are quite important in propagating action potentials in smooth muscle and cardiac muscle. In the nervous system, **chemical synapses** are found at the ends of axons where they meet their target cell; here, an action potential is converted into a chemical signal. The following steps are involved in the transmission of a signal across a chemical synapse in the nervous system (Figure 6), as well as at the junctions of neurons with other cell types, such as skeletal muscle cells:

1) An action potential reaches the end of an axon, the synaptic knob.
2) Depolarization of the presynaptic membrane opens voltage-gated calcium channels.
3) Calcium influx into the presynaptic cell causes exocytosis of neurotransmitter stored in secretory vesicles.
4) Neurotransmitter molecules diffuse across the narrow synaptic cleft (small space between cells).
5) Neurotransmitter binds to receptor proteins in the postsynaptic membrane. These receptors are ligand-gated ion channels.
6) The opening of these ion channels in the postsynaptic cell alters the membrane polarization.
7) If the membrane depolarization of the postsynaptic cell reaches the threshold of voltage-gated sodium channels, an action potential is initiated.
8) Neurotransmitter in the synaptic cleft is degraded and/or removed to terminate the signal.

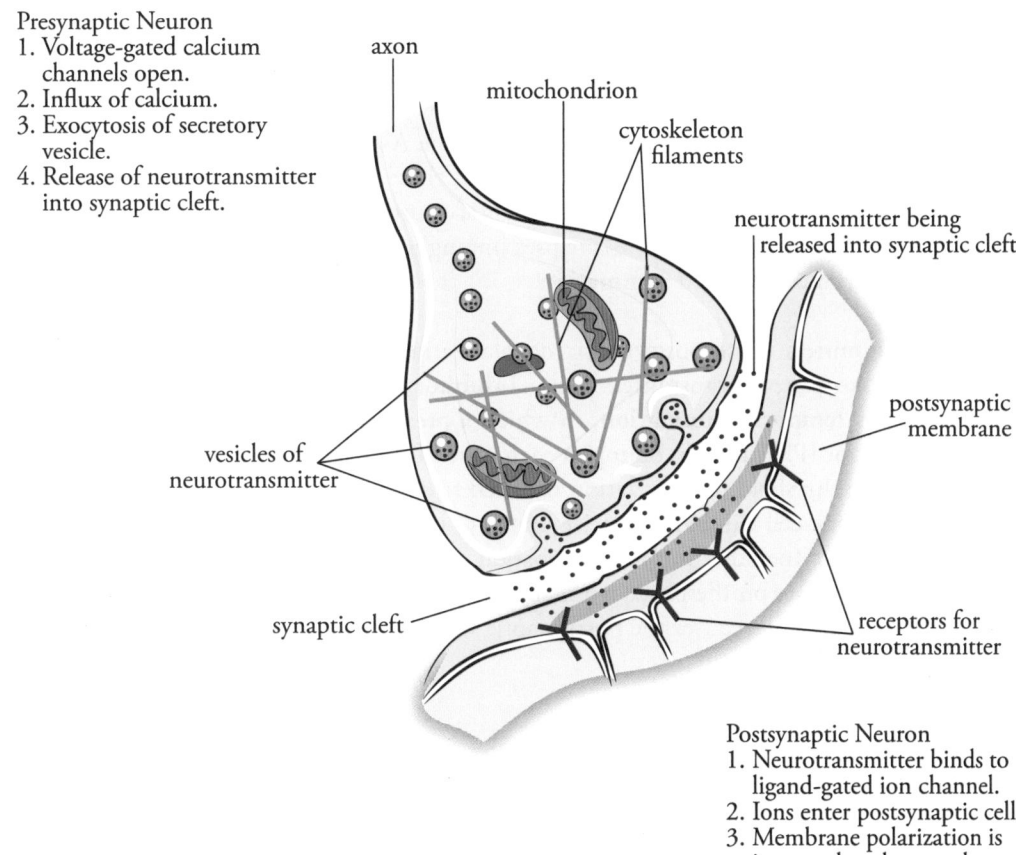

Figure 6 A typical synapse

An example of a chemical synapse that is commonly used is the **neuromuscular junction** between neurons and skeletal muscle. The neurotransmitter that is released at the neuromuscular junction is **acetylcholine (ACh)**. When an action potential reaches such a synapse, acetylcholine is released into the synaptic cleft. The acetylcholine binds to the acetylcholine receptor on the surface of the postsynaptic cell membrane. When acetylcholine binds to its receptor, the receptor opens its associated sodium channel, allowing sodium to flow down a gradient into the cell, depolarizing the postsynaptic cell membrane. Meanwhile, acetylcholine in the synaptic cleft is degraded by the enzyme **acetylcholinesterase (AChE)**.

There are several different neurotransmitters and neurotransmitter receptors. Some of the other neurotransmitters are **gamma-aminobutyric acid (GABA)**, **serotonin**, **dopamine**, and **norepinephrine**. If a neurotransmitter, such as acetylcholine, opens a channel that depolarizes the postsynaptic membrane, the neurotransmitter is termed **excitatory**. Other neurotransmitters, however, have the opposite effect, making the postsynaptic membrane potential more negative than the resting potential, or hyperpolarized. Neurotransmitters that induce hyperpolarization of the postsynaptic membrane are termed **inhibitory.** (Note, however, that ultimately it is not the *neurotransmitter* that determines the effect on the postsynaptic cell, it is the *receptor* for that neurotransmitter and its associated ion channel. The same neurotransmitter can be excitatory in some cases and inhibitory in others.) Postsynaptic neurons may have many different receptors, allowing them to respond to many different neurotransmitters.

Summation

Once an action potential is initiated in a neuron, it will propagate to the end of the axon at a speed and magnitude of depolarization that do not vary from one action potential to another. The action potential is an "**all-or-nothing**" event. The key-regulated step in the nervous system is whether or not a neuron will fire an action potential. Action potentials are initiated when the postsynaptic membrane reaches the threshold depolarization (about −50 mV) required to open voltage-gated sodium channels. The postsynaptic depolarization caused by the release of neurotransmitter by one action potential at one synapse is not generally sufficient to induce this degree of depolarization. A postsynaptic neuron has many different neurons with synapses leading to it, however, and each of these synapses can release neurotransmitters many times per second. The "decision" by a postsynaptic neuron whether to fire an action potential is determined by adding the effect of all of the synapses impinging on a neuron, both excitatory and inhibitory. This addition of stimuli is termed **summation**.

Excitatory neurotransmitters cause postsynaptic depolarization, or **excitatory postsynaptic potentials (EPSPs)**, while inhibitory neurotransmitters cause **inhibitory postsynaptic potentials (IPSPs)**. One form of summation is **temporal summation**, in which a presynaptic neuron fires action potentials so rapidly that the EPSPs or IPSPs pile up on top of each other. If they are EPSPs, the additive effect might be enough to reach the threshold depolarization required to start a postsynaptic action potential. If they are IPSPs, the postsynaptic cell will hyperpolarize, moving further and further away from threshold, effectively becoming inhibited. The other form of summation is **spatial summation**, in which the EPSPs and IPSPs from all of the synapses on the postsynaptic membrane are summed at a given moment in time. If the total of all EPSPs and IPSPs causes the postsynaptic membrane to reach the threshold voltage, an action potential will be fired.

12.3 FUNCTIONAL ORGANIZATION OF THE HUMAN NERVOUS SYSTEM

The nervous system must receive information, decide what to do with it, and cause muscles or glands to act upon that decision. Receiving information is the **sensory** function of the nervous system (carried out by the peripheral nervous system, or **PNS**), processing the information is the **integrative** function (carried out by the central nervous system, or **CNS**), and acting on it is the **motor** function (also carried out by the PNS). **Motor neurons** carry information from the nervous system toward organs which can act upon that information, known as **effectors**. Notice that "motor" neurons do not lead only "to muscle." Motor neurons, which carry information away from the central nervous system and innervate effectors, are called **efferent** neurons (remember, efferents go to effectors). **Sensory neurons**, which carry information toward the central nervous system, are called **afferent** neurons.

Reflexes

The simplest example of nervous system activity is the **reflex**. This is a direct motor response to sensory input which occurs without conscious thought. In fact, it usually occurs without any involvement of the brain at all. In the simplest example, a sensory neuron transmits an action potential to a synapse with a motor neuron in the spinal cord, which causes an action to occur. For example, in the **muscle stretch reflex**, a sensory neuron detects stretching of a muscle (Figure 7). The sensory neuron has a long dendrite and a long axon, which transmits an impulse to a motor neuron cell body in the spinal cord. The motor neuron's long axon synapses with the muscle that was stretched and causes it to contract. That is why the quadriceps (thigh) muscle contracts when the patellar tendon is stretched by tapping it with a reflex hammer. A reflex such as this one, involving only two neurons and one synapse, is known as a **monosynaptic reflex arc.**

Something else also happens when a physician taps the patellar tendon. Not only does the quadriceps *contract*, but the hamstring also *relaxes*. If it did not, the leg would not be able to extend (straighten). The sensory neuron (that detects stretch) synapses with not only a motor neuron for the quadriceps, but also with an **inhibitory interneuron**. This is a short neuron which forms an inhibitory synapse with a motor neuron innervating the hamstring muscle. When the sensory neuron is stimulated by stretch, it stimulates both the quadriceps motor neuron and the inhibitory interneuron to the hamstring motor neuron. The interneuron inhibits the motor neuron for the hamstring. As a result, the quadriceps contracts and the hamstring relaxes (note that the hamstring part of the reflex—sensory neuron to interneuron to hamstring motor neuron—involves three neurons and two synapses, hence it is known as a **disynaptic reflex arc**). An interneuron is the simplest example of the integrative role of the nervous system. Concurrent relaxation of the hamstring and contraction of the quadriceps is an example of **reciprocal inhibition**.

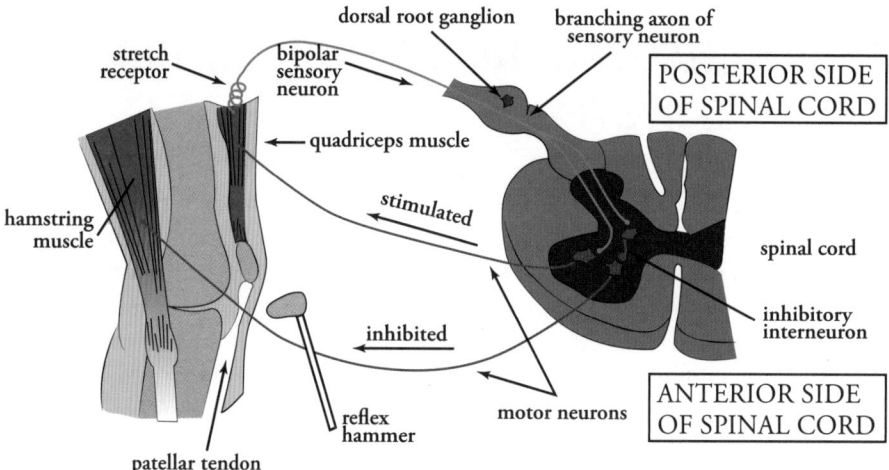

Figure 7 The muscle stretch reflex

Large-Scale Functional Organization

The peripheral nervous system can be subdivided into several functional divisions (Figure 8). The portion of this system concerned with conscious sensation and deliberate, voluntary movement of skeletal muscle is the **somatic** division. The portion concerned with digestion, metabolism, circulation, perspiration, and other involuntary processes is the **autonomic** division. The somatic and autonomic divisions both include afferent and efferent functions, although the sources of sensory input and the target of efferent nerves are different. The efferent portion of the autonomic division is further split into two subdivisions: **sympathetic** and **parasympathetic**. When the sympathetic system is activated, the body is prepared for "fight or flight." When the parasympathetic system is activated, the body is prepared to "rest and digest." Table 2 summarizes the main effects of the autonomic system. Notice that many sympathetic effects result from release of epinephrine into the bloodstream by the adrenal medulla. The parasympathetic system prepares you to rest and digest food.

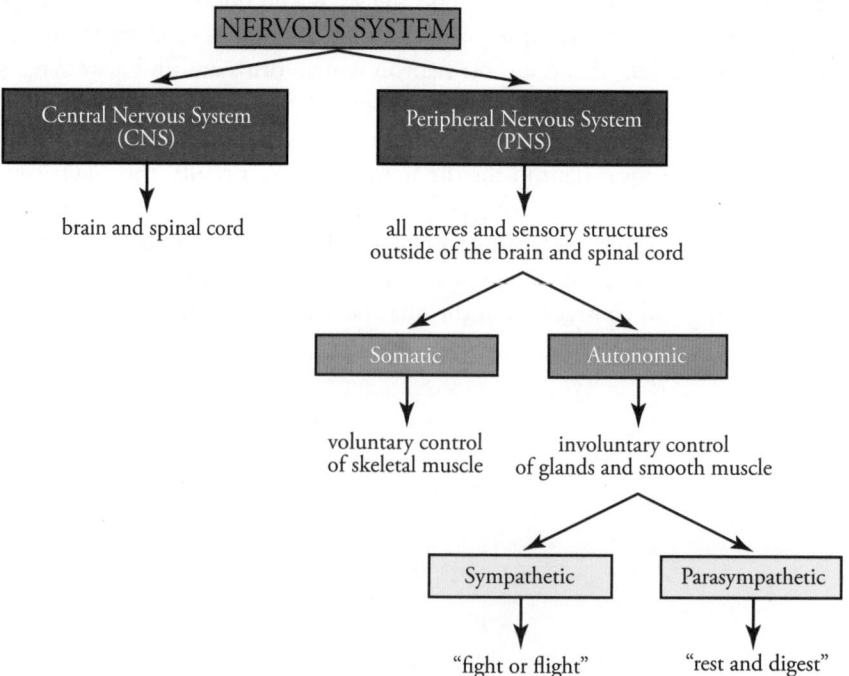

Figure 8 Overall organization of the nervous system

Table 2 Effects of the Autonomic Nervous System

Organ or System	Parasympathetic: rest and digest	Sympathetic: fight or flight
digestive system: glands	stimulation	inhibition
motility	stimulation (stimulates digestion)	inhibition (inhibits digestion)
sphincters	relaxation	contraction
urinary system: bladder	contraction (stimulates urination)	relaxation (inhibits urination)
urethral sphincter	relaxation (stimulates urination)	contraction (inhibits urination)
bronchial smooth muscle	constriction (closes airways)	relaxation (opens airways)
cardiovascular system: heart rate and contractility	decreased	increased
blood flow to skeletal muscle	—	increased
skin	—	sweating and general vasoconstriction; emotional vasodilation (blushing)
eye: pupil	constriction	dilation
muscles controlling lens	near vision accommodation	accommodation for far vision
adrenal medulla	—	release of epinephrine
genitals	erection / lubrication	ejaculation / orgasm

PNS Anatomical Organization

All neurons entering and exiting the CNS are carried by 12 pairs of **cranial nerves** and 31 pairs of **spinal nerves**. Cranial nerves convey sensory and motor information to and from the brainstem. Spinal nerves convey sensory and motor information to and from the spinal cord. The different functional divisions of the nervous system have different anatomical organizations (Figure 9).

The **vagus nerve** is an important example of a cranial nerve, and one that you should be familiar with for the MCAT. The effects of this nerve upon the heart and GI tract are to decrease the heart rate and increase GI activity; as such, it is part of the *parasympathetic division* of the autonomic nervous system. It is a bundle of axons that end in ganglia on the surface of the heart, stomach, and other visceral organs. The many axons constituting the vagus nerve are preganglionic and come from cell bodies located in the CNS. On the surface of the heart and stomach they synapse with postganglionic neurons. The detailed terminology in this paragraph will make more sense to you as you read through the next couple of sections.

Somatic PNS Anatomy

The somatic system has a simple organization:

- *All* somatic motor neurons innervate skeletal muscle cells, use ACh as their neurotransmitter, and have their cell bodies in the brain stem or the ventral (front) portion of the spinal cord.

- *All* somatic sensory neurons have a long dendrite extending from a sensory receptor toward the soma, which is located just outside the CNS in a **dorsal root ganglion**. The dorsal root ganglion is a bunch of somatic (and autonomic) sensory neuron cell bodies located just dorsal to (to the back of) the spinal cord. There is a pair of dorsal root ganglia for every segment of the spinal cord, and thus the dorsal root ganglia form a chain along the dorsal (back) aspect of the vertebral column. The dorsal root ganglia are protected within the vertebral column but are outside the **meninges** (protective sheath of the brain and cord) and thus outside the CNS. An axon extends from the somatic sensory neuron's soma into the spinal cord. In all somatic sensory neurons, the first synapse is in the CNS; depending on the type of sensory information conveyed, the axon either synapses in the cord, or stretches all the way up to the brain stem before its first synapse!

Autonomic PNS Anatomy

Anatomical organization of autonomic efferents is a bit more complex. The efferents of the sympathetic and parasympathetic systems consist of two neurons: a preganglionic and a postganglionic neuron. The **preganglionic neuron** has its cell body in the brainstem or spinal cord. It sends an axon to an autonomic ganglion, located outside the spinal column. In the ganglion, this axon synapses with a **postganglionic neuron**. The postganglionic neuron sends an axon to an effector (smooth muscle or gland). *All* autonomic preganglionic neurons release acetylcholine as their neurotransmitter. *All* parasympathetic postganglionic neurons also release acetylcholine. Nearly all sympathetic postganglionic neurons release norepinephrine (NE, also known as noradrenaline) as their neurotransmitter.

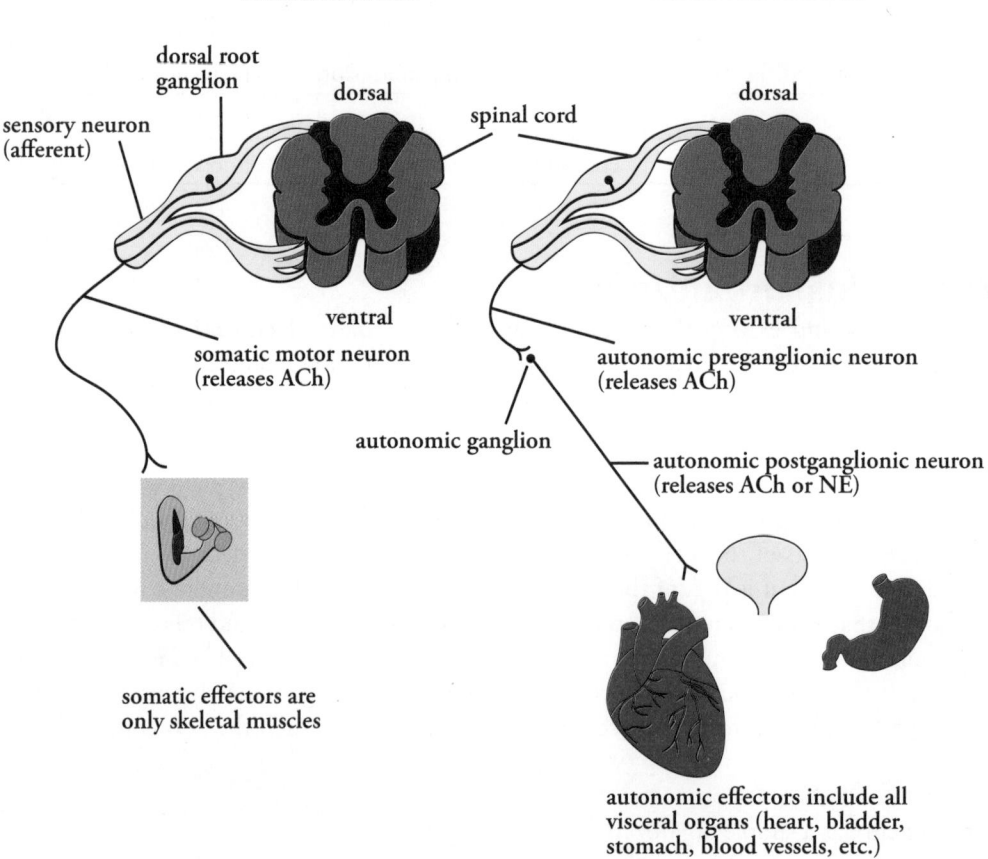

Figure 9   Anatomical organization of PNS efferents

All sympathetic preganglionic efferent neurons have their cell bodies in the thoracic (chest) or lumbar (lower back) regions of the spinal cord. Hence, the sympathetic system is also referred to as the *thoraco-lumbar system*. The parasympathetic system is known as the *craniosacral system*, because all of its preganglionic neurons have cell bodies in the brainstem (which is in the head or cranium) or in the lowest portion of the spinal cord, the sacral portion. In the sympathetic system, the preganglionic axon is relatively short, and there are only a few ganglia; these sympathetic ganglia are quite large. The sympathetic postganglionic cell sends a long axon to the effector. In contrast, the parasympathetic preganglionic neuron sends a long axon to a small ganglion which is close to the effector. For example, parasympathetic ganglia controlling the intestines are located on the outer wall of the gut. The parasympathetic postganglionic neuron has a very short axon, since the cell body is close to the target. These differences are visualized in Figure 10 and summarized in Table 3.

Autonomic Nervous System

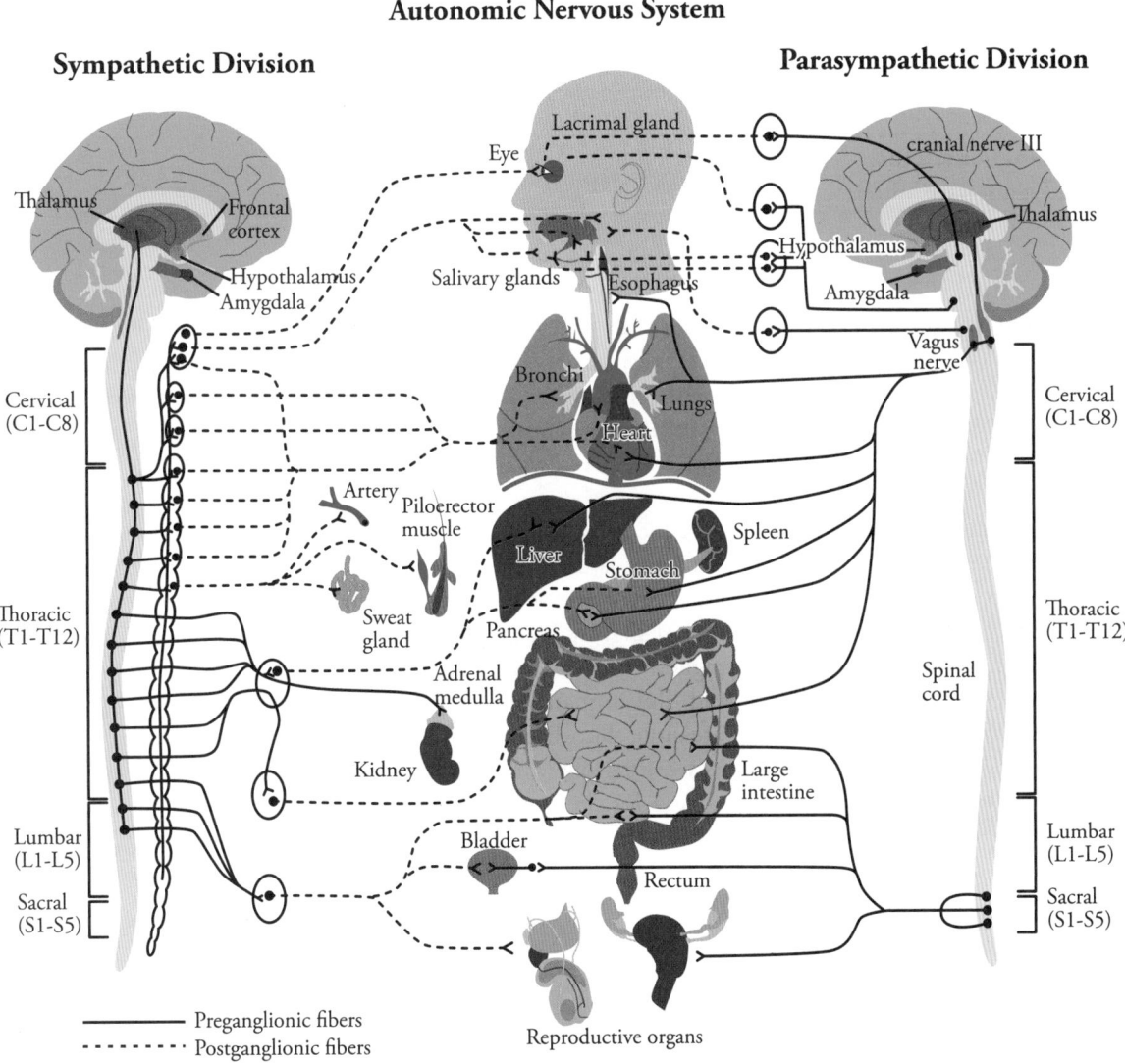

Figure 10   Pre- and post-ganglionic fibers of the autonomic nervous system

The autonomic afferent (sensory) neurons are similar to the somatic afferent neurons with one exception: they can synapse in the PNS (at the autonomic ganglia) with autonomic efferent neurons in what is known as a "short reflex." (Recall that the first synapse of somatic afferent neurons is in the CNS.)

Table 3 Sympathetic vs. Parasympathetic

	Sympathetic	Parasympathetic
General function	fight or flight, mobilize energy	rest and digest, store energy
Location of preganglionic soma	thoracolumbar = thoracic and lumbar spinal cord	craniosacral = brainstem ("cranial") and sacral spinal cord
Preganglionic axon neurotransmitter = acetylcholine (ACh)	short	long
Ganglia	close to cord, far from target	far from cord, close to target
Postganglionic axon (usual neurotransmitter)	long (norepinephrine [NE])	short (ACh)

The Adrenal Medulla

The **adrenal gland** is named for its location: "ad-" means "above" and "renal" refers to the kidney. There are two adrenal glands, one above each kidney. The adrenal has an inner portion known as the **medulla** and an outer portion known as the **cortex**. The cortex is an important endocrine gland, secreting **glucocorticoids** (the main one is cortisol), **mineralocorticoids** (the main one is aldosterone), and some sex hormones.

The **adrenal medulla,** however, is part of the sympathetic nervous system. It is embryologically derived from sympathetic postganglionic neurons and is directly innervated by sympathetic preganglionic neurons. Upon activation of the sympathetic system, the adrenal gland is stimulated to release **epinephrine**, also known as **adrenaline**. Epinephrine is a slightly modified version of *nor*epinephrine, the neurotransmitter released by sympathetic postganglionic neurons. Epinephrine is a hormone because it is released into the bloodstream by a ductless gland. But in many ways it behaves like a neurotransmitter. It elicits its effects very rapidly, and the effects are quite short-lived. Epinephrine release from the adrenal medulla is what causes the sudden flushing and sweating one experiences when severely startled. In general, epinephrine's effects are those listed in Table 4 for the sympathetic system. Stimulation of the heart is an especially important effect.

12.4 THE ENDOCRINE SYSTEM

The nervous system and endocrine system represent the two major control systems of the body. The nervous system is fast-acting with relatively short-term effects, whereas the endocrine system takes longer to communicate signals but has generally longer lasting effects. These two control systems are interconnected, as neurons can signal the release of hormones from endocrine glands. A primary connection between the nervous and endocrine systems is the **hypothalamic-pituitary axis**, which is described in more detail below.

Hormone Types: Transport and Mechanisms of Action

While the nervous system regulates cellular function from instant to instant, the endocrine system regulates physiology (especially metabolism) over a period of hours to days. The nervous system communicates via the extremely rapid action potential. The signal of the endocrine system is the **hormone**, defined as a molecule which is *secreted into the bloodstream* by an endocrine gland, and which has its effects upon *distant* target cells possessing the appropriate receptor. An **endocrine gland** is a *ductless* gland whose secretory products are picked up by capillaries supplying blood to the region. (In contrast, **exocrine glands** secrete their products into the external environment by way of ducts, which empty into the gastrointestinal lumen or the external world.) A **hormone receptor** is a polypeptide that possesses a ligand-specific binding site. Binding of ligand (hormone) to the site causes the receptor to modify target cell activity. *Tissue-specificity of hormone action is determined by whether the cells of a tissue have the appropriate receptor.*

Some signaling molecules modify the activity of the cell which secreted them; this is an **autocrine** activity (*auto-* means self). For example, a T cell secretes interleukin 2, which binds to receptors on the same T cell to stimulate increased activity.

Hormones can be grouped into one of two classes. *Hydrophilic* hormones, such as **peptides** and **amino-acid derivatives**, must bind to receptors on the cell surface, while *hydrophobic* hormones, such as the **steroid hormones**, bind to receptors in the cellular interior.

Peptide Hormones

Peptide hormones are synthesized in the rough ER and modified in the Golgi. Then they are stored in vesicles until needed, when they are released by exocytosis. In the bloodstream they dissolve in the plasma, since they are hydrophilic. Their hydrophilicity also means they cannot cross biological membranes and thus are required to communicate with the interior of the target cell by way of a second messenger cascade. To briefly review, the peptide hormone is a first messenger which must bind to a cell-surface receptor. The receptor is a polypeptide with a domain on the inner surface of the plasma membrane that contains the ability to catalytically activate a second messenger. The end result of second messenger activation is that the function of proteins in the cytoplasm is changed. A key feature of second messenger cascades is signal amplification, which allows a few activated receptors to change the activity of many enzymes in the cytoplasm.

Because peptide hormones modify the activity of existing enzymes in the cytoplasm, their effects are exerted rapidly, minutes to hours from the time of secretion. Also, the duration of their effects is brief.

There are two subgroups within the peptide hormone category: polypeptides and amino acid derivatives. An example of a polypeptide hormone is insulin, which has a complex tertiary structure involving disulfide bridges. It is secreted by the β cells of the pancreatic islets of Langerhans in response to elevated blood glucose and binds to a cell-surface receptor with a cytoplasmic domain possessing protein kinase activity. Amino acid derivatives, as their name implies, are derived from single amino acids and contain no peptide bonds. For example, tyrosine is the parent amino acid for the catecholamines (which include epinephrine) and the thyroid hormones. Despite the fact that these two classes are derived from the same precursor molecule, they have different properties. The catecholamines act like peptide hormones, while the thyroid hormones behave more like steroid hormones. Epinephrine is a small cyclic molecule secreted by the adrenal medulla upon activation of the sympathetic nervous system. It binds to cell-surface receptors to trigger a cascade of events that produces the second messenger cyclic adenosine monophosphate (cAMP) and activates protein kinases in the cytoplasm. Thyroid hormones incorporate iodine into their structure. They enter cells, bind to DNA, and activate transcription of genes involved in energy mobilization.

Steroid Hormones

Steroids are hydrophobic molecules synthesized from cholesterol in the smooth endoplasmic reticulum. Due to their hydrophobicity, steroids can freely diffuse through biological membranes. Thus, they are not stored but rather diffuse into the bloodstream as soon as they are made. If a steroid hormone is not needed, it will not be made. Steroids' hydrophobicity also means they cannot be dissolved in the plasma. Instead they journey through the bloodstream stuck to proteins in the plasma, such as albumin. The small, hydrophobic steroid hormone exerts its effects upon target cells by *diffusing through the plasma membrane to bind with a receptor in the cytoplasm*. Once it has bound its ligand, the steroid hormone-receptor complex is transported into the nucleus, where it acts as a sequence-specific regulator of transcription. Because steroid hormones must modify transcription to change the *amount* and/or *type* of proteins in the cell, their effects are exerted slowly, over a period of days, and persist for days to weeks.

Steroids regulating sexuality, reproduction, and development are secreted by the testes, ovaries, and placenta. Steroids regulating water balance and other processes are secreted by the adrenal cortex. All other endocrine glands secrete peptide hormones. (Note that although thyroid hormone is derived from an amino acid, its mechanism of action more closely resembles that of the steroid hormones.)

Table 4   Peptide vs. Steroid Hormones

	Peptides	Steroids
Structure	hydrophilic, large (polypeptides) or small (amino acid derivatives)	hydrophobic, small
Site of synthesis	rough ER	smooth ER
Regulation of release	stored in vesicles until a signal for secretion is received	synthesized only when needed and then used immediately, not stored
Transport in bloodstream	free	stuck to protein carrier
Specificity	only target cells have appropriate surface receptors (exception: thyroxine = cytoplasmic)	only target cells have appropriate cytoplasmic receptors
Mechanism of effect	bind to receptors that generate second messengers which result in modification of *enzyme activity*	bind to receptors that alter *gene expression* by regulating DNA transcription
Timing of effect	rapid, short-lived	slow, long-lasting

Organization and Regulation of the Human Endocrine System

The endocrine system has many different roles. Hormones are essential for gamete synthesis, ovulation, pregnancy, growth, sexual development, and overall level of metabolic activity. Despite this diversity of function, endocrine activity is harmoniously orchestrated. Maintenance of order in such a complex system might seem impossible to accomplish in a preplanned manner. Regulation of the endocrine system is not preplanned or rigidly structured, but is instead generally automatic. Hormone levels rise and fall as dictated by physiological needs. The endocrine system is ordered yet dynamic. This flexible, automatic orderliness is attributable to feedback regulation. The amount of a hormone secreted is controlled not by a preformulated plan but rather by changes in the variable the hormone is responsible for controlling.

Continuous circulation of blood exposes target cells to regulatory hormones and also exposes endocrine glands to serum concentrations of physiological variables that they regulate. Thus, *regulator* and that which is *regulated* are in continuous communication. Concentration of a species X in the aqueous portion of the bloodstream is denoted "serum [X]."

An example of feedback regulation is the interaction between the hormone calcitonin and serum [Ca^{2+}]. The function of calcitonin is to prevent serum [Ca^{2+}] from peaking above normal levels, and the amount of calcitonin secreted is directly proportional to increases in serum [Ca^{2+}] above normal. When serum [Ca^{2+}] becomes elevated, calcitonin is secreted. Then when serum [Ca^{2+}] levels fall, calcitonin secretion stops. The falling serum [Ca^{2+}] level (*that which is regulated*) feeds back to the cells which secrete calcitonin (*regulators*). The serum [Ca^{2+}] level is a **physiological endpoint** which must be maintained at constant levels. This demonstrates the role of the endocrine system in maintaining **homeostasis**, or physiological consistency.

An advantage of the endocrine system and its feedback regulation is that very complex arrays of variables can be controlled automatically. It's as if the variables controlled themselves. However, some integration (a central control mechanism) is necessary. Superimposed upon the hormonal regulation of physiological endpoints is another layer of regulation: hormones that regulate hormones. Such meta-regulators are known as **tropic hormones**.

For example, adrenocorticotropic hormone (ACTH) is secreted by the anterior pituitary. The role of ACTH is to stimulate increased activity of the portion of the adrenal gland called the **cortex**, which is responsible for secreting cortisol (among other steroid hormones). ACTH is a tropic hormone because it does not directly affect physiological endpoints, but merely regulates another regulator (cortisol). Cortisol regulates physiological endpoints, including cellular responses to stress and serum [glucose]. Feedback regulation applies to tropic hormones as well as to direct regulators of physiological endpoints; the level of ACTH is influenced by the level of cortisol. When cortisol is needed, ACTH is secreted, and when the serum [cortisol] increases sufficiently, ACTH secretion slows.

You may have noticed that in both of our examples the effect of feedback was *inhibitory*: the result of hormone secretion inhibits further secretion. Inhibitory feedback is called **negative feedback** or **feedback inhibition**. Most feedback in the endocrine system (and if you remember, most biochemical feedback in general) is negative. There are few examples of positive feedback which we will not discuss here.

There is yet another layer of control. Many of the functions of the endocrine system depend on instructions from the brain. The portion of the brain which controls much of the endocrine system is the **hypothalamus**, located at the center of the brain. The hypothalamus controls the endocrine system by releasing tropic hormones that regulate other tropic hormones, called **releasing and inhibiting factors** or **releasing and inhibiting hormones**.

For example (Figure 11), the hypothalamus secretes corticotropin-releasing hormone (CRH, also known as CRF, where "F" stands for factor). The role of CRH is to cause increased secretion of ACTH. Just as ACTH secretion is regulated by feedback inhibition from cortisol, CRH secretion, too, is inhibited by cortisol. You begin to see that regulatory pathways in the endocrine system can get pretty complex.

12.4

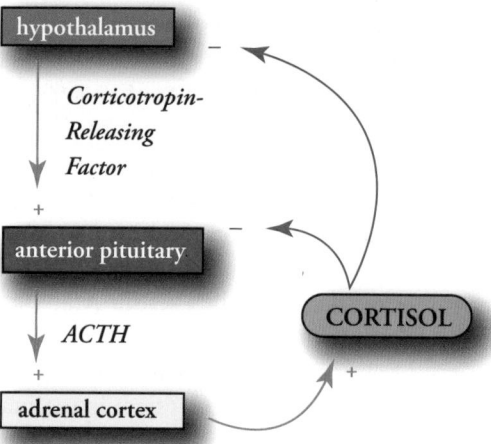

Figure 11   Feedback regulation of cortisol secretion

Understanding that the hypothalamus controls the anterior pituitary and that the anterior pituitary controls most of the endocrine system is important. Damage to the connection between the hypothalamus and the pituitary is fatal, unless daily hormone replacement therapy is given. This endocrine control center is given a special name: **hypothalamic-pituitary control axis** (Figure 12). The hypothalamus exerts its control of the pituitary by secreting its hormones into the bloodstream, just like any other endocrine gland; what's unique is that a special miniature circulatory system is provided for efficient transport of hypothalamic releasing and inhibiting factors to the anterior pituitary. This blood supply is known as the **hypothalamic-pituitary portal system**. You will also hear the term *hypothalamic-hypophysial portal system*. **Hypophysis** is another name for the pituitary gland.

A Note on Portal Systems: As a general rule, blood leaving the heart moves through only one capillary bed before returning to the heart, since the pressure drops substantially in capillaries. A portal system, however, consists of two capillary beds in sequence, allowing for direct communication between nearby structures. The two portal systems you need to understand are: the hypothalamic-pituitary portal system and the hepatic portal system (from the gastrointestinal tract to the liver).

One more bit of background information is necessary before we can delve into specific hormones. The pituitary gland has two halves: front (*anterior*) and back (*posterior*); see Figure 12. The **anterior pituitary** is also called the **adenohypophysis** and the **posterior pituitary** is also known as the **neurohypophysis**. It is important to understand the difference. The anterior pituitary is a normal endocrine gland, and it is controlled by hypothalamic releasing and inhibiting factors (essentially tropic hormones). The posterior pituitary is composed of axons which descend from the hypothalamus. These hypothalamic neurons that send axons down to the posterior pituitary are an example of **neuroendocrine cells**, neurons which secrete hormones into the bloodstream. The hormones of the posterior pituitary are ADH (antidiuretic hormone or vasopressin), which causes the kidney to retain water during times of thirst, and oxytocin, which causes milk let-down for nursing as well as uterine contractions during labor.

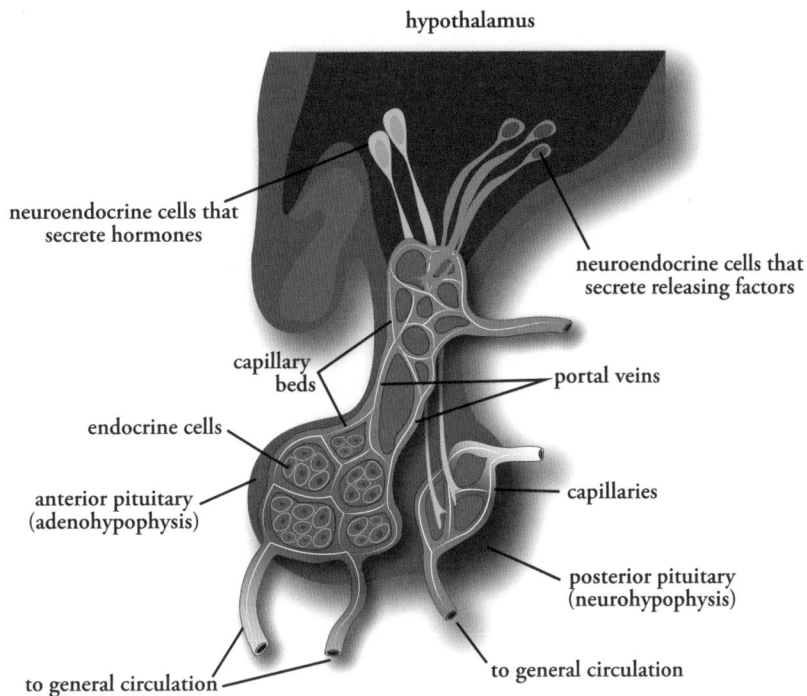

hypothalamus

neuroendocrine cells that
secrete hormones

neuroendocrine cells that
secrete releasing factors

capillary
beds

portal veins

endocrine cells

capillaries

anterior pituitary
(adenohypophysis)

posterior pituitary
(neurohypophysis)

to general circulation

to general circulation

Figure 12   The hypothalamic-pituitary control axis

Major Glands and Their Hormones

The major hormones and glands of the endocrine system are shown in Figure 13 and listed in Table 5. Many of these hormones will be discussed in detail in the MCAT Biology Review. The function of epinephrine has already been presented as part of the sympathetic nervous system response. In general, the hormones are involved in development of the body and in maintenance of constant conditions, homeostasis, in the adult.

Thyroid hormone and **cortisol** have broad effects on metabolism and energy usage. Thyroid hormone is produced from the amino acid tyrosine in the thyroid gland and comes in two forms, with three or four iodine atoms per molecule. The production of thyroid hormone is increased by thyroid stimulating hormone (TSH) from the anterior pituitary, which is regulated by the hypothalamus and the central nervous system in turn. The mechanism of action of thyroid hormone is to bind to a receptor in the cytoplasm of cells that then regulates transcription in the nucleus. The effect of this regulation is to increase the overall metabolic rate and body temperature, and, in children, to stimulate growth. Exposure to cold can increase the production of thyroid hormone. Cortisol is secreted by the adrenal cortex in response to ACTH from the pituitary. In general, the effects of cortisol tend to help the body deal with stress. Cortisol helps to mobilize glycogen and fat stores to provide energy during stress and also increases the consumption of proteins for energy. These effects are essential, since removal of the adrenal cortex can result in the death of animals exposed to even a small stress. Long-term high levels of cortisol tend to have negative effects, however, including suppression of the immune system.

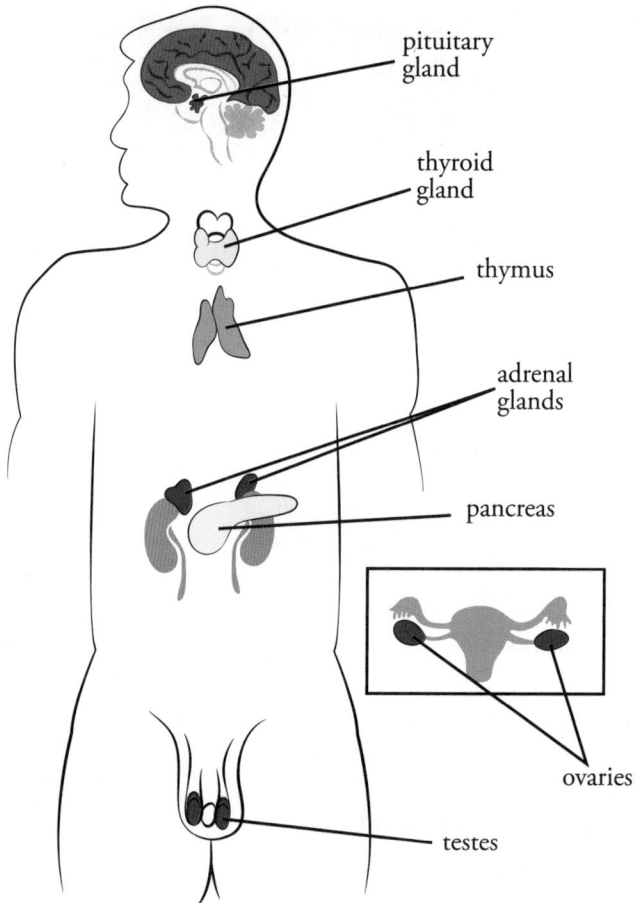

Figure 13   The major endocrine glands

Table 5 Summary of the Hormones of the Endocrine System

Gland	Hormone [class]	Target/effect
Hypothalamus	releasing and inhibiting factors (peptides)	anterior pituitary/modify activity
Anterior pituitary	growth hormone (GH) (peptide)	↑ bone & muscle growth, ↑ cell turnover rate
	prolactin (peptide)	mammary gland/milk production
tropic	thyroid stimulating hormone (TSH) (peptide)	thyroid/↑ synthesis & release of TH
	adrenocorticotropic hormone (ACTH) (peptide)	↑ growth & secretory activity of adrenal ctx
gonadotropic	luteinizing hormone (LH) (peptide)	ovary/ovulation, testes/testosterone synth.
	follicle stimulating hormone (FSH) (peptide)	ovary/follicle development, testes/spermatogenesis
Posterior pituitary	antidiuretic hormone (ADH, vasopressin) (peptide)	kidney/water retention
	oxytocin (peptide)	breast/milk let-down, uterus/contraction
Thyroid	thyroid hormone (TH, thyroxine) (modified amino acid)	child: necessary for physical & mental development; adult: ↑ metabolic rate & temp.
thyroid C cells	calcitonin (peptide)	bone, kidney; lowers serum $[Ca^{2+}]$
Parathyroids	parathyroid hormone (PTH) (peptide)	bone, kidney, small intestine/raises serum $[Ca^{2+}]$
Thymus	thymosin (children only) (peptide)	T cell development during childhood
Adrenal medulla	epinephrine (modified amino acid)	sympathetic stress response (rapid)
Adrenal cortex	cortisol ("glucocorticoid") (steroid)	longer-term stress response; ↑ blood [glucose]; ↑ protein catabolism; ↓ inflammation & immunity; many other
	aldosterone ("mineralocorticoid") (steroid)	kidney/↑ Na^+ reabsorption to ↑ b.p.
	sex steroids	not normally important, but an adrenal tumor can overproduce these, causing masculinization or feminization
Endocrine pancreas (islets of Langerhans)	insulin (β cells secrete) (peptide) —absent or ineffective in diabetes mellitus	↓ blood [glucose]/↑ glycogen & fat storage
	glucagon (α cells secrete) (peptide)	↑ blood [glucose]/↓ glycogen & fat storage
	somatostatin (SS—δ cells secrete) (peptide)	inhibits many digestive processes
Testes	testosterone (steroid)	male characteristics, spermatogenesis
Ovaries/placenta	estrogen (steroid)	female characteristics, endometrial growth
	progesterone (steroid)	endometrial secretion, pregnancy
Heart	atrial natriuretic factor (ANF) (peptide)	kidney/↑ urination to ↓ blood pressure
Kidney	erythropoietin (peptide)	bone marrow/↑ RBC synthesis

Chapter 12 Summary

- The neuron is the basic structural and functional unit of the nervous system. It has several specialized structures that allow it to transmit action potentials.

- Neurons receive incoming information via dendrites. Signals are summed by the axon hillock, and if the signal is greater than the threshold, an action potential is initiated.

- The action potential is an all-or-none signal that includes depolarization (via voltage-gated sodium channels) and repolarization (via voltage-gated potassium channels); it begins and ends at the cell's resting potential of –70 mV.

- Since action potentials are all-or-none events, signal intensity is coded by the frequency of the action potentials being fired.

- Neurons communicate with other neurons, organs, and glands at synapses. Most synapses are chemical in nature.

- The central nervous system includes the spinal cord and the brain; specialized areas control specific aspects of human behavior, movement, intelligence, emotion, and reflexes.

- The peripheral nervous system includes the somatic (voluntary) and autonomic (involuntary) subdivisions.

- The sympathetic branch of the autonomic system controls our fight-or-flight response; norepinephrine is the primary neurotransmitter of this system, and it is augmented by epinephrine from the adrenal medulla.

- The parasympathetic branch of the autonomic system controls our resting and digesting state; acetylcholine is the primary neurotransmitter of this system.

- Humans have several types of receptors (mechanoreceptors, chemoreceptors, nociceptors, thermoreceptors, electromagnetic receptors, and proprioceptors) that allow us to detect a variety of stimuli.

- The endocrine system controls our overall physiology and homeostasis by hormones that travel through the bloodstream.

- Peptide hormones are made from amino acids, bind to receptors on the cell surface, and typically affect target cells via second messenger pathways.

- Steroid hormones are derived from cholesterol, bind to receptors in the cytoplasm or nucleus, and bind to DNA to alter transcription.

CHAPTER 12 FREESTANDING PRACTICE QUESTIONS

1. A demyelinating disorder, such as multiple sclerosis, would cause all of the following symptoms EXCEPT:

A) a reduction of white matter in the central nervous system.
B) increased saltatory conduction.
C) slower propagation of signals along the axon.
D) a deficiency of sensation.

2. Which area of the brain is responsible for coordinating complex motor functions?

A) Frontal lobe
B) Occipital lobe
C) Reticular activating system
D) Cerebellum

3. All of the following brain areas are associated with the experience of emotion EXCEPT the:

A) temporal lobes.
B) amygdala.
C) hypothalamus.
D) pons.

4. Acetylcholine is stimulatory to which of the following?

   I. Skeletal muscle
  II. Postganglionic neurons
 III. Cardiac muscle

A) I only
B) I and II only
C) II and III only
D) I, II, and III

5. Cortisol has a direct inhibitory effect on:

A) the posterior pituitary.
B) the hypothalamus.
C) the adrenal cortex.
D) glycogen mobilization.

CHAPTER 12 PRACTICE PASSAGE

Long-term potentiation (LTP) involves communication between two neurons and is a major cellular mechanism underlying learning and memory processes. During LTP, a presynaptic neuron releases the neurotransmitter glutamate, which binds to receptors on the postsynaptic neuron. This leads to an influx of sodium, and ultimately calcium, followed by activation of various genes (see Figure 1). The initial receptor activated by glutamate is the AMPA receptor; the NMDA receptor is blocked by extracellular Mg^{2+} that must be displaced by a sufficient change in membrane potential before that channel will fully open.

LTP has been shown to be disrupted in neurodegenerative disorders, such as Alzheimer's disease, leading to memory deficits. In the brains of Alzheimer's patients, loss of vital neurons occurs in the hippocampus (a region of the brain involved in memory acquisition). Several mechanisms are hypothesized to lead to this neurodegeneration. One involves calcium-mediated toxicity and occurs due to excessive glutamate-induced neuronal excitation.

Another potential contributing factor to this cell loss is exposure to chronic stress, which results in elevated levels of corticosteroids that can influence neuronal activity in the brain. This has led to the formation of the "glucocorticoid hypothesis of aging." The intact hippocampus has an inhibitory effect on the stress axis (hypothalamic-pituitary-adrenal axis) that is responsible for inducing release of cortisol from the adrenal gland during times of stress. Thus, if the hippocampal region is compromised, it could lead to lack of inhibition of the stress axis and further release of cortisol, causing a feed-forward cycle of excessive release of steroids with each stressful event.

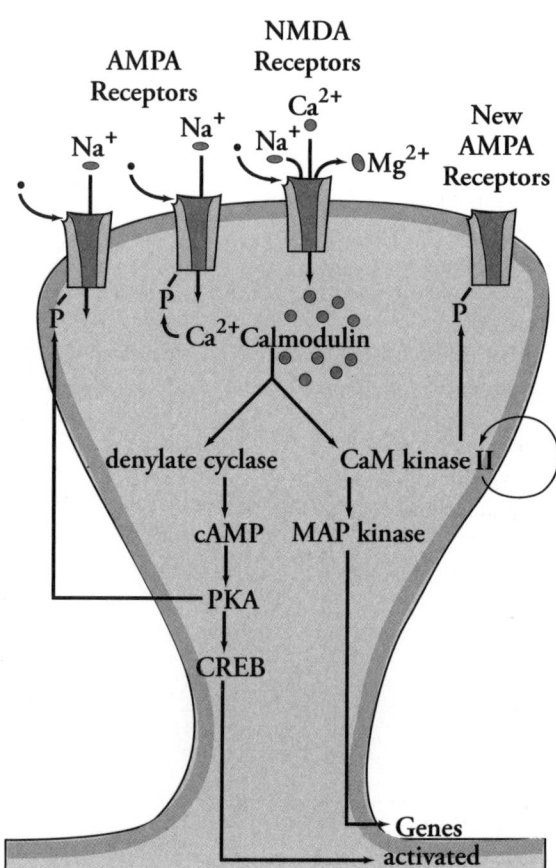

Figure 1   Synaptic transmission during LTP

1. In which region of the brain is the hippocampus located?

A) Cerebellum
B) Occipital lobe
C) Temporal lobe
D) Hypothalamus

2. One treatment for Alzheimer's disease involves a drug that blocks NMDA receptors. This treatment could lead to all of the following EXCEPT:

A) a suppression of LTP.
B) a suppression of gene expression.
C) a significant decrease in intracellular sodium.
D) a significant decrease in intracellular calcium.

3. A researcher removes the adrenal glands from a rat and then supplements the rat with baseline levels of steroids for the remainder of its lifespan. Which of the following would be expected?

   I.   Blunted sympathetic nervous system response
   II. Slowing of age-related neurodegeneration
   III. Enhancement of LTP

A) II only
B) II and III
C) I and II
D) I, II, and III

4. Which of the following statements is LEAST likely to be true?

A) Drugs that increase Cl^- influx into the postsynaptic cell could disrupt LTP.
B) Drugs that increase K^+ efflux from the postsynaptic cell would result in hyperpolarization of the cell and would increase LTP.
C) The insertion of new AMPA receptors in the postsynaptic cell membrane would increase the rate at which Mg^{2+} is displaced from NMDA receptors upon subsequent stimulation by glutamate.
D) The influx of Na^+ upon initial stimulation by glutamate depolarizes the postsynaptic cell in order to displace Mg^{2+}.

5. AMPA receptors are found throughout the central nervous system and are comprised of four different subunits. Not all AMPA receptors have all the subunits. If a knockout mouse was made deficient for the gene for one of the AMPA receptor subunits, what would be the expected outcome?

A) An observed deficit only in LTP and the mouse's ability to learn
B) Altered function in any region containing an AMPA receptor
C) No change in LTP function due to the NMDA receptor still being present and functional
D) Altered function and/or compensatory expression of other AMPA receptor subunits in regions with AMPA receptors that lack the affected subunit

6. Based on Figure 1, what is a logical function of CREB?

A) To interact with the genomic DNA to enhance transcription
B) To interact with RNA to enhance translation
C) To bind ribosomes to enhance transcription
D) To bind RNA polymerase to enhance replication

7. Symptoms of Alzheimer's disease include all of the following EXCEPT:

A) disorientation.
B) forgetfulness.
C) mood swings.
D) slow, uncoordinated fine movements.

SOLUTIONS TO CHAPTER 12 FREESTANDING PRACTICE QUESTIONS

1. **B** Myelin is an insulating sheath wrapped around the axons of neurons. White matter in the central nervous system is composed of myelinated axons; thus, a reduction in myelination would result in a decrease in white matter (choice A is a symptom and can be eliminated). Gaps in the myelin sheath (called nodes of Ranvier) allow depolarization of the axon and conduction of neuronal signals along the length of the axon. Myelination speeds the movement of the action potential along the length of the axon (choice C would be a symptom and can be eliminated), in a process called saltatory conduction; a reduction in myelination would decrease (not increase) saltatory conduction (choice B is not a symptom and is the correct answer choice). This would decrease sensation, as sensory information from the peripheral nervous system would be hindered from reaching the central nervous system (choice D is a symptom and can be eliminated).

2. **D** The cerebellum, located behind the pons and below the cerebrum, receives input from the primary motor cortex in the forebrain, and coordinates complex motor function (choice D is correct). The frontal lobe contains the primary motor cortex, which is responsible for initiating movement, but does not coordinate complex motor functions (choice A is wrong). The occipital lobe is responsible for vision (choice B is wrong), and the reticular activating system is responsible for arousal and wakefulness (choice C is wrong).

3. **D** The pons is located below the midbrain and above the medulla oblongata, and connects the brain stem and the cerebellum. Along with the medulla, the pons controls some autonomic functions and plays a role in equilibrium and posture, but it is not associated with the experience of emotion (choice D is correct). The amygdala, located in the temporal lobes, is part of the limbic system and is responsible for processing information about emotion (choices A and B are associated with emotion and can be eliminated). The hypothalamus links the nervous system to the endocrine system and also plays a role in emotion (choice C is associated with emotion and can be eliminated).

4. **B** Item I is true: acetylcholine is the neurotransmitter released by motor neurons onto skeletal muscle to cause contraction (choice C can be eliminated). Item II is true: the preganglionic neurons of both the sympathetic and parasympathetic nervous systems release acetylcholine onto the postganglionic neurons, triggering action potentials (choice A can be eliminated). Item III is false: acetylcholine on cardiac muscle is inhibitory and reduces the heart rate (choice D can be eliminated, and choice B is correct).

5. **B** The hypothalamic-pituitary axis (HPA) regulates the release of cortisol via negative feedback. The hypothalamus releases corticotropin-releasing hormone (CRH), which stimulates the anterior pituitary to release adrenocorticotropic hormone (ACTH), which in turn stimulates the adrenal cortex to release cortisol. Cortisol then inhibits the hypothalamus from releasing further CRH and the anterior pituitary from releasing more ACTH, thus having an inhibitory effect on both (choice B is correct). The posterior pituitary releases oxytocin and antidiuretic hormone; cortisol does not inhibit the posterior pituitary (choice A is wrong). Additionally, cortisol does not inhibit the adrenal cortex directly, but rather inhibits the hypothalamus and anterior pituitary from releasing the hormones that stimulate the adrenal cortex; thus cortisol has an indirect inhibitory effect on the adrenal cortex (choice C is wrong). Cortisol stimulates glycogen mobilization (choice D is wrong).

SOLUTIONS TO CHAPTER 12 PRACTICE PASSAGE

1. **C** The passage states that the hippocampus is involved in memory acquisition; thus, it is likely to be located in the temporal lobe of the cerebrum (choice C is correct). The cerebellum is involved in balance and coordination, not memory (choice A is wrong), the occipital lobe is responsible for vision (choice B is wrong), and the hypothalamus is involved in maintaining homeostasis and hormonal regulation (choice D is wrong).

2. **C** If NMDA receptor activation is necessary for LTP, then blocking this receptor would likely suppress LTP (choice A could occur and can be eliminated). Based on Figure 1, activation of the NMDA receptor triggers an influx of intracellular calcium and a cascade of events resulting in activation of gene expression; thus, blocking this receptor could lead to both a significant decrease in intracellular calcium and a suppression of gene expression (choices B and D could occur and can be eliminated). Since the NMDA receptor allows an influx of sodium, some reduction in intracellular sodium could be expected; however, this is unlikely to be significant since the AMPA receptor would still be functional and is the main source of Na^+ influx (choice C would not occur and is the correct answer choice).

3. **C** Item I is true: The adrenal glands secrete both steroid hormones (from the adrenal cortex) and epinephrine (from the adrenal medulla). If the researcher only replaces the steroids, then the sympathetic response (which relies on epinephrine) could be blunted (choices A and B can be eliminated). Since both remaining answer choices include Item II, then Item II must be true and we only need to evaluate Item III. Item III is false: based on Figure 1, corticosteroids do not seem to play an integral role in LTP. In addition, the passage only discusses their possible involvement in neuronal cell death at high concentrations. Keeping baseline levels may not lead to cell death, but would not necessarily enhance LTP (choice D can be eliminated, and choice C is correct). Note that Item II is in fact true: based on information in the passage (the glucocorticoid aging hypothesis), stress levels of corticosteroids could lead to age-related neurodegeneration. Thus, if the levels of these hormones are kept at baseline throughout the life of the animal, it is possible to attenuate age-related neurodegeneration.

4. **B** The passage states that the NMDA receptor is blocked by extracellular Mg^{2+} that must be displaced by a sufficient change in membrane potential. It is fair to assume that this change must be a depolarization, since the initial receptor activated is the AMPA receptor, and according to the figure, that receptor allows an influx of Na^+ (choice D is likely to be true and can be eliminated). Additional AMPA receptors would increase the rate of depolarization and thus the rate of Mg^{2+} displacement. This is in fact the basis for LTP; the first stimulation leads to the effects shown in the figure, including new receptors in the membrane, thus the effect of subsequent stimulation is enhanced (choice C is likely to be true and can be eliminated). Anything that would lead to a hyperpolarization of the cell would not displace Mg^{2+} and would disrupt the calcium influx and all associated events, including LTP. An increase of Cl^- influx would hyperpolarize the cell and disrupt LTP (choice A is likely to be true and can be eliminated), but an increase in K^+ efflux, while it would hyperpolarize the cell, would not increase LTP (choice B is unlikely to be true and is the correct answer choice).

5. **D** The question states essentially that AMPA receptors can be varied (have variable subunits) and are found throughout the CNS. Certainly if the gene for one of the subunits was deficient, we would expect some deficit to be present. However, because of the widespread location of these receptors, we would not expect the deficit to be limited to only the region of the brain responsible for LTP (choice A is wrong), nor would we expect the deficit to be found in ANY region with receptors, because some regions may have AMPA receptors that do not have the knocked out subunit (choice B is wrong). According to the diagram, the functions of both AMPA and NMDA receptors are required during LTP, so if one of the receptors was compromised, we might expect some alteration in LTP function (choice C is wrong). The most likely outcome is that there would be altered function or potentially compensatory expression of other AMPA receptor subunits in those regions of the CNS that contain an affected AMPA receptor (choice D is correct).

6. **A** In the diagram, CREB is located immediately before gene activation, which would suggest it has something to do with transcription (choices B and D are wrong). Ribosomes do not have anything to do with transcription (choice C is wrong, and choice A is correct). CREB stands for cAMP Response Element Binding and is a transcription factor; thus, it interacts with DNA to enhance transcription.

7. **D** Alzheimer's disease involves the loss of vital neurons throughout the cerebral cortex; symptoms include disorientation (choice A can be eliminated), forgetfulness (choice B can be eliminated), mood swings (choice C can be eliminated), and impairment of other cognitive functions like speaking, writing, thinking, reasoning, and making judgments and decisions. As the disease progresses, it can also lead to changes in personality and behavior, depression, and social withdrawal. However, Alzheimer's disease does not affect fine motor skills (choice D is correct).

Psychology and Sociology Glossary

After each entry, the section number in the *MCAT Psychology & Sociology Review* text where the term is discussed is given.

absolute poverty
The inability to meet a bare minimum of basic necessities. [Section 5.2]

acetylcholine (ACh)
The neurotransmitter used at the neuromuscular junction, throughout the parasympathetic nervous system, and by the preganglionic neurons of the sympathetic nervous system. [Section 12.2]

acetylcholinesterase
The enzyme that breaks down acetylcholine in the synaptic cleft. [Section 12.2]

achieved status
A status due largely to an individual's efforts. [Section 6.3]

acquisition
The process of learning the association between a conditioned stimulus and response. [Section 9.1]

action potential
A localized change in a neuron's membrane potential that propagates away from its point of origin. [Section 12.1]

activation-synthesis theory
The theory that dreams are simply byproducts of brain activation during REM sleep. [Section 11.5]

actor-observer bias
The tendency to blame our actions on the situation and blame the actions of others on their personalities. [Section 6.2]

addiction
A compulsion to perform an act repeatedly, often with detrimental effects on the individual. [Section 10.3]

adrenal cortex
The outer region of the adrenal gland that produces cortisol in response to long-term (chronic) stress and aldosterone in response to low blood pressure or low blood osmolarity. [Section 12.4]

adrenal medulla
The inner region of the adrenal gland that releases epinephrine (adrenaline) and norepinephrine into the bloodstream. [Section 12.3]

adrenocorticotropic hormone (ACTH)
A tropic hormone produced by the anterior pituitary gland that targets the adrenal cortex, stimulating it to release cortisol and aldosterone. ACTH is part of the stress response. [Sections 12.4 & 8.2]

affect
A person's visible emotion in the moment. [Section 8.1]

affirmative action
Policies that seek to benefit underrepresented groups in admissions or job hiring decisions. [Section 6.2]

aggregate
People who exist in the same space but do not interact or share a common sense of identity. [Section 6.2]

aggression
Behavior that is forceful, hostile, or attacking. [Section 6.3]

agnosia
The inability to recognize objects through sensory mechanisms despite intact function of the underlying sense itself. [Section 11.4]

Ainsworth, Mary
Conducted famous studies on attachment style in infants. [Section 9.3]

algorithm
A step-by-step detailing aid to problem-solving. [Section 11.4]

alpha waves
Low amplitude, high frequency brain waves present in a relaxed state. [Section 11.5]

altruistic behavior
A behavior that benefits others, possibly at the expense of the individual. [Section 6.3]

Alzheimer's disease
The most prevalent form of dementia, characterized by severe memory impairment. [Section 8.1]

amalgamation
Occurs when majority and minority groups combine to form a new group. [Section 6.1]

amygdala
Almond-shaped structure deep within the brain that orchestrates emotional experiences. [Section 10.3]

anal stage
The second of Freud's five psychosexual stages, in this stage the child seeks sensual pleasure through control of elimination. [Section 7.1]

anterograde amnesia
An inability to form new memories. [Sections 8.1 & 9.2]

antisocial personality disorder
A psychological disorder characterized by serious behavior problems beginning in adolescence, including significant aggression against people or animals, property destruction, lying, or theft. [Section 8.1]

anxiety disorder
A psychological disorder characterized by intense, frequent, and uncontrollable anxiety. [Section 8.1]

archival studies
Studies that explore historical records and search for patterns or insight. [Section 3.3]

Asch, Solomon
Conducted important research on conformity and group pressure. [Section 6.2]

ascribed status
A status that is assigned to a person by society regardless of the person's own efforts. [Section 6.3]

assimilation
The process in which an individual forsakes aspects of his or her own cultural tradition to adopt those of a different culture. [Section 6.1]

associative learning
Process of learning in which one event, object, or action is directly connected with another. Two general categories include classical and operant conditioning. [Section 9.1]

attenuation model of selective attention
Model of selective attention in which the mind has an attenuator, like a volume knob, that tunes up attended inputs and tunes down unattended inputs, rather than eliminating them. [Section 11.4]

attitude
A person's feelings and beliefs about other people or events and behavioral tendencies. [Section 7.3]

attribution theory
A theory that attempts to explain behavior by attributing it to either internal or external causes. [Section 6.2]

attrition
Occurs when participants in a study drop out before completion. [Section 3.1]

auditory cortex
The area of the temporal lobe responsible for processing sound information. [Section 11.1]

auditory tube
Functions to equalize middle ear pressure with atmospheric pressure so that pressure on both sides of the tympanic membrane is equal. [Section 11.1]

authoritarian parenting
Parents impose strict rules that are expected to be followed unconditionally. [Section 9.3]

authoritative parenting
Parents place limits on behavior and consistently follow through on consequences, but also allow for two-way communication with children. [Section 9.3]

autonomic nervous system (ANS)
The division of the peripheral nervous system that innervates and controls the visceral organs. It can be subdivided into sympathetic and parasympathetic branches. [Sections 10.3 & 12.3]

availability heuristic
Mental shortcut of making judgments on the frequency of something occurring based on how readily it is available in our memories. [Section 11.4]

avoidance learning
The process by which one learns to ensure that a negative stimulus will not occur. [Section 9.1]

avoidant personality disorder
A psychological disorder characterized by feelings of inadequacy, inferiority, and undesirability, and a preoccupation with fears of criticism. [Section 8.1]

axon
A long projection of the cell body of a neuron down which an action potential can be propagated. [Section 12.1]

back stage
In the dramaturgical perspective, this is where we can "let down our guard" and be ourselves. [Section 6.3]

Bandura, Albert
Famous for his Bobo doll studies that demonstrated observational learning. [Section 9.1]

baroreceptor
A sensory receptor that responds to changes in pressure. [Section 11.2]

basal nuclei, or basal ganglia
Structures that coordinate smooth motion by inhibiting excess movement. [Section 10.2]

basilar membrane
Membrane in the cochlea that supports the organ of Corti, which contains hearing receptors. [Section 11.1]

behavioral genetics
Study of the role of inheritance in interacting with experience to determine an individual's personality and behaviors. [Section 6.4]

behavioral therapy
This type of therapy uses conditioning to shape a client's behaviors in the desired direction. [Section 7.1]

behaviorism
The perspective that personality is a result of learned behavior patterns based on the environment. [Section 7.1]

belief bias
A tendency to draw conclusions based on what one already believes rather than sound logic. [Section 11.4]

belief perseverance
The maintenance of beliefs even in the face of evidence to the contrary. [Section 11.4]

beliefs
The convictions or principles that people within a culture hold. [Section 5.1]

beta waves
Waking EEG waves seen during alert focus with oscillations between 12.5 Hz and 30 Hz. [Section 11.5]

between-subjects design
Comparisons are made between one group and another to test for differences. [Section 3.1]

bilateral descent
A system of lineage in which the relatives on the mother's side and father's side are considered equally important. [Section 4.2]

biofeedback
Means of recording and feeding back information about autonomic responses to an individual in an attempt to train the individual to control previously involuntary responses. [Section 8.2]

biographical studies
Studies that investigate all relevant details of the life of an individual or small group. [Section 3.3]

bipolar disorder
A psychological disorder characterized by cyclic mood episodes of depression and mania. [Section 8.1]

bipolar neuron
A neuron with a single axon and a single dendrite. [Section 12.1]

borderline personality disorder
A psychological disorder characterized by enduring or recurrent instability in impulse control, mood, and image of self and others. [Section 8.1]

bottom-up processing
Sensory processing that begins with sensory receptors and works up to complex integration of information in the brain. [Section 11.2]

Broca's area
Region in the left hemisphere of the frontal lobe involved in language production. [Section 11.6]

bystander effect
The fact that a person is less likely to provide help when there are other people around. [Section 6.2]

Cannon-Bard Theory
Asserts that the physiological and cognitive aspects of emotion occur simultaneously and collectively lead to the behavioral reaction. [Section 7.4]

capitalism
An economic system in which resources and production are mainly privately owned and goods/services are produced for a profit. [Section 4.1]

case studies
Studies that make a deep and comprehensive exploration of a single individual, phenomenon, or disorder. [Section 3.3]

caste system
A closed social stratification where people remain in the category that they are born into. [Section 5.2]

category
People who share similar characteristics but are not otherwise linked as a group. [Section 6.2]

Cattell, Raymond
Psychologist who used factor analysis with hundreds of traits to identify sixteen source traits, then reduced these into five global factors. [Section 6.4]

central executive
Part of working memory that controls the visuospatial sketchpad, phonological loop, and episodic buffer. [Section 11.4]

central nervous system
The subdivision of the nervous system consisting of the brain and spinal cord. [Sections 10.2 & 12.3]

central route
Cognitive route of persuasion based on the content and deeper aspects of an argument. [Section 6.4]

cerebellum
The region of the brain that coordinates and smooths skeletal muscle activity. [Section 10.2]

cerebral cortex
A thin layer of gray matter on the surface of the cerebral hemispheres. [Section 10.2]

cerebrospinal fluid (CSF)
A clear fluid that circulates around and through the brain and spinal cord. [Section 10.2]

charismatic authority
A form of leadership where devotion is reliant upon an individual with exceptional charisma. [Section 4.2]

chemical synapse
Synapse at which a neurotransmitter is released from the axon of a neuron into the synaptic cleft, where it binds to receptors on the next structure. [Section 12.2]

chemoreceptor
A sensory receptor that responds to specific chemicals, for example, gustatory (taste) receptors, and olfactory (smell) receptors. [Section 11.1]

chunking
Memory technique in which information is organized into groups of data, allowing more information to be remembered overall. [Section 9.2]

church
A type of well-integrated religious organization that attempts to provide an all-encompassing worldview for followers. [Section 4.2]

ciliary muscle
Muscle that helps focus light on the retina by controlling the curvature of the lens of the eye. [Section 11.1]

circadian rhythm
The waxing and waning of alertness throughout the 24-hour day. [Section 11.5]

class system
A social stratification where people are grouped together by similar wealth, income, and education, but the classes are open, so people can strive to reach a higher class (or fall to a lower one). [Section 5.2]

classical conditioning
Process in which two stimuli are paired in a way that changes a response to one of them. [Section 9.1]

cochlea
The curled structure in the inner ear that contains the membranes and hair cells used to transduce sound waves into action potentials. [Section 11.1]

cocktail party effect
Phenomenon in which salient information "catches" one's attention. [Section 11.3]

coercive organizations
Organization in which members do not have a choice in joining. [Section 6.3]

cognitive behavioral therapy (CBT)
A type of therapy that addresses thoughts and behaviors that are maladaptive by using goal-oriented and systematic techniques. [Section 7.1]

cognitive dissonance theory
A theory that explains that we feel tension ("dissonance") whenever we hold two thoughts ("cognitions") that are incompatible. [Section 7.3]

cognitive psychology
Tradition of psychology that focuses on the brain, cognitions, and thoughts as mediating learning and stimulus-response behaviors. [Section 9.1]

conditioned response
Previously unlearned response that has become a learned response to a conditioned stimulus. [Section 9.1]

conditioned stimulus
An originally neutral stimulus that is paired until it can produce the conditioned response without the unconditioned stimulus. [Section 9.1]

conduction aphasia
Language dysfunction characterized by poor speech repetition despite intact comprehension and fluent speech. [Section 11.6]

cones
Photoreceptors in the retina of the eye that respond to bright light and provide color vision. [Section 11.1]

confederates
A person who is working with the experimenter and posing as a part of the experiment, but the subjects are not aware of this affiliation. [Section 6.2]

confirmation bias
A tendency to search only for information that confirms a preconceived conclusion. [Section 11.4]

conflict theory
A theory that views society as being in competition for limited resources. [Section 4.1]

conformity
The phenomenon of adjusting behavior or thinking based on the behavior or thinking of others. [Section 6.2]

confounding variables
Variables other than the research variables that would explain an experimental effect if one were found; also known as extraneous variables. [Section 3.1]

consciousness
Awareness of self, internal states, and the environment. [Section 11.5]

construct validity
The extent to which a psychometric instrument measures what it purports to. [Section 3.1]

control group
The group that does not receive the treatment in an experiment, and is used as a point of reference for the experimental group. [Section 3.1]

conversion disorder
A psychological disorder characterized by a change in sensory or motor function that has no discernible physical or physiological cause. [Section 8.1]

cornea
The clear portion of the tough outer layer of the eyeball, found over the iris and the pupil. [Section 11.1]

corpus callosum
The largest bundle of white matter (axons) connecting the two cerebral hemispheres. [Section 10.2]

correlational studies
Studies that measure the quantitative relationship between two variables. [Section 3.3]

cortisol
Steroid hormone released during chronic stress. Prolonged release of cortisol is associated with suppressed immunity and increased illness. [Sections 8.2, 10.3, & 12.4]

cross-sectional study
A study design in which data collection or survey of a population or sample occurs at a specific time. [Section 3.3]

crude birth rate
The annual number of live births per thousand people in a population. [Section 5.1]

crude death rate
The annual number of deaths per thousand people in a population. [Section 5.1]

cult
A religious organization that is far outside society's norms. [Section 4.2]

cultural capital
The non-financial social assets that promote social mobility. [Section 5.2]

cultural relativism
Judging another culture based on its own cultural standards. [Section 6.2]

cultural universals
Patterns or traits that are common to all people, such as securing food and shelter. [Section 5.1]

culture
A shared way of life, including the beliefs and practices that a social group shares. [Section 5.1]

cyclothymic disorder
A psychological disorder that is similar to bipolar disorder but the moods are less extreme. [Section 8.1]

death drive
According to psychoanalytic theory, the death instinct drives aggressive behaviors fueled by an unconscious wish to die or to hurt oneself or others. [Section 7.1]

debriefing
After participants complete a study or some part of a study, researchers thoroughly review the purpose of the study, hypotheses, and implications. [Section 3.2]

deindividuation
An explanation of people's uncharacteristic behavior when situations provide a high degree of arousal and low sense of responsibility. [Section 6.2]

delusion
A false belief that is not due to culture, and is not relinquished despite evidence that it is false. [Section 8.1]

demand characteristics
Researcher expectations that influence participant responses; often, participants subconsciously adapt their behavior and responses to fit with the research hypothesis, which they have guessed. [Section 3.2]

demography
The study of human population dynamics, including the size, structure, and distribution of a population, and changes in the population over time due to birth, death, and migration. [Section 5.1]

dendrite
A projection off the cell body of a neuron that receives nerve impulses from a different neuron and sends the impulse to the cell body. Neurons can have one or several dendrites. [Section 12.1]

dependent personality disorder
A psychological disorder characterized by a need to be taken care of by others and an unrealistic fear of being unable to take care of himself or herself. [Section 8.1]

depersonalization disorder
A psychological disorder characterized by a recurring or persistent feeling of being cut off or detached from one's body or mental processes, as if observing one's self from the outside. [Section 8.1]

depolarization
The movement of the membrane potential of a cell away from the resting potential to a more positive membrane potential. [Section 12.1]

depressant
Class of drugs that depress or slow down neural activity. [Section 11.5]

depth of processing
The idea that information that is thought about at a deeper level is better remembered. [Section 9.2]

deviance
A violation of society's standards of conduct or expectations. [Sections 6.1 & 6.2]

Diagnostic and Statistical Manual (DSM)
The universal authority on the classification and diagnosis of psychological disorders. [Section 8.1]

diencephalon
The portion of the forebrain that includes the thalamus and hypothalamus. [Section 10.2]

difference threshold
The minimum noticeable difference between any two sensory stimuli 50% of the time. [Section 11.2]

disclosure
Before participants take part in a study, researchers must give them an idea of what they will be expected to do, and reinforce the right to discontinue participation in the study at any time. [Section 3.2]

discrimination (scientific)
Occurs when the conditioned stimulus is differentiated from other stimuli. [Section 9.1]

discrimination
Unjust treatment of a group, based on group characteristics. [Sections 5.1 & 6.2]

dishabituation
The restoration to full strength of a response to a stimulus that had previously become weakened through habituation. [Section 9.1]

dissociative amnesia
A psychological disorder characterized by at least one episode of suddenly forgetting some important personal information, usually related to severe stress or trauma. [Section 8.1]

dissociative disorder
A psychological disorder characterized by a person's thoughts, feelings, or behaviors being separated from conscious awareness and control, and not explainable as mere forgetfulness. [Section 8.1]

dissociative fugue
A psychological disorder in which someone goes on a journey, during which he or she cannot recall personal history prior to the journey. [Section 8.1]

dissociative identity disorder
A psychological disorder characterized by alternating between multiple personality states. [Section 8.1]

divided attention
Focusing on multiple tasks simultaneously. [Section 11.3]

downward mobility
A decrease in social class. [Section 5.2]

dramaturgical perspective
Assumes that people are theatrical performers and that everyday life is a stage. [Section 6.3]

drive
An urge originating from a physiological discomfort such as hunger, thirst, or sleepiness. [Section 7.2]

Drive Reduction Theory
A theory that suggests that a physiological need creates an aroused state (drive) that motivates the organism to reduce that drive (satiate the need) by engaging in some behavior. [Section 7.2]

dual coding hypothesis
A hypothesis that it is easier to remember words with associated images than either words or images alone. [Section 9.2]

Durkheim, Émile
Considered the founder of sociology and a major proponent of functionalism. [Section 4.1]

dynamic equilibrium
Occurs when complex societies contain many different but interdependent parts working together to maintain stability. [Section 4.1]

dyssomnias
Disorders that involve abnormalities in the amount, quality, or timing of sleep. [Section 11.5]

dysthymic disorder
A psychological disorder characterized as a less intense, less chronic form of depression. [Section 8.1]

ecclesia
A dominant religious organization that includes most members of a society, and is recognized as the exclusive national religion. [Section 4.2]

echoic memory
Sensory memory for sound. [Section 9.2]

effector
The organ that carries out the command sent along a particular motor neuron. [Section 12.3]

efferent neurons
A neuron that carries information away from the central nervous system; a motor neuron. [Section 12.3]

egalitarian family
A family system where spouses are equals involved in negotiation when making decisions. [Section 4.2]

ego
According to Freud's psychoanalytic theory, the ego is ruled by the reality principle, and uses logical thinking and planning to control consciousness. [Section 7.1]

ego defense mechanisms
According to psychoanalytic theory, mechanisms developed to cope with anxiety and protect the ego, in a way that unconsciously denies or distorts reality. [Section 7.1]

eidetic memory
Ability found in some children to vividly recall an image after brief exposure. [Section 9.2]

elaboration likelihood model
Model that explains whether the content of an argument or some more superficial attribute is more likely to cause persuasion. [Section 6.4]

Electra complex
Occurs during the phallic stage when a female child is sexually attracted to her father and hostile toward her mother, who is seen as a rival. [Section 7.1]

electrical synapse
A type of synapse in which the cells are connected by gap junctions, allowing ions (and therefore the action potential) to spread easily from cell to cell. [Section 12.2]

electroencephalography
Low resolution functional technique that provides real-time data on brain wave synchronization at nodes spread through the scalp. [Section 10.1]

electromyogram (EMG)
Recording of skeletal muscle movements. [Section 11.5]

electrooculogram (EOG)
Recording of eye movements. [Section 11.5]

empathy
The ability to identify with others' emotions. [Section 6.3]

encoding
The process of transferring sensory information into the memory system. [Section 9.2]

endocrine gland
A ductless gland that secretes hormones into the blood. [Section 12.4]

endocrine system
A system of ductless glands that secrete chemical messengers (hormones) into the blood. [Section 12.4]

endogamy
The practice of marrying within a particular group. [Section 4.2]

environmental injustice
When people in poorer communities are more likely to be subjected to negative environmental impacts to their health and well-being. [Section 5.2]

epinephrine
A hormone produced and secreted by the adrenal medulla that prolongs and increases the effects of the sympathetic nervous system. [Section 12.3]

episodic buffer
Part of working memory that interacts with information in long-term memory. [Section 11.4]

episodic memory
Autobiographical memory for information of personal importance. [Section 9.2]

Erikson, Erik
Extended Freud's theory of developmental stages by adding social factors and adding developmental stages in adolescence and adulthood. [Section 7.1]

escape learning
Through operant conditioning, this is the process of learning to engage in a particular behavior in order to get away from a negative or aversive stimulus. [Section 9.1]

ethnicity
A socially defined concept referring to whether a large social group identifies with each other based on culture. [Section 5.1]

ethnocentrism
The tendency to judge people from another culture by the standards of one's own culture. [Section 6.2]

ethnographic studies
Studies that make a deep and comprehensive exploration of an ethnicity or culture. [Section 3.3]

excitatory postsynaptic potential (EPSP)
A slight depolarization of a postsynaptic cell, bringing the membrane potential closer to the threshold for an action potential. [Section 12.2]

executive functions
Higher order thinking processes that include planning, organizing, and decision-making. [Section 10.3]

exocrine gland
A gland, such as a sweat gland, that secretes its product into a duct, which ultimately carries the product to the surface of the body or into a body cavity. [Section 12.4]

exogamy
A requirement to marry outside a particular group, to prohibit sexual relationships between certain relatives. [Section 4.2]

experimental group
The group that receives the treatment in an experiment, in contrast to the control group. [Section 3.1]

experimental hypothesis
The hypothesis that there is an experimental effect and the treatment is responsible for the measured difference. [Section 3.1]

explicit (or declarative) memory
Memories that can be consciously recalled, such as factual knowledge. [Section 9.2]

external locus of control
The belief that outcomes in one's life are determined by outside forces. [Section 6.1]

external validity
The extent to which experimental results can be applied to real-world situations. [Section 3.2]

extinction
In classical conditioning, the unpairing of the conditioned and unconditioned stimuli. [Section 9.1]

extraneous variables
Variables other than the research variables that would explain an experimental effect if one were found; also known as confounding variables. [Section 3.1]

false consensus
Occurs when we assume that everyone else agrees with what we do (even though they may not). [Section 6.2]

false memory
Inaccurate memory created by the power of imagination or suggestion. [Sections 9.2 & 11.5]

feature detection theory
A theory of visual perception that proposes that certain neurons fire for specific features of a visual stimulus, such as shape, color, movement, etc. [Section 11.2]

feral children
Neglected or abandoned children who grow up without human contact or care. [Section 6.1]

filter model
Model of selective attention developed by Donald Broadbent that suggests that information is put through a filter that allows only selected inputs through. [Section 11.3]

Five-Factor Model
A model developed to explain personality using five overarching personality traits. [Section 7.1]

fixed-interval schedule
Reinforcement schedule in which reward is offered after a set period of time has passed. [Section 9.1]

fixed-ratio schedule
Reinforcement schedule in which reward is offered after a set number of instances of a behavior. [Section 9.1]

flashbulb memory
Intense vivid "snapshot" of an emotionally intense experience. [Section 9.2]

folkways
Norms that are more informal, yet shape everyday behavior (styles of dress, ways of greeting). [Section 6.1]

food desert
An area, typically in a highly populated lower-income urban environment, where healthy, fresh food is difficult to find. [Section 4.2]

foot-in-the-door phenomenon
A persuasion strategy that involves enticing people to take small actions, then gradually asking for larger commitments. [Section 7.3]

Freud, Sigmund
An Austrian neurologist who is considered the founder of psychoanalytic theory. [Section 7.1]

front stage
In the dramaturgical perspective, this is where we play a role and use impression management to craft the way we come across to other people. [Section 6.3]

frustration-aggression principle
This principle suggests that when someone is blocked from achieving a goal, this frustration can trigger anger, which can lead to aggression. [Section 6.3]

functional fixedness
A tendency to perceive the functions of objects as fixed and unchanging. [Section 11.4]

functionalism
A theory that conceptualizes society as a living organism with many different parts and organs, each of which has a distinct purpose. [Section 4.1]

fundamental attribution error
The tendency to underestimate the impact of the situation and overestimate the impact of a person's character or personality on their behavior. [Section 6.2]

fundamentalists
People who observe strict adherence to religious beliefs. [Section 4.2]

Gage, Phineas
Famous case of a man who suffered damage to his prefrontal cortex after a railroad tie blasted through his head. [Section 10.1]

game theory
A theory used to predict large, complex systems, such as the overall behavior of a population. [Sections 4.1 & 6.4]

ganglion
A clump of gray matter (unmyelinated neuron cell bodies) found in the peripheral nervous system. [Section 11.1]

gender bias in medicine
Occurs when women and men receive different treatment for the same disease or illness. [Section 5.2]

gender conditioning
The socialization of gender roles is also known as gender conditioning [Section 5.1].

gender schema theory
The study of how gender beliefs become socialized in society. [Section 5.1]

general fertility rate
The annual number of live births per 1000 women of childbearing age within a population. [Section 5.1]

general intelligence
Foundational base of intelligence that supports more specialized abilities. [Section 6.4]

generalization
In classical conditioning, the process by which stimuli similar to a conditioned stimulus elicit the conditioned response. [Section 9.1]

generalized anxiety disorder (GAD)
A psychological disorder characterized by tension or anxiety much of the time about many issues, but without the presence of panic attacks. [Section 8.1]

generalized other
When a person tries to imagine what is expected of them from society, they are taking on the perspective of the generalized other. [Section 6.1]

genotype
The genetic makeup of an organism. [Section 6.4]

gestalt psychology
A theory that the brain processes information in a holistic manner. [Section 11.2]

global inequality
The extent to which wealth is distributed unevenly among the world's population. [Section 5.2]

global stratification
A comparison of the wealth, economic stability, and power of various countries. [Section 5.2]

gray matter
Unmyelinated neuron cell bodies and short unmyelinated axons. [Section 10.2]

group
A collection of people (as few as two) who regularly interact and identify. [Section 6.2]

group polarization
The phenomenon where groups tend to intensify the preexisting views of their members until the average view is more extreme than it initially was. [Section 6.2]

group pressure (or peer pressure)
Pressure exerted by a group that causes one to change behaviors, values, attitudes, or beliefs. [Section 6.2]

groupthink
A phenomenon in which the desire for group harmony results in an easy consensus, even if the final decision is not the best one. [Section 6.2]

growth hormone
Hormone released by the anterior pituitary that causes whole body growth in children and adolescents, and increasing cell turnover rate in adults. [Section 12.4]

gustatory receptors
Chemoreceptors on the tongue that respond to chemicals in food. [Section 11.1]

habit
Action that is performed repeatedly until it becomes automatic. [Section 9.1]

habituation
A decrease in response to a stimulus after repeated presentations. [Section 9.1]

hair cells
Sensory receptors found in the inner ear that respond to vibrations in the cochlea caused by sound waves and changes in position and acceleration (used for balance). [Section 11.1]

hallucination
A false sensory perception that occurs while a person is conscious (not during sleep or delirium). [Section 8.1]

hallucinogens
Class of drugs that distort perceptions in the absence of any sensory input, creating hallucinations or altered sensory perceptions. [Section 11.5]

halo effect
A tendency to believe that people have inherently good or bad natures, rather than looking at individual characteristics. [Section 6.2]

Harlow, Harry and Margaret
Researchers known for their controversial experiments with isolated baby monkeys. [Section 9.3]

health care disparities
The population-specific differences in the presence of disease, health outcomes, and quality of health care across different social groups. [Section 5.2]

heritability
The extent to which a behavior is due to genetic factors. [Section 3.3]

heuristics
Mental shortcuts used for problem-solving; sometimes sacrifices accuracy for speed. [Section 11.4]

hindsight bias
Tendency to believe that an event was predictable after it has already occurred. [Section 6.2]

hippocampus
Brain structure located in the medial temporal lobe; plays a key role in forming memories. [Section 10.3]

histrionic personality disorder
A psychological disorder characterized by a strong desire to be the center of attention. [Section 8.1]

homogenous
The same throughout; often used to describe a sample in which participants have similar characteristics. [Section 3.1]

humanistic psychology
A psychological perspective that emphasizes an individual's inherent drive toward self-actualization. [Section 6.1]

hypnotism
Structured interaction in which an individual is instructed to focus attention a particular way, relax, and let go. [Section 11.5]

hypochondriasis
A psychological disorder characterized by a preoccupation with having a serious illness. [Section 8.1]

hypophysis
The pituitary gland. [Section 12.4]

hypothalamus
Brain structure that is involved in many autonomic processes including body temperature, hunger, thirst, fatigue, and sleep. [Sections 12.4]

iconic memory
The brief photographic memory for visual information, which decays in a few tenths of a second. [Section 9.2]

id
According to Freud's psychoanalytic theory, is the source of energy and instincts that seeks to gain pleasure. [Section 7.1]

ideal self
Constructed out of experiences, expectations, and role models; the person one wishes to be. [Section 6.1]

identity formation (or individuation)
Development of a distinct personality. [Section 6.1]

illusory correlation
A perceived relationship between two things, even when none exists. [Section 6.2]

implicit (or procedural) memory
Memory that involves conditioned associations and knowledge of how to do something. [Section 9.2]

impression management or self-presentation
The process whereby people attempt to manage their images by influencing others' perceptions. [Section 6.3]

in-group
A group that an individual belongs to and believes to be an integral part of who they are. [Section 6.2]

incentive theory
A theory that suggests that incentives (objects that either induce or discourage behaviors) motivate human behavior. [Section 7.2]

inclusive fitness
A theory that suggests that cooperation among organisms promotes genetic success. [Section 6.3]

incongruity
The emotional result when the real self falls short of the ideal self. [Section 6.1]

infantile amnesia
A lack of explicit memory for events that occurred before the age of roughly 3.5 years. [Section 9.3]

information-processing models
Models that use computers as an analogy for understanding cognitive processes such as attention, perception, and memory. [Section 11.4]

informational social influence
The process of complying to do the right thing because others "know something we don't know." [Section 6.2]

Inhibitory postsynaptic potential (IPSP)
Slight hyperpolarization of a postsynaptic cell, moving the membrane potential of that cell further from threshold. [Section 12.2]

insecure attachment
Category of attachment styles in which infants are less likely to explore the environment in the presence of the mother and less likely to be soothed by her. [Section 9.3]

insight learning
Sudden flash of inspiration that provides a solution to a problem. [Section 9.1]

insomnia
Most common sleep disorder, characterized by difficulty falling or staying asleep. [Section 11.5]

instinct
Behaviors that are unlearned and present in fixed patterns throughout a species. [Section 7.2]

institutional discrimination
Unjust practices employed by large organizations that have been codified into operating processes or institutional objectives. [Section 6.2]

instrumental conditioning
See operant conditioning. [Section 9.1]

intellectual disability
Classification for individuals who have an IQ below 70 and functional impairment in their everyday lives. [Section 6.4]

intelligence
The ability to learn from experience, problem-solve, and adapt to new situations. [Section 6.4]

intergenerational mobility
A change (increase or decrease) in social class between parents and children within a family. [Section 5.2]

internal locus of control
An individual's belief that they can affect outcomes through their own actions. [Section 6.1]

internal validity
How "well designed" a study is; how valid it is to draw conclusions from the research based on the way it was constructed. [Section 3.2]

interneuron
A neuron found completely within the central nervous system. [Section 12.3]

intragenerational mobility
Describes the differences in social class between different members of the same generation. [Section 5.2]

iris
A pigmented membrane found just in front of the lens of the eye. The iris regulates the diameter of the pupil in response to the brightness of light. [Section 11.1]

James-Lange Theory
Theory of emotion in which emotional experience is the result of physiological responses. [Section 7.4]

just world phenomenon
The tendency to believe that the world is fair and people get what they deserve. [Section 6.2]

justification of effort
When people modify their attitudes to match their behaviors, specifically those involving effort. [Section 7.3]

K-complex
Large and slow wave with a duration of a half second that occurs in Stage 2 sleep. [Section 11.5]

kinship
Familial relationships including blood ties, family ties, and common ancestry. [Section 4.2]

Kohlberg's stages of moral development
Six developmental stages of moral reasoning, which form the basis of ethical behavior. [Section 6.1]

language
A symbolic system that is codified for communication. [Section 11.6]

language acquisition
The process by which infants learn to understand and speak their native language. [Section 11.6]

language acquisition device
The Nativist theory proposes that there is a theoretical language acquisition device (LAD) somewhere in our brains that is responsible for learning a language during the critical period of language acquisition (before adolescence). [Section 11.6]

latent content
The unconscious drives and wishes that are difficult to express and underlie dreams. [Section 11.5]

latent functions
The unintended or less recognizable consequences or a social structure. [Section 4.1]

latent learning
Learning that takes place in the absence of any observable behavior to show that it has occurred. [Section 9.1]

learned helplessness
A condition where an individual does not act even though there are opportunities to avoid unpleasant circumstances or gain positive rewards. [Sections 6.1 & 8.2]

libido
The life instinct, which drives behaviors focused on survival, growth, creativity, pain avoidance, and seeking pleasure. [Section 7.1]

life course perspective
Sociological theory that investigates key events in a person's life and how they unfold over time and lead to a person's development. [Section 6.4]

life expectancy
The number of years that an individual at a given age can expect to live at present mortality rates. [Section 5.1]

linguistic relativity hypothesis
Asserts that the language one speaks determines their thoughts and perceptions of the world. [Section 11.6]

long-term memory
Information that is retained long-term, potentially indefinitely. [Section 9.1]

long-term potentiation
An increase in synaptic strength between two neurons following simultaneous firing. [Sections 9.1 & 10.3]

looking glass self
The idea that a person's sense of self develops from interpersonal interactions with others in society and the perceptions of others. [Section 6.1]

major depressive disorder
A psychological disorder characterized by one or more depressive episodes, in which a person has felt worse than usual for most of the day, nearly every day, for at least two weeks. [Section 8.1]

manic episode
An experience of an abnormal euphoric, unrestrained, or irritable mood. [Section 8.1]

manifest content
According to Freud, the overt storylines of dreams. [Section 11.5]

manifest functions
The intended and obvious consequences of a social structure. [Section 4.1]

marginal poverty
Poverty that is due to circumstantial conditions, such as a lack of stable employment. [Section 5.2]

Marx, Karl
Founder of Conflict Theory who argued that societies progress through class struggle between those who control production and those who provide the labor for production. [Section 4.1]

Maslow's Hierarchy of Needs
Abraham Maslow's pyramid of motivational factors from physiological needs, at the base, progressively up to higher level needs such as self-actualization that must be met in order. [Section 7.2]

master status
The status that dominates other statuses and determines an individual's position in society. [Section 6.3]

material culture
Consists of the physical objects that are particular to a culture. [Section 5.1]

matriarchy
A social system where females are the primary authority figures. [Section 4.2]

matrilineal descent
A system of lineage in which the relatives on the mother's side are considered most important. [Section 4.2]

mechanoreceptor
A sensory receptor that responds to mechanical disturbances, such as shape changes (being squashed, bent, pulled). [Section 11.1]

meditation
Mindfulness technique for training attention in a particular way. [Section 11.5]

medulla oblongata
Portion of the hindbrain that controls respiratory rate and blood pressure, and specialized digestive and respiratory functions. [Section 10.2]

melatonin
Hormone produced by the pineal gland that affects sleep/wake cycles and seasonal functions. [Section 11.5]

meninges
The protective connective tissue wrappings of the central nervous system. [Section 12.3]

mental set
A tendency to fixate on ideas and solutions that have worked in the past, even if they may not apply to the current situation. [Section 11.4]

mere exposure effect
The phenomenon where people develop a preference for things because they have been exposed to them. [Section 6.3]

mere presence
The most basic level of "interaction" between individuals; when people are simply in each other's presence. [Section 6.2]

meritocracy
An idealized social stratification in which people's social standings are judged based on merit alone. [Section 5.2]

meta-analysis
An review of many studies to combine results and find emergent patterns in an area of research. [Section 3.1]

method of loci
A memory technique that involves imagining moving through a familiar place, and leaving visual representation topics to be remembered. [Section 9.2]

midbrain
The portion of the brain responsible for visual and auditory startle reflexes. [Section 10.2]

Milgram, Stanley
Conducted research on obedience in which he asked subjects to administer a shock to what they thought was another subject (who was just an actor). [Section 6.2]

Mindfulness-based stress reduction (MBSR)
Protocol involving mindfulness meditation that reduces pain, stress, and anxiety. [Section 11.5]

mindguarding
When dissenting opinions are prevented from permeating a group by filtering out information that goes against group beliefs. [Section 6.2]

mirror neurons
Neurons that fire when a particular behavior or emotion is observed in another. [Sections 9.1 & 10.3]

misinformation effect
A tendency to misremember an event, particularly when misleading information is presented between the event and the mental encoding of the event. [Section 9.2]

mixed methods
Any two types of research methodology are combined in the same study, such as qualitative and quantitative or between-subjects and within-subjects. [Section 3.1]

mnemonic
Any memory technique use to promote the retention and retrieval of information. [Section 9.2]

modeling
Mechanism behind observational learning in which an observer sees a behavior performed, then imitates the behavior. [Section 9.1]

monogamy
A form of marriage in which two individuals are married only to each other. [Section 4.2]

mood
A person's sustained internal emotion that colors his or her view of life. [Section 8.1]

mood-dependent memory
When learning occurs during a particular emotional state, it is most easily recalled when one is again in that emotional state. [Section 9.2]

mood disorder
A psychological disorder, such as bipolar disorder, or depressive disorders, characterized by a persistent pattern of abnormal mood serious enough to cause significant personal distress. [Section 8.1]

mores
Norms that are highly important for the benefit of society and so are often strictly enforced. [Section 6.1]

mortality
The death rate in a population. [Section 5.1]

multiculturalism (also known as pluralism)
A perspective that endorses equal standing for all cultural traditions. [Section 6.1]

multipolar neuron
A neuron with a single axon and multiple dendrites. [Section 12.1]

myelin
An insulating layer of membranes wrapped around the axons of almost all neurons in the body. [Section 12.1]

narcissistic personality disorder
A psychological disorder characterized by grandiosity and inflated sense of self. [Section 8.1]

narcolepsy
Sleep disorder in which an individual experiences short bursts of periodic, overwhelming sleepiness during waking periods. [Section 11.5]

negative feedback
A biological process that maintains homeostasis by feeding back to promote the limitation of a biological product. [Sections 7.2 & 12.4]

negative punishment
The removal of a positive or rewarding stimulus that decreases the likelihood of that behavior. [Section 9.1]

negative reinforcement
The removal of a negative or aversive stimulus following a behavior. Tends to increase the frequency of that behavior. [Section 9.1]

neural plasticity
A process that refers to the malleability of the brain's pathways and synapses based on behavior, the environment, and neural processes. [Section 10.3]

neuron
The basic functional and structural unit of the nervous system. [Section 12.1]

neurotransmitter
A chemical released by a neuron that binds to receptors on the postsynaptic cell and causes it to either depolarize or hyperpolarize. [Sections 10.2, 12.1, & 12.2]

neutral stimulus
A stimulus that does not elicit any intrinsic response. [Section 9.1]

night terror
Occurs during stage 3 sleep when an individual appears terrified and may sit up or walk around. [Section 11.5]

nociceptors
Pain receptors. [Section 11.1]

nodes of Ranvier
Gaps in the myelin sheath of the axons of peripheral neurons that increases the speed of conduction. [Section 12.1]

nonassociative learning
Learning that occurs in the absence of associating specific stimuli or events. [Section 9.1]

nonverbal communication
Involves all the methods of communication that do not include words. [Section 6.3]

norepinephrine (NE)
The neurotransmitter used by the sympathetic division of the autonomic nervous system at the postganglionic (organ-level) synapse. [Section 12.2]

normative organizations
An organization where membership is based on morally relevant goals. [Section 6.3]

normative social influence
When the motivation for compliance is a desire for the approval of others and to avoid rejection. [Section 6.2]

norms
The visible and invisible rules of social conduct within a society. [Sections 5.1 & 6.1]

nucleus accumbens
Structure located in the brainstem that releases dopamine in response to many drugs, contributing to addictive behavior. [Section 10.2]

null hypothesis
The hypothesis that there is no experimental effect and any differences, if measured, are due to chance. [Section 3.1]

object permanence
The understanding that things continue to exist once they are out of sight. [Section 11.4]

observational learning
A type of learning that occurs when a person watches another person. [Section 7.1]

observational studies
A type of research characterized by minimal manipulation in an attempt to investigate phenomena in their naturalistic state. [Section 3.3]

obsessive-compulsive disorder (OCD)
A psychological disorder characterized by repeated, intrusive, uncontrollable thoughts and repeated physical behaviors that are done in response to an obsession. [Section 8.1]

Oedipus complex
This complex occurs during the phallic stage when a male child is sexually attracted to his mother and hostile toward his father, who is seen as a rival. [Section 7.1]

olfactory receptors
Chemoreceptors in the upper nasal cavity that respond to odor chemicals. [Section 11.1]

operant conditioning
A form of associative learning based on consequences, in which rewards increase the frequency of behaviors and punishments decrease their frequency. [Section 9.1]

operational definition
The specifications of experimental variables in terms that can be used by other researchers to replicate methodology. [Section 3.1]

optic disk
The "blind spot" of the eye, where axons of ganglion cells exit the retina to form the optic nerve. [Section 11.1]

optic nerve
The nerve extending from the back of the eyeball to the brain that carries visual information. [Section 11.1]

optimism bias
The belief that bad things happen to other people, but not to us. [Section 6.2]

oral stage
The first of Freud's five psychosexual stages, in this stage the child seeks sensual pleasure through oral activities such as sucking and chewing. [Section 7.1]

organ of Corti
The structure in the cochlea of the inner ear made up of the basilar membrane, the auditory hair cells, and the tectorial membrane. [Section 11.1]

organization
A large group, more impersonal than a network, that comes together to pursue particular activities and meet goals efficiently. [Section 6.3]

ossicles
The three small bones found in the middle ear (the malleus, the incus, and the stapes) that help to amplify the vibrations from sound waves. [Section 11.1]

out-group
A group that an individual does not belong to. [Section 6.2]

outer ear
The portion of the ear consisting of the pinna and the external auditory canal. [Section 11.1]

oval window
The membrane that separates the middle ear from the inner ear. [Section 11.1]

overconfidence
An overestimation of the accuracy of one's knowledge and judgments. [Section 11.4]

p-value
Numerical value that gives the probability that a measured difference occurred due to chance. [Section 3.1]

pain disorder
A psychological disorder characterized by clinically important pain affected by psychological factors. [Section 8.1]

panic disorder
A psychological disorder that is characterized by panic attacks that are cued by certain situations or occur frequently and unexpectedly. [Section 8.1]

parallel processing
A system whereby many aspects of a stimulus are processed simultaneously instead of in a step-by-step or serial fashion. [Section 11.2]

paranoid personality disorder
A psychological disorder characterized by mistrust and misinterpretation of others' motives and actions, and suspicion of harm or betrayal. [Section 8.1]

paranoid-type schizophrenia
A psychological disorder characterized by psychosis is in the form of hallucinations and/or delusions, usually relating to a certain theme. [Section 8.1]

parasomnia
Abnormal behaviors during sleep, including somnambulism and night terrors. [Section 11.5]

parasympathetic nervous system (PNS)
The division of the autonomic nervous system known as the "resting and digesting" system. It causes a general decrease in body activities such as heart rate and blood pressure. [Sections 10.2 & 12.3]

Parkinson's disease
A movement disorder caused by the death of dopamine-releasing cells. [Section 8.1]

patriarchy
A social system where males are the primary authority figures. [Section 4.2]

patrilineal descent
A system of lineage in which the relatives on the father's side are considered most important. [Section 4.2]

Pavlov, Ivan
Famous for naming and describing the process of classical conditioning by training dogs to salivate to the sound of a ringing bell. [Section 9.1]

Pearson correlation
A numerical value between −1 and 1 that indicates how two variables correlate; a negative value indicates an inverse relationship, a positive value indicates a direct relationship, and values further from zero indicate a stronger relationship. [Section 3.3]

peg word method
Mnemonic strategy that involves assigning images to a sequence of numbers. [Section 9.2]

penis envy
Occurs during the phallic stage (the third of Freud's five psychosexual stages), when a female realizes she does not have a penis. [Section 7.1]

peptide hormone
A hormone made of amino acids that is generally hydrophilic and cannot cross the plasma membranes of cells. [Section 12.4]

peripheral nervous system
All the parts of the nervous system except for the brain and spinal cord. [Sections 10.2 & 12.3]

peripheral route
Cognitive route of persuasion that involves more superficial or secondary characteristics. [Section 6.4]

permissive parenting
Parenting style that creates few rules and demands and little discipline. [Section 9.3]

person-situation controversy
A disagreement about the degree to which a person's reaction in a given situation is due to their personality or is due to the situation itself. [Section 7.1]

personal identity
A distinct sense of self, including personally-defined attributes. [Section 6.1]

personality
The nuanced and complex individual pattern of thinking, feeling, and behavior associated with each person. [Section 7.1]

personality disorder
A psychological disorder characterized by an enduring, rigid set of personality traits that deviates from cultural norms, impairs functioning, and causes distress. [Section 8.1]

personality trait
A generally stable predisposition toward a certain behavior. [Section 7.1]

phenomenological method
The use of introspection to explore the nature of phenomena, often related to perception or subjective experience. [Section 3.3]

phenotype
The observable characteristics and traits of an organism. [Section 6.4]

pheromone
A chemical signal that causes a social response in members of the same species. [Section 11.1]

phobia
A strong unreasonable fear that almost always causes either general anxiety or a full panic attack. [Section 8.1]

phonological loop
Part of working memory that allows for repetition of verbal information to aid with encoding. [Section 11.4]

photoreceptor
A receptor that responds to light. [Section 11.1]

physical attractiveness stereotype
The tendency of people to rate attractive individuals more favorably for personality traits. [Section 6.2]

Piaget, Jean
Developmental psychologist who formulated a four-stage theory of development for children. [Section 11.4]

pineal gland
Region of the brain responsible for the production of melatonin, a hormone that influences sleep/wake cycles and seasonal functions. [Section 11.5]

placebo effect
The phenomenon that if a group of participants simply believes that it has been given a treatment, this can lead to a measurable effect. [Section 3.1]

polyandry
A form of marriage in which a woman is married to more than one man. [Section 4.2]

polygamy
A form of marriage in which an individual may have multiple wives or husbands simultaneously. [Section 4.2]

polygyny
A form of marriage in which a man is married to more than one woman. [Section 4.2]

polysomnography (PSG)
Multimodal technique for measuring physiological processes during sleep, including EEG, EMG, and EOG. [Section 11.5]

positive punishment
The introduction of a negative or aversive stimulus following a behavior. Tends to decrease the likelihood of that behavior. [Section 9.1]

positive reinforcement
Reward immediately following a behavior that increases the frequency of that behavior (for example, praise). [Section 9.1]

positive transfer
When old information facilitates the learning of new information. [Section 9.2]

posttraumatic stress disorder (PTSD)
Disorder characterized by re-experiencing a traumatic event through flashbacks or nightmares. [Section 8.1]

posterior pituitary gland
Nervous tissue located at the rear of the pituitary that secretes two hormones made by the hypothalamus: oxytocin and ADH. [Section 12.4]

postganglionic neuron
In the autonomic division of the PNS, a neuron that has its cell body in an autonomic ganglion, and whose axon synapses with the target organ. [Section 12.3]

power
The ability of a study to pick up an effect if one is indeed present; this is related to factors such as large sample size and low variation. [Section 3.1]

predictive validity
The extent to which a psychometric instrument predicts results along a well-known test or in variable of interest. [Section 3.2]

prefrontal cortex
Anterior part of the frontal lobes of the brain involved in complex behaviors such as planning, sequencing, social responses, and decision making. [Sections 10.1 & 10.3]

preganglionic neuron
In the autonomic division of the PNS, neuron that has its cell body located in the CNS, and whose axon extends into the PNS to synapse with a second neuron at an autonomic ganglion. [Section 12.3]

prejudice
Thoughts, attitudes, and feelings someone holds about a group that are based on a prejudgment or biased thinking about a group and its members. [Section 6.2]

primacy effect
A tendency to better recall the first items on a list. [Section 9.2]

primary groups
Groups that play a more important role in an individual's life; these groups are usually smaller and include those with whom the individual engages with in person. [Section 6.2]

primary reinforcers
Unconditioned consequences that are innately satisfying or desirable. May be biologically driven. [Section 9.1]

priming
An effect of implicit memory whereby exposure to a given stimulus "primes" or prepares the brain to respond to a later stimulus. [Section 9.2]

principle of aggregation
The idea that an attitude affects a person's aggregate or average behavior, but cannot necessarily predict each isolated act. [Section 7.3]

proactive interference
A type of memory interference that occurs when previously learned information interferes with the recall of information learned more recently. [Section 9.2]

projection bias
Occurs when we assume others have the same beliefs we do, due to our tendency to look for similarities between ourselves and others. [Section 6.2]

proprioceptor
A receptor that responds to changes in the body position, such as stretch on a tendon, or contraction of a muscle. [Section 11.1]

prospective memory
Remembering to do something in the future. [Section 9.2]

psychoanalytic theory
According to this theory, personality is shaped by a person's unconscious thoughts, feelings, and memories. [Section 7.1]

psychoanalytic therapy
This therapy approach helps a patient become aware of his or her unconscious sources for emotional issues and conflicts that are causing difficulties. [Section 7.1]

psychological disorder
A set of behavioral and/or psychological symptoms that are not in keeping with cultural norms and are severe enough to cause significant personal distress. [Section 8.1]

psychological fixation
Occurs in psychoanalytic theory when parents either frustrate or overindulge a child's expression of sensual pleasure at a certain stage, and as an adult the individual continues to seek sensual pleasure through behaviors related to that stage. [Section 11.4]

psychometrics
The art and science of measuring psychological processes. [Section 3.1]

psychosexual stages
According to Freud's psychoanalytic theory, individuals progress through five psychosexual stages, one corresponding to the part of the body that is the focus of sensual pleasure. [Section 7.1]

punishment
In operant conditioning, a consequence that decreases the likelihood that a preceding behavior will be repeated. [Section 9.1]

pupil
A hole in the center of the iris of the eye that allows light to enter the eyeball. [Section 11.1]

qualitative
Descriptive, as opposed to numerical; often used to refer to data. [Section 3.1]

quantitative
Numerical, as opposed to descriptive; often used to describe data. [Section 3.1]

race
The biological, anthropological, or genetic origin of an individual. [Section 5.1]

racism
Prejudices and discriminatory actions that are based on race (or ethnicity), or hold that one race (or ethnicity) is inferior to another. [Sections 5.1 & 6.2]

randomized block technique
A technique used by researchers who wish to make experimental and control groups similar along a set of variables. [Section 3.1]

rapid eye movement (REM)
Bursts of quick eye movements present in the last stage of sleep. [Section 11.5]

rational-legal authority
A form of leadership that is organized around rational legal rules. [Section 4.2]

recall
Retrieving information from memory. [Sections 9.2 & 11.4]

recency effect
A tendency to recall the last items presented in a list. [Section 9.2]

reciprocal determinism
A reciprocal interaction between a person's behaviors, personal factors, and environmental factors. [Section 6.4]

recognition
Retrieving information from memory with the use of cues. [Section 9.2]

reconstructive memory
Theory that memory is constructed rather than a perfect recollection of an event. [Section 9.2]

reference group
A group that serves as a standard measure that people compare themselves to. [Section 6.2]

reflex
Automatic behaviors that occur without thinking. [Section 12.3]

reflex arc
A relatively direct connection between a sensory neuron and a motor neuron that allows an extremely rapid response to a stimulus. [Section 12.3]

rehearsal
Technique of repeating verbal information in one's phonological loop to promote the encoding of sensory information into memory. [Section 9.2]

reinforcement
A consequence that increases the likelihood that a preceding behavior will be repeated. Two types are positive and negative reinforcement. [Section 9.1]

reinforcement schedule
The frequency and regularity with which rewards are offered, based on a number of target behaviors (ratio) or on a time interval (interval). [Section 9.1]

relative poverty
An inability to meet the average standard of living within a society. [Section 5.2]

relative refractory period
The period of time following an action potential when it is possible, but difficult, for the neuron to fire a second action potential. [Section 12.1]

relearning
The process of learning material that was originally learned. [Section 9.2]

reliable
The tendency of a survey or other instrument of measurement to produce similar results under similar conditions and measure what they are purported to. [Section 3.1]

religiosity
The extent that religion influences a person's life. [Section 4.2]

REM stage
Final stage of sleep characterized by rapid eye movements (REM) and beta waves, which are seen in individuals when they are awake. [Section 11.5]

replacement fertility rate
The number of children that a woman or couple must have in order to replace the number of the people in the population who die. [Section 5.1]

replicability
Obtaining consistent results across various studies attempting to answer the same scientific question using different data and/or new statistical methods. [Section 3.1]

representativeness heuristic
A mental shortcut in which one judges the likelihood of things based on typical mental representations or examples of those things. [Section 11.4]

reproducibility
Obtaining consistent results using the same data and statistical methods as a prior study. [Section 3.1]

reproductive memory
Theory that suggests memory recall occurs through storage of the original stimulus input and subsequent recall. [Section 9.2]

resource model of attention
States that if multiple tasks exceed the limit of attention, they cannot be done simultaneously. [Section 11.3]

retention interval
The amount of time elapsed since information was learned and when it must be recalled. [Section 9.2]

reticular formation
Also known as the Reticular Activating System. Structures in the brainstem that are important for alertness and arousal (as in wakefulness). [Section 11.5]

retina
The innermost layer of the eyeball. The retina is made up of photoreceptors, bipolar cells, and a layer of ganglion cells. [Section 11.1]

retroactive interference
A type of memory interference that occurs when newly learned information interferes with the recall of information learned previously. [Section 9.2]

retrograde amnesia
Occurs when one is unable to recall information that was previously encoded. [Sections 8.1 & 9.2]

rods
Photoreceptors in the retina that respond to dim light and provide black and white vision. [Section 11.1]

Rogers, Carl
Considered the founder of humanistic psychology who pioneered the person-centered approach to therapy. [Section 6.1]

role conflict
Occurs when there is a conflict in society's expectations for multiple statuses held by the same person (for example "male" and "nurse"). [Section 6.3]

role exit
The process of disengaging from a role that has become closely tied to one's self-identity to take on a new role. [Section 6.3]

role strain
Occurs when a single status results in conflicting expectations. [Section 6.3]

saltatory conduction
A rapid form of neural conduction in which the action potential "jumps" along nodes of Ranvier. [Section 12.1]

sample size
The number of participants in a study. [Section 3.1]

sampling bias
Occurs when some individuals from a population have a greater likelihood of being selected than others. [Section 3.1]

sanctions
Rewards and punishments for behaviors that are in accord with or against norms. [Section 6.1]

scapegoat
The people or group who are unfairly blamed for something, or at whom displaced aggression is directed. [Section 6.2]

Schachter-Singer Theory
Theory of emotion that asserts that the experience of physiological arousal occurs first and is followed by a conscious cognitive interpretation that allows for identification of the emotion. [Section 7.4]

schemas
Mental frameworks or blueprints that shape and are shaped by experience. [Section 11.4]

schizoaffective disorder
A psychological disorder characterized by the combination of mood and psychotic symptoms. [Section 8.1]

schizoid personality disorder
A psychological disorder characterized by little interest or involvement in close relationships, even those with family members. [Section 8.1]

schizophrenia
A psychological disorder that is chronic and incapacitating and is characterized by psychosis and impairment in functioning. [Section 8.1]

schizophreniform disorder
A psychological disorder characterized by symptoms of schizophrenia present for a period of one to six months, during which the symptoms may or may not have interfered with functioning. [Section 8.1]

schizotypal personality disorder
A psychological disorder characterized by constricted or inappropriate affect, magical or paranoid thinking, and odd beliefs, speech, behavior, appearance, and perceptions. [Section 8.1]

Schwann cell
One of the two peripheral nervous system supporting (glial) cells. Schwann cells form the myelin sheath on axons of peripheral neurons. [Section 12.1]

sclera
The white portion of the tough outer layer of the eyeball. [Section 11.1]

secondary group
A larger and more impersonal group than a primary group, which interacts for specific reasons for relatively short periods of time. [Section 6.2]

secondary reinforcers
Conditioned reinforcers that are learned through their relationship with primary reinforcers. [Section 9.1]

sect
A religious organization that is distinct from the parent religion from which it was formed. [Section 4.2]

secure attachment
An attachment style that forms when an infant has caregivers who are sensitive and responsive to needs. [Section 9.3]

selection bias
Nonrandom processes in the selection of participants, experimental groups, or any other process that introduce potential bias into a research study. [Section 3.1]

selective attention
The process by which one input is selected out of the field of environmental stimuli. [Section 11.3]

selective priming
Predisposition to observe something because it has previously been encountered frequently. [Section 11.3]

self-actualization (or actualizing tendency)
According to humanistic psychology, individuals have an innate drive to realize their human potential. [Section 7.1]

self-concept (or self-identity)
The sum of an individual's knowledge and understanding of his- or herself. [Section 6.1]

self-consciousness
Awareness of one's self. [Section 6.1]

self-efficacy
The belief in one's own competence and effectiveness. [Section 6.1]

self-esteem
One's overall self-evaluation of one's self-worth. [Section 6.1]

self-fulfilling prophecy
When stereotypes lead a person to behave in such a way as to affirm the original stereotypes. [Section 6.2]

self-handicapping
A strategy in which people create obstacles and excuses to avoid self-blame when they do poorly. [Section 6.3]

self-reference effect
The tendency to better remember information relevant to ourselves. [Section 9.2]

self-schemas
The beliefs and ideas people have about themselves. [Section 6.1]

self-serving bias
The tendency to attribute our successes to ourselves and our failures to others or the external environment. [Section 6.2]

self verification
Social psychology theory that individuals wish to be understood in terms of their deeply held beliefs in a way that is consistent with their self-concept. [Section 6.1]

semantic memory
Memory for factual information. [Section 9.2]

semicircular canals
Three loop-like structures in the inner ear that contain sensory receptors to monitor balance. [Section 11.1]

sensitization
An increase in the strength of a response with repeated presentations of a stimulus. [Section 9.1]

sensory memory
The initial recording of sensory information in the memory system; sensory memory is a very brief snapshot that quickly decays. [Section 9.2]

serial position effect
When information is presented in a list, individuals are more likely to recall the first and last items presented. [Section 9.2]

shaping
In operant conditioning, the process of reinforcing intermediate, proximal behaviors until a final, desired behavior is achieved. [Section 9.1]

short-term memory
Memory that is limited in duration and in capacity. [Section 9.2]

signal detection theory
A theory that attempts to predict how and when someone will detect the presence of a given sensory stimulus amidst all of the other sensory stimuli in the background (considered the "noise"). [Section 11.2]

significant difference
A difference between two measurements that is unlikely to be due simply to chance, according to a predetermined threshold. [Section 3.1]

Skinner, B.F.
Founder of Behaviorism who measured the effects of reward and punishment on shaping behavior. [Section 9.1]

sleep apnea
Sleep disorder in which the individual intermittently stops breathing during sleep and may wake up gasping for breath. [Section 11.5]

sleep cycle
One progression through sleep stages 1 through 4 in sequence, followed by an ascension from 4 back to 1 and then a transition into REM sleep. Typically takes about ninety minutes. [Section 11.5]

sleep spindle
Bursts of waves present in Stage 2 sleep. [Section 11.5]

social behaviorism
The idea that the mind and self emerge through the process of communicating with others. [Section 6.1]

social capital
The potential for social networks to allow for upward social mobility. [Section 5.2]

social cognition
The ability of the brain to store and process information regarding social perception. [Section 6.2]

social cognitive perspective
According to this perspective, personality is formed by a reciprocal interaction among behavioral, cognitive, and environmental factors. [Sections 6.4 & 7.1]

social constructionism
A social mechanism or practice that is created and sustained by society. [Section 4.1]

social constructionism
A sociological theory that argues that reality is constructed, not inherent. [Section 4.1]

social cues
Verbal or nonverbal hints that guide social interactions.
[Section 7.1]

social dysfunction
A process that has undesirable consequences, and may actually
reduce the stability of society. [Section 4.1]

social epidemiology
The study of the distribution of health and disease across a
population using social concepts to explain patterns of health
and illness. [Sections 4.2 & 5.2]

social facilitation effect
The phenomenon that describes how people tend to perform
simple, well-learned tasks better when other people are present,
while difficult, novel tasks are performed more poorly in front
of others. [Section 6.2]

social facts
The elements that serve some function in society, such as the
laws, morals, values, religions, customs, rituals, and rules that
make up a society. [Section 4.1]

social identity
The social definitions of self, including race, religion, gender,
occupation, and the like. [Section 6.1]

social institutions
A complex of roles, norms, and values organized into a
relatively stable form that contributes to social order by
governing the behavior of people. [Section 4.2]

social loafing
The phenomenon where people tend to exert less effort if they
are being evaluated as a group than if they are individually
accountable. [Section 6.2]

social mobility
The ability to move up or down within the social stratification
system. [Section 5.2]

social network
A web of social relationships, including those in which a
person is directly linked as well as indirectly connected to
people. [Section 6.3]

social perception
The ability to understand others in our social world. [Section 6.2]

social phobia
An unreasonable, paralyzing fear of feeling embarrassed or
humiliated while one is watched by others. [Section 8.1]

social reproduction
The phenomenon of social inequality transmitted from one
generation to the next. [Section 5.2]

social roles
Expectations for people of a given social status. [Section 6.3]

social stratification
The way that people are categorized in society. [Section 5.2]

social support
The perception that one is cared for and part of a social
network; supportive resources can be tangible or emotional.
[Section 6.3]

socialism
An economic system where resources and production are
collectively owned. [Section 4.1]

socialization
The process through which people learn to be proficient
members of society. [Section 6.1]

society
A group of people who share a culture and live/interact with
each other within a definable area. [Section 4.1]

sociobiology
The study of how biology and evolution have affected human
social behavior. [Section 5.1]

socioeconomic status (SES)
Prestige and power associated with one's standing in society
due to income, and other factors. [Section 5.2]

sociology
The study of how individuals interact with, shape, and are
subsequently shaped by society. [Section 4.1]

soma
The cell body of a neuron. [Section 12.1]

somatization disorder
A psychological disorder characterized by a variety of physical
symptoms over an extended time period. [Section 8.1]

somatoform disorder
A psychological disorder characterized primarily by
physical symptoms and concerns, but the symptoms are
not explainable medically and do not improve with medical
treatment. [Section 8.1]

somnambulism
Sleepwalking. [Section 11.5]

source monitoring error
A specific type of error of recollection where a memory is
incorrectly attributed to the wrong source. [Section 9.2]

source traits
The factors underlying human personality and behavior.
[Section 7.1]

spatial summation
Integration by a postsynaptic neuron of inputs (EPSPs and
IPSPs) from multiple sources. [Section 12.2]

specific phobia
A persistent, strong, and unreasonable fear of a certain object
or situation. [Section 8.1]

spontaneous recovery
In classical conditioning, a reoccurrence of a previously
extinct conditioned response in the presence of a conditioned
stimulus. [Section 9.1]

spotlight model
Model for visual attention, with a spotlight representing one's
attention and its ability to move focus onto different targets.
[Section 11.3]

spreading activation theory
A theory of information retrieval that involves a search process
where specific nodes are activated, which leads to the activation
of related nodes, and so on. [Section 10.3]

state
Situational factors that can influence personality and behavior;
states are unstable, temporary, and variable. [Section 7.1]

state capitalism
A system in which companies are privately run, but work
closely with the government in forming laws and regulations.
[Section 4.2]

status
A sociological term that refers to all the socially defined
positions within a society. [Section 6.3]

stereotype threat
Refers to a self-fulfilling fear that one will be evaluated based on a
negative stereotype. [Section 6.2]

stereotypes
Oversimplified ideas about groups of people, based on
characteristics. [Section 6.2]

steroid hormone
A hormone derived from cholesterol that is hydrophobic and
can easily cross the cell membrane, thus receptors for steroids
are found intracellularly. [Section 12.4]

stigma
Extreme disapproval of a person or group based on the person
or groups actual or perceived deviance from society.
[Section 6.2]

stimulants
Class of drugs that speed up body functions and neural
activity. [Section 11.5]

stranger anxiety
Developmentally typical anxiety displayed by children aged
eight to twelve months toward strangers. [Section 9.3]

structural poverty
Poverty due to structural effects such as systemic oppression
or lack of infrastructure and reliable social institutions.
[Section 5.2]

subculture
A segment of society that shares a distinct pattern of traditions
and values that differs from that of the larger society.
[Section 6.1]

summation
The integration of input from many presynaptic neurons by
a single postsynaptic neuron, either temporally or spatially.
[Section 12.2]

superego
According to Freud's psychoanalytic theory, the superego
inhibits the id and influences the ego to follow moralistic rather
than realistic goals. [Section 7.1]

survey studies
Studies that use questionnaires to explore a research variable.
[Section 3.3]

symbolic culture
Consists of symbols that carry a particular meaning and are
recognized by people of the same culture. [Section 5.1]

symbolic interactionism
A micro-level theory in sociology which examines the
relationship between individuals and society by focusing on
communication, the exchange of information through language
and symbols. [Section 4.1]

sympathetic nervous system (SNS)
Subdivision of the autonomic nervous system directing the
"fight or flight" response to prepare the body for action. It
increases heart rate, blood pressure, and directs the adrenal
glands to release stress hormones. [Sections 8.2 & 12.4]

synapse
A neuron-to-neuron, neuron-to-organ, or muscle cell-to-
muscle cell junction. [Section 12.2]

synaptic cleft
A microscopic space between the axon of one neuron and the cell
body or dendrites of a second neuron, or between the axon of a
neuron and an organ. [Section 12.2]

telencephalon
The cerebral hemispheres. [Section 10.2]

temperament
Dispositional emotional excitability. [Section 6.4]

temporal summation
Summation by a postsynaptic cell of input from a single source over time. [Section 12.2]

thalamus
A relay station and major integrating area for sensory impulses. [Section 10.2]

thermoreceptor
A receptor that responds to changes in temperature. [Section 11.1]

theta waves
Waves of low to moderate intensity and intermediate frequency present during Stage 1 of sleep. [Section 11.5]

top-down processing
A type of information processing that occurs when the brain applies experience and expectations to interpret sensory information. [Section 11.2]

traditional authority
A form of leadership where power is due to custom, tradition, or accepted practice. [Section 4.2]

trait
Internal, stable, and enduring aspects of personality that should be consistent across most situations. [Section 7.1]

trial and error
Strategy of problem-solving that involves trying different alternatives sequentially until success is achieved. [Section 11.4]

tropic hormone
A hormone that controls the release of another hormone. [Section 12.4]

twin studies
Studies that incorporate research into different types of twins to gain insight into heritability. [Section 3.3]

tympanic membrane
The membrane that separates the outer ear from the middle ear. The tympanic membrane is also known as the eardrum. [Section 11.1]

type 1 error
Researchers incorrectly reject the null hypothesis, also known as false positive. [Section 3.1]

type 2 error
Researchers accept the null hypothesis when in fact it is false, also known as false negative. [Section 3.1]

unconditioned response
A response that automatically follows an unconditioned stimulus, without necessitating learning and conditioning to create the link. [Section 9.1]

unconditioned stimulus
A stimulus that elicits an unconditioned response automatically, without necessitating learning and conditioning to create the link. [Section 9.1]

undifferentiated-type schizophrenia
A psychological disorder characterized by the basic criteria for schizophrenia, but symptoms that do not fit into one of the other subtypes. [Section 8.1]

universal emotions
Six major emotions that appear to be universal across cultures: happiness, sadness, surprise, fear, disgust, and anger. [Section 7.4]

universal grammar
Basic rules of language, presumed to be innate, that allow the human mind to gain mastery of language from limited exposure during sensitive developmental years in early childhood. [Section 11.6]

upward mobility
An increase in social class. [Section 5.2]

urbanization
The growth of urban areas as the result of global change. Urbanization is tied to industrialization. [Section 5.1]

utilitarian organization
An organization in which members get paid for their efforts, such as businesses. [Section 6.3]

vagus nerves
Very large mixed nerves that innervate virtually every visceral organ. They are especially important in transmitting parasympathetic input to the heart and digestive smooth muscle. [Section 12.3]

values
A culture's standard for evaluating what is good or bad. [Section 5.1]

variable-interval schedule
Reinforcement schedule in which reward is offered after an unpredictable time interval. [Section 9.1]

variable-ratio schedule
Reinforcement schedule in which reward is offered after an unpredictable number of occurrences of a behavior. [Section 9.1]

visual cortex
The area of the occipital lobe responsible for processing visual information. [Section 11.1]

visuospatial sketchpad
Allows for the repetition of visuospatial information (images) to aid with encoding it into memory. [Section 11.4]

Weber, Max
Conflict theorist who modified and tempered many of Marx's ideas on society. [Section 4.1]

Weber's law
This law pertains to sensory perception and dictates that two stimuli must differ by a constant proportion in order for their difference to be perceptible. [Section 11.2]

welfare capitalism
A system in which most of the economy is private with the exception of extensive social welfare programs to serve certain needs within society. [Section 4.2]

Wernicke's area
The area of the brain, located in the posterior section of the temporal lobe, that is involved with the comprehension of speech and written language. [Section 11.6]

white matter
Myelinated axons. [Section 10.2]

withdrawal
An uncomfortable and often painful experience that may accompany the discontinuing of a drug. [Section 11.5]

within-subjects design
Comparisons are made at different time points for the same group. [Section 3.1]

working memory
Short-term memory for information in immediate awareness, consisting of four components: a central executive, a phonological loop, a visuospatial sketchpad, and an episodic buffer. [Sections 9.2 & 11.4]

Yerkes-Dodson law
Law that asserts that a moderate level of arousal creates optimal performance. Too little arousal leads to complacency and too much arousal can be overwhelming. [Section 7.4]

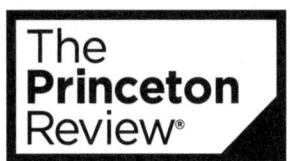

MCAT®

Critical Analysis and Reasoning Skills Review

3rd Edition

The Staff of The Princeton Review

Penguin
Random
House

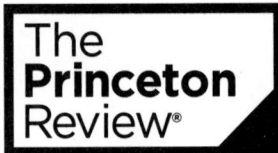

The Princeton Review
110 East 42nd St, 7th Floor

New York, NY 10017

Copyright © 2022 by TPR Education IP Holdings, LLC.
All rights reserved.

Published in the United States by Penguin Random House LLC, New York, and in Canada by Random House of Canada, a division of Penguin Random House Ltd., Toronto.

The material in this book is up-to-date at the time of publication. However, changes may have been instituted by the testing body in the test after this book was published.

If there are any important late-breaking developments, changes, or corrections to the materials in this book, we will post that information online in the Student Tools. Register your book and check your Student Tools to see if there are any updates posted there.

Every attempt has been made to obtain permission to reproduce material protected by copyright. Where omissions may have occurred the editors will be happy to acknowledge this in future printings.

ISBN: 978-0-593-51624-9
ISSN: 2332-404X

MCAT is a registered trademark of the Association of American Medical Colleges.

The Princeton Review is not affiliated with Princeton University.

Editor: Meave Shelton
Production Editor: Emma Parker, Sarah Litt
Production Artists: Deborah Weber, Shavon I. Serrano

Manufactured in China.

10 9 8 7 6 5 4 3 2 1

3rd Edition

The Princeton Review Publishing Team
Rob Franek, Editor-in-Chief
David Soto, Senior Director, Data Operations
Stephen Koch, Senior Manager, Data Operations
Deborah Weber, Director of Production
Jason Ullmeyer, Production Design Manager
Jennifer Chapman, Senior Production Artist
Selena Coppock, Director of Editorial
Aaron Riccio, Senior Editor
Meave Shelton, Senior Editor
Chris Chimera, Editor
Orion McBean, Editor
Patricia Murphy, Editor
Laura Rose, Editor
Alexa Schmitt Bugler, Editorial Assistant

Penguin Random House Publishing Team
Tom Russell, VP, Publisher
Alison Stoltzfus, Senior Director, Publishing
Brett Wright, Senior Editor
Emily Hoffman, Assistant Managing Editor
Ellen Reed, Production Manager
Suzanne Lee, Designer
Eugenia Lo, Publishing Assistant

For customer service, please contact **editorialsupport@review.com,** and be sure to include:

- full title of the book

- ISBN

- page number

CONTRIBUTORS

Jennifer S. Wooddell
    Senior Author and Editor

Edited for Production by

Judene Wright, M.S., M.A.Ed.
    National Content Director, MCAT Program, The Princeton Review

Jennifer and Judene would like to thank the following people for their contributions to this book:

Elizabeth Aamot (Fatith), John Bahling, M.D., Gary Bedford, Jessica Burstrem, M.A., Alix Claps, M.A., Cynthia Cowan, B.A., Sara Daniel, B.S., Cory Eicher, B.A., (James) Ben Gill, Jacqueline R. Giordano, Gina Granter, M.A., Corinne Harol, Christopher Hinkle, Th.D., Alison Howard, Paul Kugelmass, Jay Lee, Addie Lozjanin, Rohit Madani, B.S., Mike Matera, B.A., Ashleigh Menhadji, Katherine Montgomery, Don Osborne, Rupal Patel, B.S., Vivek Patel, Tyler Peikes, Nadia Reynolds, M.A., Maryam Shambayati, M.S., Angela Song, Kate Speiker, David Stoll, Jonathan Swirsky, Neil Thornton, Laura Tubelle de González, and David Weiskopf, M.A.

CONTENTS

Get More (Free) Content
at **PrincetonReview.com/prep**

As easy as **1·2·3**

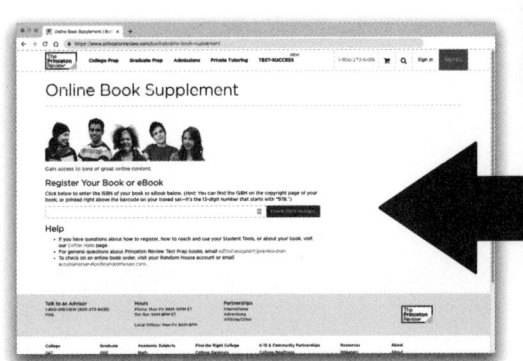

1 Go to PrincetonReview.com/prep or scan the **QR code** and enter the following ISBN for your book:

9780593516249

2 Answer a few simple questions to set up an exclusive Princeton Review account. *(If you already have one, you can just log in.)*

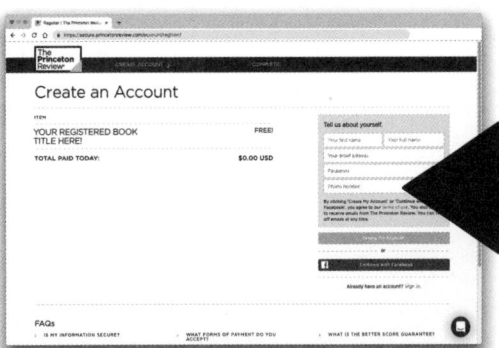

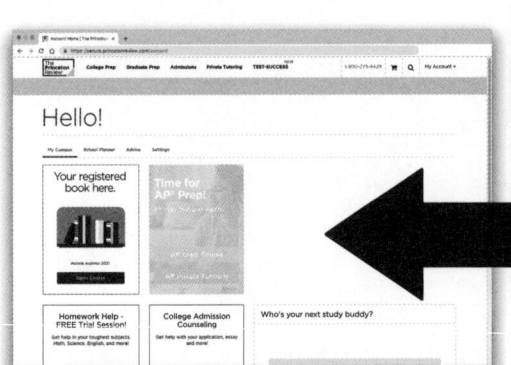

3 Enjoy access to your **FREE** content!

Once you've registered, you can...

- Take **3** full-length practice MCAT exams

- Find useful information about taking the MCAT and applying to medical school

- Check to see if there have been any corrections or updates to this edition

- Get our take on any recent or pending updates to the MCAT

Need to report a potential **content** issue?

Contact **EditorialSupport@review.com** and include:

- full title of the book
- ISBN
- page number

Need to report a **technical** issue?

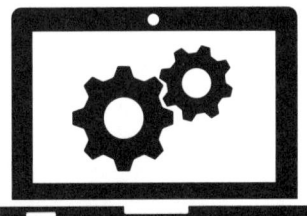

Contact **TPRStudentTech@review.com** and provide:

- your full name
- email address used to register the book
- full book title and ISBN
- Operating system (Mac/PC) and browser (Chrome, Firefox, Safari, etc.)

Chapter 1
MCAT Basics

SO YOU WANT TO BE A DOCTOR

So...you want to be a doctor. If you're like most premeds, you've wanted to be a doctor since you were pretty young. When people asked you what you wanted to be when you grew up, you always answered "a doctor." You had toy medical kits, bandaged up your dog or cat, and played hospital. You probably read your parents' home medical guides for fun.

When you got to high school you took the honors and AP classes. You studied hard, got straight As (or at least really good grades!), and participated in extracurricular activities so you could get into a good college. And you succeeded!

At college you knew exactly what to do. You took your classes seriously, studied hard, and got a great GPA. You talked to your professors and hung out at office hours to get good letters of recommendation. You were a member of the premed society on campus, volunteered at hospitals, and shadowed doctors. All that's left to do now is get a good MCAT score.

Just the MCAT.

Just the most confidence-shattering, most demoralizing, longest, most brutal entrance exam for any graduate program. At about 7.5 hours (including breaks), the MCAT tops the list...even the closest runners up, the LSAT and GMAT, are only about 4 hours long. The MCAT tests significant science content knowledge along with the ability to think quickly, reason logically, and read comprehensively, all under the pressure of a timed exam.

The path to a good MCAT score is not as easy to see as the path to a good GPA or the path to a good letter of recommendation. The MCAT is less about what you know, and more about how to apply what you know—and how to apply it quickly to new situations. Because the path might not be so clear, you might be worried. That's why you picked up this book.

We promise to demystify the MCAT for you, with clear descriptions of the different sections, how the test is scored, and what the test experience is like. We will help you understand general test-taking techniques as well as provide you with specific techniques for each section. In this book, we'll give you strategies for the Critical Analysis and Reasoning Skills (CARS) section, while our other MCAT subject books will review the science content. We'll show you the path to a good MCAT score and help you walk that path.

After all...you want to be a doctor. And we want you to succeed.

WHAT IS THE MCAT...REALLY?

Most test-takers approach the MCAT as though it were a typical college science test, one in which facts and knowledge simply need to be regurgitated in order to do well. They study for the MCAT the same way they did for their college tests, by memorizing facts and details, formulas, and equations. And when they get to the MCAT they are surprised...and disappointed.

It's a myth that the MCAT is purely a content-knowledge test. If medical school admission committees want to see what you know, all they have to do is look at your transcripts. What they really want to see is how you think, especially under pressure. That's what your MCAT score will tell them.

The MCAT is really a test of your ability to apply basic knowledge to different, possibly new, situations. It's a test of your ability to reason out and evaluate arguments. Do you still need to know your science content? Absolutely. But not at the level that most test-takers think they need to know it. Furthermore, your science knowledge won't help you on the Critical Analysis and Reasoning Skills (CARS) section. So how do you study for a test like this?

You study for the science sections by reviewing the basics and then applying them to MCAT practice questions. You study for the CARS section by learning how to adapt your existing reading and analytical skills to the nature of the test. (More information about the science sections can be found in their respective *MCAT Review* books.)

The book you are holding will teach you the strategies you need to do well on the MCAT CARS section. It includes many passages and questions designed to make you think about the material in a deeper way, along with full explanations to clarify the logical thought process needed to get to the answer. It also comes with access to three full-length online practice exams to further hone your skills. For more information on accessing those online exams, please refer to the "Get More (Free) Content" spread on page viii.

MCAT NUTS AND BOLTS

Overview

The MCAT is a computer-based test (CBT) that is *not* adaptive. Adaptive tests base your next question on whether or not you've answered the current question correctly. The MCAT is *linear*, or *fixed-form*, meaning that the questions are in a predetermined order and do not change based on your answers. However, there are many versions of the test, so that on a given test day, different people will see different versions. The following table highlights the features of the MCAT exam.

Registration	Online via www.aamc.org. Begins as early as six months prior to test date; available up until week of test (subject to seat availability).
Testing Centers	Administered at small, secure, climate-controlled computer testing rooms.
Security	Photo ID with signature, electronic fingerprint, electronic signature verification, assigned seat.
Proctoring	None. Test administrator checks examinee in and assigns seat at computer. All testing instructions are given on the computer.
Frequency of Test	Many times per year distributed over January, April, May, June, July, August, and September.
Format	Exclusively computer-based. NOT an adaptive test.
Length of Test Day	7.5 hours
Breaks	Optional 10-minute breaks between sections, with a 30-minute break for lunch.
Section Names	1. Chemical and Physical Foundations of Biological Systems (Chem/Phys) 2. Critical Analysis and Reasoning Skills (CARS) 3. Biological and Biochemical Foundations of Living Systems (Bio/Biochem) 4. Psychological, Social, and Biological Foundations of Behavior (Psych/Soc)
Number of Questions and Timing	59 Chem/Phys questions, 95 minutes 53 CARS questions, 90 minutes 59 Bio/Biochem questions, 95 minutes 59 Psych/Soc questions, 95 minutes
Scoring	Test is scaled. Several forms per administration.
Allowed/ Not allowed	No timers/watches. Noise reduction headphones available. Noteboard booklet and wet-erase marker given at start of test and taken at end of test. Locker or secure area provided for personal items.
Results: Timing and Delivery	Approximately 30 days. Electronic scores only, available online through AAMC login. Examinees can print official score reports.
Maximum Number of Retakes	The test can be taken a maximum of three times in one year, four times over two years, and seven times over the lifetime of the examinee. An examinee can be registered for only one date at a time.

Registration

Registration for the exam is completed online at www.aamc.org/students/applying/mcat/reserving. The Association of American Medical Colleges (AAMC) opens registration for a given test date at least two months in advance of the date, often earlier. It's a good idea to register well in advance of your desired test date to make sure that you get a seat.

Sections

There are four sections on the MCAT, all of which consist of multiple-choice questions:

Section	Concepts Tested	Number of Questions and Timing
Chemical and Physical Foundations of Biological Systems (Chem/Phys)	Basic concepts in chemistry and physics, including biochemistry, scientific inquiry, reasoning, research and statistics skills.	59 questions in 95 minutes
Critical Analysis and Reasoning Skills (CARS)	Critical analysis of information drawn from a wide range of social science and humanities disciplines.	53 questions in 90 minutes
Biological and Biochemical Foundations of Living Systems (Bio/Biochem)	Basic concepts in biology and biochemistry, scientific inquiry, reasoning, research and statistics skills.	59 questions in 95 minutes
Psychological, Social, and Biological Foundations of Behavior (Psych/Soc)	Basic concepts in psychology, sociology, and biology, research methods and statistics.	59 questions in 95 minutes

Most questions on the MCAT (44 in the science sections, all 53 in the CARS section) are passage-based; the science sections have 10 passages each and the CARS section has 9. A passage consists of a few paragraphs of information on which several following questions are based. In the science sections, passages often include equations or reactions, tables, graphs, figures, and experiments to analyze. CARS passages come from literature in the social sciences, humanities, ethics, philosophy, cultural studies, and population health, and do not test content knowledge in any way.

Some questions in the science sections are freestanding questions (FSQs). These questions are independent of any passage information and appear in four groups of about three to four questions, interspersed throughout the passages. 15 of the questions in the science sections are freestanding, and the remainder are passage-based.

Each section on the MCAT is separated by either a 10-minute break or a 30-minute lunch break. We recommend that you take these breaks.

Section	Time
Test Center Check-In	Variable, can take up to 40 minutes if center is busy.
Tutorial	10 minutes
Chemical and Physical Foundations of Biological Systems	95 minutes
Break (optional)	10 minutes
Critical Analysis and Reasoning Skills	90 minutes
Lunch Break (optional)	30 minutes
Biological and Biochemical Foundations of Living Systems	95 minutes
Break (optional)	10 minutes
Psychological, Social, and Biological Foundations of Behavior	95 minutes
Void Option	5 minutes
Survey (optional)	5 minutes

The survey includes questions about your satisfaction with the overall MCAT experience, including registration, check-in, etc., as well as questions about how you prepared for the test.

Scoring

The MCAT is a scaled exam, meaning that your raw score will be converted into a scaled score that takes into account the difficulty of the questions. There is no guessing penalty. All sections are scored from 118–132, with a total scaled score range of 472–528. Because different versions of the test have varying levels of difficulty, the scale will be different from one exam to the next. Thus, there is no "magic number" of questions to get right in order to get a particular score. Plus, some of the questions on the test are considered "experimental" and do not count toward your score; they are just there to be evaluated for possible future inclusion in a test.

At the end of the test (after you complete the Psychological, Social, and Biological Foundations of Behavior section), you will be asked to choose one of the following two options, "I wish to have my MCAT exam scored" or "I wish to VOID my MCAT exam." You have 5 minutes to make a decision, and if you do not select one of the options in that time, the test will automatically be scored. If you choose the VOID option, your test will not be scored (you will not now, or ever, get a numerical score for this test), medical schools will not know you took the test, and no refunds will be granted. You cannot "unvoid" your scores at a later time.

So, what's a good score? The AAMC is centering the scale at 500 (i.e., 500 will be the 50th percentile), and recommends that application committees consider applicants near the center of the range. To be on the safe side, aim for a total score of around 510. And remember that if your GPA is on the low side, you'll need higher MCAT scores to compensate, and if you have a strong GPA, you can get away with lower MCAT scores. But the reality is that your chances of acceptance depend on a lot more than just your MCAT scores. It's a combination of your GPA, your MCAT scores, your undergraduate course work, letters of recommendation, experience related to the medical field (such as volunteer work or research), extracurricular activities, your personal statement, etc. Medical schools are looking for a complete package, not just good scores and a good GPA.

GENERAL LAYOUT AND TEST-TAKING STRATEGIES

Layout of the Test

In each section of the test, the computer screen is divided vertically, with the passage on the left and the range of questions for that passage indicated above (e.g., "Passage 1 Questions 1–5"). The scroll bar for the passage text appears in the middle of the screen. Each question appears on the right, and you need to click "Next" to move to each subsequent question.

In the science sections, the freestanding questions are found in groups of 3–4, interspersed with the passages. The screen is still divided vertically; on the left is the statement "Questions [X–XX] do not refer to a passage and are independent of each other," and each question appears on the right as described above.

CBT Tools

There are a number of tools available on the test, including highlighting, strike-outs, the Flag for Review button, the Navigation and Review Screen buttons, the Periodic Table button, and of course, the noteboard booklet. All tools are available with both mouse control (buttons to click) or keyboard commands (Alt+ a letter). As everyone has different preferences, you should practice with both types of tools (mouse and keyboard) to see which is more comfortable for you personally. The following is a brief description of each tool.

1) **Highlighting:** This is done in the passage text (including table entries and some equations, but excluding figures and molecular structures), in the question stems, and in the answer choices (including Roman numerals). Select the words you wish to highlight (left-click and drag the cursor across the words), and in the upper left corner click the "Highlight" button to highlight the selected text yellow. Alternatively, press "Alt+H" to highlight the words. Highlighting can be removed by selecting the words again and in the upper left corner clicking the down arrow next to "Highlight." This will expand to show the "Remove Highlight" option; clicking this will remove the highlighting. Removing highlighting via the keyboard is cumbersome and is not recommended.

2) **Strike-outs:** This can be done on the answer choices, including Roman numeral statements, by selecting the text you want to strike out (left-click and drag the cursor across the text), then clicking the "Strikethrough" button in the upper left corner. Alternatively, press "Alt+S" to strike out the words. The strike-out can be removed by repeating these actions. Figures or molecular structures cannot be struck out, however, the letter answer choice of those structures can.

3) **Flag for Review button:** This is available for each question and is found in the upper right corner. This allows you to flag the question as one you would like to review later if time permits. When clicked, the flag icon turns yellow. Click again to remove the flag. Alternatively, press "Alt+F."

4) **Navigation button:** This is found near the bottom of the screen and is only available on your first pass through the section. Clicking this button brings up a navigation table listing all questions and their statuses (unseen, incomplete, complete, flagged for review). You can also press "Alt+N" to bring up the screen. The questions can be sorted by their statuses, and clicking a question number takes you immediately to that question. Once you have reached the end of the section and viewed the Review screen (described below), the Navigation screen is no longer available.

5) **Review Screen button:** This button is found near the bottom of the screen after your first pass through the section and, when clicked, brings up a new screen showing all questions and their statuses (either incomplete, unseen, or flagged for review). Questions that are complete are assigned no additional status. You can then choose one of three options by clicking with the mouse or with keyboard shortcuts: Review All (Alt+A), Review Incomplete (Alt+I), or Review Flagged (Alt+R); alternatively, you can click a question number to go directly back to that question. You can also end the section from this screen.

6) **Periodic Table button:** Clicking this button will open the periodic table (or press "Alt+T"). Note that the periodic table is large, covering most of the screen. However, this window can be resized to see the questions and a portion of the periodic table at the same time. The table text will not decrease, but scroll bars will appear on the window so you can center the section of the table of interest in the window.

7) **Noteboard Booklet (Scratch Paper):** At the start of the test, you will be given a spiral-bound set of four laminated 8.5″ × 14″ sheets of paper and a wet-erase black marker to use as scratch paper. You can request a clean noteboard booklet at any time during the test; your original booklet will be collected. The noteboard is only useful if it is kept organized; do not give in to the tendency to write on the first available open space! Good organization will be very helpful when/if you wish to review a question. Indicate the passage number, the range of questions for that passage, and a topic in a box near the top of your scratch work, and indicate the question you are working on in a circle to the left of the notes for that question. Draw a line under your scratch work when you change passages to keep the work separate. Do not erase or scribble over any previous work. If you do not think it is correct, draw one line through the work and start again. You may have already done some useful work without realizing it.

General Strategy for the Science Sections

Passages vs. FSQs in the Science Sections: What to Start With

Since the questions are displayed on separate screens, it is awkward and time consuming to click through all of the questions up front to find the FSQs. Therefore, go through the section on a first pass and decide whether to do the passage now or to save it for later, basing your decision on the passage text and the first question. Tackle the FSQs as you come upon them. More details are below.

Here is an outline of the procedure:

1) For each passage, write a heading on your noteboard with the passage number, the general topic, and its range of questions (e.g., "Passage 1, thermodynamics, Q 1–5" or "Passage 2, enzymes, Q 6–9"). The passage numbers do not currently appear in the Navigation or Review screens, thus having the question numbers on your noteboard will allow you to move through the section more efficiently.

2) Skim the text and rank the passage. If a passage is a "Now," complete it before moving on to the next passage (also see "Attacking the Questions" below). If it is a "Later" passage, first write "SKIPPED" in block letters under the passage heading on your noteboard and leave room for your work when you come back to complete that passage. (Note that the specific passages you skip will be unique to you; in the Bio/Biochem section, you might choose to do all Biology passages first, then come back for Biochemistry. Or in Chem/Phys you might choose to skip experiment-based or analytical passages. Know ahead of time what type of passage you are going to skip and follow your plan.)

3) Next, click on the "Navigation" button at the bottom to get to the navigation screen. Click on the first question of the next passage; you'll be able to identify it because you know the range of questions from the passage you just skipped. This will take you to the next passage, where you will repeat steps 1–3.

4) Once you have completed the "Now" passages, go to the review screen and double-click the first question for the first passage you skipped. Answer the questions, and continue going back to the review screen and repeating this procedure for other passages you have skipped.

Attacking the Questions

As you work through the questions, if you encounter a particularly lengthy question, or a question that requires a lot of analysis, you may choose to skip it. This is a wise strategy because it ensures you will tackle all the easier questions first, the ones you are more likely to get right. If you choose to skip the question (or if you attempt it but get stuck), write down the question number on your noteboard, click the Flag for Review button to flag the question in the Review screen, and move on to the next question. At the end of the passage, click back through the set of questions to complete any that you skipped over the first time through, and make sure that you have filled in an answer for every question.

General Strategy for the CARS Section

Ranking and Ordering the Passages: What to Start With

Ranking: Since the questions are displayed on separate screens, it is awkward and time consuming to click through all of the questions before ranking each passage as "Now" (an easier passage), "Later" (a harder passage), or "Killer" (a passage that you will randomly guess on). Therefore, rank the passage and decide whether or not to do it on the first pass through the section based on the passage text, by skimming the first 2–3 sentences.

Ordering: Because of the additional clicking through screens (or, use of the Review screen) that is required to navigate through the section, the "Two-Pass" system (completing the "Now" passages as you find them) is likely to be your most efficient approach. However, if you find that you are continuously making a lot of bad ranking decisions, it is still valid to experiment with the "Three-Pass" approach (ranking all nine passages up front before attempting your first "Now" passage).

Here is an outline of the basic Ranking and Ordering procedure to follow.

1) For each passage, write a heading on your scratch paper with the passage number and its range of questions (e.g., "Passage 1 Q 1–7"). The passage numbers do not currently appear in the Review screen, thus having the question numbers on your scratch paper will allow you to move through the section more efficiently.

2) Skim the first 2–3 sentences and rank the passage. If the passage is a "Now," complete it before moving on to the next. If it is a "Later" or "Killer," first write either "Later" or "Killer" and "SKIPPED" in block letters under the passage heading on your scratch paper and leave room for your work if you decide to come back and complete that passage. Then click through each question, flagging each one and filling in random guesses, until you get to the next passage.

3) Once you have completed the "Now" passages, come back for your second pass and complete the "Later" passages, leaving your random guesses in place for any "Killer" passages that you choose not to complete. Go to the Review screen and use your scratch paper notes on the question numbers. Double-click on the number of the first question for that passage to go back to that question, and proceed from there. Alternatively, if you have consistently flagged all the questions for passages you skipped in your first pass, you can use "Review Flagged" from the Review screen to find and complete your "Later" passages.

4) Regardless of how you choose to find your second pass passages, unflag each question after you complete it, so that you can continue to rely on the Review screen (and the "Review Flagged" function) to identify questions that you have not yet attempted.

Previewing the Questions

The formatting and functioning of the tools facilitates effective previewing. Having each question on a separate screen will encourage you to really focus on that question. Even more importantly, you can highlight in the question stem (but not in the answer choices).

Here is the basic procedure for Previewing the Questions:

1) Start with the first question, and if it has lead words referencing passage content, highlight them. You may also choose to jot them down on your scratch paper. Once you reach and preview the last question for the set on that passage, THEN stay on that screen and work the passage (your highlighting appears and stays on every passage screen, and persists through the whole 90 minutes).

2) Once you have worked the passage and defined the Bottom Line—the main idea and tone of the entire passage—work **backward** from the last question to the first. If you skip over any questions as you go (see "Attacking the Questions" below), write down the question number on your scratch paper. Then click **forward** through the set of questions, completing any that you skipped over the first time through. Once you reach and complete the last question for that passage, clicking "Next" will send you to the first question of the next passage. Working the questions from last to first the first time through the set will eliminate the need to click back through multiple screens to get to the first question immediately after previewing, and will also make it easier and more efficient to do the hardest questions last (see "Attacking the Questions" below).

3) Remember that previewing questions is a CARS-only technique. It is not efficient to preview questions in the science sections.

Attacking the Questions

The question types and the procedure for actually attacking each type will be discussed later. However, it is still important **not** to attempt the hardest questions first (you'll risk potentially getting stuck, wasting time, and discouraging yourself).

So, as you work the questions from last to first (see "Previewing the Questions" above), if you encounter a particularly difficult and/or lengthy question (or if you attempt a question but get stuck) write down the question number on your scratch paper (you may also choose to flag it) and move on backward to the next question you will attempt. Then click **forward** through the set and complete any that you skipped over the first time through the set, unflagging any questions that you flagged that first time through and making sure that you have filled in an answer for every question.

Pacing Strategy for the MCAT

Since the MCAT is a timed test, you must keep an eye on the timer and adjust your pacing as necessary. It would be terrible to run out of time at the end only to discover that the last few questions could have been easily answered in just a few seconds each.

In the science sections you will have about one minute and thirty-five seconds (1:35) per question, and in the CARS section you will have about one minute and forty seconds (1:40) per question (not taking into account time spent reading the passage before answering the questions).

Section	# of Questions in passage	Approximate time (including reading the passage)
Chem/Phys, Bio/Biochem, and Psych/Soc	4	6.5 minutes
	5	8 minutes
	6	9.5 minutes
CARS	5	8.5 minutes
	6	10 minutes
	7	11.5 minutes

When starting a passage in the science sections, make note of how much time you will allot for it, and the starting time on the timer. Jot down on your noteboard what the timer should say at the end of the passage. Then just keep an eye on it as you work through the questions. If you are near the end of the time for that passage, guess on any remaining questions, make some notes on your noteboard, Flag the questions, and move on. Come back to those questions if you have time.

For the CARS section, keep in mind that many people will maximize their score by *not* trying to complete every question or every passage in the section. A good strategy for test-takers who cannot achieve a high level of accuracy on all nine passages is to randomly guess on at least one passage in the section, and spend your time getting a high percentage of the other questions right. To complete all nine CARS passages, you have about ten minutes per passage. To complete eight of the nine, you have about 11 minutes per passage.

To help maximize your number of correct answer choices in any section, do the questions and passages within that section in the order *you* want to do them in. See "General Strategy" above.

Process of Elimination

Process of Elimination (POE) is probably the most useful technique you have to tackle MCAT questions. Since there is no guessing penalty, POE allows you to increase your probability of choosing the correct answer by eliminating those you are sure are wrong.

1) Strike out any choices that you are sure are incorrect or that do not address the issue raised in the question.
2) Jot down some notes to help clarify your thoughts if you return to the question.
3) Use the "Flag for Review" button to flag the question for review. (Note, however, that in the CARS section, you generally should not be returning to rethink questions once you have moved on to a new passage.)
4) Do not leave it blank! For the sciences, if you are not sure and you have already spent more than 60 seconds on that question, just pick one of the remaining choices. If you have time to review it at the end, you can always debate the remaining choices based on your previous notes. For CARS, if you have been through the choices two or three times, have reread the question stem and gone back to the passage and you are still stuck, move on. Do the remaining questions for that passage, take one more look at the question you were stuck on, then pick an answer and move on for good.
5) Special Note: if three of the four answer choices have been eliminated, the remaining choice must be the correct answer. Don't waste time pondering *why* it is correct; just click it and move on. The MCAT doesn't care if you truly understand why it's the right answer, only that you have the right answer selected.
6) More subject-specific information on techniques will be presented in the next chapter.

Guessing

Remember, there is NO guessing penalty on the MCAT. NEVER leave a question blank!

QUESTION TYPES

In the science sections of the MCAT, the questions fall into one of three main categories.

1) Memory questions: These questions can be answered directly from prior knowledge and represent about 25 percent of the total number of questions.
2) Explicit questions: These questions are those for which the answer is explicitly stated in the passage. To answer them correctly, for example, may just require finding a definition, or reading a graph, or making a simple connection. Explicit questions represent about 35 percent of the total number of questions.
3) Implicit questions: These questions require you to apply knowledge to a new situation; the answer is typically implied by the information in the passage. These questions often start "if... then..." (for example, "if we modify the experiment in the passage like this, then what result would we expect?"). Implicit style questions make up about 40 percent of the total number of questions.

In the CARS section, the questions fall into four main categories.

1) Specific questions: These either ask you for facts from the passage (Retrieval questions) or require you to deduce what is most likely to be true based on the passage (Inference questions).
2) General questions: These ask you to summarize themes (Main Idea and Primary Purpose questions) or evaluate an author's opinion (Tone/Attitude questions).
3) Reasoning questions: These ask you to describe the purpose of, or the support provided for, a statement made in the passage (Structure questions) or to judge how well the author supports his or her argument (Evaluate questions).

4) Application questions: These ask you to apply new information from either the question stem itself (New Information questions) or from the answer choices (Strengthen, Weaken, and Analogy questions) to the passage.

More detail on question types and strategies can be found in Chapter 4.

TESTING TIPS

Before Test Day

- Take a trip to the test center at least a day or two before your actual test date so that you can easily find the building and room on test day. This will also allow you to gauge traffic and see if you need money for parking or anything like that. Knowing this type of information ahead of time will greatly reduce your stress on the day of your test.
- During the week before the test, adjust your sleeping schedule so that you are going to bed and getting up in the morning at the same times as on the day before and morning of the MCAT. Prioritize getting a reasonable amount of sleep during the last few nights before the test.
- Don't do any heavy studying the day before the test. This is not a test you can cram for! Your goal at this point is to rest and relax so that you can go into test day in a good physical and mental condition.
- Eat well. Try to avoid excessive caffeine and sugar. Ideally, in the weeks leading up to the actual test you should experiment a little bit with foods and practice tests to see which foods give you the most endurance. Aim for steady blood sugar levels during the test: sports drinks, peanut-butter crackers, trail mix, etc. make good snacks for your breaks and lunch.

General Test Day Info and Tips

- On the day of the test, arrive at the test center at least a half hour prior to the start time of your test.
- Examinees will be checked into the center in the order in which they arrive.
- You will be assigned a locker or secure area in which to put your personal items. Textbooks and study notes are not allowed, so there is no need to bring them with you to the test center.
- Your ID will be checked, your palm vein will be scanned, and you will be asked to sign in.
- You will be given your noteboard booklet and wet-erase marker, and the test center administrator will take you to the computer on which you will complete the test. You may not choose a computer; you must use the computer assigned to you.
- Nothing is allowed at the computer station except your photo ID, your locker key (if provided), and a factory sealed packet of ear plugs; not even your watch.
- If you choose to leave the testing room at the breaks, you will have your palm vein scanned again, and you will have to sign in and out.
- You are allowed to access the items in your locker, except for notes and cell phones. (Check your test center's policy on cell phones ahead of time; some centers do not even allow them to be kept in your locker.)
- Don't forget to bring the snack foods and lunch you experimented with in your practice tests.
- At the end of the test, the test administrator will collect your noteboard.
- Definitely take the breaks! Get up and walk around. It's a good way to clear your head between sections and get the blood (and oxygen!) flowing to your brain.
- Ask for a clean noteboard at the breaks if you want a fresh one.

Chapter 2
Introduction to MCAT
Critical Analysis
and Reasoning Skills

GOALS

1) To understand the structure and scoring of the Critical Analysis and Reasoning Skills Section
2) To learn the fundamentals of Critical Analysis and Reasoning Skills strategies

Congratulations on choosing The Princeton Review for your MCAT preparation. You are well on your way to significantly raising your MCAT score and getting into your top-choice medical school. We understand that the Critical Analysis and Reasoning Skills (CARS) section presents many challenges to the typical MCAT student. We want our students to have every available tool, so we have devoted ourselves to developing the most rigorous CARS materials possible, based on intensive study of the MCAT itself and of the best strategies that lead to success on this test.

2.1 THE CRITICAL ANALYSIS AND REASONING SKILLS (CARS) SECTION

Structure

- CARS is the second section of the test.
- It consists of nine passages, which typically average 500–700 words each.
- Each passage is followed by 5–7 questions (with four answer choices per question), for a total of 53 questions.
- You will have 90 minutes to complete the section. You can do the questions and passages in any order that you choose within the 90-minute limit.
- You will be able to scroll up and down within the passage text. The questions are displayed one at a time on the right, with the passage (and any highlighting you have done in the passage text) always displayed on the left. Click on the Next and Previous buttons on the bottom of the screen to go back and forth between the questions and passages within the section. Clicking Next from the last question for a passage takes you to the next passage and the first question for that passage. Once the 90 minutes are up, however, you cannot go back to any of the CARS passages or questions.

Pacing

You do not necessarily need to complete all nine passages to get a competitive score. Many people will maximize their score by randomly guessing on at least one passage and focusing on getting a high percentage of the rest of the questions correct. Also, keep in mind that there is no guessing penalty. Never leave a question blank; always select a random guess for questions that you choose not to complete. You have a 25 percent chance of getting those questions right.

Content

The passages may be on any subject in the humanities and social sciences. Passage topics may include philosophy, ethics, archeology, economics, history, political science, literature and literary theory, psychology, sociology, anthropology, cultural studies, geography, population health, and art history and theory. This range of topics may seem overwhelming. However, unlike the other multiple choice sections of the test, CARS tests no outside knowledge of the subject. In fact, using your own factual knowledge or opinions of the subject can lead you to pick incorrect answers; the questions require you to use only the information provided in the passage. Clearly, you can't prepare for or approach this section of the test in the same way as physics or chemistry!

2.2 DEVELOPING YOUR CRITICAL REASONING SKILLS

The Critical Analysis and Reasoning Skills section can be intimidating for many people taking the MCAT. You have been studying hard for many years, packing your brain with lots of science knowledge and refining your memorization skills. But now, as you confront the CARS section, all those facts and mnemonics are useless, and you have to employ an entirely different approach. Even if you have taken a lot of humanities and social science courses and have been speaking and reading English for many years, you might find the CARS section to be challenging at first. This is because you need to adapt to the specific nature and requirements of this section of the MCAT.

There are many false beliefs regarding the CARS section, one of which is that your score depends on luck. That is, if you happen to get "good" passages, all is well, but if you don't, you are in trouble. However (and thankfully!), this is entirely untrue. There are ways that you can improve your CARS score regardless of the passages you happen to get on your test. BUT... to achieve this improvement, many, if not most, of you will need to fundamentally change how you read the passages and go about answering the questions. You will need to develop new skills that have little to do with memorization and everything to do with reading efficiently and thinking critically. The good news is that these are skills that everyone can develop and improve through practice and careful self-evaluation. These core skills fall into three basic categories.

Working the Passage

*   **Reading the passage efficiently:** identifying the most important points made by the author while moving quickly through the details
*   **Following the logical structure of the author's argument:** identifying such things as key shifts in direction, comparisons and contrasts, conclusions, and author's tone
*   **Synthesizing the Bottom Line of the entire passage:** identifying the author's Main Idea and Attitude

Attacking the Questions

- **Correctly identifying and translating the questions:** knowing what each question is asking you to do in order to choose the correct answer
- **Using the passage (and only the passage) as a resource:** quickly locating the relevant passage information for each question
- **Answering in your own words:** predicting what the correct answer will do before considering the answer choices
- **Using Process of Elimination (POE):** eliminating down to the "least wrong" choice rather than just picking an answer that "sounds good"

General Test Strategy

- **Time management:** getting what you need from the passage without getting bogged down in irrelevant facts or spending too much time on one question
- **Pacing and accuracy:** not going so fast that you miss a high percentage of the questions that you complete, or so slow that you overthink the questions or do not complete enough questions to reach your target score
- **Stress management:** thinking clearly and working efficiently under stressful conditions

2.3 FUNDAMENTALS: THE SIX STEPS

Based on these core skills, here are the six steps to follow when working the CARS section.

■ STEP 1: RANK AND ORDER THE PASSAGES

Ranking

The passages are not necessarily, or even usually, presented in order of difficulty. There is no reason to waste time on the hardest passage or passages, only to skip or rush through an easy passage at the end of the section. So your first step, as you reach each new passage, is to decide if it is a Now (or easier) passage, a Later (or harder) passage, or a Killer passage (one that you will simply randomly guess on, or do last). To assign a rank, skim a few sentences of the passage and see if you can easily paraphrase it. If you can, it's most likely an easier passage to understand. If not, it is likely to be a harder passage that you should either come back to later during your 90 minutes or just randomly guess on.

Ordering

If a passage is a Now passage, go ahead and work it through, completing all of the questions. If it is a Later or Killer passage, click through each question, Flag it for review and fill in a random guess, and move on to ranking the next passage. Also note the passage number on your notepad. Once you have completed the Now passages in the section, come back through the section and complete the Later passages, and make sure that you have filled in your random guesses on your Killer passage or passages. (See Chapter 6 of this book for more information on Ranking and Ordering.)

STEP 2: PREVIEW THE QUESTIONS

Knowing what topics show up in the questions will help you work the passage more quickly and effectively. Before working the passage, read through the question stems from first to last (not the answer choices), identifying and highlighting any words or phrases that indicate important passage content. Do not worry at this stage about understanding the question or identifying the question type. (See Chapter 3 of this book for more information on Previewing the Questions.)

STEP 3: WORK THE PASSAGE

Stay on the screen for the last question and work the passage from here (your highlighting will stay and appear in the passage text regardless of which question for that passage you are working on). As you read through the passage, use the highlighting function (sparingly) to annotate the most important references in the text. This would include things like: question topics, topic sentences, shifts in direction or continuations, the author's tone, different points of view, and conclusions. As you read, articulate the Main Point of each chunk of information (usually, each paragraph). Use your notepad, especially on difficult passages, to jot down these main points. As you move through the passage, think about how these chunks relate to each other; that is, track the logical structure of the author's argument in the passage. (See Chapter 3 of this book for more information on Active Reading and Annotation.)

STEP 4: BOTTOM LINE

After you have read the entire passage, sum up the Bottom Line: the main idea and tone of the entire passage. For particularly difficult passages, write this down on your notepad to make sure that you have a reasonably clear idea of the point and purpose of the passage as a whole. (See Chapter 3 for more information on finding the Bottom Line.)

STEP 5: ATTACK THE QUESTIONS

This is how the question will be formatted on the screen.

1. When an argument is inductive, that argument:

A) is necessarily less conclusive than an argument that attempts to use deductive logic.

B) is based on probability, such that the likelihood that its premises are all true is no greater than the likelihood of the truth of its conclusion.

C) seeks to find or identify causes or explanations.

D) when valid, may be based on evaluation of a representative sample of a population.

Work through the questions backwards, so that you don't need to click back to the first question for that passage. As you work through each question, follow these steps:

- Read the question word for word and identify the question type.
- Translate the question task into your own words, thinking about what the question is asking you to do with or to the passage.
- When the question stem provides a specific reference to the passage, go back to the passage before reading the answer choices and find the relevant information (reading at least five lines above and below the reference).

2.4

- Paraphrase the passage information. Then, with the question type firmly in mind, think about what the correct answer will need to do.
- As you go through the choices, use POE actively. Look for reasons to strike out incorrect choices, and select the "least wrong" of the four. (See Chapters 4 and 5 of this book for more information on identifying and answering different question types.)
- If you hit a particularly difficult question, skip over it for the moment and complete the other easier questions. Then click forward through the questions towards the next passage, completing any questions that you initially skipped.

▬ STEP 6: INSPECT THE SECTION

At or before the 5-minute mark (ideally, before you begin your last passage), double-check to make sure that you haven't left any incomplete questions. You can use the Review screen at this stage. Do NOT rethink questions you have already completed. Your goal in this step is simply to make sure that you have selected an answer for each question.

2.4 GUIDELINES FOR USING YOUR REVIEW MATERIALS

Focus on Accuracy

Whenever you're acquiring a new skill, you need to learn to do it well before learning to do it quickly. Many students feel that speed is their number one concern. This often leads them to rush through the initial "learning to do it well" phase. Unfortunately, this is entirely counterproductive and will ultimately keep you from scoring as highly as you possibly can.

As you begin working practice passages, do the passages untimed; focus on following the techniques and improving your accuracy. Once you become comfortable with these techniques, set a timer to count *up* as you do each passage (or, note your start and end times with a watch). Record how long it takes you to do a passage, but don't attempt to complete the passage within a set time limit. We will let you know when to begin using set time limits for individual passages or for full CARS sections.

Even after you have been studying for some time and have taken many practice tests, it is still useful to do some untimed passages, focusing on avoiding the types of mistakes you tend to make. Then bring that same focus into the next set of timed passages you complete or the next practice test that you take.

Build Endurance

At first, work on only a few passages at a time, developing the skills you've learned. Allowing yourself this time to practice slowly but accurately gives you a strong foundation for accurate timed practice. Always do passages at least two at a time to practice ranking and ordering them. After a couple of weeks, try to do a number of practice passages at once, and don't take any breaks between the passages. Also, at this stage, don't check your answers after every one or two passages. You need to get used to working through each new passage without the reassurance or feedback from knowing how you did on the previous passage. Build up your endurance over time, so that you can eventually maintain your concentration at its peak over the course of an entire 90-minute section. Set aside a daily time for CARS work and stick to your schedule. Keep in mind the particular strategies you should be focusing on depending on where you are in this book and in your preparation process.

Control Your Environment

Give your full attention to the passages when you practice. That is, don't do homework while watching TV or conversing with friends. However, when you take the actual MCAT, you'll be in a room full of people who are muttering to themselves, sniffling and coughing, typing loudly, standing up and sitting down at different times, and generally behaving in a distracting or annoying manner (unintentionally, we hope!). Therefore, practice working in less-than-ideal conditions. Go to a reasonably quiet coffeehouse, a room in the library where there are people moving around, or some other location with low-level distractions. Learn how to tune out what is going on around you and how to keep your focus on the passages in front of you. (Note: basic foam earplugs in a factory sealed package are allowed on the MCAT. You will also be provided with noise-reduction headphones in the testing center.)

Manage Your Stress

Managing your psychological and physical condition is just as important as studying and practicing. It doesn't do you any good to work all day every day if you are so burned out that your brain doesn't function any more. Build times for relaxation, including some kind of physical activity, into your schedule. Later in the book, we will discuss specific ways of reducing anxiety and stress as you study and on test day.

Evaluate Your Work

Constant self-evaluation is the key to continued improvement. Don't just answer the questions and tally your score at the end. Use the materials to teach yourself how to improve. What kinds of questions do you consistently miss? What kinds of passages slow you down? What kinds of answer traps do you tend to fall for? What caused you to pick the wrong answer to each question that you missed?

However, don't just think about the questions you got wrong—also analyze how you arrived at the credited response when your answers are correct. Did you avoid a common trap? Are there question types on which you are particularly strong? Did you successfully apply one of our techniques?

Use the charts and the Self-Evaluation Survey provided at the end of this chapter to identify patterns in the mistakes you are making. Only by identifying your mistakes can you learn to correct them. The next section provides you with guidance on how to use those resources.

2.5 SELF-EVALUATION

Every student has different strengths and weaknesses on the MCAT CARS section. To improve on your weaknesses, you must first recognize them. From now on, keep a log of every passage that you do (sample logs are provided later on).

The time you spend reviewing your work is just as important as the time spent working on the passages. After you complete a passage, go through each question and answer choice. Pay particular attention to those questions that you got wrong. In order to increase your score, you'll need to assess and change the way that you think. Often we continue to take the same steps or read in the same way, even when we've seen that this way is not successful. You may not even realize that you're making the same mistake over and over again until you see it logged into your chart several times. Look for patterns in your mistakes and successes; based on those patterns, define ways in which you need to change how you read and think in order to raise your score.

There are three resources provided at the end of this chapter to help you with the self-evaluation process.

I. Individual Passage Log

Fill out this log for every passage that you do, and for every question within each passage that you miss. Also fill out the log for every question that you got right but were unsure of the correct answer when you picked it (for example, you were down to two choices and then guessed).

At the end of each chapter there are two Individual Passage Logs to use on the practice passages for that chapter. To use the Individual Passage Logs on other practice materials (such as online practice passages), make clean copies of the logs or follow the same structure on notebook paper or in an Excel spreadsheet.

II. Test Assessment Log

Fill out this log for each full CARS test section that you do. Complete it as soon as you can after the test; once a few hours have passed, it will be difficult to remember why you made the choices that you did. As with the Individual Passage Log, either make multiple clean copies of the log for future use, or follow the same structure on notebook paper or in a spreadsheet.

Following the blank version of that log you will find a filled-out sample log. It doesn't correspond to any particular test; it is provided to give you an idea of how you should be filling out your own logs.

III. Self-Evaluation Survey

Complete the Self-Evaluation survey for every full CARS test section that you do. It consists of a series of questions to help you to analyze your overall performance on the section and on each question within it. It is generally best to fill out the Test Assessment Log first, while the questions are still fresh in your mind, and then use the Survey to sum up your analysis and set goals for future tests.

2.5

I. Individual Passage Log

Key for Passage Log

Passage # and Time spent on passage   Indicate the location of the passage and how long it took you to complete it (once we have instructed you to begin timing the passages).

Q # and Q type   For each question you miss in a passage, indicate the number and the type of question. Refer to the list of question types in Chapter 4.

Attractors   For the first 15 individual logs that you fill out, list what was wrong with every wrong answer, including the ones that you did not pick. After that, you can list only the wrong answers that you chose or seriously considered choosing.

Refer to the Attractors described and listed in Chapters 4 and 5.

What did you do wrong?   Describe the error that led you down the path to the wrong answer, and how you will avoid making that same mistake in the future. Below is a (non-exhaustive) list of common mistakes. Choose one or more items from this list (there may be more than one misstep involved in picking a wrong answer), or, if none fits, describe the error in your own words. If, time after time, you cannot figure out why you chose the wrong answer, it is very likely that you are working too quickly and/or too carelessly. Did you

- misread the question?
- fail to go back to the passage?
- fail to read all four of the answer choices?
- fail to read the entire answer choice?
- over-interpret the passage or the answer choice?
- forget the "EXCEPT/LEAST/NOT" in the question?
- pick an answer choice that was
    - …out of scope or not the issue?
    - …too extreme or absolute?
    - …from the wrong part of the passage?
    - …half right, half wrong?
    - …strengthening when it should have been weakening (or vice versa)?
    - …too narrow on a general question?

Using the Individual Passage Log, take the time to assess how your current thought processes led you to a tempting but wrong answer choice, and how a different way of thinking on the question would have been more successful. The log will help you to see how the test is constructed, and most importantly, how you are responding to it. **You can't change the test, but you can change your responses to it.** This process will allow you to work through the MCAT CARS section more quickly and with greater accuracy.

Individual Passage Log

2.5

Passage # _____ Time spent on passage _____

Q#	Q type	Attractors	What did you do wrong?

Revised Strategy _____

Passage # _____ Time spent on passage _____

Q#	Q type	Attractors	What did you do wrong?

Revised Strategy _____

II. Test Assessment Log

Use this worksheet to record and monitor your performance on full nine-passage sections, as well as to continue the self-evaluation process. In particular, use it to see if you are spending the time you need on the easier passages in order to get most of those questions right. Keep track of how much time you spent (roughly) on the Now passages and on the Later passages. If you find that you are spending the bulk of your 90 minutes on the harder passages with a low level of accuracy, you need to reapportion your time. You should also evaluate your ranking; are you choosing the right passages?

Now Passages

Now Passage #	Q # and Type (for questions you got wrong)	Attractors (for wrong answers you picked or seriously considered)	What did you do wrong?

Approximate time spent on Now passages _____

Total Now passages attempted _____

Total # of Qs on Now passages attempted _____

Total # of Now Qs correct _____

% correct of Now Qs attempted _____

Later Passages

Later Passage #	Q # and Type (for questions you got wrong)	Attractors (for wrong answers you picked or seriously considered)	What did you do wrong?

Approximate time spent on Later passages _____

Total Later passages attempted _____

Total # of Qs on Later passages attempted _____

Total # of Later Qs correct _____

% correct of Later Qs attempted _____

Final Analysis

Total # of passages attempted (including partially completed) _____

Total # of questions attempted _____

Total # of correct answers _____

Total % correct of attempted questions _____

Revised Strategy

Pacing	
Passage choice/ranking	
Working the Passage	
Attacking the Questions	

2.5

Sample Completed Test Assessment Log—Now Passages

Now Passage #	Q # and Type (for questions you got wrong)	Attractors (for wrong answers you picked or seriously considered)	What did you do wrong?
1	None	N/A	Spent a bit too much time—was *overly* cautious
3	Q12: Main Point	Q12 D: too narrow	Q12: got it down to two and guessed—didn't compare choices or reread the question stem
4	Q23: Inference	Q23 A: out of scope	Q23: Got it right but took too much time—should have gone back to the passage before POE (almost talked myself into an answer that was clearly wrong once I went back to passage)
7	Q39: Weaken Q41: New Information Q42: Inference	Q39 B: opposite Q41 C: opposite Q42 C: reversal	All three: shouldn't have done this passage at all—it was a killer. Didn't understand the passage at all (very abstract and confusing), and got the author's argument all turned around.
9	None!	N/A	Nothing!

Approximate time spent on Now passages **a little less than an hour**

Total Now passages attempted **5**

Total # of Qs on Now passages attempted **28**

Total # of Now Qs correct **23**

% correct of Now Qs attempted **82%**

Sample Completed Test Assessment Log—Later Passages

Later Passage #	Q # and Type (for questions you got wrong)	Attractors (for wrong answers you picked or seriously considered)	What did you do wrong?
2	Q7: Analogy Q10: New Information/ Weaken	Q7 A: half right, half wrong Q10 D: opposite	Q7: didn't read the whole choice (or the rest of the answer choices) carefully—made up my mind too fast Q10: lost track of question type—picked what would be strengthened, not weakened
5	Q26: Retrieval	Q26 B: words out of context	Q26: didn't read carefully enough when went back to passage. Easy question.
6	Q33: Evaluate Q35: Analogy Q37: Inference	Q33 A: half right, half wrong Q35 D: out of scope Q37 C: too extreme	Q33: didn't make sure that the description matched Q35: panicked and didn't think about the logic/theme of the relevant part of the passage Q37: saw the strong language but picked it anyway because was rushed
8	Q43: Inference Q44: Weaken Q46: Structure Q47: Retrieval	Q43 B: too extreme Q44 C: opposite Q46 D: right answer wrong question Q47 A: words out of context	Q43: didn't pay enough attention to strength of language Q44: forgot the question type and picked something supported by the passage (as if was answering Inference question) Q46: forgot the question type and picked answer that was supported by passage but not the purpose of the reference Q47: picked answer because sounded like what I remembered from the passage—in reality, was never mentioned Overall: was rushing, running out of time

Approximate time spent on Later passages **35 minutes**

Total Later passages attempted **4**

Total # of Qs on Later passages attempted **25**

Total # of Later Qs correct **15**

% correct of Later Qs attempted **60%**

2.5

Final Analysis

Total # of passages attempted (including partially completed)   __**9**__

Total # of questions attempted   __**53**__

Total # of correct answers   __**38/53**__

Total % correct of attempted questions   __**72%**__

Revised Strategy

Pacing	Slow down—only do 8 passages.
Passage choice/ranking	Skip over more Later/Killer passages in first pass. Take difficulty of abstract passage texts seriously—skip or do Later.
Working the Passage	Pay more attention to author's opinion, and to contrasting points of view (so that I don't mix them up later). Write down the main points and Bottom Line on harder passages.
Attacking the Questions	Read the question carefully and reread it when down to two answer choices. Go back to the passage more, and read more carefully when I do. Read THE WHOLE answer choice word for word and paraphrase it. Compare choices to each other when down to two. Pay more attention to strength of language and tone.

III.   CARS Self-Evaluation Survey

This section consists of a series of questions intended to help you evaluate your performance on each practice test.

Before answering the questions in this section, you should review your score report, go back over the questions that you missed, and fill out your Self-Evaluation Passage Logs or Test Assessment Logs. You may wish to look through the questions in this survey first and then review your exam using the score report. Finally, come back and select your answers for the survey and read the feedback corresponding to your responses.

Do this one exam at a time—i.e., answer these survey questions after each exam you take. Don't answer them for multiple exams in a group. The survey is extensive; you may even wish to break up your evaluation of a single exam into two or more chunks of time. Note that it is important to answer the survey questions, especially those regarding the reasons why you missed particular questions, as soon as possible after taking the exam, when your reasoning is fresh in your mind. Therefore, answer the questions in Part III within a day of taking the practice test. However, you can fill in your responses for Parts I and II a day or two later.

There is space under each question to list the answer choice or choices (for some of the survey questions, you may be selecting more than one choice). Compare your responses for each practice test to look for trends.

After completing the survey for each test that you take, write down at least three things that you will focus on during your next practice test, or during your next set of practice passages. Space is provided at the end of the survey for you to write down these goals.

PART I: OVERALL ACCURACY AND PACING

1. **Approximately what percentage of the 53 questions did you get correct?**

   Test 1 _____

   Test 2 _____

   Test 3 _____

   Test 4 _____

   Test 5 _____

A. 85–100%

Your accuracy is excellent. Define the strategies that led to your correct answers and apply them to the practice MCATs that you take in the future. If you missed any questions, carefully diagnose the reasons why, so that you can achieve an even higher level of accuracy in the future.

B. 70–84%

Your accuracy is reasonably good. Make a list of at least three reasons why you missed the questions that were incorrect, and focus on not making those same kinds of mistakes on the practice passages and MCATs that you take in the future. Define some of the strategies that led to correct answers, and apply those to future practice tests as well.

C. 55–69%

You need to work on improving your accuracy, especially if you are on the low end of this range. Make a list of at least three reasons why you missed the questions that were incorrect and focus on not making those same kinds of mistakes on the practice MCATs you take in the future. Compare the questions you got wrong to the questions that you got right in order to diagnose the strategies that were and were not working for you.

D. 40–54%

Your accuracy is relatively low. In the prep you do in the near future, focus on getting a higher percentage of the questions that you complete correct, even if that means slowing down for now and not answering all of the questions. Make a list of at least three reasons why you missed the questions that you got incorrect and focus on not making those same kinds of mistakes on the practice MCATs you take in the future.

Compare the questions you got wrong to the questions that you got right in order to diagnose the strategies that were and were not working for you.

E. Less than 40%

Your accuracy is low. You will need to significantly increase your percentage correct in order to get a competitive score. That will likely involve slowing down and randomly guessing on at least one passage in the section. Make a list of at least three reasons why you missed the questions that were incorrect and focus on not making those same kinds of mistakes on the practice MCATs you take in the future.

2. Is your accuracy:

Test 1 _____

Test 2 _____

Test 3 _____

Test 4 _____

Test 5 _____

A. highest in the beginning of the section and falling off toward the end?

Work on building up your endurance by studying for longer and longer periods of time. Taking as many mock MCATs as you can will also help you keep your concentration at a high level throughout a test. You may also have been lingering too long on the questions in the beginning, and then rushing the questions at the end.

Many test-takers will maximize their score by randomly guessing on a certain percentage of the questions in a CARS section. If you had to rush through many of the questions and if you got many of those questions wrong, this is an indication that, at this point in your preparation process, you should not be trying to work through all of the passages or questions.

B. highest in the middle of the section?

It is likely that it took you some time to warm up in the beginning, and then you tired out (or got impatient or rushed) at the end. Try warming up a bit by working through a passage before you take your next test. Take little 5-10 second breaks every 10-15 minutes during a test so that you can maintain your energy and focus at the end of the section.

C. highest at the end of the section?

It is likely that you gradually warmed up as you went through the test. The good news is that endurance was not a problem for you. To achieve a high level of accuracy from beginning to end, try warming up by working through a passage before you take your next practice test.

D. about the same all the way through the section?

Good work, if your accuracy was relatively good. On the MCAT, your goal is to hit the ground running and to keep your focus and energy high through the entire test.

2.5

3. For the questions that you missed, on average, what was your level of confidence as you answered those questions?

Test 1 _____

Test 2 _____

Test 3 _____

Test 4 _____

Test 5 _____

2.5

A. Fairly high

If you commonly felt very confident while picking answers that were in fact incorrect, and if you answered those questions relatively quickly, you may have been answering based on memory rather than by using the passage actively. If this is the case, in the future go back to the passage, find the relevant information, and base your answer closely on the passage text. Alternatively, you may have misread the question stem and/or answer choices, or selected a response before reading through all four choices. Look back at the questions you missed to determine if this was the case. Make a conscious effort to slow down when you read the question stem and answer choices, and read all four choices before selecting your response.

However, if you spent a great deal of time on the questions before picking the wrong answer, and if you read through the answer choices multiple times or spent a lot of time debating between two choices, you may have been overthinking the question and talking yourself into a wrong answer. In the future, limit yourself to two careful passes through the answer choices, select an answer (based on the passage information and question task), and then move on.

B. Moderate

It is normal to have a moderate level of confidence on most of the questions that you miss. If you missed quite a few questions (more than 16), however, your confidence and accuracy will increase if you read the question, the answer choices, and the relevant passage text more carefully, and if you base your answers more closely on the information in the passage. Use the feedback for your responses to the survey, especially questions 8–10, to diagnose specific reasons for your mistakes.

C. Fairly low

If you only missed a few questions, it is normal to have a low level of confidence on those questions; they were likely among the hardest questions in the test. However, if you missed many questions (more than 16), it is likely that you were not using the passage information actively enough. If you read the question stem and answer choices more carefully and go back to the passage text more consistently to find the relevant information, your level of confidence and your accuracy (and potentially your speed as well) will increase.

2.5

4. **For the questions that you got correct, what was your average level of confidence while answering the question?**

Test 1 _____

Test 2 _____

Test 3 _____

Test 4 _____

Test 5 _____

A. Fairly high

If you completed the section in the time allowed, and if you had excellent accuracy (that is, missed 8 or fewer), a high level of confidence is a sign that your approach to the questions was solid. However, if you had trouble completing the section (that is, did not get to one or more passages and/or had to rush at the end and missed many of those final questions), you may have been overly cautious. If your experience fits this scenario, don't double or triple check your answers. Once you have eliminated three of the choices and have a reasonable answer left, select that choice and move on.

B. Moderate

If your accuracy was fairly good (that is, you missed 12 or fewer), a moderate level of confidence on the questions that you got correct is normal. However, if your accuracy was significantly lower than this, it can improve through a combination of reading the passage text more carefully (at least the part that is relevant to the question), thinking through the question task more carefully, and paying attention to every word in each answer choice. Use the feedback for your responses to this survey, especially questions 8–10, to diagnose specific reasons for your mistakes.

C. Fairly low

If your accuracy was fairly good (you missed 12 or fewer questions and you completed the section), having a low level of confidence is not necessarily a bad thing. You do not need to understand every idea or detail in the passage in order to get most questions correct. If your accuracy was significantly lower, however, it most likely means that in general you may not be reading the questions carefully enough, using the passage actively enough, or reading and analyzing the answer choices closely enough. Focus on reading the question stem and answer choices word for word, as well as on finding specific information in the passage to support your response.

PART II: GENERAL TESTING STRATEGIES

5. **Did you read the question stems (not the choices) before you read the passage text?**

   Test 1 _____

   Test 2 _____

   Test 3 _____

   Test 4 _____

   Test 5 _____

A. Yes

This is an effective approach for most test-takers. When you preview the questions, don't worry about the question type. Rather, look for words in the question that relate to passage content to help you focus in on the key parts of the passage as you read it the first time through.

B. No

On the MCAT, Previewing the Questions (just the stem, not the choices) can be a very useful technique. If you haven't tried it, or if you have only tried it a few times and then abandoned the technique, it is worth practicing to see if it will pay off for you. On your next set of practice passages or practice test, try quickly reading through the question stems before reading the passage. Don't worry about the question type at that stage. Instead, pick out and highlight the words and phrases that relate to the content of the passage. This will allow you to focus on the most important parts of the passage, and to highlight words in those sections to help you go back efficiently to find the necessary information as you answer the questions.

However, if you have in fact practiced it for a month or more, and if you have implemented it on several tests without seeing a payoff in accuracy and/or speed, then not Previewing the Questions is a reasonable choice for you.

6. **Did you use notepad as you took the test?**

   Test 1 _____

   Test 2 _____

   Test 3 _____

   Test 4 _____

   Test 5 _____

A. No

Using notepad (provided by the test center on the real MCAT) is a very useful strategy. Writing down a few words to express the main point of each paragraph or big chunk of information, as well as the main point or Bottom Line of the whole passage, can help you to understand and keep track of the key parts of the author's argument, especially on the harder passages. It can also be quite helpful to keep track of your Process of Elimination on Roman numeral and EXCEPT/LEAST/NOT questions. If you are not used to using notepad, try it on several practice passages and then on at least two practice tests. Once you practice it, you will most likely find that it improves both your accuracy and your speed.

B. Yes

If you are using notepad already, the next step is to think about how you can use it even more effectively than you are now. In particular, make sure that it is well organized and that you are writing clearly. If you are writing quite a bit, work on paring it down (for example, limiting yourself to 4-5 words to express the main point of a paragraph or of the passage as a whole). You may not need to write down the main point of every paragraph for every passage. If the passage is easy to follow and understand, you might define some or all of the main points as a mental step without writing them all down. If you are making notes on the passage but never on the questions, try using it (sparingly) to write down brief notes to help you clarify and organize your thought process on difficult questions.

PART III: ATTACKING THE QUESTIONS AND POE

7. **When you went back over the questions that you missed, which of the following reactions did you often have? Select all that apply and read the feedback for those responses.**

   Test 1 _____

   Test 2 _____

   Test 3 _____

   Test 4 _____

   Test 5 _____

A. "The correct answer looks obvious in retrospect, and I don't know why I didn't pick it."

If the correct answer looks obvious in retrospect and/or if you don't remember why you made the choices that you did during the test, this is often due to going too fast and choosing based on intuition rather than on test-appropriate reasoning. Don't just pick the first answer that "sounds good." Instead, base your answer closely on the question task and the passage text.

B. "I see why the right answer could be right, but I still think the answer I picked is right too."

In MCAT CARS, many wrong answers are written to sound very good, but they have something, sometimes something fairly subtle, in them that makes them worse than the credited response. The correct answer is the "least wrong" answer. That is, it may not be perfect, but the other three are even worse. Furthermore, the correct answer must be based on the passage, not on outside knowledge or your own opinion. Go back to the questions that you missed, compare the right answers to your wrong answers, and identify the differences between them that make the credited response the best of the four choices.

C. "I see why the right answer is right and the wrong answer is wrong, but I think that I would still pick the wrong answer in the future."

A big part of maximizing your CARS score is learning the logic of the test itself. Each time you break down the logic of a question that you missed, you prepare yourself to get similar questions right in the future. Always review questions that you missed, not only to see why the right answer was right, but to diagnose what caused you to disregard it. Your ultimate goal is to get points; if you understand the logic of the test, you can begin to answer more strategically and avoid picking wrong answers in the future.

D. "I still don't get it."

Make sure to read the explanations for these questions especially carefully. Then go back through the question step by step: paraphrase what the question is really asking, identify and paraphrase the relevant information in the passage text, and go through the choices one more time, comparing them to each other and identifying differences between them. Even if this process takes some time, on most questions you will come to see the logic of the test, and questions will make more and more sense to you in the future.

> 8. **For which of the following question types did you miss two or more questions? Select all that apply and read the corresponding feedback below each response.**
>
> Test 1 _____
>
> Test 2 _____
>
> Test 3 _____
>
> Test 4 _____
>
> Test 5 _____

A. Inference and Retrieval questions

The key to getting these questions right is sticking as closely as possible to the information in the passage. Compare your wrong answers to the credited responses and identify how the right answers are better supported by the text. In the future, whenever possible, answer in your own words (based only on the passage text) before you evaluate the answer choices.

B. Main Point, Primary Purpose, and Tone/Attitude questions

The answers to these general question types must include, explicitly or implicitly, the whole passage, not just a part of it. Commonly, wrong answers for these types will be too narrow, too strong, or have a word or phrase within them that is inconsistent with the passage. Identify the Bottom Line of the passage (including the author's tone) before you go through the answer choices. Make sure to track the author's tone or attitude throughout the passage and highlight the relevant words. When you are down to two answers, look for differences in tone and scope.

2.5

2.5

C. Structure and Evaluate questions

To get these questions right, you need to identify the logical structure of the relevant part of the passage. You must see how different statements in the passage relate to each other, which includes separating the author's claims or conclusions from the support for those claims. Often, wrong answers are true based on the passage, but do not answer the question being asked. When attacking these questions, generate an answer in your own words, based not just on content but also on the logical structure of the passage, before you go through the answer choices.

D. New Information questions

These questions require you to summarize the theme of the new information in the question stem, and then apply it to the relevant information in the passage text. When you get these questions wrong, identify whether or not you correctly understood the point of the new information. If you did, see if you might have lost track of the relevant issue in the passage, and/or picked an answer that took the wrong direction (e.g., it was inconsistent with the passage, but the question asked how the author would respond). In the future, first identify the theme of the new information, then describe its relationship to the passage, including whether the question requires an answer consistent or inconsistent with the passage. Keep track of this direction as you evaluate each answer choice.

9. **For which of the following question types or formats did you miss two or more questions? Select all that apply and read the corresponding feedback below each response.**

   Test 1 _____

   Test 2 _____

   Test 3 _____

   Test 4 _____

   Test 5 _____

A. Strengthen and Weaken questions

These questions require you to accept the new information in the answer choices as true, and to find the correct answer that goes in the right direction. The answer must be strong enough to have a significant impact on the relevant part of the author's argument. Look at your wrong answers and identify if they were too weak to "most strengthen" or "most undermine" the passage, if they went in the opposite direction (for example, strengthened instead of weakened), or if they were not directly relevant to the passage. In the future, define what the correct answer needs to do before evaluating the answer choices. You may benefit from jotting this on your notepad, especially on Weaken questions.

B. Analogy questions

These questions ask you to find an answer with the same logic as the relevant part of the passage. In most cases, the correct answer will not be about the same subject matter as the passage. Look at your wrong answers to see if they match the content/topic but not the passage logic, or if they are part right/part wrong (one piece matches, another does not). In the future, describe the logic of the relevant part of the passage in generic terms before looking at the answer choices (e.g., if the passage states "increased food production led to a population explosion," you could write "an increase in A led to a large increase in B").

2.5

C. Roman Numeral questions

These questions provide you with three statements, and ask you to select the answer choice that includes all the statements that correctly answer the question and none that do not. Look at your wrong answers. Did you include too many (you were not strict enough) or too few (you eliminated statements that were not quite as good as those most obviously correct, but that were still good enough)? In the future, use your notepad to keep track of your evaluation of each statement as you go. Also, if you are sure that a statement is correct, eliminate answer choices that do not include it, and compare the remaining choices. If you are sure a statement is incorrect, eliminate choices that do include it and compare what remains.

D. EXCEPT/LEAST/NOT questions

These questions ask you to select the "worst" answer. For example, when a question asks "All of the following can be inferred EXCEPT," the three wrong answers will be supported by the passage, and the correct answer will not. Look at the questions you missed to see if you lost track of the EXCEPT, LEAST, or NOT. In the future, use your notepad to keep track of why you are eliminating each choice as you go.

10. For which of the following reasons did you miss one or more questions? Select all that apply and read the suggestions below each selection.

Test 1 _____

Test 2 _____

Test 3 _____

Test 4 _____

Test 5 _____

A. "I misunderstood the question."

Read the question stem word for word and put it into your own words before you read the answer choices.

B. "I misunderstood the passage."

If you read the passage text very quickly, slow down a bit and (at least!) pay more attention to the most important statements. When you go back to the passage while answering the question, read the relevant part carefully and paraphrase it. If you spent quite a bit of time reading the passage, however, you may have overthought it. Stick to what is explicitly stated, and don't waste time speculating about what the author might have meant.

C. "I answered from memory, and my memory was inaccurate."

Go back to the passage and read the relevant part carefully when answering the questions.

D. "I based my answer on the wrong part of the passage."

Make sure to keep track of the precise issue raised in the question stem, and to identify all the parts of the passage that may be relevant to it. Previewing the Questions before you work the passage will help you to do this most effectively and efficiently.

E. "I misunderstood or misread one or more of the answer choices."

Read each answer choice word for word the first time through. Paraphrase complicated choices to make sure that you understand what they are saying.

F. "I talked myself into the wrong answer."

The correct answer should not take a lot of effort to justify. Stick to the question task, the passage, and the exact wording of the answer choice. Use process of elimination aggressively; look for reasons to strike out choices.

G. "I got it down to two and then picked the wrong one."

This happens because there is often at least one wrong answer that is written to be very attractive. When you are down to two choices, reread the question, compare the two choices to each other, and if needed, go back to the passage again. Remember to pick the "least wrong" answer, not just the answer that "sounds best."

11. **On average, how often did you read all or part of the passage before answering a question?**

    Test 1 _____

    Test 2 _____

    Test 3 _____

    Test 4 _____

    Test 5 _____

A. Once

This is fine if you had a high level of accuracy. If you had a low level of accuracy, use the passage more actively (as if you are taking an open book test).

B. Twice

This is usually appropriate. Most of the time, you will read the passage as a whole once, and then go back at least once to the relevant section or sections as you answer each question.

C. Three times

This can be appropriate for harder questions. However, make sure that you are both reading the relevant section thoroughly enough and pausing to paraphrase it. Often, reading the appropriate part of the passage more completely and thoughtfully earlier on (during the process of answering the question) will eliminate the need to go back to it again and again. Focus more on answering the question in your own words in order to increase your efficiency and speed.

D. Four or more times

You may be reading and rereading bits and pieces of the passage out of context, which then requires you to go back and forth between the answer choices and the passage too often. Focus on reading and paraphrasing the entire relevant chunk, as well as on answering in your own words so that you can increase your efficiency and speed.

Ask yourself if you are overworking the questions, rethinking them or rereading parts of the passage over and over, even when you have a solid basis for picking an answer and moving on. If so, give yourself a limit on the number of times you can go back to the passage (for example, twice). Once you have hit that limit, select an answer and go on to the next question.

2.5

> **12. On average, how many times did you read through the set of answer choices before making a final selection?**
>
> Test 1 _____
>
> Test 2 _____
>
> Test 3 _____
>
> Test 4 _____
>
> Test 5 _____

A. Once

This was appropriate if you had a high level of accuracy (you missed 8 or fewer questions). If your accuracy was significantly lower, take two passes through the choices, at least on the more difficult questions. Eliminate the one or two most clearly wrong answers the first time through, and then compare the remaining choices before making a final selection.

B. Twice

This is usually appropriate. In most cases, you will eliminate one or two choices the first time through, and then compare the remaining answers in order to make a final decision.

C. Three times

This can be necessary on the more difficult questions. However, if you are going through the choices three times on most questions, you can increase your efficiency (and accuracy) by answering in your own words first whenever possible, and by reading the choices word for word (and paraphrasing complicated statements) the first time through.

D. Four or more times

If you are often reading through the choices four or more times, you need to work on attacking the questions more efficiently. Make it a goal to eliminate at least one or two choices on your first read through, based on the question task and the relevant passage information. Whenever possible, answer the question in your own words first so that you have more information in hand up front. When you are down to two choices, compare them to each other, reread the question, and go back to the passage rather than just rereading the choices over and over. Keep your focus on what is wrong with each choice, and on selecting the "least wrong" answer.

2.5

Goals for Test 2:

1)

2)

3)

Goals for Test 3:

1)

2)

3)

Goals for Test 4:

1)

2)

3)

Goals for Test 5:

1)

2)

3)

Goals for Real MCAT:

1)

2)

3)

2.6 STRESS MANAGEMENT

Most students feel some level of stress before an important exam. A certain level of anxiety, while uncomfortable, is beneficial: it sharpens your attention, keeps you alert, and intensifies your focus. However, if you find that your stress and anxiety gets out of control to the point where your performance suffers, there are ways to manage it and reduce it to a reasonable level. Some of these methods (see I, II, and IV below) involve scheduling your time and acclimating yourself to the experience of taking the test: these are important for everyone to implement from the beginning of your preparation. Other methods (see III below) involve reducing anxiety through relaxation and other exercises. You will find that some of these techniques work better for you than others. Try them all out, settle on some that work for you, and then use them consistently up to, and on, the day of the test.

2.6

I. Preparing for the Test

Develop and Implement a Clear Strategy

Anxiety comes in part from feeling as if you are unable to control a situation. Identify the aspects of the test, the testing conditions, and the importance of the test that instill fear in you, and do things that will help you confront and minimize those fears.

- **Build up your stamina.**
  It is difficult to maintain concentration over many hours under normal circumstances, let alone under stressful conditions. Prepare for test day by working passages over longer and longer periods with shorter and shorter breaks, until you can comfortably concentrate for a few hours at a time.

- **Take as many full practice tests as possible.**
  Experience builds confidence. Once you have practiced doing several passages at a stretch, take on doing more and more practice tests. Complete full tests in one sitting, taking breaks between sections. Don't have any food or water during the test except during the breaks. If you get cold or hot, don't put on or take off clothing unless you're on a break. That is, take your practice tests under the same conditions as the real MCAT. On test day, you can walk in to the testing center knowing that you know how to do this—this is just one more test in a long line of tests you've already completed.

- **Practice dealing with distraction.**
  Do passages or practice tests under less-than-ideal conditions. Go to a reasonably quiet coffee house, or an area of the library where people are moving around (but not talking loudly). Practice tuning out your surroundings while you work.

II. Taking the Test (including Practice Tests)

- **Take a breath.**

  The more tense we get, the more shallow our breathing becomes. Lack of oxygen can then contribute to your anxiety in a feedback loop. Stop this process as soon as you realize that your muscles are tightening or your focus is fading. Sit back in your chair and take three deep breaths. Take your eyes off the screen for 10-15 seconds, and move your arms and shoulders around to release the muscles. Don't force yourself onward to the next question if you realize that you're not working at your peak. Rather than wasting a big chunk of time getting questions wrong because you can't think straight, take a few seconds to relax and regroup, and make the most of the rest of your time.

- **Don't obsess about time.**

  Of course you are going to check the timer while you work, but checking the time constantly will distract you and make things more stressful. Doing lots of practice tests will help you develop a sense of timing while you work, so you know how long it takes you to read passages and get through questions. Only check the clock between passages; otherwise, immerse yourself in the task of working passages and attacking questions efficiently and effectively.

- **Take the breaks you are given.**

  The MCAT is designed to give you a feeling of burnout. The test makers give you as little help as possible during your test day, so make good use of what they DO give you! Just as you should use the annotation tools provided, such as highlighting and strikeout, you must also take advantage of the breaks you are offered. Use them for the basics (eating, using the restroom, etc.) but also to clear your mind, breathe deeply, get your eyes away from the screen, and shift gears for the next session.

III. Reducing Anxiety

Use Positive Reinforcement

- When we place high demands on ourselves, it's easy to fall into negative thinking at moments of frustration. You may find yourself thinking self-critical thoughts while studying or doing a practice test. Do "How could I miss that question!", "I'm so stupid!", or "I'm never going to get this!" sound familiar?

- Recognize these responses for what they are: a reaction to stress, not a representation of reality. Find words and phrases to replace the negative thoughts, such as "I know I'm smart, I'm working hard, and it will all pay off in the end." It may sound goofy, but it works.

Reward Yourself

- Don't let yourself burn out over the next month or two (or three). Yes, study and practice are crucial, but so is maintaining peace of mind. If you are so overworked and tired that you cannot concentrate on what you're doing, give yourself a break. If you can't commit to scheduling your time as extensively as recommended below, just make sure to nip feelings of being overworked in the bud as soon as you feel them coming on: set a goal (i.e., a certain number of hours of study time, or a particular number of practice passages). Once you achieve that goal, go to a movie, hang out with friends, go to the gym: do whatever you enjoy most for a few hours.

Practice Creative Visualization

2.6

- Creative visualization, if practiced over time, can offer significant long-term anxiety reduction. Lie on the floor (at home, not during the test!) on your back, with your arms and legs stretched out. Adjust your position until you feel comfortable and relaxed. Then close your eyes and picture the most wonderful, relaxing place you have ever visited or would like to visit, or a situation that makes you feel safe and at peace. It may be a tropical island, a quiet forest, a deserted beach, or a gathering at home with friends and family. See your surroundings clearly, smell the air, hear the birds, or picture the faces of the people who make you happy. When you are ready to stop, picture the most relaxing part of the scene one last time. Count to three slowly, then open your eyes. If you practice this regularly for a few weeks, especially at times when you feel tense, you should begin to feel less anxious. Then, if you do find yourself becoming anxious during the test, breathe deeply and imagine yourself back in that peaceful place. You will find yourself relaxing quickly, because you've trained yourself to respond that way.

- While creative visualization of relaxing escapes are great for managing stress, if you're going to think about the aftermath of the test, it is helpful to focus on positive outcomes, imagining success. Who will be the first person you tell about your MCAT score? How will that person react to the good news? Imagine the look on your parent's face, the hugs you will get, and the feeling of accomplishment you will have as you share news of your score. Thinking of these things as part of your goal, rather than simply focusing on the numerical score you want to achieve, can help you feel more motivated.

IV. Managing Your Time

- Just as a clear pacing strategy will help you to work more methodically and stay calm during the test, pacing yourself in your preparation will help you feel more in control and will help ensure that you still make time to relax and spend time with friends and family (and therefore maintain your sanity).

- Consider how many hours of MCAT preparation you should do in a week and create a daily schedule of the hours of the day you will dedicate to it. Be practical in your estimation of hours: you may feel like you should be studying all the time but you likely have other responsibilities and commitments, plus you need time to eat, rest, exercise, and unwind.

2.6

- Below are two sample schedules. Both are for days when you don't have to go to class or work: the first is for a day dedicated to reading and passage drills, and the second is for days on which you are taking full practice tests. Both entail 8–9 hour prep days. Notice how much time is left to do other things.

- You may only be able to manage two hours of MCAT prep if you have a heavy day with classes, work, or other commitments—set your schedule accordingly. And, if you can manage it, having one day a week that is completely, or at least significantly, free of MCAT study can be restorative (and help you to get even more out of the other six days of the week). A great benefit of creating a schedule to manage your time is that when you are not scheduled to study, you don't have to feel guilty about not studying!

- Your schedule should be personalized based on when you tend to wake, eat, sleep, and on your own individual activities. Do make sure to adjust your sleep and study schedule to correspond to the time of day you are taking the MCAT, at least in the last few weeks before your test.

Construct your own agenda for the weeks or months remaining before the MCAT, using these sample schedules as guidelines.

Sample Schedule: No Full Practice Test

6:30 A.M.–8:00 A.M.: Wake up, breakfast, quick morning walk/run or workout, shower.

8:00 A.M.–11:30 A.M.: MCAT prep (this could be half a practice test, practice questions and passages, test review, or some chapter reading for various subjects)

11:30 A.M.–1:00 P.M.: Lunch and leisure time (read a magazine, check social media news, meet with a friend, dance to your favorite song)

1:00 P.M.–4:00 P.M.: MCAT prep

4:00 P.M.–5:00 P.M.: Snack, stretch, unwind

5:00 P.M.–7:00 P.M.: MCAT prep

7:00 P.M.–10:30 P.M.: Dinner and leisure time

10:30 P.M.–11:00 P.M.: Go to bed

Sample Schedule: Full Practice Test

6:30 A.M.–7:30 A.M.: Wake up, breakfast, quick morning walk/run or workout, shower.

7:30 A.M.–9:00 A.M.: Warm up for the test (do a few practice questions and passages to get your mind going)

9:00 A.M.–4:30 P.M.: Full practice MCAT (including break times)

4:30 P.M.–6:00 P.M.: Dinner/snack, relax

6:00 P.M.–8:00 P.M.: Test review (always review your performance as soon as possible; review CARS on the same day as the test so that you can remember your thought process during the test)

8:00 P.M.–10:30 P.M.: Relax, do whatever else needs to be done

10:30 P.M.–11:00 P.M.: Go to bed

2.6

Chapter 2 Summary

Your preparation for the MCAT CARS section should include familiarization with passage structure, question types, and answer traps, as well as training in the efficient and effective use of passage information.

In addition to reading practice passages and answering the questions, smart preparation includes a careful, continuing analysis of your performance.

CHAPTER 2 PRACTICE PASSAGES

Individual Practice Drills

Do the following two passages untimed. Focus on implementing the six steps you learned in this chapter. After you have checked your answers, fill out an Individual Passage Log for each passage.

CHAPTER 2 PRACTICE PASSAGE 1

"To live as our fathers and grandfathers lived will not do. The village resident more and more feels that his life is connected by thousands of invisible threads not only with his fellow villagers, with the nearest rural township, but this connection goes much farther. He dimly perceives that he is a subject of a vast state, and that events taking place far from his place of birth can have a much greater influence on his life than some event in his village." –Petr Koropachinskii, Ufa Provincial Zemstvo Chairman, 1906

When Koropachinskii wrote these words, he viewed the "invisible threads" connecting the villager with the state as a new political consciousness gained primarily through the political mobilization of the 1905 revolution. Salient features of this mobilization, such as political parties, their programs, and a freer press, drew the attention of political actors at the time and, subsequently, of historians of late imperial Russia. We might consider these connections from another perspective, however: that of the state and the "invisible threads" it used to connect with its subjects. Furthermore, many of these connections were not so much invisible threads as paper trails—written documents found in the files of bureaucracies staffed by officials who sought to extend the regime's knowledge about its population.

[One such method,] registration through the state church, presented complications in an empire composed of many religious groups. Not all of the tsar's subjects were Orthodox. What to do about the rest? As Gérard Noiriel has pointed out, the Old Regime in France had faced a similar problem. Registration by Catholic priests left many Jews and Protestants without civil status. In 1792, the revolutionary Republic addressed this situation by secularizing registration and requiring municipal authorities to register all French citizens. This option held little attraction for the Russian state, where an autocrat ruled an empire organized by legal estates. Tsar Nicholas had no interest in creating citizens. As protector of the Orthodox Church, Nicholas I did not desire to eliminate religious registration, either.

Nonetheless, Nicholas I and his officials did seek to identify the tsar's subjects and to include them in the civic order. The tsarist regime attempted to achieve the civic inclusion of the non-Orthodox by insisting that they register with their own religious institutions. Between 1826 and 1837, the tsar decreed that Catholic priests, Muslim imams, Lutheran pastors, and Jewish rabbis must keep metrical registers. These laws did not extend civil status to all religious groups. Religious dissenters known as Old Believers, numbering as much as 10 percent of the empire's population, and animist peoples were notable exceptions. The Orthodox Church claimed Old Believers as part of its flock, but the dissenters had rejected seventeenth-century reforms in the liturgy and generally wanted nothing to do with the Orthodox clergy. Furthermore, the expansion of metrical registration came at the expense of uniformity. Muslim imams did not report estate status. Religious leaders who did not know Russian could maintain the books in their native languages—the imams could use Tatar, for instance. Nonetheless the expansion of metrical books in the 1820s and 1830s represented a major step toward the inclusion of the empire's non-Orthodox residents into legally recognized subjecthood.

[Decades later, under a different regime,] the Great Reform era brought a new governing ethos to the empire, one that changed the role of metrical registration. Reform-minded bureaucrats sought to increase the population's participation in the administration of the empire and to reduce the importance of estate distinctions. The state emancipated the peasantry, introduced a new court system, and allowed elected units of self-administration (zemstvos) a limited role in local affairs. The military service reform of 1874 marked a shift toward the equalization of male subjects in law. Before 1874, military service was an obligation for those of lower status. The military reform of 1874 made males of all estates liable for military service. A universal military obligation, with reduced burdens based on educational achievement, replaced an estate-based system. After the Great Reforms, the autocracy took the first, halting steps toward a more inclusive, less particularistic civic order.

Material used in this particular passage has been adapted from the following source:

C. Steinwedel, "Making Social Groups, One Person at a Time: The Identification of Individuals by Estate, Religious Confession, and Ethnicity in Late Imperial Russia," *Documenting Individual Identity: The Development of State Practices in the Modern World.* © 2001 by Princeton University Press.

1. Nicholas I's regime ordered inhabitants of Russia to register with their particular religious institutions because:

A) the Orthodox Church would have required registrants to convert.
B) the tsar did not want to extend civil rights to all people by having the state register them.
C) some political parties, such as the Old Believers, rejected the authority of the Catholic Church.
D) the military service reform of 1874 had not yet been enacted to equalize the status of the male population.

2. Suppose a Russian peasant in the early 20th century returning home from a day's work first told his wife of rumors from St. Petersburg that the tsar had been deposed and only later mentioned to her, as an afterthought, that the local Orthodox Church had new priest. Based on the information in the passage:

A) the peasant's conversation with his wife supports the claim that Old Believers did not value the Orthodox Clergy.
B) the tsar's hope of including subjects in the civic order through registration had been fulfilled.
C) the peasant is likely part of a minority religious group not recognized by the Orthodox Church.
D) the peasant's behavior may strengthen Koropachinskii's assertions in paragraph 1.

3. Which of the following is LEAST supported by the passage?

A) Nicholas I's new court system sought to increase the population's participation in the administration of his empire.
B) Some residents of Russia were not citizens prior to the reign of Nicholas I.
C) Nicholas I had an interest in maintaining the power of the Orthodox Church.
D) Not all Russian residents understood the official language.

4. Which of the following events, if it occurred, would most support the author's description of the changes happening in Russian society and politics in the 1870s?

A) Old Believers and animists united to oppose registration and were granted independent civil status in 1835.
B) A peasant attended university in 1880 and was then elected chairman of the zemstvo.
C) A man in early 20th century Russia had a life different from his father's.
D) The progress of the so-called Great Reform era was reversed upon Nicholas II's ascent to the throne.

5. The author's discussion of Koropachinskii's assertions most supports which of the following statements?

A) The changes Koropachinskii identified were possible only after the advent of political parties and a freer press.
B) Religion was less important in people's lives than were the affairs of government.
C) Koropachinskii did not believe the threads were actually invisible.
D) Part of the chairman's statement may not be entirely accurate.

6. The passage includes discussion of Gérard Noiriel's work in order to do all of the following EXCEPT:

A) help place events in Russia in a broader context.
B) provide a precedent for the author's analysis of Nicholas I's policies.
C) offer one solution Nicholas I declined to pursue.
D) illustrate another situation where the Orthodox Church served a majority but not all of the population.

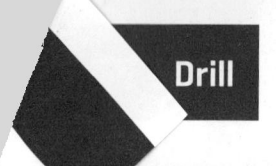

...PTER 2 PRACTICE PASSAGE 2

People's facility with numbers ranges from the aristocratic to the Ramanujanian, but it's an unfortunate fact that most are on the aristocrats' side of our old Mainer. I'm always amazed and depressed when I encounter students who have no idea what the population of the United States is, or the approximate distance from coast to coast, or roughly what percentage of the world is Chinese. I sometimes ask them as an exercise to estimate how fast human hair grows in miles per hour, or approximately how many people die on earth each day, or how many cigarettes are smoked annually in this country. Despite some initial reluctance (one student maintained that hair just doesn't grow in miles per hour), they have often improved their feel for numbers dramatically.

Without some appreciation of common large numbers, it's impossible to react with the proper skepticism to terrifying reports that more than a million American kids are kidnapped each year, or with the proper sobriety to a warhead carrying a megaton of explosive power—the equivalent of a million tons (or two billion pounds) of TNT.

And if you don't have some feeling for probabilities, automobile accidents might seem like a relatively minor problem of local travel, whereas being killed overseas by terrorists might seem to be a major risk when going overseas. As often observed, however, the 45,000 people killed annually on American roads are approximately equal to all American dead in the Vietnam War. On the other hand, the seventeen Americans killed by terrorists in 1985 were among the 28 million of us who traveled abroad that year—that's one chance in 1.6 million of becoming a victim. Compare that with these annual rates in the United States: one chance in 68,000 of choking to death; one chance in 75,000 of dying in a bicycle crash; one chance in 20,000 of drowning; and one chance in 5,300 of dying in a car crash.

Confronted with these large numbers and with the correspondingly small probabilities associated with them, the innumerate will invariably respond with the non sequitur, "Yes, but what if you're that one," and then nod knowingly, as if they've demolished your argument with their penetrating insight. This tendency to personalize is, as we'll see, a characteristic of many people who suffer from innumeracy. Equally typical is a tendency to equate the risk from obscure and exotic malady with the chances of suffering from heart and circulatory disease, from which about 12,000 Americans die each week.

There's a joke I like that is marginally relevant. An old married couple in their nineties contact a divorce lawyer, who pleads with them to stay together. "Why get divorced now after seventy years of marriage? Why not last it out? Why now?" The little old lady finally pipes up in a creaky voice: "We wanted to wait until the children were dead."

A feeling for what quantities or time spans are appropriate in various contexts is essential to getting the joke. Slipping between millions and billions or between billions and trillions should in the sense be equally funny, but it isn't, because we too often lack an intuitive feeling for these numbers. Many educated people have little grasp for these numbers and are even unaware that a million is 1,000,000; a billion is 1,000,000,000; and a trillion, 1,000,000,000,000.

A recent study by Drs. Kronlund and Phillips of the University of Washington showed that most doctors' assessments of the risks of various operations, procedures, and medications (even in their own specialties) were way off the mark, often by several orders of magnitude. I once had a conversation with a doctor who, within approximately twenty minutes, stated that a certain procedure he was contemplating (a) had a one-chance-in-a-million risk associated with it; (b) was 99 percent safe; and (c) usually went quite well. Given the fact that so many doctors seem to believe that there must be at least eleven people in the waiting room if they're to avoid being idle, I'm not surprised at this new evidence for their innumeracy.

Material used in this particular passage has been adapted from the following source:

J.A. Paulos, *Innumeracy: Mathematical Illiteracy and Its Consequences.* © 1988, 2001 by John Allen Paulos.

1. Which of the following best describes the author's primary purpose?

A) To explain the causes of innumeracy and provide options on how to prevent it
B) To demonstrate that Americans are, on the whole, undereducated
C) To provide data concerning probabilities of various causes of death
D) To describe innumeracy and some of its consequences

2. It can be inferred that, as used in paragraph 1, the term *aristocratic*:

A) describes individuals with better-than-average mathematical skill.
B) refers to the traditional ruling class.
C) represents people with only a limited facility with numbers.
D) refers to an inability to understand the difference between a million and a billion.

3. The author would most likely agree with which one of the following statements?

A) A megaton describes an unimpressive amount of explosive power.
B) It is unlikely that more than a million American children are kidnapped each year.
C) Driving an automobile is less dangerous than swimming.
D) Numbers such as a billion or a trillion are often amusing.

4. Which of the following, according to the passage, may characterize the innumerate?

   I. Inability to improve their understanding of numbers
   II. Personalizing improbable but tragic outcomes
   III. Inaccurate assessments of the probabilities of possible outcomes of medical procedures

A) I only
B) II only
C) I and III
D) II and III

5. The author most likely included the joke about the old married couple in order to:

A) provide further evidence of innumeracy in the elderly.
B) argue that couples in their nineties should not seek divorce.
C) illustrate the significance of an understanding of apt quantities based on context.
D) further support a point made in paragraph 3.

6. Which of the following is NOT included as evidence of innumeracy among doctors?

A) Personal experience in the form of an anecdote
B) Statistics regarding the frequency of death due to heart disease
C) Recent academic research
D) A humorous exaggeration of a common experience

SOLUTIONS TO CHAPTER 2 PRACTICE PASSAGE 1

1. **B**   This is an Inference question.

    A: No. The passage does not suggest that the Orthodox Church would *require* conversion.

    B: **Yes. See the end of paragraph 3 and the beginning of paragraph 4. Nicholas rejects the French solution, municipal registration, because "Nicholas had no interest in creating citizens...Nicholas I and his officials did seek to identify the tsar's subjects and to include them in the civic order. The tsarist regime attempted to achieve the civic inclusion of the non-Orthodox by insisting that they register with their own religious institutions."**

    C: No. The Catholic Church is not the church from which the Old Believers (who also aren't described as a political party) dissented—they rejected the Orthodox Church (paragraph 4).

    D: No. Even though this choice includes an accurate description of the military service reform of 1874, lack of equality is not, according to the passage, the reasoning behind Nicholas's religious registration.

2. **D**   This is a New Information question.

    A: No. The peasant and his wife were not identified as Old Believers. Furthermore, there is no suggestion in the new information that the actions of the peasant indicate anything about ideas of Old Believers regarding the value of the Orthodox Church.

    B: No. This situation doesn't specifically relate to the issue of religious registration.

    C: No. The peasant and his wife were not identified with any fringe or minority religious group.

    D: **Yes. Koropachinskii notes that a Russian villager, "dimly perceives that he is a subject of a vast state and that events taking place far from his place of birth can have a much greater influence on his life than some event in his village." The fact that the peasant reports rumors regarding the distant tsar before he reports more concrete news about his own village could support Koropachinskii's assertion.**

3. **A**   This is an Inference/EXCEPT question (for more on EXCEPT questions, see Chapter 4, page 142).

    A: **Yes. The correct answer will be the statement that is NOT supported by the passage. The author does not state that Nicholas I instituted a new court system. This came "decades later, under a different regime" (paragraph 5).**

    B: No. In paragraph 3 and paragraph 4, the author states that "Nicholas had no interest in creating citizens" through registration. Note that although the passage doesn't say that Nicholas made everyone citizens, this choice is still correct in saying that not everyone was a citizen before his reign (even if during and after his reign that may still have been the case).

    C: No. The end of paragraph 3 says, "As protector of the Orthodox Church, Nicholas I did not desire to eliminate religious registration, either." If Nicholas sought to protect a function of the Church, this suggests that he had an interest in maintaining the Church's power.

    D: No. The end of paragraph 4 states that some religious groups in Russia whose leaders "did not know Russian could maintain the books in their native languages."

4. **B** This is a Strengthen question (for more on Strengthen questions, see Chapter 4, page 132).

A: No. This would likely undermine the author's description of events; the passage indicates in paragraph 4 that Nicholas I was opposed to extending civil recognition to these groups.

B: **Yes. If a peasant had access to higher education and was then able to rise to a position of power in local government, it supports the claim in paragraph 5 that eventually measures were taken to promote a "more inclusive, less particularistic civil order."**

C: No. This is consistent with Koropachinskii's description of Russian life in paragraph 1, but the question asks you to support the author's description, not Koropachinskii's.

D: No. Ultimately, this choice is irrelevant to the author's description. The passage never argues or suggests that the changes were temporary. Furthermore, the passage never discusses the reign of Nicholas II, only that of Nicholas I.

5. **D** This is an Inference question.

A: No. The author does say that the changes Koropachinskii noted occurred as a result of shifts in 1905 that included the advent of a freer press and political parties, but the author never says that those were the *only* things that could have led to these changes. This choice is too extreme.

B: No. The author's discussion does not suggest that religion became less important than government, just that the state's actions served to make people aware that they were part of something larger than simply their individual townships.

C: No. While the author notes in paragraph 2 that "these connections were not so much invisible threads as paper trails—written documents," this is the author's belief, not Koropachinskii's.

D: **Yes. The author states in paragraph 2 that "these connections were not so much invisible threads as paper trails—written documents."**

6. **D** This is a Structure/EXCEPT question.

A: No. When the author says "the Old Regime in France had faced a similar problem," he's announcing a parallel between Old France and the events in Russia, creating a broader context.

B: No. The events in France occurred prior to the events in Russia. Therefore, the case of France can be seen as a precedent.

C: No. This choice is in line with the author's analysis of Noiriel's parallel: that the French option "held little attraction" for Nicholas (paragraph 3).

D: **Yes. The correct answer will be the statement that doesn't explain why the author cited Noiriel. The Orthodox Church was never mentioned as being in France—the only cited French religious authority is the Catholic Church (paragraph 3).**

SOLUTIONS TO CHAPTER 2 PRACTICE PASSAGE 2

1. **D** This is a Main Idea/Primary Purpose question.
   A: No. The author addresses neither the causes of innumeracy, nor any options for preventing it.
   B: No. While the passage does suggest that most Americans have a relatively poor understanding of numbers, it does not address the overall level of American education. Lack of education is not described as a cause of innumeracy, nor is innumeracy used as an example for a more general critique of the educational system.
   C: No. This choice is too narrow. The author provides data and probabilities in paragraph 3 as examples supporting the broader point of the passage. That is, the purpose of the passage as a whole is not limited to providing death statistics.
   D: Yes. The passage describes innumeracy in the first paragraph and discusses its consequences through the rest of the passage.

2. **C** This is an Inference question.
   A: No. The passage uses the term "unfortunate" to refer to the aristocrats' side of the spectrum measuring people's facility with numbers (paragraph 1), indicating that their facility with numbers is NOT better-than-average.
   B: No. There is no reference to an actual social or ruling class in the passage. Always stick to the context of the passage and beware of applying outside knowledge to MCAT questions, especially where vocabulary is concerned, since this is a common trap.
   C: Yes. The author states in paragraph 1 that "it's an unfortunate fact that most [people's facility with numbers is]...on the aristocrats' side," and then goes on to discuss students' lack of understanding of numbers.
   D: No. This answer choice is too specific. This is only one example of innumeracy; while the "aristocrats" might not understand the difference between a million and a billion, the word itself does not refer specifically to the lack of understanding of that difference.

3. **B** This is an Inference question.
   A: No. The author uses the phrase "proper sobriety" to describe the appropriate reaction to a warhead carrying a megaton of explosive power, indicating his belief that this is a serious amount of power.
   B: Yes. The author's use of the phrase "proper skepticism" provides strong support for this answer choice by indicating his opinion that such figures are likely exaggerated.
   C: No. While, in paragraph 3, the author cites statistics on the likelihood of drowning and dying in a car crash, he does not explicitly relate these to swimming or being the driver of a car.
   D: No. The passage states in paragraph 6 that slipping between millions and billions or between billions and trillions should be funny but isn't, not that the numbers themselves are funny.

4. **D** This is an Inference/Roman numeral question.
   I: False. This statement is too extreme. The last sentence of paragraph 1 states that students "have often improved their feel for numbers dramatically."
   II: True. This is discussed in paragraph 4.
   III: True. This paraphrases the findings of the recent study referenced in the last paragraph.

5. **C** This is a Structure question.
   A: No. The passage never discusses innumeracy specifically in the elderly.
   B: No. The author makes no personal judgment on whether or not people should divorce.
   C: Yes. This answer choice paraphrases the first sentence of paragraph 6, which explicitly refers to the joke.
   D: No. Paragraph 3 discusses errors in judging risks. The joke in paragraph 5 relates to understanding appropriate quantities and times, as the author indicates in the paragraph immediately following the joke itself.

6. **B** This is a Retrieval/EXCEPT question.
   A: No. The author describes a conversation he had with a doctor, which qualifies as a personal anecdote.
   B: Yes. The correct answer will contain a statement that is NOT given as an example of innumeracy among doctors. Death due to heart and circulatory disease is mentioned in paragraph 4 as an example of the tendency to "equate the risk from obscure and exotic malady" with the chances of acquiring a common disease. There is no connection made here to risk assessments made by doctors.
   C: No. The "recent study" referenced in paragraph 7 is given as an example of doctors' inaccurate risk assessments.
   D: No. The author speculates that in order to avoid being idle, doctors seek to have at least eleven people in the waiting room. The author intends this as a humorous exaggeration of the common experience of waiting in a doctor's office—the last sentence of the passage links the example to the issue of innumeracy.

Chapter 3
Active Reading

GOALS

1) To develop new—and more effective—active reading habits
2) To read for logical structure and get to the Bottom Line
3) To use annotation in order to be able to retrieve information quickly and accurately

3.1 BASIC APPROACH: THE SIX STEPS

First, here is a review of the six basic steps to approaching the CARS section that we discussed in Chapter 2. In the rest of this chapter, we will focus on steps two, three, and four.

■ STEP 1: RANK AND ORDER THE PASSAGES

Decide whether to do the passage Now, Later, or Never, based on the difficulty level of the passage text.

■ STEP 2: PREVIEW THE QUESTIONS

Read through the question stems from first to last (not the answer choices) before you read the passage. Look for and highlight words and phrases that indicate important passage content. Do not worry at this stage about identifying the question type.

■ STEP 3: WORK THE PASSAGE

As you read through the passage (staying on the screen that includes the last question of the set for that passage), use the highlighting function (sparingly) to annotate the most important references in the passage, especially words that indicate the logical structure of the author's argument and references that appeared in your preview of the questions. Notice topic sentences that help you to identify conclusions made by the author. Articulate the Main Point of each chunk of information (usually, each paragraph). Use your noteboard, especially on difficult passages, to jot down these main points. As you read, think about how these chunks relate to each other, and identify the structure of the passage.

■ STEP 4: BOTTOM LINE

After you have read the passage, sum up the Bottom Line: the main point and tone of the entire passage.

■ STEP 5: ATTACK THE QUESTIONS

Start with the last question in the set for that passage. Read the question word for word, identifying the question type and translating the question task into your own words. Go back to the passage before reading the answer choices and find the relevant information (reading at least five lines above and below the reference). Think about what the correct answer will need to do, and generate an answer to the question in your own words. Use Process of Elimination (POE) actively. Select the "least wrong" answer.

Move backwards through the set of questions. If a question looks especially difficult, skip over it the first time through, and answer it after the easier questions as you click forward through the questions towards the next passage.

■ STEP 6: INSPECT THE SECTION

At or before the 5-minute mark (ideally, before you begin your last passage), double-check to make sure that you haven't left anything blank. You can use the Review function at this stage. Do NOT rethink questions you have already completed.

3.2 ACTIVE READING: READING FOR STRUCTURE AND THE BOTTOM LINE

What Is the Bottom Line?

When you read a CARS passage for the first time, you must read it in a very different way than you would read most other texts. For example, when you are studying for a bio exam for a class, you are trying to understand and memorize every fact and detail in the course material. If you read a CARS passage in that way, however, you will not only waste a great deal of precious time, but you will also overlook the things that are really important: the main points being made by the author, and how they fit together to communicate the core idea, or Bottom Line, of the entire passage. In this chapter, we will first discuss what you are reading FOR the first time through a passage: the logical structure and core ideas of the passage. Then we will lay out HOW you should be working the passage by using your highlighter and noteboard to map out those basic aspects of the passage.

As you've no doubt noticed, MCAT CARS passages are often dense, convoluted, and full of details that you ultimately don't need to know in order to answer the questions. Such passages are impossible to read as closely as you would read a text for school, especially given the time constraint. On the MCAT, your goal is not to develop a deep understanding of every aspect of the passage; your goal is to find the information you need to answer the questions, and to pay as little attention as possible to everything else.

Therefore, do not attempt to understand or memorize every detail. This is time-consuming and counterproductive. Instead, visualize the passage as comprised of several large chunks of information. Each chunk, which may span part or all of a paragraph, has a Main Point and serves a particular function within the passage as a whole.

As you read, separate the central point of each paragraph from the evidence used to support that point. Translate the Main Point of each paragraph into your own words. What is the author trying to prove? Pay close attention to words that indicate the author's opinion or attitude. Jot down a few words or a short sentence indicating the Main Point of the chunk and/or paragraph on your noteboard. Link this theme with the Main Points of the previous paragraphs. Imagine that you are reading a mystery novel, following a twisty plot line and adding up the major clues to the story as you go.

After you have read and identified the Main Point of the last paragraph, define the main idea and tone of the passage as a whole: this is the Bottom Line of the entire passage.

How to Get the Bottom Line

In order to read the passages effectively (that is, quickly and with a reasonable degree of comprehension), you must become an *active reader*. Don't read passively; imagine yourself attacking and taking control over each passage. Think of the passage as an argument that you are breaking down into its most basic parts.

Here are the basic principles for active reading.

1) Preview the questions for content (not for question type). Predict what issues will be especially important in the passage you are about to read.
2) Note the author's tone and purpose. What side is the author on? Why is he or she writing this passage?
3) Notice pivotal words and other transitions: use them to identify the "chunks" of an argument and how those chunks relate to each other.
4) Highlight the words that indicate the logical structure of the passage—that is, how the parts of the passage relate to each other. Also highlight topics that appeared in the questions.
5) Translate the Main Point of each paragraph or chunk of information into your own words. Link it to what you've already read and predict what will come next.
6) Articulate the Bottom Line of the whole passage to yourself before answering the questions.

Reading For Structure

The structure of a passage can be identified on three levels.

- **Level 1:** The structure of individual sentences. Look for how the parts of the sentence work together, and how the words used by the author indicate the meaning of that sentence. Don't get caught up in parsing out the structure of every line of every paragraph. But, when sentences contain **indicator words** like *however, although, therefore, on one hand, for example,* etc., it is important to use those words to figure out the meaning of that sentence.

  For example, pivotal words such as *however* or *but* signal a shift in meaning or subject. When you identify a pivotal word in the sentence, ask, "What is it shifting from, and what is it shifting to? How do the two parts of a sentence (or the pair of sentences, if the indicator words come at the beginning of a sentence) relate to each other, and what does this tell me about the author's argument?" Or, if you see the word *therefore*, your immediate question should be, "What is the conclusion or claim being made and where is the evidence supporting that claim?" (especially important for answering Reasoning questions). The words *for example* should raise the question, "what larger claim is being supported by this example, and how does it connect to the author's argument in the passage as a whole?"

  By paying attention to indicator words, you can identify the sentences that will play a particularly important role in constructing the author's argument and skim over the sentences that are less important at this stage.

- **Level 2:** The structure of a paragraph or chunk of information. If you ask these questions about individual sentences, it naturally leads you to the structure and intent of the entire paragraph. Did it introduce an opposing point of view? Did it provide specific evidence and support for a conclusion drawn earlier? Does it introduce another stage of development, or continue to develop a description of a particular phase?

  Separate the paragraph into **claims** and **evidence**. The claims being made are important in understanding the main point of the paragraph, whereas the details of the evidence supporting those claims are usually important only when answering the questions.

  Look for **topic sentences.** Often (but not always) the author uses the first or last sentence of the paragraph to sum up the theme or main point of the paragraph as a whole.

- **Level 3:** The structure of the passage as a whole. The relationship between the individual paragraphs creates or constructs the logical structure of the author's argument. This leads you naturally into an understanding of the Bottom Line (the author's overall argument). Having this map of the passage in mind also helps you to quickly locate the information you need as you are answering the questions.

Some common passage structures are

- compare and contrast
- cause and effect
- thesis with evidence
- rebuttal
- narration or description
- analysis of different aspects of an issue or idea
- old and new theory
- chronology

3.3 THE MAPS OF A PASSAGE

There are four basic components to any passage that, when clearly identified and articulated, give you a firm grounding in the text and build a foundation for the process of answering the questions.

These components are the **MAPS** or

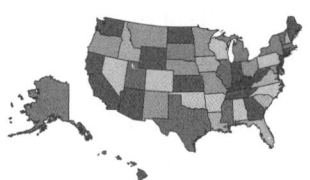

Main Point

Attitude

Purpose

Support

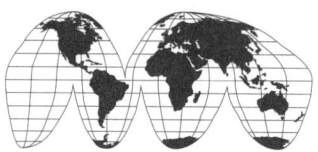

1) The **MAIN POINT** of each paragraph encapsulates the core of *what* the author is trying to communicate. It includes the main idea of each paragraph or chunk of information, and defines and delimits the scope of the passage. The **MAIN POINT** of the passage is the Bottom Line.

2) The **ATTITUDE** expresses *who* the author is through the tone of the passage. Is the author presenting himself or herself as a critic? An advocate? A neutral observer?

3) The **PURPOSE** is the intent of each chunk of the passage and of the passage as a whole. *Why* did the author write it? Was it to compare and contrast two theories? To propose a new theory? To trace the evolution of an idea? To describe a process?

4) The **SUPPORT** is the evidence the author uses to support his or her claims. *How* does the author construct the passage?

Think about a real map. It is constructed in a particular way with a particular purpose: to guide you to your destination. When you use a map, you don't need to pay attention to every street or highway or reference; you only need to find the streets and the connections between those streets which are relevant to your particular goal at that particular time. Memorizing the entire map is not only unnecessary, it's impossible. If you look at the entire picture without separating out the important from the unimportant sections, you will be lost—it's just too much information!

By breaking a passage down into MAPS, you define both Logic and Location. The Logic gives you the Bottom Line, which is crucial for all questions. Location "labels" the different parts of the passage, enabling you to use your map to find the specific information you need as you are answering each question.

So, let's look at our four MAPS components in more detail in connection to passage structure. To follow the process you actually go through as you work a passage, we will reverse the components to SPAM, starting at the lowest level and working up to the Main Point.

Support

How does the passage use evidence to support the author's larger claims?

All passages, even neutral explanatory passages, are made up of big claims and specific evidence supporting those claims. As we discussed above, your main goal the first time through a passage should be to identify the author's main points and overall purpose; the evidence or support should be skimmed or read more quickly so that you don't get bogged down in the details. So, you need to be able to identify the support used by the author in order to 1) decide to skim through it in your first read-through, as it is less important to the logic of the passage, and 2) re-locate it, if and when it becomes relevant to the questions. Many CARS questions also require you to enumerate or to characterize evidence presented in a passage. While you should not dwell on the support during your first reading of the passage, you should ask yourself, "What larger point is being supported here?"

So, how do you recognize the support?

There are many ways to support a Main Point. The following are the most common:

1) **Examples:** The author illustrates the Main Point with an example from the real world or with a hypothetical example meant to reflect the real world. Examples are often introduced with standard words or phrases that help you to identify them: *in this case, in illustration, for example.*

2) **Generalizations:** To make a point about Christmas, for example, an author might generalize about something larger—like holidays in general. Or the author might make a point about Christmas by discussing Christmas trees. In other words, a generalization supports a main idea by giving an example of something larger—or something smaller—than the subject.

3) **Steps/stages:** Many passages describe the development of an idea, a historical time line, or an evolutionary process. Generally, each paragraph will describe one of those stages. Or, a passage may describe how one thing preceded another in order to support a larger claim about cause and effect.

4) **Comparisons/contrasts:** An effective way to explain something is to compare it to, or contrast it with, something else. Through differences and similarities, the specific characteristics of an idea can be highlighted. A specific type of comparison is an *analogy*, where one situation is described in order to communicate something about another, supposedly similar situation.

5) **Statistics:** Statistics can be any type of numerical information—percentages, ratios, probabilities, populations, prices, etc. It is especially important to avoid getting bogged down in these details. You will be able to find them again later, if you need to.

6) **Studies:** The author cites studies, research, or polling data to support a conclusion.

7) **Definitions:** The author defines key terms in order to communicate something about the context or issues within which those terms are used.

8) **Quotes or citation of others:** The passage includes either direct quotes or citation of other works. It is important to ask yourself if the author is agreeing or disagreeing with these other writers or speakers.

9) **General opinion:** The author describes a past or present common belief. Authors often do this in order to introduce a different or alternative idea. Always define whether the common belief is consistent or inconsistent with the author's point of view.

10) **Anecdotes:** The author tells a story, often from his or her personal experience.

Purpose

Why was the passage written?

Purpose is closely related to structure, and it can be broken down to three levels in a similar way.

1) **W**hat is the purpose of the support provided by the author? What larger claim is being supported? Answering this question will lead you to the next level.
2) **W**hat is the purpose of the paragraph? What role does it play within the logical structure of the passage? How do the different paragraphs connect to each other? Answering this question leads you to the final level.
3) **W**hat is the purpose of the passage as a whole? Why did the author write it? What overall claim or point is being made?

The purpose of the passage as a whole includes the author's attitude. The intent of neutral passages is to describe or explain something. In a purely descriptive passage, it is likely that each paragraph will deal with a different characteristic of the thing being described.

An explanatory passage often includes both generalizations as well as specific examples as illustrations of those generalizations. Identify transition words to ascertain when the author is moving from one point to another (*additionally, also, furthermore,* etc.) or from a generalization to a specific case or illustration (*for example*).

On the other hand, evaluative, critical, or persuasive passages often present one idea or position, a contrasting idea or position, and the author's opinion, which may involve choosing one of those sides over the other or presenting a separate alternative altogether. A common purpose is to contrast old with new theories, or to present and evaluate a debate or controversy.

Keep in mind the strength of the tone and the language. For example, the author may be rejecting the validity of a claim, or may simply be raising questions about or problems with that claim. Keep track of pivotal words (*however, but, yet, conversely, although,* etc.) that indicate when the author is shifting in the discussion from one side to the other, or introducing a qualification. (Pivotal words, however, are not limited to opinionated passages, just as transitional words do not appear exclusively in neutral passages.) Difficult passages may have several such shifts.

Attitude

Who wrote the passage? What is the author's tone?

When asking yourself "who wrote the passage," don't take the question literally, and don't speculate about what kind of person the author might be in real life. Rather, connect this to the purpose of the passage and to how the author presents himself or herself through the passage text. An author may position himself or herself as a neutral observer, simply describing or explaining without expressing an opinion. The author may even describe a debate or conflicting points of view without directly entering into that debate.

In other passages, the author is more present—speculating, evaluating, criticizing, praising, or advocating. To define the attitude of the author, look for words that indicate the tone of the passage (e.g., *unfortunately, shamefully, at last, thankfully*, etc.), or statements that embody the voice or opinion of the author. If the author does have an opinion, evaluate how strongly negative or positive it is. Look out for qualifying language (e.g., *might, could, in some cases, while it is sometimes true that*, etc.) that authors often use to moderate their tone.

Occasionally, a question will directly ask for the attitude or tone of the author. However, attitude can play a role in any question type. It is particularly central to Main Point or Primary Purpose questions, to any question that asks how the author would respond to new information, and to Strengthen and Weaken questions.

Main Point

What is the passage trying to prove?

Articulating the main point or main idea (that is, the Bottom Line of the passage) is one of the most important steps you can take to maximize both your accuracy and your speed in working through the questions. A question may directly ask for the main point or central thesis. However, even if there is no such question, the main point can be used on a variety of question types to quickly eliminate answer choices that are out of scope or not the issue of the passage. The main point may be summarized in the first or last paragraph of the passage, but this is not always the case. In many passages, parts of the main point are scattered throughout, and it can be defined only by synthesizing or piecing together the main idea of each chunk of information.

Students often fall into one of two traps when attempting to identify the main point. On the one hand, they might state it too broadly, as a vague category or idea that includes—but goes beyond—the passage. On the other hand, they may define it too narrowly, focusing on only one among several of the points made by the author.

3.4   CARS EXERCISES: MAPS

3.4

Exercise 1: Separating Claims from Evidence

Read and highlight each of the following paragraphs. As you read, identify the evidence used and the claims made based on that evidence. Note the wording and/or paragraph structure used by the author to distinguish the evidence from the main point. Note any topic sentences (sentences that express the main point of the paragraph). Finally, answer the three questions following each paragraph. Answers follow at the end of the Exercise.

Paragraph 1

Drug activity was the life force of Coco's new building. There was no pretense of security: doors were propped open, and the interior hallway made for a nerve-wracking trip from the sidewalk to the hall. Pigeon droppings formed a putrid sand castle in the building's crumbling fountain. The mailboxes were bashed in, their little doors dented and askew. People snatched the light bulbs from the hallways.

1. What is the Main Point? Is it expressed in a topic sentence?

2. What is the evidence supporting that Main Point, and what is the nature of that evidence?

3. What language or paragraph structure did the author use to distinguish the evidence from the claims?

Paragraph 2

To assert, as one is tempted to, whether friendly or hostile to Nietzsche, that his results were flashes of poetic insight, or brilliant intuition, misses, I think, the real thrust and importance of his position. The fundamental intention of Nietzsche's work must be to recover and make manifest these underlying presuppositions which were the foundations of the coherence of Greek culture. It is apparent, for instance, that he does not intend a historical portrait of Greece shortly after the Cliesthenian reforms. In another context, speaking of Myerbeer's opera, he will argue that "it is *now* a matter of *indifference*" that the founders of opera were revolting against the Church, and that "it is *enough* to have perceived" that they were in fact engaged in *sub rosa* glorification of natural man.

1. What is the Main Point? Is it expressed in a topic sentence?

2. What is the evidence supporting that Main Point, and what is the nature of that evidence?

3. What language or paragraph structure did the author use to distinguish the evidence from the claims?

3.4

Paragraph 3

English serfs were not slaves—human chattels—as in the Roman Empire and American South. They had legal rights to strips of arable land of their own to work (after putting in around two-thirds of their time working the lord's personal lands, called his demesnes). The serf villagers had a right to pasturage of a modest number of domesticated animals. They could hunt for boar and rabbits (not deer, which were reserved for the ruling class) in the neighboring forests or haul fish out of a nearby stream to eat on Catholic Fridays and during Lent. They could plant vegetable gardens next to their houses. The lord had to provide in each village a mill to grind the peasant's grain for their heavily cereal diet.

1. What is the Main Point? Is it expressed in a topic sentence?

2. What is the evidence supporting that Main Point, and what is the nature of that evidence?

3. What language or paragraph structure did the author use to distinguish the evidence from the claims?

Paragraph 4

The *Nude Descending a Staircase* is now one of the most celebrated milestones of modern art, but when the show's organizers saw it, far from being dazzled, they were horrified. Their view of what Cubism was, or ought to be, centered increasingly narrowly upon the mathematics of the Golden Section. Marcel's *Nude* owed nothing to this. In fact, it was clearly influenced as much by the Futurists as the Cubists. The Futurists were concerned with speed, noise, movement: their works had been exhibited the previous month at Bernheim Jeune's gallery, an exhibition which Duchamp visited several times. He was at this time concerned not with pure form, but with the problem of describing movement on a static canvas: he said later that the idea had come from Marey's serial photographs of people and animals in movement, and described its geometry a 'sport of distortion other than Cubism.'

1. What is the Main Point? Is it expressed in a topic sentence?

2. What is the evidence supporting that Main Point, and what is the nature of that evidence?

3. What language or paragraph structure did the author use to distinguish the evidence from the claims?

Paragraph 5

3.4

The discrepancy between people who had rats and people who did not was underscored in 1959. It was a time when Americans and New Yorkers were thinking pretty highly of themselves, when people on Park Avenue felt safe from rats. It was during the Cold War, and Soviet officials were in Manhattan visiting a technology show that highlighted Soviet inventions. A headline in the *Daily News* boasted U.S. EXPERTS WANDER AT RED SHOW AND WONDER AT NOTHING. The same week, however, a three-year old baby died in Coney Island. His mother had heard him crying in the night and thought he wanted a bottle but soon discovered he was being bitten by rats.... Between January of 1959 and June 1960, 1,025 rat bites were reported in New York.... Sixty thousand buildings were identified as rat harborages by the city's health department—buildings constructed before 1902 that had been designed to house a few families and were now housing dozens. In 1964, nine hundred thousand people were reported living in forty-three thousand old tenements.

1. What is the Main Point? Is it expressed in a topic sentence?

2. What is the evidence supporting that main point, and what is the nature of that evidence?

3. What language or paragraph structure did the author use to distinguish the evidence from the claims?

Answers to Exercise 1: Separating Claims from Evidence

Paragraph 1:

1.   Topic sentence: "Drug activity was the life force of Coco's new building."
2.   The paragraph uses anecdotal evidence to illustrate the Main Point.
3.   The paragraph flows from the assertion into the description.

Paragraph 2:

1.   Topic sentence: "The fundamental intention of Nietzsche's work must be to recover and make manifest these underlying presuppositions which were the foundations of the coherence of Greek culture."
2.   The author quotes from Nietzsche's work to support his position.
3.   The author starts by contradicting the "tempting" position, then asserting his own, and supporting that assertion with evidence from Nietzsche's writings.

Paragraph 3:

1.   Topic sentence: "English serfs were not slaves…"
2.   The author lists the legal rights that the English serfs did have, as evidence that they were not outright slaves.
3.   The claim is presented in the topic sentence, and the rest of the paragraph works to support that claim.

Paragraph 4:

1.   The Main Point of this passage is that Marcel Duchamp's painting, *Nude Descending a Staircase*, was influenced by Futurism as much as, or more than, by Cubism. There is no single topic sentence in this paragraph.
2.   The author uses general evidence about the artistic philosophy of the Cubists and the Futurists to prove his point about this painting. The contrast between how the painting was seen at the time and how it is now viewed reinforces this point.
3.   The author's claim needs to be pieced together from the historical and general evidence she provides. The initial contrast between the painting's reception in its time and now introduces the point, however.

Paragraph 5:

1.   The Main Point of the passage is that rats were an identifiable city-wide problem for many people in New York in 1959. There is no single topic sentence in this paragraph.
2.   The author uses both anecdotal evidence (the baby on Coney Island) and statistical evidence to demonstrate the rat problem. He also contrasts people on Park Avenue with people living in tenements to show that some people did not have to worry about the rat problem, while others were severely affected by it.
3.   An initial contrast is suggested ("The discrepancy…"), and then developed by discussion of the complacency of many people as opposed to the rat-related suffering of others. The latter is introduced by a pivotal phrase: "The same week, however…".

Exercise 2: MAPS Exercise

Read the following passage in 3–4 minutes, and then write down the Main Point, Attitude, Purpose, and Support. Don't just think about the answers; *write them down* to ensure that you have clearly articulated each component. Explanations follow the exercise.

3.4

Race relations and racial attitudes in the United States have changed dramatically over the past quarter of a century. Although many of these changes are well documented, controversies persist about whether, in fact, race has declined in its significance as a determinant of social, economic, and political statuses and outlooks.

An intriguing argument which attempts to reconcile and make sense of the discrepant findings about the status of Blacks vis-à-vis whites is the "polarization thesis." William Julius Wilson, for example, argues that the Black community is becoming socially, politically, and economically polarized. He points out that a number of Blacks are completing college educations and moving into the kinds of prestigious jobs that provide economic security, higher standards of living, and homes in the suburbs. These Blacks, he argues, have been able to take advantage of the opportunities which emerged as a result of the civil rights movement. On the other hand, many other Blacks are trapped in inner-city ghettos where schools are poor and where opportunities for employment and advancement are limited. As the Black community becomes more socioeconomically differentiated, race becomes a less important determinant of the life chances and outlooks of individual Blacks than does socioeconomic status. Implicit in this argument is the idea that as race decreases in importance as a stratifying agent, Blacks will become more similar to non-Blacks with the same socioeconomic position than they will be to other Blacks with vastly different socioeconomic statuses.

When it was first published in 1978, Wilson's *Declining Significance of Race* touched off much controversy and debate. Critics of the book marshaled a great deal of evidence and numerous counter-arguments to undermine Wilson's declining significance of race thesis. Charles V. Willie, for example, basing his arguments on data concerning income, education, and housing, put forth the idea that not only was race not declining in its import, but it was actually increasing as a determinant of the quality of life for Blacks.

Similarly, Robert Hill argued that conditions for Blacks as a group were not improving, and on some fronts things were actually getting worse. For example, he pointed out that recessions continued to affect Blacks disproportionately. Unemployment rates for Blacks remain twice those of whites. The number of Blacks living in poverty continued to rise at the same time that the number of whites living in poverty decreased.

Recent empirical investigations have provided both support for Wilson's declining significance hypothesis and evidence against this position. For example, through the 1960s and 1970s, Blacks improved their relative standings in education, occupational status, and personal income, but failed to make substantial gains when compared with whites in such areas as family income, unemployment rates, housing patterns, and rates of poverty. To date, however, no study has indicated whether changes in stratification patterns have simultaneously led to a convergence between Blacks and non-Blacks in their social, political, and economic outlooks and a polarization among Blacks.

Material used in this particular passage has been adapted from the following source:

C. Herring, "Convergence, Polarization, or What? Racially Based Changes in Attitudes and Outlooks," *Sociological Quarterly.* © 2005, Midwest Sociological Society.

Main Point: _____

_____

_____

Attitude: _____

_____

_____

Purpose: _____

_____

_____

Support: _____

_____

_____

Analysis of the Passage

Here is one possible MAPS outline for the preceding passage.

Main Point:	Although Black people have made gains in some areas and suffered losses in others, it is difficult to know whether polarization has occurred, and if it has, what its effect might be.
Attitude:	Interested in Wilson's thesis, but not convinced without empirical evidence
Purpose:	To describe a promising theory, present critics of the theory, and suggest there is no clear resolution to date
Support:	Illustrates a controversy by citing authors on both sides, and describes how they back up their claims. Cites own evidence showing that empirical support exists for both sides.

Exercise 3: Putting It All Together

To break down and explore each of these components in more detail in the context of tracking the structure of the passage, let's visit a sample MCAT CARS Passage, which is reproduced on the following pages.

3.4

Preview the questions and work the passage. For each example provided, ask yourself why the author uses that example. Identify wording that indicates the author's tone. For each paragraph, identify how that paragraph relates to the rest of the passage. Articulate the Bottom Line of the passage.

Then answer the questions, specifically looking for how your understanding of MAPS and passage structure applies. Finally, read through the explanation that follows.

From Romania to Germany, from Tallinn to Belgrade, a major historical process—the death of communism—is taking place. The German Democratic Republic does not exist anymore as a separate state. And the former GDR will serve as the first measure of the price a post-Communist society has to pay for entering the normal European orbit. In Yugoslavia we will see whether the federation can survive without communism, and whether the nations of Yugoslavia will want to exist as a federation. (On a larger scale, we will witness the same process in the Soviet Union.)

One thing seems common to all these countries: dictatorship has been defeated and freedom has won, yet the victory of freedom has not yet meant the triumph of democracy. Democracy is something more than freedom. Democracy is freedom institutionalized, freedom submitted to the limits of the law, freedom functioning as an object of compromise between the major political forces on the scene.

We have freedom, but we still have not achieved the democratic order. That is why this freedom is so fragile. In the years of democratic opposition to communism, we supposed that the easiest thing would be to introduce changes in the economy. In fact, we thought that the march from a planned economy to a market economy would take place within the framework of the *nomenklatura* system, and that the market within the Communist state would explode the totalitarian structures. Only then would the time come to build the institutions of a civil society; and only at the end, with the completion of the market economy and the civil society, would the time of great political transformations finally arrive.

The opposite happened. First came the big political change, the great shock, which either broke the monopoly and the principle itself of Communist Party rule or simply pushed the Communists out of power. Then came the creation of civil society, whose institutions were created in great pain, and which had trouble negotiating the empty space of freedom. And only then, as the third moment of change, the final task was undertaken: that of transforming the totalitarian economy into a normal economy where different forms of ownership and different economic actors will live one next to the other.

Today we are in a typical moment of transition. No one can say where we are headed. The people of the democratic opposition have the feeling that we won. We taste the sweetness of our victory the same way the Communists, only yesterday our prison guards, taste the bitterness of their defeat. And yet, even as we are conscious of our victory, we feel that we are, in a strange way, losing. In Bulgaria the Communists have won the parliamentary elections and will govern the country, without losing their social legitimacy. In Romania the National Salvation Front, largely dominated by people from the old Communist *nomenklatura,* has won. In other countries democratic institutions seem shaky, and the political horizon is cloudy. The masquerade goes on: dozens of groups and parties are created, each announces similar slogans, each accuses its adversaries of all possible sins, and each declares itself representative of the national interest. Personal disputes are more important than disputes over values. Arguments over labels are fiercer than arguments over ideas.

1. Which of the following best expresses the main idea of the passage?

A) Communism will never completely vanish from the Earth.
B) Democracy is the highest good that any Eastern European country can ever hope to achieve.
C) Market economies do not always behave as we might predict.
D) Although many formerly Communist countries are now "free," this does not always mean that they have a democracy.

2. The author originally thought that the order of events in the transformation of society would be represented by which of the following?

A) The totalitarian structure would collapse, leaving in its wake a social structure whose task would be to change the state-controlled economy into a free market.
B) The transformation of the economy would destroy totalitarianism, after which a different social and political structure would be born.
C) The people would freely elect political representatives who would then transform the economy, which would then undermine the totalitarian structure.
D) The change to a democratic state would necessarily undermine totalitarianism, after which a new economy would be created.

3. Which of the following best represents the relationship between freedom and democracy, as it is described by the author?

A) A country can have freedom without having democracy.
B) If a country has freedom, it necessarily has democracy.
C) A country can have democracy without having freedom.
D) A country can never have democracy if it has limited freedom.

4. Which of the following best describes the author's attitude toward what has taken place in communist society?

A) He is relieved that at last the democratic order has surfaced.
B) He sees the value of returning to the old order.
C) He is disappointed with the nature of the democracy that has emerged but nevertheless pleased with the victory of freedom.
D) He is confident that a free economy will ultimately provide the basis for a true democracy.

5. When the author mentions "the same process" (paragraph 1), it can be inferred from the passage that he is most likely referring to:

A) the gradual shift away from authoritarian politics.
B) the potential disintegration of the Soviet Union.
C) the possible breakdown in the general distribution systems in the Soviet Republic.
D) the expected sale of state-owned farms to private enterprise.

3.4

6. Which of the following does the author imply has contributed to the difficulties involved in creating a new democratic order in Yugoslavia?

I. The people who existed under a totalitarian structure did not have the experience of "negotiating the empty space of freedom."
II. Mistaking the order in which political, economic, and social restructuring would occur.
III. Changes in the economy were more difficult than anticipated.

A) II only
B) I and III only
C) II and III only
D) I, II, and III

7. It can be inferred from the passage that the democratic opposition feels that it is "in a strange way, losing" (paragraph 5) because:

A) some of the old governments are still unwilling to give in to freedoms at the individual level.
B) the new governments are not strong enough to exist as a single federation.
C) newly elected officials have ties to old political parties.
D) no new parties have been created to fill the vacuum created by the victory of freedom.

Answers to Exercise 3: Putting It All Together

1. **D**
2. **B**
3. **A**
4. **C**
5. **B**
6. **B**
7. **C**

Support

This passage supports its main thesis by contrasting what *actually* happens with the expectation that formerly communist nations would evolve into democracies, and then cites specific cases in the first and last paragraphs to illustrate the point. Your paragraph-by-paragraph outline might look like this.

1) Examples of the death of communism
2) Generalization and contrast nature of freedom and democracy
3) Expected progression
4) Real progression
5) Examples of incomplete transition

Knowing where and how the author supports his claims is particularly important in answering questions 2, 5, 6, and 7.

Purpose

In this passage, the purpose is to analyze how and why sociopolitical transformation in the formerly communist nations did not follow the expected path, and to express regret that this has left their evolution into democracies incomplete.

Take a look at questions 2 and 5, and consider the role played by the Purpose of the author in each of the credited responses.

Attitude

The author is clearly present in this passage. Note the repeated use of the word "we"; the author presents as a participant (paragraph 3) as well as an informed expert (paragraph 1), not as a disinterested outsider. Note also the tone and language of the passage. Democracy is something to be "achieved," from which we can infer that it is a desirable thing. The author speaks of the "sweetness of our victory," telling us that freedom, in this sense, while limited, is greatly appreciated. Yet at the same time the author feels that "we are, in a strange way, losing." This indicates the author's discontent with the incomplete nature of the transformation.

Now take a look at question 4, which directly asks for the author's attitude. Choices A and D are too positive (and A is wrong for other reasons as well; it is inconsistent with the author's analysis). Choice B is too negative. The author appreciates the changes that have occurred, and wants the transformation to continue. Only choice C reflects the mixture of appreciation and regret that defines the author's attitude in this passage.

Main Point

In this passage, the author argues that many formerly communist nations have overthrown totalitarian regimes and achieved political freedom. However, because the transformation of the economy and civil society of these countries is as yet incomplete, true democracy does not exist. A student without a firm grasp on the driving theme and scope of the argument might incorrectly identify the main point as, "One can have freedom without democracy," which is too broad. A student who gets too caught up in one part of the passage might say the Main Point is that, "In Bulgaria and Romania, members of the old communist order still hold positions of power." A student who gets it just right, however, might say that the Main Point is something like this: "Many countries have overthrown communism and are now free, but they have not yet achieved democracy."

Now take a look in particular at questions 1, 3, and 4. Notice how useful it is to have a clear statement of the Main Point as a tool to eliminate traps and choose the correct answer.

Exercise 4: Practice MAPS

Use this log as a template to outline the MAPS for at least 8 passages from online or from other resources. **While you do not need to actually write down the MAPS of a passage during an MCAT,** by practicing this technique, you will improve your ability to characterize and evaluate the passage's central thesis, its logical structure, and the nature and strength of its claims.

MAPS Log

Passage #

MAIN POINT:

ATTITUDE:

PURPOSE:

SUPPORT:

3.5 PASSAGE ANNOTATION AND MAPPING

Now that we have broken down what you are reading for during your first time through a passage, let's get into the mechanics of working a passage. That is, what you should be doing with your pencil and the highlighter in order to keep your focus on the logic and structure of the passage, and to set up the process of answering the questions as accurately and efficiently as possible.

Why Annotate?

Annotation is a crucial part of active reading. Like any successful traveler, you need a *map* to help you navigate the passage. Intelligent annotation can help you to create this map. A smart annotation system is neither too sparse nor too elaborate.

In the course of your undergraduate studies, you may have become accustomed to highlighting large chunks of text. However, this approach is not going to help you on the MCAT. If you highlight everything that "looks important" in the passage, in the end, all you will have is some big blocks of yellow text. This won't help you to understand the logic of the argument as you read, and you will have to reread huge chunks of text to find the relevant information as you answer the questions.

You must have a specific strategy for annotating or mapping the text of the passage. While you do not need to write down all aspects of the four parts of MAPS that we discussed above, your physical mapping of the passage is based on the logical structure of the passage that you identified through reading for MAPS. Mapping is an active process that keeps you engaged with the text. It forces you to decide which points are most crucial to the author's argument, and how those points relate to each other to create the Bottom Line. It also marks the breaks between logically important chunks of the passage, which helps you locate information necessary for answering the questions.

Mapping

There are two tools you have to map the passage: *making notes on your noteboard* and *highlighting the passage*.

Making Notes

Use your noteboard to jot down the Main Point of each paragraph and the Bottom Line of the passage. Do this for every passage now; eventually, you may only need to write it down for the harder passages. Do NOT, however, use your noteboard to list every fact mentioned in each paragraph; your goal is to identify the core idea of that chunk, not to write down a detailed outline of it. Also, if there is a complicated time-line in the passage, write it down so that you can use your notes as you answer the questions. You can also use your noteboard to write down translations of difficult questions and answer choices.

What to Highlight

Question Topics   When you see words or phrases that you recognize from your preview, highlight them. However, don't jump out of the passage to answer the question at this point (you don't know yet what else the author might have to say about that subject!). By highlighting them, you make it easy to come back and find them when you do answer the question.

Transitions: Pivotal Words   Pivotal words are especially important, so let's discuss them in more detail.

MCAT CARS passages rarely contain a single point reiterated over and over again. Rather, a chain of reasoning is more likely to change direction one or more times. These turns in the overall direction of a passage are often marked by **pivotal words**. Here are some common pivotal words and phrases.

but	although	however
yet	despite	nevertheless
nonetheless	except	admittedly
in spite of the fact that	in contrast	even though

These words indicate *change* or *contrast*. Pivotal words signal that the author is about to shift the course of the argument by

- placing a condition on the argument;
- introducing an antithetical point;
- shifting from a simple to a more complex level of argument;
- making a concession to an opposing viewpoint.

Think of pivotal words as signposts that appear at crucial turns or refinements in the argument. Highlight them as you work through the passage. Highlighting pivotal words serves at least two functions.

- First, it increases the visibility of the parts of the passage that are likely to contain key ideas.
- Second, stopping to highlight a pivotal word lets you know that you need to determine *why* a transition is occurring at that point. In other words, the most valuable aspect of highlighting pivotal words—indeed, of annotating in general—is that it alerts you to the parts of the passage to which you need to pay the most attention, and it helps you track the logic of the author's argument.

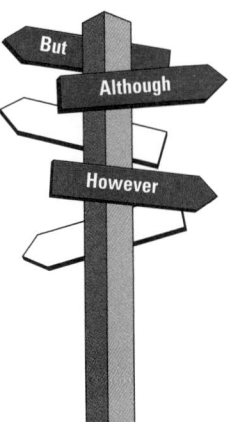

3.5

Transitions: Continuations   These words indicate that the author is further developing or explaining the point he or she has just made. Noticing and highlighting them will help you to distinguish different parts of the author's argument from each other. Here are words commonly used to indicate continuations.

furthermore
additionally
also
moreover

Conclusions   Authors use these words to sum up their Main Points. Finding and highlighting these words will help you to do the same. Here are some common conclusion indicators.

therefore	thus
so	consequently
clearly	hence
for this reason	

Opinion Indicators   One of the most important aspects of the Bottom Line is the author's tone. To accurately identify the author's point of view, look for and highlight phrases that express opinion, and words like

finally
fortunately
thankfully
unfortunately
sadly

Emphasis Words   Authors use words like these to catch your attention, because what follows is especially important. Here are some examples of emphasis words.

most important
primarily
chiefly
key
crucial

Comparisons and Contrasts   Not only are these words important to the logical structure of the passage; they also alert you to potential traps in the questions. When the passage describes two things as different, a wrong answer will describe them as similar, and vice versa. When the author discusses a change over time, wrong answers will reverse the chronology. By locating and highlighting comparison/contrast indicators, you are already helping yourself get the questions right. Here are some examples.

similarly	like
analogy	unlike
in contrast	later
the difference between	before/after

All of the categories of words discussed above indicate that something important to the Bottom Line is being discussed by the author; that is, major claims that deserve some attention on your first reading of the passage. These last three categories, however, tend to indicate details or support for those major claims. Highlight these markers to indicate location of the support, but read through what follows them in the text more quickly. You can follow your highlighting back to the relevant part of the passage if you need to as you are answering the questions.

Examples   These words tell you that what follows is an example or illustration of a larger, more important point. Highlight them so that you can find these details if they become important to the questions. These markers are especially useful for answering questions that ask you if, or how well, the author's claims are supported. What you should be *thinking* about now as you read, however, is the conclusion being supported by the example. This is what will give you the Main Point of the chunk and eventually the Bottom Line of the passage. Here are some common example indicators.

for example
because
since
in this case
in illustration

List Markers   When the author provides a string of claims or examples, it can be difficult to pull out the relevant item from that list when you are answering the questions. Highlight just the markers, not the entire list. But, just as with example indicators, define what this list is illustrating as you read: what is it a list of? List markers include

first   There are three aspects
second
thirdly

Names   Highlight names now so that you don't have to reread large chunks of text to find them when they show up in the question stems and answer choices.

3.6 CARS EXERCISES: ACTIVE READING

Exercise 1: Working the Passage

Previewing the Questions

Read through the five questions below. Identify the words and phrases that indicate the issues in the passage that will be relevant to answering these questions. Don't try to identify the question type at this stage; focus only on clues to passage content. After we preview these questions, we will move on and read the passage attached to them.

1. According to the author, which of the following constitutes a fundamental human characteristic?

2. Which of the following, based on information in the passage, would most strengthen the author's claim in paragraph 6 that the work of economists is necessary to the advancement of civilization?

3. The author claims that human beings find it difficult to survive. What explanation is offered in support of this conclusion?

4. According to the passage, why do economists have such significant influence over society?

5. It can be inferred from the passage that economists are relatively unknown because:

Summing it up: What will this passage be about? _____

_____

_____

The questions you have just previewed are about the passage (presented paragraph by paragraph) on the following pages. As you work through those paragraphs, keep in mind what you learned from these questions.

Defining the Main Points and the Bottom Line

What we have here is an entire passage. These paragraphs have already been highlighted for you, as an illustration of what you should be (and shouldn't be) highlighting. As you read, think about *why* those words have been highlighted, and what those highlighted words tell you about the important parts of the author's argument.

For each paragraph, define the Main Point of that chunk. Write down the Main Point in the space provided before you move on to the next paragraph. Don't make a list of all the information included. Focus on the claims being made, not the evidence supporting those claims. At the end, we will articulate the Bottom Line of this passage.

3.6

The very fact that man has had to depend on his fellow man has made the problem of survival extraordinarily difficult. Man is not an ant, conveniently equipped with an inborn pattern of social instincts. On the contrary, he is preeminently the creature of his will-o'-the-wisp whims, his unpredictable impulses, and his selfishness. Man is torn between a basic need for gregariousness—to coexist peaceably with his neighbors—and a pronounced tendency toward greediness. Often, his tendency to guard his own interest is at odds with his need to survive in a community. And it is to this clash and conflict that the first great economists addressed themselves.

Main Point: _____

_____

_____

One would think that in a world torn by economic problems, a world in which we constantly worry about economic affairs and talk of economic issues, the great economists would have an important place in history and be as familiar to us as the great philosophers or statesmen. Yet they seem to be only shadowy figures of the past. In the 1760s an educated traveler in England would probably have heard of Adam Smith, a professor at the University of Glasgow, but today a great many educated people do not know that this gentleman was the father of economics.

Main Point: _____

_____

_____

No economist has ever been either a national hero or a national villain. Yet what economists have done has been more decisive for history than many acts of statesmen who basked in brighter glory. Often their deeds have been more profoundly disturbing than the shuttling of armies back and forth across frontiers, more powerful for good and bad than the edicts of kings and legislatures. Since economists have shaped and swayed men's minds they have necessarily shaped and swayed the world.

Main Point: _____

_____

_____

Few economists ever lifted a finger in action. They worked, in the main, as scholars: quietly, inconspicuously, and without much regard for what the world had to say about them.

Main Point: _____

_____

_____

Economists are not well known because most people do not understand the significance of economics and believe it to be a rather uninteresting academic pursuit. But a man who thinks that economics is only a matter for professors forgets that this is the science that has sent men to their battle stations. A man who has looked into an economics textbook and concluded that economics is boring is like a man who has read a primer on logistics and decided that the study of warfare must be dull.

Main Point: _____

_____

_____

To be sure, not all the economists were titans. Adam Smith was a stunningly interesting character. But thousands of his followers wrote texts, some of them monuments of dullness, and explored minutiae with all the zeal of medieval scholars. Nonetheless, economists are the worldly philosophers, and their work is essential to the growth and continuation of advanced civilizations. Economists have sought to embrace in a scheme of philosophy the most worldly of man's activities: his drive for wealth. It is not, perhaps, the most elegant kind of philosophy, but there is no more intriguing or important[1].

Main Point: _____

_____

_____

Bottom Line of the passage as a whole: _____

_____

_____

---

[1] Material used in this particular passage has been adapted from the following source: R. L. Heilbroner, *The Worldly Philosophers.* © 1999 by Simon & Schuster Inc.

Answers for Exercise 1: Mapping the Passage

Previewing the Questions

Summing it up: What will this passage be about?

This passage will be about human nature and survival, economists and their relationship to society, and why economists are not well known.

3.6

Defining the Main Points and the Bottom Line:

NOTE: Your own notes may be briefer; these are written out in more complete terms than you may need for your own understanding.

1) Man's independence conflicts with his need to be part of a group for survival.
2) Economists surprisingly fade into the background of history.
3) Economists have great influence over history.
4) Economists are scholarly, removed from the world.
5) People don't "get" economics, and so don't know economists.
6) Economists are vital to civilization.

Bottom Line of the passage as a whole: Although they fade into history, economists are crucial to the advancement of society.

Exercise 2: Annotation and Active Reading—Putting It All Together

Read and annotate the following passage. As you read, stop and write down the Main Point of each paragraph on your noteboard. When you have read the whole passage, write down the Bottom Line. Then, turn the page and read through the sample annotations and explanation of the passage. The sample passage also indicates what sections of the passage you should skim or move through more quickly.

Passage for Annotation Exercise 2

There are two major systems of criminal procedure in the modern world—the adversarial and the inquisitorial. The former is associated with common law tradition and the latter with civil law tradition. Both systems were historically preceded by the system of private vengeance in which the victim of a crime fashioned his own remedy and administered it privately, either personally or through an agent. The vengeance system was a system of self-help, the essence of which was captured in the slogan "an eye for an eye, a tooth for a tooth." The modern adversarial system is only one historical step removed from the private vengeance system and still retains some of its characteristic features. Thus, for example, even though the right to institute criminal action has now been extended to all members of society, and even though the police department has taken over the pretrial investigative functions on behalf of the prosecution, the adversarial system still leaves the defendant to conduct his own pretrial investigation. The trial is still viewed as a duel between two adversaries, refereed by a judge who, at the beginning of the trial, has no knowledge of the investigative background of the case. In the final analysis the adversarial system of criminal procedure symbolizes and regularizes punitive combat.

By contrast, the inquisitorial system begins historically where the adversarial system stopped its development. It is two historical steps removed from the system of private vengeance. Therefore, from the standpoint of legal anthropology, it is historically superior to the adversarial system. Under the inquisitorial system the public investigator has the duty to investigate not just on behalf of the prosecutor but also on behalf of the defendant.

Additionally, the public prosecutor has the duty to present to the court not only evidence that may lead to the conviction of the defendant but also evidence that may lead to his exoneration. This system mandates that both parties permit full pretrial discovery of the evidence in their possession. Finally, in an effort to make the trial less like a duel between two adversaries, the inquisitorial system mandates that the judge take an active part in the conduct of the trial, with a role that is both directive and protective.

Fact-finding is at the heart of the inquisitorial system. This system operates on the philosophical premise that in a criminal case the crucial factor is not the legal rule but the facts of the case and that the goal of the entire procedure is to experimentally recreate for the court the commission of the alleged crime.

Material used in this particular passage has been adapted from the following source:

M. A. Glendon, *Comparative Legal Traditions in a Nutshell.* © 1982 by West Academic Publishing.

3.6

3.6

Sample Annotation (Annotation Exercise 2)

There are two major systems of criminal procedure in the modern world—the adversarial and the inquisitorial. The former is associated with common law tradition and the latter with civil law tradition. Both systems were historically preceded by the system of private vengeance in which the victim of a crime fashioned his own remedy and administered it privately, either personally or through an agent. The vengeance system was a system of self-help, the essence of which was captured in the slogan "an eye for an eye, a tooth for a tooth." The modern adversarial system is only one historical step removed from the private vengeance system and still retains some of its characteristic features. Thus, for example, even though the right to institute criminal action has now been extended to all members of society, and even though the police department has taken over the pretrial investigative functions on behalf of the prosecution, the adversarial system still leaves the defendant to conduct his own pretrial investigation. The trial is still viewed as a duel between two adversaries, refereed by a judge who, at the beginning of the trial, has no knowledge of the investigative background of the case. In the final analysis the adversarial system of criminal procedure symbolizes and regularizes punitive combat.

By contrast, the inquisitorial system begins historically where the adversarial system stopped its development. It is two historical steps removed from the system of private vengeance. Therefore, from the standpoint of legal anthropology, it is historically superior to the adversarial system. Under the inquisitorial system the public investigator has the duty to investigate not just on behalf of the prosecutor but also on behalf of the defendant. Additionally, the public prosecutor has the duty to present to the court not only evidence that may lead to the conviction of the defendant but also evidence that may lead to his exoneration. This system mandates that both parties permit full pretrial discovery of the evidence in their possession. Finally, in an effort to make the trial less like a duel between two adversaries, the inquisitorial system mandates that the judge take an active part in the conduct of the trial, with a role that is both directive and protective.

Fact-finding is at the heart of the inquisitorial system. This system operates on the philosophical premise that in a criminal case the crucial factor is not the legal rule but the facts of the case and that the goal of the entire procedure is to experimentally recreate for the court the commission of the alleged crime.

skim this section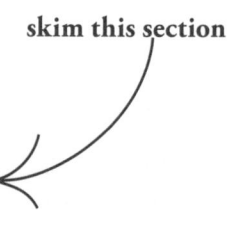

skim this section

Explanation of the Passage

This passage presents a clear argument, using detailed descriptions to support it. The trick to understanding this argument is to keep track of the three kinds of legal systems: the adversarial, the inquisitorial, and the system of private vengeance, and the differences among them.

Notice that there are three major chunks of information here. They roughly correspond to the three legal systems, but they do not correspond to the three paragraphs; paragraph 1 contains two chunks: a description of the system of private vengeance and of the adversarial system. Paragraphs 2 and 3 work together as one chunk to describe the features of the modern inquisitorial system. Your annotation and summation of the Main Points in the passage should focus on the contrast drawn by the author between the three different systems. Good annotation and "chunking" will help you to get to the Bottom Line of a passage and to find the details necessary to answer the questions.

Your understanding of the Bottom Line of the passage should be something like: "The adversarial system of criminal law is similar to the traditional system of private vengeance and is therefore less developed than the modern inquisitorial system."

On the next page is an example of what your noteboard might look like. You will notice that these notes are very brief. Remember that you may be expressing the main points and Bottom Line with just a few words; only you—no one else—needs to be able to understand your notes.

3.6

3.6

P1: *Private vengeance: self-help*

   *Adversarial came next: similar features

P2: *Inquisitorial more developed: public actors greater role*

P3: *Inquisitorial: goal of discovering facts*

BL: *Inquisitorial more developed than adversarial*

   —less like private vengeance

3.7 HABITS OF EFFECTIVE READERS

Here are some suggestions for learning to read not only faster but more efficiently, the first time through the passage.

- **Focus on big ideas and skim the details.** Don't get bogged down in long descriptions. Practice using the clues provided in the author's wording to distinguish the major claims from the (potentially irrelevant) details.
- **Hit the right pace.** If you read too fast, you won't get anything out of the passage, and will end up rereading the entire passage as you answer the questions. If you go too slowly, however, you will lose focus and/or overthink what you are reading.
- **Don't try to memorize.** Remember: this is essentially an open book test. You will be going back to the passage for the facts you need for the questions.
- **Practice reading in chunks of words.** Rather than "sounding out" each word in your mind as if you were reading out loud, think about seeing the words in groups of two or three to get a sense of what is being said. When you are answering the questions, however, always read word-for-word.
- **Push your eyes forward towards the end of the sentence.** Keep your momentum; don't linger on or ponder every word.
- **Visualize as you read.** When you hit an important point in the passage, create an image in your mind that captures the author's meaning.
- **Sit back and relax!** If you have your nose up against the screen, it is harder to think about the "big picture." You will get tired and stiff, and it will be harder to keep focused.

3.7

Outside Reading

Many MCAT students feel uncomfortable with the kind of material they encounter in the CARS section. You may not have much experience reading texts from the social sciences and humanities. To further develop your active reading skills, use some of the sources and resources listed on the next page. Use these sources not to learn more about the subject, but to practice active reading and annotation. If you are using a hard copy source, photocopy a chapter or article or two from a few different books or periodicals. Treat each page as a passage. Highlight the key words and phrases that fall into the categories we have discussed in this chapter. Articulate the Main Point of each paragraph and write it down. Think about how the paragraphs fit together logically to come up with the Bottom Line (including the author's tone) for each page or two.

Suggested Supplemental Reading List

Books

1) Wellek, Rene and Warren, Austin (1955), *Theory of Literature*
2) Bate, Walter Jackson (1991), *The Burden of the Past and the English Poet*
3) Campbell, Joseph (1949), *The Hero with a Thousand Faces*
4) Durant, Will (1935), *The Story of Civilization*
5) Giroux, Henry A. (1988), *Schooling and the Struggle for Public Life: Critical Pedagogy in the Modern Age*
6) Lakoff, George and Johnson, Mark (1980), *Metaphors We Live By*
7) Panofsky, Erwin (1955), *Meaning in the Visual Arts*
8) Bronowski, Jacob (1962), *The Western Intellectual Tradition*
9) Sontag, Susan (1983), *A Susan Sontag Reader*
10) Stanovich, Keith (2009), *How to Think Straight About Psychology*

Periodicals

Make sure to choose articles that are written at a fairly high level (that is, not a simple news article or movie review).

The New Yorker
Atlantic Monthly
The Economist
The American Scholar
Legal Affairs
Harper's
Foreign Affairs

Online Sources

If you find that you have more difficulty doing passages online than on paper, make sure to do as much of your outside reading as possible online. Many of the periodicals listed above allow some degree of free online access. There are also two websites that provide non-copyright material for free.

Gutenberg.org
Authorama.com

Make sure to choose nonfiction texts that are at a fairly high level of difficulty (that is, at MCAT CARS level). Here are some appropriate texts that will give you practice with reading challenging passage material.

1) Plato, *The Republic*
2) Friedrich Wilhelm Nietzsche, *Beyond Good and Evil*
3) Henry David Thoreau, *Walden*
4) Edward Gibbon, *The History of the Decline and Fall of the Roman Empire*
5) Ludwig Wittgenstein, *Tractatus Logico-Philosophicus*
6) Friedrich Wilhelm Nietzsche, *Thus Spake Zarathustra*
7) Adam Smith, *An Inquiry into the Nature and Causes of the Wealth of Nations*

3.8 DOS AND DON'TS FOR ACTIVE READING

Do

- Highlight key words and phrases.
- Link and predict major themes.
- Take notes on your noteboard.
- Keep it simple.
- Translate the main idea of each paragraph into your own words.
- Summarize the main point and tone of the whole passage before attacking the questions.

Don't

- Focus on the details.
- Read parts of the passage text over and over (instead, move on!).
- Memorize.
- Copy words or phrases on to your noteboard without knowing what they mean.

3.8

Chapter 3 Summary

- Read actively! Take control of the passage. Don't let the passage control you.

- Read efficiently! If a detail is important for a question, you'll find it when you go back to the passage text to answer that question. If it isn't important, don't waste your time.

- Limit your highlighting to words and phrases that relate to the logical structure of the author's argument and to your preview of the questions.

- Find the annotation style that works best for you and stick to it. It may seem to slow you down at first, but it will save you time and increase your accuracy in the long run.

CHAPTER 3 PRACTICE PASSAGES

Individual Passage Drills

Do the following two passages untimed. Separate the claims (Main Points of each chunk) from the evidence used to support them (details). Use a yellow highlighter to annotate the words and phrases that appeared in your preview of the questions or that related to the logical structure of the author's argument.

As you answer the questions, uses your annotation (notes and highlighting) actively.

Once you have completed the passages, use the Individual Passage Log to evaluate your performance. Think in particular about how, and how well, you worked the passage, and how that affected your performance on the questions. Did you miss any questions because you didn't get the Bottom Line? Could more effective annotation have helped you find the information you needed? Did you highlight too much or too little, and then didn't know where to go back to in the passage?

CHAPTER 3 PRACTICE PASSAGE 1

Nothing short of this curious sympathy could have brought into close relations two young men so hostile as Roony Lee and Henry Adams, but the chief difference between them as collegians consisted only in their difference of scholarship: Lee was a total failure; Adams a partial one. Both failed, but Lee felt his failure more sensibly, so that he gladly seized the chance of escape by accepting a commission offered him by General Winfield Scott in the force then being organized against the Mormons. He asked Adams to write his letter of acceptance, which flattered Adams's vanity more than any Northern compliment could do, because, in days of violent political bitterness, it showed a certain amount of good temper. The diplomat felt his profession.

If the student got little from his mates, he got little more from his masters. The four years passed at college were, for his purposes, wasted. Harvard College was a good school, but at bottom what the boy disliked most was any school at all. He did not want to be one in a hundred—one per cent of an education. He regarded himself as the only person for whom his education had value, and he wanted the whole of it. He got barely half of an average. Long afterwards, when the devious path of life led him back to teach in his turn what no student naturally cared or needed to know, he diverted some dreary hours of faculty-meetings by looking up his record in the class-lists, and found himself graded precisely in the middle. In the one branch he most needed—mathematics— barring the few first scholars, failure was so nearly universal that no attempt at grading could have had value, and whether he stood fortieth or ninetieth must have been an accident or the personal favor of the professor. Here his education failed lamentably. At best he could never have been a mathematician; at worst he would never have cared to be one; but he needed to read mathematics, like any other universal language, and he never reached the alphabet.

Beyond two or three Greek plays, the student got nothing from the ancient languages. Beyond some incoherent theories of free-trade and protection, he got little from Political Economy. He could not afterwards remember to have heard the name of Karl Marx mentioned, or the title of "Capital." He was equally ignorant of Auguste Comte. These were the two writers of his time who most influenced its thought. The bit of practical teaching he afterwards reviewed with most curiosity was the course in Chemistry, which taught him a number of theories that befogged his mind for a lifetime. The only teaching that appealed to his imagination was a course of lectures by Louis Agassiz on the Glacial Period and Paleontology, which had more influence on his curiosity than the rest of the college instruction altogether. The entire work of the four years could have been easily put into the work of any four months in after life.

Harvard College was a negative force, and negative forces have value. Slowly it weakened the violent political bias of childhood, not by putting interests in its place, but by mental habits which had no bias at all. It would also have weakened the literary bias, if Adams had been capable of finding other amusement, but the climate kept him steady to desultory and useless reading, till he had run through libraries of volumes which he forgot even to their title-pages. Rather by instinct than by guidance, he turned to writing, and his professors or tutors occasionally gave his English composition a hesitating approval; but in that branch, as in all the rest, even when he made a long struggle for recognition, he never convinced his teachers that his abilities, at their best, warranted placing him on the rank-list, among the first third of his class. Instructors generally reach a fairly accurate gauge of their scholars' powers. Henry Adams himself held the opinion that his instructors were very nearly right, and when he became a professor in his turn, and made mortifying mistakes in ranking his scholars, he still obstinately insisted that on the whole, he was not far wrong. Student or professor, he accepted the negative standard because it was the standard of the school.

Material used in this particular passage has been adapted from the following source:
H. Adams, *The Education of Henry Adams.* © 1918 by Houghton Mifflin Co.

1. Which of the following best characterizes the author's opinion of Adams' college experience?

A) Positive, because Harvard College was a good school
B) Negative, because the four years at college were a complete waste
C) Mixed, because while Adams learned little, there was some value to the experience
D) It cannot be determined from the passage because the opinions expressed are Adams', not the author's

2. The author's claim that in mathematics "failure was so nearly universal that no attempt at grading could have had value" is most *inconsistent* with which of the following statements also made in the passage?

A) "Instructors generally reach a fairly accurate gauge of their scholars' powers."
B) "The four years passed at college were, for his purposes, wasted."
C) "The entire work of the four years could have been easily put into the work of any four months in after life."
D) "He regarded himself as the only person for whom his education had value, and he wanted the whole of it."

3. Which of the following statements is/are supported by information in the passage?

   I. Adams was a man beholden to vanity regarding his appearance.
   II. Adams returned to teach and was motivated by instilling a new generation with useful information that was well received by his students.
   III. Adams had a predilection for politics and literature.

A) I only
B) III only
C) I and III only
D) I, II, and III

4. All of the following are suggested as occupations or interests held by Adams EXCEPT:

A) college professor.
B) paleontology.
C) chemistry.
D) military officer.

5. The author's primary purpose in the passage is to:

A) detail the academic life of a subpar college student's experience and lobby for changing the system of education.
B) argue for the necessity of a liberal arts education in order to create a well-educated citizenry.
C) critically recount Adams' college experiences.
D) recount the positive and negative experiences of students at Harvard.

CHAPTER 3 PRACTICE PASSAGE 2

A college class on the American novel is reading Alice Walker's *The Color Purple* (1982). A student raises her hand and recalls that the Steven Spielberg film version (1985) drew angry responses from many African American viewers. The discussion takes off: Did Alice Walker "betray" African Americans with her harsh depiction of Black men? Did Spielberg enhance this feature of the book or play it down? Another hand goes up: "But she *was* promoting lesbianism." "Spielberg *really* played that down!" the professor replies. A contentious voice in the back of the room: "Well I just want to know what a serious film was doing with Oprah Winfrey in it." This is answered by another student, "Dude, she does have a *book* club on her show!" Class members respond to these points, examining interrelationships among race, gender, popular culture, the media, and literature. This class is practicing cultural studies.

Cultural studies approaches generally share four goals. First, cultural studies transcends the confines of a particular discipline such as literary criticism or history. Cultural studies involves scrutinizing the cultural phenomenon of a text—for example, Italian opera, a Latino telenovela, the architectural styles of prisons, body piercing—and drawing conclusions about the changes in textual phenomena over time. Cultural studies is not necessarily about literature in the traditional sense or even about art. Henry Giroux and others write in their *Dalhousie Review* manifesto that cultural studies practitioners are "resisting intellectuals" who see what they do as "an emancipatory project" because it erodes the traditional disciplinary divisions in most institutions of higher education. For students, this sometimes means that a professor might make his or her own political views part of the instruction, which, of course, can lead to problems. But this kind of criticism, like feminism, is an engaged rather than a detached activity.

Second, cultural studies is politically engaged. Cultural critics see themselves as "oppositional," not only within their own disciplines but to many of the power structures of society at large. They question inequalities within power structures and seek to discover models for restructuring relationships among dominant and "minority" or "subaltern" discourses. Because meaning and individual subjectivity are culturally constructed they can thus be reconstructed. Such a notion, taken to a philosophical extreme, denies the autonomy of the individual, whether an actual person or a character in literature, a rebuttal of the traditional humanistic "Great Man" or "Great Book" theory, and a relocation of aesthetics and culture from the ideal realms of taste and sensibility, into the arena of a whole society's everyday life as it is constructed.

Third, cultural studies denies the separation of "high" and "low" or elite and popular culture. You might hear someone remark at the symphony or at an art museum: "I came here to get a little culture." Being a "cultured" person used to mean being acquainted with "highbrow" art and intellectual pursuits. But isn't *culture* also to be found with a pair of tickets to a rock concert? Cultural critics today work to transfer the term *culture* to include *mass culture*, whether popular, folk, or urban. Transgressing of boundaries among disciplines high and low can make cultural studies just plain fun. Think, for example, of a possible cultural studies research paper with the following title: "The Birth of Captain Jack Sparrow: An Analysis." For sources of Johnny Depp's funky performance in Disney's *Pirates of the Caribbean* movies, you could research cultural topics ranging from the trade economies of the sea two hundred years ago, to real pirates of the Caribbean such as Blackbeard and Henry Morgan, then on to memorable screen pirates, John Cleese's rendition of Long John Silver on *Monty Python's Flying Circus*, and, of course, Keith Richards's eye makeup.

Finally, cultural studies analyzes not only the cultural work, but the means of production. Marxist critics have long recognized the importance of such paraliterary questions as, Who supports a given artist? Who publishes his or her books, and how are these books distributed? Who buys books? For that matter, who is literate and who is not? These studies help us recognize that literature does not occur in a space separate from other concerns of our lives. Cultural studies thus joins *subjectivity*—that is, culture in relation to individual lives—with *engagement*, a direct approach to attacking social ills. Though cultural studies practitioners deny "humanism" of "the humanities" as universal categories, they strive for what they might call "social reason," which often (closely) resembles the goals and values of humanistic and democratic ideals.

Material used in this particular passage has been adapted from the following source:

W. Guerin et al, *A Handbook of Critical Approaches to Literature.* © 2005 by Oxford University Press.

1. Which of the following would be LEAST consistent with the author's description of cultural studies?

A) An analysis of Missourian Mark Twain's *A Connecticut Yankee in King Arthur's Court* that examined questions regarding the oppressive inequality embodied in monarchical social etiquette and regional class structures
B) A discussion of female image and intelligence as presented by reality TV dating shows such as VH1's *Rock of Love* with rock star Bret Michaels
C) An exploration of whether Steven Spielberg's absent father characters in *E.T.*, *Catch Me If You Can*, and *Indiana Jones and the Last Crusade* are a response to his own father being absent in his childhood
D) An examination of the influence of gospel hymns on the speechwriting of civil rights leaders such as Rev. Dr. Martin Luther King, Jr., and Medgar Evers

2. If a hard-line cultural studies practitioner were to conclude, after researching the text, that white supremacist Asa Earl Carter's novel *The Education of Little Tree* about the traditional upbringing of a Native American boy was written free of his opinions about non-Caucasian peoples, it would most *undermine* the author's assertion that:

A) cultural studies is not exclusively about literature or even art.
B) the oppositional nature of cultural studies, carried to an extreme, denies the sovereignty of individual will.
C) analyzing the means of production is one of the important goals of cultural studies.
D) cultural studies is politically engaged.

3. When the author quotes Henry Giroux's description of cultural studies practitioners as "resisting intellectuals" (paragraph 2), he most nearly means that:

A) professors approaching literature this way reject an overly academic approach.
B) the cultural studies movement began as an underground movement.
C) professors reveal their own opinions in class in order to provoke disagreement and discussion from students.
D) such academics take a multifarious approach to analyzing phenomena in a text.

4. The author's reference to a rock concert serves to indicate that:

A) rock music combines both highbrow and lowbrow culture.
B) music can serve political purposes.
C) culture includes musical expression.
D) popular artistic forms have not always been considered to be highly sophisticated.

5. Elsewhere the author writes, "Images of India circulated during the colonial rule of the British raj by writers like Rudyard Kipling seem innocent, but reveal an entrenched argument for white superiority and worldwide domination of other races." This, if taken as an example of cultural studies, illustrates the author's belief that such studies:

A) deny the separation between lowbrow culture like Kipling's innocent stories and highbrow culture like discussions of political power.
B) examine questions of power and influence, such as the structure of colonial society in India, and raise questions about who was circulating Kipling's writing.
C) include mass culture such as Kipling's stories "The Jungle Book" and "Rikki-Tikki-Tavi."
D) transcend historical analysis.

6. In the context of the passage as a whole, "emancipatory" (paragraph 2) most nearly means:

A) excusing from an obligation.
B) freeing from service.
C) endorsing a wider perspective.
D) promoting equality.

7. Suppose a critic were to propose a comparative analysis between Shakespeare's 16th-century play *Romeo and Juliet* and Tennessee Williams's 20th-century play *A Streetcar Named Desire*, focusing entirely on how the number of acts in each play affects the development of the main female character. Which of the following statements best represents how the author of the passage would most likely view this study and/or its author?

A) This critic is not a cultural studies practitioner because she limits her investigations to questions internal to the plays.
B) The critic is resisting historical disciplines by cutting across several centuries in her analysis.
C) The critic should include an analysis of Shakespeare's and Williams's lives and the impact of personal events on their writing.
D) Questions of who supported Shakespeare and Williams financially are irrelevant.

SOLUTIONS TO CHAPTER 3 PRACTICE PASSAGE 1

1. **C** This is a Tone/Attitude question.

   A: No. While the author does state in paragraph 2 that Harvard was a good school, the passage has a largely negative tone about Adam's experience. For example, the author states that Adams "got little more from his masters" than from his peers (paragraph 2), that in mathematics "his education failed lamentably" (paragraph 2), and that Adams got little out of his study of ancient languages, political economy, and chemistry (paragraph 3). The author also criticizes Adams' professors in paragraph 2.

   B: No. While the tone is largely negative, the author states in paragraph 4 that "Harvard College was a negative force, and negative forces have value. Slowly it weakened the violent political bias of childhood, not by putting interests in its place, but by mental habits which had no bias at all." Therefore, "complete waste" is too strong.

   C: **Yes. While the author describes the failings of Adams' education in paragraphs 2 and 3, the author also states that there was some value to the experience: "Harvard College was a negative force, and negative forces have value. Slowly it weakened the violent political bias of childhood, not by putting interests in its place, but by mental habits which had no bias at all" (paragraph 4).**

   D: No. While the passage does suggest Adams' opinion, it also clearly indicates the author's opinion of Adams as a student ("a partial [failure]" (paragraph 1)), of the professors at Harvard ("In the one branch he most needed—mathematics—barring the few first scholars, failure was so nearly universal that no attempt at grading could have had value, and whether he stood fortieth or ninetieth must have been an accident or the personal favor of the professor" (paragraph 2)), and of Adams' education as a whole, including the value Adams did get out of the experience ("Harvard College was a negative force, and negative forces have value." (paragraph 4)).

2. **A** This is a Structure question.

   Note: The correct answer will be the statement made elsewhere in the passage that most contradicts the statement cited in the question stem. If a statement in an answer choice is on a different issue, it will not be inconsistent (that is, the two statements would be consistent in that they could both be true).

   A: **Yes. Following the statement that grading could have had little value, the author states: "whether he stood fortieth or ninetieth must have been an accident or the personal favor of the professor" (paragraph 2). This suggests that grades or rankings did not in fact reflect the skill or accomplishment of the student. This would be inconsistent with the claim cited in choice A (from paragraph 4) that instructors accurately evaluate their students.**

   B: No. The claim that the four years were wasted is consistent with the author's critique of how professors graded.

   C: No. The quote in this choice is on a different issue: that Adams was interested in only a small portion of his course material (paragraph 3). Therefore the two claims are not inconsistent with each other.

   D: No. This refers to a somewhat different issue (Adams' self-centeredness (paragraph 2)), rather than the value or accuracy of the grading. Furthermore, to the extent that this statement relates to the existence of other students (who were also graded by the same standards), it is consistent (not inconsistent) with the claim in the question stem.

3. **B** This is an Inference/Roman numeral question.
    I: False. This statement is not supported by the passage. While Adams' vanity is mentioned in the first paragraph, there was no mention of Adams being vain specifically about his appearance.
    II: False. While it is correct that Adams did teach, the passage states that Adams went "back to teach in his turn what no student naturally cared or needed to know" (paragraph 2). Therefore the claim that Adams was "motivated by instilling a new generation with useful information that was well received by his students" is inconsistent with the text.
    III: True. By stating that the Harvard experience "weakened the violent political bias of childhood" (paragraph 4), the author suggests that Adams did have an interest in, or predilection towards, politics in the first place. The author also mentions in paragraph 1 that because of Lee's request, "The diplomat felt his profession." As for literature, in paragraph 4 the author states: "Rather by instinct than by guidance, he turned to writing," suggesting that Adams had some interest himself in literature.

4. **D** This is an Inference/EXCEPT question.
    A: No. Paragraph 2 states: "Long afterwards, when the devious path of life led him back to teach in his turn what no student naturally cared or needed to know, he diverted some dreary hours of faculty-meetings by looking up his record in the class-lists, and found himself graded precisely in the middle." This suggests that Adams returned to Harvard as a professor.
    B: No. Paragraph 3 states: "The only teaching that appealed to his imagination was a course of lectures by Louis Agassiz on the Glacial Period and Paleontology, which had more influence on his curiosity than the rest of the college instruction altogether." This suggests Adams had an interest in paleontology.
    C: No. Paragraph 3 states: "The bit of practical teaching he afterwards reviewed with most curiosity was the course in Chemistry, which taught him a number of theories that befogged his mind for a lifetime." Even if Adams was confused by chemistry, the passage suggests that he did have some interest in or "curiosity" about it.
    D: Yes. There is no mention of Adams having any interest in military affairs. The passage does talk of Lee accepting a military commission (paragraph 1), but not of Adams doing the same or having any interest in military affairs.

5. **C** This is a Main Point/Primary Purpose question.
    A: No. While the passage does provide some details about Adams' education, it does not explicitly lobby for, or make suggestions concerning, education.
    B: No. There is no mention of preparing well-educated citizens.
    C: Yes. The author casts a critical eye on Adams' college experiences by speaking throughout the passage in largely negative terms; the value gained in lessening Adams' political biases (paragraph 4) still came out of the negative nature of the experiences themselves.
    D: No. While one could infer that some of the experiences described applied to other students as well (e.g., how they were evaluated), the main focus of the passage is on Adams himself. Furthermore, the emphasis is on the negative experiences; even the positive outcome mentioned in the beginning of the last paragraph came out of *negative experiences*.

SOLUTIONS TO CHAPTER 3 PRACTICE PASSAGE 2

1. **C**   This is an Inference/LEAST question.

    A: No. This is consistent with the author's description of cultural studies in paragraph 2, where the author states that cultural studies transcends traditional boundaries between academic disciplines. It is also consistent with the author's discussion in paragraph 3: "Cultural critics see themselves as 'oppositional,'...to many of the power structures on society at large. They question inequalities within power structures..."

    B: No. This examination of gender depictions is consistent with the discussion of gender depictions in paragraph 1's example of cultural studies.

    C: Yes. This analysis is not consistent with any description of cultural studies laid out in the passage because it limits its scope to the artist's own life rather than the culture within which he or she created his or her movie.

    D: No. This is consistent with paragraph 2's assertion that "Cultural studies involves scrutinizing the cultural phenomenon of a text—for example, Italian opera," as well as with paragraph 4's examples of the types of cultural phenomena, including "mass culture," examined by cultural studies practitioners.

2. **B**   This is a New Information question.

    A: No. The analysis of Carter's book would be consistent with the idea that history and traditional customs are also a part of cultural studies.

    B: Yes. Someone who is extremely committed to a cultural studies approach, according to the author, would be unlikely to assert that an artist could create a text in which he or she effectively and consciously omitted all trace or influence of his or her cultural context. According to the passage, an individual author would not be seen by this type of cultural critic as having this kind of autonomy (paragraph 3).

    C: No. There is no indication, either way, whether the critic examined questions of the means of production. Thus, the new information neither strengthens nor weakens this claim of the author.

    D: No. There is no reason, based on the passage, to believe that political engagement in this case would require a hard-line cultural critic to identify racist themes within the novel itself.

3. **D**   This is an Inference question.

    A: No. While these practitioners are resisting traditional divisions in academia between disciplines (e.g., between literary criticism and history), being "academic" is not identified in the passage with respecting these divisions. Therefore, there is no evidence to support the idea that what they are rejecting is an "overly academic" approach.

    B: No. There is no evidence that cultural studies began as a secretive movement. This is taking the word "resisting" out of the context of the passage.

    C: No. This choice is wrong first because there is no evidence that professors introduce their own viewpoints *in order to* provoke disagreement, only that introduction of the professor's own political views may be part of instruction. Second, introduction of the professor's own views is given as perhaps one aspect of the "emancipatory project," but not as part of a definition of what the term "resisting intellectuals" itself means.

D: Yes. The author states that these intellectuals "see what they do as 'an emancipatory project' because it erodes the traditional disciplinary divisions" by "scrutinizing the cultural phenomenon of a text" (paragraph 2). This means that rather than studying only the text itself (or other aspects traditionally seen as "literary" issues related to it) cultural critics bring in other issues relating to the culture within which the text appears. This aligns with what the author said earlier in the paragraph, that "cultural studies transcends the confines of a particular discipline." Therefore, these academics take a multifarious or diverse approach to a text.

4. **D**   This is an Inference question.

    A: No. There is no indication rock music is *both* highbrow and lowbrow—on the contrary, the passage indicates that rock music has traditionally been considered lowbrow instead of highbrow.

    B: No. Politics is not an issue in this paragraph. In addition, to the extent that the author discusses political motivations elsewhere in the passage, the issue is the political engagement of cultural critics, not of culture itself.

    C: No. The point of the reference is not to show that culture includes music; an earlier reference to the symphony suggests that at least some forms of music are already seen as cultural expression. Furthermore, the point being made is that cultural critics deny the distinction between high (the symphony) and low (the rock concert) culture.

    D: Yes. In paragraph 4, the author writes that "cultural studies denies the separation of 'high' and 'low' or elite and popular culture...Being a 'cultured' person used to mean being acquainted with 'highbrow' art and intellectual pursuits. But isn't *culture* also to be found with a pair of tickets to a rock concert?" The change cultural studies has created from what culture "used to mean" has been to include forms (such as the rock concert) that were once considered not to be elite, intellectual, highbrow, or highly sophisticated.

5. **B**   This is a New Information question.

    A: No. Nothing indicates that Kipling's stories are or would have been considered lowbrow.

    B: Yes. This is consistent with the author's description of the second major goal of cultural studies ("They question inequalities within power structures"), as detailed in paragraph 3; it is also consistent with the author's description of the fourth major goal of cultural studies ("Marxist critics have long recognized the importance of such paraliterary questions as, Who supports a given artist? Who publishes his or her books, and how are these books distributed?") as described in paragraph 5. (Note: Marxist critics are referred to as part of the description of cultural critics.)

    C: No. Nothing indicates that Kipling's stories constitute mass culture. Note that A and C are saying basically the same thing, and they have the same problem—so you can cross them both out.

    D: No. This perspective is rooted in history, so it doesn't illustrate how cultural studies transcends, or goes beyond, history.

6. **C** This is an Inference question.

A: No. There is no indication of obligation in the passage. This choice takes the meaning of the word out of context.

B: No. There is no indication of service in the passage. As in choice A, this answer represents a common definition of emancipation, but one that does not fit in the context of the passage.

C: Yes. Paragraph 2 says cultural studies practitioners see their field "as 'an emancipatory project' because it erodes the traditional disciplinary divisions." Eroding divisions would produce a "wider perspective;" that is, one not limited by the practices or assumptions of a particular academic field.

D: No. While the author indicates in paragraph 3 that cultural critics "question inequalities," this is not the context in which the word "emancipatory" appears in paragraph 2. This choice then has two problems: it uses a common definition of the word that does not fit in the context of the relevant part of the passage, and it refers to an issue that arises elsewhere in the passage but not in this paragraph.

7. **A** This is a New Information question.

A: Yes. Because the question the critic asks is limited to the form of the plays and the development of characters within that structure, and because it does not address culture or any of the goals of cultural studies as they are outlined in the passage, the author is most likely to argue that the critic is not practicing cultural studies.

B: No. If anything, comparing texts from two different periods in history would be embracing a historical approach, not resisting it.

C: No. Examining the text in terms of the events of the author's life is not one of the goals of cultural studies.

D: No. We have no evidence the author disagrees with the fourth goal of cultural studies, as he described it in paragraph 5, which asserts the relevance of questions of finance and production.

Individual Passage Log

Passage # _____

Q#	Q type	Attractors	What did you do wrong?

Revised Strategy _____

Passage # _____

Q#	Q type	Attractors	What did you do wrong?

Revised Strategy _____

Think Like a Test-Writer: Exercise 1

THINK LIKE A TEST-WRITER: EXERCISE 1

The AAMC gives this section the fancy name "Critical Analysis and Reasoning Skills" (instead of simply calling it "Reading Comprehension") to emphasize that the CARS section tests a variety of skills that go beyond simply understanding the information in the passage text. One of those skills is the ability to follow the logical structure of the passage. One of the most effective ways to track that structure is to ask questions of the text as you read, questions such as "What new idea is being introduced here?" or "How does this statement or paragraph relate to previous statements or paragraphs?" or "Has the author made their own position on this issue clear?" or "Why is the author making this claim?" or even "What might be coming next?"

The test-writers have these same questions in mind when they create the test questions. When you ask and answer these questions, you are getting into the minds of the test-writers; you are picking up on the aspects of the passage they will use to create the questions, the right answers, and those attractive wrong answers that are sometimes so tempting. To help you develop this way of reading and thinking, we have provided you with three "Think Like a Test-Writer" Exercises.

This first exercise focuses on asking questions as you read in order to effectively track the logical structure of the passage. The second (after Chapter 4) asks you to think about what kinds of questions a test-writer might create based on that logical structure. The third exercise (after Chapter 5) adds in the challenge of thinking about not only possible passage questions but types of attractive wrong answers they might create.

For this first exercise, read the following text, tracking the author's tone and purpose in each paragraph. Pay attention to key words that indicate transitions, emphasis, and tone.

As you read, you will see questions inserted into the text [in red and in brackets] to help you focus on defining the purpose of statements within the passage, the purpose of each paragraph, and the purpose of the passage as a whole. Some of these questions can be answered at that point in the text, while others are questions that will be answered later in the passage. Jot down your response to those questions as you read; answers are provided after the passage.

Note: This text is longer than a CARS passage in order to give you practice with tracking logical structure across multiple paragraphs.

EXERCISE 1

Three circumstances have seemed to liars to provide the strongest excuse for their behavior—a crisis where overwhelming harm can be averted only through deceit; complete harmlessness and triviality to the point where it seems absurd to quibble about whether a lie has been told; and the duty to particular individuals to protect their secrets. [**Q1:** Does the author agree that these are legitimate excuses?] I have shown how lies in times of crisis can expand into vast practices where the harm to be averted is less obvious and the crisis less and less immediate; how white lies can shade into equally vast practices no longer so harmless, with immense cumulative costs; and how lies to protect individuals and to cover up their secrets can be told for increasingly dubious purposes to the detriment of all. [**Q2:** Now do we know if the author agrees? **Q3:** Why is the author referring to her previous statements?]

_____

_____

_____

When these three expanding streams [**Q4:** What "three expanding streams" is the author referring to?] flow together and mingle with yet another—a desire to advance the public good—they form the most dangerous body of deceit of all. These lies may not be justified by immediate crisis nor by complete triviality nor by duty to any one person; rather, liars tend to consider them as right and unavoidable because of the altruism that motivates them....

_____

_____

_____

Naturally, there will be large areas of overlap between these lies and those considered earlier. But the most characteristic defense for these lies is a separate one, based on the benefits they may confer and the long range harm they can avoid. The intention may be broadly paternalistic, as when citizens are deceived "for their own good," or only a few may be lied to for the benefit of the community at large. Error and self-deception mingle with these altruistic purposes and blur them; the filters through which we must try to peer at lying are thicker and more distorting than ever in these practices. But I shall try to single out, among these lies, the elements that are consciously and purposefully intended to benefit society. [**Q5:** What new idea is introduced, starting with the word "But," in this paragraph?]

_____

_____

_____

A long tradition in political philosophy endorses some lies for the sake of the public. Plato...first used the expression "noble lie" for the fanciful story that might be told to people in order to persuade them to accept class distinctions and thereby safeguard social harmony. According to this story, God himself mingled gold, silver, iron, and brass in fashioning rulers, auxiliaries, farmers, and craftsmen, intending these groups for separate tasks in a harmonious hierarchy. ... [**Q6:** What is the purpose of this discussion of Plato?]

_____

_____

_____

Rulers, both temporal and spiritual, have seen their deceits in the benign light of such social purposes. They have propagated and maintained myths played on the gullibility of the ignorant, and sought stability in shared beliefs. They have seen themselves as high minded and well bred—whether by birth or by training—and as superior to those they deceive. Some have gone so far as to claim that those who govern have a *right* to lie. The powerful tell lies believing that they have greater than ordinary understanding of what is at stake; very often, they regard their dupes as having inadequate judgment, or as likely to respond in the wrong way to truthful information. [**Q7:** Is the point of view described in this paragraph consistent or inconsistent with that of Plato?]

_____

_____

_____

At times, those who govern also regard particular circumstances as too uncomfortable, too painful, for most people to be able to cope with rationally. They may believe, for instance, that their country must prepare for long-term challenges of great importance, such as a war, an epidemic, or a belt-tightening in the face of future shortages. Yet they may fear that citizens will be able to respond only to short-range dangers. Deception at such times may seem to the government leaders as the only means of attaining the necessary results. [**Q8:** Is the author discussing a point of view shared by Plato, or is this a contrasting position?]

_____

_____

_____

The perspective of the liar is paramount in all such decisions to tell "noble" lies. If the liar considers the responses of the deceived at all, he assumes that they will, once the deceit comes to light and its benefits are understood, be uncomplaining if not positively grateful. The lies are often seen as necessary merely at one stage in the education of the public. …[**Q9:** Is there a new idea in this paragraph, or, is it simply further elaboration on the idea that some justify lying for the good of the public?]

_____

_____

_____

Some experienced public officials are impatient with any effort to question the ethics of such deceptive practices (except actions obviously taken for private ends). They argue that vital objectives in the national interest require a measure of deception to succeed in the face of powerful obstacles. Negotiations must be carried on that are best left hidden from public view; bargains must be struck that simply cannot be comprehended by a politically unsophisticated electorate. A certain amount of illusion is needed in order for public servants to be effective. Every government, therefore, has to deceive people to some extent in order to lead them. [**Q10:** Is this the author's point of view, or is she still describing someone else's argument?]

_____

_____

_____

If we assume the perspective of the deceived—those who experienced the consequences of government deception—such arguments are not persuasive. [**Q11:** What has changed in the nature of the author's argument in this part of the passage?] We cannot take for granted either the altruism or the good judgment of those who lie to us, no matter how much they intend to benefit us. We have learned that much deceit for private gain masquerades as being in the public interest. We know how deception, even for the most unselfish motive, corrupts and spreads. And we have lived through the consequences of lies told for what were believed to be noble purposes. Equally unpersuasive is the argument that there always has been government deception, and always will be, and that efforts to draw lines and set standards are therefore useless annoyances. It is certainly true that deception can never be completely absent from most human practices. But there are great differences among societies in the kinds of deceit that exist and the extent to which they are practiced, differences also among individuals in the same government and among successive governments within the same society. This strongly suggests that it is worthwhile trying to discover why such differences exist and to seek ways of raising the standards of truthfulness. ...[**Q12:** What is the purpose of the second part of this paragraph?]

_____

_____

_____

Can there be exceptions to the well-founded distrust of deception in public life? Are there times when the public itself might truly not care about possible lies, or might even prefer to be deceived? Are some white lies so trivial or so transparent that they can be ignored? And can we envisage public discussion of more seriously misleading government statements such that reasonable persons could consent to them in advance? [**Q13:** What is the author's purpose in asking this series of questions?]

_____

_____

_____

White lies, first of all, are as common to political and diplomatic affairs as they are to the private lives of most people. [**Q14:** What does the phrase "first of all" indicate about what may follow this discussion of one aspect of "white lies"?] Feigning enjoyment of an embassy gathering or a political rally, toasting the longevity of a dubious regime or an unimpressive candidate for office—these are forms of politeness that mislead few. It is difficult to regard them as threats to either individuals or communities. As with all white lies, however, the problem is that they spread so easily, and that lines are very hard to draw. Is it still a white lie for a Secretary of State to announce that he is going to one country when in reality he travels to another? Or for a president to issue a "cover story" to the effect that a cold is forcing him to return to the White House, when in reality an international crisis made him cancel the rest of his campaign trip? Is it a white lie to issue a letter of praise for a public servant one has just fired? Given the vulnerability of public trust, it is never more important than in public life to keep the deceptive element of white lies to an absolute minimum, and to hold down the danger of their turning into more widespread deceitful practices. ...[**Q15:** How does this paragraph about "white lies" answer the questions raised in the previous paragraph?]

_____

_____

_____

Another form of deception takes place when the government regards the public as frightened, or hostile, and highly volatile. In order not to create a panic, information about early signs of an epidemic may be suppressed or distorted. And the lie to a mob seeking its victim is like lying to the murderer asking where the person he is pursuing has gone. It can be acknowledged and defended as soon as the threat is over. In such cases, one may at times be justified in withholding information; perhaps, on rare occasions, even in lying. But such cases are so rare that they hardly exist for practical purposes. ...[**Q16:** How does this paragraph about "another form of deception" relate to the questions raised in the earlier paragraph? Is the author going back on her argument against lying?]

_____

_____

_____

Whenever lies to the public become routine, then, very special safeguards should be required. The test of public justification of deceptive practices is more needed than ever. It will be a hard test to satisfy, the more so the more trust is invested in those who lie and the more power they wield. Those in government and other positions of trust should be held to the highest standard. Their lies are not ennobled by their positions; quite the contrary. Some lies—notably minor white lies and emergency lies rapidly acknowledged—may be more _excusable_ than others, but only those deceptive practices which can be openly debated and consented to in advance are _justifiable_ in a democracy. [**Q17:** What is the purpose of the last paragraph of this passage? Does it add anything new, or is it simply a summation of points already made?]

_____

_____

_____

[**Q18:** What is the author's overall purpose in writing this passage?]

_____

_____

_____

—Text adapted from S. Bok, _Lying: Moral Choice in Public and Private Life._ © 1978 by Sissela Bok.

SOLUTIONS TO EXERCISE 1

1. We don't know yet if the author agrees. The phrase "have seemed to liars," however, should make you wonder if the author may in fact disagree.

2. We still do not know, although the negative tone of this portion of the passage suggests that the author may not agree. However, you need more evidence to conclusively infer that the author believes that these particular lies are illegitimate.

3. The purpose is to set the stage for her judgment regarding the three excuses for lying listed at the beginning of the passage, and to suggest that at least some kinds of lies may be hard to justify.

4. This refers to the three expanding streams listed at the end of the previous paragraph; the theme of that list is that lies may have cumulative negative effects that go beyond any harm done by the initial lie, and that altruistic motives may not be enough to justify a lie.

5. This paragraph introduces the new idea that some lies are meant to benefit society, and that it is difficult to know if they are justified. Given the negative tone of the passage so far regarding lying, it is possible that the author will eventually claim that they are not in fact justified, but you need to read further before you can make that assessment.

6. The purpose of the reference to Plato is to give an example of a justification of lying for the public good. You don't know yet, however, if the author agrees or disagrees with Plato.

7. The point of view in this paragraph is consistent with that of Plato; the purpose of the paragraph is to further elaborate on the idea that some justify lying to the public for the public's own good. Note wording such as "myths played on the gullibility of the ignorant," and "dupes." This negative language suggests that the author of the passage may reject this justification, but we still don't know for sure what the author's own position is.

8. This paragraph is discussing, and elaborating on, the point of view shared by Plato: lying to the public may be necessary to protect the public interest.

9. While this paragraph is still discussing the claim that lying to the public may be in the public's own interest, it is introducing a new idea: the liars are not seriously considering the perspective of those being lied to.

10. The author is still describing someone else's argument in this paragraph. Note the wording in the beginning of the paragraph: "Some experienced public officials are impatient with any effort to question the ethics of such deceptive practices (except actions obviously taken for private ends). They argue…" Taken in that context, the statements at the end of the paragraph are still attributed to others.

11. Here the author is finally telling us what she thinks, and that she rejects the claim that lies for the public's own good are legitimate. Now it becomes clear why the author introduced, in the previous paragraph, the idea of the perspective of the deceived. When she says "If we assume the perspective of the deceived—those who experienced the consequences of government deception—such arguments are not persuasive" she is definitively saying that this perspective must be considered, and that that it invalidates the arguments made in defense of these kinds of lies.

12. The purpose of the rest of the paragraph is to elaborate on the claim made in the beginning, and to discount a series of possible justifications for lying in the public good, At the end of the paragraph the author also calls for investigation into differences in lies and into justifications for those lies between different societies.

13. Authors usually ask rhetorical questions (questions the reader is not expected to answer for themselves) to set up the next point. Here, the author is asking if the kind of lying she has criticized in the previous paragraph might ever be justified. As the reader, you should be looking out for a potential twist: is the author going to take this in an unexpected direction and actually justify certain types of lies, or is she using these questions to further elaborate on her rejection of such justifications?

14. "First of all" indicates that there will be multiple aspects of white lies discussed, not just how common they are in public life. Noting this phrase alerts you to the need to track where each different aspect is discussed.

15. The discussion of white lies in this paragraph constitutes a rejection of one possible justification for lying raised in the previous paragraph: "Are some white lies so trivial or so transparent that they can be ignored?" The author says no.

16. Here the author is conceding that in some cases lying can be justified, especially if the lie is soon exposed. But, she goes on to say that these cases are very rare. Therefore even though the author is conceding that some lies may be justified, she is still making her case against lying overall.

17. While this last paragraph does solidify the author's position against lying, it also introduces a new idea: lying may be *excusable* in rare cases after the fact, but it is only *justifiable* in a democracy when they are consented to in advance by the public.

18. The author's purpose in the passage as a whole is to address a variety of possible justifications for lying in public life and to warn us that even seemingly innocuous or well-motivated lies may have significant negative consequences.

Chapter 4
Question Types
and Strategies

GOALS

1) To learn the types of questions that are likely to be asked and strategies for attacking them
2) To refine the use of Process of Elimination (POE)

4.1 REVIEW: THE SIX STEPS

Here, one last time, is a brief outline of the six basic steps to approaching the MCAT CARS section:

▬ STEP 1: RANK AND ORDER THE PASSAGES

Decide whether to do the passage Now, Later, or Never (Killer) based on the difficulty level of the passage text.

▬ STEP 2: PREVIEW THE QUESTIONS

Read through the question stems (not the answer choices) before you read the passage. Look for and highlight words and phrases that indicate important passage content. Do not worry at this stage about identifying the question type.

▬ STEP 3: WORK THE PASSAGE

As you read through the passage, use the highlighting function (sparingly) to annotate the most important references in the passage, especially words that indicate the logical structure of the author's argument and references that appeared in your preview of the questions. Notice topic sentences that help you to identify conclusions made by the author. Articulate the Main Point of each chunk of information (usually, each paragraph). Use your noteboard, especially on difficult passages, to jot down these main points. As you read, think about how these chunks relate to each other, and identify the structure of the passage.

▬ STEP 4: BOTTOM LINE

After you have read the passage, sum up the Bottom Line: the Main Point and tone of the entire passage.

▬ STEP 5: ATTACK THE QUESTIONS

Read the question word for word, identifying the question type and translating the question task into your own words. Go back to the passage before reading the answer choices and find the relevant information (reading at least five lines above and below the reference). Think about what the correct answer will need to do, and generate an answer to the question in your own words. Use POE actively. Select the "least wrong" answer.

▬ STEP 6: INSPECT THE SECTION

At or before the 5-minute mark (ideally before you begin your last passage), double-check to make sure that you haven't left anything blank. You can use the Review function at this stage. Do NOT rethink questions you have already completed.

In the rest of this chapter, we'll focus on **Step Five: Attack the Questions.**

4.2 ATTACKING THE QUESTIONS

In order to continue to improve your CARS skills, you will need to refine your approach to the questions. In this chapter we will discuss the five basic steps you should take in answering any question, and the specific tactics appropriate to each question type.

Five Steps For Answering Questions

1) Read the question word for word and identify the question type.
2) Translate the question into your own words: identify what the question task is asking you to do with the information in the passage.
3) Identify any key words that refer to specific parts of the passage. If key words are provided, *go back to the passage* to locate that information.
4) Answer in your own words: articulate what the correct answer will need to do based on the question type and the information in the passage.
5) Use Process of Elimination (POE), and choose the *least wrong* answer choice.

Let's look at each step in more detail.

1) **Read the question word for word; identify the question type.**
   WHY?
   - If you misread or misinterpret the question now, you may never catch your mistake. Now is not the time to skim, or to get only a vague impression of what the question is asking.
   - No matter how good your annotation and mapping of the passage, if you're headed to the wrong destination, those signposts do you no good. You could have an excellent map of the United States, but if you're supposed to get to Boston and you think your destination is Biloxi, you are in big trouble. Know your destination!
   - The MCAT writers are highly skilled at predicting likely misinterpretations and at giving you wrong answers with which you could be perfectly happy. If you've ever completed a passage, pleased with how quickly and smoothly it went, only to realize upon checking your answers that you got many questions wrong, you may be reading the questions too carelessly.
   - Different kinds of questions ask for different kinds of information. Most importantly, General questions require general answers and can usually be answered with your own statement of the Bottom Line. Specific answer choices can be very narrow and always require going back to the passage. Reasoning and Application questions will usually also require you to go back to the passage, but they also ask you to either describe the logic or structure of the author's argument, or to apply new information to it. Identifying the question type is important because that will guide the rest of the process.
   HOW?
   - Read the question as if you have never seen it before. Focus on each word rather than taking it in as a chunk.
   - Think of the question as assigning you a task: what mission do you need to accomplish in answering the question? Do you need to find information that matches the passage? Describe the author's argument in the passage (in part or the whole)? Strengthen or weaken the author's argument? Apply new information from the question stem?

2) **Translate the question into your own words; identify what the question task is asking you to do.**
WHY?

- You may have noticed by now that questions are not always phrased in an easily comprehensible way. The test-writers do this on purpose to see if you can understand difficult, complex writing and ideas.

HOW?

- When you come across a long, complex, and convoluted question, take it out of MCAT-speak and put it into your own words. You may find it useful to jot down a few words on your noteboard.
- The benefits of translation are two-fold. First, it helps you to clarify exactly what the question is asking. Second, it will enable you to remember exactly what you're looking for when you go back to the passage.

For example, a question for a passage on Abstract Expressionism may ask

1. Which of the following would be most inconsistent with Brown's claim that Jackson Pollock did not lack influence within the movement called Abstract Expressionism, as that movement and its subsequent offshoots and internal divisions are described in the passage?

When you cut away the extraneous stuff and clarify the convoluted wording, all this question is asking is

1. Which of the following answer choices indicates that Pollock had little or no influence on Abstract Expressionism?

3) **Identify any key words that refer to specific parts of the passage. If key words are provided, go back to the passage to locate that information.**
WHY?

- Going back to the passage to answer questions with specific lead words is fundamental. You simply don't have time to memorize the details. Relying on your ability to recall facts under time pressure will only get you into trouble.
- If you don't check your answers against the text, you are likely to pick a choice that contains words from the passage taken out of context, or one that is true in the real world, but not supported by the passage.
- Going back to the passage before you read the answer choices will not only increase your accuracy, but will also increase your overall speed. If you already have a solid grounding in the passage, you will more quickly recognize the correct choice, and you are much less likely to get stuck between two answers.

HOW?

- A key word or phrase is something in the question that appears only a few times in the passage, and it guides you toward the relevant sections in the passage that you'll need to reread.
- Looking again at the sample question above, the phrase "Abstract Expressionism" would not make a good key phrase if the whole passage is about Abstract Expressionism; it's likely to appear many times throughout the passage. The name Jackson Pollock, however, is likely to lead you right to the relevant sections for that particular question.
- Once you've identified the key words, *scan* the passage (using your annotations) until you locate those words, and then read a few sentences above and below until you find what you need. "Five lines above and five lines below" is a good guide. However, you should start reading where the relevant information begins, and keep reading until the passage moves on to another issue.
- Pay attention to the logical structure of the author's argument. For example, if the sixth line below begins with a word like *yet* or *additionally*, you need to keep reading. Pivotal and transitional words indicate that the author may be qualifying what he or she has just said, or adding an additional point that you need to take into account.
- Some Specific (such as, "With which of the following statements would the author be most likely to agree?") and Application questions do not give you lead words as clues. For these questions, eliminate the choices that are inconsistent with the Bottom Line (or, for a Weaken question, that are consistent with the passage), and then go back to the passage to check each of the remaining possibilities.
- For General questions, you can usually use your own articulation of the Bottom Line. You may, however, still need to go back to the passage when you are down to two choices.

4) **Answer in your own words; articulate what the correct answer will need to do, based on the question type and the information in the passage.**
WHY?

- Think of the answer choices as a minefield, full of potentially fatal missteps and pitfalls. Before you enter that minefield, you should have a detailed map of what a strong answer choice will accomplish.
- The wording of the credited response may be quite different from what you expect, but with your own answer as a guide, you will recognize it while avoiding the traps.

HOW?

- Once you've located the relevant information—and not before—articulate your own answer to the question. For particularly difficult questions, you may wish to jot this down on your noteboard.
- This does not mean, however, that you should try to predict the exact wording of the credited response. Instead, come up with a guide to what the correct answer needs to *do* (such as, in the sample question above, to show that Jackson Pollock had little or no influence).

4.3

5) **Use Process of Elimination (POE) to choose the *least wrong* answer choice.**
   WHY?
   - POE is the best friend of every strategic test-taker. Very often on the MCAT, there is no perfectly correct answer among the given choices, only better and worse choices. On particularly difficult passages, the credited response can even be a pretty bad answer. However, it will be *less bad* than the other three.
   - There are a number of standard ways in which the MCAT writers make loser choices look like winners. The answer that at first glance "looks good" may in fact be a trap. See the rest of this chapter and Chapter 5 for more information on types of wrong answers.

   HOW?
   - Use your own understanding of the question task and of what the correct choice needs to do in order to eliminate the most clearly wrong answers. This will usually take you down to two choices.
   - Reread the question and compare the choices you have left to each other. Identify what is wrong, if anything, with each choice. The winner is the choice that has the *least wrong* with it. You may not like that winner very much, but you score a point, which is all that matters in this game.
   - When you are down to two choices, actively look for the types of Attractors that commonly appear for that question type.

4.3 QUESTION TYPES AND FORMATS

There are ten basic questions types that you will encounter in an MCAT CARS section. These ten types of questions fall into four categories.

Specific
1) Retrieval
2) Inference

General
3) Main Idea/Primary Purpose
4) Tone/Attitude

Reasoning
5) Structure
6) Evaluate

Application
7) Strengthen
8) Weaken
9) New Information
10) Analogy

Specific questions ask you for the answer that is best supported by a particular part of the author's argument. General questions ask you what is true of the passage as a whole. Reasoning questions ask you to describe some aspect of the logical structure of the author's argument. Finally, Application questions require you to apply new information (provided either in the question stem or in the answer choices) to the passage.

Occasionally, there can be a variation within a category. For example, a Tone/Attitude question could refer to a particular part of the passage rather than the passage as a whole, and so qualify as a Specific question. Or, a Structure question could ask for the overall organization of the passage, which would make it a General Reasoning question.

These ten types can appear in one of three formats.

1) **Standard:** The question task is direct.
2) **EXCEPT/LEAST/NOT:** The question asks you to find the exception.
   That is, the choice that does NOT address, or that LEAST addresses, the question task (e.g., the statement that is *not* supported by the passage). The three wrong answers will in fact address the task (e.g., *will be* supported by the passage).
3) **Roman numeral:** The question offers you three items. The correct answer will include all of the items that do appropriately address the question task and none of the items that do not.

A firm knowledge of all of these types and of the common trap answers that appear in each is necessary for dealing with the questions quickly and accurately. Before you take the MCAT, you will be able to easily identify each question and know immediately what strategy you will need to employ.

As you move through the set of questions for a passage, use your understanding of question types to attack the questions in the order that works best for you. If you hit a particularly difficult question, skip over it for the moment, and continue answering the easier questions on that passage. Then click back through the set of questions one more time, answering the harder questions. Here is the most efficient approach.

1) Preview the questions from first to last.
2) Work the passage from the screen containing the last question for that passage (remember—your highlighting will not disappear).
3) Then work backwards through the questions, answering the easier ones and skipping harder ones as you go.
4) Finally, click forward through the set of questions, answering the ones you left blank the first time through.
5) Click "Next" from the last question to move on to the next passage.

In the next part of this chapter, we will go through each question type in the Standard format, as well as the EXCEPT/LEAST/NOT and Roman numeral formats. After a discussion of the basic approach to the type, you will find a sample question and a description of how to apply the Five Steps to that question. The sample questions are attached to the passage on criminal procedure that you annotated for an Active Reading Exercise in Chapter 3. The passage is reproduced here; first rework the passage so that it is fresh in your mind.

4.4   QUESTION TYPES: SAMPLE PASSAGE AND QUESTIONS

There are two major systems of criminal procedure in the modern world—the adversarial and the inquisitorial. The former is associated with common law tradition and the latter with civil law tradition. Both systems were historically preceded by the system of private vengeance in which the victim of a crime fashioned his own remedy and administered it privately, either personally or through an agent. The vengeance system was a system of self-help, the essence of which was captured in the slogan "an eye for an eye, a tooth for a tooth." The modern adversarial system is only one historical step removed from the private vengeance system and still retains some of its characteristic features. Thus, for example, even though the right to institute criminal action has now been extended to all members of society, and even though the police department has taken over the pretrial investigative functions on behalf of the prosecution, the adversarial system still leaves the defendant to conduct his own pretrial investigation. The trial is still viewed as a duel between two adversaries, refereed by a judge who, at the beginning of the trial, has no knowledge of the investigative background of the case. In the final analysis the adversarial system of criminal procedure symbolizes and regularizes punitive combat.

By contrast, the inquisitorial system begins historically where the adversarial system stopped its development. It is two historical steps removed from the system of private vengeance. Therefore, from the standpoint of legal anthropology, it is historically superior to the adversarial system. Under the inquisitorial system the public investigator has the duty to investigate not just on behalf of the prosecutor but also on behalf of the defendant. Additionally, the public prosecutor has the duty to present to the court not only evidence that may lead to the conviction of the defendant but also evidence that may lead to his exoneration. This system mandates that both parties permit full pretrial discovery of the evidence in their possession. Finally, in an effort to make the trial less like a duel between two adversaries, the inquisitorial system mandates that the judge take an active part in the conduct of the trial, with a role that is both directive and protective.

Fact-finding is at the heart of the inquisitorial system. This system operates on the philosophical premise that in a criminal case the crucial factor is not the legal rule but the facts of the case and that the goal of the entire procedure is to experimentally recreate for the court the commission of the alleged crime.

Material used in this particular passage has been adapted from the following source:

M. A. Glendon, *Comparative Legal Traditions in a Nutshell.* © 1982 by West Academic Publishing.

Type 1: Specific—Retrieval Questions

Retrieval questions test your ability to locate information in the passage. They may also involve simple paraphrasing and summarizing, but they do not require any substantial analysis or interpretation. They will include some reference to a detail in the passage (a person's name, a theory, a time period, etc.).

Retrieval questions may be phrased in the following ways:

- "According to the passage, the three components of Brown's theory are..."
- "The passage states that Brown's theory is rejected by..."
- "Which of the following statements is *not* mentioned as a characteristic of Brown's theory?" (EXCEPT/LEAST/NOT format)

Sample Question 1:

1. According to the author, the inquisitorial system is two steps removed from:

   A) the adversarial system.
   B) the system of punitive vengeance.
   C) pretrial discovery.
   D) regularized punitive combat.

1) **Read the question word for word and identify the question type.**
   The words "according to the passage" tell you that this is a Retrieval question.

2) **Translate the question into your own words: identify what the question task is asking you to do with the information in the passage.**
   Retrieval questions tend to be fairly straightforward. Here, the question is asking you to locate information in the passage about the inquisitorial system, and to find an answer choice that is best supported by that information.

3) **Identify any key words that refer to specific parts of the passage. If key words are provided, go back to the passage to locate that information.**
   The word "inquisitorial" appears in all three paragraphs. However, "two historical steps" is found only in the beginning of paragraph 2. That is where you will find the answer to this question.

4) **Answer in your own words: articulate what the correct answer will need to do, based on the question type and the information in the passage.**
   The correct answer will state what the "inquisitorial system" is two steps removed from. If you start at the beginning of paragraph 2 and read five lines down, you will see that it is "two historical steps removed from the system of private vengeance." The correct answer needs to state or paraphrase this. Also note that paragraph 1 describes the two systems that preceded the inquisitorial system; any choice that mixes up the three systems will be incorrect.

5) **Use Process of Elimination (POE) to choose the *least wrong* answer choice.**
   As we indicated earlier, each question usually has at least one trap or Attractor answer; that is, a choice that "sounds good" but in fact has some significant flaw. (See Chapter 5 for further discussion of Attractors.) Because Retrieval questions tend to be relatively easy, the MCAT writers often try to distract you from the credited response by pairing it with an answer choice that sounds very similar to the passage but *is not* directly supported by it. These Attractors

4.4

often copy words and phrases directly from the passage text, but don't capture the meaning of those words in the passage. The test-writers may also give you an answer choice that *is* directly supported by the text, but that is not an appropriate answer to that particular question. They may also change or reverse a relationship (for example, the passage says A leads to B, and the wrong answer says that B leads to A). The only way to spot and avoid these traps is to go back to the passage and reread the relevant sections.

Let's take a look at each answer choice for our sample question.

A: No. The first sentence of paragraph 2 states that "the inquisitorial system begins historically where the adversarial system stopped its development." You also know from paragraph 1 that the adversarial system followed "the system of private vengeance." Therefore, the inquisitorial system is one step, not two steps, removed from the adversarial system. This is a classic trap answer on a Retrieval question; it gives you something that is discussed in the same part of the passage, but that doesn't match the specific reference in the question task.

B: Yes. Notice that that the author uses "punitive combat" at the end of paragraph 1 to describe what came before the adversarial system (the adversarial system regularized that punitive combat). Thus "punitive vengeance" is another way of saying "private vengeance." Therefore, this choice is directly supported by the relevant part of the passage.

C: No. This choice takes words from the passage out of context and doesn't directly address the question task. Pretrial discovery is part of the inquisitorial system; it isn't something that the inquisitorial system is removed from.

D: No. This choice is tricky because it sounds a lot like choice B. But when you compare the two, you will see that choice D mentions *regularized* punitive combat. The end of paragraph 1 states that "the adversarial system…symbolizes and regularizes punitive combat." "Punitive combat" itself describes the system of private vengeance. So, this is just another way of saying "the adversarial system," and, just like choice A, it is incorrect.

Type 2: Specific—Inference Questions

Inference questions are the most common question type in the CARS section. They require you to choose the answer that is best supported by the passage. They may ask you what can be inferred or concluded, what the author would agree with, what is implied or suggested by the author, what the author assumes to be true, or what the author means by a particular word or phrase. They may also ask which answer choice would be an example of something described in the passage.

There is no such thing as being "too close" to the passage to qualify as a correct answer to an Inference question. An answer that directly paraphrases the passage may in fact be the credited response. On the other hand, the correct answer may seem debatable (that is, you could argue that it isn't literally deducible from the passage information), but it will still be better supported by the passage text than the other three choices.

To approach an Inference question, find the relevant section or sections of the passage. Check each answer choice against that information, choosing the one that has the most support. The credited response may seem like a stretch (for example, something that you think is not particularly "reasonable" to conclude), but it will be the best supported of the four. Be flexible; the correct answer may be something that you would never have come up with on your own, but there will be some solid evidence for it in the passage.

There are a variety of ways in which Inference questions can be phrased. Some of the most common phrasings are:

- "It can be inferred from the passage that…"
- "An assumption underlying the author's discussion of Brown's theory is that…"
- "The author implies that Brown's theory is most closely linked to…"
- "Implicit in the passage is the contention that Brown's theory is…"
- "By *only dimly perceived*, the author most likely means:"
- "The author suggests that…"
- "Based on information in the passage, it can be most reasonably concluded that…"
- "With which of the following statements would the author be most likely to agree?"
- "Which of the following statements is best supported by the passage?"
- "Which of the following would be an example of Surrealism, as it is described in the passage?"

Sample Question 2:

2. The passage suggests that the inquisitorial system differs from the adversarial system in that:

A) it provides the judge with information about the findings of the pretrial investigation.
B) it makes the defendant solely responsible for gathering evidence.
C) it guarantees that all defendants get a fair trial.
D) a defendant who is innocent would prefer to be tried under the inquisitorial system.

1) **Read the question word for word and identify the question type.**
   The words "The passage suggests that" identify this as an Inference question.
2) **Translate the question into your own words: identify what the question task is asking you to do with the information in the passage.**
   This question is asking you how the author contrasts the inquisitorial with the adversarial system.
3) **Identify any key words that refer to specific parts of the passage. If key words are provided, *go back to the passage* to locate that information.**
   This is where many students falter, thinking that they don't need to go back to the passage because the question is asking us to infer something (or, in this case, what is suggested). The correct answer still must be closely based on the passage text, not on your own ideas or deductions.

   The words "inquisitorial" and "adversarial" appear in multiple places. However, the words "in contrast" at the beginning of paragraph 2 indicate that this is the beginning of the author's discussion of the differences between the two systems. Your annotation should alert you to the fact that there are a variety of differences listed in this paragraph. Don't reread the whole paragraph at this point, but you will need to check the answer choices against it.

4.4

4) **Answer in your own words: articulate what the correct answer will need to do, based on the question type and the information in the passage.**

The credited response will need to not only match the description of the two systems, but will also need to correctly describe a difference between them.

5) **Use Process of Elimination (POE) to choose the *least wrong* answer choice.**

A wide variety of Attractors appear in Inference answer choices. One of the most common is a statement that puts information from the passage into overly absolutist or extreme language. For example, the passage may say that something *often* occurs, while the trap answer will say that same thing *always* occurs.

Do not, however, eliminate a choice for an Inference question only because it is narrower or more moderate than the scope or wording of the passage.

Be careful to eliminate answer choices that are out of scope; that is, answer choices which refer to issues that could be tangentially related but that are never discussed in the passage.

Just like for Retrieval questions, look out for Attractors that take words out of context, or that are supported by the passage but not relevant to the question.

Let's take a look at each answer choice from our sample question.

A: **Yes. At the end of paragraph 2, the author states (in the context of differences between the two systems) that "the judge takes an active part in the conduct of the trial that is both directive and protective." Earlier in that same paragraph, the author also states that the inquisitorial system requires "full pretrial discovery." From this you can infer that in the inquisitorial system the judge would have access to information uncovered in the pretrial investigation or discovery.**

B: No. The passage suggests that this is true of the adversarial, not the inquisitorial system.

C: No. This choice is too extreme. The passage suggests that the inquisitorial system may lead to increased fairness, but not that fairness is guaranteed.

D: No. Although many of these words appear in the passage, there is nothing to suggest which system an innocent person would prefer. While this choice makes common sense, it is too much of a stretch, especially when compared with choice A, which is directly supported by the passage text.

Type 3: General—Main Idea/Primary Purpose Questions

These questions require you to summarize claims and implications made throughout the passage in order to formulate a general statement of the central point or primary activity of the passage. Think of the passage as an argument. The Main Idea is the overall claim, supported by specific evidence in the various paragraphs, which the author wants to convince you to accept as true. The Primary Purpose is then very closely related; it will express what the author *does* in order to convey the Main Idea.

Good active reading is the key to these questions; don't wait until you encounter a Main Idea question to think about the Main Point or Bottom Line of the passage. Synthesize the major themes as you read the passage. Distill these themes into a summary of the content and tone of the author's argument or

4.4

presentation. Don't ignore the author's attitude as expressed in the passage. An answer may have the correct content and scope, but if the tone or attitude doesn't match the passage, the choice is incorrect.

Main Idea questions are often phrased in the following ways:

- "The main idea of the passage is that…"
- "The central thesis of this passage is…"

Primary Purpose questions are often phrased as follows:

- "The author's primary purpose is to explain that…"

Sample Question 3:

3. The primary purpose of the passage is to:

A) explain why the inquisitorial system is the best system of criminal justice.

B) explain how the adversarial and the inquisitorial systems of criminal justice both evolved from the system of private vengeance.

C) show how the adversarial and inquisitorial systems of criminal justice can both complement and hinder each other's development.

D) analyze two systems of criminal justice and deduce which one is more advanced.

1) **Read the question word for word and identify the question type.**
   General questions are generally very easy to identify. Here, the words "primary purpose" tip you off.

2) **Translate the question into your own words: identify what the question task is asking you to do with the information in the passage.**
   The question is asking you to summarize the author's overall goal in writing this passage. A good translation of this question would be: "Why did the author describe the two modern criminal procedure systems, as well as the pre-modern system of private vengeance?"

3) **Identify any key words that refer to specific parts of the passage. If key words are provided, *go back to the passage* to locate that information.**
   On Main Idea and Primary Purpose questions you will not usually need to go back to the passage before reading the choices. Use your original articulation of the Bottom Line to take a first pass or cut through the choices. You may, however, need to go back to the passage when you are down to two or three choices.

4) **Answer in your own words: articulate what the correct answer will need to do, based on the question type and the information in the passage.**
   For this type, the correct answer needs to include (explicitly or implicitly) all of the major themes of the passage, without going beyond the scope of the author's argument. Your own answer to this question would be something like: "The author describes the pre-modern system of private vengeance in order to set up contrast between the adversarial and inquisitorial systems; the adversarial system is closer to the system of private vengeance, and the inquisitorial system is more highly evolved."

5) **Use Process of Elimination (POE) to choose the *least wrong* answer choice.**
Common Attractors for Main Idea and Primary Purpose questions will understate or over-state the author's point. Choices that summarize the main idea of a paragraph or two but which leave out other major themes are too narrow. Vague or overly inclusive choices that go beyond the scope of the passage are too broad. Take the "Goldilocks approach": eliminate what is too big or too small, and find the one that is the best fit.

For Primary Purpose questions, focus in part on the verb in each answer choice, and elimi-nate the ones that are inappropriate; that is, too opinionated, too neutral, or that go in the opposite direction from the passage.

Eliminate choices that are too extreme. Is the author really *proving* or *disproving* a claim, or just *supporting* or *challenging* that claim? Eliminate any verb that expresses an opinion (*criti-cizing, propounding*, etc.) on a neutral passage (*explaining, describing*, etc.) and vice versa.

Be very careful to read and evaluate all parts of each answer choice. An answer choice may begin beautifully, but change halfway through to bring in something inconsistent with or irrelevant to the author's argument. If any part of the choice is wrong, the whole thing is wrong.

Let's take a look at the choices for this question.

A: No. This choice is too extreme ("the best") and too broad in scope. The passage only com-pares the inquisitorial system to the adversarial and private vengeance systems, not to all other systems of criminal justice.

B: No. This choice is too narrow in scope. The author not only explains this evolutionary con-nection, but explicitly contrasts the inquisitorial with the adversarial system in order to judge the former to be "historically superior."

C: No. This choice is out of scope. The passage never suggests that these two systems coexist, or that one would either contribute to, or get in the way of, the other.

D: **Yes. While this choice does not explicitly mention the system of private vengeance, it doesn't need to; the author discusses the pre-modern system of private vengeance in or-der to argue that the inquisitorial system is historically superior to the adversarial system (because the adversarial system is closer to the system of private vengeance).**

Type 4: General—Tone/Attitude Questions

Tone and Attitude questions ask you to evaluate whether or not the author expresses an opinion regarding the material in the passage, and if so, to judge how strongly positive or negative that opinion is. Or, the ques-tion may ask you who or what the author is most likely to be. Pure Tone or Attitude questions are fairly rare (however, Main Idea and Primary Purpose questions always involve assessing the tone of the passage).

Just as for Main Idea and Primary Purpose questions, you must identify the tone of the author through active reading before you begin any of the questions.

When pure Tone/Attitude questions do appear, they are usually general questions, as in the following:

- "In this passage, the author's tone is one of…"
- "The author's attitude can best be described as…"
- "The passage makes it clear that the author is…"

However, Tone/Attitude questions may also appear in Specific form, asking about the author's attitude towards a particular part of the passage (in which case they are Specific Tone/Attitude question), as in:

- "The author's attitude toward Brown's claim can best be described as…"
- "What is the tone of the author's response to Brown's critics?"
- "The author's attitude towards the controversy surrounding Brown's theory can best be characterized as exhibiting…"

Sample Question 4:

4. The author's attitude regarding the evolution of criminal procedure systems can best be characterized as:

A) condemnatory.
B) instructive.
C) admiring.
D) ambivalent.

1) **Read the question word for word and identify the question type.**
   The word "attitude" is a pretty clear indication of a tone question. Because the passage as a whole is about the evolution of criminal procedure systems, this is a General Attitude question.

2) **Translate the question into your own words: identify what the question task is asking you to do with the information in the passage.**
   This question is asking you what the author thinks about how criminal procedures have changed over time.

3) **Identify any key words that refer to specific parts of the passage. If key words are provided, *go back to the passage* to locate that information.**
   As with most General questions, you already have an answer, based on the passage, in mind. Therefore you may not need to go back to the passage before you begin evaluating the answer choices. However, you may well need to refer back to the passage during POE.

4) **Answer in your own words: articulate what the correct answer will need to do, based on the question type and the information in the passage.**
   The correct answer must be fairly neutral in tone. The author is describing how criminal procedure has evolved, not condemning or advocating any particular system. The author does state that the inquisitorial system is superior, but in the context of being "historically superior;" that is, more highly evolved.

4.4

5) **Use Process of Elimination (POE) to choose the *least wrong* answer choice.**
Common Attractors on Attitude and Tone questions are choices that take the author's opinion to extremes. If the passage expresses qualified or moderate admiration, for example, an Attractor may incorrectly describe the author as "enthusiastic." If the author expresses both positive and negative thoughts about a subject, incorrect answer choices may leave out the positive or ignore the negative. Also, positive and negative comments don't cancel each other out to create a neutral tone. If the passage is neutral, any choice that expresses an opinion one way or the other is incorrect.

Beware of choices that express strange attitudes rarely seen in MCAT passages. For example, if you see a choice like "obtuse ambiguity," you should be highly suspicious of it.

Let's apply POE to our sample question.

A: No. This choice is too strong—and too negative. The author does not condemn earlier criminal procedure systems; the passage only labels them as less highly evolved. The author definitely does not condemn "the evolution of criminal procedure systems" as a whole; the author says nothing negative about the inquisitorial system, which is the most highly evolved version.

B: **Yes. The author is describing this evolution in a fairly neutral tone. Thus you can say that the tone of the passage is instructive; its goal is to teach us about the evolution of criminal procedure.**

C: No. This choice is too strong and too positive. It is tempting, given that reference to "historically superior." However, the passage isn't praising the inquisitorial system, but just describing it as the most recent system. Even if you speculate that the author may have positive feelings about the inquisitorial system, this would be only speculation; "instructive," based only on passage information, is the least wrong choice.

D: No. "Ambivalent" means uncertain, or torn between multiple options. Nothing in the passage suggests that the author is torn between different opinions regarding the evolution of criminal procedure systems.

Type 5: Reasoning—Structure Questions

Structure questions ask you to describe how the author makes his or her argument. They differ from other questions in that they address the passage's construction or logical structure along with its content. This is what puts them into the category of Reasoning Questions, even though they almost always relate to one specific area of the passage. Structure questions may ask you for the purpose of a particular reference within the passage. That reference could be to an example, a conclusion, a contrasting point of view, etc. For example, the question stem may cite evidence from the passage and ask you to find the answer that describes the claim or larger point being supported by that evidence. This version of a Structure question often includes the wording "in order to," as in: "The author states X in order to...."

Alternatively, a Structure question might cite a claim from the passage and ask you how, or if, that claim is supported by the author. Similarly, the question may ask what kinds of support are not used in the passage, or what claims are not supported in a particular way; for example: "Which of the following statements is NOT supported by an example or explanation?"

To answer these questions, it is crucial to identify the Main Point of the paragraph or chunk of information in which a reference cited in the question appears, and to separate the claims made by the author from the evidence (if any is given) supporting those claims. Look for words—like *for example* or *for instance*—that indicate that what comes next is the support or evidence, and conclusion words—like *therefore, thus, so,* or *hence*—that indicate that what comes next is the claim being supported.

It is also possible for Structure questions to appear in General form, asking you to describe the organization of the passage as a whole. When answering a General Structure question, separate the choices into pieces and check for pieces that are out of order, that have an inappropriate tone, or that describe things that never happened in the passage.

Specific Structure questions may be worded as follows:

- "The author probably mentions the controversy surrounding Brown's ideas in order to…"
- "The three experiments carried out by Brown are cited in the passage as evidence that…"
- "The author describes Brown's unique methodology in order to make the point that…"

or

- "Which of the following items of information presented in the passage provides the most support for the author's claim that Brown's methodology is unique?"
- "The author's claim that Brown's methodology is unique is supported by…"
- "Which of the following claims made by the author regarding Brown's methodology is NOT supported by example or reference to authority?"

General structure questions can be phrased as:

- "Which of the following best describes the overall organization of the passage?"
- "Which of the following statements best describes the logical progression of the author's argument?"

Sample Question 5:

5. The author cites the slogan "an eye for an eye and a tooth for a tooth" (paragraph 1) in order to:

A) show how aspects of the private vengeance system persist in today's legal system.
B) criticize pre-modern systems of justice as overly violent.
C) characterize private vengeance as a system that required the victim himself to seek justice.
D) demonstrate how the legal rule rather than the facts of the case provided the foundation of the system of private vengeance.

1) **Read the question word for word and identify the question type.**
   The words "in order to" tell you that this is a Structure question.
2) **Translate the question into your own words: identify what the question task is asking you to do with the information in the passage.**
   The question is asking you to describe why the author used this phrase at this point in the passage.

3) **Identify any key words that refer to specific parts of the passage. If key words are pro-vided, *go back to the passage* to locate that information.**

The quote "An eye for an eye…" appears in paragraph 1. The author argues that it "captures the essence" of the private vengeance system, in which "the victim of a crime fashioned his own remedy and administered it privately…."

4) **Answer in your own words: articulate what the correct answer will need to do, based on the question type and the information in the passage.**

The correct answer must connect the quote to the system of private vengeance, and describe it as part of the author's explanation of how victims themselves had to administer punishments to those who had wronged them.

5) **Use Process of Elimination (POE) to choose the *least wrong* answer choice.**

For Structure questions, beware of Attractors that describe claims that are made in the passage but that are not relevant to or directly supported by the reference given in the question. Also beware of half right, half wrong choices. All parts of the correct answer choice must check out.

The correct choice must be consistent with the Main Point and tone of the relevant chunk of passage, as well as with the Bottom Line of the passage as a whole.

Let's evaluate the answer choices for our sample question.

A: No. The author argues that while the adversarial system does share some aspects with private vengeance, we have moved on to a system based on "fact-finding" where the judge directs the proceedings. Our modern inquisitorial system is "two historical steps removed from the system of private vengeance" (paragraph 2). Therefore, today's legal system is shown to be very different from the system of private vengeance.

B: No. The tone of this choice does not match the passage. While you might think of "an eye for an eye" as a violent way to mete out justice, the author does not describe it that way, or criticize it as such.

C: **Yes. The quote appears in a sentence describing private vengeance as "a system of self-help." The preceding sentence also discusses how "the victim had to fashion his own remedy and administer it privately…." This choice fits with both the content and tone of the passage and with the specific reference in the question.**

D: No. This choice takes words from the end of the passage out of context. There is no direct connection made by the author between basing a system on a legal rule, and the "eye for an eye" approach to justice.

Type 6: Reasoning—Evaluate Questions

Evaluate questions are similar to Structure questions in that you need to identify the logical structure of the author's argument. Evaluate questions, however, go a step further by asking either how well an author supports their claims *(Type 1: "Claims and Evidence")* or for a logical error or contradiction in the passage *(Type 2: "Flaw")*. That is, the question asks you to evaluate whether or not the author does a good job justifying his or her conclusions.

Type 1—"Claims and Evidence": The answers for these questions often come in two parts. One part will be some version of "strongly" or "weakly" supported. The other part will be the explanation or justification for that evaluation (for example, that it is weakly supported *because* no examples are given, or, strongly supported *because* relevant examples are provided). When choosing an answer, make sure to check that both parts of the choice are supported by the text; that is, both the judgment itself (strongly or weakly) and the justification for that judgment.

These questions may be phrased as follows:

- "The author asserts that Brown's theoretical model is 'dangerously incomplete.' The support offered for this conclusion is…"
- "Is Brown's analysis of the implications of Herrera's theoretical model well supported?"
- "The author's assertion that Brown's model is incomplete is…"

Type 2—"Flaw": This version of an Evaluate question asks you for an error or self-contradiction in the passage. Unless the question stem references a particular part of the passage, go straight into POE rather than trying to answer in your own words first. That is, use the answer choices to go back and locate the relevant parts of the passage, and then decide if that part of the author's argument is logically flawed.

These questions may be phrased as follows:

- "Which of the following represents a logical error in the passage?"
- "The author's claim regarding Brown's model is flawed in which of the following ways?"
- "Which of the following pairs of statements from the passage represent a logical contradiction?"

Sample Question 6:

6. How well supported is the author's claim that the adversarial system still retains some features of private vengeance?

A) Strongly, because the claim is inherent in the meaning of the word "adversarial"
B) Strongly, because examples of similarities between the two are provided by the author
C) Weakly, because the claim is logically inconsistent with the author's description of the inquisitorial system
D) Weakly, because no evidence is cited to bolster the claim

1) **Read the question word for word and identify the question type.**
   The question asks *how well* supported the author's claim is, which makes it an Evaluate question. Notice that it doesn't just ask *what* the author's claim is (this would be a Retrieval or Inference question).

2) **Translate the question into your own words: identify what the question task is asking you to do with the information in the passage.**
   The question is asking if there are any significant flaws or weaknesses in the author's argument about the relationship between private vengeance and the adversarial system. If so, what are those flaws? If not, why is it a strong argument?

3) **Identify any key words that refer to specific parts of the passage. If key words are provided, *go back to the passage* to locate that information.**

This question sends you back to paragraph 1. The claim cited in the question comes in the middle of the paragraph. Immediately after the claim, the author discusses particular similarities (as well as some differences) between private vengeance and the adversarial system.

4) **Answer in your own words: articulate what the correct answer will need to do, based on the question type and the information in the passage.**

Read through the examples supporting the claim: the defendant must conduct "his own pretrial investigation," and "the trial is still viewed as a duel between two adversaries." This leads the author to the conclusion that the adversarial system "symbolizes and regularizes punitive combat;" punitive combat characterizes private vengeance. Because the author gives relevant examples, and draws reasonably well-supported conclusions based on those examples, you can say that the claim is strongly supported.

5) **Use Process of Elimination (POE) to choose the *least wrong* answer choice.**

Answer choices that mischaracterize the strength of the argument are incorrect.

Once you have narrowed it down to the choices that fall on the correct side (in this case, "strongly" or "weakly") narrow it down further by analyzing precisely what is either good or bad about the author's logic.

Let's go through the answer choices for our sample question.

A: No. While the claim is in fact supported strongly, it is not because of the definition of "adversarial." Instead, it is because the author provides relevant examples.

B: **Yes. The fact that the defendant must carry out his own pretrial investigation; and that the trial is still seen as a duel, show that the adversarial system retains aspects of private vengeance, even if they are in a somewhat more symbolic or institutionalized form.**

C: No. There is no inconsistency in the logic of the author's argument (which claims that the adversarial and inquisitorial systems are in fact quite different).

D: No. Direct, relevant evidence is in fact given (note the phrase "for example" in the passage, directly following the claim cited in the question).

Type 7: Application—Strengthen Questions

A Strengthen question asks you to find the answer that most supports the passage (as opposed to Structure and Evaluate questions, which ask how, if, or how well the author has supported his or her own argument). That is, the correct answer will make the author's argument more convincing than it already was.

Notice that Strengthen questions often use the phrase, "which of the following, if true…." Take those words *if true*—whether implied or explicitly stated—seriously. Do not try to find the answer choices *in* the passage. Take each statement as if it were true and find the one that does what it needs to do *to* the relevant part of the passage. These questions are quite different from Specific, General, and Reasoning questions in that they give you new information in the answer choices; the correct answer will change (for the better), not just describe or reflect, the passage. These questions are also distinct from other question types (except for Weaken questions) in that it is impossible for an answer to be "too extreme" to be correct. You want the answer that goes the farthest in the correct direction.

Strengthen questions may be phrased as follows:

- "Which of the following, if valid, would provide the best support for the author's conclusion in the last paragraph?"
- "Which of the following, if true, would most strengthen the author's claims?"

Strengthen EXCEPT/LEAST/NOT

Strengthen questions sometimes appear in the EXCEPT/LEAST/NOT format. EXCEPT/LEAST/NOT Strengthen questions have a bit of a twist, compared to most other questions in this format; the correct answer may do the opposite (in this case, Weaken), but they may also just do nothing (have no effect or be irrelevant), or not go as far in the strengthening direction as the three wrong answers (that is, barely strengthen the passage, but less so than the other choices). It is especially crucial to compare choices to each other and pick the one that is the farthest away from strengthening as possible.

The correct answer is the one that goes the farthest to the left along this spectrum.

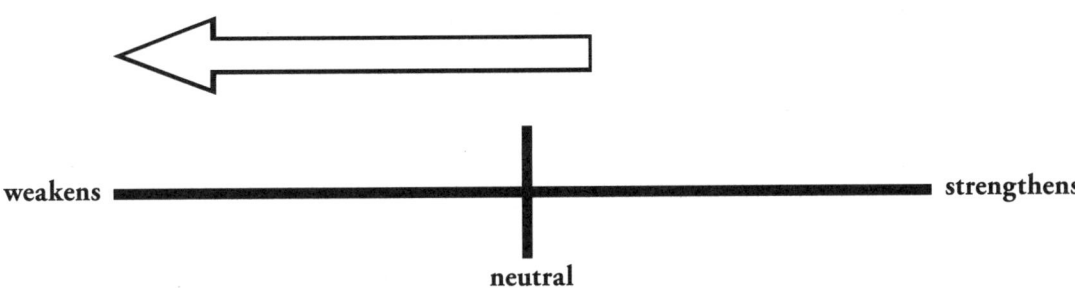

Sample Question 7:

7. Which of the following, if true, would most strengthen the author's claim that the inquisitorial system is historically superior to the adversarial system of justice?

A) Judges within the inquisitorial system are expected to be familiar with the facts of the case before a trial begins.

B) The justice systems currently used in some countries still treat a trial as a duel between two adversaries.

C) While the inquisitorial system in theory is based on fact-finding, in practice it often takes on the form of a private contest between victim and defendant.

D) In some cases tried under the adversarial system, the judge is biased towards either the defendant or the victim.

1) **Read the question word for word and identify the question type.**

   The words "most strengthen" tell you that this is a Strengthen question.

2) **Translate the question into your own words: identify what the question task is asking you to do with the information in the passage.**

   You will need to take each choice as true, rather than looking for support for the right answer in the passage. You will still need to go back to the passage, however, to pin down what is being strengthened. The question is asking you to find new evidence in the passage that makes the author's claim that the inquisitorial system is more historically developed than the adversarial system (that is, that it is even further away from the system of private vengeance) even more compelling.

3) **Identify any key words that refer to specific parts of the passage. If key words are provided, *go back to the passage* to locate that information.**

   The passage as a whole is making the argument that the inquisitorial system is more historically developed. Therefore, you can take the Bottom Line into the answer choices and look for the one that most supports this overall claim. You may, however, need to go back to the passage as you go through POE to pin down the relevance of details included in the answer choices.

4) **Answer in your own words: articulate what the correct answer will need to do, based on the question type and the information in the passage.**

   The correct answer will provide new evidence that the inquisitorial system is in fact different, along the lines discussed in the passage, from the system of private vengeance, from the adversarial system, or from both.

5) **Use Process of Elimination (POE) to choose the *least wrong* answer choice.**

   When using POE on Strengthen questions, eliminate choices that are irrelevant to the cited part or issue in the passage (that is, that are out of scope). Remember, however, that the correct answer will bring in new information: "irrelevant" is not the same thing as "never mentioned."

Do *not* eliminate choices on the basis of absolute or extreme wording. It is impossible on these questions (in contrast to Specific, General, and Reasoning questions) for an answer to be wrong solely on the basis of being too strong. The more it strengthens the passage, the better. In fact, choices on this question type may be wrong because they don't go far enough to have a significant impact on the author's argument. Also, make sure to look out for wrong answers that weaken instead of strengthen by suggesting that the inquisitorial system is less historically superior than the author claims.

Let's use POE on our sample question.

A: **Yes. The author states in the first paragraph that one reason that the adversarial system is "only one historical step removed from the private vengeance system" is that the judge has no knowledge of the background of the case as the trial begins. While the author does state in the second paragraph that "the inquisitorial system mandates that the judge take an active part in the conduct of the trial, with a role that is both directive and protective," the passage never indicates that this also means that the judge is familiar before the trial with the facts of the case. Therefore, this answer choice strengthens the author's claim by providing one more relevant way in which the inquisitorial system has evolved even further from private vengeance than the adversarial system.**

B: No. This choice has no impact on the author's argument. While the author does suggest that the adversarial system still exists in the world, this isn't relevant to his or her claim that the *qualities* of the inquisitorial system make it historically superior.

C: No. This choice does the opposite of what the question requires. It weakens, not strengthens, the author's claim by suggesting that the inquisitorial system is not as different from the adversarial system (or from the system of private vengeance) as the author claims.

D: No. While this choice is consistent with the author's argument, it doesn't go far enough to actually strengthen it, especially when compared to choice A. The author does imply that the judge plays a neutral role in the inquisitorial system. However, the fact in *some* (which could be one or two) adversarial justice systems the judge plays a biased role doesn't strongly support the author's claim that *in general* the inquisitorial system is more distinct than the adversarial system from private vengeance.

4.4

Type 8: Application—Weaken Questions

A Weaken question requires you to find the answer choice that most undermines or calls into question the claim or claims made by the author.

Notice that just like Strengthen questions, Weaken questions often use the phrase, "which of the following, if true…." Take those words *if true*—whether implied or explicitly stated—seriously. Do not try to find the answer choices *in* the passage. Take each statement as if it were true and find the one that is most *inconsistent* with the relevant part of the passage. These questions are quite different from Specific, General, and Reasoning questions in that they give you new information in the answer choices; the correct answer will change the passage by making the author's argument less convincing than it originally was. These questions are also distinct from other question types (except for Strengthen questions) in that it is impossible for an answer to be "too extreme" to be correct. You want the answer that goes the farthest in the correct direction.

Weaken questions are often phrased as follows:

- "Which of the following, if valid, would most *weaken* the author's point?"
- "Which of the following, if true, would most *undermine* the author's claims?"
- "Which of the following results, if proven to be valid, would most call into question the author's conclusion regarding Brown's methodology?"

You might also see a variation on Weaken questions that cites a statement from the passage, and asks you to decide which *answer choice* would be most weakened by that statement. For example:

- "The claims made by Brown, if true, would cast the most *doubt* on which of the following statements?"

Regardless of the wording, you are doing the same thing in answering any Weaken question in the Standard format: finding the answer choice that is *most inconsistent* with the cited part of the passage.

4.4

Weaken EXCEPT/LEAST/NOT

As with Strengthen questions, Weaken questions sometimes appear in the EXCEPT/LEAST/NOT format, as in, "Which of the following would LEAST weaken the claims made by the author?" EXCEPT/LEAST/NOT Weaken questions have the same twist as Strengthen questions in this format; the correct answer may do the opposite (Strengthen), but they may also just do nothing (have no effect or be irrelevant), or not go as far in weakening as the three wrong answers (i.e., weaken a little bit but less than the other choices). It is especially crucial to compare choices to each other and pick the one furthest along the spectrum we discussed for Strengthen EXCEPT/LEAST/NOT questions, but in this case in the opposite direction.

The correct answer is the one that goes the farthest to the right along this spectrum.

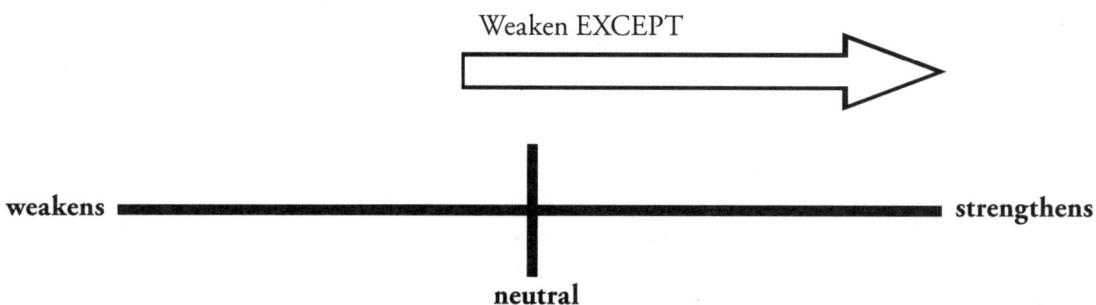

Sample Question 8:

8. Which of the following, if true, would most *undermine* the author's main argument in the passage?

A) The vengeance system did not precede all systems of criminal procedure in the world.
B) The inquisitorial and adversarial systems have many things in common.
C) The adversarial system is a system of self-help.
D) Personal vengeance is at the heart of the inquisitorial system.

1) **Read the question word for word and identify the question type.**
   The words "most undermine" identify this as a Weaken question. The question is asking you to undermine the author's central argument.

2) **Translate the question into your own words: identify what the question task is asking you to do with the information in the passage.**
   You will need to take each choice as true, rather than looking for support for the right answer in the passage. You will still need to go back to the passage, however, to pin down the credited response. You need the response that most undermines the author's argument as a whole.

3) **Identify any key words that refer to specific parts of the passage. If key words are provided,** *go back to the passage* **to locate that information.**
   Because the question asks you to weaken the author's main argument, you can use your own articulation of the Bottom Line of the passage. With that already clearly defined, you don't need to go back to the passage before you start evaluating the choices. If the question stem had asked you to weaken a particular claim within the passage, you would need to first go back and find and paraphrase that part of the author's argument.

4) **Answer in your own words: articulate what the correct answer will need to do, based on the question type and the information in the passage.**

The correct answer will suggest that the adversarial and inquisitorial systems are more similar than the author claims, and/or that the inquisitorial system is not in fact historically superior.

5) **Use Process of Elimination (POE) to choose the *least wrong* answer choice.**

For a Weaken question, the best answer will go the furthest toward making it impossible for the claim made in the passage to be true. Look for the answer choice that is most inconsistent with the relevant part of the passage.

When using POE on Weaken questions, eliminate choices that are irrelevant to the cited part or issue in the passage (that is, that are out of scope). Remember, however, that the correct answer will bring in new information: "irrelevant" is not the same thing as "never mentioned."

Do *not* eliminate choices on the basis of absolute or extreme wording. It is impossible on these questions (in contrast to all other question types except for Strengthen questions) for an answer to be wrong solely on the basis of being too strong. The more it weakens the passage, the better.

In fact, choices on this question type may be wrong because they don't go far enough to have a significant impact on the author's argument.

Finally, look out for Attractors that strengthen instead of weaken.

Let's use POE on our sample question.

A: No. The author does not claim that private vengeance was the very first system used to punish criminals. For all you know, there could have been other pre-modern systems that preceded private vengeance. This choice attacks a claim that is never made by the author; it is therefore out of scope.

B: No. The passage itself suggests some similarities: e.g., there is a judge, and there is a private investigator searching for evidence to support the prosecution (the inquisitorial system just broadens those duties to include finding evidence for the defense as well). Because the author's main argument is not founded on the assumption that there are few or no similarities between the two, this choice does not go far enough to weaken the passage.

C: No. This choice is entirely consistent with the author's depiction of the adversarial system in paragraph 1. This choice strengthens, not weakens, the author's contrast between the adversarial and inquisitorial systems.

D: **Yes. The author argues that the inquisitorial system is historically superior because it is "two historical steps removed from the system of private vengeance" (paragraph 2) and because it is based on "the facts of the case" (paragraph 3). The adversarial system, in contrast, "is only one historical step removed from the private vengeance system and still retains some of its characteristic features" (paragraph 1). If private vengeance was in fact at the heart of the inquisitorial system, this would undermine the author's argument about the historical character and evolutionary place of the inquisitorial system. Thus, choice D is the best answer.**

Type 9: Application—New Information Questions

All New Information questions have one thing in common: they provide new facts or scenarios in the question stem that are never mentioned in the passage. That said, the question may require you to do a variety of things with that new information. New Information questions break down into two general types.

Type 1: New Information/Inference questions

These questions give you new facts that are in the same general issue area of the passage and then ask what, according to the passage, is likely to be true. In essence, you're inserting the new facts into the existing passage, and then drawing an inference from both the new and the old information. Before you read the answer choices, answer the question in your own words, based on the information already in the passage and on the new facts in the question stem.

For example, the question might ask the following:

- "If China experienced an unusually rainy winter, what would also be true, based on the passage?"
- "According to the passage, what would likely happen if China experienced an unusually rainy winter?"
- "What would the author recommend as the best way to predict whether China is likely to experience an unusually rainy winter next year?"
- "If a meteorologist were to claim that China's climate can be studied in isolation, how would the author respond?"

Type 2: New Information/Strengthen/Weaken questions

These questions provide you with new facts in the question stem (as opposed to pure Strengthen or Weaken questions that give the new information only in the answer choices). They then ask you to evaluate what effect those new facts would have on the author's argument as a whole, or on one specific claim made or described in the passage.

Use the passage much like you do Strengthen, Weaken, and Structure questions. Identify the issue of the question, and go back to the passage to find the relevant sections. Pay close attention to the logical structure of the author's argument. Define what the correct answer needs to do based on the passage, the information in the question stem, and the direction (strengthen or weaken) the correct choice must take.

This type of New Information question may be phrased as follows:

- "Suppose it was shown to be true that when winters in China are unusually rainy, summers in Latin America are unusually dry. What effect would this have on the author's argument as it is described in the passage?"
- "Which of the following claims made in the passage would be most strengthened by data showing that industrialization has affected global weather patterns?"
- "Recent studies have shown that the jet stream has shifted 10 degrees in latitude over the past five years. This fact tends to *undermine* the author's claim that…"
- "El Niño has been proven to be a recurring and invariant pattern. This fact tends to support the author's claims in paragraph 2 because…"

4.4

The following sample question falls into the *Type 1* category.

Sample Question 9:

9. Suppose that in an inquisitorial system of justice a judge perceives that the prosecution is misdirecting the trial by introducing irrelevant evidence. The author would most likely advise the judge to:

A) protect the prosecution by turning a blind eye to the proceedings.
B) admonish the prosecution and get the trial back to the issues at hand.
C) call a mistrial and free the defendant.
D) refuse to participate in the trial.

1) **Read the question word for word and identify the question type.**
The word "suppose" is our first indication that this is a New Information question. What follows is a scenario that does not already appear in the passage. The question asks you what the author of the passage would advise, making this a *Type 1* question.

2) **Translate the question into your own words: identify what the question task is asking you to do with the information in the passage.**
The question is asking you to find an answer choice that is consistent both with the passage and with the new situation in the question stem; in this new scenario, the judge discovers that the prosecution is breaking the rules.

3) **Identify any key words that refer to specific parts of the passage. If key words are provided, *go back to the passage* to locate that information.**
The role of the judge in the inquisitorial system is described at the end of paragraph 2. The judge must "take an active part in the conduct of the trial, with a role that is both directive and protective."

4) **Answer in your own words: articulate what the correct answer will need to do, based on the question type and the information in the passage.**
Based on the passage, the judge in this situation must take action to protect the defense from the unfair tactics used by the prosecution, and must direct the trial in a way consistent with the system's rules.

5) **Use Process of Elimination (POE) to choose the *least wrong* answer choice.**
A common Attractor for any New Information question is an answer choice that focuses on the wrong part of the passage. Also beware of answer choices that are inconsistent with the passage (for all but the Weaken version of this question type), or that deal with irrelevant issues. This means choices that do not connect to the passage, or that are not relevant to the theme of the new information in the question.

For *Type 1* questions, beware of extreme language. The correct answer can't go too far beyond the scope and tone of the passage.

For *Type 2* questions, beware of choices that go in the opposite direction (e.g., that strengthen instead of weaken or vice versa).

Let's go through POE on our sample question.

A: No. This is inconsistent with the author's claim that in the inquisitorial system, the interests of the defense as well as of the prosecution should be protected. This is also inconsistent with the author's claim that the judge must take an active role to direct the proceedings.

B: **Yes. This is consistent with the author's claim that the judge has a protective role (protecting the rights of the defense by admonishing the prosecution) and a directive role (getting the trial back on track). This choice is relevant to the theme of the new information and is consistent with the passage (as required by the question task). Thus, it is the "least wrong" of the four choices.**

C: No. This choice is too extreme; the passage does not indicate that prosecutorial misbehavior would invalidate the trial as a whole. This choice is also out of scope; the issue of calling a mistrial arises in neither the passage nor the question stem.

D: No. As in choice A, this is inconsistent with the author's claim that judges in the inquisitorial system must play an active role.

Type 10: Application—Analogy Questions

These questions ask you to take something described in the passage, abstract or generalize it, and then apply it to an entirely new situation. They differ from New Information questions in that the new information is in the answer choices, not in the question stem. They differ from Strengthen questions in that the new information in the correct choice will not make the original argument stronger than it already was. It will be similar to it in logic, but is likely to be on a different issue or subject matter.

These questions can be tricky, as all the answers at first glance may seem to have nothing to do with the passage. However, you are matching the logic or purpose of the author's argument, not the informational content of the passage. Therefore, the correct answer can match the logic of the passage (or relevant part of the passage) while still bringing in entirely new content.

Take, for example, a passage in which the author argues the following: "Weather is the result of a global interactive system. Therefore, to understand and predict the weather in a particular region, you must analyze how the climates of all regions interact with each other, and not limit your focus to the weather patterns in that region alone."

The question might ask:

- "Which of the following approaches to educational reform would most likely be advocated by a school board member following the same logic as the author of the passage?"

To answer this question, you must *first* generalize the author's own claims to create an abstracted model that could be applied to other situations. For example, you might say, "Large interactive systems cannot be understood by looking at the parts in isolation from the whole; you must understand how those parts relate to and affect each other," or, more simply, "the whole is more than the sum of its parts."

Now, take this generalized version into the answer choices, and look for a choice that has the same theme. The school board member might place the school system within the context of larger socioeconomic forces that also affect educational performance. Or, she might argue that the school itself is a large interactive system, and that you can't improve education by addressing only one piece of the puzzle (standardized testing, for example). As you can see, a wide variety of answer choices are possible. Don't waste time coming up with specific scenarios; generalize the passage's argument as much as possible, and then match each answer choice against that abstracted model.

Remember that the correct answer must depend solely on the content of the passage, not on outside information or your own opinion!

Sample Question 10:

10. The author's discussion of the history of systems of criminal procedure is most similar to which of the following?

A) A study of the transmission of infectious diseases
B) A proposal for civil rights reforms
C) An evolutionary biologist's study of plant species
D) An architect's blueprint

1) **Read the question word for word and identify the question type.**
The phrase "most similar to" tells you that this is an Analogy question.

2) **Translate the question into your own words: identify what the question task is asking you to do with the information in the passage.**
The question is asking you to describe the overall logic and purpose of the passage in order to match it to a similar logic and purpose (but, in a different subject area) in the correct answer.

3) **Identify any key words that refer to specific parts of the passage. If key words are provided, *go back to the passage* to locate that information.**
Because this question asks you to make an analogy to the author's overall logic and purpose in the passage as a whole, you don't necessarily need to go back the passage at this point; use your own articulation of the Bottom Line and your understanding of the logical structure of the passage as a guide.

4) **Answer in your own words: articulate what the correct answer will need to do, based on the question type and the information in the passage.**
The passage describes the historical evolution of criminal procedure: how private vengeance evolved into the adversarial system, which then evolved into the inquisitorial system. Therefore, you need an answer that has this theme of evolution or change over time.

5) **Use Process of Elimination (POE) to choose the *least wrong* answer choice.**
Keep in mind that all of the answer choices may be on different topics (i.e., not on criminal procedure). The correct choice will be the one that is most similar in logic to the author's overall argument in the passage. Be careful to eliminate choices that have the wrong tone (compared to the passage).

When you are down to two, pick the choice that has the most similarities to the passage. If one of the two remaining choices has one similarity, but the other remaining choice is similar in two ways, the latter choice will be the credited response.

4.4

Let's use POE on our sample answer choices.

A: No. First of all, this choice has a negative tone that does not match the passage. While the passage does describe how the adversarial system maintained some of the characteristics of private vengeance, the author doesn't use language suggesting it was "infected" (which has an overly negative tone) by the earlier system. Furthermore, this theme of transmission of a disease from one thing to another doesn't fit with the passage's theme of difference and contrast (between the adversarial and inquisitorial systems).

B: No. The tone of this choice does not match the tone and purpose of the passage. The author describes change over time, but does not recommend further change.

C: Yes. An evolutionary biologist studying plant species would look at change over time through the succession of species. This choice is most similar to the logic and purpose of the passage, and matches the tone reasonably well.

D: No. Compare this choice to choice C. While there are some aspects of a blueprint (describing the structure a system), there is no theme in this choice of change over time. Also, the author of the passage is describing structures themselves (that already exist) not plans for structures.

Now that we have looked at the ten question types in the Standard format, let's look at examples of the other two formats: EXCEPT/LEAST/NOT and Roman numeral questions.

EXCEPT/LEAST/NOT Questions

This question type can appear in combination with most of the question tasks described above. Because of its potentially confusing structure (looking for the worst instead of the best), students often misread or misapply the question. In fact, the correct answer to this question type can be the wacky or totally irrelevant answer choice that you are used to eliminating first.

To avoid making a mistake, use your noteboard. Write down the passage number (if you haven't already) and the number of the question. Next to the question number jot down a translation of the question, including what kind of choices you will be eliminating. Do this before looking at the answer choices. For example, in a Weaken EXCEPT question, write down

eliminate what weakens, pick what strengthens or does nothing.

Also jot down the four letters. As you assess each answer choice write "W" (for "yes this weakens") next to each choice that definitely weakens, cross it off on your noteboard, and then strike it out on the screen. If an answer does not appear to weaken, either leave it as is, or give it an "N" for "No, it does not weaken." At the end, you should have three "W"s and one "N" (or one with nothing written next to it). That is, it should look something like this:

1 ~~A~~ W
   Ⓑ N
   ~~C~~ W
   ~~D~~ W

Use notation for the wrong answers that is specific to the question type; for example "S" for "Strengthen" or "T" (for true) or "I" (for inference) for Inference questions.

Sample Question 11:

11. The author would be most likely to agree with all of the following statements EXCEPT:

A) the judge actively participates in the inquisitorial system.
B) the prosecutor in the adversarial system need not disclose evidence to the defense.
C) the inquisitorial system regularizes punitive combat.
D) the vengeance system was a system of self-help.

1) **Read the question word for word and identify the question type.**
   EXCEPT/LEAST/NOT questions are quite easy to recognize. Here, the key word is "EXCEPT." This is an Inference question ("The author would be most likely to agree") in EXCEPT/LEAST/ NOT format.

2) **Translate the question into your own words: identify what the question task is asking you to do with the information in the passage.**
   This question is asking you to eliminate the choices that are supported by the passage (that is, statements that the author of the passage would accept as true), and to pick the one that is most inconsistent with the author's argument.

3) **Identify any key words that refer to specific parts of the passage. If key words are provided,** *go back to the passage* **to locate that information.**
   In this question, there is no specific reference to the passage. You will need, however, to go back to the passage as you work through the answer choices. If the question had given you a specific reference (e.g., to "the police department"), you would go back to the passage and read above and below that reference before moving on to the next step.

4) **Answer in your own words: articulate what the correct answer will need to do, based on the question type and the information in the passage.**
   The correct choice will contradict the passage in some way. The incorrect answers will be consistent with the passage information as well as consistent with the author's tone and purpose.

5) **Use Process of Elimination (POE) to choose the** *least wrong* **answer choice.**
   As you might predict, the most common Attractor is the opposite: a choice that would be the correct answer to a Standard Format question. Approach EXCEPT/LEAST/NOT questions carefully and methodically to avoid falling into this (very annoying) trap. Keep in mind that your reasons for eliminating choices on a Standard question (e.g., language that is too extreme, or a statement that mixes up two different things in the passage) now become your reasons for keeping, and perhaps selecting, an answer.

Let's take a look at our answer choices.

A: No. This choice is directly supported by the end of paragraph 1.

B: No. This choice is supported by the discussion of pretrial discovery in paragraph 2. If the inquisitorial system is different in that it does require the prosecutor to disclose its evidence to the court (and so to the defense), the author would agree that the prosecutor need not disclose it under the adversarial system.

C: Yes. This is true of the adversarial, not the inquisitorial system (see the end of paragraph 1). This choice contradicts the passage; therefore, it is the credited response.

D: No. This choice is supported by the middle of paragraph 1.

Roman Numeral Questions

Like EXCEPT/LEAST/NOT questions, Roman numeral questions can appear in combination with a variety of question tasks.

To approach these questions, evaluate numeral I (unless it appears in all four choices, in which case it must be true). If it is not an appropriate answer to the question, strike out all of the choices that include it. If it *is* appropriate, eliminate the choices that do *not* include it. (If you are not sure about a numeral, leave it and look at the next numeral before eliminating any more answer choices.) Compare the choices you have left to each other. If numeral II or III appears in all of them, read it but don't overthink it. Unless there is something terribly wrong with it, it must also be true based on the combinations you have.

Sample Question 12:

12. According to the passage, which of the following is a duty of the prosecutor in the inquisitorial system?

    I.   To present evidence that may lead to the defendant's exoneration

    II.   To disclose all evidence in his/her possession

    III.   To assume a role that is both protective and directive

A) II only
B) III only
C) I and II only
D) I and III only

1) **Read the question word for word and identify the question type.**
    This is a Retrieval question ("According to the passage") in Roman numeral format.

2) **Translate the question into your own words: identify what the question task is asking you to do with the information in the passage.**
    The question is asking which of the three statements accurately represent things that are required of a prosecutor within the inquisitorial system.

3) **Identify any key words that refer to specific parts of the passage. If key words are provided,** *go back to the passage* **to locate that information.**

The inquisitorial system is described in paragraphs 2 and 3. Prosecutor's duties are specifically mentioned in the context of pretrial discovery, in the second half of paragraph 2 (after the word "additionally," and before the word "finally").

4) **Answer in your own words: articulate what the correct answer will need to do, based on the question type and the information in the passage.**

Prosecutors in the inquisitorial system must permit full disclosure of all evidence they have uncovered, even if that evidence would help the defense. They must also comply with all of the other rules of the inquisitorial system.

5) **Use Process of Elimination (POE) to choose the** *least wrong* **answer choice.**

In some ways, you are approaching the choices just as you would for a Standard question (in our Sample, a Retrieval task). For each numeral, ask yourself if this statement accomplishes the question task (here, if it describes a prosecutor's duty in the inquisitorial system).

However, you can also often use the combinations in the answer choices to your advantage. If, for example, you are sure that numeral I is supported, and unsure about numeral III, but no choice includes both I and III, you know that numeral III is in fact not supported (as it doesn't appear in any of the possible correct answer choices).

If you tend to miss Roman numeral questions, diagnose the most common reasons for your mistakes. If you tend to pick incomplete answers that are missing one or two numerals, you may be reading the numerals too quickly, picking only the ones that are the most obvious, and missing the more subtly supported statements. If you tend to pick choices that include too many, you may not be going back to the passage enough to check your answers carefully against the text.

Let's go through POE on our sample question item by item.

I: True. This statement is supported by the author's discussion of pretrial discovery in paragraph 2. Therefore, you can eliminate choices A and B, because neither includes Roman numeral I. You are now down to choices C and D. The difference between them is that choice C includes II but not III, and choice D includes III but not II. It is now a battle between choices II and III—only one of them can be correct!

II: True. This is also supported by the author's description of pretrial discovery. Note that you essentially have the correct answer at this stage, as there is no answer that includes all three numerals.

III: False. This is the role of the judge, not of the prosecutor (see the end of paragraph 2, after the word "finally").

So, your credited response is **choice C: I and II only.**

4.4

MCAT CRITICAL ANALYSIS AND REASONING SKILLS: QUESTION TYPES			
QUESTION TYPES AND STRATEGIES			
Question	Sample Wording	Strategy Tips	Common Types of Wrong Answers
1. Specific: Retrieval	"According to the passage, what is true of 'X'?" "The author states that 'X' is:"	• Go back to the passage before POE: find and paraphrase the relevant information. • Answer in your own words.	• uses similar language as passage but changes meaning • good answer to a question on a different passage topic or to a different question type • too strong to be supported by passage • relies too much on speculation or outside knowledge
2. Specific: Inference	"The passage implies/suggests/assumes that…" "Based on the passage, it is reasonable to conclude/infer which of the following regarding 'X'?" "With which of the following statements would the author be most likely to agree?"	• Go back to passage as soon as possible to find and paraphrase relevant information. • Answer in your own words.	
3. General: Main Point/ Primary Purpose	"Which of the following best expresses the main point of the passage?" "The author's primary purpose in the passage is to:"	• Use your Bottom Line, including author's tone.	• too narrow to represent the passage as a whole • too broad/goes beyond scope of the passage • too extreme • wrong tone • part right, part wrong
4. General: Overall Tone/ Attitude	"The author's apparent attitude toward 'X' can best be described as…"	• Use your Bottom Line. • Look for tone indicators you have highlighted in passage.	• positive or negative tone for a neutral passage • opposite tone (e.g., negative instead of positive) • too strong/extreme
5. Reasoning: Structure	"The author of the passage states 'X' in order to…" "The author's claim 'X' is based on evidence that:"	• Go back to the passage before POE. • Determine if the statement is a conclusion or evidence for a conclusion. • Pay attention to context of the cited statement.	• references wrong part of the author's argument • can be inferred from the passage, but doesn't describe logical structure

4.4

MCAT CRITICAL ANALYSIS AND REASONING SKILLS: QUESTION TYPES			
QUESTION TYPES AND STRATEGIES			
Question	Sample Wording	Strategy Tips	Common Types of Wrong Answers
6. Reasoning: Evaluate	"How well supported is the author's claim that 'X'?" "Which of the following represents a logical error in the passage?"	• Go back to the passage and find the cited claim. • Use your highlighting to help locate the support, if any, given for claim. • If question asks for an error or contradiction, go straight to POE and then back to the passage as needed.	• incorrectly describes logical structure of argument • opposite evaluation (e.g., strongly rather than weakly supported) • Part of the passage that is NOT flawed or self-contradictory (for question asking for a flaw)
7. Application: Strengthen	"Which of the following, if true, most strengthens/supports the passage author's argument?"	• Go back to the passage; find and paraphrase the relevant claim. • Define the necessary issue and direction (consistent or inconsistent with passage) of the correct choice.	• opposite • not relevant to cited claim • not strong enough to have a significant impact
8. Application: Weaken	"Which of the following statements, if true, most *weakens/ undermines/calls into question* the author's argument in the passage?"		
9. Application: New Information	"Elsewhere, the author of the passage states 'X.' Given the information in the passage, this is most likely due to:"	• Summarize theme of new info. • Define the relationship of new info to relevant parts of the passage/Bottom Line.	• not relevant to new info and/or the passage • relevant only to wrong part of passage • incorrectly describes the new information's impact on or relevance to the passage.
10. Application: Analogy	"Which of the following relationships is most similar to 'X' as it is described in the passage?"	• Go back to passage; define the theme or logic of the relevant part of the passage.	• similar content but different logic • incomplete match compared to other choices • reversal or opposite of passage logic

4.5 EXERCISE 1: IDENTIFYING QUESTION TYPES

Here are 10 sample questions. Read each question carefully, and identify the question type and format. Also think about what this question type is asking you to do.

4.5

1. The author lists the duties of City Council representatives in order to:

2. If it is shown to be true that only two species of egg-laying mammals exist, the author would most likely conclude that the platypus:

3. The passage suggests which of the following to be true of the Treaty of Versailles?

4. According to passage information, the Sahara Desert:

5. Which of the following claims, if true, would most *undermine* the author's contention that most environmental regulation is counterproductive?

6. Which of the following is most similar to Professor Bybee's experimental methodology?

7. By "quarantine" the author most likely means:

8. All of the following strengthen the author's claim that caps on jury awards should be lifted EXCEPT:

9. How well is the author's criticism of deconstructionist literary theory supported?

10. Which of the following claims is NOT supported by the author's argument in the passage?

Answers for CARS Exercise 1: Identifying Question Types

1. **Structure:** What role does this list play in the author's argument?
2. **New Information *Type 1*:** What would the author say is true about the platypus, based both on the new information and on the existing information in the passage?
3. **Inference:** Which statement about the Treaty of Versailles is best supported by information in the passage?
4. **Retrieval:** Which statement about the Sahara Desert is best supported by information in the passage?
5. **Weaken:** Which answer choice goes farthest to suggest that environmental regulation *is* productive?
6. **Analogy:** Which choice most describes the same kind of methodology or process as that used, according to the passage, by Bybee?
7. **Inference:** Which definition of quarantine best fits with the author's use of that word in the passage?
8. **Strengthen EXCEPT:** Which choice either weakens that claim (by indicating caps should not be lifted) or has no effect on that claim? *Eliminate* the choices that do suggest that caps should be lifted.
9. **Evaluate:** Is the author's criticism of deconstructionist literary theory strongly or weakly supported? If strongly, then how? If weakly, then what are the flaws in the argument?
10. **Inference/NOT:** Look for the answer that is least supported by the passage. *Eliminate* the choices that are most supported by the information presented in the passage.

4.6 EXERCISE 2: FOCUS ON QUESTION TYPES— PRACTICE PASSAGES

Once you have learned the basic approach to each question type, it is time to dig in and solidify your understanding of type-specific logic and approach. The passages in this exercise will help you to accomplish this as they are specialized to include only one or two questions types. On the real MCAT, passages will include a mix of different question types. However, practicing the different types in isolation is a useful exercise; as you work each passage below, keep your focus on the logic of each type. Don't rely on the heading to tell you the type; still read the question stem word for word, and think about what type corresponds to that wording and why. Translate the question, thinking about what it is really asking you to do. As you do POE, keep your focus on predicting Attractors, and on identifying them as they come up.

Do not do these passages timed. However, do work the passage efficiently, just as you would on a test, and focus on taking the most efficient route to the correct answer.

There are six passages in this exercise, followed by explanations for each one.

PASSAGE I: SPECIFIC—RETRIEVAL QUESTIONS

4.6

For as long as they have been inhabited, Shenandoah National Park lands have been subject to direct human change. Homesteads, farms, cattle pastures, and orchards dotted the slopes of the Blue Ridge until the National Park Service took possession of the lands in 1936, and, to use the landscape architect's term, obliterated almost all traces of human history. In recent decades, the official story of Shenandoah has been one of "re-creation," of a wilderness lost to human exploitation and then restored by natural processes. But nature alone did not re-create a lost wilderness. The National Park Service and the Civilian Conservation Corps created a landscape never before seen on the Blue Ridge, through fire suppression, road construction, wildlife protection, human removal, landscaping, and engineering. Through the various stages of acquiring park lands, establishing Shenandoah, and re-creating the landscape, park officials and supporters told a variety of stories that justified both the "preservation" and the transformation of the Blue Ridge Mountains. Throughout Shenandoah's history, stories and landscapes have re-created each other.

This history of storytelling and land management in Shenandoah National Park attempts to make a contribution to the broader study of environmental history. In unveiling evidence of significant human influence in Shenandoah, it suggests that the historiography of the national parks, while focusing on how parks preserve landscapes, continues to underemphasize how these places create new landscapes. This history highlights the dynamic relationship between stories about nature and the landscapes of a national park.

Shenandoah National Park has occupied an uncomfortable position in the history of the National Park Service. The master narrative of this history, exemplified by Alfred Runte's National Parks: The American Experience, describes a progression from parks designed to preserve natural wonders and scenic grandeur to ones designed to preserve representative environments from around the country. Runte treats Shenandoah as a "transition" between the two types of preservation in the park system. He argues Shenandoah "anticipated the ecological standards of the later twentieth century" but could only "approximate the visual standards of the national park idea as originally conceived." He defines Shenandoah as a marginalized follower to the "crown jewels" of the West.

The management of landscapes and the management of stories can be woven into a single history of Shenandoah. Land management in Shenandoah has been deeply influenced by the stories that park officials have told about nature and about appropriate human relations with the environment. At the same time, the official park narrative has always reflected the contemporary condition of the environment on the Blue Ridge. Stories about Shenandoah's nature lead to management practices that in turn lead to new stories. For the last seventy-five years, Shenandoah's landscape and story have changed and have changed each other.

Every park faces a tension between what it is and what it is supposed to be; otherwise management would be unnecessary. Parks can resolve this tension in two ways: rhetorically or materially. Supporters and officials can either argue that the park meets the relevant standards or that those standards ought to be changed to include the park. Or, park managers can materially change parklands so they approach the ideal landscape. This tension between ideal and reality has motivated the evolution of stories and land management in Shenandoah.

The history of Shenandoah began when the National Park Service first proposed a park in the Southern Appalachians in 1924. To those who suggested that no place in the East could meet standards for western parks, boosters retorted that eastern scenery had its own virtues. In 1936, the Virginia lobby celebrated their success at the dedication of Shenandoah National Park. In the decade that followed, Shenandoah attempted to transform the landscape into a model of Southern Appalachian wilderness. So successful were landscape architects in both executing and veiling their efforts that the following generation of park managers described Shenandoah's re-creation entirely in terms of natural processes. This re-creation narrative is the one that presently dominates the signs, guides, and histories of Shenandoah National Park. Only recently, as Shenandoah officials have found a renewed interest in the cultural history of their park, has the narrative of Shenandoah begun to again recognize the park's landscape as a collaboration between human and natural actors.

Material used in this particular passage has been adapted from the following source:

J. Reich, *"Re-Creating the Wilderness: Shaping Narratives and Landscapes in Shenandoah National Park"* © 2001 by Forest History Society and American Society for Environmental History.

1. According to the passage, why is park management necessary?

A) To navigate the tension between what a park is and what it should be
B) To protect and preserve that natural environment
C) To manage the re-creation processes
D) To prevent human destruction and encroachment

2. According to the author, what contribution can an understanding of land management at Shenandoah National Park make to a broader study of environmental history?

A) Emphasizing the importance of preservation in national parks
B) Drawing attention to the idea that national parks create new landscapes
C) Demonstrating that eastern parks can be just as beautiful as western parks
D) Encouraging more communities to engage with wildlife

3. According to the passage:

A) because of model preservation practices, Shenandoah National Park has remained a near-pristine monument to nature in Appalachia.
B) Shenandoah National Park serves as an excellent example of how stories about nature usurp the actual natural resources the stories were originally created about in the first place.
C) Shenandoah National Park is considered by many to be the crown jewel of the East.
D) there is a cyclical relationship between Shenandoah's lore and management practices.

4. The author mentions all of the following EXCEPT:

A) the acknowledgment of human as well as natural forces in shaping Shenandoah National Park is a more recent phenomenon.
B) fire prevention played an important role in shaping Shenandoah National Park.
C) land management of Shenandoah National Park has evolved over the decades.
D) Shenandoah National Park was preserved merely as a representative of Appalachian wilderness.

5. According to Alfred Runte, Shenandoah is:

A) a marginalized victim in the competition for the best representative landscape.
B) a transition between national parks intended to protect the wilderness, and parks designed as a paradigm.
C) an important contribution to the broader study of environmental land management.
D) an example of the relationship between stories about landscapes and the actual landscapes themselves.

4.6

PASSAGE II: SPECIFIC—INFERENCE QUESTIONS

4.6

The Migratory Bird Treaty Act (MBTA) is a strict liability statute that makes it "unlawful, at any time, by any means or in any manner, to pursue, hunt, take, capture, kill, attempt to take or capture any migratory bird, or any part, nest, or egg of any such bird." The Fish and Wildlife Service (FWS) has defined the scope of the term "take" to encompass "to pursue, hunt, shoot, wound, kill, trap, capture, or collect, or attempt to pursue, hunt, shoot, wound, kill, trap, capture, or collect." Unlike the Endangered Species Act, the MBTA does not provide for "incidental take" permits. Thus, the United States may prosecute for death or other "take" of migratory birds under the MBTA even if the take occurred as part of an activity conducted under a federal permit.

Courts in the Ninth Circuit have confirmed that the MBTA does not require an intent to kill, capture, or wound a bird; the fact of killing, wounding, or capturing by the defendant would suffice. As with other similar regulatory acts, where the penalties are small and there is no "grave harm to an offender's reputation," the Supreme Court has long recognized that a different standard applies to those federal criminal statutes that are essentially regulatory. Therefore, there is no requirement that proof be offered that a defendant specifically intended to violate the MBTA, or that the defendant was aware of the violation. Accordingly, the courts have upheld convictions under the MBTA for the deaths of birds caused by electric power line, pesticide application, oil sump pumps, and oil drilling equipment.

The scope of strict liability is not unlimited, but neither is it well-defined. The Ninth Circuit and the District of California courts have found that the reach of the MBTA is limited by the overlapping requirements for the government to prove causation in fact, proximate causation, and that the defendant had some reasonable knowledge of the potential for danger. Questions abound regarding what types of predicate acts—acts which lead to the MBTA's specifically prohibited acts—can constitute a crime. Conceptually, the constitutional challenge to the criminalization of these predicate acts can be placed under a rubric of notice or causation. The inquiries regarding whether a defendant was on notice that an innocuous predicate act would lead to a crime, and whether a defendant caused a crime in a legally meaningful sense, are analytically indistinct and go to the heart of due process constraints on criminal statutes. The Ninth Circuit noted and approved the attempts of one district court to limit the MBTA's reach by holding that the defendants must "proximately cause" the MBTA violation in order to be found guilty. Specifically, the court focused on whether the government had demonstrated "proximate causation" or "legal causation beyond a reasonable doubt" by showing that trapped birds are a reasonably anticipated or foreseeable consequence

of failing to cap an exhaust stack and cover access holes to the heater. Unfortunately, the courts have not fully defined how the concept of proximate cause would limit the scope of MBTA liability in the real world. Courts have speculated in dicta that some everyday activities like driving cars or piloting aircraft would not reasonably be linked to bird death, while other (more industrial or hazardous) activities like operating power lines or oil drilling equipment would. "Because the death of a protected bird is generally not a probable consequence of driving an automobile, piloting an aircraft, maintaining an office building, or living in a residential dwelling with a picture window, such activities would not normally result in liability under the provisions of proximate cause, even if such activities would/could cause the death of protected birds. Proper application of the law to an MBTA prosecution should not lead to absurd results." When the MBTA is stretched to criminalize predicate acts that could not have been reasonably foreseen to result in a proscribed effect on birds, the statute reaches its constitutional breaking point.

Recently, a case was brought to the Ninth Circuit court regarding an environmental project entitled "Borderlands" erected near the U.S./Mexico border in California. The U.S. Attorney is bringing suit under the provisions of the MBTA on the basis that the project, consisting of a high net fence (meant to dramatize the environmental and cultural effects of the border), both blocks the migration path of various bird species and presents a clear danger to the lives of the birds that might fly into the fence.

Material used in this particular passage has been adapted from the following source:

L. Standers, "*Liability and Causation in the Migratory Bird Treaty Act*" © 2011

1. The passage indicates that the MBTA:

A) entails harsher penalties for those who violate its provisions than does the Endangered Species Act.
B) is in some ways stricter than the Endangered Species Act in regard to the activities that are allowed or disallowed under its provisions.
C) was enacted in part because it was felt that the Endangered Species Act was not strict enough in its provisions.
D) controls the hunting, capturing, wounding, or killing of endangered bird species.

2. Which of the following best represents the relationship between a predicate act and a proximate cause, in the context of the author's discussion of the MBTA?

A) A predicate act is defined by the motives of the actors, while a proximate cause directly results in the relevant effects.
B) A predicate act is behavior that precedes the harm, while proximate causation is legal responsibility for the harmful act.
C) A predicate act is innocuous, while a proximate cause is harmful.
D) A predicate act, unlike a proximate cause, does not have a foreseeable negative effect.

3. The U.S. Attorney's suit against the "Borderlands" project would be least likely to succeed if:

A) it can be shown that it is probable that migratory birds would become trapped in the net and be harmed and/or die as a result.
B) it can be shown that the project was undertaken with the intent of mitigating the negative effects of industrial activity on the health of migratory birds.
C) it can be shown that the motion of the net in the high winds that predictably occur in the area of the project can reasonably be anticipated to break the eggs of migratory birds nesting nearby.
D) it can be shown that there was no foreseeable negative effect of the project on migratory birds.

4. The passage most supports which of the following conclusions?

A) Criminalizing predicate acts that cannot reasonably be predicted to result in harm to migratory birds has a negative effect on the legitimacy of other important regulatory measures.
B) Causation is more important in determining liability than whether or not an act is a proximate cause.
C) An activity that does cause the death of migratory birds but that can be considered a normal activity that does not normally pose a threat to birds should not be prosecuted.
D) An activity undertaken without the express intent of harming migratory birds should not be prosecuted.

4.6

5. The author indicates that which of the following would qualify as "taking" a migratory bird under the provisions of the MBTA?

    I.   Damaging its eggs
    II. Wounding its leg
    III. Capturing it with a net

A) I only
B) III only
C) II and III only
D) I, II, and III

6. It can be most reasonably concluded, based on the passage, that prosecution for breaking a regulatory statute:

A) is likely to occur even if permission for the action has been granted under an "incidental take" permit.
B) is unlikely, even if successful, to cause significant harm to the reputation of the offender.
C) can result in the offender being charged with a felony rather than a misdemeanor if the offense is serious enough.
D) is carried out by the Fish and Wildlife Service.

7. The passage suggests that the author most likely believes that:

A) the role of proximate causes in defining strict liability under a statute should be clearly defined.
B) the severity of punishment for violating a regulatory statute should take the level of intent to cause harm into account as a mitigating factor.
C) the MBTA should not be used to prosecute harmful actions that are not related to industrial activity.
D) the notion of strict liability is inappropriately applied within the provisions of the MBTA.

PASSAGE III: GENERAL—MAIN POINT, PRIMARY PURPOSE, AND TONE QUESTIONS

4.6

A child and a man were one day walking on the seashore when the child found a little shell and held it to his ear. Suddenly he heard sounds—strange, low, melodious sounds, as if the shell were remembering and repeating to itself the murmurs of its ocean home. The child's face filled with wonder as he listened. Then came the man, explaining that the pearly curves of the shell simply caught a multitude of sounds too faint for human ears, and filled the glimmering hollows with the murmur of innumerable echoes. It was not a new world, but only the unnoticed harmony of the old that had aroused the child's wonder.

Some such experience as this awaits us when we begin the study of literature, which has always two aspects, one of simple enjoyment and appreciation, the other of analysis and exact description. Let a little song appeal to the ear, or a noble book to the heart, and for the moment, at least, we discover a new world, a world so different from our own that it seems a place of dreams and magic. To enter and enjoy this new world, to love good books for their own sake, is the chief thing; to analyze and explain them is a less joyous but still an important matter.... We have now reached a point where we wish to understand as well as to enjoy literature; and the first step, since exact definition is impossible, is to determine some of its essential qualities.

The first significant thing is the essentially artistic quality of all literature. All art is the expression of life in forms of truth and beauty; or rather, it is the reflection of some truth and beauty which are in the world, but which remain unnoticed until brought to our attention by some sensitive human soul, just as the delicate curves of the shell reflect sounds and harmonies too faint to be otherwise noticed. A hundred men may pass a hayfield and see only the sweaty toil and the windrows of dried grass, but there is one who pauses by a meadow, where girls are making hay and singing as they work. He looks deeper, sees truth and beauty where we see only dead grass, and reflects what he sees in a little poem in which the hay tells its own story.

The second quality of literature is its suggestiveness, its appeal to our emotions and imagination rather than to our intellect. It is not so much what it says as what it awakens in us that constitutes its charm.... When Faustus in the presence of Helen asks, "Was this the face that launched a thousand ships?" he does not state a fact or expect an answer. He opens a door through which our imagination enters a new world, a world of music, love, beauty, heroism—the whole splendid world of Greek literature. Such magic is in words.... The province of all art is not to instruct but to delight.

The third characteristic of literature, arising directly from the other two, is its permanence. The world does not willingly let any beautiful thing perish. History records deeds, outward acts largely, but every great act springs from an ideal, and to understand this we must read literature, where we find ideals recorded. When we read a history of the Anglo-Saxons, for instance, we learn that they were sea rovers, pirates, explorers, great eaters and drinkers; and we know something of their hovels and habits, and the lands which they harried and plundered. All that is interesting, but it does not tell us what most we want to know about these old ancestors of ours—not only what they did, but what they thought and felt; how they looked on life and death; what they loved, what they feared, and what they reverenced. Then we turn from history to the literature which they themselves produced, and instantly we become acquainted. These hardy people were not simply fighters and freebooters; they were people like ourselves. Their emotions awaken instant response in the souls of their descendants.

It is so with any age or people. To understand them, we must read not simply their history, which records their deeds, but their literature, which records the dreams that made their deeds possible. So Aristotle was profoundly right when he said that "poetry is more serious and philosophical than history"; and Goethe, when he explained literature as "the humanization of the whole world."

Material used in this particular passage has been adapted from the following source:

W. Long, *English Literature: Its History and Its Significance for the Life of the English-Speaking World,* 1909.

1. What is the main idea of the passage?

A) Literature's permanence allows us to better understand our ancestors.
B) Literature has three fundamental qualities that must be debated by serious students of literature.
C) Literature, in the recording of ideals rather than deeds, tells us more about the past than history can.
D) Literature calls attention to aspects of the world that would otherwise escape our notice; it appeals to emotion above reason, and it enriches our understanding of the past.

2. Which of the following statements best describes the author's tone in the passage?

A) He is enthusiastic about literature and disparaging about history.
B) He expresses his belief in the superiority of English literature over that in other languages.
C) He believes that reading literature is not only pleasurable, but fundamentally important to culture.
D) He considers contemporary literature inferior to that of the past.

3. What is the purpose of the first paragraph of the passage?

A) To illustrate that, like literature, nature can appear mysterious to a person who has not learned how to "read" it
B) To provide an analogy introducing literature's ability to delight its reader through the discovery of subtle beauty in the world
C) To introduce the author's discussion of how literature teaches us about the lives of those who produced that literature
D) To illustrate, through a narrative, the appeal of narrative literature

4. The author most likely intended this passage to be read by:

A) literary critics.
B) students.
C) historians.
D) writers.

5. What is the central theme of the passage's third paragraph?

A) Literature renders nature capable of telling its own story.
B) It takes a true artist to be able to see beauty in quotidian work.
C) Literature does not just create truth and beauty, but exposes their presence in the world.
D) All art is ostensibly based on the natural world, whose beauty transcends what the average person sees in a cursory glance.

6. Which of the following statements best describes the author's feelings about the analysis of literature?

A) He believes that it is of equal importance to the pure enjoyment of literature.
B) He feels it diminishes the joy one experiences immediately when reading a work of literature.
C) He acknowledges that while it is not the primary aspect of the experience of reading literature, it is nonetheless important.
D) He feels that those who do not wish to analyze literature beyond the simple pleasure it induces are missing out on a fundamental purpose of reading.

4.6

PASSAGE IV: REASONING—STRUCTURE AND EVALUATE QUESTIONS

4.6

If you were writing a morality play about class privilege, you couldn't do better than to dream up a glamorous ship of fools and load it with everyone from the A-list to immigrants coming to America for a better life. The class issue is one major reason the Titanic disaster has always been so ripe for dramatization…. If the indignant depictions of the class system in so many Titanic dramas coexist uneasily with their adoring depictions of upper-crust privilege, that, too, is part of the appeal: it allows us to demonstrate our liberalism even as we indulge our consumerism. In [James] Cameron's movie, you root for the steerage passenger who improbably pauses, during a last dash for a boat, to make a sardonic comment about the band as it famously played on…but you're also happy to lounge with Kate Winslet on a sunbathed private promenade deck while a uniformed maid cleans up on her hands and knees after breakfast.

Like all ships, the Titanic was a "she," and Cameron went to some lengths to push the identification between the ship and the young woman. Both are, to all appearances, "maidens" who are en route to losing their virginity; both are presented as the beautiful objects of men's possessive adoration. "She's the largest moving object ever made by the hand of man in all of history," a smug Ismay boasts to some appreciative tablemates at lunch. Later, as Rose goes in to dinner, one of Cal's fat-cat friends commends him on his fiancée as if she, too, were a prized object: "Congratulations, Hockley—she's splendid!"

All the energy spent on the mechanics, the romance, the construction, the passenger list, the endless debates about what the Californian might have done and just how many people perished…has distracted from what may, in the end, be the most obvious thing about the Titanic's story: it uncannily replicates the structure and the themes of our most fundamental myths and oldest tragedies…. The forty-six-thousand-ton liner is just the latest in a long line of lovely girl victims, an archetype of vulnerable femininity that stands at the core of the Western literary tradition.

But the Titanic embodies another strain of tragedy. This is the drama of a flawed and self-destructive hero…. The ship starts out like Oedipus: admired, idolized, hailed as different, special, exalted. Sophocles' play [*Oedipus Rex*] derives its horrible excitement from a relentless exposition of its protagonist's fall from grace. Cameron… knew that there is an ancient theatrical pleasure… in watching something beautiful fall apart.

All this is why we keep watching Cameron's movie, and why we can't stop thinking about the Titanic. The tale irresistibly conflates two of the oldest archetypes in literature…. Perhaps the most unsettling item in the immense inventory of Titanic trivia is a novel called *Futility*, by an American writer named

Morgan Robertson…. As the title suggests, the themes of this work of fiction are the old ones: the vanity of human striving, divine punishment for overweening confidence in our technological achievement, the futility of human effort in a world ruled by indifferent nature. But the writing comes to life only when Robertson focuses on the mechanical details, as in the scene of the aftermath of the collision.

> Seventy-five thousand tons—dead-weight—rushing through the fog at the rate of fifty feet per second, had hurled itself at an iceberg…. She rose out of the sea, higher and higher—until the propellers in the stern were half exposed…. The holding-down bolts of twelve boilers and three triple-expansion engines, unintended to hold such weights from a perpendicular flooring, snapped, and down through a maze of ladders, gratings, and fore-and-after bulkheads came these giant masses of steel and iron, puncturing the sides of the ship….

Down to the most idiosyncratic detail, all this is familiar…. And yet it couldn't be. Robertson published his book in 1898, fourteen years before the Titanic sailed. If she continues to haunt our imagination, it's because we were dreaming her long before the fresh spring afternoon when she turned her bows westward and, for the first time, headed toward the open sea.

Material used in this particular passage has been adapted from the following source:

D. Mendelsohn, *"Unsinkable: Why we can't let go of the Titanic,"* The New Yorker, April 16, 2012. © 2012 by Condé Nast.

1. Which of the following best describes the progression of ideas in this passage?

A) The author presents some reasons why the story of the Titanic is so compelling, and then argues that these reasons obscure the real meaning of the 1912 disaster.

B) The author discusses several interpretations of the Titanic story, and then suggests that Cameron's is the most compelling.

C) The author notes that the Titanic is a story of class privilege as well as that of an archetypal feminine vulnerability; he then moves on to suggest that it is compelling because the story has tragic themes that are among the oldest in Western literature.

D) The author notes several historical interpretations of the Titanic, and then suggests they are all undermined by Robertson's anticipation of the tragedy in his novel.

2. The author provides two quotations from Cameron's film in paragraph 2 in order to:

A) indicate that women should not be considered property.
B) express views, common at the time of the Titanic but out of fashion now, that women were little more than objects to be adored and possessed by men.
C) illustrate the similar terms by which the ship and Rose are defined.
D) give an example of Cameron's genius in film direction.

3. The author's claim that the Titanic "is the drama of a flawed and self-destructive hero" is:

A) undermined by the comparison with Oedipus.
B) not supported by any evidence in the passage.
C) supported by his claim that the ship is "an archetype of vulnerable femininity that stands at the core of the Western literary tradition."
D) supported with a reference to a play.

4. The author provides a passage from Robertson's novel primarily in order to:

A) demonstrate Robertson's skill at rendering a depiction of the fateful events leading to the Titanic's sinking.
B) note the uncanny resemblance of Robertson's prose to the story of the Titanic.
C) indicate some of the themes of Robertson's text.
D) give an example of the pleasure found in watching something beautiful fall apart.

5. The author's claim in paragraph 1 that the Titanic story "allows us to demonstrate our liberalism even as we indulge our consumerism" is best supported in the passage by:

A) the preponderance of sardonic treatments of the class issue in many interpretations of the story.
B) reference to conflicting responses the viewer of Cameron's film experiences.
C) the discussion in paragraph 2 about the parallels between the ship and Rose.
D) nothing; this is a claim made without evidence.

6. The author's claim that the story of the Titanic "conflates two of the oldest archetypes in literature" is:

A) weak: he does not indicate what either of these archetypes are.
B) strong: the paragraphs preceding this claim provide evidence supporting it.
C) weak: the author cannot claim to know what the oldest archetypes in Western literature are.
D) strong: the author supports this claim through his discussion of consumerism.

7. The author's claim that the Titanic was "admired, idolized, hailed as different, special, [and] exalted" in its time (paragraph 4) is supported by evidence in the passage about the ship's:

A) unique mechanical system.
B) absence of lower-class passengers.
C) size.
D) elaborate décor.

8. The author suggests that the viewer of Cameron's film is "happy to lounge with Kate Winslet on a sunbathed private promenade deck" in order to:

A) highlight an instance when we are tempted to indulge in upper-class fantasy even while we otherwise scorn the unfairness of the class system.
B) indicate the universal allure of Cameron's film's female protagonist.
C) criticize our hypocrisy in both appreciating and denouncing privilege.
D) express his approval of Cameron's directorial choices.

9. The author notes that the Titanic was a "she" in order to:

A) remark upon this eccentricity of assigning a gender to inanimate objects, unique to Cameron's interpretation.
B) question why all ships are assigned the feminine pronoun.
C) set up another argument for why the Titanic endures in our collective imagination.
D) indicate the sexism pervasive in the era in which the Titanic sailed.

PASSAGE V: APPLICATION—STRENGTHEN AND WEAKEN QUESTIONS

4.6

In ordinary community life, in which individuals depend on one another and yet remain divided by different interests and passions, courtesy creates possibilities for cooperation by offering an artificial code of behavior. Genuine respect and mutual affection are not required for the "false friendships" of polite society to form; courtesy offers social coordination and civil peace so long as everyone simply agrees to be well-mannered. This offer is widely accepted, in part, because most individuals are capable of only appearing to live up to community ideals. The opportunity for polite pretense is valuable in a world where people strive to keep up appearances because it permits everyone "to be better than they might be" by giving them a chance to pretend to be better than they are.

Courtesy and law are often connected in terms of symbiosis: manners mavens and legal professionals alike both argue that courtesy and law work together to maintain communal harmony. In this vein, for example, Justice Ruth Bader Ginsburg has called on fellow Supreme Court judges to avoid intemperate and abrasive language in their opinions (and especially in their dissents) in order to promote the judiciary's capacity and standing as an authoritative, dispute-resolving institution. It is by speaking in a polite "judicial voice" that courts may become more effective at performing their official duties.

Although the symbiotic view has its merits, my approach to the relationship between courtesy and law is somewhat different. Rather than examining how courtesy and law may work in combination, I wish to explore what the functioning of courtesy can tell us about the function of law. Unlike Justice Ginsburg, I do not intend to consider how the judicial voice can be made more decorous; instead, I plan to assess the ways in which judicial action may itself be a form of decorum.

To see how the dynamics that drive courtesy may also be at work in the judicial process, we should first, for the sake of analysis, accede to the proposition that the same understanding of human nature out of which courtesy grows also provides the context in which law must function. That is, we should accept, as a working premise, that differences between individuals are significant and irreducible; thus we should view disagreements as an obstinate fact of community life, never to be fully overcome but only to be more or less successfully managed. Moreover, we should accept that humans are governed by an inextricable mix of high principle and low passion. As a result, we should stipulate that most people take public moral standards seriously yet remain too filled with ambition and vanity to actually practice what they preach.

I recommend this somewhat pessimistic view of human nature, along with the understanding of courtesy that flows from it, as a way of explaining how the American judicial process works. I do not claim that this view of human nature perfectly represents how people are, nor do I claim that courtesy and law are identical. My claim is instead that an analytical model built on these ideas serves the purpose of explanation by generating new insights into how the rule of law currently operates.

What, then, does courtesy tell us about law? To begin to develop an answer to this question, consider that law, like courtesy, has often been thought to fulfill a facilitating function. A number of scholars have argued that courts effectively manage disputes by pursuing acceptable settlements without altering the fundamental factors that generate the disputes in the first place. Law, on this understanding, is an artificial medium in which otherwise opposed parties may jointly find ways of moving on.

A leading example of such thinking can be found in the classic discussion of legal reasoning by Lief Carter and Thomas Burke. Carter and Burke argue that the rule of law, in its essence, is a matter of requiring people to "look outside [their] own will for criteria of judgment." Whatever the specific features of a given political order may be, the rule of law directs individuals to adopt independent, publicly shared principles outside the sphere of personal attachments and private beliefs. Highly charged conflicts will certainly tempt people to evaluate competing claims by their own feelings and convictions. But the rule of law asks us to push beyond individual preferences....

According to Carter and Burke, one great advantage of having such independent standards of governance is that they create a highly useful language of dispute management for the courts. The rule of law sets aside the "dramatic and emotional work of poetics and theatrics" and commits the judiciary to "the logic of ideas." Unlike the world of electoral politics, in which "smart participants know that they should obfuscate, change the subject, [and] hurl mud" to achieve their goals, the rule of law requires judges to work out their arguments openly and to furnish reasons for their rulings. It is a deliberate process that relies on "elaborate mechanisms for sequencing questions" and structured frameworks that dictate how each sequenced question is to be addressed. The payoff of such "slow and steady (and often boring)" legal procedures is that they help broker community peace, channeling hotly contested questions into a forum in which they can be more easily handled.

Material used in this particular passage has been adapted from the following source:
K. Bybee, *All Judges Are Political Except When They Are Not*
© 2010 by Stanford University Press.

1. Which of the following, if true, would most challenge Justice Ginsburg's argument that judges should "avoid intemperate and abrasive language in their opinions"?

A) Some legal experts argue that the fact that few, other than legal experts, are aware of the specific nature of judicial decisions suggests that the language used in those decisions has little effect on public perceptions regarding the judiciary.

B) Professionals are especially sensitive to criticism by others in their own field, which can lead to defensiveness and unwillingness to cooperate in the future.

C) Moderation is often perceived as an indication of weakness and indecision.

D) Courtesy and law function in qualitatively different ways in society, and no relevant analogy can be drawn between them.

2. Which of the following statements, if true, would go the furthest in validating the contrast drawn in the last paragraph between the rule of law and electoral politics?

A) Candidates for office often achieve success by sticking tightly to pre-scripted talking points and repeating them by rote rather than by engaging in authentic discussion and debate.

B) Laws requiring candidates to divulge all sources of campaign donations have contributed to a healthy transparency and openness in the electoral process.

C) The level of public interest in an electoral campaign often turns on how many hotly contested issues are matters of public debate at the time.

D) Candidates for office who project a friendly and accessible image are often the most successful.

3. Which of the following, if true, would most undermine the author's suggestion that courtesy is valuable largely because it allows people to appear to be better than they really are?

A) Polite pretense, when obviously inauthentic to an extreme, can have the effect of increasing social tensions, but the effect is usually temporary.

B) The belief that aggression and dominance are prized over all other characteristics in a competitive, free-market economy is for the most part false.

C) When a person pretends for any length of time to live by certain values that he or she does not in fact hold, that person usually begins to actually believe in and live by those values.

D) Human beings do sometimes act selflessly, putting aside their own ambitions and vanity.

4. Which of the following statements, if true, would most weaken the author's central argument?

A) Human beings do sincerely value cooperation and wish, for the most part, to act in the interests of the community rather than for their own good alone.

B) Statistical studies show no correlation over the last 100 years between the level of open hostility and discourteous behavior amongst Supreme Court judges and those judges' capacity to effectively perform their judicial functions.

C) The structure provided by the rule of law allows people to compromise somewhat on their own goals and preferences without feeling that they are being taken advantage of by other individuals.

D) The facilitating function performed by the rule of law arises only when and because the existence of a stable legal structure allows community members to come to equate their own interests with those of the community; self-interest becomes one with group-interest.

5. Which of the following statements, if true, would most support the author's central argument?

A) Many studies of human decision-making have shown that fear of being taken advantage of often leads people to make choices that lead to a less-than-optimal outcome for all involved.

B) Many studies of human decision-making show that people are more highly motivated by the fear of losing than by the hope of winning.

C) Many studies in behavioral psychology show that the more time people have to consider a conflict, the more able they are to put aside emotion and consider perspectives other than their own.

D) Many psychological studies have shown that when people are bored and impatient, they often make choices based on emotion rather than on rational consideration of the pros and cons of different possible decision paths.

6. Which of the following, if true, would least weaken Carter and Burke's contention that the rule of law excludes "poetics and theatrics" from the business of the courts?

A) Legal language is often convoluted and dry due to the goal of removing any room for ambiguity, emotion, or unnecessary debate over semantics.

B) The power of the courtroom is based in large part on the ritualistic and performative aspects of a trial, rather than on the intellectual basis for those legal processes.

C) Jury members are much more likely to be swayed by appeals to the emotions of either sympathy or anger than by arguments based on the letter of the law.

D) The influence of television has led judges at all levels to base their rulings more on popular expectations of a shocking and dramatic outcome than on traditionally accepted legal rules and procedures.

4.6

PASSAGE VI: APPLICATION—NEW INFORMATION AND ANALOGY QUESTIONS

4.6

The historical roots of the civic community are astonishingly deep. Enduring traditions of civic involvement and social solidarity can be traced back nearly a millennium to the eleventh century, when communal republics were established in places like Florence, Bologna, and Genoa, exactly the communities that today enjoy civic engagement and successful government. At the core of this civic heritage are rich networks of organized reciprocity and civic solidarity—guilds, religious fraternities, and tower societies for self-defense in the medieval communes; cooperatives, mutual aid societies, neighborhood associations, and choral societies in the twentieth century.

These communities did not become civic simply because they were rich. The historical record strongly suggests precisely the opposite: They have become rich because they were civic. The social capital embodied in norms and networks of civic engagement seems to be a precondition for economic development, as well as for effective government. Development economists take note: Civics matters.

How does social capital undergird good government and economic progress? First, networks of civic engagement foster sturdy norms of generalized reciprocity: I'll do this for you now, in the expectation that down the road you or someone else will return the favor. "Social capital is akin to what Tom Wolfe called the 'favor bank' in his novel, *The Bonfire of the Vanities*, notes economist Robert Frank. A society that relies on generalized reciprocity is more efficient than a distrustful society.

Networks of civic engagement also facilitate coordination and communication and amplify information about the trustworthiness of other individuals. Students of prisoners' dilemmas and related games report that cooperation is most easily sustained through repeat play. When economic and political dealing is embedded in dense networks of social interaction, incentives for opportunism and malfeasance are reduced. This is why the diamond trade, with its extreme possibilities for fraud, is concentrated within close-knit ethnic enclaves. Dense social ties facilitate gossip and other valuable ways of cultivating reputation—an essential foundation for trust in a complex society.

Finally, networks of civic engagement embody past success at collaboration, which can serve as a cultural template for future collaboration. The civic traditions of north central Italy provide a historical repertoire of forms of cooperation that, having proved their worth in the past, are available to citizens for addressing new problems of collective action.

Sociologist James Coleman concludes, "Like other forms of capital, social capital is productive, making possible the achievement of certain ends that would not be attainable in its absence…. In a farming community…where one farmer gets his hay baled by another and where farm tools are extensively borrowed and lent, the social capital allows each farmer to get his work done with less physical capital in the form of tools and equipment." Social capital, in short, enables Hume's farmers to surmount their dilemma of collective action.

Stocks of social capital, such as trust, norms, and networks, tend to be self-reinforcing and cumulative. Successful collaboration in one endeavor builds connections and trust—social assets that facilitate future collaboration in other, unrelated tasks. As with conventional capital, those who have social capital tend to accumulate more: "them as has, gets." Social capital is what the social philosopher Albert O. Hirschman calls a "moral resource," that is, a resource whose supply increases rather than decreases through use and which (unlike physical capital) becomes depleted if not used.

Like other public goods, from clean air to safe streets, social capital tends to be underprovided by private agents. This means that social capital must often be a byproduct of other social activities. Social capital typically consists in ties, norms, and trust transferable from one social setting to another. Members of Florentine choral societies participate because they like to sing, not because their participation strengthens the Tuscan social fabric. But it does.

Material used in this particular passage has been adapted from the following source:

R. Putnam, *"The Prosperous Community"* © 1993 by *The American Prospect.*

1. Which of the following scenarios most closely demonstrates the logic of reciprocity, as described in the passage?

A) A diamond trader who pays fair prices for crude diamond ore
B) A free babysitting collective in which each parent participates in watching each other's children
C) A government that subsidizes health care and education using taxpayer money
D) A couple that signs a prenuptial agreement before their wedding

2. Which of the following is the most analogous to the relationship described by the author in the second paragraph?

A) Employees at small start-up companies often engage in after-hours collaborations and events outside of work in order to facilitate team-building and efficiency long before their companies become profitable.
B) Private universities with the largest endowments also boast the most student involvement in the academic community.
C) The wealthiest citizens are responsible for the largest private donations to charitable and community. organizations, especially to those involved in the arts.
D) Large stock market investments tend to make the most money, and, as this money is re-invested, it generates even more money.

3. Which of the following is most analogous to social capital, as it is described in the passage?

A) In long-term relationships, passionate love declines gradually as companionate love increases.
B) Positive reinforcement from peers is often more effective than parental punishment in moderating adolescent behavior.
C) Because heat is generated by electricity, electrical circuits will automatically shut down when the heat reaches a certain threshold.
D) As the temperature rises, permafrost begins to thaw, releasing carbon dioxide and methane gases into the atmosphere, which further increases the temperature.

4. Which of the following would be LEAST comparable to a network of civic engagement, as it is described in paragraph 4?

A) Businesses that are run entirely by family networks are most successful.
B) Olympic teams composed of individuals from all over the country who have not played together before tend to require much more practice than teams that have played together for years.
C) Individual consultants are routinely shuffled into new teams in order to maximize performance.
D) Prisoners tend do best when their cell mates and security personnel remain consistent.

5. Which of the following is most analogous to Florentine choral societies, as they are portrayed by the author?

A) Children who stay after school to receive tutoring in social studies, English, and math
B) Men drafted into military service during times of war
C) Community members forming a Neighborhood Watch group in an effort to reduce crime and make the neighborhood safer
D) People participating in amateur sports clubs in their free time

6. Which of the following claims made in the passage would be most strengthened by data showing a strong positive correlation between the number of Boy Scout and Girl Scout troops in a community and median income?

A) "The historical roots of the civic community are astonishingly deep."
B) "The social capital embodied in norms and networks of civic engagement seems to be a precondition for economic development."
C) "Networks of civic engagement also facilitate coordination and communication and amplify information about the trustworthiness of other individuals."
D) "Successful collaboration in one endeavor builds connections and trust—social assets that facilitate future collaboration in other, unrelated tasks."

4.6

7. Suppose that the gossip fostered by modern-day social media networks has been shown to cultivate more mistrust, bullying, and sullied reputations. Which of the following claims made in the passage is most undermined by this information?

A) Social networks are essential for effective democracy.
B) Distrustful societies are less efficient than societies built on trust.
C) Trust and repute are cultivated by gossip.
D) None; the information provided is not applicable to the information about civic engagement in the passage.

4.6

8. In the past three decades, the number of Americans who attend public meetings or political rallies has radically decreased, to less than ten percent of the total population. What might the author of this passage suggest as a possible outcome of this decline?

A) More organized protests
B) Slowing of economic progress
C) Heightened sociocultural awareness
D) Increased participation in other activities

9. If religion is the most common associational membership among people in various societies today, what is most likely true, based on the passage?

A) Government continues to rely on religion, and vice versa.
B) Active members of a religion have more social capital than those who are not religious.
C) Religious affiliation serves as a venue for modern-day civic engagement.
D) Places of worship enjoy an economic boost from high membership.

EXPLANATIONS

Passage I: Specific—Retrieval Questions

Question Type Strategies

Retrieval questions test your ability to locate and paraphrase information in the passage. Pick the answer that is best supported by the relevant part of the text. Look out for wrong answers that are supported by the passage but that are not relevant to the specific reference in the question stem, that use words from the passage out of context, or that rely on outside knowledge.

4.6

1. **A**   This is a Retrieval question.

    The term "land management" is used in several places in the passage, so it is important to narrow in on the place where the author also explains why it is necessary. In paragraph 5, the passage states: "Every park faces a tension between what it is and what it is supposed to be; otherwise management would be unnecessary.... This tension between ideal and reality has motivated the evolution of stories and land management in Shenandoah." Therefore, land management is necessary because of the tension between what a park is and what it should be.

    A: Yes. This choice is most supported by the information in paragraph 5.

    B: No. This is an "outside knowledge" Attractor; most people probably consider land management to serve this function for national parks, but this is not supported by the passage.

    C: No. The term "re-creation" is used frequently in the passage, but the author does not suggest that land management is specifically necessary for re-creation.

    D: No. This is an "outside knowledge" Attractor; most people probably consider land management to serve this function for national parks, but this is not supported by the passage.

2. **B**   This is a Retrieval question.

    In paragraph 2, the passage states: "This history of storytelling and land management in Shenandoah National Park attempts to make a contribution to the broader study of environmental history. In unveiling evidence of significant human influence in Shenandoah, it suggests that the historiography of the national parks, while focusing on how parks preserve landscapes, continues to underemphasize how these places create new landscapes. This history highlights the dynamic relationship between stories about nature and the landscapes of a national park."

    A: No. This is an "outside knowledge" Attractor; the importance of preservation is not the contribution to a broader study of environmental history.

    B: Yes. This choice is most closely supported by the information in paragraph 2.

    C: No. While this choice is supported in the final paragraph, it is not the contribution to a broader study of environmental history. This is the right answer to the wrong question.

    D: No. This choice is outside the scope of the passage and relies on outside knowledge.

4.6

3. **D**   This is a Retrieval question.

     The question stem does not provide any useful information. Therefore, translate each answer choice and determine if it is supported by information in the passage.

     A: No. The passage does not suggest that the preservation practices at Shenandoah National Park were "model," nor does it suggest that Shenandoah National Park is a "near-pristine monument to nature in Appalachia."

     B: No. The passage does not suggest that the stories about nature usurp or surpass the actual natural resources. Instead, the passage states: "Shenandoah's landscape and story have changed and have changed each other" (paragraph 4).

     C: No. This answer uses words taken out of context; the passage states: "He defines Shenandoah as a marginalized follower to the 'crown jewels' of the West" (paragraph 3). Therefore, this choice is not supported by the passage.

     D: **Yes. The passage states: "Stories about Shenandoah's nature lead to management practices that in turn lead to new stories" (paragraph 4). Therefore this choice is most directly supported by the passage.**

4. **D**   This is a Retrieval question in EXCEPT/LEAST/NOT format.

     The question stem does not provide much useful information. So, translate each answer choice and determine if it is mentioned in the passage.

     A: No. The final paragraph states: "Only recently, as Shenandoah officials have found a renewed interest in the cultural history of their park, has the narrative of Shenandoah begun to again recognize the park's landscape as a collaboration between human and natural actors." The recent acknowledgment of human forces is mentioned in the passage, so this is not the correct choice.

     B: No. The first paragraph states: "The National Park Service and the Civilian Conservation Corps created a landscape never before seen on the Blue Ridge, through fire suppression, road construction, wildlife protection, human removal, landscaping, and engineering." Therefore, fire prevention is mentioned as playing a role in shaping Shenandoah, and this is not the correct choice.

     C: No. This passage describes how land management has evolved over the decades; therefore this is not the correct choice.

     D: **Yes. The passage never mentions that Shenandoah was preserved merely as a representative of Appalachian wilderness. This, therefore, is the best choice for an EXCEPT/LEAST/NOT Retrieval question.**

5. **B**   This is a Retrieval question.

     The question is asking you specifically about Alfred Runte's take on Shenandoah; the third paragraph of this passage contains all the information that you need in order to answer this question. In the paragraph, it states there is a: "...progression from parks designed to preserve natural wonders and scenic grandeur to ones designed to preserve representative environments from around the country. Runte treats Shenandoah as a 'transition' between the two types of preservation in the park system." The best answer choice should describe this idea of transition.

     A: No. This choice is too extreme ("marginalized victim" is not in line with the passage's tone), and does not reflect Runte's description of Shenandoah; be careful not to seize on an answer simply because one word in it rings true with the passage: Runte says Shenandoah is "marginalized" but not that it is a "victim."

     B: **Yes. This choice summarizes Runte's sentiment about Shenandoah; this choice is best supported by paragraph 3.**

C: No. The contribution to the broader study of land management is described in paragraph 2, not paragraph 3. This choice, while supported by the passage, does not answer the question being asked about Runte.

D: No. This is an example of a "right answer to the wrong question" response because the information in this choice appears in the passage, but not in paragraph 3. It is mentioned at the end of paragraph 2 in a different context: "This history highlights the dynamic relationship between stories about nature and the landscapes of a national park." This idea also appears at the ends of paragraphs 4 and 5, but again, not in the context of Runte's argument.

Passage II: Specific—Inference Questions

Question Type Strategies

When attacking Inference questions, choose the answer choice that is best supported by the passage. The correct answer may be more or less stated in the text (there is no such thing as being "too close to the passage" to qualify as a correct answer for this question type). More commonly, however, the answer is not directly stated, but there is direct evidence supporting it in the passage. Occasionally, it will seem like the correct answer is a bit too much of a stretch from the passage, but, if it is better supported than the other three choices, it is the "least wrong" answer (i.e., the credited response). In particular, look out for wrong answers that are too extreme, that take words from the passage out of context, or that are supported by the passage but do not respond to the specific issue cited in the question stem.

1. **B** This is an Inference question.

   A: No. The only mention of the Endangered Species Act is in paragraph 1, and there is no direct discussion of what penalties it entails. Although the author's discussion in paragraph 2 of penalties for violations of regulatory measures may apply to the Endangered Species Act, there is no indication that those penalties are less severe than for violations of the MBTA.

   B: **Yes. In the first paragraph the author writes: "Unlike the Endangered Species Act, the MBTA does not provide for 'incidental take' permits. Thus, the United States may prosecute for death or other 'take' of migratory birds under the MBTA even if the take occurred as part of an activity conducted under a federal permit." Therefore, you can infer that the Endangered Species Act, unlike the MBTA, does allow for "incidental take" permits, and that it is in at least that way less strict. Note the moderate wording of the choice ("in some ways").**

   C: No. While the MBTA is in at least one way stricter than the Endangered Species Act (paragraph 1), the author never discusses the motivations for enacting the MBTA. This choice is out of scope and too extreme.

   D: No. This choice is half-right but half-wrong. While those activities are in fact controlled, they are controlled specifically for migratory birds, and the passage does not suggest that migratory birds are endangered.

2. **B**   This is an Inference question.

Predicate acts and proximate causes are discussed in paragraph 3. The author writes: "Questions abound regarding what types of predicate acts—acts which lead to the MBTA's specifically prohibited acts—can constitute a crime.… The Ninth Circuit noted and approved the attempts of one district court to limit the MBTA's reach by holding that the defendants must 'proximately cause' the MBTA violation in order to be found guilty. Specifically, the court focused on whether the government had demonstrated 'proximate causation' or 'legal causation beyond a reasonable doubt' by showing that trapped birds are a reasonably anticipated or foreseeable consequence of failing to cap an exhaust stack and cover access holes to the heater." By going back to this part of the passage before doing POE, you would know that predicate acts lead up to the harm, while proximate cause is legal responsibility for the harm.

A: No. This choice is half-right, half-wrong. There is no suggestion that the definition of predicate acts takes motivation into account. In fact, at least under the MBTA, motive is not a relevant factor in defining liability (paragraph 2).

B: Yes. Both parts of this answer choice correspond to the author's discussion in the passage (see explanation in the note above).

C: No. This choice takes words out of context, making the first half too extreme. For that reason the choice is half-right but half-wrong. While the author states in paragraph 3 that the "inquiries regarding whether a defendant was on notice that an innocuous predicate act would lead to a crime, and whether a defendant caused a crime in a legally meaningful sense, are analytically indistinct," she is not suggesting that all predicate acts are innocuous or harmless.

D: No. Neither term is defined by the predictability of harm. Rather, they are defined by their relative proximity to actual harm. This choice takes words out of the context of the passage.

3. **D**   This is an Inference question.

A: No. The passage suggests just the opposite. The author writes in paragraph 3 that "The Ninth Circuit noted and approved the attempts of one district court to limit the MBTA's reach by holding that the defendants must '"proximately cause"' the MBTA violation in order to be found guilty. Specifically, the court focused on whether the government had demonstrated '"proximate causation"' or '"legal causation beyond a reasonable doubt"' by showing that trapped birds are a reasonably anticipated or foreseeable consequence of failing to cap an exhaust stack and cover access holes to the heater." This indicates that a case showing proximate causation would likely succeed in the Ninth Circuit court.

B: No. The passage suggests that motivation, good or bad, is not a relevant factor in proving liability under the MBTA (paragraph 2). Therefore, this would make it neither more nor less likely that the suit would succeed.

C: No. First, the effect on the eggs of migratory birds is a relevant factor (see the definition of "take" in paragraph 1). Second, if a negative result is foreseeable, this would make the suit more, not less, likely to succeed (paragraph 2).

D: Yes. This choice is the opposite of choices A and C. According to paragraph 3, foreseeability of the harm is a major factor in the likely success of a suit under the provisions of the MBTA. If there is no predictable harm, the suit is not likely to succeed.

4. **C**   This is an Inference question.

    A: No. While this choice would strengthen the author's argument at the end of paragraph 3, it cannot be inferred from the passage: it is too extreme and out of scope. Make sure to determine if the question is asking you to support the passage (a Strengthen question), or what is supported by the passage (an Inference question).

    B: No. It is unclear in the passage what the relationship between "causation in fact" and "proximate" causation are. (The author writes in paragraph 3 that "the reach of the MBTA is limited by the overlapping requirements for the government to prove causation in fact, proximate causation, and that the defendant had some reasonable knowledge of the potential for danger.") There is no suggestion that one is or should be more important than the other in determining liability.

    C: Yes. At the end of paragraph 3, the author discusses activities that "would not normally result in liability under the provisions of proximate cause, even if such activities would/could cause the death of protected birds." The author goes on to argue that "proper application of the law to an MBTA prosecution should not lead to absurd results. When the MBTA is stretched to criminalize predicate acts that could not have been reasonably foreseen to result in a proscribed effect on birds, the statute reaches its constitutional breaking point."

    D: No. Paragraph 2 discusses how intent is not a relevant factor in determining liability under the MBTA; the author does not express any disagreement with this.

5. **D**   This is an Inference question in the Roman numeral format.

    The first step in answering this question should be to go back to paragraph 1, where the passage states that "The Migratory Bird Treaty Act (MBTA) is a strict liability statute that makes it 'unlawful, at any time, by any means or in any manner, to pursue, hunt, take, capture, kill, attempt to take or capture any migratory bird, or any part, nest, or egg of any such bird.' The Fish and Wildlife Service (FWS) has defined the scope of the term 'take' to encompass 'to pursue, hunt, shoot, wound, kill, trap, capture, or collect, or attempt to pursue, hunt, shoot, wound, kill, trap, capture, or collect.' Under this statute, any person, association, partnership, or corporation is guilty of a misdemeanor if they violate any provisions of the Act." Any item that would (1) be covered by the MBTA and (2) qualify as a "take" by this definition must be included in the correct answer.

    Numeral I: True. The MBTA covers "any part, nest, or egg of any such bird," and damage to eggs could reasonably be considered a "wound." While this may not be an intuitively obvious definition of "take," it is supported by the passage.

    Numeral II: True. The MBTA covers "any part, nest, or egg of any such bird," and "take" includes wounding. As with item I, while this may not be an intuitively obvious definition of "take," it is supported by the passage.

    Numeral III: True. The MBTA covers capturing of birds, and so does the FWS definition of "take."

6. **B**   This is an Inference question.

    A: No. First, you know from paragraph 1 that the MBTA does not grant incidental take permits. Second, while the passage does indicate that other regulatory measures, including the Endangered Species Act, do grant such permits, the passage does not indicate that prosecution is likely to occur even if a permit has been granted. This choice is too extreme.

B: Yes. This choice more or less paraphrases a statement made in the passage. In the first paragraph the author writes: "As with other similar regulatory acts, where the penalties are small and there is no 'grave harm to an offender's reputation,' the Supreme Court has long recognized that a different standard applies to those federal criminal statutes that are essentially regulatory." From this you can reasonably infer that prosecution for breaking regulatory statutes is unlikely to damage the reputation of the offender. While it is a bit ambiguous in the passage whether or not this applies to all regulatory acts, this is still the "least wrong" answer.

C: No. The passage only mentions misdemeanors (paragraph 1). Being charged with a felony is out of the scope of the passage.

D: No. While the FWS definition of a "take" is relevant to prosecution under the MBTA (paragraph 1), the passage never suggests that the FWS itself carries out prosecutions. Only "the United States" (paragraph 1) and the U.S. Attorney (paragraph 4) are mentioned as actually bringing suit or prosecuting cases.

7. **A** This is an Inference question.

A: Yes. In paragraph 3, the author states: "Unfortunately, the courts have not fully defined how the concept of proximate cause would limit the scope of MBTA liability in the real world." If the author believes that the lack of a clear definition is unfortunate in this case, you can infer that the author thinks that the role, in general, should be clearly defined.

B: No. The author never expresses disapproval of the fact that the MBTA does not take intent into account.

C: No. This choice takes words out of context, and is also too extreme. While the author states in paragraph 3 that "Courts have speculated in dicta that some everyday activities like driving cars or piloting aircraft would not reasonably be linked to bird death, while other (more industrial or hazardous) activities like operating power lines or oil drilling equipment would," the passage does not suggest that the author believes that only industrial activity should be considered liable under the MBTA.

D: No. The author never indicates that she has a problem with the fact that the MBTA is "a strict liability statute" (paragraph 1).

Passage III: General—Main Point, Primary Purpose, and Tone Questions

Question Type Strategies

Main Point and Primary Purpose questions

These questions generally ask you about the Bottom Line of the passage as a whole. Make sure to choose answers that cover all of the major themes in the passage, without going beyond its scope. Also make sure that the answer you select matches the tone (positive, negative, or neutral) of the author. A similar type of question will ask you for the main point or purpose of a paragraph. Make sure to pick an answer specific to the content, tone, and scope of that paragraph.

Tone questions

These questions directly ask you about the author's attitude toward the overall subject being discussed (General Tone questions), or toward one particular aspect of it (Specific Tone questions). Be careful to choose answers that are supported by evidence in the passage (for example, by the tone indicators that you should be highlighting); don't speculate about what the author "might" think. Beware of choices that go in the right direction but that are too extreme.

1. **D** This is a Main Point question.
    A: No. This answer choice only addresses the second-to-last paragraph of the passage; it does not go far enough in encompassing the ideas of the passage as a whole.
    B: No. While the author does discuss three qualities of literature, he does not discuss the need for debate on the part of "serious students" or anyone else. This choice is half-right but half-wrong.
    C: No. This answer choice only addresses the final two paragraphs of the passage, and is therefore too limited in scope. A common trick of MCAT questions is to feature as an Attractor the part of the passage you most recently read; you can avoid this trick by ensuring that you summarize your own Bottom Line before starting the questions.
    D: Yes. This answer choice summarizes the three qualities of literature that the author discusses, making it the best answer choice among those listed.

2. **C** This is a Tone/Attitude question.
    A: No. While the first part of this answer is correct, the second part is too strong in tone, and too negative, making this a half-right/half-wrong Attractor. While the author notes that literature can tell us things that history cannot, he does not "disparage," or harshly criticize, history.
    B: No. There is nothing in the passage to indicate that the author thinks English literature is superior to any other sort of literature; in paragraph 4, in fact, he refers to "the whole splendid world of Greek literature."
    C: Yes. In the second paragraph, the author says "...to love good books for their own sake, is the chief thing; to analyze and explain them is a less joyous but still an important matter." In the passage's final paragraph he emphasizes the seriousness and importance of literature, agreeing with Goethe that literature is "the humanization of the world." This assertion supports the strong language in this answer choice; additionally, the other answer choices all have more discernible flaws.
    D: No. The author makes no claims about contemporary literature, and does not make any comparative statements regarding the literature of the present and that of the past.

3. **B** This is a "purpose of a paragraph" question.
    A: No. The author does not explain the story in the first paragraph in terms of people who have learned how to read nature or literature versus people who have not. The author does not suggest, either, that the mystery and delight inspired by good literature is something that goes away once someone knows how to "read" it.
    B: Yes. In the first paragraph, the author describes the man's explanation of the shell: "It was not a new world, but only the unnoticed harmony of the old that had aroused the child's wonder." This relationship between the apparent newness of the world and the fact that it is in fact something that has been there all along is addressed explicitly in the third paragraph with reference to literature and the shell: "All art is the expression of life in forms of truth and beauty; or rather, it is the reflection of some truth and beauty which are in the world, but which remain unnoticed until brought to our attention by some sensitive human soul, just as the delicate curves of the shell reflect

sounds and harmonies too faint to be otherwise noticed." **This explanation by the author in terms of his opening narrative is the most concrete evidence in the passage to explain the purpose of the first paragraph, making B the best answer choice.**

C: No. This is an appealing answer that addresses things that are discussed elsewhere in the passage, but it is not the point or purpose of this particular paragraph.

D: No. The author makes no statements about narrative literature in particular; this answer choice is beyond the scope of the passage.

4. **B** This is a variation on a Tone question.

This question requires you to take the scope, tone, and subject matter into account. Eliminate choices that are not appropriate to the focus and level of the passage, for example historians (for a passage that is largely about literature) or literary critics (for a passage that is not at all technical or academic).

A: No. This discussion of literature is too basic for literary critics themselves; presumably they would know the basic qualities of literature. This answer is not supported by the passage's tone.

B: **Yes. In the second paragraph, the author says, "We have now reached a point where we wish to understand as well as to enjoy literature; and the first step, since exact definition is impossible, is to determine some of its essential qualities." This talk of a "first step" in a "wish to understand" indicates an instructive tone, making students the most likely intended audience of this passage.**

C: No. While the author mentions the difference between literature and history, there is nothing in the passage to suggest that his intended audience consists of historians.

D: No. The passage is clearly addressed to readers of literature; there is no indication that the author is addressing writers themselves.

5. **C** This is a "point of the paragraph" question.

A: No. While the author says that the poem mentioned in paragraph 3 allows the hay to tell its story, this is merely an expression, and this answer choice is therefore a good example of an Attractor that uses a word or phrase out of context. This paragraph does not support the idea that literature renders nature capable of telling its own story, but rather that literature—written by someone who sees the beauty in the mundane—reflects the truth and beauty in the world.

B: No. The author does not discuss qualities of "true" artists versus presumably lesser artists, or fakes. He notes that, in this example, there is one man who takes notice of the meadow's beauty after a hundred men have merely noted its surface appearance, but there is nothing in this statement about the particular qualities of that man and whether or not he is a true artist; the author merely notes that it is a "sensitive human soul" who regards the meadow in a different light.

C: **Yes. Paragraph 3 follows up on the idea introduced by the opening narrative. Like the shell, literature does not only reveal a new world but reveals aspects of the world that often go unnoticed in daily life. The second sentence of the third paragraph nicely paraphrases this answer choice.**

D: No. This statement is too extreme. While the author makes statements about "all art," and refers in paragraph 3 to an example involving nature, he does not make the connection that all art is based on the natural world. For example, there is no suggestion that this is true of the literature of the Anglo-Saxons discussed in paragraph 5.

6. **C**   This is a Tone/Attitude question.

A: No. While the author indicates in the second paragraph that "To enter and enjoy this new world [of literature], to love good books for their own sake, is the chief thing; to analyze and explain them is a less joyous but still an important matter." To say that analysis is "still an important matter" is not the same as saying it is an "equally important matter." That he isolates enjoyment as the "chief" thing indicates that analysis must be ranked below enjoyment.

B: No. See paragraph 2. The author indicates that analyzing literature itself is "less joyous" than entering and loving good books, but does not say that analysis itself diminishes the immediate joy of reading.

C: **Yes. This answer choice best paraphrases the author's remark in paragraph 2 that "To enter and enjoy this new world [of literature], to love good books for their own sake, is the chief thing; to analyze and explain them is a less joyous but still an important matter."**

D: No. While the author says that analysis and explanation of literature is "an important matter," he does not make such extreme statements as to say that those who do not engage in analysis and explanation "are missing out on a fundamental purpose of reading." This answer is out of scope and too extreme in tone.

4.6

Passage IV: Reasoning—Structure and Evaluate Questions

Question Type Strategies

Structure questions

These questions ask you either for the purpose of a statement or paragraph within the passage, or how a particular statement is supported by the author. They are called Structure questions because they deal with not just the content, but also the logical structure of the passage. Therefore, in choosing an answer, make sure you select a choice that not only accurately represents the content of the passage, but also the purpose of the reference (that is, how it relates to other parts of the text) or the support given for the claim (that is, what evidence the author provides to explain or justify it). A rare version of this question type is the General Structure question, which asks you to find an answer that correctly describes the progression of claims or ideas in the passage. When evaluating the answers for these General Structure questions, make sure that the different parts of the answer choice match not only the content but the ordering of the referenced parts of the passage.

Evaluate questions

Evaluate questions ask you *how well* a claim is supported by the author within the passage. When answering these questions make sure that both the judgment (usually some form of "strongly" or "weakly") and the description (of why it is strongly or weakly supported) match the passage.

1. **C**   This is a General Structure question.

A: No. This answer choice gets the tone of the passage wrong by tweaking it a bit too far toward the negative. While the author does build up to his larger points, he discusses the earlier reasons "obscuring" the "real" reasons nowhere. In paragraph 3, he merely notes that some of the reasons "distract" from what may be the "most obvious" reason. "Obscure" and "distract" are not synonyms, nor are "obvious" and "real," so this choice is an inadequate paraphrasing of passage material.

B: No. While the author makes reference to Cameron's interpretation of the Titanic story, he nowhere privileges it as the "most compelling."

C: Yes. This answer comes the closest to following the trajectory of the passage, and does not feature any changes in tone from what is found in the passage. The ordering of ideas is exactly as it occurs in the passage.

D: No. While this one gets the ordering of the passage right, the author never suggests that the interpretations of the Titanic story are undermined by Robertson's novel.

2. **C** This is a Specific Structure question.

A: No. This is not the author's purpose in using these two quotes in paragraph 2; he does not offer an explicit value judgment on the parallel between Rose and the Titanic as both female entities.

B: No. The author does not contrast the attitudes of the Titanic's era with those held today.

C: Yes. In the sentences preceding the two quotations, one of which is about the ship and the other about Rose, the author says "Both…" and lists several factors that both the ship and Rose have in common.

D: No. While Cameron's film is quoted, the author is not singling out Cameron as a genius or noting anything exceptional about his direction. This is not the purpose of using the two quotes from Cameron's film in paragraph 2.

3. **D** This is an Evaluate question.

A: No. The discussion of Oedipus supports rather than undermines the author's claim. This is the opposite of the correct answer.

B: No. The author clearly backs up his claim with reference to Oedipus, a character from Sophocles' drama.

C: No. This is in fact a claim, not support, and comes in a different paragraph (paragraph 3) from the one referenced in the question stem (paragraph 4). The author begins paragraph 4 with "But the Titanic embodies another strain of tragedy": the words in quotations (here) are ones you should have highlighted to indicate that the author was making a separate point.

D: Yes. The author discusses Oedipus from Sophocles' *Oedipus Rex* to illustrate another drama that featured a "flawed and self-destructive hero." Notice that in classic MCAT form, the more moderate answer here is preferable—as is often the case—to the more extreme answer, which in this case is A.

4. **B** This is a Specific Structure question.

A: No. This answer does not go far enough and misses the point. As with the incorrect answer choices in other questions that emphasize Cameron's strength as a director, this answer is incorrect because it valorizes Robertson rather than positions him in the context of a larger discussion of our cultural fascination with the Titanic.

B: Yes. The author quotes Robertson to note the similarity of his account with the story of the Titanic: immediately following the quote, he says, "Down to the most idiosyncratic detail, all this is familiar," only to then surprise the reader by saying Robertson's novel preceded the Titanic disaster by 14 years. In the end, his point is that even before the Titanic, our imaginations were caught up in themes present in the story of the disaster.

C: No. While the author precedes the quotation by talking about the themes of Robertson's text, the quotation itself does not address themes as much as specific details of the scene of a sinking ship. And most importantly, the author uses the quotation primarily to draw a comparison between Robertson's story and that of the Titanic.

D: No. The author does not cite this explicitly in relation to the quotation from Robertson's book. He mentions this a few paragraphs earlier as part of the theatrical appeal of the Titanic disaster, but not as a direct reference to Robertson.

5. **B** This is a Specific Structure question.

A: No. The quotation given in the question stem notes a tension or an ambivalence: we "demonstrate liberalism even as we indulge our consumerism." This answer choice only deals with the "demonstrate liberalism" aspect of the question stem. The author does note that many versions of the Titanic story feature "indignant depictions of the class system" but these "coexist uneasily with their adoring depictions of upper-crust privilege": this latter quotation addresses the "indulge our consumerism" aspect of the question stem.

B: **Yes. See the explanation for choice A above. The quotation given in the question stem notes a tension in reactions of viewers/readers to class issues in the Titanic story. The author then provides specific moments from Cameron's film as evidence to support his claims about our reactions.**

C: No. This is not relevant to the question stem; it is part of a second argument made by the author, whereas the question stem refers to the first.

D: No. As choice B explains, the author supports his claim with specific references to Cameron's film.

6. **B** This is an Evaluate question.

A: No. The author does indicate that one archetype is of feminine vulnerability, so this answer choice directly contradicts information provided in the passage.

B: **Yes. In the paragraphs preceding the claim in the question stem, the author notes the archetype of female vulnerability, and then indicates another archetype by saying "But the Titanic embodies another strain of tragedy. This is the drama of a flawed and self-destructive hero." Admittedly, the author does not use the term "archetype" in the second case, but by the time he makes his claim that the Titanic "conflates two of the oldest archetypes in literature," we have a pretty good sense of what he means. If this feels like a stretch, it at least helps to definitively rule out choice D, which is much more definitive than the words "provide evidence supporting it" in this answer choice. Process of elimination leaves choice B as the "least wrong" answer.**

C: No. This answer choice extrapolates too much on the author's credentials and focuses on something that is not really the issue here: the age of the archetypes rather than the existence of them. There is no reason to doubt the author's knowledge about Western literature: his references to Sophocles' work and Robertson's novel, for instance, illustrate that he has knowledge about literature.

D: No. The discussion of consumerism in the first paragraph is not directly tied to the author's claim about archetypes. This is the right answer to the wrong question.

7. **C** This is a Specific Structure question.

A: No. The author never mentions anything unique about the ship's mechanical system.

B: No. This information is directly refuted by the passage's first paragraph, in which the author discusses the tension between classes present in the Titanic story.

4.6

C: **Yes. In paragraph 2, the author quotes a character from Cameron's movie who says the Titanic is "the largest moving object ever made by the hand of man in all of history," and in paragraph 3 he refers to it as "the forty-six-thousand-ton liner."**

D: No. The author does not mention the ship's décor.

8. **A**   This is a Specific Structure question.

A: **Yes: This answer choice properly captures the tension that is the focus of the author in this paragraph: the tension between our liberalism and consumerism. The author provides the example of the sunbathed deck to illustrate that while we also identify with the scornful remark of the lower-class passenger to the music from the first-class section of the boat, we cannot help but enjoy the indulgence of seeing Winslet on the private deck.**

B: No. The allure, and the universal allure in particular, of the female protagonist is not something addressed in this paragraph. The allure of the sunbathed deck is more about the elitist indulgence than the attractiveness of the female enjoying it.

C: No. This choice is too extreme. The author does not suggest that this tension represents or indicates hypocrisy.

D: No: The point of this paragraph is not for the author to express his approval of Cameron's directorial choices; he does not explicitly express approval or disapproval at any point in the passage.

9. **C**   This is a Specific Structure question.

A: No. The author never suggests that the Titanic's feminine status is unique to Cameron's interpretation, but merely that "the Titanic was a 'she'" and "Cameron went to some lengths to push the identification between the ship and the young woman."

B: No. The author does not question or investigate why ships are assigned the feminine pronoun; he merely states it as fact and then explores consequences for interpretation.

C: **Yes. The author notes that the feminine pronoun used for the ship creates room for an identification between the ship and the woman in Cameron's film; this parallel leads the author to comment on the story's archetype of feminine vulnerability, which is one of his arguments for the enduring appeal of the Titanic story in our imagination.**

D: No. The author does not contrast the Titanic's era with others, and the main point of paragraph 2 is not to discuss sexism, either at that time or at any time in history.

Passage V: Application—Strengthen and Weaken Questions

Question Type Strategies

Weaken questions

First, clearly define what you are weakening (the overall argument or some part of it in the passage) based on the question stem. Next, go back to the passage to clarify the logic of the argument. You can't literally answer these questions in your own words, as the correct answer will include new information. But you do want to create a guide for yourself regarding what the direction and issue of the correct answer needs to be. As you go through POE, make sure that the answer that you choose is relevant, that it weakens rather than strengthens, and that it is strong enough to have a real impact on the passage.

Strengthen questions

First, clearly define what you are strengthening (the overall argument or some part of it in the passage) based on the question stem. Next, go back to the passage to clarify the logic of the argument. As with Weaken questions, you can't come up with an exact answer in your own words, but do create a guide for yourself based on what the direction and issue of the correct answer needs to be. As you go through POE, make sure that the answer that you choose is relevant, that it strengthens rather than weakens, and that it is strong enough to have a significant impact on the passage.

1. **C** This is a Weaken question.
    Look for the answer that provides the strongest reason to doubt Ginsburg's argument, described in paragraph 2, that judges should avoid discourteous language in order to preserve the status and effectiveness of the judiciary.

    A: No. While this answer goes in the right direction, it isn't strong enough to significantly weaken Ginsburg's claim. The fact that some (which could be only a few) experts believe something doesn't mean that it is actually true.

    B: No. This choice strengthens rather than weakens by suggesting that strong language in a dissent could undermine the functioning of the court. Note that Ginsburg states that courtesy is especially important in dissents.

    C: Yes. Ginsburg argues that it is by speaking in a "polite 'judicial voice' that courts may become more effective at performing their official duties" and preserving the status of the institution. If moderation is widely seen as a sign of weakness, however, then courteous language might undermine rather than promote the standing of the court.

    D: No. This choice is the right answer to the wrong question; it weakens the author's argument, but not Ginsburg's. Note that it is the author who argues that the law is itself a form of courtesy (see paragraph 3), whereas Ginsburg is simply calling for more courtesy within the legal system (paragraph 3).

2. **A** This is a Strengthen question.
    In the last paragraph, the author offers (and agrees with) Carter and Burke's claim that "Unlike the world of electoral politics, in which 'smart participants know that they should obfuscate, change the subject, [and] hurl mud' to achieve their goals, the rule of law requires judges to work out their arguments openly and to furnish reasons for their rulings." Look for the answer that goes the furthest in suggesting that the rule of law and electoral politics are in fact different on this basis.

    A: Yes. Sticking to scripted responses and avoiding open debate would be the opposite of "work[ing] out arguments openly and furnish[ing] reasons for their rulings." Therefore this choice does support the author's contrast between the law and politics.

    B: No. This choice weakens rather than strengthens by suggesting that politics is becoming more open, with less obfuscation (i.e., hiding things).

    C: No. This choice takes words out of context from the passage. The fact that public interest is affected by how many controversial issues are involved in a campaign doesn't tell you anything about the openness of politics as compared to the law.

    D: No. Given that you don't know how authentic this image is, this choice has no impact on the author's claim.

3.   **C**   This is a Weaken question.

The correct answer will either indicate that courtesy is not valuable, or that it is valuable largely for some reason other than that it allows people to "pretend to be better than they are."

A: No. This choice is not strong enough to most undermine the author's argument. It only indicates that courtesy can have the opposite effect in extreme cases, and for a limited amount of time.

B: No. This choice strengthens rather than weakens. If aggression and dominance are not in fact highly prized characteristics, it strengthens the claim that a "polite pretense" of cooperation and friendliness is valuable because it helps people to keep up the appearance of having good qualities ("pretend to be better than they are").

C: Yes. The author's claim rests on the assumption that the value of courtesy lies in the fact that it hides reality, since "most individuals are capable only of appearing [emphasis added] to live up to community ideals." If pretending, through courtesy, to live up to those ideals made one able to actually do so, it would undermine the author's argument by giving an alternative explanation for the value of courtesy.

D: No. The author does not claim that human beings never act selflessly; in fact, he says in paragraph 5: "I do not claim that this [pessimistic] view of human nature perfectly represents how people are...."

4.   **D**   This is a Weaken question.

The author states in paragraph 3 that while he thinks that courtesy and the law may work in symbiosis, what he really wishes to talk about is how "judicial action may itself be a form of decorum." The rest of the passage discusses reasons for this claim. Therefore, the correct answer will be the one that most undermines this claim and/or the reasoning supporting the claim.

A: No. The author does not argue that people do not want to be selfless, but rather that they are for the most part unable to do so: "most people take public moral standards seriously, yet remain too filled with ambition and vanity to actually practice what they preach" (paragraph 4). Therefore, this answer choice weakens an argument more extreme than the one that the author actually makes.

B: No. The connection between civility and the functioning of the court is made by Ginsburg (paragraph 2). While the author does not disagree with her recommendation, it is not a central part of the author's own argument.

C: No. This would do the opposite; it strengthens the author's indication in the last paragraph that the structure of the rule of law contributes to cooperation and social peace.

D: Yes. The author argues that the law, like courtesy, is an "artificial medium in which otherwise opposed parties may jointly find ways of moving on" without affecting "the fundamental factors that generate the disputes in the first place" (paragraph 3). When the author, through citation of Carter and Burke, states that the law helps us to "look outside [our] own will for criteria of judgment," he means that we act in spite of our individual preferences, not that we change those preferences. If the law acted to transform our perceptions in the way described in this answer choice, the author's argument that the law is a form of courtesy would fall apart.

5. **C**   This is a Strengthen question.

The author argues that law is a form of courtesy. Part of this argument is that the structure of the rule of law allows and directs people to look beyond their own perceptions and self-interest. The correct answer will either directly support the overall claim that one can see the law as itself a "form of decorum," or it will support the rationale given for the author's claim in the last two paragraphs.

A: No. There is no suggestion in this choice that the rule of law lessens this fear. Therefore, this choice is out of scope.

B: No. There is no suggestion in this choice of how the rule of law might relate either to this fear or to this hope. Therefore, this choice is out of scope.

C: **Yes. In the last paragraph, in the course of explaining and supporting his argument, the author cites Carter and Burke's claim that "The payoff of such 'slow and steady (and often boring)' legal procedures is that they help broker community peace." If it is the case that time is an issue, and if the more time people have to consider their options, the less likely they are to act purely on self-interest, this would support the author's argument.**

D: No. This would weaken the author's (and Carter and Burke's) argument in the last paragraph that "The payoff of such 'slow and steady (and often boring)' legal procedures is that they help broker community peace, channeling hotly contested questions into a forum in which they can be more easily handled."

6. **A**   This is a LEAST Weaken question.

For a LEAST Weaken (or Weaken EXCEPT) question, eliminate the answers that most weaken the relevant claims in the passage. The correct answer may (1) strengthen, (2) have no impact, or (3) weaken less than the other three. (The last of these three is rarely seen.) For this question, you are eliminating answers that indicate that the rule of law does NOT "set aside the 'dramatic and emotional work of poetics and theatrics'" by "commit[ting] the judiciary to the logic of ideas" (paragraph 8).

A: **Yes. This answer strengthens the relevant claim by providing more evidence that the rule of law entails excluding emotion and drama from the court.**

B: No. This would weaken the argument by suggesting that the influence of the court comes more through drama and theater than through "the logic of ideas."

C: No. This would weaken the argument by suggesting that the rule of law is unsuccessful at excluding emotion from the work of the court.

D: No. This would weaken the argument by suggesting that the rule of law is unsuccessful at committing the judiciary to the "logic of ideas," and that drama and theatrics have come to play a major role in judges' decision-making.

4.6

Passage VI: Application—New Information and Analogy Questions

Question Type Strategies

New Information questions

First, identify the theme of the new information in the question stem. Next, define if it is a New Information-Inference (Type I) or New Information-Strengthen/Weaken (Type II) question. Then define the relationship of the new information to the passage, and answer the question in your own words as best you can. Be on the lookout for wrong answers that correspond to the passage but not the new information, or that are consistent with the new information but inconsistent with the passage.

Analogy questions

First, identify the theme of the relevant part of the passage. Your goal is to generalize at this point and to get away from the precise content of the passage in order to find the more general logical theme of structure. Your goal is to find the best match in the choices; beware of answers that match the content but not the logic of the passage, or that match one part of it but not another.

1. **B**   This is an Analogy question.
   Paragraph 2 describes the logic of reciprocity as a "favor bank." That is, one person does something for another with the expectation that the favor will be returned later. The correct answer will have this theme.

   A: No. This choice is tempting because diamond trading is mentioned in the passage. Do not be fooled, however—remember that the answer choices to analogy questions will often contain new information, and they only rarely will reproduce the actual content or subject matter of the passage. Furthermore, this does not demonstrate the concept of reciprocity as described in paragraph 3: "I'll do this for you now, in the expectation that down the road you or someone else will return the favor."

   B: Yes. This choice most closely demonstrates the concept of "I'll do this for you now, in the expectation that down the road you or someone else will return the favor" (paragraph 3). Each parent who participates watches someone else's children with the expectation that they will also have their own children watched, when needed.

   C: No. This choice involves the government implementing something for the people, using the money gathered from taxing them. It does not demonstrate "I'll do this for you now, in the expectation that down the road you or someone else will return the favor."

   D: No. This choice involves two people mutually agreeing about assets before entering into marriage; as written, it does not demonstrate one of them doing something for the other now, with the expectation of payback later on.

2. **A**   This is an Analogy question.
   This question asks you to find the choice with the most similar relationship to the one established in the second paragraph: "…communities did not become civic simply because they were rich. The historical record strongly suggests precisely the opposite: They have become rich because they were civic." In other words, the best answer will demonstrate that civic engagement results in (and precedes) prosperity.

A: **Yes. This choice describes employees who were civically involved (by participating in "after-hours collaborations and events outside of work") before their companies become prosperous. Of the four choices, this is the one that comes closest to suggesting that civic engagement contributed to wealth and prosperity (through facilitating team building and efficiency).**

B: No. There is no indication in this choice whether the prosperity (large endowment) preceded the students' involvement in the community or vice versa.

C: No. This choice states that wealthy individuals donate generously to organizations; it does not demonstrate the relationship between civic engagement and wealth, as described in the second paragraph of the passage.

D: No. This choice is analogous to the relationship the author establishes about social capital in the final paragraph, not to the relationship between civic engagement and wealth as described in the second paragraph of the passage. This is an example of a "right answer, wrong question" Attractor.

3. **D** This is an Analogy question.

In the seventh paragraph, the author describes the accumulation of social capital: "Stocks of social capital, such as trust, norms, and networks, tend to be self-reinforcing and cumulative. Successful collaboration in one endeavor builds connections and trust—social assets that facilitate future collaboration in other, unrelated tasks. As with conventional capital, those who have social capital tend to accumulate more—'them as has, gets.'" Therefore, the correct answer will be a positive feedback loop (the more social capital you have, the more you get, therefore the more you will have, and so on).

A: No. This choice describes the decline of one thing (passionate love) as something else increases (companionate love); this choice does not describe a positive feedback cycle.

B: No. This choice states that peer reinforcement and parental punishment have differential impacts on adolescent behavior; this choice does not describe a positive feedback cycle.

C: No. This choice describes a negative feedback cycle: electricity generates heat, and as heat increases, it shuts off the source of the electricity, thereby reducing heat.

D: **Yes. This choice describes a positive feedback cycle: as temperature rises and permafrost thaws, carbon dioxide and methane gases are released into the atmosphere, which will further increase the temperature and increase the melting of the permafrost, releasing more gases, and so on.**

4. **C** This is an Analogy question in an EXCEPT/LEAST/NOT format.

The question asks you to take information from the fourth paragraph about how networks of civic engagement best operate and apply it to the examples given in the answers. The best choice will be the one that is least consistent with the information in paragraph 4.

A: No. Paragraph 4 states: "This is why the diamond trade, with its extreme possibilities for fraud, is concentrated within close-knit ethnic enclaves." This choice is consistent with the description of a network of civic engagement.

B: No. Paragraph 4 states: "Students of prisoners' dilemmas and related games report that cooperation is most easily sustained through repeat play." If a team is composed of people that have not played together before, it is consistent with the information in paragraph 4 that they would need more practice.

C: **Yes. Paragraph 4 suggests that repeated interaction with the same people fosters trust. However, this choice suggests the opposite—that teams of people that are frequently changed "maximizes performance." This choice is the most inconsistent with what the passage says about networks of civic engagement in paragraph 4.**

D: No. Paragraph 4 suggests that repeated interaction with the same people fosters trust; this choice implies something similar.

4.6

4.6

5.   **D**   This is an Analogy question.

At the end of the last paragraph, the author states: "Members of Florentine choral societies participate because they like to sing, not because their participation strengthens the Tuscan social fabric." Therefore, the author states that people engage in "civic participation" because they want to, not because they are consciously trying to "strengthen the…social fabric."

A: No. There is no indication that this after-school study involves group or social activities, or that the students participate because they want to.

B: No. This choice describes a situation wherein men join the military because they have no choice, not because they want to.

C: No. This choice describes people who join a civic organization with the express purpose of contributing to the community. In the passage, the beneficial impact on society was a side effect of people joining an organization for their own enjoyment. Make sure that the answer you select matches the logic and theme of the relevant part of the passage.

D: **Yes. This choice is not perfect, but it is the closest of the four in describing a situation in which people participate in something because they want to, and not for any other reason. Make sure to look for and select the "least wrong" answer.**

6.   **B**   This is a Type 2 New Information/Strengthen question.

This question provides the information that as a vehicle for civic engagement (Boy Scout and Girl Scout troops) grows, so does a community's wealth (median income). The author argues that civic engagement and wealth are positively correlated in paragraph 2.

A: No. This new information is not directly relevant to the history of civic engagement.

B: **Yes. This new information provides an example that strengthens this claim made in the second paragraph.**

C: No. This new information does not suggest that coordination and communication are increased through participation in Boy Scouts/Girl Scouts; therefore, this claim is not directly strengthened by this new information.

D: No. This new information does not suggest that trust is increased through participation in Boy Scouts/Girl Scouts or that it contributes to future endeavors; therefore, this claim is not directly strengthened by this new information.

7.   **C**   This is a Type 2 New Information/Weaken question.

This new information undermines that author's point made in the fourth paragraph that "dense social ties facilitate gossip and other valuable ways of cultivating reputation—an essential foundation for trust in a complex society."

A: No. This new information does not have any impact on democracy (a concept that is also never addressed in this passage).

B: No. While this answer choice is supported by the passage (paragraph 3: "A society that relies on generalized reciprocity is more efficient than a distrustful society"), it does not address the new information about gossip and its impact on trust and reputation. Therefore, this is not the best choice.

C: **Yes. The author states in paragraph 4: "dense social ties facilitate gossip and other valuable ways of cultivating reputation—an essential foundation for trust in a complex society." This new information essentially says the opposite (as gossip increases, trust and reputation decrease). Therefore, this is the best answer choice.**

D: No. Be wary of answer choices such as this one—the new information provided is applicable to the author's assertions about gossip in the fourth paragraph. Therefore, this is not an acceptable choice.

8. **B**   This is a Type 1 New Information question.

This new information suggests that civic engagement has decreased in the past 30 years. The author claims that civic engagement fosters economic development (paragraph 2); therefore a decline in one should result in a decline in the other.

A: No. This choice goes in the opposite direction. If anything, less civic involvement would be consistent with a decrease, not an increase, in organized protests.

B: Yes. Paragraph 2 states: "These communities did not become civic simply because they were rich. The historical record strongly suggests precisely the opposite: They have become rich because they were civic. The social capital embodied in norms and networks of civic engagement seems to be a precondition for economic development, as well as for effective government." Therefore, this is the most likely possible outcome of decreased civic engagement.

C: No. The passage never mentions "sociocultural awareness."

D: No. There is nothing to suggest that a decrease in "the number of Americans who attend public meetings or political rallies" would lead to an increase in participation in other activities. If anything, the new information would suggest that there would be a decrease in participation in other activities.

9. **C**   This is a Type 1 New Information question.

Since the passage mentions nothing about religion, this new information could be translated as saying that religious participation is the most common form of civic engagement today. Therefore, participation in religion can be viewed as "civic engagement," as described in the passage, when evaluating each answer choice.

A: No. There is no indication that civic engagement relies on government.

B: No. While participation in religion can be viewed as a form of civic engagement, which will increase social capital (according to the passage), there is not enough information in the question stem to suggest "active members of a religion have more social capital than those who are not religious." This question stem states that "religion is the most common associational membership among people;" it does not distinguish active from non-active participation, nor does it provide information about other forms of civic engagement (e.g., a non-religious person might engage in three other forms of civic engagement). This is not a logical conclusion from the new information and the passage text, and is not the best choice.

C: Yes. It is reasonable to infer, based on the passage, that membership in associations or organizations qualifies as a form of civic engagement.

D: No. Even though the author ties civic engagement to economic development, this is not a reasonable conclusion from the information provided in the question stem.

Chapter 4 Summary

Know the five steps you should take in answering any question:

1. Read the question carefully and identify the question type.

2. Translate the question into your own words.

3. Identify key words and phrases (when the question stem references a particular issue within the passage) and go back to the passage to find the relevant information.

4. Answer the question in your own words.

5. Use Process of Elimination.

Know the ten basic question types that you will encounter in MCAT CARS:

1. Retrieval

2. Inference

3. Main Idea/Primary Purpose

4. Tone/Attitude

5. Structure

6. Evaluate

7. Strengthen

8. Weaken

9. New Information

10. Analogy

Monitor your progress and improve your accuracy by keeping a Self-Evaluation Log.

CHAPTER 4 PRACTICE PASSAGES

Individual Passage Drills

Do the following two passages untimed. Use these passages to focus on answering the questions in your own words.

Get a stack of Post-it® Notes. Paste one over each set of answer choices, leaving the questions themselves visible. Work the passage as usual, but when it comes time to answer each question in your own words, write your answer on the Note. When finished answering each question in your own words, immediately lift up the Post-it® Note and use your answer as a guide, while actively using POE to eliminate choices that may sound similar but are flawed in some way.

Once you have completed the passages and checked your answers, fill out an Individual Passage Log for each passage.

In your self-evaluation, focus in particular on question types. Did you correctly identify the question type? Did you understand what the question was asking you to do? Did you apply the 5 Steps in a way that was appropriate for the question task? Which question types were easier and harder for you to complete and why? And, what kinds of Attractors did you fall for? Finally, how can you change your approach to answering questions to improve your accuracy and efficiency?

CHAPTER 4 PRACTICE PASSAGE 1

The language of efficiency, or cost-effectiveness, is all around us. We hear it everywhere, in our private lives as well as in public conversation. I recently read an advertisement in a local newspaper for a fully wired kitchen that would allow me to program my microwave and stove from the office simply by flicking a button on my handheld computer. By the time I reach home, dinner will be ready to eat. The alarm system will disengage as I reach the front door. "How efficient!" the ad proclaims in bold lettering.

But the ad misses, not by accident, I suspect, one crucial piece of information. It does not tell me *at what* this newly wired, very expensive kitchen will be efficient. At improving the quality of my food? At saving time? What, I worried, will I be expected to accomplish with the time saved? Is it legitimate to use the twenty minutes I might gain to read a novel I have been longing to read? Or am I expected to engage in "productive" work in the time I save? How will this time-saving kitchen improve my satisfaction? My welfare?

The seduction of efficiency is not restricted to the latest advances in labor-saving devices for the beleaguered working mother. The language of efficiency shapes our public as well as our private lives. Those who provide our public services are expected to do so efficiently. Physicians and nurses in the hospital where my mother was treated are expected to work efficiently. So are teachers, governments, and civil servants. They are constantly enjoined to become efficient, to remain efficient, and to improve their efficiency in the safeguarding of the public trust. Efficiency, or cost-effectiveness, has become an end in itself, a value often more important than others. But elevating efficiency, turning it into an end, misuses language, and this has profound consequences for the way we as citizens conceive of public life. When we define efficiency as an end, divorced from its larger purpose, it becomes nothing less than a cult.

Our public conversation about efficiency is misleading. Efficiency is only one part of a much larger public discussion between citizens and their governments. Efficiency is not an end, but a means to achieve valued ends. It is not a goal, but an instrument to achieve other goals. It is not a value, but a way to achieve other values. It is part of the story but never the whole.

Even when efficiency is used correctly as a means, when it is understood as the most cost-effective way to achieve our goals, much of our public discussion is fuzzy about its purpose. What does effectiveness mean? What, for example, is an effective education? To answer that question, we would first have to discuss the purposes of education, a discussion that is informed by values, and only then could we come to some understanding

of the criteria of effectiveness. At times, however, even the mention of effectiveness is absent, and the conversation slides over to focus only on costs. And when the public discussion of efficiency focuses only on costs, the cult becomes even stronger.

Yet the word "efficiency" is not only misused in public conversation as an end rather than a means. Our public conversation is not merely bedeviled by a simple technical error. The cult of efficiency, like other cults, advances political purposes and agendas. In our post-industrial age, efficiency is often a code word for an attack on the sclerotic, unresponsive, and anachronistic state, the detritus of the industrial age that fits poorly with our times. The state is branded as wasteful, and market mechanisms are heralded as the efficient alternative. This argument, we shall see, is based on a fundamental misunderstanding of the importance of the "smart" state in the global, knowledge-based economy.

Material used in this particular passage has been adapted from the following source:
J. G. Stein, *The Cult of Efficiency*. © 2001 by House of Anansi Press.

1. The author draws an important distinction between:

    A) goals and the ways those goals are accomplished.
    B) efficient and inefficient technology.
    C) representative and misleading advertising.
    D) public and private dialogues about efficiency.

2. The author suggests which of the following to be true of cults?

    A) They can influence society at large.
    B) They promote illogical and unreasonable beliefs.
    C) They are simply groups of like-minded individuals.
    D) They are usually organized around a focus on costs.

3. The author most likely supports a view of government as an institution that:

    A) finds the most cost-effective ways to provide for society's needs.
    B) is wasteful and fits poorly with our times.
    C) has an important role to play in the modern economy.
    D) is not as efficient as market mechanisms.

4. Suppose a public school board were to demand teachers use fewer hours to prepare instruction so that the school board can save money. In response, the author would most likely:

A) praise the board for striving to find more efficient ways to deliver services.
B) support the board's commitment to quality education.
C) withhold judgment and suggest the decision be considered within a larger context.
D) criticize the school board for undermining public education.

5. Which of the following assertions about language is LEAST supported by the passage?

A) Language has the power to shape how citizens think about their relationships with each other and government.
B) Language can be misused to advance political agendas.
C) Vague language sometimes leaves out important information.
D) Government uses language to mislead us in the public conversation about efficiency.

6. Elsewhere, the author writes in more detail about public hospitals in Canada. Based on the information in the passage, these hospitals are most likely:

A) offering a lower standard of care than private hospitals do.
B) unable to afford efficient, time-saving technology.
C) under pressure to provide better care without increased resources.
D) overly focused on costs rather than patient care.

7. Throughout the passage, the author suggests which of the following to be true of efficiency?

A) It is a deceptively attractive idea.
B) It is the foundation of a well-run state.
C) It is just as important to public life as to private life.
D) It is never a worthy goal.

CHAPTER 4 PRACTICE PASSAGE 2

Three basic positions have prevailed on the debate over the Voting Rights Act, distinguished largely by their different views on whether the Act should be rolled back, pushed forward, or simply maintained. Given these differences in orientation, these ideological responses to the act can be called conservative, progressive, and centrist. The conflicting claims of conservatives and progressives set the outer limits of debate, making discussion of minority representation a sharply contested and exceedingly polarized affair. In such a context of mutually exclusive assertions, the centrist attempt to strike a reasonable balance appears immediately appealing.

On the whole, while conservatives and progressives are united in their rejection of the status quo, they diverge sharply in their reasons for seeking change. Where conservatives see a politics that has been held hostage to the demands of civil rights elites, progressives describe a politics increasingly dominated by white racism and retrenchment. It is in this polarized context of claims and counterclaims that the centrists attempt to fashion a reasonable middle position. Dismissing both conservative and progressive claims as exaggerated rhetoric, centrists argue that the debate over the Voting Rights Act is actually quite narrow. While name calling and finger pointing have drawn the lion's share of attention, centrists claim that most of the disputants are actually concerned with achieving a color-blind society. Beneath the barbed polemics, controversies over minority representation amount to a disagreement over means rather than ends. Bernard Grofman and Chandler Davis suggest that the "highly abstract" mode of the current debate only breeds misunderstanding and conflict; a better approach is to be found in a "consideration of the empirical evidence of the actual consequences of the [Voting Rights Act]."

In the centrist view, then, the Voting Rights Act is neither a racially balkanizing nor a broadly empowering document. In essence, the act takes limited steps to ameliorate specific and concrete inequities. The incrementalist, case-by-case nature of voting-rights policy means that remedial measures can be crafted without raising larger issues of democratic theory. Big questions such as "What is fair minority representation?" never need to be asked because judges and other federal officials are simply correcting what is obviously wrong given the specific facts at hand.

What can be made of the centrist attempt to steer a middle course between conservative and progressive claims? Centrists make the claim for a responsive political process largely by insisting that the incrementalism of voting rights policy avoids theoretical questions. The very realism and reasonableness of the Voting Rights Act inheres in its atheoretical design. Thus, the centrist argument amounts to more than a simple

corrective of exaggerated views. If the centrists are right, the entire polarized debate between conservatives and progressives should be set aside as a distraction. We will do just fine if the country and the courts continue to muddle through the issue of minority representation a case at a time.

One could argue that so long as the Supreme Court is effectively constrained by its own canons of statutory construction, voting-rights reform need not plunge into any conceptual morass. The difficulty with such an argument is that the judiciary has historically employed a number of canons, many of which point interpretation in different directions. It is true that some legal commentators have spoken of the judge "worth his salt" or with the right "sense of the situation" who can negotiate among the various canons, consistently producing an accurate rendering of the statute's meaning or purpose. Despite such claims, widespread consensus on what should count as the proper "sense of the situation" has not emerged. Easy agreement has proved elusive because the choice between interpretive strategies itself depends on what Cass Sunstein calls "background principles" —principles that express particular visions of how government ought to operate and, thus, provide the baseline against which statutes should be understood.

In general, one can say that the process of statutory interpretation is critically concerned with normative disputes over how the government ought to operate. By stressing measurable facts and hard evidence, the centrist argument as a whole sidesteps the debate's key issue. The progressive and conservative views are not simply "mistakes" that can be corrected by a more accurate set of facts. Each of these camps anchors its claims in different conceptions of fair representation, which serve as guides for how the Voting Rights Act's promise of equal political opportunity ought to be realized. Thus, conservatives and progressives do not simply disagree on what the "facts" of the debate are. More importantly, they disagree on what the same "facts" mean in light of what fair minority representation is taken to be.

Material used in this particular passage has been adapted from the following source:

K. Bybee, *Mistaken Identity: The Supreme Court and the Politics of Minority Representation.* © 1998 by Princeton University Press.

1. Which of the following statements best expresses the main thesis of the passage?

A)   Three positions have emerged in the debate over the Voting Rights Act, which may be labeled progressive, centrist, and conservative.
B)   While imperfect, the centrist approach is the most reasonable, given that it avoids the ideological extremes embodied in the conservative and progressive positions and that it advocates a case-by-case evaluation of the impact of the Voting Rights Act.
C)   The centrist position on the Voting Rights Act, while seemingly a pragmatic middle road between two extremes, fails to address the theoretical issues that underlie questions of minority representation.
D)   While the conservative and progressive positions on the Voting Rights Act both seek significant change, the centrist position prefers a more incrementalist approach.

2. The author refers to commentators who speak of judges with the correct "sense of the situation" in order to:

A)   illustrate a way in which a common understanding of basic principles of fair representation might be reached.
B)   raise and then challenge a consideration that might be used to support the centrist approach.
C)   criticize judges for arriving at overly personal solutions to complex theoretical problems.
D)   support the claim that the Voting Rights Act turns on the contestable issue of "equal political opportunity."

3. Suppose it were shown that progressives believe fair representation of a minority group can only by achieved through electing representatives who are members of that group, while conservatives believe that minority interests are well protected by any representative who works for the good of society as a whole. If this is true, which claim described in the passage would be most *undermined*?

A)   The author's claim that background principles determine how facts are interpreted
B)   The conservative claim that the Voting Rights Act should be rolled back
C)   The centrist claim that application of the Voting Rights Act need not consider big abstract questions
D)   The progressive claim that politics is dominated by white racism

4. The author's argument in paragraph 6 that the progressive and conservative camps locate their claims in different conceptions of fair representation is supported:

A)   weakly, because no descriptions or examples of these different concepts are provided.
B)   weakly, because this claim conflicts with the centrist argument that the Voting Rights Act is atheoretical.
C)   strongly, because it is based on Sunstein's conception of "background principles."
D)   strongly, because it implies that the same facts may be interpreted in different ways by different people.

5. In the context of the passage, "incrementalism" (paragraph 4) most likely refers to a policy that:

A)   causes fundamental societal change.
B)   considers problems on a case-by-case basis.
C)   is concerned with achieving a color-blind society.
D)   takes a step-by-step approach to reaching agreement on basic theoretical principles.

6. Which of the following would be most analogous to the centrist approach, as it is described in the passage?

A)   A physicist who seeks to reconcile two competing theories by finding a middle ground that incorporates aspects of both
B)   A physicist who draws on a new field of theoretical mathematics in order to address a longstanding dispute within the field
C)   A physicist who delineates three distinct approaches to solving a problem and evaluates their relative strengths and weaknesses
D)   A physicist who suggests that a significant experimental discrepancy can be addressed without major reworking of present theories

7. Which of the following, if true, would most support the author's evaluation of the centrist position?

A)   Different ideas of what constitutes fair representation are inextricably bound up with differing ideas about the proper role of the state within society.
B)   Controversy about how to delineate electoral districts in order to ensure fair representation is often based on disagreements about population statistics.
C)   The original writers of the Voting Rights Act did not believe that the implementation of the act would require debate on abstract questions of principle.
D)   The conflicting claims set out by progressives and conservatives differ more in terms of vocabulary than on the basic ideas intended to be expressed through the rhetoric employed by each side.

SOLUTIONS TO CHAPTER 4 PRACTICE PASSAGE 1

1. **A** This is an Inference question.

   A: Yes. See paragraph 4: "Efficiency is not an end, but a means to achieve valued ends." This answer choice uses different words to refer to "ends" and "means," and this distinction is central to the author's main idea about efficiency.

   B: No. While the example of the automated kitchen in paragraph 1 does introduce the idea of efficient technology, the author does not explicitly describe a distinction between different types of technology.

   C: No. The author does suggest in paragraph 2 that the advertisement referred to in paragraph 1 is intentionally vague—"But the ad misses, not by accident, I suspect, one crucial piece of information"—but no distinction is drawn between different types of advertising.

   D: No. See paragraph 3: "The language of efficiency shapes our public as well as our private lives." This suggests our public and private views of efficiency are similar, rather than distinct.

2. **A** This is an Inference question.

   A: Yes. In paragraph 6, the author says, "The cult of efficiency, like other cults, advances political purposes and agendas." Advancing a political purpose entails making an impact on the political conversation. Cults, as the author defines them, therefore can influence society.

   B: No. Be sure to choose answers that are supported by the passage text. This choice is a common-sense view of cults that is not expressed in the passage. The author does not go so far as to call the cult of efficiency "illogical."

   C: No. The author uses the word "cult" in the context of describing how the "cult of efficiency" "misuses language" in a way that "has profound consequences for the way we as citizens conceive of public life" (paragraph 3). She also writes that the "cult of efficiency, like other cults, advances political purposes and agendas" (paragraph 6). To label cults as *simply* groups of people who agree with each other would be inconsistent with the author's tone.

   D: No. This choice uses language that is too absolute. The "cult of efficiency" may be based on a discussion of costs, but the passage does not apply this idea to other cults.

3. **C** This is an Inference question.

   A: No. The author discusses the value of government in paragraph 6, but does not say that its value lies in cost-effectiveness.

   B: No. This is the view of "the cult of efficiency" as described in paragraph 6, which the author says "is based on a fundamental misunderstanding of the importance of the 'smart' state in the global, knowledge-based economy."

   C: Yes. See paragraph 6: "The state is branded as wasteful, and market mechanisms are heralded as the efficient alternative. This argument, we shall see, is based on a fundamental misunderstanding of the importance of the 'smart' state in the global, knowledge-based economy." The author believes the state is still relevant.

   D: No. The author defends the value of the state in paragraph 6. While the passage doesn't indicate that the government is as efficient as the market (the author rejects efficiency as a valid stand-alone standard of judgment), neither does the author indicate that it is less efficient.

4. **C** This is a New Information question.

   A: No. See paragraph 4: "Efficiency...is not a goal, but an instrument to achieve other goals." The author would not necessarily see cutting costs as an important goal in its own right for the school board.

B: No. In the passage, the author argues that efficiency in and of itself does not equate with quality: "Efficiency is not an end, but a means to achieve valued ends" (paragraph 4). In paragraph 5, the author writes: "What, for example, is an effective education? To answer that question, we would first have to discuss the purposes of education, a discussion that is informed by values, and only then could we come to some understanding of the criteria of effectiveness." Therefore, the author would not automatically equate saving money with quality education (more likely, the opposite).

C: Yes. Consider paragraph 5: "Even when efficiency is used correctly as a means, when it is understood as the most cost-effective way to achieve our goals, much of our public discussion is fuzzy about its purpose. What does effectiveness mean? What, for example, is an effective education?" So, any discussion of the merits of cutting costs depends on a larger discussion of the *goals* of cutting costs. Thus, this is the author's most likely response.

D: No. The author's main idea is that efficiency should be used as a means rather than an end, but this answer takes that idea too far by implying the author is opposed to the idea of efficiency (in education) altogether.

5. **D** This is an Inference/EXCEPT question.

A: No. This assertion is supported in paragraph 3: "The language of efficiency shapes our public as well as our private lives." In paragraph 6, the author specifically discusses how the language of efficiency relates to and affects our view of the state.

B: No. This assertion is supported in paragraph 6: "Yet the word 'efficiency' is not only misused in public conversation as an end rather than a means.... The cult of efficiency, like other cults, advances political purposes and agendas." Since the former statement is the author's opinion and the latter the explanation of that opinion, it is reasonable to infer that the cult of efficiency misuses the term.

C: No. In paragraphs 1 and 2, the author states that the phrase "How efficient!" intentionally obscures "one crucial piece of information. It does not tell me *at what* this newly wired, very expensive kitchen will be efficient."

D: Yes. The passage does not suggest the government itself uses language to mislead. Thus, this is the correct choice.

6. **C** This is a New Information question.

A: No. The author does not compare public and private hospitals.

B: No. Technology is the subject of paragraphs 1 and 2, not paragraph 3 in which the author discusses the state of hospitals and other publicly funded institutions. There is no evidence in the passage that public hospitals are unable to afford any particular type of technology, only that they are under pressure to be cost-effective.

C: Yes. See paragraph 3: "Those who provide our public services are expected to do so efficiently. Physicians and nurses in the hospital where my mother was treated are expected to work efficiently.... They are constantly enjoined to become efficient, to remain efficient, and to improve their efficiency in the safeguarding of the public trust." This answer choice paraphrases the idea that hospitals and their employees are under pressure to be more efficient. We are not told what country the author is writing about in the passage; however, this choice represents a reasonable (compared to the other choices) analogy to draw, even if the author is not discussing Canada in the passage text.

D: No. The author describes the demands placed on public services from the outside. The hospital's own focus is outside the scope of the argument. This choice is also too extreme; the existence of pressure to reduce costs does not necessarily guarantee that costs have taken precedence over patient care within the hospital itself.

7.   **A**   This is an Inference question.

A: **Yes. In paragraph 1, the example of the ad illustrates that efficiency is attractive. In paragraph 2, the author then explains this promise lacks substance. In paragraph 3, she refers to this advertisement process as a "seduction," a process based on attraction.**

B: No. On one hand, the author does say efficiency is important. In paragraph 4, she says it can be "used correctly as a means...to achieve our goals." However, the author also states in the same paragraph that "Efficiency is only one part of a much larger public discussion between citizens and their governments." That is, it would be one means (perhaps among many) to a goal of a well-run state, whatever "well-run" might mean in context.

C: No. The passage makes no comparison between the importance of efficiency itself in public and private life (only that the *language* of efficiency is used in both).

D: No. This is too extreme; it is inconsistent with the author's argument that efficiency can be an important means to an end (paragraph 4).

SOLUTIONS TO CHAPTER 4 PRACTICE PASSAGE 2

1.   **C**   This is a Main Idea/Primary Purpose question.

A: No. This choice is too narrow to be the correct answer to a Main Idea question. While the statement is supported by the passage, it leaves out the heart of the author's argument, which is his evaluation of the validity (or lack thereof) of the centrist position.

B: No. This choice misrepresents the author's opinion. While the author does state that "the centrists attempt to fashion a reasonable middle position" (paragraph 2), and that their position "appears immediately appealing" (paragraph 1), the author argues in paragraphs 5–6 that this position is fundamentally flawed in its assumption that discussion and implementation of the Voting Rights Act can avoid theoretical discussion. Always make sure to take the entire passage into account for a general question and to clearly define the author's opinion.

C: **Yes. After discussing the three positions in paragraphs 1–4, the author argues that the centrists are fundamentally wrong in their assertion that the act can be understood or implemented without confronting abstract issues: for example, what constitutes fair representation. The author's tone is clear in phrases such as "The difficulty with such an argument" and "The centrist position as a whole sidesteps."**

D: No. As in choice A, this answer is supported by the passage (paragraphs 1 and 2), but is too narrow to be the main thesis of the passage. For example, it leaves out the author's negative evaluation of the centrist position.

2.   **B**   This is a Structure question.

A: No. The author suggests the opposite. He states: "Despite such claims, widespread consensus on what should count as the proper 'sense of the situation' has not emerged" (paragraph 5). Furthermore, the commentators themselves are not referring to judges who achieve a common understanding of basic principles, but rather to those who supposedly can come to an accurate understanding of the meaning or purpose of a statute (and how to apply it to a particular case).

B: Yes. A centrist might use the argument that abstract principles need not be considered by voting-rights reform because judges are able "negotiate among the various canons" to interpret and apply statutes without relying on theoretical interpretation. The author goes on to say that this is not in fact the case, because deciding how to interpret a statute requires choosing between basic principles regarding "how the government ought to operate" (paragraph 6). Notice that the author introduces the example of these judges with "it is true that," and that the following sentence begins with "Despite such claims." These phrases indicate that the point of view referenced in the question stem tends to challenge the author's overall position.

C: No. There is no criticism of the judges themselves expressed by the author. The implied criticism is of the commentators who make this argument about judges. Also, the problem identified by the author isn't that their approach is too "personal," but rather that it cannot in fact avoid theoretical issues.

D: No. This is the wrong issue. While the author does reference this argument in paragraph 5, the discussion of judges in that paragraph does not itself give evidence that the act depends or hinges on the particular contestable issue of "equal political opportunity."

3. **C** This is a New Information question.

Note: The new information suggests a disagreement about what constitutes fair representation. This, if valid, would undermine the centrist claim that "Big questions such as 'What is fair minority representation?' never need to be asked because judges and other federal officials are simply correcting what is obviously wrong given the specific facts at hand" (paragraph 3). And, by undermining the centrists, it strengthens the author's critique of the centrist position.

A: No. This new information would strengthen rather than weaken the author's position.

B: No. This new information has no impact on the conservative position. The fact that there are different conceptions of fair representation does not by itself suggest that the act is something that should be maintained or extended rather than rolled back.

C: Yes. The centrist claim that abstract questions do not need to be considered rests in part on their belief that most people agree on basic principles, and that there can be wide agreement on what is "obviously wrong given the specific facts at hand" (paragraph 3). If there is in fact disagreement on what constitutes fair representation, this would weaken or undermine the centrist position. Note that the author states in paragraph 6 that "Each of these camps anchors its claims in different conceptions of fair representation, which serve as guides for how the Voting Rights Act's promise of equal political opportunity ought to be realized." This suggests that the very different ways of conceiving of "fair representation" described in the question stem would qualify as different ends or principles, not just different means.

D: No. The new information gives no evidence one way or the other about the existence or role of white racism in the political process.

4. **A** This is an Evaluate question.

A: Yes. This statement is weakly supported. The author makes the claim but gives no supportive evidence to prove the claim. We don't know what those different conceptions are, or how significantly they might differ.

B: No. The first word of the choice is correct, but the rest of it is incorrect. The entire point of the passage is largely to disprove the centrist argument. Simply conflicting with an opposing position is not itself a weakness.

C: No. While the claim cited in the question follows from the discussion of Sunstein's idea (paragraph 5), the concept of the existence of background principles does not itself support the claim that conservatives and progressives have different concepts of fair representation.

D: No. The second part of the choice is accurate (see paragraph 6), but the evaluation ("strongly") is incorrect. This choice essentially reverses the relationship between parts of the argument. The implication of a claim (that is, the conclusion based on it) does not itself provide support for the claim.

5.   **B**   This is an Inference question.

A: No. This is the opposite of what the term expresses in the context of the centrist view. The centrists, who advocate the incrementalist view, believe that application of the act on a case-by-case basis entails simply correcting mistakes on a relatively small scale.

B: **Yes. "Incrementalism" is essentially defined in the previous paragraph: "The incrementalist, case-by-case nature of voting-rights policy means that remedial measures can be crafted without raising larger issues of democratic theory."**

C: No. This describes what the centrists believe to be true of most people (paragraph 2), but does not define incrementalism itself.

D: No. This choice is half-right but half-wrong. Yes, it is a step-by-step approach, but not to reaching agreement on theoretical principles. The centrists (who are identified with incrementalism in the passage) believe that this agreement has already been reached (see paragraph 2).

6.   **D**   This is an Analogy question.

Note: The correct answer will be the one that is most logically similar to the centrist view or approach. In the passage, the author states that according to the centrists, "the act takes limited steps to ameliorate specific and concrete inequities" (paragraph 3), that "Big questions such as 'What is fair minority representation?' never need to be asked because judges and other federal officials are simply correcting what is obviously wrong given the specific facts at hand" (paragraph 3), and that "We will do just fine if the country and the courts continue to muddle through the issue of minority representation a case at a time" (paragraph 4).

A: No. This choice is immediately attractive because it mentions a middle ground. However, the centrists aren't trying to get the progressives and conservatives to come to some new agreement through compromise. Rather, the centrists argue that there is already basic agreement or mutual understanding on what is fair, and it's just a practical issue of how to achieve that in particular cases.

B: No. The centrists do make use of any new theory or outside discipline.

C: No. Although the passage delineates three positions, the question asks for an analogy to the approach of the centrists, not of author of the passage.

D: **Yes. This choice is analogous to the author's description of the centrists as seeking to focus on a case-by-case approach that does not require engaging deep theoretical questions.**

7.   A   This is a Strengthen question.

   A: **Yes. In paragraphs 5 and 6, the author critiques the centrist position in part by arguing that agreement on how to apply statutes requires agreement on "background principles" about "how government ought to operate"(that is, the proper role of the state in society). He goes on to say that this means that because each camp has a different idea of what "fair representation" means, they disagree on abstract issues of principle regarding how to interpret "facts." The author, however, never directly states that, or explains how, the operation of government relates to fair representation. If the two are in fact fundamentally interrelated, it would support the author's critique of the centrists' claim that there is no fundamental disagreement on principles within the Voting Rights Act debate.**

   B: No. This would support the centrists themselves, by suggesting that at least some of the debate is about facts or empirical questions (here, statistics), rather than about matters of principle.

   C: No. To the extent that the intent or belief of the writers of the act is relevant, this would go against the author's interpretation.

   D: No. This would weaken the author's argument by supporting the centrist claim. This choice suggests that the disagreement between progressives and conservatives is not as stark as it may seem, and there is a fair amount of basic agreement on basic ideas.

Individual Passage Log

Passage # _____

Q#	Q type	Attractors	What did you do wrong?

Revised Strategy _____

Passage # _____

Q#	Q type	Attractors	What did you do wrong?

Revised Strategy _____

Think Like a Test-Writer: Exercise 2

THINK LIKE A TEST-WRITER: EXERCISE 2

There are certain kinds of statements in passage texts that tend to generate questions: transitions, comparisons and contrasts, expressions of the author's opinion or the opinions of others, example indicators, etc. In the passage text on the next page, some of these "question generators" are in red text and some of those are numbered. The purpose of the drill is to sensitize yourself to the kinds of things in passages that the test-writers use to create questions and the right answers to those questions (and attractive wrong answers as well). [Note: the computer-based testing tools do not allow you to change the color of the text, and there will be no red text in your MCAT passages. The red font here is only for the purpose of the drill. The questions attached to a CARS passage on the test will also not usually be presented in the order in which the relevant material appears in the test.]

First, read the entire passage. When you see red text, pay special attention to that part of the passage. Note the logical function and importance of that segment in the context of the paragraph and, as you read further, in the context of the passage as a whole. A series of numbered MCAT CARS-like questions connected to the corresponding number in the text are provided at the end of the passage. Answer the questions in your own words, going back to those parts of the passage as needed, and then check the explanations that follow.

The text on the next page is longer than a CARS passage in order to give you extra practice with these skills.

EXERCISE 2

In 1552, Francisco López de Gómara, who had been chaplain and secretary to Hernando Cortés while he lived out his old age in Spain, published an account of the conquest of Mexico. López de Gómara himself had never been to the New World, but he could envision it nonetheless. "Many [Indians] came to gape at the strange men, now so famous, and at their attire, arms and horses, and they said, "these men are gods!" [Q1] The chaplain was one of the first to claim in print that the Mexicans had believed the conquistadors to be divine. Among the welter of statements made in the Old World about inhabitants of the New, this one found particular resonance. It was repeated with enthusiasm, and soon a specific version gained credence: the Mexicans had apparently believed in a god called Quetzalcoatl, who long ago had disappeared in the east, promising to return from that direction on a certain date. In an extraordinary coincidence, Cortés appeared off the coast in that very year and was mistaken for Quetzalcoatl by the devout. Today, most educated persons in the United States, Europe, and Latin America are fully versed in this account, as readers of this piece can undoubtably affirm. In fact, however, there is little evidence that the indigenous people ever seriously believed the newcomers were gods, and there is no meaningful evidence that any story about Quetzalcoatl's returning from the east ever existed before the conquest. A number of scholars of early Mexico are aware of this, but few others are. The cherished narrative is alive and well, and in urgent need of critical attention.

In order to dismantle a construct with such a long history, it will be necessary first to explain the origins and durability of the myth and then to offer an alternate explanation of what happened in the period of conquest and what the indigenous were actually thinking. In proposing an alternative, I will make three primary assertions: first, that we must put technology in all its forms—beyond mere weaponry—front and center in our story of conquest; [Q2] second, that we can safely do this because new evidence from scientists offers us explanations for divergent technological levels that have nothing to do with differences in intelligence; and third, that the Mexicans themselves immediately became aware of the technology gap and responded to it with intelligence and savvy rather than wide-eyed talk of gods. They knew before we did, it seems, that technology was the crux. ...

Our first task must be to ask ourselves whence came the myths associated with the conquest. The simple truth is that, by the 1550s, some [Indigenous people] were themselves saying that they (or rather, their parents) had presumed the white men to be gods. ... [Q3] Numerous scholars have analyzed these words while ignoring their context. The best known such work is Tzvetan Todorov's *Conquest of America: The Question of the Other.* Although quick to say there is no "natural inferiority" (indeed, he [Q4] aptly pointed out that it is the [Indigenous people] who rapidly learn the language of the Spanish, not the other way around), he insists that it is the Spaniards' greater deftness in manipulating signs that gives them victory. While the Spanish believe in man-man communication ("What are we to do?"), the [Indigenous people] only envision man-world communication ("How are we to know?"). Thus the [Indigenous people] have a "paralyzing belief that the Spaniards are gods" and are "inadequate in a situation requiring improvisation." Popular historians have been equally quick to accept this idea of indigenous reality, often with the best intentions. Hugh Thomas's recent monumental 800-page volume is a case in point. Thomas uses apocryphal accounts as if they had been tape-recorded conversations in his portrayal of the inner workings of Moctezuma's court. ... Thomas does this, I believe, not out of naïveté but out of a genuine desire to incorporate the [Indigenous] perspective. He does not want to describe the intricate politics of the Spanish while leaving the [Indigenous] side vague, rendering it less real to his readers.

With such friends, though, perhaps the indigenous and their cultural heirs do not need enemies. A different approach is definitely needed, or the white gods will continue to inhabit our narratives. And beginning anew, let us first ask what sources we have available. We in fact have only one set of documents that were undoubtedly written at the time of conquest by someone who was certainly there—the letters of Cortés. The *Cartas* are masterful constructions [Q5], loaded with political agendas, but we are at least certain of their origin, and Cortés never wrote that he was taken for a god....

[Another] group of sources were produced by the indigenous themselves, but here is the heart of the problem: we have none that date from the years of conquest or even from the 1520s or 1530s. There are sixteen surviving pre-conquest codices (none from Mexico City itself, where the conquerors' book burning was most intense), and then, dating from the 1540s, statements written in Nahuatl using the Roman alphabet, which was then rapidly becoming accessible to educated indigenous through the school of Tlatelolco. The most famous such document about the conquest is the lengthy Book Twelve of the Florentine Codex. Although it was organized by Sahagún, and the Spanish glosses were written by him, the Nahuatl is the work of his Indian aides. [In addition,] at the end of the century, a few indigenous men wrote histories. …

These, then, are the rather limited documents we have to work with.… It is in this context that we must approach the later understanding that the Aztecs were convinced that their own omens had for years been predicting the coming of the cataclysm, [Q6] and that Cortés was recognized as Quetzalcoatl and the Europeans as gods. The most important source for all these legends is Book Twelve of the Florentine Codex. Lockhart notes that it reads very much as if it were two separate documents: the first part, covering the period from the sighting of the European sails to the Spaniards' violent attack on warrior-dancers participating in a religious festival, reads like an apocryphal fable (complete with comets as portents), while the second part, covering the period from the Aztec warriors' uprising against the Spaniards after the festival to their ultimate defeat over a year later, reads like a military archivist's record of events. Indeed, this phenomenon makes sense: the old men being interviewed in the 1550s would likely have participated as young warriors in the battles against the Spanish, or at least have been well aware of what was transpiring. On the other hand, they would most certainly not have been privy to the debates within Moctezuma's inner circle when the Spaniards arrival first became known: the king's closest advisers were killed in the conquest, and at any rate would have been older men even in 1520.

Still, the fact that the informants for the Florentine were not acquainted with the inner workings of Moctezuma's court only proves that they were unlikely to have the first part of the story straight; it tells us nothing about why they chose to say what they did. It seems likely that they retroactively sought to find particular auguries associated with the conquest. The Florentine's omens do not appear to have been commonly accepted, as

they do not appear in other Nahuatl sources. Interestingly, Fernandez-Armesto notes that the listed omens fall almost exactly in line with certain Greek and Latin texts that are known to have been available to Sahagún's students.

Why would Sahagún's assistants have been so eager to come up with a compelling narrative about omens? [Q6] We must bear in mind that they were the sons and grandsons of Tenochtitlan's most elite citizens—descendants of priests and nobles. It was their own class, even their own family members, who might have been thought to be at fault if it were true that they had had no idea that the Spaniards existed prior to their arrival. … It begins to seem not merely unsurprising, but indeed necessary, that Sahagún's elite youths should insist that their forebears had read the signs and had known what was to happen. In their version, the Truth was paralyzing and left their forebears vulnerable, even more so than they might have been.

The idea that Cortés was understood to be the god Quetzalcoatl returning from the east is also presented as fact in Book Twelve. Moctezuma sends gifts for different gods, to see which are most welcome to the newcomers, and then decides it is Quetzalcoatl who has come. There are numerous obvious problems with the story. First, Quetzalcoatl was not a particularly prominent god in the pantheon worshiped in Mexico's great city. The one city in the empire where Quetzalcoatl was prominent, Cholula, was the only one to mount a concerted attack against Cortés as he made his way to the Aztec capital. Many aspects of the usual post-conquest description of Quetzalcoatl—that he was a peace-loving god who abhorred human sacrifice, for example—are obviously European mythological constructs, thus rendering the whole story somewhat suspect. Furthermore, in the Codex itself, when the earlier explorer Juan de Grijalva lands on the coast in 1518, [Q7] he is taken to be Quetzalcoatl. So much for the explanation that Cortés happened to land in the right year, causing all the pieces to fall into place in the indigenous imagination.

—Adapted from "Burying the White Gods: New Perspectives on the Conquest of Mexico," by Camilla Townsend. *The American Historical Review,* Vol. 108, No. 3. © 2003 by Oxford University Press on behalf of the American Historical Association.

Question #1: Why does the author state that López de Gómara's account "found particular resonance" and "was repeated with enthusiasm"?

_____

_____

_____

Question #2: What can you infer from the author's statement that "we can safely [focus on the role of technology] because new evidence from scientists offers us explanations for divergent technological levels that have nothing to do with differences in intelligence"?

_____

_____

_____

Question #3: What "context" is the author referring to when she writes "Numerous scholars have analyzed these words while ignoring their context" in the third paragraph?

_____

_____

_____

Question #4: What is the author's attitude toward Todorov's work?

_____

_____

_____

Question #5: Why does the author call Cortés's letters "masterful"?

_____

_____

_____

Question #6: Suppose it were shown to be true that both the Spaniards (during their conquest of the New World) and Aztec elites (after conquest) propagated the "white god" myth. Based on the passage, could you infer that they had the same motives in promoting such similar stories?

_____

_____

_____

Question #7: Is the story of Juan de Grijalva consistent or inconsistent with the author's argument regarding the causal factors entailed in the conquest of Mexico presented earlier in the passage?

_____

_____

_____

Bonus question: What is the Primary Purpose of the passage as a whole?

_____

_____

_____

SOLUTIONS TO EXERCISE 2

1. Note that in the beginning of the passage, it at first appears that the author might agree with the story that "the Mexicans had believed the conquistadors to be divine." Remember, however, that just because the author says that other people believe something to be true doesn't by itself mean that the author agrees. Keep an open mind, read on, and you discover that the author makes these statements to indicate that this story is *widely believed, but false*. The author's true position begins to become clear with the phrase "In fact, however…" later in that same paragraph.

2. There are at least two main things that you can infer from this statement. First, and most straightforwardly, the author believes that technology, NOT belief in the divinity of the Spaniards (note the phrase "and then to offer an alternate explanation of what happened" that precedes the cited claim) played a key role in the conquest of Mexico by Spain. Secondly, the author does NOT believe that difference in intelligence played a role in that conquest; she states that we can "safely" focus on technology *because* it has "nothing to do with differences in intelligence."

3. The context being referred to here (paragraph 3) doesn't become fully clear until later in the passage. It is only in paragraph 7 that we learn that the writings of indigenous people regarding the conquest may have been affected by the desire to absolve their predecessors of blame for not understanding the threat presented by the Spaniards. Just as the author emphasizes the importance of context, you must take the full context of the passage, in this case a paragraph much later in the passage, into account when answering this question.

4. The author does say some good things about Todorov: he "*aptly* pointed out that it is the [Indigenous people] who rapidly learn the language of the Spanish…" Meaning, he was correct to do so. As with Thomas, the author does not ascribe bad motives, just the opposite: Thomas did what he did "not out of naïveté but out of a genuine desire to incorporate the [Indigenous] perspective." However, the author of the passage is using Todorov and Thomas as examples of writers who, despite their good intentions, get it wrong by buying into the story that conquest was facilitated by the Aztec's belief in the divinity of Cortés and his men. Therefore, while the author is not condemning Todorov, she is certainly critical of his claims. This negative tone is reinforced by the first sentence of the next paragraph: "With such friends, though, perhaps the indigenous and their cultural heirs do not need enemies."

5. Again, context is key. Taken by itself, the word "masterful" sounds very positive. Here, however, the author's point is that they were written at least in part for political purposes (and that Cortés did a very good job of that). The author isn't making a major point of praising Cortés's political acumen, but neither is she criticizing it. The relevant issue is that while Cortés may not have been writing with the goal of providing a fully honest portrayal of the events, his writings do have some value ("we are at least certain of their origin") as they provide more evidence that Cortés was not seen as a god by the Aztecs. You have to be careful not to over-interpret the word "masterful" or to apply it to the wrong issue in the passage.

6. Paragraphs 6-8 provide an extended discussion of indigenous sources, what they did and did not report, and how they give evidence that the Aztecs themselves asserted the truth of the "white god" explanation for their own conquest. However, while the stories are the same, the

passage indicates that their motives would be very different. The Spaniards may have promoted the story to aid in conquest of the New World, while the Aztecs told it to save or rehabilitate the reputation of their family members. Therefore, this issue represents both a comparison (same story) and a contrast (different timing and motivation).

7. The story of Juan de Grijalva is consistent with the rest of the author's argument. If read too carelessly, it may seem as if the author is contradicting herself by giving an example of a Spanish explorer who WAS seen as a god, the god Quetzalcoatl. However, when taken in context, you can see that this is yet another piece of evidence AGAINST the "white gods" story. If Juan de Grijalva, who appeared at a completely different time, was hailed as Quetzalcoatl, it is unlikely that Cortés was believed to be Quetzalcoatl returning from the east as well, or that conquest was facilitated by a crazy coincidence of Cortés appearing at just the right time to be hailed as the returning god.

Bonus question: Note the logical structure of the passage. First the author sets up the story of the Spaniards being hailed and welcomed as gods, and then she proceeds to knock that story down piece by piece, and to suggest that the superior technology of the Spaniards was the real cause. The following phrases (among others) indicate that the author's purpose is to reject the "white gods" causal story and to suggest an alternative story:

- "In fact, however, there is little evidence that the indigenous people ever seriously believed the newcomers were gods" (P1)
- "The cherished narrative is alive and well, and in urgent need of critical attention." (P1)
- "In order to dismantle a construct with such a long history, it will be necessary first to explain the origins and durability of the myth and then to offer an alternate explanation of what happened in the period of conquest" (P2)
- "three primary assertions: first, that we must put technology in all its forms—beyond mere weaponry—front and center in our story of conquest" (P2)
- "With such friends, though, perhaps the indigenous and their cultural heirs do not need enemies. A different approach is definitely needed" (P4)
- "There are numerous obvious problems with the story." (P9)

Chapter 5
The Process of
Elimination (POE)
and Attractors

GOALS

1) To learn the principles and steps of working through questions using the Process of Elimination (POE)
2) To recognize patterns in Attractors

5.1 THE PROCESS OF ELIMINATION

As we discussed in the last chapter, there are five basic steps you must take in answering any CARS question.

1) **Read the question word for word and identify the question type.**
2) **Translate the question into your own words: identify what the question task is asking you to do with the information in the passage.**
3) **Identify any key words that refer to specific parts of the passage. If key words are provided, *go back to the passage* to locate that information.**
4) **Answer in your own words: articulate what the correct answer will need to do based on the question type and the information in the passage.**
5) **Use Process of Elimination (POE), and choose the *least wrong* answer choice.**

In this chapter, we'll focus in more detail on Step 5, Process of Elimination or **POE**.

It is more effective to attack the question by eliminating the three wrong answer choices than by searching for the perfect choice. The MCAT writers are highly skilled at hiding the credited response in obscure and convoluted language, and at creating wrong answer choices that at first glance look good, but have a subtle yet fatal flaw. Your mission is to avoid the traps on your way to the correct choice.

Here are the basic steps of POE. In most cases, you will need to take two "cuts" through the choices as you narrow them down.

First Cut

Read Every Word of Every Choice Carefully.

This is not the time to skim! Once you have misinterpreted or skipped over something, it is very difficult to recognize your mistake.

Eliminate Choices Using the Bottom Line of the Passage.

Remind yourself of the Main Point and tone of the passage, and then read through each answer choice, eliminating any that violate, or directly contradict, the author's argument (unless it's a Weaken or EXCEPT/LEAST/NOT question). Understanding the passage's Bottom Line will also allow you to quickly eliminate choices that, although they may not contradict the author's points, are not relevant to the passage and thus are out of scope.

Eliminate Choices Inconsistent with Your Own Answer (When Possible, Given the Question Type).

Use your own answer to the question (which should be based closely on the passage and on the question task) as a guideline for eliminating answer choices. Do not, however, eliminate a choice just because it's not a perfect match. Be flexible.

As you gain experience predicting the answer, trust yourself more and more. Don't let an inconsistent answer make you second guess yourself. Your prediction is your life raft: don't abandon it on a whim! On the other hand, if none of the choices are consistent with your prediction, don't force a round peg into a square hole and talk yourself into one that "kind of sounds like" what you were looking for. Carefully re-read the question and go back into the passage to see what you might have missed the first time.

Second Cut

Reread the Question Stem.
Remind yourself (or improve your understanding) of the question type and issue.

Compare the Remaining Choices to Each Other.
Notice strength of language, scope, content references, and any other relevant differences between them.

Go Back to the Passage Again to Pin It Down (When Necessary).
Keep the differences between the choices in mind to help you find where you need to go.

Choose the Least Wrong Answer Choice.
When making your final choice, it's important to keep two things in mind.

1) **Be highly suspicious of absolute or extreme statements.**
   EXCEPT on Strengthen or Weaken questions, correct MCAT answer choices will rarely make an extreme claim. Do not use this test carelessly, however. Simple declarative statements (such as, *The inquisitorial system is historically superior to the adversarial system.*) are not necessarily extreme. Look for words that may indicate absolute statements such as *any, all, none, never, always, totally, must, only, exactly, impossible,* etc. Look out for statements that make extreme claims even without using any of these words.

Notice the wishy-washy or equivocal wording in the previous statement; these words *may,* not *must,* indicate statements that are too extreme for the passage. Whether or not a particular word or statement is extreme depends on how it is used within the context of the answer choice. The following phrases illustrate the difference between extreme and not so extreme statements, in the context of language that should and should not make you suspicious of answer choices.

Extreme	Not Extreme	Comments
will be	will for a time be	The phrase *will be* predicts the future, which may well be beyond the scope of the passage. The phrase *will for a time be* suggests a temporary condition, which is more moderate and therefore more likely to be supported by the text.
the greatest result	a great result	The use of the definite article *the* in combination with the suffix *-est* makes this a very strong statement. The phrase *a great result* is much less absolute, because it could be one of many great results.
kill all the roaches	kill roaches	The statement *kill roaches* sounds extreme because of the word kill, but in context the statement is not extreme or absolute. *Kill all the roaches* is in fact extreme because the statement is all-inclusive.

2) **If part of an answer choice is wrong, then it's all wrong.**

Pay attention to every word: one incorrect word or phrase will make the entire answer choice wrong. This is one reason why searching for the correct choice—instead of the three wrong choices—may lead you to an incorrect choice. Don't talk yourself into an answer just because you really like one thing about it; something really good about part of an answer can't outweigh a definitively bad part of that same answer. A wrong answer may have something attractive about it, but the credited response won't have anything incorrect in it (or will at least be the best supported of the four).

Any word can make an answer choice wrong. If the answer choice implies that something is true *all* of the time, and the passage suggests that it is true *some* (but *not all*) of the time, then the answer choice cannot be supported by the passage. Pay special attention to words of negation (such as *no, not, none, never,* etc.).

5.2 ATTRACTORS

Usually, if you understand the Bottom Line of the passage, it is easy to eliminate two of the four answer choices. But, students commonly express this lament: "I always get it down to two choices and then I pick the wrong one!" That's because the test is designed to make you do this.

For each question, there is usually at least one **Attractor**: an answer choice designed to tempt you into choosing it. It will have something attractive about it, such as words from the passage or concepts similar to those discussed by the author. If you're in too much of a hurry looking only for the "right" answer, you'll fall for an Attractor much of the time. Remember: the test-writers know how students think and what kind of logical mistakes they tend to make. Take the control away from them by predicting and avoiding the traps.

Typical Attractors

If you look for it, you'll see some patterns appear in the answer choices. The MCAT utilizes a core group of Attractors to tempt those who rush or who do not understand basic ideas presented in the passage. Here are the most common Attractors, grouped into categories. Learn them, look for them, and, thus, defend yourself against them.

Decoys

These choices are written to sound just like the passage. However, they include something that doesn't match up, either with the passage text or the question task.

- **Words out of context**

  This Attractor uses vocabulary right from the passage. It "sounds good," but the meaning of the words is changed. That is, the answer choice uses the right words but carries the wrong meaning. This is a trap in particular for people who are not going back to the passage, or who are not rereading the relevant parts of the passage carefully enough.

- **Half-right/half-wrong**

  These are "bait and switch" answers. Part or most of the choice is exactly what you are looking for, but another part is not supported by the passage (e.g., too extreme or out of scope). This is a trap set for people who make up their minds before they read the entire choice, or who try to "rehabilitate" an answer because part of it sounds so good. Remember that one word is enough to make a choice wrong.

- **Opposite/Negations**

  These choices take a sentence or idea directly from the passage, but add or remove a crucial "not" or "un." The statement therefore sounds just like the passage, but in fact directly contradicts it.

- **Reversals**

  This answer choice extracts a relationship from the passage but then reverses it to go in the opposite direction. It may flip a sequence of cause and effect, or confuse the order of events in a chronology.

- **Garbled language**

  This choice gives you some familiar words, but is difficult or impossible to understand. The test-writers are hoping that you will pick it thinking that because it is confusing it must be correct. However, another version of this trap is to put the correct choice into confusing language, with the hope that you will immediately eliminate it because it doesn't "sound good." So, when you see garbled language, don't automatically pick it, but don't automatically eliminate it either. And, don't spend five minutes trying to decipher it. Use POE aggressively: there may be a better choice, or it may be the only one left after you have eliminated the other three.

- **Right answer/wrong question**

  The statements in these Attractors, unlike in the other members of this category, are in fact directly supported by the passage. However, they aren't relevant to the question being asked. When you are down to two choices, always reread the question stem in order to avoid this trap.

- **Wrong point of view**

  This is a variation on the right answer/wrong question Attractor. If there is more than one point of view described in the passage, a wrong answer might describe a point of view different from the one referred to in the question stem.

Extremes

These choices go too far in one direction or the other.

- **Absolutes**

  This type of wrong answer uses language that is much stronger than the language in the passage. It may include extreme words such as *none, always, never, only*, etc. Keep in mind, however, that a strongly worded passage may support a strongly worded choice. Remember that a choice doesn't have to include one of the standard extreme words to be making a claim that is too extreme or absolute in its meaning.

- **Superlatives**

  These wrong answers include words like *first, last, best, most, worst, least* (or anything else ending in *–est*), or *primary*. For instance, it may describe a theory as the *first* or the *best* theory, but the author simply says that it's an important theory.

- **Judgments and recommendations**

  The choice passes judgment on whether something is good or bad, but that thing is described by the author in a neutral tone. Or, the answer choice states that a proposal should be implemented or rejected when that policy or action is merely described in the passage, or the choice may describe a moderate point of view in overly extreme terms. Finally, a wrong answer may tempt you to intuit the author's state of mind or personal beliefs in a way that is not supported by the passage text.

- **Not strong enough**

  This Attractor is specific to Strengthen and Weaken questions. Rather than being too extreme, it is too wishy-washy to significantly affect the author's argument in the passage. Always compare choices to each other; for this question type, you want the choice that goes farthest in the right direction.

Out of Scope

These answer choices introduce facts, issues, or claims that are never addressed in the passage, or, they do not match the scope of the question task.

- **Not the issue**

  This answer choice brings in ideas or facts that are not discussed in the passage. You will usually eliminate these in your first cut.

- **Outside knowledge**

  The wrong answer makes a statement that is true based on your own knowledge, but isn't directly supported by the text of the passage. Remember that the CARS section tests your ability to read actively and analyze the passage; it does not test your general knowledge.

- **Crystal ball**

  The wrong answer predicts the future (but the passage doesn't) or goes beyond the time frame of the passage.

- **No such comparison**

  This incorrect choice will take something that is mentioned in the passage and compare it to something that is not. Or, it may take two things that are mentioned by the author and compare them in a way that is not supported by the passage (often by stating that one option is better than the other).

- **Too narrow/too broad**

  The "too narrow" Attractor is typical on General questions: it mentions or contains only part of the author's argument. Keep in mind however that correct answers to Specific questions (including Inference questions) can be quite narrow. Wrong answers that are too broad have the opposite problem: they overgeneralize or go beyond the author's argument. They may describe a general category into which the topic of the passage would fit. On General questions, use the "Goldilocks Approach": eliminate any answer choices that are too narrow or too broad, and choose the one that is the best fit.

5.3 POE DOS AND DON'TS

Do

- Read and identify the question carefully—predict the traps.
- Read each answer choice word for word the first time, and consider all parts of every choice.
- Read all four answer choices carefully and with an open mind before deciding.
- Be suspicious—look for traps.
- Notice extreme or absolute wording and compare it to the passage text.
- Eliminate using the Bottom Line.
- Eliminate using your own answer.
- Compare the choices to each other.
- Go back to the passage often.

Don't

- Skim the answer choices.
- Pick the first choice that "sounds good."
- Ignore information in a choice, or add something to it, in order to make it fit. That is, don't force a square peg into a round hole.
- Eliminate choices on Strengthen or Weaken questions because of strong wording.
- Eliminate choices on Inference questions because of moderate wording.
- Pick D without reading it carefully just because you've eliminated answer choices A, B, and C.
- Answer based on memory.

5.4 THE SIX STEPS IN ACTION: MODEL PASSAGE

This exercise is intended to give you a picture of what an "ideal" process of attacking a passage looks like. One of your online CARS passages is reproduced on the next two pages.

- First, work through the passage on your own.
- Next, compare your progress through the passage to the model that follows in the book, which takes you from Previewing the Questions all the way through POE.
- The highlighting and noteboard notes in the sample passage provide a picture of what actual good highlighting and passage notes would look like and why. Keep in mind, however, that it isn't important to have matched them exactly—use the model to see if you caught and highlighted the most important things in the passage text and if you correctly understood the key parts of the author's argument. The questions that follow the highlighted passage are annotated to illustrate the thought process involved in translating the question, using the passage to generate an answer, and doing good POE.

5.4

It is strange that a novelist as superbly imaginative as John Fowles should be content to write within the canons of conventional textbook realism. Of the four stories in *The Ebony Tower*, three are simple, linear structures—situation, complication, resolution—the incidents rationally linked through the probable interactions of credible characteristics, the action and theme neatly illustrating each other. The fourth story is somewhat more open-ended and covert: a picnic in the country that ends in a disappearance and, by implication, a suicide. One has to draw the connections for oneself and see the sudden gathering storm at the end as an epiphany. But this is a technique that Joyce was practicing in *Dubliners* at the turn of the century, and it is still being practiced, from week to week, in the pages of *The New Yorker* and elsewhere.

Yet each of these stories [by Fowles] is anything but obvious or thin. However conventionally they begin and proceed, there comes a point when their issues dramatically engage and take on complexity and power—it's as though one had picked up a simple, familiar object, casually examined it, and suddenly found it shaking in one's hands. By the same token, Fowles' seemingly typecast characters—a lascivious old artist meets his decorous young critic, a timid literary scholar is ripped off by an aggressive hippie—have a way of slipping out of their mold, surprising us first as individuals and then as the strange faces that our most intense experiences tend to take on.

The popular writer turns life into clichés, the artist of realism turns clichés back into life. But why start with clichés in the first place and why tie yourself down to the restrictions and reductions of a plot? Why all this outmoded literary law and order? It's as though a brilliant playwright came upon the scene, a master of illusion, who insists upon practicing the three unities.

One may believe Fowles enjoys being so clever and also the rewards it has brought him as a writer of highly intelligent books that manage to be very popular. But judging from *The Aristos*, his "intellectual self-portrait," Fowles has more ambitious goals in view: in his quiet, detached way, just as much as Mailer does in his very different way, Fowles wants to create a revolution in the consciousness of his time. Still, if

this is so, surely he must suspect that his fiction is going about it in the wrong way. Tidy narrative structures, well-rounded characters, consistent point of view, lucid prose, accurate descriptions of times and places—aren't these the techniques at our late state of modernism, that confirm the most retrograde bourgeois tastes, that are valuable only so that they can then be superseded or, better yet, destroyed by the writer's innovations? Learn the rules so that you know what you're doing when you break them—so the young writer is told. Learn the craft so that you can then practice the art: craft being what all writers are supposed to be able to do, art being what only the individual writer can do because true art is the creation of new *forms* of consciousness, which only the individualist can achieve. Right?

Wrong. Partly wrong in theory and increasingly wrong in practice. New consciousness does not necessarily require new forms in literature any more than it does in any other field of writing. When Shakespeare wrote the "Dark Lady" sonnets, he was doing something original in love poetry, and hence for love itself, though he left the sonnet form undisturbed. And while it is true that new literary forms can provoke new consciousness, it tends more often to work the other way around. In any case, modernism, which has tended to identify individuality with formal innovation exclusively, has left the writers who still subscribe to it increasing high and dry: i.e., rarefied and empty. Or as Fowles himself put it in *The Aristos*: "There is a desperate search for the unique style, and only too often the search is conducted at the expense of content. This accounts for the enormous proliferation in styles and techniques...and for that only too characteristic coupling of exoticism, of presentation, and banality of a theme." If you don't think he is right, pick an anthology of current experimental fiction or poetry and see how much genuine new consciousness you find and how much of the same surreal solipsism, forlorn, or abrasive. Talk about conventionality.

Material used in this particular passage has been adapted from the following source:
T. Solotaroff, *A Few Good Voices in My Head: Occasional Pieces on Writing, Editing, and Reading My Contemporaries* © 1987 by Reed Business Information.

1. The author's example of Shakespeare is used to:

A) describe how Shakespeare changed the sonnet form.
B) illustrate how new forms of literature are required to bring new consciousness.
C) support the claim that writers should not necessarily learn the rules with the goal of eventually breaking them.
D) provide an example of a modernist work.

2. The author states that Joyce and other authors use plotlines similar to Fowles' fourth story in *The Ebony Tower* in order to suggest that:

A) Fowles' prose is more conventional than it seems.
B) Fowles' usage of open-ended and covert plotlines contributes to his ambition to create a revolution in consciousness.
C) the impact of Fowles' work comes more from its content than from formal innovation.
D) Fowles' work is just as good as Joyce's *Dubliners*.

3. Which of these characters or plots from novels would exemplify the author's description in paragraph 2 of Fowles' work?

   I. A private investigator falls for his client. He later discovers that she is his long-lost daughter.
   II. A suburban mother watches as her daughter is slowly dying of a mysterious illness. In the final chapter of the novel, it is revealed that the mother has been poisoning her daughter all along.
   III. The son of a small-town pastor leads the church choir to winning a national singing competition.

A) I only
B) II only
C) I and II
D) I, II, and III

4. Some literary theorists claim that the impact of a literary work is defined not by the intent of the author, but rather by the interaction between reader and text, and that different readers may have very different and at times contradictory reactions to and interpretations of the same text. If valid, what impact would this theory have on Fowles' goal of creating a revolution in consciousness?

A) It would suggest that Fowles could not succeed in his goal because for a revolution to occur there must be agreement on what new views should replace the old way of thinking.
B) It would suggest that Fowles succeeded in his goal because the popularity of his work ensured that it had impact on the thinking of a significant number of people.
C) It would suggest that Fowles misunderstood the complexity involved in creating a revolution in consciousness through literature.
D) It would suggest that achieving Fowles' goal of creating a revolution in consciousness depends on factors that go beyond using conventional forms to express original ideas.

5. What is "conventional textbook realism" as it is defined in the passage?

A) A novel with a simple story structure and believable outcome
B) Stories that are based on real-life events
C) A story based on use of stereotypical characters
D) Stories that begin conventionally and then reveal unexpected levels of complexity

6. Which of the following statements, if true, would most *undermine* the author's argument?

A) Rules are not valuable only when they are destroyed by a writer's innovative techniques.
B) Mailer's writing is often described as aggressive.
C) Literature that contributes to a transformation in consciousness is often only recognized as such many decades after it is written.
D) Fowles intended for *The Aristos* to be partially autobiographical.

5.4

Ranking the Passage

Abstract passage content + several hard question types = Later/Killer passage

5.4

Previewing the Question Stems

Below are the question stems only. The key words to note in the Preview stage are highlighted. Remember: you are only looking for references to passage content at this point in the process.

1. The author's example of Shakespeare is used to:

2. The author states that Joyce and other authors use plotlines similar to Fowles' fourth story in *The Ebony Tower* in order to suggest that:

3. Which of these characters or plots from novels would exemplify the author's description in paragraph 2 of Fowles' work?

4. Some literary theorists claim that the impact of a literary work is defined not by the intent of the author, but rather by the interaction between reader and text, and that different readers may have very different and at times contradictory reactions to and interpretations of the same text. If valid, what impact would this theory have on Fowles' goal of creating a revolution in consciousness?

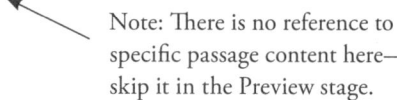

Note: When a question is this long, you may want to skip it during the Preview stage.

5. What is "conventional textbook realism" as it is defined in the passage?

6. Which of the following statements, if true, would most *undermine* the author's argument?

Note: There is no reference to specific passage content here—skip it in the Preview stage.

TONE

LIST INDICATORS—CONTRAST

QUESTION TOPICS

It is strange that a novelist as superbly imaginative as John Fowles should be content to write within the canons of conventional textbook realism. Of the four stories in *The Ebony Tower*, three are simple, linear structures—situation, complication, resolution—the incidents rationally linked through the probable interactions of credible characteristics, the action and theme neatly illustrating each other. The fourth story is somewhat more open-ended and covert: a picnic in the country that ends in a disappearance and, by implication, a suicide. One has to draw the connections for oneself and see the sudden gathering storm at the end as an epiphany. But this is a technique that Joyce was practicing in *Dubliners* at the turn of the century, and it is still being practiced, from week to week, in the pages of *The New Yorker* and elsewhere.

PIVOTAL WORD

TONE

Yet each of these stories [by Fowles] is anything but obvious or thin. However conventionally they begin and proceed, there comes a point when their issues dramatically engage and take on complexity and power—it's as though one had picked up a simple, familiar object, casually examined it, and suddenly found it shaking in one's hands. By the same token, Fowles' seemingly typecast characters—a lascivious old artist meets his decorous young critic, a timid literary scholar is ripped off by an aggressive hippie—have a way of slipping out of their mold, surprising us first as individuals and then as the strange faces that our most intense experiences tend to take on.

PIVOTAL WORDS— CONTRAST

COMPARISON

PIVOTAL WORD/ LEADING QUESTION

The popular writer turns life into clichés, the artist of realism turns clichés back into life. But why start with clichés in the first place and why tie yourself down to the restrictions and reductions of a plot? Why all this outmoded literary law and order? It's as though a brilliant playwright came upon the scene, a master of illusion, who insists upon practicing the three unities.

SUGGESTED PIVOT

ACTUAL PIVOT

COMPARISON/ CONTRAST

QUESTION TOPIC

SUGGESTED PIVOT/ LEADING QUESTION

One may believe Fowles enjoys being so clever and also the rewards it has brought him as a writer of highly intelligent books that manage to be very popular. But judging from *The Aristos*, his "intellectual self-portrait," Fowles has more ambitious goals in view: in his quiet, detached way, just as much as Mailer does in his very different way, Fowles wants to create a revolution in the consciousness of his time. Still, if this is so, surely he must suspect that his fiction is going about it in the wrong way. Tidy narrative structures, well-rounded characters, consistent point of view, lucid prose, accurate descriptions of times and places—aren't these the techniques at our late state of modernism, that confirm the most retrograde bourgeois tastes, that are valuable only so that they can then be superseded or, better yet, destroyed by the writer's innovations? Learn the rules so that you know what you're doing when you break them—so the young writer is told. Learn the craft so that you can then practice the art: craft being what all writers are supposed to be able to do, art being what only the individual writer can do because true art is the creation of new forms of consciousness, which only the individualist can achieve. Right?

AUTHOR'S/ FOWLES' POSITION

Wrong. Partly wrong in theory and increasingly wrong in practice. New consciousness does not necessarily require new forms in literature any more than it does in any other field of writing. When Shakespeare wrote the "Dark Lady" sonnets, he was doing something original in love poetry, and hence for love itself, though he left the sonnet form undisturbed. And while it is true that new literary forms can provoke new consciousness, it tends more often to work the other way around. In any case, modernism, which has tended to identify individuality with formal innovation exclusively, has left the writers who still subscribe to it increasing high and dry: i.e., rarefied and empty. Or as Fowles himself put it in *The Aristos*: "There is a desperate search for the unique style, and only too often the search is conducted at the expense of content. This accounts for the enormous proliferation in styles and techniques… and for that only too characteristic coupling of exoticism, of presentation, and banality of a theme." If you don't think he is right, pick an anthology of current experimental fiction or poetry and see how much genuine new consciousness you find and how much of the same surreal solipsism, forlorn, or abrasive. Talk about conventionality.

QUESTION TOPIC

PIVOTAL WORDS/ CONTRAST

TONE

Material used in this particular passage has been adapted from the following source:
T. Solotaroff, *A Few Good Voices in My Head: Occasional Pieces on Writing, Editing, and Reading My Contemporaries* © 1987 by Reed Business Information.

5.4

Model Noteboard Notes

This is what your noteboard for this passage might look like:

Passage [#], Q 1–6

¶ 1)   Fowles—conventional techniques
¶ 2)   But surprising complexity
¶ 3)   So why use conventions?
¶ 4)   Misguided approach?
¶ 5)   No—new form ≠ new consciousness

BL: Fowles' conventional form for new consciousness (author supports)

Attacking the Questions

The questions below are annotated to represent the thought process you would go through in answering the questions, not to represent the actual appearance of the screen. Remember: on the test, you can only strike out or select entire answer choices; partial strikeouts are not possible. The explanations to the right of each choice model a first cut through the answers: what you may have eliminated and why, and what you might have left in. The "Down to Two" explanations to the left describe the reasoning that you would use to eliminate down to the correct answer in your second cut.

5.4

1. The author's example of Shakespeare is used to:

   A) describe how Shakespeare ~~changed~~ the sonnet form. **Opposite—he didn't**

   B) illustrate how new forms of literature ~~are required~~ to bring new consciousness. **(Left it in)**

   C) support the claim that writers should not necessarily learn the rules with the goal of eventually breaking them. **(Left it in)**

   D) provide an example of a modernist work. **Words out of context—example makes larger point about literature, not just about modernism**

> **Question Type:** Structure
> **Translation:** Why does the author discuss Shakespeare?
> **Back to the Passage:** Last paragraph—Shakespeare did something original but used existing sonnet form
> **Answer:** To show that position described at end of previous paragraph is wrong

> **Down to Two—Compare:**
> B and C are opposites of each other. C fits the Bottom Line, although it is tricky—have to see relationship between paragraphs 4 and 5, and that paragraph 5 is denying validity of the position described at end of paragraph 4 ("Right? Wrong.").

> **Question Type:** Structure
> **Translation:** Why does the author state that other authors use similar plotlines?
> **Back to the Passage:** First paragraph—part of discussion of Fowles' use of conventional textbook realism (later says that issues within them are complex)
> **Answer:** To provide evidence that Fowles did not use innovative techniques to achieve his effect

2. The author states that Joyce and other authors use plotlines similar to Fowles' fourth story in *The Ebony Tower* in order to suggest that:

   A) Fowles' prose is more conventional ~~than it seems.~~ **(Left it in)**

   B) Fowles' usage of open-ended and covert plotlines contributes to his ambition to create a revolution in consciousness. **Contradicts point of the paragraph and Bottom Line—it wasn't his plotlines that did this**

   C) the impact of Fowles' work comes more from its content than from formal innovation. **(Left it in)**

   D) Fowles' work is ~~just as good as~~ Joyce's *Dubliners*. **Not the issue/No such comparison on quality**

> **Down to Two—Compare:**
> Both have idea of conventional form, but A suggests that it seemed unconventional, while passage argues the opposite. Seeing the validity of C requires connecting paragraph 1 to the Bottom Line.

3. Which of these characters or plots from novels would
exemplify the author's description in paragraph 2 of
Fowles' work?

- I. A private investigator falls for his client. He later
  discovers that she is his long-lost daughter. **Twist/
  unexpected: yes**
- II. A suburban mother watches as her daughter is
  slowly dying of a mysterious illness. In the final
  chapter of the novel, it is revealed that the mother
  has been poisoning her daughter all along. **Twist/
  unexpected: yes**
- III. The son of a small-town pastor leads the church
  choir to winning a national singing competition.
  Totally expected: No

A) I only
B) II only
C) I and II
D) I, II, and III

Eliminate anything with III. I and II
are so similar that you can't include
one without the other.

Question Type: Analogy
Translation: Which is most similar to Fowles' work as
it's described in second paragraph?
Back to the Passage: Begins conventionally, but
complex and powerful
Answer: Begins in familiar way, then surprises us with
more complexity (maybe character that does something
unexpected)

4. Some literary theorists claim that the impact of a
literary work is defined not by the intent of the author,
but rather by the interaction between reader and text,
and that different readers may have very different and
at times contradictory reactions to and interpretations
of the same text. If valid, what impact would this
theory have on Fowles' goal of creating a revolution in
consciousness?

A) It would suggest that Fowles could not succeed in his
goal because for a revolution to occur there must be
agreement on what new views should replace the old way
of thinking. **Too extreme/Out of scope**
B) It would suggest that Fowles succeeded in his goal
because the popularity of his work ensured that it had
impact on the thinking of a significant number of
people. **Too extreme/Out of scope**
C) It would suggest that Fowles misunderstood the
complexity involved in creating a revolution in
consciousness through literature. (Left it in)
D) It would suggest that achieving Fowles' goal of creating
a revolution in consciousness depends on factors that
go beyond using conventional forms to express original
ideas. (Left it in)

Question Type: New Information (Strengthen/Weaken)
Translation: If it's true that the effect of work depends
on various reader interpretations, not just author, how
would this affect Fowles' goal?
Back to the Passage: Fowles' goal most directly
discussed in paragraph 4. Passage never discusses role of
readers' interpretations.
Answer: Would have to take this additional factor into
account

Down to Two—Compare:
C indicates that Fowles was unaware of this, but we don't
know that. D only indicates that there are additional
factors. D is more moderate, and within the scope of the
passage and question stem information.

5.4

5. What is "conventional textbook realism" as it is
defined in the passage?

(A) A novel with a simple story structure and believable
outcome **(Left it in)**

B) Stories that are based on ~~real-life events~~
Out of scope/Outside "knowledge"

C) A story based on use of ~~stereotypical characters~~
Fowles' characters only *seem* typecast or stereotypical

D) Stories that begin conventionally and then ~~reveal unexpected levels of complexity~~ **(Left it in)**

Question Type: Inference

Translation: What is "conventional textbook realism," as
described in passage?

Back to the Passage: Paragraph 1—simple, linear
structure, credible, not innovative

Answer: What the passage said

Down to Two—Compare:

Both A and D describe Fowles' work, which uses
conventional realism. But only A is given as part of the
description of realism more generally, while D is specific
to Fowles' work. Choice A is a close paraphrase of the
passage description.

5.4

---

6. Which of the following statements, if true, would
most *undermine* the author's argument?

A) Rules are ~~not~~ valuable only when they are destroyed by a
writer's innovative techniques. **(Left it in)**

B) Mailer's writing is often described as aggressive.
**No effect on passage (paragraph 4—author already
says Mailer different)**

(C) Literature that contributes to a transformation in
consciousness is often only recognized as such many
decades after it is written. **(Left it in)**

D) Fowles intended for *The Aristos* to be partially
autobiographical. **Strengthens/Consistent with
"intellectual self-portrait" (paragraph 4)**

Question Type: Weaken

Translation: What would be most inconsistent with
author's claims in the passage?

Back to the Passage: Bottom Line—Fowles' conventional form for new consciousness (author supports)

Answer: Either that innovative form does/might lead to
new consciousness, or that conventional form does not

Down to Two—Compare:

A has tricky wording and connects to tricky relationship
between last two paragraphs. But when translated, it's
consistent with author's real position in last paragraph: it
strengthens, not weakens. Connection of C to passage is
less obvious, but it's inconsistent with argument in last
paragraph: it suggests that "current experimental fiction
or poetry" might eventually lead to a new consciousness.

5.5 DEALING WITH STRESS

In Chapter 2, we discussed some possible ways of dealing with the stress and anxiety that most people experience when preparing for and taking the MCAT. By now, you should have settled on a method that you can use effectively whenever anxiety or loss of concentration becomes a problem. Remember, stress won't go away, but it can be managed so that all that extra adrenaline coursing through your system can work for you, not against you.

In the table below, describe any symptoms of anxiety you may have experienced when taking a practice test or doing homework, and the method or methods you use (or will use in the future) to help manage it.

Symptoms	Management Methods

Many people use music to control and manage anxiety, and just to feel better overall. If you are a music person, create a playlist with a set of songs you can listen to whenever you find yourself feeling negative or non-productive emotions, be it anxiety and fear, or fatigue and lethargy.

5.5

When I'm feeling:	I'll listen to:

Along with stress, losing control of your pacing strategy can be a problem, especially toward the end of the test. On your next practice test or timed CARS section, monitor your pacing throughout. If you begin to panic about the time, or rush through questions without feeling reasonably secure in most of your answers, STOP and take three deep breaths. Remind yourself of the strategy and techniques you have spent so much time and effort learning. Don't let yourself lose your form at the finish line. Regain control of yourself and of the test before moving on.

Chapter 5 Summary

- Use POE aggressively.

- Know and eliminate the common Attractors.

- Read carefully—do not skim the questions or the answer choices.

- Continue to manage your stress: make it work for you, not against you!

CHAPTER 5 PRACTICE PASSAGES

Individual Passage Drills

Do this exercise *untimed* at first. Work and Annotate the passages as usual (remember to preview the questions). As you work the questions, for each answer choice you eliminate, write down the reason next to the choice, and/or highlight the word or words within the choice that make it wrong. Keep a list of Attractors nearby, and feel free to refer to it as you work. Take time to remind yourself which Attractors commonly appear on particular question types. If you cannot tell the difference between two choices and must guess between the two, note that next to the question.

When you check your answers, for each question you missed, note down in the Individual Passage Log what was wrong with the incorrect answer you chose, and what you thought was wrong with the correct answer. Look for patterns in your mistakes. Do you consistently choose the same kind of Attractor? Do you tend to eliminate the correct answer too quickly, and then talk yourself into a wrong answer choice further down the list? Do you pick the choice that sounds right, instead of eliminating the wrong answer choices and picking the least wrong choice? Devise a strategy to avoid making those same mistakes in the future.

Continue to do this exercise over the next few weeks, doing at least two passages back to back at a time. Eventually you can do the passages timed, but give yourself an extra minute or two to annotate the answer choices. Continue to monitor your progress and to diagnose any changing patterns in your performance.

CHAPTER 5 PRACTICE PASSAGE 1

The Depression yielded not only misery but also tremendous energy and radicalism. Union-organizing and reform movements of all kinds flourished as the crisis challenged Americans to abandon the constraints of the past and move forward, boldly, into the future. Recovery in the family, as in the economy, would be achieved not simply by returning to ways of the past, but by adapting to new circumstances. The economic crisis opened the way for a new type of family based on shared breadwinning and equality of the sexes.

But by the time the Depression was over and World War II had come and gone, it was clear that millions of middle-class American families would take the path toward polarized gender roles. What caused the overwhelming triumph of "traditional" roles in the "modern" home?

Although most Americans experienced some form of hardship during the Depression, it was the nation's male breadwinners—fathers who were responsible for providing economic support for their families—who were threatened or faced with the severest erosion of their identities. Those who lost income or jobs frequently lost status at home, and self-respect as well. Economic hardship placed severe strains on marriage. Going on relief may well have helped the family budget, but it would do little for the breadwinner's feelings of failure.

With the breadwinner's role undermined, other family roles shifted dramatically. Frequently wives and mothers who had never been employed took jobs to provide supplemental or even primary support for their families. Given the need for women's earnings, the widespread employment of women might have been one of the most important legacies of the Depression era. But discriminatory policies and public hostility weakened that potential. Although many families depended on the earnings of both spouses, federal policies supported unemployed male breadwinners but discouraged married women from seeking jobs. Section 213 of the Economy Act of 1932 mandated that whenever personnel reductions took place in the executive branch, married persons were to be the first discharged if married to a government employee. As a result, 1,600 married women were dismissed from their federal jobs. Many state and local governments followed suit; three out of four cities excluded married women from teaching, and eight states passed laws excluding them from state jobs. These efforts to curtail women's employment opportunities were directly related to the powerful imperative to bolster the employment of men.

If the paid labor force had been more hospitable, and if public policies had fostered equal opportunities for women, young people in the 1930s might have been less inclined to aspire to prevailing gender roles. Viable long-term job prospects for women might have prompted new ways of structuring family roles. In the face of persistent obstacles, however, that potential withered. The realities of family life combined with institutional barriers to inhibit the potential for sustained radical change among white middle-class American families.

The prevailing family ideology was gravely threatened when women and men adapted to hard times by shifting their household responsibilities. In the long run, however, these alternatives were viewed as temporary measures caused by unfortunate circumstances, rather than as positive outcomes of the crisis. Young people learned, on the one hand, to accept women's employment as necessary for the family budget; on the other hand, they saw that deviations from traditional roles often wreaked havoc in marriages. Children who grew up in economically deprived families during these years watched their parents struggle to succeed as breadwinners and homemakers, and they suffered along with their parents if those expectations proved impossible to meet. The sociologist Glen Elder, in his pioneering study of families during the Depression, found that the more a family's traditional gender roles were disrupted, the more likely the children were to disapprove of the altered balance of power in their homes.

Material used in this particular passage has been adapted from the following source:

E. T. May, "Myths and Realities of the American Family," *A History of Private Life*, Volume V. © 1991 by The Belknap Press of Harvard University Press.

1. In paragraph 1, families are compared to the economy.
    This comparison is based on:

A) a contrast between the workplace and the home.
B) the possibility of new forms of social organization.
C) the actions of radicals hoping to undermine the status quo.
D) the unfortunate results of an economic crisis.

2. The author's argument about the impact of the
    Depression on male breadwinners would be best
    supported by research that demonstrated:

A) married men were more likely to lose jobs than
    unmarried men.
B) government welfare programs helped ease financial
    hardship for the unemployed.
C) unemployment was a reliable predictor of psychological
    depression.
D) unfair wages meant many wives were unable to replace
    the breadwinner's income by entering the workforce.

3. The support for the author's view about government's
    role in the changing form of marriage is:

A) strong: the author provides several examples suggesting
    government inhibited change.
B) strong: the author supports his view thoroughly with
    relevant analogies.
C) weak: the author's examples do not effectively support
    the author's view.
D) weak: the author does not significantly address the
    government's role.

4. Which of the following best characterizes the author's
    attitude towards the effects of the Depression on
    gender roles?

A) A missed opportunity
B) A tragic development
C) An important legacy
D) A radical change

5. The author most likely feels that marriage based on
    equality of the sexes:

A) can be successful, given the right circumstances.
B) is untenable because government cannot accept women's
    equal right to work.
C) is typical in the modern home.
D) inevitably causes conflict within the family.

6. Suppose a study were to find evidence of widespread
    discrimination in employers' hiring practices during
    the Depression. Specifically, when less qualified male
    candidates and more qualified female candidates were
    in direct competition for jobs, the males were very
    frequently hired. Furthermore, the government took little
    to no action to rectify these supposed injustices. How
    would the author most likely respond?

A) This is consistent with public and government attitudes
    during the Depression: men's employment was seen as
    more important than women's.
B) Since prejudices are first shaped by family life, a radical
    change toward more equitable gender roles in marriage
    was necessary before society could reject gender
    discrimination in the workplace.
C) Public and institutional viewpoints such as these, which
    prevented women from providing supplemental or even
    primary support for their families, were unfair and
    regrettable.
D) Government's lack of response is surprising; the
    Economy Act of 1932 suggested government was
    interested in employment demographics at the time.

CHAPTER 5 PRACTICE PASSAGE 2

German anthropologists understood nature as a static system of categories that allowed them, in their study of "natural peoples," to grasp an unchanging essence of humanity, rather than the ephemeral changes historians recorded. However, the concept of nature was anything but stable in nineteenth-century Germany. Since the early part of the century there had been a deep tension between Kantian models of natural science and idealist *Naturphilosophie*, conflicts in which many anthropologists themselves were active participants. Furthermore, in nature anthropologists sought a realm free from historical change just as Darwinians began asserting that nature, like humans, did in fact change over time. The boundary between history and nature, which formed an important basis for both humanism and anthropology, came to appear more unstable than ever....

The idea of nature and natural science that informed German anthropology was based on elements from two conflicting approaches, conventionally associated with Immanuel Kant and Friedrich Schelling. The founders of German anthropology belonged to a generation of natural scientists who, in the second half of the nineteenth century, rejected Schelling's romantic *Naturphilosophie* in favor of a return to Kant's more secular and rationalist notion of nature and natural science. As is the case with so many philosophical rejections, however, anthropologists preserved as much *Naturphilosophie* as they cast off, and their understanding of nature was really a synthesis of the two philosophers' approach.

From Kant anthropologists took an idea of nature as a static and objective system that could be conclusively known by scientists. In his *Metaphysical Basis of Natural Science*, Kant had maintained that an "authentic natural science" consisted exclusively of a priori deductions of necessary laws. He thus applauded a version of Newtonian mechanics based solely on mathematics as a perfect natural science and dismissed chemistry as a "systematic art" rather than a science because its laws were derived from sensory experience of "given facts." Unlike Newton, Kant excluded theological considerations from natural science, founding a tradition in Germany of strictly separating natural science and religion, a tradition sharply distinct from British natural theology. While this law-based, objective, totally secular, and perfectly knowable nature would have appealed to anthropologists, they would not have subscribed to the Kantian notion of science as the a priori deduction of mathematical laws. Indeed, anthropology was above all a science of the given facts, which Kant had rejected as a source of natural scientific knowledge.

It was precisely over this issue of the empirical that Schelling had originally broken with Kant, and it was in their empiricist approach to nature that anthropologists retained their allegiance to Schelling. Schelling had justified experience and empirical knowledge of nature against Kant's insistence that true knowledge of nature had to be deductive, a priori, and law-like. Thus, a science of qualities, such as chemistry with its qualitatively different elements, could count as a science for Schelling but not for Kant. For Schelling, the rehabilitation of the empirical in natural knowledge was part of an idealist project to overcome the difference between theological and natural knowledge, mind and nature, and speculation and experience. When anthropologists denounced *Naturphilosophie*, it was not for its empiricism. Worse than the idealism of *Naturphilosophie* was, for anthropologists, its view of nature as becoming rather than being, a view antithetical to the concept of nature that anthropologists wanted to use against historicist humanism. Thus, Virchow asserted that, "while the facts teach that the races of humans and the species of animals are immutable," *Naturphilosophie* (wrongly, in Virchow's view) teaches that they can change. Furthermore, anthropologists separated religious and scientific questions, following Kant's rather than Schelling's understanding of the relation of natural and theological knowledge. Allowing theology and development to enter into discussions of nature would undermine the basic project of anthropology as an antihumanist science of natural peoples outside history. When they spoke of *Naturphilosophie*, anthropologists thought as much about Darwinism as about the philosophical writings of Schelling and his followers.

Anthropologists saw in the science of botany a model for their own antievolutionist synthesis of Kant's systematizing with Schelling's empiricism. There were a number of botanists active in the Berlin Anthropological Society, including the latter-day *Naturphilosoph*, Alexander Braun. Braun argued that the study of plants allowed one to observe the essence of nature relatively directly because plants do not disguise themselves with culture, as humans do. Adolf Bastian extended Braun's understanding of plants to natural peoples, whom he compared to cryptograms, flowerless plants such as algae, mosses, and ferns. As botanists had gained general knowledge about plants by studying the flowerless cryptograms, which had previously been "despised and crushed underfoot," so too would anthropologists solve the "highest questions of culture" by considering natural peoples, who lack the "flowers of culture."

Material used in this particular passage has been adapted from the following source:

A. Zimmerman, *Anthropology and Antihumanism in Imperial Germany.* © 2001 by The University of Chicago.

1. The primary purpose of the passage is most likely to:

A) describe the analogy drawn by German anthropologists between botany and anthropology.

B) criticize 19th century German anthropologists for drawing inspiration from two mutually inconsistent schools of thought regarding natural science.

C) explain the views of 19th century German anthropologists regarding the proper approach to studying human beings in the context of natural science.

D) describe how 19th century German anthropology synthesized Kant's views on theology with Schelling's belief that science consists of a priori deductions of natural laws.

2. Which of the following claims, if true, would most *undermine* the German anthropologists' view that botany is a valid model for anthropology?

A) Human beings inherently exist within a social context, and therefore there is no such thing as a people not influenced by culture.

B) Some botanists believe that the study of flowerless cryptograms can tell us little about the structure and function of flowering plants.

C) Alexander Braun abandoned *Naturphilosophie* early in his academic career, and therefore his ideas about botany have little in common with the views of that school of thought.

D) It is impossible to study theology without taking into account cultural influences.

3. Which of the following statements, based on the passage, most accurately represents a relationship between the German anthropologists' views on natural science and those of Kant and Schelling?

A) The German anthropologists accepted Kant's view that science consists of deductions from necessary laws and rejected Schelling's belief that empiricism requires combining theological and natural knowledge.

B) The German anthropologists accepted Schelling's empiricist approach and rejected Kant's belief that science consists of deductions from mathematical laws.

C) The German anthropologists rejected Kant's inclusion of theological considerations within natural science and accepted Schelling's belief that human beings are mutable.

D) The German anthropologists rejected Kant's systematizing and accepted Schelling's empiricism.

4. Which of the following, based on the passage, would be most analogous to a historicist view of anthropology?

A) A belief that physics consists of a set of unchangeable laws that govern all actions and interactions between objects.

B) A belief that chemistry is a science rather than a systematic art, given that its laws can be discovered through empirical evidence.

C) A belief that political science is the study of how different political systems create and shape, and are themselves shaped by, human beliefs and values over time.

D) A belief that economics is inherently the study of how inherent and consistent human motivations play themselves out in different contexts.

5. Elsewhere, the author of the passage writes that in 19th-century Germany the study of geology, within natural science, was divided into *Geognosie*, the study of the present-day, essential, and inherent characteristics of the earth, and *Geologie*, the study of how geological features evolve and come into being. Based on information in the passage, how would the German anthropologists most likely view these two fields of study?

A) They would accept both as related and equally essential approaches to a scientific understanding of the earth.

B) They would reject both as irrelevant to a scientific understanding of human beings.

C) They would accept *Geologie* as a scientific approach to understanding the nature of the earth, while seeing *Geognosie* as a questionable attempt to impose rigid categories on inherently changeable features.

D) They would see *Geognosie* as a more scientific approach to geology than *Geologie*.

6. With which of the following statements would the German anthropologists discussed in the passage be LEAST likely to agree?

A) Culture can obscure qualities common to all humans.

B) Nature can be described through a set of objective and unchanging categories.

C) Chemistry cannot be legitimately labeled as a science.

D) Newton erred in including theological considerations within natural science.

7. Which of the following statements made in the passage most directly supports the author's assertion that "in nature anthropologists sought a realm free from historical change" (paragraph 1)?

A) The concept of nature was unstable in 19th century Germany.

B) British natural theology combined religion with natural science.

C) According to Virchow, while *Naturphilosophie* teaches that the races of humans and species of animals can change, they are in fact immutable.

D) There was a tension between Kantian models of natural science and idealist *Naturphilosophie*.

SOLUTIONS TO CHAPTER 5 PRACTICE PASSAGE 1

1. **B** This is a Structure question.

   A: No. The author does not contrast (i.e., illustrate differences between) the workplace and the home. Rather, the author states that they are similar in that adaptation to new circumstances was needed (paragraph 1).

   B: Yes. In paragraph 1, the author states that "Recovery in the family, as in the economy, would be achieved not simply by returning to ways of the past, but by adapting to new circumstances."

   C: No. The author does mention "radicalism," but does not describe radicals hoping to make changes to the family.

   D: No. This choice is too negative. This comparison follows shortly after the sentence, "The Depression yielded not only misery but also tremendous energy and radicalism" (paragraph 1). The author also states in that paragraph that "the crisis challenged Americans to abandon the constraints of the past and move forward, boldly, into the future." Therefore, the author recognizes positive as well as negative results of the economic crisis.

2. **C** This is a Strengthen question.

   Note: The author's argument about the impact of the Depression on male breadwinners suggests breadwinners who lost their jobs were personally hurt and that this had a negative impact on families (paragraphs 3 and 6).

   A: No. This evidence would not strengthen the argument. The author's argument is about the effect of unemployment on married men on an individual and family level. Knowing that married men overall were more likely to lose their jobs would not strengthen the author's point about the impact of unemployment on individual men and their families.

   B: No. This answer choice does not strengthen the author's argument about the effects of unemployment on men. The author states in the passage that relief efforts had little impact on unemployed men's feelings (paragraph 3).

   C: Yes. Evidence that unemployment caused depression would strengthen the author's claim in the passage that loss of employment coincided with loss of identity and marriage strain.

   D: No. This choice refers to the discrimination women faced, not directly to men's experience of unemployment. According to the author, men were most affected by their perceived loss of status and identity, not just by a reduction in household income.

3. **A** This is an Evaluate question.

   A: Yes, paragraph 4 provides numerous examples in which the government tries to manipulate the job market in favor of men.

   B: No. The author does not use analogy to support her argument. The only analogy drawn is between the economy and the family (paragraph 1), but there is no direct connection between that comparison and the author's specific discussion of the role of the government.

   C: No. The examples in paragraph 4 do directly support the idea that "federal policies supported unemployed male breadwinners but discouraged married women from seeking jobs," and later, "Many state and local governments followed suit."

   D: No. The author does address government's role in paragraph 4, on a federal, state, and local level.

4.   **A**   This is a Tone/Attitude question.

    Note: This question is essentially asking about the author's overall attitude toward the events of the passage. Thus, use your sense of the author's overall purpose in writing the passage.

    A: **Yes. See paragraph 4: "Given the need for women's earnings, the widespread employment of women might have been one of the most important legacies of the Depression era. But discriminatory policies and public hostility weakened that potential." The word choice in paragraph 5 also suggests the author might have supported changes to traditional roles in marriage: "Viable long-term job prospects for women might have prompted new ways of structuring family roles. In the face of persistent obstacles, however, that potential withered."**

    B: No. While there was reason to believe the author might like to have seen more lasting change take place (see the explanation for choice A), the word "tragic" is too strong to describe the tone of the passage.

    C: No. This contradicts the author's attitude as expressed in the passage. In paragraph 4, the author states that the employment of women might have been an important legacy, but it was not allowed to take root.

    D: No. This choice represents a misreading of the main idea of the passage. The potential for radical change to gender roles in marriage did not turn into lasting change during the Depression.

5.   **A**   This is an Inference question.

    A: **Yes. The author believes external obstacles (i.e., government and social resistance) prevented family roles from changing. In paragraph 5, the author says if those obstacles were removed, we might have seen real change.**

    B: No. The use of the word "cannot" implies government still holds this view; the attitudes of government today are beyond the scope of this passage. Also, government did not discourage women from working because it "could not accept" women working, but because men's employment was seen as more important.

    C: No. This choice contradicts paragraph 2, which refers to the "overwhelming triumph of 'traditional' roles in the 'modern' home."

    D: No. This choice is too extreme. The word "inevitably" is absolute, whereas paragraph 6 says "deviations from traditional roles *often* [emphasis added] wreaked havoc in marriages."

6.   **A**   This is a New Information question.

    Note: Questions that give new information are often most relevant to a specific part of the passage. This one corresponds most closely to paragraph 4; the credited answer will reflect that.

    A: **Yes. See paragraph 4: "But *discriminatory policies and public hostility* [emphasis added] weakened that potential. Although many families depended on the earnings of both spouses, federal policies supported unemployed male breadwinners but discouraged married women from seeking jobs."**

    B: No. This answer choice puts forward a general theory—changes to the family are required for changes to the workplace—while the author suggests the opposite. That is, that government action in the workplace limited the possibility of change within the family (see paragraph 5).

    C: No. This choice suggests the author's general approach is to criticize or lament obstacles to women's progress. It would be more accurate to say the author is explaining why more equitable gender roles did not take hold at the time. Secondly, the passage suggests that women were able to provide financial support for their families at the time, at least to some extent (paragraph 4); "prevented" is too strong to be supported by the passage.

    D: No. This choice uses familiar language but is inconsistent with the passage. Government would not be expected to stop such discrimination; its inaction would not be a surprise. In fact, government institutionalized discrimination in the Economy Act of 1932 (paragraph 4).

SOLUTIONS TO CHAPTER 5 PRACTICE PASSAGE 2

1. **C**   This is a Main Idea/Primary Purpose question.

   A: No. This choice is too narrow. While the analogy described in the last paragraph is part of the author's discussion of the views of German anthropologists, it is one piece of evidence supporting the larger argument, not the main point or primary purpose of the passage as a whole.

   B: No. This choice has the wrong tone. The author is not criticizing the anthropologists, but rather is giving a neutral description of their views and of some of the sources of those views.

   C: Yes. This choice is broad enough to cover the content of the passage without going beyond its scope, and it has an appropriately neutral tone. Paragraph 1 introduces the idea that the anthropologists studied "humanity" and "natural peoples," as well as the idea that this study occurred within the larger context of natural science. The rest of the passage relates to the views of these German anthropologists, and/or sources of inspiration for those views.

   D: No. While German anthropology was based on a synthesis of views of these two men (paragraph 2), this choice partially misrepresents the pieces from each that were synthesized. The anthropologists did follow Kant's "exclu[sion] of theological considerations from natural science" (paragraph 3). However, it was Kant, not Schelling, who believed that science consists of a priori deductions of natural laws, and the passage states that the anthropologists "would not have subscribed to the Kantian notion of science as the a priori deduction of mathematical laws" (paragraph 3).

2. **A**   This is a Weaken question.

   Note: According to the last paragraph, anthropologists saw botany as a model because as botany "allowed one to observe the essence of nature relatively directly because plants do not disguise themselves with culture, as humans do," the study of so-called "natural peoples" (analogized to flowerless cryptograms) allowed anthropologists to understand culture and humanity through studying people who supposedly had no culture.

   A: Yes. The anthropologists saw botany as a model, according to the passage, largely because they believed that one could learn about an "unchanging essence of humanity" (paragraph 1) by studying people with no culture, just as botanists can learn about an "essence of nature" by studying plants with no flowers. If there is no such thing as a people without culture, however, this would significantly undermine the validity of botany as a model for anthropology.

   B: No. This choice does not go far enough to undermine the anthropologists' view. "Some botanists" could be two or three, and we don't know from the answer choice that their claim is valid. Beware of choices that are too weak to have a significant impact when answering Strengthen and Weaken questions.

   C: No. While Braun is identified as a "latter-day *Naturphilosoph*," the relevance of his views to those of the anthropologists does not depend on Braun representing that school of thought (keep in mind that the anthropologists rejected much of *Naturphilosophie* (paragraph 2)).

   D: No. This choice is not relevant to the question. The anthropologists believed that theology was not a legitimate part of natural science (paragraph 4). Therefore, even if the study of theology requires the study of culture, this has no impact on the anthropologists' views on the study of humanity within natural science.

3.   **B**   This is an Inference question.

   A: No. The first part of this choice is incorrect. The anthropologists rejected Kant's view that science consists of deductions from necessary laws (see end of paragraph 3).

   B: **Yes. Both parts of this choice are supported by the passage. The passage states in paragraph 4 that "it was in their empiricist approach to nature that anthropologists retained their allegiance to Schelling." In paragraph 3, the author writes that the anthropologists "would not have subscribed to the Kantian notion of science as the a priori deduction of mathematical laws. Indeed, anthropology was above all a science of the given facts, which Kant had rejected as a source of natural scientific knowledge."**

   C: No. This choice is accurate up until the very last word. However, it was the idea that "the facts teach that the races of humans and the species of animals are immutable" or unchangeable that the anthropologists accepted, rather than an idea that humans are mutable or changeable (an idea that Schelling did not, according to the passage, propose).

   D: No. The first part of this choice is incorrect: "Anthropologists saw in the science of botany a model for their own antievolutionist synthesis of Kant's systematizing with Schelling's empiricism" (paragraph 5). Thus, they accepted rather than rejected Kant's systematizing.

4.   **C**   This is an Analogy question.

   Note: The non-historicist view of the German anthropologists was that nature is "a static system of categories that allowed them, in their study of 'natural peoples,' to grasp an unchanging essence of humanity, rather than the ephemeral changes historians recorded" (paragraph 1). The author also states that "in nature anthropologists sought a realm free from historical change" (paragraph 1). Later in the passage the author states: "Worse than the idealism of *Naturphilosophie* was, for anthropologists, its view of nature as becoming rather than being, a view antithetical to the concept of nature that anthropologists wanted to use against historicist humanism" (paragraph 4). Therefore, a historicist view of anthropology would be based on studying changes over time rather than some unchanging "essence of humanity." To answer the question, you need to eliminate choices that would be similar to the German anthropologists' approach, and to find the answer that represents studying changes or development over time.

   A: No. This, in its study of unchanging laws, would be a non-historicist approach.

   B: No. There is no suggestion that this approach to chemistry involves studying changes over time. The reference to the discovery of empirical laws, in fact, suggests the opposite.

   C: **Yes. This approach to political science would involve studying how political systems and human beliefs and values interact and change over time, or, through history.**

   D: No. A belief in the existence of inherent and consistent human motivations (similar to an "unchanging essence of humanity") suggests consistency rather than change over time.

5.   **D**   This is a New Information question.

   Note: The German anthropologists saw nature as a "static and objective system that could be conclusively known by scientists" (paragraph 3), and believed that "Worse than the idealism of *Naturphilosophie* was…its view of nature as becoming rather than being, a view antithetical to the concept of nature that anthropologists wanted to use against historicist humanism." While the anthropologists studied human beings, they saw this study as existing within the realm of natural science. Therefore, we can infer that they would accept "*Geognosie*, the study of the present-day, essential, and inherent characteristics of the earth" as a more legitimate scientific approach than "*Geologie*, the study of how geological features evolve and come into being."

A: No. The passage suggests that they would prefer *Geognosie* over *Geologie*, as more scientific.

B: No. There is no evidence in the question stem or in the passage that the anthropologists would see either, especially *Geognosie*, as totally irrelevant.

C: No. The passage suggests that the anthropologists themselves were looking for strict categories to apply to humanity (paragraph 1). Therefore, there is no reason to infer that they would see categorization as a problem. Furthermore, the anthropologists believed natural science should look for unchanging, rather than changeable, elements.

D: Yes. *Geognosie* fits better with the anthropologists' view of legitimate natural science.

6. **C** This is an Inference/LEAST question (that is, it asks which statement is least supported by the passage).

A: No. This statement is supported by paragraph 5, where the author writes: "Braun argued that the study of plants allowed one to observe the essence of nature relatively directly because plants do not disguise themselves with culture, as humans do." Braun's ideas were part of the reason why the anthropologists saw botany as a model for their own approach.

B: No. In paragraph 1, the author states that "German anthropologists understood nature as a static [or unchanging] system of categories." In paragraph 3, the author claims: "From Kant anthropologists took an idea of nature as a static and objective system that could be conclusively known by scientists." Therefore, the anthropologists would agree with this statement.

C: Yes. While Kant believed chemistry was not a science, the anthropologists disagreed on this point. For Schelling and for the anthropologists (who followed Schelling's empirical approach), "a science of qualities, such as chemistry with its qualitatively different elements, could count as a science" (paragraph 4). Therefore the anthropologists would least agree with this statement.

D: No. In paragraph 3, the author states that "Unlike Newton, Kant excluded theological considerations from natural science" and that "this law-based, objective, totally secular, and perfectly knowable nature would have appealed to anthropologists." In paragraph 4, the passage states that "anthropologists separated religious and scientific questions, following Kant's rather than Schelling's understanding of the relation of natural and theological knowledge. Allowing theology and development to enter into discussions of nature would undermine the basic project of anthropology as an antihumanist science of natural peoples outside history." Therefore, the anthropologists would agree, not disagree, with this choice.

7. **C** This is a Structure question.

Note: All of the claims cited in the choices are in the passage. The question is, which claim is used by the author to most directly support the assertion cited in the question stem.

A: No. The existence of a debate over the concept of nature doesn't itself directly support or explain the author's claim about the anthropologists' own views. The fact that this statement appears in the same paragraph is not enough to show that it acts to logically support the assertion cited in the question.

B: No. The fact that British natural theology, unlike the anthropologists' approach to natural science, combined religion with science doesn't by itself support the author's claim about the actual content or nature of the anthropologists' views on historical change.

C: Yes. Virchow is quoted in paragraph 4, in the context of the author's explanation of the anthropologists' view that "Worse than the idealism of *Naturphilosophie* was, for anthropologists, its view of nature as becoming rather than being, a view antithetical to the concept of nature that anthropologists wanted to use against historicist humanism." (Note the word "thus" at the beginning of the next sentence, which indicates that the Virchow quote is part of the discussion of the anthropologists' view.) This is a continuation of the discussion that begins in paragraph 1 of the anthropologists' antihistorical approach. Therefore, even though Virchow's statement appears in a different paragraph, it still acts to support and explain the assertion made in paragraph 1.

D: No. While discussion of this tension is part of the author's overall argument, it doesn't itself directly support the author's claim about the specific assertion cited in the question stem. The fact that it appears in the same paragraph as the assertion doesn't guarantee that it acts to support that assertion.

Individual Passage Log

Passage # _____

Q#	Q type	Attractors	What did you do wrong?

Revised Strategy _____

Passage # _____

Q#	Q type	Attractors	What did you do wrong?

Revised Strategy _____

Think Like a Test-Writer: Exercise 3

THINK LIKE A TEST-WRITER: EXERCISE 3

Just as there are certain kinds of statements in passage texts that tend to generate questions, there are particular aspects of the logical structure of a passage text that the test-writers use to create attractive wrong answers (that is, "Attractors"). For example, if two things are compared or contrasted and a question asks what is true of one, the test-writers will likely create a wrong answer that is true of the other. If the author describes a point of view and then *disagrees* with it, a wrong answer may describe the author as *agreeing* with that point of view. If the author stakes out a moderate position, a wrong answer may describe it as much more extreme than it actually is. And, if a question asks for the main idea or primary purpose of the passage as a whole, a wrong answer may state something that is true based on the passage, but is only one theme among many in the text.

The purpose of this drill is to sensitize you to the aspects of a passage that may generate predictable wrong answers, so that you are able to predict, recognize, and eliminate them more effectively when doing a CARS passage.

In the text on the next page, you will see parts of the passage in red font. These are some of the kinds of things that test-writers may use to create attractive wrong answers. A short description of a type of Attractor this text might inspire follows, *italicized and in [brackets].*

First, read the entire passage, paying close attention to the parts in red but also tracking the author's argument in each paragraph and through the passage as a whole. Then address the questions that follow; for each question, a guide to the right answer is provided. Your task is to think about what kind of wrong answer the test-writers might create for that question, perhaps tied to a part of the passage with the text in red. You might come up with anything from a general idea about the type or category of Attractor (e.g., "the opposite of what the right answer would be") to a specific statement that could be the actual Attractor choice. Once you have completed the drill, take a look at the explanations that follow.

[Note: the computer-based testing tools do not allow you to change the color of the text, and there will be no red text in your MCAT passages. The red font here is only for the purpose of the drill. The questions attached to a CARS passage on the test will also not usually be presented in the order in which the relevant material appears in the test.]

The text on the next page is longer than a CARS passage in order to give you extra practice with these skills.

EXERCISE 3

Is it *possible* to write literary history, that is, to write that which will be both literary and a history? [*An Attractor might give the wrong answer to this rhetorical question*] Most histories of literature, it must be admitted, are either social histories, or histories of thought as illustrated in literature, or impressions and judgements on specific works arranged in more or less chronological order. [*An Attractor might mix up these views, or the views of the authors referenced next*] A glance at the history of English literary historiography will corroborate this view. Thomas Wharton, the first "formal" historian of English poetry, gave as his reason for studying ancient literature that it "faithfully records the features of the time and preserves the most picturesque and expressive representations of manners" and "transmits to posterity genuine delineations of life." Henry Morley conceived of literature as "the national biography" or the "story of the English mind." Leslie Stephen regarded literature as "a particular function of the whole social organism," "a kind of byproduct" of social change. W.J. Courthope, author of the only history of English poetry based on a unified conception of its development, defined the "study of English poetry as in effect the study of the continuous growth of our national institutions as reflected in our literature," and looked for the unity of the subject "precisely where the political historian looks for it, namely, in the life of a nation as a whole."

While these and many other historians treat literature as major document for the illustration of national or social history, those constituting another group recognize that literature is first and foremost an art, but appear unable to write history. [*An Attractor might take this overly literally or misrepresent these views on literature*] They present us with a discontinuous series of essays on individual authors, [*An Attractor might misrepresent the passage authors' criticism*] attempting to link them by "influences" but lacking any conception of real historical evolution. In his introduction to *A Short History of Modern English Literature* (1897), Edmund Gosse professed, to be sure, to show the "movement of English literature," to give a "feeling of the evolution of English literature," but he was merely paying lip service to an ideal then spreading from France. In practice, his books are a series of critical remarks on authors and some of their works, chronologically arranged.... [*An Attractor might misrepresent the nature of the passage authors' criticism*] Most leading histories of literature are either histories of civilization or collections of critical essays. One type is not a history of *art*; the other, not a *history* of art.

Why has there been no attempt, on a large scale, to trace the evolution of literature as art? One deterrent is the fact that the preparatory analysis of works of art has not been carried out in a consistent and systematic manner. Either we remain content with the old rhetorical criteria, unsatisfactory in their preoccupation with apparently superficial devices, or we have recourse to an emotive language describing the effects of a work of art upon the reader in terms incapable of real correlation with the work itself.

Another difficulty is the prejudice that no history of literature is possible save in terms of causal explanation by some other human activity. [*An Attractor might represent the passage authors' opinion as the opposite of what it really is*] A third difficulty lies in the whole conception of the development of the art of literature. Few would doubt the possibility of an internal history of painting or music. It suffices to walk through any set of art galleries arranged according to chronological order or in accordance with "schools" to see that there is a history of the art of painting quite distinct from either the history of painters or the appreciation or judgement of individual pictures. It suffices to listen to a concert in which compositions are chronologically arranged to see that there is a history of music which has scarcely anything to do with [*An Attractor might indicate that the opposite is true*] the biographies of the composers, the social conditions under which the works were produced, or the appreciation of individual pieces. Such histories have been attempted in painting and sculpture ever since Winckelmann wrote his *Geschichte der Kunst im Altertum* (1764) and most histories of music since Burney have paid attention to the history of musical forms.

Literary history has before it the analogous problem [*An Attractor might misrepresent the nature or purpose of this analogy*] of tracing the history of literature as an art, in comparative isolation from its social history, the biographies of authors, or the appreciation of individual works. Of course, the task of literary history (in this limited sense) presents its special obstacles. Compared to a painting [*An Attractor might misrepresent this comparison, or the comparison with music*], which can be seen at a glance, a literary work of art is accessible only through a time-sequence and thus is more difficult to realize as a coherent whole. But the analogy of musical form shows that a pattern as possible, even when it can be grasped only in a temporal sequence. There are, further, special problems. In literature, there is a gradual transition from simple statements to highly organized works of art, since the medium of literature, language, is also the medium of everyday communication and especially the medium of sciences. It is thus more difficult to isolate the aesthetic structure of a literary work. Yet [*An Attractor might ignore the shift indicated with this word "yet"*] an illustrative plate in a medical textbook and a military march are two examples to show that the other arts also have their borderline cases and that the difficulties in distinguishing between art and non-art in linguistic utterance are only greater quantitatively.

Theorists there are, however, who simply deny that literature has a history. W. P. Ker argued, for instance, that we do not need literary history, as its objects are always present, are "eternal," and thus have no proper history at all. T.S. Eliot also will deny the "pastness" of a work of art. "The whole of the literature of Europe from Homer," he says, "has a simultaneous existence and composes a simultaneous order." Art, one could argue with Schopenhauer, has always reached its goal. It never improves, and cannot be superseded or repeated *[An Attractor might misrepresent this claim, perhaps by taking it too literally]*…. So literary history is no proper history because it is the knowledge of the present, the omnipresent, the eternally present. One cannot deny, of course, that there is some real difference between political history and history of art. *[An Attractor might misrepresent the nature of this contrast]* There is a distinction between that which is historical and past and that which is historical and still somehow present.

As we have shown before, an individual work of art does not remain unchanged *[An Attractor might take this too literally]* through the course of history. There is to be sure a substantial identity of structure which has remained the same throughout the ages. But this structure is dynamic; it changes throughout the process of history while passing through the minds of readers, critics, and fellow artists. The process of interpretation, criticism, and appreciation has never been completely interrupted

and is likely to continue indefinitely, or at least as long as there is no complete interruption of the cultural tradition. One of the tasks of the literary historian is the description of this process. Another is the tracing of the development of works of art arranged in smaller and larger groups, according to common authorship, or genres, or stylistic types, or linguistic tradition, and finally inside a scheme of universal literature.

But the concept of the development of a series of works of art seems an extraordinarily difficult one. In a sense each work of art is, at first sight, a structure discontinuous with neighboring works of art. One can argue that there is no development from one individuality to another. One meets even with the objection that there is no history of literature, only one of men writing. Yet according to the same argument we should have to give up writing a history of language *[An Attractor might indicate that the author believes this, or the claim about "personalism" below, to be true]* because there are only men uttering words or a history of philosophy because there are only men thinking. Extreme "personalism" of this sort must lead to the view that every individual work of art is completely isolated, which in practice would mean that it would be both incommunicable and incomprehensible. We must conceive rather of literature as a whole system of works which is, with the accretion of new ones, constantly changing its relationships, growing as a changing whole.

—Adapted from Rene Wellek and Austin Warren, *Theory of Literature.* Copyright © 1956, 1949, 1942 by Houghton Mifflin Harcourt Publishing Company, renewed 1984, 1977, 1975 by Rene Wellek and Austin Warren.

Question #1: What answer to the question posed in the first sentence is suggested by the rest of the passage?

Right answer: Yes, it is possible to write a true "literary history."

Predicted Attractor: _____

_____

_____

Question #2: The authors state that Leslie Stephen believes literature to be which of the following?

Right answer: "A particular function of the whole social organism" (most likely a paraphrase of this statement).

Predicted Attractor: _____

_____

_____

Question #3: When the authors state in paragraph 2 that some writers on literature "appear unable to write history," they most likely mean that these writers:

Right answer: The authors of the passage mean that these writers may claim to be writing a literary history, but what they are really producing are assessments of individual writings with no real discussion of the evolution of literature over time, or of what links those pieces together.

Predicted Attractor: _____

_____

_____

Question #4: What can be inferred from the authors' statement in paragraph 4 that "Another difficulty is the prejudice that no history of literature is possible save in terms of causal explanation by some other human activity"?

Right answer: The authors indicate here that a history of literature CAN be written on its own terms, without reference to other aspects of human existence (for example politics or social institutions).

Predicted Attractor: _____

_____

_____

Question #5: With which of the following statements regarding the history of music would the authors be most likely to agree?

Right answer: The authors draw an analogy between literary history and musical history in paragraph 4. The authors' point is that you CAN write a history of music without reference to "the biographies of the composers, the social conditions under which the works were produced, or the appreciation of individual pieces."

Predicted Attractor: _____

_____

_____

Question #6: Which of the following would most *weaken* the passage's claim regarding the difference between literature and painting presented in paragraph 5?

Right answer: Anything that indicates that the way we perceive a work of literature and a painting is similar in a relevant way would *weaken* the contrast drawn in the passage; for example, that one DOES in some way view aspects of a painting sequentially rather than all at once "at a glance" or that we do NOT perceive a work of literature "through a time-sequence."

Predicted Attractor: _____

_____

_____

Question #7: The authors of the passage most likely refer to an illustrative plate in a medical textbook in order to:

Right answer: The authors refer to a medical illustration to suggest that (1) it may not be purely aesthetic in nature and therefore (2) literature is not unique in this way. Thus, the purpose is to (3) refute a possible objection to the authors' argument.

Predicted Attractor: _____

_____

_____

Question #8: Which of the following would be most analogous to T.S. Eliot's claim that a work of art has no true "past"?

Right answer: To understand this statement it helps to take it in the context of W. P. Ker's similar argument that the objects of literary history are "always present, are 'eternal,' and thus have no proper history at all." That is, that literature takes as its subject eternal aspects of human existence. One valid analogy, for example, might describe the field of ethics as presenting questions that are always at issue in human life and that do not fundamentally change over time.

Predicted Attractor: _____

_____

_____

Question #9: By "an individual work of art does not remain unchanged" (paragraph 7) the authors most likely mean:

Right answer: Taking this statement in the context of what follows it in the passage, the authors mean that art "changes" as others interpret it. As in, it is perceived and understood in different ways by different people in different times, and this in a sense transforms that work of art.

Predicted Attractor: _____

_____

_____

Question #10: What is the primary purpose of the passage?

Right answer: The primary purpose of this passage is to argue that it is possible to write a true evolutionary history of literature without explaining it through extraneous factors (like politics, or the author's biography or the social context in which it was written).

Predicted Attractor: _____

_____

_____

SOLUTIONS TO EXERCISE 3

1. Predicted Attractor—A wrong answer might state that no, one cannot write a true literary history, perhaps because it has not yet been accomplished, or because the two genres are supposedly mutually exclusive.

2. Predicted Attractor—A likely wrong answer would reference other views described in paragraph 1 that are not focused on change: that it "faithfully records the features of the time and preserves the most picturesque and expressive representations of manners" and "transmits to posterity genuine delineations of life" (Thomas Wharton), or that it is "the national biography" and the "story of the English mind" (Henry Morley).

3. Predicted Attractor—An answer choice that takes this statement too literally would be tempting. For example, that they are intellectually incapable of writing literary history, or that it is literally impossible to write about literature and to write history at the same time.

4. Predicted Attractor—When an author states an opposing position in order to debunk it, a wrong answer that describes the opposing position rather than the author's position often sounds great. Here, that wrong answer would suggest that literature *cannot* be explained on its own terms, and that any causal explanation would have to refer to some other human activity as well.

5. Predicted Attractor—If you got turned around in the beginning of the paragraph and thought the opposing position was the authors' position and vice versa, that mistake might carry through to this part of the paragraph as well. The test-writers know this, so they may well present the claim that you CANNOT write about music without reference to "the biographies of the composers, the social conditions under which the works were produced, or the appreciation of individual pieces" as a wrong answer.

6. Predicted Attractor—One of the most predictable Attractors on a Weaken question is something that strengthens. Add to this that one of the most predictable Attractors for a question about a contrast in the passage is something that indicates a similarity. Add those together, and the most predictable Attractor for this question would be something that *strengthens* that part of the passage by indicating that painting and literature are in fact *different* in this way.

7. Predicted Attractor—Especially given the abstract nature of this part of the passage, the test-writers know that it is hard to follow the twists and turns in the authors' argument. Therefore, they may present you with a choice that (1) indicates that the medical illustration (and the military march) are *counterexamples* to the authors' argument or that they (2) are given to support a different claim in the passage (for example the earlier argument about time sequence).

8.   Predicted Attractor—One possible way in which an answer may go wrong is to present a sce-
     nario in which something "has no past" for an opposite reason. For example, it might describe
     a technological innovation that has fundamentally changed the nature of human existence
     and that has no antecedent and therefore "no pastness."

9.   Predicted Attractor—A wrong answer may take this statement too literally, for example as
     if the authors are saying that an individual literary work may be rewritten or edited later in
     time. Or, a wrong answer may interpret the statement in the context of some other part of the
     passage; for example, as if the authors were still discussing the issue of time sequencing, or the
     possibility of tracing the evolutionary history (change over time) of literature.

10. Predicted Attractor—One of the most predictable Attractors tied to a particular question
     type is the "too narrow" answer to a general question. Here, the wrong answer could be any
     sub-point in the passage, such as "Literature, unlike a painting, cannot be perceived through
     a single glance," or "Art is always changing" or "Most histories of literature are histories of
     society or else assessment of individual works of art." These are all true according to the pas-
     sage, but none of them capture the passage as whole.

Chapter 6
Ranking and Ordering the Passages

GOALS

1) To understand the organization of the MCAT CARS section
2) To learn to assess the difficulty levels of passages
3) To learn a strategy for attacking the section as a whole

6.1 WHY RANK THE PASSAGES?

As we have discussed, to maximize your efficiency and accuracy within each passage you must take control of the material and not let the material control you. In the same way, you'll maximize your score by taking control of the section *as a whole*, working through the passages in a way that helps you get the easy questions right instead of wasting time on the most difficult questions.

This chapter outlines what you need to know about how the MCAT CARS section is organized in terms of level of difficulty and how you can assess the nine passages to design your best plan of attack.

How Are the MCAT CARS Passages Organized?

The MCAT does not follow a strict pattern in how they organize the nine passages; they are presented more or less randomly. Needless to say, the AAMC will not disclose specific information concerning how the passages are chosen, how many are at an easy, medium, or difficult level, etc. Moreover, each administration is different, and every time the test is administered there are multiple forms of the test. So, where does that leave us?

Let's begin with what we know. During the many years that we have been developing these materials, we have discovered some patterns. A lot of experience has led us to the following conclusions about the structure of the CARS section.

Passage Organization

Although one might think that the nine passages would be arranged in order of level of difficulty (that is, easy passages first, medium next, and difficult last), this is generally *not* the case. What would be the point of putting all the difficult passages at the end in a section that students sometimes don't finish? In fact, the passages are in a seemingly random order; often, the last passage in the section is an easy or medium passage that you want to be sure to complete, and the hardest passage is in the middle of the section.

Many CARS sections will have at least one passage that merits the rank of Killer, meaning it's so difficult that spending even 30 or 40 minutes wouldn't allow you to answer all—or even most of—the questions correctly. Killer passages are not worth your valuable time—guess on the questions or, at least, do them last.

Therefore, it's up to you to strategically reorganize your nine passages in order to address them most effectively.

Passage Division

Division of the nine passages generally breaks down into

- 2–3 easy passages
- 3–5 medium passages
- 1–2 difficult passages

Unless your reasonable goal is to score at the very top of the scale, you probably should be randomly guessing on at least one passage; that is, the one or two most difficult passages in the section. And if your reasonable goal is to score in the 98th or 99th percentile, you may still do best by guessing on a few of the most difficult questions you encounter.

6.2 ASSESSING DIFFICULTY LEVEL: NOW, LATER, AND KILLER

Your first objective when beginning the section is to assess the relative difficulty of the passages. A passage should be ranked Now if it seems relatively straightforward. The passages that appear to be more challenging should be ranked as Later. The most difficult passage or passages (the ones on which you may be randomly guessing) get a rank of Killer.

Although it's tempting to associate topic or subject matter with difficulty level, remember that—unlike the science sections—the CARS section of the MCAT does not test outside knowledge. Everything you need to correctly answer the questions is in the passage. In fact, bringing in outside knowledge can actually hurt your score.

Students will often want to skip easier passages simply because they're about, say, poetry or opera (or any other topic that tends to be unfamiliar). However, what really makes a passage difficult is the way it's written (and in some cases the types of questions that are asked about it). Just because a topic is boring or foreign to you doesn't mean the passage is written in an inaccessible way, and even though a topic may be interesting or familiar, the passage can be written in a dense, convoluted way.

The Passage Text

What Should You Look For?

The following criteria should be used to evaluate the difficulty of the passage text itself.

1) **Level of concreteness or abstraction:** Passages that are highly theoretical and that discuss abstract concepts will be much harder to follow than passages that are concrete and descriptive. Would you rather read a passage about the "philosophic contemplation of the Not-Self" or one on the "doubling of the cost of living in the last ten years"? And again, subject matter is not the key to difficulty. For example, an art passage that is essentially a painter's biography may be very concrete and factual, and therefore quite easy to comprehend.

2) **Language level:** While the CARS section cannot expect you to know technical language specific to a particular discipline (without defining the terms in context), difficult passages will often include esoteric language that no one really uses in everyday conversation. If the author uses many such words as *lugubrious*, *phlegmatic*, *synesthesia*, or *flagitious* in the first few sentences, she's probably not going to start using "plain English" in the next few. Lots of unfamiliar vocabulary will make the passage more difficult to understand, regardless of the topic.

3) **Sentence structure:** Extremely long, convoluted sentences are harder to read, especially under a time constraint. Short, direct sentences will be easier to follow.

How to Evaluate the Passage Text

Skim the first few sentences of the first or second paragraph. Try to paraphrase what you have just read. If your reaction is essentially "huh???," and all you can do is repeat the exact wording of the passage because the meaning of those words is so unclear, this indicates a more difficult passage. If, on the other hand, you can easily put the meaning of those lines into your own words, the passage is likely to be fairly straightforward.

Think of it this way: if, in 15 seconds, you could explain to your six-year-old sister what those two sentences are saying, then the passage will probably make sense to you, too.

Do NOT rank a passage solely on the basis of its length. The few moments it may take you to read five or six extra lines will not significantly affect your performance, but choosing a short yet difficult passage over a longer but easier passage certainly will.

The Questions

Adapting to Difficulty Level

Given that the questions are displayed one at a time, on separate screens, for most test-takers it is too cumbersome and time-consuming to click through and look at each question, evaluate the difficulty level of the set, and then incorporate that into a ranking decision. Therefore, most of your ranking decisions should be based on the apparent difficulty of the passage text.

However, once you have decided to do a passage and are Previewing the Questions, if you notice a high percentage of very difficult question types (in particular, Application and Structure-Evaluate questions) or unusually lengthy question stems and/or answer choices, you may decide at that point to skip over that passage (Flagging the questions for review, guessing on the questions and making a clear noteboard note) and move on to the next. Do not, however, employ this strategy more than once or twice during a CARS section. Otherwise, you will spend too much time previewing questions without answering them, and your efficiency and pacing will suffer.

6.3 ORDERING THE SECTION

Now that you have the criteria with which to rank your passages, let's discuss the overall ordering of the section.

The Two-Pass System

1) For the first passage, write down the passage number and question range on your noteboard (e.g., "Passage 1 Q 1-7").

2) Read the first two or three sentences of the passage and try to paraphrase. If it's a Now passage, do it now. If it's a Later or Killer passage, write "SKIPPED" under the passage heading on your noteboard, Flag for Review and randomly guess on each question, and move on to ranking the next passage. Go through the entire section in the same way: writing the passage heading on your noteboard, completing the Now passages, and noting, Flagging, and guessing on the Later or Killer passages. This is your first pass.

3) Once you've completed all the Now passages, take a second pass through the section and do all the Later passages. You can use the Review function, if necessary, to find the passages you have Flagged and guessed on.

At or before the 5-minute mark (ideally before you begin your last passage), inspect the section to make sure that you haven't left any questions blank.

If you have a few extra minutes left over for a Killer passage, quickly read the first and last sentence of each paragraph. Identify the easiest questions (especially Retrieval questions and Inference questions with paragraph references and/or lead words), and do as many as you can by going to the relevant sections of the passage text. Again, be careful to leave time to fill in random guesses for the questions you cannot complete.

6.4 CARS EXERCISES: RANKING

Exercise 1: Evaluating the Passage Text

Each of the following paragraphs represents the first two sentences of a CARS passage. Using the criteria described earlier, decide if these are likely to be Now, Later, or Killer passages. You can find answers at the end of the exercise.

Passage I

It is often argued that the attempt to regulate the behavior of corporations through legislation is at best futile and at worst deleterious; in making their argument, advocates of nonregulation assume a distinction between the morality of duty and the morality of aspiration. They argue that duties, which specify the minimum standards of human conduct, lend themselves to legal enforcement better than do aspirations, which exhort one to realize one's full potential.

Passage II

A fundamental element of the American criminal justice system is trial by impartial jury. This constitutionally protected guarantee allows the defendant to challenge prospective jurors who are clearly prejudiced in the case.

Passage III

Imagining a primal state of existence, one in which there is no notion of space or time as we know it, pushes most people's powers of comprehension to the limit.… We run up against a clash of paradigms when we try to envision a universe that is, but somehow does not invoke the concepts of space or time.

Passage IV

The KT boundary, as it is called, marks one of the most violent events ever to befall life on Earth. Sixty-five million years ago, according to the current theory, the Cretaceous period was brought to a sudden conclusion by the impact of an asteroid or comet ten kilometers in diameter.

Passage V

A satisfactory explanation of the deepest significance of the fluoridation controversy remains elusive. Despite decades of research on the topic, the persistence and the passion of the fluoridation debates are yet incompletely understood by social scientists and social philosophers.

Passage VI

Trust and its violation have intrigued sociologists for decades. Trust is no more than an attribute of individuals; trust also describes a form of social organization, and interorganizational dynamics of trust violations offer a challenge to regulatory models that are largely intercorporate and involve individual or organizational self dealing.

Passage VII

The events of the author's life as they appear in poetry cannot be taken as literally true. As we move through life, our memory of what happened in the past changes and becomes more positive; events that were full of anxiety when they occurred now seem much more enjoyable in retrospect.

Passage VIII

Mention the word "surrealism" today, and certain visual images spring immediately to mind, and these images inevitably lead to certain assumptions about Surrealism: that it was primarily concerned with the visual arts, that it was about jokes, and that it was designed with a beady eye to the market. Nothing could be further from the truth, however.

Passage IX

Punishment appears to have unintended consequences. According to social theory, for example, punishment may increase the incidence of aggression because the target may imitate the behavior of the punishing agent, and offenders who are labeled are likely to behave consistently with expectations associated with that label.

Passage X

Nietzsche sees morality in much the same way that he sees epistemology. There is a gradual emptying out of that which is living in morality.

Explanations for Exercise 1: Evaluating the Passage Text

1. **Difficult:** This paragraph includes abstract concepts such as "the morality of duty and the morality of aspiration" that are difficult to paraphrase. Also, the vocabulary level is high—"deleterious," "nonregulation," "aspiration"—and will likely remain so throughout the passage.
2. **Easy:** This passage seems straightforward and factual.
3. **Medium:** This passage is fairly abstract. "Primal state of existence" and "paradigms" are red flag phrases.
4. **Easy:** This passage seems straightforward, and it seems to have a clear viewpoint.
5. **Medium:** A passage about the "deepest significance" of a controversy is likely to be fairly abstract. This is also indicated by the fact that social scientists and philosophers are trying to understand it, meaning the passage may be a challenge for test-takers to understand as well.
6. **Difficult:** The second sentence in particular is very abstract with a complex structure that makes it difficult to follow—the passage is likely to continue in the same vein.
7. **Easy:** Even though this passage is about a perhaps unfamiliar topic (poetry), the description is straightforward and easy to follow.
8. **Easy:** Although it is about art, which is usually considered an abstract topic, the paragraph is fairly descriptive and concrete rather than being highly theoretical.
9. **Medium:** There are some fairly abstract references here (e.g., "aggression," "the target," and "the punishing agent") which may muddy up the clarity of the passage.
10. **Difficult:** Try doing the six-year-old sister test on this paragraph. The vocabulary level, the sentence structure, and the abstractness of the subject matter indicate that this will be an extremely difficult passage.

Exercise 2: Evaluating the Questions

In most cases, your passage ranking will be based only on the passage text. However, to be able to adapt your ranking, if needed, to an usually difficult set of questions during the preview stage, you need to be able to recognize what tends to make questions easier or harder. Classify each of the following CARS questions as Easy or Hard. You can find answers at the end of the exercise.

1. It can be inferred from the passage that the availability of temperature-depth records for any specific area of the United States depends primarily on the:

2. In order to support his view with respect to Wilson's *Declining Significance of Race*, Hill would be most likely to discuss which one of the following?

3. Which of the following statements would most *weaken* the author's claim that voir dire fails to ensure a jury's impartiality?

4. Suppose it was demonstrated that social media has a less significant effect on political opinion than previously thought. What impact would this have on the author's claims in the second paragraph?

5. According to the passage, which of the following was most important in creating the modern trend toward redistribution?

6. The phrase "potent political opposition" (paragraph 1) refers to:

7. The author's attitude toward insider trading can best be described as:

8. In their evaluation of the fossil record, the author states that Cutler and Behrenmeyer did all of the following EXCEPT:

9. Of the following, which would be most logically similar to the way in which a majority of fatalities from malaria occur, as the process is described in the passage?

10. The author claims that the art market rises and falls in concert with the stock market. How well is this claim supported by the author?

Explanations for Exercise 2: Evaluating the Questions

1. **Easy:** Inference questions with specific references to the passage often have straightforward answers. In this case, you would probably just need to find where these records are discussed in the passage.

2. **Hard:** This is a Strengthen question that involves two speakers—you need to keep both of their perspectives in mind and conclude what approach Hill would take to support his or her own position in comparison (or contrast) to Wilson's.

3. **Hard:** A Weaken question requires taking new information provided in the answer choices and using reasoning to apply it to the passage.

4. **Hard:** The word "suppose" indicates that this question is going to require evaluating new information in the question stem and then taking multiple steps to answer the question. Also, the question stem is quite lengthy.

5. **Easy:** This is a Retrieval question, so the answer can be found in the passage text.

6. **Easy:** This question tells you where to go to find the information you need. As long as you remember to read above and below, it should not be difficult to answer.

7. **Easy:** The author's attitude can usually be determined with little difficulty.

8. **Easy:** The wording "The author states" tells you that this is a Retrieval question. The fact that it is an "EXCEPT" question shouldn't make it significantly more difficult, as long as you keep track of the question format, and of why you are eliminating each choice.

9. **Hard:** The phrase "logically similar" indicates that this is an Analogy question, which involves a higher level of reasoning and abstraction than do most question types.

10. **Hard:** This is an Evaluate question: you will have to decide if the support given is strong or weak and why.

Exercise 3: Evaluate Your Ranking

Ranking is a skill, like any other, that needs to be learned, practiced, and refined over time. If you ever rank an easy passage as Later (or Killer), or a difficult passage as Now, review the passage to see what made it easy or difficult and how you could have evaluated it better the first time through.

6.4

Compare the ranking you gave each passage to your eventual performance (taking into account both your accuracy and your efficiency/pacing) on that passage. Determine the order of attack that would have worked best for you.

- Were there any Killer passages that you should have skipped and guessed on? How could you have known it was a Killer before you wasted any time on it?
- Did you fail to get to any easy passages lurking at the end of the section?
- How will you change your approach on the next MCAT Practice Test you take?

Chapter 6 Summary

- The nine passages in the MCAT CARS section are "organized" in a seemingly random way. The level of difficulty of each passage depends on both the reading level of the passage text and on the difficulty level of the question types.

- To maximize your score, you must attack the passages strategically. Don't waste your time on Killer passages!

CHAPTER 6 PRACTICE PASSAGES

Individual Practice Drills

Rank the two passages that follow. Do the passage that you rank as easier first. Keep track of the time you spend on each passage, but don't give yourself a set time limit.

Once you have completed the passages and checked your answers, fill out an Individual Passage Log for each passage. In particular, decide if you ranked and ordered them correctly. If not, define what you could have recognized about the passage text and/or the questions in order to rank and order the passages more accurately and effectively.

By now, you should be taking full timed CARS sections and full practice tests from online or other resources. Always evaluate your ranking after completing a CARS test section.

Don't agonize over your decisions or panic if every choice you make isn't perfect. Ranking is simply another way to gain more control over the test (and to take that control away from the test-writers).

CHAPTER 6 PRACTICE PASSAGE 1

While I would certainly not want to disparage the efforts of vegetarians to limit violence toward animals in their personal lives and in public institutions and practices involving the slaughter and consumption of animals, I think it is important also to underscore that vegetarianism is itself fundamentally deconstructible. Vegetarianism is not just a passion for other animals but a series of practices involving animals and a series of discourses about animals. And if we follow the logic of Derrida's thought on the question of the animal, then it is necessary both to support vegetarianism's progressive potential but also interrogate its limitations. I have already shown how animal ethics in general (and animal rights theory, in particular) tends to reinforce the very metaphysics of subjectivity it seeks to undercut inasmuch as animal ethicists rely on a shared subjectivity among human beings and animals to ground their theories. But there are other limitations in vegetarian and pro-animal practices that should be noted. First, no matter how rigorous one's vegetarianism might be, there is simply no way to nourish oneself in advanced, industrial countries that does not involve harm to animal life (and human life, as well) in direct and indirect forms.... Simply tracking the processes by which one's food gets to the table is enough to disabuse any consumer of the notion that a vegetarian diet is "cruelty free." As such, a vegetarian diet within the context of advanced, industrial societies is, at best, a significant challenge to dominant attitudes and practices toward animals, but it remains far from the kind of ethical idea it is sometimes purported to be. Second, there are other ethical stakes involved in eating that go beyond the effects consumption of meat and animal byproducts has on animals. All diets, even organic and vegetarian diets, have considerable negative effects on the natural environment and the human beings who produce and harvest food. Consequently, if we consider ethical vegetarianism to constitute an ethical stopping point, these other concerns will be overlooked. And it is precisely these other concerns, concerns about the other, often-overlooked forms of violence, that should *also* impassion a deconstructive approach to the question of the animal.

Although these critical points are certainly in line with the logic of a deconstructive approach to animal ethics, they do not form the focus of Derrida's analysis. Derrida draws attention, instead, to a different limitation to pro-animal ethics and politics, one that he associates with "interventionist violence" against animals. The violence at issue here takes a *symbolic* rather than literal form, and this symbolic violence against animals, Derrida seems to think, is one of the most pressing philosophical and metaphysical issues facing thought today. In view of this notion of symbolic violence, he makes the following statement: "Vegetarians, too, partake of animals, even of men. They practice a different mode of denigration." What does he mean by this? Clearly, ethical vegetarianism aims at avoiding consumption of animal flesh—and presumably human flesh, as well. So, in what manner do vegetarians partake of animals and other beings toward which they aim to be nonviolent? Derrida's remark here is part of a complicated argument about the ethical questions concerning eating, incorporation, and violence toward the Other. While Derrida, like Levinas, posits a nonviolent opening to the Other...he does not believe that a wholly nonviolent relation with the Other is possible. On his line of thought, violence is irreducible in our relations with the Other, if by nonviolence we mean a thought and practice relating to the Other that respects fully the alterity of the Other. In order to speak and think about or related to the Other, the Other must—to some extent—be appropriated and violated, even if only symbolically. How does one respect the singularity of the Other without betraying that alterity? *Any* act of identification, naming, or relation is a betrayal of and a violence toward the Other. Of course, this should not be taken to mean that such violence is immoral or that all forms of violence are equivalent.... [Within vegetarianism] the ethical question should not be "How do I achieve an ethically pure, cruelty-free diet?" but rather, "What is the best, most respectful, most grateful, and also most giving way of relating" to animals and other Others?

Material used in this particular passage has been adapted from the following source:

M. Calarco, *Zoographies: The Question of the Animal from Heidegger to Derrida.* © 2008 by Columbia University Press.

1. Which of the following assertions is/are made in the passage?

   I. Derrida believes that symbolic violence against animals is currently one of the most important issues in metaphysical thought.
   II. Symbolic violence against the Other is as bad as literal violence.
   III. Eating in an advanced industrialized society inherently entails harming others.

   A) II only
   B) I and II only
   C) I and III only
   D) I, II, and III

2. The author most likely believes that:

   A) vegetarianism is pointless since it cannot be freed from a relation of cruelty with the Other.
   B) Levinas is short-sighted in believing a non-violent relationship with the Other is possible.
   C) vegetarianism is noble in its efforts to limit violence against human and nonhuman animals, but it is not above questioning and criticism.
   D) Derrida is overly extreme in asserting that "vegetarians partake of animals, even men."

3. Suppose that a young girl rescues a formerly abused greyhound dog from an animal shelter. She names him Odysseus after the Greek explorer to honor the dog's past and celebrate his arrival in a safe and loving home. Based on information provided in the passage, how would Derrida respond to this situation?

   A) Derrida would allow that, even though the act of naming entails treating the animal as Other, the respect signified by the name balances against the violence done to the dog in the past.
   B) He would point out that even naming the Other is an act of violence, albeit a symbolic one, no matter what the intention behind the name.
   C) He would praise the girl for choosing such a historically significant and noble name, saying that this reflects her love of animals.
   D) Derrida would criticize the girl for committing an act of violence as severe as those committed by the dog's former owners.

4. What definition of the word "disabuse" (paragraph 1) best fits in the context of the passage?

   A) Treating something kindly and/or healing it after a period of abuse
   B) Chastising someone for misguided views
   C) Affirming someone's views
   D) Convincing a person that his or her views are fallacious

5. What is the primary purpose of the passage?

   A) To question the Derridian view of animals as Others to whom we owe an ethical responsibility, whether we are vegetarians or not
   B) To critique, with the help of Derrida's philosophy, the central motivations of vegetarianism and to suggest a new basis for a discussion concerning how best to treat animals
   C) To suggest that vegetarianism is fundamentally misguided since nobody can practice a completely "cruelty free" diet
   D) To interrogate the notion of "ethical purity" and argue that such a state of being is impossible

6. All of the following are claims made by the author EXCEPT:

   A) ethical vegetarianism aims to avoid the consumption of animal and human flesh.
   B) vegetarianism remains far from the ethical ideal it is purported to be.
   C) animal ethicists rely on a shared subjectivity between humans and animals to ground their theories.
   D) vegetarianism is fundamentally deconstructive.

7. The author provides the most support for which of the following claims?

   A) Derrida draws attention to a limitation of pro-animal ethics which is associated with "interventionist violence."
   B) There is simply no way to feed oneself in advanced, industrialized countries without causing some harm to animal life.
   C) All diets have considerably negative effects on the environment and on the humans who produce and harvest food.
   D) Vegetarians are not as ethically pure as vegans, who avoid all animal byproducts in their diets, thereby reducing their environmental harm.

CHAPTER 6 PRACTICE PASSAGE 2

Hispanics are the fastest growing minority in the United States. "Hispanics," "Latinos," "Chicanos," "Mexican Americans," "Puerto Ricans," "Cuban Americans," and so on, are all designations used to describe this large, heterogeneous population with different cultural, ethnic, geographic, and social backgrounds. There is still no clear definition of the term "Hispanic." The data available regarding the incidence, morbidity, and mortality from cancer in "Hispanics" are scarce, scattered, outdated, and often incomplete.

From the studies looking at the accessibility and availability of medical care to this population, few have examined in detail the variability within the entire Hispanic population. The aggregation of culturally distinct subgroups, which have resided in the United States for different periods of time, into a more inclusive "Hispanic" category assumes that all persons of Mexican, Central and South American, Cuban, and Puerto Rican extraction have similar perceptions, true or not, of cancer risks and share needs and experience similar barriers in using health services. There is, however, no clear evidence for this assumption.

On the contrary, there is evidence that each group has specific characteristics that make them different and independent from one another, despite the fact that they also share some commonalities. Recruitment of minorities, specifically Hispanics, to clinical trials has been a significant problem that can potentially be overcome by adequate protocol development and investigator education regarding specific knowledge, attitudes, and needs of minority populations. It is timely and refreshing to see a recent anthropological evaluation of the problem of cancer in (female) Hispanics. It reviews the knowledge, attitudes, and barriers (KAB) for breast and cervical cancer in four different groups of women of Hispanic/ Latino origin and compare them among themselves and against a group of physicians' KAB.

Unfortunately, there are no complete data regarding cancer in all Hispanic groups. We currently do not know the true number of cancer cases in Hispanics, nor do we have accurate morbidity, mortality, and survival data from these groups. As a result, we are not really able to fully understand or appreciate the physical, emotional, and financial impact of cancer in Hispanic patients and their families. Mortality from cancer in Hispanics is difficult to assess because of the limited data

that are available. Utilizing existing community groups and organizations and helping to create strong community bonds could improve the potential for success of minority cancer control efforts and patient recruitment to clinical trials. These programs can become networks of information with inherent trust from their respective communities. In developing these interventions, we should increase our awareness of the needs of all different Hispanic groups and assure that programs are developed together with these communities, in order to assure that they are culture- and community-sensitive, respecting and complementing the Hispanic heritage.

[The recent anthropological study reminds] us that perhaps there are no true knowledge deficits, but rather misconceptions regarding the true cancer risks. Thus, it emphasizes two facts: (1) we must get to know and understand the population(s) with whom we plan to work; and (2) there is a strong need for education, not only of the communities with whom we work but, perhaps more important, of the scientific teams (physicians, nurses, anthropologists, social workers, etc.) that will work in and with those communities. Preliminary data from our group have shown that community-based lay health educators ("Promotoras de Salud"), working together with local health departments can be successful in reaching, educating, and increasing recruitment of Hispanic (Mexican-American) women to cervical cancer screening programs and to cancer clinical trials. This program is now being piloted through the Southwest Oncology Group in San Antonio's (Texas) Hispanic community. The time has come to revise and update our sources of information and data gathering. Careful study of each Hispanic subgroup is essential in order to have a realistic picture of the overall cancer problem in the United States today. These studies must include a clearer definition of the differences among the many Hispanic subgroups with their respective problems and barriers to cancer care.

Material used in this particular passage has been adapted from the following source:

M. R. Modiano, "Breast and Cervical Cancer in Hispanic Women," *Medical Anthropology Quarterly*, © 1995, the American Anthropological Association.

1. The primary purpose of the passage is to:

A) prompt others to create a better, more accurate definition of "Hispanics."
B) promote a better understanding of Hispanic populations in order to recognize and serve their cancer health needs.
C) advocate for the term "Hispanic" to be discarded for its ineffectively inclusive description of diverse peoples.
D) educate Latino cancer patients about available resources.

2. The author characterizes Hispanics as which of the following?

A) A large, diverse minority of Spanish-speaking people in the United States with unusually strong community bonds
B) A population whose various members face similar obstacles in the health care system
C) A group whose known epidemiological cancer data may be lacking
D) A heterogeneous people who are represented well in clinical trials

3. Which of the following are limitations that exist currently, as stated by the passage?

   I.   The view of Hispanics as a culturally monolithic people
   II.   Language barriers between health care professionals and patients
   III.   Interference by medically untrained community groups

A) I only
B) I and II only
C) I and III only
D) II and III only

4. It can be inferred that the author would be in favor of a program with all of the following aspects EXCEPT:

A) a careful study of each Hispanic subgroup focusing on commonalities between them.
B) a community-based initiative that is congruent with Hispanic cultures.
C) an emphasis on cancer screening in women.
D) education of medical professionals about the populations they serve.

5. The author deems all of the following as positive aspects of the recent study discussed EXCEPT:

A) pointing out potentially helpful ways in which clinical trial recruitment can be improved.
B) separating "Hispanic" women in the study into specific groups.
C) utilizing an anthropological approach in analyzing cancer data in Hispanics.
D) gathering data on all of the different Hispanic subgroups.

6. The tone of the passage can best be described as:

A) derisive and accusatory.
B) distressed but indifferent.
C) optimistic and analytical.
D) clinical and regretful.

7. The intended audience of this passage is most likely:

A) cancer hospitals or research center administrators.
B) the American public at large.
C) Hispanic women with breast or cervical cancer.
D) the Southwest Oncology Group.

SOLUTIONS TO CHAPTER 6 PRACTICE PASSAGE 1

1. **C**   This is a Retrieval/Roman numeral question.

    I: **True. In paragraph 2, the author states: "The violence at issue here takes a *symbolic* rather than literal form, and this symbolic violence against animals, Derrida seems to think, is one of the most pressing philosophical and metaphysical issues facing thought today."**

    II: False. Near the end paragraph 2, the author states: "Of course, this should not be taken to mean that such violence is immoral or that all forms of violence are equivalent." There is no statement made that equates symbolic violence with literal violence.

    III: **True. While this answer choice may sound extreme, its language is backed up in paragraph 1, when the author says, "there is simply no way to nourish oneself in advanced, industrial countries that does not involve harm to animal life."**

2. **C**   This is an Inference question.

    A: No. This answer choice is too extreme. While the author critiques vegetarianism, he never goes so far as to dismiss it as "pointless." Note that in paragraph 1, the author states: "It is necessary both to support vegetarianism's progressive potential but also interrogate its limitations."

    B: No. The author does not evoke such critical language with regards to Levinas. Also, we don't know from the text that Levinas does in fact believe that a nonviolent relationship with the Other is possible, only that Levinas, like Derrida, "posits a nonviolent opening to the Other."

    C: **Yes. The author expresses admiration for vegetarians' efforts to limit their role in violence against animals, but spends the passage highlighting some flaws in the reasoning behind vegetarianism. See paragraph 1: "It is necessary both to support vegetarianism's progressive potential but also interrogate its limitations."**

    D: No. The author does not criticize Derrida in any way. Note that when the author asks in the middle of paragraph 2, "What does he mean by this," and goes on to say that clearly vegetarians eat neither animals nor people, he is not suggesting that this (literal consumption) is in fact what Derrida is referring to. Rather, the author goes on to explain that Derrida uses "partake" in the sense of symbolic violence towards "the Other."

3. **B**   This is a New Information question.

    A: No. Derrida believes that the act of naming "the Other" is itself an act of violence (see middle of paragraph 2). Although Derrida would most likely allow or admit that this act of violence is less severe than physical abuse, it is still (symbolic) violence. Therefore the naming adds to, rather than balances against, the violence done to the dog.

    B: **Yes. In paragraph 2, the author discusses Derridian thought and states: "*Any act of identification, naming, or relation is a betrayal of and a violence toward the Other.*" This answer choice is therefore the most appropriate one based on information from the passage.**

    C: No. There is no evidence in the passage to support this interpretation of Derrida's reaction. There is no suggestion that Derrida would care what the name is or what the intentions of the namer are.

    D: No. The author, in the context of explaining Derrida's argument, makes an effort to acknowledge that not all forms of violence are equivalent: "Of course, this should not be taken to mean that such violence is immoral or that all forms of violence are equivalent" (paragraph 2).

4. **D**   This is an Inference question.
   A: No. This answer is inappropriate given the context in which the word appears. The word is used in relation to changing one's mind about an opinion: in this case, the author is talking about exposing the reality that vegetarian diets are not in fact "cruelty free."
   B: No. This answer is too strong in tone: there is no personal chastising or reprimanding of the people who held views that vegetarian diets are "cruelty free."
   C: No. This answer choice is antithetical to the context of the word "disabuse" in the passage: disabusing is not about affirming someone's views but rather changing or eliminating them.
   D: Yes. This answer is the best fit according to the passage. The author suggests that thinking about how food gets to us is enough to convince anyone that a vegetarian diet is not in fact "cruelty free."

5. **B**   This is a Main Idea/Primary Purpose question.
   A: No. The author does not question Derrida's views about animals but rather employs them to make his analysis.
   B: Yes. This answer choice best captures the ideas presented in the passage and the purpose of the author's use of Derrida's philosophy. In paragraph 1, the author begins the discussion of vegetarianism's limitations by saying: "And if we follow the logic of Derrida's thought on the question of the animal, then it is necessary both to support vegetarianism's progressive potential but also interrogate its limitations." Paragraph 2 follows in kind, focusing on Derrida's views on the Other and how they relate to vegetarianism. The last sentence suggests a new way of approaching the issue: "[Within vegetarianism] the ethical question should not be 'How do I achieve an ethically pure, cruelty-free diet?' but rather, 'What is the best, most respectful, most grateful, and also most giving way of relating' to animals and other Others?"
   C: No. The words "fundamentally misguided" are too extreme given the tone of the passage. For example, the author states: "it is necessary...to support vegetarianism's progressive potential" as well as to look into its limitations (paragraph 1).
   D: No. This answer is too broad, since it does not address the idea of vegetarianism which is central to the passage. Furthermore, the author does not argue that ethical purity is never possible, but only that vegetarianism cannot itself be an ethically pure position (which relates back to the issue of the choice being too broad).

6. **D**   This is a Retrieval/EXCEPT question.
   A: No. This claim is made in paragraph 2: "Clearly, ethical vegetarianism aims at avoiding consumption of animal flesh—and presumably human flesh, as well."
   B: No. This statement is made in paragraph 1: "A vegetarian diet within the context of advanced, industrial societies is, at best, a significant challenge to dominant attitudes and practices toward animals, but it remains far from the kind of ethical idea it is sometimes purported to be."
   C: No. This statement is made word for word in paragraph 1 of the passage.
   D: Yes. In paragraph 1 the author states that "Vegetarianism is fundamentally deconstructible." This is different from saying it is "deconstructive," since the former term indicates that vegetarianism can be deconstructed, while the latter suggests it can deconstruct other things.

7. **A** This is an Evaluate question.

A: **Yes. After the author mentions Derrida's concept of "interventionist violence" in paragraph 2, he elaborates upon this term and defines it by means of discussion and example (i.e., naming the Other). Therefore, this, out of the four claims, is the one for which the author provides the most support within the passage.**

B: No. This claim is made in the passage (paragraph 1) but the author does not elaborate upon it by providing an explanation of how a vegetarian diet entails harm to animals. First, the following reference to the process by which food arrives at the table still does not explain what the direct or indirect harm might be. Second, the later reference to harm done to the environment hints at an explanation, but only a vague one (there is still no discussion of what that harm might be). Therefore, when comparing this choice to choice A, the statement in choice A is much more strongly supported within the passage.

C: No. This claim is made in the passage (paragraph 1) but the author does not offer specific examples or further explanation of the negative effects mentioned.

D: No. This statement is not made in the passage. The author mentions animal byproducts (second half of paragraph 1), but does not connect this to veganism (which itself is never mentioned—making this connection would require using too much outside knowledge) or suggest that people who avoid animal byproducts are more ethically pure than vegetarians.

SOLUTIONS TO CHAPTER 6 PRACTICE PASSAGE 2

1. **B** This is a Main Idea/Primary Purpose question.

A: No. The focus on simply the definition of "Hispanics" is too narrow. This answer choice ignores many of the central ideas of the text, including using community organizing and education to gain understanding about cancer information in Hispanic populations and to provide proper care.

B: **Yes. The correct answer will be the one of the four choices that best captures and covers all the major themes of the passage. The last four lines of the passage describe what the author believes is important (understanding the Hispanic populations) and the changes he believes should be made to help the affected people by creating "a realistic picture" of the situation. The rest of the passage explains why this better understanding is needed, and suggests ways in which it might be achieved.**

C: No. This choice is both too extreme and too narrow. While the author agrees that the use of the overly inclusive term "Hispanic" results in barriers to discovering important information about cancer in those populations, he never advocates discarding the term. He simply believes that each subgroup of the population should be examined separately. Furthermore, while the term "Hispanic" may be problematic in some ways, this is not the focus of the entire passage.

D: No. The passage states that education is an important facet that needs to be addressed, but the text itself does not offer much educational information regarding using cancer resources. The examples of the "Promotoras de Salud" and "Southwest Oncology Group" are only to illustrate the author's argument about the need for such organizations and programs.

2. **C** This is an Inference question.

A: No. "Hispanics" are described as a large, diverse group of people (paragraph 1). However, the author never states or suggests that Hispanics speak Spanish. Be careful not to use outside knowledge or assumptions when picking an answer choice. Furthermore, while the author does discuss measures that would help to "create strong community bonds" (paragraph 4), the passage does not suggest that Hispanics have unusually strong community bonds compared to other groups.

B: No. The passage states the opposite of this statement: the use of the "'Hispanic' category" assumes all the people "experience similar barriers" in health services (paragraph 2). However, "each group has specific characteristics that make them different and independent from one another" (paragraph 3).

C: **Yes. The last line of paragraph 1 states that "The data available regarding the incidence, morbidity, and mortality from cancer in Hispanics are scarce, scattered, outdated, and often incomplete."**

D: No. The author states that the Hispanic population is indeed heterogeneous, but notes in paragraph 3 that they are actually underrepresented in clinical trials. This is another example of an "opposite" Attractor.

3. **A** This is a Retrieval/Roman numeral question.

I: **True. The passage states that clumping together the culturally diverse groups that make up the Hispanic population results in a limited and inaccurate picture of "the physical, emotional, and financial impact of cancer in Hispanic patients and their families" (paragraph 4).**

II: False. While barriers, in general, are mentioned within the passage, specific language barriers are not addressed and are outside of the scope of the passage.

III: False. The author states that "community-based lay health educators" working with "health departments…can be successful" (paragraph 5).

4. **A** This is an Inference/EXCEPT question.

A: **Yes. The correct answer choice will have the *least* support from the passage text. While the first part of this choice is supported, the second part is not. The author calls for study and understanding of "variability" or differences between the subgroups. The author argues throughout the passage that a focus on, or assumption of, commonalities is misguided.**

B: No. Paragraph 4 emphasizes the importance of both a community-based approach and a program "complementing the Hispanic heritage."

C: No. Paragraph 5 mentions, positively, the successful "cervical cancer screening programs" carried out by community based coalitions.

D: No. Paragraph 5 highlights the importance of the education of "physicians, nurses, anthropologists, social workers, etc."

5. **D** This is an Inference/EXCEPT question.

A: No. Paragraph 3 states, "Recruitment of minorities, specifically Hispanics, to clinical trials has been a significant problem that can potentially be overcome by adequate protocol development and investigator education regarding specific knowledge, attitudes, and needs of minority populations."

B: No. In paragraph 3, the author mentions that the subjects were divided into "four different groups of women of Hispanic/Latino origin."

C: No. The author states in paragraph 3 that "it is timely and refreshing to see a recent anthropological evaluation of the problem of cancer in (female) Hispanics."

D: Yes. The correct answer choice will have the *least* support from the passage. The study in question divided the women into four categories. However, the author does not suggest that there are only four subgroups, or that the study covered all existing subgroups.

6. **C** This is a Tone/Attitude question.

A: No. While the author points out the inefficiencies of the health care system stemming in part from the inclusive term "Hispanics," he does not point fingers or accuse anybody specifically. He simply notes that the term is one with flaws: "There is still no clear definition of the term 'Hispanic'" (paragraph 1). In addition, there are no words that indicate contempt or ridicule as the word "derisiveness" would.

B: No. The author feels that there is a problem, but the word "distressed" is too extreme to describe his attitude. In addition, the author is not indifferent. He promotes ideas that he hopes will cause change. This can be noted through statements like: "The time has come to revise and update our sources of information and data gathering" (paragraph 5).

C: Yes. The author describes, in paragraph 5, progress that is occurring already, and what more improvements can be made. This indicates optimism. His explanation of the problem and situation is analytical—he discusses different aspects of the problem and provides supportive evidence.

D: No. "Clinical" does describe the relatively objective tone of the author. The text lacks passionate claims, but is, instead, professional, as the term "clinical" may indicate. However, the word "regretful" is too extreme to describe the author's attitude. While he would like the health care system to be reformed, the author does not use words that would indicate regret or disappointment. If one part of the choice is incorrect, the whole choice is wrong.

7. **A** This is an Inference question.

A: Yes. The author's intent is to encourage enactment of changes that will positively benefit Hispanics. Note wording such as "In developing these interventions, we should increase our awareness of the needs of all different Hispanic groups" (paragraph 4) or "we must get to know and understand the population(s) with whom we plan to work" (paragraph 5), which suggests that the passage is intended for people working within the field of health care. Administrators at cancer institutes or researchers have the ability to utilize his suggestions and advice, such as by carrying out useful research, or coordinating community based initiatives to reach more Hispanics.

B: No. The tone and content of the passage indicate that it is not intended for the general reader, but rather for people with a specific interest, and role to play, in this particular issue.

C: No. The primary purpose of this passage (as noted in the solution for question 1) is not to educate Hispanic women, but to create changes in our understanding of how cancer affects Hispanics and in how Hispanic people are educated, tested, and treated. While one could imagine that Hispanic women with breast or cervical cancer might be interested in this information, this group is too narrowly defined to be the "intended audience." The passage is geared towards people who would be able to carry out research, education, and treatment, rather than towards potential subjects of research, education, or treatment.

D: No. The Southwest Oncology Group already participates in the practices advocated by the author (paragraph 5). There would be little or no benefit seen by presenting the group with the information of the passage.

Individual Passage Log

Passage # _____   Time spent on passage _____

Q#	Q type	Attractors	What did you do wrong?

Revised Strategy _____

Passage # _____   Time spent on passage _____

Q#	Q type	Attractors	What did you do wrong?

Revised Strategy _____

Chapter 7
Strategy and Tactics

GOALS
1) To make the most of your time
2) To find ways to improve through self-evaluation
3) To refine your pacing strategy

7.1   MAXIMIZING YOUR PERFORMANCE

Now is the time to ask yourself a serious question: are you diligently and consistently implementing and refining a strategic approach to the test? Or, are you just doing passage after passage and taking test after test in the belief that simple repetition will continue to improve your score? If it's the latter, you must ask yourself WHY you are making the mistakes that you are and HOW you can change to improve your performance.

The Big Picture

Imagine two students. The first (say, the one who isn't using these materials) approaches the CARS section as she would any test in college. The second, a student using this book, uses the strategies she has learned. How will these students use their time on the test?

First Student, with No Specialized Test Strategy
- **On Easier Passages:** Overconfident and complacent, this student rushes through the easier passages, relying on her memory and failing to check her answer choices back to the passage text. She chooses the first answer that sounds good, and is perfectly happy with her choices, not realizing that she has fallen into all of the test-writers' traps.
- **On Harder Passages:** This student, doing the passages in the order given by the test-writers, hits a difficult passage in the middle of the section. Frustrated and confused, she slows down, reading everything three times, trying to understand exactly what the author is saying. She spends five minutes on a question, believing that she can't move on until she is sure of the correct answer. She becomes more and more anxious about the time, which makes it even harder to focus on the passage. This student tries to use sheer effort where strategy would be more effective.

Second Student, with MCAT-Appropriate Strategies
- **On Easier Passages:** Knowing that the majority of her correct answers will come from the easier passages, this student works through them with steadiness and focus. She clearly articulates the Bottom Line of the passage before answering the questions. She answers the questions in her own words before attacking the answer choices, and checks each choice against the passage.
- **On Harder Passages:** This student knows that not all passages will be completely comprehensible, and has an appropriate strategy for the harder passages. She uses POE to the fullest, remembering that she is looking for the "least wrong" choice, not an ideal answer. She asks questions of the answer choices (such as, *Is the language too extreme to be an inference? Is this choice too narrow for a Main Idea question?*) based on her knowledge of question types and common Attractors. This student gains points based on her intelligent, test-appropriate strategy.

Narrowing It Down

Let's revisit our first student. When asked why she misses questions, she responds, "I don't know. I always get it down to two choices, and then I pick the wrong one."

The second student, having done an extensive evaluation of her own performance to date, might respond, "On Inference questions, I tend to forget to look for absolute language, and I pick choices that are too extreme. Sometimes I get too impatient to define the Bottom Line, and then I pick Main Point answer choices that are too narrow. I also sometimes have too much confidence in my own memory, don't go back to the passage, and then miss easy Retrieval questions by choosing answer choices from the wrong part of the passage." The second, self-aware student knows exactly what she needs to work on over the next few weeks, and has a clear path to continued improvement. The first student will most likely continue to make the same mistakes over and over again. Remember, those who don't know and understand their own history are doomed to repeat it.

If you are identifying a bit too much with our first student, now is the time to ask yourself the following questions:

1) **Are you having trouble articulating the Bottom Line?**
   Is it difficult to locate the relevant parts of the passage when you are working the questions?
   The Diagnosis
   Both of these issues go back to articulating the main point of each paragraph or chunk, and synthesizing those themes as you read. If you don't identify the author's main points as you read, separating out the claims from the evidence, it is almost impossible to distill it down at the end to a core argument. And, if you aren't identifying the location of these different themes, the passage runs together in your mind as an undifferentiated block of information, and you will have trouble remembering and locating where different topics appeared.

   The Cure
   Review Chapter 3 on Active Reading.
   Break the argument into chunks and define the Main Points as you read; don't wait to think about it until after you have finished reading the passage. If you haven't been using your noteboard much (or at all), make yourself write down the Main Points as you go. Articulate how each new chunk logically relates to what you have already read. Preview the questions for content, so that you have some context within which to translate what you are reading, and you are alerted to some of the important issues in the passage.

2) **Do you tend to miss certain question types?**
   The Diagnosis
   Use your passage and practice test logs to identify which types give you the most trouble. Is it an overall category (e.g., Specific questions)? Is it a few particular question types or formats?

   The Cure
   Review Chapter 4 on Question Types.
   Identifying these patterns is the first step towards figuring out the exact causes of your mistakes. Here are some common problem areas and solutions.
   - Main Point/Primary Purpose: Pay attention to tone, and break down the passage by defining its logical structure. Avoid choices that are too narrow.
   - Specific questions: Keep track of the specific reference in the question stem, and go back to the passage *before* you take the first cut through the answer choices.

- Structure: Pay attention to words in the passage that distinguish claims (*therefore, thus, in conclusion*) from evidence (*for example, in illustration, in these three cases*).
- New Information: Treat the new information in the question stem like a paragraph of the passage: what is the main point of this chunk, and how does it relate to the logic of the author's argument? Use your noteboard to translate complicated questions.
- Strengthen and Weaken: Clearly define what the correct answer needs to do: what is the relevant issue, and must the correct answer be consistent or inconsistent with the passage? With what part of the passage? Keep close track of direction.
- EXCEPT/LEAST/NOT: Define not only what the right answer needs to do but what kind of choices you will be eliminating. Use your noteboard to keep track of POE.

3) **Do you tend to fall for certain types of Attractors?**
The Diagnosis
Use your logs and look for patterns!

The Cure
Review Chapter 5 on POE.
Each time you do a new passage or test section, pick out ahead of time two types of Attractors you will be on the lookout for. Define a specific tactic for recognizing and avoiding these traps, such as the following:

- Extreme wording: Look out for words like *only, most, all, must, never,* etc. Also, evaluate the strength of the statements in each choice; an answer choice can be too extreme even if it doesn't use these particular words.
- Partially correct: Force yourself to read the entire choice word for word. Actively look for that one word that can make it incorrect. Suspend all judgment on the validity of the choice until you have read every word.
- Right answer/wrong question: Always go back to the passage, with the specific reference in the question clearly in mind. Reread the question before you take your second cut through the choices.

4) **Are you going too slow or too fast?** Problems with pacing can underlie all of the above issues. So, let's move on to discuss it in more detail.

7.2 FOCUS ON PACING

By this point, you should begin timing yourself on your practice passages. If your reasonable goal is to complete eight passages with high accuracy and randomly guess on one passage, as a rule of thumb it should take you about 11 minutes per passage. If your reasonable goal is to complete all 9 (which is only reasonable if you are already scoring well), that entails taking around 10 minutes per passage. Keep in mind that this is only an approximation. A passage with seven questions will take you a bit longer than a passage of equal difficulty with only five questions, and a more difficult passage will legitimately take you a little longer to complete than an easier passage.

Here are some specific guidelines to help you to decide on an appropriate pacing plan for your target score.

Pacing Guidelines

The sections on the following pages describe the appropriate pacing for various CARS target score levels. Use your CARS score on your most recent practice test to determine which targets are most appropriate. If you are not hitting the accuracy goals for your current target level, you should not be trying to speed up or answer more questions. Once you are consistently hitting those targets, you may be ready to attempt the next level.

Current Score Level: Below Average

Target Score: Average

Pacing and Accuracy Goals: 7–8 Passage Pace

In this score range, it is critical that you identify easier (Now) passages and perform with high accuracy. Do not waste time on Killer passages, or spend too much time on Later passages. Plan to skip over at least three or four passages on your first pass through the section.

Now Passages (4):

You should spend 11–12 minutes on each of these passages. The reading should take 4–5 minutes and each question should take on average 1–1.5 minutes. Work carefully and use POE in order to avoid errors.

Accuracy Goal:

0–1 mistakes per passage.

Later Passages (3):

You should spend 13–14 minutes on each of these passages. The reading should take 3–4.5 minutes and each question should take on average 1–2 minutes. If you are taking a very long time on a question or just don't understand it, guess on that question and move on.

Accuracy Goal:

0–2 mistakes per passage.

Killer Passages (2):

You should mostly be guessing on these passages. If, after finishing the other passages, you have a few minutes left, pick another passage and read just the first and last sentences of the text. Then look for Specific questions with paragraph references or lead words. Use aggressive POE. Don't spend too much time on any one question. Make sure you have guessed on every question before time runs out.

Accuracy Goal:

At least 1 correct answer.

Current Score Level: Average

Target Score: Average-High

Pacing and Accuracy Goals: 8–9 Passage Pace

In this score range, it is critical that you not become distracted by the Later or Killer passages early in the test. Plan to skip at least two or three passages on your first pass through the test. Make sure you start with a Now passage and at your target pace.

Now Passages (5):
You should spend 10–11 minutes on each of these passages. The reading should take 3–4 minutes and each question should on average take 1–1.5 minutes. Work carefully and use POE in order to avoid errors.

Accuracy Goal:
0–1 mistakes per passage with ideally at least two perfect passages.

Later Passages (3):
You should spend 11–12 minutes on each of these passages. The reading should take 4–5 minutes and each question should on average take 1–1.5 minutes. If a question is taking a very long time, or you don't understand it at all, use aggressive POE, pick an answer, and move on. You may also choose to randomly guess on several of the hardest questions in some of the passages that you complete (see "Cherry Picking" in Section 7.5 of this chapter).

Accuracy Goal:
0–2 mistakes per passage.

Killer Passages (1):
You should be mostly guessing on one passage. If you start working on a passage early in the test and realize it is a Killer, immediately move on to easier passages. If you have time after completing the Now and Later passages, you should go to the remaining passage and read just the first and last sentence of each paragraph. Then look for Specific questions (or, if there are no Specific questions, Structure questions) with paragraph references and/or lead words from the passage. Use aggressive POE. Don't spend too much time on any single question. Make sure you have guessed on every question before time runs out.

Accuracy Goal:
At least 1 correct answer.

Current Score Level: Average-High
Target Score: High

Pacing and Accuracy Goals: 9 Passage Pace
You should only be attempting a 9–passage pace if you have consistently achieved the accuracy goals of previous levels. At this pace, plan to skip at least one or two passages on your first pass through the test. Make sure that you start with a passage that is not too difficult and to hit a good pace at the beginning.

Now Passages (6–7):
You should spend 8–9 minutes on each of these passages. The reading should take 2.5–3.5 minutes and each question should on average take 1 minute or less. Work carefully and use POE in order to avoid errors.

Accuracy Goal:
0–1 mistakes per passage with at least three perfect passages.

Later Passages (1–2):
You should spend 10–11 minutes on each of these passages. The reading should take 3.5–4.5 minutes and each question should on average take 1 minute or less. If a question is likely to take longer than 1.5 minutes or is confusing, skip it and look at it again before moving on to the next passage. You may also

choose to "cherry-pick," that is, randomly guess on 2–3 of the hardest questions in these passages (see "Cherry Picking" in Section 7.5 of this chapter). If you employ this strategy, you will need to get almost every other question correct in order to achieve the target score.

Accuracy Goal:
0–1 mistakes per passage, with at least two perfect passages.

Killer Passages (1):
Your approach to your last passage will depend on how much time you have left. To get a score at the top of the scale, you have to attack every passage and get almost all of the questions correct. However, you don't necessarily have to attempt every single question. You should not spend more time than usual reading the passage; instead keep your focus on main points and tone. Use aggressive POE and don't spend too much time on any single question. However, don't rush through all the questions if you are running out of time. Make a good attempt at most of them, and if needed, guess on one or two particularly difficult questions within the set. Make sure you have answered every question before time runs out.

Accuracy Goal:
At least 3 correct answers.

Diagnosing Pacing Problems
If you are not hitting the right pace to achieve your target score, you must

1) diagnose what is wrong with your current pace, and
2) adjust accordingly

First, let's look at four basic pacing issues.

1) **Going too fast**
   There are three signs that your score will improve if you slow down and do fewer questions.
   - If you are finishing nine passages but consistently missing two or more questions on every passage, or if you often miss more than half of the questions for a passage (that is, you do well on some passages but crash and burn on others).
   - If you realize that you often miss easy questions. This means that when you go over a test, many or most of the questions that you got wrong look obvious in retrospect. You can't imagine why you didn't pick the credited response, and you can't really remember why you liked that wrong answer so much.
   - If you are completing all nine passages and not getting a significantly above-average score.

2) **Going too slow**
   If one or more of the following describes you, increasing your speed and efficiency will improve your score:
   - You consistently answer all or almost all of the questions that you do correctly, but you are doing eight or fewer passages.
   - You spend a disproportionately high amount of time on a few passages or a few questions.
   - You spend 6 or more minutes reading the passage text the first time through.
   - You find yourself over-thinking the passage and/or the questions and spending a lot of time talking yourself into wrong answers.

7.3

3) **Getting bogged down on a Killer passage**
Let's return to our two students and compare their different approaches to the Killer passage:
- **What the first student, untrained in strategy, does with the Killer passage:**
She slows down, gets lost and distracted while reading, and spends too much time going back and rereading long sections of the passage. She gets caught up in deciphering fancy vocabulary words.

When she moves onto the questions, she goes even slower; she has spent so much time reading the passage that she feels that she has to get all of the questions right to justify it. At some point, the student realizes anxiously that too much time has passed and she guesses on the last two or three questions of the passage before moving on, stressed out and perspiring. She then speeds through the other easier passages, trying to make up for lost time, making foolish errors, and throwing away easy points.
- **What the second, trained student does with the Killer passage:**
Skips it (or does it last of all).
By randomly filling in all of the answer choices on the Killer Passage, the second student frees up at least 10–15 minutes that would have been wasted on getting questions wrong. And if she does complete it, she does it last so that it doesn't negatively affect how she does on the easier passages.

4) **Getting bogged down on a Killer question**
Even Now and Later passages can have a question that is extremely hard for you. You can't allow yourself to get sucked into that one question if doing so means you are losing the opportunity to answer two or more easier questions down the road.

7.3 REFINING YOUR PACING

Once you have decided if you need to slow down or speed up, the next question is HOW?

Slowing Down

This is not as obvious as it seems. Don't spend the time that you save by doing fewer questions or passages on excessive rereading. Also, don't sit and ponder difficult parts of the passage at great length, or come up with elaborate justifications for why a variety of answer choices might be correct. It is still important to be tightly focused and efficient, even when slowing down your pace.

Instead, invest the extra time in the following:

- translating the question and clearly identifying the question type and task,
- reading the answer choices more carefully: that is, word for word,
- comparing choices to each other and specifically looking out for common traps,
- and—most importantly—in going back to the passage to find the relevant information and defining what the correct answer needs to do.

Speeding Up

There are four common ways in which students get bogged down and lose time. To pick up your pace, focus on avoiding these traps.

1) **Reading the passage too carefully the first time through**

   If you are reading every word and highlighting the passage heavily, then you're reading the passage like a college course book rather than a CARS passage. You may feel safer going into the questions having consistently spent 6 or more minutes with the passage, but the test doesn't allow you the time to do so. Cut to the chase the first time through, and save the more careful rereading for answering the questions. (Review Chapters 3 and 7.)

2) **Not reading and translating the question carefully**

   If you go back into the passage without a clear idea of what you're looking for, you are likely to get lost and waste precious time backtracking to reread the question, or getting stuck in the answer choices because nothing fits what you first thought the question was asking. Spend a few more seconds translating the question, and the correct answers will come a lot more quickly. (Review Chapter 4.)

3) **Not aggressively using POE**

   You can waste a huge amount of time looking for a perfect answer instead of the "least wrong" answer. Trying to make a watertight case for the credited response when it is one of those "not great, but the best of what I've got" answers will not only suck up a lot of time and energy, it will also often cause you to talk yourself out of the correct choice. Maintain a critical focus through the entire POE process. (Review Chapter 5.)

4) **Overcommitting to one question or one passage**

   - Learn to recognize quickly whether you understand a test question or not. Are you rereading it over and over? Are you bouncing repeatedly (three or more times) from passage to question and back again? If so, these are clear signs that this question is not working for you (that is, it's very difficult). Many people become stubborn about seeing a question through; they think that because they have devoted some time already to the question, they can't abandon that question because doing so means they have wasted time. But spending even more time on a question that is particularly difficult means nothing more than wasting more time. You can't change the past, but you don't have to continue in an effort that is unlikely to yield a point.

   - If you doubt this logic, consider the following analogy. If you have dated someone for six months and realize that the person is a jerk, do you say, "Well, I don't want to have wasted the past six months, so I better get married to the jerk?" No! You move on, chalk up the episode to experience, and look for someone easier to get along with. Bringing it back to the world of the MCAT, in this situation use POE, take your best shot, and move on.

   - However, don't go to the opposite extreme. If you are getting it down to two and then guessing on a majority of questions, your accuracy will significantly suffer and your score will go down, not up.

   - Don't spend a high percentage of your resources on a single passage. More difficult passages should take a bit more time, but you need to keep moving. Remember that in many cases hard passages have been edited in such a way that some things are never fully explained or clarified; you could read it ten times over and still not really "get it." Luckily, in most cases you don't need to understand every aspect of the passage to get most of the questions right.

Try Pacing Exercise 1 at the end of this chapter if your accuracy is good but you need to increase your speed. Also see Section 7.5 "Variations on a Theme: Refining Your Strategy" for more specific pacing suggestions.

Avoiding KILLER Passages

Use your previous experience to refine your ranking technique. Each time you rank a passage as Now, and it turns out to be a Later or Killer, go back and re-evaluate the passage and the questions to see what made it harder than you expected, and how you could have recognized it earlier.

Conversely, every time you misidentify an easy passage as a difficult passage, do the same. Look in particular for passages with unfamiliar subject matter that you ranked as Later or Killer that were relatively easy once you got into them.

It is dangerous to rank passages on the basis of familiarity; it is really the difficulty of the language and of the question types that makes for a hard passage.

Review Chapter 6 if you are having trouble ranking passages accurately. See section 7.5 "Variations on a Theme: Refining Your Strategy," as well, for more ranking suggestions.

7.4 CARS EXERCISES: PACING AND SELF-EVALUATION

Exercise 1: Speeding Up

Do this exercise if you have excellent accuracy on the passages that you actually complete, but can only complete a limited number of passages under timed conditions. You may wish to spread this exercise out over a few days or weeks.

Do a full CARS section (or look at your most recent practice test), and note the average time spent per passage here._____

Now do four more passages back-to-back (or, an entire CARS test section), but give yourself one less minute for each passage you attempt. Use the suggestions in this chapter to diagnose areas where you may be wasting time, and to work through those areas more efficiently. If you complete those passages with good accuracy, reduce your time per passage by another 30–60 seconds and do another set of passages.

Continue this process until your accuracy begins to suffer. Note the average time spent per passage here._____

Carefully diagnose the reasons for your mistakes, and continue to work at that pace until your accuracy improves to your previous level.

Continue this exercise until you hit the appropriate pace for you.

Exercise 2: 5-Minute Drill

If you have about 5 minutes left when you've finished a passage, do not begin to carefully read the next Later or Killer passage in your ranking. If you do, you will run out of time with few or no questions answered. Instead, quickly read the first and last sentence of each paragraph. If it's a two-sentence paragraph, just read the first sentence. Next, click through the questions and pick out the easier Specific questions (such as Retrieval, and Inference questions with lead words and/or paragraph references) and do those first, going back to the passage to hunt down and read the relevant sections. You have a good chance of getting those easier questions right, even with little time remaining.

If you have time left after doing these Specific questions, take a shot at any Main Idea or Primary Purpose questions, using what you have now learned about the major themes of the passage. Be sure to rely heavily on POE, thinking actively about identifying and avoiding common Attractors. Even if you only have a minute left, you can probably at least eliminate one or two answer choices on one General question, or even a Reasoning or Application question.

So, imagine that the 5-minute warning has come up on the screen, just as you have completed a passage. Your goal now is to get what you can out of the seven questions for the passage on the next pages in the few minutes you have left.

Formal and informal reactions to crime are distinguished by whether they are administered by representatives of the state. Government officials administer formal reactions, such as penal sanctions. Informal reactions are sanctions imposed by non-state functionaries, usually ordinary citizens. These sanctions include all the detrimental consequences that convicted offenders experience that are not formally specified by law or pronounced by a judge in the disposition. To lose one's job or be ridiculed by others are examples of informal sanctions. Since equality before the law is such a symbolically important part of the criminal justice system, many investigators have examined the legal and extralegal determinants of formal sanctions. For example, the effects of offense and offender characteristics on variations in criminal sentences have been investigated extensively. By contrast, informal reactions to crime have received minimal analytic attention. This failure to explore the determinants of informal sanctions distorts understanding of the links between social structure and social control.

Position in the stratification hierarchy is one of the factors that determine susceptibility to law. Those in low positions are more susceptible to law in that, among other things, their crimes are more harshly sanctioned. The same is true for non-governmental forms of social control. Just as inequality in wealth and power influences decision-making in courtrooms, it also affects how offenders are treated in workplaces and in the community. Criminal conviction has been shown to reduce the employment opportunities of working-class defendants. Case studies of powerful corporate executives who have committed egregious offenses find that they often continue to hold respected positions in both the economic and social worlds. These studies suggest that the "stigmatizing effects" of criminal conviction are not damaging for some white-collar offenders.

Less powerful white-collar offenders may be more stigmatized by criminal conviction than business executives. For example, professionals and public-sector workers convicted of white-collar crimes lose occupational status more often than business executives convicted of similar offenses. The consequences of legal stigma may be influenced more by the offender's class position than by his or her criminal conduct.

The extent of social condemnation presumably varies directly with the seriousness of offense and severity of the criminal sentences received. In theory, those who commit minor offenses provoke little censure from the community-at-large and receive lenient treatment in the legal system. Those who commit more serious offenses do not fare as well: they may receive both stronger social condemnation and harsher punishment. Since judges supposedly deem informal sanctions, such as loss of status, sufficient punishment for white-collar offenders, they may impose less severe sentences on those who experience those sanctions. Consequently, formal and informal reactions to white-collar crime may not be consistent.

Material used in this particular passage has been adapted from the following source:

M. L. Benson, "The Influence of Class Position on the Formal and Informal Sanctioning of White-Collar Offenders," *Sociological Quarterly*. © 1989, Midwest Sociological Society.

1. It can be inferred from the passage that the courts would treat social isolation of an accused business executive as:

A) an expected consequence of public accusations but not relevant to the judicial process.
B) a more potent form of punishment than even a prison sentence.
C) a situation that, since not truly measurable, cannot be considered punitive.
D) a legitimate form of punishment that is often considered before a sentence is determined.

2. According to the passage, which of the following is a ramification of the failure to examine the determining factors of informal sanctions?

A) A misunderstanding of the relationship between the structure of society and sanctions that are used to control criminal behavior
B) A reduction of employment opportunities for working-class defendants
C) An inability to establish effective punitive measures using formal sanctions on criminal behavior
D) The ability of numerous business executives convicted of criminal offenses to maintain respectable positions

3. Which one of the following best describes the author's reaction to the two forms of sanctions discussed in the passage?

A) Frustration that class position is a factor in the severity of both formal and informal sanctions
B) Concern about the injustices frequently occurring because governmental and non-governmental sanctions against offenders are both solely determined by the hierarchy of class position
C) Advocating further study of non-governmental sanctions to address inconsistent treatment of criminal offenders
D) Favoring formal sanctions as the fairest method of punishing criminal offenders

4. The phrase "'stigmatizing effects' of criminal conviction" (paragraph 2) refers to which one of the following?

A) The severity of formal sanctions imposed upon working-class defendants after criminal convictions
B) The less severe formal sanctions received by white-collar criminals after criminal convictions
C) The informal sanctions a defendant receives as a result of being convicted of a crime
D) The inequality of treatment before the law of working-class and white collar offenders

5. Which of the following questions about the two forms of sanctions could not be answered by using the information provided in the passage?

A) What is the difference between formal and informal sanctions?
B) Why have formal sanctions received extensive analytic treatment?
C) Why have informal sanctions not received thorough investigation?
D) Why are formal and informal sanctions of white-collar crimes sometimes inconsistent?

6. Which of the following sentences would best serve as a completion to the passage?

A) As the justice system progresses, the determinants of informal sanctions should receive more investigation.
B) Accordingly, judges should not consider informal sanctions when imposing sentences on criminal offenders, regardless of their position on the social hierarchy.
C) If this trend continues, it will remain impossible for criminal defendants to receive fair sentences until more attention is paid to the study of informal sanctions.
D) It is clear that the seriousness of the offense alone should determine the formal sanctions imposed upon criminal conviction.

7. Which of the following best expresses the main idea of the passage?

A) The extent to which a person is stigmatized by criminal conviction depends in large part on their social status or class.
B) To understand how individual behavior is influenced by society, we must learn more about the effect of social stigma on criminal offenders.
C) Informal sanctions have an even greater effect than formal sanctions on those accused or convicted of crimes and so must be studied in more depth.
D) The workings of law and society cannot be studied in isolation from each other; the two are inherently intertwined in our institutions and cultural beliefs.

Answers to 5-Minute Drill

1. **D**
2. **A**
3. **C**
4. **C**
5. **C**
6. **A**
7. **B**

7.4

Exercise 3: Test Assessment Log

This Log should look familiar; there is a copy of it in Chapter 2. If you haven't been using it to evaluate your practice tests, now is the time to start.

In particular, use it to evaluate your pacing. Are you spending the time you need on the easier passages in order to get most of those questions right? Keep track of how much time you spent (roughly) on the Now passages and on the Later passages. If you find that you are spending the bulk of your 90 minutes on the harder passages with a low level of accuracy, you need to reapportion your time. At the same time, evaluate your ranking: are you choosing the right passages?

Now Passages

Now Passage #	Q # and Type (for questions you got wrong)	Attractors (for wrong answers you picked or seriously considered)	What did you do wrong?

Approximate time spent on Now passages _____

Total Now passages attempted _____

Total # of Qs on Now passages attempted _____

Total # of Now Qs correct _____

% correct of Now Qs attempted _____

7.4

Later Passages

7.4

Later Passage #	Q # and Type (for questions you got wrong)	Attractors (for wrong answers you picked or seriously considered)	What did you do wrong?

Approximate time spent on Later passages _____

Total Later passages attempted _____

Total # of Qs on Later passages attempted _____

Total # of Later Qs correct _____

% correct of Later Qs attempted _____

Final Analysis

Total # of passages attempted (including partially completed) _____

Total # of questions attempted _____

Total # of correct answers _____

Total % correct of attempted questions _____

Revised Strategy

Pacing	
Passage choice/ranking	
Working the Passage	
Attacking the Questions	

7.5 VARIATIONS ON A THEME: REFINING YOUR STRATEGY

Through your preparation you are learning a standard approach to the CARS section that has been tested and refined over decades, based in part on the experience and input of hundreds of thousands of students. However, different people process information somewhat differently. Once you have mastered the approach, you may benefit from experimenting with variations on those techniques in order to make them work optimally for you.

Unfortunately, there are no secret "tricks" to the CARS section. Making score improvements in this section requires a lot of practice, hard work, and vigilant review. It is easy to get into a rut, doing the same thing over and over without thinking about how to further improve your line of attack. This section is intended to spark, or add fuel to, that thought process.

Pacing and Accuracy

As we discussed in the previous sections, the way for many students to maximize their score is to attempt eight of the nine passages, randomly guessing on the hardest passage in the section. However, if your reasonable goal (based on your performance to date) is to score significantly above average, you will most likely need to attempt some or all of a ninth passage. And, if you are currently completing six or seven passages, unless you have close to perfect accuracy, you will need to pick up the pace in order to achieve an average or bit above-average score. The question is then, how can you speed up without a significant loss of accuracy?

Ironically, you might find that going a bit faster not only gets you through more questions, but also improves your accuracy. This may be the case if you tend to overthink the passage or the questions, by making the passage more confusing than it needs to be, or talking yourself out of correct answers.

On the other hand, if you are missing a large number of questions because you did not read carefully enough, or did not think enough about the meaning of what you read, then slowing down (especially if you are doing all nine passages) may pay off. No one really wants to randomly guess on questions (everyone would prefer to do all of the questions and get them all right); however, many students have found that once they do slow down, focusing more on accuracy and less on speed, they not only have the time to do what needs to be done, but they also think more clearly and efficiently.

Below are suggestions and variations on the standard approach that may improve your speed, your accuracy, or both. Always try new approaches on multiple passages and tests to gather enough data to see if they are really working for you. But be sure to test one new approach at a time, rather than trying to do a massive overhaul.

A. Ranking and Ordering: The Three-Pass System

Most test-takers do best with the Two-Pass system of ordering the passages; that is, doing the Now passages the first time through as you find them, then coming back for a second pass to do the Later passages. However, if you find that you struggle with separating out the Nows from the Laters from the Killers, AND that you are often making bad choices in the passages you attempt to the extent that it hurts your score, it is worth trying the Three-Pass system.

1) First Pass: Rank all nine passages Now, Later, or Killer
2) Second Pass: Do the Now passages
3) Third Pass: Do the Later passages and check the Review screen for incompletes.

The Three-Pass system may take a bit more total time than the Two-Pass system. However, if you are consistently making bad ranking decisions and wasting time struggling with difficult passages, comparing all nine passages before beginning your Nows may pay off.

B. Working the Passage
1) **Push the Pace**

a) It is comforting to read the whole passage word for word, translating and understanding every point and nuance within the author's argument. However, most questions don't require a deep understanding of the passage. And, many parts of the passage never become relevant to the questions. Try pushing yourself through the passage faster on your first reading, accepting the fact that there will be some sections that you do not fully understand. If you know what was discussed, even if you don't really get the author's meaning, you can always find it again if you need it.

b) If your reading speed is very slow and you have problems with reading comprehension, one technique to try is to read just the first and last sentence of each paragraph the first time through the passage. You may also want to try this approach if you commonly get bogged down in the passage text, losing too much time and/or comprehension.

CAUTION: This generally only works well on easier passages. This is also quite risky, as there may well be important information in the middle of the paragraph (and neither the first nor the last sentence of the paragraph is guaranteed to be a topic sentence). However, some people find that it gets them through the passage fast enough (with at least a basic comprehension of the Bottom Line and understanding of the location of different parts of the author's argument) that they can spend their time more productively on the questions. They may also get to more questions this way, and their overall percentage correct increases. This is definitely a strategy that you want to test on a wide range of passages and on multiple practice tests before you settle on it, but for a few people, it does pay off. Make sure that you evaluate your accuracy, not just the number of questions you are able to attempt. If you come out behind score-wise and in terms of overall percentage correct (taking guessing into account), this is not the strategy for you.

2) **Separate Claims From Evidence**
One way to push the pace is to vary your reading speed, paying attention to the major claims (often the main point of the paragraph or chunk) and skimming through (that is, reading faster, not word for word) the evidence supporting those claims. Look for topic sentences (if they exist) to help you make these decisions. Use "MAPS" (see Chapter 3) to help out as well. If you see data, studies, examples, descriptions, explanations, anecdotes, etc., they are highly likely to be evidence in support of a larger claim. As long as you know where they are and what they are supporting, the details are of little importance the first time through the passage.

7.5

For example, here is a sample paragraph (with highlighting).

> "Sedentarization is also having a perverse effect on the roles and
> position of women. For example, in their traditional nomadic
> state, with men away on caravans or other business, the domestic
> domain, including the tending of goat herds, education of
> children, etc., was the preserve of women. The transition from
> tent to village is being associated with a marked diminution of
> the domestic responsibilities and authority of women."

The first sentence of the paragraph sets out the main claim being made by the author. The rest of the paragraph supports that claim. If you understand that the paragraph is about the negative effects of sedentarization on women, you don't really need the rest of the details unless they appear in the questions.

3) **Write Less**

You should be writing down the main point of each paragraph (or chunk) and the Bottom Line of the passage on your noteboard for the first several weeks of your preparation. You are training yourself to read differently, and writing it all down at that stage is crucial. However, once defining those aspects of the passage comes more easily to you, and you are more and more accurate in your understanding, you can cut down the amount that you are writing to a couple of words per paragraph and for the Bottom Line. You may even find that it becomes a tool you can use on the harder passages or more confusing paragraphs only, while the rest of the time you do it as a mental step (while still highlighting within the text). This can be especially useful if you find that you usually have a good understanding of the chunks and how they relate to each other (i.e., the logical structure of the passage), but you struggle and get bogged down when putting it into your own words.

This is one area in which there is significant variation between students. Some people who consistently get high scores are writing brief notes for every paragraph and passage because it contributes both to their speed and to their accuracy, while others in the same scoring range use writing more selectively. Find what level of writing works best for you.

4) **Visualize**

a) Visualizing as you read engages a different part of your brain. When you hit an important part of the passage (especially when you go back to the passage as you answer the questions) and it isn't really making sense, create a visual image in your head. Imagine people waving signs and blocking the streets while the city stagnates around them, or elitist historians thumbing their noses at the common people, or humanists admiring Greek statues while turning a group of robed scholars away from a church, or an adult artist frowning in concentration as she paints while a carefree child spontaneously creates artwork next to her. By the way, the difficulty in visualizing an abstract argument, compared to a concrete and descriptive one, is one thing that tends to make abstract passages Laters or Killers.

b) Another way of using visualization is to create a picture in your mind of the structure of the passage. When you hit a pivotal word, imagine a detour sign. At a continuation, think of a bridge. When the author expresses an opinion, picture a smiley or frowny face. Of course, these are all things that you should also be highlighting. You may even choose to write down some quick symbols on your noteboard, such as a "+" or "–" for positive and negative tone, or a Δ (delta) for a significant shift or change. One reason students often find it harder to process a passage on the computer screen than on paper is that it is easier to have a visual map of a whole page than of a scrolled passage. If you put some effort into creating visual map markers as you read, it takes little time and can really pay off when you use them to efficiently find information in the passage as you answer the questions.

5) **To Preview or Not to Preview**

Previewing the Questions is one way of moving faster through the passage; knowing the question topics ahead of time helps you to prioritize. However, if you are spending an appropriate amount of time previewing (20–30 seconds) and still not retaining enough information to make it useful, there are a few things you can try.

a) First, make sure you are focusing on and highlighting the lead words that indicate passage content, not the question type (question types, while crucial to define as you are answering the questions, are irrelevant at this stage). Picture the lead words as little bursts of information. Focus on each burst as a distinct chunk, rather than skimming through every word of the question with equal attention. Engage your visual memory and your pattern recognition skills. You don't need to fully understand the words at this stage; you just need to fix them in your memory so that you can recognize them in the passage. And, if the question is long and complicated, or if it looks like a New Information question (which usually start with the words "Suppose" or "If"), skip over it during the preview.

b) Second, if you still can't retain the information, try jotting down a word or two for each content-containing question on your noteboard. While this will take a bit of time, if you are getting bogged down in the passage, or if you are spending an inordinate amount of time hunting for information as you work the questions, it can pay off in the long run.

c) Third, if no matter what you do, you can't make the preview work for you, then don't do it. That is, if you have practiced it for at least a month, and used it on at least three practice tests and at least 25 practice passages, and it is still not paying off, then those 20-30 seconds are better spent on answering the questions.

C. Attacking the Questions

1) **Simplify**

Even difficult questions can be amazingly straightforward when you look at them with clear eyes and a calm brain. If you are struggling with a question, stop and remind yourself that you may be overcomplicating it. Imagine a triangle connecting the question stem, the relevant part of the passage, and the correct answer. When you are stuck, ask yourself: "What was the question asking, what did the author say about it, and what answer is most closely connected to both of those things?" Staying with the geometrical theme, also ask yourself if you have left the world of the "MCAT CARS box." Are you bringing in outside knowledge? Are you speculating about what the author might think, rather than basing your answer on what the author explicitly said? Are you debating an imperfect answer, rather than asking, "Is it the least wrong of the four?" Sometimes when you just relax, use your brain, and relocate yourself within the passage and the question task, things look a lot clearer.

2) **Use Aggressive POE**

If you are going back to the passage multiple times to prove the right answer right, or cycling through the choices multiple times, remember that eliminating the other three choices is a perfectly legitimate way to get the right answer. Use the Bottom Line, tone, the main point of the relevant chunk or chunks, the strength of the language in the passage and in the answer choices, and when possible your own answer (based on the passage) to weed out what you can. If you are left with one choice still standing, a choice you can't find anything wrong with, pick it and move on, even if you aren't thrilled with it.

3) **Triage**

Some questions are not worth saving. Unless your reasonable goal is to get a perfect score, you are going to miss some questions. It can be useful to think of this as a strategy, not a failure. That is, your strategy is to allow yourself to miss some questions in order to maximize your score, rather than to try to get every single question right. If you are the kind of person who can't move on until you are 100% sure you have a question right, push yourself to take your best shot and move on (once you have been through the appropriate procedure). If you have carefully reread the question, compared the remaining choices, gone back to the passage again, looked for Attractors, and you are still stuck between two choices, pick one and move on. Even if three more minutes on that one question would produce a correct answer, it isn't worth sacrificing the two or three other questions you could have answered correctly in those three minutes.

4) **Cherry Pick**

Cherry picking is a somewhat extreme form of triage. Generally, you want to work through every question attached to a passage. Otherwise, you are wasting some of your investment of time in reading and working the passage. However, if you ALWAYS (or almost always) get the hardest question on a passage wrong no matter what you do, then take an educated guess on that question once you recognize it. If you ALWAYS (or almost always) get a particular type of Reasoning or Application question, or the longest questions, wrong, then try guessing on that type when you find it. Compare your performance on several tests, some doing eight passages working all of the questions, and others doing nine passages using cherry picking, and follow the strategy that has the best outcome.

5) **Tone Questions**

If you tend to get Tone/Attitude questions wrong, or if you miss other question types because you missed or mistook the tone of the passage, this often goes back to how you are working the passage, and to whether or not you are looking for and highlighting tone indicators as you read. However, this can also be due to how you are doing POE on questions where tone is particularly relevant. Make sure to identify the "attitude words" in each choice. For example, imagine that you have four answer choices that begin as follows:

A) To defend...
B) To recommend...
C) To show...
D) To contradict...

Make sure that you are focusing particular attention on those tone words. While you should always read all four choices carefully and fully, if you are stuck on the question and you know that the passage was entirely neutral, choice C is your best shot.

Use Exercise 1 in Section 8.2 the next chapter to work on your Attitude skills.

6) **Order the Questions Within a Passage**
If you are always doing every question in order, regardless of question difficulty, consider taking a consistent "two-pass" approach within the set of questions for a passage. As described in the Ranking and Ordering section, first preview the questions for a passage from first to last. Then, while on the last question, work the passage. Next, work backwards through the set for that passage, skipping over the harder questions and completing the easier ones. Finally, click forward through the set, completing the harder questions (and making sure that you are not leaving any blank).

D. Dealing With (or Not Dealing With) Killer Passages

Identify a set of difficult passages from your practice materials. Do at least five of them giving yourself five minutes per passage, and at least five other passages at ten minutes per passage. Compare the results.

1) If you do about the same with five or ten minutes, and your accuracy is low (that is, if you miss a majority of the questions), and if you are completing nine passages during a test without approaching your target score, that is a clear sign that you should slow down to seven and a half or eight passages. That is, your payoff on that last hard passage is very low, and you would be better off spending much or all of that time on improving your accuracy on the other passages.

2) If you do about the same on both sets and your accuracy is high (you miss on average one or zero questions per passage) and you are normally completing eight or fewer passages in a test, these are signs that you may well be able to speed up without losing accuracy.

3) If you do significantly better on a Killer passage when you have ten minutes as opposed to five minutes (getting all or almost all of the questions right in ten minutes) and you have a high level of accuracy overall, you may well want to try Cherry Picking or aggressive triage in order to get to all nine passages.

4) If you do better on hard passages when you spend five minutes than when you spend ten minutes, and you are doing eight or fewer passages, that is a very clear sign that you should try speeding up. You may well be overthinking the passages and the questions, especially the more difficult ones, and the faster pace may be forcing you to simplify and stick to the information in front of you.

Chapter 7 Summary

· Manage your 90 minutes well by maintaining a steady pace throughout the entire section. Take your time to get most of the easier questions right. Don't spend too much time on difficult passages; use POE and your knowledge of Attractors to help you through.

· Evaluate your own performance so that you can refine your pacing strategy appropriately.

· If you have an awkward amount of time left over after completing a passage (e.g., 5 minutes), shift your strategy to make sure that you can get to at least one or two easier questions on another passage. Make sure that you select random guesses for any questions that you don't have time to complete.

CHAPTER 7 PRACTICE PASSAGES

Individual Passage Drills

Complete the two passages back-to-back, timed, giving yourself a total of 22 minutes.

Once you have completed the passages and checked your answers, fill out the Individual Passage Logs. Focus in particular on the following:

1) Evaluating your pacing. Were you going too fast or too slow?
2) Identifying types of mistakes that you have also made in the past and strategizing on how to avoid making those same mistakes in the future.

CHAPTER 7 PRACTICE PASSAGE 1

No empirical studies show what proportion of the United States population would have to participate in disruptive and violent demonstrations to seriously threaten the political system. Surely the level of anti-regime violence of recent years has not been sufficient to undermine the viability of the American system. Although the actual participants in peaceful demonstrations or violent protests are far fewer in number than the individuals who approve of these activities, most Americans do not approve of either peaceful or violent protests. In both 1968 and 1972, less than one in five Americans approved of peaceful demonstrations and less than one in ten approved of violent, disruptive protests. Although the level of support for these activities did not increase between 1968 and 1972, the level of opposition declined. Increasing numbers of people seem to be willing to tolerate demonstrations and protests under some circumstances.

If the present relationships persist into the future, increasingly greater tolerance but not necessarily more widespread participation can be anticipated. Among college graduates under age thirty, more than 50 percent approve of peaceful demonstrations, and only 10 percent disapprove. These relationships suggest that as education levels increase, approval of demonstrations will increase. These attitudes suggest a growing unwillingness to be repressive against political interests expressed through peaceful demonstrations, perhaps because the claims of participants are granted some legitimacy.

In these terms, there is some uneasiness about the public support for American democracy—and perhaps for any democratic regime. It is possible to view the United States as a democratic system that has survived without a strong democratic political culture because governmental policies have gained a continual, widespread acceptance. If that satisfaction erodes, however, as it has begun to do, the public has no deep commitment to democratic values and processes that will inhibit support of anti-democratic leaders or disruptive activities.

It is argued that in the absence of insistence on particular values and procedures, democratic regimes will fail. Clearly, a mass public demanding democratic values and procedures is stronger support for a democratic system than a mass public merely willing to tolerate a democratic regime. This does not mean, however, that the stronger form of support is necessary for a democratic system, although superficially it appears desirable. Quite possibly, strong support is nearly impossible to attain, and weaker support is adequate, given other conditions.

In our view, the analysis of support for democratic regimes has been misguided by an emphasis on factors contributing to the establishment of democracy, not its maintenance. Stronger public support probably is required for the successful launching of a democracy than it is for maintaining an already established democracy. Possibly, preserving a regime simply requires that no substantial proportion of the society be actively hostile to the regime and engage in disruptive activities. In other words, absence of disruptive acts, not the presence of supportive attitudes, is crucial.

On the other hand, the positive support by leaders for a political system is essential to its existence. If some leaders are willing to oppose the system, it is crucial that there be no substantial number of followers to which the leaders can appeal. The followers' attitudes, as opposed to their willingness to act themselves, may provide a base of support for antisystem behavior by leaders. In this sense unanimous public support for democratic principles would be a more firm basis for a democratic system. The increasing levels of dissatisfaction, accompanied by a lack of strong commitment to democratic values in the American public, appear to create some potential for public support of undemocratic leaders. In this light, the public's loyalty to political parties and commitment to traditional processes that inhibit aspiring undemocratic leaders become all the more important.

Material used in this particular passage has been adapted from the following source:

W.H. Flanigan and N.H. Zingale, *Political Behavior of the American Electorate.* ©1979 by Allyn Bacon.

1. Elsewhere, the authors describe factors that led to the founding of American democracy. If their account is consistent with the information in the passage, such a discussion would most likely include which of the following?

A) Heroic descriptions of violent uprisings against the British such as the Boston Tea Party
B) Anecdotes concerning George Washington's idealistic motivations
C) Data suggesting vigorous support for democracy was widespread in America at the time
D) A suggestion that more peaceful forms of protest would have given way to a more effective democracy

2. Which of the following, if true, would most strengthen the authors' assertion that public support for peaceful protest is likely to increase over time?

A) A hunger strike by a charismatic dissident leader gains some public support
B) Clashes between protestors and police lead to increased participation in violent protests
C) Five years prior to the survey of college graduates cited by the author, 70 percent of college graduates were shown to approve of nonviolent demonstrations
D) Increased government funding will allow colleges to admit larger classes in the future

3. The authors suggest all of the following are generally necessary for a democracy to thrive EXCEPT:

A) public distaste for violent antigovernment activity.
B) leaders committed to the pursuit of democratic ideals.
C) an electorate that insists upon democratic values in government.
D) an insufficient dissident population to support an undemocratic leader.

4. The primary purpose of the passage is to:

A) contrast the relative merits of violent and nonviolent protest.
B) describe conditions in which a government would fail.
C) argue that free speech has deleterious effects.
D) consider factors that determine the stability of a certain type of political system.

5. Suppose a set of American national politicians were to renounce their loyalty to existing political parties and create a new party founded on communist ideals. Given the information in the passage, their success at creating political change would most likely depend on:

A) acceptance of their ideas among a critical mass of the populace.
B) support among more educated Americans.
C) a loyal following willing to actively campaign on their behalf.
D) a clearly delineated party platform.

6. The authors imply that between 1968 and 1972:

A) acceptance of protest increased and opposition to protest did not decline.
B) social unrest led to greater acceptance of protest as a necessary part of political life.
C) Americans' objection to certain types of protest decreased.
D) there was no change in Americans' attitudes toward protest.

7. The American populace is portrayed as generally:

A) distrustful of government and prone to take political action against its violations of democratic ideals.
B) accepting of America's long history of violence and unrest.
C) willing to passively accept a government that meets its basic requirements.
D) patriotic and unwilling to tolerate dissent.

CHAPTER 7 PRACTICE PASSAGE 2

The most famous sentence in Igor Stravinsky's autobiography reads: "Music is by its very nature powerless to express anything at all." When it appeared, this sentence surprised his audience. After all, Stravinsky had composed some of the most expressive music of the twentieth century, from the lyrical *Petrouchka* to the dramatic *Le sacre du printemps* (The Rite of Spring) to the elegiac *Symphony of Psalms*. But ever the polemicist, Stravinsky was in actuality blasting those whom he regarded as his aesthetic opponents, such as the followers of Richard Wagner; such "impurists" were always marshaling music in the service of extramusical ends, from national solidarity to religious freedom. Seeking to repair a perceived imbalance, Stravinsky portrayed the musician as a craftsman whose materials of pitch and rhythm in themselves harbor no more expression than the carpenter's beams or the jeweler's stone.

Stravinsky may have been right that in the absence of an externally imposed "program," music is simply music. He spoke of the "poetics" of music, which in its literal sense refers to the making (*poiesis*) of music. Unintentionally, however, Stravinsky vividly illustrated a different point through his own life: the extent to which the making of music is *not* possible without the externally triggered factor of politics. All creative individuals—and especially all musicians—must deal with a set of associates who not only help the creators realize their vision but also, eventually, with a wider public, determine the fate of the creators' works. Stravinsky's embroilment in personal and professional politics was extreme for an artist of any sort, yet by throwing the political aspects of creation into sharp relief, Stravinsky reveals the extent to which an artist must work with the field that regulates his chosen domain. Whether they do so well or poorly, eagerly or reluctantly, nearly all creative individuals must devote significant energies to the management of their careers.

Stravinsky's early training came in the form of an apprenticeship with Nikolay Rimsky-Korsakov, the dean of Russian composers. Rimsky-Korsakov guided Stravinsky in orchestration, teaching him how to compose for each instrument; they would each orchestrate the same passages and then compare their versions. Stravinsky was an apt pupil, whose rapid advances pleased his mentor; and, perhaps for the first time in his life, Stravinsky found himself in a milieu that fully engaged him.

A dramatic turning point in Stravinsky's career occurred shortly after his mentor's death when Stravinsky was approached by Serge Diaghilev to compose a nocturne for his theatrical project, *The Firebird*. Suddenly, instead of working alone, Stravinsky had almost daily intercourse with the ensemble—a new and heady experience for someone who had craved the companionship of individuals with whom he felt comfortable. Stravinsky turned out to be a willing pupil, one who learned quickly and reacted vividly to everything. He was sufficiently flexible, curious, and versatile to be able to work with the set designers, dancers, choreographers, and even those responsible for the business end of the enterprise. From Diaghilev young Igor learned two equally crucial lessons for ensemble work: how to meet a deadline and how to compromise on, or mediate amongst, deeply held but differing artistic visions. Yet, he may have learned Diaghilev's lessons too well. As Stravinsky gained in knowledge and confidence, he found himself engaged in strenuous disputes about characterization, choreography, and instrumentation.

The most notable creators almost always are perfectionists who have worked out every detail of their conception painstakingly and are unwilling to make further changes unless they can be convinced that such alterations are justified. Few intrepid creators are likely to cede any rights to others; and even if they are consciously tempted to do so, their unconscious sense of fidelity to an original conceptualization may prevent them from following through. Stravinsky was no exception in this, and his goals were well-defined and impassioned. Suppressing whatever revolutionary impulses may have existed in his own person and animated his earlier music, ignoring the rich emotional associations of his early masterpieces, Stravinsky stressed the importance of conventions and traditions, and the utility of self-imposed constraints. He loathed disorder, randomness, arbitrariness, the Circean lure of chaos. Music was akin to mathematical thinking and relationships, and one could discern powerful, inexorable laws at work. In the paradox-packed closing lines of *The Poetics of Music*, Stravinsky declared: "My freedom will be so much greater and more meaningful, the more narrowly I limit my field of action and the more I surround myself with obstacles. Whatever diminishes constraints, diminishes strength. The more constraints one imposes, the more one frees one's self of the chains that shackle the spirit."

Material used in this particular passage has been adapted from the following source:

H. Gardner, *Creating Minds: An Anatomy of Creativity Seen Through the Lives of Freud, Einstein, Picasso, Stravinsky, Eliot, Graham, and Gandhi.* © 1993 by Basic Books.

1. Which of Stravinsky's learning experiences or observations is most *inconsistent* with the author's statement in the last paragraph that "the most notable creators are almost always perfectionists"?

A) Orchestration techniques learned while working with Rimsky-Korsakov
B) Lessons learned from Diaghilev and involvement in the ensemble
C) The need to engage in protracted political battles
D) The observation that "the more constraints one imposes, the more one frees one's self of the chains that shackle the spirit"

2. The word "political" is used in paragraph 2 in order to refer to:

A) collaboration and artifice.
B) greed and expediency.
C) interpersonal relations.
D) cleverness and guile.

3. We can reasonably infer that the perceived imbalance that Stravinsky was seeking to repair was one of:

A) an over-dependence on inspiration rather than craftsmanship in making music.
B) some composers' tendency to inject extraneous elements into their music.
C) too great an involvement in the political side of theatrical staging and production.
D) an over-emphasis on choreography as compared to instrumentation in theatrical productions.

4. The author's discussion of Stravinsky's actions and statements suggests that which two aspects of Stravinsky's character or career may have been at odds with each other?

A) His desire to create music and his involvement with choreography and set design
B) The artistic independence expressed in *The Poetics of Music* and his dependence on others in managing his career
C) His desire to create and his inability to escape interpersonal politics
D) His desire for a strict approach to making music and his willingness to work in a highly collaborative setting

5. In the author's view, Stravinsky's collaboration with others in musical composition and theater can best be summarized as:

A) productive yet contentious.
B) accepted with reluctance.
C) onerous and ultimately destructive.
D) fruitful and harmonious.

6. According to the passage, Stravinsky believed which of the following to be a condition necessary for creativity in music?

A) A willingness to collaborate and compromise
B) Situations of total freedom
C) Openness to new and revolutionary ideas
D) Limitations to lend it structure

7. A study shows that painters who hire agents and business managers early in their careers tend to be more prolific. What effect would this information have on the author's argument regarding an artist's involvement in his own career?

A) It would be contrary to the author's claim that artists need to manage their own careers.
B) It would be relevant to evaluating the notion that the essence of Stravinsky's artistic vision was shaped by collaboration.
C) It would support the author's implication that artistic fields of endeavor are also businesses.
D) It would justify Stravinsky's engagement in strenuous disputes regarding theatrical elements.

SOLUTIONS TO CHAPTER 7 PRACTICE PASSAGE 1

1. **C** This is a New Information question.
   A: No. Nowhere do the authors suggest the conditions for starting a democracy require violence. Nor does the authors' tone suggest violence is "heroic."
   B: No. First, although the authors discuss in paragraph 6 the importance of leaders being committed to a democratic system for the existence or maintenance of democracy, this is not described as "idealism," and the motivation of those leaders is not the issue but rather their behavior. Second, this idea is not explicitly tied to the requirements for *founding* a democracy. Third, this choice, in its reference to George Washington, relies on too much outside knowledge for its relevance to the information in the question stem.
   C: Yes. In paragraph 5, the authors say, "Stronger public support probably is required for the successful launching of a democracy than it is for maintaining an already established democracy."
   D: No. The authors do not equate peaceful protest with a stronger democracy.

2. **D** This is a Strengthen question.
   A: No. An isolated incident such as this one is not enough evidence to suggest a trend will continue. Also notice the mild wording; the fact that it gained "some public support" is not enough to "most strengthen" the authors' claim.
   B: No. There is no connection made by the authors between some level (we don't know if it's a significant level) of increased participation in violent protest and increased support for peaceful protest.
   C: No. Because it suggests the number of educated people who support peaceful protest is in some level of *decline*, this answer choice would weaken the argument. Note that even if you were thinking that "more than 50 percent" could be 70 percent, this answer still gives no evidence of an increase over time, or of a likely increase in the future.
   D: Yes. The authors explain in paragraph 2 that "as education levels increase, approval of demonstrations will increase," but do not explicitly support the premise that education levels will increase. If colleges were to accept more applicants, it is fair to assume education levels would increase, thus strengthening the premise.

3. **C** This is an Inference/EXCEPT question.
   A: No. One part of the main idea of the passage is that widespread acceptance of disruptive antigovernment activity can threaten democracy (see paragraph 5). Since the question stem asks you to find an answer choice that is not a requirement for democracy, this cannot be the answer.
   B: No. See paragraph 6: "the positive support by leaders for a political system is essential to its existence."
   C: Yes. Paragraphs 4 and 5 explain that the population does not need to actively campaign for democratic ideals for democracy to work. In fact, such strong support for democratic values may be "impossible" (paragraph 4). At the end of paragraph 5, the author states that "absence of disruptive acts, not the presence of supportive attitudes, is crucial." Although paragraph 6 suggests public support for democracy is necessary when antigovernment leaders come to prominence, this is a specific situation, as opposed to the "general" view that the question stem asks for. Because this idea is not supported by the passage, it is the *correct* answer to this "EXCEPT" question.
   D: No. See paragraph 6: "If some leaders are willing to oppose the system, it is crucial that there be no substantial number of followers to which the leaders can appeal."

4. **D** This is a Main Idea/Primary Purpose question.

    A: No. The authors make no such evaluation of different forms of protest. Be sure not to be overly influenced by paragraph 1 of the passage when determining the authors' primary purpose.

    B: No. This answer uses language that is too extreme; the authors do not go so far as to assure us democracy will fail under certain circumstances.

    C: No. This answer choice is too broad. The correct answer must focus on the key issues of the passage: protest, public support, and the stability of democracies. Furthermore, this answer is too negative. While the passage does suggest that free speech is related to peaceful protest (paragraph 2), the authors don't go so far as to suggest that it has harmful effects.

    D: **Yes. Although it uses vague language to do so, this answer does address the main focus of the passage. The factors that would influence stability of a democratic political system (a "certain type of political system"), according to the passage, would be the level and type of support and/or dissent.**

5. **A** This is a New Information question.

    A: **Yes. Paragraph 6 states, "If some leaders are willing to oppose the system, it is crucial that there be no substantial number of followers to which the leaders can appeal. The followers' attitudes, as opposed to their willingness to act themselves, may provide a base of support for antisystem behavior by leaders."**

    B: No. It would be too large of an inference to take the authors' claim that educated Americans are more likely to be tolerant of protest (paragraph 2) to mean their support would be the key to such an insurgent political group's success.

    C: No. The correct answer must be supported by the passage text, rather than by common sense or real world experience. The passage says in paragraph 6 that "it is crucial that there be no substantial number of followers to which the leaders can appeal" and that the "followers' attitudes, as opposed to their willingness to act themselves, may provide a base of support for antisystem behavior by leaders." While you might think that campaigning by a loyal following would help create widespread public support for the dissidents, there is no evidence for this in the passage. Compare this answer to choice A, which does have direct support in the passage text.

    D: No. The passage gives no evidence, in paragraph 6 or elsewhere, that having a clear party platform would influence the public one way or the other.

6. **C** This is an Inference question.

    A: No. This is a reversal of the information in paragraph 1. Acceptance or support of protest stayed the same, while opposition to protest declined.

    B: No. Although this may be historically accurate, the answer must be supported by the text of the passage. There is no suggestion in the passage that social unrest lead to this kind of change in attitude.

    C: **Yes. In paragraph 1, the authors state: "Although the level of support for these activities did not increase between 1968 and 1972, the level of opposition declined."**

    D: No. Paragraph 1 clearly states there was such a change; opposition to protest declined.

7. **C** This is an Inference question.
A: No. Paragraph 1 establishes that "most Americans do not approve of either peaceful or violent protests."
B: No. The passage does not address America's history of violence or public attitudes towards it.
C: Yes. In paragraph 1, Americans are portrayed as quietly accepting the status quo. Most oppose antigovernment protest and the majority of those who tolerate dissent don't participate. Also, in paragraph 3, the authors describe the American populace as merely "satisfied": "It is possible to view the United States as a democratic system that has survived without a strong democratic political culture because governmental policies have gained a continual, widespread acceptance."
D: No. The passage does not describe Americans as patriotic. Furthermore, the authors state in paragraph 1 that "Increasing numbers of people seem to be willing to tolerate demonstrations and protests under some circumstances." Even if this is still a minority of the population, it would be too extreme to describe Americans as a whole as "unwilling to tolerate dissent."

SOLUTIONS TO CHAPTER 7 PRACTICE PASSAGE 2

1. **B** This is an Inference question.
Note: The author makes this statement in the context of discussing Stravinsky's faithfulness to his own artistic vision. The passage states that perfectionists "have worked out every detail of their conception painstakingly and are [often] unwilling to make further changes" or "cede any rights to others," and that "Stravinsky was no exception in this."
A: No. This choice may be tempting, but we have no basis for supposing compromise or acceptance of "imperfection" was required, as we're only told that they composed separately for later comparison.
B: Yes. It was from Diaghilev that Stravinsky is said to have learned "to compromise on, or mediate amongst, deeply held but differing artistic visions" (paragraph 4). The quote cited in the question stem, in the context of paragraph 5, relates to an unwillingness to "cede any rights to others" or to diverge from the artist's own "original conceptualization."
C: No. Paragraph 2 indicates that Stravinsky had to engage in political battles in order to "realize [his] vision" and to manage his career. However, there is no indication that these battles involved compromising or going against his perfectionism about the work itself.
D: No. This answer is consistent with the statement in the question stem. This observation appears in paragraph 5, in the context of the author's description of Stravinsky's dedication to realizing his own goals.

2. **C** This is an Inference question.
A: No. While "collaboration" fits, "artifice," or falsehood, does not. Be careful not to import your own associations with politics into the passage.
B: No. While "expediency" is not clearly wrong, there is no suggestion of greed. The fact that political battles were necessary in the management of an artist's career doesn't by itself show that the artists are greedy or money-hungry.
C: Yes. Paragraph 2 says, in the context of discussing the necessary role of politics, that artists "must deal with a set of associates who...help the creators realize their vision."
D: No. While "cleverness" is not clearly wrong, there is no suggestion of "guile" or deception.

3. **B**   This is an Inference question.

A: No. There is no suggestion in paragraph 1, or elsewhere in the passage, that Stravinsky discounted the importance of inspiration ("expression" is not equated with "inspiration"), or that he believed that he himself or other composers displayed insufficient craftsmanship.

B: Yes. This choice is supported by information in the lines above the reference to the "imbalance" in paragraph 1, in which the author refers to Stravinsky's intention of "blasting...his aesthetic opponents" whose goals were extra-musical, attempting to further such things as national solidarity or religious freedom.

C: No. The author does not suggest that Stravinsky tried to reduce his, or others', involvement in the political aspects specifically of presenting music or theater to an audience. Stravinsky's complaint was about injecting non-musical aspects into the music itself.

D: No. While paragraph 4 mentions Stravinsky's involvement in disputes about choreography and instrumentation, it doesn't suggest that he believed choreography had been given too much importance.

4. **D**   This is an Inference question.

A: No. Paragraph 4 suggests that his desire to create and present music and his interest in choreography and set design went hand-in-hand.

B: No. While paragraph 2 does suggest that all artists are dependent on others in realizing their vision and managing their career, this doesn't necessarily apply to artistic independence involved in making or creating the music itself.

C: No. Paragraph 2 suggests that Stravinsky believed that interpersonal politics were necessary to some aspects of the process of creation (such as career management), rather than an impediment to it.

D: Yes. Stravinsky expresses a strong attachment to making music in particular ways, untainted by extramusical intentions, and it's hinted in paragraph 5 that he would be unlikely to change his compositions. However, the discussion in paragraph 4 indicates that Stravinsky had learned to compromise artistically and to be open to differing artistic visions.

5. **A**   This is an Inference question.

A: Yes. This choice is supported by paragraph 4, where the author describes how Stravinsky benefited from the new experience of collaboration, and yet found himself "engaged in strenuous disputes."

B: No. "Reluctance" contradicts paragraph 4, which suggests that Stravinsky eagerly took on this new opportunity to collaborate, and "destructive" is too extreme to be supported by the author's mention of "strenuous disputes."

C: No. "Onerous" is unsupported; we have no evidence that Stravinsky found these disputes to be burdensome. Furthermore, "ultimately destructive" is too extreme.

D: No. This choice is half-right/half-wrong. "Fruitful" or productive is supported, but the process was not always "harmonious," as indicated in the matter of "strenuous disputes" mentioned in paragraph 4.

6. **D**   This is a Retrieval question.

A: No. This choice reflects some points made by the author in paragraphs 2 and 4, but we don't know that Stravinsky shared in this belief. The author states in paragraph 2 that Stravinsky's experience "reveals the extent to which an artist must work with the field that regulates his chosen domain," but not that Stravinsky himself expressed this idea. Note that in paragraph 2, the author states that Stravinsky's life "unintentionally" illustrates the importance of collaboration.

B: No. This choice contradicts Stravinsky's statements in paragraph 5, where he talks about the importance of constraints and obstacles.

C: No. The passage states that he eventually believed in "suppressing whatever revolutionary impulses may have existed in his own person" (paragraph 5).

D: Yes. This is explained in Stravinsky's quote in paragraph 5.

7.   **C**   This is a New Information question.

A: No. This choice may be tempting, but it takes words out of context from the passage. The author indicates in paragraph 2 that the artist must manage his or her career, but also suggests that this usually requires interaction with, and help from, other people.

B: No. This choice may also be somewhat tempting, but the study would be relevant to evaluating collaboration in the business of the artist's career, including presentation of artistic work to the public, rather than in the essence or fundamental character of the artistic vision itself.

C: Yes. The author's argument in paragraph 2 is that an artist needs to be involved with the business of his or her own career, whether personally or through agents, so a study that indicates that a business manager increases artistic productivity would support the author's argument.

D: No. A study about the effects of business management would not be directly relevant to issues of theatrical production.

Individual Passage Log

Passage # _____   **Time spent on both passages** _____

Q#	Q type	Attractors	What did you do wrong?

Revised Strategy _____

Passage # _____

Q#	Q type	Attractors	What did you do wrong?

Revised Strategy _____

Chapter 8
Refining Your Skills

GOALS

1) To continue the self-evaluation process
2) To further refine your skills
3) To prepare mentally for test day

8.1 CONTINUING THE SELF-EVALUATION PROCESS

At this point in your preparation, you have acquired a variety of tools with which to attack the passages and the CARS section as a whole. Over the remaining time leading up to MCAT day, take the opportunity to further refine those skills, taking your own individual strengths and weaknesses into account. If you don't have a clear list of those strengths and weaknesses (and if you have not been consistently filling out the Individual Passage Logs and Test Assessment Logs), *now* is the time to generate it.

It is still not too late to recognize and correct some of the persistent mistakes you may be making. There is no point in doing passage after passage if you spend little or no time evaluating your performance on those passages. You should spend at least as much time evaluating your performance as you do on doing the passage itself. If not, each passage you do reinforces rather than corrects bad habits and blind spots you may still have.

Consider some of the following things:

- Are you still trying to finish (or almost finish) the entire section and yet are missing a large number of the questions you complete? If so, think about how much time you're spending getting questions wrong. Instead, try two test sections guessing on at least one additional passage, giving yourself more time to carefully consider the questions. See how slowing down affects your overall percentage of correct answers.
- Are you defining the Main Point of each paragraph and articulating the Bottom Line of the passage before addressing the questions? This is one of your most powerful tools. Use it!
- Are you consistently going back to the passage and answering the questions in your own words before evaluating the answer choices?
- Are you actively using POE? Are you approaching the answers skeptically, looking out for traps?

8.2 REFINING YOUR SKILLS

Below are a series of exercises, focusing on the passage, the questions, and the answer choices. They will help you continue to improve your performance in each of those areas, especially on the harder passages.

EXERCISE 1: IDENTIFYING THE AUTHOR'S TONE

Below are four short passages. Read and highlight each as you would work a real MCAT CARS passage, paying close attention to tracking the author's attitude. After working each passage, answer the question or questions regarding the author's tone or attitude. Once you have completed all four, read through the explanations that follow.

1. Formalism, an approach to literary criticism, arose in the early twentieth century. The basic tenet of formalist criticism is that meaning arises from the text itself, and that the intentions of the author are essentially irrelevant. Thus, according to formalism, the appropriate approach to understanding a text relies on close reading of the structure of the work on all levels from sentence structure and grammar to the construction of the work as a whole. Formalism views a text as existing independent from the author; thus, not only the author's intent but also the cultural context within which the work was created (and possible cultural influences on the author) can be largely ignored. The only historical context that may legitimately be seen as potentially relevant is that of previous literary forms to which the given text may be seen as related. In reaction to the strict limits of formalism an alternative approach, reader-response theory, arose in the 1970s. Reader-response theory broadened the possibilities of gaining meaning from a text by examining the various ways in which different readers may interpret a given work. Reader-response theory overcame the limitations inherent in formalism by including within its purview a variety of factors that may in fact provide important insights into the meaning of a work of art. Formalists ineffectually attempted to defend the assumptions at the core of their own school of thought by claiming that while different readers may arrive at different interpretations, those interpretations are irrelevant to gaining a true understanding of the meaning of the text itself, and therefore that reader-response theory belongs in the realm of psychology, not literary criticism.

Question: What is the author's attitude toward formalism? _____

_____

2. Many people see the Denishawn dance company as the founder of modern dance in America. The Denishawn School of Dancing and Related Arts, founded in 1915, based its technique on classical ballet, but included as well influences from other cultures, in particular, India, Spain, Cambodia, and the Middle East. Ruth St. Denis and Ted Shawn, the founders of the company, also incorporated free movement into their teaching and performance; this represented a significant break from classical ballet performance and pedagogy. However others, while recognizing the ground-breaking nature of Denishawn's work, claim that one of Denishawn's students, Martha Graham, is more legitimately seen as the true founder of American modern dance. They claim that she, unlike Denishawn, truly broke with classical ballet by creating an entirely new set of movements that replaced, rather than modified, the traditional choreographical elements on which classical ballet is based.

Question: What is the author's attitude toward who deserves to be called the founder of modern dance?

_____

_____

3. Ethical practice must be fundamentally based on, and judged by, universal duties that apply in all situations. Regardless of the consequences, an action is ethical only if it conforms to these absolute duties. Consider a hypothetical case: you are the driver of a trolley car. As you are driving the car down a hill, the brakes fail and the car cannot be stopped. Ahead, standing on the track, is a group of people who will be hit and killed if you do nothing. However, you can divert the car onto a different track; standing on this track is a single person who will be killed if she is hit by the trolley. There are no other options: you must either do nothing and several people will die, or take action and a single person will be killed. One form of ethical thought, deontological ethics, holds that you have an absolute obligation to take no actions that would result in harming another human being. Therefore, you should do nothing, as taking action would result in the death of a person as a direct result of that action. Another form of ethics, utilitarianism, holds that the ethical decision is the one that results in the least amount of harm. By this way of thought, you should divert the car onto the other track, even though you will be deciding to take an action that directly results in the death of a person, as this action would save the lives of more people.

Question: Based on the passage, what would the author say the driver of the trolley should do? _____

_____

4. The role and power of the president within a political system has been analyzed in various ways. One view, propagated in particular by the political scientist James Barber, focuses on the personality of the president. Barber created a four-part typology of presidential personalities: active-positive, passive-positive, active-negative, and passive-negative. According to Barber, the biography of a president, including his or her childhood, plays a crucial role in determining presidential personality, and any analysis of the nature of a presidency (and of the office itself) must include a consideration of early influences, including family and upbringing. However, in recent decades, Barber's useful analysis has been unfairly discounted in academic fields, and Neustadt's theory based on "the power to persuade" has taken hold. Neustadt provides additional insight by arguing that the power of a president arises in part from his or her domestic and international reputation. Those who take an overly rigid interpretation of Neustadt's argument ignore the influence of formative experiences, and look only at a president's achievements and failures while in office when analyzing the nature of the office of the president as well as the efficacy of individual holders of the office.

Question: What is the author's opinion regarding Barber? _____

_____

Question: What is the author's opinion regarding Neustadt? _____

_____

Explanations for Exercise 1: Identifying the Author's Tone

1) **What is the author's attitude toward formalism?**

Negative

The author states that reader-response theory "broadened the possibilities of gaining meaning from a text" and "overcame the limitations inherent in formalism." The author also states that formalists "ineffectually" attempted to defend their assumptions.

2) **What is the author's attitude toward who deserves to be called the founder of modern dance?**

Neutral

The author discusses the debate without taking sides. Note that while the author does state Denishawn's work "represented a significant break from classical ballet performance and pedagogy," the passage does not indicate that this qualifies Denishawn as the true founder of modern dance. Nor does the author suggest that retaining aspects of classical ballet disqualifies Denishawn as the founder of modern dance, or that creating "entirely new set of movements that replaced, rather than modified, the traditional choreographical elements on which classical ballet is based" (as Graham did) is a necessary condition for being considered as such.

3) **Based on the passage, what would the author say the driver of the trolley should do?**

Stay on the track, rather than diverting in order to save more lives.

The author states at the beginning of the passage that "Ethical practice must be fundamentally based on, and judged by, universal duties that apply in all situations. Regardless of the consequences, an action is ethical only if it conforms to these absolute duties." This put the author in the deontological camp as it is described in the passage, which would hold that taking action to divert the trolley onto the other track, even if this would result in fewer deaths, would be unethical. Be careful not to use your own opinion when analyzing a passage. Even if you think that the ethical standard should be based on weighing the consequences against each other, this is not the author's opinion.

4) **What is the author's opinion regarding Barber?**

Positive

The author states that Barber's analysis is "useful" and that it has been "unfairly discounted."

What is the author's opinion regarding Neustadt?

Positive

Note that the author criticizes those that take an "overly rigid interpretation" of Neustadt's argument, not Neustadt himself. The passage states that "Neustadt provides additional insight" to Barber's analysis. Overall, the author indicates that both Barber and Neustadt have made valid contributions (and does not suggest that they are mutually exclusive, even though others might believe this to be the case).

EXERCISE 2: PARAPHRASING THE PASSAGE

Often, the more difficult passages are characterized by complex, abstract wording. To make your way through these passages with a reasonable level of comprehension (that is, enough to articulate the main point of each chunk and of the passage as a whole), you need to put the author's convoluted, obscure wording into your own clear language.

Read each of the paragraphs below, and write down the main point in the space provided. If you have difficulty with a section of a paragraph (or a paragraph as a whole), don't just go back to the beginning and read it again "harder." Often after multiple readings, a paragraph makes less, not more sense. Instead, pay attention to the structure of the sentence or paragraph. Find an "anchor," or one piece that you understand, and use it to make sense of the rest. Break the reading down into pieces, and the whole will begin to make a lot more sense.

Note: Some of these paragraphs represent the difficulty level of language found in Killer passages. Don't panic, and don't give up; just keep your focus and do the best you can. Practicing on the hardest examples will contribute to your performance on any level of passage. These are not meant to be different paragraphs from the same passage, so don't worry about finding a relationship between them. Explanations follow the exercise.

Paragraph 1

Modern medicine has fixed its own date of birth as being in the last years of the eighteenth century. Reflecting on its situation, it identifies the origin of its positivity with a return—over and above all theory—to the modest but effecting level of the perceived. In fact, this supposed empiricism is not based on a rediscovery of the absolute values of the visible, nor on the predetermined rejection of systems and all their chimeras, but on a reorganization of the manifest and secret space that opened up when a millennial gaze passed over men's sufferings. Nonetheless, the rejuvenation of medical perception, the way colors and things came to life under the illuminating gaze of the first clinicians is no mere myth. At the beginning of the nineteenth century, doctors described what for centuries had remained below the threshold of the visible and the expressible, but this did not mean that, after overindulging in speculation, they had begun to perceive once again, or that they listened to reason rather than to imagination; it meant that the relation between the visible and the invisible—which is necessary to all concrete knowledge—changed its structure, revealing through gaze and language what had previously been below and beyond their domain. A new alliance was forged between words and things, enabling one *to see* and *to say*.

Note: This is a good example of how a passage about a familiar topic (medicine) may in fact be extremely difficult. When taken as a whole, it is almost impossible to understand. Therefore, take it piece by piece. Find a sentence, or a part of a sentence, that you do understand, and use it to make some sense of the parts around it. Don't get stuck on unfamiliar vocabulary. Do you really need to know what a "chimera" or "millennial gaze" is to get the gist of the paragraph? Do, however, pay attention to the series of contrasts provided (indicated by pivotal words and phrases) to get a sense of what the author is describing.

Main Point: _____

_____

Paragraph 2

We have so far discussed the "absent person" in ads. But since this person is always signified by objects (and above all, the product) in the ad, interchangeable with them in that they represent his absence with their presence, it follows that the other side of the exchange, the product, may likewise be absent from the ad, and signified by the people in it. There is a series of lager ads on TV where the lager itself is never there. In one of these ads, two workers in a factory pick up two empty glasses from the conveyer belt and start drinking "lager" from them.… In another ad the two men come into a pub which turns out not to have this particular brand of lager when they order it. So they take two empty mugs and again "drink" the invisible lager. Although the product is actually absent in these cases, it is sufficiently signified in the ad—by the two men—by their attitude towards it, by their taste, and so on. There is also a definite place for it to fill: the surrounding presence of the mugs makes the actual presence of the lager redundant. Thus with absence in an ad, the thing meant to fill the gap is always defined, not by a simple replacement but by what is contingent: it is what surrounds the gap that determines its shape.

Note: Notice how this paragraph is organized. This structure—a claim followed by one or more examples, and then a further conclusion—is a very common one, and you can use it to help you puzzle through difficult sections of a passage. If you have difficulty with the claims, work backwards from the examples. If you have trouble understanding the examples, start with the claim.

Main Point: _____

_____

Paragraph 3

At a certain point in their historical lives, social classes become detached from their traditional parties. In other words, the traditional parties in that particular organizational form, with the particular men who constitute, represent, and lead them, are no longer recognized by their class (or fraction of a class) as its expression. When such crises occur, the immediate situation becomes delicate and dangerous, because the field is open for violent solutions, for the activities of unknown forces, represented by charismatic "men of destiny."

Note: It is always more difficult to wrap your brain around the abstract than the concrete. If the author doesn't give a specific example or illustration, imagine one of your own to help solidify your understanding of the text.

Main Point: _____

_____

Paragraph 4

As a label, "cyberpunk" is perfection. It suggests the apotheosis of postmodernism. On one hand, pure negation: of manner, history, philosophy, politics, body, will affect, anything mediated by cultural memory; on the other, pure attitude: all is power, and "subculture," and the grace of Hip negotiating the splatter of consciousness as it slams against the hard-tech future, the techno-future of artificial impermanence, where all that was once nature is simulated and elaborated by technical means, a future world-construct that is as remote from the "lessons of history" as the present mix-up is from the pitiful science fiction fantasies of the past that had tried to imagine us. The oxymoronic conceit in "cyberpunk" is so slick and global it fuses high and low, the complex and the simple, the governor and the savage, the techno-sublime and rock and roll slime.

Note: Even sentences that seem like just a cascade of words do have a structure. Try breaking up the long sentences in this paragraph into shorter, more manageable ones before trying to synthesize them into the main idea of the passage.

Main Point: _____

_____

Paragraph 5

But physiologists have also begun to see chaos as health. It has long been understood that nonlinearity in feedback processes serves to regulate and control. Simply put, a linear process, given a slight nudge, tends to remain slightly off track. A nonlinear process, given the same nudge, tends to return to its starting point.

Note: Phrases like *simply put, in other words,* or *that is to say* should be music to your ears. These phrases indicate that the author is going to say it again, in different words, in case it wasn't clear the first time. Make sure you notice and take advantage of these "second chances."

Main Point: _____

_____

Paragraph 6

Western academic philosophy may have a hard time agreeing on its own definition, but any definition must be responsible to certain facts about the application of the concept. In the Euro-American tradition nothing can count as philosophy, for example, if it does not discuss problems that have a family resemblance to those problems that have centrally concerned those we call "philosophers." And nothing that does address itself to such problems but does so in a way that bears no family resemblance to traditional philosophical methods ought to count either. And the Wittgensteinian notion of family resemblance, here, is especially appropriate because a tradition, like a family, is something that changes from one generation to the next. Just as there may be no way of seeing me as especially like my remote ancestors, even though there are substantial similarities between the members of succeeding generations, so we are likely to be able to see the continuities between Plato and Frege only if we trace steps in between.

Note: Another important tool at your disposal is the analogy. Where is an analogy used in this paragraph and what is its relationship to the author's main point?

Main Point: _____

_____

Paragraph 7

This is not to disparage the efforts of the experimenters. They are important as catalysts. For the writer is not alone is his or her endeavor, but is, rather, participating in a collaborative enterprise. The Kriges would not impress us so if it were not for the cooperation of the publishing house (which lends the nobility of its name and ensures that the cloth covers of the book are expensively textured and soberly colored), the librarian (who places the book in the anthropology shelves rather than on those reserved for science fiction) and the teacher (who secures it a place on the anthropology-class reading list). Above all, the Kriges rely on readers' skills in filling out and making sense of scientific discourse, a peculiar one in which data are presumed autonomous, interpretations are either confirmed or disconfirmed by facts that are independently specified, and the discovery of orderliness and the production of definitive accounts are normal and expected.

Note: What is it about this author's writing style that can make this paragraph difficult to read quickly? How might you deal with this "listing" tendency? How could you actually use it to your advantage?

Main Point: _____

_____

Paragraph 8

The aestheticians of painting, especially the modern ones, are the great advocates of "significant form," the movement of the line, the relations of color and tone. Of these critics, the most consistent, the clearest (and the most widely accepted), that I know is the late Mr. Bernhard Berenson. Over sixty years ago in his studies of the Italian Renaissance painters he expounded his aesthetics with refreshing clarity. The merely accurate representations of an object, the blind imitation of nature, was not art, not even if that object was what would commonly be agreed upon as beautiful, for example, a beautiful woman. There was another category of painter superior to the first. Such a one would not actually reproduce the object as it was. Being a man of visions and imagination, the object would stimulate in his impulses, thoughts, memories visually creative. These he would fuse into a whole and the result would be not so much the object as the totality of the visual image which the object had invoked in a superior mind. That too, Mr. Berenson excluded from the category of true art (and was by no means isolated in doing so): mere reproductions of objects, whether actually in existence or the product of the sublimest imaginations, was "literature" or "illustration." What then was the truly artistic? The truly artistic was a quality that existed in its own right, irrespective of the object represented.

8.2

Note: What is the importance of the sentence, "That too, Mr. Berenson excluded from the category of true art"? Were you a bit surprised, given what had come before? What role does this statement play in defining the author's main point?

Main Point: _____

_____

Explanations for Exercise 2: Paraphrasing the Passage

Notes: Many of these Main Points are wordier than yours may be (and should be). Remember that you are the only one who needs to understand your own annotation, and therefore complete sentences are unnecessary. You might have written down just a few words to represent these main points.

Paragraph 1

Main Point: Modern medicine developed at the end of the eighteenth century, with the merging of the visible and the invisible in physicians' understanding.

Paragraph 2

Main Point: Advertising sometimes uses the strategy of showing the environment in which a product exists, but not the product itself.

Paragraph 3

Main Point: When the representational party of a social class no longer accurately reflects the perceived reality of that class, violent or drastic actions may be taken.

Paragraph 4

Main Point: The word "cyberpunk" encapsulates all of the contradictory elements present in a postmodern world.

Paragraph 5

Main Point: A nonlinear feedback process can be at least as effective as a linear process, because it has the ability to self-correct.

Paragraph 6

Main Point: Western academic philosophy must trace the steps between generations of philosophical thought in order to accurately include the relevant subject matter.

Paragraph 7

Main Point: The full publication process of this textbook is defined by collaboration.

Paragraph 8

Main Point: Aestheticians of painting (such as Bernhard Berenson) do not judge a painting's beauty on the accuracy of its reproduction of reality, but on a higher level of artistry and creativity.

EXERCISE 3: PARAPHRASING THE QUESTIONS

One common characteristic of hard passages is complexly worded and structured questions. As we discussed in Chapter 4, if you don't understand the question itself, you are likely to spend a lot of time on it, only to arrive at an incorrect answer at the end. For each of the questions below, identify the question category (Specific, General, Reasoning, or Application), question type (e.g., Inference, Strengthen, Evaluate, etc.) and then translate the question into your own words, defining what this question is requiring you to do. Explanations follow the exercise.

1. The information in the passage suggests that the author would be most likely to agree with which of the following statements concerning the use of HDRs as an alternative energy in the event of a failure of other, more traditional recovery systems?

Question category: _____

_____

Question type: _____

_____

Translation: _____

_____

2. The reference to labor negotiation as an example of third party intervention is meant to illustrate which of the following theories in the context of the author's discussion of triadic and quadratic models?

Question category: _____

_____

Question type: _____

_____

Translation: _____

_____

3. The author's claim that the behavior of certain unusual stars has helped "account for previously unexplained phenomena" (paragraph 4) would be most justified by an astronomer's ability to measure the luminosity and pulsation of which of the following types of stars?

Question category: _____

_____

Question type: _____

_____

Translation: _____

_____

4. According to the passage, the author considers each of the following good advice to an owner who has arranged for fast-track construction of a building on his land EXCEPT:

Question category: _____

_____

Question type: _____

_____

Translation: _____

_____

5. The author suggests that the most valid criticism of the enactment of laws governing large corporations that encourage aspiration that has been raised by the advocates of non-regulation is which of the following?

Question category: _____

_____

Question type: _____

_____

Translation: _____

_____

6. It has been argued that when "nation" and "state" are not viewed as unrelated concepts, methodology takes a back seat to political concerns in nonacademic arenas. This claim would be LEAST inconsistent with the author's argument that:

Question category: _____

_____

Question type: _____

_____

Translation: _____

_____

7. Suppose that a veterinarian specializing in the care of large animals were to experience "differential empathy," as that term is used in the passage. This would be most similar to a lawyer who professed that:

Question category: _____

_____

Question type: _____

_____

Translation: _____

_____

8. In addressing the issue of land reform, Stunwitznow predicted that the unearned benefits accrued to landowners from prior, unregulated transactions would not, in a purely laissez-faire system, be taxed at a higher rate than earned benefits from that same classification or type of transaction given a similar absence of pre-existing regulatory jurisdiction or activity. This prediction would most undermine the author's expectation that:

Question category: _____

_____

Question type: _____

_____

Translation: _____

_____

Explanations for Exercise 3: Paraphrasing the Questions

1. Question Category: Specific
   Question Type: Inference
   Translation: What does the author think about the use of HDR as an alternative energy when traditional recovery systems fail?

2. Question Category: Reasoning
   Question Type: Structure
   Translation: Why does the author use the example of labor negotiation in the discussion of triadic and quadratic models?

3. Question Category: Application
   Question Type: Strengthen
   Translation: The luminosity and pulsation of which type of star would best prove the author's argument regarding the behavior of certain unusual stars?

4. Question Category: Specific
   Question Type: Retrieval EXCEPT
   Translation: What WOULDN'T the author recommend to the owner of land where building is being fast-tracked?

5. Question Category: Specific
   Question Type: Inference
   Translation: What is the most valid criticism raised by the advocates of non-regulation regarding these corporations?

6. Question Category: Application
   Question Type: Weaken EXCEPT (which is not exactly the same as Strengthen)
   Translation: When "nation" and "state" are viewed as related concepts, political concerns take precedence over methodology outside of academia—what part of the author's argument is this most consistent with?

7. Question Category: Application
   Question Type: New Information/Analogy
   Translation: How would "differential empathy" apply to a lawyer (like it does to a large-animal vet)?

8. Question Category: Application
   Question Type: New Information/Weaken
   Translation: Stunwitznow's prediction that the taxation of unearned benefits would be the same as that of earned benefits would undermine what expectation held by the author?

8.2

EXERCISE 4: PROCESS OF ELIMINATION

Choose a passage from your practice materials. You can use the Individual Passage Drills at the end of the last few chapters in this book or other printed passages. Put a sheet of paper over the passage, so that only the questions and answer choices are visible. Read each question carefully. Based on your knowledge of question types and common Attractors, eliminate the most suspicious choices and choose what you believe to be the most likely credited response.

For example, consider the following question:

1. The primary purpose of the passage is to:

A) urge consumers to demand quicker development of HDR resources for the production of energy.

B) denounce the federal government for its resistance to necessary changes in its long term energy policy.

C) compare and contrast the energy policies of developed and less-developed nations.

D) discuss the advantages and disadvantages of HDRs as an alternative energy source.

MCAT passage authors rarely call on the reader to take action, nor do they commonly denounce or severely criticize anybody. Thus choices A and B are likely to be inconsistent with the author's attitude and purpose. Choice C is more neutral in tone, but is it really possible to undertake such a wide-ranging study in the course of a few paragraphs? This choice is probably too broad. Choice D is more narrow than choice C, but not too narrow to describe a discussion carried out over 60–70 lines. It is also middle-of-the road in tone, as are most MCAT passages. Thus choice D is the most likely choice. (It is, in fact, the credited response.)

Of course you should never answer the questions without reading the passage on the test! However, after completing this exercise for several passages, you'll be surprised how often you do arrive at the credited response. You'll also increase your sensitivity to, and awareness of, the kinds of suspicious wording that often shows up in Attractors.

EXERCISE 5: WRITING YOUR OWN QUESTIONS

Take a passage from your practice materials. Put a piece of paper or a series of Post-It® Notes over the questions and the answer choices, so that only the passage itself is visible. Read the passage, mapping and annotating as usual. Based on what you see in the passage (for example, comparisons and contrasts, use of examples or lists, unexpected changes in direction, the author's tone or attitude, etc.), predict what questions would likely appear attached to this passage, and what kind of trap answers they will employ.

Now, write your own questions and answer choices, based on those predictions. At this point, feel free to go back to the passage and read it more carefully than you normally would the first time through. Imagine that you are an MCAT writer, trying to confuse the test-taker with complex questions or trick the test-taker into choosing Attractor answer choices. Try to write at least one question from each of the most common question types (Retrieval, Inference, Structure, Strengthen, Weaken, New Information, Main Point/Primary Purpose), but come up with as many, from any category of question, as you can. Now lift up the paper or the Post-It® Notes and work through the questions they give you. How accurately did you predict the questions? Did predicting the questions and trap answer choices help you more effectively answer their questions?

A variation on this exercise is to keep the existing questions but write your own sets of answer choices.

If you are studying with other people, exchange questions on the same passage with each other. Use your knowledge of Attractors to write questions that are defensible but difficult. See how often you fall for each other's Attractors.

You will find that by doing this exercise, you deepen your understanding of how this test is written, and that you are more able to predict and eliminate tricky wrong answers.

EXERCISE 6: QUESTION-TYPE-SPECIFIC PASSAGES

In Chapter 4, you completed a set of passages that included only particular question types. Here is another set of question-type-specific passages. As you attack each passage, keep your focus on employing the strategy appropriate for each particular category and type of question. As you review any questions that you missed, look in particular for mistakes caused by not fully understanding the question task and/or failing to employ the appropriate question strategy.

8.2

PASSAGE I: SPECIFIC—RETRIEVAL AND INFERENCE QUESTIONS

It is good anthropology to think of ballet as a form of ethnic dance. Currently, that idea is unacceptable to most Western dance scholars. This lack of agreement shows clearly that something is amiss in the communication of ideas between the scholars of dance and those of anthropology. The faults and errors of anthropologists in their approach to dance are many, but they are largely due to their hesitation to deal with something which seems esoteric and out of their field of competence. By ethnic dance, anthropologists mean to convey the idea that all forms of dance reflect the cultural traditions within which they developed. Dancers and dance scholars use this term, and the related terms *ethnologic*, *primitive*, and *folk dance*, differently and, in fact, in a way which reveals their limited knowledge of non-Western dance forms.

Despite all anthropological evidence to the contrary, however, [most] Western dance scholars set themselves up as authorities on the characteristics of non-Western (that is, non Euro-American) dance. For example, Terry describes the functions of "primitive" dance, and uses Native Americans as his model. While he writes sympathetically about Native Americans, his paternalistic feelings on the one hand, and his sense of ethnocentricity on the other, prompt him to set aside any thought that people with whom he identifies could share contemporarily those same dance characteristics, because he states "the white man's dance heritage, except for the most ancient of days, was wholly different."

Another significant obstacle to the identification of Western dancers with non-Western dance forms is the double myth that the dance grew out of some spontaneous mob action and that once formed, became frozen. Apparently it satisfies our own ethnocentric needs to believe in the uniqueness of our dance forms, and it is much more convenient to believe that so-called "primitive" dances, like Topsy, just "growed," and that "ethnological" dances are part of an unchanging tradition.

Let it be noted, once and for all, that within the various "ethnologic" dance worlds there are also patrons, dancing masters, choreographers, and performers with names woven into a very real historical fabric. The bias which those dancers have toward their own dance and artists is just as strong as ours. The difference is that they usually don't pretend to be scholars of other dance forms, nor even very much interested in them.

I have made listings of the themes and other characteristics of ballet and ballet performances, and these lists show over and over again just how "ethnic" ballet is. Consider, for example, how Western is the tradition of the proscenium stage, the usual three part performance which lasts for about two hours, our use of curtain calls and applause, and our usage of French terminology. Think how our worldview is revealed in the oft recurring themes of unrequited love, sorcery, self-sacrifice through long-suffering, mistaken identity, and misunderstandings which have tragic consequences.

Our aesthetic values are shown in the long line of lifted, extended bodies, in the total revealing of legs, of small heads and tiny feet for women, in slender bodies for both sexes, and in the coveted airy quality which is best shown in the lifts and carryings of the female. To us this is tremendously pleasing aesthetically, but there are societies whose members would be shocked at the public display of the male touching the female's thighs! So distinctive is the "look" of ballet, that it is probably safe to say that ballet dances graphically rendered by silhouettes would never be mistaken for anything else. An interesting proof of this is the ballet *Koshare* which was based on a Hopi Indian story. In silhouettes of even still photos, the dance looked like ballet and not like a Hopi dance.

The question is not whether ballet reflects its own heritage. The question is why we seem to need to believe that ballet has somehow become acultural. Why are we afraid to call it an ethnic form?

Material used in this particular passage has been adapted from the following source:

J. Kealiinohomoku, "An Anthropologist Looks at Ballet as a Form of Ethnic Dance." © 1970, *Impulse* 20: 24–33.

1. According to the passage, which of the following are aspects of the "ethnic" nature of ballet?

    I.   Common motifs that reflect the perspective of Western tradition
    II. Dance growing out of spontaneous group action
    III. The use of a specific language

A) III only
B) I and II only
C) I and III only
D) I, II, and III

2. Which of the following is implied by the author of the passage?

A) Good anthropology generally regards ethnic dance as a form of ballet.
B) Western dance academics are at odds with anthropologists' perceptions of dance.
C) Western dance scholars are not interested in non-Western dance forms.
D) Some indigenous peoples, such as Native Americans, are considered to be "Western" by dance scholars.

3. The author would most likely disagree with Terry regarding whether or not:

A) dance forms, to some extent, reflect cultural values.
B) ballet has features in common with non-Western dance forms.
C) anthropology is a valuable tool in the analysis of culture.
D) the ballet *Koshare* was based on a Hopi story.

4. Each of the following is stated to be found to be aesthetically pleasing in female ballet performers in the Western tradition EXCEPT:

A) a diminutive head.
B) the lifted body.
C) feet curled in at the toe.
D) the extension of the body.

5. The author implies which of the following to be true of the aesthetic aspects of ethnic dance?

A) They are influenced by certain cultural norms and values of the society in which the dance arose.
B) They reflect universal themes of human experience.
C) They portray the ideals that are most important to the culture in which they were generated.
D) Western and non-Western or "ethnic" dance aesthetics are inconsistent with each other, as evidenced by the failure of *Koshare* to accurately represent Hopi dance.

6. According to the passage, the problem in our understanding of "ethnological" dance forms is that this kind of dance is often incorrectly seen as:

A) shifting and growing through time.
B) deviating from an accepted norm.
C) consisting of a three-part performance.
D) unchanging once established.

7. Based on the passage, which of the following would be LEAST likely categorized as a "folk dance" by dance scholars?

A) The Hopi Powamuya or "bean dance," held in villages every February to prepare for the planting of crops
B) The African American cakewalk, created on Southern plantations before emancipation, perhaps as a way of mocking white slave-owners
C) The Maria Clara dance, done in the Philippines to portray flirtation and courtship
D) The Viennese waltz, which originated in 16th century France and was later imported into the United States, and which was at times seen as immoral because of the closeness of the partners

PASSAGE II: REASONING—STRUCTURE AND EVALUATE QUESTIONS

The notion that memory can be "distorted" assumes that there is a standard by which we can judge or measure what a veridical memory must be. If this is difficult with individual memory, it is even more complex with collective memory, where the past event or experience remembered was truly a different event or experience for its different participants. Moreover, whereas we can accept with little question that biography or the lifetime is the appropriate or "natural" frame for individual memory, there is no such evident frame for cultural memories. Neither national boundaries nor linguistic ones are as self-evidently the right containers for collective memory as the person is for individual memory.

I take the view that, in an important sense, there is no such thing as individual memory, and it is well for me to make this plain at the outset. Memory is social. It is social, first of all, because it is located in institutions rather than in individual human minds in the form of rules, laws, standardized procedures, and records, a whole set of cultural practices through which people recognize a debt to the past (including the notion of "debt" itself) or through which they express moral continuity with the past (tradition, identity, career, curriculum). These cultural forms store and transmit information that individuals make use of without themselves "memorizing" it. The individual's capacity to make use of the past piggybacks on the social and cultural practices of memory. I can move over great distances at a speed of 600 miles per hour without knowing the first thing about what keeps an airplane aloft. I benefit from a cultural storehouse of knowledge, very little of which I am obliged to have in my own head. Cultural memory, available for the use of an individual, is distributed across social institutions and cultural artifacts.

As soon as you recognize how collective memory, and even individual memory, is inextricable from social and historical processes, the notion of "distortion" becomes problematic. As the British historian Peter Burke writes, "Remembering the past and writing about it no longer seem the innocent activities they were once taken to be. Neither memories nor histories seem objective any longer. In both cases, this selection, interpretation and distortion is socially conditioned. It is not the work of individuals alone." Distortion is inevitable. Memory is distortion since memory is invariably and inevitably selective. A way of seeing is a way of not seeing, a way of remembering is a way of forgetting, too. If memory were only a kind of registration, a "true" memory might be possible. But memory is a process of encoding information, storing information, and strategically retrieving information, and there are social, psychological, and historical influences at each point.

Contest, conflict, controversy—these are the hallmark of studies of collective memory, rather than the concept of distortion. Discovering the attitudes and interests of the present becomes of much greater concern than the legitimate claims of the past upon them. Still, a focus on distortion makes sense in studies of collective or cultural memory. Even the most ardently relativist scholars among us shiver with revulsion at certain versions of the past that cry out "distortion." The most famous example is the flourishing fringe group of Holocaust revisionists who deny that there was ever a plan to exterminate the Jews or that such a plan was ever set in place. The question of what content of the past is not or cannot or should not be subject to latter-day reinterpretation haunts the papers at a 1990 conference at U.C.L.A. on "Nazism and the 'Final Solution': Probing the Limits of Representation" (Friedlander, 1992). The fascination with conflicting versions of the past and the excitement over legitimately revisionist interpretations of once settled and consensual accounts come precisely from the fact that even trained historians (or perhaps especially trained historians) retain strong beliefs in a veritable past. If interpretation were free-floating, entirely manipulable to serve present interests, altogether unanchored by a bedrock body of unshakable evidence, controversies over the past would ultimately be uninteresting. But in fact they are interesting. They are compelling. And they are gripping because people trust that a past we can to some extent know and can to some extent come to agreement about really happened.

Material used in this particular passage has been adapted from the following source:

M. Schudson, *"Dynamics in Distortion of Collective Memory,"* in *Memory Distortion: How Minds, Brains, and Societies Reconstruct the Past.* © 1995 by Harvard University Press.

1. The author provides the example of our capacity to fly in an airplane in order to:

A) indicate that some facts are not open to dispute.
B) illustrate the nature of collective memory.
C) provide a case in which individual memory exists independently of social memory.
D) demonstrate how social memory is more complex than individual memory.

2. Which of the following items of information from the passage provides the best support for the author's argument that there is such a thing as a provable historical fact?

A) It is unclear what the "natural" frame for collective memory might be.
B) A fringe group exists of people who deny that the Holocaust occurred.
C) Memory is inherently selective and therefore distorted.
D) We find controversies regarding past events to be fascinating and compelling.

3. Why does the author cite the historian Peter Burke?

A) In order to support the claim that the concept of distortion is less useful than many claim it to be
B) In order to support the contention that there is no such thing as a "true fact"
C) In order to support the claim that memory is not an entirely factual representation of reality
D) In order to support the contention that institutions encapsulate social memories and make them available to individuals

4. How well supported is the author's claim that, in a sense, individual memory is non-existent?

A) Weakly: the claim is contradicted later in the passage by the author's discussion of how individuals use collective memory
B) Weakly: the claim is simply asserted with no evidence or support
C) Strongly: the author explains with the use of an example how individual memory is shaped by social forces and institutions
D) Strongly: the author directly supports the claim through discussion of revisionist views of the Holocaust

5. Which of the following assertions made by the author is LEAST well supported?

A) The appropriate frame for individual memory is biography or lifetime.
B) Memory is inherently selective.
C) It makes sense to study distortion when considering cultural memory.
D) Our capacity to make use of the past relies on social forms of memory.

6. The author states in the last paragraph that "people trust that a past we can to some extent know and to some extent come to an agreement about really happened," while also stating in the second paragraph that "in an important sense, there is no such thing as individual memory." These two claims are:

A) consistent with each other, because they refer to different aspects of memory.
B) consistent with each other, because the claim regarding the possibility of agreeing on the past provides evidence for the claim regarding individual memory.
C) in contradiction, because it is difficult to justify the notion that historical controversies are gripping if individual memory is absent.
D) in contradiction, because the claim regarding the non-existence of individual memory is logically inconsistent with claim that we can come to agreement about historical memory.

8.2

PASSAGE III: APPLICATION—STRENGTHEN AND WEAKEN QUESTIONS

Nobody ever discovered ugliness through photographs. But many, through photographs, have discovered beauty. Except for those situations in which the camera is used to document, or to mark social rites, what moves people to take photographs is finding something beautiful. Nobody exclaims, "Isn't that ugly! I must take a photograph of it." Even if someone did say that, all it would mean is: "I find that ugly thing beautiful."

It is common for those who have glimpsed something beautiful to express regret at not having been able to photograph it. So successful has been the camera's role in beautifying the world that photographs, rather than the world, have become the standard of the beautiful. We learn to see ourselves photographically: to regard oneself as attractive is, precisely, to judge that one would look good in a photograph. Photographs create the beautiful and—over generations of picture-taking—use it up. Certain glories of nature, for example, have been all but abandoned to the indefatigable attentions of amateur camera buffs.

Many people are anxious when they're about to be photographed: not because they fear, as primitives do, being violated but because they fear the camera's disapproval. People want the idealized image: a photograph of themselves looking their best. They feel rebuked when the camera doesn't return an image of themselves as more attractive than they really are. That photographs are often praised for their candor, their honesty, indicates that most photographs, of course, are not candid. A decade after Fox Talbot's negative-positive process had begun replacing the daguerreotype (the first practical photographic process) in the mid-1840s, a German photographer invented the first technique for retouching the negative. The news that the camera could lie made getting photographed much more popular.

The consequences of lying have to be more central for photography than they ever can be for painting, because the flat, usually rectangular images which are photographs make a claim to be true that paintings can never make. A fake painting (one whose attribution is false) falsifies the history of art. A fake photograph (one which has been retouched or tampered with, or whose caption is false) falsifies reality. The history of photography could be recapitulated as the struggle between two different imperatives: beautification, which comes from the fine arts, and truth-telling, which is measured not only by a notion of value-free truth, a legacy of the sciences, but by a moralized ideal of truth-telling, adapted from nineteenth-century literary models and from the (then) new profession of independent journalism....

Freed from the necessity of having to make narrow choices (as painters did) about what images were worth contemplating, because of the rapidity with which cameras recorded anything, photographers made seeing into a new kind of project: as if seeing itself, pursued with sufficient avidity and single-mindedness, could indeed reconcile the claims of truth and the need to find the world beautiful. Once an object of wonder because of its capacity to render reality faithfully as well as despised at first for its base accuracy, the camera has ended by effecting a tremendous promotion of the value of appearances. Instead of just recording reality, photographs have become the norm for the way things appear to us, thereby changing the very idea of reality, and of realism.

The photographer was thought to be an acute but non-interfering observer—a scribe, not a poet. But as people quickly discovered that nobody takes the same picture of the same thing, the supposition that cameras furnish an impersonal, objective image yielded to the fact that photographs are evidence not only of what's there but of what an individual sees, not just a record but an evaluation of the world.

Material used in this particular passage has been adapted from the following source:

S. Sontag, *"The Heroism of Vision," On Photography.* © 1977 by Susan Sontag. Reprinted by permission of Farrar, Straus, and Giroux, LLC, and of The Wylie Agency (UK) Limited.

1. Each of the following would strengthen the author's claim that photography has been successful in beautifying the world EXCEPT:

   A) It is quite common for celebrities to have themselves photographed in new clothes before wearing them to important events to ensure that the clothes will look good for the public.

   B) Bowing to pressure from parents, many high end private schools now allow families to submit their own professionally produced and retouched yearbook photos as an alternative to having a picture taken at school.

   C) A current fad among wealthy home owners is to have a photograph of one's home actually framed on the wall inside the house, making sure that visitors can see the house's features at their best.

   D) Because of the extreme realism and the striking uses of light possible in contemporary photography, more and more art museums are devoting sections of their collections to well-known photographers.

2. Which of the following most strengthens the author's suggestion that beauty can be exhausted through overuse?

A) Although in the 1940s Ansel Adams' photographs of the Grand Canyon and of Yosemite Park captured the imagination of the art world, they now, except for their historical value, seem more appropriate to calendars than to museum walls.

B) The huge number of visitors visiting the Sistine Chapel and taking flash photographs has caused certain portions of the glorious paintings to lose their brilliancy and fade, leading officials increasingly to curb the privileges of tourists to take any pictures at all.

C) Despite the fact that almost everyone has seen multiple photographs of Michelangelo's David, seeing the enormous statue in person still generally provokes a powerful sense of awe and wonder.

D) The average career for top models has become shorter and shorter in duration, so that many models now receive top billing for only a single season before magazines and sponsors begin looking for a newer face.

3. The author's explanation of the anxiety many feel around being photographed would be most undermined by which of the following hypothetical examples?

A) After having his privacy repeatedly violated by the paparazzi, a well-known actor becomes extremely anxious and defensive about divulging details of his personal life, and hires guards to travel with him when he goes out in public.

B) A teenage boy measures his popularity, and in essence his worth as a human being, by how many photographs of him get posted online by his friends and acquaintances.

C) A new application for camera phones that automatically removes facial blemishes has the effect of decreasing the value generally placed on photos, as the application provides clear evidence that the accuracy of a photograph cannot be trusted.

D) Confined to a hospital bed, an elderly woman becomes upset when her visiting grandchildren try to take pictures of her, insisting that she doesn't want to be seen looking sick.

4. Which of the following contrasts, if valid, would most weaken the author's claim that there is a significant difference between painting and photography?

A) Unlike a painting, in which the author may portray the subject with total freedom, a photograph is highly limited by the reality of the subject matter.

B) The speed with which one can take a photograph is so much greater than the speed with which one can paint that, viewed from the perspective of the artist, the two practices have essentially nothing in common.

C) To fake a painting is less morally relevant than to fake a photograph, because a counterfeit painting, although a crime against the artist, does not ultimately undermine our collective trust in the accounts we receive of real-world events.

D) Unlike photography, which seeks to achieve both beauty and truth, the only fundamental goal of painting is to portray beauty.

5. Which of the following hypothetical reviews of a photography exhibition would most contribute to the claim that this exhibition has succeeded in the photographic project described in paragraph 5?

A) It is the shadows, the dark spaces in these images, that truly allow the creative imagination of the observer to bring an individual and higher truth, the essence of art.

B) The particular achievement of these photographs is in allowing the eye truly to enjoy the deception brought about through shifts in perspective and clever illusion.

C) The rhythm visible in this succession of images imparts to the viewer a sense of motion much richer than that possible through mere verbal description.

D) In bringing out the subtle hues of moving water, these photographs train our eyes to see water differently, as more varied and more valued than we previously knew.

6. Which of the following statements, if justified, would most undermine a claim that the typical photographer is more "scribe" than "poet" as those terms are used in the passage?

A) Just as different authors describe the same scene in different ways, so different photographers will take pictures of the same scene from different angles.

B) Individual photographer's particular techniques and choices often function as a kind of signature, making his or her photographs instantly recognizable regardless of the subject of the photograph.

C) Tourists at a famous site will frequently observe one another, as each attempts to choose what to photograph based on what, according to his peers, seems the most important or the most beautiful.

D) It is only the rare artist who brings to the practice of photography the vision and skill necessary to reveal in his photographs any meaningful aesthetic decisions or distinctive qualities.

PASSAGE IV:
APPLICATION—NEW INFORMATION AND ANALOGY QUESTIONS

"One Journalism" defines good journalism as the kind of journalism produced at the top of corporate pyramids—the networks and the major national and regional newspapers. This means that journalists address the particular problems and needs of a community in an artificial journalistic context, created and driven from other places. But people practice democratic government in specific locations, in the municipalities and states where they seek to answer the question, "What shall we do?" through deliberation. That process requires shared information and some common values—above all the value of democratic deliberation is the best way to express and experience public life, and that all citizens have a personal responsibility to take part in that process.

The reflexive, value-neutral techniques of One Journalism do not promote democratic deliberation. Rather, their skewed definitions of sources and issues systematically exclude people from democratic deliberation and generate much irrelevant information that does not advance that essential deliberation. One Journalism determines, for instance, that we define "balance" as "both sides" when in fact most issues have multiple sides. It insures the high value we put on conflict as the ultimate illuminator of political discussion. It makes it inevitable that the world we present one day seems disconnected from the world we present the next day. Meanwhile, the culture of detachment denies any journalistic concern or responsibility for what happens, if anything. When citizens see reflected in newspapers and broadcasts a politics of polar extremes that excludes them, when the machinations of experts and absolutists seem beyond their reach, they withdraw into private concerns. They abandon public life. This is a direct threat to journalism, for if people are not involved in public life, they have no need for journalists.

Journalism's authority—its right to be attended to—is disappearing in a cloud of cynicism and loss of credibility brought on by the routine and detached way we go about business. But public journalism offers a solution to this problem. At its core, public journalism suggests a close examination of the alleged overriding value of detachment and seeks to develop more useful journalistic reflexes. Its objective is to find ways for journalism to serve a purpose beyond—but not in place of—telling the news: the purpose of reinvigorating public life by re-engaging people in it. This requires both a change in the perspective of journalists and a change in what they do. It means learning to report and write about public life beyond traditional politics; to write about political issues in ways that reflect the true array of choices; to report the very important news of civic life—including civic successes—that

now occurs outside our pinched definition of news. This can only be done if journalists think of the people by their efforts not as an audience to be entertained or as spectators at an event, but as citizens capable of action.

This response to the decline in public life and journalism conflicts sharply with One Journalism's guiding axiom of detachment. A key tenet of public journalism is that the "line" of detachment defined by One Journalism is a false construct. Traditional journalists speak of "crossing the line" as if three questionable things were true: that a single line defines all possible points of moral, ethical and professional concerns; that every journalist understands precisely where that line lies; and that anything on one side of the line is "good journalism" and everything on the other side is something else.

Think of the line not as a boundary, but as a continuum that runs between two points. One point defines total detachment or non-involvement in what we cover. The other defines total involvement. Journalists exploring public journalism accept the construct of a continuum and seek to operate somewhere beyond total involvement. Precisely where their activity falls is determined by their consciences, their judgment and the needs of their communities. Public journalism is the antithesis of One Journalism.

Public journalism is openly based on broad values as: This should be a better place to live, and people should determine what that means by taking responsibility for what goes on around them. Public life, according to the values of public journalism, requires shared information and shared deliberation; people participate in answering democracy's fundamental question of "What shall we do?" Public journalism opens the possibility that journalists can serve their communities in truly useful ways that go beyond telling the news. It also offers us a chance to regain our lost credibility.

Material used in this particular passage has been adapted from the following source:
D. Merritt, *"Public Journalism—Defining a Democratic Art," Media Studies Journal: Media and Democracy.* ©1995.

1. Suppose that a political analyst wrote the following: "Framing political issues as a conflict between mutually exclusive extremes is the most useful narrative device for engaging the interest of the citizenry in public policy." What would most likely be the passage author's reaction to such a statement?

A) Opposition, because the author believes that a focus on conflict dissuades people from taking an interest in politics
B) Opposition, because the author believes that a focus on conflict undermines the value-neutral stance necessary for good journalism
C) Support, because the author believes that a healthy discussion regarding different policy options is necessary for true democratic deliberation to occur
D) Support, because the author believes that the survival of journalism requires re-engaging the public by presenting the news in an entertaining fashion

2. Suppose that several national surveys showed that the proliferation of different points of view on political issues offered by the spread of blogs and other forms of social media confuses and discourages the public by making politics seem overly complicated. Which of the following claims made in the passage would be most undermined by this information?

A) "One Journalism" defines a balanced story as one that presents two different sides of the issue.
B) Democratic deliberation requires shared information and shared values.
C) The reinvigoration of public life requires that citizens be presented with a true array of options rather than with a dichotomous choice.
D) A culture of journalistic detachment denies that news reporters bear any responsibility for events.

3. Research has shown that under repressive political regimes in which the public has little role in policymaking, people tend to disregard journalistic reports, assuming that news reporters will only present events from a single officially sanctioned point of view. This favors the author's thesis in the passage by suggesting that:

A) the "culture of detachment" fostered by One Journalism discourages engagement in public life.
B) lack of widespread engagement in public life endangers the vitality and relevance of journalism.
C) reporting on positive political outcomes is one way of reengaging people in public life.
D) "good reporting" is defined in part by the motives of the journalist and the relevance of the information to the needs of the community.

4. Which of the following pairs would be most analogous, respectively, to the role of citizens in One Journalism on one hand, and in public journalism on the other?

A) People attending a movie vs. people attending a play
B) People doing their own research into investment opportunities vs. people unquestioningly taking the advice of a financial advisor
C) People investing their own money vs. people investing other people's money
D) People viewing works hanging in a museum vs. audience members going on stage and playing roles within a performance art event

5. Which of the following would be LEAST logically similar to the author's discussion of the correct way to distinguish good from bad journalism?

A) Judging the culpability of a criminal defendant through taking into account her motives, whether or not her actions were reasonable in the situation, and the amount of harm her actions caused to others
B) Judging the artistic merit of a poem by defining whether or not it conforms to clearly defined compositional rules
C) Judging the policies carried out by a mayor by considering the intended and actual effects of the policy on the city
D) Judging the moral character of a historical figure by taking into account the reasonableness of his or her actions within the cultural context in which he or she lived as well as the personal motivations behind his or her actions

6. Which of the following hypothetical examples most closely illustrates the perspective embodied and encouraged by public journalism, as it is described in the passage?

A) A documentary examining the traditional values of detachment and neutrality in the news, detailing how local news stations are trying to change this traditional approach to reporting
B) A magazine article about small town life, written by a national news reporter in New York City
C) An expose on the subversive involvement of corporations in democratic political systems
D) A local newspaper article about a successful community service initiative that cleaned up a polluted town lake

SOLUTIONS TO PASSAGE I: SPECIFIC— RETRIEVAL AND INFERENCE QUESTIONS

1. **C**   This is a Retrieval/Roman Numeral question.

   I. **True. Different characteristics of ballet and evidence that ballet is ethnic are discussed in the fifth and sixth paragraphs and different examples are provided. The author mentions "oft recurring themes" such as one-sided love, suffering, and tragedy as examples of things that reveal the Western worldview.**

   II. False. Start with this numeral, as it appears in exactly two answer choices. The idea of dance growing out of spontaneous group action is discussed in the fourth paragraph in the context of myths regarding so-called "primitive" dance, not as part of the discussion of ethnic characteristics of ballet. Hence, it does not answer the question. Strike through this numeral and eliminate any answers that contain it: choices B and D.

   III. **True. The usage of French terminology is specifically referenced as a tradition found in Western ballet (paragraph 5).**

2. **B**   This is an Inference question.

   A: No. This answer is a reversal of passage information and takes the words out of their original context. The passage says that "good anthropology...[thinks] of ballet as a form of ethnic dance" (paragraph 1), meaning that ballet is a specific type of ethnic dance. This does not allow the reverse to be inferred: we don't know that ethnic dance is a specific form of ballet. For Inference questions, be careful to not just match up words from the passage, but instead to look at the meaning as well.

   B: **Yes. The first paragraph references the view anthropology has of ballet as dance, and that dance scholars in the West view this as "unacceptable." In addition, the passage states that there is a "lack of agreement" that shows "something is amiss" between these two groups.**

   C: No. The author indicates that Western dance scholars ARE interested in non-Western dance forms. For example, the author states at the beginning of paragraph 2 that "Western dance scholars set themselves up as authorities on the characteristics of non-Western dance." The problem, according to the passage, is that they misunderstand and misrepresent non-Western dance.

   D: No. The author indicates the opposite to be true. The passage suggests in paragraph 2 that the dance scholar Terry sees Native Americans as performing "non-Western dance."

3. **B**   This is an Inference question.

   A: No. The author of the passage would agree with this statement (paragraph 6) and there is no evidence that Terry would disagree. Terry may or may not belief that ballet reflects any cultural values, but he may agree that some "ethnic" dances do. Therefore, we do not have enough evidence that they would disagree on this point.

   B: **Yes. According to the author, Terry views things from an ethnocentric perspective and "set[s] aside any thought that people with whom he identifies could share contemporarily those same dance characteristics" (paragraph 2). Later, in the third paragraph, the author mentions "double myth[s]" that prevent Western dancers being associated with non-Western dance forms. This suggests that the author believes it possible that ethnic dances (which the author believes includes ballet) can have things in common with other dances including non-Western dances, whereas Terry views Western and non-Western dances as completely different.**

C: No. Although Terry sets himself up as an expert on non-Western dance in opposition to anthropological evidence on the topic, this does not mean that Terry would think that anthropology has no value in studying different cultures.

D: No. The author states that the *Koshare* was indeed based on a Hopi narrative in the second-last paragraph. However, there is no indication in the passage that Terry might disagree with this specific fact.

4. **C** This is a Retrieval/EXCEPT question.

A: No. The sixth paragraph discusses the aesthetically pleasing aspects of the ballet. Small heads are mentioned as an example.

B: No. The author twice explicitly references the lifted body in the sixth paragraph as something pleasing.

C: **Yes. Though feet are mentioned as aesthetically pleasing, it's only in reference to their size ("tiny feet for women"), not the shape of the foot. If anything, the passage suggests the elongated form is more pleasing, not a form that curls inward.**

D: No. The author refers to the long line of the extended body in the sixth paragraph.

5. **A** This is an Inference question.

A: **Yes. The author argues for example that the "lifts and carryings of the female" to us are aesthetically pleasing, but that there are societies whose members would be shocked at the public display of the male touching the female's thighs" (paragraph 6). This indicates that the values of a society can affect what is considered aesthetically pleasing in that society.**

B: No. The author suggests the opposite, that at least some dances reflect the values of particular societies, not values shared by all peoples. For example, ballet, rather than being "acultural" (paragraph 7), reflects the values of "our" society but not all others. The author writes: "Our aesthetic values are shown in the long line of lifted, extended bodies, in the total revealing of legs, of small heads and tiny feet for women, in slender bodies for both sexes, and in the coveted airy quality which is best shown in the lifts and carryings of the female. To us this is tremendously pleasing aesthetically, but there are societies whose members would be shocked at the public display of the male touching the female's thighs" (paragraph 6).

C: No. This choice is too extreme. While the author would say that dance does reflect certain cultural values, the passage does not go so far as to indicate those values are the *most important* values in that culture.

D: No. While the author might say that some Western and some non-Western societies have different values and different "ethnic" dances, the author does not suggest that they are always mutually exclusive. The point made in the discussion of *Koshare* is not that Hopi society was incapable of expressing itself through ballet, but rather that *Koshare* as presented was aesthetically "Western" rather than incorporating true Hopi dance forms.

6. **D**   This is a Retrieval question.

    A: No. The author indicates the opposite to be true; that is, this is a correct view, not a misconception (paragraphs 3 and 4).

    B: No. This is out of scope. The passage does not provide any discussion of moving away from an accepted norm. Deviation would also suggest change, which is the opposite of what the author describes as the myth of ethnological dance.

    C: No. Three parts of a dance are referenced in the sixth paragraph, where the author discusses common Western dance traditions, but not the incorrect assumptions related to ethnological dance.

    D: Yes. In the fourth paragraph, the author discusses the double myth that pertains to so-called primitive dance and ethnological dance. The author says this myth is that "once formed, [it] became frozen" and that ethnological dances are "part of an unchanging tradition." It's implied that this is incorrect, since it's referred to as a myth that we tell ourselves to fulfill our ethnocentric view of how unique the dance is.

7. **D**   This is an Inference question.

    Note: In paragraph 1 the author indicates that dance scholars use the terms "ethnic," "ethnologic," "primitive," and "folk dance" more or less interchangeably. In paragraph 2 the author indicates that "non-Western" is equivalent to "non Euro-American" dance. In that same paragraph, the author also indicates that Terry (presented by the author as representative of the views of dance scholars) draws a clear line between "ethnic" and "white-man's" dance. Therefore, the right answer will be the form of dance that as described in the answer choice is least "ethnic" (as that term is used by dance scholars like Terry) and the most "Euro-American."

    A: No. Although a Hopi dance, the *Koshare*, inspired a ballet, the answer choice describes this dance as performed by the Hopi themselves. Therefore, a dance scholar WOULD consider this to be a folk dance.

    B: No. There is no European aspect or influence described here. Also, the dance scholar Terry distinguishes between the dance heritage of the "white man" and that of ethnic dances. Therefore, a dance scholar likely WOULD call this a folk dance.

    C: No. There is nothing "Euro-American" about the Maria Clara, as described in the answer choice. Therefore, a dance scholar likely WOULD call this a folk dance.

    D: Yes. This dance as described had a European origin and was then brought to the United States. That is, it is a "Euro-American" dance form. There is also nothing in the answer choice that excludes the waltz from the "white-man's dance heritage." Therefore, a dance scholar would most likely NOT call the waltz a folk dance.

SOLUTIONS TO PASSAGE II:
REASONING—STRUCTURE AND EVALUATE QUESTIONS

1. **B** This is a Structure question

    A: No. This is the right answer to the wrong question. While the author does indicate at the end of the passage that there are historical facts that can in fact be proven, this is not the author's point in this part of the passage. This choice is also attractive based on outside knowledge. It is indisputable that flight in airplanes is possible (and the author would agree that this is true), but again, showing this is not the author's purpose. Rather, the author uses the possibility of flight to illustrate the nature of social memory. When answering Structure questions, make sure to choose an answer that accurately represents not only the passage content, but also the author's purpose in the relevant part of the passage.

    B: Yes. The author argues in the beginning of the passage that "in an important sense, there is no such thing as individual memory" and that "Memory is social." The author then goes on to describe how forms of collective memory make information useful without individuals themselves having to "memorize" it; the example of air flight illustrates how we can travel in a plane without actually knowing how or why flight is possible. Be careful not to impose your own definitions on terms used by the author; you might not think of a flight as a form of memory, but the author describes it as such.

    C: No. This choice contradicts the passage. The author states in paragraph 2 that "in an important sense, there is no such thing as individual memory." The rest of the paragraph, including the example of air travel, is intended to illustrate the social, not individual, nature of memory.

    D: No. As with choice A, this is the right answer to the wrong question. In paragraph 1 the author argues that finding a standard by which to judge the truth of a memory is especially complex when dealing with collective memory. Aside from the fact that it is judging the truthfulness of a social memory, not social memory itself, that is "even more complex," in paragraph 2 the author moves on to a different issue: the social nature of all memory. This is the point being illustrated by the example cited in the question.

2. **D** This is a Structure question

    Note: In this form of a Structure question, all the answer choices will generally be paraphrases of statements actually made in the passage (if the statement is not even supported by the passage, the choice is wrong for that reason). The correct answer will be the statement that is offered as direct evidence for the claim cited in the question stem.

    A: No. The author states this in paragraph 1 in support of the claim that judging the truth of a collective memory is even more complicated than judging the truth of an individual memory. This is a different issue than the argument cited in the question stem.

    B: No. This choice is attractive, as the existence of Holocaust deniers is part of the author's argument in the relevant part of the passage (paragraph 4). However, it is not the existence of Holocaust deniers that supports the author's claim about provable facts, but rather the fact that we find such controversies to be fascinating. If Holocaust deniers existed and no one really cared, there would be no support for the author's claim about a provable past.

    C: No. The claim you need to find support for is that there is such a thing as a knowable past exists. The statement in this answer choice is about the other side of the coin; that is, how coming to agreement is challenging because of the inherently distorted nature of memory.

    D: Yes. In the last paragraph the author gives the example of those who deny the Holocaust, and states that we are fascinated by "conflicting versions of the past." Then, at the end of the passage, the author argues that if there was no such thing as a "veritable" or provable fact, "controversies over the past would be ultimately uninteresting." But, such controversies are interesting to us; therefore, there must be some aspects of the past that are in fact provable.

3. **C**   This is a Structure question

A: No. This choice contradicts the passage. Make sure to take the author's statement that "the notion of 'distortion' becomes problematic" (paragraph 3) in context. When you continue to read paragraphs 3 and 4, you see that the author is not denying that distortion is an important concept. Rather, the author is arguing that distortion is unavoidable, and so presents a problem that should be addressed. For example, directly after the quote from Burke the author states: "Distortion is inevitable. Memory is distortion since memory is invariable and inevitably selective."

B: No. Facts are different from memory, according to the passage. The author indicates at the end of the passage that there are true facts; the author cites Burke in paragraph 3 in order to make the argument that memory inherently distorts factual reality.

C: **Yes. First, note the wording used by the author to introduce the quote; when the author says "As the British historian Peter Burke writes," the word "as" indicates that the author agrees with Burke. According to Burke, and as therefore also according to the author, "Neither memories nor histories seem objective any longer." The author goes on to make the point even more strongly directly after the quote: "Distortion is inevitable. Memory is distortion since memory is invariably and inherently selective."**

D: No. This is the right answer to the wrong question. While this statement is supported by the second paragraph (where the author discusses the institutional nature of social memory), it is not the claim being supported by the quote from Burke (which is about the inaccuracy of memory). To the extent that the two claims are related, their relationship is reversed; it is in part the social (including institutional) nature of memory that distorts it (given that memory "is inextricable from social and historical processes (paragraph 3)), rather than the distortion of memory that makes it institutional.

4. **C**   This is an Evaluate question

A: No. The author's discussion of how individuals use collective memory (paragraph 2) supports rather than undermines the claim. When answering an Evaluate question, make sure that the answer choice correctly describes the logic and direction of the author's argument.

B: No. The author provides extensive explanation for the claim in the second paragraph, including the use of an example (air travel). Make sure to read above and below the relevant passage reference, and take into account how other parts of the paragraph and passage as a whole relate to the cited claim.

C: **Yes. The second paragraph provides a detailed discussion of why the author believes that individual memory is always essentially shaped by institutions and social practices.**

D: No. While the claim is strongly supported, the purpose of the Holocaust example is not to support the claim about individual vs. social memory, but rather to bolster the case for taking the concept of distortion of memory seriously. When answering an Evaluate question, make sure that all parts of the answer choice are consistent with the content and logical structure of the passage.

5. **A**   This is an Evaluate question

A: **Yes. The author states this in the first paragraph, but never supports or explains it; the passage immediately moves on to discuss the greater complexity of collective memory.**

B: No. The author goes on to explain that "memory is a process of encoding information, storing information, and strategically retrieving information, and there are social, psychological, and historical influences on this process."

C: No. The much of the last paragraph, including the example of revisionist versions of history and our interest in them, supports this claim.

D: No. The example of how we can fly in a plane without understanding how a plane actually works directly supports this claim.

6. **A** This is an Evaluate question

A: **Yes. When the author argues in the second paragraph that individual memory does not exist, he means that all memory is essentially shaped by social forces and institutions, not that individuals literally have no memory or knowledge of the past. The author's point in the last paragraph is that historical facts do exist, and it seems that there must be some way within our collective memory of coming to an "agreement about what really happened."**

B: No. The answer choice reverses the relationship between the two statements in the passage. The author's claim that individual memory does not exist is based on the argument that all memory is collective or social. This supports the claim (rather than being supported by) at the end of the passage that there appears to be some way of coming to agreement about history based on our collective memory. When answering any Reasoning question, make sure that the answer you choose accurately represents the logical relationship between the relevant points in the passage.

C: No. There is no inconsistency between the two claims. The author argues in the second paragraph that all memory, including so-called individual memory, is shaped by social forces. In the last paragraph, the author claims that because historical controversies are gripping, we must believe that there is a knowable past within our social memory. In sum, the "absence" (that is, the social nature) of individual memory is part of, not inconsistent with, the author's argument in the last paragraph.

D: No. This choice has the same problem as choice C. If individual memory is non-existent because all memory is essentially social or collective, and if it is within or through our social memory that we can come to some agreement about the past, the two claims cited in the question stem are consistent, not in contradiction, with each other.

SOLUTIONS TO PASSAGE III:
APPLICATION—STRENGTHEN AND WEAKEN QUESTIONS

1. **D** This is a Strengthen question in the EXCEPT/LEAST/NOT format

Note: The incorrect answers to this question type and format will Strengthen the relevant part of the passage. The correct answer will weaken it, or have no impact on it, or strengthen it less than the other three choices.

A: No. The author explains the claim that photography beautifies the world by asserting that photography determines for us what qualifies as beauty and that we measure beauty according to our ability to see it in photographs. Photographing clothes to determine whether they are sufficiently attractive would strengthen this claim.

B: No. The author explains the claim that photography beautifies the world by asserting that photography determines for us what qualifies as beauty and that we measure beauty according to our ability to see it in photographs. Increasing significance being attributed to attractive yearbook photos would strengthen this claim.

C: No. The author explains the claim that photography beautifies the world by asserting that photography determines for us what qualifies as beauty and that we measure beauty according to our ability to see it in photographs. The idea that seeing a photograph of the house (in addition to the actual house) will impress visitors would certainly strengthen this claim.

D: **Yes. The author explains the claim that photography beautifies the world by asserting that photography determines for us what qualifies as beauty and that we measure beauty according to our ability to see it in photographs. Although the photographs in museums may be beautiful, there is no indication here that they are altering the way anyone perceives reality. So this answer choice does not strengthen the claim.**

2. **A**   This is a Strengthen question.

  A: **Yes. The idea that beauty can be exhausted through overuse suggests that after seeing too many photographic representations of something, one's capacity to find it beautiful will fade. The example of these Grand Canyon photos shows that images once seen as fresh and beautiful have, after years of public attention, come to seem more mundane and amateurish. This does strengthen the claim.**

  B: No. The idea that beauty can be exhausted through overuse suggests that after seeing too many photographic representations of something, one's capacity to find it beautiful will fade. The fading described in the Sistine Chapel example is a physical change, not a change in perception, through the influence of light rather than of over-exposure.

  C: No. This choice is the opposite. The idea that beauty can be exhausted through overuse suggests that after seeing too many photographic representations of something, one's capacity to find it beautiful will fade. The David example would weaken the claim, suggesting that in this case much exposure has not caused the experience of beauty to fade.

  D: No. The idea that beauty can be exhausted through overuse suggests that after seeing too many photographic representations of something, one's capacity to find it beautiful will fade. The passage describes this process as one that happens over generations, not over a single season. The magazine example suggests a pursuit of novelty but not necessarily the idea that familiar models are not regarded as beautiful.

3. **C**   This is a Weaken question.

  A: No. The author attributes contemporary anxiety towards being photographed to a fear of looking bad in the picture (the camera's disapproval). It is loss of privacy, not a fear of looking unattractive that troubles this actor.

  B: No. The author attributes contemporary anxiety towards being photographed to a fear of looking bad in the picture (the camera's disapproval). The boy in this example is concerned with the frequency of pictures, not with their quality or his appearance.

  C: **Yes. The author attributes contemporary anxiety towards being photographed to a fear of looking bad in the picture (the camera's disapproval). This application might, accordingly, be expected to reduce anxiety. However the answer choice says that it causes dissatisfaction, weakening the claim that people want photographs to look better than reality.**

  D: No. The author attributes contemporary anxiety towards being photographed to a fear of looking bad in the picture (the camera's disapproval). This grandmother fears having a poor appearance in a picture, so this answer choice strengthens rather than weakens the claim.

4. **A**   This is a Weaken question.

  A: **Yes. In paragraph 4 (and first sentence of paragraph 5) the author contrasts photography with painting, claiming that for the former "lying" is more important because reality itself is at stake. This answer choice contradicts the passage and weakens that claim in suggesting that photography cannot deceive as readily as can painting.**

  B: No. This choice is consistent with the author's argument. The author describes quicker speed of photography in paragraph 5, and suggests that this represents an important difference between photography and painting.

  C: No. This choice strengthens rather than weakens the author's argument. In paragraph 4 (and first sentence of 5) the author contrasts photography with painting, claiming that for the former "lying" is more important because reality itself is at stake. This answer choice strengthens the claim that photography and painting are different by emphasizing that the distinction the author describes, between reality and the history of art, is indeed a real and an important one.

D: No. This choice is not inconsistent with the passage. The author herself argues that photography is concerned with both truth and beauty (paragraph 4). While the author does not discuss painting's concerns, the claim in this choice that painting is only concerned with truth supports a contrast between painting and photography.

5.   **D**   This is a Strengthen question.
   A: No. The project, as described in the passage, is to reconcile the claims of truth and beauty with the effect of changing how we actually view reality. Truth, as portrayed in this context, refers to the accurate portrayal of reality. There is nothing in this answer choice to suggest that the photographs are accurate; rather, they are obscure. There is also nothing to suggest that the photograph affects our view of reality.
   B: No. The project, as described in the passage, is to reconcile the claims of truth and beauty. Focused on deception, the photographs in this answer choice do not appear to value truth, nor do they affect our view of reality.
   C: No. The project, as described in the passage, is to reconcile the claims of truth and beauty. The contrast between image and word in this answer choice perhaps hints at the scribe vs. poet contrast in the passage, but there is nothing in this answer choice that directly relates to truth or beauty.
   D: Yes. The project, as described in the passage, is to reconcile the claims of truth and beauty. According to the author, this entails "changing the very idea of reality, and of realism." The description in this choice suggests that the photographs capture "true" (unaltered) images of water but impart to it a new beauty, and by so doing change our vision of the real nature of water.

6.   **B**   This is a Weaken question.
   Note: The author herself rejects this claim in the last paragraph. She writes: "The photographer was thought [emphasis added] to be an acute, but non-interfering observer—a scribe, not a poet. But as people quickly discovered that nobody takes the same picture of the same thing, the supposition that cameras furnish an impersonal, objective image yielded to the fact that photographs are evidence not only of what's there but of what an individual sees, not just a record but an evaluation of the world."

   The correct answer will be consistent with the view we have come to have of photography by indicating that the photographer is not necessarily just a scribe, but can also be a poet.

   A: No. This choice, while tempting, doesn't go far enough to weaken the claim. The fact that different photographers choose different angles does not by itself indicate that they are not just recording reality.
   B: Yes. The scribe, as described in the passage, is a non-interfering observer and recorder of "what's there," whereas the poet brings artistry and self-expression. The fact that many photographers have a distinctive style that separates them from all others indicates that these photographers are not simply recording, but are interpreting or evaluating, reality.
   C: No. The scribe, as described in the passage, is a non-interfering observer, whereas the poet brings artistry and self-expression. This answer choice suggests that amateur photographers make their choices based on other people rather than on an artistic vision. This choice provides no reason to believe that photographers go beyond recording "what's there."
   D: No. The scribe, as described in the passage, is a non-interfering observer, whereas the poet expresses a personal and subjective view of the world. The statement in this answer choice suggests that most photographers do not express a unique aesthetic vision, which is consistent with the view that the typical photographer is a mere scribe.

8.2

SOLUTIONS TO PASSAGE IV:
APPLICATION—NEW INFORMATION AND ANALOGY QUESTIONS

1. **A** This is a New Information question

    A: **Yes. The author argues in paragraph 2 that placing a high value on conflict disengages the public from journalism and from public life.**

    B. No. This choice is half-right but half-wrong. While the author would oppose the political analyst's claim—the author argues in paragraph 2 against focusing on conflict— the author also opposes the idea that journalism should take a value-neutral stance (paragraph 2).

    C: No. This choice is half-right but half-wrong. On one hand, the author would most likely agree that healthy discussion is necessary for democratic deliberation in the service of answering the question "What shall we do?" (paragraphs 1 and 6). On the other hand, however, the author believes that a focus on conflict between polar extremes dissuades people from taking part in that discussion (paragraph 2).

    D: No. Both parts of this answer choice are wrong. The author would oppose the statement; the passage argues that conflict, and framing issues in terms of opposing extremes, discourages people from paying attention to public concerns (paragraph 2). Furthermore, the author argues at the end of paragraph 3 that people can be reengaged in public life only if "journalists think of people by their efforts not as an audience to be entertained or as spectators at an event, but as citizens capable of action."

2. **C** This is a New Information/Weaken question

    A: No. The effect of social media (which would not, by the author's description in the passage, qualify as part of "One Journalism") has no relevance to this part of the author's definition of One Journalism.

    B: No. The new information in the question stem is relevant to whether or not public journalism would encourage public engagement in democratic deliberation, not to the necessary conditions for the deliberation itself.

    C: **Yes. The author claims in the passage that the limited range of information and points of view offered through One Journalism discourages engagement in public life (paragraph 2), and that presenting "the true array of choices" would reengage the public (paragraph 3). If credible evidence exists that the public is confused and discouraged by the presentation of multiple options and ideas, it would undermine this part of the author's argument in the passage.**

    D: No. The new information in the question stem is not directly relevant to the author's argument about responsibility. It is possible for both claims to be true; that is, that public journalism confuses people, and One Journalism denies journalistic responsibility.

3. **B** This is a New Information/Strengthen question

    A: No. The author describes the "culture of detachment" as the supposed value-neutral and "balanced" nature of One Journalism (paragraph 2). However, the reporting described in the question stem is anything other than value-neutral. Rather, it presents only one value or point of view (that of the political regime). Therefore, the new information and the passage information are describing two significantly different factors that would discourage public interest in journalism.

B: Yes. The author argues in paragraph 2 that when citizens feel excluded from the life reported in the news, they "withdraw into private concerns" and that this is a "direct threat to journalism." The new information in the question stem describes a different cause of exclusion from public life, but that exclusion has the same result—people see journalism as irrelevant. Therefore, the new information would strengthen the causal connection drawn by the author between engagement in public life and the perceived relevance of journalism.

C: No. The new information in the question stem describes a form of "positive" reporting that discourages, not encourages, engagement in public life. Furthermore, the successes discussed by the author are "civic successes" that occur "outside our pinched definition of the news" (paragraph 3); that is, the successes brought about by active citizens (not a by repressive regime).

D: No. While the journalism described in the question stem might not qualify as good journalism or reporting by the author's standards, it has no impact on the validity of the author's discussion in paragraphs 4 and 5 of how to evaluate what constitutes good reporting.

4. **D** This is an Analogy question

   Note: The author indicates that within One Journalism, people play a passive role "as an audience to be entertained or as spectators at an event," whereas public journalism treats the public as "citizens capable of action" (paragraph 3). Therefore, the correct answer will show a contrast between a passive viewer or consumer on one hand, and an active participant on the other. Look out for wrong answers that reverse the relationship ("respectively" in the question stem means in the same order), or that show no contrast between the two sides.

   A: No. Both parts of this choice describe a passive audience.

   B: No. This choice reverses the relationship; doing one's own research would be more active, while taking advice without question would be more passive.

   C: No. In both cases people are actively involved; there is no reason to think that investing someone else's money would entail more active involvement than investing one's own money.

   D: **Yes. In the first case, people are passively viewing art with no role in actually creating the art. In the second case, the audience members become an active part of the performance.**

5. **B** This is an Analogy question in the EXCEPT/LEAST/NOT format

   Note: The author discusses distinguishing good from bad journalism in paragraphs 4 and 5. The author rejects the method used by One Journalism, which is to draw a clear line between good and bad. According to One Journalism, if you cross that clearly defined line, you are creating bad journalism, and if not, you are writing good journalism. The author argues that instead we should judge journalists in terms of where their work lies along a spectrum, taking into account a variety of factors such as "their consciences, their judgment, and the needs of their communities" (paragraph 5). The correct answer will be most similar to the unitary standard used by One Journalism, or at least significantly different from the author's approach, while the wrong answers will be more similar to the author's proposed method of evaluation.

   A: No. This method of judgment takes a variety of factors into account, including the motives or conscience and the judgment of the defendant, and the effect of her actions on others (which would be comparable to considering the needs of the community). Therefore, this case is similar to the standard of judgment proposed by the author.

   B: **Yes. This method of evaluation assumes that a clear standard (compositional rules) exists, and does not take a variety of factors into account. Therefore, this case out of the four choices is the least similar to the author's proposed method.**

C: No. In this case, a variety of factors are taken into account and weighed against each other, including the effect on the community and the mayor's intentions. Unlike in choice B, there is no suggestion of the existence of a single clear standard or line that can be used to evaluate the merit of the mayor's decisions.

D: No. There is no suggestion in this choice of a single line or standard that can be used to judge a person. Instead, a variety of factors are taken into account including how reasonable his or her actions were within a particular historical context, and his or her motivations (which could include judgment and conscience).

6.   **D**   This is an Analogy question

Note: This is a twist on a standard Analogy question. It has aspects of an Inference question in that the answer choices are all about the same topic as the passage. However, the answer choices also include new information that is or is not logically similar to what is described in the relevant part of the passage.

The author states in the passage that the objective of public journalism is reengage people in public life and to "find ways for journalism to serve a purpose beyond—but not in place of—telling the news." This includes reporting on "the very important news of civic life—including civic successes—that now occurs outside our pinched definition of news" and treating people as "citizens capable of action" (paragraph 3). The correct answer will be the closest among the four choices to this description.

A: No. While this story reports on the actions of journalists trying to change how reporting is done, there is no indication of citizen involvement or civic successes.

B: No. The author states in paragraph 1 that One Journalism addresses "the particular problems and needs of a community in an artificial journalistic context, created and driven from other places." Therefore, while this article is about small town life, the fact that it is written by a national news reporter in New York puts this closer to One Journalism than to public journalism.

C: No. This choice jumbles together a variety of words and concepts from the passage (including corporations and democracy) but does not suggest that the story represents or encourages citizen involvement or civic successes.

D: **Yes. This locally written story depicts a civic success achieved through active involvement of the citizenry. Therefore, of the four choices, it is the most logically similar to the perspective encouraged by public journalism.**

8.3   MANAGING STRESS:
PREPARING FOR THE DAY OF THE TEST

There are a variety of things you can do in the time remaining to make the day of the MCAT as comfortable and familiar as possible.

- Make peace with your anxiety. Everyone experiences it, including the highest scorers. Feel free to be nervous on test day and the several days (or weeks) before. Even if you don't sleep well the night before the test, you'll be fine. Nervousness can be a good thing; adrenaline intensifies your ability to concentrate intensely.
- Let go of the need to be perfect. You don't need to complete every question, or get every question that you complete correct, to get a high CARS score.
- This is not the time to quit smoking (do that *after* the MCAT) or give up caffeine, but take care of your health. Keep eating well and exercising up until the test date. And, don't turn to drugs or alcohol for stress management, and definitely don't start experimenting with black-market ADHD drugs! Maintain a habit of 7–8 hours of sleep (per night, not per week).
- Get up roughly at the same time each morning as you will on test day, and go to bed at the same time that you will the night before the test. If you are in the habit of staying up until 2 A.M., but need to go to bed at 10 P.M. in order to get a reasonable amount of sleep the night before the test, you won't be able to magically change your sleeping habits at the last minute. Get into a good sleep schedule at least the week or two before the test, and you will thank yourself on test day!
- Whenever possible, practice CARS at the same time of day as the real test.
- Make a plan for getting to your testing site, and practice it. What time will you get up? What will you eat? What route will you take to the test site? Make sure that you plan to leave in plenty of time to get there a little early. Travel to the site at the same time as you will on the day of the test to see how long it takes you.
- Visualize success. Elite athletes, before each competition, visualize themselves going through each step of a successful performance. This both calms their nerves and focuses them on the task at hand. Remember a time in which you worked through a passage or set of passages with good results, and mentally run through the steps you took. Recall the sense of control and confidence you have when you stay calm and focused, use the techniques you've learned, and take charge of the material. If you begin to feel stress or anxiety, close your eyes and remember that feeling.

Chapter 8 Summary

- Continue to evaluate your performance and diagnose reasons for mistakes. Focus on correcting bad habits, rather than on doing as many practice passages as possible.

- Continue to hone your skills in the three basic areas: working the passage, translating the questions, and POE.

- Monitor your stress level and find ways to relax. Don't wait to feel overwhelmed; build "vacations" into your weekly study schedule.

CHAPTER 8 PRACTICE PASSAGES

Individual Passage Drills

You may wish to use these passages for Exercises 3 and 4 from this chapter. If not, do them back-to-back, timed, at the pace you have determined works best for you (for most people, this will be approximately 10–11 minutes per passage).

Once you have completed the passages and checked your answers, fill out the Individual Passage Logs. Focus in particular on identifying continuing patterns in the mistakes you are making, as well as identifying times when you successfully implemented appropriate strategies.

CHAPTER 8 PRACTICE PASSAGE 1

We all start out as animists, as toddlers vaguely uncertain about whether our beloved doll or pull-toy puppy might be a living being. When I was a child, my favorite cartoons were those that played in to that confusion, films in which toasters or teapots or slippers sprouted legs and faces and revealed their true natures as menacing agents of mayhem and chaos.

In time, we learn to distinguish the creature from the object, and, later, consumer society conditions us to detach ourselves from our stuff so effectively that we can dedicate ourselves to the perpetual quest for nicer stuff and embrace the necessity of regularly exchanging older models for newer ones. But some vestige of the child remains, evidenced by the tenacious hold material things have over us, as objects of desire and, more mysteriously, as personal mementos and totems—as clues to our secret selves and as signposts along the circuitous route that has taken us from the past into the present. Objects survive because we need them, or because we are convinced that we need them. The unreconstructed animist will see a Darwinian triumph in the rapidity with which a crumpled boarding pass evolves into an all-important and indispensable detail in the narrative of some meaningful chapter in our lives.

One such chapter is the subject of *Important Artifacts and Personal Property from the Collection of Lenore Doolan and Harold Morris, Including Books, Street Fashion, and Jewelry*. A series of captioned photographs, Leanne Shapton's ingenious book does a deadpan imitation of the auction catalogues that often accompany the sale of an estate or private collection, catalogues that constitute a peculiar genre in themselves. Typically, the detritus of dead movie stars and the obsessions of rich eccentrics crowd the pages of these paperbound volumes designed to persuade potential bidders that the auction is a purely professional, emotionally neutral transaction, and not, as one might suspect, a thinly disguised *memento mori*, an indication that something has ended—a life, someone's fiscal solvency, or, in the best case, an acquisitive passion.

Shapton presents and describes the artifacts that once belonged to a couple, now broken up. Someone (one or both of the lovers) is jettisoning everything (or almost everything; some lots have been removed from the sale, for unspecified reasons) that the pair possessed or acquired over a relationship that lasted four years, more or less. There are cake stands, blankets, sports equipment, snapshots, T-shirts, clippings, hand-lettered menus from celebratory dinners for two, unopened bottles of wine — and many of these humble items will turn out to signal a plot turn in the history of a romance.

A slightly charred backgammon set, a souvenir of a summer the lovers spend in the country, precedes a handwritten message from Hal: "I want this to work, but there are sides to you I just can't handle sometimes. Chucking the backgammon board into the fire was the last straw." The phone number of a couples' therapist appears on the back of a business card, and we realize that the crisis has escalated when we see a photo of Morris's white-noise machine, which appears to be smashed by a hammer.

Just as the concept of *Important Artifacts* is amusing in itself, so is its central conceit: Although the bidding estimates assigned to the lots fall well within the range that a provident auction house might term "sensibly" or "reasonably" priced, the fact is that a large percentage of what is being auctioned off is basically crap that no sensible person would want, not even for free. The seriousness beneath the joke is that these scraps of paper, used clothes, and borderline garbage were formerly objects of incalculable worth; indeed, they once meant everything to this fictional couple.

Reading the final pages of *Important Artifacts*, I found myself reflecting that the cartoonists whose work I so loved as a child might have been right about the potentially subversive or maniacal ways that objects would behave, if only they could. It may not be true that the furious teapot is plotting to grab a soup spoon and chase us around the house, but it seems inarguable that the deceptively innocent tea cozy could say far more than we would ever want strangers—or anyone, really—to know about who we are, what we did, what was done to us, and how we felt when it happened.

Material used in this particular passage has been adapted from the following source:

F. Prose, *"Love for Sale: Appraising the Relics of a Relationship," Harper's Magazine,* © 2009, Francine Prose.

1. All of the following items are listed in the passage as relics of Doolan and Morris's relationship EXCEPT:

A) a white-noise machine.
B) bottles of wine.
C) a crumpled boarding pass.
D) T-shirts.

2. The author's attitude toward Shapton's book is:

A) predominantly critical but balanced.
B) effusive with praise and superficial.
C) approving and contemplative.
D) disparaging and plaintive.

3. Which of the following statements best summarizes the author's central purpose?

A) To express her appreciation of *Important Artifacts* and to explain how it gave her an elevated awareness of the meaning of objects
B) To praise Shapton's defense of animism inherent in the pages of *Important Artifacts*
C) To laugh at the irony that the objects that once meant so much to Doolan and Morris as a couple become, after their breakup, objects of little to no worth
D) To heighten the reader's awareness of everyday objects and those objects' potential to speak for us and tell stories of the events of our lives

4. Why does the author present the example of the backgammon set in paragraph 5?

A) To provide proof of Lenore Doolan's bad temper as the reason for the decline of the couple's relationship
B) As a piece of evidence for her claim that objects photographed for the book signal plot turns in the couple's relationship
C) To support her point that worthless objects acquire sentimental value when people are in relationships and are therefore invaluable
D) To suggest that objects only acquire meaning after they are altered in some form

5. The author most likely believes that:

A) her toaster is plotting grand schemes to reveal her darkest secrets.
B) it was not right of Shapton to expose a couple's private life the way she does in her book.
C) Doolan and Morris' relationship was doomed to failure.
D) we turn certain objects into significant and necessary documents of memorable parts of our lives.

6. According to the author, auction catalogues are generally designed to create what sort of impression for potential bidders?

A) A belief that the lives of movie stars and rich eccentrics are more fascinating than our own
B) An acknowledgment that something has ended—a life, someone's fiscal solvency, or an acquisitive passion
C) A wistful imagining of the stories and secrets those objects can potentially reveal
D) An appearance of impartiality and professionalism

CHAPTER 8 PRACTICE PASSAGE 2

One difficulty in following Adam Smith's account of self-interest is that he had discussed the matter thoroughly in the *Theory of Moral Sentiments*, and he assumed that the reader of the *Wealth of Nations* would not think that he, Smith, considered self-interest the only or even the main motive, or virtue, of humanity. His teacher, Hutchenson, indeed, had taught that the only virtue was benevolence; but Smith, while agreeing that this was the major virtue and the one which aimed "at the greatest possible good," felt strongly that the system of benevolent ethics was too simple and left no room for the "inferior virtues." Therefore he devoted himself to a more naturalistic theory of morals, in which man's nature was accepted as it was.

In the *Wealth of Nations*, Smith combined the two doctrines: God's providential benevolence and man's earthly self-interest. The result is his famous "invisible hand" theory in which the individual, intending only his own gain, is led "to promote an end which was no part of his intention," the well-being of society. The view that personal self-interest is the best regulator of public affairs had been put forward before: it is expressed in Bernard de Mandeville's, *Private Vices, Public Benefits*. When Smith wrote, this view was already familiar to eighteenth-century thinkers. What Smith did was to give it a reasoned economic exposition which made it acceptable and, so to speak, respectable. From then on, the inevitable benefits of self-interest become a doctrine to which rising manufacturers and owners of newly enclosed land constantly appealed. However, he was constantly inveighing against the farmers, the workers, the manufacturers, and the banks, complaining that they did not understand their own particular interests. He chided the mercantilists that their very cupidity, by imposing a heavy duty on certain goods, called into being a smuggling of the goods which ruined their business. Country gentlemen were told that in their demand for a bounty on corn "they did not act with that complete comprehension of their own interest" which should have directed their efforts.

Smith's method was to form out of experience an abstract principle, to state this as a general rule and to give evidence and examples to support it. Thus, he and his science of economics could show "how" and "in what manner." In order to discover such a science of economics, however, Smith had to posit a faith in the orderly structure of nature, underlying appearances and accessible to man's reason. This, in our judgment, is what Smith really meant by the "invisible hand"; that, so to speak, an "order of nature" or a "structure of things" existed which permitted self-interest, if enlightened, to work for mankind's good.

Man's task, therefore, was to understand the nature or structure of things and to adjust himself harmoniously to the necessary results of this structure. On one level, this might mean the acceptance of a "natural" price of things (reached when the supply, whether of goods or of labor, exactly equaled the demand). On another level, Smith applied his faith in a structure of things when he said: "A nation of hunters can never be formidable to the civilized nations in their neighbourhood. A nation of shepherds may." This is true, he thought, because the nature of hunting is such that large numbers cannot indulge in it; the game would be exterminated. On the other hand, shepherds can grow in number as their flocks grow: and can carry war into the hearts of civilized nations because they carry with them their food supply.

What effect did Smith's work actually have? First, it gave the rising manufacturers and merchants a rationale for their desire to change existing government policy. (Existing policy, as we have pointed out, favored the older trades, methods, and classes against the new "Lunar Society" type of individual and enterprise.) Thus, for example, it helped Pitt to pass a free-trade agreement, the Eden Treaty of 1786 with France, through Parliament.

The second effect of Smith's work was in the shaping of thought. His influence in introducing historical method into political economy was far-reaching. He made the foundation of all subsequent economics the notion that wealth was created by labor. But, more than any of these things, he introduced science into the study of economics. Although he talked much about the "invisible hand" and the "natural course of things," Smith really freed man from the tyranny of chance by forming for him the analytical tools with which he might learn to control his economic activities.

Material used in this particular passage has been adapted from the following source:

J. Bronowski and B. Mazlish, *The Western Intellectual Tradition.* ©1960 by HarperCollins Publishers.

1. The authors state that Smith draws which of the following relationships between nature and economics?

A) Humans are selfish and always take as much from the marketplace as they can.
B) Humans are inherently communal beings and share all their resources.
C) Humans fundamentally act in their own interest.
D) Humans are generous and act in defense of others.

2. Which of the following statements, if true, would most *undermine* the authors' characterization of Smith?

A) Smith extrapolated his theories from real-life observations.
B) Smith's work was wholly theoretical.
C) Smith based part of his work on an older idea.
D) Smith's theory influenced the work of later economists.

3. Which of the following items of information from the passage most supports the authors' claim that Smith believed that the economy can be not only studied but influenced by human actions?

A) Smith felt that the system of benevolent ethics was too simple and left no room for the "inferior virtues."
B) Smith combined two doctrines to create his "invisible hand" theory.
C) Smith introduced a historical method into the study of economy.
D) Smith criticized businessmen who did not act in their own best interest.

4. According to the information provided, the attitude of the authors toward Smith's theories can best be described as:

A) exuberant support.
B) informed approval.
C) qualified praise.
D) inexplicable disappointment.

5. A reasonable supposition from passage information about Smith and de Mandeville is that they agreed that:

A) individual motivation can provide a benefit to society.
B) benevolence is the only virtue.
C) a naturalist theory of morals would prove the most accurate.
D) economics is a science.

6. The term "invisible hand" in Smith's economic theory is most defined by the principle that:

A) there is a "natural" price of things.
B) individual action can influence society.
C) economics can be quantified through analytical tools.
D) manufacturers can change existing government policy.

7. According to the authors, Smith's most important contribution to economics was:

A) identifying benevolence as man's only virtue.
B) identifying the role of nature in economics.
C) identifying self-interest as the best regulator of public affairs.
D) identifying a method by which to analyze economic activity.

SOLUTIONS TO CHAPTER 8 PRACTICE PASSAGE 1

1. **C**   This is a Retrieval question.

   A: No. This item is mentioned in paragraph 5.

   B: No. This item is mentioned in paragraph 4.

   C: Yes. While a crumpled boarding pass is mentioned in paragraph 2, this is a hypothetical example and not tied explicitly to the relationship.

   D: No. This item is mentioned in paragraph 4.

2. **C**   This is a Tone/Attitude question.

   A: No. Nowhere in the passage does the author say anything critical about the book.

   B: No. While the author praises Shapton's book at a few points in the course of the passage, "effusive with praise" is too extreme. Also, the opening and closing ruminations on the relationship of objects to people's lives mean the author is not superficial in her treatment of the subject matter.

   C: Yes. This comes closest to capturing the author's tone. She calls the book "ingenious" in paragraph 3, and in paragraph 6, she calls the book's concept and central concept "amusing." The author clearly enjoys the book and has given its ideas some thought (which supports "contemplative") as evidenced by the first and last paragraphs.

   D: No. This is overly negative. The author never criticizes or disparages the book. Also, there is no mournfulness about, or lamenting of, anything regarding the book, which invalidates "plaintive."

3. **A**   This is a Main Idea/Primary Purpose question.

   A: Yes. While the author does not mention Shapton's book immediately, her early discussion about objects leads into a discussion and appreciation of *Important Artifacts*; the last paragraph shows the author's elevated understanding of the meaning of objects after reading the book.

   B: No. While the author mentions animism in paragraph 1, she does not indicate that Shapton's book explicitly deals with this concept.

   C: No. This choice puts too negative a spin on the author's tone. While the author is interested in the difference between the dollar value and the emotional investment in objects (paragraph 6), she is not discussing these things to laugh at Doolan and Morris or their possessions.

   D: No. While this answer contains correct information, it makes no reference to Shapton's book, which is central to the author's understanding and explanation of the relationship between people and objects.

4. **B**   This is a Structure question.

   A: No. The author is not interested in analyzing the reasons for the decline of the relationship; she is only interested in how the objects that belonged to the couple tell the story of their romance. Also, the word "proof" is too strong.

   B: Yes. At the end of paragraph 4, the author suggests that objects signal plot turns in the couple's relationship. The backgammon example immediately following is illustrative, along with Hal's note, of this point, since it is evidence of a negative turn for the couple. This is furthered by the author's assertion in paragraph 5 that the smashed white-noise machine helps us "realize the crisis has escalated."

   C: No. This is a point made in paragraph 6 where the author discusses the central conceit of the book. The example of the backgammon set is given to support a different idea in paragraph 5: the connection between changes in the couple's relationship and these objects.

   D: No. The author does not suggest that things must be altered in order to acquire significance.

5. **D** This is an Inference question.

A: No. This takes the reference in paragraph 1 out of context. While the author mentions cartoons she watched as a child in which objects would sprout limbs and move, and in the final paragraph she suggests that a tea cozy may have a lot to say about one's personal life, she would not go so far as to believe her toaster capable of plotting schemes. Note in the final paragraph she says "if only they could," referring to the fact that objects are unable to enact or consider plots on their own.

B: No. The author makes no negative judgment about Shapton; besides, the author mentions that the couple is fictional (paragraph 6), so real lives are not actually being exposed.

C: No. The author does not weigh in on whether the relationship had chances of survival or not; she is merely interested in how the objects from that relationship tell its story.

D: Yes. See the final sentences of paragraph 2. This answer fits well with the author's assertion that objects become "all-important and indispensable" details in the narratives of chapters of our lives.

6. **D** This is a Retrieval question.

A: No. There is nothing in the passage that contrasts the lives of famous people with those of regular people in terms of fascination.

B: No. This choice directly contradicts the passage. In paragraph 3, the author states that the catalogues are not designed to give "an indication that something has ended."

C: No. See paragraph 3. While the author herself expresses this attitude, she does not suggest that the catalogues do so.

D: Yes. In paragraph 3 the author says, "Typically, the detritus of dead movie stars and the obsessions of rich eccentrics crowd the pages of these paperbound volumes designed to persuade potential bidders that the auction is a purely professional, emotionally neutral transaction."

SOLUTIONS TO CHAPTER 8 PRACTICE PASSAGE 2

1. **C** This is a Retrieval question.

A: No. This overstates Smith's contention that self-interest is the primary motivation of humans. While one might call acting in one's self interest "selfish," the authors do not indicate that self-interest always involves taking as much as one can. For example, in the second half of paragraph 2 the authors suggest that self-interest is more complex.

B: No. Although the passage mentions benevolence (paragraph 1) and Smith's acceptance of it as "the major virtue," this answer choice misrepresents how Smith saw human nature as fundamentally self-interested (paragraphs 1 and 2).

C: Yes. The authors most directly discuss the relationship between nature and economics in paragraph 3: "In order to discover such a science of economics, however, Smith had to posit a faith in the orderly structure of nature...This...is what Smith really meant by 'the invisible hand'; that...an 'order of nature' or a 'structure of things' existed which permitted self-interest, if enlightened, to work for mankind's good." Also, in paragraph 1 and the beginning of paragraph 2 the authors discuss how Smith believed that humans are motivated by their own self-interest, which grows out of man's very nature.

D: No. Despite the mention of benevolence in paragraph 1, the passage does not indicate that humans are fundamentally generous, nor that they act in defense of others as a general rule.

2. **B** This is a Weaken question.

A: No. The authors characterize Smith as forming an abstract principle out of real-life experience (paragraph 3.) Therefore, this choice is consistent, not inconsistent, with the passage.

B: **Yes. The authors stress the real-life evidence formulating Smith's theories, and the real-life impact they had (see paragraph 2 for examples). Therefore this statement, if true, would undermine the authors' characterization of Smith.**

C: No. Smith did base his work in part on the work of Hutchenson and de Mandeville (see paragraphs 1 and 2). This choice is consistent with the passage.

D: No. The authors state that Smith's work laid the foundation of all subsequent economic studies (see paragraph 6). This choice is consistent with the passage.

3. **D** This is a Structure question.

Note: This question asks you to decide which of the four statements cited in the choices is most directly used within the passage as support for the authors' claim that Smith believed the economy can be influenced.

A: No. This statement represents the inspiration for Smith's theory, but does not demonstrate that Smith feels that the economy can be influenced.

B: No. The fact that the "invisible hand" theory combines two different elements (the doctrines of "God's providential benevolence and man's earthly self-interest" (paragraph 2) does not show that Smith feels that the economy can be influenced. These are two separate issues in the passage.

C: No. This answer speaks to how the economy is now studied (paragraph 6), but has no direct relevance to whether or not the economy can actually be influenced.

D: **Yes. The fact that Smith actively tried to get farmers, workers, and manufacturers to act in their own best interest (and not just their perception of it) clearly indicates that by changing their behavior, he feels that he can change the marketplace (see paragraph 2). Therefore, out of the four choices (all of which are from the passage), this information most acts to give support for the claim cited in the question stem.**

4. **B** This is a Tone/Attitude question.

A: No. This answer is too extreme. The authors do give Smith's work credit, but in a balanced manner.

B: **Yes. The authors provide concrete reasons for their support of Smith's work.**

C: No. There is no qualification of, or stepping back from, the praise that the authors have for Smith's work.

D: No. The passage is complimentary towards Smith and gives no indication of disappointment.

5. **A** This is an Inference question.

A: **Yes. As we can see in paragraph 2, they both believe that "personal self-interest is the best regulator of public affairs."**

B: No. This is Hutchenson's idea, not de Mandeville's. Also, we know from paragraph 1 that Smith does not agree with this idea, because his work is based on a modification of it.

C: No. We are not told how de Mandeville (mentioned only in paragraph 2) would feel about such a statement.

D: No. According to the passage, it was Smith who "introduced science into the study of economics" (paragraph 6); we have no way of knowing whether de Mandeville would agree or not.

6. **B**   This is an Inference question.

    A: No. While Smith does believe in the possibility of a "natural" price of things (see paragraph 4), this is not the primary principle underlying his "invisible hand" theory. The idea of the "natural" price level creates a backdrop within which Smith's "invisible hand" (human self-interest) may act.

    B: Yes. Smith believes that people acting in self-interest will have an inadvertent effect on the "well-being of society" (see paragraph 2). This is at the heart of Smith's theory of the "invisible hand."

    C: No. Although Smith did introduce analytical tools to the study of economics (paragraph 6), the idea of quantification is not presented as an underlying principle of the "invisible hand" theory.

    D: No. While paragraph 5 explains that Smith's theory provides manufacturers a rationale for desiring change in government policy, the authors do not present this very specific possibility as an underlying principle (nor do we know that the manufacturers were successful).

7. **D**   This is a Retrieval question.

    A: No. This was Hutchenson, not Smith (see paragraph 1).

    B: No. Smith used the term "nature" but the passage does not suggest that he was the first to connect human nature (or the nature of things in general) to economics, or that this was the most important aspect of Smith's work.

    C: No. This was an aspect of his contribution, but the author specifically describes the "science" that Smith provides as his most important contribution to the study of economics (paragraph 6).

    D: Yes. The authors stress that his lasting and most important contribution was introducing a scientific methodology to economics (paragraph 6).

Individual Passage Log

Total time spent _____

Passage # _____

Q#	Q type	Attractors	What did you do wrong?

Revised Strategy _____

Passage # _____

Q#	Q type	Attractors	What did you do wrong?

Revised Strategy _____

Chapter 9
Final Preparation

GOAL

- To stay relaxed and focused

9.1 MENTAL PREPARATION

Yes, the MCAT is very important to your future. Medical schools put a lot of emphasis on the MCAT score and therefore you're likely to feel a great deal of pressure and anxiety about the test. We know this. You know this.

More importantly, however, the AAMC knows this. In fact, they are counting on it to "standardize" you. They want you to become nervous about finishing, to wonder how well you are doing compared to the person next to you, and to start watching the clock, rushing, and re-thinking your strategy.

However, having completed your entire CARS preparation with us, you will be much better prepared for the test than most of your peers. Nobody else will have had a more rigorous experience. You've learned about how the test is put together, you've practiced the types of reading strategies needed for the exam, you've evaluated your strengths and weaknesses, and you have un-learned the habits the AAMC is counting on to standardize you. In other words, you are as well-prepared as humanly possible to beat the odds and to score well on the MCAT.

Take time to prepare mentally also. Visualize yourself calm and confident on the day of the exam. See yourself alert and rested. Imagine beginning the test with confidence because you have seen and practiced on dozens of tests just like it.

Your main job in the last week before the exam is to keep yourself relaxed and focused. Don't burn yourself out at the end. Taper off the hours you spend per day on homework as you approach the test day. Continue to practice your stress reduction techniques. Make time for some enjoyable activities.

Here are some suggestions for the day before—and of—the MCAT.

- Do not study the day before the test. Try to do some light exercise (don't overdo it), eat well, watch a funny movie, and get to bed at your regular set time.
- Don't rush. Make sure that you set your alarm—or better still, alarms!—to ensure that you have time to eat a good breakfast, take a shower, and do what you need to do before you leave the house. Most importantly, NO CRAMMING! Aside from doing a quick warm-up (see below), don't open your MCAT books on the day of the test, and don't bring any books or notes with you to the test center.
- Warm up before the test. Get your mind working in the right direction before you leave home. That could mean just reading through some MCAT-like material, or doing a passage or two (best to redo passages you have already done) untimed. You are not trying to learn anything new; you just want to get your mind into "MCAT mode."

- Use music to set a good tone. Have a playlist selected ahead of time. As you get ready to leave the house, or as you make your way to the testing center, use music to either calm down or rev up.
- While waiting to be seated, if other test-takers are gathered together talking frantically about their fears or, on the other hand, about their superior preparation, step away. Don't let anyone make you nervous or negatively influence your calm, confident state of mind.
- Once the test begins, follow the strategy that you have outlined for yourself. Work calmly and methodically. Do not re-think your strategy or your career choice at this point! If you feel that the test is very hard and that you do not have enough time to finish it, then you are doing it correctly—this is not a reason to panic.
- During the test, take the breaks you are given. You have a long testing day ahead of you. If you power through the first couple of sections without taking advantage of your rest periods, you will burn out at some point. Use the breaks to eat and hydrate, but also to clear your mind, refresh your eyes, and shift gears for the next section.
- Put things into perspective—do not overestimate the importance of the results of this particular test. It is not the only thing in your admissions packet. Yes, the test is a big deal, but schools look at a large array of things when evaluating candidates.
- Plan to reward yourself after the test. Make plans with friends or family to do something that you like to do. You deserve a reward!

CHAPTER 9 PRACTICE PASSAGES

Individual Passage Drill

On the following pages are two final individual passages. Do them timed, but with an intense focus on maximizing both your accuracy and your efficiency. After completing the passages and checking your answers, fill out the Individual Passage Logs.

Identify continuing patterns in the mistakes you are making, as well as identifying times when you successfully implemented appropriate strategies.

PASSAGE 1

Basketball, a game of constant movement and a thousand actions, is a difficult game to remember; Leonard Koppett makes this and other excellent points in *All About Basketball*. Football is a series of set plays, as clear in our minds as moves in chess; and the high drama of a baseball game is often distilled in a single pitch, catch, throw, or hit. We remember baseball and football actions as though the players were etched upon our minds like figures on a distant green. In basketball, by contrast, we remember movement, style, flair, but only occasionally a single play. Perhaps we recall the seventh game of the Lakers-Knicks playoff on May 8, 1970, after the Lakers had pounded the Knicks in the sixth game. Willis Reed was injured and out, it seemed, for the season; and we may remember Reed walking stiffly to the floor for that final game just minutes before warm-ups were concluded; remember the sustained ovation; remember his stiff jumps as he put the first two shots of the game through and then had to leave the game in pain; remember that the Knicks, lifted high by his courage, went on to win game seven, bringing to New York basketball a new perspective. But it is hardly ever, even here, individual plays one remembers. A basketball game plays past like a river, like a song.

In basketball as in no other sport, Koppett also notes, the referee is part of the drama. Decisions of the scorer and the timer are critical and affect the outcomes of countless games every year. But the referee is an agent, an actor; he affects the changing tissue of the drama every instant. He cannot call every infraction, but he must control the game. He needs to gain the players' and the crowds' attention, respect, and emotional cohesion. Thus, referees like Pat Kennedy, Sid Borgia, and Mendy Rudolph in the NBA became better known than many of the players. Each blew the whistle in a range of different tones and styles; each had a repertoire of operatic gestures; each had an energy and physical exuberance that added to the total drama. All won respect for coolness under withering emotion.

Basketball players are visible in every action, Koppett notes, and easily singled out by the spectators as football players are not. They handle the ball scores of times and are physically involved in every moment of offense and defense, as baseball players are not. They are subject to many more flukes than baseball or football players, for they pass and run at high speed constantly, forcing dozens of errors, breaks, and opportunities. "Don't shoot!" the coach screams in despair, his voice trailing off to "Nice shot" as he sits down.

Teams move in patterns, in rhythms, at high velocity; one must watch the game abstractly, not focusing on any single individual alone, but upon, as it were, the blurred and intricate designs woven by the paths through which all five together cast a spell upon an opposition. The eye watches five men at once, delighting in their unity, groaning at their lapses of concentration. Yet basketball moves so rapidly and so depends on the versatility of each individual in escaping from the defense intended to contain him that the game cannot be choreographed in advance. Twelve men are constantly in movement (counting two referees), the rebounds of the ball are unpredictable, the occasions for passing or dribbling or shooting must be decided instantaneously; basketball players must be improvisers. They have a score, a melody; each team has its own appropriate tempo, a style of game best suited to its talents; but within and around that general score, each individual is free to elaborate as the spirit moves him. Basketball is jazz: improvisatory, free, individualistic, corporate, sweaty, fast, exulting, screeching, torrid, explosive, exquisitely designed for letting first the trumpet, then the sax, then the drummer, then the trombonist soar away in virtuosic excellence.

The point to stress is the mythic line of basketball: a game of fake and feint and false intention; a game of run, run, run; a game of feet, of swift decision, instantaneous reversal, catlike "moves", cool accuracy, spring and jump. The pace is hot. The rhythm of the game beats with the seconds: a three-second rule, a ten-second rule, a rule to shoot in twenty-four seconds. Only when the ball goes out of bounds, or a point is scored, or a foul is called does the clock stop; the play flows on. Teams do not move by timeless innings as in baseball, nor by set, formal, single plays as in football. Even when a play is called or a pattern is established, the game flows on until a whistle blows, moving relentlessly as lungs heavy and legs weary. It is like jazz.

Material used in this particular passage has been adapted from the following source:

M. Novak, *The Joy of Sports.* © 1955 by Madison Books, Incorporated.

1. We can justifiably infer from this passage that the appearance of Willis Reed at the seventh game of the Lakers-Knicks playoff in 1970:

   A) brought New Yorkers a new perspective on the significance of physical injury.
   B) played some part in the Knicks' victory.
   C) was at the insistence of his coach.
   D) was necessary to the Knick's victory.

2. As it is used in the context of the passage, word "operatic" in paragraph 2 most nearly means:

   A) classical.
   B) musical.
   C) comedic.
   D) histrionic.

3. Which of the following would most *undermine* Koppett's position on the difference between basketball and other sports like football and baseball?

   A) Days after a basketball game, commentators cite a memorable play made in the third quarter.
   B) After a football game, commentators cite a memorable play made in the last few moments of the game.
   C) Following a basketball game, commentators discuss the contrasting playing styles of team members.
   D) After a basketball game, commentators discuss a particular team member's strengths and weaknesses.

4. The author most likely compares basketball to jazz primarily in order to:

   A) claim that because of the fast-paced and unpredictable nature of the sport, basketball players are among the most skilled athletes.
   B) suggest that, like jazz, basketball allows for flexibility and individual excellence within a set format.
   C) assert that basketball is a newer and more dynamic sport than football or baseball.
   D) indicate that basketball requires athletes to be fast.

5. The primary purpose of the passage is most nearly:

   A) to describe the unique characteristics and challenges of the sport of basketball.
   B) to defend the ideas offered in Leonard Koppett's *All About Basketball* against his critics.
   C) to compare and contrast basketball players and musicians.
   D) to describe the crucial role of the referee in a basketball game.

6. The role of the individual athlete during a basketball game as described by the author is most analogous to:

   A) the role of the solo instrumentalist in an orchestra.
   B) the role of the director of a film.
   C) the role of a member of a selective think-tank in a brainstorming session.
   D) the role of an average student in a class.

7. The author describes the reaction of the coach in paragraph 3 in order to do all of the following EXCEPT:

   A) provide an illustration of the various emotions that can be inspired by the game.
   B) contrast the limited role of the coach with the central role of the referee.
   C) indicate a limitation on the role of the coach during the game.
   D) communicate the unpredictable nature of the game.

CHAPTER 9 PRACTICE PASSAGE 2

It is not easy to define Benjamin Franklin's religious and moral beliefs; yet it is important to do so, because they are representative of a large body of men of his time, whose worldly success certainly derived from their beliefs. D. H. Lawrence, who was angered by all success, treats Franklin as a hypocrite who found the rules which lead to success and turned them into a religion. This analysis is certainly false, but even if it were true, it would not take us far enough. For it would not tell us what made Franklin respected by men as different as his American friends, his English enemies, and his French admirers. There was something in Franklin's beliefs which had a symbolic quality for them all.

The charge that Franklin was a hypocrite can be presented simply. He advocated many virtues at a time when he undoubtedly lapsed into some vices. He began his marriage in 1730 by bringing an illegitimate son into the house. Indeed, he may never have been very vigorous in resisting the temptations of the flesh. These lapses from the conventions of family life would not have outraged D. H. Lawrence if they had not been coupled with a certain priggishness in many of the household maxims which Franklin popularized. In 1732, Franklin began publishing *Poor Richard's Almanac*, which was by far the most successful work that he wrote, and in some ways the most influential. Like other almanacs, this is stuffed with those plums of wisdom which most people like to taste and few to digest—"hunger never saw bad bread," and "well done is better than well said." It is these crystallized plums, so eminently homely and homemade, which have made Franklin's beliefs seem commonplace.

But this criticism confuses the manner in which Franklin expressed himself—and expressed himself at all times—with the content of his thought. Franklin had a special gift for putting a thought into a simple and earthy sentence. This is a gift of expression: a rare gift, but Franklin had it to perfection. The gift has a drawback, however. In this form, Franklin's isolated thoughts do indeed wear a simple and sometimes a commonplace air. But it is a crude error to suppose therefore that the totality of Franklin's thoughts, the system into which the isolated thoughts lock and combine, is commonplace. In this respect, the simplicity of Franklin's sentences is as deceptive as the simplicity of Bertrand Russell's, and the outlook which they make up all together is equally complex.

The informality with which Franklin wrote and spoke is, however, just to his thought in one respect: he was opposed to formality and rigidity of belief. It is not merely that he did not care for the fine points of dogma; he thought it wrong in principle to wish to formulate religion in fine points. He did

not acknowledge any sectarian monopoly of truth. For example, when, at the age of 83, he stated his belief in God, he coupled it with another belief, "that the most acceptable service we render Him is doing good to His other children."

At bottom, it is this tolerance in Franklin's make-up which we must understand. He was tolerant of others because he recognized in them the same humanity that he knew in himself. He never hid his motives from himself, but neither did he belittle the motives of others. We should recognize him as honest because he judges others exactly as he judges himself, with a realistic and generous sense of what can be expected of human beings. Sustained by humanity, he could gain the respect of those as religiously diverse as the anticlerical Tom Paine and the evangelist George Whitefield.

Material used in this particular passage has been adapted from the following source:
J. Bronowski and Bruce Mazlish, *The Western Intellectual Tradition.* ©1960 by HarperCollins Publishers.

1. Which of the following statements best expresses the main point of the passage?

A) Benjamin Franklin's writings were distinctive in his day for arguing against religious dogma and in favor of tolerance, thereby attracting much criticism from other authors.
B) The simplicity of Benjamin Franklin's writing, although somewhat at odds with the sophistication of his thought, was connected to the broad-mindedness that gained him the respect of many of his contemporaries.
C) Despite being accused of hypocrisy, Benjamin Franklin became successful because of his gift for simple speech and to his impressive tolerance.
D) Benjamin Franklin's deep insights into moral and religious questions, although gaining him the respect of many, contrasted sharply with the simplicity of his writing style.

2. It is reasonable to infer from the passage that D. H. Lawrence:

A) was more critical of Franklin's writings than of his behavior.
B) upheld in his own household and writings the accepted conventions of family life.
C) was envious of Benjamin Franklin's wealth and popularity.
D) believed that successful religions are usually hypocritical.

3. In the context of the passage, the word "vigorous" most nearly signifies:

A) healthy.
B) vociferous.
C) diligent.
D) tolerant.

4. According the passage, the relationship of Franklin's writing style to his ideas is most analogous to which of the following?

A) A symphony which alternates between fast and slow sections.
B) An intricate painting composed entirely of basic geometric shapes.
C) A novel advocating virtues that the author does not uphold in his own personal life.
D) A movie showing the same events from different perspectives, each of which is equally valid.

5. The authors probably quote Franklin in paragraph 2 in order to:

A) illustrate his simple and unpretentious style.
B) contrast Franklin's and Lawrence's moral outlook.
C) deride the trite expressions common to his more popular writings.
D) emphasize his preference for action over speech.

6. Which of the following statements, if true, would most call into question the authors' characterization of Benjamin Franklin's attitude towards religion?

A) Although Franklin often attended religious services, he did not claim formal membership in any religious institution.
B) Like D. H. Lawrence, Franklin was greatly intrigued by Eastern religions, helping to bring Buddhist and Hindu lecturers to Boston and Philadelphia.
C) Franklin was influential in removing "sacred and undeniable" from Thomas Jefferson's first draft of the Declaration of Independence and in replacing these words with "self-evident."
D) Active with the Freemasons, Franklin published pamphlets denouncing the beliefs of the Catholic Church.

7. It may be inferred from the passage that each of the following describes Benjamin Franklin's writings EXCEPT:

A) they attracted some readership outside the United States.
B) they at times addressed controversial religious topics.
C) they were notable for their somewhat commonplace style.
D) their style reflected in a certain fashion Franklin's attitude towards religion.

SOLUTIONS TO CHAPTER 9 PRACTICE PASSAGE 1

1. **B**   This is an Inference question.
    A: No. While the author does ask us to "remember that the Knicks, lifted high by his courage, went on to win game seven, bringing to New York basketball a new perspective," choice A goes too far by appending the idea of "physical injury" to that new perspective.
    B: Yes. The author says in paragraph 1 that "the Knicks, lifted high by his courage, went on to win game seven."
    C: No. This choice goes too far, since we do not know from the passage what Reed's motive was, or whether or not the coach was involved in his decision to play.
    D: No. The word "necessary" makes this choice too strong. Remember that when dealing with inferences, it is best to stick with answers that do not stray too far from the passage. It is impossible to say with certainty that the Knicks would have lost had it not been for Reed's appearance. This makes B a better supported answer than choice D.

2. **D**   This is a an Inference question.
    A: No. While "classical" as in classical music or as in traditional or elegant (which are other possible interpretations of the word "classical") may come to your mind when you think of opera, there is nothing in the passage to support this interpretation of the word.
    B: No. As in choice A, this may fit your own interpretation of "operatic," but there isn't anything in this part of the passage to suggest a connection or relationship to music.
    C: No. "Comedic" does not fit the author's description of the referees as respected, cool under pressure, and dramatic. It also doesn't fit the author's relatively serious tone in this passage.
    D: Yes. Be careful not to eliminate a word just because you don't know what it means. "Histrionic" is a synonym for "dramatic" and thus best fits the author's context.

3. **A**   This is a Weaken question.
    A: Yes. Koppett posits in paragraph 1 that "basketball, a game of constant movement and a thousand actions, is a difficult game to remember" and that "it is hardly ever...individual plays that one remembers." Because it is fast-paced and relies on action from multiple players, the author of the passage points out, fewer single plays stick out in our minds. In order to weaken Koppett's position, our credited response should describe a memorable singular moment. Choice A does this. While this choice doesn't destroy Koppett's argument, it is the only one of the four answers that is at all inconsistent with it.
    B: No. Choice B describes a memorable moment in a football game, in a way that is consistent with Koppett's claim about the difference between basketball and football.
    C: No. This answer actually strengthens Koppett's position, since the passage points out that we remember the "movement, style, [and] flair" of basketball players (paragraph 1).
    D: No. As in choice C, this answer is consistent, not inconsistent. According to paragraph 4, "the versatility of each individual" is crucial, and "each individual is free to elaborate as the spirit moves him." Therefore, a discussion of an individual's strengths and weaknesses would fit with Koppett's position.

4. **B**   This is a Structure question.
    A: No. This choice goes too far, since the author never tells us baseball and football are not challenging in their own way.
    B: Yes. The author tells us that "basketball players must be improvisers. They have a score, a melody; each team has its own appropriate tempo, a style of game best suited to its talents; but within and around that general score, each individual is free to elaborate as the spirit moves him" (paragraph 4). This answer choice is the best paraphrase of this idea.

C: No. This option takes the metaphor too literally and is too judgmental in tone towards football and baseball. Furthermore, nothing in the passage suggests that basketball is a newer sport.

D: No. While the author does mention speed in paragraph 4, this is not the primary purpose of the metaphor, but only one of many aspects within it. The main theme of the comparison is how basketball, like jazz, relies on individual action and creativity within the context of a group or team endeavor.

5.   **A**   This is a Main Idea/Primary Purpose question.

A: **Yes. This choice can include all of the author's major points, without going beyond the scope of the passage.**

B: No. This option is too narrow; also, the author never makes mention of any critics of Koppett's ideas.

C: No. This answer might be tempting, since so much of the passage is devoted to comparing basketball and jazz. But since the answer frames it in terms of "comparing and contrasting basketball players and musicians," it misrepresents the focus of the passage, which is on the sport of basketball itself not just the players.

D: No. This choice is too narrow. Referees are discussed only in paragraphs 2 and 4, and the rest of the passage isn't written in support of the author's claims about referees in those paragraphs.

6.   **C**   This is an Analogy question.

A: No. The soloist may be virtuosic, but not an equal member of a team. This choice also fails to capture the theme of constant interaction in the passage.

B: No. The director of a film is in charge of the other "players" rather than being on equal footing with the rest of the team.

C: **Yes. Novak describes basketball players as all being virtuosic in their own way, but working together, all players being equally necessary to success. A member of a think tank involved in a brainstorming session would play a similar role, including the constant interaction and responsiveness to new scenarios that is described in the passage.**

D: No. We don't have any indication in this choice that an average student would be virtuosic in his or her own way, and yet in constant interaction with the rest of the class, improvising as the class progressed in unpredictable ways.

7.   **B**   This is a Structure/EXCEPT question.

A: No. This choice is supported by the passage. The coach's reaction demonstrates varied emotions in response to the unexpected twists and turns of the game.

B: **Yes. This choice is not supported by the passage, and so is the correct answer to an EXCEPT question. This answer is too extreme; we don't know from the passage that the coach's role overall is limited, just that at times the coach's instructions are invalidated by rapid changes in the game as it plays out. Also, the there is no suggestion in the passage that the purpose of the reference is to contrast the role of the coach with that of the referee in terms of their relative importance.**

C: No. This statement is supported by the passage. While we don't know that the coach plays a limited role overall, his or her role during the game is constrained, such that the command "Don't shoot" is invalidated by the rapidly changing nature of play on the court.

D: No. This statement is supported by the passage. The coach's scream of "Don't shoot" is contradicted by an unpredictable shift in the game which leads to a successful shot.

SOLUTIONS TO CHAPTER 9 PRACTICE PASSAGE 2

1. **B** This is a Main Idea/Primary Purpose question.

   A: No. This choice may be eliminated because, although Franklin and Lawrence are contrasted, the passage makes no general claim that Franklin's writings were distinctive or much criticized. In fact, paragraph 1 suggests that his beliefs were shared by a wide range of other people.

   B: Yes. Both paragraphs 1 and 5 address the respect with which Franklin was viewed. Franklin's simple writing style also relates to the tolerance (paragraph 4) which the authors describe as central to his character.

   C: No. The only reference to Franklin's success is in paragraph 1, which suggests that his worldly success derived from his beliefs. While tolerance may have been one of these beliefs, the passage as a whole is not about the reasons for his success in life, but about the beliefs themselves, and how they related to his style of writing.

   D: No. This choice is attractive in appearing to draw on many components of the passage. However, the authors do not claim that Franklin had deep insights into religious and moral questions. Complexity of thought (paragraph 3) is not necessarily the same as deep insight. Furthermore, this answer choice says nothing about Franklin's tolerance, which is a major theme in the passage. Finally, it was this complexity, not the deepness of his insight, which contrasted with Franklin's simple writing style.

2. **A** This is an Inference question.

   A: Yes. Paragraph 2 emphasizes that D. H. Lawrence was not outraged by Franklin's behavior but by the apparent hypocrisy of his publications, which the authors describe as described as "priggish" and "commonplace" in paragraph 2.

   B: No. We know nothing of Lawrence's own family life.

   C: No. Like choice B, this reaches beyond the available information since, although Lawrence was angered by success, there is nothing in the passage to indicate envy.

   D: No. This answer may be attractive because it draws on language in paragraph 1. However, Lawrence believed Franklin was hypocritical in his success; we don't know how Lawrence felt about "successful religions" in general.

3. **C** This is an Inference question.

   A: No. "Healthy" may be one literal definition of "vigorous," but it doesn't fit in the context of the passage, which is about Franklin's lack of will rather than his health.

   B: No. "Vociferous" means outspoken. The issue in the passage is about Franklin's behavior, not his expressed opinions (which were at odds with his behavior).

   C: Yes. The authors suggest that Franklin's lapses were somewhat common and that Franklin did not make any great effort to uphold family norms.

   D: No. Tolerance is not discussed until paragraph 5, and it is not directly relevant to this discussion of Franklin's failures to live up to his own standards of virtue in his private life.

4. **B** This is an Analogy question.

   A: No. There is no alternation or back and forth (that is, first one, then the other, then back again to the first) between Franklin's style and ideas.

   B: Yes. The principle relationship (paragraph 3) is that Franklin's simple words, taken singly, may deceptively mask the complexity of his overall thought.

C: No. This choice is attractive because it points to the charge of hypocrisy brought against him in paragraph 2. However, the question asks about the relationship between Franklin's style and his beliefs, not about a relationship between his beliefs and his private life.

D: No. While this choice may reflect Franklin's tolerance towards other beliefs (paragraphs 4 and 5), it doesn't match the relationship between his writing style and his beliefs.

5.   **A**   This is a Structure question.

   A: Yes. These words make Franklin's beliefs seem commonplace or simple.

   B: No. There is no reference to different moral positions in this paragraph.

   C: No. While the authors do say that Franklin's maxims show a certain "priggishness" and commonplace nature, the passage goes on in paragraph 3 to show that the simple and commonplace nature of Franklin's individual statements hides to some extent the true complexity of his thought. Therefore, the authors are not deriding or mocking his expressions, or calling them "trite" or trivial.

   D: No. Although this is a paraphrase of the second maxim, it does not relate to the authors' purpose in including the quotation, which is to illustrate the simplicity of Franklin's sayings.

6.   **D**   This is a Weaken question.

   A: No. The authors make no claim concerning Franklin's formal affiliation. The passage's characterization of Franklin's attitude toward religion, or of his self-professed "belief in God," doesn't rest on an assumption that Franklin was affiliated with a particular church.

   B: No. This choice would strengthen, not weaken, the authors' claim that Franklin was tolerant towards other religious beliefs.

   C: No. This answer is consistent with the authors' claim that Franklin denied any "sectarian monopoly of truth" and that he resisted dogma (paragraph 4).

   D: Yes. The authors characterize Franklin's attitude as tolerant of other beliefs. As part of this argument, the authors state that Franklin, because of his tolerance, was respected by other diverse religious figures (paragraph 5). If Franklin denounced the beliefs of the Catholic Church, this would significantly undermine the authors' characterization. Notice the difference between choice C and choice D. Choice C involves resistance to incorporating language that suggests religious dogma into the Declaration, but does not involve criticizing any particular beliefs themselves.

7.   **B**   This is an Inference/EXCEPT question.

   A: No. Paragraph 1 demonstrates that Franklin's work was known internationally.

   B: Yes. Although Franklin spoke of God (paragraph 4), there is no evidence that his writings addressed religious topics, especially controversial religious topics. Also, the fact that D.H. Lawrence claimed that Franklin "found the rules which lead to success and turned them into a religion" (paragraph 1) can't be interpreted to mean that Franklin literally wrote about religion itself. Because you cannot infer this answer to be true based on the passage, it is the correct answer to an EXCEPT question.

   C: No. Their commonplace style is discussed in paragraphs 2 and 3. Note the more moderate wording of this choice as compared to choice B.

   D: No. This is a paraphrase of the first sentence of paragraph 4. Note the difference between choice B and choice D. Choice D says that the style of Franklin's writings reflected religious attitudes, but choice B states that his writings directly addressed religious topics.

Individual Passage Log

Passage # _____   Time spent on passage _____

Q#	Q type	Attractors	What did you do wrong?

Revised Strategy _____

Passage # _____   Time spent on passage _____

Q#	Q type	Attractors	What did you do wrong?

Revised Strategy _____

CARS Appendix

A.1 APPLYING CARS TECHNIQUES TO THE SCIENCE PASSAGES

The challenges posed by the science sections of the MCAT differ in a number of important ways from those posed by the CARS section. Indeed, the differences must seem all too obvious. Most striking is the amount of information you need to bring with you to the test; even the brightest and most alert reader would be lost in Physics or Biology without an understanding of the basic scientific principles and a good grasp of the fundamental definitions and nomenclature. It's also the case that you must engage in a lot more problem-solving for the sciences than you do for CARS, where your primary task is to *find* answers rather than to calculate them. CARS passages tell you almost everything you need to know, while the science passages require you to know much more before you read them.

Nevertheless, there's a great deal of overlap in the skills required to do well on these apparently dissimilar sections. *You will not score very high in the sciences if you merely try to plug numbers into formulas or to spit back information that you've stuffed into your memory; you also need to be able to draw inferences from the passages, to extrapolate answers from the information provided to you.* You need to work quickly, wasting no time on calculating answers that can be taken directly from the text—or, conversely, on searching a passage for information that isn't there. Most important, you need to mobilize your scientific "common sense," your intuitive understanding of what is and isn't likely to be true for any described scenario involving the physical world. You also need to apply that common sense to the answer choices, eliminating those that are not likely ever to be true. For all of these tasks—looking for specific information, drawing inferences, evaluating the plausibility of answer choices—your CARS skills will be invaluable.

In short, to do well on the MCAT, you need to think both scientifically *and* strategically. Many people feel that they *must* work out the answer to every last question. There is something very noble in this endeavor, but it is not smart test-taking. Remember: you don't get extra points for the tougher questions. Use your knowledge of the test to help you find the correct answers.

For one thing, you should know when the passage information can help you and when it cannot. There are, broadly speaking, three types of MCAT science questions.

1) **Memory ("Pure Science") Questions**
   These are based entirely on information that you bring with you to the test; there is nothing in the passage that will help you solve them, or, there is no passage attached to the questions.
2) **Explicit ("Retrieval") Questions**
   Less common than the other two question types, these require only that you *find* an answer in the passage.
3) **Implicit ("Application") Questions**
   The most common question type, these require you to apply your scientific knowledge to the information in the passage.

Recognizing the question types will affect your solution strategy. You should answer all Explicit/Retrieval questions. Their answers are right in the passage; just use the same techniques you would for CARS Retrieval questions, checking your final answer choice to make sure that it matches the information in the passage.

Implicit/Application questions will vary in difficulty, depending on the amount and type of outside information involved. Some will require that you apply a quite basic principle; for example, that gases expand as they warm. Others call for more precise knowledge of, say, the function of a particular endocrine gland. Most questions will be Implicit or a hybrid of Implicit and Explicit (even Explicit/Retrieval questions require some knowledge to recognize the answer). Your strategy here is to determine how much help the passage will give you, and to pass quickly over those questions for which you lack sufficient outside knowledge.

Finally, Memory/"Pure Science" questions are freestanding, or they deal with the passage *topic* but refer only nominally to the passage itself. You can skip a pure science question if you cannot work out the answer, coming back to it at the end of the section if you have time. Such a strategy doesn't work for CARS, because the questions are so closely based on the passages, and because once you've left a passage, you will most likely forget most of it. Pure Science questions, however, don't rely on context and can be solved at any point.

Solutions to Some Sample Passages

The following pages contain four passages from General Chemistry, Physics, Biology, and Psychology/Sociology and outline the ways in which you can use CARS strategies to tackles these types of passages. Note that these techniques are less useful for Organic Chemistry passages, which tend to have much less text, often consisting of little more than a few chemical equations. Solutions to all four passages can be found at the end of this Appendix.

MCAT G-Chem Drill: Solubility

Oxygen is transported from the lungs to the capillaries where it is released into the tissues. The oxygen in the circulatory system of mammals is bound to hemoglobin, a protein found in red blood cells.

Hemoglobin has a complex quaternary structure since it is composed of four separate polypeptide chains. Each polypeptide serves as a giant ligand for the single iron(II)-heme unit, the location of oxygen fixation. The oxygen-binding strength of the heme unit and transport efficiency are directly related to blood pH level.

Unlike oxygen, the carbon dioxide which is released into the capillaries by the surrounding tissue is transported by two different mechanisms. Foremost, carbon dioxide is rather soluble in water due to the following equilibria:

$$(1) \quad CO_2 + H_2O \rightleftharpoons H_2CO_3$$

$$(2) \quad H_2CO_3 \rightleftharpoons H^+ + HCO_3^-$$

Therefore, some carbon dioxide immediately dissolves into the blood plasma and is transported to the lungs as bicarbonate ion. Most mammals have an enzyme, carbonic anhydrase, to catalyze Reaction (1), because under normal conditions, CO_2 and carbonic acid cannot reach equilibrium fast enough for efficient transport.

In the second mechanism, CO_2 may react with the N-terminus of the protein chains of hemoglobin, forming a carbamate functional group:

$$(3) \; Hb-NH_2 = CO_2 \rightleftharpoons Hb-NHCOO^- + H^+$$

Once in the lungs, the Hb-carbamate decomposes to release CO_2, and Hb NH_2 is restored.

1. Carbon dioxide is much more soluble in water than is oxygen. Why?

A) Oxygen has a greater dipole moment.
B) Carbon dioxide has a greater dipole moment than oxygen.
C) Carbon dioxide is a polar molecule.
D) Carbon dioxide is reactive to nucleophilic attack.

2. The expiration of CO_2 from the bloodstream in the lungs:

A) increases blood pH.
B) decreases blood pH.
C) decreases the oxygen content of the blood.
D) None of the above

3. Acidosis—a condition characterized by a decrease in blood pH—rapidly develops after cardiac arrest because tissues continue to load the capillary plasma with more and more CO_2. If the blood pH is not buffered (reset to normal), the patient may die, even after cardiac revival. Why?

A) Too much CO_2 can cause a cell's lipid bilayer to decompose.
B) High concentrations of bicarbonate can cause insoluble salts to precipitate out of the plasma.
C) The nervous system can no longer function properly.
D) Hemoglobin cannot effectively transport O_2.

4. If the enzyme carbonic anhydrase were added to a glass of soda pop which had been allowed to reach equilibrium with the atmosphere, it would:

A) produce a large number of carbon dioxide bubbles.
B) produce a large amount of oxygen.
C) form more carbonic acid.
D) have no effect on the equilibrium.

5. Which one of the following will decrease the solubility of CO_2 in water?

A) Increasing the external pressure of CO_2
B) Increasing the temperature of the water
C) Increasing the pH of the water
D) None of the above

6. What is the electron configuration of the iron(II) ion?

A) $[Ar] \, 3d^6$
B) $[Ar] \, 4s^2 \, 3d^4$
C) $[Ar] \, 4s^2 \, 3d^6$
D) $[Ar] \, 4s^2 \, 3p^{10}$

CARS Strategies for MCAT G-Chem Drill: Solubility

This passage deals with aspects of oxygen transport in the blood. It consists of four paragraphs, two of which include chemical reactions. Although it begins by referring to hemoglobin (paragraphs 1 and 2), the bulk of the questions have to do with plasma CO_2.

1) Oxygen/hemoglobin introduction
2) Structure and functionality of hemoglobin
3) Chemical reactions re: CO_2 solubility (especially re: carbonic acid)
4) CO_2/hemoglobin reaction

1. Nominally, a **Memory** question—but you can make a good guess by treating this as a Retrieval question. See 3: "Foremost, carbon dioxide is rather soluble in water *because of* the following equilibrium reactions…" [emphasis added]. Since the passage states that the solubility of carbon dioxide is due to a chemical reaction, look for an answer choice that refers to a chemical reaction. This leads you to the correct answer, which is D.

2. An unusual example of an **Explicit** question: the answer is really in the next question! You are asked what happens to the blood when CO_2 is expired by the lungs. Question 3 tells you that when plasma CO_2 goes up, blood pH goes down. Hence, when CO_2 goes down (via the lungs), blood pH must go up. This gives you A, the correct answer.

3. See paragraph 2: O_2 binding and transport is proportional to blood pH. Thus low pH = low oxygen transport = a dead person (answer choice D, in other words). This is mostly an **Explicit** question.

4. See paragraph 3: **Apply** your knowledge of what "equilibrium" means to the information that carbonic anhydrase speeds up the reaction—until it reaches equilibrium.

5. **Memory:** The answer comes only from your own outside knowledge, not from passage information.

6. **Memory:** The answer comes only from your own outside knowledge, not from passage information.

MCAT Physics Drill: Force

Near the surface of the earth, the density of air is approximately 1.2 kg/m³. A hot-air balloon with total mass M (including passengers) and volume V will float motionless if there is no wind and the buoyant force (magnitude F_B) due to the air is equal to the weight of the balloon and passengers: $F_B = Mg$, where g is the magnitude of the acceleration due to gravity near the surface of the Earth.

The strength of the buoyant force may be altered by heating the air inside the balloon, thereby changing its volume. The total weight of the balloon may be decreased by equipping the balloon with sandbags that can be dropped to the ground.

Many hot-air balloons are equipped with propellers that drive air backward and allow the balloon to travel horizontally. All balloons have a maximum achievable volume which depends on the extent to which the air inside can be heated as well as on the elastic limits of the material used to construct the balloon.

1. A balloon, moving upward and eastward, casts a shadow that moves along the ground at a speed of 10 m/s. What is the balloon's total speed if its velocity vector makes an angle of 60° with the horizontal?

A) 5 m/s
B) 17 m/s
C) 20 m/s
D) 34 m/s

2. A balloon of total mass M sits motionless 40 m above the ground. A sandbag of mass m is dropped out of the balloon. What is then the net force on the balloon?

A) Mg
B) $(M - m)g$
C) mg
D) $(M + m)g$

3. Two unladen hot-air balloons are weighed and measured. Their masses and volumes are as follows:

   Balloon I: Mass = 1200 kg; Volume = 1600 m³

   Balloon II: Mass = 1100 kg; Volume = 1200 m³

   Which of these balloons could be used to carry four people whose average mass is 100 kg each?

A) I only
B) II only
C) I and II
D) Neither balloon could carry such a load.

4. Which of the following best illustrates the flow of air inside a closed-top balloon as the air is heated by a flame directly beneath the opening at the base of the balloon?

A)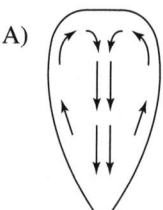

B)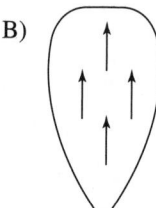

C)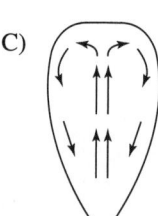

D)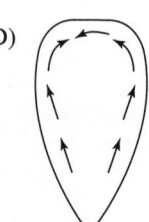

5. A balloon is moving upward at constant velocity. Which one of the following equations involved the magnitudes of the gravitational force, F_G, the drag forces due to air resistance, F_D, and the buoyant force of the air, F_B, is correct?

A) $F_D + F_B > F_G$
B) $F_D + F_B = F_G$
C) $F_D + F_G < F_B$
D) $F_D + F_G = F_B$

6. A balloon for a county fair is designed to carry four 100-kg passengers when it is expanded to its maximum volume. The designers assumed the balloon would operate in ordinary spring temperatures. If, on the day of the fair, the temperature reaches a record-breaking maximum:

A) the balloon will not be able to achieve its maximum volume.
B) more sandbags will be needed for proper operation of the balloon.
C) the total weight the balloon is able to carry will be reduced.
D) once in flight, the balloon cannot be lowered until the ambient temperature drops.

7. A balloon has a mass of 1500 kg with no passengers. A typical passenger weighs 100 kg. A balloon with 5 passengers is floating motionless high above the ground when a 2 kg pelican lands on the balloon. Making which of the following adjustments would allow the balloon to remain floating motionless?

A) Increase the volume of the balloon by 0.1%
B) Slightly cool the air in the balloon
C) Drop a 4-kg sandbag from the balloon
D) None of the above

8. Four 100-kg people are holding a 1200-kg inflated balloon by means of four ropes. Three people let go and the balloon accelerates upward at 2 m/s^2. What is the tension in the rope that the last person is holding?

A) 200 N
B) 400 N
C) 800 N
D) 1200 N

CARS Strategies for MCAT Physics Drill: Force

Three short paragraphs about hot-air balloons. Notice that almost all of the useful information is contained in paragraph 1.

1) Useful stuff: density of air, forces acting on the balloon, etc.
2) How to make a balloon go up (gee, Toto…)
3) Balloon propellers, elasticity

1. **Memory.** It doesn't matter if it's a balloon, a pelican, or the space shuttle that's moving upward and eastward; just mobilize your math here.

2. **Implicit.** Use your understanding of "net force" and apply it to paragraph 1. If it's motionless, there's no net force. If you dump a sandbag of mass m, what has changed?

3. **Implicit/Explicit.** Be canny about this one. You're given the density of air. You aren't given any other information (e.g., the mass of air *inside* the balloon, the temperature of the air inside or outside of the balloon, etc.). Don't panic, thinking this is one of those questions where you need to remember some complicated physics formula or something. With what you've been given, you must be able to answer this one by calculating the mass of air displaced by the balloon, and then seeing if it's more or less than the combined mass of the balloon and the passengers.

4. **Memory.** Or pure common sense: where is the hot air going to go? And what is it going to do when it gets there? As for A, what would make the stream of hot air split into two? As for D, why would the air circulate counterclockwise as opposed to clockwise?

5. **Implicit.** See paragraph 1 and note that answer choices A and B can't be right because F_G and F_D have to go on the same side of the equation.

6. **Implicit.** Use your knowledge of what happens to air when it gets hot (it expands and its density decreases) to answer this one.

7. **Implicit**—but a little common sense would help, too. B makes no sense; you know what happens to balloons as they cool and shrink. C makes no sense because the pelican only weighs 2 kg. As often happens, you're left with two plausible answer choices—and, in a time crunch, you might want to abandon the calculations and figure that there *is* a way to adjust to one crummy bird landing on the balloon, so answer choice D is rather unlikely.

8. **Memory.** The answer cannot be found in the passage.

MCAT Biology Drill: Embryology

The events that contribute to successful fertilization have been intensively studied in the soil nematode *Caenorhabditis elegans*. This organism has several advantages for developmental biology. First, at 1 mm in length, it is small enough to easily culture, and yet the embryos are large enough to see under a compound microscope. Second, its three-day life cycle makes it ideal for genetic studies. Third, *C. elegans* is a self-fertilizing hermaphroditic species—its two sexes are 1) male and 2) self-replicating hermaphrodite. Heterozygous mutations can easily be made homozygous by allowing the hermaphrodites to self-fertilize. Finally the males are missing an X chromosome, and can thus be crossed to normal XX hermaphrodites, facilitating genetic studies.

The entire developmental process from fertilization to adulthood can be observed under the compound microscope. Fertilization takes place in the hermaphrodites as the oocyte passes through the spermatheca, which is where the sperm are stored. If the embryos are collected at this point, the following events can be observed in the light microscope: After the entry of the sperm into the posterior end of the egg, the oocyte nucleus, having been suspended in diakinesis of meiotic prophase I, now completes the meiotic divisions. The excess genetic material is extruded as polar bodies, and the eggshell is secreted, forming an impermeable barrier that protects the developing embryo. The cytoplasmic rearrangements that follow begin with the female pronucleus migrating toward the male pronucleus. A pseudocleavage is observed, where a cleavage furrow appears but disappears without cell division. The pronuclei fuse in the posterior end of the cell, rotate, then move toward the center. At this point, the nucleus of the embryo is formed. Finally, the first division occurs, producing a smaller posterior (P) cell and a larger anterior cell (AB).

Another event that can be observed is the migration of granules from the cytoplasm of the fertilized embryo into the P cell — hence their name, P-granules. As the zygote develops by mitosis into a full organism, the P-granules become sequestered by the cells destined to become the germ line. The function of the P-granules is not known. Exposing the developing embryos to microtubule inhibitors (such as colcemid) blocks the migration of the pronuclei, but does not affect P-granule movement. The inhibitor of actin polymerization, cytochalasin B, has the opposite effect, preventing P-granule segregation, but allowing pronuclei to migrate. The entire process of fertilization, from entry of the sperm to the first cell division, takes about 35 minutes.

Material used in this particular passage has been adapted from the following source:

W.B. Wood, *The Nematode, Caenorhabditis elegans,* (Cold Spring Harbor Monograph Series 17), © 1988 by Cold Spring Harbor Laboratory Press.

1. Which of the following would be the least appropriate organism for studying developmental processes such as fertilization and the ensuing cell divisions?

A) The bacterium, *Escherichia coli*
B) The fruit fly, *Drosophila melanogaster*
C) The African clawed toad, *Xenopus laevis*
D) The human being, *Homo sapiens*

2. Since male nematodes arise as a result of nondisjunction in the XX hermaphrodite, what is their genotype?

A) XY
B) XXX
C) XO
D) XYY

3. What is the ploidy of the fertilized egg?

A) *n*
B) 2*n*
C) 3*n*
D) 4*n*

4. The spermatheca is where:

A) the progenitor cells of the sperm enter meiosis.
B) sperm are stored in the hermaphrodite.
C) sperm received their protein coat.
D) sperm are stored in the males.

5. Which one of the following accurately describes pseudocleavage?

A) The embryo divides into two cells, which then fuse.
B) A cleavage furrow forms then disappears.
C) A cell membrane begins to form then disappears.
D) Polar bodies are formed.

6. When the pronuclei fuse, which of the following event(s) must occur for cell division to proceed?

    I.   Homologous chromosomes pair
    II.   Recombination events occur
    III. Nuclear membranes are reorganized

A) I only
B) I and II only
C) III only
D) I, II, and III

7. The effects of colcemid and cytochalasin B on the embryo suggest that:

    I.   Microfilaments are involved in P-granule migration.
    II.   Microfilaments are involved in pronuclear migrations.
    III. Microtubules are involved in pronuclear migrations.
    IV. Microtubules are involved in P-granules migration.

A) I and III only
B) I and IV only
C) II and III only
D) II and IV only

CARS Strategies for MCAT Biology Drill: Embryology

This passage is long and dense; let's map it. There are only three paragraphs here, but each is long and filled with detail. Annotate this passage so that you can find where important categories of information begin and end.

1) Nematode sex
   Research advantages:
   - size
   - 3-day life cycle
   - self-fertilizing hermaphrodite
   - males missing X chromosome
2) Development from fertilization to adulthood
   Map separate events after *oocyte* passes through *spermatheca*
3) Migration of P-granules
   (Note: "P cell" is defined at the end of paragraph 2)

1. **Memory.** Don't sweat this one: how much fertilizing do bacteria do?

2. **Explicit.** See paragraph 1: the hermaphrodite is XX, and the male is missing an X chromosome; $2 - 1 = ?$

3. **Implicit.** Apply your knowledge of the meaning of "ploidy" and "diakinesis of meiotic prophase I" to the information in paragraph 2.

4. **Explicit.** You can read the definition of "spermatheca" exactly from paragraph 2.

5. **Explicit.** "pseudocleavage" is defined in paragraph 2.

6. **Implicit.**

7. **Implicit/Explicit.** See paragraph 3: everything is spelled out for you except the role of microfilaments in pronuclear migration.

MCAT Psychology/Sociology Drill: Global Health Trends

Across the globe, income and health outcomes are positively correlated. As gross domestic product (GDP) increases, so do certain standard measures of a population's health (such as longevity), while others (such as infant mortality) decrease. Taking multiple standard measures into account, each country is assigned an overall health score, meant to use aggregate health data to reflect the population's general health (or, as a predictor of any given individual's health). The wealthiest countries consistently receive the highest overall health scores, while the poorest countries consistently receive the lowest. This can also be seen at the individual level; as a general rule, the lower a person or family's income, the more likely they are to develop certain health problems and the less likely they are to have access to care for these problems.

Obesity is one of the few measures that defies this global health trend. In recent years, obesity rates have been skyrocketing in the countries with the highest GDPs. The most extreme example of this is the United States, which has an obesity rate that far exceeds every other country (Figure 1). Many experts predict that by the year 2020, obesity (and obesity-related health problems) will trump cancer and heart disease as the number one risk factor for premature death in the U.S. And in almost all cases, obesity is completely preventable.

Country	GDP per capita in thousands (converted to U.S. dollars)	% population with BMI > 30 in 2012
United States	55.6	31.5
Canada	46.0	19.4
Sweden	40.4	12.3
Belgium	38.3	15.8
South Africa	10.1	20.6
China	6.5	10.3
India	1.5	9.3

Figure 1 Prosperity (measured by Gross Domestic Product or GDP in U.S. dollars) and obesity (measured by percent of the population exceeding a BMI of 30) in selected countries in 2012

Body Mass Index (BMI) is used as a rough, non-invasive way to assess body fat. BMI is calculated using weight and height, and is a fairly reliable indicator of body fat for most people. For U.S. adults, a BMI of less than 18.5 corresponds to "underweight status;" between 18.5 and 24.9 corresponds

to "normal weight status;" between 25.0 and 29.9 corresponds to "overweight status;" and a BMI over 30 is considered obese. The U.S. National Health Statistics Center conducted a 30-year longitudinal study of BMI rates for adults and children per state based on a representative sample of the total population for each state. These data were also used to calculate national averages. The state with the highest rate of adult and childhood obesity is Mississippi, and the state with the lowest rate of adult and childhood obesity is Colorado (Figure 2).

Percentage of population with BMI >30 from 1980 to 2010

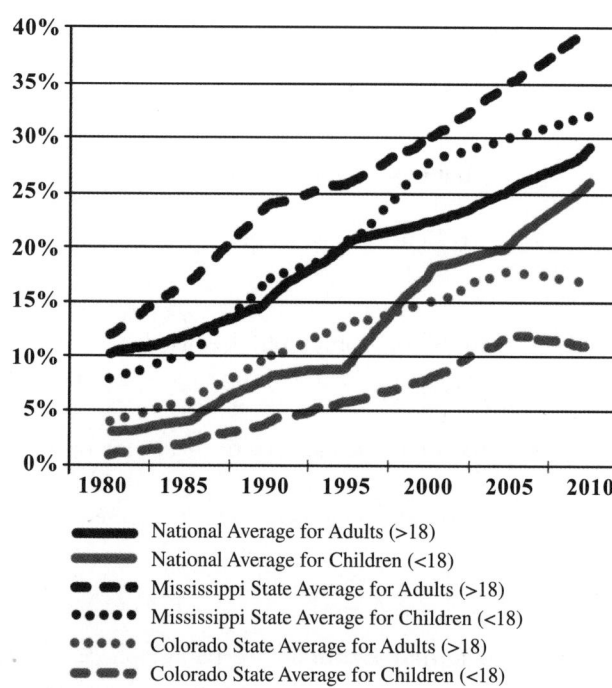

Figure 2 Percentage of the population with a BMI over 30 for the state with the highest rates of obesity (Mississippi), lowest rates of obesity (Colorado), and the national averages, from 1980 to 2010.

Based on this study, the Mississippi Department of Health implemented mandatory health screenings for third graders and eighth graders in 2011. Preliminary data suggest that third graders are more than twice as likely to be diagnosed with type-II diabetes, and about three times as likely to be diagnosed with other hormonal imbalances, when compared to national health statistics for children the same age. Eighth graders are almost four times as likely to be diagnosed with type-II diabetes and over five times as likely to be diagnosed with other hormonal imbalances compared to national health statistics for children the same age. Based on these preliminary results, the state of Mississippi is considering implementing new laws concerning school-based activity minimums and school lunch calorie maximums.

1. Catecholamine derivatives that act as agonists for a specific neuronal receptor have been shown to help prevent obesity in many severely overweight patients. These derivatives also promote neuroprotection from Parkinson's disease. What is a possible mechanism of action for this process?

A) For people suffering from a food addiction, eating excessive high fat food triggers the dopamine reward system in the brain (similar to a drug addict). The catecholamine derivative acts as an agonist for dopamine, thus stimulating the dopamine reward center without the presence of food, and leading to a decrease in overeating.

B) Catecholamine derivatives stimulate the parasympathetic nervous system, thus increasing the activity of the gut. Therefore, despite consuming a highly caloric diet, food is processed more quickly, leading to weight loss.

C) Acetylcholine is responsible for muscular contractions. Since catecholamine derivatives are the precursors to acetylcholine, the presence of these derivatives in the body stimulates the musculoskeletal system, thus burning additional calories and leading to weight loss.

D) Catecholamine derivatives block the release of cortisol, a known contributor to stress-related over eating and weight gain.

2. Obesity is considered a marker of poor health. According to Figure 1, which country most aligns with the general global health trend described in the first paragraph concerning the relationship between GDP and population health?

A) Canada
B) South Africa
C) China
D) India

3. Which of the following is NOT a known environmental risk factor for developing obesity in individuals below the poverty line in the U.S.?

A) Limited access to health care
B) Presence of "food deserts" (areas where healthy food is hard to find)
C) Genetic predisposition
D) Lack of green space for exercise or other physical activity

4. Which of the following weight-loss strategies would a neobehaviorist most endorse?

A) A combination of group therapy and prescription medication to help people lose as much weight as possible in a short time frame.
B) For every five pounds a person loses, they are given a non-food reward such as money or praise/attention from others.
C) Whenever a person gains weight they are publicly criticized by others.
D) A group exercise class where the exercises become increasingly more difficult over time.

5. Which of the following does NOT demonstrate how social networks can influence weight?

A) Research shows that joining an online weight-loss community is successful at helping people lose weight.
B) Kids who participate in group sports are less likely to be obese than those who prefer solitary activities, such as reading or playing video games.
C) Teenage girls who report having at least one friend with an eating disorder are more than twice as likely to also experiment with disordered eating behaviors such as binging and purging or extreme calorie restriction.
D) Multiple studies have shown that people eat roughly the same amount when they are dining out as they do when dining alone at home.

CARS Strategies for MCAT Psychology/Sociology Drill: Global Health Trends

The passage includes four paragraphs and two figures relating to the relationship between GDP and health and to national and state trends in obesity. Here is the map of the passage.

1) Positive correlation between health and wealth of nation—also individual level
2) Obesity is exception—opposite relationship
3) BMI: categories and study results
4) Mississippi: children's poor health, state response

And here are the questions.

1. **Memory.** For this question, you really do have to know something about catecholamine neurotransmitters, the parasympathetic nervous system, and Parkinson's disease.

2. **Explicit.** Once you define what the question is asking for—high GDP + low obesity/better health or vice versa—all you need to do is use the data in Figure 1. Make sure to read the question carefully; you are not looking for the relationship discussed in paragraph 2, which tells you that high GDP is correlated with high levels of obesity.

3. **Implicit.** While the question appears to require you to use your knowledge of specific environmental risk factors to eliminate choices B and D, and to use either your own knowledge or information from paragraph 1 to eliminate choice A, all you really need to do is read the question stem carefully. Once you see that it is asking which is NOT a known environmental risk factor, look for a non-environmental factor in the answer choices.

4. **Memory.** For this question, you do need to know the basics of neobehaviorism.

5. **Memory.** Even if you don't know much about social networks, this question is doable if you just read the question stem carefully. It asks which answer does NOT demonstrate how social networks influence weight. Look for any choice that either does not discuss social/group influence on behavior, or that suggests that social factors do not play a causal role.

Final Notes

In general, using CARS techniques on the science passages will increase your speed and accuracy, and help you to make the most of your scientific knowledge. The MCAT does not demand an exhaustive understanding of biology, chemistry, and physics; rather, it requires you to have a sound basic knowledge of chemical and physical principles, and of the ways in which organisms function. Combine your scientific common sense with your critical reading skills to raise your science scores.

Use your understanding of the three types of science questions (Memory, Implicit, and Explicit) to shape your solution strategies; make the information in the passages work for you. Don't waste your time working out a solution that the passage spells out for you; conversely, don't bother to search a passage for information that your map indicates isn't there.

Solutions to MCAT G-Chem Drill: Solubility

1. **D** The first three choices are false. O_2 and CO_2 are nonpolar (i.e., have no dipole). As a consequence of the electronegativity of the oxygen atoms, the carbon in carbon dioxide has a slight positive charge and is therefore attracted to any atom with a negative charge. Organic chemists use the term electrophile for an atom or molecule which has some positive charge and nucleophile for an atom or molecule with a negative charge. The oxygen in water is a mild nucleophile.

2. **A** Based upon the first two equilibrium reactions in the passage, if the concentration of CO_2 were decreased, the first equilibrium would shift to the left. The subsequent reduction in the concentration of H_2CO_3 would cause the second equilibrium to also shift to the left, hence the concentration of H^+ would decrease and blood pH would increase.

3. **D** The last sentence of paragraph 2 indicates that the transport efficiency of O_2 is directly related to the blood pH. Therefore, as blood pH decreases, so too does the ability of hemoglobin to transport oxygen. Choice A is incorrect because lipid bilayers are only unstable under extreme conditions. If this statement were true, drinking a glass of soda would be a painful experience. Bicarbonate is one of the most soluble anions, so choice B is not plausible. The passage does not provide any insight as to how the nervous system (choice C) would be impacted by acidosis.

4. **D** A catalyst increases the rate at which a reaction reaches equilibrium. The addition of a catalyst to a system that is already at equilibrium, like this one, will have no effect.

5. **B** The solubility of a gas in a liquid decreases with increasing temperature (as illustrated by the fact that CO_2 readily erupts from a bottle of warm soda). Choices A and C will increase the solubility of CO_2 gas in water.

6. **A** Whenever dealing with electron configuration questions, first eliminate any choices that have the wrong number of electrons. A neutral Fe atom has twenty-six electrons, so Fe^{2+} must have twenty-four electrons. Choices C and D are eliminated because they account for twenty-six and thirty electrons, respectively. Choice A is the correct answer because transition metal elements always lose their valence s electrons (here the $4s$ electrons) before losing any d electrons (choice B is eliminated).

Solutions to MCAT Physics Drill: Force

1. **C** The question says that the horizontal component of velocity, $v_x = v \cos \theta$, is 10 m/s. Since $\cos 60° = 1/2$, the total velocity v must be 20 m/s.

2. **C** As explained in the passage, dropping a sandbag does not change the buoyant force, but it does change the gravitational force. When the sandbag is dropped the gravitational force drops by mg while the buoyant force stays the same. Since the two forces originally balanced, the buoyant force is now bigger by mg. Note that the buoyant force is a constant Mg pointing up, while the gravitational force is originally Mg pointing down and then $(Mg - mg)$ pointing down after the sandbag is dropped.

3. **A** For a balloon to float, its density has to be less than that of air. So if the mass in kg divided by the volume in m³ is less than 1.2 (the density of air), then the balloon floats. If you add the mass of the four people (total = 400 kg) to the mass of the balloon and divide by the volume, you get a value of less than 1.2 for Balloon I only.

4. **C** The upward buoyant force (acting along the central axis of the balloon, directly above the flame) on the warmer, less dense air propels it upward. When it reaches the closed top of the balloon, it will be deflected downward. As the warmed air makes its journey, it cools, returns downward, and the cycle repeats.

5. **D** The buoyant force makes it go up; gravity and the drag force hold it back. The net force is zero since its velocity is constant ($a = 0$), so the upward forces are equal to the downward forces, as stated in choice D.

6. **C** Warmer air is less dense than cooler air. Less dense air will give a smaller buoyant force and the balloon will be able to carry less weight.

7. **A** The pelican is 2 kg added on to 2000 kg for the balloon and passengers. This is a 0.1% increase in mass and therefore a 0.1% increase in gravitational force. Increasing the volume by 0.1% will result in a compensating increase in the buoyant force (which is $\rho g V$, where ρ is the density of the air).

8. **D** The rope is pulling a 100-kg person at an acceleration of 2 m/s², so the tension (the force on the person exerted by the rope) is just $T = m(g + a) = 100(10 + 2) = 1200$ N.

Solutions to MCAT Biology Drill: Embryology

1. **A** Since bacteria are unicellular and reproduce asexually through binary fission, they do not undergo fertilization, and would not be appropriate organisms to study that process. All the other organisms listed reproduce sexually; they can be (and have been!) used for developmental studies (choices B, C, and D can be eliminated).

2. **C** The question states that the males are the result of nondisjunction in the hermaphrodite. Nondisjunction is the failure of the chromosomes to separate properly during cell division. Since the hermaphrodite has two X chromosomes and no Y chromosomes, and the male arises from the hermaphrodite, the males cannot contain Y chromosomes (choices A and D are wrong; do not always assume male organisms have Y chromosomes). Furthermore, the passage states that the males are missing an X chromosome, not that they have gained one (choice B is wrong).

3. **C** The sperm nucleus is $1n$ (choice A is wrong), and because the oocyte has not yet completed meiosis I (it is suspended in prophase I), its nucleus is $2n$ (choice B is wrong). Therefore, the ploidy of the fertilized egg is $3n$ ($1n$ sperm + $2n$ oocyte, choice D is wrong).

4. **B** The passage states that sperm are stored in the spermatheca (choices A and C are wrong) and that this is found in the hermaphrodite (choice D is wrong).

5. **B** The passage describes pseudocleavage as an event where a cleavage furrow appears, then disappears without cell division (choice A is wrong). Formation of a cleavage furrow does not require the formation of a cell membrane (the existing membrane simply pinches inward, choice C is wrong), and polar bodies are formed during the meiotic division of the oocyte following fertilization (choice D is wrong).

6. **C** The cell division that occurs after fusion of the pronuclei is mitosis. Pairing of homologous chromosomes (numeral I) and recombination events (numeral II) occur during meiosis, so these statements are false (choices A, B, and D can be eliminated). Only numeral III is true; nuclear membranes must be reorganized both when the pronuclei fuse and when the (now) embryonic nucleus disintegrates during prophase.

7. **A** The passage states cytochalasin B inhibits actin polymerization (actin filaments are also called microfilaments) and prevents P-granule movement, thus movement of the P-granules must depend on microfilaments; numeral I is true (choices C and D can be eliminated). However, cytochalasin B does not affect migration of the pronuclei, so that process must not depend on microfilaments; numeral II is false. The passage also states that colcemid inhibits microtubules and prevents migration of the pronuclei, thus migration must depend on microtubules; numeral III is true (choice B can be eliminated). However, colcemid does not affect P-granules movement, so that process must not depend on microtubules; numeral IV is false.

Solutions to MCAT Psychology/Sociology Drill: Global Health Trends

1. **A** The catecholamine neurotransmitters are dopamine, norepinephrine, and epinephrine. Therefore, a catecholamine derivative that acts as an agonist would somehow act on a pathway involving one of these three neurotransmitters (choices C and D are wrong). The primary neurotransmitter of the parasympathetic nervous system is acetylcholine, so choice B is also wrong. In Parkinson's disease, neurons in the brain that make dopamine and control muscle movement begin to die. Therefore, even without necessarily knowing which of the catecholamine neurotransmitters is involved in obesity, the most reasonably correct answer is choice A.

2. **B** The first paragraph describes a relationship where high GDP correlates to better public health and low GDP correlates to worse public health. The only country in Figure 1 that roughly reflects this relationship and that also appears in the answer choices is South Africa; with the second highest percentage of the population with a BMI above 30 (reflecting worse public health) and a relatively low GDP, this is the only country where a low GDP corresponds to worse health (choice B is correct). Canada has a high GDP and a moderately high percentage of the population with a BMI above 30 (indicating poor health, choice A is wrong), and China and India both have low GDPs and low percentages of the population with a BMI above 30 (indicating better health, choices C and D are wrong).

3. **C** Genetic predisposition to obesity is not an environmental risk factor for developing obesity, it's a biological risk factor (choice C is the correct answer choice); for those living below the poverty line in the U.S., limited access to health care (choice A), limited access to healthy food (choice B), and a lack of green space to exercise (choice D) are all environmental risk factors contributing to the development of obesity. Therefore, choices A, B, and D can all be eliminated.

4. **B** Neobehaviorists believe that behavior can be modified by rewards or punishments. Therefore, if someone exhibits a desired behavior, providing a reward after that behavior will encourage the behavior to happen again (positive reinforcement). When a person exhibits an undesirable behavior, the application of a punishment will discourage that behavior from happening again (positive punishment). Choice A is wrong because it does not describe any type of reward or punishment. Choice B describes positive reinforcement, and choice C describes positive punishment; neobehaviorists believe that the most effective way to modify behavior is with positive reinforcement. Therefore, choice B is right and choice C is wrong. Choice D seems to be describing the implementation of a punishment (exercises getting harder) in response to a desired behavior (exercise). This would be the opposite of a strategy that a neobehaviorist would endorse, and choice D is incorrect.

5. **D** Social networks involve an individual and any of the various other individuals, groups, or organizations that an individual might interact with; by definition, social networks will influence the behavior of the individual in some way. Since the question asks which choice does NOT demonstrate the influence of social networks on weight, all of the answer choices that demonstrate that an individual is somehow influenced by others should be eliminated (choices A, B, and C indicate that weight is somehow influenced by groups or individuals, and can be eliminated). Choice D, however, indicates that there is no difference between eating around others and eating alone (choice D does not demonstrate how social networks can influence weight and is the correct answer choice).

A.2 INTERVIEW AND PERSONAL STATEMENT PREPARATION QUESTIONS

The following list of questions will help prepare you for your interviews and inspire your personal statements. Try to answer a few each week. Answers that are written out will be the most fully formed and the ones you are likely to remember.

1) Where did you grow up and go to school? What was your town/community like? How did this shape your views?
2) What was your family life like? What do your parents do?
3) How is your relationship with your parents and siblings now? How did your family life shape you as a person?
4) Was one particular person an inspiration to you in your life? Why?
5) Why did you choose your undergraduate major?
6) How have you tried to achieve breadth in your undergraduate education?
7) How has your undergraduate research experience, if any, better prepared you for a medical career?
8) If you get into medical school, you will be making a huge time commitment. What *won't* you give up in order to be successful in your medical career?
9) How have the jobs, volunteer opportunities, or extracurricular experiences that you have had made you better prepared for the responsibilities of being a physician?
10) How do you envision using your medical school education?
11) You have stated many humanistic and socially responsible ideals in your essays. What have you done so far to demonstrate those ideals in practice?

12) How would you describe yourself in terms of your greatest strengths and weaknesses?

13) In the broad sense, what travels have you taken, and what exposure to cultures other than your own have you had?

14) Thinking of examples from your recent past, how would you assess your empathy and compassion?

15) What excites you about medicine in general?

16) What do you know about the current trends in our nation's health care system?

17) Tell me what you believe to be the most pressing health issues today. Why?

18) What do you feel are the social responsibilities of a physician?

19) What is the most important social problem facing the United States today, and why?

20) How do you think national health insurance might affect physicians, patients, and society?

21) In what manner and to what degree do you stay in touch with current events?

22) What books, films, or other media come to mind as having been particularly important to your non-science education?

23) What is "success," in your opinion? After practicing medicine for 20 years, what kind of "successes" do you hope to have achieved?

24) What qualities do you look for in a physician? Can you provide an example of a physician who exemplifies these ideals? How does he or she do this?

25) What kind of experiences have you had working with sick people? What have you learned from these experiences?

26) If you could invite four people from the past to dinner, who would they be, and why? What would you talk to them about?

27) Do you have any "blemishes" on your academic record? If so, explain the circumstances.

28) If you are a minority candidate, how do you feel your background uniquely prepares you to be, and will influence you as, a physician?

29) If you are not a minority, how do you feel prepared to meet the diverse needs of a multiethnic, multicultural patient population?

30) To what extent do you feel that you owe a debt to humanity? To what extent do you owe a debt to those less fortunate than you?

31) Who has been influential in your decision to pursue a medical career?

32) What special qualities do you feel you possess that would set you apart from other medical school candidates? What makes you unique or different as a medical school candidate?

33) What sort of expectations will you hold for your classmates?

34) What are the three most important properties you think the ideal medical student should have?

35) What kind of medical schools are you applying to, and why?

36) Pick any specific medical school that you are applying to, and tell the interviewer about it. What goes on there, and what makes it particularly desirable to you?

37) What general and specific skills would you hope an "ideal" medical school experience would give you? How might your ideal school achieve that result?

38) When did you decide to become an MD, and why?

39) Why did you decide to choose medicine and not some other field where you can help others, such as nursing, physical therapy, pharmacology, psychology, education, or social work?

40) How have you tested your motivation to become an MD? Please explain.

41) Where do you see yourself in five years? In ten years?

42) Have you decided what to specialize in? How did you reach this decision?

43) What will you do if you are not accepted to medical school this year? Do you have an alternative career plan?

44) Is there anything else we have not covered that you feel the interviewer should know about you or your interest in becoming a physician?

GOOD LUCK ON THE MCAT AND IN MEDICAL SCHOOL!

Passage Permissions Information

Adapted from "Love for Sale: Appraising the Relics of a Relationship," by Francine Prose. © 2009 Francine Prose. First appeared in *Harper's Magazine*. Reprinted with permission of the Denise Shannon Literary Agency, Inc. All rights reserved.

J.A. Paulos, *Innumeracy: Mathematical Illiteracy and its Consequences*. © 1988, 2001 by John Allen Paulos. Reprinted with permission of Macmillan Publishers.

Robert L. Heilbroner, *The Worldly Philosophers: The Lives, Times And Ideas Of The Great Economic Thinkers,* Seventh Edition. © 1999 Simon & Schuster Inc.

Mary Ann Glendon, *Comparative Legal Traditions in a Nutshell*. © 1982 West Academic Publishing. Reprinted with permission.

H. Adams, *The Education of Henry Adams*. © 1918 Houghton Mifflin Co.

Keith Bybee, *Mistaken Identity: The Supreme Court and the Politics of Minority Representation*. © 1998 Princeton University Press. Reprinted with permission of Princeton University Press.

Excerpt from E. T. May, "Myths and Realities of the American Family," from *A History of Private Life, Volume V: Riddles of Identity in Modern Times,* edited by Antoine Prost and Gérard Vincent, translated by Arthur Goldhammer, Cambridge, Mass.: The Belknap Press of Harvard University Press, Copyright © 1991 by the President and Fellows of Harvard College. Used by permission. All rights reserved.

Andrew Zimmerman, *Anthropology and Antihumanism in Imperial Germany*. © 2001 by The University of Chicago. Reprinted with permission of the University of Chicago Press.

Excerpt from *Theory of Literature*, New Revised Edition by Rene Wellek and Austin Warren. Copyright © 1956, 1949, 1947, 1942 by Houghton Mifflin Harcourt Publishing Company, renewed 1984, 1977, 1975 by Rene Wellek and Austin Warren. Reprinted by permission of Mariner Books, an imprint of HarperCollins Publishers. All rights reserved.

Ruth Brandon, *Surreal Lives: The Surrealists 1917-1945*. © 1999 Ruth Brandon, Grove/Atlantic Inc.

Tracy B. Strong, *Friedrich Nietzsche and the Politics of Transfiguration*. © 1988 the Regents of the University of California, the University of California Press.

M.R. Modiano, "Breast and Cervical Cancer in Hispanic Women," *Medical Anthropology Quarterly*, © 1995. Reproduced with permission of the American Anthropological Association from Medical Anthropology Quarterly Volume 9(1), 1995. Not for sale or further reproduction.

Matthew Calarco, *Zoographies: The Question of the Animal from Heidegger to Derrida*. © 2008 Columbia University Press.

Adrian Nicole LeBlanc, *Random Family: Love, Drugs, Trouble, and Coming of Age in the Bronx*. © 2004 Scribner.

Norman F. Cantor, *In the Wake of the Plague: The Black Death and the World it Made*. © 2002 Harper Perennial.

Robert Sullivan, *Rats: Observations on the History and Habitat of the City's Most Unwanted Inhabitants*. © 2004 Bloomsbury USA.

Cedric Herring, "Convergence, Polarization, or What? Racially Based Changes in Attitudes and Outlooks." *Sociological Quarterly,* Volume 30, Issue 2, pgs. 267–281. Published online on April 21, 2005. Copyright © Midwest Sociological Society, reprinted by permission of Taylor & Francis Ltd, http://www.tandfonline.com, on behalf of Midwest Sociological Society, http://www.themss.org.

Janice Gross Stein, *The Cult of Efficiency.* © 2001 Janice Gross Stein. Reproduced with permission of House of Anansi Press, Toronto.

W. Guerin et al., *A Handbook of Critical Approaches to Literature.* © 2005 Oxford University Press. Reproduced with permission of the Licensor through PLSclear.

Excerpt(s) from *Lying: Moral Choice in Public and Private Life* by Sissela Bok, copyright © 1978 by Sissela Bok. Used by permission of Pantheon Books, an imprint of the Knopf Doubleday Publishing Group, a division of Penguin Random House LLC. All rights reserved.

Michael L. Benson, "The Influence of Class Position on the Formal and Informal Sanctioning of White-Collar Offenders," *The Sociological Quarterly,* Volume 30, Issue 3, pgs. 465–479. Copyright © Midwest Sociological Society, reprinted by permission of Taylor & Francis Ltd, http://www.tandfonline.com on behalf of Midwest Sociological Society, http://www.themss.org.

W.H. Flanigan and N.H. Zingale, *Political Behavior of the American Electorate.* © 1979 Allyn Bacon. Copyright © 2018 by CQ Press, an imprint of SAGE Publications, Inc. CQ Press is a registered trademark of Congressional Quarterly, Inc.

Howard E. Gardner, *Creating Minds: An Anatomy of Creativity Seen Through the Lives of Freud, Einstein, Picasso, Stravinsky, Eliot, Graham, and Gandhi.* © 1993. Reprinted by permission of Basic Books, an imprint of Hachette Book Group, Inc.

Michel Foucault, *The Birth Of The Clinic: An Archaeology Of Medical Perception.* © 1973 Tavistock Publications Limited.

Istvan Csicsery-Ronay Jr., "Cyberpunk and Neuromanticism" in *Storming The Reality Studio: A Casebook Of Cyberpunk And Postmodern Science* by Larry McCaffery, © 1991 Duke University Press.

C.L.R. James, *Beyond A Boundary.* © 1983 Pantheon.

C. Steinwedel, "Making Social Groups, One Person at a Time: The Identification of Individuals by Estate, Religious Confession, and Ethnicity in Late Imperial Russia," from *Documenting Individual Identity: The Development of State Practices in the Modern World,* edited by Jane Caplan and John Torpey. © 2001 Princeton University Press.

Jacob Bronowski and Bruce Mazlish, *The Western Intellectual Tradition: From Leonardo to Hegel,* pgs. 350–362. © 1960 Jacob Bronowski and Bruce Mazlish. Reprinted with permission of HarperCollins Publishers.

Michael Novak, The Joy of Sports: End Zones, Bases, Baskets, Balls, and the Consecration of the American Spirit, © 1955, 1993 Madison Books, Incorporated. Reprinted with permission of Rowman & Littlefield Publishing Group, Inc.

Joann Kealiinohomoku, "An Anthropologist Looks at Ballet as a Form of Ethnic Dance." © 1970, *Impulse* 20: 24–33.

NOTES

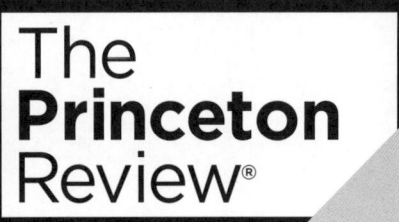
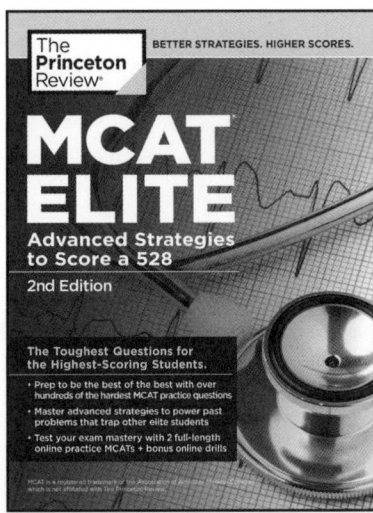
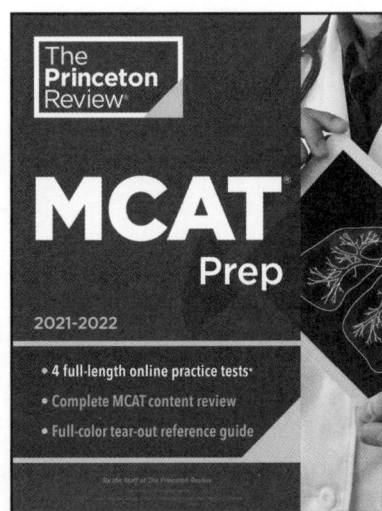
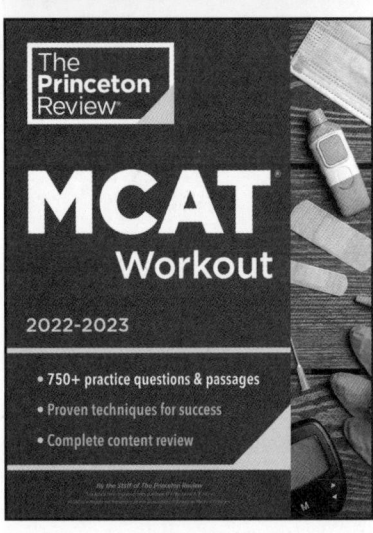
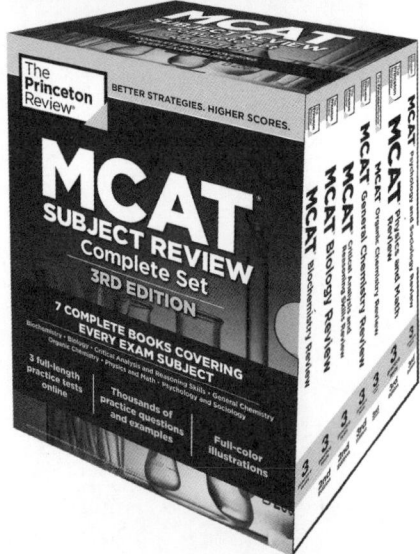

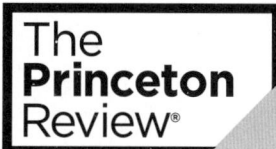

MCAT®

General Chemistry Review

4th Edition

The Staff of The Princeton Review

Penguin
Random
House

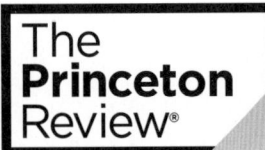

The Princeton Review
110 E. 42nd Street
New York, NY 10017

Published in the United States by Penguin Random House LLC, New York, and in Canada by Random House of Canada, a division of Penguin Random House Ltd., Toronto.

Terms of Service: The Princeton Review Online Companion Tools ("Student Tools") for retail books are available for only the two most recent editions of that book. Student Tools may be activated only once per eligible book purchased, for a total of 24 months of access. Activation of Student Tools more than once per book is in direct violation of these Terms of Service and may result in discontinuation of access to Student Tools Services.

The material in this book is up-to-date at the time of publication. However, changes may have been instituted by the testing body in the test after this book was published.

If there are any important late-breaking developments, changes, or corrections to the materials in this book, we will post that information online in the Student Tools. Register your book and check your Student Tools to see if there are any updates posted there.

ISBN: 978-0-593-51625-6
ISSN: 2150-8879

MCAT is a registered trademark of the Association of American Medical Colleges.

The Princeton Review is not affiliated with Princeton University.

Editor: Orion McBean
Production Artist: Lindsey Cleworth
Production Editors: Ali Landreau and Chris Stobart

Manufactured in China.

10 9 8 7 6 5 4 3 2 1

4th Edition

The Princeton Review Publishing Team

Rob Franek, Editor-in-Chief
David Soto, Senior Director, Data Operations
Stephen Koch, Senior Manager, Data Operations
Deborah Weber, Director of Production
Jason Ullmeyer, Production Design Manager
Jennifer Chapman, Senior Production Artist
Selena Coppock, Director of Editorial
Aaron Riccio, Senior Editor
Meave Shelton, Senior Editor
Chris Chimera, Editor
Orion McBean, Editor
Patricia Murphy, Editor
Laura Rose, Editor
Alexa Schmitt Bugler, Editorial Assistant

Random House Publishing Team

Tom Russell, VP, Publisher
Alison Stoltzfus, Senior Director, Publishing
Brett Wright, Senior Editor
Emily Hoffman, Associate Managing Editor
Ellen Reed, Production Manager
Suzanne Lee, Designer
Eugenia Lo, Publishing Assistant

For customer service, please contact **editorialsupport@review.com,** and be sure to include:

- full title of the book

- ISBN

- page number

CONTRIBUTORS

Steven A. Leduc
    Senior Author
Kendra Bowman
    Ph.D., Senior Author

TPR MCAT G-Chem Development Team:
Catherine Chow, M.Sc., Senior Editor, Lead Developer
Brad Hutnick, B.S.

Edited for Production by:
Judene Wright, M.S., M.A.Ed.
    National Content Director, MCAT Program, The Princeton Review

The TPR MCAT G-Chem Team and Judene would like to thank the following people for their contributions to this book :

Patrick Abulencia, Ph.D., Kashif Anwar, M.D., M.M.S., Bethany Blackwell, M.S., Argun Can, Brian Cato, Nita Chauhan, H.BSc, MSc, William Ewing, Ph.D., Rob Fong, M.D., Ph.D., Chris Fortenbach, B.S., Neil Maluste, B.S., Chris Manuel, M.P.H., Douglas K. McLemore, B.S., Marion-Vincent L. Mempin, B.S., Donna Memran, Brian Mikolasko, M.D., M.BA, Katherine Miller, Ph.D., Steven Rines, Ph.D., Andrew Snyder, Danish Vaiyani, Christopher Volpe, Ph.D.

PERIODIC TABLE OF THE ELEMENTS

1																	18
1 **H** 1.0	2												13	14	15	16	17	2 **He** 4.0
3 **Li** 6.9	4 **Be** 9.0												5 **B** 10.8	6 **C** 12.0	7 **N** 14.0	8 **O** 16.0	9 **F** 19.0	10 **Ne** 20.2
11 **Na** 23.0	12 **Mg** 24.3	3	4	5	6	7	8	9	10	11	12	13 **Al** 27.0	14 **Si** 28.1	15 **P** 31.0	16 **S** 32.1	17 **Cl** 35.5	18 **Ar** 39.9
19 **K** 39.1	20 **Ca** 40.1	21 **Sc** 45.0	22 **Ti** 47.9	23 **V** 50.9	24 **Cr** 52.0	25 **Mn** 54.9	26 **Fe** 55.8	27 **Co** 58.9	28 **Ni** 58.7	29 **Cu** 63.5	30 **Zn** 65.4	31 **Ga** 69.7	32 **Ge** 72.6	33 **As** 74.9	34 **Se** 79.0	35 **Br** 79.9	36 **Kr** 83.8
37 **Rb** 85.5	38 **Sr** 87.6	39 **Y** 88.9	40 **Zr** 91.2	41 **Nb** 92.9	42 **Mo** 95.9	43 **Tc** (98)	44 **Ru** 101.1	45 **Rh** 102.9	46 **Pd** 106.4	47 **Ag** 107.9	48 **Cd** 112.4	49 **In** 114.8	50 **Sn** 118.7	51 **Sb** 121.8	52 **Te** 127.6	53 **I** 126.9	54 **Xe** 131.3
55 **Cs** 132.9	56 **Ba** 137.3	57 ***La** 138.9	72 **Hf** 178.5	73 **Ta** 180.9	74 **W** 183.9	75 **Re** 186.2	76 **Os** 190.2	77 **Ir** 192.2	78 **Pt** 195.1	79 **Au** 197.0	80 **Hg** 200.6	81 **Tl** 204.4	82 **Pb** 207.2	83 **Bi** 209.0	84 **Po** (209)	85 **At** (210)	86 **Rn** (222)
87 **Fr** (223)	88 **Ra** (226)	89 **†Ac** (227)	104 **Rf** (267)	105 **Db** (268)	106 **Sg** (271)	107 **Bh** (270)	108 **Hs** (269)	109 **Mt** (278)	110 **Ds** (281)	111 **Rg** (282)	112 **Cn** (285)	113 **Nh** (286)	114 **Fl** (289)	115 **Mc** (289)	116 **Lv** (293)	117 **Ts** (294)	118 **Og** (294)

*Lanthanoids

58 **Ce** 140.1	59 **Pr** 140.9	60 **Nd** 144.2	61 **Pm** (145)	62 **Sm** 150.4	63 **Eu** 152.0	64 **Gd** 157.3	65 **Tb** 158.9	66 **Dy** 162.5	67 **Ho** 164.9	68 **Er** 167.3	69 **Tm** 168.9	70 **Yb** 173.0	71 **Lu** 175.0

†Actinoids

90 **Th** 232.0	91 **Pa** (231)	92 **U** 238.0	93 **Np** (237)	94 **Pu** (244)	95 **Am** (243)	96 **Cm** (247)	97 **Bk** (247)	98 **Cf** (251)	99 **Es** (252)	100 **Fm** (257)	101 **Md** (258)	102 **No** (259)	103 **Lr** (266)

MCAT GENERAL CHEMISTRY CONTENTS

MCAT MATH FOR GENERAL CHEMISTRY

Get More (Free) Content
at **PrincetonReview.com/prep**

As easy as 1·2·3

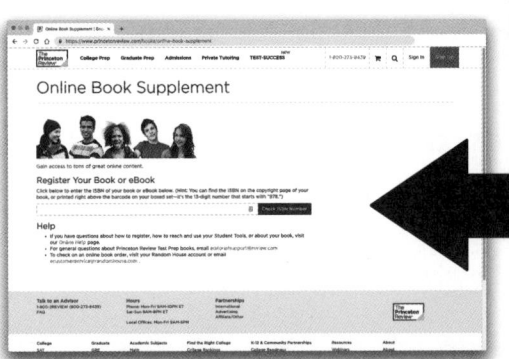

1 Go to PrincetonReview.com/prep or scan the **QR code** and enter the following ISBN for your book:
9780593516256

2 Answer a few simple questions to set up an exclusive Princeton Review account. *(If you already have one, you can just log in.)*

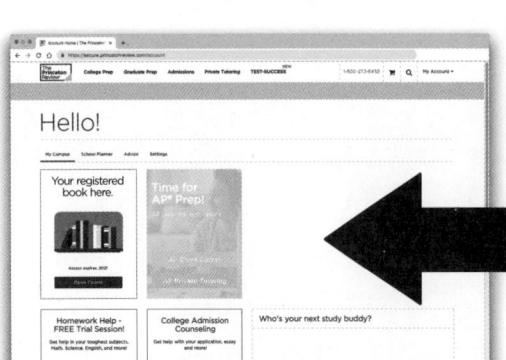

3 Enjoy access to your **FREE** content!

Once you've registered, you can...

- Take **3** full-length practice MCAT exams

- Find useful information about taking the MCAT and applying to medical school

- Check to see whether there have been any corrections or updates to this edition

- Get our take on any recent or pending updates to the MCAT

Need to report a potential **content** issue?

Contact **EditorialSupport@review.com** and include:

- full title of the book
- ISBN
- page number

Need to report a **technical** issue?

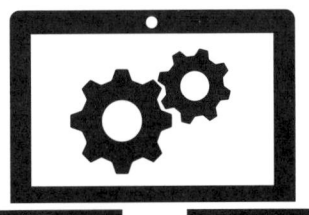

Contact **TPRStudentTech@review.com** and provide:

- your full name
- email address used to register the book
- full book title and ISBN
- Operating system (Mac/PC) and browser (Chrome, Firefox, Safari, etc.)

Chapter 1
MCAT Basics

SO YOU WANT TO BE A DOCTOR

So...you want to be a doctor. If you're like most premeds, you've wanted to be a doctor since you were pretty young. When people asked you what you wanted to be when you grew up, you always answered "a doctor." You had toy medical kits, bandaged up your dog or cat, and played "hospital." You probably read your parents' home medical guides for fun.

When you got to high school you took the honors and AP classes. You studied hard, got straight A's (or at least really good grades!), and participated in extracurricular activities so you could get into a good college. And you succeeded!

At college you knew exactly what to do. You took your classes seriously, studied hard, and got a great GPA. You talked to your professors and hung out at office hours to get good letters of recommendation. You were a member of the premed society on campus, volunteered at hospitals, and shadowed doctors. All that's left to do now is get a good MCAT score.

Just the MCAT.

Just the most confidence-shattering, most demoralizing, longest, most brutal entrance exam for any graduate program. At about 7.5 hours (including breaks), the MCAT tops the list. Even the closest runners up, the LSAT and GMAT, are only about 4 hours long. The MCAT tests significant science content knowledge along with the ability to think quickly, reason logically, and read comprehensively, all under the pressure of a timed exam.

The path to a good MCAT score is not as easy to see as the path to a good GPA or the path to a good letter of recommendation. The MCAT is less about what you know, and more about how to apply what you know...and how to apply it quickly to new situations. Because the path might not be so clear, you might be worried. That's why you picked up this book.

We promise to demystify the MCAT for you, with clear descriptions of the different sections, how the test is scored, and what the test experience is like. We will help you understand general test-taking techniques as well as provide you with specific techniques for each section. We will review the science content you need to know as well as give you strategies for the Critical Analysis and Reasoning Skills (CARS) section. We'll show you the path to a good MCAT score and help you walk the path.

After all...you want to be a doctor. And we want you to succeed.

WHAT IS THE MCAT...REALLY?

Most test-takers approach the MCAT as though it were a typical college science test, one in which facts and knowledge simply need to be regurgitated in order to do well. They study for the MCAT the same way they did for their college tests: by memorizing facts and details, formulas and equations. And when they get to the MCAT they are surprised...and disappointed.

It's a myth that the MCAT is purely a content-knowledge test. If medical-school admission committees want to see what you know, all they have to do is look at your transcripts. What they really want to see is how you *think*, especially under pressure. *That's* what your MCAT score will tell them.

The MCAT is really a test of your ability to apply basic knowledge to different, possibly new, situations. It's a test of your ability to reason out and evaluate arguments. Do you still need to know your science content? Absolutely. But not at the level that most test-takers think they need to know it. Furthermore, your science knowledge won't help you on the Critical Analysis and Reasoning Skills (CARS) section. So how do you study for a test like this?

You study for the science sections by reviewing the basics and then applying them to MCAT practice questions. You study for the CARS section by learning how to adapt your existing reading and analytical skills to the nature of the test (more information about the CARS section can be found in the *MCAT Critical Analysis and Reasoning Skills Review*).

The book you are holding will review all the relevant MCAT General Chemistry content you will need for the test, and a little bit more. It includes hundreds of questions designed to make you think about the material in a deeper way, along with full explanations to clarify the logical thought process needed to get to the answers. It also comes with access to three full-length online practice exams to further hone your skills. For more information on accessing those online exams, please refer to the "Register Your Book Online!" spread on page x.

MCAT NUTS AND BOLTS

Overview

The MCAT is a computer-based test (CBT) that is *not* adaptive. Adaptive tests base your next question on whether or not you've answered the current question correctly. The MCAT is *linear*, or *fixed-form*, meaning that the questions are in a predetermined order and do not change based on your answers. However, there are many versions of the test, so that on a given test day, different people will see different versions. The following table highlights the features of the MCAT exam.

Registration	Online via www.aamc.org. Begins as early as six months prior to test date; available up until week of test (subject to seat availability).
Testing Centers	Administered at small, secure, climate-controlled computer testing rooms.
Security	Photo ID with signature, electronic fingerprint, electronic signature verification, assigned seat.
Proctoring	None. Test administrator checks examinee in and assigns seat at computer. All testing instructions are given on the computer.
Frequency of Test	Many times per year distributed over January, April, May, June, July, August, and September.
Format	Exclusively computer-based. NOT an adaptive test.
Length of Test Day	7.5 hours
Breaks	Optional 10-minute breaks between sections, with a 30-minute break for lunch.
Section Names	1. Chemical and Physical Foundations of Biological Systems (Chem/Phys) 2. Critical Analysis and Reasoning Skills (CARS) 3. Biological and Biochemical Foundations of Living Systems (Bio/Biochem) 4. Psychological, Social, and Biological Foundations of Behavior (Psych/Soc)
Number of Questions and Timing	59 Chem/Phys questions, 95 minutes 53 CARS questions, 90 minutes 59 Bio/Biochem questions, 95 minutes 59 Psych/Soc questions, 95 minutes
Scoring	Test is scaled. Several forms per administration.
Allowed/ Not allowed	No timers/watches. Noise reduction headphones available. Noteboard booklet and wet-erase marker given at start of test and taken at end of test. Locker or secure area provided for personal items.
Results: Timing and Delivery	Approximately 30 days. Electronic scores only, available online through AAMC login. Examinees can print official score reports.
Maximum Number of Retakes	The test can be taken a maximum of three times in one year, four times over two years, and seven times over the lifetime of the examinee. An examinee can be registered for only one date at a time.

Registration

Registration for the exam is completed online at www.aamc.org/students/applying/mcat/reserving. The AAMC opens registration for a given test date at least two months in advance of the date, often earlier. It's a good idea to register well in advance of your desired test date to make sure that you get a seat.

Sections

There are four sections on the MCAT, all of which consist of multiple-choice questions:

Section	Concepts Tested	Number of Questions and Timing
Chemical and Physical Foundations of Biological Systems (Chem/Phys)	Basic concepts in chemistry and physics, including biochemistry, scientific inquiry, reasoning, research, and statistics skills.	59 questions in 95 minutes
Critical Analysis and Reasoning Skills (CARS)	Critical analysis of information drawn from a wide range of social science and humanities disciplines.	53 questions in 90 minutes
Biological and Biochemical Foundations of Living Systems (Bio/Biochem)	Basic concepts in biology and biochemistry, scientific inquiry, reasoning, research and statistics skills.	59 questions in 95 minutes
Psychological, Social, and Biological Foundations of Behavior (Psych/Soc)	Basic concepts in psychology, sociology, and biology, research methods, and statistics.	59 questions in 95 minutes

Most questions on the MCAT (44 in each of the science sections, all 53 in the CARS section) are passage-based; the science sections have 10 passages each and the CARS section has 9. A passage consists of a few paragraphs of information on which several following questions are based. In the science sections, passages often include equations or reactions, tables, graphs, figures, and experiments to analyze. CARS passages come from literature in the social sciences, humanities, ethics, philosophy, cultural studies, and population health, and do not test content knowledge in any way.

Some questions in the science sections are freestanding questions (FSQs). These questions are independent of any passage information and appear in four groups of about three to four questions, interspersed throughout the passages. 15 of the questions in each of the sciences sections are freestanding, and the remainder are passage-based.

Each section on the MCAT is separated by either a 10-minute break or a 30-minute lunch break. We recommend that you take these breaks.

Section	Time
Test Center Check-In	Variable, can take up to 40 minutes if center is busy.
Tutorial	10 minutes
Chemical and Physical Foundations of Biological Systems	95 minutes
Break (optional)	10 minutes
Critical Analysis and Reasoning Skills	90 minutes
Lunch Break (optional)	30 minutes
Biological and Biochemical Foundations of Living Systems	95 minutes
Break (optional)	10 minutes
Psychological, Social, and Biological Foundations of Behavior	95 minutes
Void Option	5 minutes
Survey (optional)	5 minutes

The survey includes questions about your satisfaction with the overall MCAT experience, including registration, check-in, etc., as well as questions about how you prepared for the test.

Scoring

The MCAT is a scaled exam, meaning that your raw score will be converted into a scaled score that takes into account the difficulty of the questions. There is no guessing penalty. All sections are scored from 118–132, with a total scaled score range of 472–528. Because different versions of the test have varying levels of difficulty, the scale will be different from one exam to the next. Thus, there is no "magic number" of questions to get right in order to get a particular score. Plus, some of the questions on the test are considered "experimental" and do not count toward your score; they are just there to be evaluated for possible future inclusion in a test.

At the end of the test (after you complete the Psychological, Social, and Biological Foundations of Behavior section), you will be asked to choose one of the following two options, "I wish to have my MCAT exam scored" or "I wish to VOID my MCAT exam." You have five minutes to make a decision, and if you do not select one of the options in that time, the test will automatically be scored. If you choose the VOID option, your test will not be scored (you will not now, or ever, get a numerical score for this test), medical schools will not know you took the test, and no refunds will be granted. You cannot "unvoid" your scores at a later time.

So, what's a good score? The AAMC is centering the scale at 500 (i.e., 500 will be the 50th percentile), and recommends that application committees consider applicants near the center of the range. To be on the safe side, aim for a total score of around 510. Remember that if your GPA is on the low side, you'll need higher MCAT scores to compensate, and if you have a strong GPA, you can get away with lower MCAT scores. But the reality is that your chances of acceptance depend on a lot more than just your MCAT scores. It's a combination of your GPA, your MCAT scores, your undergraduate coursework, letters of recommendation, experience related to the medical field (such as volunteer work or research), extracurricular activities, your personal statement, etc. Medical schools are looking for a complete package, not just good scores and a good GPA.

GENERAL LAYOUT AND TEST-TAKING STRATEGIES

Layout of the Test

In each section of the test, the computer screen is divided vertically, with the passage on the left and the range of questions for that passage indicated above (such as "Passage 1, Questions 1–5"). The scroll bar for the passage text appears in the middle of the screen. Each question appears on the right, and you need to click "Next" to move to each subsequent question.

In the science sections, the freestanding questions are found in groups of 3–4, interspersed with the passages. The screen is still divided vertically; on the left is the statement "Questions [X–XX] do not refer to a passage and are independent of each other" and each question appears on the right as described above.

CBT Tools

There are a number of tools available on the test, including highlighting, strike-outs, the Flag for Review button, the Navigation and Review Screen buttons, the Periodic Table button, and of course, the noteboard booklet. All tools are available with both mouse control (buttons to click) or keyboard commands (Alt+ a letter). As everyone has different preferences, you should practice with both types of tools (mouse and keyboard) to see which is more comfortable for you personally. The following is a brief description of each tool.

1) **Highlighting:** This is done in the passage text (including table entries and some equations, but excluding figures and molecular structures), in the question stems, and in the answer choices (including Roman numerals). Select the words you wish to highlight (left-click and drag the cursor across the words), and in the upper left corner click the "Highlight" button to highlight the selected text yellow. Alternatively, press "Alt+H" to highlight the words. Highlighting can be removed by selecting the words again and in the upper left corner clicking the down arrow next to "Highlight." This will expand to show the "Remove Highlight" option; clicking this will remove the highlighting. Removing highlighting via the keyboard is cumbersome and is not recommended.

2) **Strike-outs:** This can be done on the answer choices, including Roman numeral statements, by selecting the text you want to strike out (left-click and drag the cursor across the text), then clicking the "Strikethrough" button in the upper left corner. Alternatively, press "Alt+S" to strike out the words. The strike-out can be removed by repeating these actions. Figures or molecular structures cannot be struck out; however, the letter answer choices of those structures can.

3) **Flag for Review button:** This is available for each question and is found in the upper right corner. This allows you to flag the question as one you would like to review later if time permits. When clicked, the flag icon turns yellow. Click again to remove the flag. Alternatively, press "Alt+F."

4) **Navigation button:** This is found near the bottom of the screen and is only available on your first pass through the section. Clicking this button brings up a navigation table listing all questions and their statuses (unseen, incomplete, complete, flagged for review). You can also press "Alt+N" to bring up the screen. The questions can be sorted by their statuses, and clicking a question number takes you immediately to that question. Once you have reached the end of the section and viewed the Review screen (described below), the Navigation screen is no longer available.

5) **Review Screen button:** This button is found near the bottom of the screen after your first pass through the section, and when clicked, brings up a new screen showing all questions and their statuses (either incomplete, unseen, or flagged for review). Questions that are complete are assigned no additional status. You can then choose one of three options by clicking with the mouse or with keyboard shortcuts: Review All (Alt+A), Review Incomplete (Alt+I), or Review Flagged (Alt+R); alternatively, you can click a question number to go directly back to that question. You can also end the section from this screen.

6) **Periodic Table button:** Clicking this button will open a periodic table (or press "Alt+T"). Note that the periodic table is large, covering most of the screen. However, this window can be resized to see the questions and a portion of the periodic table at the same time. The table text will not decrease, but scroll bars will appear on the window so you can center the section of the table of interest in the window.

7) **Noteboard Booklet (Scratch Paper):** At the start of the test, you will be given a spiral-bound set of four laminated 8.5"×14" sheets of paper and a wet-erase black marker to use as scratch paper. You can request a clean noteboard booklet at any time during the test; your original booklet will be collected. The noteboard is only useful if it is kept organized; do not give in to the tendency to write on the first available open space! Good organization will be very helpful when/if you wish to review a question. Indicate the passage number, the range of questions for that passage, and a topic in a box near the top of your scratch work, and indicate the question you are working on in a circle to the left of the notes for that question. Draw a line under your

scratch work when you change passages to keep the work separate. Do not erase or scribble over any previous work. If you do not think it is correct, draw one line through the work and start again. You may have already done some useful work without realizing it.

General Strategy for the Science Sections

Passages vs. FSQs in the Science Sections: What to Start With

Since the questions are displayed on separate screens, it is awkward and time consuming to click through all of the questions up front to find the FSQs. Therefore, go through the section on a first pass and decide whether to do the passage now or to save it for later, basing your decision on the passage text and the first question. Tackle the FSQs as you come upon them. More details are below.

Here is an outline of the procedure:

1) For each passage, write a heading on your scratch paper with the passage number, the general topic, and its range of questions (e.g. "Passage 1, thermodynamics, Q 1–5" or "Passage 2, enzymes, Q 6–9"). The passage numbers do not currently appear in the Navigation or Review screen; thus having the question numbers on your noteboard will allow you to move through the section more efficiently.

2) Skim the text and rank the passage. If a passage is a "Now," complete it before moving on to the next passage (also see "Attacking the Questions" below). If it is a "Later" passage, first write "SKIPPED" in block letters under the passage heading on your noteboard and leave room for your work when you come back to complete that passage. (Note that the specific passages you skip will be unique to you; in the Bio/Biochem section, you might choose to do all Biology passages first, then come back for Biochemistry. Or in Chem/Phys you might choose to skip experiment-based or analytical passages. Know ahead of time what type of passage you are going to skip and follow your plan.)

3) Next, click on the "Navigation" button at the bottom to get to the navigation screen. Click on the first question of the next passage; you'll be able to identify it because you know the range of questions from the passage you just skipped. This will take you to the next passage, where you will repeat steps 1–3.

4) Once you have completed the "Now" passages, go to the Review screen and click the first question for the first passage you skipped. Answer the questions, and continue going back to the Review screen and repeating this procedure for other passages you have skipped.

Attacking the Questions

As you work through the questions, if you encounter a particularly lengthy question, or a question that requires a lot of analysis, you may choose to skip it. This is a wise strategy because it ensures you will tackle all the easier questions first, the ones you are more likely to get right. If you choose to skip the question (or if you attempt it but get stuck), write down the question number on your noteboard, click the Flag for Review button to flag the question in the Review screen, and move on to the next question. At the end of the passage, click back through the set of questions to complete any that you skipped over the first time through, and make sure that you have filled in an answer for every question.

General Strategy for the CARS Section

Ranking and Ordering the Passages: What to Start With

Ranking: Since the questions are displayed on separate screens, it is awkward and time consuming to click through all of the questions before ranking each passage as "Now" (an easier passage), "Later" (a harder passage), or "Killer" (a passage that you will randomly guess on). Therefore, rank the passage and decide whether or not to do it on the first pass through the section based on the passage text, skimming the first 2–3 sentences.

Ordering: Because of the additional clicking through screens (or, use of the Review screen) that is required to navigate through the section, the "Two-Pass" system (completing the "Now" passages as you find them) is likely to be your most efficient approach. However, if you find that you are continuously making a lot of bad ranking decisions, it is still valid to experiment with the "Three-Pass" approach (ranking all nine passages up front before attempting your first "Now" passage).

Here is an outline of the basic Ranking and Ordering procedure to follow.

1) For each passage, write a heading on your noteboard with the passage number and its range of questions (e.g. "Passage 1, Q 1–7"). The passage numbers do not currently appear in the Navigation or Review screen; thus having the question numbers on your noteboard will allow you to move through the section more efficiently.

2) Skim the first 2–3 sentences and rank the passage. If the passage is a "Now," complete it before moving on to the next. If it is a "Later" or "Killer," first write either "Later" or "Killer" and "SKIPPED" in block letters under the passage heading on your noteboard and leave room for your work if you decide to come back and complete that passage. Then click through each question, flagging each one and filling in random guesses, until you get to the next passage.

3) Once you have completed the "Now" passages, come back for your second pass and complete the "Later" passages, leaving your random guesses in place for any "Killer" passages that you choose not to complete. Go to the Review screen and use your noteboard notes on the question numbers. Click on the number of the first question for that passage to go back to that question, and proceed from there. Alternatively, if you have consistently flagged all the questions for passages you skipped in your first pass you can use "Review Flagged" from the Review screen to find and complete your "Later" passages.

4) Regardless of how you choose to find your second pass passages, unmark each question after you complete it, so that you can continue to rely on the Review screen (and the "Review Flagged" function) to identify questions that you have not yet attempted.

Previewing the Questions

The formatting and functioning of the tools facilitates effective previewing. Having each question on a separate screen will encourage you to really focus on that question. Even more importantly, you can highlight in the question stem and in the answer choices.

Here is the basic procedure for previewing the questions:

1) Start with the first question, and if it has lead words referencing passage content, highlight them. You may also choose to jot them down on your noteboard. Once you reach and preview the last question for the set on that passage, THEN stay on that screen and work the passage (your

highlighting appears and stays on every passage screen, and persists through the whole 90 minutes).

2) Once you have worked the passage and defined the Bottom Line—the main idea and tone of the entire passage—work **backward** from the last question to the first. If you skip over any questions as you go (see "Attacking the Questions" below), write down the question number on your noteboard. Then click **forward** through the set of questions, completing any that you skipped over the first time through. Once you reach and complete the last question for that passage, clicking "Next" will send you to the first question of the next passage. Working the questions from last to first the first time through the set will eliminate the need to click back through multiple screens to get to the first question immediately after previewing, and will also make it easier and more efficient to do the hardest questions last (see "Attacking the Questions" below).

3) Remember that previewing questions is a CARS-only technique. It is not efficient to preview questions in the science sections.

Attacking the Questions

The question types and the procedure for actually attacking each type will be discussed later. However, it is still important **not** to attempt the hardest questions first (potentially getting stuck, wasting time, and discouraging yourself).

So, as you work the questions from last to first (see "Previewing the Questions" above), if you encounter a particularly difficult and/or lengthy question (or if you attempt a question but get stuck) write down the question number on your noteboard (you may also choose to flag it) and move on backward to the next question. Then click **forward** through the set and complete any that you skipped over the first time through the set, unflagging any questions that you flagged that first time through and making sure that you have filled in an answer for every question.

Pacing Strategy for the MCAT

Since the MCAT is a timed test, you must keep an eye on the timer and adjust your pacing as necessary. It would be terrible to run out of time at the end to discover that the last few questions could have been easily answered in just a few seconds each.

In the science sections you will have about one minute and thirty-five seconds (1:35) per question, and in the CARS section you will have about one minute and forty seconds (1:40) per question (not taking into account time spent reading the passage before answering the questions).

Section	# of Questions in passage	Approximate time (including reading the passage)
Chem/Phys, Bio/Biochem, and Psych/Soc	4	6.5 minutes
	5	8 minutes
	6	9.5 minutes
CARS	5	8.5 minutes
	6	10 minutes
	7	11.5 minutes

When starting a passage in the science sections, make note of how much time you will allot for it, and the starting time on the timer. Jot down on your noteboard what the timer should say at the end of the passage. Then just keep an eye on it as you work through the questions. If you are near the end of the time for that passage, guess on any remaining questions, make some notes on your noteboard, flag the questions, and move on. Come back to those questions if you have time.

For the CARS section, keep in mind that many people will maximize their score by *not* trying to complete every question or every passage in the section. A good strategy for test takers who cannot achieve a high level of accuracy on all nine passages is to randomly guess on at least one passage in the section, and spend your time getting a high percentage of the other questions right. To complete all nine CARS passages, you have about ten minutes per passage. To complete eight of the nine, you have about 11 minutes per passage.

To help maximize your number of correct answer choices in any section, do the questions and passages within that section in the order *you* want to do them in. See "General Strategy" above.

Process of Elimination

Process of elimination (POE) is probably the most useful technique you have to tackle MCAT questions. Since there is no guessing penalty, POE allows you to increase your probability of choosing the correct answer by eliminating those you are sure are wrong.

1) Strike out any choices that you are sure are incorrect or that do not address the issue raised in the question.
2) Jot down some notes to help clarify your thoughts if you return to the question.
3) Use the "Flag for Review" button to flag the question for review. (Note, however, that in the CARS section, you generally should not be returning to rethink questions once you have moved on to a new passage.)
4) Do not leave it blank! For the sciences, if you are not sure and you have already spent more than 60 seconds on that question, just pick one of the remaining choices. If you have time to review it at the end, you can always debate the remaining choices based on your previous notes. For CARS, if you have been through the choices two or three times, have re-read the question stem and gone back to the passage, and you are still stuck, move on. Do the remaining questions for that passage, take one more look at the question you were stuck on, then pick an answer and move on for good.
5) Special Note: if three of the four answer choices have been eliminated, the remaining choice must be the correct answer. Don't waste time pondering *why* it is correct, just click it and move on. The MCAT doesn't care if you truly understand why it's the right answer, only that you have the right answer selected.
6) More subject-specific information on techniques will be presented in the next chapter.

Guessing

Remember, there is NO guessing penalty on the MCAT. NEVER leave a question blank!

QUESTION TYPES

In the science sections of the MCAT, the questions fall into one of three main categories.

1) Memory questions: These questions can be answered directly from prior knowledge and represent about 25 percent of the total number of questions.

2) Explicit questions: These questions are those for which the answer is explicitly stated in the passage. To answer them correctly, for example, may just require finding a definition, or reading a graph, or making a simple connection. Explicit questions represent about 35 percent of the total number of questions.

3) Implicit questions: These questions require you to apply knowledge to a new situation; the answer is typically implied by the information in the passage. These questions often start "if…then…" (for example, "if we modify the experiment in the passage like this, then what result would we expect?"). Implicit style questions make up about 40 percent of the total number of questions.

In the CARS section, the questions fall into four main categories:

1) Specific questions: These either ask you for facts from the passage (Retrieval questions) or require you to deduce what is most likely to be true based on the passage (Inference questions).

2) General questions: These ask you to summarize themes (Main Idea and Primary Purpose questions) or evaluate an author's opinion (Tone/Attitude questions).

3) Reasoning questions: These ask you to describe the purpose of, or the support provided for, a statement made in the passage (Structure questions) or to judge how well the author supports his or her argument (Evaluate questions).

4) Application questions: These ask you to apply new information from either the question stem itself (New Information questions) or from the answer choices (Strengthen, Weaken, and Analogy questions) to the passage.

More detail on question types and strategies can be found in Chapter 2.

TESTING TIPS

Before Test Day

- Take a trip to the test center at least a day or two before your actual test date so that you can easily find the building and room on test day. This will also allow you to gauge traffic and see whether you need money for parking or anything like that. Knowing this type of information ahead of time will greatly reduce your stress on the day of your test.

- During the week before the test, adjust your sleeping schedule so that you are going to bed and getting up in the morning at the same times as on the day before and morning of the MCAT. Prioritize getting a reasonable amount of sleep during the last few nights before the test.

- Don't do any heavy studying the day before the test. This is not a test you can cram for! Your goal at this point is to rest and relax so that you can go into test day in good physical and mental condition.

- Eat well. Try to avoid excessive caffeine and sugar. Ideally, in the weeks leading up to the actual test you should experiment a little bit with foods and practice tests to see which foods give you the most endurance. Aim for steady blood sugar levels during the test: sports drinks, peanut-butter crackers, trail mix, etc. make good snacks for your breaks and lunch.

General Test Day Info and Tips

- On the day of the test, arrive at the test center at least a half hour prior to the start time of your test.
- Examinees will be checked in to the center in the order in which they arrive.
- You will be assigned a locker or secure area in which to put your personal items. Textbooks and study notes are not allowed, so there is no need to bring them with you to the test center.
- Your ID will be checked, your palm vein will be scanned, and you will be asked to sign in.
- You will be given your noteboard booklet and wet-erase marker, and the test center administrator will take you to the computer on which you will complete the test. You may not choose a computer; you must use the computer assigned to you.
- Nothing is allowed at the computer station except your photo ID, your locker key (if provided), and a factory sealed packet of ear plugs; not even your watch.
- If you choose to leave the testing room at the breaks, you will have your palm vein scanned again, and you will have to sign in and out.
- You are allowed to access the items in your locker, except for notes and cell phones. (Check your test center's policy on cell phones ahead of time; some centers do not even allow them to be kept in your locker.)
- Don't forget to bring the snack foods and lunch you experimented with in your practice tests.
- At the end of the test, the test administrator will collect your noteboard.
- Definitely take the breaks! Get up and walk around. It's a good way to clear your head between sections and get the blood (and oxygen!) flowing to your brain.
- Ask for a clean noteboard at the breaks if you want a fresh one.

Chapter 2
General Chemistry
Strategy for the MCAT

2.1 SCIENCE SECTIONS OVERVIEW

There are three science sections on the MCAT:

- Chemical and Physical Foundations of Biological Systems
- Biological and Biochemical Foundations of Living Systems
- Psychological, Social, and Biological Foundations of Behavior

The Chemical and Physical Foundations of Biological Systems section (Chem/Phys) is the first section on the test. It includes questions from General Chemistry (about 30%), Physics (about 25%), Organic Chemistry (about 15%), Biochemistry (about 25%), and Biology (about 5%). Further, the questions often test chemical and physical concepts within a biological setting: for example, pressure and fluid flow in blood vessels. A solid grasp of math fundamentals is required (arithmetic, algebra, graphs, trigonometry, vectors, proportions, and logarithms); however, there are no calculus-based questions.

The Biological and Biochemical Foundations of Living Systems section (Bio/Biochem) is the third section on the test. Approximately 65% of the questions in this section come from biology, approximately 25% come from biochemistry, and approximately 10% come from Organic and General Chemistry. Math calculations are generally not required on this section of the test; however, a basic understanding of statistics as used in biological research is helpful.

The Psychological, Social, and Biological Foundations of Behavior section (Psych/Soc) is the fourth and final section on the test. About 65% of the questions will be drawn from Psychology (and about 5% of these will be Biological Psychology), about 30% from Sociology, and about 5% from Biology. As with the Bio/Biochem section, calculations are generally not required; however, a basic understanding of statistics as used in research is helpful.

Most of the questions in each science section (44 of the 59) are passage-based, and each section has ten passages. Passages consist of a few paragraphs of information and include equations, reactions, graphs, figures, tables, experiments, and data. Four to six questions will be associated with each passage.

The remaining 25% of the questions (15 of 59) in each science section are freestanding questions (FSQs). These questions appear in approximately four groups interspersed between the passages. Each group contains three to four questions.

There are 95 minutes allotted to each of the science sections. This breaks down to approximately one minute and 35 seconds per question.

2.2 GENERAL SCIENCE PASSAGE TYPES

The passages in the science sections fall into one of three main categories: Information and/or Situation Presentation, Experiment/Research Presentation, or Persuasive Reasoning.

Information and/or Situation Presentation

These passages either present straightforward scientific information or they describe a particular event or occurrence. Generally, questions associated with these passages test basic science facts or ask you to predict outcomes given new variables or new information. Here is an example of an Information/Situation Presentation passage:

> Figure 1 shows a portion of the inner mechanism of a typical home smoke detector. It consists of a pair of capacitor plates which are charged by a 9-volt battery (not shown). The capacitor plates (electrodes) are connected to a sensor device, D; the resistor R denotes the internal resistance of the sensor. Normally, air acts as an insulator and no current would flow in the circuit shown. However, inside the smoke detector is a small sample of an artificially produced radioactive element, americium-241, which decays primarily by emitting alpha particles, with a half-life of approximately 430 years. The daughter nucleus of the decay has a half-life in excess of two million years and therefore poses virtually no biohazard.

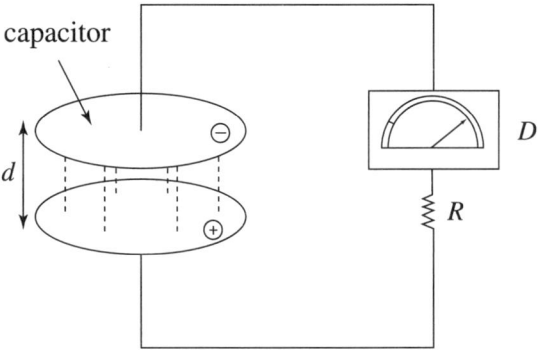

Figure 1   Smoke detector mechanism

> The decay products (alpha particles and gamma rays) from the ^{241}Am sample ionize air molecules between the plates and thus provide a conducting pathway which allows current to flow in the circuit shown in Figure 1. A steady-state current is quickly established and remains as long as the battery continues to maintain a 9-volt potential difference between its terminals. However, if smoke particles enter the space between the capacitor plates and thereby interrupt the flow, the current is reduced, and the sensor responds to this change by triggering

the alarm. (Furthermore, as the battery starts to "die out," the resulting drop in current is also detected to alert the homeowner to replace the battery.)

$$C = \varepsilon_0 \frac{A}{d}$$

Equation 1

where ε_0 is the universal permittivity constant, equal to 8.85×10^{-12} $C^2/(N \cdot m^2)$. Since the area A of each capacitor plate in the smoke detector is 20 cm^2 and the plates are separated by a distance d of 5 mm, the capacitance is 3.5×10^{-12} F = 3.5 pF.

Experiment/Research Presentation

These passages present the details of experiments and research procedures. They often include data tables and graphs. Generally, questions associated with these passages ask you to interpret data, draw conclusions, and make inferences. Here is an example of an Experiment/Research Presentation passage:

The development of sexual characteristics depends upon various factors, the most important of which are hormonal control, environmental stimuli, and the genetic makeup of the individual. The hormones that contribute to the development include the steroid hormones estrogen, progesterone, and testosterone, as well as the pituitary hormones FSH (follicle-stimulating hormone) and LH (luteinizing hormone).

To study the mechanism by which estrogen exerts its effects, a researcher performed the following experiments using cell culture assays.

Experiment 1:

Human embryonic placental mesenchyme (HEPM) cells were grown for 48 hours in Dulbecco's Modified Eagle Medium (DMEM), with media change every 12 hours. Upon confluent growth, cells were exposed to a 10 mg per mL solution of green fluorescent-labeled estrogen for 1 hour. Cells were rinsed with DMEM and observed under confocal fluorescent microscopy.

Experiment 2:

HEPM cells were grown to confluence as in Experiment 1. Cells were exposed to Pesticide A for 1 hour, followed by the 10 mg/mL solution of labeled estrogen, rinsed as in Experiment 1, and observed under confocal fluorescent microscopy.

Experiment 3:

Experiment 1 was repeated with Chinese Hamster Ovary (CHO) cells instead of HEPM cells.

Experiment 4:

CHO cells injected with cytoplasmic extracts of HEPM cells were grown to confluence, exposed to the 10 mg/mL solution of labeled estrogen for 1 hour, and observed under confocal fluorescent microscopy.

The results of these experiments are given in Table 1.

Table 1 Detection of Estrogen (+ indicates presence of Estrogen)

Experiment	Media	Cytoplasm	Nucleus
1	+	+	+
2	+	+	+
3	+	+	+
4	+	+	+

After observing the cells in each experiment, the researcher bathed the cells in a solution containing 10 mg per mL of a red fluorescent probe that binds specifically to the estrogen receptor only when its active site is occupied. After 1 hour, the cells were rinsed with DMEM and observed under confocal fluorescent microscopy. The results are presented in Table 2.

The researcher also repeated Experiment 2 using Pesticide B, an estrogen analog, instead of Pesticide A. Results from other researchers had shown that Pesticide B binds to the active site of the cytosolic estrogen receptor (with an affinity 10,000 times greater than that of estrogen) and causes increased transcription of mRNA.

Table 2 Observed Fluorescence and Estrogen Effects (G = green, R = red)

Experiment	Media	Cytoplasm	Nucleus	Estrogen effects observed?
1	G only	G and R	G and R	Yes
2	G only	G only	G only	No
3	G only	G only	G only	No
4	G only	G and R	G and R	Yes

Based on these results, the researcher determined that estrogen had no effect when not bound to a cytosolic, estrogen-specific receptor.

Persuasive Reasoning

These passages typically present a scientific phenomenon along with a hypothesis that explains the phenomenon, and may include counter-arguments as well. Questions associated with these passages ask you to evaluate the hypothesis or arguments. Persuasive Reasoning passages in the science sections of the MCAT tend to be less common than Information Presentation or Experiment-based passages. Here is an example of a Persuasive Reasoning passage:

Two theoretical chemists attempted to explain the observed trends of acidity by applying two interpretations of molecular orbital theory. Consider the pK_a values of some common acids listed along the conjugate base of each acid:

acid	pK_a	conjugate base
H_2SO_4	< 0	HSO_4^-
H_2CrO_4	5.0	$HCrO_4^-$
H_2PO_4	2.1	$H_2PO_4^-$
HF	3.9	F^-
HOCl	7.8	ClO^-
HCN	9.5	CN^-
HIO_3	1.2	IO_3^-

Recall that acids with a $pK_a < 0$ are called strong acids, and those with a $pK_a > 0$ are called weak acids. The arguments of the chemists are given below.

Chemist #1:

"The acidity of a compound is proportional to the polarization of the H—X bond, where X is some nonmetal element. Complex acids, such as H_2SO_4, $HClO_4$, and HNO_3 are strong acids because the H—O bonding electrons are strongly drawn towards the oxygen. It is generally true that a covalent bond weakens as its polarization increases. Therefore, one can conclude that the strength of an acid is proportional to the number of electronegative atoms in that acid."

Chemist #2:

"The acidity of a compound is proportional to the number of stable resonance structures of that acid's conjugate base. H_2SO_4, $HClO_4$, and HNO_3 are all strong acids because their respective conjugate bases exhibit a high degree of resonance stabilization."

Mapping a Passage

"Mapping a passage" refers to the combination of on-screen highlighting and noteboard notes that you take while working through a passage. Typically, good things to highlight include the overall topic of a paragraph, unfamiliar terms, unusual terms, italicized terms, numerical values, hypotheses, and experimental results. Noteboard notes can be used to summarize the paragraphs and to jot down important facts and connections that are made when reading the passage. More details on passage mapping will be presented in Section 2.5.

2.3 GENERAL SCIENCE QUESTION TYPES

Questions in the science sections are generally one of three main types: Memory, Explicit, or Implicit.

Memory Questions

These questions can be answered directly from prior knowledge, with no need to reference the passage or question text. Memory questions represent approximately 25 percent of the science questions on the MCAT. Usually, Memory questions are found as FSQs, but they can also be tucked into a passage. Here's an example of a Memory question:

Which of the following acetylating conditions will convert diethylamine into an amide at the fastest rate?

A) Acetic acid/HCl
B) Acetic anhydride
C) Acetyl chloride
D) Ethyl acetate

2.3

Explicit Questions

Explicit questions can be answered primarily with information from the passage, along with prior knowledge. They may require data retrieval, graph analysis, or making a simple connection. Explicit questions make up approximately 35–40 percent of the science questions on the MCAT; here's an example (taken from the Information/Situation Presentation passage above):

The sensor device *D* shown in Figure 1 performs its function by acting as:

A) an ohmmeter.
B) a voltmeter.
C) a potentiometer.
D) an ammeter.

Implicit Questions

These questions require you to take information from the passage, combine it with your prior knowledge, apply it to a new situation, and come to some logical conclusion. They typically require more complex connections than do Explicit questions, and may also require data retrieval, graph analysis, etc. Implicit questions usually require a solid understanding of the passage information. They make up approximately 35–40 percent of the science questions on the MCAT; here's an example (taken from the Experiment/Research Presentation passage above):

If Experiment 2 were repeated, but this time exposing the cells first to Pesticide A and then to Pesticide B before exposing them to the green fluorescent-labeled estrogen and the red fluorescent probe, which of the following statements would most likely be true?

A) Pesticide A and Pesticide B would bind to the same site on the estrogen receptor.
B) Estrogen effects would be observed.
C) Only green fluorescence would be observed.
D) Both green and red fluorescence would be observed.

The Rod of Asclepius

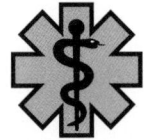

You may notice this Rod of Asclepius icon as you read through the book. In Greek mythology, the Rod of Asclepius is associated with healing and medicine; the symbol continues to be used today to represent medicine and healthcare. You won't see this on the actual MCAT, but we've used it here to call attention to medically related examples and questions.

2.4 GENERAL CHEMISTRY ON THE MCAT

Although general chemistry is sometimes remembered as a daunting topic from college, the MCAT does not test the fine details of general chemistry. Rather, the focus of this section is on having a strong knowledge of chemistry fundamentals, and manipulating that knowledge to adapt to different scenarios presented in passages and questions. The passages often contain information that recapitulates basic chemistry knowledge, and may present additional information that builds on fundamental concepts.

The majority of the G-Chem questions will not be based on rote memory, but will require you to retrieve information from the passage and use some deductive reasoning skills. Thus, in order to succeed in this section, you not only need solid knowledge of fundamental principles of chemistry, but also strong critical reasoning and reading comprehension skills. These three components may be stressed differently depending on the passage type.

The science sections of the MCAT each have 10 passages and 15 freestanding questions (FSQs). General Chemistry will make up about a third of the questions in the Chemical and Physical Foundations of Biological Systems section. The remaining questions will be on Physics (25%), Organic Chemistry (15%), and Biochemistry (25%). In addition, about 5% of the questions on the Biological and Biochemical Foundations of Living Systems section will be General Chemistry.

2.5 PASSAGE TYPES AS THEY APPLY TO GENERAL CHEMISTRY

Information/Situation Presentation: G-Chem

These passages assume knowledge of basic scientific concepts, and also present new information that builds on these basic concepts. The new information may be presented in a way that is very similar to how it would appear in a textbook or other scientific reference. The questions may be about basic scientific facts that you already know, but often the passage will present topics or subtopics with which you are unfamiliar. Information/Situation Presentation passages can be intimidating, as they often explore topics in a greater level of detail than the scope of your MCAT preparation. However, keep in mind that the whole point of these types of passages is to force you to use critical reasoning and apply your basic scientific knowledge to new topics. It is not to see how much advanced scientific coursework you have memorized. Therefore, it is important when you see a passage on, say, molecular orbital theory, that you don't think to yourself, "Oh no!! I forgot to study molecular orbital theory!!!" Rather, look at the information in the passage, and consider how your knowledge about more basic chemical concepts, such as electron configurations, can be applied in order to answer the questions. The new information in the passage can supplement your basic knowledge.

This type of passage may also present information in the context of a specific situation, such as the results of a research study or an experiment. In this case, the questions may ask you to distinguish between data that supports and data that refutes the result being presented. In some passages, an apparently contradictory or erroneous result is presented and questions may ask what mistakes could have been made over the course of the experiment to cause such a result. Thus, these passages require you to think critically about the importance of each chemical and physical element of an experiment. Note however, that they do not present the steps of an experiment in great detail; that style is reserved for Experiment/Research Presentation passages.

Experiment/Research Presentation: G-Chem

These passages present an experimental set up in great detail; they describe the rationale behind an experiment, how it is set up and executed, and its results. In these passages you are often asked to analyze data given in the form of charts and graphs. In addition, questions may ask you how the results of the experiment would differ if a certain variable were changed; this requires you to think critically about the role of each element of the experiment. In this passage type, be careful not to gloss over important experimental details as you retrieve information from the passage. Be aware that details such as units can make the difference between answering a question correctly and incorrectly, and be vigilant about these experimental details as you work through the questions and look back to the passage.

Persuasive Argument: G-Chem

In a Persuasive Argument passage, two perspectives on a problem are presented. It may be different researchers putting forth two different methodologies for conducting an experiment, or two different explanations for an experimental result or phenomenon.

The questions may ask how the authors came to develop different perspectives, or ask you to evaluate the credibility of each of their arguments. Persuasive Argument passages are the least common passage type in G-Chem.

Reading a General Chemistry Passage

Reading a G-Chem passage is not like reading a scientific paper or a textbook. That is, you are not reading thoroughly and trying to understand the relevance of each sentence, as the passage will likely contain details beyond the scope of the questions.

Instead, your goal is to take no more than 60 seconds and skim the passage in order to determine the general topic area being tested and create a brief passage map before moving on to the questions. To do this as efficiently as possible, focus on the first sentence of each paragraph and any bolded or italicized words. In addition, chemical equations and figures may provide insight as to the general topic of the passage. For example, if you see a titration curve, it is likely that the passage will test acid-base chemistry.

G-Chem passages often include complex graphs and data tables. Avoid the temptation to analyze this data on your first pass through the passage. Rather, wait until you find a question that requires the use of the data in the graph or table, then analyze the data in the context of that question. This approach is more efficient and productive than trying to preemptively interpret data.

The bottom line: You can always go back and reread more details from the passage. Furthermore, not all of the details from the passage are necessary to answer the questions. Therefore, it is a waste of your time to read and attempt to thoroughly understand the passage the first time you read it.

Mapping a G-Chem Passage

As you skim through a G-Chem passage to get a feel for the type of questions that might follow, take note of the general location of information within the passage. The highlighting tool is a useful way to visually note a few key words that relate to the general topic of the passage or some unusual or new term that is introduced. Highlight sparingly, and use the noteboard to make more detailed notes. An example of a highlighted passage is shown below. This is an Information Presentation passage:

The batteries that start an automobile or power flashlights are devices that convert chemical energy into electrical energy. These devices use spontaneous oxidation-reduction reactions (called half-reactions) that take place at the electrodes to create an electric current. The strength of the battery, or electromotive force, is determined by the difference in electric potential between the half cells, expressed in volts. This voltage depends on which reactions occur at the anode and the cathode, the concentrations of the solutions in the cells, and the temperature. The cell voltage, E, at a temperature of 25°C and nonstandard conditions, can be calculated from the Nernst equation, where $E°$ is the standard potential, n denotes the number of electrons transferred in the balanced half reaction, and Q is the reaction quotient.

$$E = E° - \frac{0.0592}{n} \log_{10} Q$$

Equation 1

The lead storage battery used in automobiles is composed of six identical cells joined in series. The anode is solid lead, the cathode is lead dioxide, and the electrodes are immersed in a solution of sulfuric acid. As each cell discharges during normal operation, the sulfate ion is consumed as it is deposited in the form of lead sulfate on both electrodes, as shown in Reaction 1:

Reaction 1:

$$Pb(s) + PbO_2(s) + 4 H^+(aq) + 2 SO_4^{2-}(aq)$$
$$\downarrow$$
$$2 PbSO_4(s) + 2 H_2O(l)$$

Each cell produces 2 V, for a total of 12 V for the typical car battery. Unlike many batteries, however, the lead storage battery can be recharged by applying an external voltage. Because the redox reaction in the battery consumes sulfate ions, the degree of discharge of the battery can be checked by measuring the density of the battery fluid with a hydrometer. The fluid density in a fully charged battery is 1.2 g/cm^3.

Table 1 Standard Reduction Potentials at T = 25°C

Half-reaction	$E°$ (V)
$F_2(g) + 2e^- \rightarrow 2F^-(aq)$	+2.87
$Cl_2(g) + 2e^- \rightarrow 2Cl^-(aq)$	+1.36
$Cu^+(aq) + e^- \rightarrow Cu(s)$	+0.52
$Cu^{2+}(aq) + 2e^- \rightarrow Cu(s)$	+0.34
$Zn^{2+}(aq) + 2e^- \rightarrow Zn(s)$	−0.76
$Al^{3+}(aq) + 3e^- \rightarrow Al(s)$	−1.66
$Li^+(aq) + e^- \rightarrow Li(s)$	−3.05

Note that only a few words are highlighted. In the first paragraph, "batteries" and "spontaneous oxidation-reduction" relate to the general topic of the passage, and serve as a reminder that batteries contain a spontaneous redox reaction. The second paragraph identifies the two electrodes in the battery and, in the last paragraph, the voltage and density of a car battery are highlighted. Since these are specific and unusual pieces of information, they might come up in a question.

Rather than highlighting large portions of the passage as you skim it, use your noteboard to create a simple passage map to help organize where different types of information are in the passage. Scratch paper is only useful if it is kept organized! Make sure that your notes for each passage are clearly delineated and marked with the passage number and range of questions. This will allow you to easily read your notes when you come back to review a flagged question. Resist the temptation to write in the first available blank space, as this makes it much more difficult to refer back to your work.

As you skim the passage, note the subject of each paragraph and any key words or values. A well-constructed passage map makes it easier and more efficient to go back and retrieve specific information as you work through the questions. Here is an example of a passage map for the passage shown above:

P1 – Batteries, general information, background
P2 – Automobile batteries, more specific information about them
P3 – Recharging car battery, Reduction Potentials in Table 1

As you can see, your passage map does not need to be particularly detailed, nor should it be, as reading and mapping the passage should only take a minute of your time. However, this does provide a valuable framework for efficiently locating information within the passage.

Let's look at another passage and how to map it. This is an Experiment/Research Presentation passage:

2.5

Two cube-shaped compartments, X and Y, each with a volume of one cubic meter, were used in several experiments to study the properties of gases. Compartment X was fitted with a piston of negligible mass which fit snugly against the walls of the container. The compartments were connected by a pinhole which could be opened or closed at will (see Figure 1). The pressure and temperature could be measured in either compartment. At the start of each experiment, Compartment X contained equal molar quantities of four gases (helium, oxygen, nitrogen, and carbon dioxide), the temperature in Compartment X was 25°C and the pressure was 1 atm. Initially, Compartment Y was evacuated. The behavior of all the gases can be assumed to be ideal. (Note: 1 atm ≈ 105 Pa.)

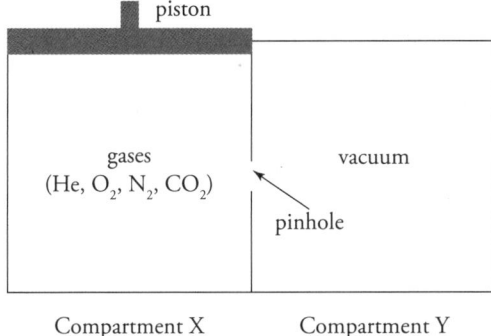

Figure 1   Experimental apparatus

Experiment 1:

With the pinhole closed, the temperature of the gases in Compartment X was gradually increased to 50°C, and the pressure of the gas inside the compartment was measured.

Experiment 2:

With the pinhole closed, the piston was gradually lowered into Compartment X until it had dropped a distance of 0.5 m. The pressure of the gas in the container was then measured.

Experiment 3:

The pinhole was opened, and the pressure change in each compartment was measured until equilibrium was reached.

Here, the highlighter tool can be used to emphasize that this passage is about the behavior of gases. Any time a passage is about gases, it's useful to know whether the gas behaves in a real or ideal manner;

therefore the phrase "assumed to be ideal" is also highlighted. In experimental passages, if important details jump out at you on your initial skim of the passage, it's useful to highlight them. For example, Figure 1 makes it fairly obvious that compartment X contains four gases, while compartment Y is a vacuum with no gas, however the "equal molar quantities" of the four gases in compartment X is a useful detail to highlight. Here's how you might map this passage on your noteboard:

> *P1 – Experimental setup*
> *E1 – Temp change, constant volume*
> *E2 – Pressure change*
> *E3 – Pressure change, equilibrium*

As was true of our last passage map, the main purpose is to create an outline so that it will be easier to retrieve necessary information as you work through the questions. Since this is an Experiment Presentation passage, the map points out the locations of the main experimental details. Note that on the first pass, it is not important to note all the specific details of each individual experiment on your noteboard, though quickly highlighting new experimental conditions, like temperature, etc. can be helpful. If possible, however, it may be helpful to note the general variable being changed.

Let's look at one more example of passage mapping. This passage is a Persuasive Argument Passage:

Two theoretical chemists attempted to explain the observed trends of acidity by applying two interpretations of molecular orbital theory. Consider the pK_a values of some common acids listed along with the conjugate base of each acid:

acid	pK_a	conjugate base
H_2SO_4	< 0	HSO_4^-
H_2CrO_4	5.0	$HCrO_4^-$
H_3PO_4	2.1	$H_2PO_4^-$
HF	3.9	F^-
HOCl	7.8	ClO^-
HCN	9.5	CN^-
HIO_3	1.2	IO_3^-

Recall that acids with a $pK_a < 0$ are called strong acids, and those with a $pK_a > 0$ are called weak acids. The arguments of the chemists are given below.

Chemist #1:

"The acidity of a compound is proportional to the polarization of the H—X bond, where X is some nonmetal element. Complex acids, such as H_2SO_4, $HClO_4$, and HNO_3 are strong acids because the H—O bonding electrons are strongly drawn towards the oxygen. It is generally true that a covalent bond weakens as its polarization increases. Therefore, one can conclude that the strength of an acid is proportional to the number of electronegative atoms in that acid."

Chemist #2:

"The acidity of a compound is proportional to the number of stable resonance structures of that acid's conjugate base. H_2SO_4, $HClO_4$, and HNO_3 are all strong acids because their respective conjugate bases exhibit a high degree of resonance stabilization."

For a Persuasive Argument passage, the goal of passage mapping and highlighting is to identify the issue being addressed, and the main points of each of the opposing lines of reasoning. This can be accomplished using the highlighter tool to emphasize that the passage is about "trends of acidity," and that Chemist #1 attributes the behavior of acids to "polarization of the H—X bond," while Chemist #2 focuses on "number of stable resonance structures."

In this case, a passage map would be very similar to the results achieved by highlighting. However, keep in mind that the very act of writing things down helps clarify it in your head:

P1/Main issue: Trends of acidity, using MO theory
Chemist #1: acidity $\propto$ # of EN atoms; polarization of H—X bond
Chemist #2: # of res. struct. for conj. base

As you can see from the examples above, effective passage-mapping requires a combination of highlighting and jotting down notes in an organized fashion on your noteboard. The best way to improve your passage mapping, and to determine which combination of these skills works best for you, is to practice, practice, practice.

2.6   TACKLING THE QUESTIONS

In general, G-Chem questions require a combination of basic knowledge, passage retrieval, and critical reasoning. The more difficult G-Chem questions tend to weigh the last two skills more heavily. Therefore, if you have a sound basis in the fundamental principles of General Chemistry, it is safe to assume that a tough question will be best addressed by looking back to the passage for information that is either explicitly stated or implied.

In the section on passage mapping, we reviewed an Information/Situation Presentation passage on batteries and redox reactions. We will draw on questions from this passage in order to illustrate the different question types.

G-Chem Memory Questions

These questions test background knowledge and require you to recall a specific definition or relationship. Memory questions are most often freestanding questions that appear on their own, without a passage associated with them. Memory questions are less frequently associated with passages on the MCAT, but when they are, they will help you complete a passage more quickly, since there is no information retrieval required that will slow you down. For example, a question from the car battery passage shown above asked:

If the reaction in a concentration cell is spontaneous in the reverse direction, then:

A) $Q < K$, ΔG for the forward reaction is negative, and the cell voltage is positive.

B) $Q < K$, ΔG for the forward reaction is positive, and the cell voltage is negative.

C) $Q > K$, ΔG for the forward reaction is negative, and the cell voltage is positive.

D) $Q > K$, ΔG for the forward reaction is positive, and the cell voltage is negative.

In order to answer this question correctly, you need to know the connection between ΔG and spontaneity. A spontaneous reaction has a negative ΔG, and a nonspontaneous reaction has a positive ΔG. Since the reaction is spontaneous in the reverse direction, it must be nonspontaneous in the forward direction. Therefore, the ΔG of the forward reaction is positive, eliminating choices A and C. Alternatively, you could know that cell voltage applies to the forward direction, and that a nonspontaneous cell has a negative voltage, also eliminating choices A and C.

To distinguish between choices B and D, you must have a fundamental understanding of equilibrium and Le Châtelier's Principle. The reaction quotient, Q, always approaches the equilibrium constant, K, and if $Q > K$ the reaction will be pushed in the reverse direction, toward the reactants side of the equilibrium, in order to decrease the value of Q. Thus, since the question says the reaction is spontaneous in the reverse direction, Q must be greater than K. This makes choice D the best answer.

Also, note that this question asks about concentration cells, which are not mentioned in the passage, and therefore this problem is essentially a free-standing question.

G-Chem Explicit Questions

Explicit questions require direct retrieval of information from the passage. Sometimes, the answers to Explicit questions are definitions or relationships that are clearly stated in the passage. However, these types of questions may also require some background knowledge or a simple step of logical reasoning. Here is another example from the car battery redox passage shown above:

Of the following, which is the best reducing agent?

A) Li^+

B) Li

C) Cl^-

D) F^-

2.6

To answer this question, you must have fundamental knowledge of redox definitions and relationships, but you also need to retrieve information from the passage. The best reducing agent is the species that has the highest oxidizing potential, and Table 1 gives the reduction potentials for these reagents. However, you also need the knowledge that the oxidation potential is the same as the reduction potential, but with the opposite sign. Since the oxidation of Li has the highest positive potential (3.05 V), Li is the strongest reducing agent.

The best way to approach Explicit questions is to refer to your passage map to find the location of the information you need. Then, go back to the passage and read that section in greater detail. There are two instances when retrieval of information for Explicit questions can be especially tricky. First, in research study passages, be cautious when retrieving information from tables and graphs. Rather than simply pulling data directly from the figures, be sure to read the text just before and after the figures as well, as it may contain important information that changes the way the data should be interpreted. Second, when a passage goes into greater detail about a subject that you already have fundamental knowledge of, avoid the temptation to answer questions directly from memory. Often, these types of passages will provide some obscure detail or anomalous situation that will be tested in the questions, and require you to retrieve information from the passage in order to select the correct answer.

G-Chem Implicit Questions

Implicit questions require you to work through two or more steps of critical reasoning based on your background knowledge and information given in the passage. In other words, the answer is not directly stated in the passage, but is implied by the information provided. The distinction between an Implicit and an Explicit question can be subtle, as both require you to retrieve information from the passage, and Explicit questions may also require you to make a simple critical reasoning decision. The difference is that in Implicit questions, the reasoning step required is not as direct or obvious, and more than one step is usually required. For example:

> When a lead storage battery recharges, what happens to
> the density of the battery fluid?
>
> A)   It decreases to 1.0 g/cm^3.
> B)   It increases to 1.0 g/cm^3.
> C)   It decreases to 1.2 g/cm^3.
> D)   It increases to 1.2 g/cm^3.

First, information on the density of the battery fluid must be retrieved from the passage. Our passage map tells us that specific information on car batteries can be found in paragraphs two and three, and reviewing the highlighted text reveals that the third paragraph of the passage states that the density of fluid in a fully charged battery is 1.2 g/cm^3. Therefore, as the battery is recharging, its density is approaching this value, eliminating choices A and B.

The difference between choices C and D is whether the density of the solution is increasing or decreasing to 1.2 g/cm^3 during recharge. To determine this, we can look for additional information in the passage that may relate to changing density of the battery fluid. The second paragraph of the passage states that as

2.6

the battery discharges, sulfate ions are consumed and deposited in the form of lead sulfate. The removal of ions from solution implies that the amount of mass in the solution is going down, and therefore its density is also decreasing. Therefore, density is decreasing during discharge, and increasing during recharge. This makes choice D the best answer.

The key step here is focusing on the differences among the answer choices. What can be difficult about approaching implicit questions is that it is often hard to determine which information is supposed to "imply" something about the answer. Zeroing in on differences among the answer choices can help you determine which information from the passage is most relevant, and may help you rephrase what the question is really asking. Also, note that the first step of our analysis, eliminating the choices with 1.0 g/cm³ density, was basically just answering an explicit question via direct passage retrieval. Many implicit questions begin this way, and it is much easier to eliminate answer choices first based on explicit information than it is to try to make a decision based on implicit information.

2.7   SUMMARY OF THE APPROACH TO GENERAL CHEMISTRY

How to Map the Passage and Use the Noteboard

1) The passage should not be read as you'd read textbook material, with the intent of learning something from every sentence (science majors especially will be tempted to read this way). Skim through the paragraphs to get a feel for the type of questions that will follow, and to get a general idea of the location of information within the passage.

2) Highlighting—Use this tool sparingly, or you will end up with a passage that is completely covered in yellow highlighter! Highlighting in a General Chemistry passage should be used to draw attention to a few words that demonstrate one of the following:

   - The main theme of a paragraph
   - Important predictions or conclusions about an experiment
   - Any unusual or unfamiliar terms that are defined specifically for that passage (such as something that is italicized)

3) Pay brief attention to equations, figures, and experiments, noting only what information they deal with (i.e., read titles, axes, and column/row headings). Do not spend a lot of time analyzing at this point, as you can come back and look more closely at this information if a question requires it.

4) The noteboard is only useful if it is kept organized! Make sure that your notes for each passage are clearly delineated and marked with the passage number and range of questions on your scratch paper. This will allow you to easily read your notes when you come back to review a marked question. Resist the temptation to write in the first available blank space, as this makes it much more difficult to refer back to your work.

General Chemistry Question Strategies

1) Remember that Process of Elimination is paramount! The strike-out tool allows you to eliminate answer choices; this will improve your chances of guessing the correct answer if you are unable to narrow it down to one choice.

2) Answer the straightforward questions first. Leave questions that require analysis of experiments and graphs for later. Take the test in the order YOU want. Make sure to use your noteboard to indicate questions you skipped.

3) Make sure that the answer you choose actually answers the question, and isn't just a true statement.

4) Roman numeral questions: Whenever possible, start by evaluating the Roman numeral item that shows up in exactly two answer choices. This allows you to quickly eliminate two wrong answer choices regardless of whether the item is true or false. Typically then, you will only have to assess one of the other Roman numeral items to determine the correct answer. Always work between the I-II-III items and the answer choices. Once an item is found to be true (or false) strike out answer choices which do not contain (or do contain) that item number. Make sure to strike out the actual Roman numeral item as well, and highlight those items that are true.

5) LEAST/EXCEPT/NOT questions: Don't get tricked by these questions that ask you to pick the answer that doesn't fit (the incorrect or false statement). It's often good to use your noteboard and write 'A B C D' with a T or F next to each answer choice. The one that stands out as different is the correct answer. Don't forget that you can also highlight information in the question stem, so draw attention to the LEAST/EXCEPT/NOT in the question so you don't forget!

6) 2 x 2 style questions: These questions require you to know two pieces of information to get the correct answer, and are easily identified by their answer choices, which commonly take the form A because X, B because X, A because Y, B because Y. Tackle one piece of information at a time, which should allow you to quickly eliminate two answer choices.

7) Ranking questions: When asked to rank items, look for an extreme—either the greatest or the smallest item—and eliminate answer choices that do not have that item shown at the correct end of the ranking. This is often enough to eliminate one to three answer choices. Based on the remaining choices, look for the other extreme at the other end of the ranking and use POE again.

8) If you read a question and do not know how to answer it, look to the passage for help. It is likely that the passage contains information pertinent to answering the question, either within the text or in the form of experimental data.

9) If a question requires a lengthy calculation, flag it and return to it later, particularly if you are slow with arithmetic or dimensional analysis.

10) Again, don't leave any question blank, and when randomly guessing, choose the same letter for every question unless you have already eliminated it.

2.7

A Note About Flashcards

For most of the exams you've taken previously, flashcards were likely very helpful. This was because those exams mostly required you to regurgitate information, and flashcards are pretty good at helping you memorize facts. However, the most challenging aspect of the MCAT is not that it requires you to memorize the fine details of content knowledge, but that it requires you to apply your basic scientific knowledge to unfamiliar situations: flashcards alone may not help you there.

Flashcards can be beneficial if your basic content knowledge is deficient in some area. For example, if you don't know the strong acids and bases, flashcards can certainly help you memorize these facts. Or, maybe you are unsure of some of the molecular geometries and shapes from the VSEPR theory. You might find that flashcards can help you memorize these. But unless you are trying to memorize basic facts in your personal weak areas, you are better off doing and analyzing practice passages than carrying around a stack of flashcards.

2.7

Chapter 3
Chemistry Fundamentals

3.1 METRIC UNITS

Before we begin our study of chemistry, we will briefly go over metric units. Scientists use the *Système international d'unités* (the International System of Units), abbreviated SI, to express measurements of physical quantities. The six MCAT-relevant **base units** of SI are given below:

SI Base Unit	Abbreviation	Measures
meter	m	length
kilogram	kg	mass
second	s	time
mole	mol	amount of substance
kelvin	K	temperature
ampere	A	electric current

The units of any physical quantity can be written in terms of the SI base units. For example, the SI unit of speed is meters per second (m/s), the SI unit of energy (the joule) is kilograms times meters^2 per second^2 (kg $\cdot$ m^2/s^2), and so forth.

Multiples of the base units that are powers of ten are often abbreviated and precede the symbol for the unit. For example, m is the symbol for milli-, which means 10^{-3} (one thousandth). So, one thousandth of a second, 1 millisecond, would be written as 1 ms. The letter M is the symbol for mega-, which means 10^6 (one million); a distance of one million meters, 1 megameter, would be abbreviated as 1 Mm. Some of the most common power-of-ten prefixes are given in the list below:

Prefix	Symbol	Multiple
nano-	n	10^{-9}
micro-	μ	10^{-6}
milli-	m	10^{-3}
centi-	c	10^{-2}
kilo-	k	10^3
mega-	M	10^6

Two other units, ones that are common in chemistry, are the liter and the angstrom. The liter (abbreviated L) is a unit of volume equal to 1/1000 of a cubic meter:

$$1000 \text{ L} = 1 \text{ m}^3$$

$$1 \text{ L} = 1000 \text{ cm}^3$$

The standard SI unit of volume, the cubic meter, is inconveniently large for most laboratory work. The liter is a smaller unit. Furthermore, the most common way of expressing solution concentrations, **molarity** (**M**), uses the liter in its definition: M = moles of solute per liter of solution.

In addition, you will see the milliliter (mL) as often as you will see the liter. A simple consequence of the definition of a liter is the fact that one milliliter is the same volume as one cubic centimeter:

$$1 \text{ mL} = 1 \text{ cm}^3 = 1 \text{ cc}$$

While the volume of any substance can, strictly speaking, be expressed in liters, you rarely hear of a milliliter of gold, for example. Ordinarily, the liter is used to express the volumes of liquids and gases, but not solids.

The **angstrom**, abbreviated Å, is a unit of length equal to 10^{-10} m. The angstrom is convenient because atomic radii and bond lengths are typically around 1 to 3 Å.

Example 3-1: By how many orders of magnitude is a centimeter longer than an angstrom?

Solution: An **order of magnitude** is a factor of ten. Since 1 cm = 10^{-2} m and 1 Å = 10^{-10} m, a centimeter is 8 factors of ten, or 8 orders of magnitude, greater than an angstrom.

3.2 DENSITY

The **density** of a substance is its mass per volume:

$$\text{Density: } \rho = \frac{\text{mass}}{\text{volume}} = \frac{m}{V}$$

In SI units, density is expressed in kilograms per cubic meter (kg/m^3). However, in chemistry, densities are more often expressed in grams per cubic centimeter (g/cm^3). This unit of density is convenient because most liquids and solids have densities of around 1 to 20 g/cm^3. Here is the conversion between these two sets of density units:

$$\text{g/cm}^3 \rightarrow \text{multiply by 1000} \rightarrow \text{kg/m}^3$$

$$\text{g/cm}^3 \leftarrow \text{divide by 1000} \leftarrow \text{kg/m}^3$$

For example, water has a density of 1 g/cm^3 (it varies slightly with temperature, but this is the value the MCAT will expect you to use). To write this density in kg/m^3, we would multiply by 1000. The density of water is 1000 kg/m^3. As another example, the density of copper is about 9000 kg/m^3, so to express this density in g/cm^3, we would divide by 1000: The density of copper is 9 g/cm^3.

Example 3-2: Diamond has a density of 3500 kg/m^3. What is the volume, in cm^3, of a 1 3/4-carat diamond (where, by definition, 1 carat = 0.2 g)?

Solution: If we divide mass by density, we get volume, so, converting 3500 kg/m^3 into 3.5 g/cm^3, we find that

$$V = \frac{m}{\rho} = \frac{1.75(0.2\,\text{g})}{3.5\ \text{g/cm}^3} = \frac{0.35\,\text{g}}{3.5\ \text{g/cm}^3} = 0.10\,\text{cm}^3$$

3.3 MOLECULAR FORMULAS

When two or more atoms form a covalent bond they create a **molecule**. For example, when two atoms of hydrogen (H) bond with one atom of oxygen (O), the resulting molecule is H_2O, water. A compound's **molecular formula** gives the identities and numbers of the atoms in the molecule. For example, the formula $C_4H_4N_2$ tells us that this molecule contains four carbon atoms, four hydrogen atoms, and two nitrogen atoms.

Example 3-3: What is the molecular formula of *para*-nitrotoluene?

A) $C_6H_5NO_2$
B) $C_7H_7NO_2$
C) $C_7H_8NO_2$
D) $C_7H_9NO_2$

Solution: There are a total of seven carbon atoms, seven hydrogen atoms, one nitrogen atom, and two oxygen atoms, so choice B is the correct answer.

3.4 EMPIRICAL FORMULAS

Let's look again at the molecule $C_4H_4N_2$. There are four atoms each of carbon and hydrogen, and half as many (two) nitrogen atoms. Therefore, the smallest whole numbers that give the same *ratio* of atoms (carbon to hydrogen to nitrogen) in this molecule are 2:2:1. If we use *these* numbers for the atoms, we get the molecule's **empirical formula**: C_2H_2N. In general, to reduce a molecular formula to the empirical formula, divide all the subscripts by their greatest common factor. Here are a few more examples:

Molecular Formula	Empirical Formula
$C_6H_{12}O_6$	CH_2O
$K_2S_2O_8$	KSO_4
$Fe_4Na_8O_{35}P_{10}$	$Fe_4Na_8O_{35}P_{10}$
$C_{30}H_{27}N_3O_{15}$	$C_{10}H_9NO_5$

Example 3-4: What is the empirical formula for ethylene glycol, $C_2H_6O_2$?

A) CH_3O
B) CH_4O
C) CH_6O
D) $C_2H_6O_2$

Solution: Dividing each of the subscripts of $C_2H_6O_2$ by 2, we get CH_3O, choice A.

3.5   POLYATOMIC IONS

You should also be familiar with a handful of common polyatomic ions for the MCAT. Those in the table below are the ones you're most likely to come across.

Ammonium	NH_4^+
Hydronium	H_3O^+
Acetate (AcO$^-$)	$CH_3CO_2^-$
Bicarbonate	HCO_3^-
Cyanide	CN^-
Hydroxide	OH^-
Nitrate	NO_3^-
Nitrite	NO_2^-
Perchlorate	ClO_4^-
Carbonate	CO_3^{2-}
Sulfate	SO_4^{2-}
Sulfite	SO_3^{2-}
Phosphate	PO_4^{3-}

3.6   FORMULA AND MOLECULAR WEIGHT

If we know the chemical formula, we can figure out the **formula weight**, which is the sum of the atomic weights of all the atoms in the molecule. The unit for atomic weight is the **atomic mass unit**, abbreviated **amu**. (Note: Although *weight* is the popular term, it should really be *mass*.) One atomic mass unit is, by definition, equal to exactly 1/12 the mass of an atom of carbon-12 (^{12}C), the most abundant naturally occurring form of carbon. The periodic table lists the atomic mass of each element, which is actually a weighted average of the atomic masses of all its naturally occurring forms (isotopes) based on their relative abundance. To calculate the formula weight of the compound in question, refer to the periodic table. The atomic mass of carbon is 12.0 amu, that of hydrogen is 1.0 amu, and that of nitrogen as 14.0 amu. Therefore, the formula weight for $C_4H_4N_2$ is

$$4(12) + 4(1) + 2(14) = 80$$

(The unit *amu* may not be explicitly included.) When a compound exists as discrete molecules, the term **molecular weight** (**MW**) is usually used instead of formula weight. For example, the molecular weight of water, H_2O, is $2(1) + 16 = 18$. The term formula weight is usually used for *ionic* compounds, such as NaCl. The formula weight of NaCl is $23 + 35.5 = 58.5$.

Example 3-5: What is the formula weight of calcium phosphate, $Ca_3(PO_4)_2$?

A)   310 amu
B)   350 amu
C)   405 amu
D)   450 amu

Solution: The masses of the elements are Ca = 40 amu, P = 31 amu, and O = 16 amu. Therefore, the formula weight of calcium phosphate is

$$3(40\text{ amu}) + 2(31\text{ amu}) + 8(16\text{ amu}) = 310\text{ amu}$$

Choice A is the answer.

3.7   THE MOLE

A **mole** is simply a particular number of things, like a dozen is any group of 12 things. One mole of anything contains 6.02×10^{23} entities. A mole of atoms is a collection of 6.02×10^{23} atoms; a mole of molecules contains 6.02×10^{23} molecules, and so on. This number, 6.02×10^{23}, is called **Avogadro's number**, denoted by N_A (or N_0). What is so special about 6.02×10^{23}? The answer is based on the atomic mass unit, which is defined so that the mass of a carbon-12 atom is exactly 12 amu. *The number of carbon-12 atoms in a sample of mass of 12 grams is 6.02×10^{23}.* Avogadro's number is the link between atomic mass units and grams. For example, the periodic table lists the mass of sodium (Na, atomic number 11) as 23.0. This means that 1 atom of sodium has a mass of 23 atomic mass units, or that 1 *mole* of sodium atoms has a mass of 23 *grams*.

Since 1 mole of a substance has a mass in grams equal to the mass in amus of 1 formula unit of the substance, we have the following formula:

$$\# \text{ moles} = \frac{\text{mass in grams}}{\text{molecular weight (MW)}}$$

Example 3-6:

a)   Which has the greater formula weight: potassium dichromate ($K_2Cr_2O_7$) or lead azide $Pb(N_3)_2$?

b)   Which contains more formula units: a 1-mole sample of potassium dichromate or a 1-mole sample of lead azide?

Solution:

a)   The formula weight of potassium dichromate is

$$2(39.1) + 2(52) + 7(16) = 294.2$$

and the formula weight of lead azide is

$$207.2 + 6(14) = 291.2$$

Therefore, potassium dichromate has the greater formula weight.

b)   Trick question. Both samples contain the same number of formula units, namely 1 mole of them. (Which weighs more: a pound of rocks or a pound of feathers?)

Example 3-7: How many molecules of hydrazine, N_2H_4, are in a sample with a mass of 96 grams?

Solution: The molecular weight of N_2H_4 is $2(14) + 4(1) = 32$. This means that 1 mole of N_2H_4 has a mass of 32 grams. Therefore, a sample that has a mass of 96 grams contains 3 moles of molecules, because the formula above tells us that

$$n = \frac{96 \text{ g}}{32 \text{ g/mol}} = 3 \text{ moles}$$

To calculate the number of molecules, multiply the number of moles by Avogadro's number:

$$3 \times (6.02 \times 10^{23}) \approx 1.8 \times 10^{24} \text{ molecules}$$

3.8   PERCENTAGE COMPOSITION BY MASS

A molecule's molecular or empirical formula can be used to determine the molecule's percent mass composition. For example, let's find the mass composition of carbon, hydrogen, and nitrogen in $C_4H_4N_2$. Using the compound's empirical formula, C_2H_2N, will give us the same answer but the calculations will be easier because we'll have smaller numbers to work with. The empirical molecular weight is $2(12) + 2(1) + 14 = 40$, so each element's contribution to the total mass is

$$\%C = \frac{2(12)}{40} = \frac{12}{20} = \frac{60}{100} = 60\%, \quad \%H = \frac{2(1)}{40} = \frac{1}{20} = \frac{5}{100} = 5\%, \quad \%N = \frac{14}{40} = \frac{7}{20} = \frac{35}{100} = 35\%$$

We can also use information about the percentage composition to determine a compound's empirical formula. Suppose a substance is analyzed and found to consist, by mass, of 70 percent iron and 30 percent oxygen. To find the empirical formula for this compound, the trick is to start with 100 grams of the substance. We choose 100 grams since percentages are based on parts in 100. One hundred grams of this substance would then contain 70 g of Fe and 30 g of O. Now, how many *moles* of Fe and O are present in this 100-gram substance? Since the atomic weight of Fe is 55.8 and that of O is 16, we can use the formula given above in Section 3.6 and find

$$\text{\# moles of Fe} = \frac{70 \text{ g}}{55.8 \text{ g/mol}} \approx \frac{70}{56} = \frac{5}{4} \quad \text{and} \quad \text{\# moles of O} = \frac{30 \text{ g}}{16 \text{ g/mol}} = \frac{15}{8}$$

Because the empirical formula involves the ratio of the numbers of atoms, let's find the ratio of the amount of Fe to the amount of O:

$$\text{Ratio of Fe to O} = \frac{5/4 \text{ mol}}{15/8 \text{ mol}} = \frac{5}{4} \cdot \frac{8}{15} = \frac{2}{3}$$

Since the ratio of Fe to O is 2:3, the empirical formula of the substance is Fe_2O_3.

Example 3-8: What is the percent composition by mass of each element in sodium azide, NaN_3?

- A) Sodium 25%; nitrogen 75%
- B) Sodium 35%; nitrogen 65%
- C) Sodium 55%; nitrogen 45%
- D) Sodium 65%; nitrogen 35%

Solution: The molecular weight of this compound is 23 + 3(14) = 65. Therefore, sodium's contribution to the total mass is

$$\%\text{Na} = \frac{23}{65} \approx \frac{1}{3} \approx 33\%$$

Without even calculating nitrogen's contribution, we already see that choice B is best.

Example 3-9: What is the percent composition by mass of carbon in glucose, $C_6H_{12}O_6$?

- A) 40%
- B) 50%
- C) 67%
- D) 75%

Solution: The empirical formula for this compound is CH_2O, so the empirical molecular weight is 12 + 2(1) + 16 = 30. Therefore, carbon's contribution to the total mass is

$$\%\text{C} = \frac{12}{30} = 40\%$$

So choice A is the answer. We would have found the same answer using the molecular formula, but the numbers would have been messier:

$$\%\text{C} = \frac{6(12)}{6(12) + 12(1) + 6(16)} = \frac{72}{180} = 40\%$$

Example 3-10: What is the empirical formula of a compound that is, by mass, 90 percent carbon and 10 percent hydrogen?

A) CH_2
B) C_2H_3
C) C_3H_4
D) C_4H_5

Solution: A 100-gram sample of this compound would contain 90 g of C and 10 g of H. Since the atomic weight of C is 12 and that of H is 1, we have

$$\text{\# moles of C} = \frac{90 \text{ g}}{12 \text{ g/mol}} = \frac{15}{2} \quad \text{and} \quad \text{\# moles of H} = \frac{10 \text{ g}}{1 \text{ g/mol}} = 10$$

Therefore, the ratio of the amount of C to the amount of H is

$$\frac{15/2 \text{ mol}}{10 \text{ mol}} = \frac{3}{4}$$

Because the ratio of C to H is 3:4, the empirical formula of the compound is C_3H_4, and choice C is the answer.

Example 3-11: What is the percent by mass of water in the hydrate $MgCl_2 \cdot 5H_2O$?

A) 27%
B) 36%
C) 49%
D) 52%

Solution: The formula weight for this hydrate is 24.3 + 2(35.5) + 5[2(1) + 16] = 185.3. Since water's total molecular weight in this compound is 5[2(1) + 16] = 90, we see that water's contribution to the total mass is %H_2O = 90/185.3, which is a little *less* than one half (50 percent). Therefore, the answer is C.

3.8

3.9 CONCENTRATION

Molarity (*M*) expresses the concentration of a solution in terms of moles of solute per volume (in liters) of solution:

$$\text{Molarity } (M) = \frac{\text{\# moles of solute}}{\text{\# liters of solution}}$$

Concentration is denoted by enclosing the solute in brackets. For instance, "[Na⁺] = 1.0 *M*" indicates a solution in which the concentration is equivalent to 1 mole of sodium ions per liter of solution.

Mole fraction simply expresses the fraction of moles of a given substance (which we'll denote here by S) relative to the total moles in a solution:

$$\text{mole fraction of S} = X_S = \frac{\text{\# moles of substance S}}{\text{total \# moles in solution}}$$

Mole fraction is a useful way to express concentration when more than one solute is present, and is often used when discussing the composition of a mixture of gases.

3.10 CHEMICAL EQUATIONS AND STOICHIOMETRIC COEFFICIENTS

The equation

$$2 \text{ Al} + 6 \text{ HCl} \rightarrow 2 \text{ AlCl}_3 + 3 \text{ H}_2$$

describes the reaction of aluminum metal (Al) with hydrochloric acid (HCl) to produce aluminum chloride (AlCl₃) and hydrogen gas (H₂). The **reactants** are on the left side of the arrow, and the **products** are on the right side. A chemical equation is **balanced** if, for every element represented, the number of atoms on the left side of the arrow is equal to the number of atoms on the right side. This illustrates the **Law of Conservation of Mass** (or of **Matter**), which says that the amount of matter (and thus mass) does not change in a chemical reaction. For a *balanced* reaction such as the one above, the coefficients (2, 6, 2, and 3) preceding each compound—which are known as **stoichiometric coefficients**—tell us in what proportion the reactants react and in what proportion the products are formed. For this reaction, 2 atoms of Al react with 6 molecules of HCl to form 2 formula units of AlCl₃ and 3 molecules of H₂. The equation also means that 2 *moles* of Al react with 6 *moles* of HCl to form 2 *moles* of AlCl₃ and 3 *moles* of H₂.

The stoichiometric coefficients give the ratios of the number of molecules (or moles) that apply to the combination of reactants and the formation of products. They do *not* give the ratios by mass.

Balancing Equations

Balancing most chemical equations is simply a matter of trial and error. It's a good idea to start with the most complex species in the reaction. For example, let's look at the reaction above:

$$Al + HCl \rightarrow AlCl_3 + H_2 \text{ (unbalanced)}$$

Start with the most complex molecule, $AlCl_3$. The total number of atoms, or moles of atoms, is calculated by multiplying the coefficient in front of a compound times the subscript within the formula. To get 3 atoms of Cl on the product side, we need to have 3 atoms of Cl on the reactant side; therefore, we put a 3 in front of the HCl:

$$Al + 3 HCl \rightarrow AlCl_3 + H_2 \text{ (unbalanced)}$$

We've now balanced the Cl's, but the H's are still unbalanced. Since we have 3 H's on the left, we need 3 H's on the right to accomplish this, so we put a coefficient of 3/2 in front of the H_2:

$$Al + 3 HCl \rightarrow AlCl_3 + 3/2 H_2$$

Notice that we put a 3/2 (*not* a 3) in front of the H_2, because a hydrogen molecule contains 2 hydrogen atoms. All the atoms are now balanced—we see 1 Al, 3 H's, and 3 Cl's on each side. Because it's customary to write stoichiometric coefficients as whole numbers, we simply multiply through by 2 to get rid of the fraction and write

$$2 Al + 6 HCl \rightarrow 2 AlCl_3 + 3 H_2$$

3.10

Example 3-12: Balance each of these equations:

a) $NH_3 + O_2 \rightarrow NO + H_2O$
b) $CuCl_2 + NH_3 + H_2O \rightarrow Cu(OH)_2 + NH_4Cl$
c) $C_3H_8 + O_2 \rightarrow CO_2 + H_2O$
d) $C_8H_{18} + O_2 \rightarrow CO_2 + H_2O$

Solution:

a) $4 NH_3 + 5 O_2 \rightarrow 4 NO + 6 H_2O$
b) $CuCl_2 + 2 NH_3 + 2 H_2O \rightarrow Cu(OH)_2 + 2 NH_4Cl$
c) $C_3H_8 + 5 O_2 \rightarrow 3 CO_2 + 4 H_2O$
d) $2 C_8H_{18} + 25 O_2 \rightarrow 16 CO_2 + 18 H_2O$

3.11 STOICHIOMETRIC RELATIONSHIPS IN BALANCED REACTIONS

Once the equation for a chemical reaction is balanced, the stoichiometric coefficients tell us the relative amounts of the reactant species that combine and the relative amounts of the product species that are formed. For example, recall that the reaction

$$2 \text{ Al} + 6 \text{ HCl} \rightarrow 2 \text{ AlCl}_3 + 3 \text{ H}_2$$

tells us that 2 moles of Al react with 6 moles of HCl to form 2 moles of AlCl_3 and 3 moles of H_2.

Example 3-13: If 108 grams of aluminum metal are consumed, how many grams of hydrogen gas will be produced?

Solution: Because the stoichiometric coefficients give the ratios of the number of moles that apply to the combination of reactants and the formation of products—not the ratios by mass—we first need to determine how many *moles* of Al react. Since the molecular weight of Al is 27, we know that 27 grams of Al is equivalent to 1 mole. Therefore, 108 grams of Al is 4 moles. Now we use the stoichiometry of the balanced equation: for every 2 moles of Al that react, 3 moles of H_2 are produced. So, if 4 moles of Al react, we'll get 6 moles of H_2. Finally, we convert the number of moles of H_2 produced to grams. The molecular weight of H_2 is 2(1) = 2. This means that 1 mole of H_2 has a mass of 2 grams. Therefore, 6 moles of H_2 will have a mass of 6(2 g) = 12 grams.

Example 3-14: Consider the following reaction:

$$\text{CS}_2 + 3 \text{ O}_2 \rightarrow \text{CO}_2 + 2 \text{ SO}_2$$

How much carbon disulfide must be used to produce 64 grams of SO_2?

A) 38 g
B) 57 g
C) 76 g
D) 114 g

Solution: Since the molecular weight of SO_2 is 32.1 + 2(16) ≈ 64, we know that 64 grams of SO_2 is equivalent to 1 mole. From the stoichiometry of the balanced equation, we see that for every 1 mole of CS_2 that reacts, 2 moles of SO_2 are produced. Therefore, to produce just 1 mole of SO_2, we need 1/2 mole of CS_2. The molecular weight of CS_2 is 12 + 2(32.1) ≈ 76, so 1/2 mole of CS_2 has a mass of 38 grams. The answer is A.

3.12   THE LIMITING REAGENT

Let's look again at the reaction of aluminum with hydrochloric acid:

$$2\ Al + 6\ HCl \rightarrow 2\ AlCl_3 + 3\ H_2$$

Suppose that this reaction starts with 4 moles of Al and 18 moles of HCl. We have enough HCl to make 6 moles of $AlCl_3$ and 9 moles of H_2. *However,* there's only enough Al to make 4 moles of $AlCl_3$ and 6 moles of H_2. There isn't enough aluminum metal (Al) to make use of all the available HCl. As the reaction proceeds, we'll run out of aluminum. This means that aluminum is the **limiting reagent** here, because we run out of this reactant *first*, so it limits how much product the reaction can produce.

Now suppose that the reaction begins with 4 moles of Al and 9 moles of HCl. There's enough Al metal to produce 4 moles of $AlCl_3$ and 6 moles of H_2. But there's only enough HCl to make 3 moles of $AlCl_3$ and 4.5 moles of H_2. There isn't enough HCl to make use of all the available aluminum metal. As the reaction proceeds, we'll find that all the HCl is consumed before the Al is consumed. In this situation, HCl is the limiting reagent. Notice that we had more moles of HCl than we had of Al and the initial mass of the HCl was greater than the initial mass of Al. Nevertheless, the limiting reagent in this case was the HCl. The limiting reagent is the reactant that is consumed first, not necessarily the reactant that's initially present in the smallest amount.

Example 3-15:   Consider the following reaction:

$$2\ ZnS + 3\ O_2 \rightarrow 2\ ZnO + 2\ SO_2$$

If 97.5 grams of zinc sulfide undergoes this reaction with 32 grams of oxygen gas, what will be the limiting reagent?

A)   ZnS
B) O_2
C)   ZnO
D) SO_2

Solution: Since the molecular weight of ZnS is 65.4 + 32.1 = 97.5 and the molecular weight of O_2 is 2(16) = 32, this reaction begins with 1 mole of ZnS and 1 mole of O_2. From the stoichiometry of the balanced equation, we see that 1 mole of ZnS would react completely with $\frac{3}{2}$ = 1.5 moles of O_2. Because we have only 1 mole of O_2, the O_2 will be consumed first; it is the limiting reagent, and the answer is B. Note that choices C and D can be eliminated immediately, because a limiting reagent is always a reactant.

3.13 SOME NOTATION USED IN CHEMICAL EQUATIONS

In addition to specifying what atoms or molecules are involved in a chemical reaction, an equation may contain additional information. One type of additional information that can be written right into the equation specifies the **phases** of the substances in the reaction, i.e., whether each substance is a solid, liquid, or gas. Another common condition is that a substance may be dissolved in water when the reaction proceeds. In this case, we'd say the substance is in aqueous solution. These four "states" are abbreviated and written in parentheses as follows:

Solid	(s)
Liquid	(l)
Gas	(g)
Aqueous	(aq)

These immediately follow the chemical symbol for the reactant or product in the equation. For example, the reaction of sodium metal with water, which produces sodium hydroxide and hydrogen gas, could be written like this:

$$2\ Na(s) + 2\ H_2O(l) \rightarrow 2\ NaOH(aq) + H_2(g)$$

In some cases, the reactants are heated to produce the desired reaction. To indicate this, we write a "Δ"—or the word "heat"—above (or below) the reaction arrow. For example, heating potassium nitrate produces potassium nitrite and oxygen gas:

$$2\ KNO_3(s) \xrightarrow{\Delta} 2\ KNO_2(aq) + O_2(g)$$

Some reactions proceed more rapidly in the presence of a **catalyst**, which is a substance that increases the rate of a reaction without being consumed. For example, in the industrial production of sulfuric acid, an intermediate step is the reaction of sulfur dioxide and oxygen to produce sulfur trioxide. Not only are the reactants heated, but they are combined in the presence of V_2O_5. We indicate the presence of a catalyst by writing it below the arrow in the equation:

$$2\ SO_2 + O_2 \xrightarrow[V_2O_5]{\Delta} 2\ SO_3$$

3.14 OXIDATION STATES

An atom's **oxidation state** (or **oxidation number**) is meant to indicate how the atom's "ownership" of its valence electrons changes when it forms a compound. For example, consider the formula unit NaCl. The sodium atom will transfer its valence electron to the chlorine atom, so the sodium's "ownership" of its valence electron has certainly changed. To indicate this, we'd say that the oxidation state of sodium is now +1 (or 1 *less* electron than it started with). On the other hand, chlorine accepts ownership of that 1 electron, so its oxidation state is –1 (that is, 1 *more* electron than it started with). Giving up ownership results in a more positive oxidation state; accepting ownership results in a more negative oxidation state.

This example of NaCl is rather special (and easy) since the compound is **ionic**, and we consider ionic compounds to involve the complete transfer of electrons. But what about a non-ionic (that is, a **covalent)** compound? *The oxidation state of an atom is the "charge" it would have if the compound were ionic.* Here's another way of saying this: the oxidation state of an atom in a molecule is the charge it would have if all the shared electrons were completely transferred to the more electronegative element. Note that for covalent compounds, this is not a real charge, just a bookkeeping trick.

The following list gives the rules for assigning oxidation states to the atoms in a molecule. If following one rule in the list causes the violation of another rule, the rule that is higher in the list takes precedence.

Rules for Assigning Oxidation States
1) The oxidation state of any element in its standard state is 0.
2) The sum of the oxidation states of the atoms in a neutral molecule must always be 0, and the sum of the oxidation states of the atoms in an ion must always equal the ion's charge.
3) Group 1 metals have a +1 oxidation state, and Group 2 metals have a +2 oxidation state.
4) Fluorine has a −1 oxidation state.
5) Hydrogen has a +1 oxidation state in most compounds, unless it is bound to a metal. In that case, it has an oxidation state of −1.
6) Oxygen has a −2 oxidation state.
7) The rest of the halogens have a −1 oxidation state, and the atoms of the oxygen family have a −2 oxidation state.

It's worth noting a common exception to Rule 6: In peroxides (such as H_2O_2 or Na_2O_2), oxygen is in a −1 oxidation state (which is consistent with Rules 3 and 5 having a higher priority than rule 6).

As we will discuss later, the order of electronegativities of some elements can be remembered with the mnemonic FONClBrISCH (pronounced "fawn-cull-brish"). This lists the elements in order from the most electronegative (F) to the least electronegative (H). Hence, bonds from H to anything found in the list will give hydrogen a +1 oxidation state, and bonds from H to anything *not* found in the list will give H a −1 oxidation state.

Let's find the oxidation number of manganese in $KMnO_4$. By Rule 3, K is +1, and by Rule 6, O is −2. Therefore, the oxidation state of Mn must be +7 in order for the sum of all the oxidation numbers in this electrically-neutral molecule to be zero (the unbreakable Rule 2).

Like many other elements, transition metals can assume different oxidation states, depending on the compound they're in. (Note, however, that a metal will never assume a negative oxidation state!) For example, iron has an oxidation number of +2 in $FeCl_2$ but an oxidation number of +3 in $FeCl_3$. The oxidation number of a transition metal is given as a Roman numeral in the name of the compound. Therefore, $FeCl_2$ is iron(II) chloride, and $FeCl_3$ is iron(III) chloride.

3.14

Example 3-16: Determine the oxidation state of the atoms in each of the following molecules:

a) NO_3^-

b) HNO_2

c) O_2

d) SF_4

Solution:

a) By Rule 6, the oxidation state of O is –2; therefore, by Rule 2, the oxidation state of N must be +5.

b) By Rule 5, the oxidation state of H is +1, and by Rule 6, O has an oxidation state of –2. Therefore, by Rule 2, N must have an oxidation state of +3 in this molecule.

c) By Rule 1 (which is higher in the list than Rule 5 and thus takes precedence), each O atom in O_2 has an oxidation state of 0.

d) By Rule 4, F has an oxidation state of –1. So, by Rule 2, S has an oxidation state of +4.

3.14

Chapter 4
Atomic Structure
and Periodic Trends

PERIODIC TABLE OF THE ELEMENTS

1																	18
1 **H** 1.0	2											13	14	15	16	17	2 **He** 4.0
3 **Li** 6.9	4 **Be** 9.0											5 **B** 10.8	6 **C** 12.0	7 **N** 14.0	8 **O** 16.0	9 **F** 19.0	10 **Ne** 20.2
11 **Na** 23.0	12 **Mg** 24.3	3	4	5	6	7	8	9	10	11	12	13 **Al** 27.0	14 **Si** 28.1	15 **P** 31.0	16 **S** 32.1	17 **Cl** 35.5	18 **Ar** 39.9
19 **K** 39.1	20 **Ca** 40.1	21 **Sc** 45.0	22 **Ti** 47.9	23 **V** 50.9	24 **Cr** 52.0	25 **Mn** 54.9	26 **Fe** 55.8	27 **Co** 58.9	28 **Ni** 58.7	29 **Cu** 63.5	30 **Zn** 65.4	31 **Ga** 69.7	32 **Ge** 72.6	33 **As** 74.9	34 **Se** 79.0	35 **Br** 79.9	36 **Kr** 83.8
37 **Rb** 85.5	38 **Sr** 87.6	39 **Y** 88.9	40 **Zr** 91.2	41 **Nb** 92.9	42 **Mo** 95.9	43 **Tc** (98)	44 **Ru** 101.1	45 **Rh** 102.9	46 **Pd** 106.4	47 **Ag** 107.9	48 **Cd** 112.4	49 **In** 114.8	50 **Sn** 118.7	51 **Sb** 121.8	52 **Te** 127.6	53 **I** 126.9	54 **Xe** 131.3
55 **Cs** 132.9	56 **Ba** 137.3	57 ***La** 138.9	72 **Hf** 178.5	73 **Ta** 180.9	74 **W** 183.9	75 **Re** 186.2	76 **Os** 190.2	77 **Ir** 192.2	78 **Pt** 195.1	79 **Au** 197.0	80 **Hg** 200.6	81 **Tl** 204.4	82 **Pb** 207.2	83 **Bi** 209.0	84 **Po** (209)	85 **At** (210)	86 **Rn** (222)
87 **Fr** (223)	88 **Ra** (226)	89 **†Ac** (227)	104 **Rf** (267)	105 **Db** (268)	106 **Sg** (271)	107 **Bh** (270)	108 **Hs** (269)	109 **Mt** (278)	110 **Ds** (281)	111 **Rg** (282)	112 **Cn** (285)	113 **Nh** (286)	114 **Fl** (289)	115 **Mc** (289)	116 **Lv** (293)	117 **Ts** (294)	118 **Og** (294)

*Lanthanoids	58 **Ce** 140.1	59 **Pr** 140.9	60 **Nd** 144.2	61 **Pm** (145)	62 **Sm** 150.4	63 **Eu** 152.0	64 **Gd** 157.3	65 **Tb** 158.9	66 **Dy** 162.5	67 **Ho** 164.9	68 **Er** 167.3	69 **Tm** 168.9	70 **Yb** 173.0	71 **Lu** 175.0
†Actinoids	90 **Th** 232.0	91 **Pa** (231)	92 **U** 238.0	93 **Np** (237)	94 **Pu** (244)	95 **Am** (243)	96 **Cm** (247)	97 **Bk** (247)	98 **Cf** (251)	99 **Es** (252)	100 **Fm** (257)	101 **Md** (258)	102 **No** (259)	103 **Lr** (266)

4.1 ATOMS

The smallest unit of any element is one **atom** of the element. All atoms have a central **nucleus**, which contains **protons** and **neutrons**, known collectively as **nucleons**. Each proton has an electric charge of +1 elementary unit; neutrons have no charge. Outside the nucleus, an atom contains electrons, and each **electron** has a charge of –1 elementary unit.

In every neutral atom, the number of electrons outside the nucleus is equal to the number of protons inside the nucleus. The electrons are held in the atom by the electrostatic attraction of the positively charged nucleus.

The number of protons in the nucleus of an atom is called its **atomic number**, Z. The atomic number of an atom uniquely determines what element the atom is, and Z may be shown explicitly by a subscript before the symbol of the element. For example, every beryllium atom contains exactly four protons, and we can write this as $_4$Be.

A proton and a neutron each have a mass slightly more than one atomic mass unit (1 amu = 1.66×10^{-27} kg), and an electron has a mass that's only about 0.05 percent of the mass of either a proton or a neutron. So, virtually all the mass of an atom is due to the mass of the nucleus.

The number of protons plus the number of neutrons in the nucleus of an atom gives the atom's **mass number**, A. If we let N stand for the number of neutrons, then $A = Z + N$.

In designating a particular atom of an element, we refer to its mass number. One way to do this is to write A as a superscript. For example, if a beryllium atom contains 5 neutrons, then its mass number is $4 + 5 = 9$, and we would write this as $_4^9$Be or simply as ^{9}Be. Another way is simply to write the mass number after the name of the elements, with a hyphen; ^{9}Be is beryllium-9 or Be-9.

4.2 ISOTOPES

If two atoms of the same element differ in their numbers of neutrons, then they are called **isotopes**. The atoms shown below are two different isotopes of the element beryllium. The atom on the left has 4 protons and 3 neutrons, so its mass number is 7; it's ^{7}Be (or beryllium-7). The atom on the right has 4 protons and 5 neutrons, so it's ^{9}Be (beryllium-9).

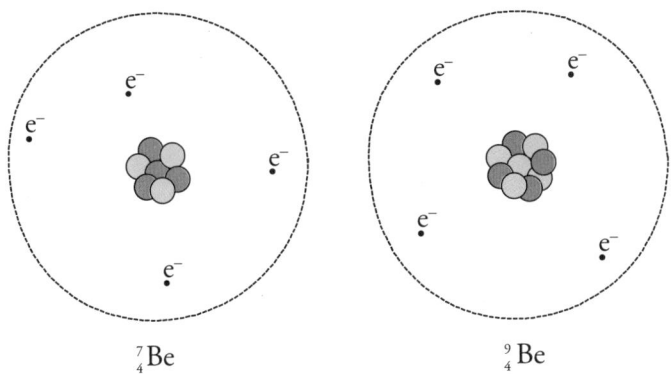

$$^7_4\text{Be} \qquad\qquad ^9_4\text{Be}$$

(These figures are definitely not to scale. If they were, each dashed circle showing the "outer edge" of the atom would literally be about 1500 m—almost a mile across! The nucleus occupies only the *tiniest* fraction of an atom's volume, which is mostly empty space.) Notice that these atoms—like all isotopes of a given element—*have the same atomic number but different mass numbers.*

Example 4-1: An atom with 7 neutrons and a mass number of 12 is an isotope of what element?

A) Boron
B) Nitrogen
C) Magnesium
D) Potassium

Solution: If $A = 12$ and $N = 7$, then $Z = A - N = 12 - 7 = 5$. The element with an atomic number of 5 is boron. Therefore, choice A is the answer.

Atomic Weight

Elements exist naturally as a collection of their isotopes. The **atomic weight of an element** is a *weighted average* of the masses of its naturally occurring isotopes. For example, boron has two naturally occurring isotopes: boron-10, with an atomic mass of 10.013 amu, and boron-11, with an atomic mass of 11.009 amu. Since boron-10 accounts for 20 percent of all naturally occurring boron, and boron-11 accounts for the other 80 percent, the atomic weight of boron is

$$(20\%)(10.013 \text{ amu}) + (80\%)(11.009 \text{ amu}) = 10.810 \text{ amu}$$

and this is the value listed in the periodic table. (Recall that the atomic mass unit is defined so that the most abundant isotope of carbon, carbon-12, has a mass of precisely 12 amu.)

4.3 IONS

When a neutral atom gains or loses electrons, it becomes charged, and the resulting atom is called an **ion**. For each electron it gains, an atom acquires a charge of –1 unit, and for each electron it loses, an atom acquires a charge of +1 unit. A negatively charged ion is called an **anion**, while a positively charged ion is called a **cation**.

We designate how many electrons an atom has gained or lost by placing this number as a superscript after the chemical symbol for the element. For example, if a lithium atom loses 1 electron, it becomes the lithium cation Li^{1+}, or simply Li^+. If a phosphorus atom gains 3 electrons, it becomes the phosphorus anion P^{3-}, or phosphide.

Example 4-2: An atom contains 16 protons, 17 neutrons, and 18 electrons. Which of the following best indicates this ion?

A) $^{33}Cl^-$
B) $^{34}Cl^-$
C) $^{33}S^{2-}$
D) $^{34}S^{2-}$

Solution: Any nucleus that contains 16 protons is sulfur, so we can eliminate choices A and B immediately. Now, because $Z = 16$ and $N = 17$, the mass number, A, is $Z + N = 16 + 17 = 33$. Therefore, the answer is C.

Example 4-3: Of the following atoms/ions, which one contains the greatest number of neutrons?

A) $^{60}_{28}Ni$
B) $^{64}_{29}Cu^+$
C) $^{64}_{30}Zn$
D) $^{64}_{30}Zn^{2+}$

Solution: To find N, we just subtract Z (the subscript) from A (the superscript). The atom in choice A has $N = 60 - 28 = 32$; the ion in choice B has $N = 64 - 29 = 35$, and the atom and ion in choices C and D, respectively, have $N = 64 - 30 = 34$. Therefore, of the choices given, the ion in choice B contains the greatest number of neutrons.

4.4 NUCLEAR STABILITY AND RADIOACTIVITY

The protons and neutrons in a nucleus are held together by a force called the **strong nuclear force**. It's stronger than the electrical force between charged particles, since for all atoms besides hydrogen, the strong nuclear force must overcome the electrical repulsion between the protons. In fact, of the four fundamental forces of nature, the strong nuclear force is the most powerful even though it only works over extremely short distances, as seen in the nucleus.

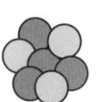

radioactive
beryllium
nucleus

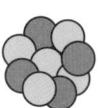

stable
beryllium
nucleus

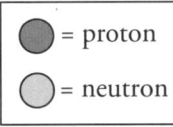

Unstable nuclei are said to be **radioactive**, and they undergo a transformation to make them more stable, altering the number and ratio of protons and neutrons or just lowering their energy. Such a process is called **radioactive decay**, and we'll look at three types: **alpha**, **beta** and **gamma**. The nucleus that undergoes radioactive decay is known as the **parent**, and the resulting more stable nucleus is known as the **daughter**.

Alpha Decay

When a large nucleus wants to become more stable by reducing the number of protons and neutrons, it emits an alpha particle. An **alpha particle**, denoted by $_2^4\alpha$, consists of 2 protons and 2 neutrons:

alpha particle

This is equivalent to a helium-4 nucleus, so an alpha particle can also be denoted by $_2^4\text{He}$. Alpha decay reduces the parent's atomic number by 2 and the mass number by 4. For example, polonium-210 is an α-emitter. It undergoes alpha decay to form the stable nucleus lead-206:

$$_{84}^{210}\text{Po} \rightarrow \underbrace{_{82}^{206}\text{Pb}}_{\text{daughter}} + \underbrace{_{2}^{4}\alpha}_{\text{ejected}}$$

parent

Although alpha particles are emitted with high energy from the parent nucleus, this energy is quickly lost as the particle travels through matter or air. As a result, the particles do not typically travel far, and can be stopped by the outer layers of human skin or a piece of paper.

Beta Decay

There are actually three types of beta decay: β⁻, β⁺, and electron capture. Each type of beta decay involves the conversion of a neutron into a proton (along with some other particles that are beyond the scope of the MCAT), or vice versa, through the action of the **weak nuclear force**.

Beta particles are more dangerous than alpha particles since they are significantly less massive. They therefore have more energy and a greater penetrating ability. However, they can be stopped by aluminum foil or a centimeter of plastic or glass.

β⁻ Decay

When an unstable nucleus contains too many neutrons, it may convert a neutron into a proton and an electron; the electron is subsequently ejected and is also known as a β⁻ **particle**. The atomic number of the resulting daughter nucleus is 1 greater than the radioactive parent nucleus, but the mass number remains the same. The isotope carbon-14, the decay of which is the basis of radiocarbon dating of archaeological artifacts, is an example of a radioactive nucleus that undergoes β⁻ decay:

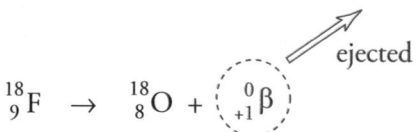

$$^{14}_{6}C \rightarrow \ ^{14}_{7}N + \ ^{0}_{-1}\beta$$

β⁻ decay is the most common type of beta decay, and when the MCAT mentions "beta decay" without any further qualification, it means β⁻ decay.

β⁺ Decay (or Positron Emission)

When an unstable nucleus contains too few neutrons, it converts a proton into a neutron and a positron, which is ejected. This is known as β⁺ **decay**. The positron is the electron's *antiparticle*; it's identical to an electron except its charge is positive. The atomic number of the resulting daughter nucleus is 1 less than the radioactive parent nucleus, but the mass number remains the same. The isotope fluorine-18, which can be used in medical diagnostic bone scans in the form Na¹⁸F, is an example of a positron emitter:

$$^{18}_{9}F \rightarrow \ ^{18}_{8}O + \ ^{0}_{+1}\beta$$

Electron Capture

Another way for an unstable nucleus to increase its number of neutrons is to capture an electron from the closest electron shell (the $n = 1$ shell) and use it in the conversion of a proton into a neutron. Just like positron emission, **electron capture** causes the atomic number to be reduced by 1 while the mass number remains the same. The nucleus chromium-51 is an example of a radioactive nucleus that undergoes electron capture, becoming the stable nucleus vanadium-51:

$$^{51}_{24}\text{Cr} + {}^{0}_{-1}\text{e}^- \rightarrow {}^{51}_{23}\text{V}$$

Gamma Decay

A nucleus in an excited energy state—which is usually the case after a nucleus has undergone alpha or any type of beta decay—can "relax" to its ground state by emitting energy in the form of one or more photons of electromagnetic radiation. These photons are called **gamma photons** (symbolized by γ) and have a very high frequency and energy. Gamma photons (or gamma rays) have neither mass nor charge, and can therefore penetrate matter most effectively. A few inches of lead or about a meter of concrete will stop most gamma rays. Their ejection from a radioactive atom changes neither the atomic number nor the mass number of the nucleus. For example, after silicon-31 undergoes β^- decay, the resulting daughter nucleus then undergoes gamma decay:

$$^{31}_{14}\text{Si} \xrightarrow{\beta^- \text{ decay}} {}^{31}_{15}\text{P}^* \xrightarrow{\gamma \text{ decay}} {}^{31}_{15}\text{P} + {}^{0}_{0}\gamma \quad \text{emitted}$$

indicates nucleus
is in an excited
energy state

Notice that alpha and beta decay change the identity of the nucleus, but gamma decay does not. Gamma decay is simply an expulsion of energy.

4.4

Summary of Radioactive Decay

$\boxed{N\downarrow \quad Z\downarrow}$	Alpha Decay	Decreases the number of neutrons *and* protons in large nucleus
		Subtracts 4 from the mass number
		Subtracts 2 from the atomic number
		$^A_Z X \xrightarrow{\alpha} {}^{A-4}_{Z-2} Y + {}^4_2 \alpha$

$\boxed{N\downarrow \quad Z\uparrow}$	Beta$^-$ Decay	Decreases the number of neutrons, increases the number of protons
		Adds 1 to the atomic number
		$^A_Z X \xrightarrow{\beta^-} {}^A_{Z+1} Y + {}^{\;0}_{-1} \beta$

$\boxed{N\uparrow \quad Z\downarrow}$	Positron Emission	Increases the number of neutrons, decreases the number of protons
		Subtracts 1 from the atomic number
		$^A_Z X \xrightarrow{\beta+} {}^A_{Z-1} Y + {}^{\;0}_{+1} \beta$

$\boxed{N\uparrow \quad Z\downarrow}$	Electron Capture	Increases the number of neutrons, decreases the number of protons
		Subtracts 1 from the atomic number
		$^A_Z X + {}^{\;0}_{-1} e^- \xrightarrow{EC} {}^A_{Z-1} Y$

	Gamma Decay	Brings an excited nucleus to a lower energy state
		Doesn't change mass number or atomic number
		$^A_Z X* \xrightarrow{\gamma} {}^A_Z Y + {}^0_0 \gamma$

Example 4-4: Radioactive calcium-47, a known β^- emitter, is administered in the form of $^{47}CaCl_2$ by I.V. as a diagnostic tool to study calcium metabolism. What is the daughter nucleus of ^{47}Ca?

A) ^{46}K
B) ^{47}K
C) $^{47}Ca^+$
D) ^{47}Sc

Solution: Since β^- decay will always change the identity of an element, eliminate choice C. The β^- decay of ^{47}Ca is described by this nuclear reaction:

$$^{47}_{20}Ca \rightarrow {}^{47}_{21}Sc + {}^{\;0}_{-1}\beta$$

Therefore, the daughter nucleus is scandium-47, choice D.

Example 4-5: Americium-241 is used to provide intracavitary radiation for the treatment of malignancies. This radioisotope is known to undergo alpha decay. What is the daughter nucleus?

A) ^{237}Np
B) ^{241}Pu
C) ^{237}Bk
D) ^{243}Bk

Solution: Alpha decay will reduce the mass by 4, to 237, so eliminate choices B and D. It will reduce the nuclear charge by 2 from 95 to 93, so choose A. The α decay of ^{241}Am is described by this nuclear reaction:

$$^{241}_{95}Am \rightarrow {}^{237}_{93}Np + {}^{4}_{2}\alpha$$

Example 4-6: Vitamin B_{12} can be prepared with *radioactive* cobalt (^{58}Co), a known β^+ emitter, and administered orally as a diagnostic tool to test for defects in intestinal vitamin B_{12} absorption. What is the daughter nucleus of ^{58}Co?

A) ^{57}Fe
B) ^{58}Fe
C) ^{59}Co
D) ^{59}Ni

Solution: All types of β^+ decay leave the mass of the daughter and parent elements the same, thus the mass must be 58, making choice B the only option. The β^+ decay of ^{58}Co is described by this nuclear reaction:

$$^{58}_{27}Co \rightarrow {}^{58}_{26}Fe + {}^{0}_{+1}\beta$$

Example 4-7: A certain radioactive isotope is administered orally as a diagnostic tool to study pancreatic function and intestinal fat absorption. This radioisotope is known to undergo β^- decay, and the daughter nucleus is xenon-131. What is the parent radioisotope?

A) ^{131}Cs
B) ^{131}I
C) ^{132}I
D) ^{132}Xe

Solution: Eliminate choices C and D since the mass number should remain the same for all forms of β^- decay. The β^- decay that results in ^{131}Xe is described by this nuclear reaction:

$$^{131}_{53}I \rightarrow {}^{131}_{54}Xe + {}^{0}_{-1}\beta$$

Therefore, the parent nucleus is iodine-131, choice B.

Example 4-8: Which of these modes of radioactive decay causes a change in the mass number of the parent nucleus?

A) α
B) β^-
C) β^+
D) γ

Solution: Gamma decay causes no changes in the number of protons or neutrons, so we can eliminate choice D. Beta decay (β^-, β^+, and EC) changes both N and Z by 1, but always such that the change in the sum $N + Z$ (which is the mass number, A) is zero. Therefore, we can eliminate choices B and C. The answer is A.

Example 4-9: One of the naturally occurring radioactive series begins with radioactive ^{238}U. It undergoes a series of decays, one of which is: alpha, beta, beta, alpha, alpha, alpha, alpha, alpha, beta, beta, alpha, beta, alpha, beta. What is the final resulting nuclide of this series of decays?

A) ^{204}Pb
B) ^{204}Pt
C) ^{206}Pb
D) ^{206}Pt

Solution: Since there are so many individual decays, let's find the final daughter nucleus using a simple shortcut: For every alpha decay, we'll subtract 4 from the mass number (the superscript) and subtract 2 from the atomic number (the subscript); for every beta decay, we'll add 0 to the mass number and 1 to the atomic number. Since there are a total of 8 alpha-decays and 6 beta-decays, we get

$$^{238}_{92}\text{U} \xrightarrow{8\alpha} {}^{238\ -8(4)}_{92\ -8(2)} \xrightarrow{6\beta^-} {}^{+6(0)}_{+6(1)} = {}^{206}_{82}\text{Pb}$$

Therefore, the final daughter nucleus is lead-206, choice C.

Half-Life

Different radioactive nuclei decay at different rates. The **half-life**, which is denoted by $t_{1/2}$, of a radioactive substance is the time it takes for one-half of some sample of the substance to decay. Thus, the shorter the half-life, the faster the decay. The amount of a radioactive substance decreases exponentially with time, as illustrated in the following graph.

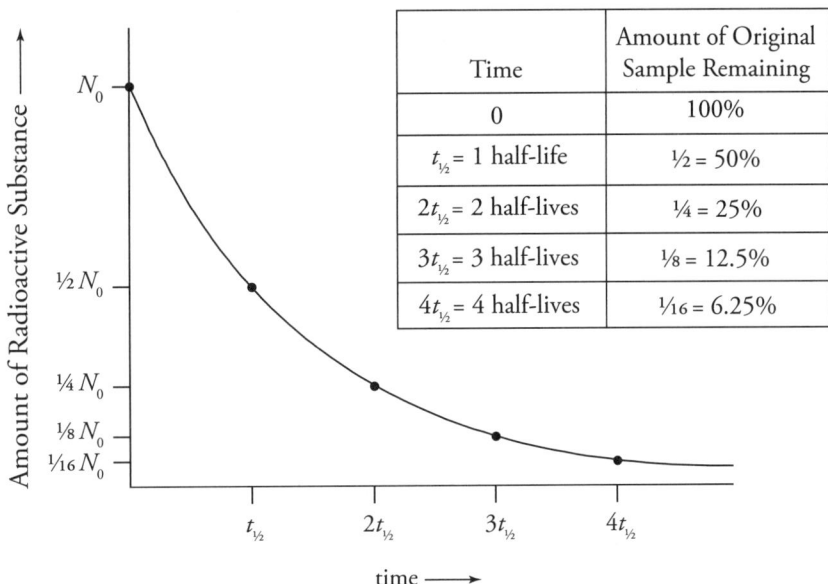

For example, a radioactive sample with an initial mass of 80 grams and a half-life of 6 years will decay as follows:

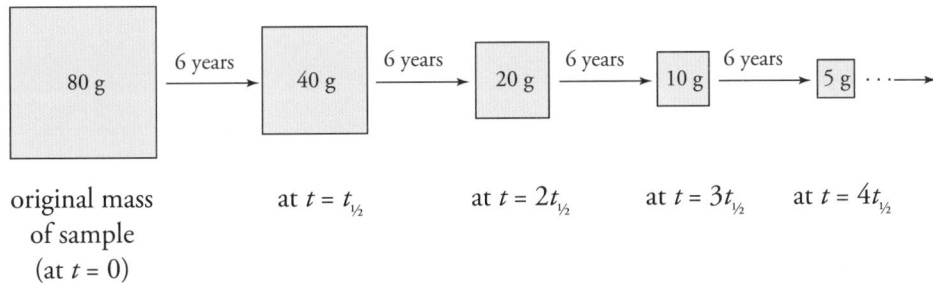

The equation for the exponential decay curve shown above is often written as $N = N_0 e^{-kt}$, but a simpler—and much more intuitive way—is

$$N = N_0 (1/2)^{T/t_{1/2}}$$

where $t_{1/2}$ is the half-life and T is the total time the sample has decayed. For example, when $T = 3t_{1/2}$, the number of radioactive nuclei remaining, N, is $N_0(1/2)^3 = 1/8 N_0$, just what we expect. If the form $N_0 e^{-kt}$ is used, the value of k (known as the **decay constant**) is inversely proportional to the half-life: $k = (\ln 2)/t_{1/2}$. The shorter the half-life, the greater the decay constant, and the more rapidly the sample decays.

Example 4-10: Cesium-137 has a half-life of 30 years. How long will it take for only 0.3 g to remain from a sample that had an original mass of 2.4 g?

A) 60 years
B) 90 years
C) 120 years
D) 240 years

Solution: Since 0.3 grams is 1/8 of 2.4 grams, the question is asking how long it will take for the radio-isotope to decrease to 1/8 its original amount. We know that this requires 3 half-lives, since 1/2 × 1/2 × 1/2 = 1/8. So, if each half-life is 30 years, then 3 half-lives will be 3(30) = 90 years, choice B.

Example 4-11: Radiolabeled vitamin B_{12} containing radioactive cobalt-58 is administered to diagnose a defect in a patient's vitamin-B_{12} absorption. If ^{58}Co has a half-life of 72 days, approximately what percentage of the radioisotope will still remain in the patient a year later?

A) 3%
B) 5%
C) 8%
D) 10%

Solution: One year is approximately equal to 5 half-lives of this radioisotope, since 5 × 72 = 360 days ≈ 1 year. After 5 half-lives, the amount of the radioisotope will drop to $(1/2)^5$ = 1/32 of the original amount administered. Because 1/32 ≈ 3/100 = 3%, the best answer is choice A.

Example: 4-12: Iodinated oleic acid, containing radioactive iodine-131, is administered orally to study a patient's pancreatic function. If ^{131}I has a half-life of 8 days, how long after the procedure will the amount of ^{131}I remaining in the patient's body be reduced to 1/5 its initial value?

A) 19 days
B) 32 days
C) 40 days
D) 256 days

Solution: Although the fraction 1/5 is not a whole-number power of 1/2, we do know that it's between 1/4 and 1/8. If 1/4 of the sample were left, we'd know that 2 half-lives had elapsed, and if 1/8 of the sample were left, we'd know that 3 half-lives had elapsed. Therefore, because 1/5 is between 1/4 and 1/8, we know that the amount of time will be between 2 and 3 half-lives. Since each half-life is 8 days, this amount of time will be between 2(8) = 16 days and 3(8) = 24 days. Of the choices given, only choice A is in this range.

Nuclear Binding Energy

Every nucleus that contains protons *and* neutrons has a **nuclear binding energy**. This is the energy that was released when the individual nucleons (protons and neutrons) were bound together by the strong force to form the nucleus. It's also equal to the energy that would be required to break up the intact nucleus into its individual nucleons. The greater the binding energy per nucleon, the more stable the nucleus.

When nucleons bind together to form a nucleus, some mass is converted to energy, so the mass of the combined nucleus is *less* than the sum of the masses of all its nucleons individually. The difference, Δm, is called the **mass defect**, and its energy equivalent *is* the nuclear binding energy. For a stable nucleus, the mass defect,

$$\Delta m = \text{(total mass of separate nucleons)} - \text{(mass of nucleus)}$$

will always be positive.

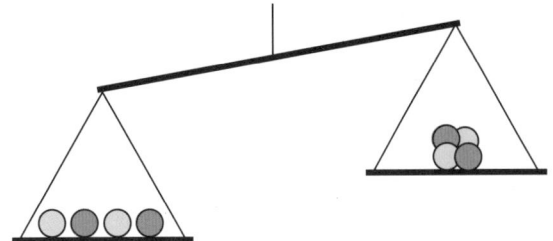

The nuclear binding energy, E_B, can be found from the mass defect using **Einstein's equations for mass-energy equivalence**: $E_B = (\Delta m)c^2$, where c is the speed of light (3×10^8 m/s). If mass is measured in kilograms and energy in Joules, then 1 kg $\leftrightarrow$ 9×10^{16} J. But in the nuclear domain, masses are often expressed in atomic mass units (1 amu $\approx 1.66 \times 10^{-27}$ kg), and energy is expressed in **electronvolts** (1 eV $\approx 1.6 \times 10^{-19}$ J). In terms of these units, the equations for the nuclear binding energy, $E_B = (\Delta m)c^2$, can be written as E_B (in eV) = [Δm(in amu)] $\times$ 931.5 MeV.

Example 4-13: The mass defect of a helium nucleus is 5×10^{-29} kg. What is its nuclear binding energy?

Solution: The equation $E_B = (\Delta m)c^2$ implies that 1 kg $\leftrightarrow$ 9×10^{16} J, so a mass defect of 5×10^{-29} kg is equivalent to an energy of $(5 \times 10^{-29}$ kg$)(9 \times 10^{16}$ J$) = 4.5 \times 10^{-12}$ J. (For practice, check that this binding energy is approximately equal to 30 MeV.)

Example 4-14: The mass defect of a triton (the nucleus of a tritium, $_1^3$H) is about 0.009 amu. What is its nuclear binding energy, in electronvolts?

Solution: In terms of amus and electronvolts, the equation for the nuclear binding energy is E_B(in eV) = [Δm(in amu)] $\times$ 931.5 MeV. Therefore, for the tritium nucleus, we have
$$E_B = (0.009) \times (931.5 \text{ MeV}) \approx 8.4 \text{ MeV}$$

4.5 ATOMIC STRUCTURE

Emission Spectra

Imagine a glass tube filled with a small sample of an element in gaseous form. When electric current is passed through the tube, the gas begins to glow with a color characteristic of that particular element. If this light emitted by the gas is then passed through a prism—which will separate the light into its component wavelengths—the result is the element's **emission spectrum**.

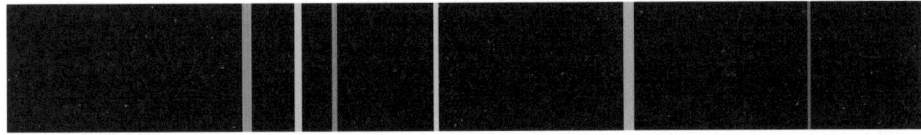

An atom's emission spectrum gives an energetic "fingerprint" of that element because it consists of a unique sequence of *bright* lines that correspond to specific wavelengths and energies. The energies of the photons, or particles of light that are emitted, are related to their frequencies, *f*, and wavelengths, λ, by the equation

$$E_{photon} = hf = h\frac{c}{\lambda}$$

where *h* is a universal constant called **Planck's constant** (6.63×10^{-34} J·s) and *c* is the speed of light. For the following discussion, a general understanding of the electromagnetic spectrum will be useful. More detail on this topic can be found in Section 13.1 of the *MCAT Physics Review*.

The Bohr Model of the Atom

In 1913 the Danish physicist Niels Bohr realized that the model of atomic structure of his time was inconsistent with emission spectral data. In order to account for the limited numbers of lines that are observed in the emission spectra of elements, Bohr described a new model of the atom. In this model that would later take his name, he proposed that the electrons in an atom orbited the nucleus in circular paths, much as the planets orbit the sun in the solar system. Distance from the nucleus was related to the energy of the electrons; electrons with greater amounts of energy orbited the nucleus at greater distances. However, the electrons in the atom cannot assume any arbitrary energy, but have *quantized* energy states, and thereby only orbit at certain allowed distances from the nucleus.

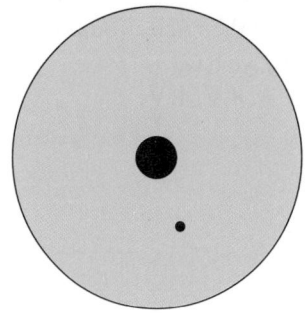
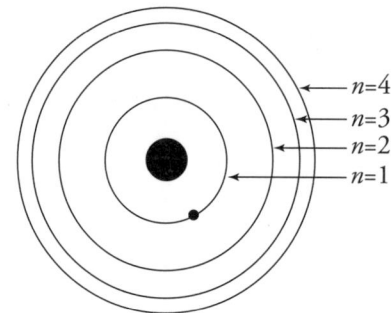

Pre-Bohr Model
Electrons assume arbitrary energies

Bohr Model
Electrons assume discrete energies

If an electron absorbs energy that's exactly equal to the difference in energy between its current level and that of an available higher level, it "jumps" to that higher level. The electron can then "drop" to a lower energy level, emitting a photon with an energy exactly equal to the difference between the levels. This model predicted that elements would have line spectra instead of continuous spectra, as would be the case if transitions between all possible energies could be expected. An electron could only gain or lose very specific amounts of energy due to the quantized nature of the energy levels. Therefore, only photons with certain energies are observed. These specific energies corresponded to very specific wavelengths, as seen in the emission line spectra.

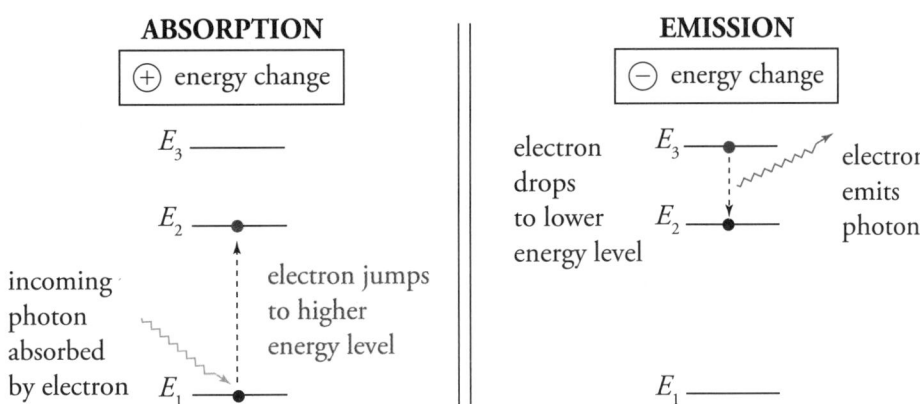

In the transition depicted below, an electron is initially in its **ground state** ($n = 1$), or its lowest possible energy level. When this electron absorbs a photon it jumps to a higher energy level, known as an **excited state** (in this case $n = 3$). Electrons excited to high energy don't always relax to the ground state in large jumps, rather they can relax in a series of smaller jumps, gradually coming back to the ground state. From this excited state the electron can relax in one of two ways, either dropping into the $n = 2$ level, or directly back to the $n = 1$ ground state. In the first scenario, we can expect to detect a photon with energy corresponding to the difference between $n = 3$ and $n = 2$. In the latter case we'd detect a more energetic photon of energy corresponding to the difference between $n = 3$ and $n = 1$.

Note: Distances between energy levels are not drawn to scale.

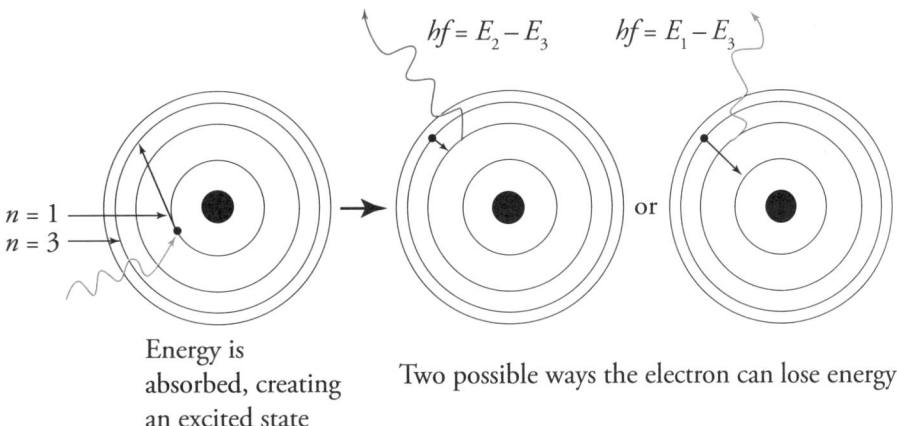

Two possible ways the electron can lose energy

The energies of these discrete energy levels were given by Bohr in the following equation, which only accurately predicted the behavior of atoms or ions containing one electron, now known as Bohr atoms. The value n in this case represents the energy level of the electron.

$$E_n = \frac{(-2.178 \times 10^{-18}\,\text{J})}{n^2}$$

Since we can calculate the energies of the levels of a Bohr atom, we can predict the wavelengths of photons emitted or absorbed when electrons transition between any two energy levels. To do this we calculate the energy differences between discrete levels by subtracting the initial energy of the electron from the final energy of the electron. We can find the energies of the two possible emitted photons shown above as follows:

$$\Delta E_{3\to 2} = \frac{(-2.178 \times 10^{-18}\,\text{J})}{(2)^2} - \frac{(-2.178 \times 10^{-18}\,\text{J})}{(3)^2}$$

$$\Delta E_{3\to 2} = -3.025 \times 10^{-19}\,\text{J}$$

$$\Delta E_{3\to 1} = \frac{(-2.178 \times 10^{-18}\,\text{J})}{(1)^2} - \frac{(-2.178 \times 10^{-18}\,\text{J})}{(3)^2}$$

$$\Delta E_{3\to 1} = -1.936 \times 10^{-18}\,\text{J}$$

Note that both energies calculated above are negative, indicating that energy is being released by the electron as it falls from its excited state to a lower energy level. For electron transitions from the ground state to an excited state, the ΔE values will be positive, indicating energy is absorbed by the electron.

Once the energy is calculated, the wavelength of the photon can be found by employing the relation $\Delta E = h\dfrac{c}{\lambda}$. Not all electron transitions produce photons we can see with the naked eye, but all transitions in an atom will produce photons either in the ultraviolet, visible, or infrared region of the electromagnetic spectrum.

Example 4-15: Which of the following is NOT an example of a Bohr atom?

A) H
B) He^+
C) Li^{2+}
D) H^+

Solution: A Bohr atom is one that contains only one electron. Since H^+ has a positive charge from losing the one electron in the neutral atom, thereby having no electrons at all, choice D is the answer.

Example 4-16: The first four electron energy levels of an atom are shown at the right, given in terms of electron volts. Which of the following gives the energy of a photon that could NOT be emitted by this atom?

A) 14 eV
B) 40 eV
C) 44 eV
D) 54 eV

——— $E_4 = -18$ eV

——— $E_3 = -32$ eV

——— $E_2 = -72$ eV

——— $E_1 = -288$ eV

Solution: The difference between E_4 and E_3 is 14 eV, so a photon of 14 eV would be emitted if an electron were to drop from level 4 to level 3; this eliminates choice A. Similarly, the difference between E_3 and E_2 is 40 eV, so choice B is eliminated, and the difference between E_4 and E_2 is 54 eV, so choice D is eliminated. The answer must be C; no two energy levels in this atom are separated by 44 eV.

Example 4-17: Consider two electron transitions. In the first case, an electron falls from $n = 4$ to $n = 2$, giving off a photon of light with a wavelength equal to 488 nm. In the second transition, an electron moves from $n = 3$ to $n = 4$. For this transition, we would expect that:

A) energy is emitted, and the wavelength of the corresponding photon will be shorter than the first transition.

B) energy is emitted, and the wavelength of the corresponding photon will be longer than the first transition.

C) energy is absorbed, and the wavelength of the corresponding photon will be shorter than the first transition.

D) energy is absorbed, and the wavelength of the corresponding photon will be longer than the first transition.

Solution: Since the electron is moving from a lower to higher energy level, we would expect that the atom absorbs energy (eliminating choices A and B). Since the electron transitions between energy levels that are closer together, the ΔE between levels is smaller. By the $\Delta E = h\dfrac{c}{\lambda}$ relationship, we know that energy and wavelength are inversely related. Therefore with a smaller energy change, the wavelength of the associated light will be longer. Choice D is the correct answer.

The Quantum Model of the Atom

While one-electron atoms produce easily predicted atomic spectra, the Bohr model does not do a good job of predicting the atomic spectra of many-electron atoms. This shows that the Bohr model cannot describe the electron-electron interactions that exist in many-electron atoms. The quantum model of the atom was developed to account for these differences. Bohr's model suggested, and we still hold to be true, that electrons held by an atom can exist only at discrete energy levels—that is, electron energy levels are quantized. This quantization is described by a unique "address" for each electron, consisting of four quantum numbers designating the shell, subshell, orbital, and spin. While the details of quantum numbers are beyond the scope of the MCAT, it is still useful to understand the conceptual basis of the quantum model.

The Energy Shell

The energy shell (n) of an electron in the quantum model of the atom is analogous to the circular orbits in the Bohr model of the atom. An electron in a higher shell has a greater amount of energy and a greater average distance from the nucleus. For example, an electron in the third shell ($n = 3$) has higher energy than an electron in the second shell (where $n = 2$), which has more energy than an electron in the first shell ($n = 1$).

The Energy Subshell

In the quantum model of the atom, however, we no longer describe the paths of electrons around the nucleus as circular orbits, but focus on the probability of finding an electron somewhere in the atom. Loosely speaking, an **orbital** describes a three-dimensional region around the nucleus in which the electron is most likely to be found.

A subshell in an atom is comprised of one or more orbitals, and is denoted by a letter (*s, p, d,* or *f*) that describes the shape and energy of the orbital(s). The orbitals in the subshells get progressively more complex and higher in energy in the order listed above. Each energy shell has one or more subshells, and each higher energy shell contains one additional subshell. For example, the first energy shell contains the *s* subshell, while the second energy shell contains both the *s* and *p* subshells, etc.

The Orbital Orientation

Each subshell contains one or more orbitals of the same energy (also called degenerate orbitals), and these orbitals have different three-dimensional orientations in space. The number of orientations increases by two in each successive subshell. For example, the *s* subshell contains one orientation and the *p* subshell contains three orientations.

You should be able to recognize the shapes of the orbitals in the *s* and *p* subshells. Each *s* subshell has just one spherically symmetrical orbital.

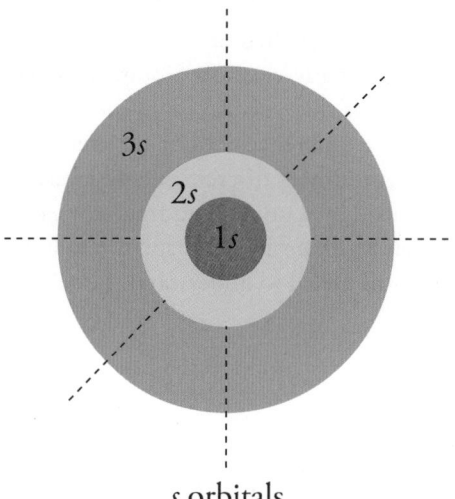

s orbitals

Each p subshell has three orbitals, each depicted as a dumbbell, with different spatial orientations.

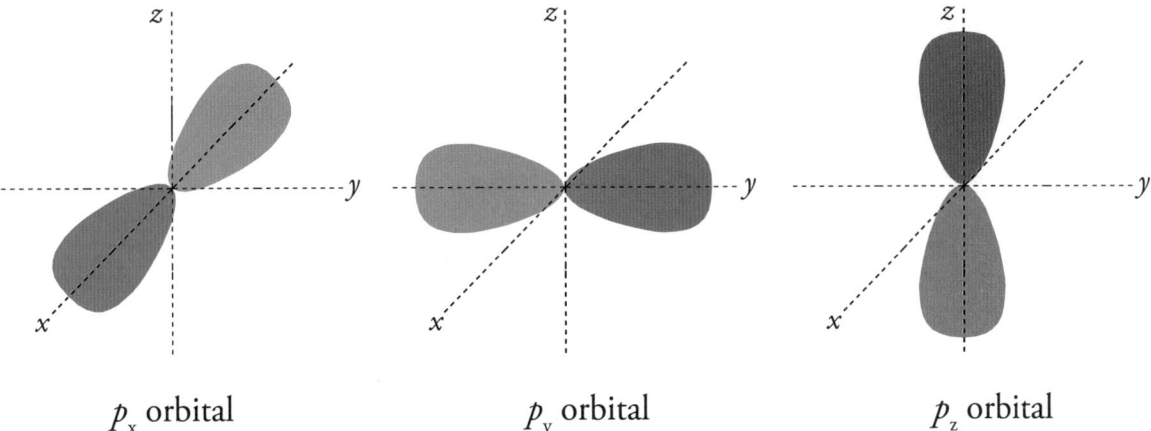

p_x orbital $\qquad$ p_y orbital $\qquad$ p_z orbital

4.6

The Electron Spin

Every electron has two possible spin states, which can be considered the electron's intrinsic magnetism. Because of this, every orbital can accommodate a maximum of two electrons, one spin-up and one spin-down. If an orbital is full, we say that the electrons it holds are "spin-paired."

4.6 ELECTRON CONFIGURATIONS

Now that we've described the modern quantum model of the atom, let's see how this is represented as an electron configuration. There are three basic rules:

1) *Electrons occupy the lowest energy orbitals available.* (This is the **Aufbau principle**.) Electron subshells are filled in order of increasing energy. The periodic table is logically constructed to reflect this fact, and therefore one can easily determine shell filling for specific atoms based on where they appear on the table. We will detail this in the next section on "Blocks."

2) *Electrons in the same subshell occupy available orbitals singly, before pairing up.* (This is known as **Hund's rule**.)

3) *There can be no more than two electrons in any given orbital.* (This is the **Pauli exclusion principle**.)

For example, let's describe the locations for all the electrons in an oxygen atom, which contains eight electrons. Beginning with the first, lowest energy shell, there is only one subshell (s) and only one orientation in that subshell, and there can only be two electrons in that one orbital. Therefore, these two electrons fill the only orbital in the $1s$ subshell. We write this as $1s^2$, to indicate that there are two electrons in the $1s$ subshell.

We still have six electrons left, so let's move on to the second, next highest, energy shell. There are two subshells (s and p). Since the s subshell is lower in energy than the p subshell, the next two electrons go in the $2s$ subshell, that is, $2s^2$.

For the remaining four electrons, there would be three orientations of orbitals in the p subshell. According to Hund's rule, we place one spin up electron in each of these three orbitals. The eighth electron now pairs up with an electron in one of the $2p$ orbitals. So, the last four electrons go in the $2p$ subshell: $2p^4$ (or more explicitly, $2p_x^2 2p_y^1 2p_z^1$).

The complete electron configuration for oxygen can now be written like this:

$$\text{Oxygen} = 1s^2 2s^2 2p^4$$

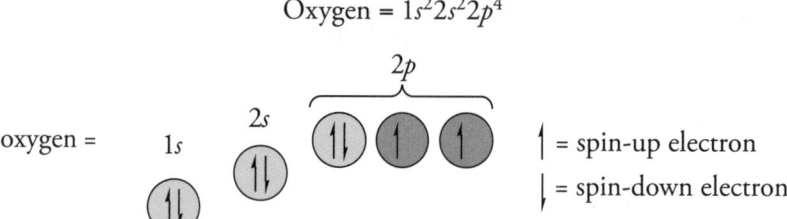

Here are the electron configurations for the first ten elements:

Z			1s
1	Hydrogen	$1s^1$	⬆
2	Helium	$1s^2$	⬆⬇

			1s	2s
3	Lithium	$1s^2 2s^1$	⬆⬇	⬆
4	Beryllium	$1s^2 2s^2$	⬆⬇	⬆⬇

			1s	2s	2p		
5	Boron	$1s^2 2s^2 2p^1$	⬆⬇	⬆⬇	⬆		
6	Carbon	$1s^2 2s^2 2p^2$	⬆⬇	⬆⬇	⬆	⬆	
7	Nitrogen	$1s^2 2s^2 2p^3$	⬆⬇	⬆⬇	⬆	⬆	⬆
8	Oxygen	$1s^2 2s^2 2p^4$	⬆⬇	⬆⬇	⬆⬇	⬆	⬆
9	Fluorine	$1s^2 2s^2 2p^5$	⬆⬇	⬆⬇	⬆⬇	⬆⬇	⬆
10	Neon	$1s^2 2s^2 2p^6$	⬆⬇	⬆⬇	⬆⬇	⬆⬇	⬆⬇

Example 4-18: What's the maximum number of electrons that can go into any s subshell? Any p subshell? Any d? Any f?

Solution: An s subshell has only one possible orbital orientation. Since only two electrons can fill any given orbital, an s subshell can hold no more than $1 \times 2 = 2$ electrons.

A p subshell has three possible orbital orientations (two more than an s subshell). Since again only two electrons can fill any given orbital, a p subshell can hold no more than $3 \times 2 = 6$ electrons.

A d subshell has five possible orbital orientations (two more than a p subshell). Since there are two electrons per orbital, a d subshell can hold no more than $5 \times 2 = 10$ electrons.

Finally, an f subshell has seven possible orbital orientations (two more than a d subshell). Since there are two electrons per orbital, an f subshell can hold no more than $7 \times 2 = 14$ electrons.

Example 4-19: Write down the electron configuration of argon (Ar, atomic number 18).

Solution: We have 18 electrons to successively place in the proper subshells, as follows:

$1s$: 2 electrons
$2s$: 2 electrons
$2p$: 6 electrons
$3s$: 2 electrons
$3p$: 6 electrons

Therefore,

$$[\text{Ar}] = 1s^2 2s^2 2p^6 3s^2 3p^6$$

Notice that the $3s$ and $3p$ subshells have their full complement of electrons. In fact, the **noble gases** (those elements in the last column of the periodic table) all have their outer 8 electrons in filled subshells: 2 in the ns subshell plus 6 in the np. (The lone exception, of course, is helium; but its one and only subshell, the $1s$, is filled—with 2 electrons.) Because their 8 valence electrons are in filled subshells, we say that these atoms—Ne, Ar, Kr, Xe, and Rn—have a complete **octet**, which accounts for their remarkable chemical stability, and lack of reactivity.

Diamagnetic and Paramagnetic Atoms

An atom that has all of its electrons spin-paired is referred to as **diamagnetic**. For example, helium, beryllium, and neon are diamagnetic. A diamagnetic atom must contain an even number of electrons and have all of its occupied subshells filled. Since all the electrons in a diamagnetic atom are spin-paired, the individual magnetic fields that they create cancel, leaving no net magnetic field. Such an atom will be *repelled* by an externally produced magnetic field.

If an atom's electrons are not all spin-paired, it is said to be **paramagnetic**. Paramagnetic atoms are *attracted* into externally produced magnetic fields.

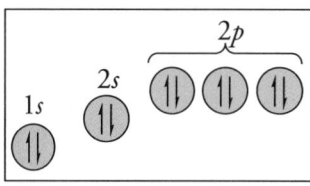

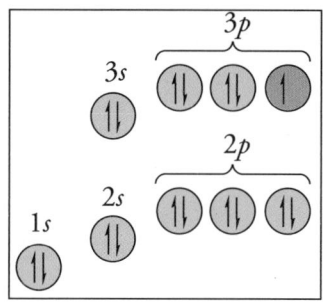

Neon	Chlorine
all electrons spin-paired	not all electrons spin-paired
∴ diamagnetic	∴ paramagnetic
repelled from a magnetic field	attracted into a magnetic field

Example 4-20: Which of the following elements is diamagnetic?

A) Sodium
B) Sulfur
C) Potassium
D) Calcium

Solution: First, a diamagnetic atom must contain an *even* number of electrons, because they all must be spin-*paired*. So, we can eliminate choices A and C, since sodium and potassium each contain an odd number of electrons (11 and 19, respectively). The electron configuration of sulfur is [Ne] $3s^23p^4$; by Hund's rule, the 4 electrons in the $3p$ subshell will look like this:

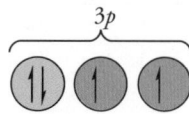

They're not all spin-paired, so sulfur is not diamagnetic. The answer must be D, calcium, because its configuration is [Ar] $4s^2$, and all of its electrons are spin-paired.

4.6

Blocks in the Periodic Table

s block →

p block →

d block

f block →

*Lanthanide Series:

†Actinide Series:

4.6

The periodic table can be divided into blocks, as shown above. The name of the block (*s, p, d,* or *f*) indicates the highest-energy subshell containing electrons in the ground-state of an atom within that block. For example, carbon is in the *p* block, and its electron configuration is $1s^2 2s^2 2p^2$; the highest-energy subshell that contains electrons (the $2p$) is a *p* subshell. In addition, each horizontal row in the periodic table is called a **period**, and each vertical column is called a **group** (or **family**). The bold numbers next to the rows on the left indicate the period number; for example, potassium (K, atomic number 19) is in Period 4.

How do we use this block diagram to write electron configurations? To illustrate, let's say we want to write the configuration for chlorine ($Z = 17$). To get to $Z = 17$, imagine starting at $Z = 1$ (hydrogen) and filling up the subshells as we move along through the rows to $Z = 17$. (Notice that helium has been moved over next to hydrogen for purposes of this block diagram.) We'll first have $1s^2$ for the 2 atoms in Period 1, *s* block ($Z = 1$ and $Z = 2$); the $2s^2$ for the next 2 atoms, which are in Period 2, *s* block ($Z = 3$ and $Z = 4$); then $2p^6$ for the next 6 atoms, which are in Period 2, *p* block ($Z = 5$ through $Z = 10$); the $3s^2$ for the next 2 atoms, which are in Period 3, *s* block ($Z = 11$ and $Z = 12$); then, finally, $3p^5$ for the atoms starting with aluminum, Al, in Period 3, *p* block and counting through to chlorine, Cl. So, we've gone through the rows and blocks from the beginning and stopped once we hit the atom we wanted, and along the way we obtained $1s^2 2s^2 2p^6 3s^2 3p^5$. This is the electron configuration of chlorine.

The noble gases are often used as starting points, because they are at the ends of the rows and represent a shell being completely filled; all that's left is to count over in the next row until the desired atom is reached. We find the closest noble gas that has an atomic number less than that of the atom for which we want to find an electron configuration. In the case of chlorine ($Z = 17$), the closest noble gas with a smaller atomic number is neon ($Z = 10$). Starting with neon, we have 7 additional electrons to take care of. To get to $Z = 17$, we go through the 2 atoms in the *s* block of Period 3 ($3s^2$), then notice that Cl is the fifth element in the *p* block, giving us $3p^5$. Therefore, the electron configuration of chlorine is the same as that of neon plus $3s^2 3p^5$, which we can write like this: Cl = [Ne] $3s^2 3p^5$.

The simple counting through the rows and blocks works as long as you remember this simple rule: Whenever you're in the *d* block, *subtract 1 from the period number.* For example, the first row of the *d* block ($Z = 21$ through $Z = 30$) is in Period 4, but instead of saying that these elements have their outermost (or **valence**) electrons in the 4*d* subshell, we subtract 1 from the period number and say that these elements put their valence electrons in the 3*d* subshell.

In summary: The block in the table tells us in which subshell the outermost (valence) electrons of the atom will be. The period (row) gives the shell, *n*, as long as we remember the following fact about the atoms in the *d* block: electrons for an atom in the *d* block of Period *n* go into the subshell $(n − 1)d$. For example, the electron configuration for scandium (Sc, atomic number 21) is [Ar] $4s^2 3d^1$. (Note: if you ever need to write the electron configuration for an element in the *f* block, the rule is: *In the f block, subtract 2 from the period number.*)

Example 4-21: Which of the following gives the electron configuration of an aluminum atom?

A) $1s^2 2s^2 2p^1$
B) $1s^2 2s^2 2p^2$
C) $1s^2 2s^2 2p^6 3s^2 3p^1$
D) $1s^2 2s^2 2p^6 3s^2 3p^2$

Solution: Since aluminum (Al) has atomic number 13, a neutral aluminum atom must have 13 electrons. This observation alone eliminates choices A, B, and D (which indicate a total of 5, 6, and 14 electrons, respectively), so the answer must be C.

Example 4-22: What is the maximum number of electrons that can be present in the $n = 3$ shell?

A) 6
B) 9
C) 12
D) 18

Solution: Every new energy level (*n*) adds a new subshell. That means that in the first energy level we have only the *s* subshell, while when $n = 2$ we have both *s* and *p* subshells, and when $n = 3$, there are *s*, *p*, and *d* subshells. Since there are 1, 3, and 5 *s*, *p*, and *d* orbitals, respectively, for a total of 9 orbitals, and since the maximum number of electrons in an orbital is 2, there can be a maximum of 18 electrons in the $n = 3$ shell. Choice D is correct.

Example 4-23: What's the electron configuration of a zirconium atom ($Z = 40$)?

A) [Kr] $4d^4$
B) [Kr] $5s^2 4d^2$
C) [Kr] $5s^2 5p^2$
D) [Kr] $5s^2 5d^2$

Solution: Zirconium (Zr) is in the *d* block of Period 5. After krypton (Kr, atomic number 36), we'll have $5s^2$ for the next 2 atoms in the Period 5, *s* block ($Z = 37$ and $Z = 38$). Then, remembering the rule that electrons for an atom in the *d* block of Period *n* go into the subshell $(n − 1)d$, we know that the last two electrons will go in the 4*d* (not the 5*d*) subshell. Therefore, the answer is B.

Some Anomalous Electron Configurations

The process described above (reading across the periodic table, from top to bottom and left to right, using the blocks as a tool for the order of filling of subshells) to determine an atom's electron configuration works quite well for a large percentage of the elements, but there are a few atoms for which the anticipated electron configuration is not the actual configuration observed.

In a few instances, atoms can achieve a lower energy state (or a higher degree of stability) *by having a filled, or half-filled, d subshell*. For example, consider chromium (Cr, $Z = 24$). On the basis of the block diagram, we'd expect its electron configuration to be [Ar] $4s^2 3d^4$. Recalling that a d subshell can hold a maximum of 10 electrons, it turns out that chromium achieves a more stable state by filling its d subshell with 5 electrons (*half-filled*) rather than leaving it with 4. This is accomplished by promoting one of its $4s$ electrons to the $3d$ subshell, yielding the electron configuration [Ar] $4s^1 3d^5$. As another example, copper (Cu, $Z = 29$) has an expected electron configuration of [Ar] $4s^2 3d^9$. However, a copper atom obtains a more stable, lower-energy state by promoting one of its $4s$ electrons into the $3d$ subshell, yielding [Ar] $4s^1 3d^{10}$ to give a *filled d* subshell.

Other atoms that display the same type of behavior with regard to their electron configuration as do chromium and copper include molybdenum (Mo, $Z = 42$, in the same family as chromium), as well as silver and gold (Ag and Au, $Z = 47$ and $Z = 79$, respectively, which are in the same family as copper).

Example 4-24: What is the electron configuration of an atom of silver?

Solution: As mentioned above, silver is one of the handful of elements with atoms that actually achieve greater overall stability by promoting one of its electrons into a higher subshell in order to make it filled. We'd expect the electron configuration for silver to be [Kr] $5s^2 4d^9$. But, by analogy with copper, we'd predict (correctly) that the actual configuration of silver is [Kr] $5s^1 4d^{10}$, where the atom obtains a more stable state by promoting one of its $5s$ electrons into the $4d$ subshell, to give a *filled d* subshell.

Electron Configurations of Ions

Recall that an ion is an atom that has acquired a nonzero electric charge. An atom with more electrons than protons is negatively charged and is called an anion; an atom with fewer electrons than protons is positively charged and is called a cation.

Atoms that gain electrons (anions) accommodate them in the first available orbital, the one with the lowest available energy. For example, fluorine (F, $Z = 9$) has the electron configuration $1s^2 2s^2 2p^5$. When a fluorine atom gains an electron to become the fluoride ion, F$^-$, the additional electron goes into the $2p$ subshell, giving the electron configuration $1s^2 2s^2 2p^6$, which is the same as the configuration of neon. For this reason, F$^-$ and Ne are said to be **isoelectronic**.

In order to write the electron configuration of an ion for an element in the s or p blocks, we can use the blocks in the periodic table as follows. If an atom becomes an anion—that is, if it acquires one or more additional electrons—then we move to the *right* within the table by a number of squares equal to the number of electrons added in order to find the atom with the same configuration as the ion.

If an atom becomes a cation—that is, if it loses one or more electrons—then we move to the *left* within the table by a number of squares equal to the number of electrons lost in order to find the atom with the same configuration as the ion.

Example 4-25: What's the electron configuration of P^{3-}? Of Sr^+?

Solution: To find the configuration of P^{3-}, we locate phosphorus (P, Z = 15) in the periodic table and move 3 places to the *right* (because we have an anion with charge of 3–); this lands us on argon (Ar, Z = 18). Therefore, the electron configuration of the anion P^{3-} is the same as that of argon: $1s^2 2s^2 2p^6 3s^2 3p^6$.

To find the configuration of Sr^+, we locate strontium (Sr, Z = 38) in the periodic table and move 1 place to the *left* (because we have a cation with charge 1+), thus landing on rubidium (Rb, Z = 37). Therefore, the electron configuration of the cation Sr^+ is the same as that of rubidium: [Kr] $5s^1$.

Electrons that are removed (*ionized*) from an atom always come from the valence shell (the highest n level), and the highest energy orbital within that level. For example, an atom of lithium, Li ($1s^2 2s^1$), becomes Li^+ ($1s^2$) when it absorbs enough energy for an electron to escape. However, recall from our discussion above that **transition metals** (which are the elements in the d block) have both ns and $(n-1)d$ electrons. To form a cation, atoms will always lose their valence electrons first, and since $n > n-1$, transition metals lose s electrons *before* they lose d electrons. Only after *all* s electrons are lost do d electrons get ionized. For example, the electron configuration for the transition metal titanium (Ti, Z = 22) is [Ar] $4s^2 3d^2$. We might expect that the electron configuration of the ion Ti^+ to be [Ar] $4s^2 3d^1$ since the d electrons are slightly higher in energy. However, the *actual* configuration is [Ar] $4s^1 3d^2$, and the valence electrons (the ones from the highest n level) are ALWAYS lost first. Similarly, the electron configuration of Ti^{2+} is not [Ar] $4s^2$—it's actually [Ar] $3d^2$.

Example 4-26: Which one of the following ions has the same electron configuration as the noble gas argon?

A) Na^+
B) P^{2-}
C) Al^{3+}
D) Cl^-

Solution: Na^+ (choice A) has the same electron configuration as the noble gas *neon*, not argon, since one element to the left of Na is Ne. The ion P^{2-} has the same electron configuration as Cl, which is two elements to the right of P. Al^{3+}, like Na^+, has the same configuration as Ne. Of the choices given, only Cl^- (choice D) has the same configuration as Ar, since Ar is one element to the right of Cl.

Example 4-27: What's the electron configuration of Cu^+? Of Cu^{2+}? Of Fe^{3+}?

Solution: Copper (Cu, Z = 29) is a transition metal, so it will lose its valence s electrons before losing any d electrons. Recall the anomalous electron configuration of Cu (to give it a filled $3d$ subshell): [Ar] $4s^1 3d^{10}$. Therefore, the configuration of Cu^+ (the *cuprous* ion, Cu(I)) is [Ar] $3d^{10}$, and that of Cu^{2+} (the *cupric* ion, Cu(II)) is [Ar] $3d^9$. Since the electron configuration of iron (Fe, Z = 26) is [Ar] $4s^2 3d^6$, the configuration of Fe^{3+} (the *ferric* ion, Fe(III)) is [Ar] $3d^5$, since the transition metal atom Fe first loses both of its valence s electrons, and then once they're ionized, one of its d electrons.

Excited State vs. Ground State

Assigning electron configurations as we've just discussed is aimed at constructing the *most probable* location of electrons, following the Aufbau principle. These configurations are the most probable because they are the lowest in energy, or as they are often termed, the ground state.

Any electron configuration of an atom that is *not* as we would assign it, provided it doesn't break any physical rules (no more than $2e^-$ per orbital, no assigning nonexistent shells such as $2d$, etc....) is an excited state. The atom has absorbed energy, so the electrons now inhabit states we wouldn't predict as the most probable ones.

Example 4-28: Which of the following could be the electron configuration of an excited oxygen atom?

A) $1s^2 2s^2 2p^4$
B) $1s^2 2s^2 2p^5$
C) $1s^2 2s^2 2p^3 3s^1$
D) $1s^2 2s^2 2p^4 3s^1$

Solution: An oxygen atom contains 8 electrons; when excited, one (or more) of these electrons will jump to a higher energy level. Choice A is the configuration of a ground-state oxygen atom, and choices B and D show the placement of 9 electrons, not 8, so all of these may be eliminated. The answer must be C; one of the $2p$ electrons has jumped to the $3s$ subshell. (Note carefully that an excited atom is not an ion; electrons are not lost or gained; they simply jump to higher energy levels within the atom.)

4.7   GROUPS OF THE PERIODIC TABLE AND THEIR CHARACTERISTICS

We will use the electron configurations of the atoms to predict their chemical properties, including their reactivity and bonding patterns with other atoms.

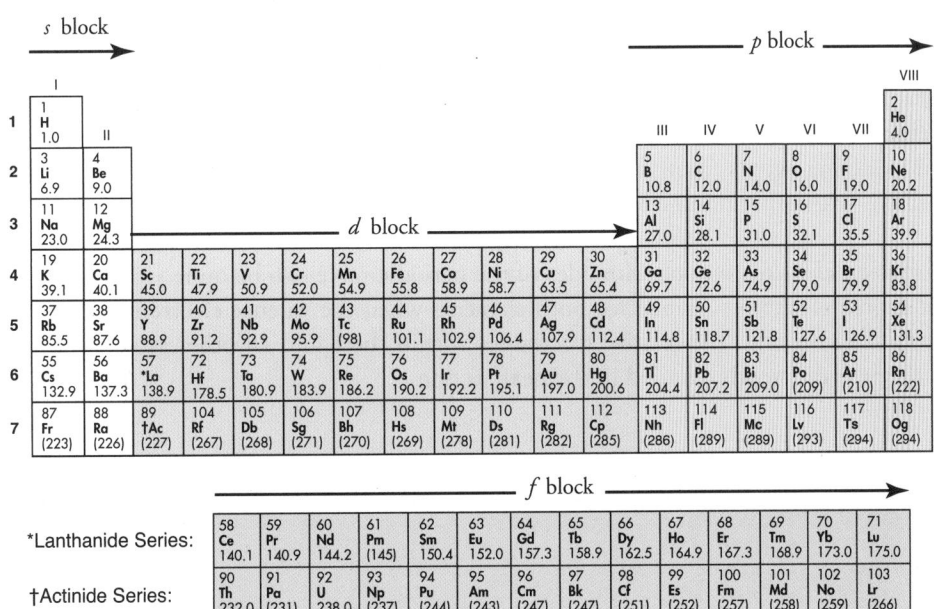

Recall that each horizontal row in the periodic table is called a **period**, and each vertical column is called a **group** (or **family**). Within any group in the periodic table, all of the elements have the same number of electrons in their outermost shell. For instance, the elements in Group II all have two electrons in their outermost shell. Electrons in an atom's outermost shell are called **valence** electrons, and it's the valence electrons that are primarily responsible for an atom's properties and chemical behavior.

Some groups (families) have special names.

Group	Name	Valence-Shell Configuration
Group I	*Alkali metals*	ns^1
Group II	*Alkaline earth metals*	ns^2
Group VII	*Halogens*	ns^2np^5
Group VIII	*Noble gases*	ns^2np^6
The *d* Block	*Transition metals*	
The *s* and *p* Blocks	*Representative elements*	
The *f* Block	*Rare earth metals*	

The valence-shell electron configuration determines the chemical reactivity of each group in the table. For example, in the noble gas family each element has eight electrons in its outermost shell (ns^2np^6). Such a closed-shell (fully-filled valence shell) configuration is called an octet and results in great stability (and therefore low reactivity) for an atom. For this reason, noble gases do not generally undergo chemical reactions, so most group VIII elements are inert. Helium is inert as well, but has a closed shell with a stable duet ($1s^2$) of electrons.

Other elements experience similar increases in stability upon reaching this stable octet electron configuration, and most chemical reactions can be regarded as the quest for atoms to achieve such closed-shell stability. The alkali metals and alkaline earth metals, for instance, possess one (ns^1) or two (ns^2) electrons in their valence shells, respectively, and behave as reducing agents (i.e., lose valence electrons) in redox reactions in order to obtain a stable octet, generally as an M^+ or M^{2+} cation.

Similarly, the halogens (ns^2np^5) require only a single electron to achieve a stable octet. To achieve this state in their elemental form, halogens naturally exist as diatomic molecules (e.g., F_2) where one electron from each atom is shared in a covalent bond. When combined with other elements, the halogens behave as powerful oxidizing agents (that is, gain electrons); they can become stable either as X^- anions or by sharing electrons with other nonmetals (more on bonding in Ch. 5).

Reactions between elements on opposite sides of the periodic table can be quite violent. This occurs due to the great degree of stability gained for both elements when the valence electrons are transferred from the metal to the nonmetal. The relative reactivities within these and all other groups can be further explained by the periodic trends detailed in the next section.

Example 4-29: Which of the following could describe an ion with the same electron configuration as a noble gas?

A) An alkali metal that has gained an electron
B) A halogen that has lost an electron
C) A transition metal that has gained an electron
D) An alkaline earth metal that has lost two electrons

Solution: Choice A is wrong, since it says "gained" rather than "lost." Choice B is incorrect, since it says "lost" rather than "gained." Choice C is also incorrect, because no element in the d block could acquire a noble-gas configuration by gaining a single electron. The answer must be D. If an element in Group II loses two electrons, it can acquire a noble-gas electron configuration. (For example, Mg^{2+} has the same configuration as Ne, and Ca^{2+} has the same configuration as Ar.)

4.8 PERIODIC TRENDS

Shielding

Each filled shell between the nucleus and the valence electrons shields—or "protects"—the valence electrons from the full effect of the positively charged protons in the nucleus. This is called **nuclear shielding** or the **shielding effect**. As far as the valence electrons are concerned, the electrical pull by the protons in the nucleus is reduced by the negative charges of the electrons in the filled shells in between; the result is an effective reduction in the positive elementary charge, from Z to a smaller amount denoted by Z_{eff} (for *effective nuclear charge*).

Example 4-30: The electrons in a solitary He atom are under the influence of two forces, one attractive and one repulsive. What are these forces?

A) Electrostatic attraction between the electrons and the nuclear protons, and electrostatic repulsion between the electrons and nuclear neutrons
B) Electrostatic attraction between the electrons and the nuclear protons, and electrostatic repulsion between the electrons
C) Gravitational attraction between the electrons and the nuclear protons, and frictional repulsion between the electrons
D) Gravitational attraction between the electrons and the entire nucleus, and frictional repulsion between the electrons

Solution: Compared to the magnitude of electrostatic forces in an atom, gravitational forces between the electrons and nucleons of an atom are negligible, so choices C and D are eliminated. Furthermore, neutrons have no charge and thus do not participate in electrostatic forces, so choice A is eliminated. Remember that opposite charges attract and like charges repel. The best choice is B.

Atomic and Ionic Radius

With progression across any period in the table, the number of protons increases, and hence their total pull on the outermost electrons increases, too. New shells are initiated only at the beginning of a period. So, as we go across a period, electrons are being added, but new shells are not; therefore, the valence electrons are more and more tightly bound to the atom because they feel a greater effective nuclear charge. Therefore, as we move from left to right across a period, **atomic radius** *decreases*.

However, with progression down a group, as new shells are added with each period, the valence electrons experience increased shielding. The valence electrons are less tightly bound, since they feel a smaller effective nuclear charge. Therefore, as we go down a group, atomic radius *increases* due to the increased shielding.

If we form an ion, the radius will decrease as electrons are removed (because the ones that are left are drawn in more closely to the nucleus), and the radius will increase as electrons are added. So, in terms of radius, we have $X^+ < X < X^-$; that is, cation radius < neutral-atom radius < anion radius.

Ionization Energy

Because the atom's positively charged nucleus is attracted to the electrons in the atom, it takes energy to remove an electron. The amount of energy necessary to remove the least tightly bound electron from an isolated atom is called the atom's (**first**) **ionization energy** (often abbreviated **IE** or IE_1). As we move from left to right across a period, or up a group, the ionization energy *increases* since the valence electrons are more tightly bound. The ionization energy of any atom with a noble-gas configuration will always be very large. (For example, the ionization energy of neon is 4 times greater than that of lithium.) The **second ionization energy** (IE_2) of an atom, X, is the energy required to remove the least tightly bound electron from the cation X^+. Note that IE_2 will always be greater than IE_1.

Electron Affinity

The energy associated with the addition of an electron to an isolated atom is known as the atom's **electron affinity** (often abbreviated **EA**). If energy is *released* when the electron is added, the usual convention is to say that the electron affinity is negative; if energy is *required* in order to add the electron, the electron affinity is positive. The halogens have large negative electron affinity values, since the addition of an electron would give them the much desired octet configuration. So they readily accept an electron to become an anion; the increase in stability causes energy to be released. On the other hand, the noble gases and alkaline earth metals have positive electron affinities, because the added electron begins to fill a new level or sublevel and destabilizes the electron configuration. Therefore, anions of these atoms are unstable. Electron affinities typically become more negative as we move to the right across a row or up a group (noble gases excepted), but there are anomalies in this trend.

Electronegativity

Electronegativity is a measure of an atom's ability to pull electrons to itself when it forms a covalent bond; the greater this tendency to attract electrons, the greater the atom's electronegativity. Electronegativity generally behaves as does ionization energy; that is, as we move from left to right across a period, electronegativity increases. As we go down a group, electronegativity decreases. You should know the order of electronegativity for the nine most electronegative elements:

$$F > O > N \approx Cl > Br > I > S > C \approx H$$

Acidity

Acidity is a measure of how well a compound donates protons, accepts electrons, or lowers pH in a chemical system. A binary acid has the structure HX, and can dissociate in water in the following manner: $HX \rightarrow H^+ + X^-$. Stronger acids have resulting X^- anions that are likely to separate from H^+ because they are stable once they do. Generally speaking, the ease with which an acid (HX) donates its H^+ is directly related to the stability of the conjugate base (X^-). With respect to the *horizontal* periodic trend for acidity, the more electronegative the element bearing the negative charge is, the more stable the anion will be. Therefore acidity increases from left to right across a period. However, the *vertical* trend for acidity depends on the size of the anion. The larger the anion, the more the negative charge can be delocalized and stabilized. Therefore, acidity increases down a group or family in the periodic table.

Summary of Periodic Trends

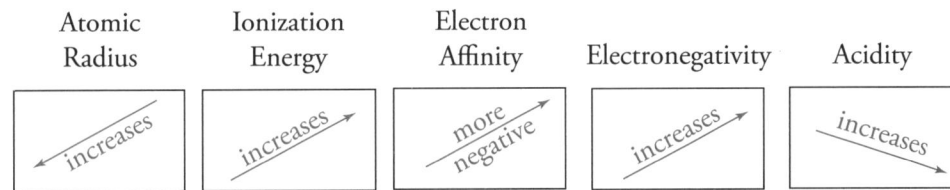

Example 4-31: Compared to calcium, beryllium is expected to have:

A) greater electronegativity and ionization energy.
B) smaller electronegativity and ionization energy.
C) greater electronegativity and smaller ionization energy.
D) smaller electronegativity and larger ionization energy.

Solution: Beryllium and calcium are in the same group, but beryllium is higher in the column. We therefore expect beryllium to have greater ionization energy and a greater electronegativity than calcium (choice A), since both of these periodic trends tend to increase as we go up within a group.

Example 4-32: Which of the following will have a greater value for phosphorus than for magnesium?

 I. Atomic radius
 II. Ionization energy
III. Electronegativity

A) I only
B) I and II only
C) II and III only
D) I, II, and III

Solution: Magnesium and phosphorus are in the same period (row), but phosphorus is farther to the right. We therefore expect phosphorus to have a smaller atomic radius, making Roman numeral I false. This allows us to eliminate choices A, B, and D, leaving C as the correct answer. This is also consistent, as we expect phosphorus to have a greater ionization energy and a greater electronegativity than magnesium, since both of these periodic trends tend to increase as we move to the right across a row. However, we expect the atomic radius of phosphorus to be smaller than that of magnesium, since atomic radii tend to *decrease* as we move to the right across a row. Therefore, the answer is C.

Example: 4-33: Of the following, which has the most negative electron affinity?

A) Barium
B) Bromine
C) Phosphorus
D) Chlorine

Solution: Barium is in Group II and therefore has a large positive electron affinity, so we can eliminate choice A immediately. Because electron affinity values tend to become more negative as we go to the right across a row or up within a column, we'd expect chlorine to have a more negative electron affinity than phosphorus or bromine. Therefore, choice D is the answer.

Example 4-34: Of the following, which has the smallest atomic radius?

A) Sodium
B) Oxygen
C) Calcium
D) Silicon

Solution: The atoms with the *smallest* atomic radius are those in the *upper right* portion of the periodic table, since atomic radius tends to increase as we move to the left or down a column. We can therefore eliminate choices A and C; these elements are in Groups I and II, respectively, at the far left end of the table. To decide between the remaining choices, we notice that oxygen is farther to the right *and* in a higher row than silicon, so we'd expect an oxygen atom to have a smaller radius than a silicon atom. Choice B is the best answer.

Example 4-35: Of the following, which is the strongest acid?

A) H_2O
B) H_2S
C) HCl
D) HBr

Solution: For binary acids, we expect acidity to increase with increasing stability of the conjugate base. When comparing anions in a period, those that are more electronegative are more stable. Since chloride is more electronegative than sulfide, choice B can be eliminated. In addition, when comparing anions in a family, those that are larger are more stable, so choices A and C can also be eliminated, making choice D the best answer.

Chapter 4 Summary

- The nucleus contains protons and neutrons. Their sum corresponds to the mass number (A).

- The number of protons corresponds to the atomic number (Z).

- An overabundance of either protons or neutrons can result in unstable nuclei, which decay via the emission of various particles.

- For nuclear decay reactions, the sum of all mass and atomic numbers in the products must equal the sum of these same numbers in the reactants.

- The rate of nuclear decay is governed by a species' half-life.

- Electrons exist in discrete energy levels within an atom. Emission spectra are obtained from energy emitted as excited electrons fall from one level to another.

- The periodic table is organized into blocks based on the architecture of electron orbitals. Therefore, valence electron configurations can be determined based on an element's location in the table.

- In their ground state, electrons occupy the lowest energy orbitals available, and occupy subshell orbitals singly before pairing.

- Atoms and ions are most stable when they have an octet of electrons in their outer shell.

- The d subshell is always backfilled: for an atom in the d block of period n, the d subshell will have a principal quantum number of $n - 1$.

- A half-filled (d^5) or filled (d^{10}) d subshell is exceptionally stable.

- Transition metals ionize from their valence s subshell before their d subshell.

- Atomic radius increases to the left and down the periodic table; for charged species, cation radius < neutral-atom radius < anion radius for a given element; for isoelectronic ions, the species with more protons will have the smaller radius.

- Ionization energy, electron affinity, and electronegativity increase up and to the right on the periodic table, while acidity increases to the right and down the periodic table.

- The relative electronegativities of common atoms in decreasing order are F O N $\approx$ Cl Br I S C $\approx$ H.

CHAPTER 4 FREESTANDING PRACTICE QUESTIONS

1. When an atom of plutonium-239 is bombarded with an alpha particle, this element along with one free neutron is created:

   A) Californium-240.
   B) Californium-241.
   C) Curium-242.
   D) Curium-243.

2. Which of the following represents the correct ground state electronic configuration for ferrous ion, Fe^{2+}?

   A) $[Ar]\ 4s^23d^6$
   B) $[Ar]\ 4s^23d^4$
   C) $[Ar]\ 3d^6$
   D) $[Ar]\ 4s^23d^2$

3. Which atom has three unpaired electrons in its valence energy level?

   A) Li
   B) Be
   C) C
   D) N

4. Which of the following elements would be most strongly attracted to a magnetic field?

   A) Mg
   B) Ca
   C) Cr
   D) Zn

5. Which of the following colors would appear as a bright band in an emission spectrum of a yellow sodium vapor lamp?

   A) Yellow, indicating a lesser wavelength than ultraviolet light
   B) Yellow, indicating a greater wavelength than ultraviolet light
   C) Blue, indicating a lesser wavelength than ultraviolet light
   D) Blue, indicating a greater wavelength than ultraviolet light

6. Which of the following atoms/ions has electrons in the subshell of highest energy?

   A) Cl^-
   B) Ca^{2+}
   C) Cr^+
   D) As

7. Of the following metallic elements, which has the lowest second ionization energy?

   A) Na
   B) K
   C) Mg
   D) Ca

8. Which of the following has the smallest atomic or ionic radius?

   A) Cl^-
   B) Ar
   C) K^+
   D) Ca^{2+}

9. Metallic character results from an element's ability to lose electrons. On the periodic table it is expected that metallic character increases:

   A) from left to right, because the decrease in electronegativity would make it easier to lose electrons.
   B) from left to right, because the decrease in atomic radius would result in more stable positive ions.
   C) from right to left, because the decrease in ionization energy would make it easier to lose electrons.
   D) from right to left, because the decrease in electron affinity would result in more stable positive ions.

CHAPTER 4 PRACTICE PASSAGE

The term "first ionization energy" is the minimum amount of energy that an atom in the gaseous state must absorb to release its outermost electron, thereby creating an ion with a charge of +1. The "second ionization energy" is the amount of energy necessary to cause the removal of the second outermost electron (after the first electron has already been removed), thereby creating an ion with a charge of +2. If an atom loses enough electrons to leave the resulting ion with a "stable octet" noble-gas electron configuration, the energy necessary to remove yet another electron will greatly exceed that which was needed to remove any of the previously displaced electrons.

A series of experiments is conducted involving the apparatus shown in Figure 1. It consists of an evacuated glass tube with an electrode situated at each end. Intake and exhaust valves are located along the upper surface of the tube so that gas may be introduced into the tube and removed.

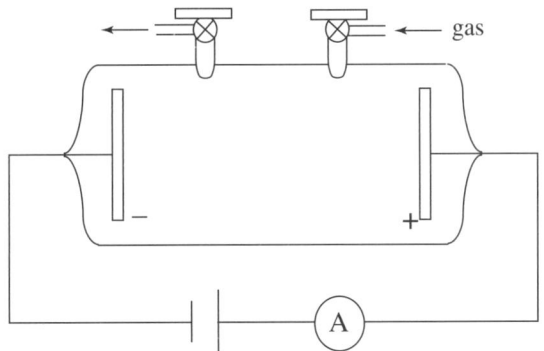

Figure 1

For each experiment, an *elemental* gas is introduced via the intake valve. While the gas remains in the glass tube the potential difference (voltage) across the electrode plates is gradually increased. As the voltage increases, it ultimately reaches a level high enough to provide the gas atoms with energy equal to their first ionization energy. In such an experimental situation the voltage that corresponds to the first ionization energy is termed the "ionization potential." When the voltage is raised to a level equal to the ionization potential, gas ions are formed and a sudden surge of current flow within the tube is noted and recorded.

For a variety of properties, including electron affinity and ionization energy, the elements follow well established periodic trends. For any given element these trends are significant to chemical behavior and reactivity. Table 1 records measured ionization energies for several elements.

Element	First Ionization Energy (eV/atom)	Second Ionization Energy (eV/atom)
Hydrogen	13.6	
Helium	24.6	
Lithium	5.4	
Nitrogen	14.5	
Neon	21.6	
Sodium	5.1	
Magnesium	7.6	
Titanium	6.8	13.6
Iron	7.9	16

Table 1

1. Which of the following represent the likely values of the first ionization energies of K and Cs (in eV), respectively?

   A) K = 5.2; Cs = 4.3
   B) K = 4.3; Cs = 5.2
   C) K = 4.3; Cs = 3.8
   D) K = 3.8; Cs = 4.3

2. Although the second ionization energies for Na and Mg do not appear in Table 1, it is most likely that the second ionization energy of Na will be:

   A) less than that of Mg, because its first ionization energy is also less.
   B) less than that of Mg, because Na^+ has a smaller effective nuclear charge than Mg^+.
   C) greater than that of Mg, because Na^{2+} is more stable than Mg^{2+}.
   D) greater than that of Mg, because the valence electron of Na^+ is in a $2p$ orbital, whereas that of Mg^+ is in a $3s$ orbital.

3. The voltage in the tube is adjusted to provide the circulating gas atoms with energy equal to 10 eV. Which of the following species can undergo ionization?

A) H, He, and Li
B) H, He, and N
C) Mg, Ti, and Fe⁺
D) Na, Mg, and Ti

4. Without information like that provided in Table 1, the experimental device shown in Figure 1 would fail to aid a researcher in identifying a tested elemental gas because the researcher would lack which of the following?

A) A control against which to compare the electrochemical events within the glass tube and the hypotheses on which the experiment is based
B) A rational basis on which to draw conclusions because the electrochemical event could not be associated with the phenomenon of ionization
C) A reference standard from which to draw conclusions based on the voltage magnitude at which the apparatus experiences a current surge
D) A scientifically designed experimental model since any appropriately controlled study requires a pre-existing data base as its premise

5. When the same setup was used to measure gaseous H_2 and N_2, ionization energies of 15.6 and 15.5 eV, respectively, were recorded. Which of the following correctly rationalizes the discrepancy between these values and the energies found for the elemental gases?

A) The electrons in the σ and π bonds of H_2 and N_2 are diffuse about the molecular surface, and hence more weakly held than in the elemental gases.
B) Nitrogen is more stable in its −3 oxidation state, and hydrogen in its +1 oxidation state, than in their neutral atomic states.
C) Bonding arrangements necessarily increase the stability of the electrons involved in any atom.
D) Large dipoles in molecules act to increase the ionization energy of electrons constituting the molecule.

SOLUTIONS TO CHAPTER 4 FREESTANDING PRACTICE QUESTIONS

1. **C** The process described is transmutation, and the new nucleus can be determined by writing a balanced nuclear equation. The preliminary equation to balance is this:

$$^{239}_{94}Pu + ^{4}_{2}\alpha \rightarrow ^{1}_{0}n + ^{A}_{Z}?$$

where the question mark stands for the new element formed. Balancing mass number gives $239 + 4 = 1 + A$, where $A = 242$; balancing the atomic number gives $94 + 2 = 0 + Z$, where $Z = 96$. Therefore, element number 96 is curium (eliminate choices A and B), and the appropriate isotope has a mass number of 242.

2. **C** When answering electron configuration questions, the first step is to eliminate all answer choices that do not display the correct number of electrons. In this case, ferrous ion possesses six electrons beyond those represented by [Ar] (eight for elemental iron minus two to generate the +2 cation). Thus, choices A and D can be eliminated. To choose between B and C, recall that when transition metals ionize, it is the outermost and therefore least tightly held electrons that are removed first. In this case, the $4s$ electrons are further from the nucleus and are less tightly held ($n = 4$ represents a greater radial distance from the nucleus than $n = 3$). Thus they are the first to be removed.

3. **D** Since Li has only one valence electron and Be has only two, neither choice A nor B can be correct. To choose between C and D, note that the valence configuration of C is $2s^2 2p^2$. Thus the $2s$ electrons are paired, leaving only two unpaired p electrons. Nitrogen has a valence configuration of $2s^2 2p^3$, and by Hund's rule, the three p electrons will singly occupy the p_x, p_y, and p_z levels, rather than pairing up, to avoid electron repulsion.

4. **C** Diamagnetic atoms are repelled by magnetic fields and paramagnetic atoms are attracted to magnetic fields. Paramagnetic atoms have unpaired electrons in their valence orbitals. Mg and Ca are in the same group and have the same valence configuration, so both cannot be the right answer. Zn is at the end of the d block and has a valence shell with all of its electrons paired. Cr only has five electrons in its $3d$ subshell, resulting in five unpaired electron orbitals. Cr is the only choice that is paramagnetic and would be attracted to a magnetic field.

5. **B** All visible light has a greater wavelength than ultraviolet, eliminating choices A and C. The sodium lamp glows yellow and would therefore emit a yellow band on a dark background. If the question asked where dark bands would have been in an absorption spectrum, several lines would be seen in regions other than yellow, since those colors are absorbed.

6. **D** Electron energy level is determined by the first two quantum numbers. Given $Cl^- = [Kr]$, $Ca^{2+} = [Ar]$, $Cr^+ = [Ar]\, 3d^5$, and $As = [Ar]\, 4s^2 3d^{10} 4p^3$, arsenic contains electrons in the highest energy subshell, $4p$.

7. **D** After their first ionizations, Na^+ and K^+ both have octet electron configurations, so a second ionization to remove another electron would require a very high amount of energy. This eliminates choices A and B. Ionization energy decreases down a group, due to increased nuclear shielding, so it is easier to remove electrons from Ca than Mg, making choice D the answer.

8. **D** All four answer choices have the same number of electrons and the same electron configuration. Ca^{2+} has the most protons pulling on these electrons, so it will be the smallest.

9. **C** Choice A is eliminated because electronegativity increases from left to right on the periodic table. Choice B is eliminated because the stability of positive ions increases as you go up and to the left on the periodic table. Finally, choice D is eliminated since electron affinity is the energy released upon gaining an electron and does not relate to the stability of a positive ion. Choice C is the correct answer because ionization energy, or the energy required to remove an electron, decreases from right to left due to a decrease in effective nuclear charge.

SOLUTIONS TO CHAPTER 4 PRACTICE PASSAGE

1. **C** As shown in Table 1, the trend in ionization energy within group I is decreasing from H (13.6 eV) at the top to Na (5.1 eV) at the bottom and Li in the middle, with an intermediate value of 5.4 eV. Potassium follows in this sequence after Na and Cs is two more rows down. Therefore, no ionization energies for these two elements should be any higher than 5.1 eV, eliminating choices A and B. Choice D shows Cs as having a greater ionization energy than K, which is the reverse of the observed trend, so it can be eliminated.

2. **D** It will require much more energy to remove an electron from Na^+ than from Mg^+, since Na^+ has a noble-gas configuration, while Mg^+ does not.

3. **D** Those species with an ionization energy less than 10 eV/atom can be ionized. According to Table 1, hydrogen has an ionization energy of 13.6 eV, so choices A and B are eliminated, and Fe^+ has an ionization energy of 16 eV, so choice C is eliminated.

4. **C** Table 1 affords the researcher the opportunity to compare data collected to previously measured, known gases. Only with such reference data can the researcher identify an unknown elemental gas. Choices A, B, and D have nothing to do with the identification of an unknown sample by comparing its properties to those of known samples.

5. **C** The greater stability (higher ionization potential) of the diatomic gases as compared to the elemental gases may be explained by the use of the most energetic electrons in the molecular gas to form bonds, thereby stabilizing them in the molecule. If the formation of bonds did not increase the electronic stability of the molecule, they would not form. A bonding arrangement that is higher in energy than its constitutive atoms would simply fly apart, decreasing the energy of the system. This is what choice C postulates. Choice A may be eliminated as it supposes that the electrons in the elemental gases are more stable than in the diatomic forms of the element, which is inconsistent with the data in Table 1. Choice B is irrelevant, as the oxidation state of H and N in their diatomic forms is still 0, and hence the same as in the elemental gases. Choice D may be eliminated as neither H_2 nor N_2 have a dipole moment.

Chapter 5
Bonding and
Intermolecular Forces

The physical properties of a substance are determined at the molecular level, and the chemistry of molecules is dominated by the reactivity of covalent and ionic bonds. An understanding of the fundamentals of bonding can provide the intuitive grasp necessary to answer a wide range of questions in both general and organic chemistry. This chapter will briefly outline some basic principles that, when mastered, will help lay a strong foundation for many chemistry concepts you will encounter on the MCAT.

5.1 LEWIS DOT STRUCTURES

Each dot in the picture below represents one of fluorine's valence electrons. Fluorine is a halogen, with a general valence-shell configuration of ns^2np^5, so there are $2 + 5 = 7$ electrons in its valence shell. We simply place the dots around the symbol for the element, one on each side, and, if there are more than 4 valence electrons, we just start pairing them up. So, for fluorine, we'd have:

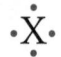

unpaired electron

This is known as a **Lewis dot symbol**. Here are some others:

K·   ·Mg·   ·B·   ·Si·   :P·   :O: :Cl: :Ne:

(*Note*: Electrons in *d* subshells are not considered valence electrons for transition metals since valence electrons are in the highest *n* level.)

Example 5-1: Consider this Lewis dot symbol:

·X·

Among the following, X could represent:

A) carbon.
B) nitrogen.
C) sulfur.
D) argon.

Solution: Since there are four dots in the Lewis symbol, X will be an element in Group 4 of the periodic table. Of the choices given, only carbon (choice A) is in Group 4.

Lewis dot structures are one type of model we use to represent what compounds look like at the molecular level. Since it's the valence electrons that are responsible for creating bonds in molecules, a Lewis dot structure that accounts for the number and location of all valence electrons gives us a sense of how molecules are held together and helps us understand their reactivity.

To create a Lewis dot structure for a molecule, we begin to pair up electrons from two separate atoms since two electrons are required to form a single bond. By sharing a pair of electrons to form a bond, each atom may acquire an octet configuration, thereby stabilizing both atoms. (Atoms with unpaired valence electrons are called **free radicals**, and are very reactive.) For example, each of the fluorine atoms below can donate its unpaired valence electron to form a bond and give the molecule F_2. The shared electrons are attracted by the nuclei of *both* atoms in the bond, which hold the atoms together.

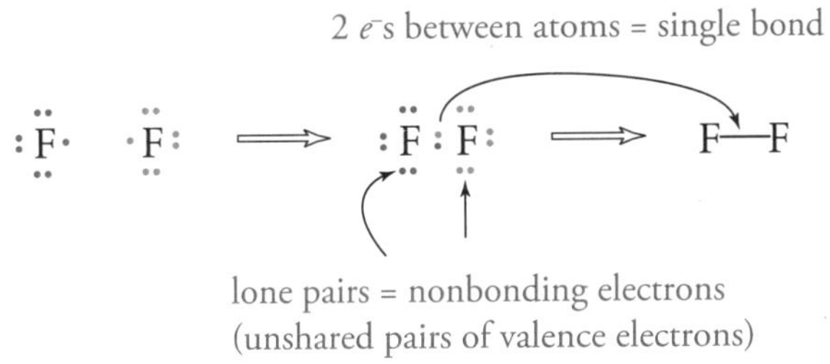

Note that in addition to the **single bond** (a bond formed from two electrons) between the fluorine atoms, each fluorine atom has three pairs of electrons that are not part of a bond. They help satisfy the octets of the F atoms and are known as "lone pairs" of electrons. We'll see in a bit how these lone pairs are important for determining physical properties of compounds, so don't forget to write these out too.

We can also use Lewis dot structures to show atoms that form multiple bonds—**double bonds** use four electrons while **triple bonds** require six. Here are a couple of examples:

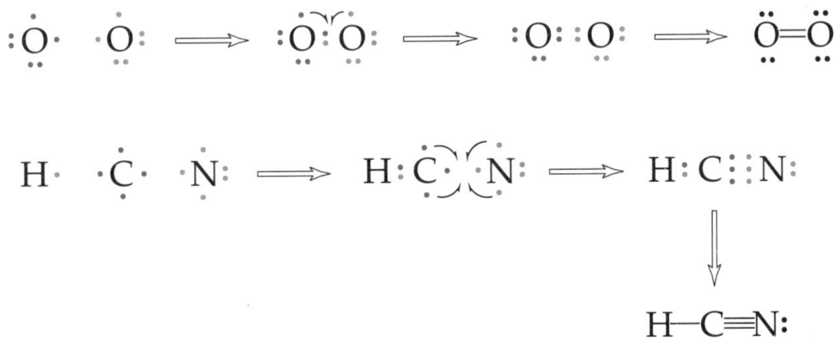

Formal Charge

The last Lewis dot structure shown above for the molecule consisting of 1 atom each of hydrogen, carbon, and nitrogen was drawn with C as the central atom. However, it could have been drawn with N as the central atom, and we could have still achieved closed-shell configurations for all the atoms:

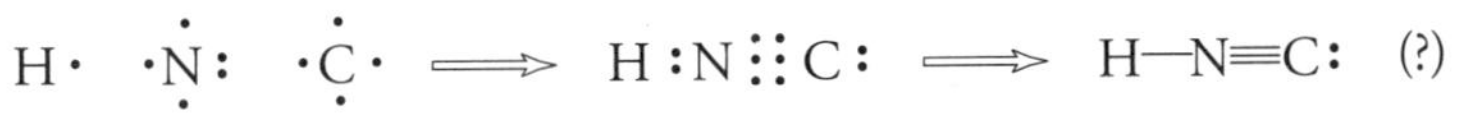

The problem is this doesn't give the correct structure for this molecule. The nitrogen atom is not actually bonded to the hydrogen. A helpful way to evaluate a proposed Lewis structure is to calculate the **formal charge** of each atom in the structure. These formal charges won't give the actual charges on the atoms; they'll simply tell us if the atoms are sharing their valence electrons in the "best" way possible, which will happen when the formal charges are all zero (or at least as small as possible). The formula for calculating the formal charge of an atom in a covalent compound is:

$$\text{Formal charge (FC)}= V - \frac{1}{2}B - L$$

where V is the number of valence electrons, B is the number of bonding electrons, and L is the number of lone-paired (non-bonding) electrons. We'll show the calculations of the formal charges for each atom in both Lewis structures:

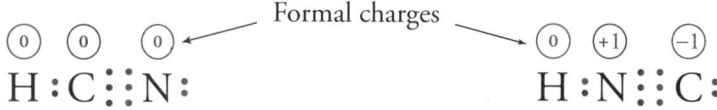

Formal charge on H = $1 - \frac{1}{2}(2) - 0 = 0$ Formal charge on H = $1 - \frac{1}{2}(2) - 0 = 0$

Formal charge on C = $4 - \frac{1}{2}(8) - 0 = 0$ Formal charge on N = $5 - \frac{1}{2}(8) - 0 = +1$

Formal charge on N = $5 - \frac{1}{2}(6) - 2 = 0$ Formal charge on C = $4 - \frac{1}{2}(6) - 2 = -1$

The best Lewis structures have an octet of electrons and a formal charge of zero on all the atoms. (Sometimes, this simply isn't possible, and then the best structure is the one that *minimizes* the magnitudes of the formal charges.) The fact that the HCN structure has formal charges of zero for all the atoms, but the HNC structure does not, tells us right away that the HCN structure is the better one. For dot structures that must contain formal charges on one or more atoms, the best structures have negative formal charges on the more electronegative element.

Example 5-2: What's the formal charge on each atom in phosgene, $COCl_2$?

Solution:

FC = $6 - \frac{1}{2}(4) - 4 = 0$

:O:
‖
:Cl — C — Cl:

FC = $4 - \frac{1}{2}(8) - 0 = 0$

each Cl:
FC = $7 - \frac{1}{2}(2) - 6 = 0$

Example 5-3: Which of the following is the best Lewis structure for CH_2O?

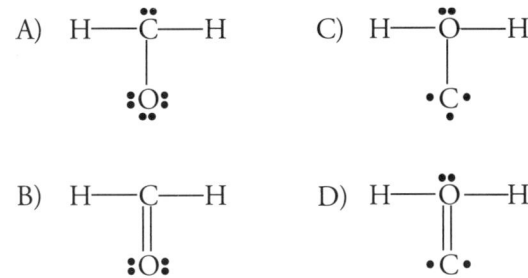

Solution: When faced with a question like this on the MCAT (and they're rather common), the first thing you should do is simply count the electrons. The correct structure for the molecule CH_2O must account for $4 + 2(1) + 6 = 12$ valence electrons. The structure in choice A has 14 and the structure in choice C has 11. Answer choices B and D both have 12 valence electrons. However, in choice D, oxygen is surrounded by 10 total electrons. This is not possible because oxygen, like all elements in the second row of the periodic table, cannot violate the octet rule and exceed 8 valence electrons. Choice B, then, with 12 valence electrons and the least electronegative atom as the central atom, is the best choice.

Resonance

Recall that Lewis dot structures are a model that we use to help us understand where the valence electrons are in a molecule. All models, being simplifications of reality, have limitations, and Lewis dot structures are no exception. Sometimes it is impossible for one structure to accurately represent the reality of a molecule's electron distribution. To account for this complexity, we need two or more structures, called **resonance structures**, to accurately depict the bonding in a molecule. These structures are often needed when there are double or triple bonds in molecules along with one or more lone pairs of electrons.

Let's draw the Lewis structure for sulfur dioxide.

$$:\ddot{O}-\ddot{S}=\ddot{O}$$

formal charges -----> (-1) $(+1)$ (0)

We could also draw the structure like this:

$$\ddot{O}=\ddot{S}-\ddot{O}:$$

(0) $(+1)$ (-1) <----- formal charges

In either case, there's one S—O single bond and one S=O double bond. This would imply that the double-bonded O would be closer to the S atom than the single-bonded O (see Section 5.2, Bond Length and Bond Dissociation Energy). Experiment, however, reveals that the bond lengths are the same. Therefore, to describe this molecule, we say that it's an "average" (or, technically, a **resonance hybrid**) of the equivalent Lewis structures shown:

$$\left[:\ddot{O}-\ddot{S}=\ddot{O} \longleftrightarrow \ddot{O}=\ddot{S}-\ddot{O}: \right]$$

We can also symbolize the resonance hybrid with a single picture, like this:

$$O \text{----} \ddot{S} \text{----} O$$

The dotted lines in the structure above indicate some double bond character for both S—O bonds, more of a "bond and a half." A molecule may be a resonance hybrid of more than two equivalent Lewis structures; for example, consider the carbonate ion, $CO_3{}^{2-}$:

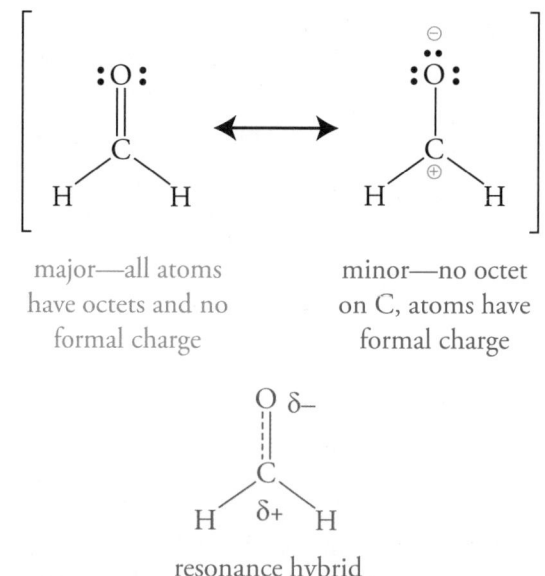

or, more simply,

In addition, a molecule may have two or more non-equivalent resonance structures, and the resonance hybrid is then a weighted average of them, as shown with formaldehyde below:

major—all atoms
have octets and no
formal charge

minor—no octet
on C, atoms have
formal charge

resonance hybrid

Example 5-4: Resonance structures are two or more structures where:

A) only atoms may move around.
B) only bonding electrons may move around.
C) only nonbonding electrons may move around.
D) only nonbonding electrons, double bonds, and triple bonds may move around.

Solution: Choice D is the correct answer. (This definition is particularly important in organic chemistry.)

5.2 BOND LENGTH AND BOND DISSOCIATION ENERGY

While the term *bond length* makes good intuitive sense (the distance between two nuclei that are bonded to one another), **bond dissociation energy (BDE)** is not quite as intuitive. Bond dissociation energy is the energy required to break a bond *homolytically*. In **homolytic bond cleavage**, one electron of the bond being broken goes to each fragment of the molecule. In this process two radicals form. This is *not* the same thing as **heterolytic bond cleavage** (also known as *dissociation*). In heterolytic bond cleavage, both electrons of the electron pair that make up the bond end up on the same atom; this forms both a cation and an anion.

These two processes are very different and hence have very different energies associated with them. Here, we will only consider homolytic bond dissociation energies.

When one examines the relationship between bond length and bond dissociation energy for a series of similar bonds, an important trend emerges: For similar bonds, *the higher the bond order, the shorter and stronger the bond.* Bond order is defined as the number of bonds between adjacent atoms, so a single bond has a bond order of 1 while a triple bond has a bond order of 3. The following table, which lists the bond dissociation energies (BDE, in kcal/mol) and the bond lengths (r, in angstroms, where $1 \text{ Å} = 10^{-10}$ m) for carbon-carbon and carbon-oxygen bonds, illustrates this trend:

	C—C	C=C	C≡C	C—O	C=O	C≡O
BDE (in kcal/mol)	83	144	200	86	191	256
r (in Å)	1.54	1.34	1.20	1.43	1.20	1.13

An important caveat arises because of the varying atomic radii: *bond length/BDE comparisons should only be made for similar bonds.* Thus, carbon-carbon bonds should be compared only to other carbon-carbon bonds; carbon-oxygen bonds should be compared only to other carbon-oxygen bonds, and so on.

Recall the shapes of atomic orbitals: *s* orbitals are spherical about the atomic nucleus, while *p* orbitals are elongated "dumbbell"-shaped about the atomic nucleus.

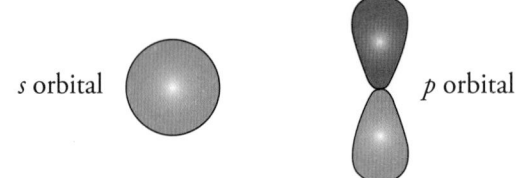

s orbital   *p* orbital

When comparing the same types of bonds, the greater the *s* character in the hybrid orbitals, the shorter the bond (because *s*-orbitals are closer to the nucleus than *p*-orbitals). A greater percentage of *p* character in the hybrid orbital also leads to a more directional hybrid orbital that is farther from the nucleus and thus a longer bond (see section 5.5 for all the details on hybridization). In addition, when comparing the same types of bonds, *the longer the bond, the weaker it is; the shorter the bond, the stronger it is.* In the following diagram, compare all the C—C bonds and all the C—H bonds:

Bond	Bond length	Bond	Bond length
C—C (*sp–sp*)	1.21 Å	C–H (*sp–s*)	1.06 Å
C—C (*sp–sp³*)	1.46 Å	C–H (*sp³–s*)	1.10 Å

5.3 TYPES OF BONDS

Covalent Bonds

A **covalent bond** is formed between atoms when each contributes one or more of its unpaired valence electrons. The electrons are *shared* by both atoms to help complete both octets. There are minor variations in how the electrons are shared, however, so there are several classes of covalent bonds.

Polarity of Covalent Bonds

Recall that electronegativity refers to an atom's ability to attract another atom's valence electrons when it forms a bond. Electronegativity, in other words, is a measure of how much an atom will "hog" the electrons that it's sharing with another atom.

Consider the Lewis dot structures of hydrogen fluoride and fluorine:

$$H\!\!-\!\!\ddot{\underset{\cdot\cdot}{F}}\!: \quad \text{vs.} \quad :\!\ddot{\underset{\cdot\cdot}{F}}\!\!-\!\!\ddot{\underset{\cdot\cdot}{F}}\!:$$

Fluorine is more electronegative than hydrogen (remember the order of electronegativity?), so the electron density will be greater near the fluorine than near the hydrogen in HF. That means that the H—F molecule is partially negative (denoted by δ^-) on the fluorine side and partially positive (denoted by δ^+) on the hydrogen side. We refer to this as **polarity** and say that the molecule has a **dipole moment**. A bond is **polar** if the electron density between the two nuclei is uneven. This occurs if there is a difference in electronegativity of the bonding atoms, and the greater the difference, the more uneven the electron density and the greater the dipole moment.

A bond is **nonpolar** if the electron density between the two nuclei is even. This occurs when there is little to no difference in electronegativity between the bonded atoms, generally when two atoms of the same element are bonded to each other, as we see in F_2.

electron density

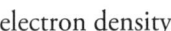

$\delta^+ \quad\quad \delta^-$
$H\!\!-\!\!\ddot{\underset{\cdot\cdot}{F}}\!: \quad\quad H\!\!-\!\!\ddot{\underset{\cdot\cdot}{F}}\!:$ POLAR

electron density

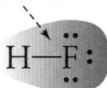

$:\!\ddot{\underset{\cdot\cdot}{F}}\!\!-\!\!\ddot{\underset{\cdot\cdot}{F}}\!: \quad\quad :\!\ddot{\underset{\cdot\cdot}{F}}\!\!-\!\!\ddot{\underset{\cdot\cdot}{F}}\!:$ NONPOLAR

Coordinate Covalent Bonds

Sometimes, one atom will donate *both* of the shared electrons in a bond. That is called a **coordinate covalent bond**. For example, the nitrogen atom in NH_3 donates both electrons in its lone pair to form a bond to the boron atom in the molecule BF_3 to give the coordinate covalent compound F_3BNH_3:

coordinate covalent bond

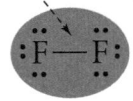

Since the NH_3 molecule donates a pair of electrons, it is known as a **Lewis base.** A Lewis base can act as a ligand, or a nucleophile (nucleus-loving), and so all three terms are synonymous. Since the BF_3 molecule accepts a pair of electrons, it's known as a **Lewis acid** or **electrophile** (electron loving). When a coordinate covalent bond breaks, the electrons that come from the ligand will leave *with* that ligand.

Example 5-5: Identify the Lewis acid and the Lewis base in the following reaction, which forms a **coordination complex**:

$$4\ NH_3 + Zn^{2+} \rightarrow Zn(NH_3)_4{}^{2+}$$

Solution: Each of the NH_3 molecules donates its lone pair to the zinc atom, thus forming four coordinate covalent bonds. Since the zinc ion accepts these electron pairs, it's the Lewis acid; since each ammonia molecule donates an electron pair, they are Lewis bases (or ligands):

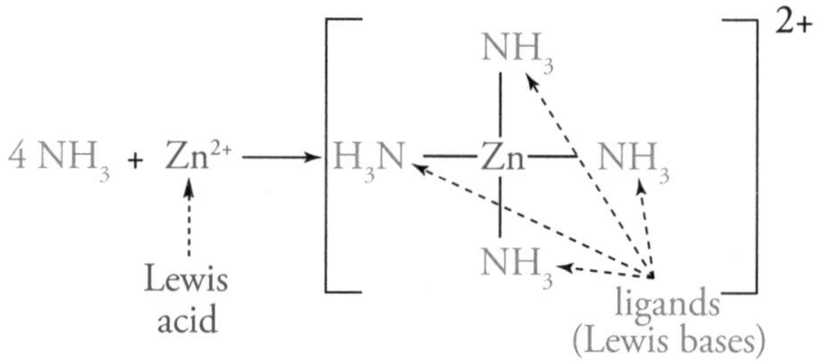

Example 5-6: Which one of the following anions *cannot* behave as a Lewis base/ligand?

A) F^-
B) OH^-
C) $NO_3{}^-$
D) $BH_4{}^-$

Solution: A Lewis base/ligand is a molecule or ion that donates a pair of nonbonding electrons. So, in order to even be a candidate Lewis base/ligand, a molecule must have a pair of nonbonding electrons in the first place. The ion in choice D does not have any nonbonding electrons.

Example 5-7: Carbon atoms with nonbonding electrons are excellent Lewis bases/ligands. Therefore, which of the following molecules is *not* a potential Lewis base/ligand?

A) CO_2
B) CO
C) CN^-
D) $CH_3{}^-$

Solution: The Lewis structures for the given molecules/ions are as follows:

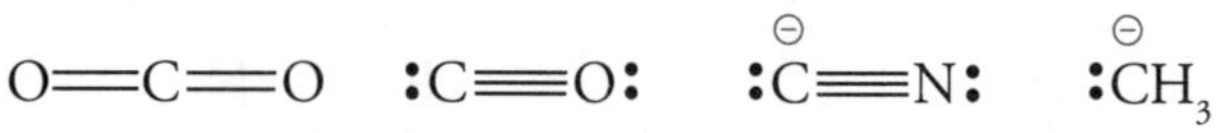

Therefore, choice A (carbon dioxide) is not a good ligand and is the correct answer here.

Ionic Bonds

While sharing valence electrons is one way atoms can achieve the stable octet configuration, the octet may also be obtained by gaining or losing electrons. For example, a sodium atom will give its valence electron to an atom of chlorine. This results in a sodium cation (Na^+) and a chloride anion (Cl^-), which form sodium chloride. They're held together by the electrostatic attraction between a cation and anion; this is an **ionic bond**.

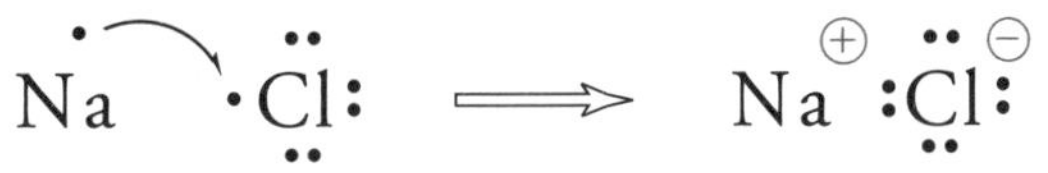

For an ionic bond to form between a metal and a non-metal, there has to be a big difference in electronegativity between the two elements. Generally speaking, the strength of the bond is proportional to the charges on the ions, and it decreases as the ions get farther apart, or as the ionic radii increase. We can use this to estimate the relative strength of ionic systems. For example, consider MgS and NaCl. For MgS, the magnesium ion has a +2 charge and the sulfide ion has a –2 charge, while for NaCl, the charges are +1 for sodium and –1 for chloride. Therefore, the MgS "bond" is expected to be about four times stronger than the NaCl "bond," assuming the sizes of the ions are very nearly the same.

Example 5-8: Which of the following is most likely an ionic compound?

A) NO
B) HI
C) ClF
D) KBr

Solution: A diatomic compound is ionic if the electronegativities of the atoms are very different. Of the atoms listed in the choices, those in choice D have the greatest electronegativity difference (K is an alkali metal, and Br is a halogen); K will give up its lone valence electron to Br, forming an ionic bond.

5.4 VSEPR THEORY

The shapes of simple molecules are predicted by **valence shell electron-pair repulsion (VSEPR) theory**. There's one rule: Since electrons repel one another, electron pairs, whether bonding or nonbonding, attempt to move as far apart as possible.

For example, the bonding electrons in beryllium hydride, BeH_2, repel one another and attempt to move as far apart as possible. In this molecule, two pairs of electrons point in opposite directions:

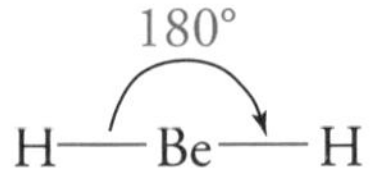

The angle between the bonds is 180°. A molecule with this shape is said to be linear.

5.4

As the BeH_2 example shows, the total number of electron groups on the central atom of a molecule determines its bond angles and *orbital geometry*. Electron groups are defined as any type of bond (single, double, triple) and lone pairs of electrons. Double and triple bonds each count only as one electron group, even though they involve two and three pairs of electrons, respectively. To illustrate, the number of electron groups and orbital geometries of the central atom are shown for some example molecules:

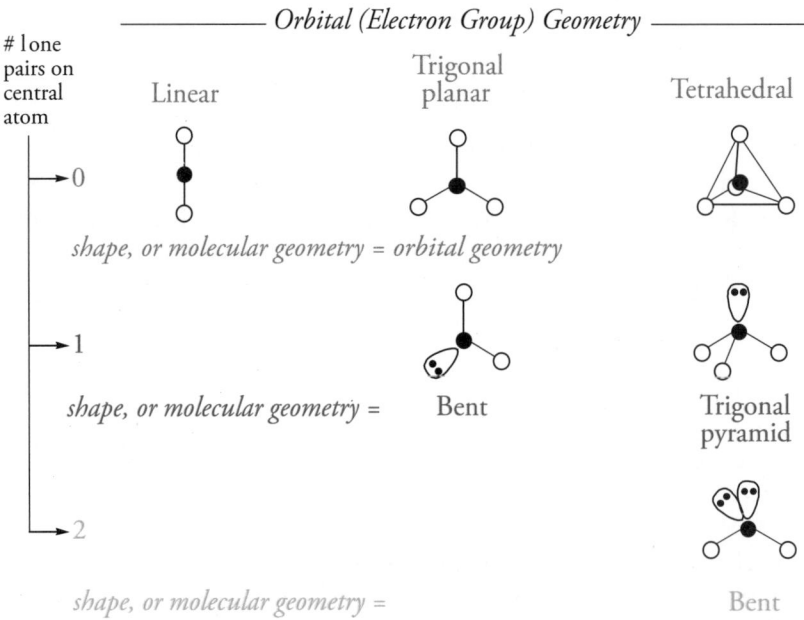

The shape of a molecule (also referred to as the **molecular geometry**) is also a function of the location of the nuclei of its constituent atoms. Therefore, when lone electron pairs are present on the central atom of a molecule, as in NH_3 above, the shape is not the same as the orbital geometry. The table below shows how the presence of lone pairs determines the shape of a molecule:

Example 5-9: Determine the orbital geometry and predict the shape of each of the following molecules or ions:

a) H_2O

b) SO_2

c) NH_4^+

d) PCl_3

e) CO_3^{2-}

Solution:

a)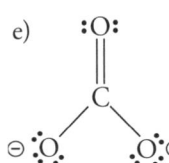

orbital geometry: *tetrahedral*
shape: *bent*

b)

orbital geometry: *trigonal planar*
shape: *bent*

c)

orbital geometry: *tetrahedral*
shape: *tetrahedral*

d)

orbital geometry: *tetrahedral*
shape: *trigonal pyramid*

e)

orbital geometry: *trigonal planar*
shape: *trigonal planar*

5.5 HYBRIDIZATION

In order to rationalize observed chemical and structural trends, chemists developed the concept of orbital hybridization. In this model, one imagines a mathematical combination of atomic orbitals centered on the same atom to produce a set of composite, **hybrid** orbitals. For example, consider an *s* and a *p* orbital on an atom.

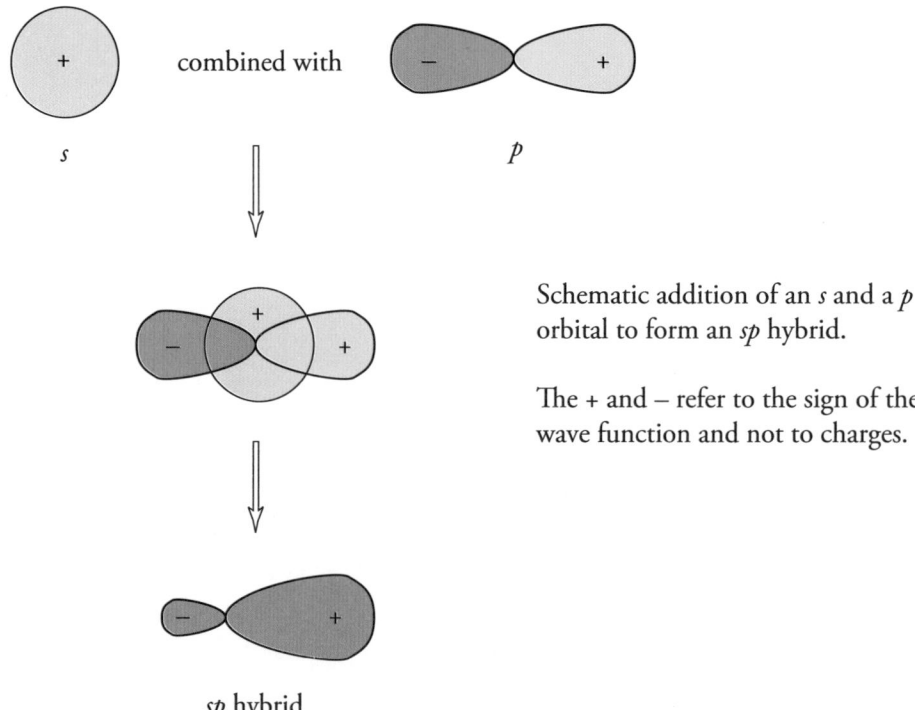

Schematic addition of an *s* and a *p* orbital to form an *sp* hybrid.

The + and – refer to the sign of the wave function and not to charges.

Notice that the new orbital is highly directional; this allows for better overlap when bonding.

There will be two such *sp* hybrid orbitals formed because two orbitals (the *s* and the *p*) were originally combined; that is, the total number of orbitals is conserved in the formation of hybrid orbitals. For this reason, the number of hybrid orbitals on a given atom of hybridization sp^x is $1 + x$ (1 for the *s*, *x* for the *p*'s), where *x* may be either 1, 2, or 3.

The percentages of the *s* character and *p* character in a given sp^x hybrid orbital are listed below:

sp^x hybrid orbital	*s* character	*p* character
sp	50%	50%
sp^2	33%	67%
sp^3	25%	75%

To determine the hybridization for most atoms in simple molecules, add the number of attached atoms to the number of non-bonding electron pairs (localized) and use the brief table on the next page (which also gives the ideal bond angles and orbital geometry). The number of attached atoms plus the number of lone pairs is equal to the number of orbitals combined to make the new hybridized orbitals.

Electron Groups [# atoms + # lone pairs]	Hybridization	Bond Angles (ideal)	Orbital Geometry
2	sp	180°	linear
3	sp^2	120°	trigonal planar
4	sp^3	109.5°	tetrahedral

5.5

sp hybridization:

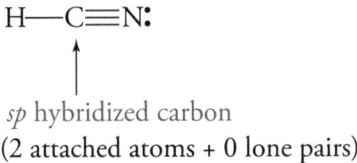

sp hybridized carbon
(2 attached atoms + 0 lone pairs)

sp² hybridization:

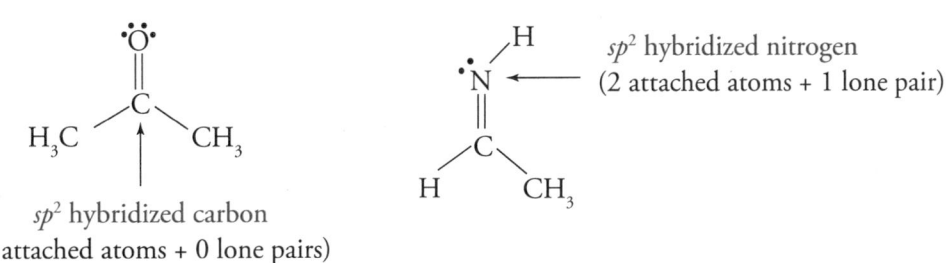

sp^2 hybridized carbon
(3 attached atoms + 0 lone pairs)

sp^2 hybridized nitrogen
(2 attached atoms + 1 lone pair)

sp³ hybridization:

sp^3 hybridized carbon
(4 attached atoms + 0 lone pairs)

sp^3 hybridized nitrogen
(3 attached atoms + 1 lone pair)

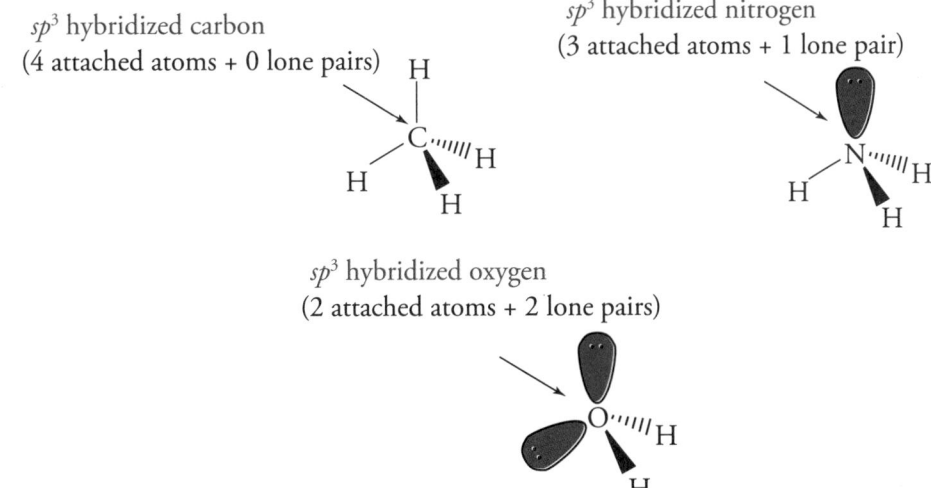

sp^3 hybridized oxygen
(2 attached atoms + 2 lone pairs)

Example 5-10: Determine the hybridization of the central atom in each of the following molecules or ions from the previous example:

a) H_2O
b) SO_2
c) NH_4^+
d) PCl_3
e) CO_3^{2-}

Solution:

a) Hybridization of O is sp^3.
b) Hybridization of S is sp^2.
c) Hybridization of N is sp^3.
d) Hybridization of P is sp^3.
e) Hybridization of C is sp^2.

Sigma (σ) Bonds

A **σ bond** consists of two electrons that are localized between two nuclei. It is formed by the end-to-end overlap of one hybridized orbital (or an *s* orbital in the case of hydrogen) from each of the two atoms participating in the bond. Below, we show the σ bonds in ethane, C_2H_6:

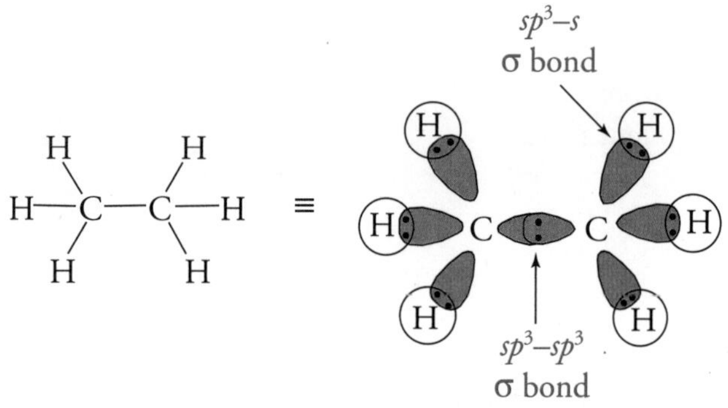

Remember that an sp^3 carbon atom has four sp^3 hybrid orbitals, which are derived from one *s* orbital and three *p* orbitals.

Example 5-11: Label the hybridization of the orbitals comprising the σ bonds in the molecules shown below:

a)

b)

c)

d)

Solution:

a) Bonds to H are sp^3—s σ bonds. The C—O bond is an sp^3—sp^3 σ bond.
b) The bonds to H are sp^2—s σ bonds. The C=O bond contains an sp^2—sp^2 σ bond. (It's also composed of a π bond, which we'll discuss in the next section.)
c) All C—C bonds are sp^3—sp^3 σ bonds, while all C—H bonds are sp^3—s σ bonds.
d) All bonds to H are sp^3—s σ bonds. The C—N bond is an sp^3—sp^3 σ bond.

Pi (π) Bonds

A **π bond** is composed of two electrons that are localized to the region that lies on opposite sides of the plane formed by the two bonded nuclei and immediately adjacent atoms, not directly between the two nuclei as with a σ bond. A π bond is formed by the proper, parallel, side-to-side alignment of two unhybridized p orbitals on adjacent atoms. (An sp^2 hybridized atom has three sp^2 orbitals—which come from one s and two p orbitals—plus one p orbital that remains unhybridized.) Below, we show the π bonds in ethene, C_2H_4:

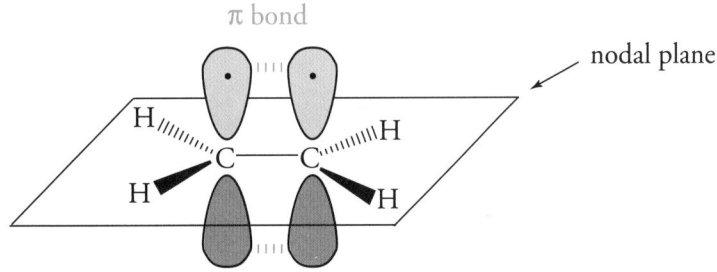

In any multiple bond, *there is only one σ bond; the remainder are π bonds.* Therefore:

a single bond: composed of 1 σ bond
a double bond: composed of 1 σ bond and 1 π bond
a triple bond: composed of 1 σ bond and 2 π bonds

Example 5-12: Count the number of σ bonds and π bonds in each of the following molecules. (Don't forget to count all of the C–H σ bonds!)

a)

b)

c)

d) H—C≡N

e)

f)

Solution:

a)   14 σ, 1 π
b)   9 σ, 1 π
c)   12 σ, 2 π
d)   2 σ, 2 π
e)   27 σ, 4 π
f)   24 σ, 7 π

5.6 MOLECULAR POLARITY

A molecule as a whole may also be polar or nonpolar. If a molecule contains no polar bonds, it cannot be polar. In addition, if a molecule contains two or more symmetrically oriented polar bonds, the bond dipoles effectively cancel each other out, evenly distributing the electron density over the entire molecule. However, if the polar bonds in a molecule are not symmetrically oriented around the central atom (generally, though not always, due to the presence of a lone pair of electrons on the central atom), the individual bond dipoles will not cancel. Therefore, there will be an uneven distribution of electron density over the entire molecule, and this results in a polar molecule.

Example 5-13: For each of the molecules N_2, OCS, and CCl_4, describe the polarity of each bond and of the molecule as a whole.

5.6

Solution:

- The $N\equiv N$ bond is nonpolar (since it's a bond between two identical atoms), and since this *is* the molecule, it's nonpolar, too; no dipole moment.
- For the molecule O=C=S, each bond is polar, since it connects two different atoms of unequal electronegativities. Furthermore, the O=C bond is more polar than the C=S bond, because the difference between the electronegativities of O and C is greater than the difference between the electronegativities of C and S. Therefore, the molecule as a whole is polar (that is, it has a dipole moment):

polar bonds   polar molecule

- For the molecule CCl_4, each bond is polar, since it connects two different atoms of unequal electronegativities. However, the bonds are symmetrically arranged around the central C atom, leaving the molecule as a whole nonpolar, with no dipole moment:

polar bonds   non-polar molecule

5.7 INTERMOLECULAR FORCES

Liquids and solids are held together by intermolecular forces, such as dipole-dipole forces and London dispersion forces. **Intermolecular forces** are the relatively weak interactions that take place between neutral molecules.

Polar molecules are attracted to ions, producing **ion-dipole** forces. **Dipole-dipole forces** are the attractions between the positive end of one polar molecule and the negative end of another polar molecule. (Hydrogen bonding [which we will look at more closely below] is the strongest dipole-dipole force.) A permanent dipole in one molecule may induce a dipole in a neighboring nonpolar molecule, producing a momentary **dipole-induced dipole force**.

Finally, an instantaneous dipole in a nonpolar molecule may induce a dipole in a neighboring nonpolar molecule. The resulting attractions are known as **London dispersion forces**, which are very weak and transient interactions between the instantaneous dipoles in nonpolar molecules. They are the weakest of all intermolecular interactions, and they're the "default" force; all an atom or molecule needs to experience them is electrons. In addition, as the size (molecular weight) of the molecule increases, so does its number of electrons, which increases its polarizability. As a result, the partial charges of the induced dipoles get larger, so the strength of the dispersion forces increases.

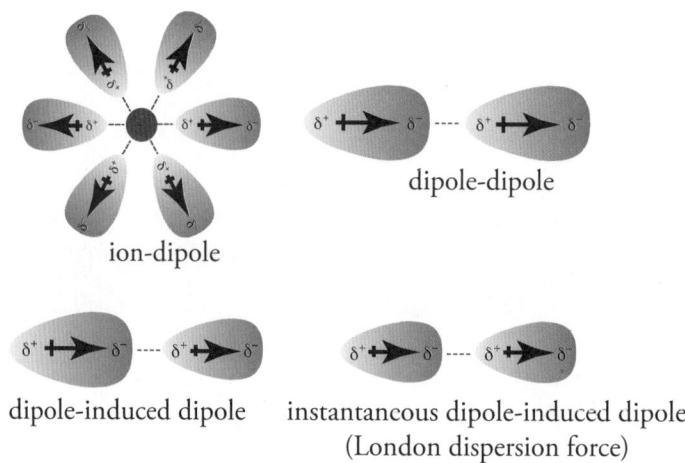

ion-dipole

dipole-dipole

dipole-induced dipole

instantaneous dipole-induced dipole
(London dispersion force)

Despite being weak, all intermolecular forces, including London dispersion forces, can have a profound impact on the physical properties of a particular molecule. Specifically, substances with stronger intermolecular forces will exhibit greater melting points, greater boiling points, greater viscosities, and lower vapor pressures (more on this below) than similar compounds with weaker intermolecular forces. For example, many substances that experience only dispersion forces, like fluorine (F_2) and chlorine (Cl_2), exist as gases under standard conditions (1 atm and 25°C). However, bromine (Br_2) is a liquid and iodine (I_2) is a solid because the strength of the dispersion forces increase as atomic size increases.

A final note: Dipole forces, hydrogen bonding, and London forces are *all* collectively known as **van der Waals forces**. However, you may sometimes see the term "van der Waals forces" used to mean only London dispersion forces.

Hydrogen Bonding

Hydrogen bonding is the strongest type of intermolecular force between neutral molecules. In order for a hydrogen bond to form, two very specific criteria must be fulfilled: 1) a molecule must have a covalent bond between H and either N, O, or F, and 2) another molecule must have a lone pair of electrons on an N, O, or F atom. A very common example of a substance that experiences hydrogen bonding is water:

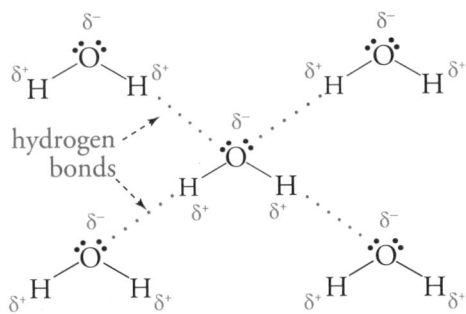

One of the consequences of hydrogen bonding is the high boiling points of compounds such as NH_3, H_2O, and HF. The boiling points of these hydrogen-containing compounds are higher than those of the hydrogen-containing compounds of other elements from Groups V, VI, and VII (the groups where N, O, and F reside). For example, the boiling point of H_2S is approximately $-50°C$, while that of H_2O is (of course) $100°C$.

Example 5-14: Identify the mixture of compounds that *cannot* experience hydrogen bonding with each other:

A) NH_3/H_2O
B) H_2O/HF
C) HF/CO_2
D) H_2S/HCl

Solution: Hydrogen bonding occurs when an H covalently bonded to an F, O, or N electrostatically interacts with another F, O, or N (which doesn't need to have an H). Therefore, choices A, B, and C can all experience hydrogen bonding. Choice D, however, cannot, and this is the answer.

Vapor Pressure

One of the physical properties determined by the strength of the intermolecular forces of a substance is its vapor pressure. **Vapor pressure** is the pressure exerted by the gaseous phase of a liquid that evaporated from the exposed surface of the liquid. The weaker a substance's intermolecular forces, the higher its vapor pressure and the more easily it evaporates. For example, if we compare diethyl ether ($H_5C_2OC_2H_5$) and water, we notice that while water undergoes hydrogen bonding, diethyl ether does not, so despite its greater molecular mass, diethyl ether will vaporize more easily and have a higher vapor pressure than water. Easily vaporized liquids—liquids with *high* vapor pressures—like diethyl ether are said to be **volatile**.

5.7

While a substance's vapor pressure is determined in part by its intermolecular forces, vapor pressure is also temperature dependent and increases with the temperature of the substance. Increasing the average kinetic energy of the particles (which is proportional to temperature), allows them to overcome the intermolecular forces holding them together and increases the proportion of particles that can move into the gas phase. As a result, the vapor pressure of a substance is indirectly related to its boiling point, a topic we'll discuss in more detail in Chapter 7.

Example 5-15: An understanding of intermolecular forces is of critical importance because they govern so many physical properties of a substance. The property *least* likely to be influenced by intermolecular force strength is:

A) color.
B) melting point.
C) solubility.
D) vapor pressure.

Solution: Any physical property that involves separating molecules from one another will very much depend upon the strength of intermolecular forces. Molecules are spread out during melting (choice B), dissolving (choice C), and evaporation (choice D). Choice A is therefore the best choice here.

5.8   TYPES OF SOLIDS

Ionic Solids

An **ionic solid** is held together by the electrostatic attraction between cations and anions in a lattice structure. The bonds that hold all the ions together in the crystal lattice are the same as the bonds that hold each pair of ions together. Ionic bonds are strong, and most ionic substances (like NaCl and other salts) are solid at room temperature. As discussed previously, the strength of the bonds is primarily dependent on the magnitudes of the ion charges, and to a lesser extent, the size of the ions. The greater the charge, the stronger the force of attraction between the ions. The smaller the ions, the more they are attracted to each other.

Network Solids

In a **network solid**, atoms are connected in a **lattice** of covalent bonds, meaning that all interactions between atoms are covalent bonds. As in an ionic solid, in a network solid the *inter*molecular forces are identical to the *intra*molecular forces. You can think of a network solid as one big molecule; in a network solid there are only intramolecular forces. As a result, network solids are very strong, and tend to be very hard solids at room temperature. Diamond (one of the allotropes of carbon) and quartz (a form of silica, SiO_2) are examples of network solids.

Metallic Solids

A sample of metal can be thought of as a covalently bound lattice of nuclei and their inner shell electrons, surrounded by a "sea" or "cloud" of electrons. At least one valence electron per atom is not bound to any one particular atom and is free to move throughout the lattice. These freely roaming valence electrons are called **conduction electrons**. As a result, metals are excellent conductors of electricity and heat, and are malleable and ductile. Metallic bonds vary widely in strength, but almost all metals are solids at room temperature.

Molecular Solids

The particles at the lattice points of a crystal of a molecular solid are molecules. These molecules are held together by one of three types of *inter*molecular interactions—hydrogen bonds, dipole-dipole forces, or London dispersion forces. Since these forces are *significantly* weaker than ionic, network, or metallic bonds, molecular compounds typically have much lower melting and boiling points than the other types of solids above. Molecular solids are often liquids or gases at room temperature, and are more likely to be solids as the strength of their intermolecular forces increase.

Example 5-16: Of the following, which one will have the lowest melting point?

A) MgO
B) CH_4
C) Cr
D) HF

Solution: Almost all ionic compounds are solids at room temperature. Therefore, choice A is eliminated. Similarly, all metals except for mercury (Hg) are solids at room temperature, so eliminate choice C. Both answers B and D will be molecular solids. Hydrogen fluoride is able to hydrogen bond and will therefore have stronger intermolecular interactions than the nonpolar methane. Since choice B has the weakest intermolecular forces (London dispersion), it will be easiest to melt.

5.8

Chapter 5 Summary

- The best Lewis dot or resonance structures have 1) octets around all atoms, 2) minimized formal charge, and 3) negative charges on more electronegative elements.

- Covalent bonds form between elements with similar electronegativities (two non-metals).

- Nonpolar bonding means equal electron sharing; polar bonding means unequal electron sharing, and electron density is higher around the more electronegative element.

- Coordinate covalent bonds form between a Lewis base (e^- pair donor) and a Lewis acid (e^- pair acceptor); electrons are shared.

- Ionic bonds form between elements with large differences in electronegativity (metals + nonmetals), and the strength of that bond depends on the charge and the size of the ions. Larger charges and smaller ions make the strongest ionic bonds.

- VSEPR theory predicts the shapes of molecules; angles between electron groups around the central atom are maximized for greatest stability.

- The hybridization of an atom is dependent on the number of electron groups on the atom (two e^- groups = sp, three e^- groups = sp^2, four e^- groups = sp^3).

- Sigma (σ) bonds generally form through the end-on-end overlap of hybrid orbitals; pi (π) bonds form through the side-to-side overlap of unhybridized p orbitals.

- If bond dipoles are symmetrically oriented in a molecule, the molecule as a whole is nonpolar; if the dipoles are asymmetrical, the molecule will be polar.

- Intermolecular forces are cohesive, and determine the physical properties (melting and boiling points, solubility, vapor pressure, etc.) of a compound based on relative strengths.

- While all molecules have London dispersion forces, they are the predominant intermolecular force that holds nonpolar molecules together. Dipole-dipole forces are the predominant intermolecular force that holds polar molecules together.

- Molecules with an H—F, H—O, or H—N bond and an N, O, or F with a lone electron pair can hydrogen bond.

CHAPTER 5 FREESTANDING PRACTICE QUESTIONS

1. Which of these molecules has the strongest dipole moment?

A) PBr_3O
B) PF_5
C) CCl_4
D) SF_6

2. A pure sample of which of the following ions/molecules will participate in intermolecular hydrogen bonding?

   I. CH_3CO_2H
   II. CO_2
   III. H_2S

A) I only
B) III only
C) I and II
D) I and III

3. Which of the following best describes the intramolecular bonding present within a cyanide ion (CN^-)?

A) Ionic bonding
B) Covalent bonding
C) Van der Waals forces
D) Induced dipole

4. All of the following would be categorized as having tetrahedral orbital geometry EXCEPT:

A) NH_3
B) NH_4^+
C) CO_2
D) CH_4

5. Rank the following from highest to lowest boiling point:

   I. H_2SO_4
   II. NH_3
   III. CO_2
   IV. H_2O

A) I > IV > II > III
B) II > I > IV > III
C) I > III > IV > II
D) IV > III > I > II

6. Liquid helium is used to cool magnets in MRI scanners. Which of the following forces is most specifically responsible for maintaining helium in this state?

A) Hydrogen bonding
B) Strong nuclear forces
C) Metallic bonding
D) London dispersion forces

7. In the following reaction, which of the following most accurately describes the type of bond formed?

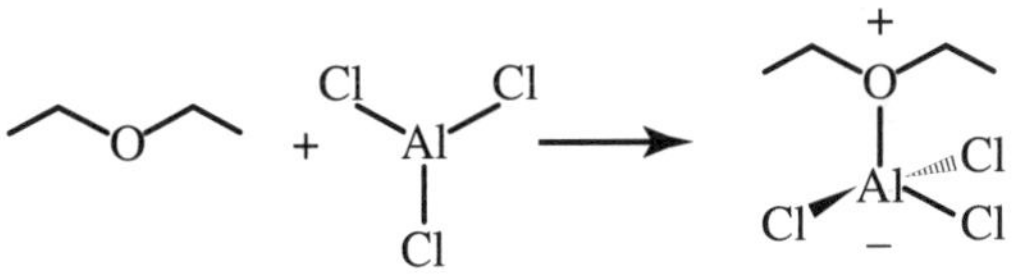

A) Covalent
B) Electrostatic
C) Metallic
D) Coordinate covalent

CHAPTER 5 PRACTICE PASSAGE

Metallic mercury, mercury salts, and organometallic mercury compounds are now recognized as critical toxins, but have historically been introduced into the environment through a number of industrial processes. The noted neurotoxicity of the element stems in part from its inhibition of cellular mechanisms that control oxidative damage. The brain is particularly sensitive to these effects, as the amount of oxygen consumed in the organ is large and thus the potential for oxidative damage is high.

Many standard elemental testing procedures for mercury, such as flame atomic absorption spectroscopy, are unable to differentiate between the three aforementioned types of mercury (metallic, ionic, organometallic). Since biological effects of each form are different, especially in acute dosages, a process has been developed for the separation of the three varieties of mercury (Figure 1), and is used primarily for detection of mercury in soil samples.

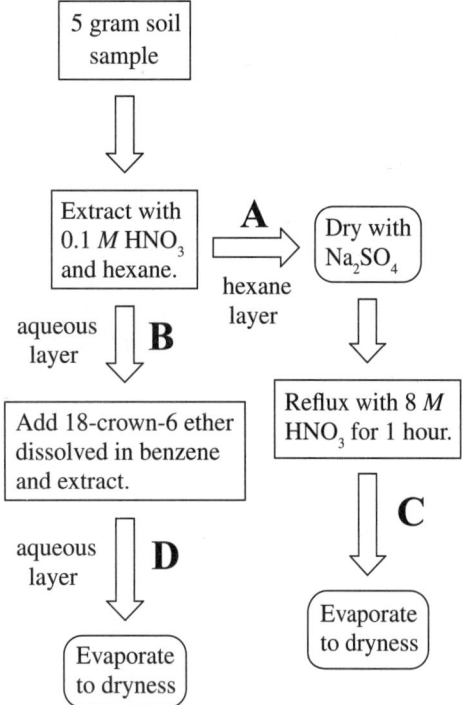

Figure 1 Test for organic and inorganic mercury

The first step is to extract a 5-gram soil sample with 50 mL of hexane and 50 mL of dilute nitric acid. The organic layer is removed, dried, and then refluxed with a 1:1 mixture of *conc.* HNO_3 and water. The water layer is removed, evaporated to dryness, and then quantitatively analyzed using AA (Atomic Absorption Spectroscopy).

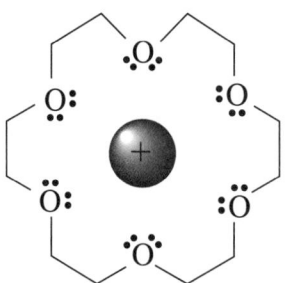

Structure of 18-crown-6 ether with chelated cation

The aqueous layer in the first extract is treated with 0.5 gram of a crown ether dissolved in benzene. The purpose of the crown ether is to chelate large radius cations present in solution (such as sodium, potassium, calcium, and barium) and carry them into the organic layer. The crown ether 18-crown-6, so named as it consists of an 18-membered ring with 6 oxygen atoms, was found to be ideal for the chelation of the large mercury cation. This bilayer solution is shaken and then separated. The aqueous layer is evaporated to dryness, and then analyzed via AA.

1. Assume that the cation in the crown ether is a potassium ion. What is the charge of the crown ether–K$^+$ complex?

   A) −1
   B) 0
   C) +1
   D) Greater than zero but less than one

2. In which solution(s) would you find $(CH_3)_2Hg$?

   A) Solution A only
   B) Solutions A and C
   C) Solution B only
   D) Solutions B and D

3. Based upon information presented in the passage, which of the following statements is NOT true?

A) The ionic radius of mercury is not equal to the radius of K^+.
B) Insoluble mercury salts have a greater solubility in solutions of nitric acid.
C) Crown ethers increase the organic solubility of cations by encapsulating the ion with a relatively nonpolar shell.
D) Mercury salts are highly volatile.

4. Which of the following methods might be used to separate ionic Zn^{2+} contamination from the Hg-containing material in the aqueous layer after extraction step B?

A) Add 15-crown-5 ether and extract with an organic phase.
B) Fractionally distill Zn from the solution.
C) Add a strong alkylating agent, such as $LiCH_3$ and extract with an organic phase.
D) Add 21-crown-7 ether and extract with an organic phase.

5. What is the purpose of refluxing the hexane solution with 8 M nitric acid for one hour?

A) To reduce all organometallic compounds to methane and metal
B) To oxidize all organometallic compounds to CO_2, water, and metal ions
C) To nitrate (i.e., create $R–NO_2$ groups in) the organometallic compounds
D) To increase the hydrophobic nature of organometallic compounds

SOLUTIONS TO CHAPTER 5 FREESTANDING PRACTICE QUESTIONS

1. **A**   A bond has a dipole moment when the two atoms involved in the bond differ in electronegativity. However, an entire molecule can only have a dipole if it contains bond dipoles and is asymmetrical. Choice A is tetrahedral and not all four substituents are the same. Therefore, it is asymmetrical and has a small negative dipole in the direction of the most electronegative substituent, oxygen. The remaining choices are trigonal bipyramidal, tetrahedral, and octahedral respectively. All have identical substituents, are symmetrical, and have no net dipole moment.

2. **A**   In order to participate in intermolecular hydrogen bonding, a molecule must be able to act as both a hydrogen bond donor and acceptor. In order to act as a hydrogen bond donor, a molecule must possess a hydrogen (H) atom covalently bound to a nitrogen (N), oxygen (O), or fluorine (F) atom. In order to act as a hydrogen bond acceptor, a molecule must have an oxygen, nitrogen, or fluorine atom with an unshared pair of electrons. CH_3CO_2H meets both of these requirements, and is therefore a valid choice. CO_2 does not possess any hydrogen atoms and is therefore an invalid option. While H_2S may seem like an enticing choice, sulfur is not sufficiently electronegative to produce hydrogen bonding when covalently bound to hydrogen atoms.

3. **B**   Van der Waals forces and induced dipoles are both examples of intermolecular forces, not intramolecular bonding, therefore choices C and D can be eliminated. The disparity in electronegativities between the carbon (C) and nitrogen (N) atoms in cyanide is not sufficient to produce ionic bonding, therefore choice B, covalent bonding, is the best answer.

4. **C**   In choice A the central atom, N, possesses three bonding electron groups and one lone pair of electrons. NH_3 therefore has tetrahedral orbital geometry.

In choice B the central atom, N, possesses four bonding electron groups and zero lone pairs. NH_4^+ therefore has tetrahedral geometry.

In choice C the central atom, C, possesses two bonding electron groups and zero lone pairs. Recall that double bonds each count as a single electron group. CO_2 therefore has linear geometry.

$$\ddot{O} = C = \ddot{O}$$

In choice D the central atom, C, possesses four bonding electron groups and zero lone pairs. CH_4 therefore has tetrahedral geometry.

$$
\begin{array}{c}
H \\
| \\
C \\
/ \ \backslash\ \ H \\
H\quad H
\end{array}
$$

5. **A** When answering ranking questions, it is best to determine the extremes and eliminate answer choices. Of the four molecules, only H_2O and H_2SO_4 are liquids at room temperature, and therefore would have higher boiling points than the two gases. Both experience strong hydrogen bonding, but the H_2SO_4 molecule is substantially larger, and, aside from this, has more sites to accept H-bonds from surrounding molecules. Therefore, H_2SO_4 should have the highest boiling point, eliminating answer choices B and D. Both NH_3 and CO_2 are gases at room temperature. However, NH_3 experiences hydrogen bonding, and therefore its boiling point would be higher than that of CO_2, eliminating choice C and making choice A the correct answer.

6. **D** For helium to form a liquid, there must be intermolecular forces holding the atoms in relatively fixed positions. Hydrogen bonding requires the presence of hydrogen atoms, which are not present in a sample of helium; choice A can be eliminated. The strong nuclear force holds nucleons together in the nucleus, and acts only within the nucleus; choice B can be eliminated. Metallic bonding exists between metal atoms, but helium is a noble gas, so choice C can be eliminated. (Metallic helium is postulated to exist in the high-pressure interior of Jupiter, but this question remains firmly on the surface of the Earth.) Choice D is correct. The only intermolecular force experienced by the helium atoms is London dispersion forces.

7. **D** This is an example of a Lewis acid-base reaction. In this type of reaction, one species accepts an electron pair from another species and a coordinate covalent bond is formed. One member of the bond donates *both* electrons in the bond. Whereas a coordinate covalent bond is a type of covalent interaction, the questions asks for the best answer, and coordinate covalent is more specific (eliminate choice A). Therefore, choice D is correct. An electrostatic bond is an ionic bond (eliminate choice B), and a metallic bond involves long-range delocalization of valence electrons, which is not the case in the product molecule (eliminate choice C).

SOLUTIONS TO CHAPTER 5 PRACTICE PASSAGE

1. **C**   By giving the structure, the passage indicates that the crown ether molecule is neutral. Since the charge of the potassium ion is +1, than the total charge of the complex is 0 + (+1) = +1.

2. **A**   Dimethyl mercury is a nonpolar molecule. So in the very first extraction, it will preferentially dissolve in the hexane solution (solution A). However, later, this solution is refluxed with nitric acid, a powerful oxidizing agent, which oxidizes dimethyl mercury into CO_2, H_2O, and Hg^{2+} (as the nitrate). Like other metal nitrates, mercuric nitrate is water soluble and is then found in the aqueous portion of the solution (solution C). (This is why you keep the aqueous layer for the analysis!) So dimethyl mercury will only be found in solution A.

3. **D**   Choices A, B, and C are all correct statements.

   A: The radius of Hg^{2+} is much smaller than that of K^+ because of ion contraction—2+ ions contract more than 1+ ions do. However, you should have been able to reason that the sizes of the potassium and mercury ions had to be different because 18-crown-6 ether, a polydentate ligand, will chelate any metal ion which snugly fits within the ring. 18-crown-6 ether chelated potassium ions, but evidently left the mercuric ions in the aqueous phase.

   B: The soil sample was extracted with 0.1 M HNO_3 for this reason. Since most soils are frequently washed through rainfall, almost all soluble salts are leached out of the soil. Hence, any mercury salts which remain in the soil must be of the insoluble type. So through the addition of HNO_3, these salts are solubilized.

   C: This is how and why crown ethers act to carry highly hydrophilic cations into hydrophobic solvents. Thus, crown ethers can be extremely toxic because of their ability to deposit toxic, heavy metal ions in bad places (just as outlined in the explanation of question 2 above).

   D: This is not true. Almost all ionic compounds are solids at room temperature, and have extremely low volatilities.

4. **A**   The meaning behind the naming scheme for crown ethers is given in the passage. 18-Crown-6 ether is an 18-membered ring with 6 oxygen atoms, and is stated as being the ideal fit for the very large mercury ion. 15-Crown-5 ether, a 15 membered ring with 5 oxygens, is smaller, and as it is less ideal for mercury it might be safely assumed it is better for smaller cations, such as Zn^{2+}. Extraction with this smaller ether should preferentially complex zinc, leaving the mercury behind in the aqueous phase. Choice D suggests using a larger ether to remove a smaller cation, which does not make sense (eliminate choice D). Fractional distillation of Zn salts from an aqueous solution is not viable, as salts have an insignificant vapor pressure at reasonably achievable temperatures (eliminate choice B). A strong alkylating agent would be expected to make both organozinc and organomercury compounds, which would both favor an organic phase (eliminate choice C).

5. **B**   Choice A is not true; nitric acid, one of the grand masters of oxidizing agents, will never reduce anything! Choice C is not so bad since HNO_3 is actually used to nitrate alcohols and electrophilic functional groups such as aromatic rings and alkenes. Unfortunately for this choice, there are none of these functionalities in dimethyl mercury. Choice D is wrong and is contrary to the fact that the mercury is found in the aqueous solution after this process. Any highly reduced molecule, such as organometallic compounds, are readily oxidized by hot nitric acid.

Chapter 6
Thermodynamics

6.1 SYSTEM AND SURROUNDINGS

Why does anything happen? Why does a creek flow downhill, a puddle of water evaporate after it rains, a chemical reaction proceed? It's all **thermodynamics:** the transformation of energy from one form to another. The laws of thermodynamics underlie any event in which energy is transformed.

The Zeroth Law of Thermodynamics

The Zeroth Law is often conceptually described as follows: If two systems are both in thermal equilibrium with a third system, then the two initial systems are in thermal equilibrium with one another.

Thus, the Zeroth Law establishes a definition of thermal equilibrium. When systems are in thermal equilibrium with one another, their temperatures must be the same. When bodies of different temperatures are brought into contact with one another, heat will flow from the body with the higher temperature into the body with lower temperature in order to achieve equilibrium at the same temperature value. This means that devices (thermometers) may be designed to achieve thermal equilibrium with their surroundings, and give a quantified, relative value of the temperature at this equilibrium.

In this way, the Zeroth Law defines what we call temperature, and is the logical basis for the subsequent thermodynamic laws that rely on it. It also establishes the link between heat and temperature. An important practical application of the Zeroth Law is calorimetry, which will be discussed in more detail in Chapter 7.

The First Law of Thermodynamics

The First Law states that *the total energy of the universe is constant.* Energy may be transformed from one form to another, but it cannot be created or destroyed.

An important result of the First Law is that an isolated system has a constant energy—no transformation of the energy is possible. When systems are in contact, however, energy is allowed to flow, and thermal equilibrium can be attained. In addition, the First Law also establishes that work can be put into a system to increase its overall energy. This may or may not occur with a corresponding change in temperature. The concept of work and its effects on physical thermodynamics can be examined more closely in the *MCAT Physics and Math Review*.

Conventions Used in Thermodynamics

In thermodynamics we have to designate a "starting line" and a "finish line" to be able to describe how energy flows in chemical reactions and physical changes. To do this we use three distinct designations to describe energy flow: the system, the surroundings, and the thermodynamic universe (or just universe).

The system is the thing we're looking at: a melting ice cube, a solid dissolving into water, a beating heart, anything we want to study. Everything else: the table the ice cube sits on and the surrounding air, the beaker that holds the solid and the water, the chest cavity holding the heart, is known collectively as the surroundings. The system and the surroundings taken together form the thermodynamic universe.

We need to define these terms so that we can assign a direction—and therefore a sign, either (+) or (–)—to energy flow. For chemistry (and for physics), we define everything in terms of what's happening to the *system*.

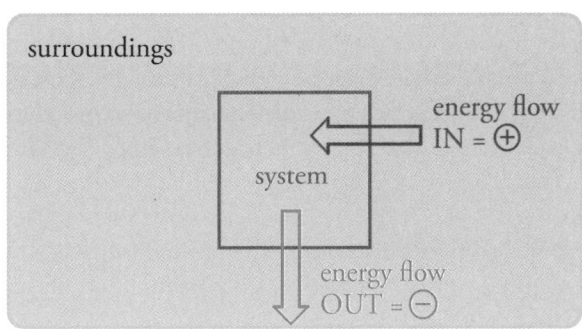

Consider energy flowing from the surroundings into the system, like the heat flowing from the table to the ice cube that's sitting on it. What is happening in the system? As energy flows in (here it's heat), the molecules in the system absorb it and start to jiggle faster. Eventually enough energy is absorbed to cause the ice to melt. Overall, the energy of the system *increased*, and we therefore give it a (+) sign. What about water when it freezes? Here energy (once again, heat) leaves the water (our system), and the jiggling of the water molecules slows down. The energy of the system has *decreased*, and we therefore assign a (–) sign to energy flow. Finally, energy that flows into the system flows out of the surroundings, and energy that flows out of the system flows into the surroundings. Therefore, we can make these statements:

1) When energy flows into a system from the surroundings, the energy of the system increases and the energy of the surroundings decreases.
2) When energy flows out of a system into the surroundings, the energy of the system decreases and the energy of the surroundings increases.

Keep this duality in mind when dealing with energy.

6.2 ENTHALPY

Enthalpy is a measure of the heat energy that is released or absorbed when bonds are broken and formed during a reaction that's run at constant pressure. The symbol for enthalpy is **H**. Some general principles about enthalpy prevail over all reactions:

- When a bond is formed, energy is released. $\Delta H < 0$.
- Energy must be put into a bond in order to break it. $\Delta H > 0$.

In a chemical reaction, energy must be put into the reactants to break their bonds. Once the reactant bonds are broken, the atoms rearrange to form products. As the product bonds form, energy is released. The enthalpy of a reaction is given by the difference between the enthalpy of the products and the enthalpy of the reactants.

$$\Delta H = H_{products} - H_{reactants}$$

The enthalpy change, ΔH, is also known as the **heat of reaction**.

If the products of a chemical reaction have stronger bonds than the reactants, then more energy is released in the making of product bonds than was put in to break the reactant bonds. In this case, energy is released overall from the system, and the reaction is **exothermic**. The products are in a lower energy state than the reactants, and the change in enthalpy, ΔH, is negative, since heat flows out of the system. If the products of a chemical reaction have weaker bonds than the reactants, then more energy is put in during the breaking of reactant bonds than is released in the making of product bonds. In this case, energy is absorbed overall and the reaction is **endothermic**. The products are in a higher energy state than the reactants, and the change in enthalpy, ΔH, is positive, since heat had to be added to the system from the surroundings.

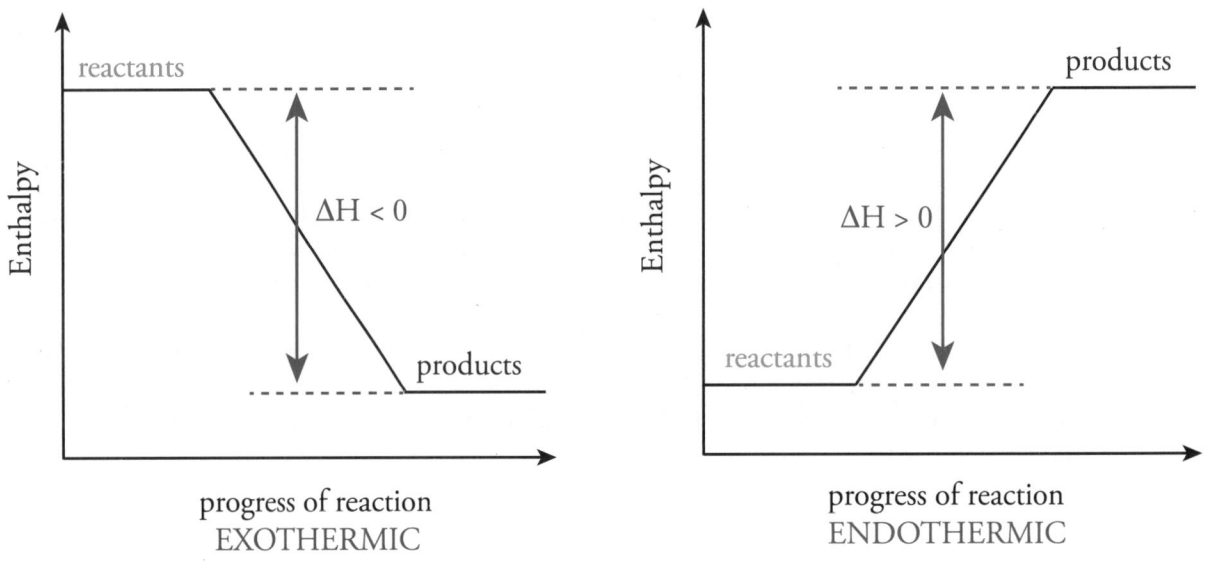

Example 6-1: The combustion of methanol is given by this reaction:

$$2\ CH_3OH(g) + 3\ O_2(g) \rightarrow 2\ CO_2(g) + 4\ H_2O(g) \qquad \Delta H = -1352\ kJ$$

a)   How much heat is produced when 16 g of oxygen gas reacts with excess methanol?
b)   Is the reaction exothermic or endothermic?
c)   How many moles of carbon dioxide are produced when 676 kJ of heat is produced?

Solution:

a) The molecular weight of O_2 is $2(16) = 32$ g/mol, so 16 g represents one-half mole. If 1352 kJ of heat is released when 3 moles of O_2 react, then just $(1/6)(1352 \text{ kJ}) = 225$ kJ of heat will be released when one-half mole of O_2 reacts.

b) Because ΔH is negative, the reaction is exothermic. And since 6 moles of gaseous products are being formed from just 5 moles of gaseous reactants, the disorder (entropy) has increased.

c) The stoichiometry of the given balanced reaction tells us that 2 moles of CO_2 are produced when 1352 kJ of heat is produced. So, half as much CO_2 (that is, 1 mole) is produced when half as much heat, 676 kJ, is produced.

Example 6-2: Which one of the following processes does NOT contribute to the change in enthalpy, ΔH_{rxn}, of a chemical reaction?

A) Phase change
B) Formation of stronger intermolecular forces
C) Breaking covalent bonds
D) The presence of a heterogeneous catalyst

Solution: A catalyst lowers the activation energy, but does not affect an equilibrium constant, enthalpy, entropy, or free energy in any way. Choice D is the answer. The other choices do fall under the umbrella of enthalpy.

6.3 CALCULATION OF ΔH_{rxn}

The heat of reaction (ΔH_{rxn}) can be calculated in a number of ways. Each of these will lead to the same answer given accurate starting values. The three most important methods to be familiar with are the use of standard heats of formation ($\Delta H°_f$), Hess's law of heat summation, and the summation of average bond enthalpies.

Standard Conditions

Scientists have a convention called the *standard state* for which most constants, heats of formation, enthalpies, and so on are determined. Solids and liquids in the standard state are assumed to be pure. Gases are assumed to behave ideally, and have a pressure of 1 atm. Solutions have a concentration of 1 *M*. Values that have been determined for chemicals in the standard state are designated by a ° superscript : $\Delta H°$, for example. While temperature does not appear in the formal definition of standard state, most reference works give values which have been measured at 25°C, or 298 K. This temperature has become the *de facto* standard when referring to "standard conditions." Be careful not to confuse *standard conditions* with *standard temperature and pressure* (STP). STP is 0°C, while standard conditions refers to 25°C.

Heat of Formation

The **standard heat of formation**, ΔH°_f, is the amount of energy required to make one mole of a compound *from its constituent elements in their natural or standard state,* which is the way the element exists under standard conditions. The convention is to assign elements in their standard state forms a ΔH°_f of zero. For example, the ΔH°_f of $C(s)$ (as graphite) is zero. Diatomic elements, such as O_2, H_2, Cl_2 and so on are also assigned a ΔH°_f of zero, rather than their atomic forms (such as O, Cl, etc.), because the diatomic state is the *natural* state for these elements at standard conditions. For example, $\Delta H^\circ_f = 0$ for O_2, but for O, $\Delta H^\circ_f = 249$ kJ/mol at standard conditions, because it takes energy to break the O=O double bond.

When the ΔH°_f of a compound is positive, then an input of heat is required to make that compound from its constituent elements. When ΔH°_f is negative, making the compound from its elements gives off energy.

You can calculate the ΔH° of a reaction if you know the heats of formation of the reactants and products:

$$\Delta H^\circ_{rxn} = (\Sigma n \times \Delta H^\circ_{f,\,products}) - (\Sigma n \times \Delta H^\circ_{f,\,reactants})$$

In the above equation "n" denotes the stoichiometric coefficient applied to each species in a chemical reaction as written. ΔH°_f of a given compound is the heat needed to form one mole, and as such if two moles of a molecule are needed to balance a reaction one must double the corresponding ΔH°_f in the enthalpy equation. If only half a mole is required one must divide the ΔH°_f by 2.

Example 6-3: Which of the following substances does NOT have a heat of formation equal to zero at standard conditions?

- A) $F_2(g)$
- B) $Cl_2(g)$
- C) $Br_2(g)$
- D) $I_2(s)$

Solution: Heat of formation, ΔH°_f, is zero for a pure element in its natural phase at standard conditions. All of the choices are in their standard state, except for bromine, which is a liquid, not a gas, at standard conditions. The correct answer is C.

Example 6-4: What is ΔH° for the following reaction under standard conditions if the ΔH°_f of $CH_4(g) = -75$ kJ/mol, ΔH°_f of $CO_2(g) = -393$ kJ/mol, and ΔH°_f of $H_2O(l) = -286$ kJ/mol?

$$CH_4(g) + 2\,O_2(g) \rightarrow CO_2(g) + 2\,H_2O(l)$$

Solution: Using the equation for ΔH°_{rxn}, we find that

$$\Delta H^\circ_{rxn} = (\Delta H^\circ_f CO_2 + 2\,\Delta H^\circ_f H_2O) - (\Delta H^\circ_f CH_4 + 2\,\Delta H^\circ_f O_2)$$

$$= (-393 \text{ kJ/mol} + 2(-286) \text{ kJ/mol}) - (-75 \text{ kJ/mol} + 0 \text{ kJ/mol})$$

$$= -890 \text{ kJ/mol}$$

Hess's Law of Heat Summation

Hess's law states that if a reaction occurs in several steps, then the sum of the energies absorbed or given off in all the steps will be the same as that for the overall reaction. This is due to the fact that enthalpy is a state function, which means that changes are independent of the pathway of the reaction. Therefore, ΔH is independent of the pathway of the reaction.

For example, we can consider the combustion of carbon to form carbon monoxide to proceed by a two-step process:

1) $C(s) + O_2(g) \rightarrow CO_2(g)$ $\qquad \Delta H_1 = -394 \text{ kJ}$
2) $CO_2(g) \rightarrow CO(g) + 1/2\ O_2(g)$ $\qquad \Delta H_2 = +283 \text{ kJ}$

To get the overall reaction, we add the two steps:

$$C(s) + \ 1/2\ O_2(g) \rightarrow CO(g)$$

So, to find ΔH for the overall reaction, we just add the enthalpies of each of the steps:

$$\Delta H_{rxn} = \Delta H_1 + \Delta H_2 = -394 \text{ kJ} + 283 \text{ kJ} = -111 \text{ kJ}$$

It's important to remember the following two rules when using Hess's law:

1) *If a reaction is reversed, the sign of ΔH is reversed too.*
   For example, for the reaction $CO_2(g) \rightarrow C(s) + O_2(g)$, we'd have $\Delta H = +394 \text{ kJ}$.

2) *If an equation is multiplied by a coefficient, then ΔH must be multiplied by that same value.*
   For example, for $1/2\ C(s) + \ 1/2\ O_2(g) \rightarrow 1/2\ CO_2(g)$, we'd have $\Delta H = -197 \text{ kJ}$.

Summation of Average Bond Enthalpies

Enthalpy itself can be viewed as the energy stored in the chemical bonds of a compound. Bonds have characteristic enthalpies that denote how much energy is required to break them homolytically (often called the bond dissociation energy, or BDE; see Section 5.2).

As indicated at the start of this section, an important distinction should be made here in the difference in sign of ΔH for making a bond versus breaking a bond. One must, necessarily, infuse energy into a system to break a chemical bond. As such the ΔH for this process is positive, making it endothermic. On the other hand, creating a bond between two atoms must have a negative value of ΔH. It therefore gives off heat and is exothermic. If this weren't the case it would indicate that the bonded atoms were higher in energy than they were when unbound; such a bond would be unstable and immediately dissociate.

Therefore we have a very important relation that can help you on the MCAT:

> Energy is needed to break a bond.
>
> Energy is released in making a bond.

From this we come to the third method of determining ΔH_{rxn}. If a question provides a list of bond enthalpies, ΔH_{rxn} can be determined through the following equation:

$$\Delta H_{rxn} = \Sigma \text{ (BDE bonds broken)} - \Sigma \text{ (BDE bonds formed)}$$

One can see that if stronger bonds are being formed than those being broken, then ΔH_{rxn} will be negative. More energy is released than supplied and the reaction is exothermic. If the opposite is true and breaking strong bonds takes more energy than is regained through the making of weaker product bonds, then the reaction is endothermic.

Example 6-5: Given the table of average bond dissociation energies below, calculate ΔH_{rxn} for the combustion of methane given in Example 6-4.

Bond	Average Bond Dissociation Energy (kJ/mol)
C—H	413
O—H	467
C=O	799
C≡N	615
H—Cl	427
O=O	495

A) 824 kJ/mol
B) 110 kJ/mol
C) −824 kJ/mol
D) −110 kJ/mol

Solution: First determine how many of each type of bond are broken in the reactants and formed in the products based on the stoichiometry of the balanced equation. Then using the bond dissociation energies we can calculate the enthalpy change:

$$\Delta H_{rxn} = \sum (\text{BDE bonds broken}) - \sum (\text{BDE bonds formed})$$

$$\Delta H_{rxn} = (4(\text{C—H}) + 2(\text{O=O})) - (2(\text{C=O}) + 4(\text{O—H}))$$

$$= (4(413) + 2(495)) - (2(799) + 4(467))$$

$$= -824 \text{ kJ/mol}$$

The correct answer is C. You may notice that the two methods of calculating the reaction enthalpy for the same reaction did not produce exactly the same answer. This is due to the fact that bond energies are reported as the average of many examples of that type of bond, whereas heats of formation are determined for each individual chemical compound. The exact energy of a bond will be dependent not only on the two atoms bonded together but also the chemical environment in which they reside. The average bond energy gives an approximation of the strength of an individual bond, and as such, the summation of bond energies gives an approximation of ΔH_{rxn}.

6.4 ENTROPY

The Second Law of Thermodynamics

There are several different ways to state the **second law of thermodynamics**, each appropriate to the particular system under study, but they're all equivalent. One way to state this law is that the disorder of the universe increases in a spontaneous process. For this to make sense, let's examine what we mean by the term *spontaneous*. For example, water will spontaneously splash and flow down a waterfall, but it will not spontaneously collect itself at the bottom and flow up the cliff. A bouncing ball will come to rest, but a ball at rest will not suddenly start bouncing. If the ball is warm enough, it's got the energy to start moving, but heat—the disorganized, random kinetic energy of the constituent atoms—will not spontaneously organize itself and give the ball an overall kinetic energy to start it moving. From another perspective, heat will spontaneously flow from a plate of hot food to its cooler surroundings, but thermal energy in the cool surroundings will not spontaneously concentrate itself and flow into the food. None of these processes would violate the first law, but they do violate the second law.

Nature has a tendency to become increasingly disorganized, and another way to state the second law is that *all processes tend to run in a direction that leads to maximum disorder*. Think about spilling milk from a glass. Does the milk ever collect itself together and refill the glass? No, it spreads out randomly over the table and floor. In fact, it needed the glass in the first place just to have any shape at all. Likewise, think about the helium in a balloon: It expands to fill its container, and if we empty the balloon, the helium diffuses randomly throughout the room. The reverse doesn't happen. Helium atoms don't collect themselves from the atmosphere and move into a closed container. The natural tendency of *all* things is to increase their disorder.

We measure disorder or randomness as **entropy**. The greater the disorder of a system, the greater is its entropy. Entropy is represented by the symbol S, and the change in entropy during a reaction is represented by the symbol ΔS. The change in entropy is determined by the equation

$$\Delta S = S_{products} - S_{reactants}$$

If randomness increases—or order decreases—during the reaction, then ΔS is positive for the reaction. If randomness decreases—or order increases—then ΔS is negative. For example, let's look at the decomposition reaction for carbonic acid:

$$H_2CO_3 \rightleftharpoons H_2O + CO_2$$

In this case, one molecule breaks into two molecules, and disorder is increased. That is, the atoms are less organized in the water and carbon dioxide molecules than they are in the carbonic acid molecule. The entropy is increasing for the forward reaction. Let's look at the reverse process: If CO_2 and H_2O come together to form H_2CO_3, we've decreased entropy because the atoms in two molecules have become more organized by forming one molecule.

In general, entropy is predictable in many cases:

- Liquids have more entropy than solids.
- Gases have more entropy than solids or liquids.
- Particles in solution have more entropy than undissolved solids.
- Two moles of a substance have more entropy than one mole.
- The value of ΔS for a reverse reaction has the same magnitude as that of the forward reaction, but with opposite sign: $\Delta S_{reverse} = -\Delta S_{forward}$.

While the overall drive of nature is to increase entropy, reactions can occur in which entropy decreases, but we must either put in energy or gain energy from making more stable bonds. (We'll explore this further when we discuss Gibbs free energy.)

Example 6-6: Which of the following processes would have a negative ΔS?

A) The evaporation of a liquid
B) The freezing of a liquid
C) The melting of a solid
D) The sublimation of a solid

Solution: Only the change described in choice B involves a decrease in randomness—the molecules of a solid are more ordered and organized than those in a liquid. So this process would have a negative change in entropy.

Example 6-7: Of the following reactions, which would have the greatest positive entropy change?

A) $2 NO(g) + O_2(g) \rightarrow 2 NO_2(g)$
B) $2 HCl(aq) + Mg(s) \rightarrow MgCl_2(aq) + H_2(g)$
C) $2 H_2O(g) + Br_2(g) + SO_2(g) \rightarrow 2 HBr(g) + H_2SO_4(aq)$
D) $2 I^-(aq) + Cl_2(g) \rightarrow I_2(s) + 2 Cl^-(aq)$

6.4

Solution: The reactions in choices A, C, and D all describe processes involving a decrease in randomness, that is, an increase in order. However, the process in choice B has a highly ordered solid on the left, but a highly disordered gas on the right, so we'd expect this reaction to have a positive entropy change.

Example 6-8: For the endothermic reaction

$$2 CO_2(g) \rightarrow 2 CO(g) + O_2(g)$$

which of the following is true?

A) ΔH is positive, and ΔS is positive.
B) ΔH is positive, and ΔS is negative.
C) ΔH is negative, and ΔS is positive.
D) ΔH is negative, and ΔS is negative.

Solution: Since we're told that the reaction is endothermic, we know that ΔH is positive. This eliminates choices C and D. Now, what about ΔS? Has the disorder increased or decreased? On the reactant side, we have one type of gas molecule, while on the right we have two. The reaction increases the numbers of gas molecules, so this describes an increase in disorder. ΔS is positive, and the answer is A.

Example 6-9: A gas is observed to undergo condensation. Which of the following is true about the process?

A) ΔH is positive, and ΔS is positive.
B) ΔH is positive, and ΔS is negative.
C) ΔH is negative, and ΔS is positive.
D) ΔH is negative, and ΔS is negative.

Solution: Condensation is the phase change from gas to liquid, which *releases* heat (since the reverse process, vaporization, requires an input of heat). Therefore, ΔH is negative, and choices A and B are eliminated. Now, because the change from gas to liquid represents an increase in order—since gases are so highly disordered—this process will have a negative change in entropy. The answer is therefore D.

The Third Law of Thermodynamics

The Third Law defines absolute zero to be a state of zero-entropy. At absolute zero, thermal energy is absent and only the least energetic thermodynamic state is available to the system in question. If only one state is possible, then there is no randomness to the system and $S = 0$. In this way, the Third Law describes the least thermally energetic state, and therefore the lowest achievable temperature. Kelvin defined the temperature at this state as 0 on his temperature scale.

6.5 GIBBS FREE ENERGY

The magnitude of the change in **Gibbs free energy**, ΔG, is the energy that's available (free) to do useful work from a chemical reaction. The spontaneity of a reaction is determined by changes in enthalpy and in entropy, and G includes both of these quantities. Now we have a way to determine whether a given reaction will be spontaneous. In some cases—namely, when ΔH and ΔS have different signs—it's easy. For example, if ΔH is negative and ΔS is positive, then the reaction will certainly be spontaneous (because the products have less energy and more disorder than the reactants; there are two tendencies for a spontaneous reaction: to decrease enthalpy and/or to increase entropy). If ΔH is positive and ΔS is negative, then the reaction will certainly be nonspontaneous (because the products would have more energy and less disorder than the reactants).

But what happens when ΔH and ΔS have the *same* sign? Which factor—enthalpy or entropy—will dominate and determine the spontaneity of the reaction? The sign of the single quantity ΔG will dictate whether or not a process is spontaneous, and we calculate ΔG from this equation:

Change in Gibbs Free Energy

$$\Delta G = \Delta H - T\Delta S$$

---

where T is the absolute temperature (in kelvins). We can then say this:

- $\Delta G < 0 \;\rightarrow\;$ spontaneous in the forward direction
- $\Delta G = 0 \;\rightarrow\;$ reaction is at equilibrium
- $\Delta G > 0 \;\rightarrow\;$ nonspontaneous in the forward direction

If ΔG for a reaction is positive, then the value of ΔG for the *reverse* reaction has the same magnitude but is negative. Therefore, the reverse reaction is spontaneous.

ΔG and Temperature

The equation for ΔG shows us that the entropy term ($T\Delta S$) depends directly on temperature. At low temperatures, the entropy doesn't have much influence on the free energy, and ΔH is the dominant factor in determining spontaneity. But as the temperature increases, the entropy term becomes more significant relative to ΔH and can dominate the value for ΔG. In general, the universe tends towards increasing disorder (positive ΔS) and stable bonds (negative ΔH), and a favorable combination of these will make a process spontaneous. The following chart summarizes the combinations of ΔH and ΔS that determine ΔG and spontaneity.

ΔH	ΔS	ΔG	Reaction is...?
–	+	–	spontaneous
+	+	– at sufficiently high T + at low T	spontaneous nonspontaneous
–	–	+ at high T – at sufficiently low T	nonspontaneous spontaneous
+	–	+	nonspontaneous

6.5

Important note: While values of ΔH are usually reported in terms of kJ, values of ΔS are usually given in terms of J. When using the equation $\Delta G = \Delta H - T\Delta S$, make sure that your ΔH and ΔS are expressed *both* in kJ or *both* in J.

Example 6-10: What must be true about a spontaneous, endothermic reaction?

A) ΔH is negative.
B) ΔG is positive.
C) ΔS is positive.
D) ΔS is negative.

Solution: Since the reaction is spontaneous, we know that ΔG is negative, and since we know the reaction is endothermic, we also know that ΔH is positive. The equation $\Delta G = \Delta H - T\Delta S$ then tells us that ΔS must be positive, choice C.

Example 6-11: If it's discovered that a certain nonspontaneous reaction becomes spontaneous if the temperature is lowered, then which of the following must be true?

A) ΔS is negative and ΔH is positive.
B) ΔS is negative and ΔH is negative.
C) ΔS is positive and ΔH is positive.
D) ΔS is positive and ΔH is negative.

Solution: If the temperature at which the reaction takes place has an impact on the spontaneity of the reaction, that means that the signs of ΔH and ΔS must both be either positive or negative (eliminate choices A and D). Lowering the temperature term makes the $T\Delta S$ term a smaller value in magnitude, and changes the sign of ΔG from positive to negative. That must mean that the ΔH is a negative value, as its impact is now more obvious at the new lower temperature, making choice B the correct answer.

6.6 REACTION ENERGY DIAGRAMS

A chemical reaction can be graphed as it progresses in a reaction energy diagram. True to its name, a reaction energy diagram plots the free energy of the total reactions versus the conversion of reactants to products.

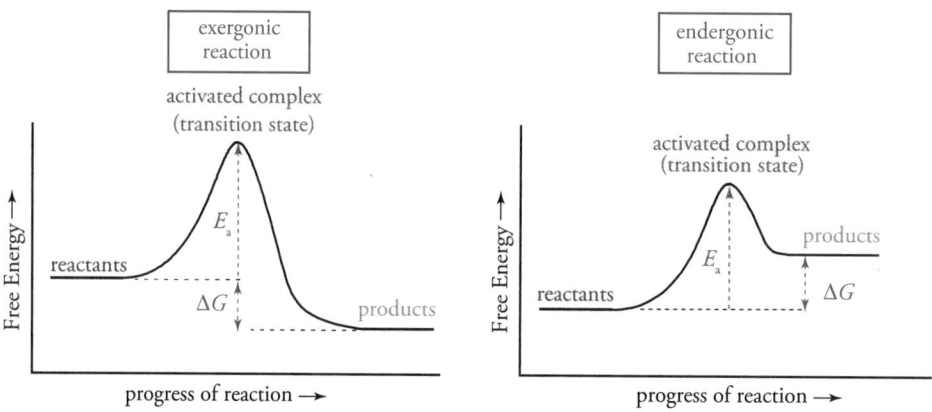

The ΔG of the overall reaction is the difference between the energy of the products and the energy of the reactants: $\Delta G_{rxn} = G_{products} - G_{reactants}$. When the value of $T\Delta S$ is very small, then ΔG can approximate ΔH, with the difference between the energy of products and reactants being very close to the heat of reaction, ΔH.

The activation energy, E_a, is the extra energy the reactants required to overcome the activation barrier, and determines the kinetics of the reaction. The higher the barrier, the slower the reaction proceeds towards equilibrium; the lower the barrier, the faster the reaction proceeds towards equilibrium. However, E_a does *not* determine the equilibrium, and an eternally slow reaction (very big E_a) can have a very favorable (large) K_{eq}. Many more details of both kinetics and equilibrium will be discussed in Chapters 9 and 10, respectively.

Kinetics vs. Thermodynamics

Just because a reaction is thermodynamically favorable (i.e., *spontaneous*), does not automatically mean that it will be taking place rapidly. **Do not confuse kinetics with thermodynamics** (this is something the MCAT will *try* to get you to do many times!). They are separate realms. *Thermodynamics predicts the spontaneity (and the equilibrium) of reactions, not their rates*. If you had a starting line and a finish line, thermodynamics tells you how far you will go, while kinetics tells you how quickly you will get there. A classic example to illustrate this is the formation of graphite from diamond. Graphite and diamond are two of the several different forms (**allotropes**) of carbon, and the value of $\Delta G°$ for the reaction $C_{(diamond)} \rightarrow C_{(graphite)}$ is about –2900 J/mol. Because $\Delta G°$ is negative, the formation of graphite is favored under standard conditions, but it's *extremely* slow. Even diamond heirlooms passed down through many generations are still in diamond form.

Reversibility

Reactions follow the principle of microscopic reversibility: The reverse reaction has the same magnitude for all thermodynamic values (ΔG, ΔH, and ΔS) but of the opposite sign, and the same reaction pathway, but in reverse. This means that the reaction energy diagram for the reverse reaction can be drawn by simply using the mirror image of the forward reaction. The incongruity you should notice is that E_a is different for the forward and reverse reactions. Coming from the products side towards the reactants, the energy barrier will be the difference between $G_{products}$ and the energy of the activated complex.

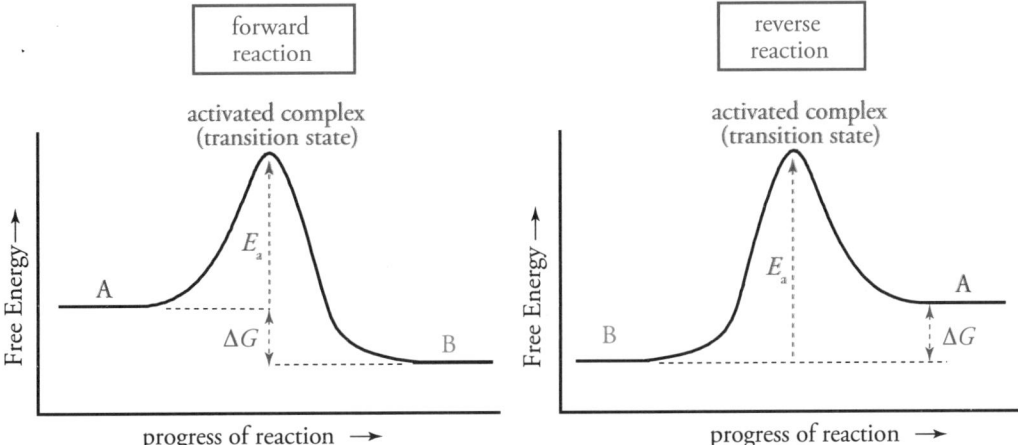

6.6

Chapter 6 Summary

- The Zeroth Law of Thermodynamics states that energy will flow from a body at a higher temperature to a body at a lower temperature until both bodies have the same temperature.

- Energy flow into a system has a positive sign. Energy flow out of a system has a negative sign.

- The First Law of Thermodynamics states that energy cannot be created or destroyed.

- The internal energy of an object is proportional to its temperature.

- The Second Law of Thermodynamics states that all processes tend toward maximum disorder, or entropy (S).

- Enthalpy (H) is a measure of the energy stored in the bonds of molecules.

- Breaking bonds requires energy ($+\Delta H$), while forming bonds releases energy ($-\Delta H$).

- Standard conditions are 1 atm pressure and 1 M concentrations. Temperature is usually taken to be 298 K. Standard conditions are denoted by a superscript "°".

- An endothermic reaction has a $\Delta H > 0$. An exothermic reaction has a $\Delta H < 0$.

- $\Delta H_{reaction} = H_{products} - H_{reactants}$. This equation can also be applied to ΔG and ΔS.

- ΔG, the Gibbs free energy, is the amount of energy in a reaction available to do chemical work.

- For a reaction under any set of conditions, $\Delta G = \Delta H - T\Delta S$.

- If $\Delta G < 0$, the reaction is spontaneous in the forward direction. If $\Delta G > 0$, the reaction is nonspontaneous in the forward direction. If $\Delta G = 0$, the reaction is at equilibrium.

CHAPTER 6 FREESTANDING PRACTICE QUESTIONS

1. During the electrolysis of liquid water into hydrogen and oxygen gas at standard temperature and pressure, energy is:

A) absorbed during the breaking of H—H bonds and the reaction is spontaneous.
B) released during the formation of H—H bonds and the reaction is nonspontaneous.
C) absorbed during the formation of O=O bonds and the reaction is spontaneous.
D) released during the breaking of O—H bonds and the reaction is nonspontaneous.

2. At standard conditions, the following reaction is endothermic, and non-spontaneous:

$$2 NH_3(g) \rightarrow N_2(g) + 3 H_2(g)$$

What change could make the reaction spontaneous?

A) Adding a catalyst
B) Increasing temperature
C) Decreasing temperature
D) The reaction will always be non-spontaneous

3. Which of the following should have the highest enthalpy of vaporization?

A) N_2
B) Br_2
C) Hg
D) Al

4. A 36 gram sample of water requires 93.4 kJ to sublime. What are the heats of fusion (ΔH_{fus}) and vaporization (ΔH_{vap}) for water?

A) ΔH_{fus} = −20 kJ/mol, ΔH_{vap} = 66.7 kJ/mol
B) ΔH_{fus} = 40.7 kJ/mol, ΔH_{vap} = 6.0 kJ/mol
C) ΔH_{fus} = 6.0 kJ/mol, ΔH_{vap} = 40.7 kJ/mol
D) ΔH_{fus} = 12.0 kJ/mol, ΔH_{vap} = 81.4 kJ/mol

5. Given the standard enthalpies of formation ($\Delta H_f°$) at 298 K for the compounds below, all of the following reactions are exothermic EXCEPT:

Compound	$\Delta H_f°$ (kJ/mol)
$C_2H_5OH(l)$	−238.86
$CH_3CHO(l)$	−77.80
$CH_3COOH(l)$	−484.50
$H_2O(l)$	−285.83

A) $CH_3COOH(l) \rightarrow CH_3CHO(l) + ½ O_2(g)$
B) $C_2H_5OH(l) + ½ O_2(g) \rightarrow CH_3CHO(l) + H_2O(l)$
C) $CH_3CHO(l) + ½ O_2(g) \rightarrow CH_3COOH(l)$
D) $C_2H_5OH(l) + O_2(g) \rightarrow CH_3COOH(l) + H_2O(l)$

6. The citric acid cycle consists of reactions that break down acetate into carbon dioxide. Given that some steps are thermodynamically unfavorable, why does the cycle proceed in the forward direction overall?

A) The rate constant for the unfavorable reactions is very large.
B) The cycle contains exergonic reactions that drive the endergonic reactions forward.
C) The endothermically unfavorable reactions also have a negative entropy change.
D) The activation energies of the unfavorable reactions are lowered by catalysts.

7. The $\Delta H_f°$ of ozone, O_3, is 142.7 kJ/mol. Which of the following statements is true for the decomposition of ozone into oxygen, shown below?

$$2 O_3(g) \rightarrow 3 O_2(g)$$

A) The reaction is always spontaneous.
B) The reaction is never spontaneous.
C) The reaction is only spontaneous at low temperatures.
D) The reaction is only spontaneous at high temperatures.

CHAPTER 6 PRACTICE PASSAGE

The extent to which a salt dissolves in water can be quantified by its solubility product constant, (K_{sp}) which is defined, for a hypothetical salt X_aY_b, as shown in Equation 2. The greater the value of K_{sp}, the more soluble the compound. The K_{sp} of a salt is related to the free energy of dissolution by the equation $\Delta G^\circ_{diss} = -RT\ln(K_{sp})$. Table 1 lists the K_{sp} values for some insoluble salts.

$$X_aY_b(s) \rightleftharpoons a\ X^{b+}(aq) + b\ Y^{a-}(aq)$$

Equation 1

$$K_{sp} = [X^{b+}]^a\ [Y^{a-}]^b$$

Equation 2

Salt	K_{sp}
$PbCl_2$	1.2×10^{-5}
$MgCO_3$	6.8×10^{-6}
$BaSO_4$	1.1×10^{-10}
$AgCl$	5.4×10^{-13}

Table 1 K_{sp} values for select insoluble salts

When a solid completely dissolves, solute particles are separated and encapsulated by solvent molecules. This process requires several steps: 1) breaking all solute-solute interactions, 2) disrupting some solvent-solvent interactions, and 3) forming new solute-solvent interactions. The combination of these processes determines the overall enthalpy change for the dissolution, which can be either exothermic or endothermic regardless of the solubility of the salt. Table 2 shows the enthalpies of dissolution for several soluble salts.

Salt	ΔH_{diss} (kJ/mol)
$LiCl$	–37.03
KCH_3CO_2	–15.33
$NaCl$	3.87
NH_4NO_3	25.69
$KClO_4$	41.38

Table 2 Dissolution enthalpies for some soluble salts

As solids are low entropy materials, their dissolution entails an increase in entropy. The size of ΔS_{diss} is dependent on the organization of solvent molecules in the solvation sphere of the dissolved ions.

1. Which of the following species is isoelectronic with the silver ion in AgCl?

    A) Rh^+
    B) Pd
    C) Cd^{2+}
    D) In^-

2. Given that the dissolution of sodium chloride is spontaneous below the saturation concentration, which of the following statements must be true?

    A) Forming solute-solvent interactions requires energy, while breaking solute-solute and solvent-solvent interactions releases energy.
    B) The increase in entropy must outweigh the enthalpy change of dissolution to create a negative Gibbs free energy.
    C) Sodium chloride is only soluble at high temperatures.
    D) All ionically-bound materials are substantially soluble in water.

3. Which one of the salts in Table 1 has the smallest value of ΔG°_{diss}?

    A) $PbCl_2$
    B) $MgCO_3$
    C) $BaSO_4$
    D) $AgCl$

4. Which of the following is consistent with the differences in $\Delta H°_{diss}$ for NaCl and LiCl?

A) The electrostatic forces in solid LiCl are much stronger than in solid NaCl, while coordination of water is equivalent for both salts.

B) The electrostatic forces in the two solids are approximately equivalent, while water molecules coordinate much more effectively to Na^+ than Li^+.

C) The electrostatic forces in solid LiCl are weaker than in solid NaCl, while water cannot effectively coordinate to the very small Li^+ cation.

D) The electrostatic forces in solid NaCl are slightly weaker than in solid LiCl, while water far more efficiently coordinates Li^+ than Na^+.

5. The transfer of heat to or from a solution changes the temperature of the solution according to the equation $q = mc\Delta T$ where q is the heat transferred, m is the mass of solvent, and c is the specific heat of the solvent. If a 1 g sample of a salt was dissolved in 20 mL of water (specific heat = 4.18 J/g°C) in an insulated beaker and the temperature was found to decrease by 4°C, which of the following salts was used? Assume no phase change for the water.

A) LiCl
B) KCH_3CO_2
C) NH_4NO_3
D) NaCl

SOLUTIONS TO CHAPTER 6 FREESTANDING PRACTICE QUESTIONS

1. **B** Electrolysis requires energy. Water will not split into hydrogen and oxygen gas spontaneously at standard temperature and pressure, which eliminates choices A and C. When bonds are broken, energy is absorbed (eliminates choice D). Energy is released when bonds are formed.

2. **B** Choice A is eliminated because catalysts only change the rates of the reactions, not their overall spontaneity. The question implies that the process has a positive ΔH. Since the reaction involves changing two moles of gas to four moles of gas, the entropy of the reaction increases, so it will have a positive ΔS. Using the equation $\Delta G = \Delta H - T\Delta S$, a reaction with a positive ΔH and ΔS will be spontaneous only at sufficiently high temperatures. Therefore, choices C and D can be eliminated, making choice B correct.

3. **D** Enthalpy of vaporization is the heat energy required per mole to change from the liquid to gas phase. N_2 is a gas at room temperature, Br_2 and Hg are both liquids at room temperature, and Al is a solid at room temperature. Therefore, it is expected that Al will have the highest enthalpy of vaporization, making choice D correct.

4. **C** Both fusion (melting) and vaporization (boiling) require energy and are endothermic, eliminating choice A. Comparing both processes, vaporization takes substantially more energy. During vaporization, intermolecular forces are essentially completely overcome, and gaseous molecules separate widely due to their increased kinetic energy. Choice B is therefore eliminated. A 36 gram sample of water is 2 moles, so the heat of sublimation of 1 mole is half of 93.4 kJ, or 46.7 kJ/mol. This eliminates choice D. Examining the fusion and vaporization of water and adding their enthalpies by Hess's law gives choice C as the correct answer:

$$H_2O(s) \rightarrow H_2O(l) \qquad \Delta H_{fus} = X \ (6.0 \text{ kJ/mol})$$

$$H_2O(l) \rightarrow H_2O(g) \qquad \Delta H_{vap} = Y \ (40.7 \text{ kJ/mol})$$

$$H_2O(s) \rightarrow H_2O(g) \qquad \Delta H_{vap} = X + Y = 46.7 \text{ kJ/mol}$$

5. **A** The change in enthalpy (ΔH) for a reaction is equal to the sum of ΔH_f° for products minus the sum of ΔH_f° for reactants: $\Delta H = \Sigma \ \Delta H_{f \ (products)} - \Sigma \ \Delta H_{f \ (reactants)}$. For choice A, the lone reduction reaction, $\Delta H = (-77.8 \text{ kJ/mol}) - (-484.50 \text{ kJ/mol})$. This is a positive value indicating that enthalpy is absorbed and the reaction is endothermic. Note that the heat of formation of diatomic oxygen gas or any element in its naturally occurring form is defined as 0. The other answer choices, which are all oxidation reactions, will yield negative values indicating they are exothermic.

6. **B** The question is asking about thermodynamic principles, so answer choices A and D that involve kinetics can be eliminated. Reactions with a positive ΔH and a negative ΔS are never spontaneous according to $\Delta G = \Delta H - T\Delta S$, eliminating choice C. If the sum of all reactions is more exergonic ($-\Delta G$) than endergonic ($+\Delta G$), the net release of free energy will drive the cycle forward, making choice B the best answer.

7. **A** In order to determine the spontaneity of the reaction, the equation $\Delta G = \Delta H - T\Delta S$ must be used. Entropy increases (positive ΔS) in the reaction, since the number of moles of gas increases. The decomposition of ozone represents the reverse reaction of the formation of ozone, represented by the ΔH_f° value; therefore, the decomposition reaction has a negative ΔH. This combination of a negative ΔH and a positive ΔS gives a ΔG which is negative at all temperatures, so the reaction is always spontaneous. Choice A is correct.

SOLUTIONS TO CHAPTER 6 PRACTICE PASSAGE

1. **C** Isoelectronic species have the same electron configurations, and hence the same number of electrons. Ag^+ has 46 electrons, eliminating choices A and D because they have 44 and 50 electrons, respectively. The electron configuration of Ag^+ is [Kr] $4d^{10}$. The electron configuration of Pd is [Kr] $5s^2 3d^8$ (eliminate choice B). The electron configuration of Cd^{2+} is [Kr] $4d^{10}$, which is isoelectronic with Ag^+.

2. **B** Similar to bond formation, forming solute-solvent interactions is exothermic, meaning energy is released, not required; similarly breaking solute-solute or solvent-solvent interactions is endothermic (requires energy), like bond breaking (eliminate choice A). In addition, sodium chloride is soluble at room temperature (eliminate choice C). Salts are held together by ionic bonds, but Table 1 shows through the small K_{sp} values that not all of them are substantially soluble (eliminate choice D). For the dissolution of sodium chloride to be spontaneous, the increase in entropy must outweigh the endothermic process (note that NaCl has a positive enthalpy of dissolution from Table 2), yielding a negative Gibbs free energy.

3. **A** The important relationship between the standard state Gibbs free energy of dissolution and the solubility product constant is given in the passage:

$$\Delta G^\circ_{diss} = -RT\ln K_{sp}$$

Since the question asks for an extreme, first eliminate the two choices for K_{sp} in Table 1 that are the middle values (choices B and C). The ln function is similar to the log function, and can be thought of in the same way when judging relative magnitudes of ΔG°_{diss} in the equation above. For values of $K_{sp} > 1$, the ΔG° value will be negative, and for values of $K_{sp} < 1$, the ΔG° value will be positive. Therefore, the larger value of K_{sp} for $PbCl_2$ will give the smallest value for ΔG°.

4. **D** Effective dissolution involves the endothermic step of overcoming the electrostatic charges holding the solid salts together and the exothermic step of coordinating solvents to the separated ions. A negative value of $\Delta H°_{diss}$ likely indicates relatively weak electrostatic forces in the solid (small endothermic step), and effective solvation by water (large exothermic step). Table 2 shows that LiCl has a much more negative value of $\Delta H°_{diss}$ than NaCl. Choice A, stronger electrostatic forces in LiCl and no difference in solvation, would lead to a more negative $\Delta H°_{diss}$ for NaCl. Choice B would also result in a more negative value of $\Delta H°_{diss}$ for NaCl, as it indicates that electrostatics are equivalent while Na^+ has stronger interactions with water. Choice C is incorrect because a large negative value of $\Delta H°_{diss}$ would be difficult to achieve if water were unable to coordinate Li^+. Choice D includes a viable combination of slightly weaker attractive forces in NaCl but much better solvation for Li^+.

5. **C** Since the question states that the temperature of the solution decreased, the salts with exothermic dissolution enthalpies (choices A and B) can be eliminated. Using the calorimetry equation given in the question stem ($q = mc\Delta T$), we can estimate:

$$20 \text{ g} \times \sim4 \text{ J/g°C} \times 4°C \approx 320 \text{ J} \approx 0.32 \text{ kJ} = q$$

Since this heat is associated with 1 g of salt, in order to compare to the $\Delta H°_{diss}$ in Table 2, convert this energy to a per mole basis by multiplying by the molar mass of the salt.

For choice C (NH_4NO_3, MW = 80 g/mol), this yields:

$$\sim0.3 \text{ kJ/1 g } NH_4NO_3 \times 80 \text{ g } NH_4NO_3/\text{mol} = 24 \text{ kJ/mol}$$

which is close to the given 25.69 kJ/mol in the table. The comparable calculation for NaCl yields:

$$\sim0.3 \text{ kJ/1 g NaCl} \times \sim60 \text{ g NaCl/mol} = 18 \text{ kJ/mol}$$

so choice D can be eliminated.

Chapter 7
Phases

7.1 PHYSICAL CHANGES

Matter can undergo physical changes as well as chemical changes. Melting, freezing, and boiling are all examples of physical changes. A key property of a physical change is that no *intra*molecular bonds are made or broken; a physical change affects only the *inter*molecular forces between molecules or atoms. For example, ice melting to become liquid water does not change the molecules of H_2O into something else. Melting reflects the disruption of the attractive interactions between the molecules.

Every type of matter experiences intermolecular forces such as dispersion forces, dipole interactions, and hydrogen bonding. All molecules have some degree of attraction towards each other (dispersion forces at least), and it's the intermolecular interactions that hold matter together as solids or liquids. The strength and the type of intermolecular forces depend on the identity of the atoms and molecules of a substance and vary greatly. For example, NaCl(*s*), $H_2O(l)$ and $N_2(g)$ all have different kinds and strengths of intermolecular forces, and these differences give rise to their widely varying melting and boiling points.

Phase Transitions

Physical changes are closely related to temperature. What does temperature tell us about matter? Temperature is a measure of the amount of internal kinetic energy (the energy of motion) that molecules have. The average kinetic energy of the molecules of a substance directly affects its **state** or **phase**: whether it's a **solid, liquid,** or **gas.** Kinetic energy is also related to the degree of disorder, or **entropy.** In general, the higher the average kinetic energy of the molecules of a substance, the greater its entropy.

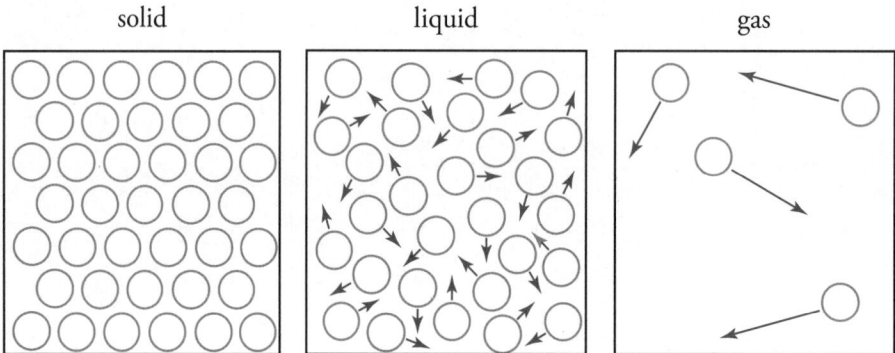

If we increase the temperature at a given pressure, a solid typically transforms into liquid and then into gas. What causes the phase transitions as the temperature increases? Phase changes are simply the result of breaking (or forming) intermolecular interactions. At low temperatures, matter tends to exist as a solid and is held together by intermolecular interactions. The molecules in a solid may jiggle a bit, but they're restricted to relatively fixed positions and form an orderly array, because the molecules don't have enough kinetic energy to overcome the intermolecular forces. Solids are the most ordered and least energetic of the phases. As a solid absorbs heat its temperature increases, meaning the average kinetic energy of the molecules increases. This causes the molecules to move around more, loosening the intermolecular interactions and increasing the entropy. When enough energy is absorbed for the molecules to move freely around one another, the solid melts and becomes liquid. At the molecular level, the molecules in a liquid are still in contact and interact with each other, but they have enough kinetic energy to escape fixed positions. Liquids have more internal kinetic energy and greater entropy than solids. If enough heat is absorbed by the liquid, the kinetic energy increases until the molecules have enough speed to escape intermolecular forces and vaporize into the gas phase. Molecules in the gas phase move freely of one another and experience very few, if any, effects of intermolecular forces. Gases are the most energetic and least ordered of the phases.

To illustrate these phase transitions, let's follow ice through the transitions from solid to liquid to gas. Ice is composed of highly organized H_2O molecules held rigidly by hydrogen bonds. The molecules have limited motion. If we increase the temperature of the ice, the molecules will eventually absorb enough heat to move around, and the organized structure of the molecules will break down as fixed hydrogen bonds are replaced with hydrogen bonds in which the molecules are *not* in fixed positions. We observe the transition as ice melting into liquid water. If we continue to increase the temperature, the kinetic energy of the molecules eventually becomes great enough for the individual molecules to overcome all hydrogen bonding and move freely. This appears to us as vaporization, or boiling of the liquid into gas. At this point the H_2O molecules zip around randomly, forming a high-entropy, chaotic swarm. All the phase transitions are summarized here.

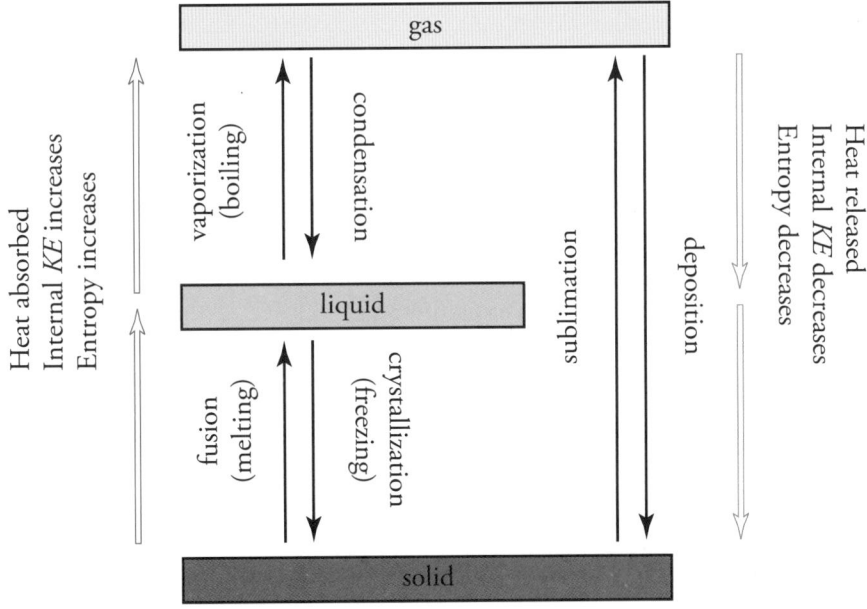

Example 7-1: Which of these phase changes releases heat energy?

A) Melting
B) Fusion
C) Condensation
D) Sublimation

Solution: Phase changes that bring molecules together (*condensation, freezing, deposition*) release heat, while phase changes that spread molecules out (*melting/fusion, vaporization, sublimation*) absorb heat. Choice C is the correct answer. (Note also that choices A and B are identical, so you know they have to be wrong no matter what.)

7.2 HEATS OF PHASE CHANGES

When matter undergoes a phase transition, energy is either absorbed or released. The amount of energy required to complete a transition is called the **heat of transition,** symbolized ΔH. For example, the amount of heat that must be absorbed to change a solid into a liquid is called the **heat of fusion**, and the energy absorbed when a liquid changes to a gas is the **heat of vaporization**. Each substance has a specific heat of transition for each phase change, and the magnitude is directly related to the strength and number of the intermolecular forces that substance experiences.

The amount of heat required to cause a change of phase depends on two things: the type of substance and the amount of substance. For example, the heat of fusion for H_2O is 6.0 kJ/mol. So, if we wanted to melt a 2 mol sample of ice (at 0°C), 12 kJ of heat would need to be supplied. The heat of vaporization for H_2O is about 41 kJ/mol, so vaporizing a 2 mol sample of liquid water (at 100°C) would require 82 kJ of heat. If that 2 mol sample of steam (at 100°C) condensed back to liquid, 82 kJ of heat would be released. In general, the amount of heat, q, accompanying a phase transition is given by

$$q = n \times \Delta H_{\text{phase change}}$$

where n is the number of moles of the substance. If ΔH and q are positive, heat is absorbed; if ΔH and q are negative, heat is released.

Example 7-2: The melting point of iron is 1530°C, and its heat of fusion is 64 cal/g. How much heat would be required to completely melt a 50 g chunk of iron at 1530°C?

Solution: Since the heat of transition is given in units of cal/g, we can simply multiply it by the given mass

$$q = m \times \Delta H_{\text{fusion}} = 50 \text{ g} \times 64 \text{ cal/g} = 3200 \text{ cal}$$

By the way, a **calorie** is, by definition, the amount of heat required to raise the temperature of 1 gram of water by 1°C. The SI unit of heat (and of all forms of energy) is the **joule**. Here's the conversion between joules and calories: 1 cal ≈ 4.2 J. (The popular term *calorie*—the one most of us are concerned with day to day when we eat—is actually a kilocalorie [10^3 cal] and is sometimes written as Calorie [with a capital C]).

Example 7-3: What happens when a container of liquid water (holding 100 moles of H_2O) at 0°C completely freezes? (Note: $\Delta H_{\text{fusion}} = 6$ kJ/mol, and $\Delta H_{\text{vap}} = 41$ kJ/mol.)

A) 600 kJ of heat is absorbed.
B) 600 kJ of heat is released.
C) 4100 kJ of heat is absorbed.
D) 4100 kJ of heat is released.

Solution: In order for ice to melt, it must absorb heat; therefore, the reverse process—water freezing into ice—must *release* heat. This eliminates choices A and C. The heat of transition from liquid to solid is $-\Delta H_{\text{fusion}}$, so in this case the heat of transition is $q = (100 \text{ mol})(-6 \text{ kJ/mol}) = -600$ kJ, so choice B is the answer.

7.3 CALORIMETRY

In between phase changes, matter can absorb or release energy without undergoing transition. We observe this as an increase or a decrease in the temperature of a substance. When a sample is undergoing a phase change, it absorbs or releases heat *without* a change in temperature, so when we talk about a temperature change, we are considering only cases where the phase doesn't change. One of the most important facts about physical changes of matter is this (and it will bear repeating):

> When a substance absorbs or releases heat, one of two things can happen: either its temperature changes *or* it will undergo a phase change *but not both at the same time.*

The amount of heat absorbed or released by a sample is proportional to its change in temperature. The constant of proportionality is called the substance's **heat capacity, C**, which is the product of its **specific heat**, c, and its mass, m; that is, $C = mc$. We can write the equation $q = C\Delta T$ in this more explicit form:

$$q = mc\Delta T$$

where

q = heat added to (or released by) a sample
m = mass of the sample
c = specific heat of the substance
ΔT = temperature change

A substance's specific heat is an *intrinsic* property of that substance and tells us how resistant it is to changing its temperature. For example, the specific heat of liquid water is 1 calorie per gram·°C. (This is actually the definition of a **calorie**: the amount of heat required to raise the temperature of 1 gram of water by 1°C.) The specific heat of copper, however, is much less: 0.09 cal/g·°C. So, if we had a 1 g sample of water and a 1 g sample of copper and each absorbed 10 calories of heat, the resulting changes in the temperatures would be

$$\Delta T_{water} = \frac{q}{mc_{water}} \qquad \Delta T_{copper} = \frac{q}{mc_{copper}}$$

$$= \frac{10 \text{ cal}}{(1 \text{ g})(1\frac{\text{cal}}{\text{g·}^\circ\text{C}})} \qquad = \frac{10 \text{ cal}}{(1 \text{ g})(0.09\frac{\text{cal}}{\text{g·}^\circ\text{C}})}$$

$$= 10^\circ\text{C} \qquad\qquad = 111^\circ\text{C}$$

That's a big difference! So, while it's true that the temperature change is proportional to the heat absorbed, it's *inversely* proportional to the substance's heat capacity. A substance like water, with a relatively high specific heat, will undergo a smaller change in temperature than a substance (like copper) with a lower specific heat.

A few notes:

1) The specific heat of a substance also depends upon phase. For example, the specific heat of ice is different from that of liquid water.
2) The SI unit for energy is the joule, not the calorie. You may see specific heats (and heat capacities) given in terms of joules rather than calories. Remember, the conversion between joules and calories is: 1 cal ≈ 4.2 J.
3) Specific heats may also be given in terms of kelvins rather than degrees Celsius; that is, you may see the specific heat of water, say, given as 4.2 J/g·K rather than 4.2 J/g·°C. However, since the size of a Celsius degree is the same as that of a kelvin (that is, if two temperatures differ by 1°C, they also differ by 1 K), the numerical value of the specific heat won't be any different if kelvins are used.

Example 7-4: The specific heat of tungsten is 0.03 cal/g·°C. If a 50-gram sample of tungsten absorbs 100 calories of heat, what will be the change in temperature of the sample?

Solution: From the equation $q = mc\Delta T$, we find that

$$\Delta T = \frac{q}{mc} = \frac{100 \text{ cal}}{(50 \text{ g})(0.03 \text{ cal/g·°C})} = \frac{2}{3/100} \,°C \approx 67\,°C$$

Example 7-5: Equal amounts of heat are absorbed by 10 g solid samples of four different metals, aluminum, lead, tin, and iron. Of the four, which will exhibit the *smallest* change in temperature?

A) Aluminum (specific heat = 0.9 J/g·K)
B) Lead (specific heat = 0.13 J/g·K)
C) Tin (specific heat = 0.23 J/g·K)
D) Iron (specific heat = 0.45 J/g·K)

Solution: Since q and m are constant, ΔT is inversely proportional to c. So, the substance with the greatest specific heat will undergo the smallest change in temperature. Of the metals listed, aluminum (choice A) has the greatest specific heat.

Example 7-6: A researcher attempts to determine the specific heat of a substance by gradually heating a sample of it over time and measuring the temperature change. His first trial fails because it produces no significant change in temperature. Which changes to his experimental procedure would be most effective in producing a larger temperature change in his second trial?

A) Increasing the mass of the sample and increasing the heat input
B) Increasing the mass of the sample and decreasing the heat input
C) Decreasing the mass of the sample and increasing the heat input
D) Decreasing the mass of the sample and decreasing the heat input

Solution: Since $\Delta T = q/mc$, to increase ΔT, the researcher should increase q and decrease m. (Intuitively, adding more heat to a smaller sample should result in a greater temperature increase.) Therefore, the answer is C.

Example 7-7: Molecules that experience strong intermolecular forces tend to have high specific heats. Of the following molecules, which one is likely to have the highest specific heat?

A) CH_4
B) $(CH_3)_4Si$
C) CO
D) CH_3OH

Solution: We're looking for the molecule with the strongest intermolecular forces. Choices A and B are eliminated because these are nonpolar molecules that only experience weak London dispersion forces. Methanol (choice D) is a better choice than carbon monoxide (choice C), because methanol will experience hydrogen bonding while carbon monoxide experiences only weak dipole forces. Therefore, choice D is the answer.

7.4 PHASE TRANSITION DIAGRAM/HEATING CURVE

Let's consider the complete range of phase changes from solid to liquid to gas. The process in this direction requires the input of heat. As heat is added to the solid, its temperature increases until it reaches its melting point. At that point, absorbed heat is used to change the phase to liquid, not to increase the temperature. Once the sample has been completely melted, additional heat again causes its temperature to rise, until the boiling point is reached. At that point, absorbed heat is used to change the phase to gas, not to increase the temperature. Once the sample has been completely vaporized, additional heat again causes its temperature to rise. We can summarize all this with a **phase transition diagram,** also known as a **heating curve,** which plots the temperature of the sample versus the amount of heat absorbed. The figure below is a typical heating curve.

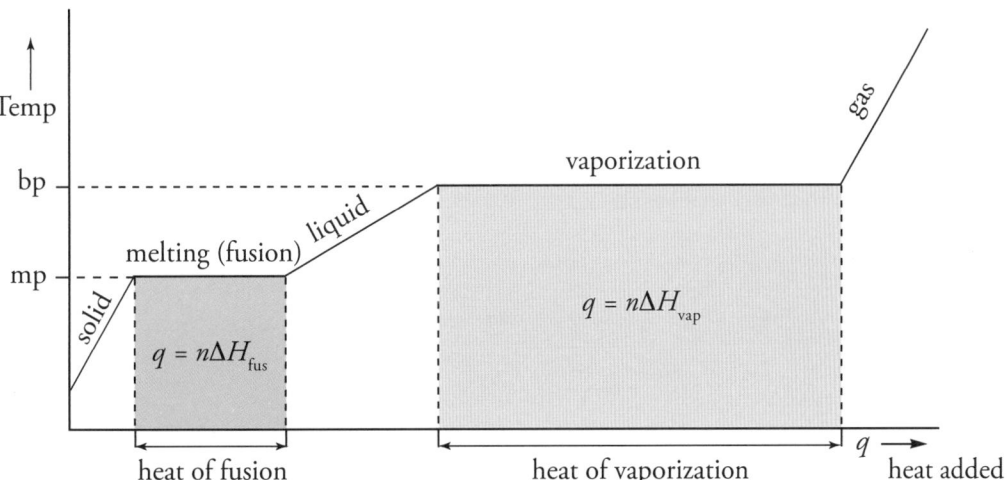

7.4

The horizontal axis represents the amount of heat added, and the vertical axis is the corresponding temperature of the substance. Notice the flat lines when the substance reaches its melting point (mp) and boiling point (bp). *During a phase transition, the temperature of the substance does not change.* Also, the greater the value for the heat of transition, the longer the flat line. A substance's heat of vaporization is always greater than its heat of fusion. The sloped lines show how the temperature changes (within a phase) as heat is added. Since $\Delta T = q/C$, the slopes of the non-flat lines are equal to $1/C$, the reciprocal of the substance's heat capacity in that phase.

Example 7-8: How much heat (in calories) is necessary to raise the temperature of 2 g of solid H_2O from $0°C$ to $85°C$? (*Note:* Heat of fusion for water = 80 cal/g and the specific heat of water is 1 cal/g·°C.)

A) 85 cal
B) 165 cal
C) 170 cal
D) 330 cal

Solution: There are two steps here: (1) melt the ice at $0°C$ to liquid water at $0°C$, and (2) heat the water from $0°C$ to $85°C$.

$$
\begin{aligned}
q_{total} &= q_1 + q_2 \\
&= m\Delta H_{fusion} + mc_{water}\Delta T \\
&= (2 \text{ g})(80 \text{ cal/g}) + (2 \text{ g})(1 \text{ cal/g}°C)(85°C) \\
&= (160 \text{ cal}) + (170 \text{ cal}) \\
&= 330 \text{ cal}
\end{aligned}
$$

The correct answer is D.

Example 7-9: Given that each of the following solutions is at equilibrium with its environment, which solution should have the lowest temperature at 1 atm?

A) A solution that is 1% ice and 99% liquid water
B) A solution that is 50% ice and 50% liquid water
C) A solution that is 99% ice and 1% liquid water
D) All these solutions will have the same temperature

Solution: As long as there is any amount of ice and liquid water coexisting at equilibrium, the temperature must be $0°C$ at 1 atm. Therefore, D is the answer.

Phase Diagrams

The phase of a substance doesn't depend just on the temperature; it also depends on the pressure. For example, even at high temperatures, a substance can be squeezed into the liquid phase if the pressure is high enough, and at low temperature, a substance can enter the gas phase if the pressure is low enough. A substance's **phase diagram** shows how its phases are determined by temperature and pressure. The figure below is a generic example of a phase diagram.

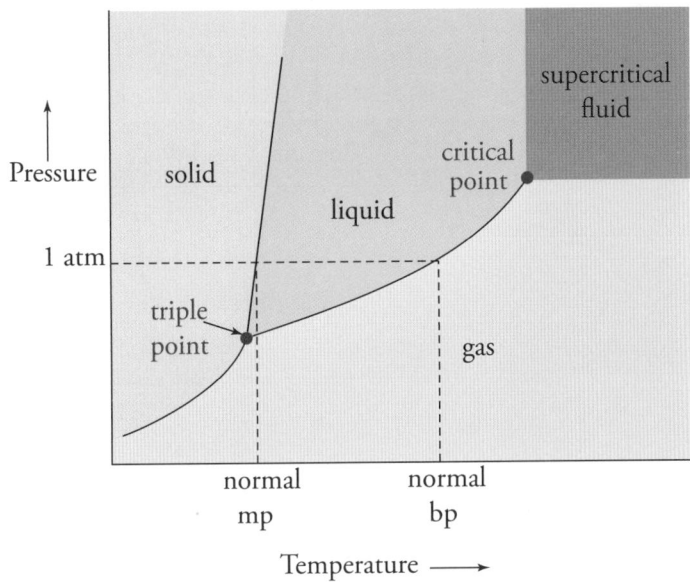

The boundary lines between phases represent points at which the two phases are in equilibrium. For example, a glass of liquid water at 0°C containing ice cubes is a two-phase system, and if its temperature and pressure were plotted in a phase diagram, it would be on the solid-liquid boundary line. Crossing a boundary line implies a phase transition. Notice that the solid phase is favored at low temperatures and high pressures, while the gas phase is favored at high temperatures and low pressures.

If we draw a horizontal line at the "1 atm" pressure level, the temperature at the point where this line crosses the solid-liquid boundary is the substance's **normal melting point**, and the temperature at the point where the line crosses the liquid-gas boundary is the **normal boiling point**.

The **triple point** is the temperature and pressure at which all three phases exist simultaneously in equilibrium, and therefore all phase changes are happening simultaneously.

The **critical point** marks the end of the liquid-gas boundary. Beyond this point, the substance displays properties of both a liquid (such as high density) and a gas (such as low viscosity). If a substance is in this state—where the liquid and gas phases are no longer distinct—it's called a **supercritical fluid**, and no amount of increased pressure can force the substance back into its liquid phase.

The Phase Diagram for Water

Water is the most common of a handful of substances that are denser in the liquid phase than in the solid phase. As a result, the solid-liquid boundary line in the phase diagram for water has a slightly *negative* slope, as opposed to the usual positive slope for most other substances. Compare these diagrams:

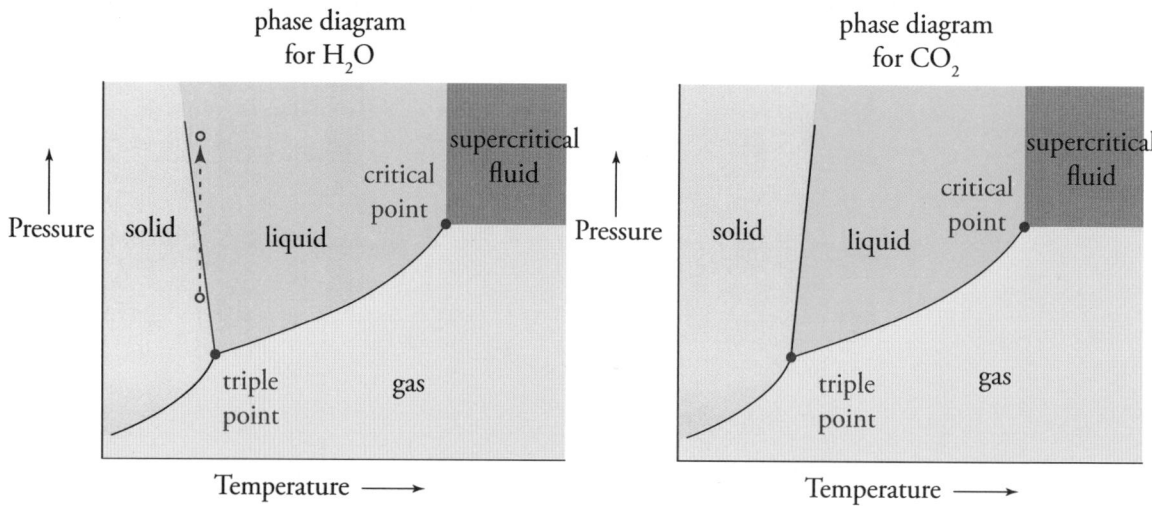

For H_2O, an increase in pressure at constant temperature can favor the *liquid* phase, not the solid phase as would be the case for most other substances (like CO_2, for example). You are probably already familiar with the following phenomenon: as the blade of an ice skate bearing all of the weight of the skater contacts the ice, the pressure increases, melting the ice under the blade and allowing the skate to glide over the liquid water. (The dashed arrow in the phase diagram for water above depicts this effect.) As the skater moves across the ice, each blade continually generates a thin layer of liquid water that refreezes as the blade passes. (This is also the reason why glaciers move.) The properties of CO_2 don't allow for skating because solid CO_2 will never turn to liquid when the pressure is increased. (And now you know why solid CO_2 is called *dry ice!*)

7.4

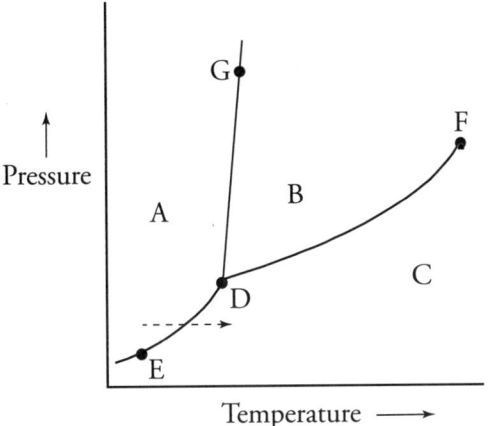

Example 7-10: In which region of the diagram above is the substance in the gas phase?

A) A
B) B
C) C
D) G

Solution: The gas phase is favored at high temperatures and low pressure, so we know that region C represents the gas phase.

Example 7-11: In which part of the diagram is gas in equilibrium with liquid?

A) Along the curve between E and D
B) Along the curve between D and G
C) Along the curve between D and F
D) In region B

Solution: The liquid phase is represented by region B and the gas phase by region C. Therefore, an equilibrium between liquid and gas phases is represented by a point on the boundary between regions B and C. This boundary is the curve between points D and F, choice C.

Example 7-12: The dashed arrow in the diagram indicates what type of phase transition?

A) Evaporation
B) Crystallization
C) Deposition
D) Sublimation

Solution: The arrow shows a substance in the solid phase (region A) moving directly to the gaseous phase (region C) without melting first. The phase transition from solid to gas is called sublimation, choice D.

Chapter 7 Summary

- Changes in pressure and/or temperature of a substance can induce changes in phase.

- The three important phases are (in order of low-to-high entropy and low-to-high internal energy) solid, liquid, and gas.

- Specific heat (c) is an intrinsic property that defines how resistant a substance is to temperature change.

- The change in temperature associated with the input or extraction of heat when phase is unchanged is given by $q = mc\Delta T$, where c is the specific heat of a substance and m is the amount (either mass or moles, depending on c).

- Heat capacity (C) is given by $C = mc$, where m is the mass of the sample. Heat capacity is a proportionality constant that defines how much heat is required to change the temperature of a sample by 1°C.

- A substance cannot simultaneously undergo a phase change and a temperature change.

- The heat associated with a phase change is given by $q = n\Delta H_{phase\ change}$, where n is the number of moles of substance (or mass if ΔH is given in energy/mass).

- Boundaries on a phase diagram correspond to equilibria between phases and phase transitions. The intersection of all three boundaries on a phase diagram is known as the triple point, and represents equilibrium between all three phases.

- The phase diagram of water is unusual in that its solid/liquid equilibrium line has a negative slope. This accounts for the fact that ice melts under increased pressure, and for why the density of ice is less than that of liquid water.

CHAPTER 7 FREESTANDING PRACTICE QUESTIONS

1. Which of the following correctly describe(s) the physical properties of water?

   I.   The hydrogen bonds in water result in a lower boiling point than H_2S.
   II. Water has a high specific heat due to the hydrogen bonding between molecules.
   III. As pressure increases liquid water is favored over solid water.

   A) II only
   B) III only
   C) II and III only
   D) I, II and III

2. As a substance goes from the gas phase to the solid phase, heat is:

   A) absorbed, internal energy decreases, and entropy decreases.
   B) released, internal energy increases, and entropy decreases.
   C) released, internal energy decreases, and entropy decreases.
   D) released, internal energy decreases, and entropy increases.

3. In the following phase transition diagram, Substance X is in the solid phase during Segment A and in the gas phase during Segment C. What process is occurring during Segment B?

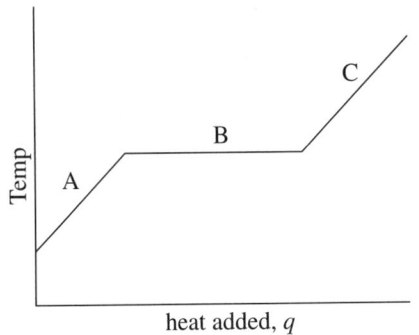

   A) The substance is warming.
   B) The substance is cooling.
   C) Sublimation
   D) Condensation

4. Denver is at a higher altitude than Los Angeles and therefore the atmospheric pressure is lower in Denver than in Los Angeles. Compared to Los Angeles, the melting point of water in Denver will be:

   A) higher.
   B) lower.
   C) the same.
   D) undetermined from the information given.

5. At 1 atm, deionized water can remain a liquid at temperatures down to –42°C. If a foreign body is added to the supercooled liquid, it will immediately turn into ice. Which of the following is true about this process?

   A) The reaction is exothermic.
   B) Tap water could also be supercooled to –42°C.
   C) The transformation of a supercooled fluid to a solid is nonspontaneous.
   D) Water's unique phase diagram allows it to be supercooled.

6. A pot containing 0.5 L of water at sea level is brought to 100°C. It is insulated around its sides to minimize heat loss to the environment, and heat is applied at the bottom of the container at a rate of 6 kJ/min over 3 minutes. What is the resulting temperature of the water?
   (ΔH_{vap} = 40.7 kJ/mol; $c(g)$ = 1.9 kJ/kg · °C; $c(l)$ = 4.2 kJ/kg · °C)

   A) 115°C
   B) 108°C
   C) 104°C
   D) 100°C

CHAPTER 7 PRACTICE PASSAGE

Lyophilization, or freeze drying, is a technique used to remove water from samples. Lyophilization uses sublimation to convert frozen, solid water directly to water vapor. This technique offers advantages over liquid-solvent removal techniques in that it can be performed at low temperatures, resulting in minimal damage to heat-sensitive samples.

A chamber containing the sample solution is attached to the lyophilizer, which freezes the sample at a temperature less than 0°C and then applies a vacuum, generally holding a pressure less than 0.006 atm. Under these conditions the frozen water sublimes and water vapor is pulled from the sample chamber into a condenser held at −50°C, where it is refrozen and held immobile.

The phase diagram for water is shown below, with its unique negatively sloped equilibrium line between the solid and liquid phases. At low pressures the solid phase of water is favored as long as any solute in the water is reasonably dilute. However, the freezing point of water decreases as the concentration of solute is increased. If concentrated enough, the sample can melt instead of sublime when pressure is decreased. In addition, volatile solvents often cannot be removed from the chamber by the condenser, as their freezing point at low pressures is below −50°C. Volatile solvents remaining in the gaseous environment can compound the impurity of the remaining water, favoring the liquid phase even more.

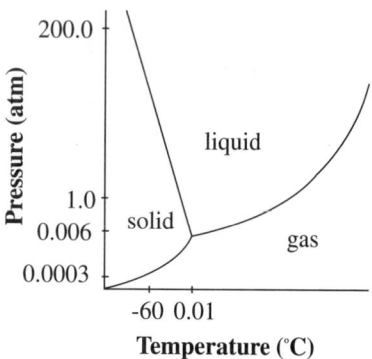

Figure 1 Phase diagram of water

1. The addition of which of the following substances is most likely to result in the melting of a sample during lyophilization?

   A) $(CH_3)_2CHOH$
   B) CH_3CH_2COOH
   C) $CH_3CH_2OCH_2CH_3$
   D) $CH_3(CH_2)_4OH$

2. If the temperature inside the chamber is −60°C, what pressure must the chamber be at in order for the sublimation reaction to be at equilibrium?

   A) 3×10^{-4} atm
   B) 3×10^{-3} atm
   C) 1 atm
   D) 125 atm

3. Lyophilization would most likely be employed industrially in which of the following separations?

   A) Salicylic acid dissolved in methanol
   B) An enzyme in aqueous solution
   C) NaCl in water
   D) A small molecular drug dissolved in dichloromethane

4. Sublimation of water inside the sample chamber causes the temperature of the chamber to:

   A) increase.
   B) decrease.
   C) stay the same.
   D) change in a manner dependent on the identity of the solvent.

5. The heat of sublimation of water is 46 kJ/mol. If heat is transferred to the sample by the environment at a rate of 0.1 kJ/min, approximately how long will it take to lyophilize 40 cm³ of frozen water (density = 0.91 g/mL)?

   A) 7.7 hours
   B) 15.3 hours
   C) 77.0 hours
   D) 153.0 hours

SOLUTIONS TO CHAPTER 7 FREESTANDING PRACTICE QUESTIONS

1. **C**   Since water experiences hydrogen bonding, more energy is required to boil water compared with SH_2, which leads to a higher boiling point, making Item I false and eliminating choice D. Since temperature is a measure of molecular motion, and hydrogen bonds bind molecules together, making this motion more difficult, hydrogen-bonded materials will require more energy to increase T and thus have high specific heats. Item II is true and choice B can be eliminated. The negative slope of the line between the solid and liquid phase on the phase diagram of water indicates that at higher pressures, liquid water is favored over solid, making Item III correct and C the best answer choice.

2. **C**   As a substance undergoes deposition, it becomes a much more ordered substance, decreasing entropy (eliminate choice D). In addition, heat will be released (eliminate choice A) because the potential energy of the substance decreases (eliminate choice B).

3. **C**   Substance X is changing from a solid to a gas during Segment B. This is an example of sublimation. Note that choices A and B cannot be correct answer choices because the temperature of Substance X remains constant during Segment B. Condensation occurs when a gas becomes a liquid, so choice D is eliminated.

4. **A**   On a P vs. T phase diagram of water, the solid-liquid equilibrium line has a negative slope for water. Water's melting point increases with decreasing external pressure. Therefore, in Denver the melting point of water is higher than in Los Angeles.

5. **A**   Upon nucleation with a foreign body, supercooled water will transition from liquid to solid phase. This phase transition (crystallization) requires heat to be released since intermolecular interactions are formed. Choice B is eliminated because tap water contains many dissolved particles that can serve as sites of nucleation. Choice C is incorrect because the supercooled fluids are only kinetically stabilized against freezing, and their transformation to a solid form is thermodynamically spontaneous. Since pressure remains constant, the negative sloped solid-liquid equilibrium line in water's phase diagram does not play a role in supercooling, eliminating Choice D.

6. **D**   The addition of 6 kJ/min for three minutes imparts 18 kJ of heat to the sample. However, since the ΔH_{vap} of water is 40.7 kJ/mol, and 0.5 L is roughly 28 mol (1 L of $H_2O \approx 55$ mol), there is nowhere near enough heat provided to vaporize the entire sample. As such, all the heat given to the sample is going toward vaporization and not toward increasing temperature. The temperature will remain constant at 100°C.

SOLUTIONS TO CHAPTER 7 PRACTICE PASSAGE

1. **C** The passage states that volatile chemicals cannot be used in samples subjected to lyophilization because they will hinder sublimation and favor the liquid phase through melting. This is because these compounds have a high vapor pressure and cannot be removed from the system by the condenser. Choices A, B, and D are all hydrogen donors and acceptors. Choice C, diethyl ether, can only act as a hydrogen bond acceptor. Therefore, it has the weakest intermolecular forces and is the most volatile.

2. **A** On a *P* vs. *T* diagram, sublimation equilibrium is indicated by the line separating the solid and vapor phases. On the graph in Figure 1, it is shown that at –60°C, the solid/gas line is at P = 0.0003 or 3×10^{-4} atm.

3. **B** Both dichloromethane and methanol are removed as liquids at reasonably low temperatures and have freezing points far lower than water. This eliminates choices A and D. The passage states that one of the major advantages to lyophilization is that it can be performed at low temperatures, and therefore preserve the activity of heat-sensitive samples. NaCl is a salt that is stable at high temperatures, whereas enzymes are proteins that denature at high temperatures. Therefore, lyophilization is best suited as a means to remove water from aqueous protein solutions.

4. **B** Sublimation is an endothermic reaction, requiring heat input. As this reaction removes heat from the surroundings, it lowers the temperature of the surroundings, in this case, the reaction chamber. This is very similar to sweat cooling the body as it evaporates off of the skin (also an endothermic process).

5. **B** 40 cm^3 of ice is 36 g or 2 moles of water. The heat required to sublimate this sample is 46 kJ/mol(2 mol) = 92 kJ. If heat is transferred at 0.1 kJ/min, then 920 minutes are required. Dividing 920 min by 60 min/hour gives just over 15 hours. Overall:

$$\textit{Time} = (40\,\text{cm}^3)\left(\frac{0.91\,\text{g}}{\text{mL}}\right)\left(\frac{\text{mol}\,\text{H}_2\text{O}}{18\,\text{g}}\right)\left(\frac{46\,\text{kJ}}{\text{mol}}\right)\left(\frac{\text{min}}{0.1\,\text{kJ}}\right)\left(\frac{\text{hour}}{60\,\text{min}}\right)$$

$$\textit{Time} \approx (40\,\text{cm}^3)\left(\frac{0.9\,\text{g}}{\text{mL}}\right)\left(\frac{\text{mol}\,\text{H}_2\text{O}}{18\,\text{g}}\right)\left(\frac{45\,\text{kJ}}{\text{mol}}\right)\left(\frac{\text{min}}{0.1\,\text{kJ}}\right)\left(\frac{\text{hour}}{60\,\text{min}}\right)$$

$$\textit{Time} \approx 15 \text{ hours}$$

PHARMACEUTICAL COCRYSTALS OF DIFLUNISAL AND DICLOFENAC WITH THEOPHYLLINE

Artem O. Surov, Alexander P. Voronin, Alex N. Manin, Nikolay G. Manin, Lyudmila G. Kuzmina, Andrei V. Churakov, and German L. Perlovich

INTRODUCTION

The development of pharmaceutical cocrystals is one of the hot topics in the field of crystal engineering nowadays as cocrystals can fine-tune relevant physicochemical properties of active pharmaceutical ingredients (API). All pharmaceutical cocrystals can be conventionally divided into two groups: with cocrystal formers (coformers) appearing on the Generally Recognized as Safe (GRAS) list and the so-called "drug–drug" cocrystals which consist of different API molecules.

In this paper, we report new cocrystals of nonsteroidal anti-inflammatory drugs (NSAID) diflunisal (DIF) and diclofenac (DIC) with theophylline (THP) (Figure 1).

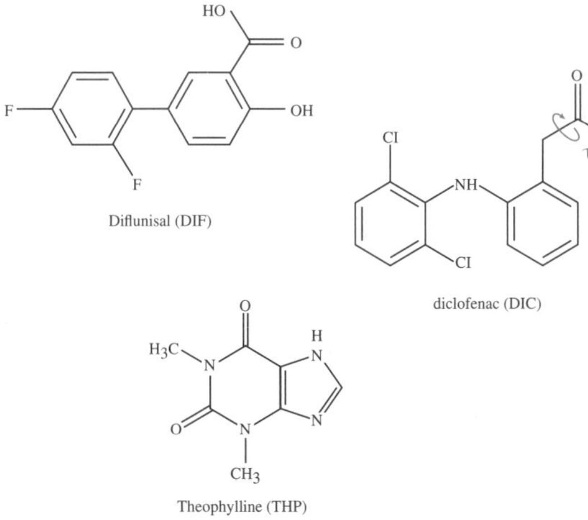

Figure 1. Molecular structures of diflunisal, diclofenac acid, and theophylline. For diclofenac acid, flexible torsion angle is indicated by τ_1.

In this study, theophylline was employed as a model cocrystal former with DIC and DIF. Theophylline is known to have good potential for cocrystal formation due to the presence of donor and acceptor sites of hydrogen bonding in the molecule. Being well soluble in water, THP is able to improve the aqueous solubility of DIC and DIF to obtain novel solid-state forms of the API with enhanced physicochemical properties. In addition, a set of data has been reported suggesting the anti-inflammatory, antiarthritic, and anti-hyperalgesia effects of theophylline. Therefore, THP cocrystals with NSAIDs are of considerable interest because of its potential application in a combination drug therapy. The cocrystals are characterized by single-crystal X-ray diffraction, differential scanning calorimetry (DSC), and solution calorimetry. In addition, analysis of crystal lattice energies of the cocrystals was done using the PIXEL approach. Pharmaceutically relevant properties such as aqueous dissolution and intrinsic dissolution rate are also reported.

MATERIAL AND METHODS

Cocrystal Preparation

Solvent-drop grinding experiments were performed using a Fritsch planetary micromill. The experiments were carried out with stoichiometric amounts of diflunisal or diclofenac and theophylline and a few drops of solvent (methanol or acetonitrile) added with a micropipette.

Crystallization Procedure

[DIF + THP] (1:1)
Equimolar amounts of diflunisal and theophylline were dissolved in an acetonitrile–methanol–water mixture (2:1:1 v:v:v) and stirred at room temperature. The resulting clear solution was filtered and allowed to evaporate slowly. Diffraction quality crystals were grown over a week.

[DIC + THP] (1:1)
Diclofenac and theophylline in a 3:1 molar ratio were dissolved in hot methanol. The obtained clear solution was slowly cooled, covered by parafilm perforated with a few small holes, and allowed to evaporate slowly. Diffraction quality crystals were obtained over few days.

X-ray Diffraction Experiments

Single-crystal X-ray diffraction data were collected on a Bruker SMART APEX II diffractometer using graphite-monochromated Mo Kα radiation (λ = 0.71073 Å).

DSC Experiments

Thermal analysis was carried out employing a DSC 204 F1 Phoenix differential scanning heat flux calorimeter (NETZSCH, Germany) with a high sensitivity μ-sensor. The sample was heated at the rate of 10 K·min^{-1} in an argon atmosphere and cooled with gaseous nitrogen.

Aqueous Dissolution and Intrinsic Dissolution Rate Experiments

Dissolution measurements were carried out by the shake-flask method at 25.0 ± 0.1 °C. The samples were suspended in 10 mL of pH 7.4 phosphate buffer in Pyrex glass tubes. The amount of DIC or DIF and the cocrystals dissolved was measured by taking aliquots of 1 mL of the respective media. The concentration was determined by HPLC. The results are stated as the average of at least three replicated experiments.

For IDR experiments, approximately 200 mg of pure DIC or DIF and the cocrystals were compressed by a hydraulic press for 5 min to form a nonporous compact of 8 mm diameter. The intrinsic attachment with the sample was rotated at 120 rpm in 500 mL of pH 7.4 phosphate buffer preheated to 37.0 °C. The cumulative amount dissolved per unit surface area was determined by taking aliquots of 1 mL of the respective media every 5–6 min with the volume replacement and concentration measured by HPLC. The slope of the plot of mass dissolved per unit surface area vs time gives the intrinsic dissolution rate in appropriate units, e.g., mg min^{-1} cm^{-2}.

Solution Calorimetry Experiments

Enthalpies of solution were measured by using an ampule-type isoperibolic calorimeter with a 50 cm^3 titanium reaction vessel.

A minimum of four measurements were made for each of the analyzed samples.

The enthalpy of formation, $\Delta H_f^T(AB)$, of a cocrystal with 1:1 stoichiometry can be calculated as $\Delta H_f^T(AB) = \Delta H_{sol}^T(A)_B + \Delta H_{sol}^T(B)_A - \Delta H_{sol}^T(AB)_B$ where $\Delta H_{sol}^T(A)_B$ and $\Delta H_{sol}^T(B)_A$ are the solution heat values for solid A in a solution containing B and solid B in a solution containing A, respectively. It is essential to consider that the solution enthalpy of one of the pure solid coformers may be affected by the presence of the other coformer in the solution. Thus, it is necessary to measure the solution heat in the presence of the second coformer. This ensures that the same solute A–solute B interactions that occur during cocrystal dissolution are accounted for in the calculation of the formation enthalpy. All experiments were conducted at T = 298.15 K.

Computational Procedure

Intermolecular interaction energies were calculated using the PIXEL approach developed by Gavezzotti.

RESULTS AND DISCUSSION

Crystal Structures

In each structure, the asymmetric unit contains API and THP molecules connected by O–H⋯N hydrogen bonds involving the carboxylic acid of the API and an unsaturated N atom of the imidazole ring of THP (acid–imidazole heterosynthon) (Figure 2). In addition, the API forms the C–H⋯O contacts with the neighboring THP molecule. The THP molecules are connected to each other by N–H⋯O hydrogen bonds to form centrosymmetric dimers that may be described in graph set notation as $R_2^2(10)$. In the [DIF + THP] crystal, DIF molecules also form dimer motifs through O–H⋯O hydrogen bonds between the hydroxyl and carboxylic groups ($R_2^2(12)$) (Figure 2b). Furthermore, the hydroxyl group of DIF accepts the C–H⋯O contacts from the neighboring THP molecule and participates in intramolecular hydrogen bond formation.

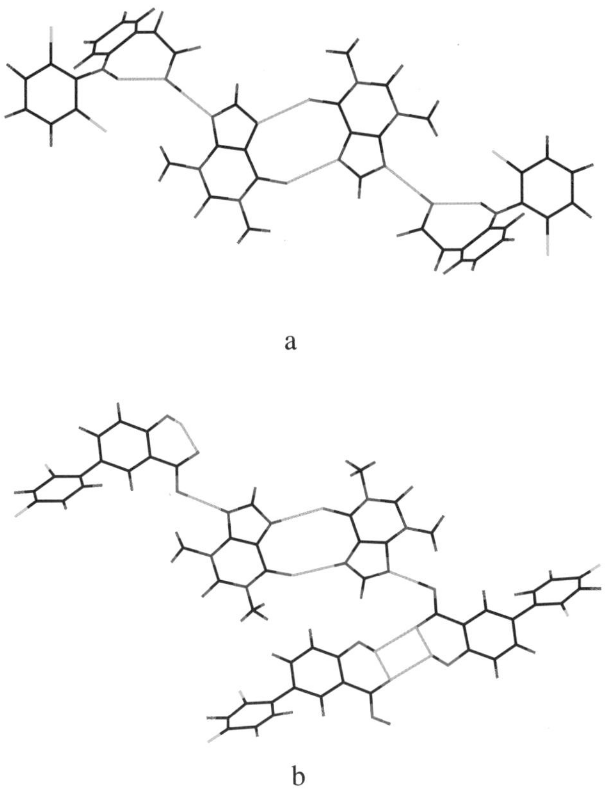

a

b

Figure 2. Hydrogen bonded supramolecular units in the crystal structures of (a) [DIC + THP] and (b) [DIF + THP].

The carboxylic group in the [DIC + THP] cocrystal is rotated by approximately 180° compared to pure DIC. A similar rotation effect of the carboxylic group in the DIC molecule is also observed in DIC cocrystals with isonicotinamide and 2-aminopyrimidine. Probably, this reflects the relatively low energy barrier for rotation of the COOH group due to the decrease in the conjugation effect and attenuation of the intramolecular hydrogen bond energy. The conformational flexibility of the COOH group promotes the most efficient hydrogen bonding between DIC and coformer molecules in a crystal.

In contrast to the [DIC + THP] cocrystal, the conformational state of DIF in [DIF + THP] is comparable to that in the known polymorphs and solvates of pure DIF. As was mentioned above, both cocrystals have a similar organization of intermolecular hydrogen bonds to form a four-component supramolecular unit which consists of a THP centrosymmetric dimer and two API molecules. It can be assumed that formation of this supramolecular

unit must be energy-profitable because of efficient crystal packing.

Crystal Lattice Energy Calculations

Table 1. Results of PIXEL Calculations: Lattice Energies (E_{latt}), Coulombic Energies (E_{coul}), Polarization Energies (E_{pol}), Dispersion Energies (E_{disp}), and Repulsion (E_{rep}) Terms in kJ·mol^{-1}

	E_{coul}	E_{pol}	E_{disp}	E_{rep}	E_{latt}
[DIC + THP]	−104.9	−50.0	−140.6	156.0	−139.6
[DIF + THP]	−108.4	−54.1	−120.9	159.4	−124.1

Calculations show that the lattice energy value obtained for [DIC + THP] is ca. 15 kJ·mol^{-1} lower than the one for [DIF + THP]. It is evident that the packing energy gain for the [DIC + THP] cocrystal is derived only from the dispersion energy which dominates the structures of the cocrystals, while the Coulombic, the polarization, and the repulsion terms are comparable. Table 3 shows sums of the intermolecular interaction energies between the different types of molecules calculated using the PIXEL method. The main energy difference is observed in API–API interactions, but the API–THP and THP–THP interactions have closely comparable total energies. Therefore, the crystal lattice energy gain for the [DIC + THP] compared to [DIF + THP] is accompanied by an increase in the energy of dispersion interactions due to more effective packing of the DIC molecules in the cocrystal. In both cases, the API–THP interactions provide the largest contribution to the lattice energy (more than 40%). The THP–THP interactions comprise approximately a quarter of the total energy, while in [DIF + THP], the contributions of the THP–THP and API–API interactions are comparable.

Table 2. Sums of the Intermolecular Interaction Energies (kJ·mol^{-1}) between the Different Types of Molecules Calculated Using the PIXEL Method

	API–API	API–THP	THP–THP	total
[DIC + THP]	−47.6	−57.0	−34.9	−139.6
	(34.1%)	(40.8%)	(25.0%)	
[DIF + THP]	−34.3	−56.5	−33.3	−124.1
	(27.7%)	(45.5%)	(26.8%)	

Thermal Analysis and Solution Calorimetry

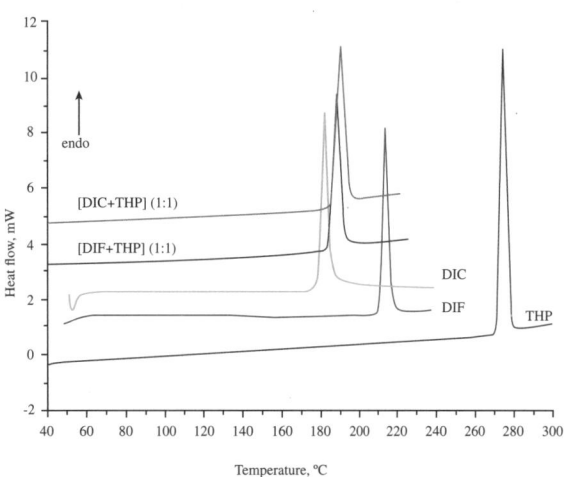

Figure 3. DSC curves of the cocrystals, diclofenac acid, diflunisal, and theophylline recorded at 10 °C·min^{-1} heating rate.

Table 3. Thermophysical Data for the Cocrystals, Compared to DIC, DIF, and THP

	T_{fus}, °C (onset)	ΔH_{fus}, kJ mol^{-1}	ΔS_{fus}, J mol^{-1} K^{-1}
[DIC + THP]	186.9 ± 0.3	70.6 ± 2.0	153.4
[DIF + THP]	184.8 ± 0.4	61.5 ± 2.0	134.2
DIC	179.8 ± 0.2	40.9 ± 0.7	90.2
DIF	211.8 ± 0.2	36.0 ± 0.5	74.3
THP	271.3 ± 0.2	29.6 ± 0.5	65.2

DSC thermograms show only one major endotherm for the cocrystals which corresponds to the melting process, whereas other phase transitions are not observed. The difference in the melting temperatures between different APIs is equal to ca. 38 °C, while the difference in T_{fus} between APIs and THP is more than 70 °C. However, the cocrystals' melting points are closely comparable. As it is seen, the melting temperature of [DIC + THP] is higher than that of pure API. In the case of [DIF + THP], the cocrystal formation decreases the melting temperature compared to the pure DIF. It seems that the intermolecular interactions (including hydrogen bonds), which are responsible for the thermal stability of the pure DIC crystal, are energetically comparable to those in the [DIC + THP] cocrystal. For DIF, however, change of the supramolecular

surroundings leads to formation of intermolecular contacts, which are less thermally stable. In spite of the marginal difference in the melting temperatures (ca. 2 °C), the cocrystal fusion enthalpies are distinguishable (ca. 9 kJ mol^{-1}), indicating a greater stability of [DIC + THP], which is qualitatively consistent with the PIXEL calculations.

Table 4. Solution Enthalpies, ΔH_{sol}^{0}, (in Methanol) and Calculated Enthalpies of Formation, ΔH_{f}^{0}, at 298 K (kJ mol^{-1})

	ΔH_{sol}° (API + THP^{ab})	ΔH_{sol}° (API)$_{THP}$a	ΔH_{sol}° (THP)$_{API}$b	ΔH_{f}° (API + THP^{ab})
[DIC + THP]	46.3 ± 0.5	17.2 ± 0.2	24.2 ± 0.2	−4.8 ± 0.9
[DIF + THP]	47.1 ± 0.2	14.5 ± 0.3	21.4 ± 0.2	−11.2 ± 0.7

a Heat of solution of APIs in the presence of THP.
b Heat of solution of THP in the presence of APIs.

In contrast to the fusion enthalpies, the solution enthalpies of the cocrystals coincide within experimental error, which seems to be a likely influence of the solvation effects. It should be noted that the formation enthalpy is an integral parameter which incorporates the sum of energetic and structural changes of the system. Such important interactions in a crystal as hydrogen bonds make a significant contribution to the formation enthalpies. In this case, however, small values of the formation enthalpies indicate that a large portion of that contribution was used to compensate for the breaking of the lattice energy of the original components. In fact, cocrystal formation between APIs and THP leads to considerable changes in the supramolecular surroundings for both components compared to their initial state. The experimental formation enthalpies suggest that energies of hydrogen bonds in the cocrystals and pure components are comparable, and the packing energy gain is obtained mainly from weak van der Waals forces.

Solubility and Intrinsic Dissolution Rate (IDR)

It is known that solubility and dissolution rate in aqueous media are key parameters among other physicochemical properties for pharmaceutical cocrystals.

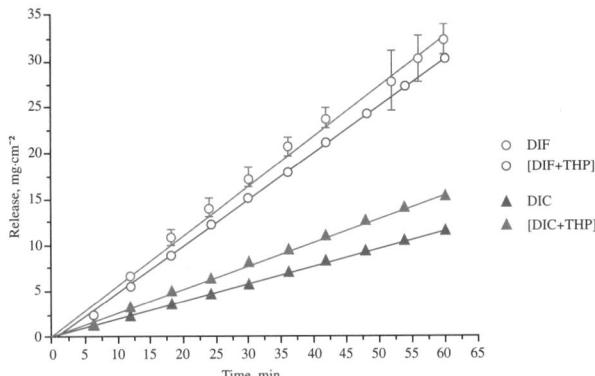

Figure 4. Intrinsic dissolution rates of the cocrystals and APIs in pH 7.4 phosphate buffer at 37.0 °C. The results are expressed as mean ± SD, n = 3.

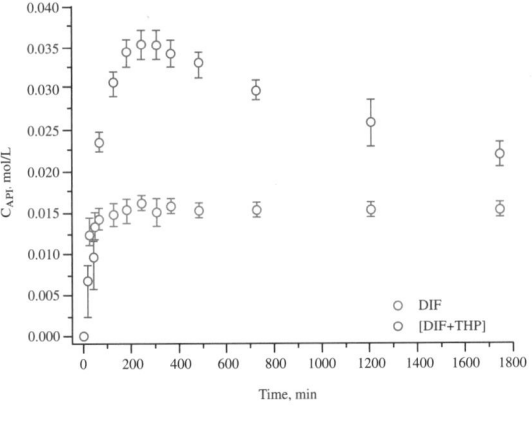

a

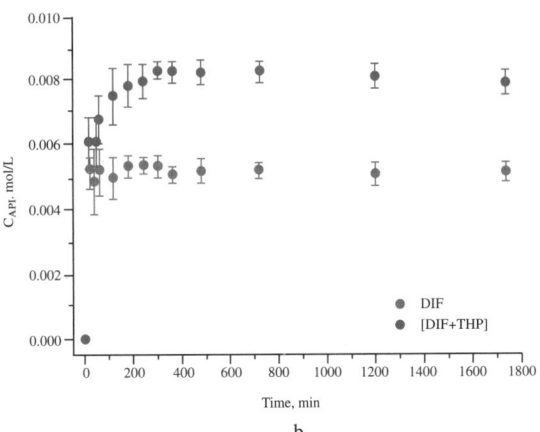

b

Figure 5. Dissolution profiles for (a) DIF and [DIF + THP] and (b) DIC and [DIC + THP] in pH 7.4 phosphate buffer at 25.0 °C. The results are expressed as mean ± SD, n = 3.

Figure 4 shows that the intrinsic dissolution rate of [DIF + THP] is comparable to that of pure DIF. In the case of [DIC + THP], the dissolution rate of the cocrystal form is found to be ca. 1.3 times higher compared to the initial API. Therefore, in the pH 7.4 phosphate buffer under consideration, the cocrystallization of DIF and DIC with THP has almost no influence on the intrinsic dissolution rate of the pure APIs. It should be noted that similar results have been reported for various pharmaceutical cocrystals with THP.

In the case of a longer-term dissolution experiment, the cocrystals behave differently compared to a relatively short-time IDR study. Figure 5a shows that, after ca. 300 min (5 h) of [DIF + THP] dissolution, the amount of DIF reaches the maximum concentration, which is higher by a factor of 2.3 compared to the pure DIF solubility. As is seen, the dissolution profile for [DIF + THP] demonstrates a classical so-called "spring and parachute" behavior. This concept has been introduced to describe the dissolution process of cocrystals in aqueous media. (1d, 1e, 1h, 35) For the [DIF + THP] cocrystal, a 5 h time period corresponds to the "spring" phase. This is followed by a longer-term "parachute" phase, when slow crystallization and precipitation of the unstable DIF species occurs. The latter process lasts the following 25 h. In the case of the [DIC + THP] system (Figure 5b), the "spring" effect is not so evident. After 5–6 h of dissolution, the concentration of [DIC + THP] cocrystal is equal to ca. 1.6 times the solubility of pure DIC. It should be noted that the enhanced concentration level of DIC remains stable for quite a long time (at least 25 h), which indicates a greater stability of [DIC + THP] in aqueous media compared to [DIF + THP]. It has been established in the literature that an increase in the cocrystal solubility of a poorly soluble API is effectively correlated with an enhancement of its oral bioavailability. Therefore, the results of the dissolution experiments suggest that a bioavailability of DIC and DIF can be increased by cocrystallization of the drugs with THP.

CONCLUSIONS

Pharmaceutical cocrystals of nonsteroidal anti-inflammatory drugs diflunisal and diclofenac with theophylline were obtained, and their crystal structures were determined. Both cocrystals show a similar organization of intermolecular hydrogen bonds to form a four-component supramolecular unit, which consists of a centrosymmetric THP dimer and two API molecules. PIXEL calculations reveal that the crystal lattice energy of

[DIC + THP] is higher than that of [DIF + THP] on account of increased dispersion energy between the DIC molecules. The cocrystal formation enthalpies are small. It suggests that energies of hydrogen bonds in the cocrystals and pure components are comparable, and the packing energy gain is obtained mainly from weak van der Waals forces. The intrinsic dissolution studies show that [DIF + THP] IDR is comparable to that of pure DIF. In the case of [DIC + THP], the cocrystal form dissolution rate is found to be ca. 1.3 times higher compared to the initial API. The aqueous dissolution profile of [DIF + THP] demonstrates a classical "spring and parachute" shape, while for [DIC + THP] the "spring" effect cannot be easily seen. The cocrystals show the enhanced apparent solubility compared to the corresponding pure APIs.

JOURNAL ARTICLE EXERCISE 1

The science sections on the MCAT include a significant number of passages with experiments. Questions for these passages often ask you to analyze data, read charts and graphs, and come to some reasonable conclusion based on the information they give you. If you don't know how to extract information efficiently and analyze data effectively, you will be at a distinct disadvantage.

There are three "Journal Article Exercises" in this book. In this first exercise, we'll show you the type of information you should be able to extract from the article and the sorts of things to pay attention to in the data. In the subsequent exercise, you'll do more of that on your own, and in the final exercise we'll show you how that article might get turned into an MCAT-style passage.

When analyzing an experiment, you should be able to:

- identify the controls.
- extract information from graphs and data tables.
- determine how the experimental groups change relative to the control.
- come to a reasonable conclusion about WHY the results were observed.
- consider potential weaknesses in the study.
- decide what the next most logical experiment or study should be.

The goal of these exercises is NOT to learn content from the articles, just to get a little more comfortable reading and extracting information from them.

For the (abridged) article on pages 157–162, try to summarize the purpose of the experiment and the methods in 4–5 sentences. Consider the following questions:

1. What is being studied? Why is it important?
2. What is new about these results?
3. What was measured?
4. How are the results presented?
5. What (if anything) was the experimental group compared to?
6. Are any of the results unexpected?

Try interpreting the data on your own before reading the results/discussion section. When you do read the discussion, consider:

7. How are the conclusions of the authors supported by the data?
8. What potential weaknesses or flaws do you see in the experimental design? Are these addressed in the discussion section?
9. What would be the next most logical experiment?

SOLUTIONS TO JOURNAL ARTICLE EXERCISE 1

Let's answer those questions for the article on the previous pages.

1. **What is being studied? Why is it important?**

   Physical properties of diflunisal/theophylline cocrystals and diclofenac/theophylline cocrystals were studied. Cocrystallization can alter physical properties of pharmaceuticals, which might make them more stable or more bioavailable.

2. **What is new about these results?**

   Theophylline has been used as a coformer for other drugs, but not these ones.

3. **What was measured?**

   Crystal structures, crystal lattice energy (by calculation), melting point, ΔH_{fus}, ΔS_{fus}, ΔH_{soln}, solubility, dissolution rate humidities

4. **How are the results presented?**

   Crystal structures: figure. Crystal lattice energy (by calculation): table. Melting point: graph, table. ΔH_{fus}, ΔS_{fus}: table. ΔH_{soln}: table. Solubility: graph. Dissolution rate: Graph.

5. **What (if anything) was the experimental group compared to?**

   The measured properties of the DIC-THP and DIF-THP cocrystals were compared to each other, as well as to those of pure DIC, pure DIF, and pure THP.

6. **Are any of the results unexpected?**

   The increase in the mp of DIC-THP cocrystal relative to pure DIC is surprising: impurities usually disrupt the crystal lattice and lower the melting point. Also, the "spring and parachute" dissolution behavior of DIF is interesting—the solution becomes supersaturated before the concentration drops off.

7. **How are the conclusions of the authors supported by the data?**

   The authors synthesize data from empirical sources (single-crystal diffraction structures, calorimetry) as well as calculations to support their statements about the contributions made by hydrogen bonding and dispersion forces to cocrystal stability. The authors tested both short- and long-term dissolution behavior of the cocrystals.

8. **What potential weaknesses or flaws do you see in the experimental design? Are these addressed in the discussion section?**

   Solubility tested at only one pH. This was not discussed in the discussion section.

9. **What would be the next most logical experiment?**

   Extend pH range of solubility tests, test thermal stability of cocrystals, and test cocrystals *in vitro* or *in vivo* to see whether enhanced bioavailability is maintained.

Summary of experiment and results:

- In order to explore the effect of cocrystallization on diclofenac and diflunisal, the authors grew diclofenac-theophylline (DIC-THP) and diflunisal-theophylline (DIF-THP) cocrystals. Single-crystal X-ray diffraction studies revealed several similarities in the cocrystal structures. Calculations suggest that the (DIC-THP) cocrystal displays a greater crystal lattice energy due to stronger dispersion forces in the (DIC-THP) cocrystal. Cocrystallization with THP does not seem to affect the dissolution rate of DIF. However, the (DIC-THP) cocrystal has an increased dissolution rate compared to pure DIC. Both cocrystals exhibit enhanced water solubility relative to the pure drugs.

Chapter 8
Gases

8.1 GASES AND THE KINETIC-MOLECULAR THEORY

Unlike the condensed phases of matter (solids and liquids), **gases** have no fixed volume. A gas will fill all the available space in a container. Gases are *far* more compressible than solids or liquids, and their densities are very low (roughly 1 kg/m³ at standard temperature and pressure), about three to four orders of magnitude less than those of solids and liquids. But the most striking difference between a gas and a solid or liquid is that the molecules of a gas are free to move over large distances.

The most important properties of a gas are its **pressure, volume,** and **temperature**. How these macroscopic properties are related to each other can be derived from some basic assumptions concerning the *microscopic* behavior of gas molecules. These assumptions are the foundation of the **kinetic-molecular theory**.

Kinetic-molecular theory, a model for describing the behavior of gases, is based on the following assumptions:

1) The molecules of a gas are so small compared to the average spacing between them that the molecules themselves take up essentially no volume.

2) The molecules of a gas are in constant motion, moving in straight lines at constant speeds and in random directions between collisions. The collisions of the molecules with the walls of the container define the **pressure** of the gas (the average force exerted per unit area), and all collisions—molecules striking the walls and each other—are *elastic* (that is, the total kinetic energy is the same after the collision as it was before).

3) Since each molecule moves at a constant speed between collisions and the collisions are elastic, the molecules of a gas experience no intermolecular forces.

4) The molecules of a gas span a distribution of speeds, and the average kinetic energy of the molecules is directly proportional to the absolute temperature (the temperature in kelvins) of the sample: $KE_{avg} \propto T$.

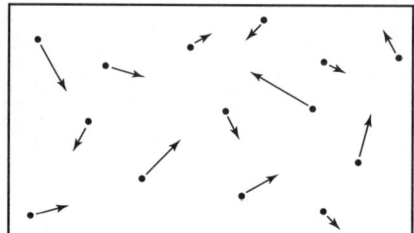

A gas that satisfies all these requirements is said to be an **ideal gas.** Most real gases behave like ideal gases under ordinary conditions, so the results that follow from the kinetic-molecular theory can be applied to real gases.

Units of Volume, Temperature, and Pressure

Volume

The SI unit for volume is the cubic meter (m³), but in chemistry, the **cubic centimeter (cm³** or **cc)** and **liter (L)** are commonly used. One cubic meter is equal to one thousand liters.

$$1 \text{ cm}^3 = 1 \text{ cc} = 1 \text{ mL} \quad \text{and} \quad 1 \text{ m}^3 = 1000 \text{ L}$$

Temperature

Temperature may be expressed in degrees Fahrenheit, degrees Celsius, or in kelvins (not degrees Kelvin). In scientific work, the Celsius scale is popular: in it water freezes at 0°C and boils at 100°C (at standard atmospheric pressure). However, the "proper" unit for expressing temperatures is the kelvin (K), and this is the one we use when talking about gases (because of assumption #4 stated above for the kinetic-molecular theory). The relationship between kelvins and degrees Celsius is simple:

$$T \text{ (in K)} = T \text{ (in °C)} + 273.15$$

When dealing with gases, the best unit for expressing temperature is the kelvin (K). This is an absolute temperature scale whereby zero kelvin (0 K) defines a point of zero entropy (see Chapter 6) where molecular motion is at a minimum. From a practical perspective, this avoids the issue of calculations involving negative temperatures, so all of the gas laws equations on the MCAT require the use of absolute temperatures.

Pressure

Since pressure is defined as force per unit area, the SI unit for pressure is the **pascal** (abbreviated **Pa**), where $1 \text{ Pa} = 1 \text{ N/m}^2$. The unit is inconveniently small for normal calculations involving gases (for example, a nickel sitting on a table exerts about 140 Pa of pressure), so several alternative units for pressure are usually used.

At sea level, atmospheric pressure is about 101,300 pascals (or 100 kPa for MCAT math); this is 1 **atmosphere** (1 **atm**). Related to the atmosphere is the **torr**, where 1 atm = 760 torr. (Therefore, 1 torr is about the same as the pressure exerted by a nickel sitting on a table.) At 0°C, 1 torr is equal to 1 **mm Hg** (**millimeter of mercury**), so we generally just take 1 atm to equal 760 mm Hg:

$$1 \text{ atm} = 760 \text{ torr} = 760 \text{ mm Hg} = 101.3 \text{ kPa}$$

Standard Temperature and Pressure

Standard Temperature and Pressure (STP) means a temperature of 0°C (273.15 K) and a pressure of 1 atm.

Example 8-1: A temperature of 273°C is equivalent to:

A) −100 K.
B) 0 K.
C) 100 K.
D) 546 K.

Solution: Choice A is eliminated, because negative values are not permitted when using the Kelvin temperature scale. Since $T \text{ (in K)} = T \text{ (in °C)} + 273$, we have

$$T \text{ (in K)} = 273 + 273 = 546 \text{ K}$$

Therefore, choice D is the answer.

8.2 THE IDEAL GAS LAW

The volume, temperature, and pressure of an ideal gas are related by a simple equation called the **ideal gas law**. Most real gases under ordinary conditions act very much like ideal gases, so the ideal gas law applies to most gas behavior:

Ideal Gas Law

$$PV = nRT$$

---

where

P = the pressure of the gas in atmospheres
V = the volume of the container in liters
n = the number of moles of the gas
R = the universal gas constant, 0.0821 L·atm/K·mol
T = the absolute temperature of the gas (that is, T in kelvins)

Questions on gas behavior typically take one of two forms. The first type of question simply gives you some facts, and you use $PV = nRT$ to determine a missing variable. In the second type, "before" and "after" scenarios are presented for which you determine the effect of changing the volume, temperature, or pressure. In this case, you apply the ideal gas law twice, once for each scenario. We'll solve a typical example of each type of question.

1. If two moles of helium at 27°C fill a 3 L balloon, what is the pressure?

Take the ideal gas law, solve it for P, then substitute the numbers (and don't forget to convert the temperature in °C to kelvin!):

$$PV = nRT$$

$$P = \frac{nRT}{V}$$

$$P = \frac{(2 \text{ mol})(0.082 \text{ L·atm/K·mol})(300 \text{ K})}{3 \text{ L}}$$

$$P = 16 \text{ atm}$$

2. Argon, at a pressure of 2 atm, fills a 100 mL vial at a temperature of 0°C. What would the pressure of the argon be if we increase the volume to 500 mL, and the temperature is 100°C?

We're not told how much argon (the number of moles, n) is in the vial, but it doesn't matter since it doesn't change. Since R is also a constant, the ratio of PV/T, which is equal to nR, remains constant. Therefore,

$$\frac{P_1 V_1}{T_1} = \frac{P_2 V_2}{T_2} \quad \Rightarrow \quad P_2 = P_1 \frac{V_1}{V_2}\frac{T_2}{T_1}$$

$$P_2 = (2\ \text{atm})\left[\frac{0.1\ \text{L}}{0.5\ \text{L}}\right]\left[\frac{373\ \text{K}}{273\ \text{K}}\right]$$

$$P_2 = 0.55\ \text{atm}$$

P-V-T Gas Laws in Systems Where n Is Constant

As we saw in answering Question 2 above, the amount of gas often remains the same, and the n drops out (we make this assumption in the equations that follow). Our work can be simplified even further if the pressure, temperature, or volume is also held constant. (And remember: when working with the gas laws, *temperature* always means *absolute temperature* [that is, T in kelvins].)

- If the pressure is constant, $V/T = k$ (where k is a constant). Therefore, the volume is proportional to the temperature: $V \propto T$

This is known as **Charles's law**. If the pressure is to remain constant, then a gas will expand when heated and contract when cooled. If the temperature of the gas is increased, the molecules will move faster, hitting the walls of the container with more force; in order to keep the pressure the same, the frequency of the collisions would need to be reduced. This is accomplished by expanding the volume. With more available space, the molecules strike the walls less often in order to compensate for hitting them harder.

- If the temperature is constant, $PV = k$ (where k is a constant). Therefore, the pressure is inversely proportional to the volume: $P \propto 1/V$

This is known as **Boyle's law**. If the volume decreases, the molecules have less space to move around in. As a result, they'll collide with the walls of the container more often, and the pressure increases. On the other hand, if the volume of the container increases, the gas molecules have more available space and collide with the walls less often, resulting in a lower pressure.

- If the volume is constant, $P/T = k$ (where k is a constant). Therefore, the pressure is proportional to the temperature: $P \propto T$

If the temperature goes up, so does the pressure. This should make sense when you consider the origin of pressure. As the temperature increases, the molecules move faster. As a result, they strike the walls of the container surface more often and with greater speed.

Since each of the two-variable relationships reviewed above are equal to a constant as described, this means that the product or quotient will not change if we meet the specified assumptions (hold the other variables constant). This allows us to generate equations where we compare properties of a gas under two different conditions:

In a system with constant n:

At constant P: $\dfrac{V_1}{T_1} = \dfrac{V_2}{T_2}$

At constant T: $P_1V_1 = P_2V_2$

At constant V: $\dfrac{P_1}{T_1} = \dfrac{P_2}{T_2}$

If only n (which tells us the amount of gas) stays constant, we can combine Boyle's Law and Charles's Law to get the **combined gas law** (which we used to answer Question 2 above):

Combined Gas Law (constant n)

$$\frac{P_1V_1}{T_1} = \frac{P_2V_2}{T_2}$$

Example 8-2: Helium, at a pressure of 3 atm, occupies a 16 L container at a temperature of 30°C. What would be the volume of the gas if the pressure were increased to 5 atm and the temperature lowered to –20°C?

Solution: We use the combined gas law after remembering to convert the given temperatures to kelvin:

$$\frac{P_1V_1}{T_1} = \frac{P_2V_2}{T_2} \;\Rightarrow\; V_2 = V_1\frac{P_1}{P_2}\frac{T_2}{T_1} = (16\text{ L})\left(\frac{3\text{ atm}}{5\text{ atm}}\right)\left(\frac{253\text{ K}}{303\text{ K}}\right) \approx (16\text{ L})\left(\frac{3}{5}\right)\left(\frac{250\text{ K}}{300\text{ K}}\right) = 8\text{ L}$$

All of these laws follow from the ideal gas law and can be derived easily from it. They tell us what happens when n and P are constant, when n and T are constant, when n and V are constant, and in the case of the combined gas law, when n alone is constant. But what about n when P, V, and T are constant? That law of gases was proposed by Avogadro:

- If two equal-volume containers hold gas at the same pressure and temperature, then they contain the same number of particles (regardless of the identity of the gas).

Avogadro's law can be restated more broadly as **$V/n = k$** (where k is a constant). We can also determine the **standard molar volume** of an ideal gas at STP, which is the volume that one mole of a gas—any *ideal* gas—would occupy at 0°C and 1 atm of pressure:

$$V = \frac{nRT}{P} = \frac{(1\text{ mol})(0.0821\,\text{L·atm/K·mol})(273\text{ K})}{1\text{ atm}} = 22.4\text{ L}$$

To give you an idea of how much this is, 22.4 L is equal to the total volume of three basketballs.

Avogrado's law and the **standard molar volume** of a gas can be used to simplify some gas law problems. Consider the following questions:

> **3.** Given the Haber process, $3 H_2(g) + N_2(g) \rightarrow 2 NH_3(g)$, if you start with 5 L of $H_2(g)$ and 4 L of $N_2(g)$ at STP, what will the volume of the three gases be when the reaction is complete?

We can answer this question by using the ideal gas law, or we can recognize that the only thing changing is n (the number of moles of each gas) and use the standard molar volume. If we further recognize that the standard molar volume is the same for all three gases, and it is this value that we'd use to convert each given volume into moles (and then vice versa), we can use the balanced equation to quickly determine the answer.

Since we need 3 L of H_2 for every 1 L of N_2, and we have 4 L of N_2 but only 5 L of H_2, H_2 will be the limiting reagent, and its volume will be zero at the end of the reaction. Since 1 L of N_2 is needed for every 3 L of H_2, we get

$$5 \text{ L of } H_2 \times \frac{1 \text{ L of } N_2}{3 \text{ L of } H_2} = 1.7 \text{ L of } N_2$$

So the amount of N_2 remaining will be $4 - 1.7 = 2.3$ L. The volume of NH_3 produced is

$$5 \text{ L of } H_2 \times \frac{2 \text{ L of } NH_3}{3 \text{ L of } H_2} = 3.3 \text{ L of } NH_3$$

Example 8-3: Three moles of oxygen gas are present in a 10 L chamber at a temperature of 25°C. Which one of the following expressions is equal to the pressure of the gas (in atm)?

A) (3)(0.08)(10)/25
B) (3)(0.08)(25)/10
C) (3)(0.08)(10)/298
D) (3)(0.08)(298)/10

Solution: Since 25°C = 298 K, the ideal gas law gives

$$P = \frac{nRT}{V} = \frac{(3)(0.08)(298)}{10} \text{ atm}$$

The answer is D.

Example 8-4: An ideal gas at 2 atm occupies a 5-liter tank. It is then transferred to a new tank of volume 12 liters. If temperature is held constant throughout, what is the new pressure?

Solution: Since n and T are constants, we can use Boyle's law to find

$$P_1V_1 = P_2V_2 \quad \Rightarrow \quad P_2 = P_1\frac{V_1}{V_2} = (2 \text{ atm})\frac{5 \text{ L}}{12 \text{ L}} = \frac{5}{6} \text{ atm}$$

Example 8-5: A 6-liter container holds $H_2(g)$ at a temperature of 400 K and a pressure of 3 atm. If the temperature is increased to 600 K, what will be the pressure?

Solution: Since n and V are constants, we can write

$$\frac{P_1}{T_1} = \frac{P_2}{T_2} \quad \Rightarrow \quad P_2 = P_1 \frac{T_2}{T_1} = (3 \text{ atm}) \frac{600 \text{ K}}{400 \text{ K}} = 4.5 \text{ atm}$$

Example 8-6: How many atoms of helium are present in 11.2 liters of the gas at $P = 1$ atm and $T = 273$ K?

- A) 3.01×10^{23}
- B) 6.02×10^{23}
- C) 1.20×10^{24}
- D) Cannot be determined from the information given

Solution: $P = 1$ atm and $T = 273$ K define STP, so 1 mole of an ideal gas would occupy 22.4 L. A volume of 11.2 L is exactly half this so it must correspond to a 0.5 mole sample. Since 1 mole of helium contains 6.02×10^{23} atoms, 0.5 mole contains half this many: 3.01×10^{23} (choice A).

8.3 DEVIATIONS FROM IDEAL-GAS BEHAVIOR

Let's review two of the assumptions that were listed for the kinetic-molecular theory:

1) The particles of an ideal gas experience no intermolecular forces.
2) The volume of the individual particles of an ideal gas is negligible compared to the volume of the gas container.

Under some conditions, namely high pressures and low temperatures, these assumptions don't hold up very well, and the laws for ideal gases don't rigorously apply to real gases.

To determine the effect of non-ideality on gases on a macroscopic level, work though the following thought experiments, which examine each assumption above independently:

1) *No intermolecular forces:*

   Imagine blowing up a balloon to a given volume with an ideal gas. Now, fix the volume of the container and allow the gas to behave as a real gas with strongly attractive intermolecular forces (e.g., like water vapor would have). How will the pressure change? Remember that the number of collisions gas particles have with the container walls (and their momentum) determines pressure. While the particles in a real gas have attractive intermolecular forces, they do not have the same attractive forces with the walls. Increased particle interactions therefore lead to fewer collisions with the walls of the container, and the collisions that do occur will involve a smaller transfer of momentum than they would have if the gas were ideal and all collisions perfectly elastic. The resulting pressure of the real gas is therefore smaller than if the gas were ideal, or $P_{real} < P_{ideal}$.

2) *Volumeless particles:*

Imagine blowing up a balloon with an ideal gas somewhere half-way through the atmosphere of Jupiter (with its high pressures), then fix the pressure of the ideal gas system after it equilibrates with external pressure. Now, instead of the ideal volumeless particles, give the individual gas particles finite volumes. How does the volume of the gas change? The tricky part here is that the volume of a gas is defined as the free space the particles have in which to move around. For an ideal gas this volume is simply the volume of the container, since there is no volume taken up by individual particles. However, at high pressures the volume occupied by each gas particle becomes a greater proportion of the gas sample, so it is no longer negligible, and reduces the free space available for particle movement. The overall effect is to decrease the volume, making $V_{real} < V_{ideal}$.

From these two thought experiments we see that the attractive forces between particles cause a decrease in pressure if the volume of the container is fixed, and accounting for particle volume causes a decrease in free space (system volume) if the pressure is fixed. As these two variables interact with many others in a real system, we can sometimes see deviations from the general principles outlined here, especially at exceedingly high pressures.[1] However, complex situations like this are beyond the scope of the MCAT, so we will focus our analysis on the deviations as described above.

To make accurate predictions about the deviations real gases show from ideal-gas behavior, the ideal gas law must be altered. The **van der Waals equation** includes terms to account for the differences in the observed behavior of real gases and calculated properties of ideal gases:

$$P_{real} = \left(\frac{nRT}{V - nb} \right) - \left(\frac{an^2}{V^2} \right)$$

This equation can be rearranged to maintain the same form as the ideal gas law:

van der Waals Equation

$$\left(P_{real} + \frac{an^2}{V^2} \right)(V - nb) = nRT$$

The an^2/V^2 term serves as a correction for the intermolecular forces that generally result in lower pressures for real gases, while the nb term corrects for the physical volume that the individual particles occupy in a real gas. Both a and b are known as van der Waals constants and are generally larger for gases that experience greater intermolecular forces (a) and have larger molecular weights, and therefore volumes (b).

To illustrate the impact of intermolecular forces on real gas pressure, let's compare the pressures of two moles of oxygen and two moles of water, each in separate 5 L containers at a moderate temperature (500 K). Using the ideal gas law, we predict the following:

$$P_{ideal} = \frac{nRT}{V} = \frac{2 \text{ moles} \times 0.0821 \text{ L·atm/mol·K} \times 500 \text{ K}}{5 \text{L}} = 16.4 \text{ atm}$$

---

[1] For example, at pressures > 300 atm, gas particles are pushed so close together that they begin to repel one another, which can result in an increase in the volume of real gases over what would be predicted by the ideal gas law.

Now, using the van der Waals equation to solve for the pressure of oxygen (where $a = 1.34$ atm·L^2/mol^2 and $b = 0.0318$ L/mol):

$$P_{O_2} = \left(\frac{2 \text{ mol} \times 0.0821 \text{ L·atm/mol·K} \times 500\,\text{K}}{5\,\text{L} - 2\text{ mol} \times 0.0318 \text{ L/mol}} \right) - \left(\frac{1.34 \text{ atm·L}^2/\text{mol}^2 \times (2 \text{ mol})^2}{(5\,\text{L})^2} \right)$$

$$= 16.6 \text{ atm} - 0.2 \text{ atm} = 16.4 \text{ atm}$$

Notice that the pressure, due to oxygen's lack of substantial intermolecular forces, is effectively the same as was predicted by the ideal gas law. If we select a gas with significantly stronger intermolecular forces, the deviation from ideal gas behavior becomes more pronounced. For instance, the van der Waals a constant for water is significantly higher than that of oxygen due to water's ability to hydrogen bond ($a = 5.47$ atm·L^2/mol^2 and $b = 0.0305$ L/mol).

$$P_{H_2O} = \left(\frac{2 \text{ mol} \times 0.0821 \text{ L·atm/mol·K} \times 500 \text{ K}}{5\,\text{L} - 2\text{ mol} \times 0.0305 \text{ L/mol}} \right) - \left(\frac{5.47 \text{ atm·L}^2/\text{mol}^2 \times (2 \text{ mol})^2}{(5\,\text{L})^2} \right)$$

$$= 16.6 \text{ atm} - 0.9 \text{ atm} = 15.7 \text{ atm}$$

This represents a 4% decrease in pressure from that predicted by the ideal gas law.

To underscore the concept that gases behave more ideally at higher temperatures, if we increase the temperature of the system for any gas, the first term in the van der Waals equation approaches the pressure of the ideal gas while the second term remains unchanged. For example, if the temperature of our systems above is increased by 100 K (to 600 K), two moles of an ideal gas would exert 19.7 atm of pressure, while the van der Waals equation predicts pressures of 19.7 atm and 19.1 atm for oxygen and water, respectively. Therefore, we can see that at increased temperature the real gas (H_2O) behaves more ideally since it now deviates by only 3% from the pressure predicted by the ideal gas law.

So conceptually, why do higher pressures and lower temperatures cause larger deviations from ideal behavior? As pressure increases, gas particles become closer to one another. This accentuates the effects of attractive intermolecular forces, causing a decrease in observed pressure ($P_{real} < P_{ideal}$). Similarly, at low temperatures, intermolecular forces become more important, and when taken to an extreme, cause condensation to occur. Liquids aren't very ideal gases. In addition, when gas particles are packed closer to one another at high pressures, particle volume of the gas itself begins to limit the free space in which the gas particles can move ($V_{real} < V_{ideal}$). However, under extremely high pressure, these particles can begin to repel one another, leading to an increase in volume.

To summarize and focus on MCAT-relevance, those gases that behave most ideally have the weakest intermolecular forces and the smallest molecular weights (and volumes). Furthermore, by maintaining conditions of high temperature and low pressure, the potential interactions between particles are minimized and particle volume remains insignificant compared to the container size, helping to favor more ideal behavior for all gases.

Example 8-7: Of the following, which gas would likely *deviate* the most from ideal behavior at high pressure and low temperature?

A) $He(g)$
B) $H_2(g)$
C) $O_2(g)$
D) $H_2O(g)$

Solution: Since H_2O molecules will experience hydrogen bonding, they feel significantly stronger intermolecular forces than the other gases do. Therefore, of the choices given, $H_2O(g)$ will deviate the most from ideal behavior at high pressure and low temperature.

Example 8-8: Of the following, which gas would behave most like an ideal gas if all were at the same temperature and pressure?

A) $O_2(g)$
B) $CH_4(g)$
C) $Ar(g)$
D) $Cl_2(g)$

Solution: The molecules of a perfect (ideal) gas take up zero volume, so the gas in this list that will behave most like an ideal gas will be the one that takes up the smallest volume. O_2, CH_4, and Cl_2 are all polyatomic molecules that occupy more space than atomic argon. Therefore, choice C is the answer.

Example 8-9: Of the following, which gas would behave most like an ideal gas if all were at the same temperature and pressure?

A) $H_2O(g)$
B) $CH_4(g)$
C) $HF(g)$
D) $NH_3(g)$

Solution: The molecules of a perfect (ideal) gas experience no intermolecular forces, so the gas in this list that will behave most like an ideal gas will be the one that has the weakest intermolecular forces. H_2O, HF, and NH_3 experience hydrogen-bonding, while CH_4 experiences only weak dispersion forces. Therefore, choice B is the answer.

8.4 DALTON'S LAW OF PARTIAL PRESSURES

Consider a mixture of, say, three gases in a single container.

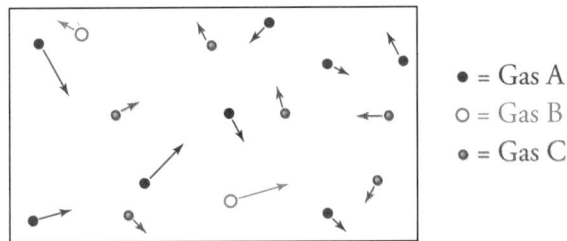

● = Gas A
○ = Gas B
● = Gas C

The total pressure is due to the collisions of all three types of molecules with the container walls. The pressure that the molecules of Gas A alone exert is called the **partial pressure** of Gas A, denoted by p_A. Similarly, the pressure exerted by the molecules of Gas B alone and the pressure exerted by the molecules of Gas C alone are p_B and p_C.

Dalton's law of partial pressures says that the total pressure is simply the sum of the partial pressures of all the constituent gases. In this case, then, we'd have

Dalton's Law

$$P_{tot} = p_A + p_B + p_C$$

So, if we know the partial pressures, we can determine the total pressure. We can also work backward. Knowing the total pressure, we can figure out the individual partial pressures. All that is required is the mole fraction. For example, in the diagram above, there are a total of 16 molecules: 8 of Gas A, 2 of Gas B, and 6 of Gas C. Therefore, the mole fraction of Gas A is $X_A = 8/16 = 1/2$, the mole fraction of Gas B is $X_B = 2/16 = 1/8$, and the mole fraction of Gas C is $X_C = 6/16 = 3/8$. *The partial pressure of a gas is equal to its mole fraction times the total pressure.* For example, if the total pressure in the container above is 8 atm, then

$$p_A = X_A P_{tot} = \frac{1}{2} P_{tot} = \frac{1}{2} (8 \text{ atm}) = 4 \text{ atm}$$

$$p_B = X_B P_{tot} = \frac{1}{8} P_{tot} = \frac{1}{8} (8 \text{ atm}) = 1 \text{ atm}$$

$$p_C = X_C P_{tot} = \frac{3}{8} P_{tot} = \frac{3}{8} (8 \text{ atm}) = 3 \text{ atm}$$

Example 8-10: A mixture of neon and nitrogen contains 0.5 mol Ne(g) and 2 mol N$_2$(g). If the total pressure is 20 atm, what is the partial pressure of the neon?

Solution: The mole fraction of Ne is

$$X_{Ne} = \frac{n_{Ne}}{n_{Ne} + n_{N_2}} = \frac{0.5}{(0.5 + 2)} = \frac{0.5}{2.5} = \frac{1}{5}$$

Therefore,

$$p_{Ne} = X_{Ne} P_{tot} = \frac{1}{5} P_{tot} = \frac{1}{5} (20 \text{ atm}) = 4 \text{ atm}$$

Example 8-11: A vessel contains a mixture of three gases: A, B, and C. There is twice as much A as B and half as much C as A. If the total pressure is 300 torr, what is the partial pressure of Gas C?

A) 60 torr
B) 75 torr
C) 100 torr
D) 120 torr

Solution: The question states that there is twice as much A as B, and it also says (backward) there is twice as much A as C. So the amounts of B and C are the same, and each is half the amount of A. Since this is a multiple choice question, instead of doing algebra we'll just plug in the choices and find the one that works. The only one that works is choice B, so that p_A = 150 torr, p_B = 75 torr, and p_C = 75 torr, for a total of 300 torr.

Example 8-12: If the ratio of the partial pressures of a pair of gases mixed together in a sealed vessel is 3:1 at 300 K, what would be the ratio of their partial pressures at 400 K?

A) 3:1
B) 4:1
C) 4:3
D) 12:1

Solution: Remember that the partial pressure of a gas is the way that we talk about the amount of gas in a mixture. The question states that the ratio of partial pressures of two gases is 3:1. That just means there's three times more of one than the other. Regardless of the temperature, if the vessel is sealed, then there will always be three times more of one than the other. Choice A is the correct answer.

8.5   GRAHAM'S LAW OF EFFUSION

The escape of a gas molecule through a very tiny hole (comparable in size to the molecules themselves) into an evacuated region is called **effusion**:

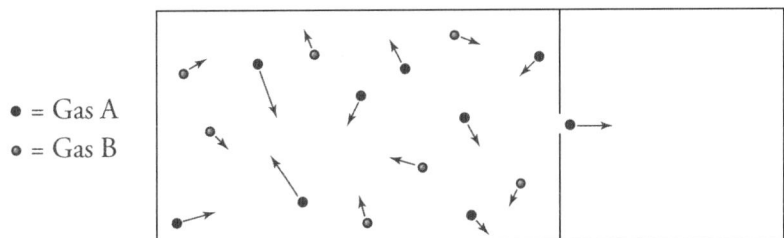

The gases in the left-hand container are at the same temperature, so their average kinetic energies are the same. If Gas A and Gas B have different molar masses, the heavier molecules will move, on average, slower than the lighter ones will. We can be even more precise. The average kinetic energy of a molecule of Gas A is $\frac{1}{2}m_A(v_A^2)_{avg}$, and the average kinetic energy of a molecule of Gas B is $\frac{1}{2}m_B(v_B^2)_{avg}$. Setting these equal to each other, we get

$$\frac{1}{2}m_A(v_A^2)_{avg} = \frac{1}{2}m_B(v_B^2)_{avg} \quad \Rightarrow \quad \frac{(v_A^2)_{avg}}{(v_B^2)_{avg}} = \frac{m_B}{m_A} \quad \Rightarrow \quad \frac{rms\ v_A}{rms\ v_B} = \sqrt{\frac{m_B}{m_A}}$$

(The abbreviation **rms** stands for *root-mean-square*; it's the square root of the mean [average] of the square of speed. Therefore, rms v is a convenient measure of the average speed of the molecules.) For example, if Gas A is hydrogen gas (H_2, molecular weight = 2) and Gas B is oxygen gas (O_2, molecular weight = 32), the hydrogen molecules will move, on average,

$$\sqrt{\frac{m_B}{m_A}} = \sqrt{\frac{32}{2}} = \sqrt{16} = 4$$

times faster than the oxygen molecules.

This result—which follows from one of the assumptions of the kinetic-molecular theory (namely that the average kinetic energy of the molecules of a gas is proportional to the temperature)—can be confirmed experimentally by performing an effusion experiment. Which gas should escape faster? The rate at which a gas effuses should depend directly on how fast its molecules move; the faster they travel, the more often they'd "collide" with the hole and escape. So we'd expect that if we compared the effusion rates for Gases A and B, we'd get a ratio equal to the ratio of their average speeds (if the molecules of Gas A travel 4 times faster than those of Gas B, then Gas A should effuse 4 times faster). Since we just figured out that the ratio of their average speeds is equal to the reciprocal of the square root of the ratio of their masses, we'd expect the ratio of their effusion rates to be the same. This result is known as **Graham's law of effusion**:

Graham's Law of Effusion

$$\frac{\text{rate of effusion of Gas A}}{\text{rate of effusion of Gas B}} = \sqrt{\frac{\text{molar mass of Gas B}}{\text{molar mass of Gas A}}}$$

Let's emphasize the distinction between the relationships of temperature to the kinetic energy and to the speed of the gas. The molecules of two different gases at the same temperature have the same average kinetic energy. But the molecules of two different gases at the same temperature don't have the same average *speed*. Lighter molecules travel faster, because the kinetic energy depends on both the mass and the speed of the molecules.

Also, it's important to remember that not all the molecules of the gas in a container—even if there's only one type of molecule—travel at the same speed. Their speeds cover a wide range. What we *can* say is that as the temperature of the sample is increased, the *average* speed increases. In fact, since $KE \propto T$, the root-mean-square speed is proportional to $\sqrt{T}$. The figure below shows the distribution of molecular speeds for a gas at three different temperatures. Notice that the rms speeds increase as the temperature is increased.

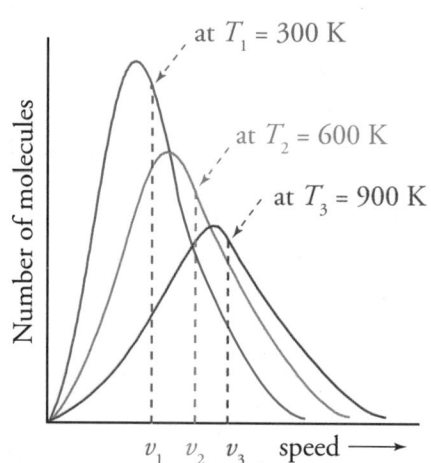

Example 8-13: A container holds methane (CH_4) and sulfur dioxide (SO_2), at a temperature of 227°C. Let v_M denote the rms speed of the methane molecules and v_S the rms speed of the sulfur dioxide molecules. Which of the following best describes the relationship between these speeds?

A) $v_S = 16\, v_M$
B) $v_S = 2\, v_M$
C) $v_M = 2\, v_S$
D) $v_M = 16\, v_S$

8.5

Solution: The molecular weight of methane is $12 + 4(1) = 16$, and the molecular weight of sulfur dioxide is $32 + 2(16) = 64$. Therefore

$$\frac{v_M}{v_S} = \sqrt{\frac{m_S}{m_M}} = \sqrt{\frac{64}{16}} = \sqrt{4} = 2 \quad \Rightarrow \quad v_M = 2v_S$$

So, choice C is the answer.

Example 8-14: In a laboratory experiment, Chamber A holds a mixture of four gases: 1 mole each of chlorine, fluorine, nitrogen, and carbon dioxide. A tiny hole is made in the side of the chamber, and the gases are allowed to effuse from Chamber A into an empty container. When 2 moles of gas have escaped, which gas will have the greatest mole fraction in Chamber A?

A) $Cl_2(g)$
B) $F_2(g)$
C) $N_2(g)$
D) $CO_2(g)$

Solution: The gas with the greatest mole fraction remaining in Chamber A will be the gas with the *slowest* rate of effusion. This is the gas with the highest molecular weight. Of the gases in the chamber, Cl_2 has the greatest molecular weight. Therefore, the answer is A.

Example 8-15: A container holds methane (CH_4) and sulfur dioxide (SO_2) at a temperature of 227°C. Let KE_M denote the average kinetic energy of the methane molecules and KE_S the average kinetic energy of the sulfur dioxide molecules. Which of the following best describes the relationship between these energies?

A) $KE_S = 4\, KE_M$
B) $KE_S = 3\, KE_M$
C) $KE_M = KE_S$
D) $KE_M = 4\, KE_S$

Solution: Since both gases are at the same temperature, the average kinetic energies of their molecules will be the *same* (remember: $KE_{avg} \propto T$). Thus, the answer is C.

Example 8-16: The temperature of neon gas in a glass tube is increased from 10°C to 160°C. As a result, the average kinetic energy of the neon atoms will increase by a factor of:

A) less than 2.
B) 2.
C) 4.
D) 16.

Solution: We use the fact that $KE_{avg} \propto T$. However, don't fall for the trap of thinking that the temperature has increased by a factor of 16. Calculations involving the gas laws (and that includes the proportionality between KE_{avg} and T from kinetic-molecular theory) must be done with temperatures expressed in *kelvins*. The temperature here increased from 283 K to 433 K, which is less than a factor of 2 increase. Therefore, KE_{avg} will also increase by a factor of less than 2 (choice A).

Chapter 8 Summary

- The pressure of a gas is due to the collisions gas particles have with the container walls.

- The ideal gas law states that $PV = nRT$.

- Standard temperature and pressure (STP) conditions are at 1 atm and 273 K. Under these conditions, 1 mol of any gas will occupy 22.4 L of space.

- Particles of an ideal gas take up no volume and experience no intermolecular forces. They also have elastic collisions with each other and the walls of their container.

- Real gases approach ideal behavior under most conditions, but deviate most from ideal behavior under conditions of high pressure and low temperature.

- Real gases can be quantified using the van der Waals equation:

$$\left(P + \frac{an^2}{V^2}\right)(V - nb) = nRT$$

- Dalton's law of partial pressures states that the total pressure inside a container is equal to the sum of the partial pressures of each constituent gas. The partial pressure of a gas divided by the total pressure of all gases is equal to its mole fraction within the gaseous mixture.

- Temperature is a measure of the average kinetic energy of molecules within a sample.

- Graham's law of effusion states that the rate of effusion of a gas is inversely pro-portional to its molecular weight. In other words, lighter gases effuse more quickly than heavier gases.

CHAPTER 8 FREESTANDING PRACTICE QUESTIONS

1. A sample of nitrogen gas is heated in a sealed, rigid container. The pressure inside the container increases because the added energy causes:

A) some of the nitrogen molecules to split, so more particles contribute to increase the pressure.
B) the molecules of gas to move faster, increasing the frequency of intermolecular collisions.
C) the molecules of gas to move faster, increasing the frequency of collisions with the container.
D) the molecules of gas to stick together in clusters that have a greater momentum.

2. Two identical balloons are filled with different gases at STP. Balloon A contains 0.25 moles of neon, and balloon B contains 0.25 moles of oxygen. Which of the following properties would be greater for balloon B?

A) Density
B) Volume
C) Number of particles
D) Average kinetic energy

3. The figure below depicts the relative sizes and mole fractions of two monatomic gases in a closed container.

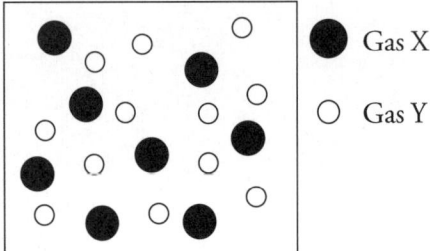

Gas X

Gas Y

Which of the following is true about the gas mixture after a small hole is punched in the container and the gases are allowed to completely effuse?

A) The partial pressure of Gas X will never equal the partial pressure of Gas Y.
B) The partial pressure of Gas Y will decrease faster than the partial pressure of Gas X.
C) The partial pressure of Gas Y will increase because the mole fraction of Gas Y will increase.
D) The partial pressures of each gas will remain unchanged.

4. There are an unknown number of moles of argon in a steel container. A chemist injects two moles of nitrogen into the container. The temperature and volume do not change, but the pressure increases by ten percent. Originally the container held:

A) 16 moles of Ar.
B) 18 moles of Ar.
C) 20 moles of Ar.
D) 22 moles of Ar.

5. Which of the following gases will deviate most from ideal behavior?

A) NO_2
B) CO_2
C) CS_2
D) N_2O

6. Which of the following is true for a closed flask containing both 1 mole of ideal Gas X and 1 mole of real Gas Y?

A) The total energy of X is equal to the total energy of Y.
B) The average kinetic energy of X is equal to the average kinetic energy of Y.
C) The total volume available to the gases is the same as the total volume of the flask.
D) Gases X and Y are at different temperatures.

7. Given the following combustion reaction, calculate the mole fraction of hydrocarbon in the reactant mixture before combustion. Assume both starting materials are present in stoichiometric amounts; neither is limiting.

$$Z\ C_xH_y(g) + 8\ O_2(g) \rightarrow 5\ CO_2(g) + 6\ H_2O(l)$$

A) 1/8
B) 1/9
C) 2/9
D) 1/3

CHAPTER 8 PRACTICE PASSAGE

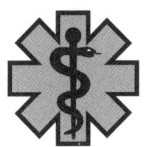

As a part of ongoing human metabolism, oxygen combines with fuels to yield ATP, CO_2, and H_2O. Hence the tissues tend constantly to reduce the blood's oxygen concentration and increase its carbon dioxide concentration. The lungs serve to replenish the blood's oxygen supply and to empty it of accumulated carbon dioxide via the process of passive diffusion. The lungs are also the delivery organ for gas phase pharmacological agents, the absorption of which is a characteristic trait of the specific drug compound.

During inspiration, contraction of the diaphragm produces negative pressure change in the lungs, and air therefore moves from the atmosphere into the lungs. At the level of the alveoli, carbon dioxide continuously moves from capillary blood into the lungs, and oxygen moves from the lungs into the blood. The net result is that the partial pressure of oxygen in the lungs is 100 torr, which is 59 torr less than the partial pressure of oxygen in the atmosphere. Partial pressure of carbon dioxide in the lungs is 40 torr greater than in the atmosphere.

The total pressure of gases in the lungs is the sum of the partial pressures of each of the individual gases. Equation 1 below shows the result of substituting values for partial pressures into the ideal gas law equation. P_t represents the total pressure of the gases, and the n's denote the numbers of moles of the individual, nonreactive gases. As air passes from the atmosphere to the alveoli, the partial pressures of both nitrogen and oxygen decrease (although nitrogen is not absorbed by the alveoli to any appreciable extent).

$$P_t = (n_1 + n_2 + n_3 + \ldots)RT/V$$

Equation 1

| Gas | Pressure (torr) | | |
	Atmosphere	Inspired air	Alveolar air
N_2	595	564	573
O_2	159	149	100
H_2O	6	47	47
CO_2	0	0	40

Table 1

Inhaled bioactive compounds, such as anesthetics, must be present in concentrations sufficient for the absorption of a biologically relevant concentration, but not so much that large amounts of the compounds are exhaled and wasted. The alveolar concentration of a particular anesthetic required to prevent movement (motor response) in response to surgical (pain) stimulus is known as the compound's MAC (minimum alveolar concentration).

1. Which of the following causes the exchange of oxygen and carbon dioxide between the lungs and bloodstream?

A) Concentration gradients
B) Different values for the gas constant
C) Greater permeability of oxygen
D) Decreased volumes of gases in the bloodstream

2. Between the time it is inhaled from the atmosphere and the time it is exhaled, air experiences a greater decrease in molar quantity of which gas: oxygen or nitrogen?

A) Oxygen, because nitrogen is less reactive than oxygen in the gaseous state
B) Oxygen, because it diffuses from lung to capillary
C) Nitrogen, because nitrogen is not soluble in the bloodstream
D) Nitrogen, because the proportionally lesser partial pressure decrease corresponds to a proportionally greater decrease in molar quantity

3. The relationship between the partial pressure of a gas (P) and the number of moles of that gas (n) is best represented by which of the following graphs?

A)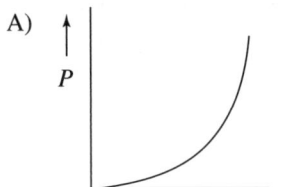

C)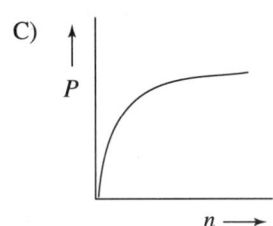

B)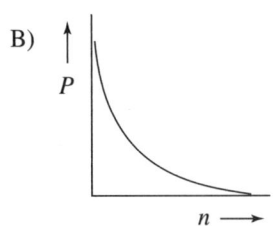

D)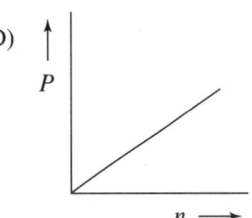

4. Which one of the following expressions can be used to compare atmospheric air and alveolar air and calculate the reduction in the number of moles of oxygen present in the alveoli?

A) $(V/RT)(100)$
B) $(V/RT)(149 - 100)$
C) $(V/RT)(159 - 100)$
D) $(V/RT)(159 - 149)$

5. If the MAC of the anesthetic Sevoflurane is 2.1 vol%, what is the partial pressure of Sevoflurane that must be maintained in the alveoli to ensure anesthetic potency?

A) 16 torr
B) 32 torr
C) 87 torr
D) 160 torr

SOLUTIONS TO CHAPTER 8 FREESTANDING PRACTICE QUESTIONS

1. **C** According to kinetic molecular theory, pressure is defined by the frequency of collisions between gas particles and the walls of their container. While increasing the temperature of the gas will cause more collisions between particles as well, these collisions do not define pressure (eliminate choice B). In addition, collisions between particles are elastic, so unless the particles are highly polar and have a strong attraction for each other (the gas is behaving non-ideally), they will not stick together. Since N_2 is non-polar it should behave ideally, so choice D can be eliminated. Finally, nitrogen is a very stable diatomic element, and heating a sample of nitrogen is not likely to break the strong triple bond between nitrogen atoms, eliminating choice A.

2. **A** Since both balloons contain the same number of moles of gas under identical pressure and temperature conditions (STP), they should have the same volume (in this case 5.6 L since 1 mol = 22.4 L). Eliminate choice B. An identical amount of each gas is added to each balloon, so they should also contain the same number of gas particles (0.25 mol × 6.02 × 10^{23} particles/mol), eliminating choice C. Since the gases are at the same temperature they will have the same average kinetic energy, so by process of elimination, A must be the correct answer. Density is mass/volume. Since the two gases have the same volume, oxygen, with a larger molar mass (O_2 = 32 g/mol vs. Ne = 20 g/mol), will have the greater density.

3. **B** After a hole is punched in the container and the gases begin to escape, the total pressure of the container will decrease, and the individual partial pressures of the gases will therefore also decrease. Eliminate choices C and D. According to Graham's law, the lighter the gas molecule, the faster its rate of effusion through a small hole. Gas Y will effuse faster than Gas X, so its partial pressure will decrease at a faster rate. The gases are allowed to completely effuse and the figure indicates that the mole fraction of Y is slightly larger than X. Therefore there will most likely be a moment in time when the partial pressures of both gases are equal (and this will definitely be the case when the container is finally empty), eliminating choice A.

4. **C** At constant V and T, the pressure of an ideal gas reflects the number of particles (regardless of their identity). It is a simplification of the ideal gas law from $PV = nRT$ to $P \propto n$. So, if the addition of two moles of N_2 into the chamber results in an increase in P of 10 percent, then the moles added must be 10 percent of the initial number of Ar moles. Two moles are 10 percent of 20 moles.

5. **C** The most ideal gases are those that have the smallest molecular volumes and the weakest intermolecular forces. The compounds in choices A, B, and D are made of elements in the second period, making them very similar in size, whereas CS_2 (choice C) has two sulfur atoms, which are in the third period. Carbon disulfide therefore has a significantly larger molecular volume than the others, and relatively strong London dispersion forces as a result. Choice C therefore deviates the most from ideal behavior.

6. **B** Temperature is a measure of average kinetic energy. If gases X and Y are in the same flask they must be at the same temperature, eliminating choice D and making choice B correct. The total energy of a gas is equal to its kinetic energy plus its potential energy. Since Gas Y is a real gas and experiences intermolecular forces, it has potential energy, whereas ideal Gas X does not. Therefore, choice A is eliminated. Real gas molecules occupy some volume in the container, whereas ideal gases have no molecular volume. Since the flask contains a real gas, the total volume available to the gases is slightly less than the total volume of the flask, eliminating choice C.

7. **B** First, balance the equation:

$$C_5H_{12}(g) + 8\ O_2(g) \rightarrow 5\ CO_2(g) + 6\ H_2O(l)$$

The hydrocarbon must be C_5H_{12} and the coefficient Z is 1. Since the question indicates that neither reactant is limiting, there must be a 1:8 molar ratio of hydrocarbon to oxygen present in the reaction flask, so the mole fraction (X) of hydrocarbon in the reactant solution before combustion is calculated by:

$$X = \text{(moles hydrocarbon)/(total moles)}$$

$$X = 1/(1+8) = 1/9$$

SOLUTIONS TO CHAPTER 8 PRACTICE PASSAGE

1. **A** The passage states that gases move by passive diffusion. Molecules undergo passive diffusion due to concentration gradients (they diffuse from high to low concentrations).

2. **B** According to the data in Table 1, oxygen experiences the greater decrease in partial pressure (this eliminates choices C and D). This drop is due to the binding of oxygen to hemoglobin in the capillaries.

3. **D** Partial pressure is proportional to the number of moles of the gas. The graph of a proportion is a straight line through the origin: the graph in choice D.

4. **C** Since $n = (V/RT)P$, we have $\Delta n = (V/RT)\Delta P = (V/RT)(159\text{ torr} - 100\text{ torr})$ from Table 1.

5. **A** The overall pressure in the alveoli must be equal to atmospheric pressure (760 torr), which is confirmed by summing the values in Table 1. Assuming at least a rough ideal gas behavior, a volume percentage is equivalent to a molar percentage and therefore the percentage of partial pressure associated with it by Equation 1. The pressure representing 2.1% of 760 torr can be quickly ascertained by realizing that 1% is 7.6 torr, meaning 2% is 15.2 torr. As such, 2.1% is roughly 16 torr.

Chapter 9
Kinetics

9.1 REACTION MECHANISM: AN ANALOGY

Chemical **kinetics** is the study of how reactions take place and how fast they occur. (Kinetics tells us nothing about the *spontaneity* of a reaction, however!)

Consider this scenario: A group of people are washing a pile of dirty dishes and stacking them up as clean, dry dishes. Our "reaction" has dirty dishes as starting material, and clean, dry dishes as the product:

$$\text{dirty dish} \rightarrow \text{clean-and-dry dish}$$

But what about a *soapy* dish? We know it's part of the process, but the equation doesn't include it. When we break down the pathway of a dirty dish to a clean-and-dry dish, we realize that the reaction happens in several steps, a sequence of **elementary** steps that show us the reaction **mechanism:**

1) dirty dish $\rightarrow$ soapy dish
2) soapy dish $\rightarrow$ rinsed dish
3) rinsed dish $\rightarrow$ clean-and-dry dish

The soapy and rinsed dishes are reaction **intermediates**. They are necessary for the conversion of dirty dishes to clean-and-dry dishes, but don't appear either in the starting material or products. If you add up all the reactants and products, the intermediates cancel out, and you'll have the overall equation.

In the same way, we write chemical reactions as if they occur in a single step:

$$2\,NO + O_2 \rightarrow 2\,NO_2$$

But in reality, things are a little more complicated, and reactions often proceed through intermediates that we don't show in the chemical equation. The truth for the reaction above is that it occurs in two steps:

1) $2\,NO \rightarrow N_2O_2$
2) $N_2O_2 + O_2 \rightarrow 2\,NO_2$

The N_2O_2 comes and goes during the reaction, but isn't part of the starting material or products. N_2O_2 is a reaction intermediate.

Just as the soapy dishes and rinsed dishes are produced and then consumed, we can identify an **intermediate** in a series of elementary steps as a substance that is produced in one elementary step and then consumed in a subsequent step. Although the two elementary steps don't need to be sequential, they often are. As above, note that intermediates will not be part of the overall balanced chemical reaction. Depending on the rate of the elementary step that consumes the intermediate, the concentration of the intermediate will vary in solution. As the consuming elementary step becomes faster, the steady-state concentration of the intermediate becomes smaller, and it becomes harder to detect the intermediate.

Rate-Determining Step

What determines the rate of a reaction? Consider our friends doing the dishes.

1) dirty dish → soapy dish   Bingo washes at 5 dishes per minute.

2) soapy dish → rinsed dish   Ringo rinses at 8 dishes per minute.

3) rinsed dish → clean-and-dry dish   Dingo dries at 3 dishes per minute.

What will be the rate of the overall reaction? Thanks to Dingo, the dishes move from dirty to clean-and-dry at only 3 dishes a minute. It doesn't matter how fast Bingo and Ringo wash and rinse; the dishes will pile up behind Dingo. The **rate-determining step** is Dingo's drying step, and true to its name, it determines the overall rate of reaction.

The slowest step in a process determines the overall reaction rate.

This applies to chemical reactions as well. For our chemical reaction given above, we have

$$2\ NO \rightarrow N_2O_2 \quad \text{(fast)}$$

$$N_2O_2 + O_2 \rightarrow 2\ NO_2 \quad \text{(slow)}$$

The second step is the slower, and it will determine the overall rate of reaction. No matter how fast the first step moves along, the intermediates will "pill up" in front of the second step as it plods along. The slow step dictates the rate of the overall reaction.

Once again, there's an important difference between our dishes analogy and a chemical reaction: While the dishes pile up behind Dingo, in a chemical reaction the intermediates will not actually pile up. Rather they will shuttle back and forth between reactants and products until the slow step takes it forward. This would be like taking a rinsed dish and getting it soapy again, until Dingo is ready for it!

Example 9-1: Which of the following is the best example of a rate?

A)   Rate = $\Delta[A]/\Delta t$
B)   Rate = $\Delta[A]/\Delta[B]$
C)   Rate = $\Delta[A]\Delta[B]$
D)   Rate = $\Delta[A]^2$

Solution: Regardless of the topic, rate is always defined as change in something over change in time. Choice A is the answer.

9.2 REACTION RATE

The **rate** of a reaction indicates how fast reactants are being consumed or how fast products are being formed. The **collision theory model** explains how the reaction rate depends on several factors. Since the reactant molecules must collide and interact in order for old bonds to be broken and new ones to be formed to generate the product molecules, anything that affects these collisions and interactions will affect the reaction rate. The reaction rate is determined by the following:

1) How frequently the reactant molecules collide
2) The orientation of the colliding molecules
3) Their energy

Activation Energy

Every chemical reaction has an **activation energy** (E_a), or the minimum energy required of reactant molecules during a molecular collision in order for the reaction to proceed to products. If the reactant molecules don't possess this much energy, their collisions won't be able to produce the products and the reaction will not occur. If the reactants possess the necessary activation energy, they can reach a high-energy (and short-lived!) **transition state**, also known as the **activated complex**. For example, if the reaction is $A_2 + B_2 \rightarrow 2\,AB$, say, the activated complex might look something like this:

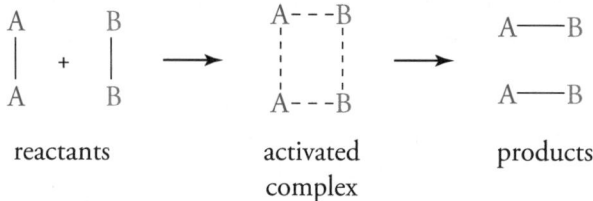

Now that we have introduced all species that might appear throughout the course of a chemical reaction, we can illustrate the energy changes that occur as a reaction occurs in a **reaction coordinate diagram**. Consider the following two-step process and its reaction coordinate graph below:

$$\text{Step 1:} \quad A \rightarrow X$$
$$\text{Step 2:} \quad X \rightarrow B$$
$$\overline{\text{Overall reaction:} \quad A \rightarrow B}$$

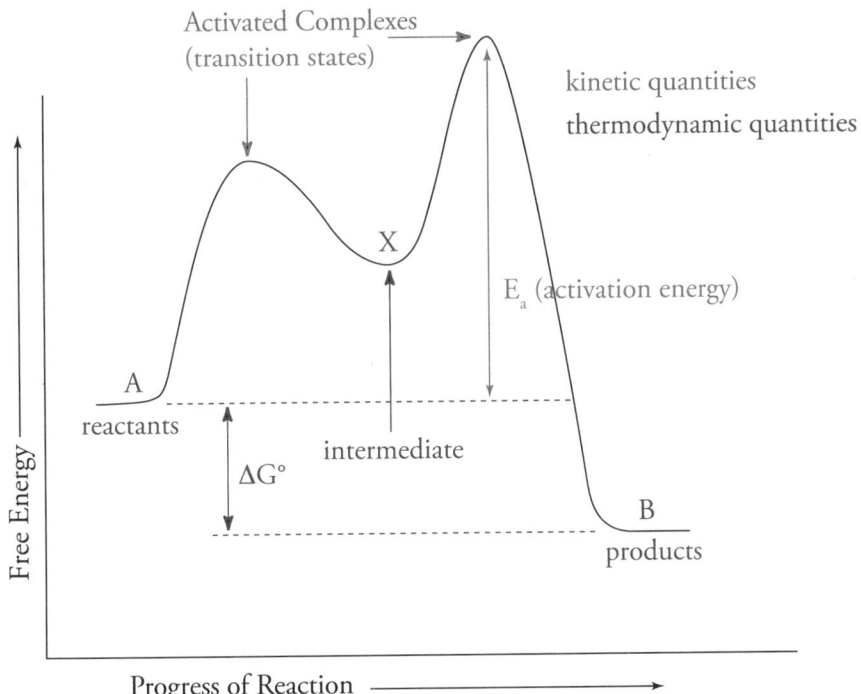

Notice that the transition state is always an energy maximum, and is therefore distinct from an intermediate. Remember that reaction intermediates (shown as X in this case) are produced in an early step of the mechanism, and are later used up so they do not appear as products of the overall reaction. The intermediate is shown here as a local minimum in terms of its energy, but has more energy than either the reactants or products. The high energy intermediate is therefore highly reactive, making it difficult to isolate.

Since the progress of the reaction depends on the reactant molecules colliding with enough energy to generate the activated complex, we can make the following statements concerning the reaction rate:

1) *The lower the activation energy, the faster the reaction rate.* The reaction coordinate diagram above suggests that the second step of the mechanism will therefore be the slow step, or the rate-determining step, since the second "hill" of the diagram is higher.

2) *The greater the concentrations of the reactants, the faster the reaction rate.* Favorable collisions are more likely as the concentrations of reactant molecules increase.

3) *The higher the temperature of the reaction mixture, the faster the reaction rate.* At higher temperatures, more reactant molecules have a sufficient energy to overcome the activation-energy barrier, and molecules collide at a higher frequency, so the reaction can proceed at a faster rate.

Notice in the reaction coordinate diagram above that the $\Delta G°$ of the reaction has no bearing on the rate of the reaction, and vice versa. Thermodynamic factors and kinetic factors *do not affect each other* (a concept the MCAT loves to ask about).

9.3 CATALYSTS

Catalysts provide reactants with a different route, usually a shortcut, to get to products. A **catalyst** will almost always make a reaction go faster by either speeding up the rate-determining step or providing an optimized route to products. A catalyst that accelerates a reaction does so *by lowering the activation energy of the rate-determining step*, and therefore the energy of the highest-energy transition state:

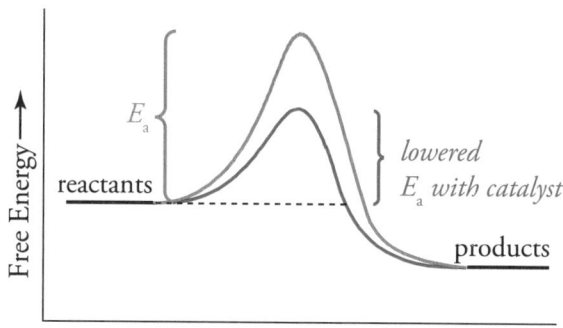

The key difference between a reactant and a catalyst is that the reactants are converted to products, but *a catalyst remains unchanged at the end of a reaction*. A catalyst can undergo a temporary change during a reaction, but it is always converted back to its original state. Like reaction intermediates, catalysts aren't included in the overall reaction equation.

Our dish crew could use a catalyst. Picture Dingo walking to pick up each wet dish, drying it on both sides, and walking back to place it in the clean dish stack. Now imagine a helper, Daisy, who takes the wet dish from Ringo, then walks it over to Dingo, and while he dries and stacks, she returns with another wet dish. This way, Dingo can dry 5 dishes a minute instead of 3, and the overall dish-cleaning rate increases to 5 dishes a minute. Daisy is the catalyst, but the chain of events in the overall reaction remains the same.

In the same way, chemical reactions can be catalyzed. Consider the decomposition of ozone:

$$O_3(g) + O(g) \rightarrow 2\ O_2(g)$$

This reaction actually takes place in two steps and is catalyzed by nitric oxide (NO):

1) $NO(g) + O_3(g) \rightarrow NO_2(g) + O_2(g)$
2) $NO_2(g) + O(g) \rightarrow NO(g) + O_2(g)$

$NO(g)$ is necessary for this reaction to proceed at a noticeable rate, and even undergoes changes itself during the process. But $NO(g)$ remains unchanged at the end of the reaction and makes the reaction occur much faster than it would in its absence. $NO(g)$, a product of automobile exhaust, is a catalyst in ozone destruction.

It is important to note that the addition of a catalyst will affect the rate of a reaction, but not the equilibrium or the thermodynamics of the reaction. A catalyst provides a different pathway for the reactants to get to the products, and lowers the activation energy, E_a. But a catalyst does not change any of the thermodynamic quantities such as ΔG, ΔH, and ΔS of a reaction.

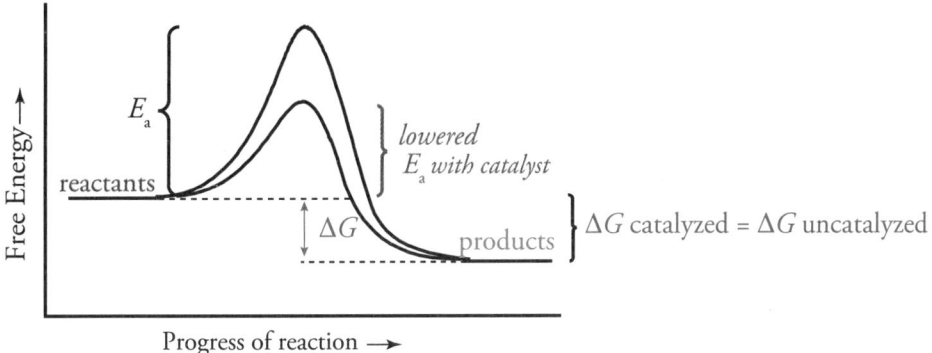

Example 9-2: Which of the following statements is true?

A) Catalysts decrease the activation energy of the forward reaction only.
B) Catalysts decrease the activation energy of the reverse reaction only.
C) Catalysts decrease the activation energy of both the forward and reverse reactions.
D) Catalysts decrease the activation energy of the forward reaction and increase the activation energy of the reverse reaction.

Solution: Catalysts decrease the activation energy of the forward reaction and reverse reaction—that's why they have no net effect on a system that's already at equilibrium. Choice C is the correct choice.

Example 9-3: Which of the following is true about the hypothetical two-step reaction shown below?

1) $A + 2\,B \rightarrow C + 2\,D$ (fast)
2) $C \rightarrow A + E$ (slow)

A) A is a catalyst, and C is an intermediate.
B) A is a catalyst, and D is an intermediate.
C) B is a catalyst, and A is an intermediate.
D) B is a catalyst, and C is an intermediate.

Solution: C is an intermediate; it's formed in one step and consumed in the other. This eliminates choices B and C. Now, is A or B the catalyst? Notice that B is consumed but not reformed; therefore, it cannot be the catalyst. The answer is A.

Example 9-4: A reaction is run without a catalyst and is found to have an activation energy of 140 kJ/mol and a heat of reaction, ΔH, of 30 kJ/mol. In the presence of a catalyst, however, the activation energy is reduced to 120 kJ/mol. What will be the heat of reaction in the presence of the catalyst?

A) –10 kJ/mol
B) 10 kJ/mol
C) 30 kJ/mol
D) 50 kJ/mol

Solution: Catalysts affect only the kinetics of a reaction, not the thermodynamics. The heat of the reaction will be the same with or without a catalyst. The answer is C.

9.4 RATE LAWS

On the MCAT, you might be given data about the rate of a particular reaction and be asked to derive the **rate law**. The data for rate laws are determined by the *initial rates* of reaction and typically are given as the **rate at which the reactant disappears**. You'll rarely see products in a rate law expression: usually only reactants. What does a rate law tell us? Although a reaction needs all the reactants to proceed, *only those that are involved in the rate-determining step (the slow step) are part of the rate law expression*. Some reactants may not affect the reaction rate at all, and so they won't be a part of the rate law expression.

Let's look at a generic reaction, $a\,A + b\,B \rightarrow c\,C + d\,D$, and its rate law:

$$\text{rate} = k[A]^x[B]^y$$

where

x = the **order** of the reaction with respect to A

y = the **order** of the reaction with respect to B

$(x + y)$ = the **overall order** of the reaction

k = the rate constant

The rate law can only be determined *experimentally*. You *can't* get the orders of the reactants, not to mention the rate constant k, just by looking at the balanced equation. The exception to this rule is for an *elementary step* in a reaction mechanism. The rate law is first order for a unimolecular elementary step and second order for a **bimolecular** elementary step. The individual order of the reactants in a rate law will follow from their stoichiometry in the rate-determining step (similar to the way they're included in an equilibrium constant).

Let's look at a set of reaction rate data and see how to determine the rate law for the reaction

$$A + B + C \rightarrow D + E$$

Experiment	[A]	[B]	[C]	Initial reaction rate (M/s)
1	0.2 M	0.1 M	0.05 M	1×10^{-3}
2	0.4 M	0.1 M	0.05 M	2×10^{-3}
3	0.2 M	0.2 M	0.05 M	4×10^{-3}
4	0.2 M	0.1 M	0.10 M	1×10^{-3}

From the experimental data, we can determine the orders with respect to the reactants—that is, the exponents x, y, and z in the equation

$$\text{rate} = k[A]^x[B]^y[C]^z$$

and the overall order of the reaction, $x + y + z$.

Let's first find the order of the reaction with respect to Reactant A. As we go from Experiment 1 to Experiment 2, only [A] changes, so we can use the data to figure out the order of the reaction with respect to Reactant [A]. We notice that the value of [A] doubled, and the reaction rate doubled. Therefore, the reaction rate is proportional to [A], and $x = 1$.

Next, let's look at [B]. As we go from Experiment 1 to Experiment 3, only [B] changes. When [B] is doubled, the rate is quadrupled. Therefore, the rate is proportional to $[B]^2$, and $y = 2$.

Finally, let's look at [C]. As we go from Experiment 1 to Experiment 4, only [C] changes. When [C] is doubled, the rate is unaffected. This tells us that the reaction rate does not depend on [C], so $z = 0$.

Therefore, the rate law has the form

$$\text{rate} = k[A][B]^2$$

The reaction is first order with respect to [A], second order with respect to [B], zero order with respect to [C], and third order overall. In general, if a reaction rate increases by a factor f when the concentration of a reactant increases by a factor c, and $f = c^x$, then we can say that x is the order with respect to that reactant.

The Rate Constant

From the experimental data, you can also calculate the rate constant, k. For the reaction we looked at above, we found that the rate law is given by: rate $= k[A][B]^2$. Solving this for k, we get

$$k = \frac{\text{rate}}{[A][B]^2}$$

Now, just pick any experiment in the table. For example, using the results of Experiment 1, you'd find that

$$k = \frac{\text{rate}}{[A][B]^2} = \frac{1 \times 10^{-3}}{(0.2)(0.1)^2} = 0.5$$

Any of the experiments will give you the same value for k because it's a constant for any given reaction at a given temperature. That is, each reaction has its own rate constant, which takes into account such factors as the frequency of collisions, the fraction of the collisions with the proper orientation to initiate the desired bond changes, and the activation energy. This can be expressed mathematically with the **Arrhenius equation**:

$$k = Ae^{-(E_a/RT)}$$

Here, A is the Arrhenius factor (which takes into account the orientation of the colliding molecules), E_a is the activation energy, R is the gas-law constant, and T is the temperature in kelvins. If we rewrite this equation in the form $\ln k = \ln A - (E_a/RT)$, we can more clearly see that *adding a catalyst* (thus decreasing

E_a) or *increasing the temperature* will increase k. In either case, the expression E_a/RT decreases, and subtracting something smaller gives a greater result, so ln k (and thus k itself) will increase. (By the way, a rough rule of thumb is that the rate will increase by a factor of about 2 to 4 for every 10-degree [Celsius] increase in temperature.)

The units of the rate constant are not necessarily uniform from one reaction to the next. Reactions of different orders will have rate constants bearing different units. In order to obtain the units of the rate constant one must keep in mind that the rate, on the left side of the equation, must always have units of M/s as it measures the change in concentration of a species in the reaction over time. The units given to the rate constant must, when combined with the units of the concentrations in the rate equation, provide M/s.

Below is a generic second order rate equation.

$$\text{Rate} = k[A][B]$$

Assuming that the concentrations of both A and B are in molarity (M), then in order to give the left side of the equation units of M/s, the units of the rate constant must be $M^{-1}s^{-1}$. If the rate were third order, the units would be $M^{-2}s^{-1}$, or if first order then simply s^{-1}.

Experiment	[A]	[B]	Initial reaction rate [M/s]
1	0.01 M	0.01 M	4.0×10^{-3}
2	0.01 M	0.02 M	8.0×10^{-3}
3	0.02 M	0.02 M	1.6×10^{-2}
4	0.04 M	0.02 M	3.2×10^{-2}

Example 9-5: Based on the data given above, determine the rate law for the reaction A + B → C.

A) Rate = $k[B]$
B) Rate = $k[A][B]$
C) Rate = $k[A]^2[B]$
D) Rate = $k[A][B]^2$

Solution: Comparing Experiments 1 and 2, we notice that when [B] doubled (and [A] remained unchanged), the reaction rate doubled. Therefore, the reaction is first order with respect to [B]; this eliminates choice D. Now, comparing Experiments 3 and 4, we notice that when [A] doubled (and [B] remained unchanged), the reaction rate also doubled. This means that the reaction is first order with respect to [A] as well. Therefore, the answer is B.

Example 9-6: Which of the following gives the form of the rate law for the balanced reaction shown below?

$$4\,A + 2\,B \;\rightarrow\; C + 3\,D$$

A)   Rate = $k[A]^4[B]^2$
B)   Rate = $k[A]^2[B]$
C)   Rate = $k[C][D]^3/[A]^4[B]^2$
D)   Cannot be determined from the information given

Solution: Unless the given reaction is the rate-determining, elementary step, we have no way of knowing what the rate law is. The answer is D.

Experiment	[A]	[B]	Initial reaction rate [M/s]
1	0.1 M	0.2 M	2.0×10^{-5}
2	0.2 M	0.3 M	1.2×10^{-4}
3	0.1 M	0.4 M	4.0×10^{-5}
4	0.2 M	0.4 M	1.6×10^{-4}

Example 9-7: Using the data given above, determine the numerical value of the rate constant for the reaction $A + B \rightarrow C$.

Solution: First, let's find the rate law. Comparing Experiments 3 and 4, we notice that when [A] doubled (and [B] remained unchanged), the reaction rate increased by a factor of 4. This means the reaction is second order with respect to [A]. Comparing Experiments 1 and 3, we notice that when [B] doubled (and [A] remained unchanged), the reaction rate increased by a factor of 2. This means the reaction is first order with respect to [B]. Therefore, the rate law is $rate = k[A]^2[B]$. Finally, using any of the experiments, we can solve for k; using the data in Experiment 1, say, we find that

$$k = \frac{rate}{[A]^2[B]} = \frac{2 \times 10^{-5}\,M/s}{2 \times 10^{-3}\,M^3} = 10^{-2}\,M^{-2}\,s^{-1} = 0.01\,M^{-2}\,s^{-1}$$

Chapter 9 Summary

- Kinetics is the study of how quickly a reaction occurs, but does not determine *whether or not* a reaction will occur.

- All rates are experimentally determined by measuring a change in the concentration of a reactant or product compared to a change in time (often given in M/s).

- Molecules must collide in order to react, and the frequency and energy of these collisions determines how fast the reaction occurs.

- Increasing the concentration of reactants *often* increases the reaction rate due to an increased number of collisions.

- Increasing the temperature of a reaction *always* increases the reaction rate since molecules move faster and collide more frequently; the energy of collisions also increases.

- Activation energy (E_a) is the minimum energy required to start a reaction and decreases in the presence of a catalyst, thereby increasing the reaction rate.

- Transition states are at energy maxima, while intermediates are at local energy minima along a reaction coordinate.

- A reaction mechanism must agree with experimental data, and suggests a possible pathway by which reactants and intermediates might collide in order for a chemical reaction to occur.

- The sum of all elementary steps of a mechanism will add to give the overall chemical reaction.

- The slow step of the mechanism is the rate limiting step, and determines the rate of the overall reaction.

- A rate law can only be determined from experimental data or if given a mechanism, and has the general form: Rate $= k[\text{reactants}]^x$, where x is the order of the reaction with respect to the given reactant, and k is the rate constant.

- The overall order of a reaction is the sum of all exponents in the rate law.

- The value of the rate constant, k, depends on temperature and activation energy, and its units will vary depending on the reaction order.

- Coefficients of the reactants in the rate limiting step of a mechanism can be used to determine the order of a reaction in the rate law; coefficients from the overall reaction alone CANNOT be used to find the order of a reaction.

CHAPTER 9 FREESTANDING PRACTICE QUESTIONS

1. In the reaction A + 2 B → C, the rate law is experimentally determined to be rate = $k[B]^2$. What happens to the initial rate of reaction when the concentration of A is doubled?

A) The rate doubles.
B) The rate quadruples.
C) The rate is halved.
D) The rate is unchanged.

2. Which of the following statements is always true about the kinetics of a chemical reaction?

A) The rate law includes all reactants in the balanced overall equation.
B) The overall order equals the sum of the reactant coefficients in the overall reaction.
C) The overall order equals the sum of the reactant coefficients in the slow step of the reaction.
D) The structure of the catalyst remains unchanged throughout the reaction progress.

3. Which of the following is represented by a localized minimum in a reaction coordinate diagram?

A) Transition state
B) Product
C) Activated complex
D) Intermediate

4. Which factor always affects both thermodynamic and kinetic properties?

A) Temperature
B) Transition state energy level
C) Reactant coefficients of the overall reaction
D) No single factor always affects both thermodynamics and kinetics.

5. Which of the following best describes the role of pepsin in the process of proteolysis?

A) It stabilizes the structure of the amino acid end products.
B) It lowers the energy requirement needed for the reaction to proceed.
C) It increases the K_{eq} of proteolysis.
D) It lowers the free energy of the peptide reactant.

6. Based on the reaction mechanism shown below, which of the following statements is correct?

$$2 NO + O_2 \rightarrow 2 NO_2$$

1) $2 NO \rightarrow N_2O_2$ (fast)
2) $N_2O_2 + O_2 \rightarrow 2 NO_2$ (slow)

A) Step 1 is the rate-determining step and the rate of the overall reaction is $k[N_2O_2]$.
B) Step 1 is the rate-determining step and the rate of the overall reaction is $k[NO]^2$.
C) Step 2 is the rate-determining step and the rate of the overall reaction is $k[NO_2]^2$.
D) Step 2 is the rate-determining step and the rate of the overall reaction is $k[N_2O_2][O_2]$.

7. When table sugar is exposed to air it undergoes the following reaction:

$$C_{12}H_{22}O_{11} + 12 O_2 \rightarrow 12 CO_2 + 11 H_2O$$

$$(\Delta G = -5693 \text{ kJ/mol})$$

When this reaction is observed at the macroscopic level, it appears as though nothing is happening, yet one can detect trace amounts of CO_2 and H_2O being formed. These observations are best explained by the fact that the reaction is:

A) thermodynamically favorable but not kinetically favorable.
B) kinetically favorable but not thermodynamically favorable.
C) neither kinetically nor thermodynamically favorable.
D) both kinetically and thermodynamically favorable.

CHAPTER 9 PRACTICE PASSAGE

One way to determine a rate law is to look at the slowest elementary step in a reaction mechanism. The rate law is equal to the rate constant times the initial concentrations of the reactants in the slowest step raised to the power of their coefficients in the balanced equation. If a chemical appears in the rate law raised to the X power, we say the reaction is X order for that chemical.

In cases where the slow step is not the first step, the rate law will likely depend on the concentration of intermediate species. This is experimentally inconvenient, since the concentration of intermediates is not as straightforward to control as starting materials. As such, rate laws are often rewritten substituting terms consisting solely of starting materials, when possible. For example, consider the decomposition of nitramide:

$$O_2NNH_2(aq) \rightarrow N_2O(g) + H_2O(l)$$

Reaction 1

This reaction consists of three elementary steps (shown below), with step 2 as the slow step.

Step 1 (fast equilibrium):
$$O_2NNH_2(aq) \rightleftharpoons O_2NNH^-(aq) + H^+(aq)$$

Step 2 (slow):
$$O_2NNH^-(aq) \rightarrow N_2O(g) + OH^-(aq)$$

Step 3 (fast):
$$H^+(aq) + OH^-(aq) \rightarrow H_2O(l)$$

One could write a valid rate law for this reaction of the form:

$$\text{rate} = k[O_2NNH^-]$$

However, the inclusion of the intermediate term is not ideal. The fast equilibrium in Step 1 allows the substitution of $[O_2NNH^-]$ according to the equilibrium condition:

$$K_{eq} = \frac{[O_2NNH^-][H^+]}{[O_2NNH_2]}$$

Solving for $[O_2NNH^-]$, and substituting into the rate law gives an equally valid expression, detailing how the rate may be altered by varying the concentration of starting material and the pH of the reaction mixture:

$$\text{rate} = k\left(\frac{K_{eq}[O_2NNH_2]}{[H^+]}\right)$$

The mechanism for this reaction consists of three elementary steps. The first step is an equilibrium reaction with a significant back reaction and the last step is an equilibrium reaction lying so far to the right that we consider it to go to completion:

1. What is the order of the decomposition of nitramide in water with respect to H^+?

   A) Negative first order
   B) One half order
   C) First order
   D) Second order

2. If Step 1 were simply a fast reaction and not a fast equilibrium, what would be the expected rate law for the decomposition of nitramide in water?

   A) $\text{Rate} = k[O_2NNH_2]$

   B) $\text{Rate} = k[O_2NNH^-]$

   C) $\text{Rate} = k[H^+][OH^-]$

   D) $\text{Rate} = k\dfrac{[O_2NNH_2]}{[H^+]}$

3. If separately synthesized $Na^+[O_2NNH^-]$ were added to a reaction in progress (assuming total solubility of the salt), what effect would this have on the rate?

   A) No reaction would be observed.
   B) The rate of the reaction would decrease.
   C) The rate of the reaction would increase.
   D) It is impossible to tell without experimental data.

4. If the $[H^+]$ goes up by a factor of four, the reaction rate will:

   A) increase by a factor of four.
   B) increase by a factor of two.
   C) decrease by a factor of two.
   D) decrease by a factor of four.

5. Considering Step 1 in isolation, if a known amount of O_2NNH_2 is dissolved in water, which of the following plays a role in determining how fast the reaction reaches equilibrium?

    A) The pH of the solution
    B) The reaction temperature
    C) The magnitude of the equilibrium constant
    D) The stability of O_2NNH_2 compared to O_2NNH^- and H^+

6. What is true regarding the enthalpy and entropy changes for Step 3 of the mechanism?

    A) $\Delta H > 0, \Delta S > 0$
    B) $\Delta H > 0, \Delta S < 0$
    C) $\Delta H < 0, \Delta S > 0$
    D) $\Delta H < 0, \Delta S < 0$

SOLUTIONS TO CHAPTER 9 FREESTANDING PRACTICE QUESTIONS

1. **D** Since the rate law is independent of [A], (i.e., rate is only dependent on the concentration of B), changing the amount of A will have no effect on the rate.

2. **C** Choice A is incorrect because rate laws are dependent on the slowest step. If a reactant does not participate in the slow step, it will not be included in the overall rate law. Choice B is incorrect because rate laws of overall reactions can only be determined experimentally. Choice D is incorrect because while it is true that a catalyst comes out of a reaction unchanged, it can undergo temporary transformations during the reaction and revert back into its original form at the end. Choice C is the best option because rate laws can be determined from elementary steps of a reaction mechanism by simply raising the reactants to their respective coefficients.

3. **D** It should be noted that choices A and C are the same and should therefore be eliminated. Additionally, transition states are localized maximums, not minimums. Choice B is incorrect because the product for a spontaneous reaction is the absolute minimum and not a localized minimum. Intermediates are formed and then used. They have a certain lifespan represented by a local minimum on the reaction coordinate diagram.

4. **A** Choice B is purely a kinetic factor and can be eliminated. Choice C is eliminated because it dictates the thermodynamic quantity K_{eq} but not necessarily the kinetics of the overall reaction (only of the rate limiting step). Gibbs free energy, a thermodynamic property, is defined as $\Delta G = \Delta H - T\Delta S$, and the Arrhenius equation defines the rate constant k, a kinetic property, as $k = Ae^{(-E_a/RT)}$. Both equations contain the T variable representing temperature. Therefore, choice A is correct and choice D must be incorrect.

5. **B** Pepsin is an enzyme, a biological catalyst. Catalysts lower the activation energy by providing the correct orientation of reactants for a reaction to proceed. Enzymes make a reaction go faster and affect the kinetics of the reaction, making choice B the best answer. Stability of the products, K_{eq}, and free energy of the reactants are all thermodynamic properties, so choices A, C, and D are eliminated.

6. **D** The rate-determining step (RDS) of a reaction mechanism is the slowest step of that mechanism, eliminating choices A and B. The rate law of an elementary step can be determined from the coefficients of the reactants in the elementary step. Because Step 2 is the RDS, the overall rate law will be equivalent to the rate law for the RDS. Therefore, rate = $k[N_2O_2][O_2]$.

7. **A** Given the very negative ΔG value, this is a very thermodynamically favorable, spontaneous chemical reaction (eliminate choice B and C). It is important to make the distinction in this case between kinetics and thermodynamics. The reason only trace amounts of products are formed is that the reaction proceeds at an incredibly slow rate (therefore NOT kinetically favorable) due to a high activation energy.

SOLUTIONS TO CHAPTER 9 PRACTICE PASSAGE

1. **A** The passage states that if a chemical is raised to the X power, the reaction is X order with respect to that chemical. The rate law can be written as Rate = $k[O_2NNH_2][H^+]^{-1}$, so the reaction is negative first order with respect to H^+.

2. **B** If the first step was simply a fast step, then we would be able to make the normal assumptions about elementary steps and rate laws. More specifically, the rate law could be determined by the stoichiometry of the slow Step 2, which would yield the rate law in choice B.

3. **C** Recall that re-writing the rate law in terms of observable starting conditions does not make the rate including $[O_2NNH^-]$ invalid. The two rate laws are equivalent to one another. As such, increasing the concentration of $[O_2NNH^-]$ will increase the reaction rate.

4. **D** Since $[H^+]$ is in the denominator of the rate law expression and raised to the first power, if $[H^+]$ goes up by a factor of four, the rate will go down by a factor of four.

5. **B** The question requires an answer related to the kinetics of the reaction. Choices A, C, and D are not kinetic factors. The temperature of a reaction is factored into the rate constant ($k = Ae^{-(E_a/RT)}$), so it will play a role in determining the speed of progress to equilibrium.

6. **D** Neutralization reactions release large amounts of heat, so ΔH must be less than zero, eliminating choices A and B. From the point of view of entropy, two molecules become one, increasing the order of the system. Moreover, two aqueous species turning into a pure liquid increases order. Therefore, disorder decreases and ΔS must be less than zero.

FIBRIL NUCLEATION KINETICS OF A PHARMACEUTICAL PEPTIDE: THE ROLE OF CONFORMATION STABILITY, FORMULATION FACTORS, AND TEMPERATURE EFFECT

Jingtao Zhang, Xinpei Mao, and Wei Xu

Physical instability, such as aggregation, can pose a significant risk for the pharmaceutical development of peptides. Amyloid fibril formation corresponds to the conversion of the peptide from its native conformation into long-range-ordered aggregates, which are mostly β-sheet conformations assembled as intertwined fibers. The resulting aggregates are irreversible and would not dissolve or dissociate by dilution, gentle heat, or pH treatment. Their formation can lead to a number of issues in drug quality, ranging from poor processability to loss of drug efficacy as well as immunogenicity concerns. Therefore, strategies to stabilize against fibril formation are critical to the formulation development of fibril-prone peptide drugs.

The key to formulation stabilization is to minimize the aggregation rate. It is noted that the shelf life of a peptide product is determined from the long-term real time measurement of aggregation kinetics, which typically becomes available during late stage development. In contrast, during early stage development, kinetics studies under accelerated or stressed conditions are frequently leveraged to forecast risks of the compound, and they help to make decisions on the viability of compound or formulation options.

Amyloid fibril aggregation typically follows nucleated polymerization kinetics, frequently characterized as nucleation, growth, and plateau phases. The nucleation phase corresponds to the formation of the "critical fibril nucleus", which serves as the initiation template for the rapid physical polymerization of fibrils in the growth phase. The nucleation phase is characterized by lag phase, with the time spent in this phase commonly referred to as lag time, due to the apparent absence of aggregates during this period of time. The growth phase corresponds to chain propagation, transfer, reinitiation, etc. and is characterized by the rapid loss of soluble peptide. Eventually, the depletion of soluble peptide leads to the end of the growth phase and chain termination, while aggregation reaches a plateau.

However, from a formulation development perspective, the ability to measure and predict the lag time of the formulation is of utmost importance, since this is the region where the formulation is considered to be metastable, and the stability of the formulation is justified (as shelf life). Therefore, the present research is focused on studying the factors that impact the lag time and the approaches that can permit the prediction of the lag time of formulations at the intended storage conditions.

Past studies have investigated the factors that influence peptide fibril aggregation kinetics, although the majority of the systems or conditions are not pharmaceutically relevant. Despite these investigations, studies on the correlation between accelerated kinetics and real-time performance are very limited. Furthermore, the majority of the kinetics study investigating the impact of temperature was conducted on peptides that do not have native folding. The presence of folding in peptides will introduce an additional unfolding energy barrier in the activation energy.

MATERIALS

Peptide A was supplied with greater than 97% purity according to a reverse phase HPLC analysis. The molecular weight is 3824 Da, and the isoelectric point (pI) is 3.8. Solubility of the peptide is pH dependent and is >5 mg/mL when pH is above 6.

Circular Dichroism

Circular dichroism (CD) measurement was performed on a Jasco J-810 CD spectrometer (Tokyo, Japan) to study the conformation stability of the peptide. CD spectra were presented as an average of three consecutive measurements.

Soluble Peptide Concentration by HPLC Analysis

The soluble peptide amount was determined from the sample supernatant after a 10 min 14,000 rpm centrifugation (~18 000g). Peptide concentration was then determined by gradient reverse-phase high-performance liquid chromatography. The peptide amount was determined using peak areas at a wavelength of 214 nm in the UV spectrum and calculated from an external peptide A standard curve.

Fluorescence Measurement of Peptide Fibril Amount by Thioflavin T

The fluorescence signal increase upon thioflavin T (ThioT) binding to the peptide fibril was used to track the aggregation kinetics of peptide A.

Aggregation Kinetics Study from Microplate Fluorimeter

Before measurement, ThioT working solution was added to the peptide solution to reach 5 μM concentration. Typically, a glass coated 96-well polypropylene microplate (Thermo Scientific) was used for the experiment. To determine the impact of solid substrate interface, polypropylene, polystyrene, or polystyrene low binder plates (Corning, Kennebunk, ME) were used in the study.

Turbidity Measurement To Determine the Lag Time of Peptide A

Crystal 16 (Technobis, Netherland) was used to assess the temperature-dependent aggregation kinetics under stirring conditions. The cells in the instrument were first equilibrated to the study temperature. Light transmission reading from the vials was recorded every minute immediately after stirring started. The relative turbidity value was calculated by subtracting the percentage of light transmission from 100. For each temperature, 3–5 replicate vials were studied simultaneously; the reported lag time was the average of these measurements.

Lag Time Analysis Method

The aggregation kinetics data from ThioT kinetics and Crystal 16 turbidity measurement were analyzed by one of two ways to determine the lag time, curve fitting using sigmoidal function or onset point determination. In general, GraphPad Prism 7.0 and a sigmoidal function, as shown in eq 1, were used to fit the ThioT kinetics curve. The lag time was then determined using eq 2. It is noted, that for the determination of activation energy, the apparent nucleation rate was defined as the inverse of lag time.

$$F = F_0 + B \times t + \frac{C + D \times t}{1 + e^{\left(\frac{t_0 - t}{\tau}\right)}} \qquad (1)$$

$$\text{Lag time} = t_0 - 2 \times \tau \qquad (2)$$

F represents the measured signal as a function of t, while F_0, B, C, D, τ, and t_0 are the fitted parameters.

RESULTS

Conformation Stability of Peptide A

CD was utilized to evaluate the secondary structure and conformation stability of the peptide. As shown in Figure 1, peptide A adopts an α-helical secondary structure at 5 °C, as evidenced by the double minima at wavelengths 208 and 222 nm, and a maximum at around 192 nm. At elevated temperatures, a gradual loss of the α-helical feature was observed, suggesting the conversion to random coil. We further evaluated the reversibility of the folding by comparing the peptide CD signal after cooling the thermal melt solution back to 5 °C. Samples returning back to 5 °C after a heating cycle have identical spectra compared to the sample that did not undergo a prior thermal denaturation (data not shown). This shows that the folding of the peptide is reversible. Comparison of peptide CD spectra in different pH buffer (pH 6–9) shows no significant differences, suggesting that peptide conformation at 5 °C is not significantly affected by pH.

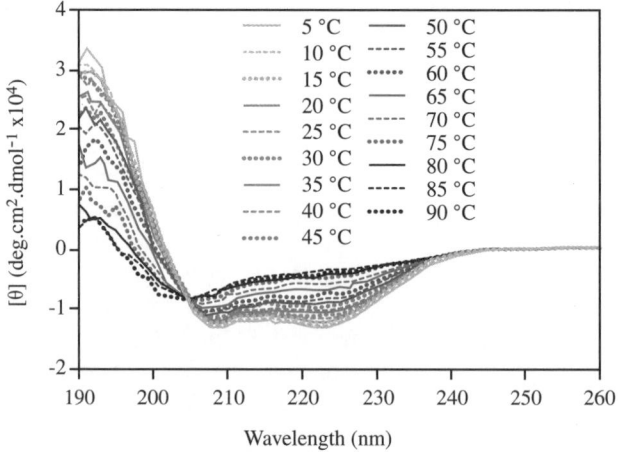

Figure 1. (A) CD spectra of 0.2 mg/mL peptide A at temperatures ranging from 5 to 90 °C. Peptide A was in 20 mM pH 7.2 NaPO$_4$ formulation.

Peptide A Can Form β-Sheet Fibril with Nucleated Polymerization Aggregation Kinetics

During the formulation development of peptide A, it was observed that the initially clear peptide solution would convert to either transparent gel or turbid suspension upon extended incubation at 25 or 40 °C. Both events corresponded to the loss of soluble peptide in the solution. Due to the similarity of these observations to amyloid fibrils, it was thus suspected that β-sheet self-assembly could be responsible for the behavior of peptide A. Indeed, CD spectra on a clear gel of the 40 °C-incubated peptide showed β-sheet spectra.

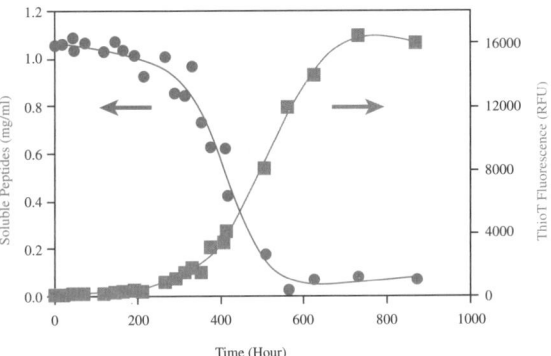

Figure 2. Soluble peptide A concentration and ThioT signal of a peptide A formulation (1 mg/mL, pH 6.5) during the static incubation at 25 °C. ThioT was added to the sample at each time point, and the fluorescence signal is determined from the admixture. Soluble peptide content was assessed by the amount of peptide in the supernatant after a 14 000 rpm centrifugation. The data were fitted using a sigmoidal equation to determine the lag time.

To determine fibril aggregation kinetics, quantitative methods that could correlate with the amount of aggregated peptide were used to monitor the formulation during the stability study. ThioT was a frequently used fluorescent dye for fibril detection. Its fluorescence value will increase significantly upon binding to the hydrophobic pocket in the β-sheet fibril, partly due to its reduced quenching upon binding. We sampled the formulation at predefined intervals and measured the fluorescence of the admixture immediately after the addition of ThioT. It is noted, that the ThioT fluorescence value could be potentially affected by fibril polymorphism and the availability of binding sites in the β-sheet fibril. Therefore, in addition to the ThioT fluorescence, soluble peptide content was also measured at each time point prior to the addition of ThioT. Figure 2 showed the aggregation kinetics of a 1 mg/mL peptide A formulation while being incubated at 25 °C under static

conditions. It is shown that both ThioT fluorescence and the amount of soluble peptide followed three stage processes, lag phase, growth phase, and plateau phase. During the lag phase, no loss of soluble peptide and change of ThioT fluorescence were observed. During the growth phase, a rapid growth of the ThioT fluorescence correlated with the loss of soluble peptide. This type of profile is highly consistent with the nucleated polymerization kinetic profile commonly observed for other peptide fibrils.

High-Throughput Experiments To Evaluate Factors Affecting the Lag Time of Peptide Fibril Aggregation Kinetics

Formulation development of biologics formulation utilizes excipient factors, such as pH, buffer, ionic strength, polymers, surfactants, etc. to stabilize against product degradation. Other formulation factors, such as agitation, stirring, and substrates, are also known to play important roles in the aggregation of protein-based formulations. We sought to evaluate how these factors affect the lag time of peptide A. Although the addition of ThioT can potentially affect the aggregation kinetics of the peptide, it is expected that the consistent change still permits the ability to determine the effect of formulation factors on the aggregation kinetics. For example, Figure 3 showed the aggregation kinetics from a peptide A formulation monitored by the high-throughput ThioT method. Overall, a three phase kinetics profile similar to those generated in the absence of ThioT was apparent.

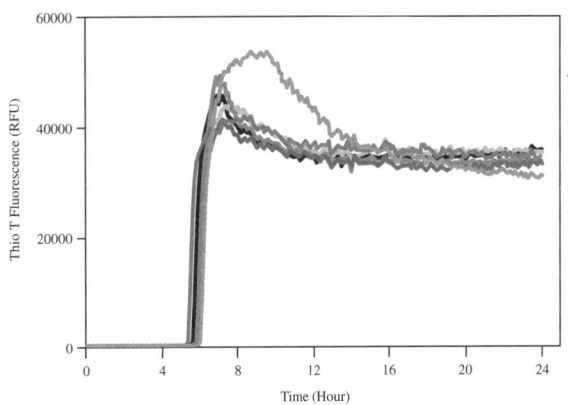

Figure 3. Aggregation kinetics of a 1 mg/mL peptide A formulation at 40 °C. The results corresponded to 6 replicate measurements of the same sample. The formulation was in pH 7 20 mM $NaPO_4$ buffer. ThioT was added at the beginning of the experiment to the formulation. The fluorescence value was monitored every 5 min. The samples were shaken between measurements inside a microplate reader.

To evaluate the impact of the initial peptide A concentration on the aggregation kinetics, we measured the lag time for peptide A in the concentration range of 0.2–20 mg/mL (Figure 4). Lag time was shown to decrease with the increases in the initial peptide concentration. However, when the initial concentration is above 6 mg/mL (1.6 mM), there is no further significant decrease in lag time. Although lower concentration can be used to increase the lag time of the formulation, the formulation needs to be >0.5 mg/mL to provide sufficient dose. Hence, the concentration of subsequent formulations was set at 1 mg/mL.

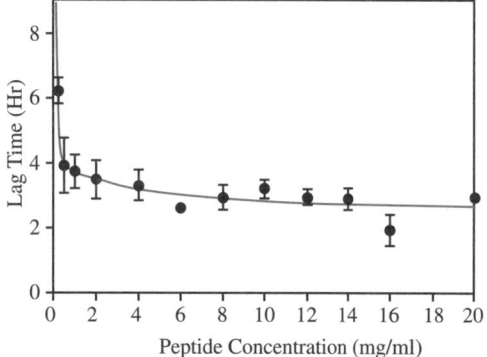

Figure 4. Lag time of peptide A formulations of different initial concentration at 40 °C. The formulations are in pH 6.5 20 mM NaPO$_4$ buffer. ThioT was added at the beginning of the experiment to the formulation. The fluorescence value was monitored every 5 min. The samples were shaken between measurements inside a microplate reader. A fitting line was used to guide the data reading.

To evaluate the impact of pH and buffer on the aggregation kinetics, we measured the lag time for the peptide in the pH region between 6 and 9 (Figure 5A). Several buffers were compared at the same pH to decouple the effect of pH and buffer species. It is found that pH plays a very significant role in determining the aggregation lag time of peptide A. For example, the lag time roughly increases exponentially with the increase of pH. In fact, lag time increases ~3-fold for every pH unit increase. This suggests that protonation or deprotonation of the peptide strongly impacts the fibril nucleation rate. Due to the pI 4.3, peptide A maintains a net negative charge between pH 6 and 9. It is likely that increasing the negative charge at higher pH leads to more repulsion between the peptide, and therefore less productive strand alignment for fibril nucleus formation. To assess this hypothesis, we evaluated the lag time of formulations with increasing NaCl concentration (Figure 5B). For formulations at the same pH, it was found

that the addition of NaCl can greatly reduce the lag time of the formulation, consistent with the above hypothesis. Interestingly, despite the large difference in lag time between pH 8 and 9 samples at low NaCl concentration, the lag time of these formulations reach similar values when NaCl concentration is above 500 mM. Taken together, the results suggest that charge repulsion as affected by pH or ionic strength could be one of the major approaches for stabilization of peptide fibril formulation.

A

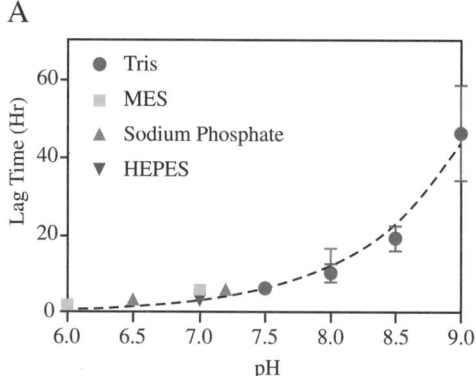

B

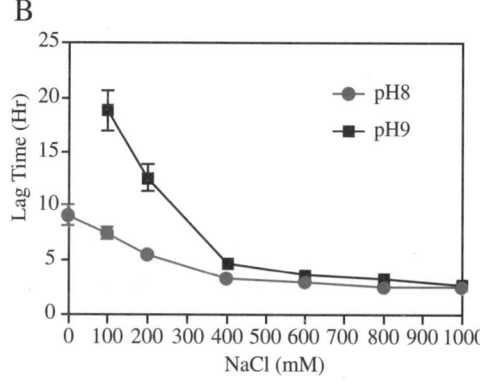

Figure 5. Lag time of 1 mg/mL peptide A formulation at different pH (A) or NaCl concentration (B). Lag time was determined from the high throughput ThioT kinetics measurement at 40 °C. All buffers were 20 mM in buffer concentration. An exponential fitting equation was used to guide the data reading in (A).

Impact of Temperature on Peptide Fibril Aggregation Lag Time

The effect of temperature on peptide fibril aggregation kinetics was studied under three different conditions. First, a high-throughput ThioT fluorescence method was used to evaluate the aggregation kinetics under a gentle shaking condition. Due to the limit of the fluorescence plate reader, the study temperature was limited between 25 and 50 °C.

Three formulations at different pH values (pH 6.5, 7.2 and 8.0) were chosen to evaluate the impact of temperature on lag time. For formulations at the same pH, it is shown that lag time decreases nonlinearly with the increase in temperature (Figure 6A). Further study was focused on the pH 6.5 formulation, where kinetics can be studied within a reasonable study time. For the pH 6.5 formulation, the lag time was further converted to an apparent nucleation rate (1/lag time) to produce the Arrhenius plot according to eq 3 (Figure 6B). It is shown, that ln(apparent nucleation rate) is linearly correlated to the inverse of the absolute temperature (1/T). It is noted, that the narrow temperature range (25–50 °C) preclude from concluding on the Arrhenius nature of the nucleation kinetics since non-Arrhenius behavior is frequently observed at refrigerated conditions, and non-Arrhenius behavior could be modeled as Arrhenius in a narrow temperature range. Next, the turbidity-based detection system from Crystal 16 was used to determine the lag time of peptide fibril aggregation under a wider temperature range (5–70 °C). It is noted, that the formulations were stirred at 800 rpm during the study. Interestingly, it is shown, that a similarly linear relationship can be found between ln(apparent nucleation rate) and the inverse of temperature spanning this wide temperature range (Figure 6B). This strongly suggests that the nucleation rate for fibril formation follows Arrhenius-like behavior at least in the temperature range of 5–70 °C. Finally, to provide a direct assessment of peptide aggregation kinetics under simulated shelf storage conditions, we investigated the aggregation kinetics under static conditions. Four temperatures (5, 25, 40, and 60 °C) were evaluated for the real time aggregation kinetics, which was determined by a combination of soluble peptide content analysis and ThioT fluorescence of samples assessed at each time interval. It is found that an Arrhenius-like behavior is also observed between 5–60 °C for the formulation under static incubation conditions (Figure 6B). Table 1 lists the activation energy calculated from the three different kinetics experiments. Interestingly, it is shown, that despite the large difference observed in the apparent nucleation rate, these kinetics experiments share very similar activation energies. This suggests that the increase in nucleation rate under stirring and shaking conditions is not due to the change in the activation energy of the rate limiting steps but rather due to the increase in the productive collision events for the nucleation step (i.e., pre-exponential factor). A is the pre-exponential factor indicating the productive attempt frequency for nucleation, and E_a is the activation energy for the rate limiting step.

$$\ln(k) = \ln(A) - \frac{E_a}{RT} \qquad (3)$$

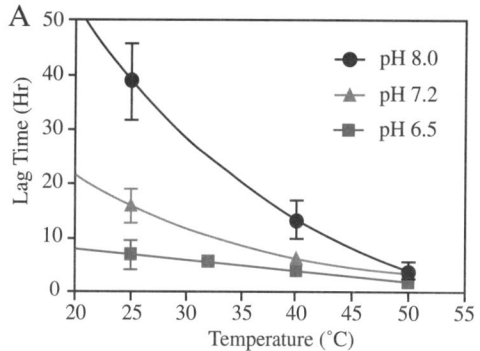

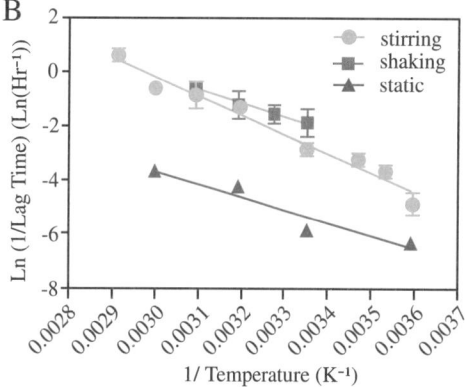

Figure 6. (A) Impact of temperature on the lag time of 1 mg/mL peptide A formulations (pH 6.5, 7.2, or 8.0). Lag time was determined from the high-throughput ThioT kinetics measurement under gentle shaking conditions. All buffers were 20 mM NaPO$_4$. An exponential fitting equation was used to guide the data reading. (B) Arrhenius plot of the apparent nucleation rate (1/lag time) versus the inverse of temperature of 1 mg/mL peptide A formulation. The formulation was in pH 6.5 20 mM NaPO$_4$ buffer. Activation energies were determined from the slope of the fitting curves (eq 3).

Table 1. Activation Energy of the Fibril Nucleation of 1 mg/mL Peptide A Formulations under Different Formulations and Stressed Conditions

stress conditions	activation energy (kcal/mol)		
	pH 6.5	pH 7.2	pH 8.0
stirring	14.1 ± 1.0	N.D.	N.D.
shaking	9.6 ± 0.9	11.9 ± 0.5	17.5 ± 3.1
static	9.5 ± 1.9	N.D.	N.D.

Data are presented as fitted value ± standard error.

DISCUSSION

A key requirement for a pharmaceutical product is to maintain drug stability during manufacturing, storage, and in use. This ensures the quality and consistency of the drug, and safeguards patients from harmful exposure to untested or under-tested substances. From a commercial perspective, 18 months is frequently the minimally acceptable shelf life due to the time required for production, packaging, and distribution. During this period of time, minimal degradation or active loss is permitted.

Similar to proteins, peptides can form both reversible and irreversible high-molecular weight (HMW) aggregates. The formation of an irreversible HMW aggregate is of most concern due to the permanent loss of the active and the increased risk in immunogenicity. Formation of peptide fibrils will generally lead to a loss of soluble peptide. Structural characterization shows that it has an α-helical fold when initially dissolved in solution (Figure 1). The solution will gradually convert to gel or precipitate upon extended incubation. It was shown, that the fibril formed is composed of β-sheets and fibers in nature, with concomitant loss of soluble peptide during the process. The conversion of peptide A can lead to 100% loss of the active peptide, which poses a great challenge for formulation development (Figure 2). While fibril risk is clearly outlined from accelerated stress studies, two outstanding questions need to be answered to understand the commercial viability of this candidate: (1) What are the formulation factors that will influence the stability of the candidate? (2) Is greater than 18 month stability at designated shelf conditions (e.g., 5 °C) achievable through a practical formulation approach? These questions hinge on the understanding of aggregation kinetics as well as how to define the developability criteria for peptide fibril kinetics.

Peptide A aggregates through classic nucleated polymerization kinetics, consisting of nucleation, growth, and plateau phases (Figure 2). For pharmaceutical development, the nucleation phase is of the utmost importance since it signifies a metastable state, and minimal degradation occurs during this period of time. Hence, we define the time in the nucleation phase, lag time, as the critical parameter of interest for the kinetics study. The apparent nucleation rate constant for amyloids is inversely correlated to lag time and is calculated as 1/lag time.

It is further noted, that lag time is defined by the lack of aggregation during the nucleation phase according to analytical methods. Hence, the measurement of lag time is inherently limited by the sensitivity of the analytical tools used.

Peptide A fibril aggregating kinetics show strong dependence on a variety of formulation factors. Peptide A lag time increases with the increase in pH and the decrease in ionic strength (Figure 5). This suggests that high pH and low ionic strength will be the preferred formulation conditions. It is noted that peptides typically will have significant chemical degradation at elevated alkaline conditions. Hence, selection of the final pH conditions for the formulation needs to balance the gain in lag time vs the loss in chemical degradation. Peptide A lag time decreases significantly in the presence of agitation (shaking or stirring) and hydrophobic interfaces. This is consistent with the thought that hydrophobic force is the driving force for fibril formation. It also suggests that the use of surfactant, which will interact through hydrophobic interaction, will likely be beneficial for extending the lag time of fibril aggregation.

Defining developability criteria for peptide fibril kinetics requires the ability to predict real-time kinetics from accelerated kinetic studies. Indeed, in the absence of direct correlation between accelerated and real-time kinetics, only the real-time study can be used to inform the developability of the formulation candidates. The most frequently used approach to predict kinetics is through the Arrhenius equation by investigating the temperature dependent behavior of kinetics (eq 3). As described by the equation, ln(reaction rate constant) is inversely proportional to the temperature of the reaction. This simple relationship allows for the prediction of the reaction rate from a short high temperature study to a long low temperature study.

Figure 6 shows that ln(apparent nucleation rate) is linearly proportional to $1/T$, showing that nucleation of peptide

A does follow Arrhenius relationship. Interestingly, the nucleation under different stress conditions appears to share the same activation energy as static conditions (Table 1). This observation suggests that the presence of shaking or stirring did not impact the nucleation rate by altering the energetics in the rate limiting step. Instead, it might impact the kinetics by increasing the success rate of collision required for nucleation. It is also noted, that the activation energy of the aggregation nucleation step for peptide A is in the range of 10–20 kcal/mol. This value is similar to the nucleation activation energy of other natively unfolded proteins and polypeptides, and it is much smaller than those observed for large proteins. This suggests that peptide A will not have large temperature-dependent aggregation kinetics like large proteins.

The Arrhenius behavior in the apparent nucleation rate shows that the lag time of the peptide at 5 °C static conditions (i.e., pseudo storage conditions) can be directly extrapolated from the lag time studies determined at several higher temperatures.

It is noted, that current study was conducted on the peptide under relatively simple solution conditions. Except buffer, pH, and NaCl excipients, no other excipients, such as surfactants, were tested in the study. Under most of these conditions, it is expected that aggregation kinetics is mostly governed by peptide itself due to the lack of strong peptide–excipient interaction. For formulations where surfactants or other stabilizing excipients are present, the anticipated peptide–excipient interaction will introduce additional complexities to the temperature-dependent aggregation kinetics, since the interaction will likely alter the rate limiting step or contribute significantly to the activation energy. Indeed, our preliminary evaluation on fibril stabilizing excipients has shown that the presence of other stabilizers, especially those based on hydrophobic interactions, appears to show non-Arrhenius behavior due to potentially weaker hydrophobic interaction under refrigerated conditions. Hence, further study needs to be done to evaluate the role of stabilizing excipients and their impact on aggregation kinetics for the practical development of fibril-stabilizing formulations. Nevertheless, the present study serves as the foundation for these ongoing studies and remains critically important for the studies where the peptide alone system is primarily concerned (e.g., discovery compound risk assessment).

CONCLUSION

Peptide fibrillation is a significant risk for the development of peptide pharmaceuticals. Thorough understanding of the fibrillation kinetics, especially the nucleation phase, is fundamental to the development of the risk mitigation strategy to address this challenge. Motivated by the need to predict real time kinetics of the peptide fibril from an accelerated kinetics study, a helical 29 mer peptide A was chosen as the model peptide system. It can form β-sheet fibril when incubated in solution. It was found that the lag time of peptide A fibrillation is most significantly influenced by pH, ionic strength, temperature, and agitation. Conditions that favor electrostatic repulsion could be most effective in stabilizing the peptide against fibril formation. It was also found, that the peptide A nucleation rate follows Arrhenius kinetics in the range of 5–70 °C in buffers between pH 6.5 and 8, regardless of the presence of agitation or not. Interestingly, the activation energy for the nucleation process appears to be in the range of 10–20 kcal/mol for all conditions assessed. The consistent activation energy and Arrhenius kinetics show that an accelerated kinetics study at elevated temperature can be leveraged to predict the real time nucleation kinetics at the intended storage temperature when the peptide and simple buffer conditions are involved. The present findings suggest that peptides behave differently from proteins, which frequently demonstrate non-Arrhenius aggregation kinetics. Hence, care should be taken to develop developability criteria and formulation strategies that are appropriate for peptide drugs.

JOURNAL ARTICLE EXERCISE 2

Remember that the science sections on the MCAT include a significant number of passages with experiments. You'll need to be able to extract information efficiently and analyze data effectively in order to do well on these passages.

This is the second of three "Journal Article Review Exercises" in this book. In the first exercise, we showed you the type of information you should be able to extract from the article and the sorts of things to pay attention to in the data. In this exercise, you'll do more of that on your own, and in the final exercise we'll show you how that article might get turned into an MCAT-style passage.

As a reminder, when analyzing an experiment, you should be able to:

- identify the controls.
- extract information from graphs and data tables.
- determine how the experimental groups change relative to the control.
- come to a reasonable conclusion about WHY the results were observed.
- consider potential weaknesses in the study.
- decide what the next most logical experiment or study should be.

Again, the goal of these exercises is NOT to learn content from the articles, just to get a little more comfortable reading and extracting information from them. See whether you can formulate answers to the following questions based on the (abridged) article presented on pages 205–211.

1. What is being studied? Why is it important?
2. What is new about these results?
3. What was measured?
4. How are the results presented?
5. What (if anything) was the experimental group compared to?
6. Are any of the results unexpected?
7. How are the conclusions of the authors supported by the data?
8. What potential weaknesses or flaws do you see in the experimental design? Are these addressed in the discussion section?
9. What would be the next most logical experiment?

Write brief responses to the questions below:

1. What is being studied? Why is it important?

    _____

    _____

    _____

2. What is new about these results?

    _____

    _____

    _____

3. What was measured?

    _____

    _____

    _____

4. How are the results presented?

    _____

    _____

    _____

5. What (if anything) was the experimental group compared to?

    _____

    _____

    _____

6. Are any of the results unexpected?

    _____

    _____

    _____

7. How are the conclusions of the authors supported by the data?

    _____

    _____

    _____

8. What potential weaknesses or flaws do you see in the experimental design? Are these addressed in the discussion section?

    _____

    _____

    _____

9. What would be the next most logical experiment?

    _____

    _____

    _____

Summary of experiment and results:

    _____

    _____

    _____

    _____

    _____

    _____

    _____

SOLUTIONS TO JOURNAL ARTICLE EXERCISE 2

1. **What is being studied? Why is it important?**

   Fibril formation is a specific example of peptide aggregation, which can deactivate peptide-based drugs. To better understand this phenomenon, a model peptide was used to study factors affecting the kinetics of fibril formation. The researchers analyzed the effects of pH, ionic strength of the solution, temperature, and agitation of the solution. The effects of changing these parameters on the lag time of fibril formation were studied. The results of the study can be used both to predict long-term results from accelerated, short-term studies, as well as to suggest methods of preventing aggregation in drug formulations.

2. **What is new about these results?**

   Few studies have been performed under pharmaceutically-relevant conditions. The peptides used in previous studies did not exhibit native folded states.

3. **What was measured?**

   Secondary structure of Peptide A via circular dichroism, lag time of fibril formation via three methods: ThioT fluorescence, soluble peptide, and turbidity measurements

4. **How are the results presented?**

   Secondary structure: in-text, Figure 1. Aggregation kinetics: Figure 2, Figure 3. Effect of Peptide A concentration on lag time: Figure 4. Effect of pH on lag time: Figure 5a. Effect of ionic strength on lag time: Figure 5b. Effect of temperature on lag time: Figure 6a. Effect of agitation on lag time: Figure 6b. Activation energy of fibril nucleation: Table 1.

5. **What (if anything) was the experimental group compared to?**

   No comparisons to other peptides were made; the study focuses only on the behavior of Peptide A under varying conditions. Effect of Peptide A concentration on lag time: lag time decreases with increased concentration. Effect of pH on lag time: lag time increases with increased pH. Effect of ionic strength on lag time: lag time decreases with increased NaCl concentration. Effect of temperature on lag time: lag time decreases with increased temperature. Effect of agitation on lag time: lag time decreases with agitation.

6. **Are any of the results unexpected?**

   There seem to be some threshold effects. For example, the lag time reaches a lower limit at 6 mg/mL concentration. There is a significant difference between pH 8 and pH 9 lag time at low NaCl concentration, but this difference disappears at a high NaCl concentration. The difference in the rate of fibril nucleation when the peptide is shaken or stirred seems to be due to a change in the pre-exponential factor, A, rather than the activation energy.

7. **How are the conclusions of the authors supported by the data?**

   Aggregation kinetics were measured via three different methods, which are consistent with each other. Most measurements are replicated. The Arrhenius behavior of aggregation is supported by the linear relationship between ln(1/lag time) and $1/T$.

8. **What potential weaknesses or flaws do you see in the experimental design? Are these addressed in the discussion section?**

    The detection of fibrils or other aggregates is limited by the analytical techniques that are used. The authors conceded that the conditions tested were limited. Other chemicals, such as surfactants, could be added to stabilize the peptide, but those were not tested in this study. Only a single peptide (29 mer) was used in this experiment. Some of the conclusions may not apply to larger proteins, which could behave differently.

9. **What would be the next most logical experiment?**

    Examine the lag time in the presence of other chemicals; test other peptides to see whether the results from this study are more widely applicable.

Summary of Experiment and Results:

*   Peptides are prone to aggregation, which is undesirable for drugs. The formation of aggregates, such as fibrils, during storage would likely decrease the effectiveness of a peptide drug. The authors of this study studied the aggregation kinetics of a model 29 residue peptide by measuring the lag time: the amount of time that the peptide remains soluble, before fibrils are formed. For this peptide, lag time could be increased by decreasing the concentration, increasing the pH, decreasing the ionic strength of the solution, and decreasing the temperature. They also investigated whether results from accelerated studies could be used predict results of longer-term studies. Unlike proteins, the peptide in this study exhibited Arrhenius-like behavior, suggesting that data from accelerated studies could be used to model long-term storage conditions.

Chapter 10
Equilibrium

10.1 EQUILIBRIUM

Many reactions are reversible, and situations can occur in which the forward and reverse reactions come into a balance called **equilibrium**. How does equilibrium come about? Before any bonds are broken or made, the reaction flask contains only reactants and no products. As the reaction proceeds, products begin to form and eventually build up, and some of them begin to revert to reactants. That is, once products are formed, both the forward and reverse reactions will occur. Ultimately, the reaction will come to equilibrium, a state at which both the forward and reverse reactions occur at the same constant rate. At equilibrium, the overall concentration of reactants and products remains the same, but at the molecular level, they are continually interconverting. Because the forward and reverse processes balance one another perfectly, we don't observe any net change in concentrations.

> *When a reaction is at equilibrium (and only at equilibrium), the rate of the forward reaction is equal to the rate of the reverse reaction.*

Equilibria occur for *closed systems* (which means no new reactants, products, or other changes are imposed).

The Equilibrium Constant

Each reaction will tend towards its own equilibrium and, for a given temperature, will have an **equilibrium constant, K_{eq}**. For the generic, balanced reaction

$$a\,A + b\,B \rightleftharpoons c\,C + d\,D$$

the **equilibrium expression** is given by:

$$K_{eq} = \frac{[C]^c [D]^d}{[A]^a [B]^b}$$

This is known as the **mass-action ratio**, where the square brackets represent the molar concentrations at equilibrium.

The constant K is often given a subscript to indicate the type of reaction it represents. For example, K_a (for acids), K_b (for bases), and K_{sp} (for solubility product) are all equilibrium constants. The equilibrium expression is derived from the ratio of the concentration of products to reactants at equilibrium, as follows:

1) Products are in the numerator, and reactants are in the denominator. They are in brackets because the equilibrium expression comes from the *concentrations* (at equilibrium) of the species in the reaction. For two or more reactants or products, multiply the concentrations of each species together.

2) The coefficient of each species in the reaction becomes an exponent on its concentration in the equilibrium expression.

3) Solids and pure liquids are *not* included, because their concentrations don't change. (A substance that's a solid or pure liquid in the reaction is often indicated by an "(s)" or "(l)" subscript, respectively. We're also allowed to omit solvents in dilute solutions because the solvents are in vast excess and their concentrations do not change.)

4) Aqueous dissolved particles are included.

5) If the reaction is gaseous, we can use the partial pressure of each gas as its concentration. The value of the equilibrium constant determined with pressures will be different than with molar concentrations because of their different units. The constant using partial pressures is often termed K_p.

The value of K_{eq} is constant at a given temperature for a particular reaction, no matter what ratio of reactants and products are given at the beginning of the reaction. That is, any closed system will proceed towards its equilibrium ratio of products and reactants even if you start with all products, or a mixture of some reactants and some products. You can even open the flask and add more of any reactant or product, and the system will change until it has reached the K_{eq} ratio. We'll discuss this idea in detail in just a moment, but right now focus on this:

The value of K_{eq} for a given reaction is a constant at a given temperature.

If the temperature changes, then a reaction's K_{eq} value will change.

The value of K_{eq} tells you the direction the reaction favors:

$K_{eq} < 1 \rightarrow$ reaction favors the reactants (i.e., there are more reactants than products at equilibrium)

$K_{eq} = 1 \rightarrow$ reaction has roughly equal amounts of reactants and products

$K_{eq} > 1 \rightarrow$ reaction favors the products (i.e., there are more products than reactants at equilibrium)

Example 10-1: Which of the following expressions gives the equilibrium constant for this reaction:

$$2\ NO \rightleftharpoons N_2 + O_2$$

A) $[N_2][O_2]/[2\ NO]$
B) $[N_2][O_2]/[NO]^2$
C) $[NO]/[N_2][O_2]$
D) $[NO]^2/[N_2][O_2]$

Solution: The mass-action ratio is products over reactants, so we can immediately eliminate choices C and D. Stoichiometric coefficients become exponents on the concentrations, not coefficients inside the square brackets. Therefore the coefficient of 2 for the reactant NO means the denominator will be $[NO]^2$, so the answer is B.

Example 10-2: A certain reversible reaction comes to equilibrium with high concentration of products and low concentration of reactants. Of the following, which is the most likely value of the equilibrium constant for this reaction?

A) $K_{eq} = -1 \times 10^{-5}$
B) $K_{eq} = 1 \times 10^{-5}$
C) $K_{eq} = 1$
D) $K_{eq} = 1 \times 10^{5}$

Solution: First, eliminate choice A since equilibrium constants are never negative. If the concentration of products is high and the concentration of reactants is low at equilibrium, then the ratio "products over reactants" will have a large value certainly greater than 1. Therefore, choice D is the answer.

Example 10-3: When the reaction $2\,A + B \rightleftharpoons 2\,C$ reaches equilibrium, $[A] = 0.1\,M$ and $[C] = 0.2\,M$. If the value of K_{eq} for this reaction is 8, what is $[B]$ at equilibrium?

A) $0.1\,M$
B) $0.2\,M$
C) $0.4\,M$
D) $0.5\,M$

Solution: The expression for K_{eq} is $\dfrac{[C]^2}{[A]^2[B]}$. We now solve for $[B]$ and substitute in the given values:

$$K_{eq} = \frac{[C]^2}{[A]^2[B]} \rightarrow [B] = \frac{[C]^2}{[A]^2 K_{eq}} = \frac{(0.2)^2}{(0.1)^2(8)} = \frac{2^2}{8} = 0.5$$

The answer is D.

Example 10-4: Which of the following illustrates a chemical system that is at equilibrium?

I. Bubbles forming in solution
II. A solution saturated with solute
III. The ratio of products to reactants remains constant

A) I only
B) II only
C) I and II only
D) II and III only

Solution: *Equilibrium* means that the system no longer changes with time. Both II and III illustrate this; therefore, choice D is best.

10.2   THE REACTION QUOTIENT

The equilibrium constant expression is a ratio: the concentration of the products divided by those of the reactants, each raised to the power equal to its stoichiometric coefficient in the balanced equation. If the reaction is not at equilibrium, the same expression is known simply as the **reaction quotient, Q**. For the generic, balanced reaction

$$a A + b B \rightleftharpoons c C + d D$$

the reaction quotient is given by:

$$Q = \frac{[C]^c[D]^d}{[A]^a[B]^b}$$

where the square brackets represent the molar concentrations of the species. The point now is that the concentrations in the expression Q do *not* have to be the concentrations at equilibrium. (If the concentrations are the equilibrium concentrations, the Q will equal K_{eq}.)

Comparing the value of Q to K_{eq} tells us in what direction the reaction will proceed. The reaction will strive to reach a state in which $Q = K_{eq}$. So, if Q is less than K_{eq}, then the reaction will proceed in the forward direction (in order to increase the concentration of the products and decrease the concentration of the reactants) to increase Q to the K_{eq} value. On the other hand, if Q is greater than K_{eq}, then the reaction will proceed in the reverse direction (in order to increase the concentrations of the reactants and decrease the concentrations of the products) to reduce Q to K_{eq}.

K_{eq} is the condition the reaction will try to achieve.
If $Q = K_{eq}$, the reaction is at equilibrium.

$Q \Longrightarrow K_{eq} \Longleftarrow Q$

If $Q < K_{eq}$,
reaction proceeds in
the **forward** direction
so Q gets closer to K_{eq}.

If $Q > K_{eq}$,
reaction proceeds in
the **reverse** direction
so Q gets closer to K_{eq}.

Example 10-5: The value of the equilibrium constant for the reaction

$$2 COF_2(g) \rightleftharpoons CO_2(g) + CF_4(g)$$

is $K_{eq} = 2$. If a 1 L reaction container currently holds 1 mole each of CO_2 and CF_4 and 0.5 mole of COF_2, then:

A)   the reaction is at equilibrium.
B)   the forward reaction will be favored.
C)   the reverse reaction will be favored.
D)   no prediction can be made without knowing the pressure of the container.

Solution: The expression for Q is $\dfrac{[CO_2][CF_4]}{[COF_2]^2}$. Therefore, the value of Q is:

$$\frac{(1)(1)}{(0.5)^2} = 4$$

Since $Q > K_{eq}$, the reverse reaction will be favored (choice C).

10.3   LE CHÂTELIER'S PRINCIPLE

Le Châtelier's principle states that a system at equilibrium will try to neutralize any imposed change (or stress) in order to reestablish equilibrium. For example, if you add more reactant to a system that is at equilibrium, the system will react by favoring the forward reaction in order to consume that reactant and reestablish equilibrium.

To illustrate, let's look at the Haber process for making ammonia:

$$N_2(g) + 3\,H_2(g) \rightleftharpoons 2\,NH_3(g) + heat$$

Let's assume the reaction is at equilibrium, and see how it reacts to disturbances to the equilibrium by changing the concentrations of the species, the pressure, or the temperature.

Adding Ammonia

If we add ammonia, the system is no longer at equilibrium, and there is an excess of product. How can the reaction reestablish equilibrium? By consuming some of the added ammonia, the ratio of products to reactants would decrease towards the equilibrium ratio, so the reverse reaction will be favored (we say the system "shifts to the left"), converting ammonia into nitrogen and hydrogen, until equilibrium is restored.

You can see how this follows from comparing the reaction quotient of the disturbed system to the equilibrium constant. If we add ammonia to the reaction mixture, then $[NH_3]$ increases, and the reaction quotient, Q, becomes greater than K_{eq}. As a result, the reaction will proceed in the reverse direction in order to reduce Q to K_{eq}.

Removing Ammonia

If we remove the product, ammonia, then the forward reaction will be favored—the reaction "shifts to the right"—in order to reach equilibrium again. Again, you can see how this follows from comparing the reaction quotient of the disturbed system to the equilibrium constant. If we remove ammonia from the reaction mixture, then $[NH_3]$ decreases, and the reaction quotient, Q, becomes less than K_{eq}. As a result, the reaction will proceed in the forward direction in order to increase Q to K_{eq}.

Adding Hydrogen

If we add some reactant, say $H_2(g)$, then the forward reaction will be favored—the reaction "shifts to the right"—in order to reach equilibrium again. This follows from comparing the reaction quotient of the disturbed system to the equilibrium constant. If we add hydrogen to the reaction mixture, the $[H_2]$ increases, and the reaction quotient, Q, becomes less than K_{eq}. As a result, the reaction will proceed in the forward direction in order to increase Q to K_{eq}.

Removing Nitrogen

If we remove some reactant, say $N_2(g)$, then the reverse reaction will be favored—the reaction "shifts to the left"—in order to reach equilibrium again. Again, this follows from comparing the reaction quotient of the disturbed system to the equilibrium constant. If we remove nitrogen from the reaction mixture, then $[N_2]$ decreases, and the reaction quotient, Q, becomes greater than K_{eq}. As a result, the reaction will proceed in the reverse direction in order to decrease Q to K_{eq}.

Changing the Volume of the Reaction Container

The Haber process is a gaseous reaction, so a change in volume will cause the partial pressures of the gases to change. Specifically, a decrease in volume of the reaction container will cause the partial pressures of the gases to increase; an increase in volume reduces the partial pressures of the gases in the mixture. If the number of moles of gas on the left side of the reaction does not equal the number of moles of gas on the right, then a change in pressure due to a change in volume will disrupt the equilibrium ratio, and the system will react to reestablish equilibrium.

How does the system react? Let's first assume the volume is reduced so that the pressure increases. Look back at the equation for the Haber process: There are 4 moles of gas on the reactant side (3 of H_2 plus 1 of N_2) for every 2 moles of NH_3 gas formed. If the reaction shifts to the right, four moles of gas can be condensed into 2 moles, reducing the pressure to reestablish equilibrium. On the other hand, if the volume is increased so that the pressure decreases, the reaction will shift to the left, increasing the pressure to reestablish equilibrium.

To summarize: Consider a gaseous reaction (at equilibrium) with unequal numbers of moles of gas of reactants and products. If the volume is reduced, increasing the pressure, a net reaction occurs favoring the side with the smaller total number of moles of gas. If the volume is expanded, decreasing the pressure, a net reaction occurs favoring the side with the greater total number of moles of gas. (This is only true for reactions involving gases.)

Changing the Temperature of the Reaction Mixture

Heat can be treated as a reactant or a product just like all the chemical reactants and products. Adding or removing heat (by increasing or decreasing the temperature) is like adding or removing any other reagent. Exothermic reactions release heat (which we note on the right side of the equation like a product), and the ΔH will be negative. Endothermic reactions consume heat (which we note on the left side of the equation like a reactant), and the ΔH will be positive.

The Haber process is an exothermic reaction. So, if you increase the temperature at which the reaction takes place once it's reached equilibrium, the reaction will shift to the left in order to consume the extra heat, thereby producing more reactants. If you decrease the temperature at which the reaction takes place once it's reached equilibrium, the reaction will shift to the right in order to produce extra heat, thereby producing more product.

Since the reverse of an exothermic reaction is an endothermic one (and vice versa), every equilibrium reaction involves an exothermic reaction and an endothermic reaction. We can then say this: *Lowering* the temperature favors the *exothermic* reaction, while *raising* the temperature favors the *endothermic* one. Keep in mind that, unlike changes in concentration or pressure, changes in temperature *will* affect the reaction's K_{eq} value, depending on the direction the reaction shifts to reestablish equilibrium.

Note that the above changes are specific to the system *once it is at equilibrium*. The kinetics of the reaction are a different matter. Remember, all reactions proceed faster when the temperature is increased, and this is true for the Haber process. Indeed, in industry this reaction is typically run at around 500°C, despite the fact that the reaction is exothermic. The reason is that a fast reaction with a 10 percent yield of ammonia may end up being better overall than a painfully slow reaction with a 90 percent yield of ammonia. Heating a reaction gets it to equilibrium faster. Once it's there, adding or taking away heat will affect the equilibrium as predicted by Le Châtelier's principle.

Adding an Inert (or Non-Reactive) Gas

What if we injected some helium into a constant volume reaction container? This inert gas doesn't participate in the reaction (and for the MCAT, inert gases don't participate in *any* reaction), so it will change neither the partial pressure nor the concentration of the products or reactants. If neither of these values change, then there is no change in equilibrium.

However, if we inject some helium into a constant pressure container, like one with a movable piston, the extra gas particles will push against the piston, raising it to increase the volume and equilibrate the internal pressure of the gases with external pressure. Since the volume increases, the partial pressures of the gases involved in the reversible reaction will change, thereby causing a shift in the equilibrium as described above for volume changes.

Adding a Catalyst

Adding a catalyst to a reaction that's already at equilibrium has no effect. Because it increases the rate of both the forward and reverse reactions equally, the equilibrium amounts of the species are unchanged. So, the introduction of a catalyst would cause no disturbance. Remember that a catalyst increases the reaction rate but does *not* affect the equilibrium.

Example 10-6: Nitrogen dioxide gas can be formed by the endothermic reaction shown below. Which of the following changes to the equilibrium would *not* increase the formation of NO_2?

$$N_2O_4(g) \rightleftharpoons 2\ NO_2(g) \qquad \Delta H = +58 \text{ kJ}$$

A) An increase in the temperature
B) A decrease in the volume of the container
C) Adding additional N_2O_4
D) Removing NO_2 as it is formed

Solution: Since ΔH is positive, this reaction is endothermic, and we can think of heat as a reactant. So if we increase the temperature (thereby "adding a reactant," namely heat), the equilibrium would shift to the right, thus increasing the formation of NO_2. This eliminates choice A. Adding reactant (choice C) or removing product (choice D) would also shift the equilibrium to the right. The answer must be B. A decrease in the volume of the container would increase the pressure of the gases, causing the equilibrium to shift in favor of the side with the fewer number of moles of gases; in this case, that would be to the left.

Example 10-7: If the following endothermic reaction is at equilibrium in a rigid reaction vessel,

$$CH_4(g) + H_2O(g) \rightleftharpoons CO(g) + 3\ H_2(g)$$

which one of the following changes would cause the equilibrium to shift to the right?

A) Adding $Ne(g)$
B) Removing some $H_2O(g)$
C) Increasing the pressure
D) Increasing the temperature

Solution: Choice A would have no effect, since neon is an inert gas and the question states the reaction vessel is rigid, therefore the volume does not change. Removing some reactant (choice B) would shift the equilibrium to the left. An increase in pressure (choice C) would cause the equilibrium to shift in favor of the side with the fewer number of moles of gases; in this case, that would be to the left. The answer must be D. Increasing the temperature of an endothermic reaction will shift the equilibrium toward the products.

Example 10-8: If the reaction

$$2\ NO(g) + O_2(g) \rightleftharpoons 2\ NO_2(g) \qquad \Delta H = -120\ kJ$$

is at equilibrium, which one of the following changes would cause the formation of additional $NO_2(g)$?

A) Increasing the temperature
B) Adding a catalyst
C) Reducing the volume of the reaction container
D) Removing some $NO(g)$

Solution: First, eliminate choice B; adding a catalyst to a reaction that's already at equilibrium has no effect. Now, because ΔH is negative, the reaction is exothermic (that is, we can consider heat to be a product). Increasing the temperature would therefore shift the equilibrium to the left; this eliminates choice A. Also, choice D can be eliminated, since removing a reactant shifts the equilibrium to the left. The answer is C: reducing the volume of the reaction container will increase the pressure, and the equilibrium responds to this stress by favoring the side with the fewer number of moles of gas. In this case, that would mean a shift to the right.

Example 10-9: The Haber process takes place in a container of fixed volume and is at equilibrium:

$$N_2(g) + 3\ H_2(g) \rightleftharpoons 2\ NH_3(g) + heat$$

The amounts of the gases present are measured and recorded. Some additional $N_2(g)$ is then injected into the container, and the system is allowed to return to equilibrium. When it does:

A) the amount of H_2 will be smaller than before, and the amounts of N_2 and NH_3 will be greater than before.

B) the amount of N_2 will be smaller than before, and the amounts of H_2 and NH_3 will be greater than before.

C) the amount of NH_3 will be smaller than before, and the amounts of N_2 and H_2 will be greater than before.

D) the amounts of all three gases will be the same as before.

Solution: The system will respond to this change by shifting to the right to reestablish equilibrium. The added N_2 will mean there's more N_2 in the reaction container, even after equilibrium has been reestablished. Also, the shift toward the product side means there'll be more NH_3 than before as well. And in the shifting of the equilibrium in an attempt to reestablish equilibrium, some of the H_2 got used. As a result, we'd expect that the amount of H_2 will be smaller than before, while the amounts of N_2 and NH_3 are greater than before the injection of the extra N_2 (choice A).

10.4 SOLUTIONS AND SOLUBILITY

Solutions

A **solution** forms when one substance **dissolves** into another, forming a *homogeneous* mixture. The process of dissolving is known as **dissolution**. For example, sugar dissolved into iced tea is a solution (though so is unsweetened tea). A substance present in a relatively smaller proportion is called a **solute**, and a substance present in a relatively greater proportion is called a **solvent**. The process that occurs when the solvent molecules surround the solute molecules is known as **solvation**; if the solvent is water, the process is called **hydration**.

Solutions can involve any of the three phases of matter. For example, you can have a solution of two gases, of a gas in a liquid, of a solid in a liquid, or of a solid in a solid (an **alloy**). However, most of the solutions with which you're familiar have a liquid as the solvent. Salt water has solid salt (NaCl) dissolved into water, seltzer water has carbon dioxide gas dissolved in water, and vinegar has liquid acetic acid dissolved in water. In fact, most of the solutions that you commonly see have water as the solvent: lemonade, tea, soda pop, and corn syrup are examples. When a solution has water as the solvent, it is called an **aqueous** solution.

How do we know which solutes are soluble in which solvents? Well, that's easy:

Like dissolves like.

Solutes will dissolve best in solvents where the intermolecular forces being broken in the solute are being replaced by equal (or stronger) intermolecular forces between the solvent and the solute.

Electrolytes

When ionic substances dissolve, they **dissociate** into ions. Free ions in a solution are called **electrolytes** because the solution can conduct electricity. Some salts dissociate completely into individual ions, while others only partially dissociate (that is, a certain percentage of the ions will remain paired, sticking close to each other rather than being independent and fully surrounded by solvent). Solutes that dissociate completely (like ionic substances) are called **strong electrolytes**, and those that remain ion-paired to some extent are called **weak electrolytes**. (Covalent compounds that don't dissociate into ions are **non-electrolytes**.) Solutions of strong electrolytes are better conductors of electricity than those of weak electrolytes.

Different ionic compounds will dissociate into different numbers of particles. Some won't dissociate at all, and others will break up into several ions. The **van't Hoff** (or **ionizability**) **factor** (*i*) tells us how many ions one unit of a substance will produce in a solution. For example,

- $C_6H_{12}O_6$ is non-ionic, so it does not dissociate. Therefore, $i = 1$.
  (Note: The van't Hoff factor for almost all biomolecules—hormones, proteins, steroids—is 1.)
- NaCl dissociates into Na^+ and Cl^-. Therefore, $i = 2$.
- HNO_3 dissociates into H^+ and NO_3^-. Therefore, $i = 2$.
- $CaCl_2$ dissociates into Ca^{2+} and 2 Cl^-. Therefore, $i = 3$.

Example 10-10: Of the following, which is the *weakest* electrolyte?

A) NH_4I
B) LiF
C) AgBr
D) H_2O_2

Solution: All ionic compounds, whether soluble or not, are defined as strong electrolytes, so choices A, B, and C are eliminated. Choice D, hydrogen peroxide, is a covalent compound that does not produce an appreciable number of ions upon dissolution and thus is a weak electrolyte. Choice D is the best answer.

The **concentration** of a solution tells you how much solute is dissolved in the solvent (see Section 3.9). A **concentrated** solution has a greater amount of solute per unit volume than a solution that is **dilute**. A **saturated** solution is one in which no more solute will dissolve. At this point, we have reached the **molar solubility** of the solute for that particular solvent, and the reverse process of dissolution, called **precipitation**, occurs at the same rate as dissolving. Both the solid form and the dissolved form of the solute are said to be in **dynamic equilibrium**.

Solubility

Solubility refers to the amount of solute that will saturate a particular solvent. Solubility is specific for the type of solute and solvent. For example, 100 mL of water at 25°C becomes saturated with 40 g of dissolved NaCl, but it would take 150 g of KI to saturate the same volume of water at this temperature. And both of these salts behave differently in methanol than in water. Solubility also varies with temperature, increasing or decreasing with temperature depending upon the solute and solvent as outlined in the first set of solubility rules below.

There are two sets of solubility rules that show up time and time again on the MCAT. The first set governs the general solubility of solids and gases in liquids, as a function of the temperature and pressure. These rules below should be taken as just rules of thumb because they are only 95 percent reliable (still not bad). Memorize the following:

Phase Solubility Rules

1. The solubility of solids in liquids tends to increase with increasing temperature.
2. The solubility of gases in liquids tends to decrease with increasing temperature.
3. The solubility of gases in liquids tends to increase with increasing pressure.

Keep in mind, the solubility of a gas in a liquid is also a function of the partial pressure of that gas above the liquid and the Henry's law constant (Solubility = kP). As partial pressure increases, the quantity of dissolved gas necessarily increases as the equilibrium constant remains unchanged.

The second set governs the solubility of salts in water. Memorize the following too:

Salt Solubility Rules

1. All Group I (Li^+, Na^+, K^+, Rb^+, Cs^+) and ammonium (NH_4^+) salts are *soluble*.

2. All nitrate (NO_3^-), perchlorate (ClO_4^-), and acetate ($C_2H_3O_2^-$) salts are *soluble*.

3. All silver (Ag^+), lead (Pb^{2+}/Pb^{4+}), and mercury (Hg_2^{2+}/Hg^{2+}) salts are *insoluble, except* for their nitrates, perchlorates, and acetates.

Example 10-11: Which of the following salts is expected to be *insoluble* in water?

A) CsOH
B) NH_4NO_3
C) $CaCO_3$
D) $AgClO_4$

Solution: According to the solubility rules for salts in water, choices A, B, and D are expected to be soluble. Choice C is therefore the best answer.

Example 10-12: Which of the following acids could be added to an unknown salt solution and NOT cause precipitation?

A) HCl
B) HI
C) H_2SO_4
D) HNO_3

Solution: According to the solubility rules for salts, all nitrate (NO_3^-) salts are soluble. Therefore, only the addition of nitric acid guarantees that any new ion combination would be soluble. Choice D is the correct answer.

Example 10-13: Which one of the following observations is *inconsistent* with the solubility rules given above?

A)   More sugar dissolves in a pot of hot water than in a pot of cold water.

B)   Boiler scales are caused by the precipitation of $CaCO_3$ inside plumbing when hot water heaters heat up cold well water.

C)   After breathing compressed air at depth, scuba divers that ascend to the surface too quickly risk having air bubbles in their body.

D)   Boiling the water before making ice cubes out of it results in clear ice cubes that have no trapped air bubbles.

Solution: Choice A is consistent with phase solubility rule 1, so it is eliminated. Choice C is consistent with phase solubility rule 3, so it is eliminated as well. And finally, choice D is consistent with the second solubility rule 2, so it is also eliminated. Although choice B is a true statement, it is one of those few examples that runs counter to our phase solubility rule 1. Choice B is the correct answer.

Solubility Product Constant

All salts have characteristic solubilities in water. Some, like NaCl, are very soluble, while others, like AgCl, barely dissolve at all. The extent to which a salt will dissolve in water can be determined from its **solubility product constant, K_{sp}**. The solubility product is simply another equilibrium constant, one in which the reactants and products are just the undissolved and dissolved salts.

For example, let's look at the dissolution of magnesium hydroxide in water:

$$Mg(OH)_2(s) \rightleftharpoons Mg^{2+}(aq) + 2 \, OH^-(aq)$$

At equilibrium, the solution is *saturated*; the rate at which ions go into solution is equal to the rate at which they precipitate out. The equilibrium expression is

$$K_{sp} = [Mg^{2+}][OH^-]^2$$

Notice that we leave the $Mg(OH)_2$ out of the equilibrium expression because it's a pure solid. (The "concentration of a solid" is meaningless when discussing the equilibrium between a solid and its ions in a saturated aqueous solution.)

Solubility Computations

Let's say you know the K_{sp} for a solid, and you're asked to find out just how much of it can dissolve into water; that is, you're asked to determine the salt's **molar solubility**, the number of moles of that salt that will saturate a liter of water.

To find the solubility of $Mg(OH)_2$, we begin by figuring out how much of each type of ion we'll have once we have x moles of the salt. Since each molecule dissociates into one magnesium ion and two hydroxide ions, if x moles of this salt have dissolved, the solution contains x moles of Mg^{2+} ions and $2x$ moles of OH^- ions:

$$Mg(OH)_2(s) \rightleftharpoons Mg^{2+}(aq) + 2\ OH^-(aq)$$

$$x \rightleftharpoons x + 2x$$

So, if x stands for the number of moles of $Mg(OH)_2$ that have dissolved per liter of saturated solution (which is what we're trying to find), then $[Mg^{2+}] = x$ and $[OH^-] = 2x$. Substituting these into the solubility product expression gives us

$$K_{sp} = [Mg^{2+}][OH^-]^2$$

$$= x(2x)^2 = x(4x^2) = 4x^3$$

It is known that K_{sp} for $Mg(OH)_2$ at 25°C is about 1.6×10^{-11}. So, if we set this equal to $4x^3$, we can solve for x. We get $x \approx 1.6 \times 10^{-4}$. This means that a solution of $Mg(OH)_2$ at 25°C will be saturated at a $Mg(OH)_2$ concentration of $1.6 \times 10^{-4}\ M$.

Example 10-14: The value of the solubility product for copper(I) chloride is $K_{sp} = 1.2 \times 10^{-6}$. Under normal conditions, the maximum concentration of an aqueous CuCl solution will be:

A) less than $10^{-6}\ M$.
B) greater than $10^{-6}\ M$ and less than $10^{-4}\ M$.
C) greater than $10^{-4}\ M$ and less than $10^{-2}\ M$.
D) greater than $10^{-2}\ M$ and less than $10^{-1}\ M$.

Solution: The equilibrium is $CuCl(s) \rightleftharpoons Cu^+(aq) + Cl^-(aq)$. If we let x denote $[Cu^+]$, then we also have $x = [Cl^-]$. Therefore, $K_{sp} = x \times x = x^2$; setting this equal to 1.2×10^{-6}, we find that x is $1.1 \times 10^{-3}\ M$. Therefore, the answer is C.

Example 10-15: The solubility product for lithium phosphate, Li_3PO_4, is $K_{sp} = 2.7 \times 10^{-9}$. How many moles of this salt would be required to form a saturated, 1 L aqueous solution?

Solution: The equilibrium is $Li_3PO_4(s) \rightleftharpoons 3Li^+(aq) + PO_4^{3-}(aq)$. If we let x denote $[PO_4^{3-}]$, then we have $[Li^+] = 3x$. Therefore, $K_{sp} = (3x)^3 \times x = 27x^4$; setting this equal to $2.7 \times 10^{-9} = 27 \times 10^{-10}$ we find that

$$27x^4 = 27 \times 10^{-10} \quad \rightarrow \quad x = (10^{-10})^{1/4} = 10^{-2.5} = 10^{0.5} \times 10^{-3} \approx 3.2 \times 10^{-3}$$

Therefore, 3.2×10^{-3} mol will be required.

10.5 ION PRODUCT

The **ion product** is the reaction quotient for a solubility reaction. That is, while K_{sp} is equal to the product of the concentrations of the ions in solution when the solution is saturated (that is, *at equilibrium*), the ion product—which we'll denote by Q_{sp}—has exactly the same form as the K_{sp} expression, but the concentrations don't have to be those at equilibrium. The reaction quotient allows us to make predictions about what the reaction will do:

$$Q_{sp} < K_{sp} \rightarrow \text{more salt can be dissolved}$$
$$Q_{sp} = K_{sp} \rightarrow \text{solution is saturated}$$
$$Q_{sp} > K_{sp} \rightarrow \text{excess salt will precipitate}$$

For example, let's say we had a liter of solution containing 10^{-4} mol of barium chloride and 10^{-3} mol of sodium sulfate, both of which are soluble salts:

$$BaCl_2(s) \rightarrow Ba^{2+}(aq) + 2\ Cl^-(aq)$$

$$Na_2SO_4(s) \rightarrow 2\ Na^+(aq) + SO_4^{2-}(aq)$$

When you mix two salts in solution, ions can recombine to form new salts, and you have to consider the new salt's K_{sp}. Barium sulfate, $BaSO_4$, is a slightly soluble salt, and at 25°C, its K_{sp} is 1.1×10^{-10}. Its dissolution equilibrium is

$$BaSO_4(s) \rightleftharpoons Ba^{2+}(aq) + SO_4^{2-}(aq)$$

Its ion product is $Q_{sp} = [Ba^{2+}][SO_4^{2-}]$, so in this solution, we have $Q_{sp} = (10^{-4})(10^{-3}) = 10^{-7}$, which is much greater than its K_{sp}. Since $Q_{sp} > K_{sp}$, the reverse reaction would be favored, and $BaSO_4$ would precipitate out of solution.

10.6 THE COMMON-ION EFFECT

Let's consider again a saturated solution of magnesium hydroxide:

$$Mg(OH)_2(s) \rightleftharpoons Mg^{2+}(aq) + 2\ OH^-(aq)$$

What would happen if we now added some sodium hydroxide, NaOH, to this solution? Since NaOH is very soluble in water, it will dissociate completely:

$$NaOH(s) \rightarrow Na^+(aq) + OH^-(aq)$$

The addition of NaOH has caused the amount of hydroxide ion—the **common ion**—in the solution to increase. This disturbs the equilibrium of magnesium hydroxide; since the concentration of a product of that equilibrium is increased, Le Châtelier's principle tells us that the system will react by favoring the reverse reaction, producing solid $Mg(OH)_2$, which will precipitate. Therefore, the molar solubility of the slightly soluble salt [in this case, $Mg(OH)_2$] is decreased by the presence of another solute (in this case, NaOH) that supplies a common ion. This is the **common-ion effect**.

10.5

Example 10-16: Barium chromate solid ($K_{sp} = 1.2 \times 10^{-10}$) is at equilibrium with its dissociated ions in an aqueous solution. If calcium chromate ($K_{sp} = 7.1 \times 10^{-4}$) is introduced into the solution, it will cause the molar quantity of:

A) solid barium chromate to increase and barium ion to decrease.
B) solid barium chromate to increase and barium ion to increase.
C) solid barium chromate to decrease and barium ion to decrease.
D) solid barium chromate to decrease and barium ion to increase.

Solution: The answer is A. The introduction of additional chromate ion (CrO_4^{2-})—the common ion—will cause the amount of barium ion in solution to decrease (since the solubility equilibrium of $BaCrO_4$ will be shifted to the left, consuming Ba^{2+}). And, as a result, the amount of solid barium chromate will increase, because some will precipitate.

Example 10-17: A researcher wishes to prepare a saturated solution of a lead compound that contains the greatest concentration of lead(II) ions. Of the following, which should she use?

A) $Pb(OH)_2$ ($K_{sp} = 2.8 \times 10^{-16}$)
B) $PbCl_2$ ($K_{sp} = 1.7 \times 10^{-5}$)
C) PbI_2 ($K_{sp} = 8.7 \times 10^{-9}$)
D) $PbBr_2$ ($K_{sp} = 6.3 \times 10^{-6}$)

Solution: Since the equilibrium had the form $PbX_2(s) \rightleftharpoons Pb^{2+}(aq) + 2\,X^-(aq)$, we have $K_{sp} = [Pb^{2+}][X^-]^2$. Therefore, to maximize $[Pb^{2+}]$, the researcher would want to maximize K_{sp}. Of the choices given, $PbCl_2$ (choice B) has the largest K_{sp} value.

10.7 COMPLEX ION FORMATION AND SOLUBILITY

Complex ions consist of metallic ions surrounded by generally two, four, or six ligands, also known as Lewis bases. Complexed metal ions may have extremely different solubility properties than the "naked," hydrated metal ions. Therefore, the addition of ligands may substantially alter the solubility of simple metal salts. For example, as described by the solubility rules in Section 10.4 above, silver chloride (AgCl) is largely insoluble in water as is evident by its extremely low K_{sp} (1.8×10^{-10}). However, addition of AgCl to an aqueous solution containing ammonia (NH_3) results in greater solubility, owing to the formation of the complex ion $[Ag(NH_3)_2]^+$. The overall effect is described by the equations below:

$$AgCl(s) \;\rightleftharpoons\; Ag^+(aq) + Cl^-(aq) \qquad\qquad K_{sp} = 1.8 \times 10^{-10}$$

$$Ag^+(aq) + 2\,NH_3(aq) \;\rightleftharpoons\; [Ag(NH_3)_2]^+\,(aq) \qquad\qquad K_{eq} = 1.5 \times 10^7$$

Overall: $\qquad AgCl(s) + 2\,NH_3(aq) \;\rightleftharpoons\; [Ag(NH_3)_2]^+\,(aq) + Cl^-(aq) \qquad K_{overall} \approx 10^{-3}$

The inclusion of ammonia in the system greatly increases the propensity of the AgCl(s) to exist as ions in solution. While the final value of K (10^{-3}) is still less than 1, it is several orders of magnitude greater than the initial K_{sp} of AgCl. The dissolution of the initial silver salt can be favored even more by taking advantage of Le Châtelier's Principle through the simple addition of excess ammonia.

One biological application of complex ion formation is metal-chelation therapy; one of the most commonly used metal chelation agents, ethylenediaminetetraacetic acid (EDTA) is approved by the FDA for the treatment of acute lead poisoning. After the administration of EDTA (generally as a mixed calcium/sodium salt), an equilibrium is established, sequestering the toxic Pb^{2+} ions in the patient's system in a very stable EDTA complex. The following reaction demonstrates the association of fully deprotonated EDTA and Pb^{2+} to form the complex ion:

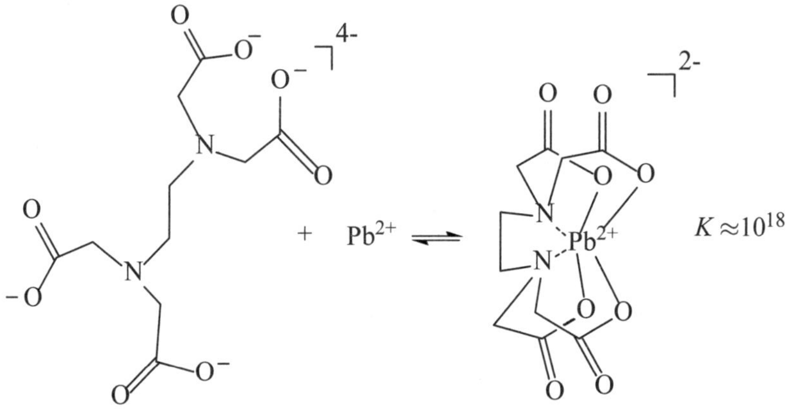

The extremely high equilibrium constant for the formation of the complexed Pb^{2+} ensures that it is prevented from further deleterious interactions with other biological functionalities, and allows its speedy excretion from the body.

10.8 THERMODYNAMICS AND EQUILIBRIUM

In Section 6.5 on Gibbs Free Energy, we saw that if ΔG was negative we could expect a reaction to proceed spontaneously in the forward direction, with the opposite being true for the case in which ΔG is positive. When a system proceeds in one direction or another there is necessarily a change in the relative values of products and reactants that redefine ΔG, and the reaction proceeds until ΔG is equal to 0 and equilibrium is achieved. Therefore, there must be a relationship between ΔG and the reaction quotient Q, as well as the equilibrium constant K_{eq}. This relationship is given in the following equation.

$$\Delta G = \Delta G^\circ + RT \ln Q$$

As the superscript denotes, ΔG° is the Gibbs free energy for a reaction under standard conditions. You may recall from Section 10.2 that when $Q = K$ the reaction is at equilibrium. Since ΔG is always equal to zero at equilibrium we can change the equation to

$$0 = \Delta G^\circ + RT \ln K_{eq}$$

or

$$\Delta G^\circ = -RT \ln K_{eq}$$

It is important to draw the distinction between ΔG and $\Delta G°$. Whereas ΔG is a statement of spontaneity of a reaction in one direction or another, $\Delta G°$ is, as seen in its relation to K_{eq}, a statement of the relative proportions of products and reactants present at equilibrium. The standard state $\Delta G°$ for a reaction only describes a reaction at one specific temperature, pressure, and set of concentrations, whereas ΔG changes with changing reaction composition until it reaches zero. From the above relationship, we can surmise the following:

$\Delta G° < 0$; $K_{eq} > 1$, products are favored at equilibrium

$\Delta G° = 0$; $K_{eq} = 1$, products and reactants are present in roughly equal amounts at equilibrium

$\Delta G° > 0$; $K_{eq} < 1$, reactants are favored at equilibrium

The difference between the heights of the reactants and products on any reaction coordinate diagram is $\Delta G°$. As we know from analyzing these plots, if the reactants are higher than the products, we expect the products to be favored. This would give us the expected negative value of $\Delta G°$, and likewise a value of K_{eq} greater than 1.

10.8

Chapter 10 Summary

- The equilibrium constant dictates the relative ratios of products to reactants when a system is at equilibrium.

- For $aA + bB \rightarrow cC + dD$: $K_{eq} = [[C]^c[D]^d]/[[A]^a[B]^b]$

- Pure solids and liquids are not included in the equilibrium expression.

- If $K > 1$, products are favored. If $K < 1$ reactants are favored.

- The reaction quotient, Q, is a ratio of products and reactants with the same form as K, but can be used when the reaction isn't at equilibrium. If $Q < K$, the reaction will proceed in the forward reaction; if $Q > K$, the reaction will proceed in the reverse direction until equilibrium is achieved.

- The only factor that changes the equilibrium constant is temperature.

- Changing the concentrations of the products or reactants of a reaction at equilibrium will force the system to shift according to Le Châtelier's principle.

- Increasing the temperature of a system at equilibrium favors the products in an endothermic reaction and the reactants in an exothermic reaction. Decreasing the temperature will have the opposite effect on both types of reactions.

- In a gaseous reaction, increasing the pressure by decreasing the volume favors the side of the reaction with fewer moles of gas. Decreasing the pressure has the opposite effect.

- An electrolyte is a solute that produces free ions in solution. Strong electrolytes produce more ions in solution than weak electrolytes.

- The van't Hoff (or ionizability) factor, i, tells us how many ions one unit of a substance will produce in solution.

- All Group I, ammonium, nitrate, perchlorate, and acetate salts are completely soluble. All silver, lead, and mercury salts are insoluble, except when they are paired with nitrate, perchlorate, or acetate.

- The solubility of solids in liquids increases with increasing temperature.

- The solubility of gases in liquids decreases with increasing temperature and increases with increasing pressure.

- The amount of a salt that can be dissolved in a solute is given by its solubility product constant (K_{sp}).

- For a reaction at equilibrium under standard conditions, $\Delta G° = -RT\ln K_{eq}$.

- For a reaction under non-standard conditions, ΔG can be calculated using $\Delta G = \Delta G° + RT\ln Q$.

CHAPTER 10 FREESTANDING PRACTICE QUESTIONS

1. Which of the following manipulations is capable of changing the K_{eq} of the reaction shown below?

$$N_2(g) + 3\,H_2(g) \rightleftharpoons 2\,NH_3(g)$$

A) Doubling the concentrations of $N_2(g)$, $H_2(g)$, and $NH_3(g)$
B) Tripling the volume of the reaction container
C) Increasing the pressure from 1 to 2 atm
D) Decreasing the temperature to from 298 K to 273 K

2. A group of scientists is studying the dynamics of the acetic acid dissociation below. They bring the process to equilibrium under standard conditions. If the scientists then add 35 g of sodium acetate to the reaction container, which of the following will be true?

$$CH_3COOH(aq) \rightleftharpoons CH_3COO^-(aq) + H^+ (aq)$$

A) $Q > K_{eq}$ and the reaction will move in reverse.
B) $Q < K_{eq}$ and the reaction will move forward.
C) $Q > K_{eq}$ and the reaction will move forward.
D) $Q < K_{eq}$ and the reaction will move in reverse.

3. Given the following equilibrium:

$$N_2(g) + 3\,H_2(g) \rightleftharpoons 2\,NH_3(g) \quad \Delta H = -91.8\,kJ$$

How would an increase in temperature affect the concentration of N_2 at equilibrium?

A) The concentration of N_2 will increase because of an increase in K_{eq}.
B) The concentration of N_2 will decrease because of an increase in K_{eq}.
C) The concentration of N_2 will increase because of a decrease in K_{eq}.
D) The concentration of N_2 will remain unchanged.

4. Na_2SO_4 is soluble in water. If $NaCl(s)$ is added to a solution of $Na_2SO_4(aq)$ so that the concentration of Na^+ doubles, then the:

A) solubility constant of Na_2SO_4 increases while that of NaCl decreases.
B) solubility constants of Na_2SO_4 and NaCl both decrease.
C) solubility of Na_2SO_4 and NaCl both decrease.
D) solubility of Na_2SO_4 decreases while that of NaCl increases.

5. Which of the following salts is least soluble in water?

A) PbI_2 ($K_{sp} = 7.9 \times 10^{-9}$)
B) $Mg(OH)_2$ ($K_{sp} = 6.3 \times 10^{-10}$)
C) $Zn(IO_3)_2$ ($K_{sp} = 3.9 \times 10^{-6}$)
D) SrF_2 ($K_{sp} = 2.6 \times 10^{-9}$)

6. The water solubility of $MgSO_4$ is approximately 25 g/100 mL at 20°C. Compared to a 0.25 g/mL solution of $MgSO_4$ prepared at 20°C, a 0.25 g/mL solution prepared at 37°C will:

A) dissolve faster and have the same concentration of ions in solution.
B) dissolve faster and have a higher concentration of ions in solution.
C) dissolve slower and have a lower concentration of ions in solution.
D) dissolve slower and have the same concentration of ions in solution.

7. If the K_{sp} of KI is 1.45×10^{-6} in propanol at 25°C, what would the K_{sp} of KI be in propane at the same temperature?

A) 1.84
B) 2.90×10^{-3}
C) 1.81×10^{-6}
D) 7.56×10^{-23}

8. The K_{sp} of NaCl in water is 35.9 at 25°C. If 500 mL of 12 M NaOH(aq) and 500 mL of 12 M HCl(aq) solution both at 25°C are combined, what would best describe the resulting solution?

A) A small amount of NaCl(s) would precipitate.
B) There will be a 6 M aqueous solution of NaCl.
C) Enthalpy and entropy would increase.
D) The resulting solution would be slightly basic.

CHAPTER 10 PRACTICE PASSAGE

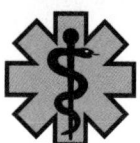 Although the mechanisms of anesthetic action are not well-understood, the behavior of anesthetics can be characterized in several ways. The minimal alveolar concentration (MAC) is the concentration of anesthetic in the alveoli at which 50% of patients stay immobile in response to a pain stimulus. The blood/gas partition coefficient ($\lambda_{B/G}$) is the ratio of the concentration of the anesthetic in the blood to its concentration in the gas above the surface of the blood (Equation 1). The oil/gas partition coefficient ($\lambda_{O/G}$) is similarly defined as the ratio of the concentration of the anesthetic in dissolved in oil to the concentration in the gas phase. The potency of an anesthetic can be correlated to its $\lambda_{O/G}$.

$$B/G = \frac{[\text{Anesthetic}]_{blood}}{[\text{Anesthetic}]_{gas}}$$

Equation 1

	MAC (% vol)	$\lambda_{B/G}$	$\lambda_{O/G}$
Halothane	0.75	2.3	224
Isoflurane	1.15	1.4	98
Sevoflurane	2.10	0.68	47

Table 1 Properties of Volatile General Anesthetics in Humans

These properties have also been measured in animals. The $\lambda_{B/G}$ of three inhalational anesthetics were measured in horses. Blood samples were taken from the jugular vein, then placed into a tonometer, where they were equilibrated with the gaseous anesthetic. The concentration of the anesthetic was 1 MAC in the carrier gas, and equilibration was performed for 10 minutes at a flow rate of 500 mL/min. A sample of the equilibrated blood was then extracted with a syringe, injected into an empty vial, and allowed to come to equilibrium in a water bath at 37°C for 30 minutes. Gas chromatography of the gases in the headspace at the top of the vial was used to determine the mole fraction of the anesthetic in the gas phase, and ultimately the $\lambda_{B/G}$ for each anesthetic.

	$\lambda_{B/G}$
Halothane	1.66 (0.06, $n = 8$)
Isoflurane	0.92 (0.04, $n = 8$)
Sevoflurane	0.47 (0.03, $n = 8$)

Table 2 Blood/Gas Partition Coefficients in Horses (standard deviations in parentheses)

Adapted from: Bergadano, A. *et al. British Journal of Anaesthesia* **91** (2): 276-8 (2003).

1. Which anesthetic is the least soluble in blood?

A) Halothane
B) Isoflurane
C) Sevoflurane
D) Cannot be determined from the information given

2. If the blood/oil partition coefficient for sevoflurane in horses was measured, which of the following values would be the closest?

A) 0.01
B) 22
C) 48
D) 100

3. Which of the following changes would most likely cause the $\lambda_{O/G}$ of an anesthetic to increase?

A) An increase in the temperature
B) A decrease in the temperature
C) Increasing the concentration of the anesthetic in the oil
D) Decreasing the concentration of the anesthetic in the oil

4. The relative values of $\lambda_{B/G}$ and $\lambda_{O/G}$ for the anesthetics suggest that:

A) none of the anesthetics are hydrophilic.
B) all the anesthetics are hydrophilic.
C) only halothane and isoflurane are hydrophilic.
D) only sevoflurane is hydrophilic.

5. How would the results of the experiment be different if the concentration of anesthetic during the tonometer equilibration was 2 MAC? Assume no other changes were made to the procedure.

A) The measured $\lambda_{B/G}$ would decrease, because there would be more anesthetic in the headspace of the sampling vial.

B) The measured $\lambda_{B/G}$ would increase, because the blood will absorb more anesthetic during the tonometer equilibration.

C) The measured $\lambda_{B/G}$ would increase, because there would be more anesthetic in the headspace of the sampling vial.

D) The measured $\lambda_{B/G}$ would not change.

6. What is the approximate molar concentration of halothane at its MAC, given a temperature of 37°C and a pressure of 760 mmHg?

A) 7.5 mmol/L
B) 0.30 mmol/L
C) 0.075 mmol/L
D) 0.0030 mmol/L

SOLUTIONS TO CHAPTER 10 FREESTANDING PRACTICE QUESTIONS

1. **D** Equilibrium constants are specific to a single temperature and standard state free energy change according to: $\Delta G° = -RT\ln K$. Altering temperature is the only answer choice that can change the reaction's K_{eq}.

2. **A** K_{eq} = [products]/[reactants] when both reactant and product concentrations are those at equilibrium. Q = [products]/[reactants] regardless of whether reactant and product concentrations are those at equilibrium. The addition of sodium acetate essentially translates into the addition of acetate ion, a product in this equilibrium. As a result of such an addition, $Q > K_{eq}$ and products are present in excess of equilibrium values. Le Châtelier's principle states that net reverse movement is created when the concentration of products is increased in an equilibrium system.

3. **C** Since the reaction is exothermic, an increase in temperature will shift the equilibrium to the left, and the concentration of N_2 will increase, eliminating choices B and D. For exothermic reactions, an increase in temperature will decrease the K_{eq}, eliminating choice A and making choice C the correct answer.

4. **C** Solubility constants, like all equilibrium constants, are functions of temperature only. This eliminates choices A and B. Given the equilibria:

$$Na_2SO_4(s) \rightleftharpoons 2\,Na^+\,(aq) + SO_4^{2-}\,(aq)$$
$$NaCl(s) \rightleftharpoons Na^+\,(aq) + Cl^-\,(aq)$$

Na^+ is a common ion to both systems. Increasing Na^+ concentration will decrease the solubility of both salts, eliminating choice D and making choice C the best answer.

5. **B** All of the compounds are composed of one cation and two anions, so comparing K_{sp} values will give relative solubility. Since the question asks for an extreme, the middle values of the variable cannot be correct, eliminating choices A and D. The compound with the lowest K_{sp} value will have the lowest solubility because for all the compounds, K_{sp} = [cation][anion]^2. Therefore, choice B is correct.

6. **A** This is a two-by-two problem. First, consider rate. Any time temperature is increased, the reaction kinetics increase. In this case, the salt will dissolve faster, eliminating choices C and D. An increase in temperature generally causes an increase in the solubility of solids in liquids. However, both solutions contain the same amount of $MgSO_4$ that does not exceed the maximum solubility at either temperature. Therefore, the concentrations of ions will be the same, eliminating choice B.

7. **D** The golden rule of solubility is "like dissolves like." Potassium iodide is a salt held together by ionic forces and therefore comprised of charged ions. A salt will dissolve in a polar solvent better than a non-polar solvent. Propanol has a polar –OH group whereas propane is completely non-polar. Therefore, KI must have a smaller K_{sp} in propane than in propanol. The only answer that has a smaller K_{sp} value is choice D.

8. **B** Neutralizations are exothermic and form salt and water. The starting 500 mL solutions contain 6 moles each of NaOH and HCl. The final solution will be 1 L of 6 M NaCl(aq):

$$6\ HCl(aq) + 6\ NaOH(aq) \rightarrow 6\ NaCl(aq) + 6\ H_2O(l)$$

Although the reaction quotient of NaCl in this resulting solution will slightly exceed K_{sp}:

$$Q = [Na^+][Cl^-] = [6][6] = 36$$

the temperature will be significantly increased, allowing more NaCl to dissolve (K_{sp} will increase with temperature), eliminating choice A. Choice C is eliminated because enthalpy significantly decreases as heat is given off in this exothermic reaction. Choice D is eliminated because NaCl is a neutral salt.

SOLUTIONS TO CHAPTER 10 PRACTICE PASSAGE

1. **C** Choice D can be eliminated, since the $\lambda_{B/G}$ values in the table are an indication of solubility. From the information in the table, isoflurane (choice B) can be eliminated right away; its values are intermediate to the other anesthetics. The passage states that the $\lambda_{B/G}$ is the "ratio of the concentration of the anesthetic in the blood to its concentration in the gas"; therefore, the higher the $\lambda_{B/G}$, the more anesthetic is dissolved in the blood. Choice C is correct; it has the lowest $\lambda_{B/G}$ of the three anesthetics.

2. **A** By analogy to the blood/gas partition coefficient presented in the passage, a blood/oil partition coefficient would be calculated as follows:

$$\frac{[\text{Anesthetic}]_{blood}}{[\text{Anesthetic}]_{oil}}$$

Such a value could be determined by multiplying the $\lambda_{B/G}$ by the reciprocal of the $\lambda_{O/G}$ value:

$$\frac{[\text{Anesthetic}]_{blood}}{[\text{Anesthetic}]_{gas}} \times \frac{[\text{Anesthetic}]_{gas}}{[\text{Anesthetic}]_{oil}}$$

Since $(0.47) \times \left(\frac{1}{47}\right) = 0.01$, choice A is correct.

3. **B** The $\lambda_{O/G}$ is an equilibrium constant, so changing the concentration of the anesthetic in the oil will not affect the $\lambda_{O/G}$ (choices C and D can be eliminated). However, a change in temperature would. The solubility of gases in liquids generally increases when the temperature is decreased; therefore, choice A can be eliminated, and choice B is correct.

4. **A**   For each anesthetic, the $\lambda_{O/G}$ value is greater than the $\lambda_{B/G}$ value, so either all of them are hydrophilic, or none of them are hydrophilic (choices C and D can be eliminated). Since the $\lambda_{O/G}$ values are higher, this suggests that anesthetics have greater solubility in the oil than in blood, suggesting that they are hydrophobic, not hydrophilic (eliminate choice B, choice A is correct.)

5. **D**   The equilibration of the blood with anesthetic in the tonometer saturates the blood with dissolved anesthetic, so an increase in the concentration of the anesthetic in the gas will not make an overall difference to the amount of anesthetic dissolved in the blood by that step (eliminate choice B). Since there is no change in the amount of anesthetic dissolved in the blood, there can be no change in the amount of anesthetic found in the headspace (eliminate choices A and C). Choice D is correct.

6. **B**   In a gas mixture behaving ideally, the volume percent concentration will be equal to the mole percent concentration. In other words, 0.75% by volume can be expressed as 0.0075 mol/1 mol. At STP, 1 mol of gas has a volume of 22.4 L. While the pressure in the question is the same as at STP (760 mmHg = 1 atm), the temperature is higher than STP. Therefore, 22.4 L will be an underestimate of the molar volume at this temperature; however, a volume of 22.4 L (and judicious rounding) can still be used for a quick estimate. (Coincidentally, the molar volume of an ideal gas at 1 atm and 37°C is about 25.4 L.)

$$\frac{0.0075 \text{ mol}}{22.4 \text{ L}} \approx \frac{0.0075 \text{ mol}}{25 \text{ L}} = 0.0003 \frac{\text{mol}}{\text{L}} = 0.3 \frac{\text{mmol}}{\text{L}}$$

Chapter 11
Acids and Bases

11.1 DEFINITIONS

Svante Arrhenius proposed the first modern definition of acids and bases. Acids are chemicals than increase the concentration of H^+ in aqueous solution, while bases are chemicals which increase the concentration of OH^- in solution. However, this definition has been supplanted by more general ones. There are two important definitions of acids and bases you should be familiar with for the MCAT.

Brønsted-Lowry Acids and Bases

Brønsted and Lowry offered the following definitions:

Acids are proton (H^+) donors.
Bases are proton (H^+) acceptors.

While the often seen hydroxide ions qualify as Brønsted-Lowry bases, many other compounds fit this definition as well. Since a Brønsted-Lowry base is any substance that is capable of accepting a proton, any anion or any neutral species with a lone pair of electrons can function as a base.

If we consider the reversible reaction below:

$$H_2CO_3 + H_2O \rightleftharpoons H_3O^+ + HCO_3^-$$

then according to the Brønsted-Lowry definition, H_2CO_3 and H_3O^+ are acids and HCO_3^- and H_2O are bases. The Brønsted-Lowry definition of acid and bases is the most important one for MCAT General Chemistry.

Lewis Acids and Bases

Lewis's definitions of acids and bases are broader:

Lewis acids are electron-pair acceptors.
Lewis bases are electron-pair donors.

If we consider the reversible reaction below:

$$AlCl_3 + H_2O \rightleftharpoons (AlCl_3OH)^- + H^+$$

then according to the Lewis definition, $AlCl_3$ and H^+ are acids because they accept electron pairs; H_2O and $(AlCl_3OH)^-$ are bases because they donate electron pairs. Lewis acid/base reactions frequently result in the formation of coordinate covalent bonds, as discussed in Chapter 5. For example, in the reaction above, water acts as a Lewis base since it donates both of the electrons involved in the coordinate covalent bond between OH^- and $AlCl_3$. $AlCl_3$ acts as a Lewis acid, since it accepts the electrons involved in this bond.

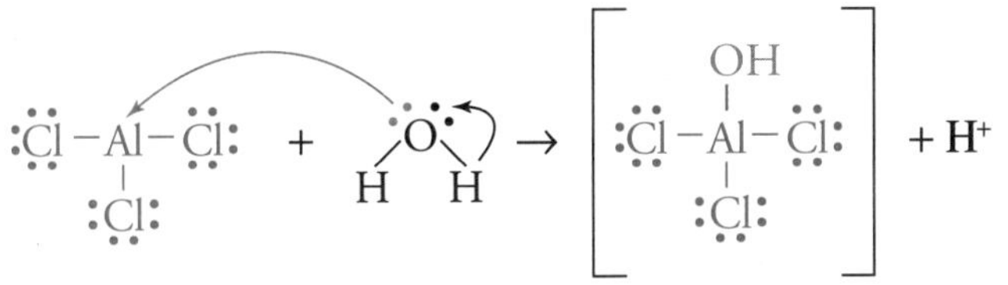

11.2 CONJUGATE ACIDS AND BASES

When a Brønsted-Lowry acid donates an H^+, the remaining structure is called the **conjugate base** of the acid. Likewise, when a Brønsted-Lowry base bonds with an H^+ in solution, this new species is called the **conjugate acid** of the base. To illustrate these definitions, consider this reaction:

acid–base conjugates

$$NH_3 + H_2O \rightleftharpoons NH_4^+ + OH^-$$

acid–base conjugates

Considering only the forward direction, NH_3 is the base and H_2O is the acid. The products are the conjugate acid and conjugate base of the reactants: NH_4^+ is the conjugate acid of NH_3, and OH^- is the conjugate base of H_2O:

acid ------------> conjugate base

$$NH_3 + H_2O \rightleftharpoons NH_4^+ + OH^-$$

base ------------> conjugate acid

Now consider the reverse reaction in which NH_4^+ is the acid and OH^- is the base. The conjugates are the same as for the forward reaction: NH_3 is the conjugate base of NH_4^+, and H_2O is the conjugate acid of OH^-:

conjugate base <------------ acid

$$NH_3 + H_2O \rightleftharpoons NH_4^+ + OH^-$$

conjugate acid <---------- base

The difference between a Brønsted-Lowry acid and its conjugate base is that the base is missing an H^+. The difference between a Brønsted-Lowry base and its conjugate acid is that the acid has an extra H^+.

forming conjugates:

$$\text{acid} \underset{+H^+}{\overset{-H^+}{\rightleftharpoons}} \text{base}$$

11.3

Example 11-1: Which one of the following can behave as a Brønsted-Lowry acid but not a Lewis acid?

A) CF_4
B) $NaAlCl_4$
C) HF
D) Br_2

Solution: A Brønsted-Lowry acid donates an H^+, while a Lewis acid accepts a pair of electrons. Since a Brønsted-Lowry acid must have an H in the first place, only choice C can be the answer.

Example 11-2: What is the conjugate base of HBrO (hypobromous acid)?

A) H^+
B) H_2BrO_2
C) H_2BrO^+
D) BrO^-

Solution: To form the conjugate base of an acid, simply remove an H^+. Therefore, the conjugate base of HBrO is BrO^-, choice D.

11.3 THE STRENGTHS OF ACIDS AND BASES

Brønsted-Lowry acids can be placed into two big categories: *strong* and *weak*. Whether an acid is strong or weak depends on how completely it ionizes in water. A **strong** acid is one that dissociates completely (or very nearly so) in water; hydrochloric acid, HCl, is an example:

$$HCl(aq) + H_2O(l) \rightarrow H_3O^+(aq) + Cl^-(aq)$$

This reaction goes essentially to completion.

On the other hand, hydrofluoric acid, HF, is an example of a **weak** acid, since its dissociation in water,

$$HF(aq) + H_2O(l) \rightleftharpoons H_3O^+(aq) + F^-(aq)$$

does not go to completion; most of the HF remains undissociated.

If we use HA to denote a generic acid, its dissociation in water has the form

$$HA(aq) + H_2O(l) \rightleftharpoons H_3O^+(aq) + A^-(aq)$$

The strength of the acid is directly related to how much the products are favored over the reactants. The equilibrium expression for this reaction is

$$K_a = \frac{[H_3O^+][A^-]}{[HA]}$$

This is written as K_a, rather than K_{eq}, to emphasize that this is the equilibrium expression for an acid-dissociation reaction. In fact, K_a is known as the **acid-ionization** (or **acid-dissociation**) **constant** of the acid (HA). If $K_a > 1$, then the products are favored, and we say the acid is strong; if $K_a < 1$ then the reactants are favored and the acid is weak. We can also rank the relative strengths of acids by comparing their K_a values: The larger the K_a value, the stronger the acid; the smaller the K_a value, the weaker the acid.

The acids for which $K_a > 1$—the strong acids—are so few that you should memorize them:

Common Strong Acids	
Hydroiodic acid	HI
Hydrobromic acid	HBr
Hydrochloric acid	HCl
Perchloric acid	$HClO_4$
Sulfuric acid	H_2SO_4
Nitric acid	HNO_3

The values of K_a for these acids are so large that most tables of acid ionization constants don't even list them. On the MCAT, you may assume that any acid that's not in this list is a weak acid. (Other acids that fit the definition of *strong* are so uncommon that it's very unlikely they'd appear on the test. For example, $HClO_3$ has a K_a of 10, and could be considered strong, but it is definitely one of the weaker strong acids and is not likely to appear on the MCAT.)

Example 11-3: In a 1 M aqueous solution of boric acid (H_3BO_3, $K_a = 5.8 \times 10^{-10}$), which of the following species will be present in solution in the greatest quantity?

A) H_3BO_3
B) $H_2BO_3^-$
C) HBO_3^{2-}
D) H_3O^+

Solution: The equilibrium here is $H_3BO_3(aq) + H_2O(l) \rightleftharpoons H_3O^+(aq) + H_2BO_3^-(aq)$. Boric acid is a weak acid (it's not on the list of strong acids), so the equilibrium lies to the left (also, notice how small its K_a value is). So, there'll be very few H_3O^+ or $H_2BO_3^-$ ions in solution but plenty of undissociated H_3BO_3. The answer is A.

Example 11-4: Of the following, which statement best explains why HF is a weak acid, but HCl, HBr, and HI are strong acids?

A) F has a greater ionization energy than Cl, Br, or I.
B) F has a larger radius than Cl, Br, or I.
C) F^- has a larger radius than Cl^-, Br^-, I^-.
D) F^- has a smaller radius than Cl^-, Br^-, I^-.

Solution: F is smaller than Cl, Br, or I (eliminating choices B and C). Ionization energy is associated with forming a cation from a neutral atom, and has no bearing here. Choice D is therefore correct. The more stable an acid's conjugate base is, the stronger the acid. Larger anions are better able to spread out their negative charge, making them more stable. HF is the weakest of the H-X acids because it has the least stable conjugate base due to its size.

Example 11-5: Of the following acids, which one would dissociate to the greatest extent (in water)?

A)   HCN (hydrocyanic acid), $K_a = 6.2 \times 10^{-10}$
B)   HNCO (cyanic acid), $K_a = 3.3 \times 10^{-4}$
C)   HClO (hypochlorous acid), $K_a = 2.9 \times 10^{-8}$
D)   HBrO (hypobromous acid), $K_a = 2.2 \times 10^{-9}$

Solution: The acid that would dissociate to the greatest extent would have the greatest K_a value. Of the choices given, HNCO (choice B) has the greatest K_a value.

We can apply the same ideas as above to identify strong and weak *bases*. If we use B to denote a generic base, its dissolution in water has the form

$$\text{B}(aq) + \text{H}_2\text{O}(l) \rightleftharpoons \text{HB}^+(aq) + \text{OH}^-(aq)$$

The strength of the base is directly related to how much the products are favored over the reactants. If we write the equilibrium constant for this reaction, we get:

$$K_b = \frac{[\text{HB}^+][\text{OH}^-]}{[\text{B}]}$$

This is written as K_b, rather than K_{eq}, to emphasize that this is the equilibrium expression for a base-dissociation reaction. In fact, K_b is known as the **base-ionization** (or **base-dissociation**) **constant**. We can rank the relative strengths of bases by comparing their K_b values: The larger the K_b value, the stronger the base; the smaller the K_b value, the weaker the base.

For the MCAT and general chemistry, you should know about the following strong bases that may be used in aqueous solutions:

Common Strong Bases
Group 1 hydroxides (For example, NaOH)
Group 1 oxides (For example, Li$_2$O)
Some group 2 hydroxides (Ba(OH)$_2$, Sr(OH)$_2$, Ca(OH)$_2$)
Metal amides (For example, NaNH$_2$)

Weak bases include ammonia (NH_3) and amines, as well as the conjugate bases of many weak acids, as we'll discuss below.

The Relative Strengths of Conjugate Acid–Base Pairs

Let's once again look at the dissociation of HCl in water:

$$HCl(aq) + H_2O(l) \rightarrow H_3O^+(aq) + Cl^-(aq)$$

no basic properties

The chloride ion (Cl⁻) is the conjugate base of HCl. Since this reaction goes to completion, there must be no reverse reaction. Therefore, Cl⁻ has no tendency to accept a proton and thus does not act as a base. The conjugate base of a strong acid has no basic properties in water.

On the other hand, hydrofluoric acid, HF, is a weak acid since its dissociation is not complete:

$$HF(aq) + H_2O(l) \rightleftharpoons H_3O^+(aq) + F^-(aq)$$

Since the reverse reaction does take place to a significant extent, the conjugate base of HF, the fluoride ion, F⁻, *does* have some tendency to accept a proton, and so behaves as a weak base. The conjugate base of a weak acid is a weak base.

In fact, the weaker the acid, the more the reverse reaction is favored, and the stronger its conjugate base. For example, hydrocyanic acid (HCN) has a K_a value of about 5×10^{-10}, which is much smaller than that of hydrofluoric acid ($K_a \approx 7 \times 10^{-4}$). Therefore, the conjugate base of HCN, the cyanide ion, CN⁻, is a stronger base than F⁻.

The same ideas can be applied to bases:

1) The conjugate acid of a strong base has no acidic properties in water. For example, the conjugate acid of LiOH is Li⁺, which does not act as an acid in water.
2) The conjugate acid of a weak base is a weak acid (and the weaker the base, the stronger the conjugate acid). For example, the conjugate acid of NH_3 is NH_4^+, which is a weak acid.

Example 11-6: Of the following anions, which is the strongest base?

A) I⁻
B) CN⁻
C) NO_3^-
D) Br⁻

Solution: Here's another way to ask the same question: Which of the following anions has the weakest conjugate acid? Since HI, HNO_3, and HBr are all strong acids, while HCN is a weak acid, CN⁻ (choice B) has the weakest conjugate acid, and is thus the strongest base.

Example 11-7: Of the following, which acid has the weakest conjugate base?

A) $HClO_4$
B) HCOOH
C) H_3PO_4
D) H_2CO_3

Solution: Here's another way to ask the same question: Which of the following acids is the strongest? Thought about this way, the answer's easy. Perchloric acid, choice A, is the only strong acid in the list.

Amphoteric Substances

Take a look at the dissociation of carbonic acid (H_2CO_3), a weak acid:

$$H_2CO_3(aq) + H_2O(l) \rightleftharpoons H_3O^+(aq) + HCO_3^-(aq) \quad (K_a = 4.5 \times 10^{-7})$$

The conjugate base of carbonic acid is HCO_3^-, which also has an ionizable proton. Carbonic acid is said to be **polyprotic**, because it has more than one proton to donate.

Let's look at how the conjugate base of carbonic acid dissociates:

$$HCO_3^-(aq) + H_2O(l) \rightleftharpoons H_3O^+(aq) + CO_3^{2-}(aq) \quad (K_a = 4.8 \times 10^{-11})$$

In the first reaction, HCO_3^- acts as a base, but in the second reaction it acts as an acid. Whenever a substance can act as either an acid or a base, we say that it is **amphoteric**. The conjugate base of a weak polyprotic acid is always amphoteric, because it can either donate or accept another proton. Also notice that HCO_3^- is a weaker acid than H_2CO_3; in general, every time a polyprotic acid donates a proton, the resulting species will be a weaker acid than its predecessor.

11.4   THE ION-PRODUCT CONSTANT OF WATER

Water is amphoteric. It reacts with itself in a Brønsted-Lowry acid-base reaction, one molecule acting as the acid, the other as the base:

$$H_2O(l) + H_2O(l) \rightleftharpoons H_3O^+(aq) + OH^-(aq)$$

This is called the autoionization (or self-ionization) of water. The equilibrium expression is

$$K_w = [H_3O^+][OH^-]$$

This is written as K_w, rather than K_{eq}, to emphasize that this is the equilibrium expression for the autoionization of water; K_w is known as the ion-product constant of water. Only a very small fraction of the water molecules will undergo this reaction, and it's known that at 25°C,

$$K_w = 1.0 \times 10^{-14}$$

(Like all other equilibrium constants, K_w varies with temperature; it increases as the temperature increases. However, because 25°C is so common, this is the value you should memorize.) Since the number of H_3O^+ ions in pure water will be equal to the number of OH^- ions, if we call each of their concentrations x, then $x^2 = K_w$, which gives $x = 1 \times 10^{-7}$. That is, the concentration of both types of ions in pure water is 1×10^{-7} M. (In addition, K_w is constant at a given temperature, regardless of the H_3O^+ concentration.)

If the introduction of an acid increases the concentration of H_3O^+ ions, then the equilibrium is disturbed, and the reverse reaction is favored, decreasing the concentration of OH^- ions. Similarly, if the introduction of a base increases the concentration of OH^- ions, then the equilibrium is again disturbed; the reverse reaction is favored, decreasing the concentration of H_3O^+ ions. However, in either case, the product of $[H_3O^+]$ and $[OH^-]$ will remain equal to K_w.

For example, suppose we add 0.002 moles of HCl to water to create a 1-liter solution. Since the dissociation of HCl goes to completion (it's a strong acid), it will create 0.002 moles of H_3O^+ ions, so $[H_3O^+] =$ 0.002 M. Since H_3O^+ concentration has been increased, we expect the OH^- concentration to decrease, which it does:

$$[OH^-] = \frac{K_w}{[H_3O^+]} = \frac{1 \times 10^{-14}}{2 \times 10^{-3}} = 5 \times 10^{-12} \, M$$

11.5 pH

The pH scale measures the concentration of H^+ (or H_3O^+) ions in a solution. Because the molarity of H^+ tends to be quite small and can vary over many orders of magnitude, the pH scale is logarithmic:

$$pH = -\log[H^+]$$

This formula implies that $[H^+] = 10^{-pH}$. Since $[H^+] = 10^{-7} \, M$ in pure water, the pH of water is 7. At 25°C, this defines a pH neutral solution. If $[H^+]$ is greater than $10^{-7} \, M$, then the pH will be less than 7, and the solution is said to be acidic. If $[H^+]$ is less than $10^{-7} \, M$, the pH will be greater than 7, and the solution is basic (or alkaline). Notice that a *low* pH means a *high* $[H^+]$ and the solution is *acidic*; a *high* pH means a *low* $[H^+]$ and the solution is basic.

pH > 7	basic solution
pH = 7	neutral solution
pH < 7	acidic solution

The range of the pH scale for most solutions falls between 0 and 14, but some strong acids and bases extend the scale past this range. For example, a 10 M solution of HCl will fully dissociate into H^+ and Cl^-. Therefore, the $[H^+] = 10 \, M$, and the pH = –1.

An alternate measurement expresses the acidity or basicity in terms of the hydroxide ion concentration, $[OH^-]$, by using pOH. The same formula applies for hydroxide ions as for hydrogen ions.

$$pOH = -\log[OH^-]$$

This formula implies that $[OH^-] = 10^{-pOH}$.

Acids and bases are inversely related: the greater the concentration of H^+ ions, the lower the concentration of OH^- ions, and vice versa. Since $[H^+][OH^-] = 10^{-14}$ at 25°C, the values of pH and pOH satisfy a special relationship at 25°C:

$$pH + pOH = 14$$

So, if you know the pOH of a solution, you can find the pH, and vice versa. For example, if the pH of a solution is 5, then the pOH must be 9. If the pOH of a solution is 2, then the pH must be 12.

On the MCAT, it will be helpful to be able to figure out the pH even in cases where the H^+ concentration isn't exactly equal to the whole-number power of 10. In general, if y is a number between 1 and 10, and you're told that $[H^+] = y \times 10^{-n}$ (where n is a whole number) then the pH will be between $(n - 1)$ and n. For example, if $[H^+] = 6.2 \times 10^{-5}$, then the pH is between 4 and 5.

Relationships Between Conjugates

pK_a and pK_b

The definitions of pH and pOH both involve a negative logarithm. In general, "p" of something is equal to the $-\log$ of that something. Therefore, the following definitions won't be surprising:

$$pK_a = -\log K_a$$

$$pK_b = -\log K_b$$

Because H^+ concentrations are generally very small and can vary over such a wide range, the pH scale gives us more convenient numbers to work with. The same is true for pK_a and pK_b. Remember that the larger the K_a value, the stronger the acid. Since "p" means "take the negative log of…," the *lower* the pK_a value, the stronger the acid. For example, acetic acid (CH_3COOH) has a K_a of 1.75×10^{-5}, and hypochlorous acid (HClO) has a K_a of 2.9×10^{-8}. Since the K_a of acetic acid is larger than that of hypochlorous acid, we know this means that more molecules of acetic acid than hypochlorous acid will dissociate into ions in aqueous solution. In other words, acetic acid is stronger than hypochlorous acid. The pK_a of acetic acid is 4.8, and the pK_a of hypochlorous acid is 7.5. The acid with the lower pK_a value is the stronger acid. The same logic applies to pK_b: the lower the pK_b value, the stronger the base.

K_a and K_b

Let's now look at the relationship between the K_a and the K_b for an acid-base conjugate pair by working through an example question. Let K_a be the acid-dissociation constant for formic acid (HCOOH) and let K_b stand for the base-dissociation constant of its conjugate base (the formate ion, $HCOO^-$). If K_a is equal to 5.6×10^{-11}, what is $K_a \times K_b$?

The equilibrium for the dissociation of HCOOH is

$$HCOOH(aq) + H_2O(l) \rightleftharpoons H_3O^+(aq) + HCOO^-(aq)$$

so

$$K_a = \frac{[H_3O^+][HCOO^-]}{[HCOOH]}$$

The equilibrium for the dissociation of $HCOO^-$ is

$$HCOO^-(aq) + H_2O(l) \rightleftharpoons HCOOH(aq) + OH^-(aq)$$

so

$$K_b = \frac{[HCOOH][OH^-]}{[HCOO^-]}$$

Therefore,

$$K_a K_b = \frac{[H_3O^+][HCOO^-]}{[HCOOH]} \times \frac{[HCOOH][OH^-]}{[HCOO^-]} = [H_3O^+][OH^-]$$

We now immediately recognize this product as K_w, the ion-product constant of water, whose value (at 25°C) is 1×10^{-14}.

This calculation wasn't special for HCOOH; we can see that the same thing will happen for any acid and its conjugate base. So, for any acid-base conjugate pair, we'll have

$$K_a K_b = K_w = 1 \times 10^{-14}$$

This gives us a way to quantitatively relate the strength of an acid and that of its conjugate base. For example, the value of K_a for HF is about 7×10^{-4}; therefore, the value of K_b for its conjugate base, F^-, is about 1.4×10^{-11}. For HCN, $K_a \approx 5 \times 10^{-10}$, so K_b for CN^- is 2×10^{-5}.

It also follows from our definitions and logarithm algebra that for an acid-base conjugate pair at 25°C, we'll have

$$pK_a + pK_b = 14$$

Example 11-8: Of the following liquids, which one contains the lowest concentration of H_3O^+ ions?

A) Lemon juice (pH = 2.3)
B) Blood (pH = 7.4)
C) Seawater (pH = 8.5)
D) Coffee (pH = 5.1)

Solution: Since pH = $-\log [H_3O^+]$, we know that $[H_3O^+] = 1/10^{pH}$. This fraction is smallest when the pH is greatest. Of the choices given, seawater (choice C) has the highest pH.

Example 11-9: What is the pH of a solution at 25°C whose hydroxide ion concentration is 1×10^{-4} M?

Solution: Since pOH = $-\log[OH^-]$, we know that pOH = 4. Therefore, the pH is 10.

Example 11-10: Orange juice has a pH of 3.5. What is its $[H^+]$?

Solution: Because pH = $-\log[H^+]$, we know that $[H^+] = 10^{-pH}$. For orange juice, then, we have $[H^+] = 10^{-3.5} = 10^{0.5-4} = 10^{0.5} \times 10^{-4} = \sqrt{10} \times 10^{-4} \approx 3.2 \times 10^{-4}$ M.

Example 11-11: If 99% of the H_3O^+ ions are removed from a solution whose pH was originally 3, what will be its new pH?

Solution: If 99% of the H_3O^+ ions are removed, then only 1% remain. This means that the number of H_3O^+ ions is now only 1/100 of the original. If $[H_3O^+]$ is decreased by a factor of 100, then the pH is *increased* by 2—to pH 5 in this case—since log 100 = 2.

Example 11-12: Given that the self-ionization of water is endothermic, what is the value of the sum pH + pOH at 50°C?

$$H_2O(l) + H_2O(l) \rightleftharpoons H_3O^+(aq) + OH^-(aq)$$

A) Less than 14
B) Equal to 14
C) Greater than 14
D) Cannot determine from the information given

Solution: This is a Le Châtelier's principle question in disguise. Imagine we start at equilibrium at 25°C; which way would the self-ionization reaction shift if we increase the temperature to 50°C? Since the question tells us this reaction is endothermic, we can consider heat as one of the reactants, and therefore an increase in temperature would cause the system to shift to the right. Shifting to the right means that at equilibrium, $[H^+]$ and $[OH^-]$ will increase. So pH and pOH will both be *lower* than 7 at 50°C, and the sum of pH and pOH will be less than 14 at 50°C. Choice A is the correct answer.

pH Calculations

For Strong Acids

Strong acids dissociate completely, so the hydrogen ion concentration will be the same as the concentration of the acid. That means that you can calculate the pH directly from the molarity of the solution. For example, a 0.01 M solution of HCl will have $[H^+] = 0.01$ M and pH = 2.

For Weak Acids

Weak acids come to equilibrium with their dissociated ions. In fact, for a weak acid at equilibrium, the concentration of undissociated acid will be much greater than the concentration of hydrogen ion. To get the pH of a weak acid solution, you need to use the equilibrium expression.

Let's say you add 0.2 mol of HCN (hydrocyanic acid, a weak acid) to water to create a 1-liter solution, and you want to find the pH. Initially, [HCN] = 0.2 M, and none of it has dissociated. If x moles of HCN are dissociated at equilibrium, then the equilibrium concentration of HCN is 0.2 – x. Now, since each molecule of HCN dissociates into one H^+ ion and one CN^- ion, if x moles of HCN have dissociated, there'll be x moles of H^+ and x moles of CN^-:

	HCN	$\rightleftharpoons$	H^+	+	CN^-
initial:	0.2 M		0 M		0 M
at equilibrium:	(0.2 – x) M		x M		x M

(Actually, the initial concentration of H^+ is 10^{-7} M, but it's so small that it can be neglected for this calculation.) Our goal is to find x, because once we know [H^+], we'll know the pH. So, we set up the equilibrium expression:

$$K_a = \frac{[H^+][CN^-]}{[HCN]} = \frac{x^2}{0.2 - x}$$

It's known that the value of K_a for HCN is 4.9×10^{-10}. Because the K_a is so small, not that much of the HCN is going to dissociate. (This assumption, that x added to or subtracted from a number is negligible, is always a good one when $K < 10^{-4}$ [the usual case found on the MCAT].) That is, we can assume that x is going to be a very small number, insignificant compared to 0.2; therefore, the value (0.2 – x) is almost exactly the same as 0.2. By substituting 0.2 for (0.2 – x), we can solve the equation above for x:

$$\frac{x^2}{0.2} \approx 4.9 \times 10^{-10}$$
$$x^2 \approx 1 \times 10^{-10}$$
$$\therefore x \approx 1 \times 10^{-5}$$

Since [H^+] is approximately 1×10^{-5} M, the pH is about 5.

We simplified the computation by assuming that the concentration of hydrogen ion [H^+] was insignificant compared to the concentration of undissociated acid [HCN]. Since it turned out that [H^+] $\approx 10^{-5}$ M, which is much less than [HCN] = 0.2 M, our assumption was valid. On the MCAT, you should always simplify the math wherever possible.

Example 11-13: If 0.7 mol of benzoic acid (C_6H_5COOH, $K_a = 6.6 \times 10^{-5}$) is added to water to create a 1-liter solution, what will be the pH?

Solution: Initially $[C_6H_5COOH] = 0.7 \ M$, and none of it has dissociated. If x moles of C_6H_5COOH are dissociated at equilibrium, then the equilibrium concentration of C_6H_5COOH is $0.7 - x$. Now, since each molecule of C_6H_5COOH dissociates into one H^+ ion and one $C_6H_5COO^-$ ion, if x moles of C_6H_5COOH have dissociated, there'll be x moles of H^+ and x moles of $C_6H_5COO^-$:

	C_6H_5COOH	$\rightleftharpoons$	H^+	$+$	$C_6H_5COO^-$
initial:	$0.7 \ M$		$0 \ M$		$0 \ M$
at equilibrium:	$(0.7 - x) \ M$		$x \ M$		$x \ M$

(Again, the initial concentration of H^+ is $10^{-7} \ M$, but it's so small that it can be neglected.) Our goal is to find x, because once we know $[H^+]$, we'll know the pH. So, we set up the equilibrium expression:

$$K_a = \frac{[H^+][C_6H_5COO^-]}{[C_6H_5COOH]} = \frac{x^2}{0.7 - x} \approx \frac{x^2}{0.7}$$

and then solve the equation for x:

$$\frac{x^2}{0.7} \approx 6.6 \times 10^{-5}$$
$$x^2 \approx 4.6 \times 10^{-5} = 46 \times 10^{-6}$$
$$\therefore x \approx 7 \times 10^{-3}$$

Since $[H^+]$ is approximately $7 \times 10^{-3} \ M \approx 10^{-2} \ M$, the pH is a little more than 2, say 2.2.

11.6 NEUTRALIZATION REACTIONS

When an acid and a base are combined, they will react in what is called a **neutralization reaction**. Oftentimes this reaction will produce a salt and water. Here's an example:

$$\begin{array}{ccccccc} HCl & + & NaOH & \rightarrow & NaCl & + & H_2O \\ \text{acid} & & \text{base} & & \text{salt} & & \text{water} \end{array}$$

This type of reaction takes place when, for example, you take an antacid to relieve excess stomach acid. The antacid is a weak base, usually carbonate, that reacts in the stomach to neutralize acid.

If equimolar amounts of a strong acid and strong base react (as in the example above), the resulting solution will be pH neutral. However, if the reaction involves a weak acid or weak base, the resulting solution will not be pH neutral.

No matter how weak an acid or base is, when mixed with an equimolar amount of a strong base or acid, we can expect complete neutralization. It has been found experimentally that all neutralizations have the same exothermic "heat of neutralization," the energy released from the reaction that is the same for all neutralizations: $H^+ + OH^- \rightarrow H_2O$.

As you can see from the reaction above, equal molar amounts of HCl and NaOH are needed to complete the neutralization. To determine just how much base (B) to add to an acidic solution (or how much acid (A) to add to a basic solution) in order to cause complete neutralization, we just use the following formula:

$$a \times [A] \times V_A = b \times [B] \times V_B$$

where a is the number of acidic hydrogens per formula unit and b is a constant that tells us how many H^+ ions the base can accept.

For example, let's calculate how much 0.1 M NaOH solution is needed to neutralize 40 mL of a 0.3 M HCl solution:

$$V_B = \frac{a \times [A] \times V_A}{b \times [B]} = \frac{1 \times (0.3\,M) \times (40\text{ mL})}{1 \times (0.1\,M)} = 120\text{ mL}$$

Example 11-14: Binary mixtures of equal moles of which of the following acid-base combinations will lead to a complete (99+%) neutralization reaction?

  I.   HCl and NaOH
  II.   HF and NH_3
 III. HNO_3 and $NaHCO_3$

  A)   I only
  B)   I and II only
  C)   II and III only
  D)   I, II, and III

Solution: Remember, regardless of the strengths of the acids and bases, all neutralization reactions go to completion. Choice D is the correct answer.

11.7   HYDROLYSIS OF SALTS

A **salt** is an ionic compound, consisting of a cation and an anion. In water, the salt dissociates into ions, and depending on how these ions react with water, the resulting solution will be either acidic, basic, or pH neutral. To make the prediction, we notice that there are essentially two possibilities for both the cation and the anion in a salt:

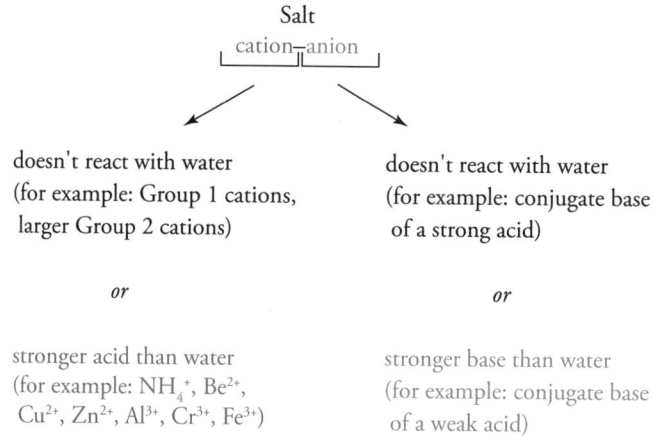

Whether the salt solution will be acidic, basic, or pH neutral depends on which combination of possibilities (four total) from the diagram above applies. The reaction of a substance—such as a salt or an ion—with water is called a hydrolysis reaction, a more general use of the term since the water molecule may not be split. Let's look at some examples.

If we dissolve NaCl in water, Na^+ and Cl^- ions go into solution. Na^+ ions are Group 1 ions and do not react with water. Since Cl^- is the conjugate base of a strong acid (HCl), it also doesn't react with water. These ions just become hydrated (surrounded by water molecules). Therefore, the solution will be pH neutral.

How about NH_4Cl? In solution it will break into NH_4^+ and Cl^-. The ammonium ion is a stronger acid than water (it's the conjugate acid of NH_3, a weak base), and Cl^- will not react with water. As a result, a solution of this salt will be acidic (note the formation of hydronium ions as products), and have a pH less than 7. NH_4Cl is called an acidic salt.

$$NH_4^+(aq) + H_2O(l) \rightleftharpoons NH_3(aq) + H_3O^+(aq)$$

Now let's consider sodium acetate, $Na(CH_3COO)$. In solution it will break into Na^+ and CH_3COO^-. Na^+ is a Group 1 cation and does not react with water. However, CH_3COO^- is a stronger base than water since it's the conjugate base of acetic acid (CH_3COOH), a weak acid. Therefore, a solution of the salt will be basic (note the formation of hydroxide ions as products), and have a pH greater than 7. $NaCH_3COO$ is a basic salt.

$$CH_3COO^-(aq) + H_2O(l) \rightleftharpoons CH_3COOH(aq) + OH^-(aq)$$

Finally, let's consider NH_4CN. In solution it will break into NH_4^+ and CN^-. NH_4^+ is a stronger acid than water, and CN^- is a stronger base than water (it's the conjugate base of HCN, a weak acid). So, which one wins? In a case like this, we need to know the K_a value for the reaction of the cation with water with the K_b value for the reaction of the anion with water and compare these values. Since

$$NH_4^+(aq) + H_2O(l) \rightleftharpoons NH_3(aq) + H_3O^+(aq) \quad (K_a = 6.3 \times 10^{-10})$$

$$CN^-(aq) + H_2O(l) \rightleftharpoons HCN(aq) + OH^-(aq) \quad (K_b = 1.6 \times 10^{-5})$$

we see that in this case K_b of $CN^- > K_a$ of NH_4^+, so the forward reaction of the second reaction will dominate the forward reaction of the first reaction, and the solution will be basic. It is highly unlikely that the level of analysis required for this final example will be required on the MCAT, but you *should* be able to *qualitatively* predict the pH of any salt solution the MCAT throws at you.

11.7

Example 11-15: Which of the following salts will produce a basic solution when added to pure water?

A) KCl
B) NaClO
C) NH_4Cl
D) $MgBr_2$

Solution: NaClO (choice B) will dissociate into Na^+ and ClO^-. Na^+ is a Group 1 cation, so it has no effect on the pH. However, ClO^-, the hypochlorite ion, is the conjugate base of a weak acid, HClO (hypochlorous acid). Therefore, the solution will be basic. The salt in choice A will have no effect on the pH, and the salts in choices C and D will leave the solution acidic (since NH_4^+ is the conjugate acid of a weak base, NH_3, and Mg^{2+} will react with water to form the weak base $Mg(OH)_2$).

Example 11-16: Which of the following is an acidic salt?

A) KNO_3
B) $SrCl_2$
C) $CuCl_2$
D) $Ba(CH_3COO)_2$

Solution: Cu^{2+} is a stronger acid than water, so $CuCl_2$ (choice C) is an acidic salt. The salts in choices A and B are neither acidic nor basic, and choice D is a basic salt.

11.8 BUFFER SOLUTIONS

A **buffer** is a solution that resists changing pH when a small amount of acid or base is added. The buffering capacity comes from the presence of a weak acid and its conjugate base (or a weak base and its conjugate acid) in roughly equal concentrations.

One type of buffer is made from a weak acid and a salt of its conjugate base. To illustrate how a buffer works, let's look at a specific example and add 0.1 mol of acetic acid (CH_3COOH) and 0.1 mol of sodium acetate ($NaCH_3COO$) to water to obtain a 1-liter solution. Since acetic acid is a weak acid ($K_a = 1.75 \times 10^{-5}$), it will partially dissociate to give some acetate (CH_3COO^-) ions. However, the salt is soluble and will dissociate completely to give plenty of acetate ions. The addition of this common ion will shift the acid dissociation to the left, so the equilibrium concentrations of undissociated acetic acid molecules and acetate ions will be essentially equal to their initial concentrations, 0.1 M.

$$CH_3COOH + H_2O \rightleftharpoons H_3O^+ + CH_3COO^-$$

Since buffer solutions are designed to resist changes in pH, let's first figure out the pH of this solution. Writing the expression for the equilibrium constant gives

$$K_a = \frac{[H_3O^+][CH_3COO^-]}{[CH_3COOH]}$$

which we can solve for $[H_3O^+]$:

$$[H_3O^+] = \frac{K_a[CH_3COOH]}{[CH_3COO^-]} \qquad \text{(Equation 1)}$$

Since the equilibrium concentrations of both CH_3COOH and CH_3COO^- are 0.1 M, this equation tells us that

$$[H_3O^+] = \frac{K_a[CH_3COOH]}{[CH_3COO^-]} = \frac{K_a(0.1\,M)}{0.1\,M} = 1.75 \times 10^{-5}$$

and pH = $-\log[H_3O^+]$, so

$$pH = -\log(1.75 \times 10^{-5})$$
$$pH = 4.76$$

Okay, now let's see what happens if we add a little bit of strong acid—HCl, for example. If we add, say, 0.005 mol of HCl, it will dissociate completely in solution into 0.005 mol of H^+ ions and 0.005 mol of Cl^- ions. The Cl^- ions will have no effect on the equilibrium, but the added H^+ (or H_3O^+) ions will. Adding a product shifts the equilibrium to the left, and the acetate ions react with the additional H_3O^+ ions to produce additional acetic acid molecules. As a result, the concentration of acetate ions will drop by 0.005, from 0.1 M to 0.095 M; the concentration of acetic acid will increase by 0.005, from 0.1 M to 0.105 M. Let's now use Equation (1) above to find the new pH:

$$[H_3O^+] = \frac{K_a[CH_3COOH]}{[CH_3COO^-]} = \frac{K_a(0.105\,M)}{0.095\,M} = 1.75 \times 10^{-5}(1.105) = 1.93 \times 10^{-5}$$

and

$$pH = -\log(1.93 \times 10^{-5})$$
$$pH = 4.71$$

Notice that the pH dropped from 4.76 to 4.71, a decrease of just 0.05. If we had added this HCl to a liter of pure water, the pH would have dropped from 7 to 2.3, a *much* larger decrease! The buffer solution we created was effective at resisting a large drop in pH because it had enough base (in the form of acetate ions in this case) to neutralize the added acid.

Now let's see what happens if we add a little bit of strong base—KOH, for example. If we add, say, 0.005 mol of KOH, it will dissociate completely in solution into 0.005 mol of K^+ ions and 0.005 mol of OH^- ions. The K^+ ions will have no effect, but the added OH^- ions will shift the equilibrium to the right, since they'll react with acetic acid molecules to produce more acetate ions ($CH_3COOH + OH^- \rightarrow CH_3COO^- + H_2O$). As a result, the concentration of acetic acid will drop by 0.005, from 0.1 M to 0.095 M; the concentration of acetate ions will increase by 0.005, from 0.1 M to 0.105 M. Let's again use Equation (1) above to find the new pH:

$$[H_3O^+] = \frac{K_a[CH_3COOH]}{[CH_3COO^-]} = \frac{K_a(0.095\ M)}{0.105\ M} = 1.75 \times 10^{-5}(0.905) = 1.58 \times 10^{-5}$$

and

$$pH = -\log(1.58 \times 10^{-5})$$
$$pH = 4.80$$

Notice that the pH increased from 4.76 to 4.80, an increase of just 0.04. If we had added this KOH to a liter of pure water, the pH would have increased from 7 to 11.7, a much larger increase! The buffer solution we created was effective at resisting a large rise in pH because it had enough acid to neutralize the added base.

If we generalize Equation (1) to any buffer solution containing a weak acid and a salt of its conjugate base, we get $[H_3O^+] = K_a([\text{weak acid}]/[\text{conjugate base}])$. Taking the –log of both sides give us the

Henderson-Hasselbalch Equation (for acid)

$$pH = pK_a + \log\left(\frac{[\text{conjugate base}]}{[\text{weak acid}]}\right)$$

To design a buffer solution, we choose a weak acid whose pK_a is as close to the desired pH as possible. An ideal buffer would have [weak acid] = [conjugate base], so pH = pK_a. If no weak acid has the exact pK_a needed, just adjust the initial concentrations of the weak acid and conjugate base accordingly.

11.8

We can also design a buffer solution by choosing a weak base (and a salt of its conjugate acid) such that the pK_b value of the base is as close to the desired pOH as possible. The version of the Henderson-Hasselbalch equation in this situation looks like this:

Henderson-Hasselbalch Equation (for base)

$$pOH = pK_b + \log\left(\frac{[\text{conjugate acid}]}{[\text{weak base}]}\right)$$

Example 11-17: Which of the following compounds could be added to a solution of HCN to create a buffer?

A) HNO_3
B) $CaCl_2$
C) NaCN
D) NaCl

11.9

Solution: HCN is a weak acid, so we'd look for a salt of its conjugate base, CN^-. Choice C, NaCN, is such a salt.

11.9 INDICATORS

An **indicator** is a weak acid that undergoes a color change when it's converted to its conjugate base. Let HA denote a generic indicator. In its non-ionized form, it has a particular color, which we'll call color #1. When it has donated a proton to become its conjugate base, A^-, it has a different color, which we'll call color #2.

Indicator

$$HA + H_2O \rightleftharpoons H_3O^+ + A^-$$

color #1   **color #2**

Under what conditions would an indicator change its color? What if an indicator were added to an acidic solution—that is, one whose pH were quite low due to a high concentration of H_3O^+ ions? Then according to Le Châtelier, the indicator's equilibrium would shift to the left, and the indicator would display color #1. Conversely, if the indicator were added to a basic solution (that is, one with plenty of OH^- ions), the amount of H_3O^+ would decrease, and the indicator's equilibrium would be shifted to the right, causing it to display color #2. We can make this discussion a little more precise.

Take the expression for the indicator's equilibrium constant, $K_a = [H_3O^+][A^-]/[HA]$ and easily rearrange it into

$$\frac{[H_3O^+]}{K_a} = \frac{[HA]}{[A^-]}$$

Written this way, we can see that

- If $[H_3O^+] \gg K_a$, then $[HA] \gg [A^-]$, so we'd see color #1.
- If $[H_3O^+] \approx K_a$, then $[HA] \approx [A^-]$, so we'd see a mix of colors #1 & #2.
- If $[H_3O^+] \ll K_a$, then $[HA] \ll [A^-]$, so we'd see color #2.

Note that the indicator changes color within a fairly short pH range, about 2 units:

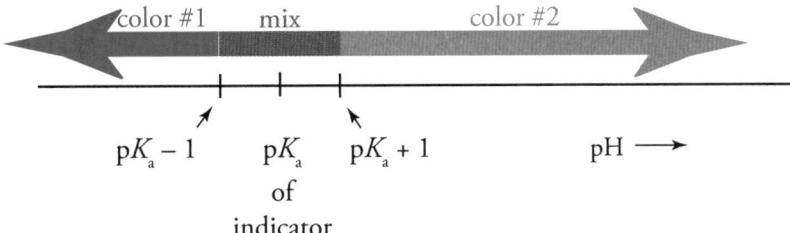

Therefore, if we want our indicator to be useful, we need to select one whose pK_a value is convenient for our purposes. For example, phenolphthalein is an indicator with a pK_a value of about 9.0. When added to a solution whose pH is less than 8, it remains colorless. However, if the solution's pH is above 10, it will turn a deep magenta. (For 8 < pH < 10, the solution will be a paler pink.) Thus, phenolphthalein can be used to differentiate between a solution whose pH is, say, 7 from one whose pH is 11. However, the indicator methyl orange could not distinguish between two such solutions: It would be yellow at pH 7 and yellow at pH 11. Methyl orange has a pK_a of about 3.8, so it changes color around pH 4.

Note: The $pK_a \pm 1$ range for an indicator's color change is convenient and typical, but it's not a hard-and-fast rule. Some indicators (like methyl orange) have a color-change range of only 1.2 (rather than 2) pH units. Also, some indicators have more than just two colors. Polyprotic indicators, like thymol blue and bromocesol green, can change color more than once, and can therefore exhibit more than two distinct colors.

11.10 ACID-BASE TITRATIONS

An **acid-base titration** is an experimental technique used to determine the identity of an unknown weak acid (or weak base) by determining its pK_a (or pK_b). Titrations can also be used to determine the concentration of *any* acid or base solution (whether it be known or unknown). The procedure consists of adding a strong acid (or a strong base) of *known* identity and concentration—the **titrant**—to a solution containing the unknown base (or acid). (One never titrates an acid with an acid or a base with a base.) While the titrant is added in small, discrete amounts, the pH of the solution is recorded (with a pH meter).

If we plot the data points (the pH value vs. the volume of titrant added), we obtain a graph called a titration curve. Let's consider a specific example: the titration of HF (a weak acid) with NaOH (a strong base).

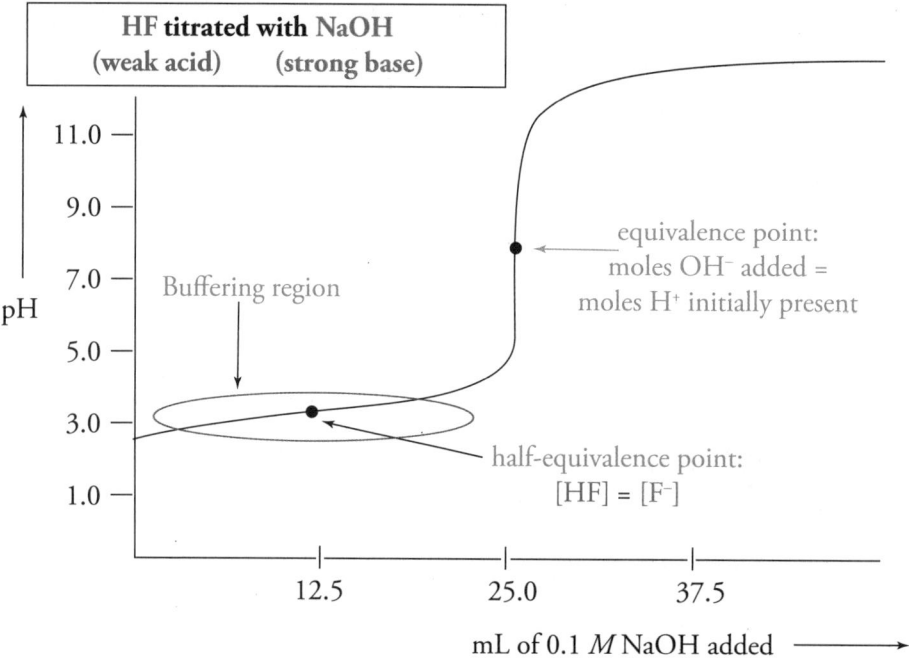

When the amount of titrant added is 0, the pH is of course just the pH of the original, pure solution of HF. Then, as NaOH is added, an equivalent amount of HF will be neutralized according to the reaction

$$NaOH \; + \; HF \; \rightarrow \; Na^+ \; + \; F^- \; + \; H_2O$$

As HF is neutralized, the pH will increase. But from the titration curve, we can see that the pH is certainly not increasing very rapidly as we add the first 20 or so mL of NaOH. This should tell you that at the beginning of this titration the solution is behaving as a buffer. As HF is being converted into F^-, we are forming a solution that contains a weak acid and its conjugate base. This section of the titration curve, where the pH changes very gradually, is called the **buffering domain** (or **buffering region**).

Now, as the experiment continues, the solution suddenly loses its buffering capability and the pH increases dramatically. At some point during this drastic increase, all HF is neutralized and no acid remains in solution. Every new ion of OH^- that is added remains in solution. Therefore, the pH continues to increase rapidly until the OH^- concentration in solution is not that much different from the NaOH concentration in the titrant. From here on, the pH doesn't change very much and the curve levels off.

There is a point during the drastic pH increase at which just enough NaOH has been added to completely neutralize all the HF. This is called the **acid-base equivalence point**. At this point, we simply have Na^+ ions and F^- ions in solution. Note that the solution should be *basic* here. In fact, from what we know about the behavior of conjugates, we can state the following facts about the equivalence point of different titrations:

- For a weak acid (titrated with a strong base), the equivalence point will occur at a pH > 7.
- For a weak base (titrated with a strong acid), the equivalence point will occur at a pH < 7.
- For a strong acid (titrated with a strong base) or for a strong base (titrated with a strong acid), the equivalence point will occur at pH = 7.

11.10

Therefore, by just looking at the pH at the equivalence point of our titration, we can tell whether the acid (or base) we were titrating was weak or strong.

Recall the purpose of this titration experiment: to determine the pK_a (or pK_b) of the unknown weak acid (or weak base). From the titration curve, determine the volume of titrant added at the equivalence point; call it $V_{at\ equiv}$. A key question is this: What's in solution when the volume of added titrant is $1/2\ V_{at\ equiv}$? Let's return to our titration of HF by NaOH. We can read from its titration curve that $V_{at\ equiv}$ = 25 mL. When the amount of NaOH added was $1/2\ V_{at\ equiv}$ = 12.5 mL, the solution consisted of equal concentrations of HF and F⁻, i.e., enough NaOH was added to convert 1/2 of the HF to F⁻. (After all, when the amount of titrant added was twice as much, $V_{at\ equiv}$ = 25 mL, *all* of the HF had been converted to F⁻. So naturally, when 1/2 as much was added, only 1/2 was converted.) Therefore, at this point—called the **half-equivalence point**—we have

$$[HF]_{at\ half\text{-}equiv} = [F^-]_{at\ half\text{-}equiv}$$

The Henderson-Hasselbalch equation then tells us that

$$pH_{at\ half\text{-}equiv} = pK_a + \log\left(\frac{[F^-]_{at\ half\text{-}equiv}}{[HF]_{at\ half\text{-}equiv}}\right) = pK_a + \log 1 = pK_a$$

The pK_a of HF equals the pH at the half-equivalence point. **For our curve, we see that this occurs around** pH 3.2, so we conclude that the pK_a of HF is about 3.2.

11.10

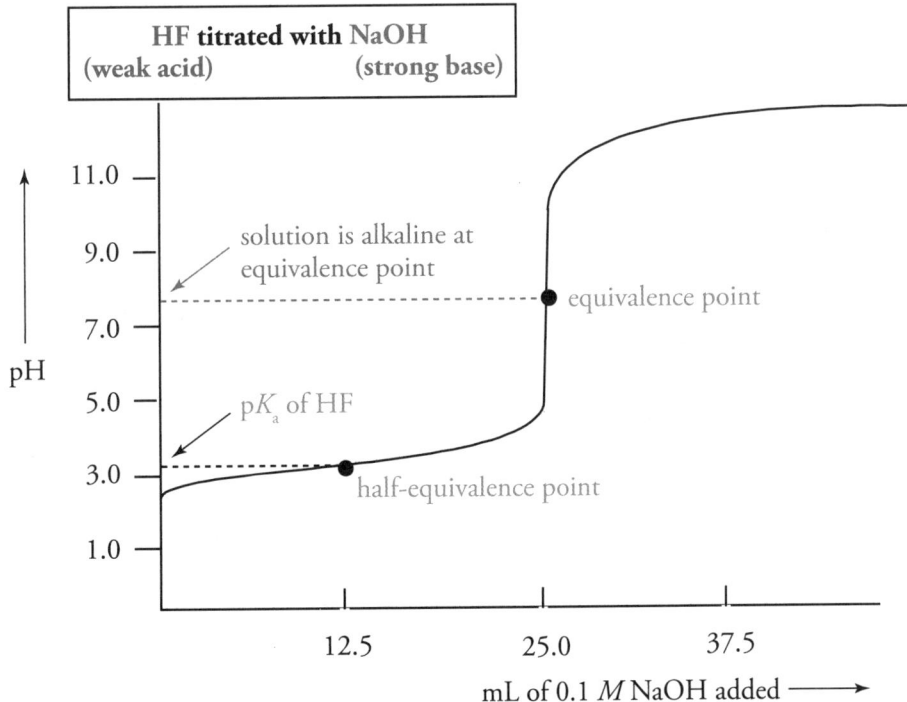

Compare the sample titration curves for a weak base titrated with a strong acid to the one for a weak acid titrated with a strong base (like the one we just looked at). Note the pH at the equivalence point (relative to pH 7) for each curve.

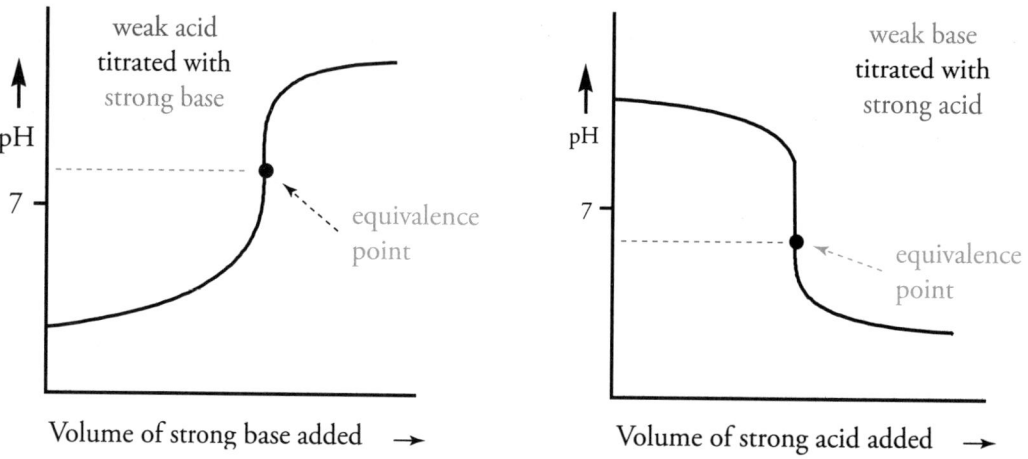

As mentioned above, the titration curve for a strong acid-strong base titration would have the equivalence point at a neutral pH of 7, as shown below.

11.10

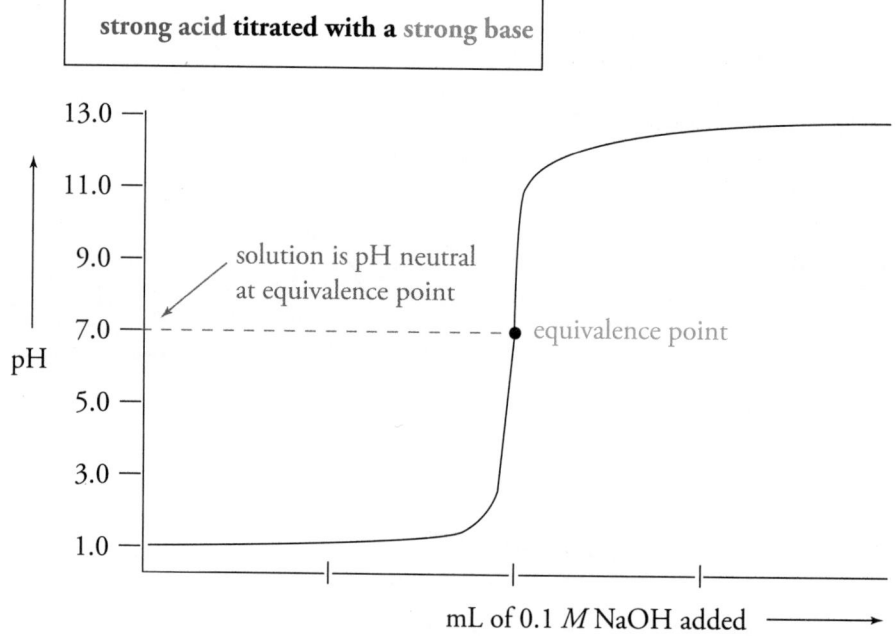

The titration curve for the titration of a polyprotic acid (like H_2CO_3 or an amino acid) will have more than one equivalence point. The number of equivalence points is equal to the number of ionizable hydrogens the acid can donate.

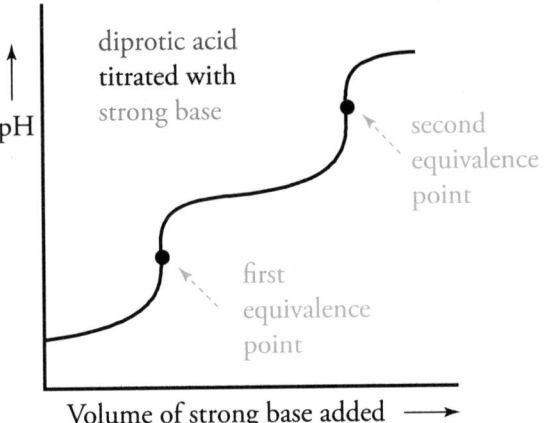

Example 11-18: A fifty mL solution of HCOOH (formic acid) is titrated with 0.2 M NaOH. The equivalence point is reached when 40 mL of the NaOH solution has been added. What was the original concentration of the formic acid solution?

Solution: Using our formula $a \times [A] \times V_A = b \times [B] \times V_B$, we find that

$$[A] = \frac{b \times [B] \times V_B}{a \times V_A} = \frac{1 \times (0.2\ M) \times (40\ \text{mL})}{1 \times (50\ \text{mL})} = 0.16\ M$$

Example 11-19: Methyl red is an indicator that changes from red to yellow in the pH range 4.4–6.2. For which of the following titrations would methyl red be useful for indicating the equivalence point?

A)   HCN titrated with KOH
B)   NaOH titrated with HI
C) C_6H_5COOH (benzoic acid) titrated with LiOH
D) $C_6H_5NH_2$ (aniline) titrated with HNO_3

Solution: Since methyl red changes color in a range of *acidic* pH values, it would be an appropriate indicator for a titration whose equivalence point occurs at a pH less than 7. For a weak base titrated with a strong acid, the equivalence point occurs at a pH less than 7. Only choice D describes such a titration.

11.10

Chapter 11 Summary

- Acids are proton donors and electron acceptors; bases are proton acceptors and electron donors.

- Strong acids completely dissociate in water ($K_a > 1$). You should memorize the list of strong acids and bases.

- The higher the K_a (lower the pK_a), the stronger the acid. The higher the K_b (lower the pK_b), the stronger the base.

- For any conjugate acid and base pair, $K_a K_b = K_w$. Therefore, it follows that the stronger the acid, the weaker its conjugate base. Conjugates of strong acids and bases have no acid/base properties in water.

- Amphoteric substances may act as either acids or bases.

- Water is amphoteric, and autoionizes into OH^- and H_3O^+. The equilibrium constant for the autoionization of water is $K_w = [OH^-][H_3O^+]$. At 25°C, $K_w = 1 \times 10^{-14}$.

- $pH = -\log[H_3O^+]$. For a concentration of H_3O^+ given in a 10^{-x} M notation, simply take the negative exponent to find the pH. The same is true for the relationship between $[OH^-]$ and pOH, K_a and pK_a, and K_b and pK_b.

- At 25°C, $pK_a + pK_b = 14$.

- If a salt is dissolved in water and the cation is a stronger acid than water, the resulting solution will have a pH < 7. If the anion is a base stronger than water, the resulting solution will have a pH > 7.

- Buffers resist pH change upon the addition of a small amount of strong acid or base. A higher concentration of buffer resists pH change better than a lower concentration of buffer (that is, the solution has a higher buffering capacity).

- A buffer consists of approximately equal molar amounts of a weak acid and its conjugate base, and maintains a pH close to its pK_a.

- The Henderson-Hasselbalch equation can be used to determine the pH of a buffer solution.

- Indicators are weak acids that change color upon conversion to their conjugate bases. An indicator changes color in the range +/− 1 pH unit from its pK_a.

· In a titration, the equivalence point is the point at which all of the original acid or base has been neutralized.

· When a strong acid is titrated against a weak base, the pH at the equivalence point is < 7. When a strong base is titrated against a weak acid, the pH at the equivalence point is > 7. When a strong base is titrated against a strong acid, the pH at the equivalence point is = 7.

· At the half equivalence point of a titration of a weak plus a strong acid or base, the solution has equal concentrations of acid and conjugate base, and pH = pK_a.

CHAPTER 11 FREESTANDING PRACTICE QUESTIONS

1. The pH of a CH_3COOH solution is < 7 because when this compound is added to water:

   A) CH_3COOH donates H^+, making $[H^+] > [OH^-]$.
   B) CH_3COOH loses OH^-, making $[H^+] < [OH^-]$.
   C) CH_3COO^- deprotonates H_2O, increasing $[OH^-]$.
   D) CH_3COOH dissociation increases $[H^+]$, thereby increasing K_w.

2. All of the following are amphoteric EXCEPT:

   A) HCO_3^-.
   B) $H_2PO_4^-$.
   C) SO_4^{2-}.
   D) $HOOCCOO^-$.

3. A graph depicting a titration of a weak acid with a strong base will start at a:

   A) high pH and slope downwards with an equivalence pH equal to 7.
   B) high pH and slope downwards with an equivalence pH below 7.
   C) low pH and slope upwards with an equivalence pH equal to 7.
   D) low pH and slope upwards with an equivalence pH above 7.

4. List the following compounds by increasing pK_a:

   I. H_2SO_4
   II. NH_3
   III. CH_3CH_2COOH
   IV. HF

   A) $I < III < II < IV$
   B) $I < IV < III < II$
   C) $III < I < IV < II$
   D) $II < III < IV < I$

5. The amino and carboxyl terminals of alanine lose protons according to the following equilibrium:

   Which of the following indicators would be best used to determine the second equivalence point when alanine is titrated with sodium hydroxide?

   A) Methyl violet ($pK_b = 13.0$)
   B) Methyl yellow ($pK_b = 10.5$)
   C) Thymol blue ($pK_b = 12.0$)
   D) Phenolphthalein ($pK_b = 4.9$)

6. The K_a of HSCN is equal to 1×10^{-4}. The pH of a HSCN solution:

   A) will be approximately 4.
   B) will be approximately 10.
   C) will increase as [HSCN] increases.
   D) cannot be determined from the information given.

7. A 25.0 mL solution of 0.2 M acetic acid ($pK_a = 4.76$) is mixed with 50 mL of 1.0 M sodium acetate ($pK_b = 9.24$). What is the final pH?

   A) 4.8
   B) 5.8
   C) 9.2
   D) 10.2

8. The pK_a of formic acid is 3.75. If 0.1 M formic acid is titrated with NaOH, then the pH of the titration will be closest to 4 at:

   A) the beginning of the titration.
   B) the half-equivalence point.
   C) the equivalence point.
   D) It is impossible to determine this without the molarity of the NaOH.

CHAPTER 11 PRACTICE PASSAGE

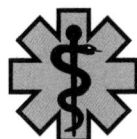

Blood pH homeostasis is the result of several systems operating within the bloodstream. They collectively maintain blood plasma pH at 7.4, since a drop in pH below 6.8 or rise above 7.8 may result in death.

One component of this system is the enzyme *carbonic anhydrase*, which catalyzes the conversion of CO_2 in the blood to carbonic acid. Carbonic acid, in turn, ionizes to form the carbonic acid-bicarbonate buffer. The interdependence of these reactions is shown below in Equation 1.

$$CO_2(g) + H_2O(l) \rightleftharpoons H_2CO_3(aq) \rightleftharpoons H^+(aq) + HCO_3^-(aq)$$

Equation 1

Uncatalyzed blood CO_2 and H^+ can be found binding to hemoglobin after oxygen liberation in peripheral tissues. As the blood reaches the lungs these actions reverse themselves; hemoglobin binds with oxygen, releasing the CO_2 and H^+ ions. The exchange of gases between the lungs and the blood and other tissues in the body is a physiologic process known as respiration.

A second system, the phosphoric acid buffer, plays a minor role compared to the carbonic acid-bicarbonate buffer. Phosphoric acid (H_3PO_4), the primary reactant of this system, is a triprotic acid, which can ionize three protons. This three-step process is illustrated below:

	Reaction	K_a
1	$H_3PO_4(aq) \rightleftharpoons H^+(aq) + H_2PO_4^-(aq)$	$K_{a1} = 7.5 \times 10^{-3}$
2	$H_2PO_4^-(aq) \rightleftharpoons H^+(aq) + HPO_4^{2-}(aq)$	$K_{a2} = 6.2 \times 10^{-8}$
3	$HPO_4^{2-}(aq) \rightleftharpoons H^+(aq) + PO_4^{3-}(aq)$	$K_{a3} = 1.7 \times 10^{-12}$

1. Carbonic acid is best described as:

A) amphoteric.
B) polyprotic.
C) a strong acid.
D) the conjugate acid for CO_2.

2. If CO_2 gas is bubbled continuously in a beaker of water to form carbonic acid, which of the following would be true?

I. Addition of carbonic anhydrase will increase the K_{eq} of the reaction.
II. Carbonic acid will increase in concentration until K_{eq} is reached.
III. Addition of bicarbonate will increase the pH of the system.

A) I only
B) II only
C) III only
D) II and III

3. All of the following statements are true regarding human respiration EXCEPT:

A) when a person's breathing is hampered by conditions such as asthma or emphysema, the blood $[H^+]$ increases.
B) exercise stimulates deeper and more rapid breathing, which increases blood plasma pH.
C) slow, shallow breathing allows CO_2 to accumulate in the blood.
D) hyperventilation can result in the loss of too much CO_2, causing the accumulation of bicarbonate ions.

4. In the dissociation of phosphoric acid, the trend $K_{a1} > K_{a2} > K_{a3}$ is predominantly due to:

A) an equilibrium shift towards the reactants side in Reactions 2 and 3 due to the release of H^+ in Reaction 1.
B) a smaller radius in the H^+ liberated in Reaction 1 compared to that in Reactions 2 and 3.
C) a slower rate of reaction after subsequent ionizations.
D) an increasing influence of the anion after subsequent ionizations.

5. What is the relationship between the K_{a1} value for phosphoric acid and the K_{b1} value for dihydrogen phosphate?

   A) K_{a1} and K_{b1} are inversely related through the dissociation constant for water, K_w.
   B) K_{a1} and K_{b1} are directly related through the dissociation constant for water, K_w.
   C) The K_{a1} is less than the K_{b1}.
   D) There is no relationship between K_{a1} and K_{b1}.

6. What would be the pH of a solution made from combining 50 mL of 0.030 M acetic acid ($K_a = 1.8 \times 10^{-5}$) and 10 mL of 0.15 M sodium acetate?

   A) pH = 1.6
   B) pH = 2.5
   C) pH = 3.3
   D) pH = 4.7

SOLUTIONS TO CHAPTER 11 FREESTANDING PRACTICE QUESTIONS

1. **A** CH_3COOH is acetic acid, a common organic, carboxylic acid. It will dissociate in water to produce H^+ and CH_3COO^-, eliminating choice B. An acidic solution (pH < 7) has more H^+ ions in solution than OH^- ions, making choice A the best answer. Choice C can be eliminated because if $[OH^-]$ were to increase, the pH of the solution would be greater than 7, rather than less than 7. Choice D can be eliminated because the only thing that changes the value of K_w, or any equilibrium constant, is temperature.

2. **C**   An amphoteric substance is one that can act as both an acid and a base. This definition fits choices A, B, and D because they can all donate or accept a proton. Choice C has no protons for donation and cannot be acidic.

3. **D**   A graph showing the titration of a weak acid will start at a low pH and slope upwards as the titrant (in this case a strong base) is added. Therefore, choices A and B cannot be true. As the weak acid and titrant (strong base) react, water and salt are formed as products. The salt will determine the pH at the equivalence point. The conjugate acid of a strong base has no acidic properties and will be neutral in solution. However, the conjugate base of the weak acid will be weakly basic. Because of this, the pH at the equivalence point will be above 7.

4. **B**   A higher pK_a means a weaker acid, while a lower pK_a means a stronger acid. Since this is a ranking question, start with the extremes. Compound I is a strong acid and will have the lowest pK_a, eliminating choices C and D. Compound II is the only base so it will have the largest pK_a and choice A can be eliminated.

5. **D**   Alanine is a neutral amino acid with an isoelectric point close to 7. Therefore, the second equivalence point represents when all the ammonium residue of the zwitterion (the middle structure shown in the question) is deprotonated. This must occur at a basic pH. An appropriate indicator will change color if its pK_a is ±1 of the pH at this equivalence point. Therefore, the desired indicator should have a $pK_a > 7$, or $pK_b < 7$, making choice D the best answer. Another approach to this question is to recognize that no numerical data are provided and choice D is the only indicator for a basic region. There would be no other reasonable way to choose between choices A, B, and C.

6. **D**   The K_a of an acid is a measure of its ability to dissociate in water, not the pH of a solution (the smaller the K_a the weaker the acid). If we know the $[H^+]$ of a solution we can find the pH by finding $-\log[H^+]$, but we cannot find the pH of a weak acid solution from only the K_a. We must also know the concentration of the acid. Choice A is a trap answer if you confuse pK_a with pH. The greater the concentration of an acid, the more H^+ ions will be in solution. However, this will *decrease* the pH of the solution, not increase it (choices B and C can be eliminated). By process of elimination, choice D is the best answer.

7. **B** The sodium acetate solution will be completely ionized:

$$NaC_2H_3O_2 \rightarrow Na^+ + C_2H_3O_2^-$$

However, acetic acid will have negligible dissociation in solution:

$$HC_2H_3O_2 \rightleftharpoons H^+ + C_2H_3O_2^- \ (K_a \approx 1 \times 10^{-5})$$

Therefore, for the combined solution, it is reasonable to assume that all of the $HC_2H_3O_2$ is contributed from the acid solution, and all of the $C_2H_3O_2^-$ is contributed from the salt solution:

$$(0.2 \ M \ HC_2H_3O_2)(0.025 \ L) = 5 \times 10^{-3} \ mol \ HC_2H_3O_2$$

$$(1 \ M \ NaC_2H_3O_2)(0.05 \ L) = 5 \times 10^{-2} \ mol \ C_2H_3O_2^-$$

The new volume of 0.075 L cancels out when solving for the pH using the Henderson-Hasselbalch equation:

$$pH = pK_a + \log\frac{[C_2H_3O_2^-]}{[HC_2H_3O_2]}$$

$$pH = 4.76 + \log\frac{\left(\dfrac{5 \times 10^{-2} \ mol}{0.075 \ L}\right)}{\left(\dfrac{5 \times 10^{-3} \ mol}{0.075 \ L}\right)}$$

$$pH = 4.76 + \log(10) = 5.76$$

8. **B** There are two points in a weak acid-strong base titration for which you should be able to predict the pH quickly. At the equivalence point, the pH will be higher than 7, since only formate, the conjugate base of formic acid, will exist in solution. Choice C can be eliminated. At the half-equivalence point, the pH should be equal to the pK_a of the weak acid, so the pH at the half-equivalence point should be close to 3.75. Choice B is correct. This is true regardless of the molarity of the NaOH (choice D is incorrect.) At the beginning of the titration, the formic acid solution has a pH close to 2.40. Choice A is incorrect.

SOLUTIONS TO CHAPTER 11 PRACTICE PASSAGE

1. **B** Even though the bicarbonate ion is amphoteric and can donate and accept a proton, carbonic acid cannot (eliminate choice A). Choice C is eliminated because carbonic acid is not one of the six strong acids you should know for the MCAT (HI, HBr, HCl, $HClO_4$, H_2SO_4, HNO_3). Choice D is false because carbon dioxide and carbonic acid cannot be a conjugate acid-base pair since they differ by more than one H^+. Choice B is correct because carbonic acid has the ability to donate two protons, making it polyprotic.

2. **D** Addition of a catalyst (such as the enzyme carbonic anhydrase) will simply increase the rate of a reaction. It plays no role in shifting the equilibrium, or changing the equilibrium constant, making Item I false (eliminate choice A). As carbon dioxide is bubbled through, carbonic acid will form until its equilibrium concentration is attained, making Item II valid (eliminate choice C). Finally, addition of bicarbonate will shift the carbonic acid equilibrium to the reactant side, consuming H^+ in the process. Since the concentration of H^+ will decrease, pH will increase, making Item III valid (eliminate choice B).

3. **D** Choices A and C can be eliminated because they create the same effect. A decrease in breathing rate causes less CO_2 to exchange, leading to an increase in CO_2 remaining in the blood (i.e., increased CO_2 concentration). Consequently, this shifts the equilibria shown in Equation 1 to the right, which results in increased H^+ concentration, and decreased pH. Choice B is the opposite effect. Deeper, more rapid breathing expels more CO_2, decreasing the CO_2 in the blood and increasing pH. Hyperventilation may involve the loss of too much CO_2. This loss will shift the equilibria shown in Equation 1 to the left. Loss of bicarbonate ions will result, making choice D the only statement that is NOT true.

4. **D** Generation of H^+ in Reaction 1 is coupled with a release of $H_2PO_4^-$. Both the product and reactant sides of Reaction 2 are increased proportionally, causing no shift in equilibrium (eliminate choice A). Atomic radius is a function of an atom's position in the periodic table. Thus, the radius of H^+ is the same in all three reactions, eliminating choice B. Equilibrium constants have no relationship to reaction rates, so choice C can be eliminated. The K_a values progressively decrease when removing a proton from a polyprotic acid because it is more difficult to remove a proton from an anion compared to a neutral molecule. In subsequent ionizations, the anion becomes more negative, resulting in greater difficulty liberating a positively charged H^+ ion.

5. **A** The relationship between the K_a value of an acid and the K_b value of its conjugate base is through the dissociation constant of water, where $K_w = (K_a)(K_b)$. Therefore, the relationship between K_{a1} and K_{b1} is $K_{a1} = K_w/K_{b1}$; an inverse relationship.

6. **D** The final solution is composed of (50 mL)(0.03 M) = 1.5 mmol of $HC_2H_3O_2$ and (10 mL) (0.15 M) = 1.5 mmol of $NaC_2H_3O_2$ (or 1.5 mmol of $C_2H_3O_2^-$). The total volume will be 60 mL and the starting concentration of acetic acid will be the same as the starting concentration of its conjugate base. Since acetic acid is a weak acid, any subsequent dissociation will be relatively insignificant and the equilibrium concentrations of acid and base will remain approximately the same. When the concentration of the two species in a conjugate pair are equal, the $pK_a = $ pH from the Henderson-Hasselbalch equation: pH = pK_a + log [conjugate base]/[acid]. The pK_a of acetic acid ($K_a = 1.8 \times 10^{-5}$) is approximately 4.7.

Chapter 12
Electrochemistry

12.1 OXIDATION-REDUCTION REACTIONS

Recall that the **oxidation number** (or **oxidation state**) of each atom in a molecule describes how many electrons it is donating or accepting in the overall bonding of the molecule. Many elements can assume different oxidation states depending on the bonds they make. A reaction in which the oxidation numbers of any of the reactants change is called an **oxidation-reduction** (or **redox**) reaction.

In a redox reaction, atoms gain or lose electrons as new bonds are formed. The total number of electrons does not change, of course; they're just redistributed among the atoms. When an atom loses electrons, its oxidation number increases; this is **oxidation**. When an atom gains electrons, the oxidation number decreases; this is **reduction**. A mnemonic device is helpful:

LEO the lion says GER

LEO: Lose Electrons = Oxidation

GER: Gain Electrons = Reduction

An atom that is oxidized in a reaction loses electrons to another atom. We call the oxidized atom a **reducing agent** or **reductant**, because by giving up electrons, it reduces another atom that gains the electrons. On the other hand, the atom that gains the electrons has been **reduced**. We call the reduced atom an **oxidizing agent** or **oxidant**, because it oxidizes another atom that loses the electrons. (You may want to review Section 3.14 on Oxidation States.)

Example 12-1: In an oxidation-reduction, the oxidation number of an aluminum atom changes from 0 to +3. The aluminum atom has been:

- A) reduced, and is a reducing agent.
- B) reduced, and is an oxidizing agent.
- C) oxidized, and is a reducing agent.
- D) oxidized, and is an oxidizing agent.

Solution: Since the oxidation number has increased, the atom's been oxidized. And since it's been oxidized, it reduced something else and thus acted as a reducing agent. Therefore, the answer is C.

Take a look at this redox reaction:

$$Fe + 2\ HCl\ \rightarrow\ FeCl_2 + H_2$$

The oxidation state of iron changes from 0 to +2. The oxidation state of hydrogen changes from +1 to 0. (The oxidation state of chlorine remains at –1.) So, iron has lost two electrons, and two protons (H^+) have gained one electron each. Therefore, the iron has been oxidized, and the hydrogens have been reduced. In order to better see the exchange of electrons, a redox reaction can be broken down into a pair of **half-reactions** that show the oxidation and reduction separately. These **ion-electron** equations show only the actual oxidized or reduced species—and the electrons involved—in an electron-balanced reaction. For the redox reaction shown above, the ion-electron half-reactions are:

$$\text{oxidation:} \qquad Fe \rightarrow Fe^{2+} + 2e^-$$
$$\text{reduction:} \qquad 2\ H^+ + 2e^- \rightarrow H_2$$

Example 12-2: For the redox reaction

$$3 MnO_2 + 2 Al \rightarrow 2 Al_2O_3 + 3 Mn$$

which of the following shows the oxidation half-reaction?

A) $Mn^{4+} + 4e^- \rightarrow Mn$
B) $Mn^{2+} + 2e^- \rightarrow Mn$
C) $Al \rightarrow Al^{3+} + 3e^-$
D) $Al^{4+} \rightarrow Al^{6+} + 6e^-$

Solution: First, eliminate choices A and B since they're *reduction* half-reactions. We can then eliminate choice D for two reasons: First, Al^{4+} is not the species of aluminum on the reactant side; second, it's not balanced electrically. The answer must be C.

12.2   GALVANIC CELLS

Because a redox reaction involves the transfer of electrons, and the flow of electrons constitutes an electric current that can do work, we can use a spontaneous redox reaction to generate an electric current. A device for doing this is called a **galvanic** (or **voltaic**) **cell**, the main features of which are shown in the figure below.

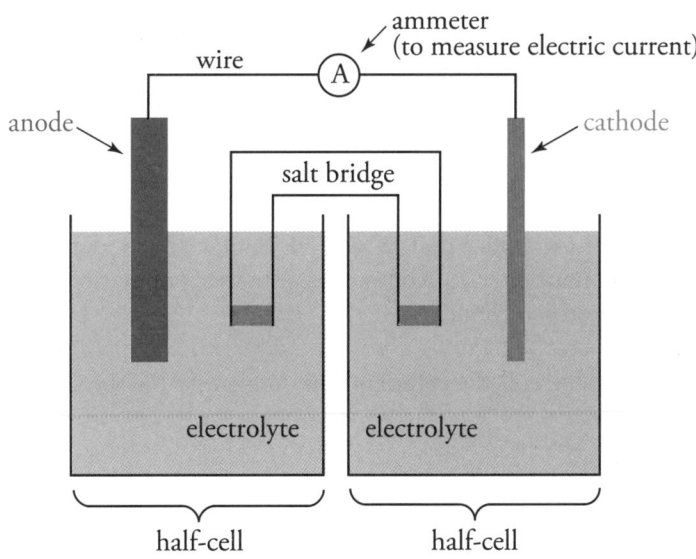

One **electrode**, generally composed of a metal (labeled the **anode**) gets oxidized, and the electrons its atoms lose travel along the wire to a second metal electrode (labeled the **cathode**). It is at the cathode that reduction takes place. In this way, the anode acts as an electron source, while the cathode acts as an electron sink. Electrons always flow through the conducting wire from the anode to the cathode. This electron flow is the electric current that is produced by the spontaneous redox reaction between the electrodes.

Let's look at a specific galvanic cell, with the anode made of zinc, and the cathode made of copper. The anode is immersed in a $ZnSO_4$ solution, the cathode is immersed in a $CuSO_4$ solution, and the half cells are connected by a **salt bridge** containing an aqueous solution of KNO_3. When the electrodes are connected by a wire, zinc atoms in the anode are oxidized ($Zn \rightarrow Zn^{2+} + 2e^-$), and the electrons travel through the wire to the cathode. There, the Cu^{2+} ions in solution pick up these electrons and get reduced to copper metal ($Cu^{2+} + 2e^- \rightarrow Cu$), which accumulates on the copper cathode. The sulfate anions balance the charge on the Zn^{2+}, but do not participate in any redox reaction, and are therefore known as spectator ions.

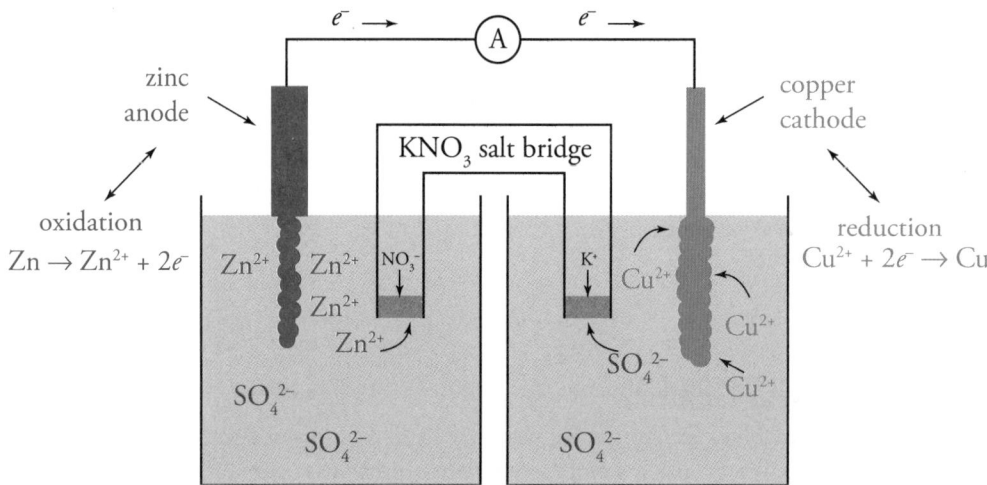

The Zn^{2+} ions that remain in the solution in the zinc half-cell attract NO_3^- ions from the salt bridge, and K^+ ions in the salt bridge are attracted into the copper half-cell. Notice that anions in solution travel from the right cell to the left cell—and cations travel in the opposite direction—using the salt bridge as a conduit. This movement of ions completes the circuit and allows the current in the wire to continue, until the zinc strip is consumed. Remember that anions from the salt bridge go to the anode and cations from the salt bridge go to the cathode.

Notice that the anode is always the site of oxidation, and the cathode is always the site of reduction. One way to help remember this is just to notice that "a" and "o" (anode and oxidation) are both vowels, while "c" and "r" (cathode and reduction) are both consonants. Another popular mnemonic is "an ox, red cat" for "anode = oxidation, reduction = cathode."

We often use a shorthand notation, called a **cell diagram**, to identify the species present in a galvanic cell. Cell diagrams are read as follows:

Anode | Anodic solution (concentration) | | Cathodic solution (concentration) | Cathode

If the concentrations are not specified in the cell diagram, you should assume they are 1 M.

Example 12-3: In the electrochemical cell described by the following cell diagram, what reaction occurs at the anode?

$$Zn(s) \mid Zn^{2+}(aq) \mid\mid Cl^-(aq) \mid Cl_2(g)$$

A) $Zn \rightarrow Zn^{2+} + 2e^-$
B) $Zn^{2+} + 2e^- \rightarrow Zn$
C) $2\ Cl^- \rightarrow Cl_2 + 2e^-$
D) $Cl_2 + 2e^- \rightarrow 2\ Cl^-$

Solution: For any electrochemical cell, oxidation occurs at the anode, and reduction occurs at the cathode. Therefore, we're looking for an oxidation, and choices B and D are eliminated. Since Zn is present at the anode, the answer is A.

Example 12-4: In the absence of a salt bridge, charge separation develops. The anode develops a positive charge and the cathode develops a negative charge, quickly halting the flow of electrons. In this state, the battery resembles:

A) a resistor.
B) a capacitor.
C) a transformer.
D) an inductor.

Solution: The question tells us that the result of removing a salt bridge is charge separation. In physics, we learned that a capacitor is a device that stores electrical energy due to the separation of charge on adjacent surfaces. Thus, choice B is the correct choice.

12.3 STANDARD REDUCTION POTENTIALS

To determine whether the redox reaction of a cell is spontaneous and can produce an electric current, we need to figure out the cell voltage. Each half-reaction has a potential (E), which is the cell voltage it would have if the other electrode were the standard reference electrode. (*Note*: We usually consider cells at standard conditions: 25°C, 1 atm pressure, aqueous solutions at 1 M concentrations, and with substances in their standard states. To indicate standard conditions, we use a ° superscript on quantities such as E and ΔG.) By definition, the standard reference electrode is the site of the redox reaction $2\ H^+ + 2e^- \rightarrow H_2$, which is assigned a potential of 0.00 volts. By adding the half-reaction potential for a given pair of electrodes, we get the cell's overall voltage. Tables of half-reaction potentials are usually given for reductions only. Since each cell has a reduction half-reaction and an oxidation half-reaction, we get the potential of the oxidation by simply reversing the sign of the corresponding reduction potential.

For example, the standard reduction potential for the half-reaction $Cu^{2+} + 2e^- \rightarrow Cu$ is +0.34 V. The standard reduction potential for the half-reaction $Zn^{2+} + 2e^- \rightarrow Zn$ is –0.76 V. Reversing the zinc reduction to an oxidation, we get $Zn \rightarrow Zn^{2+} + 2e^-$, with a potential of +0.76 V. Therefore, the overall cell voltage for the zinc-copper cell is (+0.76 V) + (+0.34 V) = +1.10 V:

oxidation:	$Zn \rightarrow Zn^{2+} + 2e^-$	$E° = +0.76$ V
reduction:	$Cu^{2+} + 2e^- \rightarrow Cu$	$E° = +0.34$ V
	$Zn + Cu^{2+} \rightarrow Zn^{2+} + Cu$	$E° = +1.10$ V

The free-energy change, $\Delta G°$, for a redox reaction in which cell voltage is $E°$ is given by the equation

$$\Delta G° = -nFE°$$

where n is the number of moles of electrons transferred and F stands for a **faraday** (the magnitude of the charge of one mole of electrons, approximately 96,500 coulombs). Since a reaction is spontaneous if $\Delta G°$ is negative, this equation tells us that the redox reaction in a cell will be spontaneous if the cell voltage is positive. Since the cell voltage for our zinc-copper cell was +1.10 V, we know the reaction will be spontaneous and produce an electric current that can do work.

> If the cell voltage is positive, then the reaction is spontaneous.
>
> If the cell voltage is negative, then the reaction is nonspontaneous.

Let's do another example and consider what would happen if the zinc electrode in our cell above were replaced by a gold electrode, given that the **standard reduction potential** for the reaction $Au^{3+} + 3e^- \rightarrow$ Au is $E° = +1.50$ V. The redox reaction that we're investigating is

$$Au + Cu^{2+} \rightarrow Au^{3+} + Cu$$

Let's first break this down into half-reactions:

$Au \rightarrow Au^{3+} + 3e^-$	$E° = -1.50$ V
$Cu^{2+} + 2e^- \rightarrow Cu$	$E° = +0.34$ V

The overall reaction is not electron balanced; but by multiplying the first half-reaction by 2 and the second half-reaction by 3, we get

$2\,Au \rightarrow 2\,Au^{3+} + 6e^-$	$E° = -1.50$ V
$3\,Cu^{2+} + 6e^- \rightarrow 3\,Cu$	$E° = +0.34$ V
$2\,Au + 3\,Cu^{2+} \rightarrow 2\,Au^{3+} + 3\,Cu$	$E° = -1.16$ V

The final equation is now electron balanced. Notice that although we multiplied the half-reactions by stoichiometric coefficients, we did *not* multiply the potentials by those coefficients. You never multiply the potential by a coefficient, even if you multiply a half-reaction by a coefficient to get the balanced equation for the reaction. This is because the potentials are *intrinsic* to the identities of the species involved and do not depend on the number of moles of the species.

Because the cell voltage is negative, this reaction would not be spontaneous. However, it would be spontaneous in the other direction; that is, if copper were the *anode* and gold the *cathode*, then the potential of the cell would be +1.16 V, which implies a spontaneous reaction.

Oxidizing and Reducing Agents

We can also use reduction potentials to determine whether reactants are good or poor oxidizing or reducing agents. For example, let's look again at the half-reactions in our original zinc-copper cell. The half-reaction $Zn^{2+} + 2e^- \rightarrow Zn$ has a standard potential of -0.76 V, and the half-reaction $Cu^{2+} + 2e^- \rightarrow Cu$ has a standard potential of $+0.34$ V. The fact that the reduction of Zn^{2+} is nonspontaneous means that the oxidation of Zn is spontaneous, so Zn would rather give up electrons. If it does, this means that Zn acts as a reducing agent because in giving up electrons it reduces something else. The fact that the reduction of Cu^{2+} has a positive potential tells us that this reaction would be spontaneous at standard conditions. In other words, Cu^{2+} is a good oxidizing agent because it's looking to accept electrons, thereby oxidizing something else. So, in general, if a reduction half-reaction has a large negative potential, then the product is a good reducing agent. On the other hand, if a reduction half-reaction has a large positive potential, then the reactant is a good oxidizing agent. Now, whether something is a "good" oxidizing or reducing agent depends on what it's being compared to. So, to be more precise, we should say this:

> The more negative the reduction potential, the weaker the reactant is as an oxidizing agent, and the stronger the product is as a reducing agent.
>
> The more positive the reduction potential, the stronger the reactant is as an oxidizing agent, and the weaker the product is as a reducing agent.

For example, given that $Pb^{2+} + 2e^- \rightarrow Pb$ has a standard potential of -0.13 V, and $Al^{3+} + 3e^- \rightarrow Al$ has a standard potential of -1.67 V, what could we conclude? Well, since Al^{3+} has a large negative reduction potential, the product, aluminum metal, is a good reducing agent. In fact, because the reduction potential of Al^{3+} is more negative than that of Pb^{2+}, we'd say that aluminum is a stronger reducing agent than lead.

Example 12-5: A galvanic cell is set to operate at standard conditions. If one electrode is made of magnesium and the other is made of copper, then the magnesium electrode will serve as the:

A) anode and be the site of oxidation.
B) anode and be the site of reduction.
C) cathode and be the site of oxidation.
D) cathode and be the site of reduction.

Reaction	$E°$ (volts)
$Li^+ + e^- \rightarrow Li$	-3.05
$Mg^{2+} + 2e^- \rightarrow Mg$	-2.36
$Al^{3+} + 3e^- \rightarrow Al$	-1.67
$Zn^{2+} + 2e^- \rightarrow Zn$	-0.76
$Fe^{2+} + 2e^- \rightarrow Fe$	-0.44
$Pb^{2+} + 2e^- \rightarrow Pb$	-0.13
$2 H^+ + 2e^- \rightarrow H_2$	0.00
$Cu^{2+} + 2e^- \rightarrow Cu$	0.34
$Ag^+ + e^- \rightarrow Ag$	0.80
$Pd^{2+} + 2e^- \rightarrow Pd$	0.99
$Pt^{2+} + 2e^- \rightarrow Pt$	1.20
$Au^{3+} + 3e^- \rightarrow Au$	1.50
$F_2 + 2e^- \rightarrow 2 F^-$	2.87

Solution: First, eliminate choices B and C since the anode is always the site of oxidation and the cathode is always the site of reduction. From the table, we see that the reduction of Mg^{2+} is nonspontaneous, whereas the reduction of Cu^{2+} is spontaneous. Therefore, the copper electrode will serve as the cathode and be the site of reduction, and the magnesium electrode will serve as the anode and be the site of oxidation (choice A).

Example 12-6: For the reaction below, which of the following statements is true?

$$2\ Au + 3\ Fe^{2+} \rightarrow 2\ Au^{3+} + 3\ Fe$$

A) The reaction is spontaneous, because its cell voltage is positive.
B) The reaction is spontaneous, because its cell voltage is negative.
C) The reaction is not spontaneous, because its cell voltage is positive.
D) The reaction is not spontaneous, because its cell voltage is negative.

Solution: First, eliminate choices B and C. Even without looking at the table of reduction potentials, these choices can't be correct. If the cell voltage $E°$ is negative, then the reaction is nonspontaneous, and if $E°$ is positive, then the reaction is spontaneous. The half-reactions are

$$2(Au \rightarrow Au^{3+} + 3e^-) \qquad E° = -1.50\ V$$
$$3(Fe^{2+} + 2e^- \rightarrow Fe) \qquad E° = -0.44\ V$$

Notice again that the question is really asking only about $E°$, and the potentials of the half-reactions are *not* affected by stoichiometric coefficients (2 and 3, in this case). Since each of these half-reactions has a negative value for $E°$, the cell voltage (obtained by adding them) will also be negative, so the answer is D.

Example 12-7: Of the following, which is the strongest reducing agent?

A) Zn
B) Fe
C) Pd
D) Pd^{2+}

Solution: Remember the rule: The more negative the reduction potential, the stronger the product is as a reducing agent. Zn (choice A) is the product of a redox half-reaction whose potential is -0.76 V. Fe (choice B) is the product of a redox half-reaction whose potential is -0.44 V. So, we know we can eliminate choice B. Pd (choice C) is the product of a redox half-reaction whose potential is $+0.99$ V, so C is eliminated. Finally, in order for Pd^{2+} to be a reducing agent, it would have to be oxidized—that is, lose more electrons. A cation getting further oxidized? Not likely, especially when there's a neutral metal (choice A) that is happier to do so.

Example 12-8: Of the following, which is the strongest oxidizing agent?

A) Al^{3+}
B) Ag^+
C) Au^{3+}
D) Cu^{2+}

Solution: Remember the rule: The more positive the reduction potential, the stronger the reactant is as an oxidizing agent. Al^{3+} (choice A) is the reactant of a redox half-reaction whose potential is negative, so we can probably eliminate choice A right away. Ag^+ (choice B) is the reactant of a redox half-reaction whose potential is +0.80 V. (Now we know that A can be eliminated). Au^{3+} (choice C) is the reactant of a redox half-reaction whose potential is +1.50 V, so now B is eliminated. Finally, Cu^{2+} (choice D) is the reactant of a redox half-reaction whose potential is only +0.34 V, so choice C is better.

Example 12-9: Which of the following best approximates the value of $\Delta G°$ for this reaction:

$$2\ Al + 3\ Cu^{2+} \rightarrow 2\ Al^{3+} + 3\ Cu?$$

A) $-(12)(96,500)$ J
B) $-(6)(96,500)$ J
C) $+(6)(96,500)$ J
D) $+(12)(96,500)$ J

Solution: The half-reactions are

$$2(Al \rightarrow Al^{3+} + 3e^-) \qquad E° = +1.67\ V$$
$$3(Cu^{2+} + 2e^- \rightarrow Cu) \qquad E° = 0.34\ V$$

so the overall cell voltage is $E° = 2.01\ V \approx 2\ V$. Because the number of electrons transferred is $n = 2 \times 3 = 6$, the equation $\Delta G° = -nFE°$ tells us that choice A is the answer:

$$\Delta G° = -(6)(96,500)(2)\ J = -(12)(96,500)\ J$$

12.4   NONSTANDARD CONDITIONS

All the previous discussion of potentials assumed the conditions to be standard state, meaning that all aqueous reactants in the mixture were 1 M in concentration. So long as this is true, the tabulated values for reduction potentials apply to each half reaction.

However, since conditions are not always standard we must have a way to alternatively, and more generally, describe the voltage of an electrochemical reaction. To do this we use the Nernst equation.

Recall the following relationship:

$$\Delta G = \Delta G° + RT \ln Q$$

If we substitute ΔG and $\Delta G°$ with their respective relation to E and $E°$, we arrive at

$$-nFE = -nFE° + RT \ln Q$$

or

$$E = E° - \left(\frac{RT}{nF}\right) \ln Q$$

This is the **Nernst equation**. It describes how deviations in temperature and concentration of reactants can alter the voltage of a reaction under nonstandard conditions. As in the standard chemical systems previously discussed, the concentrations of products and reactants will change until $Q = K_{eq}$, and $E = 0$.

Concentration Cells

A **concentration cell** is a galvanic cell that has identical electrodes but which has half-cells with different ion concentrations. Since the electrodes and relevant ions in the two beakers have the same identities, the *standard* cell voltage, $E°$, would be zero. But, such a cell is *not* standard because both electrolytic solutions in the half-cells are not 1 M. So even though the electrodes are the same, in a concentration cell there *will* be a potential difference between them, and an electric current will be produced. For example, let's say both electrodes are made of zinc, and the $[Zn^{2+}]$ concentrations in the electrolytes are 0.1 M and 0.3 M, respectively. We'd expect electrons to be induced to flow through the conducting wire to the half-cell with the higher concentration of these positive ions. So, the zinc electrode in the 0.1 M solution would serve as the anode, with the liberated electrons flowing across the wire to the zinc electrode in the 0.3 M solution, which serves as the cathode. When the concentrations of the solutions become equal, the reaction will stop.

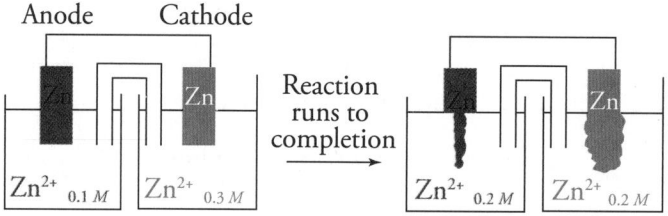

12.5 REDOX TITRATIONS

Just as the titration of an acid with a strong base of known concentration can provide information about the initial acid solution (most notably the concentration and pK_a), titration of a redox active species with a strong oxidant or reductant can be used to determine similar unknowns.

Most redox titrations involve the use of a redox indicator. Much like an indicator in acid/base chemistry, a redox indicator uses a change in color to determine the **endpoint**. However, in a redox reaction, this change in color is due to a change in oxidation state rather than loss or gain of a proton. One commonly used redox indicator is the Ce^{4+} ion, a strong oxidant according to the equation below:

$$Ce^{4+} + 1e^- \rightarrow Ce^{3+} \qquad E° \approx 1.5 \text{ V (1 } M \text{ HCl solution)}$$

The Ce^{4+} ion is bright yellow in solution, whereas the reduced Ce^{3+} is colorless. This color change, along with the comparatively high redox potential, make Ce^{4+} an ideal indicator for the determination of the concentration of solutions of oxidizable species.

For example, cerium is known to oxidize secondary alcohols to ketones in aqueous solution. As such, titration with Ce^{4+} is an appropriate method for the determination of alcohol concentration in solution, or for the determination of the number of secondary hydroxyl groups present in a chemical species. As long as the Ce^{4+} added to the solution is consumed, the solution will remain colorless. However, the solution will turn yellow immediately after all oxidizable hydroxyls have been consumed. Knowledge of the concentration of the Ce^{4+} titrant allows for the determination of initial alcohol concentration.

A redox titration curve, similar to an acid-base titration curve, can be plotted for any such redox titration. An example is given below where a generic reductant is titrated with Ce^{4+}.

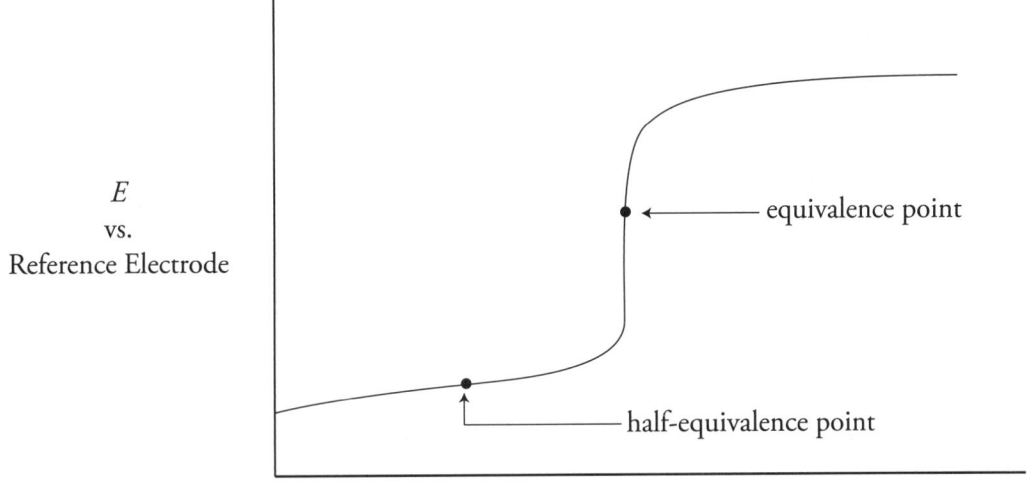

The equivalence point on the plot above will coincide with the solution turning yellow, indicating the completion of the redox reaction and the total consumption of the reductant as described by the system's balanced redox equation. The significance of the half-equivalence point can be seen in the Nernst equation:

$$E = E° - (RT/nF) \ln Q$$

In this case, Q refers to the ratio of oxidized and non-oxidized reactant. At the half-equivalence point these two quantities are equal and $Q = 1$. Since $\ln(1) = 0$, at the half equivalence point the value of E (measured against whichever reference electrode one chooses) is equal to the value of $E°$ for the redox couple being titrated.

12.6   ELECTROLYTIC CELLS

Unlike a galvanic cell, an **electrolytic cell** *uses* an external voltage source (such as a battery) to *create an electric current* that forces a nonspontaneous redox reaction to occur. This is known as **electrolysis**. A typical example of an electrolytic cell is one used to form sodium metal and chlorine gas from molten NaCl.

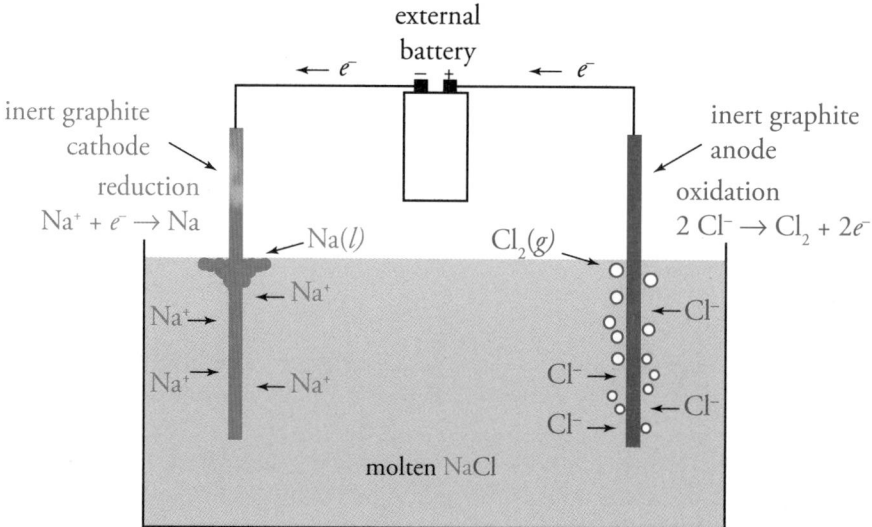

The half-reactions for converting molten Na^+Cl^- into sodium and chlorine are:

$$Na^+ + e^- \rightarrow Na(l) \qquad E° = -2.71 \text{ V}$$
$$2\,Cl^- \rightarrow Cl_2(g) + 2e^- \qquad E° = -1.36 \text{ V}$$

The standard voltage for the overall reaction is −4.07 V, which means the reaction is *not* spontaneous. The electrolytic cell shown above uses an external battery to remove electrons from chloride ions and forces sodium ions to accept them. In so doing, the sodium ions are reduced to sodium metal, and the chloride ions are oxidized to produce chlorine gas, which bubbles out of the electrolyte.

Electrolytic cells are also used for plating a thin layer of metal on top of another material, a process known as **electroplating**. If a fork is used as the cathode in an electrolytic cell whose electrolyte contains silver ions, silver will precipitate onto the fork, producing a silver-plated fork. Other examples of metal plating include gold-plated jewelry, and plating tin or chromium onto steel (for tin cans and car bumpers).

Galvanic vs. Electrolytic Cells

Notice that in both galvanic cells and electrolytic cells, the anode is the site of oxidation and the cathode is the site of reduction. Furthermore, electrons in the external circuit always move from the anode to the cathode. The difference, of course, is that a galvanic cell uses a spontaneous redox reaction to create an electric current, whereas an electrolytic cell uses an electric current to force a nonspontaneous redox reaction to occur.

It follows that in a galvanic cell, the anode is negative and the cathode is positive, since electrons are spontaneously moving from a negative to a positive charge. However, in an electrolytic cell the anode is positive and the cathode is negative, since electrons are being forced to move where they don't want to go.

Galvanic	Electrolytic
Reduction at cathode Oxidation at anode Electrons flow from anode to cathode Anions migrate to anode Cations migrate to cathode	
Spontaneously generates electrical power ($\Delta G° < 0$)	Nonspontaneous, requires an external electric power source ($\Delta G° > 0$)
Total $E°$ of reaction is positive	Total $E°$ of reaction is negative
Anode is negative	Anode is positive
Cathode is positive	Cathode is negative

Example 12-10: The final products of the electrolysis of aqueous NaCl are most likely:

A)   Na(s) and Cl$_2$(g).
B)   HOCl(aq) and Na(s).
C)   Na(s) and O$_2$(g).
D)   NaOH(aq) and HOCl(aq).

Solution: This is a little tricky, but it provides a good example of using the process of elimination. We're not expected to be able to answer this question outright, since there is virtually no information provided. Instead, realize that choices A, B and C list metallic sodium as a final product. That's a problem because we're in an aqueous medium, and we know that sodium metal reacts violently in water to form NaOH and hydrogen gas and fire. So after eliminating these choices, we're left with choice D.

Common Rechargeable Batteries

One particularly useful galvanic cell uses two different oxidation states of Pb for its constitutive electrodes and sulfuric acid as an electrolyte. Often referred to as lead-acid batteries, these cells constitute the oldest type of rechargeable batteries, and are perhaps most commonly employed as automobile batteries.

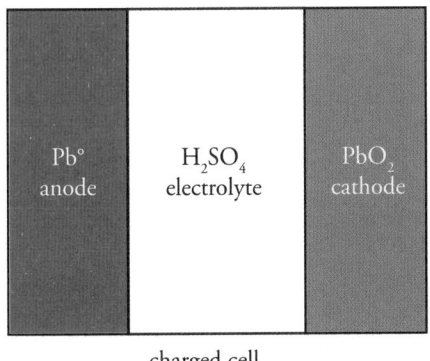

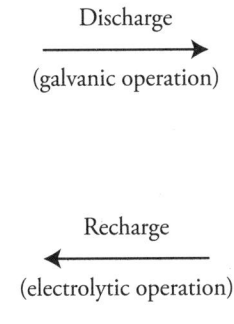

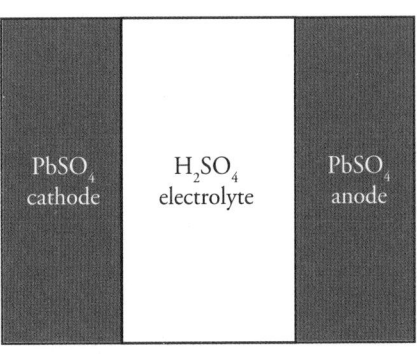

charged cell   discharged cell

As depicted in the simplified figure above, fully charged lead acid batteries utilize $Pb°$ as an anodic electrode and a cathode consisting of PbO_2. As the battery discharges, $Pb°$ undergoes a two-electron oxidation to $PbSO_4$, while PbO_2 is reduced to the same species, as described by the following equations.

$$Pb° + HSO_4^- \rightarrow PbSO_4 + H^+ + 2e^-$$

$$PbO_2 + HSO_4^- + 3H^+ + 2e^- \rightarrow PbSO_4 + 2H_2O$$

Recharging the battery involves reversing the electron flow of discharge with applied voltage, as an electrolytic cell. The oxidation of $PbSO_4$ back to PbO_2, along with the regeneration of $Pb°$ by the reduction of $PbSO_4$, restores the initial potential of the cell.

Nickel-cadmium batteries, or NiCad batteries, are another common type of rechargeable battery. These cells utilize a metallic $Cd°$ anode and a nickel oxide hydroxide $(NiO(OH))$ cathode. The redox reactions involved in the discharge of the battery are given below. To facilitate these reactions, NiCad cells contain an alkaline KOH electrolyte.

$$Cd° + 2OH^- \rightarrow Cd(OH)_2 + 2e^-$$

$$2NiO(OH) + 2H_2O + 2e^- \rightarrow 2Ni(OH)_2 + 2OH^-$$

Recharging spent NiCad batteries, as one might expect, involves applying a voltage to run these two reactions in reverse (typical electrolytic-cell behavior).

12.7 FARADAY'S LAW OF ELECTROLYSIS

We can determine the amounts of sodium metal and chlorine gas produced at the electrodes in the electrolytic cell shown in Section 12.6 using Faraday's law of electrolysis:

> ### Faraday's Law of Electrolysis
> The amount of chemical change is proportional to the amount of electricity that flows through the cell.

For example, let's answer this question: If 5 amps of current flowed in the NaCl electrolytic cell for 1930 seconds, how much sodium metal and chlorine gas would be produced?

Step 1: First determine the amount of electricity (in coulombs, C) that flowed through the cell.
We use the equation $Q = It$ (that is, charge = current × time) to find that

$$Q = (5 \text{ amps})(1930 \text{ sec}) = 9650 \text{ coulombs}$$

Step 2: Use the faraday, F, to convert Q from Step 1 to moles of electrons.
The faraday is the magnitude of the charge on 1 mole of electrons; it's a constant equal to $(1.6 \times 10^{-19} \text{ C}/e^-)(6.02 \times 10^{23} \ e^-/\text{mol}) \approx 96{,}500$ C/mol. So, if 9650 C of charge flowed through the cell, this represents

$$9650 \text{ C} \times \frac{1 \text{ mol } e^-}{96{,}500 \text{ C}} = 0.1 \text{ mol } e^-$$

Step 3: Use the stoichiometry of the half-reactions to finish the calculation.
   a) From the stoichiometry of the reaction $Na^+ + e^- \rightarrow Na$, we see that 1 mole of electrons would give 1 mole of Na. Therefore, 0.1 mol of electrons gives 0.1 mol of Na. Since the molar mass of sodium is 23 g/mol, we'd get $(0.1)(23 \text{ g}) = 2.3$ g of sodium metal deposited onto the cathode.
   b) From the stoichiometry of the reaction $2 \text{ Cl}^- \rightarrow Cl_2(g) + 2e^-$, we see that for every 1 mole of electrons lost, we get 0.5 mole of $Cl_2(g)$. Since Step 2 told us that 0.1 mol of electrons were liberated at the anode, 0.05 mol of $Cl_2(g)$ was produced. Because the molar mass of Cl_2 is $2(35.5 \text{ g/mol}) = 71$ g/mol, we'd get $(0.05 \text{ mol})(71 \text{ g/mol}) = 3.55$ g of chlorine gas.

Example 12-11: A piece of steel is the cathode in a hot solution of chromic acid (H_2CrO_4) to electroplate it with chromium metal. How much chromium would be deposited onto the steel after 48,250 C of electricity was forced through the cell?

A) $\dfrac{1}{12}$ mol

B) $\dfrac{1}{6}$ mol

C) $\dfrac{1}{4}$ mol

D) 3 mol

Solution: First, we notice that 48,250 C of electricity is equal to $\dfrac{1}{2}$ faraday (F = 96,500 C/mol). This is equivalent to $\dfrac{1}{2}$ mole of electrons. In the molecule H_2CrO_4, chromium is in a +6 oxidation state. So, from the stoichiometry of the reaction $Cr^{6+} + 6e^- \rightarrow Cr$, we see that for every 6 moles of electrons gained, we get 1 mole of Cr metal. Another way of looking at this is to say that for every 1 mole of electrons gained, we get just $\dfrac{1}{6}$ mole of Cr metal. Therefore, if we have a supply of $\dfrac{1}{2}$ mol of electrons, we'll produce $(\dfrac{1}{6})(\dfrac{1}{2}) = \dfrac{1}{12}$ mol of Cr, choice A.

12.7

Chapter 12 Summary

- Oxidation is electron loss; reduction is electron gain (remember "OIL RIG").

- A species that is oxidized is a reducing agent, and a species that is reduced is an oxidizing agent.

- In all electrochemical cells, oxidation occurs at the anode and reduction occurs at the cathode.

- Electrons always flow from the anode to the cathode.

- Salt bridge anions always migrate toward the anode, and cations always migrate toward the cathode.

- The free energy of an electrochemical cell can be calculated from its potential based on $\Delta G° = -nFE°$.

- A galvanic cell spontaneously generates electrical power ($-\Delta G$, $+E$).

- An electrolytic cell consists of nonspontaneous reactions and requires an external electrical power source ($+\Delta G$, $-E$).

- In a galvanic cell, electrons spontaneously flow from the negative ($-$) terminal to the positive ($+$) terminal. Therefore, it follows that in a galvanic cell the anode is negatively charged ($-$) and the cathode is positively charged ($+$).

- In an electrolytic cell, electrons are forced from the positive ($+$) terminal to the negative ($-$) terminal, and therefore the anode is positively charged ($+$) and the cathode is negatively charged ($-$).

- Standard reduction and oxidation potentials are intrinsic values and therefore should not be multiplied by molar coefficients in balanced half reactions.

- For a given reduction potential, the reverse reaction, or oxidation potential, has the same magnitude of E but the opposite sign.

- Faraday's law of electrolysis states that the amount of chemical change is proportional to the amount of electricity that flows through the cell.

- Under nonstandard conditions, the potential of an electrochemical cell can be calculated using the Nernst equation: $E = E° - [\frac{RT}{nF}]\ln Q$.

CHAPTER 12 FREESTANDING PRACTICE QUESTIONS

1. Typical dry cell batteries contain a zinc anode and a carbon cathode and produce a potential difference of 1.5 V. Given that many electronic devices require additional voltage, which of the following would result in an overall increase in voltage?

    I.   Doubling the quantity of Zn(s)
    II. Placing two batteries in parallel
    III. Replacing Zn(s) with Na(s)

A) I only
B) III only
C) I and II only
D) II and III only

2. Given the following reactions:

$$Pb^{2+} + 2e^- \rightarrow Pb(s) \quad E° = -0.13 \text{ V}$$
$$Fe(s) \rightarrow Fe^{2+} + 2e^- \quad E° = 0.45 \text{ V}$$

Which one of the following is true?

A) Pb(s) is a better reductant than Fe(s).
B) Fe(s) is a worse reductant than Pb(s).
C) Fe^{2+} is a better oxidant than Pb^{2+}.
D) Pb^{2+} is a better oxidant than Fe^{2+}.

3. Which of the following best characterizes the spontaneous half-reaction below under standard conditions?

$$Pd^{2+} + 2e^- \rightarrow Pd$$

A) $\Delta G° > 0$ and $E° < 0$
B) $\Delta G° < 0$ and $E° < 0$
C) $\Delta G° > 0$ and $E° > 0$
D) $\Delta G° < 0$ and $E° > 0$

4. High valent metals (those with large, positive oxidation states) are often used as strong oxidizing agents. Which of the following compounds would have the most positive reduction potential vs. a standard hydrogen electrode?

A) $FeCl_3$
B) OsO_4
C) $Zn(NO_3)Cl$
D) $W(CO)_6$

5. Which of the following best describes the difference between a galvanic cell and an electrolytic cell?

A) In a galvanic cell, the anode is the site of oxidation, whereas in an electrolytic cell the anode is the site of reduction.
B) In a galvanic cell, the cathode is the negative electrode, whereas in an electrolytic cell the cathode is the positive electrode.
C) In a galvanic cell, spontaneous reactions generate a current, whereas in an electrolytic cell a current forces nonspontaneous reactions to occur.
D) In a galvanic cell, the electrons flow from anode to cathode, whereas in an electrolytic cell the electrons flow from cathode to anode.

6. To give "white gold" a white appearance, it is plated with rhodium by immersion in a rhodium sulfate solution $(Rh_2(SO_4)_3(aq))$. Provided with a current of 2.0 A, how long must a 3.0 g white gold broach be immersed to plate 3.0×10^{-5} g of rhodium? (Faraday's constant = 96,500 C/mol e^-)

A) 0.0009 s
B) 0.0098 s
C) 0.042 s
D) 0.56 s

7. A galvanic cell is constructed from two half-cells of platinum and iron. The half-reactions for these two elements are provided as follows:

$$Pt^{2+}(aq) + 2e^- \rightarrow Pt(s) \qquad E° = +1.20 \text{ V}$$
$$Fe^{3+}(aq) + 3e^- \rightarrow Fe(s) \qquad E° = -0.036 \text{ V}$$

Which of the following statements is true about the galvanic cell?

A) $E° = 1.164$ V, and Pt^{2+} is the reducing agent.
B) $E° = 1.164$ V, and Fe^{3+} is the reducing agent.
C) $E° = 1.236$ V, and Pt^{2+} is the oxidizing agent.
D) $E° = 1.236$ V, and Fe^{3+} is the oxidizing agent.

8. An electrochemical cell is constructed using two inert electrodes in one chamber with an inert electrolyte. The binary compound ICl is dissolved in the electrolyte, current is applied, and I_2 and Cl_2 are produced. Which of the following statements is true?

A) Cl_2 was produced by reduction at the cathode.
B) I_2 was produced by oxidation at the cathode.
C) Cl_2 was produced by oxidation at the cathode.
D) I_2 was produced by reduction at the cathode.

CHAPTER 12 PRACTICE PASSAGE

A student performed an extensive experiment to determine the relative rates of corrosion of various metals with a variety of strong acids. The experimental procedure involved immersing three sets of ten 1.0-gram metal samples into three different acid baths, and then quantifying the reaction's spontaneity based upon the vigor of gas evolution. Reactions were designated as being either *violent* (X), *vigorous* (V), *moderate* (M), *sluggish* (S), or *nonspontaneous* (OO). The reactions were performed in a Styrofoam calorimeter. Gas evolution was monitored visually, and the heat evolved in the bath C reactions (data not given here) was measured with a calibrated thermometer. All reactions in bath C were allowed to go to completion.

Metal	Bath A	Bath B	Bath C
Magnesium	V	V	X
Lead	OO	OO	V
Iron	M	S	X
Aluminum	V	M	X
Copper	OO	OO	V
Silver	OO	OO	M
Zinc	V	V	X
Cobalt	M	M	X
Tin	M	M	V
Mercury	OO	OO	M

Table 1 Rates of gas evolution

Reagents:
Bath A contained hydrochloric acid (12 *M*)
Bath B contained sulfuric acid (18 *M*)
Bath C contained nitric acid (16 *M*)

Based upon his observations, the student constructed two linear rankings of the reduction potentials of the acids and the metals. The first ranking was based solely upon the qualitative rates of gas evolution as listed above, and the second ranking was based solely upon his quantitative Bath C heat data.

He found that his first table was in general agreement with previously published reductions tables, although pairs of metals with similar reduction potentials were in reversed order half of the time. Yet surprisingly, his second table had no correlation with any accepted work. It assigned Al and Mg with potentials far too high (negative 10 and 12 volts), and gave mercury, silver, and lead values much smaller than what they should have been.

1. Based upon his first reduction potential table, the student correctly listed the metal with the highest (most positive) reduction potential as:

A) silver.
B) copper.
C) magnesium.
D) lead.

2. Which of the following statements is inconsistent with the *student's* data?

A) The nitrate ion has a higher reduction potential than H^+.
B) The nitrate ion is a better oxidizing agent than H^+.
C) The sulfate ion is a better oxidizing agent than H^+.
D) H^+, Cl^- and SO_4^{2-} must all have lower reduction potentials than lead, silver, copper, and mercury.

3. Not surprisingly, the student's thermodynamic data failed to produce the accepted reduction potential table because he made some fundamental mistakes in this portion of his experiment. Which one of the following did NOT contribute to the huge experimental error?

A) In measuring and contrasting the heats of reactions of several compounds with differing molecular weights, the student should have used equal moles of reactants, not equal masses.
B) The acids in the immersion baths should have been the same concentration.
C) For reactions in which gaseous products are generated, one should use a sealed calorimeter with an airtight lid.
D) The specific heats of each of the systems were not taken into account, and may have differed.

4. As noted in the passage, the data in columns A and B are similar, but different from the data in column C. Which of the following acids would most likely re-create the data found in column C?

A) HBr
B) H_3PO_4
C) HF
D) $HClO_4$

SOLUTIONS TO CHAPTER 12 FREESTANDING PRACTICE QUESTIONS

1. **B** Increasing reagent quantity has no effect on voltage (Item I is incorrect, eliminating choices A and C), and placing batteries in parallel would leave the voltage unchanged (Item II is incorrect, eliminating choice D). Oxidation of zinc takes place at the anode, and sodium is a better reducing agent than zinc due to its lower ionization energy and tendency to give up an electron (Item III would result in an increase in voltage; the correct answer is choice B).

2. **D** *Oxidant* and *reductant* are synonymous with *oxidizing agent* and *reducing agent*, respectively. Choices A and B are saying the same thing, so both can be eliminated. To compare the relative strengths of the ions as oxidizing agents, reverse the half reaction for Fe so that it reads as a reduction:

$$Pb^{2+} + 2e^- \rightarrow Pb(s) \quad E° = -0.13 \text{ V}$$
$$Fe^{2+} + 2e^- \rightarrow Fe(s) \quad E° = -0.45 \text{ V}$$

   Note that the sign of $E°$ is reversed in this process. Pb^{2+} has a greater reduction potential than Fe^{2+}, making it the better oxidant.

3. **D** This question is asking about two factors (a two-by-two question): $\Delta G°$ and $E°$, which are related by $\Delta G° = -nFE°$. For any spontaneous reaction, the change in Gibbs free energy ($\Delta G°$) is always less than 0 (eliminate choices A and C). As shown in the equation above, the standard reduction potential ($E°$) must be positive when $\Delta G°$ is negative, so eliminate choice B.

4. **B** A large, positive reduction potential indicates a strong tendency to be reduced, and hence the ability to act as an oxidizing agent. The question states that high-valent metals act as strong oxidizing agents. Examining the oxidation states of the metals in question, we see that Fe = +3, Os = +8, Zn = +2, and W = 0. Therefore, since Os bears the largest positive oxidation state, we know that it is the strongest oxidizing agent.

5. **C** The anode is always the site of oxidation and the cathode is always the site of reduction; therefore, electrons always flow from the anode (oxidation) to the cathode (reduction) regardless of the kind of cell (choices A and D are wrong). In a galvanic cell, a spontaneous reaction liberates electrons and they flow freely to the positive electrode, which in this case would be the cathode. However, in an electrolytic cell the current is forcing the electrons to flow where they don't want to go: the negative electrode. In this case the cathode would be the negative electrode (choice B is wrong).

6. **C** Since current (I) = charge(Q)/time(t) we can set up and solve the following equation, keeping in mind that the rhodium reduction in question is $Rh^{3+} + 3e^- \rightarrow Rh(s)$.

$$t = \frac{Q}{I} = \frac{(3 \times 10^{-5} \text{ g})\left(\dfrac{1 \text{ mol Rh}}{102.9 \text{ g}}\right)\left(\dfrac{3 \text{ mol } e^-}{1 \text{ mol Rh}}\right)\left(\dfrac{9.65 \times 10^4 \text{ C}}{1 \text{ mol } e^-}\right)}{2.0 \text{ A}}$$

$$t \approx \frac{(3 \times 10^{-5} \text{ g})\left(\dfrac{1 \text{ mol Rh}}{100 \text{ g}}\right)\left(\dfrac{3 \text{ mol } e^-}{1 \text{ mol Rh}}\right)\left(\dfrac{1.0 \times 10^5 \text{ C}}{1 \text{ mol } e^-}\right)}{2.0 \text{ A}} \approx \frac{9 \times 10^{-2} \text{ C}}{2.0 \text{ A}} \approx 0.045 \text{ s}$$

7. **C** The half-reaction with the *less positive* reduction potential (in this case, $Fe^{3+}(aq) + 3e^- \rightarrow$ $Fe(s)$) should be reversed in order to combine the half-reactions to obtain an $E^o > 0$ and create a galvanic cell. When the Fe half-reaction is reversed, the sign of the potential must be reversed. Combining the two half-reactions then gives: $3\ Pt^{2+}(aq) + 2\ Fe(s) \rightarrow 2\ Fe^{3+}(aq) +$ $3\ Pt(s)$ with an $E^o = 1.236$ V (eliminate choices A and B). Since Fe^{3+} is the product of the reaction, it cannot be the oxidizing agent (eliminate choice D). However, Pt^{2+} is reduced (it gains electrons from the Fe that is oxidized), so it is therefore the oxidizing agent.

8. **D** In the compound ICl, I has an +1 oxidation state, and Cl has a –1 oxidation state owing to the greater electronegativity of Cl. Therefore, production of Cl_2 must be an oxidation, and production of I_2 must be a reduction, eliminating choices A and B. Moreover, reduction always takes place at the cathode, eliminating choice C.

SOLUTIONS TO CHAPTER 12 PRACTICE PASSAGE

1. **A** A metal with a high reduction potential will not be easily oxidized by the H^+ in the acid. The student's data indicated that choices B, C, and D were more reactive with acids than choice A.

2. **C** Of all the strong acids in the passage, only nitric acid and sulfuric acid have conjugate bases with positive reduction potentials. Choices A and B are correct: nitric acid is more corrosive than sulfuric and hydrochloric acid because the nitrate ion has a higher reduction potential (is a better oxidizing agent) than H^+. This is supported by data in the table. Choice D is also correct because the ions present in Bath A and Bath B were unable (had a lower reduction potential) to oxidize lead, silver, copper, and mercury—the student observed no reaction. If choice C were correct, sulfuric acid should be more corrosive than HCl, but this was not observed in the data set.

3. **B** Choices A, C, and D would be serious errors. Since the metal samples were the limiting reagent, not the acids themselves, the concentration of the acids is irrelevant.

4. **D** HCl, H_2SO_4 and HNO_3 are all strong acids, and may undergo reduction through their H^+ entity resulting in the formation of H_2. However, the fact that the three columns are not the same indicates another mechanism of reduction. In this case, the highly oxidized nitrogen in the NO_3^- anion (formally N^{+5}) is capable of extracting electrons and forming nitrogen oxides with lower oxidation states. The most similar acid listed in this regard is $HClO_4$, which contains a highly oxidized formal Cl^{+7}. The remaining three acids may be expected, to one degree or another, to show reduction to H_2 in the presence of reducing equivalents, but none of these have such highly unstable electronegative elements in highly positive oxidation states. The phosphorous atom in H_3PO_4 is in a +5 state, but is much more like the S^{+6} atom in the stable SO_4^{2-} (column B) than the N^{+5} in NO_3^-.

HEME/COPPER ASSEMBLY MEDIATED NITRITE AND NITRIC OXIDE INTERCONVERSION

Shabnam Hematian, Maxime A. Siegler, and Kenneth D. Karlin

Nitrogen oxides (NO_x) are components of great interest in both biological and environmental sciences. Nitric oxide (NO) is an important cellular signaling molecule and a powerful vasodilator involved in many physiological and pathological processes. Nitrite (NO_2^-) is the one-electron-oxidized product of endogenous NO metabolism. Recent studies indicate that nitrite plays a critical biological role by serving as a biochemical circulating reservoir for NO, in particular under conditions of physiologic hypoxia (low O_2 tensions; see also below) and ischemia. Suggested conserved roles for the NO_2^-/NO pool in cellular processes include oxygen sensing and oxygen-dependent modulation of intermediary metabolism. It is now considered that in order to stimulate NO signaling, nitrite reductase activity occurs widely in differing cellular environments and is effected by a variety of proteins/enzymes, including hemes, those with molybdenum, and what draws our current interest, cytochrome c oxidases (CcO's).

The link between nitrite/NO redox interconversion and O_2 sensing is thought to occur in mitochondria at the CcO binuclear heme$_{a3}$/Cu$_B$ center; CcO is the terminal enzyme of the mitochondrial respiratory chain. Here, molecular oxygen consumption (i.e., O_2 reduction to water) is down-regulated in hypoxia by increased NO generation via CcO nitrite reductase activity, as reduced heme/Cu centers dominate when the O_2 concentration is low. The NO thus generated inhibits CcO activity by reversibly binding to heme$_{a3}$ in place of O_2, resulting in cellular O_2 accumulation (Figure 1).

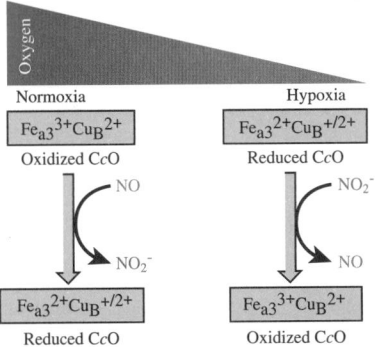

Figure 1. Cytochrome c oxidase (CcO) functioning in nitrite (NO_2^-)/nitric oxide (NO) interconversion as part of its role in regulation of O_2 balance. The availability of O_2 influences the redox state of the CcO containing the heme$_{a3}$/Cu$_B$ binuclear center.

In turn, in normoxia, high local O_2 concentrations do not allow nitrite to compete as an oxidant at the CcO binuclear center; thus, NO/O_2 binding is noncompetitive, and heme$_{a3}$/Cu$_B$ oxidizes NO back to nitrite (Figure 1) to rejoin the storage pool. NO is thought to first attack oxidized Cu$_B$, formally giving Cu^I–NO$^+$; the latter hydrolyzes to nitrite.

In this report, we describe a chemical system involving a heme/Cu assembly-mediated interconversion of these important nitrogen oxides. A partially reduced/oxidized state, with reduced heme and oxidized copper ion (i.e., $Fe^{II}\cdots Cu^{II}$) efficiently converts nitrite to NO. When a fully oxidized $Fe^{III}\cdots Cu^{II}$ heme/Cu complex is employed, NO is readily oxidized to nitrite. The overall reactions are represented by eqs 1 and 2:

$$(P)Fe^{II}Cu^{II} + NO_2^- \rightarrow (P)Fe^{III}-O-Cu^{II} + NO \qquad (1)$$

$$(P)Fe^{III}-O-Cu^{II} + NO \rightarrow (P)Fe^{II}Cu^{II} + NO_2^- \qquad (2)$$

The nitrite reductase chemistry, here however in a heme/Cu chemical system, consisted of the iron(II) complex (F$_8$) Fe^{II} [F$_8$ ≡ tetrakis(2,6-difluorophenyl)porphyrinate(2–)] and a preformed copper(II)–nitrito complex [(tmpa) Cu^{II}(NO$_2$)][B(C$_6$F$_5$)$_4$] [tmpa ≡ tris(2-pyridylmethyl)amine].

When 2 equiv of (F$_8$)Fe^{II} were mixed with 1 equiv of [(tmpa)Cu^{II}(NO$_2$)]$^+$ under a N$_2$ atmosphere in acetone at room temperature (RT), a reaction ensued, and on the basis of UV–vis, electron paramagnetic resonance (EPR), and IR spectroscopies, a 1:1 mixture of the heme–nitrosyl species (F$_8$)Fe^{II}(NO) and the μ-oxo complex [(F$_8$)Fe^{III}–O–Cu^{II}(tmpa)]$^+$ were produced. To determine whether the heme or the copper ion is the reductant in this one-electron process ($NO_2^- \rightarrow NO$), we also carried out the reaction in which nitrite was added to the oxidized heme complex [(F$_8$)Fe^{III}]SbF$_6$ (binding of nitrite to the ferric heme was indicated by a large UV–vis change) and then the reduced complex [(tmpa)Cu^I(MeCN)]$^+$ was added. In this case there was no reaction (Scheme 1), even over a period of days. Control experiments showed that nitrite reacts only very slowly with (F$_8$)Fe^{II} and not at all with [(tmpa) Cu^I(MeCN)]$^+$. Moreover, no nitrite reductase activity was observed for the fully reduced metal combination, nitrite plus (F$_8$)Fe^{II} and [(tmpa)Cu^I(MeCN)]$^+$.

These observations indicate that the heme is the reductant in this heme/Cu nitrite reductase chemistry. The need for 2 equiv of $(F_8)Fe^{II}$ is due to the well-known high affinity of NO to bind ferrous hemes. The initially formed NO reacts very rapidly with $(F_8)Fe^{II}$; thus, if the reaction were carried out with equimolar quantities of $(F_8)Fe^{II}$ and $[(tmpa)Cu^{II}(NO_2)]^+$, only half of the iron would be available to reduce nitrite, and the rest would trap the NO as $(F_8)Fe^{II}(NO)$. The role of the Cu^{II} ion appears to be to provide a Lewis acid interaction with nitrite, facilitating NO_2^- (N–O) bond cleavage and stabilization of the resulting oxo anion via eventual formation of $[(F_8)Fe^{III}–O–Cu^{II}(tmpa)]^+$.

To demonstrate that heme/copper assemblies can mediate NO oxidation to nitrite, as occurs biologically in order to remove excess NO when it is not needed and return it to the nitrite pool (see above), we employed $[(F_8)Fe^{III}–O–Cu^{II}(tmpa)]^+$. Addition of NO to this fully oxidized heterobinuclear complex led to rapid reaction (Scheme 1) and formation of nitrite, which bound to Cu(II); the $(F_8)Fe^{II}$ formed in this redox reaction was trapped by a second equivalent of NO to give $(F_8)Fe^{II}(NO)$. UV–vis (Figure 2) and IR (ν_{NO} = 1688 cm^{-1}) spectroscopies directly indicated nitrosyl complex formation.

EPR spectroscopy confirmed that a copper(II)–nitrito complex was produced (Figure 2).

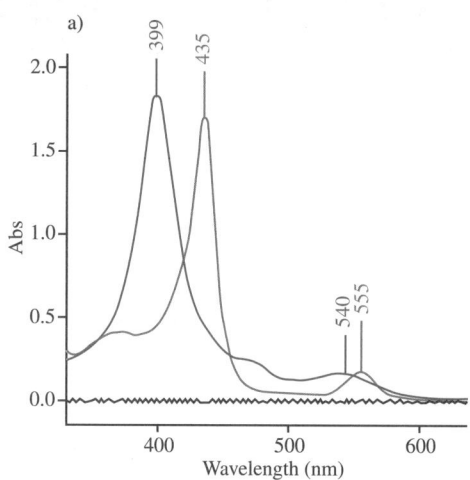

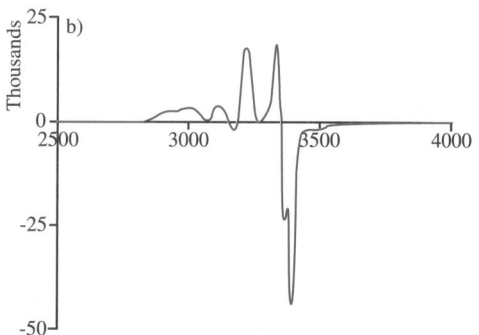

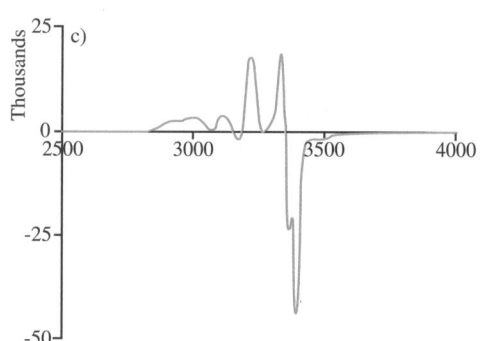

Figure 2. (a) UV–vis spectra of $(F_8)Fe^{III}–O–Cu^{II}(tmpa)][B(C_6F_5)_4]$ (**1**) (blue) and $(F_8)Fe^{II}(NO)$ generated from **1** + NO(g) (12 μM in acetone at RT) (red). (b, c) EPR spectra of (b) the products of the reaction of $(F_8)Fe^{III}–O–Cu^{II}(tmpa)][B(C_6F_5)_4]$ and NO (red) and (c) an authentic sample of a 1:1 mixture of $F_8Fe^{II}(NO)$ and $[(tmpa)Cu(NO_2)][B(C_6F_5)_4]$ (green). The EPR spectra were recorded at 20 K (1 mM in MeTHF).

Scheme 1. Heme/Copper Assembly-Mediated Oxidation of Nitric Oxide to Nitrite

We also tested the μ-hydroxo complex $[(F_8)Fe^{III}-(OH)-Cu^{II}(tmpa)]^{2+}$ for "NO oxidase" chemistry, but upon addition of NO, there was no nitrite production (Scheme 1). Instead, very slow (hours) reductive nitrosylation occurred, and all of the heme present was converted to $(F_8)Fe^{II}(NO)$. It is thus clear that the μ-oxo complex $([(F_8)Fe^{III}-O-Cu^{II}(tmpa)]^+$ is efficient or at least special in its ability to effect a redox reaction (formally $Fe^{III} \rightarrow Fe^{II}$) that includes oxo transfer.

In summary, this report has described new chemistry with heme/Cu assemblies and nitrogen oxide interconversion: nitrite reduction to nitric oxide can readily be effected with our heme/copper chemistry. The reduced heme is the source of the one electron required. The presence of Cu^{II} ion as a Lewis acid is crucial.

It appears that the transformation with heme/Cu synthetic complexes has not been examined to date. We have shown here that both heme and Cu are required, at least in our system. It is notable that the heme is the reductant on the basis of the observed products; however, cyclic voltammetric determination of the redox potentials for the separate complexes $(F_8)Fe$ (–0.20 V vs Fc^+/Fc) and $Cu(tmpa)$ (–0.42 V vs Fc^+/Fc) indicate the latter is a better reductant. For CcO, the opposite appears to be the case, as the heme$_{a3}$ has a lower redox potential than does Cu_B.

Further investigations will include our probing of the mechanisms of the reactions described in this report. As our heme and Cu centers have switched redox capabilities compared with CcO, we also wish to change the heme or the Cu ligand to make the Cu center a better oxidant than the heme.

Reprinted with permission from Molecular Pharmaceutics. Copyright © 2012 American Chemical Society.

JOURNAL ARTICLE EXERCISE 3

The science sections on the MCAT include a significant number of passages with experiments. Questions for these passages often ask you to analyze data, read charts and graphs, and come to some reasonable conclusion based on the information they give you. If you don't know how to extract information efficiently and analyze data effectively, you will be at a distinct disadvantage.

There are three "Journal Article Review Exercises" in this book. In this final exercise, you'll read and extract information from the article, then complete an MCAT passage based on this article. After that, we'll show you the "correct" information to pull out and the answers to the passage.

As before, when analyzing an experiment, you should be able to:

- identify the controls.
- extract information from graphs and data tables.
- determine how the experimental groups change relative to the control.
- come to a reasonable conclusion about WHY the results were observed.
- consider potential weaknesses in the study.
- decide what the next most logical experiment or study should be.

And, as before, the goal of these exercises is NOT to learn content from the articles, just to get a little more comfortable reading and extracting information from them. When you read the article, consider:

1. What is being studied? Why is it important?
2. What is new about these results?
3. What was measured?
4. How are the results presented?
5. What (if anything) was the experimental group compared to?
6. Are any of the results unexpected?
7. How are the conclusions of the authors supported by the data?
8. What potential weaknesses or flaws do you see in the experimental design? Are these addressed in the discussion section?
9. What would be the next most logical experiment?

In this exercise, see whether you can formulate answers to the questions based on the (abridged) article presented on pages 297–299.

Write brief responses to the questions below:

1. What is being studied? Why is it important?

_____

_____

_____

2. What is new about these results?

_____

_____

_____

3. What was measured?

_____

_____

_____

4. How are the results presented?

_____

_____

_____

5. What (if anything) was the experimental group compared to?

_____

_____

_____

6. Are any of the results unexpected?

_____

_____

_____

7. How are the conclusions of the authors supported by the data?

_____

_____

_____

8. What potential weaknesses or flaws do you see in the experimental design? Are these addressed in the discussion section?

_____

_____

_____

9. What would be the next most logical experiment?

_____

_____

_____

Summary of experiment and results:

_____

_____

_____

_____

_____

_____

JOURNAL ARTICLE EXERCISE 3 PASSAGE

Nitric oxide (NO) is a biologically-important signaling molecule. It can be synthesized in the body from L-arginine via nitric oxide synthase, or from nitrite (NO_2^-) via cytochrome c oxidase, CcO. As the terminal acceptor in the mitochondrial electron transport chain, CcO reduces O_2 to water, but can also reduce NO_2^- to NO. The balance between NO and NO_2^- is linked to local O_2 concentrations. At high O_2 concentrations, the Fe/Cu center in CcO is in the oxidized state, and tends to oxidize NO to NO_2^-; the opposite is true at low O_2 concentrations.

Researchers synthesized a Fe/Cu system as a model for the active site of O_2 and NO_2^- reduction in CcO. The iron complex used was a synthetic heme, (P)Fe^{II} ((P) = a synthetic porphyrin), and the copper complex used was (tmpa)Cu^{II} (tmpa = a tetradentate amine ligand). They found that the reaction of two equivalents of (P)Fe^{II} with one equivalent of (tmpa) Cu^{II}(NO_2) led to the formation of a bimetallic Fe-Cu species with a bridging oxo ligand, (P)Fe^{III}—O—Cu^{II}(tmpa), and (P) Fe^{II}(NO), thus demonstrating the ability of such a system to reduce NO_2^- to NO (Reaction 1). The results of investigations are summarized in the table below.

Table 1   Summary of nitrite reduction chemistry with (P)Fe^{II} and (tmpa)Cu^{II}

Reaction	Fe center	Cu center	Additional reaction conditions	Result
1	2 equiv. (P)Fe^{II}	1 equiv. (tmpa) Cu^{II}(NO_2)	n/a	Formation of (P)Fe^{III}—O—Cu^{II}(tmpa) and (P) Fe^{II}(NO)
2	1 equiv. (P)Fe^{III}(NO_2)	1 equiv. (tmpa) Cu^{I}(MeCN)	n/a	No reaction
3	1 equiv. (P)Fe^{II}	1 equiv. (tmpa) Cu^{I}(MeCN)	2 equiv. NO_2^-	No reaction

Note: (MeCN) is a weakly coordinating ligand; all reactions were performed in acetone under an anaerobic N_2 atmosphere.

Adapted from: Hematian, S. et al. "Heme/Copper Assembly Mediated Nitrite and Nitric Oxide Interconversion." J. Am. Chem. Soc. 2012, 134, 46, 18912–18915.

1. Based on the experimental data, what is the reducing agent in the conversion of NO_2^- to NO?

A) Cu^{II}
B) Fe^{II}
C) O_2
D) N_2

2. What are the oxidation states of the nitrogen atoms in NO_2^- and NO, respectively?

A) −1 and 0
B) +2 and +2
C) −3 and −2
D) +3 and +2

3. NO is known to strongly coordinate to Fe^{II} heme complexes. If only one equivalent of (P)Fe^{II} were used in Reaction 1, what would have been the likely result?

A) Only half of the NO_2^- would have been reduced, because half of the available iron would be used for the reduction, and the other half would bind to the NO product.
B) No reduction of NO_2^- would have occurred, because this is the same experiment as Reaction 3.
C) No reduction of NO_2^- would have occurred, because a collision between two iron complexes and one copper complex is required for the reaction to occur.
D) There would have been no change in the experimental results.

4. What additional experiments should the researchers do to confirm a binuclear system is required to reduce NO_2^-?

   I.   React (P)Fe^{II} with NO_2^-
   II. React (P)Fe^{III} with NO_2^-
   III. React (tmpa)Cu^{I} with NO_2^-

A) I only
B) II only
C) I and III only
D) II and III only

SOLUTIONS TO JOURNAL ARTICLE EXERCISE 3

1. **What is being studied? Why is it important?**

   Nitric oxide, NO, is an important signaling molecule and can be generated in the body via arginine and nitric oxide synthase, or by the reduction of nitrite (NO_2^-). This study looks at a synthetic heme/copper system which can cause the same transformation.

2. **What is new about these results?**

   The reduction of nitrite to nitric oxide in the heme/copper system described in this study has not been studied before.

3. **What was measured?**

   Three things: (a) the products of the reaction between $(F_8)Fe^{II}$ and $[(tmpa)Cu^{II}(NO_2)]^+$ via UV-Vis, EPR, and IR spectroscopies: reduction of NO_2 to NO, (b) the products of the reaction between $[(F_8)Fe^{III}—O—Cu^{II}(tmpa)]^+$ and 2 equiv NO via UV-Vis, IR, and EPR: oxidation of 1 equivalent of NO to NO_2 (bound to Cu^{II}), and (c) the products of the reaction between $[(F_8)Fe^{III}—OH—Cu^{II}(tmpa)]^+$ and 2 equiv NO via UV-Vis, IR, and EPR: slow reductive nitrosylation.

4. **How are the results presented?**

   All reactions are described in the text of the article. Reaction (1) is drawn in Scheme 1. Reaction (2) is drawn in Scheme 1, and UV-Vis and EPR data are displayed in Figure 2.

5. **What (if anything) was the experimental group compared to?**

   No comparisons to systems other than the one under study were made. The reaction between $(F_8)Fe^{II}$ and $[(tmpa)Cu^{II}(NO_2)]^+$, which resulted in the reduction of NO_2^-, was compared to: (a) $(F_8)Fe^{III}$ and $[(tmpa)Cu^I(MeCN)]^+$ (reversed oxidation states, no reaction), (b) $(F_8)Fe^{II}$ and $[(tmpa)Cu^I(MeCN)]^+ + NO_2^-$ (reduced ions, no reaction), (c) $(F_8)Fe^{II} + NO_2^-$ (very slow reaction), and (d) $[(tmpa)Cu^I(NO_2)]^+$ (no reaction).

6. **Are any of the results unexpected?**

   Two equivalents of either the heme complex or NO were required for some reactions because of the iron complex's high affinity for NO. The binding of NO to the iron center prevented the iron from participating in a redox reaction. The analogous hydroxo complex cannot affect the nitrite/nitric oxide transformations despite having the metals in a similar oxidation state. CV data suggest that the isolated copper complex is a better reducing agent than the isolated iron complex; however, the products suggest that the heme acted as the reducing agent.

7. **How are the conclusions of the authors supported by the data?**

   The various spectroscopic methods used (UV-Vis, IR, EPR) are consistent with one another.

8. **What potential weaknesses or flaws do you see in the experimental design? Are these addressed in the discussion section?**
The authors suggest that their system is similar to cytochrome c oxidase (which also contains iron and copper); however, in the system studied, heme appears to be the reducing agent, while it is known to be the copper in cytochrome c oxidase.

9. **What would be the next most logical experiment?**
A study of the mechanism of nitrite reduction by this system could clarify which metal acts as the reducing agent. Changing the ligands on the metal may change the redox potentials of the metal ions so that they are more in line with cytochrome c oxidase.

Summary of experiment and results:
- Cytochrome c oxidase can reduce nitrite to nitric oxide. The authors of this study investigated a synthetic Fe/Cu system which catalyzes the conversion of nitrite to nitric oxide, as well as the reverse process. In this synthetic system, the iron acts as the reducing agent, but the presence of the Cu^{2+} ion is also required.

SOLUTIONS TO JOURNAL ARTICLE EXERCISE 3 PASSAGE

1. **B**   A reducing agent becomes oxidized in a redox reaction, since it reduces another chemical. Choice C can be eliminated, since the note beneath the table states that the experiments were performed in anaerobic (oxygen-free) conditions. Additionally, O_2 is a good oxidizing agent, not a good reducing agent. Choice D can also be eliminated, since N_2 is used to provide an inert (non-reactive) atmosphere for these experiments. From looking at Table 1, it can be deduced that Fe^{II} is the reducing agent, since Cu^{II} does not appear to change in the reaction (eliminate choice A, choice B is correct). One of the Fe^{II} centers gets oxidized to Fe^{III} in the product. Additionally, Reaction 2 demonstrates that even when the copper ion is in the reduced form, it is unable to reduce nitrite.

2. **D**   Since NO is a reduction product of NO_2^-, the oxidation number of nitrogen in NO must be lower than in NO_2^- (choices B and C can be eliminated). It is more straightforward to calculate the oxidation number of nitrogen in NO; since oxygen is always –2, nitrogen must be +2 in this neutral molecule. Choice D is correct. In NO_2^-, the oxidation state of nitrogen can be calculated by solving for x in $x + 2(-2) = -1$; $x = +3$. (Do not confuse the overall charge on a species with the oxidation state of an atom; this is basis for choice A, a trap answer.)

3. **A**   Use process of elimination for this question. Choice B is incorrect; the copper reactant in Reaction 3 is Cu^I, not Cu^{II}, so the reactions are not identical. Choice C is also incorrect; there is no information in the passage to support this assertion, and termolecular collisions involving three molecules are rare. Finally, choice D is also incorrect; it is impossible to balance the reaction $(P)Fe^{II} + (tmpa)Cu^{II}(NO_2) \rightarrow (P)Fe^{III}—O—Cu^{II}(tmpa) + (P)Fe^{II}(NO)$. There are too many Fe atoms and (P) ligands on the product side. Choice A is correct. One equivalent of Fe^{II} is required to reduce the NO_2^-, and the second equivalent reacts immediately with the NO product. The balanced reaction for the scenario described in choice A would be:

$$(P)Fe^{II} + (tmpa)Cu^{II}(NO_2) \rightarrow$$
$$0.5\ (P)Fe^{III}—O—Cu^{II}(tmpa) + 0.5\ (P)Fe^{II}(NO) + 0.5\ (tmpa)Cu^{II}(NO_2)$$

4. **C**   For this Roman numeral question, all items appear exactly twice in the choices, so you can begin with any of the items. All the items describe investigations into the possibility of reductions of NO_2^- mediated by a single metal center. Item I is true: it describes the iron complex used in Reaction 1 in the passage. $(P)Fe^{II}$ should be tested alone to see whether its presence in the absence of Cu^{II} is sufficient to reduce NO_2^- (choices B and D can be eliminated). From the remaining answer choices, only Item III needs further consideration. Item III is true: it is the reduced form of the copper ion used in Reaction 1; such an ion could act as a reducing agent, and should also be tested (choice A can be eliminated and choice C is correct). Note that Item II is in fact false: the iron center in item II is the Fe^{III} ion, which is unlikely to act as a reducing agent for NO_2^-, since it is already oxidized.

Glossary

absolute zero
The temperature (−273.15°C or 0 K) at which the volume and pressure of an ideal gas extrapolate to zero according to the ideal gas law. **[Section 6.4]**

acid
See *Arrhenius acid*, *Brønsted-Lowry acid*, and *Lewis acid*. **[Section 11.1]**

acid-base indicator
A weak acid and conjugate base pair, such as litmus or phenolphthalein, that changes color with changes in solution pH. **[Section 11.9]**

acid-dissociation constant (K_a)
A measure of the extent of dissociation of an acid, HA. K_a is defined as $K_a = [H_3O^+][A^-]/[HA]$. **[Section 11.3]**

activation energy, E_a
The energy required by the reactants in a chemical reaction to reach a transition state from which the products of the reaction can form. **[Section 6.6]**

alkali metal
One of the metal elements in Group I (Li, Na, K, Rb, Cs, and Fr). **[Section 4.7]**

alkaline earth metal
One of the metal elements in Group II (Be, Mg, Ca, Sr, Ba, and Ra). **[Section 4.7]**

allotropes
Forms of a pure element with different structures and therefore different chemical and physical properties, such as O_2 and O_3 or $carbon_{(diamond)}$ and $carbon_{(graphite)}$. **[Section 6.6]**

alloy
A blend of two or more metallic elements. Bronze, for example, is an alloy of copper and tin. **[Section 10.4]**

alpha (α) particle
A positively charged particle consisting of two protons and two neutrons emitted during alpha decay. An alpha particle is identical to a helium-4 nucleus. **[Section 4.4]**

amphoteric
An ion or molecule, such as H_2O or HCO_3^-, that can act as either a Brønsted-Lowry acid or base. **[Section 11.3]**

anhydrous
A substance that is devoid of water. Used, for example, to differentiate between liquid (anhydrous) ammonia at temperatures below its boiling point (−33°C) and solutions of ammonia dissolved in water.

anion
A negatively charged ion, such as F⁻. **[Section 4.3]**

anode
The site of oxidation in a galvanic or electrolytic cell. Also, the electrode towards which anions flow through a salt bridge. **[Section 12.2]**

aqueous
Solutions of substances where water is the primary solvent. **[Section 10.4]**

Arrhenius acid
A compound that dissociates when it dissolves in water to give the H⁺ ion. **[Section 11.1]**

Arrhenius base
A compound that dissociates when it dissolves in water to give the OH⁻ ion. **[Section 11.1]**

Arrhenius equation
The equation for the rate constant (k) of a chemical reaction, in terms of the temperature (T), activation energy (E_a), and collision frequency/steric orientation factor (A):
$k = Ae^{-E_a/RT}$. **[Section 9.4]**

atomic mass unit (amu, u)
The unit of mass most convenient for individual subatomic particles, atoms, and molecules. **[Section 3.6]**

atomic number (Z)
The number of protons in the nucleus of an atom. **[Section 4.1]**

atomic orbital
A region in space where electrons of an atom are most probably found. **[Section 4.5 and 5.2]**

atomic radius
The size of an atom equal to the volume of space carved out by the outermost (valence) electrons. **[Section 4.8]**

atomic weight
The weighted average of the atomic masses of the different isotopes of an element. A single ^{12}C atom, for example, has a mass of 12 amu, but naturally occurring carbon also contains 1.1% ^{13}C. The atomic weight of carbon is therefore 12.011 amu. **[Section 4.2]**

Aufbau principle
The principle that atomic orbitals are filled one at a time, starting with the orbital that has the lowest energy and then filling upwards. **[Section 4.6]**

Avogadro's number
The number of items that make up one mole, approximately 6.02×10^{23}. **[Section 3.7]**

Avogadro's Law
The hypothesis that equal volumes of different gases at the same temperature and pressure contain the same number of particles. **[Section 8.2]**

base
See *Arrhenius base*, *Brønsted-Lowry base*, and *Lewis base*. **[Section 11.1]**

base-dissociation constant (K_b)
A measure of the extent of dissociation of a base, B: $K_b = [HB^+][OH^-]/[B]$. **[Section 11.3]**

battery
A set of electrochemical cells connected in series or parallel. **[Section 12.6]**

beta (β) decay
A nuclear reaction in which an electron (e^-) or positron (β^+) is absorbed by or emitted from the nucleus of an atom. **[Section 4.4]**

beta (β) particle
An electron or a positron. **[Section 4.4]**

bimolecular
A step in a chemical reaction in which two molecules collide to form products. **[Section 9.4]**

Bohr model
A model of the distribution of electrons in an atom based on the assumption that the electron in a hydrogen atom is in one of a limited number of circular orbits. **[Section 4.5]**

Bohr atom
An atom or ion that has just one electron, such as H, He$^+$, Li^{2+}, etc. **[Section 4.5]**

boiling point
The temperature at which the vapor pressure of a liquid is equal to the external or atmospheric pressure. **[Section 7.4]**

bond dissociation energy/enthalpy
The energy needed to homolytically break an X—Y bond to give X and Y atoms in the gas phase. **[Section 5.2]**

bonding electrons
A pair of electrons, always the outermost (valence) electrons, used to form a covalent bond between adjacent atoms. **[Section 5.1]**

Boyle's law
A statement of the relationship between the pressure and volume of a constant amount of gas at constant temperatures: $P \propto 1/V$. **[Section 8.2]**

Brønsted-Lowry acid
Any molecule or ion that can donate an H$^+$ (proton) to a base. **[Section 11.1]**

Brønsted-Lowry base
Any molecule or ion that can accept an H$^+$ (proton) from an acid. **[Section 11.1]**

buffer
A mixture of a weak acid (HA) and its conjugate base (A$^-$), which should be present in roughly equal amounts. Buffers resist a change in the pH of a solution according to Le Châtelier's principle when small amounts of acid or base are added. **[Section 11.8]**

buffer capacity
The amount of acid or base a buffer solution can absorb without significant changes in pH. **[Section 11.8]**

calorie
The heat needed to raise the temperature of 1 gram of water by 1°C. **[Section 7.2]**

calorimeter
An insulated apparatus used to measure the heat absorbed/released in a chemical reaction.

catalyst
A substance that increases the rate of a chemical reaction without being consumed in the reaction.
A substance that lowers the activation energy for a chemical reaction by providing an alternate pathway for the reaction. **[Section 9.3]**

cathode
The site of reduction in a galvanic or electrolytic cell. Also, the electrode in an electrochemical cell towards which cations flow through a salt bridge. **[Section 12.2]**

cation
A positively charged ion, such as Na$^+$. **[Section 4.3]**

cell potential
A measure of the driving force behind an electrochemical reaction, reported in volts. **[Section 12.3]**

Charles's law
A statement of the relationship between the temperature and volume of a constant amount of gas at constant pressure: $V \propto T$. **[Section 8.2]**

collision theory model
A model used to explain the rates of chemical reactions, which assumes that molecules must collide in order to react. **[Section 9.2]**

common-ion effect
The decrease in the solubility of a salt that occurs when the salt is dissolved in a solution that contains another source of one of its ions. Just another form of Le Châtelier's principle. **[Section 10.6]**

complex ion
An ion in which a ligand is bound to a metal via a coordinate covalent bond. An ion formed when a Lewis acid such as the Co^{2+} ion reacts with a Lewis base such as NH_3 to form an acid-base complex such as the $Co(NH_3)_4^{2+}$ ion. **[Section 10.7]**

compound
A substance with a constant composition that contains two or more elements. **[Section 3.10]**

concentration
A measure of the ratio of the amount of solute in a solution to the amount of either solvent or solution. Frequently expressed as molarity (units of moles of solute per liter of solution). **[Section 3.9]**

concentration cell
A type of electrochemical cell that has identical reactants in each half reaction, but at different concentrations, thus driving a weak electrical current. **[Section 12.4]**

conjugate acid-base pair
Two substances related by the gain or loss of a proton. An acid (such as HBr) and its conjugate base (Br^-), or a base (such as NH_3) and its conjugate acid (NH_4^+) are examples of conjugate acid-base pairs. **[Section 11.2]**

coordinate covalent bond
A covalent bond formed as a result of a Lewis acid-base reaction, most often formed between a metal atom and a nonmetal atom. **[Section 5.3]**

coordination complex
A compound in which one or more ligands are coordinated to a metal atom. **[Section 5.3]**

corrosion
A process in which a metal is destroyed by a chemical reaction. When the metal is iron, the process is called rusting.

covalent bond
A bond between two atoms formed by the sharing of at least one pair of electrons. **[Section 5.3]**

covalent compound
A compound, such as water (H_2O), composed of neutral molecules in which the atoms are held together by covalent bonds. **[Section 5.3]**

critical point
The temperature and pressure at which two phases of a substance that are in equilibrium (usually the gas and liquid phases) become identical and form a single phase. **[Section 7.4]**

crystal
A three-dimensional solid formed by regular repetition of the packing of atoms, ions, or molecules. **[Section 5.8]**

Dalton's law of partial pressures
A statement of the relationship between the total pressure of a mixture of gases and the partial pressures of the individual components: $P_{total} = p_1 + p_2 + p_3 + ...$ **[Section 8.4]**

daughter nucleus
The product nucleus after a nuclear reaction. **[Section 4.4]**

density
The mass of a sample divided by its volume. **[Section 3.2]**

deposition
A process in which a gas goes directly to the solid state without passing through an intermediate liquid state. **[Section 7.1]**

diamagnetic
A substance in which the electrons are all paired. **[Section 4.6]**

dilution
The process by which more solvent is added to decrease the concentration of a solution.

dimer
A compound (such as B_2H_6) produced by combining two smaller identical molecules (such as BH_3).

dipole
Anything with two equal but opposite electrical charges, such as the positive and negative ends of a polar bond or molecule. **[Section 5.6]**

diprotic acid
An acid, such as H_2SO_4, that can lose two H^+. **[Section 11.10]**

diprotic base
A base, such as the O^{2-} ion, that can accept two H^+. **[Section 11.10]**

dissolution
The process in which a bulk solid or liquid breaks up into individual molecules or ions and diffuses throughout a solvent. **[Section 10.4]**

ductile
Capable of being drawn into thin sheets or wires without breaking; a property of metals. **[Section 5.8]**

effusion
The process by which a gas escapes through a pinhole into a region of lower pressure. [**Section 8.5**]

elastic collision
A collision in which no kinetic energy is lost. [**Section 8.1**]

electrolyte
A substance that increases the electrical conductivity of water by dissociating into ions. [**Section 10.4**]

electrolysis
A process in which an electric current is used to drive a nonspontaneous chemical reaction. [**Section 12.6**]

electrolytic cell
A nonspontaneous electric cell in which electrolysis is done. [**Section 12.6**]

electron
A subatomic particle with a mass of only about 0.0005 amu and a charge of –1 that surrounds the nucleus of an atom. [**Section 4.1**]

electron affinity
The energy given off when a neutral atom in the gas phase picks up an electron to form a negatively charged ion. [**Section 4.8**]

electron capture
A type of beta decay where the nucleus of an atom captures an electron and converts a nuclear proton into a neutron. [**Section 4.4**]

electron configuration
The arrangement of electrons in atomic orbitals; for example, $1s^2 2s^2 2p^3$. [**Section 4.6**]

electronegativity
The tendency of an atom to draw or polarize bonding electrons toward itself. [**Section 4.8**]

element
A substance that cannot be decomposed into a simpler substance by a chemical reaction. A substance composed of only one kind of atom. [**Section 4.1**]

empirical formula
The formula for a compound in which the number of atoms of each element in the compound are represented by the lowest whole number ratio.[**Section 3.4**]

endergonic
A process that leads to an increase in the free energy of a system and is therefore not spontaneous: ΔG_{rxn} is positive. [**Section 6.6**]

endothermic
A chemical reaction that absorbs heat from the surroundings: ΔH_{rxn} is positive. [**Section 6.2**]

endpoint
The point at which the indicator of an acid-base titration changes color. [**Section 12.5**]

enthalpy (H)
The total potential energy in a substance due to intermolecular forces and covalent bonds. [**Section 6.2**]

enthalpy of reaction (ΔH_{rxn})
The change in the enthalpy that occurs during a chemical reaction. The difference between the sum of the enthalpies of the products and the reactants. [**Section 6.2**]

entropy (S)
A measure of the disorder in a system. Increasing disorder yields a positive ΔS. [**Section 6.4**]

equilibrium (dynamic)
The point at which there is no longer a change in the concentrations of the reactants and the products of a chemical reaction. The point at which the rates of the forward and reverse reactions are equal: ΔG_{rxn} = 0. [**Section 10.4**]

equilibrium constant (K_{eq})
The product of the concentrations (or partial pressures) of the products of a reaction at equilibrium divided by the product of the concentrations (or partial pressures) of the reactants. [**Section 10.1**]

equilibrium expression
The expression used to calculate the equilibrium constant for a reaction that takes the form [products]/[reactants]. [**Section 10.1**]

equivalence point
The point in an acid-base titration at which the number of moles of H_3O^+ in solution equals the number of moles of OH^- in solution. [**Section 11.10**]

excited state configuration
One of an infinite number of electron configurations of an energized atom where at least one electron occupies an orbital of higher energy than that dictated by Hund's rule and/or the Aufbau principle. [**Section 4.6**]

exergonic
A process that leads to a decrease in the free energy of the system and is therefore spontaneous: ΔG_{rxn} is negative. [**Section 6.6**]

exothermic

A chemical reaction that releases energy to the surroundings: ΔH_{rxn} is negative. [**Section 6.2**]

family

A vertical column of elements in the periodic table, such as the elements Li, Na, K, etc. [**Section 4.7**]

Faraday's law of electrolysis

A statement of the relationship between the amount of electric current that passes through an electrolytic cell and the amount of product formed during electrolysis. The amount of chemical change is proportional to the amount of electric current that flows through the cell. [**Section 12.7**]

first ionization energy

The energy needed to remove the valence electron from a neutral atom in the gas phase. [**Section 4.8**]

first law of thermodynamics

The total energy in the universe is conserved: energy is neither created nor destroyed, but may change from one form to another. [**Section 6.1**]

first-order reaction

A reaction in which the rate is proportional to the concentration of a single reactant raised to the first power: rate = $k[A]$. [**Section 9.4**]

formal charge

The theoretical charge on an atom in a molecule, calculated by $V - \frac{1}{2}B - L$, where V is the number of valence electrons, B is the number of bonding electrons, and L is the number of lone-pair electrons. [**Section 5.1**]

free energy, Gibbs (G)

The energy associated with a chemical reaction that can be used to do work. The change in free energy of a system is calculated by the formula $\Delta G = \Delta H - T\Delta S$, where G is the free energy, H is enthalpy, T is temperature (in kelvins), and S is entropy. [**Section 6.5**]

free radical

An atom or molecule that contains an unpaired electron. [**Section 5.2**]

freezing point

The temperature at which the solid and liquid phases of a substance are in equilibrium. [**Section 7.1**]

fusion

The melting of a solid to form a liquid. [**Section 7.1**]

galvanic cell

An electrochemical cell that uses a spontaneous chemical reaction to do work. Synonymous with *voltaic cell*. [**Section 12.2**]

gamma ray (γ)

A high energy, short wavelength form of electromagnetic radiation emitted by the nucleus of an atom that carries off some of the energy generated in a nuclear reaction. [**Section 4.4**]

Gibbs free energy

See *free energy*. [**Section 6.5**]

Graham's law

The relationship between the rate at which a gas diffuses or effuses and its molecular weight: rate $\propto 1/(MW)^{1/2}$. [**Section 8.5**]

ground state configuration

The most stable arrangement of electrons in an atom that satisfies Hund's rule and the Aufbau principle. [**Section 4.5**]

group

A vertical column, or family, of elements in the periodic table. [**Section 4.7**]

half-life

The time required for the amount of a decaying substance to decrease to half its initial value. [**Section 4.4**]

halogen

Elements of Group VII: F, Cl, Br, I, and At. [**Section 4.7**]

heat (q)

Thermal energy in transit from a hotter system to a colder one. [**Section 6.1**]

heat of fusion

The heat that must be absorbed to melt a unit quantity of a solid. [**Section 7.2**]

heat of reaction

The change in the enthalpy of the system that occurs when a reaction is run at constant pressure. Synonymous with *enthalpy of reaction*, ΔH_{rxn}. [**Section 6.2**]

heat of vaporization

The heat that must be absorbed to boil a unit quantity of a liquid. [**Section 7.2**]

heat capacity

The amount of heat required to raise the temperature of a given amount of a substance by one degree. Not to be confused with *specific heat*. Heat capacity is typically the product of mass and specific heat. [**Section 7.3**]

Hess's law
The heat given off or absorbed in a chemical reaction does not depend on whether the reaction occurs in a single step or in many steps. [**Section 6.3**]

homonuclear diatomic molecule
A molecule, such as O_2 or F_2, that contains two atoms of the same element.

Hund's rule
Rule for placing electrons in equal-energy orbitals, which states that electrons are added with parallel spins until each of the orbitals has one electron, before a second electron is placed in a given orbital. [**Section 4.6**]

hybrid orbitals
Orbitals formed by mixing two or more atomic orbitals. [**Section 5.5**]

hybridization
A process in which things are mixed. A resonance hybrid is a mixture, or average, of two or more Lewis structures. Hybrid orbitals are formed by mixing two or more atomic orbitals. [**Section 5.5**]

hydride
The species H^-. [**Section 5.4**]

hydrogen bonding
A strong dipole-dipole interaction that occurs between a hydrogen atom covalently bonded to an F, O, or N that electrostatically interacts with a lone pair of electrons on another F, O, or N atom. [**Section 5.7**]

hydrophilic
"Water loving"; attracted or compatible with water (for example, ions that are soluble in water).

hydrophobic
"Water fearing"; repelled by or incompatible with water (for example, lipids that are insoluble in water).

ideal gas
A gas that obeys all the postulates of the kinetic-molecule theory and has properties that can be predicted by the ideal gas law. [**Section 8.1**]

ideal gas law
The relationship between the pressure, volume, temperature, and amount of an ideal gas: $PV = nRT$. [**Section 8.2**]

indicator
See *acid-base indicator*. [**Section 11.9**]

induced dipole
A short-lived separation of charge, or dipole, of a nonpolar atom or molecule caused by the electrostatic influence of a nearby polar atom or ion. [**Section 5.7**]

inert
Unreactive. Used to describe compounds that do not undergo chemical reactions. [**Section 4.7**]

insoluble
Used to describe a substance that does not noticeably dissolve in a solvent. [**Section 10.4**]

intermolecular forces
Attractive electrostatic forces, the strength of which determine a compound's phase, vapor pressure, melting point, boiling point, solubility, and viscosity. From strongest to weakest, the main categories of intermolecular forces are: *ionic, dipole-dipole* (with H-bonds the strongest), and *London dispersion forces*. [**Section 5.7**]

intramolecular bonds
Synonym for covalent bonds. There are three primary types: normal covalent bonds, metallic covalent bonds, and coordinate covalent bonds. [**Section 7.1**]

ion product (Q_{sp})
The product of the concentrations of the ions in a solution at any moment. [**Section 10.5**]

ion-product constant of water (K_w)
The product of the equilibrium concentration of the H_3O^+ and OH^- ions in an aqueous solution at 25°C: $K_w = 1.0 \times 10^{-14}$. [**Section 11.4**]

ionic bond
Misappropriation of the term *bond*. Simply the strong electrostatic attraction between two oppositely charged ions; there is no electron sharing. [**Section 5.3**]

ionic compound
A compound made up of ions (synonymous with *salt*). [**Section 3.6**]

ionizability factor (i)
The number of individual particles formed when an individual solute dissolves. Synonymous with *van't Hoff factor*. [**Section 10.4**]

ionization
A process in which an ion is created from a neutral atom or molecule by adding or removing one or more electrons. [**Section 4.8**]

ionization energy
See *first ionization energy*. [**Section 4.8**]

isoelectronic
Atoms or ions that have the same number of electrons and therefore the same electron configuration, such as O^{2-}, F^-, Ne, and Na^+. [**Section 4.6**]

isotopes
Nuclides of the same element, but with differing numbers of neutrons, such as ^{12}C, ^{13}C, and ^{14}C. Isotopes have nearly identical chemical properties. [**Section 4.2**]

joule
A unit of measurement for both heat and work in the SI system. 1 J = 4.184 cal. [**Section 3.1**]

kinetic energy
The energy associated with motion. The kinetic energy of an object is equal to one-half the product of its mass and the square of its speed: $KE = \frac{1}{2}mv^2$. [**Section 8.5**]

kinetic-molecular theory
The theory that states heat is associated with the thermal motion of particles, taking into account the important assumptions that individual gas molecules take up no volume and collisions between gas molecules are perfectly elastic. [**Section 8.1**]

Le Châtelier's principle
A principle that describes the effect of changes in the temperature, pressure, or concentration of one of the reactants or products of a reaction at equilibrium. It states that when a system at equilibrium is subjected to a stress, it will shift in the direction that minimizes the effect of this stress. [**Section 10.3**]

Lewis acid
An atom or molecule that accepts a pair of electrons to form a new coordinate covalent bond. Almost always a metal atom, positively charged ion, or both. [**Section 11.1**]

Lewis base
An atom or molecule that donates a pair of electrons to form a new coordinate covalent bond. Almost always a nonmetal with a pair of nonbonding electrons. Synonymous with *ligand* and *chelator*. [**Section 11.1**]

ligand
See *Lewis base*. [**Section 11.1**]

limiting reagent
The reactant in a chemical reaction that is exhausted first, thus limiting the amount of product that can be formed. [**Section 3.12**]

London dispersion forces
Intermolecular forces that arise from interactions between an instantaneous dipole/induced dipole pair. Typically, these are the weakest of all intermolecular forces. However LDFs are additive, and nonpolar molecules with large, flat surface areas can experience moderate LDFs. [**Section 5.7**]

malleable
Something that can be hammered, pounded, or pressed into different shapes without breaking (a common property of metals). [**Section 5.8**]

mass number (*A*)
The total number of protons and neutrons in the nucleus of an atom. [**Section 4.1**]

melting point
The temperature at which the solid and liquid phases of a substance are in equilibrium at a particular external pressure. [**Section 7.4**]

metal
An element that is solid, has a metallic luster, is malleable and ductile, and conducts both heat and electricity. [**Section 4.7**]

metalloid
An element with properties that fall between the extremes of metals and nonmetals. [**Section 4.7**]

mixture
A substance that contains two or more elements or compounds that retain their chemical identities and can be separated by a physical process. For example, the mixture of N_2 and O_2 in the atmosphere. [**Section 3.9**]

molarity (*M*)
The number of moles of a solute in a solution divided by the volume of the solution in liters. [**Section 3.1**]

mole
6.02×10^{23} of anything. [**Section 3.7**]

mole fraction (*X*)
The fraction of the total number of moles in a mixture due to one component of the mixture. The mole fraction of a solute, for example, is the number of moles of solute divided by the total number of moles of solute plus solvent. [**Section 3.9**]

mole ratio
The ratio of the moles of one reactant or product to the moles of another reactant or product in the balanced equation for a chemical reaction.

molecular formula
The formula representing the number and types of constituent atoms in a compound. [**Section 3.3**]

molecular geometry
The arrangement of atoms surrounding a central atom of a small molecule. Molecular geometry (or the shape of a molecule) and orbital geometry are identical only when the central atom possesses no lone pairs of electrons. [Section 5.4]

molecular weight
The weight of the molecular formula, calculated from a table of atomic weights. Note that atomic weights are a weighted average of masses of isotopes as they occur in nature. [Section 3.6]

molecule
The smallest particle that has any of the chemical or physical properties of a compound. [Section 3.3]

monoprotic acid (HA)
An acid, such as HF or HOCl, that can lose only one H^+. [Section 11.3]

negative electrode
The electrode in an electrochemical cell that carries a negative charge. In a galvanic cell, it is the anode; in an electrolytic cell, it is the cathode. [Section 12.2]

Nernst equation
Used to calculate or track the voltage of an electrochemical cell under *nonstandard* conditions: $E = E° - (RT/nF) \ln Q$. [Section 12.4]

network solid
A solid, such as diamond, in which every atom is covalently bonded to its nearest neighbors to form an extended array of atoms rather than individual molecules. [Section 5.8]

neutron
A subatomic particle with a mass of about 1 amu and no charge. [Section 4.1]

noble gases
The elements in the last column of the periodic table that are chemically unreactive. [Section 4.7]

nonbonding electrons
Electrons in the valence shell of an atom that are not used to form covalent bonds. [Section 5.1]

nonmetal
An element that lacks the properties generally associated with metals. These elements are found in the upper right of the periodic table. [Section 4.7]

nonpolar
Used to describe a compound that has a homogenous electron distribution and thus does not carry a permanent dipole moment. [Section 5.3]

nonspontaneous
A reaction in which the products are not favored, implying that the reverse reaction would be favored: ΔG_{rxn} is positive (and E_{cell} is negative). [Section 6.5]

nucleon
Generic term for a proton or neutron. [Section 4.1]

nuclide
The generic term for any particular isotope of an element, such as the ^{13}C nuclide.

octet rule
The tendency of main-group elements to react in order to possess eight valence-shell electrons in their compounds. [Section 4.6]

orbital geometry
The arrangement of electron clouds surrounding a central atom of a small molecule. Orbital geometry is a consequence of hybridization. Not to be confused with *shape,* or *molecular geometry.* [Section 5.4]

orbitals
Regions in space where electrons have a high probability of existing. [Section 4.5]

order
Used to describe the relationship between the rate of a step in a chemical reaction and the concentration of one of the reactants consumed in that step. Essentially just the value of the exponent found in a reactant term in the rate law. [Section 9.4]

oxidation
A process in which an atom, ion, or molecule loses one or more electrons. [Section 3.14]

oxidation number
Synonymous with *oxidation state.* It is the hypothetical charge that would be present on each atom if a molecule was shattered into its individual constituent atoms with bonding electrons ending up with the atom of the bond having the higher electronegativity. [Section 3.14]

oxidation-reduction reaction
A chemical reaction involving the exchange of electrons such that oxidation numbers of reactants change. [Section 12.1]

oxidizing agent / oxidant
An atom, ion, or molecule that undergoes reduction by gaining electrons, thereby oxidizing something else. **[Section 12.1]**

pH
A measure of acidity ranging from about −1.5 to 15.5 in aqueous media, defined as −log [H_3O^+]. **[Section 11.5]**

pOH
The complement of pH, defined as −log [OH^-]. **[Section 11.5]**

paramagnetic
A compound that contains one or more unpaired electrons and is attracted into a magnetic field. **[Section 4.6]**

parent nucleus
The initial nucleus prior to a nuclear reaction. **[Section 4.4]**

partial pressure
The fraction of the total pressure of a mixture of gases that is due to one component of the mixture. As molarity is the primary way of expressing the amount of solute in a solution, so partial pressure is the primary way to report the quantity of a gas in a mixture of gases. **[Section 8.4]**

Pauli exclusion principle
The maximum number of electrons in any given orbital is two, and they must have the opposite spin. **[Section 4.6]**

period
A horizontal row in the periodic table. **[Section 4.6]**

polar covalent bond
A covalent bond between atoms with differing electronegativities such that electrons spend more time in the vicinity of one atom than the other. **[Section 5.3]**

polar
Used to describe a molecule that has a dipole moment because it consists of a positive pole and a negative pole. **[Section 5.3]**

polyatomic ion
An ion that contains more than one atom, such as CO_3^{2-} or SO_4^{2-}. **[Section 3.5]**

polyprotic acid
An acid, such as H_2SO_4 or H_3PO_4, that can lose more than one H^+. **[Section 11.3]**

polyprotic base
A base, such as the PO_4^{3-} ion, that can accept more than one H^+. **[Section 11.3]**

positive electrode
The electrode in an electrochemical cell that carries a positive charge. In a galvanic cell, it is the cathode; in an electrolytic cell, it is the anode. **[Section 12.2]**

positron (β⁺)
The antiparticle of the electron. A positron has the same mass as an electron but is positively charged. Contact between an electron and positron results in instant annihilation and emission of two high energy gamma rays. **[Section 4.4]**

positron emission
A mode of beta decay where a positron is emitted as a consequence of the conversion of a nuclear proton to a neutron. **[Section 4.4]**

potential
A measure of the driving force behind an electrochemical reaction that is reported in units of volts. **[Section 12.3]**

precipitation
A process in which dissolved ions combine to form a solid salt in solution. **[Section 10.4]**

precision
A measure of the extent to which individual measurements of the same phenomenon agree.

pressure
The force exerted perpendicular to a surface divided by the area of the surface. **[Section 8.1]**

proton
A subatomic particle that has a charge of +1 and a mass of about 1 amu. (Synonymous with H^+.) **[Section 4.1]**

quantized
A property or quality that appears only in certain discrete amounts, such as electric charge. **[Section 4.5]**

radioactivity
The spontaneous disintegration of an unstable nuclide by a first-order rate law. Synonymous with *nuclear decay*. **[Section 4.4]**

rate of reaction
The change in the concentration of a compound divided by the amount of time necessary for this change to occur: rate = $\Delta[X]/\Delta t$. **[Section 9.2]**

rate constant (*k*)
The proportionality constant in the equation that describes the relationship between the rate of a step in a chemical reaction and the product of the concentrations of the reactants consumed in that step. **[Section 9.4]**

rate law
An equation that describes how the rate of a chemical reaction depends on the concentrations of the reactants consumed in that reaction, along with the rate constant that takes into account temperature, activation energy, and collision frequency/steric effects. **[Section 9.4]**

rate-determining step
The slowest step in a chemical reaction. **[Section 9.1]**

reaction quotient (Q)
The quotient obtained when the concentrations (or partial pressures) of the products of a reaction are multiplied and the result is divided by the product of the concentrations (or partial pressures) of the reactants. Basically, putting nonequilibrium values into an equilibrium expression yields a reaction quotient instead of the equilibrium constant. **[Section 10.2]**

real gas
A gas that deviates from the behavior predicted by the ideal gas law. Real gases differ from the expected behavior of an ideal gas (e.g., lower V and P) for two reasons: (1) the forces of attraction between the particles in a gas are not zero and (2) the volume of the particles in a gas is not zero. **[Section 8.3]**

redox
An abbreviation for oxidation-reduction. **[Section 12.1]**

reducing agent / reductant
An atom, ion, or molecule that is oxidized by giving up electrons, thereby reducing something else. **[Section 12.1]**

reduction
A process in which an atom, ion, or molecule gains one or more electrons. **[Section 12.1]**

resonance structures
Two or more Lewis dot structures that differ only by the placement of electrons in the molecule. Taken together as an average (a resonance hybrid), they best approximate the electron distribution and types of bonds in the molecule better than any one structure can alone. **[Section 5.1]**

salt
Synonymous with *ionic compound*. **[Section 5.8]**

salt bridge
An ion-rich junction between the anodic and cathodic chambers of an electrochemical cell that prevents charge separation that would otherwise stop the cell from functioning. Anions always migrate toward the anode, and cations always migrate toward the cathode of any cell. **[Section 12.2]**

saturated solution
A solution that contains as much solute as possible. **[Section 10.4]**

second ionization energy
The energy needed to remove an electron from a +1 cation in the gas phase. **[Section 4.8]**

second law of thermodynamics
Processes that increase the entropy in the universe are spontaneous. **[Section 6.4]**

second-order reaction
A reaction in which rate is proportional to the concentration of a single reactant raised to the second power: rate = $k[A]^2$, or two reactants each raised to the first power: rate = $k[A][B]$. **[Section 9.4]**

shielding
The masking and weakening of the electrostatic attraction between the nucleus and outer electrons by inner electrons. **[Section 4.8]**

solubility
The ratio of the maximum amount of solute to the volume of solvent in which this solute can dissolve. Often expressed in units of grams of solute per 100 g of water, or in moles of solid per liter of solution. **[Section 10.4]**

solubility equilibria
Equilibria that exist in a saturated solution, in which additional solid dissolves at the same rate that particles of solution come together to precipitate more solid. **[Section 10.4]**

solubility product (K_{sp})
The product of the equilibrium concentrations of the ions in a saturated solution of a salt. **[Section 10.4]**

solute
The substance that dissolves in a solvent to form a solution. **[Section 10.4]**

solution
A homogeneous mixture of one or more solutes dissolved in a solvent. **[Section 10.4]**

solvent
The substance in which a solute dissolves. **[Section 10.4]**

specific heat
The amount of heat required to raise the temperature of 1 g of a substance by 1°C (or 1 K). (Do not confuse with *heat capacity*). **[Section 7.2]**

spontaneous reaction
A reaction in which the products are favored: ΔG_{rxn} is negative (and E_{cell} is positive). [**Section 6.5**]

standard cell potential
The potential, $E°_{cell}$, of a cell measured under standard-state conditions. [**Section 12.3**]

standard heat of formation ($\Delta H_f°$)
The change in the enthalpy that occurs during a chemical reaction that leads to the formation of one mole of a compound from its elements in their standard states at standard conditions. [**Section 6.3**]

standard state/conditions
State in which T = 298 K (25°C), P = 1 atm, and all concentrations are 1 M. Not to be confused with *STP*. [**Section 6.3**]

standard temperature and pressure (STP)
State in which T = 273 K (0°C) and P = 1 atm. Generally used when referring to gases. Not to be confused with *standard state* or *standard conditions*. [**Section 6.3**]

state
1. One of the three states of matter: gas, liquid, or solid.

2. A set of physical properties that describe a system. [**Section 3.13**]

state function
A quantity whose value depends only on the state of the system and not its history; X is a state function if and only if the value of ΔX does not depend on the path used to go from the initial to the final state of the system. [**Section 6.3**]

stoichiometry
The study of the quantitative relationships between the reactants and the products of a balanced chemical reaction. [**Sections 3.10–3.12**]

strong acid
An acid that dissociates completely in water. [**Section 11.3**]

strong base
A base that dissociates completely in water. [**Section 11.3**]

sublimation
The process in which a solid goes directly to the gas phase without passing through an intermediate liquid state. [**Section 7.1**]

supercooled liquid
A substance that is a liquid even though its temperature is below its freezing point.

supercritical fluid
A substance that displays properties of both a liquid and a gas and exists under conditions of high temperature and pressure. If a substance is in this state—where the liquid and gas phases are no longer distinct—no amount of increased pressure can force the substance back into its liquid phase. [**Section 7.4**]

surface tension
The perpendicular force per unit length of liquid surface that acts to reduce the surface area of a liquid, resulting from intermolecular forces below the surface.

surroundings
In thermodynamics, the part of the universe not included in the system. [**Section 6.1**]

system
In thermodynamics, that small portion of the universe in which we are interested at the moment. [**Section 6.1**]

thermal conductor
A substance or object that readily conducts heat (metals, for example). [**Section 5.8**]

thermal insulator
An object, such as a blanket or a fur coat, that tends to slow down the rate at which heat is transferred from one object to another.

titrant
The strong acid or base reagent added to the unknown solution in a titration experiment. [**Section 11.10**]

titration
A technique used to determine the concentration and/or the chemical identity of a solute in a solution. [**Section 11.10**]

torr
A unit of pressure equal to the pressure exerted by a column of mercury 1 millimeter tall. By definition, 1 torr = 1 mm Hg. [**Section 8.1**]

transition metal
Metals in the block of elements that serve as a transition between the two columns on the left side of the periodic table, where *s* orbitals are filled, and the six columns on the right, where *p* orbitals are filled. [**Section 4.6**]

triple point
The unique pressure and temperature at which the three phases of a substance (gas, liquid, and solid) can all coexist in equilibrium. [**Section 7.4**]

unimolecular
Describes a step in a reaction mechanism in which only one reactant molecule is present. [**Section 9.4**]

valence electrons
Electrons in the outermost or highest-energy level or shell of an atom. The electrons that are gained, shared, or lost in a chemical reaction. [**Section 3.14**]

van der Waals equation
An equation that accounts for deviations from ideal behavior in gaseous systems due to interactions between gas particles and particle volume. [**Section 8.3**]

van't Hoff factor (i)
See *ionizability factor*. [**Section 10.4**]

vapor pressure
The partial pressure of the gas molecules over the surface of a liquid that originate from the surface of a liquid. [**Section 5.7**]

voltaic cell
An electrochemical cell in which a spontaneous chemical reaction is used to create electricity. Synonymous with *galvanic cell*. [**Section 12.2**]

volatile
The physical characteristic of having a high vapor pressure at standard conditions. [**Section 5.7**]

VSEPR theory
A model in which the repulsion between pairs of valence electrons is used to predict the shape of a molecule. [**Section 5.4**]

weak acid
An acid that only partially dissociates in water. [**Section 11.3**]

weak base
A base that only partially dissociates in water. [**Section 11.3**]

zero-order reaction
A reaction in which rate is not proportional to the concentration of any of the reactants.

MCAT G-Chem Formula Sheet

Stoichiometry

Avogadro's number: $N_A = 6.02 \times 10^{23}$

$$\text{\# moles} = \frac{\text{mass in grams}}{\text{MW}}$$

$$\text{\% composition by mass of } X = \frac{\text{mass of X}}{\text{mass of molecule}} \times 100\%$$

Mole fraction: $X_S = \dfrac{\text{moles of S}}{\text{total moles}}$ Molarity: $M = \dfrac{\text{moles of solute}}{\text{L of solution}}$

Nuclear and Atomic Chemistry

N_A amu (u) = 1 gram $\qquad E_{photon} = hf = hc/\lambda$

electron energy: $E_n = \dfrac{(-2.178 \times 10^{-18}\,\text{J})}{n^2}$ for any 1-electron (Bohr) atom

Z = # of protons = atomic number, N = # of neutrons

$A = Z + N$ = mass number

Decay	Description	ΔZ	ΔN	ΔA
α	eject $\alpha = {}^4_2\text{He}$	−2	−2	−4
β^-	$n \rightarrow p + e^-$	+1	−1	0
β^+	$p \rightarrow n + e^+$	−1	+1	0
EC	$p + e^- \rightarrow n$	−1	+1	0
γ	$X^* \rightarrow X + \gamma$	0	0	0

Bonding and Intermolecular Forces

formal charge: $FC = V - (\frac{1}{2}B + L)$

V = (# of valence e^-s)

B = (# of bonding e^-s)

L = (# of lone-pair e^-s)

VSEPR Theory

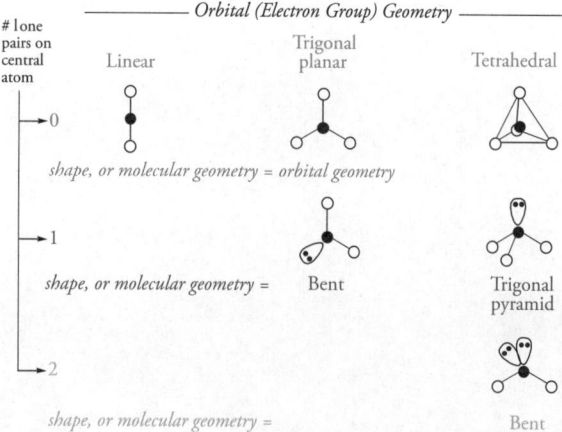

Intermolecular forces

intermolecular forces (D=dipole, I=induced, i=instantaneous):

ion–ion > ion–D > H-bonds > D–D > D–ID > iD–ID (London dispersion)

Periodic Trends

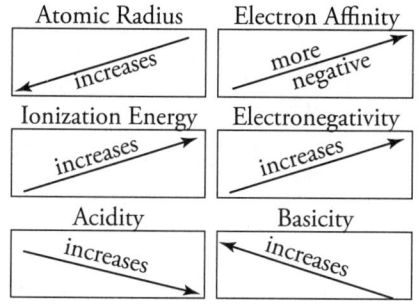

electronegativity of some common atoms:

F > O > (N ≈ Cl) > Br > (I ≈ S ≈ C) > H

Thermodynamics

T (in K) = $T_{°C}$ + 273, 1 cal ≈ 4.2 J, q = heat

$q = mc\Delta T = C\Delta T$ (if no phase changes)

$q = n\Delta H_{\text{phase change}}$ ($\Delta T = 0$ during phase change)

enthalpy change: ΔH = heat of rxn at const P

$\Delta H < 0 \Leftrightarrow$ exothermic, $\Delta H > 0 \Leftrightarrow$ endothermic

standard state: 1 M, 25°C, 1 atm

$\Delta H°_{\text{rxn}} = \sum n\Delta H°_{\text{f, products}} - \sum n\Delta H°_{\text{f, reactants}}$

Laws of Thermodynamics (E = energy, S = entropy):

1) E_{universe} is constant. $\Delta E_{\text{system}} = Q - W$.

2) Spontaneous rxn $\Rightarrow \Delta S_{\text{universe}} > 0$

3) $S = 0$ for pure crystal at $T = 0$ K

Gibbs Free Energy: $\Delta G = \Delta H - T\Delta S$ [const. T]

$\Delta G < 0 \Leftrightarrow$ forward reaction is spontaneous

$\Delta G = 0 \Leftrightarrow$ at equilibrium

$\Delta G > 0 \Leftrightarrow$ reverse reaction is spontaneous

$$\Delta G° = -RT \ln K \approx -2.3RT \log K$$

Gases

STP: T = 0 °C = 273 K, P = 1 atm = 760 torr = 760 mmHg

Avogadro's Law: $V \propto n$

$$V_{\text{at STP}} = n(22.4 \text{ L})$$

Boyle's Law: $V \propto 1/P$ (at constant T)

Charles's Law: $V \propto T$ (at constant P)

Combined Gas Law: $P_1V_1/T_1 = P_2V_2/T_2$

Ideal Gas Law: $PV = nRT$

van der Waals: $\left(P_{real} + \dfrac{an^2}{V^2}\right)(V - nb) = nRT$

Dalton's law of partial pressures: $P_{tot} = \sum p_i$

Graham's law of effusion:

$$v_{2,\,rms} = v_{1,\,rms}\sqrt{\dfrac{m_1}{m_2}} \Rightarrow \dfrac{\text{rate of effusion of gas 2}}{\text{rate of effusion of gas 1}} = \sqrt{\dfrac{m_1}{m_2}}$$

Kinetics

Concentration rate $= -\dfrac{\Delta[\text{reactant}]}{\text{time}}$ or $+\dfrac{\Delta[\text{product}]}{\text{time}}$

Reaction rate $= -\dfrac{1}{\text{coeff}}\dfrac{\Delta[\text{reactant}]}{\text{time}}$ or $+\dfrac{1}{\text{coeff}}\dfrac{\Delta[\text{product}]}{\text{time}}$

Rate law for rate-determining step:

$$\text{rate} = k[\text{reactant}_1]^{\text{coeff}_1}\ldots$$

Arrhenius equation: $k = Ae^{-E_a/RT}$

Equilibrium

For generic balanced reaction

$a\text{A} + b\text{B} \rightleftharpoons c\text{C} + d\text{D}$,

equilibrium constant: $K_{eq} = \dfrac{[\text{C}]_{at\,eq}^c[\text{D}]_{at\,eq}^d}{[\text{A}]_{at\,eq}^a[\text{B}]_{at\,eq}^b}$ (excluding pure solids and liquids)

(gas rxns use partial pressures in K_p expression)

K_{eq} is a constant at a given temperature

$K_{eq} < 1 \Leftrightarrow$ equilibrium favors reactants

$K_{eq} > 1 \Leftrightarrow$ equilibrium favors products

Reaction quotient: $Q = \dfrac{[\text{C}]^c[\text{D}]^d}{[\text{A}]^a[\text{B}]^b}$

Le Châtelier's Principle

$Q < K_{eq} \Leftrightarrow$ rxn proceeds in a forward direction

$Q = K_{eq} \Leftrightarrow$ rxn at equilibrium

$Q > K_{eq} \Leftrightarrow$ rxn proceeds in a reverse direction

Acids and Bases

$pH = -\log[\text{H}^+] = -\log[\text{H}_3\text{O}^+]$

$pOH = -\log[\text{OH}^-]$

$K_w = [\text{H}^+][\text{OH}^-] = 1 \times 10^{-14}$ at 25 °C

$pH + pOH = 14$ at 25 °C

$K_a = \dfrac{[\text{H}^+][\text{A}^-]}{[\text{HA}]}$ $\qquad$ $K_b = \dfrac{[\text{OH}^-][\text{HB}^+]}{[\text{B}]}$

$pK_a = -\log K_a$ $\qquad\qquad$ $pK_b = -\log K_b$

$K_aK_b = K_w =$ ion-product constant for water

Henderson-Hasselbalch equations:

$$pH = pK_a + \log\dfrac{[\text{conjugate base}]}{[\text{weak acid}]} = pK_a - \log\dfrac{[\text{weak acid}]}{[\text{conjugate base}]}$$

$$pOH = pK_b + \log\dfrac{[\text{conjugate acid}]}{[\text{weak base}]} = pK_b - \log\dfrac{[\text{weak base}]}{[\text{conjugate acid}]}$$

acid-base neutralization: $a \times [\text{A}] \times V_A = b \times [\text{B}] \times V_B$

Redox and Electrochemistry

Rules for determining oxidation state (OS):[*]

1) OS of pure element = 0

2) sum of OS's = 0 in neutral molecule

   sum of OS's = charge on ion

3) Group 1 metals: $OS = +1$

   Group 2 metals: $OS = +2$

4) OS of F = -1

5) OS of H = $+1$

6) OS of O = -2

7) OS of halogens = -1 of O family = -2

If one rule contradicts another, rule higher in list takes precedence.

$F =$ faraday $= 96{,}500$ C/mol e^-

$\Delta G = -nFE_{cell}$

$E_{cell} > 0 \Leftrightarrow$ spontaneous

$E_{cell} < 0 \Leftrightarrow$ reverse rxn is spontaneous

Nernst equation: $E = E° - \dfrac{0.06}{n}\log Q$

Faraday's Law of Electrolysis:

The amount of chemical charge is proportional to the amount of electricity that flows through the cell.

---

[*] These rules work 99 percent of the time.

MCAT Math for General Chemistry

PREFACE

The MCAT is primarily a conceptual exam, with little actual mathematical computation. Any math that is on the MCAT is fundamental: just arithmetic, algebra, and trigonometry (and there is virtually no trigonometry in General Chemistry). There is absolutely no calculus. The purpose of this section of the book is to go over some math topics (as they pertain to General Chemistry) on which you may feel a little rusty[1].

This text is intended for reference and self-study. Therefore, there are lots of examples, all completely solved. Practice working through these examples and master the fundamentals!

---

[1] For a complete discussion of all the math found on the MCAT, see our book *MCAT Physics and Math Review*.

Chapter 13
Arithmetic, Algebra, and Graphs

13.1 THE IMPORTANCE OF APPROXIMATION

Since you aren't allowed to use a calculator on the MCAT, you need to practice doing arithmetic calculations by hand again. Fortunately, the amount of calculation you'll have to do is small, and you'll also be able to approximate. For example, let's say you were faced with performing the following calculation:

$$\begin{array}{r} 23.6 \\ \times\ 72.5 \\ \hline 1180 \\ 472\ \ \ \\ 1652\ \ \ \ \\ \hline 1711.00 \end{array}$$

Your first inclination would be to reach for your calculator, but...you don't have one available. Now what? Realize that on the Chemical and Physical Foundations of Biological Systems section of the MCAT, you have roughly a minute and twenty-five seconds per question, so there simply cannot be questions requiring lengthy, complicated computation. Instead, we'll figure out a reasonably accurate (and fast) approximation of the value of the expression above:

$$\begin{array}{r} 25 \\ \times\ \ 70 \\ \hline 1750 \end{array}$$

So, if the answer to an MCAT question was the value of the expression above, and the four answer choices were, say, 1324, 1617, 1711, and 1856, we'd know right away that the answer was 1711. The choices are far enough apart that even with our approximations, we were still able to tell which choice was the correct one. Just as importantly, we didn't waste time trying to be more precise; it was unnecessary, and it would have decreased the amount of time we had to spend on other questions.

If you find yourself writing out lengthy calculations on your noteboard when you're working through MCAT questions that contain some mathematical calculation, it's important that you recognize that you're not using your time efficiently. Say to yourself, "I'm wasting valuable time trying to get a precise answer, when I don't need to be precise."

Try this one: What's 1583 divided by 32.1? (You have five seconds. Go.)

For the previous practice exercise, you should have written (or done in your head): $\dfrac{1500}{30} = 50$

13.2 SCIENTIFIC NOTATION, EXPONENTS, AND RADICALS

It's well known that very large or very small numbers can be handled more easily when they're written in **scientific notation**, that is, in the form $\pm m \times 10^n$, where $1 \leq m < 10$ and n is an integer. For example:

$$602{,}000{,}000{,}000{,}000{,}000{,}000{,}000 = 6.02 \times 10^{23}$$
$$-35{,}000{,}000{,}000 = -3.5 \times 10^{10}$$
$$0.000000004 = 4 \times 10^{-9}$$

Quantities like these come up all the time in physical problems, so you must be able to work with them confidently. Since a power of ten (the term 10^n) is part of every number written in scientific notation, the most important rules for dealing with such expressions are the Laws of Exponents:

Laws of Exponents		
		Illustration (with $b = 10$ or a power of 10)
Law 1	$b^p \times b^q = b^{p+q}$	$10^5 \times 10^{-9} = 10^{5+(-9)} = 10^{-4}$
Law 2	$b^p/b^q = b^{p-q}$	$10^5/10^{-9} = 10^{5-(-9)} = 10^{14}$
Law 3	$(b^p)^q = b^{pq}$	$(10^{-3})^2 = 10^{(-3)(2)} = 10^{-6}$
Law 4	$b^0 = 1$ (if $b \neq 0$)	$10^0 = 1$
Law 5	$b^{-p} = 1/b^p$	$10^{-7} = 1/10^7$
Law 6	$(ab)^p = a^p b^p$	$(2 \times 10^4)^3 = 2^3 \times (10^4)^3 = 8 \times 10^{12}$
Law 7	$(a/b)^p = a^p/b^p$	$[(3 \times 10^{-6})/10^2]^2 = (3 \times 10^{-6})^2/(10^2)^2 = 9 \times 10^{-16}$

Example 13-1: Simplify each of the following expressions, writing your answers in scientific notation:

a) $(4 \times 10^{-3})(5 \times 10^9)$
b) $(4 \times 10^{-3})/(5 \times 10^9)$
c) $(3 \times 10^{-4})^3$
d) $[(1 \times 10^{-2})/(5 \times 10^{-7})]^2$

Solution:

a) $(4 \times 10^{-3})(5 \times 10^9) = (4)(5) \times 10^{-3+9} = 20 \times 10^6 = 2 \times 10^7$
b) $(4 \times 10^{-3})/(5 \times 10^9) = (4/5) \times 10^{-3-9} = 0.8 \times 10^{-12} = 8 \times 10^{-13}$
c) $(3 \times 10^{-4})^3 = 3^3 \times (10^{-4})^3 = 27 \times 10^{-12} = 2.7 \times 10^{-11}$
d) $[(1 \times 10^{-2})/(5 \times 10^{-7})]^2 = (1 \times 10^{-2})^2/(5 \times 10^{-7})^2 = (1 \times 10^{-4})/(25 \times 10^{-14}) = (1/25) \times 10^{-4-(-14)}$
    $= (4/100) \times 10^{10} = 4 \times 10^8$

Another important skill involving numbers written in scientific notation involves changing the power of 10 (and compensating for this change so as not to affect the original number). The approximation carried out in the very first example in this chapter is a good example of this. To find the square root of 5×10^{-7}, it is much easier to first rewrite this number as 50×10^{-8}, because then the square root is easy:

$$\sqrt{50 \times 10^{-8}} = \sqrt{50} \times \sqrt{10^{-8}} \approx 7 \times 10^{-4}$$

Other examples of this procedure are found in Example 13-1 above; for instance,

$$20 \times 10^6 = 2 \times 10^7$$
$$0.8 \times 10^{-12} = 8 \times 10^{-13}$$
$$27 \times 10^{-12} = 2.7 \times 10^{-11}$$

In writing $\sqrt{50 \times 10^{-8}} = \sqrt{50} \times \sqrt{10^{-8}} \approx 7 \times 10^{-4}$, I used a familiar law of square roots, that the square root of a product is equal to the product of the square roots. Here's a short list of rules for dealing with radicals:

Laws of Radicals		
		Illustration
Law 1	$\sqrt{ab} = \sqrt{a} \cdot \sqrt{b}$	$\sqrt{9 \times 10^{12}} = \sqrt{9} \times \sqrt{10^{12}} = 3 \times 10^6$
Law 2	$\sqrt{a/b} = \sqrt{a}/\sqrt{b}$	$\sqrt{(4 \times 10^{-6})/10^{-18}} = \sqrt{(4 \times 10^{-6})}/\sqrt{10^{-18}} =$ $(2 \times 10^{-3})/10^{-9} = 2 \times 10^6$
Law 3	$\sqrt[q]{a^p} = a^{p/q}$	$\sqrt[3]{(8 \times 10^6)^2} = (8 \times 10^6)^{2/3} = 8^{2/3} \times 10^{(6)(2/3)} = 4 \times 10^4$

A couple of remarks about this list: First, Laws 1 and 2 illustrate how to handle square roots, which are the most common. However, the same laws are true even if the index of the root is not 2. [The **index** of a root (or radical) is the number that indicates the root that's to be taken; it's indicated by the little q in front of the radical sign in Law 3. Cube roots are index 3 and written $\sqrt[3]{}$; fourth roots are index 4 and written $\sqrt[4]{}$; and square roots are index 2 and written $\sqrt[2]{}$, although we hardly ever write the little 2.] Second, Law 3 provides the link between exponents and radicals.

Example 13-2: Approximate each of the following expressions, writing your answer in scientific notation:

a) $\sqrt{3.5 \times 10^9}$

b) $\sqrt{8 \times 10^{-11}}$

c) $\sqrt{\dfrac{1.5 \times 10^{-5}}{2.5 \times 10^{-17}}}$

Solution:

a) $\sqrt{3.5 \times 10^9} = \sqrt{35 \times 10^8} = \sqrt{35} \times \sqrt{10^8} \approx \sqrt{36} \times \sqrt{10^8} = 6 \times 10^4$

b) $\sqrt{8 \times 10^{-11}} = \sqrt{80 \times 10^{-12}} = \sqrt{80} \times \sqrt{10^{-12}} \approx \sqrt{81} \times \sqrt{10^{-12}} = 9 \times 10^{-6}$

c) $\sqrt{\dfrac{1.5 \times 10^{-5}}{2.5 \times 10^{-17}}} = \dfrac{\sqrt{1.5 \times 10^{-5}}}{\sqrt{2.5 \times 10^{-17}}} = \dfrac{\sqrt{15 \times 10^{-6}}}{\sqrt{25 \times 10^{-18}}} \approx \dfrac{\sqrt{16} \times \sqrt{10^{-6}}}{\sqrt{25} \times \sqrt{10^{-18}}} = \dfrac{4 \times 10^{-3}}{5 \times 10^{-9}} = 0.8 \times 10^6 = 8 \times 10^5$

Example 13-3: Approximate each of the following expressions, writing your answer in scientific notation:

a)   The mass (in grams) of 4.7×10^{24} molecules of CCl_4:
$$\frac{(4.7 \times 10^{24})(153.8)}{6.02 \times 10^{23}}$$

b)   The electrostatic force (in newtons) between the proton and electron in the ground state of hydrogen:
$$\frac{(8.99 \times 10^{9})(1.6 \times 10^{-19})^2}{(5.3 \times 10^{-11})^2}$$

Solution:

a) $\dfrac{(4.7 \times 10^{24})(153.8)}{6.02 \times 10^{23}} \approx \dfrac{5(150)}{6} \times 10^{24-23} = 5(25) \times 10 = 1.25 \times 10^{3}$

b) $\dfrac{(8.99 \times 10^{9})(1.6 \times 10^{-19})^2}{(5.3 \times 10^{-11})^2} \approx \dfrac{9(1.6)^2 \times 10^{9+(-19)(2)}}{(5.3)^2 \times 10^{(-11)(2)}} \approx \dfrac{(9)3 \times 10^{-29}}{27 \times 10^{-22}} = 1 \times 10^{-7}$

13.3   FRACTIONS, RATIOS, AND PERCENTS

A **fraction** indicates a division; for example, 3/4 means 3 divided by 4. The number above (or to the left of) the fraction bar is the numerator, and the number below (or to the right) of the fraction bar is called the denominator.

$$\frac{3}{4} \begin{array}{l} \longleftarrow \text{ numerator} \\ \longleftarrow \text{ denominator} \end{array} \quad 3/4$$

Our quick review of the basic arithmetic operations on fractions begins with the simplest rule: the one for multiplication:

$$\frac{a}{b} \times \frac{c}{d} = \frac{ac}{bd}$$

In words, just multiply the numerators and then, separately, multiply the denominators.

Example 13-4: What is 4/9 times 2/5?

Solution:

$$\frac{4}{9} \times \frac{2}{5} = \frac{4 \times 2}{9 \times 5} = \frac{8}{45}$$

The rule for dividing fractions is based on the reciprocal. If $a \neq 0$, then the **reciprocal** of a/b is simply b/a; that is, to form the reciprocal of a fraction, just flip it over. For example, the reciprocal of 3/4 is 4/3; the reciprocal of –2/5 is –5/2; the reciprocal of 3 is 1/3; and the reciprocal of –1/4 is –4. (The number 0 has no reciprocal.) As a result of this definition, we have the following basic fact: The product of any number and its reciprocal is 1.

13.3

Example 13-5: Find the reciprocal of each of these numbers:

    a)   2.25

    b) 5×10^{-4}

    c) 4×10^{5}

Solution:

    a)   2.25 is equal to 2 + (1/4), which is 9/4. The reciprocal of 9/4 is 4/9.

    b) $$\frac{1}{5 \times 10^{-4}} = \frac{1}{5} \times \frac{1}{10^{-4}} = 0.2 \times 10^{4} = 2 \times 10^{3}$$

    c) $$\frac{1}{4 \times 10^{5}} = \frac{1}{4} \times \frac{1}{10^{5}} = 0.25 \times 10^{-5} = 2.5 \times 10^{-6}$$

Now, in words, the rule for dividing fractions reads: *multiply by the reciprocal of the divisor.* That is, flip over whatever you're dividing by, and then multiply:

$$\frac{a}{b} \div \frac{c}{d} = \frac{a}{b} \times \frac{d}{c}$$

Example 13-6: What is 4/9 divided by 2/5?

Solution:

$$\frac{4}{9} \div \frac{2}{5} = \frac{4}{9} \times \frac{5}{2} = \frac{4 \times 5}{9 \times 2} = \frac{20}{18} = \frac{10}{9}$$

Finally, we turn to addition and subtraction. In elementary and junior high school, you were probably taught to find a common denominator (preferably, the *least* common denominator, known as the LCD), rewrite each fraction in terms of this common denominator, then add or subtract the numerators. If a common denominator is easy to spot, this may well be the fastest way to add or subtract fractions:

$$\frac{1}{2} + \frac{3}{4} = \frac{2}{4} + \frac{3}{4} = \frac{2+3}{4} = \frac{5}{4}$$

However, it's now time to learn the grown-up way to add or subtract fractions:

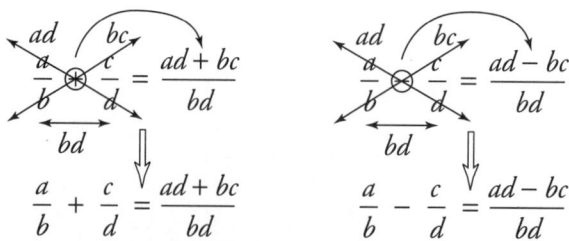

Here's what the arrows in the top line represent: "Multiply *up* (*d* times *a* gives *ad*), multiply *up* again (*b* times *c* gives *bc*), do the adding or subtracting of these products, and place the result over the product of the denominators (*bd*)." The length of this last sentence hides the simplicity of the rule, but it describes the recipe to follow. For example,

$$\frac{4}{9} + \frac{2}{5} = \frac{20+18}{45} = \frac{38}{45} \qquad\qquad \frac{4}{9} - \frac{2}{5} = \frac{20-18}{45} = \frac{2}{45}$$

Example 13-7:

a) Approximate the sum $\dfrac{1}{2.4 \times 10^5} + \dfrac{1}{6 \times 10^4}$

b) What is the reciprocal of this sum?

c) Simplify: $\dfrac{1}{2 \times 10^{-8}} - \dfrac{2}{5 \times 10^{-7}}$

Solution:

a) Using the rule illustrated above, we find that

$$\frac{1}{2.4 \times 10^5} + \frac{1}{6 \times 10^4} = \frac{(6 \times 10^4) + (2.4 \times 10^5)}{(2.4 \times 10^5)(6 \times 10^4)} = \frac{(6 \times 10^4) + (24 \times 10^4)}{(2.4 \times 10^5)(6 \times 10^4)} = \frac{(6+24) \times 10^4}{(2.4)(6) \times 10^{5+4}} \approx \frac{30 \times 10^4}{15 \times 10^9} = 2 \times 10^{-5}$$

b) The reciprocal of this result is $\dfrac{1}{2 \times 10^{-5}} = \dfrac{1}{2} \times \dfrac{1}{10^{-5}} = 0.5 \times 10^5 = 5 \times 10^4$.

c) $\dfrac{1}{2 \times 10^{-8}} - \dfrac{2}{5 \times 10^{-7}} = \dfrac{(5 \times 10^{-7}) - (2 \times 10^{-8})(2)}{(2 \times 10^{-8})(5 \times 10^{-7})} = \dfrac{(50 \times 10^{-8}) - (4 \times 10^{-8})}{(2)(5) \times 10^{-8+(-7)}} = \dfrac{(50-4) \times 10^{-8}}{10 \times 10^{-15}} = 46 \times 10^6$

$$= 4.6 \times 10^7$$

Let's now move on to ratios. A **ratio** is simply another way of saying *fraction*. For example, the ratio of 3 to 4, written 3:4, is equal to the fraction 3/4. Here's an illustration using isotopes of chlorine: The statement *the ratio of ^{35}Cl to ^{37}Cl is 3:1* means that there are 3/1 = 3 times as many ^{35}Cl atoms as there are ^{37}Cl atoms.

A particularly useful way to interpret a ratio is in terms of parts of a total. A ratio of *a:b* means that there are *a* + *b* total parts, with *a* of them being of the first type and *b* of the second type. Therefore, *the ratio of ^{35}Cl to ^{37}Cl is 3:1* means that if we could take all ^{35}Cl and ^{37}Cl atoms, we could partition all them into 3 + 1 = 4 equal parts such that 3 of these parts will all be ^{35}Cl atoms, and the remaining 1 part will all be ^{37}Cl atoms. We can now restate the original ratio as a ratio of these parts to the total. Since ^{35}Cl atoms account for 3 parts out of the 4 total, the ratio of ^{35}Cl atoms to all Cl atoms is 3:4; that is, 3/4 of all Cl atoms are ^{35}Cl atoms. Similarly, the ratio of ^{37}Cl atoms to all Cl atoms is 1:4, which means that 1/4 of all Cl atoms are ^{37}Cl atoms.

Example 13-8: The formula for the compound TNT (trinitrotoluene) is $C_7H_5N_3O_6$.

   a)   What fraction of the atoms in this compound are nitrogen atoms?

   b)   If the molar masses of C, H, N, and O are 12 g, 1 g, 14 g, and 16 g, respectively, what is the ratio of the mass of all the nitrogens to the total mass?

Solution:

   a)   There are a total of 7 + 5 + 3 + 6 = 21 atoms per molecule. The ratio of N atoms to the total is 3:21, or, more simply, 1:7. Therefore, 1/7 of the atoms in this compound are nitrogen atoms.

   b)   The desired ratio of masses is calculated like this:

$$\frac{\text{mass of all N atoms}}{\text{total mass of molecule}} = \frac{3(14)}{7(12) + 5(1) + 3(14) + 6(16)} = \frac{42}{227} \approx \frac{40}{220} = \frac{2}{11}$$

Example 13-9: In a simple hydrocarbon (molecular formula C_xH_y), the ratio of C atoms to H atoms is 5:4, and the total number of atoms in the molecule is 18. Find x and y.

Solution: Since the ratio of C atoms to H atoms is 5:4, there are 5 parts C atoms and 4 parts H atoms, for a total of 9 equal parts. These 9 equal parts account for 18 total atoms, so each part must contain 2 atoms. Thus, C (which has 5 parts) has 5 × 2 = 10 atoms, and H (which has 4 parts) has 4 × 2 = 8 atoms. Therefore, $x = 10$ and $y = 8$.

Example 13-10: The ratio of O atoms to C atoms in each molecule of triethylene glycol is 2:3, and the ratio of O atoms to the total number of C atoms and H atoms is 1:5. If there are 24 atoms (C, H, and O only) per molecule, find the formula for this compound.

Solution: The ratio of O to C atoms is 2:3, which tells us there are 2 parts O atoms and 3 parts C atoms, for a total of 5 parts C and O. Since the ratio of O to (C *and* H) atoms is 1:5, there are 5 times as many C and H atoms as there are O atoms. But, we have found that there are 2 parts O atoms, so C and H must account for 5 times as many: 10 parts. And, because there are 3 parts C atoms, there must be 10 – 3 = 7 parts H atoms. We therefore have 2 + 3 + 7 = 12 parts total, accounting for 24 atoms, which means 2 atoms per part. So, there must be 2 × 2 = 4 O atoms, 3 × 2 = 6 C atoms, and 7 × 2 = 14 H atoms. The formula is $C_6H_{14}O_4$.

The word **percent**, symbolized by %, is simply an abbreviation for the phrase "out of 100". Therefore, a percentage is represented by a fraction whose denominator is 100. For example, 60% means 60/100, or 60 out of 100. The three main question types involving percents are as follows:

   1)   What is y % of z?

   2) x is what percent of z?

   3) x is y % of what?

Fortunately, all three question types fit into a single form and can all be answered by one equation. Translating the statement *x is y % of z* into an algebraic equation, we get

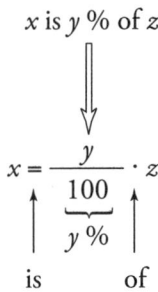

So, if you know any two of the three quantities x, y, and z, you can use the equation above to figure out the third.

Example 13-11:

a)   What is 25% of 200?
b)   30 is what percent of 150?
c)   400 is 80% of what?

Solution:

a)   Solving the equation $x = (25/100) \times 200$, we get $x = 25 \times 2 = 50$.
b)   Solving the equation $30 = (y/100) \times 150$, we get $y = (30/150) \times 100 = (1/5) \times 100 = 20$.
c)   Solving the equation $400 = (80/100) \times z$, we get $z = (100/80) \times 400 = 100 \times 5 = 500$.

It's also helpful to think of a simple fraction that equals a given percent, which can be used in place of $y/100$ in the equation above. For example, 25% = 1/4, 50% = 1/2, and 75% = 3/4. Other common fractional equivalents are: 20% = 1/5, 40% = 2/5, 60% = 3/5, and 80% = 4/5; 33 1/3% = 1/3 and 66 2/3% = 2/3; and 10n% = n/10 (for example, 10% = 1/10, 30% = 3/10, 70% = 7/10, and 90% = 9/10).

Example 13-12:

a)   What is 60% of 35?
b)   12 is 75% of what?
c)   What is 70% of 400?

Solution:

a)   Since 60% = 3/5, we find that $x = (3/5) \times 35 = 3 \times 7 = 21$.
b)   Because 75% = 3/4, we solve the equation $12 = (3/4) \times z$, and find $z = 12 \times (4/3) = 16$.
c)   Since 70% = 7/10, we find that $x = (7/10) \times 400 = 7 \times 40 = 280$.

Example 13-13:

a)   What is the result when 50 is increased by 50%?
b)   What is the result when 80 is decreased by 40%?

Solution:

a)   "Increasing 50 by 50%" means adding (50% of 50) to 50. Since 50% of 50 is 25, increasing 50 by 50% gives us 50 + 25 = 75.
b)   "Decreasing 80 by 40%" means subtracting (40% of 80) from 80. Since 40% of 80 is 32, decreasing 80 by 40% gives us 80 − 32 = 48.

Example 13-14:

a)   What is 250% of 60?
b)   2400 is what percent of 500?

Solution:

a)   Solving the equation $x = (250/100) \times 60$, we get $x = 25 \times 6 = 150$.
b)   Solving the equation $2400 = (y/100) \times 500$, we get $2400 = 5y$, so $y = 2400/5 = 480$.

Example 13-15: There are three stable isotopes of magnesium: ^{24}Mg, ^{25}Mg, and ^{26}Mg. The relative abundance of ^{24}Mg is 79%. Consider a sample of natural magnesium containing a total of 8×10^{24} atoms.

a)   About how many atoms in the sample are ^{24}Mg atoms?
b)   If the number of ^{25}Mg atoms in the sample is 8×10^{23}, what is the relative abundance (as a percentage) of ^{25}Mg?
c)   What's the relative abundance of ^{26}Mg?

Solution:

a)   Since the question is asking, *What is 79% of 8×10^{24}?*, we have

$$x = \frac{79}{100} \times (8 \times 10^{24}) \approx \frac{80}{100} \times (8 \times 10^{24}) = 6.4 \times 10^{24}$$

b)   The question is asking, *8×10^{23} is what percent of 8×10^{24}?*, so we write

$$8 \times 10^{23} = \frac{y}{100} \times (8 \times 10^{24}) \Rightarrow \frac{y}{100} = \frac{8 \times 10^{23}}{8 \times 10^{24}} = \frac{1}{10} \Rightarrow y = 10 \Rightarrow \text{ relative abundance} = 10\%$$

c)   Assuming that these three isotopes account for all naturally occurring magnesium, the sum of the relative abundance percentages should be 100%. Therefore, we need only solve the equation $79\% + 10\% + Y\% = 100\%$, from which we find that $Y = 11$.

Example 13-16: What is the percentage by mass of carbon in $C_7H_5N_3O_6$? (Given: Molar mass of compound = 227 g.)

A) 26%
B) 37%
C) 49%
D) 62%

Solution: Once the fraction of the total molar mass of the compound that's contributed by carbon is calculated, we obtain a percentage by multiplying this fraction by 100%. Since the molar mass of carbon is 12 g, and the molecule contains 7 C atoms, we have

$$\text{\%C, by mass } = \frac{7(12)}{227} = \frac{84}{227} \approx \frac{100}{250} = \frac{2}{5} = \frac{2}{5} \times 100\% = 40\%$$

Therefore, choice B is best.

13.4 EQUATIONS AND INEQUALITIES

You may have several questions on the MCAT that require you to solve—or manipulate—an algebraic equation or inequality. Fortunately, these equations and inequalities won't be very complicated.

When manipulating an algebraic equation, there's basically only one rule to remember: *Whatever you do to one side of the equation, you must do to the other side.* (Otherwise, it won't be a valid equation anymore.) For example, if you add 5 to the *left*-hand side, then add 5 to the *right*-hand side; if you multiply the *left*-hand side by 2, then multiply the *right*-hand side by 2, and so forth.

Inequalities are a little more involved. While it's still true that whatever you do to one side of an inequality you must also do to the other side, there are a couple of additional rules, both of which involve flipping the inequality sign—that is, changing > to < (or vice versa) or changing ≥ to ≤ (or vice versa).

1) *If you multiply both sides of an inequality by a negative number, then you must flip the inequality sign.*

 For example, let's say you're given the inequality $-2x > 6$. To solve for x, you'd multiply both sides by $-1/2$. Since this is a negative number, the inequality sign must be flipped: $x < -3$.

2) *If both sides of an inequality are positive quantities, and you take the reciprocal of both sides, then you must flip the inequality sign.*

 For example, let's say you're given the inequality $2/x \leq 6$, where it's known that x must be positive. To solve for x, you can take the reciprocal of both sides. Upon doing so, the inequality sign must be flipped: $x/2 \geq 1/6$, so $x \geq 1/3$.

Example 13-17:

a) Solve for T: $PV = nRT$
b) Solve for v: $KE = (1/2)mv^2$
c) Solve for x (given that x is positive): $4x^2 = 2.4 \times 10^{-11}$
d) Solve for B: $h = k + \log(B/A)$
e) If $F = q_1 q_2 / r^2$ and r is positive, solve for r in terms of F, q_1, and q_2.
f) Solve for x: $3(2 - x) < 18$
g) Find all positive values of λ that satisfy

$$\frac{2 \times 10^{-25}}{\lambda} \geq 4 \times 10^{-19}$$

Solution:

a) Dividing both sides by nR, we get $T = PV/(nR)$.

b) Multiply both sides $2/m$, then take the square root: $v = \sqrt{\dfrac{2KE}{m}}$.

c) $4x^2 = 2.4 \times 10^{-11} \Rightarrow x^2 = 6 \times 10^{-12} \Rightarrow x = \sqrt{6} \times 10^{-6} \approx 2.5 \times 10^{-6}$

d) $h = k + \log \dfrac{B}{A} \Rightarrow \log \dfrac{B}{A} = h - k \Rightarrow 10^{h-k} = \dfrac{B}{A} \Rightarrow B = 10^{h-k} A$ [see Chapter 15]

e) $F = \dfrac{q_1 q_2}{r^2} \Rightarrow r^2 = \dfrac{q_1 q_2}{F} \Rightarrow r = \sqrt{\dfrac{q_1 q_2}{F}}$

f) $3(2 - x) < 18 \Rightarrow 2 - x < 6 \Rightarrow -x < 4 \Rightarrow x > -4$

g) $\dfrac{2 \times 10^{-25}}{\lambda} \geq 4 \times 10^{-19} \Rightarrow \dfrac{\lambda}{2 \times 10^{-25}} \leq \dfrac{1}{4 \times 10^{-19}} \Rightarrow \lambda \leq \dfrac{2 \times 10^{-25}}{4 \times 10^{-19}} = 0.5 \times 10^{-6} \Rightarrow \lambda \leq 5 \times 10^{-7}$

13.5   THE *x-y* PLANE, LINES, AND OTHER GRAPHS

The figure below shows the familiar *x-y* **plane**, which we use to plot data and draw lines and curves showing how one quantity is related to another one:

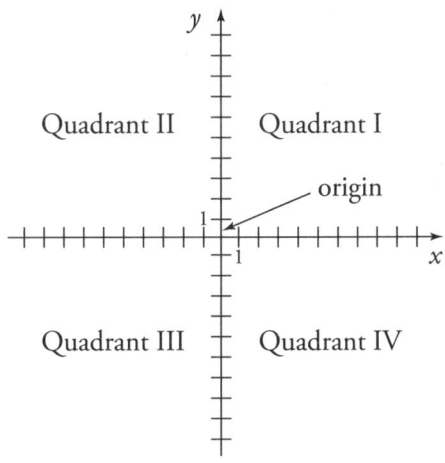

The *x-y* plane is formed by intersecting two number lines perpendicularly at the origins. The horizontal axis is generically referred to as the ***x*-axis** (although the quantity measured along this axis might be named by some other letter, such as time, *t*), and the vertical axis is generically known as the ***y*-axis**. The axes split the plane into four **quadrants**, which are numbered consecutively in a counterclockwise fashion. Quadrant I is in the upper right and represents all points (x, y) where x and y are both positive; in Quadrant II, x is negative and y is positive; in Quadrant III, x and y are both negative; and in Quadrant IV, x is positive and y is negative.

Suppose that two quantities, x and y, were related by the equation $y = 2x^2$. We would consider x the **independent variable**, and y the **dependent variable**, since for each value of x we get a unique value of y (that is, y *depends* uniquely on x). The independent variable is plotted along the horizontal axis, while the dependent variable is plotted along the vertical axis. Constructing a graph of an equation usually consists of plotting specific points (x, y) that satisfy the equation—in this case, examples include $(0, 0)$, $(1, 2)$, $(2, 8)$, $(-1, 2)$, $(-2, 8)$, etc.—and then connecting these points with a line or other smooth curve. The first coordinate of each point—the x coordinate—is known as the **abscissa**, and the second coordinate of each point—the y coordinate—is known as the **ordinate**.

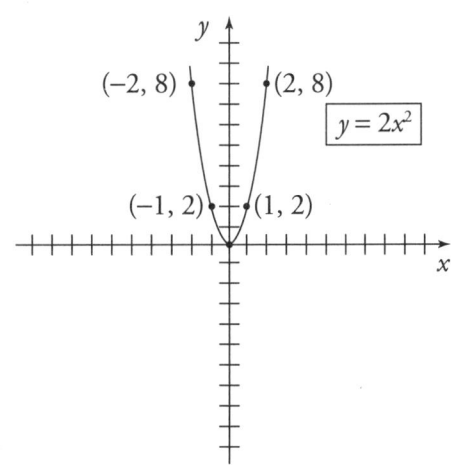

Lines

One of the simplest and most important graphs is the (straight) **line**. A line is determined by its slope—its steepness—and one specific point on the line, such as its intersection with either the x- or y-axis. The **slope** of a line is defined to be a change in y divided by the corresponding change in x ("rise over run"). Lines with positive slope rise to the right; those with negative slope fall to the right. And the greater the magnitude (absolute value) of the slope, the steeper the line.

13.5

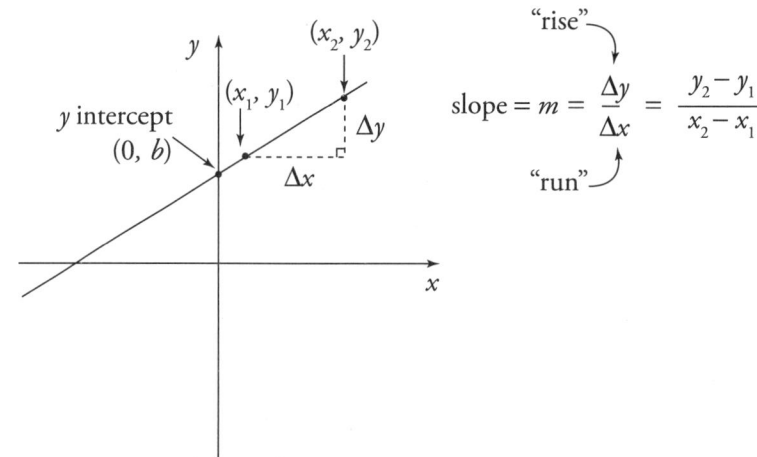

Perhaps the simplest way to write the equation of a line is in terms of its slope and the y-coordinate of the point where it crosses the y-axis. If the slope is m and the y-intercept is b, the equation of the line can be written in the form

$$y = mx + b$$

The only time this form doesn't work is when the line is vertical, since vertical lines have an undefined slope and such a line either never crosses the y-axis (no b) or else coincides with the y-axis. The equation of every vertical line is simply $x = a$, where a is the x-intercept.

Example 13-18:

a) Where does the line $y = 3x - 4$ cross the y-axis? the x-axis? What is its slope?
b) Find the equation of the line that has slope -2 and crosses the y-axis at the point $(0, 3)$.
c) Find the equation of the line that has slope 4 and crosses the y-axis at the origin.
d) A *linear* function is a function whose graph is a line. Let's say it's known that some quantity p is a linear function of x. If $p = 50$ when $x = 0$ and $p = 250$ when $x = 20$, find an equation for p in terms of x. Then use the equation to find the value of p when $x = 40$.

Solution:

a) The equation $y = 3x - 4$ matches the form $y = mx + b$ with $m = 3$ and $b = -4$. Therefore, this line has slope 3 and crosses the y-axis at the point $(0, -4)$. To find the x-intercept, we set y equal to 0 and solve for x: $0 = 3x - 4$ implies that $x = 4/3$. Therefore, this line crosses the x-axis at the point $(4/3, 0)$.
b) We're given $m = -2$ and $b = 3$, so the equation of the line is $y = -2x + 3$.
c) We're given $m = 4$ and $b = 0$, so the equation of the line is $y = 4x$.
d) Since p is a linear function of x, it must have the form $p = mx + b$ for some values of m and b. Because $p = 50$ when $x = 0$, we know that $b = 50$, so $p = mx + 50$. Now, since $p = 250$ when

$x = 20$, we have $250 = 20m + 50$, so $m = 10$. Thus, $p = 10x + 50$. Finally, substituting $x = 40$ into this formula, we find that the value of p when $x = 40$ is $(10)(40) + 50 = 450$.

Example 13-19: An insulated 50 cm³ sample of water has an initial temperature of $T_i = 10°C$. If Q calories of heat are added to the sample, the temperature of the water will rise to T, where $T = kQ + T_i$. When the graph of T vs. Q is sketched (with Q measured along the horizontal axis), it's found that the point $(Q, T) = (200, 14)$ lies on the graph.

a) What is the value of k?
b) How much heat is required to bring the water to 20°C?
c) If $Q = 2200$ cal, what will be the value of T?

Solution:
a) The equation $T = kQ + T_i$ matches the form $y = mx + b$, so k is the slope of the line. To find the slope, we evaluate the *rise-over-run* expression—which in this case is $\Delta T/\Delta Q$—for two points on the line. Using $(Q_1, T_1) = (0, 10)$ and $(Q_2, T_2) = (200, 14)$, we find that

$$k = \text{slope} = \frac{\Delta T}{\Delta Q} = \frac{T_2 - T_1}{Q_2 - Q_1} = \frac{14 - 10}{200 - 0} = \frac{1}{50}$$

b) We set T equal to 20 and solve for Q:

$$T = kQ + T_i \Rightarrow T = \frac{1}{50}Q + 10 \Rightarrow 20 = \frac{1}{50}Q + 10 \Rightarrow Q = 500 \text{ (cal)}$$

c) Here we set $Q = 2200$ and evaluate T:

$$T = kQ + T_i \Rightarrow T = \frac{1}{50}Q + 10 \Rightarrow T = \frac{1}{50}(2200) + 10 = 44 + 10 = 54 \text{ (°C)}$$

(*Technical note:* The equation for the temperature of the water, $T = kQ + T_i$, is valid as long as no phase change occurs.)

Besides lines, there are a few other graphs and features you should be familiar with.

The equation $y = kx^2$, where $k \neq 0$, describes the basic **parabola**, one whose turning point (**vertex**) is at the origin. It has a U shape, and opens upward if k is positive and downward if k is negative. The graph of the related equation $y = k(x - a)^2$ is obtained from the basic parabola by shifting it horizontally so that its vertex is at the point $(a, 0)$. The graph of the equation $y = kx^2 + b$ is obtained from the basic parabola by shifting it vertically so that its vertex is at the point $(0, b)$. Finally, the graph of the equation $y = k(x - a)^2 + b$ is obtained from the basic parabola in two shifting steps: First, shift the basic parabola horizontally so that its vertex is at the point $(a, 0)$; next, shift this parabola vertically so that the vertex is at the point (a, b). These parabolas are illustrated below for positive a, b, k, and x:

13.5

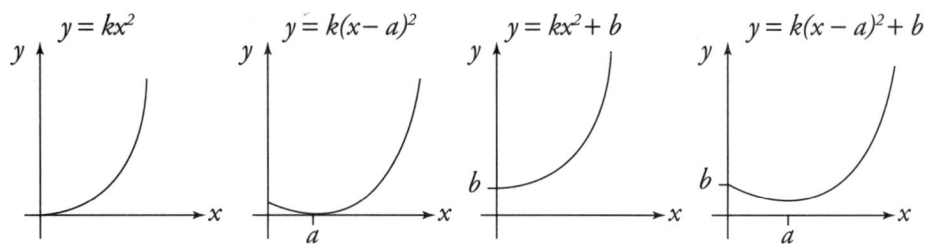

The equation $y = k/x$, where $k \neq 0$, describes a **hyperbola**. It is the graph of an inverse proportion (see Section 14.2). For small values of x, the values of y are large; and for large values of x, the values of y are small. Notice that the graph of a hyperbola approaches—but never touches—both the x- and y-axes. These lines are therefore called **asymptotes**.

The equation $y = k/x^2$, where $k \neq 0$, has a graph whose shape is similar to a hyperbola but it approaches its asymptotes faster than a hyperbola does (because of the square in the denominator).

The graph of the equation $y = Ae^{-kx}$ (where k is positive) is an **exponential decay curve**. It intersects the y axis at the point $(0, A)$, and, as x increases, the value of y decreases. Here, the x-axis is an asymptote.

The graph of the equation $y = A(1 - e^{-kx})$, where k is positive, contains the origin, and as x increases, the graph rises to approach the horizontal line $y = A$. This line is an asymptote.

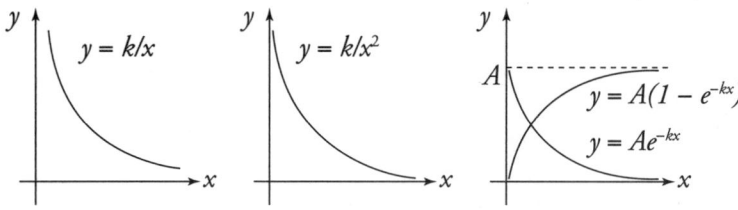

Chapter 14
Proportions

The concept of proportionality is fundamental to analyzing the behavior of many physical phenomena and is a common topic for MCAT questions.

14.1 DIRECT PROPORTIONS

If one quantity is always equal to a constant times another quantity, we say that the two quantities are **proportional** (or **directly proportional**, if emphasis is desired). For example, if k is some nonzero constant and the equation $A = kB$ is always true, then A and B are proportional, and k is called the **proportionality constant**. We express this fact mathematically by using this symbol: $\propto$, which means *is proportional to*. So, if $A = kB$, we'd write $A \propto B$. Of course, if $A = kB$, then $B = (1/k)A$, so we could also say that $B \propto A$.

Here are a few examples:

Example 14-1: Energy is equal to Planck's constant times frequency, $E = hf$. Therefore $E \propto f$.

Example 14-2: The ideal gas law states that $PV = nRT$. If n, V, and R are constant, $P \propto T$.

Example 14-3: The rate law for a chemical reaction that is first order with respect to reactant A is rate = $k[A]$. Assuming k is constant, rate $\propto [A]$.

The most important fact about direct proportions is this:

> *If $A \propto B$, and B is multiplied by a factor of b, then A will also be multiplied by a factor of b.*

After all, if $A = kB$, then $bA = k(bB)$.

Example 14-4: Since the energy of a photon is proportional to its frequency, $E \propto f$, then, if the frequency is doubled, so is the energy. If the frequency is reduced by half, so is the energy. If the frequency is tripled, so is the energy.

Example 14-5: Since the pressure inside a system is proportional to its temperature when volume and the number of moles present are constant, $P \propto T$, when the temperature is quadrupled, the pressure is quadrupled. When the pressure is decreased by a factor of 3, the temperature is also decreased by a factor of 3.

Example 14-6: Since the rate of a first order chemical reaction is proportional to the concentration of reactant A, [rate] $\propto [A]$, if $[A]$ is increased by a factor of 2, the rate also increases by a factor of 2. If $[A]$ is decreased by a factor of 4 (same as multiplying by ¼), the rate of reaction is ¼ of what it was originally.

It's important to notice that the actual numerical value of the proportionality constant was irrelevant in the statements made above. For example, the fact that h is the proportionality constant in the equation $E = hf$ did not affect the conclusions made above. If E and f were some other quantities and E happened to always be equal to $(17,000)f$, we'd still say $E \propto f$, and all the conclusions made in Example 14-4 above would still be correct.

Graphically, proportions are easy to spot. If the horizontal and vertical axes are labeled linearly (as they usually are), then *the graph of a proportion is a straight line through the origin*. Be careful not to make the common mistake of thinking that any straight line is the graph of a proportion. If the line doesn't go through the origin, then it's *not* the graph of a proportion.

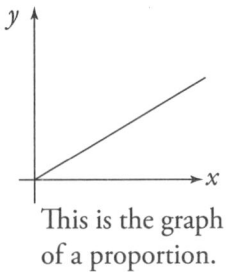

This is the graph of a proportion.

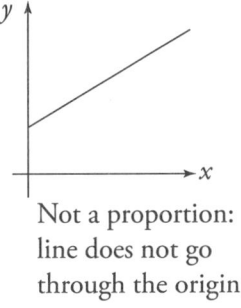

Not a proportion: line does not go through the origin.

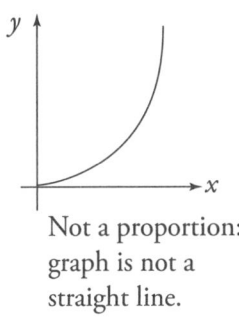

Not a proportion: graph is not a straight line.

The examples we've seen so far have been the equations $E = hf$, $PV = nRT$, and $rate = k[A]$. Notice that in all of these equations, all the variables are present to the first power. But what about an equation like this: $KE = \frac{1}{2}mv^2$? This equation gives the kinetic energy of an object of mass m moving with speed v. So, if m is constant, KE is proportional to v^2. Now, what if v were multiplied by, say, a factor of 3, what would happen to KE? Because $KE \propto v^2$, if v increases by a factor of 3, then KE will increase by a factor of 3^2, which is 9. (By the way, this does not mean that if we graph KE versus v, we'll get a straight line through the origin. KE is not proportional to v; it's proportional to v^2. If we were to graph KE vs. v^2, *then* we'd get a straight line through the origin.) Here's another example using the same proportion, $KE \propto v^2$: If v were decreased by a factor of 2, then KE would decrease by a factor of $2^2 = 4$.

Here is one more example:

Example 14-7: The reaction quotient Q for a reaction is described by $Q = [A][B]^3$. Therefore, Q is proportional to the concentration of $[B]^3$: $Q \propto [B]^3$. So, for example, if $[B]$ were doubled, Q would increase by a factor $2^3 = 8$.

14.2 INVERSE PROPORTIONS

If one quantity is always equal to a nonzero constant *divided* by another quantity (that is, if $A = k/B$, where k is some constant), we say that the two quantities are **inversely proportional**. Here are two equivalent ways of saying this:

(i)　　If the product of two quantities is a constant ($AB = k$), then the quantities are inversely proportional.

(ii)　　If A is proportional to $1/B$ [that is, if $A = k(1/B)$], then A and B are inversely proportional.

In fact, we'll use this final description to symbolize an inverse proportion. That is, if A is inversely proportional to B, then we'll write $A \propto 1/B$. (There's no commonly accepted single symbol for *inversely proportional to*.) Of course, if $A = k/B$, then $B = k/A$, so we could also say that $B \propto 1/A$.

Here are a couple of examples:

Example 14-8: The pressure P and volume V of a sample containing n moles of an ideal gas at a fixed temperature T is given by the equation $PV = nRT$, where R is a constant. Therefore, the pressure is inversely proportional to the volume: $P \propto 1/V$.

Example 14-9: For electromagnetic waves traveling through space, the wavelength λ and frequency f are related by the equation $\lambda f = c$, where c is the speed of light (a universal constant). Therefore, wavelength is inversely proportional to frequency: $\lambda \propto 1/f$.

The most important fact about inverse proportions is this:

> *If $A \propto 1/B$, and B is multiplied by a factor of b, then A will be multiplied by a factor of $1/b$.*

After all, if $A = k/B$, then $(1/b)A = k/(bB)$. Intuitively, if one quantity is *increased* by a factor of b, the other quantity will *decrease* by the same factor, and vice versa. Look at a few more examples:

Example 14-10: Since the pressure of an ideal gas at constant temperature is inversely proportional to the volume, $P \propto 1/V$, then if the volume is doubled, the pressure is reduced by a factor of 2. If the volume is quadrupled, the pressure is reduced by a factor of 4. If the volume is divided by 3 (which is the same as saying it's multiplied by 1/3), then the pressure will increase by a factor of 3.

Example 14-11: Because for electromagnetic waves traveling through space, the wavelength is inversely proportional to frequency, $\lambda \propto 1/f$, if f is increased by a factor of 10, λ will decrease by a factor of 10. If the frequency is decreased by a factor of 2, the wavelength will increase by a factor of 2.

The graph of an inverse proportion is a *hyperbola*. In the graph below, $xy = k$, so x and y are inversely proportional to each other.

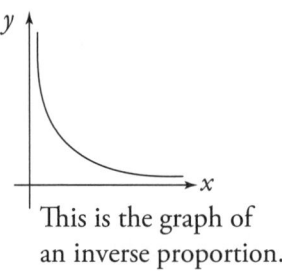

This is the graph of
an inverse proportion.

The examples we've seen so far have been cases in which one quantity is inversely proportional to the first power of another quantity. But what about an equation like this:

$$F = \frac{q_1 q_2}{r^2}$$

This equation gives the electrostatic force between two point charges of magnitude q_1 and q_2 separated by a distance r. So, if q_1 and q_2 are constant, F is inversely proportional to r^2. Now, if r were increased by, say, a factor of 3, what would happen to F? Because $F \propto 1/r^2$, if r increases by a factor of 3, then F will decrease by a factor of 3^2, which is 9. Here's another example using the same proportion, $F \propto 1/r^2$: If r were decreased by a factor of 2, then F would increase by a factor of $2^2 = 4$.

Example 14-12: Graham's law of effusion states that

$$\frac{\text{rate of effusion of Gas 1}}{\text{rate of effusion of Gas 2}} = \sqrt{\frac{m_2}{m_1}},$$

where m_2 is the molecular mass of Gas 2 and m_1 is the molecular mass of Gas 1. Therefore, the rate of effusion of Gas 1 is inversely proportional to the square root of its molecular mass: rate of effusion of Gas 1 $\propto \sqrt{\frac{1}{m_1}}$. So, if Gas 1 were changed to a molecule whose mass was 4 times greater, the rate of effusion of Gas 1 would decrease by a factor of 2.

Example 14-13: The kinetic energy of an object of mass m traveling with speed v is given by the formula $KE = mv^2/2$.
   a)   If v is increased by a factor of 6, what happens to KE?
   b)   In order to increase KE by a factor of 6, what must happen to v?

Solution:
   a)   Since $KE \propto v^2$, if v increases by a factor of 6, then KE increases by a factor of $6^2 = 36$.
   b)   Since $KE \propto v^2$, it follows that $\sqrt{KE} \propto v$. So, if KE is to increase by a factor of 6, then v must be increased by a factor of $\sqrt{6}$.

Chapter 15
Logarithms

15.1   THE DEFINITION OF A LOGARITHM

A **logarithm** (or just **log**, for short) is an exponent.

For example, in the equation $2^3 = 8$, 3 is the exponent, so 3 is the logarithm. More precisely, since 3 is the exponent that gives 8 when the base is 2,

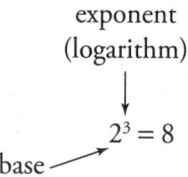

we say that the base-2 log of 8 is 3, symbolized by the equation $\log_2 8 = 3$.

Here's another example: Since $10^2 = 100$, the base-10 log of 100 is 2; that is, $\log_{10} 100 = 2$. The logarithm of a number to a given base is the exponent the base needs to be raised to give the number. What's the log, base 3, of 81? It's the exponent we'd have to raise 3 to in order to give 81. Since $3^4 = 81$, the base-3 log of 81 is 4, which we write as $\log_3 81 = 4$.

The exponent equation $2^3 = 8$ is equivalent to the log equation $\log_2 8 = 3$; the exponent equation $10^2 = 100$ is equivalent to the log equation $\log_{10} 100 = 2$; and the exponent equation $3^4 = 81$ is equivalent to the log equation $\log_3 81 = 4$. For every exponent equation, $b^x = y$, there's a corresponding log equation: $\log_b y = x$, and vice versa. To help make the conversion, use the following mnemonic, called the *two arrows method*:

$$\log_2 8 = 3 \iff 2^3 = 8$$

$$\log_b y = x \iff b^x = y$$

You should read the log equations with the two arrows like this:

$$\log_2 8 = 3 \iff 2 \longrightarrow 3 \longrightarrow 8 \iff 2^3 = 8$$

equals to the equals to the

$$\log_b y = x \iff b \longrightarrow x \longrightarrow y \iff b^x = y$$

equals to the equals to the

Always remember: The log is the exponent.

15.2 LAWS OF LOGARITHMS

There are only a few rules for dealing with logs that you'll need to know, and they follow directly from the rules for exponents (given earlier, in 13.2). After all, logs *are* exponents.

In stating these rules, we will assume that in an equation like $\log_b y = x$, the base b is a positive number that's different from 1, and that y is positive. (Why these restrictions? Well, if b is negative, then not every number has a log. For example, $\log_{-3} 9$ is 2, but what is $\log_{-3} 27$? If b were 0, then only 0 would have a log; and if b were 1, then every number x could equal $\log_1 y$ if $y = 1$, and *no* number x could equal $\log_1 y$ if $y \neq 1$. And why must y be positive? Because if b is a positive number, then b^x [which is y] is always positive, no matter what real value we use for x. Therefore, only positive numbers have logs.)

Laws of Logarithms	
Law 1	The log of a product is the sum of the logs: $\log_b (yz) = \log_b y + \log_b z$
Law 2	The log of a quotient is the difference of the logs: $\log_b (y/z) = \log_b y - \log_b z$
Law 3	The log of (a number to a power) is that power times the log of the number: $\log_b (y^z) = z \log_b y$

We could also add to this list that *the log of 1 is 0*, but this fact just follows from the definition of a log: Since $b^0 = 1$ for any allowed base b, we'll always have $\log_b 1 = 0$.

For the MCAT, the two most important bases are $b = 10$ and $b = e$. Base-10 logs are called **common** logs, and the "10" is often not written at all:

$$\log y \text{ means } \log_{10} y$$

The base-10 log is useful because we use a *decimal* number system, which is based (pun intended) on the number 10. For example, the number 273.15 means $(2 \times 10^2) + (7 \times 10^1) + (3 \times 10^0) + (1 \times 10^{-1}) + (5 \times 10^{-2})$. In physics, the formula for the decibel level of a sound uses the base-10 log. In chemistry, the base-10 log has many uses, such as finding values of the pH, pOH, pK_a, and pK_b.

Base-e logs are known as **natural** logs. Here, e is a particular constant, approximately equal to 2.7. This may seem like a strange number to choose as a base, but it makes calculus run smoothly—which is why it's called the *natural* logarithm—because (and you don't need to know this for the MCAT) the only numerical value of b for which the function $f(x) = b^x$ is its own derivative is $b = e = 2.71828\ldots$. Base-e logs are often used in the mathematical description of physical processes in which the rate of change of some quantity is proportional to the quantity itself; radioactive decay is a typical example. The notation "ln" (the abbreviation, in reverse, for **n**atural **l**ogarithm) is often used to mean $\log_e$:

$$\ln y \text{ means } \log_e y$$

The relationship between the base-10 log and the base-e log of a given number can be expressed as $\ln y \approx 2.3 \log y$. For example, if $y = 1000 = 10^3$, then $\ln 1000 \approx 2.3 \log 1000 = 2.3 \times 3 = 6.9$. You may also find it useful to know the following approximate values:

$$\log 2 \approx 0.3 \qquad \ln 2 \approx 0.7$$
$$\log 3 \approx 0.5 \qquad \ln 3 \approx 1.1$$
$$\log 5 \approx 0.7 \qquad \ln 5 \approx 1.6$$

Example 15-1:
a) What is $\log_3 9$?
b) Find $\log_5 (1/25)$.
c) Find $\log_4 8$.
d) What is the value of $\log_{16} 4$?
e) Given that $\log 5 \approx 0.7$, what's $\log 500$?
f) Given that $\log 2 \approx 0.3$, find $\log (2 \times 10^{-6})$.
g) Given that $\log 2 \approx 0.3$ and $\log 3 \times 0.5$, find $\log (6 \times 10^{23})$.

Solution:
a) $\log_3 9 = x$ is the same as $3^x = 9$, from which we see that $x = 2$. So, $\log_3 9 = 2$.
b) $\log_5 (1/25) = x$ is the same as $5^x = 1/25 = 1/5^2 = 5^{-2}$, so $x = -2$. Therefore, $\log_5 (1/25) = -2$.
c) $\log_4 8 = x$ is the same as $4^x = 8$. Since $4^x = (2^2)^x = 2^{2x}$ and $8 = 2^3$, the equation $4^x = 8$ is the same as $2^{2x} = 2^3$, so $2x = 3$, which gives $x = 3/2$. Therefore, $\log_4 8 = 3/2$.
d) $\log_{16} 4 = x$ is the same as $16^x = 4$. To find x, you might notice that the square root of 16 is 4, so $16^{1/2} = 4$, which means $\log_{16} 4 = 1/2$. Alternatively, we can write 16^x as $(4^2)^x = 4^{2x}$ and 4 as 4^1. Therefore, the equation $16^x = 4$ is the same as $4^{2x} = 4^1$, so $2x = 1$, which gives $x = 1/2$.
e) $\log 500 = \log (5 \times 100) = \log 5 + \log 100$, where we used Law 1 in the last step. Since $\log 100 = \log 10^2 = 2$, we find that $\log 500 \approx 0.7 + 2 = 2.7$.
f) $\log (2 \times 10^{-6}) = \log 2 + \log 10^{-6}$, by Law 1. Since $\log 10^{-6} = -6$, we find that $\log (2 \times 10^{-6}) \approx 0.3 + (-6) = -5.7$.
g) $\log (6 \times 10^{23}) = \log 2 + \log 3 + \log 10^{23}$, by Law 1. Since $\log 10^{23} = 23$, we find that $\log (6 \times 10^{23}) \approx 0.3 + 0.5 + 23 = 23.8$.

Example 15-2: In each case, find y.
a) $\log_2 y = 5$
b) $\log_2 y = -3$
c) $\log y = 4$
d) $\log y = 7.5$
e) $\log y = -2.5$
f) $\ln y = 3$

Solution:
a) $\log_2 y = 5$ is the same as $2^5 = y$, so $y = 32$.
b) $\log_2 y = -3$ is the same as $2^{-3} = y$, which gives $y = 1/2^3 = 1/8$.
c) $\log y = 4$ is the same as $10^4 = y$, so $y = 10,000$.
d) $\log y = 7.5$ is the same as $10^{7.5} = y$. We'll rewrite 7.5 as $7 + 0.5$, so $y = 10^{7+(0.5)} = 10^7 \times 10^{0.5}$. Because $10^{0.5} = 10^{1/2} = \sqrt{10}$, which is approximately 3, we find that $y \approx 10^7 \times 3 = 3 \times 10^7$.
e) $\log y = -2.5$ is the same as $10^{-2.5} = y$. We'll rewrite -2.5 as $-3 + 0.5$, so $y = 10^{-3+(0.5)} = 10^{-3} \times 10^{0.5}$. Because $10^{0.5} = 10^{1/2} = \sqrt{10}$, which is approximately 3, we have that $y \approx 10^{-3} \times 3 = 0.003$.
f) $\ln y = 3$ means $\log_e y = 3$; this is the same as $y = e^3$ (which is about 20).

Example 15-3: The definition of the pH of an aqueous solution is

$$pH = -\log [H_3O^+] \text{ (or, simply, } -\log [H^+])$$

where $[H_3O^+]$ is the hydronium ion concentration (in M).

Part I: Find the pH of each of the following solutions:
  a) coffee, with $[H_3O^+] = 8 \times 10^{-6} M$
  b) seawater, with $[H_3O^+] = 3 \times 10^{-9} M$
  c) vinegar, with $[H_3O^+] = 1.3 \times 10^{-3} M$

Part II: Find $[H_3O^+]$ for each of the following pH values:
  d) pH = 7
  e) pH = 11.5
  f) pH = 4.7

Solution:
  a) $pH = -\log (8 \times 10^{-6}) = -[\log 8 + \log (10^{-6})] = -\log 8 + 6$. We can now make a quick approximation by simply noticing that log 8 is a little less than log 10; that is, log 8 is a little less than 1. Let's say it's 0.9. Then $pH \approx -0.9 + 6 = 5.1$.
  b) $pH = -\log (3 \times 10^{-9}) = -[\log 3 + \log (10^{-9})] = -\log 3 + 9$. We now make a quick approximation by simply noticing that log 3 is about 0.5 (after all, $9^{0.5}$ *is* 3, so $10^{0.5}$ is close to 3). This gives $pH \approx -0.5 + 9 = 8.5$.
  c) $pH = -\log (1.3 \times 10^{-3}) = -[\log 1.3 + \log (10^{-3})] = -\log 1.3 + 3$. We can now make a quick approximation by simply noticing that log 1.3 is just a little more than log 1; that is, log 1.3 is a little more than 0. Let's say it's 0.1. This gives $pH \approx -0.1 + 3 = 2.9$.

> **Note 1:**
> We can generalize these three calculations as follows: If $[H_3O^+] = m \times 10^{-n} M$, where $1 \le m < 10$ and n is an integer, then the pH is between $(n - 1)$ and n; it's closer to $(n - 1)$ if $m > 3$ and it's closer to n if $m < 3$. (We use 3 as the cutoff since $\log 3 \approx 0.5$.)

  d) If pH = 7, then $-\log [H_3O^+] = 7$, so $\log [H_3O^+] = -7$, which means $[H_3O^+] = 10^{-7} M$.
  e) If pH = 11.5, then $-\log [H_3O^+] = 11.5$, so $\log [H_3O^+] = -11.5$, which means $[H_3O^+] = 10^{-11.5} = 10^{(0.5)-12} = 10^{0.5} \times 10^{-12} \approx 3 \times 10^{-12} M$.
  f) If pH = 4.7, then $-\log [H_3O^+] = 4.7$, so $\log [H_3O^+] = -4.7$, which means $[H_3O^+] = 10^{-4.7} = 10^{(0.3)-5} = 10^{0.3} \times 10^{-5} \approx 2 \times 10^{-5} M$. [$10^{-0.3} \approx 2$ follows from the fact that log 2 $\approx$ 0.3.]

> **Note 2:**
> We can generalize these last two calculations as follows: If pH = $n.m$, where n is an integer and m is a digit from 1 to 9, then $[H_3O^+] = y \times 10^{-(n+1)} M$, where y is closer to 1 if $m > 3$ and closer to 10 if $m < 3$. (We take $y = 5$ if $m = 3$.)

Example 15-4: The definition of the pK_a of a weak acid is
$$pK_a = -\log K_a$$

where K_a is the acid's ionization constant.

Part I: Approximate the pK_a of each of the following acids:

a)   HBrO, with $K_a = 2 \times 10^{-9}$
b) HNO_2, with $K_a = 7 \times 10^{-4}$
c)   HCN, with $K_a = 6 \times 10^{-10}$

Part II: Approximate K_a for each of the following pK_a values:

d) $pK_a = 12.5$
e) $pK_a = 2.7$
f) $pK_a = 9.2$

Solution:

a) $pK_a = -\log (2 \times 10^{-9}) = -[\log 2 + \log (10^{-9})] = -\log 2 + 9$. We can now make a quick approximation by remembering that log 2 is about 0.3. Then $pK_a \approx -0.3 + 9 = 8.7$. Because the formula to find pK_a from K_a is exactly the same as the formula for finding pH from $[H^+]$, we could also make use of Note 1 in the solution to Example 15-3. If $K_a = m' \times 10^{-n} M$, where $1 \leq m < 10$ and n is an integer, then the pK_a is between $(n-1)$ and n; it's closer to $(n-1)$ if $m > 3$ and it's closer to n if $m < 3$. In this case, $m = 2$ and $n = 9$, so the pK_a is between $(n-1) = 8$ and $n = 9$. And, since $2 < 3$, the pK_a will be closer to 9 (which is just what we found, since we got the value 8.7). Given a list of possible choices for the pK_a of this acid, just recognizing that it's a little less than 9 will be sufficient.

b)   With $K_a = 7 \times 10^{-4}$, we have $m = 7$ and $n = 4$. Therefore, the pK_a will be between $(n-1) = 3$ and $n = 4$. Since $m = 7$ is greater than 3, the value of pK_a will be closer to 3 (around, say, 3.2).

c)   With $K_a = 6 \times 10^{-10}$, we have $m = 6$ and $n = 10$. Therefore, the pK_a will be between $(n-1) = 9$ and $n = 10$. Since $m = 6$ is greater than 3, the value of pK_a will be closer to 9 (around, say, 9.2).

d)   If $pK_a = 12.5$, then $-\log K_a = 12.5$, so $\log K_a = -12.5$, which means $K_a = 10^{-12.5} = 10^{(0.5)-13} = 10^{0.5} \times 10^{-13} \approx 3 \times 10^{-13}$. We could also make use of Note 2 in the solution to Example 15-3. If $pK_a = n.m$, where n is an integer and m is a digit from 1 to 9, then $K_a = y \times 10^{-(n+1)} M$, where y is closer to 1 if $m > 3$ and y is closer to 10 if $m < 3$. In this case, with $pK_a = 12.5$, we have $n = 12$ and $m = 5$, so the K_a value is $y \times 10^{-(12+1)} = y \times 10^{-13}$, with y closer to 1 (than to 10) since $m = 5$ is greater than 3 (this agrees with what we found, since we calculated that $K_a \approx 3 \times 10^{-13}$).

e)   With $pK_a = 2.7$, we have $n = 2$ and $m = 7$. Therefore, the K_a value is $y \times 10^{-(2+1)} = y \times 10^{-3}$, with y close to 1 since $m = 7$ is greater than 3. We can check this as follows: If $pK_a = 2.7$, then $-\log K_a = 2.7$, so $\log K_a = -2.7$, which means $K_a = 10^{-2.7} = 10^{(0.3)-3} = 10^{0.3} \times 10^{-3} \approx 2 \times 10^{-3}$.

f)   With $pK_a = 9.2$, we have $n = 9$ and $m = 2$. Therefore, the K_a value is $y \times 10^{-(9+1)} = y \times 10^{-10}$, with y closer to 10 (than to 1) since $m = 2$ is less than 3. We can say that $K_a \approx 6 \times 10^{-10}$.

Example 15-5:

a)   If y increases by a factor of 100, what happens to log y?
b)   If y decreases by a factor of 1000, what happens to log y?
c)   If y increases by a factor of 30,000, what happens to log y?
d)   If y is reduced by 99%, what happens to log y?

Solution:

a)   If y changes to $y' = 100y$, then the log increases by 2, since

$$\log y' = \log (100\, y) = \log 100 + \log y = \log 10^2 + \log y = 2 + \log y$$

b) If y changes to $y' = y/1000$, then the log decreases by 3, since

$$\log y' = \log \left(\frac{y}{1000}\right) = \log y - \log 1000 = \log y - \log 10^3 = \log y - 3$$

c) If y changes to $y' = 30{,}000y$, then the log increases by about 4.5, since

$$\log y' = \log (30000\ y) = \log 3 + \log 10000 + \log y \approx 0.5 + 4 + \log y = 4.5 + \log y$$

d) If y is reduced by 99%, that means we're subtracting $0.99y$ from y, which leaves $0.01y = y/100$. Therefore, y has decreased by a factor of 100. And if y changes to $y' = y/100$, then the log decreases by 2, since

$$\log y' = \log \left(\frac{y}{100}\right) = \log y - \log 100 = \log y - \log 10^2 = \log y - 2$$

Example 15-6: A radioactive substance has a half-life of 70 hours. For each of the fractions below, figure out how many hours will elapse until the amount of substance remaining is equal to the given fraction of the original amount.
   a)   1/4
   b)   1/8
   c)   1/3

Solution:
   a) After one half-life has elapsed, the amount remaining is 1/2 the original (by definition). After another half-life elapses, the amount remaining is now 1/2 of 1/2 the original amount, which is 1/4 the original amount. Therefore, a decrease to 1/4 the original amount requires 2 half-lives, which in this case is 2(70 hr) = 140 hr.
   b) The fraction 1/8 is equal to 1/2 of 1/2 of 1/2; that is, $1/8 = (1/2)^3$. In terms of half-lives, a decrease to 1/8 the original amount requires 3 half-lives, which in this case is equal to 3(70 hr) = 210 hr. *In general, a decrease to $(1/2)^n$ the original amount requires n half-lives.*
   c) The fraction 1/3 is not a whole-number power of 1/2, so we can't directly apply the fact given in the italicized sentence in the solution to part (b). However, 1/3 is between 1/2 and 1/4, so the time to get to 1/3 the original amount is between 1 and 2 half-lives. Since one half-life is 70 hr, the amount of time is between 70 and 140 hours; the middle of this range (since 1/3 is roughly in the middle between 1/2 and 1/4) is about 110 hours. The most general formula for calculating the elapsed time involves a logarithm: If $x < 1$ is the fraction of a radioactive substance remaining after a time t has elapsed, then

$$t = \frac{\log \frac{1}{x}}{\log 2} \times t_{1/2}$$

where $t_{1/2}$ is the half-life. (If you want to use this formula, remember that $\log 2 \approx 0.3$.)

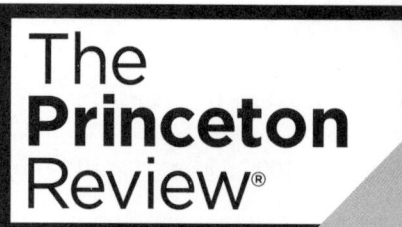
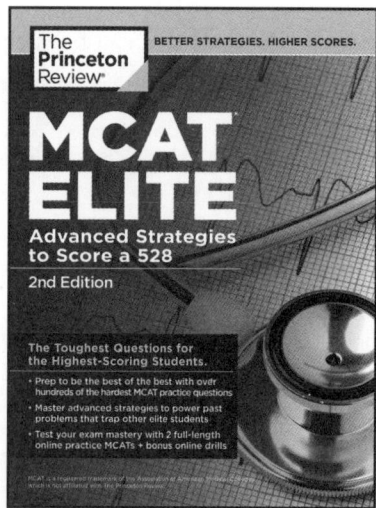
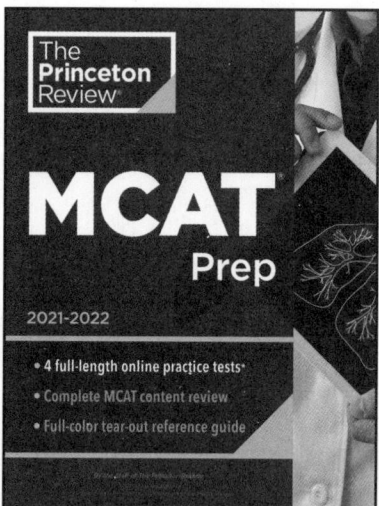
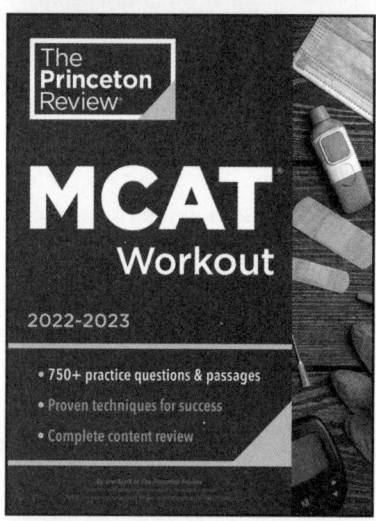
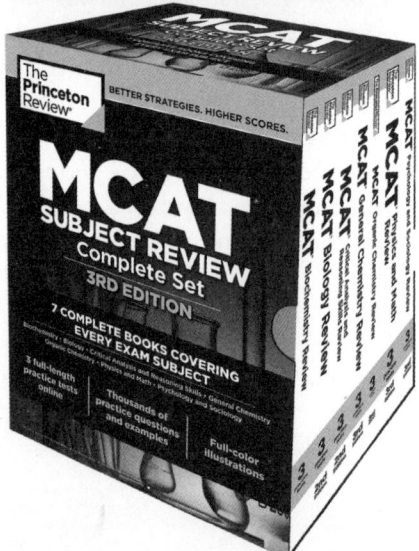

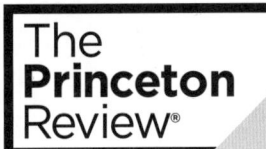
The Princeton Review®

MCAT®

Biochemistry Review

2nd Edition

The Staff of The Princeton Review

Penguin
Random
House

The Princeton Review
110 E. 42nd Street, 7th Floor
New York, NY 10017

Published in the United States by Penguin Random House
LLC, New York, and in Canada by Random House of Canada,
a division of Penguin Random House Ltd., Toronto.

Terms of Service: The Princeton Review Online Companion
Tools ["Student Tools"] for retail books are available for only
the two most recent editions of that book. Student Tools
may be activated only once per eligible book purchased
for a total of 24 months of access. Activation of Student
Tools more than once per book is in direct violation of these
Terms of Service and may result in discontinuation of
access to Student Tools Services.

ISBN: 978-0-593-51621-8
ISSN: 2380-7741

MCAT is a registered trademark of the Association of
American Medical Colleges.

The Princeton Review is not affiliated with Princeton
University.

The material in this book is up-to-date at the time of publication. However, changes may have been instituted by the
testing body in the test after this book was published.

If there are any important late-breaking developments,
changes, or corrections to the materials in this book, we
will post that information online in the Student Tools.
Register your book and check your Student Tools to see if
there are any updates posted there.

Every attempt has been made to obtain permission to
reproduce material protected by copyright. Where
omissions may have occurred the editors will be happy
to acknowledge this in future printings.

Permission has been granted to reprint portions of the
following

The Princeton Review Publishing Team
Rob Franek, Editor-in-Chief
David Soto, Senior Director, Data Operations
Stephen Koch, Senior Manager, Data Operations
Deborah Weber, Director of Production
Jason Ullmeyer, Production Design Manager
Jennifer Chapman, Senior Production Artist
Selena Coppock, Director of Editorial
Aaron Riccio, Senior Editor
Meave Shelton, Senior Editor
Chris Chimera, Editor
Orion McBean, Editor
Patricia Murphy, Editor
Laura Rose, Editor
Alexa Schmitt Bugler, Editorial Assistant

Random House Publishing Team
Tom Russell, VP, Publisher
Alison Stoltzfus, Senior Director, Publishing
Brett Wright, Senior Editor
Emily Hoffman, Assistant Managing Editor
Ellen Reed, Production Manager
Suzanne Lee, Designer
Eugenia Lo, Publishing Assistant

For customer service, please contact
editorialsupport@review.com,
and be sure to include:

- full title of the book

- ISBN

- page number

Editor: Chris Chimera
Production Editors: Kathy Carter and Lyssa Mandel
Production Artist: Jason Ullmeyer

Manufactured in China.

10 9 8 7 6 5 4 3 2 1

2nd Edition

CONTRIBUTORS

Daniel J. Pallin, M.D.
     Senior Author
Judene Wright, M.S., M.A.Ed.
     Senior Author

TPR MCAT Biology and Biochemistry Development Team:

Jessica Adams, Ph.D.
Britney McMurren, B.H.Sc., M.Sc.
Judene Wright, M.S., M.A.Ed., Senior Editor, Lead Developer
Sarah Woodruff, B.S., B.A.

Edited for Production by:

Judene Wright, M.S., M.A.Ed.
     National Content Director, MCAT Program, The Princeton Review

The TPR MCAT Biology and Biochemistry Team and Judene would like to thank the following people for their contributions to this book:

Kashif Anwar, M.D., M.M.S., John Bahling, M.D., Kristen Brunson, Ph.D., Phil Carpenter, Ph.D., Khawar Chaudry, B.S., Nita Chauhan, H.BSc, MSc, Dan Cho, M.P.H., Glenn E. Croston, Ph.D., Nathan Deal, M.D., Ian Denham, B.Sc., B.Ed., Joshua Dilworth, M.D., Ph.D., Annie Dude, Rob Fong, M.D., Ph.D., Chris Fortenbach, B.S., Kirsten Frank, Ph.D., Isabel L. Jackson, B.S., Erik Kildebeck, George Kyriazis, Ph.D., Ben Lee, Heather Liwanag, Ph.D., Travis MacKoy, B.S., Joey Mancuso, M.S., D.O., Evan Martow, BMSc, Brian Mikolasko, M.D., M.BA, Abhisehk Mohapatra, B.A., Christopher Moriates, M.D., Stephen L. Nelson, Jr., Ph.D., Rupal Patel, B.S., Mary Qiu, Ina C. Roy, M.D., Jayson Sack, M.D., M.S., Will Sanderson, Jeanine Seitz-Partridge, M.S., Oktay Shuminov, B.S., Andrew D. Snyder, M.D., Preston Swirnoff, Ph.D., M.S.,Jenkang Tao, B.S., B.A., Rhead Uddin, Jia Wang.

PERIODIC TABLE OF THE ELEMENTS

1																	18
1 **H** 1.0	2																**2** **He** 4.0
3 **Li** 6.9	**4** **Be** 9.0											13	14	15	16	17	**10** **Ne** 20.2
												5 **B** 10.8	**6** **C** 12.0	**7** **N** 14.0	**8** **O** 16.0	**9** **F** 19.0	
11 **Na** 23.0	**12** **Mg** 24.3	3	4	5	6	7	8	9	10	11	12	**13** **Al** 27.0	**14** **Si** 28.1	**15** **P** 31.0	**16** **S** 32.1	**17** **Cl** 35.5	**18** **Ar** 39.9
19 **K** 39.1	**20** **Ca** 40.1	**21** **Sc** 45.0	**22** **Ti** 47.9	**23** **V** 50.9	**24** **Cr** 52.0	**25** **Mn** 54.9	**26** **Fe** 55.8	**27** **Co** 58.9	**28** **Ni** 58.7	**29** **Cu** 63.5	**30** **Zn** 65.4	**31** **Ga** 69.7	**32** **Ge** 72.6	**33** **As** 74.9	**34** **Se** 79.0	**35** **Br** 79.9	**36** **Kr** 83.8
37 **Rb** 85.5	**38** **Sr** 87.6	**39** **Y** 88.9	**40** **Zr** 91.2	**41** **Nb** 92.9	**42** **Mo** 95.9	**43** **Tc** (98)	**44** **Ru** 101.1	**45** **Rh** 102.9	**46** **Pd** 106.4	**47** **Ag** 107.9	**48** **Cd** 112.4	**49** **In** 114.8	**50** **Sn** 118.7	**51** **Sb** 121.8	**52** **Te** 127.6	**53** **I** 126.9	**54** **Xe** 131.3
55 **Cs** 132.9	**56** **Ba** 137.3	**57** ***La** 138.9	**72** **Hf** 178.5	**73** **Ta** 180.9	**74** **W** 183.9	**75** **Re** 186.2	**76** **Os** 190.2	**77** **Ir** 192.2	**78** **Pt** 195.1	**79** **Au** 197.0	**80** **Hg** 200.6	**81** **Tl** 204.4	**82** **Pb** 207.2	**83** **Bi** 209.0	**84** **Po** (209)	**85** **At** (210)	**86** **Rn** (222)
87 **Fr** (223)	**88** **Ra** (226)	**89** **†Ac** (227)	**104** **Rf** (267)	**105** **Db** (268)	**106** **Sg** (271)	**107** **Bh** (270)	**108** **Hs** (269)	**109** **Mt** (278)	**110** **Ds** (281)	**111** **Rg** (282)	**112** **Cn** (285)	**113** **Nh** (286)	**114** **Fl** (289)	**115** **Mc** (289)	**116** **Lv** (293)	**117** **Ts** (294)	**118** **Og** (294)

*Lanthanoids	**58** **Ce** 140.1	**59** **Pr** 140.9	**60** **Nd** 144.2	**61** **Pm** (145)	**62** **Sm** 150.4	**63** **Eu** 152.0	**64** **Gd** 157.3	**65** **Tb** 158.9	**66** **Dy** 162.5	**67** **Ho** 164.9	**68** **Er** 167.3	**69** **Tm** 168.9	**70** **Yb** 173.0	**71** **Lu** 175.0
†Actinoids	**90** **Th** 232.0	**91** **Pa** (231)	**92** **U** 238.0	**93** **Np** (237)	**94** **Pu** (244)	**95** **Am** (243)	**96** **Cm** (247)	**97** **Bk** (247)	**98** **Cf** (251)	**99** **Es** (252)	**100** **Fm** (257)	**101** **Md** (258)	**102** **No** (259)	**103** **Lr** (266)

CONTENTS

Get More (**Free**) Content
at **PrincetonReview.com/prep**

As easy as **1·2·3**

1 Go to PrincetonReview.com/prep or scan the **QR code** and enter the following ISBN for your book: **9780593516218**

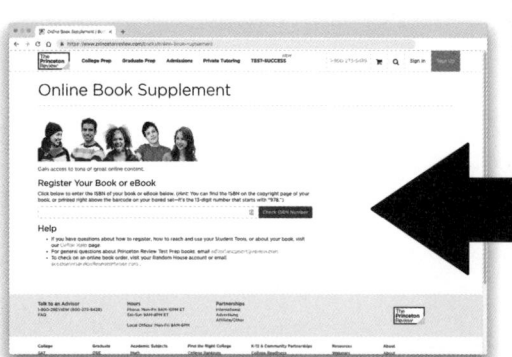

2 Answer a few simple questions to set up an exclusive Princeton Review account. *(If you already have one, you can just log in.)*

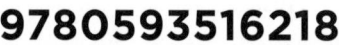

3 Enjoy access to your **FREE** content!

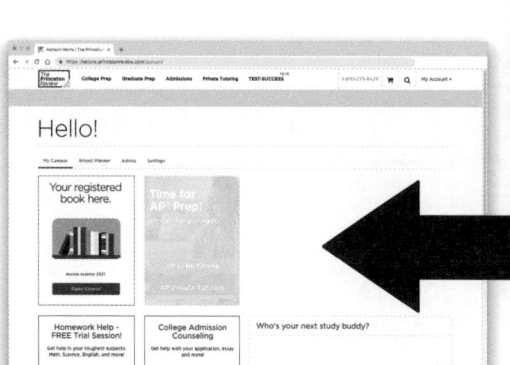

Once you've registered, you can...

- Take **3** full-length practice MCAT exams

- Find useful information about taking the MCAT and applying to medical school

- Check to see if there have been any corrections or updates to this edition

- Get our take on any recent or pending updates to the MCAT

Need to report a potential **content** issue?

Contact **EditorialSupport@review.com** and include:

- full title of the book
- ISBN
- page number

Need to report a **technical** issue?

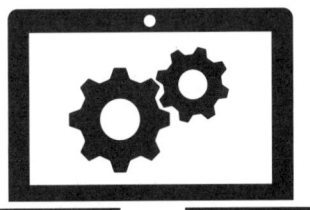

Contact **TPRStudentTech@review.com** and provide:

- your full name
- email address used to register the book
- full book title and ISBN
- Operating system (Mac/PC) and browser (Chrome, Firefox, Safari, etc.)

Chapter 1
MCAT Basics

SO YOU WANT TO BE A DOCTOR

So...you want to be a doctor. If you're like most premeds, you've wanted to be a doctor since you were pretty young. When people asked you what you wanted to be when you grew up, you always answered "a doctor." You had toy medical kits, bandaged up your dog or cat, and played "hospital." You probably read your parents' home medical guides for fun.

When you got to high school you took the honors and AP classes. You studied hard, got straight A's (or at least really good grades!), and participated in extracurricular activities so you could get into a good college. And you succeeded!

At college you knew exactly what to do. You took your classes seriously, studied hard, and got a great GPA. You talked to your professors and hung out at office hours to get good letters of recommendation. You were a member of the premed society on campus, volunteered at hospitals, and shadowed doctors. All that's left to do now is get a good MCAT score.

Just the MCAT.

Just the most confidence-shattering, most demoralizing, longest, most brutal entrance exam for any graduate program. At about 7.5 hours (including breaks), the MCAT tops the list...even the closest runners up, the LSAT and GMAT, are only about 4 hours long. The MCAT tests significant science content knowledge along with the ability to think quickly, reason logically, and read comprehensively, all under the pressure of a timed exam.

The path to a good MCAT score is not as easy to see as the path to a good GPA or the path to a good letter of recommendation. The MCAT is less about what you know, and more about how to apply what you know...and how to apply it quickly to new situations. Because the path might not be so clear, you might be worried. That's why you picked up this book.

We promise to demystify the MCAT for you, with clear descriptions of the different sections, how the test is scored, and what the test experience is like. We will help you understand general test-taking techniques as well as provide you with specific techniques for each section. We will review the science content you need to know as well as give you strategies for the Critical Analysis and Reasoning Skills (CARS) section. We'll show you the path to a good MCAT score and help you walk the path.

After all...you want to be a doctor. And we want you to succeed.

WHAT IS THE MCAT...REALLY?

Most test-takers approach the MCAT as though it were a typical college science test, one in which facts and knowledge simply need to be regurgitated in order to do well. They study for the MCAT the same way they did for their college tests, by memorizing facts and details, formulas and equations. And when they get to the MCAT, they are surprised...and disappointed.

It's a myth that the MCAT is purely a content-knowledge test. If medical-school admission committees want to see what you know, all they have to do is look at your transcripts. What they really want to see is how you think, especially under pressure. That's what your MCAT score will tell them.

The MCAT is really a test of your ability to apply basic knowledge to different, possibly new, situations. It's a test of your ability to reason out and evaluate arguments. Do you still need to know your science content? Absolutely. But not at the level that most test-takers think they need to know it. Furthermore, your science knowledge won't help you on the Critical Analysis and Reasoning Skills (CARS) section. So how do you study for a test like this?

You study for the science sections by reviewing the basics and then applying them to MCAT practice questions. You study for the CARS section by learning how to adapt your existing reading and analytical skills to the nature of the test (more information about the CARS section can be found in *MCAT Critical Analysis and Reasoning Skills Review*).

The book you are holding will review all the relevant MCAT Biochemistry content you will need for the test and a little bit more. It includes hundreds of questions designed to make you think about the material in a deeper way, along with full explanations to clarify the logical thought process needed to get to the answer. It also comes with access to three full-length online practice exams to further hone your skills. For more information on accessing those online exams, please refer to the "Get More (Free) Content" spread on page viii.

MCAT NUTS AND BOLTS

Overview

The MCAT is a computer-based test (CBT) that is *not* adaptive. Adaptive tests base your next question on whether or not you've answered the current question correctly. The MCAT is *linear*, or *fixed-form*, meaning that the questions are in a predetermined order and do not change based on your answers. However, there are many versions of the test, so that on a given test day, different people will see different versions. The following table highlights the features of the MCAT exam.

Registration	Online via www.aamc.org. Begins as early as six months prior to test date; available up until week of test (subject to seat availability).
Testing Centers	Administered at small, secure, climate-controlled computer testing rooms.
Security	Photo ID with signature, electronic fingerprint, electronic signature verification, assigned seat.
Proctoring	None. Test administrator checks examinee in and assigns seat at computer. All testing instructions are given on the computer.
Frequency of Test	Many times per year distributed over January, April, May, June, July, August, and September.
Format	Exclusively computer-based. NOT an adaptive test.
Length of Test Day	7.5 hours
Breaks	Optional 10-minute breaks between sections, with a 30-minute break for lunch.
Section Names	1. Chemical and Physical Foundations of Biological Systems (Chem/Phys) 2. Critical Analysis and Reasoning Skills (CARS) 3. Biological and Biochemical Foundations of Living Systems (Bio/Biochem) 4. Psychological, Social, and Biological Foundations of Behavior (Psych/Soc)
Number of Questions and Timing	59 Chem/Phys questions, 95 minutes 53 CARS questions, 90 minutes 59 Bio/Biochem questions, 95 minutes 59 Psych/Soc questions, 95 minutes
Scoring	Test is scaled. Several forms per administration.
Allowed/ Not allowed	No timers/watches. Noise reduction headphones available. Noteboard booklet and wet-erase marker given at start of test and taken at end of test. Locker or secure area provided for personal items.
Results: Timing and Delivery	Approximately 30 days. Electronic scores only, available online through AAMC login. Examinees can print official score reports.
Maximum Number of Retakes	The test can be taken a maximum of three times in one year, four times over two years, and seven times over the lifetime of the examinee. An examinee can be registered for only one date at a time.

Registration

Registration for the exam is completed online at www.aamc.org/students/applying/mcat/reserving. The AAMC opens registration for a given test date at least two months in advance of the date, often earlier. It's a good idea to register well in advance of your desired test date to make sure that you get a seat.

Sections

There are four sections on the MCAT exam: Chemical and Physical Foundations of Biological Systems (Chem/Phys), Critical Analysis and Reasoning Skills (CARS), Biological and Biochemical Foundations of Living Systems (Bio/Biochem), and Psychological, Social, and Biological Foundations of Behavior (Psych/Soc). All sections consist of multiple-choice questions.

Section	Concepts Tested	Number of Questions and Timing
Chemical and Physical Foundations of Biological Systems	Basic concepts in chemistry and physics, including biochemistry, scientific inquiry, reasoning, research and statistics skills.	59 questions in 95 minutes
Critical Analysis and Reasoning Skills	Critical analysis of information drawn from a wide range of social science and humanities disciplines.	53 questions in 90 minutes
Biological and Biochemical Foundations of Living Systems	Basic concepts in biology and biochemistry, scientific inquiry, reasoning, research and statistics skills.	59 questions in 95 minutes
Psychological, Social, and Biological Foundations of Behavior	Basic concepts in psychology, sociology, biology, research methods, and statistics.	59 questions in 95 minutes

Most questions on the MCAT (44 in the science sections, all 53 in the CARS section) are passage-based; the science sections have 10 passages each, and the CARS section has 9. A passage consists of a few paragraphs of information on which several following questions are based. In the science sections, passages often include equations or reactions, tables, graphs, figures, and experiments to analyze. CARS passages come from literature in social sciences, humanities, ethics, philosophy, cultural studies, and population health, and do not test content knowledge in any way.

Some questions in the science sections are freestanding questions (FSQs). These questions are independent of any passage information and appear in four groups of about three to four questions, interspersed throughout the passages. In the science sections, 15 of the question are freestanding, and the remainder are passage-based.

Each section on the MCAT is separated by either a 10-minute break or a 30-minute lunch break. We recommend that you take these breaks.

Section	Time
Test Center Check-In	Variable, can take up to 40 minutes if center is busy.
Tutorial	10 minutes
Chemical and Physical Foundations of Biological Systems	95 minutes
Break (optional)	10 minutes
Critical Analysis and Reasoning Skills	90 minutes
Lunch Break (optional)	30 minutes
Biological and Biochemical Foundations of Living Systems	95 minutes
Break (optional)	10 minutes
Psychological, Social, and Biological Foundations of Behavior	95 minutes
Void Option	5 minutes
Survey (optional)	5 minutes

The survey includes questions about your satisfaction with the overall MCAT experience, including registration, check-in, etc., as well as questions about how you prepared for the test.

Scoring

The MCAT is a scaled exam, meaning that your raw score will be converted into a scaled score that takes into account the difficulty of the questions. There is no guessing penalty. All sections are scored from 118–132, with a total scaled score range of 472–528. Because different versions of the test have varying levels of difficulty, the scale will be different from one exam to the next. Thus, there is no "magic number" of questions to get right in order to get a particular score. Plus, some of the questions on the test are considered "experimental" and do not count toward your score; they are just there to be evaluated for possible future inclusion in a test.

At the end of the test (after you complete the Psychological, Social, and Biological Foundations of Behavior section), you will be asked to choose one of the following two options, "I wish to have my MCAT exam scored" or "I wish to VOID my MCAT exam." You have five minutes to make a decision, and if you do not select one of the options in that time, the test will automatically be scored. If you choose the VOID option, your test will not be scored (you will not now, or ever, receive a numerical score for this test), medical schools will not know you took the test, and no refunds will be granted. You cannot "unvoid" your scores at a later time.

So, what's a good score? The AAMC is centering the scale at 500 (i.e., 500 will be the 50th percentile), and recommends that application committees consider applicants near the center of the range. To be on the safe side, aim for a total score of around 510. Remember that if your GPA is on the low side, you'll need higher MCAT scores to compensate, and if you have a strong GPA, you can get away with lower MCAT scores. But the reality is that your chances of acceptance depend on a lot more than just your MCAT scores. It's a combination of your GPA, your MCAT scores, your undergraduate coursework, letters of recommendation, experience related to the medical field (such as volunteer work or research), extracurricular activities, your personal statement, etc. Medical schools are looking for a complete package, not just good scores and a good GPA.

GENERAL LAYOUT AND TEST-TAKING STRATEGIES

Layout of the Test

In each section of the test, the computer screen is divided vertically, with the passage on the left and the range of questions for that passage indicated above (e.g., "Passage 1 Questions 1–5"). The scroll bar for the passage text appears in the middle of the screen. Each question appears on the right, and you need to click "Next" to move to each subsequent question.

In the science sections, the freestanding questions are found in groups of 3–4, interspersed with the passages. The screen is still divided vertically; on the left is the statement "Questions [X–XX] do not refer to a passage and are independent of each other," and each question appears on the right as described above.

CBT Tools

There are a number of tools available on the test, including highlighting, strike-outs, the Flag for Review button, the Navigation and Review Screen buttons, the Periodic Table button, and of course, the noteboard booklet. All tools are available with both mouse control (buttons to click) or keyboard commands (Alt+ a letter). As everyone has different preferences, you should practice with both types of tools (mouse and keyboard) to see which is more comfortable for you personally. The following is a brief description of each tool.

1) **Highlighting:** This is done in the passage text (including table entries and some equations, but excluding figures and molecular structures), in the question stems, and in the answer choices (including Roman numerals). Select the words you wish to highlight (left-click and drag the cursor across the words), and in the upper left corner click the "Highlight" button to highlight the selected text yellow. Alternatively, press "Alt+H" to highlight the words. Highlighting can be removed by selecting the words again and in the upper left corner clicking the down arrow next to "Highlight." This will expand to show the "Remove Highlight" option; clicking this will remove the highlighting. Removing highlighting via the keyboard is cumbersome and is not recommended.

2) **Strike-outs:** This can be done on the answer choices, including Roman numeral statements, by selecting the text you want to strike out (left-click and drag the cursor across the text) and then clicking the "Strikethrough" button in the upper left corner. Alternatively, press "Alt+S" to strike out the words. The strike-out can be removed by repeating these actions. **Figures or molecular structures cannot be struck out; however, the letter answer choice of those structures can.**

3) **Flag for Review button:** This is available for each question and is found in the upper right corner. This allows you to flag the question as one you would like to review later if time permits. When clicked, the flag icon turns yellow. Click again to remove the flag. Alternatively, press "Alt+F."

4) **Navigation button:** This is found near the bottom of the screen and is available only on your first pass through the section. Clicking this button brings up a navigation table listing all questions and their statuses (unseen, incomplete, complete, flagged for review). You can also press "Alt+N" to bring up the screen. The questions can be sorted by their statuses, and clicking a question number takes you immediately to that question. Once you have reached the end of the section and viewed the Review screen (described below), the Navigation screen is no longer available.

5) **Review Screen button:** This button is found near the bottom of the screen after your first pass through the section. When the button is clicked, it brings up a new screen showing all questions and their statuses (either incomplete, unseen, or flagged for review). Questions that are complete are assigned no additional status. You can then choose one of three options by clicking with the mouse or with keyboard

shortcuts: Review All (Alt+A), Review Incomplete (Alt+I), or Review Flagged (Alt+R); alternatively, you can click a question number to go directly back to that question. You can also end the section from this screen.

6) **Periodic Table button:** Clicking this button will open a periodic table (or press "Alt+T"). Note that the periodic table is large, covering most of the screen. However, this window can be resized to see the questions and a portion of the periodic table at the same time. The table text will not decrease, but scroll bars will appear on the window so you can center the section of the table of interest in the window.

7) **Noteboard Booklet (Scratch Paper):** At the start of the test, you will be given a spiral-bound set of four laminated 8.5"×14" sheets of paper and a wet-erase black marker to use as scratch paper. You can request a clean noteboard booklet at any time during the test; your original booklet will be collected. The noteboard is useful only if it is kept organized; do not give in to the tendency to write on the first available open space! Good organization will be very helpful when/if you wish to review a question. Indicate the passage number, the range of questions for that passage, and a topic in a box near the top of your scratch work, and indicate the question you are working on in a circle to the left of the notes for that question. Draw a line under your scratch work when you change passages to keep the work separate. Do not erase or scribble over any previous work. If you do not think it is correct, draw one line through the work and start again. You may have already done some useful work without realizing it.

General Strategy for the Science Sections

Passages vs. FSQs in the Science Sections: What to Start With

Since the questions are displayed on separate screens, it is awkward and time consuming to click through all of the questions up front to find the FSQs. Therefore, go through the section on a first pass and decide whether to do the passage now or to save it for later, basing your decision on the passage text and the first question. Tackle the FSQs as you come upon them. More details are below.

Here is an outline of the procedure:

1) For each passage, write a heading on your noteboard with the passage number, the general topic, and its range of questions (e.g., "Passage 1, thermodynamics, Q 1–5" or "Passage 2, enzymes, Q 6–9"). The passage numbers do not currently appear in the Navigation or Review screens; thus having the question numbers on your noteboard will allow you to move through the section more efficiently.

2) Skim the text and rank the passage. If a passage is a "Now," complete it before moving on to the next passage (also see Attacking the Questions below). If it is a "Later" passage, first write "SKIPPED" in block letters under the passage heading on your noteboard and leave room for your work when you come back to complete that passage. (Note that the specific passages you skip will be unique to you; in the Bio/Biochem section, you might choose to do all Biology passages first and then come back for Biochemistry. Or in Chem/Phys you might choose to skip experiment-based or analytical passage. Know ahead of time what type of passage you are going to skip and follow your plan.)

3) Next, click on the "Navigation" button at the bottom to get to the Navigation screen. Click on the first question of the next passage; you'll be able to identify it because you know the range of questions from the passage you just skipped. This will take you to the next passage, where you will repeat steps 1–3.

4) Once you have completed the "Now" passages, go to the Review screen and click the first question for the first passage you skipped. Answer the questions, and continue going back to the Review screen and repeating this procedure for other passages you have skipped.

Attacking the Questions

As you work through the questions, if you encounter a particularly lengthy question, or a question that requires a lot of analysis, you may choose to skip it. This is a wise strategy because it ensures you will tackle all the easier questions first, the ones you are more likely to get right. If you choose to skip the question (or if you attempt it but get stuck), write down the question number on your noteboard, click the Flag for Review button to flag the question in the Review screen, and move on to the next question. At the end of the passage, click back through the set of questions to complete any that you skipped over the first time through, and make sure that you have filled in an answer for every question.

General Strategy for the CARS Section

Ranking and Ordering the Passages: What to Start With

Ranking: Since the questions are displayed on separate screens, it is awkward and time consuming to click through all of the questions before ranking each passage as "Now" (an easier passage), "Later" (a harder passage), or "Killer" (a passage that you will randomly guess on). Therefore, rank the passage and decide whether or not to do it on the first pass through the section based on the passage text, skimming the first 2–3 sentences.

Ordering: Because of the additional clicking through screens (or, use of the Review screen) that is required to navigate through the section, the "Two-Pass" system (completing the "Now" passages as you find them) is likely to be your most efficient approach. However, if you find that you are continuously making a lot of bad ranking decisions, it is still valid to experiment with the "Three-Pass" approach (ranking all nine passages up front before attempting your first "Now" passage).

Here is an outline of the basic Ranking and Ordering procedure to follow.

1) For each passage, write a heading on your noteboard with the passage number and its range of questions (e.g. "Passage 1, Q 1–7"). The passage numbers do not currently appear in the Navigation or Review screens, thus having the question numbers on your noteboard will allow you to move through the section more efficiently.
2) Skim the first 2–3 sentences and rank the passage. If the passage is a "Now," complete it before moving on to the next. If it is a "Later" or "Killer," first write either "Later" or "Killer" and "SKIPPED" in block letters under the passage heading on your noteboard and leave room for your work if you decide to come back and complete that passage. Then click through each question, flagging each one and filling in random guesses, until you get to the next passage.
3) Once you have completed the "Now" passages, come back for your second pass and complete the "Later" passages, leaving your random guesses in place for any "Killer" passages that you choose not to complete. Go to the Review screen and use your noteboard notes on the question numbers. Click on the number of the first question for that passage to go back to that question, and proceed from there. Alternatively, if you have consistently flagged all the questions for passages you skipped in your first pass you can use "Review Flagged" from the Review screen to find and complete your "Later" passages.
4) Regardless of how you choose to find your second pass passages, unflag each question after you complete it, so that you can continue to rely on the Review screen (and the "Review Flagged" function) to identify questions that you have not yet attempted.

Previewing the Questions

The formatting and functioning of the tools facilitates effective previewing. Having each question on a separate screen will encourage you to really focus on that question. Even more importantly, you can highlight in the question stem and in the answer choices.

Here is the basic procedure for previewing the questions:

1) Start with the first question, and if it has lead words referencing passage content, highlight them. You may also choose to jot them down on your noteboard. Once you reach and preview the last question for the set on that passage, THEN stay on that screen and work the passage (your highlighting appears and stays on every passage screen, and persists through the whole 90 minutes).

2) Once you have worked the passage and defined the Bottom Line—the main idea and tone of the entire passage—work **backward** from the last question to the first. If you skip over any questions as you go (see Attacking the Questions below), write down the question number on your noteboard. Then click **forward** through the set of questions, completing any that you skipped over the first time through. Once you reach and complete the last question for that passage, clicking "Next" will send you to the first question of the next passage. Working the questions from last to first the first time through the set will eliminate the need to click back through multiple screens to get to the first question immediately after previewing, and it will also make it easier and more efficient to do the hardest questions last (see Attacking the Questions below).

3) Remember that previewing questions is a CARS-only technique. It is not efficient to preview questions in the science sections.

Attacking the Questions

The question types and the procedure for actually attacking each type will be discussed later. However, it is still important **not** to attempt the hardest questions first (potentially getting stuck, wasting time, and discouraging yourself).

So, as you work the questions from last to first (see Previewing the Questions above), if you encounter a particularly difficult and/or lengthy question (or if you attempt a question but get stuck), write down the question number on your noteboard (you may also choose to Flag it) and move on to the next question. Then click **forward** through the set and complete any that you skipped over the first time through the set, unflagging any questions that you flagged that first time through and making sure that you have filled in an answer for every question.

Pacing Strategy for the MCAT

Since the MCAT is a timed test, you must keep an eye on the timer and adjust your pacing as necessary. It would be terrible to run out of time at the end only to discover that the last few questions could have been easily answered in just a few seconds each.

In the science sections, you will have about one minute and thirty-five seconds (1:35) per question, and in the CARS section you will have about one minute and forty seconds (1:40) per question (not taking into account time reading the passage before answering the questions).

Section	# of Questions in Passage	Approximate Time (including reading the passage)
Chem/Phys, Bio/Biochem, and Psych/Soc	4	6.5 minutes
	5	8 minutes
	6	9.5 minutes
CARS	5	8.5 minutes
	6	10 minutes
	7	11.5 minutes

When starting a passage in the science sections, make note of how much time you will allot for it and the starting time on the timer. Jot down on your noteboard what the timer should say at the end of the passage. Then just keep an eye on it as you work through the questions. If you are near the end of the time for that passage, guess on any remaining questions, make some notes on your noteboard, Flag the questions, and move on. Come back to those questions if you have time.

For the CARS section, keep in mind that many people will maximize their score by *not* trying to complete every question or every passage in the section. A good strategy for test takers who cannot achieve a high level of accuracy on all nine passages is to randomly guess on at least one passage in the section, and spend your time getting a high percentage of the other questions right. To complete all nine CARS passages, you have about 10 minutes per passage. To complete eight of the nine, you have about 11 minutes per passage.

To help maximize your number of correct answer choices in any section, do the questions and passages within that section in the order *you* want to do them (see General Strategy).

Process of Elimination

Process of Elimination (POE) is probably the most useful technique you have to tackle MCAT questions. Since there is no guessing penalty, POE allows you to increase your probability of choosing the correct answer by eliminating those you are sure are wrong.

1) Strike out any choices that you are sure are incorrect or that do not address the issue raised in the question.
2) Jot down some notes to help clarify your thoughts if you return to the question.
3) Use the "Flag for Review" button to flag the question for review. (Note, however, that in the CARS section, you generally should not be returning to rethink questions once you have moved on to a new passage.)
4) Do not leave it blank! For the sciences, if you are not sure and you have already spent more than 60 seconds on that question, just pick one of the remaining choices. If you have time to review it at the end, you can always debate the remaining choices based on your previous notes. For CARS, if you have been through the choices two or three times, have reread the question stem and gone back to the passage and you are still stuck, move on. Do the remaining questions for that passage, take one more look at the question you were stuck on, then pick an answer and move on for good.

5) Special Note: If three of the four answer choices have been eliminated, the remaining choice must be the correct answer. Don't waste time pondering *why* it is correct, just click it and move on. The MCAT doesn't care if you truly understand why it's the right answer, only that you have the right answer selected.

6) More subject-specific information on techniques will be presented in the next chapter.

Guessing

Remember, there is NO guessing penalty on the MCAT. NEVER leave a question blank!

QUESTION TYPES

In the science sections of the MCAT, the questions fall into one of three main categories.

1) Memory questions: These questions can be answered directly from prior knowledge and represent about 25 percent of the total number of questions.

2) Explicit questions: These questions are those for which the answer is explicitly stated in the passage. To answer them correctly, for example, may just require finding a definition, reading a graph, or making a simple connection. Explicit questions represent about 35 percent of the total number of questions.

3) Implicit questions: These questions require you to apply knowledge to a new situation; the answer is typically implied by the information in the passage. These questions often start "if…then…." (For example, "If we modify the experiment in the passage like this, then what result would we expect?") Implicit style questions make up about 40 percent of the total number of questions.

In the CARS section, the questions fall into four main categories:

1) Specific questions: These either ask you for facts from the passage (Retrieval questions) or require you to deduce what is most likely to be true based on the passage (Inference questions).

2) General questions: These ask you to summarize themes (Main Idea and Primary Purpose questions) or evaluate an author's opinion (Tone/Attitude questions).

3) Reasoning questions: These ask you to describe the purpose of, or the support provided for, a statement made in the passage (Structure questions) or to judge how well the author supports his or her argument (Evaluate questions).

4) Application questions: These ask you to apply new information to the passage—information from either the question stem itself (New Information questions) or from the answer choices (Strengthen, Weaken, and Analogy questions).

More detail on question types and strategies can be found in Chapter 2.

TESTING TIPS

Before Test Day

- Take a trip to the test center at least a day or two before your actual test date so that you can easily find the building and room on test day. This will also allow you to gauge traffic and see if you need money for parking or anything like that. Knowing this type of information ahead of time will greatly reduce your stress on the day of your test.
- During the week before the test, adjust your sleeping schedule so that you are going to bed and getting up in the morning at the same times as on the day before and morning of the MCAT. Prioritize getting a reasonable amount of sleep during the last few nights before the test.
- Don't do any heavy studying the day before the test. This is not a test you can cram for! Your goal at this point is to rest and relax so that you can go into test day in a good physical and mental condition.
- Eat well. Try to avoid excessive caffeine and sugar. Ideally, in the weeks leading up to the actual test you should experiment a little bit with foods and practice tests to see which foods give you the most endurance. Aim for steady blood sugar levels during the test: sports drinks, peanut-butter crackers, trail mix, etc. make good snacks for your breaks and lunch.

General Test Day Info and Tips

- On the day of the test, arrive at the test center at least a half hour prior to the start time of your test.
- Examinees will be checked in to the center in the order in which they arrive.
- You will be assigned a locker or secure area in which to put your personal items. Textbooks and study notes are not allowed, so there is no need to take them with you to the test center.
- Your ID will be checked, a scan of your palm will be taken, and you will be asked to sign in.
- You will be given a noteboard booklet and a wet-erase marker. The test center administrator will take you to the computer on which you will complete the test. You may not choose a computer; you must use the computer assigned to you.
- Nothing, not even your watch, is allowed at the computer station except your photo ID, your locker key (if provided), and a factory sealed packet of ear plugs.
- If you choose to leave the testing room at the breaks, you will have your palm scanned again, and you will have to sign in and out.
- You are allowed to access the items in your locker, except for notes and cell phones. (Check your test center's policy on cell phones ahead of time; some centers do not even allow them to be kept in your locker.)
- Don't forget to take the snack foods and lunch you experimented with during your practice tests.
- At the end of the test, the test administrator will collect your noteboard and clean off your notes.
- Definitely take the breaks! Get up and walk around. It's a good way to clear your head between sections and get the blood (and oxygen!) flowing to your brain.
- Ask for a clean noteboard at the breaks if you want a fresh one.

Chapter 2
Biochemistry
Strategy for the MCAT

2.1 SCIENCE SECTIONS OVERVIEW

There are three science sections on the MCAT:

- Chemical and Physical Foundations of Biological Systems
- Biological and Biochemical Foundations of Living Systems
- Psychological, Social, and Biological Foundations of Behavior

The Chemical and Physical Foundations of Biological Systems section (Chem/Phys) is the first section on the test. It includes questions from General Chemistry (about 30%), Physics (about 25%), Organic Chemistry (about 15%), Biochemistry (about 25%), and Biology (about 5%). Further, the questions often test chemical and physical concepts within a biological setting: for example, pressure and fluid flow in blood vessels. A solid grasp of math fundamentals is required (arithmetic, algebra, graphs, trigonometry, vectors, proportions, and logarithms); however, there are no calculus-based questions.

The Biological and Biochemical Foundations of Living Systems section (Bio/Biochem) is the third section on the test. Approximately 65% of the questions in this section come from Biology, approximately 25% come from Biochemistry, and approximately 10% come from Organic and General Chemistry. Math calculations are generally not required on this section of the test; however, a basic understanding of statistics as used in biological research is helpful.

The Psychological, Social, and Biological Foundations of Behavior section (Psych/Soc) is the fourth and final section on the test. About 65% of the questions will be drawn from Psychology (and about 5% of these will be Biological Psychology), about 30% from Sociology, and about 5% from Biology. As with the Bio/Biochem section, calculations are generally not required; however a basic understanding of statistics as used in research is helpful.

Most of the questions in the science sections (44 of the 59) are passage-based, and each section has 10 passages. Passages consist of a few paragraphs of information and include equations, reactions, graphs, figures, tables, experiments, and data. Four to six questions will be associated with each passage.

The remaining 25% of the questions (15 of 59) in each science section are freestanding questions (FSQs). These questions appear in approximately four groups interspersed between the passages. Each group contains three to four questions.

You are allowed 95 minutes to complete each of the science sections. This breaks down to approximately one minute and 35 seconds per question.

2.2 SCIENCE PASSAGE TYPES

The passages in the science sections fall into one of three main categories: Information and/or Situation Presentation, Experiment/Research Presentation, or Persuasive Reasoning.

Information and/or Situation Presentation

These passages either present straightforward scientific information or they describe a particular event or occurrence. Generally, questions associated with these passages test basic science facts or ask you to predict outcomes given new variables or new information. Here is an example of an Information/Situation Presentation passage:

Figure 1 shows a portion of the inner mechanism of a typical home smoke detector. It consists of a pair of capacitor plates which are charged by a 9-volt battery (not shown). The capacitor plates (electrodes) are connected to a sensor device, D; the resistor R denotes the internal resistance of the sensor. Normally, air acts as an insulator and no current would flow in the circuit shown. However, inside the smoke detector is a small sample of an artificially produced radioactive element, americium-241, which decays primarily by emitting alpha particles, with a half-life of approximately 430 years. The daughter nucleus of the decay has a half-life in excess of two million years and therefore poses virtually no biohazard.

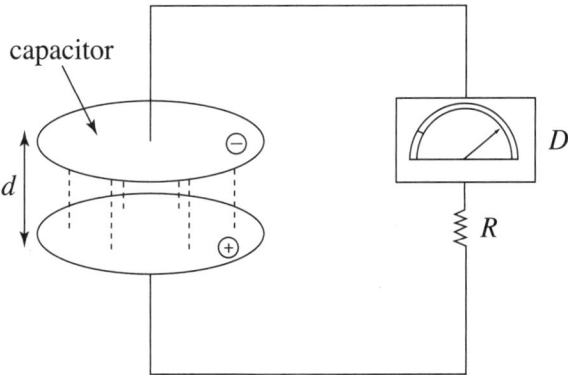

Figure 1 Smoke detector mechanism

The decay products (alpha particles and gamma rays) from the [241]Am sample ionize air molecules between the plates and thus provide a conducting pathway which allows current to flow in the circuit shown in Figure 1. A steady-state current is quickly established and remains as long as the battery continues to maintain a 9-volt potential difference between its terminals. However, if smoke particles enter the space between the capacitor plates and thereby interrupt the flow, the current is reduced, and the sensor responds to this change by triggering

the alarm. (Furthermore, as the battery starts to "die out," the resulting drop in current is also detected to alert the homeowner to replace the battery.)

$$C = \varepsilon_0 \frac{A}{d}$$

Equation 1

where ε_0 is the universal permittivity constant, equal to 8.85 $\times 10^{-12}$ $C^2/(N\ m^2)$. Since the area A of each capacitor plate in the smoke detector is 20 cm^2 and the plates are separated by a distance d of 5 mm, the capacitance is 3.5×10^{-12} F = 3.5 pF.

Experiment/Research Presentation

These passages present the details of experiments and research procedures. They often include data tables and graphs. Generally, questions associated with these passages ask you to interpret data, draw conclusions, and make inferences. Here is an example of an Experiment/Research Presentation passage:

The development of sexual characteristics depends upon various factors, the most important of which are hormonal control, environmental stimuli, and the genetic makeup of the individual. The hormones that contribute to the development include the steroid hormones estrogen, progesterone, and testosterone, as well as the pituitary hormones FSH (follicle-stimulating hormone) and LH (luteinizing hormone).

To study the mechanism by which estrogen exerts its effects, a researcher performed the following experiments using cell culture assays.

Experiment 1:

Human embryonic placental mesenchyme (HEPM) cells were grown for 48 hours in Dulbecco's Modified Eagle Medium (DMEM), with media change every 12 hours. Upon confluent growth, cells were exposed to a 10 mg per mL solution of green fluorescent-labeled estrogen for 1 hour. Cells were rinsed with DMEM and observed under confocal fluorescent microscopy.

Experiment 2:

HEPM cells were grown to confluence as in Experiment 1. Cells were exposed to Pesticide A for 1 hour, followed by the 10 mg/mL solution of labeled estrogen, rinsed as in Experiment 1, and observed under confocal fluorescent microscopy.

Experiment 3:

Experiment 1 was repeated with Chinese Hamster Ovary (CHO) cells instead of HEPM cells.

Experiment 4:

CHO cells injected with cytoplasmic extracts of HEPM cells were grown to confluence, exposed to the 10 mg/mL solution of labeled estrogen for 1 hour, and observed under confocal fluorescent microscopy.

The results of these experiments are given in Table 1.

Table 1 Detection of Estrogen (+ indicates presence of Estrogen)

Experiment	Media	Cytoplasm	Nucleus
1	+	+	+
2	+	+	+
3	+	+	+
4	+	+	+

After observing the cells in each experiment, the researcher bathed the cells in a solution containing 10 mg per mL of a red fluorescent probe that binds specifically to the estrogen receptor only when its active site is occupied. After 1 hour, the cells were rinsed with DMEM and observed under confocal fluorescent microscopy. The results are presented in Table 2.

The researcher also repeated Experiment 2 using Pesticide B, an estrogen analog, instead of Pesticide A. Results from other researchers had shown that Pesticide B binds to the active site of the cytosolic estrogen receptor (with an affinity 10,000 times greater than that of estrogen) and causes increased transcription of mRNA.

Table 2 Observed Fluorescence and Estrogen Effects (G = green, R = red)

Experiment	Media	Cytoplasm	Nucleus	Estrogen effects observed?
1	G only	G and R	G and R	Yes
2	G only	G only	G only	No
3	G only	G only	G only	No
4	G only	G and R	G and R	Yes

Based on these results, the researcher determined that estrogen had no effect when not bound to a cytosolic, estrogen-specific receptor.

2.2

Persuasive Reasoning

These passages typically present a scientific phenomenon along with a hypothesis that explains the phenomenon, and may include counter-arguments as well. Questions associated with these passages ask you to evaluate the hypothesis or arguments. Persuasive Reasoning passages in the science sections of the MCAT tend to be less common than Information Presentation or Experiment/Research Presentation passages. Here is an example of a Persuasive Reasoning passage:

Two theoretical chemists attempted to explain the observed trends of acidity by applying two interpretations of molecular orbital theory. Consider the pK_a values of some common acids listed along with the conjugate base:

acid	pK_a	conjugate base
H_2SO_4	< 0	HSO_4^-
H_2CrO_4	5.0	$HCrO_4^-$
H_3PO_4	2.1	$H_2PO_4^-$
HF	3.9	F^-
HOCl	7.8	ClO^-
HCN	9.5	CN^-
HIO_3	1.2	IO_3^-

Recall that acids with a $pK_a < 0$ are called strong acids, and those with a $pK_a > 0$ are called weak acids. The arguments of the chemists are given below.

Chemist #1:

"The acidity of a compound is proportional to the polarization of the H—X bond, where X is some nonmetal element. Complex acids, such as H_2SO_4, $HClO_4$, and HNO_3 are strong acids because the H—O bonding electrons are strongly drawn towards the oxygen. It is generally true that a covalent bond weakens as its polarization increases. Therefore, one can conclude that the strength of an acid is proportional to the number of electronegative atoms in that acid."

Chemist #2:

"The acidity of a compound is proportional to the number of stable resonance structures of that acid's conjugate base. H_2SO_4, $HClO_4$, and HNO_3 are all strong acids because their respective conjugate bases exhibit a high degree of resonance stabilization."

Mapping a Passage

"Mapping a passage" refers to the combination of on-screen highlighting and noteboard notes that you take while working through a passage. Typically, good things to highlight include the overall topic of a paragraph, unfamiliar terms, italicized terms, unusual terms, numerical values, any hypothesis, and experimental results. Noteboard notes can be used to summarize the paragraphs and to jot down important facts and connections that are made when reading the passage. More details on passage mapping will be presented in Section 2.5.

2.3 SCIENCE QUESTION TYPES

Questions in the science sections are generally one of three main types: Memory, Explicit, or Implicit.

Memory Questions

These questions can be answered directly from prior knowledge, with no need to reference the passage or question text. Memory questions represent approximately 25 percent of the science questions on the MCAT. Usually, Memory questions are found as FSQs, but they can also be tucked into a passage. Here's an example of a Memory question:

Which of the following acetylating conditions will convert diethylamine into an amide at the fastest rate?

A) Acetic acid / HCl
B) Acetic anhydride
C) Acetyl chloride
D) Ethyl acetate

2.3

Explicit Questions

Explicit questions can be answered primarily with information from the passage, along with prior knowledge. They may require data retrieval, graph analysis, or making a simple connection. Explicit questions make up approximately 35–40 percent of the science questions on the MCAT; here's an example (taken from the Information/Situation Presentation passage):

The sensor device *D* shown in Figure 1 performs its function by acting as:

A)   an ohmmeter.
B)   a voltmeter.
C)   a potentiometer.
D)   an ammeter.

Implicit Questions

These questions require you to take information from the passage, combine it with your prior knowledge, apply it to a new situation, and come to some logical conclusion. They typically require more complex connections than do Explicit questions, and they may also require data retrieval, graph analysis, etc. Implicit questions usually require a solid understanding of the passage information. They make up approximately 35–40 percent of the science questions on the MCAT; here's an example (taken from the Experiment/Research Presentation passage):

If Experiment 2 were repeated, but this time exposing the cells first to Pesticide A and then to Pesticide B before exposing them to the green fluorescent-labeled estrogen and the red fluorescent probe, which of the following statements will most likely be true?

A)   Pesticide A and Pesticide B bind to the same site on the estrogen receptor.
B)   Estrogen effects would be observed.
C)   Only green fluorescence would be observed.
D)   Both green and red fluorescence would be observed.

The Rod of Asclepius

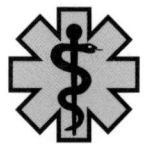

You may notice this Rod of Asclepius icon as you read through the book. In Greek mythology, the Rod of Asclepius is associated with healing and medicine; the symbol continues to be used today to represent medicine and healthcare. You won't see this on the actual MCAT, but we've used it here to call attention to medically related examples and questions.

2.4 BIOCHEMISTRY ON THE MCAT

The science sections of the MCAT all have 59 questions: 10 passages (with 44 total questions) and 15 freestanding questions. Biochemistry makes up a sizable chunk of two different sections of the MCAT. 25% of the Chemical and Physical Foundations of Biological Systems section, and 25% of the Biological and Biochemical Foundations of Living Systems section are made up of Biochemistry passages and questions. This means that in both sections approximately 15 of the 59 questions will be biochemistry based, and likely 2–3 of the passages will have a biochemistry theme. The application of this material can be anything from the details of some biochemical pathway, to the complexities of an experiment on a novel drug, to the subtleties of a condition caused by a missing or malfunctioning enzyme.

2.5 TACKLING A BIOCHEMISTRY PASSAGE

Generally speaking, time is not an issue in the Bio/Biochem section of the MCAT. Because students have a stronger background in biology and biochemistry than in other subjects, the passages seem more understandable; in fact, readers sometimes find themselves getting caught up and interested in the passage. Often, students report having about 5 to 10 minutes "left over" after completing the section. This means that an additional minute or so can potentially be spent on each passage, thinking and understanding.

Passage Types as They Apply to Biochemistry

Experiment/Research Presentation: Biochemistry

This is the most common type of Biochemistry passage. It typically presents the details behind an experiment along with data tables, graphs, and figures. Often these are the most difficult passages to deal with because they require an understanding of the reasoning behind the experiment, the logic to each step, and the ability to analyze the results and form conclusions. A basic understanding of biometry (basic statistics as they apply to biology and biochemistry research) is necessary.

Information/Situation Presentation: Biochemistry

This is the second most common type of Biochemistry passage on the MCAT. These passages generally appear as one of two variants: either a basic concept with additional levels of detail included (for example, all the detail you ever wanted to know about the electron transport chain), or a novel concept with ties to basic information (for example, a rare inborn error of metabolism and its effect on the body). Either way, Biochemistry passages are notorious for testing concepts in unusual contexts. The key to dealing with these passages is to, first, not become anxious about all the stuff you might not know, and second, figure out how the basics you do know apply to the new situation. For example, you might be presented with a passage that introduces hormones you never heard of or novel drugs to combat diseases you didn't know existed. First, don't panic. Second, look for how these new things fit into familiar categories: for example, "peptide vs. steroid" or "competitive inhibitor." Then answer the questions with these basics in mind.

That said, you have to know your basics. This will increase your confidence in answering freestanding questions, as well as increase the speed with which to find the information in the passage. The astute MCAT student will never waste time staring at a question thinking, "Should I know this?" Instead, because she has a solid understanding of the necessary core knowledge, she'll say, "No, I am NOT expected to know this, and I am going to look for it in the passage."

Persuasive Reasoning: Biochemistry

This is the least common passage type in Biochemistry. It typically describes some biological or biochemical phenomenon and offers one or more theories to explain it. Questions in Persuasive Reasoning passages ask you to determine support for one of the theories or present new evidence and ask which theory is now contradicted.

One last thought about Biochemistry passages in general: because the array of topics is so vast, passages in these sections of the test often pull questions from multiple areas of biology and/or biochemistry into a single, general topic. Consider, for example, a passage on hemoglobin. Question topics could include basics about enzymes and cooperative binding, protein structure, DNA mutations, effects of sickle cell disease, regulation of expression of the hemoglobin genes, and the data from an experiment done on sickle cell patients.

Reading a Biochemistry Passage

Although tempting, try not to get bogged down reading all the little details in a passage. Again, because most premeds have an inherent interest in biology and the mechanisms behind disease, it's very easy to get lost in the science behind the passages. In spite of having that "extra" time, you don't want to use it all up reading what isn't necessary. Each passage type requires a slightly different style of reading.

Information/Situation Presentation passages require the least reading. These should be skimmed to get an idea of the location of information within the passage. These passages include a fair amount of detail that you might not need, so save the reading of these details until a question comes up about them. Then go back and read for the finer nuances.

Experiment/Research Presentation passages require the most reading. You are practically guaranteed to get questions that ask you about the details of the experiment, why a particular step was carried out, why the results are what they are, how to interpret the data, or how the results might change if a particular variable is altered. It's worth spending a little more time reading to understand the experiment. However, because there will be a fair number of questions unrelated to the experiment, you might consider answering these first and then going back for the experiment details.

Persuasive Argument passages are somewhere in the middle. You can skim them for location of information, but you also want to spend a little time reading the details of and thinking about the arguments presented. It is extremely likely that you will be asked a question about them.

Advanced Reading Skills

To improve your ability to read and glean information from a passage, you need to practice. Be critical when you read the content; watch for vague areas or holes in the passage that aren't explained clearly. Remember that information about new topics will be woven throughout the passage; you may need to piece together information from several paragraphs and a figure to get the whole picture.

After you've read, highlighted, and mapped a passage (more on this in a bit), stop and ask yourself the following questions:

2.5

- What was this passage about? What was the conclusion or main point?
- Was there a paragraph that was mostly background?
- Were there paragraphs or figures that seemed useless?
- What information was found in each paragraph? Why was that paragraph there?
- Are there any holes in the story?
- What extra information could I have pulled out of the passage? What inferences or conclusions could I make?
- If something unique was explained or mentioned, what might be its purpose?
- What am I *not* being told?
- Can I summarize the purpose and/or results of the experiment in a few sentences?
- Were there any comparisons in the passage?

This takes awhile at first, but eventually it will become second nature and you'll start doing it as you read the passage. If you have a study group you are working with, consider doing this as an exercise with your study partners. Take turns asking and answering the questions above. Having to explain something to someone else not only solidifies your own knowledge, but helps you see where you might be weak.

Mapping a Biochemistry Passage

Mapping a Biochemistry passage is a combination of highlighting and noteboard notes that can help you organize and understand the passage information.

Resist the temptation to highlight everything! (Everyone has done this: you're reading a textbook with a highlighter, and then look back and realize that the whole page is yellow!) Restrict your highlighting to a few things:

- the main theme of a paragraph
- an unusual or unfamiliar term that is defined specifically for that passage (e.g., something that is italicized)
- statements that either support the main theme or contradict the main theme
- list topics: sometimes lists appear in paragraph form within a passage. Highlight the general topic of the list.
- relationships (how one thing changes relative to another thing)

The noteboard should be organized. Make sure the passage number appears at the top of your noteboard notes. For each paragraph, note "P1," "P2," etc., on the noteboard, and jot down a few notes about that paragraph. Try to translate biology/biochemistry jargon into your own words using everyday language (this is particularly useful for experiments). Also, make sure to note down simple relationships (e.g., the relationship between two variables).

Pay attention to equations, figures, and the like to see what type of information they deal with. Don't spend a lot of time analyzing at this point, but do jot down on your noteboard "Fig 1" and a brief summary of the data. Also, if you've discovered a list in the passage, note its topic and location on your noteboard.

Let's take a look at how we might highlight and map a passage. Below is a passage on the pentose phosphate pathway.

The pentose phosphate pathway (PPP) produces ribose-5-phosphate from glucose-6-phosphate and generates NADPH, which is used by the cell in biosynthetic pathways (such as fatty acid biosynthesis) as a reducing agent. Ribose-5-phosphate is converted to 5-phosphoribosyl-1-pyrophosphate (PRPP) by the enzyme ribose phosphate pyrophosphokinase. PRPP is an essential precursor in the biosynthesis of all nucleotides. Ribose phosphate pyrophosphokinase is inhibited by both ADP and GDP nucleotides.

The committed step in purine nucleotide synthesis is catalyzed by the enzyme amidophosphoribosyl transferase, which uses glutamine and PRPP as substrates. This enzyme is inhibited by AMP and GMP and is activated by high concentrations of PRPP. An intermediate in purine biosynthesis is inosine monophosphate (IMP). The conversion of IMP to AMP is inhibited by AMP, and the conversion of IMP to GMP is inhibited by GMP. An essential precursor in pyrimidine biosynthesis is carbamoyl phosphate, which is generated by the enzyme carbamoyl phosphate synthase. This enzyme is inhibited by UTP and activated by ATP and PRPP. The production of CTP from UTP is inhibited by CTP. These reactions are summarized in Figure 1.

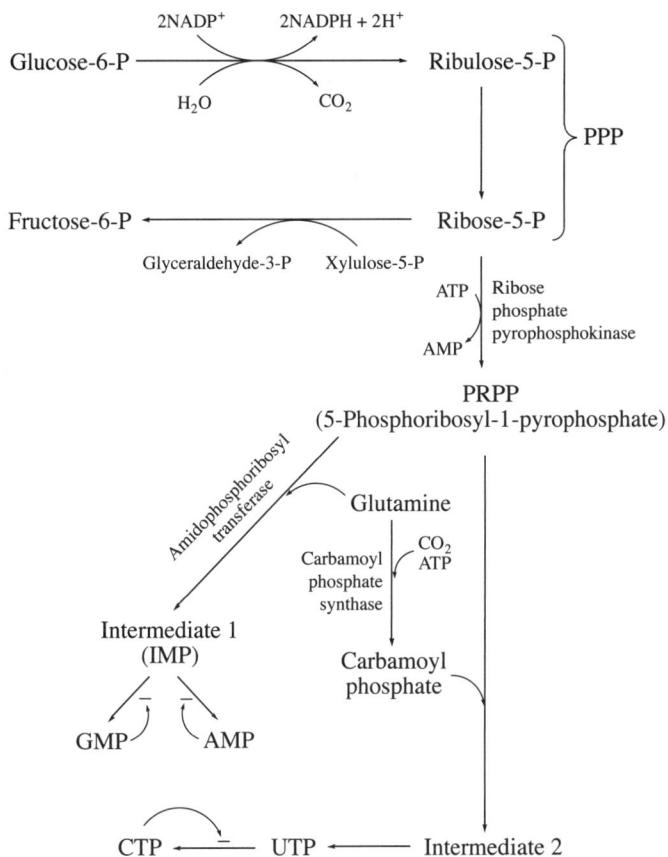

Figure 1 Biosynthetic pathway

Analysis and Passage Map

This passage is an Information Presentation passage and starts out with a paragraph about the pentose phosphate pathway. This is primarily a background paragraph and can be skimmed quickly, with a few words highlighted.

The second paragraph goes into more detail about the steps in purine and pyrimidine biosynthesis and specifically discusses some of the enzymes and their inhibitors. This paragraph presents information that is beyond what you are expected to know about the pentose phosphate pathway for the MCAT. Figure 1 shows some of the details of the pathway.

Here's what your passage map might look like:

> *P1 – pentose phosphate pathway, products and their uses*
> *P2 – committed step purines, enzyme and inhib.*
>   *precursor to pyrim., enzyme, and inhib.*
>   *Fig 1 = details of pathway*

Let's take a look at a different passage. Below is an Experiment/Research Presentation passage.

In times of fasting, the body relies more heavily on catabolism of amino acids to produce either ketone bodies (in the case of ketogenic amino acids) or precursors of glucose (in the case of glucogenic amino acids) through a series of interactions involving an α-ketoacid intermediate. A representative reaction is shown in Figure 1.

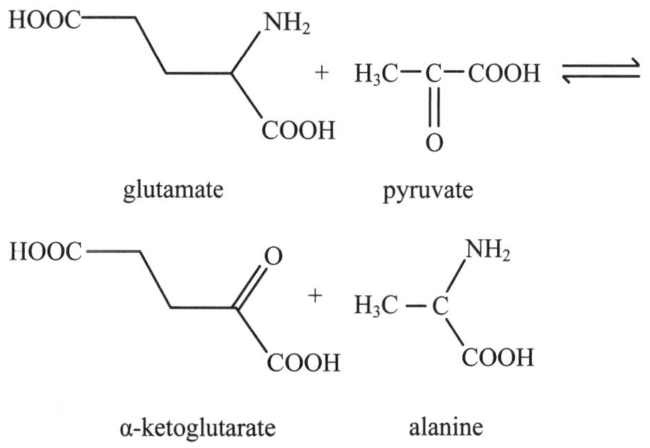

glutamate   pyruvate

α-ketoglutarate   alanine

Figure 1   Interconversion of pyruvate and alanine

"Low carb" diets capitalize on this feature of metabolism to achieve a ketogenic state in which the body is chronically deprived of carbohydrate sources of energy and thus forced to produce ketone bodies from either fat or amino acids to obtain energy. Interested in changes in the makeup of energy molecules in blood during this ketogenic state, researchers measure the levels of ketone bodies, glucose, insulin, glucagon, and fatty acids at various time points after a participant begins a ketogenic diet. Their findings are shown below.

	After normal meal	Overnight fasting	2 days after starting diet	5 days after starting diet
Insulin	↑	↓	↓	↓
Glucagon	↓	↑	↑	↑
Glucose	Normal	Normal	Normal	Normal
Fatty Acids	↑	↓	↑	↑ ↑ ↑
Ketones	↓	↓	↑	↑ ↑ ↑

Figure 2   Results of experiment

Adapted from Harvey, R. A., & Ferrier, D. R. (2011). *Lippincott's illustrated reviews, biochemistry* (5th ed.). Philadelphia: Wolters Kluwer Health.

Analysis and Passage Map

This passage starts out by describing the effects of fasting on the body and how it turns to amino acid catabolism to generate ketones or glucose precursors. It mentions the involvement of an α-ketoacid intermediate; Figure 1 shows this reaction.

The second paragraph describes how "low carb" diets can lead to ketogenesis. It also describes the experiment and refers us to Figure 2 for the results of the experiment.

Here's how your map might look:

P1 – fasting, a.a. catabolism → ketones, glu precursors
P2 – low carb diet effects, desc. of experiment
Fig 2 – keto diet causes ↑ glucagon, fats, and ketones and ↓ insulin

One last thought about passages: as with all sections on the MCAT, you can do the passages in the order *you* want to. There are no extra points for taking the test in order. Generally, passages in the Bio/Biochem section will fall into one of four main subject groups:

- biochemistry
- other non-physiology
- physiology
- organic/general chemistry

Figure out which group you are most comfortable with and do those passages first. See Chapter 1 for general strategies for moving through each of the sections efficiently.

2.5

2.6 TACKLING THE QUESTIONS

Questions in the Bio/Biochem section mimic the three typical questions of the science sections in general: Memory, Explicit, and Implicit.

Question Types as They Apply to Biochemistry

Biochemistry Memory Questions

Memory questions are exactly what they sound like: they test your knowledge of some specific fact or concept. While Memory questions are typically found as freestanding questions, they can also be tucked into a passage. These questions, aside from requiring memorization, do not generally cause problems for students because they are similar to the types of questions that appear on a typical college biochemistry exam. Below is an example of a freestanding Memory question:

> ACE inhibitors are a class of drugs frequently prescribed to treat hypertension. Captopril, a compound that is structurally similar to angiotensin I, was developed in 1975 as the first ACE inhibitor. When patients take Captopril, which of the following is true about the kinetics of their ACE?
>
> A) V_{max} decreases, K_m remains the same.
> B) V_{max} remains the same, K_m increases.
> C) Both V_{max} and K_m increase.
> D) Both V_{max} and K_m remain the same.

The correct answer to the question above is choice B. Here's another example. This question is from a passage:

> GAPDH converts an aldehyde into a carboxylic acid in order to change NAD^+ to NADH. Which of the following is true regarding this reaction in humans?
>
> A) The aldehyde is reduced.
> B) NAD^+ is oxidized.
> C) NAD^+ gains 2 e^- and one proton.
> D) The carboxylic acid ($pK_a = 2.19$) is mostly in its protonated form.

The question asks you to draw on your knowledge of oxidation/reduction reactions. The correct answer is choice C.

There is no specific "trick" to answering Memory questions; either you know the answer or you don't.

If you find that you are missing a fair number of Memory questions, it is a sure sign that you don't know the content well enough. Go back and review.

Biochemistry Explicit Questions

True, pure Explicit questions are rare in the Bio/Biochem section. A purely Explicit question can be answered only with information in the passage. Below is an example of a pure Explicit question taken from the previous pentose phosphate pathway passage:

> Which of the following are products of the pentose phosphate pathway?
>
> I. NADPH
> II. Glycolytic intermediates
> III. Ribose-5-phosphate
>
> A) I only
> B) II only
> C) I and III only
> D) I, II, and III

2.6

The map for this passage indicates that information about the products of the pathway are in paragraph 1 and Figure 1. Paragraph 1 states that NADPH and ribose 5-phosphate are both products, and Figure 1 shows that both fructose 6-P and glyceraldehyde 3-P are glycolytic intermediates. The correct answer is choice D.

However, more often in this section, Explicit questions are more of a blend of Explicit and Memory; they require not only retrieval of passage information, but also recall of some relevant fact. They usually do not require a lot of analysis or connections. Here's an example of the more common type of Explicit question, taken from the ketogenesis passage on page 28:

> Which of the following enzymes in the liver is most active five days after someone starts a ketogenic diet?
>
> A) Hexokinase
> B) Phosphofructokinase I
> C) HMG-CoA synthase
> D) Glycogen phosphorylase

To answer this question, you first need to retrieve information from the passage about the substances that are elevated in the blood after five days on a ketogenic diet. From Figure 2 you know that fatty acids, ketones, and glucagon are elevated. You also need to remember the metabolic pathways in which the enzymes in the answer choices participate. Hexokinase and phosphofructokinase I are glycolytic enzymes, and fats and ketones are not products of glycolysis. Thus it is unlikely that these enzymes would be very active (choices A and B can be eliminated). Glycogen phosphorylase breaks down glycogen. Fats and ketones are not the products of glycogen breakdown, so it is unlikely that glycogen phosphorylase would be very active. The correct answer is HMG-CoA synthase, choice C.

Graph interpretation questions comprise a final subgroup in the Explicit question category. These fall into one of two types: those that ask you to take graphical information from the passage and convert it to a text answer, or those that take text from the passage and ask you to convert it to a graph. On the following page is an example of the latter type.

Which of the following represents the Lineweaver-Burk plot of an enzyme alone (solid line) and in the presence of an inhibitor that binds exclusively to the enzyme active site (dashed line)?

A)

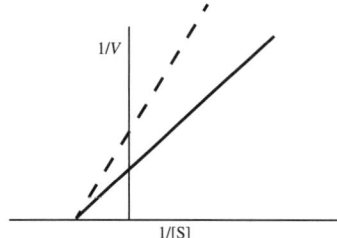

B)

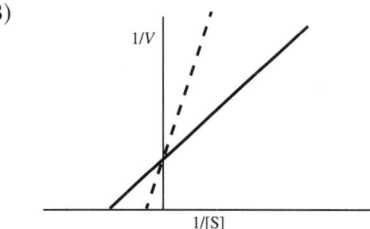

C)

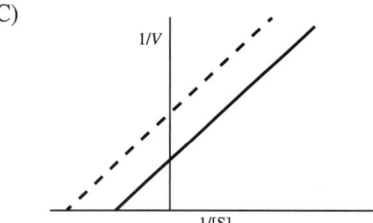

D)

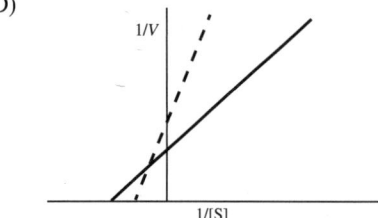

The passage for this question describes how a Lineweaver-Burk plot is generated. You have to combine that information with your knowledge about enzyme inhibitors and how they affect V_{max} and K_m. The correct answer for this question is choice B.

If you find that you are missing Explicit questions, practice your passage mapping. Make sure you aren't missing the critical items in the passage that lead you to the right answer. Slow down a little; take an extra 15 to 30 seconds per passage to read or think about it more carefully.

Biochemistry Implicit Questions

Implicit questions require the most thought. These require recall not only of biochemistry information but also information gleaned from the passage and a more in-depth analysis of how the two relate. Implicit questions require more analysis and connections to be made than Explicit questions. Often they take the form "If...then...." Below is an example of a classic Implicit question, taken from the ketogenesis passage shown earlier.

> If the researchers observed on Day 6 that the levels of fatty acids and ketones decreased while the level of insulin increased, which of the following could be assumed?
>
> A) Protein and amino acid catabolism has increased in this participant.
> B) The participant consumed a meal containing carbohydrates.
> C) An increase in Krebs cycle activity would also be observed.
> D) Glucagon levels would be unchanged from their levels five days after starting the ketogenic diet.

To answer this question, conclusions have to be drawn from the experiments described in the passage, and new conclusions have to be predicted based on the new circumstance. You must make many more connections than when you are answering an Explicit question. From the passage, you need to realize that the low insulin levels on Day 5, combined with high fatty acid and ketone levels in the blood, indicate that the participant is in ketosis, i.e, is burning fat as fuel. If insulin levels suddenly rise while fats and ketones fall, the participant must have eaten some carbohydrates. Protein and amino acid catabolism can result in ketone body production, according to the passage. If protein and amino acid catabolism had increased, you would expect if anything, to see an increase in ketone bodies, not a decrease (choice A is false). There is no reason to assume that Krebs cycle activity would increase; Krebs generally runs well during ketogenesis because of the acetyl CoA from fat breakdown. If the levels of fats are decreased on Day 6, then Krebs cycle activity would likely decrease as well (choice C is false). Insulin and glucagon are opposing hormones; insulin is released when blood sugar levels increase, and glucagon is released when blood sugar levels fall. If insulin is elevated, the glucagon will be decreased (choice D is false).

If you find that you are missing a lot of Implicit questions, first make sure that you are using POE aggressively. Second, go back and review the explanations for the correct answer to figure out where your logic went awry. Did you miss an important fact in the passage? Did you forget the relevant Biochemistry content? Did you follow the logical train of thought to the right answer? Once you figure out where you made your mistake, you will know how to correct it.

2.7 SUMMARY OF THE APPROACH TO BIOCHEMISTRY

2.7

How to Map the Passage and Use the Noteboard

1) The passage should not be read like textbook material, with the intent of learning something from every sentence (science majors especially will be tempted to read this way). Passages should be read to get a feel for the type of questions that will follow and to get a general idea of the location of information within the passage.

2) Highlighting—Use this tool sparingly, or you will end up with a passage that is completely covered in yellow highlighter! Highlighting in a Biochemistry passage should be used to draw attention to a few words that demonstrate one of the following:
   - the main theme of a paragraph
   - an unusual or unfamiliar term that is defined specifically for that passage (e.g., something that is italicized)
   - statements that either support the main theme or counteract the main theme
   - list topics (see below)
   - relationships`

3) Pay brief attention to equations, figures, and experiments, noting only what information they deal with. Do not spend a lot of time analyzing at this point.

4) For each passage, start by noting the passage number, the general topic, and the range of questions on your noteboard. You can then work between your noteboard and the Review screen to easily get to the questions you want (see Chapter 1).

5) For each paragraph, note "P1," "P2," etc. on the noteboard and jot down a few notes about that paragraph. Try to translate biochemistry jargon into your own words using everyday language. Especially note down simple relationships (e.g., the relationship between two variables).

6) Lists—Whenever a list appears in paragraph form, jot down on the noteboard the paragraph and the general topic of the list. It will make returning to the passage more efficient and help to organize your thoughts.

7) The noteboard is useful only if it is kept organized! Make sure that your notes for each passage are clearly delineated and marked with the passage number and question range. This will allow you to easily read your notes when you come back to a review a flagged question. Resist the temptation to write in the first available blank space as this makes it much more difficult to refer back to your work.

Biochemistry Question Strategies

1) Remember that the amount of potential content in Biochemistry is significant, so don't panic if something seems completely unfamiliar. Understand the basic content well, find the basics in the unfamiliar topic, and apply them to the question.

2) Process of Elimination is paramount! The strikeout tool allows you to eliminate answer choices; this will improve your chances of guessing the correct answer if you are unable to narrow it down to one choice.

3) Answer the straightforward questions first (typically the memory questions). Leave questions that require analysis of experiments and graphs for later. Take the test in the order YOU want. Make sure to use your noteboard to indicate questions you skipped.

4) Make sure that the answer you choose actually answers the question and isn't just a true statement.

5) Try to avoid answer choices with extreme words such as "always," "never," etc. In biology, there is almost always an exception and answers are rarely black-and-white.

6) Roman numeral questions: whenever possible, start by evaluating the Roman numeral item that shows up in exactly two answer choices. This allows you to quickly eliminate two wrong answer choices regardless of whether the item is true or false. Typically then, you will have to assess only one of the other Roman numeral items to determine the correct answer. Always work between the I-II-III items and the answer choices. Once an item is found to be true (or false), strike out answer choices which do not contain (or do contain) that item number. Make sure to strike out the actual Roman numeral item as well, and highlight those items that are true.

7) LEAST/EXCEPT/NOT questions: don't get tricked by these questions that ask you to pick that answer that doesn't fit (the incorrect or false statement). Make sure to highlight the words "LEAST," "EXCEPT," OR "NOT" in the question stem. It's often good to use your noteboard and write "A B C D" with a T or F next to each answer choice. The one that stands out as different is the correct answer!

8) Again, don't leave any question blank.

A Note About Flashcards

For most of the exams you've taken previously, flashcards were likely very helpful. This was because those exams mostly required you to regurgitate information, and flashcards are pretty good at helping you memorize facts. However, the most challenging aspect of the MCAT is not that it requires you to memorize the fine details of content knowledge, but that it requires you to apply your basic scientific knowledge to unfamiliar situations: flashcards alone may not help you there.

Flashcards can be beneficial if your basic content knowledge is deficient in some area. For example, if you don't know the amino acids and their 1- and 3-letter abbreviations, flashcards can certainly help you memorize these facts. Or, maybe you are unsure of the functions of the different types of enzymes. You might find that flashcards can help you memorize these. But unless you are trying to memorize basic facts in your personal weak areas, you are better off doing and analyzing practice passages than carrying around a stack of flashcards.

2.7

Chapter 3
Biochemistry Basics

The notion of life refers to both the activities and the physical structures of living organisms. Both the storage/utilization of energy and the synthesis of structures depend on a large number of chemical reactions that occur within each cell. Fortunately, these reactions do not proceed on their own spontaneously, without regulation. If they did, each cell's energy would rapidly dissipate and total disorder would result. Most reactions are slowed by a large barrier known as the activation energy (E_a), discussed below. The E_a is a bottleneck in a reaction, like a nearly closed gate. The role of the enzyme is to open this chemical gate. In this sense, the enzyme is like a switch. When the enzyme is on, the gate is open (low E_a) and the reaction accelerates. When the enzyme is off, the gate closes and the reaction slows. Before we discuss how enzymes work, we must digress a bit to review the basics of thermodynamics. Then we can review some of the major metabolic pathways in the cell.

3.1 THERMODYNAMICS

Thermodynamics is the study of the energetics of chemical reactions. There are two relevant forms of energy in chemistry: kinetic energy (movement of molecules) and potential energy (energy stored in chemical bonds). [What is the most important potential energy storage molecule in all cells?[1]] The **first law of thermodynamics,** also known as the **law of conservation of energy,** states that the energy of the universe is constant. It implies that when the energy of a system *decreases,* the energy of the rest of the universe (the **surroundings**) must *increase,* and vice versa. The **second law of thermodynamics** states that the disorder, or **entropy,** of the universe tends to increase. Another way to state the second law is as follows: spontaneous reactions tend to increase the disorder of the universe. The symbol for entropy is S, and "a change in entropy" is denoted ΔS, where $\Delta S = S_{final} - S_{initial}$. [If the ΔS of a system is negative, has the disorder of that system increased or decreased?[2]]

A practical way to discuss thermodynamics is the mathematical notion of **free energy (Gibbs free energy),** defined by Josiah Gibbs as follows:[3]

$$\textbf{Eq. 1} \quad \Delta G = \Delta H - T\Delta S$$

T denotes temperature, and H denotes **enthalpy,** which is defined by another equation:

$$\textbf{Eq. 2} \quad \Delta H = \Delta E + P\Delta V$$

Here E represents the bond energy of products or reactants in a system, P is pressure, and V is volume. [Given that cellular reactions take place in the liquid phase, how is H related to E in a cell?[4]] ΔG increases with increasing ΔH (bond energy) and decreases with increasing entropy.

- Given the second law of thermodynamics and the mathematical definition of ΔG, which reaction will be favorable: one with a decrease in free energy ($\Delta G < 0$) or one with an increase in free energy ($\Delta G > 0$)?[5]

The change in the Gibbs free energy of a reaction determines whether the reaction is favorable (**spontaneous,** ΔG negative) or unfavorable (**nonspontaneous,** ΔG positive). In terms of the generic reaction

$$A + B \rightarrow C + D$$

the Gibbs free energy change determines whether the reactants (denoted A and B) will stay as they are or be converted to products (C and D).

---

[1] ATP, which stores energy in the ester bonds between its phosphate groups.

[2] If ΔS is negative, then the system lost entropy, which means that disorder decreased.

[3] As in ΔS, the Greek letter Δ (delta) indicates "the change in." For example, $\Delta G_{rxn} = G_{products} - G_{reactants}$.

[4] $H \approx E$, since the change in volume is negligible ($\Delta V \approx 0$).

[5] Favorable reactions have $\Delta G < 0$. We can deduce this from the second law and Equation 1 because the second law states that increasing entropy is favorable, and the equation has ΔG directly related to $-T\Delta S$.

Spontaneous reactions, ones that occur without a net addition of energy, have $\Delta G < 0$. They occur with energy to spare. Reactions with a negative ΔG are **exergonic** (energy *exits* the system); reactions with a positive ΔG are **endergonic**. Endergonic reactions occur only if energy is added. In the lab, energy is added in the form of heat; in the body, endergonic reactions are driven by reaction coupling to exergonic reactions (more on this later). Reactions with a negative ΔH are called **exothermic** and liberate heat. Most metabolic reactions are exothermic (which is how homeothermic organisms such as mammals maintain a constant body temperature). Reactions with a positive ΔH require an input of heat and are referred to as **endothermic**. (Thermodynamics will be discussed in more detail in *MCAT General Chemistry Review* and *MCAT Physics and Math Review*.)

The signs of thermodynamic quantities are assigned from the point of view of *the system*, not the surroundings or the universe. Thus, a negative ΔG means that the system goes to a lower free energy state, and a system will always move in the direction of the lowest free energy. As an analogy, visualize a spinning top as the system. What happens to the top? Does it spin faster and faster? No. It moves towards the lowest energy state. Let's expand the analogy, using an equation:

$$\text{motionless top} \;\rightarrow\; \text{spinning top}$$

Here the "reactant" is the motionless top, and the "product" is the spinning top. Which is lower: the free energy of product or reactant? The reactant. Is the reaction "spontaneous" as written? No; in fact, the reverse reaction is spontaneous. Therefore,

$$G_{\text{spinning}} > G_{\text{motionless}}$$

and thus,

$$\Delta G_{\text{reaction as written (motionless to spinning; left to right)}} > 0$$

So the reaction is nonspontaneous. In other words, *it requires energy input*, namely, energy from your muscles as you spin the top. [If the products in a reaction have more entropy than the reactants and the enthalpy (H) of the reactants and the products are the same, can the reaction occur spontaneously?[6]]

The value of ΔG depends on the concentrations of reactants and products, which can be variable in the body. Therefore, to compare reactions, chemists calculate a standard free energy change, denoted $\Delta G°$, with all reactants and products present at 1 M concentration. Under physiological conditions, however, the hydrogen ion concentration is far from 1 M, so biochemists use an even more standardized ΔG, with 1 M concentration for all solutes except H^+ and a pH of 7; this is denoted $\Delta G°'$.

$\Delta G°'$ is related to the equilibrium constant for a reaction by the following equation:

$$\textbf{Eq. 3}\quad \Delta G°' = -RT \ln K'_{eq}$$

---

6   Yes. If $\Delta S > 0$ and $\Delta H = 0$, then according to the second law of thermodynamics, the reaction is spontaneous; see Equation 1.

where R is the gas constant (which would be given on the MCAT, along with the entire equation), and K'_{eq} is the ratio of products to reactants at equilibrium:

$$K'_{eq} = \frac{[C]_{eq}[D]_{eq}}{[A]_{eq}[B]_{eq}}$$

K'_{eq} is the ratio of products to reactants when enough time has passed for equilibrium to be reached [When $K'_{eq} = 1$, what is $\Delta G^{\circ\prime}$?[7]]

But what if we wanted to calculate ΔG for a reaction in the body? In this case, we need one more equation:

Eq. 4 $\Delta G = \Delta G^{\circ\prime} + RT \ln Q$, where $Q = \dfrac{[C][D]}{[A][B]}$

Here, Q is calculated using the actual concentrations of A, B, C, and D (for example, the concentrations in the cell). Equation 4 is simply a conversion from $\Delta G^{\circ\prime}$ (the laboratory standard ΔG with initial concentrations at 1 M) to the real-life here-and-now ΔG. Note that if we put 1 M concentrations of A, B, C, and D into a beaker (at pH 7), we have recreated the laboratory standard initial set-up: $Q = 1$, so $\ln Q = 0$, which means $\Delta G = \Delta G^{\circ\prime}$.

Remember that Q and K_{eq} are not the same. Q is the ratio of products to reactants in any given set-up; K_{eq} is the ratio *at equilibrium*. **Equilibrium** is defined as the point at which the rate of reaction in the forward direction equals the rate of reaction in the reverse direction. At equilibrium, there is constant product and reactant turnover as reactants form products and vice versa, but overall concentrations stay the same. Theoretically (given enough time), all reactant/product systems in a closed system will eventually reach this point.

While all reactions will eventually reach an equilibrium defined by the constant above, we can disturb this balance with the addition or removal of a reactant or product. This causes a change in Q but not K_{eq}, and the reaction will proceed in the direction necessary to reestablish equilibrium. (The shift to restore equilibrium is a demonstration of Le Châtelier's principle which will be discussed in further detail in *MCAT General Chemistry Review*.) Using this principle, a reaction which favors reactants at equilibrium can be driven to generate additional products (such strategies are employed frequently in cellular respiration).

- You are studying a particular reaction. You find the reaction in a book and read $\Delta G^{\circ\prime}$ from a table. Can you calculate ΔG for this reaction in a living human being without any more information?[8]

---

[7] Equation 3 says that $\Delta G^{\circ\prime} = 0$ when $K'_{eq} = 1$ since $\ln 1 = 0$. Note: for more information about MCAT Math, see *MCAT Physics and Math Review*.

[8] No. You need to know the concentrations of A, B, C, and D in the human cell. For example, $\Delta G^{\circ\prime}$ might be +14.8 kcal/mol, indicating that the reaction is very unfavorable under standard conditions and has a $K < 1$, which means that at equilibrium there are more reactants than products. If, however, the ratio of reactants to products is made to be higher than that established at equilibrium, the Q for the reaction becomes less than K, and the forward reaction is spontaneous under these conditions, since ΔG will be less than zero (even though $\Delta G^{\circ\prime}$ will not change). The significance of Q as an independent variable in Equation 4 is that it accounts for Le Châtelier's principle. If a system at equilibrium has reactants added to it, $Q < K$ and $\Delta G < 0$, so the high concentration of reactants will drive the reaction forward to reestablish equilibrium. If a system at equilibrium has products added to it, $Q > K$ and $\Delta G > 0$, so the high concentration of products will drive the reaction backward to reestablish equilibrium. All reactions at equilibrium will respond to these stresses in the same way, regardless of the sign of their $\Delta G^{\circ\prime}$.

- How can ΔG be negative if $\Delta G^{\circ\prime}$ is positive (which indicates that the reaction is unfavorable at standard conditions)?[9]
- Does K_{eq} indicate the rate at which a reaction will proceed?[10]
- When K_{eq} is large, which has lower free energy: products or reactants?[11]
- When Q is large, which has lower free energy: products or reactants?[12]
- Which direction, forward or backward, will be favored in a reaction if $\Delta G = 0$? (*Hint*: What does Equation 4 look like when $\Delta G = 0$?)[13]
- Radiolabeled chemicals are often used to trace constituents in biochemical reactions. The following reaction with $\Delta G = 0$ is in aqueous solution:

$$A \rightleftharpoons B + C, \quad K_{eq} = \frac{[B][C]}{[A]}$$

A small amount of radiolabeled B is added to the solution. After a period of time, where will the radiolabel most likely be found: in A, in B, or in both?[14]

In summary, then, there are two factors that determine whether a reaction will occur spontaneously (ΔG negative) in the cell:

1) The intrinsic properties of the reactants and products (K_{eq})
2) The concentrations of reactants and products ($RT \ln Q$)

(In the lab there is third factor: temperature. If $\ln Q$ is negative and the temperature is high enough, ΔG will be negative, regardless of the value of $\Delta G^{\circ\prime}$.)

---

[9] The reaction may be favorable ($\Delta G < 0$) if the ratio of the concentrations of reactants to products is sufficiently large to drive the reaction forward (that is, if $RT \ln Q$ is more negative than $\Delta G^{\circ\prime}$ is positive, which would make their sum (which, by Equation 4, is ΔG) negative).

[10] K_{eq} indicates only the relative concentrations of reagents once equilibrium is reached, not the reaction rate (how fast equilibrium is reached).

[11] A large K_{eq} means that more products are present at equilibrium. Remember that equilibrium tends toward the lowest energy state. Hence, when K_{eq} is large, products have lower free energy than reactants.

[12] The size of Q says nothing about the properties of the reactants and products. Q is calculated from whatever the initial concentrations happen to be. It is K_{eq} that says something about the nature of reactants and products, since it describes their concentrations after equilibrium has been reached.

[13] If ΔG is 0, then neither the forward nor the reverse reaction is favored. Look at Equations 3 and 4. Note that when $\Delta G = 0$, Equation 4 reduces to Equation 3, and thus $Q = K_{eq}$ (which means Q at this moment is the same as K_{eq}, measured after the reaction system is allowed to reach equilibrium). When $Q = K_{eq}$, we are by definition at equilibrium. Understand and memorize the following: when $\Delta G = 0$, you are at equilibrium; forward reaction rate equals back reaction rate, and the net concentrations of reactants and products do not change.

[14] The reaction is in dynamic equilibrium where reactions are occurring in both directions, but at an equal rate. Because $\Delta G = 0$, we know that the forward reaction and the reverse reaction proceed at equal rates, even though we don't know the actual value. Therefore, after a period of time, the radiolabel will be present in both A and B.

Thermodynamics vs. Reaction Rates

The term *spontaneous* is used to describe a reaction system with $\Delta G < 0$. This can be misleading, since the common usage of the word *spontaneous* has a connotation of *rapid rate*; this is not what spontaneous means in the context of chemical reactions. For example, many reactions have a negative ΔG, indicating that they are "spontaneous" from a thermodynamic point of view, but they do not necessarily occur at a significant rate. Spontaneous means that a reaction is energetically favorable, *but it says nothing about the rate of reaction.*

Thermodynamics will tell you where a system starts and finishes but nothing about the path traveled to get there. The difference in free energy in a reaction is only a function of the nature of the reactants and products. Thus, ΔG does not depend on the pathway a reaction takes or the rate of reaction; it is only a measurement of the difference in free energy between reactants and products.

3.2 KINETICS AND ACTIVATION ENERGY (E_A)

The reason some spontaneous (i.e., *thermodynamically favorable*) reactions proceed very slowly or not at all is that a large amount of energy is required to get them going. For example, the burning of wood is spontaneous, but you can stare at a log all day and it won't burn. Some energy (heat) must be provided to kick-start the process.

The study of reaction rates is called **chemical kinetics**. All reactions proceed through a **transition state** **(TS)** that is unstable and takes a great deal of energy to produce. The transition state exists for a very, very short time, either moving forward to form products or breaking back down into reactants. The energy required to produce the transition state is called the **activation energy** (E_a). This is the barrier that prevents many reactions from proceeding even though the ΔG for the reaction may be negative. The match you use to light your fireplace provides the activation energy for the reaction known as burning. It is the activation energy barrier that determines the kinetics of a reaction. [How would the rate of a spontaneous reaction be affected if the activation energy were lowered?[15]]

The concept of E_a is key to understanding the role of enzymes, so let's spend some time on it. To illustrate, take this reaction:

$$\text{Bob}_{\text{without a job}} + \text{job} \rightarrow \text{Bob}_{\text{with a job}}$$

Is this a favorable reaction, i.e., will the universe be better off, with less total (nervous) energy, if Bob gets the job? Will things settle down? Let's assume yes. However, between the two states (without/with), there is a temporary state, namely, $\text{Bob}_{\text{applying for job}}$. So the reaction will look this way:

$$\text{Bob}_{\text{without a job}} + \text{job} \rightarrow [\text{Bob}_{\text{applying for job}}]^{\ddagger} \rightarrow \text{Bob}_{\text{with a job}}$$

---

[15] The rate would be increased, since lowering E_a is tantamount to reducing the energy required to achieve the transition state. The more transition state products that are formed, the greater the amount of product produced, i.e., the more rapid the rate of reaction.

The middle term is the transition state, traditionally written in square brackets with a double-cross symbol: [TS]‡. The energy required for Bob to be job hunting is much higher than the energy of Bob with a job *or* Bob without a job. As a result, he may not go job hunting, even though he'd be happier in the long run if he did. In this model, we can describe the E_a as the energy necessary to get Bob to apply for a job.

A **catalyst** lowers the E_a of a reaction *without changing the* ΔG. The catalyst lowers the E_a by *stabilizing the transition state*, making its existence less thermodynamically unfavorable. The second important characteristic of a catalyst is that it is not consumed in the reaction; it is *regenerated* with each reaction cycle.

In our model, an example of a catalyst would be a career planning service (CPS). Adding a CPS won't make Bob$_{without\ a\ job}$ any happier or sadder, nor will it make Bob$_{with\ a\ job}$ happier or sadder. But it will make it much easier for Bob to move between the two states: without a job versus with a job. The traditional way to represent a reaction system like this is using a *reaction coordinate* graph, as shown in Figure 1. This is just a way to look at the energy of the reaction system as compared to the three possible states of the system: 1) reactants, 2) [TS]‡, and 3) products. The *x*-axis plots the physical progress of the reaction system (the "reaction coordinate"), and the *y*-axis plots energy.

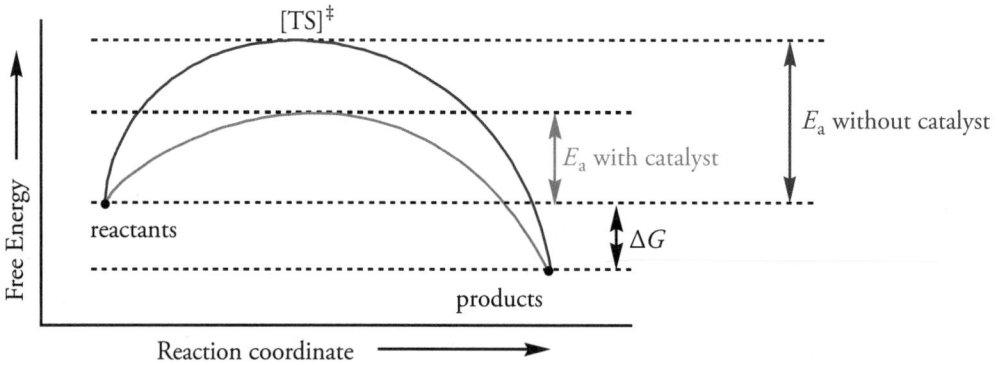

Figure 1   The Reaction Coordinate Graph

Enzymes are biological catalysts. They increase the rate of a reaction by lowering the reaction's activation energy, but they *do not affect* ΔG between reactants and products. As catalysts, enzymes have a kinetic role, *not* a thermodynamic one. [Will an enzyme alter the concentration of reagents at equilibrium?[16]] Enzymes may alter the rate of a reaction enormously: a reaction that would take a hundred years to reach equilibrium without an enzyme may occur in just seconds with an enzyme. More information on enzymes can be found in Chapter 4.

---

[16] No. It will affect only the rate at which the reactants and products reach equilibrium.

3.3 OXIDATION AND REDUCTION

Energy Metabolism and the Definitions of Oxidation and Reduction

Where does the energy in foods come from? How do we make use of this energy? Why do we breathe? The answers begin with **photosynthesis**, the process by which plants store energy from the sun in the bond energy of carbohydrates. Plants are **photoautotrophs** because they use energy from light ("photo") to make their own ("auto") food. We are **chemoheterotrophs**, because we use the energy of chemicals ("chemo") produced by other ("hetero") living things, namely plants and other animals. Plants and animals store chemical energy in reduced molecules such as carbohydrates and fats. These reduced molecules are oxidized to produce CO_2 and ATP. The energy of ATP is used in turn to drive the energetically unfavorable reactions of the cell. That's the basic energetics of life; all the rest is detail.

In essence, the production and utilization of energy boil down to a series of oxidation/reduction reactions. **Oxidation** is a chemical term meaning the loss of electrons. **Reduction** means the opposite, the gain of electrons. Molecules can gain or lose electrons depending on the other atoms that they are bound to. There are three common ways to identify oxidation/reduction reactions on the MCAT, and it is important for you to know them:

Recognizing Oxidation Reactions:

1) gain of oxygen atoms
2) loss of hydrogen atoms
3) loss of electrons

Recognizing Reduction Reactions (just the opposite):

1) loss of oxygen atoms
2) gain of hydrogen atoms
3) gain of electrons

Though you should memorize this, it is not a subject worthy of philosophizing. If you can answer questions like the following, you're set: is changing CH_3CH_3 to $H_2C=CH_2$ an oxidation, a reduction, or neither?[17] What about changing Fe^{3+} to Fe^{2+}?[18] What about this: $O_2 \rightarrow H_2O$?[19] You can also identify oxidation/reduction reactions visually by looking at the structure of the molecules. Is the formation of a disulfide bond (Figure 2) an oxidation or a reduction reaction?[20]

---

[17] It's an oxidation, because hydrogens have been removed.

[18] It's a reduction, because an electron has been added.

[19] It's a reduction, because hydrogens have been added to the oxygen molecule.

[20] It's an oxidation, because hydrogens have been removed.

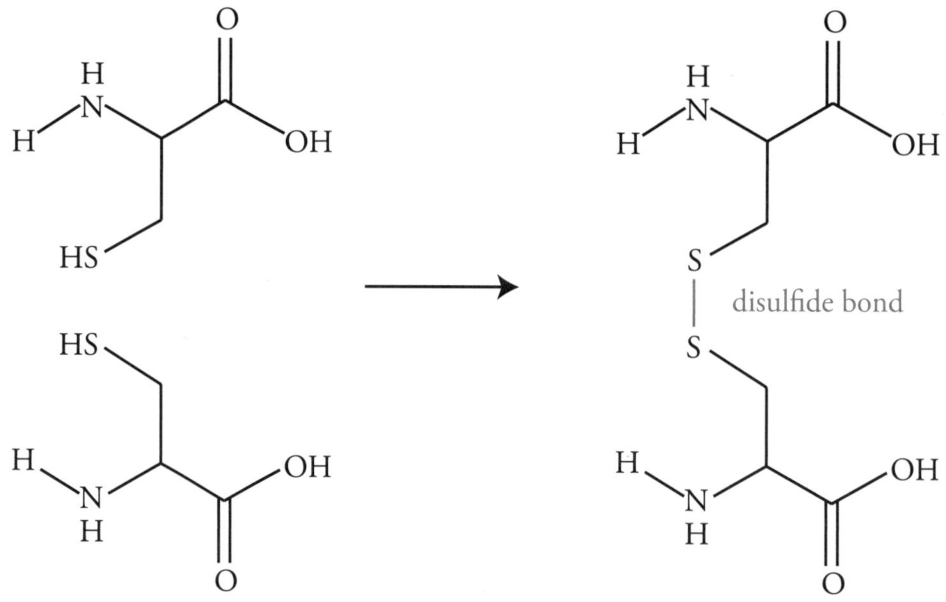

Figure 2 Formation of a Disulfide Bond

Here is one other important fact about oxidation and reduction: when one atom gets reduced, another one *must* be oxidized; hence the term ***redox pair***. As you study the process of glucose oxidation, you will see that each time an oxidation reaction occurs, a reduction reaction occurs too.

Catabolism is the process of breaking down molecules. The opposite is **anabolism**, which is "building-up" metabolism.[21] For example, the way we extract energy from glucose is by **oxidative catabolism**. We break down the glucose by oxidizing it. The stoichiometry of glucose oxidation looks like this:

$$C_6H_{12}O_6 + 6\,O_2 \;\rightarrow\; 6\,CO_2 + 6\,H_2O$$

- What are the two members of the redox pair in this reaction?[22]

As we oxidize foods, we release the stored energy plants received from the sun. But we don't make use of that energy right away. Instead, we store it in the form of ATP. Alternatively, we can use the energy in ATP to generate storage molecules such as glycogen and fatty acids. Fatty acids are generated by successive reductions of a carbon chain, thus anabolic processes are generally reductive.

---

[21] The mnemonics are *cata* = breakdown, as in catastrophe, and *ana* = buildup, sounds like "add-a." (Think of anabolic steroids, which weightlifters use to bulk up.)

[22] The carbons in the sugar are oxidized (to CO_2), and oxygen is reduced (to H_2O).

3.4 ACIDS AND BASES

There are two important definitions of acids and bases you should be familiar with for biochemistry on the MCAT.

Brønsted-Lowry Acids and Bases

Brønsted and Lowry offered the following definitions:

> *Acids are proton (H^+) donors.*
> *Bases are proton (H^+) acceptors.*

While the often seen hydroxide ions qualify as Brønsted-Lowry bases, many other compounds fit this definition as well. Since a Brønsted-Lowry base is any substance that is capable of accepting a proton, any anion or any neutral species with a lone pair of electrons can function as a base.

If we consider the reversible reaction below:

$$H_2CO_3 + H_2O \rightleftharpoons H_3O^+ + HCO_3^-$$

then according to the Brønsted-Lowry definition, H_2CO_3 and H_3O^+ are acids and HCO_3^- and H_2O are bases. The Brønsted-Lowry definition of acids and bases is the most important one for the MCAT.

Lewis Acids and Bases

Lewis's definitions of acids and bases are broader:

> *Lewis acids are electron-pair acceptors.*
> *Lewis bases are electron-pair donors.*

If we consider the reversible reaction below:

$$AlCl_3 + H_2O \rightleftharpoons (AlCl_3OH)^- + H^+$$

then according to the Lewis definition, $AlCl_3$ and H^+ are acids because they accept electron pairs; H_2O and $(AlCl_3OH)^-$ are bases because they donate electron pairs. Lewis acid/base reactions frequently result in the formation of coordinate covalent bonds. For example, in the reaction above, water acts as a Lewis base, since it donates both of the electrons involved in the coordinate covalent bond between OH^- and $AlCl_3$. $AlCl_3$ acts as a Lewis acid, since it accepts the electrons involved in this bond.

3.4

The binding of an oxygen molecule to the iron atom in a heme group is a great biological example of a coordinate covalent bond formed between a Lewis acid and base:

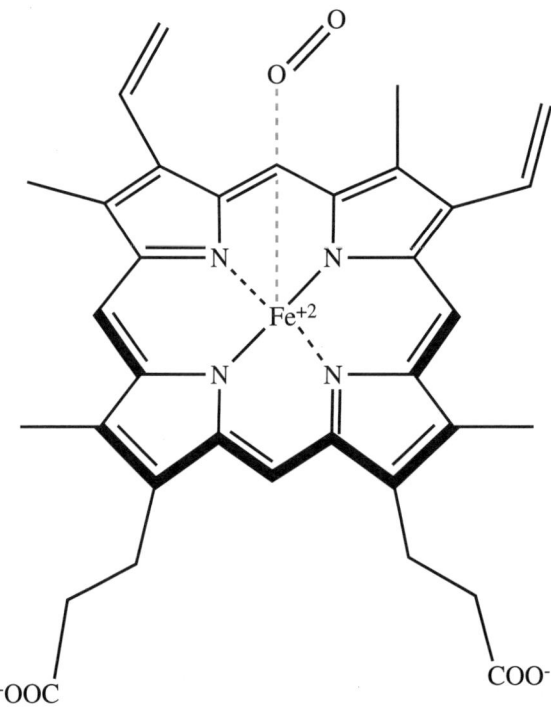

Figure 3   Example of a Coordinate Covalent Bond

- Is oxygen the Lewis acid or Lewis base in the heme group?[23]

Conjugate Acids and Bases

When a Brønsted-Lowry acid donates an H⁺, the remaining structure is called the **conjugate base** of the acid. Likewise, when a Brønsted-Lowry base bonds with an H⁺ in solution, this new species is called the **conjugate acid** of the base. To illustrate these definitions, consider this reaction:

acid–base conjugates

$$NH_3 + H_2O \rightleftharpoons NH_4^+ + OH^-$$

acid–base conjugates

---

[23] Oxygen is donating a pair of electrons to the Fe^{2+} ion and is therefore the Lewis base.

Considering only the forward direction, NH_3 is the base and H_2O is the acid. The products are the conjugate acid and conjugate base of the reactants: NH_4^+ is the conjugate acid of NH_3, and OH^- is the conjugate base of H_2O:

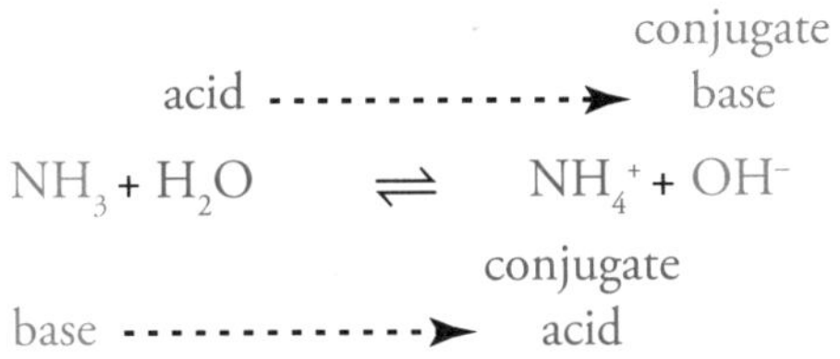

Now consider the reverse reaction in which NH_4^+ is the acid and OH^- is the base. The conjugates are the same as for the forward reaction: NH_3 is the conjugate base of NH_4^+, and H_2O is the conjugate acid of OH^-:

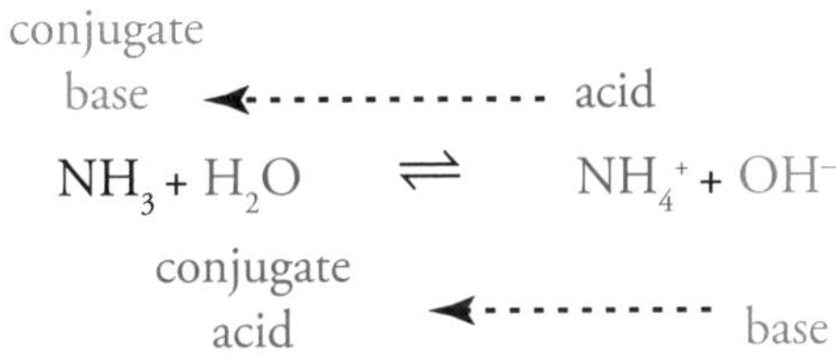

The difference between a Brønsted-Lowry acid and its conjugate base is that the base is missing an H^+. The difference between a Brønsted-Lowry base and its conjugate acid is that the acid has an extra H^+.

forming conjugates:

$$\text{acid} \underset{+\,H^+}{\overset{-\,H^+}{\rightleftharpoons}} \text{base}$$

The Strengths of Acids and Bases

If we use HA to denote a generic acid, its dissociation in water has the form

$$HA(aq) + H_2O(l) \rightleftharpoons H_3O^+(aq) + A^-(aq)$$

The strength of the acid is directly related to how much the products are favored over the reactants. The equilibrium expression for this reaction is

$$K_a = \frac{[H_3O^+][A^-]}{[HA]}$$

This is written as K_a, rather than K_{eq}, to emphasize that this is the equilibrium expression for an <u>a</u>cid-dissociation reaction. In fact, K_a is known as the **acid-ionization** (or **acid-dissociation**) **constant** of the acid (HA). We can rank the relative strengths of acids by comparing their K_a values: the larger the K_a value, the stronger the acid; the smaller the K_a value, the weaker the acid.

- Of the following acids, which one would dissociate to the greatest extent (in water)?[24]
  A) HCN (hydrocyanic acid), $K_a = 6.2 \times 10^{-10}$
  B) HNCO (cyanic acid), $K_a = 3.3 \times 10^{-4}$
  C) HClO (hypochlorous acid), $K_a = 2.9 \times 10^{-8}$
  D) HBrO (hypobromous acid), $K_a = 2.2 \times 10^{-9}$

We can apply the same ideas as above to identify the strength of *bases*. If we use B to denote a generic base, its dissolution in water has the form

$$B(aq) + H_2O(l) \rightleftharpoons HB^+(aq) + OH^-(aq)$$

Similar to acids, the strength of the base is directly related to how much the products are favored over the reactants. If we write the equilibrium constant for this reaction, we get:

$$K_b = \frac{[HB^+][OH^-]}{[B]}$$

This is written as K_b, rather than K_{eq}, to emphasize that this is the equilibrium expression for a <u>b</u>ase-dissociation reaction. In fact, K_b is known as the **base-ionization** (or **base-dissociation**) **constant**. We can rank the relative strengths of bases by comparing their K_b values: the larger the K_b value, the stronger the base; the smaller the K_b value, the weaker the base.

Amphoteric Substances

Take a look at the dissociation of carbonic acid (H_2CO_3), a weak acid:

$$H_2CO_3(aq) + H_2O(l) \rightleftharpoons H_3O^+(aq) + HCO_3^-(aq) \quad (K_a = 4.5 \times 10^{-7})$$

The conjugate base of carbonic acid is HCO_3^-, which also has an ionizable proton. Carbonic acid is said to be **polyprotic**, because it has more than one proton to donate.

---

[24] **B.** The acid that would dissociate to the greatest extent would have the greatest K_a value. Of the choices given, HNCO (choice B) has the greatest K_a value.

Let's look at how the conjugate base of carbonic acid dissociates:

$$HCO_3^-(aq) + H_2O(l) \rightleftharpoons H_3O^+(aq) + CO_3^{2-}(aq) \quad (K_a = 4.8 \times 10^{-11})$$

In the first reaction, HCO_3^- acts as a base, but in the second reaction, it acts as an acid. Whenever a substance can act as either an acid or a base, we say that it is **amphoteric**. The conjugate base of a weak polyprotic acid is always amphoteric, because it can either donate or accept another proton. Also notice that HCO_3^- is a weaker acid than H_2CO_3; in general, every time a polyprotic acid donates a proton, the resulting species will be a weaker acid than its predecessor. Amino acids, which will be discussed in more detail in the next chapter, are all also amphoteric compounds and very important for the MCAT.

pH

The pH scale measures the concentration of H^+ (or H_3O^+) ions in a solution. Because the molarity of H^+ tends to be quite small and can vary over many orders of magnitude, the pH scale is logarithmic:

$$pH = -\log[H^+]$$

This formula implies that $[H^+] = 10^{-pH}$. Since $[H^+] = 10^{-7} M$ in pure water, the pH of water is 7. At 25°C, this defines a pH neutral solution. If $[H^+]$ is greater than $10^{-7} M$, then the pH will be less than 7, and the solution is said to be acidic. If $[H^+]$ is less than $10^{-7} M$, the pH will be greater than 7, and the solution is basic (or alkaline). Notice that a *low* pH means a *high* $[H^+]$ and the solution is *acidic*; a *high* pH means a *low* $[H^+]$ and the solution is basic.

pH > 7	basic solution
pH = 7	neutral solution
pH < 7	acidic solution

The range of the pH scale for most solutions falls between 0 and 14, but some strong acids and bases extend the scale past this range. For example, a 10 M solution of HCl will fully dissociate into H^+ and Cl^-. Therefore, the $[H^+] = 10 M$, and the pH = -1.

An alternate measurement expresses the acidity or basicity in terms of the hydroxide ion concentration, $[OH^-]$, by using pOH. The same formula applies for hydroxide ions as for hydrogen ions.

$$pOH = -\log[OH^-]$$

This formula implies that $[OH^-] = 10^{-pOH}$.

Acids and bases are inversely related: the greater the concentration of H^+ ions, the lower the concentration of OH^- ions, and vice versa. Since $[H^+][OH^-] = 10^{-14}$ at 25°C, the values of pH and pOH satisfy a special relationship at 25°C:

$$pH + pOH = 14$$

So, if you know the pOH of a solution, you can find the pH, and vice versa. For example, if the pH of a solution is 5, then the pOH must be 9. If the pOH of a solution is 2, then the pH must be 12.

Relationships Between Conjugates

pK_a and pK_b

The definitions of pH and pOH both involve a negative logarithm. In general, "p" of something is equal to the −log of that something. Therefore, the following definitions won't be surprising:

$$pK_a = -\log K_a$$

$$pK_b = -\log K_b$$

Because H^+ concentrations are generally very small and can vary over such a wide range, the pH scale gives us more convenient numbers to work with. The same is true for pK_a and pK_b. Remember that the larger the K_a value, the stronger the acid. Since "p" means "take the negative log of…," the *lower* the pK_a value, the stronger the acid. For example, lactic acid has a K_a of 1.3×10^{-4}, and uric acid has a K_a of 2.5×10^{-6}. Since the K_a of lactic acid is larger than that of uric acid, more molecules of lactic acid than uric acid will dissociate into ions in aqueous solution. In other words, lactic acid is stronger than uric acid. The pK_a of lactic acid is 3.9, and the pK_a of uric acid is 5.6. **The acid with the lower pK_a value is the stronger acid. The same logic applies to pK_b: the lower the pK_b value, the stronger the base.** Memorize this!

- Of the following liquids, which one contains the lowest concentration of H_3O^+ ions?[25]
    A) Lemon juice (pH = 2.3)
    B) Blood (pH = 7.4)
    C) Seawater (pH = 8.5)
    D) Coffee (pH = 5.1)

- Which of the following compounds is the least acidic?[26]
    A) CH_3COOH, acetic acid (pK_a = 4.76)
    B) H_2CO_3, carbonic acid (pK_a = 6.35)
    C) H_3PO_4, phosphoric acid (pK_a = 2.15)
    D) HCO_3^-, bicarbonate (pK_a = 10.33)

---

[25] **C.** Since pH = − log $[H_3O^+]$, we know that $[H_3O^+]$ = 1/10 pH. This fraction is smallest when the pH is greatest. Of the choices given, seawater has the highest pH.

[26] **D.** The compound with the highest pK_a is the least acidic. Bicarbonate has the highest pK_a of all the answer choices.

Buffer Solutions

A **buffer** is a solution that resists changing pH when a small amount of acid or base is added. The buffering capacity comes from the presence of a weak acid and its conjugate base (or a weak base and its conjugate acid) in roughly equal concentrations.

Buffers are extremely important because nearly every biological process in the human body is pH-dependent. The H^+ ion commonly functions as a reactant, product, or catalyst in chemical reactions in metabolic pathways. In addition, there are many sources of acids and bases in the body that can cause significant changes in the pH if it weren't for our buffer systems.

The most important buffer system in our blood plasma (and for the MCAT) is the bicarbonate buffer system. This buffer consists of carbonic acid (H_2CO_3) and its conjugate base, bicarbonate (HCO_3^-):

$$\textbf{Reaction 1} \qquad H_2CO_3 \rightarrow H^+ + HCO_3^-$$

This buffer system is particularly complex because of how carbonic acid is formed in the body. During cellular respiration, an activity that is constantly occurring in our body, our cells produce carbon dioxide (CO_2) as a byproduct. The carbon dioxide can then react in a reversible fashion with water to form carbonic acid:

$$\textbf{Reaction 2} \qquad CO_2 + H_2O \rightarrow H_2CO_3$$

To understand how this buffer system works, we can consider the following scenario. Let's say you go on a run, causing your muscle tissue to produce lactic acid. The lactic acid would seek to increase the concentration of H^+ ions in your body and thus decrease the pH. As discussed earlier, a drop in pH is problematic; it can severely impact our metabolic processes. However, when the lactic acid produces H^+ ions, Reaction 1 shifts to the left by Le Châtelier's principle, reducing the amount of free H^+ ions. While this shift does not completely prevent the pH from falling, it significantly reduces the degree to which the pH falls.

Chapter 3 Summary

- ΔG, the Gibbs free energy, is the amount of energy in a reaction available to do chemical work.

- For a reaction under any set of conditions, $\Delta G = \Delta H - T\Delta S$.

- If $\Delta G < 0$, the reaction is spontaneous in the forward direction. If $\Delta G > 0$, the reaction is nonspontaneous in the forward direction. If $\Delta G = 0$, the reaction is at equilibrium.

- Kinetics is the study of how quickly a reaction occurs, but it does not determine *whether or not* a reaction will occur.

- Activation energy (E_a) is the minimum energy required to start a reaction and decreases in the presence of a catalyst, thereby increasing the reaction rate.

- Acids are proton donors and electron acceptors; bases are proton acceptors and electron donors.

- The higher the K_a (lower the pK_a), the stronger the acid. The higher the K_b (lower the pK_b), the stronger the base.

- Amphoteric substances may act as either acids or bases.

- $pH = -\log[H^+]$. For a concentration of H^+ given in a $10^{-x}\,M$ notation, simply take the negative exponent to find the pH. The same is true for the relationship between $[OH^-]$ and pOH, K_a and pK_a, and K_b and pK_b.

- Buffers resist pH change upon the addition of a small amount of acid or base. The key buffer system in the body is the bicarbonate buffer system.

CHAPTER 3 FREESTANDING PRACTICE QUESTIONS

1. Which of the following best describes the function of enzymes?

A) By decreasing the E_a, enzymes increase both the reaction rate and the total amount of product formed.
B) By making the ΔG of the reaction more negative, enzymes increase the amount of product formed per unit time.
C) By decreasing the energy of the transition state, enzymes increase the amount of product formed per unit time.
D) By making the ΔG of the reaction more positive, enzymes increase the total amount of product formed.

2. Malate dehydrogenase is a key enzyme in TCA cycle, which catalyzes the following reaction, which is unfavorable under standard conditions:

$$C_4H_6O_5 + NAD^+ \rightarrow C_4H_4O_5 + NADH + H^+$$

Which of the following corresponds to the compound that is most likely to be oxidized under standard conditions?

A) $C_4H_6O_5$
B) NAD^+
C) $C_4H_4O_5$
D) NADH

3. All of the following are examples of oxidation-reduction reactions EXCEPT:

  I. $C_3H_7O_6P + NAD^+ + P_i \rightarrow C_3H_8O_{10}P_2 + NADH + H^+$
  II. $C_6H_{12}O_6 + 6\ O_2 \rightarrow 6\ CO_2 + 6\ H_2O$
  III. $C_6H_{14}O_{12}P_2 \rightarrow 2\ C_3H_7O_6P$

A) II only
B) III only
C) I and II only
D) I and III only

4. An acidic Glu residue in a protein (neutral in its protonated form) has a pK_a value of 2.3 in the wild-type protein and is found near a neutral Ile residue. What will be the effect on the pK_a of the Glu residue if a mutation substitutes a positively charged Lys residue for the Ile residue?

A) The pK_a will decrease due to favorable ionic interactions between the deprotonated Glu and Lys residues.
B) The pK_a will decrease due to unfavorable ionic interactions between the deprotonated Glu and Lys residues.
C) The pK_a will increase due to favorable ionic interactions between the deprotonated Glu and Lys residues.
D) The pK_a will increase due to unfavorable ionic interactions between the deprotonated Glu and Lys residues.

5. Which of the following best orders the relative basicity of the side chains of Glu (pK_a = 4.1), Cys (pK_a = 8.3), and Lys (pK_a = 10.8)?

A) Cys > Glu > Lys
B) Lys > Glu > Cys
C) Lys > Cys > Glu
D) Glu > Cys > Lys

6. The cells in your body are constantly undergoing cellular respiration, producing CO_2 as a byproduct. What would happen to the pH of your blood if you were to hold your breath?

A) It would increase.
B) It would be the same.
C) It would decrease.
D) It cannot be determined with the information provided.

CHAPTER 3 PRACTICE PASSAGE

The complexity of hemoglobin's function is exemplified by its chemical structure. Multiple factors are believed to affect the kinetics of oxygen binding to the molecule's active sites. It has been proposed that the binding of oxygen (Figure 1) reduces strain on the heme protein superstructure by counterbalancing the pull of the proximal imidazole. Similarly, increasing basicity of the proximal imidazole (e.g., through loss of a hydrogen atom) is believed to exert additional strain on the heme protein in the deoxygenated state by inducing a dome-shaped molecular structure. Because the binding of oxygen relieves this strain, increasing basicity of the proximal imidazole increases the affinity of the heme for oxygen. The hydrophobic pocket created by hydrocarbon-like residues from adjacent heme proteins are also believed to facilitate oxygenation, though it has been proposed steric hindrance may provide an antagonistic effect. The distal imidazole shown below may inhibit dissociation by stabilizing the oxygen molecule in place.

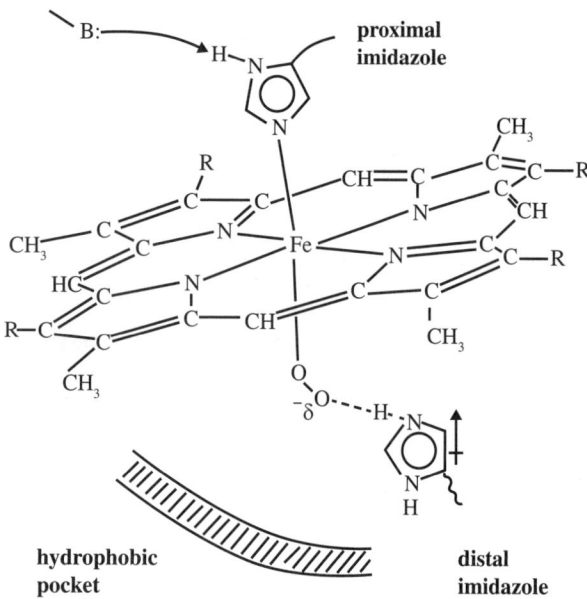

Figure 1 Summary schematic of selected stereoelectronic factors in oxygen affinity of heme

The net effect of these and other factors affecting oxygen dissociation from hemoglobin can be expressed kinetically:

Equation 1 $\text{Heme} + O_2 \underset{k}{\overset{k'}{\rightleftharpoons}} \text{Heme-}O_2$

A single heme molecule will associate with O_2 to form a heme-O_2 complex with rate constant k'; in a reverse reaction, oxygen will dissociate from the heme-O_2 complex with rate constant k. One study examined the kinetics of association of oxygen at different oxygen-bound states as well as the

implied equilibrium constants (K_{O_2}) for each stage of oxygen association (Table 1).

Heme	k' $(M^{-1}\ sec^{-1} \times 10^{-7})$	$k\ (sec^{-1})$	K'_{O_2} $(M^{-1} \times 10^{-6})$
Hb	0.20	1079	0.0019
Hb(O_2)	0.39	245	0.016
Hb(O_2)$_2$	0.35	30	0.12
Hb(O_2)$_3$	4.00	47	0.85

Table 1 Kinetic data pertaining to oxygen association with hemoglobin

Another study examined the thermodynamics of the association of hemoglobin dimers ($\alpha\beta$) to form the tetrameric hemoglobin protein.

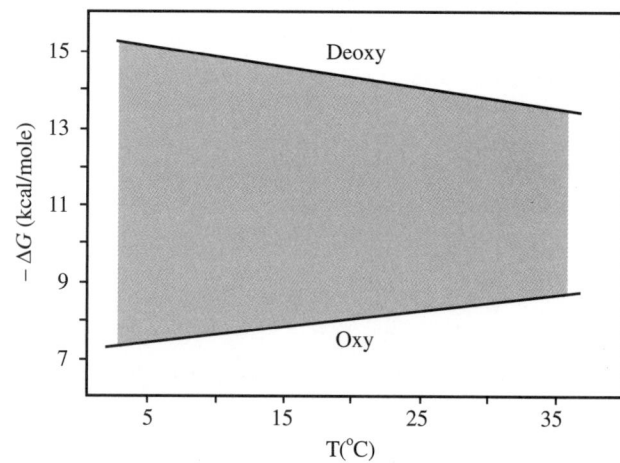

Figure 2 Free energy coupling for dimer-tetramer association in deoxygenated and oxygenated hemoglobin

Extrapolating from the respective linear models depicted in Figure 2, specific data for free energy as well as enthalpy and entropy at body temperature (310 K) are shown in Table 2.

Ligation state	Enthalpy ΔH (kcal/mol)	ΔS (cal/mol-K)	ΔG (kcal/mol)
Oxygenated	4.0	40	−8.4
Deoxygenated	−29.0	−50.1	−13.5

Table 2 Thermodynamic parameters for dimer-tetramer association of hemoglobin at 310 K

Adapted from Chang, C. K., and Traylor, T. G. *Kinetics of oxygen and carbon monoxide binding to synthetic analogs of the myoglobin and hemoglobin active sites;* Ip, S. H. C., and Ackers, G. K. *Thermodynamic studies on subunit assembly in human hemoglobin.*

1. Based on information presented in the passage, which of the following most likely describes the outcome of replacing the distal imidazole with a nonpolar amino acid residue?

A) The bond between iron and oxygen would be stabilized, decreasing the rate at which oxygen dissociates from hemoglobin.

B) The bond between iron and oxygen would be stabilized, increasing the rate at which oxygen dissociates from hemoglobin.

C) The bond between iron and oxygen would be destabilized, decreasing the rate at which oxygen dissociates from hemoglobin.

D) The bond between iron and oxygen would be destabilized, increasing the rate at which oxygen dissociates from hemoglobin.

2. What is the most likely effect of the addition of acid to the solution in which hemoglobin is suspended?

A) The structure of deoxyhemoglobin would become relatively less strained, reducing affinity for oxygen.

B) The structure of deoxyhemoglobin would become relatively less strained, increasing affinity for oxygen.

C) The structure of deoxyhemoglobin would become relatively more strained, reducing affinity for oxygen.

D) The structure of deoxyhemoglobin would become relatively more strained, increasing affinity for oxygen.

3. Which of the following would be most likely to bind oxygen the fastest in the pulmonary vasculature?

A) Hb

B) $Hb(O_2)$

C) $Hb(O_2)_2$

D) $Hb(O_2)_3$

4. Thermodynamic data for the formation of the hemoglobin tetramer (i.e., association of hemoglobin dimer subunits) provide insight into the "cooperativity" of hemoglobin binding of oxygen. Which of the following statements is most likely to be true based on information in the passage?

A) The positive ΔH for oxyhemoglobin suggests that tetramer association occurs spontaneously at body temperature.

B) The difference in sign between oxygenated and deoxygenated ΔS values suggests that deoxyhemoglobin may be stabilized by increased hydrophobic interactions in the dimer-dimer contact region.

C) The similarity in magnitude of ΔS values supports the idea that the effect of oxygen on the overall order of hemoglobin is incident only at the fourth oxygen binding event.

D) The relatively lesser magnitude of the negative ΔG suggests that oxyhemoglobin dimers will associate more readily than deoxyhemoglobin.

5. At body temperature, which of the following statements is likely true based on the data shown in Table 2?

A) Formation of the deoxygenated hemoglobin tetramer is favored due to more favorable heat of formation.

B) Formation of the deoxygenated hemoglobin tetramer is favored due to more favorable entropy.

C) Formation of the oxygenated hemoglobin tetramer is favored due to more favorable heat of formation.

D) Formation of the oxygenated hemoglobin tetramer is favored due to more favorable entropy.

SOLUTIONS TO CHAPTER 3 FREESTANDING PRACTICE QUESTIONS

1. **C** Enzymes are biological catalysts that affect the kinetics of biological reactions. By lowering the energy of the transition state, enzymes decrease the E_a of biological reactions and increase the amount of product formed per unit time (choice C is correct). ΔG is a thermodynamic quantity and will be unaffected by the addition of an enzyme (choices B and D are wrong). The total amount of product formed once the reaction has reached equilibrium is determined by thermodynamic factors, whereas the amount of product formed in a given time period is determined by kinetic factors (choice A is wrong).

2. **D** Given that the question stem indicates that the reaction is unfavorable under standard conditions, it is likely to proceed in the reverse direction under standard conditions. NADH loses a hydrogen atom in forming NAD^+ in the reverse reaction and is thereby oxidized (choice D is correct). Both $C_4H_6O_5$ and NAD^+ are more likely to be the product, rather than the reactant, of this redox reaction under standard conditions (choices A and B are wrong). Because $C_4H_4O_5$ gains hydrogen atoms in generating $C_4H_6O_5$, it is reduced, not oxidized (choice C is wrong).

3. **B** Item I is false: NAD^+ gains a hydrogen atom and is reduced to NADH, and $C_3H_7O_6P$ must therefore be oxidized. This is an example of a redox reaction and is therefore not an exception (choices C and D can be eliminated). Item II is false: O_2 is in its standard state, giving it a zero oxidation state. It is reduced to have a -2 oxidation state in the products. The O to H ratio is substantially increased in generating CO_2 from $C_6H_{12}O_6$, which indicates $C_6H_{12}O_6$ has been oxidized. This is an example of a redox reaction and is therefore not an exception (choice A can be eliminated, and choice B is correct). Item III is true: this reaction simply splits $C_6H_{12}O_6$ into two three-carbon molecules, while maintaining the O to H ratio. It is not a redox reaction and is therefore the exception.

4. **A** The substitution of a positively charged lysine for a neutral isoleucine would help stabilize Glu in its deprotonated, negatively-charged state (choices B and D can be eliminated). Because it would be more stable, it is more likely to give up its proton (i.e., it becomes more acidic), and the pK_a would decrease (choice C is wrong, and choice A is correct).

5. **C** pK_a is a measure of acid strength. The lower the pK_a, the more acidic the functional group. The question, however, is asking about basicity. Logically, the more acidic the functional group, the less basic it is. Therefore, the most basic group is the one with the highest pK_a, and the least basic is the one with lowest pK_a. Of the three amino acids, the side chain of Lys has the highest pK_a (choices A and D can be eliminated), and the side chain of Glu has the lowest pK_a (choice B can be eliminated, and choice C is correct).

6. **C** When you hold your breath, the CO_2 concentration in your blood increases. The increase in CO_2 will increase the formation of carbonic acid, H_2CO_3, in your blood, which will decrease the pH (choice C is correct; choices A, B, and D are wrong).

SOLUTIONS TO CHAPTER 3 PRACTICE PASSAGE

1. **D** In its protonated form, the distal imidazole forms a hydrogen bond with the oxygen molecule, stabilizing its position with respect to the iron. Introducing a nonpolar amino acid residue in place of this imidazole would remove the hydrogen bond, destabilizing the interaction between iron and oxygen (choices A and B are wrong). If the interaction between iron and oxygen is destabilized, this would likely result in an increase in the rate at which oxygen dissociates from heme (choice D is correct, and choice C is wrong).

2. **A** Increasing the acidity of the buffer in which hemoglobin is suspended would effectively *decrease* the basicity of the proximal imidazole by maximizing the chance that H^+ will remain bound to the five-member ring. As a result, the proximal imidazole would exert less strain on the deoxygenated state of hemoglobin (choices C and D can be eliminated). According to the passage, increased basicity of the proximal imidazole this would increase the affinity of the heme for oxygen; therefore, decreased basicity would decrease the affinity for oxygen (choice B can be eliminated, and choice A is correct). Indeed, while there are numerous effects of increasing acidity (decreasing pH) on the heme molecule, the commonly depicted oxygen dissociation curve below demonstrates a relative decrease in heme affinity for oxygen with increasing acidity; higher pO_2 is required for the same oxyhemoglobin saturation.

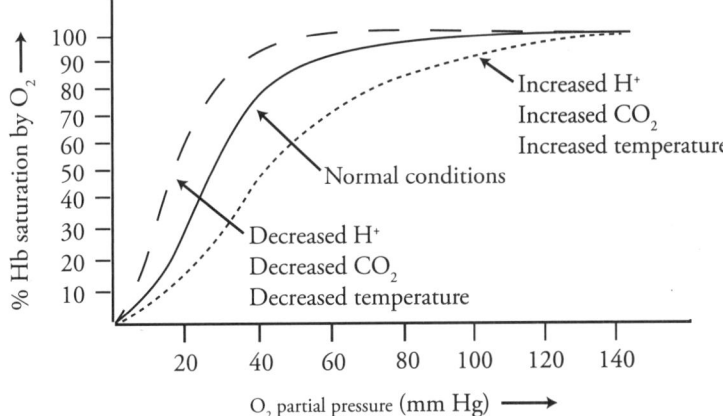

3. **D** Table 1 demonstrates that $Hb(O_2)_3$ has the highest k' (rate constant for association) of all the oxygen-bound states of hemoglobin; thus, it can be said that this state would bind oxygen the fastest (choice D is correct). This conclusion is most consistent with the concept of "cooperativity" in binding oxygen to hemoglobin; up to a total of four oxygen molecules, each act of association with oxygen induces structural changes in the heme protein that result in a tendency to increase the rate at which oxygen binds according to the sigmoidal curve shown above in the answer to question 2. All other less-oxygenated states of hemoglobin bind additional oxygen less quickly than $Hb(O_2)_3$ (choices A, B, and C are wrong).

4. **B** ΔS indicates a change in overall disorder consistent with sign; a positive sign indicates increasing disorder, while a negative ΔS indicates an increase in order. Deoxyhemoglobin, with its negative ΔS, thus experiences an increase in order on tetramer association; one reason for this could be increased hydrophobic interactions at the dimer-dimer contact site (i.e., increased stability; choice B is correct). A positive ΔH value implies that the reaction

is *endothermic*, indicating that it requires investment of energy from the surrounding system in order to proceed; while the negative ΔG value indicates that tetramer association is spontaneous for oxyhemoglobin, the positive ΔH actually "works against" this reaction (choice A is wrong). While the fourth oxygen-binding event may be the most rapid per data in Table 1, it is unlikely that previous oxygen-binding events would have had little effect on the overall order of the molecule. Consistent with the "cooperativity" phenomenon of each of these binding events, it is likely that each binding event increases overall *dis*order of the tetramer association reaction incrementally (choice C is wrong). A more negative ΔG indicates increasing spontaneity of the tetramer association; thus tetramer association occurs more spontaneously for deoxyhemoglobin ($\Delta G = -13.5$) than for oxyhemoglobin ($\Delta G = -8.4$; choice D is wrong).

5. **A** While formation of both the deoxygenated and oxygenated hemoglobin molecules is favored as indicated by negative Gibbs free energy for both reactions, the formation of the deoxygenated tetramer has a more negative ΔG, meaning that this reaction is favored over the formation of a tetramer from oxygenated dimers (choices C and D can be eliminated). Additionally, considering the calculation of Gibbs free energy ($\Delta G = \Delta H - T\Delta S$), the key driver in this case is the change in enthalpy (ΔH), which is negative for the formation of the deoxygenated tetramer. The negative change in entropy (ΔS) for the deoxygenated tetramer actually works against formation, since a negative ΔS indicates an increase in order (decrease in disorder; choice B can be eliminated, and choice A is correct). Note, however, that the magnitude of this spontaneity-decreasing factor is reduced dramatically by the fact that its units include *cal* (not *kcal*) in the numerator position; thus change in entropy is not the driving factor in the spontaneity of tetramer formation for this question.

Chapter 4
Amino Acids and Proteins

The biological macromolecules are grouped into four classes of molecules that play important roles in cells and in organisms as a whole. All of them are polymers, strings of repeated units (monomers).

This chapter discusses amino acids and proteins from a biological perspective: what they are made of, how they are put together, and what their roles are in the body. These molecules are also discussed in *MCAT Organic Chemistry Review* from an organic chemistry perspective: nomenclature, chirality, etc.

4.1 AMINO ACIDS

Proteins are biological macromolecules that act as enzymes, hormones, receptors, channels, transporters, antibodies, and support structures inside and outside cells. Proteins are composed of 20 different amino acids linked together in polymers. The composition and sequence of amino acids in the polypeptide chain is what makes each protein unique and able to fulfill its special role in the cell. Here, we will start with amino acids, the building blocks of proteins, and work our way up to three-dimensional protein structure and function.

Amino Acid Structure and Nomenclature

Understanding the structure of amino acids is key to understanding both their chemistry and the chemistry of proteins. The generic formula for all 20 amino acids is shown below.

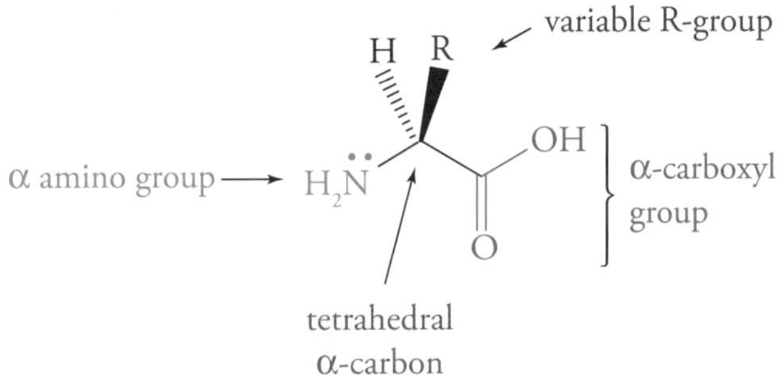

Figure 1   Generic Amino Acid Structure

All 20 amino acids share the same nitrogen-carbon-carbon backbone. The unique feature of each amino acid is its **side chain** (variable R-group), which gives it the physical and chemical properties that distinguish it from the other 19.

Classification of Amino Acids

Each of the 20 amino acids is unique because of its side chain, but many of them are similar in their chemical properties. You should be very familiar with the side chains, and it is important to understand the chemical properties that characterize them, such as their varying *shape, ability to hydrogen bond, and ability to act as acids or bases (which determines their charge at physiological pH).*

As you study the 20 amino acids, do so by organizing them into four broad categories: ACIDIC, BASIC, NONPOLAR, and POLAR amino acids. Each amino acid has a three-letter abbreviation and a one-letter abbreviation, which are both important to know for the MCAT.

Acidic Amino Acids

Aspartic acid and glutamic acid are the only amino acids with carboxylic acid functional groups ($pK_a \approx 4$) in their side chains, thereby making the side chains acidic. Thus, there are three functional groups in these amino acids that may act as acids—the two backbone groups and the R-group. You may hear the terms aspart*ate* and glutam*ate*—these simply refer to the anionic (deprotonated) form of each molecule, which is how these amino acids are observed at physiological pH.

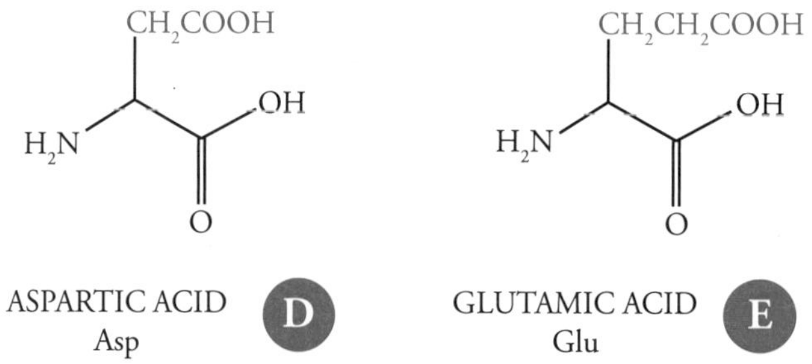

Figure 2   Acidic Amino Acids

Basic Amino Acids

Lysine, arginine, and histidine have basic R-group side chains. The pK_a values for the side chains in these amino acids are 10 for Lys, 12 for Arg, and 6.5 for His. Both Lys and Arg are cationic (protonated) at physiological pH, but histidine is unique in having a side chain with a pK_a close to physiological pH. At pH 7.4, histidine may be either protonated or deprotonated—we put it in the basic category, but it often acts as an acid too. This makes it a readily available proton acceptor or donor, explaining its prevalence at protein active sites. A mnemonic is "His goes both ways." This contrasts with amino acids containing –COOH or –NH$_2$ side chains, which are *always* anionic (RCOO⁻) or cationic (RNH$_3^+$) at physiological pH. [By the way, *histamine* is a small molecule that has to do with allergic responses, itching, inflammation, and other processes. (You've heard of antihistamine drugs, for example.) It is not an amino acid; don't confuse it with *histidine*.]

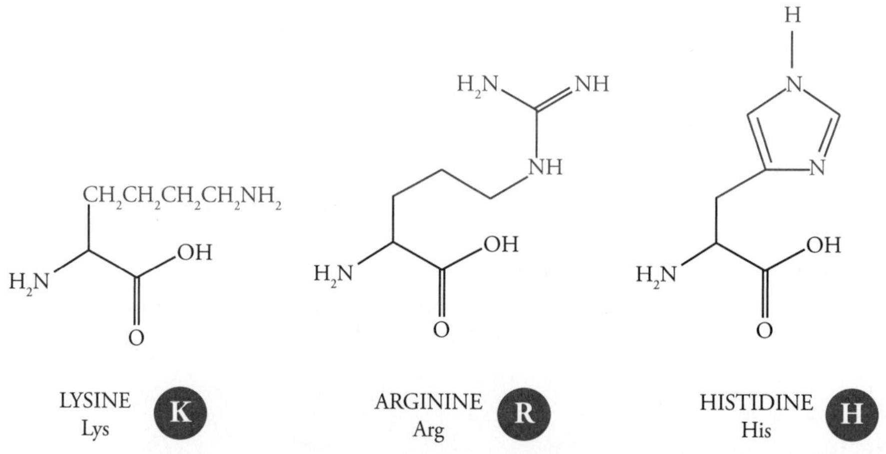

Figure 3   Basic Amino Acids

Hydrophobic (Nonpolar) Amino Acids

Hydrophobic amino acids have either aliphatic (alkyl) or aromatic side chains. Amino acids with aliphatic side chains include glycine, alanine, valine, leucine, and isoleucine. Amino acids with aromatic side chains include phenylalanine, tryptophan, and tyrosine (though the latter is a polar amino acid). Hydrophobic residues tend to associate with each other rather than with water, and therefore are found on the interior of folded globular proteins, away from water. The larger the hydrophobic group, the greater the hydrophobic force repelling it from water.

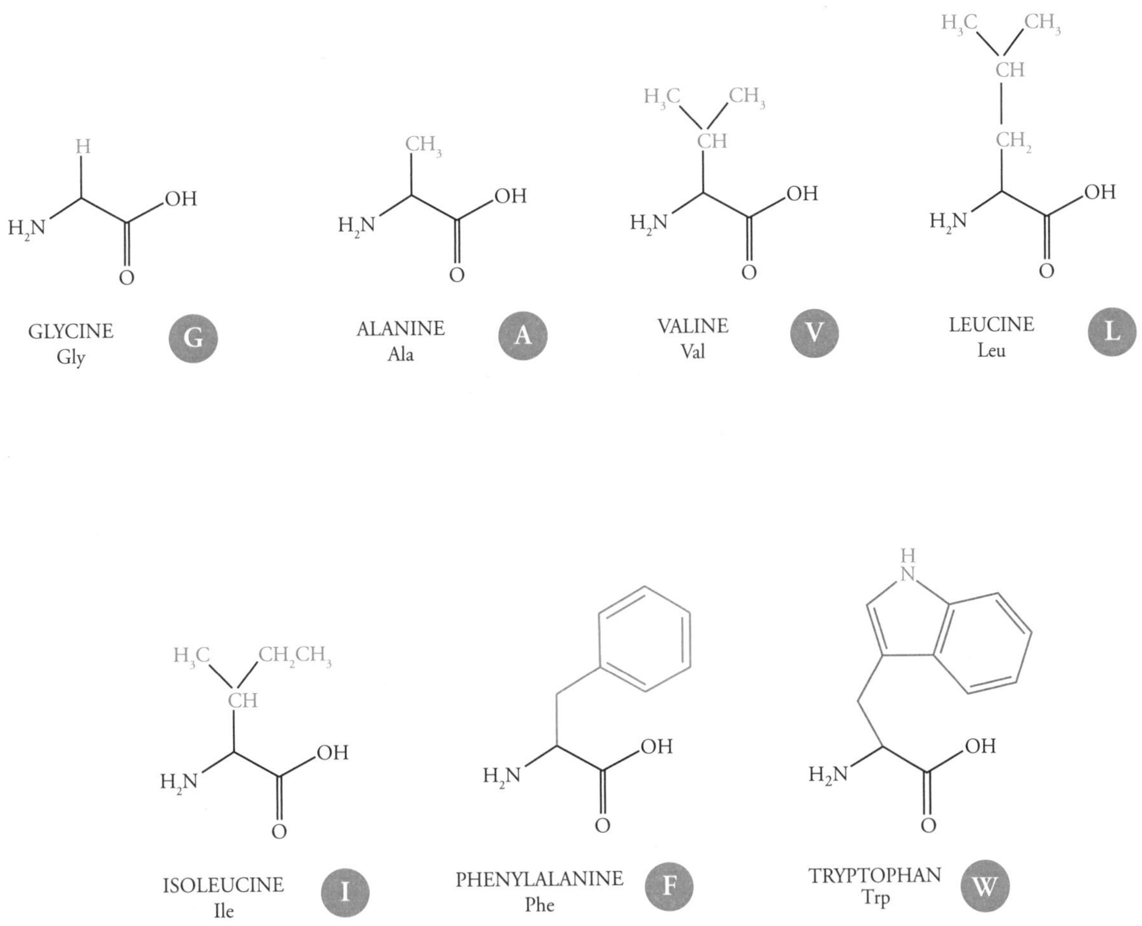

Figure 4   Nonpolar Amino Acids

Polar Amino Acids

These amino acids are characterized by an R-group that is polar enough to form hydrogen bonds with water but which does not act as an acid or base. This means they are hydrophilic and will interact with water whenever possible. The hydroxyl groups of serine, threonine, and tyrosine residues are often modified by the attachment of a phosphate group by a regulatory enzyme called a kinase. The result is a change in structure due to the very hydrophilic phosphate group. This modification is an important means of regulating protein activity. This category also includes the amide derivatives of aspartic acid and glutamic acid, which are named asparagine and glutamine, respectively.

SERINE
Ser **S**

THREONINE
Thr **T**

TYROSINE
Tyr **Y**

ASPARAGINE
Asn **N**

GLUTAMINE
Gln **Q**

Figure 5   Polar Amino Acids

Sulfur-Containing Amino Acids

Amino acids with sulfur-containing side chains include cysteine and methionine. Cysteine, which contains a thiol (also called a sulfhydryl—like an alcohol that has an S atom instead of an O atom), is fairly polar, and methionine, which contains a thioether (like an ether that has an S atom instead of an O atom), is fairly nonpolar.

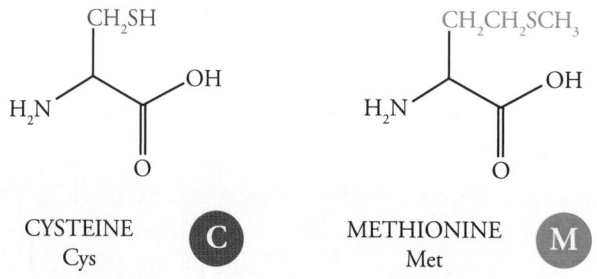

CYSTEINE
Cys **C**

METHIONINE
Met **M**

Figure 6   Sulfur-Containing Amino Acids

Proline

Proline is unique among the amino acids in that its amino group is covalently bound to its nonpolar side chain, creating a secondary α-amino group and a distinctive ring structure. This unique feature of proline has important consequences for protein folding (see Section 4.3).

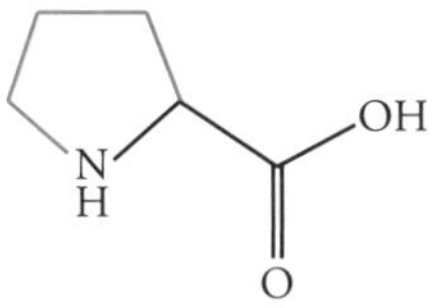

PROLINE
Pro

Hydrophilic			Hydrophobic
ACIDIC	BASIC	POLAR	NONPOLAR
Aspartic acid	Lysine*	Serine	Glycine
Glutamic acid	Arginine	Cysteine	Alanine
	Histidine*	Tyrosine	Valine*
		Threonine*	Leucine*
		Asparagine	Isoleucine*
		Glutamine	Phenylalanine*
			Tryptophan*
			Methionine*
			Proline
*Denotes one of the **nine essential** amino acids, those that cannot be synthesized by adult humans and must be obtained from the diet.			

Table 1 Summary Table of Amino Acids

- Which of the following amino acids is most likely to be found on the exterior of a protein at pH 7.0?[1]
    A) Leucine
    B) Alanine
    C) Serine
    D) Isoleucine

---

[1] Leucine, alanine, and isoleucine are all hydrophobic residues more likely to be found on the interior than the exterior of proteins. Serine (choice **C**), which has a hydroxyl group that can hydrogen bond with water, is the correct answer.

4.2 AMINO ACID REACTIVITY

Since amino acids are composed of an acidic group (the carboxylic acid) and a basic group (the amine), we must be sure to understand the acid/base chemistry of amino acids.

Reviewing the Fundamentals of Acid/Base Chemistry

Recall from the previous chapter that amino acids are **amphoteric**, which means that amino acids can act as acids or bases. This should make sense since an amino acid contains the acidic carboxylic acid group and the basic amino group.

Carboxyl groups of amino acids generally have a pK_a of about 2 (stronger acid), while the ammonium groups generally have a pK_a of 9 or 10 (weaker acid).

The mathematical formula that describes the relationship between pH, pK_a, and the position of equilibrium in an acid-base reaction is known as the **Henderson–Hasselbalch** equation:

$$pH = pK_a + \log \frac{[A^-]}{[HA]} = pK_a + \log \frac{[\text{base form}]}{[\text{acid form}]}$$

Given the pH and the pK_a, we can calculate the ratio of the base and acid forms of a compound at equilibrium. You will go through this equation much more thoroughly in *MCAT General Chemistry Review*. Don't worry too much about doing any calculations here; just make sure you memorize the following rules:

- When the pH of the solution is less than the pK_a of an acidic group, the acidic group will mostly be in its protonated form.
- When the pH of the solution is greater than the pK_a of an acidic group, the acidic group will mostly be in its deprotonated form.

- Which functional group of amino acids has a stronger tendency to donate protons: carboxyl groups (pK_a = 2.0) or ammonium groups (pK_a = 9)? Which group will donate protons at the lowest pH?[2]

---

[2] A high pK_a indicates a weak acid. Acids with a low pK_a tend to deprotonate more easily. Therefore, ammonium groups have a stronger tendency to keep their protons, and carboxyl groups will donate protons at the lowest pH (highest $[H^+]$).

Application of Fundamental Acid/Base Chemistry to Amino Acids

All amino acids contain an amino group that acts as a base and a carboxyl group ($pK_a \approx 2$) that acts as an acid. In its protonated, or acidic, form, the amine is called an **ammonium group**, and it has a pK_a between 9–10. For example:

$$-NH_3^+ \rightleftharpoons -NH_2 + H^+ \qquad pK_a \approx 9$$

$$-COOH \rightleftharpoons -COO^- + H^+ \qquad pK_a \approx 2$$

- Assuming a pK_a of 2, will a carboxylate group be protonated or deprotonated at pH 1.0?[3]
- Will the amino group be protonated or deprotonated at pH 1.0?[4]
- Glycine is the simplest amino acid, with only hydrogen as its R-group. Its only functional groups are the backbone groups discussed above (amino and carboxyl). What will be the net charge on a glycine molecule at pH 12?[5]
- At pH 6.0, between the pK_as of the ammonium and carboxyl groups, what will be the net charge on a molecule of glycine?[6]

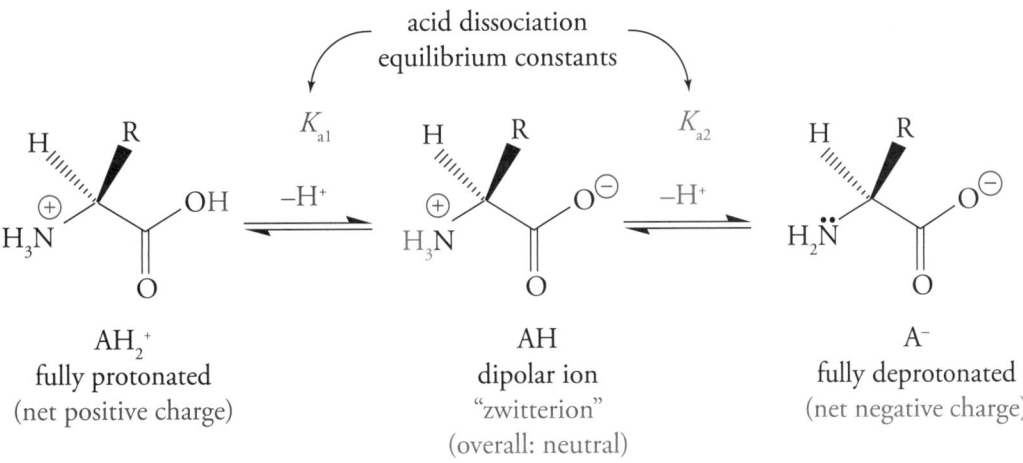

Figure 7 Important Amino Acid Conjugate Acid/Base Pairs

The Isoelectric Point of Amino Acids

There is a pH for every amino acid at which it has no overall net charge (the positive and negative charges cancel). A molecule with positive and negative charges that balance is referred to as a dipolar ion or **zwitterion**. The pH at which a molecule is uncharged (zwitterionic) is referred to as its **isoelectric point** (pI). "Zwitter" is German for "hybrid," implying that an amino acid at its pI has both (+) and (–) charges.

---

[3] The pH is less than the pK_a here, so protonation wins over dissociation, and the group will be protonated. The correct answer is –COOH.

[4] The pH is much lower than the pK_a for the ammonium group, so the amino group is protonated: NH_3^+.

[5] Since pH 12 represents a very low $[H^+]$, both groups will become deprotonated (COO^- and NH_2), creating a net charge of –1 per glycine molecule.

[6] The carboxyl group will be deprotonated (COO^-) with a charge of –1, and the amino group will be protonated (NH_3^+) with a charge of +1, creating a net charge of 0 per glycine molecule.

It is possible to calculate the pI of an amino acid—in other words, to figure out the pH value at which (+) and (−) charges balance (that's the definition of pI). For a molecule with two functional groups, such as glycine, the calculation is simple: just *average the pK$_a$s of the two functional groups*. The pI of more complex molecules can also be calculated, but the math is complex. For the MCAT, you should know how to calculate the pI of a molecule with two functional groups (with no acidic or basic functional groups in the side chain). Another important thing to know for the MCAT is how to compare the pH of a solution to the pK$_a$ of a functional group of an amino acid and determine if a site is mostly protonated or deprotonated. If the pH is higher than the pK$_a$, the site is mostly deprotonated; if the pH is lower than the pK$_a$, the site is mostly protonated. This can be illustrated in the titration curve (titrations will be discussed in more detail in *MCAT General Chemistry Review*) for glycine:

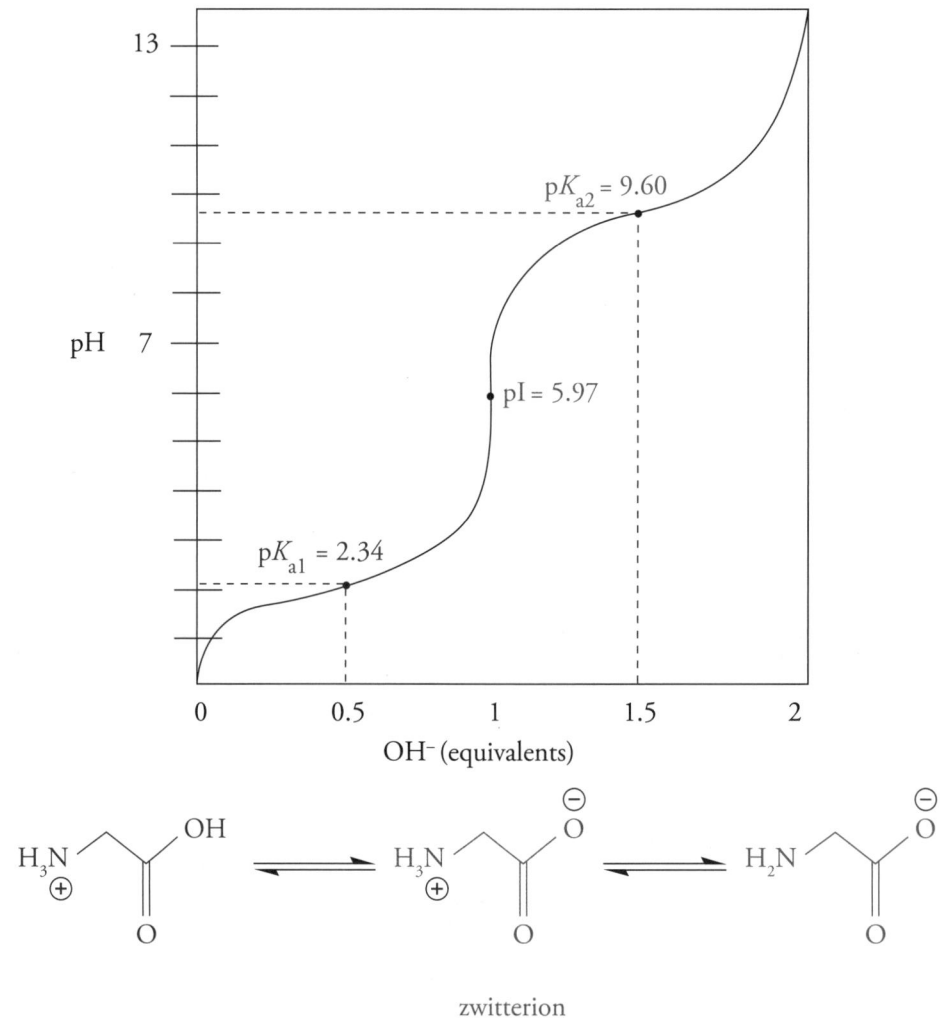

zwitterion

- What is the pI of glycine?[7]

---

[7] To calculate the pI, just average the pK$_a$s of the two functional groups: (9.60 + 2.34)/2 = 5.97, or roughly 6 (this will be discussed in more detail in *MCAT Organic Chemistry Review*).

4.3 PROTEIN STRUCTURE

There are two common types of covalent bonds between amino acids in proteins: the **peptide bonds** that link amino acids together into polypeptide chains and **disulfide bridges** between cysteine R-groups.

The Peptide Bond

Polypeptides are formed by linking amino acids together in peptide bonds. A peptide bond is formed between the carboxyl group of one amino acid and the α-amino group of another amino acid with the loss of water. The figure below shows the formation of a dipeptide from the amino acids glycine and alanine.

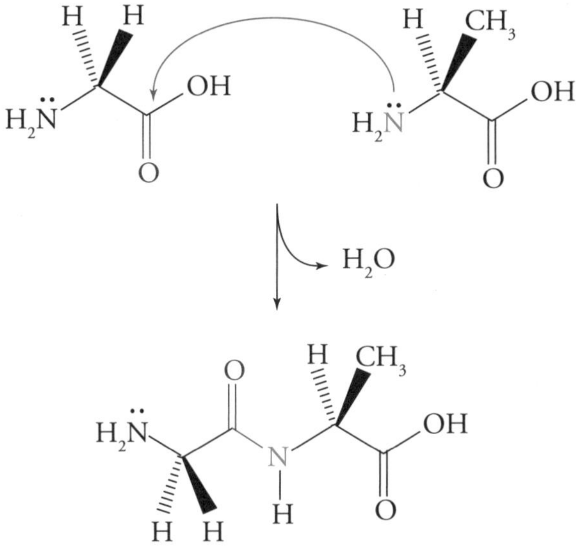

Figure 8   Peptide Bond (Amide Bond) Formation

In a polypeptide chain, the N–C–C–N–C–C pattern formed from the amino acids is known as the **backbone** of the polypeptide. An individual amino acid is termed a **residue** when it is part of a polypeptide chain. The amino terminus is the first end made during polypeptide synthesis, and the carboxy terminus is made last. Hence, by convention, the amino-terminal residue is also always written first.

- In the oligopeptide Phe-Glu-Gly-Ser-Ala, state the number of acid and base functional groups, which residue has a free α-amino group, and which residue has a free α-carboxyl group. (Refer to the beginning of the chapter for structures.)[8]
- How many unique dipeptides (made from linking two amino acids) can be synthesized using only alanine and glycine residues?[9]

---

[8] As stated above, the amino end is always written first. Therefore, the oligopeptide begins with an exposed Phe amino group and ends with an exposed Ala carboxyl; all the other backbone groups are hitched together in peptide bonds. Out of all the R-groups, there is only one acidic or basic functional group, the acidic glutamate R-group. This R-group plus the two terminal backbone groups gives a total of three acid/base functional groups.

[9] Four (Gly-Gly, Ala-Ala, Gly-Ala, Ala-Gly). Note that Ala-Gly and Gly-Ala are not identical peptides. In Ala-Gly, the N-terminus is Ala and the C-terminus is Gly. In Gly-Ala, the N-terminus is Gly and the C-terminus is Ala.

- Thermodynamics states that free energy must decrease for a reaction to proceed spontaneously and that such a reaction will spontaneously move toward equilibrium. The diagram below shows the free energy changes during peptide bond formation. At equilibrium, which is thermodynamically favored: the dipeptide or the individual amino acids?[10]

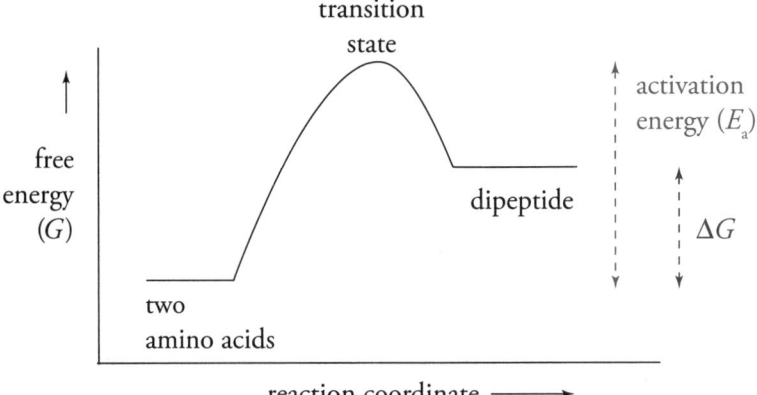

- In that case, how are peptide bonds formed and maintained inside cells?[11]

Hydrolysis of a protein by another protein is called **proteolysis** or **proteolytic cleavage**, and the protein that does the cutting is known as a **proteolytic enzyme** or **protease**. Proteolytic cleavage is a specific means of cleaving peptide bonds. Many enzymes only cleave the peptide bond adjacent to a specific amino acid. For example, the protease trypsin cleaves on the carboxyl side of the positively charged (basic) residues arginine and lysine, while chymotrypsin cleaves adjacent to large hydrophobic residues such as phenylalanine. (Do *not* memorize these examples.)

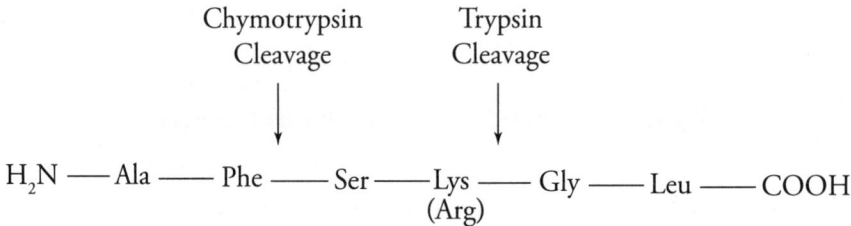

Figure 9 Specificity of Protease Cleavage

- Based on the above, if the following peptide is cleaved by trypsin, what amino acid will be on the new N-terminus and how many fragments will result: Ala-Gly-Glu-Lys-Phe-Phe-Lys?[12]

---

[10] The dipeptide has a higher free energy, so its existence is less favorable. In other words, existence of the chain is less favorable than existence of the isolated amino acids.

[11] During protein synthesis, stored energy is used to force peptide bonds to form. Once the bond is formed, even though its destruction is thermodynamically favorable, it remains stable because the activation energy for the hydrolysis reaction is so high. In other words, hydrolysis is thermodynamically favorable but kinetically slow.

[12] Trypsin will cleave on the carboxyl side of the Lys residue, with Phe on the N-terminus of the new Phe-Phe-Lys fragment. There will be two fragments after trypsin cleavage: Phe-Phe-Lys and Ala-Gly-Glu-Lys.

The Disulfide Bond

Cysteine is an amino acid with a reactive thiol (sulfhydryl, SH) in its side chain. The thiol of one cysteine can react with the thiol of another cysteine to produce a covalent sulfur-sulfur bond known as a disulfide bond, as illustrated below. The cysteines forming a disulfide bond may be located in the same or different polypeptide chain(s). The disulfide bridge plays an important role in stabilizing tertiary protein structure; this will be discussed in the section on protein folding. Once a cysteine residue becomes disulfide-bonded to another cysteine residue, it is called *cystine* instead of cysteine.

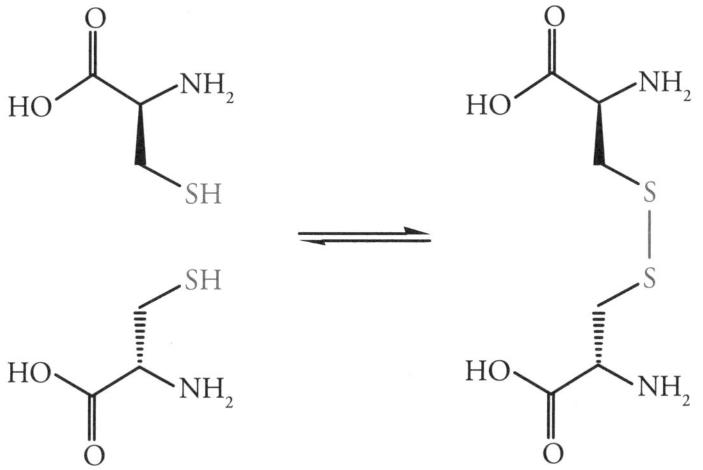

Figure 10   Formation of the Disulfide Bond

- Which is more oxidized, the sulfur in *cysteine* or the sulfur in *cystine*?[13]
- The inside of cells is known as a reducing environment because cells possess antioxidants (chemicals that prevent oxidation reactions). Where would disulfide bridges be more likely to be found, in extracellular proteins, under oxidizing conditions, or in the interior of cells, in a reducing environment?[14]

Protein Structure in Three Dimensions

Each protein folds into a unique three-dimensional structure that is required for that protein to function properly. Improperly folded, or **denatured**, proteins are nonfunctional. There are four levels of protein folding that contribute to their final three-dimensional structure. Each level of structure is dependent upon a particular type of bond, as discussed in the following sections.

---

[13] In forming cystine from two cysteine residues, hydrogen atoms are removed (an oxidation reaction), indicating that the sulfur in cystine is more oxidized.

[14] In a reducing environment, the S-S group is reduced to two SH groups. Disulfide bridges are found only in extracellular polypeptides, where they will not be reduced. Examples of protein complexes held together by disulfide bridges include antibodies and the hormone insulin.

4.3

Denaturation is an important concept. It refers to the **disruption of a protein's shape without breaking peptide bonds**. Proteins are denatured by *urea* (which disrupts hydrogen bonding interactions), by *extremes of pH*, by extremes of *temperature,* and by *changes in salt concentration (tonicity).*

Primary (1°) Structure: The Amino Acid Sequence

The simplest level of protein structure is the order of amino acids bonded to each other in the polypeptide chain. This linear ordering of amino acid residues is known as primary structure. **Primary structure** is the same as **sequence**. The bond which determines 1° structure is the peptide bond, simply because this is the bond that links one amino acid to the next in a polypeptide.

Secondary (2°) Structure: Hydrogen Bonds Between Backbone Groups

Secondary structure refers to the initial folding of a polypeptide chain into shapes stabilized by hydrogen bonds between backbone NH and CO groups. Certain motifs of secondary structure are found in most proteins. The two most common are the α-**helix** and the β-**pleated sheet**.

All α-helices have the same well-defined dimensions that are depicted below with the R-groups omitted for clarity. The α-helices of proteins are always right-handed, 5 angstroms in width, with each subsequent amino acid rising 1.5 angstroms. There are 3.6 amino acid residues per turn with the α-carboxyl oxygen of one amino acid residue hydrogen-bonded to the α-amino proton of an amino acid three residues away. (*Don't* memorize these numbers, but *do* try to visualize what they mean.)

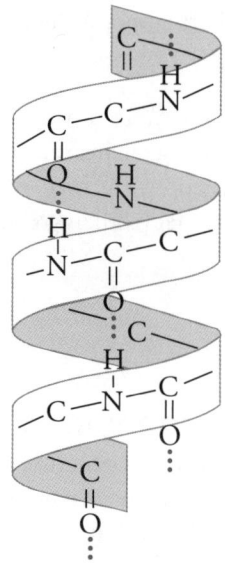

Figure 11   An α-Helix

The unique side chain of proline causes two problems in polypeptide chains:

1. The formation of a peptide bond with proline (shown below) eliminates the only hydrogen atom on the nitrogen atom of proline. The absence of the N-H bond disrupts the backbone hydrogen bonding in the polypeptide chain.
2. The unique structure of proline forces it to kink the polypeptide chain.

For both reasons, proline residues never appear within the α-helix.

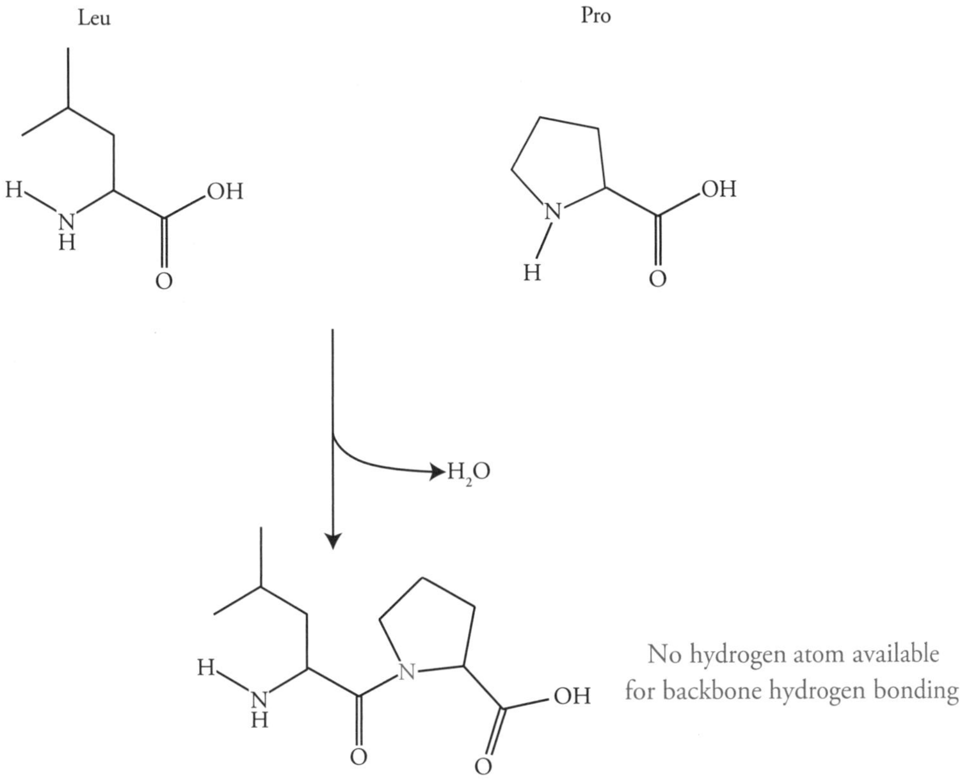

No hydrogen atom available for backbone hydrogen bonding

Figure 12 Proline

Proteins such as hormone receptors and ion channels are often found with α-helical transmembrane regions integrated into the hydrophobic membranes of cells. The α-helix is a favorable structure for a hydrophobic transmembrane region because all polar NH and CO groups in the backbone are hydrogen-bonded to each other on the inside of the helix, and thus don't interact with the hydrophobic membrane interior. α-Helical regions that span membranes also have hydrophobic R-groups, which radiate out from the helix, interacting with the hydrophobic interior of the membrane.

β-pleated sheets are also stabilized by hydrogen bonding between NH and CO groups in the polypeptide backbone. In β-sheets, however, hydrogen bonding occurs between residues distant from each other in the chain or even on separate polypeptide chains. Also, the backbone of a β-sheet is extended, rather than coiled, with side groups directed above and below the plane of the β-sheet. There are two types of β-sheets, one with adjacent polypeptide strands running in the *same* direction (**parallel** β-pleated sheet) and another in which the polypeptide strands run in *opposite* directions (**antiparallel** β-pleated sheet).

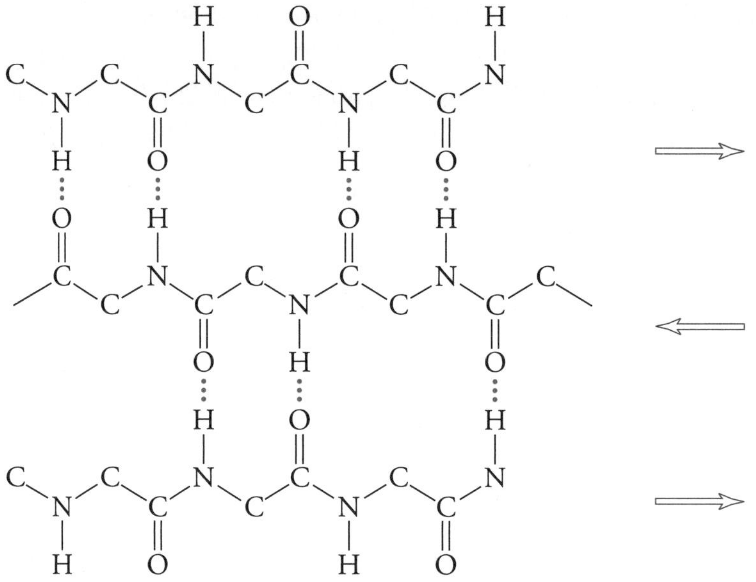

Figure 13 A β-Pleated Sheet

- If a single polypeptide folds once and forms a β-pleated sheet with itself, would this be a parallel or antiparallel β-pleated sheet?[15]
- What effect would a molecule that disrupts hydrogen bonding, such as urea, have on protein structure?[16]

Tertiary (3°) Structure: Hydrophobic/Hydrophilic Interactions

The next level of protein folding, tertiary structure, concerns interactions between amino acid residues located more distantly from each other in the polypeptide chain. These interactions may include van der Waals forces between nonpolar side chains, hydrogen bonds between polar side chains, disulfide bonds between cysteine residues, and electrostatic interactions between acidic and basic side chains. The folding of secondary structures such as α-helices into higher order tertiary structures is driven by interactions of R-groups with each other and with the solvent (water). Hydrophobic R-groups tend to fold into the interior of the protein, away from the solvent, and hydrophilic R-groups tend to be exposed to water on the surface of the protein (shown for the generic globular protein). This is called the **hydrophobic effect.**

---

[15] It would be antiparallel because one participant in the β-pleated sheet would have a C to N direction, while the other would be running N to C.

[16] Putting a protein in a urea solution will disrupt H-bonding, thus disrupting secondary structure (and possibly tertiary and quaternary) by unfolding α-helices and β-sheets. It would not affect primary structure, which depends on the much more stable peptide bond. Disruption of 2°, 3°, or 4° structure without breaking peptide bonds is *denaturation.*

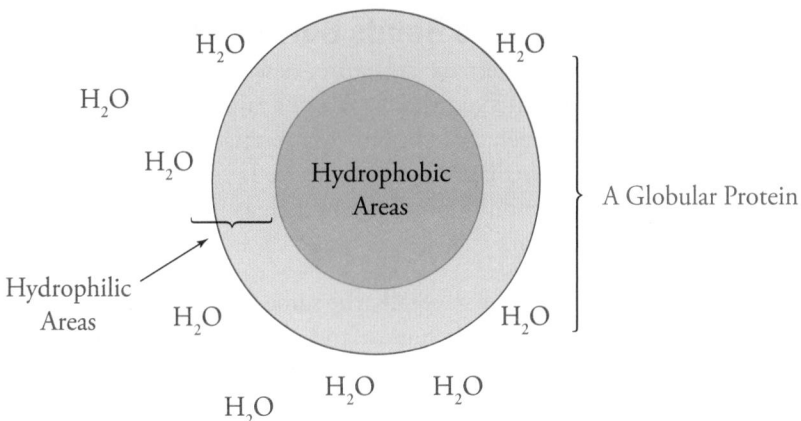

Figure 14   Folding of a Globular Protein in Aqueous Solution

Under the right conditions, the forces driving hydrophobic avoidance of water and hydrogen bonding will fold a polypeptide spontaneously into the correct conformation, the lowest energy conformation. In a classic experiment by Christian Anfinsen and coworkers, the effect of a denaturing agent (urea) and a reducing agent (β-mercaptoethanol) on the folding of a protein called ribonuclease was examined. In the following questions, you will reenact their thought processes. Try to answer the questions before reading the footnotes.

- Ribonuclease has eight cysteines that form four disulfides bonds. What effect would a reducing agent have on its tertiary structure?[17]
- If the disulfides serve only to lock into place a tertiary protein structure that forms first on its own, then what effect would the reducing agent have on correct protein folding?[18]
- Would a protein end up folded normally if you (1) first put it in a reducing environment, (2) then denatured it by adding urea, (3) next removed the reducing agent, allowing disulfide bridges to reform, and (4) finally removed the denaturing agent?[19]
- What if you did the same experiment but in this order: 1, 2, 4, 3?[20]
- Which of the following may be considered an example of tertiary protein structure?[21]
  - I.   van der Waals interactions between two Phe R-groups located far apart on a polypeptide
  - II. Hydrogen bonds between backbone amino and carboxyl groups
  - III. Covalent disulfide bonds between cysteine residues located far apart on a polypeptide

---

[17] The disulfide bridges would be broken. Tertiary structure would be less stable.

[18] The shape should not be disrupted if breaking disulfides is the only disturbance. It's just that the shape would be less sturdy—like a concrete wall without the rebar.

[19] No. If you allow disulfide bridges to form while the protein is still denatured, it will become locked into an abnormal shape.

[20] You should end up with the correct structure. In step 1, you break the reinforcing disulfide bridges. In step 2, you denature the protein completely by disrupting H-bonds. In step 4, you allow the H-bonds to reform; as stated in the text, normally the correct tertiary structure will form spontaneously if you leave the polypeptide alone. In step 3, you reform the disulfide bridges, thus locking the structure into its correct form.

[21] **Item I is true:** this is a good example of 3°. Item II is false: this describes 2°, not 3° structure. **Item III is true:** this describes the disulfide bond, which is another example of tertiary structure.

Quaternary (4°) Structure: Various Bonds Between Separate Chains

The highest level of protein structure, quaternary structure, describes interactions between polypeptide subunits. A **subunit** is a single polypeptide chain that is part of a large complex containing many subunits (a **multisubunit complex**). The arrangement of subunits in a multisubunit complex is what we mean by quaternary structure. For example, mammalian RNA polymerase II contains 12 different subunits. The interactions between subunits are instrumental in protein function, as in the cooperative binding of oxygen by each of the four subunits of hemoglobin.

The forces stabilizing quaternary structure are generally the same as those involved in tertiary structure—van der Waals forces, hydrogen bonds, disulfide bonds, and electrostatic interactions. It is key to understand, however, that there is one bond that may not be involved in quaternary structure—the peptide bond—because this bond defines sequence (1° structure).

- What is the difference between a disulfide bridge involved in quaternary structure and one involved in tertiary structure?[22]

4.4 PROTEINS AS ENZYMES

Enzymes are biological catalysts. They increase the rate of a reaction by lowering the reaction's activation energy, but they *do not affect* ΔG between reactants and products. As catalysts, enzymes have a kinetic role, *not* a thermodynamic one. Enzymes may alter the rate of a reaction enormously: a reaction that would take a hundred years to reach equilibrium without an enzyme may occur in just seconds with an enzyme.

Given that thousands of enzymes have been discovered, scientists frequently classify them based upon reaction type. Table 2 lists several examples but note that enzymes cannot control the direction in which a reaction proceeds; it is common to see enzymes in a given class function in reverse.

Enzyme Class	Reaction
Hydrolase	hydrolyzes chemical bonds (includes ATPases, proteases, and others)
Isomerase	rearranges bonds within a molecule to form an isomer
Ligase	forms a chemical bond (e.g., DNA ligase)
Lyase	breaks chemical bonds by means other than oxidation or hydrolysis (e.g., pyruvate decarboxylase)
Kinase	transfers a phosphate group to a molecule from a high energy carrier, such as ATP (e.g., phosphofructokinase [PFK])
Oxidoreductase	runs redox reactions (includes oxidases, reductases, dehydrogenases, and others)
Polymerase	polymerization (e.g., addition of nucleotides to the leading strand of DNA by DNA polymerase III)
Phosphatase	removes a phosphate group from a molecule
Phosphorylase	transfers a phosphate group to a molecule from inorganic phosphate (e.g., glycogen phosphorylase)
Protease	hydrolyzes peptide bonds (e.g., trypsin, chymotrypsin, pepsin, etc.)

Table 2 Enzyme Classes

[22] Quaternary disulfides are bonds that form between chains that aren't linked by peptide bonds. Tertiary disulfides are bonds that form between residues in the same polypeptide.

ATP as an Energy Source: Reaction Coupling

Enzymes increase the rate of reactions that have a negative ΔG. These reactions would occur on their own without an enzyme (they are spontaneous) but far more slowly than with one. However, there are many reactions in the body that occur which have a positive ΔG. The biosynthesis of macromolecules such as DNA and protein is not spontaneous ($\Delta G > 0$), but clearly these reactions *do* take place (or we wouldn't be here). How can this be? Thermodynamically unfavorable reactions in the cell can be driven forward by **reaction coupling**. In reaction coupling, one very favorable reaction is used to drive an unfavorable one. This is possible because *free energy changes are additive*. [What is the favorable reaction that the cell can use to drive unfavorable reactions?[23]] In the lab, the $\Delta G^{\circ\prime}$ for the hydrolysis of one phosphate group from ATP is –7.3 kcal/mol, so it is a very favorable reaction. In the cell, ΔG is about –12 kcal/mol, so in the cell it is even more favorable. [What's the difference between the situation *in vitro* (lab) under standard conditions and *in vivo* (cell) under nonstandard conditions?[24]]

How does ATP hydrolysis drive unfavorable reactions? There are many ways. One example is by causing a conformational change in a protein; in this way ATP hydrolysis can be used to power energy-costly events like transmembrane transport. Another example is by transfer of a phosphate group from ATP to a substrate. Take the unfavorable reaction A + B → C. Let's say that Reactant A must proceed through an intermediate, APO_4^{2-}, in order to participate. Let's say $\Delta G = +7$ kcal/mol for the overall reaction. What if the two partial reactions have ΔGs as follows:

$$A + PO_4^{2-} \rightarrow APO_4^{2-} \qquad \Delta G = \quad +2 \text{ kcal/mol}$$

$$\underline{APO_4^{2-} + B \rightarrow C + PO_4^{2-} \qquad \Delta G = \quad +5 \text{ kcal/mol}}$$

$$\textit{Total} \quad \Delta G = \quad +7 \text{ kcal/mol}$$

These reactions will not proceed because the overall ΔG will be +7 kcal/mol. What will be the *overall* ΔG if we *couple* the reaction A + B → C to the hydrolysis of one ATP? All we have to do is add up all the ΔG values, as follows:

$$ATP \rightarrow ADP + PO_4^{2-} \qquad \Delta G = \quad -12 \text{ kcal/mol}$$

$$A + PO_4^{2-} \rightarrow APO_4^{2-} \qquad \Delta G = \quad +2 \text{ kcal/mol}$$

$$\underline{APO_4^{2-} + B \rightarrow C + PO_4^{2-} \qquad \Delta G = \quad +5 \text{ kcal/mol}}$$

$$\textit{Total} \quad \Delta G = \quad -5 \text{ kcal/mol}$$

Now the overall reaction, shown below, is thermodynamically favorable. We have *coupled* the unfavorable reaction A + B → C to the highly favorable hydrolysis of ATP:

$$A + B + ATP \rightarrow C + ADP + PO_4^{2-} \quad \Delta G = -5 \text{ kcal/mol}$$

---

[23] ATP hydrolysis!

[24] $Q_{(cell)} \neq K_{eq}$. This means that the relative concentrations of ATP and ADP + P_i are not at equilibrium levels in the cell. Actually, $Q_{(cell)} \ll K_{eq}$ because the cell keeps a high concentration of ATP around.

Note that we first stated that the enzyme has only a kinetic role (influencing rate only), not a thermo-dynamic one (determining favorability). Then we went on to discuss reaction coupling, which allows enzymes to promote otherwise unfavorable reactions. There is no contradiction, however. The only dif-ference is viewing reactions in an isolated manner or in the complex series of linked reactions more com-monly found in the body. The same rule applies in either case: ΔG must be negative for either a single reaction or a series of linked reactions to occur spontaneously.   In summary:

- One reaction in a test tube—the enzyme is a catalyst with a kinetic role only. It influences the rate of the reaction, but not the outcome.
- Many "real-life" reactions in the cell—enzyme controls outcomes by selectively promoting unfavorable reactions via reaction coupling.

4.5 ENZYME STRUCTURE AND FUNCTION

Most enzymes are proteins that must fold into specific three-dimensional structures to act as catalysts. (Some enzymes are RNA or contain RNA sequences with catalytic activity. Most catalyze their own splic-ing, and the rRNA in ribosomes helps in peptide-bond formation.) An enzyme may consist of a single polypeptide chain or several polypeptide subunits held together in a ____[25] (primary? secondary? etc.) structure. The reason for the importance of folding in enzyme function is the proper formation of the **active site**, the region in an enzyme's three-dimensional structure that is directly involved in catalysis. [What shape are enzymes more likely to have: fibrous/elongated or globular/spherical?[26]] The reactants in an enzyme-catalyzed reaction are called **substrates**. (Products have no special name; they're just "prod-ucts.") What is the role of the active site, that is, how do enzymes work? The **active site model**, com-monly referred to as the "lock and key hypothesis," states that the substrate and active site are perfectly complementary. This differs from the **induced fit model,** which asserts that the substrate and active site differ slightly in structure and that the binding of the substrate induces a conformational change in the enzyme. The induced fit model has gained greater acceptance in recent years, but regardless of the model, enzymes accelerate the rate of a given reaction by helping to *stabilize the transition state*. For example, if a transition state intermediate possesses a transient negative charge, what amino acid residues might be found at the active site to stabilize the transition state?[27] This lowers the activation energy barrier between reactants and products. In our previous example of Bob looking for a job, the use of a career planning service would function as an enzyme by making the process of job hunting easier.

- Is it possible that amino acids located far apart from each other in the primary protein sequence may play a role in the formation of the same active site?[28]
- If, during an enzyme-catalyzed reaction, an intermediate forms in which the substrate is covalently linked to the enzyme via a serine residue, can this occur at any serine residue or must it occur at a specific serine residue?[29]

---

[25] quaternary

[26] Globular. Structural proteins such as collagen tend to be fibrous, but proteins that act as catalysts tend to be roughly spherical to form an active site in a cleft in the sphere.

[27] A positive charge would stabilize the negative charge in the intermediate. Such a charge might be contributed by His, Arg, or Lys. Alterna-tively, the hydrogen of the $-NH_2$ group in glutamine or asparagine could hydrogen bond with the negative charge.

[28] Yes, the amino acids at the active site may be distant from each other in a polypeptide's primary sequence but be near each other in the final folded protein. This is why protein folding is crucial for enzyme function.

[29] It must occur at a particular serine residue which sticks out into the active site.

- Compound A converts into Compound B in solution: $A \rightleftharpoons B$. The reaction has the following equilibrium constant: $K_{eq} = [B]_{eq}/[A]_{eq} = 1,000$. If pure A is dissolved in water at 298 K, will ΔG for the reaction $A \rightleftharpoons B$ be positive or negative? Is it possible to answer this question without knowing $\Delta G^{\circ\prime}$?[30]

- Regarding the reaction described in the previous question, if pure B is put into solution in the presence of an enzyme that catalyzes the reaction between A and B, which one of the following will be true?[31]

    A) All the B will be converted into A, until there is 1,000 times more A than B.

    B) All of the B will remain as B, since B is favored at equilibrium.

    C) The enzyme will have no effect, since enzymes act on the transition state and there is no transition state present.

    D) The reaction that produces A will predominate until $\Delta G = 0$.

The active site for enzymes is generally highly specific in its substrate recognition, including stereospecificity (the ability to distinguish between stereoisomers). For example, enzymes which catalyze reactions involving amino acids are specific for D or L amino acids, and enzymes catalyzing reactions involving monosaccharides may distinguish between stereoisomers as well. [Which configurations are found in animals?[32]]

Many **proteases** (protein-cleaving enzymes) have an active site with a serine residue whose OH group can act as a nucleophile, attacking the carbonyl carbon of an amino acid residue in a polypeptide chain. Examples are trypsin, chymotrypsin, and elastase. These enzymes also usually have a **recognition pocket** near the active site. This is a pocket in the enzyme's structure which attracts certain residues on substrate polypeptides. The enzyme always cuts polypeptides at the same site, just to one side of the recognition residue. For example, chymotrypsin always cuts on the carboxyl side of one of the large hydrophobic or aromatic residues Tyr, Trp, Phe, and Met. Enzymes that act on hydrophobic substrates have hydrophobic amino acids in their active sites, while hydrophilic/polar amino acids will comprise the active site of enzymes with hydrophilic substrates.

Given the importance of the active site, it becomes clear that small alterations in its structure can drastically alter enzymatic activity. Therefore, both temperature and pH play a critical role in enzymatic function. As temperature increases, the thermal motion of the peptide and surrounding solution destabilize its structure. If the temperature rises sufficiently, the protein **denatures** and loses its orderly structure. The pH of the surrounding medium also impacts protein stability; several amino acids possess ionizable –R groups that change charge depending on pH. This can decrease the affinity of a substrate for the active site and, if the pH deviates sufficiently, the protein can denature.

---

[30] You don't need to calculate $\Delta G^{\circ\prime}$; all you need to know is that with a K_{eq} of 1,000, there will be 1,000 times more B than A in solution at equilibrium. If we create a solution with only A, the reaction must move spontaneously toward B.

[31] If only B exists in solution, then the back-reaction producing A will predominate until equilibrium is reached ($\Delta G = 0$), regardless of the presence or absence of enzyme (choice **D** is correct, and choice B is wrong). According to the K_{eq} given, at equilibrium there will be 1,000 times more B than A, not the other way around (choice A is wrong). Note that enzymes do not act on the transition state; they act to produce the transition state (choice C is wrong).

[32] L amino acids and D sugars. Remember the L in aLanine.

- The transition state for a reaction possesses a transient negative charge. The active site for an enzyme catalyzing this reaction contains a His residue to stabilize the intermediate. If the His residue at the active site is replaced by a glutamate that is negatively charged at pH 7.0, what effect will this have on the reaction, assuming that the reactants are present in excess compared to the enzyme?[33]

  A) The repulsion caused by the negative charge in the glutamate at the altered active site will increase the activation energy and make the reaction proceed more slowly than it would in a solution without enzyme.
  B) The rate of catalysis will be unaffected, but the equilibrium ratio of products and reactants will change, favoring reactants.
  C) The transition state intermediate will not be stabilized as effectively by the altered enzyme, lowering the rate relative to the rate with catalysis by the normal enzyme.
  D) The rate of catalysis will decrease, and the equilibrium constant will change.

Enzymatic function can also depend upon the association of additional molecules. **Cofactors**, which are metal ions or small molecules (not themselves a protein), are required for activity in many enzymes. In fact, the majority of the vitamins in our diet serve as precursors for cofactors (e.g., niacin [B3] is ultimately transformed into NAD^+). When a cofactor is an organic molecule, it is referred to as a **coenzyme**; these often bind to the substrate during the catalyzed reaction. One prime example of a coenzyme, which we will focus on later in the chapter, is coenzyme A (CoA).

4.6 REGULATION OF ENZYME ACTIVITY

Metabolic pathways in the cell are not all continually on, but must be tightly regulated to maintain health. For example, if glycogen synthesis and breakdown occur in the same cell at the same time, a great deal of energy will be wasted without accomplishing anything. Therefore, the activity of key enzymes in metabolic pathways is usually regulated in one or more of the following ways:

1) **Covalent modification.** Proteins can have several different groups covalently attached to them, and this can regulate their activity, lifespan in the cell, and/or cellular location. The addition of a phosphoryl group from a molecule of ATP by a protein **kinase** to the hydroxyl of serine, threonine, or tyrosine residues is the most common example. Phosphorylation of these different sites on an enzyme can either activate or inactivate the enzyme. Protein **phosphorylases** also phosphorylate proteins, but use free-floating inorganic phosphate (P_i) in the cell instead of ATP. Protein phosphorylation can be reversed by protein **phosphatases**.

2) **Proteolytic cleavage.** Many enzymes (and other proteins) are synthesized in inactive forms (zymogens) that are activated by cleavage by a protease.

---

[33] Beware of long, complex-sounding questions! They may not be as bad as they look; for instance, the phrase "assuming that the reactants are present in excess compared to the enzyme" adds nothing to the substance of this question. If His (which is positive or neutral at pH 7) is replaced by Glu (negatively charged at pH 7), this could decrease the effectiveness of—or destroy altogether—the active site of the enzyme. This means the transition state would not be effectively stabilized, and the rate of the reaction would simply reduce to that of the uncatalyzed reaction (choice **C** is correct). The rate would not proceed more slowly than the uncatalyzed reaction (i.e., "in solution without enzyme"; choice A is wrong), and remember that enzymes do not alter reaction equilibria (K_{eq} will be unaffected; choices B and D are wrong).

3) **Association with other polypeptides.** Some enzymes have catalytic activity in one polypeptide subunit that is regulated by association with a separate regulatory subunit. For example, there are some proteins that demonstrate continuous rapid catalysis if their regulatory subunit is removed; this is known as **constitutive activity** (*constitutive* means continuous or unregulated). There are other proteins that require association with another peptide in order to function. Still other proteins can bind many regulatory subunits. There are numerous examples of this in the cell, and many of them have diverse and complex regulatory mechanisms that all revolve around the theme of "associations with other polypeptides can affect enzyme activity."

4) **Allosteric regulation.** The modification of active-site activity through interactions of molecules with other specific sites on the enzyme (called **allosteric sites**). Let's look at this in a little more detail.

4.6

Allosteric Regulation

If the cell is to make use of the enzyme as a biochemical switch, there must be a way to turn the enzyme *on* or *off*. One mechanism of regulation is the binding of small molecules to particular sites on an enzyme that are distinct from the active site; this is allosteric regulation. This name comes from the fact that the particular spot on the enzyme which can bind the small molecule is *not* the active site; *allo* means "other," and *steric* refers to a location in space (as in "steric hindrance"), so *allosteric* means "at another place." The binding of the allosteric regulator to the allosteric site is generally noncovalent and reversible. When bound, the allosteric regulator can alter the conformation of the enzyme to increase or decrease catalysis, even though it may be bound to the enzyme at a site distant from the active site or even on a separate polypeptide.

Feedback Inhibition

Enzymes usually act as part of pathways, not alone. Rather than regulate every enzyme in a pathway, usually there are one or two key enzymes that are regulated, such as the enzyme that catalyzes the first irreversible step in a pathway. The easiest way to explain this is with an example. Three enzymes (E1, E2, and E3) catalyze the three steps required to convert Substrate A to Product D. When plenty of D is around, it would be logical to shut off E1 so that excess B, C, and D are not made. This would conserve A and would also conserve energy. Commonly, an end-product such as D will shut off an enzyme early in the pathway, such as E1. This is called **negative feedback**, or **feedback inhibition**.

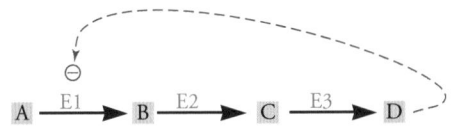

Figure 15 Feedback Inhibition

There are examples of positive feedback ("feedback *stimulation*"), but negative feedback is by far the most common example of feedback regulation. On the other hand, *feedforward stimulation* is common. This involves the stimulation of an enzyme by its substrate or by a molecule used in the synthesis of the substrate. For example, in Figure 15, A might stimulate E3. This makes sense because when lots of A is around, we want the pathway for utilization of A to be active.

Allosteric regulation can be quite complex. It is possible for more than one small molecule to be capable of binding to an allosteric site. For example, imagine a reaction pathway from A through Z, in which each step (A → B, B → C, etc.) is catalyzed by an enzyme. Let's say that an allosteric enzyme called E15 catalyzes the reaction O → P. It would be possible for A to allosterically activate E15 (feedforward stimulation) and for Z to allosterically inhibit E15 (feedback inhibition). This may sound complex, but it's quite logical. What it means is that when lots of A is around, E15 will be stimulated to use the molecules made from A (B, C, D, etc.) to make P, which could then be used to make Q, R, S, etc., all the way up to Z. On the other hand, if a lot of excess Z built up, it would inhibit E15, thereby conserving the supply of A, B, C, etc. and preventing more build-up of Z, Y, X, etc. Therefore, in addition to acting as switches, enzymes act as *valves*, because they regulate the flow of substrates into products.

4.7 ENZYME KINETICS

Enzyme kinetics is the study of the rate of formation of products from substrates in the presence of an enzyme. The **reaction rate** (V, for velocity) is the amount of product formed per unit time, in moles per second (mol/s). It depends on the concentration of substrate, [S], and enzyme.[34] If there is only a little substrate, then the rate V is directly proportional to the amount of substrate added: double the amount of substrate and the reaction rate doubles, triple the substrate and the rate triples, and so forth. But eventually there is so much substrate that the active sites of the enzymes are occupied much of the time, and adding more substrate doesn't increase the reaction rate as much, that is, the slope of the V vs. [S] curve decreases. Finally, there is so much substrate that every active site is continuously occupied, and adding more substrate doesn't increase the reaction rate at all. At this point, the enzyme is said to be **saturated**. The reaction rate when the enzyme is saturated is denoted V_{max} (see Figure 16). This is a property of each enzyme at a particular concentration of enzyme. You can look it up in a book for the common ones. [If a small amount of enzyme in a solution is acting at V_{max} and the substrate concentration is doubled, what is the new reaction rate?[35]]

Another commonly used parameter on these enzyme kinetics graphs is the Michaelis constant K_m. K_m is the substrate concentration at which the reaction velocity is half its maximum. To find K_m on the enzyme kinetics graph, mark the V_{max} on the y-axis; then divide this distance in half to find $V_{max}/2$. K_m is found by drawing a horizontal line from $V_{max}/2$ to the curve and then a vertical line down to the x-axis. K_m is unique for each enzyme-substrate pair and gives information on the affinity of the enzyme for its substrate. If an enzyme-substrate pair has a low K_m, it means that not very much substrate is required to get the reaction rate to half the maximum rate; thus, the enzyme has a high affinity for this particular substrate.

---

[34] Usually the concentration of enzyme is kept fixed, and [S] is taken as the only independent variable (the one the rate depends on). This is applicable to biological systems, where substrate concentrations change much more than enzyme concentrations.

[35] If the enzyme is acting at V_{max}, it is saturated with substrate; adding more substrate will not increase the reaction rate; the rate is still V_{max}.

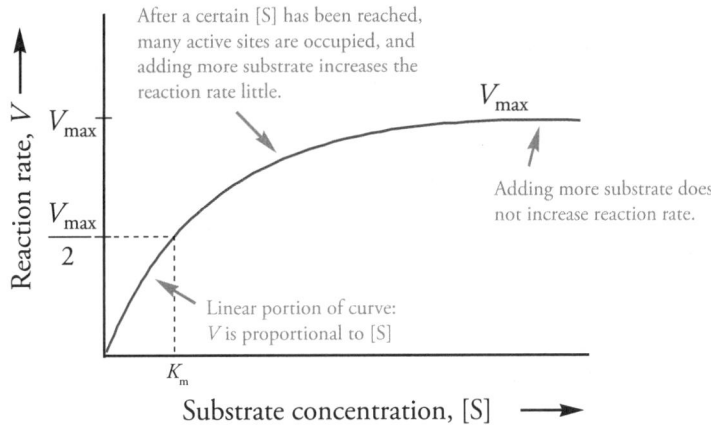

Figure 16   Saturation Kinetics

Cooperativity

Many multisubunit enzymes do not behave in the simple kinetic manner described above. In such enzymes, the binding of substrate to one subunit modulates the affinity of other subunits for substrate. Such enzymes are said to bind substrate cooperatively. There are two types of cooperativity: positive and negative. In positive cooperativity, the binding of a substrate to one subunit increases the affinity of the other subunits for substrate. The conformation of the enzyme prior to substrate binding, with low substrate affinity, is sometimes termed "tense," and the conformation of enzyme with increased affinity is termed "relaxed"[36] (Figure 17). Negative cooperativity (which is less important for the MCAT) is the opposite: the binding of a substrate to one subunit reduces the affinity of the other subunits for substrate. Cooperative enzymes must have more than one active site. They are usually multisubunit complexes, composed of more than one protein chain held together in a quaternary structure. They may also be a single-subunit enzyme with two or more active sites.

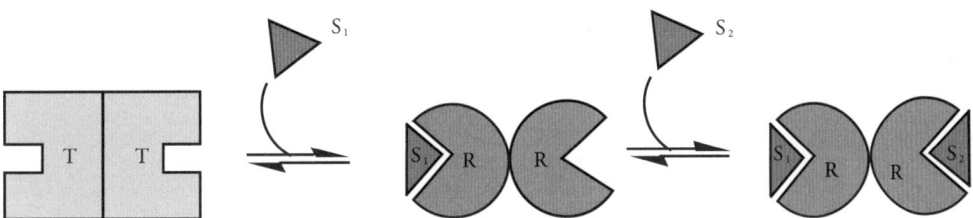

Figure 17   Positive Enzyme Cooperativity

---

[36] Imagine a group of people who can't get any dates. They are all depressed about it, and they keep each other depressed, which makes it even less likely that any will get a date. They are tense, "turned off," and inactive. Then one of the depressed group gets a date and gets so excited about it that all the other friends in the group get so enthusiastic that they get dates too. They are "turned on," relaxed, hip, groovy, and active.

A sigmoidal curve results from positive cooperative binding. In Figure 18 below, the flat part at the bottom left (Region 1) is explained by the notion that at low [S] the enzyme complex has a low affinity for substrate (is in the tense state), and adding more substrate increases the rate little. The steep part in the middle of the curve (Region 2) represents the range of substrate concentrations in which adding substrate greatly increases the reaction rate, because the enzyme complex is in the relaxed state. [The leveling off at the upper right part of the curve (Region 3) represents what?[37]]

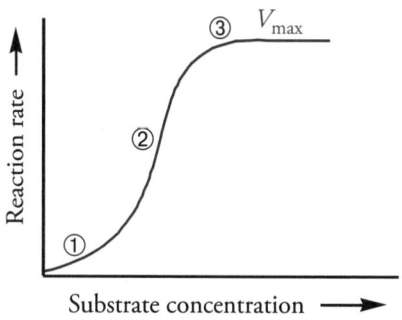

Figure 18   Sigmoidal Kinetics of Positive Cooperativity

Cooperativity does not apply just to catalytic enzymes. For example, hemoglobin (Hb) is a protein complex made of four polypeptide subunits, each of which contains a heme prosthetic group with a single O_2-binding site. (So one Hb has four hemes and four binding sites.) Hb is a carrier (of oxygen), not a catalyst of any reaction (not an enzyme). It exhibits positively cooperative O_2 binding. This is why the Hb-O_2 dissociation curve is sigmoidal. [What is the relationship between the two notions *allosteric* and *cooperative*?[38]]

---

[37] Saturation, just as in the case of a noncooperative enzyme.

[38] Cooperativity is a special kind of allosteric interaction. One active site acts like an allosteric regulatory site for the other active sites. Secondly, cooperative enzyme complexes are often allosterically regulated also. Hb is an excellent example. Not only does O_2 binding to one subunit increase the other subunits' affinities, but also several other molecules can bind to various sites to change the affinity of the complex. For example, CO_2 stabilizes tense Hb, causing each of the four binding sites to have a lower affinity for oxygen. As a result, in the presence of CO_2, Hb tends to give up whatever O_2 it has bound. The most important thing to remember, though, is that the binding in cooperativity takes place at the active site, while the binding in allosteric regulation takes place at "other sites."

4.8 INHIBITION OF ENZYME ACTIVITY

Enzyme inhibitors can reduce enzyme activity by a few different mechanisms, including **competitive inhibition, noncompetitive inhibition, uncompetitive inhibition,** and **mixed-type inhibition. Competitive inhibitors** are molecules that *compete* with substrate for binding at the active site. [You can predict that structurally, competitive inhibitors resemble what?[39]] The key thing to remember about competitive inhibitors is that their inhibition can be overcome by adding more substrate; if the substrate concentration is high enough, the substrate can *outcompete* the inhibitor. Hence, V_{max} is not affected. You can get to the same V_{max}, but it takes more substrate (see Figure 19). Therefore, the K_m of the reaction to which a competitive inhibitor has been added is increased compared to the K_m of the uninhibited reaction. [If an enzyme has a reaction rate of 1 μmole/min at a substrate concentration of 50 μ*M* and a rate of 10 μmole/min at a substrate concentration of 100 μ*M*, does this indicate the presence of a competitive inhibitor?[40]]

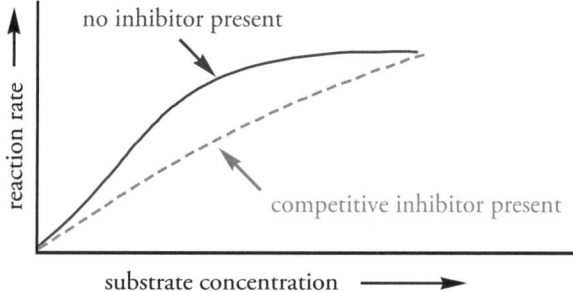

Figure 19   Competitive Inhibition

Noncompetitive inhibitors bind at an allosteric site, not at the active site. No matter how much substrate you add, the inhibitor will not be displaced from its site of action (see Figure 20). Hence, noncompetitive inhibition *does* diminish V_{max}. Remember that V_{max} is always calculated at the same enzyme concentration, since adding more enzyme will increase the measured V_{max}. Addition of a noncompetitive inhibitor changes the V_{max} and $V_{max}/2$ of the reaction, but typically does not alter K_m. This is because the substrate can still bind to the active site, but the inhibitor prevents the catalytic activity of the enzyme.

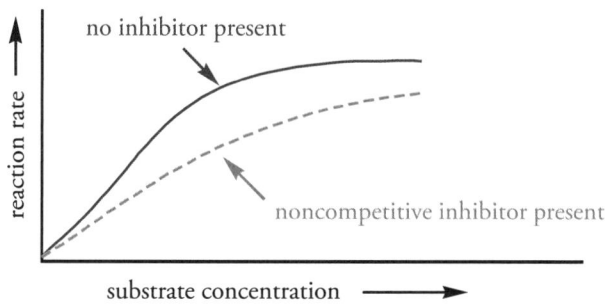

Figure 20   Noncompetitive Inhibition

---

[39] Structurally, competitive inhibitors must at least resemble the substrate; however, the most effective competitive inhibitors resemble the transition state that the active site normally stabilizes.

[40] No. The rate increase is greater than linear, indicating that the effect is caused by cooperativity.

- Carbon dioxide is an allosteric inhibitor of hemoglobin. It dissociates easily when Hb passes through the lungs, where the CO_2 can be exhaled. Carbon *mon*oxide, on the other hand, binds at the oxygen-binding site with an affinity 300 times greater than oxygen; it can be displaced by oxygen, but only when there is much more O_2 than CO in the environment. Which of the following is/are correct?[41]

  - I.   Carbon monoxide is an irreversible inhibitor.
  - II. CO_2 is a reversible inhibitor.
  - III. CO_2 is a noncompetitive inhibitor.

- In the figure below, the kinetics of an enzyme are plotted. In each case, an inhibitor may be present or absent. Which one of the following statements is true?[42]

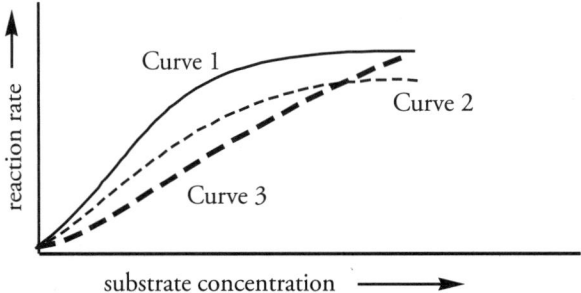

- A) Curve 3 represents noncompetitive inhibition of the enzyme.
- B) Curve 1 represents noncompetitive inhibition of the enzyme.
- C) The V_{max} values of Curve 2 and Curve 3 are the same.
- D) Curve 3 represents competitive inhibition of the enzyme, and the enzyme is uninhibited in Curve 1.

If an inhibitor is only able to bind to the enzyme-substrate complex (that is, it cannot bind before the substrate has bound), it is referred to as an **uncompetitive inhibitor**. Uncompetitive inhibitors, like non-competitive inhibitors, bind to allosteric sites. This effectively decreases V_{max} by limiting the amount of available enzyme-substrate complex which can be converted to product. By sequestering enzyme bound to substrate, this increases the apparent affinity of the enzyme for the substrate as it cannot readily dissociate (decreasing K_m).

---

[41] Item I: False. The question states that CO can be displaced by oxygen. **Item II: True.** The question states that it dissociates easily. **Item III: True.** The question states it binds allosterically, which means "at another site" (not the active site).

[42] Since Curve 3 and Curve 1 have the same V_{max}, but Curve 3 has a reduced rate of product formation, it suggests that Curve 3 represents competitive inhibition of the enzyme in Curve 1 (choice **D** is correct). If Curve 3 represented noncompetitive inhibition, its V_{max} would be reduced compared to Curve 1 (choice A is wrong), and in no case would an inhibitor have a higher V_{max} than an uninhibited reaction (choice B is wrong). Lastly, it can be seen on the graph that Curve 2 has a reduced V_{max} compared to Curve 3 (choice C is wrong).

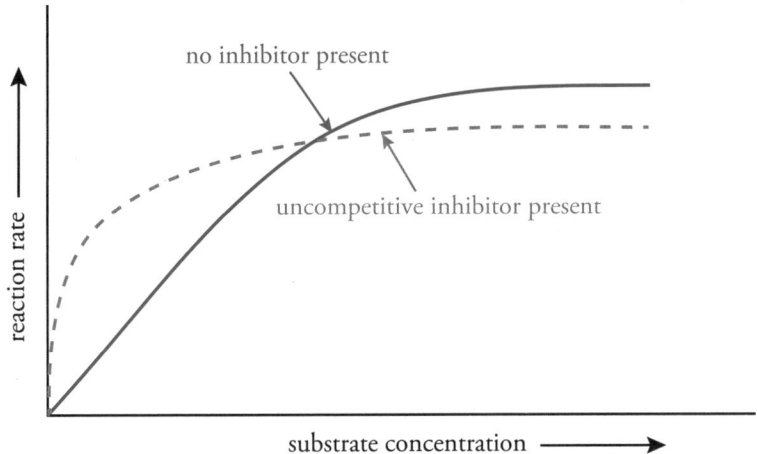

Figure 21 Uncompetitive Inhibition

Mixed-type inhibition occurs when an inhibitor can bind to either the unoccupied enzyme or the enzyme-substrate complex. If the enzyme has greater affinity for the inhibitor in its free form, the enzyme will have a lower affinity for the substrate similar to competitive inhibition (K_m increases). If the enzyme-substrate complex has greater affinity for the inhibitor, the enzyme will have an apparently greater affinity (K_m decreases) for the substrate similar to what we saw in uncompetitive inhibition. On the rare occasion when it displays equal affinity in both forms, it would actually be a noncompetitive inhibitor (many textbooks list noncompetitive inhibition as an example of mixed-type inhibition). In each of these situations, the inhibitor binds to an allosteric site and additional substrate cannot overcome inhibition (V_{max} decreases).

Inhibition Type	$V_{max, app}$	$K_{m, app}$
Competitive	no change	↑
Noncompetitive	↓	no change
Uncompetitive	↓	↓
Mixed-type	↓	varies

Table 3 Changes in the Apparent V_{max} and K_m in Response to Various Types of Inhibition

4.9 LINEWEAVER-BURK PLOT

The Lineweaver-Burk plot is a graphical representation of enzyme kinetics using the Lineweaver-Burk Equation:

$$\frac{1}{V} = \left(\frac{K_m}{V_{max}}\right)\left(\frac{1}{[S]}\right) + \frac{1}{V_{max}}$$

The equation may appear intimidating but can be interpreted as a simple linear equation of the form: $y = mx + b$. The graph is called a double reciprocal plot because the y-axis is the inverse of the reaction rate $\left(\frac{1}{V}\right)$ and the x-axis is the inverse of the substrate concentration $\left(\frac{1}{[S]}\right)$. The key aspects you need to know about the Lineweaver-Burk plot are the following:

1) The slope of the graph is $\dfrac{K_m}{V_{max}}$.

2) The y-intercept of the graph is $\dfrac{1}{V_{max}}$.

3) The x-intercept of the graph is $\dfrac{-1}{K_m}$.

Recall that increasing the substrate concentration ([S]) increases the reaction rate V up to a point. An increase in substrate concentration, however, is a *decrease* in the inverse of the substrate concentration $\left(\frac{1}{[S]}\right)$. Thus, an interesting aspect of the Lineweaver-Burk plot is that an increase in substrate concentration means a decrease in the value along the x-axis. Similarly, an increase in the reaction rate V is a *decrease* in the inverse of the reaction rate $\left(\frac{1}{V}\right)$. Thus, as the reaction rate increases, the value along the y-axis decreases.

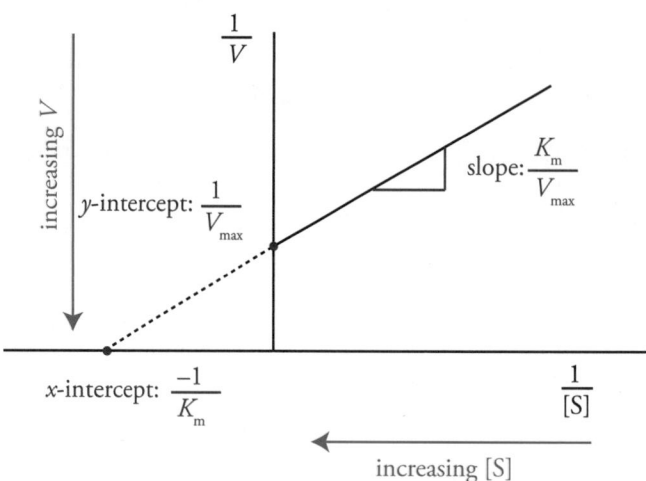

Figure 22 Lineweaver-Burk Plot

- How would the Lineweaver-Burk plot change when a noncompetitive inhibitor is added?[43]

---

[43] A noncompetitive inhibitor does not affect the K_m (so the x-intercept is unchanged) but does decrease the V_{max} (so the y-intercept increases and the slope increases).

Chapter 4 Summary

- Amino acids (AAs) consist of a tetrahedral α-carbon connected to an amino group, a carboxyl group, and a variable R-group, which determines the AA's properties.

- The isoelectric point of an AA is the pH at which the net charge on the molecule is zero; this structure is referred to as the zwitterion.

- Proteins consist of amino acids linked by peptide bonds, which are very stable. The primary structure of a protein consists of its amino acid sequence.

- The secondary structure of proteins (α-helices and β-sheets) is formed through hydrogen bonding interactions between atoms in the backbone of the molecule.

- The most stable tertiary protein structure generally places polar AAs on the exterior and nonpolar AAs on the interior of the protein. This minimizes interactions between nonpolar AAs and water, while optimizing interactions between side chains inside the protein.

- Proteins have a variety of functions in the body including (but not limited to) enzymes, structural roles, hormones, receptors, channels, antibodies, and transporters.

- Enzymes are biological catalysts that increase the rate of a reaction by lowering the activation energy.

- Unfavorable reactions in the cell are performed by coupling them to favorable reactions (such as ATP hydrolysis).

- Enzyme activity can be controlled via covalent modification, proteolytic cleavage, associations, or allosteric regulation.

- Competitive inhibitors bind at the active site of an enzyme, do not affect V_{max} but increase K_m.

- Noncompetitive inhibitors bind at an allosteric site of an enzyme, decrease V_{max} but do not change K_m.

- Uncompetitive inhibitors bind to the enzyme-substrate complex and reduce both K_m and V_{max}.

- Mixed-type inhibitors can bind to either the enzyme alone or the enzyme-substrate complex. They reduce V_{max} but have variable effects on K_m.

- The Lineweaver-Burk plot is a linear graph used to extrapolate the V_{max} and K_m of an enzyme. It is a visual aid that can be used to identify inhibitor type.

CHAPTER 4 FREESTANDING PRACTICE QUESTIONS

1. If a mutation changed an Arg residue in the protein interior to a Leu residue, what would be the likely effect on the ΔG of protein folding?

A) ΔG would become more positive.
B) ΔG would become more negative.
C) ΔG would remain unchanged.
D) The effect on ΔG cannot be determined without additional information.

2. Some inhibitors bind irreversibly to enzymes by covalent attachment. Would the kinetics seen under these conditions (V vs. [S] curve) be similar to those seen with a reversible noncompetitive inhibitor?

A) Yes, because it would reduce the K_m of the reaction.
B) Yes, because the net effect would be a loss of active enzyme available for the reaction.
C) No, because if enough substrate binds to the active site, the reaction will reach V_{max}.
D) No, because K_m will increase and V_{max} will stay the same, similar to competitive inhibition.

3. Some enzymes can modify their substrate, and by this means, regulate its activity. In many instances, these modifications are not permanent since other enzymes can reverse them. Which of the following category of enzymes will irreversibly modify their substrate?

A) A kinase
B) A protease
C) A phosphatase
D) An acetylase

4. Which of the following would have the LEAST effect on the ability of an enzyme to bind its substrate?

A) Placing an enzyme that optimally functions at pH 7 in a pH 5 solution
B) Increasing the temperature of the enzyme's surroundings
C) Mutating the Glu and Asp residues in the active site to Lys and His
D) Changing the substrate from a tripeptide to a disaccharide

5. For a given enzyme concentration at a low substrate concentration, how does reaction rate change as the substrate concentration increases?

A) Logarithmically
B) Linearly
C) Exponentially
D) Indirectly

6. Both hemoglobin and myoglobin are proteins that carry oxygen in the human body. Hemoglobin exhibits cooperativity and is found in red blood cells, whereas myoglobin is not cooperative and is found in muscle cells. Which of the following is likely true regarding these oxygen-carrying proteins?

A) The O_2 saturation curve will be sigmoidal for myoglobin, but not hemoglobin.
B) Hemoglobin has a lower binding affinity for oxygen than myoglobin.
C) Hemoglobin is used to tightly bind oxygen in the body, while myoglobin is used to deliver oxygen to body cells.
D) Hemoglobin most likely consists of multiple protein subunits, whereas myoglobin may or may not consist of multiple protein subunits.

7. Which of the following will be true of the Lineweaver-Burk plot of an enzyme in the presence of increasing concentrations of a competitive inhibitor?

A) It will be a series of lines that intersect along the y-axis.
B) It will be a series of lines that intersect along the x-axis.
C) It will be a series of parallel lines.
D) It will be a series of lines that will intersect, but neither on the y- or x-axis.

CHAPTER 4 PRACTICE PASSAGE

The Michaelis-Menten equation expresses the relationship between reaction velocity (V) and substrate concentration ([S]) for enzymatic reactions involving a single substrate.

$$V = V_{max}[S] / (K_m + [S])$$

Equation 1

Equation 1 yields a hyperbolic curve when V is plotted against [S] (Figure 1). Prior to the availability of computer programs that were able to perform non-linear regression, it was difficult to curve fit V vs. [S] data accurately to obtain values for K_m and V_{max}. To overcome this problem, multiple strategies were developed to represent the Michaelis-Menten equation in a linear form. One of the most commonly employed was the Lineweaver-Burk formulation (Equation 2), in which taking the reciprocal of Equation 1 yields a relationship that can be represented by a linear plot of $1/V$ vs. $1/[S]$ (Figure 1):

$$1/V = (K_m/V_{max}) \times 1/[S] + 1/V_{max}$$

Equation 2

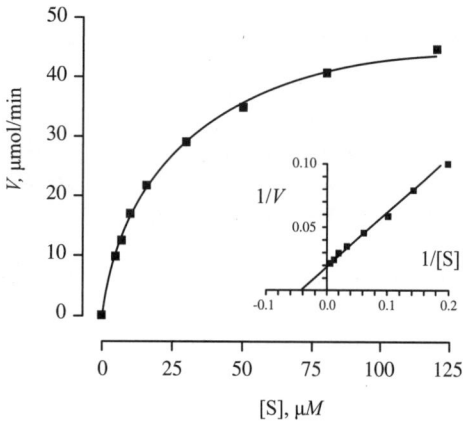

Figure 1 Sample V vs. [S] plot with Lineweaver-Burk representation (inset)

Despite the advantages of this linear representation of enzymatic rate data, the Lineweaver-Burk plot introduces greater error when used to determine V_{max} and K_m. Thus, it is not recommended when highly accurate values of these kinetic parameters are desired. Instead, the continued utility of the Lineweaver-Burk plot lies in its ability to clearly differentiate modes of enzyme inhibition.

Many organisms employ enzymes related to complexes in the mitochondrial electron transport chain for oxidative transformation of environmental toxins. NADH oxidoreductase, isolated from *Methylococcus capsulatus*, is an example of such an enzyme that participates in the oxidative conversion of methane into methanol. In an experiment whose results are shown below in Figure 2, a researcher tested the ability of two different inhibitors to affect the activity of NADH oxidoreductase at two different concentrations. The results are displayed as Lineweaver-Burk plots.

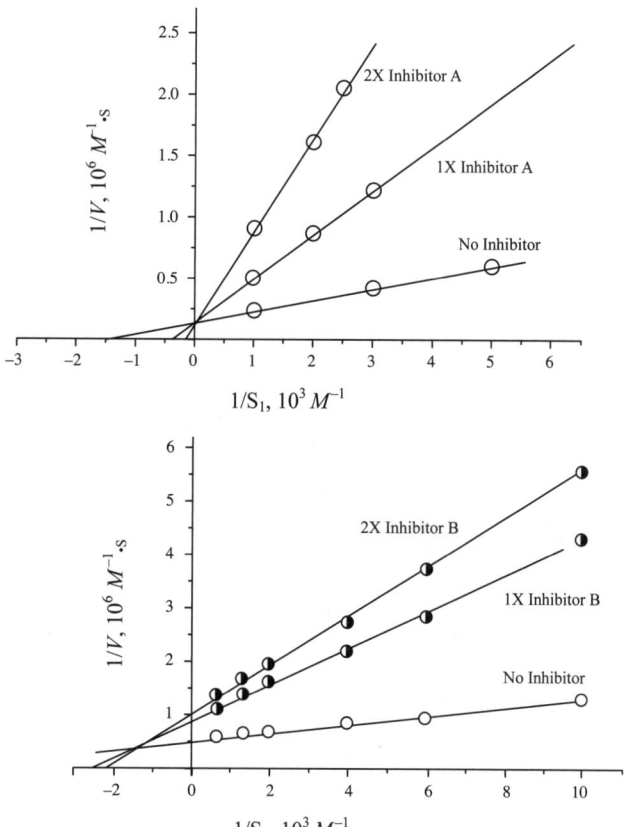

Figure 2 Inhibition of NADH oxidoreductase by two different inhibitors

Adapted from Saratovskikh, EA. *Kinetics and Mechanism of Inhibition of Oxidation Enzymes by Herbicides.* In Herbicides, Advances in Research. Edited by Price A and Kelton J. 2013

1. Which of the following is the best estimate for the V_{max} of the enzyme represented by Figure 1?

   A) 0.02 µmol / min
   B) 23 µmol / min
   C) 44 µmol / min
   D) 52 µmol / min

2. Which of the following represent possible sources of error when estimating K_m and V_{max} from a Lineweaver-Burk plot?

   I. The inability to obtain negative values of 1/[S] often requires extrapolation of the linear fit over a long stretch lacking data points in order to determine the x-intercept.
   II. Errors in the data obtained at low substrate concentration have a disproportionate impact on the determination of the best linear fit.
   III. Visual estimation of K_m and V_{max} is more challenging from a linear plot as compared to the hyperbolic plot of V vs. [S].

   A) I only
   B) II only
   C) I and II only
   D) I, II, and III

3. Which of the following is true concerning the slope of a Lineweaver-Burk plot in the presence of a competitive versus a noncompetitive inhibitor?

   A) The slope changes in the presence of both a competitive and noncompetitive inhibitor.
   B) The slope changes in the presence of a competitive inhibitor only.
   C) The slope changes in the presence of a noncompetitive inhibitor only.
   D) The slope does not change in the presence of either type of inhibitor.

4. Reductive detoxification of reactive oxygen intermediates is critical to the survival of aerobic organisms. Which of the following is most directly involved in this process in humans?

   A) NADH produced by the pentose phosphate pathway
   B) NADH produced by gluconeogenesis
   C) NADPH produced by the pentose phosphate pathway
   D) NADPH produced by gluconeogenesis

5. All of the following are true concerning Inhibitor A EXCEPT:

   A) its effect on enzyme activity can be overcome by increasing the substrate concentration.
   B) its effect on enzyme activity is equivalent to that of decreasing the concentration of the uninhibited enzyme.
   C) it is unable to bind to the enzyme at the same time that substrate is bound.
   D) its effect on enzyme activity is equivalent to that of decreasing the enzyme-substrate binding affinity.

6. Which of the following represents the Lineweaver-Burk plot of an enzyme alone (solid line) and in the presence of a noncompetitive inhibitor (dashed line)?

   A)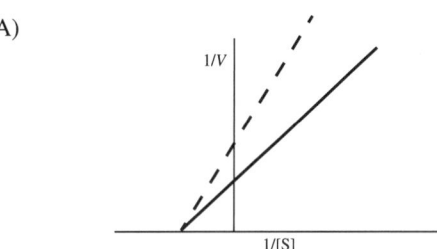

   B)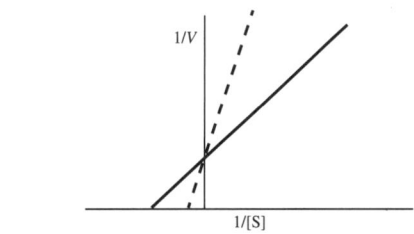

   C)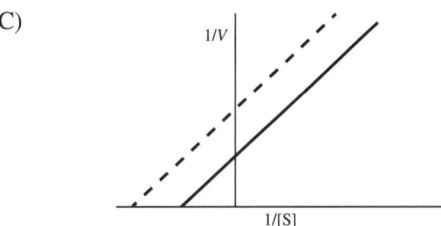

   D)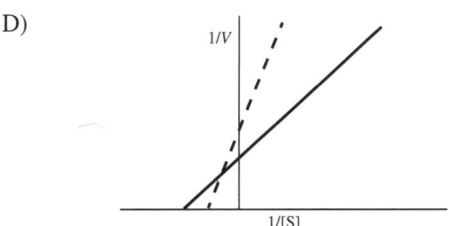

SOLUTIONS TO CHAPTER 4 FREESTANDING PRACTICE QUESTIONS

1. **D**   Although the hydrophobic effect is a major driving force in protein folding, the favorability of protein folding is also determined by the favorability of amino acid interactions. Generally, the positively charged Arg residue would not be favored in the nonpolar protein interior, relative to the nonpolar Leu residue. The Arg residue, however, may be favorably interacting with an acidic residue in the protein interior. As such, without additional information about other interactions the Arg is involved in, the effect on ΔG cannot be reasonably predicted (choices A, B, and C are wrong, and choice D is correct).

2. **B**   An irreversible inhibitor (regardless of where it binds) will permanently deactivate some enzyme, reducing effective enzyme concentration. If the enzyme concentration is effectively lowered, V_{max} will be reduced (choices C and D are wrong). This is similar to what is seen in noncompetitive inhibition, in which the inhibitor binds to an allosteric site and turns the enzyme off. Even if the noncompetitive inhibitor is reversible, because at any given time some enzyme is "off," the effective enzyme concentration is lowered and V_{max} is reduced. If K_m were affected, it would increase, not decrease; an increase in K_m indicates that the substrate-enzyme interaction has been compromised in some way (choice A is wrong).

3. **B**   Proteases are enzymes that cleave their substrates at specific sites, permanently removing a part of the protein. This modification is practically irreversible—there are no enzymes that can reconnect proteins split by a protease. Choices A, C, and D are wrong because these categories of enzymes can reversibly modify their substrates. A kinase adds a phosphate to its substrate, but this modification can be reversed by a phosphatase that will remove the phosphate. An acetylase will add an acetyl group, while a deacetylase will remove it.

4. **B**   Increasing the temperature of an enzyme's surroundings may or may not affect the likelihood of an enzyme binding its substrate. Increasing temperature will increase the kinetic energy of the substrate and make it more likely to enter the active site, unless the temperature is increased beyond the temperature of denaturation; since the question is not specific as to the magnitude of the temperature change, this is the choice that would likely have the LEAST effect (choice B is correct). Changing the pH of the solution to a non-optimal value will likely affect the charge of the protein side chains and enzyme function (choice A is wrong). Mutating acidic residues to basic residues will change the charge of the active site substantially and likely affect the substrate's ability to bind to the active site (choice C is wrong). Significantly altering the shape and size of the substrate will decrease its ability to effectively bind to the active site (choice D is wrong).

5. **B**   At low substrate concentrations, the reaction rate increases linearly as the substrate concentration increases (see curve below). At or near saturation levels, the reaction rate begins to level off and does not change regardless of how much substrate it added. This is called the maximum velocity of reaction rate or V_{max}.

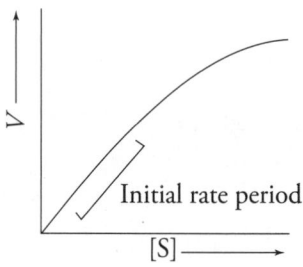

6.   **D**   In order to exhibit cooperativity, a protein must be composed of multiple protein subunits that are able to interact with one another (or, less likely, it should have multiple active sites within the same protein); thus, it is likely that hemoglobin is composed of multiple subunits. Since myoglobin does not exhibit cooperativity, it may either be composed of one subunit or multiple non-cooperative subunits (choice D is correct). Cooperative enzymes usually exhibit sigmoidal curves; hemoglobin would be expected to exhibit a sigmoidal curve, but not myoglobin (choice A is wrong). Cooperativity is a phenomenon involving changes in binding affinity when a substrate is bound; thus, binding affinity between a cooperative protein and a non-cooperative protein is not directly comparable (choice B is wrong). Note, however, that at the typical oxygen concentration found in tissues (e.g., muscle), myoglobin would have to have the higher affinity in order to be able to "steal" oxygen from hemoglobin and store it. Since hemoglobin is found in red blood cells, it must be the delivery protein, while myoglobin in muscle cells is the storage protein (choice C is wrong).

7.   **A**   In a Lineweaver-Burk plot, the y-intercept represents $1/V_{max}$, and the x-intercept represents $-1/K_m$. Because competitive inhibitors do not change the V_{max} and instead increase the K_m value, a Lineweaver-Burk plot with differing concentrations of competitive inhibitor will show intersecting lines that share a common y-intercept (choice A is correct). A common x-intercept would be indicative of an unchanged K_m value, as in the case of noncompetitive inhibition (choice B is wrong). A series of parallel lines is indicative of uncompetitive inhibition (choice C is wrong). A series of lines with any common intersection point not on the axes is indicative of mixed-type inhibition (choice D is wrong).

SOLUTIONS TO CHAPTER 4 PRACTICE PASSAGE

1.   **D**   This question highlights a main advantage of the Lineweaver-Burk plot. If Equation 2 is considered in $y = mx + b$ form, it is clear that the y-intercept (b) represents $1/V_{max}$. Looking at the hyperbolic curve that we are all used to, in which V_{max} is approached asymptotically, choices A and B are clearly wrong. In particular, choice A is too small a number, and it represents the y-intercept of the Lineweaver-Burk plot, which is $1/V_{max}$, not V_{max}. Choices C and D both seem in reasonable range when looking at the hyperbolic graph, but estimation is difficult, as it has not completely leveled off at the highest shown substrate concentration. In the linear plot, this ambiguity is resolved as we are looking for the y-axis intercept. In this case, it occurs at just less than 0.02, so V_{max} is just greater than 1/0.02 or 50 µmol/min.

2.   **C**   Item I is true: as it is impossible to have negative substrate concentrations, a Lineweaver-Burk plot will never have data points in negative x-axis (1/[S]) territory. As such, extrapolation of the line back to the x-axis will occur over a stretch of graph lacking data points (choice B can be eliminated). Item II is true: data obtained at low substrate concentration (and thus higher 1/[S]; in effect, the points at upper right of the graph), which are likely to have more measurement error, have a larger role in determining the slope of the linear fit (choice A can be eliminated). Item III is false: the passage suggests that the impetus for creating the Lineweaver-Burk formulation was the lack of computer programs that could accurately perform non-linear regression (fitting the hyperbola of a V vs. [S] graph). Clearly, drawing a straight line through points is easier (choice D can be eliminated, and choice C is correct).

3. **A** This question requires recognition of the meaning of the slope of a Lineweaver-Burk plot. Equation 2 is conveniently written in $y = mx + b$ format, in which the dependent variable (y) is $1/V$, the independent variable (x) is $1/[S]$, the y-intercept (b) is $1/V_{max}$, and the slope (m) is K_m/V_{max}. Competitive inhibition increases K_m, while non-competitive inhibition reduces V_{max}. As both K_m and V_{max} contribute to the slope, both modes of inhibition will engender a change in slope of the Lineweaver-Burk plot.

4. **C** NADPH is not generated by gluconeogenesis, and NADH is not generated by the pentose phosphate pathway (choices A and D can be eliminated). While our cells use NAD⁺ as an electron acceptor in the oxidative metabolism of nutrients, they employ NADPH as the electron donor in reductive biosynthesis and in the process of detoxification of reactive oxygen species. Production of NADPH by the pentose phosphate pathway is one of the important functions of this pathway for the cell. The other is generating ribose for nucleotide biosynthesis.

5. **B** If you evaluate the linear plot in Figure 2 in the presence of Inhibitor A, you can see that the y-intercept ($1/V_{max}$) is not affected by the inhibitor, while the slope (K_m/V_{max}) increases. Thus, you conclude that the effect of this inhibitor is to increase K_m while leaving V_{max} unchanged. This is the signature of a competitive inhibitor, which competes with the substrate for binding to the active site (choice C is true and can be eliminated). Because they compete, increasing the concentration of the substrate will overcome the effect of the inhibitor on the enzyme (choice A is true and can be eliminated). As K_m is a measure of binding affinity of the enzyme for the substrate, the increase in K_m caused by this inhibitor is functionally equivalent to a decrease in affinity of the enzyme for its substrate (choice D is true and can be eliminated). However, since V_{max} depends on enzyme concentration, and since this inhibitor does not affect V_{max}, choice B is a false statement and the correct answer choice.

6. **A** A non-competitive inhibitor binds to an allosteric site on the enzyme, effectively turning the enzyme off, but it does not affect the ability of the enzyme to bind substrate. Thus, V_{max} will be decreased and K_m will remain the same. On the Lineweaver-Burk plot, a decrease in V_{max} is represented by an increase in the y-intercept (if V decreases, $1/V$ increases; choice B can be eliminated). K_m is represented by the x-intercept; since K_m is the same, there should be no change in the x-intercept (choices C and D can be eliminated, and choice A is correct).

COMPLEX II SUBUNIT SDHD IS CRITICAL FOR CELL GROWTH AND METABOLISM, WHICH CAN BE PARTIALLY RESTORED WITH A SYNTHETIC UBIQUINONE ANALOG

Aloka B. Bandara, Joshua C. Drake & David A. Brown

BMC Molecular and Cell Biology volume 22, Article number: 35 (2021)

BACKGROUND

Mitochondria generate the majority of adenosine triphosphate (ATP) through the electron transport chain (ETC). Succinate dehydrogenase (Complex II) uniquely serves as a component of both the Krebs cycle and the ETC. As a component of the Krebs Cycle, Complex II catalyzes oxidation of succinate to fumarate, whereas in the ETC, it is one of two entry points for electrons, acquiring electrons from succinate and donating them to ubiquinone (CoQ). Thus, impairments in Complex II function can have severe consequences for maintaining energetic homeostasis. Mutations in Complex II subunits have been found in patients with mitochondrial respiratory deficiency, as well as a number of cancers. Therefore, an in-depth understanding of Complex II in energetic homeostasis and its viability as a target for treatment is warranted.

Complex II carries four protein subunits, all of which are encoded by nuclear genes. Two subunits, SDHA and SDHB, are localized on the matrix side of the inner membrane, and carry the binding site for succinate, three FeS clusters, as well as a flavoprotein bound to an FAD cofactor. The two remaining subunits, SDHC and SDHD, are hydrophobic and anchor the complex to the inner-membrane. Subunits SDHC and SDHD form the CoQ binding site of Complex II and serve as terminal electron transfers from Complex II to CoQ. In particular, mutation of SDHD has been noted in patients with paragangliomas and pheochromocytomas. Therefore, given the particular role of SDHD in anchoring Complex II to the inner-membrane, passaging electrons to CoQ, and noted pathologies, modeling SDHD dysfunction could be a valuable tool for understanding the role of Complex II in metabolism and developing novel therapeutics. To date, however, suitable models for molecular examinations of any Complex II subunit do not exist.

We successfully used a CRISPR/cas9 approach to mutate the SDHD subunit of Complex II in HEK293 cells, and characterized its requirement for mitochondrial respiration, ATP synthesis, and cell growth in vitro. Furthermore, we demonstrate the efficacy of the mitochondrial therapeutic idebenone to improve mitochondrial dysfunction in cells with SDHD mutation. Our results demonstrate the necessity of SDHD for energetic homeostasis and suggests it as a viable target for therapies aimed to improve mitochondrial function.

RESULTS

Construction of mutant HEK293Δ*SDHD*

The single guide RNA (sgRNA) sequences were designed based on the 609 bp long *SDHD* nucleotide sequence of *Homo sapiens*. A 118-bp site of the forward strand of *SDHD* was predicted as the most reliable for mutation. The guide strand predicted was TCTGTTGCTTCGAACTCCAG (Fig. 1a). The constructed mutant HEK293Δ*SDHD* was validated by Western immunoblotting. The predicted molecular weight of SDHD is approximately 17 kDa. Nevertheless, the antibody used for mutant validation was anticipated to produce an additional band of about 29 kDa as well on the blot from parent cells. Our mutant HEK293Δ*SDHD* was found missing both 17 kDa and 29 kDa protein bands (Fig. 1b).

A. GTTCGTTGCAACAAATTGATGAGCAATGCTTTTTTTATAATGCC
AACTTTGTACAAAAAAGTTGGCATGGCGGTTCTCTGGAGGCTG
AGTGCCGTTCCGGTGCCCTAGGAGGCCGAGCTCTGTTGCTTC
GAACTCCAGTGGTCAGACCTGCTCATATCTCAGCATTTCTTCA
GGACCGACCTATCCCAGAATGGTGTGGAGTGCAGCACATACAC
TTGTCACCGAGCCACCATTCTGGCTCCAAGGTGCATCTCTCC
ACTGGACTAGCGAGAGGGTTGTCAGTGTTTGCTCCTGGGTCT
GCTTCCGGCTGTTATTTGAATCCTTGCTCTGCGATGGACTAT
TCCCTGGCTGCAGCCCTCACTCTTCATGGTCATGGGGCCTTG
GACAAGTTGTTACTGACTATGTTCATGGGGATGCCTTGCAGAA
AGCTGCCAAGGCAGGGTTTTGGCACTTTCAGCTTTAACCTTT
GCTGGGCTTTGTATTTCAACTATCACGATGTGGACATCTGCA
AAGCTGTTGCCATGCTGTGGAAGCTCTGCCCAACTTTCTTGTA
CAAAGTTGGCATTATAAGAAAGCATTGCTTATCAATTTGTTGC
AACGAAC

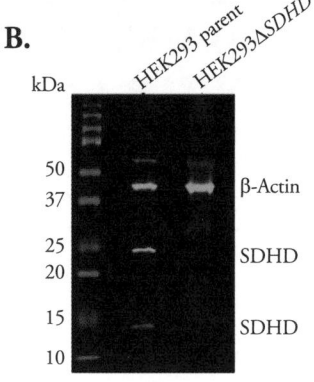

B.

C.

Parent: AGCTCTGTTGCTTCGAACTCCAGTGGTCAGACCTGCTCATA

Bases C and A have been deleted | Base G has been inserted

Mutant: AGCTCTGTTGCTTCGAACTCGGTGGTCAGACCTGCTCATA

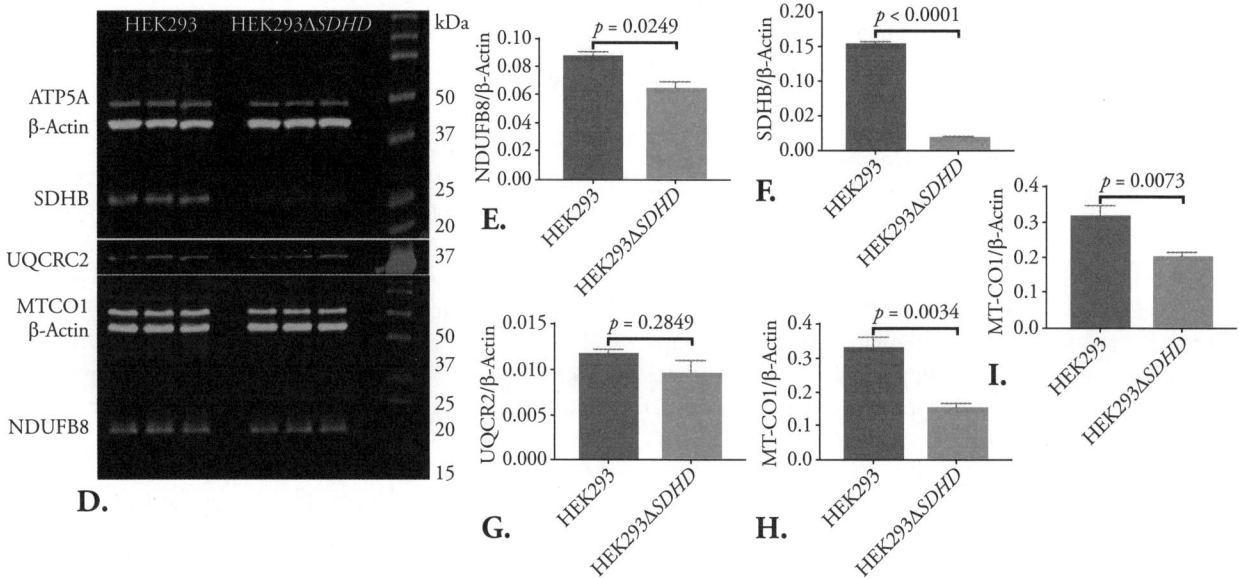

Figure 1 Construction of the SDHD mutant. The gene sequence of SDHD with CRISPR targeting sites is shown **a**. Expression of SDHD protein is shown **b**. The protein extracts reacted with rabbit polyclonal antibodies to SDHD and rabbit polyclonal antibodies to β-Actin are shown. The DNA level recombination events in the genome of the mutant are illustrated **c**. Expression of representative subunits from all five ETC complexes are shown **d-i**. The expression of NDUFB8 (complex **i**; **d** and **e**), SDHB (complex II; **d** and **f**), UQCRC2 (complex III; **d** and **g**), MTCO1 (complex IV; **d** and **h**) and ATP5A (complex V; **d** and **i**) were normalized to the expression of β-Actin

We then PCR amplified and sequenced the *SDHD* region encompassing the CRISPR targeting site (at 118-bp) of the mutant. The results indicated that an INDEL mutation has been generated at a site two bases upstream of the GTT PAM sequence. Two bases (a C and an A) have been deleted from this site and one base (a G) has been inserted at the deletion site (Fig. 1c). As a result, the whole amino acid sequence downstream of this INDEL site has been altered. Moreover, a stop codon has been inserted 180 bases downstream of the GTT PAM sequence.

Using the online CRISPR prediction site of the Integrated DNA Technologies, we identified the top three potential off-target sites. The DNA regions encompassing these sites were PCR amplified and sequenced and were identical to those of the parent cell line indicating absence of any off-target genetic alterations in the genome of the mutant.

We then investigated whether mutation in *SDHD* altered the expression of other subunits of the five ETC complexes. Expression of complex II subunit SDHB (Fig. 1d and f) decreased significantly in the mutant ($p < 0.0001$) suggesting that SDHD expression has direct impact on expression of other subunits of the complex II. Moreover, expression of complex I subunit NDUFB8 (Fig. 1d and e), complex IV subunit MT-CO1 (Fig. 1d and h), and complex V subunit ATP5A (Fig. 1d and i) decreased significantly in the mutant ($p = 0.0249$, 0.0034, and 0.0073, respectively) suggesting an association in protein expression between complexes II and other ETC complexes. The expression of complex III subunit UQCRC2 (Fig. 1d and g) was not different between the parent and the mutant suggesting that mutation did not impact expression of this subunit/complex.

Loss of SDHD increases apoptosis and necrosis

Compared to the parent HEK293, the mutant HEK293Δ*SDHD* produced significantly increased amount of ROS at 0 h (immediately after addition of the substrate to the reaction; $p = 0.0128$; Fig. 2a). Nevertheless, the mutant produced significantly decreased ROS amounts at 24 h ($p = 0.0035$) and 72 h ($p < 0.0001$) after addition of the substrate. These observations suggest that disruption of *SDHD* results in subsequent decrease of ROS generation over time. At all the time points, the mutant displayed significantly increased apoptosis ($p < 0.0001$, < 0.0001, < 0.0001, and $= 0.0043$ respectively at 0, 2, 24, and 72 h post-incubation; Fig. 2b). The mutant also showed significantly increased necrosis ($p < 0.0001$ for each time point; Fig. 2c).

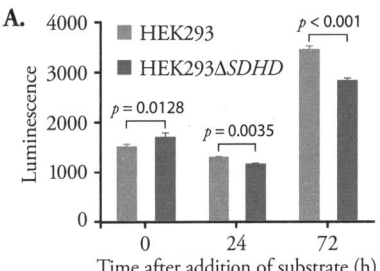

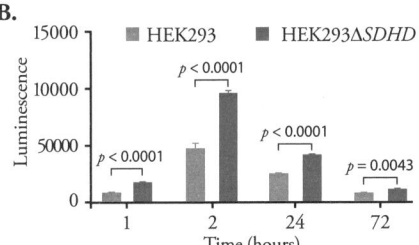

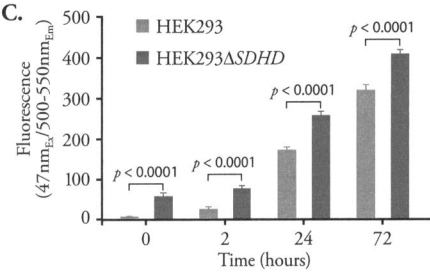

Fig. 2 ROS production, apoptosis, and necrosis of cell lines. ROS generation measured using ROS-Glo H_2O_2 Assay of parent HEK293 and the mutant HEK293Δ*SDHD* is shown (**A**). The measurements are expressed as total luminescence per 15,000 cells measured at 0, 24, and 72 hours after addition of substrate to the reaction. Apoptosis (**B**) and necrosis (**C**) per 15,000 cells measured using RealTime-Glo Annexin V Apoptosis and Necrosis Assay at 0, 2, 24 and 72 hours of incubation are shown. The apoptosis measurements are expressed as total luminescence, whereas necrosis measurements expressed as total fluorescence. Error bars represent the SE of the mean

Loss of SDHD impairs growth

After 4 days of incubation in growth media, the number of cells recovered from the mutant HEK293Δ*SDHD* culture was ~73% less than the amount recovered from parent HEK293 culture ($p = 0.0002$; Fig. 3a). The doubling of mutant over 4 days was significantly slower compared to that of the parent during the same duration of growth ($p = 0.0008$; Fig. 3b), suggesting that SDHD is vital for cell growth.

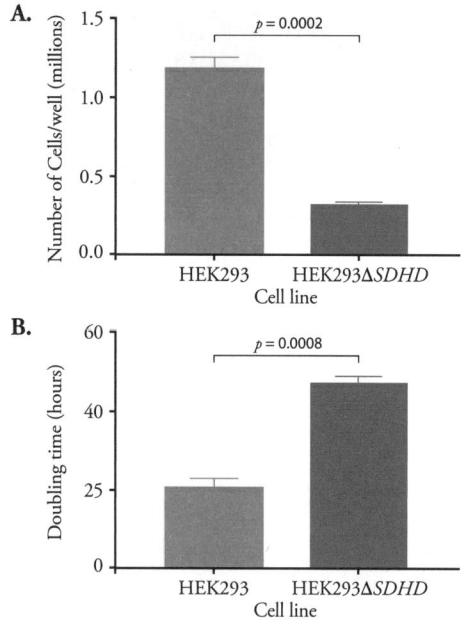

A.

B.

Fig. 3 Growth of cell lines. The number of cells harvested from the parent HEK293 and the mutant HEK293ΔSDHD cells after four days of the culture (**A**) and doubling times of cells (**B**) are shown. Error bars represent the SE of the mean

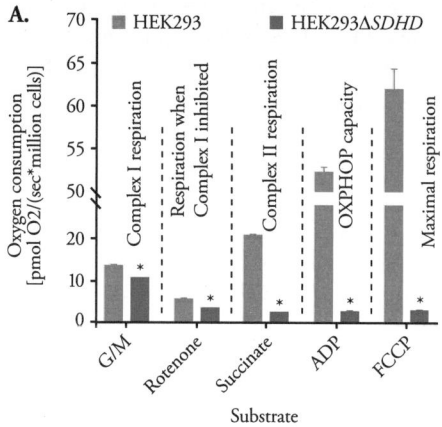

A.

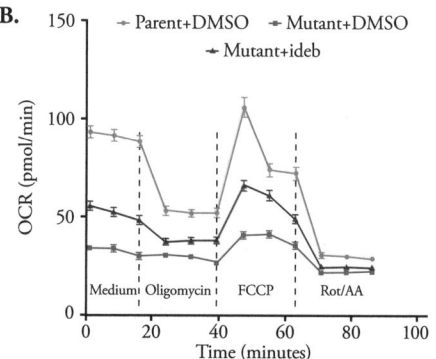

B.

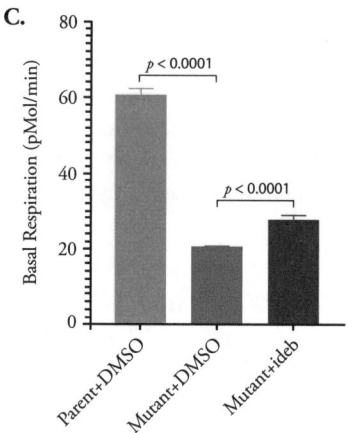

C.

Loss of SDHD impairs mitochondrial respiration

Mutation in SDHD decreased oxygen consumption all along the ETC (Fig. 4a). Complex I respiration was significantly decreased in mutant cells compared to parent ($p = 0.0019$). Subsequent to rotenone treatment, oxygen consumption of both parent and mutant decreased, but the oxygen consumption of mutant cells was significantly less than that of parent cells ($p = 0.0101$). In response to treatment with succinate, Complex II-mediated oxygen consumption was significantly repressed in mutant cells compared to parent cells ($p = 0.0002$), further confirming the effect SDHD mutation. The mutant also had decreased OXPHOS capacity ($p = 0.0002$) and maximal respiration ($p = 0.0017$). Oxygen consumption of permeabilized cells was also assessed (Fig. 4b). In the mutant, basal respiration ($p < 0.0001$; Fig. 4c), reserve respiratory capacity ($p < 0.0001$; Fig. 4d), and maximal respiratory capacity ($p < 0.0001$; Fig. 4e) decreased significantly. These assays collectively indicate a severe impairment of cellular respiration due to SDHD disruption.

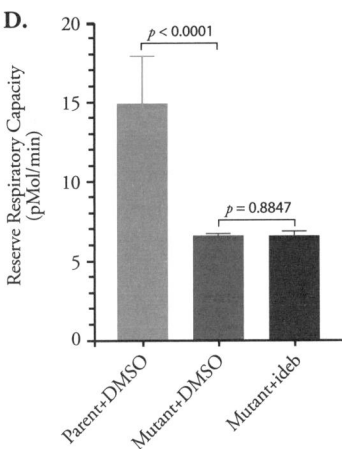

D.

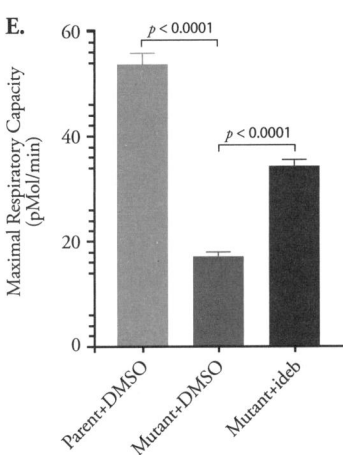

E.

Loss of SDHD impairs glycolytic capacity and ATP synthesis of cell lines

Extracellular Acidification Rate (ECAR) of intact cells was determined (Fig. 5a). Both glycolysis ($p < 0.0001$; Fig. 5b) and glycolytic capacity ($p < 0.0001$; Fig. 5c) decreased significantly in mutant cells. The findings indicate an association between SDHD function and glycolysis. The mutant cells produced significantly less ATP than parent cells at two different cell densities ($p < 0.0001$ when 3500 or 10,000 cells/well were used; Fig. 5d). Impaired ATP synthesis was consistent with suppressed mitochondrial and glycolytic metabolism.

A.

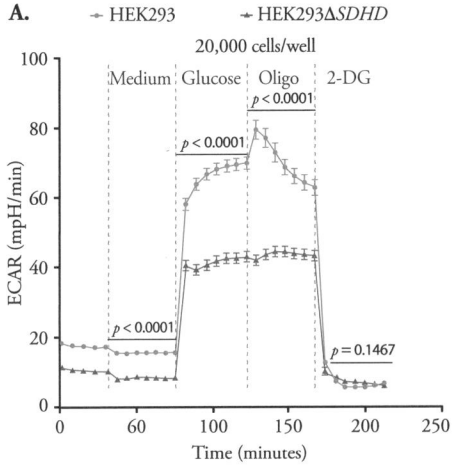

B.

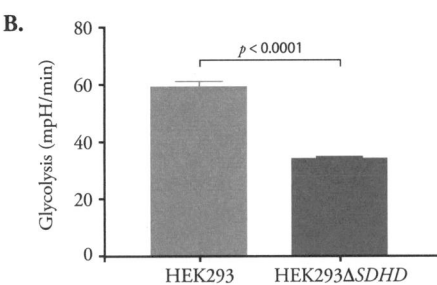

C.

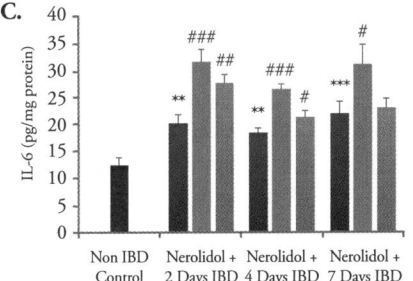

Fig. 4 Respiration, of cell lines. Oxygen consumption rates in response to treatment with glutamate-malate (G/M), rotenone, succinate, ADP, and FCCP (**A**) are shown. The mean oxygen consumption rates were compared between the parent HEK293 and the mutant HEK293Δ*SDHD*. The *p* values for the differences between the mean values were 0.0019, 0.0101, 0.0002, 0.0002 and 0.0017, respectively for Complex I respiration, rotenone treatment, Complex II respiration, OXPHOS capacity, and maximal respiration. Oxygen consumption rate (OCR) was measured of parent cells treated DMSO (Parent + DMSO), mutant cells treated DMSO (Mutant + DMSO), and mutant cells treated 1μM idebenone (Mutant + Ideb). OCR per 20,000 permeabilized cells (**B**), and the calculated basal respiration (**C**), reserve respiratory capacity (**D**) and maximal respiratory capacity (**E**) are shown. The mean OCR values were compared between the parent versus the mutant or DMSO treatment versus idebenone treatment. Error bars represent the SE of the mean.

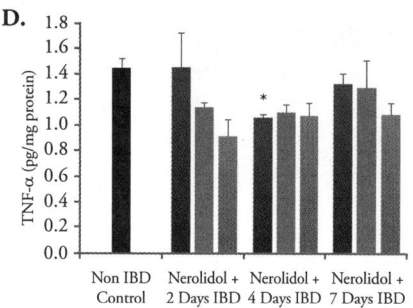

D.

Fig. 5 Glycolysis and ATP synthesis of cell lines. ECAR measured using 20,000 live cells/well (**A**), and calculated glycolysis (**B**) and glycolytic capacity (**C**) are shown. The mean values were compared between the parent HEK293 and the mutant HEK293Δ*SDHD*. ATP synthesis of parent and mutant cells measured using Mitochondrial ToxGlo Assay (**D**) is shown. The measurements are expressed as total luminescence per 3500 or 10,000 cells. Error bars represent the SE of the mean

Improved respiration and growth of HEK293Δ*SDHD* mutant cells treated with mitochondrial therapeutic idebenone

Idebenone is a short-chain benzoquinone with greater hydrophilicity, which has shown promise as a therapeutic for mitochondrial dysfunction. We tested whether idebenone modified oxygen consumption of mutant HEK293Δ*SDHD* cells. Treatment of permeabilized mutant cells with 1 µM idebenone significantly increased basal respiration ($p<0.0001$; Fig. 4c) and maximal respiratory capacity ($p<0.0001$; Fig. 4e), but not reserved respiratory capacity ($p=0.8847$; Fig. 4d). In O2k respirometry assay, in the presence of succinate, idebenone was incrementally added 10 min apart, with concentrations of 1 µM, following by three subsequent injections of 5 µM each (Fig. 6a). Compared to vehicle (DMSO), 1 µM idebenone elicited a non-statistically significant increase in oxygen consumption ($p=0.1250$; Fig. 6a). Subsequent dose of 5 µM idebenone significantly increased oxygen consumption compared to vehicle in mutant cells ($p=0.0119$), which peaked after the second dose of 5 µM idebenone ($p=0.0508$; Fig. 6a). After the final injection of 5 µM idebenone, OXPHOS capacity was measured by adding ADP. Idebenone treated mutant cells had significantly improved OXPHOS capacity compared to the DMSO treated cells ($p=0.0148$) (Fig. 6a). We next investigated whether long-term idebenone treatment would influence cell growth. Due to the slow growth of HEK293Δ*SDHD* cells (Fig. 6b), cells were grown for 10 days in growth media where either 1, 5, or 10 µM idebenone was added to

the media. After 10 days, 25.4% more cells were recovered from cells treated with 1 µM idebenone compared to the DMSO control ($p=0.00959$; Fig. 6b). However, treatment with 5 µM idebenone did not improve growth of the mutant ($p=0.9433$; Fig. 6b), whereas treatment with 10 µM idebenone caused cell death (not shown).

A.

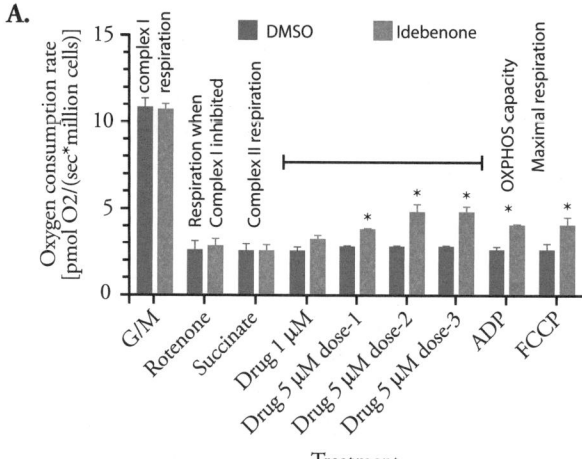

B.

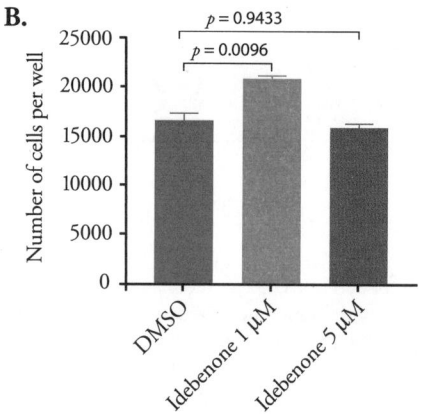

Fig. 6 Restoring the defects of the mutant with use of the mitochondrial therapeutic idebenone. The oxygen consumption rates of permeabilized cells treated with DMSO or idebenone are shown (**A**). The rates per million cells in response to injection of substrates, inhibitor, or drug are depicted. The mean oxygen consumption values were compared between the idebenone treatment and DMSO control. The *p* values for the differences between the mean values of DMSO control versus idebenone treatment were 0.8689, 0.7605, 0.9394, 0.1250, 0.0119, 0.0508, 0.0323, 0.0148, and 0.1084 respectively for G/M, rotenone, succinate, 1 µM idebenone, 1st dose of 5 µM idebenone, 2nd dose of 5 µM idebenone, 3rd dose of 5 µM idebenone, ADP, and FCCP. The number of cells recovered from the mutant cultures treated with 1 µM idebenone or DMSO are shown (**B**). Error bars represent the SE of the mean.

DISCUSSION

We successfully used a CRISPR/Cas9 approach to mutate *SDHD*, a Complex II subunit in the inner-membrane region, in HEK293 cells, generating the first such model to study the role of this essential Complex II subunit. The INDEL recombination events at the 118-bp site disrupted or altered the whole amino acid sequence downstream of the PAM site. And, mutagenesis procedure did not create any detectable off-target genetic alterations. In agreement with the observed alteration of the *SDHD* DNA sequence, amino acid level expression of the protein SDHD was totally disrupted in the mutant. Moreover, as a result of the *SDHD* mutation, expression of another complex II subunit (SDHB) decreased significantly suggesting interdependency in expression among different subunits of this complex. Quite interestingly, the expression of a complex I subunit (NDUFB8), a complex IV subunit (MT-CO1), and a complex V subunit (ATP5A) also decreased significantly in the mutant suggesting an association in protein expression between complex II and other complexes. Nevertheless, the SDHD mutation did not alter expression of the complex III subunit UQCRC2 suggesting independency of this complex from complex II in terms of protein expression.

Mutation in *SDHD* disrupted respiration all along the ETC, suppressed glycolysis and overall ATP synthesis, as well as limited cellular growth. Importantly, acute treatment with the synthetic ubiquinone analog idebenone was sufficient to improve Complex II-mediated mitochondrial respiration, OXPHOS capacity, and cell proliferation.

Predictably, mutation of SDHD inhibited Complex II-mediated respiration. Interestingly, however, mutation in SDHD significantly reduced Complex I-mediated respiration as well. Since Complex II drives Krebs cycle in a clock-wise direction by converting succinate to fumarate, we hypothesize that mutation of SDHD slowed and/or disrupted Krebs cycle production of NADH, the substrate for Complex I. Mutation in SDHD also impaired OXPHOS capacity, maximal respiration, and ATP synthesis. Taken together, impairment in the SDHD subunit of Complex II is sufficient to impair overall ETC energy production.

Glycolysis, as determined by ECAR, was significantly reduced in HEK293ΔSDHD compared to parent cells. Reduced glycolysis may reflect a lower demand for pyruvate due to disrupted Krebs cycle as a result of mutation in SDHD, representing a potential negative feedback on glycolysis. Also, inhibition of mitochondrial respiration with oligomycin did not elicit a change in glycolysis in mutant cells, further reflecting impaired mitochondrial respiration. In addition to the suppressed metabolism, we also noted significantly slower growth in mutant cells compared to parent cells in culture media, which is likely reflective of the metabolic impairment in mutant cells.

Mutation of SDHD increased apoptosis and necrosis. The impaired glycolysis and mitochondrial respiration may have weakened the cell and cell membrane of the mutant making the cells more apoptotic and susceptible to necrosis. Quite interestingly, the long-term ROS generation declined as a result of SDHD mutation. In general, electrons that do not follow the normal order of the ETC pathway and instead leaked out are eventually transferred directly to O_2 to generate ROS. In our SDHD mutant, it is possible that impairment of clock-wise direction of Krebs cycle may have decreased the synthesis of NADH and $FADH_2$, the two electron donors to the ETC. Thus, limited donation of electrons may have led decreased electron transport through the ETC as well as decreased electron leakage out of the ETC giving rise to decreased ROS generation.

Finally, we explored whether SDHD mutation could be bypassed to improve some of the phenotypes observed. Idebenone, is a short-chain benzoquinone that is more hydrophilic than ubiquinone, and has potential as a therapeutic for conditions associated with oxidative stress and mitochondrial dysfunction. Treatment with varying concentrations of idebenone improved Complex II-mediated oxygen consumption and OXPHOS capacity, suggesting that the ubiquinone analog idebenone is able to substitute for Complex II as an electron donor to improve ETC function. Interestingly, long-term treatment with $1\,\mu M$ of idebenone increased cell proliferation in HEK293ΔSDHD cells whereas $5\,\mu M$ did not. Idebenone is known to have cell-type specific effects on cell proliferation. While an increase in cell proliferation in our mutant HEK293ΔSDHD cells with idebenone is likely a result of improved substrate utilization, cell type should be taken into consideration for mitochondrial targeted therapies as to how other process may be influenced.

CONCLUSIONS

We generated a novel mutant of the Complex II subunit SDHD via CRISPR/Cas9 that resulted in severe augmentation to mitochondrial respiration and cell metabolism as well as suppressed growth. This novel tool could be valuable for testing potential mitochondrial-focused therapeutics as well as elucidating other mechanisms regulated by Complex II function.

METHODS

Cell lines and culture conditions

Human embryonic kidney cell line 293 (HEK293) were maintained in Dulbecco's Modified Eagle's medium (DMEM) supplemented with 10% (by volume) fetal bovine serum and 1% penicillin-streptomycin. Cells were sustained in a humidified incubator at 37 °C and 5% CO_2. *Escherichia coli* were used for constructing the mutagenesis plasmid. Bacteria carrying the plasmids were maintained in Luria Bertani agar or broth, and sustained in a humidified incubator at 37 °C.

Construction and validation of *SDHD* mutant

Disruption of SDHD synthesis was validated by Western Immuno-blotting using rabbit polyclonal antibody SDHD (1:1000 in blocking buffer) and rabbit polyclonal antibodies to β-Actin (1:10,000). A clone missing the protein bands representing SDHD was chosen for further work and designated as HEK293Δ*SDHD* (Fig. 1).

The DNA regions encompassing the top three off-targets were PCR amplified and sequenced.

Expression of protein subunits representative to each of the five ETC complexes was examined by Western immunoblotting.

Cell growth and metabolism

Aliquots of 100,000 cells of the parent HEK293 and the mutant HEK293Δ*SDHD* were introduced into 75 cm² flasks each carrying 25 ml growth media. After 4 days of incubation, cell numbers were quantified in triplicates.

Restoring the impaired growth and respiration of the mutant

Effectiveness of the potential mitochondrial therapeutic idebenone in restoring the growth defects of the mutant HEK293Δ*SDHD* was evaluated. In this procedure, mutant cells were cultured on 6-well plates at 2000 cells/well in DMEM medium supplemented 1, 5, or 10 μM of idebenone. Fresh media containing the drug was added on days 3, 6 and 9, and the cell counts in wells of triplicates was determined following 10 days incubation. Efficacy of idebenone in improving respiration of permeabilized mutant cells was measured by O2k respirometry.

Statistical analyses

Student's t-tests were performed. Mean differences between groups were considered statistically significant at $p < 0.05$.

Abbreviations

ETC: Electron transport chain
SDHD: Succinate dehydrogenase subunit D
OXPHOS: Oxidative phosphorylation
ATP: Adenosine triphosphate
CRISPR/Cas9:   Clustered regularly interspaced short palindromic repeats/CRISPR-associated protein 9
DMSO: dimethyl sulfoxide
ROS: Reactive oxygen species
OCR: Oxygen consumption rate

JOURNAL ARTICLE EXERCISE 1

The science sections on the MCAT include a significant number of passages with experiments. Questions for these passages often ask you to analyze data, read charts and graphs, and come to certain conclusions based on the information they give you. If you don't know how to extract information efficiently and analyze data effectively, you will be at a distinct disadvantage.

There are three "Journal Article Exercises" in this book. In this first exercise, we'll show you the type of information you should be able to extract from the article and the sorts of things to pay attention to in the data. In the subsequent exercise, you'll do more of that on your own, and in the final exercise we'll show you how that article might get turned into an MCAT-style passage.

When analyzing an experiment, you should be able to:

- identify the control group(s).
- extract information from graphs and data tables.
- determine how the experimental group(s) change relative to the control.
- determine if the results are statistically significant.
- come to a reasonable conclusion about WHY the results were observed.
- consider potential weaknesses in the study.
- determine how to increase the power of the study.
- decide what the next most logical experiment or study should be.

The goal of these exercises is NOT to learn content from the articles, just to get more comfortable reading and extracting information from them.

For the (abridged) article on the pages 99–106, try to summarize the purpose of the experiment and the methods in four to five sentences. Consider the following mnemonic: Oh ouR Car Won't Start (ORCWS).

- **O = Organism and Organization**: is the research being conducted on humans or on animals or on bacteria, or something else? What is being done to these organisms? Are there any unique qualities to these organisms? Are there multiple groups? Is the study conducted over a long period of time with multiple data points, or is it a short-term study? Does it have a large or small n?
- **R = Results**: where and how are the results presented? Is it a graph? A data table? Figures and images? What is/are the independent variable(s)? What is/are the dependent variable(s)? Do the results show correlation or cause and effect, or both? Describe.
- **C = Control and Comparison**: is there a control group? How does it differ from the experimental group? Is it given a placebo or nothing at all? Is it held under different conditions? If there are multiple experimental groups, how do they differ from one another? Is it a blinded study? If so, double-blind or single-blind?
- **W = Weirdness**: does anything or do any of the results stand out as unexpected?
- **S = Statistics**: was any sort of statistical analysis done? How is it presented? Are there error bars on a graph? Standard errors around a mean? Are there p-values? Is there an asterisk indicating statistical significance? Is there any data that is not statistically significant?

Try interpreting the data on your own before reading the results/discussion section. When you do read the discussion, consider:

- What are the conclusions of the study?
- How are the conclusions supported by the data?
- What potential weaknesses or flaws do you see in the experimental design? Are these addressed in the discussion section?
- How might this study be potentially biased?
- How might this study be improved?
- What would be the next most logical experiment?

SOLUTIONS TO JOURNAL ARTICLE EXERCISE 1

Let's answer the above questions for the article on pages 99–106.

1. **O = Organism and Organization:**
    - Is the research being conducted on humans or on animals or on bacteria, or something else? *Human cell line – human embryonic kidney, HEK293*
    - What is being done to these organisms? *The gene for Complex II SDHD (succinate dehydrogenase complex subunit D) is knocked out and mitochondrial respiration is measured in comparison to parent cell line.*
    - Are there any unique qualities to these organisms? *The knockout cell line was created via CRISPR-Cas9.*
    - Are there multiple groups? *Two: HEK293 cells and HEK293ΔSDHD cells*
    - Is the study conducted over a long period of time with multiple data points, or is it a short-term study? *Short-term study (72 hours)*
    - Does it have a large or small n? *Large n: just over one million HEK293 cells, just under 0.5 million HEK293ΔSDHD cells*

2. **R = Results:**
    - Where and how are the results presented? Is it a graph? A data table? Figures and images? *Graphs, images of sequences, and images of gels*
    - What is/are the independent variable(s)? *Time, presence/absence of SDHD*
    - What is/are the dependent variable(s)? *Cell growth, ROS levels, apoptosis, necrosis, oxygen consumption, glycolysis, ATP synthesis*
    - Do the results show correlation or cause and effect, or both? Describe. *Both. Correlation: Decreased cell numbers and increased doubling time for mutant HEK293ΔSDHD cells over parent HEK cells; Cause and effect: HEK293ΔSDHD cells demonstrated less ROS but more apoptosis and necrosis than HEK cells.*

3. **C = Control and Comparison:**
    - Is there a control group? *Yes*
    - How does it differ from the experimental group? Is it given a placebo or nothing at all? Is it held under different conditions? *HEK cells have SDHS intact*
    - If there are multiple experimental groups, how do they differ from one another? *Only one experimental group, HEK293ΔSDHD cells*
    - Is it a blinded study? If so, double blind or single blind? *Not a blinded study*

4. **W = Weirdness:**
    - Does anything or do any of the results stand out as unexpected? *It seemed unexpected that the 5 μM idebenone treatment was less effective than the 1μM.*

5. **S = Statistics:**
    - Was any sort of statistical analysis done? *Yes*
    - How is it presented? Are there error bars on a graph? Standard errors around a mean? Are there p-values? Is there an asterisk indicating statistical significance? *P-values, error bars, asterisks*
    - Is there any data that is not statistically significant? *Yes, difference in Complex III between HEK293 and HEK293ΔSDHD cells, difference between treatment with DMSO and 5 μM idebenone.*

6. **Interpreting the data:**
    *   What are the conclusions of the study? *Mutations in Complex II can augment mitochondrial respiration and impair cell growth. As done in cell culture, this model could be used to test therapeutics for mitochondrial disorders and/or further explore the regulation of Complex II.*
    *   How are the conclusions supported by the data? *The data shows significant differences in cell numbers over time between the mutated and control cultures. Additionally, measurements of cellular respiration show statistical differences between the mutated and control cell lines.*
    *   What potential weaknesses or flaws do you see in the experimental design? Are these addressed in the discussion section? *Study represents an in vitro model that can isolate SDHD from Complex II and measure the isolated effect of its knockout but does not provide an in vivo comparison for this knockout.*
    *   How might this study be potentially biased? *Sample bias: the study was conducted on one cell line and its knockout.*
    *   How might this study be improved? *Repeated on a broader range of human cell lines*
    *   What would be the next most logical experiment? *Determine a method to simulate knockout conditions in a small animal model.*

7. **Final Summary of Experiment and Results:**
    *   *In this journal article the impact of Complex II's SDHD on mammalian cell growth and metabolism was explored using HEK parent cells and a knockout strain, HEK293ΔSDHD. Cell growth of both strains was measured with the doubling time of the knockout showing significant increase along with its rates of apoptosis and necrosis. Additionally, multiple measures of cellular respiration were taken including but not limited to oxygen consumption and ATP synthesis with the knockout again being found to be significantly impaired. Treatment with mitochondrial therapeutics negated this effect in the knockout and could be scaled for greater bioenergetic capacity.*

Chapter 5
Carbohydrates and Carbohydrate Metabolism

Carbohydrates can be broken down to CO_2 in a process called **oxidation**. Because the process releases large amounts of energy, carbohydrates generally serve as the principle energy source for cellular metabolism. Glucose can be stored as the polymer glycogen in animals and as the polymer starch in plants. Glucose in the form of the polymer cellulose is the building block of wood and cotton. Understanding the nomenclature, structure, and chemistry of carbohydrates is essential to understanding cellular metabolism. This chapter will also help you understand key facts such as why we can eat potatoes and cotton candy but not wood and cotton T-shirts, and why milk makes some adults flatulent.

5.1 MONOSACCHARIDES AND DISACCHARIDES

A single carbohydrate molecule is called a **monosaccharide** (meaning "single sweet unit"), also known as a **simple sugar**. Monosaccharides have the general chemical formula $C_nH_{2n}O_n$.

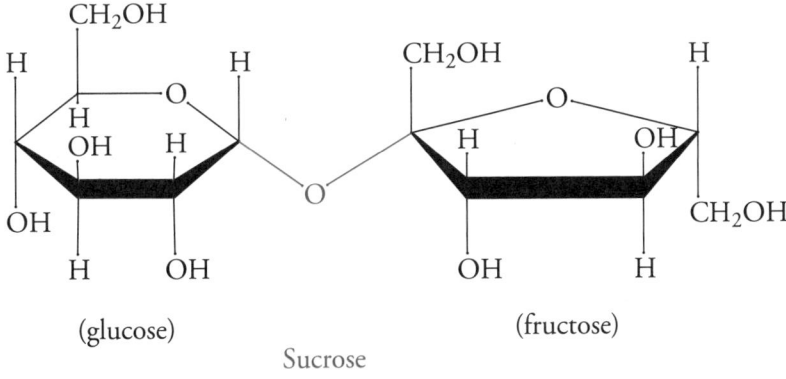

Fructose   Glucose   Ribose

Figure 1   Some Metabolically Important Monosaccharides

Two monosaccharides bonded together form a **disaccharide**, a few form an oligosaccharide, and many form a polysaccharide. The bond between two sugar molecules is called a **glycosidic linkage**. This is a covalent bond, formed in a dehydration reaction that requires enzymatic catalysis.

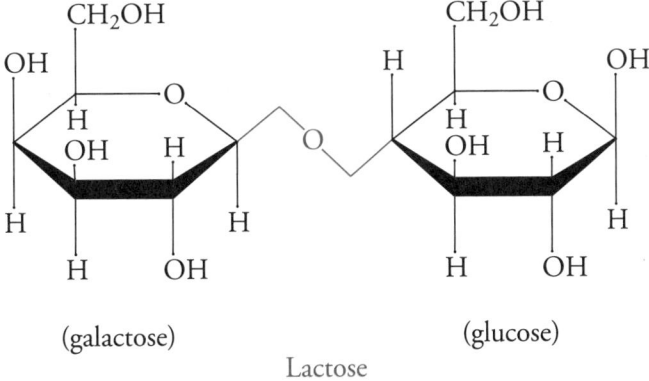

(glucose)   (fructose)

Sucrose

(galactose)   (glucose)

Lactose

Figure 2   Disaccharides and the α- or β-Glycosidic Bond

Glycosidic linkages are named according to which carbon in each sugar comprises the linkage. The configuration (α or β) of the linkage is also specified. For example, lactose (milk sugar) is a disaccharide joined in a galactose-β-1,4-glucose linkage (above). Sucrose (table sugar) is also shown above, with a glucose unit and a fructose unit.

- Does sucrose contain an α- or β-glycosidic linkage?[1]

Some common disaccharides you might see on the MCAT are sucrose (Glc-α-1,2-Fru), lactose (Gal-β-1,4-Glc), maltose (Glc-α-1,4-Glc), and cellobiose (Glc-β-1,4-Glc). However, you should NOT try to memorize these linkages.

5.2 POLYSACCHARIDES

Polymers (polysaccharides) made from the common disaccharides listed above form important biological macromolecules. Glycogen serves as an energy storage carbohydrate in animals and is composed of thousands of glucose units joined in α-1,4 linkages; α-1,6 branches are also present. Starch is the same as glycogen (except that the branches are a little different), and it serves the same purpose in plants. Cellulose is a polymer of cellobiose; but note that cellobiose does not exist freely in nature. It exists only in its polymerized, cellulose form. The β-glycosidic bonds allow the polymer to assume a long, straight, fibrous shape. Wood and cotton are made of cellulose.

Hydrolysis of Glycosidic Linkages

The hydrolysis of polysaccharides into monosaccharides is favored thermodynamically. Hydrolysis is essential in order for these sugars to enter metabolic pathways (e.g., glycolysis) and be used for energy by the cell. However, this hydrolysis does not occur at a significant rate without enzymatic catalysis. Different enzymes catalyze the hydrolysis of different linkages. The enzymes are named for the sugar they hydrolyze. For example, the enzyme that catalyzes the hydrolysis of maltose into two glucose monosaccharides is called **maltase**. Each enzyme is highly specific for its linkage.

This specificity is a great example of the significance of stereochemistry. Consider cellulose. A cotton T-shirt is pure sugar. The only reason we can't digest it is that mammalian enzymes generally can't break the β-glycosidic linkages found in cellulose. Cellulose is actually the energy source in grass and hay. Cows are mammals, and all mammals lack the enzymes necessary for cellulose breakdown. To live on grass, cows depend on bacteria that live in an extra stomach called a rumen to digest cellulose for them. If you're really on the ball, here's your next question: Humans are mammals, so how can we digest lactose, which has a β linkage? The answer is that we have a specific enzyme, **lactase**, which can digest lactose. This is an exception to the rule that mammalian enzymes cannot hydrolyze β-glycosidic linkages. People without lactase are **lactose malabsorbers**, and any lactose they eat ends up in the colon. There it may cause gas and diarrhea, if certain bacteria are present; people with this problem are said to be **lactose intolerant**. People produce lactase as children so that they can digest mother's milk, but most adults naturally stop making this enzyme, and thus become lactose malabsorbers and sometimes intolerant.

---

[1] The oxygen on the anomeric carbon of glucose is pointing down, which means the linkage is α-1,2. So, sucrose is Glc-α-1,2-Fru.

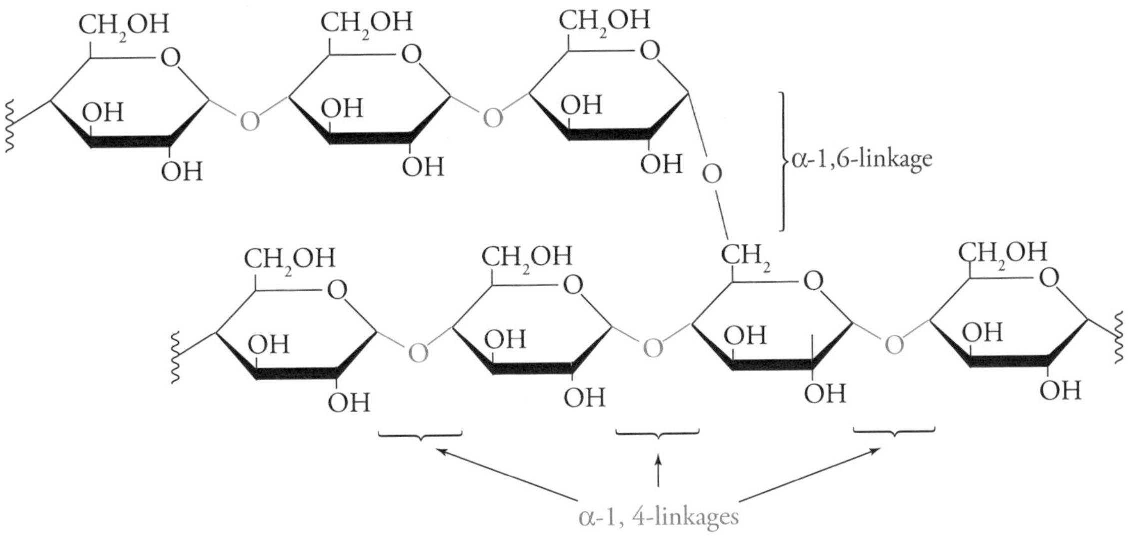

Figure 3 The Polysaccharide Glycogen

- Which requires net energy input: polysaccharide synthesis or hydrolysis?[2]
- If the activation energy of polysaccharide hydrolysis were so low that no enzyme was required for the reaction to occur, would this make polysaccharides better for energy storage?[3]

5.3 INTRODUCTION TO CELLULAR RESPIRATION

When glucose is oxidized to release energy, very little ATP is generated directly. Instead, the oxidation of glucose is accompanied by the reduction of high-energy electron carriers, nicotinamide adenine dinucleotide (**NAD$^+$**) and flavin adenine dinucleotide (**FAD**). Each of these carriers accepts high-energy electrons during redox reactions (forming **NADH** and **FADH$_2$**) and are later oxidized when they deliver the electrons to the electron transport chain. This generates the proton gradient that is used to generate ATP. Both of these carriers can serve as enzymatic cofactors and fulfill diverse roles in biological processes. For instance, NAD$^+$ is required for activation of adenylate cyclase by cholera toxin, and FAD can associate with a protein to become a **flavoprotein**. Dozens of flavoproteins have been characterized and are commonly involved in redox reactions (e.g., amino acid metabolism).

Glucose is oxidized to produce CO_2 and ATP in a four-step process: glycolysis, the pyruvate dehydrogenase complex (PDC), the Krebs cycle, and electron transport/oxidative phosphorylation. The first stage is **glycolysis** ("glucose splitting"). Here, glucose is partially oxidized while it is split in half, into two identical **pyruvic acid** molecules. [How many carbon atoms does pyruvic acid have?[4]] Glycolysis produces a

---

[2] Because hydrolysis of polysaccharides is thermodynamically favored, energy input is required to drive the reaction toward polysaccharide synthesis.

[3] No, because then polysaccharides would hydrolyze spontaneously (they'd be unstable). The high activation energy of polysaccharide hydrolysis allows us to use enzymes as gatekeepers—when we need energy from glucose, we open the gate of glycogen hydrolysis.

[4] The text states that glucose is split in half in the formation of pyruvate. Since glucose has six carbons, pyruvate must have three.

small quantity of ATP and a small quantity of NADH. Glycolysis occurs in the cytoplasm and does not require oxygen.

In the second stage (the **pyruvate dehydrogenase complex**), the pyruvate produced in glycolysis is decarboxylated to form an acetyl group. The acetyl group is then attached to **coenzyme A**, a carrier that can transfer the acetyl group into the Krebs cycle. A small amount of NADH is produced.

In the third stage, the **Krebs cycle** (also known as the **tricarboxylic acid cycle (TCA cycle)** or the **citric acid cycle**), the acetyl group from the PDC is added to oxaloacetate to form citric acid. The citric acid is then decarboxylated and isomerized to regenerate the original oxaloacetate. A modest amount of ATP, a large amount of NADH, and a small amount of $FADH_2$ are produced. Note that although the PDC and the Krebs cycle occur only when oxygen is available to the cell, *neither uses oxygen directly*. Rather, oxygen is necessary for stage four, in which NADH and $FADH_2$ generated throughout cellular respiration are reconverted into NAD^+ and FAD. The PDC and the Krebs cycle occur in the innermost compartment of the mitochondria: the **matrix**.

In stage four of energy harvesting, **electron transport/oxidative phosphorylation**, the high-energy electrons carried by NADH and $FADH_2$ are oxidized by the **electron transport chain** in the inner mitochondrial membrane. The reduced electron carriers dump their electrons at the beginning of the chain, and oxygen is reduced to H_2O at the end. (The word *oxidative* in "oxidative phosphorylation" refers to the use of oxygen to oxidize the reduced electron carriers NADH and $FADH_2$.) The electron energy liberated by the transport chain is used to pump protons out of the innermost compartment of the mitochondrion. The protons are allowed to flow back into the mitochondrion, and the energy of this proton flow is used to produce the high-energy triphosphate group in ATP.

Glycolysis

Glycolysis is an extremely old pathway, having evolved several billion years ago. It is the universal first step in glucose metabolism, the extraction of energy from carbohydrates. All cells from *all domains* (a domain is the highest taxonomic category) possess the enzymes of this pathway. In glycolysis, a glucose molecule is oxidized and split into two pyruvate molecules, producing a net surplus of 2 ATP (from ADP + P_i) and producing 2 NADH (from NAD^+ + H^+):

$$\text{Glucose} + 2\text{ ADP} + 2\text{ P}_i + 2\text{ NAD}^+ \rightarrow 2\text{ Pyruvate} + 2\text{ ATP} + 2\text{ NADH} + 2\text{ H}_2\text{O} + 2\text{ H}^+$$

Of course, it's not quite that simple. Glycolysis involves several reactions, each of which is catalyzed by a different enzyme (see Figure 4). The general strategy is to first put phosphorylate glucose on both ends and then split it into two 3-carbon units that can go on to the PDC and Krebs cycle. In the first step of glycolysis, a phosphate is taken from ATP and used to phosphorylate glucose, producing glucose 6-phosphate (G6P). This is isomerized to fructose 6-phosphate (F6P), which is then phosphorylated on carbon #1 (with the phosphate again taken from ATP) to produce fructose-1,6-bisphosphate (F1,6bP). This is split into two 3-carbon units that are oxidized to pyruvate, producing 2 ATP and 1 NADH per pyruvate, or 4 ATP and 2 NADH per glucose (since we get two 3-carbon units from each glucose). Don't forget that *each* glucose gives rise to *two* 3-carbon units that pass through the second part of glycolysis and into the Krebs cycle.

- An extract of yeast contains all of the enzymes required for glycolysis, ADP, P_i, Mg^{2+}, NAD^+, and glucose, but when these are all combined, none of the glucose is consumed. Provided that there are no enzyme inhibitors present, why doesn't the reaction proceed?[5]

Hexokinase catalyzes the first step in glycolysis, the phosphorylation of glucose to G6P. G6P feedback-inhibits hexokinase.

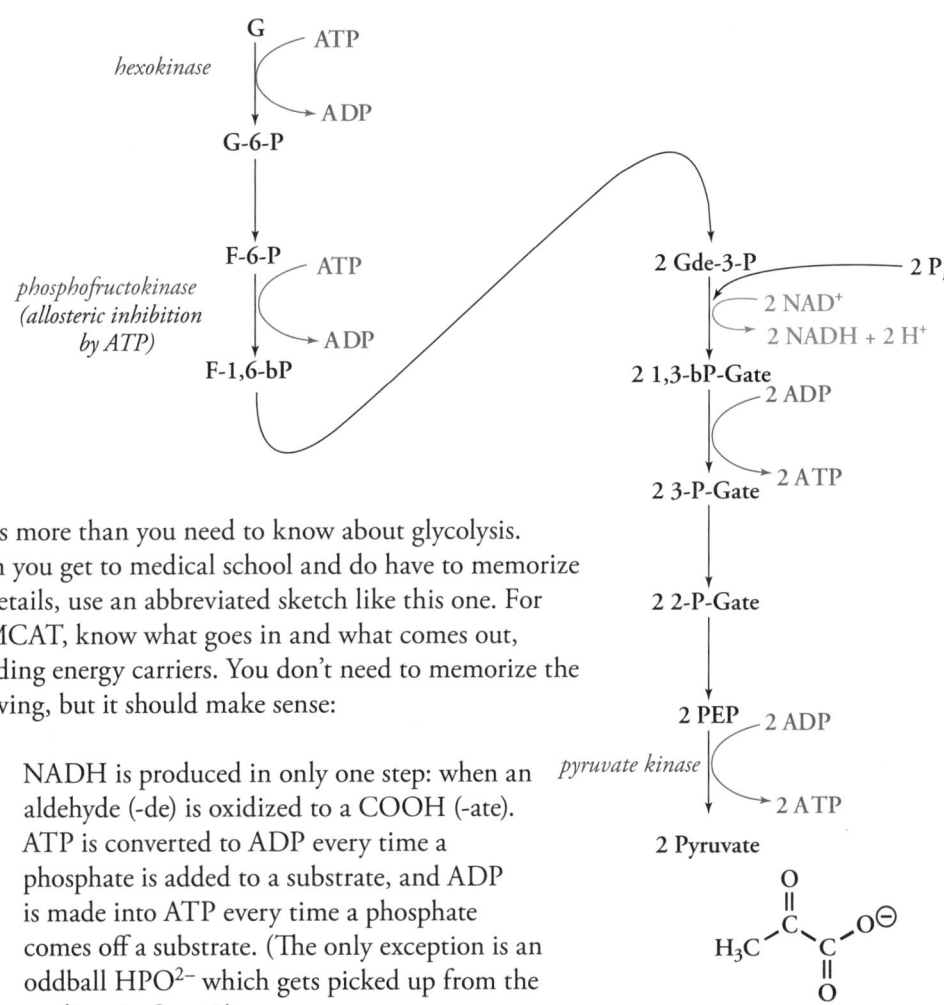

This is more than you need to know about glycolysis. When you get to medical school and do have to memorize the details, use an abbreviated sketch like this one. For the MCAT, know what goes in and what comes out, including energy carriers. You don't need to memorize the following, but it should make sense:

1) NADH is produced in only one step: when an aldehyde (-de) is oxidized to a COOH (-ate).
2) ATP is converted to ADP every time a phosphate is added to a substrate, and ADP is made into ATP every time a phosphate comes off a substrate. (The only exception is an oddball HPO^{2-} which gets picked up from the medium in Step 5.)

Figure 4 The 9 Reactions (Steps) of Glycolysis

---

[5] Although glycolysis results in a net ATP production, ATP is initially required to drive the reaction forward in the phosphorylation of glucose to glucose-6-phosphate and the phosphorylation of fructose-6-phosphate to fructose-1,6-bisphosphate. Without ATP to "prime the pump," there is no way to start the pathway. In case you're wondering about the Mg^{2+}, it's necessary for all reactions involving ATP.

Phosphofructokinase (PFK) catalyzes the third step: the transfer of a phosphate group from ATP to fructose-6-phosphate to form fructose-1,6-bisphosphate (F1,6bP). This is an important step because the reaction catalyzed by PFK is thermodynamically very favorable ($\Delta G \ll 0$), so it's practically irreversible. Also, G6P can be shunted to various pathways, but F1,6bP can react only in glycolysis. So once you light the PFK fire, you're committed to glycolysis. Therefore, PFK is the key biochemical valve controlling the flow of substrate to product in glycolysis, and the conversion of F6P to F1,6bP is known as a **committed step**. In the remainder of glycolysis, F1,6bP is split into two 3-carbon molecules that are converted to pyruvate, with the production of NADH and ATP. Very favorable steps in enzymatic pathways (those with a large negative ΔG) are practically irreversible (because the back-reaction is so unfavorable). These reactions are the ones that are usually subject to allosteric regulation. Another generalization about what steps get regulated is this: early steps in a long pathway tend to be regulated. This makes sense; if you're going from A to Z, it's more practical to regulate the A $\rightarrow$ B reaction than the W $\rightarrow$ X one.

For example, the enzyme PFK is a key regulatory point in glycolysis. PFK is allosterically regulated by ATP. [What effect would you think a high concentration of ATP would have on PFK activity?[6]]

Two molecules of NAD$^+$ are reduced in glycolysis per glucose catabolized, forming 2 NADH. As discussed above, NADH is an electron carrier, a molecule that is responsible for shuttling energy in the form of **reducing power** (i.e., reduction potential). Remember, these high-energy electron carriers are not used directly as an energy source, but are used later to generate ATP through electron transport and oxidative phosphorylation.

Fermentation

Under **aerobic** conditions (that is, in the presence of oxygen), the pyruvate produced in glycolysis enters the PDC and Krebs cycle to be oxidized completely to CO_2. The NADH produced in glycolysis and the PDC, as well as NADH and $FADH_2$ produced in the Krebs cycle, are all reoxidized in electron transport, where O_2 is the final electron acceptor. In **anaerobic** conditions (without oxygen), electron transport cannot function, and the limited supply of NAD$^+$ becomes entirely converted to NADH. [Would a limiting supply of NAD$^+$ stimulate or inhibit glycolysis?[7]]

Fermentation has evolved to regenerate NAD$^+$ in anaerobic conditions, thereby allowing glycolysis to continue in the absence of oxygen. Fermentation uses pyruvate as the acceptor of the high energy electrons from NADH (see Figure 5). Two examples of this process are (1) the reduction of pyruvate to ethanol (yeast do this in the making of beer, wine, etc.) and (2) the reduction of pyruvate to lactate in human muscle cells. Lactate is thought to contribute to the "burn" that athletes encounter during anaerobic exertion, such as sprinting, when the cardiovascular system fails to deliver enough oxygen to keep the electron transport chain running in muscle cells.

---

[6] When energy (ATP) is abundant, the cell should slow glycolysis. High concentrations of ATP inhibit PFK activity by binding to an allosteric regulatory site. It is interesting to note that since ATP is a reactant in the reaction catalyzed by PFK, you would expect a high concentration of ATP to increase the rate of the reaction (Le Châtelier's principle). However, the inhibitory allosteric effects of ATP on PFK outweigh this thermodynamic consideration. So lowering the concentration of ATP will increase the reaction rate, even though ATP is a reactant. Of course, if the ATP level went too low, the reaction could not proceed at all.

[7] If NAD$^+$ has all been converted to NADH, then the step in glycolysis that produces NADH (catalyzed by glyceraldehyde 3-phosphate dehydrogenase) cannot occur because it requires NAD$^+$ as a substrate. Thus, a lack of NAD$^+$ will *inhibit* glycolysis.

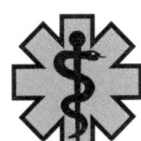

Figure 5   Anaerobic Pathways for Regeneration of NAD$^+$ from NADH

The NAD$^+$ produced by reducing pyruvate anaerobically is available for reuse in the glycolytic pathway, so more ATP can be produced. There is a limit to the use of anaerobic glycolysis as an energy source, however. The ethanol or lactate that is produced builds up, having no other use in the cell, and acts as a poison at high concentrations. Wine yeast die when the ethanol concentration reaches about 12 percent, and lactic acid is damaging at high concentrations in our tissues as well.

- What happens to the lactate in human muscle cells after a period of strenuous exercise?[8]

The Pyruvate Dehydrogenase Complex

The pyruvate produced in glycolysis in the cytoplasm is transported into the mitochondrial matrix, where it will be entirely oxidized to CO_2. Pyruvate does not enter the Krebs cycle directly, however. First it is oxidatively decarboxylated by the pyruvate dehydrogenase complex (PDC; Figure 6). **Oxidative decarboxylation** is a reaction repeated again in the Krebs cycle, in which a molecule is oxidized to release CO_2 and produce NADH. In oxidative decarboxylation, pyruvate is changed from a 3-carbon molecule to a __, while __ is given off and __ is produced.[9] The PDC changes pyruvate into an activated acetyl unit. An acetyl unit is [(CH$_3$)(O=C–)], and *activated* means the acetyl is not floating around freely but rather is attached to a carrier, namely **coenzyme A.** This coenzyme is basically a long handle with a sulfur at the end, abbreviated CoA-SH. It is used in many reaction systems to pass acetyl units around (e.g., fatty

---

[8] The lactate is exported from the muscle cell to the liver. When oxygen becomes available, the liver cell will convert the lactate back to pyruvate, while making NADH from NAD$^+$. Then the liver will utilize this excess NADH to make ATP in oxidative phosphorylation. This pyruvate can enter gluconeogenesis or the Krebs cycle in the liver, or it can be sent back to the muscle. (This cycle, whereby the liver deals with lactate from muscle, is known as the Cori Cycle.)

[9] Pyruvate is converted to a 2-carbon molecule, CO_2 is given off, and NADH is made from NAD$^+$. You can figure all of this out based on your knowledge of oxidative decarboxylation. Also, note the name of the enzyme, "dehydrogenase." To remove a hydrogen (*dehydrogenate*) is to oxidize. So the name of the enzyme also tells us that pyruvate is oxidized.

acid and cholesterol synthesis and degradation). When loaded with an acetyl unit, CoA-SH is abbreviated acetyl-CoA. The bond between sulfur and the acetyl group is high energy, making it easy for acetyl-CoA to transfer the acetyl fragment into the Krebs cycle for further oxidation. Regulation of the PDC is crucial. [AMP (adenosine monophosphate) is a low-energy molecule produced by the hydrolysis of ATP during metabolism. What effect would you predict a high level of AMP to have on the activity of pyruvate dehydrogenase?[10] The PDC is composed of three different enzymes. Why might a complex of three enzymes be more efficient than three independent enzymes?[11]]

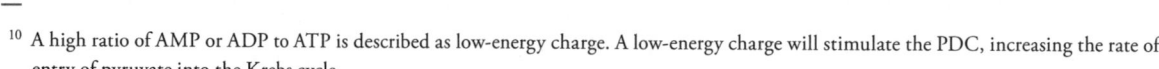

Figure 6 Oxidation of Pyruvate by Pyruvate Dehydrogenase

Many enzymes require additional non-protein compounds for their biological activity. These molecules are called **cofactors**. Cofactors can be small (such as a zinc or magnesium ion) or they can be larger (such as a more complex organic molecule like NAD^+). If the cofactor is very tightly or covalently bound to the enzyme it is referred to as a **prosthetic group**. The PDC contains a thiamine pyrophosphate (TPP) prosthetic group at one of its active sites. The α-ketoglutarate dehydrogenase complex, which catalyzes the third step in the Krebs cycle, is very similar to the PDC; it has a TPP prosthetic group and catalyzes an oxidative decarboxylation. The **thiamine** in thiamine pyrophosphate is vitamin B_1. Vitamins often serve as cofactors or prosthetic groups.

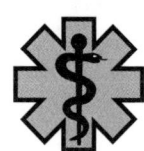

- Beriberi is a disease caused by thiamine deficiency, which frequently results from a diet of white rice in underdeveloped nations. Which of the following would best describe the effect of thiamine deficiency on cellular metabolism in humans?[12]
  A) The rate of glycolysis would increase.
  B) Glycolysis would proceed anaerobically to maintain ATP production at normal levels.
  C) Glucose consumption would slow, and ATP production would increase.
  D) Acetyl-CoA would be provided by fatty acid metabolism, so the Krebs cycle would proceed uninhibited.

---

[10] A high ratio of AMP or ADP to ATP is described as low-energy charge. A low-energy charge will stimulate the PDC, increasing the rate of entry of pyruvate into the Krebs cycle.

[11] Simply because intermediates are passed directly from active site to active site, without having to diffuse.

[12] Thiamine deficiency would effectively shut down both the PDC and the Krebs cycle (choice D is wrong), since both of these processes require thiamine in their TPP prosthetic group. In the absence of PDC and Krebs, the amount of NADH and $FADH_2$ provided to the electron transport chain would be reduced, and ATP production would fall (choice C is wrong). In order to compensate and maintain ATP levels as close to normal as possible, the rate of glycolysis would increase (choice **A** is correct). Note that this would not happen anaerobically, as conditions are not anaerobic (choice B is wrong).

The Krebs Cycle

The **Krebs cycle** is a group of reactions which take the 2-carbon acetyl unit from acetyl-CoA, combine it with oxaloacetate, and release two CO_2 molecules. NADH and $FADH_2$ are generated in the process. The figure below shows an overview of the process; note that many of the names are not necessary to know and have intentionally been left out.

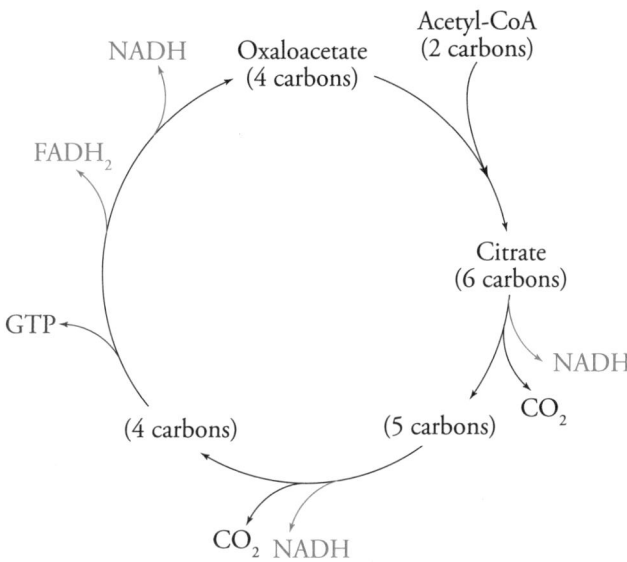

Figure 7   Overview of the Krebs Cycle

These reduced electron carriers (NADH and $FADH_2$) go on to generate ATP in electron transport and oxidative phosphorylation. Two other names for the Krebs cycle are the **tricarboxylic acid cycle** (**TCA cycle**) and the **citric acid cycle**. Citrate is the first intermediate produced in the cycle, as soon as the acetyl unit is supplied. Citrate possesses three carboxylic acid functional groups, hence the term "tricarboxylic acid." We will now break the multistep cycle down into three general stages. The reactions are shown for conceptual understanding only; there is no need to memorize structures or details. At most, you might choose to memorize the names.

Krebs Stage 1: The two carbons in the acetate fragment of acetyl-CoA are condensed with the 4-carbon compound **oxaloacetate** (OAA; the name is worth remembering), producing **citrate**; see Figure 8. As you will see, the OAA is derived from the previous round of the Krebs cycle; it is recycled each time. [How many chiral carbons are present in citrate?[13] If pyruvate is radiolabeled on its number one (most oxidized) carbon, where will the labeled carbon end up in the Krebs cycle?[14]]

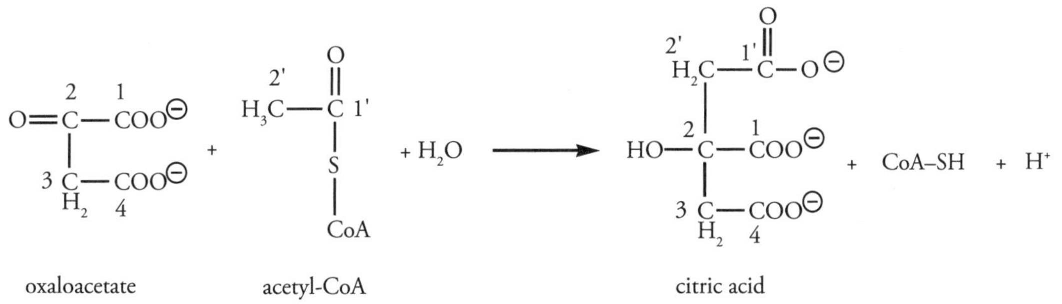

$$O=\overset{2}{C}-COO^{\ominus} \qquad H_3\overset{2'}{C}-\overset{1'}{C}\overset{O}{\parallel} \qquad + H_2O \longrightarrow \qquad HO-\overset{1}{\underset{3}{C}}-COO^{\ominus} \qquad + \text{CoA-SH} \quad + \text{H}^+$$

oxaloacetate   acetyl-CoA   citric acid

Figure 8   The Entry of Acetyl-CoA into the Krebs Cycle

---

[13] None, since none of the six carbons has four unique substituents.

[14] It will not end up in the Krebs cycle. Pyruvate's most oxidized carbon is a carboxylic acid, which is removed as CO^2 by the PDC.

Krebs Stage 2: Citrate is further oxidized (twice!) to release CO_2 and to produce NADH from NAD^+ with each oxidative decarboxylation (Figure 9). The two carbons that leave as CO_2 during these reactions are not the same ones that entered the cycle as acetate. Thus, the two original acetyl carbons remain within the Krebs cycle. They will be lost as CO_2 in later cycles. [How many carbons from the CoA component of acetyl-CoA enter into the Krebs cycle?[15]]

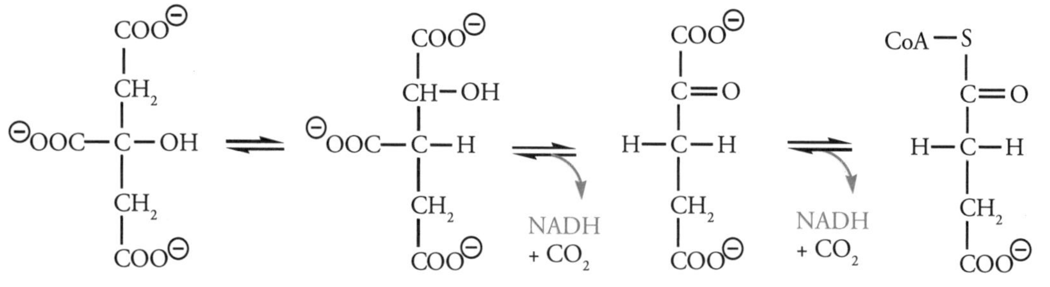

citrate (6 carbons) | isocitrate (6 carbons) | α-ketoglutarate (5 carbons) | succinyl-CoA (4 carbons)

Figure 9 Oxidation of Citric Acid to Succinate

Krebs Stage 3: OAA is regenerated so that the cycle can continue. In the process, reducing power is stored in 1 NADH and 1 $FADH_2$, and a high-energy phosphate bond is produced directly as GTP. Here GTP plays the role normally reserved for ATP. This GTP will eventually transfer its high-energy phosphate bond to ADP, converting it into ATP. $FADH_2$ is similar to NADH, but ultimately results in the production of less ATP.

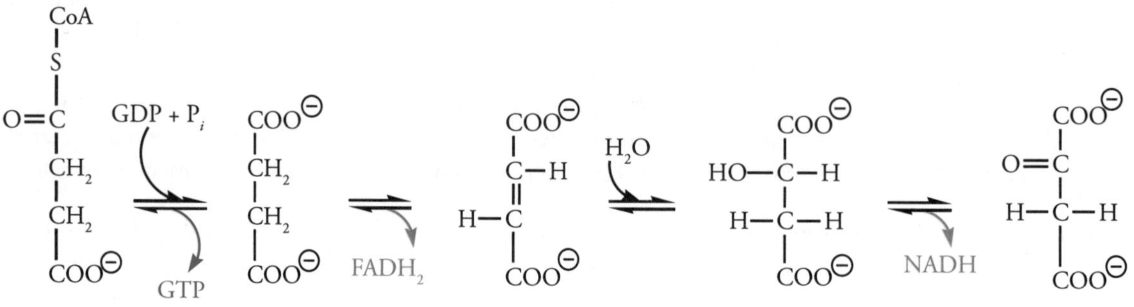

succinate | fumarate | malate | oxaloacetate

Figure 10 Succinyl CoA to OAA

To review, the oxidation of glucose has so far created:

1) 2 ATP and 2 NADH per glucose molecule in glycolysis
2) Pyruvate Dehydrogenase: 2 NADH per glucose (one per pyruvate)
3) Krebs cycle: 6 NADH, 2 $FADH_2$, and 2 GTP per glucose

Thus, most of the energy of glucose is not extracted directly as ATP (or GTP) but in high-energy electron carriers. We will see how ATP is generated from NADH and $FADH_2$ in electron transport/oxidative phosphorylation.

—

[15] None. CoA assists in catalysis, which means that it is not consumed in the reaction, but regenerated as CoA-SH.

Compartmentalization of Glucose Catabolism in Eukaryotes: The Mitochondria

To understand oxidative phosphorylation, you must know the structure of the mitochondrion (Figure 11). The mitochondrion contains two membranes, an **outer membrane** and an **inner membrane**, each composed of a lipid bilayer. The outer membrane is smooth and contains large pores formed by **porin** proteins. The inner membrane is impermeable, even to very small items like H^+, and is densely folded into structures termed **cristae**. The cristae extend into the **matrix**, which is the innermost space of the mitochondrion. The space between the two membranes, the **intermembrane space**, is continuous with the cytoplasm due to the large pores in the outer membrane. The enzymes of the Krebs cycle and the pyruvate dehydrogenase complex are located in the matrix, and those of the electron transport chain and ATP synthase involved in oxidative phosphorylation are bound to the inner mitochondrial membrane.

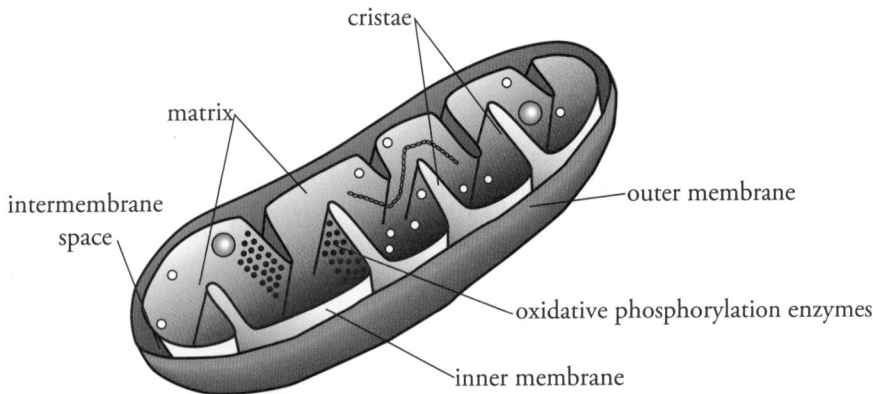

Figure 11 The Mitochondrion

The two goals of electron transport/oxidative phosphorylation are to:

1) reoxidize all the electron carriers reduced in glycolysis, PDC, and the Krebs cycle, and
2) store energy in the form of ATP in the process.

Where are all the reduced electron carriers located? Per each glucose catabolized, two NADH are created by glycolysis in the cytoplasm; the electrons from these NADH will have to be transported into the mitochondria before they can be passed along the electron transport chain. All the other NADHs and $FADH_2$s were produced inside the mitochondrial matrix, so they are in the right place to donate electrons to the electron transport chain.

The situation in prokaryotes is a bit different: all of the reduced electron carriers are located in the cytoplasm. In fact, everything is located in the cytoplasm, since there are *no membrane-bound organelles at all* in prokaryotes (no mitochondria, no nucleus, no lysosomes—everything just floats around in the cytoplasm). Since they have no mitochondria, can bacteria perform oxidative phosphorylation? *Yes, they can!* The way the process works is that a proton gradient must be created and then used to power ATP synthesis by the membrane-bound **ATP synthase**. So all that's required is a membrane impermeable to protons. Eukaryotes use the inner mitochondrial membrane; bacteria just use their cell membrane. The end result of this difference is that when eukaryotes perform aerobic respiration, they have to shuttle the electrons from cytosolic NADH into the mitochondrial matrix (at the cost of some energy), but bacteria do not. So, all things considered, prokaryotes get two more high-energy phosphate bonds from aerobic respiration than eukaryotes do (this will be discussed in more detail in just a bit). From this point forward, we will discuss the eukaryotic system. Remember that it's the same in prokaryotes except that they do it on the cell membrane instead of on the inner mitochondrial membrane.

Electron Transport and Oxidative Phosphorylation

Oxidative phosphorylation is the oxidation of the high-energy electron carriers NADH and $FADH_2$ coupled to the phosphorylation of ADP to produce ATP. The energy released through oxidation of NADH and $FADH_2$ by the electron transport chain is used to pump protons out of the mitochondrial matrix and into the intermembrane space. This proton gradient is the source of energy used to drive the phosphorylation of ADP to ATP. The **electron-transport chain** is a group of five electron carriers (Figure 12). Each member of the chain reduces the next member down the line. All five are named for their redox roles. Three of them are large protein complexes found embedded in the inner mitochondrial membrane. They are classified as **cytochromes** due to the presence of a heme group, a porphyrin ring containing a tightly bound iron atom. The other two members of the electron transport chain are small mobile electron carriers. The chain is organized so that the first large carrier receives electrons (reducing power) from NADH; the NADH is thus oxidized to NAD^+. Hence, the first large carrier in the e^- transport chain ("A" in the figure) is called **NADH dehydrogenase**. It passes its electrons to one of the small carriers in the transport chain, called **ubiquinone**, also known as **coenzyme Q.**[16] NADH dehydrogenase is also known as **coenzyme Q reductase**.

Cytoplasm

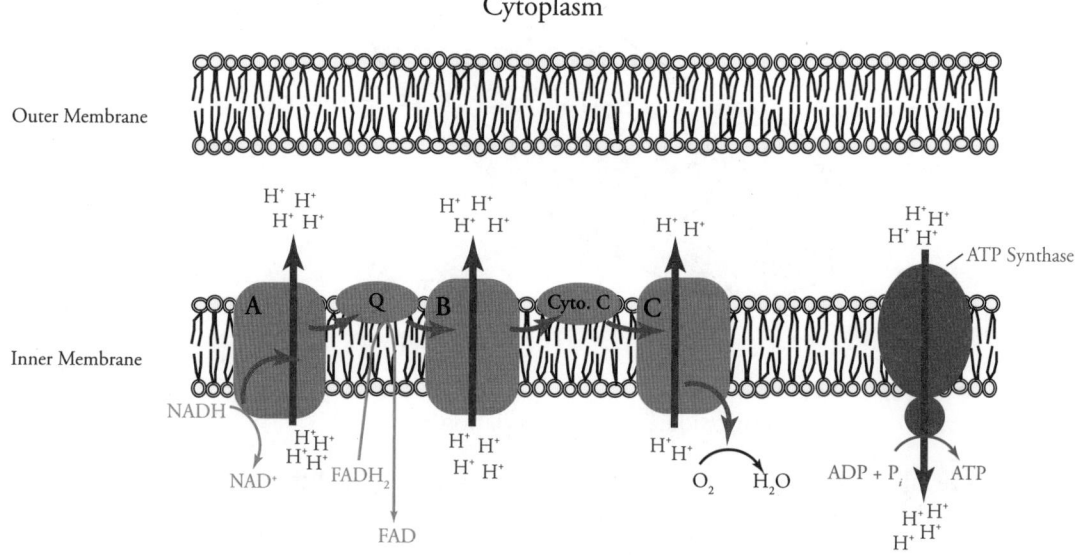

Figure 12 The Electron Transport Chain

Ubiquinone then passes its electrons to the second large membrane-bound complex in the chain ("B"), known as **cytochrome C reductase**. From this name, you can guess what the next carrier in the chain is called; it is **cytochrome C**, a small hydrophilic iron-containing protein bound loosely to the inner mitochondrial membrane. The last member of the electron transport chain ("C") is simply called **cytochrome C oxidase**. [Where does it pass its electrons to?[17]]

Each of the three large membrane-bound proteins in the electron transport chain pumps protons across the inner mitochondrial membrane every time electrons flow past. Protons are pumped out of the matrix, into the intermembrane space. The inner mitochondrial membrane is highly impermeable to protons. As a result, the electron transport chain creates a large proton gradient, with the pH being much ___[18] (higher/lower) inside the matrix than in the rest of the cell.

---

[16] A quinone is a particular type of aromatic molecule, and the prefix "ubi" indicates that this molecule is ubiquitous, i.e., present in all cells.

[17] If it's the last member of the chain, it must pass its reducing power to O_2, reducing it to H_2O, an end product of electron transport. This is the only reason we breathe and the only reason we evolved with lungs, RBCs, etc.

[18] higher (remember, high pH = low $[H^+]$)

What does this have to do with ATP synthesis? Well, there is one more very important protein embedded in the inner mitochondrial membrane: **ATP synthase**. It is a large protein complex which contains a proton channel that spans the inner membrane. The passage of protons from the intermembrane space through the ATP synthase channel causes it to synthesize ATP from ADP + P_i. Thus, ATP production is dependent on a **proton gradient**. The overall process of electron transport and ATP production is said to be *coupled* by the proton gradient. Together, electron transport and ATP production are known as **oxidative phosphorylation**. Make sure you understand these questions:

- Dinitrophenol (DNP) is an uncoupler: It destroys the proton gradient by allowing protons to flow into the matrix. Which one of the following processes does it inhibit first?[19]
  - A) Pyruvate decarboxylation by the PDC
  - B) The TCA cycle
  - C) Electron transport
  - D) Muscular contraction

- Which one of the following processes has a positive ΔG under normal aerobic conditions in the cell?[20]
  - A) ATP hydrolysis
  - B) The pumping of protons to form a pH gradient
  - C) The oxidation of NADH by NADH dehydrogenase
  - D) The folding of a protein into its correct tertiary structure

- The reason cyanide is a poison is that it inactivates cytochrome C oxidase by binding to its active site with high affinity. When a person is exposed to cyanide[21]
  - A) the difference in pH inside and outside the matrix is already as large as it can become, so no more electrons can be pumped against the gradient.
  - B) anaerobic glycolysis depletes pyruvate, thereby slowing the Krebs cycle and the electron transport chain and slowing the rate of proton pumping.
  - C) the electron transport chain ceases to transport electrons and therefore ceases to pump protons.
  - D) NADH becomes fully oxidized by the Krebs cycle and therefore cannot reduce NADH dehydrogenase, so no protons are pumped.

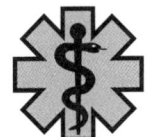

---

[19] If the proton gradient is destroyed, the processes in A, B, and C will continue unabated, because NADH will be reoxidized to NAD^+ at a normal rate, or perhaps faster than normal. The problem will be that without a proton gradient no ATP will get made from all this glucose breakdown. The answer is choice **D** because this will be the first problem encountered from running out of ATP.

[20] Choices A, C, and D are all thermodynamically favorable processes that occur spontaneously without any external energy input. Thus, all of these processes have a negative ΔG. However, the large positive ΔG of the process in choice **B** makes undoing it favorable enough for it to power ATP synthesis. Creation of the proton gradient is dependent upon the very negative ΔG of electron transport.

[21] If the active site of cytochrome C oxidase is occupied with cyanide, then oxygen cannot bind there to be reduced to water; in other words, cytochrome C oxidase will be unable to get rid of its electrons and will remain reduced. Therefore, it will be unable to accept electrons from cytochrome C, which will be unable to accept electrons from cytochrome C reductase, which will be unable to accept electrons from coenzyme Q, and so on, all the way back up the electron transport chain. The end result will be a cessation of all electron transport chain activity (choice **C** is correct). Note that protons, not electrons, are pumped against their gradient (choice A is wrong), and this will stop completely, not just be slowed down (choice B is wrong). Also, NAD^+ is reduced to NADH in the Krebs cycle, not the other way around (choice D is wrong).

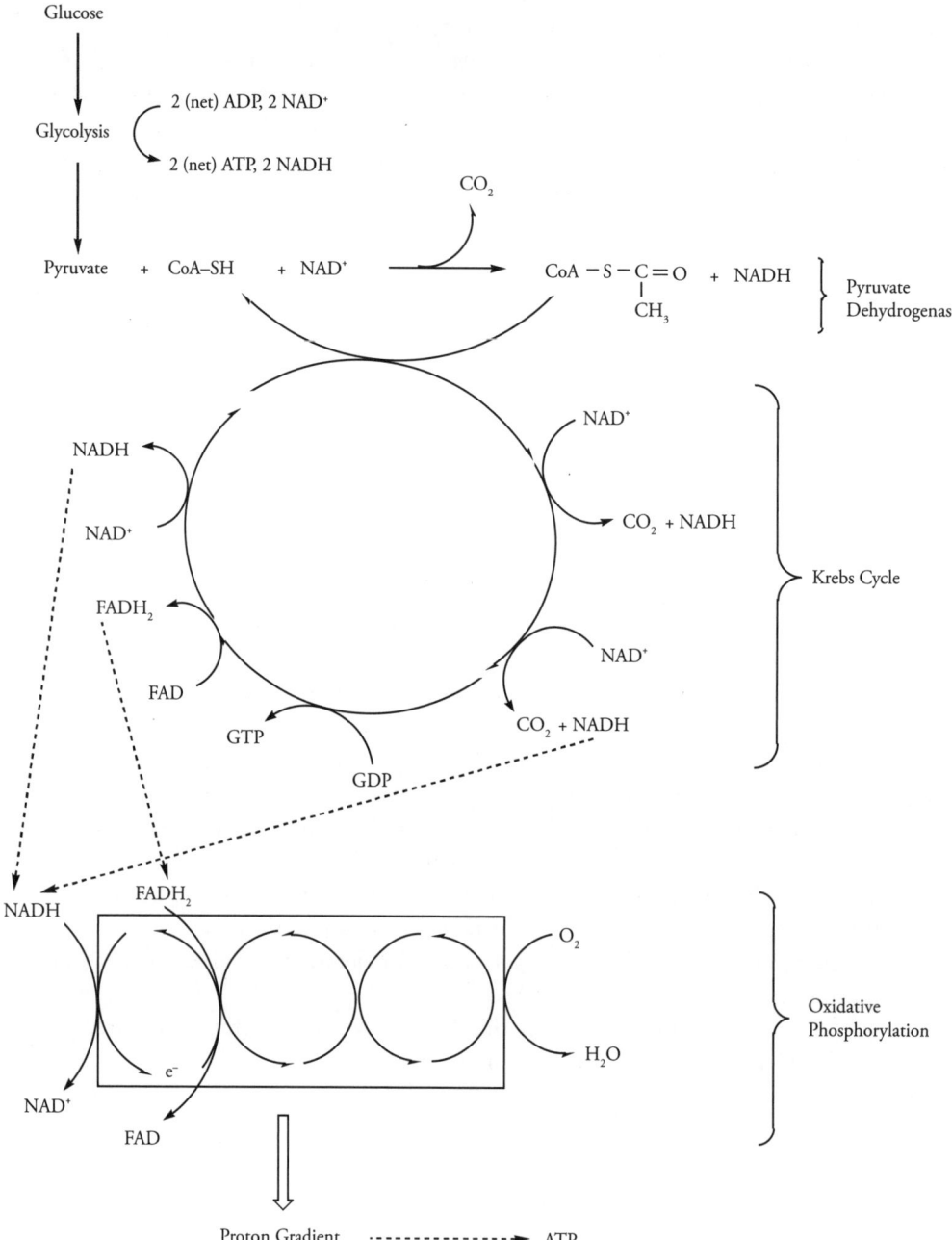

Figure 13 Cellular Respiration

Energetics of Glucose Catabolism

How is electron transport quantitatively connected to ATP synthesis? For every NADH that is oxidized to NAD$^+$, the three large electron transport proteins pump about 10 protons across the inner mitochondrial membrane, into the intermembrane space. The ATP synthase requires three protons to generate a molecule of ATP from ADP and P$_i$; however, an additional proton is required to bring P$_i$ into the matrix. This brings the "cost" of ATP synthesis up to four protons per molecule of ATP. Since NADH is responsible for the pumping of 10 protons, each molecule of NADH provides the energy to produce approximately 2.5 ATP molecules.

Even though NADH and $FADH_2$ have similar functions, their fates are a little different. $FADH_2$ gives its electrons to ubiquinone instead of to NADH dehydrogenase. By bypassing the first proton pump, $FADH_2$ is only responsible for the pumping of six protons across the inner membrane.

- How many ATP are made every time an $FADH_2$ is reoxidized to FAD?[22]

As mentioned earlier, the PDC, the Krebs cycle, and oxidative phosphorylation all occur in mitochondria in eukaryotes, while glycolysis occurs in the cytoplasm. The electrons from the NADH generated in glycolysis must be transported into the mitochondria before they can enter the electron transport chain. In most cells, they are transported by a pathway termed the **glycerol phosphate shuttle**. This shuttle delivers the electrons directly to ubiquinone (just like $FADH_2$ does), bypassing NADH dehydrogenase, and results in the production of only 1.5 molecules of ATP per cytosolic NADH, rather than the 2.5 normally formed from matrix NADH.[23] Bacteria, because they lack cellular organelles, do not need to transport cytosolic electrons across any membranes; hence the discrepancy in Table 1 in how much ATP is yielded from each NADH from glycolysis in eukaryotes compared to prokaryotes. All values in the following table are per glucose molecule catabolized.

Process	Molecules Formed/Used	ATP Equivalents
Glycolysis	–2 ATP 4 ATP 2 NADH	–2 ATP 4 ATP 3 ATP (eukaryotes) 5 ATP (prokaryotes)
Pyruvate Dehydrogenase Complex	2 NADH	5 ATP
Krebs Cycle	6 NADH 2 $FADH_2$ 2 GTP	15 ATP 3 ATP 2 ATP
Total		**30 ATP (eukaryotes)** **32 ATP (prokaryotes)**

Table 1   Theoretical ATP Yield from Cellular Respiration

Notes:

1) These numbers are an estimate of the theoretical maximum amount of ATP that can be produced from a single molecule of glucose. As the proton gradient is used to transport other molecules into or out of the matrix, the actual yield may differ depending on the number of protons (i.e., the gradient) available for ATP synthesis.
2) These numbers reflect the most recent understanding of ATP synthesis, and as such, may not appear in some textbooks that still cling to the previously established counts of 36 ATP per glucose in eukaryotes and 38 ATP per glucose in prokaryotes.

---

[22] Only 1.5 ATP are made as a result of the reoxidation of $FADH_2$. Six protons divided by four protons per ATP equals 1.5 ATP.

[23] Some high energy-requiring tissues (such as liver and cardiac muscle cells) utilize a different shuttle (the malate-aspartate shuttle) to bring the electrons to NADH hydrogenase, thus getting the full 2.5 ATP from those electrons. But this is the exception, and generally the MCAT does not test exceptions.

5.4 GLUCONEOGENESIS

Gluconeogenesis occurs when dietary sources of glucose are unavailable and when the liver has depleted its stores of glycogen and glucose (more on glycogen metabolism in a bit). This process occurs primarily in the liver (and to a lesser extent in the kidneys), and it involves converting non-carbohydrate precursor molecules (such as lactate, pyruvate, Krebs cycle intermediates, and the carbon skeletons of most amino acids) into intermediates of the above pathways where they ultimately become glucose. Gluconeogenesis is an 11-step pathway that uses many of the same enzymes as glycolysis. In simplified terms, it can be thought of as "glycolysis-in-reverse," in which those enzymes catalyzing the irreversible reactions (hexokinase, phosphofructokinase, and pyruvate kinase) have been replaced.

In Figure 14, starting from the bottom and working toward the top (i.e., starting with pyruvate), the first reaction of gluconeogenesis adds CO_2 to pyruvate, converting it to oxaloacetate. This step requires ATP hydrolysis and is run by the enzyme **pyruvate carboxylase**. In the very next step, oxaloacetate is decarboxylated and phosphorylated to form phosphoenolpyruvate (PEP); this step is run by **phosphoenolpyruvate carboxykinase (PEPCK)**. While this might seem odd (add CO_2 to then remove CO_2), oxidative decarboxylation is a favorable process, and it is often used to drive less favorable reactions. This same process is used in fatty acid synthesis as well (see Chapter 6).

The next several steps are run by the same enzymes as in glycolysis (PEP to fructose-1,6-bisphosphate). However, the phosphorylation of fructose-6-P to form fructose-1,6-bisP in glycolysis is essentially irreversible ($\Delta G \ll 0$), so it will require an enzyme other than PFK to reverse it. **Fructose-1,6-bisphosphatase** catalyzes the removal of a phosphate group from fru-1,6-bisP to form fru-6-P. This is then isomerized to glu-6-P and dephosphorylated by the final enzyme, **glucose-6-phosphatase** (as with fru-1,6-bisP, the reaction to form glucose-6-P in glycolysis is irreversible; therefore, its dephosphorylation must be run by an enzyme other than hexokinase). Furthermore, the dephosphorylation of glu-6-P is required in order for glucose to be released from liver cells into the bloodstream. Phosphorylated glucose is charged and cannot cross the cell membrane. This "newly-made" glucose can now travel to other cells in the body so that they can take it up and use it for energy.

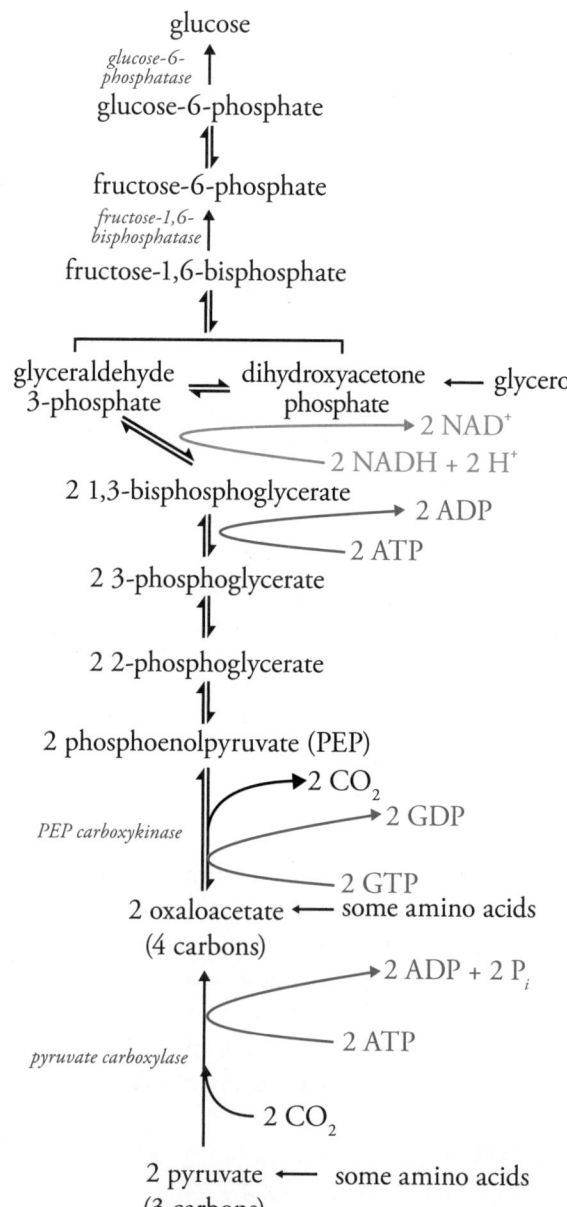

Figure 14 Gluconeogenesis

Altogether then, gluconeogenesis requires six high-energy phosphate bonds (four ATP and two GTP) and two reduced electron carriers (two NADH).

- As discussed previously, glycolysis is a thermodynamically favorable process with an overall $\Delta G < 0$. How is it possible for gluconeogenesis, which is seemingly the reverse process of glycolysis, to also be thermodynamically favorable?[24]

Note that while the majority of the intermediates discussed in cellular respiration can take part in gluconeogenesis, acetyl-CoA cannot. This helps explain why free fatty acids cannot be converted to glucose during periods of starvation, while the glycerol backbone of a triglyceride can.

5.5 REGULATION OF GLYCOLYSIS AND GLUCONEOGENESIS

Pathways that serve opposing roles (e.g., glycolysis and gluconeogenesis) must be tightly regulated to prevent the net loss of energy due to **futile cycling** (running both pathways at the same time). Therefore, **reciprocal control** in response to current cellular needs is critical. In reciprocal control, the same molecule regulates two enzymes in opposite ways.

As we already know, glycolysis and gluconeogenesis utilize many of the same enzymes. Attempts to regulate any one of these would fail to isolate a single pathway, so regulation must focus on those enzymes catalyzing irreversible reactions. Two such heavily regulated enzymes are **phosphofructokinase (PFK)** and **fructose-1,6-bisphosphatase (F-1,6-BPase)**. These enzymes serve opposing roles in glycolysis and gluconeogenesis, respectively. Both enzymes are allosterically regulated by glycolytic intermediates that activate one enzyme while inhibiting the other. For instance, in energy-starved states, elevated cellular AMP levels activate PFK while inhibiting F-1,6-BPase, resulting in enhanced glycolysis activity and a suppression of gluconeogenesis.

Another metabolic intermediate that exerts reciprocal control on these two enzymes is **fructose-2,6-bisphosphate (F-2,6-BP)**. Its intracellular concentration is set by a single large protein that functions as two separate enzymes: one that synthesizes F-2,6-BP and one that breaks it down. **Insulin** and **glucagon** help control the concentration of intracellular F-2,6-BP by regulating the activity of this large protein. Note that F-2,6-BP stimulates PFK (thus stimulating glycolysis) and inhibits fructose-1,6-bisphosphatase (thus inhibiting gluconeogenesis). To better illustrate how this works, let us consider an example. When blood glucose levels are high, insulin is released from the pancreas. Insulin stimulates the formation of F-2,6-BP, leading to the stimulation of PFK and activation of the glycolytic pathway. Simultaneously, the F-2,6-BP inhibits fructose-1,6-bisphosphatase, turning off gluconeogenesis so that these opposing pathways do not run at the same time. The reverse situation occurs when blood glucose levels are low; under these conditions, glucagon (also released from the pancreas) triggers the breakdown of F-2,6-BP. The drop in F-2,6-BP levels stops the stimulation of PFK, thus inhibiting glycolysis, and stops the inhibition of fructose-1,6-bisphosphatase, thus stimulating gluconeogenesis.

---

[24] There are three major steps in glycolysis with a $\Delta G < 0$ (the other steps have a ΔG close to 0). In gluconeogenesis, these same steps would have a $\Delta G > 0$. However, they are made thermodynamically favorable ($\Delta G < 0$) by coupling the reactions to the hydrolysis of the high energy phosphate bonds of GTP and ATP ($\Delta G \ll 0$).

- Following a high carb meal, the blood concentration of insulin _____ and glucagon _____.[25]

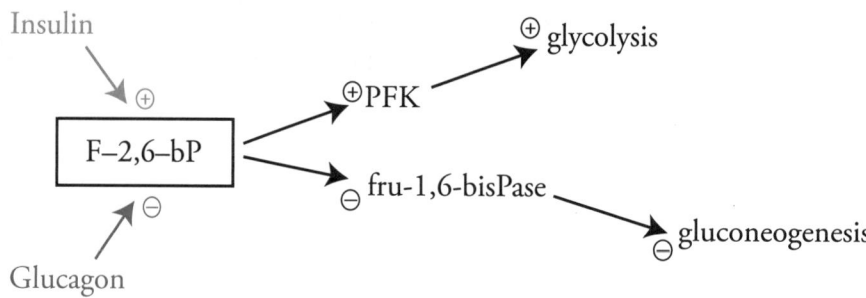

Figure 15   Hormonal Regulation of Glycolysis and Gluconeogenesis

Overview

In order to meet the varied metabolic demands of the cell, many additional forms of regulation occur beyond the limited examples outlined here. The following general principles, however, allow for reasonable predictions of the activity of a given pathway in response to cellular conditions:

1) In a pathway, those enzymes which catalyze irreversible (i.e., exergonic) reactions are frequently sites of regulation.
2) Increased concentrations of intermediates in a pathway generally serve to decrease the activity of that pathway (e.g., citrate decreases the activity of PFK in glycolysis).
3) Each pathway responds to the energy state of the cell. Cellular respiration is stimulated by energy deficits (e.g., high ADP:ATP or NAD^+:NADH ratios) and inhibited by energy surpluses (e.g., high ATP:ADP or NADH:NAD^+ ratios).

The table below outlines some of the regulatory steps described in this chapter.

Pathway	Enzyme	Positive Regulators	Negative Regulators
Glycolysis	Phosphofructokinase	Fructose-2,6-bisphosphate	ATP
		AMP	
Gluconeogenesis	Fructose-1,6-bisphosphatase	ATP	Fructose-2,6-bisphosphate
			AMP

Table 2   Summary of Metabolic Regulation

---

[25] Following a high-carb meal, the blood concentration of insulin increases and glucagon decreases. If you have a lot of carbs in your blood, you don't need to make any more!

5.6   GLYCOGEN METABOLISM

Glycogen is a polymer of glucose that is found in muscle and liver cells, and it is the main form of carbohydrate storage in animals. Glycogenesis, the formation of glycogen, starts with glucose-6-phosphate. The molecule is isomerized in a reversible reaction to glucose-1-phosphate by the enzyme phosphoglucomutase. Glu-1-P is activated with UTP to form UDP-glucose, which is added to the growing glycogen polymer by glycogen synthase.

Glycogenolysis starts with the phosphorylation and removal of one glucose unit at the end of the polymer, producing glucose-1-P. This is isomerized to glu-6-P, which can then reenter the glycolytic pathway. As in gluconeogenesis, in order to release the glucose into the bloodstream it must be dephosphorylated with glucose-6-phosphatase.

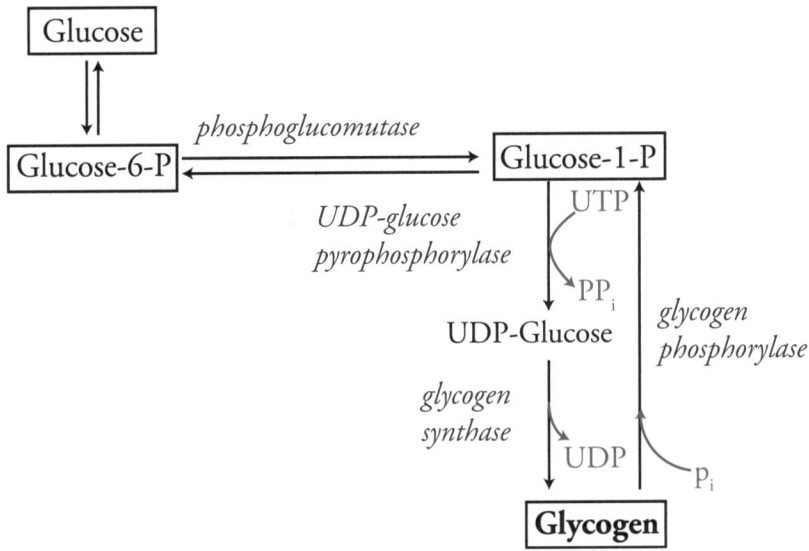

Figure 16   Glycogen Metabolism

Glycogenesis and glycogenolysis occur in both the liver and in skeletal muscle. Liver glycogen is broken down to maintain blood glucose levels during fasting states, while skeletal muscle glycogen is broken down to supply the skeletal muscle with glucose during exercise. Thus, skeletal muscle lacks glucose-6-phosphatase; the absence of this enzyme keeps the glucose phosphorylated and unable to leave the muscle cell.

Glycogenesis and glycogenolysis are opposing processes, controlled by the hormones that regulate blood sugar levels and energy. Insulin, released when blood glucose is high, stimulates glycogenesis. At first this seems paradoxical, as insulin was discussed above as a positive regulator of glycolysis (i.e., glucose breakdown), and it is not immediately apparent why breakdown and storage would be stimulated by the same hormone. However, it makes sense when you consider that it's unnecessary for all of the food just consumed to be immediately turned into energy, just as you don't necessarily need to spend your entire paycheck the moment you get it. You might spend some and put the rest in the bank. So insulin stimulates glycolysis (spending some of your paycheck) as well as glycogenesis (putting the rest in the bank).

Glycogenolysis occurs in response to glucagon, when blood sugar levels are low. It results in glucose being released from the liver into the blood where it can then be taken up by cells and enter glycolysis.

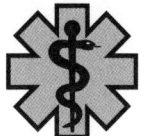

- Patients with Von Gierke's disease have a deficiency in the enzyme glucose-6-phosphatase. What would you expect these patients' blood glucagon and insulin levels to be?[26]

5.7 PENTOSE PHOSPHATE PATHWAY

The **pentose phosphate pathway** (PPP, also known as the hexose monophosphate shunt) diverts glucose-6-phosphate from glycolysis in order to form NADPH, ribose-5-phosphate, and glycolytic intermediates. This cytoplasmic pathway is composed of an irreversible oxidative phase followed by a non-oxidative phase consisting of a series of reversible reactions. NADPH and ribulose-5-P (from which ribose-5-P is derived) are made in the oxidative phase, ribose-5-P and the glycolytic intermediates are formed in the non-oxidative phase.

NADPH, although sharing much of its structure with NADH, has a different cellular role and serves as an important reducing agent in many anabolic processes (most notably, fatty acid synthesis). It also aids in the neutralization of reactive oxygen species. Ribose-5-P is used to synthesize nucleotides, while the other carbohydrate intermediates can be returned to glycolysis. Therefore, the "shunt" part of hexose monophosphate shunt...glucose can be shunted out of glycolysis to generate NADPH and ribose-5-P when necessary, and the glycolytic intermediates shunted back in.

- In order for NADPH to be an effect reducing agent, should the ratio of NADPH to NADP+ in the cell be high or low?[27]

---

[26] Without glucose-6-phosphatase, patients with von Gierke's disease are unable to produce free glucose from glycogen (and gluconeogenesis). As a result, these patients would have low blood-glucose levels, leading to chronically high levels of glucagon and low levels of insulin.

[27] A reducing agent is a substance that causes other molecules to be reduced (and is itself oxidized). As NADPH is the reduced form of NADP+, you would want a high NADPH to NADP+ ratio. This would favor the oxidation of NADPH in order for other molecules to be reduced.

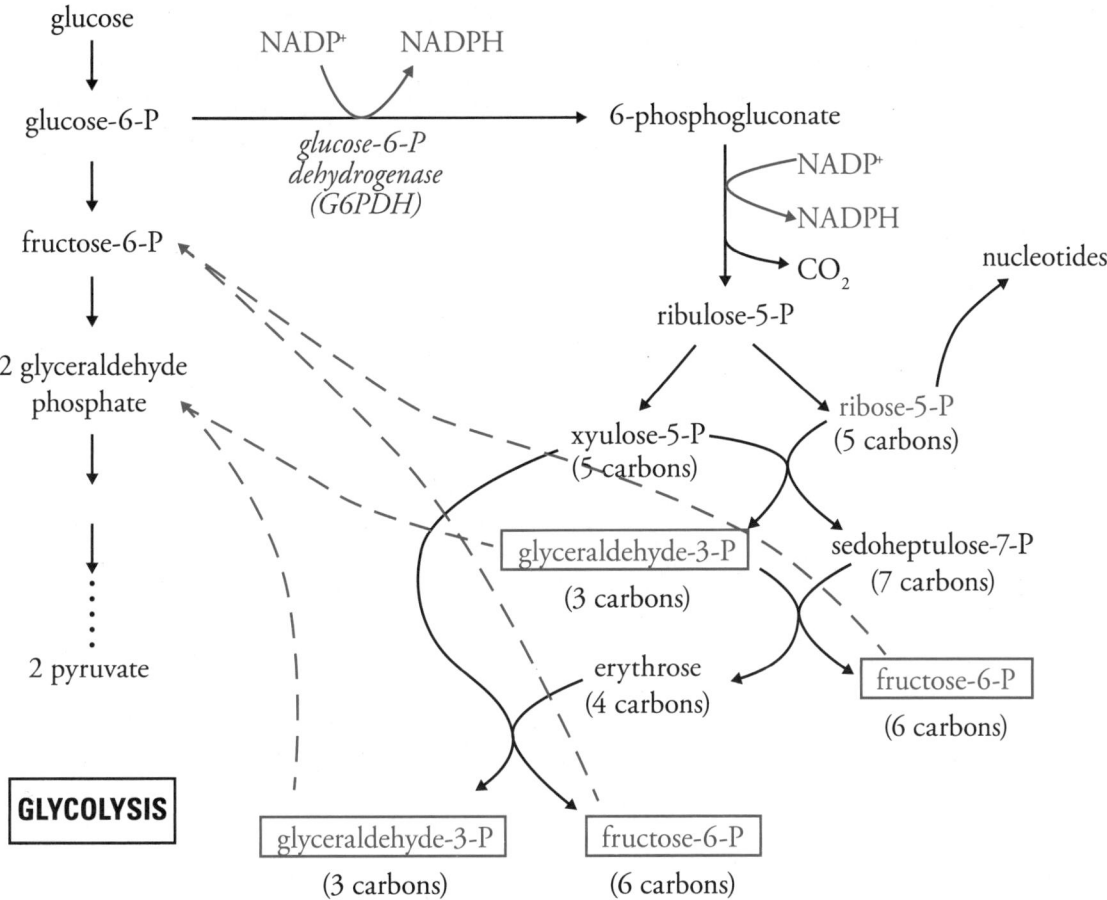

PENTOSE PHOSPHATE PATHWAY

Figure 17   Pentose Phosphate Pathway

The first enzyme in the PPP, **glucose-6-phosphate dehydrogenase (G6PDH)**, is the primary point of regulation. Its product, NADPH, acts via negative feedback to inhibit G6PDH. The two successive oxidations in this part of the pathway (thus the name "oxidative phase") generate 2 NADPH. A deficiency of this enzyme (which is a common heritable disease) limits the ability of red blood cells to eliminate reactive oxygen species; this can lead to cell death and potential renal and hepatic complications.

Chapter 5 Summary

- Cellular respiration is the oxidation of carbohydrates, reduction of electron carriers, and generation of ATP.

- Glycolysis occurs in the cytoplasm and generates two pyruvate molecules: two ATP and two NADH per glucose.

- Under anaerobic conditions, the cell performs fermentation to regenerate NAD^+ so that glycolysis can continue.

- The pyruvate dehydrogenase complex (PDC) functions in the mitochondrial matrix, converts pyruvate into acetyl-CoA, and generates an NADH.

- The Krebs cycle in the mitochondrial matrix generates six NADH, two $FADH_2$, and two GTP per glucose.

- The electron transport chain in the inner mitochondrial membrane starts with the oxidation of the electron carriers NADH and $FADH_2$ and ends with the reduction of oxygen and the generation of a proton gradient across the inner mitochondrial membrane.

- ATP synthase in the inner mitochondrial membrane uses the proton gradient to generate ATP (2.5 ATP per NADH from the mitochondrial matrix, 1.5 ATP per NADH from the cytoplasm, and 1.5 ATP per $FADH_2$).

- Both eukaryotes and prokaryotes perform cellular respiration, but prokaryotes use their plasma membrane for the electron transport chain and generate two more ATP per glucose than eukaryotes.

- Gluconeogenesis generates "new" glucose from precursors such as pyruvate, oxaloacetate, amino acids, and glycerol.

- In reciprocal regulation, a single molecule controls two different enzymes in opposite ways. This helps prevent futile cycles (opposite pathways running at the same time).

- Glycogenesis stores glucose as a glycogen polymer. This occurs in the liver and the skeletal muscle.

- During times of starvation, glycogenolysis in the liver produces glucose that can be released into the blood. When the glycogen is depleted, gluconeogenesis can generate glucose from precursors such as pyruvate, lactate, and Krebs cycle intermediates.

- The pentose phosphate pathway generates ribose-5-phosphate (necessary for nucleotide synthesis) and NADPH (necessary as a reducing agent during anabolic pathways).

CHAPTER 5 FREESTANDING PRACTICE QUESTIONS

1. In eukaryotes, the ultimate yield of ATP from NADH is lower when the NADH is produced by:

A) glycolysis.
B) pyruvate dehydrogenase complex (PDC).
C) the Krebs cycle.
D) electron transport and oxidative phosphorylation.

2. Glycogen is a polysaccharide of glucose molecules with α1→4 connections and α1→6 branches. Amylose, a glucose-storing polysaccharide in plants, contains identical linkages, yet is hydrolyzed more slowly than glycogen. Which of the following explains this difference?

A) Glycogen adopts a tighter conformation than amylose does *in vivo*.
B) Plant digestive enzymes are specific to β linkages and therefore digest the α linkages in amylose at a decreased rate.
C) Glycogen contains α1→6 branches every 8–12 monomers, whereas amylose contains α1→6 branches every 12–20 monomers.
D) Amylose's α1→6 branches require more energy to hydrolyze than those present in glucose.

3. Which of the following changes would lead to a long-term increase in intracellular glucose levels in liver cells?

A) Decreased production of glycogen phosphorylase
B) Type 1 diabetes mellitus, caused by destruction of the beta cells of the pancreas
C) Expression of an overactive isoform of the pyruvate dehydrogenase complex (PDC)
D) Overexpression of pyruvate carboxylase

4. Salicylic acid (aspirin), if taken in excess, may act as an *uncoupling agent*. Uncoupling agents increase the permeability of the inner mitochondrial membrane, resulting in the dissipation of the proton gradient. Which of the following would most likely be true in the presence of an uncoupling agent?

A) Electron transport at the inner mitochondrial membrane would cease.
B) The energy from the proton-motive force would likely be dissipated as heat rather than in producing ATP from ADP.
C) H^+ ions would flow through the inner membrane into the intermembrane space.
D) There would be an increase in biosynthesis.

5. Which of the following is FALSE regarding the pentose phosphate pathway?

A) A decrease in the $NADPH:NADP^+$ ratio will activate the pentose phosphate pathway.
B) The pentose phosphate pathway would be upregulated during fatty acid synthesis.
C) The pentose phosphate pathway is most active during the M phase of the cell cycle.
D) A decrease in the pentose phosphate pathway activity may cause hemolytic anemia (premature destruction of red blood cells).

6. Glycogen metabolism is regulated by different hormones that activate reciprocal pathways. After several hours of fasting, a person eats a large meal. Which of the following statements is correct?

A) Elevated glucagon levels deactivate glycogen phosphorylase and activate glycogen synthase.
B) Elevated insulin levels deactivate glycogen phosphorylase and activate glycogen synthase.
C) Elevated glucagon levels activate glycogen phosphorylase and deactivate glycogen synthase.
D) Elevated insulin levels activate glycogen phosphorylase and deactivate glycogen synthase.

7. Which of the following is a product of the pentose phosphate pathway?

A) NADH
B) NADPH
C) Succinyl-CoA
D) Fructose-1,6-bisphosphate

CHAPTER 5 PRACTICE PASSAGE

Glycogen storage diseases (GSDs) result from the inappropriate synthesis or breakdown of glycogen. There are numerous types of GSDs caused by the production of dysfunctional or nonfunctional enzymes involved in glycogen metabolism. GSD V, commonly referred to as McArdle's disease, is caused by a deficiency in muscle glycogen phosphorylase, a key enzyme used in glycogenolysis. Patients with GSD V typically exhibit elevated levels of myoglobin in the urine and experience fatigue during the first 15 minutes of exercise followed by a sudden increase in the tolerance of exercise known as the "second wind" phenomenon.

Various tests are performed on patients with McArdle's disease to confirm the diagnosis. In addition to checking creatine kinase levels, patients will often undergo an ischemic (or non-ischemic) forearm exercise test. During an ischemic forearm exercise test, a blood pressure cuff is placed on the patient's upper arm and inflated to a pressure greater than systolic pressure, stopping blood flow to the lower arm. The patient then repeatedly clenches and unclenches their fist until they fatigue. Ammonia and lactate levels from the exercised arm are taken prior to exercise and at regular intervals after the forearm fatigues. For the non-ischemic forearm exercise test, the same procedure is used without the blood pressure cuff.

A patient complaining of low exercise tolerance and muscle cramps was also experiencing episodes of dark urine after exertion. A diagnosis of GSD V was suspected and diagnostic tests were performed. The person's creatine kinase levels were found to be four times the normal level. The results of an ischemic forearm test are presented in Figure 1.

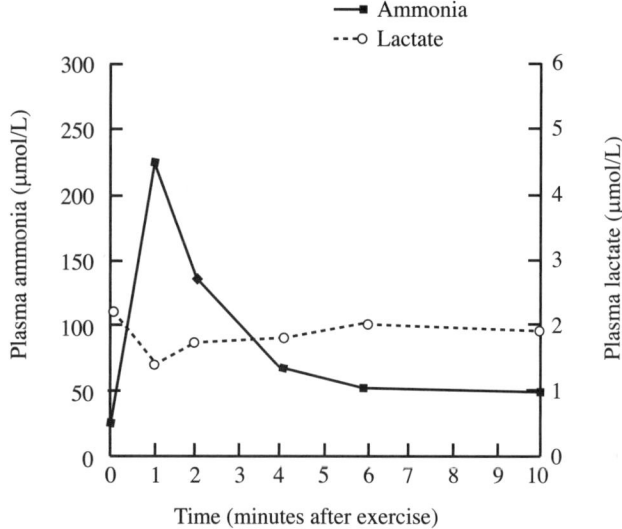

Figure 1   Ischemic Forearm Exercise Test

Adapted from Park H, Shin H, Cho Y, Kim S, Choi Y. *The Significance of Clinical and Laboratory Features in the Diagnosis of Glycogen Storage Disease Type V: A Case Report.* JKMS: 2014; 7:1021-1024.

1. Which of the following best explains the changes in lactate levels after the first minute of the ischemic forearm test shown in Figure 1?

A) Depletion of NAD⁺
B) Depletion of glycogen stores
C) Depletion of glucose
D) Depletion of ADP

2. Which of the following is/are expected be elevated in the muscle cells of a patient with GSD V?

    I.   Glycogen
   II.   Glucose
  III.   Lactate

A) I only
B) III only
C) I and II only
D) I and III only

3. The purpose of preventing blood flow to the forearm during the ischemic exercise test is most likely to:

A) encourage anaerobic respiration.
B) decrease blood pressure in the forearm.
C) prevent the delivery of glycogen to the forearm.
D) decrease the level of lactate in the forearm.

4. Would the results of the ischemic forearm test in Figure 1 contribute to a diagnosis of GSD V for the patient?

A) No, increased glycogenolysis should result in increased lactate levels.
B) No, muscle fatigue should result in decreased ammonia levels.
C) Yes, decreased glycogenesis will lead to increased ammonia levels.
D) Yes, decreased glycogenolysis will lead to decreased lactate levels.

5. Given that the generation of creatine phosphate from ATP and creatine occurs spontaneously under standard conditions, which of the following is true regarding creatine phosphate metabolism in the human body?

A) Under resting conditions, the generation of creatine phosphate is favored.
B) During strenuous exercise, the generation of creatine phosphate is favored.
C) The generation of creatine phosphate is not favored in the human body.
D) In the presence of low concentrations of ATP, the generation of creatine phosphate is favored.

SOLUTIONS TO CHAPTER 5 FREESTANDING PRACTICE QUESTIONS

1. **A** In order for the NADH produced during glycolysis to be utilized by the electron transport chain (ETC) in ATP formation, the electrons must be shuttled into the mitochondria (remember, glycolysis occurs in the cytosol and the ETC along the inner mitochondrial membrane). When shuttled in, the electrons are typically used to reduce coenzyme Q and bypass NADH dehydrogenase. This results in the pumping of fewer protons out of the mitochondrial matrix, and thus, ultimately, in fewer ATP being formed. The NADH produced by the PDC or Krebs cycle is energetically equivalent because both occur in the mitochondrial matrix. Thus, this NADH is immediately accessible to the ETC (choices B and C are wrong). Finally, note that the ETC regenerates NAD^+ rather than producing NADH (choice D is wrong).

2. **C** Because glycogen contains more $\alpha1 \rightarrow 6$ branches, glycogen is a more branched polymer than amylose. The increase in the number of branches provides ends for hydrolysis, resulting in an elevated rate of digestion relative to amylose (choice C is correct). If glycogen were to adopt a tighter conformation, its glucose monomers would be more difficult to access, and it would likely be digested more slowly than amylose (choice A is wrong). If plant enzymes were specific to β linkages, they would be completely unable to digest α linkages, rather than show slowed digestion rates (choice B is wrong). Since both glycogen and amylose contain identical linkages, there is no expected energy difference of hydrolysis (choice D is wrong).

3. **D** Pyruvate carboxylase is responsible for the conversion of pyruvate to oxaloacetate in the first step of gluconeogenesis. Over-expression of pyruvate carboxylase would increase the rate of gluconeogenesis, causing increased intracellular glucose levels (choice D is correct). If glycogen phosphorylase production were decreased, glycogenolysis would decrease, leading to decreased glucose production (choice A is wrong). Destruction of the beta cells of the pancreas would lead to insulin deficiency, a hallmark of Type 1 diabetes mellitus. The absence of insulin would prevent the cellular uptake of glucose, leading to lower intracellular glucose levels (choice B is wrong). An overactive PDC would decrease pyruvate levels, driving glycolysis forward and causing decreased rates of gluconeogenesis. This would lower intracellular glucose (choice C is wrong).

4. **B** The proton gradient obtained by the electron transport chain (which pumps H^+ ions across the inner membrane into the intermembrane space) is necessary in order to create ATP at the ATP synthase. This enzyme allows the protons to move through its channel back into the matrix, and thus harnesses the energy created by the gradient to create ATP from ADP + P_i. If the inner membrane was made more permeable by uncoupling agents, then the H^+ ions would naturally move down their gradient, from the intermembrane space back to the mitochondrial matrix (choice C is wrong). This unharnessed energy would be dissipated as heat (known as non-exercise activity thermogenesis [NEAT]), and since the ions would not pass through the ATP synthase, less ATP would be created (choice B is correct). Although the utility of the electron transport chain would be compromised, the uncoupling agent would not inhibit electron transport itself (choice A is wrong); in fact this would lead to the rapid oxidation of Krebs cycle substrates and would promote the mobilization of carbohydrates and fats. Since the energy is lost as heat, biosynthesis is not promoted (choice D is wrong), and weight loss can be dramatic. Experimental uncoupling agents have been used in the past as effective diet pills; however, their use is very dangerous and thankfully this practice has fallen out of use.

5. **C**   The pentose phosphate pathway is used to generate nucleotide precursors for DNA synthesis and is therefore most active during the S phase of the cell cycle, not the M phase (choice C is a false statement and the correct answer choice). An increase in $NADP^+$, corresponding to a decrease in the $NADPH:NADP^+$ ratio, will activate the pentose phosphate pathway (choice A is true and can be eliminated). The pentose phosphate pathway (PPP) also creates NADPH, which is used as reducing power in fatty acid synthesis and also to limit oxidative stress; we would expect it to be upregulated during fatty acid synthesis (choice B is true and can be eliminated). Further, deficiencies in the PPP may increase oxidative stress in red blood cells, leading to cell lysis and hemolytic anemia (choice D is true and can be eliminated).

6. **B**   Insulin levels are elevated when blood glucose levels rise, such as after consuming a large meal. Glucagon levels are elevated during fasting (choices A and C can be eliminated). Insulin allows cells to take up glucose and activates the pathways that store it as glycogen (as well as those that convert it into energy). Therefore, high insulin levels would lead to activation of the enzyme that synthesizes glycogen, glycogen synthase, and deactivation of the enzyme that breaks glycogen down, glycogen phosphorylase (choice D can be eliminated, and choice B is correct).

7. **B**   The pentose phosphate pathway produces ribose, which acts as a backbone for nucleotide synthesis as well as NADPH (choice B is correct). NADH is made in catabolic reactions, such as glycolysis and the Krebs cycle (choice A is wrong). Succinyl-CoA is an intermediate product of the Krebs cycle, not the pentose phosphate pathway (choice C is wrong). Fructose-1,6-bisphosphate is one of the intermediate products of glycolysis (choice D is wrong).

SOLUTIONS TO CHAPTER 5 PRACTICE PASSAGE

1. **C**   During the ischemic forearm test, blood flow is cut off from the patient's arm, reducing the delivery of oxygen to the muscles. Without oxygen, the muscle cells cannot undergo aerobic respiration and thus must undergo anaerobic respiration, producing lactate as a byproduct. Patients with GSD V have a deficiency in glycogen phosphorylase, an enzyme required to break down glycogen. As they are unable to break down glycogen, these patients will quickly consume all the glucose freely available and will not be able to produce lactic acid from anaerobic respiration (choice C is correct). Depletion of NAD^+ should not have an effect on lactate levels because NAD^+ is a byproduct of lactic acid production (the oxidation of NADH drives the reduction of pyruvate to lactate). In other words, the drop in lactic acid could explain a depletion in NAD^+, but a drop in NAD^+ cannot explain a drop in lactic acid (choice A is wrong). As glycogen cannot be broken down, the glycogen stores would also not be depleted (choice B is wrong). A drop in ADP would indicate more ATP production which is not enhanced in an ischemic state (choice D is wrong).

2. **A** Since Item III appears in exactly two answer choices, start by evaluating it; whether it is true or false you'll be able to eliminate half the answers. Item III is false: decreased levels of glucose in the muscle cells would decrease the rate of glycolysis as well as the rate of lactic acid fermentation (choices B and D can be eliminated). Since both remaining answer choices include Item I it must be true and you can evaluate Item II. Item II is false: with decreased glycogen breakdown, there will be lower levels of glucose in the muscle cells (choice C can be eliminated and choice A is correct). Note that Item I is in fact true: because patients with GSD V lack glycogen phosphorylase, they are unable to regularly break down glycogen into glucose. As a result, these patients are expected to have elevated levels of glycogen.

3. **A** The passage indicates that the purpose of the ischemic forearm test is to monitor levels of lactate and ammonia following exercise to confirm the diagnosis of McArdle's disease. In order to promote the production of lactate, anaerobic conditions must be favored. Without blood flow, limited oxygen will reach the forearm, creating the anaerobic environment necessary for this test (choice A is correct). Although decreased blood flow to the forearm will decrease its blood pressure, decreasing the blood pressure does not help in the diagnosis of McArdle's disease (choice B is incorrect). Generally, glycogen is not delivered to muscle via the bloodstream, but it is rather generated via glycogenesis in the muscle itself (choice C is incorrect). Preventing blood flow to the forearm may lead to decreased delivery of lactate from other parts of the body, but the purpose of stopping blood flow is to encourage the production of lactic acid, not decrease the level of lactic acid in the forearm (choice D is incorrect).

4. **D** Patients with GSD V lack a crucial enzyme needed for glycogenolysis. As a result, these patients would exhibit decreased glycogenolysis, and glucose levels would drop. This would decrease the rate of glycolysis and lactic acid fermentation and decrease the levels of lactate in the body (choice D is correct, and choice A is wrong). Although glycogenesis may be decreased in individuals with GSD V due to the presence of excess glycogen stores, this would not be expected to substantially affect ammonia levels (choice C is wrong). In fact, the increased ammonia levels in patients with GSD V following the ischemic forearm test is primarily due to the increased breakdown of amino acids for fuel as the muscle fatigues (choice B is wrong).

5. **A** The question stem states that under standard conditions (1 *M* concentration of starting materials and products), the formation of creatine phosphate is favored. Under resting conditions, ATP levels in the body are high, which favors the formation of creatine phosphate by mass action (choice A is correct, and choice C is wrong). During strenuous exercise, ATP levels drop in the body, favoring the degradation of creatine phosphate to generate more ATP (choices B and D are wrong).

Chapter 6
Lipids

The biological macromolecules are grouped into four classes of molecules that play important roles in cells and in organisms as a whole. All of them are polymers; strings of repeated units (monomers).

This chapter discusses the lipids from a biological perspective: what they are made of, how they are put together, and what their roles are in the body. These molecules are also discussed in *MCAT Organic Chemistry Review* from an organic chemistry perspective: nomenclature, chirality, etc.

6.1 INTRODUCTION TO LIPIDS

Lipids are oily or fatty substances that play three primary physiological roles, summarized here and discussed below.

1) In adipose cells, triglycerides (fats) store energy.
2) In cellular membranes, phospholipids constitute a barrier between intracellular and extracellular environments.
3) Cholesterol is a special lipid that serves as the building block for the hydrophobic steroid hormones.

The cardinal characteristic of the lipid is its **hydrophobicity**. *Hydrophobic* means "water-fearing." It is important to understand the significance of this. Since water is very polar, polar substances dissolve well in water; these are known as "water-loving," or **hydrophilic** substances. Carbon-carbon bonds and carbon-hydrogen bonds are nonpolar. Hence, substances that contain only carbon and hydrogen will not dissolve well in water. Here are some examples: table sugar dissolves well in water, but cooking oil floats in a layer above water or forms many tiny oil droplets when mixed with water. Cotton T-shirts become wet when exposed to water because they are made of glucose polymerized into cellulose, but a nylon jacket does not become wet because it is composed of atoms covalently bound together in a nonpolar fashion. A synonym for *hydrophobic* is **lipophilic** (which means "lipid-loving"); a synonym for *hydrophilic* is **lipophobic**. We return to these concepts below.

Fatty Acid Structure

Fatty acids are composed of long unsubstituted alkanes that end in a carboxylic acid. The chain is typically 14 to 18 carbons long, and because they are synthesized two carbons at a time from acetate, predominantly *even-numbered* fatty acids are made in human cells. A fatty acid with no carbon-carbon double bonds is said to be **saturated** with hydrogen because every carbon atom in the chain is covalently bound to the maximum number of hydrogens. **Unsaturated** fatty acids have one or more double bonds in the tail. These double bonds are almost always (*Z*) (or *cis*).

Saturated fatty acid

Unsaturated fatty acid

*   How does the shape of an unsaturated fatty acid differ from that of a saturated fatty acid?[1]
*   If fatty acids are mixed into water, how are they likely to associate with each other?[2]

---

[1] An unsaturated fatty acid is bent, or "kinked," at the *cis* double bond.

[2] The long hydrophobic chains will interact with each other to minimize contact with water, exposing the charged carboxyl group to the aqueous environment.

Figure 1 illustrates how free fatty acids interact in an aqueous solution; they form a structure called a **micelle**. The force that drives the tails into the center of the micelle is called the **hydrophobic interaction**. The hydrophobic interaction is a complex phenomenon. In general, it results from the fact that water molecules must form an orderly **solvation shell** around each hydrophobic substance. The reason is that H_2O has a dipole that "likes" to be able to share its charges with other polar molecules. A solvation shell allows for the most water-water interaction and the least water-lipid interaction. In the case of the fatty acid micelle, water forms a shell around the spherical micelle with the result being that water interacts with polar carboxylic acid head groups while hydrophobic lipid tails hide inside the sphere.

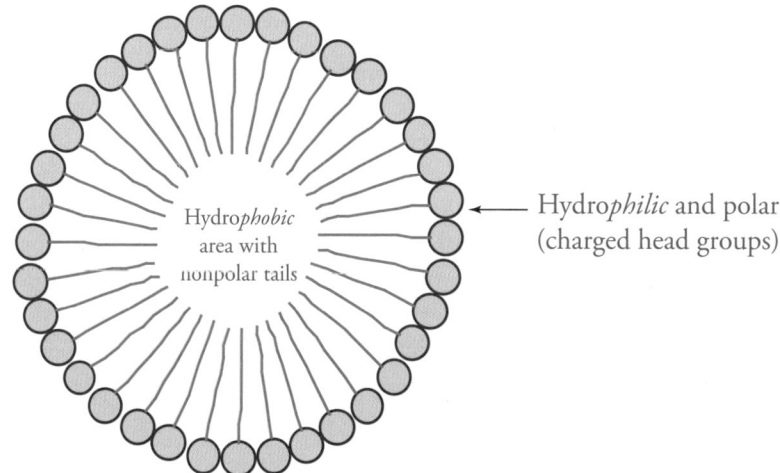

Hydro*phobic* area with nonpolar tails

Hydro*philic* and polar (charged head groups)

Figure 1   A Fatty Acid Micelle

- How does soap help to remove grease from your hands?[3]

6.2   TRIACYLGLYCEROLS (TG)

The storage form of the fatty acid is fat. The technical name for fat is **triacylglycerol** or **triglyceride** (see Figure 2). The triglyceride is composed of three fatty acids esterified to a glycerol molecule. Glycerol is a three-carbon triol with the formula $HOCH_2–CHOH–CH_2OH$. As you can see, it has three hydroxyl groups that can be esterified to fatty acids. It is necessary to store fatty acids in the relatively inert form of fat because free fatty acids are reactive chemicals.

---

[3]   Grease is hydrophobic. It does not wash off easily in water because it is not soluble in water. Scrubbing your hands with soap causes micelles to form around the grease particles.

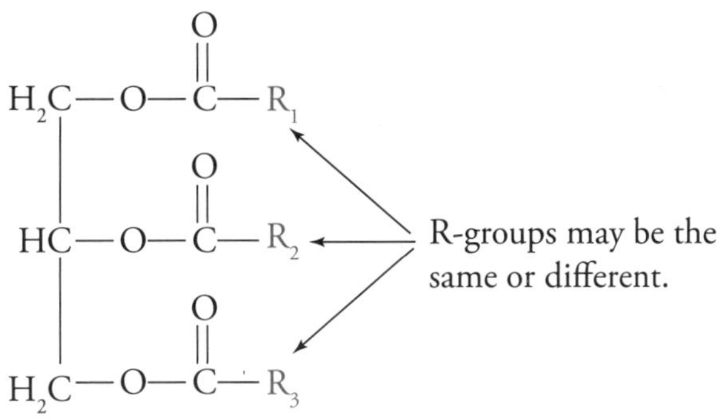

Figure 2 A Triglyceride (Fat)

The triacylglycerol undergoes reactions typical of esters, such as base-catalyzed hydrolysis. Soaps are the sodium salts of fatty acids (RCOO–Na$^+$). They are **amphipathic**, which means they have both hydrophilic and hydrophobic regions. Soap is economically produced by base-catalyzed hydrolysis of triglycerides from animal fat into fatty acid salts (soaps). This reaction is called **saponification** and is illustrated in Figure 3.

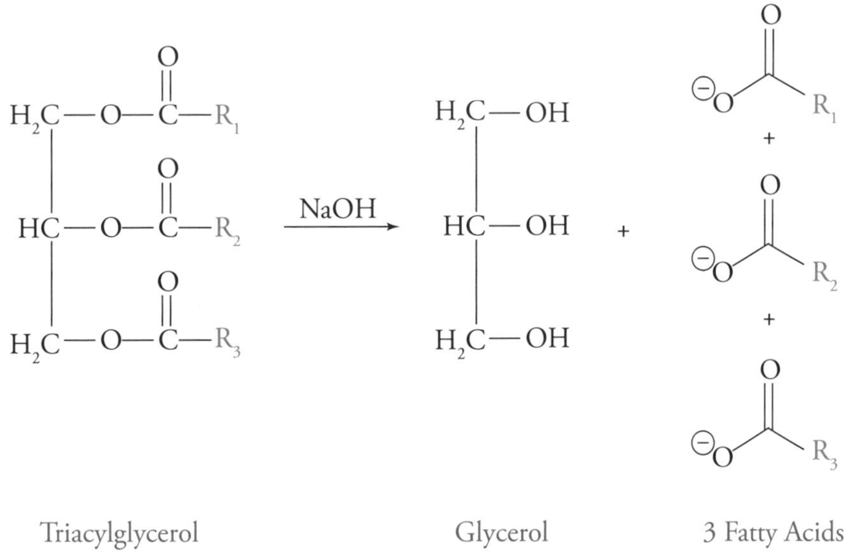

Triacylglycerol   Glycerol   3 Fatty Acids

Figure 3 Saponification

Lipases are enzymes that hydrolyze fats. Triacylglycerols are stored in fat cells as an energy source. Fats are more efficient energy storage molecules than carbohydrates for two reasons: packing and energy content.

1) **Packing:** Their hydrophobicity allows fats to pack together much more closely than carbohydrates. Carbohydrates carry a great amount of water-of-solvation (water molecules hydrogen-bonded to their hydroxyl groups). In other words, the amount of carbon per unit area or unit weight is much greater in a fat droplet than in dissolved sugar. If we could store sugars in a dry powdery form in our bodies, this problem would be obviated.

2) **Energy content:** All packing considerations aside, fat molecules store much more energy than carbohydrates. In other words, regardless of what you dissolve it in, a fat has more energy carbon-for-carbon than a carbohydrate. The reason is that fats are much more reduced. Remember that energy metabolism begins with the oxidation of foodstuffs to release energy. Since carbohydrates are more oxidized to start with, oxidizing them releases less energy. Animals use fat to store most of their energy, storing only a small amount as carbohydrates (glycogen). Plants such as potatoes commonly store a large percentage of their energy as carbohydrates (starch).

6.3 PHOSPHOLIPIDS AND LIPID BILAYER MEMBRANES

Membrane lipids are **phospholipids** (also called phosphatides) derived from diacylglycerol phosphate or DG-P. Often the phosphate group has even bigger polar molecules attached to it, such as choline (phosphatidylcholine), ethanolamine (phosphatidylethanolamine), and inositol (phosphatidylinositol). For example, phosphatidylcholine is a phospholipid formed by the esterification of a choline molecule $[HO(CH_2)_2N^+(CH_3)_3]$ to the phosphate group of DG-P. Phosphatidylcholine and phosphatidylethanolamine are the most common phospholipids in eukaryotic cells. Beyond its role as a membrane lipid, phosphatidylcholine is a major lipid component of lung surfactant (important in reducing surface tension inside lung alveoli), and phosphatidylinositol plays a role in signal transmission across cell membranes.

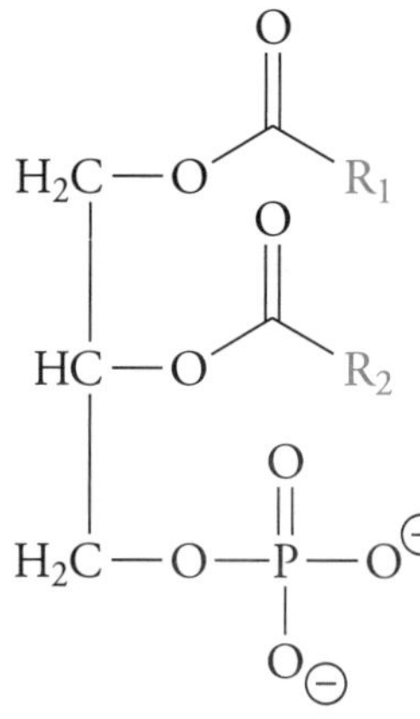

Figure 4   A Phosphoglyceride (Diacylglycerol Phosphate, or DG-P)

We saw above how fatty acids spontaneously form micelles. Phospholipids also minimize their interactions with water by forming an orderly structure—in this case, it is a **lipid bilayer** (Figure 5). Hydrophobic interactions drive the formation of the bilayer, and once formed, it is stabilized by van der Waals forces between the long tails.

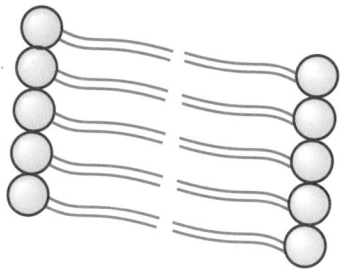

Figure 5 A Small Section of a Lipid Bilayer Membrane

- Would a saturated or an unsaturated fatty acid residue have more van der Waals interactions with neighboring alkyl chains in a bilayer membrane?[4]

A more precise way to give the answer to the question above is to say that double bonds (unsaturation) in phospholipid fatty acids *tend to increase membrane fluidity*. Unsaturation prevents the membrane from solidifying by disrupting the orderly packing of the hydrophobic lipid tails. The right amount of fluidity is essential for function. Decreasing the *length* of fatty acid tails also increases fluidity. The steroid **cholesterol** (discussed a bit later) is a third important modulator of membrane fluidity. At low temperatures, it increases fluidity in the same way as kinks in fatty acid tails; hence, it is known as *membrane antifreeze*. At high temperatures, however, cholesterol attenuates (reduces) membrane fluidity. Don't ponder this paradox too long; just remember that cholesterol keeps fluidity at an *optimum level*. Remember, the structural determinants of membrane fluidity are degree of saturation, tail length, and amount of cholesterol.

The lipid bilayer acts like a barrier surrounding the cell in the sense that it separates the interior of the cell from the exterior. However, the cell membrane is much more complex than a simple barrier; it is a dynamic structure that regulates what comes into and goes out of the cell and transmits extracellular signals to the interior of the cell. Proteins embedded in the plasma membrane play a big role in this. Since the plasma bilayer membrane surrounding cells is impermeable to charged particles such as Na^+, protein gateways such as ion channels are required for ions to enter or exit cells. Further, certain hormones (peptides) cannot pass through the cell membrane due to their charged nature; instead, protein **receptors** in the cell membrane bind these hormones and transmit a signal into the cell in a **second messenger cascade** (see *MCAT Biology Review* for more details about the plasma membrane).

6.4 TERPENES AND STEROIDS

A terpene is a member of a broad class of compounds built from isoprene units (C_5H_8) with a general formula $(C_5H_8)_n$.

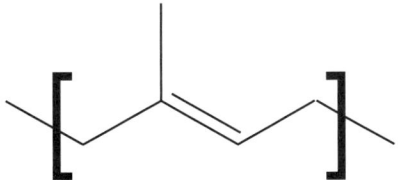

Figure 6 Isoprene Unit

---

[4] The bent shape of the unsaturated fatty acid means that it doesn't fit in as well and has less contact with neighboring groups to form van der Waals interactions. Phospholipids composed of saturated fatty acids make the membrane less fluid.

Terpenes may be linear or cyclic, and they are classified by the number of isoprene units they contain. For example, monoterpenes consist of two isoprene units, sesquiterpenes consist of three, and diterpenes contain four.

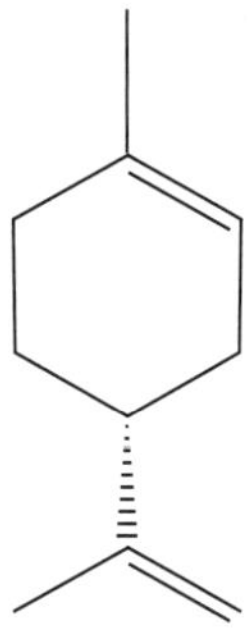

limonene
$C_{10}H_{16}$
(a monoterpene)

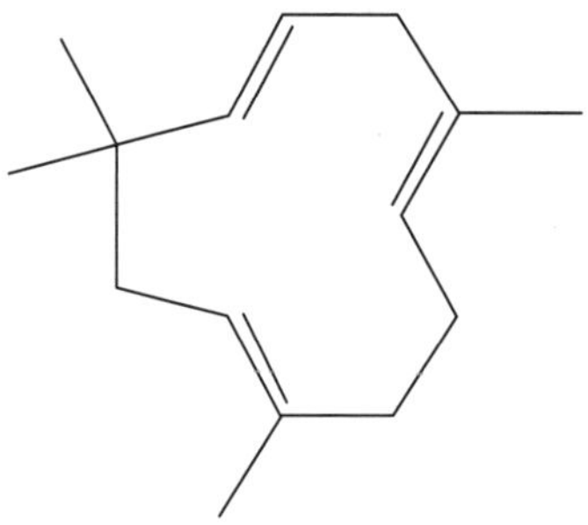

humulene
$C_{15}H_{24}$
(a sesquiterpene)

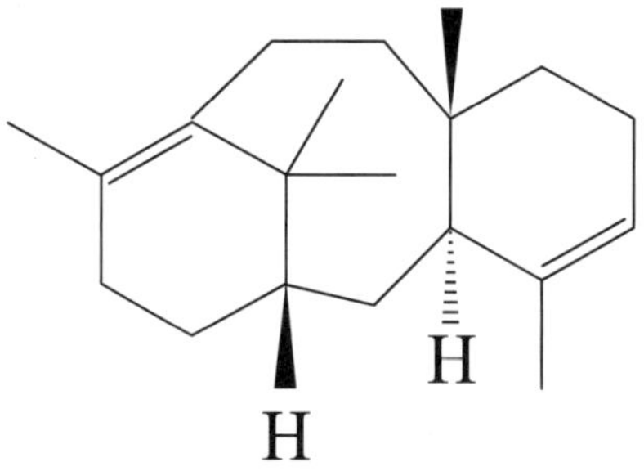

taxadiene
$C_{20}H_{32}$
(a diterpene)

Figure 7 Terpene Structures

Squalene is a triterpene (made of six isoprene units), and it is a particularly important compound, as it is biosynthetically utilized in the manufacture of steroids. Squalene is also a component of earwax.

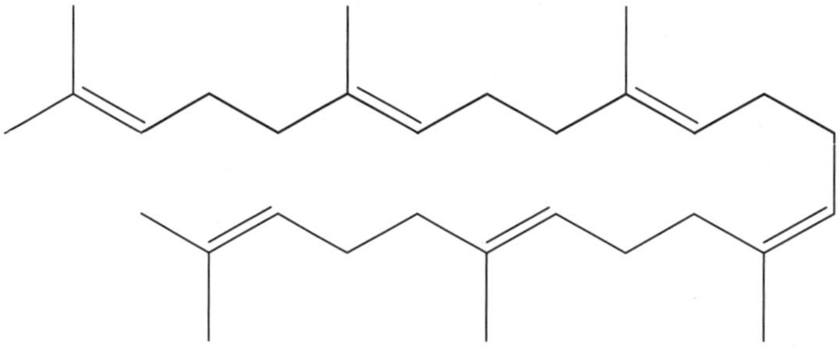

Figure 8 Squalene

Whereas a terpene is formally a simple hydrocarbon, there are a number of natural and synthetically derived species that are built from an isoprene skeleton and functionalized with other elements (O, N, S, etc.). These functionalized-terpenes are known as *terpenoids*. Vitamin A ($C_{20}H_{30}O$) is an example of a terpenoid.

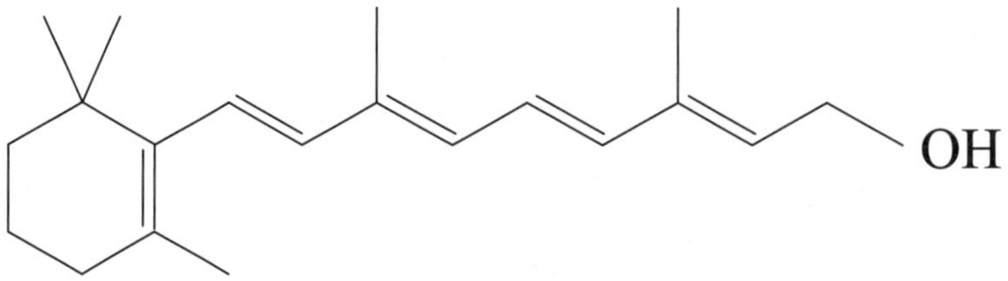

Figure 9 Vitamin A

Steroids

Steroids are included here because of their hydrophobicity, and, hence, similarity to fats. Their structure is otherwise unique. All steroids have the basic tetracyclic ring system (Figure 10), based on the structure of **cholesterol**, a polycyclic amphipath. (Polycyclic means several rings, and amphipathic means displaying both hydrophilic and hydrophobic characteristics.)

As discussed earlier, the steroid cholesterol is an important component of the lipid bilayer. It is both obtained from the diet and synthesized in the liver. It is carried in the blood packaged with fats and proteins into **lipoproteins**. One type of lipoprotein has been implicated as the cause of atherosclerotic vascular disease, which refers to the build-up of cholesterol "plaques" on the inside of blood vessels.

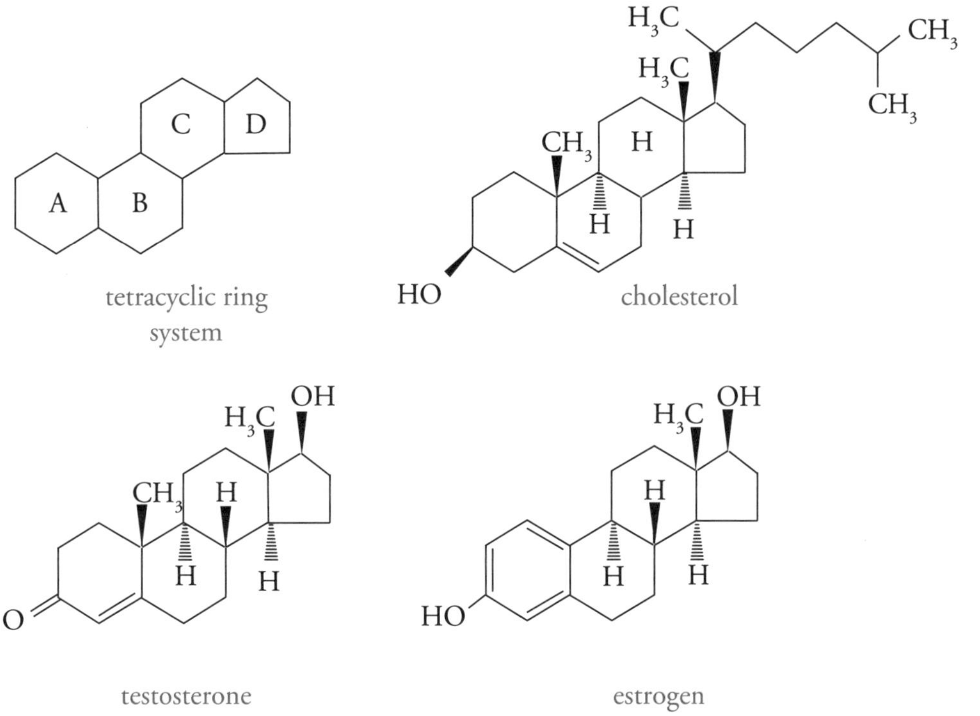

tetracyclic ring
system

cholesterol

testosterone

estrogen

Figure 10   Cholesterol-Derived Hormones

Steroid hormones are made from cholesterol. Two examples are **testosterone** (an androgen, or male sex hormone) and **estradiol** (an estrogen, or female sex hormone). There are no receptors for steroid hormones on the surface of cells; because steroids are highly hydrophobic, they can diffuse right through the lipid bilayer membrane into the cytoplasm. The receptors for steroid hormones are located within cells rather than on the cell surface. This is an important point! You must be aware of the contrast between *peptide* hormones, such as insulin, which exert their effects by binding to receptors at the cell-surface, and *steroid* hormones, such as estrogen, which diffuse into cells to find their receptors.

6.5 OTHER LIPIDS

Beyond fatty acids, triglycerides, phospholipids, terpenes, cholesterol, and steroids, there are a few other lipids with which you should be familiar for the MCAT.

Sphingolipids

Sphingolipids are structured in a similar manner as phospholipids, except that the backbone is sphingosine instead of glycerol. The only significant sphingolipid in humans is sphingomyelin, an important component of the myelin sheath around neurons.

sphingosine

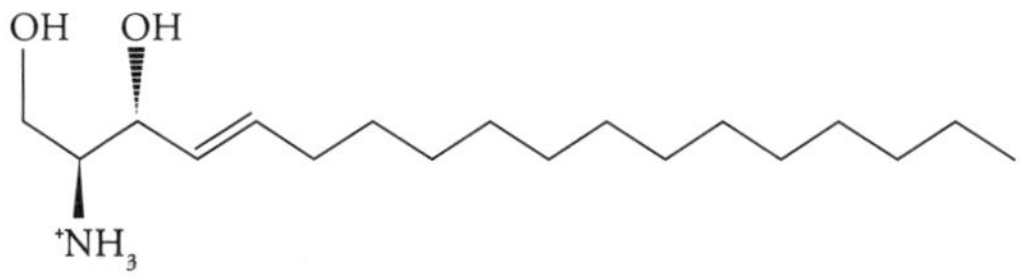

a ceramide

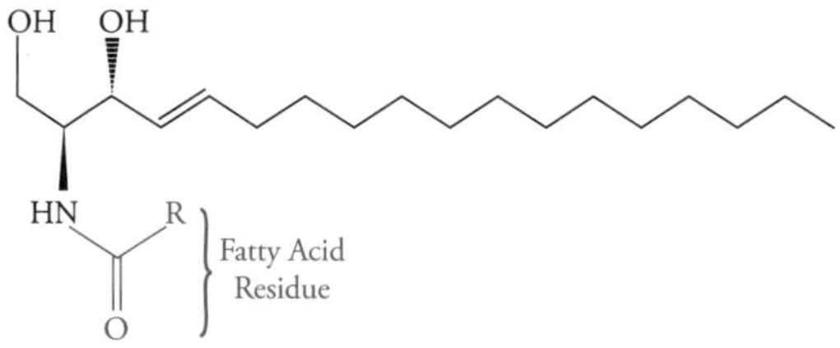

a sphingomyelin (phosphatidylcholine)

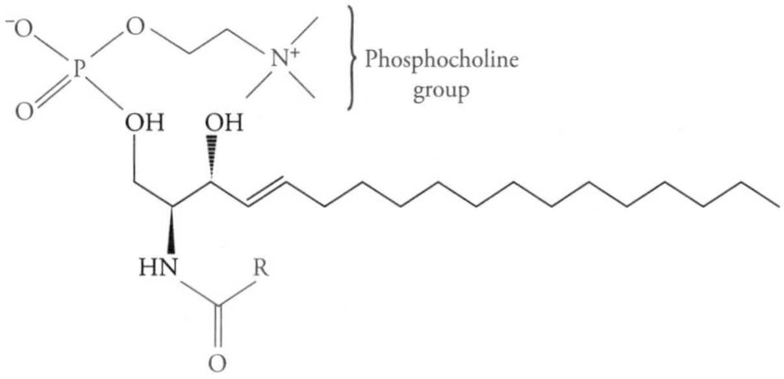

a sphingomyelin (phosphatidylethanolamine)

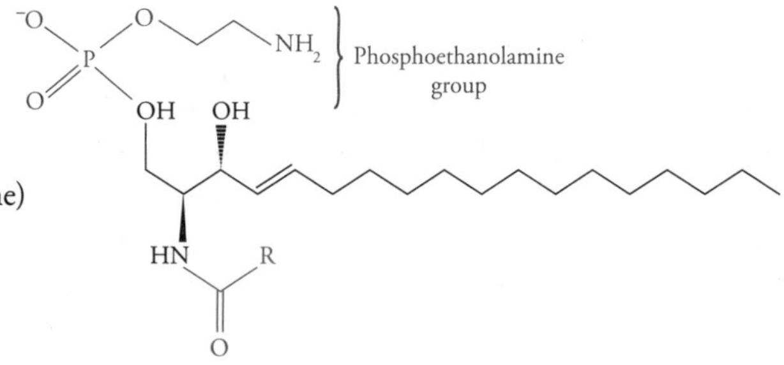

Figure 11 Sphingolipids

Waxes

Waxes are long chain fats esterified to long chain alcohols. They are extremely hydrophobic and often form waterproof barriers, most notably in plants. Animals also use waxes to form a protective barrier (e.g., earwax).

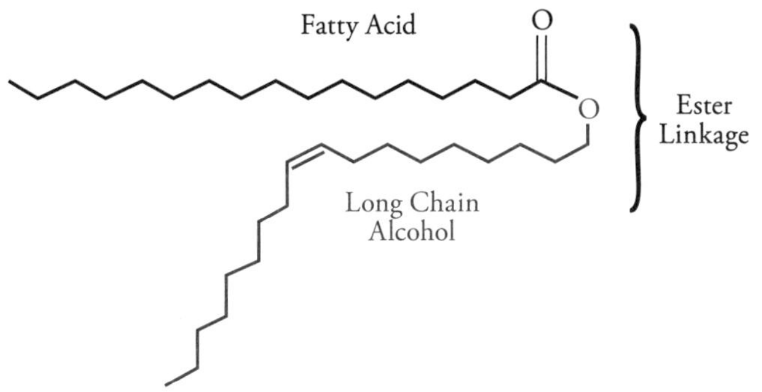

Figure 12   Wax

Fat-Soluble Vitamins

Fat-soluble vitamins are absorbed with dietary fat and stored in adipose tissue and in the liver. The four fat-soluble vitamins are vitamins A, D, E, and K; all of them have ring structures. Vitamin A is a terpenoid (mentioned earlier) essential for vision, growth, epithelial maintenance, and immune function. Vitamin D is derived from cholesterol (it is a steroid) important in regulating blood levels of calcium and phosphate. Vitamin E is actually a group of compounds, called **tocopherols** (methylated phenols), that are important as antioxidants. α-Tocopherol is the most active vitamin E. Vitamin K serves as an important coenzyme in the activation of clotting proteins.

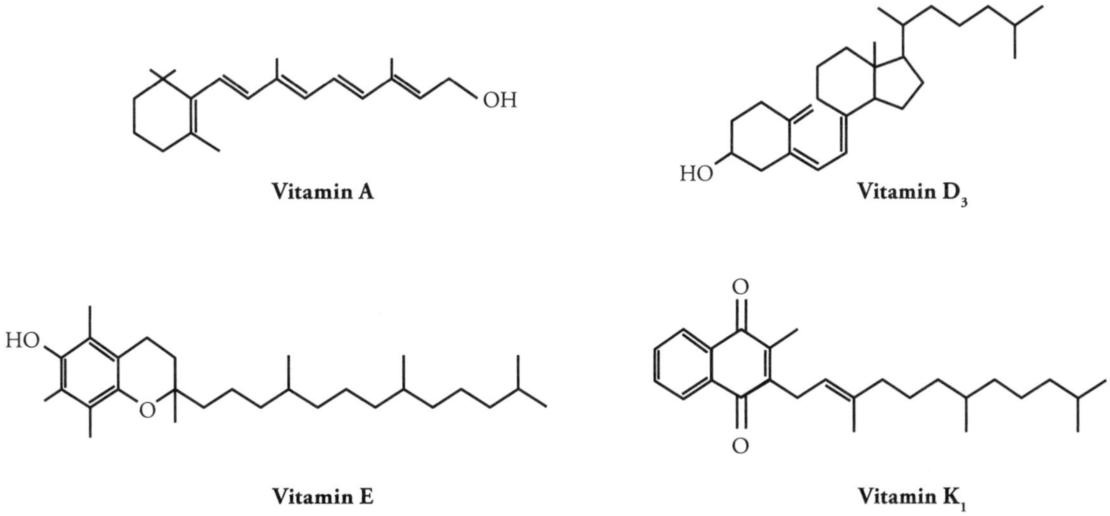

Figure 13   Fat-Soluble Vitamins

Prostaglandins

Prostaglandins belong to a group of molecules known as eicosanoids, derived from 20-carbon fatty acids (the prefix *eicosa* means "20"). They have vastly different roles in different tissues, depending on the receptor to which they bind. Their roles include regulating smooth muscle contraction in the intestines and uterus, regulating blood vessel diameter, maintaining gastric integrity (by decreasing acid secretion and increasing mucus secretion), among others. They all have the same general structure, including a five-membered ring. See Figure 14.

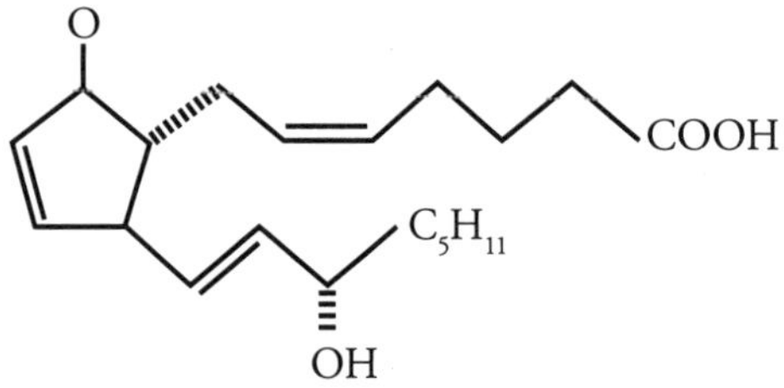

6.5

Prostaglandin A$_2$

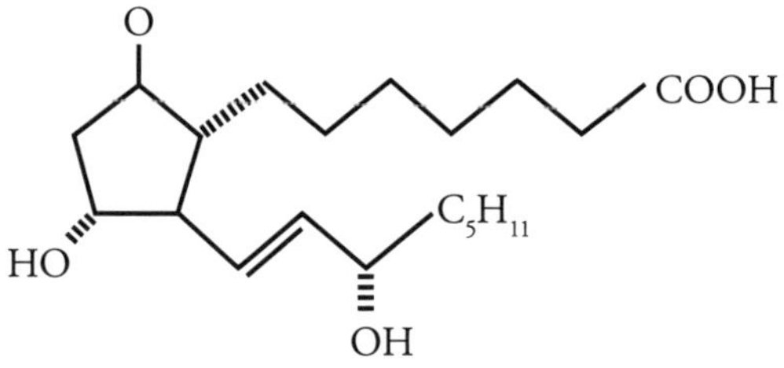

Prostaglandin E$_1$

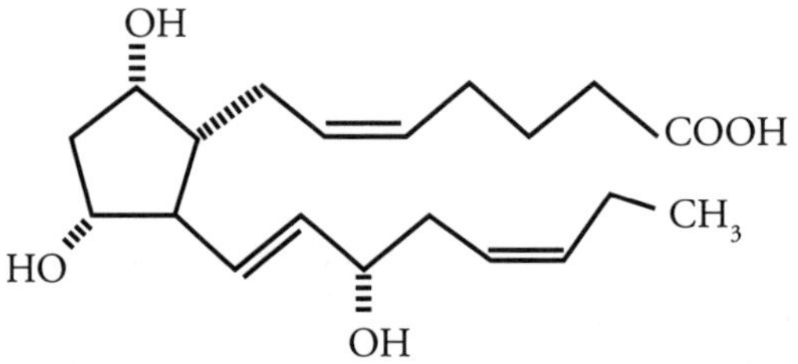

Prostaglandin E$_{3\alpha}$

Figure 14　Prostaglandins

6.6 FATTY ACID METABOLISM

Fatty Acid Oxidation

Following the initial steps in fat digestion, **chylomicrons** composed of fat and lipoprotein are transported via the lymphatic system and bloodstream to the liver, heart, lungs, and other organs. This dietary fat, or triacylglycerol, is then hydrolyzed to liberate free fatty acids which can then undergo β-**oxidation**. This process begins at the outer mitochondrial membrane with the activation of the fatty acid. This reaction, catalyzed by **acyl-CoA synthetase,** requires the investment of two ATP equivalents to generate a fatty acyl-CoA which is then transported into the mitochondrion.

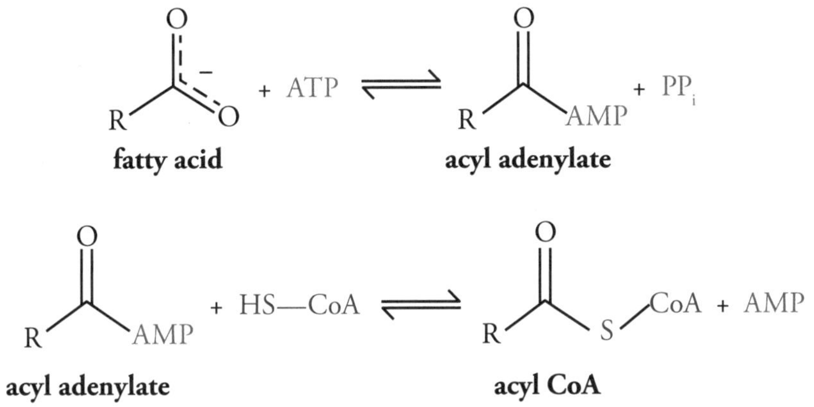

Figure 15   Fatty Acid Activation

Once in the matrix, the fatty acyl-CoA undergoes a repeated series of four reactions which cleave the bond between the alpha and beta carbons to liberate an acetyl-CoA in addition to generating one $FADH_2$ and NADH.

6.6

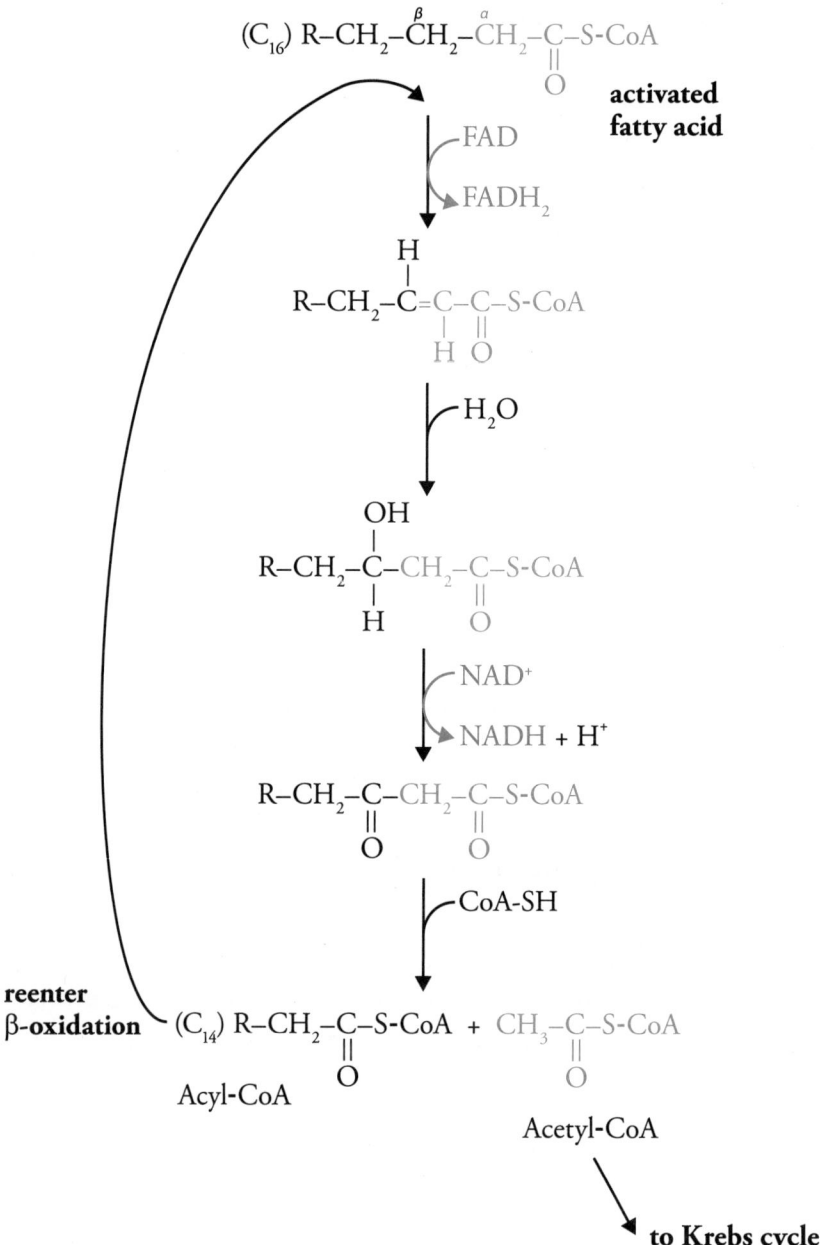

Figure 16   Fatty Acid (β) Oxidation

Each round of β-oxidation cleaves a two-carbon acetyl-CoA from the molecule; however, the final round cleaves a four-carbon fatty acyl-CoA to generate two acetyl-CoA. For instance, the complete β-oxidation of lauric acid (a 12-carbon saturated fatty acid) involves the following: an investment of two ATP equivalents to convert it to a fatty acyl-CoA and then *five* rounds of β-oxidation. This generates five $FADH_2$, five NADH, and *six* acetyl-CoA which can then enter the Krebs cycle. When these six acetyl-CoA go through the Krebs cycle, they will generate an additional 18 NADH, 6 $FADH_2$, and 6 GTP. We then have a grand total of 11 $FADH_2$ (five from β-oxidation and six from the Krebs cycle), 23 NADH (five from β-oxidation and 18 from the Krebs cycle), and six ATP equivalents (from the Krebs cycle). After the electron transport chain (and subtracting the two ATP equivalents required at the beginning of β-oxidation), we obtain 78 ATP from lauric acid.

The oxidation of unsaturated fatty acids (those containing double bonds) requires additional steps. For a monounsaturated fatty acid, β-oxidation proceeds normally, cleaving two-carbon subunits from the fatty acid, until the double bond is encountered. An isomerase then moves the double bond (if necessary) and allows the fatty acid to continue in its oxidation. If the fatty acid contains several double bonds, both the isomerase and a reductase are required to allow the fatty acid to continue through β-oxidation.

Ketogenesis

During periods of starvation, glycogen stores become exhausted and blood glucose falls significantly. To help supply the central nervous system with energy when glucose is in short supply, the liver generates **ketone bodies** via a process in the mitochondrial matrix known as **ketogenesis**. The ketone bodies are generated from acetyl-CoA and include acetone, acetoacetate, and β-hydroxybutyrate. These molecules can cross the blood-brain barrier and be converted back to acetyl-CoA once they arrive at their target organ; the acetyl-CoA can then enter the Krebs cycle (see Figure 17).

6.6

6.6

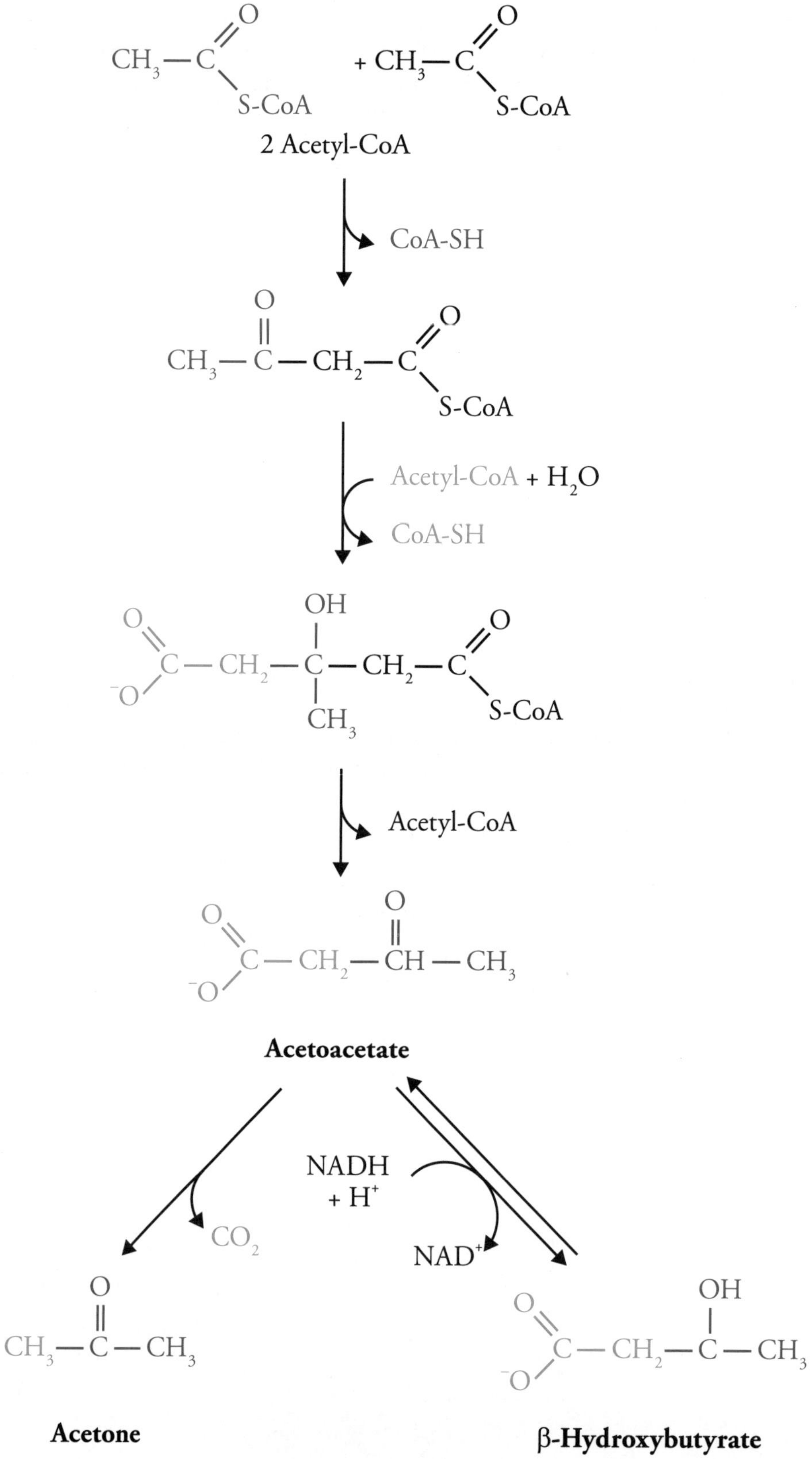

Figure 17 Ketogenesis

In some circumstances, ketogenesis can take place when adequate glucose is present in the blood but cannot enter the cell. This can occur, for example, when a patient suffering from type I diabetes does not receive an insulin injection for a prolonged period of time. Without insulin, glucose cannot enter cells in order to be used for energy, and the patient relies exclusively on fatty acid oxidation for the acetyl-CoA to turn the Krebs cycle. However, because the levels of acetyl-CoA are so high, many of them get converted into ketone bodies. Ketone bodies are acidic, and this can result in diabetic ketoacidosis, which is a potentially life-threatening condition. Patients commonly experience fatigue, confusion, and fruity-scented breath due to the acetone (which is very volatile) present in their blood. This combination of symptoms has even led to patients being mistakenly classified as intoxicated and arrested for driving under the influence.

Fatty Acid Synthesis

The *de novo* synthesis of fatty acids is reminiscent of β-oxidation with several notable exceptions. While fatty acid catabolism occurs in the mitochondrial matrix, anabolism takes place in the cytoplasm. This compartmentalization allows for easier regulation, since the enzymes required for synthesis and breakdown are separated. Much as β-oxidation involved the removal of two-carbon subunits from a fatty acid chain, the synthesis of a fatty acid involves the repeated addition of two-carbon subunits. Rather than building the nascent fatty acid directly with acetyl-CoA, acetyl-CoA is first activated in a carboxylation reaction. The activation is the committed step in fatty acid synthesis and requires the investment of ATP; it is facilitated by **acetyl-CoA carboxylase** to generate **malonyl-CoA**.

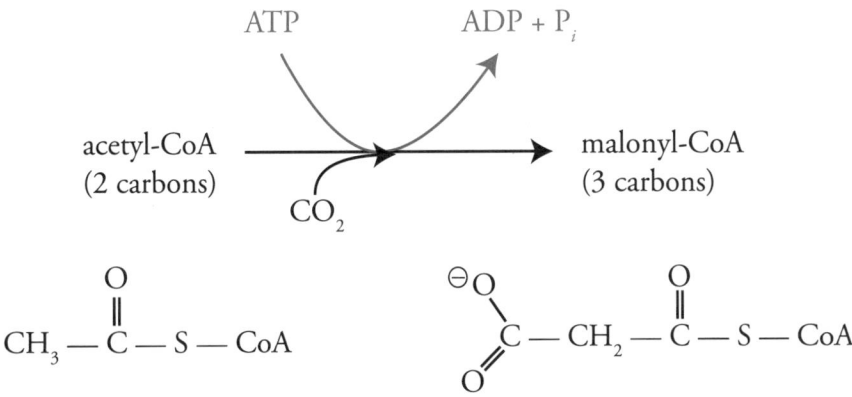

Figure 18   Synthesis of Malonyl-CoA

Fatty acid synthase is a large enzyme with multiple catalytic domains. Acetyl-CoA first binds to a domain known as the **acyl carrier protein (ACP)**. It is then shifted to another domain on the enzyme with a cysteine residue, and malonyl-CoA binds to the ACP. The acetyl group condenses with the malonyl group as the malonyl is decarboxylated. (Recall that the successive addition, then removal of CO_2 can drive unfavorable reactions; this same process occurs in gluconeogenesis with the carboxylation of pyruvate to oxaloacetate, and the subsequent decarboxylation of oxaloacetate to PEP.) The ACP domain now holds a four-carbon unit, which undergoes two reductions. This process requires the reducing power of NADPH, which is generally obtained from the pentose phosphate pathway (see Chapter 5). The saturated four-carbon acyl unit is shifted to the domain with the cysteine residue, and another malonyl-CoA binds to the ACP. The process then repeats: the four-carbon unit condenses with malonyl as CO_2 is lost, two successive reductions occur, and the now six-carbon chain is shifted to the cysteine residue.

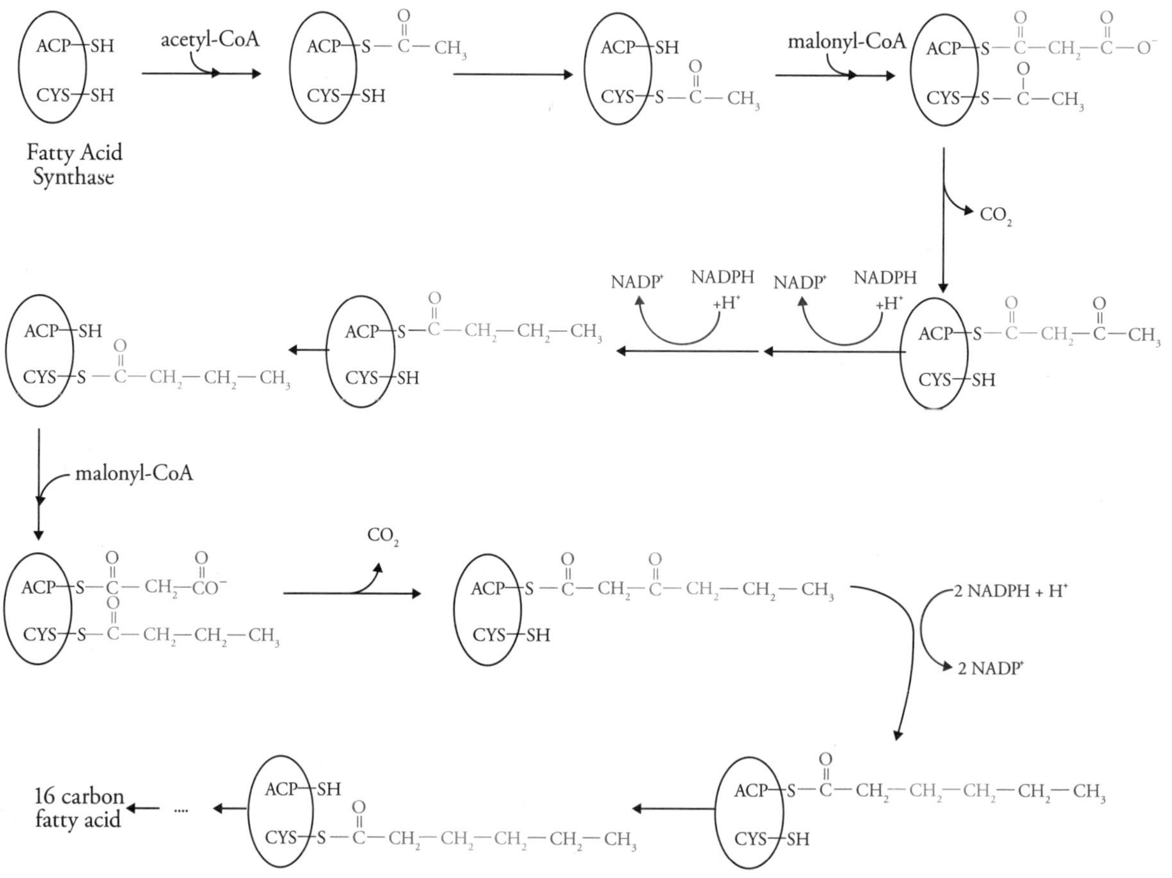

Figure 19   Fatty Acid Synthesis

Once a 16-carbon long fatty acid is generated, additional enzymes aid in further modification of the fatty acid (e.g., addition of functional groups and elongation). Note that this process requires no template (nor does glycogen or amino acid synthesis), which means that nothing is "read" to generate the products. This differs from the template-based syntheses of polypeptides (mRNA is "read" to generate an amino acid sequence) and nucleic acids (DNA is "read" to generate DNA during replication and RNA during transcription; for more information on these processes, see *MCAT Biology Review*).

6.7 AMINO ACID CATABOLISM AND METABOLIC SUMMARY

We discussed amino acid structure and protein structure and function in Chapter 4, but we haven't yet really touched on the idea of proteins as fuel. Proteins in cells are constantly being made, kept for a certain period of time (minutes to weeks), and then degraded back into amino acids. In addition, humans absorb amino acids from dietary proteins. These free amino acids can be catabolized via several pathways. They can be taken up by cells and used to make cellular proteins. The amino group can be removed and either used to synthesize nitrogenous compounds, such as nucleotide bases, or it can be converted into urea for excretion. The remaining carbon skeleton (also called an α-keto acid) can either be broken down into water and CO_2, or it can be converted to glucose (glucogenic amino acids) or acetyl-CoA (ketogenic amino acids).

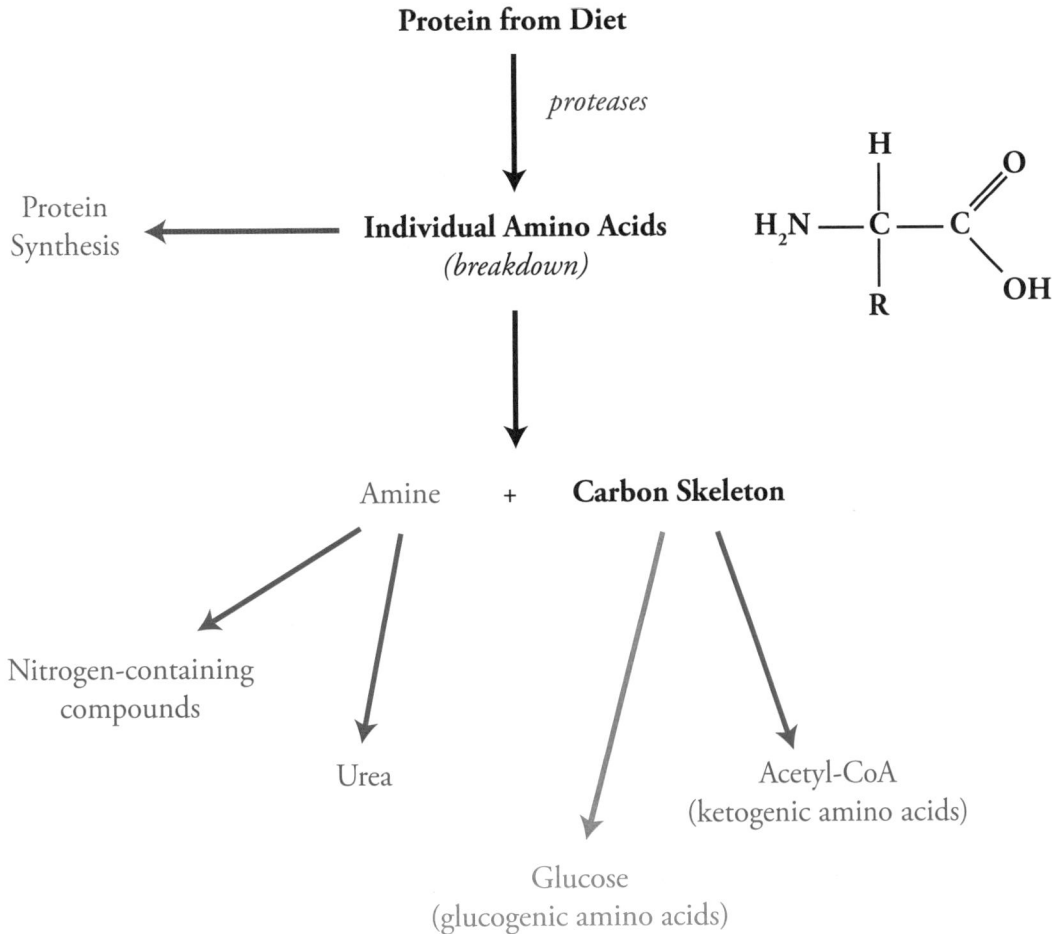

Figure 20   Protein Breakdown

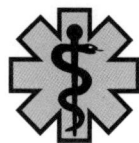

Metabolism Summary

Generally speaking, cells prefer to use carbohydrates as fuel. When blood sugar is high, cells will take up glucose and make ATP via glycolysis. Liver and muscle cells will also store glucose as glycogen (glycogenesis), and the liver can also take some of the acetyl-CoA generated by the pyruvate dehydrogenase complex to make fatty acids (fatty acid synthesis). These are converted into triglycerides and stored in adipose tissue. These pathways are shown in black in Figure 21.

When blood sugar levels fall (starved state), the liver will break down the stored glycogen (glycogenolysis) and release glucose into the bloodstream. It will also begin the process of gluconeogenesis to synthesize "new" glucose that can also be released into the bloodstream. This glucose can be taken up by other body cells and used in glycolysis to generate ATP. These pathways are shown in green in Figure 21.

If the starved state continues past the point at which all glycogen stores are used (12–24 hours), then fatty acid breakdown will occur. Triglycerides from adipose tissue are broken down into free fatty acids and glycerol that are released into the bloodstream. Cells will take up the fatty acids and run β-oxidation. The liver can use the glycerol to generate glucose in gluconeogenesis. Some of the acetyl-CoA made in β-oxidation is used to turn the Krebs cycle, and some is converted into ketone bodies (ketogenesis). These pathways are shown in red in Figure 21.

Finally, proteins and amino acids can be used as fuel. The carbon skeleton of the amino acids can be used in gluconeogenesis (glucogenic amino acids) or to make acetyl-CoA and ketone bodies (ketogenic amino acids).

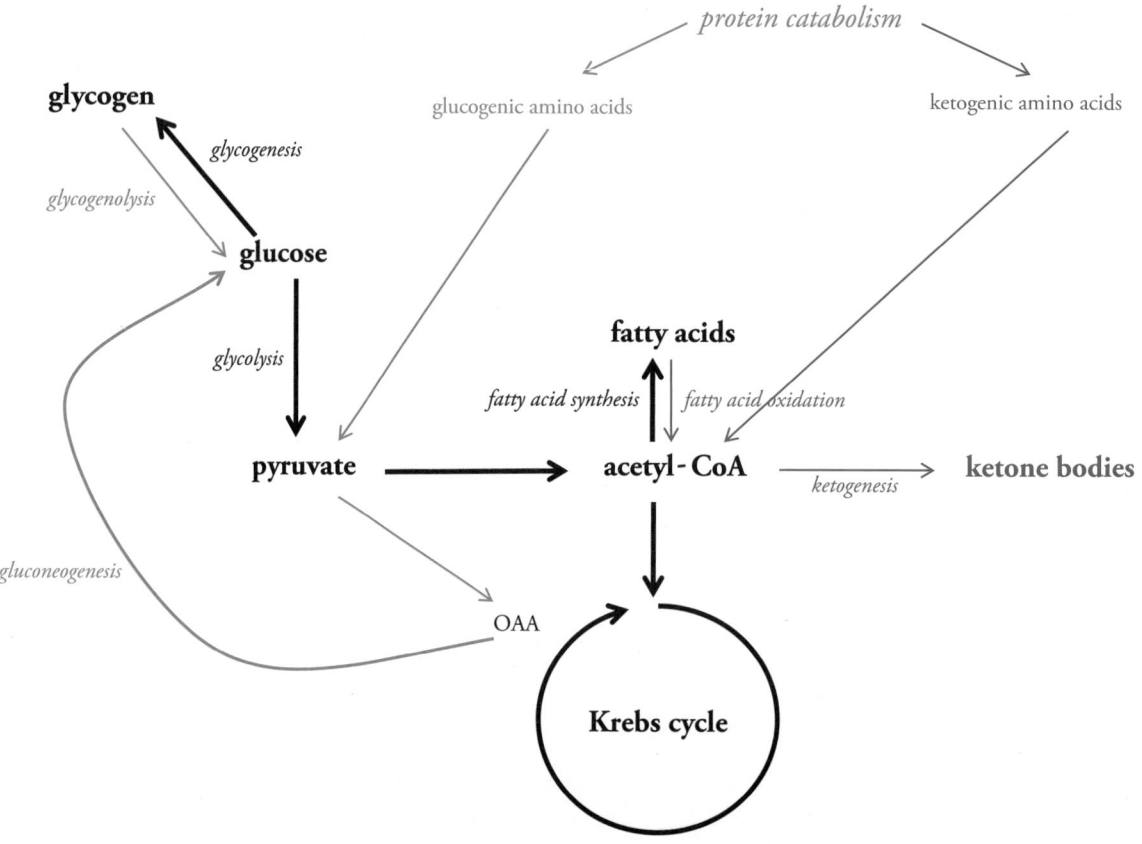

Figure 21 Summary of Metabolism

Chapter 6 Summary

- Lipids are found in several forms in the body, including (but not limited to) triglycerides, phospholipids, cholesterol and steroids, and terpenes. Triglycerides and phospholipids are linear, while cholesterol and steroids have a ring structure.

- Lipids are hydrophobic. Triglycerides are used for energy storage, phospholipids form membranes, and cholesterol is the precursor to the steroid hormones.

- Other lipids include sphingolipids, waxes, fat-soluble vitamins, and prostaglandins.

- The only significant sphingolipid is sphingomyelin, found in the myelin sheath of neurons.

- Waxes are long-chain fats esterified to long-chain alcohols and act as very hydrophobic protective barriers.

- Fat-soluble vitamins include vitamins A, D, E, and K. Vitamin A is necessary for vision, vitamin D is essential for bone structure and calcium regulation, vitamin E is an antioxidant, and vitamin K is important for blood clotting.

- Fatty acid (or beta) oxidation is the repetitive removal of 2-carbon units as acetyl-CoA from the fatty acid. Each round of fatty acid oxidation yields 1 $FADH_2$ and 1 NADH. The acetyl units can enter the Krebs cycle or be converted to ketone bodies.

- Fatty acid synthesis requires high amounts of ATP and NADPH. Fats are synthesized by the successive addition of 2-carbon units to the fatty acid chain until a 16-carbon fat is produced.

- During starvation, acetyl-CoA from fatty acid oxidation can be converted into ketone bodies (acetone, acetoacetate, and β-hydroxybutyrate). The ketone bodies can easily travel through the blood and supply energy to the brain (all can be reconverted to acetyl-CoA), but can also lower blood pH.

- When the body is in a well-fed state (e.g., blood glucose levels are high), glycolysis, glycogenesis, and fatty acid synthesis are favored. When the body is in a starved state (e.g., blood glucose levels are low), glycogenolysis, gluconeogenesis, and fatty acid oxidation are favored.

CHAPTER 6 FREESTANDING PRACTICE QUESTIONS

1. Which property of lipids contributes most to their higher energy density per carbon in comparison to carbohydrates?

A) Lipids can contain more double bonds in existing carbon chains than carbohydrates can in cyclic structures.
B) Carbohydrates exist in a more oxidized state, while lipids are more reduced.
C) Carbohydrates are absorbed more easily than lipids by the digestive system.
D) Lipids can contribute more isoprenes to the Krebs cycle than carbohydrates.

2. Artemisinin, a drug used as part of a multi-valent approach to treating malaria, is a sesquiterpene now being produced in yeast. The biosynthesis of sesquiterpenes requires how many isoprene units?

A) 1
B) 2
C) 3
D) 4

3. Fatty acid synthesis requires all of the following EXCEPT:

    I.   ACP
    II. ADP
    III. NADPH

A) I only
B) II only
C) I and III only
D) II and III only

4. An inhibitor of isomerases in fatty acid oxidation would most hinder the catabolism of:

A) terpenes.
B) saturated fatty acids.
C) phospholipids.
D) unsaturated fatty acids.

5. Increasing the amount of cholesterol in a plasma membrane would lead to an increase in:

A) permeability.
B) atherosclerotic plaques.
C) melting temperature.
D) freezing temperature.

6. Stearic acid is a 16-carbon saturated fatty acid. Including those made in the Krebs cycle, how many NADH and $FADH_2$ would be produced by the complete oxidation of stearic acid?

A) 15 $FADH_2$ and 15 NADH
B) 16 $FADH_2$ and 16 NADH
C) 15 $FADH_2$ and 31 NADH
D) 16 $FADH_2$ and 32 NADH

CHAPTER 6 PRACTICE PASSAGE

Some lipid molecules in the plasma membrane display asymmetry in membrane distribution. For example, glycolipids are found exclusively in the noncytosolic side of the lipid bilayer. This means that the cell surface is covered in carbohydrates, which can be covalently linked to other biological macromolecules. The plasma membrane can contain glycoproteins, glycosaminoglycans, and glycosphingolipids (GSLs).

GSLs consist of a lipid molecule called *ceramide*, linked to carbohydrates; this is a diverse group of macromolecules with over 300 members. The diversity hinges on the carbohydrate chains and variation in glycan buildup. Catalysis of glycan addition is directed by a range of proteins involved in biosynthesis. Of this enzyme family, glycosyltransferases are well studied and the mechanism of action for many glycosyltransferase enzymes has been determined and published.

Glycolipids tend to associate together in the plasma membranes, forming microdomains and lipid rafts. These associations are likely to facilitate glycolipid function, which can include immune cell development, protection of the cell against harsh conditions, facilitating cell to cell interactions, maintaining plasma membrane integrity, cell signaling, and membrane transport.

Globotriaosylceramide (GL3) is a glycosphingolipid and is formed by alpha linkage of galactose to lactosylceramide. Biosynthesis of lactosylceramide includes expansion of the monosaccharide chain by adding a galactose unit to monoglucosylceramide. Lactosylceramide is found in small amounts in most tissues. In contrast, ceramides are found in high concentrations within the cell membrane of most eukaryotic cells. A ceramide is composed of sphingosine and a fatty acid. A recent study examined the levels of GL3 in specific human cell types (Figure 1). Four biopsies of metastatic cancers were also tested for GL3 levels (Figure 2).

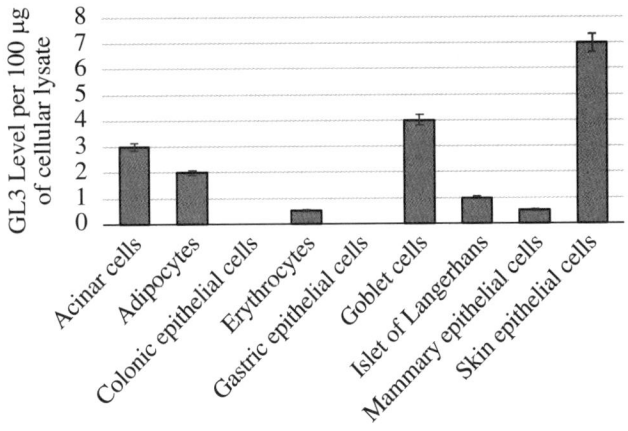

Figure 1 GL3 levels in some human cell types

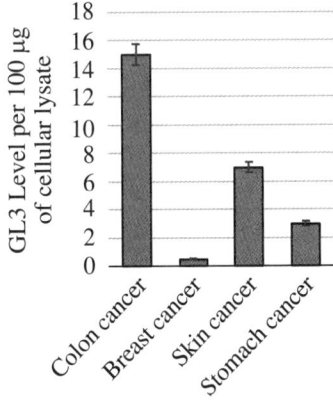

Figure 2 GL3 levels in metastatic cancer biopsy samples

1. Which of the following is true of glycosyltransferases?

A) They function in the Golgi apparatus and transfer carbohydrate groups to lipid molecules.

B) These enzymes are made of ceramide linked to carbohydrates.

C) They function outside the cell and transfer carbohydrate groups to lipid molecules.

D) They are enzymes and proteins, but their mechanism of action is unknown.

2. Accumulation of GL3 has been implicated in a metabolic disease. Which of the following would be the best way to inhibit this accumulation?

A) Activation of lactosylceramide 4-α-galactosyltransferase, which synthesizes globotriaosylceramide.
B) Activation of β-1,4-galactosyltransferase, which synthesizes lactosylceramide.
C) Activation of α-galactosidase, which degrades globotriaosylceramide.
D) Competitive inhibition of α-galactosidase, which degrades globotriaosylceramide.

3. Globotriaosylsphingosine (lyso-Gb3) is a GL3 metabolite and could be a promising secondary screening biomarker for:

    I.   colon cancer.
    II. skin cancer.
    III. stomach cancer.

A) I only
B) II and III only
C) I and III only
D) I, II, and III

4. Based on the known functions of glycolipids, which of the following can be inferred?

A) Glycolipids associate with other biological macromolecules, such as proteins.
B) Glycolipids are isolated in lipid rafts and do not associate with proteins.
C) Lipids rafts are made of protein clusters and do not include lipids.
D) At least 30% of human cells must express appreciable levels of glycolipids.

5. Based on the data presented in the passage, all of the following are true EXCEPT:

A) expression of GL3 in colonic epithelial cells is a good indicator that the cells have become cancerous.
B) since it is expressed in all four types of metastatic cancer cells, GL3 is a good screening marker for all four types of metastatic cancer.
C) the expression of GL3 in stomach cancer cells is a better indicator that the cells might metastasize than the expression of GL3 in breast cancer cells.
D) there is a significant difference in the expression of GL3 between goblet cells and acinar cells.

6. Globotriaosylceramide contains:

A) two monosaccharides linked to the intracellular side of a ceramide lipid in the plasma membrane
B) two monosaccharides linked to the extracellular side of a ceramide lipid in the plasma membrane
C) three monosaccharides linked to the intracellular side of a ceramide lipid in the plasma membrane
D) three monosaccharides linked to the extracellular side of a ceramide lipid in the plasma membrane

SOLUTIONS TO CHAPTER 6 FREESTANDING PRACTICE QUESTIONS

1. **B** Energy production in cells is essentially based on oxidation. Since carbohydrates are more oxidized per carbon and lipids are more reduced, the catabolism of lipids can produce more energy (choice B is correct). While an unsaturated fatty acid would have double bonds, this does not address the question of why, on a per-carbon basis, lipids in general yield more energy than carbohydrates (choice A is wrong). The ease of absorption has nothing to do with energy density per carbon (choice C is wrong). Isoprenes are not utilized by the Krebs cycle (choice D is wrong).

2. **C** The prefix *sesqui-* means "one and a half," so a sesquiterpene is made up of one and a half terpenes. A terpene is at minimum two isoprene units, so a sesquiterpene, one and a half terpenes, would be made up of three isoprene units (choice C is correct). One isoprene unit creates to a hemiterpene (half a terpene; choice A is wrong), two isoprene units creates a monoterpene (choice B is wrong), and four isoprene units creates a diterpene (choice D is wrong).

3. **B** Item I is false: ACP, acyl-carrier protein, is a subunit of the fatty acid synthase enzyme and replaces coenzyme A on both acetyl-CoA and malonyl-CoA as part of the activation steps of fatty acid synthesis (ACP is required for fatty acid synthesis, so choices A and C can be eliminated). Since both of the remaining choices include Item II, it must be true and we can go directly to Item III. Item III is false: NADPH is used during the elongation steps of fatty acid synthesis as reducing power (NADPH is required for fatty acid synthesis; choice D can be eliminated, and choice B is correct). Note that Item II is true: ADP is not used in fatty acid synthesis. Instead, ATP is needed to convert acetyl-CoA and bicarbonate into malonyl-CoA. Of the three given items, ADP is the only one not required for fatty acid synthesis.

4. **D** Isomerases are used during β-oxidation of unsaturated fatty acids to ensure correct placement of a carbon-carbon double bond for the process to begin (choice D is correct). Terpenes are specialized fats (such as squalene) and phospholipids are membrane lipids, neither of which go through β-oxidation (choices A and C are wrong), and the β-oxidation of saturated fats does not require isomerase (choice B is wrong).

5. **C** Plasma membranes can be up to 50% composed of sterols. Sterols help stabilize the membrane at both spectrums of the temperature. At low temperatures, they increase fluidity because the ring structure of cholesterol does not allow for tight phospholipid tail packing. This decreases the temperature at which the membrane would freeze (choice D is wrong). At high temperatures, cholesterol decreases membrane fluidity (the OH group of cholesterol prevents phospholipid dispersion) and permeability (by filling in the "holes" between the fatty acid tails; choice A is wrong), thus increasing the temperature at which membranes would melt (choice C is correct). The formation of atherosclerotic plaques, while related to cholesterol, is due to high levels of blood cholesterol, not membrane cholesterol (choice B is wrong).

6. **C** A 16-carbon fatty acid will require 7 turns of β-oxidation to produce 8 acetyl CoA, which will subsequently go through the Krebs cycle. Each turn of the β-oxidation cycle produces 1 $FADH_2$ and 1 NADH, and each turn of the Krebs cycle produces 1 $FADH_2$ and 3 NADH. 7 $FADH_2$ + 7 NADH + 8 $FADH_2$ + 24 NADH = 15 $FADH_2$ and 31 NADH (choice C is correct, and choices A, B, and D are wrong).

SOLUTIONS TO CHAPTER 6 PRACTICE PASSAGE

1. **A**   According to the passage, glycosyltransferases are enzymes that catalyze the addition of sugar groups to lipids. Most enzymes are proteins, and so are made of amino acids (eliminate choice B). The passage also says glycosyltransferases are well studied and the mechanism of action for many glycosyltransferase enzymes has been determined and published (eliminate choice D). This leaves options A and C as the potential answer. These answer choices differ in where glycosyltransferases function. While the carbohydrate portions of glycolipids are found on the extracellular surface of the plasma membrane, there is no information in the passage to support that glycosyltransferases function outside of the cell (eliminate choice C). The Golgi apparatus is involved in macromolecule trafficking to the plasma membrane and contains enzymes that modify carbohydrate groups on many macromolecules. It is more likely that glycosyltransferases function in the Golgi apparatus than outside the cell (choice A is correct).

2. **C**   The question stem tells you that GL3 accumulation is causing a metabolic disease. The best treatment for this disease would be one that blocks or inhibits this accumulation. Activation of the enzyme that synthesizes GL3 would lead to even more GL3; this is the opposite of what you're looking for (eliminate choice A). Lactosylceramide is a building block of GL3. Activating the enzyme that makes lactosylceramide would not decrease GL3 levels (eliminate choice B). Both choices C and D discuss the enzyme that catabolizes (or breaks down) GL3. A good way to decrease GL3 accumulation would be to activate the enzyme that breaks it down; competitive inhibition of that enzyme would reduce its function (eliminate choice D, choice C is correct).

3. **C**   Since this is a Roman numeral question, start by analyzing the item that appears in exactly two answer choices; whether it is true or false you'll be able to eliminate half the answers. In this case, Item II is found in exactly two choices. Item II is false: first, from the information in the question stem, lyso-Gb3 is a metabolite of GL3. This means that if a tissue type has high GL3, it may have high lyso-Gb3 as well. Based on Figure 2, skin cancer cells express GL3, but from Figure 1, so do normal skin cells, and at the same level of skin cancer cells. Thus, lyso-Gb3 is not a good secondary screening biomarker for skin cancer (choices B and D can be eliminated). Since both remaining choices include Item I it must be true and we can focus on Item III. Item III is true: stomach cancer cells express some GL3 (Figure 2), but normal stomach (gastric) epithelial cells do not (Figure 1), so lyso-Gb3 could be a good secondary screening marker for stomach cancer (choice A can be eliminated and choice C is correct). Note that Item I is in fact true: similar to stomach cancer cells, colon cancer cells express GL3 at high levels (Figure 2), but normal colon epithelial cells do not (Figure 1), so lyso-Gb3 could be a good secondary screening marker for colon cancer.

4. **A**   The passage says that glycolipids function in cell signaling and membrane transport. Based on this, it is highly likely they associate and cooperate with membrane proteins (choice A is correct; eliminate choice B). The passage says that lipid rafts contain glycolipids (eliminate choice C). There is no way to know if answer choice D is true or not based on information in the passage. This very specific statement is not supported (eliminate choice D).

5. **B**   Make sure to highlight the word "EXCEPT" and write "A B C D" on your noteboard. Evaluate each answer choice, writing "T" if it is true and "F" if it is false. Since GL3 is expressed at a very high level in metastatic colonic cancer cells, and not at all in normal colonic cells, the expression of GL3 is a good indicator of colon cancer (write "T" next to "A" on the noteboard). Although GL3 is expressed in all four types of cancer, the level of expression in breast cancer cells and skin cancer cells is exactly the same as the level of expression in normal mammary and skin cells. While GL3 might be a good screening marker for colon and stomach cancer, it would likely not be a good screening marker for breast and skin cancer (write "F" next to "B" on the noteboard). Similar to choice A, metastatic stomach cancer cells express GL3 at a much higher level than normal gastric cells, while breast cancer cells and normal mammary cells express GL3 at the same level. While breast cancer cells can still metastasize (and do), the presence of GL3 in those cells is not as good an indicator of the likelihood for metastasis as the presence of GL3 in stomach cancer cells (write "T" next to "C" on the noteboard). Both goblet cells and acinar cells express GL3, with goblet cells having a higher level of expression than acinar cells. Since the error bars do not overlap for these two cell types, it can be said that the difference in expression is significant (write "T" next to "D" on the noteboard). Since choice B stands out with an "F" instead of a "T," it the correct answer choice.

6. **D**   The passage says that the carbohydrate groups of glycolipids are expressed on the extracellular surface of the cell (eliminate choices A and C). The last paragraph of the passage says that a fatty acid and a sphingosine join to form a ceramide. A glucose is added to form monoglucosylceramide. A galactose is added to form lactosylceramide. Another galactose is added to form globotriaosylceramide. This means that GL3 is made of a ceramide lipid with three carbohydrate groups (eliminate choice B, choice D is correct).

NEROLIDOL, A SESQUITERPENE, ATTENUATES OXIDATIVE STRESS AND INFLAMMATION IN ACETIC ACID-INDUCED COLITIS IN RATS

Salim M. A. Bastaki[1], Naheed Amir[1], Ernest Adeghate[2], Shreesh Ojha[1]

Received: 5 September 2020 / Accepted: 29 January 2021 / Published online: 17 May 2021

INTRODUCTION

Inflammatory bowel disease (IBD) is an incurable chronic intestinal disorder of the gastrointestinal (GI) tract. The principal types of IBD are ulcerative colitis and Crohn's disease (CD), which are characterized by chronic inflammation of the intestine with alternating relapses and remissions and requires long-term treatment. Although it is considered a group of complex heterogeneous gastrointestinal disease that involves genetic variations, intestinal microbiota, immunological factors, and environmental factors, which interact with an inherent genetic predisposition, the underlying mechanism remains unknown. The inappropriate immune response to environment changes and the gut microbiota are among the main causes of intestinal inflammation in IBD. Experimental models and clinical studies data suggest that oxidative signaling through multiple functional levels is the major underlying mechanism in the pathogenesis of IBD. The products of oxidative stress along with rising inflammation caused by induction and release of pro-inflammatory cytokines contribute to damages of the mucosal layer in the GI tract, bacterial invasion, which in turn triggers immune response and eventually cell death. Thus, targeting inflammation and oxidative stress represents an important therapeutic target for IBD.

The available therapies for IBD are not very satisfactory for the majority of the patients who require continuous medication to keep the disease under control. In addition, the currently used agents including aminosalicylates, corticosteroids, immunomodulators, and biological agents often elicit variable responses with side effects and a diminishing therapeutic benefit over time. Aside from radical surgery for refractory ulcerative colitis, there is no cure or preventive measures available. Various treatment strategies have been shown initially to exert beneficial effects for the treatment of IBD, but prolonged treatments resulted in severe side effects. An ideal agent would prevent relapses and maintain remission with minimal adverse effects and lesser variation in therapeutic effects.

The use of many plants in therapeutics is based on traditional consumption in diets for health benefits since ancient times. In recent years, numerous plant-derived bioactive compounds known as phytochemicals and also referred to as phytobiotics or phytogenics have raised interest for their therapeutic potential in IBD due to multiple pharmacological properties. These bioactive compounds have been shown to ameliorate intestinal inflammation through reduction of inflammatory cytokines and modulation of intracellular signaling transduction pathways. To date, many novel dietary compounds of natural origin, belonging to different classes of phytochemicals such as glycosides, alkaloids, terpenes, saponins, and flavonoids, have been shown to be effective in experimental models of colitis by targeting oxidative stress and immune-inflammatory cascade.

Among different classes, the terpenes commonly found in essential oils of edible plants have generated immense interest due to their favorable pharmacological properties and therapeutic effects in gastrointestinal diseases. One of the dietary bioactive phytochemicals, nerolidol (NRD), a naturally occurring aliphatic sesquiterpene alcohol has garnered attention for its therapeutic potential in human diseases along with its dietary and cosmetic use. It is widely present in ornamental as well as edible plants including *Oplopanax horridus* and *Thymus alternans* and has been found to be beneficial to health. It is widely

Salim M. A. Bastaki

[1] Department of Pharmacology and Therapeutics, College of Medicine and Health Sciences, United Arab Emirates University, PO Box 17666, Al Ain, Abu Dhabi, United Arab Emirates

[2] Department of Anatomy, College of Medicine and Health Sciences, United Arab Emirates University, PO Box 17666, Al Ain, Abu Dhabi, United Arab Emirates

used as flavor enhancer, in a traditional semi-oxidized Chinese tea known as Oolong tea and Portuguese Madeira wines. It has been included in the list of safe compounds by the US Food and Drug Administration (USFDA) for its use in the food industry as a preservative and flavoring agent. NRD has been shown to possess neuroprotective, hepatoprotective, cardioprotective, genoprotective, anti-nociceptive and wound-healing properties, which is mainly attributed to its action in reducing inflammation. Studies have shown that NRD ameliorates drug- and toxicant-induced oxidative stress and inflammatory events in body organs such as brain, kidney, liver, heart, lungs, testes, eye, stomach, and uterus. Despite the potent antioxidant and anti-inflammatory roles in various organs, there are no reports available on its role in colonic tissues to demonstrate its therapeutic potential in colitis.

NRD is a lipophilic and highly bioavailable agent that makes it able to achieve required concentration for its therapeutic effect and restores redox balance by abolishing oxidative stress and subsequent inflammatory responses involving many pathways. In a preliminary study, NRD was shown to have a protective effect against ethanol-, indomethacin-, and stress-induced gastric ulcer and to significantly inhibit ulcer formation. Additionally, NRD has been shown to inhibit cell growth and proliferation and to induce cell death in colon cancer (SW-480, and HCT-116 cells). Integrating therapeutic roles of NRD in gastric tissues and colon cancer along with its property of inhibiting ROS inflammation, it was thought worthwhile to evaluate the therapeutic eff of NRD in experimental model of colitis.

Therefore, the aim of the present study was to investigate the effect of NRD on Acetic acid (AA) induced IBD and underlying antioxidant and anti-inflammatory mechanisms in the rat model. In addition, the effects of NRD on colonic macroscopic and microscopic changes were also investigated. Furthermore, the suppression of free radical formation by the endogenous antioxidant defense system and the levels of inflammatory mediators such as cytokines and calprotectin were also measured in AA-induced IBD in rats.

MATERIALS AND METHODS

Experimental animals

Adult male albino Wistar rats weighing 225–240 g were maintained at the experimental animal research facility housed in polycarbonate cages lined with husk (replaced every 24 h), under standard laboratory conditions required for animal house viz. photoperiod of 12-h light–dark cycle, room temperature at 22 °C, and humidity at 55%. The rodent chow diet was obtained commercially and water was available to the animals ad libitum. The animals were randomly divided into different groups and acclimatized for a week before commencing the experiments. They were fasted for 24 h prior to the induction of colitis by intrarectal administration of 1 ml of 4% AA at 8 cm proximal to the anus for 30 s under the influence of light anesthesia with ether after overnight fasting. The rats were kept in Trendelenburg position during rectal instillation and for 1 min after instillation to prevent leakage of the solution. To flush the colon, 1 ml of phosphate-buffered saline (PBS) was also administered in similar conditions.

Experimental design

The dose of NRD 50 mg/kg was chosen based on a dose–response pilot study in our laboratory and the basis of results published from our labs and other previous studies on antioxidant and anti-inflammatory properties. NRD was administered under two different regimens: (1) therapeutic regimen wherein the effect of NRD was tested for 1 week after the induction of IBD and (2) prophylactic, wherein NRD was administered 3 days before the induction of IBD and continued for 7 days after IBD induction. In summary, for each treatment modality, rats were divided into pre-IBD NRD-treated (n = 18) and post-IBD NRD-treated groups (n = 18). NRD 50 mg/kg in olive oil was adminis-tered orally 30 min after the induction of IBD (post-treated groups) daily. Control animals received olive oil alone using the same technique. The animals were weighed at 0, 2, 4, and 7 days after IBD and colon samples from control and post- and pretreatment groups were collected in liquid nitrogen and 4% neutral buffered formalin.

Assessment of macroscopic ulcer score

To examine the extent of colonic inflammation by mac-roscopic and microscopic analysis, histological samples were collected at selected time points (0 day and after 2, 4, and 7 days of IBD with or without NRD treatment). On the 7th day after IBD, the rats were euthanized by cervical dislocation and the colons were excised 2 cm above the anal margin, opened longitudinally, and washed with saline. Macroscopic damage was assessed by a previously described and well-established scoring method, which takes into account the area of inflammation and the presence or absence of ulcers. The criteria for assessing macroscopic damage were based on a semi-quantitative scoring system where features are graded as follows: 0, no ulcer, no inflammation; 1, no ulcer, local hyperemia; 2, ulceration without hyperemia; 3, ulceration and inflammation at one site only; 4, two or more sites of ulceration and inflammation; and 5, ulceration extending more than 2 cm.

Assessment of microscopic ulcer score

After macroscopic observation, samples of the colon were subsequently excised and processed for microscopic observation according to a previously described method.

Preparation of colon tissue homogenate

Samples of 8 cm portion of distal colon were cut longitudinally to open and washed with ice-cold PBS. The tissue was weighed and homogenized with complete protease inhibitor cocktail. The resulting homogenates, after 30 min incubation on ice, were centrifuged at 15,000 rpm for 30 min at 4 °C. The obtained supernatant was stored at –40 °C until ELISA. Protein concentration was determined in each sample by a commercially available kit following BCA method.

Determination of myeloperoxidase activity in colon

Myeloperoxidase (MPO) was measured by sandwich ELISA according to manufacturer's protocols.

Determination of calprotectin in colon

Enzyme immunoassay of calprotectin, in distal colon protein samples, was performed by using commercially available sandwich ELISA kit.

Measurements of glutathione content in colon

The glutathione (GSH) content in colon homogenate was estimated following manufacturer's protocol of the assay kit. Briefly, the kinetic assay method was used to measure in which catalytic amounts (nmoles) of GSH cause a continuous reduction of 5,5-dithiobis (2-nitrobenzoic acid) to nitrobenzoic acid (TNB), and the glutathione disulfide (GSSG) formed was recycled by glutathione reductase and NADPH.

Determination of catalase activity in colon

Catalase (CAT) activity was measured by catalase assay kit which utilized the peroxidation function of CAT for determination of enzyme activity. The method was based on the reaction of the enzyme with methanol in the presence of an optimal concentration of H_2O_2. The formaldehyde produced was measured spectrophotometrically.

Determination of superoxide dismutase (SOD) in colon

Superoxide dismutase (SOD) activity was determined by SOD assay kit following the manufacturer's protocol. This colorimetric assay utilized the tetrazolium salt for detection of superoxide radicals generated by xanthine oxidase and hypoxanthine.

Measurement of malondialdehyde

The lipid peroxidation product, malondialdehyde (MDA), in the colon homogenate from each group, was measured using MDA assay kit. The assay is based on the reaction of MDA with thiobarbituric acid (TBA) to form an adduct MDA-TBA that absorbs strongly at 532 nm.

Determination of Inflammatory cytokines TNF-α, IL-1β, IL-6, and IL-23 in colon

Enzyme immunoassay of TNFα, IL-1β, IL-6, and IL-23 in colon homogenate was performed by using commercial sandwich duo set ELISA kit.

Table 1 Effect of nerolidol (NRD) on body weight (g) in IBD rat model

Day	Non-IBD control	IBD control	IBD post-nerolidol-treated	Pre-IBD nerolidol-treated
Day 0	220 ± 2.00	221 ± 5.00	224 ± 6.00	216 ± 2.00
Day 2	231 ± 4.00	209 ± 3.30***	214 ± 5.00##	237 ± 4.60###
Day 4	240 ± 3.50	213 ± 5.00***	217 ± 7.00#	240 ± 4.60###
Day 7	250 ± 3.00	206 ± 3.40***	224 ± 5.00##	240 ± 4.57###

***$P < 0.001$ day 0 non IBD control group vs IBD control group; #$P < 0.05$, ##$P < 0.01$, ###$P < 0.001$, IBD control group vs post/pre-treatment

Statistical analysis

SPSS 23.0 software was used for statistical analyses of the data which are presented as mean ± standard error of mean (SEM). Independent t-test was used for data analyses and to determine the significance of the mean between the groups. Values of $P < 0.05$ were considered significant.

RESULTS

Effect of nerolidol on mean body weight (BW) in acetic acid-induced IBD

Table 1 shows the mean BW of rats treated with NRD either 3 days before or after the induction of IBD, by gastric gavage at doses of 50 mg/kg per day. The mean BW of rats was significantly reduced by IBD ($P < 0.001$). After the induction of IBD, administration of NRD at a dose of 50 mg/kg orally and continued for 7 days, significantly ($P < 0.05$-$P<0.01$) decreased the mean BW. The mean BW of Pre-IBD NRD treated was significantly ($P < 0.001$) increased.

Effect of nerolidol on mean macroscopic ulcer score in acetic acid-induced IBD

Figures 1a and b show the effect of oral administration of NRD on macroscopic changes and mean macroscopic ulcer score (MAUS) in rats, respectively, after AA-induced IBD. The colonic mucosa of control (untreated) rats showed marked ulceration and hyperemia (Fig. 1a). After the induction of IBD, there was a significant ($P < 0.001$) increase in mean MAUS (Fig. 1b). Administration of 50 mg/kg NRD produced a significant ($P < 0.05$-$P < 0.001$) decrease in mean MAUS when administered either 3 days before or 30 min post IBD when compared to control (IBD, untreated, $n = 6$) (Fig. 1b). Mean MAUS reduces, when compared

to control (IBD, untreated) (Fig. 1b). Similarly, when NRD was administered post-IBD, there was a significant ($P < 0.05$, $P < 0.01$, $n=6$) reduction in the mean MAUS (Fig. 1b).

Effect of nerolidol on mean microscopic ulcer score in AA-induced IBD

Figures 2a and b show the effect of oral administration of NRD on light microscopic (histological) changes and mean microscopic ulcer score (MiUS) in rats, respectively, after AA-induced IBD. There was a significant ($P < 0.001$) increase in microscopic ulcer score (MiUS) after the induction of IBD (Fig. 2b). Administration of NRD 3 days before the induction of IBD at a dose of 50 mg/kg, resulted in a non-significant reduction in MiUS on all the days tested (Fig. 2b). NRD administered orally at a dose of 50 mg/kg after the induction of IBD in rats significantly ($P < 0.05$, $P < 0.01$, $n=6$) reduced MiUS (Fig. 2b).

a: Effect of nerolidol on colon macroscopic ulcer score in acetic acid-induced IBD

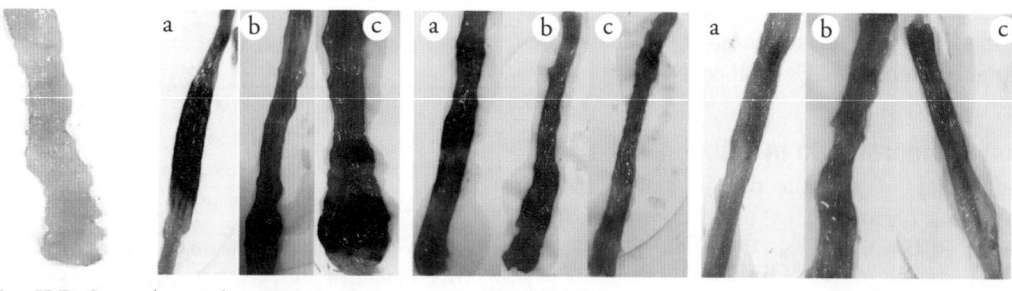

Non IBD Control 2 days IBD 4 days IBD 7 days IBD

a: IBD Control (no Nerolidol); b: Post IBD Nerolidol treatment; c: Pre IBD Nerolidol treatment

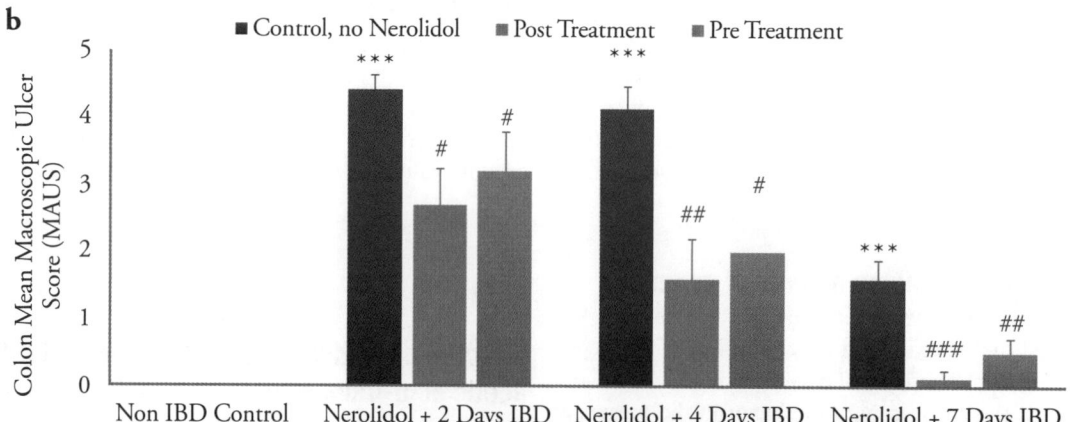

Fig. 1 Effect of nerolidol on macroscopic image (a), ulcer score (b) in IBD rat model. Data are mean ± SEM. *Significant difference between nerolidol-treated and non-IBD control. #Significant difference between nerolidol-treated and IBD control. ***$P < 0.001$; #$P < 0.05$, ##$P < 0.01$, ###$P < 0.001$

Administration of NRD to rats after the induction of IBD also reduced lymphatic infiltration in the colon (Fig. 2a). Fig. 2a shows the effect of NRD on microscopic structure in the colonic mucosa of treated and untreated rats. Figures 2a-B1, 2C1, 2D1, showed a colonic mucosa which was severely inflamed and necrotic with inflammatory cell infiltration, edema, hyperemia and goblet cell hyperplasia. As shown in Fig. 2a, cross section histopathological screening of the rat's colon tissue, revealed normal looking mucosal epithelium with neither necrosis nor inflammation in the control group. Pre- (Figures 2b-B2, C2, D2) and post-treatment (Figures 2a-B3, C3, D3) with NRD resulted in healing of the mucosal epithelium, a reduction in inflammatory edema, and a reduction in necrotic tissues and eroded surfaces. Hyperemia was not observed in NRD-treated groups.

Effect of nerolidol on mean calprotectin levels in acetic acid-induced IBD

Figure 3 shows the effect of NRD treatment on calprotectin, a marker of bowel inflammation in colon tissues, administered either 3 days before or 30 min after the induction of IBD in rats and continued for 7 days. There was a significant ($P < 0.01$, $P < 0.001$, $n = 6$) increase in calprotectin levels 2 and 7 days after the induction of IBD. Colonic calprotectin levels were unaffected after 4 days of IBD. Administration of NRD, 30 min after the induction of IBD significantly ($P < 0.001$, $n=6$) decreased colon calprotectin levels on days 2 of IBD, but was non-significant on days 4 and 7 of IBD. Administration of NRD 3 days before the induction of IBD, caused significant ($P < 0.05$, $P < 0.01$, $n = 6$) reduction in colonic calprotectin levels on days 2 and 7 of IBD. Colonic calprotectin levels were unaffected by NRD after 4 days of IBD.

Effect of nerolidol on mean glutathione levels in acetic acid-induced IBD

Fig. 4a shows the effect of NRD on mean colonic tissue levels of glutathione (GSH) in rats. GSH in control (no IBD, no NRD) was 35.50 ± 3.66 μM ($n = 6$) of colonic tissue levels. IBD significantly ($P < 0.05$, $n = 6$) decreased mean colonic tissue levels of GSH to 22.34 ± 3.20 μM on day 4 of IBD. There was a non-significant reduction in mean colonic tissue levels of GSH on days 2 and 7 of IBD. Administration of NRD 30 minutes after the induction of IBD, significantly ($P < 0.05$, $P < 0.01$) increased mean GSH colonic levels on days 4 and 7, respectively. After 2 days of IBD, there was a non-significant increase in mean colonic tissue levels of GSH. There was a significant ($P < 0.05$, $n = 6$) increase in mean colonic tissue levels of GSH, after

oral administration of NRD for 3 days before the induction of IBD. There was an increase in mean colonic tissue levels of GSH on day 4 but increased non-significantly after 2 and 7 days of IBD.

Effect of nerolidol on catalase activity in acetic acid-induced IBD

In order to examine the protective effect of NRD against oxidative stress, we measured colonic catalase (CAT) tissue levels after the administration of NRD either 3 days before or 30 min after the induction of IBD in rats (Fig. 4b). Catalase is an antioxidative enzyme located in peroxisomes that safely decomposes superoxide anions and thus protects against oxidative stress. Before the induction of IBD, colonic tissue catalase activity level in the untreated control group (no IBD, no NRD) was 2.13 ± 0.20 nmol/min/mg protein. There was a significant ($P < 0.001$, no NRD, $n = 6$) increase in mean colonic tissue catalase activity after the induction of IBD on all the days tested. NRD had a non-significant ($P > 0.05$) effect on catalase colonic tissue activity, when administered orally 30 min after the induction of IBD, on all the days tested. However, administration of NRD 3 days before the induction of IBD, significantly ($P < 0.001$, $n = 6$) increased the catalase colonic tissue activity only on day 7, from 6.60 ± 0.31 (no NRD) to 10.24 ± 0.48 nmol/min/mg of protein. NRD had no effect on colonic catalase tissue activity on days 4 and 7 of IBD.

Effect of nerolidol on mean superoxide dismutase activity in acetic acid-induced IBD

Superoxide dismutase (SOD), a metal ion cofactor-requiring enzyme, is an antioxidant enzyme that protects against oxidative stress. To test whether NRD has any effect on SOD, it was administered either 3 days pre- or 30 min post-IBD in rats (Fig. 4c). There was a significant ($P < 0.05$, IBD, no NRD, $n=6$) increase in mean colonic superoxide dismutase activity 4 days post-IBD. The activity level of superoxide dismutase was unaffected on days 2 and 7 of IBD. Administration of NRD after the induction of IBD, significantly ($P < 0.05$, $n = 6$) increased mean colonic SOD activity level on days 2 and 7 of IBD, respectively. The activity level of SOD was unaffected by NRD on day 4 of IBD. There was a significant ($P < 0.05$, $n = 6$) increase in SOD activity level when NRD was administered before IBD. Pre-treated NRD had no effect on the superoxide dismutase activity on day 4 of IBD.

Effect of nerolidol on mean malondialdehyde levels in acetic acid-induced IBD

Malondialdehyde (MDA), a highly reactive compound generated by peroxidation of membrane polyunsaturated fatty acids, is a marker for oxidative stress. In order to measure the effects of NRD on mean MDA levels in the colonic tissues, it was administered either 3 days pre- or 30 min post-IBD and continued for 7 days in rats (Fig. 4d). There was a significant ($P < 0.001$, $n=6$) increase in mean colonic tissue levels of MDA after the IBD induction, on day 2. IBD had no effect on the MDA levels on days 4 and 7. Post-IBD administration of NRD significantly ($P < 0.01$, $n = 6$) deceased MDA levels on day 2 of IBD. The mean colonic tissue levels of MDA were unaffected by NRD after 4 and 7 days of IBD. Administration of NRD 3 days before IBD, significantly ($P < 0.001$, $n = 6$) decreased MDA levels on day 2 but had no effect on MDA levels on days 4 and 7 of IBD.

a

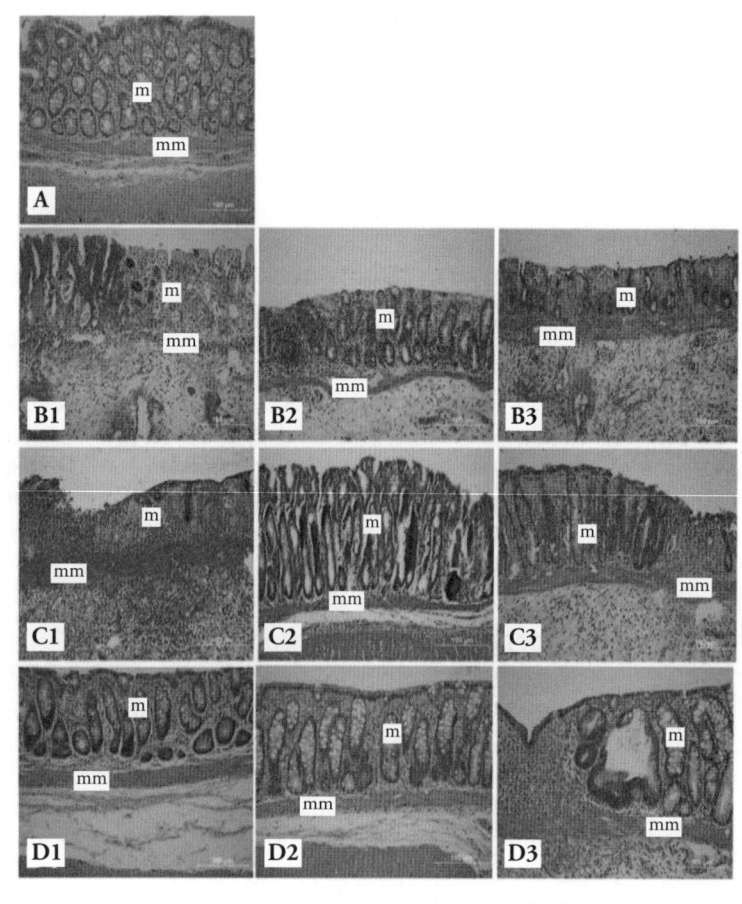

b

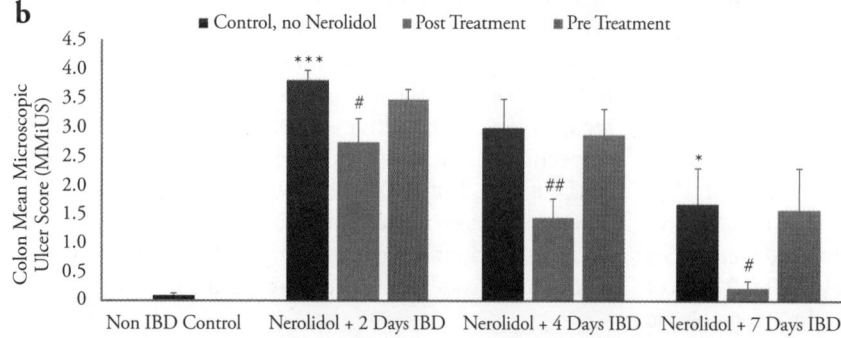

Fig. 2 (a) Light micrographs of the colon of rats showing the effects of nerolidol on IBD-induced lesions. **A**: Naïve (control); (**B**) 1: 2-day IBD control—no nerolidol, 2: 2-day IBD, post-treated with nerolidol, 3: 2-day IBD (pretreated). (**C**) 1: 4-day IBD control – no nerolidol, 2: 4-day IBD, post-treated with nerolidol 3: 4-day IBD (pretreated). (**D**) 1: 7-day IBD control – no nerolidol, 2: 7-day IBD, post-treated with nerolidol, 3: 7-day IBD (pretreated). (**b**) Effect of nerolidol on microscopic Ulcer score in IBD rat model. Data are presented as mean ± SEM. *Significant difference between nerolidol-treated and non-IBD control. #Significant difference between nerolidol-treated and IBD control. * $P< 0.05$, ***$P < 0.001$ vs. non-IBD control group; #$P < 0.05$, ##$P < 0.01$ vs. relative IBD control group

Effect of nerolidol on interleukin-1 (IL-1β) levels in acetic acid-induced IBD

Interleukin-1 (IL-1β), also known as leukocyte pyrogen or leukocyte endogenous factor, is a cytokine protein and a mediator of colonic inflammation. To examine whether the administration of NRD has any effects on colonic tissue levels of interleukin-1 (IL-1β), after it was administered either pre- or post-IBD in rats (Fig. 5a). There was a significant ($P < 0.05$, $P < 0.001$, $n=6$) increase in colonic tissue levels of IL-1β levels after IBD after 2 and 4 days of IBD, respectively. Mean colonic tissue IL-1β levels were unaffected by NRD on day 7 of IBD. However, post-IBD administration of NRD resulted in a significant ($P < 0.05$, $P < 0.001$, $n = 6$) reduction in mean colonic tissue levels of IL-1β levels 2 and 4 days after the induction of IBD, respectively. After 7 days of IBD, colonic tissue levels of IL-1β were seen unaffected by administration of NRD. Pre-IBD administration of NRD significantly ($P < 0.05$, $P < 0.001$, $n = 6$) reduced the colonic tissue levels of IL-1β in untreated group (IBD, no NRD), as well as 2 and 4 days after the induction of IBD, respectively. Pre-IBD administration of NRD had no effect on colonic tissue levels of IL-1β after 7 days of IBD.

Effect of nerolidol on interleukin-23 levels in acetic acid-induced IBD

Interleukin-23 (IL-23) is the key mediator of intestinal inflammation. To determine whether NRD has any effect on mean colonic tissue levels of IL-23, NRD was administered either 3 days before or 30 min after the induction of IBD (Fig. 5b). In the control group (no IBD, no NRD), IL-23 level was 14.19 ± 2.21 pg/mg of protein. After 2 days of IBD induction, there was a non-significant increase in IL-23 colonic tissue levels on day 2 but a significant increase ($P < 0.05$, $P < 0.01$) after 4 and 7 days of IBD (control, No NRD). Administration of NRD after the induction of IBD had a significant ($P < 0.05$, $n = 6$) effect on colonic tissue levels of IL-23 only after 4 days but no effect on days 2

and 7 of IBD. There was a significantly ($P < 0.05$, $P < 0.01$, $n = 6$) reduction in the colonic tissue levels of IL-23 when NRD was administered pre-IBD on days 4 and 7. NRD had no effect on mean colonic IL-23 tissue levels on day 2 of IBD.

Effect of nerolidol on interleukin-6 levels in acetic acid-induced IBD

Interleukin-6 (IL-6), is a pro-inflammatory cytokine in the intestine but anti-inflammatory myokine in skeletal muscles. In order to study the effect of NRD on IL-6, it was administered either 3 days pre- or 30 min post-IBD (Fig. 5c). Mean colonic tissue levels of IL-6 was significantly ($P < 0.01$, $P < 0.001$, $n = 6$) increased by IBD. Moreover, there was a significant ($P < 0.05$, $P < 0.001$, $n = 6$) increase in mean colonic tissue levels of IL-6 when NRD was administered post-IBD. Administration of NRD 3 days pre-IBD, significantly ($P < 0.05$, $P < 0.01$, $n = 6$) increased the mean colonic tissue levels of IL-6 in the untreated group (IBD, no NRD), as well as after 2 and 4 days of IBD, respectively. Colonic tissue levels of IL-6 on day 7 was unaffected by NRD administered 3 days before IBD.

Effect of nerolidol on mean TNF-α levels in acetic acid-induced IBD

Tumor necrosis factor-α (TNF-α) is a cell signaling protein involved in systemic inflammation and is one of the cytokines that make up the acute phase reaction. To measure its involvement in AA-induced inflammation, NRD was administered either 3 days pre- or 30 min post-IBD in rats (Fig. 5d). There was a significant ($P < 0.05$, $n=6$) decrease in mean colonic levels of TNF-α (IBD, no NRD) on day of IBD. It decreased only on day 4. IBD had no effect on mean colonic TNF-α levels after days 2 and 7. Mean colonic levels of TNF-α were unaffected by the administration of NRD either pre- or post-IBD, on all the days tested.

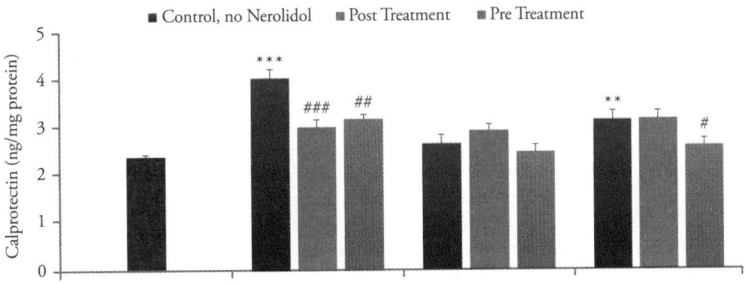

Fig. 3 Effect of nerolidol on calprotectin levels in colon. Data are presented as mean ± SEM. *Significant difference between nerolidol-treated and non-IBD control. #Significant difference between nerolidol-treated and IBD control. *$P < 0.05$, ***$P < 0.001$; ##$P < 0.01$, ###$P < 0.001$

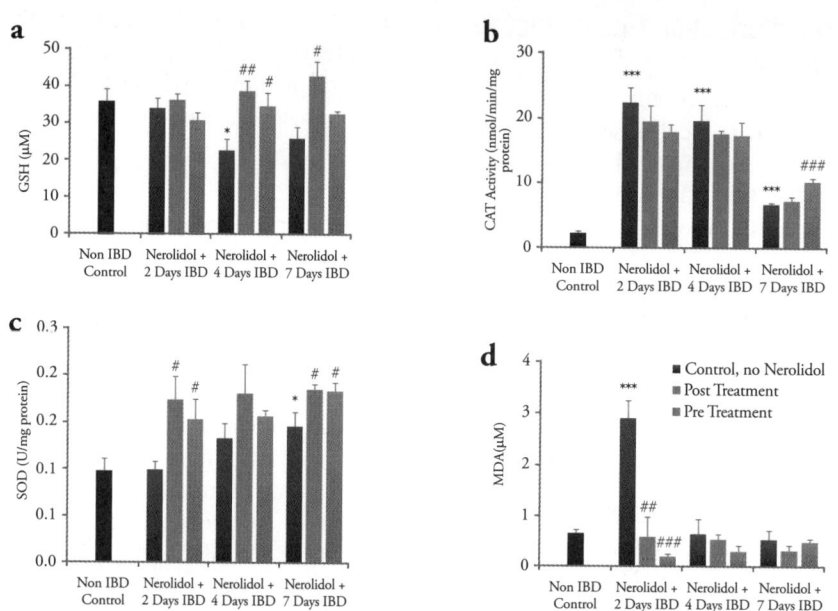

Fig. 4 Effect of nerolidol on a GSH, b catalase, c SOD and d MDA in colon. Data are presented as mean ± SEM. *Significant difference between nerolidol-treated and non-IBD control. #Significant difference between nerolidol-treated and IBD control. *$P < 0.05$, **$P < 0.01$, *** $P < 0.001$; #$P < 0.05$, ##$P < 0.01$, ###$P < 0.001$

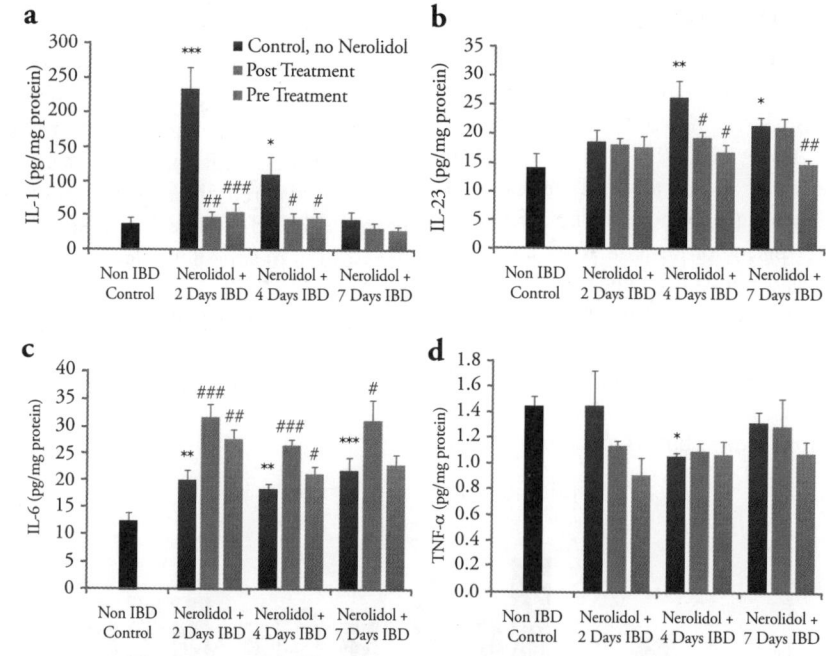

Fig. 5 Effect of nerolidol on pro-inflammatory cytokines a IL-1β, b IL-23, c Il-6 and d TNF-α in colon. Data are presented as mean ± SEM. *Significant difference between nerolidol-treated and non-IBD control. # Significant difference between nerolidol-treated and IBD control. *$P < 0.05$, **$P < 0.01$ ***$P < 0.001$; #$P < 0.05$, ##$P < 0.01$, ###$P < 0.001$

Dose (mg/kg)	Non-IBD control	IBD control	IBD post-nerolidol-treated	Pre-IBD nerolidol-treated
Day 0 Control	24.30 ± 7.72			
Day 2		45686.36 ± 9180.63***	2958 ± 784.93##	3149.64 ± 892.25##
Day 4		462.45 ± 133.86**	159.57 ± 1.46#	191.29 ± 21.56#
Day 7		117.80 ± 30.03***	89.03 ± 15.29	54.05 ± 3.81

***$P < 0.001$ day 0 non IBD control group vs IBD control group; #$P < 0.05$, ##$P < 0.01$, ###$P < 0.001$, IBD control group vs post/pre-treatment

Effect of nerolidol on mean myeloperoxidase (MPO) activity in acetic acid-induced IBD

Myeloperoxidase (MPO) is a heme-enzyme localized in lysosomes of neutrophils, macrophages and monocytes. Increased activity is also found in inflamed mucosa in ulcerative colitis. Therefore, to measure its activity in colonic tissues and the extent of neutrophil migration to the site of inflammation, NRD was administered either 3 days pre- or 30 min post-IBD (Table 2). There was a significant ($P < 0.01$, $P < 0.001$) increase in colonic tissue activity of MPO in control group (IBD, no NRD) on days 2, 4 and 7 of IBD, respectively. However, there was a significant ($P < 0.05$, $P < 0.01$, $n = 6$) reduction in colonic tissue activity of MPO when NRD was administered post-IBD. NRD had no effect on mean colonic tissue activity of MPO on day 7 of IBD. Moreover, mean colonic tissue activity of MPO was significantly ($P < 0.05$, $P < 0.01$, $n = 6$) reduced when NRD was administered 3 days Pre-IBD. Mean colonic tissue activity of MPO was unaffected by NRD on day 7 of IBD.

DISCUSSION

The result of our study shows that NRD effectively improved body weight, colonic length by attenuating oxidative stress, and inflammation. Furthermore, the preservation and protection of colonic mucosa by NRD clearly show its usefulness in AA-induced colitis in rats.

Recent insights into the role of oxidative stress in IBD have shed light in improving therapy in IBD, particularly the health benefits of plants as well as plant-derived phytochemicals due to their antioxidant and anti-inflammatory properties. These natural antioxidants are believed to impede the progression of disease, as well as rescue patients from the disease. The results of the present findings also suggest that NRD could be a useful agent in the treatment of IBD. This is the first report to demonstrate the protective eff of NRD on acetic acid-induced in rats in line with various other terpene compounds such as geraniol, carvacrol, menthol, betulinic acid, celastrol, and eucalyptol by suppressing inflammatory process in animal models of IBD.

The rat model of AA-induced colitis used in the present study is a widely used animal model for testing the effectiveness of different agents that target inflammation and oxidative stress. This model mimics the pathogenesis of clinical IBD. The result of the present study showed that IBD altered the epithelial integrity and colonic injury by modulating the mucosal immune system following neutrophil and macrophage infiltrations. Despite the mucoprotective barrier of the epithelial layer, ingested materials or pathogens activate the mucosal epithelium, polymorphonuclear neutrophils, and macrophages to produce pro-inflammatory cytokines and other mediators that affect colon mucosa integrity. In the present study, induction of IBD by 4% AA caused a high degree of inflammation, loss of goblet cell, and colon tissue injury due to infiltration of the surface epithelium by leucocytes, which is well supported by the histopathology observations. The reduction in body weight and changes in the length of the colon tissue in rats are sensitive indicators of the extent and severity of inflammatory responses. In the present study, improved body weight, colon length, and reduced diarrhea following treatment with NRD illustrate its usefulness in ulcerative colitis and the possibility of other terpene compounds for possible use as therapeutic agents in colitis.

Treatment with NRD attenuated the macroscopic and microscopic injury in the colonic tissue of rat as observed histologically. The preservation of epithelial goblet cells, which produce mucin, is the main reason for reduced tissue damage. Vascular mechanisms and mucin, a glucoprotein, play an important role in the protection and healing of gut mucosa. Studies have shown that low mucosal blood flow predisposes to injury, whereas increase in blood flow protects against noxious agents. The mechanism of protection involves supply of oxygen and bicarbonate (HCO^-_3) and the prevention of deleterious agents entering the mucosa. Alteration in the balance between the production of ROS and detoxification by endogenous antioxidant defense system are factors that lead to intestinal damage in IBD. In normal physiological circumstances, the colonic mucosa keeps the level of endogenous antioxidant enzymes activity balanced in such a precise manner that it is enough to keep the levels of ROS low. In situation where there is an increased level of ROS (H_2O_2) due to decrease in its removal, an alternative reaction occurs which results in increased levels of cellular hydroxyl radical (OH$^{\bullet}$) or hypochlorous acid (HOCl) which lead to impaired epithelial cell integrity, impeding mucosal recovery, and increasing intestinal mucosal permeability. This results in reduced barrier function and host defense leading to the infiltration of bacteria and microorganisms, which in turn releases a large amount of reactive oxygen metabolites. Endogenous antioxidant enzymes such as SOD and CAT and a non-enzymatic antioxidant, GSH, protect cells and organisms from cytotoxic reactive oxygen and reactive nitrogen species. SODs are metal ion cofactor-requiring enzymes that catalyzes the dismutation of $O2^{\bullet-}$ into O_2 and H_2O_2. The uncharged H_2O_2 in the cytosol is further converted into water by CAT, a heme-enzyme located in peroxisomes, or enzymes of the glutathione redox cycle, a component of endogenous antioxidant defense system.

The present study showed that NRD, by increasing the tissue levels of SOD and CAT, prevented excessive free radical generation and reduced the formation of lipid peroxides and aldehyde, MDA, in AA-induced colitis. GSH, a tripeptide with a reactive sulphydryl group, plays an important role in detoxification by inhibiting ROS, facilitating the synthesis and repair of DNA, thus reducing the risk of colon cancer, enhances the promotion of the recycling of endogenous anti-oxidants, and subsequently improves vitamin C antioxidant activity and enhances amino acids transport. Despite being a substrate for antioxidant enzyme, GPx, GSH scavenges several reactive oxygen metabolites including $O2^{\bullet-}$, OH$^{\bullet}$, peroxynitrite, and hydroperoxides. During its function as an antioxidant, reduced GSH is converted to its oxidized state. Subsequently, it is reduced back to GSH by glutathione reductase. A reduced level of GSH in colonic tissues indicates occurrence of oxidative stress and enhanced level of GSH following treatment with NRD demonstrate its antioxidant properties in colitis. NRD has been shown to interfere with ROS production and restore the levels of GSH bioavailability leading to a reduction of ethanol- and indomethacin-induced mucosal damage, stress-induced gastric ulcer, as well as in heart, brain and lungs.

In addition to reduced antioxidant defense, there was an increased formation of lipid peroxides following lipid peroxidation of membranes which was characterized by increased colonic tissue levels of malondialdehyde (MDA) in AA-challenged animals. This explains its usage as an indicator of oxidative stress in cells and tissues besides myeloperoxidase (MPO). MDA is a naturally occurring product of lipid peroxidation; it can also be generated during prostaglandin biosynthesis in cells. An increase in free

radical causes overproduction of MDA. Lipid peroxidation is a process under which oxidants such as free radicals inflict direct damage on membrane lipids containing carbon–carbon double bonds, especially polyunsaturated fatty acids (PUFAs). It also affects other lipids, proteins, and DNA. ROS initiates lipid peroxidation by removing a hydrogen atom. Previous studies have shown that MDA levels are elevated in IBD peroxidation. Furthermore, there has been an increased report of lipid peroxidation in AA-induced tissue injuries, which is similar to the findings of the present study. Therefore, substances which prevent the formation ROS or potentiate the endogenous enzymatic or non-enzymatic anti-oxidant systems can have beneficial effects in reducing intestinal inflammation and damage in ulcerative colitis. Similarly, NRD has been shown to enhance antioxidant enzymes, inhibit lipid peroxidation, and bring a reduction in the infiltration of inflammatory cells (neutrophils) in various other tissues.

Under normal conditions, there is a tight-control in the balance between pro-inflammatory (IL-1β, IL-6, IL-8, IL-17, IL-23, and TNF-α) and anti-inflammatory (IL-5, IL-10, IL-11, and TGF-β) cytokines in the mucosa of the gastrointestinal (GI) tract. The secretion of pro-inflammatory cytokines is initiated by macrophages and neutrophils, which activate the adaptive immune system. This results in the disruption of the balance between T-helper (Th) cells and intolerant regulatory T cells, leading to initiation and progression of inflammation in colonic tissues. Crohn's disease is characterized by Th1 cell-mediated inflammation of the colonic mucosa with increased level of IL-12, IL-17, and IL-23 cytokines while ulcerative colitis is influenced by IL-4, IL-5, IL-10, and IL-13 produced by Th2- type T cells. Increased colonic tissue level of IL-1β, IL-23, and TNF-α is often used as a biomarker for the severity of colitis. IL-1β is made mainly by monocytes, tissue macrophages, and various other cells, are involved in myriad immunological responses spanning both innate and adaptive immunity. IL-1β production, which is synthetized in inactive form and activated by caspase-1, is initiated by cyclooxygenase type 2, phospholipase A, and iNOS. In contrast to other cytokines, IL-6 is a pleiotropic cytokine that acts both as pro-inflammatory cytokine and an anti-inflammatory myokine. Recent evidence has suggested that IL-6 may play an important role in driving chronic inflammation, autoimmunity, endothelial dysfunction by activated macrophages, and colon epithelial cells to secrete inflammatory cytokines. TNF-α, released mainly from activated macrophages, disrupts intestinal epithelial barrier, induces apoptosis of epithelial cells, promotes ROS production, activates neutrophils, and plays an important role in the pathogenesis of IBD. TNF-α is a critical cytokine that facilitates the generation of superoxides in colon epithelial cells by activating NOX1 and NADPH oxidase organizer 1 (NOXO1). Activation of NOX1, and ROs generation are all involved in activating NF-kB by TNF-α. Activation of NOX1, ROs generation, and IkBa are all involved in activating NF-kB through TNF-α. Research has shown that oxidative stress is involved in activation of NF-κB signaling in IBD which can elevate the transcription of different types of genes that are instrumental in the pathogenesis of IBD.

NRD has been shown to have anti-inflammatory effects by downregulating the expression of inflammatory mediators and signaling pathways such as inhibition of LOX-1/ IL-1β and TLR4/NF-κB signaling and AMPK/ Nrf-2/ HO-1 pathway. The anti-inflammatory activities observed in the present study are in line with previous reports wherein NRD showed potent anti-inflammatory activity by inhibiting the release and secretion of proinflammatory cytokines in brain, kidney, liver, heart, lungs, testes, uterus, stomach, and ocular tissues. Based on the results of the present study and studies conducted by other workers, NRD is found to be beneficial in IBD and like other herbal anti-inflammatory agents, NRD does not cause gastrointestinal adverse effects and appears safer than conventional anti-inflammatory drugs.

Polymorphonuclear infiltration of the colonic tissue was reduced when the rats were treated with NRD, which was evidenced by microscopic examination and significant reduction in MPO activity. NRD appears to inhibit leukocyte and neutrophil migration and, in addition, inhibits the rolling and adhesion of leukocytes in colon tissues. Neutrophil and macrophage infiltrate into AA-induced damaged sites in colon tissues and the degree of tissue infiltration depends on the activity of MPO. This enzyme is mainly found in primary granules of neutrophils in humans and to a lesser extent in monocytes and macrophages. The degree of MPO activity serves as the bases for quantitative assay for acute inflammation of the intestine, which is a measure of neutrophil infiltration. The primary granules of neutrophils release MPO, a heme-containing enzyme, during inflammation which catalyzes H_2O_2-dependent peroxidation of Cl^-, HOCl, which exert antimicrobial properties. The reactive oxygen species formed in this process are responsible for intracellular damages to host cells targeting carbohydrates, proteins, nucleic acids, and lipids. Neutrophils and macrophages exhibit prominent roles during mucosal inflammation by producing superoxide and nitric oxide (NO) by activating NOX and iNOS, respectively, leading to barrier dysfunction and tissue necrosis.

Furthermore, in this study, decreased calprotectin following NRD treatment demonstrated the protective effects of NRD on colonic tissues. Calprotectin is associated with inflammation and is derived from neutrophils and studies have shown an increased tissue levels of calprotectin in patients with IBD and fetal calprotectin accurately predicts relapse. Wide margin of safety and negligible adverse effects of NRD indicates its safety and the beneficial effect following oral route of administration further indicates its convenient dosage form for therapeutic and nutritional use in humans.

There is a clear evidence for the protective role of NRD on AA-induced colitis in rats by macroscopic and biochemical observations, which is well supported by the histopathological studies. In the present study, AA, administered rectally, resulted in severe inflammation and necrosis of the colonic mucosa, reduced colonic length, increased inflammatory cell infiltration with edema, and caused occasional hyperemia and goblet cell hyperplasia as observed in the histopathological studies. These observations, which characterize IBD, are consistent with our studies done previously using similar animal model. NRD treatment remarkably improved the colonic histoarchitecture by preserving microscopic and macroscopic structures of colon and preventing depletion of colonic wall mucosa. Pretreatment with NRD resulted in reduction of the histological signs of inflammation, namely leukocyte infiltration, edema, and tissue injury. The observation of the present study wherein NRD protects against AA-induced colitis is in support of other studies done with ethanol, NSAIDs such as indomethacin, and stress-induced gastric lesion where the mean gastric lesion area was significantly reduced.

Integrating the anticancer activity in cancer cells of the colon by suppressing cell growth, cell proliferation, and induction of apoptosis without affecting the integrity of normal cells as well as antiulcer, antioxidant, and anti-inflammatory potential, NRD appears to be a promising molecule for its therapeutic potential in colitis, a risk factor of colon cancer. Additionally, the results of our study also provide scientific validation of traditional claims of plants containing NRD for the treatment of diseases of the gastrointestinal tract.

This study reveals the potent antioxidant and anti-inflammatory effects of NRD in an acute colon inflammation model induced by AA. Considering the safety of NRD and demonstrated efficacy of NRD in gastric as well as colon tissues, the results of the present study provide a foundation for further investigations on molecular mechanism and it can be a promising phytochemical agent for nutraceutical or development of pharmaceuticals in IBD.

JOURNAL ARTICLE EXERCISE 2

Remember that the science sections on the MCAT include a significant number of passages with experiments. You'll need to be able to extract information efficiently and analyze data effectively in order to do well on these passages.

This is the second of three "Journal Article Exercises" in this book. In the first exercise, we showed you the type of information you should be able to extract from the article and the sorts of things to pay attention to in the data. In this exercise, you'll do more of that on your own, and in the final exercise we'll show you how that article might get turned into an MCAT-style passage.

As a reminder, when analyzing an experiment, you should be able to:

- identify the control group(s).
- extract information from graphs and data tables.
- determine how the experimental group(s) change relative to the control.
- determine if the results are statistically significant.
- come to a reasonable conclusion about WHY the results were observed.
- consider potential weaknesses in the study.
- determine how to increase the power of the study.
- decide what the next most logical experiment or study should be.

Again, the goal of these exercises is NOT to learn content from the articles, just to get a little more comfortable reading and extracting information from them.

For the (abridged) article on pages 171–181, try to summarize the purpose of the experiment and the methods in 4–5 sentences. Consider the following mnemonic: Oh ouR Car Won't Start (ORCWS).

- **O = Organism and Organization**: is the research being conducted on humans or on animals or on bacteria, or something else? What is being done to these organisms? Are there any unique qualities to these organisms? Are there multiple groups? Is the study conducted over a long period of time with multiple data points, or is it a short-term study? Does it have a large or small n?
- **R = Results**: where and how are the results presented? Is it a graph? A data table? Figures and images? What is/are the independent variable(s)? What is/are the dependent variable(s)? Do the results show correlation or cause and effect, or both? Describe.
- **C = Control and Comparison**: is there a control group? How does it differ from the experimental group? Is it given a placebo or nothing at all? Is it held under different conditions? If there are multiple experimental groups, how do they differ from one another? Is it a blinded study? If so, double-blind or single-blind?
- **W = Weirdness**: does anything or do any of the results stand out as unexpected?
- **S = Statistics**: was any sort of statistical analysis done? How is it presented? Are there error bars on a graph? Standard errors around a mean? Are there p-values? Is there an asterisk indicating statistical significance? Is there any data that is not statistically significant?

Try interpreting the data on your own before reading the results/discussion section. When you do read the discussion, consider:

- What are the conclusions of the study?
- How are the conclusions supported by the data?
- What potential weaknesses or flaws do you see in the experimental design? Are these addressed in the discussion section?
- How might this study be potentially biased?
- How might this study be improved?
- What would be the next most logical experiment?

Answer these questions for the article on pages 171–181.

1. O = Organism and Organization:

- Is the research being conducted on humans or on animals or on bacteria in a petri dish, or something else?

_____

_____

- What is being done to these organisms?

_____

_____

- Are there any unique qualities to these organisms?

_____

_____

- Are there multiple groups?

_____

_____

- Is the study conducted over a long period of time with multiple data points, or is it a short-term study?

_____

_____

- Does it have a large or small n?

_____

_____

2. R = Results:

- Where and how are the results presented? Is it a graph? A data table? Figures and images?

_____

_____

- What is/are the independent variable(s)?

_____

_____

- What is/are the dependent variable(s)?

_____

_____

- What are the results of the study?

_____

_____

- Do the results show correlation or cause and effect, or both? Describe.

  _____

  _____

3. **C = Control and Comparison:**
   - Is there a control group?

     _____

     _____

   - How does it differ from the experimental group? Is it given a placebo or nothing at all? Is it held under different conditions?

     _____

     _____

   - If there are multiple experimental groups, how do they differ from one another?

     _____

     _____

   - Is it a blinded study? If so, double blind or single blind?

     _____

     _____

4. **W = Weirdness:**
   - Does anything or do any of the results stand out as unexpected?

     _____

     _____

5. **S = Statistics:**
   - Was any sort of statistical analysis done?

     _____

     _____

   - How is it presented? Are there error bars on a graph? Standard errors around a mean? Are there p-values? Is there an asterisk indicating statistical significance?

     _____

     _____

   - Is there any data that is not statistically significant?

     _____

     _____

6. **Interpreting the data:**
   - What are the conclusions of the study?

     _____

     _____

- How are the conclusions supported by the data?

  _____

  _____

- What potential weaknesses or flaws do you see in the experimental design? Are these addressed in the discussion section?

  _____

  _____

- How might this study be potentially biased?

  _____

  _____

- How might this study be improved?

  _____

  _____

- What would be the next most logical experiment?

  _____

  _____

7. **Final Summary of Experiment and Results:**

  _____

  _____

  _____

  _____

  _____

  _____

  _____

SOLUTIONS TO JOURNAL ARTICLE EXERCISE 2

1. **O = Organism and Organization:**
   - Is the research being conducted on humans or on animals or on bacteria in a petri dish, or something else? *Rats.*
   - What is being done to these organisms? *Colitis is induced and the effect of nerolidol (a terpene found in tea) is assessed (both as a treatment and as a preventative).*
   - Are there any unique qualities to these organisms? *No.*
   - Are there multiple groups? *Yes. Control, pre-colitis treatment, and post-colitis treatment*
   - Is the study conducted over a long period of time with multiple data points, or is it a short-term study? *Short term (7–10 days), several data points within those 7–10 days*
   - Does it have a large or small *n*? *small n: 18 animals per group.*

2. **R = Results:**
   - Where and how are the results presented? Is it a graph? A data table? Figures and images? *Photos and graphs*
   - What is/are the independent variable(s)? *Nerolidol*
   - What is/are the dependent variable(s)? *Ulceration (severity of colitis), body weight, calprotectin levels, glutathione levels, catalase activity, superoxide dismutase activity, malondioaldehyde levels, interleukin levels, tumor necrosis factor levels, myeloperoxidase activity.*
   - What are the results of the study? *The rats treated with nerolidol, both after induction of colitis and as a pretreatment, showed less tissue damage, less oxidative damage, and lower levels of inflammatory markers.*
   - Do the results show correlation or cause and effect, or both? Describe. *Cause and effect: treatment of rats with nerolidol reduced the effects of the induced colitis.*

3. **C = Control and Comparison:**
   - Is there a control group? *Yes*
   - How does it differ from the experimental group? Is it given a placebo or nothing at all? Is it held under different conditions? *There were two control groups: one that was not induced to colitis and one that was induced to colitis and not treated with nerolidol.*
   - If there are multiple experimental groups, how do they differ from one another? *There were two experimental groups, one that was pretreated with nerolidol before induction of colitis and one that was treated with nerolidol after induction of colitis.*
   - Is it a blinded study? If so, double blind or single blind? *Not a blinded study*

4. **W = Weirdness:**
   - Does anything or do any of the results stand out as unexpected? *Not all inflammatory cytokine levels are reduced. Il-6 was increased in nerolidol treated rats.*

5. **S = Statistics:**
   - Was any sort of statistical analysis done? *Yes*
   - How is it presented? Are there error bars on a graph? Standard errors around a mean? Are there *p*-values? Is there an asterisk indicating statistical significance? *P values, error bars, asterisks*
   - Is there any data that is not statistically significant? *There are a few measures that are not statistically significant, e.g., IL-23 levels 2 days after induction of colitis. TNF-α levels are generally not statistically significant.*

6. **Interpreting the data:**
   - What are the conclusions of the study? *Generally speaking, treatment with nerolidol reduces tissue damage and levels of inflammatory markers, while increasing levels of antioxidant enzymes.*
   - How are the conclusions supported by the data? *Data on tissue damage and levels of inflammatory markers and antioxidant enzymes show significant differences between treated and untreated groups.*
   - What potential weaknesses or flaws do you see in the experimental design? Are these addressed in the discussion section? *Treatment was on animals; results do not always transfer to humans.*
   - How might this study be potentially biased? *These studies were done previously with similar animal models; the researchers may have been biased in looking for/expecting positive results.*
   - How might this study be improved? *No obvious ways to improve the study.*
   - What would be the next most logical experiment? *Repeat the experiment, but compare treatment with nerolidol to treatment with other anti-inflammatory agents. Study the effects of nerolidol treatment in humans with IBD or ulcerative colitis.*

7. **Final Summary of Experiment and Results:**
   - *In this study, colitis was induced in rats by the application of acetic acid. Some rats were treated prophylactically with nerolidol prior to induction of colitis, and some rats were treated with nerolidol after induction of colitis. In all cases, tissue damage and inflammation were reduced by nerolidol. No adverse effects of nerolidol treatment occurred. This points to nerolidol, a plant compound, as a reasonable treatment for IBD and colitis in humans.*

Chapter 7
Nucleic Acids

The biological macromolecules are grouped into four classes of molecules that play important roles in cells and in organisms as a whole. All of them are polymers—strings of repeated units (monomers).

This chapter discusses the nucleic acids from a biological perspective: what they are made of, how they are put together, and what their roles are in the body. These molecules are also discussed in *MCAT Organic Chemistry Review* from an organic chemistry perspective: nomenclature, chirality, etc.

7.1 PHOSPHORUS-CONTAINING COMPOUNDS

Phosphoric acid is an *inorganic* acid (it does not contain carbon) with the potential to donate three protons. The pK_as for the three acid dissociation equilibria are 2.1, 7.2, and 12.4. Therefore, at physiological pH, phosphoric acid is significantly dissociated, existing largely in anionic form. The most common species (approximately 60% in extracellular fluid) is hydrogen phosphate (HPO_4^{-2}), and the second most common (approximately 40%) is dihydrogen phosphate ($H_2PO_4^-$).

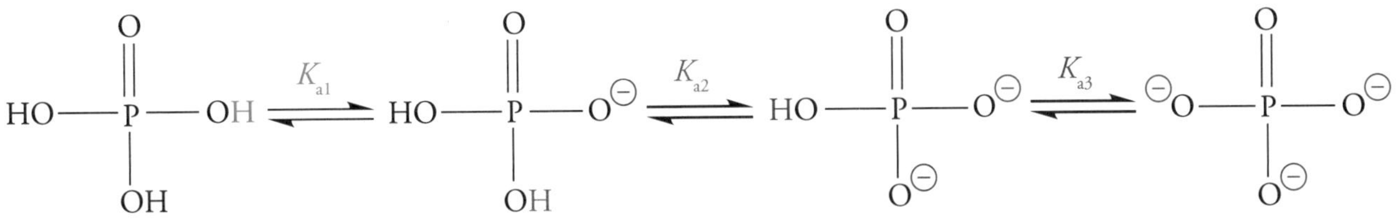

Figure 1   Phosphoric Acid Dissociation

Phosphate is also known as orthophosphate. Two orthophosphates bound together via an **anhydride linkage** form **pyrophosphate**. The P–O–P bond in pyrophosphate is an example of a **high-energy phosphate bond**. This name is derived from the fact that the hydrolysis of pyrophosphate is thermodynamically extremely favorable. The $\Delta G°$ for the hydrolysis of pyrophosphate is about –7 kcal/mol. This means that it is a very favorable reaction. The actual ΔG in the cell is about –12 kcal/mol, which is even more favorable. How is this possible?[1]

There are three reasons that phosphate anhydride bonds store so much energy:

1) When phosphates are linked together, their negative charges repel each other strongly.
2) Orthophosphate has more resonance forms and thus a lower free energy than linked phosphates.
3) Orthophosphate has a more favorable interaction with the biological solvent (water) than linked phosphates.

The details are not crucial. What is essential is that you fix the image in your mind of linked phosphates acting like compressed springs, just waiting to fly open and provide energy for an enzyme to catalyze a reaction.

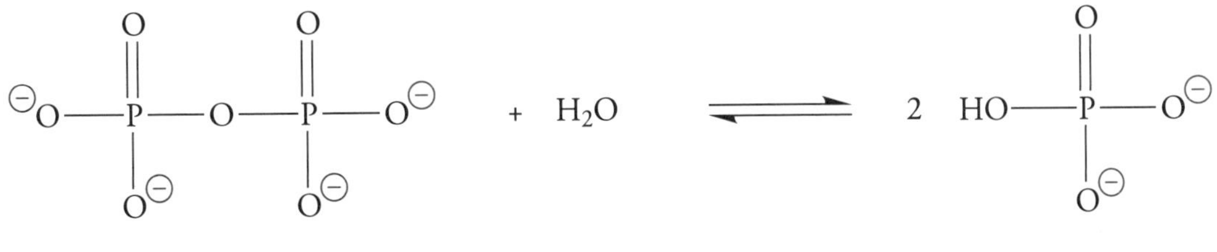

Figure 2   The Hydrolysis of Pyrophosphate

---

[1] Remember from Chapter 3 that $\Delta G°$ is the free energy change at standard conditions. The concentrations of reactants and products inside the cell are not at standard conditions. In fact, the cell maintains a concentration of ATP much higher than that of ADP and phosphate, which makes ATP hydrolysis so much more favorable.

Nucleotides

Nucleotides are the building blocks of nucleic acids (RNA and DNA). Each nucleotide contains a **ribose** (or **deoxyribose**) **sugar** group; a **purine** or **pyrimidine base** joined to carbon number one of the ribose ring; and one, two, or three phosphate units joined to carbon five of the ribose ring. The nucleotide **a**denosine **trip**hosphate (ATP) plays a central role in cellular metabolism in addition to being an RNA precursor. Significantly more information about the function of the nucleic acids RNA and DNA will be provided in *MCAT Biology Review*.

ATP is the universal short-term energy storage molecule. It is a ribonucleotide (ribose is the sugar, as opposed to deoxyribose). Energy extracted from the oxidation of foodstuffs is immediately stored in the phospho-anhydride bonds of ATP. This energy is used to power cellular processes, and as we have already seen, it may also be used to synthesize glucose or fats, which are longer-term energy storage molecules. This applies to *all* living organisms, from bacteria to humans. Even some viruses carry ATP with them outside the host cell, though viruses cannot make their own ATP.

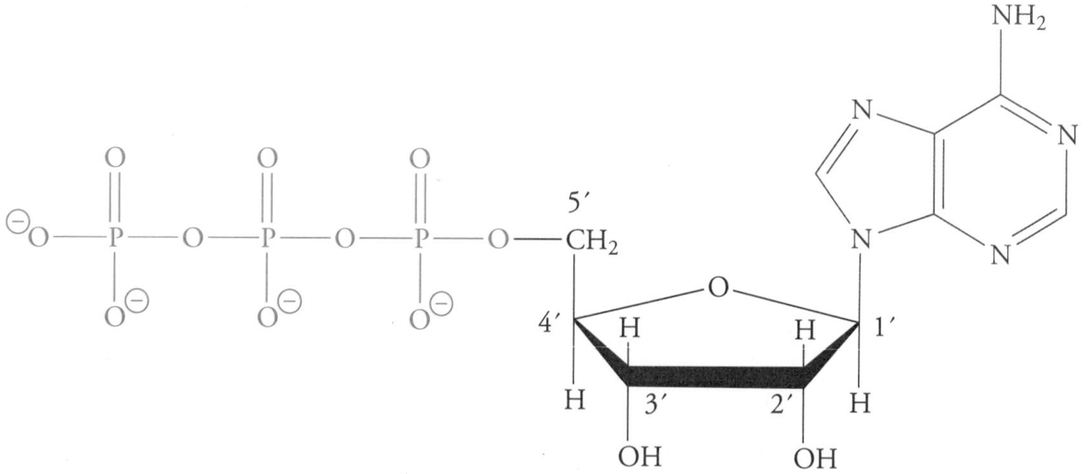

Figure 3   Adenosine Triphosphate (ATP)

The other nucleotides can also be used as energy (high-energy phosphate is high-energy phosphate, after all!), but they are used for this purpose far less often. GTP is used for energy in protein synthesis, and UTP is used to activate glucose-1-P in glycogenesis.

7.2 DNA STRUCTURE

General Overview

Understanding the structure of DNA provides great insight into its function, so let's start at the smallest level and work our way up. DNA is short for deoxyribonucleic acid. DNA and RNA (ribonucleic acid) are called **nucleic acids** because they are found in the nucleus and possess many acidic phosphate groups.

The building block of DNA is the deoxyribonucleoside 5′ triphosphate (dNTP, where N represents one of the four basic nucleosides). Deoxyadenosine 5′ triphosphate (dATP) is shown in Figure 4. Deoxyribonucleotides are built from three components. The first is a simple monosaccharide, deoxyribose. [How does the structure of deoxyribose compare with that of ribose?[2]] In a dNTP, carbons on the ribose are referred to as 1′, 2′, and so on. The next component of the dNTP is an aromatic, nitrogenous base, namely **adenine** (A), **guanine** (G), **cytosine** (C), or **thymine** (T); see Figure 5. (Don't mix up the DNA base thymine with vitamin B_1, thiamine.) These aromatic molecules are bases because they contain several nitrogens which have free electron pairs capable of accepting protons. G and A are derived from a precursor called purine, so they are referred to as the **purines** and have a double-ring structure (a six-membered ring and a five-membered ring). C and T are the **pyrimidines**; they have single six-membered ring structure.[3]

A **nucleo***side* is ribose (a deoxynucleoside is deoxyribose) with a purine or pyrimidine linked to the 1′ carbon in a β-N-glycosidic linkage. [In the β-N-glycosidic linkage of a nucleoside, is the aromatic base above or is it below the plane of ribose in a Haworth projection?[4]] The nucleosides are named as follows: A-ribose = adenosine, G-ribose = guanosine, C-ribose = cytidine, T-ribose = thymidine, and U-ribose = uridine. Both purines and pyrimidines have abundant hydrogen bonding potential. [Will adenine and thymine H-bond with each other in dilute aqueous solution (0.1 *M*, for example)?[5]]

The final component of the deoxyribonucleotide building block of DNA is a phosphate group. **Nucleo***tides* are phosphate esters of nucleosides, with one, two, or three phosphate groups joined to the ribose ring by the 5′ hydroxy group. When nucleotides contain three phosphate residues, they may also be referred to as **deoxynucleoside triphosphates**; they are abbreviated **dNTP**, where d is for *deoxy* and N is for *nucleoside*. In individual nucleotides, N is replaced by A, G, C, T, or U. Because they contain acidic phosphates, the nucleotides may also be referred to by a name ending in "ylate." For example, TTP is thymidylate. The ubiquitous energy molecule, ATP, is a nucleotide which may be called adenylate (it's not deoxy).

---

[2] The 2′ OH is missing in deoxyribose.

[3] A mnemonic for this is: Pyramids (pyrimidines) have sharp edges, so they CUT. The U stands for *uracil*, which is a pyrimidine found in RNA instead of T. Another mnemonic is CUT the Py.

[4] A beta linkage indicates that the anomeric carbon has a configuration with the attached group (a nitrogen of the aromatic ring of a purine or pyrimidine base) drawn *above* the plane of the ribose ring. Remember, it's better to β up!

[5] No. In dilute solution they will be H-bonded to water. However, H-bonds are the key determinant of the double-stranded structure of DNA; in DNA, the bases do not interact with water because DNA coiling places them inside the tube-like structure of the double helix, where they interact with each other.

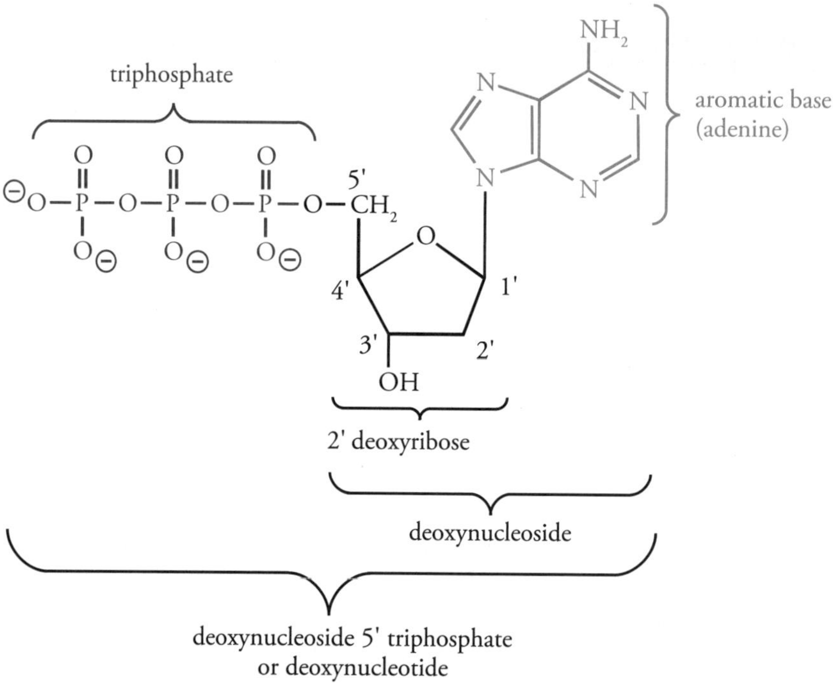

Figure 4 Deoxyadenosine Triphosphate (dATP)

The sugar-phosphate portion of the nucleotide is referred to as the **backbone** of the nucleic acid because it is invariant. The base is the variable portion of the building block. Thus, there are four different dNTPs, and they differ only in the aromatic base. [What is the backbone in protein, and what is the variable portion of the amino acid?[6] If an enzyme binds to a specific sequence of nucleotides in DNA, will the binding specificity be derived from interactions of portions of the polypeptide enzyme with the ribose and phosphate groups or with the purine and pyrimidine bases?[7]]

---

[6] Peptide bonds with a carbon between them are the backbone, and the R-group attached to the α carbon is the variable portion.

[7] Since the backbone is the same regardless of the nucleotide sequence, the specificity in binding must be derived from interactions with bases.

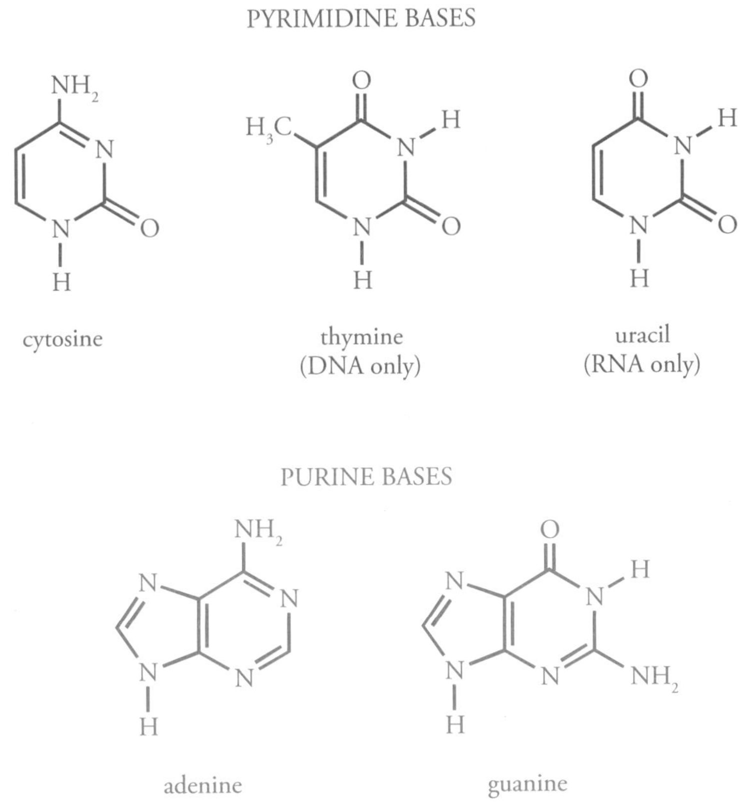

PYRIMIDINE BASES

cytosine

thymine
(DNA only)

uracil
(RNA only)

PURINE BASES

adenine

guanine

Figure 5 Aromatic Bases of DNA and RNA

Polynucleotides

Nucleotides in nucleic acids are covalently linked by **phosphodiester bonds** between the 3′ hydroxy group of the sugar in one nucleotide and the 5′ phosphate group of the sugar in the next nucleotide (Figure 6). [Which reaction is more thermodynamically favorable: the polymerization of nucleoside monophosphates, or the polymerization of nucleoside triphosphates?[8]] A polymer of several nucleotides linked together is termed an *oligo*nucleotide, and a polymer of many nucleotides is a *poly*nucleotide. Since the only unique part of the nucleotide is the base, the sequence of a polynucleotide can be abbreviated by simply listing the bases attached to each nucleotide in the chain. The end of the chain with a free 5′ phosphate group is written first in a polynucleotide, with other nucleotides in the chain indicated in the 5′ to 3′ direction. [Which of the nucleotides in the oligonucleotide ACGT has a free 3′ hydroxy group?[9]]

---

[8] During polymerization of nucleoside triphosphates, pyrophosphate is released and hydrolyzed, driving the polymerization reaction forward. Hydrolysis of the high-energy pyrophosphate molecule makes the polymerization of nucleoside triphosphates more energetically favorable.

[9] The T is written last and is therefore the 3′ nucleotide, or the nucleotide with the free 3′ hydroxy group.

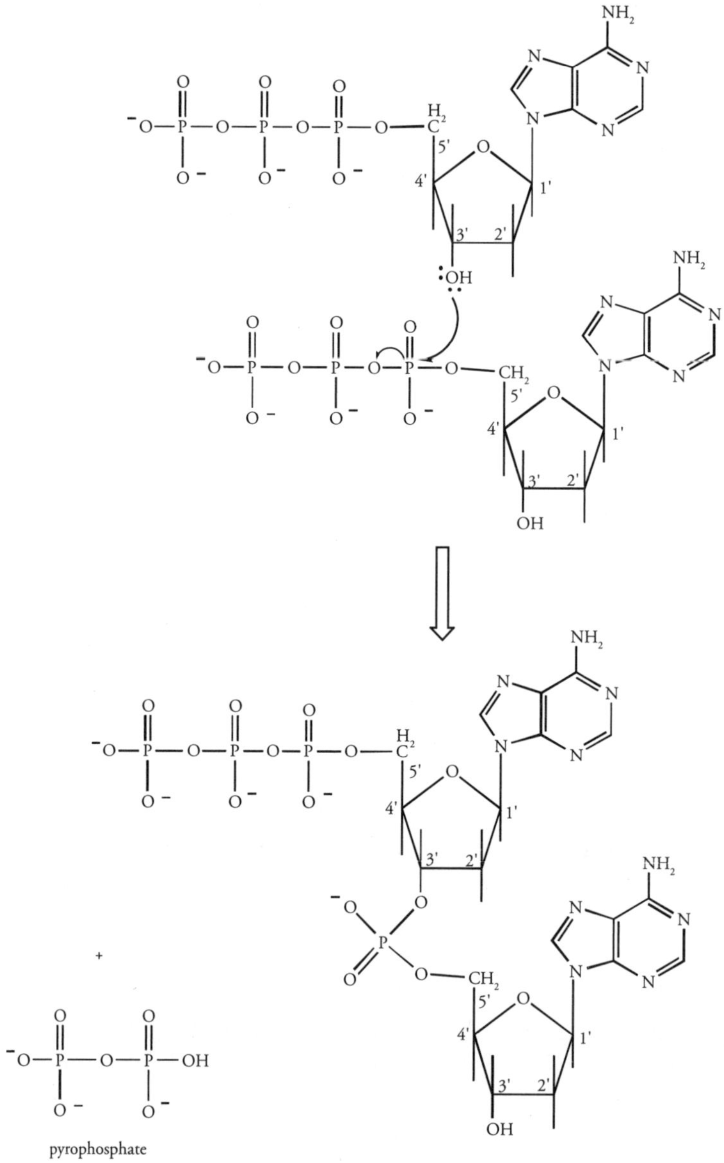

Figure 6 The Polymerization of Nucleotides

The Watson-Crick Model of DNA Structure

James Watson and Francis Crick (with the help of Maurice Wilkins and Rosalind Franklin) developed a model of the structure of DNA in the cell. According to the **Watson-Crick model**, cellular DNA is a right-handed double helix held together by hydrogen bonds and hydrophobic forces between bases. It is important to understand each facet of this model.

In the cell, DNA does not exist in the form of a single long polynucleotide. Instead, the DNA found in the nucleus is double-stranded (**ds**). In ds-DNA, two very long polynucleotide chains are hydrogen-bonded together in an **antiparallel orientation**. Antiparallel means the 5′ end of one chain is paired with the 3′ end of the other. [What common protein structure often depends on H-bonds between antiparallel chains?[10]] The H-bonds in ds-DNA are between the bases on adjacent chains. This H-bonding is very specific: A is always H-bonded to T, and G is always H-bonded to C (Figure 7). Note that this means an H-bonded pair always consists of a *purine plus a pyrimidine*.[11] Thus, both types of base pairs (AT or GC) take up the same amount of room in the DNA double helix. The GC pair is held together by three hydrogen bonds, the AT pair by two. Two chains of DNA are said to be complementary if the bases in each strand can hydrogen bond when the strands are oriented in an antiparallel fashion. If we are talking about ds-DNA 100 nucleotides long, we would say it is 100 base pairs (bp) long. A kbp (kilobase pair) is ds-DNA 1,000 nucleotides long.

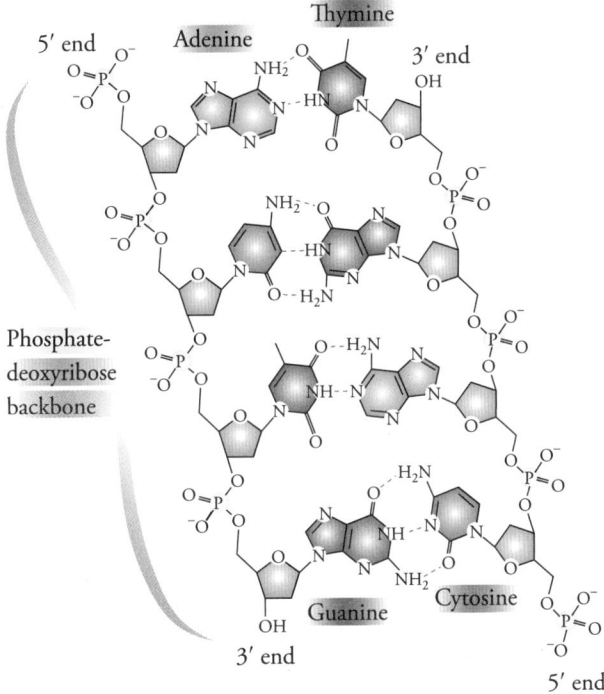

Figure 7   Base Pairing

The binding of two complementary strands of DNA into a double-stranded structure is termed **annealing**, or **hybridization**. The separation of strands is termed **melting**, or **denaturation**. The temperature at which a solution of DNA molecules is 50 percent melted is termed the T_m. [Would the T_m of ATTATCAT and its complementary strand be higher than, lower than, or equal to the melting temperature of AGTCGCAT and its complementary strand?[12] If you attached methyl groups to all the acidic phosphate oxygens along the length of a DNA double helix, would the chain have a higher or lower T_m than normal DNA?[13]]

---

[10] Antiparallel H-bonding is reminiscent of the β-pleated sheet, which is a common secondary structure (it can be quaternary, when two separate chains come together to form a sheet).

[11] This fact has a fringe benefit: we can calculate the number of purines if we know the number of pyrimidines. We can actually calculate several variables. Chargoff's rule states that [A] = [T] and [G] = [C]; and [A] + [G] = [T] + [C].

[12] The T_m of the first oligonucleotide pair would be lower because it contains more AT pairs. A and T form only two hydrogen bonds while G and C form three. Thus, it takes less kinetic energy to disrupt A-T rich ds-DNA than G-C rich ds-DNA.

[13] The charged phosphates electrostatically repel each other in normal DNA. Methyl esters will not be charged. The lack of electrostatic repulsion between the methyl ester backbones will increase the T_m, meaning that more kinetic energy will be required to melt the oligonucleotides.

- Which of the following is/are true about ds-DNA?[14]
  - I. If the amount of G in a double helix is known, the amount of C can be calculated.
  - II. If the fraction of purine nucleotides and the total molecular weight of a double helix are known, the amount of cytosine can be calculated.
  - III. The two chains in a piece of ds-DNA containing mostly purines will be bonded together more tightly than the two chains in a piece of ds-DNA containing mostly pyrimidines.
  - IV. The oligonucleotide ATGTAT is complementary to the oligonucleotide ATACAT.

There is another important detail about DNA structure: not only is it double stranded, it is also *coiled*. In ds-DNA, the two hydrogen-bonded antiparallel DNA strands form a **right-handed double helix** (meaning it corkscrews in a clockwise motion) with the bases on the interior and the ribose/phosphate backbone on the exterior. The double helix is stabilized by van der Waals interactions between the bases, which are stacked upon each other. Hydrophobic interactions between the bases are also very important in stabilizing the double helix. [But wait a minute. "Hydro*phobic* interactions between *bases*?" Isn't that a contradiction in terms? How can a *base* be hydro*phobic*?[15]] The bases lie in a plane, perpendicular to the length of the DNA molecule, stacked 3.4 angstroms (Å) apart from each other. The helix pattern repeats itself (i.e., completes a full turn) once every *34 angstroms*, which is every *10 base pairs*. While the length of a DNA double helix may vary enormously, from a few Å in an oligonucleotide to macroscopic lengths in a chromosome, the width is always 20 Å. [If a human chromosome has 9×10^7 base pairs, how long would the chromosome be if it were stretched out completely?[16]]

---

[14] **Item I: True.** For every G, there is a C, and for every A there is a T. Item II: False. The ratio of purines to pyrimidines is always the same (50:50) since each purine is paired with a pyrimidine. In order to calculate the amount of any one base, you have to know the ratio of AT to GC pairs. Item III: False. Again, the ratio of purines to pyrimidines is always the same—50:50. However, two chains containing mostly GC pairs will bond more tightly than two chains containing mostly AT pairs, since GC pairs are held together by 3 H-bonds, while AT pairs have only 2. **Item IV: True.** Remember, the strands are antiparallel: A and T pair, G and C pair, and the 5' end is always written first.

[15] Once a purine is H-bonded to a pyrimidine, most of the polar nature of the individual bases disappears because the charge dipoles are occupied in H-bonds.

[16] Since one angstrom is 10^{-10} meter, the length is $(3.4 \times 10^{-10}$ meters/base pair$)(9 \times 10^7$ base pairs$) = 30 \times 10^{-3}$ meters = 30 millimeters.

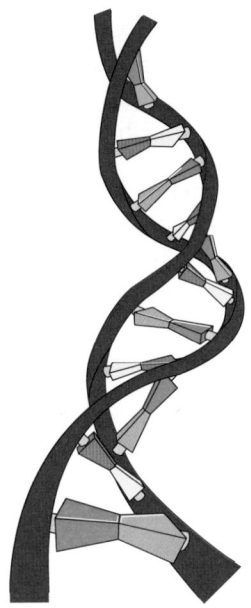

Figure 8   A Small Section of a DNA Double Helix

Chromosome Structure and Packing

The sum total of an organism's genetic information is called its **genome**. Eukaryotic genomes are composed of several large pieces of linear ds-*DNA*; each piece of ds-DNA is called a **chromosome**. Humans have 46 chromosomes, 23 of which are inherited from each parent. Prokaryotic (bacterial) genomes are composed of a **single circular chromosome**. Viral genomes may be linear or circular DNA or RNA. The human genome consists of over 10^9 base pairs, while bacterial genomes contain only 10^6 base pairs. But there is no direct correlation between genome size and evolutionary sophistication, since the organisms with the largest known genomes are amphibians. Much of the size difference in higher eukaryotic genomes is the result of repetitive DNA that has no known function.

If the DNA remained as a simple double helix floating free in the cell, it would be very bulky and fragile. Prokaryotes have a distinctive mechanism for making their single circular chromosome more compact and sturdy. An enzyme called **DNA gyrase** uses the energy of ATP to twist the gigantic circular molecule. Gyrase functions by breaking the DNA and twisting the two sides of the circle around each other. The resulting structure is a twisted circle that is composed of ds-DNA. As discussed above, the two strands are already coiled, forming a helix. The twists created by DNA gyrase are called **supercoils**, since they are coils of a structure that is already coiled.

Since eukaryotes have even more DNA in their genome than prokaryotes, the eukaryotic genome requires denser packaging to fit within the cell (Figure 9). To accomplish this, eukaryotic DNA is wrapped around globular proteins called **histones**. After being wrapped around histones, but before being completely packed away, DNA has the microscopic appearance of beads on a string. The beads are called **nucleosomes**; they are composed of DNA wrapped around an octamer of histones (a group of eight). The octamer is composed of two units of each of the histone proteins H2A, H2B, H3, and H4. The string between the beads is a length of double-helical DNA called linker DNA and is bound by a single linker histone. Fully packed DNA is called **chromatin**; it is composed of closely stacked nucleosomes. [Based on your knowledge of the interactions of macromolecules and the chemical composition of DNA, do you suppose that histones are mostly basic or mostly acidic?[17]]

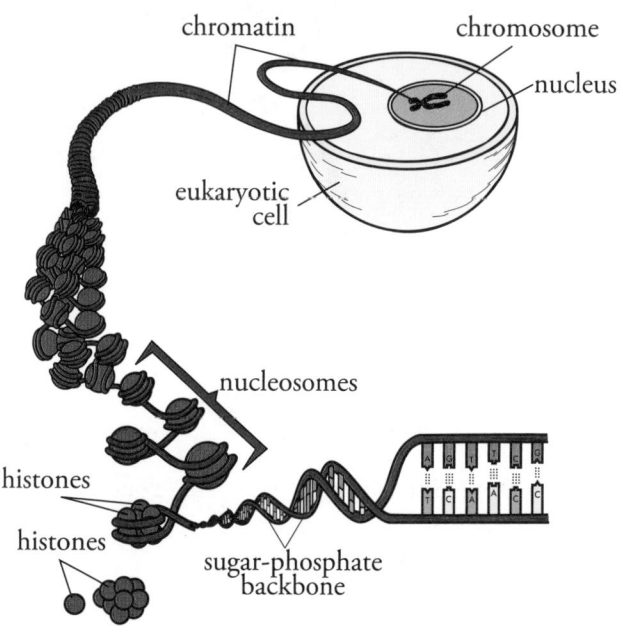

Figure 9 DNA Packaging

The following flow summarizes the structure of DNA in the nucleus: **Deoxyribose** → *add base* → **nucleoside** → *add three phosphates* → **nucleotide** → *polymerize with loss of two phosphates* → **oligonucleotide** → *continue polymerization* → **single-stranded polynucleotide** → *two complete chains H-bond in antiparallel orientation* → **ds DNA chain** → *coiling occurs* → **ds helix** → *wrap around histones* → **nucleosomes** → *complete packaging* → **chromatin**.

To look for patterns and morphology, chromosomes can be stained with chemicals. Usually, condensed metaphase chromosomes are used, as they are compact and easier to see. When chromosomes are treated, distinct light and dark regions become visible. The darker regions are denser, and are called **heterochromatin**. Heterochromatin is rich in repeats (see below). The lighter regions are less dense and are called **euchromatin**. Density gives a sense of DNA coiling or compactness, and these patterns are constant and heritable. It's now known that the lighter regions have higher transcription rates and therefore higher gene activity. The looser packing makes DNA accessible to enzymes and proteins.

Giemsa stain can also be used, and it produces what are called "G-banding patterns." Here too, darker staining regions are more dense than lighter staining regions. Chromosome bands are constant and specific to each chromosome, which means they can be used for diagnostic purposes (where cytologists look at chromosome structure). Banding patterns have also been linked to DNA replication, as it's been shown that lighter staining regions start replication earlier than darker staining regions. Again, this is likely due to accessibility of the DNA. Giemsa stains are most often used to produce karyotypes, as shown in Figure 10.

---

[17] They're mostly basic, since they must be attracted to the acidic exterior of the DNA double helix. This basicity is supplied by the amino acids arginine and lysine, which are unusually abundant in histones.

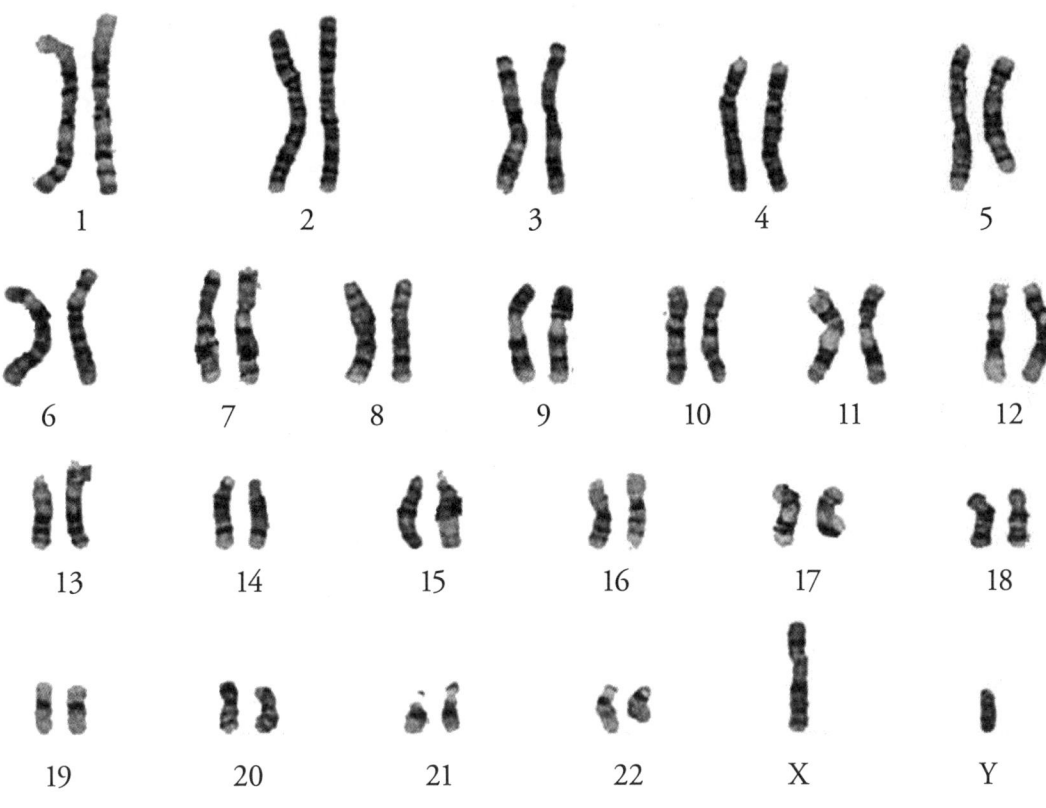

Figure 10   Giemsa Stain (a karyotype)

Centromeres

A centromere is the region of the chromosome to which spindle fibers attach during cell division. The fibers attach via **kinetochores**, multiprotein complexes that act as anchor attachment sites for spindle fibers. Other protein complexes also bind the centromere after DNA replication to keep sister chromatids attached to each other. Centromeres are made of heterochromatin and repetitive DNA sequences. Chromosomes have p (short) and q (long) arms, and the centromere position defines the ratio between the two (Figure 11).

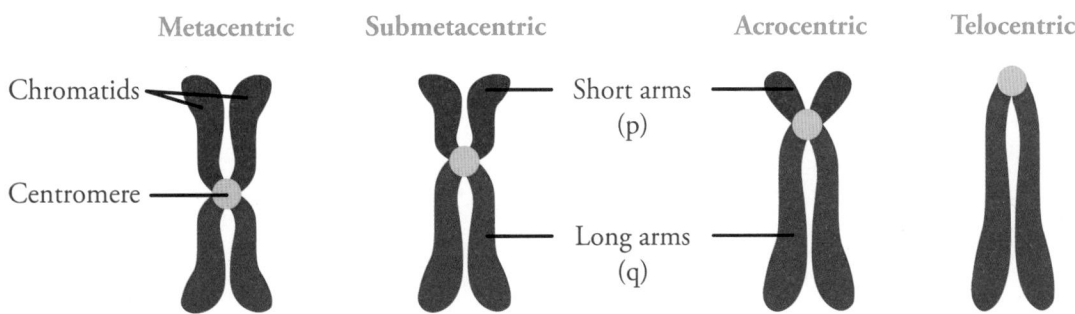

Figure 11   Centromere Positions

Telomeres

The ends of linear chromosomes are called **telomeres**. At the DNA level, these regions are distinguished by the presence of distinct nucleotide sequences repeated 50 to several hundred times. The repeated unit is usually 6–8 base pairs long and guanine-rich. Many vertebrates (including humans and mice) have the same repeat: 5'-TTAGGG-3'. Telomeres are composed of both single- and double-stranded DNA. Single-stranded DNA is found at the very end of the chromosome and is about 300 base pairs in length. It loops around to form a knot, held together by many telomere-associated proteins. This stabilizes the end of the chromosome; specialized telomere cap proteins distinguish telomeres from double-stranded breaks, and this prevents activation of repair pathways.

Telomeres function to prevent chromosome deterioration and also prevent fusion with neighboring chromosomes. They function as disposable buffers, blocking the ends of chromosomes. Since most prokaryotes have circular genomes, their DNA does not contain telomeres.

7.3 CHARACTERISTICS OF RNA

RNA is chemically distinct from DNA in three important ways:

1) RNA is **single-stranded**, except in some viruses.
2) RNA contains **uracil** instead of thymine.
3) The pentose ring in RNA is **ribose** rather than 2' deoxyribose.

As a result of this last difference, the RNA polymer is less stable, because the 2' hydroxyl can nucleophilically attack the backbone phosphate group of an RNA chain, causing hydrolysis when the remainder of the chain acts as leaving group. This cannot occur in DNA because there is no 2' hydroxyl. [Why is the stability of RNA relatively unimportant?[18] Anticancer drugs often seek to block growth of rapidly dividing cells by inhibiting production of thymine. Why is this an attractive target for cancer therapy?[19]] This chemical property has a big impact in molecular biology labs, where DNA samples are stable at a range of temperatures for a relatively long period of time, but high quality RNA is difficult to extract and is only stable for a short time.

There are several different types of RNA, each with a unique role.

Coding RNA

You are already familiar with **messenger RNA** (mRNA), the only type of coding RNA. This molecule carries genetic information to the ribosome, where it can be translated into protein (more information about translation can be found in *MCAT Biology Review*).

---

[18] Because a cell's DNA is necessary for the cell's entire life. RNA is a transient molecule that is transcribed, translated, and destroyed. As a matter of fact, the reason RNA contains uracil also has to do with the reduced need for fidelity in transcription as compared to replication. Without getting into the details, thymine is easier for DNA repair systems to work with, while uracil is much less energy-costly to make. So RNA has uracil, DNA has thymine.

[19] All cells require RNA production, even if they are not growing, in order to continually replenish degraded RNA. RNA contains the bases cytosine, guanine, uracil, and adenine, but only DNA contains thymine. Thus, if thymine production is blocked, only DNA *replication* will be inhibited and only rapidly dividing cells such as cancer cells will be affected. Unfortunately, some normal cells in the body normally divide a lot (such as lining cells of the gut and hair follicles), explaining the side effects of chemotherapy.

Messenger RNA is constantly produced and degraded, according to the cell's need for the protein encoded by each piece of mRNA. In fact, this is the principal means by which cells regulate the amount of each particular protein they synthesize. Note that in eukaryotes, the first RNA transcribed from DNA is an immature or precursor to mRNA called **heterogeneous nuclear RNA** (hnRNA). Processing events (such as addition of a cap and tail and splicing) are required for hnRNA to become mature mRNA. Since prokaryotes do not process their primary transcripts, hnRNA is found only in eukaryotes.

Non-Coding RNA

Non-coding RNA (ncRNA) is a functional RNA that is not translated into a protein. The human genome codes for thousands of ncRNAs, and there are several types. The two major types to know for the MCAT are transfer RNA (tRNA) and ribosomal RNA (rRNA).

Transfer RNA (tRNA) is responsible for translating the genetic code. Transfer RNA carries amino acids from the cytoplasm to the ribosome to be added to a growing protein. The structure of tRNA and how it does its job is discussed in *MCAT Biology Review*. [Estimate how many different tRNAs there are.[20]]

Ribosomal RNA (rRNA) is the major component of the ribosome. Humans have only four different types of rRNA molecules (18S, 5.8S, 28S, and 5S), though almost all of the RNA made in a given cell is rRNA. All rRNAs serve as components of the ribosome, along with many polypeptide chains. One rRNA provides the catalytic function of the ribosome, which is a little odd. In most other cases, enzymes are made from polypeptides. Catalytic RNAs are also called **ribozymes** (or ribonucleic acid enzymes), since they are capable of performing specific biochemical reactions, similar to protein enzymes.

Some other interesting non-coding RNAs include the following:

- **Small nuclear RNA** (snRNA) molecules (150 nucleotides) associate with proteins to form snRNP (small nuclear ribonucleic particles) complexes in the spliceosome.
- **MicroRNA** (miRNA) and **small interfering RNA** (siRNA) function in RNA interference (RNAi), a form of post-transcriptional regulation of gene expression. Both can bind specific mRNA molecules to either increase or decrease translation.
- **Long ncRNAs** are longer than 200 nucleotides. They help control the basal transcription level in a cell by regulating initiation complex assembly on promoters. They also contribute to many types of post-transcriptional regulation, by controlling splicing and translation, and they function in imprinting and X-chromosome inactivation.

---

[20] Each tRNA must recognize a codon on mRNA and respond by delivering the appropriate amino acid to the ribosome. There are 20 different amino acids, so there at least 20 different tRNAs. However, there are 61 possible codons, so there could be as many as 61 different tRNAs. The actual number is between 20 and 61, because the third nucleotide of the codon is often not needed for specificity of the amino acid.

Chapter 7 Summary

- DNA is the fundamental unit of inheritance in cells.

- DNA and RNA are polymers, made of nucleotide monomers. A nucleotide contains phosphate group(s), a sugar (either deoxyribose for DNA or ribose for RNA), and a nitrogenous base, either a purine (adenine or guanine) or a pyrimidine (thymine, cytosine, or uracil).

- In DNA, adenine always pairs with thymine via two hydrogen bonds, and cytosine always pairs with guanine via three hydrogen bonds.

- Uracil replaces thymine in RNA, and the ribose in RNA has an OH group on carbon 2.

- DNA is supercoiled in prokaryotes and packaged around histone proteins in eukaryotes.

- Eukaryotic DNA is divided into several linear chromosomes which have unique structures including the long (q) and short (p) arms, centromere and telomeres on the ends.

- There are several types of RNA that do not encode proteins. Some are directly involved in translation (rRNA and tRNA), while others play a role in gene expression (snRNA, miRNA, siRNA).

CHAPTER 7 FREESTANDING PRACTICE QUESTIONS

1. A chromosome in metaphase is stained to look for patterns in gene expression. Both light and dark regions on the chromosome appear. All of the following are true of the lightly stained region EXCEPT that:

A) it is likely to contain genes that are being actively transcribed.

B) it is called euchromatin, and is densely wrapped around histone proteins.

C) it contains an octamer of histones, composed of 2 units each of H2A, H2B, H3 and H4.

D) it consists of double-helical DNA bound by a single histone between nucleosomes.

2. Why is the 2′ OH group removed from ribose in order to form the monosaccharide component of DNA?

A) It ensures proper purine-purine pairing.

B) It converts a nucleoside into a nucleotide.

C) It sets up a phosphodiester bond.

D) It creates greater stability in the molecule.

3. High temperatures and some chemicals can separate (denature) two strands of antiparallel, complementary DNA. Which of the following accounts for the separation of double-stranded DNA after applying heat?

A) Disruption of the hydrogen bonds between pyrimidines and purines

B) Breakage of the phosphodiester bond between pyrimidines and purines

C) Disruption of the antiparallel nature of DNA strands

D) Disturbance in the hydrophobic forces between bases

4. Which of the following accurately describes the function of the centromere?

A) It is an attachment point for the synaptonemal complex during mitosis.

B) It is a cytoplasmic organelle that serves as an organizing center for microtubules.

C) It directly binds homologous chromosomes during meiosis.

D) It is an attachment point for spindle fibers via kinetochores.

5. DNA helicase is an enzyme that uses ATP to separate two complementary DNA strands during the replication process. Which of the following strands of DNA would require the most energy to separate from its complementary strand?

A) ATATATATAT

B) CCCGTAAAAT

C) CCGGCGTATA

D) ATCGATCGAT

6. What is a defining characteristic of heterogeneous nuclear RNA (hnRNA)?

A) It has a methylated guanine cap on the 5′ end.

B) It has a sequence containing introns and exons.

C) It contains uracil.

D) It has a poly A sequence on the 3′ end.

7. Shelterin is a protein complex involved in stabilizing the loop formed by the last approximately 300 bp of DNA at the end of eukaryotic chromosomes. A cell is found with mutations in the genes that code for shelterin. The most likely direct effect(s) of these mutations would be:

I. activation of DNA repair pathways due to exposure of single-stranded DNA.

II. an increase in double-stranded TTAGGG repeats.

III. deletion of genes in the telomere regions.

A) I only

B) II and III only

C) I and III only

D) I, II and III

CHAPTER 7 PRACTICE PASSAGE

Antibiotic resistance presents an increasingly concerning problem for infectious disease management around the world. Perhaps one of the more disappointing recent trends is an increase in resistance to fluoroquinolone antibiotics. Well-tolerated with a minimal side effect profile, drugs from this class have been widely-prescribed for numerous infections, ranging from pneumonias to urinary tract infections. The main action of this class drug focuses on inhibiting DNA gyrase, an enzyme found in bacteria, but not humans. More specifically, the mechanism of action focuses on disruption of DNA replication by inhibiting the DNA topoisomerase II gyrase and ligase domains, while leaving nuclease activity intact. Acquisition of resistance to fluoroquinolones is typically associated with mutations, leading to structural changes in these proteins, increased expression of porins associated with decreased drug accumulation, as well as genes encoding peptides that directly block fluoroquinolone action.

In bacteria, gyrase utilizes the energy from ATP hydrolysis to relieve strain on the DNA double helix, while helicase unwinds it. The enzyme accomplishes this goal by generating double-stranded breaks with subsequent chiral wrapping of the strands to form a negative supercoil. Gyrase also relaxes any positive supercoils, allowing for unidirectional coiling across the whole DNA strand. Positive supercoiling is characterized by additional twisting and coiling in the same direction as the helix, whereas negative supercoiling are twists in the opposite direction. When able to bind to DNA topoisomerase II, fluoroquinolones disrupt these functions, resulting in the accumulation of positive supercoiling and increased strain on the DNA strand. Similarly, additional inhibition of the ligase domain by fluoroquinolones prevents DNA topoisomerase from repairing any breaks, further compromising the structure of the double-stranded molecule.

The structure of DNA gyrase consists of an A_2B_2 tetramer whose A and B subunits are encoded by the *gyrA* and *gyrB* genes. Generally speaking, the A subunit is responsible for inducing double-stranded breaks, while the B subunit facilitates the ATPase activity. Shown in Figure 1, the general mechanism of action by which supercoiling is induced involves creating a break in the first DNA strand (G) by forming a transient "gate" through which the second (T) strand can be "transported." It is generally accepted that fluoroquinolones inhibit DNA gyrase activity directly by forming a ternary complex with the enzyme that stabilizes it and prevents it from religating the broken DNA strands. The resulting fragmentation of chromosomal DNA ultimately leads to cell death.

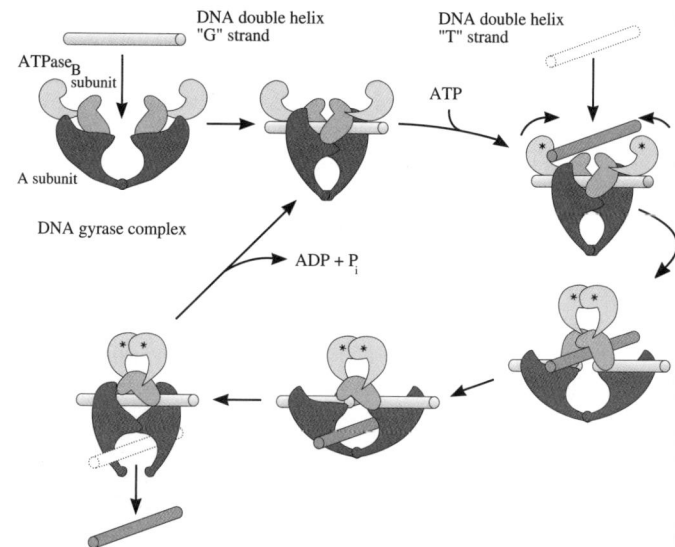

Figure 1   Schematic of DNA gyrase structure and function

Microbiologists examining the genetic origins of fluoroquinolone resistance in *Mycobacterium tuberculosis* looked at the relative effect of multiple different mutations in the *gyrA* and *gyrB* genes on (1) the minimum inhibitory concentration (MIC) and (2) the resistance to ofloxacin, a second generation fluoroquinolone. The data pertaining to one potentially important instance are shown in Table 1.

gyrA mutation	*gyrB* mutation	MIC (mg/L)	Susceptibility
D89N	None	5	Resistant
None	N533T	1	Susceptible
None	None	4	Resistant

Table 1   Select MIC and susceptibility data for mutant and wild-type *Mycobacterium tuberculosis*

The MIC is characterized as the lowest concentration of antibiotic that will inhibit measurable bacterial growth after incubation.

Adapted from: Fabrega, A., et al. *Mechanism of action of and resistance to quinolones* and van Groll, A., et al. *Fluoroquinolone resistance in Mycobacterium tuberculosis and mutations in gyrA and gyrB.*

1. Which of the following bonds in DNA is the most likely target of DNA gyrase?

A) Hydrogen bond between aromatic bases
B) 5′–3′ phosphodiester bond between nucleotides
C) 4′ C–O covalent bond in deoxyribose
D) 1′ C–N covalent bond between deoxyribose and base

2. Based on information presented in the passage, which of the following statements is most likely to be true?

A) The hydrolysis of ATP is required to cut and religate the DNA double helix.
B) The toxicity of fluoroquinolones in humans is likely to be high due to an increased number of double-stranded breaks resulting from inhibition of DNA gyrase activity.
C) The formation of chromatin in bacteria is likely to be inhibited by fluoroquinolones due to characteristic disruption of orderly supercoiling.
D) The overall efficiency with which DNA is stored in the bacterial genome is disrupted by the action of fluoroquinolone antibiotics.

3. Which of the following is LEAST likely to be a driver of fluoroquinolone resistance in bacteria?

A) Adaptation characterized by increased expression of cell membrane efflux pumps
B) Mutations that lead to downregulation of the nuclease activity of topoisomerase
C) Mutations inducing structural changes in DNA gyrase
D) Transmission of code for direct fluoroquinolone inhibitor protein by plasmid

4. Which of the following conclusions is NOT supported by the data shown in Table 1?

A) Structural changes in any of the *gyr* genes result in increased fluoroquinolone resistance.
B) D89N mutation in the *gyrA* gene may result in a structural change that prevents fluoroquinolone binding.
C) N533T mutation in the *gyrB* gene may result in a structural change that further stabilizes the gyrase-DNA complex.
D) Not all mutations in the *gyr* genes result in increased fluoroquinolone resistance.

5. Which of the following graphs most accurately represents the effects of fluoroquinolones with increasing drug concentration?

A)
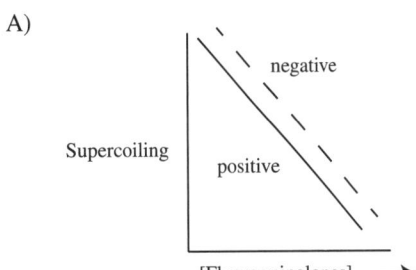

B)
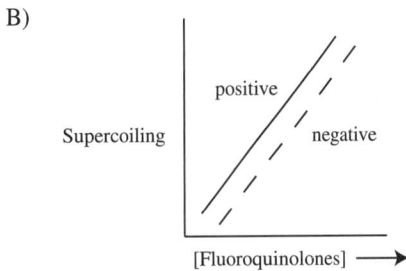

C)
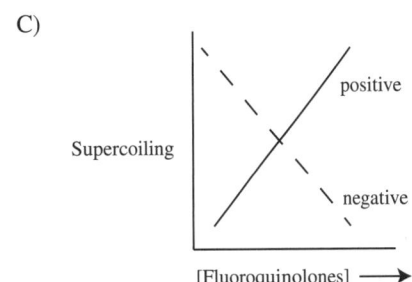

D)
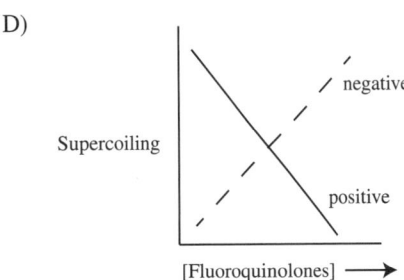

SOLUTIONS TO CHAPTER 7 FREESTANDING PRACTICE QUESTIONS

1. **B** Make sure to highlight the word "EXCEPT" and write "A B C D" on your noteboard. Then evaluate each answer choice, writing "T" if it is true or "F" if it is false. The lightly stained regions of the chromosome are called euchromatin, which is thought to contain genes that are being actively transcribed into RNA (write "T" next to "A" on the noteboard). This is because the DNA is loosely wrapped around histone proteins, making it more accessible for transcription machinery (write "F" next to "B" on the noteboard). Chromatin is wrapped around eight histone proteins (write "T" next to "C" on the noteboard), called a nucleosome, and is punctuated by regions of ds-DNA between each nucleosome (write "T" next to "D" on the noteboard). Since choice B stands out with an "F" instead of a "T", it is the correct answer choice.

2. **D** Using deoxyribose (a ribose with the 2' OH removed) generates greater stability in DNA, which is important because DNA, rather than RNA, is the primary form of long-term storage for genomes; certain viruses are a notable exception (choice D is correct). The OH group is not involved in base pairing, and, in any case, purines are meant to pair with pyrimidines (choice A is wrong). A nucleoside becomes a nucleotide when the phosphate is attached (choice B is wrong). The phosphodiester bond is formed between nucleotides using the phosphate backbone, not the 2' OH group (choice C is wrong).

3. **A** Two strands of antiparallel and complementary DNA are held together in a helix by hydrogen bonding between pyrimidines and purines. As per the question stem, high temperatures can lead to the separation of strands, therefore the disruption of the hydrogen bonds. Phosphodiester bonds hold together the nucleotide backbone in a single strand of DNA, and are broken by nucleases rather than heat (choice B is wrong). Heat would not affect the propensity for a 5'-3' DNA strands to bind with a complementary strand in 3'-5' orientation (choice C is wrong). While heat does affect hydrophobic forces between bases, these forces serve to stabilize the DNA double helix, rather than directly bind the two strands together (choice D is wrong).

4. **D** The centromere is a region on the chromosome between sister chromatids. The synaptonemal complex is formed during meiosis, when there is pairing of homologous chromosomes, not mitosis (choice A is wrong). The cytoplasmic organelle that serves as an organizing center for microtubules is the centrosome, made up of two centrioles, not the centromere (choice B is false). Pairs of homologous chromosomes are held together by the synaptonemal complex proteins that anchor to the centromere, rather than the centromere binding the pairs directly (choice C is false). Centromeres serve as an attachment point for spindle fibers to mediate cell division (choice D is correct).

5. **C** There are three hydrogen bonds between cytosine (C) and guanine (G) base pairs, and only two hydrogen bonds between adenine (A) and thymine (T) pairs. Thus the strand with the most C:G base pairs will require the most energy to separate it from its complementary strand (choices A, B and D are incorrect; choice C is the answer).

6. **B** Heterogeneous nuclear RNA (hnRNA) is a precursor to mature RNA sequences that have had introns removed and exons spliced together; thus it can contain both types of sequence (choice B is correct). The presence of a methylated guanine cap indicates a fully modified transcript (choice A is wrong), as does the presence of poly-A tail (choice D is wrong). Uracil is a nucleotide used in all types of RNA and is not specific to hnRNA (choice C is wrong).

7. **A** Since this is a Roman numeral question, start by analyzing the Roman numeral item that appears in exactly two answer choices (in this case Item II); whether it is true or false you can eliminate half the answers. Item II is false: while telomere regions do contain TTAGGG repeats, active telomerase is responsible for adding these nucleotides. Not all cells express telomerase, and in any case this would not be affected by mutations shelterin (choices B and D can be eliminated). Since both remaining answer choices include Item I, it must be true and you can focus on Item III. Item III is false: there are no genes in the telomere regions, just many repeats of TTAGGG (choice C can be eliminated and choice A is correct). Note that Item I is in fact true: the very end segment of eukaryotic telomeres contains single-stranded DNA that forms a loop, which is stabilized by shelterin proteins, as per the question stem. If the shelterin complex is disrupted, it is likely that DNA repair pathways would be activated due to exposure of single-stranded DNA.

SOLUTIONS TO CHAPTER 7 PRACTICE PASSAGE

1. **B** The transient double-stranded breaks introduced by DNA gyrase involve the phosphodiester bonds that comprise the linkage between nucleotides. The breakage of none of the other bonds included in the answer choices would allow for one double helix to "pass through" another, as shown in Figure 1 (choice B is correct). Since the two strands of the double helix are not being separated, hydrogen bonds between bases will not be affected (choice A is wrong). Breakages of a single covalent bond within the deoxyribose ring or between deoxyribose and a base would not only be difficult and likely energetically unfavorable, it also wouldn't allow for the creation of the "gate" needed for DNA gyrase function (choices C and D are wrong).

2. **D** One major impact on the bacterial genome caused by the introduction of fluoroquinolones is the disruption of the uniform, orderly supercoiling process described in the passage; because this process is essential for efficient packaging and storage of bacterial DNA, its disruption would certainly reduce efficiency of storage of DNA in the bacterial genome (choice D is correct). As shown in Figure 1, hydrolysis of ATP comes after the helices have been cut and religated; the energy from ATP hydrolysis is most likely used to "reset" the enzyme to its original state after it has accomplished the cut/ligate action (choice A is wrong). Though there are some side effects in humans associated with fluoroquinolone administration, the main action of fluoroquinolone antibiotics focuses on disrupting the function of DNA gyrase, an enzyme not found in humans (choice B is wrong). Bacterial DNA is stored in the form of supercoiled circular DNA molecules, not the more complex chromatin-histone complexes found in eukaryotes (choice C is wrong).

3. **B** The increased expression of efflux pumps would likely reduce the intracellular concentration of an antibiotic, reducing its effect on gyrase activity and driving resistance (choice A is a driver of resistance and can be eliminated). The passage states that mutations in the code for DNA gyrase that result in structural alterations can lead to fluoroquinolone resistance (choice C is a driver in resistance and can be eliminated). Transmission of genetic code via plasmid is a commonly cited mechanism for transferring adaptive characteristics in bacteria (choice D is a driver of resistance and can be eliminated). However, simply downregulating the nuclease activity of DNA topoisomerase is unlikely to affect resistance. There is no reason to assume the drug can't bind just because the activity of the enzyme is slowed (choice B is least likely to drive resistance and is the correct answer).

4. **A** The data presented in Table 1 provides an important example that not all mutations in the *gyr* genes result in fluoroquinolone resistance; the *gyrB* mutation shown may actually increase susceptibility of the strain tested (choice A is not supported by the data and is the correct answer choice). While the increase in MIC for the D89N mutated strain is modest (5 mg/L) with respect to that for the non-mutated strain (4 mg/L), it is certainly possible that this mutation prevents fluoroquinolone binding. If the drug can't bind, the organism would be resistant (choice B is supported and can be eliminated). The passage states that fluoroquinolones stabilize the DNA-gyrase complex, and the table shows that the N533T mutation leads to a relative decrease in MIC, indicating increased susceptibility to the drug. Thus, it might be concluded that this mutation helps to stabilize the complex, thereby helping the action of the fluoroquinolones (choice C is supported and can be eliminated). This data does support the conclusion that not all mutations in *gyr* genes confer fluoroquinolone resistance; based on this data alone, it appears that some mutations may actually increase susceptibility (choice D is supported and can be eliminated).

5. **C** The passage states that fluoroquinolones disrupt the ability of DNA gyrase to introduce negative supercoils; therefore, the number of negative supercoils should decrease (choices B and D can be eliminated). This would lead to an accumulation of positive supercoils (choice A can be eliminated, and choice C is correct).

JOURNAL ARTICLE 3

A HIGHLY DURABLE RNAi THERAPEUTIC INHIBITOR OF PCSK9

Kevin Fitzgerald, Ph.D., Suellen White, B.S.N., Anna Borodovsky, Ph.D., Brian R. Bettencourt, Ph.D., Andrew Strahs, Ph.D., Valerie Clausen, Ph.D., Peter Wijngaard, Ph.D., Jay D. Horton, M.D., Jorg Taubel, M.D., Ashley Brooks, M.B., Ch.B., Chamikara Fernando, M.B., B.S., Robert S. Kauffman, M.D., Ph.D., David Kallend, M.D., Akshay Vaishnaw, M.D., and Amy Simon, M.D.

This article was published on November 13, 2016, at NEJM.org.

N Engl J Med 2017;376:41-51. DOI: 10.1056/NEJMoa1609243 Copyright © 2016 Massachusetts Medical Society.

An elevated level of low-density lipoprotein (LDL) cholesterol is a major risk factor for cardiovascular disease. Despite the use of statin therapy, alone or in combination with other lipid-lowering medications, many at-risk patients continue to have elevated levels of LDL cholesterol. Hence, there is a need for additional treatment options for lowering of the LDL cholesterol level to reduce cardiovascular risk.

Proprotein convertase subtilisin–kexin type 9 (PCSK9) is a recently identified but well-validated target for LDL cholesterol–lowering therapy. This serine protease, which is expressed and secreted into the bloodstream predominantly by the liver, binds LDL receptors both intracellularly and extracellularly and promotes the lysosomal degradation of these receptors in hepatocytes, thereby increasing the circulating LDL cholesterol levels. *PCSK9* loss-of-function mutations are associated with low circulating LDL cholesterol levels and diminished cardiovascular risk with no apparent negative health consequences.

PCSK9-blocking antibodies, administered once or twice monthly, reduce circulating PCSK9 levels and lower LDL cholesterol levels. Preliminary data suggest that long-term treatment with such antibodies is associated with a lower incidence of cardiovascular events than placebo. However, PCSK9 antibodies have a short duration of effect, necessitating frequent subcutaneous injections.

A recently discovered means of decreasing PCSK9 levels is the administration of small interfering RNA (siRNA) molecules. The siRNA molecules engage the natural pathway of RNA interference (RNAi) by binding intracellularly to the RNA-induced silencing complex (RISC), enabling it to cleave messenger RNA (mRNA) molecules encoding PCSK9 specifically. The cleaved mRNA is degraded and thus unavailable for protein translation, which results in decreased levels of the PCSK9 protein. A single siRNA-bound RISC is catalytic and cleaves many transcripts. This characteristic may be important during use of statins, which are known to up-regulate the production of PCSK9, potentially limiting the effectiveness of the drugs. The lipid nanoparticle ALN-PCS, an intravenous formulation of siRNA that inhibits PCSK9 synthesis, has been shown in a small phase 1 study to reduce the levels of both PCSK9 and LDL cholesterol in adult volunteers.

Inclisiran (ALN-PCSsc) is a long-acting, subcutaneously delivered, synthetic siRNA directed against PCSK9 that is conjugated to triantennary *N*-acetylgalactosamine carbohydrates. These carbohydrates bind to abundant liver-expressed asialoglycoprotein receptors, leading to inclisiran uptake specifically into hepatocytes. The siRNA was modified with a combination of phosphorothioate, 2′-*O*-methyl nucleotide, and 2′-fluoronucleotide modifications to improve molecular stability. In preclinical studies involving nonhuman primates, doses of more than 3 mg per kilogram of body weight resulted in reductions of more than 80% in plasma PCSK9 levels and approximately 60% lowering of the serum LDL cholesterol level, with peak effects lasting more than 30 days, with a very slow return to baseline levels over a period of 90 to 120 days after administration (unpublished data). This phase 1 study assessed the safety, side-effect profile, and pharmacodynamic effects of inclisiran when it was administered subcutaneously in single or multiple doses in healthy volunteers who had an LDL cholesterol level of at least 100 mg per deciliter (2.60 mmol per liter) and in a small number of participants taking a stable dose of statin cotherapy.

METHODS

Study Design and Oversight

We conducted this randomized, single-blind, placebo-controlled study in two stages — a single-dose phase (with ascending doses for sequential cohorts of patients), followed by a multiple-dose phase.

The study was performed at two contract research sites in the United Kingdom (Richmond Pharmacology and Covance). Data were collected by the investigators and analyzed by Covance and Alnylam Pharmaceuticals.

Participants

Men and women (18 to 60 years of age in the single-dose phase and 18 to 75 years of age in the multiple-dose phase) who had a serum LDL cholesterol level of at least 100 mg per deciliter and a fasting triglyceride level of less than 400 mg per deciliter (4.5 mmol per liter) were eligible. Participants taking statin therapy had to have been receiving a stable statin dose and regimen for at least 30 days before screening and had to have no planned changes during the study. Participants were not specifically instructed to maintain a stable dietary pattern. Participants with a history of cardiovascular disease, cerebrovascular disease, or diabetes mellitus were excluded except for those who were taking statins; such patients could be enrolled if they had noninsulindependent diabetes mellitus or controlled hypertension.

Randomization and Study Treatment

In the single-dose phase, six cohorts (with four participants each) were included. Participants in each cohort were randomly assigned in a 3:1 ratio to receive a subcutaneous injection of either inclisiran at a dose of 25, 100, 300, 500, or 800 mg (two cohorts for the 800-mg dose) or placebo.

In the multiple-dose phase, the participants in six cohorts (with four to eight participants each) were randomly assigned in a 3:1 ratio with the use of block sizes of four to receive inclisiran or placebo. One cohort received a dose of 125 mg once per week for 4 weeks, one cohort received a dose of 250 mg once every 2 weeks for 4 weeks, two cohorts (one of which was receiving statin therapy) received a dose of 300 mg once per month for 2 months, and two cohorts (one of which was receiving statin therapy) received a dose of 500 mg once per month for 2 months.

In the two phases, the first dose was administered on the day of randomization (day 0). Inclisiran or placebo (administered in sterile 0.9% normal saline) was injected subcutaneously into one or more sites of the abdomen; dose volumes of more than 1.5 ml were administered in two to three injections of equal volume. Inclisiran was supplied at a dose of 200 mg per milliliter of sterile solution. Participants were unaware of the assigned treatment because of syringe masking. No participant was included in more than one cohort.

Evaluations

Participants were monitored as inpatients for 3 days, with day −1 considered to be the day before initial administration. Participants underwent randomization and treatment commenced on day 0. Participants were evaluated as outpatients for safety, side-effect profile, and pharmacodynamic end points at specified times throughout the study period (56 days for the single-dose phase, and ≤84 days for the multiple-dose phase). Pharmacodynamic end points were evaluated for an additional month after the completion of the safety and side-effect profile assessments.

Participants were considered to have completed the trial according to the protocol after their final planned safety and pharmacodynamic follow-up visit. If at that visit the most recent three LDL cholesterol levels averaged less than 80% of the baseline value, pharmacodynamic monitoring continued every 2 weeks for 1 month, and then every 4 weeks, until the more recent three LDL cholesterol measurements averaged 80% or more of the baseline value or until 180 days after the last dose of inclisiran or placebo, whichever came sooner.

The safety evaluation included clinical laboratory tests (hematologic, biochemical, coagulation, and urinalysis tests), vital signs (oral body temperature, blood pressure, heart rate, and respiration rate), physical examination, 12-lead electrocardiography (ECG), and adverse-event monitoring.

Pharmacodynamic monitoring included plasma PCSK9 and serum LDL cholesterol measurements. The exploratory biomarkers that were evaluated included levels of total cholesterol, high-density lipoprotein (HDL) cholesterol, non-HDL cholesterol (total cholesterol level minus the HDL cholesterol level), apolipoprotein B, lipoprotein(a), and triglycerides.

Statistical Analysis

In each study phase, data from the participants in the placebo group were combined across cohorts for analysis. The mean percent reductions in the plasma PCSK9 level, as compared with baseline, at day 84 after the first dose of the study regimen were compared with those in the placebo group by means of a repeated-measures analysis of covariance (ANCOVA), including the baseline PCSK9 level as a covariate, and treatment-by-time interaction. The model used an autoregressive first-order covariance structure. This method was also used for the lipid data. A nominal P value of less than 0.05 was considered to indicate statistical significance.

RESULTS

Participants

The characteristics of the participants at baseline, according to study phase and assigned group, in the safety population are shown in Table 1.

Safety and Side-Effect Profile

All the adverse events were mild or moderate (grade 1 or 2) in severity. There were no treatment discontinuations that were due to adverse events, and no serious adverse events were reported.

PCSK9 Levels

In the single-dose phase, inclisiran at a dose of 300 mg or more was associated with reductions from baseline in the PCSK9 level that were significant, as compared with placebo, at day 84 (Table 2 and Fig. 1A). The magnitudes of the reduction in the PCSK9 level were similar across the dose range of 300 to 800 mg (least-squares mean change, 69.9 to 74.5%); the largest reduction, 74.5%, occurred in the group that was treated with 300 mg of inclisiran. PCSK9 levels had returned to baseline values by day 180 after the receipt of the dose in the 25-mg and 100-mg cohorts. For inclisiran doses of 300 mg or more, the PCSK9 levels remained reduced, as compared with baseline, at day 180 after receipt of the dose (Fig. 1A).

In the multiple-dose phase, all the inclisiran regimens were associated with reductions from baseline in the PCSK9 level that were significant, as compared with placebo, at day 84 after receipt of the first dose (Table 3 and Fig. 1B). The magnitude of the reductions in the PCSK9 level were similar across all the inclisiran cohorts, with the least-squares mean change from baseline ranging from 71.8 to 83.8% at day 84 after receipt of the first dose; the largest reduction, 83.8%, was observed in the group that received 500 mg of inclisiran once per month for 2 months as well as statin cotherapy. Levels of PCSK9 remained reduced, as compared with baseline, in all the inclisiran cohorts at day 196 after receipt of the first dose (Fig. 1B).

LDL Cholesterol Levels

In the single-dose phase, reductions from baseline in the LDL cholesterol level that were significant, as compared with placebo, were observed at day 84 after receipt of inclisiran doses of 100 mg or more (Table 2 and Fig. 2A). At these doses, the least-squares mean reductions in the LDL cholesterol level ranged from 36.7 to 50.6%; the largest reduction, 50.6%, was observed in the group that received 500 mg of inclisiran. The LDL cholesterol levels returned toward baseline values at 180 days after receipt of the dose in the 25-mg and 100-mg cohorts, whereas the levels remained reduced, as compared with baseline, until at least 180 days after receipt of inclisiran doses of 300 mg or more (Fig. 2A).

In the multiple-dose phase, reductions in the LDL cholesterol level that were significant, as compared with placebo, were observed at day 84 after receipt of the first dose for all inclisiran regimens except for the cohort that received 125 mg weekly for 4 weeks. Reductions ranged from a least-squares mean change of 45.1 to 59.7%, with the largest reduction, 59.7%, occurring in the group that received 300 mg of inclisiran monthly for 2 months (Table 3 and Fig. 2B). The LDL cholesterol levels remained reduced, as compared with baseline, in all the inclisiran cohorts at day 196 after receipt of the first dose (Fig. 2B).

Exploratory Analyses

In both the single-dose and multiple-dose phases, decreases in the levels of total cholesterol, non-HDL cholesterol, and apolipoprotein B were noted in participants treated with inclisiran (Tables 2 and 3). The reductions in these variables from baseline to day 84 after receipt of the first dose were significant, as compared with placebo, for single or multiple doses of 250 mg or more.

Table 1 Demographic and Clinical Characteristics of the Participants at Baseline (Safety Population)*

| Characteristic | Single-Dose Phase | | Multiple-Dose Phase | | | |
| | | | Placebo | | Inclisiran | |
	Placebo (N = 6)	Inclisiran (N = 18)	with statin (N = 4)†	without statin (N = 8)	with statin (N = 9)‡	without statin (N = 24)
Age — yr	48 ± 14	46 ± 10	58 ± 3	51 ± 14	54 ± 16	51 ± 12
Male sex —no. (%)	2 (33)	17 (94)	2 (50)	6 (75)	4 (44)	17 (71)
Race —no. (%)						
White	4 (67)	12 (67)	4 (100)	7 (88)	6 (67)	19 (79)
Other	2 (33)	6 (33)	0	1 (12)	3 (33)	5 (21)
Weight —kg	70.6 ± 12.0	77.1 ± 7.7	74.3 ± 5.1	77.6 ± 10.3	77.7 ± 17.0	74.7 ± 11.7
Height —cm	168 ± 11	173 ± 6	168 ± 10	171 ± 9	171 ± 12	171 ± 8
LDL cholesterol —mg/dl	131.5 ± 19.3	163.0 ± 32.9	143.1 ± 89.7	131.5 ± 20.9	143.4 ± 29.8	139.3 ± 32.3
Triglycerides —mg/dl	70.9 ± 12.4	135.5 ± 55.7	150.6 ± 46.9	124.0 ± 38.1	116.3 ± 64.3	123.4 ± 82.9
PCSK9 —µg/liter	279.0 ± 99.5	275.4 ± 58.2	460.7 ± 56.3	276.2 ± 58.7	451.8 ± 132.2	317.1 ± 66.8

* Plus–minus values are means ±SD.

† Three participants were taking simvastatin at a dose of 40 mg per day, and one was taking pravastatin at a dose of 20 mg per day.

‡ Four participants were taking atorvastatin at a dose of 40 mg per day, two at a dose of 20 mg per day, and one at a dose of 10 mg per day; one participant was taking simvastatin at a dose of 40 mg per day and one at a dose of 20 mg per day.

Table 2 Least-Squares Mean Percent Change from Baseline in Pharmacodynamic Variables at Day 84 in the Single-Dose Phase (Pharmacodynamic Population)*

| Variable | Placebo (N = 6) | Inclisiran | | | | |
		25 mg (N = 3)	100 mg (N = 3)	300 mg (N = 3)	500 mg (N = 3)	800 mg (N = 6)
PCSK9						
Percent change (95% CI)	0.6 (−24.2 to 30.4)	46.6 (−65.4 to −17.8)†	32.0 (−52.5 to −2.7)	74.5 (−82.1 to −63.6)‡	69.9 (−78.9 to −57.0)‡	73.1 (−79.1 to −65.4)‡
LDL cholesterol						
Percent change (95% CI)	10.9 (−26.0 to 7.1)	21.5 (−41.3 to 5.0)	36.7 (−50.2 to −19.4)†	50.0 (−60.7 to −36.3)‡	50.6 (−61.3 to −36.9)‡	43.4 (−52.5 to −32.4)‡
Total cholesterol						
Percent change (95% CI)	4.4 (−15.9 to 8.7)	12.0 (−30.1 to 10.8)	17.7 (−30.0 to −3.4)	30.9 (−41.2 to −18.9)¶	27.1 (−38.2 to −14.0)†	29.1 (−36.8 to −20.6)¶
HDL cholesterol						
Percent change (95% CI)	13.6 (−9.2 to 42.1)	7.3 (−22.0 to 47.7)	17.9 (−9.2 to 53.1)	36.8 (2.9 to 82.0)	7.4 (−17.4 to 39.8)	0.1 (−16.8 to 20.5)
Non-HDL cholesterol						
Percent change (95% CI)	11.7 (−23.7 to 2.3)	19.8 (−36.1 to 0.6)	28.4 (−40.8 to −13.5)	48.9 (−57.8 to −38.2)‡	36.3 (−47.4 to −22.9)¶	37.0 (−44.9 to −28.0)¶
Apolipoprotein B						
Percent change (95% CI)	15.3 (−31.4 to 4.6)	11.3 (−36.8 to 24.5)	26.5 (−43.3 to −4.7)	47.1 (−59.0 to −31.9)¶	39.9 (−53.9 to −21.7)†	37.5 (−47.7 to −25.2)†
Lipoprotein (a)						
Percent change (95% CI)	3.6 (−28.6 to 50.2)	14.0 (−55.1 to 64.6)	20.8 (−51.0 to 28.0)	44.5 (−65.7 to −10.4)†	35.5 (−60.1 to 4.3)	21.3 (−45.0 to 12.6)

Differences shown in the inclisiran groups are with the placebo group. CI denotes confidence interval, and HDL high-density lipoprotein.

† P<0.05 for the pairwise comparison with placebo.

‡ P<0.001 for the pairwise comparison with placebo.

§ The group nadir was defined as the largest mean percent reduction from the baseline value during the study.

¶ P < 0.01 for the pairwise comparison with placebo.

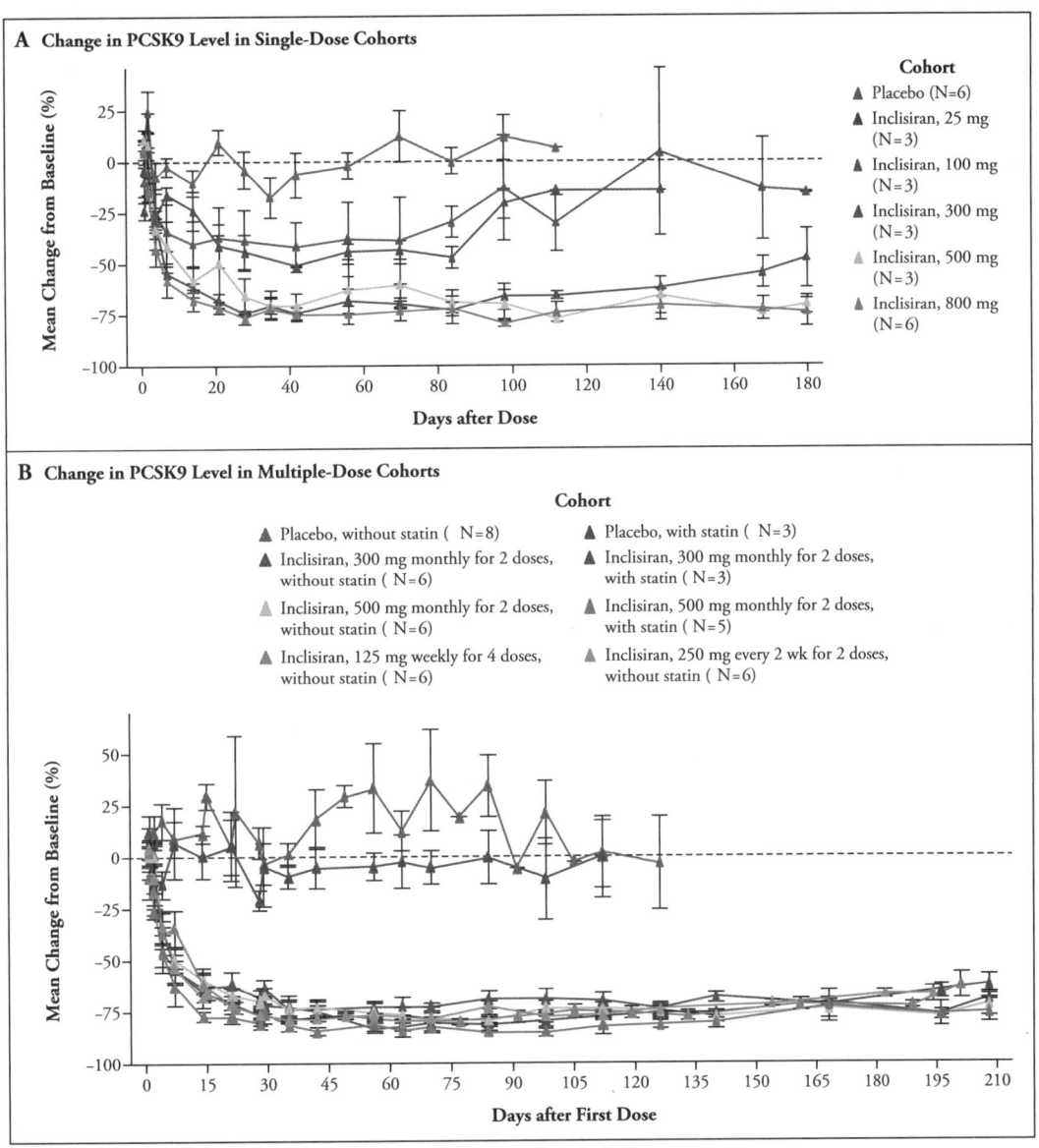

Figure 1. Change in Plasma Levels of Proprotein Convertase Subtilisin–Kexin Type 9 (PCSK9), According to Study Group and Dose Cohort. Shown are the effects (mean percentage changes from baseline) of single or multiple doses of inclisiran or placebo on plasma levels of PCSK9 over time. Baseline values were the average of all the study measurements obtained before the first dose.

Table 3 Least-Squares Mean Percent Change from Baseline in Pharmacodynamic Variables at Day 84 after the First Dose in the Multiple-Dose Phase (Pharmacodynamic Population)*

Variable	Placebo (N = 11)	Inclisiran					
		300 mg with Statin (N = 3)	300 mg without Statin (N = 6)	500 mg with Statin (N = 5)	500 mg without Statin (N = 6)	125 mg without Statin (N = 6)	250 mg without Statin (N = 6)
PCSK9							
Percent change (95% CI)	16.9 (−2.4 to 40.0)	−79.9 (−85.4 to −72.5)†	−71.8 (−77.4 to −64.8)†	−83.8 (−87.3 to −79.3)†	−81.5 (−85.2 to −76.9)†	−77.4 (−81.9 to −71.8)†	−75.7 (−80.5 to −69.6)†
LDL cholesterol							
Percent change (95% CI)	−14.2 (−30.2 to 5.5)	−45.1 (−61.6 to −21.4)‡	−59.7 (−68.7 to −48.1)†	−53.2 (−64.5 to −38.3)§	−51.7 (−62.5 to −37.8)§	−39.8 (−51.1 to −25.9)	−52.2 (−62.9 to −38.4)§
Total cholesterol							
Percent change (95% CI)	−7.6 (−15.5 to 1.0)	−24.9 (−35.8 to −12.0)‡	−40.4 (−46.7 to −33.4)†	−30.4 (−38.4 to −21.3)†	−27.0 (−34.7 to −18.3)§	−23.8 (−31.9 to −14.7)	−34.5 (−41.4 to −26.7)†
HDL cholesterol							
Percent change (95% CI)	0.6 (−6.0 to 7.6)	10.8 (−1.5 to 24.6)	11.7 (2.7 to 21.4)	5.3 (−3.9 to 15.3)	12.8 (3.8 to 22.6)‡	12.9 (3.8 to 22.7)	12.9 (−4.2 to 13.1)
Non-HDL cholesterol							
Percent change (95% CI)	−10.6 (−21.3 to 1.6)	−35.7 (−48.7 to −19.3)‡	−56.9 (−63.3 to −49.4)†	−46.2 (−54.9 to −35.8)†	−45.1 (−53.3 to −35.5)†	−36.9 (−46.3 to −25.9)	−45.3 (−53.4 to −35.8)†
Apolipoprotein B							
Percent change (95% CI)	−12.8 (−23.2 to −1.0)	−37.2 (−49.8 to −21.4)‡	−52.4 (−59.4 to −44.2)†	−41.8 (−51.1 to −30.7)†	−46.4 (−54.3 to −37.2)†	−33.3 (−43.1 to −21.8)	−46.5 (−54.3 to −37.3)†
Lipoprotein (a)							
Percent change (95% CI)	−6.0 (−26.7 to 20.4)	−30.7 (−54.3 to 5.1)	−19.2 (−40.0 to 8.8)	−42.7 (−59.7 to −18.4)‡	−27.4 (−45.8 to −2.7)	−22.7 (−28.4 to −16.5)‡	−28.1 (−46.4 to −3.4)

Differences shown in the inclisiran groups are with the placebo group.

† P<0.001 for the pairwise comparison with placebo.

‡ P<0.05 for the pairwise comparison with placebo.

§ P<0.01 for the pairwise comparison with placebo.

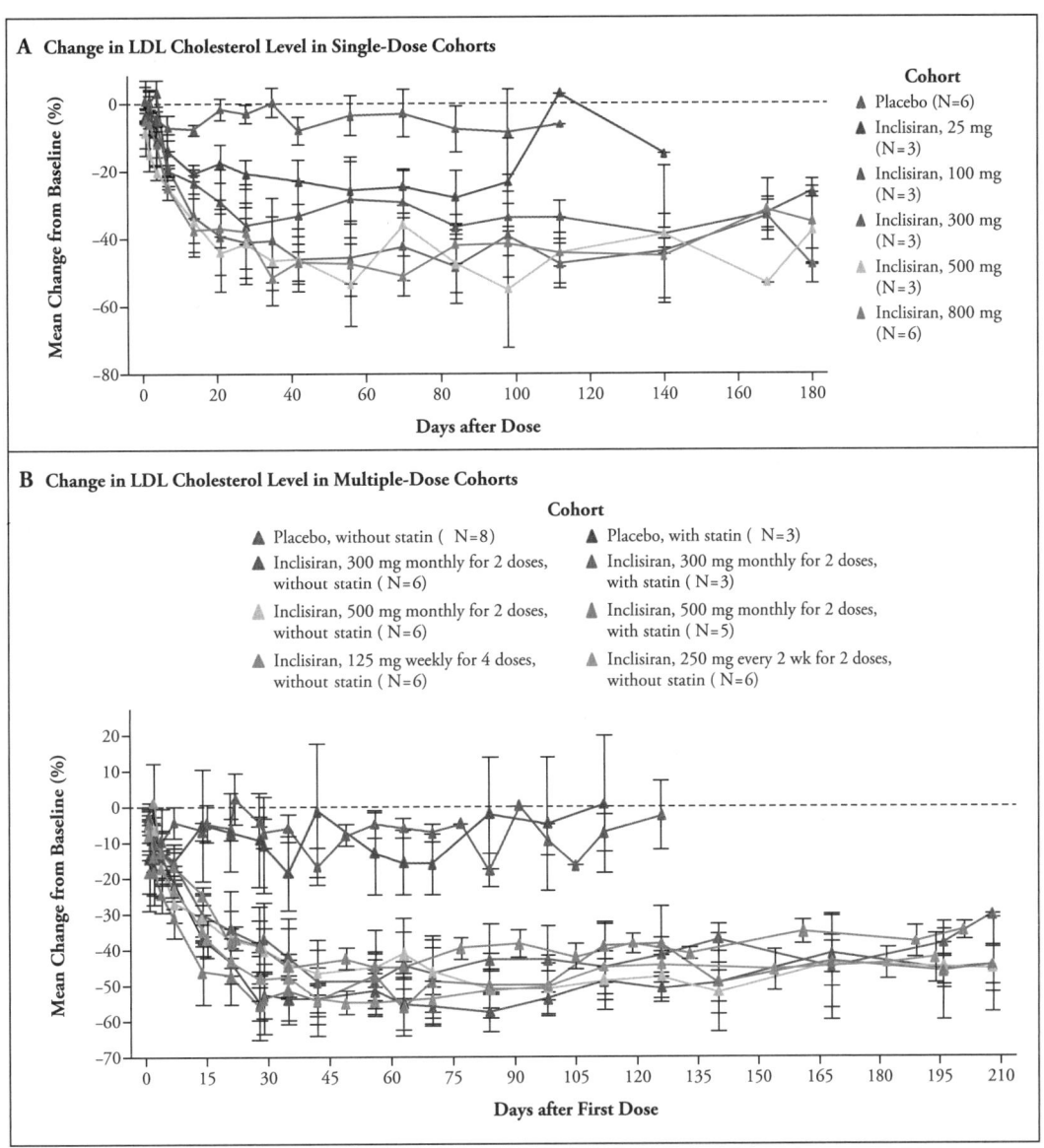

Figure 2. Effects on Serum Levels of Low-Density Lipoprotein (LDL) Cholesterol, According to Study Group and Dose Cohort. Shown are the effects (mean percentage changes from baseline) of inclisiran or placebo on the serum levels of LDL cholesterol over time. Baseline values were the average of all the study measurements taken before the first dose.

DISCUSSION

In this study, treatment with inclisiran, a subcutaneously administered RNAi therapeutic agent targeting PCSK9 to reduce LDL cholesterol levels, resulted in no treatment discontinuations due to adverse events and no serious adverse events at the doses we studied. All the adverse events were mild or moderate in severity.

Single doses of inclisiran of 300 mg or more and all the multiple-dose regimens that we studied were associated with reductions of circulating levels of both PCSK9 and LDL cholesterol at 84 days after receipt of the first dose. We observed reductions in the PCSK9 level of up to 83.8% and in the LDL cholesterol level of up to 59.7%. We also observed lowering of the serum LDL cholesterol level when inclisiran was administered to patients taking stable doses of statin therapy. These findings add to previous nonclinical and clinical evidence that supports the ability of RNAi therapeutic agents in general to inhibit the synthesis of liver-derived target proteins.

The results of this study also add to the clinical evidence from anti-PCSK9 antibody trials that supports PCSK9 as a therapeutic target for significant lowering of the LDL cholesterol level. The magnitude of the lowering of the LDL cholesterol level that we found with inclisiran was generally similar to that observed previously with anti-PCSK9 antibodies or intensive statin therapy. However, inclisiran differs mechanistically from anti-PCSK9 antibodies. Whereas anti-PCSK9 antibodies bind to extracellular PCSK9 (produced from any tissue) and prevent its interaction with the LDL receptor, inclisiran inhibits the synthesis of PCSK9 protein specifically in the liver.

The pharmacodynamic profile of inclisiran also differs substantially from that of the anti-PCSK9 antibodies that have been studied to date. The effect on the PCSK9 and LDL cholesterol levels persisted for at least 180 days after the initiation of treatment, with little variation over the 6-month period after the receipt of the first dose. Our data suggest that inclisiran has the potential to provide effective management of hypercholesterolemia with administration every 3 or 6 months, as compared with the recommended regimens of administration once or twice monthly for the currently approved antibodies.

The limitations of the study should be considered carefully. First, although the trial was randomized and placebo-controlled, it was a singleblind trial and included only a limited number of participants in order to obtain an initial assessment of safety and pharmacodynamics. Therefore, the results must be regarded as preliminary and be confirmed in larger clinical trials of longer duration. Second, the sample included mainly healthy participants with relatively normal lipid profiles, albeit with a baseline LDL cholesterol level of at least 100 mg per deciliter. A limited number of patients taking statins were enrolled, and the coadministration of nonstatin LDL cholesterol–lowering agents was not investigated. In addition, in the multiple-dose phase, subsequent doses of inclisiran were administered well within the period of maximal pharmacodynamic activity of the first dose. Also, the cumulative doses of the multiple-dose regimens (500 to 1000 mg) were similar to the most effective single doses studied (300 to 800 mg). This situation may explain the apparently moderate incremental effects of increasing doses on the levels of PCSK9 and LDL cholesterol.

In conclusion, in this small phase 1 study, single or multiple doses of inclisiran, an RNAi therapeutic agent targeting PCSK9, were administered over a 1-month period. No serious adverse events occurred, and consistent, sustained reductions in the circulating PCSK9 and LDL cholesterol levels were observed.

JOURNAL ARTICLE EXERCISE 3

The science sections on the MCAT include a significant number of passages with experiments. Questions for these passages often ask you to analyze data, read charts and graphs, and come to some reasonable conclusion based on the information they give you. If you don't know how to extract information efficiently and analyze data effectively, you will be at a distinct disadvantage.

There are three "Journal Article Exercises" in this book. In this final exercise, you'll read and extract information from the article and then complete an MCAT passage based on this article. After that, we'll show you the "correct" information to pull out and the answers to the passage.

As before, when analyzing an experiment, you should be able to:

- identify the control group(s).
- extract information from graphs and data tables.
- determine how the experimental group(s) change relative to the control.
- determine if the results are statistically significant.
- come to a reasonable conclusion about WHY the results were observed.
- consider potential weaknesses in the study.
- determine how to increase the power of the study.
- decide what the next most logical experiment or study should be.

And, as before, the goal of these exercises is NOT to learn content from the articles, just to get a little more comfortable reading and extracting information from them.

For the (abridged) article pages 211–218. summarize the purpose of the experiment and the methods in a few sentences. Remember the mnemonic: Oh ouR Car Won't Start (ORCWS).

- O = Organism and Organization
- R = Results
- C = Control and Comparison
- W = Weirdness
- S = Statistics

Try interpreting the data on your own before reading the results/discussion section. When you do read the discussion, consider:

- What are the conclusions of the study?
- How are the conclusions supported by the data?
- What potential weaknesses or flaws do you see in the experimental design? Are these addressed in the discussion section?
- How might this study be potentially biased?
- How might this study be improved?
- What would be the next most logical experiment?

Answer these questions for the article on pages 211–218.

1. **O = Organism and Organization:**
   - Is the research being conducted on humans or on animals or on bacteria in a petri dish, or something else?

   _____

   _____

   - What is being done to these organisms?

   _____

   _____

   - Are there any unique qualities to these organisms?

   _____

   _____

   - Are there multiple groups?

   _____

   _____

   - Is the study conducted over a long period of time with multiple data points, or is it a short-term study?

   _____

   _____

   - Does it have a large or small n?

   _____

   _____

2. **R = Results:**
   - Where and how are the results presented? Is it a graph? A data table? Figures and images?

   _____

   _____

   - What is/are the independent variable(s)?

   _____

   _____

   - What is/are the dependent variable(s)?

   _____

   _____

   - What are the results of the study?

   _____

   _____

- Do the results show correlation or cause and effect, or both? Describe.

  _____

  _____

3. **C = Control and Comparison:**
   - Is there a control group?

     _____

     _____

   - How does it differ from the experimental group? Is it given a placebo or nothing at all? Is it held under different conditions?

     _____

     _____

   - If there are multiple experimental groups, how do they differ from one another?

     _____

     _____

   - Is it a blinded study? If so, double-blind or single-blind?

     _____

     _____

4. **W = Weirdness:**
   - Does anything or do any of the results stand out as unexpected?

     _____

     _____

5. **S = Statistics:**
   - Was any sort of statistical analysis done?

     _____

     _____

   - How is it presented? Are there error bars on a graph? Standard errors around a mean? Are there p-values? Is there an asterisk indicating statistical significance?

     _____

     _____

   - Is there any data that is not statistically significant?

     _____

     _____

6. **Interpreting the data:**
   - What are the conclusions of the study?

     _____

     _____

- How are the conclusions supported by the data?

  _____

  _____

- What potential weaknesses or flaws do you see in the experimental design? Are these addressed in the discussion section?

  _____

  _____

- How might this study be potentially biased?

  _____

  _____

- How might this study be improved?

  _____

  _____

- What would be the next most logical experiment?

  _____

  _____

7. **Final Summary of Experiment and Results:**

  _____

  _____

  _____

  _____

  _____

  _____

JOURNAL ARTICLE EXERCISE 3 PASSAGE

Low density lipoproteins (LDLs) transport cholesterol made by the liver to cells that require it as source material for steroid hormones, a component of cell plasma membranes, or other similar functions. However, elevated LDL levels, typically characterized as above 100 mg/dL, present a clinical risk; at these higher levels, additional circulating cholesterol carried by LDLs may become attached to the walls of blood vessels, both forming plaques and contributing to arteries becoming hardened as part of coronary artery disease.

Hepatocytes and other body cells have receptors that can bind LDLs to limit their distribution in the body. Those receptors can be destroyed by serine proteases; one example is proprotein convertase subtilisin–kexin type 9 (PCSK9), which triggers lysosomal degradation of LDL receptors. Therapeutic approaches to dealing with high LDL levels have sought to target the lipoprotein itself as well as enzymes like PCSK9 to help manage the overall lipid profile in the body.

A new therapeutic, inclisiran, acts as a small interfering RNA (siRNA) and is thought to limit expression of PCSK9. Researchers aimed to determine if administration of inclisiran lowered circulating levels of LDL, in part by helping to maintain the receptors that can bind it. A limited clinical trial of the drug was launched in which subjects were either given a single dose of inclisiran (N = 3 for each dose level), or a placebo (N = 6), then tracked for six months, or given two doses per month (or a placebo) and tracked for seven months. All subjects were tracked for several months. Those in the multidose group were also divided such that some participants in both the treatment and placebo groups were also given a statin, a class of drugs that helps remove cholesterol from plaques attached to blood vessels (N < 8 for all multidose groups). Measures of PCSK9 and LDL were taken throughout the study and results are presented in Figures 1 and 2.

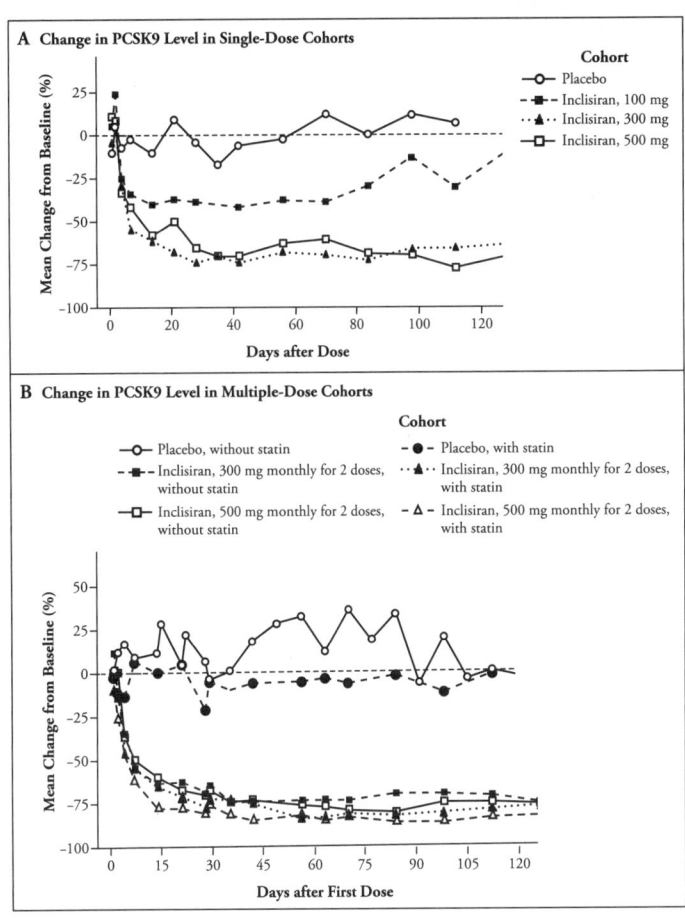

Figure 1 Change in plasma levels of PCSK9 as mean percentage changes from baseline. All cohorts compared to placebo. At day 84, single-dose cohorts, $p < 0.001$; multiple-dose cohorts without statin, $p < 0.01$; multiple-dose cohorts with statin, $p < 0.001$.

Figure 2 Changes in serum levels of LDL cholesterol as mean percentage changes from baseline. All cohorts compared to placebo. At day 84, single-dose cohorts, $p < 0.001$; multiple-dose cohorts without statin, $p < 0.01$; multiple-dose cohorts with statin, $p < 0.001$.

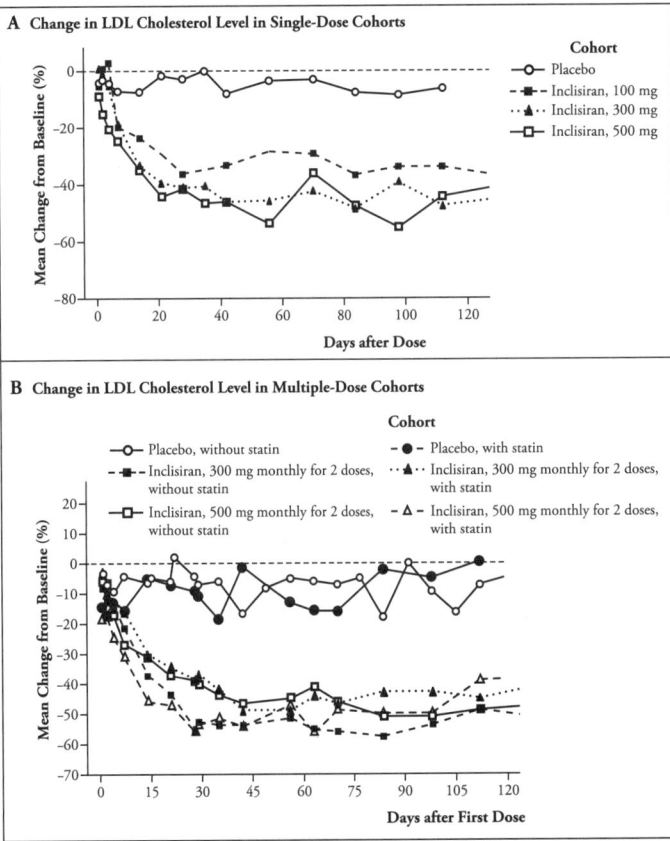

Adapted from Fitzgerald, K., White, S., Borodovsky, A. *et al.* A Highly Durable RNAi Therapeutic Inhibitor of PCSK9. *N Engl J Med* **376** (2017).

1. Based on the experimental data at approximately two months, which treatment might be interpreted as most effective?

A) Multiple doses of placebo paired with a statin
B) Single 100 mg dose of inclisiran
C) Multiple 500 mg doses of inclisiran not paired with a statin
D) Multiple 500 mg doses of inclisiran paired with a statin

2. It is most likely that inclisiran will have what effect on treated cells?

A) RNA polymerase will be prevented from binding promoter sequences for the targeted genes.
B) Transcripts for the targeted genes will be broken down before they are translated.
C) Post-transcriptional modification will be prevented as methylated guanine is blocked from binding the 5′ end of the transcript.
D) The sense strand of the DNA helix will be transcribed instead of the anti-sense strand.

3. According to the data in Figures 1 and 2, what conclusion about PCSK9 and LDL is best suppported?

A) Compared to placebo, multiple doses of inclisiran with statin have a statistically significant effect on the level of PCSK9, but not on the level of LDL.
B) Statically speaking, multiple doses of inclisiran given without additional statin have the same effect on the level of PCSK9 and the level of LDL.
C) The single dose protocol of inclisiran only shows a statistically significant effect when paired with statin treatment.
D) Compared to placebo, the single dose protocol of inclisiran has a statistically significant effect on the level of PCSK9 and LDL.

4. If LDL levels remain above 100 mg/dL for an extended period, the amount of oxygen supplied to the cardiac muscle will:

A) decrease due to increased stiffness in coronary blood vessels and decreased flow due to plaque blockage.
B) decrease due to hardening in the vessels involved in external respiration in the lungs
C) increase due to the stabilizing effect produced with hardening of blood vessels.
D) increase due to a higher respiratory rate resulting from the stress of coronary artery disease.

5. Based on the available experimental data, what limitation is evident in the design of the protocol?

A) The small number of different doses of inclisiran that were included in both
B) Statins were not tested on their own
C) Small sample size (N) restricts the power of the experiment
D) Statistical analysis requires calculation of both p values and standard deviation

SOLUTIONS TO JOURNAL ARTICLE EXERCISE 3

1. **O = Organism and Organization:**
    - Is the research being conducted on humans or on animals or on bacteria in a petri dish, or something else? *Humans (21 women, 48 men)*
    - What is being done to these organisms? *They are being treated with either inclisiran (a drug) or a placebo to see if the drug will lower the levels of low density lipoproteins (LDLs).*
    - Are there any unique qualities to these organisms? *A requirement for the study was subjects having an LDL level of 100 or higher.*
    - Are there multiple groups? *Yes, one group receives inclisiran in a single dose, and one group receives inclisiran as a multidose process. The multidose group was also split into those receiving a statin drug versus those not taking a statin.*
    - Is the study conducted over a long period of time with multiple data points, or is it a short-term study? *Long-ish. The single-dose group was followed for approximately six months while the multidose group was followed for approximately seven months.*
    - Does it have a large or small *n*? *The n for the study is relatively small, but it is still reasonable given the challenges in recruiting human subjects.*

2. **R = Results:**
    - Where and how are the results presented? Is it a graph? A data table? Figures and images? *The results are presented in tables and graphs.*
    - What is/are the independent variable(s)? *Time, inclisiran versus placebo, statin versus no statin*
    - What is/are the dependent variable(s)? *Measurement of LDL levels and proprotein convertase subtilisin–kexin type 9 (PCSK9), a serine protease that can raise LDL levels by destroying its receptors.*
    - What are the results of the study? *Single-dose treatment with inclisiran generated a statistically significant reduction in LDL and PCSK9 at doses of 300 mg or higher as did each level of the multidose treatment protocol.*
    - Do the results show correlation or cause and effect, or both? Describe. *The results are causative; both the single-dose and multidose versions of the protocol used a placebo group and the effect seen in those receiving inclisiran was not seen in the placebo subjects.*

3. **C = Control and Comparison:**
    - Is there a control group? *Yes*
    - How does it differ from the experimental group? Is it given a placebo or nothing at all? Is it held under different conditions? *Yes, both the single-dose and multidose groups have subsets of subjects receiving a placebo instead of inclisiran.*
    - If there are multiple experimental groups, how do they differ from one another? *The single-dose group had one dose administered, the dose ranging from 25 mg to 800 mg. The multidose group had a smaller number of dose sizes being tested, but also included an additional variant as to whether or not the subject received a statin drug along with the inclisiran.*
    - Is it a blinded study? If so, double blind or single blind? *Yes, single-blinded*

4. **W = Weirdness:**
    - Does anything or do any of the results stand out as unexpected? *The effectiveness of the single-dose protocol was demonstrated starting at 300 mg and for the multidose protocol, all doses were found to be effective, but the lowest total dose in the multidose protocol was 250 mg, which was less than the effective amount in the single-dose protocol.*

5. **S = Statistics:**
    - Was any sort of statistical analysis done? *Yes*
    - How is it presented? Are there error bars on a graph? Standard errors around a mean? Are there p-values? Is there an asterisk indicating statistical significance? *P-values, standard errors reported on means, error bars on graphs*
    - Is there any data that is not statistically significant? *The placebo branches for both the single-dose and multidose versions of the protocol did not have a statistically significant effect.*

6. **Interpreting the data:**
    - What are the conclusions of the study? *Treatment with inclisiran could be effective at reducing LDL levels for those with LDL levels above 100 mg per deciliter, with or without the accompanying use of a statin.*
    - How are the conclusions supported by the data? *The conclusions are supported based on the statistically significant drop both in the measure of LDL in treated groups as well as the drops in PCSK9.*
    - What potential weaknesses or flaws do you see in the experimental design? Are these addressed in the discussion section? *The protocol worked to recruit across a range of ages, but the study population was mostly male and mostly white. The number of subjects would need to be larger and their selection would need to represent a broader range of demographics.*
    - How might this study be potentially biased? *This study may be biased based on the composition of its patient population.*
    - How might this study be improved? *A larger N with a broader range of demographics represented*
    - What would be the next most logical experiment? *An additional trial with a larger pool of subjects run at more than two centers*

7. **Final Summary of Experiment and Results:**
    - *In this journal article, the effect of inclisiran on both LDL levels and the levels of PCSK9 (an enzyme that can cause elevations in LDL) was evaluated in a population with elevated LDL. Subjects were given either a single dose of the drug or a placebo, across a range of doses; some subjects received multiple doses across a smaller range of doses. The multidose group was split into those receiving a statin drug or not. All subjects receiving at least 300 mg in the single-dose trial, and all subjects in the multidose trial (starting at two doses of 125 mg), showed a significant decrease in both LDL and PCSK9.*

SOLUTIONS TO JOURNAL ARTICLE EXERCISE 3 PASSAGE

1. **D** Two months is approximately 60 days so examine that time point on each of the graphs. The placebo in all cases is less effective than any other treatment (choice A can be eliminated). A single 100 mg dose triggered an approximate 30% decrease in both measures; however, other treatment protocols available in the answer choices did better (choice B can be eliminated). Multiple doses at 500 mg but lacking a statin reduced PCSK9 levels by about 75% and LDL levels by about 40%, while multiple doses at 500 mg with a statin similarly lowered PCSK9 levels but reduced LDL levels even further (almost 60%; choice C can be eliminated and choice D is correct).

2. **B** The passage states that inclisiran as an siRNA; these trigger post-transcriptional destruction of mRNA transcripts, preventing them from being translated and preventing expression of the associated proteins (choice B is correct). siRNAs do not interact with the RNA polymerases (choice A is wrong) nor do they prevent binding of the 5′ methylated guanine cap necessary for a transcript to continue with translation in eukaryotic cells (choice C is wrong). This form of RNA acts post-transcriptionally and does not change which strand of the DNA helix is transcribed in the first place (choice D is wrong).

3. **D** Since the graph captions contain information on p values, this would be the best source to assess statistical significance. The multidose protocol that includes statin has $p < 0.001$ for both PCSK9 and LDL, indicating that both effects are statistically significant (choice A is eliminated). The multidose protocol that does not include statin has a p value less than 0.001 for PCSK9, but less than 0.01 for LDL; while both are significant, they are not necessarily the same as each other (choice B is eliminated). The single dose protocol is not run with statin treatment, so this experimental group cannot be evaluated (choice C is eliminated). However, the single dose protocol has a p value less than 0.001 for both PCSK9 and LDL, showing statistical significance for both (choice D is correct).

4. **A** The passage describes LDL levels above 100 mg/dL as a clinical concern due to the increased level of plaques found in blood vessels and their link to coronary artery disease. Blocking these vessels would physically limit oxygenated blood flow (choices C and D can be eliminated). The passage states that arteries (the vessels delivering oxygen to the heart) are hardened, not the capillary beds around the lungs where external respiration occurs (choice B can be eliminated and choice A is correct).

5. **C** The graphs report on the number of subjects in each treatment arm and these numbers are fairly small; this will limit the power of the study overall (choice C is correct). There is a range of doses represented and not enough information is present to evaluate whether this is sufficient or if there really should be more; without more support, this cannot be evaluated (choice A can be eliminated). The statins are tested on their own; the multidose cohorts include a group that was administered a placebo plus statin, effectively testing the statin on its own (choice B can be eliminated). Standard deviation analysis is often useful, but is not required if p values are reported (choice D can be eliminated).

Appendix
Some Lab Techniques

The material in this section is not *strictly* MCAT material; it is presented in this appendix as a reference source. In other words, you don't need to memorize it, but do read it for familiarity. The MCAT is a test of your ability to deal with new material like this, presented on the exam in passage form.

A.1 ENZYME-LINKED IMMUNO-SORBENT ASSAY (ELISA)

As the name suggests, an ELISA is a biochemical technique that utilizes antigen-antibody interactions ("immuno-sorbency") to determine the presence of either

- antigens (like proteins or cytokines), or
- specific immunoglobulins (antibodies)

in a sample (such as cells recovered from a tumor biopsy or a patient's serum). Figure 1 illustrates the basic protocol when testing for the presence of a specific antigen.

Step 1: The experimental wells are coated with antibodies that are specific for the target antigen.

Step 2: A sample of serum or cell extract is added to the wells.

Step 3: The antibodies immobilize the antigen by binding to it (if it is present in the sample).

Step 4: Any unbound proteins remaining in the sample are washed away.

Step 5: An enzyme-linked antibody that also recognizes the target protein is added to the wells.

Step 6: The wells are filled with a solution that changes color in the presence of the detection enzyme (the one linked to the antibody added in Step 5). A color change indicates the target protein was present in the sample; no color change means the protein was absent.

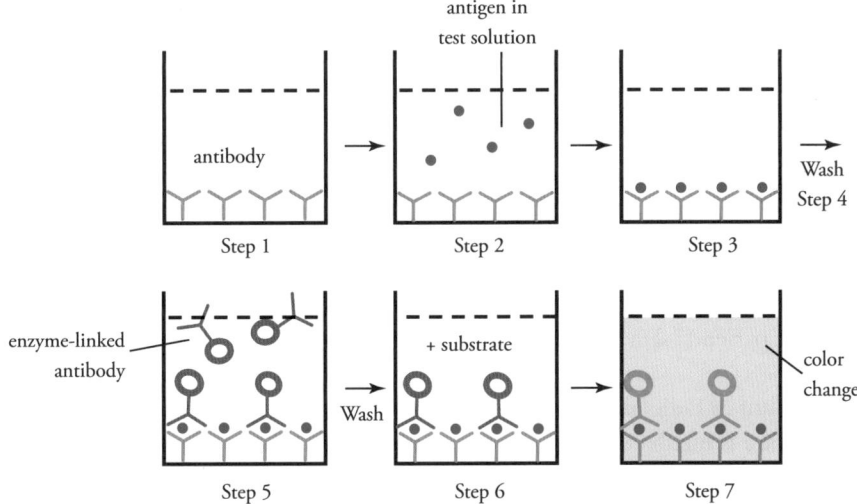

Figure 1 Testing for the Presence of Antigen

When testing for the presence of a specific antibody in a sample, the *antigen* (for which the antibody is specific) is first allowed to adhere directly to the wells. The sample is added as above, and then mixed with enzyme-linked antibodies (see Figure 2).

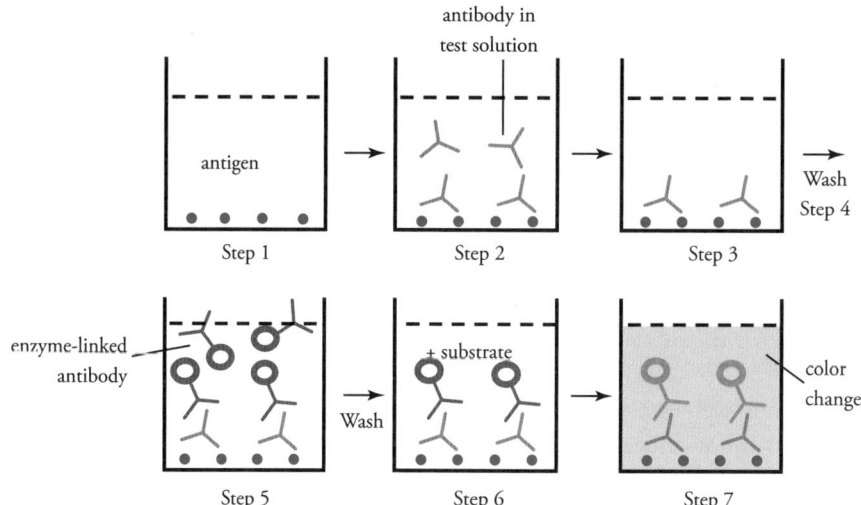

Figure 2   Testing for the Presence of Antibody

ELISA can be used to screen patients for viral infections. For example, serum from a patient suspected to be infected with HIV is loaded into wells that are coated with HIV coat proteins. If the serum contains anti-HIV antibodies (indicating infection), the antibodies will adhere to the proteins on the wells, bind enzyme-linked antibodies, and effect a color change.

A.2   RADIOIMMUNOASSAY (RIA)

RIAs are similar to ELISAs but use radiolabeled antibodies rather than enzyme-linked antibodies. Thus, the presence of target proteins or antibodies is assayed by measuring the amount of radioactivity instead of a color change. RIAs are more extensively used in the medical field to measure the relative amounts of hormones or drugs in patients' sera (see Figure 3).

Step 1: A known amount of radiolabeled antigen (for example, insulin that was synthesized with ^{125}I-labeled tyrosines) is incubated with a known amount of antibody that is specific to the antigen.

Step 2: The insulin:antibody complexes are isolated.

Step 3: The total amount of radioactivity is measured.

Step 4: Unlabeled insulin (also called *cold insulin*) is mixed into the solution in increasing amounts. The cold insulin competes with the labeled insulin (*hot insulin*) for the antibody. As more cold insulin is added, less total radioactivity is recovered and measured. This competition assay helps formulate a standard curve (see Figure 4).

Step 5: Steps 1–3 are repeated using patient serum instead of the cold insulin. The standard curve is used to extrapolate the amount of insulin that is circulating in a patient's serum.

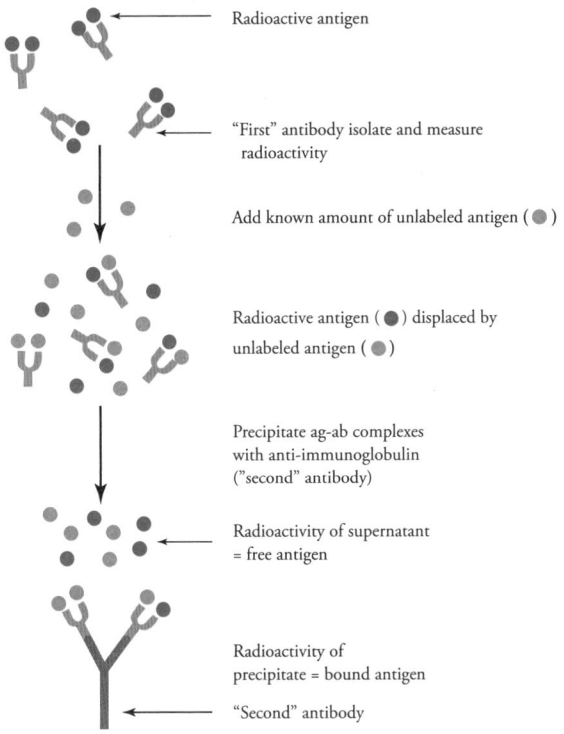

Radioactive antigen

"First" antibody isolate and measure radioactivity

Add known amount of unlabeled antigen (●)

Radioactive antigen (●) displaced by unlabeled antigen (●)

Precipitate ag-ab complexes with anti-immunoglobulin ("second" antibody)

Radioactivity of supernatant = free antigen

Radioactivity of precipitate = bound antigen

"Second" antibody

Figure 3   Radioimmunoassay (RIA)

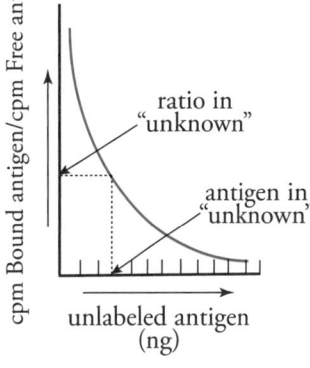

ratio in "unknown"

antigen in "unknown"

cpm Bound antigen/cpm Free antigen

unlabeled antigen (ng)

Figure 4   Standard Curve

A.3   ELECTROPHORESIS

Electrophoresis is a means of separating things by size (for example, nucleic acids or proteins) or by charge (for example, proteins or individual amino acids). A "gel" is made out of either acrylamide or agarose by solubilizing the acrylamide or agarose, pouring it into a rectangular mold, and then allowing it to cool and solidify. Acrylamide and agarose form "nets" as they solidify; the more acrylamide or agarose used in the initial solution, the smaller the pores in the nets.

The mold used to pour the gel creates wells in the gel into which samples can be loaded. An electrical current is applied such that the end of the gel with the wells is negatively charged and the opposite end is positively charged. This causes the samples to migrate toward the positive pole, according to size; smaller things migrate faster (because they fit more easily through the pores of the gel) and larger things migrate more slowly.

For example, here are the steps for separating DNA fragments by size.

Step 1:   Isolate the sample DNA from cells.
Step 2:   Expose the DNA to enzymes called **restriction endonucleases** (see Section A.5), which cleave the strands of DNA into smaller fragments of varying size. This may not be necessary in some cases.
Step 3:   Add a loading dye to the DNA sample. This makes the sample visible as it is being loaded into the gel. Loading dye also contains a chemical to help inhibit DNA degradation. Finally, glycerol in the loading dye makes the sample more dense than the surrounding buffer, which means the DNA sample sinks to the bottom of the gel wells.

Step 4: Load the mixture of fragments into the gel wells and apply the electrical current (this is called "running a gel"). Each strand of DNA (negatively charged!) migrates toward the positive end of the gel, but the smaller fragments migrate more quickly, so they are found farther from the wells at any point in the experiment. You run the samples alongside a "standard" lane, which contains fragments of known size (this helps identify the size of the unknowns).

Step 5: Visualize the bands of DNA in the gel. This is done using a dye that binds to nucleic acids and fluoresces when exposed to UV light. This dye is typically added to the gel when it is being made, but it can also be applied after the gel is run. The size of each DNA band can be approximated by comparing it to the ladder.

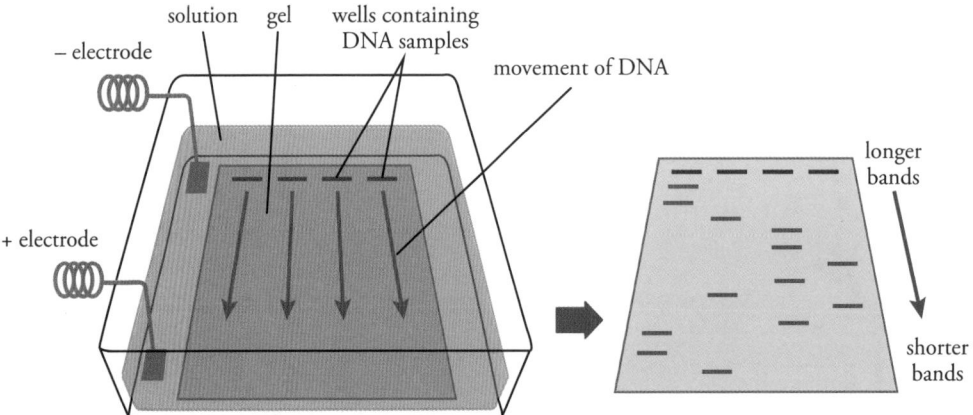

Figure 5 Agarose Gel Electrophoresis of DNA

In addition to determining their sizes, fragments of DNA (or RNA) in an electrophoresed gel can be transferred to a more solid and stable membrane in a process called "blotting." There are several types of blots used in biology laboratories.

A.4 BLOTTING

Simply put, blotting is the transfer of DNA or proteins from an electrophoresis gel to a nitrocellulose of PVDF membrane. Once transferred, further experiments can be run to isolate or detect a particular nucleic acid fragment or protein (called "probing"). Blotting is classified by the type of molecule being probed.

Southern Blotting

Southern blotting allows you detect the presence of specific sequences within a heterogeneous sample of DNA. This process also allows you to isolate and purify target sequences of DNA for further study.

Step 1: Separate the DNA fragments on an electrophoresis gel.

Step 2: Transfer the fragments to a nitrocellulose membrane.

Step 3: "Probe" the filter for the target DNA sequence. Hybridization probes are short single-stranded sequences of nucleic acid (usually DNA) that have two important features:

- They are complementary to (and thus will base-pair with) a portion of the target DNA sequence.
- They are constructed with radiolabeled nucleotides, which allows the visualization of the target sequence with special film.

Probes are often engineered to complement mutations or certain gene rearrangements, making Southern blotting a useful diagnostic tool.

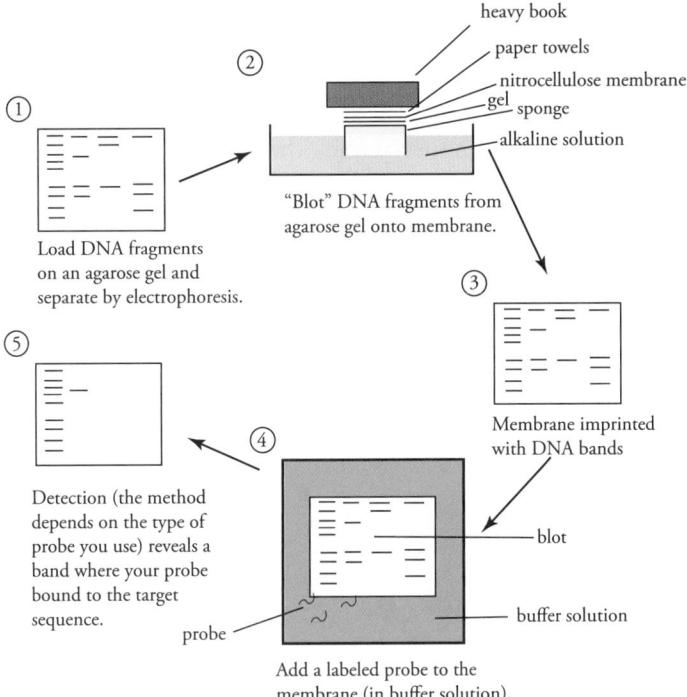

Figure 6 Southern Blotting

Northern Blotting

Northern blotting is almost identical to Southern blotting, except that RNA is separated via gel electrophoresis instead of DNA. The rest of the process is the same; once the RNA has been separated on a gel, it is transferred to a nitrocellulose membrane and detected via radiolabeled nucleic acid probe. This technique allows you to determine whether specific gene products (normal or pathologic) are being expressed (if their mRNA is present in a cell, they are probably being translated to protein).

Western Blotting

Western blotting allows you to detect the presence of certain proteins within a sample and also serves as a diagnostic tool. You are able to determine, for example, whether cancer cells express certain tumor-promoting growth receptors on their surface. Here are the steps.

Step 1: Cells are collected and solubilized in detergent to release their cytoplasmic contents.

Step 2: Cell lysates, which contain hundreds of different proteins, are denatured (meaning they lose their secondary and tertiary structures). Lysates and a ladder are loaded onto a gel. Similar to nucleic acid gel electrophoresis, a ladder is used so protein size can be compared to a standard.

Step 3: An electric current is applied. Because of the detergent used, the proteins are all negatively charged. Therefore, they migrate toward the positive electrode, with the smaller proteins migrating the farthest from the wells.

Step 4: The separated proteins from the gel are transferred to a nitrocellulose or PVDF membrane.

Step 5: The membrane is probed for the target protein. Probing for proteins in Western blotting differs from probing in Southern or Northern blotting in that antibodies are used as the probes rather than nucleic acids. This is similar to the technique in ELISA; a primary antibody is used first, which will recognize only the target protein via its antigen-binding portions. Then, an enzyme-linked secondary antibody is used that recognizes the constant region of the primary antibody. The enzyme on the secondary antibody will fluoresce when a detection substrate is added, and this light can be photographed with special film. The target protein will show up as a band with an intensity that is proportional to the abundance of the protein in the sample (see Figure 7).

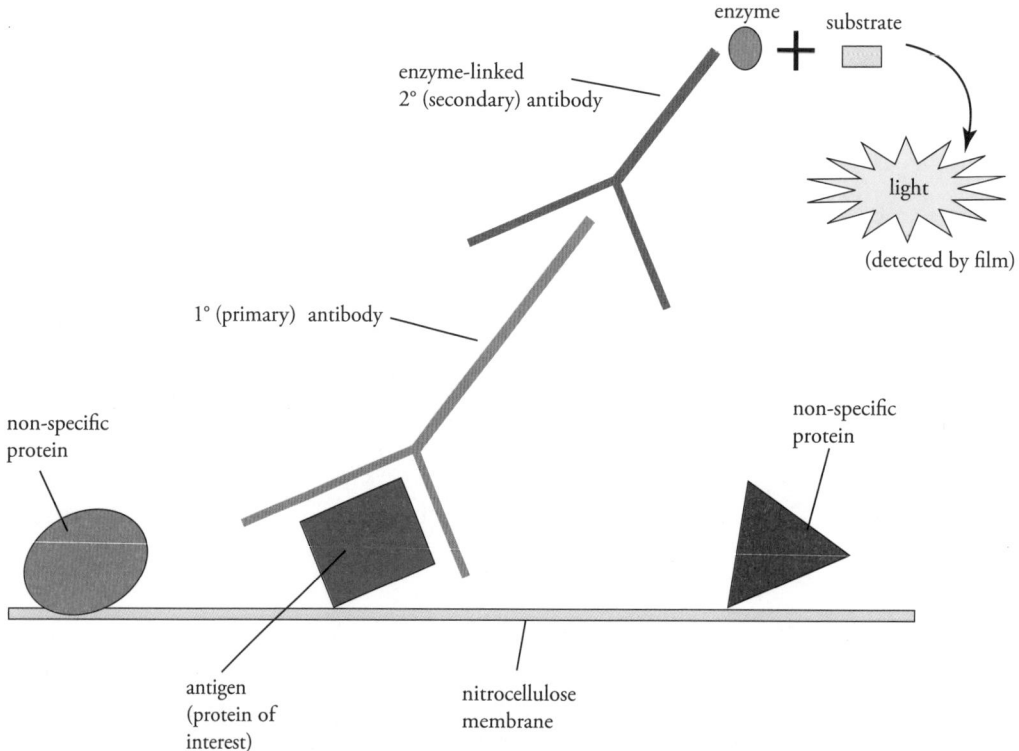

Figure 7   Western Blotting Detection

Eastern Blotting

Several variations of Eastern blotting have been reported, but these tests are not commonly used in molecular biology labs. Eastern blots are used to analyze post-translational modification of peptides, such as the addition of lipids or carbohydrates. The details of this protocol depend on the specifics of the experiment.

A.5 RECOMBINANT DNA

In the past 20 years, a major change has occurred in biology that has allowed it to not only describe the mechanisms of life, but also to manipulate living organisms. The cloning and sequencing of genes, production of recombinant DNA, and the subsequent production of recombinant proteins for use as therapeutic agents in medicine have now become commonplace procedures. A **recombinant protein** is one which has been obtained by transcribing and translating a novel combination of DNA (**recombinant DNA**) from different organisms. For example, the gene for human insulin can be placed in a bacterial **plasmid** (described below). Bacteria with the plasmid will then produce insulin that can be used to treat diabetes. To a large extent, these advances are due to the development of new technologies for the handling of DNA, such as the discovery of restriction endonucleases that cleave particular DNA sequences.

Restriction endonucleases are bacterial enzymes that recognize specific sequences of DNA and cut the double-stranded molecule in two pieces. A **nuclease** is an enzyme that cuts nucleic acids. An **_endo_nuclease** cuts in the middle of a DNA chain (contrast with **_exo_nucleases**, which nibble nucleotides from the ends of DNA chains). They are isolated from bacteria and used in the lab. Their natural role in the bacterium is to destroy viral DNA that gets injected into the cell; thus, they _restrict_ the reproduction of hostile viruses.

Restriction enzymes have found great use in molecular biology, where they have permitted manipulation of genes to create recombinant DNA. For example, in Figure 8 below, the cutting-specificity of a restriction enzyme known as _Eco_RI is shown (other restriction enzymes cut at different sequences). The free ends of the DNA molecule that were complementary are known as **sticky ends** since they are able to base pair with other DNA molecules with similar sequences.

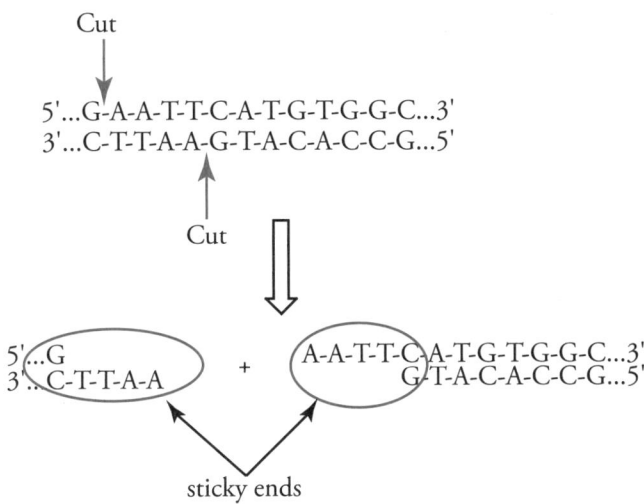

Figure 8   Restriction Digestion of DNA by _Eco_RI

Study the sequence shown in Figure 8. Notice anything in particular? If you read the top strand from left to right (5' to 3'), it begins GAATTC. Now read the bottom strand from right to left (still 5' to 3'), but only read the six nucleotides on the _left_ side of the chain. It says GAATTC (same as above)! Just looking at these six nucleotides, we see that the chain possesses **two-fold rotational symmetry**. The six 5' nucleotides of the top chain are the same as the six 3' nucleotides of the bottom one. Sequences with two-fold rotational symmetry are known as **palindromes**. Many restriction enzymes recognize palindromic sequences.

When a fragment of double-stranded DNA is created by cutting with a restriction endonuclease, it can be inserted into DNA from any source that was also digested by the same restriction endonuclease. For example, *Eco*RI-generated DNA fragments from a human can be isolated, mixed with *Eco*RI-digested DNA from a bacterial plasmid, and then joined by the enzyme DNA ligase. Hybrid DNA produced in this fashion is referred to as recombinant DNA.

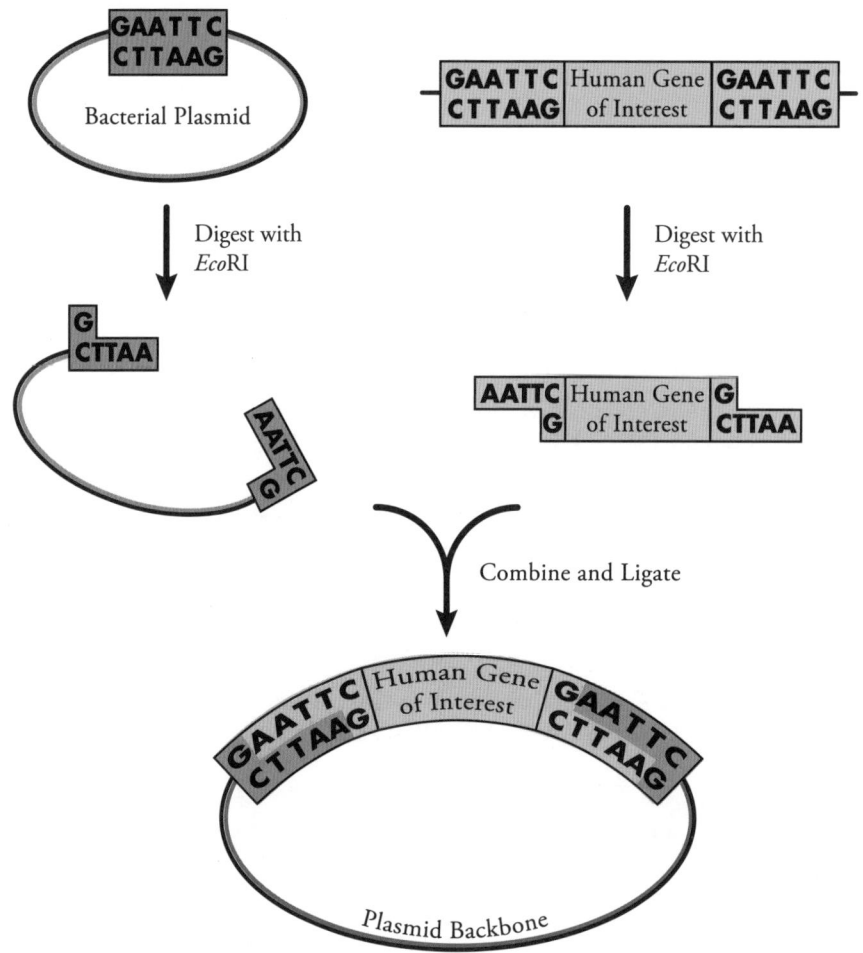

Figure 9 Cloning DNA Using a Sticky-End Restriction Enzyme

Some restriction enzymes generate DNA with blunt ends rather than sticky ends. That is, the 3' and 5' ends at the cut site are even, with no overhanging bases. Ligating blunt ends together is less specific, and restriction sites may or may not be retained. For example, if the same blunt-cutting restriction enzyme is used on both pieces of DNA, the restriction site will be maintained after ligation. If different blunt-cutting enzymes are used, the products can be ligated together but neither restriction site will be maintained. In Figure 10, a bacterial plasmid was digested with the restriction enzyme *Sma*I (which is a blunt cutter and recognizes the restriction site CCCGGG). A human gene of interest was digested with the restriction enzyme *Eco*RV (which is a blunt cutter and recognizes the sequence GATATC). Notice that both these restriction sites are six base pair palindromes. Because both enzymes generate blunt ends, these products can be ligated together. However, the recombinant DNA has lost the restriction sites for both enzymes. The DNA that remains is a combination of the two blunt sites (CCCATC and GATGGG), and it cannot be digested with either *Sma*I or *Eco*RV.

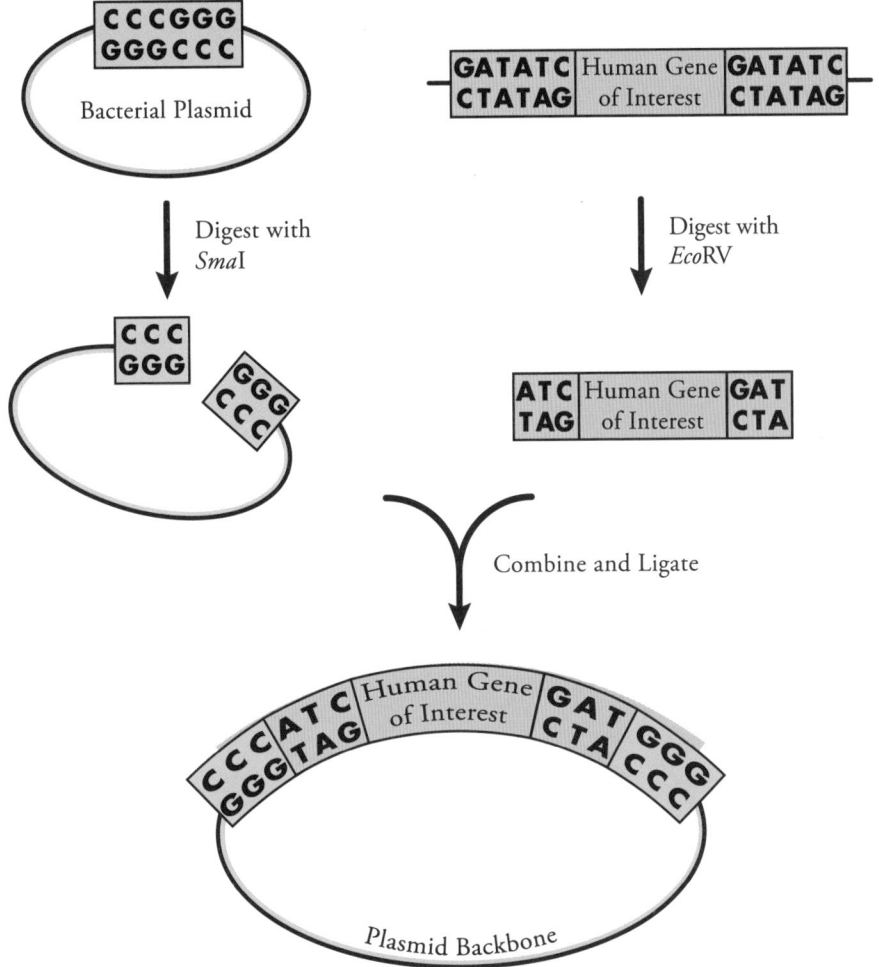

Figure 10 Cloning DNA Using Two Blunt-End Restriction Enzymes

Plasmids

Plasmids are small circular ds-DNA molecules found in bacteria that are capable of autonomous replication (replication that is independent of chromosome replication). Plasmid replication still requires an origin of replication (ORI), and this affects the copy number of the plasmid. Some plasmids have strong ORIs, leading to hundreds of plasmid copies per cell. Other ORIs are less efficient, leading to only a few copies of the plasmid per cell. In addition, plasmid segregation during binary fission is not regulated. For high copy plasmids, both daughter cells will most likely end up with copies of the plasmid. For lower copy plasmids, one daughter cell could get all copies of the plasmid, while the other daughter cell gets none. Plasmids used in laboratories are almost always high copy plasmids. The presence of a large number of copies is convenient, since it allows for isolation of a large amount of plasmid DNA with identical sequences.

Plasmids have been manipulated by recombinant techniques to propagate and express foreign genes in bacteria. In addition to an ORI, they also contain a multiple cloning site, which has restriction sites for dozens of restriction enzymes. This means the plasmid can be digested and any desired sequence with complementary ends can be ligated into the plasmid. Furthermore, plasmids have a drug resistance gene that helps select and isolate bacteria possessing the plasmid from other bacteria. For example, bacteria containing a plasmid with the ampicillin-resistance gene are able to grow in the presence of the antibiotic ampicillin (and are AmpR, or resistant), while bacteria that do not possess the plasmid will die in the presence of ampicillin (and are AmpS, or sensitive). By growing all bacteria in the presence of ampicillin, only those bacteria that possess and express the plasmid can grow and maintain colonies (see Figure 11). Tetracycline, penicillin, and streptomycin are other commonly used prokaryotic selection agents.

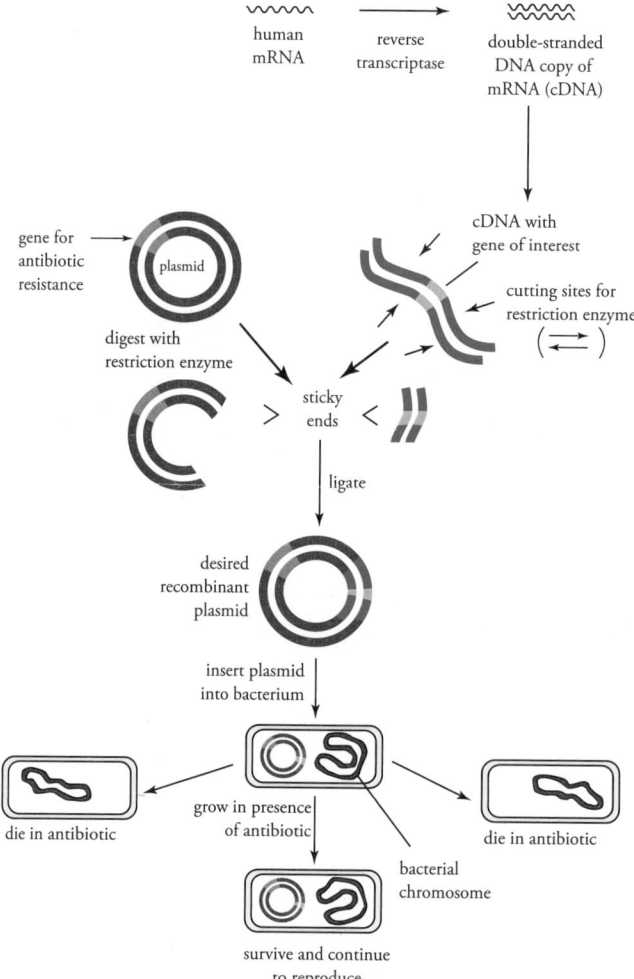

Figure 11   Expression of a Human Gene in Bacteria

Bacterial expression plasmids need extra components. A prokaryotic promoter and start site allow expression of an inserted gene in the bacterial host. The promoter can be either constitutively active or inducible upon addition of a chemical.

Bacterial Transformation

Plasmids can be easily reintroduced into bacterial cells via transformation. Transformation is a naturally occurring process, but only a very small percentage of bacteria are naturally willing to accept pieces of DNA floating around in their environment. These "competent" bacteria express special machinery that translocates the hydrophilic DNA across the lipid membrane. More often, the bacteria (or other cell types) must be coaxed to take up the plasmid. There are several ways to do this; the cells may be cooled in calcium chloride and then heat shocked to facilitate plasmid uptake. In another (called electroporation), an electric field is applied and this pokes holes in the membrane, which allows the plasmid to diffuse into the cell.

Once inside the bacteria, the plasmid will be exposed to the host's replication machinery, which replicates the plasmid (remember, it has its own origin of replication). If you are working with an expression plasmid, the DNA is also exposed to bacterial transcription machinery (remember, the plasmid contains the proper promoters and start signals). Newly synthesized mRNA can then access host ribosomes, which translate the encoded protein; on completion of translation, the cells are lysed to release the protein.

If the plasmid remains within the cytosol of the bacterium, the transformation is referred to as transient. In contrast, some plasmids are constructed to integrate within the host's genome. These stable transformations allow the plasmid to be replicated each time the bacterium replicates its own genome.

Complementary DNA

Many applications of DNA technology involve expressing eukaryotic genes in prokaryotic cells such as *E. coli*. This is conceptually simple: all you have to do is get eukaryotic DNA into a plasmid and get the plasmid into a bacterium, and the bacterium should express the gene. However, there are two main problems that need to be overcome. First, prokaryotes lack the equipment necessary for splicing out introns. Second, many eukaryotic genes are extremely long, making them hard to work with. One way to overcome these obstacles is to work with eukaryotic complementary DNA.

Complementary DNA (or cDNA) is produced from fully spliced eukaryotic mRNA. This is accomplished by a special enzyme you have encountered before: reverse transcriptase, obtained from retroviruses. This enzyme reads an RNA template and builds complementary DNA. Therefore, RNA can be isolated from a eukaryotic cell and converted into cDNA by the addition of reverse transcriptase, some generic primers and dNTP building blocks in buffer. cDNAs carry the complete coding sequences for genes, but they lack introns (and thus are smaller than the genomic sequence of the gene). Once a cDNA is ligated into a bacterial plasmid and bacteria are transformed with this plasmid, they can produce the protein encoded by the cDNA.

cDNA libraries are also commonly generated. This is where each of the thousands of mRNAs being generated by a given cell type or tissue are converted into cDNAs. Each cDNA is then cloned into a plasmid. This generates thousands of plasmids (the library), with each one containing one cDNA molecule. cDNA libraries can be compared across tissue types of a certain organism (brain versus liver, for example) to study tissue-specific gene expression.

Artificial Chromosomes

Plasmids can carry inserts only up to a certain size. If large inserts are required, artificial chromosomes can be used. Bacterial artificial chromosomes (BACs) typically carry inserts of 100 to 350 kilobase pairs (kb), while yeast artificial chromosomes (YACs) can carry inserts between 100 and 3,000 kb. In other words, BACs can easily carry up to 350,000 base pairs of DNA, and YACs can contain up to 3 million base pair inserts!

BACs contains sequences to allow replication and regulation of copy number, partition genes that promote their even distribution after bacterial cell division, and a selectable marker for antibiotic resistance. BACs that express inserted sequences also contain promoter regions.

YACs contain a centromere, telomeres, and sequences that function as replication origins. They also typically contain a gene that allows tryptophan or pyrimidine biosynthesis, allowing for selection of auxotrophic cells that contain the artificial chromosome. This system works similarly to antibiotic selection in bacteria.

BACs can be used to study inherited diseases that involve complex genes with several regulatory sequences and promoters upstream of the coding sequence. The entire gene can be cloned into a BAC, and this can be used to model genetic diseases in mice. For example, both Alzheimer's disease and Down syndrome have been studied in this way. BACs have also been used to clone the entire genome of some viruses, such as herpesviruses, poxviruses, and coronaviruses. These infective BACs initiate viral infection in the host cell and have facilitated research on these viruses.

Both BACs and YACs were initially used in the Human Genome Project, to help make chromosome maps. However, YACs were eventually abandoned because they are less stable than BACs. Despite this, they do have one major advantage: because yeast cells are eukaryotic, YACs can be used to express and study proteins that require post-translational modification.

Eukaryotic Plasmids

Eukaryotic plasmids also exist. They require many of the same components as bacterial plasmids. Eukaryotes use different selection agents, usually either puromycin or neomycin. They also require different promoters in expression plasmids, as well as a poly-adenylation signal downstream of the inserted gene, to terminate transcription.

Eukaryotic plasmids can be introduced into mammalian host cells via transfection. Similar to transformation, there are several experimental options for transfection. Cells can be chemically transfected, usually using calcium phosphate precipitates or plasmid packaging in liposomes. These lipid vesicles mask the plasmid, but they deliver it to the interior of the cell by fusing with the plasma membrane. Non-chemical options for transfection include electroporation, optical transfection with lasers, or shooting the DNA coupled to a gold nanoparticle into a cell nucleus using a gene gun.

Viruses can also deliver DNA into eukaryotic cells, a process called viral transduction. Transduced cells can express genes carried by the viral vector.

A.6 POLYMERASE CHAIN REACTION

Polymerase chain reaction (PCR) is a very quick and inexpensive method for detecting and amplifying specific DNA sequences, screening hereditary and infectious diseases, cloning genes, and fingerprinting DNA. Designed to generate myriad copies of a single template sequence, PCR allows the amplification and subsequent analysis of very small samples of DNA.

Let's say that PCR is to be used to determine whether a certain viral gene has been integrated within a bacterial host genome. A nuclear extract of the bacteria is obtained. Then primers are carefully constructed that will help locate the viral gene (if it is present within the host). Primers are engineered DNA oligonucleotides (~15 bases of single stranded DNA) that will recognize and base pair with specific DNA sequences; in this example, the primers will each recognize a 15-base stretch of the viral gene. Two primers, which will flank a total of ~10 kb of DNA, are used. The "forward primer" will recognize a 15-base stretch at the 3' end of the antisense strand, and the "reverse primer" will recognize a 15-base stretch at the 3' end of the sense strand. When base-paired to their respective gene sequences, the primers will bookend (on opposite sides) the intervening target gene segment (see Figure 12).

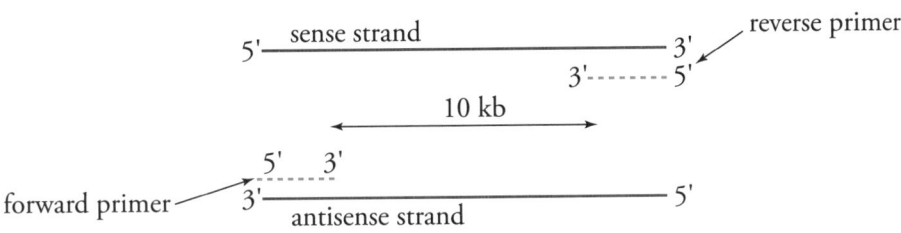

Figure 12 PCR Primers

The primers have free 3' hydroxyl groups to which dNTPs can be added in a 5' to 3' direction. This will allow the elongation of complementary strands of DNA. The bacterial DNA is mixed with multiple copies of the forward and reverse primers, lots of dNTP bases, a heat-sensitive DNA polymerase, and ions into a buffer. The mixture is then placed into a PCR machine, which will carry out three basic steps (see Figure 13):

Step 1: Initialization. The sample is heated to ~95°C. Heating the sample "melts" the hydrogen bonds that hold the ds-DNA together, which creates single-stranded DNA.

Step 2: Annealing. The sample is cooled to ~55°C. At this temperature, the primers base-pair with the template strands.

Step 3: Elongation. The sample is heated to ~72°C. Using the primers as starting points, the heat-sensitive DNA polymerase (usually *Taq* polymerase isolated from algae that thrive in hot springs) elongates strands of DNA that are complementary to each of the template strands. Each strand is polymerized in the 5' to 3' direction. Any mismatched primers will dissociate from the template strands and will not be extended (this helps ensure the purity of the PCR product). Longer DNA targets take longer to synthesize, so the length of the elongation step depends on the length of the product DNA.

A.6

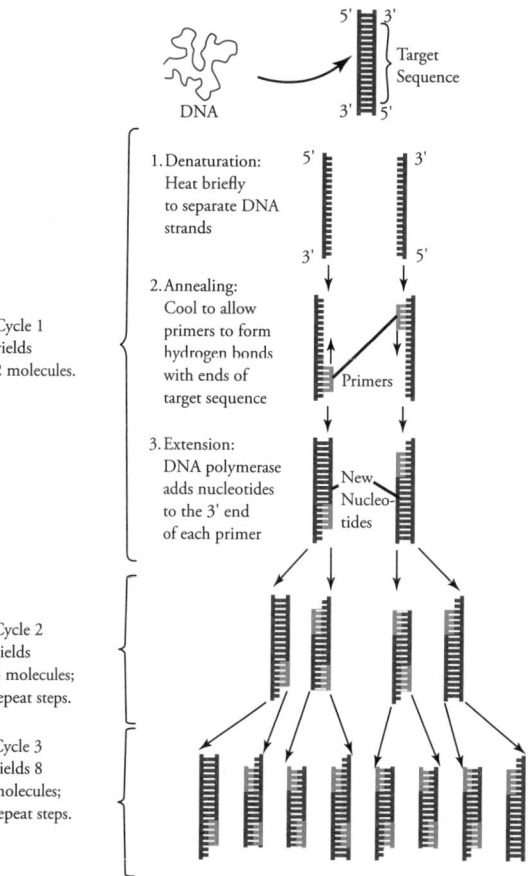

Figure 13 PCR Steps

Each cycle of three steps takes between 0.5 and 5 minutes, depending on the length of the target DNA product (and subsequent length of the elongation step). Because two new complementary strands are synthesized for each template strand in the sample, the PCR product grows at an exponential rate, yielding over a billion copies in just 30 cycles. The sample of DNA is separated via electrophoresis and stained to visualize the products, including the amplified viral gene segment (if present).

Reverse Transcriptase-Polymerase Chain Reaction (RT-PCR)

This is an extension of classic PCR and is used to detect the relative expression of specific gene products. While RT-PCR does not measure the actual expression or abundance of proteins, the technique provides a gauge of gene transcription by measuring the relative amount of target mRNAs. To conduct an RT-PCR experiment, all of the mRNAs from within a cell population are first isolated and then converted into complementary DNA (cDNA) using the enzyme reverse transcriptase. This "library" of cDNAs is then subjected to PCR, using primers specific for a certain gene of interest. If the gene was actively transcribed at the time of harvest, its mRNA will have yielded a cDNA, which will be amplified by the PCR reaction and visualized on a gel.

Quantitative Polymerase Chain Reaction (qPCR)

In quantitative PCR (qPCR, also called real-time PCR), the PCR product is both detected and quantified, either as an absolute number of copies or as a relative amount normalized to a control. The amplified DNA is detected in "real time," as the reaction progresses. The detection process can either use a dye that is fluorescent and binds DNA or a fluorescent oligonucleotide probe which hybridizes to the sequence of interest. qPCR can be performed on either DNA or cDNA templates, meaning it can give information on the presence and abundance of a particular DNA sequence in samples (if DNA is the template) or on gene expression (if the template is cDNA).

A.7   DNA SEQUENCING AND GENOMICS

DNA sequencing is a method by which scientists can determine gene sequences. This provides the basis for investigating the genetics of health and disease. Knowing gene sequences is also a critical component of other experimental techniques, for example, when constructing primers for PCR reactions.

The most widely used DNA sequencing method (the Sanger technique) hinges on a simple yet important structural characteristic of DNA molecules. The ringed ribose of a dNTP has various substituents attached to its carbons: a nitrogenous base at the 1' carbon, a hydrogen at the 2' carbon (recall that a hydroxyl group occupies this site in RNA), a hydroxyl group at the 3' carbon, and a string of three phosphates at the 5' carbon. The 3' carbon hydroxyl group serves as the binding site for another dNTP. Without a free 3' carbon hydroxyl group, dNTPs could not be linked together, and DNA synthesis would not be possible. The Sanger technique utilizes a modified dNTP, which lacks the 3' carbon hydroxyl group. These dideoxynucleotide triphosphates (ddNTPs) maintain their 5' carbon triphosphate moiety and can be incorporated normally into a growing DNA molecule; however, because they are lacking the 3' carbon hydroxyl group, no further bases can be added to them. Thus, these ddNTPs terminate stand elongation at the point of their insertion. The basic protocol is as follows (see Figure 14):

Step 1: Obtain a sample of DNA to sequence.

Step 2: Denature the DNA into single strands.

Step 3: Mix the sample of DNA with radiolabeled primers, DNA polymerase, and a mixture of dCTP, dTTP, dGTP, dATP, and ddATP (with the dideoxy form making up 1 percent of the adenine base population). This step of the assay will yield a population of newly synthesized DNA fragments, varying in length, each complimentary to the template strand and covalently bonded to a radiolabeled primer at the 5' end (this will aid in the detection of the newly synthesized fragments later). The variety in length of the fragments results from the random insertion of a ddATP into the growing chain.

Step 4: Conduct three more separate reactions as in the previous step, using each of the three other bases in dideoxy form (ddCTP, ddGTP, and ddTTP).

Step 5: Separate the fragments via gel electrophoresis, running each reaction from Steps 3 and 4 in a separate lane.

Step 6: Transfer the fragments to a membrane and visualize them with radio-sensitive film.

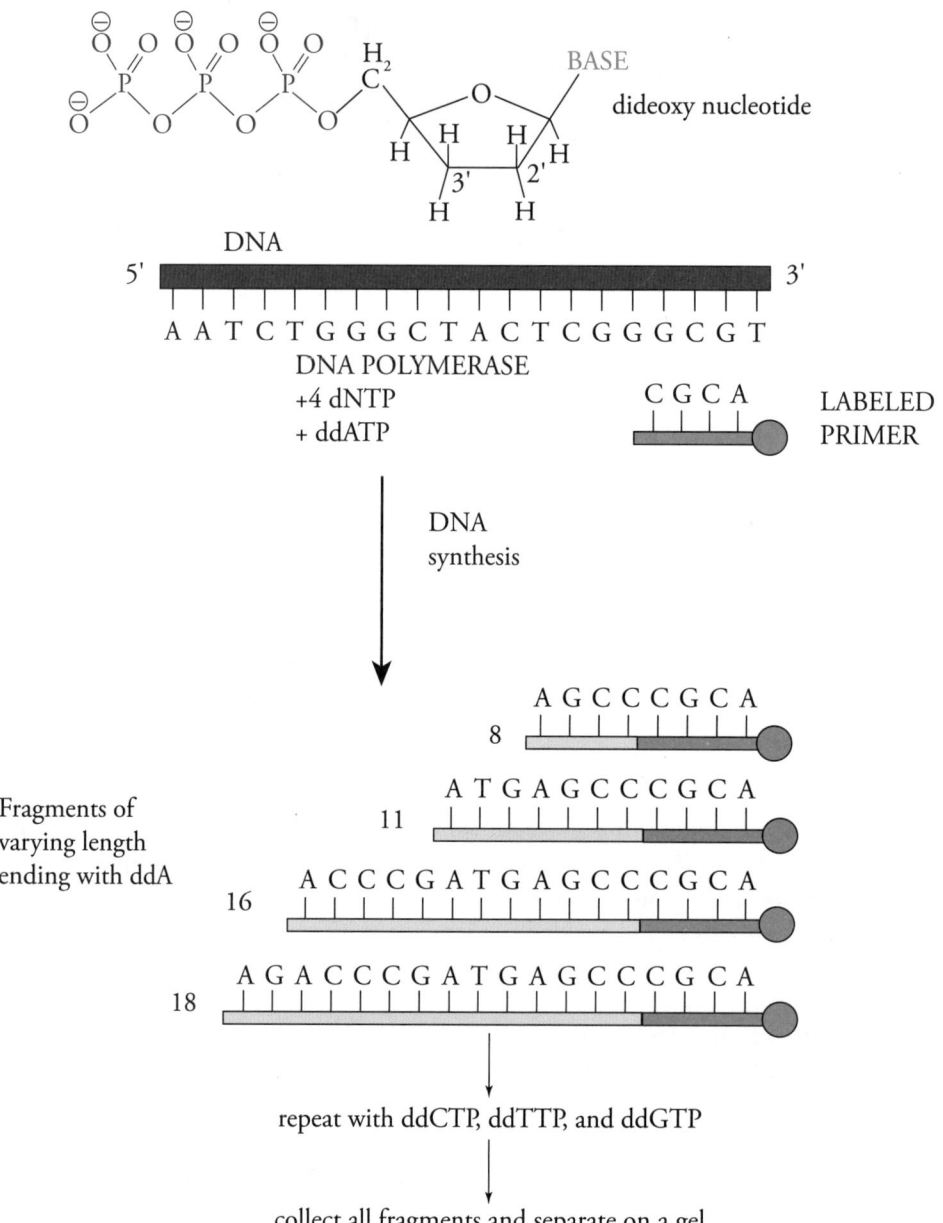

Figure 14   DNA Sequencing Reactions

The smallest fragment (i.e., the fragment that migrates the farthest from the well) is a primer with only a single ddNTP attached to it. The lane it ran in corresponds to the first base incorporated into the strand which is the first base of the sequence of the complimentary strand. The second smallest fragment is a primer with two bases attached; this fragment ran in the lane corresponding to the base at the second position in the complimentary strand (see Figure 15). Reading the membrane from bottom (farthest from the wells) to top (closest to the wells) indicates the sequence (in the 5' to 3' direction) of the complimentary strand. Remembering the simple rules of base-pairing (A:T and C:G), you can easily extrapolate the sequence of the template strand.

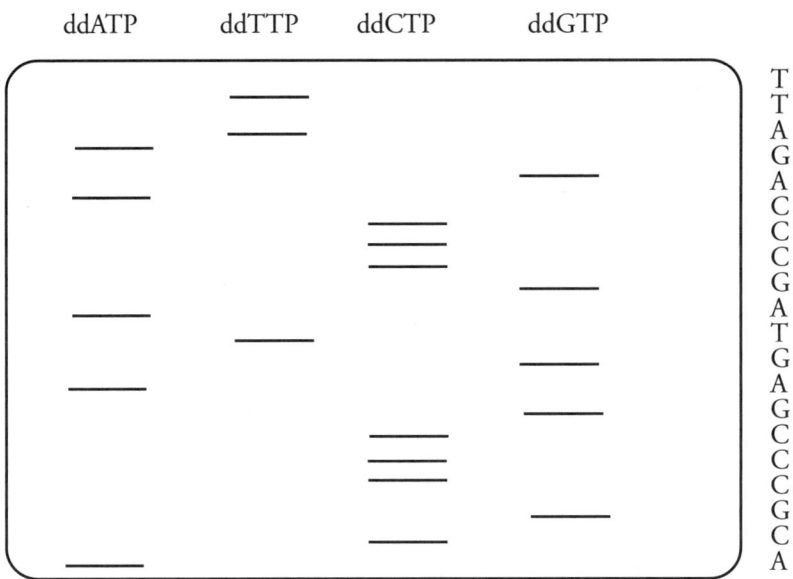

DNA sequence can be read from bottom of gel up

Figure 15   DNA Sequencing Gel

Genomics

The genome of the bacterium *Haemophilus influenzae* was the first to be sequenced and published in 1995. Since then, the genomes of hundreds of organisms have been sequenced and published, including humans and model organisms commonly used in biology laboratories (e.g., *E. coli*, *D. melanogaster*, etc.). Researchers and clinicians have recently started sequencing the genome of many cancers, which allows comparative studies between different types and subtypes of cancer, as well as a better understanding of how the cancer genome is different from a normal one.

Genomic sequencing is generally done in two ways, which can be complementary. The first strategy is to generate a genetic linkage map, with several hundred markers per chromosome. This map is then refined to a physical map by preparing YAC or BAC libraries containing large chromosomal fragments. The library is put in order and then gradually cloned into libraries containing smaller and smaller fragments. Each of these small fragments is eventually sequenced and assembled into an overall sequence.

The second strategy is a whole-genome shotgun approach, in which chromosomes are cut into small fragments, which are cloned and sequenced. This strategy skips generating maps, and because of this, requires much more extensive analysis of sequencing data by computers in order to align fragments.

Genomic data can lead to predictions on how many genes there are in a certain organism, where they are located, how expression is controlled, and how the genome is organized. It also supports larger questions, like how evolution and speciation occur. Finally, genomic data can be used to study genetic variation within and across species. Tools for analysis of genomic data have been developed and are always being refined. Researchers can now submit several different gene or protein sequences and receive a report that predicts how related the sequences are from an evolutionary point of view. There are also tools to align multiple sequences so we can study how similar and different they are.

A.8 DNA FINGERPRINTING

Much like visualizing subtle differences in the whorl pattern of a thumbprint, DNA fingerprinting allows scientists (and police departments!) to detect sequence variations that make each individual's DNA unique. The ability to appreciate subtle differences within different individuals' DNA comes in handy when matching a DNA sample from a murder suspect to the DNA in a drop of blood found at a crime scene, or when screening for disease-causing genes, or when doing paternity testing. Since the DNA of any two people is more than 99 percent identical, DNA fingerprinting exploits stretches of repetitive and highly variable DNA called **polymorphisms**. These intervening 2–100 base-pair sequences of DNA are structurally variable with respect to their sequence, length, multiplicity, and location within the genome. Two of the several methods of fingerprinting are described below, **restriction fragment length polymorphism** (RFLP) analysis and **short tandem repeat** (STR) analysis.

Restriction Fragment Length Polymorphism (RFLP) Analysis

Step 1: This method uses restriction endonucleases to cut 10–100 base-pair stretches of polymorphic DNA (called minisatellites) into small fragments. Because of the size variations inherent in this DNA, the resulting DNA fragments (now referred to as RFLPs) also vary in size and are unique to an individual.

Step 2: The RFLPs are separated via gel electrophoresis and transferred to a membrane. Southern blotting techniques are used to analyze the sample. The membrane is probed with radiolabeled DNA oligonucleotides that base-pair with specific RFLP sequences, and the membrane is visualized with special film. Polymorphic DNA, even though recovered from the same chromosomal region, will yield unique band distributions for each person. When RFLPs are recovered from DNA sequences within genes, mutations can be detected. For example, sickle cell disease is caused by a single base substitution in the beta chain of hemoglobin. The substituted valine at the sixth position (normally, glutamic acid is present) will introduce a novel restriction site within the gene. When cut with restriction endonucleases, the point mutation generates a different sized RFLP (when compared to the normal gene cut with the same enzymes) and will yield an anomalous banding pattern (see Figure 16).

Short Tandem Repeat (STR) Analysis

Step 1: This method uses PCR to amplify 5–10 base-pair stretches of highly polymorphic and repetitive DNA located within noncoding (introns) regions of the genome. These STRs vary with respect to the sequence and number of repeats found at each locus. To profile an individual, a sample of DNA is obtained and the polymorphic DNA is amplified with PCR.

Step 2: The amplified STRs are separated via electrophoresis and analyzed with Southern blotting.

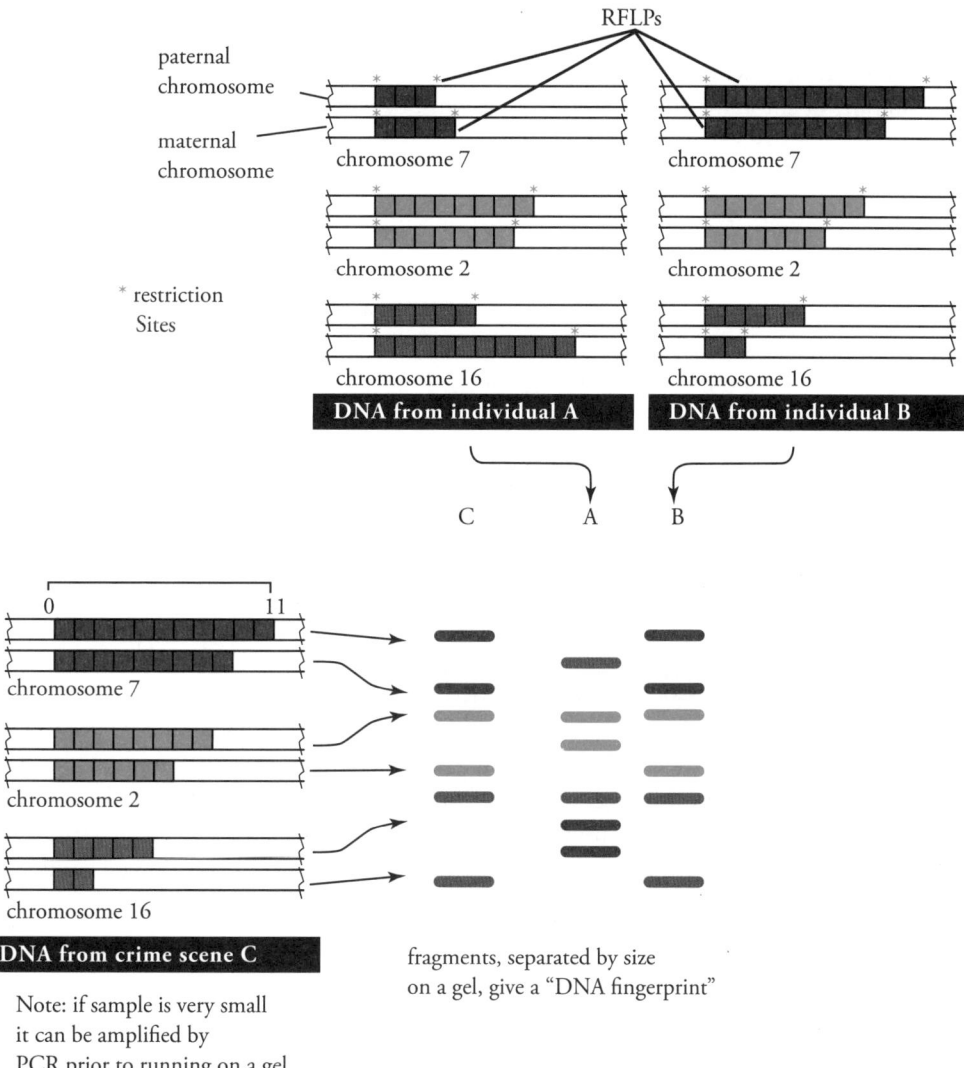

Figure 16 RFLP Analysis

A.9 ADDITIONAL METHODS TO STUDY THE GENOME

Genomic sequencing is the ultimate study of the genome. However, it is very costly and takes a long time. Depending on the experiment, one of the following methods may be better suited to answering a biological question.

Exome and Targeted Sequencing

Instead of sequencing the entire genome, scientists can target only certain regions of interest. Exome sequencing involves sequencing only the exons of the genome. On a smaller scale, individual genes can be sequenced. These selective techniques involve enriching the DNA of interest (by amplification for example), followed by standard sequencing.

Karyotyping

When generating a karyotype, scientists order all the chromosomes from 1 to 22 plus the sex chromosomes, for a genome-wide view of genetic information. Chromosomes are stained (using Giemsa stain) to highlight structural features. Major genetic changes (involving millions of base pairs), aneuploidy (when a cell contains an abnormal number of chromosomes), and some insertions, deletions, or translocations can be revealed.

Fluorescence *in situ* Hybridization

Fluorescence *in situ* hybridization (FISH) uses fluorescently labeled probes to locate the positions of specific DNA sequences on chromosomes. This detects and localizes the presence or absence of specific DNA sequences on chromosomes. Fluorescence microscopy is used to find out where the fluorescent probe is bound to the chromosomes. For example, large chromosomal translocations have been found in several types of cancer. A translocation between chromosomes 2 and 3 is often found in follicular thyroid carcinoma. This translocation produces a fusion gene that contains the promoter from one gene and the coding sequence of another. FISH analysis using chromosome 2 and 3 probes can detect and diagnose this translocation.

A.10   ANALYZING GENE EXPRESSION

Many of the techniques discussed above give information about gene expression. For example, RT-PCR and qPCR give information on which genes are being transcribed in a given cell population. Western blot analysis can directly test protein expression, and it is limited only by the amount of starting lysate and the availability of antibodies specific for the protein being studied. Additional methods have been developed to study gene expression. Each of these techniques can be used to study a certain gene and gather information about its expression and function, or they can be used to study certain cells and gain information on which genes they are expressing and how they grow and survive.

Microarrays

Microarrays can be used to study relative RNA amounts between two samples or to compare RNA levels in one sample to a normal reference. The two samples of RNA (either two different experimental samples being compared to each other, or one sample and a control) are reverse-transcribed into cDNA and labeled with fluorescent dyes of different colors, then mixed and applied to an array chip. This chip contains binding sites for every known gene, which act as probes to determine transcript levels in the samples. For example, in Figure 17, gene expression is being compared between two tissue samples (A and B) using a hybridization microarray. The cDNA generated from sample A is labeled red, and cDNA generated from sample B is labeled green. Samples are mixed and applied to the chip. Genes 1 and 5 are more highly expressed in Sample A, since these sites on the chip are red. Genes 2 and 4 are more highly expressed in Sample B, since these sites on the chip are green. Gene 3 is expressed in both samples in approximately equal amount resulting in yellow. Microarray data is quantitative, and actual fold-changes can be calculated based on color and intensity.

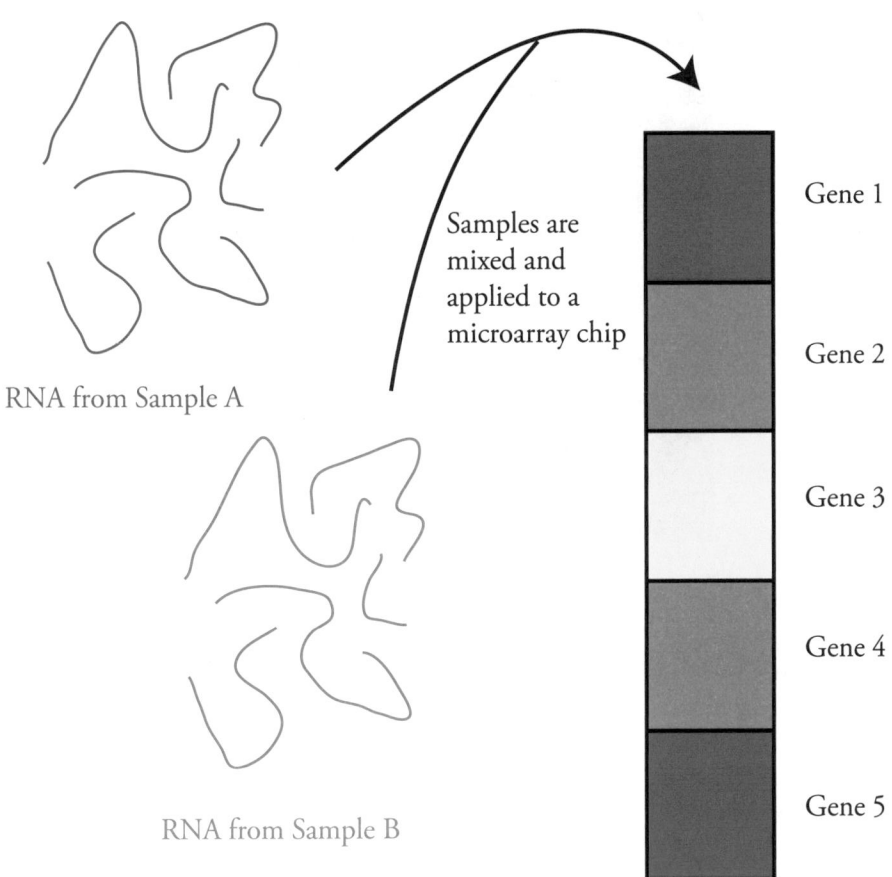

Figure 17   Transcriptional Profiling via Microarray

In situ Hybridization

In situ hybridization (ISH) can be used to determine expression of a gene of interest in a tissue, or in an embryo. A very thin slice (or "section") of a tissue sample is mounted onto a microscope slide. The tissue is fixed to keep transcripts in place, and then it is permeabilized to open the cell membrane. A labeled probe, which is specific for the transcript of interest, is added to the section and binds to the transcript being studied. An enzyme-linked antibody is added and binds to the probe. When a substrate for the enzyme is added, the target transcript-probe-antibody complex is detected. In this way, it can be determined when and where transcripts are expressed on a multicellular level.

Immunohistochemistry

This technique is similar to ISH, but it is specific for proteins instead of nucleic acids. As such, it gives a direct report on protein expression in a tissue. Immunohistochemistry (IHC) requires an antibody against a known protein. This antibody is recognized by a secondary antibody, which is either linked to an enzyme or a fluorescent molecule. IHC is commonly used in the clinic. For example, breast cancer biopsies from women are stained for the estrogen receptor (ER), the progesterone receptor (PR), and a plasma membrane receptor called HER2. Breast tumors are then classified as ER$^+$ or ER$^-$, PR$^+$ or PR$^-$, and HER2$^+$ or HER2$^-$. These classifications affect which therapy the patient is given.

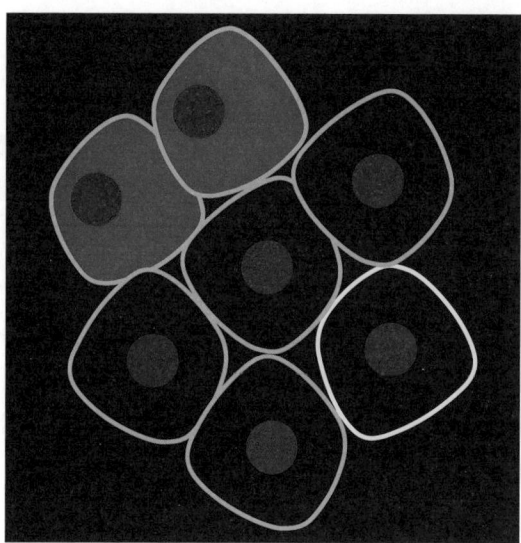

Figure 18   Using Immunofluorescence to Determine Subcellular Protein Expression

In Figure 18, cells were stained with three different markers: the plasma membrane was labeled in green, the nucleus was labeled in blue, and the protein of interest was labeled in red. Four different staining patterns are observed. The two cells at the top express the protein of interest in the cytoplasm. The three cells in the middle do not express the protein of interest. The cell on the bottom left expresses the protein of interest in the nucleus; the blue nuclear stain and red protein of interest stain are overlapping to make the nucleus purple. In the bottom right cell, the protein of interest is expressed on the plasma membrane. Co-expression of the green plasma membrane marker and the red protein of interest cause yellow staining of the plasma membrane.

Flow Cytometry

Flow cytometry again uses many of the same principles already discussed. Here, single cells (either from lab cultures or tissue samples) are stained for certain protein markers using specific antibodies. The antibodies are then linked to a fluorescent tag. Next, the labeled cells are suspended in a fluid stream and passed through a beam of light. Light detectors are found on the other side of, and perpendicular to, the laser. As the labeled cells pass through the light, the beam scatters and the fluorescent tag(s) on the cells can emit light. This combination of scattered and emitted light is measured to give information on cell size and how many cells in the sample express each of the markers that were labeled. Flow cytometers can have over a dozen different light channels, so many labeled antibodies can be added to one experimental sample. In addition to being analyzed, cells can also be sorted as they go through the machine (a technique called fluorescence-activated cell sorting, or FACS). In this way, a heterogeneous mixture of cells can be sorted based on expression of markers.

For example, the earliest (or least differentiated) thymocytes in the thymus express neither CD4 nor CD8; therefore, they are classed as double-negative ($CD4^-CD8^-$) cells. As these cells progress through their development, they become double-positive thymocytes ($CD4^+CD8^+$), and they finally mature to single-positive ($CD4^+CD8^-$ helper T-cells, or $CD4^-CD8^+$ killer T-cells) thymocytes that are then released from the thymus to peripheral tissues. Each of these four cell populations could be studied using flow cytometry (to determine their relative amounts for example) and could be isolated from each other using FACS.

A.11 PROTEIN QUANTIFICATION

A good understanding of genomics has led to the field of **proteomics**, the systematic and large-scale study of protein structure and function. This is usually done in a particular context, such as in a certain biochemical pathway, organelle, cell, tissue, or organism. Often, this involves quantitative analysis of proteins. This means measuring amounts of different proteins from a functional standpoint, looking at how the amount, state, or location of a protein changes. Here are some examples.

- It's been hypothesized that a particular protein under study functions in G_1 of the cell cycle, but not the other phases. A biochemist tags the protein with a fluorescent molecule, and observes live and cycling cells under a fluorescent microscope. He finds that the cells have high levels of fluorescence in G_1, but very low levels of fluorescence in the other cell phases. This suggests the protein under study is expressed at high levels in G_1 and then is degraded at the beginning of S phase.

- A biochemist is studying the function of an unknown protein, which has been shown to have important functions when a specific transcription factor is mutated. The biochemist obtains two cell lines. One has a mutation in the transcription factor, and the other doesn't. She generates lysate samples from the two cell lines. [This means she collects and lyses cells, releasing cellular proteins. Other macromolecules (such as lipid bilayers, DNA and RNA) are cleared or degraded by enzymes.] She then examines the two lysate samples, looking specifically at the protein of interest. She finds it is not phosphorylated in the cell line without the transcription factor mutation, but is phosphorylated in the cell line with the mutation.

- A biochemist has a culture of actively growing cells and applies a drug that is being tested for its therapeutic use. The drug targets a protein normally found in the nucleus of the cell. Addition of the drug causes the protein to be transported out of the nucleus and into the cytoplasm. A quantitative protein experiment measured the total amount of protein in different parts of the cell before and after treatment. It found 90% of the protein in the nucleus before drug treatment, and only 15% was in the nucleus after drug treatment.

Many different techniques can help with studying proteins quantitatively. Some of these look at proteins in a cell, either alive (FACS, labeling a protein and looking and subcellular location) or not (immunohistochemistry, flow cytometry). Others measure proteins harvested from a cell (ELISA, Western blotting, immunoprecipitation). All of these techniques are discussed earlier in this in Appendix.

It's common for proteins to be grown in a biological system and then extracted and studied. Often, protein levels in lysates or purified samples must be quantified before an experiment can be started. For example, before performing a Western blot, biochemists typically measure protein concentrations in each sample being studied, to make sure the same amount of lysate is loaded into each well of the gel.

A.11

The most commonly used quantification method is Bradford Quantification, using UV-Vis spectrophotometers designed for biochemical analysis. This method uses a Bradford reagent containing a blue pigment called Coomassie blue. When proteins bind the pigment, it shifts the absorption peak of the sample (Figure 19). Absorption is measured at 600 nm. This technique is very simple and has good sensitivity.

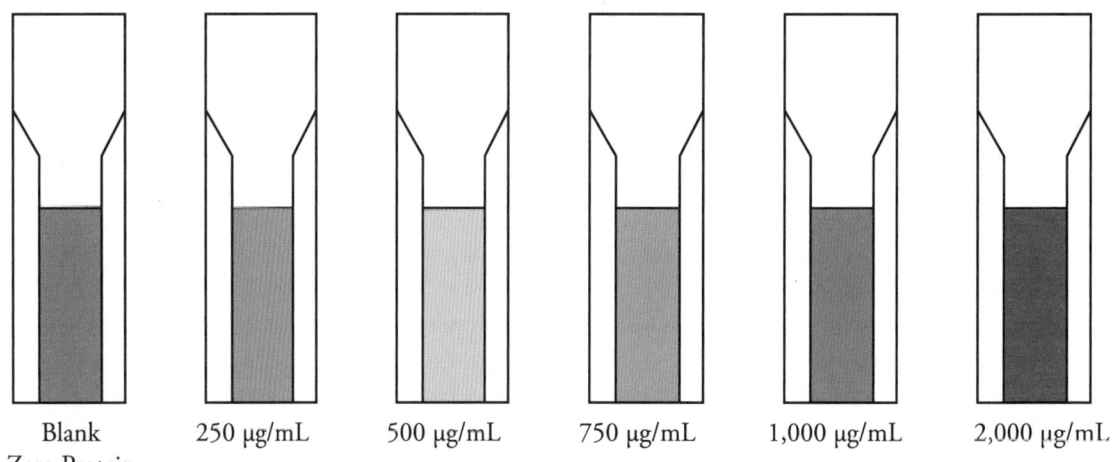

| Blank Zero Protein | 250 µg/mL | 500 µg/mL | 750 µg/mL | 1,000 µg/mL | 2,000 µg/mL |

Figure 19 Bradford Quantification of Proteins

To perform quantification, first, the negative control sample is put in the spectrophotometer, to set the zero value. Next, the samples with known concentration are applied, and the spectrophotometer generates a concentration curve. This relates absorbance of the sample with protein concentration. A new curve should be made every time proteins are being quantified. Next, the samples are put in the machine one by one. The spectrophotometer applies light in the visible and adjacent (near-UV and near-infrared) ranges. Absorbance is determined and compared to the calibration curve, and the machine usually reports both the absorbance and the subsequent protein concentration.

A.12

A.12   AFFINITY CHROMATOGRAPHY

Affinity chromatography, which is used to separate biochemical mixtures, is based on highly specific interactions between macromolecules. While affinity chromatography is most commonly used to purify proteins, it can also be used on other macromolecules (such as nucleic acids). It uses many of the same principles described above: you start with a heterogeneous mixture of molecules (such as cell lysate, growth media or blood). To isolate a protein of interest, you can either use an antibody or tag the protein with an affinity tag. (For example, His-tagged proteins can be purified with nickel-based resins and slightly basic conditions; the bound proteins are eluted by adding imidazole or by lowering the pH.) The target molecule is trapped on a stationary phase due to specific binding, and the stationary phase is washed to increase purity. The target protein is then released (or eluted) off the solid phase, in a highly purified state.

Biochemistry Glossary

After each definition, the section number in *MCAT Biochemistry Review* where the term is discussed is given.

acetyl-CoA
The first substrate in the Krebs cycle, produced primarily from the oxidation of pyruvate by the pyruvate dehydrogenase complex; however acetyl-CoA is also produced during fatty acid oxidation and protein catabolism. [**Section 5.3**]

activation energy (E_a)
The amount of energy required to produce the transition state of a chemical reaction. If the activation energy for a reaction is very high, the reaction occurs very slowly. Enzymes (and other catalysts) increase reaction rates by reducing activation energy. [**Section 3.2**]

active site
The three-dimensional site on an enzyme where substrates (reactants) bind and a chemical reaction is facilitated. [**Section 4.5**]

active site model
Also called the "lock and key" model, this states that the active site of an enzyme and its substrate are perfectly complementary. [**Section 4.5**]

adenine
One of the four aromatic bases found in DNA and RNA; also a component of ATP, NADH, and $FADH_2$. Adenine is a purine; it pairs with thymine (in DNA) and with uracil (in RNA). [**Section 7.2**]

allosteric regulation
The modification of enzyme activity through interaction of molecules with specific sites on the enzyme other than the active site (called allosteric sites). [**Section 4.6**]

amino acids
The building blocks (monomers) of proteins. There are 20 different amino acids. [**Section 4.1**]

amphoteric substance
A substance that can act as either an acid or a base; e.g., the conjugate base of a weak polyprotic acid. [**Section 3.4**]

anabolism
The process of building complex structures out of simpler precursors (for example, synthesizing proteins from amino acids). [**Section 3.3**]

antiparallel orientation
The normal configuration of double-stranded DNA in which the 5' end of one strand is paired with the 3' end of the other. [**Section 7.2**]

ATP synthase
A protein complex found in the inner membrane of the mitochondria. It is essentially a channel that allows H^+ ions to flow from the intermembrane space to the matrix (down the gradient produced by the enzyme complexes of the electron transport chain); as the H^+ ions flow through the channel, ATP is synthesized from ADP and P_i. [**Section 5.3**]

blotting
The transfer of DNA or proteins from an electrophoresis gel to a nitrocellulose filter. [**Section A.4**]

Brønsted-Lowry acid/base
Brønsted-Lowry acids are proton donors; Brønsted-Lowry bases are proton acceptors. [**Section 3.4**]

buffer solution
A solution that resists changes in pH when acids or bases are added; it is usually made up of a weak acid and its conjugate base. [**Section 3.4**]

catabolism
The process of breaking down large molecules into smaller precursors (e.g. digestion of starch into glucose). [**Section 3.3**]

catalyst
Something that increases the rate of a chemical reaction by reducing the activation energy for that reaction. The ΔG of the reaction remains unchanged. [**Section 3.2**]

centromere
A structure near the middle of eukaryotic chromosomes to which the fibers of the mitotic spindle attach during cell division. [**Section 7.2**]

cholesterol
A large, ring-shaped lipid found in cell membranes. Cholesterol is the precursor for steroid hormones and is used to manufacture bile salts. [**Sections 3.4 and 7.3**]

chromatin
DNA that is densely packed around histone proteins. The genes in heterochromatin are generally inaccessible to enzymes and are turned off. [**Section 7.2**]

chromosome
A single piece of double-stranded DNA; part of the genome of an organism. Prokaryotes have circular chromosomes, and eukaryotes have linear chromosomes. [**Section 7.2**]

citric acid cycle
See "Krebs cycle." [**Section 5.3**]

coenzyme

An organic molecule that associates non-covalently with an enzyme; it is required for the proper functioning of the enzyme. [**Section 4.6**]

coenzyme Q (ubiquinone)

A small non-protein electron carrier in the electron transport chain. [**Section 5.3**]

cofactor

An inorganic molecule that associates non-covalently with an enzyme; it is required for the proper functioning of the enzyme. [**Section 4.6**]

competitive inhibitor

An enzyme inhibitor that competes with substrate for binding at the active site of the enzyme. When the inhibitor is bound, no product can be made. [**Section 4.8**]

cooperativity

A type of substrate binding to a multi-active site enzyme, in which the binding of one substrate molecule modulates the binding of subsequent substrate molecules. If the substrate affinity of the other subunits increases, it is positive cooperativity. If the substrate affinity of the other subunits decreases, it is negative cooperativity. A graph of reaction rate vs. substrate concentration appears sigmoidal. Note that cooperativity can be found in other situations as well; for example, hemoglobin binds oxygen with positive cooperativity. [**Section 4.7**]

cristae

The folds of the inner membrane of a mitochondrion. [**Section 5.3**]

cytochrome C

A small, iron-containing protein in the electron transport chain. [**Section 5.3**]

cytosine

One of the four aromatic bases found in DNA and RNA. Cytosine is a pyrimidine; it pairs with guanine. [**Section 7.2**]

denaturation

To lose three-dimensional structure, as when a protein is exposed to high temperatures. [**Section 4.3**]

disaccharide

A molecule formed by joining two monosaccharides. Common disaccharides are maltose, sucrose, and lactose. [**Section 5.1**]

disulfide bridge

A covalent sulfur-sulfur bond between the side chains of two cysteine residues; it can be in the same peptide or between two different peptides. [**Section 4.3**]

electron transport chain

A series of enzyme complexes found along the inner mitochondrial membrane. NADH and $FADH_2$ are oxidized by these enzymes; the electrons are shuttled down the chain and are ultimately passed to oxygen to produce water. The electron energy is used to pump H^+ out of the mitochondrial matrix; the resulting H^+ gradient is subsequently used to drive the production of ATP. [**Section 5.3**]

electrophoresis

A means of separating things by size (for example, nucleic acids or proteins) or by charge (for example, proteins). [**Section A.3**]

ELISA

A biochemical technique that utilizes antigen-antibody interactions to determine the presence of either antigens (such as proteins or cytokines), or specific immunoglobulins (antibodies) in a sample (such as cells recovered from a tumor biopsy or a patient's serum). [**Section A.1**]

enzyme

A physiological catalyst. Enzymes are usually proteins, although some RNAs have catalytic activity. [**Sections 3.2 and 4.4**]

euchromatin

DNA that is loosely packed around histones. This DNA is more accessible to enzymes, and the genes in euchromatin can be activated if needed. [**Section 7.2**]

$FADH_2$

The reduced form (carries electrons) of FAD (flavin adenine dinucleotide). This is the other main electron carrier in cellular respiration (NADH is the most common). [**Section 5.3**]

fatty acid

A long chain hydrocarbon with a carboxylic acid functional group. [**Section 6.1**]

fatty acid oxidation

Also called beta-oxidation; the breakdown of fatty acids into acetyl-CoA molecules. [**Section 6.6**]

fatty acid synthase

The enzyme that synthesizes fatty acids from 2-carbon units derived from malonyl-CoA. This enzyme requires the reducing power of NADPH, obtained from the pentose phosphate pathway. [**Section 6.6**]

feedback inhibition
Also called *negative feedback*, the inhibition of an early step in a series of events by the product of a later step in the series. This has the effect of stopping the series of events when the products are plentiful and the series is unnecessary. Feedback inhibition is the most common form of regulation in the body, controlling such things as enzyme reactions, hormone levels, blood pressure, body temperature, and so on. [**Section 4.6**]

fermentation
The reduction of pyruvate to either ethanol or lactate in order to regenerate NAD⁺ from NADH. Fermentation occurs in the absence of oxygen and allows glycolysis to continue under those conditions. [**Section 5.3**]

flavoproteins
A protein associated with FAD that is commonly involved in redox reactions. [**Section 5.3**]

fructose-1,6-bisphosphatase
Dephosphorylates fru-1,6-bisP in gluconeogenesis. [**Section 5.5**]

futile cycling
The simultaneous activation of metabolic pathways with opposing roles, e.g., running glycolysis and gluconeogenesis at the same time. The tight regulation of metabolic pathways exists to prevent futile cycling. [**Section 5.5**]

gene
A portion of DNA that codes for some product, usually a protein, including all regulatory sequences. Some genes code for rRNA and tRNA, which are not translated. [**Section 7.2**]

genome
All the genetic information in an organism; all of an organism's chromosomes. [**Section 7.2**]

Gibbs free energy
The energy in a system that can be used to drive chemical reactions. If the change in free energy of a reaction (ΔG, the free energy of the products minus the free energy of the reactants) is negative, the reaction will occur spontaneously. [**Section 3.1**]

glucagon
A peptide hormone produced and secreted by the α cells of the pancreas. It targets primarily the liver, stimulating the breakdown of glycogen, thus increasing blood glucose levels. [**Section 5.5**]

gluconeogenesis
A metabolic pathway that synthesizes glucose from non-carbohydrate precursors. It occurs in the liver when dietary stores of glucose are unavailable and the liver has depleted its stores of glycogen and glucose. [**Section 5.4**]

glucose-6-phosphate dehydrogenase (G6PDH)
The enzyme that catalyzes the first step in the oxidative phase of the pentose phosphate pathway; it decarboxylates glucose-6-P to form ribulose-5-P and forms NADPH in the process. [**Section 5.7**]

glucose-6-phosphatase
The enzyme that decarboxylates glu-6-P in gluconeogenesis. This step is important so that glucose can exit the liver cell and enter the bloodstream. [**Section 5.5**]

glycogen phosphorylase
The enzyme that catalyzes the phosphorylation and subsequent removal of one glucose monomer at the end of a glycogen polymer. [**Sections 4.4 and 5.6**]

glycogen synthase
The enzyme that catalyzes the addition of glucose monomers to the glycogen polymer. [**Section 5.6**]

glycogenolysis
A term for glycogen breakdown. [**Section 5.6**]

glycolysis
The anaerobic splitting of a glucose molecule into 2 pyruvic acid molecules, producing two net ATP molecules and two NADH molecules. This is the first step in cellular respiration. [**Section 5.3**]

glycosidic linkage
The bond holding two monosaccharides together. [**Section 5.1**]

guanine
One of the four aromatic bases found in DNA and RNA. Guanine is a purine; it pairs with cytosine. [**Section 7.2**]

heterochromatin
Densely packed, tightly coiled DNA that is generally inactive (not being transcribed). [**Section 7.2**]

hexokinase
The enzyme that catalyzes the phosphorylation of glucose to form glucose-6-phosphate in the first step of glycolysis. This is one of the main regulatory steps of this pathway. Hexokinase is feedback-inhibited by glucose-6-P. [**Section 5.3**]

histones
Globular proteins that assist in DNA packaging in eukaryotes. Histones form octamers around which DNA is wound to form a nucleosome. [**Section 7.2**]

hydrolase
A generic term for an enzyme that hydrolyzes chemical bonds (ATPases, proteases, etc.). [**Section 4.4**]

induced fit model
This model of enzyme-substrate interaction asserts that the active site and the substrate differ slightly in structure/shape and that binding of the substrate induces a conformational change in the enzyme. [**Section 4.5**]

insulin
A peptide hormone produced and secreted by the β-cells of the pancreas. Insulin targets all cells in the body, especially the liver and muscle, and allows them to take glucose out of the blood (thus lowering blood glucose levels). [**Section 5.5**]

isoelectric point
The pH at which an amino acid has no overall charge. [**Section 4.2**]

isomerase
An enzyme that rearranges bonds within a molecule. [**Section 4.4**]

ketogenesis
The production of ketone bodies from fats and protein during times of starvation; it occurs in the liver. [**Section 6.6**]

ketone bodies
Produced from acetyl-CoA under starvation conditions. Ketone bodies can cross the blood brain barrier to act as a fuel source for the brain. [**Section 6.6**]

kinase
An enzyme that transfers a phosphoryl group from ATP to other compounds. Kinases are frequently used in regulatory pathways, phosphorylating other enzymes. [**Sections 4.4 and 4.6**]

K_a
The acid-dissociation constant. The larger the K_a value, the stronger the acid. [**Section 3.4**]

K_b
The base-dissociation constant. The larger the K_b value, the stronger the base. [**Section 3.4**]

K_m
The substrate concentration required to reach $1/2\ V_{max}$; a measure of an enzyme's affinity for its substrate. [**Section 4.7**]

Krebs cycle
The third stage of cellular respiration, in which acetyl-CoA is combined with oxaloacetate to form citric acid. The citric acid is then decarboxylated twice and isomerized to recreate oxaloacetate. In the process, 3 molecules of NADH, 1 molecule of $FADH_2$, and 1 molecule of GTP are formed. [**Section 5.3**]

lactic acid
Produced in muscle cells from the reduction of pyruvate (under anaerobic conditions) to regenerate NAD^+ so that glycolysis can continue. A rise in lactic acid levels usually accompanies an increase in physical activity. [**Section 3.4**]

Le Châtelier's Principle
A principle that describes the effect of changes in the temperature, pressure, or concentration of one of the reactants or products of a reaction at equilibrium. It states that when a system at equilibrium is subjected to a stress, it will shift in the direction that minimizes the effect of this stress. [**Section 3.1**]

Lewis acid/base
Lewis acids are electron-pair acceptors; Lewis bases are electron-pair donors. [**Section 3.4**]

lipoproteins
Large conglomerations of protein, fats, and cholesterol that transport lipids in the bloodstream. [**Section 6.4**]

lipid
A hydrophobic molecule, usually formed from long hydrocarbon chains. The most common forms in which lipids are found in the body are as triglycerides (energy storage), phospholipids (cell membranes), and cholesterol (cell membranes and steroid synthesis). [**Section 6.1**]

lyase
An enzyme that breaks chemical bonds by means other than oxidation or hydrolysis (e.g., pyruvate decarboxylase). [**Section 4.4**]

matrix
The interior of a mitochondrion (the region bounded by the inner membrane). The matrix is the site of action of the pyruvate dehydrogenase complex and the Krebs cycle. [**Section 5.3**]

mitochondrion
An organelle surrounded by a double-membrane (two lipid bilayers) where ATP production takes place. The interior (matrix) is where PDC and the Krebs cycle occur, and the inner membrane contains the enzymes of the electron transport chain and ATP synthase. [**Section 5.3**]

mixed-type inhibition
An enzyme inhibitor that can bind to the enzyme either in its free form or as enzyme-substrate complex. [**Section 4.8**]

NADH
The reduced form (carries electrons) of NAD^+ (nicotinamide adenine dinucleotide). This is the most common electron carrier in cellular respiration. [**Section 5.3**]

negative feedback
See "feedback inhibition." [**Section 4.6**]

non-coding RNA
RNA that is not translated into protein, includes tRNA and rRNA (both involved in protein synthesis), and snRNA, miRNA, and siNRA (that help regulate gene expression). [**Section 7.3**]

noncompetitive inhibitor
An enzyme inhibitor that binds at a site other than the active site of an enzyme (i.e., binds at an *allosteric site*). This changes the three-dimensional shape of the enzyme such that it can no longer catalyze the reaction. [**Section 4.8**]

nucleoside
A structure composed of a ribose molecule linked to one of the aromatic bases. In a deoxynucleoside, the ribose is replaced with deoxyribose. [**Section 7.2**]

nucleosome
A structure composed of two coils of DNA wrapped around an octet of histone proteins. The nucleosome is the primary form of packaging of eukaryotic DNA. [**Section 7.2**]

nucleotide
A nucleoside with one or more phosphate groups attached. Nucleoside triphosphates (NTPs) are the building blocks of RNA and are also used as energy molecules, especially ATP. Deoxynucleoside triphosphates (dNTPs) are the building blocks of DNA; in these molecules, the ribose is replaced with deoxyribose. [**Section 7.2**]

oxaloacetate
A four-carbon molecule that binds with the two-carbon acetyl unit of acetyl-CoA to form citric acid in the first step of the Krebs cycle. [**Section 5.3**]

oxidation
A process that attaches oxygen, removes hydrogen, or removes electrons from a molecule. [**Section 3.3**]

oxidative phosphorylation
The oxidation of high-energy electron carriers (NADH and FADH$_2$) coupled to the phosphorylation of ADP, producing ATP. In eukaryotes, oxidative phosphorylation occurs in the mitochondria. [**Section 5.3**]

oxidoreductase
A class of enzymes that runs redox reactions; this class includes oxidases, reductases, dehydrogenases, etc. [**Section 4.4**]

pentose phosphate pathway (PPP)
A metabolic pathway that diverts glucose-6-P from glycolysis in order to form ribose-5-P, which can be used to synthesize nucleotides. It also produces NADPH, which can be used as reducing power in fatty acid synthesis. [**Section 5.7**]

PEPCK
Phosphoenolpyruvate carboxykinase; decarboxylates and phosphorylates oxaloacetate to form phosphoenolpyruvate in the second step of gluconeogenesis. [**Section 5.4**]

pH
The negative log of [H$^+$]; the lower the pH the more acidic the solution. [**Section 3.4**]

phosphatase
An enzyme that dephosphorylates (or removes a phosphoryl group) from a compound. [**Section 4.4**]

phosphofructokinase (PFK)
The enzyme that catalyzes the phosphorylation of fructose-6-phosphate to form fructose-1-6-bisphosphate in the third step of glycolysis. This is the main regulatory step of glycolysis. PFK is feedback-inhibited by ATP. [**Section 5.3**]

phospholipid
The primary membrane lipid. Phospholipids consist of a glycerol molecule esterified to two fatty acid chains and a phosphate molecule. Additional, highly hydrophilic groups are attached to the phosphate, making this molecule extremely amphipathic. [**Section 6.3**]

phosphorylase
An enzyme that transfers a free-floating inorganic phosphate to another molecule. [**Section 4.4**]

pK_a
The negative log of the K_a value. The lower the pK_a, the stronger the acid. [**Section 3.4**]

pK_b
The negative log of the K_b value. The lower the pK_b, the stronger the base. [**Section 3.4**]

pOH
The negative log of [OH$^-$]; the lower the pOH, the more basic the solution. [**Section 3.4**]

polyprotic acid
An acid with more than one ionizable proton. [**Section 3.4**]

polysaccharides
Multiple monosaccharides joined in a large polymer. Polysaccharides are often storage molecules for glucose (glycogen, starch) or structural molecules (cellulose). [**Section 5.2**]

primary structure
The amino acid sequence of a protein. [**Section 4.3**]

prostaglandins
Eicosanoids derived from 20-carbon fatty acids, prostaglandins have different roles in different tissues, such as regulating smooth muscle contraction, increasing mucus secretion, regulating blood vessel diameter, etc. [**Section 6.5**]

prosthetic group
A non-protein, but organic, molecule (such as a vitamin) that is covalently bound to an enzyme as part of the active site. [**Section 5.3**]

protease
A class of enzymes that hydrolyzes peptide bonds (e.g., trypsin and pepsin). [**Section 4.3**]

purine bases
Aromatic bases found in DNA and RNA that are derived from purine. They have a double-ring structure and include adenine and guanine. [**Section 7.1**]

pyrimidine bases
Aromatic bases found in DNA and RNA that have a single-ring structure. They include cytosine, thymine, and uracil. [**Section 7.1**]

pyruvate dehydrogenase complex
A group of three enzymes that decarboxylates pyruvate, creating an acetyl group and carbon dioxide. The acetyl group is then attached to coenzyme A to produce acetyl-CoA, a substrate in the Krebs cycle. In the process, NAD^+ is reduced to NADH. The pyruvate dehydrogenase complex is the second stage of cellular respiration. [**Section 5.3**]

pyruvate carboxylase
An enzyme that adds CO_2 to pyruvate to form oxaloacetate in the first step of gluconeogenesis. [**Section 5.4**]

pyruvate kinase
An enzyme that catalyzes the final step in glycolysis, the conversion of PEP into pyruvate. [**Section 5.3**]

pyruvic acid
The product of glycolysis; 2 pyruvic acid (pyruvate) molecules are produced from a single glucose molecule. In the absence of oxygen, pyruvic acid undergoes fermentation and is reduced to either lactic acid or ethanol; in the presence of oxygen, pyruvic acid is oxidized to produce acetyl-CoA, which can enter the Krebs cycle. [**Section 5.3**]

quaternary structure
A level of protein structure that involves interactions between side chains of amino acids in separate peptides of a multisubunit protein. [**Section 4.4**]

reaction coupling
Using the energy released by a spontaneous reaction to drive a non-spontaneous reaction; the most often coupled reaction is ATP hydrolysis. [**Section 4.4**]

reciprocal control
The tight regulatory control exerted over opposing metabolic pathways in order to avoid futile cycling. [**Section 5.5**]

reduction
A process that removes oxygen, adds hydrogen, or adds electrons to a molecule. [**Section 3.3**]

replication
The duplication of DNA. [**Section 7.2**]

secondary structure
Hydrogen bonding between the backbone atoms of amino acids in a protein; includes alpha helices and beta pleated sheets. [**Section 4.3**]

sphingolipid
A molecule similar to a phospholipid, except that the backbone is sphingosine instead of glycerol. [**Section 6.5**]

substrate(s)
The reactants in an enzyme-catalyzed reaction. Substrate binds at the active site of an enzyme. [**Section 4.5**]

telomere
A specialized region at the ends of eukaryotic chromosomes that contains several repeats of a particular DNA sequence. These ends are maintained (in some cells) with the help of a special DNA polymerase called *telomerase*. In cells that lack telomerase, the telomeres slowly degrade with each round of DNA replication; this is thought to contribute to the eventual death of the cell. [**Section 7.2**]

terpenes
A member of a broad class of compounds built from isoprene units (C_5H_8). [**Section 6.4**]

tertiary structure
A level of protein structure that involves side chain interactions between amino acids in a protein; produces the three-dimensional shape of the protein. [**Section 4.3**]

thymine
One of the four aromatic bases found in DNA. Thymine is a pyrimidine; it pairs with adenine. [**Section 7.2**]

transcription
The enzymatic process of reading a strand of DNA to produce a complementary strand of RNA. [**Section 6.6**]

transition state (TS)
A high-energy, temporary compound produced during a chemical reaction. The energy required to produce TS (the activation energy) determines the rate of the reaction. [**Section 3.2**]

translation
The process of reading a strand of mRNA to synthesize protein. Protein translation takes place on a ribosome. [**Section 7.3**]

tricarboxylic acid (TCA) cycle
See "Krebs cycle." [**Section 5.3**]

triglyceride
Three fatty acids bound to a glycerol molecule. This is an energy storage molecule for the body. [**Section 6.2**]

uncompetitive inhibition
An enzyme inhibitor that can bind to the enzyme only after its substrate has bound. Uncompetitive inhibitors appear to increase the affinity an enzyme has for its substrate because it effectively locks the two together. [**Section 4.8**]

uracil
One of four aromatic bases found in RNA. Uracil is pyrimidine; it pairs with adenine. [**Section 7.3**]

waxes
Long-chain fats esterified to long-chain alcohols. Waxes form waterproof barriers. [**Section 6.5**]

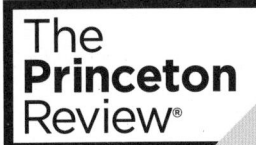

MCAT®

Biology Review

3rd Edition

The Staff of The Princeton Review

Penguin
Random
House

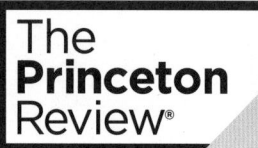

The Princeton Review
110 E. 42nd Street
New York, NY 10017

ISBN: 978-0-593-51623-2
ISSN: 2770-453X

The MCAT is a registered trademark of the Association of American Medical Colleges.

The Princeton Review is not affiliated with Princeton University.

Editor: Aaron Riccio
Production Artist: John Stecyk
Production Editor: Liz Dacey, Sarah Litt

Manufactured in China.

10 9 8 7 6 5 4 3 2 1

3rd Edition

The Princeton Review Publishing Team
Rob Franek, Editor-in-Chief
David Soto, Senior Director, Data Operations
Stephen Koch, Senior Manager, Data Operations
Deborah Weber, Director of Production
Jason Ullmeyer, Production Design Manager
Jennifer Chapman, Senior Production Artist
Selena Coppock, Director of Editorial
Aaron Riccio, Senior Editor
Meave Shelton, Senior Editor
Chris Chimera, Editor
Orion McBean, Editor
Patricia Murphy, Editor
Laura Rose, Editor
Alexa Schmitt Bugler, Editorial Assistant

Random House Publishing Team
Tom Russell, VP, Publisher
Alison Stoltzfus, Senior Director, Publishing
Brett Wright, Senior Editor
Emily Hoffman, Assistant Managing Editor
Ellen Reed, Production Manager
Suzanne Lee, Designer
Eugenia Lo, Publishing Assistant

For customer service, please contact
editorialsupport@review.com,
and be sure to include:

- full title of the book

- ISBN

- page number

CONTRIBUTORS

Daniel J. Pallin, M.D.
    Senior Author
Judene Wright, M.S., M.A.Ed.
    Senior Author

TPR MCAT Biology and Biochemistry Development Team:

Jessica Adams, Ph.D.
Britney McMurren, B.H.Sc., M.Sc.
Judene Wright, M.S., M.A.Ed., Senior Editor, Lead Developer
Sarah Woodruff, B.S., B.A.

Edited for Production by:

Judene Wright, M.S., M.A.Ed.
    National Content Director, MCAT Program, The Princeton Review

The TPR MCAT Biology and Biochemistry Team and Judene would like to thank the following people for their contributions to this book :

Kashif Anwar, M.D., M.M.S., John Bahling, M.D., Kristen Brunson, Ph.D., Phil Carpenter, Ph.D., Khawar Chaudry, B.S., Nita Chauhan, H.BSc, MSc, Dan Cho, M.P.H., Glenn E. Croston, Ph.D., Nathan Deal, M.D., Ian Denham, B.Sc., B.Ed., Joshua Dilworth, M.D., Ph.D., Annie Dude, Rob Fong, M.D., Ph.D., Chris Fortenbach, B.S., Kirsten Frank, Ph.D., Isabel L. Jackson, B.S., Erik Kildebeck, George Kyriazis, Ph.D., Ben Lee, Heather Liwanag, Ph.D., Travis MacKoy, B.S., Joey Mancuso, M.S., D.O., Evan Martow, BMSc, Brian Mikolasko, M.D., M.BA, Abhisehk Mohapatra, B.A., Christopher Moriates, M.D., Stephen L. Nelson, Jr., Ph.D., Rupal Patel, B.S., Mary Qiu, Ina C. Roy, M.D., Jayson Sack, M.D., M.S., Will Sanderson, Jeanine Seitz-Partridge, M.S., Oktay Shuminov, B.S., Andrew D. Snyder, M.D., Preston Swirnoff, Ph.D., M.S., Jenkang Tao, B.S., B.A., Rhead Uddin, Jia Wang.

PERIODIC TABLE OF THE ELEMENTS

1																	18
1 **H** 1.0	2												13	14	15	16	17	2 **He** 4.0
3 **Li** 6.9	4 **Be** 9.0												5 **B** 10.8	6 **C** 12.0	7 **N** 14.0	8 **O** 16.0	9 **F** 19.0	10 **Ne** 20.2
11 **Na** 23.0	12 **Mg** 24.3	3	4	5	6	7	8	9	10	11	12	13 **Al** 27.0	14 **Si** 28.1	15 **P** 31.0	16 **S** 32.1	17 **Cl** 35.5	18 **Ar** 39.9
19 **K** 39.1	20 **Ca** 40.1	21 **Sc** 45.0	22 **Ti** 47.9	23 **V** 50.9	24 **Cr** 52.0	25 **Mn** 54.9	26 **Fe** 55.8	27 **Co** 58.9	28 **Ni** 58.7	29 **Cu** 63.5	30 **Zn** 65.4	31 **Ga** 69.7	32 **Ge** 72.6	33 **As** 74.9	34 **Se** 79.0	35 **Br** 79.9	36 **Kr** 83.8
37 **Rb** 85.5	38 **Sr** 87.6	39 **Y** 88.9	40 **Zr** 91.2	41 **Nb** 92.9	42 **Mo** 95.9	43 **Tc** (98)	44 **Ru** 101.1	45 **Rh** 102.9	46 **Pd** 106.4	47 **Ag** 107.9	48 **Cd** 112.4	49 **In** 114.8	50 **Sn** 118.7	51 **Sb** 121.8	52 **Te** 127.6	53 **I** 126.9	54 **Xe** 131.3
55 **Cs** 132.9	56 **Ba** 137.3	57 ***La** 138.9	72 **Hf** 178.5	73 **Ta** 180.9	74 **W** 183.9	75 **Re** 186.2	76 **Os** 190.2	77 **Ir** 192.2	78 **Pt** 195.1	79 **Au** 197.0	80 **Hg** 200.6	81 **Tl** 204.4	82 **Pb** 207.2	83 **Bi** 209.0	84 **Po** (209)	85 **At** (210)	86 **Rn** (222)
87 **Fr** (223)	88 **Ra** (226)	89 **†Ac** (227)	104 **Rf** (267)	105 **Db** (268)	106 **Sg** (271)	107 **Bh** (270)	108 **Hs** (269)	109 **Mt** (278)	110 **Ds** (281)	111 **Rg** (282)	112 **Cn** (285)	113 **Nh** (286)	114 **Fl** (289)	115 **Mc** (289)	116 **Lv** (293)	117 **Ts** (294)	118 **Og** (294)

*Lanthanoids	58 **Ce** 140.1	59 **Pr** 140.9	60 **Nd** 144.2	61 **Pm** (145)	62 **Sm** 150.4	63 **Eu** 152.0	64 **Gd** 157.3	65 **Tb** 158.9	66 **Dy** 162.5	67 **Ho** 164.9	68 **Er** 167.3	69 **Tm** 168.9	70 **Yb** 173.0	71 **Lu** 175.0
†Actinoids	90 **Th** 232.0	91 **Pa** (231)	92 **U** 238.0	93 **Np** (237)	94 **Pu** (244)	95 **Am** (243)	96 **Cm** (247)	97 **Bk** (247)	98 **Cf** (251)	99 **Es** (252)	100 **Fm** (257)	101 **Md** (258)	102 **No** (259)	103 **Lr** (266)

CONTENTS

Get More
(Free) Content
at PrincetonReview.com/prep

As easy as 1·2·3

1 Go to PrincetonReview.com/prep or scan the **QR code** and enter the following ISBN for your book:
9780593516232

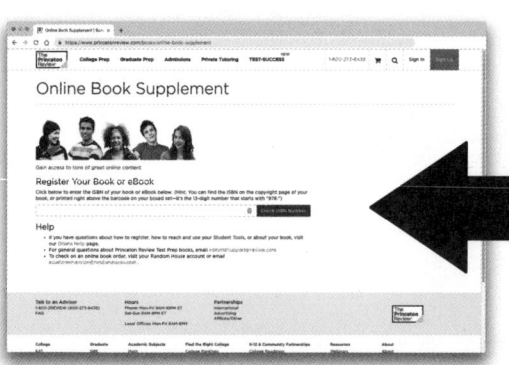

2 Answer a few simple questions to set up an exclusive Princeton Review account. *(If you already have one, you can just log in.)*

3 Enjoy access to your **FREE** content!

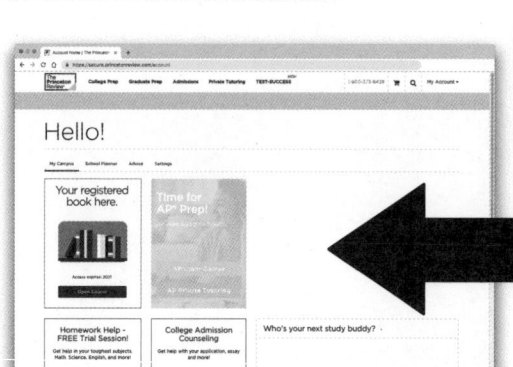

Once you've registered, you can...

- Take **3** full-length practice MCAT exams

- Find useful information about taking the MCAT and applying to medical school

- Check to see if there have been any corrections or updates to this edition

- Get our take on any recent or pending updates to the MCAT

Need to report a potential **content** issue?

Contact **EditorialSupport@review.com** and include:

- full title of the book
- ISBN
- page number

Need to report a **technical** issue?

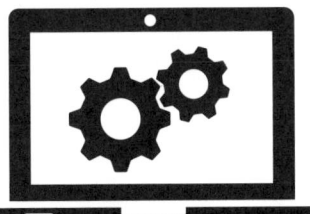

Contact **TPRStudentTech@review.com** and provide:

- your full name
- email address used to register the book
- full book title and ISBN
- Operating system (Mac/PC) and browser (Chrome, Firefox, Safari, etc.)

Chapter 1
MCAT Basics

SO YOU WANT TO BE A DOCTOR

So...you want to be a doctor. If you're like most premeds, you've wanted to be a doctor since you were pretty young. When people asked you what you wanted to be when you grew up, you always answered "a doctor." You had toy medical kits, bandaged up your dog or cat, and played "hospital." You probably read your parents' home medical guides for fun.

When you got to high school you took the honors and AP classes. You studied hard, got straight A's (or at least really good grades!), and participated in extracurricular activities so you could get into a good college. And you succeeded!

At college you knew exactly what to do. You took your classes seriously, studied hard, and got a great GPA. You talked to your professors and hung out at office hours to get good letters of recommendation. You were a member of the premed society on campus, volunteered at hospitals, and shadowed doctors. All that's left to do now is get a good MCAT score.

Just the MCAT.

Just the most confidence-shattering, most demoralizing, longest, most brutal entrance exam for any graduate program. At about 7.5 hours (including breaks), the MCAT tops the list...even the closest runners up, the LSAT and GMAT, are only about 4 hours long. The MCAT tests significant science content knowledge along with the ability to think quickly, reason logically, and read comprehensively, all under the pressure of a timed exam.

The path to a good MCAT score is not as easy to see as the path to a good GPA or the path to a good letter of recommendation. The MCAT is less about what you know, and more about how to apply what you know...and how to apply it quickly to new situations. Because the path might not be so clear, you might be worried. That's why you picked up this book.

We promise to demystify the MCAT for you, with clear descriptions of the different sections, how the test is scored, and what the test experience is like. We will help you understand general test-taking techniques as well as provide you with specific techniques for each section. We will review the science content you need to know as well as give you strategies for the Critical Analysis and Reasoning Skills (CARS) section. We'll show you the path to a good MCAT score and help you walk the path.

After all...you want to be a doctor. And we want you to succeed.

WHAT IS THE MCAT...REALLY?

Most test-takers approach the MCAT as though it were a typical college science test, one in which facts and knowledge simply need to be regurgitated in order to do well. They study for the MCAT the same way they did for their college tests, by memorizing facts and details, formulas and equations. And when they get to the MCAT, they are surprised...and disappointed.

It's a myth that the MCAT is purely a content-knowledge test. If medical-school admission committees want to see what you know, all they have to do is look at your transcripts. What they really want to see is how you *think*, especially how you think under pressure. That's what your MCAT score will tell them.

The MCAT is really a test of your ability to apply basic knowledge to different, possibly new, situations. It's a test of your ability to reason out and evaluate arguments. Do you still need to know your science content? Absolutely. But not at the level that most test-takers think they need to know it. Furthermore, your science knowledge won't help you on the Critical Analysis and Reasoning Skills (CARS) section. So how do you study for a test like this?

You study for the science sections by reviewing the basics and then applying them to MCAT practice questions. You study for the CARS section by learning how to adapt your existing reading and analytical skills to the nature of the test. (More information about the CARS section can be found in *MCAT Critical Analysis and Reasoning Skills Review*.)

The book you are holding will review all the relevant MCAT Biology content you will need for the test, and a little bit more. It includes hundreds of questions designed to make you think about the material in a deeper way, along with full explanations to clarify the logical thought process needed to get to the answer. It also comes with access to three full-length online practice exams to further hone your skills. For more information on accessing those online exams, please refer to the "Get More (Free) Content" spread on pages x–xi.

MCAT NUTS AND BOLTS

Overview

The MCAT is a computer-based test (CBT) that is *not* adaptive. Adaptive tests base your next question on whether or not you've answered the current question correctly. The MCAT is *linear*, or *fixed-form*, meaning that the questions are in a predetermined order and do not change based on your answers. However, there are many versions of the test, so that on a given test day, different people will see different versions. The following table highlights the features of the MCAT exam.

Registration	Online via www.aamc.org. Begins as early as six months prior to test date; available up until week of test (subject to seat availability).
Testing Centers	Administered at small, secure, climate-controlled computer testing rooms.
Security	Photo ID with signature, electronic fingerprint, electronic signature verification, assigned seat.
Proctoring	None. Test administrator checks examinee in and assigns seat at computer. All testing instructions are given on the computer.
Frequency of Test	Many times per year distributed over January, April, May, June, July, August, and September.
Format	Exclusively computer-based. NOT an adaptive test.
Length of Test Day	7.5 hours
Breaks	Optional 10-minute breaks between sections, with a 30-minute break for lunch.
Section Names	1. Chemical and Physical Foundations of Biological Systems (Chem/Phys) 2. Critical Analysis and Reasoning Skills (CARS) 3. Biological and Biochemical Foundations of Living Systems (Bio/Biochem) 4. Psychological, Social, and Biological Foundations of Behavior (Psych/Soc)
Number of Questions and Timing	59 Chem/Phys questions, 95 minutes 53 CARS questions, 90 minutes 59 Bio/Biochem questions, 95 minutes 59 Psych/Soc questions, 95 minutes
Scoring	Test is scaled. Several forms per administration.
Allowed/ Not allowed	No timers/watches. Noise reduction headphones available. Noteboard booklet and wet-erase marker given at start of test and taken at end of test. Locker or secure area provided for personal items.
Results: Timing and Delivery	Approximately 30 days. Electronic scores only, available online through AAMC login. Examinees can print official score reports.
Maximum Number of Retakes	The test can be taken a maximum of three times in one year, four times over two years, and seven times over the lifetime of the examinee. An examinee can be registered for only one date at a time.

Registration

Registration for the exam is completed online at www.aamc.org/students/applying/mcat/reserving. The AAMC opens registration for a given test date at least two months in advance of the date, often earlier. It's a good idea to register well in advance of your desired test date to make sure that you get a seat.

Sections

There are four sections on the MCAT, all of which consist of multiple-choice questions:

Section	Concepts Tested	Number of Questions and Timing
Chemical and Physical Foundations of Biological Systems	Basic concepts in chemistry and physics, including biochemistry; scientific inquiry; reasoning; research and statistics skills.	59 questions in 95 minutes
Critical Analysis and Reasoning Skills	Critical analysis of information drawn from a wide range of social science and humanities disciplines.	53 questions in 90 minutes
Biological and Biochemical Foundations of Living Systems	Basic concepts in biology and biochemistry, scientific inquiry, reasoning, and research and statistics skills.	59 questions in 95 minutes
Psychological, Social, and Biological Foundations of Behavior	Basic concepts in psychology, sociology, and biology; research methods; and statistics.	59 questions in 95 minutes

Most questions on the MCAT (44 in the science sections, all 53 in the CARS section) are passage-based; the science sections have 10 passages each and the CARS section has 9. A passage consists of a few paragraphs of information on which several following questions are based. In the science sections, passages often include equations or reactions, tables, graphs, figures, and experiments to analyze. CARS passages come from literature in social sciences, humanities, ethics, philosophy, cultural studies, and population health, and they do not test content knowledge in any way.

Some questions in the science sections are freestanding questions (FSQs). These questions are independent of any passage information and appear in four groups of about three to four questions, interspersed throughout the passages. Fifteen of the questions in the science sections are freestanding, and the remainder are passage-based.

Each section on the MCAT is separated by either a 10-minute break or a 30-minute lunch break. We recommend that you take these breaks.

Section	Time
Test Center Check-In	Variable, can take up to 40 minutes if center is busy.
Tutorial	10 minutes
Chemical and Physical Foundations of Biological Systems	95 minutes
Break (optional)	10 minutes
Critical Analysis and Reasoning Skills	90 minutes
Lunch Break (optional)	30 minutes
Biological and Biochemical Foundations of Living Systems	95 minutes
Break (optional)	10 minutes
Psychological, Social, and Biological Foundations of Behavior	95 minutes
Void Option	5 minutes
Survey (optional)	5 minutes

The survey includes questions about your satisfaction with the overall MCAT experience, including registration, check-in, etc., as well as questions about how you prepared for the test.

Scoring

The MCAT is a scaled exam, meaning that your raw score will be converted into a scaled score that takes into account the difficulty of the questions. There is no guessing penalty. All sections are scored from 118–132, with a total scaled score range of 472–528. Because different versions of the test have varying levels of difficulty, the scale will be different from one exam to the next. Thus, there is no "magic number" of questions to get right in order to get a particular score. Plus, some of the questions on the test are considered "experimental" and do not count toward your score; they are just there to be evaluated for possible future inclusion in a test.

At the end of the test (after you complete the Psychological, Social, and Biological Foundations of Behavior section), you will be asked to choose one of the following two options, "I wish to have my MCAT exam scored" or "I wish to VOID my MCAT exam." You have five minutes to make a decision, and if you do not select one of the options in that time, the test will automatically be scored. If you choose the VOID option, your test will not be scored (you will not now, or ever, get a numerical score for this test), medical schools will not know you took the test, and no refunds will be granted. You cannot "unvoid" your scores at a later time.

So, what's a good score? The AAMC is centering the scale at 500 (i.e., 500 will be the 50th percentile), and recommends that application committees consider applicants near the center of the range. To be on the safe side, aim for a total score of around 510. Remember that if your GPA is on the low side, you'll need higher MCAT scores to compensate, and if you have a strong GPA, you can get away with lower MCAT scores. But the reality is that your chances of acceptance depend on a lot more than just your MCAT scores. It's a combination of your GPA, your MCAT scores, your undergraduate coursework, letters of recommendation, experience related to the medical field (such as volunteer work or research), extracurricular activities, your personal statement, etc. Medical schools are looking for a complete package, not just good scores and a good GPA.

GENERAL LAYOUT AND TEST-TAKING STRATEGIES

Layout of the Test

In each section of the test, the computer screen is divided vertically, with the passage on the left and the range of questions for that passage indicated above (e.g., "Passage 1 Questions 1–5"). The scroll bar for the passage text appears in the middle of the screen. Each question appears on the right, and you need to click "Next" to move to each subsequent question.

In the science sections, the freestanding questions are found in groups of 3–4, interspersed with the passages. The screen is still divided vertically; on the left is the statement "Questions [X–XX] do not refer to a passage and are independent of each other," and each question appears on the right as described above.

CBT Tools

There are a number of tools available on the test, including highlighting, strike-outs, the Flag for Review button, the Navigation and Review Screen buttons, the Periodic Table button, and of course, the noteboard booklet. All tools are available with both mouse control (buttons to click) or keyboard commands (Alt+ a letter). As everyone has different preferences, you should practice with both types of tools (mouse and keyboard) to see which is more comfortable for you personally. The following is a brief description of each tool.

1) **Highlighting:** This is done in the passage text (including table entries and some equations, but excluding figures and molecular structures), in the question stems, and in the answer choices (including Roman numerals). Select the words you wish to highlight (left-click and drag the cursor across the words), and in the upper left corner click the "Highlight" button to highlight the selected text yellow. Alternatively, press "Alt+H" to highlight the words. Highlighting can be removed by selecting the words again and in the upper left corner clicking the down arrow next to "Highlight." This will expand to show the "Remove Highlight" option; clicking this will remove the highlighting. Removing highlighting via the keyboard is cumbersome and is not recommended.

2) **Strike-outs:** This can be done on the answer choices, including Roman numeral statements, by selecting the text you want to strike out (left-click and drag the cursor across the text), then clicking the "Strikethrough" button in the upper left corner. Alternatively, press "Alt+S" to strikeout the words. The strike-out can be removed by repeating these actions. Figures or molecular structures cannot be struck out, however, the letter answer choice of those structures can.

3) **Flag for Review button:** This is available for each question and is found in the upper right corner. This allows you to flag the question as one you would like to review later if time permits. When clicked, the flag icon turns yellow. Click again to remove the flag. Alternatively, press "Alt+F."

4) **Navigation button:** This is found near the bottom of the screen and is only available on your first pass through the section. Clicking this button brings up a navigation table listing all questions and their statuses (unseen, incomplete, complete, flagged for review). You can also press "Alt+N" to bring up the screen. The questions can be sorted by their statuses, and clicking a question number takes you immediately to that question. Once you have reached the end of the section and viewed the Review screen (described below), the Navigation screen is no longer available.

5) **Review Screen button:** This button is found near the bottom of the screen after your first pass through the section, and when clicked, brings up a new screen showing all questions and their statuses (either incomplete, unseen, or flagged for review). Questions that are complete are assigned no additional status. You can then choose one of three options by clicking with the mouse or with keyboard shortcuts: Review All (Alt+A), Review Incomplete (Alt+I), or Review Flagged (Alt+R); alternatively, you can click a question number to go directly back to that question. You can also end the section from this screen.

6) **Periodic Table button:** Clicking this button will open a periodic table (or press "Alt+T"). Note that the periodic table is large, covering most of the screen. However, this window can be resized to see the questions and a portion of the periodic table at the same time. The table text will not decrease, but scroll bars will appear on the window so you can center the section of the table of interest in the window.

7) **Noteboard Booklet (Scratch Paper):** At the start of the test, you will be given a spiral-bound set of four laminated 8.5"×14" sheets of paper and a wet-erase black marker to use as scratch paper. You can request a clean noteboard booklet at any time during the test; your original booklet will be collected. The noteboard is only useful if it is kept organized; do not give in to the tendency to write on the first available open space! Good organization will be very helpful when/if you wish to review a question. Indicate the passage number, the range of questions for that passage, and a topic in a box near the top of your scratch work, and indicate the question you are working on in a circle to the left of the notes for that question. Draw a line under your scratch work when you change passages to keep the work separate. Do not erase or scribble over any previous work. If you do not think it is correct, draw one line through the work and start again. You may have already done some useful work without realizing it.

General Strategy for the Science Sections

Passages vs. FSQs in the Science Sections: What to Start With

Since the questions are displayed on separate screens, it is awkward and time consuming to click through all of the questions up front to find the FSQs. Therefore, go through the section on a first pass and decide whether to do the passage now or to save it for later, basing your decision on the passage text and the first question. Tackle the FSQs as you come upon them. More details are below.

Here is an outline of the procedure:

1) For each passage, write a heading on your noteboard with the passage number, the general topic, and its range of questions (e.g., "Passage 1, thermodynamics, Q 1–5" or "Passage 2, enzymes, Q 6–9"). The passage numbers do not currently appear in the Navigation or Review screens, thus having the question numbers on your noteboard will allow you to move through the section more efficiently.

2) Skim the text and rank the passage. If a passage is a "Now," complete it before moving on to the next passage (also see Attacking the Questions below). If it is a "Later" passage, first write "SKIPPED" in block letters under the passage heading on your noteboard and leave room for your work when you come back to complete that passage. (Note that the specific passages you skip will be unique to you; in the Bio/Biochem section, you might choose to do all Biology passages first, then come back for Biochemistry. Or in Chem/Phys you might choose to skip experiment-based or analytical passage. Know ahead of time what type of passage you are going to skip and follow your plan.)

3) Next, click on the "Navigation" button at the bottom to get to the Navigation screen. Click on the first question of the next passage; you'll be able to identify it because you know the range of questions from the passage you just skipped. This will take you to the next passage, where you will repeat steps 1–3.

4) Once you have completed the "Now" passages, go to the Review screen and click the first question for the first passage you skipped. Answer the questions, and continue going back to the Review screen and repeating this procedure for other passages you have skipped.

Attacking the Questions

As you work through the questions, if you encounter a particularly lengthy question, or a question that requires a lot of analysis, you may choose to skip it. This is a wise strategy because it ensures you will tackle all the easier questions first, the ones you are more likely to get right. If you choose to skip the question (or if you attempt it but get stuck), write down the question number on your noteboard, click the Flag for Review button to flag the question in the Review screen, and move on to the next question. At the end of the passage, click back through the set of questions to complete any that you skipped over the first time through, and make sure that you have filled in an answer for every question.

General Strategy for the CARS Section

Ranking and Ordering the Passages: What to Start With

Ranking: Since the questions are displayed on separate screens, it is awkward and time consuming to click through all of the questions before making a "Now," "Later," or "Killer" decision. Therefore, rank the passage and decide whether or not to do it on the first pass through the section based on the passage text, skimming the first 2–3 sentences.

Ordering: Because of the additional clicking through screens (or, use of the Review screen) that is required to navigate through the section, the "Two-Pass" system (completing the "Now" passages as you find them) is likely to be your most efficient approach. However, if you find that you are continuously making a lot of bad ranking decisions, it is still valid to experiment with the "Three-Pass" approach (ranking all nine passages up front before attempting your first "Now" passage).

Here is an outline of the basic Ranking and Ordering procedure to follow.

1) For each passage, write a heading on your noteboard with the passage number and its range of questions (e.g., "Passage 1 Q 1–7"). The passage numbers do not currently appear in the Navigation or Review screens, thus having the question numbers on your noteboard will allow you to move through the section more efficiently.
2) Skim the first 2–3 sentences and rank the passage. If the passage is a "Now," complete it before moving on to the next. If it is a "Later" or "Killer," first write either "Later" or "Killer" and "SKIPPED" in block letters under the passage heading on your noteboard and leave room for your work if you decide to come back and complete that passage. Then click through each question, flagging each one and filling in random guesses, until you get to the next passage.
3) Once you have completed the "Now" passages, come back for your second pass and complete the "Later" passages, leaving your random guesses in place for any "Killer" passages that you choose not to complete. Go to the Review screen and use your noteboard notes on the question numbers; click on the number of the first question for that passage to go back to that question and proceed from there. Alternatively, if you have consistently flagged all the questions for passages you skipped in your first pass you can use "Review Flagged" from the Review screen to find and complete your "Later" passages.
4) Regardless of how you choose to find your second pass passages, unflag each question after you complete it, so that you can continue to rely on the Review screen (and the "Review Flagged" function) to identify questions that you have not yet attempted.

Previewing the Questions

The formatting and functioning of the tools facilitates effective previewing. Having each question on a separate screen will encourage you to really focus on that question. Even more importantly, you can highlight in the question stem and in the answer choices.

Here is the basic procedure for previewing the questions:

1) Start with the first question, and if it has lead words referencing passage content, highlight them. You may also choose to jot them down on your noteboard. Once you reach and preview the last question for the set on that passage, THEN stay on that screen and work the passage (your highlighting appears and stays on every passage screen, and persists through the whole 90 minutes).

2) Once you have worked the passage and defined the Bottom Line—the main idea and tone of the entire passage—work **backward** from the last question to the first. If you skip over any questions as you go (see Attacking the Questions below), write down the question number on your noteboard. Then click **forward** through the set of questions, completing any that you skipped over the first time through. Once you reach and complete the last question for that passage, clicking "Next" will send you to the first question of the next passage. Working the questions from last to first the first time through the set will eliminate the need to click back through multiple screens to get to the first question immediately after previewing, and will also make it easier and more efficient to do the hardest questions last (see Attacking the Questions below).

3) Remember that previewing questions is a CARS-only technique. It is not efficient to preview questions in the science section.

Attacking the Questions

The question types and the procedure for actually attacking each type will be discussed later. However, it is still important **not** to attempt the hardest questions first (potentially getting stuck, wasting time, and discouraging yourself).

So, as you work the questions from last to first (see Previewing the Questions above), if you encounter a particularly difficult and/or lengthy question (or if you attempt a question but get stuck), write down the question number on your noteboard (you may also choose to Flag it) and move on backward to the next question. Then click **forward** through the set and complete any that you skipped over the first time through the set, unflagging any questions that you flagged that first time through and making sure that you have filled in an answer for every question.

Pacing Strategy for the MCAT

Since the MCAT is a timed test, you must keep an eye on the timer and adjust your pacing as necessary. It would be terrible to run out of time at the end only to discover that the last few questions could have been easily answered in just a few seconds each.

In the science sections you will have about one minute and thirty-five seconds (1:35) per question, and in the CARS section you will have about one minute and forty seconds (1:40) per question (not taking into account time reading the passage before answering the questions).

Section	# of Questions in Passage	Approximate Time (including reading the passage)
Chem/Phys, Bio/Biochem, and Psych/Soc	4	6.5 minutes
	5	8 minutes
	6	9.5 minutes
CARS	5	8.5 minutes
	6	10 minutes
	7	11.5 minutes

When starting a passage in the science sections, make note of how much time you will allot for it and the starting time on the timer. Jot down on your noteboard what the timer should say at the end of the passage. Then just keep an eye on it as you work through the questions. If you are near the end of the time for that passage, guess on any remaining questions, make some notes on your noteboard, Flag the questions, and move on. Come back to those questions if you have time.

For the CARS section, keep in mind that many people will maximize their score by *not* trying to complete every question or every passage in the section. A good strategy for test-takers who cannot achieve a high level of accuracy on all nine passages is to randomly guess on at least one passage in the section, and spend your time getting a high percentage of the other questions right. To complete all nine CARS passages, you have about ten minutes per passage. To complete eight of the nine, you have about 11 minutes per passage.

To help maximize your number of correct answer choices in any section, do the questions and passages within that section in the order *you* want to do them in.

Process of Elimination

Process of Elimination (POE) is probably the most useful technique you have to tackle MCAT questions. Since there is no guessing penalty, POE allows you to increase your probability of choosing the correct answer by eliminating those you are sure are wrong.

1) Strike out any choices that you are sure are incorrect or that do not address the issue raised in the question.
2) Jot down some notes to help clarify your thoughts if you return to the question.
3) Use the "Flag for Review" button to flag the question for review. (Note, however, that in the CARS section, you generally should not be returning to rethink questions once you have moved on to a new passage.)
4) Do not leave it blank! For the sciences, if you are not sure and you have already spent more than 60 seconds on that question, just pick one of the remaining choices. If you have time to review it at the end, you can always debate the remaining choices based on your previous notes. For CARS, if you have been through the choices two or three times, have re-read the question stem and gone back to the passage and you are still stuck, move on. Do the remaining questions for that passage, take one more look at the question you were stuck on, then pick an answer and move on for good.

5) Special Note: If three of the four answer choices have been eliminated, the remaining choice must be the correct answer. Don't waste time pondering *why* it is correct, just click it and move on. The MCAT doesn't care if you truly understand why it's the right answer, only that you have the right answer selected.

6) More subject-specific information on techniques will be presented in the next chapter.

Guessing

Remember, there is NO guessing penalty on the MCAT. NEVER leave a question blank!

QUESTION TYPES

In the science sections of the MCAT, the questions fall into one of three main categories.

1) Memory questions: These questions can be answered directly from prior knowledge and represent about 25 percent of the total number of questions.

2) Explicit questions: These questions are those for which the answer is explicitly stated in the passage. To answer them correctly, for example, may just require finding a definition, reading a graph, or making a simple connection. Explicit questions represent about 35 percent of the total number of questions.

3) Implicit questions: These questions require you to apply knowledge to a new situation; the answer is typically implied by the information in the passage. These questions often start "if…then…." (For example, "If we modify the experiment in the passage like this, then what result would we expect?") Implicit style questions make up about 40 percent of the total number of questions.

In the CARS section, the questions fall into four main categories:

1) Specific questions: These either ask you for facts from the passage (Retrieval questions) or require you to deduce what is most likely to be true based on the passage (Inference questions).

2) General questions: These ask you to summarize themes (Main Idea and Primary Purpose questions) or evaluate an author's opinion (Tone/Attitude questions).

3) Reasoning questions: These ask you to describe the purpose of, or the support provided for, a statement made in the passage (Structure questions) or to judge how well the author supports his or her argument (Evaluate questions).

4) Application questions: These ask you to apply new information from either the question stem itself (New Information questions) or from the answer choices (Strengthen, Weaken, and Analogy questions) to the passage.

More detail on question types and strategies can be found in Chapter 2.

TESTING TIPS

Before Test Day

- Take a trip to the test center at least a day or two before your actual test date so that you can easily find the building and room on test day. This will also allow you to gauge traffic and see if you need money for parking or anything like that. Knowing this type of information ahead of time will greatly reduce your stress on the day of your test.
- During the week before the test, adjust your sleeping schedule so that you are going to bed and getting up in the morning at the same times as on the day before and morning of the MCAT. Prioritize getting a reasonable amount of sleep during the last few nights before the test.
- Don't do any heavy studying the day before the test. This is not a test you can cram for! Your goal at this point is to rest and relax so that you can go into test day in a good physical and mental condition.
- Eat well. Try to avoid excessive caffeine and sugar. Ideally, in the weeks leading up to the actual test, you should experiment a little bit with foods and practice tests to see which foods give you the most endurance. Aim for steady blood sugar levels during the test: sports drinks, peanut-butter crackers, trail mix, etc. make good snacks for your breaks and lunch.

General Test Day Info and Tips

- On the day of the test, arrive at the test center at least a half hour prior to the start time of your test.
- Examinees will be checked in to the center in the order in which they arrive.
- You will be assigned a locker or secure area in which to put your personal items. Textbooks and study notes are not allowed, so there is no need to bring them with you to the test center.
- Your ID will be checked, a scan of your palm will be taken, and you will be asked to sign in.
- You will be given a noteboard booklet and a wet-erase marker, and the test center administrator will take you to the computer on which you will complete the test. You may not choose a computer; you must use the computer assigned to you.
- Nothing, not even your watch, is allowed at the computer station except your photo ID, your locker key (if provided), and a factory sealed packet of ear plugs.
- If you choose to leave the testing room at the breaks, you will have your palm scanned again, and you will have to sign in and out.
- You are allowed to access the items in your locker, except for notes and cell phones. (Check your test center's policy on cell phones ahead of time; some centers do not even allow them to be kept in your locker.)
- Don't forget to bring the snack foods and lunch you experimented with during your practice tests.
- At the end of the test, the test administrator will collect your noteboard and clean off your notes.
- Definitely take the breaks! Get up and walk around. It's a good way to clear your head between sections and get the blood (and oxygen!) flowing to your brain.
- Ask for a clean noteboard at the breaks if you want a fresh one.

Chapter 2
Biology Strategy
for the MCAT

2.1 SCIENCE SECTIONS OVERVIEW

There are three science sections on the MCAT:

- Chemical and Physical Foundations of Biological Systems
- Biological and Biochemical Foundations of Living Systems
- Psychological, Social, and Biological Foundations of Behavior

The Chemical and Physical Foundations of Biological Systems section (Chem/Phys) is the first section on the test. It includes questions from General Chemistry (about 30%), Physics (about 25%), Organic Chemistry (about 15%), Biochemistry (about 25%), and Biology (about 5%). Further, the questions often test chemical and physical concepts within a biological setting: for example, pressure and fluid flow in blood vessels. A solid grasp of math fundamentals is required (arithmetic, algebra, graphs, trigonometry, vectors, proportions, and logarithms); however, there are no calculus-based questions.

The Biological and Biochemical Foundations of Living Systems section (Bio/Biochem) is the third section on the test. Approximately 65% of the questions in this section come from biology, approximately 25% come from biochemistry, and approximately 10% come from Organic and General Chemistry. Math calculations are generally not required on this section of the test; however, a basic understanding of statistics as used in biological research is helpful.

The Psychological, Social, and Biological Foundations of Behavior section (Psych/Soc) is the fourth and final section on the test. About 65% of the questions will be drawn from Psychology (and about 5% of these will be Biological Psychology), about 30% from Sociology, and about 5% from Biology. As with the Bio/Biochem section, calculations are generally not required, however, a basic understanding of statistics as used in research is helpful.

Most of the questions in the science sections (44 of the 59) are passage-based, and each section has ten passages. Passages consist of a few paragraphs of information and include equations, reactions, graphs, figures, tables, experiments, and data. Four to six questions will be associated with each passage.

The remaining 25% of the questions (15 of 59) in each science section are freestanding questions (FSQs). These questions appear in approximately four groups interspersed between the passages. Each group contains three to four questions.

There are 95 minutes allotted to each of the science sections. This breaks down to approximately one minute and 35 seconds per question.

2.2 SCIENCE PASSAGE TYPES

The passages in the science sections fall into one of three main categories: Information and/or Situation Presentation, Experiment/Research Presentation, or Persuasive (or Scientific) Reasoning.

Information and/or Situation Presentation

These passages either present straightforward scientific information or they describe a particular event or occurrence. Generally, questions associated with these passages test basic science facts or ask you to predict outcomes given new variables or new information. Here is an example of an Information/Situation Presentation passage:

Figure 1 shows a portion of the inner mechanism of a typical home smoke detector. It consists of a pair of capacitor plates which are charged by a 9-volt battery (not shown). The capacitor plates (electrodes) are connected to a sensor device, D; the resistor R denotes the internal resistance of the sensor. Normally, air acts as an insulator and no current would flow in the circuit shown. However, inside the smoke detector is a small sample of an artificially produced radioactive element, americium-241, which decays primarily by emitting alpha particles, with a half-life of approximately 430 years. The daughter nucleus of the decay has a half-life in excess of two million years and therefore poses virtually no biohazard.

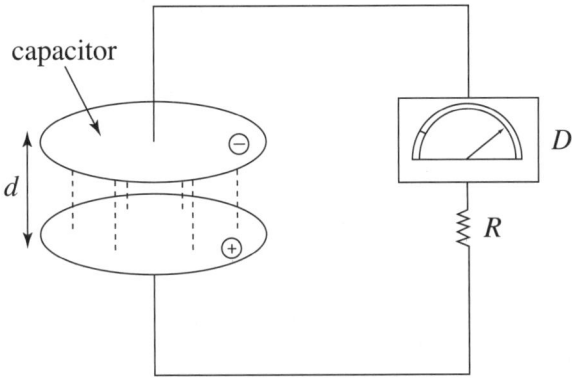

Figure 1   Smoke detector mechanism

The decay products (alpha particles and gamma rays) from the ^{241}Am sample ionize air molecules between the plates and thus provide a conducting pathway which allows current to flow in the circuit shown in Figure 1. A steady-state current is quickly established and remains as long as the battery continues to maintain a 9-volt potential difference between its terminals. However, if smoke particles enter the space between the capacitor plates and thereby interrupt the flow, the current is reduced, and the sensor responds to this change by triggering

the alarm. (Furthermore, as the battery starts to "die out," the resulting drop in current is also detected to alert the homeowner to replace the battery.)

$$C = \varepsilon_0 \frac{A}{d}$$

Equation 1

where ε_0 is the universal permittivity constant, equal to 8.85×10^{-12} $C^2/(N\ m^2)$. Since the area A of each capacitor plate in the smoke detector is 20 cm^2 and the plates are separated by a distance d of 5 mm, the capacitance is 3.5×10^{-12} F = 3.5 pF.

Experiment/Research Presentation

These passages present the details of experiments and research procedures. They often include data tables and graphs. Generally, questions associated with these passages ask you to interpret data, draw conclusions, and make inferences. Here is an example of an Experiment/Research Presentation passage:

The development of sexual characteristics depends upon various factors, the most important of which are hormonal control, environmental stimuli, and the genetic makeup of the individual. The hormones that contribute to the development include the steroid hormones estrogen, progesterone, and testosterone, as well as the pituitary hormones FSH (follicle-stimulating hormone) and LH (luteinizing hormone).

To study the mechanism by which estrogen exerts its effects, a researcher performed the following experiments using cell culture assays.

Experiment 1:

Human embryonic placental mesenchyme (HEPM) cells were grown for 48 hours in Dulbecco's Modified Eagle Medium (DMEM), with media change every 12 hours. Upon confluent growth, cells were exposed to a 10 mg per mL solution of green fluorescent-labeled estrogen for 1 hour. Cells were rinsed with DMEM and observed under confocal fluorescent microscopy.

Experiment 2:

HEPM cells were grown to confluence as in Experiment 1. Cells were exposed to Pesticide A for 1 hour, followed by the 10 mg/mL solution of labeled estrogen, rinsed as in Experiment 1, and observed under confocal fluorescent microscopy.

Experiment 3:

Experiment 1 was repeated with Chinese Hamster Ovary (CHO) cells instead of HEPM cells.

Experiment 4:

CHO cells injected with cytoplasmic extracts of HEPM cells were grown to confluence, exposed to the 10 mg/mL solution of labeled estrogen for 1 hour, and observed under confocal fluorescent microscopy.

The results of these experiments are given in Table 1.

Table 1 Detection of Estrogen (+ indicates presence of Estrogen)

Experiment	Media	Cytoplasm	Nucleus
1	+	+	+
2	+	+	+
3	+	+	+
4	+	+	+

After observing the cells in each experiment, the researcher bathed the cells in a solution containing 10 mg per mL of a red fluorescent probe that binds specifically to the estrogen receptor only when its active site is occupied. After 1 hour, the cells were rinsed with DMEM and observed under confocal fluorescent microscopy. The results are presented in Table 2.

The researcher also repeated Experiment 2 using Pesticide B, an estrogen analog, instead of Pesticide A. Results from other researchers had shown that Pesticide B binds to the active site of the cytosolic estrogen receptor (with an affinity 10,000 times greater than that of estrogen) and causes increased transcription of mRNA.

Table 2 Observed Fluorescence and Estrogen Effects (G = green, R = red)

Experiment	Media	Cytoplasm	Nucleus	Estrogen effects observed?
1	G only	G and R	G and R	Yes
2	G only	G only	G only	No
3	G only	G only	G only	No
4	G only	G and R	G and R	Yes

Based on these results, the researcher determined that estrogen had no effect when not bound to a cytosolic, estrogen-specific receptor.

Persuasive (Scientific) Reasoning

These passages typically present a scientific phenomenon, along with a hypothesis that explains the phenomenon, and may include counterarguments as well. Questions associated with these passages ask you to evaluate the hypothesis or arguments. Persuasive Reasoning passages in the science sections of the MCAT tend to be less common than Information Presentation or Experiment-based passages. Here is an example of a Persuasive Reasoning passage:

Two theoretical chemists attempted to explain the observed trends of acidity by applying two interpretations of molecular orbital theory. Consider the pK_a values of some common acids listed along with the conjugate base:

acid	pK_a	conjugate base
H_2SO_4	< 0	HSO_4^-
H_2CrO_4	5.0	$HCrO_4^-$
H_2PO_4	2.1	$H_2PO_4^-$
HF	3.9	F^-
HOCl	7.8	ClO^-
HCN	9.5	CN^-
HIO_3	1.2	IO_3^-

Recall that acids with a $pK_a < 0$ are called strong acids, and those with a $pK_a > 0$ are called weak acids. The arguments of the chemists are given below.

Chemist #1:

"The acidity of a compound is proportional to the polarization of the H—X bond, where X is some nonmetal element. Complex acids, such as H_2SO_4, $HClO_4$, and HNO_3 are strong acids because the H—O bonding electrons are strongly drawn towards the oxygen. It is generally true that a covalent bond weakens as its polarization increases. Therefore, one can conclude that the strength of an acid is proportional to the number of electronegative atoms in that acid."

Chemist #2:

"The acidity of a compound is proportional to the number of stable resonance structures of that acid's conjugate base. H_2SO_4, $HClO_4$, and HNO_3 are all strong acids because their respective conjugate bases exhibit a high degree of resonance stabilization."

Mapping a Passage

"Mapping a passage" refers to the combination of on-screen highlighting and noteboard notes that you take while working through a passage. Typically, good things to highlight include the overall topic of a paragraph, unfamiliar terms, italicized terms, unusual terms, numerical values, hypothesis, and experimental results. Noteboard notes can be used to summarize the paragraphs and to jot down important facts and connections that are made when reading the passage. More details on passage mapping will be presented in Section 2.5.

2.3 SCIENCE QUESTION TYPES

Questions in the science sections are generally one of three main types: Memory, Explicit, or Implicit.

Memory Questions

These questions can be answered directly from prior knowledge, with no need to reference the passage or question text. Memory questions represent approximately 25 percent of the science questions on the MCAT. Usually, Memory questions are found as FSQs, but they can also be tucked into a passage. Here's an example of a Memory question:

Which of the following acetylating conditions will convert diethylamine into an amide at the fastest rate?

A) Acetic acid / HCl
B) Acetic anhydride
C) Acetyl chloride
D) Ethyl acetate

2.3

Explicit Questions

Explicit questions can be answered primarily with information from the passage, along with prior knowledge. They may require data retrieval, graph analysis, or making a simple connection. Explicit questions make up approximately 35–40 percent of the science questions on the MCAT; here's an example (taken from the Information/Situation Presentation passage):

> The sensor device D shown in Figure 1 performs its function by acting as:
>
> A) an ohmmeter.
> B) a voltmeter.
> C) a potentiometer.
> D) an ammeter.

Implicit Questions

These questions require you to take information from the passage, combine it with your prior knowledge, apply it to a new situation, and come to some logical conclusion. They typically require more complex connections than do Explicit questions, and they may also require data retrieval, graph analysis, etc. Implicit questions usually require a solid understanding of the passage information. They make up approximately 35–40 percent of the science questions on the MCAT; here's an example (taken from the Experiment/Research Presentation passage):

> If Experiment 2 were repeated, but this time exposing the cells first to Pesticide A and then to Pesticide B before exposing them to the green fluorescent-labeled estrogen and the red fluorescent probe, which of the following statements will most likely be true?
>
> A) Pesticide A and Pesticide B bind to the same site on the estrogen receptor.
> B) Estrogen effects would be observed.
> C) Only green fluorescence would be observed.
> D) Both green and red fluorescence would be observed.

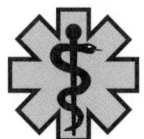

The Rod of Asclepius

You may notice this Rod of Asclepius icon as you read through the book. In Greek mythology, the Rod of Asclepius is associated with healing and medicine; the symbol continues to be used today to represent medicine and healthcare. You won't see this on the actual MCAT, but we've used it here to call attention to medically related examples and questions.

2.4 BIOLOGY ON THE MCAT

Biology is by far the most information-dense section on the MCAT. MCAT Biology topics span six different semester-length courses (molecular biology, cell biology, microbiology, genetics, anatomy, and physiology). Further, the application of this material is potentially vast; passages can discuss anything from the details of some viral life cycle to the complexities of genetic studies, to the nuances of an unusual disease. Fortunately, biology is the subject that MCAT students typically find the most interesting, and the one they have the most background in. People who want to go to medical school have an inherent interest in biology; thus this subject, although vast, seems more manageable than all the others on the MCAT.

The science sections of the MCAT have 10 passages and 15 freestanding questions (FSQs). The Biological and Biochemical Foundations of Living Systems section (Bio/Biochem) is primarily biology (65%) and biochemistry (25%). The remaining 10% are General and Organic Chemistry questions. Further, Biology questions can show up in the Psychological, Social, and Biological Foundations of Behavior section (about 10%) and in the Chemical and Physical Foundations of Biological Systems section (about 5%). Note also that about 25% of the Chem/Phys section is Biochemistry, and frequently the passages and questions are biology-based.

2.5 TACKLING A BIOLOGY PASSAGE

Generally speaking, time is not an issue in the Bio/Biochem section of the MCAT. Because students have a stronger background in biology than in other subjects, the passages seem more understandable; in fact, readers sometimes find themselves getting caught up and interested in the passage. Often, students report having about 5 to 10 minutes "left over" after completing the section. This means that an additional minute or so can potentially be spent on each passage, thinking and understanding.

Passage Types as They Apply to Biology

Experiment/Research Presentation: Biology

This is the most common type of Biology passage. It typically presents the details behind an experiment along with data tables, graphs, and figures. Often these are the most difficult passages to deal with because they require an understanding of the reasoning behind the experiment, the logic to each step, and the ability to analyze the results and form conclusions. A basic understanding of biometry (basic statistics as they apply to biology and biology research) is necessary.

Information/Situation Presentation: Biology

This is the second most common type of Biology passage on the MCAT. These passages generally appear as one of two variants: either a basic concept with additional levels of detail included (for example, all the detail you ever wanted to know about the electron transport chain), or a novel concept with ties to basic information (for example, a rare demyelinating disease). Either way, Biology passages are notorious for testing concepts in unusual contexts. The key to dealing with these passages is to, first, not become anxious about all the stuff you might not know, and second, figure out how the basics you do know apply to the new situation. For example, you might be presented with a passage that introduces hormones you never heard of or novel drugs to combat diseases you didn't know existed. First, don't panic. Second, look for how these new things fit into familiar categories: for example, "peptide vs. steroid" or "sympathetic antagonist." Then answer the questions with these basics in mind.

2.5

That said, you have to know your basics. This will increase your confidence in answering freestanding questions, as well as increase the speed with which to find the information in the passage. The astute MCAT student will never waste time staring at a question thinking, "Should I know this?" Instead, because she has a solid understanding of the necessary core knowledge, she'll say, "No, I am NOT expected to know this, and I am going to look for it in the passage."

Persuasive Reasoning: Biology

This is the least common passage type in Biology. It typically describes some biological phenomenon and then offers one or more theories to explain it. Questions in Persuasive Reasoning passages ask you to determine support for one of the theories, or present new evidence and ask which theory is now contradicted.

One last thought about Biology passages in general: because the array of topics is so vast, Biology passages often pull questions from multiple areas of biology into a single, general topic. Consider, for example, a passage on renal function. Question topics could include basics about the kidney, transmembrane transport, autonomic control, blood pressure, hormones, biochemical energy needs, or a genetics question about a rare kidney disease.

Reading a Biology Passage

Although tempting, try not to get bogged down reading all the little details in a passage. Again, because most premeds have an inherent interest in biology and the mechanisms behind disease, it's very easy to get lost in the science behind the passages. In spite of having that "extra" time, you don't want to use it all up reading what isn't necessary. Each passage type requires a slightly different style of reading.

Information/Situation Presentation passages require the least reading. These should be skimmed to get an idea of the location of information within the passage. These passages include a fair amount of detail that you might not need, so save the reading of these details until a question comes up about them. Then go back and read for the finer nuances.

Experiment/Research Presentation passages require the most reading. You are practically guaranteed to get questions that ask you about the details of the experiment, why a particular step was carried out, why the results are what they are, how to interpret the data, or how the results might change if a particular variable is altered. It's worth spending a little more time reading to understand the experiment. However, because there will be a fair number of questions unrelated to the experiment, you might consider answering these first and then going back for the experiment details.

Persuasive Argument passages are somewhere in the middle. You can skim them for location of information, but you also want to spend a little time reading the details of and thinking about the arguments presented. It is extremely likely that you will be asked a question about them.

Advanced Reading Skills

To improve your ability to read and glean information from a passage, you need to practice. Be critical when you read the content; watch for vague areas or holes in the passage that aren't explained clearly. Remember that information about new topics will be woven throughout the passage; you may need to piece together information from several paragraphs and a figure to get the whole picture.

After you've read, highlighted, and mapped a passage (more on this in a bit), stop and ask yourself the following questions:

- What was this passage about? What was the conclusion or main point?
- Was there a paragraph that was mostly background?
- Were there paragraphs or figures that seemed useless?
- What information was found in each paragraph? Why was that paragraph there?
- Are there any holes in the story?
- What extra information could I have pulled out of the passage? What inferences or conclusions could I make?
- If something unique was explained or mentioned, what might be its purpose?
- What am I *not* being told?
- Can I summarize the purpose and/or results of the experiment in a few sentences?
- Were there any comparisons in the passage?

This takes a while at first, but eventually it will become second nature and you'll start doing it as you read the passage. If you have a study group you are working with, consider doing this as an exercise with your study partners. Take turns asking and answering the questions above. Having to explain something to someone else not only solidifies your own knowledge, but helps you see where you might be weak.

Mapping a Biology Passage

Mapping a Biology passage is a combination of highlighting and noteboard notes that can help you organize and understand the passage information.

Resist the temptation to highlight everything! (Everyone has done this: You're reading a biology textbook with a highlighter, and then look back and realize that the whole page is yellow!) Restrict your highlighting to a few things:

- the main theme of a paragraph
- an unusual or unfamiliar term that is defined specifically for that passage (e.g., something that is italicized)
- statements that either support the main theme or contradict the main theme
- general topics of a list that appears in paragraph form within a passage
- relationships (how one thing changes relative to another thing)

The noteboards should be organized. Make sure the passage number appears at the top of your noteboard notes. For each paragraph, note "P1," "P2," etc., on the noteboard, and jot down a few notes about that paragraph. Try to translate biology jargon into your own words using everyday language (this is particularly useful for experiments). Also, make sure to note down simple relationships (e.g., the relationship between two variables).

Pay attention to equations, figures, and the like to see what type of information they deal with. Don't spend a lot of time analyzing at this point, but do jot down on your noteboard "Fig 1" and a brief summary of the data. Also, if you've discovered a list in the passage, note its topic and location down on your noteboard.

Let's take a look at how we might highlight and map a passage. Below is a passage on eye physiology.

The wall of the human eye is composed of three layers of tissue, an outer layer of tough connective tissue, a middle layer of darkly pigmented vascular tissue, and an inner layer of neural tissue. The outer layer is subdivided into the sclera, the white portion, and the cornea, the clear portion. The inner layer is more commonly known as the *retina* and contains several types of cells.

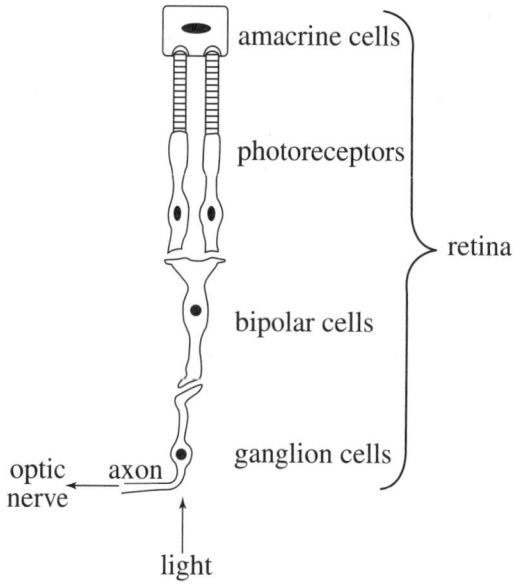

Figure 1   Retina Structure

The photoreceptors of the retina include rods and cones which respond to light under different circumstances. Rods are more sensitive to light but cannot distinguish color; cones are less sensitive to light overall, but can respond to different wavelengths. Response to light involves visual pigments, which in all cases consist of a light-absorbing molecule called *retinal* (derived from vitamin A) bound to a protein called *opsin*. The type of opsin in the visual pigment determines the wavelength specificity of the retinal. The specific visual pigment in rod cells is called *rhodopsin*.

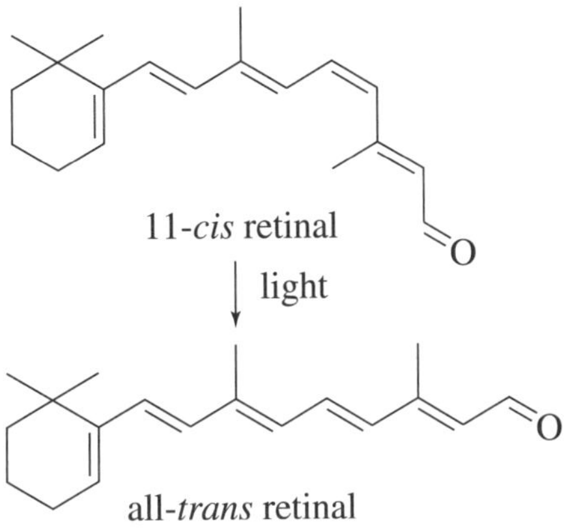

Figure 2   The Two Forms of Retinal

In the absence of light, Na^+ channels in the membranes of rod cells are kept open by cGMP. The conformational change in retinal upon light absorption causes changes in opsin as well; this triggers a pathway by which phosphodiesterase (PDE) is activated. Active PDE converts cGMP to GMP, causing it to dissociate from the Na^+ channel and the channel to close. Until retinal regains its bent shape (helped by enzymes), the rod is unable to respond further to light.

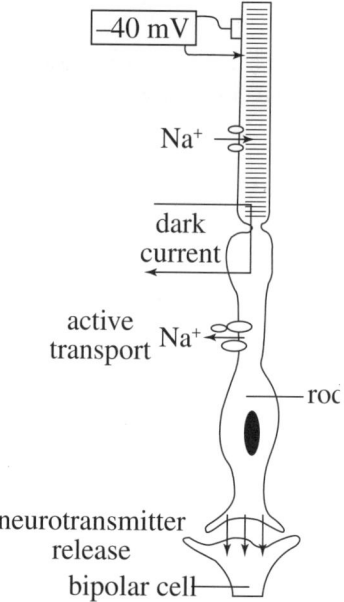

Figure 3 Rod Cell in Darkness

Visual defects can be caused by abnormal visual pigments or by misshapen eyeballs; for example, myopia (nearsightedness) is due to an eyeball that is too long, causing light rays from distant objects to focus in front of the retina so the image appears blurry.

Analysis and Passage Map

This passage is an Information Presentation passage and starts out with a paragraph about the structure of the eye and its layers. This is primarily a background paragraph and can be skimmed quickly, with a few words highlighted. Figure 1 shows the detail of the retina.

The second paragraph goes into more detail about the photoreceptors, and specifically compares the functions of rods and cones. There are few more italicized terms; this paragraph is presenting information that is beyond what you are expected to know about the eye for the MCAT. Figure 2 shows the conversion between the two forms of retinal.

The third paragraph presents details about rod cells, and in particular, points out a unique feature of rod cells: that their Na$^+$ channels are typically open in the absence of light. On stimulation by light, they close. This is unusual behavior in the nervous system, since it is the opposite of what typically occurs. Figure 3 confirms this, as the cell in darkness appears to be resting at −40 mV, 30 mV more positive than typical neurons rest at.

The final paragraph is a brief description of visual defects. Like paragraph 1, it only needs to be skimmed briefly. Here's what your passage map might look like:

> P1 – 3 layers of eyeball, Fig 1 retina detail
> P2 – photoreceptors
> > rods no color, more sensitive
> > cones less sensitive, respond to different colors
> > details on vis pigments. Fig 2 convert retinal
> P3 – rod function. WEIRD Na⁺ channels open in dark, close in light.
> > depol in dark, hyperpol in light
> P4 – visual defects

Let's take a look at a different passage. Below is an Experiment/Research Presentation passage.

The development of sexual characteristics depends upon various factors, the most important of which are hormonal control, environmental stimuli, and the genetic makeup of the individual. The hormones that contribute to the development include the steroid hormones estrogen, progesterone, and testosterone, as well as the pituitary hormones FSH (follicle-stimulating hormone) and LH (luteinizing hormone).

To study the mechanism by which estrogen exerts its effects, a researcher performed the following experiments using cell culture assays.

Experiment 1:

Human embryonic placental mesenchyme (HEPM) cells were grown for 48 hours in Dulbecco's Modified Eagle Medium (DMEM), with media change every 12 hours. Upon confluent growth, cells were exposed to a 10 mg per mL solution of green fluorescent-labeled estrogen for 1 hour. Cells were rinsed with DMEM and observed under confocal fluorescent microscopy.

Experiment 2:

HEPM cells were grown to confluence as in Experiment 1. Cells were exposed to Pesticide A for 1 hour, followed by the 10 mg/mL solution of labeled estrogen, rinsed as in Experiment 1, and observed under confocal fluorescent microscopy.

Experiment 3:

Experiment 1 was repeated with Chinese Hamster Ovary (CHO) cells instead of HEPM cells.

2.5

Experiment 4:

CHO cells injected with cytoplasmic extracts of HEPM cells were grown to confluence, exposed to the 10 mg/mL solution of labeled estrogen for 1 hour, and observed under confocal fluorescent microscopy.

The results of these experiments are given in Table 1.

Table 1 Detection of Estrogen
(+ indicates presence of estrogen)

Experiment	Media	Cytoplasm	Nucleus
1	+	+	+
2	+	+	+
3	+	+	+
4	+	+	+

After observing the cells in each experiment, the researcher bathed the cells in a solution containing 10 mg/mL of a red fluorescent probe that binds specifically to the estrogen receptor only when its active site is occupied. After 1 hour, the cells were rinsed with DMEM and observed under confocal fluorescent microscopy. The results are presented in Table 2.

The researcher also repeated Experiment 2 using Pesticide B, an estrogen analog, instead of Pesticide A. Results from other researchers had shown that Pesticide B binds to the active site of the cytosolic estrogen receptor (with an affinity 10,000 times greater than that of estrogen) and causes increased transcription of mRNA.

Table 2 Observed Fluorescence and Estrogen Effects
(G = green, R = red)

Experiment	Media	Cytoplasm	Nucleus	Estrogen effects observed?
1	G only	G and R	G and R	Yes
2	G only	G only	G only	No
3	G only	G only	G only	No
4	G only	G and R	G and R	Yes

Based on these results, the researcher determined that estrogen had no effect when not bound to a cytosolic, estrogen-specific receptor.

Analysis and Passage Map

This passage starts out with a very general background paragraph. Not much to do here, but it does tell us that estrogen is going to be the hormone of focus.

The next few paragraphs are short descriptions of four different experiments. These should be read to understand not only what's happening in each experiment but also what the differences in the experiments are. Note this on your noteboard.

Table 1 shows the results of the four experiments. It should jump out at you that estrogen is found everywhere; in other words, it is not restricted from any area of the cell.

After Table 1, the passage describes two modifications to the experiments. As with the original experiments, it's worth taking a little time to read and understand what's going on. The first big difference is that the researchers aren't just looking for the presence of estrogen, but also want to know when it's bound to its receptor. The second big difference is the testing of an estrogen analog, Pesticide B.

Table 2 shows the results of when estrogen is bound and when it isn't. These results could be combined with the experiment description results on your map:

> *P1 – hormones that contribute to development, estrogen*
> *E1 – HEPM cells exposed to estrogen, green + red = estrogen effects*
> *E2 – Pesticide A, green only, must inhibit binding of estrogen to recept.*
> *E3 – CHO cells, green only, no recept.*
> *E4 – CHO cells + HEPM cytoplasm, green + red, recept is in cytoplasm*
> *Table 1 – estrogen is not restricted from anywhere in the cell*
> *Further exp'ts – red probe for bound active site, and Pesticide B (estrogen analog w/higher affinity)*

One last thought about passages: Remember that, as with all sections on the MCAT, you can do the passages in the order *you* want to. There are no extra points for taking the test in order. Generally, passages will fall into one of four main subject groups:

- biochemistry
- other non-physiology
- physiology
- organic/general chemistry

Figure out which group you are most comfortable with, and do those passages first. (See Chapter 1 for general strategies for moving around in the sections efficiently.)

2.6 TACKLING THE QUESTIONS

Questions in the Biology section mimic the three typical questions of the science sections in general: Memory, Explicit, and Implicit.

Question Types as They Apply to Biology

Biology Memory Questions

Memory questions are exactly what they sound like: they test your knowledge of some specific fact or concept. While Memory questions are typically found as freestanding questions, they can also be tucked into a passage. These questions, aside from requiring memorization, do not generally cause problems for students because they are similar to the types of questions that appear on a typical college biology exam. Below is an example of a freestanding Memory question:

Regarding embryogenesis, which of the following sequence of events is in correct order?

A) Implantation—cleavage—gastrulation—neurulation—blastulation
B) Blastulation—implantation—cleavage—neurulation—gastrulation
C) Implantation—blastulation—gastrulation—cleavage—neurulation
D) Cleavage—blastulation—implantation—gastrulation—neurulation

The correct answer to the question above is choice D. Here's another example. This question is from a passage:

The genital organs of the *guevedoche* that develop at puberty are derivatives of the mesodermal germ layer. Which of the following is/are also derivatives of the mesodermal germ layer?

I. Skeletal muscle
II. Liver
III. Kidney

A) I only
B) II only
C) I and III only
D) II and III only

Note that this question includes an additional, unnecessary sentence at the beginning, but it is a Memory question all the same. You don't need to know anything about the *guevedoche* to answer the question, and the information in that first sentence does not help you in any way. The correct answer is choice C.

There is no specific "trick" to answering Memory questions; either you know the answer or you don't.

If you find that you are missing a fair number of Memory questions, it is a sure sign that you don't know the content well enough. Go back and review.

Biology Explicit Questions

True, pure Explicit questions are rare in the Biology section. A purely Explicit question can be answered only with information in the passage. Below is an example of a pure Explicit question taken from the eye passage above:

> The middle layer of the eyeball wall most likely contains:
>
> A) bipolar cells.
> B) photoreceptors.
> C) blood vessels.
> D) collagen fibers.

Referring back to the map for this passage, it indicates that information about the layers of the eyeball are in paragraph 1. It states that the middle layer is a "darkly pigmented vascular layer," meaning that it contains blood vessels. The correct answer is choice C.

However, more often in the biology section, Explicit questions are more of a blend of Explicit and Memory; they require not only retrieval of passage information, but also recall of some relevant fact. They usually do not require a lot of analysis or connections. Here's an example of the more common type of Explicit question:

> Pesticide A most likely functions as:
>
> A) an agonist.
> B) an inhibitor.
> C) a lipase.
> D) a receptor.

To answer this question, you first need to retrieve information from the passage about the effects of Pesticide A. From Table 2 we know that it prevents estrogen from binding to its receptor (and we noted this on our passage map). You also need to remember the definitions of the terms in the answer choices (agonists cause similar effects, inhibitors prevent effects, lipases break down lipids, and receptors bind ligands to cause effects). Based on our known definitions, choices A and D can be eliminated, and while Pesticide A could be functioning as a lipase that breaks down estrogen, "inhibitor" is a more accurate term (choice B is better than choice C and is the correct answer).

A final subgroup in the Explicit question category are graph interpretation questions. These fall into one of two types: those that ask you to take graphical information from the passage and convert it to a text answer, or those that take text from the passage and ask you to convert it to a graph. On the following page is an example of the latter type:

Which of the following graphs would best illustrate the binding of estrogen (E) to its receptor in the presence of its analog, Pesticide B?

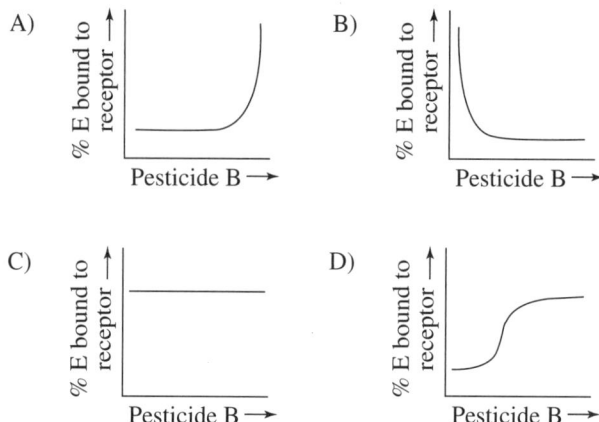

From our passage map, we know that information about Pesticide B is found near the end of the passage, where it describes "further experiments." The passage states that Pesticide B functions as an estrogen analog that binds to the estrogen receptor with a much higher affinity than does estrogen. In other words, if Pesticide B is around, the receptor will preferentially bind it, and not estrogen. So as the concentration of Pesticide B rises, the amount of estrogen bound to the receptor should fall. This is shown in choice B.

If you find that you are missing Explicit questions, practice your passage mapping. Make sure you aren't missing the critical items in the passage that lead you to the right answer. Slow down a little; take an extra 15 to 30 seconds per passage to read or think about it more carefully.

Biology Implicit Questions

Implicit questions require the most thought. These require recall of not only biology information but also information gleaned from the passage and a more in-depth analysis of how the two relate. Implicit questions require more analysis and connections to be made than Explicit questions. Often they take the form "If…then…." Below is an example of a classic Implicit question, taken from the Experiment passage shown earlier.

If Experiment 2 were repeated, but this time exposing the cells first to Pesticide A and then to Pesticide B before exposing them to the green fluorescent-labeled estrogen and the red fluorescent probe, which of the following statements will most likely be true?

A) Pesticide A and Pesticide B bind to the same site on the estrogen receptor.
B) Estrogen effects would be observed.
C) Only green fluorescence would be observed.
D) Both green and red fluorescence would be observed.

To answer this question, conclusions have to be drawn from the experiments described in the passage, and new conclusions have to be predicted based on the new circumstance. Many more connections need to be made than when answering an Explicit question. From the passage, we need to figure out that Pesticide A is an inhibitor. We also have to figure out that it does not bind at the active site of the receptor (data from Table 2). We have to know what green fluorescence and red fluorescence imply. We have to draw on the information provided about Pesticide B to know that it is an analog and that it binds to the active site of the estrogen receptor. We have to combine all of this together and come to a logical conclusion: since Pesticide A is an inhibitor, it would prevent the binding of Pesticide B and thus prevent estrogen effects (choice B can be eliminated). If Pesticide B cannot bind, we would only see green fluorescence (choice D can be eliminated, and choice C is probably correct). Since Pesticide A by itself does not produce red fluorescence, it must not be binding at the active site, which is where Pesticide B binds, (choice A can be eliminated, and choice C is definitely correct).

Here's another example of an Implicit question, drawn from the same passage:

> When the researcher performed Experiment 2 using Pesticide B instead of Pesticide A, which of the following fluorescence and estrogen effects did the researcher most likely observe?

A) *Media*: green and red
   Cytoplasm: green and red
   Nucleus: green and red
   Estrogen effects: no

B) *Media*: green only
   Cytoplasm: green and red
   Nucleus: green and red
   Estrogen effects: no

C) *Media*: green only
   Cytoplasm: green and red
   Nucleus: green and red
   Estrogen effects: yes

D) *Media*: green only
   Cytoplasm: green and red
   Nucleus: green only
   Estrogen effects: no

To answer this question, we again must combine passage information with logical inference and working memory. Since red fluorescence indicates binding of the receptor, and since the receptor is never in the media, there can never be red fluorescence in the media (choice A can be eliminated). We know from the passage that Pesticide B binds at the active site of the receptor, and we know that the receptor is found in the cytoplasm. We also know from the passage that Pesticide B causes increased mRNA transcription, and we know from memory that to induce mRNA transcription, the receptor must move into the nucleus. Thus, red fluorescence must be observed in the nucleus as well (choice D can be eliminated). Since Pesticide B is defined as an "estrogen analog," and since we know from memory that analogs cause similar effects, it is likely that estrogen effects will be observed. The fact that increased mRNA transcription occurs supports this idea (choice B can be eliminated, and choice C is correct). Again, many more connections need to be made to answer Implicit questions; Process of Elimination is typically the best approach.

If you find that you are missing a lot of Implicit questions, first make sure that you are using POE aggressively. Second, go back and review the explanations for the correct answer to figure out where your logic went awry. Did you miss an important fact in the passage? Did you forget the relevant Biology content? Did you follow the logical train of thought to the right answer? Once you figure out where you made your mistake, you will know how to correct it.

2.7 SUMMARY OF THE APPROACH TO BIOLOGY

How to Map the Passage and Use the Noteboard

1) The passage should not be read like textbook material, with the intent of learning something from every sentence (science majors especially will be tempted to read this way). Passages should be read to get a feel for the type of questions that will follow and to get a general idea of the location of information within the passage.

2) Highlighting—Use this tool sparingly, or you will end up with a passage that is completely covered in yellow highlighter! Highlighting in a Biology passage should be used to draw attention to a few words that demonstrate one of the following:
   - the main theme of a paragraph
   - an unusual or unfamiliar term that is defined specifically for that passage (e.g., something that is italicized)
   - statements that either support the main theme or counteract the main theme
   - list topics (see below)
   - relationships

3) Pay brief attention to equations, figures, and experiments, noting only what information they deal with. Do not spend a lot of time analyzing at this point.

4) For each passage, start by noting the passage number, the general topic, and the range of questions on your noteboard. You can then work between your noteboard and the Review screen to easily get to the questions you want to (see Chapter 1).

5) For each paragraph, note "P1," "P2," etc. on the noteboard and jot down a few notes about that paragraph. Try to translate biology jargon into your own words using everyday language. Especially note down simple relationships (e.g., the relationship between two variables).

6) Lists—Whenever a list appears in paragraph form, jot down on the noteboard the paragraph and the general topic of the list. It will make returning to the passage more efficient and help to organize your thoughts.

7) The noteboard is only useful if it is kept organized! Make sure that your notes for each passage are clearly delineated and marked with the passage number and question range. This will allow you to easily read your notes when you come back to review a flagged question. Resist the temptation to write in the first available blank space as this makes it much more difficult to refer back to your work.

Biology Question Strategies

1) Remember that the content in Biology is vast, so don't panic if something seems completely unfamiliar. Understand the basic content well, find the basics in the unfamiliar topic, and apply them to the question.

2) Process of Elimination is paramount! The strikeout tool allows you to eliminate answer choices; this will improve your chances of guessing the correct answer if you are unable to narrow it down to one choice.

3) Answer the straightforward questions first (typically the memory questions). Leave questions that require analysis of experiments and graphs for later. Take the test in the order YOU want. Make sure to use your noteboard to indicate questions you skipped.

4) Make sure that the answer you choose actually answers the question and isn't just a true statement.

5) Try to avoid answer choices with extreme words such as "always," "never," etc. In biology, there is almost always an exception and answers are rarely black-and-white.

6) Roman numeral questions: Whenever possible, start by evaluating the Roman numeral item that shows up in exactly two answer choices. This allows you to quickly eliminate two wrong answer choices regardless of whether the item is true or false. Typically then, you will only have to assess one of the other Roman numeral items to determine the correct answer. Always work between the I-II-III items and the answer choices. Once an item is found to be true (or false), strike out answer choices which do not contain (or do contain) that item number. Make sure to strike out the actual Roman numeral item as well, and highlight those items that are true.

7) LEAST/EXCEPT/NOT questions: Don't get tricked by these questions that ask you to pick that answer that doesn't fit (the incorrect or false statement). Make sure to highlight the words "LEAST," "EXCEPT," or "NOT" in the question stem. It's often good to use your noteboard and write "A B C D" with a T or F next to each answer choice. The one that stands out as different is the correct answer!

8) Again, don't leave any question blank.

A Note About Flashcards

For most of the exams you've taken previously, flashcards were likely very helpful. This was because those exams mostly required you to regurgitate information, and flashcards are pretty good at helping you memorize facts. However, the most challenging aspect of the MCAT is not that it requires you to memorize the fine details of content knowledge, but that it requires you to apply your basic scientific knowledge to unfamiliar situations: flashcards alone may not help you there.

Flashcards can be beneficial if your basic content knowledge is deficient in some area. For example, if you don't know the hormones and their effects in the body, flashcards can certainly help you memorize these facts. Or, maybe you are unsure of the functions of the different brain regions. You might find that flashcards can help you memorize these. But unless you are trying to memorize basic facts in your personal weak areas, you are better off doing and analyzing practice passages than carrying around a stack of flashcards.

Chapter 3
Biologically Important Molecules

The biological macromolecules are grouped into four classes of molecules that play important roles in cells and in organisms as a whole. All of them are polymers, strings of repeated units (monomers).

This chapter discusses the biomolecules from a biological perspective: what they are made of, how they are put together, and what their roles are in the body. These molecules are also discussed in *MCAT Biochemistry Review* in more detail, as well as in *MCAT Organic Chemistry Review* from an organic chemistry perspective: nomenclature, chirality, etc.

3.1 PROTEIN BUILDING BLOCKS

Proteins are biological macromolecules that act as enzymes, hormones, receptors, channels, transporters, antibodies, and support structures inside and outside cells. Proteins are composed of twenty different amino acids linked together in polymers. The composition and sequence of amino acids in the polypeptide chain is what makes each protein unique and able to fulfill its special role in the cell.

Amino Acid Structure and Nomenclature

Understanding the structure of amino acids is key to understanding both their chemistry and the chemistry of proteins. The generic formula for all twenty amino acids is shown below.

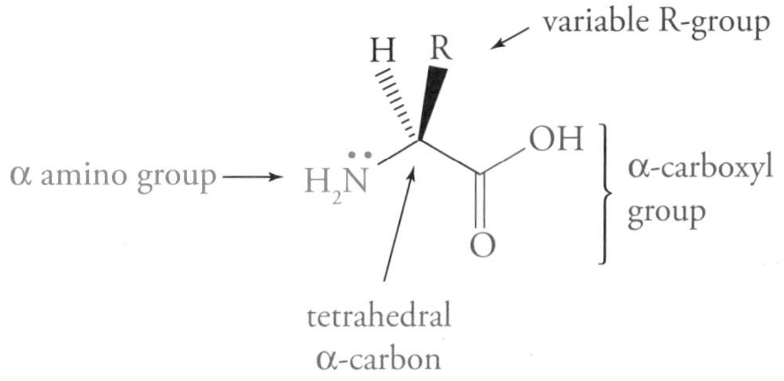

Figure 1   Generic Amino Acid Structure

All twenty amino acids share the same nitrogen-carbon-carbon backbone. The unique feature of each amino acid is its **side chain** (variable R-group), which gives it the physical and chemical properties that distinguish it from the other nineteen. Much more detail about amino acid structure, including their chemical properties, can be found in *MCAT Biochemistry Review.*

3.2 PROTEIN STRUCTURE

There are two common types of covalent bonds between amino acids in proteins: the **peptide bonds** that link amino acids together into polypeptide chains and **disulfide bridges** between cysteine R-groups.

The Peptide Bond

Polypeptides are formed by linking amino acids together in peptide bonds. A peptide bond is formed between the carboxyl group of one amino acid and the α-amino group of another amino acid with the loss of water. The figure below shows the formation of a dipeptide from the amino acids glycine and alanine.

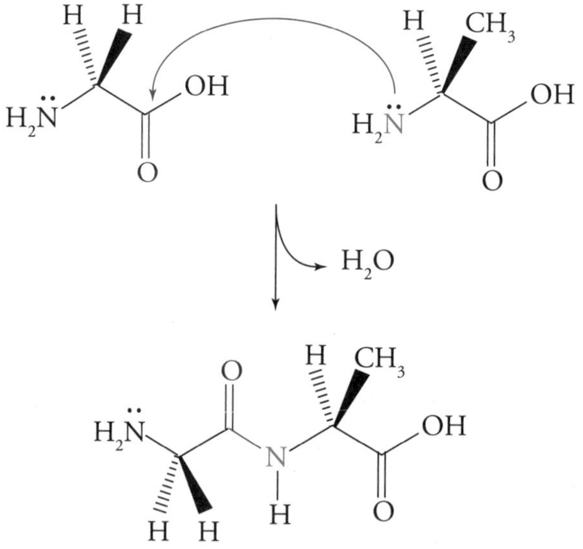

Figure 2   Peptide Bond (Amide Bond) Formation

In a polypeptide chain, the N–C–C–N–C–C pattern formed from the amino acids is known as the **backbone** of the polypeptide. An individual amino acid is termed a **residue** when it is part of a polypeptide chain. The amino terminus is the first end made during polypeptide synthesis, and the carboxy terminus is made last. Hence, by convention, the amino-terminal residue is also always written first.

- In the oligopeptide Phe-Glu-Gly-Ser-Ala, which residue has a free α-amino group, and which residue has a free α-carboxyl group? (Refer to the beginning of the chapter for structures.)[1]

---

[1]   As stated above, the amino end is always written first. Therefore, the oligopeptide begins with an exposed Phe amino group and ends with an exposed Ala carboxyl; all the other backbone groups are hitched together in peptide bonds.

Hydrolysis of a protein by another protein is called **proteolysis** or **proteolytic cleavage**, and the protein that does the cutting is known as a **proteolytic enzyme** or **protease**. Proteolytic cleavage is a specific means of cleaving peptide bonds. Many enzymes only cleave the peptide bond adjacent to a specific amino acid. For example, the protease trypsin cleaves on the carboxyl side of the residues arginine and lysine, while chymotrypsin cleaves adjacent to hydrophobic residues such as phenylalanine. (Do *not* memorize these examples.)

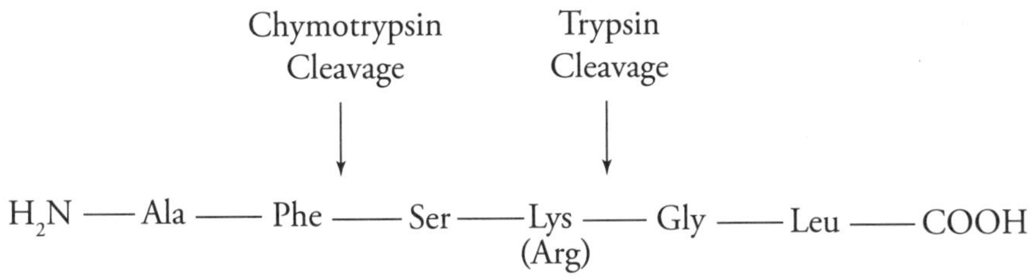

Figure 3   Specificity of Protease Cleavage

- Based on the above, if the following peptide is cleaved by trypsin, what amino acid will be on the new N-terminus and how many fragments will result: Ala-Gly-Glu-Lys-Phe-Phe-Lys?[2]

The Disulfide Bond

Cysteine is an amino acid with a reactive thiol (sulfhydryl, SH) in its side chain. The thiol of one cysteine can react with the thiol of another cysteine to produce a covalent sulfur-sulfur bond known as a disulfide bond, as illustrated below. The cysteines forming a disulfide bond may be located in the same or different polypeptide chain(s). The disulfide bridge plays an important role in stabilizing tertiary protein structure; this will be discussed in the section on protein folding. Once a cysteine residue becomes disulfide-bonded to another cysteine residue, it is called *cystine* instead of cysteine.

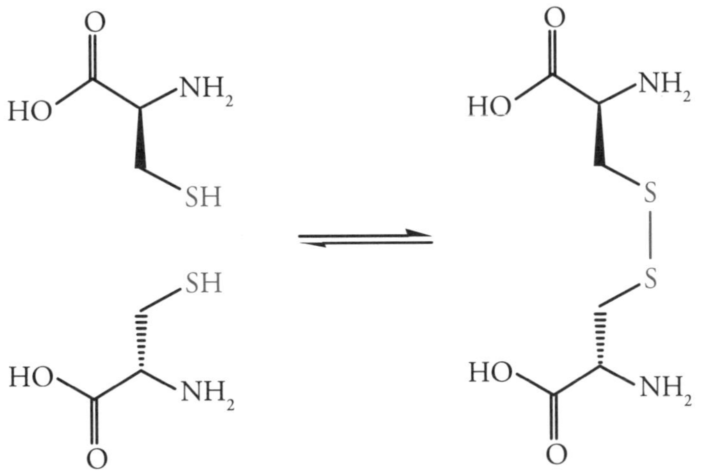

Figure 4   Formation of the Disulfide Bond

---

[2]   Trypsin will cleave on the carboxyl side of the Lys residue, with Phe on the N-terminus of the new Phe-Phe-Lys fragment. There will be two fragments after trypsin cleavage: Phe-Phe-Lys and Ala-Gly-Glu-Lys.

Protein Structure in Three Dimensions

Each protein folds into a unique three-dimensional structure that is required for that protein to function properly. Improperly folded, or **denatured**, proteins are non-functional. There are four levels of protein folding that contribute to their final three-dimensional structure. Each level of structure is dependent upon a particular type of bond, as discussed in the following sections.

Denaturation is an important concept. It refers to the **disruption of a protein's shape without breaking peptide bonds**. Proteins are denatured by *urea* (which disrupts hydrogen bonding interactions), by *extremes of pH*, by extremes of *temperature,* and by *changes in salt concentration (tonicity).*

Primary [1°] Structure: The Amino Acid Sequence

The simplest level of protein structure is the order of amino acids bonded to each other in the polypeptide chain. This linear ordering of amino acid residues is known as primary structure. Primary structure is the same as **sequence**. The bond which determines 1° structure is the peptide bond, simply because this is the bond that links one amino acid to the next in a polypeptide.

Secondary [2°] Structure: Hydrogen Bonds Between Backbone Groups

Secondary structure refers to the initial folding of a polypeptide chain into shapes stabilized by hydrogen bonds between backbone NH and CO groups. Certain motifs of secondary structure are found in most proteins. The two most common are the α-**helix** and the β-**pleated sheet**.

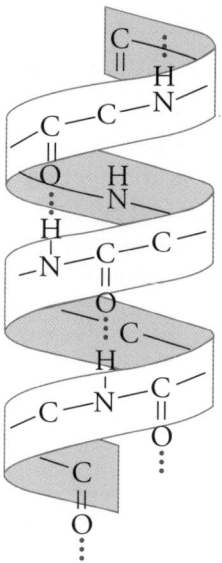

Figure 5   An α Helix

There are two types of β-sheets: one with adjacent polypeptide strands running in the *same* direction (**parallel** β-pleated sheet) and another in which the polypeptide strands run in *opposite* directions (**antiparallel** β-pleated sheet), as shown in Figure 6.

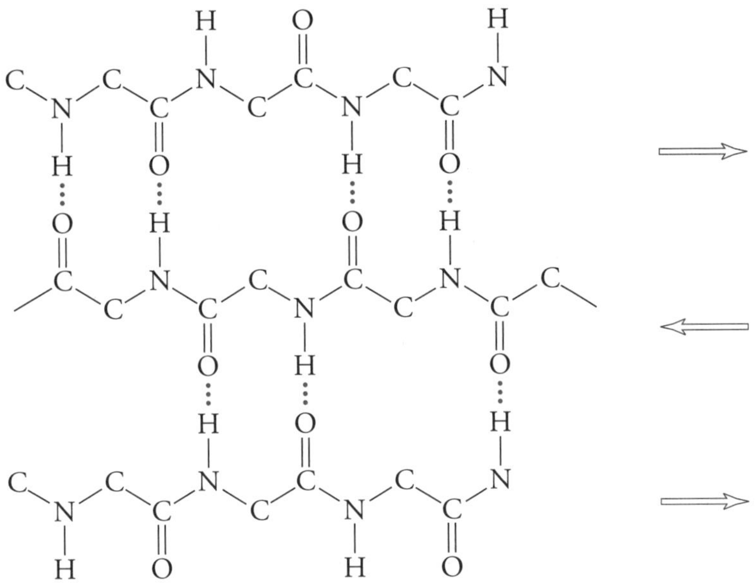

Figure 6 A β-Pleated Sheet

- If a single polypeptide folds once and forms a β-pleated sheet with itself, would this be a parallel or antiparallel β-pleated sheet?[3]

Tertiary (3°) Structure: Hydrophobic/Hydrophilic Interactions

The next level of protein folding, tertiary structure, concerns interactions between amino acid residues located more distantly from each other in the polypeptide chain. The folding of secondary structures such as α-helices into higher order tertiary structures is driven by interactions of R-groups with each other and with the solvent (water). Hydrophobic R-groups tend to fold into the interior of the protein, away from the solvent, and hydrophilic R-groups tend to be exposed to water on the surface of the protein (shown for the generic globular protein).

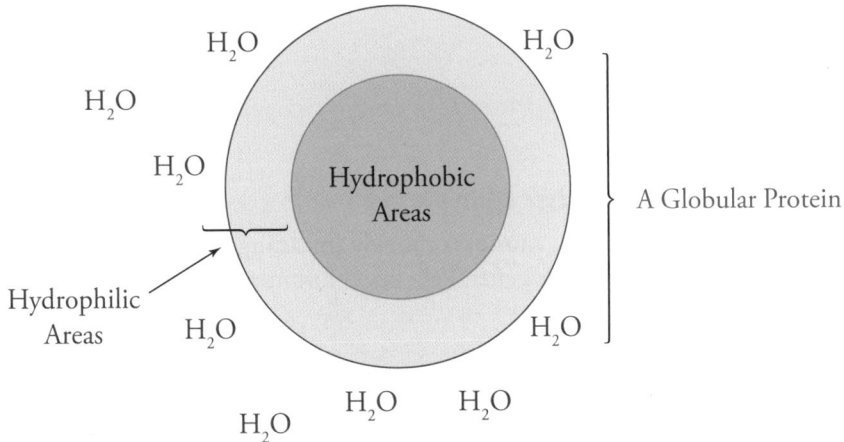

Figure 7 Folding of a Globular Protein in Aqueous Solution

---

[3] It would be antiparallel because one participant in the β-pleated sheet would have a C to N direction, while the other would be running N to C.

Under the right conditions, the forces driving hydrophobic avoidance of water and hydrogen bonding will fold a polypeptide spontaneously into the correct conformation, the lowest energy conformation.

- Which of the following may be considered an example of tertiary protein structure?[4]
  - I. van der Waals interactions between two Phe R-groups located far apart on a polypeptide
  - II. Hydrogen bonds between backbone amino and carboxyl groups
  - III. Covalent disulfide bonds between cysteine residues located far apart on a polypeptide

Quaternary (4°) Structure: Various Bonds Between Separate Chains

The highest level of protein structure, quaternary structure, describes interactions between polypeptide subunits. A **subunit** is a single polypeptide chain that is part of a large complex containing many subunits (a **multisubunit complex**). The arrangement of subunits in a multisubunit complex is what we mean by quaternary structure. For example, mammalian RNA polymerase II contains twelve different subunits. The interactions between subunits are instrumental in protein function, as in the cooperative binding of oxygen by each of the four subunits of hemoglobin.

The forces stabilizing quaternary structure are generally the same as those involved in tertiary structure—non-covalent interactions, van der Waals forces, hydrogen bonds, disulfide bonds, and electrostatic interactions. It is key to understand, however, that there is one bond that may not be involved in quaternary structure—the peptide bond—because this bond defines sequence (1° structure).

- What is the difference between a disulfide bridge involved in quaternary structure and one involved in tertiary structure?[5]

3.3   CARBOHYDRATES

Carbohydrates can be broken down to CO_2 in a process called **oxidation**, which is also known as burning or combustion. Because this process releases large amounts of energy, carbohydrates generally serve as the principle energy source for cellular metabolism. Glucose in the form of the polymer cellulose is also the building block of wood and cotton.

Monosaccharides and Disaccharides

A single carbohydrate molecule is called a **monosaccharide** (meaning "single sweet unit"), also known as a **simple sugar**. Monosaccharides have the general chemical formula $C_nH_{2n}O_n$.

---

[4] **Item I is true:** this is a good example of 3° structure. Item II is false: this describes 2°, not 3°, structure. **Item III is true:** this describes the disulfide bridge, which is considered to be tertiary.

[5] Quaternary disulfides are bonds that form between chains that aren't linked by peptide bonds. Tertiary disulfides are bonds that form between residues in the same polypeptide.

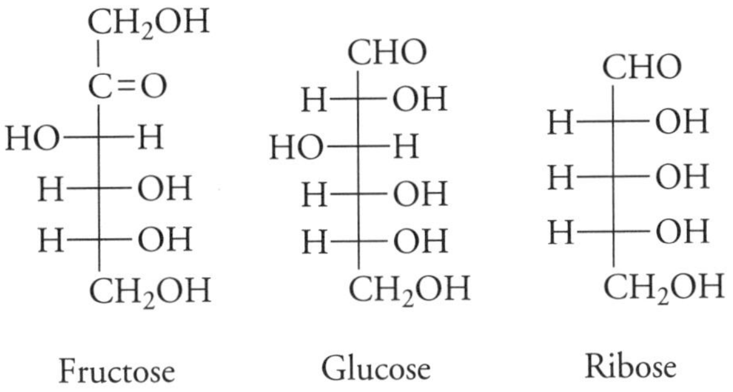

Figure 8   Some Metabolically Important Monosaccharides

Two monosaccharides bonded together form a disaccharide, a few form an oligosaccharide, and many form a polysaccharide. The bond between two sugar molecules is called a **glycosidic linkage**. This is a covalent bond, formed in a dehydration reaction that requires enzymatic catalysis.

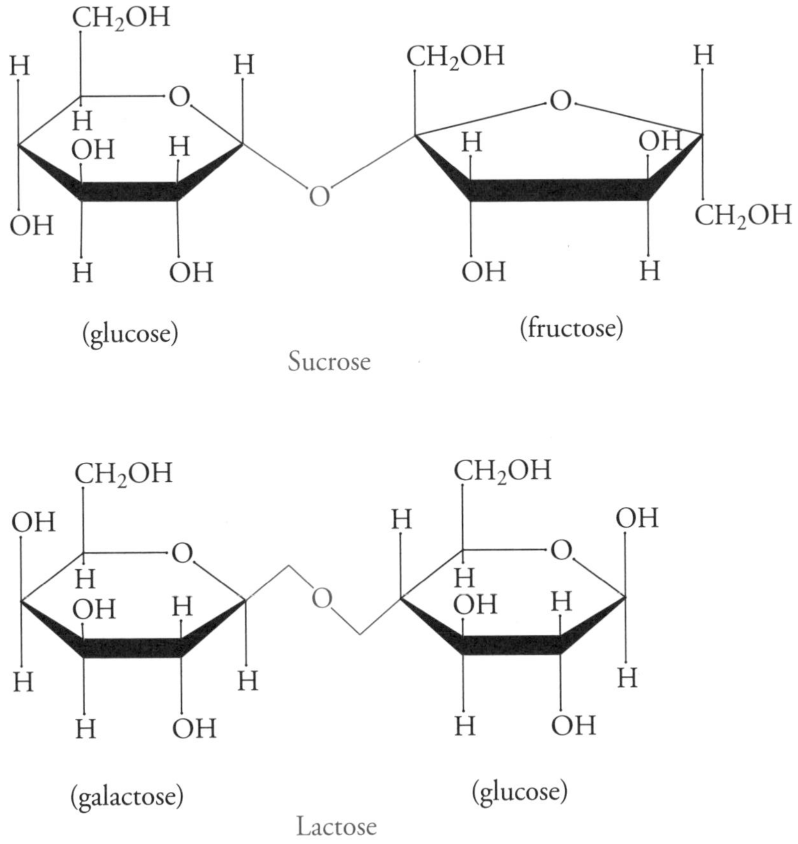

Figure 9   Disaccharides and the α- or β-Glycosidic Bond

Some common disaccharides you might see on the MCAT are sucrose (Glc-α-1,2-Fru), lactose (Gal-β-1,4-Glc), maltose (Glc-α-1,4-Glc), and cellobiose (Glc-β-1,4-Glc). However, you should NOT try to memorize these linkages.

Polymers made from these disaccharides form important biological macromolecules. Glycogen serves as an energy storage carbohydrate in animals and is composed of thousands of glucose units. Starch is the same as glycogen (except that the branches are a little different), and serves the same purpose in plants. Cellulose is a polymer of cellobiose; but note that cellobiose does not exist freely in nature. It exists only in its polymerized, cellulose form. The glycosidic bonds allow the polymer to assume a long, straight, fibrous shape. Wood and cotton are made of cellulose.

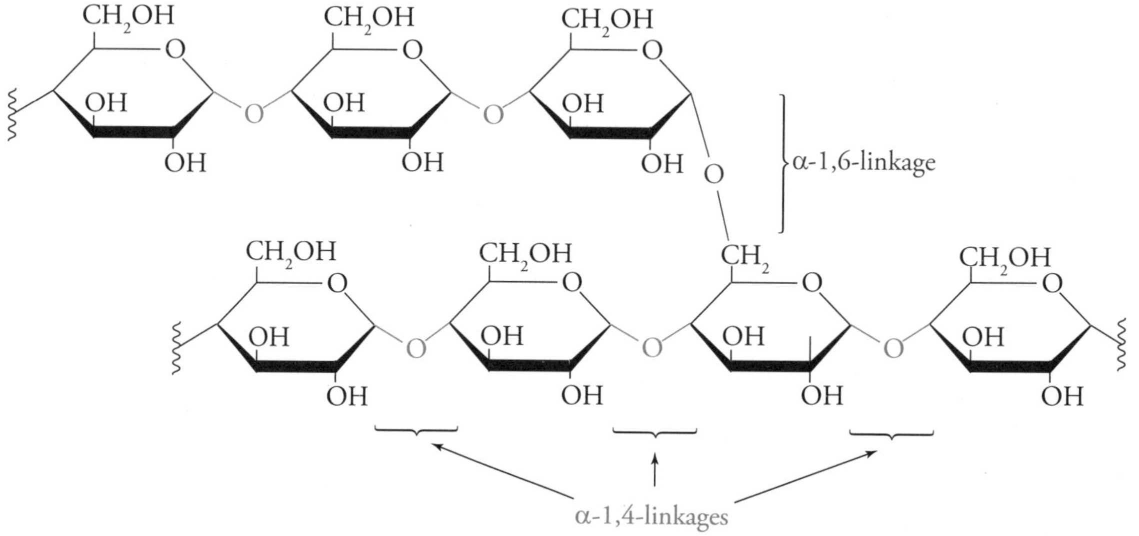

Figure 10   The Polysaccharide Glycogen

3.4   LIPIDS

Lipids are oily or fatty substances that play three physiological roles, summarized here and discussed below.

1)   In adipose cells, triglycerides (fats) store energy.
2)   In cellular membranes, phospholipids constitute a barrier between intracellular and extracellular environments.
3)   Cholesterol is a special lipid that serves as the building block for the hydrophobic steroid hormones.

The cardinal characteristic of the lipid is its **hydrophobicity**. *Hydrophobic* means "water-fearing." It is important to understand the significance of this. Since water is very polar, polar substances dissolve well in water; these are known as "water-loving," or **hydrophilic** substances. Carbon-carbon bonds and carbon-hydrogen bonds are nonpolar. Therefore, substances that contain only carbon and hydrogen will not dissolve well in water. Here are some examples: Table sugar dissolves well in water, but cooking oil floats in a layer above water or forms many tiny oil droplets when mixed with water. Cotton T-shirts become wet when exposed to water because they are made of glucose polymerized into cellulose; a nylon jacket does not become wet because it is composed of atoms covalently bound together in a nonpolar fashion. A synonym for hydrophobic is **lipophilic** (which means "lipid-loving"); a synonym for hydrophilic is **lipophobic**. We return to these concepts below.

Fatty Acid Structure

Fatty acids are composed of long unsubstituted alkanes that end in a carboxylic acid. The chain is typically 14 to 18 carbons long, and because they are synthesized two carbons at a time from acetate, only *even-numbered* fatty acids are made in human cells. A fatty acid with no carbon-carbon double bonds is said to be **saturated** with hydrogen because every carbon atom in the chain is covalently bound to the maximum number of hydrogens. **Unsaturated** fatty acids have one or more double bonds in the tail. These double bonds are almost always (Z) (or *cis*).

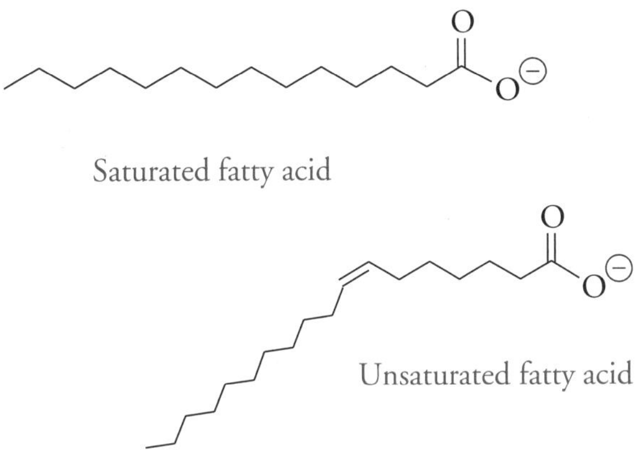

Saturated fatty acid

Unsaturated fatty acid

Figure 11   Fatty Acid Structure

- How does the shape of an unsaturated fatty acid differ from that of a saturated fatty acid?[6]
- If fatty acids are mixed into water, how are they likely to associate with each other?[7]

Figure 12 illustrates how free fatty acids interact in an aqueous solution; they form a structure called a **micelle**. The force that drives the tails into the center of the micelle is called the **hydrophobic interaction**.

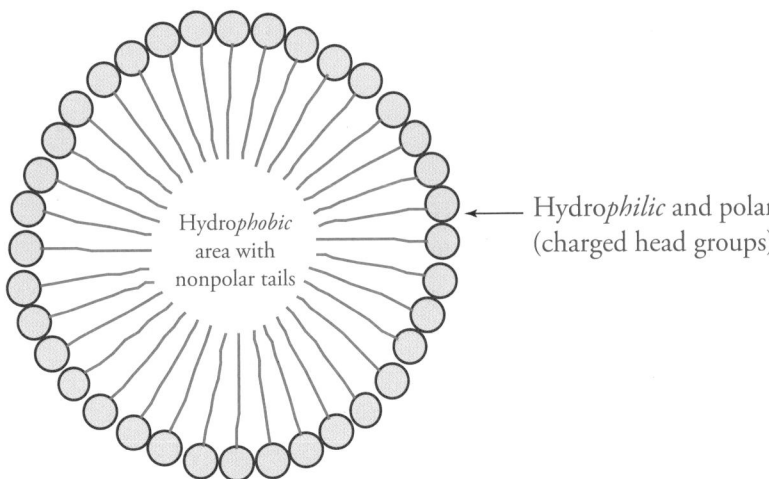

Hydro*phobic* area with nonpolar tails

Hydro*philic* and polar (charged head groups)

Figure 12   A Fatty Acid Micelle

---

[6]   An unsaturated fatty acid is bent, or "kinked," at the *cis* double bond.

[7]   The long hydrophobic chains will interact with each other to minimize contact with water, exposing the charged carboxyl group to the aqueous environment.

Triacylglycerols (TG)

The storage form of the fatty acid is fat. The technical name for fat is **triacylglycerol** or **triglyceride** (shown below). The triglyceride is composed of three fatty acids esterified to a glycerol molecule. Glycerol is a three-carbon triol with the formula $HOCH_2-CHOH-CH_2OH$. As you can see, it has three hydroxyl groups that can be esterified to fatty acids. It is necessary to store fatty acids in the relatively inert form of fat because free fatty acids are reactive chemicals.

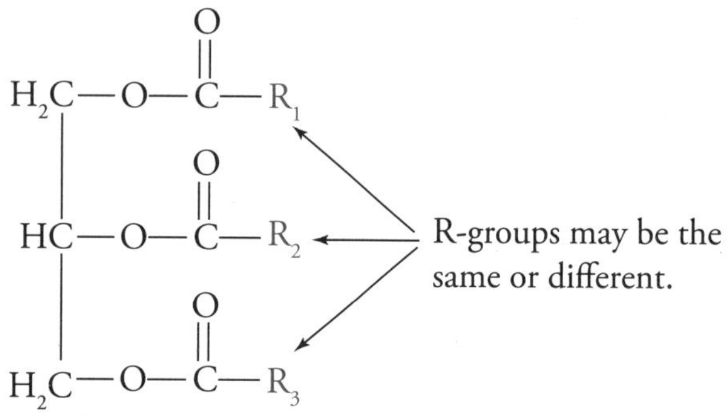

Figure 13 A Triglyceride (Fat)

Lipases are enzymes that hydrolyze fats. Triacylglycerols are stored in fat cells as an energy source. Fats are more efficient energy storage molecules than carbohydrates for two reasons: packing and energy content.

1) **Packing:** Their hydrophobicity allows fats to pack together much more closely than carbohydrates. Carbohydrates carry a great amount of water-of-solvation (water molecules hydrogen-bonded to their hydroxyl groups).
2) **Energy content:** All packing considerations aside, fat molecules store much more energy than carbohydrates. In other words, regardless of what you dissolve it in, a fat has more energy carbon-for-carbon than a carbohydrate.

Introduction to Lipid Bilayer Membranes

Membrane lipids are **phospholipids** derived from diacylglycerol phosphate or DG-P.

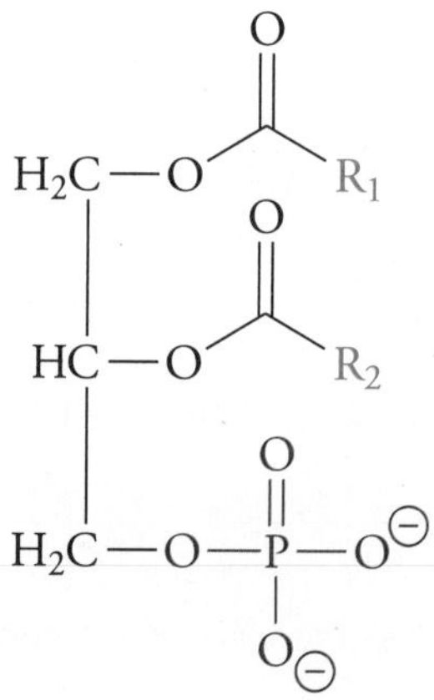

Figure 14 A Phosphoglyceride (Diacylglycerol Phosphate, or DGP)

We saw above how fatty acids spontaneously form micelles. Phospholipids also minimize their interactions with water by forming an orderly structure—in this case, it is a **lipid bilayer** (below). Hydrophobic interactions drive the formation of the bilayer, and once formed, it is stabilized by van der Waals forces between the long tails.

3.4

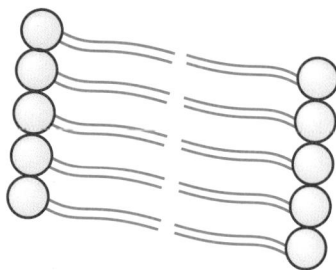

Figure 15   A Small Section of a Lipid Bilayer Membrane

- Would a saturated or an unsaturated fatty acid residue have more van der Waals interactions with neighboring alkyl chains in a bilayer membrane?[8]

A more precise way to give the answer to the question above is to say that double bonds (unsaturation) in phospholipid fatty acids *tend to increase membrane fluidity*. Unsaturation prevents the membrane from solidifying by disrupting the orderly packing of the hydrophobic lipid tails. The right amount of fluidity is essential for function. Decreasing the *length* of fatty acid tails also increases fluidity. The steroid **cholesterol** (discussed a bit later) is a third important modulator of membrane fluidity. At low temperatures, it increases fluidity in the same way as kinks in fatty acid tails; therefore, it is known as *membrane antifreeze*. At high temperatures, however, cholesterol attenuates (reduces) membrane fluidity. Don't ponder this paradox too long; just remember that cholesterol keeps fluidity at an *optimum level*. Remember, the structural determinants of membrane fluidity are: degree of saturation, tail length, and amount of cholesterol.

Terpenes

A terpene is a member of a broad class of compounds built from isoprene units (C_5H_8) with a general formula $(C_5H_8)_n$.

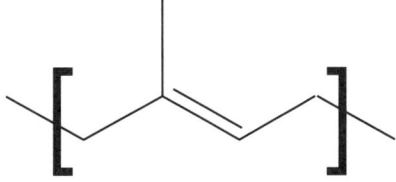

Figure 16   Isoprene Unit

---

[8]   The bent shape of the unsaturated fatty acid means that it doesn't fit in as well and has less contact with neighboring groups to form van der Waals interactions. Phospholipids composed of saturated fatty acids make the membrane more solid.

Terpenes may be linear or cyclic, and are classified by the number of isoprene units they contain. For example, monoterpenes consist of two isoprene units, sesquiterpenes consist of three, and diterpenes contain four.

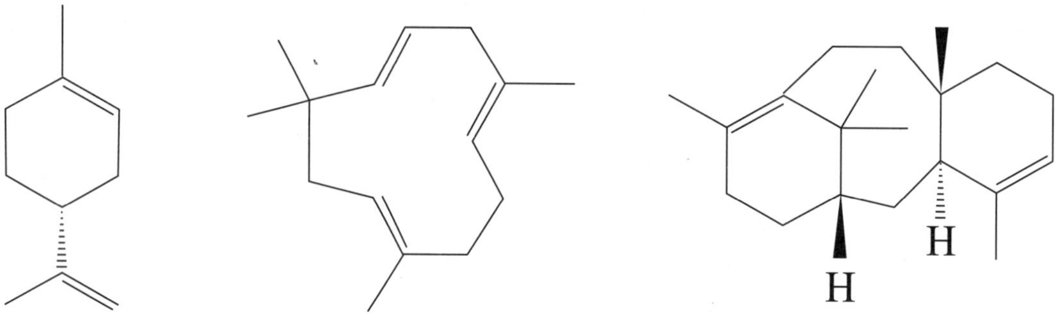

limonene
$C_{10}H_{16}$
(a monoterpene)

humulene
$C_{15}H_{24}$
(a sesquiterpene)

taxadiene
$C_{20}H_{32}$
(a diterpene)

Figure 17   Terpene Structures

Squalene is a triterpene (made of six isoprene units) and a particularly important compound, as it is biosynthetically utilized in the manufacture of steroids. Squalene is also a component of earwax.

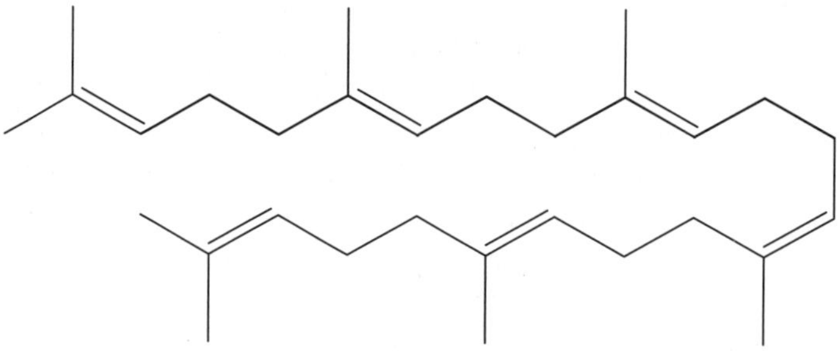

Figure 18   Squalene

Whereas a terpene is formally a simple hydrocarbon, there are a number of natural and synthetically derived species that are built from an isoprene skeleton and functionalized with other elements (O, N, S, etc.). These functionalized-terpenes are known as *terpenoids*. Vitamin A ($C_{20}H_{30}O$) is an example of a terpenoid.

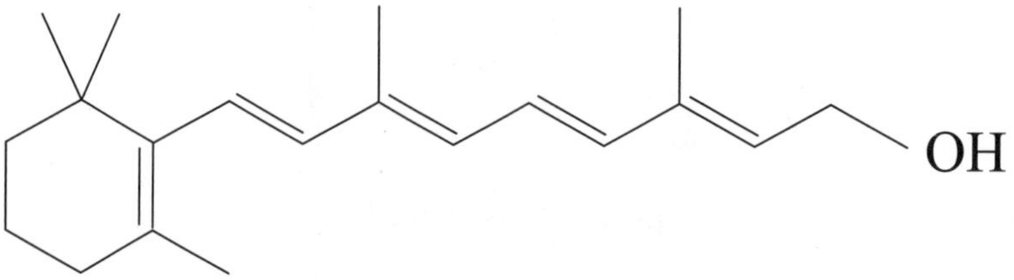

Figure 19   Vitamin A

Steroids

Steroids are included here because of their hydrophobicity, and, hence, similarity to fats. Their structure is otherwise unique. All steroids have the basic tetracyclic ring system (see below) based on the structure of **cholesterol**.

As discussed earlier, the steroid cholesterol is an important component of the lipid bilayer. It is both obtained from the diet and synthesized in the liver. It is carried in the blood packaged with fats and proteins into **lipoproteins**. One type of lipoprotein has been implicated as the cause of atherosclerotic vascular disease, which refers to the build-up of cholesterol "plaques" on the inside of blood vessels.

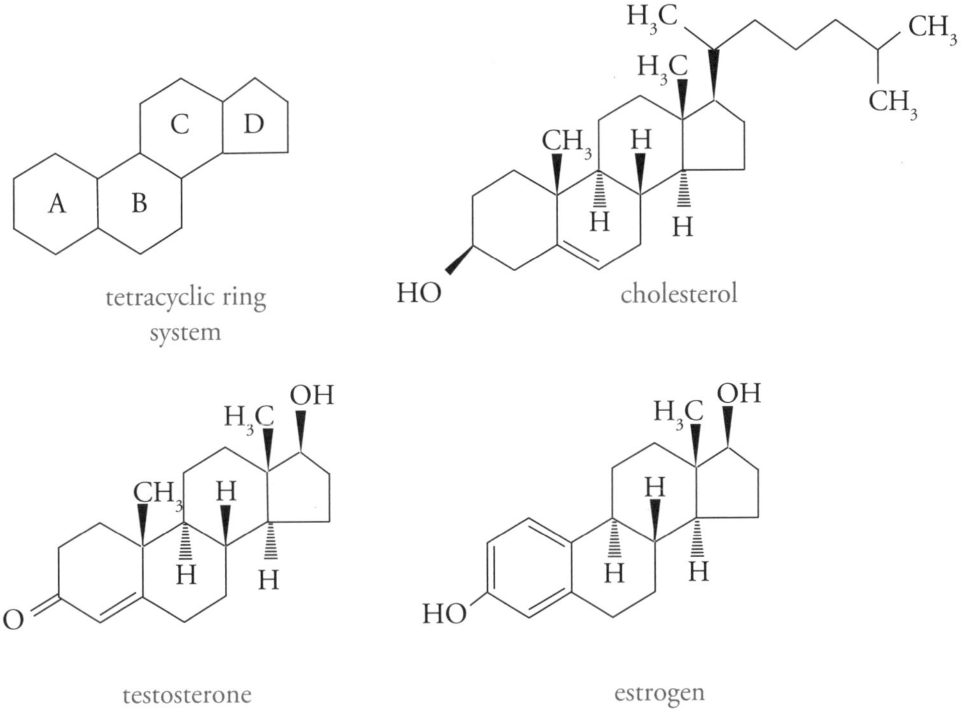

Figure 20   Cholesterol-Derived Hormones

Steroid hormones are made from cholesterol. Two examples are **testosterone** (an androgen or male sex hormone) and **estradiol** (an estrogen or female sex hormone).

3.5 PHOSPHORUS-CONTAINING COMPOUNDS

Phosphoric acid is an *inorganic* acid (it does not contain carbon) with the potential to donate three protons. The pK_as for the three acid dissociation equilibria are 2.1, 7.2, and 12.4. Therefore, at physiological pH, phosphoric acid is significantly dissociated, existing largely in anionic form.

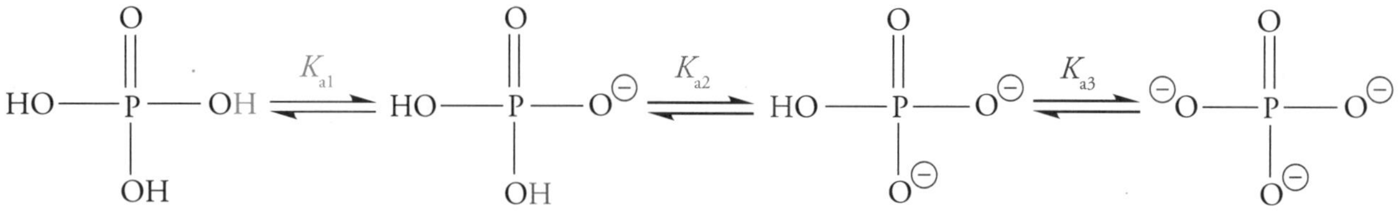

Figure 21   Phosphoric Acid Dissociation

Phosphate is also known as orthophosphate. Two orthophosphates bound together via an **anhydride linkage** form **pyrophosphate**. The P–O–P bond in pyrophosphate is an example of a **high-energy phosphate bond**. This name is derived from the fact that the hydrolysis of pyrophosphate is extremely favorable.

There are three reasons that phosphate anhydride bonds store so much energy:

1) When phosphates are linked together, their negative charges repel each other strongly.
2) Orthophosphate has more resonance forms and thus a lower free energy than linked phosphates.
3) Orthophosphate has a more favorable interaction with the biological solvent (water) than linked phosphates.

The details are not crucial. What is essential is that you fix the image in your mind of linked phosphates acting like compressed springs, just waiting to fly open and provide energy for an enzyme to catalyze a reaction.

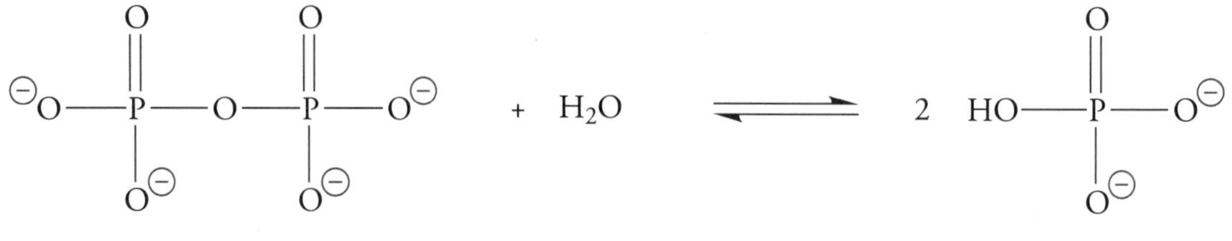

Figure 22   The Hydrolysis of Pyrophosphate

Nucleotides

Nucleotides are the building blocks of nucleic acids (RNA and DNA). Each nucleotide contains a **ribose** (or **deoxyribose**) **sugar** group; a **purine** or **pyrimidine base** joined to carbon number one of the ribose ring; and one, two, or three phosphate units joined to carbon five of the ribose ring. The nucleotide **a**denosine **t**ri**p**hosphate (ATP) plays a central role in cellular metabolism in addition to being an RNA precursor. Significantly more information about the structure of the nucleic acids can be found in *MCAT Biochemistry Review*. More information on the function of the nucleic acids will be provided in Chapter 4 of this book.

ATP is the universal short-term energy storage molecule. Energy extracted from the oxidation of foodstuffs is immediately stored in the phosphoanhydride bonds of ATP. This energy will later be used to power cellular processes; it may also be used to synthesize glucose or fats, which are longer-term energy storage molecules. This applies to *all* living organisms, from bacteria to humans. Even some viruses carry ATP with them outside the host cell, though viruses cannot make their own ATP.

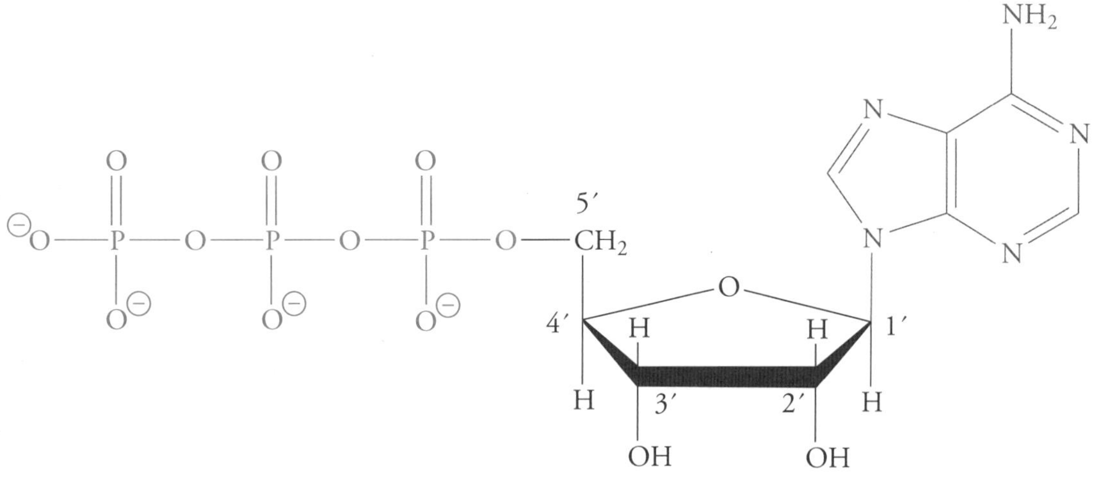

Figure 23 Adenosine Triphosphate (ATP)

Chapter 3 Summary

- Amino acids (AAs) consist of a tetrahedral α-carbon connected to an amino group, a carboxyl group, and a variable R-group, which determines the AA's properties.

- Proteins consist of amino acids linked by peptide bonds, which are very stable. The primary structure of a protein consists of its amino acid sequence.

- The secondary structure of proteins (α-helices and β-sheets) is formed through hydrogen-bonding interactions between atoms in the backbone of the molecule.

- The most stable tertiary protein structure generally places polar AAs on the exterior and non-polar AAs on the interior of the protein. This minimizes interactions between nonpolar AAs and water, while optimizing interactions between side chains inside the protein.

- Proteins have a variety of functions in the body including (but not limited to) enzymes, structural roles, hormones, receptors, channels, antibodies, transporters, etc.

- The monomer for a carbohydrate is a monosaccharide (simple sugar), with the molecular formula $C_nH_{2n}O_n$. The common monosaccharides are glucose, fructose, galactose, ribose, and deoxyribose.

- Two monosaccharides joined with a glycosidic linkage form a disaccharide. The common disaccharides are maltose, sucrose, and lactose. Mammals can digest α glycosidic linkages, but generally not β linkages.

- Polysaccharides consist of many monosaccharides linked together. Glycogen (animals) and starch (plants) are storage units for glucose and can be broken down for energy. Cellulose is also a glucose polymer, but the beta linkage prevents digestion. It forms wood and cotton.

- Lipids are found in several forms in the body, including triglycerides, phospholipids, cholesterol and steroids, and terpenes. Triglycerides and phospholipids are linear, while cholesterol and steroids have a ring structure.

- Lipids are hydrophobic. Triglycerides are used for energy storage, phospholipids form membranes, and cholesterol is the precursor to the steroid hormones.

- The building blocks of nucleic acids (DNA and RNA) are nucleotides, which are comprised of a pentose sugar, a purine or pyrimidine base, and 2-3 phosphate units.

CHAPTER 3 FREESTANDING PRACTICE QUESTIONS

1. Why is ATP known as a "high energy" structure at neutral pH?

A) It exhibits a large decrease in free energy when it undergoes hydrolytic reactions.
B) The phosphate ion released from ATP hydrolysis is very reactive.
C) It causes cellular processes to proceed at faster rates.
D) Adenine is the best energy storage molecule of all the nitrogenous bases.

2. Which of the following best describes the secondary structure of a protein?

A) Various folded polypeptide chains joining together to form a larger unit
B) The amino acid sequence of the chain
C) The polypeptide chain folding upon itself due to hydrophobic/hydrophilic interactions
D) Peptide bonds hydrogen-bonding to one another to create a sheet-like structure

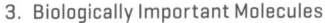

3. Phenylketonuria (PKU) is an autosomal recessive disorder that results from a deficiency of the enzyme phenylalanine hydroxylase. This enzyme normally converts phenylalanine into tyrosine. PKU results in intellectual disability, growth retardation, fair skin, eczema, and a distinct musty body odor. Which of the following is most likely true?

A) Treatment should include a decrease in tyrosine in the diet.
B) The musty body odor is likely caused by a disorder in aromatic amino acid metabolism.
C) Patients with PKU should increase the amount of phenylalanine in their diet.
D) PKU can be acquired by consuming too much aspartame (an artificial sweetener that contains high levels of phenylalanine).

4. A genetic regulator is found to contain a lysine residue that is important for its binding to DNA. If a mutation were to occur such that a different amino acid replaces the lysine at that location, which of the following resulting amino acids would likely be the least harmful to its ability to bind DNA?

A) Glycine
B) Glutamate
C) Aspartate
D) Arginine

5. Increasing the amount of cholesterol in a plasma membrane would lead to an increase in:

A) membrane permeability.
B) atherosclerotic plaques.
C) membrane fluidity at low temperatures but a decrease in membrane fluidity at high temperatures.
D) membrane fluidity at high and low temperatures.

6. A human space explorer crash-lands on a planet where the native inhabitants are entirely unable to digest glycogen, but are able to digest cellulose. Consequently, they make their clothing out of glycogen-based material. The starving space explorer eats one of the native inhabitants' shirts and the natives are amazed. Based on this information, which of the following is/are true?

   I.   The explorer can digest α-glycosidic linkages.
   II. The native inhabitants can digest α-glycosidic linkages.
   III. The native inhabitants can digest starch.

A) I only
B) I and III only
C) II and III only
D) I, II, and III

CHAPTER 3 PRACTICE PASSAGE

Photosynthesis is the process plants use to derive energy from sunlight and is associated with a cell's chloroplasts. The energy is used to produce carbohydrates from carbon dioxide and water. Photosynthesis involves light and dark phases. Figure 1 represents two initial steps associated with the light phase.

The light phase supplies the dark phase with NADPH and a high-energy substrate.

A researcher attempted to produce a photosynthetic system outside the living organism according to the following protocols:

- Chloroplasts were extracted from green leaves and ruptured, and their membranes were thereby exposed, then a solution of hexachloroplatinate ions carrying a charge of −2 was added.

- The structure of the composite was analyzed, and the amount of oxygen produced by the system was measured.

The researcher concluded that the ions were bound to the membrane's Photosystem 1 site by the attraction of opposite charges. The resulting composite is shown in Figure 2. It was found that the hexachloroplatinate-membrane composite was photosynthetically active.

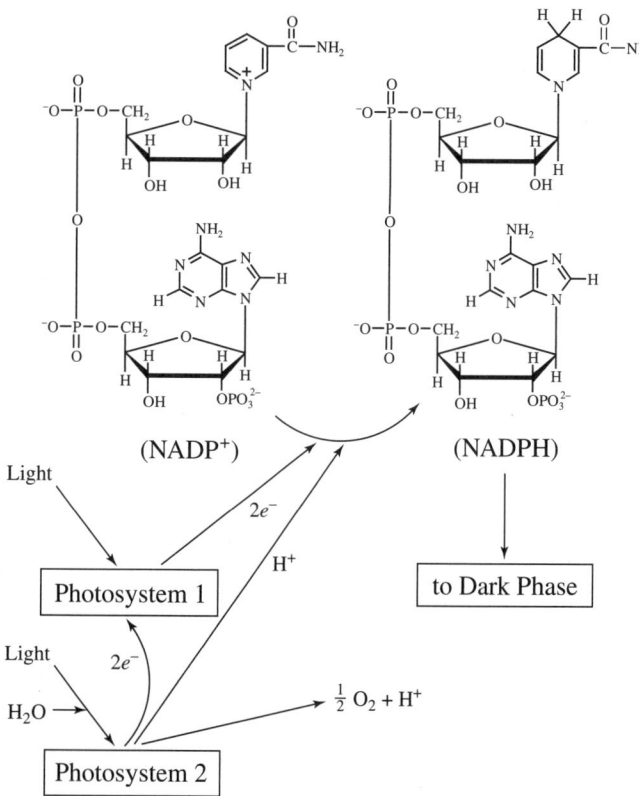

Figure 1

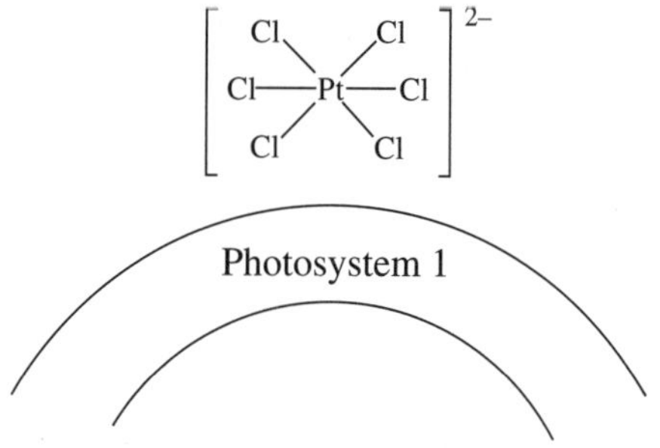

Figure 2

1. In concluding that the hexachloroplatinate ions were bound to Photosystem 1 due to the attraction of opposite charges, the researchers apparently assumed that the structure of the membrane was:

A) determined solely by hydrophobic bonding.
B) positively charged.
C) covalently bound to the platinate.
D) negatively charged.

2. Figure 1 indicates that:

A) photoactivation of the chloroplast membrane results in the reduction of the anhydride-containing molecule $NADP^+$.
B) electrons are lost from Photosystem 1 through the conversion of NADPH to $NADP^+$, and are replaced by electrons from Photosystem 2.
C) there is a net gain of electrons by the system.
D) electrons are lost from Photosystem 1 through the conversion of $NADP^+$ to NADPH, but are not replaced by electrons from Photosystem 2.

3. If $NADP^+$ is fully hydrolyzed to its component bases, phosphates, and sugars, what type of monosaccharide would result?

A) A three-carbon triose
B) A hexose
C) A pentose
D) An α-D-glucose

4. If in a given cell the photosynthetic dark phase were artificially arrested while the light phase proceeded, the cell would most likely experience:

A) decreased levels of NADPH.
B) increased levels of NADPH.
C) increased levels of carbohydrate.
D) increased photoactivation of the chloroplast.

5. To determine the primary structure of the protein portion of Photosystem 1, a series of cleavage reactions was undertaken. To break apart the protein, the most logical action to take would be to:

A) decarboxylate free carboxyl groups.
B) hydrolyze peptide bonds.
C) repolymerize peptide bonds.
D) hydrolyze amide branch points.

6. A researcher examined a sample of the principal substance produced by the photosynthetic dark phase and concluded that he was working with a racemic mixture of glucose isomers. Which of the following experimental findings would be *inconsistent* with such a conclusion?

A) The sample is composed of carbon, hydrogen, and oxygen only.
B) The sample consists of an aldohexose.
C) The sample rotates the plane of polarized light to the left.
D) The sample is optically inactive.

SOLUTIONS TO CHAPTER 3 FREESTANDING PRACTICE QUESTIONS

1. **A** Choice A is the best answer because it directly addresses the energetics of ATP hydrolysis. Choice B discusses the reactivity of the released phosphate ion and not the structure of ATP itself, so it can be eliminated. Choice C can be eliminated because it describes the rate of cellular processes, not the energy of ATP. Choice D can be eliminated because the structure of adenine is not related to why ATP is a good energy storage molecule.

2. **D** The secondary structure of proteins is the initial folding of the polypeptide chain into α-helices or β-pleated sheets. Choice A can be eliminated because it describes the formation of a quaternary protein, choice B can be eliminated because it describes the primary protein structure, and choice C can be eliminated because it describes the tertiary protein structure.

3. **B** A defect in phenylalanine hydroxylase (or the THB cofactor) would result in a build-up of phenylalanine. This would lead to an excess of phenylalanine byproducts such as phenyl-acetate, phenyllactate, and phenylpyruvate, and a decrease in tyrosine. Therefore, patients with PKU should increase the amount of tyrosine in their diet (it becomes an essential amino acid in this condition; choice A is wrong), as well as eliminate phenylalanine from their diet (choice C is wrong). PKU is a genetically acquired disorder (autosomal recessive), as mentioned in the passage, and thus it is not acquired by consuming too much phenyl-alanine (choice D is wrong). It is true that phenylalanine and its derivatives are aromatic amino acids and that the high levels of these compounds lead to the distinct musty body odor (choice B is correct). Process of Elimination (POE) is probably the best method to use in answering this question since it is unclear (without prior knowledge of PKU) what the underlying mechanism of the body odor would be.

4. **D** While knowing the structures of the different amino acids is unlikely to be important for the MCAT, knowing which of the amino acids are basic (histidine, arginine, lysine) and which are acidic (glutamate, aspartate) is likely to be relevant. In this case, since lysine is basic (and therefore best at binding the negatively charged DNA), one can assume that a mutation resulting in another basic amino acid would cause the least change in its ability to bind DNA. Therefore, a mutation from lysine to arginine would cause the least harm (choice D is correct). A mutation from lysine to glutamate or aspartate (both acidic) would likely cause the most harm to its ability to bind DNA (choices B and C are wrong). Glycine is a neutral amino acid (choice A is wrong).

5. **C** Plasma membranes can be up to 50% composed of sterols. Sterols help stabilize the mem-brane at both spectrums of the temperature. At low temperatures, cholesterol increases flu-idity because the ring structure of cholesterol does not allow for tight phospholipid tail packing. At high temperatures, cholesterol decreases membrane fluidity (the OH group of cholesterol prevents phospholipid dispersion; choice C is correct, and choice D is wrong). Cholesterol decreases the permeability of membranes by filling in the "holes" between the fatty acid tails (choice A is wrong). The formation of atherosclerotic plaques, while related to cholesterol, is due to high levels of blood cholesterol, not membrane cholesterol (choice B is wrong).

6. **A** Item I is true: humans can digest α-glycosidic linkages, such as those found in glycogen. If the natives' shirts are made of glycogen, the space explorer should have no trouble consuming and digesting them (choice C can be eliminated). Item II Is false: cellulose contains β-glycosidic linkages. If the natives can digest cellulose, but not glycogen, then they cannot digest α-glycosidic linkages (choice D can be eliminated). Item III is false: starch also contains a α-glycosidic linkages. If the natives cannot digest glycogen, then they likely cannot digest starch either (choice B can be eliminated, and choice A is true).

SOLUTIONS TO CHAPTER 3 PRACTICE PASSAGE

1. **B** The passage states that the ion is attracted to Photosystem 1 by the attraction of opposite charges (positively charged photosystem and negatively charged hexachloroplatinate ion).

2. **A** The main result of the light phase, as depicted in Figure 1, is the reduction of $NADP^+$ to make NADPH (choice A is correct). Choice B is wrong since $NADP^+$ is converted into NADPH, not vice versa. Choice C is incorrect since in any system, mass and charge are conserved. Electrons move from one molecule to another, but they are not created or destroyed in a chemical reaction. Choice D can be eliminated since Figure 1 depicts electrons moving from Photosystem 2 to Photosystem 1.

3. **C** NADPH contains ribose, a pentose. Choice C is correct.

4. **B** The light phase makes NADPH, and the dark phase consumes it. In the absence of the dark phase, NADPH will continue to be produced, but none will be consumed, making NADPH levels rise (choice B is correct). Choice C is wrong since the dark phase is responsible for biosynthesis, such as carbohydrate production, so this will decrease, not increase. Choice D can be eliminated since the amount of light and photoactivation should remain the same.

5. **B** Proteins are composed of amino acid residues which are joined together by peptide bonds during the translation process. To split the protein into smaller pieces, proteases and chemical reagents act to hydrolyze the peptide bond, reversing the biosynthetic process.

6. **C** A racemic mixture is one which contains equal quantities of two stereoisomers that rotate plane-polarized light in opposite directions. Since there are equal quantities of both, racemic mixtures are optically inactive. Thus, choice C, which states that the sample rotates light, is inconsistent with the conclusion that the sample is racemic and is the correct answer choice. All other choices are consistent with the conclusion that the sample is a racemic mixture of glucose. Carbohydrates, of which glucose is one, are made of only carbon, hydrogen, and oxygen (choice A is consistent and can be eliminated). Glucose, with six carbons and a carbonyl group on the 6th carbon, is an aldohexose (choice B is consistent and can be eliminated), and racemic mixtures do not rotate light (choice D is consistent and can be eliminated).

Chapter 4
Molecular Biology

It was once thought that simple living organisms were generated spontaneously from nonliving matter. When a steak went bad and became infested with larvae, it was because the decomposing meat actually became squirming worms. Most religions have traditional explanations for the origin of human life, too. Children are derived from adults due to the will of a deity; the original adults were placed on the Earth by that deity. But as empiricism developed during the Enlightenment, rigorous experiments were used to explain life, resulting in "scientific" models that gradually replaced more traditional explanations.

One early conclusion was that simple organisms were derived not from decomposing matter but from parental organisms. Subsequently, it was found that some organisms are too small to be seen with the naked eye. These "germs" were eventually implicated as the cause of most major diseases. Gradually, the scientific community came to the conclusion that all life was derived from other life. The patterns of inheritance and evolution were elucidated by a chain of scientists, from Mendel through Darwin. But the mechanism remained a mystery. Finally, cellular biology advanced to the point that scientists were aware of two substances found in cells that seemed appropriate vehicles for the transmission of inherited information: DNA and protein. The extreme length and orderly arrangement of repeating units in DNA and protein made it seem very likely that they could contain information. Researchers had waded through a chemical ocean of alphabet soup and suddenly come upon long strings of what looked like letters.

This is where biology stood in the early 1940s. In the '40s and '50s, two monumental achievements in microbiology finally clarified the gears in the clock of evolution and how they turn. One was the elucidation of the structure of DNA by Watson and Crick. The other was the proof by Avery, Herriott, Hershey, Chase, and their coworkers that DNA was the fundamental unit of genetic inheritance in microorganisms. In the following discussion, we will summarize the wealth of information that has been built upon these two prescient cornerstones.

4.1 DNA STRUCTURE

General Overview

Significant detail about the structure of DNA and RNA is provided in *MCAT Biochemistry Review;* here we will give a brief overview of this topic. DNA is short for **d**eoxyribo**n**ucleic **a**cid. DNA and RNA (**ri**bo**n**ucleic **a**cid) are called **nucleic acids** because they are found in the nucleus and possess many acidic phosphate groups.

The building block of DNA is the **d**eoxyribo**n**ucleoside 5' **tri**phosphate (dNTP, where N represents one of the four basic nucleosides). Deoxyadenosine 5' triphosphate (dATP) is shown in Figure 1; the other bases are shown in Figure 2. Nucleotides are built from three components: a sugar (deoxyribose for DNA, ribose for RNA), an aromatic, nitrogenous base, and 1-3 phosphate groups. The bases G and A are derived from a precursor called purine, so they are referred to as **the purines**. C, T, and U are **the pyrimidines**.[1]

A nucleo*side* is ribose or deoxyribose with a purine or pyrimidine linked to the 1' carbon; nucleo*tides* are phosphate esters of nucleosides, with one, two, or three phosphate groups joined to the ribose ring by the 5' hydroxy group. When nucleotides contain three phosphate residues, they are also referred to as **nucleoside triphosphates**, abbreviated **NTP** (if the sugar is deoxyribose, they are abbreviated **dNTP**). In individual nucleotides, N is replaced by A, G, C, T, or U.

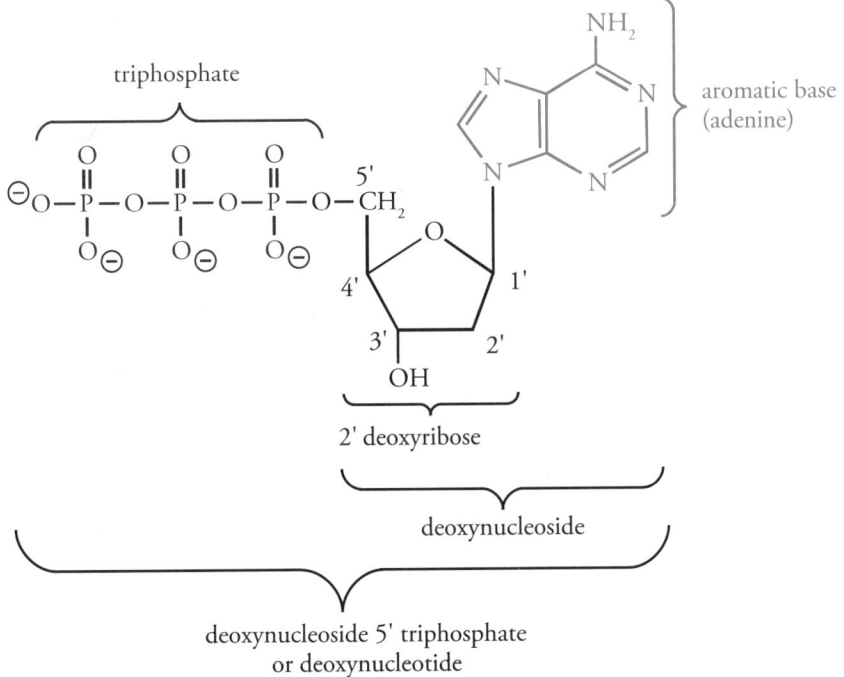

Figure 1 Deoxyadenosine Triphosphate (dATP)

---

[1] A mnemonic for this is Pyramids (pyrimidines) have sharp edges, so they CUT. Another mnemonic is CUT the Py.

The sugar + phosphate portion of the nucleotide is referred to as the **backbone** of DNA, because it is invariant. The base is the variable portion of the building block.

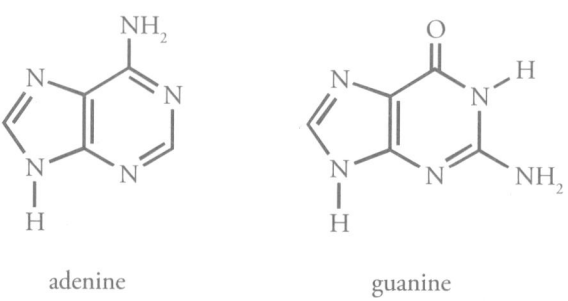

Figure 2 shows PYRIMIDINE BASES (cytosine, thymine (DNA only), uracil (RNA only)) and PURINE BASES (adenine, guanine).

Figure 2   Aromatic Bases of DNA and RNA

Polynucleotides

Nucleotides in the DNA chain are covalently linked by **phosphodiester bonds** between the 3' hydroxy group of one deoxyribose and the 5' phosphate group of the next deoxyribose (Figure 3). A polymer of several nucleotides linked together is termed an *oligo*nucleotide, and a polymer of many nucleotides is a *poly*nucleotide. Since the only unique part of the nucleotide is the base, the sequence of a polynucleotide can be abbreviated by simply listing the bases attached to each nucleotide in the chain. The end of the chain with a free 5' phosphate group is written first in a polynucleotide, with other nucleotides in the chain indicated in the 5' to 3' direction.

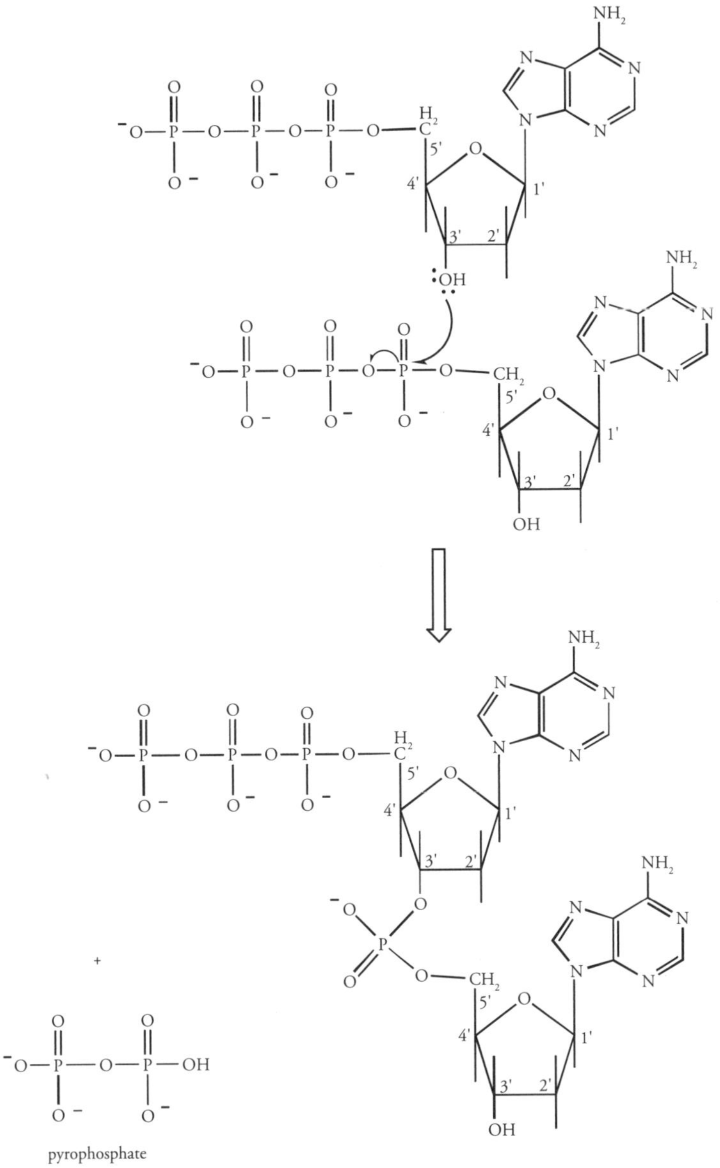

Figure 3 The Polymerization of Nucleotides

The Watson-Crick Model of DNA Structure

James Watson and Francis Crick (with the help of Maurice Wilkins and Rosalind Franklin) developed a model of the structure of DNA in the cell. According to the **Watson-Crick model**, cellular DNA is a right-handed double helix held together by hydrogen bonds between bases. It is important to understand each facet of this model.

In the cell, DNA does not exist in the form of a single long polynucleotide. Instead, the DNA found in the nucleus is double-stranded (**ds**). In ds-DNA, two very long polynucleotide chains are hydrogen-bonded together in an **antiparallel** orientation. Antiparallel means the 5' end of one chain is paired with the 3' end of the other. The H-bonds in ds-DNA are between the bases on adjacent chains. This H-bonding is very specific: A is always H-bonded to T, and G is always H-bonded to C (Figure 4). Note that this means an H-bonded pair always consists of a *purine plus a pyrimidine.*[2] Thus, both types of base pairs (AT or GC) take up the same amount of room in the DNA double helix. The GC pair is held together by three hydrogen bonds, the AT pair by two. Two chains of DNA are said to be complementary if the bases in each strand can hydrogen bond when the strands are oriented in an antiparallel fashion. If we are talking about ds-DNA 100 nucleotides long, we would say it is 100 base pairs (bp) long. A kbp (kilobase pair) is ds-DNA 1000 nucleotides long.

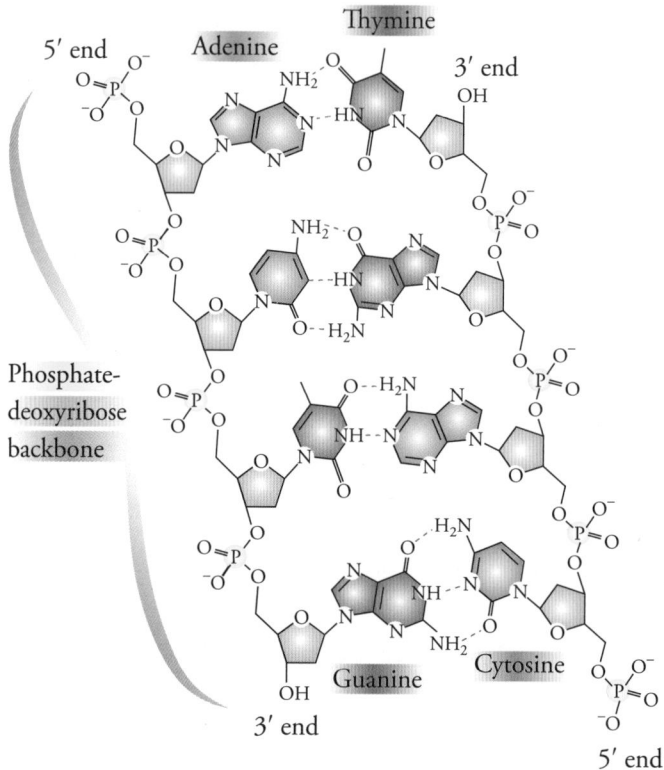

Figure 4   Base Pairing

The binding of two complementary strands of DNA into a double-stranded structure is termed **annealing**, or **hybridization**. The separation of strands is termed **melting**, or **denaturation**.

- Which of the following is/are true about ds-DNA?[3]
    I. If the amount of G in a double helix is known, the amount of C can be calculated.
    II. If the fraction of purine nucleotides and the total molecular weight of a double helix are known, the amount of cytosine can be calculated.
    III. The two chains in a piece of ds-DNA containing mostly purines will be bonded together more tightly than the two chains in a piece of ds-DNA containing mostly pyrimidines.
    IV. The oligonucleotide ATGTAT is complementary to the oligonucleotide ATACAT.

---

[2] This fact has a fringe benefit: we can calculate the number of purines if we know the number of pyrimidines. We can actually calculate several variables. Chargaff's Rule rule states that [A] = [T] and [G] = [C]; and [A] + [G] = [T] + [C].

[3] **Item I: True.** For every G, there is a C; and for every A there is a T. Item II: False. The ratio of purines to pyrimidines is always the same (50:50) since each purine is paired with a pyrimidine. In order to calculate the amount of any one base, you have to know the ratio of AT to GC pairs. Item III: False. Again, the ratio of purines to pyrimidines is always the same; 50:50. However, two chains containing mostly GC pairs will bond more tightly than two chains containing mostly AT pairs, since GC pairs are held together by 3 H-bonds while AT pairs have only 2. **Item IV: True.** Remember: the strands are antiparallel, A and T pair, G and C pair, and the 5' end is always written first.

There is another important detail about DNA structure: not only is it double-stranded, it is also *coiled*. In ds-DNA, the two hydrogen-bonded antiparallel DNA strands form a **right-handed double helix** (meaning it corkscrews in a clockwise motion) with the bases on the interior and the ribose/phosphate backbone on the exterior. The double helix is stabilized by van der Waals interactions between the bases, which are stacked upon each other.

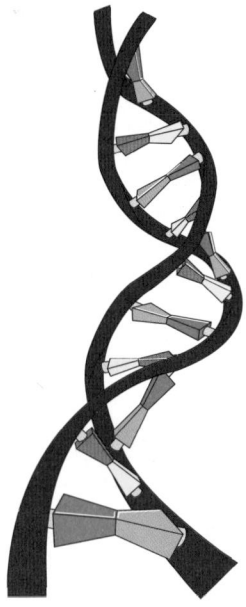

Figure 5   A Small Section of a DNA Double Helix

Chromosome Structure and Packing

The sum total of an organism's genetic information is called its **genome**. Eukaryotic genomes are composed of several large pieces of linear ds-DNA; each piece of ds-DNA is called a **chromosome**. Humans have 46 chromosomes, 23 of which are inherited from each parent. Prokaryotic (bacterial) genomes are composed of a **single circular chromosome**. Viral genomes may be linear or circular DNA or RNA. The human genome consists of over 10^9 base pairs, while bacterial genomes contain only 10^6 base pairs. But there is no direct correlation between genome size and evolutionary sophistication, since the organisms with the largest known genomes are amphibians. Much of the size difference in higher eukaryotic genomes is the result of repetitive DNA that has no known function.

If the DNA remained as a simple double helix floating free in the cell, it would be very bulky and fragile. Prokaryotes have a distinctive mechanism for making their single circular chromosome more compact and sturdy. An enzyme called **DNA gyrase** uses the energy of ATP to twist the gigantic circular molecule. Gyrase functions by breaking the DNA and twisting the two sides of the circle around each other. The resulting structure is a twisted circle that is composed of ds-DNA. As discussed earlier, the two strands are already coiled, forming a helix. The twists created by DNA gyrase are called **supercoils**, since they are coils of a structure that is already coiled.

Since eukaryotes have even more DNA in their genome than prokaryotes, the eukaryotic genome requires denser packaging to fit within the cell (Figure 6). To accomplish this, eukaryotic DNA is wrapped around globular proteins called **histones**. After being wrapped around histones, but before being completely packed away, DNA has the microscopic appearance of beads on a string. The beads are called **nucleosomes**; they are composed of DNA wrapped around an octamer of histones (a group of eight). The string between the beads is a length of double-helical DNA called linker DNA and is bound by a single linker histone. Fully packed DNA is called **chromatin**; it is composed of closely stacked nucleosomes.

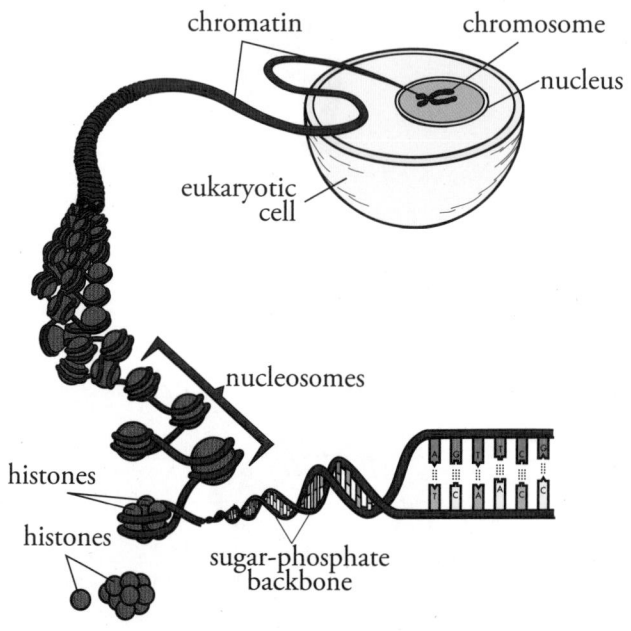

Figure 6   DNA Packaging

To look for patterns and morphology, chromosomes can be stained with chemicals. Usually, condensed metaphase chromosomes are used, as they are compact and easier to see. When chromosomes are treated, distinct light and dark regions become visible. The darker regions are denser and are called **heterochromatin**. Heterochromatin is rich in repeats; the lighter regions are less dense and are called **euchromatin**. Density gives a sense of DNA coiling or compactness, and these patterns are constant and heritable. It's now known that the lighter regions have higher transcription rates and therefore higher gene activity. The looser packing makes DNA accessible to enzymes and proteins.

Centromeres

A centromere is the region of the chromosome to which spindle fibers attach during cell division. The fibers attach via **kinetochores**, multiprotein complexes that act as anchor attachment sites for spindle fibers. Other protein complexes also bind the centromere after DNA replication to keep sister chromatids attached to each other. Centromeres are made of heterochromatin and repetitive DNA sequences. Chromosomes have p (short) and q (long) arms, and centromere position defines the ratio between the two (Figure 7).

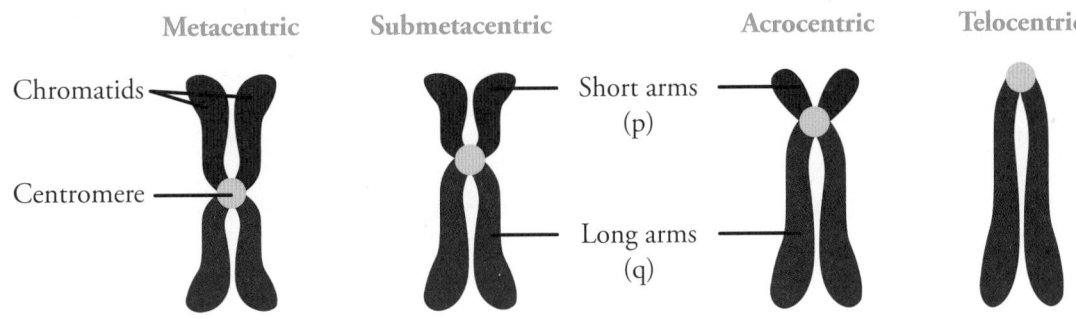

Figure 7   Centromere Positions

Telomeres

The ends of linear chromosomes are called **telomeres**. At the DNA level, these regions are distinguished by the presence of distinct nucleotide sequences repeated 50 to several hundred times. The repeated unit is usually 6–8 base pairs long and guanine-rich. Many vertebrates (including humans and mice) have the same repeat: 5'-TTAGGG-3'. Telomeres are composed of both single- and double-stranded DNA. Single stranded DNA is found at the very end of the chromosome and is about 300 base pairs in length. It loops around to form a knot, held together by many telomere-associated proteins. This stabilizes the end of the chromosome; specialized telomere cap proteins distinguish telomeres from double-stranded breaks (Section 4.4), and this prevents activation of repair pathways.

Telomeres function to prevent chromosome deterioration and also prevent fusion with neighboring chromosomes. They function as disposable buffers, blocking the ends of chromosomes. DNA replication of telomeres represents a special challenge to cellular machinery (see Section 4.4). Since most prokaryotes have circular genomes, their DNA does not contain telomeres.

4.2   GENOME STRUCTURE AND GENOMIC VARIATIONS

The human genome contains 24 different chromosomes (22 autosomes, plus two different sex chromosomes), 3.2 billion base pairs, and codes for about 21,000 genes. The sequence of the human genome was reported by two independent groups in 2001 (the publicly funded Human Genome Project lead by Dr. Francis Collins, and Dr. J. Craig Venter and his firm Celera Genomics).

The human genome has numerous regions with high transcription rates, separated by long stretches of intergenic space. **Intergenic regions** are composed of noncoding DNA; they may direct the assembly of specific chromatin structures and can contribute to the regulation of nearby genes, but many have no known function. Tandem repeats and transposons are major components of intergenic regions.

Genomic regions with high transcription rates are rich in genes. A gene is a DNA sequence that encodes a gene product. It includes both regulatory regions (such as promoters and transcription stop sites), and a region that codes for either a protein or a non-coding RNA.

Nucleotide Variation

Small-scale and large-scale variation across a genome is common. For example, one person could have the sequence CCCGGG, while another has CCTGGG. It's been predicted that there are single nucleotide changes once in every 1,000 base pairs in the human genome. These variations are called **single nucleotide polymorphisms** (SNPs, pronounced "snips") and are essentially mutations. [If the size of the human genome is just over 3 billion base pairs, approximately how many human SNPs are there?[4]] These SNPs occur most frequently in noncoding regions of the genome; however, some SNPs can lead to specific traits and phenotypes. For example, about 70% of people taste phenylthiocarbamide (PTC) as very bitter, and the remaining 30% don't taste PTC at all. You may have done this test yourself, as PTC response is commonly used as an example in genetics classes. This ability is a dominant genetic trait and is determined by a gene on chromosome 7. Three SNPs in this gene determine PTC taste sensitivity.

Copy-Number Variation

Copy-number variations (CNVs) are structural variations in the genome that lead to different copies of DNA sections. Large regions of the genome (10^3 to 10^6 base pairs) can be duplicated (increasing copy number) or deleted (decreasing copy number). The specific mechanism by which this occurs is not clear, but it may be due to misalignment of repetitive DNA sequences during synapsis of homologous chromosomes in meiosis. These changes therefore apply to much larger regions of the genome compared to SNPs. They are a normal part of our genome (0.4% of the genome can have CNV), but have also been associated with cancer and other diseases. Genes involved in immune system function, as well as brain development and activity, are often enriched in CNVs.

Repeated Sequences: Tandem Repeats

Much of our genome is single copy, meaning there is one copy of the gene in a haploid set of the genome. This is true for most eukaryotic genes that code for proteins. However, genomes also have regions of **tandem repeats**, where short sequences of nucleotides are repeated one right after the other, from as little as three to over 100 times. The human genome has over a thousand regions of tandem repeats. Repeats can be unstable, when the repeating unit is short (such as di- or trinucleotides) or when the repeat itself is very long. Unstable tandem repeats can lead to chromosome breaks and some have been implicated in disease. Tandem repeats often show variations in length between individuals, which can be useful in DNA fingerprinting. Heterochromatin, centromeres, and telomeres are all rich in repeats.

4.3 THE ROLE OF DNA

DNA encodes and transmits the genetic information passed down from parents to offspring. Before 1944 it was generally believed that protein, rather than DNA, carried genetic information, since proteins have an "alphabet" of 20 letters (the amino acids), while DNA's "alphabet" has only 4 letters (the four nucleotides). But in that year, Oswald Avery showed that DNA was the active agent in bacterial transformation. In short, this means he proved that pure DNA from one type of *E. coli* bacteria could transform *E. coli* of another type, causing it to acquire the genetic nature of the first type. Later Hershey and Chase proved that DNA was the active chemical in the infection of *E. coli* bacteria by bacteriophage T2.[5] These experiments will be discussed in more detail in Chapter 7.

---

[4] 3×10^9 base pairs × 1 SNP/1000 base pairs = 3×10^6 SNPs, or approximately 3 million human SNPs.

[5] Transformation and bacteriophage will be discussed in Chapter 5.

The Genetic Code

DNA does not directly exert its influence on cells, but merely contains sequences of nucleotides known as **genes** that serve as **templates** for the production of another nucleic acid known as RNA. The process of reading DNA and writing the information as RNA is termed **transcription**. This can generate either a final gene product (as in the case of all non-coding RNAs, discussed below), or a messenger molecule. The messenger RNA (mRNA) is then read, and the information is used to construct protein. The synthesis of proteins using RNA as a template is termed **translation** and is accomplished by the **ribosome**, which is a massive enzyme composed of many proteins and pieces of RNA (known as ribosomal RNA or rRNA).[6]

The overall process looks like this: DNA → RNA → protein. This unidirectional flow equation represents the **Central Dogma** (fundamental law) of molecular biology. This is the mechanism whereby inherited *information* is used to create actual *objects*, namely enzymes and structural proteins.

This language used by DNA and mRNA to specify the building blocks of proteins is known as the **Genetic Code**. The alphabet of the genetic code contains only four letters (A, T, G, C). How can four letters specify the ingredients of the multitude of proteins in every cell? [What is the smallest "word" size that would allow this four-letter alphabet to encode twenty different amino acids?[7]] A number of experiments confirmed that the genetic code is written in three-letter words, each of which codes for a particular amino acid. A nucleic acid word (3 nucleotide letters) is referred to as a **codon**.

The genetic code is represented in Figure 8, on the next page. The first nucleotide in a codon is given at the left, the second on top, and the third on the right. At the intersection of these three nucleotides is the amino acid called for by that codon. [Why is uracil (U) shown in the chart, and why is thymine (T) absent?[8] The codon GTG in DNA is transcribed in RNA as __, which the ribosome translates into what amino acid?[9]]

---

[6] To *transcribe* a letter is to listen to spoken words and write them down as printed text. The message doesn't change, and the language doesn't change. To *translate* a letter is to change it from one language to another. Cellular transcription is the process whereby a code is read from a nucleic acid (DNA) and written in the language of another nucleic acid (RNA), so the language is the same. In cellular translation, nucleic acids are read and polypeptides are written, so here the language does change.

[7] With four nucleotides, if a "word" (codon) is two nucleotides long, there are $4^2 = 16$ possible codons; too few to specify 20 unique amino acids. However, there are $4^3 = 64$ possible 3-letter "words," and 64 is more than enough different codons to specify 20 unique amino acids. Thus, three nucleotides is the minimum codon size.

[8] RNA is the nucleic acid that actually encodes protein during translation. RNA has U instead of T.

[9] The RNA codon transcribed from the DNA will be CAC, coding for histidine.

1st Position (5' End)	2nd Position				3rd Position (3' End)
	U	**C**	**A**	**G**	
U	Phe	Ser	Tyr	Cys	U
	Phe	Ser	Tyr	Cys	C
	Leu	Ser	**Stop**	**Stop**	A
	Leu	Ser	**Stop**	Trp	G
C	Leu	Pro	His	Arg	U
	Leu	Pro	His	Arg	C
	Leu	Pro	Gln	Arg	A
	Leu	Pro	Gln	Arg	G
A	Ile	Thr	Asn	Ser	U
	Ile	Thr	Asn	Ser	C
	Ile	Thr	Lys	Arg	A
	Met	Thr	Lys	Arg	G
G	Val	Ala	Asp	Gly	U
	Val	Ala	Asp	Gly	C
	Val	Ala	Glu	Gly	A
	Val	Ala	Glu	Gly	G

Figure 8   The Genetic Code

- The genetic code was studied by experimenters using a cell-free protein synthesis system. All of the materials necessary for protein synthesis (ribosomes, amino acids, tRNA, GTP, ATP) were purified and placed in a beaker. Then synthetic RNA was added, and protein was translated from this template. For example, when synthetic RNA containing only cytosine (CCCCC…) was added, polypeptides containing only proline (polyproline) resulted. What kind of synthetic RNA would give rise to a mixture of polyproline, polyhistidine, and polythreonine?[10]

There are 64 codons. Sixty-one of them specify amino acids; the remaining three are called **stop codons**. Their function is to notify the ribosome that the protein is complete and cause it to stop reading the mRNA (see Section 4.5). Stop codons are also called **nonsense codons**, since they don't code for any amino acid. Note that most of the twenty amino acids can be coded for by more than one codon. Often, all four of the codons with the same first two nucleotides (e.g., CU_) encode the same amino acid. [If the last nucleotide in the codon CUU is changed in a gene that codes for a protein, will the protein be affected?[11]] Two or more codons coding for the same amino acid are known as **synonyms**. Because it has such synonyms, the genetic code is said to be **degenerate**. However, it is very important to realize that though an amino acid may be specified by several codons, *each codon specifies only a single amino acid*. This means that each piece of DNA can be interpreted only one way: the code has no **ambiguity**.

---

[10] The RNA would have to be CCACCACCACCACCACCACCAC…. This would yield polyproline if read as CCA, CCA, CCA. But if it were read as CAC, CAC, CAC, it would give rise to polyhistidine. If it were read ACC, ACC, ACC, it would encode polythreonine.

[11] No, since CUN codes for leucine, regardless of what N is. Notice that switching the third nucleotide in the majority of codons will have no effect.

The code in Figure 8 is the standard genetic code and is used by most organisms. However, some protists use an alternate genetic code, and the mitochondrial genome of many organisms (including humans and many other vertebrates) uses a slightly different code.

Beyond the Central Dogma

There are several aspects of molecular biology that aren't explicitly stated in the Central Dogma.

- Some viruses (retroviruses) make DNA from RNA using the enzyme reverse transcriptase.
- Information can also be transferred in other ways. For example, DNA methylation and post-translational modification of proteins can alter gene expression and convey information, despite the fact that neither is directly included in the Central Dogma.
- Many final gene products are not proteins but are RNAs instead.

4.4 DNA REPLICATION

The DNA genome is the control center of the cell. When mitosis produces two identical daughter cells from one parental cell, each daughter must have the same genome as the parent. Therefore, cell division requires duplication of the DNA, known as **replication**. This is an enzymatic process, just as the Krebs cycle and glycolysis are enzymatic processes. It occurs during **S** (synthesis) **phase** in interphase of the cell cycle (Chapter 6). Let's go through the process of replication, stopping to add essential facts to a list of things to memorize. But before we get bogged down with details, we should have a look at the big picture.

There is only one logical way to make a new piece of DNA that is identical to the old one: copy it. The old DNA is called **parental** DNA, and the new is called **daughter** DNA. What is the relationship between parental and daughter DNA after replication? There are several possibilities (Figure 9 on the next page). In other words, where do the atoms from the parent go when the daughters are made?

Experiments done by Meselson and Stahl in 1958 aimed to determine if DNA replication is semiconservative, conservative, or dispersive (Figure 9 on the next page). In *conservative* replication, the parental ds-DNA would remain as-is while an entirely new double-stranded genome was created. The *dispersive* theory said that both copies of the genomes were composed of scattered pieces of new and old DNA. Meselson and Stahl showed that replication is semiconservative; after replication, one strand of the new double helix is parental (old) and one strand is newly synthesized daughter DNA.

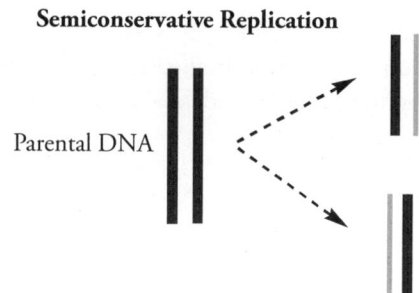

Semiconservative Replication

Parental DNA

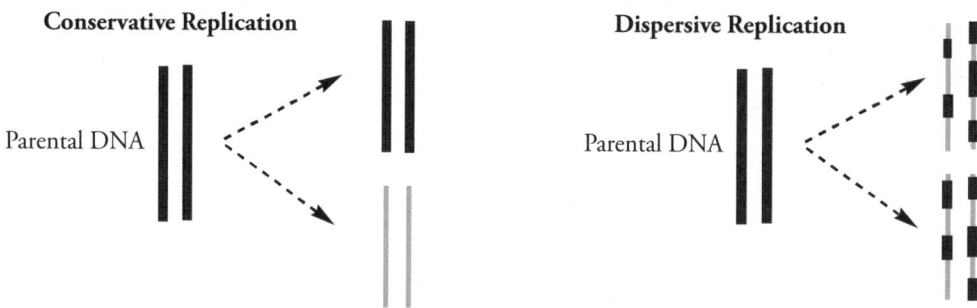

Conservative Replication

Parental DNA

Dispersive Replication

Parental DNA

Figure 9   Meselson-Stahl Experiments

Let's begin the list of things to memorize here:

1) **DNA replication is semiconservative.**
   Individual strands of the double-stranded parent are pulled apart, and then a new daughter strand is synthesized using the parental DNA as a template to copy from.[12] Each new daughter chain is perfectly __[13] to its template or parent.

Now we'll look at replication at the molecular level. When it is not being replicated, DNA is tightly coiled. The replication process cannot begin unless the double helix is uncoiled and separated into two single strands. The enzyme that unwinds the double helix and separates the strands is called helicase. [Would you expect helicase to use the energy of ATP hydrolysis to do its job?[14]] The place where the helicase begins to unwind is not random. It is a specific location (sequence of nucleotides) on the chromosome called the **origin of replication** (abbreviated ORI). This sequence is found by proteins with tertiary structures to specifically recognize a particular pattern of nucleotides. They scan along the chromosome (like a train on a track) until they find the right spot; then they call in helicase and other enzymes to initiate DNA replication. In prokaryotes, a protein called DnaA finds the ORI to initiate DNA replication. In eukaryotes, three proteins cooperate to find the ORI, two of which are synthesized during M and G_1 phases of the cell cycle (see Chapter 6) but rapidly destroyed once the S phase begins. This means these two proteins link DNA replication to the cell cycle, ensuring DNA replication doesn't initiate during other phases of the cell cycle.

---

[12] A template is something that is copied. The metal plates used in printing presses are an example.

[13] complementary

[14] Yes. Separating the strands requires the breaking of many H-bonds.

When helicase unwinds the helix at the origin of replication, the helix gets wound more tightly upstream and downstream from this point.[15] The chromosome would get tangled and eventually break, except that enzymes called **topoisomerases** cut one or both of the strands and unwrap the helix, releasing the excess tension created by the helicases. Another potential problem is that single-stranded DNA is much less stable than ds-DNA. **Single-strand binding proteins (SSBPs)** protect DNA that has been unpackaged in preparation for replication and help keep the strands separated. The separated strands are referred to as an **open complex**. Replication may now begin.

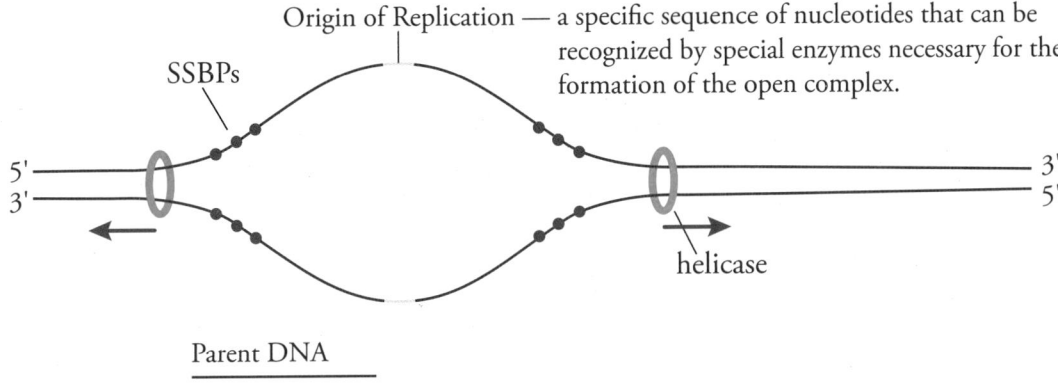

Figure 10 Initiation—The Open Complex

An RNA primer must be synthesized for each template strand. This is accomplished by a set of proteins called the primosome, of which the central component is an RNA polymerase called **primase**. Primer synthesis is important because the next enzyme, DNA polymerase, cannot start a new DNA chain from scratch. It can only add nucleotides to an existing nucleotide chain. The RNA primer is usually 8–12 nucleotides long, and is later replaced by DNA.

Daughter DNA is created as a growing polymer. **DNA polymerase** (DNA pol) catalyzes the elongation of the daughter strand using the parental template, and elongates the primer by adding dNTPs to its 3' end. In fact, the 3' hydroxyl group acts as a nucleophile in the polymerization reaction to displace 5' pyrophosphate from the dNTP to be added. [The template strand is read in what direction?[16]] DNA pol is part of a large complex of proteins called the replisome. Other accessory proteins in this complex help DNA polymerase and allow it to polymerize DNA quickly. The prokaryotic replisome contains 13 components, and the eukaryotic replisome contains 27 proteins; additional complexity in the eukaryotic system is required because replication machinery must also unwind DNA from histone proteins.

Rapid elongation of the daughter strands follows. Since the two template strands are antiparallel, the two primers will elongate toward opposite ends of the chromosome. After a while it looks like this:

---

[15] Imagine two long ropes wound around each other. What happens if you pull them apart in the middle?

[16] If the daughter is made 5' to 3', and the two strands have to end up antiparallel, the template must be read 3' to 5'.

4.4

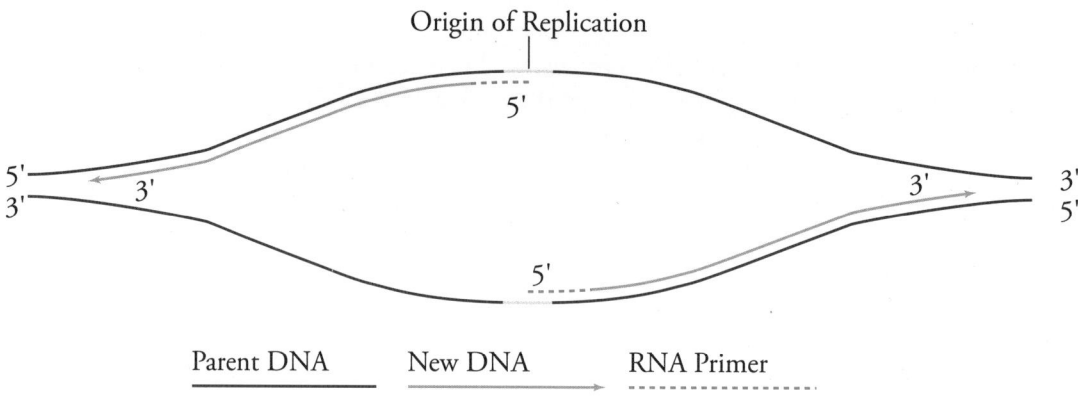

Figure 11   Elongation

DNA polymerase checks each new nucleotide to make sure it forms a correct base-pair before it is incorporated in the growing polymer. The thermodynamic driving force for the polymerization reaction is the removal and hydrolysis of pyrophosphate ($P_2O_7^{4-}$) from each dNTP added to the chain. Here are some more replication rules to memorize:

2) **Polymerization occurs in the 5' to 3' direction, without exception.** This means the existing chain is always lengthened by the addition of a nucleotide to the 3' end of the chain. There is never 3' to 5' polymerase activity.

3) **DNA pol requires a *template*.** It cannot make a DNA chain from scratch but must copy an old chain. This makes sense because it would be pretty useless if DNA pol just made a strand of DNA randomly, without copying a template.

4) **DNA pol requires a *primer*.** It cannot start a new nucleotide chain.

• Can DNA polymerase make the following partially double-stranded structure completely double stranded in the presence of excess nucleotides, using the top strand as a primer?[17]

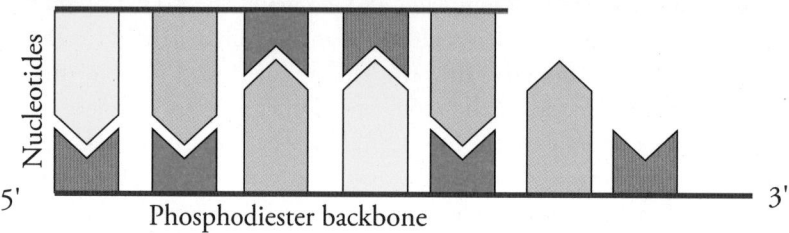

---

[17] No. The DNA strands are antiparallel, meaning that the upper strand would have to be extended in a 3' to 5' direction, which is impossible. Note that the phrase "in the presence of excess nucleotides" is extraneous. It just means there are plenty of building blocks around. Typical MCAT smokescreen.

Replication proceeds along in both directions away from the origin of replication. Both template strands are read 3' to 5' while daughter strands are elongated 5' to 3'. The areas where the parental double helix continues to unwind are called the **replication forks.** Let's split Figure 11 and look at an enlargement of the right side:

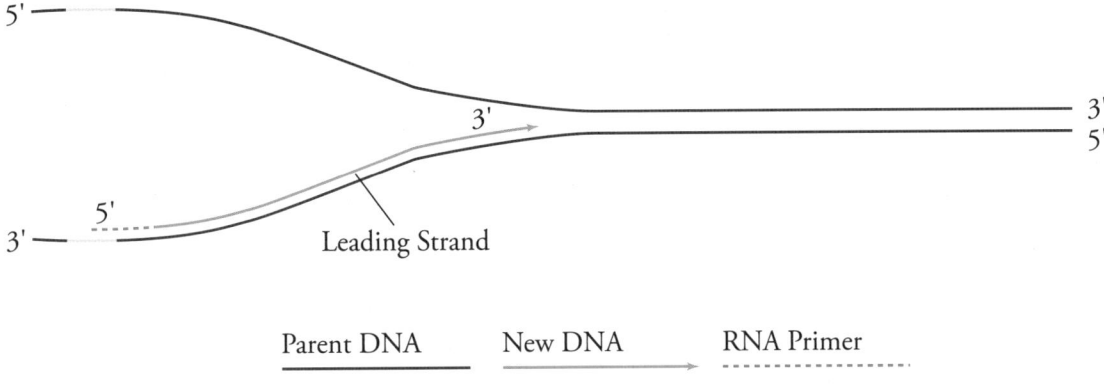

Figure 12   Leading Strand

See how it looks like a big fork? In examining these pictures, you have probably become aware of a problem. It seems like only half of each template strand will be replicated (in Figure 12, the right half of the bottom strand and the left half of the top strand). The problem is that chain elongation can only proceed in one direction, 5' to 3', but in order to replicate the right half of the top chain and the left half of the bottom one continuously, we would have to go in the opposite direction. Here's the solution:

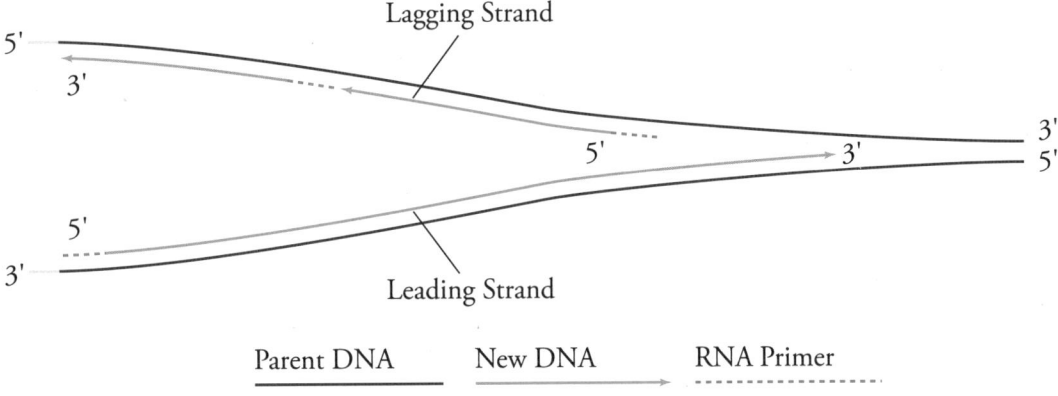

Figure 13   Leading and Lagging Strands

The solution to this problem involves building strands of DNA on opposite sides of the ORI using different methods. As the bottom chain on the right is elongated continuously, the replication fork widens. After a good bit of the top template chain becomes exposed, primase comes in and lays down a primer, which DNA pol can elongate. Then, when the replication fork widens again and more of the top template becomes exposed, these events are repeated. The bottom daughter on the right side, and the top daughter on the left side are called the **leading strands** because they elongate continuously right into the widening replication fork. The top daughter on the right, and the bottom daughter on the left are called the **lagging strands** because they must wait until the replication fork widens before beginning to polymerize.

The small chunks of DNA comprising the lagging strand are called **Okazaki fragments**, after their discoverer. [As the replication forks grow, does helicase have to continue to unwind the double helix and separate the strands?[18]] Let's continue our memorization list:

5) **Replication forks grow away from the origin in both directions.** Each replication fork contains a **leading strand** and a **lagging strand**.

6) Replication of the leading strand is **continuous** and leads into the replication fork, while replication of the lagging strand is **discontinuous**, resulting in Okazaki fragments.

7) Eventually **all RNA primers are replaced by DNA**, and the **fragments are joined by an enzyme called DNA ligase.**

DNA Polymerase

DNA polymerase can rapidly build DNA and is able to add tens of thousands of nucleotides before falling off the template. It is therefore said to be *processive.*

Eukaryotes have several different DNA polymerase enzymes, and their mechanisms of action are complex. You do not need to worry about this complexity.

Prokaryotes, on the other hand, have five types of DNA polymerases, called DNA polymerase I, II, III, IV, and V. You should definitely know the functions of DNA pol III and DNA pol I:

1) **DNA pol III** is responsible for the super-fast, super-accurate elongation of the leading strand. In other words, it has high processivity. It has 5' to 3' polymerase activity as well as 3' to 5' exonuclease[19] activity. This is when the enzyme moves backward to chop off the nucleotide it just added if it was incorrect; the ability to correct mistakes in this way is known as **proofreading function**. It has no known function in repair, and so is considered a replicative enzyme.

2) **DNA pol I** starts adding nucleotides at the RNA primer; this is 5' to 3' polymerase activity. Because of its poor processivity (it can only add 15-20 nucleotides per second), DNA pol III usually takes over about 400 base pairs downstream from the ORI. DNA pol I is also capable of 3' to 5' exonuclease activity (proofreading). DNA pol I removes the RNA primer via 5' to 3' exonuclease activity, while simultaneously leaving behind new DNA in __[20] activity. Finally, DNA pol I is important for excision repair.

The functions of DNA pol II, IV, and V are less important to know for the MCAT:

3) DNA pol II has 5' to 3' polymerase activity, and 3' to 5' exonuclease proofreading function. It participates in DNA repair pathways and is used as a backup for DNA pol III.

4) DNA pol IV and DNA pol V have similar characteristics. They are error prone in 5' to 3' polymerase activity, but function to stall other polymerase enzymes at replication forks when DNA repair pathways have been activated. This is an important part of the prokaryotic checkpoint pathway.

---

[18] Yes.

[19] **Exonuclease** means "cutting a nucleic acid chain at the end." An **endonuclease** will cut a polynucleotide acid chain in the middle of the chain, usually at a particular sequence. Two important types of endonucleases are: **repair enzymes** that remove chemically damaged DNA from the chain, and **restriction enzymes**, which are endonucleases found in bacteria. Their role is to destroy the DNA of infecting viruses, thus restricting the host range of the virus.

[20] 5' to 3' polymerase; remember, all polymerization is 5' to 3'.

If a bacterium possesses a mutation in the gene for DNA polymerase III, resulting in an enzyme without the 3' to 5' exonuclease activity, will mutations occur more often than in bacteria with a normal DNA polymerase gene?[21]

Prokaryotic vs. Eukaryotic Replication

Prokaryotes have only one chromosome, and this one chromosome has only one origin. Because the chromosome is circular, as replication proceeds the partially duplicated genome begins to look like the Greek letter θ (theta). Hence the replication of prokaryotes is said to proceed by the **theta mechanism** and is referred to as **theta replication** (see Figure 14).

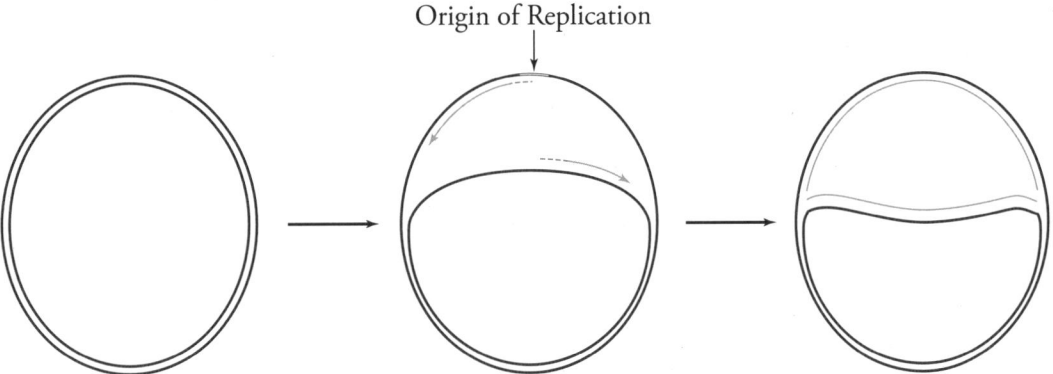

Figure 14   Theta (θ) Replication

In eukaryotic replication, each chromosome has several origins. This is necessary because eukaryotic chromosomes are so huge that replicating them from a single origin would be too slow. As the many replication forks continue to widen, they create an appearance of bubbles along the DNA strand, so they are referred to as "replication bubbles." Eventually the replication forks meet, and the many daughter strands are ligated together.

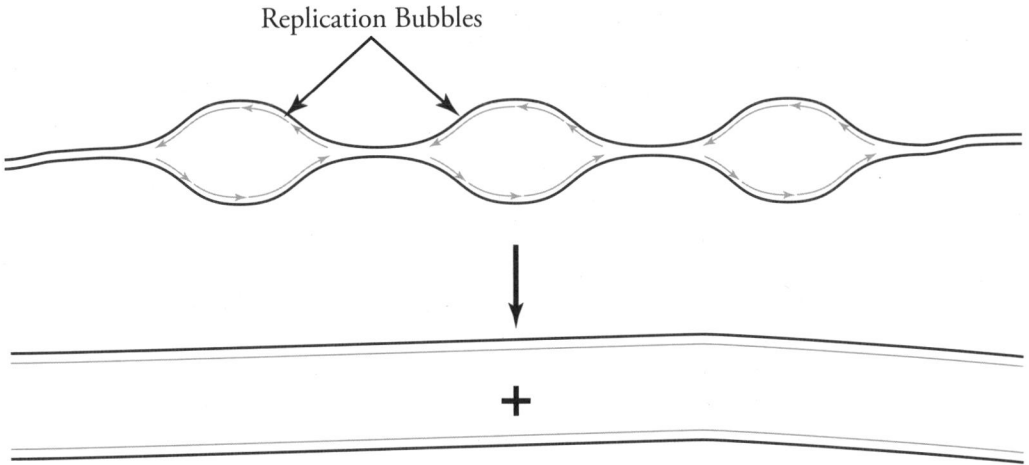

Figure 15   Eukaryotic Replication

---

[21] Yes. The 3' to 5' exonuclease activity is the polymerase's way of editing its work. Without this editing function, many more point mutations would occur due to the incorporation of wrong nucleotides. The normal polymerase is remarkably adept at sensing correct base pairing and removing bases that don't belong.

Replicating Telomeres in Eukaryotes

DNA polymerase can only build DNA in one direction (5' to 3'), and it requires both a template and a primer. These requirements lead to a roadblock at chromosome ends. Eventually there will be no place on the lagging strand to lay down a primer, and primers close to the end of DNA cannot be replaced with DNA because there is nothing on the other side (DNA polymerase usually uses a previous length of upstream DNA to replace the primer, but this isn't available at the end of a chromosome). This means that DNA replication machinery is unable to replicate sequences at the very ends of chromosomes, and after each round of the cell cycle and DNA replication, the ends of chromosomes shorten. **Telomeres** are disposable repeats at the end of chromosomes. They are consumed and shorten during cell division, becoming between 50 and 200 base pairs shorter.

When telomeres become *too* short, they reach a critical length where the chromosome can no longer replicate. As a consequence, cells can activate DNA repair pathways, enter a senescent state (where they are alive but not dividing), or activate apoptosis (pre-programmed cell death). The *Hayflick limit* is the number of times a normal human cell type can divide until telomere length stops cell division. Many age-related diseases are linked to telomere shortening.

Telomerase is an enzyme that adds repetitive nucleotide sequences to the ends of chromosomes and therefore lengthens telomeres. Telomerase is a ribonucleoprotein complex, containing an RNA primer and reverse transcriptase enzyme. Reverse transcriptases read RNA templates and generate DNA. In humans, the RNA template is 3' CCCAAUCCC 5', and this allows for chromosome extension, one DNA repeat (5'-TTAGGG-3') at a time (Figure 16). The telomerase complex continuously polymerizes, then translocates, allowing extension of six-nucleotide telomere repeats.

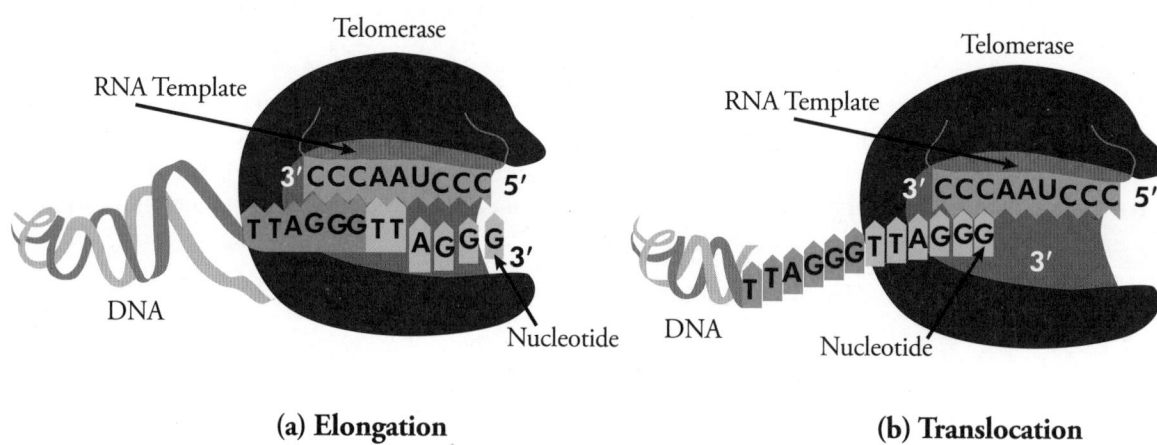

(a) Elongation　　　　　　　　　　**(b) Translocation**

Figure 16　Telomerase and Telomere Lengthening

In most organisms, telomerase is only expressed in the germ line, embryonic stem cells, and some white blood cells. However, cancer cells can also express telomerase, which can help the cells immortalize. Telomere extension allows the cells to bypass senescence and apoptosis, and can therefore contribute to their transformation to a pre-cancerous state.

4.5 GENETIC MUTATION

Genetic mutation refers to any alteration of the DNA sequence of an organism's genome. These can be inherited or acquired throughout life. Mutations that can be passed onto offspring are called germline mutations, since they occur in the germ cells (which give rise to gametes). Somatic mutations occur in somatic (non-gametic) cells and are not passed onto offspring. In other words, somatic mutations can have a major effect on an individual, but will not be passed on to future individuals in that population. Our cells have evolved elaborate repair pathways to help deal with mutations, and these will be discussed in the next section.

Causes of Mutation

There are many causes of mutation. Most are induced by an environmental or chemical factor; however, they can also occur spontaneously.

Physical Mutagens

Ionizing radiation (such as X-rays, alpha particles, and gamma rays) can cause DNA breaks. If these only occur on one strand (Figure 17, left), they can be easily patched up because the DNA helix is still held together in one piece. However, if both backbones are broken close to each other on a segment of DNA, a double-strand break (DSB) occurs (Figure 17, right). Here, the chromosome has been split into two pieces and it's much more difficult to piece them back together.

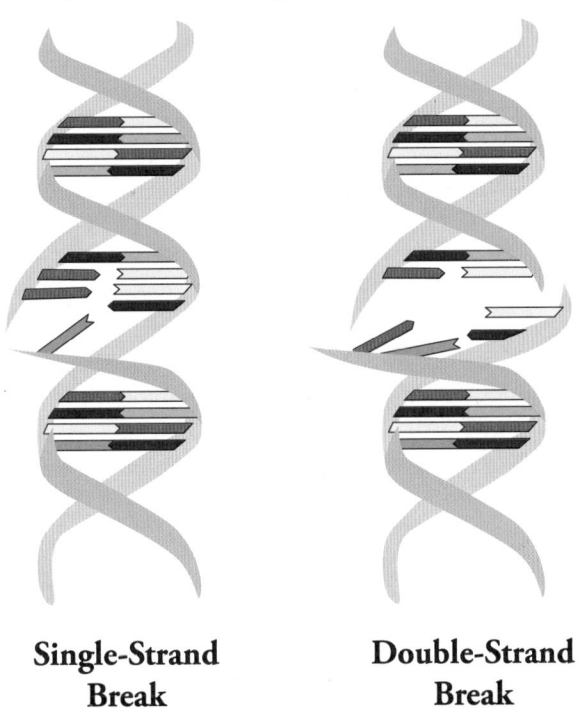

**Single-Strand
Break**

**Double-Strand
Break**

Figure 17   Single- and Double-Strand Breaks in DNA

UV light causes photochemical damage to DNA. For example, if two pyrimidines (two Cs or two Ts) are beside each other on a DNA backbone, UV light can cause them to become covalently linked. These pyrimidine dimers distort the DNA backbone (Figure 18) and can cause mutations during DNA replication if they are not repaired.

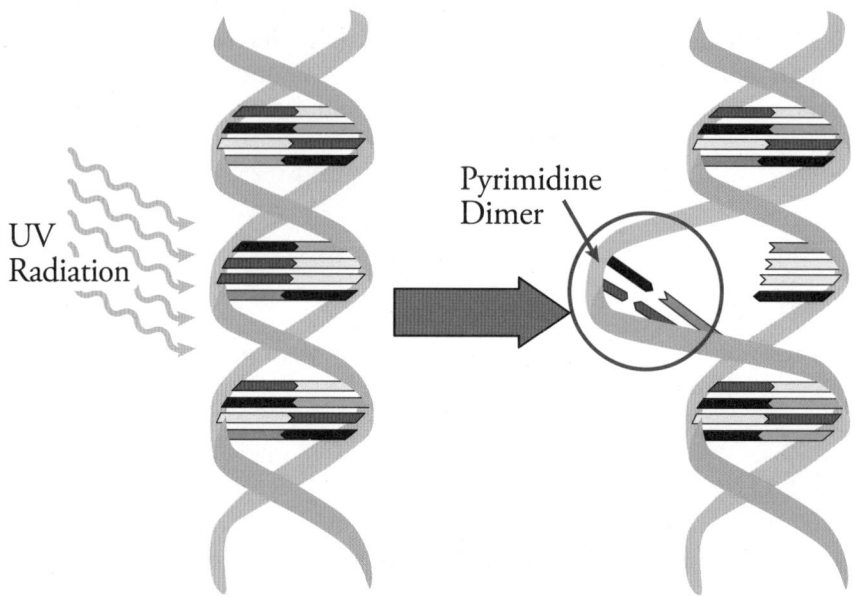

Figure 18   Pyrimidine Dimers in the DNA Helix

Reactive Chemicals

Many chemicals interact directly with DNA, and many others turn into damaging agents as they're being processed by a cell. Chemicals can covalently alter bases or can cause cross-linking or strand breaks. Cross-links are abnormal covalent bonds between different parts of DNA. Any compound that can cause mutations is called a **mutagen**.

Compounds that look like purines and pyrimidines (with large flat aromatic ring structures) cause mutations by inserting themselves between base pairs, or *intercalating*, thereby causing errors in DNA replication. Ethidium bromide is often used to visualize nucleic acids during gel electrophoresis in molecular biology labs. This chemical is used because it is planar (and therefore intercalates with the DNA ladder), and glows orange when exposed to UV light (meaning nucleic acids in a gel can be easily visualized). However, because it intercalates with DNA, is also distorts the structure and can therefore disrupt DNA replication and transcription. Thus, ethidium bromide is a mutagen.

Biological Agents

Biological agents can also cause mutations. For example, although DNA polymerase has proofreading and correction abilities, it can still make a mistake. An incorrect base pair may be repaired (see Section 4.6), but if not, it will be passed on to all daughter cells. In this case, there is no mutagen. The mistake is spontaneous. Viruses can also affect DNA. Lysogenic viruses insert into the genome of the host cell (see Chapter 5), and this can cause mutations and disrupt genetic function. Some viruses can cause cancer because of this function. And finally, transposons can induce mutations. This will be described in the next section.

Types of Mutations

Based on structure, there are seven kinds of mutations:

1) Point mutations
2) Insertions
3) Deletions
4) Inversions
5) Amplifications
6) Translocations and rearrangements
7) Loss of heterozygosity

Point mutations are single base pair substitutions (A in place of G, for example). Point mutations can be *transitions* (substitution of a pyrimidine for another pyrimidine or substitution of a purine for another purine) or *transversions* (substitution of a purine for a pyrimidine or vice versa). There are three types of point mutations:

1) **Missense mutation**: This causes one amino acid to be replaced with a different amino acid. This may not be serious if the amino acids are similar. [How can this occur?[22]]
2) **Nonsense mutation**: A stop codon replaces a regular codon and prematurely shortens the protein.
3) **Silent mutation**: A codon is changed into a new codon for the same amino acid, so there is no change in the protein's amino acid sequence.

Insertion refers to the addition of one or more extra nucleotides into the DNA sequence, and deletion is the removal of nucleotides from the sequence. Both of these mutations can cause a shift in the reading frame. For example, AAACCCACC is read as AAA, CCC, ACC. It would code for Lys-Pro-Thr. Inserting an extra G into the first codon could produce this: AGAACCCACC. This would be read AGA, ACC, CAC, C. It now codes for Arg-Thr-His (plus there's an extra C). Not only has the first codon and amino acid changed, the whole gene will be read differently and all amino acids in the protein from that point on will change. Mutations that cause a change in the reading frame are called **frameshift mutations**. Generally speaking, frameshift mutations are very serious. Note that a frameshift can lead to premature termination of translation (yielding an incomplete polypeptide) if it results in the presence of an abnormal stop codon. [Are all insertions and deletions frameshift mutations?[23] If the following oligonucleotide is mutated by inserting a G between the fifth and sixth codons, what effect will this have on the oligopeptide it encodes: AUG AAG GGG CCC UUU AAA UGA CCC?[24] For each type of mutation, does it involve a change in the genotype, the phenotype, or both?[25]]

---

[22] For example, substituting a small hydrophobe such as valine for another small hydrophobe like leucine will probably cause little disruption of protein structure. Another way of defining conservative mutations is that they cause changes in primary structure but do not affect secondary, tertiary, or quaternary structure.

[23] No. If you insert or delete one whole codon or several whole codons, you add or remove amino acids to the polypeptide without changing the reading frame.

[24] The original RNA codes for Met-Lys-Gly-Pro-Phe-Lys. After the insertion, the oligonucleotide will code for Met-Lys-Gly-Pro-Phe-Glu-Met-Thr. Note that this contains different amino acids and it's longer. The extra length is due to the fact that a stop codon, UGA, changed by the frameshift.

[25] By definition, all mutations involve a change in the genotype. Most mutations also cause a change in the phenotype, but in the case of conservative mutations, it is a very subtle change that would be hard to detect.

In addition to mutations at individual nucleotides, larger-scale mutations are also common. Insertions and deletions can involve thousands of bases. An **inversion** is when a segment of a chromosome is reversed end-to-end. The chromosome undergoes breakage and rearrangement within itself (Figure 19). Insertions, deletions, and inversions can be caused by transposons (see below).

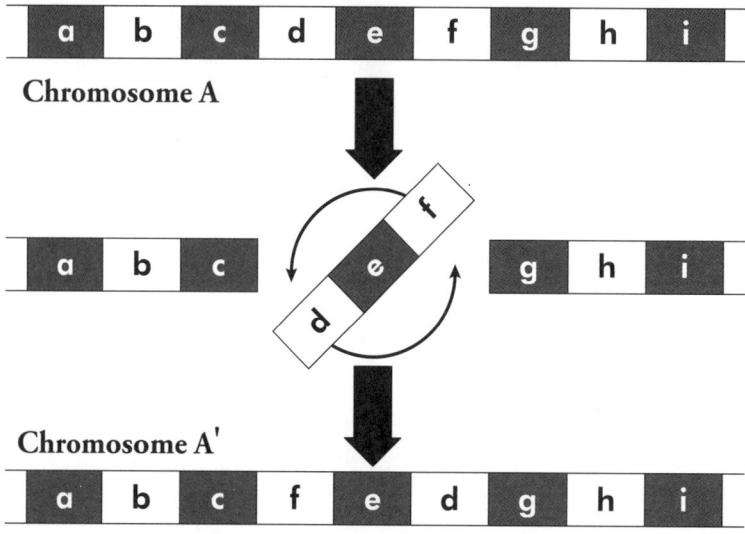

Figure 19   Chromosome Inversion

Chromosome amplification is when a segment of a chromosome is duplicated. **Translocations** result when recombination occurs between nonhomologous chromosomes (Figure 20). This can create a gene fusion, where a new gene product is made from parts of two genes that were not previously connected. This is a common occurrence in many types of cancer. Translocations can be balanced (where no genetic information is lost), or unbalanced (where genetic information is lost or gained).

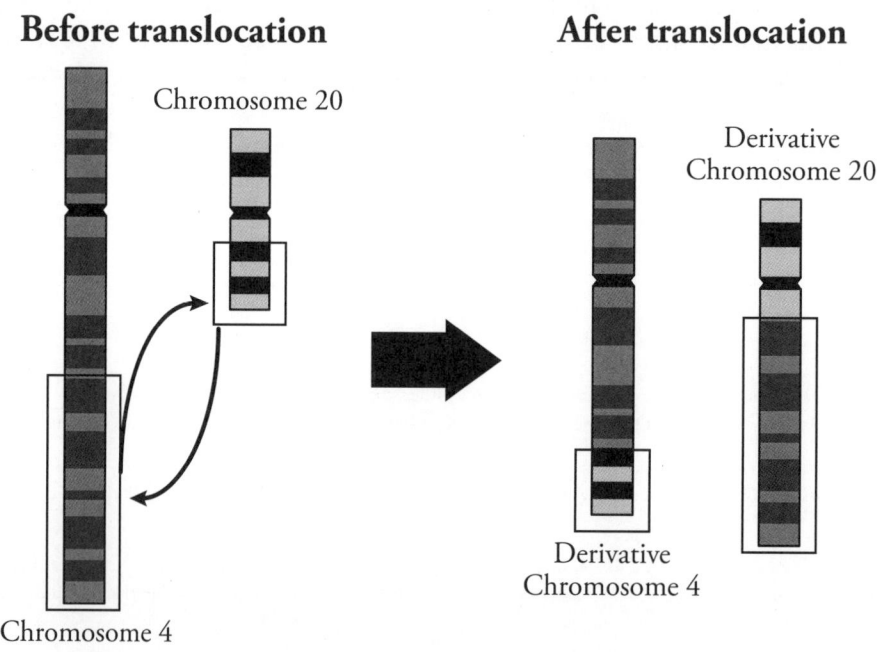

Figure 20   Chromosome Translocation

Transposons

Both prokaryotes and eukaryotes have mobile genetic elements in their genomes, called transposable elements or **transposons**. It is thought that many eukaryotic transposons are degenerate (old and defective) retroviruses. "Genetic mobility" means that these short segments can jump around the genome. Transposons can cause mutations and chromosome changes such as inversions, deletions, and rearrangements.

There are three common types of transposons, each with a different structure. The first type is the simplest and is called an IS element (Figure 21, top). It is composed of a transposase gene (discussed below), flanked by inverted repeat sequences. The structure of an example inverted repeat is shown in Figure 22. Some transposons are more complex, in that they also contain additional genes (Figure 21, middle). For example, some transposons contain genes for antibiotic resistance. Finally, composite transposons have two similar or identical IS elements with a central region in between (Figure 21, bottom).

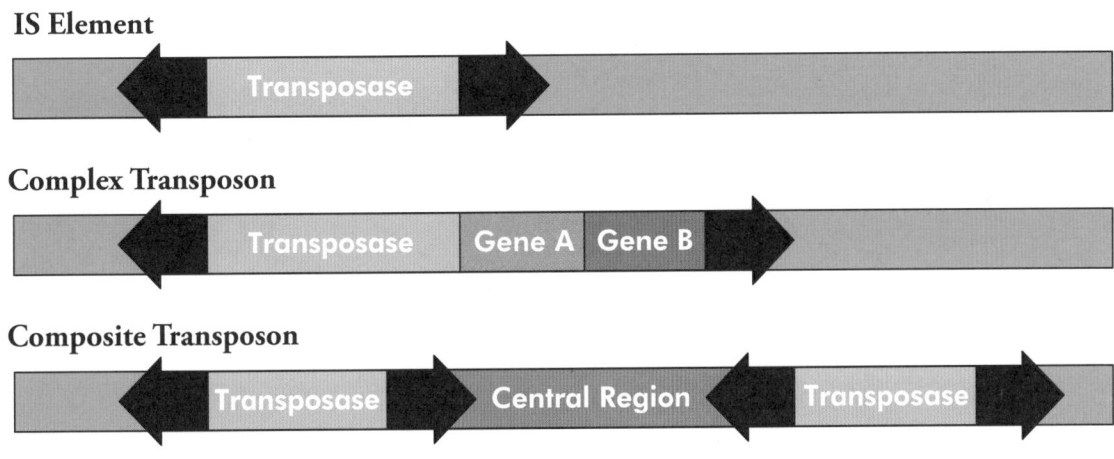

Figure 21   Transposon Structure

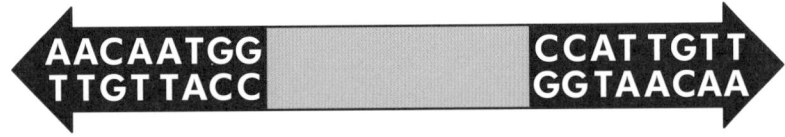

Figure 22   Inverted Repeats

All transposons contain a gene that codes for a protein called **transposase**. This enzyme has "cut and paste" activity, where it catalyzes mobilization of the transposon (excision from the donor site) and integration into a new genetic location (the acceptor site). Sometimes the transposon sequence is completely excised and moved, and sometimes it is duplicated and moved while still maintained at the original location (Figure 23, next page). The inverted repeats are important for this mobilization.

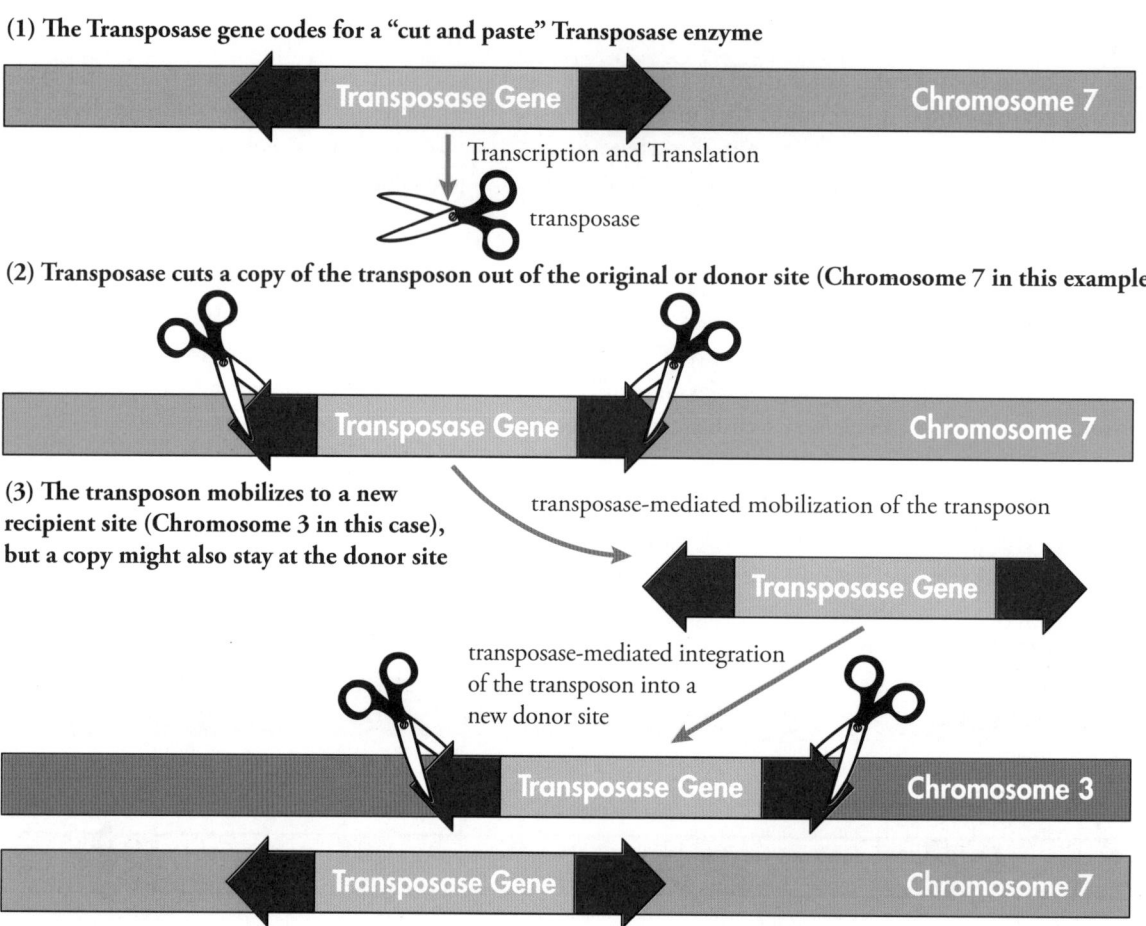

(1) The Transposase gene codes for a "cut and paste" Transposase enzyme

Transposase Gene   Chromosome 7

Transcription and Translation

transposase

(2) Transposase cuts a copy of the transposon out of the original or donor site (Chromosome 7 in this example)

Transposase Gene   Chromosome 7

(3) The transposon mobilizes to a new recipient site (Chromosome 3 in this case), but a copy might also stay at the donor site

transposase-mediated mobilization of the transposon

Transposase Gene

transposase-mediated integration of the transposon into a new donor site

Transposase Gene   Chromosome 3

Transposase Gene   Chromosome 7

Figure 23   The Mechanism of Transposon Mobilization

Many mobilizations have no effect because the transposon inserts into a relatively unimportant part of the genome. However, transposons can cause mutations if they jump into an important part of the genome.

When transposons are mobilized, they can insert in any part of the genome, and this can affect gene expression or cause mutations. They can jump into a promoter and turn gene expression off. They can jump into a protein-coding region and disrupt (or mutate) the sequence. They can also jump into regulatory parts of the genome and ramp up gene expression at a nearby site.

In addition to jumping around the genome, transposons can cause structural changes to chromosomes when they work in pairs. Directionality of the transposon is important here, as it determines what happens to the chromosome. If a chromosome has two transposons with the same direction (Figure 24), the transposons can line up beside each other, so they are parallel. This causes the chromosomal segment between them to loop around. Recombination occurs between the transposons, and this causes deletion of the DNA between the two transposons. The original chromosome therefore completely loses the DNA segment between the transposons (a deletion). The segment of DNA that is lost takes one transposon with it, meaning it can actually jump back into the genome somewhere else, causing chromosome rearrangement: one chunk of a chromosome has moved to a new location in the genome.

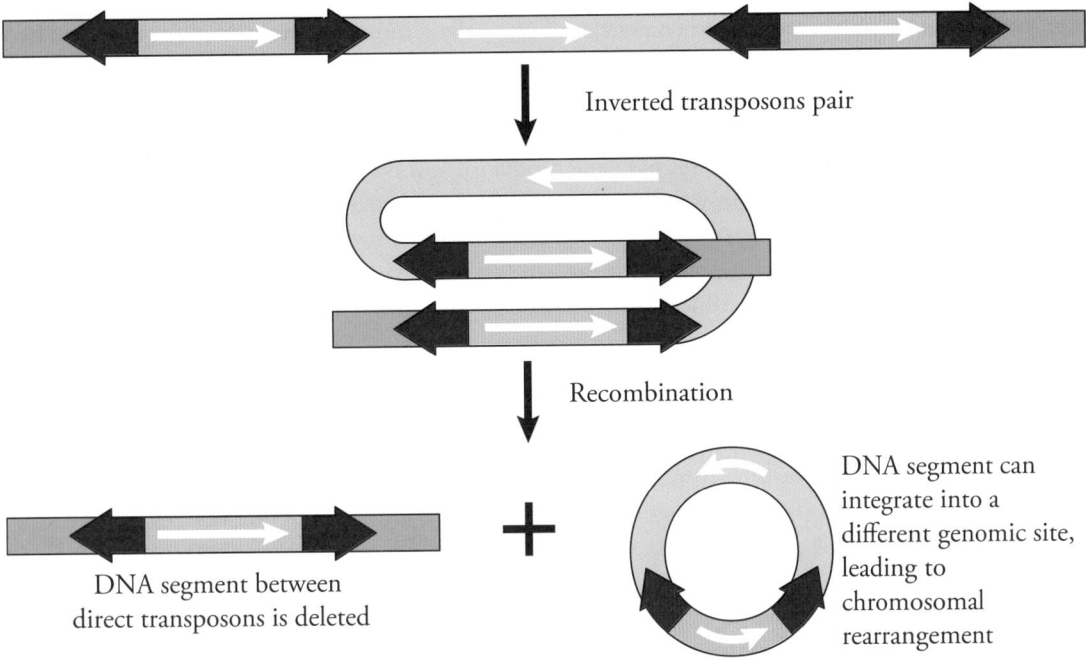

Figure 24   Deletion and Chromosomal Rearrangements via Transposons

If a chromosome has two transposons with inverted orientations (Figure 25), they can again pair and align with each other. After recombination, the sequence of DNA between the two transposons ends up inverted.

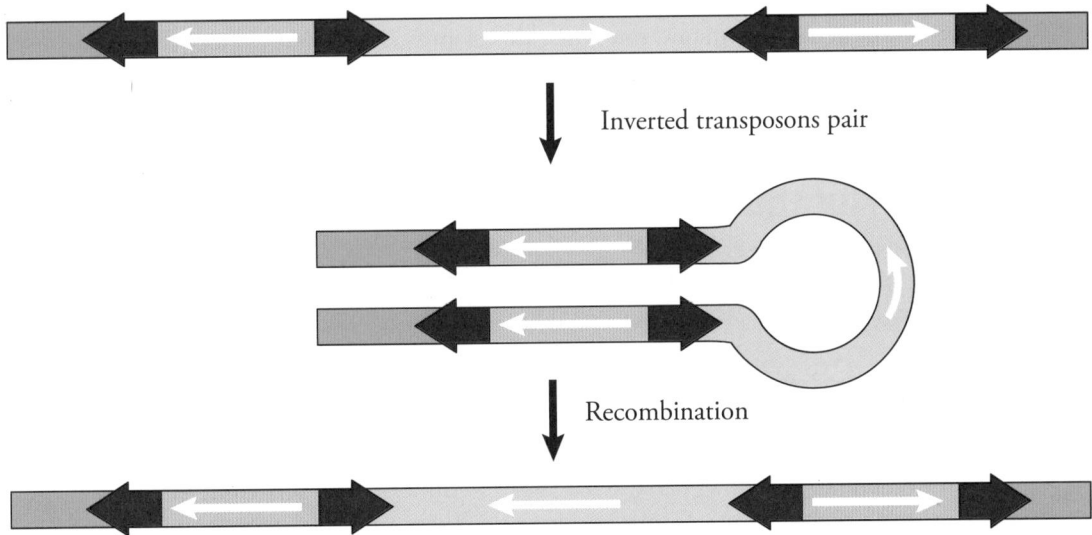

DNA segment between inverted transposons is inverted

Figure 25   Chromosome Inversion via Transposons

Diploid organisms have two copies of each gene, and generally a mutation in one copy is tolerated as long as the other copy of the gene is normal. However, if a deletion removes the normal copy of the gene, the only remaining copy is the mutated version. This is referred to as **loss of heterozygosity**. This makes the locus **hemizygous**: there is only one gene copy in the diploid organism. If the remaining allele is mutant or defective, all gene expression of the normal gene product is lost. For example, hereditary retinoblastoma is a type of retinal cancer common in young children. It occurs when a child receives a flawed copy of the tumor suppressor Rb1 from one parent, and a loss of heterozygosity event leads to loss of the normal allele (from the other parent). With no functional Rb protein (due to having only one copy of Rb1, and it being a flawed or mutant copy), the child almost invariably develops retinoblastoma.

Effects of Mutations

There are many mechanisms by which mutations can exert their effects on the cell. A single amino acid change can affect protein activity, localization, degradation, half-life, or interactions, or, it may have no effect at all. The outcome of a mutation on a protein depends on where the mutation occurs. Mutations on sex chromosomes typically have a greater effect than mutations on autosomes since autosomes are present in double copies. Males have only one X chromosome and one Y chromosome, with no back-up copy of either. Similarly, most females only express one of their X chromosomes (see Section 4.9), and so they, too, often don't have a back-up copy. Haploid expression in a diploid organism is **hemizygosity**, and this can lead to an increased effect of mutations on these chromosomes.

Gain-of-function mutations increase the activity of a certain gene product, or change it such that it gains a new and abnormal function. Loss-of-function mutations are the opposite; they result in the gene product having less or no function. In **haploinsufficiency**, a diploid organism has only a single functional copy of a gene, and this single copy is not enough to support a normal state. Haploinsufficiency highlights the importance of gene dose: many times, just expressing a gene is not enough. You must express *enough* of the gene to maintain good health.

Good and Bad Mutations

Despite the bad reputation they have, not all mutations are bad. Many mutations are neutral, and have no effect. Evolution is based on mutations and selection, and some mutations are beneficial. Those that confer a survival advantage will be selected for in a population.

There are examples of beneficial mutations in humans:

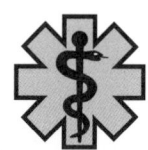

- Sickle-cell anemia is caused by mutations in the gene for hemoglobin (Hb). One of the most common mutations allows deoxygenated Hb to dimerize and form long chains, which distorts the red blood cell shape, causing it to sickle. These deformed cells cannot function properly and are prematurely destroyed, leading to anemia. However, people who carry this gene also have an advantage in that they are more resistant to malaria. In areas where malaria is common, this is an important benefit.

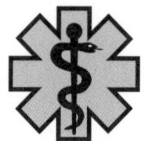

- Some humans are missing 32 base pairs in a gene called CCR5. This deletion confers HIV resistance to homozygotes and delays AIDS onset in heterozygotes. This mutation may have also conferred resistance to diseases in the past (such as the bubonic plague or smallpox), explaining its prevalence in populations of European descent, where these diseases were prevalent.

Mutations can also be disease *causing*. In some cases, one mutation is sufficient to induce a diseased state. In other cases, many mutations have to cooperate and occur together to cause a disease.

Inborn errors of metabolism are a huge group of genetic diseases that involve disorders of metabolism. Most of these are due to a single mutation in a single gene that codes for some sort of metabolic enzyme. Symptoms are caused by either the build-up of a toxic compound that can't be broken down or by the deficiency of an essential molecule that cannot be synthesized. Because cellular metabolism is crucial, many symptoms are possible and a wide range of systems can be affected. Inborn errors of metabolism are typically organized into groups of disorders, depending on what type of metabolic pathways they affect: carbohydrate, amino acid, urea cycle, organic acids, fatty acid oxidation, mitochondrial, porphyrin, purine or pyrimidine, steroid, peroxisomal function, or lysosomal storage.

Cancer is driven by mutation accumulation. These mutations can either be inherited or can be caused by carcinogen exposure. A carcinogen is a mutagen that is directly involved in causing cancer. Tumors typically have hundreds of mutations, ranging from point mutations to massive chromosomal changes. These mutations are often in oncogenes and tumor suppressors. An oncogene is a gene that can cause cancer when it is mutated or expressed at high levels. Tumor suppressors are the opposite in that their deletion (or expression at decreased levels) can cause cancer. Some mutations will drive tumor growth and are highly selected for. These mutations are the most promising targets for developing cancer treatments, as the cancer cells rely on these mutations for growth.

4.6 DNA REPAIR

Cells have developed several mechanisms to deal with DNA damage. First, cell cycle checkpoints are activated, and arrest cell cycle progression. In eukaryotes, checkpoint pathways function at phase boundaries (such as the G_1/S transition, and the G_2/M transition), and can also be activated within some phases. Extensive DNA damage can induce apoptosis in eukaryotes, but before this happens, cells try to repair the DNA damage. This is important so that defective DNA isn't passed on to daughter cells. There are several types of DNA repair.

Direct Reversal

Many types of DNA damage are irreversible and require repair pathways to fix the damage. However, a few can be directly reversed. For example, some enzymes can repair UV-induced pyrimidine photodimers using visible light. This process is called photoreactivation, and directly repairs the UV damage to DNA. This is commonly performed by bacteria and many plants. If pyrimidine dimers are not directly reversed, nucleotide excision repair can be used instead. Nucleotide excision repair is the main mechanism of repair in humans, but it can introduce a mutation when trying to complete the repair. If left unrepaired, pyrimidine dimers in humans may lead to melanoma, a type of very dangerous and malignant skin tumor.

Homology-Dependent Repair

One of the benefits of DNA structure is the presence of a back-up copy; because DNA is double stranded, mutations on one strand of DNA can be repaired using the undamaged, complementary information on the other strand. Repair pathways that rely on this characteristic of DNA are called **homology-dependent repair pathways**. These can be divided into repair that happens before DNA replication (**excision repair**), or repair that happens during and after DNA replication (**post-replication repair**).

Excision Repair

Excision repair involves removing defective bases or nucleotides and replacing them. If these bases are not repaired, they can induce mutations during DNA replication, since replication machinery cannot pair them properly.

Post-Replication Repair

The **mismatch repair pathway** (MMR) targets mismatched Watson-Crick base pairs that were not repaired by DNA polymerase proofreading during replication. To do this, mispaired bases must be identified and fixed, but the crucial question is: which base is the correct one and which is the mistake? For example, if DNA contains an AC base pair, is the adenine correct and C should be removed and replaced with T? Or is the cytosine correct and A should be removed and replaced with G?

Some bacteria use genome methylation to help differentiate between the older DNA template strand and the newly synthesized daughter strand. Methylation takes a while to complete, which means that shortly after DNA synthesis, the parental template strand will be labeled with methylated bases and the new daughter strand will not. Bacterial machinery can read these methyl tags and know which base is the correct one (the one on the older strand) and which needs to be replaced (the newer one).

Other prokaryotes and most eukaryotes use a different system, where the newly synthesized strand is recognized by the free 3'-terminus on the leading strand, or by the presence of gaps between Okazaki fragments on the lagging strand.

Double-Strand Break Repair

DNA double-strand breaks (DSBs) can be caused by reactive oxygen species, ionizing radiation, UV light or chemical agents. Cells have two pathways to help in DSB repair: homologous recombination and nonhomologous end-joining. The goal of both is to reattach and fuse chromosomes that have come apart because of DSB. If done incorrectly, this can lead to deletions (where genetic information is lost) or translocations (where chromosome segments move to other chromosomes).

Homologous Recombination

After DNA replication, the genome contains identical sister chromatids. Homologous recombination is a process where one sister chromatid can help repair a DSB in the other. First, the DSB is identified and trimmed at 5' ends to generate single-stranded DNA (Figure 26). This is done by nucleases (which break phosphodiester bonds) and helicase (to unwind the DNA). Many proteins bind these ends and start a search of the genome to find a sister chromatid region that is complementary to the single-stranded DNA. Once found, the complementary sequences are used as a template to repair and connect the broken

4.6

chromatid. This requires a "joint molecule," where damaged and undamaged sister chromatids cross over. DNA polymerase and ligase build a corrected DNA strand.

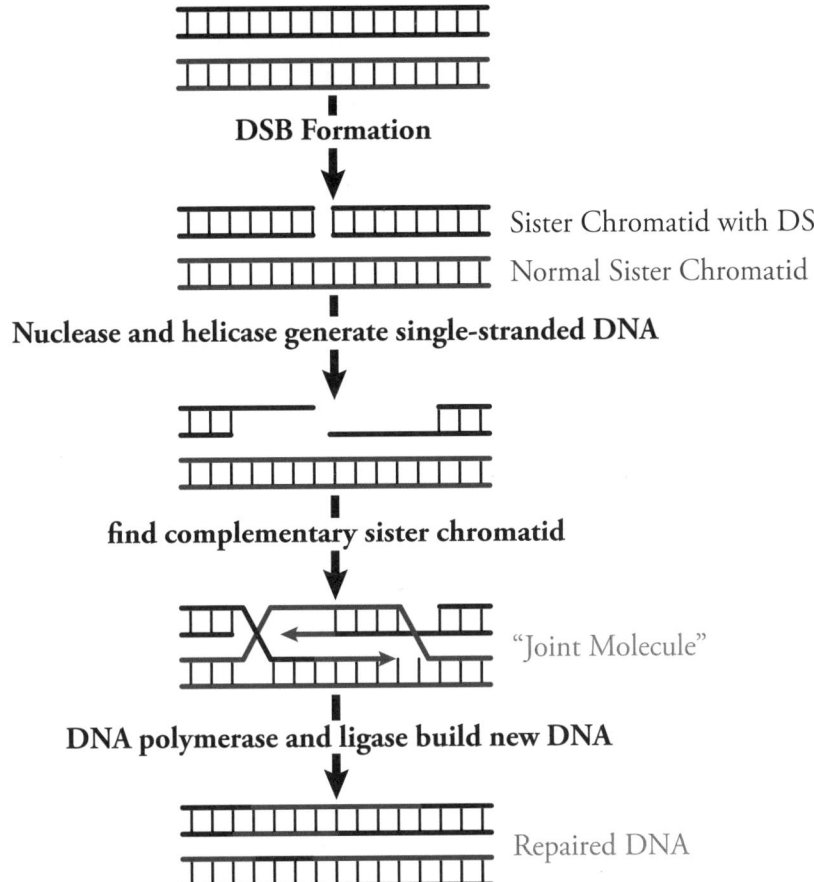

Figure 26 Homologous Recombination to Repair Double-Strand Breaks

Nonhomologous End Joining

Cells that aren't actively growing or cycling through the cell cycle don't have the option of using sister chromatids to repair DSBs in an error-free way. Since DNA replication isn't happening, there is no chromosome backup to use. In this case, even a poorly repaired chromosome is better than one with a DSB, since chromosome breaks can lead to rearrangements.

Nonhomologous end joining is used to accomplish repair in this case. This process is common in eukaryotes but relatively uncommon in prokaryotes. First, broken ends are stabilized and processed, then DNA ligase connects the fragments. Nothing about this process requires specificity; the goal is just to reconnect broken chromosomes. Often this can result in base pairs being lost or chromosomes being connected in an abnormal way.

4.7 GENE EXPRESSION: TRANSCRIPTION

Gene expression refers to the process whereby the information contained in genes begins to have effects in the cell. The Central Dogma tells us that genetic information must be written in the form of RNA (i.e., it must be **transcribed**); and then it must be expressed as protein (i.e., it must be **translated**). Therefore, the logical place to begin our discussion of gene expression is with the nature of RNA and transcription.

Characteristics of RNA

RNA is chemically distinct from DNA in three important ways:

1) RNA is **single-stranded**, except in some viruses.
2) RNA contains **uracil** instead of thymine.
3) The pentose ring in RNA is **ribose** rather than 2' deoxyribose.

There are several different types of RNA, each with a unique role.

Coding RNA

You are already familiar with **messenger RNA** (mRNA), the only type of coding RNA. This molecule carries genetic information to the ribosome, where it can be translated into protein; each unique polypeptide is created according to the sequence of codons on a particular piece of mRNA, which was transcribed from a particular gene. To allow for this, each mRNA has several regions. The 5' region is not translated into protein (so it's called the 5' untranslated region, or **5'UTR**), but it is important in initiation and regulation. Following the 5'UTR is the region that codes for a protein. This starts at a start codon and ends at a stop codon, and it is called the **open reading frame** (ORF). The 3' end of the mRNA (after the stop codon) isn't translated into protein, but it often contains regulatory regions that influence post-transcriptional gene expression (see Section 4.9).

Eukaryotic mRNA is usually **monocistronic** and obeys the "one gene, one protein" principle. This means that each piece of mRNA encodes only one polypeptide (and so contains one ORF). Hence, there are as many different mRNAs as there are proteins. Because each mRNA can be read many times, each transcript can be used to make many copies of its polypeptide. There are a few exceptions to the "one gene, one protein" principle; recently, some polycistronic eukaryotic mRNAs have been discovered, and these will be discussed below.

In contrast, prokaryotic mRNA often codes for more than one polypeptide and is termed **polycistronic**. Different open reading frames on the same polycistronic mRNA are generally related in function.[26] Translation termination and initiation sequences are found between the ORFs. The termination information helps finish the previous peptide chain, and initiation information helps start translation of the next open reading frame on the transcript.

---

[26] For instance, if five enzymes are necessary for the synthesis of a particular molecule, then all five enzymes might be encoded on a single piece of mRNA.

Messenger RNA is constantly produced and degraded, according to the cell's need for the protein encoded by each piece of mRNA. In fact, this is the principal means whereby cells regulate the amount of each particular protein they synthesize. This is an important point that will be emphasized later. Note that in eukaryotes, the first RNA transcribed from DNA is an immature or precursor to mRNA called **heterogeneous nuclear RNA** (hnRNA). Processing events (such as addition of a cap and tail, and splicing) are required for hnRNA to become mature mRNA. Since prokaryotes do not process their primary transcripts, hnRNA is only found in eukaryotes.

Non-Coding RNA

Non-coding RNA (ncRNA) is a functional RNA that is not translated into a protein. The human genome codes for thousands of ncRNAs, and there are several types. The two major types to know for the MCAT are transfer RNA (tRNA) and ribosomal RNA (rRNA).

Transfer RNA (tRNA) is responsible for translating the genetic code. Transfer RNA carries amino acids from the cytoplasm to the ribosome to be added to a growing protein. The structure of tRNA and how it does its job will be discussed in Section 4.8. [Estimate how many different tRNAs there are.[27]]

Ribosomal RNA (rRNA) is the major component of the ribosome. Humans have only four different types of rRNA molecules (18S, 5.8S, 28S and 5S), although almost all the RNA made in a given cell is rRNA. All rRNAs serve as components of the ribosome, along with many polypeptide chains. One rRNA provides the catalytic function of the ribosome, which is a little odd. In most other cases, enzymes are made from polypeptides. Catalytic RNAs are also called **ribozymes** (or ribonucleic acid enzymes), since they are capable of performing specific biochemical reactions, similar to protein enzymes. There are additional examples of ribozymes, including snRNA (discussed below) and some introns that are self-splicing.

Some other interesting non-coding RNAs are:

- **Small nuclear RNA** (snRNA) molecules (150 nucleotides) associate with proteins to form snRNP (small nuclear ribonucleic particles) complexes in the spliceosome.
- **MicroRNA** (miRNA) and **small interfering RNA** (siRNA) function in RNA interference (RNAi), a form of post-transcriptional regulation of gene expression. Both can bind specific mRNA molecules to either increase or decrease translation. This will be discussed more in Section 4.9.
- **Long ncRNAs** are longer than 200 nucleotides. They help control the basal transcription level in a cell by regulating initiation complex assembly on promoters. They also contribute to many types of post-transcriptional regulation by controlling splicing and translation, and they function in imprinting and X-chromosome inactivation (see Section 4.9).

4.7

---

[27] Each tRNA must recognize a codon on mRNA and respond by delivering the appropriate amino acid to the ribosome. There are 20 different amino acids, so there at least 20 different tRNAs. However, there are 61 possible codons, so there could be as many as 61 different tRNAs. The actual number is between 20 and 61, because the third nucleotide of the codon is often not needed for specificity of the amino acid.

Replication vs. Transcription

Transcription is the synthesis of RNA (usually mRNA, tRNA, or rRNA) using DNA as the template. The word *transcription* indicates that in the process of reading and writing information, the language does not change. Information is transferred from one polynucleotide to another. This should lead you to expect transcription to be fairly similar to replication. And it is.

Both replication and transcription involve **template-driven polymerization**. [Because of this, the RNA transcript produced in transcription is __ [28] to the DNA template, just as the daughter strand produced in replication was.] The *driving force* for both processes is the removal and subsequent hydrolysis of pyrophosphate from each nucleotide added to the chain, with the existing chain acting as nucleophile. [Transcription, like replication, can occur only in the __ [29] direction. Do the polymerase enzymes in both replication and transcription require a primer?[30]] Another important difference between transcription and DNA replication is that RNA polymerase has not been shown to possess the ability to remove mismatched nucleotides (it lacks exonuclease activity); in other words, it cannot correct its errors. Thus, transcription is a lower fidelity process than replication. [A virus possessing an RNA genome relies on RNA polymerase rather than DNA polymerase to replicate its genome. Will this virus have a higher or a lower rate of spontaneous mutation than organisms with ds-DNA genomes?[31]]

Another similarity is that transcription, like replication, begins at a specific spot on the chromosome. The name of the site where transcription starts (the **start site**) is different from the name of the place where replication begins, __.[32] The sequence of nucleotides on a chromosome that activates RNA polymerase to begin the process of transcription is called the **promoter**, and the point where RNA polymerization actually *starts* is called the start site. In fact, from this point forward, just about every event in transcription is given a different name from the events in replication.

Reference Points in Transcription

Before we discuss the mechanics of transcription, we need to clarify a few reference points (see Figure 27). We noted previously that the chromosome is referred to as the *template*, not *parent*. What about the individual strands of the chromosome? Are they both templates for the same mRNA? Let's answer with a thought experiment. Say there is a strand of DNA which has the sequence AAAAAAAAA. If we transcribe this strand, the resulting mRNA will look like: UUUUUUUUU. When it is translated, this mRNA will result in an oligopeptide with this primary structure: Phe-Phe-Phe. (Refer to the genetic code table in Section 4.3.) Now, what if we transcribe the other strand of the chromosome? What is its DNA sequence? What will the transcript look like? And the oligopeptide?[33] Our conclusion is that only one of the strands of the DNA template encodes a particular mRNA molecule. But it makes sense: paired DNA

---

[28] complementary

[29] 5' to 3'

[30] No, RNA pol does not require a primer. Remember, the primer in replication is a piece of RNA, made by an RNA polymerase.

[31] The virus will have a very high rate of mutation. It is a general law that most mutations are harmful. Hence, individual viruses will be far less likely to survive than organisms with DNA genomes. However, the high mutation rate will allow the entire species of virus to evolve very rapidly, making it very successful as a parasite (since it will evade host defense systems).

[32] the origin

[33] The DNA strand must be complementary to the first strand we discussed. So the sequence must be TTTTTTTTT. Thus, the transcript will have to be AAAAAAAAA. Because AAA codes for lysine, the oligopeptide would be Lys-Lys-Lys.

strands are *complementary*, not *identical*. The strand which is actually transcribed is called the **template**, **non-coding**, **transcribed**, or **antisense strand**; it is complementary to the transcript. The other DNA strand is called the **coding** or **sense strand**; it has the same sequence as the transcript (except it has T in place of U). It is customary to say that transcription starts at a point and proceeds **downstream**, which means toward the 3' end of the coding strand and transcript. **Upstream** means toward the 5' end of the coding strand, beyond the 5' end of the transcript. Upstream nucleotide sequences are referred to using negative numbers, and downstream sequences are referred to using positive numbers. The first nucleotide on the template strand which is actually transcribed is called the start site. The corresponding nucleotide on the coding strand is given the number +1. As we'll see below, regulatory sequences on the chromosome are referred to by where they occur on the coding strand.

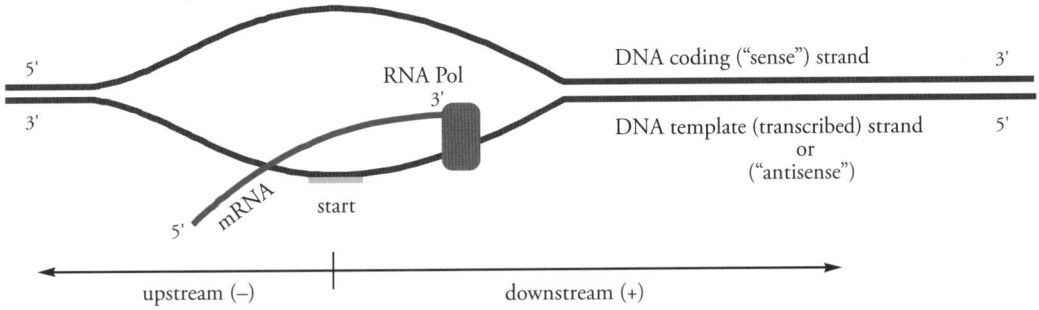

Figure 27   Reference Points in Transcription

- The figure above labels the transcript "mRNA." Is this accurate in all life forms? (Hint: in eukaryotes, is the initial transcript mature mRNA ready to be translated?)[34]

Prokaryotic Transcription

It is important to understand all the vocabulary and general principles presented above. In this section and the next, we will present some more detailed information.

In bacteria (prokaryotes), all types of RNA are made by the same RNA polymerase. Prokaryotic RNA polymerase is a large enzyme complex consisting of five subunits: two alpha subunits, a beta subunit, a beta' subunit, and an omega subunit ($\alpha_2\beta\beta'\omega$). This is the **core enzyme** responsible for rapid elongation of the transcript. However, the core enzyme alone cannot initiate transcription. An additional subunit termed the **sigma factor** (σ) is required to form what is sometimes referred to as the **holoenzyme** (*holo* = complete), which is responsible for initiation.

Transcription occurs in three stages: **initiation**, **elongation**, and **termination**. Initiation occurs when RNA polymerase holoenzyme binds to a promoter. The typical bacterial promoter contains two primary sequences: the **Pribnow box** at –10 and the **–35 sequence**. Holoenzyme scans along the chromosome like a train on a railroad track until it recognizes a promoter and then stops, forming a **closed complex**. The RNA polymerase must unwind a portion of the DNA double helix before it can begin to synthesize

---

[34] No, it is accurate for prokaryotes only. In eukaryotes, the RNA transcript must be processed (spliced) and transported out of the nucleus before it can be translated. We will discuss this in-depth later in the chapter.

RNA. The RNA polymerase bound at the promoter with a region of single-stranded DNA is termed the **open complex**. Once the open complex has formed, transcription can begin.

The sigma factor plays two roles in helping the polymerase find promoters. The first is to greatly increase the ability of RNA polymerase to recognize promoters. The second is to decrease the nonspecific affinity of holoenzyme for DNA. Once the open complex and several phosphodiester bonds have been formed, the sigma factor is no longer necessary and leaves the RNA polymerase complex.

The core enzyme elongates the RNA chain *processively*, with one polymerase complex synthesizing an entire RNA molecule. As the core enzyme elongates the RNA, it moves along the DNA downstream in a **transcription bubble** in which a region of the DNA double helix is unwound to allow the polymerase to access the complementary DNA template. When a termination signal is detected, in some cases with the help of a protein called rho, the polymerase falls off of the DNA, releases the RNA, and the transcription bubble closes.

Comparing Prokaryotic and Eukaryotic Transcription

Eukaryotic and prokaryotic transcription are similar, but you need to be aware of four major differences. Differences in location, RNA polymerases, and primary transcripts are discussed here. Regulation of transcription is another major difference and is discussed in Section 4.9.

Location

Eukaryotic means "true-kernelled." Prokaryotic means "before-the-kernel." The **karyon** (kernel) is, of course, the nucleus. The fact that prokaryotes have no nucleus means transcription occurs free in the cytoplasm, in the same compartment where translation occurs, and transcription and translation can occur *simultaneously*. Eukaryotes must transcribe their mRNA in the nucleus, modify it (see below), and then transport it across the nuclear membrane to the cytoplasm where it can be translated. Transcription and translation in eukaryotes *do not* occur simultaneously.

Another important difference between prokaryotic and eukaryotic gene expression is that the primary transcript in prokaryotes is mRNA. In other words, the product of transcription by prokaryotic RNA polymerase is ready to be translated. In fact, translation of prokaryotic mRNA begins before transcription is completed!

In contrast, the eukaryotic primary transcript (hnRNA made by RNA pol II, see below for info on eukaryotic RNA polymerases) is modified extensively before translation (Figure 30). The most important example is **splicing**. Eukaryotic DNA has non-coding sequences intervening between the segments that actually code for proteins. Sometimes these intervening sequences contain enhancers or other regulatory sequences and they can be quite long. The average size of a mammalian intron, for example, is about 2,000 nucleotides. _Int_ervening sequences in the RNA are called **introns**. Note that introns are intragenic regions (and not intergenic space, discussed in Section 4.2). Protein-coding regions of the RNA are termed **ex**ons because they actually get _ex_pressed. Before the RNA can be translated, introns must be removed and exons joined together; this is accomplished via splicing.

Splicing is mediated by the **spliceosome**, a complex that contains over 100 proteins and 5 small nuclear RNA (snRNA) molecules. About half the proteins stably bind snRNAs, and these form three small nuclear ribonucleic particles (snRNPs). Each snRNP is therefore made of proteins and snRNAs. The spliceosome assembles around each intron that needs to be removed. This happens in a series of steps, where different snRNP components are recruited and released as the reaction proceeds.

To catalyze the splicing reaction, snRNPs recognize and hydrogen bond to conserved nucleotides in the intron: typically GU at the 5' end, AG at the 3' end, and an adenine 15–45 bases upstream of the 3' splice site. This aligns the hnRNA such that the splicing mechanism can take place (Figure 28). Two splicing reactions are catalyzed by the spliceosome. The first reaction attaches one end of the intron to the conserved adenine. This causes the intron to form a looped structure, then the second reaction joins the two exons (Figure 28) and releases the loop. The five conserved nucleotides necessary for this reaction (GU, A and AG) are found in all genes and across all eukaryotic species.

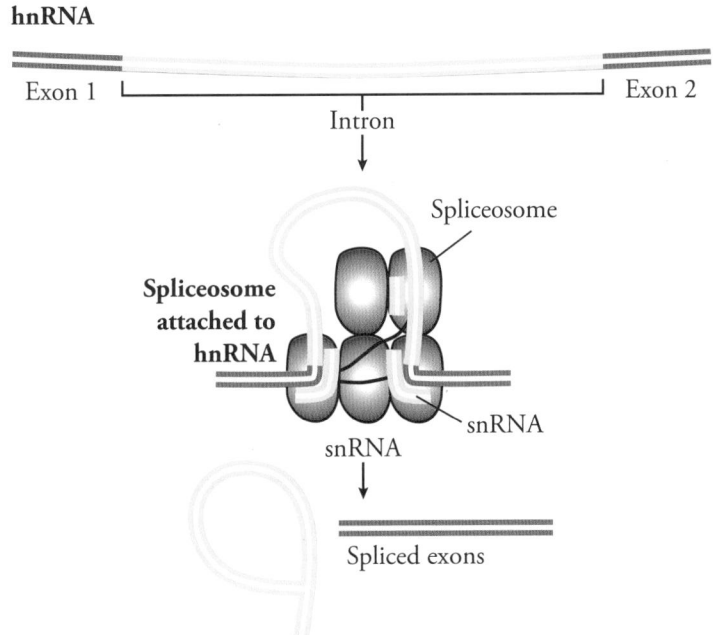

Figure 28   Mechanism of Splicing

For a given gene, there are often different options or patterns of splicing, a phenomenon called **alternative splicing**. One gene could have different promoters in the 5' region, which can change where/how the RNA begins. There can be alternative 5' exons or 3' exons, which can affect either end of the RNA. In the middle, too, some exons can be included or skipped. Finally, there could be mutually exclusive exons, where sometimes one is included and sometimes the other is kept. This leads to different mRNAs being made from one DNA gene sequence; the mRNAs can be different in length and sequence. Shuffling exons in this way is one way to increase the complexity of gene expression (Figure 29 on the following page).

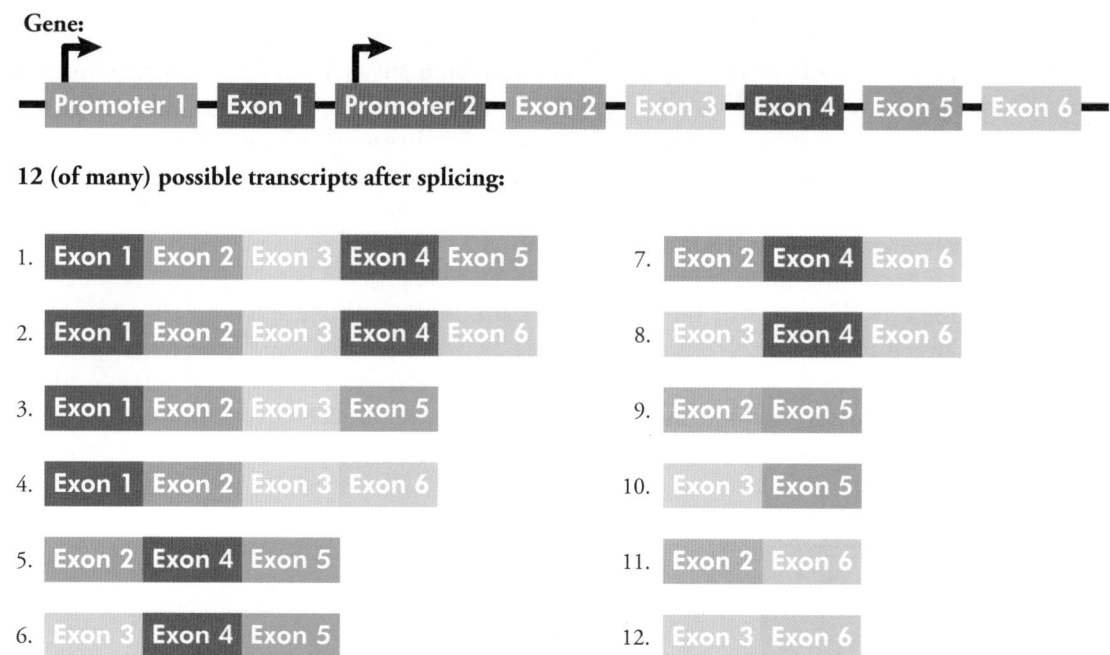

Figure 29 An Example of Alternative Splicing

Alternative splicing is mediated by introns and exons, as well as by the proteins that can bind to these sequences. There are almost 200,000 introns in the human genome, with an average of about seven per gene. It was initially thought that introns were unimportant and had no function, but the current picture of introns is a little more complicated than first believed.

Eukaryotic hnRNA must be modified in two other ways before translation can occur. A tag is added to each end of the molecule: a **5' cap** and a **3' poly-A tail**. The 5' cap is a methylated guanine nucleotide stuck on the 5' end [which is the end made __ (first or last?)[35]]. The poly-A tail is a string of several hundred adenine nucleotides. The cap is essential for translation, while both the cap and the poly-A tail are important in preventing digestion of the mRNA by exonucleases that are free in the cell.

---

[35] It is made first, since transcription proceeds from 5' to 3'.

- Why would active exonucleases be floating free in the cell?[36]

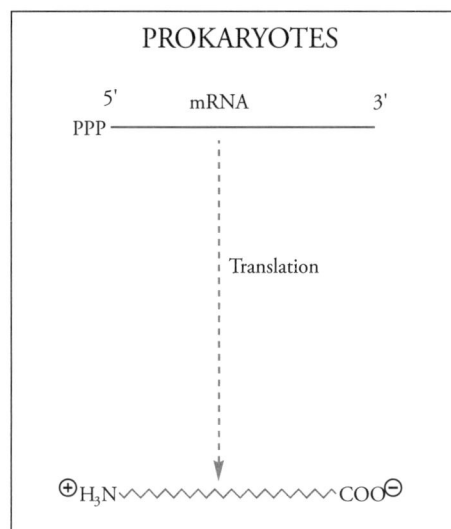 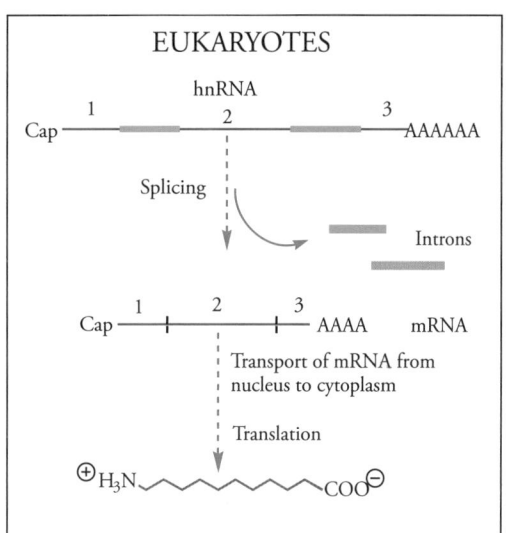

Figure 30 Comparison of Prokaryotic and Eukaryotic Gene Expression

- One piece of RNA isolated from a human cell is found to produce two different polypeptides when added to a cell-free protein synthesis system containing all the enzymes necessary for eukaryotic gene expression. When the two polypeptides are separated and digested with trypsin, they produce fragments of the following molecular weights:
  Polypeptide 1: 5 kD, 8 kD, 12 kD, and 14 kD
  Polypeptide 2: 3 kD, 5 kD, 8 kD, 10 kD, 12 kD, and 14 kD
How can we explain the synthesis of two different polypeptides from one piece of RNA?[37]

RNA Polymerase

In prokaryotes, all RNA is made by the $\alpha_2\beta\beta'\omega\sigma$ RNA polymerase complex. In eukaryotes, there are many different RNA polymerases:

- **RNA polymerase I transcribes most rRNA**
- **RNA polymerase II transcribes hnRNA** (so ultimately mRNA), most snRNA, and some miRNA
- **RNA polymerase III transcribes tRNA**, long ncRNA, siRNA, some miRNA, and a subset of rRNA

Please note: In our discussion of replication, you learned about many *prokaryotic DNA* polymerases. In contrast, here you learned about many eukaryotic RNA polymerases. Don't get mixed up!

---

[36] Two conceivable reasons: 1) *mRNA has a very short lifespan;* it is degraded rapidly, and more must be made if the protein is still needed. Note that this is consistent with the idea that regulation of gene expression occurs primarily at the transcriptional level since this is more efficient. 2) Viruses may inject RNA into the cell. If it does not have the correct cap and tail modifications, exonucleases will destroy it.

[37] Here is an example of the use of splicing for the regulation of gene expression. The piece of RNA must have been hnRNA. In the cell-free system it underwent **differential splicing** to produce one of two different mRNA molecules. Apparently, Polypeptide 1 came from an mRNA which had more material spliced out than the mRNA coding for Polypeptide 2.

4.8 GENE EXPRESSION: TRANSLATION

Translation is the synthesis of polypeptides according to the amino acid sequence dictated by the sequence of codons in mRNA. During translation, an mRNA molecule attaches to a ribosome at a specific codon, and the appropriate amino acid is delivered by a tRNA molecule. Then the second amino acid is delivered by another tRNA. Then the ribosome binds the two amino acids together, creating a dipeptide. This process is repeated until the polypeptide is complete, at which point the ribosome drops the mRNA and the new polypeptide departs.

Transfer RNA (tRNA)

Each tRNA is composed of a single transcript produced by RNA polymerase III. The tertiary structure of every tRNA molecule is similar. tRNAs have a stem-and-loop structure stabilized by hydrogen bonds between bases on neighboring segments of the RNA chain (Figures 31 and 32). Several modified nucleotides are found in tRNA (e.g., dihydrouridine). One end of the structure is responsible for recognizing the mRNA codon to be translated. This is the **anticodon**, a sequence of three ribonucleotides which is complementary to the mRNA codon the tRNA translates. A key step in translation is *specific base pairing between the tRNA anticodon and the mRNA codon*. It is this specificity that dictates which amino acid of the twenty will be added to a growing polypeptide chain by the ribosome. [Is it likely that the three nucleotides of the anticodon contribute to the tertiary structure of tRNA by base-pairing with other nucleotides in the chain?[38]] The other end of the tRNA molecule has the **amino acid acceptor site**, which is where the amino acid is attached to the tRNA. [If you analyzed a thousand tRNA molecules, which region would you expect to vary the most?[39]] Since there is a tRNA for each codon, each tRNA is specific for one amino acid, while each amino acid may have several tRNAs. Each tRNA can be named according to the amino acid it's specific for. For example, a tRNA for valine would be written $tRNA_{Val}$. When the amino acid is attached, the tRNA is written this way: $Val\text{-}tRNA_{Val}$.

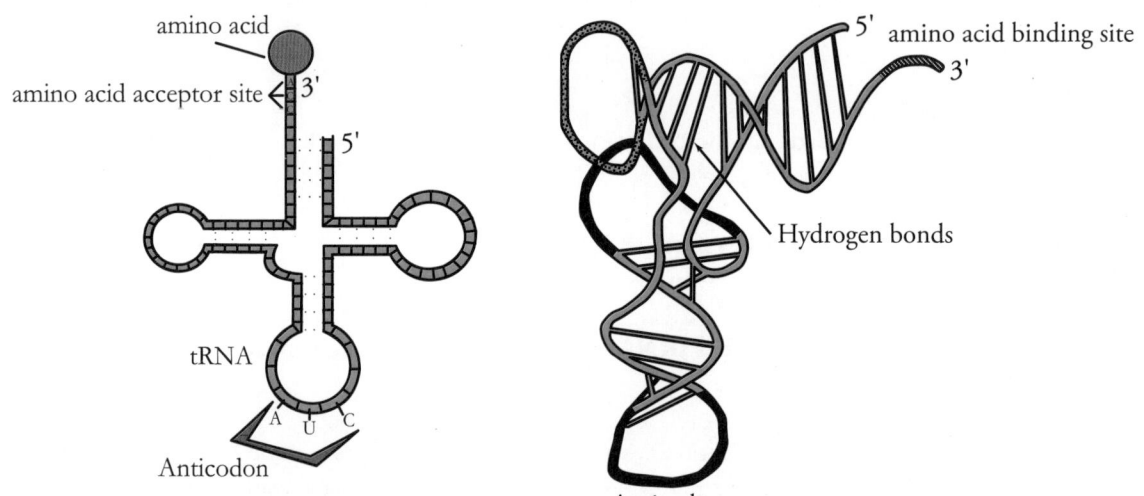

Figure 31 Cloverleaf (Two-Dimensional) Structure of tRNA

Figure 32 Three-Dimensional Structure of tRNA

---

[38] No. They must be available for base pairing with the codon.

[39] The anticodon is different for each of the different tRNA molecules. Part of the rest of the molecule varies from one tRNA to the next, but about 60 percent is constant. The amino acid binding site is always the same: CCA (at the 3' end of the tRNA molecule).

tRNA molecules often contain nitrogenous bases in many positions that have been covalently modified. Base methylation is particularly common. Some specific examples are inosine (derived from adenine), pseudouridine (derived from uracil), or lysidine (derived from cytosine). Inosine in particular plays an important role in wobble base pairing.

The Wobble Hypothesis

Using the standard genetic code, you would guess that organisms have 61 distinct tRNA molecules to recognize the 61 amino acid-coding codons possible in mRNA. In actual fact, most organisms have fewer than 45 different types of tRNAs, meaning some anticodons must pair with more than one codon. Francis Crick's **Wobble Hypothesis** explains this and states that the first two codon-anticodon pairs obey normal base pairing rules, but the third position is more flexible (Figure 33). This allows for non-traditional pairing and explains why a smaller number of tRNAs are possible.

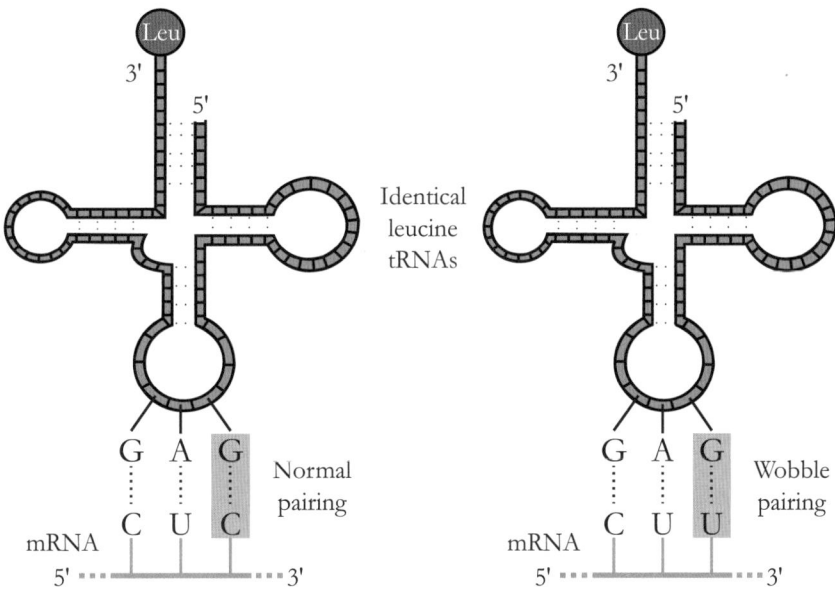

Figure 33   Wobble Base Pairing Between a tRNA Anticodon and an mRNA Codon

A modified inosine base (I) at the 5' end of the anticodon is particularly wobbly, as it can bond to three different codon bases (A, U, or C). Some common wobble pairing combinations are:

5' Base in Anticodon (tRNA)	3' Base in Codon (mRNA)
G	C (Watson-Crick base) or U (wobble base)
C	G
A	U
U	A (Watson-Crick base) or G (wobble base)
I	A, U, or C (all wobble bases)

In other words, the most common wobble base pairs are guanine-uracil, inosine-uracil, inosine-adenine, and inosine-cytosine (G-U, I-U, I-A, and I-C). Both the wobble base pair and the normal Watson-Crick base pair have similar thermodynamic stabilities.

Amino Acid Activation

Peptide bond formation during protein synthesis is a process that requires a lot of energy because the peptide bond has unfavorable thermodynamics ($\Delta G > 0$) and slow kinetics (high activation energy). Reaction coupling is used to power the process: two high-energy phosphate bonds are hydrolyzed to provide the energy to attach an amino acid to its tRNA molecule. This process is called **tRNA loading** or **amino acid activation**, and it is useful because breaking the aminoacyl-tRNA bond will drive peptide bond formation forward. Amino acid activation occurs in several steps:

1) An amino acid is attached to AMP to form *aminoacyl* AMP. In this reaction, the nucleophile is the acidic oxygen of the amino acid, and the leaving group is PP_i.
2) The pyrophosphate leaving group is hydrolyzed to 2 orthophosphates. This reaction is highly favorable ($\Delta G \ll 0$).
3) tRNA loading, an unfavorable reaction, is driven forward by the destruction of the high-energy aminoacyl—AMP bond created in Step 1.

4.8

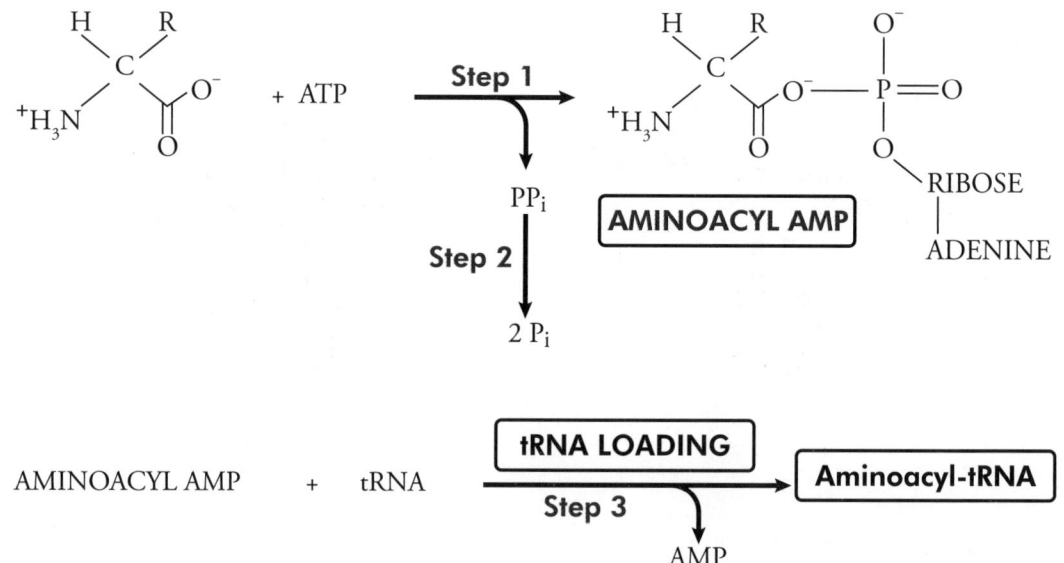

Figure 34   Amino Acid Activation as an Example of Reaction Coupling
Note: water as a reactant has been left out of all reactions in this figure.

Overall, amino acid activation requires 2 ATP equivalents because it uses two high-energy bonds. An ATP equivalent is a single high-energy phosphate bond. You can get 2 ATP equivalents by hydrolyzing 2 ATP to 2 ADP + 2 P_i or by hydrolyzing 1 ATP to AMP + 2 P_i.

Eventually, the bond between the amino acid and the tRNA molecule will be broken. This hydrolysis will power peptide bond formation: the nitrogen of another amino acid will nucleophilically attack the carbonyl carbon of this amino acid, and tRNA will be the leaving group.

Aminoacyl-tRNA Synthetases

We have stated that incorporation of the appropriate amino acid in a growing polypeptide depends on the delivery of the correct amino acid by a specific tRNA. But we also noted that the amino acid acceptor sites of all tRNA molecules are the same. How is the attachment of the appropriate amino acid to each tRNA molecule accomplished? **Aminoacyl-tRNA synthetase enzymes** are specific to each amino acid, and there is at least one aminoacyl-tRNA synthetase for every amino acid. This family of enzymes recognizes both the tRNA and the amino acid based on their three-dimensional structures. They are highly specific, which is important because joining the wrong amino acid to a tRNA would result in the wrong amino acid being incorporated into a polypeptide. Given that some amino acids differ only by a single methyl group, this specificity is quite amazing. Aminoacyl-tRNA synthetases also function with a very low error rate. [If there is a 1/1000 error rate in amino acid incorporation, what percentage of polypeptides that are 500 amino acid residues long will not contain any errors?[40]]

Overall then, **amino acid activation** serves two functions. One is specific and accurate amino acid delivery, and the other is thermodynamic activation of the amino acid.

- A bacterial strain with a point mutation in the gene for hexokinase is not able to metabolize glucose. The mutation causes a substitution of arginine for serine. These bacteria are used to test whether chemicals are mutagenic. The chemical is added to a culture of bacteria with glucose as the only carbon source. Any bacteria that grow must have undergone a mutation which remedied the problem (this is called *suppression* of the original mutation). When a particular hair spray ingredient is tested, several colonies grow on the glucose-only medium. Which one of the following might act as a suppressor of the first mutation?[41]
    A) A point mutation during replication of a tRNA gene
    B) A mutation in RNA polymerase that increases the rate of promoter recognition
    C) A base pair deletion in the hexokinase gene
    D) A point mutation during transcription of a tRNA molecule

The Ribosome

The ribosome is composed of many polypeptides and rRNA chains held together in a massive quaternary structure. Ribosomes float around in the cytoplasm, and each has a small subunit and a large subunit. The unit of measurement is the Svedberg, or S, unit. Svedbergs are a measure of sedimentation rate, that is, how quickly something will sink in a gradient during centrifugation, thus the sum of the small and large subunits' S values is not the same as the S value of the whole ribosome.

---

[40] The easiest way to calculate this is to figure out the probability of getting *all* amino acids in the protein correct, in other words, we must use the *non*-error rate for our calculation, not the error rate. If the error rate is 1/1000, then the non-error rate is 999/1000. The probability of having no errors is $.999^n$, where n = the number of amino acid residues. In other words, a single amino acid has .999 probability, or 99.9% probability of being correct. Two amino acids correct in a row have a $.999 \times .999$ probability $(.999^2)$, or .998, or 99.8% probability of happening. Continuing in this manner, a 500-amino acid protein has a $.999^{500}$ probability of being entirely correct, or .606, approximately a 60% probability. Longer proteins have a higher chance of containing errors.

[41] A single base change in the anticodon of the tRNA for arginine could cause it to recognize the codon for serine. If that happened in the mutant bacteria, problems might ensue, but one good result would be that the correct amino acid would be incorporated at the mutated site in hexokinase (choice **A** is correct; note that point mutations in tRNA genes are actually a common means of suppression in bacteria). Increasing the rate at which RNA polymerase recognizes the promoter might increase the rate of transcription, but it would not fix a mutant enzyme (choice **B** is wrong), and a base pair deletion in the hexokinase gene would cause a frameshift mutation and a serious significant change in protein structure and function (choice **C** is wrong). A point mutation during transcription of a tRNA molecule might have a temporary effect on a single bacterium, but it would not be passed on to its progeny; remember than only DNA mutations have lasting effects and errors made during transcription are generally insignificant (choice **D** is wrong).

The prokaryotic ribosome sediments in a gradient at a rate of 70S, so it is referred to as the **70S ribosome**. It is composed of a 30S small subunit and a 50S large subunit. Eukaryotes have an **80S ribosome**. It also has a small and large subunit. The large subunit sediments in a gradient at a rate of 60S. The small subunit sediments in a gradient at a rate of 40S. The large and small subunits of both prokaryotic and eukaryotic ribosomes are made up of many smaller peptides and several rRNA molecules (see Figure 35). The ribozymic activity of both prokaryotic and eukaryotic ribosomes is found in the large subunit and is associated with the rRNAs.

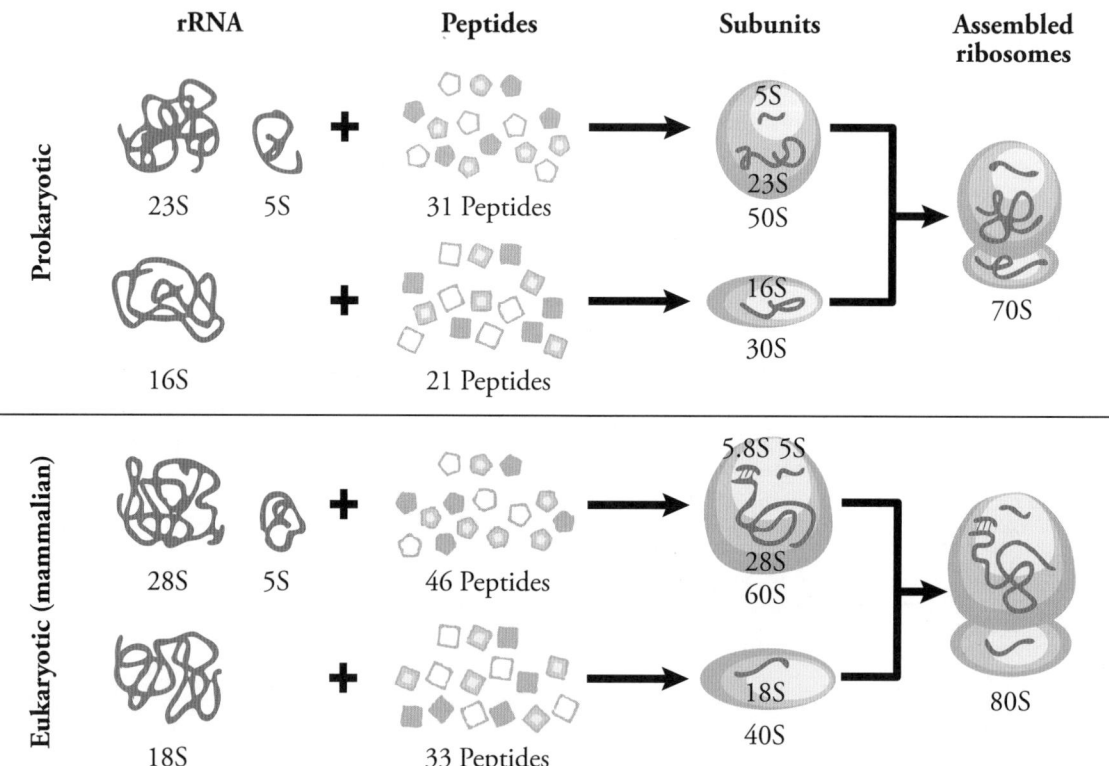

Figure 35 Ribosome Components

In both prokaryotes and eukaryotes, the complete ribosome (both subunits together) has three special binding sites. The **A site** (*a*minoacyl-tRNA site) is where each new tRNA delivers its amino acid. The **P site** (*p*eptidyl-tRNA site) is where the growing polypeptide chain, still attached to a tRNA, is located during translation. The **E site** (*e*xit-tRNA site) is where a now-empty tRNA sits prior to its release from the ribosome. [During translation, the next codon to be translated is exposed in the __[42].] tRNAs move through the sites from **A → P → E.**

---

[42] A site, since this is where the next amino acid to be added must bind.

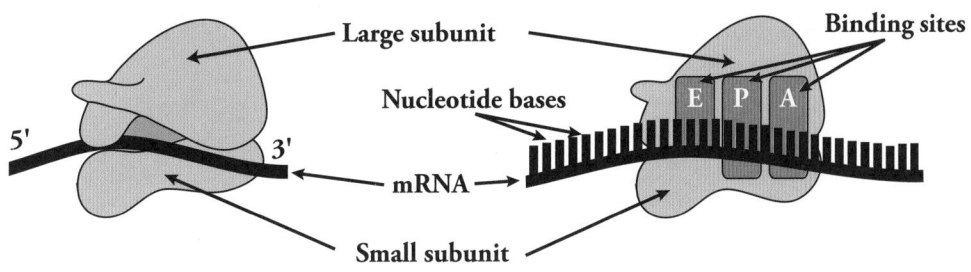

Figure 36 The Ribosome

Prokaryotic Translation

In prokaryotes, translation occurs in the same compartment and at the same time as transcription. In other words, *while the mRNA is being made*, ribosomes attach and begin translating it. [Does this mean that the first end of the mRNA to be translated is 5' or 3'?[43]] Note that it says ribosome**s** above. Several ribosomes attach to the mRNA and translate it simultaneously (see Figure 37; you may hear the term *polyribosome* used to describe this arrangement; polyribosomes are seen in both prokaryotes and eukaryotes). [You figured out the direction of translation on the mRNA from what you already know. Do you have any previous knowledge that would help you answer this: Does translation always begin at the 5' end of the mRNA, or somewhere up the chain?[44]]

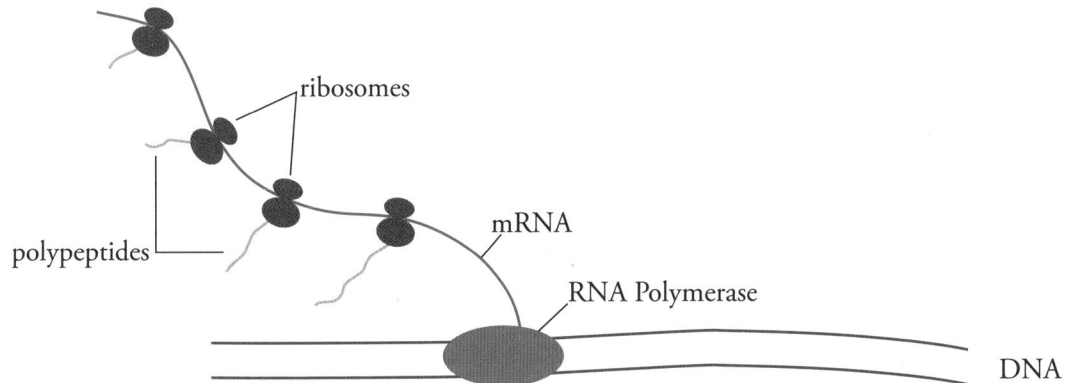

Figure 37 A Prokaryotic Polyribosome

Because prokaryotes often have polycistronic mRNAs, their ribosomes can also start translation in the middle of the chain. This means termination and initiation sequences are found between each ORF. Even for the first open reading frame on a transcript, translation doesn't begin right at the 5' end. An upstream regulatory sequence is essential for initiation, just as in transcription. Here, instead of a promoter, we have a **ribosome binding site**, also known as the **Shine-Dalgarno sequence**, located at −10 (ten ribonucleotides upstream, or on the 5' side of the start codon). The Shine-Dalgarno sequence is complementary to a pyrimidine-rich region on the small subunit, and thus helps position the initiation machinery on the transcript.

---

[43] 5' first, since the mRNA is made 5' end first. Transcription and translation go in the same direction on mRNA.

[44] It does not always occur at the very end. You can deduce this from the fact that mRNA is polycistronic. If there are more than one translation start sites on the mRNA, they can't all be at the 5' end.

Like transcription, translation has three distinct stages: initiation, elongation, and termination. Many antibiotics function by inhibiting a particular stage.[45]

Initiation starts with the small ribosomal subunit (30S) binding two initiation proteins. This complex then binds the mRNA transcript. Next, the first aminoacyl-tRNA joins, along with a third initiation factor, which is also bound to one GTP. Finally, the 50S subunit completes the complex. This process is powered by the hydrolysis of one GTP molecule.[46] The first aminoacyl-tRNA is special; it is called the **initiator tRNA**, abbreviated **fMet-tRNA$_{fMet}$**. The "fMet" stands for *formylmethionine*, which is a modified methionine used as the first amino acid in all prokaryotic proteins.[47] The initiator tRNA sits in the P site of the 70S ribosome, hydrogen-bonded with the **start codon**. [What is the start codon? Does this codon initiate translation wherever it appears?[48]] Before elongation, all initiation factors dissociate from the complex.

Elongation, a three-step cycle, may now begin. In the first step, the second aminoacyl-tRNA enters the A site and hydrogen bonds with the second codon. This process requires the hydrolysis of one phosphate from GTP. This is done by an elongation factor protein, which is a GTPase. In the second step, the **peptidyl transferase** activity of the large ribosomal subunit catalyzes the formation of a peptide bond between fMet and the second amino acid. The amino group of amino acid #2 acts as nucleophile, and tRNA$_{fMet}$ is the leaving group; it dissociates from the ribosome. A new dipeptide is now attached to tRNA #2. Now you can figure out the direction of translation from the point of view of the polypeptide; you won't have to memorize it.[49] The third step is **translocation**, in which tRNA #1 (now empty) moves into the E site, tRNA #2 (holding the growing peptide) moves into the P site, and the next codon to be translated moves into the A site. An elongation factor helps with translocation, and this process costs one GTP. The new dipeptide is still attached to tRNA #2, and tRNA #2 is still H-bonded to codon #2. The presence of tRNA #1 in the E site (still H-bonded to codon #1), is thought to help maintain the reading frame of the mRNA (disruption of tRNA binding to the E site results in an increase in the number of frameshift mutations in the resulting protein). [Does the ribosome move relative to the mRNA during translocation?[50]] These three steps repeat over and over again, connecting amino acids in the order their codons appear along the mRNA strand (and thus appear in the A site).

Termination occurs when a stop codon appears in the A site. Instead of a tRNA, a **release factor** now enters the A site. This causes the peptidyl transferase to hydrolyze the bond between the last tRNA and the completed polypeptide. Prokaryotes have three release factor proteins, two of which recognize stop codons and one that works with the other two to help terminate translation. Finally, the ribosome separates into its subunits and releases both mRNA and polypeptide.

---

[45] For example, streptomycin and tetracycline bind to the 30S subunit of the prokaryotic ribosome. Chloramphenicol and erythromycin bind to the 50S subunit.

[46] This may seem odd, as ATP is normally the energy molecule. But a high-energy phosphate is a high-energy phosphate. Another example is the GTP produced in the Krebs cycle.

[47] In fact, cells of our immune system release cytotoxins when they sniff out fMet, because this chemical is a sure sign that bacteria are busily translating.

[48] Refer to the genetic code table. The codon for methionine is AUG; that's the start codon. It only initiates translation when it is preceded by a Shine-Dalgarno sequence (prokaryotes).

[49] The direction of synthesis is N → C, since the N of amino acid #2 binds to the C of #1. As the polypeptide elongates, its N terminus will come snaking out of the ribosome.

[50] It must, if the tRNA remains H-bonded to the mRNA while moving to another spot in the ribosome.

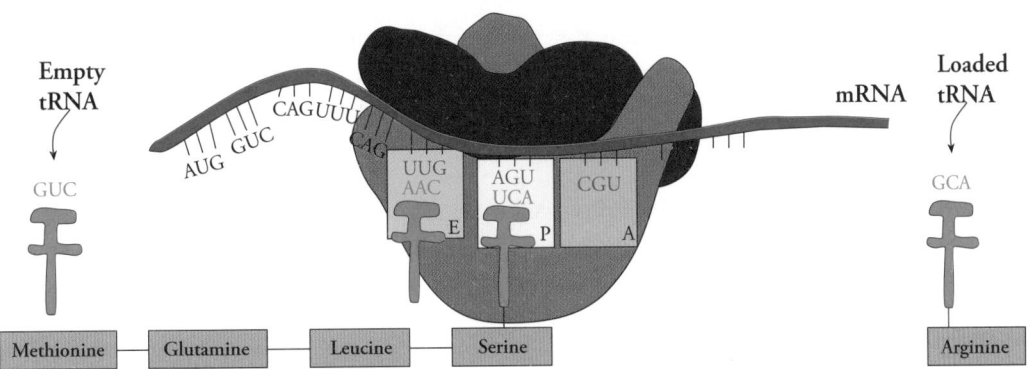

Figure 38 Translation Elongation

Let's focus for a moment on the energetics of translation. Why doesn't peptide bond formation require GTP hydrolysis, like the other steps in translation?[51] You should be able to answer questions like this: How many high-energy phosphate bonds are required to make a 50 amino acid polypeptide chain, including the energy used to activate amino acids to aminoacyl-tRNAs?[52]

Eukaryotic Translation

There are several differences between eukaryotic and prokaryotic translation. Many of these have already been mentioned: the ribosome is larger (80S) and has different components than the prokaryotic ribosome, the mRNA must be processed before it can be translated (spliced, with cap and tail added), and the N-terminal amino acid is different (Met instead of fMet). Also remember that eukaryotic mRNA must not only be spliced, capped, and tailed, but it also requires transport from nucleus to cytoplasm, thus transcription and translation *cannot* proceed simultaneously.

Eukaryotes do not use the Shine-Dalgarno sequence to initiate translation. There are 5' UTR sequences in eukaryotes that function in starting translation; a common one is the *Kozak sequence*, which is a consensus sequence typically located a few nucleotides before the start codon.

Eukaryotic translation begins with formation of the initiation complex. The assembled complex is recruited to the 5' capped end of the transcript, by an initiation complex of proteins. Additional proteins are recruited (such as a poly-A tail binding protein) and the initiation complex starts scanning the mRNA from the 5' end, looking for a start codon. Once the start codon has been found, the large ribosomal subunit (60S) is recruited and translation can begin.

---

[51] Because the bond between each amino acid and its tRNA is a high-energy bond whose hydrolysis drives peptide bond formation. Remember that the aminoacyl-tRNA bond was formed using the energy of two phosphate bonds from ATP.

[52] There are two phosphate bonds hydrolyzed per amino acid to make the aminoacyl-tRNAs, or 100 for the 50 amino acid polypeptide. Two phosphate bonds are required for each elongation step, one for the entrance of each new aminoacyl-tRNA into the ribosomal A site and the other for translocation. Since there are 49 elongation steps for a 50-amino acid protein, 98 high-energy bonds are hydrolyzed during elongation. Finally, one GTP is hydrolyzed during initiation to position the first tRNA and mRNA on the ribosome, and one GTP is hydrolyzed in termination. Thus, a total of 200 high-energy bonds are required for the translation of a 50-amino acid protein. In other words, it costs 4n high-energy bonds to make a peptide chain, where n is the number of amino acids in the chain.

The order in which the initiation complex is formed is different in eukaryotes. [Are the nascent (newly formed) polypeptide chains emerging from a polyribosome in a eukaryote all the same?[53]] Eukaryotic translation termination involves two release factors, that, like their prokaryotic counterparts, recognize stop codons and work together to end translation and release the completed polypeptide.

- Which one of the following pairs of processes may occur simultaneously on the same RNA molecule in a eukaryotic cell?[54]
  - A) Translation and transcription
  - B) Transcription and splicing
  - C) Splicing and translation
  - D) Messenger RNA degradation and transcription

4.8

Cap-Independent Translation

It was long thought that all eukaryotic translation started at the 5' end of an mRNA. In other words, all eukaryotic transcripts were assumed to be monocistronic, and coded for only one polypeptide chain. It is true that this mechanism is by far the major one in eukaryotic cells. Because of the important role of 5' mRNA cap recognition, it's called **cap-dependent translation**.

However, it's recently been discovered that eukaryotes are sometimes capable of starting translation in the middle of an mRNA molecule, a process called **cap-independent translation** (because the beginning of translation doesn't require the 5' cap of the mRNA). To do this, the transcript must have an internal ribosome entry site, or IRES. This is a specialized nucleotide sequence, and was first discovered in viruses. Since then, IRESs have been found in a number of eukaryotic transcripts. Most code for proteins that help the cell deal with stress, or help activate apoptosis. In other words, the IRESs found so far make sure the cell can make essential proteins when under sub-optimal growth conditions. Cells under stress generally inhibit translation (via inhibiting translation initiation), and cap-independent translation allows the cell to make proteins when doing so is crucial for survival or programmed cell death. Activation of translation using an IRES requires different proteins than normal initiation.

Additional nucleotide sequences have been identified, which allow cap-independent translation in eukaryotes. While some of these are used in molecular biology labs, it's unclear how or if they function in normal eukaryotic cells.

---

[53] In eukaryotes, the answer is: yes, always, because eukaryotic mRNA is monocistronic. In prokaryotes, however, different polypeptides may be translated from a single piece of mRNA, since prokaryotic mRNA is polycistronic.

[54] In order for processes in eukaryotes to occur simultaneously, they must occur in the same compartment. Transcription and splicing both occur in the nucleus and could therefore occur simultaneously (choice **B** is correct). Translation occurs in the cytoplasm, while transcription and splicing occur in the nucleus, thus translation cannot occur at the same time as either of these processes (choices A and C are wrong). mRNA degradation and transcription cannot occur at the same time; if this were true, no mRNA molecules would survive to be translated (choice D is wrong).

4.9 CONTROLLING GENE EXPRESSION

Adult humans have over 220 different types of cells, all with the same genome, but with different attributes such as morphology, lifespan, function, ability to secrete, response to signaling molecules, mobility, etc. These changes are due to differences in gene expression and protein function. In each cell type, some genes are expressed and others are silenced; further, genes that are expressed can have different levels of expression, where in one cell type the gene is expressed at a high level (to produce lots of ncRNA or protein), and in a different cell type the same gene is expressed at a low level. They can also have varying activity, stability, and half-life. These variations in gene expression can be altered using many different mechanisms:

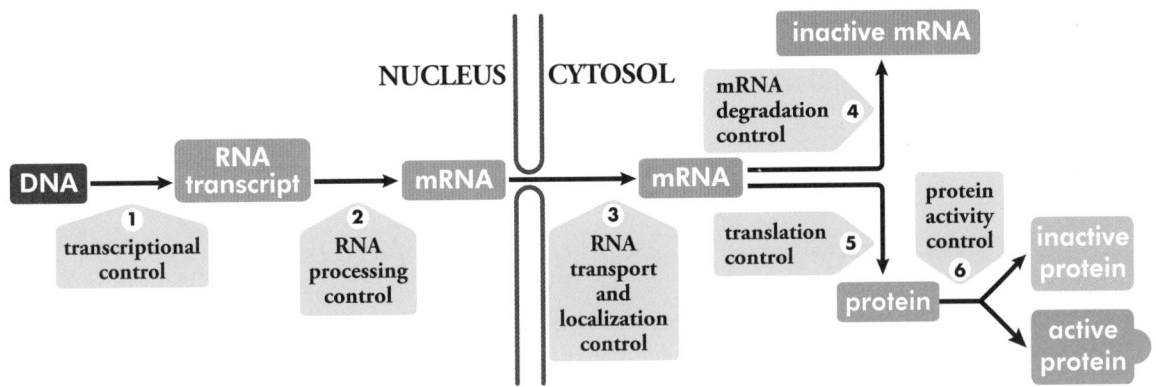

Figure 39   Mechanisms of Controlling Gene Expression in Eukaryotes

Transcription is the principle site of the regulation of gene expression in both eukaryotes and prokaryotes. This means that the amount of each protein made in every cell is affected by the amount of mRNA that gets transcribed. Gene expression can also be controlled epigenetically. Broadly speaking, **epigenetics** focuses on changes in gene expression that are not due to changes in DNA sequences, but are either heritable or have a long-term effect. The three most commonly studied areas in this field are DNA methylation, chromatin remodeling, and RNA interference. Let's look at the regulation of gene expression, starting with DNA and working down toward proteins.

Controlling Gene Expression at the DNA Level

DNA Methylation and Chromatin Remodeling

Both prokaryotic and eukaryotic DNA can be covalently modified by adding a methyl group. Bacteria methylate new DNA shortly after synthesis, and the brief delay is useful in mismatch repair pathways (see above). Methylation can also control gene expression in prokaryotes, either by promoting or inhibiting transcription.

Eukaryotic DNA methylation has been found in every vertebrate genome studied so far. Broadly speaking, it plays an important role in controlling gene expression (especially during embryonic development), and has also been implicated in several diseases.

DNA methylation turns off eukaryotic gene expression two ways:

1) Methylation physically blocks the gene from transcriptional proteins.
2) Certain proteins bind methylated CpG groups and recruit chromatin remodeling proteins that change the winding of DNA around histones.

- Regulation of a gene is examined *in vitro* in the presence and absence of chromatin assembly, and in the presence and absence of a sequence-specific regulator of transcription. Transcription is quantitated after the experiment and the following results are obtained:

	Sequence-Specific Factor	DNA	Relative Amount of Transcription
1.	None	unpackaged	0.74
2.	None	packaged	0.07
3.	Present	unpackaged	1.0
4.	Present	packaged	0.59

Which one of the following conclusions can be drawn from this experiment?[55]

A) The degree of activation by the sequence-specific factor is greater in the presence of chromatin assembly than in its absence.
B) The sequence-specific factor acts to repress transcription.
C) The histones increase the rate of transcription.
D) The sequence-specific factor increases the rate of transition from a closed complex to an open complex.

Gene Dose

One way to increase gene expression is to increase the copy number of a gene by amplification. Increasing gene dose will allow a cell to make large quantities of the corresponding protein. Similarly, gene deletion causes a decrease in gene expression. Both are examples of copy number variation, discussed earlier in Section 4.2.

Imprinting

Genomic imprinting is when only one allele of a gene is expressed. In some situations, the maternal allele is expressed, and in others, the paternal allele is expressed. Imprinted genes tend to be clustered together on chromosomes. Imprinting is a dynamic process and can change from generation to generation. In other words, a gene that is imprinted in an adult may be "unimprinted" and expressed in that adult's offspring. This observation led to the notion that imprinting is an epigenetic process. Silencing of a certain gene involves DNA methylation, histone modification, and binding of long ncRNAs. These epigenetic marks are established in the germline and are maintained throughout life and mitotic divisions.

---

[55] A quick glance at the data indicates that transcription is increased in the presence of the sequence-specific factor (compare lines 1 and 2 with lines 3 and 4; choice B is wrong), and that histones decrease the rate of transcription (packaged DNA has a lower rate of transcription than unpackaged; choice C is wrong). Looking closer, it appears that the sequence specific factor causes an approximate 8-fold increase in the transcription rate of packaged DNA (compare lines 2 and 4), but it doesn't even double the rate of transcription of unpackaged DNA (compare lines 1 and 3). It might be that this occurs because the factor increases the rate of transition to an open complex, but there is no data to support this (choice **A** is a better answer than choice D). Don't confuse "open complex" (which means separated DNA strands) with "unpackaged" (which means not wrapped around histones).

X Chromosome Inactivation

Female mammals have two X chromosomes, one of which is active (called Xa) and one of which is silenced, or inactive (and is called Xi). In humans, X-inactivation occurs early in development, at the blastocyst stage (Chapter 13). Each cell in the inner cell mass randomly inactivates an X chromosome, and this decision is irreversible. This means every cell derived from each cell in the inner cell mass will have the same X chromosome inactivated, however, because each cell makes its own decision, an adult can have different X chromosomes inactivated in different tissues and cells. Because of X-inactivation, all humans have the same number of gene products for the X chromosome; males have only one X chromosome, and females have only one *active* X chromosome. Not all animals behave the same when it comes to X-inactivation. Some animals (such as marsupials) consistently silence one X chromosome; in the case of marsupials, the paternally derived X chromosome is inactivated and the maternal X chromosome is active. Xi is very condensed, and packaged in heterochromatin. It has high levels of DNA methylation.

Controlling Gene Expression at the RNA Level: Regulation of Transcription in Prokaryotes

4.9

Regulation of transcription is the primary method of regulation of gene expression in prokaryotes. One simple mechanism of transcriptional regulation in bacteria is that some promoters are simply stronger than others. The problem with this mechanism of regulation is that it is "pre-set" and cannot respond to changing conditions within the cell. Bacteria also possess far more complex regulatory mechanisms, which activate or suppress transcription depending on current needs for specific gene products. For example, bacteria only produce the enzyme β-galactosidase and other proteins required for lactose catabolism when lactose is present. [Assuming these protein products do not have a harmful effect on the cell, what advantage might there be in turning off the genes when the protein products are not required?[56]]

- Are the terms *polypeptide enzyme* and *gene product* synonymous? Or are there gene products that are not polypeptide enzymes? Are there polypeptides which are not enzymes?[57]

Enzymes involved in anabolism (biosynthesis) should be produced when the item they help make (their product) is scarce. Enzymes involved in catabolism (degradative metabolism) should be produced when the item they help break down (their substrate) is abundant, such as food. Thus, there are two basic ways we can imagine how transcription is regulated. The transcription of enzymes involved in biosynthetic pathways should be inhibited by their product. The transcription of enzymes involved in catabolic pathways should be automatically inhibited whenever the substrate is not around, and activated when it is. That is in fact exactly what happens. Anabolic enzymes whose transcription is inhibited in the presence of excess amounts of product are **repressible**. Catabolic enzymes whose transcription can be stimulated by the abundance of a substrate are called **inducible enzymes**.[58]

---

[56] It takes a great deal of ATP to synthesize RNA and protein, so it's more energy-efficient to transcribe and translate only the proteins that are needed.

[57] They are not synonymous. All polypeptides are gene products, but some gene products are not polypeptides and some polypeptides are not enzymes. Transfer RNA and rRNA are gene products, but not polypeptides. Microfilaments and other elements of the cytoskeleton, as well as collagen and many other polypeptides, are not enzymes.

[58] So note: the default for repressible systems is "ON"; for inducible systems the default is "OFF."

There are two common examples of this. The **lac operon** is inducible, since the enzymes it codes for are part of lactose catabolism, and the **trp operon** is repressible, since the enzymes it codes for mediate tryptophan biosynthesis or anabolism. An operon has two components, a coding sequence for enzymes, and upstream regulatory sequences or control sites. Operons may also include genes for regulatory proteins, such as repressors or activators, but they don't have to. These genes can be located elsewhere in the genome and typically have their own promoters.

The Lac Operon

The lac operon contains several components:

1) P region: the promoter site on DNA to which RNA polymerase binds to initiate transcription of *Y*, *Z*, and *A* genes
2) O region: the operator site to which the Lac repressor binds
3) *Z* gene: codes for the enzyme β-galactosidase, which cleaves lactose into glucose and galactose
4) *Y* gene: codes for permease, a protein which transports lactose into the cell
5) *A* gene: codes for transacetylase, an enzyme which transfers an acetyl group from acetyl-CoA to β-galactosides (note that this function is not required for lactose metabolism)

4.9

Additionally, there are two genes, each with their own promoter, that code for proteins important in the regulation of the lac operon:

1) *crp* gene: located at a distant site, this gene codes for a catabolite activator protein (CAP) and helps couple the lac operon to glucose levels in the cell
2) *I* gene: located at a distant site, this gene codes for the Lac repressor protein

So overall, there are five protein coding genes and two regulatory sequences. Both *crp* and *I* have their own promoters. The protein products of these two genes control gene expression of *Z*, *Y*, and *A*.

Bacterial cells preferentially use glucose as an energy source. This means that in the presence of glucose, the lac operon will be off, or expressed at low amounts (see Figures 40 and 41). This is mediated by the CAP and repressor proteins. Glucose levels control adenylyl cyclase, which converts ATP to cAMP. In high glucose conditions, adenylyl cyclase is inactivated and cAMP levels are very low. In low glucose conditions, the opposite is true: adenylyl cyclase is activated and cAMP levels are high. CAP binds cAMP and this complex binds the promoter of the lac operon (Figure 42). This helps activate RNA polymerase at the lac operon and contributes to the operon being turned on when glucose levels are low.

The *I* gene codes for a repressor protein, which binds the operator of the lac operon. This prevents RNA pol from binding the promoter and transcribing *Z*, *Y*, and *A* genes, thereby blocking transcription of the operon when lactose is absent (Figure 40). The repressor protein can also bind lactose, and this blocks its activity on the operator. This binding is allosteric, and it causes a conformational change in the tertiary structure of the repressor protein, such that it is no longer capable of binding to the operator. As a consequence, it falls off the DNA (Figures 41 and 42).

High transcription of *Z*, *Y*, and *A* genes occurs when glucose is absent and lactose is present (Figure 42, page 116). Low glucose results in an increased amount of cAMP, which binds to CAP and helps activate RNA polymerase activity at the lac operon. Lactose presence means the Lac repressor protein is unable to bind the lac operator and negatively regulate transcription; thus, the polycistronic mRNA is transcribed at high levels. When the supply of lactose becomes very scarce, there isn't enough to bind to the repressors, and most of the repressor proteins return to their original structure. They now rebind to the operator, decreasing transcription of *Z*, *Y*, and *A* genes.

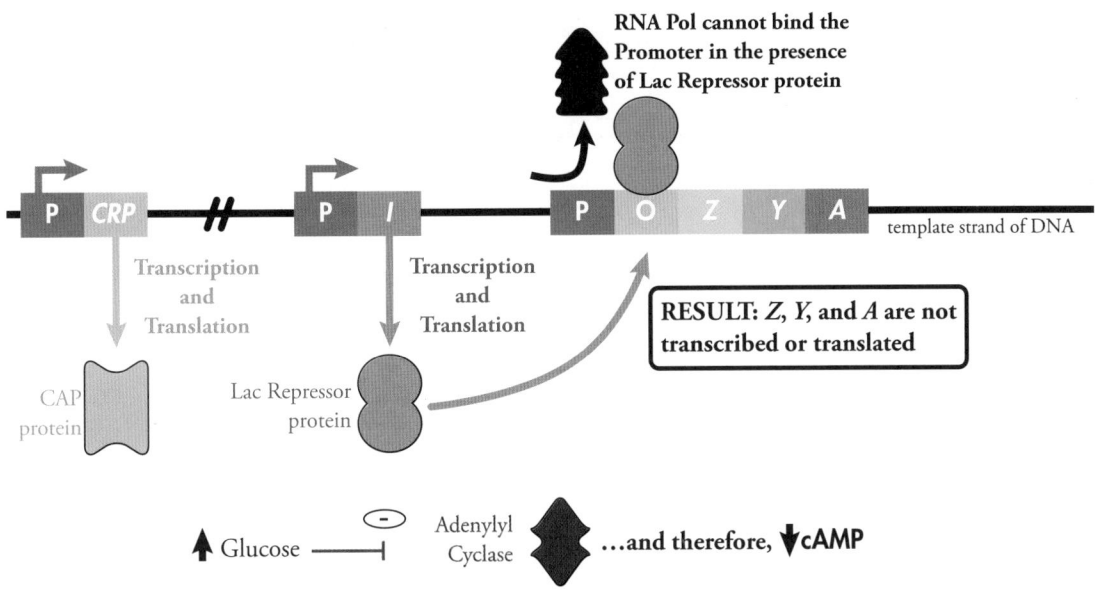

Figure 40   The Lac Operon in the Presence of Glucose and Absence of Lactose

4.9

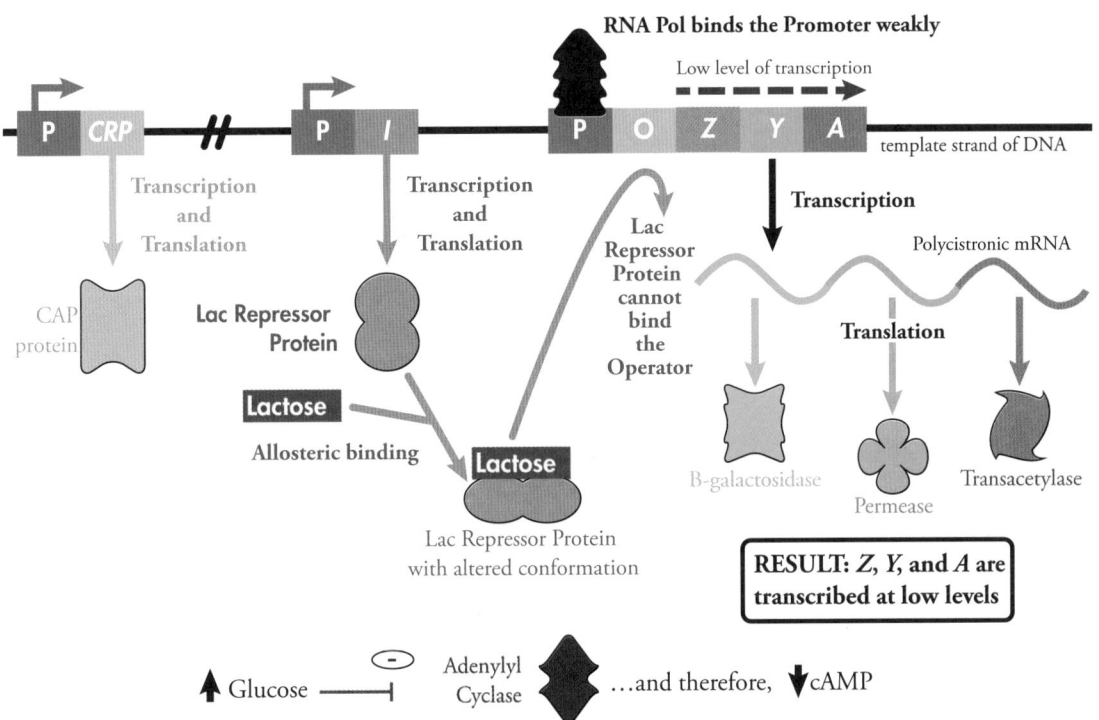

Figure 41   The Lac Operon in the Presence of both Glucose and Lactose

4.9

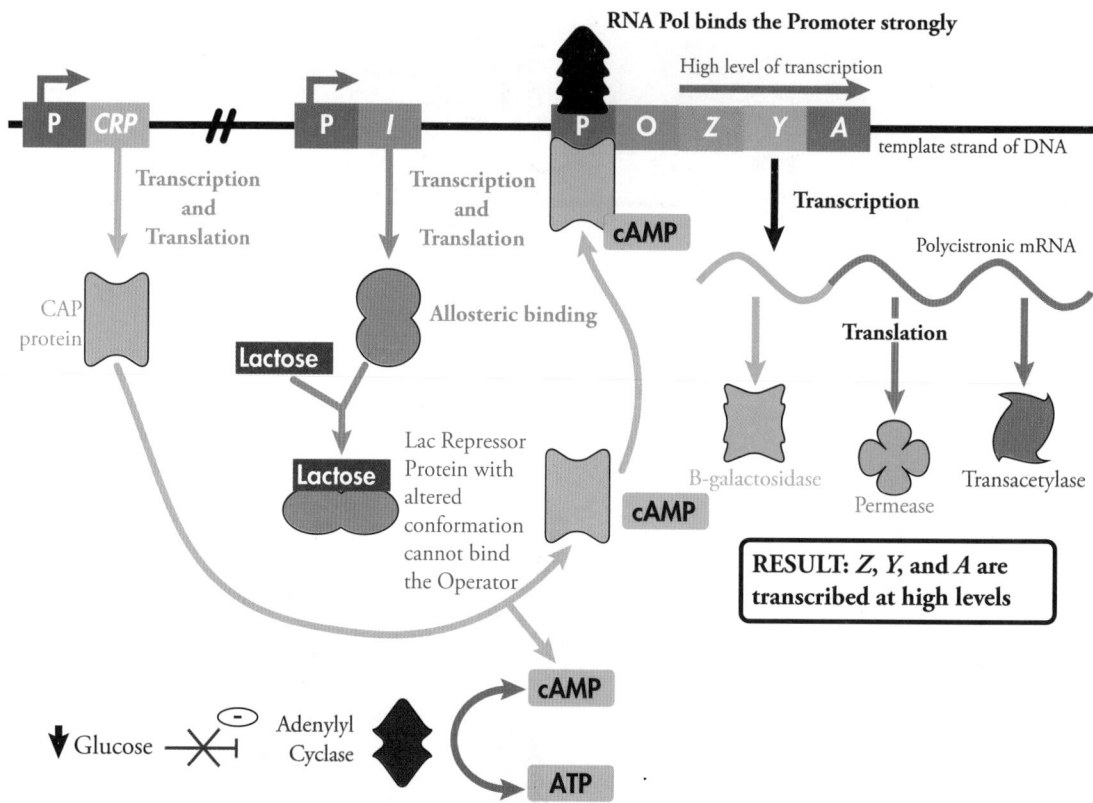

Figure 42 The Lac Operon in the Absence of Glucose and Presence of Lactose

- If the operator is mutated so that the lac repressor can no longer bind, what effect will this have on transcription?[59]

    A) Transcription of the *Z* gene will be activated, and the *Y* and *A* genes will not be affected.
    B) None of the genes will be transcribed, regardless of the presence or absence of lac repressor.
    C) Transcription will still be activated by lactose.
    D) All three genes will be expressed constitutively, regardless of the presence of lactose.

The Trp Operon

Bacteria use a five enzyme synthetic pathway to make the amino acid tryptophan from chorismic acid. In the presence of tryptophan, there is little point in making these enzymes, so the repressor protein is coded by the *trpR* gene (Figure 43). The repressor binds tryptophan when it is present, and the two together then bind the operator to turn off transcription of the other five trp genes.

---

[59] If the repressor cannot bind to the operator, nothing will prevent RNA polymerase from transcribing all the genes on the operon in an unregulated, constitutive (or continuous) fashion (choice **D** is true and choice B is false). All genes on the operon are expressed or repressed together (choice A is false), and lactose will no longer have any effect (the expression of the genes is unregulated, so choice C is false).

With no tryptophan present, the repressor protein cannot bind the operator. Without this block, RNA polymerase transcribes the five genes in the trp operon, and the five gene products allow the cell to make tryptophan. This is an example of anabolic repressible transcription.

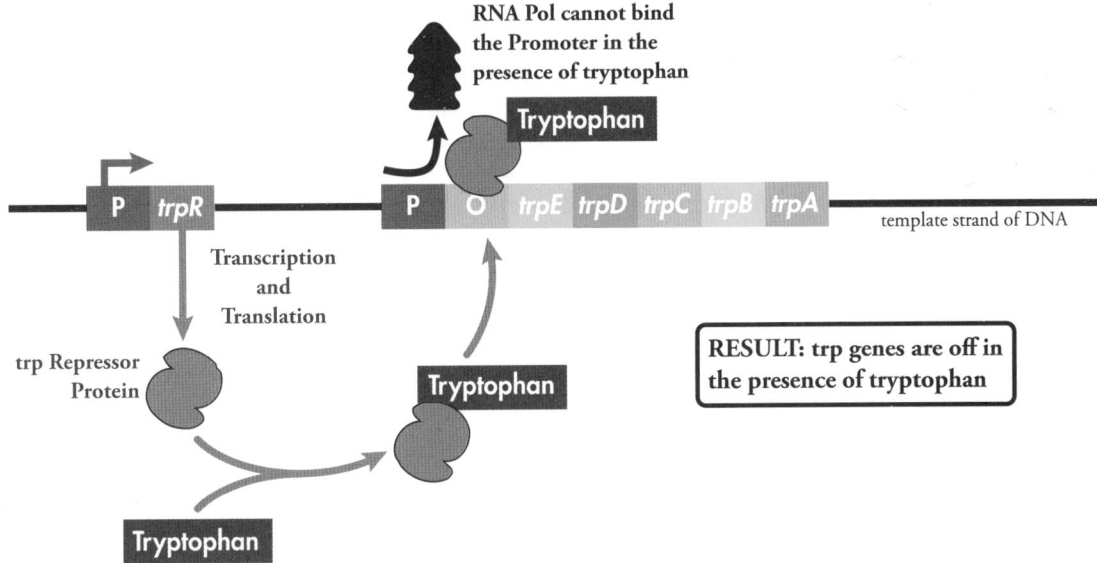

Figure 43 The Trp Operon in the Presence of Tryptophan

Control of Gene Expression at the RNA Level: Regulation of Transcription in Eukaryotes

Given the complexity of eukaryotes compared to prokaryotes, it is not surprising that the regulation of eukaryotic transcription is also more complex. Most of this regulation happens at initiation.

For protein-coding genes, there are upstream control elements (UCEs), usually about 200 bases upstream of the initiation site, a core promoter containing binding sites for the basal transcription complex and RNA polymerase II (about 50 bases upstream of the transcription start site), and a TATA box at –25. The TATA box is a highly conserved DNA recognition sequence for the TATA box binding protein (TBP). Binding of TBP to the TATA box initiates transcription complex assembly at the promoter.

Enhancer sequences in DNA are bound by **activator proteins**, and this is another kind of transcriptional regulation. The enhancer may be located many thousands of base pairs away from a promoter (either upstream or downstream) and still regulate transcription. This is likely done by DNA looping so enhancers and their activator proteins can get close to transcriptional machinery.

Eukaryotes also have **gene repressor proteins**, which inhibit transcription; this can also be done by modifying chromatin structure. *Transcription factors* have DNA-binding domains and are crucial in transcription regulation. They can bind promoters or other regulatory sequences. In fact, in many cases, transcription levels in eukaryotes are controlled by huge committees of proteins. This produces a combinatorial effect, where each protein contributes to regulation, and can itself be regulated. These complex networks help link transcription to cell signaling and status. The binding of transcriptional machinery to DNA is often regulated by extracellular signals. For example, steroid hormones bind to receptors in the cell, and this sends the receptor to the nucleus. The complex binds DNA to regulate transcription. [If a mutation in a eukaryotic fat cell reduces the level of several proteins related to fat metabolism, does this mean the proteins are encoded by the same mRNA?[60]]

Beyond regulating the initiation of transcription, eukaryotes employ several other methods of transcriptional regulation, including:

- **RNA Translocation**: mRNA transcripts must be exported from the nucleus to the cytoplasm and can also be transported to different areas of the cell. They are translationally silent while this is happening. This system is especially important in cells that have a high level of polarity, where one area or end of the cell is distinctly different from the other. For example, neurons have polarity, and some transcripts are transported to the dendrites, while others stay in the soma. This is a way of controlling gene expression: mRNA transcripts aren't translated into proteins until they are localized properly in the cell.
- **mRNA Surveillance**: Cells closely monitor mRNA molecules to ensure that only high-quality mRNA transcripts are read by the ribosome. Defective transcripts (such as those with premature stop codons, or those without stop codons at all) and stalled transcripts (where the ribosome is stalled in translation) are degraded.
- **RNA Interference**: RNA interference (RNAi) is a way to silence gene expression after a transcript has been made. It is mediated by miRNA and siRNA (Section 4.7). Molecular biology labs often use the RNAi system experimentally, as a way to decrease protein expression (see Appendix). Generally speaking, the siRNAs bind complementary sequences on mRNAs, and this ds-RNA is then degraded. The amount of transcript in the cell decreases, and gene expression is thus negatively regulated.

Control of Gene Expression at the Protein Level: Translation Initiation

We've already discussed the complex process of assembling translational machinery. In both prokaryotes and eukaryotes, this is a highly regulated process that links protein synthesis with upstream signaling pathways. Otherwise there is little control at the level of translation.

Post-Translational Modification

Newly synthesized proteins released from the ribosome are rarely able to function. They need to be correctly folded, modified, or processed, and transported to where they function in the cell. These modifications are called post-translational events, since they occur after protein synthesis.

---

[60] No, it does not. *Eukaryotic mRNA is monocistronic.* A more likely explanation is that a number of different genes located throughout the genome have related regulatory sequences that bind the same sequence-specific transcription factors. This is the means used by eukaryotes to achieve coordinated expression of genes. Related proteins are clumped together on the same piece of mRNA in prokaryotes only.

Protein Folding

First, the newly synthesized nascent protein is folded into its correct three-dimensional shape. This is accomplished by a family of proteins called **chaperones**. If folded correctly, the protein is said to be in its native conformation. If the protein is unfolded or misfolded, it's said to be in its non-native state. Chaperone proteins are found across all types of organisms (from bacteria to plants to mammals), and also function in assembly or folding of other macromolecular structures. For example, chaperone proteins assist in nucleosome assembly from folded histones and DNA. In eukaryotic cells, chaperones are found in many subcellular compartments.

Covalent Modification

Many proteins are covalently modified. Some have hydrophobic groups added to facilitate membrane localization. For example, the addition of a fatty acid can target a protein to a membrane (either the plasma membrane or an organelle membrane).

Smaller chemical groups can also be added. For example, proteins can be:

- Acetylated: addition of an acetyl group ($-C(O)CH_3$), usually at the N-terminus of a protein, or at a lysine amino acid
- Formylated: addition of a formyl group ($-C(O)H$)
- Alkylated: addition of an alkyl group (such as methyl, ethyl, etc.). Methylation is a common post-translational modification, and is usually done to lysine or arginine amino acids.
- Glycosylated: addition of a glycosyl group to arginine, asparagine, cysteine, serine, threonine, tyrosine, or tryptophan amino acids. A glycosyl group is the substituent form of a cyclic mono- , di-, or oligosaccharide. This results in a glycoprotein.
- Phosphorylated: addition of a phosphate group (PO_4^{3-}) to a serine, threonine, tyrosine, or histidine amino acid
- Sulphated: addition of a sulphate group (SO_4^{2-}) to a tyrosine amino acid

Proteins can also be linked to other proteins. For example, in ubiquitination, proteins are covalently linked to ubiquitin.

There are many other examples of protein covalent modification. Overall, these modifications can have many effects on a protein and its function. They can change protein subcellular localization, target a protein for degradation, change interactions between proteins and other molecules, activate or inhibit enzyme activity, or change enzyme affinity for substrates. These modifications are typically studied in the lab using mass spectrometry (see *MCAT Organic Chemistry Review*), western blotting, or eastern blotting (see Appendix).

Processing

Many proteins require cleavage of some sort to become mature or functional. Cleavage can occur at either end of a peptide chain, or in the middle. Protein precursors are often used when the mature protein may be dangerous to the organism. Because the precursor is already made, it allows large quantities of mature protein to be available on short notice. Enzyme precursors are called **zymogens** or **proenzymes**.

A well-known example of post-translational processing is insulin. Insulin is made from a prohormone (Figure 44, next page); preproinsulin is the primary translational product of the human *INS* gene. This peptide is 110 amino acids in length. To form proinsulin, an N-terminus signal peptide is removed and disulphide bonds form in the endoplasmic reticulum. Three cleavage events are necessary to process proinsulin: the C peptide is removed by a family of enzymes called proprotein convertases, and a dipeptide fragment is removed from the C-terminus of the B chain peptide by a carboxypeptidase. These cleavage events occur in a secretory vesicle. The biological effects of insulin are well known, but it's recently been shown that peptide C also has signaling properties.

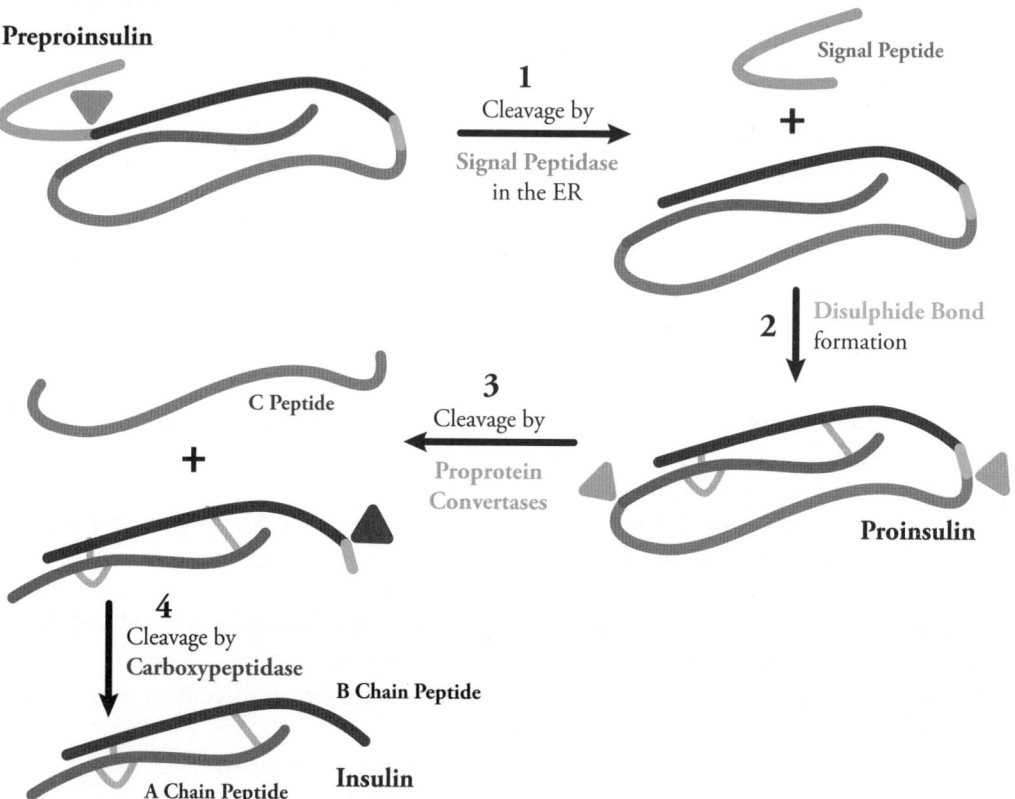

Figure 44   Insulin Processing: An Example of Post-Translational Modification

4.10 RETURN TO GENE STRUCTURE: A SUMMARY

Now that we have been through all the processes that a cell uses to turn a gene into a protein, and control this process, let's review the components once again (Figure 45). Transcription begins at a start site but needs a promoter upstream of this. It ends at a termination signal. The RNA transcript contains the open reading frame (which goes from start codon to stop codon), as well as both 5' and 3' regulatory regions.

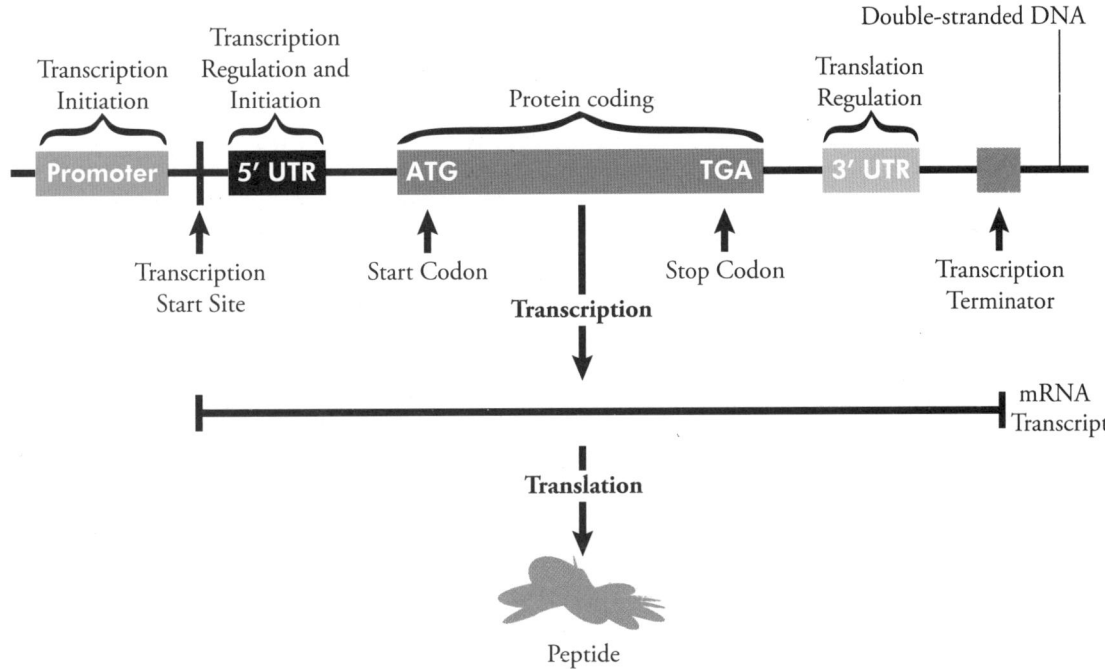

Figure 45 Gene Structure and Protein Expression

DNA replication, transcription, and translation have many similarities and some differences, and these are summarized in Table 1.

Table 1   A Review of Molecular Biology Processes

	DNA Replication	Transcription	Translation
Signal to get ready	ORI	Promoter	• Shine-Dalgarno (prok) • Kozak sequence (euk) • these are found in 5'UTR (untranslated region)
Signal to start	ORI	Start site	AUG start codon
Key synthesis enzyme	DNA polymerase	RNA polymerase	Ribosome (made of rRNA and peptides)
Other important enzymes	Helicase Topoisomerase SSBPs Primase Ligase Telomerase	Spliceosome machinery	Aminoacyl tRNA synthetases Initiation factors Elongation factors Release factors
Template molecule	DNA	DNA	mRNA
Read direction	3' to 5' on the DNA template	3' to 5' on the DNA template	5' to 3' on the RNA template
Molecule synthesized	DNA	RNA (mRNA in prok, hnRNA in euk)	Peptides
Build direction	5' to 3'	5' to 3'	N-terminus to C-terminus
Prokaryotic location	Cytoplasm	Cytoplasm	Cytoplasm
Eukaryotic location	Nucleus	Nucleus	Cytoplasm
Signal to stop	When the replication bubbles or newly synthesized strands meet and are ligated together	Transcription stop sequence or poly-A sequence	Stop codon (UAG, UGA, UAA)

4.10

Chapter 4 Summary

- DNA is the fundamental unit of inheritance in cells.

- DNA and RNA are polymers, made of nucleotide monomers. A nucleotide contains phosphate group(s), a sugar (either deoxyribose for DNA or ribose for RNA), and a nitrogenous base, either a purine (adenine or guanine) or a pyrimidine (thymine, cytosine, or uracil).

- In DNA, adenine always pairs with thymine via two hydrogen bonds, and cytosine always pairs with guanine via three hydrogen bonds.

- Uracil replaces thymine in RNA, and the ribose in RNA has an OH group on carbon 2.

- DNA is supercoiled in prokaryotes and packaged around histone proteins in eukaryotes.

- Eukaryotic DNA is divided into several linear chromosomes which have unique structures, including the long (q) and short (p) arms, centromere and telomeres on the ends.

- Genomes have extensive variation, including single nucleotide polymorphisms and copy number variation; transposons are mobile genetic elements which also contribute to genomic variation.

- Mutations can occur spontaneously, or can be caused by environmental factors (such as ionizing radiation), chemicals, or biological agents.

- Point mutations are classified based on their effect on the DNA (transition/transversion) or their effect on the amino acid sequence (missense, nonsense, or silent).

- Frameshift mutations are caused by insertions or deletions in the DNA base sequence that affect the reading frame of a gene. These are generally very serious mutations because they affect every amino acid codon from the point of the mutation on.

- Other types of mutations include inversions, translocations, and rearrangements.

- Transposons are mobile genetic elements that can "jump" from chromosome to chromosome. This can lead to deletions, insertions, and mutations. They consist of two inverted repeats flanking the gene for transposase and may include other genes as well.

- DNA replication occurs in the S-phase of the cell cycle and is semiconservative in nature.

- Several enzymes are involved in DNA replication. Helicases unwind the parental DNA at the origin of replication. Primases synthesize an RNA primer. DNA polymerase synthesizes new DNA, proofreads, and replaces the RNA primer. DNA ligase attaches the Okazaki fragments in the lagging strand.

- Cells have developed several ways to fix mutations, including: direct reversal, homology-dependent repair pathways (such as excision repair and post-replication repair), double-strand break repair (such as homologous recombination and nonhomologous end joining), and SOS repair.

- Transcription is the first part of protein synthesis; it is the creation of an RNA transcript by an RNA polymerase that reads the DNA template. Translation is the second part of protein synthesis; it is the creation of a polypeptide chain by ribosomes that read the mRNA transcript.

- There are several types of RNA that do not encode proteins. Some are directly involved in translation (rRNA and tRNA), while others play a role in gene expression (snRNA, miRNA, siRNA).

- Key info about prokaryotes: theta replication, genome is a single circular piece of DNA, three different DNA polymerases, one RNA polymerase, no mRNA processing, polycistronic mRNA, simultaneous transcription/translation, smaller ribosomes.

- Key info about eukaryotes: replication bubbles, genome is several linear pieces of DNA, one DNA polymerase, three RNA polymerases, capping, tailing, and splicing of mRNA prior to translation, monocistronic mRNA, transcription in nucleus, translation in cytosol, larger ribosomes.

CHAPTER 4 FREESTANDING PRACTICE QUESTIONS

1. A competitive inhibitor of eukaryotic RNA polymerase III would have the greatest effect on:

A) replication.
B) reverse transcription.
C). translation.
D) mutation.

2. In the lac operon, transcription is regulated by a repressor protein and only takes place in the presence of lactose. Which of the following statements is correct?

A) The repressor protein binds to the promoter site to inhibit transcription.
B) Lactose binds to the promoter site to initiate transcription.
C) Lactose binds to the repressor protein to inhibit transcription.
D) The repressor protein binds the operator site to inhibit transcription.

3. Which of the following could not be caused by a single point mutation in the DNA?

A) Ala-Gln-Cys-Asp-Leu → Ala-Gln
B) Ala-Gln-Cys-Asp-Leu → Ala-Gln-Cys-Asp-Leu
C) Ala-Gln-Cys-Asp-Leu → Ala-Gln-Cys-His-Lys
D) Ala-Gln-Cys-Asp-Leu → Ala-Gln-Cys-His-Leu

4. Which of the following is/are true with respect to eukaryotic mRNA?

  I.   Monocistronic
  II. Transcription stops at the stop codon
  III. Has the same sequence as the template DNA that it was transcribed from

A) I only
B) I and II
C) II and III
D) I, II, and III

5. Which of the following is NOT a similarity between replication and transcription?

A) Both processes occur with the same fidelity.
B) Polymerization in both processes is based on reading a template.
C) A pyrophosphate is removed from every nucleotide as polymerization occurs.
D) Both processes occur in the 5' to 3' direction.

6. Which of the following functions is NOT typically attributed to small nuclear RNA (snRNA)?

A) Processing of pre-mRNA
B) Regulation of transcription factors
C) Coordinating amino acid addition in translation
D) Maintaining telomeres

7. Organisms with a higher degree of complexity do not necessarily have more diverse genomes than less complex organisms, in spite of the need for a greater diversity of proteins. Post-translational modification is one method used by more complex organisms to produce proteins that serve a wider variety of distinct functions. Which of the following explains this phenomenon?

A) The genome itself is manipulated by the agents responsible for post-translational modification in order to yield an increase in the number of transcriptional products.
B) Post-translational modification alters the structures and functions of proteins produced from a relatively smaller number of genes.
C) hnRNA is modified by the actions of post-transcriptional agents to provide increased variety in the mRNA used for translation.
D) Post-translational modifications enhance the ability of the ribosome to produce distinct protein products.

CHAPTER 4 PRACTICE PASSAGE

Protein synthesis involves a number of complex steps, from transcription of the gene through to translation and post-translational modification. After mRNA is transcribed in eukaryotes, it must be processed (capped, poly-A tailed, and spliced) before it can be translated. Prokaryotes do not need to process their mRNA.

Due to the exonuclease activity of DNA polymerase, DNA replication is generally a high-fidelity process. Random errors occasionally occur and these mutations are classified as *frameshift mutations* (insertions or deletions in the base sequence) or *point mutations* (a single base pair change). Any mutation is subject to natural selection, with advantageous mutations preserved and the most deleterious mutations eliminated quickly. Thus, areas of the genome that appear to evolve very slowly (i.e., have a slower rate of mutation than other areas) do not actually have a slower rate; rather, that area is highly critical to normal functioning of the organism involved.

Point mutations can be further classified by their final effect on the mature protein. Because of the redundancy of the genetic code, some mutations do not alter the final amino acid sequence of the protein and are referred to as *silent mutations*. However, it was discovered that all redundant codons are not equal; some are used preferentially to enhance the speed or accuracy of protein translation. tRNAs corresponding to redundant codons are not found equally in the cell; some tRNAs are more common than others. Silent mutations can cause phenotypic changes by altering mRNA stem-and-loop folding, half-life, and splicing sites. Thus, mutations formerly considered "silent" have now been implicated in a number of different disorders, such as Marfan syndrome, phenylketonuria, Seckel syndrome, and increased pain sensitivity.

1st Position (5' End)	2nd Position				3rd Position (3' End)
	U	C	A	G	
U	Phe	Ser	Tyr	Cys	U
	Phe	Ser	Tyr	Cys	C
	Leu	Ser	Stop	Stop	A
	Leu	Ser	Stop	Trp	G
C	Leu	Pro	His	Arg	U
	Leu	Pro	His	Arg	C
	Leu	Pro	Gln	Arg	A
	Leu	Pro	Gln	Arg	G
A	Ile	Thr	Asn	Ser	U
	Ile	Thr	Asn	Ser	C
	Ile	Thr	Lys	Arg	A
	Met	Thr	Lys	Arg	G
G	Val	Ala	Asp	Gly	U
	Val	Ala	Asp	Gly	C
	Val	Ala	Glu	Gly	A
	Val	Ala	Glu	Gly	G

Figure 1   The Genetic Code

1. Based on information in the passage, genes coding for particularly abundant proteins in a cell would have all of the following EXCEPT:

A) codons corresponding to abundant tRNAs.
B) equal use of redundant codons.
C) greater use of preferential codons.
D) high-fidelity replication.

2. Which of following could account for the changes brought on by silent mutations in both eukaryotes and prokaryotes?

    I.   Decrease in mRNA half-life
    II.   Disruption of splicing sites
    III. Changes in mRNA folding

A) I and II only
B) II and III only
C) I and III only
D) I, II, and III

3. Researchers studying a gene associated with breast cancer found that regions where silent mutations occur ("silent sites") in this gene evolve very slowly compared to other regions within this gene. Comparisons were made between mice and humans. Which of the following is most likely true about this gene?

A) Mutations at other sites are more detrimental to the health of the organism than mutations at the silent sites.
B) Mutations at the silent sites increase the accuracy of mRNA splicing.
C) Mutations within the silent sites often lead to the death of the organism.
D) The silent sites are less critical to overall function than the other sites.

4. Researchers studying the DNA polymerase activity in several different organisms discovered a mutant *E. coli* polymerase that retained almost 100% of wild-type activity. Which of the following active-site missense mutations is LEAST likely to affect enzyme activity?

A) A → D
B) V → L
C) R → G
D) L → W

5. Point mutations are found in three subclasses: nonsense mutations, missense mutations, and silent mutations. Which of the following represents a silent mutation?

A) UGC to UGA
B) UUA to CUA
C) CAC to CAA
D) CAU to CUU

6. How could changing the half-life of an mRNA lead to phenotypic changes?

A) A shorter mRNA half-life would lead to a truncated protein.
B) A longer mRNA half-life would increase the amount of time the mRNA stays bound to the template strand of DNA, and reduce the amount of protein translated.
C) Differences in mRNA folding could alter the rates of translation.
D) More or less of the protein encoded by that mRNA would be translated.

SOLUTIONS TO CHAPTER 4 FREESTANDING PRACTICE QUESTIONS

1. **C** RNA polymerase III transcribes transfer RNA (tRNA), which then carries amino acids to ribosomes for use in translation. This polymerase plays no role in replication (choice A is wrong), and reverse transcription uses a DNA polymerase (in any case, it is not carried out by eukaryotes; choice B is wrong). Blocking the action of this enzyme would not alter the base sequence, so mutation would not be affected (choice D is wrong).

2. **D** The lac operon includes an operator site to which a repressor protein binds (choice A is wrong). The operator site is located between the promoter region and the start transcription site. When the repressor is bound, RNA polymerase (which binds to the promoter site; choice B is wrong) cannot move forward to the start site; thus, transcription is inhibited (choice D is correct). Lactose binds to the repressor protein at an allosteric site, causing a conformational change so that the repressor protein can no longer bind to the operator. When this happens, RNA polymerase can move forward to the start site and transcription will occur (choice C is wrong).

3. **C** A point mutation is a single base pair substitution. There are few possibilities that can result if a single base is substituted. If the new codon is now a stop codon, then the polypeptide will be truncated (choice A could result from a point mutation and can be eliminated). If the new codon codes for the same amino acid as before the mutation, then a silent point mutation has occurred and no change will be seen in the amino acid sequence (choice B could result from a point mutation and can be eliminated). If the mutation leads to a single new amino acid, then a missense point mutation has occurred (choice D could result from a point mutation and can be eliminated). However, if more than one base was changed, or bases were added/deleted (a frameshift mutation), this would lead to multiple new amino acids (choice C could not result from a point mutation and is the correct answer choice).

4. **A** Item I is true: Eukaryotic mRNA is monocistronic, meaning that only one protein is transcribed from each mRNA (choice C can be eliminated). Item II is false: transcription does not stop at a stop codon; *translation* stops at a stop codon (choices B and D can be eliminated, and choice A is the correct answer). Transcription stops when a termination signal is reached. Item III is also false: when mRNA is transcribed, it is complementary to the template strand, not identical to it.

5. **A** Fidelity refers to accuracy. Because RNA polymerases do not proofread, transcription is less accurate (i.e., a lower-fidelity process; choice A is not a similarity and is the correct answer choice). Both replication and transcription use DNA as a template (choice B is a similarity and can be eliminated). In both cases, the removal of pyrophosphate provides the energy for polymerization to occur (choice C is a similarity and can be eliminated). Lastly, although RNA polymerase (in transcription) and DNA polymerase (in replication) move along the parent chain in the 3' → 5' direction, the new chain is made in the 5' → 3' direction.

6. **C** Transfer RNA (tRNA), not snRNA, is typically involved in the process of coordinating the amino acids that are added to a growing protein during translation (choice C is not a function of snRNA and is the correct answer choice). It should also be noted that translation is NOT taking place in the nucleus, which is the location of snRNA. Processing of

pre-mRNA, regulation of transcription factors, and maintenance of telomeres are all functions typically attributed to snRNA and take place in the nucleus (choices A, B, and D are all functions that include snRNAs and can be eliminated).

7. **B** Post-translational modification is, by definition, the manipulation of protein products after translation; the primary purpose of these modifications is to allow for a large increase in the number of possible protein products from a relatively small genome (choice B is correct). The genome itself is not changed during post-translational modification (choice A is wrong). hnRNA is processed in the nucleus after transcription to yield a variety of mRNA transcripts (and this is the other primary way that protein diversity can be achieved), but the question specifically asks about post-translational modification, not post-transcriptional effects (choice C is wrong). The ribosome is essentially a factory that reads the code on an mRNA and links amino acids together, and that's it. Ribosomes create the primary protein structure; this IS translation. Post-translational modification happens after this step (choice D is wrong).

SOLUTIONS TO CHAPTER 4 PRACTICE PASSAGE

1. **B** Proteins that are abundant require speed and accuracy during translation, and the passage states that this can be accomplished by using preferential codons (choice C is true and can be eliminated; choice B is false and the correct answer choice). Likewise, codons corresponding to abundant tRNAs would be used instead of those corresponding to the more rare tRNAs (choice A is true and can be eliminated). Choice D is true of all genes, abundant proteins or not (choice D can be eliminated).

2. **C** The passage states that silent mutations can lead to all three of the Roman numeral items listed; however, prokaryotes do not undergo mRNA splicing. Thus, Item I is true for both eukaryotes and prokaryotes (choice B can be eliminated), Item II is only true for eukaryotes (choices A and D can be eliminated), and Item III is true for both.

3. **C** According to the passage, areas of the genome that appear to evolve very slowly are highly critical to normal functioning of the organism. Thus, mutations in these areas most likely disrupt function in a major way, leading to the death of the organism and thus the loss of the mutation (hence the reason it appears to evolve very slowly; choice C is correct, and choice D is wrong). If other sites appear to evolve more quickly, mutations at those sites must be less detrimental (choice A is wrong). If mutations at the silent sites increase the accuracy of mRNA splicing, this would be beneficial and thus preserved (choice B is wrong). Note that the information on breast cancer and humans versus mice is not necessary to answer the question and is there solely to distract you. Focus on what the question is asking you.

4. **B** In order for a mutation to have a minimal effect on enzyme activity, it must be a relatively conservative mutation. Both valine (V) and leucine (L) are nonpolar amino acids; the substitution of L for V is not likely to have a significant effect on enzyme activity (choice B is correct). Alanine (A) is nonpolar, and aspartic acid (D) is acidic (and polar). The substitution of D for A would likely be disruptive (choice A is wrong). Arginine (R) is basic (polar)

and glycine (G) is nonpolar; the substitution of G for R would likely be disruptive (choice C is wrong). Leucine (L) is nonpolar, as is tryptophan (W); however, the structure of tryptophan is significantly different than leucine. Tryptophan has a large double-ring side chain, while the side chain of leucine is a short hydrocarbon, $-CH_2CH(CH_3)_2$, very similar to valine, $-CH(CH_3)_2$. The substitution of leucine for valine is likely to be much better tolerated than the substitution of tryptophan for leucine (choice B is better than choice D).

5. **B**   Nonsense mutations convert a codon for an amino acid into a stop codon, missense mutations lead to amino acid substitutions, and silent mutations do not affect the amino acid sequence of a protein. To answer this question, you must use the genetic code in Figure 1. UGC codes for cysteine and UGA is a STOP codon, making this a nonsense mutation (choice A is wrong). The codons UUA and CUA both code for leucine, making this a silent mutation (choice B is correct). CAC codes for histidine and CAA codes for glutamine; this is a missense mutation (choice C is wrong). CAU codes for histidine and CUU codes for leucine; this is also a missense mutation (choice D is wrong).

6. **D**   If the half-life of an mRNA is increased, it will stay in the cell longer and more of the protein would be translated. Likewise, if the mRNA's half-life is decreased, it will be eliminated from the cell more quickly, and less of the protein would be translated. The mRNA half-life has nothing to do with the length of the protein; protein size is dictated by the length of the open reading frame on the mRNA molecule and the number of codons in the translated region (choice A is wrong). mRNA does not stay bound to the DNA template strand for any length of time, regardless of half-life. As mRNA is transcribed, the DNA helix reforms immediately behind it, releasing the mRNA from the transcription bubble as it is synthesized (choice B is wrong). Choice C is a true statement but does not address the question of half-life (choice C is wrong).

Chapter 5
Microbiology

A milestone in microbiology was the demonstration by Louis Pasteur in 1861 that microbes do not spontaneously arise in boiled broth; they must arrive there by contamination. This put the last nail in the coffin of the idea of spontaneous generation of life. Another major contribution to the golden age of microbiology was the isolation of the bacteria responsible for anthrax in 1876 by a physician named Robert Koch. This and other experiments led to the germ theory of disease, the idea that disease was not caused by bad air ("malaria"), but by microorganisms. In this chapter, we will examine three major groups of disease-causing organisms, beginning with the smallest (viruses) and ending with the largest (fungi—which are often not microscopic at all but visible with the naked eye).

5.1   VIRUSES

With the identification of bacteria as the cause of anthrax and other diseases, medical science appeared in the late 1800s to be headed toward explanation of all infectious disease. Researchers soon found, however, that some infectious agents could not be trapped by passage through filters in the same manner as bacteria. These agents also proved invisible to the light microscope, unlike bacteria. With the advent of electron microscopy, the tiny infectious agents known as **viruses** were finally visualized. Today, molecular biology has shed great light onto viruses, down to the nucleotide sequence of entire viral genomes. However, viruses such as HIV still remain one of the most serious threats to health, indicating there is still much to learn.

Viruses infect all life forms on Earth, including plants, animals, protists, and bacteria. A virus is an **obligate intracellular parasite**. As such, they are only able (*obligated*) to reproduce within (*intra*) cells. While within cells, viruses have some of the attributes of living organisms, such as the ability to reproduce; but outside cells, viruses are without activity. Viruses on their own are unable to perform any of the chemical reactions characteristic of life, such as synthesis of ATP and macromolecules.[1] *Viruses are not cells or even living organisms.* To reproduce, they commandeer the cellular machinery of the host they infect and use it to manufacture copies of themselves. In the final analysis, a virus is nothing more than a package of nucleic acid that says: "Pick me up and reproduce me." Remember this crucial definition: a virus is an obligate intracellular parasite that relies on host machinery whenever possible. In the following sections, we will look at some of the variations on this basic theme.

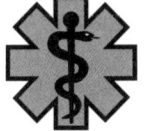

- Cyanide (an inhibitor of the electron transport chain) is added to a culture of virus-infected mammalian cells. The virus has none of the components of electron transport or any other proteins that are inhibited by cyanide. Which one of the following best describes the effect of cyanide?[2]
    - A) The mammalian cells will die, and all viruses will be destroyed as well, regardless of their stage of development.
    - B) Mammalian cells are killed, and viral replication halted, but the culture remains infectious.
    - C) Mammalian cells stop growing, and viral replication is unaffected.
    - D) Mammalian cells continue to grow, but viral replication is halted.

Viral Structure and Function

The structure of viruses reflects their life cycle. In general, all viruses possess a nucleic acid genome packaged in a protein shell. The exterior protein packaging helps to convey the genome from one cell to infect other cells. Once in a cell, the viral genome directs the production of new copies of the genome and of the

---

[1] Note, however, that some viruses store some ATP in their capsids. They acquired this ATP from the previous host and typically use it to power penetration (see below).

[2] The mammalian cells are directly dependent on the ATP generated by the electron transport chain, so if cyanide inhibits the electron transport chain, the mammalian cells will die (choice D is wrong). The viruses are dependent on the mammalian cells for the ATP and enzymes needed for replication, so if the mammalian cells die, viral replication will stop (choice C is wrong). However, any viruses that had already completed the replication process when the cyanide was added will not be affected, and will remain infectious (choice **B** is correct, and choice A is wrong).

protein packaging needed to produce more virus. However, the nature of the genome, the protein packaging, and the viral life cycle vary tremendously between different viruses.

A viral genome may consist of either DNA *or* RNA that is either single- *or* double-stranded and is either linear *or* circular. Viruses utilize virtually every conceivable form of nucleic acid as their genome. However, a given type of virus can have only one type of nucleic acid as its genome, and a mature virus does not contain nucleic acid other than its genome.[3] [If the ratio of adenine to thymine in a DNA virus is not one to one, what can be said about the genome of this virus?[4] A disease agent that is isolated from a human cannot reproduce on its own in cell-free broth but can reproduce in a culture of human cells. In its pure form, it possesses both RNA and DNA. Is it possible that the disease agent is a virus?[5]]

A factor that influences all viral genomes, regardless of the form of the nucleic acid used as genome, is size as a limiting factor. Viruses are much smaller than the hosts they infect, both prokaryotic and eukaryotic. Figure 1 depicts the relative size of a **bacteriophage** (a virus that infects bacteria) and its host.

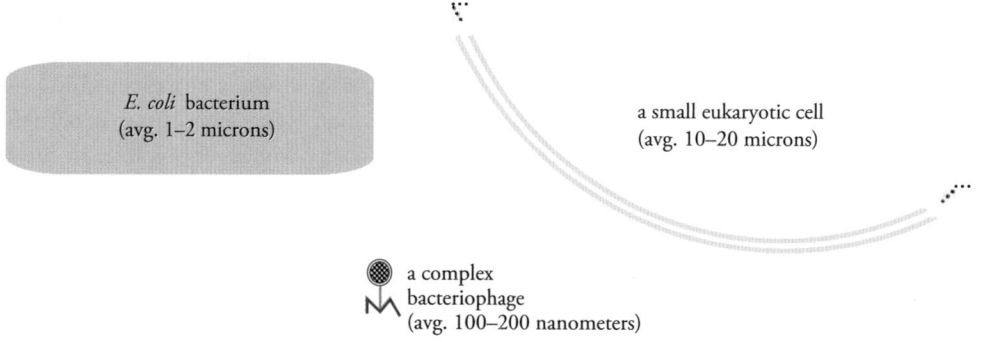

Figure 1   The Relative Size of a Virus

Not only are viruses small, but the exterior protein shell of a virus is typically a rigid structure of fixed size that cannot expand to accommodate a larger genome. [What is the likely result if a viral genome is tripled in size?[6]] To adapt to this size constraint, viral genomes have evolved to be extremely economical. One adaptation is for the viral genome to carry very few genes and for the virus to rely on host-encoded proteins for transcription, translation, and replication. [How do ribosomes used to translate viral proteins compare to host ribosomes?[7]] Another adaptation found in viral genomes is the ability to encode more than one protein in a given length of genome. A virus can accomplish this feat by utilizing more than one reading frame within a piece of DNA so that genes may overlap with each other.

---

[3] There are exceptions. For example, it has recently been discovered that the Hepatitis B virus has a circular DNA genome which is part single-stranded and part double-stranded. The take-home point here is that when a virus is not inside a host cell, it contains only its genome, which is always the same (except in special situations such as when a piece of host genome accidentally becomes incorporated in the viral genome). In contrast, a true cell contains not only its genome, but also mRNA, rRNA, and tRNA.

[4] Adenine base pairs with thymine in double-stranded DNA. Thus, for every A, there should be one T, for a one to one ratio of A to T. If the ratio differs from this, the genome must be single-stranded DNA, or RNA, which has no T.

[5] No, it cannot be a virus. Viruses possess only one kind of nucleic acid. The disease agent is another kind of obligate intracellular parasite (certain bacteria can only reproduce inside host cells, e.g., *Chlamydia*).

[6] The viral genome will probably no longer fit within the normal viral structure, and the genome will therefore not be packaged into infectious viral particles.

[7] Viruses use host ribosomes. Viral and host proteins are translated by the same ribosomes.

- A 1000 base pair region of viral genome is found to encode two polypeptides unrelated in amino acid sequence during infection of eukaryotic cells. If one of these polypeptides is 250 amino acids in length and the other is 300, what is the best explanation for this?[8]
  - A) A missense mutation
  - B) Viruses use a different genetic code than eukaryotes do
  - C) Overlapping multiple reading frames
  - D) The polypeptides are splicing variants

Surrounding the viral nucleic acid genome is a protein coat called the **capsid**. The capsid provides the external morphology that is used to classify viruses. It is made from a repeating pattern of only a few protein building blocks. *Helical* capsids are rod-shaped, while *polyhedral* capsids are multiple-sided geometric figures with regular surfaces. Complex viruses may contain a mixture of shapes. For example, the T4 bacteriophage has a helical sheath and a polyhedral head (Figure 2). This virus is commonly used in research; its host is the bacterium *E. coli*. The genome is located within the capsid **head**. Other parts of the capsid are used during infection of the host. The **tail fibers** attach to the surface of the host cell, as does the **base plate**. The **sheath** contracts using the energy of stored ATP, injecting the genome into the host. [Why might a bacteriophage inject its DNA, while animal viruses do not?[9]]

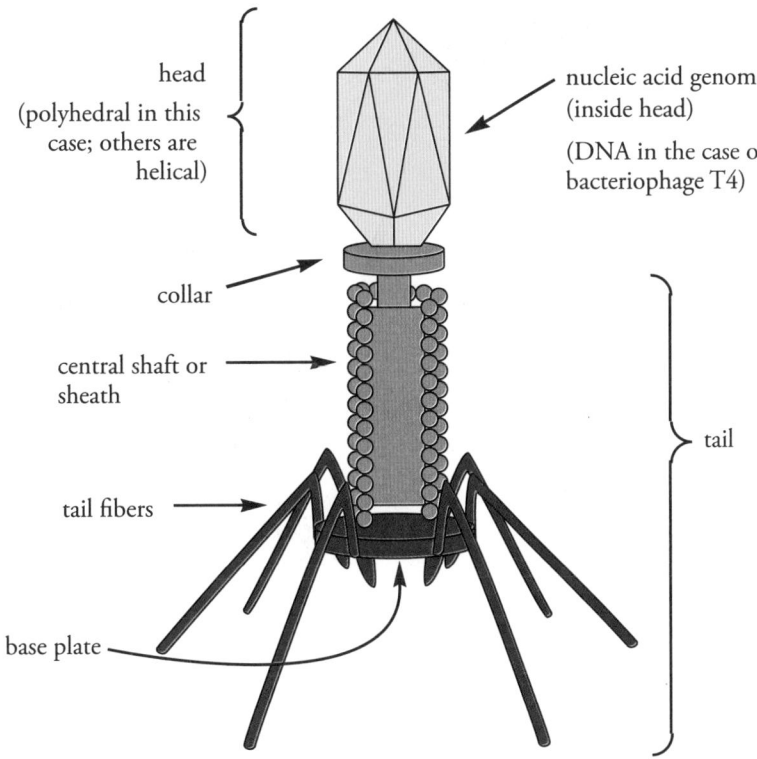

head
(polyhedral in this case; others are helical)

nucleic acid genome
(inside head)
(DNA in the case of bacteriophage T4)

collar

central shaft or sheath

tail

tail fibers

base plate

Figure 2   Bacteriophage T4

---

[8]   The problem is that the virus must contain at least 750 bp (250 amino acids) and 900 bp (300 amino acids) of genetic information for unrelated polypeptides in 1000 bp of DNA. The only way to do this is overlapping multiple reading frames (choice **C**).

[9]   Phage must puncture the bacterial cell wall, while animal viruses can be internalized whole into animal cells (since they do not have a cell wall).

The most important thing to understand is that the entire viral capsid is composed of protein, while the viral genome is composed of nucleic acid (DNA or RNA). Most viruses are not as structurally complex as the bacteriophage shown in Figure 2. See Figure 3 for more examples.

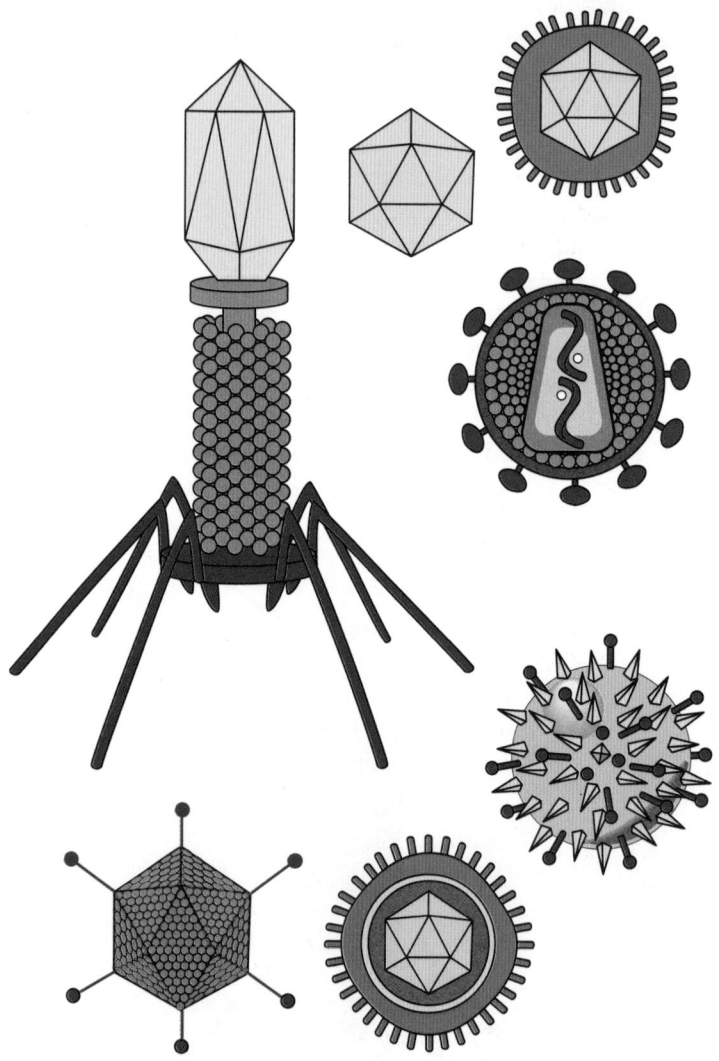

Figure 3   A Variety of Viruses

Many animal viruses also possess an **envelope** that surrounds the capsid. This is a membrane on the exterior of the virus derived from the membrane of the host cell. It contains phospholipids, proteins, and carbohydrates from the host membrane, in addition to proteins encoded by the viral genome. Enveloped viruses acquire this covering by **budding** through the host cell membrane. To infect a new host, some enveloped viruses fuse their envelope with the host's plasma membrane, which leaves the de-enveloped capsid inside the host cell. Viruses which do not have envelopes are called **naked viruses**. All phages and plant viruses are naked. [Can you imagine why this might be true?[10]]

---

[10]   Remember: viruses acquire envelopes by budding through host membranes. Phages and plant viruses infect hosts that possess cell walls. When viruses begin to exit the cell, the cell wall is destroyed, and host membranes rupture. Thus, there is no membrane through which the remaining viruses must bud; they simply escape in a lytic explosion.

Whether enveloped or naked, the surface of a virus determines what host cells it can infect. Viral infection is not a random process, but highly specific. A virus binds to a specific receptor on the cell surface as the first step in infection. After binding, the virus will be internalized, either by fusion with the plasma membrane or by receptor-mediated endocytosis. Only cells with a receptor that matches the virus will become infected, explaining why only specific species or specific cell types are susceptible to infection. The viral surface is also important for recognition by our immune system. [If antibodies to a viral capsid protein are ineffective in blocking infection, what might this indicate about the virus?[11]]

Bacteriophage Life Cycles

Since viruses lack the ability to produce energy and replicate on their own, they use the machinery of the cell they infect to carry out these processes. The viral genome contains genes that redirect the infected cell to produce viral products. The first step is binding to the exterior of a bacterial cell in a process termed **attachment** or **adsorption**. The next step is injection of the viral genome into the host cell in a process termed **penetration** or **eclipse**. It is called "eclipse" because the capsid remains on the outer surface of the bacterium while the genome disappears into the cell, removing infectious virus from the media. From this point forward, a phage follows one of two different paths: it enters either the **lytic cycle** or the **lysogenic cycle**.

The Lytic Cycle of Phages

As soon as the phage genome has entered the host cell, host polymerases and/or ribosomes begin to rapidly transcribe and translate it. One of the first viral gene products made is sometimes an enzyme called **hydrolase**, a hydrolytic enzyme that degrades the entire host genome. (Hydrolase is an example of an **early gene**; one of a group of genes that are expressed immediately after infection and which includes any special enzymes required to express viral genes.) Then multiple copies of the phage genome are produced (using the dNTPs resulting from degradation of the host genome), as well as an abundance of capsid proteins. Next, each new capsid automatically assembles itself around a new genome. Finally, an enzyme called **lysozyme** is produced. An example of a **late gene**, lysozyme is also present in human tears and saliva. It destroys the bacterial cell wall. Because osmotic pressure is no longer counteracted by the protection of the cell wall, the host bacterium bursts ("lyses," hence the name *lytic*), releasing about 100 progeny viruses, which can begin another round of the cycle (see Figure 4 on the next page). [If lysozyme were an early gene, would this be advantageous to the virus?[12]]

---

[11] It suggests that the virus is enveloped, so the antibody cannot reach its epitope on the capsid surface in infectious virus.

[12] No. The host cell would lyse before the phage had time to replicate and assemble.

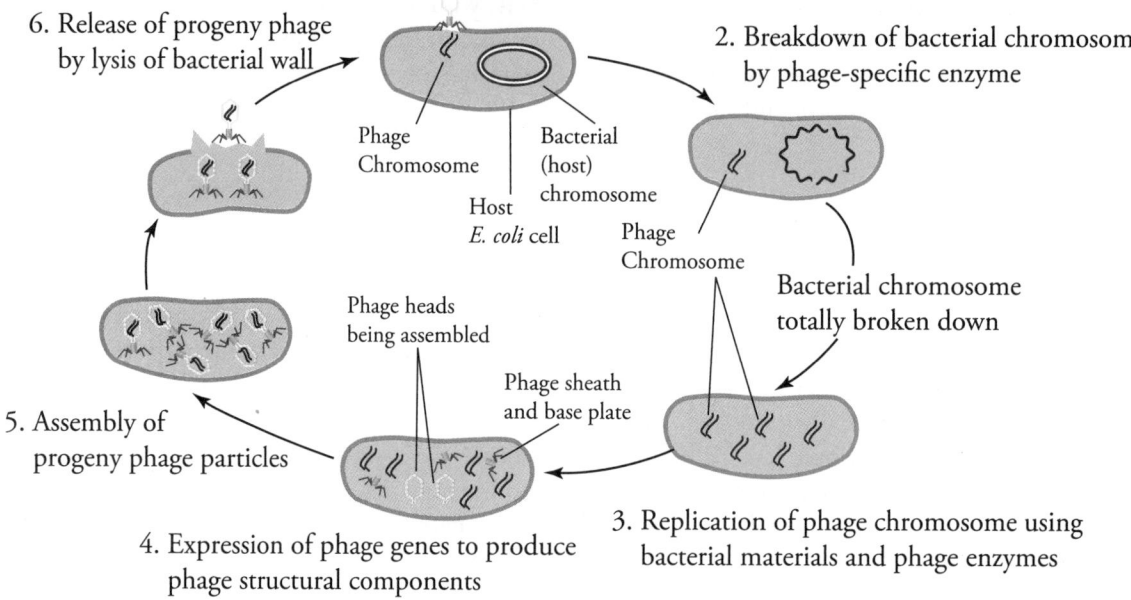

Figure 4 The Lytic Cycle

- When phage are first added to a bacterial culture, the number of infective viruses initially decreases before it later increases. Why does this occur?[13]
- Bacteria cultured in the presence of ^{35}S-labeled cysteine and ^{32}P-labeled phosphates are infected with phage T4. When phage from this culture are used to infect a new nonradiolabeled bacterial culture, which of the isotopes will be found in the interior of the newly infected bacteria?[14]
- A bacteriophage with an important capsid gene deleted infects the same cell as another virus with a normal copy of the same gene. At the time of host-cell lysis:[15]
  - A) all released viruses will be capable of infecting new hosts, but only some of these new infections will give rise to phage capable of infecting new hosts.
  - B) no infective viruses will be released.
  - C) each individual virus that is released will produce a mixture of infective and noninfective viruses in subsequent infections.
  - D) only normal viruses will be released.

---

[13] The initial decrease is due to the simple fact that many phage have injected their genomes into hosts and are no longer infectious.

[14] The ^{35}S cysteine will be incorporated into viral coat proteins and the ^{32}P phosphate will be incorporated into the viral nucleic acid genome in newly released viral particles. (Proteins contain no P and nucleic acids contain no S.) When these viruses infect bacteria, their nucleic acids are injected into the bacteria while the capsid proteins remain on the exterior, which means that only the ^{32}P will be found in the interior of the newly infected cells.

[15] When two viruses infect the same cell, it is called co-infection. Some normal viruses will result, and some genomes from defective viruses will get packaged into capsids made from proteins encoded by the normal virus. The latter will be capable of infecting new hosts, but when they do, their progeny will not survive due to the capsid abnormality. Choice **A** is correct, and choices B and D are wrong. Think about it: where did the phage with the deleted capsid gene come from?! The deficient virus must have come from a co-infection such as this. The deficient phage can only infect host cells and reproduce with the help of normal viruses. Note that because a single virus carries only a single genome, it can produce only one type of progeny (choice C is wrong).

The Lysogenic Cycle of Phages

The lytic cycle is an efficient way for a virus to rapidly increase its numbers. It presents a problem though: all host cells are destroyed. This is an evolutionary disadvantage. Some viruses are cleverer: they enter the **lysogenic cycle**. Upon infection, the phage genome is incorporated into the bacterial genome and is now referred to as a **prophage**; the host is now called a **lysogen** (Figure 5). The prophage is silent; its genes are not expressed, and viral progeny are not produced. This dormancy is due to the fact that transcription of phage genes is blocked by a phage-encoded repressor protein that binds to specific DNA elements in phage promoters (operators). The cleverness of the lysogenic cycle lies in the fact that every time the host cell reproduces itself, the prophage is reproduced too. Eventually, the prophage becomes activated. It now removes itself from the host genome (in a process called **excision**) and enters the lytic cycle.

One potential consequence of the lysogenic cycle is that when the viral genome activates, excising itself from the host genome, it may take part of the host genome along with it. When the virus replicates, the small piece of host genome will be replicated and packaged with the viral genome. In subsequent infections, the virus will integrate the "stolen" host DNA along with its own genome into the new host's genome. The presence of the new DNA will become evident if it codes for a trait that the newly infected host did not previously possess, such as the ability to metabolize galactose. This process is called **transduction**. [Why would a bacterial gene, carried with a virus and integrated with viral genes into a new bacterial genome, not be repressed along with the viral genes during lysogeny?[16]]

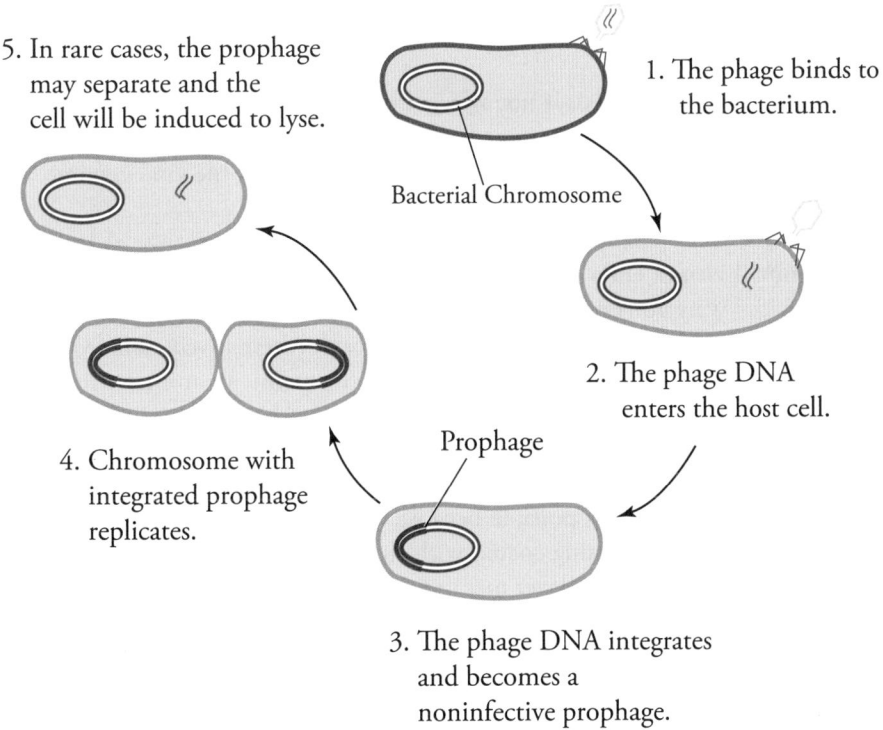

5. In rare cases, the prophage may separate and the cell will be induced to lyse.

1. The phage binds to the bacterium.

Bacterial Chromosome

2. The phage DNA enters the host cell.

4. Chromosome with integrated prophage replicates.

Prophage

3. The phage DNA integrates and becomes a noninfective prophage.

Figure 5   The Lysogenic Cycle

---

[16] Prophage latency results from a viral repressor protein binding to viral DNA in a sequence-specific manner. The specific DNA sequence to which the repressor binds is present in the viral genes but not in the bacterial genes, so the bacterial gene can be expressed while the viral genes are repressed.

Replication of Animal Viruses

There are a number of differences between phages and viruses which infect animal cells. (Animal viruses don't have a special name like "phage.") The general outline of the viral life cycle, however, remains the same. The virus must specifically bind to a proper host cell, release its genetic material into the host, take over host machinery, replicate its genome, synthesize capsid components, assemble itself, and finally escape to infect a new cell.

Animal cells have proteins on the surface of their plasma membranes that serve as specific receptors for viruses. These receptors play a role in normal cellular function; they do not exist simply for the benefit of the virus. Part of the tissue-specificity of animal viruses is due to the distribution of receptors necessary for adsorption. For example, the binding of the HIV virus protein gp120 to a T cell membrane protein termed CD4 is one of the first steps in HIV infection.

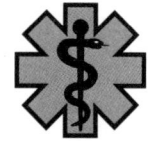

- Would treatment of an HIV-infected person with a soluble form of CD4 protein affect the infectivity of the virus?[17]
- Mutation of the cell-surface receptor that viruses attach to would be a means for an organism to become resistant to viral infection. Why is this mechanism not common?[18]
- Treatment of an enveloped animal virus with a mild detergent solubilizes several proteins from the virus, although the genome does not become accessible. Which one of the following is consistent with this scenario?[19]
  - A) Some of the proteins that are released by detergent may be encoded by the genome of the infected cell.
  - B) The infectivity of the virus is not affected by detergent treatment.
  - C) The proteins released by detergent are capsid proteins.
  - D) All the proteins released by the detergent are encoded by the viral genome.

The next step in the infection of an animal cell is penetration into the cell, just as in bacterial infection by a phage. Many animal viruses enter cells by **endocytosis** (a process whereby the host cell engulfs the virus and internalizes it). [Why don't phages enter their hosts by endocytosis?[20]] Once inside the host, the viral genome is *uncoated*, meaning it is released from the capsid. Alternatively, some viruses fuse with the plasma membrane to release virus into the cytoplasm. From this point, an animal virus may enter either a lytic cycle, a lytic-like cycle called the productive cycle, or a lysogenic cycle.

The lytic cycle in animal viruses is the same as in phages. The **productive cycle** is similar to the lytic cycle but does not destroy the host cell. It is possible because enveloped viruses exit the host cell by *budding through the host's cell membrane*, becoming coated with this membrane in the process. Budding does not necessarily destroy a cell since the lipid bilayer membrane can reseal as the virus leaves. Finally, in the animal virus lysogenic cycle the dormant form of the viral genome is called a **provirus** (analogous to a prophage). For example, Herpes simplex I is the virus that causes oral herpes. After infection, it may remain dormant as a provirus for an indefinite period of time. Then one day, usually when the host encounters stress (e.g., lack of sleep, upcoming professional school entrance exams), the virus reactivates.

---

[17] Yes, it would. The soluble CD4 protein would bind to the virus's CD4 receptor (gp120) and block attachment of the virus to the T cells.

[18] Two reasons: 1) The receptor has a specific role in the normal physiology of the host, which a mutation might compromise. 2) Viruses generally evolve so rapidly that they can keep up with any changes in the host, but this is not an absolute rule. Cells of our immune system keep us alive by keeping up with most microorganisms' tricks.

[19] The detergent solubilized the viral envelope (choice C is wrong). As stated in the text, some envelope proteins are encoded by the virus and some are derived from the host's membranes during budding (choice **A** is correct, and choice D is wrong). Removal of envelope proteins will impair viral adsorption and reduce infectivity (choice B is wrong).

[20] Bacteria do not perform endocytosis, in part because they have a rigid cell wall that does not permit them to.

Viral Genomes

Many factors determine the uniqueness of each virus. The type of genome, possession or lack of an envelope, nature of cell-surface proteins, and type of life cycle are examples. All of these parameters are used in the classification of viruses, and all are potential targets for therapeutic intervention. The nature of the genome is perhaps the most important of these and has important consequences for how infection by each virus proceeds. In the following discussion, we will look at a few viral genomes with an eye to *what proteins the virus must encode or actually carry in its capsid based on its genome type.* Our purpose is not to provide new information, but rather to demonstrate what conclusions can be drawn from what you already know (typical MCAT passage material). Do not memorize, but rather read for comprehension. We will not discuss ds-RNA or ss-DNA genomes, but by the end of this section, you should be able to imagine components they might require.

(+) RNA Viruses
—must *encode* RNA-dependent RNA pol (and do not have to carry it).

A (+) RNA virus, with a single-stranded RNA genome, is the simplest imaginable type of viral genome. (A piece of single-stranded viral RNA which serves as mRNA is called (+) RNA.) As soon as the (+) RNA genome is in the host cell, host ribosomes begin to translate it, creating viral proteins. The viral genome acts directly as mRNA. The technical way to describe this scenario is to say the genome is **infective**, meaning injecting an isolated genome into the host cell will result in virus production. In order for the virus to replicate itself, one of the proteins it encodes must be an **RNA-dependent RNA polymerase**, the role of which is __?[21] (+) RNA viruses cause the common cold, polio, and rubella. [Will an infectious virus be produced if the genome of an enveloped (+) strand RNA virus is added to an extract prepared from the cytoplasm of eukaryotic cells that retains translational activity but lacks DNA replication or transcription of host genes?[22] If a viral genome is (+) strand RNA, what is used as a template by the RNA-dependent RNA polymerase?[23]]

(−) RNA Viruses
—must *carry* RNA-dependent RNA pol (and, of course, encode it too).

The genome of a (−) RNA virus is *complementary* to the piece of RNA that encodes viral proteins. In other words, the genome of a (−) RNA virus is the template for viral mRNA production. If host ribosomes translate (−) RNA, useless polypeptides will be made. Hence, the virus must not only encode an RNA-dependent RNA polymerase, it must actually carry one with it in the capsid. When the virus enters the host cell, this enzyme will create a (+) strand from the (−) genome. Then the viral life cycle can proceed. (−) RNA viruses cause rabies, measles, mumps, and influenza. [Do (−) strand RNA viruses use host enzymes to catalyze RNA production in transcription or in replication of the genome?[24]]

---

[21] to copy the RNA genome for viral replication; the host never makes RNA from RNA.

[22] No. The (+) strand RNA virus will be able to produce viral genome and proteins, but progeny will not be able to acquire the envelope they need to be infectious.

[23] To make (+) strand copies of the genome, the virus needs the complementary strand as a template: the (−) strand RNA. Thus, the RNA-dependent RNA polymerase produces a (−) strand intermediate before generating new (+) strand genomes.

[24] Neither. Viral RNA-dependent RNA polymerase first makes (+) strand as mRNA and then uses the (+) strand as the template to replicate new (−) strand genomes.

Retroviruses
—must *encode* reverse transcriptase.

HIV, the virus that causes AIDS, and HTLV (Human T cell Leukemia Virus) are examples of retroviruses. These are (+) RNA viruses that undergo lysogeny. In other words, they integrate into the host genome as proviruses. In order to integrate into our double-stranded DNA genome, a viral genome must also be composed of double-stranded DNA. Since these viral genomes enter the cell in an RNA form, they must undergo **reverse transcription** to make DNA from an RNA template. This snubbing of the central dogma is accomplished by an **RNA-dependent DNA polymerase** (*reverse transcriptase*) encoded by the viral genome. Retroviruses are theoretically not required to carry this enzyme, only to encode it. [Why?[25]] The three main retroviral genes are *gag* (codes for viral capsid proteins), *pol* (polymerase codes for reverse transcriptase), and *env* (envelope codes for viral envelope proteins). [After integration of a retrovirus into the cellular genome, a reverse transcriptase inhibitor is added to the cell. Will the production of new viruses be blocked?[26]]

Double-Stranded DNA Viruses
—often *encode* enzymes required for dNTP synthesis and DNA replication.

These viruses often have large genomes that include genes for enzymes involved in deoxyribonucleotide synthesis (which we do whenever we make DNA) and DNA replication. [Given the limited information that viruses may contain in their genomes, why carry around genes for an enzyme possessed by the host?[27] Why don't RNA viruses do this?[28] What is a factor likely to limit the size of RNA genomes?[29] Some DNA viruses induce infected host cells to enter mitosis and may even override cellular inhibition of cell division so strongly that the cell becomes cancerous; what is the advantage to the virus of inducing host-cell division?[30]]

---

[25] Because the viral RNA genome can be translated by host ribosomes; thus, reverse transcriptase may be made after the viral genome enters the host. It just so happens that HIV does carry its reverse transcriptase within its capsid. You should understand why this is not a theoretical necessity.

[26] No, it will not. Reverse transcriptase is required for only one phase of the retrovirus life cycle: the copying of the viral RNA genome into DNA so that it can integrate into the host genome and be transcribed. Once the viral genome has integrated, transcription to produce viral mRNA and new viral RNA genomes does not involve reverse transcriptase. It can proceed with the normal host-cell enzymes.

[27] The host cell will only make dNTPs in preparation for replication. If the virus wants to reproduce without waiting for the host to do so, it must encode its own enzymes for the synthesis of DNA building blocks.

[28] Transcription is always occurring in all cells, so NTPs (not dNTPs) are always present.

[29] The error rate in RNA synthesis is much higher than in DNA synthesis, in part because there are mechanisms to proofread and correct errors in DNA synthesis (but not in RNA synthesis). If an RNA genome were too large, every copy of the viral genome synthesized would suffer from so many errors that no infectious virus would be produced.

[30] To replicate, the DNA virus must either provide all of the necessary components (such as dNTPs) itself, infect a cell that is already dividing, or induce the cell it infects to enter mitosis and produce the ingredients for DNA synthesis.

- Adenoviruses have a single linear ds-DNA genome which contains a number of different promoters that are regulated during infection. Although transcription is carried out by cellular RNA polymerase, the viral E1A gene product is required for transcription of most viral genes. If the E1A gene is deleted from the virus or if the gene product is inactivated, viral infection is unable to proceed. Adenoviruses also encode much of their own replication machinery, including DNA polymerase. If two different adenoviruses infect the same cell, one with a deleted E1A gene and another with a deleted DNA polymerase gene, will successful infection of the cell result?[31]

5.2 SUBVIRAL PARTICLES

Some infectious agents are even smaller and simpler than viruses and are termed **subviral particles**. These include prions and viroids.

Prions

As infectious agents, prions do not strictly follow the Central Dogma because they are self-replicating proteins [Why does this violate the Central Dogma?[32]]. The prion itself is a misfolded version of a protein that already exists (see Figure 6).

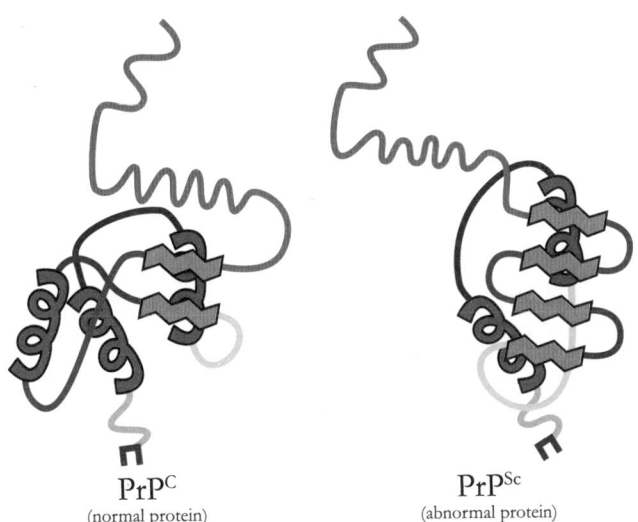

PrP^C
(normal protein)

PrP^Sc
(abnormal protein)

Figure 6 Comparison of the PrP^C structure to the PrP^Sc structure

---

[31] Yes, thanks to complementation. The mutant viruses will complement each other, one providing the E1A protein and the other providing DNA polymerase. Note that this had to have happened before; how else could defective viruses such as these exist? One virus which complements another is called a helper virus.

[32] The Central Dogma states that information flows in its nucleotide form from DNA to RNA (transcription), and then in its amino acid form from RNA to protein (translation). Prions take both transcription and translation out of the process and have proteins being shaped based on other proteins, hence the term "self-replicating."

When the normally folded protein (designated PrP^C) comes into contact with the prion (designated PrP^{Sc}), the prion acts as a template; the shape of the normal protein is altered and it too becomes infectious. Prions are responsible for a class of diseases in mammals referred to as the **transmissible spongiform encephalopathies** (TSEs). These diseases cause degeneration in the nervous system, especially the brain where characteristic holes develop, and are always fatal. The misfolded proteins are found in the nervous tissues and are very resistant to degradation by chemicals or heat, making them hard to destroy. Bovine spongiform encephalopathy (BSE, commonly called *mad cow disease*) is the prion disease found in cows; this was originally transmitted to cows from sheep because all types of tissue from sheep, including the brain and spinal cord, were used as a supplement in the feed for other farm animals. (Since this was discovered, strict rules have been put in place about which specific organs can be used to supplement animal feed, and those organs most likely to transmit prion disease are banned.) Though much less common, the disease *kuru* follows a similar transmission path in humans; it is only found in a limited number of tribes where consumption of the body, particularly of the brain, is part of honoring the dead (since identification of the transmission route, this practice has stopped and kuru has virtually disappeared).

However, prion diseases can also be genetically linked through mutations in the gene that codes for the prion protein. For example, fatal familial insomnia (FFI) is an autosomal dominant condition inherited on chromosome 20, and Creutzfeldt-Jakob disease (CJD) is also inherited. It is also possible for these diseases to arise spontaneously (through mutation) in someone with no prior family history. In general, however, prion diseases are very rare, striking only 1–2 people per million.

Whether transmitted, inherited, or spontaneously arising, prion diseases are characterized by their very long incubation periods, which can be several months to years in animals and several years to decades in humans. The misfolded proteins cause the destruction of neurons, particularly in the central nervous system, leading to loss of coordination, dementia, and death. Diagnosis is difficult, in part because of the long incubation periods and in part because the symptoms can be indicative of other conditions.

Viroids

Viroids consist of a short piece of circular, single-stranded RNA (200–400 bases long) with extensive self-complementarity (i.e., it can base-pair with itself to create some regions that are double-stranded; see Figure 7). Generally they do not code for proteins and they lack capsids. Some viroids are catalytic ribozymes, while others, when replicated, produce siRNAs that can silence normal gene expression.

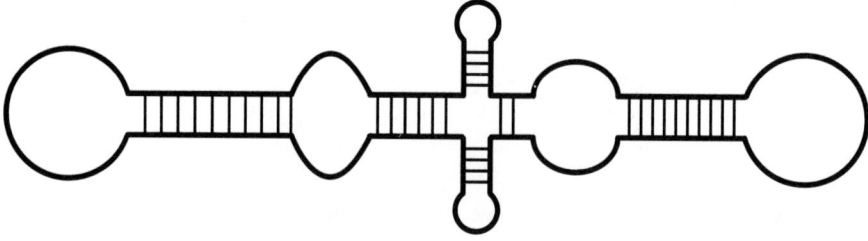

Figure 7   Structure of a Viroid Showing Double-Stranded Regions

Replication of some viroids shares similarity to the replication of RNA viruses. A viroid RNA-dependent RNA polymerase synthesizes a (–) strand, which is circularized by an RNA ligase derived from the host;

this is then used as the round, rolling template to make more (+) copies that match the original RNA viroid sequence. An alternative to this mechanism leaves the (–) stand in a more linear state where it can still act as a template for (+) strand creation and then become circularized. In other cases, viroids somehow hijack the cell's DNA dependent RNA polymerase and direct it to read RNA templates. This mechanism is not well understood.

Most of the diseases caused by viroids are found in plants. The only human disease linked to viroids is Hepatitis D. The Hepatitis D viroid can only enter hepatocytes (liver cells) if it is contained in a capsid with a binding protein; since viroids do not have capsids, successful Hepatitis D infection required coinfection with Hepatitis B, from which it derives its capsid.

5.3 PROKARYOTES (DOMAIN BACTERIA)

Cell Theory

Advances in microbiology have been made possible by advancing technologies in magnification. Once humans were able to utilize basic, if crude, microscopy, the cell as the monomer of tissues and organs could be studied. In 1655, this led the English scientist, Robert Hooke, to define the Cell Theory based on his studies of cork. Its tenets are as follows:

1) All living organisms are composed of one or more cells and their products.
2) Cells are the monomer for any organism.
3) New cells arise from pre-existing, living cells.

Though these basic principles are still true, more modern extensions of Cell Theory also include the idea that no matter what the species, the chemical composition of cells is similar, that DNA is the source of hereditary programming information passed from cell to cell, that an organism's activity is determined by the total activity of its cells, and that biochemical energy flow occurs within cells. These additional principles have been explored and verified due to vast improvements both in microscopy as well as biochemical and genetic testing.

All living organisms (which does not include viruses) can be classified as either **prokaryotes** or **eukaryotes**. The classification of organisms into these groups is based on examination of their internal cellular structure. Representatives from both groups are able to carry out the basic biochemical processes of photosynthesis, the Krebs cycle, and oxidative phosphorylation to produce ATP. The primary feature of prokaryotes that distinguishes them from eukaryotes is that they do not contain **membrane-bound organelles** (nucleus, mitochondria, lysosomes, etc.). *Prokaryote* means "before the nucleus," and the lack of a nucleus indicates that prokaryotes are evolutionarily the oldest domains. Unlike viruses, however, prokaryotes possess all of the machinery required for life. They are true cells; true living organisms. The prokaryotes include **bacteria**, **archaea** (extremophiles), and **blue-green algae** (cyanobacteria).

5.3

The classification of living organisms, **taxonomy**, is an important part of biology because it is used to determine the evolutionary relationship of organisms to one another. The largest taxonomic division is the **domain**. There are three recognized domains: Bacteria, Archaea, and Eukarya. Domains Bacteria and Archaea include prokaryotic organisms, and Domain Eukarya includes eukaryotic organisms. Each domain can be further subdivided into **kingdoms**. Currently there are three well-recognized eukaryotic kingdoms (Animalia, Plantae, and Fungi), and great debate over the number of kingdoms that should be present in the other prokaryotic domains and in the single-celled eukaryotes (protists).

In this section, we will begin to study the most basic and ancient of organisms, the prokaryotes.

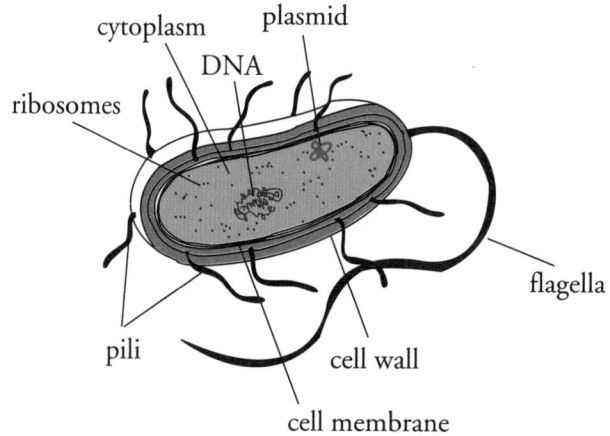

Figure 8   A Prokaryote

Bacterial Structure and Classification

Contents of the Cytoplasm

Unlike a eukaryotic cell, there are *no membrane-bound organelles* in prokaryotic cells (note that ribosomes, which are *not* membrane-bound, *are* found in bacteria). The prokaryotic genome is a single double-stranded circular DNA chromosome.[33] It is not located in a nucleus, and it is not associated with histone proteins as the eukaryotic genome is. In bacteria, transcription and translation occur in the same place at the same time. Ribosomes begin to translate mRNA before it is completely transcribed. Many ribosomes translating a single piece of mRNA form a structure known as a **polyribosome**.

[In Figure 9 on the next page, is the free end of the mRNA the 3' or the 5' end? Which end of the nascent polypeptides is the free end?[34]] Remember that the bacterial ribosome is structurally different from the eukaryotic ribosome, though both function the same way. The differences allow us to prescribe various antibiotics which interfere with bacterial translation without disrupting our own. (Examples are strepto-mycin and tetracycline, which bind only to bacterial ribosomes.)

---

[33] There are a few exceptions to this (e.g., bacteria with more than one chromosome and/or linear chromosomes), but you do not have to know them for the MCAT.

[34] The 5' end of the mRNA polymer is free, since elongation of mRNA proceeds 5' to 3'. Proteins are made N to C, so the free end of the polypeptides is the N terminus.

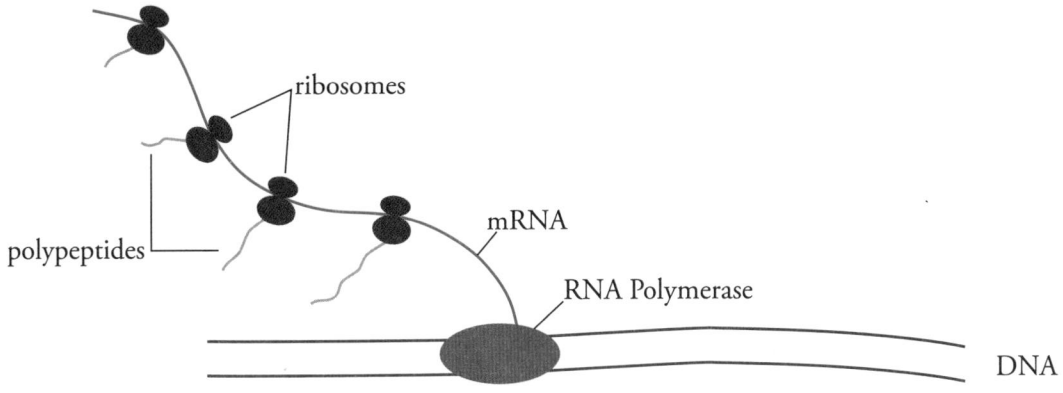

Figure 9 A Prokaryotic Polyribosome

One last genetic element that can be found in prokaryotic cells is the **plasmid**. This is a circular piece of double-stranded DNA which is much smaller than the genome. Plasmids are referred to as **extrachromosomal genetic elements**. They often encode gene products which may confer an advantage upon a bacterium carrying the plasmid. For example, plasmids frequently carry antibiotic-resistance genes (genes that encode proteins which can break down antibiotics). Many plasmids are capable of autonomous replication, which means that a single plasmid molecule within a bacterial cell may cause itself to be replicated into many copies. Plasmids are important not only because they may encode advantageous gene products, but also because they orchestrate bacterial exchange of genetic information, or **conjugation**, which is discussed below.

Bacterial Shape

Bacteria are often classified according to their shape. The three shapes and their proper names are organized in the following table:

Table 1 Bacterial Classification by Shape

Shape	Proper name (plural)	Proper name (singular)
round	cocci	coccus
rod-shaped	bacilli	bacillus
spiral-shaped	spirochetes or spirilla	spirochete, spirillum

The Cell Membrane and the Cell Wall

The bacterial cytoplasm is bounded by a lipid bilayer which is similar to our own plasma membrane. Outside the lipid bilayer is a rigid cell wall. It provides support for the cell, preventing lysis due to osmotic pressure. The bacterial cell wall is composed of **peptidoglycan**, a complex polymer unique to prokaryotes. It contains cross-linked chains made of sugars and amino acids, including D-alanine, which is not found in animal cells (our amino acids have the L configuration). The bacterial cell wall is the target of many antibiotics, such as penicillin. The enzyme *lysozyme*, which is found in tears and saliva and made by lytic viruses, destroys the peptidoglycan in the bacterial cell wall, resulting in an osmotically fragile structure called a **protoplast**. [Would a protoplast moved from salt water to fresh water shrivel or burst?[35]]

---

[35] It would burst, since water would flow into the cell by osmosis.

5.3

Gram Staining of the Cell Wall

As part of our tour of the bacterial cell, we will say a word about classification of bacteria according to two different types of cell wall. The method of classification is derived from the extent to which bacteria turn color in a procedure termed **Gram staining**. The two groupings are **Gram-positive**, which stain strongly (a dark purple color) and **Gram-negative** bacteria, which stain weakly (a light pink color).

Gram-positive bacteria have a thick peptidoglycan layer outside of the cell membrane and no other layer beyond this. Gram-negative bacteria have a thinner layer of peptidoglycan in the cell wall but have an additional outer layer containing lipopolysaccharide. The intermediate space in Gram-negative bacteria between the cell membrane and the outer layer is termed the **periplasmic space**, in which are sometimes found enzymes that degrade antibiotics (see Figure 10). The increased protection of Gram-negative bacteria from the environment is reflected in their weak staining, as well as in their increased resistance to antibiotics. [Which bacteria would be more susceptible to lysis when treated with lysozyme: Gram-positive or Gram-negative?[36]]

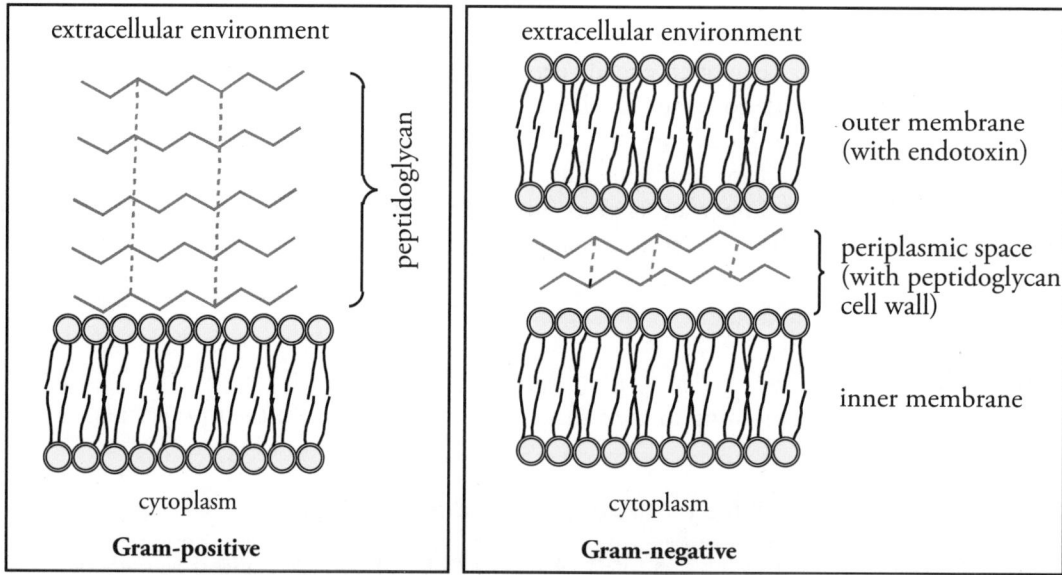

Figure 10   Gram-positive vs. Gram-negative Bacteria

---

[36] Lysozyme hydrolyzes linkages in peptidoglycan to weaken the cell wall. The peptidoglycan in Gram-positive cells is more accessible, since these cells do not possess an additional outer layer; therefore, Gram-positive cells will lyse more easily when treated with lysozyme.

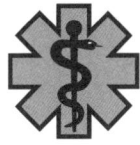

Endotoxins vs. Exotoxins

Endotoxins are normal components of the outer membrane of Gram-negative bacteria that aren't inherently poisonous. However, they cause our immune system to have such an extreme reaction that we may die as a result. Endotoxins cause the most trouble when many bacteria die and their disintegrated outer membranes are released into the circulation. When this occurs, cells of the immune system release so many chemicals that the patient goes into what is called septic shock, in which much of the aqueous portion of the blood is leaked into the tissues, causing a drop in blood pressure, and other problems, which may be fatal. Endotoxins can have various chemical structures, including lipopolysaccharide, which contains sugars bound to lipids.

Exotoxins are very toxic substances secreted by both Gram-negative and Gram-positive bacteria into the surrounding medium. Exotoxins help the bacterium compete with other bacterial species, such as normal inhabitants of the mammalian gut. Some diseases that are caused by exotoxins are botulism, diptheria, tetanus, and toxic shock syndrome.

The Capsule

Another attribute which only some bacteria have is the **capsule** or **glycocalyx**. This is a sticky layer of polysaccharide "goo" surrounding the bacterial cell and often surrounding an entire colony of bacteria. It makes bacteria more difficult for immune system cells to eradicate. It also enables bacteria to adhere to smooth surfaces such as rocks in a stream or the lining of the human respiratory tract.

Flagella

Another item only some bacteria have are long, whip-like filaments known as **flagella**, which are involved in bacterial motility. [Can viruses move via flagellar propulsion to find host cells?[37]] A bacterium which possesses one or more flagella is said to be **motile**, because flagella are the only means of bacterial locomotion. Bacteria may be **monotrichous** (meaning they have a flagellum located at only one end), **amphitrichous** (meaning they have a flagellum located at both ends), or **peritrichous** (meaning that they have multiple flagella). The following is which?[38]

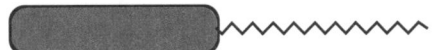

The structure of the flagellum is fairly complicated, with components encoded by over 35 genes, but it can be broken down into a few major components: the **filament**, the **hook**, and the **basal structure** (Figure 11 on the next page). The basal structure contains a number of rings that anchor the flagellum to the inner and outer membrane (for a Gram-negative bacterium) and serve to rotate the **rod** and the rest of the attached flagellum in either a clockwise or counterclockwise manner. The most important thing to remember about the prokaryotic flagellum is that its structure is different from the eukaryotic one (which contains a "9 + 2" arrangement of microtubules, discussed in Chapter 6).

---

[37] No. Viruses lack any means of energy production on their own and any means of active movement. They rely on diffusion to find host cells.

[38] Monotrichous

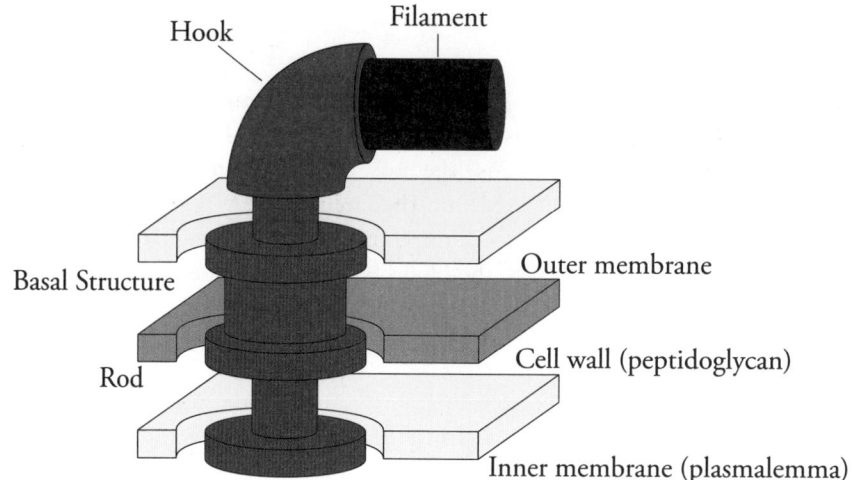

Figure 11 The Prokaryotic Flagellum

The rotation of the rod is powered by the diffusion of H^+ down the proton gradient generated across the inner membrane by electron transport. Bacterial motion can be directed toward attractants, such as food, or away from toxins, such as acid, in a process termed **chemotaxis**. The connection between chemotaxis and flagellar propulsion is dependent upon **chemoreceptors** on the cell surface that bind attractants or repellents and transmit a signal that influences the direction of flagellar rotation. The response of flagellar rotation to chemical attractants (or repellents) is not dependent on an *absolute* concentration, but to a *change* in the concentration over time. Thus, as the bacterium moves through the solution, it is able to detect whether it is moving toward or away from the highest concentration and respond accordingly.

Pili

Pili are long projections on the bacterial surface involved in attaching to different surfaces. The **sex pilus** is a special pilus attaching F^+ (male) and F^- (female) bacteria which facilitates the formation of **conjugation bridges** (discussed below). **Fimbriae** are smaller structures that are not involved in locomotion or conjugation but are involved in adhering to surfaces. [What other bacterial structure is involved in adhering to surfaces? Is it possible that the fimbriae play a role in infection by pathogenic organisms?[39]]

---

[39] The capsule, or glycocalyx is also involved in adherence. And yes, fimbriae do play a role in infection, by facilitating adhesion to cells so that the bacteria can colonize a tissue.

Bacterial Growth Requirements and Classification

Temperature

Another characteristic of bacteria used to categorize them is their ability to tolerate environmental variables, such as temperature. Though bacteria as a group can grow at a wide range of temperatures, each species has an optimal growth temperature. If the temperature is too high or too low, bacteria fail to grow and may be killed, hence the use of boiling to kill bacteria and refrigeration to slow bacterial growth and prevent food spoilage. Most bacteria favor mild temperatures similar to the ones that humans and other organisms favor (30°C); they are called **mesophiles** (moderate temperature lovers). **Thermophiles** (heat lovers) can survive at temperatures up to 100°C in boiling hot springs or near geothermal vents in the ocean floor. Bacteria that thrive at very low temperatures (near 0°C) are termed **psychrophiles** (cold lovers). [How might a decrease in temperature increase the bacterial growth rate?[40]]

Nutrition

Bacteria can be classified according to their *carbon source* and their *energy source*. "**Troph**" is a Latin root meaning "eat." **Autotrophs** utilize CO_2 as their carbon source. **Heterotrophs** rely on organic nutrients (glucose, for example) created by other organisms. **Chemotrophs** get their energy from chemicals. **Phototrophs** get their energy from light; not only plants but also some bacteria do this. Each bacterium is either a chemotroph or a phototroph and is either an autotroph or a heterotroph. There are thus four types of bacteria:

1) **Chemoautotrophs** build organic macromolecules from CO_2 using the energy of chemicals. They obtain energy by oxidizing inorganic molecules like H_2S.
2) **Chemoheterotrophs** require organic molecules such as glucose made by other organisms as their carbon source and for energy. (We are chemoheterotrophs.)
3) **Photoautotrophs** use only CO_2 as a carbon source and obtain their energy from the Sun. (Plants are photoautotrophs.)
4) **Photoheterotrophs** are odd in that the get their energy from the Sun, like plants, but require an organic molecule made by another organism as their carbon source.

- A bacterium that causes an infection in the bloodstream of humans is most likely to be classified as which one of the following?[41]
    A) Chemoautotroph
    B) Photoautotroph
    C) Chemoheterotroph
    D) Photoheterotroph

---

[40] Normally, you expect decreasing temperature to decrease the rate of all chemical, biochemical, and biological processes, since reactions accelerate when kinetic energy increases. However, bacteria that have evolved to live at low temperatures (psychrophiles) possess enzymes that may be optimally active at a low temperature, leading to better growth.

[41] Since there's no sunlight in the bloodstream, choices B and D are out. If it's a parasite, it most likely uses some of our chemicals, so it must be a heterotroph, which eliminates choice A. The answer is choice **C**.

- Which one of the following categories best describes an organism which uses sunlight to drive ATP production but cannot incorporate carbon dioxide into sugars?[42]
  - A) Chemoautotroph
  - B) Photoautotroph
  - C) Chemoheterotroph
  - D) Photoheterotroph

Growth Media

The environment in which bacteria grow is the **medium** (plural: **media**). In the lab, the most common solid medium is agar, a firm transparent gel made from seaweed. Bacteria live in the agar but do not metabolize it. The agar is usually kept in a clear plastic plate called a **Petri dish**, and the process of putting bacteria on such a plate is called **plating**. When one bacterium is plated onto a dish, if it grows, it will eventually give rise to many progeny in an isolated spot called a **colony**. **Minimal medium** contains nothing but glucose (in addition to the agar). More key terms: a **wild-type** bacterium (or a wild-type strain) is one which possesses all the characteristics normal to that particular species. The dense growth of bacteria seen in laboratory Petri dishes is known as a bacterial **lawn**. A **plaque** is a clear area in the lawn. Plaques result from death of bacteria and are caused by lytic viruses or toxins.

Bacteria can reproduce very rapidly, provided that the conditions of their environment are favorable and nutrients are abundant. The **doubling time** is the amount of time required for a population of bacteria to double its number. It ranges from a minimum of 20 minutes for *E. coli* to a day or more for slow growers, such as the bacteria responsible for tuberculosis and leprosy. The doubling time of a bacterial species will vary, depending upon the availability of nutrients and other environmental factors.

One other important term in bacterial nutrition is **auxotroph** (don't confuse this term with *auto*troph). This is a bacterium which cannot survive on minimal medium because it can't synthesize a molecule it needs to live. Therefore, it requires an *aux*iliary *troph*ic substance to live. For instance, a bacterium which is auxotrophic for arginine won't form a colony when plated onto minimal medium, but if the medium is supplemented with arginine, a colony will form. This arginine auxotrophy is denoted arg⁻. Auxotrophy results from a mutation in a gene coding for an enzyme in a synthetic pathway.

Bacteria can be differentiated not only by what substances they require, but also by what substances they are capable of metabolizing for energy. For instance, a strain of bacteria may be capable of surviving on minimal medium that has the disaccharide lactose as the only carbon source (no glucose). This would be denoted lac⁺. Mutation in a gene for the enzyme lactase would impair the bacterium's ability to survive on lactose-only medium. A bacterial strain incapable of growing with lactose as its only carbon source would be denoted lac⁻. Genetic exchange between bacteria by means of conjugation, transduction, or transformation (discussed below) can remedy these disabilities.

Oxygen Utilization and Tolerance

Oxygen metabolism is *aerobic* metabolism. Bacteria which require oxygen are called **obligate aerobes**. Bacteria which do not require oxygen are called **anaerobes**. There are three subcategories: **facultative anaerobes** will use oxygen when it's around, but they don't need it. [How much more ATP can they

---

[42] The ability to use sunlight indicates that the organism is a phototroph, and the inability to use carbon dioxide as a carbon source indicates that it is a heterotroph—it must use organic molecules as a carbon source. The answer is choice **D**.

make per glucose molecule when O_2 is present?[43]] **Tolerant anaerobes** can grow in the presence or absence of oxygen but do not use it in their metabolism. **Obligate anaerobes** are poisoned by oxygen. This is because they lack certain enzymes necessary for the detoxification of free radicals which form spontaneously whenever oxygen is around.[44] Obligate anaerobes commonly infect wounds.

- If a bacterium cannot use oxygen as an electron acceptor, is it an obligate anaerobe, a tolerant anaerobe, or a facultative anaerobe, or is it not possible to distinguish based on the information given?[45]

- A sample of bacteria is evenly mixed into a cool liquid agar nutrient mix in the absence of oxygen and then poured into a glass-walled tube that is open to the atmosphere on top. When the agar mix cools, it solidifies, and bacterial growth is observed as shown below. How would you classify the bacteria in terms of oxygen utilization and tolerance? (*Note*: Agar is practically impermeable to oxygen.)[46]

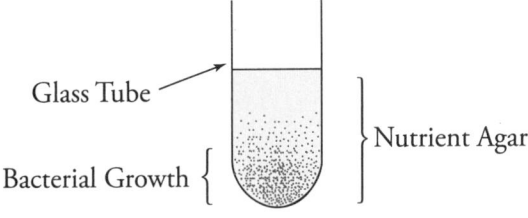

Fermentation vs. Respiration

Respiration is glucose catabolism with use of an inorganic electron acceptor such as oxygen. In contrast, fermentation is glucose catabolism which does not use an electron acceptor such as O_2; instead, a reduced by-product of glucose catabolism such as lactate or ethanol is given off as waste. [Why is fermentation necessary whenever an external electron acceptor is not used?[47]]

Anaerobic Respiration

This is not a contradiction in terms! It refers to glucose metabolism with electron transport and oxidative phosphorylation relying on an external electron acceptor *other than* O_2. For example, instead of reducing O_2 to H_2O, some anaerobic bacteria reduce SO_4^{2-} to H_2S, or CO_2 to CH_4. Nitrate (NO_3^-) is another possible electron acceptor.

---

[43] Sixteen times as much. For more on this topic, see *MCAT Biochemistry Review*.

[44] The enzymes include superoxide dismutase (converts O_2^- to H_2O_2) and catalase (converts H_2O_2 to $H_2O + O_2$). An example of a harmful O_2 by-product is superoxide anion, O_2^-.

[45] The bacterium cannot be a facultative anaerobe, since the question states it cannot use O_2. It could be either an obligate or a tolerant anaerobe depending on its ability to neutralize harmful oxygen-free radicals.

[46] Since the bacteria grew only at the bottom of the tube, farthest away from any oxygen, this indicates that they could only grow in the absence of oxygen. Thus, they are obligate anaerobes.

[47] Because NAD^+ must be regenerated from NADH for glycolysis to continue. In fermentation, the electrons are passed from NADH to a molecule other than O_2, such as pyruvic acid.

- In an experiment, facultative anaerobic bacteria that are growing on glucose in air are shifted to anaerobic conditions. If they continue to grow at the same rate while producing lactic acid, then the rate of glucose consumption will:[48]
  - A) increase 16 fold.
  - B) decrease 16 fold.
  - C) decrease 2 fold.
  - D) not change.

Bacterial Life Cycle

Bacteria reproduce asexually. In asexual reproduction, there is no meiosis, no meiotic generation of haploid gametes, and no fusion of gametes to form a new individual organism. Instead, each bacterium grows in size until it has synthesized enough cellular components for two cells rather than one, replicates its genome, then divides in two. This process in bacteria is also known as **binary fission** (fission means "to split"). [In prokaryotes, does reproduction increase genetic diversity?[49] If a eukaryote reproduces strictly by asexual reproduction, how will this affect the genetic diversity of a population?[50] How is asexual reproduction in a eukaryote different from asexual reproduction in a prokaryote?[51]] Although bacteria do not reproduce sexually, they do possess a mechanism, termed **conjugation**, for exchanging genetic information (more on this later).

Growth of bacterial populations is described in stages (see Figure 12). Under ideal conditions, bacterial population growth is exponential, meaning that the number of bacterial cells increases exponentially with time. This also means the log of the population size grows linearly with time, hence the name **log phase.** [If 10 bacteria in log phase are placed in ideal growth conditions and the doubling time is 20 minutes, how many bacteria will there be after four hours?[52]]

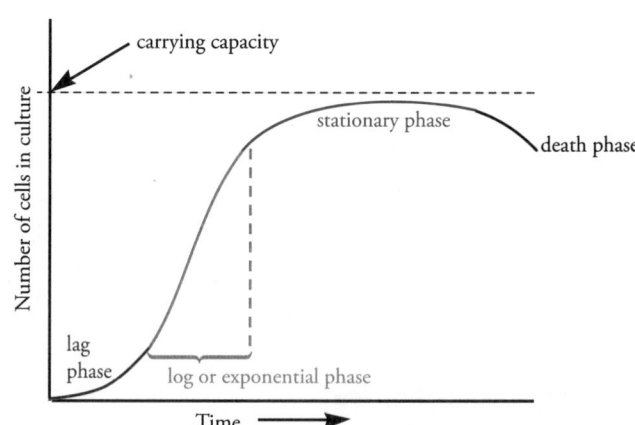

Figure 12 Bacterial Reproduction

---

[48] Aerobic respiration produces 32 ATP per glucose in prokaryotes compared to only 2 ATP per glucose in fermentation. If the rate of growth is to remain the same, the rate of ATP production must remain the same to drive biosynthetic pathways forward. Since fermentation produces 1/16 the amount of ATP per glucose, the rate of glucose consumption must increase sixteen fold to maintain the rate of growth at the same level. The answer is choice **A**. (In reality the growth rate would probably decrease.)

[49] No. Each daughter cell is identical to the parent cell (assuming no mutation took place).

[50] Many eukaryotes reproduce asexually. Sexual reproduction allows for generation of new allelic combinations through meiotic recombination and random union of gametes. Without this, diversity will decrease over time.

[51] In eukaryotes, asexual reproduction occurs through mitosis. Prokaryotes do not go through mitosis.

[52] Since four hours is equal to 240 minutes, the bacteria will divide twelve times. Therefore, one bacterium will produce $2^{12} = 4,096$ bacteria after 12 divisions. Since there are 10 bacteria initially, the total after four hours will be $10 \times 2^{12} = 40,960$.

Prior to achieving exponential growth, bacteria that were not previously growing undergo a **lag phase**, during which cell division does not occur even if the growth conditions are ideal.

- If growth conditions are ideal, why wouldn't cell division occur immediately?[53]
- Will bacteria that are transferred from a culture that is in log phase to a fresh new culture show a lag phase?[54]

As metabolites in the growth medium are depleted, and metabolic waste products accumulate, the bacterial population passes from log phase to **stationary phase**, in which cells cease to divide for lack of nutrients. The maximum population at the stationary phase is referred to as the **carrying capacity** for that environment. In the last stages of the stationary phase, cell death may occur as a result of the medium's inability to support growth. [If bacteria are grown in a medium with glucose as the main source of energy, when will the glycolytic pathway be more active: during the lag phase or during the stationary phase?[55]]

Endospore Formation

Some types of Gram-positive bacteria, such as the bacteria responsible for botulism, form **endospores** under unfavorable growth conditions. Endospores have tough, thick external shells comprised of peptidoglycan. Within the endospore are found the genome, ribosomes, and RNA which are required for the spore to become metabolically active when conditions become favorable. Endospores are able to survive temperatures above 100°C, which is why autoclaves or pressure cookers are required to completely sterilize liquids and substances that cannot be heated sufficiently in a dry oven. The metabolic reactivation of an endospore is termed **germination**. A single bacterium is able to form only one spore per cell. Thus, bacteria cannot increase their population through spore formation. [When are bacteria most likely to form endospores: during lag phase, log phase, or stationary phase? Is endospore formation a means for bacteria to reproduce?[56]]

Genetic Exchange Between Bacteria

Bacteria reproduce asexually, but genetic exchange is evolutionarily favorable because it fosters genetic diversity. Bacteria have three mechanisms of acquiring new genetic material: **transduction**, **transformation**, and **conjugation**. Note that none of these has anything to do with reproduction! Transduction was discussed in Section 5.1; it is the transfer of genomic DNA from one bacterium to another by a lysogenic phage. Transformation refers to a peculiar phenomenon: if pure DNA is added to a bacterial culture, the bacteria internalize the DNA in certain conditions and gain any genetic information in the DNA. Conjugation appears most likely to be related to normal bacterial function, however.

---

[53] Cells that are not growing are not actively producing components that are needed for cell division, such as dNTPs. The lag period is a time when biosynthetic pathways are very actively producing new cellular components so that cells can then begin to divide.

[54] No, since they will have all the gear necessary for population growth at the ready.

[55] The bacteria will use glucose during the lag phase to produce ATP and cellular machinery. During this period, glucose is abundant, and the cell is actively performing biosynthesis, so glycolysis is very active. During the stationary phase, however, the glucose will be depleted, and the rate of metabolism will have slowed dramatically, so the rate of glycolysis will decrease as well.

[56] Stationary. Forming an endospore is like hibernating, not reproducing. Bacteria do it in order to sleep through the bad times.

Conjugation

5.3

Although bacteria reproduce asexually, they have developed conjugation to exchange genetic information. In conjugation, bacteria make physical contact and form a bridge between the cells. One cell copies DNA, and this copy is transferred through the bridge to the other cell. A key to bacterial conjugation is an extrachromosomal element known as the **F (fertility) factor**. Bacteria that have the F factor are **male**, or **F⁺**, and will transfer the F factor to female cells. Bacteria that do not contain the F factor are **female**, **F⁻**, and will receive the F factor from male cells to become male. [If all cells in a population are F⁺, will conjugation occur?[57]]

The F factor is a single circular DNA molecule. Although much smaller than the bacterial chromosome, the F factor contains several genes, many of which are involved in conjugation itself. [Which cell will produce sex pili: the male cell or the female cell?[58]] After the male cell produces sex pili and the pili contact a female cell, a **conjugation bridge** forms. The F factor is replicated and transferred from the F⁺ to the F⁻ cell. DNA transfer between F⁺ and F⁻ cells is unidirectional; it occurs in one direction only (see Figure 13).

Although the F factor is an extrachromosomal element, it does sometimes become integrated into the bacterial chromosomes through recombination. A cell with the F factor integrated into its genome is called an **Hfr (high frequency of recombination) cell**. [Will an Hfr cell undergo conjugation with an F⁻ cell?[59]] When an Hfr cell performs conjugation, replication of the F factor DNA occurs as in F⁺ cells with the extra chromosomal F factor. Since the F factor DNA is integrated in the bacterial genome in Hfr cells, replication of F factor DNA continues into bacterial genes, and these too can be transferred into the F⁻ cell (see Figure 13).

- If bacteria contain only one copy of the bacterial genome, how can recombination occur?[60]
- If the F factor in an Hfr strain integrates near a gene required for lactose metabolism, is it likely that other genes involved in lactose metabolism will be transferred during conjugation at the same time?[61]

---

[57] No. Conjugation occurs only between F+ (male) and F⁻ (female).

[58] The male cell contains the F factor that encodes the genes for pili production and will produce pili.

[59] Yes. All of the genes of the F factor are still present and expressed normally in the Hfr cell.

[60] When an Hfr cell conjugates with an F⁻ cell and transfers a portion of the bacterial chromosomes, the F⁻ cell will have two copies of some genes, and recombination can occur between the two copies.

[61] Yes. Genes for proteins of related functions are often adjacent to each other in prokaryotes (in operons) and so will transfer to an F⁻ cell together.

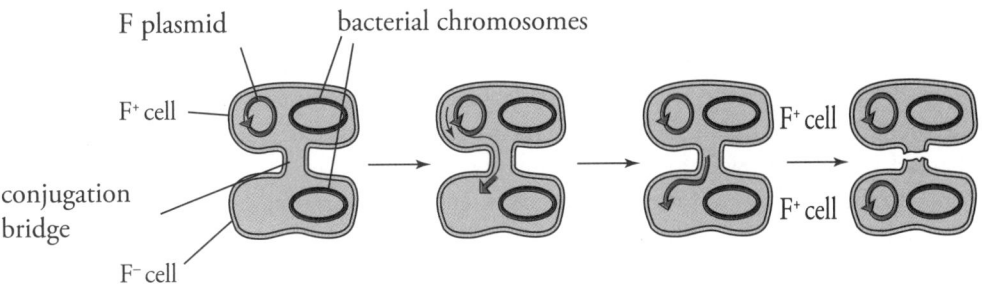

a) Conjugation and transfer of an F plasmid from an F⁺ donor to an F⁻ recipient

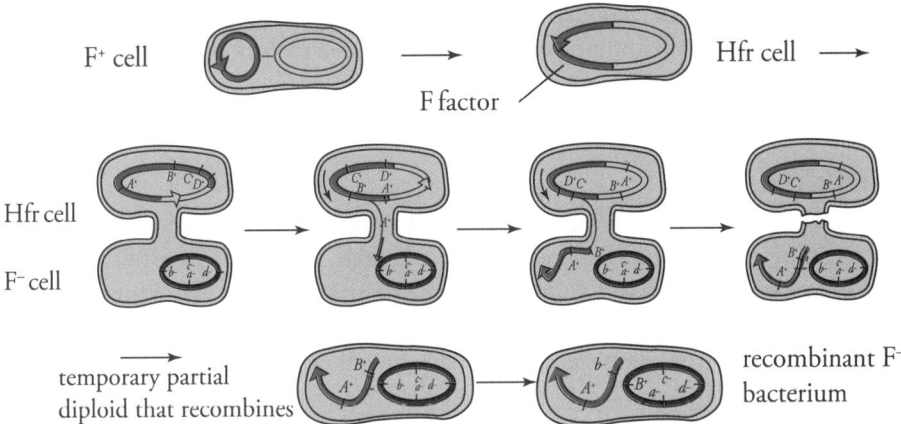

b) Conjugation and transfer of part of the bacterial chromosome from an Hfr donor to an F⁻ recipient, resulting in recombination

Figure 13 Conjugation

Conjugation Mapping

Hfr bacteria provide a mechanism of mapping the bacterial genome. By allowing Hfr cells to conjugate in the lab and stopping the conjugation process after different time intervals, researchers can figure out the order of the genes on the bacterial chromosome by analyzing recipient cells to see what genes were transferred.

For example, you have two strains of *E. coli*. One is a normal Hfr bacterium. The other is F⁻ and auxotrophic for arginine, leucine, and histidine (F⁻ Arg⁻ Leu⁻ His⁻). You allow conjugation to begin and stop it after 2 minutes. You find that all the recipients are now F⁻ Arg⁻ Leu⁻ His⁺. Then you take another bunch of bacteria and allow conjugation to proceed for 5 minutes. Now all the recipients are F⁻ Arg⁺ Leu⁻ His⁺. You do the experiment a third and final time, allowing 8 minutes of conjugation, and find the recipients to be F⁻ Arg⁺ Leu⁺ His⁺.

- What is the arrangement on the genome of the enzymes responsible for synthesis of each amino acid, relative to the site of F plasmid integration?[62]

---

[62] The experiments showed that the ability to make histidine was transferred in a short time. After a slightly longer time, the ability to make both histidine and arginine was transferred. Lastly, the ability to make leucine were transferred. So the arrangement on the genome (the map) must be: His-Arg-Leu-plasmid integration site.

Domain Archaea

Though all bacteria are prokaryotes, not all prokaryotes are equal. Certain prokaryotes belong to the domain *Archaea*, to be distinguished from the more "typical" bacteria (or eubacteria) which we have just discussed. The Archaea are the organisms that live in the world's most extreme environments, including hot springs, thermal vents, and hypersaline environments (although they can also be found in less extreme environments, such as soil, water, the human colon, etc.). Structurally, they differ from other bacteria because their cell wall lacks peptidoglycan. Genetically, they share traits with eukaryotes including the presence of introns and the use of many similar mRNA sequences. However, since they are single celled, they do reproduce via fission or budding. [What does this mean for their ability to increase their genetic diversity?[63]]

Since Archaea have to produce enzymes that can function in extreme environments, they are of great use in industrial applications, such as food processing and sewage treatment. The development of applications for products from these cells is an ongoing area of research.

Parasitic Bacteria

Parasitic bacteria can either be *obligate*, meaning that they must be inside a host cell to replicate, or *facultative*, meaning that they can live and replicate inside or outside of a host cell. In either case, the designation as a **parasite** means that damage is being done to the host cell. However, in order to ensure a continued supply of energy and cellular materials needed to survive and reproduce, parasitic bacteria need to modulate the course of that damage. [How is this model similar to viruses?[64]]

T cells (lymphocytes involved in immunity; see Chapter 9) are responsible for monitoring cellular contents; people who are T cell deficient have a hard time fighting off these types of bacterial infections, just as they would also struggle with viral infections. *Mycobacteria*, the genus of bacteria which encompasses the cause of tuberculosis as well as other diseases, has members which are obligate and others which are facultative, whereas the sexually transmitted disease chlamydia is caused solely by an obligate parasitic bacteria.

Symbiotic Bacteria

Symbiotic bacteria coexist with a host, where both the bacterial cell and the host cell derive a benefit. An example of this would be the *Rhizobia* genus, which is responsible for the fixing of nitrogen in the nodules that exist on the roots of legumes. Without these bacteria the legume plants would not be able to grow, as they would be unable to derive the necessary nitrogen from the soil on their own. Similarly, *Cyanobacteria* are responsible for nitrogen fixing in marine environments. Some of the bacterial flora in the human gut is also composed of symbionts which aid the human body in defending against other pathogenic strains. [What other functions do the bacteria in the gut have?[65]] Due to their close relationship with their host cells, these bacteria often have smaller genomes with a more limited number of cellular products that are made, since the host cells can provide some of what the bacteria need. This can often mean that the symbiotic bacteria do not survive long outside of the host environment.

---

[63] Archaea would need to use separate strategies to increase their genetic diversity, just like eubacteria. The ability to become more genetically diverse would not be built into reproduction as it is in humans, in part because meiosis is not occurring.

[64] Viruses are obligate intracellular parasites. They do not have the option to replicate outside of a host cell, but must also balance the damage that is done to the host cell against what is needed for more virus to be made.

[65] The gut flora is responsible for the production of vitamin K, which is necessary for blood clotting and in feeding off of undigested material from what humans have consumed; they are one of the final stages in processing our solid waste for excretion.

Chapter 5 Summary

- All viruses are made up of nucleic acids (either RNA or DNA) surrounded by a protein coat (capsid). They are obligate intracellular parasites and must rely on other cells to reproduce.

- Animal viruses may also have an envelope (lipid bilayer) surrounding the capsid. The envelope is derived from the host cell and is acquired by budding through the host cell membrane.

- Viral infection is specific; molecules on the viral surface determine which type of host cell it will infect.

- Viruses replicate via two major life cycles, the lytic cycle (in which more virus is made very quickly) and the lysogenic cycle (in which the virus goes dormant by integrating into the host cell genome). Viruses in the lysogenic cycle can excise from the genome and enter the lytic cycle.

- Animal viruses can also participate in a third life cycle, the productive cycle. This is very similar to the lytic cycle, but the new viruses escape by budding instead of by lysing the host.

- Lysogenic viruses can take pieces of the host DNA with them when they excise and transfer it to the next host. This is called transduction.

- RNA viruses require special virus-derived enzymes (RNA dependent RNA polymerases) in order to replicate their genomes.

- Prions and viroids are subviral particles that can cause disease and infection. They are unique in that prions are simply abnormal proteins (with no genetic material) and viroids are small pieces of RNA with no associated capsid, that do not code for proteins.

- The primary difference between prokaryotes and eukaryotes is that prokaryotes have no membrane-bound organelles (e.g., nucleus, mitochondria, etc.), thus all cellular processes occur in the cytosol.

- The shapes of bacteria can be used to classify them (round = coccus, rod = bacillus, spiral = spirochete).

- Bacteria have cell walls made out of peptidoglycan that can bind crystal violet (a purple stain used in Gram stain). Gram-positive bacteria have thick cell walls and stain a dark purple. Gram-negative bacteria have thinner cell walls and an outer membrane; they stain a light pink.

- Some bacteria can be classified by the presence or absence of flagella. Bacterial flagella are used for motility and are distinct from eukaryotic flagella in structure.

- Preferred growth temperature, nutrition, and oxygen use/tolerance are means of characterizing bacteria and can be used to select for growth of a particular bacteria.

- Binary fission is a means of asexual bacterial reproduction that increases the population size exponentially, but it does not increase the genetic diversity of the population.

- Conjugation is a means of increasing genetic diversity in a bacterial population by exchanging DNA (plasmid or genomic) via a conjugation bridge.

- Bacteria in Domain Archaea are sometimes classified as extremophiles because they can live in harsh, extreme environments, like hot springs, thermal vents, extreme acids/bases, and hyper-saline environments.

- Parasitic bacteria can live inside or outside of host cells and harm the host cells. Symbiotic bacteria coexist with host cells, but provide the host cells with a benefit; for example, the gut bacteria provide us with vitamin K.

CHAPTER 5 FREESTANDING PRACTICE QUESTIONS

1. A researcher has an agar plate covered with a lawn of *E. coli*. She adds a drop of a substance, and the next day there is a clear spot on the plate where the substance was added. This substance could be:

    I.   a virus undergoing the lytic cycle.
    II. a virus undergoing the productive cycle.
    III. a chemical that is toxic to prokaryotes.

A) I only
B) III only
C) I and III
D) I, II, and III

2. A lab technician grows a liquid bacterial culture overnight, in media without any antibiotics. The next morning, the culture is cloudy. She takes a small amount of this culture and puts it into new media containing tetracycline. The next day, she checks the culture and the media is not cloudy. What happened?

A) The bacterial culture grew the first night but not the second night.
B) The bacteria were resistant to the antibiotic tetracycline.
C) The bacteria were in the lag phase after the first night of growth.
D) The bacteria were in the stationary phase after the second night of growth.

3. Which of the following is associated with prokaryotes and does NOT introduce new genetic material?

A) Mitosis
B) Binary fission
C) Transformation
D) Transduction

4. Which of the following statements concerning viruses is true?

A) The productive cycle is the most efficient infective cycle for phages.
B) Viruses that infect human cells must have an envelope.
C) Genetic information can be transferred between hosts via transfection.
D) A lytic virus with an RNA genome must code for an RNA-dependent RNA polymerase.

5. A researcher is trying to characterize a novel prokaryotic organism that has been found in the Indian Ocean. When Gram stained, the cells are a light pink color under the microscope. When exposed to antibiotics commonly used in the lab, the bacteria are able to enter the log growth phase in a manner similar to *E. coli* grown in media lacking ampicillin. A reasonable explanation is that:

A) this is a Gram-positive bacterium with an additional lipopolysaccharide layer that increases their resistance to antibiotics.
B) this is a Gram-positive bacterium with a cell membrane outside its peptidoglycan layer that increases their resistance to antibiotics.
C) this is a Gram-negative bacterium with an additional lipopolysaccharide layer that increases their resistance to antibiotics.
D) this is a Gram-negative bacterium with a peptidoglycan layer outside the cell membrane that increases their resistance to antibiotics.

6. Which of the following is true regarding prokaryotic flagella?

A) It is the predominant form of bacterial locomotion.
B) It is made of microtubules connected by dynein proteins.
C) It allows viruses to maneuver between host cells.
D) It can only be located on one end of a bacterium and this defines the polarity of the cell.

7. In prion diseases like Creutzfeldt-Jakob disease (CJD), the characteristic misfolded proteins are notoriously resistant to degradation. As a result, abnormal proteins accumulate in the endosomes and lysosomes of the cell, eventually leading to cellular dysfunction and death through a chronic, neurodegenerative process. Which of the following is the most likely explanation for the unusual resistance of these proteins to breakdown?

A) Accelerated rate of protein biosynthesis leads to early cell lysis
B) Excessive amount of protein accumulation results in cellular dysfunction
C) Aberrant protein function leads to disruption of normal cellular processes
D) Abnormal protein secondary structure results in poor binding with innate lysosomal proteases

CHAPTER 5 PRACTICE PASSAGE

Laboratory tests are a useful diagnostic tool for determining the cause of illness. One such test is the complete blood count or, CBC, as it is commonly called. In an infected individual, the white blood cell count can increase from a normal range of 4000–10,000 cells/μL to 15,000 to 20,000 cells/μL. Circulating neutrophils have a short lifespan upon release from the bone marrow (generally about ten hours); however, the demand for phagocytic cells during an infection increases markedly. The result is the release of immature neutrophils called band cells. In a differential white blood cell count, the presence of band cells is referred to as a *shift to the left*. A decrease in the number of neutrophils (neutropenia) can also occur as a result of inflammation or severe infection, when the removal of the neutrophils from the circulation outpaces their production. Neutropenia is also seen in certain blood cancers, such as leukemia and lymphomas, as the neutrophil precursor cells are crowded out by the cancerous cells.

The type of microorganism responsible for an infection can often be determined by changes identified in the population of white blood cells. For example, an increase in neutrophils is commonly seen in bacterial infections. An increase in eosinophils frequently accompanies parasitic infections, as well as allergic responses. A decrease in neutrophils with an increase in lymphocytes (lymphocytosis) can signify a viral infection. All types of infections can result in inflammation (fever, swelling, redness, pain).

An emergency room saw patients presenting with respiratory complaints and fever. One symptom was cough, either productive and mucus-producing, or non-productive. The fevers were mild to severe. A blood sample was obtained from each patient; a CBC was ordered on each and each sample was cultured for any infection-causing bacteria. Standard growth media providing sufficient nutrients for a wide range of bacteria was used. The following results were obtained:

Table 1 Bacterial Culture Results in Four Different Patients

Patient	Growth in culture
1	No
2	Yes
3	No
4	Yes

Table 2 WBC Counts in Four Different Patients

Patient	Elevated eosinophils	Elevated neutrophils	Elevated lymphocytes
1	Yes	No	No
2	No	No	Yes
3	No	No	Yes
4	No	Yes	No

1. If placed on a course of antibiotic therapy, which of the following patients would feel significantly improved after approximately 1–2 days?

A) Patient 1
B) Patient 2
C) Patient 3
D) Patient 4

2. Why did the culture performed on the sample obtained from Patient 3 not yield any growth?

A) The bacteria causing the infection in Patient 3 is a uracil auxotroph.
B) Patient 3 has a bacterial infection.
C) Patient 3 is suffering from allergic symptoms.
D) A different growth medium was required.

3. To determine the most appropriate type of antibiotic to prescribe, which of the following additional tests could be performed on a patient sample for classification purposes?

A) Phage-typing
B) Gram-staining
C) Fermentation
D) Transduction

4. Which of the following bacterial types are LEAST likely to cause a respiratory infection?

A) Tolerant anaerobe
B) Obligate aerobe
C) Facultative anaerobe
D) Obligate anaerobe

5. If a patient's symptoms included neutropenia and elevated lymphocyte counts, which of the following diagnoses could be possible?

I. Allergies

II. Leukemia/lymphoma

III. Viral infection

A) I only
B) II only
C) I and III only
D) II and III only

6. An experimental therapy to treat patients with multiple antibiotic-resistant bacteria involves introduction of a highly specific bacteriophage to the infected patient's bloodstream. Which of the following bacteriophage types would be the LEAST useful for this type of therapy?

A) A lytic bacteriophage
B) A lysogenic bacteriophage
C) An RNA virus
D) An enveloped virus

SOLUTIONS TO CHAPTER 5 FREESTANDING PRACTICE QUESTIONS

1. **C**   A clear spot on a plate (known as a *plaque*) indicates that the *E. coli* are dead. This could be due to the addition of a lytic virus (Item I is true, and choice B can be eliminated) or toxin (Item III is true, and choice A can be eliminated). However, only animal viruses can go through the productive cycle because viruses cannot bud out of a cell with a cell wall, such as bacteria (Item II is false; choice D can be eliminated, and choice C is correct).

2. **A**   Cloudy cultures are usually in the stationary phase and clear cultures are either not growing or still in the lag phase. Since the culture was cloudy on the first morning, bacteria had grown overnight and were most likely in stationary phase (choice A is correct, and choice C is wrong). The culture on the second morning was clear, indicating minimal growth (choice D is wrong). Since the first overnight culture did not contain tetracycline and the second overnight culture did, it is possible that the strain was sensitive to tetracycline, not resistant (choice B is wrong).

3. **B**   Binary fission is the means by which bacteria divide and reproduce. It produces two progeny cells that are genetically identical to the parent; no new genetic information is introduced (choice B is correct). Although mitosis also does not introduce new genetic information, it is a process undergone by eukaryotic cells, not prokaryotes (choice A is wrong). Both transformation and transduction are associated with prokaryotes, but both involve the introduction of new genetic material. Transformation is the uptake of genetic material (plasmids or chromosomal DNA) from the extracellular environment (choice C is wrong), and transduction is the transfer of genetic information from one bacteria to another via a lysogenic phage (choice D is wrong).

4. **D**   In order to replicate its genome, a lytic RNA virus must code for an RNA-dependent RNA polymerase; this enzyme will create a new strand of RNA by reading a template strand of RNA. Viral host cells will not express these enzymes naturally; they have no need to make RNA by reading RNA. Host cells normally produce RNA using DNA as a template (choice D is correct). Note also that lysogenic RNA viruses do not need an RNA-dependent RNA polymerase either, because they are not replicating their RNA genome. They first convert it to DNA using an RNA-dependent DNA polymerase (reverse transcriptase), then insert the DNA version of their genome into the host genome. New copies of the viral RNA genome can be made by simply transcribing (using host RNA polymerases) new copies of the viral genome. Phages only infect bacteria and can only undergo the lytic and lysogenic cycles; the productive cycle involves budding through cell membrane and cannot occur in hosts with cell walls, such as bacteria (choice A is wrong). Although viruses with an envelope (lipid bilayer coating) are restricted to infecting animal cells, the outer membrane is not required (choice B is wrong). Genetic information can indeed be transferred between hosts, but this process is called *transduction*, not *transfection* (choice C is wrong).

5. **C**   The answer options all start with Gram positive or Gram negative, and the light pink staining in the question stem indicates that this bacteria is Gram negative. Gram-positive bacteria have a peptidoglycan layer outside the cell membrane and therefore stain a dark purple (choices A and B are wrong). Gram-negative bacteria have a lipopolysaccharide layer outside

the peptidoglycan layer. This additional outer layer prevents dark staining (thus the light pink color) and increases resistance to antibiotics (choice C is correct, and choice D is wrong).

6. **A** Prokaryotic flagella are the predominant means of bacterial locomotion (choice A is correct). Only eukaryotic flagella are made of microtubules and dynein; bacterial flagella have a different structure and are made of the protein flagellin (choice B is wrong). Viruses rely on diffusion to maneuver between host cells, not flagella (choice C is wrong). Bacteria can have flagella on one end (monotrichous), both ends (amphitrichous), or in multiple places (peritrichous; choice D is wrong).

7. **D** Typically in a cell, abnormal proteins are targeted to proteasomes in the cytosol for degradation or to the lysosomes for digestion. The accumulation of the abnormal prions in the lysosomes suggests that they are somehow resistant to the lysosomal enzymes, and this could be due to their abnormal structure that prevents efficient binding at the active sites of the lysosomal digestive enzymes (choice D is correct). CJD and other prion diseases do not involve accelerated protein biosynthesis; normal prion proteins are produced at their typical rate, but are converted after translation into the abnormal prion version (choice A is wrong). While the accumulation of misfolded proteins likely contributes to cellular dysfunction, and while prions could (and likely do) lead to disruption of normal cellular processes, neither of these explain why the abnormal proteins are resistant to breakdown (choice D is a better choice than either B or C).

SOLUTIONS TO CHAPTER 5 PRACTICE PASSAGE

1. **D** Antibiotics only treat bacterial infections. Table 1 shows that Patients 2 and 4 have positive cultures, confirming a bacterial infection (choices A and C can be eliminated). However, from Table 2, only Patient 4 has elevated neutrophils, which the passage states is indicative of a bacterial infection, making this patient a candidate for antibiotic therapy. Patient 2 has elevated lymphocytes (not neutrophils), which indicates a concomitant viral infection; the lack of elevated neutrophils in this patient is most likely the result of overwhelming infection. While the bacterial infection of Patient 2 would begin to subside by 1–2 days, the viral infection would take longer to eradicate, and therefore this patient would still be feeling poorly at this point (choice D is better than choice B).

2. **D** From Table 2, Patient 3 has elevated lymphocytes, indicating a viral infection (choices A, B, and C can be eliminated); no growth would occur on standard growth media. Viruses are obligate intracellular parasites and require special growth media containing live cells for reproduction. According to the passage, standard growth media for bacterial culturing was used. Note that if the patient had elevated neutrophils and normal lymphocyte levels (indicating a bacterial infection), choice A would be the best answer, since uracil was not added to the culture media.

3. **B** Determination of Gram status can aid in antibiotic selection. Phage typing applies to bacteriophage, not bacteria (choice A can be eliminated). Fermentation refers to metabolic activity (choice C can be eliminated). Transduction is not a classification method (choice D can be eliminated).

4. **D** The lungs are a high oxygen environment that is unfavorable to obligate anaerobes. Tolerant anaerobes, obligate aerobes, and facultative anaerobes can all survive in the presence of oxygen (choices A, B, and C can be eliminated).

5. **D** Item I is false: the passage states that elevated eosinophil counts (not lymphocytes) accompany allergic reactions (choices A and C can be eliminated). Note that both remaining answer choices include Item II, so it must be true: the passage states that neutropenia and elevated lymphocyte counts are seen in lymphoma and leukemia (blood cancers). Item III is true: neutropenia and lymphocytosis are seen in viral infections (choice B can be eliminated, and choice D is correct).

6. **D** Enveloped viruses infect only animal cells and would not be useful in eliminating bacteria from a human patient. The most useful type of virus would attack the infecting bacteria and cause the bacteria to lyse, eradicating the patient's infection (choice A would be useful and can be eliminated), and this virus could have either an RNA or a DNA genome (choice C could be useful and can be eliminated). A virus that incorporates itself into the bacterial genome and then goes dormant (a lysogenic virus) would not be as helpful as a lytic virus in eradicating an infection; however, it would still be more useful than a virus that cannot infect bacteria at all (choice B would be more useful than choice D).

Chapter 6
Eukaryotic Cells

The first cells were prokaryotes. They consisted of a cell membrane and a cell wall surrounding the cytoplasm or cell fluid. All of the structures necessary for survival and reproduction floated in the cytoplasm, including the double-stranded circular DNA genome, ribosomes, the enzymes of aerobic and anaerobic metabolism, etc. As evolution proceeded, cell complexity increased. The greatest landmark in the evolution of the cell was the development of membrane-bound compartments within the cytoplasm known as organelles. These served to organize the cytoplasm, with each membrane acting to seal its compartment. The most important organelle is the control center of the cell: the nucleus. In fact, *eukaryotic* is from the Greek *karyon*, meaning "kernel" or "nucleus," plus the prefix "eu," meaning "true." *Prokaryotic* means "before the nucleus" and also implies "before organelles." All true living organisms are either prokaryotes or eukaryotes. There are three well-defined kingdoms within Domain Eukarya (Plantae, Animalia, and Fungi), and one group of organisms for whom the kingdom classifications are under debate (single-celled eukaryotes—the Protists).

6.1 INTRODUCTION

It would be impossible to understand medicine without sound knowledge of the eukaryotic cell. In this chapter, we will examine each of the principal organelles, beginning with the nucleus. Next we will focus on the plasma membrane, then the cytoskeleton, and finally we will finish with a discussion of the cell cycle. You should be able to explain the function of each item labeled in Figure 1 below. Our discussion will be based on the animal cell; fungi, plants, and protists are not covered on the MCAT.

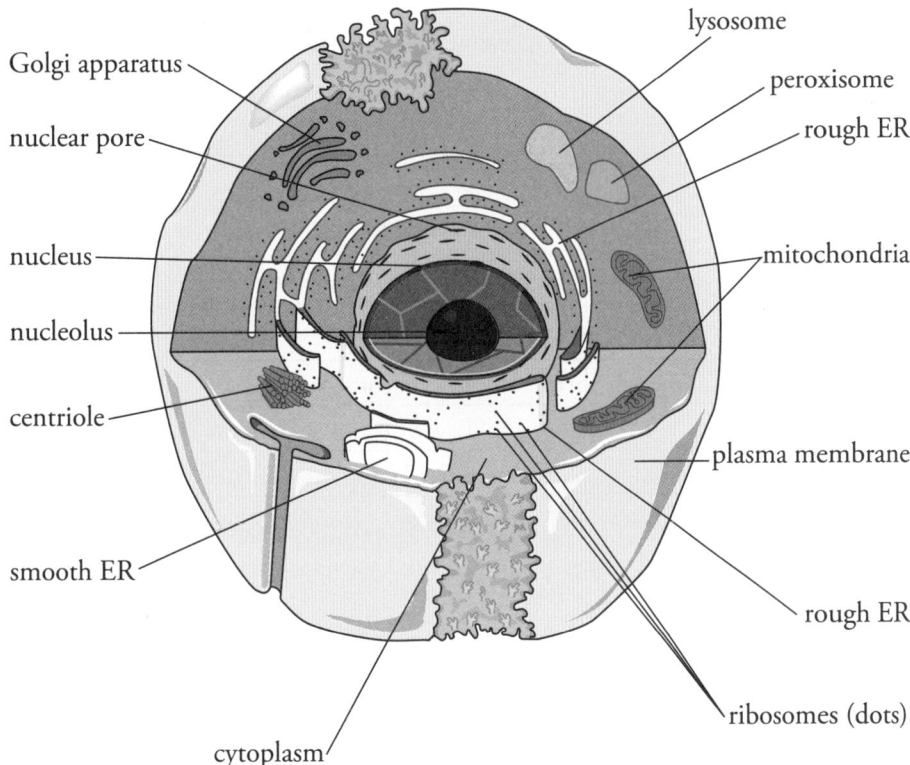

Figure 1 The Eukaryotic Cell

6.2 THE ORGANELLES

An **organelle** is a small structure within a cell that carries out specific cellular functions. Most organelles are bounded by their own lipid bilayer membrane. The membrane acts like a plastic bag to seal off the contents of the organelle from the rest of the cytoplasm and control what enters and exits. A summary of the major animal cell organelles is given in the table below:

Table 1 Animal Cell Organelles

Organelle	Function [number of membranes surrounding]
nucleus	contain and protect DNA; transcription; partial assembly of ribosomes (2)
mitochondria	produce ATP via the Krebs cycle and oxidative phosphorylation (2)
ribosomes	synthesize proteins (0)
RER	location of synthesis/modification of secretory, membrane-bound, and organelle proteins (1)
SER	detoxification and glycogen breakdown in liver; steroid synthesis in gonads (1)
Golgi apparatus	modification and sorting of protein, some synthesis (1)
lysosomes	contain acid hydrolases that digest various substances (1)
peroxisomes	metabolize lipids and toxins using H_2O_2 (1)

The Nucleus

One of the primary features of eukaryotic cells distinguishing them from prokaryotic cells is the **nucleus**. The nucleus contains the genome surrounded by the **nuclear envelope** that separates the contents of the nucleus into a distinct compartment, isolated from other organelles and from the cytoplasm. In prokaryotes the genome may be localized in the cell, but without a nuclear envelope to form a separate compartment, the genome remains accessible to the cytoplasm. In prokaryotes, replication, transcription and translation, and everything else all happens in the same compartment (the cytoplasm). In eukaryotes, replication, transcription, and splicing occur in the nucleus, while translation occurs in the cytoplasm.

- If an enzyme that degrades mRNA is injected into the cytoplasm of a cell and all translation ceases, is the cell prokaryotic or eukaryotic?[1]
- When an enzyme that degrades DNA (DNase) is incubated with intact DNA isolated from an organism, the DNA is degraded. But when DNase is injected into the cytoplasm of cells from the same organism, no effect on the genome is observed. Which one of the following is the best explanation for this?[2]
  - A) The cell is a prokaryote; therefore, the genome is inaccessible to cytoplasmic enzymes.
  - B) The cell is a prokaryote; therefore, the circular genome is resistant to DNase.
  - C) The cell is a eukaryote; therefore, the genome is inaccessible to cytoplasmic enzymes.
  - D) The cell is a eukaryote; therefore, the linear genome is resistant to DNase.

---

[1] It could be either. mRNA and translation are found in the cytoplasm of both prokaryotes and eukaryotes, so the cell could be either.

[2] The isolated genome and the genome in the cell respond differently, so the key is not the circular or linear nature of the genome (choices B and D are wrong). The key is that in prokaryotes the injected cytoplasmic DNase will have access to the genome to degrade since they are in the same compartment, while in eukaryotes the DNase will not have access to the genome unless it enters the nucleus (choice **C** is the best answer).

The Genome

The eukaryotic genome was discussed in Chapter 4, so we will not repeat that material. The large size of the typical eukaryotic genome appears to make it necessary to split the genome into pieces, each a separate linear DNA molecule, termed a **chromosome**. Yeast have 4 different chromosomes, while there are 23 different human chromosomes. Since humans and most adult animals are diploid, they have two copies of each chromosome (except for the sex chromosomes; see Chapter 7).

Within each chromosome is also a portion of the many thousands of genes in the genome as a whole. Genes can be mapped genetically and physically to the chromosome they reside on and to a specific location on that chromosome, a **locus**.

Finally, the nucleus is not a loose membrane bag with DNA floating inside. If nuclei are treated with DNase and with detergent, an insoluble mesh of protein, known as the **nuclear matrix** or **nuclear scaffold**, is left behind. The role of the nuclear matrix may be in part analogous to the role of the cytoskeleton in the cytoplasm: to support and provide overall structure. The matrix may also play a role in regulating gene expression. The DNA in chromosomes is attached to the matrix at specific sites, and these (in some cases) appear to be involved in regulating gene expression or in limiting the effects of promoters and enhancers to discrete chromosomal regions known as domains. The role of the nuclear matrix is an area of ongoing research.

The Nucleolus

The **nucleolus** ("little nucleus") is a region within the nucleus which functions as a ribosome factory. There is no membrane separating the nucleolus from the rest of the nucleus. It consists of loops of DNA, RNA polymerases, rRNA, and the protein components of the ribosome. [Would you expect the nucleolus to be larger in cells that are actively synthesizing protein, or in quiescent cells?[3] What role would the loops of DNA in the nucleolus play?[4]]

The nucleolus is the site of transcription of rRNA by RNA pol I. Transcription of mRNA and tRNA is performed by other polymerases in other areas of the nucleus. [Does a similar "division of labor" exist in the prokaryotic cell?[5]] The ribosome is partially assembled while still in the nucleolus. The protein components of the ribosome are not produced in the nucleolus; they are transported into the nucleus from the cytoplasm (remember that *all* translation takes place in the cytoplasm). After partial assembly, the ribosome is exported from the nucleus, remaining inactive until assembly is completed in the cytoplasm. This may serve to prevent translation of hnRNA.

---

[3] The nucleolus is largest in cells that are producing large amounts of protein. The increased size reflects increased synthesis of ribosomes.

[4] The DNA will serve as template for ribosomal RNA production.

[5] No. Bacteria have only a single kind of RNA pol which is responsible for all transcription.

The Nuclear Envelope

Surrounding the nucleus and separating it from the cytoplasm is the **nuclear envelope**, composed of two lipid bilayer membranes. The inner nuclear membrane is the surface of the envelope facing the nuclear interior, and the outer nuclear membrane faces the cytoplasm. The membrane of the endoplasmic reticulum is at points continuous with the outer nuclear membrane, making the interior of the ER (the **lumen** of the ER) contiguous with the space between the two nuclear membranes. [Is the space between the inner and outer membranes contiguous with the cytoplasm?[6]]

The nuclear envelope is punctuated with large **nuclear pores** that allow the passage of material into and out of the nucleus (see Figures 2 and 3). Molecules that are smaller than 60 kilodaltons, including small proteins, can freely diffuse from the cytoplasm into the nucleus through the nuclear pores. Larger proteins cannot pass freely through nuclear pores and are excluded from the nuclear interior unless they contain a sequence of basic amino acids called a **nuclear localization sequence**. Proteins with a nuclear localization sequence are translated on cytoplasmic ribosomes and then imported into the nucleus by specific transport mechanisms. It also appears likely that RNA is transported out of the nucleus by a specific transport system rather than freely diffusing into the cytoplasm. [If a 15 kD protein has a nuclear localization sequence that is then deleted from its gene, will the mutated protein still be found in the nucleus?[7]]

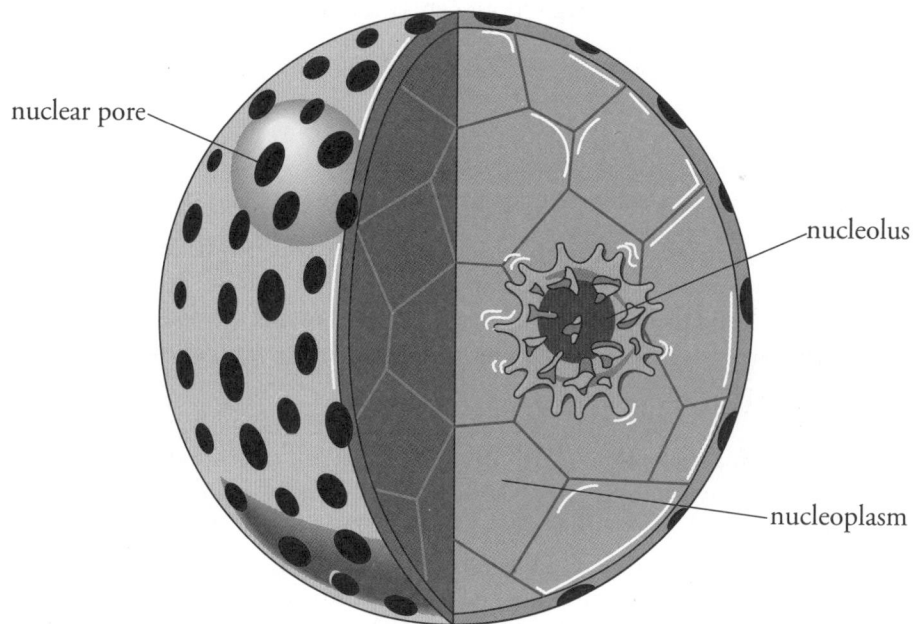

Figure 2 The Nucleus, Showing Pores

---

[6] No, it is not. The space between the nuclear membranes is contiguous with the ER lumen, which is isolated from the cytoplasm.

[7] Yes. The protein is small enough that it can still pass through the nuclear pores by diffusion even without a nuclear localization sequence.

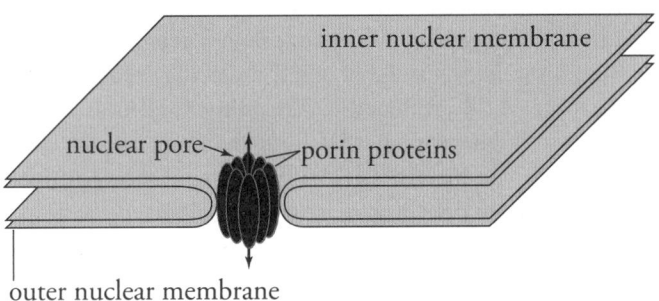

Figure 3   A Nuclear Pore Close-Up

- Which one of the following proteins would NOT be found within the nucleus?[8]
  - A) A protein component of the large ribosomal subunit
  - B) A factor required for splicing
  - C) A histone
  - D) An aminoacyl tRNA synthetase

- A researcher injects tiny gold beads into a cell and waits an hour. Then she examines the cell and finds gold beads in the cytoplasm and in the nucleus. When she injects larger gold beads, they are not found in the nucleus. However, when she binds the larger beads to a nuclear localization sequence, she finds that they end up in the nucleus. One can conclude that:[9]
  - A) the nuclear localization sequence is lysine-rich.
  - B) gold beads have an inherent import signal.
  - C) the nuclear localization mechanism is nonspecific enough to confer nuclear import on gold beads.
  - D) nuclear import relies primarily on simple diffusion.

Mitochondria

Mitochondria are the site of oxidative phosphorylation. The interior of mitochondria, the **matrix**, is bounded by the inner and outer mitochondrial membranes (see Figure 4, next page). The matrix contains pyruvate dehydrogenase and the enzymes of the Krebs cycle. The inner membrane is the location of the electron transport chain and ATP synthase and is the site of the proton gradient used to drive ATP synthesis by ATP synthase. The inner membrane is impermeable to the free diffusion of polar substances,

---

[8] Aminoacyl tRNA synthetases are enzymes that function in the cytoplasm to attach amino acids to their respective tRNAs. They are never needed in the nucleus and would not be found there (choice **D** is correct). The protein components of ribosomes are synthesized in the cytoplasm and then imported into the nucleus to be assembled in the nucleolus (choice A would be found in the nucleus and can be eliminated). Splicing occurs in the nucleus, so anything involved in splicing would be found there (choice B can be eliminated). Histones are used for DNA packaging and would be found in the nucleus (choice C can be eliminated).

[9] Gold beads are not normally found in cells, so there cannot be an existing mechanism for moving them. However, since the cell is capable of moving them when the localization signal is attached, the localization signal must be somewhat nonspecific (choice **C** is correct). It is true that the nuclear localization signal is lysine-rich, but this cannot be concluded based on the given information (true, but it doesn't answer the question; choice A is wrong). If gold beads had an inherent import signal, then they would be transported into the nucleus on their own, without the researcher having to bind them to the localization sequence (choice B is wrong). If simple diffusion were the primary means of moving things into the nucleus, no import signal would be needed (choice D is wrong).

like protons, and is folded into the matrix in projections called **cristae**. The outer membrane is smooth and contains large pores that allow free passage of small molecules. The space between the membranes is called the intermembrane space. ATP produced within mitochondria is transported out into the cytoplasm to drive a great variety of cellular processes. [Why is the inner membrane folded into cristae?[10] Are the enzymes of glycolysis found in the matrix?[11] If the inner membrane is impermeable, how does pyruvate get into the matrix where pyruvate dehydrogenase is located?[12]]

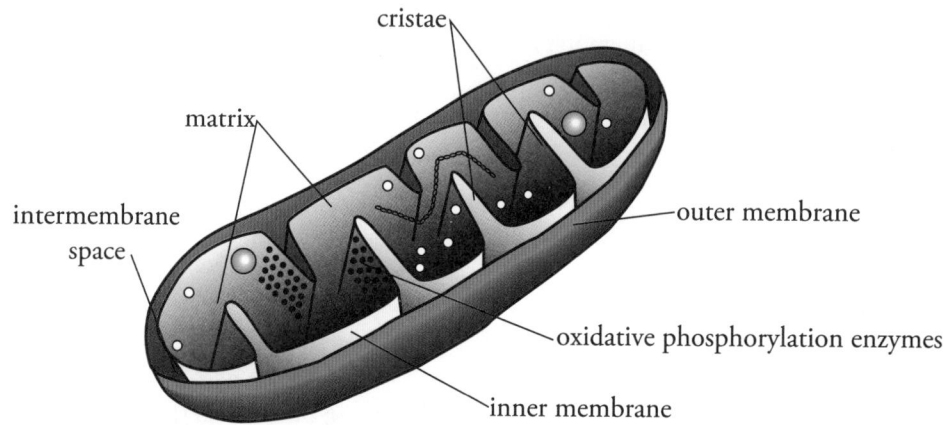

Figure 4   The Mitochondrion

Mitochondria possess their own genome which is far smaller than the cellular genome and consists of a single circular DNA molecule. (Sound familiar?) It encodes rRNA, tRNA, and several proteins, including some components of the electron transport chain and parts of the ATP synthase complex although most mitochondrial proteins are encoded by nuclear genes. Even more curious, mitochondria use a different system of transcription and translation than nuclear genes do. This includes a unique genetic code and unique RNA polymerases, DNA replication machinery, ribosomes, and aminoacyl-tRNA synthetases. In order to explain the fact that mitochondria possess a second system of inheritance, investigators have postulated that mitochondria originated as independent unicellular organisms living within larger cells. This is known as the **endosymbiotic theory** of mitochondrial evolution (*endo* = within; *symbiotic* = living together). In fact, if you compare a mitochondrion to a Gram-negative bacterium, you'll note that they look pretty similar. Pay attention to where the enzymes of electron transport are located and the genome shape.[13] Because many unique mitochondrial polypeptides are encoded by the cellular genome and not the mitochondrial genome, it has been suggested that the genes coding for these proteins may have been transferred to the nuclear genome over time. [What difficulty may be encountered in translation of a mitochondrial gene moved to the nucleus?[14]]

---

[10] The folding of the membrane increases its surface area and allows for increased electron transport and ATP synthesis per mitochondrion. (Folding is used elsewhere to increase surface area, such as in the kidney tubules and the lining of the small intestine.)

[11] No, in the cytoplasm.

[12] Pyruvate is transported through the inner mitochondrial membrane by a specific protein in the membrane.

[13] Remember that bacterial electron transport depends on a proton gradient across the cell membrane. In a Gram-negative bacterium, this membrane would correspond to the mitochondrial inner membrane.

[14] The coding system of the cellular genome is different from that of the mitochondrial genome. One might wonder how our transcription and translation machinery could sensibly produce mitochondrial gene products.

Mitochondria exhibit **maternal inheritance**. This means that mitochondria are inherited only from the mother, since the cytoplasm of the egg becomes the cytoplasm of the zygote. (The sperm contributes only genomic [nuclear] DNA.) Maternal inheritance departs from the rules of Mendelian genetics, which state that traits are inherited from both parents (see Chapter 7). If a woman has a disease caused by an abnormality in her mitochondrial genome, what are the chances that her children will have the disease (assuming her mate does not have the disease)?[15]

Endoplasmic Reticulum (ER)

The **endoplasmic reticulum** (**ER**) is a large system of folded membrane accounting for over half of the membrane of some cells. There are two types of ER (see Figure 5): **rough ER** and **smooth ER**, each with distinct functions. The rough ER is called rough due to the large number of ribosomes bound to its surface; it is the site of protein synthesis for proteins targeted to enter the secretory pathway. The smooth ER is not actively involved in protein processing but can contain enzymes involved in steroid hormone biosynthesis (gonads) or in the degradation of environmental toxins (liver). The membrane of the endoplasmic reticulum is joined with the outer nuclear membrane in places, meaning that the space within the nuclear membranes is continuous with the interior of the ER (the ER **lumen**). The rough ER plays a key role directing protein traffic to different parts of the cell.

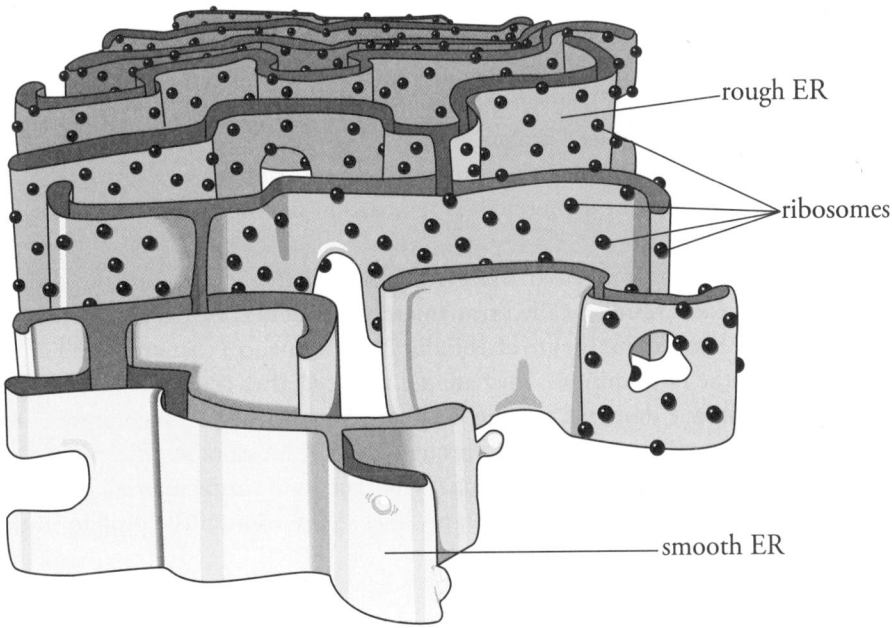

Figure 5   The ER

The Rough ER and the Secretory Pathway

There are two sites of protein synthesis in the eukaryotic cell: either on ribosomes free in the cytoplasm or on ribosomes bound to the surface of the rough ER. Proteins translated on free cytoplasmic ribosomes

---

[15] All of her children will have it, since they will inherit mitochondria exclusively from her. For a maternally inherited trait, it doesn't matter whether the father has it or not.

are headed toward peroxisomes, mitochondria, the nucleus, or will remain in the cytoplasm. Proteins synthesized on the rough ER will end up either 1) secreted into the extracellular environment, 2) as integral plasma membrane proteins, or 3) in the membrane or interior of the ER, Golgi apparatus, or lysosomes. Membrane-bound vesicles pass between these cellular compartments. Since the membranes of these organelles communicate through the traffic of vesicles, the interior of the ER, the Golgi apparatus, lysosomes, and the extracellular environment are in a sense contiguous. Proteins synthesized on the rough ER are transported in vesicles that bud from the ER to the Golgi apparatus, then to the plasma membrane or lysosome. A secreted protein that enters the ER lumen is separated by a membrane from the cytoplasm until the protein leaves the cell.

Whether a protein is translated on the rough ER is determined by the sequence of the protein itself. All proteins start translation in the cytoplasm; however, some proteins (secreted proteins and lysosomal proteins) have an amino acid sequence at their N-terminus called a **signal sequence.** The signal sequence of a nascent polypeptide is recognized by the **signal recognition particle** (**SRP**), which binds to the ribosome. The rough ER has SRP receptors that dock the ribosome-SRP complex on the cytoplasmic surface (along with the nascent polypeptide and mRNA). Translation then pushes the polypeptide, signal peptide first, into the ER lumen. After translation is complete, the signal peptide is removed from the polypeptide by a signal peptidase in the ER lumen. For secreted proteins, once the signal sequence is removed, the protein is transported in the interior of vesicles through the Golgi apparatus to the plasma membrane, where it is released by exocytosis into the extracellular environment.

- The mRNA for a secreted protein encodes a longer protein than is actually observed in the cellular exterior. Why?[16]
  - A) The protein was cleaved by a cytoplasmic protease.
  - B) The mRNA was not spliced properly.
  - C) The gene encoding the protein contained a nonsense mutation.
  - D) The signal sequence of the protein was removed in the rough ER.

Integral membrane proteins are processed slightly differently. Integral membrane proteins have sections of hydrophobic amino acid residues called **transmembrane domains** that pass through lipid bilayer membranes. The transmembrane domains are essentially signal sequences that are found in the interior of the protein (that is, not at the N-terminus). They are *not* removed after translation. A single polypeptide can have several transmembrane domains passing back and forth through a membrane. During translation, the transmembrane domains are threaded through the ER membrane. The protein is then transported in vesicles to the Golgi apparatus and plasma membrane in the same manner as a secreted protein (see Figure 6). [For a protein in the plasma membrane, does the portion of the protein in the ER lumen end up facing the cytoplasm or the cellular exterior?[17]]

Additional functions of the rough ER include the initial post-translational modification of proteins. Although glycosylation (the addition of saccharides to proteins) is usually associated with the Golgi apparatus, some glycosylation occurs in the lumen of the ER. Disulfide bond formation also occurs in the ER lumen.

---

[16] The only way a protein can be smaller than would be expected from its mRNA would be if some post-translational modification were to occur (choice **D** is correct). Choices B and C are pre-translational modifications and would not account for a size difference between mRNA and protein, and since secreted proteins are synthesized on the rough ER, they are inaccessible to cytoplasmic proteases (so choice A is wrong).

[17] The cellular exterior

Two last notes about protein traffic throughout the cell: First, the default target for proteins that go through the secretory path is the plasma membrane. **Targeting signals** are needed if a protein going through that path needs to end up elsewhere (e.g., the Golgi, the ER, the lysosome). Second, proteins that are made in the cytoplasm but need to be sent to an organelle that is not part of the secretory path (e.g., the nucleus, mitochondria, or peroxisomes) require sequences called **localization signals**. Table 2 summarizes protein traffic.

Table 2   Summary of Cellular Protein Traffic

Protein Final Destination	Signal Sequence?	Localization Signal?	Transmembrane Domains?	Targeting Signal?	Example
Secreted	Yes	No	No	No	Antibodies, neurotransmitters, peptide hormones
Plasma Membrane	Yes	No	Yes	No	Receptors, channels
Lysosome	Yes	No	No	Yes	Acid hydrolases
Rough ER	Yes	No	No	Yes	Enzymes required for protein modification
Smooth ER	Yes	No	No	Yes	Enzymes required for lipid synthesis
Golgi Apparatus	Yes	No	No	Yes	Enzymes required for protein modification
Cytoplasm	No	No	No	No	Glycolysis enzymes
Nucleus	No	Yes	No	No	Histones, DNA/RNA polymerase
Mitochondria	No	Yes	No	No	PDC/Krebs cycle enzymes
Peroxisome	No	Yes	No	No	Catalase

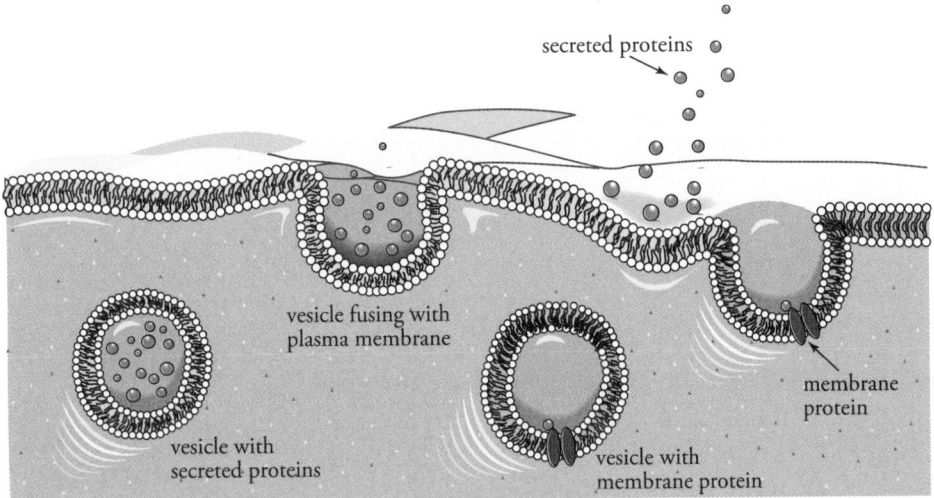

Figure 6   The Secretory Pathway—Secreted Proteins and Integral Membrane Proteins

- Disulfide bridges are found in extracellular proteins because the cytoplasm is a reducing environment that changes cystine to two cysteines. Given this fact, does it make sense that disulfide bridges are formed in the ER lumen?[18]
- Can mRNA coding for a protein destined to be embedded in the plasma membrane associate with rough ER prior to the initiation of translation?[19]

The Golgi Apparatus

The Golgi apparatus is a group of membranous sacs stacked together like collapsed basketballs (see Figure 7). It has the following functions: 1) Modification of proteins made in the RER; especially important is the modification of oligosaccharide chains. 2) Sorting and sending proteins to their correct destinations. 3) The Golgi also synthesizes certain macromolecules, such as polysaccharides, to be secreted.

The vesicle traffic to and from the Golgi apparatus is mostly unidirectional; the membrane-bound or secreted proteins which are to be sorted and modified enter at one defined region and exit at another. (Traffic is said to be *mostly* unidirectional because on occasion, proteins that are supposed to reside in the ER accidentally escape, and must be returned to the ER from the Golgi. This is called "retrograde traffic.") Each region of the Golgi has different enzymes and a different microscopic appearance. The portion of the Golgi nearest the rough ER is called the *cis* stack, and the part farthest from the rough ER is the *trans* stack. The *medial* stack is in the middle.[20] Vesicles from the ER fuse with the *cis* stack. The proteins in these vesicles are then modified and transferred to the *medial* stack, where they are further modified before passing to the *trans* stack. Proteins leave the Golgi at the *trans* face in transport vesicles. [If vesicle fusion with the *cis* Golgi was inhibited, could plasma membrane proteins still reach the cell surface?[21]] The route taken by a protein is determined by signals within the protein that determine which vesicle a protein is sorted into in the *trans* Golgi.

---

[18] Yes. Remember, the ER lumen is equivalent to (contiguous with) the extracellular space.

[19] No. It is the signal peptide in the nascent polypeptide that is recognized and bound by SRP and taken to receptors on the surface of the rough ER. The signal is an amino acid sequence on the nascent polypeptide, not a nucleotide sequence on mRNA.

[20] Note that *cis* means "near," as in a *cis* double bond. *Trans* means "far." *Medial* means "in the middle." Also note that the order is alphabetical: *cis-medial-trans*.

[21] No. Secretory proteins must proceed via a specific path: from the ER to the *cis* Golgi to the medial and *trans* Golgi and from there to the cell surface.

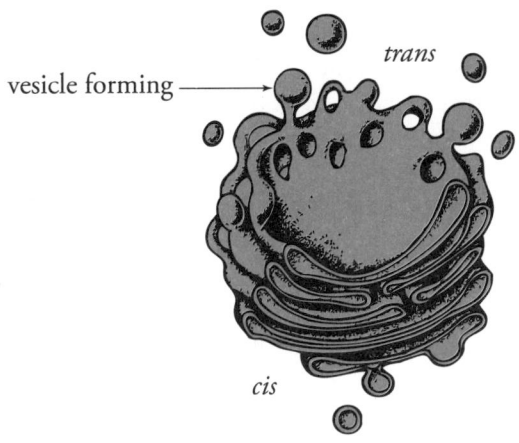

Figure 7 The Golgi Apparatus

When a vesicle moves from the *trans* Golgi toward the cell surface, it fuses with the cell membrane. As a result, the contents of the vesicle are released into the extracellular environment in a process termed *exocytosis*. Alternatively, if the vesicle contains proteins anchored to its membrane, these proteins will remain attached to the cell as cell-surface proteins. Some proteins are sent in vesicles from the Golgi immediately to the cell surface, in the **constitutive secretory pathway**. *Constitutive* connotes *continuous* or *unregulated*. In contrast, specialized secretory cells (such as pancreatic cells, B cells of the immune system, etc.) store secretory proteins in **secretory vesicles** and release them only at certain times, usually in response to a change in (or signal from) the extracellular environment. This is a **regulated secretory pathway**.

Lysosomes

Lyse means cut. The **lysosome** is a membrane-bound organelle that is responsible for the degradation of biological macromolecules by hydrolysis. Lysosome proteins are made in the RER, modified in the Golgi, and released in their final form from the *trans* face of the Golgi. Organelles such as mitochondria that have been damaged or are no longer functional may be degraded in lysosomes in a process termed **autophagy** (self-eating). Lysosomes also degrade large particulate matter engulfed by the cell by **phagocytosis** (cell eating). For example, **macrophages** of the immune system engulf bacteria and viruses. The particle or microorganism ends up in a **phagocytic vesicle**, which will fuse with a lysosome. Finally, **crinophagy** refers to lysosomal digestion of unneeded (excess) secretory products. After hydrolysis, the lysosome will release molecular building blocks into the cytoplasm for reuse.

The enzymes responsible for degradation in lysosomes are called **acid hydrolases**. This name reflects the fact that these enzymes only hydrolyze substrates when they are in an acidic environment. This is a safety mechanism. The pH of the lysosome is around 5, so the acid hydrolases are active. But the pH of the cytoplasm is 7.4. If a lysosome ruptures, its enzymes will not damage the cell because the acidic fluid will be diluted, and the acid hydrolases will be inactivated. However, if many lysosomes rupture at once, the cell may be destroyed.

Peroxisomes

Peroxisomes are small organelles that perform a variety of metabolic tasks. The peroxisome contains enzymes that produce hydrogen peroxide (H_2O_2) as a by-product. They are essential for lipid breakdown in many cell types. In the liver they assist in detoxification of drugs and chemicals. H_2O_2 is a dangerous chemical, but peroxisomes contain an enzyme called **catalase** which converts it to $H_2O + O_2$. Separating these activities into the peroxisomes protects the rest of the cell from damage by peroxides or oxygen radicals.

6.3   THE PLASMA MEMBRANE

The evolution of life most likely began with a separation of "inside" from "outside." Once this had occurred, processes in the cell could increase their orderliness despite the entropic chaos of the surroundings. An alternate hypothesis is that life began with self-replicating RNA floating free in the ocean. As it grew more complex, this early genome would require protection. In any case, the separation of the cytoplasm from the extracellular environment was a major milestone in evolution. Bacteria, plants, and fungi accomplish this by forming a cell membrane and a cell wall (made of peptidoglycan, cellulose, and chitin, respectively). Eukaryotic animal cells have no cell wall and thus rely on the cell membrane as the only boundary between inside and outside. And they must devise another means of structural support: just as chordates have a bony endoskeleton instead of the primitive exoskeleton arthropods have, animal cells rely on an internal cytoskeleton instead of an external cell wall. Further problems arise in multicellular eukaryotes. Not only must each cell maintain its structural integrity, but it must also interact with its neighbors in an organized fashion. In the following discussion, we will study how each of these goals is accomplished.

Membrane Structure

All of the membranes of the cell are composed of **lipid bilayer** membranes. The three most common lipids in eukaryotic membranes are **phospholipids**, **glycolipids**, and **cholesterol**, of which phospholipids are the most abundant. An example of a phospholipid is *phosphatidyl choline* (see Figure 8) with two long hydrophobic fatty acids esterified to glycerol, along with a charged phosphoryl choline group. Thus, phospholipids have portions that are distinctly hydrophilic and hydrophobic. Glycolipids, with fatty acids groups and carbohydrate side chains, also have hydrophilic and hydrophobic regions. When fatty acids or phospholipids are mixed with water, they spontaneously arrange themselves with the hydrophobic tails facing the interior to avoid contact with water and the hydrophilic regions facing outward toward water (see Figure 9). Fatty acids form small micelles, but, due to steric hindrance, phospholipids arrange themselves spontaneously into **lipid bilayer membranes**. Since the lipid bilayer is the lowest energy state for these molecules, the bilayer membrane can reseal and repair itself if a small portion of membrane is removed. [Does the formation of a lipid bilayer when phospholipids are mixed with water have a positive or a negative ΔG (change in free energy)?[22]]

The interior of the lipid bilayer membrane is very hydrophobic, with water largely excluded. Hydrophilic molecules such as ions, carbohydrates, and amino acids are not soluble in this environment, making the membrane a barrier to the passage of these molecules. Nonpolar molecules such as CO_2, O_2, and steroid hormones can cross the membrane easily. Water can also pass through the membrane but does so through specialized protein channels.

---

[22] Lipid bilayers form spontaneously, as the lowest energy state, without external energy input. This describes a process with a negative ΔG.

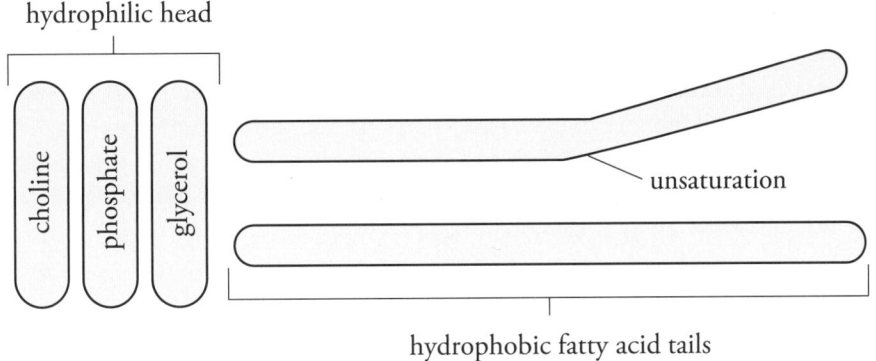

Figure 8   Phosphatidyl Choline, a Phospholipid

• Which one of the following statements best describes the physical characteristics of phospholipids?[23]
   A) Negatively charged at pH 7 and therefore entirely hydrophilic
   B) Hydrophobic
   C) Partially hydrophilic and partially hydrophobic
   D) Positively charged at pH 7 and therefore entirely hydrophilic

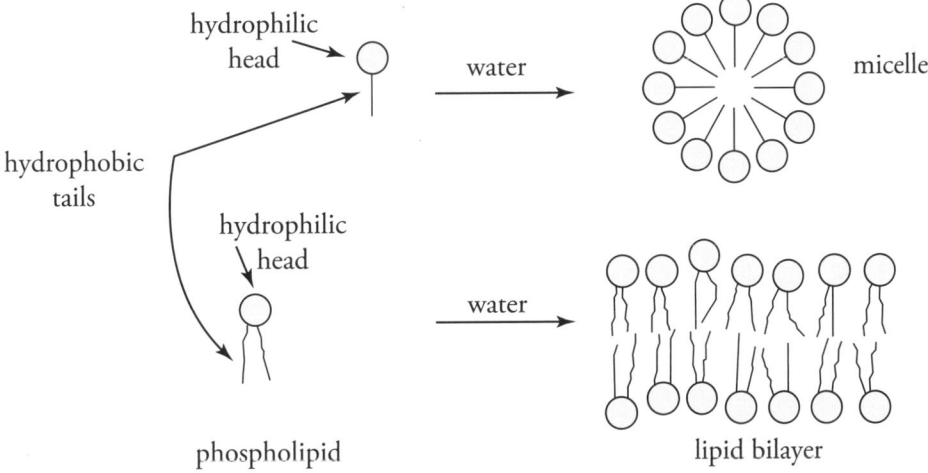

Figure 9   Lipid Behavior in an Aqueous Solvent

In addition to lipids, proteins are a major component of membranes. In some cases, such as the mitochondrial inner membrane, there is a higher protein than lipid concentration. Some proteins act to mediate interactions of the cell with other cells. Other proteins called **cell-surface receptors** bind extracellular signaling molecules such as hormones and relay these signals into the cell so that it can respond accordingly. **Channel proteins** selectively allow ions or molecules to cross the membrane. Each of these types of membrane protein is discussed below.

---

[23] Choice **C.** Phospholipids have hydrophobic components (fatty acid acyl chains) and hydrophilic components (phosphate and choline, for example, in phosphatidyl choline).

In general, membrane proteins are classified as peripheral or integral (see Figure 10). **Integral membrane proteins** are actually embedded in the membrane, held there by hydrophobic interactions. Membrane-crossing regions are called **transmembrane domains** (see Figure 11). Integral membrane proteins may have a complex pattern of transmembrane domains and portions not within the membrane. [At which point in the secretory pathway would the insertion of transmembrane domains into the membrane occur?[24]] **Peripheral membrane proteins** are not embedded in the membrane at all, but rather are stuck to integral membrane proteins, held there by hydrogen bonding and electrostatic interactions.

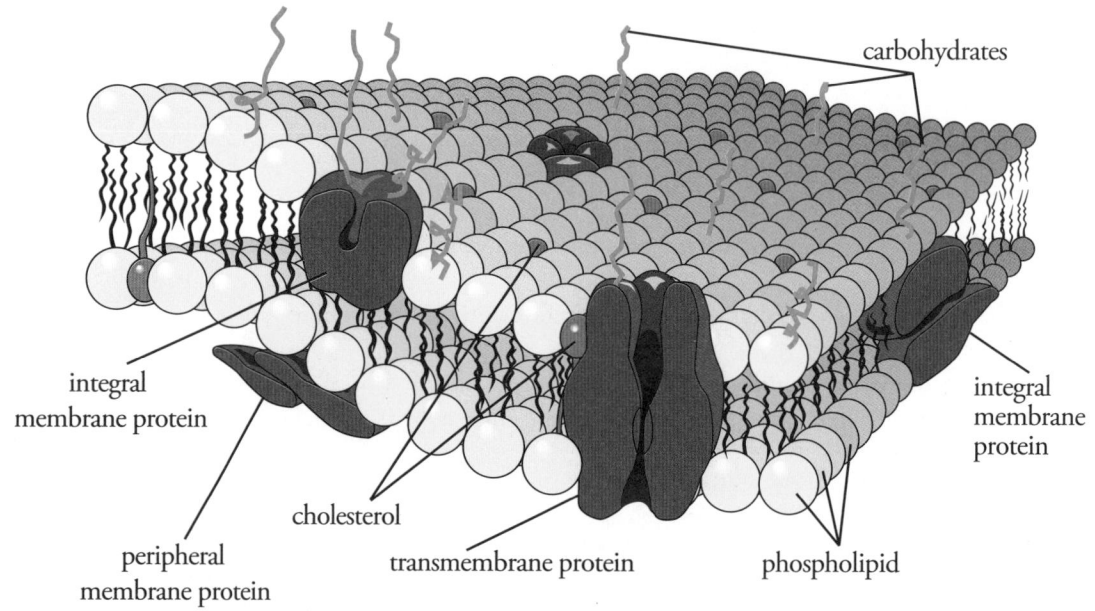

Figure 10 Membrane Proteins

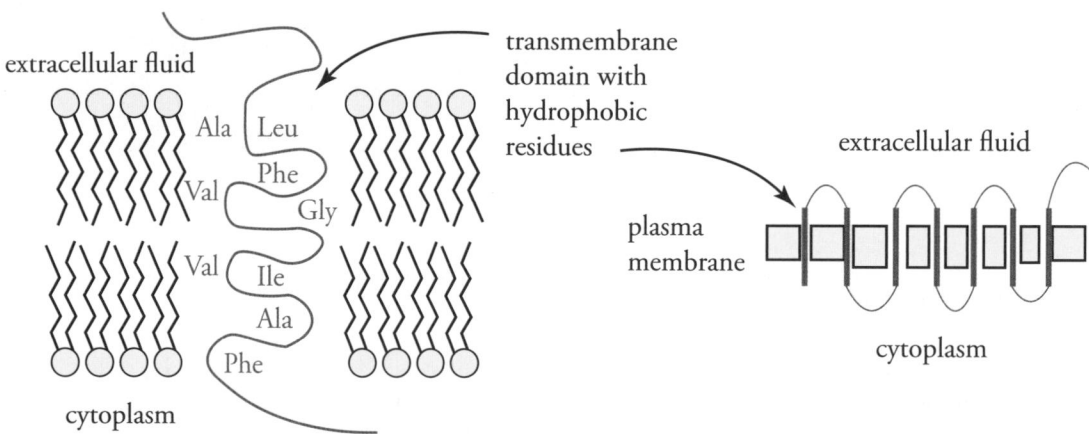

Figure 11 Transmembrane Domains

The current understanding of membrane dynamics is termed the **fluid mosaic model**, because the membrane is seen as a mosaic of lipids and proteins that are free to move back and forth fluidly. According to

---

[24] It occurs in the rough ER as the protein is translated and threaded across the ER membrane.

this model, lipids and proteins are free to diffuse laterally, in two dimensions, but are **not free to flip-flop**. Phospholipid head groups and hydrophilic protein domains are restricted from entering the hydrophobic membrane interior just as hydrophilic molecules in the extracellular space are. Thus, the membrane is said to have **polarity**. This just means that the inside face and the outside face remain different. We have already discussed one such difference: all glycosylations are found on the extracellular face. So the "fluid" in "fluid mosaic" means that things are free to move back and forth, but in two dimensions only. One exception is that some proteins are anchored to the cytoskeleton and thus cannot move in any direction.

- Phospholipids can be covalently attached to a fluorescent tag and then integrated into a lipid bilayer. If one cell has a red fluorescent tagged lipid in its plasma membrane and another cell has a green fluorescent tagged lipid in its membrane, what will happen if the two cells are fused together?[25]

The fluidity of a membrane is affected by the composition of lipids in the membrane (see Figure 12). The hydrophobic van der Waals interactions between the fatty acid side chains are a major determinant of membrane fluidity. Saturated fatty acids, lacking any double bonds, have a very straight structure and pack tightly in the membrane, with strong van der Waals forces between side chains. Unsaturated fatty acids, with one or more double bonds, have a kinked structure and pack in the membrane interior more loosely. Cholesterol also plays a key role in maintaining optimal membrane fluidity by fitting into the membrane interior. [If the percentage of unsaturated fatty acids in a membrane is increased, will membrane fluidity increase or decrease at body temperature?[26]]

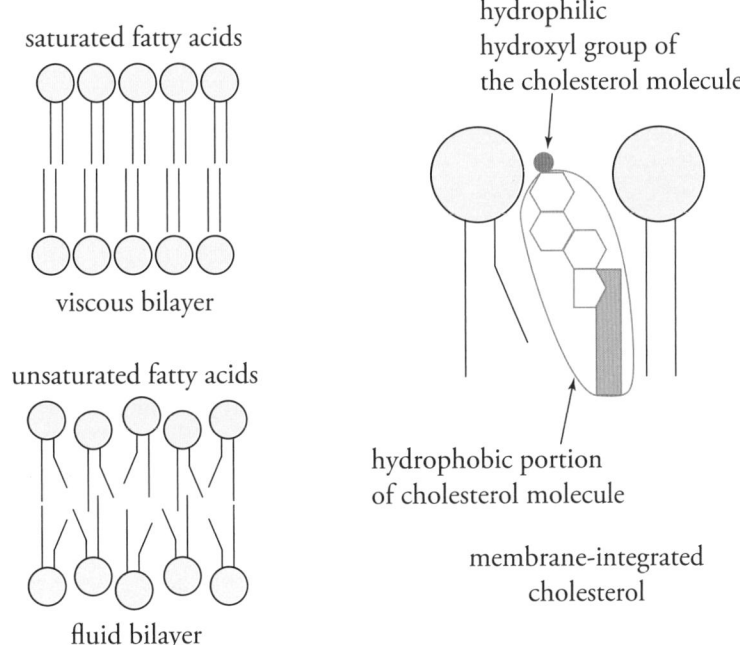

Figure 12 Factors Affecting Membrane Fluidity

---

[25] After a short period of time, the red and green tagged lipids will diffuse laterally and mix. An even distribution of the tags will be seen across the surface of the new hybrid cell.

[26] Unsaturated fatty acids, with a kinked structure, have fewer van der Waals interactions, and therefore allow a more fluid membrane structure. Increasing the unsaturated fatty acids will increase membrane fluidity.

6.4 TRANSMEMBRANE TRANSPORT

The cell requires membranes to act as barriers to diffusion but also requires the transport of many different substances across membranes. Integral membrane proteins transport material through membranes that cannot diffuse on their own across membranes. Transport across a membrane can be either **passive** (does not require cellular energy) or **active** (requires cellular energy). Before we discuss movements across membranes, let's review basic rules about concentration, ionizability, colligative properties, and diffusion and osmosis.

Concentration Measurements

Molarity (*M*) expresses the concentration of a solution in terms of moles of solute per volume (in liters) of solution:

$$\text{Molarity } (M) = \frac{\text{\# moles of solute}}{\text{\# liters of solution}}$$

Concentration is denoted by enclosing the solute in brackets. For instance, "$[Na^+] = 1.0\ M$" indicates a solution whose concentration is equivalent to 1 mole of sodium ions per liter of solution.

Molality (*m*) expresses concentration in terms of moles of solute per *mass* (in kilograms) of solvent:

$$\text{Molality } (m) = \frac{\text{\# moles of solute}}{\text{\# kg of solvent}}$$

Molality is particularly useful when measuring properties that involve temperature because, unlike molarity, molality does not change with temperature. And, since a liter of water has a mass of one kilogram, the molar and molal concentrations of dilute aqueous solutions are nearly the same. This is particularly true in biological systems, where the volume (essentially a cell) is very small and the solvent is always water.

Mole fraction simply expresses the fraction of moles of a given substance (which we'll denote here by S) relative to the total moles in a solution:

$$\text{mole fraction of S} = X_S = \frac{\text{\# moles of substance S}}{\text{total \# moles in solution}}$$

Mole fraction is a useful way to express concentration when more than one solute is present.

Electrolytes

When ionic substances dissolve, they **dissociate** into ions. Free ions in a solution are called **electrolytes** because the solution can conduct electricity. Some salts dissociate completely into individual ions, while others only partially dissociate (that is, a certain percentage of the ions will remain paired, sticking close to each other rather than being independent and fully surrounded by solvent). Solutes that dissociate completely (like ionic substances) are called **strong electrolytes**, and those that remain ion-paired to some extent are called **weak electrolytes**. (Covalent compounds that don't dissociate into ions are **non-electrolytes**.) Solutions of strong electrolytes are better conductors of electricity than those of weak electrolytes.

Different ionic compounds will dissociate into different numbers of particles. Some won't dissociate at all, and others will break up into several ions. The **van't Hoff** (or **ionizability**) **factor** (*i*) tells us how many ions one unit of a substance will produce in a solution. For example,

- $C_6H_{12}O_6$ is non-ionic, so it does not dissociate. Therefore, $i = 1$.
  (Note: The van't Hoff factor for almost all biomolecules—hormones, proteins, steroids, etc.—is 1.)
- NaCl dissociates into Na^+ and Cl^-. Therefore, $i = 2$.
- HNO_3 dissociates into H^+ and NO_3^-. Therefore, $i = 2$.
- $CaCl_2$ dissociates into Ca^{2+} and $2Cl^-$. Therefore, $i = 3$.

Colligative Properties

Colligative properties depend on the *number* of solute particles in the solution rather than the *type* of particle. For example, when any solute is dissolved into a solvent, the boiling point, freezing point, and vapor pressure of the solution will be different from those of the pure solvent. For colligative properties, *the identity of the particle is not important.* That is, for a 1 *M* solution of *any* solute, the change in a colligative property will be the same no matter what the size, type, or charge of the solute particles. Remember to consider the van't Hoff factor when accounting for particles: one mole of sucrose ($i = 1$) will have the same number of particles *in solution* as 0.5 mol of NaCl ($i = 2$), and therefore will have the same effect on a colligative property. Thus, we can consider the effective concentration to be the product *iM* (or *im*); this is the concentration of particles present.

The four colligative properties we'll study for the MCAT are vapor-pressure depression, boiling-point elevation, freezing-point depression, and osmotic pressure.

Vapor-Pressure Depression

Think about being at the ocean or a lake in the summer. The air is always more humid (moist) than in the middle of a parking lot. Why? Because some of the water molecules gain enough energy to get into the gas phase, so we see a dynamic equilibrium setup between the molecules in the liquid phase and the molecules in the gas (vapor) phase.

Vapor pressure is the pressure exerted by the gaseous phase of a liquid that evaporated from the exposed surface of the liquid. The weaker a substance's intermolecular forces, the higher its vapor pressure and the more easily it evaporates. For example, if we compare diethyl ether, $H_5C_2OC_2H_5$, and water, we notice that while water undergoes hydrogen bonding, diethyl ether does not, so despite its greater molecular mass, diethyl ether will vaporize more easily and have a higher vapor pressure than water. Easily vaporized liquids—liquids with *high* vapor pressure—like diethyl ether are said to be **volatile.**

Now let's think about what happens to vapor pressure when the liquid contains a dissolved solute. The solute molecules are attached to solvent molecules and act as "anchors." As a result, more energy is required to enter the gas phase since the solvent molecules need to break away from their interactions with the solute before they can enter the gas phase. In fact, the boiling point of a liquid is defined as the temperature at which the vapor pressure of the solution is equal to the atmospheric pressure over the solution. Thus, at sea level, where the atmospheric pressure is 760 torr, the solution must have a vapor pressure of 760 torr in order to boil. Adding more solute to the same solution will decrease its vapor pressure. Boiling will still take place when vapor pressure is 760 torr, but more heat will have to be supplied to reach this vapor pressure, and thus the solution will boil at a higher temperature. For example, salted water (say, for cooking spaghetti) boils at a higher temperature than unsalted water.

Boiling-Point Elevation

When a liquid boils, the molecules in the liquid acquire enough energy to overcome the intermolecular forces and break free into the gas phase. The liquid molecules escape as a vapor at the surface between the liquid and air. But what happens when a non-volatile solute is added to the liquid? As described before, the solute particles are attached to solvent molecules and act as "anchors." As a result, more energy is required since you not only have to convert the solvent into the gas phase, but you first have to break the interaction with the solute. What happens to the boiling point? In order for the molecules to escape, they need more energy than they did without the solute. This translates into an elevation of the boiling point. The increase in boiling point is directly related to the number of particles in solution and the type of solvent. For a given solvent (again, in biological systems this is always water), the more solute particles, the greater the boiling-point elevation. Also, you have to consider that some compounds dissociate when they dissolve, so the equation for boiling-point elevation includes the van't Hoff factor, i:

Boiling-Point Elevation

$$\Delta T_b = k_b i m$$

In this equation, k_b is the solvent's boiling-point elevation constant, i is the solute's van't Hoff factor, and m is the molal concentration of the solution. For water, $k_b \approx 0.5°C / m$.

Freezing-Point Depression

What happens when we add a solute to a liquid, then try to freeze the solution? Solids are held together by attractive intermolecular forces. During freezing, the molecules in a liquid will assemble into an orderly, tightly packed array. However, the presence of solute particles will interfere with efficient arrangement of the solvent molecules into a solid lattice. As a result, a liquid will be less able to achieve a solid state when a solute is present, and the freezing point of the solution will decrease. (Or, equivalently, the melting point of a solid containing a solute is decreased.) The good news is that the formula for freezing-point depression has exactly the same form as the formula for boiling-point elevation, except that the temperature is going down instead of up (that is, the equation for freezing-point *depression* has a *minus* sign whereas the equation for boiling-point *elevation* has a *plus* sign).

Freezing-Point Depression

$$\Delta T_f = -k_f im$$

In this equation, k_f is the solvent's freezing-point depression constant, i is the solute's van't Hoff factor, and m is the molal concentration of the solution. For water, $k_f \approx 1.9°C/m$.

- Addition of concentrated sulfuric acid to pure water will result in:[27]
  - A) vapor-pressure depression.
  - B) boiling-point elevation.
  - C) freezing-point depression.
  - D) all of the above.

Review of Diffusion and Osmosis

Diffusion is the tendency for liquids and gases to fully occupy the available volume (Figure 13, next page). Particles in the liquid or gas phase are in constant motion, depending on temperature. If all particles are concentrated in one portion of a container, we have an orderly situation, which is unfavorable according to the second law of thermodynamics (law of entropy). The constant thermal motion of particles in the cell leads to their spreading out to occupy all available space, which maximizes entropy.[28] A solute will always diffuse *down its concentration gradient*, which means *from high to low concentration*. Diffusion continues until the solute is evenly distributed throughout the available volume. At this point, movement of solute back and forth continues, but no net movement occurs.

Osmosis is a special type of diffusion in which solvent diffuses rather than solute (Figure 13). For example, if a chamber containing water and a chamber containing a solution of sucrose are connected directly, sucrose will diffuse throughout the entire volume until a uniform concentration is reached. However, if the two chambers are separated by a **semipermeable membrane** that allows water but not sucrose to cross, then diffusion of sucrose between the chambers cannot occur. In this case, osmosis draws water into the sucrose chamber to reduce the sucrose concentration as well as the volume in the water chamber. Ignoring

---

[27] The addition of a solute to a liquid always results in the effects of all the colligative properties simultaneously. Therefore, choice **D** is the answer.

[28] Remember, $\Delta G = \Delta H - T\Delta S$, so increasing ΔS decreases ΔG, indicating a thermodynamically favorable process.

gravity, water will flow into the sucrose chamber until the concentration is the same across the membrane. The plasma membrane of the cell is a semipermeable membrane that allows water—but not most polar solutes—to cross by osmosis. [If a cell is placed in a hypotonic solution (solute concentration lower than in the cell), what will happen to the cell?[29]]

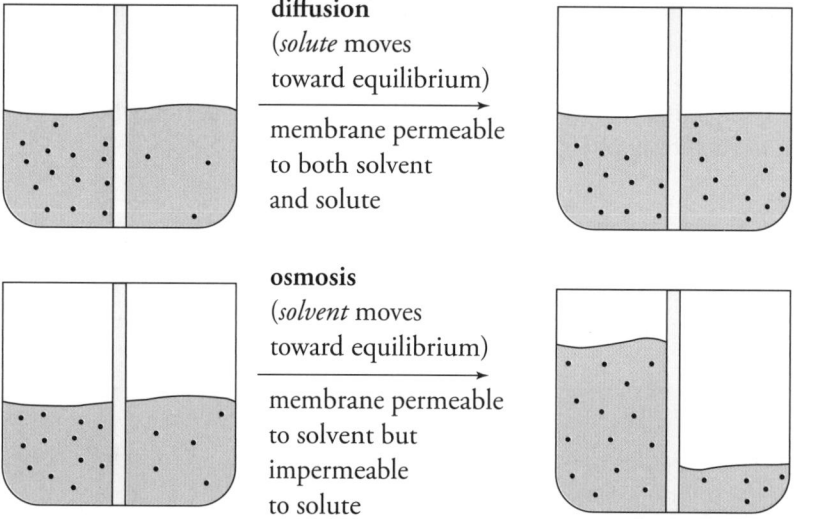

diffusion
(*solute* moves toward equilibrium)
membrane permeable to both solvent and solute

osmosis
(*solvent* moves toward equilibrium)
membrane permeable to solvent but impermeable to solute

In both diffusion and osmosis, the final result is that solute concentrations are the same on both sides of the membrane. The only difference is that in diffusion the membrane is permeable to solute and in osmosis it is not.

Figure 13   Diffusion and Osmosis

The term **tonicity** is used to describe osmotic gradients. If the environment is **isotonic** to the cell, the solute concentration is the same inside and outside. A **hypertonic** solution has more total dissolved solutes than the cell, a **hypotonic** solution has less. You may also hear the terms **isoosmotic**, **hyperosmotic**, and **hypoosmotic**. The tendency of water to move down its concentration gradient (into cells) can be a powerful force, able to cause cells to explode. This tendency (of water to move to where there are more particles), along with the inability of those particles to cross the membrane, is what accounts for the difference in fluid levels in the beaker at the bottom right-hand corner of Figure 13. The large difference in fluid levels may be a rather extreme example, but it is conceptually accurate: just as osmotic forces can cause a cell to rupture, they can overcome gravity, as shown.

Osmotic Pressure

Osmosis describes the net movement of water across a semipermeable membrane from a region of low solute concentration to a region of higher solute concentration in an effort to dilute the higher concentration solution. The semipermeable membrane prohibits the transfer of solutes, but allows water to transverse through it. In the following figure, the net movement of water will be to the right.

---

[29] Water will flow into the cell through the plasma membrane until the cell volume increases to the point that the cell bursts.

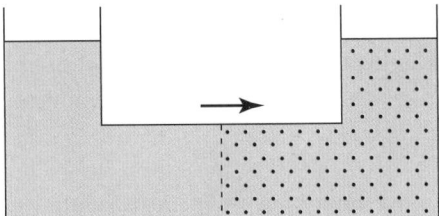

Osmotic pressure (Π) can be defined as the pressure it would take to *stop* osmosis from occurring. If a pressure gauge were added to the same system, osmotic pressure could be measured.

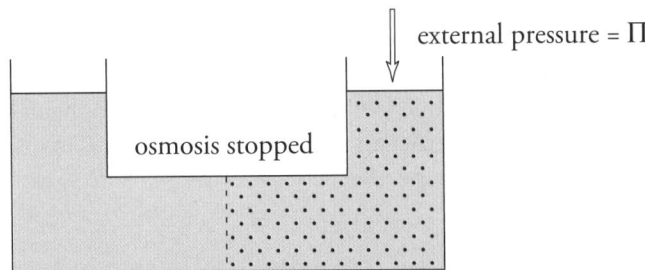

external pressure = Π

osmosis stopped

The osmotic pressure of a solution is given by the **van't Hoff equation**:

$$\Pi = MiRT$$

where Π is osmotic pressure in atm, M is the molarity of the solution, i is the van't Hoff factor, R is the universal gas constant (0.0821 L-atm/K-mol), and T is the temperature in kelvins.

Again, changes in osmotic pressure are affected only by the number of particles in solution (taking into account the van't Hoff factor), not by the identity of those particles.

Now, let's continue the discussion on movements across the cell membrane.

Passive Transport

Passive transport is a biochemical term that means diffusion. It refers to *any thermodynamically favorable movement of solute across a membrane*. Another way to phrase this is to say that passive transport is any movement of solute *down a gradient*. No energy is required since the concentration gradient drives movement of the solute. There are two types of passive transport: simple diffusion and facilitated diffusion.

6.4

Simple Diffusion

Simple diffusion is diffusion of a solute through a membrane without help from a protein. For example, steroid hormones are free to move back and forth across the membrane by simple diffusion as pushed by concentration gradients, thanks to their ___.[30]

However, lipid bilayer membranes are impermeable to most solutes; that is one of the main functions of membranes. The plasma membrane is a barrier to the free movement of all large and/or hydrophilic solutes. **Facilitated diffusion** is the movement of a solute across a membrane, down a gradient, when the membrane itself (the pure lipid bilayer) is intrinsically impermeable to that solute. Specific integral membrane proteins allow material to cross the plasma membrane down a gradient in facilitated diffusion. For example, red blood cells require glucose, which they get from the bloodstream. However, glucose is a bulky hydrophilic molecule that cannot cross the RBC lipid bilayer. Instead, it must be shuttled across by a particular protein in the RBC plasma membrane. There are two well-characterized types of proteins that serve this sort of function: **channel proteins** and **carrier proteins**. Channels and carriers give the membrane its essential feature of **selective permeability**: permeability to *some* things despite impermeability to *most* things.

Facilitated Diffusion: Channels

Channel proteins in the plasma membrane allow material that cannot pass through the membrane by simple diffusion to flow through the plasma membrane down a concentration gradient. Channels do this by forming a narrow opening in the membrane surrounded by the protein. Channels are very selective in what passes through the opening in the membrane. There are many kinds of ion channels, each of which allows the passage of only one type of ion through the channel down a gradient (see Figure 14). All cells have potassium ion channels, for example, that allow only potassium (and not sodium) to flow through the plasma membrane down a gradient. Ion channels are said to be **gated** if the channel is open in response to specific environmental stimuli. A channel that opens in response to a change in the electrical potential across the membrane is called a **voltage-gated** ion channel. One that opens in response to binding of a specific molecule like a neurotransmitter is called a **ligand-gated** ion channel. The regulation of membrane potential by gated ion channels plays a key role in the nervous system. [Can ion channels move ions against an electrochemical gradient?[31]]

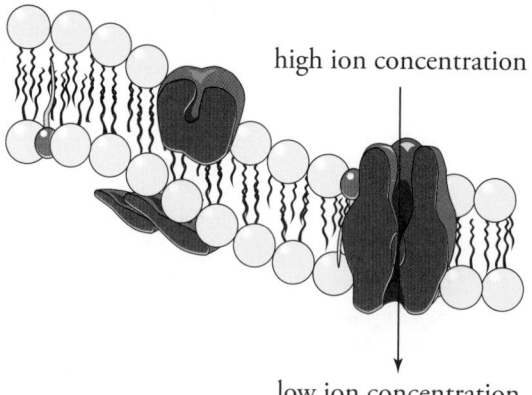

high ion concentration

low ion concentration

Figure 14 An Ion Channel

---

[30] hydrophobicity

[31] No. Ion channels are only involved in facilitated diffusion, the movement of molecules down an electrochemical gradient with the help of a protein.

Facilitated Diffusion: Carriers

Carrier proteins also can transport molecules through membranes by facilitated diffusion, but they do so by a mechanism different from that of ion channels. Carrier proteins do not form a tunnel through membranes like ion channels do. Instead, carriers appear to bind the molecule to be transported at one side of the membrane and then undergo a conformational change to move the molecule to the other side of the membrane. Some carriers, called **uniports**, transport only one molecule across the membrane at a time (see Figure 15). Other carriers termed **symports** carry two substances across a membrane in the same direction. **Antiports**, on the other hand, carry two substances in opposite directions.

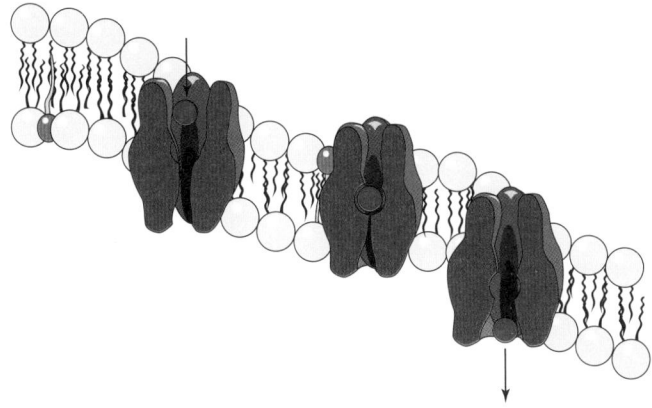

Figure 15   A Uniport

Pores and Porins

A **pore** is a tube through the membrane which is so large that it is *not selective* for any particular molecule. Rather, all molecules below a certain size may pass. (Also, a molecule which is just barely small enough to cross may not cross if it has the wrong charge on its surface.) Pores are formed by polypeptides known as **porins**. You are already familiar with several examples of pores. We have studied pores in the double nuclear membrane, the outer mitochondrial membrane, and the Gram-negative bacterial outer membrane. The eukaryotic plasma membrane does not have pores, because pores destroy the barrier function of the membrane, allowing solutes in the cytoplasm to freely diffuse out of the cell. [Are porins and ion channels found in the same membranes?[32]]

Kinetic Concerns

Simple diffusion can be distinguished from all forms of facilitated diffusion by the kinetics of the process. The rate of simple diffusion is limited only by the surface area of the membrane and the size of the driving force (gradient). Facilitated diffusion, however, depends on a finite number of integral membrane proteins. Hence, it exhibits saturation kinetics. Increasing the driving force for facilitated diffusion increases the rate of diffusion (the **flux**), but only to a point. Then all the transport proteins become saturated, and no further increase in flux is possible (Figure 16 on the following page).

---

[32] No. Porins are large holes, and ion channels are small, usually regulated channels. If porins and ion channels were found in the same membrane, the ion channels would be useless, because ions would flow in an unregulated manner through the pores.

6.4

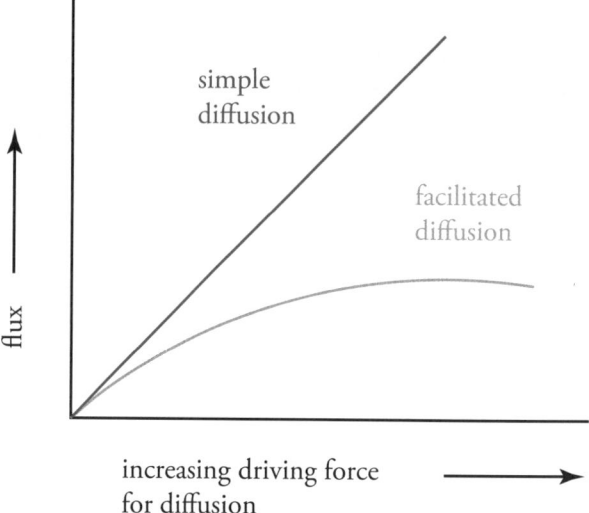

Figure 16   Saturation Kinetics of Facilitated Diffusion

Active Transport

Active transport is the movement of molecules through the plasma membrane against a gradient. Active transport requires energy input, since it is working against a gradient, and always involves a protein. Another way of saying that active transport requires energy input is to say that the transport process is coupled to a process which is thermodynamically favorable ($\Delta G < 0$). The gradient being pumped against is not necessarily just a concentration gradient, but for charged molecules, like ions, it can also involve electric potentials that form a combined electrochemical gradient that must be pumped against. The form of energy input used to drive movement of molecules against an electrochemical gradient varies. In **primary active transport**, the transport of a molecule is coupled to ATP hydrolysis. In **secondary active transport**, the transport process is not coupled *directly* to ATP hydrolysis. Instead, ATP is first used to create a gradient, then the potential energy in that gradient is used to drive the transport of some other molecule across the membrane. Since ATP is not used in the actual transport of the "other" molecule, the ATP use is described as *indirect*. For example, the transport of glucose into some cells is driven *against the glucose* concentration gradient by the cotransport of sodium ions *down the sodium* electrochemical gradient, previously established by an ATPase pump (see below). A common mechanism driving secondary active transport of many different molecules involves coupling transport to the flow of sodium ions down a gradient.

- If a protein moves sodium ions across the plasma membrane down an electrochemical gradient, what form of transport is this?[33]
  - A) Simple diffusion
  - B) Facilitated diffusion
  - C) Primary active transport
  - D) Secondary active transport

---

[33] Facilitated diffusion is the movement of molecules down a gradient with the help of a protein (choice **B** is correct). Membrane proteins are not required for simple diffusion (choice A is wrong), and active transport involves moving things *against* their gradients (choices C and D are wrong). Note also that in secondary active transport, the ion movement down its gradient must be coupled to the movement of some other molecule against *its* gradient.

The Na⁺/K⁺ ATPase and the Resting Membrane Potential

The Na⁺/K⁺ ATPase is a transmembrane protein in the plasma membrane of all cells in the body. The activity provided by this protein is to pump 3 Na⁺ out of the cell, 2 K⁺ into the cell, and to hydrolyze one ATP to drive the pumping of these ions against their gradients (Figure 17. next page). [The pumping of sodium and potassium by the Na⁺/K⁺ ATPase is an example of what form of transport?[34]] The sodium that is pumped out of the cell stays outside, since the plasma membrane is impermeable to sodium ions. Some of the potassium ions which are pumped into the cell are able to leak back out, however, through **potassium leak channels**. Potassium flows down its concentration gradient out of the cell through leak channels. The movement of ions out of the cell helps the cell to maintain osmotic balance with its surroundings. As potassium leaves the cell through the leak channels, the movement of positive charge out of the cell creates an electric potential across the plasma membrane with a net negative charge on the interior of the cell. This potential created by the Na⁺/K⁺ ATPase is known as the **resting membrane potential**. (The resting membrane potential will be examined again in Chapter 8 in relation to action potentials in neurons). The concentration gradient of high sodium outside of the cell established by the Na⁺/K⁺ ATPase is the driving force behind **secondary active transport** of many different molecules, including sugars and amino acids. To summarize, the activity of the Na⁺/K⁺ ATPase is important in three ways:

1) To maintain osmotic balance between the cellular interior and exterior
2) To establish the resting membrane potential
3) To provide the sodium concentration gradient used to drive secondary active transport

- If an inhibitor of Na⁺/K⁺ ATPase is added to cells, which of the following may occur?[35]
  - A) The cell will shrink and lose water.
  - B) The interior of the cell will become less negatively charged.
  - C) Secondary active transport processes will compensate for the loss of primary active transport.
  - D) The cell will begin to proliferate.

---

[34] The pumping of ions against a gradient which is coupled to ATP hydrolysis is primary active transport.

[35] The Na⁺/K⁺ ATPase is required to establish the resting membrane potential in which the cellular interior has a negative charge. It pumps out one net positive ion. If this net positive ion stays inside the cell, the resting potential becomes less negative (choice **B** is correct). Since the interior of the cell is now more charged, the cell will have a tendency to take on water by osmosis and will swell (choice A is wrong). Secondary active transport depends on the gradient established by primary active transport (the Na⁺/K⁺ pump). If the pump is shut down, the gradient won't be established, and secondary active transport will also stop (choice C is wrong). The Na⁺/K⁺ ATPase has nothing to do with cellular proliferation (choice D is wrong).

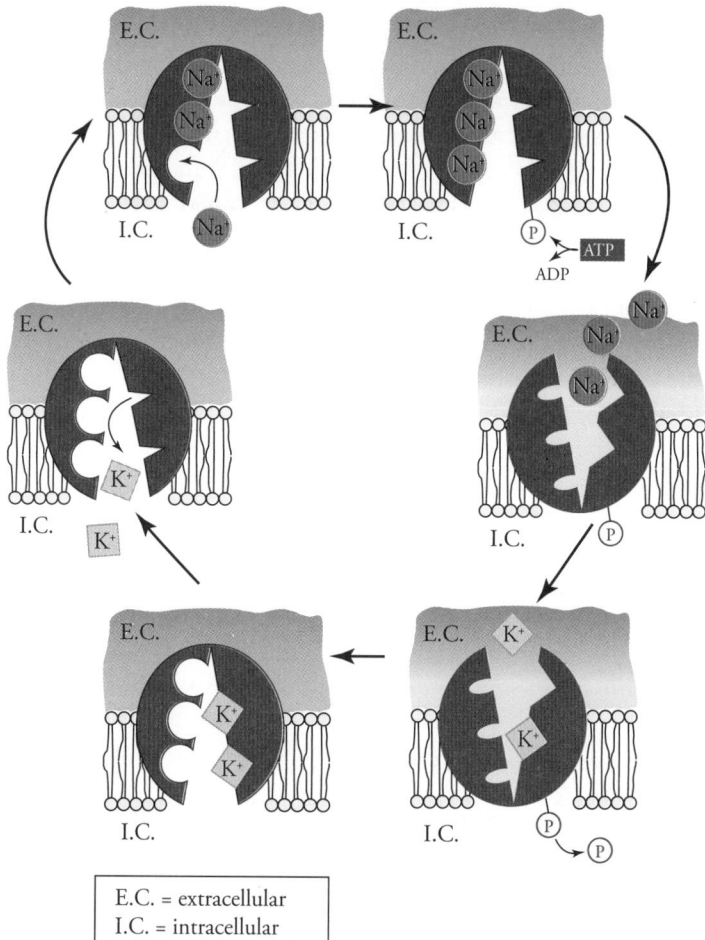

Figure 17   The Na⁺/K⁺ ATPase

How do we know exactly how the resting membrane potential is generated? For instance, how can we state with confidence that the electrogenicity of the Na⁺/K⁺ pump is far less important than the passive efflux of potassium in the generation of the RMP? The answer, given in the next two paragraphs, is not core MCAT material for memorization, but it is just the sort of thing that could show up in a passage.

The answers were determined using experiments. An artificial cell with no pumps and no channels in its membrane would have identical concentrations and charges inside and outside. An artificial cell with potassium leak channels but no active transporters would also obviously have no gradients across its membrane.

What about an artificial cell with Na⁺/K⁺ ATPase pumps and normal cellular concentrations of ATP and ADP + P_i but no potassium leak channels? Here is where experimentation was necessary. In this situation, the resting membrane potential is determined only by the electrogenicity of the Na⁺/K⁺ pump. The RMP in such a system turns out to be about −10 mV. [Why is it necessary to specify normal cellular concentrations of ATP and ADP + P_i? For example, what would happen if there were much, much more ADP + P_i

than ATP, as well as very high extracellular Na^+ concentration and very high intracellular K^+ concentration, in the artificial cell?[36]]

When K^+ leak channels are added to the membrane (in addition to the Na^+/K^+ ATPase pumps and normal cellular concentrations of ATP and ADP + P_i), the RMP is measured at the normal cellular level, around –70 mV.

The following table gives the concentrations of Na^+, K^+, and Cl^- inside and outside the cell. (Know trends; don't memorize numbers.) You already know why the Na^+ and K^+ concentrations are as they are. [Why is chloride so concentrated outside the cell?[37]] A useful mnemonic is to remember that life evolved in the ocean, which has very high concentrations of NaCl; thus the concentrations of Na^+ and Cl^- are high outside the cell and low inside.

Table 3   Concentrations of Ions Inside/Outside Cell

Ion	Intracellular Conc. (mM)	Extracellular Conc. (mM)
Na^+	10	142
K^+	140	4
Cl^-	4	110
Ca^{2+}	0.0001	2.4

Endocytosis and Exocytosis

Another mechanism used to transport material through the plasma membrane is within membrane-bound vesicles that fuse with the membrane (see Figure 18 on the next page). **Exocytosis** is a process to transport material outside of the cell in which a vesicle in the cytoplasm fuses with the plasma membrane, and the contents of the vesicle are expelled into the extracellular space. The materials released are products secreted by the cell, such as hormones and digestive enzymes.

Endocytosis is the opposite of exocytosis: generally, materials are taken into the cell by an invagination of a piece of the cell membrane to form a vesicle. Again, the cytoplasm is not allowed to mix with the extracellular environment. The new vesicle which is formed is called an **endosome**. There are three types of endocytosis:

1) Phagocytosis
2) Pinocytosis
3) Receptor-mediated endocytosis

---

[36] The pump would run backward! Remember: all active transporters are reversible.

[37] The cell contains millions of negative charges on macromolecules (e.g., nucleic acids). For the charge to be "approximately" balanced on both sides of the membrane, some negatively charged substance must be more concentrated outside. Chloride serves this role. Why did we say "approximately" balanced? Remember: the cell is a bit more negative on the inside; that's the RMP.

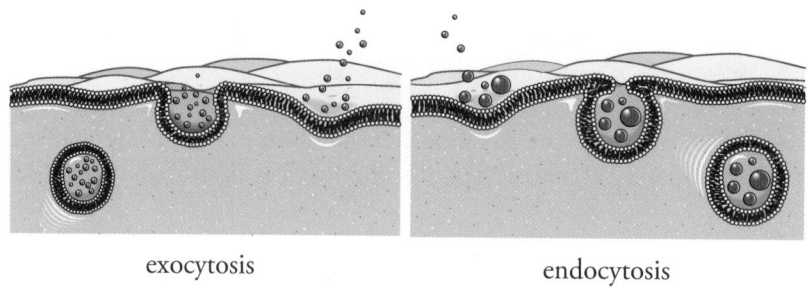

exocytosis   endocytosis

Figure 18   Endo- and Exocytosis

Phagocytosis means "cell eating." It refers to the nonspecific uptake of large particulate matter into a phagocytic vesicle, which later merges with a lysosome. Thus, the phagocytosed material will be broken down. The prime example of phagocytic human cells are macrophages ("big eaters") of the immune system, which engulf and destroy viruses and bacteria. (*Note:* This is *not* an invagination.)

Pinocytosis ("cell drinking") is the nonspecific uptake of small molecules and extracellular fluid via invagination. Primitive eukaryotic cells obtain nutrition in this manner, but virtually all eukaryotic cells participate in pinocytosis.

Receptor-mediated endocytosis, on the other hand, is very specific. The site of endocytosis is marked by pits coated with the molecule **clathrin** (inside the cell) and with **receptors** that bind to a specific molecule (outside the cell). An important example is the uptake of cholesterol from the blood. Cholesterol is transported in the blood in large particles called lipoproteins. Cells obtain some of the cholesterol they require by receptor-mediated endocytosis of these lipoproteins. If they are not removed from the blood, cholesterol accumulates in the bloodstream, sticking to the inner walls of arteries. This results in **atherosclerosis** (a buildup of plaque on the walls of the arteries). [Does clathrin recognize and bind to lipoproteins?[38]] When the receptor-lipoprotein complex internalizes, it is taken into a vesicle that is termed an endosome. Lipoproteins are taken from the endosome to a lysosome where the cholesterol is released from the lipoprotein and the lipoprotein is degraded. The lipoprotein receptor is returned to the cell surface where it may again bind a lipoprotein. [How is receptor-mediated endocytosis similar to and different from active transport?[39]]

---

[38] No. Clathrin is a fibrous protein inside the cell that associates with the cytoplasmic portions of the cell-surface receptors that bind lipoproteins.

[39] Both import a particular substance. One difference is that in endocytosis the substance ends up sealed in an endosome, whereas in active transport the substance is just dumped into the cytoplasm.

6.5 OTHER STRUCTURAL ELEMENTS OF THE CELL

Cell-Surface Receptors

Receptors form an important class of integral membrane proteins that transmit signals from the extracellular space into the cytoplasm. Each receptor binds a particular molecule in a highly specific lock-and-key interaction. The molecule that serves as the key for a given receptor is termed the **ligand**. The ligand is generally a hormone or a neurotransmitter. The binding of a ligand to its receptor on the extracellular surface of the plasma membrane triggers a response within the cell, a process termed **signal transduction**. Many cancers result from mutant cell-surface receptors which constitutively relay their signal to the cytoplasm, whether ligand is present or absent. For example, a growth factor exerts its effects by binding to a cell-surface receptor, and constitutive activity of a receptor for the growth factor causes uncontrolled growth of the cell. There are three main types of signal-transducing cell-surface receptors: ligand-gated ion channels, catalytic receptors, and G-protein-linked receptors.

Ligand-gated ion channels in the plasma membrane open an ion channel upon binding a particular neurotransmitter. An example is the ligand-gated sodium channel on the surface of the muscle cell at the neuromuscular junction. When the neurotransmitter acetylcholine binds to this receptor, the receptor undergoes a conformational change and becomes an open Na^+ channel. The result is a massive influx of sodium down its electrochemical gradient, which depolarizes the muscle cell and causes it to contract.

Catalytic receptors have an enzymatic active site on the cytoplasmic side of the membrane. Enzyme activity is initiated by ligand binding at the extracellular surface. Generally, the catalytic role is that of a protein **kinase**, which is an enzyme that covalently attaches phosphate groups to proteins. Proteins can be modified with phosphate on the side chain hydroxyl of serine, threonine, or tyrosine. The insulin receptor is an example of a tyrosine kinase. Modification of proteins with phosphates regulates their activity.

A **G-protein-linked receptor** does not directly transduce its signal, but transmits it into the cell with the aid of a **second messenger**. This is a chemical signal that relays instructions from the cell surface to enzymes in the cytoplasm. The most important second messenger is **cyclic AMP (cAMP)**. It is known as a "universal hunger signal" because it is the second messenger of the hormones epinephrine and glucagon, which cause energy mobilization (glycogen and fat breakdown). Second messengers such as cAMP allow a much greater signal than receptor alone produces (see Figure 19, next page). An epinephrine molecule activates one G-protein-linked receptor which activates many G-proteins, each G-protein activates many adenylyl cyclase enzymes, each adenylyl cyclase makes lots of cAMP from ATP, each cAMP activates many cAMP-dPK, and each cAMP-dPK phosphorylates many enzymes. Some of these enzymes will be activated, and others inactivated by phosphorylation, with the end result that the entire cell harmoniously works toward the same goal: energy mobilization.

6.5

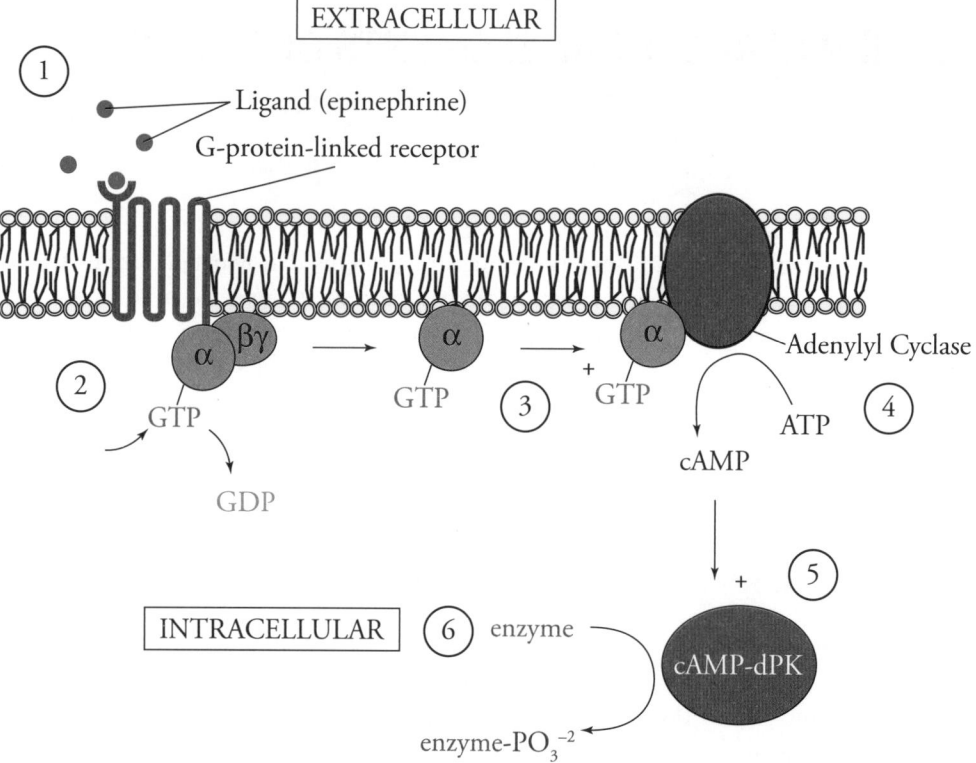

Figure 19 G-Protein Mediated Signal Transduction Stimulated by Epinephrine

1) Epinephrine arrives at the cell surface and binds to a specific G-protein-linked receptor.
2) The cytoplasmic portion of the receptor activates G-proteins, causing GDP to dissociate and GTP to bind in its place.
3) The activated G-proteins diffuse through the membrane and activate adenylyl cyclase.
4) Adenylyl cyclase makes cAMP from ATP.
5) cAMP activates cAMP-dependent protein kinases (cAMP-dPK) in the cytoplasm.
6) cAMP-dPK phosphorylates certain enzymes, with the end result being mobilization of energy. For example, enzymes necessary for glycogen breakdown will be activated, while enzymes necessary for glycogen synthesis will be inactivated, by cAMP-dPK phosphorylation.

There are different types of G-protein-linked receptors. The one depicted above is a **s**timulatory one. Its G-protein would be denoted G_s. Inhibitory G-protein-linked receptors activate **i**nhibitory G-proteins (G_i) which serve to *inactivate* adenylyl cyclase instead of activating it. In this way different hormones can modulate each other's effects.

There are also G-protein-linked receptors which have nothing to do with cAMP. Instead, their G-proteins activate an enzyme called phospholipase C, initiating a different second messenger cascade, which results in an increase in cytoplasmic Ca^{2+} levels. The common theme shared by all G-protein-based signal transduction systems is their reliance on a G-protein, which is a signaling molecule that binds GTP. You should understand these key notions: cAMP as a second messenger, signal transduction, and signal amplification. The remaining details are not important for the MCAT; read for concepts, not memory.

The Cytoskeleton

The animal cell **cytoskeleton** provides the structural support supplied by the cell wall in bacteria, plants, and fungi. It also allows movement of the cell and its appendages (cilia and flagella) and transport of substances within the cell. Animal cells have an internal cytoskeleton composed of three types of proteins: **microtubules**, **intermediate filaments**, and **microfilaments** (see Figure 20). Microtubules are the thickest, microfilaments the thinnest. All three are composed of noncovalently polymerized proteins; in other words, they are a massive example of quaternary protein structure.

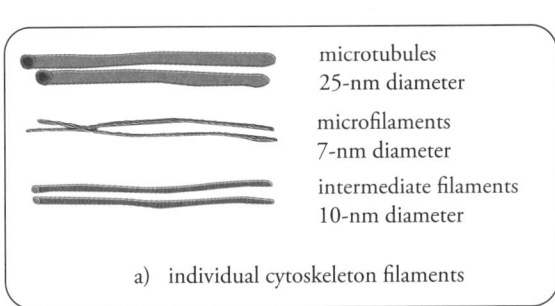

microtubules
25-nm diameter

microfilaments
7-nm diameter

intermediate filaments
10-nm diameter

a) individual cytoskeleton filaments

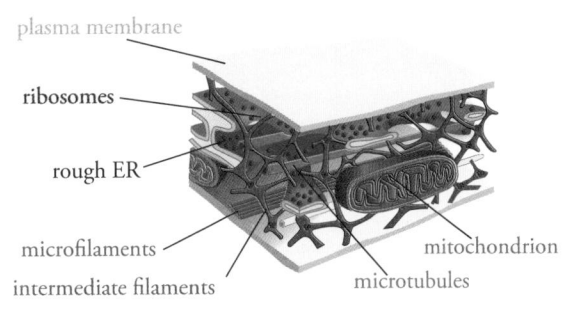

plasma membrane

ribosomes

rough ER

microfilaments

intermediate filaments

mitochondrion

microtubules

b) a portion of a cell showing the cytoskeleton

Figure 20   Cytoskeleton

Microtubules

The **microtubule** is a hollow rod composed of two globular proteins: **α-tubulin** and **β-tubulin**, polymerized noncovalently. First, α-tubulin and β-tubulin form an αβ-tubulin dimer. Then many dimers stick to one another noncovalently to form a sheet, which rolls into a tube. Once formed, the microtubule can elongate by adding αβ-tubulin dimers to one end. The other end cannot elongate, because it is anchored to the **microtubule organizing center** (**MTOC**), located near the nucleus. Microtubules are dynamic and can get longer or shorter by adding or removing tubulin monomers from the end.

Within the MTOC is a pair of **centrioles** (see Figure 21, next page). Each centriole is composed of a ring of nine microtubule triplets. When cell division occurs, the centrioles duplicate themselves, and then one pair moves to each end of the cell. During mitosis, microtubules radiating out from the centrioles attach to the replicated chromosomes and pull them apart so that one copy of each chromosome (one chromatid) moves to each end of the cell. The resulting daughter cells each get a full copy of the genome plus a centriole pair. The microtubules that radiate out from the centrioles during mitosis are called the **aster**, because they are star-shaped. The microtubules connecting the chromosomes to the aster are **polar fibers**. The whole assembly is called the **mitotic spindle**. The centromere of each chromosome contains a **kinetochore** which is attached to the spindle by tiny microtubules called **kinetochore fibers**. Refer to the figure in the upcoming section on mitosis.

6.5

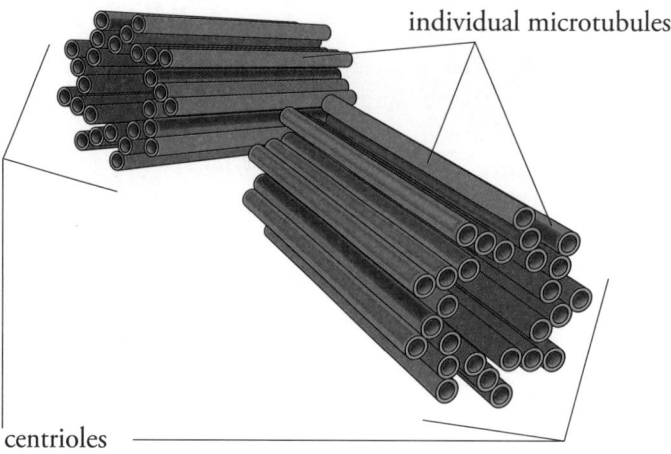

individual microtubules

centrioles

Figure 21 A Pair of Centrioles

In mitosis, the MTOC is essential, but the centrioles are not. There are two major pieces of evidence for this: 1) Plant cells lack centrioles but still undergo mitosis; 2) Experimenters have succeeded in removing the centrioles from animal cells, and the cells were still able to undergo mitosis.

Microtubules also mediate transport of substances within the cell. In nerve cells, materials are transported from the cell body to the axon terminus on a microtubule railroad. The transport process is driven by proteins that hydrolyze ATP and act as molecular motors along the microtubule.

Eukaryotic Cilia and Flagella

Cilia are small "hairs" on the cell surface which move fluids past the cell surface. For example, cilia on lining cells of the human respiratory tract continually sweep mucus toward the mouth in a mechanism termed the **mucociliary escalator**. A **flagellum** is a large "tail" which moves the cell by wiggling. The only human cell which has a flagellum is the ___.[40] Cilia are small and flagella are long, but they have the same structure, with a "**9 + 2**" arrangement of microtubules (see Figure 22). Nine pairs of microtubules form a ring around two lone microtubules in the center. Each microtubule is bound to its neighbor by a contractile protein called **dynein** which causes movement of the filaments past one another. The cilium or flagellum is anchored to the plasma membrane by a **basal body**, which has the same structure as a centriole (a ring of nine triplets of microtubules). Remember that the prokaryotic flagellum is different in structure, and its motion is driven by a different mechanism.

---

[40] sperm

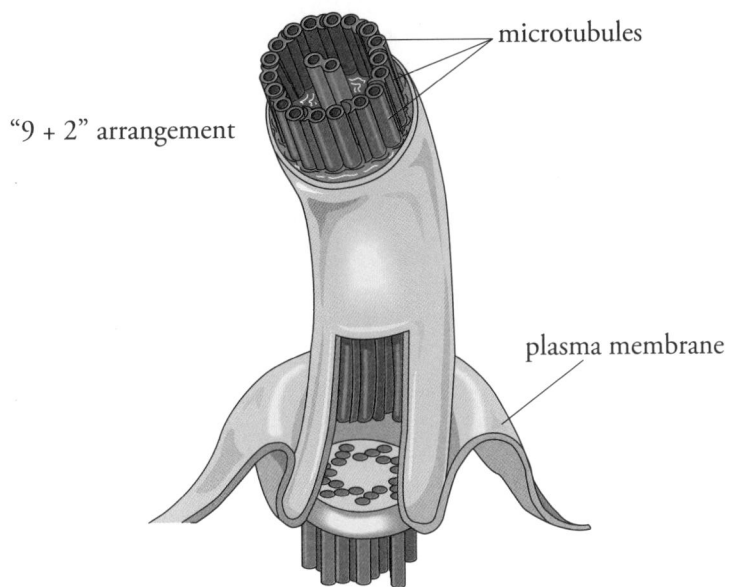

Figure 22 The Base of a Cilium or Flagellum

Microfilaments

Microfilaments are rods formed in the cytoplasm from polymerization of the globular protein **actin**. Actin monomers form a chain, and then two chains wrap around each other to form an actin filament. Microfilaments are dynamic and are responsible for gross movements of the entire cell, such as pinching the dividing parent cell into two daughters during cell division, and **amoeboid movement**. Amoeboid movement involves changes in the cytoplasmic structure which cause cytoplasm and the rest of the cell to flow in one direction.

Intermediate Filaments

Intermediate filaments are named for their thickness, which is between that of microtubules and microfilaments. Unlike microtubules and microfilaments, intermediate filaments are heterogeneous, composed of a wide range of polypeptides. Another difference is that intermediate filaments are more permanent, whereas microfilaments and microtubules are often disassembled and reassembled as needed by the cell. Intermediate filaments appear to be involved in providing strong cell structure, such as in resisting mechanical stress.

Cell Adhesion and Cell Junctions

In some tissues, cells are tightly bound to one another. For example, the intestinal wall is lined with a type of tissue called **epithelium**.[41] The layer of epithelial cells in the gut forms a tight seal, preventing items from moving freely between the intestinal lumen and the body; this is accomplished by **tight**

---

[41] An epithelial cell layer is a layer of cells which lies "upon nipples" of a type of extracellular connective tissue called *basement membrane* (*epi-* means "upon," and *-thele* means "nipple," in the sense of small bump). The basement membrane is a strong molecular sheet made of collagen. Under the microscope the basement membrane under epithelial cells has "bumps" which make epithelial cell layers easy to recognize.

junctions. Epithelial cells in the skin are held together tightly but do not form a complete seal; this is accomplished by **desmosomes**. Some specialized cell types, such as heart muscle cells, are connected by holes called **gap junctions** that allow ions to flow back and forth between them. We discuss each of these structures (see Figure 23) in the following paragraphs.

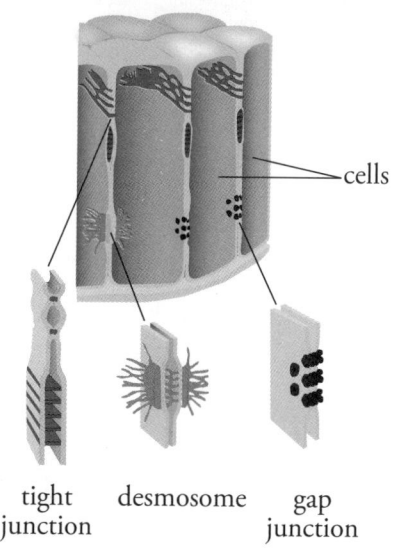

tight   desmosome   gap
junction   junction

Figure 23   Cell Junctions

Tight junctions are also termed *occluding junctions* because they do not just join cells at one point, but form a seal between the membranes of adjacent cells that blocks the flow of molecules across the entire cell layer. They are not spots where cells are stuck together, but rather bands running all the way around the cells. Intestinal epithelial cells are involved in the active transport of glucose and other molecules from one side of epithelium to the other. A tight seal between these cells is required to prevent the two compartments from mixing. Tight junctions also block the flow of molecules within the plane of the plasma membrane. For example, the surface of the plasma membrane facing the intestinal lumen, termed the **apical** surface, has different membrane proteins than the plasma membrane on the other side of the cell facing the tissues beneath, called the **basolateral** surface. [Will a transmembrane protein inserted into the apical surface of an intestinal epithelial cell diffuse in the plane of the plasma membrane to reach the basolateral surface of the cell?[42]]

Desmosomes do not form a seal, but merely hold cells together; they are also known as *spot desmosomes* because they are concise points, not bands all the way around the cell. The desmosome is composed of fibers that span the plasma membranes of two cells. Inside each cell, the desmosome is anchored to the plasma membrane by a plaque formed by the protein **keratin**. Intermediate filaments of the cytoplasm attach to the inside of the desmosome. Desmosomes do not freely diffuse in the plane of the plasma membrane, as suggested by the fluid mosaic model, because they are anchored in place by intermediate filaments of the cytoskeleton. As you can see, the fluid mosaic model is an idealization describing the plasma membrane in pure form. In the real cell membrane, things are highly organized.

Gap junctions form pore-like connections between adjacent cells, allowing the two cells' cytoplasms to mix. The connection is large enough to permit the exchange of solutes such as ions, amino acids, and carbohydrates, but not polypeptides and organelles. Gap junctions in smooth muscle and cardiac muscle allow the membrane depolarization of an action potential to pass directly from one cell to another.

---

[42] No. It is free to move around on the apical surface, but the tight junctions prevent it from diffusing to the basolateral surface.

6.6 THE CELL CYCLE AND MITOSIS

Our cells must reproduce themselves in order to replace lost or damaged cells and so that tissues can grow. Cells reproduce themselves by first doubling everything in the cytoplasm and the genome and then splitting in half. Some cells continually go through a cycle of growth and division, which is traditionally discussed in four phases (see Figure 24). **S (synthesis)** phase is when the cell actively replicates its genome, as described in Chapter 7. **M phase** includes **mitosis** and **cytokinesis**. Mitosis is the partitioning of cellular components (genes, organelles, etc.) into two halves. Cytokinesis is the physical process of cell division. Between M phase and S phase, there are two "gap" phases, G_1 and G_2. The gap phases plus S phase together form the part of the cell cycle between divisions, known as *interphase*.

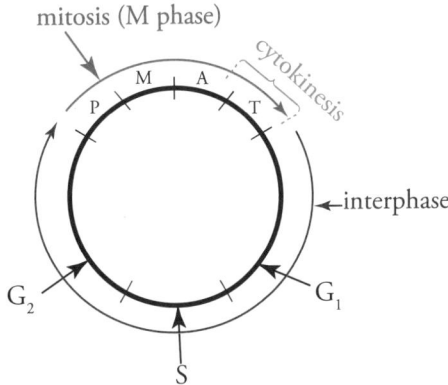

Figure 24 The Cell Cycle

The cell spends most of its time in interphase, busily metabolizing and synthesizing materials. Some cells are permanently stuck in interphase (G_0). In fact, the more specialized a cell becomes, the less likely it is to remain capable of reproducing itself. Examples are neurons, blood cells, and cells on the surface of the skin. They must be replenished by reproduction of less specialized precursor cells called **stem cells**. All the blood cells, for example, are derived from a single type of stem cell found in the bone marrow.

During interphase, the genome is spread out in a form that is not visible with a light microscope without special stains, and DNA is accessible to the enzymes of replication. By the end of S phase, the nucleus contains two complete copies of the genome. The cell now has twice the normal amount of DNA.

Mitosis is divided into four phases: **prophase, metaphase, anaphase,** and **telophase.**[43] The first sign of prophase is that the genome becomes visible upon condensing into densely packed chromosomes, instead of diffuse chromatin. [Why do the chromosomes condense?[44]] Observing a human cell under the light microscope at the beginning of prophase, one can see 46 differently shaped chromosomes. Upon closer observation, one notes that each chromosome actually consists of two identical particles joined at a centromere. These two particles are the two copies of a chromosome, known as **sister chromatids**. When mitosis is complete, each new daughter cell will have 46 chromosomes, each consisting of a single chromatid, separated from its sister. Spending a little more time staring at the nucleus, you might notice that the jumble of 46 chromatid pairs actually consists of 23 **homologous pairs** of identical-appearing sister chromatid pairs (23 pairs of pairs). Homologous chromosomes are different copies of the same chromosome, one from your mother and the other from your father. (Also refer to Chapter 7.) To repeat:

---

[43] A mnemonic is "I Pee on the MAT," where I is for interphase.

[44] Presumably so that they can be separated without tangling.

Sister chromatids are identical copies of a chromosome, attached to each other at the centromere. Homologous chromosomes are equivalent but nonidentical and do not come anywhere near each other during mitosis.

Other important events occur during prophase. The nucleolus disappears, the spindle and kinetochore fibers appear, and the centriole pairs begin to move to opposite ends of the cell. So now the cell has two MTOCs, called **asters** (stars) because of the star-like appearance of microtubules radiating out. Also at the end of prophase, the nuclear envelope converts itself into many tiny vesicles.[45]

Metaphase is simple: all the chromosomes line up at the center of the cell, forming the **metaphase plate**. The chromosomes line up in the center of the cell because the kinetochore of each sister chromatid is attached to spindle fibers that attach to MTOC at opposite ends of the cell. So each member of a pair of chromatids is pulled toward the opposite pole of the cell.

During anaphase, the spindle fibers shorten, and the centromeres of each sister chromatid pair are pulled apart. The cell elongates, and cytokinesis begins with the formation of a **cleavage furrow**, which is accomplished by __.[46]

In telophase (*telos* is Greek for "end"), a nuclear membrane forms around the bunch of chromosomes at each end of the cell, the chromosomes decondense, and a nucleolus becomes visible within each new daughter nucleus. Each daughter nucleus has $2n$ chromosomes. Cytokinesis is complete, and the cell is split in two (see Figure 25).

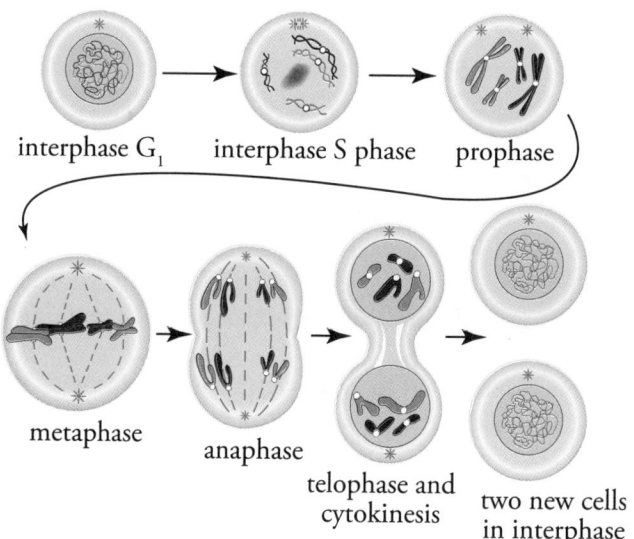

interphase G₁   interphase S phase   prophase

metaphase   anaphase   telophase and cytokinesis   two new cells in interphase

Figure 25   The Phases of Mitosis

---

[45] This stage of prophase is also referred to as **prometaphase.** It is the last event in prophase and is rather dramatic; once the nuclear membrane is disintegrated into vesicles, the spindle fibers can attach to the centromeres of the chromosomes and the cell can enter metaphase.

[46] a ring of microfilaments encircling the cell and contracting

The **karyotype** is a display of an organism's genome (see Figure 26). A cell is frozen during metaphase, its chromosomes are stained, and a photograph is taken. The micrograph is enlarged, and each chromosome is cut out of the picture with an artist's blade. Then all homologues are paired, and the entire genome is examined for abnormalities.

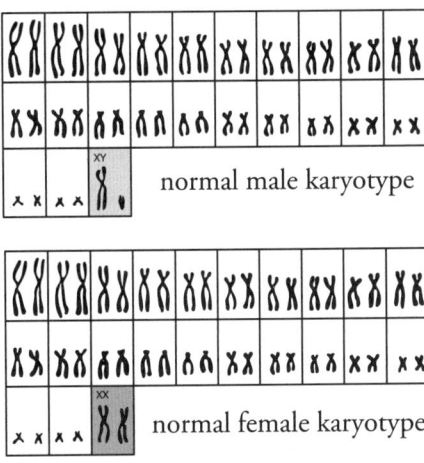

normal male karyotype

normal female karyotype

Figure 26   A Genetic Karyotype

- Eukaryotic chromosomes generally have only one of which of the following?[47]
  - A) Reading frame
  - B) Origins of replication
  - C) Promoter
  - D) Centromere

---

[47] If a chromosome had more than one centromere, it could be pulled toward different ends of the cell simultaneously and be torn (choice **D** is correct). Each eukaryotic gene has only one reading frame, but since there are many genes per chromosome there are different reading frames too. Note that the total number of possible reading frames is only 3, since a codon is only 3 nucleotides long (choice A is wrong). Eukaryotic chromosomes are so large that they must have more than one origin of replication to finish replication of the genome in a reasonable time period (choice B is wrong), and each gene has its own promoter, and there are many genes per chromosome (choice C is wrong).

6.7 CANCER, ONCOGENES, AND TUMOR SUPPRESSORS

Inappropriate cell division (i.e., cells that have lost control of the cell cycle) can have disastrous consequences. A mutation in a protein that is normally involved in regulating progression through the cell cycle can result in unregulated cell division and cancer. Cancer means "crab," as in the zodiac sign. The name derives from the observation that malignant tumors grow into the surrounding tissue, embedding themselves like clawed crabs.

- In normal eukaryotic cells, mitosis will not begin until the entire genome is replicated. If this inhibition is removed so that mitosis begins during S-phase, which one of the following would occur?[48]
  A) The cells would grow more quickly.
  B) The genome would become fragmented and incomplete.
  C) The cells would display unregulated, cancerous growth.
  D) The genome would be temporarily incomplete in each daughter cell, but DNA repair will fill in the missing gaps.

Cancers can present as malignant solid tumors or in a more diffuse cellular state, such as leukemia, a cancer occurring in the bone marrow where improper leukocytes are formed and circulated.

Mutated genes that induce cancer are termed **oncogenes** ("onco-" is a prefix denoting cancer). Normally, these genes are required for proper growth of the cell and regulation of the cell cycle. Oncogenes, then, are genes that can convert normal cells into cancerous cells. Sometimes these are abnormal versions of standard cellular growth genes. Sometimes the genes enter the cell because of a viral infection. In fact, the first identified oncogene, labeled *src*, was isolated from a retrovirus found in chickens; the oncogene contributes to sarcomas, cancers of the bone, cartilage, adipose, muscular, vascular, or hematopoietic tissues. [*Teratomas* are tumors with formed tissues from multiple germ layers. What steps might lead to their formation?[49]]

Protooncogenes are the normal versions of the genes that allow for regular growth patterns, but can be converted into oncogenes under the right circumstances. Conversion may be due to mutation or because of exposure to a mutagen. Ultraviolet radiation (such as sunlight or light from tanning booths) and various chemicals (such as benzene) are both examples of common mutagens.

Tumor suppressor genes produce proteins that are the inherent defense system to prevent the conversion of cells into cancer cells. The two primary means of cancer prevention are to (a) detect damage to the genome and halt cell growth and division until the damage can be repaired, or (b) to trigger programmed cell death if the damage is too severe to be repaired. **p53** is an example of a product of a common tumor suppressor gene. Though normally at low levels in cells, its production is scaled up when genetic damage or oncogene activity is detected, and if sufficient repair is not possible, p53 will cause the cell to die in a process referred to as **apoptosis**.

---

[48] If the genome is not completely replicated and condensed prior to mitosis, it will be torn during cell division. Each daughter cell will receive only pieces of the genome rather than the complete genome and will not be able to survive (choice **B** is correct, and choice A and C are wrong). DNA repair systems can only repair sequence errors or minor structural problems; this problem would be too large to fix (choice D is wrong).

[49] Teratomas form when oncogenes cause certain tissues to dedifferentiate (lose their specific function and regress), and then redifferentiate to become something different. This is why teratomas can contain tissues such as teeth and hair.

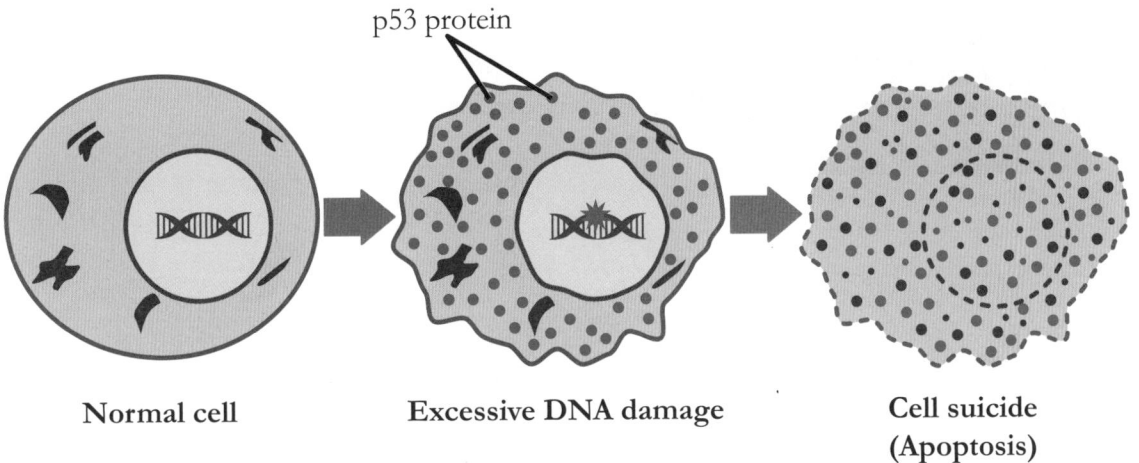

Figure 27   Representation of p53 triggering apoptosis

Apoptosis

Apoptosis, or programmed cell death, allows a cell to shrink and die while simultaneously minimizing damage to neighboring cells and limiting the exposure of other cells to its cytosolic contents. The death of a cell is triggered by a stressor which may be external (such as nitric oxide, a toxin, or cytokines) or internal (such as when the level of the p53 tumor suppressor protein reaches a critical level).

The process of apoptosis begins with the shrinking of the cell and the disassembly of the cytoskeleton. While the cellular infrastructure is taken apart, the nuclear envelope breaks down and the genome is broken into pieces. A different profile of cell surface proteins emerges, thus signaling various phagocytic cells, including macrophages, to finish deconstructing and clearing away the dead cell.

A family of proteases, referred to as **caspases**, is responsible for carrying out the events of apoptosis. They have a cysteine in their active site and they cleave their target proteins at aspartic acid sites, hence their name (*c-asp*-ases). Caspases, like all potentially damaging enzymes, are produced in their inactive form as *procaspases*. Twelve different caspases have been identified in humans, and they are generally grouped into two categories, initiators and effectors. **Initiator caspases** respond to extra- or intracellular death signals by clustering together; this clustering allows them to activate each other. The activation of the initiators leads to the activation of the effector caspases in a cascade of activation. **Effector caspases** then cleave a variety of cellular proteins to trigger apoptosis.

6.7

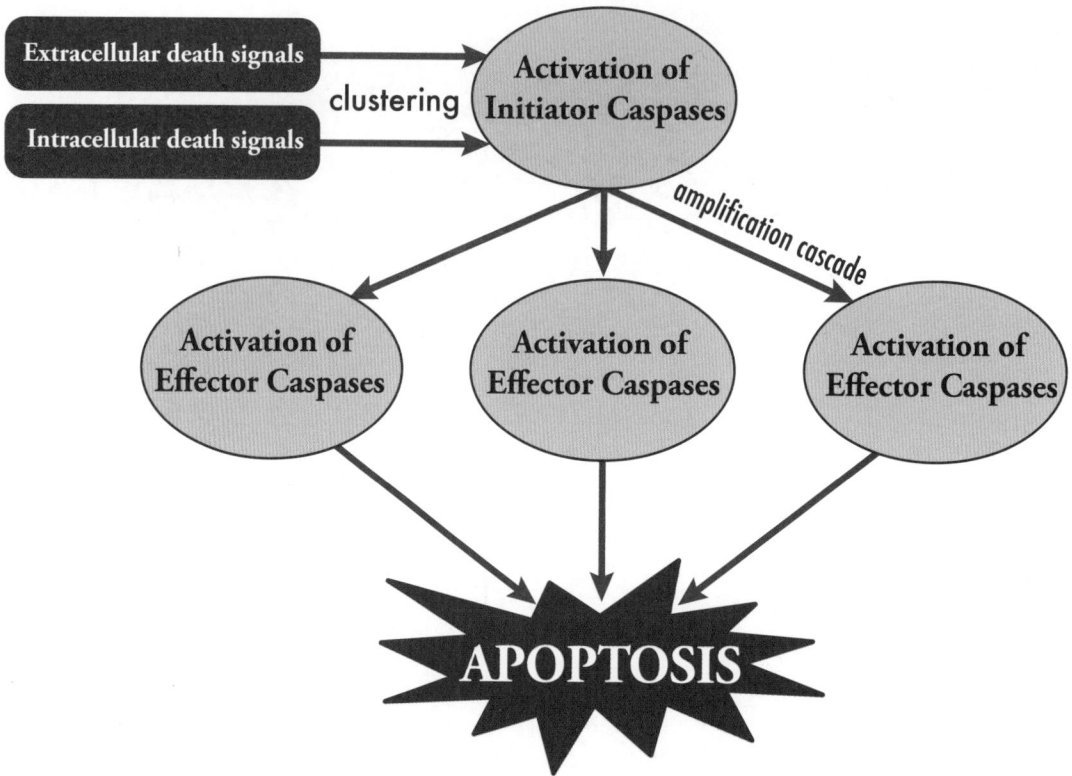

Figure 28   Caspase Activation and Cascade

Oxidative Stress

Oxidative stress occurs when the level of production of reactive oxygen species outstrips the cell's ability to detoxify them. This can include increased levels of peroxides or free oxygen, which then generates radicals. While reactive oxygen species are normally produced as part of metabolism, at high untreated levels they can damage DNA, cellular proteins, and even lipid bilayers. As such, oxidative stress is linked to cancer, since the damage it can cause sets up conditions in the cell to allow oncogenes to become active and cell growth to be impacted.

Though the potential for damage exists, creating oxidative stress is also a component of the immune system. Activated phagocytes may produce nitric oxide or superoxide (O_2^-) in order to broadly kill pathogens. The effect on foreign cells needs to be balanced against the damage being caused to host tissues.

Regenerative Capacity

The ability to restore damaged tissues is an important survival strategy, and depends on how stem cells are maintained in the body of an organism. Planarians (simple flatworms) have collections of stem cells throughout their bodies that can migrate to areas of damage and rebuild necessary tissues. Newts or lizards that lose a limb have cells that dedifferentiate and then redifferentiate to grow back all the components of that limb. Within mammals, however, the regenerative capacity is considerably more limited. The multipotent stem cells within the bone marrow are constantly regenerating the cellular components of the blood and immune system. Hepatocytes in the liver divide to produce more cells, but this process is much slower; these cells are described as being unipotent. Some cells, like neurons, do not regenerate, though inducing them to do so is an active area of research so as to better address injuries and damage caused by neurological degrading illnesses. [The benefits of having regenerative capacity are clear, but if it does not proceed properly, what could be the outcome?[50]]

Senescence

Senescence describes the process of biological aging which occurs at both the cellular and the organismal level. For eukaryotic cells, the length of the telomeres on the ends of chromosomes are a measure of cellular age; the longer the telomeres, the younger the cell. These sequences are meant to be maintained by the enzyme telomerase (Chapter 4). Research is being pursued as to whether the biological age of a cell can be reset if telomerases are manipulated to maintain the length of the telomeres. Additionally, as cells age they become prone to apoptosis. Though stressors can induce apoptosis earlier than expected, this mechanism of programmed cell death is also how organisms destroy and disassemble cells that need to be removed due to age.

The cumulative effects of cellular senescence lead to the aging of the entire organism. The functioning of organs is affected to the point where the body stops working and death occurs. These effects can be hastened based on environmental exposures and behavioral factors, but even without additional stressors, senescence is inevitable for organisms.

6.7

---

[50] Since regenerative capacity involves cell growth, dedifferentiation and redifferentiation, the possibility exists for the process to go awry and for cancerous growth to then be stimulated. Regeneration needs to be tightly regulated in order for it to proceed correctly.

Chapter 6 Summary

- For the MCAT, you should know the structures and functions of the following key eukaryotic organelles: nucleus, mitochondria, ribosomes, rough ER, smooth ER, Golgi apparatus, lysosomes, and peroxisomes.

- The rough ER is the site of translation of proteins to be either secreted from the cell, inserted into the membrane, or targeted to the lysosomes, ER, or Golgi apparatus.

- Signal sequences are specific amino acid sequences that direct proteins in translation to the rough ER and the secretory pathway (rough ER → Golgi apparatus → final location).

- Post-translational modification can occur in the rough ER or in the Golgi apparatus.

- All cellular membranes are composed of lipid bilayers with distinct hydrophobic and hydrophilic regions. The membranes act as selective barriers that regulate which molecules can cross.

- An electrolyte is a solute that produces free ions in solution. Strong electrolytes produce more ions in solution than weak electrolytes.

- The van't Hoff (or ionizability) factor, i, tells us how many ions one unit of a substance will produce in solution.

- Colligative properties depend on the number of particles in solution. Colligative properties include vapor pressure depression, boiling point elevation, freezing point depression, and osmotic pressure.

- Molecules naturally want to move from regions of higher concentration to regions of lower concentration (with respect to that particular molecule). Diffusion is the movement of particles down their concentration gradient, and osmosis is the movement of water down *its* concentration gradient.

- Hydrophobic molecules (e.g., O_2, CO_2, and steroids) cross the membrane by simple diffusion, while hydrophilic, polar molecules (e.g., ions, glucose, and water) must cross the membrane with the help of a special membrane protein (a channel or a carrier). This is called facilitated diffusion.

- Active transport uses energy to move molecules against their concentration gradients (from low concentration areas to higher concentration areas). Primary active transport uses ATP directly, while secondary active transport relies on gradients previously established by a primary active transporter.

- The Na^+/K^+ ATPase is a primary active transporter that moves three Na^+ ions out of the cell for every two K^+ ions it moves into the cell. This helps establish the resting membrane potential of the cell, helps maintain osmotic balance in the cell, and sets up a Na^+ gradient that can be used for secondary active transport.

- G-proteins help transduce signals from extracellular ligands across the membrane. They change the level of cAMP or calcium (second messengers) in the cell, which changes the metabolic enzyme pathways active in the cell.

- Microtubules form centrioles, cilia, and eukaryotic flagella, while microfilaments participate in contractile activity.

- Tight junctions help form a seal between cells so that the flow of molecules across the entire cell layer is regulated. Desmosomes form general adhesions between cells. Gap junctions form connections between cells that allow the flow of cytoplasm from cell to cell.

- During the cell cycle, DNA replication occurs during the S-phase of interphase, and cell division occurs during mitosis (M-phase).

- Mitosis is comprised of four major phases (prophase, metaphase, anaphase, and telophase) and results in two daughter cells that are identical to each other and identical to the original parent cell.

- Protooncogenes can be mutated to form oncogenes, which can lead to cancer. Tumor suppressor genes can prevent cancer by halting the cell cycle until damaged DNA is repaired or by inducing apoptosis (cell suicide).

- Apoptosis is triggered by a cascade of activation of enzymes called caspases. Caspases can be activated by extracellular or intracellular signals.

CHAPTER 6 FREESTANDING PRACTICE QUESTIONS

1. *Kartegener's syndrome* is a rare genetic disorder that results in immotile cilia. The immotile cilia cause infertility, bronchiectasis (permanent dilation of the bronchi) and recurrent sinusitis (due to the inability to "push out" bacteria and particles from the sinuses). The genetic defect causes a deficiency of a protein primarily involved in which of the following structures?

A) Microfilament
B) Intermediate filament
C) Microtubule
D) Plasma membrane

2. Different proteins have been found to be involved in vesicular trafficking. Specific proteins are responsible for specific pathways; for instance, COP-I is responsible for retrograde transmission of vesicles, while COP-II is involved in anterograde transmission. Clathrin is involved in receptor-mediated endocytosis. Vesicles on which of the following pathways would be expected to have COP-I proteins on its surface?

A) RER → *cis* Golgi
B) RER → *trans* Golgi
C) *cis* Golgi → RER
D) Nucleus → RER

3. The steroid hormones produced by the smooth endoplasmic reticulum would be stored in which of the following organelles?

A) Secretory vesicles, so the hormones could be released when needed.
B) Peroxisomes, so the hormones could aid in lipid breakdown.
C) Lysosomes, so the hormones could aid in the destruction of excess secretory products.
D) Steroid hormones are not stored, as they are able to diffuse through lipid bilayers.

4. Which of the following gives the correct order for the signals leading to the formation of cyclic AMP? (GPCR = G-Protein Coupled Receptor)

A) Epinephrine → G-proteins → GPCR → adenylyl cyclase → cAMP
B) Epinephrine → GPCR → G-proteins → adenylyl cyclase → cAMP
C) Epinephrine → GPCR → adenylyl cyclase → G-proteins → cAMP
D) Epinephrine → adenylyl cyclase → cAMP → GPCR → G-proteins

5. The nuclear membrane is absent in which of the following phases of mitosis?

   I. Anaphase
   II. Telophase
   III. Metaphase

A) I
B) I and II
C) I and III
D) II and III

6. Both the Golgi complex and rough endoplasmic reticulum contribute to protein modification through all of the following EXCEPT:

A) phosphorylation.
B) creation of disulfide bridges.
C) glycosylation.
D) creation of peptide bonds.

7. Tumor suppressor genes like *BRCA1/2* promote anticancer processes like DNA repair. When these genes are disabled via mutation, the risk for developing cancer later in life increases dramatically. A female who inherits a single mutation in *BRCA2* has a 50% and 20% chance of developing breast and ovarian cancer, respectively. Which of the following best explains why these respective chances are not 100%?

A) Individuals who are homozygous for the *BRCA2* mutation do not have a functional allele.
B) Individuals who are homozygous for the *BRCA2* mutation can still rely on other DNA repair mechanisms.
C) Individuals who are heterozygous for the *BRCA2* mutation still have a functional allele.
D) Individuals who are heterozygous for the *BRCA2* mutation can still rely on other DNA repair mechanisms.

CHAPTER 6 PRACTICE PASSAGE

Apoptosis is the most studied form of programmed cell death. It is limited to multicellular organisms and is a process that involves cells being dismantled from within. When a cell is undergoing apoptosis, it has several characteristic morphological traits; for example, the cells retract and become rounded as they detach from the extracellular matrix and neighboring cells. In addition, the plasma membrane starts blebbing, and apoptotic bodies (similar to vesicles) are pinched off the plasma membrane.

There are several stimuli that could induce apoptotic pathways in a cell. For example, there are receptor-mediated or extrinsic signals that trigger a cell to initiate apoptosis (Figure 1).

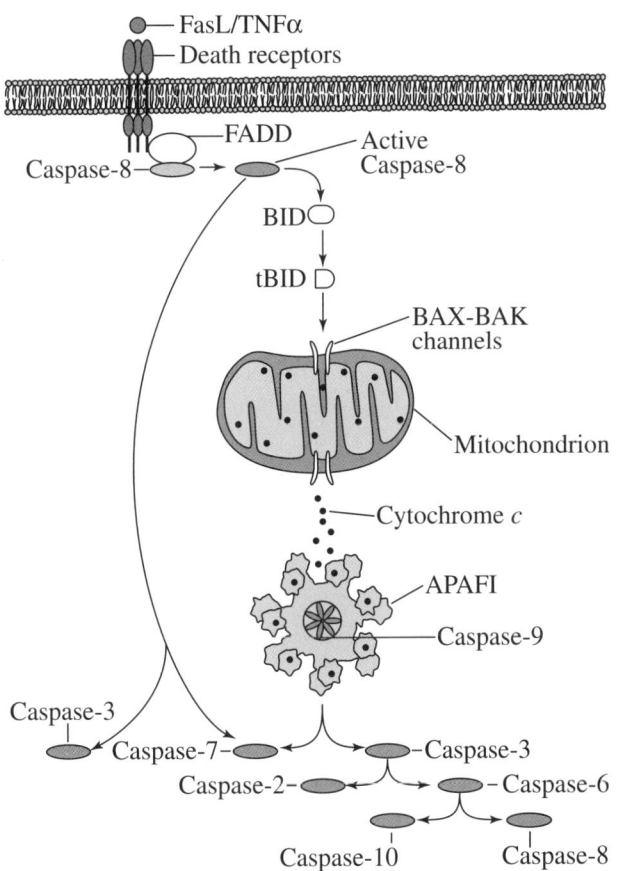

Figure 1   The Extrinsic Apoptosis Pathway

In this case, a death receptor ligand such as FasL or TNFα binds to a death receptor on the surface of the cell. This causes recruitment of adaptor proteins to the plasma membrane. The adaptor proteins serve as docking sites for other proteins, most commonly caspase 8, which is recruited to the plasma

membrane and activated. Active caspase 8 is a protease and cleaves other members of the caspase family along with a protein called BID. The cleaved form of BID (tBID) promotes the release of cytochrome c from mitochondria, and downstream activation of other caspase family members. These proteins dismantle the cytoskeleton and cause nuclear fragmentation, detachment from the surrounding environment, genome degradation, and fragmentation of organelles. After termination of the demolition phase, phagocytes are recruited to the apoptotic cell to clean up the cellular debris.

Autophagy is also a self-destructive process, but does not necessarily lead to cell death. When cells are under stress, parts of the cytoplasm and intracellular organelles are sequestered in specialized double-membrane organelles called autophagosomes. These vacuoles ultimately fuse with lysosomes and the acid hydrolases in the lysosome degrade the contents, which are then recycled to the cell to provide the missing or limited nutrients.

If the degradation of cellular material does not alleviate the stress that induced autophagy, the cell will switch to apoptosis. It is known that autophagy protein Atg5 is essential to autophagy induction and in the regulation of apoptosis. For example, Atg5 generally induces autophagy by promoting autophagosome and autolysosome formation. Atg5 also enhances the susceptibility of cancer cells to apoptosis. It has been found that the full-length Atg5 protein induces autophagy, but with lethal stress, the full-length Atg5 is proteolytically cleaved to generate a 24 kDa pro-apoptotic protein that promotes cytochrome c release and mitochondrial permeabilization.

1. p53 is a tumor suppressor protein that is commonly mutated or deleted in aberrantly growing cancer cells. Which of the following is the most likely function of p53?

A) It is a transcription factor that induces expression of pro-apoptotic proteins.
B) It indirectly induces autophagy to supply the cell with biomacromolecules.
C) It stimulates phospholipid synthesis in the smooth ER.
D) It induces cell cycle progression in response to genome stability, as part of the G_2-M checkpoint pathway.

2. Which of the following are NOT examples of enzymes found in lysosomes?

A) Phosphatases and nucleases
B) Phospholipase C and adenylyl cyclase
C) Proteases and peptidases
D) Glucosidases and lipases

3. Which of the following would NOT induce autophagy?

A) Increase in inner mitochondrial membrane permeability
B) Accumulation of incorrectly folded proteins in the ER lumen
C) Incomplete genome replication
D) Decreased intracellular metabolite concentrations

4. A researcher adds the BAX-BAC channel inhibitor Bci1 to a plate of cells in the lab. Which of the following is observed?

A) Retention of cytochrome c in the inner mitochondrial membrane
B) Inhibition of BAX-BAC channel formation in the inner mitochondrial membrane
C) Rounded cells and blebbing of the plasma membrane
D) A rapid increase in the amount of cellular autophagy

5. Monophosphate Atg13 initiates autophagosome formation and mTOR phosphorylates three amino acids on Atg13 simultaneously. Which of the following is true?

A) mTOR is anti-autophagic and functions as a kinase.
B) mTOR activates Atg13 and functions as a phosphatase.
C) Rapamycin, an mTOR inhibitor, represses autophagy.
D) In cells that are undergoing autophagy, Atg13 is phosphorylated on three amino acids.

6. Which of the following is true of Atg5?

A) Southern blot analysis of proteins from healthy cells would show a 24 kDa Atg5.
B) Calpain, the protease that cleaves Atg5, is activated in cells that have bound FasL.
C) Western blot analysis of proteins from cells undergoing autophagy would show a 19 kDa Atg5.
D) Healthy cells and autophagic cells have alternative splicing of Atg5 to generate two different proteins.

SOLUTIONS TO CHAPTER 6 FREESTANDING PRACTICE QUESTIONS

1. **C**   Cilia and flagella are both made up of microtubules; thus, a defect causing immotile cilia would likely involve a protein associated with microtubules (choice C is correct). In fact, *Kartegener's syndrome* is a defect in the dynein protein, which is an ATPase that links the peripheral 9 doublets of the cilium (remember that eukaryotic cilia and flagella both have a 9 + 2 arrangement of microtubules) and causes bending (motion) of the cilium by differential sliding of the doublets. Microfilaments are composed of the protein actin and are responsible for contractile motility and changing of cell shape, specifically, muscle contraction, leukocyte motility, and cytokinesis (choice A is wrong). Intermediate filaments are primarily responsible for the cytoskeletal structure of cells (choice B is wrong). The plasma membrane is composed of phospholipids and cholesterol, although it does include many different proteins. However, the proteins of the plasma membrane are not responsible for cilia motility (choice D is wrong).

2. **C**   The question stem states that COP-I proteins are involved in retrograde, or "backward," vesicular trafficking. Therefore, these vesicles would be traveling in the reverse pathway. Choice C (*cis* Golgi to RER) is the only correct option listed. The anterograde, or "forward," pathway in cells involves vesicles traveling from the RER to the cis Golgi (choice A is wrong), the *medial* Golgi, the *trans* Golgi and then to the cell membrane or other target site within the cell. Vesicles do not normally travel from the RER to the *trans* Golgi (choice B is wrong). Also vesicles are not involved in transport from the nucleus (choice D is wrong).

3. **D**   Because steroid hormones are made from cholesterol as lipid derivatives, they cannot be stored by lipid bilayers. Since secretory vesicles, peroxisomes, and lysosomes are membrane-bound, they cannot store steroids (choices A, B, and C are wrong). Note also that peptide hormones are stored in secretory vesicles (choice A would be true of a peptide hormone, but not of a steroid hormone). Be careful to differentiate between answer choices that are simply true versus answer choices that actually address the question. Though choices A, B, and C all describe the general function of their particular organelle, only choice D addresses the issue specific to steroids.

4. **B**   Since the question is asking about the formation of cAMP, it should be the last step in the sequence (choice D can be eliminated). G-protein coupled receptors receive the signal from ligand binding (in this example, epinephrine), and affect G-proteins. Therefore, GPCR must come before G-protein in the sequence (choice A can be eliminated). GPCRs activate G-proteins, which then affect the enzyme adenylyl cyclase (choice B is correct, and choice C is wrong). Remember also that some GPCRs activate adenylyl cyclase and others inhibit it. This depends on the cell, the ligand, and many other factors.

5. **C**   Item I is true: the nuclear membrane is degraded by the end of prophase so that the chromosomes can be appropriately separated into the daughter cells. It is therefore absent in anaphase (choice D can be eliminated). Item II is false: the nuclear membrane reforms after cytokinesis in telophase (choice B can be eliminated). Item III is true: since the membrane does not reform until telophase, it must be absent in metaphase (choice A can be eliminated).

6. **D** Phosphorylation, formation of disulfide bridges, and glycosylation are all types of protein modification and can occur in both the Golgi apparatus and the rough ER (choices A, B, and C can be eliminated). Peptide bond formation occurs during translation, prior to any protein modification (choice D is not a type of protein modification and is the correct answer choice).

7. **C** A female who inherits a single mutation still has an allele which can produce functional proteins (choice C is correct) and is heterozygous, not homozygous (choices A and B are wrong). While an individual who is heterozygous for the mutation can rely on other DNA repair mechanisms, this is not the primary reason why these individuals will not have a 100% chance of developing breast or ovarian cancer (choice C is better than choice D).

SOLUTIONS TO CHAPTER 6 PRACTICE PASSAGE

1. **A** The key to answering this question is decoding the question stem: *If p53 is commonly defective in cancer cells, it must normally have some sort of protective role.* In other words, p53 loss is beneficial for cancer cells. If p53 normally induces apoptosis and becomes mutant or lost, then it would no longer cause cell death in aberrant conditions. This could be a benefit for cancer cells, and in fact could lead to the rapid cell proliferation and tumor growth that is typically seen in cancer (choice A is correct). The passage says that autophagy can help the cell deal with times of stress, including nutrient deprivation. Since cancer cells grow quickly, they have high metabolic demands, which are accommodated in part using autophagy to supply macromolecules. If p53 normally helped the cell supply macromolecules, p53 loss would not help the growth of cancer cells (choice B can be eliminated). Similarly, if cancer cells are growing quickly, they will need lots of phospholipids. If p53 normally stimulated phospholipid synthesis, its loss would not be beneficial for the cancer cell (choice C can be eliminated). Finally, if p53 normally pushed the cell cycle forward, its loss would arrest the cell cycle. This is clearly not the case in "aberrantly growing cancer cells" (choice D is wrong).

2. **B** The passage says that the lysosome contains acid hydrolases, which degrade the contents of the autophagosomes. Since the autophagosomes contain cellular and organelle material, it is possible that they would contain proteins (which would be broken down by proteases and peptidases; choice C can be eliminated), nucleic acids (which would be broken down by nucleases; choice A can be eliminated), carbohydrates (which would be broken down by glucosidases), and lipids (which would be broken down by lipases; choice D can be eliminated). However, phospholipase C and adenylyl cyclase are both involved in cell signaling pathways, downstream of ligands binding receptors. Neither of these would function in macromolecule degradation (choice B would not be found in lysosomes and is the correct answer choice). Note that phosphatases remove the phosphate group from molecules, and in many cases, this is part of degradation.

3. **C** The passage says that autophagy is induced when cells are under nutrient stress, reactive oxygen stress, or organelle stress. Decreased intracellular metabolite concentrations would be an example of nutrient stress (choice D would induce autophagy and can be eliminated). An increase in mitochondrial permeability and an accumulation of incorrectly folded proteins in the ER lumen are examples of organelle stress (autophagy degrades broken or sickly organelles; choices A and B could induce autophagy and can be eliminated). While incomplete genome replication in the S phase is a problem for cells, there is no information to indicate that this would induce autophagy. Also, the effects of autophagy as described in the passage (break down of cytoplasmic and organelle material) would not solve this problem since the genome cannot be degraded (there is only one, after all). In fact, incomplete genome replication is detected by cell cycle checkpoint pathways to halt cell cycle progression and allow time for DNA replication and repair (choice C would not induce autophagy and is the correct answer choice).

4. **A** According to the figure, BAX proteins form channels in the mitochondrial membrane and this facilitates cytochrome *c* release. If Bci1 inhibits these channels, it would cause cytochrome *c* to remain in the inner mitochondrial membrane (choice A is correct). This would prevent apoptosis (and thus rounded cells and blebbing; choice C is wrong). While choice B might be tempting, just because Bci1 inhibits BAX channels doesn't mean it has to inhibit channel formation (although this is certainly possible). We can be sure about the end result, though (retention of cytochrome *c*), even if we aren't sure of the mechanism (choice A is better than choice B). Note that BAX functions in apoptosis, not autophagy (choice D is wrong).

5. **A** Note that there is no information about Atg13 in the passage, so this question must be answered based entirely on information in the question. The question text states that when Atg13 is phosphorylated on one amino acid, it initiates autophagy by inducing autophagosome formation (choice D is wrong). If mTOR phosphorylates Atg13 on three amino acids, it is acting as a kinase and is inhibiting Atg13 function and autophagy (choice A is correct, and choice B is wrong). If rapamycin inhibits mTOR, it is inhibiting an inhibitor of autophagy. In other words, rapamycin would induce autophagy (choice C is wrong).

6. **B** The passage says that Atg5 cleavage (from a longer precursor protein to a shorter 24 kDa protein) is involved in the switch from autophagy to apoptosis. If cells have bound FasL (a death receptor ligand), they are undergoing apoptosis, or will be soon. Since Atg5 cleavage induces apoptosis, choice B is very likely. Southern blot analysis is a lab technique used to study DNA, not proteins (choice A is wrong). While western blot analysis is the correct lab technique to study proteins, in cells undergoing autophagy (not apoptosis), Atg5 would be in the longer, nontruncated form (the 24 kDa protein, not the 19 kDa protein; choice C is wrong). The passage describes proteolytic cleavage as the mechanism for generating differently sized Atg5, not alternative splicing (choice D is wrong).

GUT MICROBIOME FERMENTATION DETERMINES THE EFFICACY OF EXERCISE FOR DIABETES PREVENTION

Yan Liu, Yao Wang, Yueqiong Ni, Cynthia K. Y. Cheung, Karen S. L. Lam, Yu Wang, Zhengyuan Xia, Dewei Ye, Jiao Guo, Michael Andrew Tse, Gianni Panagiotou, and Aimin Xu

Cell Metabolism 31, 77-91 January 7, 2020 © 2019 Elsevier Inc. https://doi.org/10.1016/j.cmet.2019.11.001

INTRODUCTION

Exercise is a cost-effective lifestyle intervention for the prevention and treatment of obesity, type 2 diabetes (T2D) and its complications, which are the leading causes of morbidity and mortality worldwide. Despite the well-recognized benefits of exercise on metabolic homeostasis, the biomarkers and molecular transducers conferring its pleotropic effects remain poorly understood. Clinical implementation of exercise for diabetes management is still in its infancy, in part due to the high variability in physiological response to standardized exercise regimen. A large proportion of individuals, ranging from 7% to 69%, do not respond (non-responders) or even respond adversely to exercise in terms of insulin sensitivity and glucose homeostasis. Though genetic predispositions and epigenetic modifications have been proposed to be potential contributors, neither the pathomechanisms nor potential predictors for the heterogeneity of exercise responsiveness have been clarified so far.

A growing body of evidence suggests that dysbiosis of gut microbiota plays an important role in the pathogenesis of insulin resistance and T2D through multiple mechanisms. Compositional and functional changes of gut microbiota have been observed in individuals with T2D and prediabetes, whereas fecal microbial transplantation from healthy donors into patients with metabolic syndrome results in increased microbial diversity and improved glycemic control, as well as insulin sensitivity.

Recently, a modulatory effect of exercise on gut microbiota in both humans and animals has been observed. The microbiome of professional athletes exhibits higher diversity and more favorable metabolic capacity compared to sedentary counterparts. Mice receiving exercise training also display favorable changes in the composition of gut microbiota, including reduced *Bacteroidetes*, but augmented *Firmicutes* and *Proteobacteria*. However, whether and how alterations in gut microbiota are functionally involved in the metabolic benefits of exercise remain obscure.

To address the above questions, we conducted a well-controlled exercise intervention in medication-naive overweight men with prediabetes, followed by comprehensive metagenomics and metabolomics analysis, and a functional interrogation in mice using fecal microbial transplantation to explore the roles of differentially shaped gut microbiota by exercise in glucose metabolism and insulin sensitivity.

RESULTS AND DISCUSSION

Heterogeneous Glycemic Responses of Individuals with Prediabetes to High-Intensity Training

Eligible participants were randomized to either sedentary control or 12-week supervised exercise training, in which exercise responsiveness was further evaluated (Figure 1A). All participants were recommended to maintain their diet routine during the study period, which was closely monitored to ensure that no significant difference existed among all these subjects (Table S1).

After exercise intervention, a modest but significant reduction in body weight and adiposity, together with obvious improvements in insulin sensitivity, lipid profiles, cardiorespiratory fitness, and levels of adipokines functionally related to insulin sensitivity had been achieved in the whole exercise group (Table S1). However, in contrast to a homogenous change in body compositions (Figures 1B–1D), a high interpersonal variability in the alterations of fasting glucose, insulin, and the homeostatic model assessment of insulin resistance (HOMA-IR) was observed (Figures 1E–1G), suggesting a highly heterogeneous response of the cohort with respect to glucose homeostasis and insulin sensitivity. Therefore, we

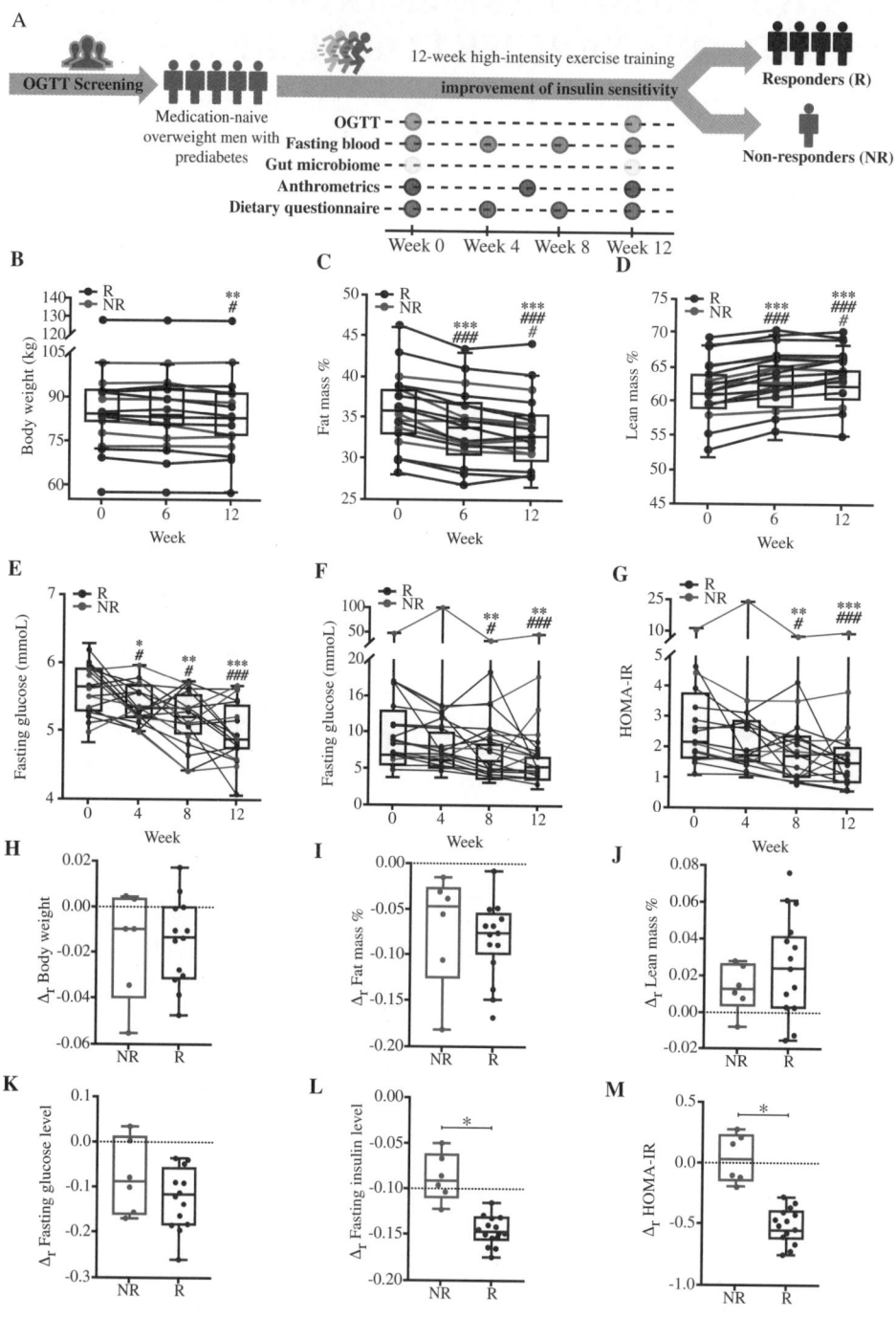

Figure 1 High Interpersonal Variability in the Improvement of Insulin Sensitivity
(A) Schematic diagram of the study design. (B–G) Boxplots (with median) showing the dynamic changes of (B) body weight and (C) fat mass and (D) lean mass body compositions at 0, 6, and 12 weeks of exercise intervention, as well as (E) fasting glucose, (F) fasting insulin and (G) HOMA-IR at 0, 4, 8, and 12 weeks of exercise, respectively. Lines connect the same subject at different time points. #$p < 0.05$ and ###$p < 0.001$ by repeated-measures ANOVA within Responders or non-responders; and *$p < 0.05$, **$p < 0.01$ and ***$p < 0.001$ by repeated-measures ANOVA within all subjects. (H–M) The relative change of (H) body weight, (I) fat mass and (J) lean mass body compositions, (K) fasting glucose, (L) fasting insulin, and (M) HOMA-IR over 12 weeks of exercise intervention. Data were shown as mean ± SEM.
*$p < 0.05$ by repeated-measures two-way ANOVA.

Table S1 Summary of clinical characteristics of the exercise group and sedentary control, Related to Figure 1

Variables	Sedentary control			Exercise group			Between group difference (p value)	
	0-week	12-week	p value[*]	0-week	12-week	p value[*]	0-week[#]	12-week[§]
Age (years)	44.94 ± 2.43	NA	NA	42.80 ± 2.55	NA	NA	0.549	NA
Weight (kg)	83.63 ± 1.96	83.46 ± 1.85	0.965	85.50 ± 3.16	84.22 ± 3.21	0.003	0.760	0.897
BMI (Kg/m^2)	29.40 ± 0.72	29.32 ± 0.85	0.807	29.09 ± 0.90	28.95 ± 0.91	0.192	0.625	0.623
WHR	0.92 ± 0.02	0.91 ± 0.02	0.852	0.95 ± 0.01	0.93 ± 0.01	2.00E-06	0.157	0.276
Fat mass%	34.79 ± 1.28	34.64 ± 0.78	0.742	35.95 ± 0.98	33.74 ± 0.91	1.00E-06	0.470	0.855
Lean mass%	61.79 ± 1.50	60.53 ± 1.48	0.745	61.22 ± 0.91	63.38 ± 0.83	1.88E-06	0.736	0.612
Fasting glucose (mM)	5.79 ± 0.25	5.94 ± 0.28	0.758	5.61 ± 0.08	4.99 ± 0.09	3.00E-06	0.943	0.022
2h glucose (mM)	8.79 ± 0.42	9.12 ± 0.46	0.182	8.30 ± 0.32	6.30 ± 0.30	1.00E-06	0.376	1.70E-05
Fasting insulin (μU/mL)	9.83 ± 1.04	8.86 ± 0.81	0.393	12.10 ± 2.17	9.10 ± 2.19	0.026	0.474	0.806
HOMA-IR	2.86 ± 0.31	2.58 ± 0.19	0.464	2.98 ± 0.49	1.99 ± 0.45	0.031	0.847	0.042
Triglycerides (mM)	2.53 ± 0.44	2.40 ± 0.39	0.992	2.33 ± 0.17	1.90 ± 0.14	0.016	0.803	0.741
Total cholesterol (mM)	5.10 ± 0.25	4.68 ± 0.25	0.256	5.37 ± 0.23	4.98 ± 0.21	0.027	0.434	0.349
HDL-c (mM)	1.15 ± 0.06	1.08 ± 0.56	0.429	1.16 ± 0.04	1.21 ± 0.43	0.301	0.859	0.260
LDL-c (mM)	3.57 ± 0.20	3.68 ± 0.20	0.669	3.55 ± 0.20	3.29 ± 0.17	0.054	0.926	0.425
Systolic blood pressure (mmHg)	133.75 ± 5.10	132.28 ± 4.39	0.790	130.79 ± 3.64	128.37 ± 3.12	0.375	0.632	0.493
Diastolic blood pressure (mmHg)	83.75 ± 2.03	85.88 ± 2.95	0.587	80.42 ± 1.93	77.37 ± 2.22	0.131	0.245	0.025
Resting heart rate (bpm)	76.83 ± 2.65	77.83 ± 3.72	0.475	77.53 ± 2.18	73.74 ± 2.04	0.028	0.743	0.711
hs-CRP (mg/L)	3.59 ± 0.75	3.72 ± 0.82	0.912	3.60 ± 0.41	2.55 ± 0.29	0.002	0.662	0.440
Total energy (Kcal/d)	1648 ± 90.05	1646.97 ± 59.86	0.988	1656.67 ± 49.45	1655.32 ± 43.61	0.983	0.935	0.904
Carbohydrate (g)	267.15 ± 14.92	257.96 ± 11.26	0.625	266.02 ± 7.16	260.08 ± 7.69	0.483	0.945	0.965
% of Energy intake	63.21 ± 1.25	61.11 ± 1.11	0.215	64.40 ± 1.05	63.55 ± 1.03	0.601	0.469	0.098

Table 2 Changes in Clinical Parameters of Prediabetic Individuals in Response to 12-Week Exercise Intervention

Characteristics	0-Week			12-Week			p Value$_c$
	Responders	Non-responders	p Value$_a$	Responders	Non-responders	p Value$_b$	Between Group Difference in Relative Change
Age (years)	43.29 ± 3.27	36.00 ± 4.55	0.228	—	—	—	—
BMI	28.78 ± 1.08	29.82 ± 1.75	0.603	28.65 ± 1.09	29.66 ± 1.78	0.850	0.613
Fat mass%	36.13 ± 1.33	35.78 ± 1.22	0.878	33.82 ± 1.22	33.53 ± 1.22	0.888	0.882
Lean mass%	60.98 ± 1.24	61.57 ± 1.10	0.776	63.26 ± 1.11	63.67 ± 1.09	0.856	0.799
WHR	0.95 ± 0.02	0.94 ± 0.01	0.730	0.93 ± 0.02	0.92 ± 0.01	0.761	0.702
Fasting glucose (mM)	5.65 ± 0.09	5.51 ± 0.13	0.426	4.95 ± 0.11	5.08 ± 0.21	0.311	0.980
2-h glucose (mM)	8.24 ± 0.33	8.46 ± 0.81	0.757	6.15 ± 0.39	6.64 ± 0.45	0.578	0.578
Fasting insulin (μU/mL)	10.37 ± 1.31	16.12 ± 6.67	0.522	5.70 ± 0.77	17.04 ± 6.26	3.84E−04	0.030
Matsuda index	5.83 ± 1.09	3.24 ± 0.78	0.097	11.01 ± 1.91	3.81 ± 0.78	0.002	0.017
Triglycerides (mM)	2.30 ± 0.21	2.41 ± 0.30	0.690	1.91 ± 0.19	1.86 ± 0.21	0.859	0.807
Total cholesterol (mM)	5.26 ± 0.31	5.60 ± 0.27	0.524	4.76 ± 0.26	5.49 ± 0.24	0.103	0.247
Systolic blood pressure (MmHg)	130.54 ± 4.74	131.33 ± 5.84	0.923	128.31 ± 4.47	128.50 ± 2.67	0.956	0.944
Diastolic blood pressure (MmHg)	80.00 ± 2.71	81.33 ± 2.04	0.759	78.08 ± 2.77	75.83 ± 3.94	0.452	0.912
Resting heart rate (bpm)	75.00 ± 2.02	83.00 ± 4.91	0.087	70.46 ± 1.92	80.83 ± 3.65	0.081	0.024
VO$_{2\,Max}$ (mL/kg/min)	25.27 ± 1.30	26.83 ± 1.38	0.485	31.42 ± 1.20	31.03 ± 1.85	0.861	0.755
Leg press (kg)	239.23 ± 11.79	226.67 ± 15.85	0.547	282.69 ± 17.97	270.83 ± 14.52	0.894	0.608
Chest press (kg)	32.46 ± 2.17	34.40 ± 3.41	0.642	38.92 ± 2.30	39.50 ± 2.97	0.886	0.546
hs-CRP (mg/L)	3.68 ± 0.46	3.39 ± 0.94	0.565	2.53 ± 0.32	2.59 ± 0.67	0.461	0.880
Total energy (Kcal/d)	1,694.74 ± 59.99	1,567.84 ± 82.97	0.250	1,685.20 ± 51.93	1,585.59 ± 79.62	0.308	0.137
Carbohydrate (g)	270.21 ± 8.94	256.26 ± 11.69	0.386	266.96 ± 9.64	244.04 ± 10.55	0.178	0.177
Protein (g)	70.51 ± 3.57	69.01 ± 4.52	0.813	70.24 ± 2.30	71.81 ± 4.65	0.738	0.933
Fat (g)	35.76 ± 3.00	33.31 ± 2.86	0.629	39.86 ± 2.63	37.43 ± 5.80	0.663	0.490
Fiber (g)	9.30 ± 0.85	8.23 ± 1.32	0.500	9.25 ± 0.56	8.10 ± 0.54	0.235	0.238

BMI, body mass index; HDL-c, high-density lipoprotein cholesterol; hs-CRP, high-sensitive C-reactive protein; LDL-c, low-density lipoprotein cholesterol; WHR, waist-hip ratio. Responders ($n = 14$) and Non-responders ($n = 6$). Data are shown as means ± SEM.

a   Determined by independent Student's t test.

b   Determined by ANCOVA model controlling for baseline measurements.

c   Determined by repeated-measures two-way ANOVA.

further classified the participants into responders (n = 14) and non-responders (n = 6), depending on whether they could demonstrate a decrease of HOMA-IR greater than 2-fold technical error, which is a threshold for true physiological adaptation. Notably, despite a homogeneous baseline characteristic (Table 1) and a similar degree of reduction in body weight and fat percentage between these two sub-groups (Figures 1H–1J), responders showed a remarkable 42.70% and 49.60% decrease in fasting insulin and HOMA-IR index, respectively (Figures 1L and 1M), as well as a striking 116.29% increase of Matsuda index (a comprehensive evaluation of both hepatic and peripheral insulin sensitivity derived from oral glucose tolerance test), whereas no obvious improvement or even deterioration in glucose homeostasis and insulin sensitivity was observed in non-responders (Table 1; Figures 1K–1M). Considering the important role of the gut microbiota in regulating glucose homeostasis and insulin sensitivity, we next explored whether it was involved in the heterogeneous metabolic effects of exercise in our cohort.

A Modest but Distinguishable Change of Gut Microbiota by Exercise Intervention in All Participants

We performed shotgun metagenome sequencing of fecal samples collected before and after the 12-week exercise regimen. We performed a compositional analysis and found that the relative abundances of 6 species, belonging to *Firmicutes*, *Bacteroidetes*, and *Proteobacteria*, respectively, were significantly altered after exercise (Figure 2A). Moreover, species falling into the *Bacteroides* genus and *Clostridiales* order, most of which are involved in the production of SCFAs, underwent a significant strain-level genomic variation by exercise (Figure 2B). Importantly, none of the alterations observed above could be detected in sedentary controls sharing similar metabolic characteristics (Table S1; Figure 3). In addition, the number of positive connections among those butyrate-producing genera within *Firmicutes* was obviously promoted, the decreased abundance of which is reported to be associated with obesity and T2D.

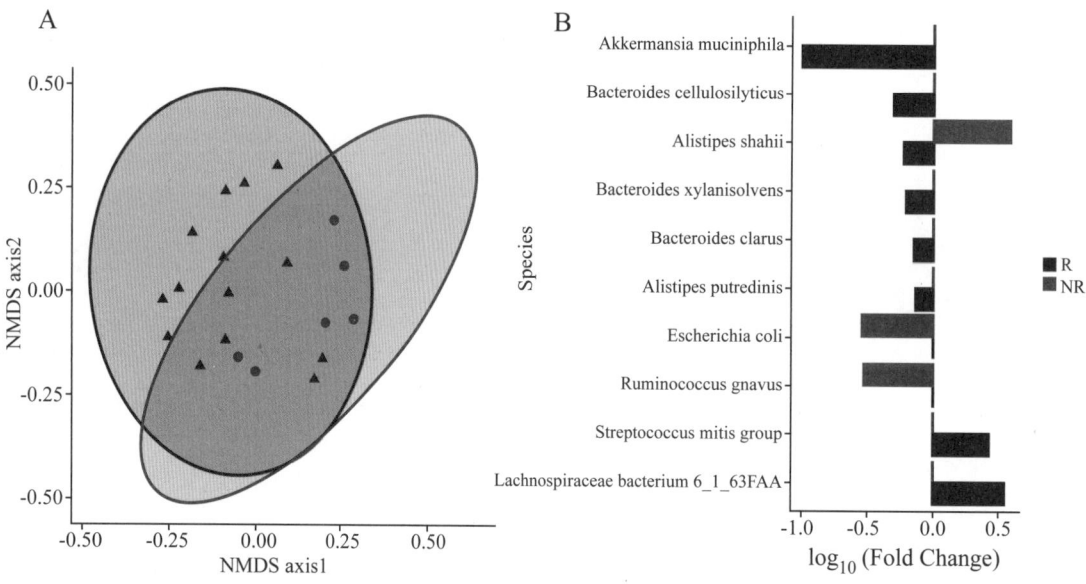

Figure 2 Exercise Promotes Differential Alteration of Gut Microbiota in Responders and Non-responders
(A and B) Participants were further classified into responders (R, blue) and non-responders (NR, red) based on the relative improvement of HOMA-IR. (A) Non-metric multidimensional scaling analysis plot of taxonomic variation induced by exercise training in R and NR, respectively. p = 0.008 by ADONIS test between R and NR. (B) Significantly altered species (p < 0.05) caused by exercise intervention in R and NR, respectively. Fold change was defined as the ratio of relative microbial abundance after exercise to those at baseline and the log fold changes were set to zero if not statistically significant.

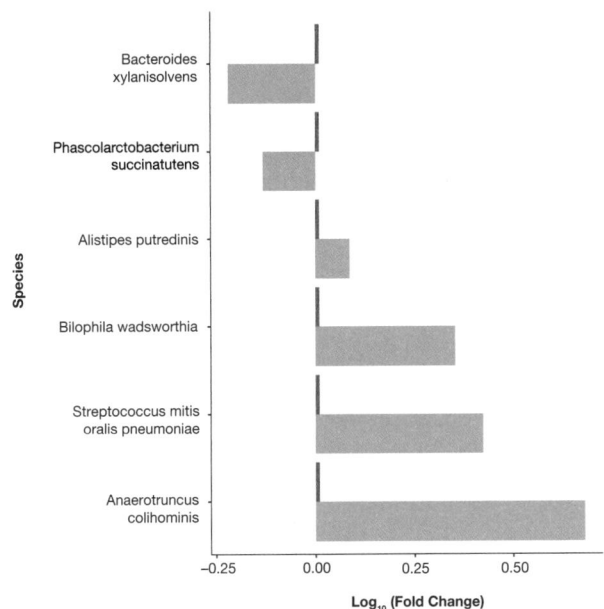

Figure 3 None of the exercise-induced microbial alterations can be detected in sedentary controls, Related to Figure 2. Green and purple indicate exercise and sedentary control respectively. Fold change was defined as the ratio of relative microbial abundance at 12-week to that at baseline (0-week).

Differential Alterations of Gut Microbiota between Exercise Responders and Non-responders

As there was a high interpersonal variability in the alteration of gut, we next interrogated whether the heterogeneous responses to exercise in glucose homeostasis and insulin sensitivity were related to differential changes in gut microbiota between responders and non-responders. We observed a significant segregation of dynamic alterations of gut microbiota between the two sub-groups (Figure 2D). Compared to responders, the microbial profiles of non-responders after 12-week exercise training shared more similarity with those of the sedentary controls (p < 0.0 01), suggesting a maladaptation of gut microbiota in non-responders. Notably, we observed that the significant decrease of *Bacteroides xylanisolvens* and increase of *Streptococcus mitis* group found in all participants only occurred in responders, but not non-responders. Contrary

to an increase of *Alistipes putredinis* in the whole group, this bacterium was found to be reduced in responders (Figure 2E). In addition, responders were characterized by a 3.5-fold increase of *Lanchospiraceae bacterium* (a butyrate-producer), whereas non-responders were featured by nearly a 70% decrease in *Ruminococcus gnavus*, which has been reported to alleviate growth and metabolic impairments caused by transplanting microbiota from undernourished donors. Moreover, *Alistipes shahii*, previously reported to be associated with inflammation and enriched in obese Japanese, decreased by 43% in responders, but increased by 3.88-fold in non-responders (Figure 2E). When taking the growth dynamics of bacteria into consideration, responders were characterized by a decreased replication rate of *Prevotella copri*, a main bacterium responsible for the production of BCAAs and a contributor to insulin resistance, as well as an increased growth rate of several species in *Bacteroides* genus, most of which are propionate producers. Collectively, these findings suggest that exercise intervention exerts differential modulatory effects on microbial compositions in responders and non-responders.

Exercise-Conditioned Microbiota from Responders Ameliorate Glucose Intolerance and Insulin Resistance in Obese Mice

To further examine the causal relationship between differentially shaped microbiota and changes in glucose metabolism and insulin sensitivity by exercise intervention, conventional antibiotics-treated mice were transplanted with microbiota from two responders and two non-responders collected at both baseline and after exercise intervention (Figure 4A). A number of microbial species, such as *Alistipes shahii*, *Alistipes putredinis* and *Ruminococcus gnavus*, demonstrated a similar trend of changes between recipient mice and human donors (Figure S7). Mice colonized with microbiota from responders and non-responders after exercise displayed a similar trend of changes in body composition, oxygen consumption, and respiratory exchange ratio compared to those receiving microbiota from the same donors taken at baseline (Figures 4B–4D). On the other hand, significant reductions in glucose and insulin levels were observed only in mice transplanted with microbiota from responders, but not non-responders after exercise training (Figures 4E–4F).

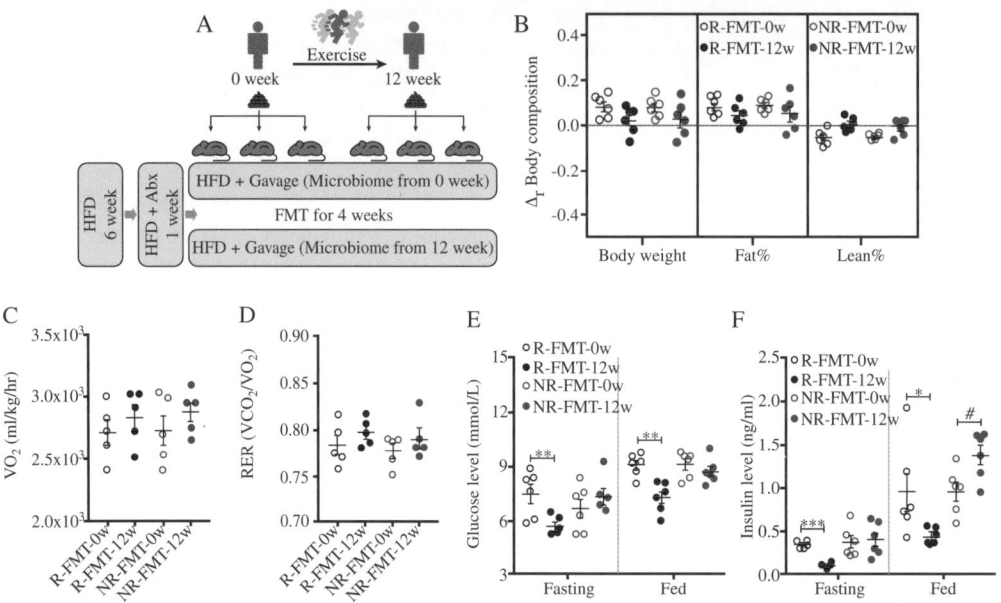

Figure 4 Transplantation of Human Fecal Microbiota into Mice Mimics the Effect of Exercise on Glucose Homeostasis and Insulin Sensitivity

(A) Schematic diagram showing the study design for fecal microbial transplantation. (B) Relative changes of body compositions. (C and D) Recipient mice were subjected to indirect calorimetry analysis for the determination of (C) oxygen consumption and (D) respiratory exchange ratio after 4 weeks of microbial colonization. (E and F) Glucose (E) and insulin (F) levels at both fasting and fed status. Data were expressed as mean ± SEM (n = 6 mice/group). *$p < 0.05$, **$p < 0.01$, and ***$p < 0.001$ between R-FMT-0w and R-FMT-12w; #$p < 0.05$ between NR-FMT-0w and NR-FMT-12w by unpaired Student's t test. Dots with different colors represent individual mice receiving FMT from different human donors.

In this well-controlled interventional study conducted in medication-naïve individuals with prediabetes, we showed that gut microbiota was an important mediator conferring the effect of exercise on glucose metabolism and insulin sensitivity. The high interpersonal variability in the adaptive changes upon exercise intervention was attributed to divergent functional alterations of gut microbiota, leading to production of distinct sets of microbial metabolites. These findings were further strengthened by animal studies showing that exercise-induced differential changes in glucose homeostasis, insulin sensitivity, and metabolites in responders and non-responders can be transferred into mice by FMT.

Although there was no obvious difference in baseline microbial structures between responders and non-responders, we were able to establish a model based on the microbiome signatures before exercise to accurately predict the exercise outcomes with respect to glycemic control and insulin sensitivity, raising the possibility of screening for individuals with high likelihood of exercise resistance using gut microbiota, so that personalized adjustments

can be implemented in time to maximize the efficacy of exercise intervention. These findings uncover the diversity of gut microbiota as a key determinant for the variability of glycemic control after dietary and exercise intervention. However, how exercise imposes such a differential impact on the composition and function of gut microbiota remains unclear and warrants further investigation. We speculate that exercise may amplify subtle difference of gut microbiota at baseline by remodeling the intestinal microenvironment (such as inflammatory and oxidative status and local immunity) critical for microbial growth and interaction, which ultimately lead to a divergent response of glycemic control to exercise intervention.

In conclusion, our study uncovers gut microbiota and its metabolism as key molecular transducers to the heterogeneous adaption to exercise intervention on glucose metabolism and insulin sensitivity. This finding, together with our demonstration of the predictive value of baseline microbial signatures for individualized responsiveness to exercise, may facilitate clinical implementation of personalized lifestyle intervention for diabetes management.

Limitations of Study

The main limitation of the current study is a relatively small sample size and rigid inclusion criteria for our study participants, which constrains the applicability of this result. Though limited only to Chinese males, these results demonstrate the adequacy of this non-invasive proxy measurement in the prediction of exercise responsiveness. Considering the regional and ethnic variations in gut microbiota, the wide applicability of our findings and prediction model needs further validation in larger and more diverse populations.

MATERIALS AND METHODS

Study Participants

Inclusion criteria were: (i) non-smoking and male Chinese aged between 20 and 60 years; (ii) weight stable (<5% weight change over last 3 months) and overweight/obese as defined by Asian criteria BMI>23 kg/m^2; (iii) pre-diabetes as defined by impaired glucose tolerance (7.8 mmol/L $\leq$ 2-h blood glucose $\leq$ 11.0 mmol/L after a 75-g oral glucose challenge) and/or impaired fasting glucose (5.6 mmol/L $\leq$ fasting blood glucose $\leq$ 6.9 mmol/L) following the American Diabetes Association practice guidelines; (iv) absence of any systemic, metabolic and cardiovascular diseases, as well as infections within the previous month; and (v) absence of any diet or medication that might interfere with glucose homeostasis and gut microbiota, especially antibiotics and probiotics.

Exclusion criteria were: (i) acute illness or current evidence of acute or chronic inflammatory or infective diseases; (ii) any neurological, musculoskeletal or cardio-respiratory conditions, which will put them at risk during exercise or inhibit their ability to adapt to an exercise program; (iii) participation in regular exercise and/or diet program more than 2 times per week in the latest 3 months prior to recruitment; and (iv) mental illness rendering them unable to understand the nature, scope, and possible consequences of the study.

Subject Recruitment and General Design

Overweight/obese subjects were recruited from our local community. Oral glucose tolerance test (OGTT) was used to screen for potential participants who met the inclusion criterion of prediabetes. Eligible subjects were randomly assigned to exercise or sedentary group. Aside from exercise training, all participants recruited were instructed to continue their normal routine and not make any changes to their habitual physical activity and diet. One-to-one interview with a validated questionnaire including nutritional intakes and physical activity was conducted every month to assess their adherence. Fecal samples were collected at baseline and 12 weeks after exercise training while fasting plasma samples were collected every 4 weeks. All examinations were conducted at 48-72 h from the final exercise session to control for the acute effects of exercise.

High-Intensity Exercise Training Protocol

The 12-week exercise program consisted of three sessions per week on non-consecutive days at the Active Health Clinic, supervised by certified exercise specialists in a one-to-one manner. Compliance in the exercise session was highly encouraged and participants were required to take part in at least 85% of all the exercise sessions for inclusion into the analysis for responsiveness. The exercise program consisted of a combination of aerobic and strength training, which was selected for its superior effectiveness in the alleviation of insulin resistance. The 70-min high-intensity combined aerobic and resistance interval training sessions including high-intensity treadmill intervals, high-intensity resistance and calisthenics exercises intervals, and high-intensity stationary bike intervals, with 3–4 min recovery. Participants wore a wireless heart rate telemetry sensor to monitor their heart rate (HR) and to ensure that they were working at the appropriate intensity level. The intensity was adjusted according to the real-time HR telemetry and the subjects were encouraged to work at 80-95% HR_{max}. The intensity of this resistance and calisthenics intervals was progressed during the 12-week training to keep the exercises challenging and also to provide adequate work to rest ratio to stimulate high intensity interval training-based resistance intervals.

Collection of Dietary and Clinical Data

Dietary data were collected by means of food frequency questionnaire administered by a nutritionist.

Definition of Responders and Non-responders

The distribution of exercise responsiveness in our cohort exhibits a two-sided shape, ranging from high responders to adverse responders with respect to changes in insulin sensitivity (data not shown). According to previous interventional surveys, the inter-individual variability in response was evaluated by technical error (TE), a parameter that captures the totality of the variance among laboratories or laboratory technicians and the normal day-to-day biological variation of a trait. It is defined as the within-subject standard deviation as derived from repeated measures (or assays) over a given period of time. A change greater than 2 times the TE means that there is a high probability that this response is a true physiological adaptation rather than a technical and/or biological variability. Therefore, non-response to exercise intervention was defined as a failure to demonstrate a decrease of HOMA-IR (levels at 12-week against those at 0-week) that was greater than 2-fold TE from zero.

Excerpted from Cell Metabolism, Volume 31, Issue 1, Yan Liu, Yao Wang, Yueqiong Ni, Cynthia K. Y. Cheung, Karen S. L. Lam, Yu Wang, Zhengyuan Xia, Dewei Ye, Jiao Guo, Michael Andrew Tse, Gianni Panagiotou, and Aimin Xu, Gut Microbiome Fermentation Determines the Efficacy of Exercise for Diabetes Prevention, Pages 77–91.E5. Copyright 2020, with permission from Elsevier.

Fecal Microbial Transplantation in Mice

500 mg of fresh stools obtained from donors before and after 12-week exercise intervention were suspended in 5 mL of PBS buffer containing 0.5 g/L cysteine as reducing agent. Two donors from exercise responders and non-responders respectively were randomly selected from each subgroup to perform fecal microbial transplantation. Fecal slurry from each donor was transferred into 3 conventional antibiotics-treated mice. Mice were randomized to receive fecal slurry from the same responder donors or non-responder donors collected at both baseline and after exercise training. Mice receiving FMT from responders after exercise with sterile tap water and mice receiving sterile PBS were included as controls. All the mice were fed with high fat diet (40% kcal fat) for 6 weeks to induce obesity before and during the 4-week period of colonization.

JOURNAL ARTICLE EXERCISE 1

The science sections on the MCAT include a significant number of passages with experiments. Questions for these passages often ask you to analyze data, read charts and graphs, and come to some reasonable conclusion based on the information they give you. If you don't know how to extract information efficiently and analyze data effectively, you will be at a distinct disadvantage.

There are three "Journal Article Exercises" in this book. In this first exercise, we'll show you the type of information you should be able to extract from the article and the sorts of things to pay attention to in the data. In subsequent exercises, you'll do more of that on your own, and in the final exercise we'll show you how that article might get turned into an MCAT-style passage.

When analyzing an experiment, you should be able to:

- identify the control group(s)
- extract information from graphs and data tables
- determine how the experimental group(s) change relative to the control
- determine if the results are statistically significant
- come to a reasonable conclusion about WHY the results were observed
- consider potential weaknesses in the study
- determine how to increase the power of the study
- decide what the next most logical experiment or study should be

The goal of these exercises is NOT to learn content from the articles, just to get a little more comfortable reading and extracting information from them.

For the (abridged) article on pages 219–226, try to summarize the purpose of the experiment and the methods in 4–5 sentences. Consider the following mnemonic: Oh ouR Car Won't Start (ORCWS).

- O = Organism and Organization: Is the research being conducted on humans or on animals or on bacteria in a petri dish, or something else? What is being done to these organisms? Are there any unique qualities to these organisms? Are there multiple groups? Is the study conducted over a long period of time with multiple data points, or is it a short-term study? Does it have a large or small n?
- R = Results: Where and how are the results presented? Is it a graph? A data table? Figures and images? What is/are the independent variable(s)? What is/are the dependent variable(s)? What are the results? Do the results show correlation or cause and effect, or both? Describe.
- C = Control and Comparison: Is there a control group? How does it differ from the experimental group? Is it given a placebo or nothing at all? Is it held under different conditions? If there are multiple experimental groups, how do they differ from one another? Is it a blinded study? If so, double blind or single blind?
- W = Weirdness: Does anything or do any of the results stand out as unexpected?
- S = Statistics: Was any sort of statistical analysis done? How is it presented? Are there error bars on a graph? Standard errors around a mean? Are there p-values? Is there an asterisk indicating statistical significance? Is there any data that is not statistically significant?

Try interpreting the data on your own before reading the results/discussion section. When you do read the discussion, consider:

- What are the conclusions of the study?
- How are the conclusions supported by the data?
- What potential weaknesses or flaws do you see in the experimental design? Are these addressed in the discussion section?
- How might this study be potentially biased?
- How might this study be improved?
- What would be the next most logical experiment?

Let's answer the above questions for the article on pages 219–226.

SOLUTIONS TO JOURNAL ARTICLE EXERCISE 1

1. O = Organism and Organization:
   - Is the research being conducted on humans or on animals or on bacteria in a petri dish, or something else? *Humans.*
   - What is being done to these organisms? *They are subjected to 12 weeks of exercise and gut microbiome assessed.*
   - Are there any unique qualities to these organisms? *All volunteers were diabetic men, no medication.*
   - Are there multiple groups? *Not initially, but they were ultimately divided into two groups.*
   - Is the study conducted over a long period of time with multiple data points, or is it a short-term study? *Long time (12 weeks) with multiple data points over that 12-week period.*
   - Does it have a large or small *n*? *Small n: 39 total subjects, 19 control, 20 experimental (6 non-responders and 14 responders).*

2. R = Results:
   - Where and how are the results presented? Is it a graph? A data table? Figures and images? *Graphs and data tables.*
   - What is/are the independent variable(s)? *Time and exercise regimen, gut microbes.*
   - What is/are the dependent variable(s)? *Body weight, fat mass, lean mass, fasting glucose, fasting insulin, insulin resistance.*
   - What are the results of the study? *As a whole, the exercise group showed reduction in body weight, fat mass, lean mass, fasting glucose, fasting insulin, and insulin resistance compared to controls. Within that group there were significant differences in fasting insulin and insulin resistance in "responders" and "nonresponders." There were also significant differences in gut microbiomes between responders and nonresponders. Obese mice transplanted with fecal samples from responders showed similar microbiomes and results as responders, whereas mice transplanted with fecal samples from nonresponders did not show these results.*
   - Do the results show correlation or cause and effect, or both? Describe. *Both. Correlation: exercise responders show gut microbe populations similar to that of professional athletes and different from those of sedentary controls; exercise non-responders show gut microbe populations similar to sedentary controls. Cause and effect: fecal transplant of responder gut microbes into obese mice result in the same types of changes in mice as seen in the humans.*

3. C = Control and Comparison:
   - Is there a control group? *Yes.*
   - How does it differ from the experimental group? Is it given a placebo or nothing at all? Is it held under different conditions? *Control group did not participate in the exercise regimen.*
   - If there are multiple experimental groups, how do they differ from one another? *Only one experimental group.*
   - Is it a blinded study? If so, double blind or single blind? *Not a blinded study.*

4. W = Weirdness:
   - Does anything or do any of the results stand out as unexpected? *I found the fact that some people responded differently to exercise unexpected.*

5. S = Statistics:
   - Was any sort of statistical analysis done? *Yes.*
   - How is it presented? Are there error bars on a graph? Standard errors around a mean? Are there *p*-values? Is there an asterisk indicating statistical significance? *P-values, error bars, asterisks.*
   - Is there any data that is not statistically significant? *Yes, initial characteristics of the responders and non-responders (weight, age, etc.) are not statistically different. Changes in body weight, fat mass, lean mass, and fasting glucose are not statistically significant.*

6. Interpreting the data:
   - What are the conclusions of the study? *Some individuals respond better to exercise (in terms of insulin levels and sensitivity) than others, and this is likely due to differences in their gut microbiomes.*
   - How are the conclusions supported by the data? *Data on fasting insulin and insulin resistance show significant differences between responders and nonresponders. These two groups also show significant differences in the makeup of their gut bacteria. Transplantation of fecal bacteria from responders into obese mice produced similar changes.*
   - What potential weaknesses or flaws do you see in the experimental design? Are these addressed in the discussion section? *Small, very select group of subjects. Maybe dietary intake. The small sample size was discussed.*
   - How might this study be potentially biased? *Sample bias: it was only conducted on Chinese males.*
   - How might this study be improved? *Bigger sample size, more diversity in subjects, include women.*
   - What would be the next most logical experiment? *Repeat the exercise intervention using different groups (women, non-Chinese origin).*

7. Final Summary of Experiment and Results:
   - *In this study a group of approximately 40 overweight diabetic Chinese men were divided into two groups, one sedentary control group and one exercise experimental group. Some of the exercisers showed significant changes in insulin sensitivity and other markers associated with a reduction in diabetic symptoms (called responders), and some of them did not (called nonresponders). The gut microbes of the responders were significantly different than those of the nonresponders, and matched the gut microbes of professional athletes. Transplantation of responder microbes into obese mice produced similar changes in insulin sensitivity and other markers.*

Chapter 7
Genetics and Evolution

The nature of the fundamental unit of inheritance, the gene, has been agreed upon by scientists only since the mid-nineteenth century. Aristotle believed that traits were passed on in the form of "pangenes," particles derived from all parts of the body and distilled into eggs and sperm. In the seventeenth century, different theorists believed that all genetic information was passed by either the father or the mother. Finally, early in the nineteenth century, people began to see that characteristics are passed from both parents; this led to the idea that parental characteristics were evenly mixed in offspring, in a process termed "blending." The notion that some characteristics were inherited in an either-or fashion, while others were in fact blended, remained unconceived.

The proponents of these early theories cannot be faulted for their lack of electron microscopes and other modern tools and techniques. But one is tempted to criticize their ideas for their obvious irrelevance to reality. One didn't need a Cray supercomputer to figure out that both parents contributed to a child's makeup. Why did researchers fail to arrive at this seemingly obvious hypothesis? Probably for two reasons: methods and dogma.

First, their approach to discovery was not empirical, but rather *a priori*. They believed knowledge could be derived by speculation alone, and that to perform experiments in the physical world was to dirty one's hands. And second, the prevailing religious dogma strongly censored empirical exploration, since it threatened the metaphysical tenets of the church.

What is different today is the approach to discovery known as the scientific method. Modern scientists know that only through careful, sober consideration of a question, formulation of a tentative answer, and testing of that hypothesis can new knowledge be uncovered. In this chapter, we will examine what is now considered to be the truth about genetics and evolution, all the way back to the origin of life.

We challenge you to attack this knowledge in the way its discoverers did. This is difficult material. Spend time thinking about the in-text questions before reading the answers. If you have trouble with a topic, stop and take out a fresh piece of paper. Write down all the facets of your current understanding, and look for internal inconsistencies and fallacies. Make up your own Punnett squares, pedigrees, and sketches of chromosomes during meiosis if the ones we present aren't sufficient. And finally, as you review, ask yourself which of the modern "truths" will one day be looked back on as preposterous ponderings of blindfolded pseudo-scientists.

7.1 INTRODUCTION TO GENETICS

Genetics is the science that describes the inheritance of traits from one generation to another. At the origin of genetics, patterns of inheritance were observed to follow certain predictable patterns, as described by Mendel's laws. The reasons for these patterns of inheritance were to remain a mystery until the nature of DNA as the genetic material was known. Today we can use our knowledge of DNA and the cell to understand Mendel's laws at the molecular level.

DNA as the Genetic Information of the Cell

Gregor Mendel described the basic principles of heredity (see Section 7.3), but not the molecular foundations. It wasn't until years later that DNA was shown to be the building block of cellular genetics. Mitosis and meiosis were actively studied in the late nineteenth century, and this paved the way for the chromosome theory of inheritance, which indicated that genes are located on chromosomes. Thomas Hunt Morgan associated a specific gene and its subsequent phenotype (eye color in the fruit fly) with a specific chromosome (the X chromosome). However, chromosomes are composed of both DNA and protein. It wasn't until an important series of experiments, which started in the 1920s, that DNA was accepted as the genetic material of the cell.

First, Frederick Griffith showed that cell extracts can transform bacteria, indicating biological macromolecules carry hereditary information. This work made use of two strains of *Streptococcus pneumoniae*. One strain is lethal in mice and is characterized by a smooth (S) appearance under the microscope due to the presence of a polysaccharide capsule. The other strain is less virulent and does not kill mice. It lacks the capsule and so has a rough (R) appearance under the microscope. When heat-killed S bacteria were injected into mice, the animals survived. However, when heat-killed S strain was mixed with live R strain and then injected together, the mice died. This suggested that the cell extract of dead S strain was capable of conferring virulence to the R strain. In addition, it was found that live S strain *S. pneumoniae* could be isolated from the dead mice (Figure 1).

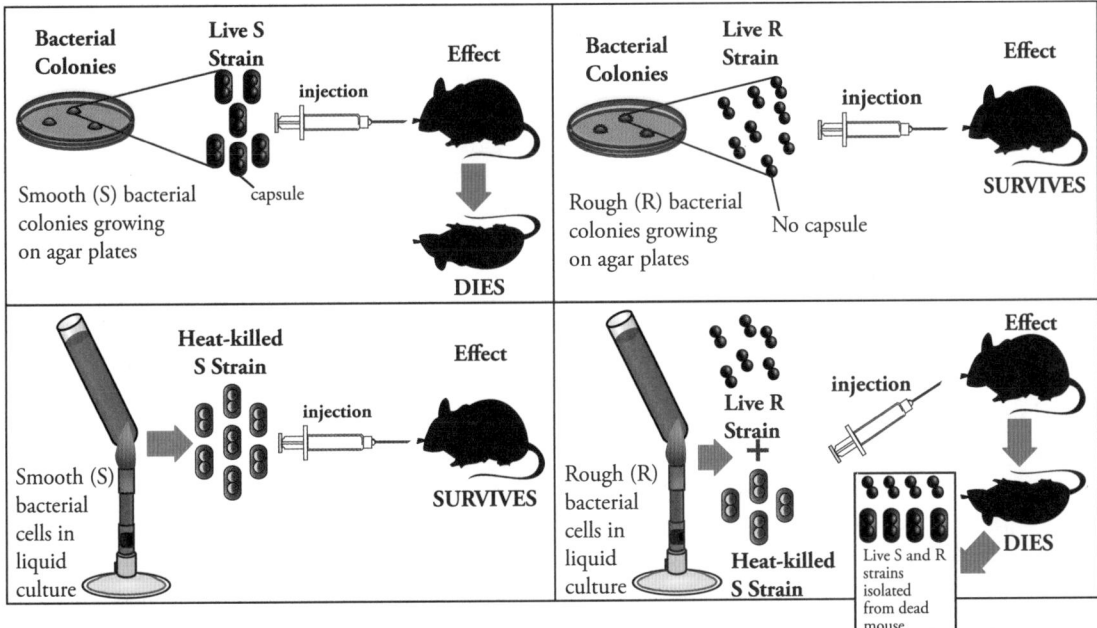

Figure 1 The Griffith Experiment

However, it still wasn't clear how the R strain was obtaining virulence. To figure this out, Oswald Avery, Colin MacLeod, and Maclyn McCarty systematically and chemically destroyed each biological macromolecule in the extracts from dead S strain *S. pneumoniae*. These treated extracts were then injected into mice with live R strain. Since the two strains were phenotypically different because of a polysaccharide coat, an obvious hypothesis was that virulence was being transferred via a polysaccharide. However, when polysaccharides were destroyed, virulence was still transferred from the dead S bacteria to the live R bacteria. Indeed, this was the case for all macromolecules save one: DNA (Figure 2). When DNase was added to S strain extracts, virulence was not conferred to the R strain. This suggested that DNA was able to transform bacteria, and was the molecule of heritability that scientists had been looking for.

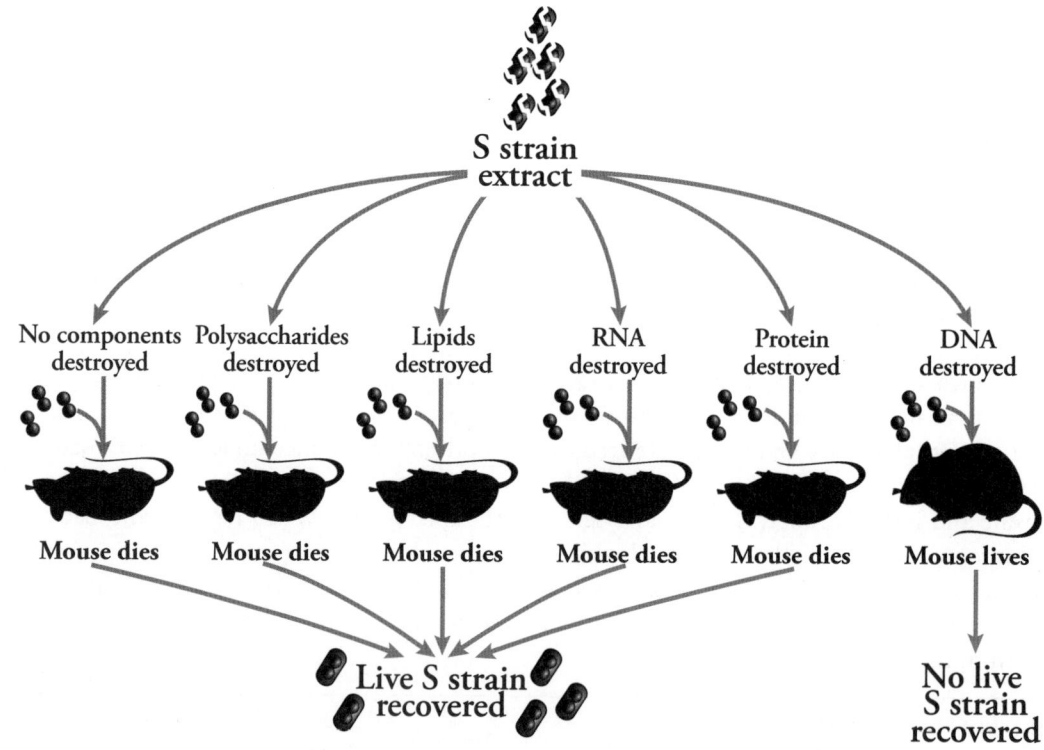

Figure 2   The Avery-MacLeod-McCarty Experiment

Still, there were scientists who didn't believe DNA contained cellular genetic information. How could a molecule with only four monomers (A, C, G and T) be the basis of such extensive genetic diversity? Wouldn't proteins (with twenty amino acid monomer building blocks) be more suited to this job?

Definitive experiments were done by Alfred Hershey and Martha Chase. The model organism here was the phage T2, a virus that infects bacteria. Hershey and Chase grew two parallel cultures of phages in bacterial hosts. One contained ^{32}P, a radioactive isotope of phosphorus. Phages made in this culture contained radioactively labeled DNA, since DNA contains phosphorus in backbone phosphate groups. The second culture contained ^{35}S, a radioactive isotope of sulphur. In this culture, phages with radioactive protein capsids were made (since amino acids such as methionine and cysteine contain sulphur atoms). The two labeled phage samples were then used to infect new cultures of unlabeled bacteria. Later, the cultures were centrifuged (spun at high speeds); this caused the bacterial cells to settle into a pellet at the bottom of the tube. The liquid layer (called the supernatant) contained growth media and phage ghosts (capsid particles without internal nucleic acids). Hershey and Chase found that for phages grown in ^{32}P, the radioactive label was transferred to bacteria host cells in the pellet. This confirmed that DNA was being transferred and was therefore the hereditary material. ^{35}S was not transferred to the bacterial cells, indicating that capsid proteins remained outside the host cell (in the supernatant) and therefore do not contribute to heritability.

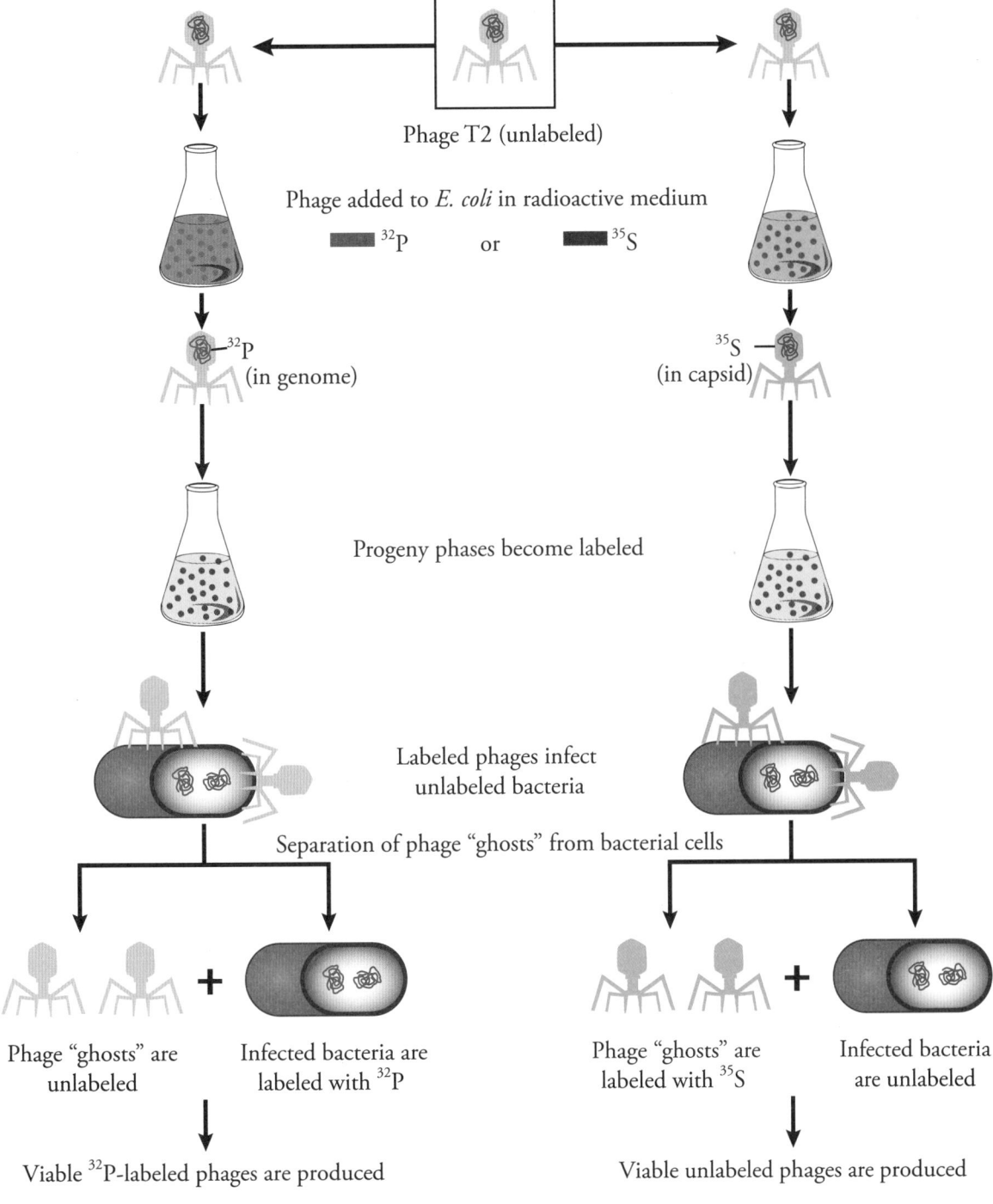

Figure 3 The Hershey-Chase Experiment

In addition to these three seminal projects, some additional evidence supports the fact that DNA carries genetic information of the cell:

- The total amount of DNA in a given cell (and species) is constant, and work by Erwin Chargaff suggested that each species has a consistent make-up of DNA; human DNA for example is 30.9% adenine, 29.4% thymine, 19.9% guanine, and 19.8% cytosine.
- Matthew Meselson and Franklin Stahl showed that DNA replication is semiconservative; cellular DNA is copied during each cell cycle, and is therefore self-perpetuating and consistent (see Chapter 4).
- In quiescent (resting) cells, macromolecules such as carbohydrates and proteins have a relatively short half-life and are constantly recycled and replaced. DNA is not broken down.
- Studies involving mutagens showed that DNA-altering chemicals induce phenotypic mutations, as do wavelengths of light that are absorbed by DNA.

Genes and Alleles

One of the basic tenets of genetics is that children inherit traits from both parents. Humans have a life cycle in which life begins with a diploid cell, the zygote. Diploid organisms (or cells) have two copies of the genome in each cell, while haploid cells have one copy of the genome. In sexual reproduction, the diploid zygote is produced by fusion of two haploid gametes: a haploid ovum from the mother and a haploid spermatozoon from the father. The zygote then goes through many mitotic divisions to develop into an adult, with half of the genetic material in each cell from each parent. The adult, male or female, produces haploid gametes by meiotic cell division to repeat the life cycle once again.

The development of a zygote into an adult and the maintenance of adult cells and tissues requires many thousands of different gene products. All of these gene products are encoded in the genome and inherited from mother and father. The **gene**, a length of DNA coding for a particular gene product, is the fundamental unit of inheritance. [Are gene products always proteins?[1]] The genes are distributed among the chromosomes that compose the genome, and every gene can be pinpointed to a specific location called the **locus** (plural: **loci**) on a specific chromosome. [Can all physical traits of an organism be mapped to a single locus?[2]]

The human genome is split into 24 different chromosomes: 22 of these are autosomes (non-sex chromosomes) and 2 are sex chromosomes (or allosomes, X and Y). Each human has 23 pairs of chromosomes (22 autosomes and a sex chromosome), for a total of 46 chromosomes. One chromosome of each pair is from the mother and one is from the father. The two nonidentical copies of a chromosome are called **homologous chromosomes**. Although these two copies look the same when examined at the crudest level under a microscope, and although they contain the same genes, the copies of the genes in the two homologous chromosomes may differ in their DNA sequence. Different versions of a gene, called **alleles**, may carry out the gene's function differently. Since a person carries two copies of every gene, one on each homologous chromosome, a person could potentially carry two different alleles. Individuals carrying

---

[1] No. tRNA and rRNA genes, as well as other small nuclear RNA genes, do not encode polypeptides.

[2] No. Every gene is located at a specific locus, but physical traits, particularly complex traits, like weight or height, can be controlled by many different genes and therefore do not map to a single locus, but to many.

different alleles of a gene will often have traits that allow the inheritance of alleles to be followed. [Is it possible for there to be more than two different alleles of a specific gene?[3]]

- Which one of the following is true if an individual has two different alleles at a given locus?[4]
  A) The individual has two phenotypes, e.g., one brown eye and one blue.
  B) There are two alleles in one place on one particular chromosome.
  C) Two siblings have different appearances.
  D) There is a different allele on each of the two members of a homologous pair.

Genotype vs. Phenotype

The **genotype** is the DNA sequence of the alleles a person carries. A person carrying two different alleles at a given locus is called a **heterozygote**, while an individual carrying two identical alleles is called a **homozygote**. The expression of alleles often is different in heterozygotes and homozygotes.

The **phenotype** is the physical expression of the genotype. For example, the phenotype of a gene involved in hair color may be brown or blond. Since there are many different kinds of alleles, there are different ways these alleles can be expressed in the phenotype. If an allele is the one expressed in the phenotype, regardless of what the second allele carried is, the expressed allele is referred to as **dominant**. An allele that is not expressed in the heterozygous state is referred to as **recessive**. For example, consider a heterozygous organism in which one allele encodes the functional version of an enzyme, while the second allele encodes an inactive version of that enzyme. Upon observation, it is noted that the organism's enzymes are all functional; then the functional-enzyme allele is *dominant* and the inactive-enzyme allele is *recessive*. Since recessive alleles are not expressed in heterozygotes, it is not always possible to tell the genotype of an individual based solely on the phenotype. [Can a haploid organism like an adult fungus have recessive alleles?[5]]

There are certain conventions used in denoting genotypes in genetics that are useful to know. The alleles of a gene are usually denoted by letters. For example, for a gene called "curly," a dominant allele may be denoted by the capital letter *C* and a recessive allele may be denoted by the lower case letter *c*. A heterozygote is referred to as *Cc*, while homozygotes would be either *CC* or *cc*. More complex situations require more complex conventions, but most questions probably only involve two alleles at a locus. [If the dominant allele for curly (*C*) results in curly hair and the recessive allele (*c*) causes straight hair, what are the phenotypes of *CC*, *Cc* and *cc* individuals?[6]]

---

[3] Yes, there can be many versions (alleles) of a particular gene. Under normal circumstances, however, one individual cannot have more than two of those different alleles, since they have only two copies of a gene (one on each homologous chromosome). An exception is when an individual is polyploid for a certain chromosome (i.e., they have more than two homologous chromosomes, for example, in Down syndrome and Klinefelter syndrome).

[4] An individual with two different alleles at a given locus has one allele on one chromosome and the other allele on its homologous partner (so choice **D** is correct and choice B is not possible). While choice A may be possible, it is an exceedingly complex phenomenon and not discernible from the information given. The question discusses a single individual, not a pair of siblings (eliminating choice C).

[5] No. If there is only one copy of a gene, then that is the copy which determines the phenotype.

[6] *CC* and *Cc* individuals have curly hair, and *cc* individuals have straight hair. Only homozygous recessive individuals express recessive traits. In the heterozygote, the presence of the recessive allele is masked by the dominant allele, so there are only two different phenotypes, although there are three different genotypes. This type of interaction between alleles is called **classical dominance**.

7.2 MEIOSIS

Mitotic cell division produces two daughter cells that are identical to the parent. However, the production of haploid cells such as gametes from a diploid cell requires a type of cell division that reduces the number of copies of each chromosome from two to one; this method of cell division is called **meiosis**. In males, meiosis occurs in the testes with haploid spermatozoa as the end result; in females, meiosis in the ovaries produces ova. (*Note*: This is not always the case, and while meiosis begins in the ovaries, it is completed only after fertilization; see Chapter 13 for a further discussion on oogenesis.) Specialized cells termed **spermatogonia** in males and **oogonia** in females undergo meiosis. Spermatogenesis and oogenesis share the same basic features of meiosis but differ in many of the specific features of gamete production. Meiosis itself will be discussed in this chapter, while the specifics of spermatogenesis and oogenesis will be discussed in Chapter 13.

Mitosis and meiosis are similar in many respects. Mitosis and meiosis are both preceded by one round of replication of the genome (S phase), leaving a diploid cell with four copies of the genome (Figure 4). The different phases in cell division are referred to by the same names (prophase, metaphase, anaphase, and telophase) in both meiosis and mitosis and are mechanistically very similar. The primary difference between meiosis and mitosis is that replication of the genome is followed by one round of cell division in mitosis and two rounds of cell division in meiosis, **meiosis I** and **meiosis II** (Figure 5). Another important difference is that in meiosis, recombination occurs between homologous chromosomes.

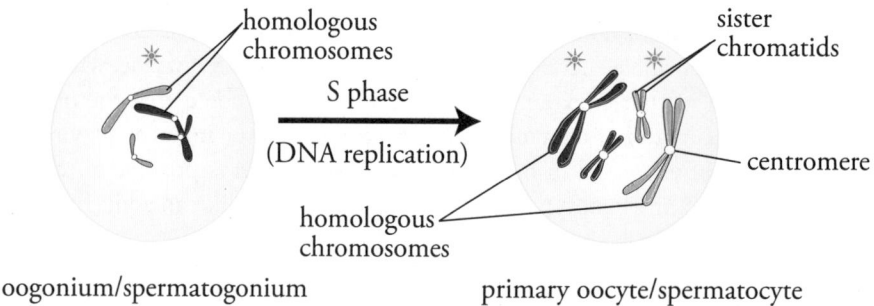

Figure 4 S Phase

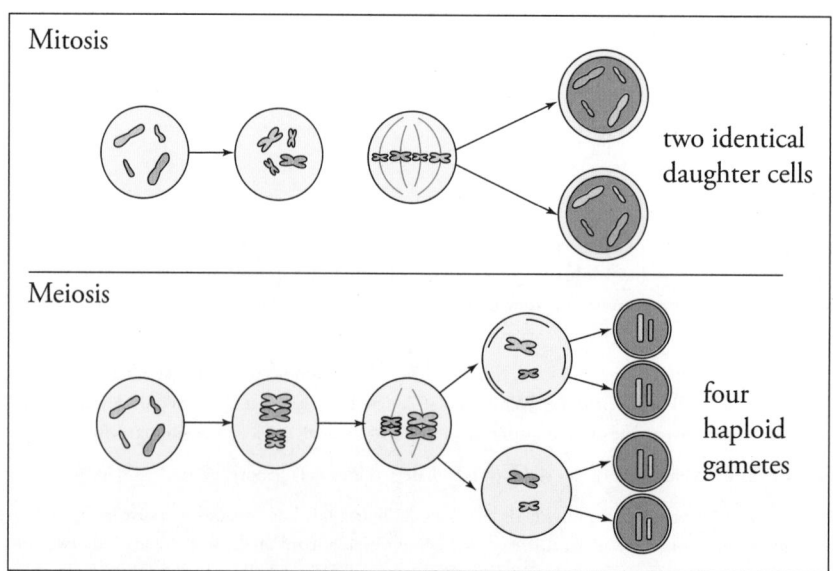

Figure 5 Mitosis vs. Meiosis

The first step in meiosis is **prophase I** (Figure 6). To depict meiosis, we will use a hypothetical model organism with a diploid genome with two different (nonhomologous) chromosomes (Figures 6–10).

- How many chromosomes are present in a cell from this organism during prophase I of meiosis?[7]

As in mitotic prophase, chromosomes condense in meiotic prophase I, and then the nuclear envelope breaks down. Unlike mitosis, however, homologous chromosomes pair with each other during meiotic prophase I in **synapsis**. Homologous chromosomes align themselves very precisely with each other in synapsis, with the two copies of each gene on two different chromosomes brought closely together. The paired homologous chromosomes are called a **bivalent** or **tetrad**.

When the DNA is aligned properly, it can then be cut precisely at the same location on homologous chromosomes. Genes are then swapped between the pair, and the chromosomes are religated (Figure 6). This process is known as **crossing over** or **recombination** (Figure 7, next page). Due to the extreme complexity of crossing over, meiotic prophase takes the most time in meiosis, days sometimes. Recombination during meiosis is an important source of genetic variation during sexual reproduction.

- Does crossing over change the number of genes on a chromosome?[8]
- Does recombination create combinations of alleles on a chromosome that are not found in the parent?[9]

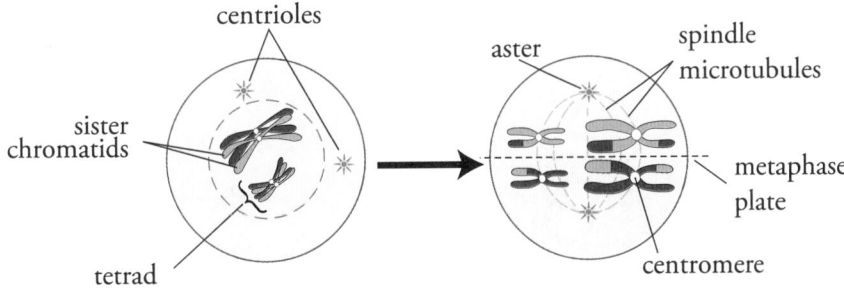

Figure 6   Prophase I and Metaphase I

---

[7]   The organism is diploid normally, with two copies of two chromosomes, or four chromosomes total. After DNA synthesis, during prophase I, the cell still has four chromosomes; however, the chromosomes are replicated and held together at the centromere. Thus, each chromosome consists of two sister chromatids, and the cell has a total of eight sister chromatids.

[8]   Not if it is done correctly. Error-free recombination involves a one-for-one swap of DNA between homologous chromosomes.

[9]   Yes. Although each chromosome contains the same genes after crossing over, it may contain different alleles of some genes that were not present on the same chromosome previously.

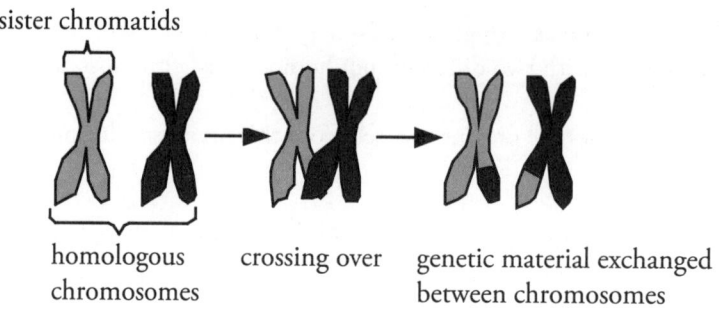

sister chromatids

homologous chromosomes   crossing over   genetic material exchanged between chromosomes

Figure 7   Crossing Over (Recombination)

Since precision is crucial in chromosome swapping, formation of the tetrad is highly regulated. Synapsis is mediated by a protein structure called the **synaptonemal complex** (SC). This structure starts to form early in meiotic prophase I. First, proteins named SYCP2 and SYCP3 attach to each of the two homologous chromatin structures that are to be paired (Figure 8). This makes up the lateral elements of the SC. The lateral regions then align and attach via a central region (made of SYCP1 and many other proteins). Both the lateral and central regions together form the SC, and essentially work like a zipper to connect homologous chromosomes.

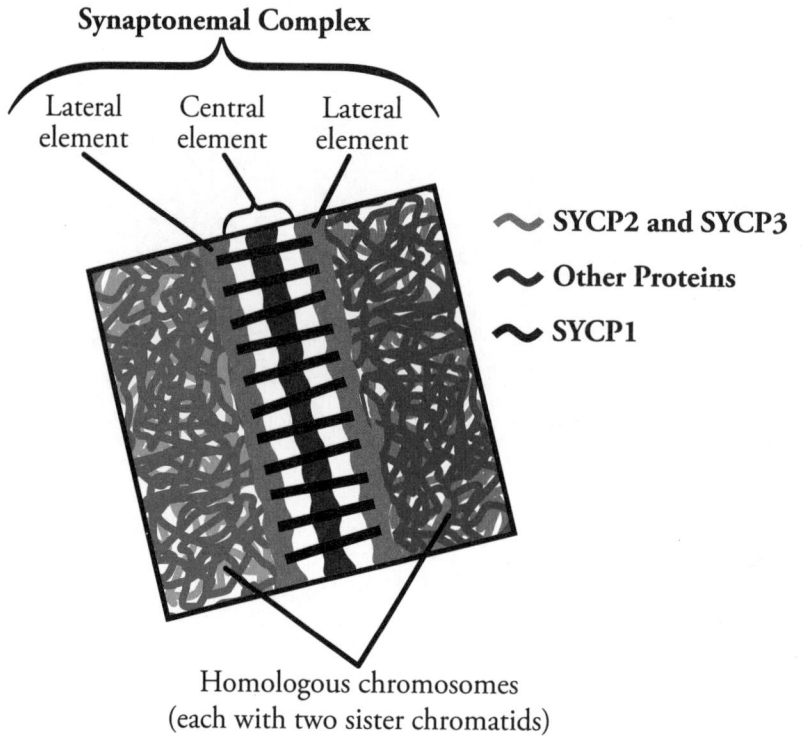

Synaptonemal Complex

Lateral element   Central element   Lateral element

∿ **SYCP2 and SYCP3**
∿ **Other Proteins**
∿ **SYCP1**

Homologous chromosomes
(each with two sister chromatids)

Figure 8   The Synaptonemal Complex

While no physical connection has yet been shown between the synaptonemal complex and recombination machinery, it's been demonstrated that SC formation and recombination are interdependent. Both happen around the same time of meiosis, and work on mice with defective synaptonemal complex formation or recombination shows that these two processes rely on one another. When synaptonemal complex formation is inhibited, recombination is disturbed, and vice versa.

After prophase I is **metaphase I**. In meiotic metaphase I, alignment along the metaphase plate occurs, as in mitosis. The difference is that in meiotic metaphase I, the *tetrads* are aligned at the center of the cell (the metaphase plate), whereas in mitosis, *sister chromatids* are aligned on the metaphase plate. In **anaphase I**, homologous chromosomes separate, and sister chromatids remain together (Figure 9). The cell then divides into two cells during **telophase I** (Figure 10). *It is important to note that at this point the cells are considered to be haploid.* Each cell has a single set of chromosomes. The chromosomes, however, are still replicated (still exist as a pair of sister chromatids). The whole point to the second set of meiotic divisions is to separate the sister chromatids so that each cell has a single set of unreplicated chromosomes.

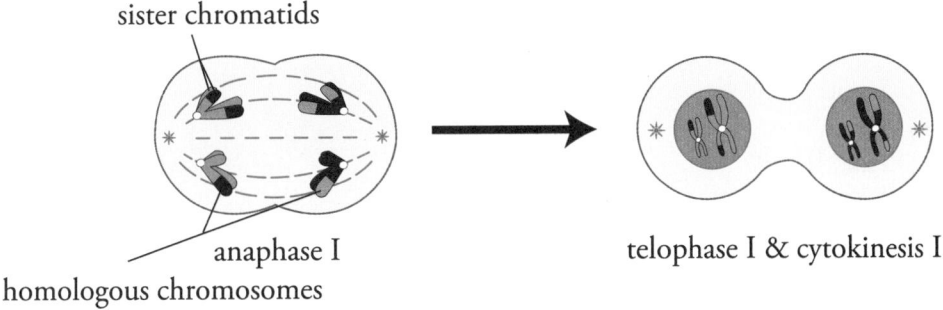

Figure 9   Anaphase I, Telophase I, and Cytokinesis I

In some species, meiosis II begins immediately after telophase I, while in other species there is a period of time before meiosis II begins. In either case, there is no further replication of the DNA before the second set of divisions. The movements of the chromosomes during meiosis II are identical to the movements in mitosis, with the sole difference being that in meiosis II there is a haploid number of chromosomes, while in mitosis there is a diploid number. The sister chromatids are separated during anaphase II, and after telophase II is complete, four haploid cells have been produced from a single diploid parent cell (Figure 10).

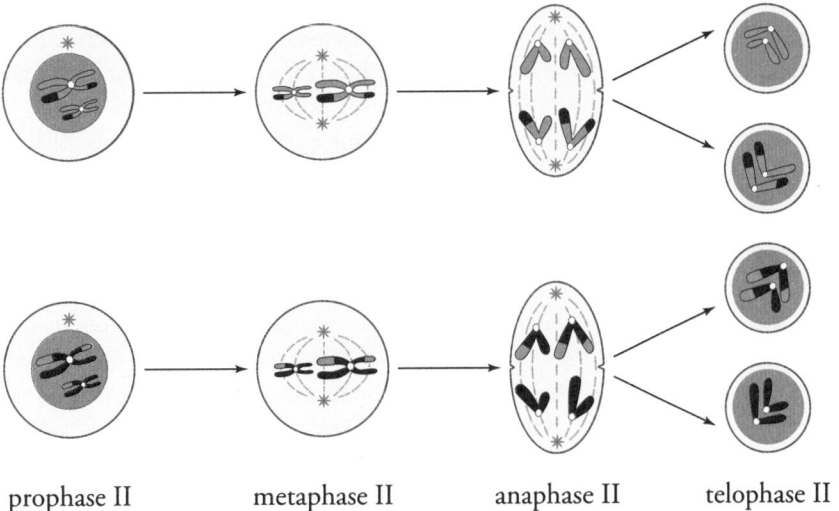

Figure 10   Meiosis II

- When homologous chromosomes separate, do all paternal and maternal chromosomes stay together in the daughter cells?[10]

- Are the sister chromatids that separate during meiotic anaphase II identical in their DNA sequence?[11]

- Which of the following occur in meiosis but NOT in mitosis?[12]
    I.   Separation of sister chromatids on microtubules
    II. Pairing of homologous chromosomes
    III. Recombination between sister chromatids

    A) I only
    B) II only
    C) I and II
    D) II and III

- If cells are blocked in meiotic metaphase II and prevented from moving on in meiosis, which one of the following will be prevented?[13]
    A) Crossing over
    B) Separation of homologous chromosomes
    C) Separation of sister chromatids
    D) Breakdown of the nuclear envelope

Nondisjunction

Sometimes during meiosis I homologous chromosomes fail to separate, and sometimes during meiosis II sister chromatids fail to separate. Such a failure of chromosomes to separate correctly during meiosis is called **nondisjunction**. [A gamete normally contains how many copies of each chromosome?[14] If two homologous chromosomes of chromosome #12 fail to separate during meiosis I, how many copies of chromosome #12 will the resulting gametes have?[15]] Gametes resulting from nondisjunction will have

---

[10] No. Homologous chromosomes separate (segregate) randomly. This is one aspect of meiosis that increases genetic variation during sexual reproduction.

[11] The sister chromatids *would* be identical, except that recombination with homologous chromosomes occurred earlier in meiosis, during prophase I, altering the sister chromatids.

[12] Item I is false: the spindle separates sister chromatids during both (choices A and C can be eliminated). Note that both remaining answer choices include Item II, so Item II must be true. **Item II is true**: only meiosis involves pairing and recombination between homologous chromosomes. Item III is false: meiotic recombination occurs between homologous chromosomes, not sister chromatids (choice D can be eliminated, and choice **B** is correct).

[13] Crossing over occurs during prophase I, separation of homologous chromosomes occurs during anaphase I, and nuclear envelope breakdown occurs during prophase I and sometimes prophase II (choices A, B, and D are false). Only separation of sister chromatids occurs after metaphase II, in anaphase II. Answer: **C**.

[14] Normal gametes have one copy of each chromosome; this is the definition of haploid.

[15] If the homologous chromosomes do not separate in meiosis I, then one daughter cell from this division will have four copies of this chromosome and the other cell will have none. In meiosis II, sister chromatids will separate, leaving two gametes with two copies of the chromosome and two gametes with no copies of the chromosome.

two copies or no copies of a given chromosome. Such a gamete can fuse with a normal gamete to create a zygote with either three copies of a chromosome (**trisomy**) or one copy of a chromosome (**monosomy**).

The genetic defect caused when an entire chromosome is either added or removed is usually so great that a zygote with either trisomy or monosomy cannot develop into a normal individual. There are examples in which nondisjunction is not lethal in humans, although it results in significant developmental abnormalities. Trisomy of chromosome #21 results in Down syndrome, with intellectual disability and abnormal growth. Nondisjunction of the sex chromosomes is also generally not lethal during development. Individuals who have only one X chromosome and no Y, for example, have Turner syndrome, with external female appearance but underdeveloped ovaries and sterility. Individuals with nondisjunction of the sex chromosomes will develop to have male appearance if they have at least one Y, no matter how many X chromosomes are present, and will have female genitalia if only X chromosomes are present. Most will be sterile, however, and many will suffer intellectual disability. [In an individual with Down syndrome, are the defects in development caused by an absence of genetic information?[16] If not, why does trisomy of this chromosome or other chromosomes have such dramatic effects?[17]]

7.3   MENDELIAN GENETICS

Gregor Mendel described the statistical behavior of the inheritance of traits in pea plants long before the nature of DNA and chromosomes was known. Unlike Mendel, however, we are now familiar with the molecular basis of genetics in meiosis and genes, and the laws of genetics that Mendel formulated can now be presented with insight based on this knowledge. Although Mendelian genetics generally only involves the simplest patterns of inheritance, it forms the foundation for understanding more complicated situations.

Mendel observed that traits were governed by pairs of hereditary material (alleles). The first of Mendel's laws, the **law of segregation**, states that the two alleles of an individual are separated and passed on to the next generation singly. [At what stage during meiosis are different alleles of a gene separated?[18]] Mendel's second law, the **law of independent assortment**, states that the alleles of one gene will separate into gametes independently of alleles for another gene. We will illustrate these principles using the garden pea plant, but the principles apply equally well to humans.

A trait that can be studied in the pea plant is the color of the pea. We can call *G* the allele for green color, while *g* is the allele for yellow pea color. Mating between plants, a **cross**, is used as a tool in genetics to discern genotypes by looking at the phenotypes of progeny from a cross. A **pure-breeding strain** of yellow or green peas consistently yields progeny of the same color when mated within the strain. For example, if mating yellow plants with yellow plants always produces yellow progeny, yellow is a pure-breeding

---

[16] There is no information missing in a person with trisomy. All of the chromosomes are present, and there is no reason to believe that any of the genes on these chromosomes are deleted or mutated to render them inactive.

[17] The problem with trisomy appears not to be that genetic information is missing, but that there is *too much* present. A mechanism involved might be gene dosage. Genes are regulated to produce the right amount of each gene product. In trisomy, many genes are present in one more copy than usual, resulting in greater quantities of the gene products encoded on this chromosome. The extra quantities of so many gene products, even if they are normal in sequence, can have dramatic consequences.

[18] During meiosis I, at the time when homologous chromosomes separate.

strain. [Can anything be deduced about the genotype of the pure-breeding strain of yellow peas?[19] If a pure-breeding yellow and pure-breeding green strain are crossed, and all of the progeny are green, what does this indicate about the expression of the yellow and green alleles?[20]] Let's assume that G is the dominant allele of the color gene, and g is the recessive allele. [Is it possible to deduce the genotype of a pea plant at the color gene if it is green?[21]] If a green plant is encountered, a **testcross** can be performed to deduce the genotype of the plant. A testcross is when one individual is crossed to another individual that has a homozygous (or pure-breeding) recessive genotype. The presence of all recessive alleles in one parent allows alleles from the other parent to be displayed phenotypically. The progeny of a testcross are called the F_1 **generation**. [If a green plant is testcrossed with a pure-breeding yellow strain, and some of the F_1 generation are yellow while others are green, what is the genotype of the original green plant?[22]] The results of a testcross are dependent on statistics and follow Mendel's laws.

The principle of segregation can be illustrated with the color gene described above for the pea. If a pea is heterozygous Gg, its gametes will contain either the G allele or the g allele, but never both. [If a gamete contained both G and g, what occurred during meiosis?[23]] The probability that a gamete in the heterozygote will contain one allele or the other is 50%, completely random. [Would the principle of segregation apply to a gene on the X chromosome in a woman?[24]] To illustrate the law of independent assortment, we need to introduce a second gene, one that controls the shape of the pea. W is the dominant allele, resulting in wrinkled peas, while w is the recessive allele, resulting in smooth peas in homozygous ww plants. According to the law of independent assortment, the genes for the color of peas and the shape of peas are passed from one generation to another independently. [If the color gene and the shape gene are right next to each other on a chromosome, will they display independent assortment?[25]] The nature of the shape gene in a given gamete does not depend on and is not influenced by the color gene, if independent assortment is true. [If an individual is heterozygous at the color gene, Gg, and heterozygous at the shape gene, Ww, what are the chances that a gamete containing the G allele will also contain the W allele?[26]]

The Punnett Square

It is possible to predict the results of a cross between two individuals using the laws of segregation and independent assortment. Determining the result can be complex, however, so a visual tool called the **Punnett square** is often employed to make the process simpler. Let's use a simple square first, with only one trait involved (Figure 11); we will then tackle a more complicated problem with two different traits (Figure 12, page 246).

---

[19] If a strain always produces the same trait when mated with itself, it is likely to be homozygous for the trait. The pure-breeding yellow pea is homozygous for the yellow allele g of the color gene.

[20] The two strains were both pure-breeding and could only produce gametes containing one type of allele. All of the progeny would be the Gg genotype. If all progeny are green, then the green allele is dominant and the yellow allele is recessive.

[21] No. A green plant could either be heterozygous Gg or homozygous GG.

[22] The original pea is heterozygous Gg.

[23] The gamete must be the result of nondisjunction.

[24] Yes. The principles are the same for human genes as for pea genes, as long as an organism is diploid and goes through sexual reproduction.

[25] No, they would not. They would display an important exception to independent assortment, linkage, which is discussed later.

[26] According to independent assortment, the segregation of one gene does not depend on segregation of another. The chances of a gamete containing the W allele are 50%, regardless of the identity of the color allele.

Possible gametes: Male (*Gg*)

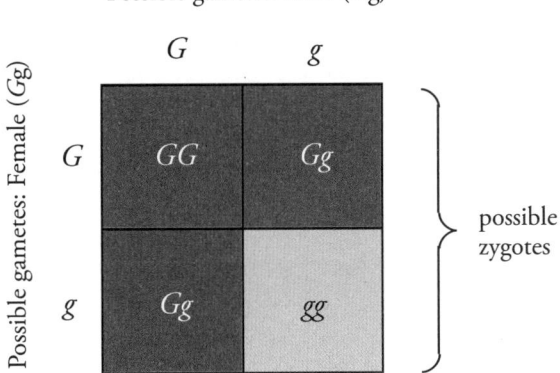

Figure 11   A Punnett Square Involving One Gene

In Figure 11, a Punnett square depicts a cross between two pea plants that are heterozygous for the color gene, with *G* the dominant green allele and *g* the recessive yellow allele. To draw a Punnett square, the following steps are involved:

Step 1: Determine the gametes that are possible from each parent in the cross.
Step 2: Draw a square with the possible gametes from each parent on two sides.
Step 3: Fill in the square with the zygote genotypes that would result from each possible combination of gamete.
Step 4: Determine the phenotype of each genotype.
Step 5: Find the probability of each genotype and each phenotype.

- In the situation shown in Figure 11, which one of the following will be true?[27]
  - A) 25% of the offspring will be green, and 75% will be yellow.
  - B) 50% of the offspring will be green, and 50% will be yellow.
  - C) 75% of the offspring will be green, and 25% will be yellow.
  - D) 100% of the offspring will be green.

A more complicated Punnett square is needed to look at two traits during a cross. In Figure 12, a cross is performed between Plant 1, heterozygous at the color gene (*Gg*), and Plant 2, also heterozygous at the color gene. Plant 1 is also homozygous for the dominant allele of the shape gene (wrinkled peas) while Plant 2 is homozygous for the recessive allele (smooth). [What are the phenotypes of the plants being crossed?[28]] The same steps are followed to construct the Punnett square in Figure 12 as the one in Figure 11. First, determine the possible gametes for each pea plant being crossed. (In this case, there are really two possible gamete types from each parent, so the box could be simplified to have only two gametes on a side). Then, determine the possible combinations of gametes that could join to form zygotes and the phenotypes and frequencies of the F$_1$ generation. [What percentage of the F$_1$ generation will have smooth

---

[27] If *G* (green allele) is dominant, then both *GG* homozygotes and *Gg* heterozygotes will be green, while only *gg* homozygotes will be yellow. 25% of the offspring in Figure 11 will be *GG* homozygotes, and 50% will be *Gg* heterozygotes, so a total of 75% of the offspring will be green (choice **C**).

[28] Plant 1 has green wrinkled peas, while Plant 2 has green smooth peas.

peas?[29] What percentage of peas will be green and wrinkled?[30] Yellow and wrinkled?[31] The cross depicted in Figure 12 was performed and produced 77 green wrinkled plants and 20 yellow wrinkled plants; why do these results not agree exactly with the ratios predicted in the Punnett square?[32]] Independent assortment and the principle of segregation are assumptions built into this Punnett square.

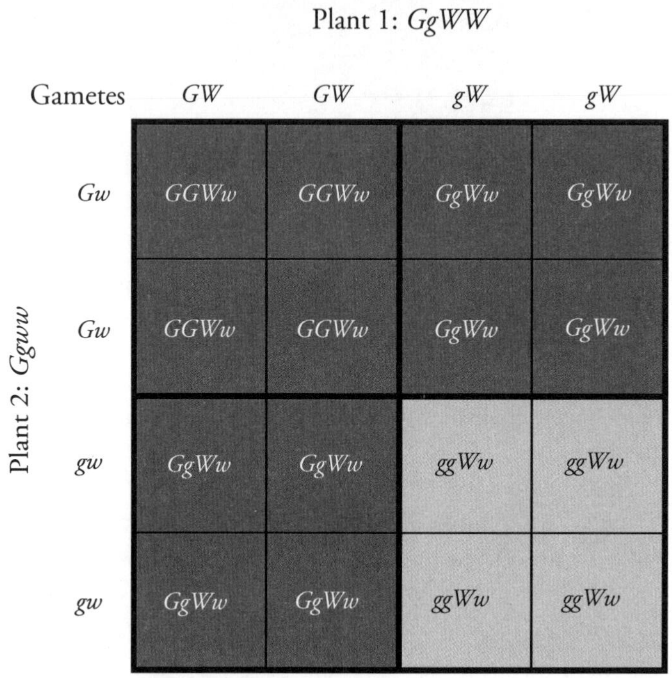

Plant 1: *GgWW*

Gametes	*GW*	*GW*	*gW*	*gW*
Gw	*GGWw*	*GGWw*	*GgWw*	*GgWw*
Gw	*GGWw*	*GGWw*	*GgWw*	*GgWw*
gw	*GgWw*	*GgWw*	*ggWw*	*ggWw*
gw	*GgWw*	*GgWw*	*ggWw*	*ggWw*

Plant 2: *Ggww*

Figure 12   A Punnett Square Depicting a Cross with Two Traits Involved

- In the cross depicted in Figure 12, how does the shape gene affect inheritance of the alleles for the color gene?[33]
  - A) The percentage of green peas is increased by the shape gene.
  - B) The shape gene has no effect on the inheritance of the alleles for the color gene.
  - C) The percentage of green peas is decreased by the shape gene.
  - D) The shape gene prevents segregation of the alleles for the color gene.

---

[29] All peas receive one *w* allele and one *W* allele, so all are wrinkled *Ww* heterozygotes (i.e., 0% are smooth).

[30] All F_1 peas are wrinkled and 75% are green, so 75% are green and wrinkled.

[31] All F_1 peas are wrinkled and 25% are yellow, so 25% are yellow and wrinkled.

[32] The results obtained in reality rarely agree exactly with the predicted result. If the results differ slightly from the prediction, the most likely explanation is statistical variability. The more progeny from the cross, the closer the result should be to the prediction.

[33] Independent assortment and the principle of segregation are inherent in the Punnett square. There is no reason to believe that these are not followed, making choice **B** the best response. Choices A, C, and D all assume that either independent assortment or segregation did not occur.

- If a green wrinkled plant from the F$_1$ generation in Figure 12 is crossed with a pure-breeding yellow smooth pea plant, what phenotypes are possible?[34]
- If any yellow smooth progeny are observed in this testcross, what does this indicate about the genotype of the F$_1$ plant?[35]

The Rules of Probability

Punnett squares are only one way to determine the probability of an outcome in a cross. Another way involves using statistical rules called the *rule of multiplication* and the *rule of addition*. The **rule of multiplication** states that the probability of both of two independent events happening can be found by multiplying the odds of either event alone. For example, if the probability of being struck by lightning is 1 in a million (10^{-6}) and the probability of winning the lottery is 10^{-7}, then the probability of both happening is the product: $10^{-6} \times 10^{-7} = 10^{-13}$.

The **rule of addition** can be used to calculate the chances of *either* of two events happening. The chance of either A or B happening is equal to the probability of A added to the probability of B, minus the probability of A and B occurring together. For example, the chance of either getting hit by lightning *or* winning the lottery is $10^{-6} + 10^{-7} = 1.1 \times 10^{-6}$. (*Note*: The product of 10^{-6} and 10^{-7} is so small that it can be neglected from the equation.) These rules can be a shortcut to using a Punnett square in some problems.

- A man that is homozygous for eye color, *bb*, is married to a woman who is heterozygous at the same gene: *Bb*. What are the chances that a child will have the *Bb* genotype and be a boy?[36]

Other Biostatistical Methods

Biologists use many other statistical methods in genetics, and many other areas. The chi-square test is used to compare observed and expected data, and *t*-tests are used to compare two data sets. Data is often summarized using mean, median and mode. Finally, standard deviation and standard error give an indication of how spread out a dataset is. Each of these is reviewed in an appendix of our *MCAT Physics and Math Review* book.

---

[34] There are two different genotypes possible for the green wrinkled phenotype in the F$_1$ generation: *GGWw* or *GgWw*. The best way to determine all possible phenotypes in the cross is to draw a Punnett square for both of these potential genotypes:

If the F$_1$ plant is *GGWw*:

	GW	GW	Gw	Gw
gw	GgWw	GgWw	Ggww	Ggww

Two genotypes are produced in equal ratios:
50% *GgWw* = green wrinkled phenotype
50% *Ggww* = green smooth

If the F$_1$ plant is *GgWw*:

	GW	Gw	gW	gw
gw	GgWw	Ggww	ggWw	ggww

Four genotypes are produced:
25% *GgWw* = green wrinkled phenotype
25% *Ggww* = green smooth
25% *ggWw* = yellow wrinkled
25% *ggww* = yellow smooth

[35] If yellow smooth progeny are observed, the F$_1$ plant must be *GgWw*.

[36] Without drawing a Punnett square, it is possible to see that all children must receive at least one *b* allele (from the father), and that 50% of the children will receive the *B* allele from the mother; thus, 50% of the children will be *Bb*. The odds of a boy are 50%. Therefore, the odds a child is both a boy and has the *Bb* genotype are, by the rule of multiplication, $0.5 \times 0.5 = 0.25$, or 25%.

7.4 EXTENDING MENDELIAN GENETICS

Mendel first started his work using mice, but abandoned rodents (either because of the mess involved, or because of the questionable ethics of a monk studying breeding schemes). In picking pea plants instead, he made a fortuitous decision. The traits he chose to study are (for the most part) controlled by a single gene with two alleles each. These two alleles have one completely dominant to the other, and therefore a simple relationship between genotype and phenotype. Although Mendel's peas all displayed very simple patterns of inheritance, the inheritance of traits is often more complicated.

Incomplete Dominance

Some alleles of genes display neither dominant nor recessive patterns of expression. If the phenotype of a heterozygote is a blended mix of both alleles, this is called **incomplete dominance**, and the alleles for that trait are given different, upper-case letters. For example, if a gene for flower color has two incompletely dominant alleles, R could be used to indicate the allele for red color and W to indicate the allele for white color. [If a gene for flower color has two alleles, R (red) and r (white), and R is dominant while r is recessive, what is the phenotype of Rr heterozygotes?[37] If R and W display incomplete dominance, what is the phenotype of RW heterozygotes?[38] How many phenotypes are possible if R and W display incomplete dominance?[39]]

Codominance

Codominance is a slightly different situation, in which two alleles are both expressed but are not blended. For example, the alleles of the gene for ABO blood group antigens that are found on the surface of red blood cells display codominance. Each of the alleles is expressed on red blood cells, regardless of the second allele in the cell. There are three alleles for the ABO blood group antigens: I^A, I^B, and i. The alleles I^A and I^B are codominant and will be expressed regardless of the second allele, while i is recessive to both I^A and I^B. The alleles I^A and I^B cause type A or type B antigens to be expressed, while i does not cause antigen expression.

- What is the phenotype of an individual heterozygous for the I^A and I^B alleles?[40]
- What is the phenotype of an individual heterozygous for I^B and i?[41]
- If a woman heterozygous for type A blood marries a man who is heterozygous for type B blood, what are the possible genotypes (and blood types) of their children?[42]

---

[37] Rr heterozygotes will have the phenotype of the dominant allele: red.

[38] In this case, RW heterozygotes will be neither red nor white, but a blend of the two: pink.

[39] Three phenotypes and three genotypes: RR (red), RW (pink), and WW (white).

[40] The red blood cells will express both type A and type B antigens, so the blood type will be AB.

[41] The red blood cells will express type B antigen only, and the blood type will be B.

[42] Because they are both heterozygous, the woman's genotype is $I^A i$ and the man's genotype is $I^B i$. Thus, their children could be $I^A I^B$ (type AB), $I^A i$ (type A), $I^B i$ (type B), or ii (type O).

The other main antigen used in blood typing is the Rh (rhesus) factor. The expression of this antigen follows a classically dominant pattern; $Rh^D Rh^D$ and $Rh^D Rh^d$ (also seen as *RR* and *Rr*) genotypes lead to the expression of this protein on the surface of the red cell (Rh positive), and the $Rh^d Rh^d$ (or *rr*) genotype leads to the absence of the protein (Rh negative).

Although Mendel's peas all displayed very simple patterns of inheritance, there are often many complications in the inheritance of traits. For example:

Pleiotropism: A gene is said to have pleiotropic effects if its expression alters many different, seemingly unrelated aspects of the organism's total phenotype. For example, a mutation in a gene may cause altered development of heart, bone, and inner ears.

Polygenism: Complex traits that are influenced by many different genes are called polygenic. These traits tend to display a range of phenotypes in a continuous distribution. For example, height is polygenic and is influenced by genes for growth factors, receptors, hormones, bone deposition, muscle development, energy utilization, and so on. As a consequence, there is a wide range of normal heights for adult humans; we are not just "tall" and "short," like Mendel's peas. Skin color and mouse fur color are additional examples of mammalian polygenic traits.

Penetrance: Penetrance describes the likelihood that a person with a given genotype will express the expected phenotype. While many traits are completely penetrant (all individuals with a given allele or mutation display the phenotype), there is a spectrum of options: alleles or mutations can also have high, incomplete, or low penetrance. The root cause of penetrance depends on the allele. Some have age-related penetrance, where the phenotype is displayed more frequently in mutation-carrying individuals as they age. The penetrance of other alleles depends on environmental and lifestyle modifiers. For example, women who carry a certain mutation that increases their risk of breast cancer display variable rates of breast cancer, depending on their diet, if they smoke, if they have had children and breast fed, etc. Finally, many alleles have genetic modifiers that affect penetrance; since several human traits are polygenic, alleles at different loci can affect penetrance.

Epistasis: This refers to a situation where expression of alleles for one gene is dependent on a different gene. For example, a gene for curly hair cannot be expressed if a different gene causes baldness.

Recessive Lethal Alleles: Some mutant alleles can cause death of an organism when present in a homozygous manner. These are called **recessive lethal alleles**, and they typically code for essential gene products. In diploid organisms, these alleles can be studied by maintaining heterozygous stocks, which are then mated together to form a homozygous recessive offspring. Embryonic development studies can shed light on when this organism dies and possibly why. Studying recessive lethal alleles in haploid organisms is much harder. Here, a conditional system is usually used where the allele is normal (or permissive) under certain conditions, allowing survival of the organism. The mutant allele can be induced under different conditions (such as a different temperature), to study effects of the allele.

- 100 people are homozygous for an allele that is implicated in cancer, but only 20 develop cancer. What are potential explanations for why only some people express a gene out of a broader population with the same genotype?[43]
- In one strain of mouse, homozygotes for an allele of a gene develop heart defects, while in another strain of mouse, homozygotes with the same allele develop normally. Heterozygotes develop normally in both strains. What is the most likely explanation for the difference between the two strains?[44]

    A) The allele is recessive.
    B) The development of the heart defect is influenced by more than one locus.
    C) The allele has pleiotropic effects on development.
    D) The allele is codominant.

The Sex Chromosomes

Early in the twentieth century it was observed that women have 23 pairs of chromosomes that are homologous, while men have only 22 pairs of chromosomes that match in appearance. The two chromosomes in men that did not match each other were termed the **X** and the **Y chromosomes** because of their appearance during mitosis (Figure 13). Males have an X and a Y, while females have two X chromosomes. The presence of a Y chromosome in humans (genotype XY) is a key factor in the determination of the gender of an embryo, and subsequent development into a male. The absence of a Y (genotype XX) results in a female as the default developmental pathway. During meiosis, females generate gametes that contain an X chromosome; males generate gametes with either an X or a Y chromosome, meaning that it is the *male* gamete that determines the sex of an embryo (Figure 14).

This is an X chromosome during interphase. (Note that it doesn't look like an "X" at all.)

This is a condensed X chromosome after S phase (replication). The X is formed by the two sister chromatids.

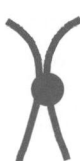

This is a Y chromosome after S phase.

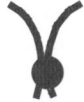

Figure 13   The Sex Chromosomes

[43] The trait of cancer development is probably polygenic, so it does not display simple patterns of inheritance. Cancer development is also influenced by the environment, such as exposure to carcinogens, further complicating the penetrance of the genotype.

[44] The key variable must not lie within the allele itself, since this remains the same (so choices A and D are wrong). The genetic background of the two different strains of mice must affect whether or not the heart defect phenotype is expressed. Further, only one defect is observed (so it can't be pleitropic; choice C is wrong). Therefore, the heart defect phenotype must be influenced by some other locus that is different in the two strains of mice, making choice **B** the best answer.

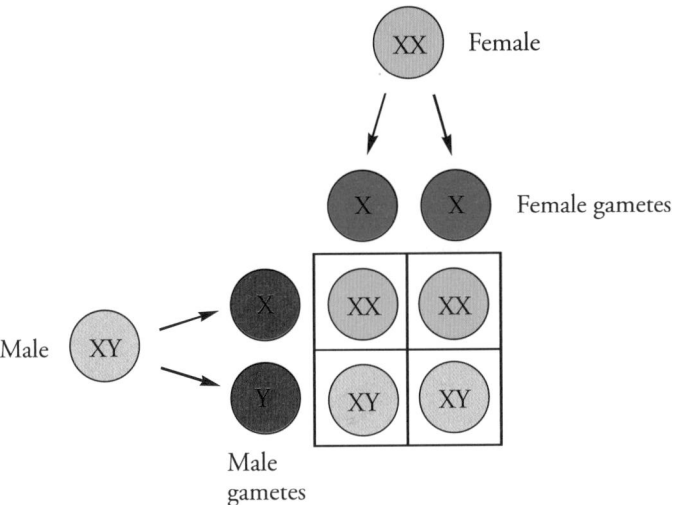

Figure 14   Determination of the Zygote's Sexual Genotype

The sex chromosomes also play a key role in the inheritance of other traits that are not directly involved in sexual development. Much of what has been discussed about inheritance was dependent on the assumption that there are two copies of every chromosome and therefore two copies of every gene in each cell. This is true for genes found on every pair of chromosomes except for one pair: the sex chromosomes. Genes that lie on the X chromosome will be present in two copies in females but only in one copy in males. [What pattern of expression will a recessive allele on the X chromosome display in males?[45]] Traits that are determined by genes on the X or Y chromosome are called **sex-linked traits** because of their unique patterns of expression and inheritance. The inheritance of traits coded by genes on sex chromosomes will be covered in Section 7.6.

7.5   LINKAGE

The traits that Mendel studied and based the law of independent assortment on were located on separate chromosomes. Genes that are located on the *same* chromosome may not display independent assortment, however. The failure of genes to display independent assortment is called **linkage**.

- If eye color is controlled by a gene on chromosome #11 and the hair color locus is located on chromosome #14, do these genes assort independently?[46]
- If the portion of chromosome #14 containing the hair color gene is translocated onto chromosome #11, will these genes still assort independently?[47]

If genes are located very close to each other on the same chromosome, then they will probably *not* be inherited independently of each other. Let's illustrate this with a pea gene for height and two alleles of the

---

[45] In males, recessive alleles on the X chromosome are always expressed, since no other allele is present that can mask the recessive allele.

[46] Yes, they will. Assortment of nonhomologous chromosomes into gametes is random during meiosis.

[47] A translocation occurs when a piece of one chromosome is moved onto another chromosome. The two genes are then found on the same chromosome and may not assort independently.

height gene, tall (*T*) and short (*t*), with the *T* allele dominant and the *t* allele recessive. If the height gene and the color gene are very near each other on the same chromosome, then the alleles of these genes on a specific chromosome will probably assort together into gametes during meiosis (Figure 15). This limits the possible combinations of the alleles in the gametes.

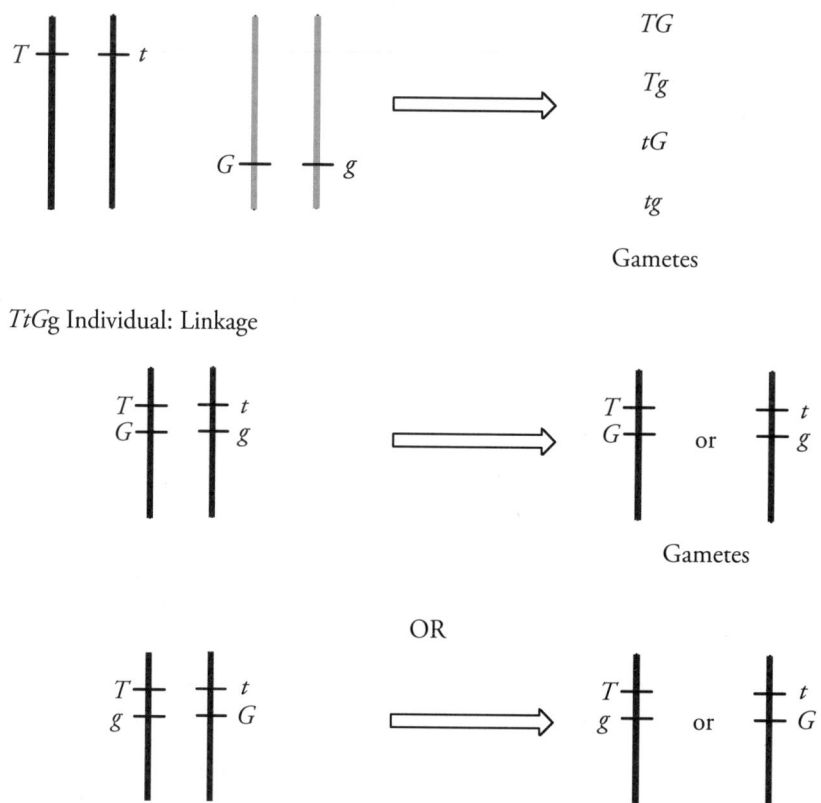

Figure 15   Linkage of Alleles during Meiosis

- If the color gene and the height gene display linkage, is it possible to predict the possible gametes of a *TTgg* individual?[48] Of a *TtGg* individual?[49]

To know how alleles that display linkage assort during meiosis, it may be necessary to know which alleles were on a chromosome together. As seen in Figure 15, there are two possible ways the height and color genes could be linked. The dominant alleles of two different genes can be linked together on the same chromosome (*TG*), the recessive alleles of two different genes can be linked (*tg*), or one dominant and one recessive allele can be linked (*Tg* and *tG*).

With genes that are found on the same chromosome, the design of a Punnett square is slightly different. The possible gametes are limited since they cannot assort independently. Consider a cross between a homozygous *ttgg* pea plant and a double-heterozygous plant with both dominant alleles on one

---

[48] Yes. A *TTgg* individual can only make *Tg* gametes, regardless of whether the genes are on the same chromosome or not.

[49] No. To predict how these traits will assort, it is necessary to know which alleles are present together on the same chromosome.

chromosome and both recessive alleles located together on another chromosome. They can only make a limited number of different gametes, not the four possible combinations of alleles that would be found if the genes were on different chromosomes. A Punnett square will help to illustrate linkage in this example (Figure 16).

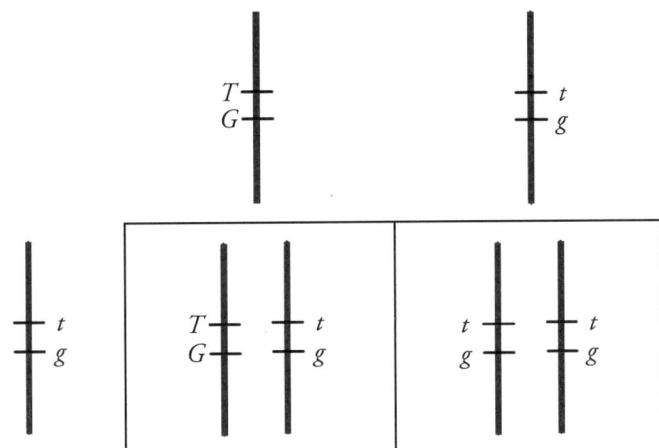

Figure 16   Assortment of Linked Genes

- What are the phenotypes of the F$_1$ progeny in the cross in Figure 16?[50]
- If a tall green pea from the F$_1$ progeny is crossed with a pure-breeding short yellow plant, what phenotypes will be observed and in what ratios?[51]
- If height and color genes were not linked, what ratios of phenotypes would be observed in a cross between a *TtGg* and a *ttgg* individual?[52]
- Assume all of the characteristics already introduced for the height, color, and shape pea genes that have been used as examples. The height and color genes are located near each other on the same chromosome and display complete linkage, but the shape gene is located on a different chromosome. If an individual with a *TtGgWw* genotype and the *T* and *g* alleles on the same chromosome is crossed with a *ttGgWw* individual, what result will be observed?[53]
  - A) All tall peas will be wrinkled.
  - B) All wrinkled peas will be tall.
  - C) All yellow peas will be tall.
  - D) All tall peas will be yellow.

---

[50] There are only two phenotypes: 50% tall green and 50% short yellow.

[51] The pure-breeding short yellow plant can only have *tg* gametes. The tall green plant can make only two types of alleles, the same gametes shown for its parent. The results of the backcross will be the same as for the original cross in Figure 16, with 50% tall green and 50% short yellow plants.

[52] The *ttgg* individual can make only *tg* gametes. The *TtGg* individual can make four different types of gametes if the genes are not linked: *TG*, *Tg*, *tG*, and *tg*. The genotypes and phenotypes of the cross will be 25% *TtGg* (tall green), 25% *Ttgg* (tall yellow), 25% *ttGg* (short green), and 25% *ttgg* (short yellow).

[53] The gene for shape (wrinkled versus smooth) is on a different chromosome than the other two genes, so there is no correlation between the wrinkled trait and the other traits (eliminating choices A and B). To be yellow, a pea must be homozygous *gg*. One of the *g* alleles must come from the chromosome with *T* and *g* together, making all yellow plants tall (choice **C** is correct). Some of the *Tg* gametes will join with *tG* gametes from the *ttGg* individual, meaning that some plants are tall and green (choice D is wrong). Drawing a Punnett Square can help to solve this problem.

Linkage and Recombination

Linkage is the exception to the law of independent assortment. When genes are located on the same chromosome, they will display linkage and will not assort independently. Meiotic recombination provides the exception to linkage. During the formation of gametes, meiotic recombination between homologous chromosomes can separate alleles that were located on the same chromosome. In the example in Figure 17, three genes are located on the same chromosome. Prior to recombination, *ABC* were found on one chromosome and *abc* were found on the homologous chromosome. [What combinations of alleles will be found in gametes in the absence of recombination?[54]] Recombination produces new combinations of alleles not found in the parent and also allows genes located on the same chromosome to assort independently.

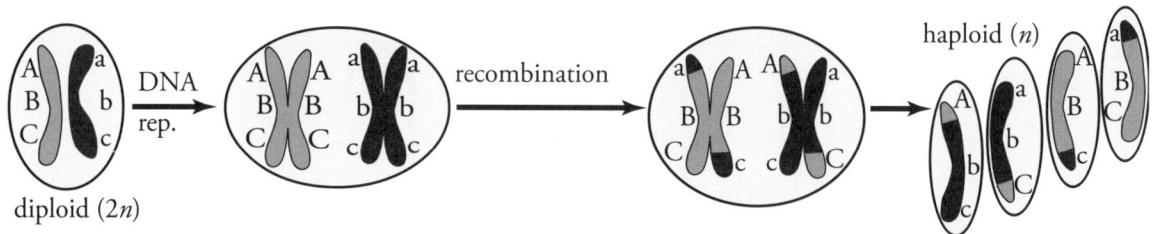

Figure 17   Recombination—Another Look

The example of the height and color genes in pea plants will help to illustrate linkage and the effects of recombination on patterns of inheritance. As before, the height and color genes are located on the same chromosome. There are two alleles of the height gene, dominant *T* (tall) and recessive *t* (short) and two alleles of the color gene, dominant *G* (green) and recessive *g* (yellow). The following cross is performed: a pure-breeding tall green plant is crossed with a pure-breeding short yellow plant. [What phenotypes are predicted in this cross if linkage is complete?[55]] A pea plant from this cross is then self-pollinated (crossed with itself) to produce an F_2 generation. [If linkage is complete, what genotypes and phenotypes will be observed in the F_2 generation?[56] If the genes assort completely randomly, what genotypes and phenotypes will be observed in the F_2 generation?[57]] The F_2 generation in this cross was observed to have the following plants: 30 tall green plants, 9 short yellow plants, 2 tall yellow plants, and 1 short green plant. [Which of these phenotypes are recombinant phenotypes?[58]] Often in a cross involving genes on the same chromosome, the result will be intermediate between independent assortment and complete linkage. The reason for this is that recombination occurs between the genes during meiosis of *some* of the gametes but not *all* of the gametes. [If it is known that two genes are located on the same chromosome but during a cross they assort completely randomly, how can this be?[59]]

---

[54] *ABC* or *abc* genotypes

[55] Only one phenotype. The F_1 generation will all receive a *TG* chromosome from the pure-breeding tall green parent and a *tg* chromosome from the pure-breeding short yellow parent.

[56] 75% tall green and 25% short yellow. Try a Punnett square to verify this result, remembering to assort alleles together into gametes.

[57] 9:3:3:1 of tall green, tall yellow, short green, and short yellow, respectively. This is a classical Mendelian ratio observed when heterozygotes at two alleles are crossed.

[58] The tall yellow and short green phenotypes would not be observed if linkage was complete (as in #56). The only way to produce these phenotypes is if a small number of gametes received chromosomes in which the *TG* and *tg* alleles were separated from each other by recombination, so these are the recombinant phenotypes.

[59] If the genes are on the same chromosome, but are far apart from one another, then recombination occurs frequently. The genes will assort randomly during meiosis and will not display any linkage even though they are on the same chromosome.

The frequency of recombination between two genes on a chromosome is proportional to the physical distance between the genes along the linear length of the DNA molecule. [Does recombination occur between genes more frequently if they are near each other or far apart?[60]] The farther apart two genes are on a chromosome, the more likely recombination will occur between the genes during meiosis. If the genes are located far enough apart, recombination will occur so frequently between the genes that they will no longer display linkage and will assort as independently as if they were on separate chromosomes. The **frequency of recombination** is given as the *number of recombinant phenotypes* resulting from a cross *divided by the total number of progeny*.

$$RF = \text{recombination frequency} = \frac{\text{number of recombinants}}{\text{total number of offspring}}$$

Since the frequency of recombination is proportional to the physical distance of genes from each other, it can be used as a tool to map genes in relation to each other on chromosomes.

Example: The height and color gene in pea plants are on the same chromosome as a third gene for big or small flowers. The alleles of flower size are a dominant B (big) and a recessive b (small). The color gene (G, green or g, yellow) is studied in relation to the flower size gene. In the first cross, pure-breeding homozygous $BBGG$ plants are crossed with $bbgg$ plants. [What is the phenotype of the F_1 progeny?[61] If a small flower green plant is observed in the F_1 generation, was recombination responsible?[62]] An F_1 progeny is then crossed with a $bbgg$ plant and the following phenotypes observed: 44 big flower green plants, 40 small flower yellow plants, 8 big flower yellow plants, and 8 small flower green plants.

- Which of these are recombinant phenotypes?[63]
- What is the frequency of recombination between the genes?[64]
- What is the maximal frequency of recombination?[65]
- In another cross, the frequency of recombination between the flower size and height genes is examined and found to be 10 recombinant plants out of 100 progeny. Is the height gene or the color gene closer to the flower size gene?[66]
- If the recombination frequencies are 0.16 between the height and color genes, 0.10 between the height and flower size genes, and 0.26 between the flower size and color genes, what is the order of the genes on the chromosome?[67]

---

[60] The farther two genes are away from each other, the greater the odds that recombination will occur between them.

[61] The F_1 progeny are all $BbGg$ genotype and therefore are big flower green plants.

[62] The small flower green phenotype could not be produced by recombination. These alleles do not exist together in either parent and so could not be recombined together in the gametes. This must be the result of mutation.

[63] Big flower yellow plants and small flower green plants can only be produced through recombination between the flower size and color genes.

[64] The frequency of recombination is 16 recombinant phenotypes out of 100 progeny = 16%.

[65] The maximal frequency of recombination would be when there was no linkage and the genes assorted independently. In this case, there would be 25% big flower yellow plants and 25% small flower green plants, or 50% maximal frequency of recombination.

[66] There is less recombination between the height and flower size genes (10% frequency) than between the color and flower size genes (16%), so the height gene is closer to the flower size gene than the color gene is.

[67] The flower size and color genes have the most recombination between them, so they must be farthest apart, with the height gene in the middle.

7.6

- Is it possible to map the distance between genes on the same chromosome even if they are so far apart that they assort independently?[68]
- Assume that hair color in humans is determined by a gene for which there are two alleles: *B* or brown, which is dominant, and *b* or blond, which is recessive. The hair color gene is located on the same chromosome as another gene that determines the strength of bones, and the two genes are very close together. The alleles of the bone strength gene are *S*, the dominant sturdy bone allele, and *s*, the recessive fragile bone allele. Jose and Tonya have dark hair and sturdy bones. One of their children has brown hair and fragile bones. One grandparent of Jose and one grandparent of Tonya had fragile bones and blond hair, while the remaining grandparents were homozygous for brown hair and sturdy bones. Which of the following is/are true?[69]

  I.   The child of Jose and Tonya represents a recombinant phenotype.
  II. All of the children of Jose and Tonya must have fragile bones.
  III. Jose and Tonya may have other children with blond hair and fragile bones.

  A) I only
  B) II only
  C) I and III only
  D) II and III only

7.6   INHERITANCE PATTERNS

There are six inheritance patterns that you should be familiar with: autosomal recessive, autosomal dominant, mitochondrial, Y-linked, X-linked recessive, and X-linked dominant. In this section, each will be described and then a summary table will be presented.

Autosomal traits are caused by genetic variation on the autosomes (the 22 pairs of non-sex chromosomes in humans). These traits can be **autosomal dominant** (in which case a single copy of the allele will confer the trait or disease phenotype) or **autosomal recessive** (in which case two copies of the allele are required for the affected phenotype). Both tend to affect males and females equally; in other words, there is no sex bias for these traits.

There is a small, haploid DNA genome inside the mitochondria and humans inherit this genome from their mothers. This is because the sperm contributes only nuclear chromosomes to the zygote; the ovum contributes nuclear chromosomes and the rest of the cellular material including the organelles. There are some traits that are inherited via the mitochondrial genome, although these **mitochondrial traits** are rare. Luckily, they are fairly easy to spot because affected females have all affected offspring (sons and daughters). Affected individuals must have an affected mother, and affected males cannot have any

---

[68] Yes, but it requires one or more genes located between the two genes. The distance between the two genes could not be mapped directly by measuring the frequency of recombination between them, but if the distance from both of them to a gene in the middle can be mapped, then the overall distance between the genes can be mapped. Whole chromosomes can be mapped this way.

[69] **Item I is true:** the simplest explanation is that the grandparent on each side passed on the fragile allele and the blond allele, but recombination occurred, so that the fragile and blond alleles assorted independently. Item II is false: Jose and Tonya both have the dominant sturdy bone gene in at least one copy, so some children are likely to have sturdy bones. **Item III is true:** both Jose and Tonya may have one chromosome with the blond allele and the fragile bone allele linked. If so, a nonrecombinant phenotype would be blond/fragile. The answer is choice **C**.

affected offspring. An individual cannot inherit mitochondrial traits from their father. Mitochondrial traits (like Y-linked traits and X-linked traits in human males) are an example of **hemizygosity**; the individual only has one copy of the chromosome in a diploid organism. Because of this, there is only one allele to keep track of for each individual. Genes encoded by the mitochondrial genome are usually given the prefix **mt** (for example, mt-*Atp6* is encoded in the mitochondrial genome and codes for a subunit of the ATP synthase). When working with inheritance patterns though, it is best to define the allele letters you are going to use and then use one letter per individual. For example, you could assign "*a*" as a normal individual and "*A*" as an affected individual. The assignment here is arbitrary since one allele is not dominant to the other (they are mutually exclusive since humans only have one mitochondrial genome). The key is to be consistent.

Traits that are determined by genes located on the X or Y chromosome are called **sex-linked traits** and display unusual patterns of inheritance. Traits encoded by genes on the Y chromosome (Y-linked traits) would only be passed from male parents to male children. [Would it be possible for a father to pass a Y-linked trait to female children?[70] Can males be carriers of recessive Y-linked traits without expressing them?[71]] Y-linked traits are quite rare, because the Y chromosome is small and contains a relatively small number of genes. Many of the genes on the Y-chromosome function in sex determination.

X-linked traits are observed quite frequently and can be X-linked recessive or X-linked dominant. There are several well-studied examples of X-linked recessive traits that are common in the human population; hemophilia is an example. Women are often carriers of X-linked recessive alleles but will only express recessive X-linked traits when they are homozygous. Men are hemizygous for X-linked traits; they have only one copy of genes on the X chromosome. As a result, males *always* express recessive X-linked alleles. [From which parent do males receive X-linked traits?[72]] These traits tend to affect males more than females.

Red-green colorblindness, an X-linked trait, is caused by a defect in a visual pigment gene on the X chromosome. The allele that is responsible for colorblindness is a pigment gene that does not produce functional protein. [Is the colorblindness allele recessive or dominant?[73]] The colorblindness allele, like many recessive traits carried in the population, is not expressed in heterozygotes. Colorblindness is unusual in women but fairly common in men. Females have two copies of the gene, so will not express the trait if they are heterozygotes, while males have only one X chromosome and so will always express the allele whenever they receive it. [A man is colorblind, and his wife is homozygous normal for genes encoding visual pigment proteins. What will be the phenotypes and genotypes of sons and of daughters of this couple?[74]]

X-linked dominant traits are harder to identify. A female will display an X-linked dominant phenotype if she has one or two copies of the allele on her X chromosomes. A male will express the phenotype if

---

[70] No. Females never have a Y chromosome and so can never carry or express a Y-linked trait.

[71] No. Y-linked traits are carried in only one copy, since there is only one Y chromosome per cell. If a male carries a recessive Y-linked trait, he will express it.

[72] Since males receive their X chromosome from their mother (and their Y chromosome from their father), they receive X-linked traits from their mother.

[73] An allele that encodes inactive protein or no protein is generally recessive, since the gene's function can be compensated for by the remaining normal copy of the gene.

[74] Sons will have a normal phenotype and carry one copy of the normal gene. Daughters will carry one normal gene and one recessive colorblindness allele and will have the normal phenotype.

he inherited the affected allele from his mother. While these traits still tend to affect males more than females, this trend is less obvious than for X-linked recessive traits.

Table 1 summarizes the six inheritance patterns you should be familiar with, and lists some strategies you can use to distinguish between them.

Inheritance Pattern	Identification Techniques	Unaffected Genotypes	Affected Genotypes
Autosomal recessive	• Can skip generations (affected individuals can have unaffected parents) • Number of affected males is usually equal to the number of affected females	*AA* *Aa*	*aa*
Autosomal dominant	• Does not skip generations (affected individuals must have an affected parent) • Number of affected males is usually equal to number of affected females • An affected parent passes the trait to either all or half of offspring	*aa*	*AA* *Aa*
Mitochondrial	• Maternal inheritance • Affected female has all affected children • Affected male cannot pass the trait onto his children • Unaffected female cannot have affected children	*a*	*A*
Y-linked	• Affects male only; females never have the trait • Affected father has all affected sons • Unaffected father cannot have an affected son	XY^a	XY^A
X-linked recessive	• Can skip generations (affected individuals can have unaffected parents) • Tend to affect males more than females • Unaffected females can have affected sons • Affected female has all affected sons, but can have both affected and unaffected daughters	$X^A X^A$ $X^A X^a$ $X^A Y$	$X^a X^a$ $X^a Y$
X-linked dominant	• Hardest to identify • Does not skip generations (affected individuals must have an affected parent) • Usually affects males more than females • Affected fathers have all affected daughters • Affected mothers can have unaffected sons (and unaffected daughters), and pass the trait equally to sons and daughters	$X^a X^a$ $X^a Y$	$X^A X^A$ $X^A X^a$ $X^A Y$

Table 1 Summary of Inheritance Patterns

7.6

- Two mouse genes located on the X chromosome are being studied. The alleles of the genes are:

Fuzzy hair: *F*, dominant (normal hair) and *f*, recessive (fuzzy hair)

Extra toes: *E*, dominant (extra toes), and *e*, recessive (normal toes)

A female with normal hair and extra toes is crossed with a male with normal hair and extra toes. The progeny have the following phenotypes:

Phenotype	Male	Female
Normal hair, extra toes	46	100
Normal hair, normal toes	4	0
Fuzzy hair, extra toes	5	0
Fuzzy hair, normal toes	45	0

7.7

Which one of the following is true concerning this experiment?[75]

A) Males have a higher rate of recombination than females do.

B) In the absence of recombination, all males would have normal hair and extra toes.

C) The rate of recombination on the X chromosome is the same in males and females.

D) Both males and females have recombinant genotypes, but only males have recombinant phenotypes.

7.7 POPULATION GENETICS

Mendelian genetics describes the inheritance of traits in the progeny of specific individuals. For the purposes of large topics such as natural selection and evolution, however, the more relevant issue is not the inheritance of traits from individuals but in a whole population from one generation to another. **Population genetics** describes the inheritance of traits in populations over time. The word *population* has a specific meaning in this setting: *a population consists of members of a species that mate and reproduce with each other.* [If a group of sea turtles lives most of the year dispersed over a large area of ocean without contact with one another but congregate once a year to reproduce, is this group a population?[76]] To a population geneticist, each individual is merely a temporary carrier of the alleles in a population.

In population genetics, the units of genetic inheritance are alleles of genes, just as in Mendelian genetics. However, in population genetics alleles are examined across the entire population rather than in individuals. The sum total of all genetic information in a population is called the **gene pool**. [For an autosomal

---

[75] The genotype of the male parent must be $X^{FE}Y$. The predominance of the normal hair-extra toes and fuzzy hair-normal toes phenotypes in the F_1 generation indicates that the female parent must have one X chromosome with both dominant alleles together, and one X chromosome with both recessive alleles together, in other words, her genotype must be $X^{FE}X^{fe}$. The fuzzy hair-extra toes and normal hair-normal toes phenotypes are much less common and must be the result of recombination in the female parent, producing X^{Fe} and X^{fE} chromosomes. Note that recombination between the X and Y chromosomes in males is not possible due to the fact that the X and Y carry different genes (choices A and C are wrong). If recombination had not occurred in the female parent, all F_1 males would have received either X^{FE} or X^{fe}, giving both normal hair-extra toes and fuzzy hair-normal toes phenotypes (choice B is wrong). Choice **D** is the correct answer: the F_1 females must also have recombinant genotypes on the X chromosomes they received from their mother, but every F_1 female also received both dominant alleles on the X chromosome they received from their father. Thus, only the dominant phenotypes are seen in the F_1 females.

[76] Yes. A population does not need to live with one another, only to reproduce sexually with one another.

gene in a population of 2,000 individuals, how many copies of the gene are present in the gene pool?[77]] The frequency of an allele in a population is a key variable used to describe the gene pool. [If there are 5,000 hippos in a population, out of which there are 100 homozygotes of an autosomal allele *h* and 400 heterozygotes, what is the frequency of the *h* allele in the population?[78] If 20% of the population is heterozygous for an allele *Q* and 10% is homozygous, what will be the frequency of the allele in the population?[79]]

Hardy-Weinberg in Population Genetics

Population genetics does not simply describe the gene pool of a population but attempts to predict the gene pool of a population in the future. The **Hardy-Weinberg law** states that the *frequencies of alleles in the gene pool of a population will not change over time*, provided that a number of assumptions are true:

1) There is no mutation.
2) There is no migration.
3) There is no natural selection.
4) There is random mating.
5) The population is sufficiently large to prevent random drift in allele frequencies.

What Hardy-Weinberg means at the molecular level is that segregation of alleles, independent assortment, and recombination during meiosis can alter the combinations of alleles in gametes but cannot increase or decrease the frequency of an allele in the gametes of one individual or the gametes of the population as a whole.

- If 100 homozygous green pea plants and 100 homozygous yellow pea plants are crossed, 1,000 green pea plants are produced. Does this mean that the yellow alleles disappeared from the population?[80]
- What is the frequency of the yellow allele in the gene pool of the progeny?[81]
- If the green peas from the F_1 generation are allowed to mate randomly within the population, and there is no mutation, migration, natural selection, or random drift, what will be the frequency of the yellow allele in the population after four generations?[82]
- If two genes are closely linked on the same chromosome, will Hardy-Weinberg still apply to these genes?[83]

---

[77] There are two copies of the gene in each of the 2,000 individuals, for a total of 4,000 copies in the gene pool.

[78] The allele frequency is the number of copies of a specific allele divided by the total number of copies of the gene in the population. If there are 5,000 hippos, and each has 2 copies of the gene, there are 10,000 copies of the gene in the population. There are 100 homozygotes of the *h* allele, each with 2 copies of it, and 400 heterozygotes with one *h* allele, for a total of 600 *h* alleles in the population. Thus, the frequency of the *h* allele is 600/10,000 = 0.06.

[79] In this case, the number of individuals in the population is not provided, but it is not needed. The total number of alleles is 100%. The frequency of the allele is 0.5 × (20% heterozygotes) + 10% homozygotes = 20%.

[80] The yellow alleles are still there (but in the heterozygous state), so they do not appear in the phenotype.

[81] The frequency of the yellow allele will be 50%, just as it was in the parents. None of the alleles in a population were destroyed, so the frequency is the same as in the parental generation.

[82] According to Hardy-Weinberg, there will be no change in the frequency of the allele. The frequency of the yellow allele will still be 50% after four generations.

[83] Yes. Independent assortment is not a requirement of Hardy-Weinberg. Allele frequencies for the genes will still remain constant, regardless of the extent of recombination between the genes, as long as the assumptions of Hardy-Weinberg hold true.

- According to Hardy-Weinberg, what will happen to the frequency of the yellow allele if predation occurs on yellow plants, but yellow plants attract bees more successfully?[84]

The Hardy-Weinberg law has also been translated into mathematical terms. Assuming that there are two alleles of a gene in a population, the letter p is used to represent the frequency of the dominant allele, and the letter q is used to represent the frequency of the recessive allele. Since there are only two alleles, the following fundamental equation must be true:

$$p + q = 1$$

Based on allele frequency, it is possible to calculate the proportion of genotypes in a population. Take a situation where the frequency of a dominant allele, G, equals p and the frequency of a recessive allele, g, equals q. If the equation above is squared on both sides, it becomes:

$$(p + q)^2 = 1$$

$$p^2 + 2pq + q^2 = 1$$

where

$$p^2 = \text{the frequency of the } GG \text{ genotype}$$

$$2pq = \text{the frequency of the } Gg \text{ genotype}$$

$$q^2 = \text{the frequency of the } gg \text{ genotype}$$

- If the frequency of the G allele is 0.25 in a population of 1,000 mice, determine the number of individuals who are Gg heterozygotes if there is random mating but no migration, mutation, random drift, or natural selection.[85]
- If allele frequencies in a population are constant, and genotype frequencies can be calculated from allele frequencies, how will genotype frequencies vary over time?[86]

After one generation, a population will reach **Hardy-Weinberg equilibrium**, in which allele frequencies no longer change. Since allele frequencies do not change, and genotype frequencies can be calculated from allele frequencies, it follows that genotype frequencies also do not change over time. [If 100 green peas (GG) and 100 yellow peas (gg) are allowed to mate randomly, will the genotype frequencies in the next generation (F_1) be the same?[87] If not, why not?[88] If the plants are allowed to mate randomly for another generation (F_2), will the genotype frequencies in the F_1 and F_2 generations be the same?[89]]

---

[84] Hardy-Weinberg says nothing about this situation. Once the assumptions no longer hold true, Hardy-Weinberg no longer applies.

[85] If the frequency of the G allele (p) is 0.25, then the frequency of the g allele (q) must be 0.75, since $p + q = 1$. The frequency of the heterozygotes in the population will be $2pq = 2(0.25)(0.75) = 0.375$. Therefore, the number of individuals in this population who are heterozygotes will be $0.375 \times 1000 = 375$.

[86] Genotype frequencies as well as allele frequencies will remain constant according to Hardy-Weinberg.

[87] No. The next generation will include GG, Gg, and gg genotypes.

[88] The population was not at Hardy-Weinberg equilibrium to start out.

[89] Yes. A population reaches Hardy-Weinberg equilibrium after one generation. The F_2 generation (and all generations after that) will have the same genotype frequencies as the F_1 generation.

7.7

Hardy-Weinberg in the Real World

Hardy-Weinberg requires a number of assumptions in order to be true. The assumptions, as presented earlier, are that in a population there is random mating and no mutation, migration, natural selection, or random drift. Thus, Hardy-Weinberg describes a highly idealized set of conditions required to prevent alleles from being added or removed from a population. In reality, it is not possible for a population to meet all of the conditions required by Hardy-Weinberg.

1) **Mutation**: Mutation is inevitable in a population. Even if there are no chemical mutagens or radiation, inherent errors by DNA polymerase would over time cause mutations and introduce new alleles in a population.

2) **Migration**: If migration occurs, animals leaving or entering the population will carry alleles with them and disturb the Hardy-Weinberg equilibrium.

3) **Natural Selection**: For there to be no natural selection, there would have to be unlimited resources, no predation, no disease, and so on. This is not a set of conditions encountered in the real world.

4) **Non-random Mating**: If individuals pick their mates preferentially based on one or more traits, alleles that cause those traits will be passed on preferentially from one generation to another.

5) **Random Drift**: If a population becomes very small, it cannot contain as great a variety of alleles. In a very small population, random events can alter allele frequencies significantly and have a large influence on future generations.

7.8 EVOLUTION BY NATURAL SELECTION

At one time, life on Earth was generally viewed as static and unchanging, but we now know that this is not the case. Over the geologic span of Earth's history, many species have arisen, changed over millions of years, given rise to new species, and died out. These changes in life on Earth are called **evolution**. Although he did not arrive at his theory alone, Charles Darwin played an important role in shaping modern thought by proposing natural selection as the mechanism that drives evolution. **Natural selection** is an interaction between organisms and their environment that causes differential reproduction of different phenotypes and thereby alters the gene pool of a population. In essence, the theory of evolution by natural selection is this:

1) In a population, there are heritable differences between individuals.

2) Heritable traits (alleles of genes) produce traits (phenotypes) that affect the ability of an organism to survive and have offspring.

3) Some individuals have phenotypes that allow them to survive longer, be healthier, and have more offspring than others.

4) Individuals with phenotypes that allow them to have more offspring will pass on their alleles more frequently than those with phenotypes that have fewer offspring.

5) Over time, those alleles that lead to more offspring are passed on more frequently and become more abundant, while other alleles become less abundant in the gene pool.

6) Changes in allele frequency are the basis of evolution in species and populations.

To put it simply, evolution occurs when natural selection acts on genetic variation to drive changes in the genetic composition of a population. A key term in evolution is **fitness**. In evolutionary terms, fitness is not how well an animal is physically adapted to a niche in the environment, or how well it can feed itself, but how successful it is in passing on its alleles to future generations. The way to have greater fitness is by having more offspring that pass on their alleles to future generations of the population. Some species achieve greater fitness through sheer numbers of progeny produced, who are then left to fend for themselves. Other species have fewer progeny, but protect and nurture the young to maturity.

- If an allele of a gene causes cancer in elderly polar bears after their reproductive years have passed, how will it affect the fitness of bears carrying the allele?[90]
- If a recessive allele causes sterility in homozygotes, how will it affect the fitness of heterozygotes?[91]
- A group of mice are infected with recombinant virus in bone marrow cells that allows the mice to live longer. The mice are then released into a wild population. Will natural selection act to increase the life span of the population?[92]
- Which of the following will have greater fitness: A fish that has two offspring and protects and nurtures its young to maturity, or a fish that has 10 offspring and abandons them, resulting in the death of 8 young fish before maturity?[93]
- The recessive allele that causes cystic fibrosis is strongly selected against in modern society, since individuals with this disease often die before sexual maturity. However, the frequency of the allele takes many generations to decrease in the population. Why?[94]
- A certain genetic disease is caused by a recessive allele. In the absence of effective therapy, homozygous individuals with this allele generally die before reaching sexual maturity. The allele also protects heterozygous individuals against several life-threatening viral diseases. If a medicine is found that provides a complete remedy for the disease, allowing individuals with the disease to live an entirely normal life, which of the following statements describes what will happen to the frequency of the allele in the population after that time?[95]
  - A) The frequency of the allele will decrease.
  - B) The frequency of the allele will remain constant.
  - C) The frequency of the allele will increase.
  - D) It is not possible to predict the future frequency of the allele.

Sources of Genetic Diversity

Natural selection acts on the genetic diversity in a population to alter allele frequencies, causing evolution. Genetic diversity in a population is a requirement for natural selection to occur. [If a population of sea otters contains only one allele of a gene that protects against cold, can natural selection drive evolution of

---

[90] The allele will not affect fitness. The bears will only be affected at a time when they can no longer have offspring, so it will not affect the ability of bears to transmit their alleles to future generations.

[91] If the allele is truly recessive, it will not affect fitness at all. Natural selection can act only on phenotypes, not genotypes.

[92] No. Natural selection only acts on heritable traits. Infected bone marrow cells will not be passed on in the germ line to the next generation and so the long life span of these mice is not a heritable trait.

[93] The fish will technically have the same fitness, since both will contribute to the gene pool of future generations equally.

[94] Natural selection acts on phenotypes, not genotypes. Even if the allele is lethal in homozygotes, heterozygotes will not be selected against if the allele is not expressed. It takes many generations for deleterious recessive alleles to decrease in frequency in a population.

[95] The correct answer is choice **C**. Homozygotes have low fitness in the absence of medicine, while heterozygotes have increased fitness due to their resistance to viral disease. In the absence of the medicine, natural selection tends to reduce the frequency of the allele by removing individuals who are homozygous but tends to increase the frequency of the allele through the higher fitness of heterozygotes. Over time these opposing selection pressures can be balanced to keep the allele at a relatively constant frequency. If medicine removes the selection against homozygotes, then the heterozygotes with the increased fitness cause to allele frequency to increase over time.

this trait?[96] Can natural selection cause new alleles to appear in the population?[97]] Natural selection does not introduce genetic diversity, however; it can act only on existing diversity to alter allele frequencies.

There are two sources of genetic variation in a population: *new alleles* and *new combinations of existing alleles*. New alleles are the result of mutations in the genome. New combinations of alleles are generated during sexual reproduction as a result of independent assortment, recombination and segregation during meiosis. By increasing and maintaining genetic variation in a population, sexual reproduction allows for greater capacity for adaptation of a population to changing environmental conditions.

- Do new alleles in a population generally confer greater or lesser fitness on an individual carrying them?[98]
- If a mutation occurs in a muscle cell of an individual who then has many progeny, does this mutation increase genetic variation in the population?[99]
- Does mitosis contribute to the genetic variation in a population?[100]
- If a population of flowers loses the ability to reproduce sexually and reproduces only asexually, how will this affect natural selection in the population?[101]
- Plants that are pollinated by insects sometimes have physical features of the flower that prevent self-pollination. What is the advantage to the plant of preventing self-pollination?[102]
- Which one of the following can create new alleles in a population?[103]
    A) Non-random mating
    B) Random drift
    C) Recombination
    D) Deletion

---

[96] If there is only one allele, then there is no variability that natural selection can act on, and no way that allele frequencies can change to cause evolution.

[97] No. Natural selection can only alter the frequency of existing alleles, not create new alleles.

[98] New alleles caused by mutation generally render gene products less active or even inactive. Animals have adapted over long periods of time to have most gene products function in the optimal manner, so most changes are harmful rather than beneficial.

[99] No. Mutation must occur in the germ line to introduce a new allele into a population. A mutation in a somatic cell cannot be passed on to the next generation.

[100] No. Mitosis can only copy a cell into an identical cell; it is not involved in creating new combinations of alleles in the same manner as meiosis.

[101] If the flowers can only reproduce asexually, then they have lost the ability of meiosis to generate new combinations of alleles and new genetic variation for natural selection to act on.

[102] Self-pollination reduces genetic variability. More variability is maintained in the population if different individuals mate, making new combinations of alleles.

[103] Nonrandom mating and random drift will alter allele frequencies but do not create new alleles (choices A and B are incorrect). Recombination will not alter allele frequencies or create new alleles, but create new combinations of alleles (choice C is wrong). The correct answer is choice **D**. Only mutation of the genome can create new alleles. A deletion can create a new allele, even if the new allele is a truncated gene product or does not express any gene product at all.

Modes of Natural Selection

Natural selection can occur in many different manners and have different effects in a population. The following are a few examples:

1) **Directional Selection:** Polygenic traits often follow a bell-shaped curve of expression, with most individuals clustered around the average and some members of a population trailing off in either direction away from the average. If natural selection removes those at one extreme, the population average over time will move in the other direction. Example: Giraffes get taller as all short giraffes die for lack of food.

2) **Divergent Selection:** Rather than removing the extreme members in the distribution of a trait in a population, natural selection removes the members near the average, leaving those at either end. Over time divergent selection will split the population in two and perhaps lead to a new species. Example: Small deer are selected for because they can hide, and large deer are selected because they can fight, but mid-sized deer are too big to hide and too small to fight.

3) **Stabilizing Selection:** Both extremes of a trait are selected against, driving the population closer to the average. Example: Birds that are too large or too small are eliminated from a population because they cannot mate.

4) **Artificial Selection:** Humans intervene in the mating of many animals and plants, using artificial selection to achieve desired traits through controlled mating. Example: The pets and crop plants we have are the result of many generations of artificial selection.

5) **Sexual Selection:** Animals often do not choose mates randomly, but have evolved elaborate rituals and physical displays that play a key role in attracting and choosing a mate. Example: Some birds have bright plumage to attract a mate, even at the cost of increased predation.

6) **Kin Selection:** Natural selection does not always act on individuals. Animals that live socially often share alleles with other individuals and will sacrifice themselves for the sake of the alleles they share with another individual. Example: A female lion sacrifices herself to save her sister's children.

7.9 THE SPECIES CONCEPT AND SPECIATION

A **species** is a group of organisms which are capable of reproducing with each other sexually. (Other criteria, such as morphology, are used to classify species that only reproduce asexually.) [What's the difference between a population and a species?[104]] Two individuals are not members of the same biological species if they cannot mate and produce fit offspring. [When a horse mates with a donkey a mule is born. Mules are healthy animals with long life spans, but they are sterile. Are horses and donkeys members of the same species?[105]] **Reproductive isolation** keeps existing species separate. There are two types of reproductive isolation: **prezygotic** and **postzygotic**.

Prezygotic barriers prevent the formation of a hybrid zygote. Such barriers may be:

• Ecological: individuals who could otherwise mate live in different habitats, and thus cannot access each other

---

[104] Members of a species *can* mate and produce fit offspring. Members of a population *do*. Remember it this way: a population is a subset of a species.

[105] No, since their offspring are unfit (unable to reproduce).

- Temporal: individuals mate at different times of the day, season, or year
- Behavioral: some species require special rituals or courtship behaviors before mating can occur
- Mechanical: reproductive structures or genital organs of two individuals are not compatible (even if they court and attempt copulation)
- Gametic: sperm from one species cannot fertilize the egg of a different species due incompatibilities in the sperm-egg recognition system, discussed in Chapter 13

Postzygotic barriers to hybridization prevent the development, survival, or reproduction of hybrid individuals (those that arise from a mating between two different species), and thus prevent gene flow if fertilization between two different species does occur. There are three types of postzygotic barriers:

- Hybrid inviability: hybrid offspring do not develop or mature normally, and normally die in the embryonic stage
- Hybrid sterility: a hybrid individual is born and develops normally, but does not produce normal gametes, and thus is incapable of breeding (e.g., a mule, offspring of a mating between a horse and a donkey, is sterile)
- Hybrid breakdown: when two hybrids mate successfully to produce a hybrid offspring, but this second generation hybrid is somehow biologically defective

7.9

The creation of new species is known as **speciation**. An important premise in modern biology is that all species come from pre-existing species. *Cladogenesis* is branching speciation (*clado* is from the Greek for branch), where one species diversifies and becomes two or more new species. *Anagenesis* is when one biological species simply becomes another by changing so much that if an individual were to go back in time, it would be unable to reproduce sexually with its ancestors. One type of cladogenesis, *allopatric isolation*, is initiated by geographical isolation. Over time, geographical isolation leads to reproductive isolation. *Sympatric* speciation occurs when a species gives rise to a new species in the same geographical area, such as through divergent selection.

Cladogenesis has left traces which taxonomists use to classify organisms. **Homologous structures** are physical features shared by two different species as a result of a common ancestor. For example, bird wings have five bony supports which resemble distorted human fingers, and dog paws also resemble distorted human hands. The explanation is that dogs, birds, and people all have a common ancestor which had five-toed feet. **Analogous structures** serve the same function in two different species, but *not* due to common ancestry. The flagellum of the human sperm and bacterial flagella are an example; they have entirely different structures from different organisms yet play the same role in motility. **Convergent evolution** is when two different species come to possess many analogous structures due to similar selective pressures. For example, bats and birds appear very similar even though bats are mammals. The opposite of convergent evolution is **divergent evolution**, in which divergent selection causes cladogenesis. **Parallel evolution** describes the situation in which two species go through similar evolutionary changes due to similar selective pressures. For example, in an ice age, all organisms would be selected for their ability to tolerate cold.

7.10 TAXONOMY

Taxonomy is the science of biological classification, originated by Carolus Linnaeus in the eighteenth century. He devised the **binomial classification** system we use today, in which each organism is given two names: genus and species. The binomial name of an organism is written in italics (or is underlined) with the genus capitalized and the species not, as in *Homo sapiens* (man the wise). There are eight principal taxonomic categories: **domain**, **kingdom**, **phylum**, **class**, **order**, **family**, **genus**, and **species**.[106] You should know how humans are classified and the defining characteristics of each kingdom. Table 2 below provides a general summary.

Domain	Bacteria	Archaea	Eukarya			
Kingdom	Eubacteria	Archaea	Protista	Fungi	Plantae	Animalia
Cell wall	peptidoglycan	polysaccharides and proteins, but no peptidoglycan	optional and varied	chitin	cellulose	none
Organelles	none	none	Typical eukaryotic organelles such as: nucleus, RER, SER, Golgi, peroxisome, lysosomes, chloroplasts, vacuoles, mitochondria, etc.			
Chromosomes	1 circular ds DNA	1 circular ds DNA	several linear ds DNA chromosomes			
Life cycle	asexual repro. (binary fission)	asexual repro. (binary fission)	varied (sexual and asexual)	varied (sexual and asexual)	mostly sexual reproduction	mostly sexual reproduction
Ploidy and Cellularity	Unicellular	Unicellular	Mostly unicellular	Mostly multi-cellular and mostly haploid	Multicellular, alternates between haploid and diploid	Multicellular and diploid
Cellular motility	flagella	flagella	amoeboid or flagellar	non-motile	some flagellated sperm	amoeboid or flagellar
Cilia/flagella	unique structure	unique structure	characteristic 9 + 2 arrangement of microtubules			
Nutrition	varied, absorptive	varied, absorptive	varied	chemohetero., absorptive	most photo-auto. w/chlorophyll	chemohetero., ingestive
Glycolysis/ ATP	All living organisms perform glycolysis and use ATP. All kingdoms contain at least some members which perform oxidative phosphorylation.					
Examples	bacteria and blue-green algae	Archaea (extremophiles)	*Plasmodium* plankton, algae, kelp, seaweed	yeasts, molds, mushrooms, truffles	trees, flowers, mosses, ferns	sponges, worms, mollusks, insects, reptiles, birds, mammals

Table 2 Taxonomic Characteristics

---

[106] A mnemonic goes: "Dumb King Philip Came Over From Greece Sunday" (or "Dumb King Phil Came Over For Great...").

Domain Bacteria and Domain Archaea were both previously classified into Kingdom Monera. Because of huge diversity in these organisms, they have since been separated into two domains, and for these organisms, the kingdom and domain are the same.

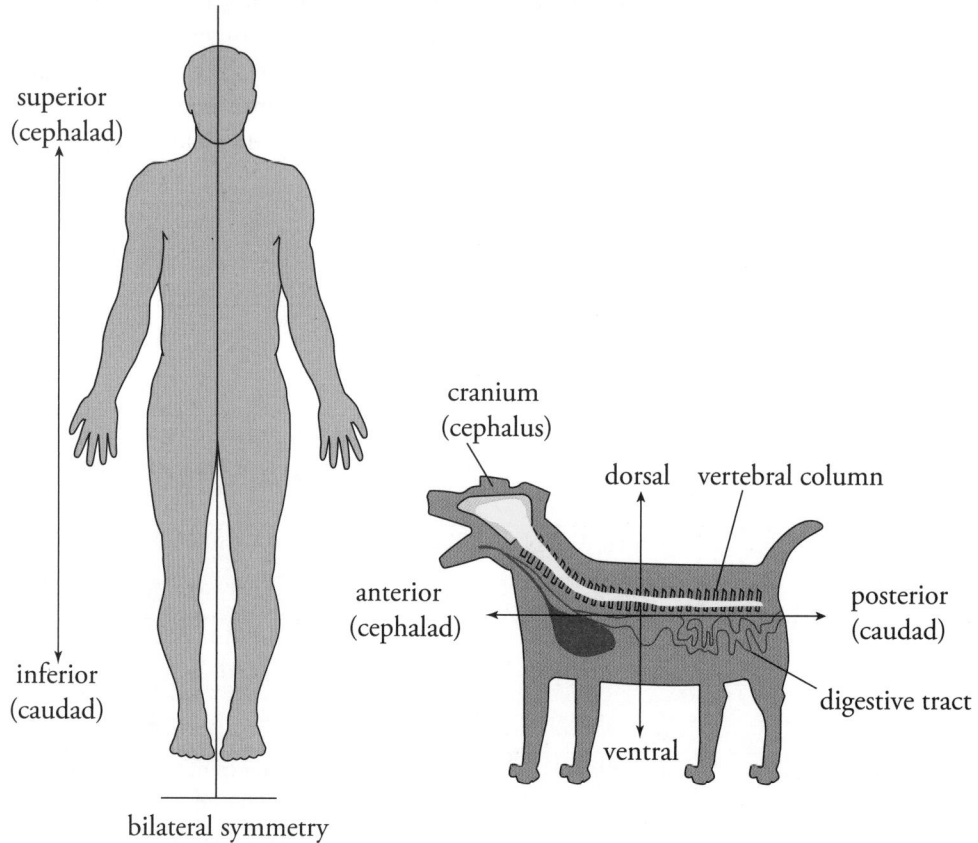

7.10

Figure 18 Bilateral Symmetry and the Anatomical Axes

Anatomists describe bodies with reference to axes such as the dorsal-ventral axis and the anterior-posterior axis (Figure 18). These are imaginary planes through the body. **Anterior** means "front-facing"; **posterior** is the opposite. **Dorsal** means "on top." A shark has a "dorsal fin," and the spines of dogs and humans are considered dorsal as well. **Ventral** is the opposite of dorsal. The belly button is a ventral structure in dogs and humans. In humans, **superior** is used to indicate "toward the head." **Inferior** means "toward the feet." Another way to say "toward the head" is **cephalad**. (Cephalus is Latin for head.) The opposite is **caudad**, meaning "toward the tail." [Does the axis of bilateral symmetry in vertebrates run parallel or perpendicular to the dorsal-ventral axis?[107]]

—

[107] The dorsal-ventral axis slices the body in half, separating front from back. The axis of symmetry separates left from right. So the two axes are perpendicular. Remember, the axes are planes, not lines.

7.11 THE ORIGIN OF LIFE

Based on radioisotope dating, the Earth is thought to be 4.5 billion years old. All life evolved from pro-karyotes. The oldest fossils are 3.5 billion-year-old outlines of primitive prokaryotic cell walls found in stromatolites (layered mats formed by colonies of prokaryotes). Even older life forms certainly existed, but lacked cell walls and thus left no fossil record (at least none have yet been discovered). Therefore, life on Earth is older than 3.5 billion years, nearly as old as the planet itself.

The atmosphere of the young Earth was different from today's atmosphere. The predominant gases then were probably H_2O, CO, CO_2, and N_2. The most important thing to note here is the absence of O_2. It is thought that the early atmosphere was a **reducing environment**, where electron donors were prevalent (see Chapter 3). Oxygen is an electron acceptor, and as such tends to break organic bonds. In this early world, simple organic molecules, or monomers ("single units") could form spontaneously. The energy for this synthesis was provided by lightning, radioactive decay, volcanic activity, or the Sun's radiation, which was more intense than it is today due to the thinner atmosphere. Laboratory recreations of the early envi-ronment result in the spontaneous formation of amino acids, carbohydrates, lipids, and ribonucleotides, as well as other organic compounds.

Spontaneous polymerization of these monomers can also be observed in the lab (including spontaneous polymerization of ribonucleotides). No enzymes were present when this was occurring for the first time in nature, but it is thought that metal ions on the surface of rocks and especially clay acted as catalysts. This is known as **abiotic synthesis**. Polypeptides made in this way are called **proteinoids**.

Proteinoids in water spontaneously form droplets called **microspheres**. When lipids are added to the solution **liposomes** form, with lipids forming a layer on the surface of proteins. A more complex particle known as a **coacervate** includes polypeptides, nucleic acids, and polysaccharides. Coacervates made with pre-existing enzymes are capable of catalyzing reactions. Microspheres, liposomes, and coacervates are collectively referred to as **protobionts**.

Protobionts resemble cells in that they contain a protected inner environment and perform chemical reactions. They can also reproduce to a certain extent: when they grow too large they split in half. What is lacking, however, is an organized mechanism of heredity. This was first provided by RNA. As noted previously, RNA chains form spontaneously in the appropriate solution. Even more interesting is the observation that single-stranded RNA chains can be self-replicating. A daughter chain lines up on the parent by base pairing and then spontaneously polymerizes with a surprisingly low error rate. A non-specific catalyst such as a metal ion can further increase the efficiency of RNA self-replication. Further-more, it is now known that RNA has catalytic activity in modern cells. For example, in primitive eukary-otes, introns are spliced out of the mRNA by **ribozymes**, which are RNA enzymes.

Somehow a mechanism evolved for polypeptides to be copied from early RNA genes. You already know about the inherent tendency for phospholipids to form lipid bilayers. Given all this information, it's not too hard to imagine true cells evolving from a primordial soup at the dawn of time. The last step in the evolution of the earliest cells would have been the switch from RNA to DNA as the genetic material. DNA is more stable due to its 2'-deoxy structure and also due to the fact that it spontaneously forms a compact double-stranded helix.

7.11

Chapter 7 Summary

- Organisms express phenotypes (physical characteristics) according to their genotypes (combinations of alleles).

- From a single diploid precursor cell, meiosis generates four haploid cells (gametes) with a random mix of alleles. This is due to crossing over in prophase I and separation of homologous chromosomes in anaphase I. Nondisjunction is a failure to separate the DNA properly during meiosis, and it can result in gametes with improper numbers of chromosomes.

- The Punnett square or the rules of probability can be used to determine the genotypes and phenotypes of offspring from given crosses, or the probability of having offspring with certain traits.

- The rule of multiplication states that the probability of A and B occurring is equal to the probability of A multiplied by the probability of B.

- The rule of addition states that the probability of A or B occurring is equal to the probability of A plus the probability of B, minus the probability of A and B together.

- Classical dominance occurs when a phenotype or trait is determined by one gene with two alleles, and one allele is dominant (expressed) and the other is recessive (silent). There are several exceptions to classical dominance, including incomplete dominance, codominance, epistasis, pleiotropism, polygenism, and penetrance.

- Incomplete dominance occurs when two different alleles for a single trait result in a blended phenotype. Codominance occurs when two different alleles for a single trait are expressed simultaneously, but independently (no blending).

- Epistasis occurs when the expression of one gene depends on the expression of another.

- Pleitropic genes affect many different aspects of the overall phenotype, while polygenic traits are affected by many different genes.

- Penetrance refers to the likelihood that a particular genotype will result in a given phenotype. Penetrance can be affected by several factors including age, environment, and lifestyle.

- Linkage occurs when two genes are close together on the same chromosome; it leads to alleles being inherited together (less recombination) instead of independently.

- The Hardy-Weinberg law can be used to study population genetics. It assumes classical dominance with only two alleles and unchanging allele frequencies. It is based on five assumptions: no mutation, no natural selection, no migration, large populations, and totally random mating.

- Natural selection drives evolution by allowing individuals with random, beneficial mutations to survive and pass those beneficial mutations on to their offspring.

- Homologous structures are the result of divergent evolution to form new species, and analogous structures are the result of convergent evolution, in which different start species must meet similar environmental challenges.

CHAPTER 7 FREESTANDING PRACTICE QUESTIONS

1. A woman is phenotypically normal but had a brother who had an autosomal recessive disorder that resulted in death during infancy. What is the probability that this woman is a carrier for the disorder that afflicted her brother?

A) 1/4
B) 1/3
C) 1/2
D) 2/3

2. A set of inherited traits show a phenotypic ratio of 9:3:3:1 among offspring of a given mating. A possible explanation for this observation is a two locus–two allele system where each locus exhibits:

A) independent assortment.
B) linkage.
C) epistasis.
D) incomplete dominance.

3. If a woman is a carrier for an X-linked recessive disorder and mates with a normal, unaffected male, what is the probability her grandson has the disorder? Assume she has a normal son and a daughter, and they both have homozygous normal partners.

A) 0
B) 1/4
C) 1/2
D) 3/4

4. In fruit flies, the gene that produces white eyes is X-linked recessive (red eyes are dominant to white). Two autosomal genes determine body color and leg length; a brown body is dominant to ebony and long legs are dominant to short. Assume dominant alleles are considered wild-type. A white-eyed male is mated to an ebony colored, short-legged female. The resulting F_1 males are all wild type. If these males are backcrossed to the female parent, what is the probability that an F_2 offspring will be a wild-type male?

A) 0
B) 1/2
C) 1/4
D) 1/8

5. A geneticist is analyzing a family tree, where mothers affected by the trait under study pass the trait on to 100% of their offspring, both sons and daughters. Fathers affected by the trait pass it on to 0% of their offspring. All affected individuals have an affected mother. What is the inheritance pattern of this trait?

A) Y-linked
B) Autosomal dominant
C) Autosomal recessive
D) Mitochondrial

6. A purebred long-tailed cat with long whiskers (*TTww*) is mated to a purebred short-tailed cat with short whiskers (*ttWW*). The kittens will be:

A) 100% long-tailed with long whiskers.
B) 100% long-tailed with short whiskers.
C) 100% short-tailed with short whiskers.
D) 50% long-tailed cat with long whiskers, 50% short-tailed cat with short whiskers.

7. A homozygous white bull is mated to a homozygous cow with a red coat. The offspring all have a roan coat color, which is composed of a mix of white hairs and red hairs. Which of the following is true?

A) Coat color in cattle is an example of codominance.
B) White hair is recessive to red hair.
C) Coat color in cattle is an example of incomplete dominance.
D) White hair is dominant over red hair.

8. If the genes for ear size (*E* or *e*) and aggressiveness (*A* or *a*) in mice are linked and 25 mu apart, what is the probability of getting a large-eared aggressive pup (*EeAa*) from a mating between a small-eared aggressive female (*eeAA*) and a large-eared nonaggressive male (*EEaa*)?

A) 12.5%
B) 25%
C) 75%
D) 100%

CHAPTER 7 PRACTICE PASSAGE

The fruit fly, *Drosophila melanogaster*, is an ideal organism on which to study genetic mechanisms. This organism has simple food requirements, occupies little space, and the reproductive life cycle is complete in about 12 days at room temperature, allowing for quick analysis of test crosses. In addition, fruit flies produce large numbers of offspring, which allows for sufficient data to be collected quickly. Many *Drosophila* genes are homologous to human genes, and are studied to gain a better understanding of what role these proteins have in humans.

To understand the inheritance patterns of certain genes in *Drosophila*, the following experiments were carried out. Assume that the alleles for red eyes, brown body, and normal wings are dominant and the alleles for white eyes, ebony body, and vestigial wings are recessive.

Experiment 1:

A red-eyed female and a white-eye male were crossed. The subsequent generation of flies was also crossed. The phenotypic results of both generations are shown below:

Generation	Red-eyed female	White-eyed female	Red-eyed male	White-eyed male
Parental	1	0	0	1
F_1	9	0	13	0
F_2	27	0	12	14

Experiment 2:

Five of the red-eyed female *Drosophila* from the F_1 generation of Experiment 1 were crossed with white-eyed males. The result of this cross is shown below:

Generation	Red-eyed female	White-eyed female	Red-eyed male	White-eyed male
F_1	5	0	0	10
F_2	8	8	9	8

Experiment 3:

The white-eyed females from Experiment 2 were crossed with red-eyed males. The result of this cross is shown below:

Generation	Red-eyed female	White-eyed female	Red-eyed male	White-eyed male
Parental	0	8	7	0
F_1	9	0	0	10

Experiment 4:

A male heterozygous for body color and wing type is crossed with an ebony, vestigial-winged female. The results of the cross are shown below:

Phenotype	Male	Female
Brown body, normal wings	32	30
Brown body, vestigial wings	2	1
Ebony body, normal wings	1	3
Ebony body, vestigial wings	28	33

1. What is the most likely mode of inheritance for white eye color?

A) X-linked recessive
B) X-linked dominant
C) Autosomal recessive
D) Autosomal dominant

2. What ratio of white-eyed to red-eyed females would be expected if the F_1 generation of Experiment 3 were crossed?

A) White-eyed females would not be present.
B) Red-eyed females would not be present.
C) 1:1
D) 1:2

3. Approximately how many of the red-eyed females of the F_2 generation of Experiment 2 are homozygous dominant?

A) 0
B) 2
C) 4
D) 8

4. Which of the following statements is/are true with regard to the results obtained from Experiment 4?

   I. The genes for body color and wing type are on the same chromosome.
  II. Recombination occurred.
 III. The heterozygous male had a dominant and recessive allele on each homologous chromosome.

A) I only
B) I and II
C) I and III
D) II only

5. What is the recombination frequency shown by the results of Experiment 4?

A) Recombination did not occur.
B) 5%
C) 50%
D) 95%

6. If the frequency of vestigial wings in a population of *Drosophila* ($n = 1500$) is 4%, how many flies would be heterozygous with regard to wing type? Assume random mating, but no migration, mutation, random drift, or natural selection.

A) 60
B) 240
C) 480
D) 960

SOLUTIONS TO CHAPTER 7 FREESTANDING PRACTICE QUESTIONS

1. **D**   If the woman's brother was affected with this autosomal recessive disorder, both of her parents must have been carriers for the trait. Since it is lethal in infancy, you know both parents must have been heterozygous. The mating between two heterozygotes produces the following genotypic ratio in their offspring: 25% homozygous recessive, 50% heterozygous, 25% homozygous dominant. Since the woman is phenotypically normal, she must not have the disorder, so she is not in the 25% homozygous recessive group. She is either in the 25% homozygous dominant group or the 50% heterozygous group, so the chance she is a carrier is 2/3 (choice D is correct).

2. **A**   If two heterozygous parents are mated (for example, $AaBb \times AaBb$), the expected F_1 phenotype ratio if the two traits are assorting independently is 9:3:3:1 (choice A is correct). If linkage were occurring, this ratio would be skewed after the mating of two double heterozygotes, since alleles would be preferentially inherited together. Since the ratio is not skewed, linkage is not occurring (choice B can be eliminated). This is not a case where one gene is silencing another, or controlling the expression of the other, as this would also lead to a skewed ratio (choice C can be eliminated). Incomplete dominance of two alleles leads to a blended heterozygous phenotype; thus, if it occurs at a single locus, it produces three different phenotypes. If it were to occur at two different loci (as in this case), there would be nine possible phenotypes (3 possible phenotypes at the first locus times 3 possible phenotypes at the second locus = $3^2 = 9$). In this case there are only four different phenotypes (choice D can be eliminated).

3. **B**   If we assign "A" as the normal allele and "a" as the affected allele, the woman is $X^A X^a$ and her mate is $X^A Y$. The question stem says that she has a normal son, who must have the genotype $X^A Y$; he received the X^A from his mother and his Y chromosome from his father. There is no probability associated with this that must be factored into the solution, because this is the only way the couple could have a normal son. If this son mates with a homozygous normal female, he will pass his Y chromosome onto his son(s), which means there is zero chance of having an affected son. In other words, an $X^A Y \times X^A X^A$ mating cannot generate $X^a Y$ sons. Next, let's work with the daughter of the woman in the question stem. The question says she has a normal phenotype. She must receive an X^A from her father. There is a 50% probability she will receive an X^a from her mother. If the daughter is $X^A X^a$ (remember there is a 50% chance of this) and her mate is $X^A Y$, there is a 50% chance their son will be affected. Overall, then, the probability that a grandson is affected is $0 + (1/2)(1/2)$, or 1/4. Therefore, choice B is correct.

4. **D**   Assign X^R = red eyes (dominant and wild-type), X^r = white eyes, B = brown body color (dominant and wild-type), b = ebony body color, S = long legs (dominant and wild-type), and s = short legs. Since all the male offspring from the first cross are wild-type, then the male parent must have been homozygous for body color and leg length, and the female parent must have been homozygous for eye color; thus, the first cross is $X^r Y BBSS \times X^R X^R bbss$. The male F_1 offspring will be $X^r Y BbSs$. Next, this male was backcrossed to the female parent ($X^R Y BbSs \times X^R X^R bbss$), and you are asked for the probability of a wild-type male. This is equal to the probability of a male (1/2), multiplied by the probability that it will have brown

body color (1/2), multiplied by the probability that it will have long legs (1/2). Therefore, the probability of a wild-type male is = 1/2 × 1/2 × 1/2 = 1/8 (choice D is correct). Notice that you do not have to factor in the probability of the F_2 being red-eyed because this is guaranteed given the genotype of their mother.

5. **D**   Females are not affected by Y-linked traits (choice A is wrong). If the trait was autosomal dominant, affected fathers would pass the trait to at least some of their offspring (choice B is wrong). Autosomal recessive traits do not demonstrate the sex bias that is described in the question stem (choice C is incorrect). By Process of Elimination, this trait must be inherited via the mitochondrial genome. All humans inherit their mitochondrial genome from their mothers; during fertilization, the sperm only contributes 23 chromosomes but the ovum contributes 23 chromosomes along with all other cellular organelles and cytoplasm (choice D is correct).

6. **B**   The offspring will be 100% *TtWw* and will display the dominant phenotype for each trait. Since each parent has a dominant and a recessive phenotype, the kittens will not have the phenotype of either parent (choice B is correct, and choices A, C, and D are wrong).

7. **A**   Since the offspring are neither red nor white, this trait is not inherited via simple Mendelian genetics, and neither trait is dominant or recessive (choices B and D are wrong). The individual hairs on the F_1 cattle are either red or white, which means that both alleles are being expressed. This best matches the definition of codominance (choice A is correct). If the individual hairs were a blend of white and red, the best answer would have been incomplete dominance (choice C is wrong).

8. **D**   The pups will get *eA* from their mom and *Ea* from their dad. All the pups will be *eA/Ea*, so the answer must be choice D. Note that the linkage information was not useful in answering this question.

SOLUTIONS TO CHAPTER 7 PRACTICE PASSAGE

1. **A**   The passage states that the allele for red eyes is dominant and the allele for white eyes is recessive (choices B and D are wrong). The results from Experiment 1 suggest that the gene for eye color is X-linked. If it were autosomal, all F_1 flies from that experiment would be heterozygous, and there would be an equal distribution of both genders and colors in the F_2 generation. Remember that a gender bias in the phenotype of a trait usually indicates that you're working with a sex-linked trait.

2. **C**   The passage states that the red allele is dominant and the white allele is recessive; further eye color is a sex-linked trait (see the explanation for Question 1). For Experiment 3, the female parental genotype must be homozygous recessive (X^cX^c), and the male parental genotype must be X^CY. Thus, the F_1 generation consists of heterozygous females (X^CX^c) and males with the recessive white-eyed allele (X^cY). If these two were mated with each other, the female progeny of this generation would consist of homozygous recessive (X^cX^c) and heterozygous (X^CX^c) females in an approximate 1:1 ratio (choice C is correct).

3. **A** Experiment 2 is a cross between an F_1 female and a white-eyed male. The genotype of the F_1 females from Experiment 1 is $X^C X^c$; they have red eyes, so they must have X^C, and they are female, so they inherited X^c from their white-eyed father. If these $X^C X^c$ females are crossed with $X^c Y$ (white-eyed) males, the females generated in the F_2 must be 50% $X^C X^c$ (red-eyed) and 50% $X^c X^c$ (white-eyed). If the father has white eyes, it is impossible to generate homozygous red-eyed females in the F_2 (choice A is correct).

4. **B** There is no sex bias in the results from Experiment 4, so you can assume the alleles are autosomal. The passage states that the alleles for brown bodies and normal wings are dominant, and the alleles for ebony bodies and vestigial wings are recessive. Let's assign B = brown and b = ebony for body color, and W = normal and w = vestigial for wing phenotype. Thus, the cross in Experiment 4 is $BbWw \times bbww$. Item I is true: if the genes for body color and wing type were on separate chromosomes, one would expect the law of independent assortment to hold true and the phenotypic ratio of the progeny would be expected to be 1:1:1:1. However, this is not the case. Two of the phenotypes predominate, indicating that the genes are close together on the same chromosome, or are linked (choice D can be eliminated). Item II is also true: the recombinant phenotypes, although rare, are nonetheless seen. Recombination between homologous chromosomes is the best explanation for this observation (choices A and C can be eliminated, and choice B is correct). Note that Item III is false: the double heterozygous *Drosophila* must have both dominant alleles on one chromosome and both recessive alleles on the other to account for the results seen. In other words, the cross performed was $BW/bw \times bw/bw$. The parental combinations of alleles are BW and bw (more frequent), and the recombinant combinations of alleles (less frequent) are Bw and bW.

5. **B** Recombination did in fact occur (see explanation for Question 4; choice A is wrong). Recombination frequency = number of recombinants/total number of offspring. In this case, the total number of recombinants is 7 and the total number of offspring is 130. 7/130 = 0.05 or 5% recombination frequency (choice B is correct, and choices C and D are wrong). Note that choice D is the frequency of non-recombination, and choice C would be correct if the genes were not linked.

6. **C** Using the Hardy-Weinberg equations for allele frequency and genotype, the frequency of the vestigial wing allele (q) must be equal to $\sqrt{0.04}$, or 0.20. Therefore, the frequency of the normal wing allele (p) is 0.80 and the frequency of the heterozygous genotype (pq and qp) is equal to $2 \times 0.2 \times 0.8$, or 0.32. The actual number of *Drosophila* that would have this genotype would be 480 (0.32 × 1500).

Chapter 8
The Nervous and Endocrine Systems

The nervous and endocrine systems are presented in the same chapter since their functions are related: they both provide communication, integrating, and coordinating the activities of the tissues and organs of the body. The means of communication by the two systems are quite different (although complementary) in many ways. The nervous system communicates through electrochemical signals (action potentials), while the endocrine system uses chemical messengers carried in the blood (hormones). The nervous system in general regulates rapid responses such as those of skeletal muscle or smooth muscle, while the endocrine system takes longer to have an effect and regulates longer-term responses such as metabolism and homeostasis. The two systems are interconnected, with two of the primary endocrine glands—the pituitary and the adrenals—regulated by the nervous system, and with the endocrine system feeding back to modulate the nervous system.

8.1 NEURONAL STRUCTURE AND FUNCTION

Neurons are specialized cells that transmit and process information from one part of the body to another. This information takes the form of electrochemical impulses known as **action potentials**. The action potential is a localized area of depolarization of the plasma membrane that travels in a wave-like manner along an axon. When an action potential reaches the end of an axon at a synapse, the signal is transformed into a chemical signal with the release of neurotransmitter into the synaptic cleft, a process called **synaptic transmission** (Section 8.2). The information of many synapses feeding into a neuron is integrated to determine whether that neuron will in turn fire an action potential. In this way the action of many individual neurons is integrated to work together in the nervous system as a whole.

Structure of the Neuron

The basic functional and structural unit of the nervous system is the **neuron** (Figure 1 on the next page). The structure of these cells is highly specialized to transmit and process **action potentials**, the electrochemical signals of the nervous system (Figure 3, page 283). Neurons have a central cell body, the **soma**, which contains the nucleus and is where most of the biosynthetic activity of the cell takes place. Slender projections, termed **axons** and **dendrites**, extend from the cell body. Neurons have only one axon (as long as a meter in some cases), but most possess many dendrites. Neurons with one dendrite are termed **bipolar**; those with many dendrites are **multipolar**. Neurons generally carry action potentials in one direction, with dendrites receiving signals and axons carrying action potentials away from the cell body. Axons can branch multiple times and terminate in **synaptic knobs** that form connections with target cells. When action potentials travel down an axon and reach the synaptic knob, chemical messengers are released and travel across a very small gap called the **synaptic cleft** to the target cell. The nature of the action potential and the transmission of signals across the synaptic cleft are key aspects of nervous system function. [In Figure 1, in what direction does an action potential travel in the axon shown?[1] What's the difference between a neuron and a nerve?[2]]

---

[1] Action potentials travel from the cell body down the axon, or from left to right in Figure 1.

[2] A neuron is a single cell. A nerve is a large bundle of many different axons from different neurons.

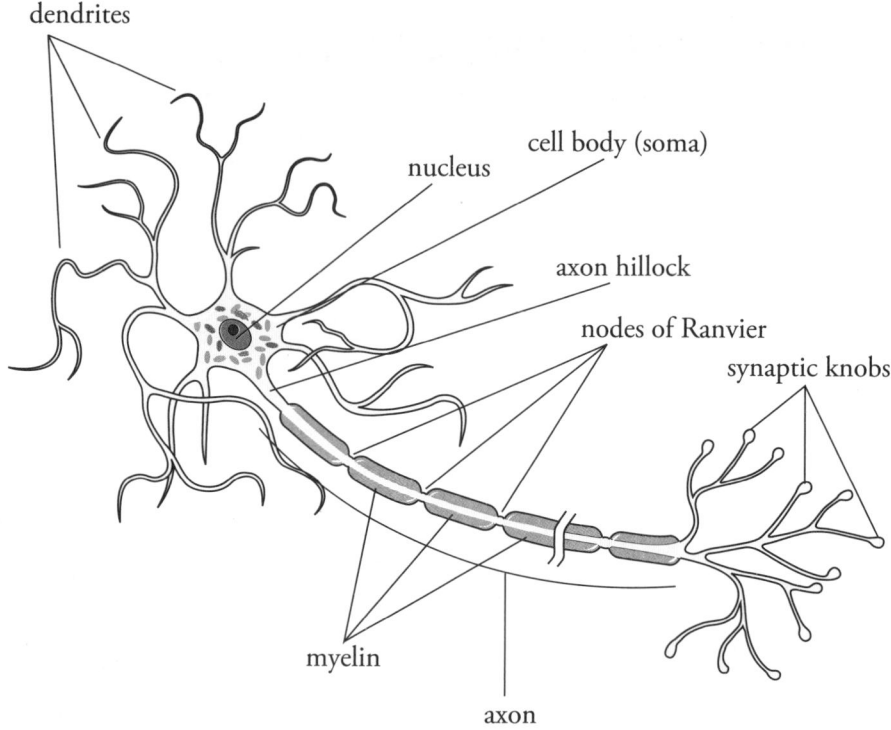

Figure 1   A Multipolar Neuron

- A motor protein called *kinesin* is one of several different proteins that drive movement of vesicles and organelles along microtubules in axons. Kinesin specifically drives anterograde movement (movement from the soma toward the axon terminus). If a kinesin inhibitor is added to neurons in culture, what is the likely result?[3]
    - A) Spontaneous action potentials
    - B) Cell division
    - C) Accumulation of material in the synaptic knob
    - D) Atrophy of axons

The Action Potential

The Resting Membrane Potential

The **resting membrane potential** is an electric potential across the plasma membrane of approximately −70 millivolts (mV), with the interior of the cell negatively charged with respect to the exterior of the cell.

---

[3] A large amount of biosynthetic activity takes place in the cell body, and materials are transported from the cell body down the axon to its end by kinesin. The correct answer is choice **D**. If material cannot be transported through the axon from the cell body, the axon will atrophy. Note that although this may not immediately be apparent, choices A, B, and C should have been easily eliminated; kinesin has nothing to do with action potentials, neurons in general do not divide (and inhibiting kinesin should not change this), and the inhibition of kinesin would prevent materials from accumulating at the synaptic knobs.

Two primary membrane proteins are required to establish the resting membrane potential: the Na$^+$/K$^+$ ATPase and the potassium leak channels. The **Na$^+$/K$^+$ ATPase** pumps three sodium ions out of the cell and two potassium ions into the cell with the hydrolysis of one ATP molecule. [What form of transport is carried out by the Na$^+$/K$^+$ ATPase?[4]] The result is a sodium gradient with high sodium outside of the cell and a potassium gradient with high potassium inside the cell. **Leak channels** are channels that are open all the time, and that simply allow ions to "leak" across the membrane according to their gradient. Potassium leak channels allow potassium, but no other ions, to flow down their gradient out of the cell. The combined loss of many positive ions through Na$^+$/K$^+$ ATPases and the potassium leak channels leaves the interior of the cell with a net negative charge, approximately 70 mV more negative than the exterior of the cell; this difference is the resting membrane potential. Note that there are very few sodium leak channels in the membrane (the ratio of K$^+$ leak channels to Na$^+$ leak channels is about 100:1), so the cell membrane is virtually impermeable to sodium.

- Are neurons the only cells with a resting membrane potential?[5]
- If the potassium leak channels are blocked, what will happen to the membrane potential?[6]
- What would happen to the membrane potential if sodium ions were allowed to flow down their concentration gradient?[7]

The resting membrane potential establishes a negative charge along the interior of axons (along with the rest of the neuronal interior). Thus, the cells can be described as **polarized**; negative on the inside and positive on the outside. An action potential is a disturbance in this membrane potential, a wave of **depolarization** of the plasma membrane that travels along an axon. Depolarization is a change in the membrane potential from the resting membrane potential of approximately –70 mV to a less negative, or even positive, potential. After depolarization, **repolarization** returns the membrane potential to normal. The change in membrane potential during the passage of an action potential is caused by movement of ions into and out of the neuron through ion channels. The action potential is therefore not strictly an electrical impulse, like electrons moving in a copper telephone wire, but an electro*chemical* impulse.

Depolarization

Key proteins in the propagation of action potentials are the **voltage-gated sodium channels** located in the plasma membrane of the axon. In response to a change in the membrane potential, these ion channels open to allow sodium ions to flow down their gradient into the cell and depolarize that section of membrane. [What is the effect of opening the voltage-gated sodium channels on the membrane potential?[8]] These channels are opened by depolarization of the membrane from the resting potential of –70 mV to a **threshold potential** of approximately –50 mV. Once this threshold is reached, the channels are opened fully, but below the threshold they are closed and do not allow the passage of any ions through the channel. When the channels open, sodium flows into the cell, down its concentration gradient, depolarizing that

---

[4] The Na$^+$/K$^+$ ATPase uses ATP to drive transport against a gradient; this is primary active transport.

[5] No. All cells have the resting membrane potential. Neurons and muscle tissue are unique in using the resting membrane potential to generate action potentials.

[6] The flow of potassium out of the cell makes the interior of the cell more negatively charged. Blocking the potassium leak channels would reduce the magnitude of the resting membrane potential, making the interior of the cell less negative.

[7] Sodium ions would flow into the cell and reduce the potential across the plasma membrane, making the interior of the cell less negative and even relatively positive if enough ions flow into the cell.

[8] Sodium (positively charged) flows into the cell, down its concentration gradient, making the interior of the cell less negatively charged, or even positively charged.

section of the membrane to about +35 mV before inactivating. Some of the sodium ions flow down the interior of the axon, slightly depolarizing the neighboring section of membrane. When the depolarization in the next section of membrane reaches threshold, those voltage-gated sodium channels open as well, passing the depolarization down the axon (Figure 2). [If an action potential starts at one end of an axon, can it run out of energy and not reach the other end?[9]]

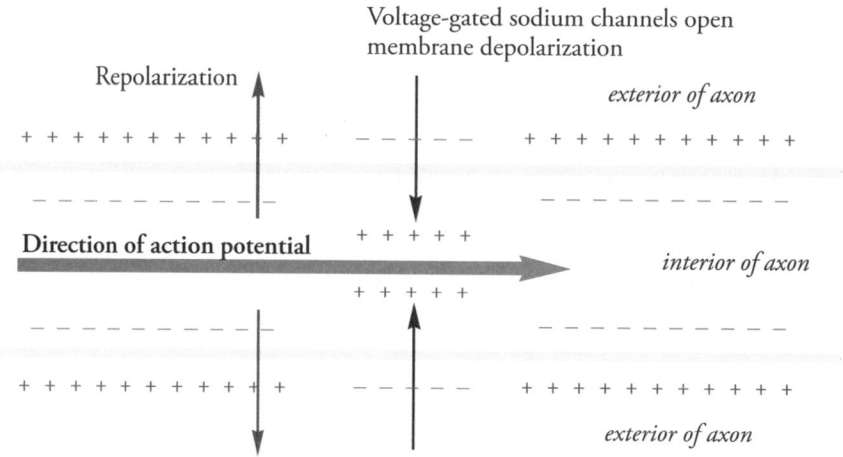

Figure 2   The Action Potential is a Wave of Membrane Depolarization

- Which one of the following can cause the interior of the neuron to have a momentary positive charge?[10]
    A) Opening of potassium leak channels
    B) Activity of the Na+/K+ ATPase
    C) Opening of voltage-gated sodium channels
    D) Opening of voltage-gated potassium channels

- Given the above description, which of the following best describes the response of voltage-gated sodium channels to a membrane depolarization from –70 mV to –60 mV?[11]
    A) All of the channels open fully.
    B) 50% of the channels open fully.
    C) All of the channels open 50%.
    D) None of the channels open.

---

[9]   No, it cannot. Action potentials are continually renewed at each point in the axon as they travel. Assuming there are enough voltage-gated channels, once an action potential starts, it will propagate without a change in amplitude (size) until it reaches a synapse.

[10]   Choices A, B, and D all make the interior of the cell more negative. Choice **C** is the answer. Voltage-gated sodium channels can make the interior of the cell momentarily positive during passage of an action potential.

[11]   Voltage-gated sodium channels require a threshold depolarization to open. A depolarization below the threshold will produce essentially no response, while a depolarization greater than or equal to the threshold will cause all of the channels to open fully. This is called an **all-or-none** response. The correct answer is choice **D**. The depolarization is less than the threshold, so there is no response.

Repolarization

With the opening of voltage-gated sodium channels, sodium flows into the cell and depolarizes the membrane to positive values. As the wave of depolarization passes through a region of membrane, however, the membrane does not remain depolarized (Figure 3).

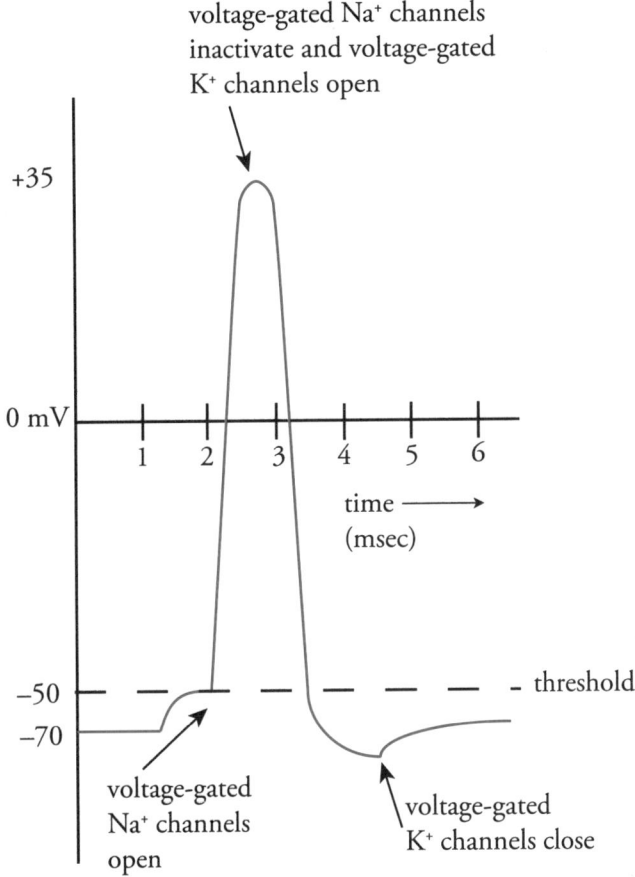

Figure 3   The Action Potential at a Single Location

After depolarization, the membrane is **repolarized**, re-establishing the original resting membrane potential. A number of factors combine to produce this effect:

1)   Voltage-gated sodium channels **inactivate** very quickly after they open, shutting off the flow of sodium into the cell. The channels remain inactivated until the membrane potential nears resting values again.

2)   Voltage-gated potassium channels open more slowly than the voltage-gated sodium channels and stay open longer. Voltage-gated potassium channels open in response to membrane depolarization. As potassium leaves the cell down its concentration gradient, the membrane potential returns to negative values, actually overshooting the resting potential by about 20 mV (to about −90 mV). At this point the voltage-gated potassium channels close.

3)   Potassium leak channels and the Na^+/K^+ ATPase continue to function (as they always do) to bring the membrane back to resting potential. These factors alone would repolarize the membrane potential even without the voltage-gated potassium channels, but it would take a lot longer.

- If a toxin prevents voltage-gated sodium channels from closing, which of the following will occur?[12]
    - I. Voltage-gated potassium channels will open but not close.
    - II. The membrane will not repolarize to the normal resting membrane potential.
    - III. The Na⁺/K⁺ ATPase will be inactivated.

    A) I only
    B) II only
    C) I and II only
    D) II and III only

Saltatory Conduction

The axons of many neurons are wrapped in an insulating sheath called **myelin** (Figure 4). The myelin sheath is not created by the neuron itself, but by cells called **Schwann cells**[13], a type of glial cell, that exist in conjunction with neurons, wrapping layers of specialized membrane around the axons. No ions can enter or exit a neuron where the axonal membrane is covered with myelin. [Would an axon be able to conduct action potentials if its entire length were wrapped in myelin?[14]] There is no membrane depolarization and no voltage-gated sodium channels in regions of the axonal plasma membrane that are wrapped in myelin. There are periodic gaps in the myelin sheath however, called **nodes of Ranvier** (Figures 1, 4, and 5). Voltage-gated sodium and potassium channels are concentrated in the nodes of Ranvier in myelinated axons. Rather than impeding action potentials, the myelin sheath dramatically speeds the movement of action potentials by forcing the action potential to jump from node to node. This rapid jumping conduction in myelinated axons is termed **saltatory conduction**.

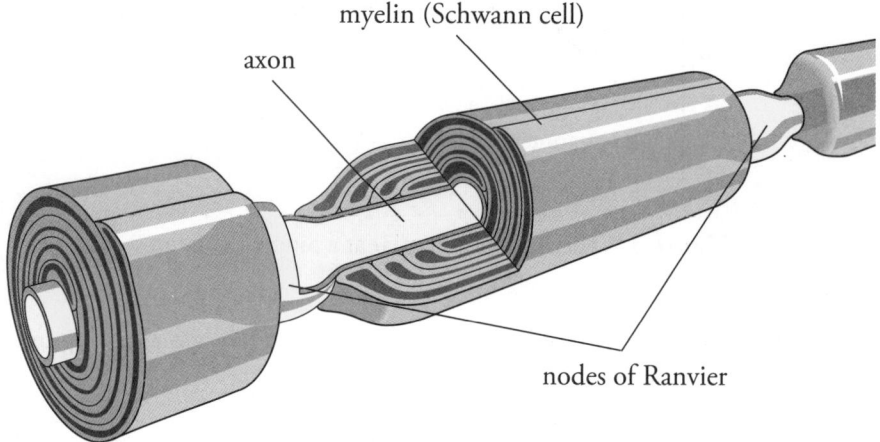

Figure 4 A Schwann Cell Wrapping an Axon with Myelin

---

[12] **Item I is true:** voltage-gated potassium channels are normally closed by the repolarization of the membrane, so if the membrane is not repolarized, they will not close. **Item II is true:** sodium ions will continue to flow into the cell, even as the Na⁺/K⁺ ATPase works to pump them out. This will prevent the repolarization of the membrane. Item III is false: the Na⁺/K⁺ ATPase will work harder than ever. The answer is choice **C**.

[13] Schwann cells are found in the peripheral nervous system (PNS). In the central nervous system (CNS) myelination of axons is accomplished via similar cells called oligodendrocytes.

[14] No. The action potential requires the movement of ions across the plasma membrane to create a wave of depolarization.

- • Which one of the following is true concerning myelinated and unmyelinated axons?[15]
  - A) The amount of energy consumed by the Na⁺/K⁺ ATPase is much less in myelinated axons than in unmyelinated axons.
  - B) Myelinated axons can conduct many more action potentials per second than can unmyelinated axons.
  - C) The size of action potential depolarization is much greater in myelinated axons than in unmyelinated axons.
  - D) Voltage-gated potassium channels do not play a role in repolarization in unmyelinated axons.

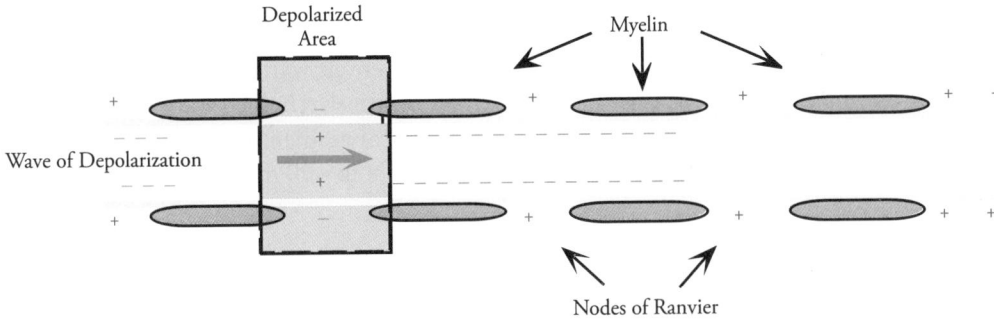

Figure 5   Propagation of the AP in a Myelinated Axon (cross section)

Glial Cells

As mentioned above, the myelin sheath is formed by a type of glial cell called a Schwann cell. However, Schwann cells are not the only type of glial cell. **Glial cells** are specialized, non-neuronal cells that typically provide structural and metabolic support to neurons (Table 1). Glia maintain a resting membrane potential but do not generate action potentials.

Table 1   Types of Glial Cells and Their Functions

Cell Type	Location	Primary Functions
Schwann cells	PNS	Form myelin—increase speed of conduction of APs along axon
Oligodendrocytes	CNS	Form myelin—increase speed of conduction of APs along axon
Astrocytes	CNS	Guide neuronal development Regulate synaptic communication via regulation of neurotransmitter levels
Microglia	CNS	Remove dead cells and debris
Ependymal cells	CNS	Produce and circulate cerebrospinal fluid

---

[15] Since the area of membrane that is conducting is much less in myelinated axons, Na⁺/K⁺ ATPase only works to maintain the resting potential in the nodes of Ranvier, whereas in unmyelinated axons the Na⁺/K⁺ ATPase hydrolyzes ATP to maintain the resting potential across the entire membrane (choice **A** is correct). The length of the refractory period (and hence the frequency of action potentials) is based on the characteristics of the voltage-gated sodium and potassium channels, which do not change (choice B is false). The size of depolarization in an action potential does not vary greatly; action potentials are an all-or-nothing response (choice C is false). Voltage-gated potassium channels are the same in both neurons (choice D is false).

Equilibrium Potentials

During the action potential, the movement of Na⁺ and K⁺ ions across the membrane through the voltage-gated channels is *passive*; driven by gradients. The **equilibrium potential** is the membrane potential at which this driving force (the gradient) does not exist; in other words, there would be no net movement of ions across the membrane. Note that the equilibrium potential is specific for a particular ion. For example, the Na⁺ equilibrium potential is *positive*, approximately +50 mV. Na⁺ ions are driven inward by their concentration gradient. However, if the interior of the cell is too positive, the positively charged ions are repelled; in other words, the *electrical* gradient would drive sodium *out*. These forces, the chemical gradient driving sodium in and the electrical gradient driving sodium out balance each other at about +50 mV, so this is the equilibrium potential for Na⁺.

K⁺, however, has a *negative* equilibrium potential. K⁺ ions are driven outward by their concentration gradient. However, if the interior of the cell is too negative, the positively charged ions cannot escape the attraction; the electrical gradient drives potassium *in*. The chemical gradient driving potassium out and the electrical gradient driving potassium in balance each other at about –90 mV, so this is the equilibrium potential for K⁺.

The equilibrium potential for any ion is based on the electrochemical gradient for that ion across the membrane, and can be predicted by the **Nernst equation**:

$$E_{ion} = \frac{RT}{zF} \ln \frac{[X]_{outside}}{[X]_{inside}}$$

where E_{ion} is the equilibrium potential for the ion, R is the universal gas constant, T is the temperature (in Kelvin), z is the valence of the ion, F is Faraday's constant, and $[X]$ is the concentration of the ion on each side of the plasma membrane. Note that the relative concentrations of the ion on each side of the membrane create the *chemical* gradient, while the valence (charge of the ion) helps determine the electrical gradient.

Note that the fact that the resting membrane potential is –70 mV reflects both the differences in the equilibrium potentials for Na⁺ and K⁺, and also the relative numbers of leak channels for these two ions. If the cell were completely permeable to K⁺, the resting potential would be about –90 mV. The fact that the resting potential is *very close* to the K⁺ equilibrium potential indicates that there are a large number of K⁺ leak channels in the membrane; the cell at rest is almost completely permeable to potassium. However, the resting potential is slightly more positive than –90 mV, indicating that there are a few Na⁺ leak channels allowing Na⁺ in. Not very many Na⁺ leak channels, though, or the resting potential would be much more positive; closer to the Na⁺ equilibrium potential. (This is in fact what we see when the cell *does* become completely permeable to Na⁺ at the beginning of the action potential; the membrane potential shoots upward to +35 mV.)

The Refractory Period

Action potentials can pass through a neuron extremely rapidly, thousands each second, but there is an upper limit to how soon a neuron can conduct an action potential after another has passed. The passage of one action potential makes the neuron nonresponsive to membrane depolarization and unable to transmit another action potential, or **refractory**, for a short period of time. There are two phases of the refractory period, caused by two different factors. During the **absolute refractory period**, a neuron will not fire another action potential no matter how strong a membrane depolarization is induced. During this time, the voltage-gated sodium channels have been *inactivated* (not the same as *closed*) after depolarization. They will not be able to be opened again until the membrane potential reaches the resting potential and the Na$^+$ channels have returned to their "closed" state. During the **relative refractory period**, a neuron can be induced to transmit an action potential, but the depolarization required is greater than normal because the membrane is **hyperpolarized**. When repolarization occurs, there is a brief period in which the membrane potential is more negative than the resting potential (Figure 3), caused by voltage-gated potassium channels that have not closed yet. Because it is further from threshold, a greater stimulus is required to open the voltage-gated sodium channels to start an action potential. [If a fruit fly mutant is found that has voltage-gated potassium channels that shut more quickly after repolarization, how would this affect the refractory period in the fly?[16]]

8.2 SYNAPTIC TRANSMISSION

A **synapse** is a junction between the axon terminus of a neuron and the dendrites, soma, or axon of a second neuron. It can also be a junction between the axon terminus of a neuron and an organ. There are two types of synapses: electrical and chemical. **Electrical synapses** occur when the cytoplasms of two cells are joined by gap junctions. If two cells are joined by an electrical synapse, an action potential will spread directly from one cell to the other. Electrical synapses are not common in the nervous system although they are quite important in propagating action potentials in smooth muscle and cardiac muscle. In the nervous system, **chemical synapses** are found at the ends of axons where they meet their target cell; here, an action potential is converted into a chemical signal. The following steps are involved in the transmission of a signal across a chemical synapse in the nervous system (Figure 6 on the next page), as well as at the junctions of neurons with other cell types, such as skeletal muscle cells:

1) An action potential reaches the end of an axon, the synaptic knob.
2) Depolarization of the presynaptic membrane opens voltage-gated calcium channels.
3) Calcium influx into the presynaptic cell causes exocytosis of neurotransmitter stored in secretory vesicles.
4) Neurotransmitter molecules diffuse across the narrow synaptic cleft (small space between cells).
5) Neurotransmitter binds to receptor proteins in the postsynaptic membrane. These receptors are ligand-gated ion channels.
6) The opening of these ion channels in the postsynaptic cell alters the membrane polarization.
7) If the membrane depolarization of the postsynaptic cell reaches the threshold of voltage-gated sodium channels, an action potential is initiated.
8) Neurotransmitter in the synaptic cleft is degraded and/or removed to terminate the signal.

---

[16] The absolute refractory period would not be altered, since this is due to the inability of voltage-gated sodium channels to open. However, the relative refractory period would be decreased.

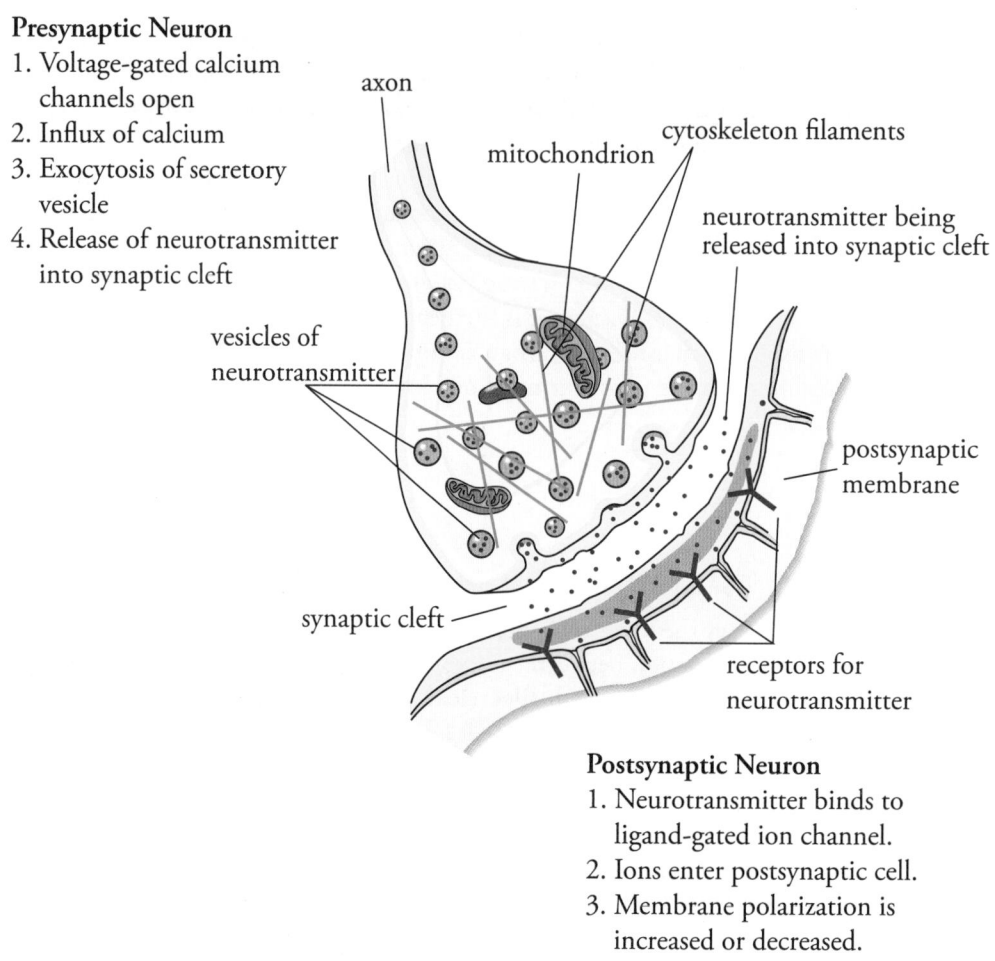

Presynaptic Neuron
1. Voltage-gated calcium channels open
2. Influx of calcium
3. Exocytosis of secretory vesicle
4. Release of neurotransmitter into synaptic cleft

axon

mitochondrion

cytoskeleton filaments

neurotransmitter being released into synaptic cleft

vesicles of neurotransmitter

postsynaptic membrane

synaptic cleft

receptors for neurotransmitter

Postsynaptic Neuron
1. Neurotransmitter binds to ligand-gated ion channel.
2. Ions enter postsynaptic cell.
3. Membrane polarization is increased or decreased.

Figure 6   A Typical Synapse

An example of a chemical synapse that is commonly used is the **neuromuscular junction** between neurons and skeletal muscle. The neurotransmitter that is released at the neuromuscular junction is **acetylcholine (ACh)**. When an action potential reaches such a synapse, acetylcholine is released into the synaptic cleft. The acetylcholine binds to the acetylcholine receptor on the surface of the postsynaptic cell membrane. When acetylcholine binds to its receptor, the receptor opens its associated sodium channel, allowing sodium to flow down a gradient into the cell, depolarizing the postsynaptic cell membrane. Meanwhile, acetylcholine in the synaptic cleft is degraded by the enzyme **acetylcholinesterase (AChE)**.

There are several different neurotransmitters and neurotransmitter receptors. Some of the other neurotransmitters are **gamma-aminobutyric acid (GABA)**, **serotonin**, **dopamine**, and **norepinephrine**. If a neurotransmitter, such as acetylcholine, opens a channel that depolarizes the postsynaptic membrane, the neurotransmitter is termed **excitatory**. Other neurotransmitters, however, have the opposite effect, making the postsynaptic membrane potential more negative than the resting potential, or hyperpolarized. Neurotransmitters that induce hyperpolarization of the postsynaptic membrane are termed **inhibitory**. (Note, however, that ultimately it is not the *neurotransmitter* that determines the effect on the postsynaptic cell, it is the *receptor* for that neurotransmitter and its associated ion channel. The same neurotransmitter can be excitatory in some cases and inhibitory in others.) Postsynaptic neurons may have many different receptors, allowing them to respond to many different neurotransmitters.

- If a neurotransmitter causes the entry of chloride into the postsynaptic cell, is the neurotransmitter excitatory or inhibitory?[17]

- If an inhibitor of acetylcholinesterase is added to a neuromuscular junction, then the postsynaptic membrane will:[18]
  A) be depolarized by action potentials more frequently.
  B) be depolarized longer with each action potential.
  C) be resistant to depolarization.
  D) spontaneously depolarize.

- Signals can be sent in only one direction through synapses such as the neuromuscular junction. Which of the following best explains unidirectional signaling at synapses between neurons?[19]
  A) The neurotransmitter is always degraded by the postsynaptic cell or in the synaptic cleft.
  B) Only the presynaptic cell has vesicles of neurotransmitter.
  C) Axons can propagate action potentials in only one direction.
  D) Only the postsynaptic cell has a resting membrane potential.

Summation

Once an action potential is initiated in a neuron, it will propagate to the end of the axon at a speed and magnitude of depolarization that do not vary from one action potential to another. The action potential is an **"all-or-nothing"** event. The key regulated step in the nervous system is whether or not a neuron will fire an action potential. Action potentials are initiated when the postsynaptic membrane reaches the threshold depolarization (about −50 mV) required to open voltage-gated sodium channels. The postsynaptic depolarization caused by the release of neurotransmitter by one action potential at one synapse is not generally sufficient to induce this degree of depolarization. A postsynaptic neuron has many different neurons with synapses leading to it, however, and each of these synapses can release neurotransmitter many times per second. The "decision" by a postsynaptic neuron whether to fire an action potential is determined by adding the effect of all of the synapses impinging on a neuron, both excitatory and inhibitory. This addition of stimuli is termed **summation**.

---

[17] Chloride ions are negatively charged. The entry of chloride ions into the cell will make the postsynaptic potential more negative, or hyperpolarized, so the neurotransmitter is inhibitory.

[18] Choice **B** is the correct answer. If acetylcholinesterase is inhibited, acetylcholine will remain in the synaptic cleft longer, and acetylcholine-gated sodium channels will remain open longer with each action potential that reaches the synapse. If the sodium channels are open longer, the depolarization of the postsynaptic membrane will last longer.

[19] Signaling is unidirectional because only the presynaptic cell has vesicles of neurotransmitter that are released in response to action potentials, and only the postsynaptic neuron has receptors that bind neurotransmitter to either depolarize or hyperpolarize the cell (choice **B** is correct). The degradation of neurotransmitter is irrelevant to the direction of signal propagation (choice A is wrong), axons are capable of propagating action potentials in both directions (even though this is not what they normally do; choice C is wrong), and all cells have a resting membrane potential (choice D is wrong).

8.3

Excitatory neurotransmitters cause postsynaptic depolarization, or **excitatory postsynaptic potentials** (**EPSPs**), while inhibitory neurotransmitters cause **inhibitory postsynaptic potentials** (**IPSPs**). One form of summation is **temporal summation**, in which a presynaptic neuron fires action potentials so rapidly that the EPSPs or IPSPs pile up on top of one another. If they are EPSPs, the additive effect might be enough to reach the threshold depolarization required to start a postsynaptic action potential. If they are IPSPs, the postsynaptic cell will hyperpolarize, moving further and further away from threshold, effectively becoming inhibited. The other form of summation is **spatial summation**, in which the EPSPs and IPSPs from all of the synapses on the postsynaptic membrane are summed at a given moment in time. If the total of all EPSPs and IPSPs causes the postsynaptic membrane to reach the threshold voltage, an action potential will be fired.

- In which one of the following ways can a presynaptic neuron increase the intensity of signal it transmits?[20]
    - A) Increase the size of presynaptic action potentials
    - B) Increase the frequency of action potentials
    - C) Change the type of neurotransmitter it releases
    - D) Change the speed of action potential propagation

8.3 FUNCTIONAL ORGANIZATION OF THE HUMAN NERVOUS SYSTEM

The nervous system must receive information, decide what to do with it, and cause muscles or glands to act upon that decision. Receiving information is the **sensory** function of the nervous system (carried out by the peripheral nervous system, or **PNS**), processing the information is the **integrative** function (carried out by the central nervous system, or **CNS**), and acting on it is the **motor** function (also carried out by the PNS).[21] **Motor neurons** carry information from the nervous system toward organs which can act upon that information, known as **effectors**. [What are the two types of effectors?[22]] Notice that "motor" neurons do not lead only "to muscle." Motor neurons, which carry information away from the central nervous system and innervate effectors, are called **efferent** neurons (remember, efferents go to effectors). **Sensory neurons**, which carry information toward the central nervous system, are called **afferent** neurons.

---

[20] A neuron cannot change the size of action potentials it transmits, but it can increase the *number* of action potentials it transmits in a given amount of time (the *frequency* of action potentials). The increased frequency of action potentials will add up through temporal summation in the postsynaptic cell to produce an increased response (choice **B** is correct). Action potentials are all-or-nothing once they are started. The magnitude of membrane depolarization during propagation of the action potential does not change (choice A is wrong). A neuron does not change the neurotransmitter it releases (choice C is wrong), and the speed of propagation cannot be varied from one action potential to the next (choice D is wrong).

[21] More detailed information about the anatomy and functions of the CNS and PNS will be presented later in this chapter.

[22] Muscles and glands

Reflexes

The simplest example of nervous system activity is the **reflex**. This is a direct motor response to sensory input which occurs without conscious thought. In fact, it usually occurs without any involvement of the brain at all. In the simplest example, a sensory neuron transmits an action potential to a synapse with a motor neuron in the spinal cord, which causes an action to occur. For example, in the **muscle stretch reflex**, a sensory neuron detects stretching of a muscle (Figure 7). The sensory neuron has a long dendrite and a long axon, which transmits an impulse to a motor neuron cell body in the spinal cord. The motor neuron's long axon synapses with the muscle that was stretched and causes it to contract. That is why the quadriceps (thigh) muscle contracts when the patellar tendon is stretched by tapping it with a reflex hammer. A reflex such as this one, involving only two neurons and one synapse, is known as a **monosynaptic reflex arc.**

Something else also happens when a physician taps the patellar tendon. Not only does the quadriceps *contract*, but the hamstring also *relaxes*. If it did not, the leg would not be able to extend (straighten). The sensory neuron (that detects stretch) synapses with not only a motor neuron for the quadriceps, but also with an **inhibitory interneuron**. This is a short neuron which forms an inhibitory synapse with a motor neuron innervating the hamstring muscle. When the sensory neuron is stimulated by stretch, it stimulates both the quadriceps motor neuron and the inhibitory interneuron to the hamstring motor neuron. The interneuron inhibits the motor neuron for the hamstring. As a result, the quadriceps contracts and the hamstring relaxes (note that the hamstring part of the reflex—sensory neuron to interneuron to hamstring motor neuron—involves three neurons and two synapses, hence it is known as a **disynaptic reflex arc**). An interneuron is the simplest example of the integrative role of the nervous system. Concurrent relaxation of the hamstring and contraction of the quadriceps is an example of **reciprocal inhibition**.

- If a reflex occurs without the involvement of the brain, how are we aware of the action?[23]

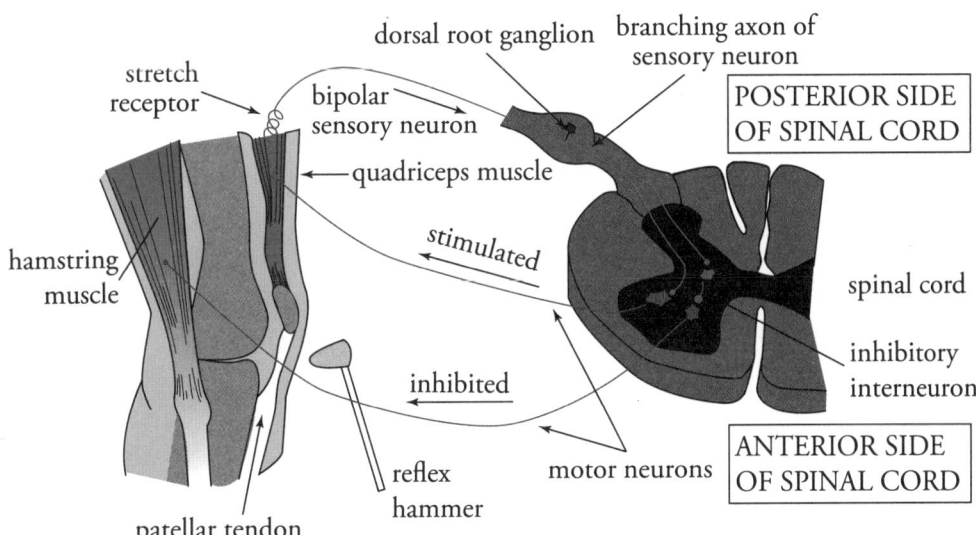

Figure 7 The Muscle Stretch Reflex

---

[23] Two ways: first, the sensory neuron also branches to form a synapse with a neuron leading to the brain. Second, other sensory information is received after the action is taken.

Large-Scale Functional Organization

The peripheral nervous system can be subdivided into several functional divisions (Figure 8). The portion of this system concerned with conscious sensation and deliberate, voluntary movement of skeletal muscle is the **somatic** division. The portion concerned with digestion, metabolism, circulation, perspiration, and other involuntary processes is the **autonomic** division. The somatic and autonomic divisions both include afferent and efferent functions, though the sources of sensory input and the target of efferent nerves are different. The efferent portion of the autonomic division is further split into two subdivisions: **sympathetic** and **parasympathetic**. When the sympathetic system is activated, the body is prepared for "fight or flight." When the parasympathetic system is activated, the body is prepared to "rest and digest." Table 2 summarizes the main effects of the autonomic system. Notice that many sympathetic effects result from release of epinephrine[24] into the bloodstream by the adrenal medulla. The parasympathetic system prepares you to rest and digest food.

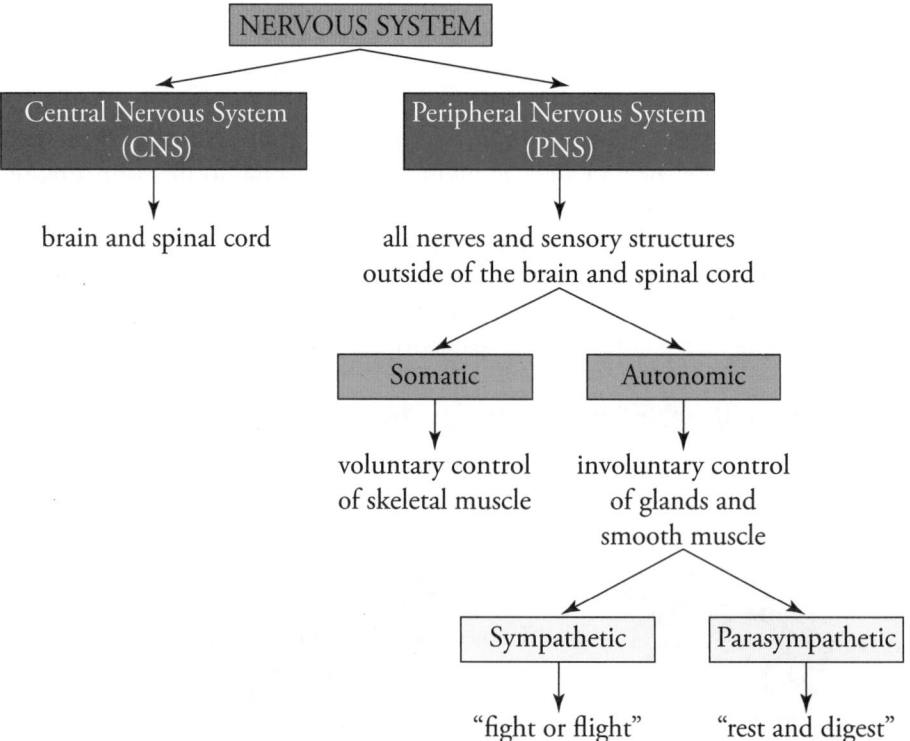

Figure 8 Overall Organization of the Nervous System

---

[24] In Greek, "epi" means upon or on top of, and "nephr" refers to the kidney (as in nephron, the microscopic functional unit of the kidney); thus epinephrine is "the hormone secreted by the gland on top of the kidney." Another name for epinephrine is adrenaline. In Latin, "ad" also means upon, and "renal" likewise refers to the kidney. The gland which secretes epinephrine is the adrenal gland.

Table 2 Effects of the Autonomic Nervous System

Organ or System	Parasympathetic: rest and digest	Sympathetic: fight or flight
digestive system: glands	stimulation	inhibition
motility	stimulation (stimulates digestion)	inhibition (inhibits digestion)
sphincters	relaxation	contraction
urinary system: bladder	contraction (stimulates urination)	relaxation (inhibits urination)
urethral sphincter	relaxation (stimulates urination)	contraction (inhibits urination)
bronchial smooth muscle	constriction (closes airways)	relaxation (opens airways)
cardiovascular system heart rate and contractility	decreased	increased
blood flow to skeletal muscle	—	increased
skin	—	sweating and general vasoconstriction
eye: pupil	constriction	dilation
muscles controlling lens	accommodation for near vision	accommodation for far vision
adrenal medulla	—	release of epinephrine
genitals	erection / lubrication	ejaculation / orgasm

8.4 ANATOMICAL ORGANIZATION OF THE NERVOUS SYSTEM

The main anatomical division of the nervous system is between the **central nervous system** (**CNS**) and the **peripheral nervous system** (**PNS**). The central nervous system is the brain and spinal cord. The peripheral nervous system includes all other axons, dendrites, and cell bodies. Bundles of myelinated axons in both the CNS and PNS is referred to as **white matter**; specifically, white matter in the brain is called a **tract**, white matter in the spinal cord is called a **tract** or a **column**, and white matter in the PNS is called a **nerve**. Unmyelinated neuronal cell bodies in both the CNS and PNS are referred to as **grey matter**; specifically, grey matter deep in the brain is called a **nucleus**, grey matter on the surface of the brain is called **cortex**, grey matter in the spinal cord is called a **horn**, and grey matter in the PNS is a **ganglion**.

CNS Anatomical Organization

The CNS includes the **spinal cord** and the brain. The brain has three subdivisions: the **hindbrain** (or the rhombencephalon), the **midbrain** (or the mesencephalon), and the **forebrain** (or the prosencephalon). These four regions of the CNS (which will be discussed individually below) perform increasingly complex functions. The entire CNS (brain and spinal cord) floats in **cerebrospinal fluid** (**CSF**), a clear liquid that serves various functions such as shock absorption and exchange of nutrients and waste with the CNS.

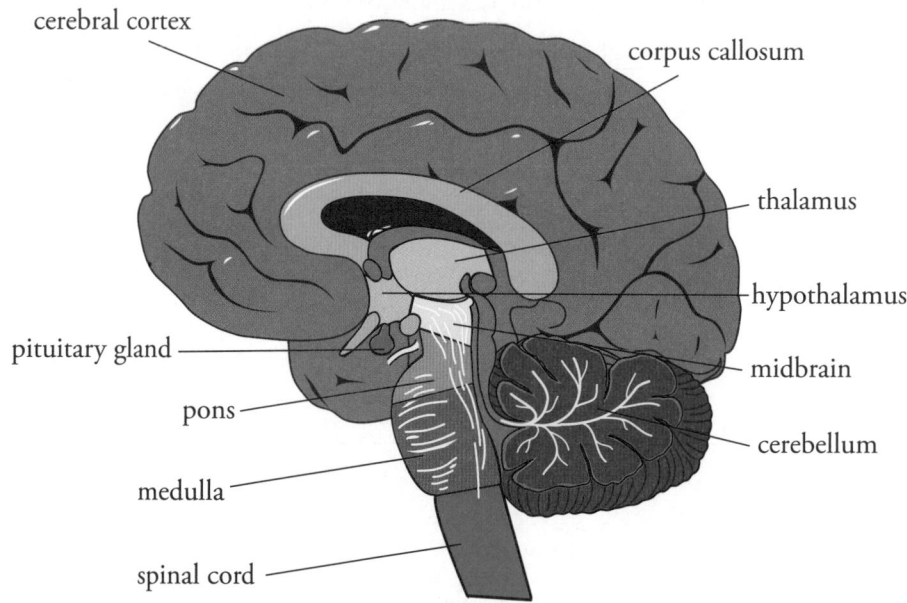

Figure 9   Organization of the CNS (cross-section of the brain)

1) The spinal cord is connected to the brain and is protected by the CSF and the vertebral column. It is a pathway for information to and from the brain. Most sensory data is relayed to the brain for integration, but the spinal cord is also a site for information integration and processing. The spinal cord is responsible for simple spinal reflexes (like the muscle stretch reflex) and is also involved in primitive processes such as walking, urination, and sex organ function.

2) The hindbrain includes the medulla, the pons, and the cerebellum.

   - The **medulla** (or medulla oblongata) is located below the pons and is the area of the brain that connects to the spinal cord. It functions in relaying information between other areas of the brain and regulates vital autonomic functions such as blood pressure and digestive functions (including vomiting). Also, the respiratory rhythmicity centers are found here.

   - The **pons** is located below the midbrain and above the medulla oblongata. It is the connection point between the brain stem and the cerebellum (see below). The pons controls some autonomic functions and coordinates movement; it plays a role in balance and antigravity posture.

   - The **cerebellum** (or "little brain") is located behind the pons and below the cerebral hemispheres. It is an integrating center where complex movements are coordinated. An instruction for movement from the forebrain must be sent to the cerebellum, where the billions of decisions necessary for smooth execution of the movement are made. Damage to the cerebellum results in poor hand-eye coordination and balance. Both the cerebellum and the pons receive information from the vestibular apparatus in the inner ear, which monitors acceleration and position relative to gravity.

3) The midbrain is a relay for visual and auditory information and contains much of the reticular activating system (RAS), which is responsible for arousal or wakefulness.

Another term you should be familiar with is **brainstem**. Together, the medulla, pons, and midbrain constitute the brainstem, which contains important processing centers and relays information to or from the cerebellum and cerebrum.

4) The forebrain includes the **diencephalon** and the **telencephalon**.
   a) The diencephalon includes the thalamus and hypothalamus:
   - The thalamus is located near the middle of the brain below the cerebral hemispheres and above the midbrain. It contains relay and processing centers for sensory information.
   - The hypothalamus interacts directly with many parts of the brain. It contains centers for controlling emotions and autonomic functions, and has a major role in hormone production and release. It is the primary link between the nervous and the endocrine systems, and by controlling the pituitary gland is the fundamental control center for the endocrine system (discussed later in this chapter).
   b) All parts of the CNS up to and including the diencephalon form a single symmetrical stalk, but the telencephalon consists of two separate cerebral hemispheres. Generally speaking, the areas of the left and right hemispheres have the same functions. However, the left hemisphere primarily controls the motor functions of the right side of the body, and the right hemisphere controls those of the left side. Also, in most people, the left side of the brain is said to be dominant. It is generally responsible for speech. The right hemisphere is more concerned with visual-spatial reasoning and music.
   - The **cerebral hemispheres** are connected by a thick bundle of axons called the **corpus callosum**. A person with a cut corpus callosum has two independent cerebral cortices and to a certain extent two independent minds![25]
   - The **cerebrum** is the largest region of the human brain and consists of the large, paired cerebral hemispheres. The hemispheres of the cerebrum consist of the **cerebral cortex** (an outer layer of gray matter) plus an inner core of white matter connecting the cortex to the diencephalon.[26] The gray matter is composed of trillions of somas; the white matter is composed of myelinated axons. (Most axons in the CNS and PNS are myelinated.) The cerebral hemispheres are responsible for conscious thought processes and intellectual functions. They also play a role in processing somatic sensory and motor information. The cerebral cortex is divided into four pairs of lobes, each of which is devoted to specific functions:
     i) The **frontal lobes** initiate all voluntary movement and are involved in complex reasoning skills and problem solving.
     ii) The **parietal lobes** are involved in general sensations (such as touch, temperature, pressure, vibration, etc.) and in gustation (taste).
     iii) The **temporal lobes** process auditory and olfactory sensation and are involved in short-term memory, language comprehension, and emotion.
     iv) The **occipital lobes** process visual sensation.

---

[25] Anyone interested in reading about jaw-dropping neurological cases should begin with Oliver Sacks' *The Man Who Mistook His Wife for a Hat*. You will *not* be sorry if you buy this book.

[26] The word *cortex* means "outside layer"; for example, an orange peel may be called the cortex of the orange; the outside layer of a gland is also known as its cortex.

Figure 10 shows some of the more important cortical areas.

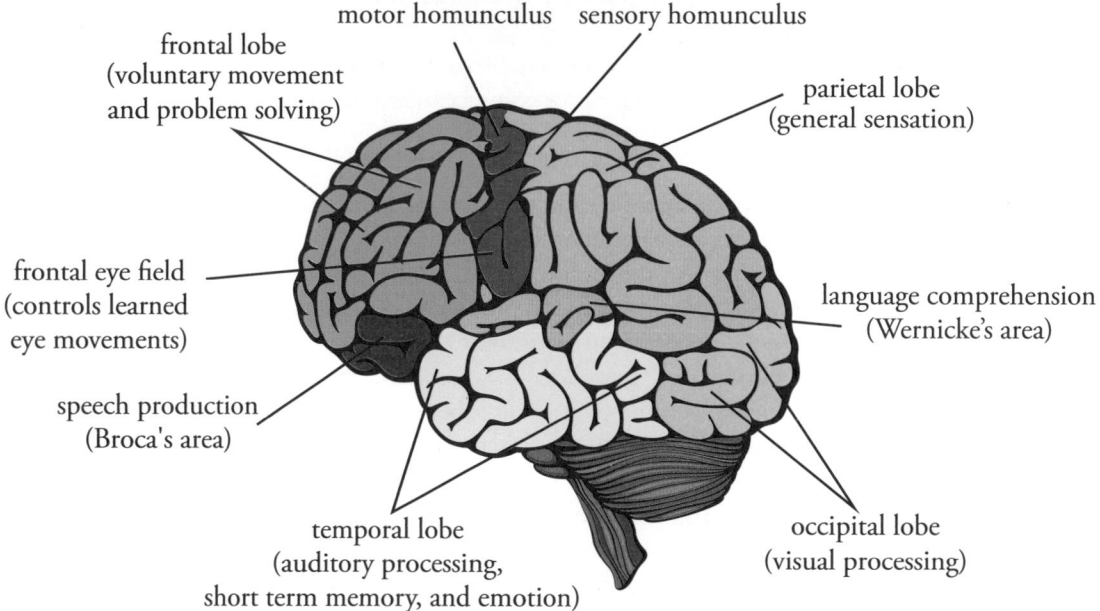

Figure 10   Principal Areas of the Cerebral Cortex

Two last regions of the brain deserve mention:

- The **basal nuclei** (also called the "cerebral nuclei," and previously known as the basal ganglia) are composed of gray matter and are located deep within the cerebral hemispheres. They include several functional subdivisions, but broadly function in voluntary motor control and procedural learning related to habits. The basal nuclei and cerebellum work together to process and coordinate movement initiated by the primary motor cortex; the basal nuclei are inhibitory (preventing excess movement), while the cerebellum is excitatory.
- The **limbic system** is located between the cerebrum and the diencephalon. It includes several substructures (such as the amygdala, the cingulate gyrus, and the hippocampus) and works closely with parts of the cerebrum, diencephalon, and midbrain. The limbic system is important in emotion and memory.

The information above describes the general functions of each region of the brain. Table 3 summarizes the brain functions and provides a little more specific detail for each region.

Table 3   Summary of Brain Functions

Structure	General Function	Specific Functions
Spinal cord	Simple reflexes	• controls simple stretch and tendon reflexes • controls primitive processes such as walking, urination, and sex organ function
Medulla	Involuntary functions	• controls autonomic processes such as blood pressure, blood flow, heart rate, respiratory rate, swallowing, vomiting • controls reflex reactions such as coughing or sneezing • relays sensory information to the cerebellum and the thalamus

Structure	General Function	Specific Functions
Pons	Relay station and balance	• controls antigravity posture and balance • connects spinal cord and medulla with upper regions of brain • relays information to the cerebellum and thalamus
Cerebellum	Movement coordination	• integrating center • coordination of complex movement, balance and posture, muscle tone, spatial equilibrium
Midbrain	Eye movement	• integration of visual and auditory information • visual and auditory reflexes • wakefulness and consciousness • coordinates information on posture and muscle tone
Thalamus	Integrating center and relay station	• relay center for somatic (conscious) sensation (except olfactory sensory input) • relays information between spinal cord and cerebral cortex
Hypo-thalamus	Homeostasis and behavior	• controls homeostatic functions (such as temperature regulation, fluid balance, appetite) through both neural and hormonal regulation • controls primitive emotions such as anger, rage, and sex drive • controls the pituitary gland
Basal nuclei	Movement	• regulate body movement and muscle tone • coordination of learned movement patterns • general pattern of rhythmic movements (such as controlling the cycle of arm and leg movements when walking) • subconscious adjustments of conscious movements
Limbic system	Emotion, memory, and learning	• controls emotional states • links conscious and unconscious portions of the brain • helps with memory storage and retrieval
Cerebral cortex	Perception, skeletal muscle movement, memory, attention, thought, language, and consciousness	• divided into four lobes (frontal, parietal, temporal, and occipital) with specialized subfunctions • perception and processing of the special senses (vision, hearing, smell, taste, touch) • conscious thought processes and planning, awareness, and sensation • intellectual function (intelligence, learning, reading, communication) • abstract thought and reasoning • memory storage and retrieval • initiation and coordination of voluntary movement • complex motor patterns • language (speech production and understanding) • personality
Corpus callosum	Connection	• connects the left and right cerebral hemispheres

The motor and sensory regions of the cortex are organized such that a particular small area of cortex controls a particular body part. A larger area is devoted to a body part which requires more motor control or more sensation (Figure 11). For example, more cortex is devoted to the lips than to the entire leg. The body parts represented on the cortex can be sketched. The drawing looks like a distorted person, known as a **homunculus** (little man).

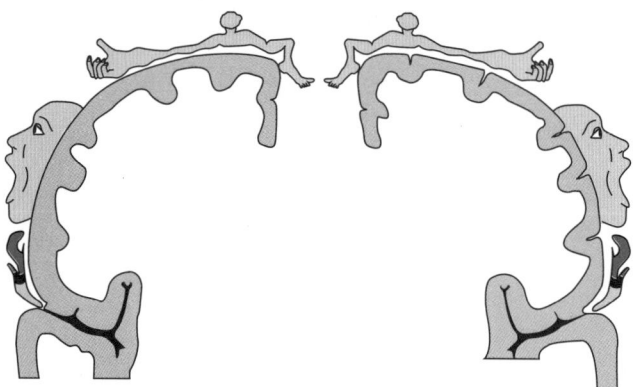

Figure 11   The Sensory Homunculus

PNS Anatomical Organization

All neurons entering and exiting the CNS are carried by 12 pairs of **cranial nerves** and 31 pairs of **spinal nerves**. Cranial nerves convey sensory and motor information to and from the brainstem. Spinal nerves convey sensory and motor information to and from the spinal cord. The different functional divisions of the nervous system have different anatomical organizations (Figure 12).

The **vagus nerve** is an important example of a cranial nerve, and one that you should be familiar with for the MCAT. The effects of this nerve upon the heart and GI tract are to decrease the heart rate and increase GI activity; as such it is part of the *parasympathetic division* of the autonomic nervous system. It is a bundle of axons that end in ganglia on the surface of the heart, stomach, and other visceral organs. The many axons constituting the vagus nerve are preganglionic and come from cell bodies located in the CNS. On the surface of the heart and stomach they synapse with postganglionic neurons. The detailed terminology in this paragraph will make more sense to you as you read through the next couple of sections.

Somatic PNS Anatomy

The somatic system has a simple organization:

- *All* somatic motor neurons innervate skeletal muscle cells, use ACh as their neurotransmitter, and have their cell bodies in the brain stem or the ventral (front) portion of the spinal cord.

- *All* somatic sensory neurons have a long dendrite extending from a sensory receptor toward the soma, which is located just outside the CNS in a **dorsal root ganglion**. The dorsal root ganglion is a bunch of somatic (and autonomic) sensory neuron cell bodies located just dorsal to (to the back of) the spinal cord. There is a pair of dorsal root ganglia for every segment of the spinal cord, and thus the dorsal root ganglia form a chain along the dorsal (back) aspect of the vertebral column. The dorsal root ganglia are protected within the vertebral column but are outside the **meninges** (protective sheath of the brain and cord) and thus outside the CNS. An axon extends from the somatic sensory neuron's soma into the spinal cord. In all somatic sensory neurons, the first synapse is in the CNS; depending on the type of sensory information conveyed, the axon either synapses in the cord, or stretches all the way up to the brain stem before its first synapse!

Autonomic PNS Anatomy

Anatomical organization of autonomic efferents is a bit more complex.[27] The efferents of the sympathetic and parasympathetic systems consist of two neurons: a preganglionic and a postganglionic neuron. The **preganglionic neuron** has its cell body in the brainstem or spinal cord. It sends an axon to an autonomic ganglion, located outside the spinal column. In the ganglion, this axon synapses with a **postganglionic neuron**. The postganglionic neuron sends an axon to an effector (smooth muscle or gland). *All* autonomic preganglionic neurons release acetylcholine as their neurotransmitter. *All* parasympathetic postganglionic neurons also release acetylcholine. Nearly all sympathetic postganglionic neurons release norepinephrine (NE, also known as noradrenaline) as their neurotransmitter.

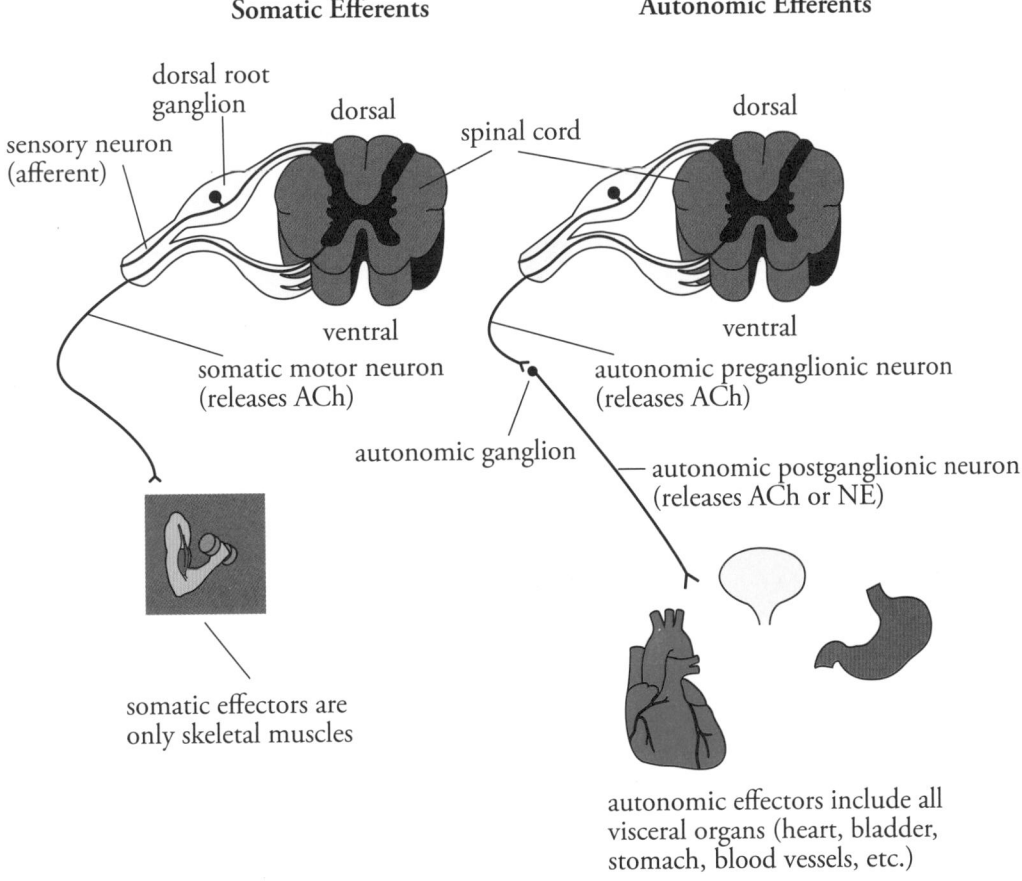

Figure 12   Anatomical Organization of PNS Efferents

---

[27] The anatomy of autonomic sensory neurons (afferents) is poorly defined and will not be on the MCAT.

All sympathetic preganglionic efferent neurons have their cell bodies in the thoracic (chest) or lumbar (lower back) regions of the spinal cord. Hence the sympathetic system is also referred to as the *thoracolumbar system*. The parasympathetic system is known as the *craniosacral system*, because all of its preganglionic neurons have cell bodies in the brainstem (which is in the head or cranium) or in the lowest portion of the spinal cord, the sacral portion. In the sympathetic system, the preganglionic axon is relatively short, and there are only a few ganglia; these sympathetic ganglia are quite large. The sympathetic postganglionic cell sends a long axon to the effector. In contrast, the parasympathetic preganglionic neuron sends a long axon to a small ganglion which is close to the effector. For example, parasympathetic ganglia controlling the intestines are located on the outer wall of the gut. The parasympathetic postganglionic neuron has a very short axon, since the cell body is close to the target.[28] These differences are visualized in Figure 13 and summarized in Table 4.

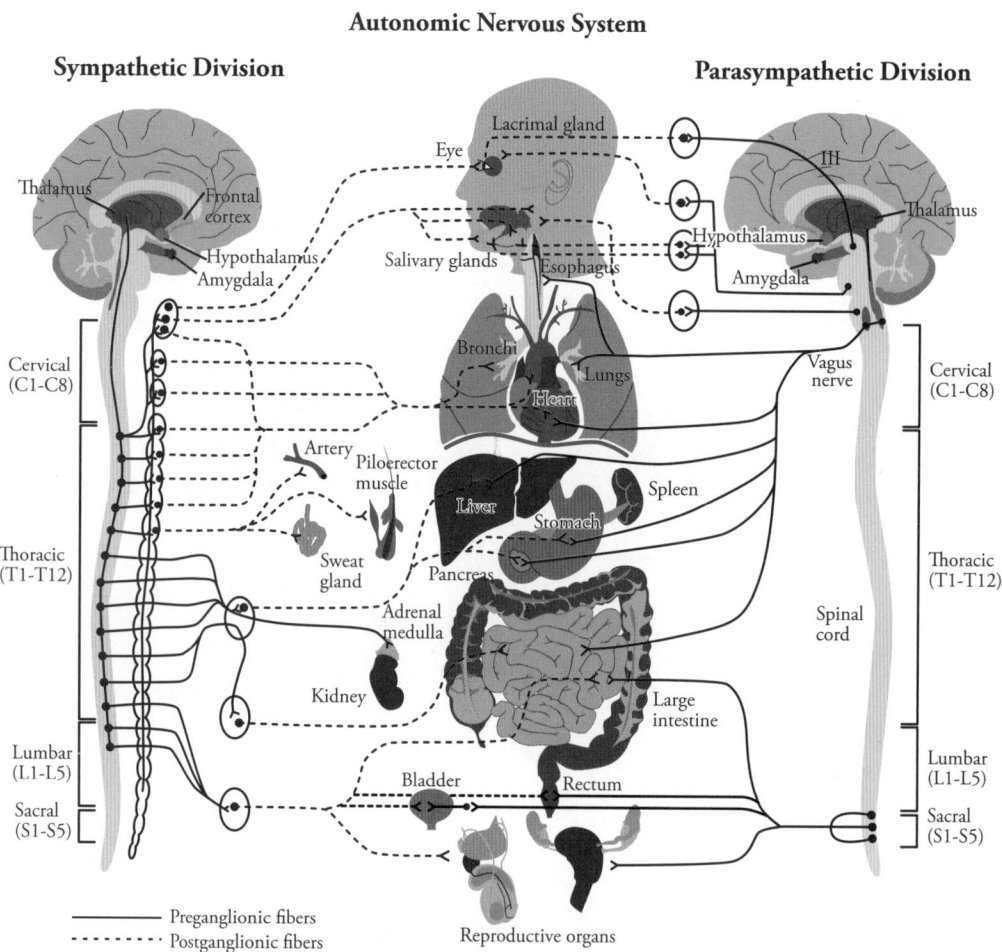

Figure 13 Pre- and Post-Ganglionic Fibers of the Autonomic Nervous System

The autonomic afferent (sensory) neurons are similar to the somatic afferent neurons with one exception: they can synapse in the PNS (at the autonomic ganglia) with autonomic efferent neurons in what is known as a "short reflex." (Recall that the first synapse of somatic afferent neurons is in the CNS.)

---

[28] The mnemonic "*para* long *pre*" will help you in med school.

Table 4 Sympathetic vs. Parasympathetic

	Sympathetic	Parasympathetic
General function	fight or flight, mobilize energy	rest and digest, store energy
Location of preganglionic soma	thoracolumbar = thoracic and lumbar spinal cord	craniosacral = brainstem ("cranial") and sacral spinal cord
Preganglionic axon neurotransmitter = acetylcholine (ACh)	short	long
Ganglia	close to cord, far from target	far from cord, close to target
Postganglionic axon (usual neurotransmitter)	long (norepinephrine [NE])	short (acetylcholine [ACh])

The Adrenal Medulla

The **adrenal gland** is named for its location: "Ad-" connotes "above," and "renal" refers to the kidney. There are two adrenal glands, one above each kidney. The adrenal has an inner portion known as the **medulla** and an outer portion known as the **cortex**. The cortex is an important endocrine gland, secreting **glucocorticoids** (the main one is cortisol), **mineralocorticoids** (the main one is aldosterone), and some sex hormones.

The adrenal medulla, however, is part of the sympathetic nervous system. It is embryologically derived from sympathetic postganglionic neurons and is directly innervated by sympathetic preganglionic neurons. Upon activation of the sympathetic system, the adrenal gland is stimulated to release **epinephrine**, also known as **adrenaline**. Epinephrine is a slightly modified version of *nor*epinephrine, the neurotransmitter released by sympathetic postganglionic neurons. Epinephrine is a hormone because it is released into the bloodstream by a ductless gland. But in many ways it behaves like a neurotransmitter. It elicits its effects very rapidly, and the effects are quite short-lived. Ongoing release of epinephrine from the adrenal medulla during fight-or-flight situations prolongs and enhances the effects of the sympathetic neurons. In general, epinephrine's effects are those listed in Table 2 for the sympathetic system. Stimulation of the heart is an especially important effect.

8.5 SENSATION AND PERCEPTION

Sensation is the process by which we receive information from the world around us. Sensory receptors detect data, both internally (from within the body) and externally (from the environment), and send this information to the central nervous system for processing. Sensation is the act of receiving information, while perception is the act of organizing, assimilating, and interpreting the sensory input into useful and meaningful information.

Types of Sensory Receptors

Sensory receptors are designed to detect one type of stimulus from either the interior of the body or the external environment. Each sensory receptor receives only one kind of information and transmits that information to sensory neurons, which can in turn convey it to the central nervous system. [How does the brain know the difference between stimulation of visual receptors and olfactory receptors?[29]] Sensory receptors that detect stimuli from the outside world are **exteroceptors** and receptors that respond to internal stimuli are **interoceptors**. A more important distinction between sensory receptors is based on the type of stimulus they detect. The types of sensory receptors are listed below.

1) **Mechanoreceptors** respond to mechanical disturbances. For example, **Pacinian corpuscles** are pressure sensors located deep in the skin. The Pacinian corpuscle is shaped like an onion. It is composed of concentric layers of specialized membranes. When the corpuscular membranes are distorted by firm pressure on the skin, the nerve ending becomes depolarized and the signal travels up the dendrite (note that these are graded potential changes—*not* action potentials). Another important mechanoreceptor is the **auditory hair cell**. This is a specialized cell found in the cochlea of the inner ear. It detects vibrations caused by sound waves. **Vestibular hair cells** are located within special organs called semicircular canals, also found in the inner ear. Their role is to detect acceleration and position relative to gravity. An example of an autonomic mechanoreceptor would be a receptor detecting stretch of the intestinal wall.

2) **Chemoreceptors** respond to particular chemicals. For example, **olfactory receptors** detect airborne chemicals and allow us to smell things. Taste buds are **gustatory receptors**. Autonomic chemoreceptors in the walls of the carotid and aortic arteries respond to changes in arterial pH, PCO_2, and PO_2 levels.

3) **Nociceptors** are pain receptors.[30] They are stimulated by tissue injury. Nociceptors are the simplest type of sensory receptor, generally consisting of a free nerve ending that detects chemical signs of tissue damage. (In that sense the nociceptor is a simple chemoreceptor.) Nociceptors may be somatic or autonomic. Autonomic pain receptors do not provide the conscious mind with clear pain information, but they frequently give a sensation of dull, aching pain. They may also create the illusion of pain on the skin, when their nerves cross paths with somatic afferents from the skin. This phenomenon is known as **referred pain**.

4) **Thermoreceptors** are stimulated by changes in temperature. There are autonomic and somatic examples. Peripheral thermoreceptors fall into three categories: cold-sensitive, warm-sensitive, and thermal nociceptors, which detect painfully hot stimuli.

5) **Electromagnetic receptors** are stimulated by electromagnetic waves. In humans, the only examples are the rod and cone cells of the retina of the eye (also termed **photoreceptors**). In other animals, electroreceptors and magnetoreceptors are separate. For example, some fish can detect electric fields with electroreceptors, and magnetoreceptors allow animals to sense the Earth's magnetic field, which can help them navigate during migration.

Encoding of Sensory Stimuli

All sensory receptors need to encode relevant information regarding the nature of the stimulus being detected. There are four properties that need to be communicated to the CNS:

1) Stimulus **modality** is the type of stimulus. As mentioned above, the CNS determines the stimulus modality based on which type of receptor is firing.

---

[29] Both signals are received in the brain as action potentials from sensory neurons. The brain distinguishes the sensory stimuli based on which sensory neurons are signaling.

[30] *Noci-* is from the Latin *nocuus*, meaning harmful, as in *noxious*.

2) Stimulus **location** is communicated by the receptive field of the sensory receptor sending the signal. Localization of a stimulus can be improved by overlapping receptive fields of neighboring receptors. This works like a Venn diagram, and allows the brain to localize a stimulus activating neighboring receptors to the area in which their receptive fields overlap. Discrimination between two separate stimuli can be improved by lateral inhibition of neighboring receptors.

3) Stimulus **intensity** is coded by the frequency of action potentials. The *dynamic range*, or range of intensities that can be detected by sensory receptors, can be expanded by range fractionation—including multiple groups of receptors with limited ranges to detect a wider range overall. One example of this phenomenon is human cone cells responding to different but overlapping ranges of wavelengths to detect the full visual spectrum of light.

4) Stimulus **duration** may or may not be coded explicitly. *Tonic receptors* fire action potentials as long as the stimulus continues. However, these receptors are subject to adaptation, and the frequency of action potentials decreases as the stimulus continues at the same level (see below). *Phasic receptors* only fire action potentials when the stimulus begins, and do not explicitly communicate the duration of the stimulus. These receptors are important for communicating changes in stimuli, and essentially adapt immediately if a stimulus continues at the same level.

The ability to adapt to a stimulus is an important property of sensory receptors. This allows the brain to tune out unimportant information from the environment. **Adaptation** is a decrease in firing frequency when the intensity of a stimulus remains constant. For example, if you walk into a kitchen where someone is baking bread, the bread odor molecules stimulate your olfactory receptors to a great degree and you smell the bread baking. But if you remain in the kitchen for a few minutes, you stop smelling the bread; the continuous input to the olfactory receptors causes them to stop firing even though the odor molecules are still present. This is what allows us to "get used to" certain environments and situations, for example, cold pool water, loud background noise, etc. The receptors don't stop being *able* to respond; they can be retriggered if the stimulus intensity increases. For example, if you open up the oven door, you will smell the bread again. Likewise, if you are used to the background noise in a restaurant, but someone drops a plate, you'll hear it. In other words: the nervous system is programmed to respond to *changing stimuli* and not so much to constant stimuli, because for the most part, constant stimuli are not a threat, whereas changing stimuli might need to be dealt with. (Note that nociceptors *do not adapt* under any circumstance. We can learn to ignore them, but pain is something that the nervous system wants us to *do* something about since it is an indication that something is wrong.)

Proprioceptors

This is a broad category including many different types of receptors. **Proprioception** refers to awareness of self (i.e., awareness of body part position) and is also known as your **kinesthetic sense**.[31] An important example of a proprioceptor is the **muscle spindle**, a mechanoreceptor. This is a sensory organ specialized to detect muscle stretch. You are already familiar with it because it is the receptor that senses muscle stretch in the deep tendon reflex. Other proprioceptors include **Golgi tendon organs**, which monitor tension in the tendons, and **joint capsule receptors**, which detect pressure, tension, and movement in the joints. By monitoring the activity of the musculoskeletal system, the proprioceptive component of the somatic sensory system allows us to know the positions of our body parts. This is most important during activity, when precise feedback is essential for coordinated motion. [What portion of the CNS would you expect to require input from proprioceptors?[32]]

---

[31] *Proprio-* means *of or pertaining to the self*, as in "proprietary."

[32] The cerebellum, which is responsible for motor coordination

Gustation and Olfaction

Taste and smell are senses that rely on chemoreceptors in the mouth and nasal passages. **Gustation** is taste, and **olfaction** is smell. Much of what is assumed to be taste is actually smell. (Try eating with a bad head cold.) In fact, taste receptors (known as **taste buds**) can only distinguish five flavors: sweet (glucose), salty (Na^+), bitter (basic), sour (acidic), and umami (amino acids and nucleotides). Each taste bud responds most strongly to one of these five stimuli. The taste bud is composed of a bunch of specialized epithelial cells, shaped roughly like an onion. In its center is a **taste pore**, with **taste hairs** that detect food chemicals. Information about taste is transmitted by cranial nerves to an area of the brain's parietal lobe.

Olfaction is accomplished by olfactory receptors in the roof of the **nasopharynx** (nasal cavity). The receptors detect airborne chemicals that dissolve in the mucus covering the nasal membrane. Humans can distinguish thousands of different smells. Olfactory nerves project directly to the **olfactory bulbs** of the brain. The olfactory bulbs are located in the temporal lobe of the brain near the limbic system, an area important for memory and emotion (which may explain why certain smells can bring back vivid memories and feelings).

Interestingly, the perception of a smell as "good" or "bad" is entirely learned, based on experiences with those smells. There is no smell that is universally noxious to people (though the military has tried to find one in order to develop a "stink" bomb), because different smells can be associated with good or bad experiences based on culture and upbringing.

Pheromones are chemical signals that cause a social response in members of the same species. Though not well understood in humans, pheromones have been studied extensively in insects, particularly those species with complex social structures (such as bees and ants). Pheromones are an important means of communicating information; for example, alarm pheromones will alert the rest of the beehive of danger, food-trail pheromones allow ants to follow a trail to a promising food source, and sex pheromones play an important role in mating between most species. In humans, pheromones are much harder to study.

Hearing and the Vestibular System

Structure of the Ear

The **auricle** or **pinna** and the external **auditory canal** comprise the **outer ear**. The **middle ear** is divided from the outer ear by the **tympanic membrane** or eardrum. The middle ear consists of the **ossicles**, three small bones called the **malleus** (hammer), the **incus** (anvil), and the **stapes** (stirrup). The stapes attaches to the **oval window**, a membrane that divides the middle and **inner ear**. Structures of the inner ear include the **cochlea**, the **semicircular canals**, the **utricle**, and the **saccule**. The semicircular canals together with the utricle and saccule are important to the sense of balance. The **round window** is a membrane-covered hole in the cochlea near the oval window. It releases excess pressure. The **Eustachian tube** (also known as the **auditory tube**) is a passageway from the back of the throat to the middle ear. It functions to equalize the pressure on both sides of the eardrum and is the cause of the "ear popping" one experiences at high altitudes or underwater.

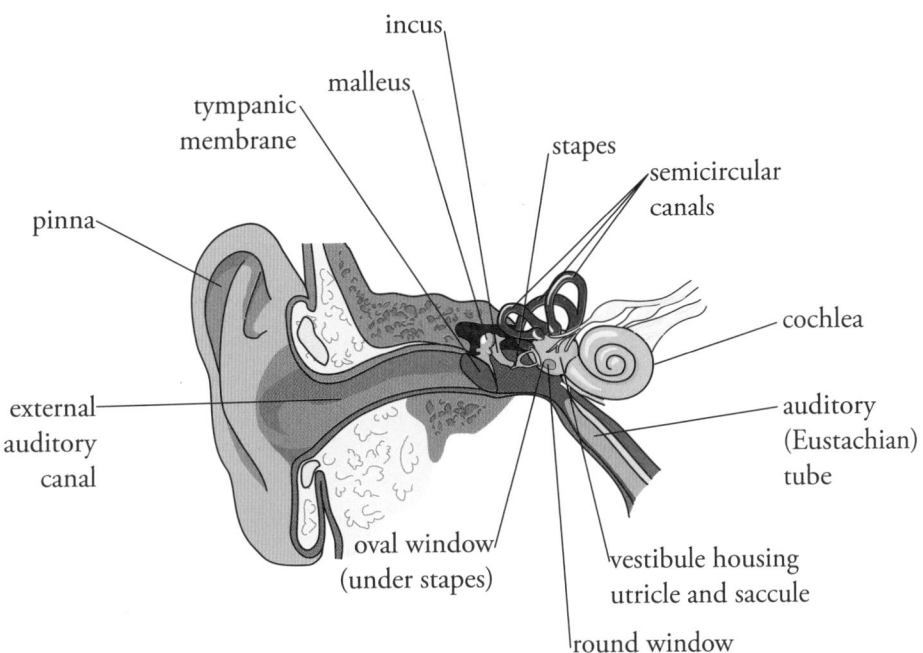

Figure 14 The Ear

Mechanism of Hearing

Sound waves enter the external ear to pass into the auditory canal, causing the eardrum to vibrate. The malleus attached to the eardrum receives the vibrations, which are passed on to the incus and then to the stapes. The bones of the middle ear are arranged in such a way that they amplify sound vibrations passing through the middle ear. The stapes is the innermost of the three middle-ear bones, contacting the oval window. Vibration of the oval window creates pressure waves in the **perilymph** and **endolymph**, the fluids in the cochlea. Note that sound vibrations are first conveyed through air, next through bone, and then through liquid before being sensed. The pressure waves in the endolymph cause vibration of the **basilar membrane**, a thin membrane extending throughout the coiled length of the cochlea. The basilar membrane is covered with the auditory receptor cells known as **hair cells**. These cells have **cilia** (hairs) projecting from their apical (top) surfaces (opposite the basilar membrane). The hairs contact the **tectorial membrane** (tectorial means "roof"), and when the basilar membrane moves, the hairs are dragged across the tectorial membrane and they bend. This displacement opens ion channels in the hair cells, which results in neurotransmitter release. Dendrites from bipolar auditory afferent neurons are stimulated by this neurotransmitter, and thus sound vibrations are converted to nerve impulses. The basilar membrane, hair cells, and tectorial membrane together are known as the **organ of Corti**. The outer ear and middle ear convey sound waves to the cochlea, and the organ of Corti in the cochlea is the primary site at which auditory stimuli are detected.

Summary: From Sound to Hearing

sound waves → auricle → external auditory canal → tympanic membrane → malleus → incus → stapes → oval window → perilymph → endolymph → basilar membrane → auditory hair cells → tectorial membrane → neurotransmitters stimulate bipolar auditory neurons → brain → perception

---

Pitch (frequency) of sound is distinguished by which *regions* of the basilar membrane vibrate, stimulating different auditory neurons. The basilar membrane is narrow, thick, and sturdy near the oval window and gradually becomes wider, thin, and floppy near the apex of the cochlea. Low frequency (long wavelength) sounds stimulate hair cells at the apex of the cochlear duct, farthest away from the oval window, while high-pitched sounds stimulate hair cells at the base of the cochlea, near the oval window. **Loudness** of sound is distinguished by the *amplitude* of vibration. Larger vibrations cause more frequent action potentials in auditory neurons.

Locating the source of sound is also an important adaptive function. Having two ears allows for stereophonic (or three-dimensional) hearing. The auditory system can determine the source of a sound based on the difference detected between the two ears. For example, if a horn blasts to your right, your right ear will receive the sound waves slightly sooner and slightly more intensely than your left ear. Sound stimuli are processed in the **auditory cortex**, located in the temporal lobe of the brain.

In humans, audition is highly adaptive. While we are able to hear a wide range of sounds, those sounds with frequencies within the range corresponding to the human voice are heard best, and we are able to differentiate variations among human voices. For example, when answering the phone, you will recognize your mom's voice within a fraction of a second.

- If a sensory neuron leading from the ear to the brain fires an action potential more rapidly, how will the brain perceive this change?[33]
- In some cases of deafness, sound can still be detected by conduction of vibration through the skull to the cochlea. If the auditory nerve is severed, can sound still be detected by conductance through bone?[34]
- If the bones of the middle ear are unable to move, would this impair the detection of sound by conductance through bone?[35]

Equilibrium and Balance

The vestibular complex is made up of the three **semicircular canals**, the **utricle**, the **saccule**, and the **ampullae**. All are essentially tubes filled with endolymph, and like the cochlea, they contain hair cells that detect motion. However, their function is to detect not sound, but rather rotational acceleration of the head. They are innervated by afferent neurons which send balance information to the pons, cerebellum, and other areas. The vestibular complex monitors both static equilibrium and linear acceleration, which contribute to your sense of balance.

Vision: Structure and Function

The eye is the structure designed to detect visual stimuli. The structures of the eye first form an image on the retina, which detects light and converts the stimuli into action potentials to send to the brain. Light enters the eye by passing through the **cornea**, the clear portion at the front of the eye. Light is bent or

---

[33] More rapid firing of a cochlear neuron indicates an increase in volume of sound. If the pitch changed, a different set of neurons would fire action potentials.

[34] Conductance through bone allows some hearing by causing the cochlea to vibrate, which stimulates action potentials that pass through the auditory nerve to the brain. However, if the auditory nerve is severed, no hearing of any kind is possible.

[35] The bones of the middle ear serve to conduct vibration from the outer ear to the liquid within the cochlea but are not involved directly in detecting sound. Bone conductance can still stimulate the cochlea and result in hearing if the middle ear is nonfunctional.

refracted as it passes through the cornea (which is highly curved and thus acts as a lens), since the refractive index of the cornea is higher than that of air. The cornea is continuous at its borders with the white of the eye, the **sclera**. Beneath the sclera is a layer called the **choroid**. It contains darkly pigmented cells; this pigmentation absorbs excess light within the eye. Beneath the choroid is the **retina**, the surface upon which light is focused.

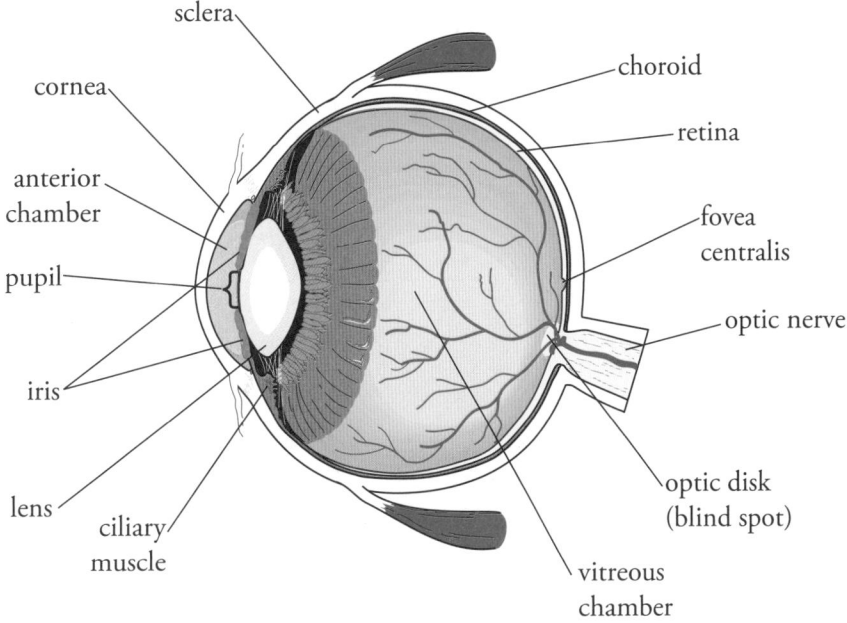

Figure 15   The Eye

Just inside the cornea is the **anterior chamber** (front chamber), which contains a fluid termed **aqueous humor**. At the back of the anterior chamber is a membrane called the **iris** with an opening called the **pupil**. The iris is the colored part of the eye, and muscles in the iris regulate the diameter of the pupil. Just behind the iris is the **posterior chamber**, also containing aqueous humor. In the back part of the posterior chamber is the **lens**. Its role is to fine-tune the angle of incoming light, so that the beams are perfectly focused upon the retina. The curvature of the lens (and thus its refractive power) is varied by the **ciliary muscle**.

Light passes through the **vitreous chamber** en route from the lens to the retina. This chamber contains a thick, jelly-like fluid called **vitreous humor**. The retina is located at the back of the eye. It contains electromagnetic receptor cells (photoreceptors) known as **rods** and **cones** which are responsible for detecting light. The rods and cones synapse with nerve cells called **bipolar cells**. In accordance with the name "bipolar," these cells have only one axon and one dendrite. The bipolar cells in turn synapse with **ganglion cells**, whose axons comprise the **optic nerve**, which travels from each eye toward the occipital lobe of the brain where complex analysis of a visual image occurs. In Figure 16 on the next page, you may notice that light has to pass through two layers of neurons before it can reach the rods and cones. The neurons are fine enough to not significantly obstruct incoming rays.

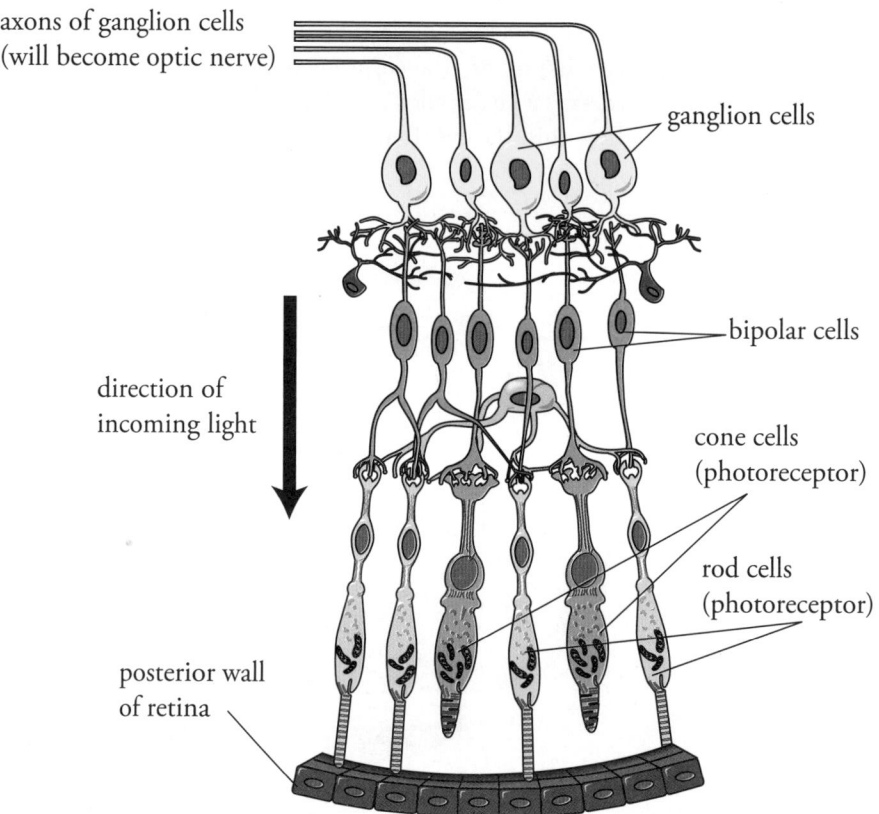

axons of ganglion cells
(will become optic nerve)

ganglion cells

bipolar cells

direction of
incoming light

cone cells
(photoreceptor)

rod cells
(photoreceptor)

posterior wall
of retina

Figure 16   Organization of the Retina

The point on the retina where many axons from ganglion cells converge to form the optic nerve is the **optic disk**. It is also known as the **blind spot** (Figure 17) because it contains no photoreceptors. Another special region of the retina is the **macula**. In the center of the macula is the **fovea centralis** (focal point), which contains only cones and is responsible for extreme visual acuity. When you stare directly at something, you focus its image on the fovea.

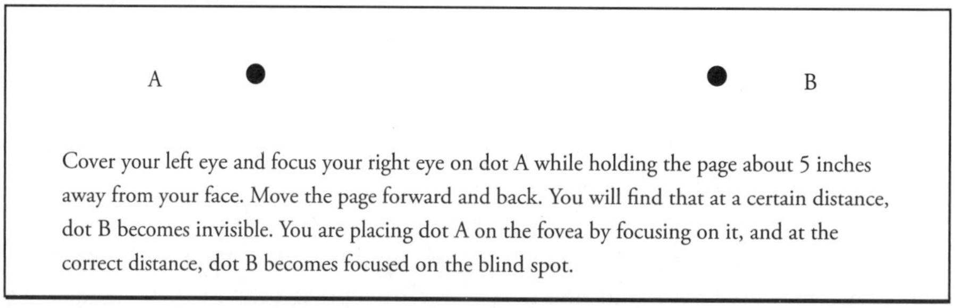

A   ●   ●   B

Cover your left eye and focus your right eye on dot A while holding the page about 5 inches away from your face. Move the page forward and back. You will find that at a certain distance, dot B becomes invisible. You are placing dot A on the fovea by focusing on it, and at the correct distance, dot B becomes focused on the blind spot.

Figure 17   Demonstrating the Blind Spot

The Photoreceptors: Rods and Cones

Rods and cones, named because of their shapes, contain special pigment proteins that change their tertiary structure upon absorbing light. Each protein, called an **opsin**, is bound to one molecule of **retinal**, which is derived from vitamin A. In the dark, when the rods and cones are resting, retinal has several *trans* double bonds and one *cis* double bond. In this conformation, retinal and its associated opsin keep a sodium channel open. The cell remains depolarized. Upon absorbing a photon of light, retinal is converted to the **all-trans form**. This triggers a series of reactions that ultimately closes the sodium channel, and the cell hyperpolarizes.

Rods and cones synapse on bipolar cells. Because of their depolarization in the dark, both types of photoreceptors release the neurotransmitter **glutamate** onto the bipolar cells. Upon the absorption of a photon of light and subsequent hyperpolarization, the photoreceptors release less glutamate, or stop releasing it altogether.

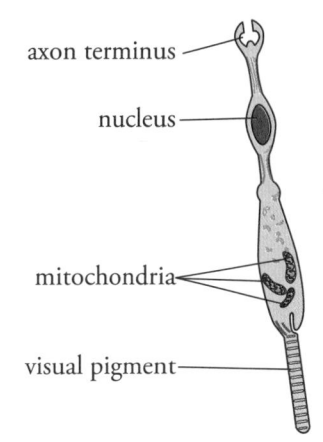

Figure 18   Rod Cell Structure

The effect on the bipolar cells varies. Some bipolar cells are "on center" and are inhibited by glutamate. This means that when the photoreceptor is in the dark and releasing glutamate, the on-center bipolar cell releases very little or no neurotransmitter. However, when the photoreceptor is in the light (light is ON the center), and stops releasing glutamate, the inhibition of the on-center bipolar cell stops, and the bipolar cell increases its release of neurotransmitter. "Off center" bipolar cells work in the opposite manner; they are stimulated by the glutamate released when the photoreceptor is in the dark, and inhibited when glutamate stops being released in the light.

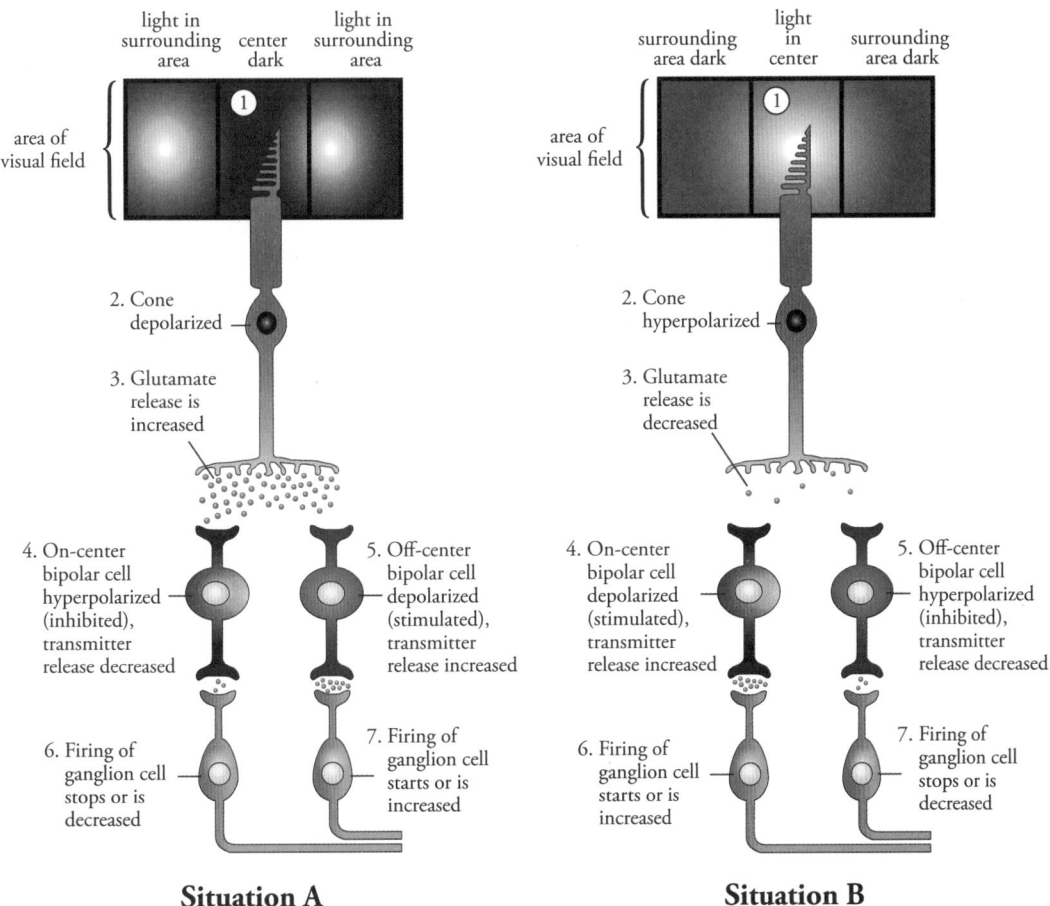

Figure 19   On-Center Off-Center Bipolar Cells

Night vision is accomplished by the rods, which are more sensitive to dim light and motion and are more concentrated in the periphery of the retina. Cones require abundant light and are responsible for color vision and high-acuity vision, and hence are more concentrated in the fovea.[36] Color vision depends on the presence of three different types of cones. One is specialized to absorb blue light, one absorbs green, and one absorbs red. [What physical difference allows this functional difference?[37]] The brain perceives hues by integrating the relative input of these three basic stimuli.

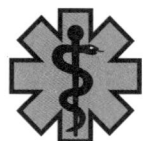

Defects in Visual Acuity

Normal vision is termed **emmetropia**. Too much or too little curvature of the cornea or lens results in visual defects. Too much curvature causes light to be bent too much and to be focused in front of the retina. The result is **myopia**, or nearsightedness. Myopia can be corrected by a concave (diverging) lens, which will cause the light rays to diverge slightly before they reach the cornea. **Hyperopia**, farsightedness, results from the focusing of light behind the retina. Hyperopia can be corrected by a convex (converging) lens, which causes light rays to converge before reaching the cornea. **Presbyopia** is an inability to **accommodate** (focus). It results from loss of flexibility of the lens, which occurs with aging.

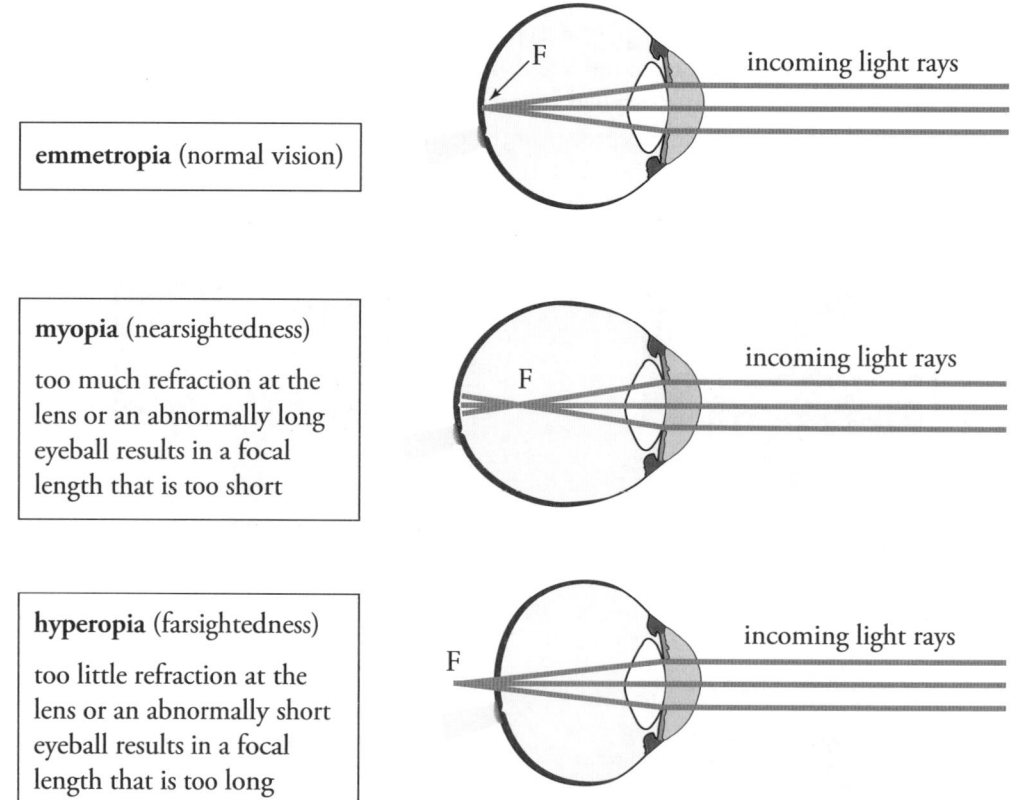

Figure 20   Defects in Visual Acuity ("F" denotes the focal point)

---

[36] Remember: *Cones—Color—aCuity.*

[37] Each type of cone makes a particular pigment protein which is specialized to change conformation when light of the appropriate frequency strikes it.

Vision: Information Processing

For humans, vision is the primary sense; even if other information (such as sound or smell) counters visual information, we are more likely to "believe our eyes." The processing of visual information is extremely complex, and highly reliant on expectations and past experience. Neurons in the **visual cortex** fire in response to very specific information; feature detecting neurons are specific neurons in the brain that fire in response to particular visual features, such as lines, edges, angles, and movement. This information is then passed along to other neurons that begin to assimilate these distinct features into more complex objects, and so on. Therefore, **feature detection theory** explains why a certain area of the brain is activated when looking at a face, a different area is activated when looking at the letters on this page, etc. In order to process vast amounts of visual information quickly and effectively, our brain employs **parallel processing**, whereby many aspects of a visual stimulus (such as form, motion, color, and depth) are processed simultaneously instead of in a step-by-step or serial fashion. [Note: parallel processing is also employed for other stimuli as well.] The occipital lobe constructs a holistic image by integrating all of the separate elements of an object, in addition to accessing stored information. For example, the brain is simultaneously processing the individual features of an image, while also accessing stored information, to rapidly come to the conclusion that you are not only viewing a face, but you are specifically viewing your mom's face. All of this requires a tremendous amount of resources; in fact, the human brain dedicates approximately 30% of the cortex to processing visual information, while only 8% is devoted to processing touch information, and a mere 3% processes auditory information!

Table 5 Summary of Sensory Modalities

Modality	Receptor	Receptor type	Organ	Stimulus
Vision	• rods and cones	• electromagnetic	• retina	• light
Hearing	• auditory hair cells	• mechanoreceptor	• organ of Corti	• vibration
Olfaction	• olfactory nerve endings	• chemoreceptor	• individual neurons	• airborne chemicals
Taste	• taste cells	• chemoreceptor	• taste bud	• food chemicals
Touch (a few examples)	• Pacinian corpuscles • free nerve endings • temperature receptors	• mechanoreceptor • nociceptor • thermoreceptor	• skin	• pressure • pain • temperature
Interoception (two examples)	• aortic arch baroreceptors • pH receptors	• baroreceptor • chemoreceptor	• aortic arch • aortic arch / medulla oblongata	• blood pressure • pH

General Sensory Processing

Absolute Thresholds

We are very sensitive to certain types of stimuli. The minimum stimulus intensity required to activate a sensory receptor 50% of the time (and thus detect the sensation) is called the **absolute threshold**. In other words, for each special sense, the 50% recognition point defines the absolute threshold. (Note that

8.5

this threshold can vary between individuals and different organisms—the absolute smell threshold for a human and a dog differs greatly.) Absolute thresholds also vary with age. For example, as we age, we gradually lose our ability to detect higher-pitched sounds. [What is the anatomical reason for this?[38]]

Difference Thresholds

Absolute thresholds are important for detecting the presence or absence of stimuli, but the ability to determine the change or difference in stimuli is also vital. The **difference threshold** (also called the *just noticeable difference*, or JND) is the minimum noticeable difference between any two sensory stimuli, 50% of the time. The magnitude of the initial stimulus influences the difference threshold; for example, if you lift a one pound weight and a two pound weight, the difference will be obvious, but if you lift a 100 pound weight and 101 pound weight, you probably won't be able to tell the difference. Indeed, **Weber's law** dictates that two stimuli must differ by a constant *proportion* in order for their difference to be perceptible. Interestingly, the exact proportion varies by stimulus; but for humans, two objects must differ in weight by 2% [in the weight example above, what is the minimum weight needed to detect a difference between it and the 100 pound weight?[39]], two lights must differ in intensity by 8%, and two tones must differ in frequency by 0.3%.

Signal Detection Theory

Detecting sensory stimuli not only depends on the information itself, but also on our psychological state, including alertness, expectation, motivation, and prior experience. **Signal detection theory** attempts to predict how and when someone will detect the presence of a given sensory stimulus (the "signal") amidst all of the other sensory stimuli in the background (considered the "noise"). There are four possible outcomes: a hit (the signal is present and was detected), a miss (the signal was present but not detected), a false alarm (the signal was not present but the person thought it was), and a correct rejection (the signal was not present and the person did not think it was). Signal detection can have important life-or-death consequences—imagine how crucial it is for doctors to be able to detect the signal (perhaps a tumor on a CT scan) from the noise.

Gestalt Psychology

Gestalt is the German word for "whole." Gestalt psychologists believe that the whole exceeds the sum of its parts; in other words, when humans perceive an object, rather than seeing lines, angles, colors, and shadows, they perceive the whole—a face or a table or a dog. Beyond merely registering the individual pieces, the human brain perceives the whole. **Bottom-up processing** begins with the sensory receptors and works up to the complex integration of information occurring in the brain. **Top-down processing** occurs when the brain applies experience and expectations to interpret sensory information; note that the brain in fact uses a combination of the two: information is received in a bottom-up fashion from sensory receptors while the brain is superimposing assumptions in a top-down manner.

---

[38] Loud sounds can mechanically harm the hair cells, causing them to die. When this occurs, the hair cell can no longer send sound signals to the brain. In people, once a hair cell dies, it will never regrow. The hair cells that detect higher frequency sounds are the smallest and the most easily damaged; therefore, as people age and more hair cells are damaged and lost, hearing loss occurs. Since the smallest hair cells are the ones most likely lost, loss of sensitivity to high-pitched sounds is common in older people.

[39] 102 pounds, which is 2% heavier than 100 pounds

8.6 THE ENDOCRINE SYSTEM

The nervous system and endocrine system represent the two major control systems of the body. The nervous system is fast-acting with relatively short-term effects, whereas the endocrine system takes longer to communicate signals but has generally longer lasting effects. These two control systems are interconnected, as neurons can signal the release of hormones from endocrine glands. [What is one such connection in the sympathetic nervous system?[40]] A primary connection between the nervous and endocrine systems is the *hypothalamic-pituitary axis*, which is described in more detail below.

Hormone Types: Transport and Mechanisms of Action

While the nervous system regulates cellular function from instant to instant, the endocrine system regulates physiology (especially metabolism) over a period of hours to days. The nervous system communicates via the extremely rapid action potential. The signal of the endocrine system is the **hormone**, defined as a molecule which is *secreted into the bloodstream* by an endocrine gland, and which has its effects upon *distant* target cells possessing the appropriate receptor. An **endocrine gland** is a *ductless* gland whose secretory products are picked up by capillaries supplying blood to the region. (In contrast, **exocrine glands** secrete their products into the external environment by way of ducts, which empty into the gastrointestinal lumen or the external world.) A **hormone receptor** is a polypeptide that possesses a ligand-specific binding site. Binding of ligand (hormone) to the site causes the receptor to modify target cell activity. *Tissue-specificity of hormone action is determined by whether the cells of a tissue have the appropriate receptor.*

Some signaling molecules modify the activity of the cell which secreted them; this is an **autocrine** activity (*auto-* means self). For example, a T cell secretes interleukin 2, which binds to receptors on the same T cell to stimulate increased activity.

Hormones can be grouped into one of two classes. *Hydrophilic* hormones, such as **peptides** and **amino-acid derivatives**, must bind to receptors on the cell surface, while *hydrophobic* hormones, such as the **steroid hormones**, bind to receptors in the cellular interior.

Peptide Hormones

Peptide hormones are synthesized into the rough ER and modified in the Golgi. Then they are stored in vesicles until needed, when they are released by exocytosis. In the bloodstream they dissolve in the plasma, since they are hydrophilic. Their hydrophilicity also means they cannot cross biological membranes and thus are required to communicate with the interior of the target cell by way of a ____,[41] discussed in Chapter 6. To briefly review, the peptide hormone is a first messenger which must bind to a cell-surface receptor. The receptor is a polypeptide with a domain on the inner surface of the plasma membrane that contains the ability to catalytically activate a second messenger. The end result of second messenger activation is that the function of proteins in the cytoplasm is changed. A key feature of second messenger cascades is signal amplification, which allows a few activated receptors to change the activity of many enzymes in the cytoplasm.

---

[40] The sympathetic nervous system directly innervates the adrenal medulla to stimulate the release of epinephrine.

[41] second messenger cascade

Because peptide hormones modify the activity of existing enzymes in the cytoplasm, their effects are exerted rapidly, minutes to hours from the time of secretion. Also, the duration of their effects is brief.

There are two subgroups within the peptide hormone category: polypeptides and amino acid derivatives. An example of a polypeptide hormone is insulin, which has a complex tertiary structure involving disulfide bridges. It is secreted by the β cells of the pancreatic islets of Langerhans in response to elevated blood glucose and binds to a cell-surface receptor with a cytoplasmic domain possessing protein kinase activity. Amino acid derivatives, as their name implies, are derived from single amino acids and contain no peptide bonds. For example, tyrosine is the parent amino acid for the catecholamines (which include epinephrine) and the thyroid hormones. Despite the fact that these two classes are derived from the same precursor molecule, they have different properties. The catecholamines act like peptide hormones, while the thyroid hormones behave more like steroid hormones. Epinephrine is a small cyclic molecule secreted by the adrenal medulla upon activation of the sympathetic nervous system. It binds to cell-surface receptors to trigger a cascade of events that produces the second messenger cyclic adenosine monophosphate (cAMP) and activates protein kinases in the cytoplasm. Thyroid hormones incorporate iodine into their structure. They enter cells, bind to DNA, and activate transcription of genes involved in energy mobilization.

Steroid Hormones

Steroids are hydrophobic molecules synthesized from cholesterol in the smooth endoplasmic reticulum. Due to their hydrophobicity, steroids can freely diffuse through biological membranes. Thus, they are not stored but rather diffuse into the bloodstream as soon as they are made. If a steroid hormone is not needed, it will not be made. Steroids' hydrophobicity also means they cannot be dissolved in the plasma. Instead they journey through the bloodstream stuck to proteins in the plasma, such as albumin. [What holds the steroid bound to a plasma protein?[42]] The small, hydrophobic steroid hormone exerts its effects upon target cells by *diffusing through the plasma membrane to bind with a receptor in the cytoplasm*. Once it has bound its ligand, the steroid hormone-receptor complex is transported into the nucleus, where it acts as a sequence-specific regulator of transcription. Because steroid hormones must modify transcription to change the *amount* and/or *type* of proteins in the cell, their effects are exerted slowly, over a period of days, and persist for days to weeks.

Steroids regulating sexuality, reproduction, and development are secreted by the testes, ovaries, and placenta. Steroids regulating water balance and other processes are secreted by the adrenal cortex. All other endocrine glands secrete peptide hormones. (Note that although thyroid hormone is derived from an amino acid, its mechanism of action more closely resembles that of the steroid hormones.)

---

[42] No bond—just hydrophobic interactions

Table 6 Peptide vs. Steroid Hormones

	Peptides	**Steroids**
Structure	hydrophilic, large (polypeptides) or small (amino acid derivatives)	hydrophobic, small
Site of synthesis	rough ER	smooth ER
Regulation of release	stored in vesicles until a signal for secretion is received	synthesized only when needed and then used immediately, not stored
Transport in bloodstream	free	stuck to protein carrier
Specificity	only target cells have appropriate surface receptors (exception: thyroxine = cytoplasmic)	only target cells have appropriate cytoplasmic receptors
Mechanism of effect	bind to receptors that generate second messengers which result in modification of *enzyme activity*	bind to receptors that alter *gene expression* by regulating DNA transcription
Timing of effect	rapid, short-lived	slow, long-lasting

Organization and Regulation of the Human Endocrine System

The endocrine system has many different roles. Hormones are essential for gamete synthesis, ovulation, pregnancy, growth, sexual development, and overall level of metabolic activity. Despite this diversity of function, endocrine activity is harmoniously orchestrated. Maintenance of order in such a complex system might seem impossible to accomplish in a preplanned manner. Regulation of the endocrine system is not preplanned or rigidly structured, but is instead generally automatic. Hormone levels rise and fall as dictated by physiological needs. The endocrine system is ordered yet dynamic. This flexible, automatic orderliness is attributable to feedback regulation. The amount of a hormone secreted is controlled not by a preformulated plan but rather by changes in the variable the hormone is responsible for controlling. Continuous circulation of blood exposes target cells to regulatory hormones and also exposes endocrine glands to serum concentrations of physiological variables that they regulate. Thus, *regulator* and that which is *regulated* are in continuous communication. Concentration of a species X in the aqueous portion of the bloodstream is denoted "serum [X]."

An example of feedback regulation is the interaction between the hormone calcitonin and serum $[Ca^{2+}]$. The function of calcitonin is to prevent serum $[Ca^{2+}]$ from peaking above normal levels, and the amount of calcitonin secreted is directly proportional to increases in serum $[Ca^{2+}]$ above normal. When serum $[Ca^{2+}]$ becomes elevated, calcitonin is secreted. Then when serum $[Ca^{2+}]$ levels fall, calcitonin secretion stops. The falling serum $[Ca^{2+}]$ level (*that which is regulated*) feeds back to the cells which secrete calcitonin (*regulators*). The serum $[Ca^{2+}]$ level is a **physiological endpoint** which must be maintained at constant levels. This demonstrates the role of the endocrine system in maintaining **homeostasis**, or physiological consistency.

An advantage of the endocrine system and its feedback regulation is that very complex arrays of variables can be controlled automatically. It's as if the variables controlled themselves. However, some integration (a central control mechanism) is necessary. Superimposed upon the hormonal regulation of physiological endpoints is another layer of regulation: hormones that regulate hormones. Such meta-regulators are known as **tropic hormones**.

For example, adrenocorticotropic hormone (ACTH) is secreted by the anterior pituitary. The role of ACTH is to stimulate increased activity of the portion of the adrenal gland called the **cortex**, which is responsible for secreting cortisol (among other steroid hormones). ACTH is a tropic hormone because it does not directly affect physiological endpoints, but merely regulates another regulator (cortisol). Cortisol regulates physiological endpoints, including cellular responses to stress and serum [glucose]. Feedback regulation applies to tropic hormones as well as to direct regulators of physiological endpoints; the level of ACTH is influenced by the level of cortisol. When cortisol is needed, ACTH is secreted, and when the serum [cortisol] increases sufficiently, ACTH secretion slows.

You may have noticed that in both of our examples the effect of feedback was *inhibitory*: the result of hormone secretion inhibits further secretion. Inhibitory feedback is called **negative feedback or feedback inhibition**. Most feedback in the endocrine system (and if you remember, most biochemical feedback) is negative. There are few examples of positive feedback, which we will not discuss here. A key example will be discussed in Chapter 13 with the reproductive systems.

There is yet another layer of control. Many of the functions of the endocrine system depend on instructions from the brain. The portion of the brain which controls much of the endocrine system is the **hypothalamus**, located at the center of the brain. The hypothalamus controls the endocrine system by releasing tropic hormones that regulate other tropic hormones, called **releasing and inhibiting factors** or **releasing and inhibiting hormones**.

For example (Figure 21), the hypothalamus secretes corticotropin releasing hormone (CRH, also known as CRF, where "F" stands for factor). The role of CRH is to cause increased secretion of ACTH. Just as ACTH secretion is regulated by feedback inhibition from cortisol, CRH secretion, too, is inhibited by cortisol. You begin to see that regulatory pathways in the endocrine system can get pretty complex.

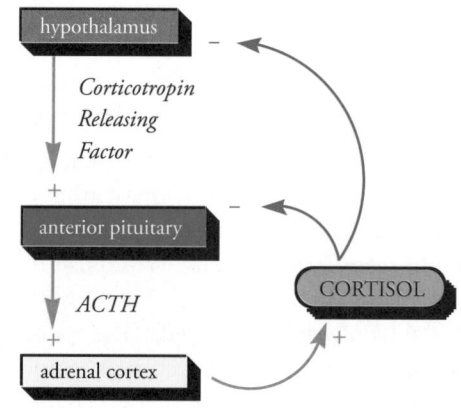

Figure 21   Feedback Regulation of Cortisol Secretion

Understanding that the hypothalamus controls the anterior pituitary and that the anterior pituitary controls most of the endocrine system is important. Damage to the connection between the hypothalamus and the pituitary is fatal, unless daily hormone replacement therapy is given. This endocrine control center is given a special name: **hypothalamic-pituitary control axis** (Figure 22). The hypothalamus exerts its control of the pituitary by secreting its hormones into the bloodstream, just like any other endocrine gland; what's unique is that a special miniature circulatory system is provided for efficient transport of hypothalamic releasing and inhibiting factors to the anterior pituitary. This blood supply is known as the **hypothalamic-pituitary portal system**. You will also hear the term *hypothalamic-hypophysial portal system*. **Hypophysis** is another name for the pituitary gland.

A Note on Portal Systems: As a general rule, blood leaving the heart moves through only one capillary bed before returning to the heart, since the pressure drops substantially in capillaries. A portal system, however, consists of two capillary beds in sequence, allowing for direct communication between nearby structures. The two portal systems you need to understand are: the hypothalamic-pituitary portal system and the hepatic portal system (from the gastrointestinal tract to the liver, which you can read more about in Chapter 10).

One more bit of background information is necessary before we can delve into specific hormones. The pituitary gland has two halves: front (*anterior*) and back (*posterior*); see Figure 22. The **anterior pituitary** is also called the **adenohypophysis** and the **posterior pituitary** is also known as the **neurohypophysis**. It is important to understand the difference. The anterior pituitary is a normal endocrine gland, and it is controlled by hypothalamic releasing and inhibiting factors (essentially tropic hormones). The posterior pituitary is composed of axons which descend from the hypothalamus. These hypothalamic neurons that send axons down to the posterior pituitary are an example of **neuroendocrine cells**, neurons which secrete hormones into the bloodstream. The hormones released by the posterior pituitary are ADH (antidiuretic hormone or vasopressin), which causes the kidney to retain water during times of thirst, and oxytocin, which causes milk let-down for nursing as well as uterine contractions during labor. [Are these hormones made by axon termini in the posterior pituitary or by somas in the hypothalamus?[43]]

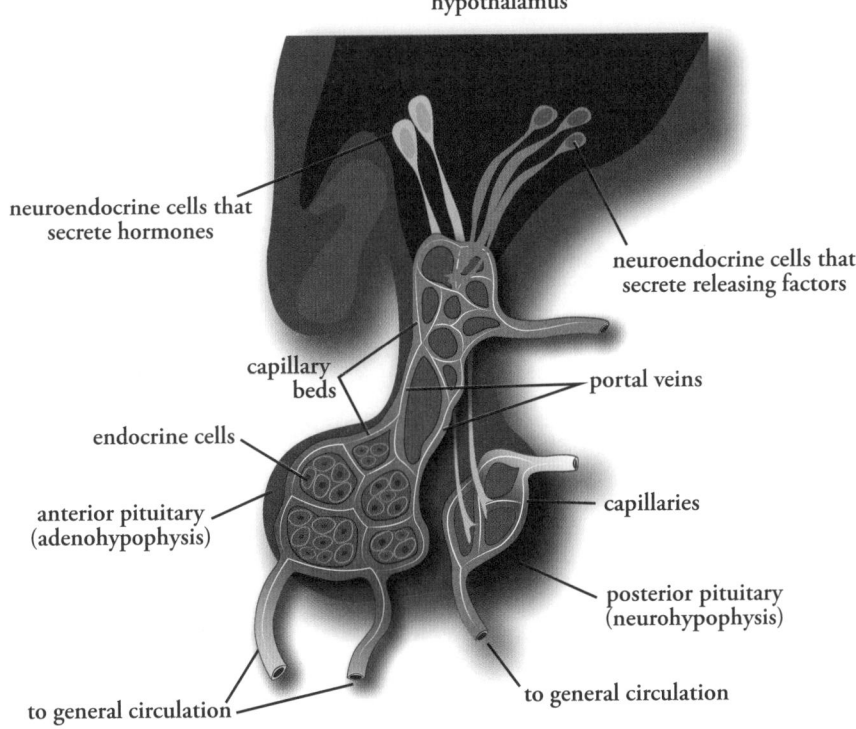

hypothalamus

neuroendocrine cells that secrete hormones

neuroendocrine cells that secrete releasing factors

capillary beds

portal veins

endocrine cells

anterior pituitary (adenohypophysis)

capillaries

posterior pituitary (neurohypophysis)

to general circulation

to general circulation

Figure 22 The Hypothalamic-Pituitary Control Axis

Major Glands and Their Hormones

The major hormones and glands of the endocrine system are listed in Table 7 on page 119. Many of these hormones will be discussed in detail in later chapters. Insulin and glucagon will be discussed in the chapter on digestion and energy metabolism (Chapter 10). Testosterone, estrogen, progesterone, FSH, and LH will be presented in the chapter on reproductive biology (Chapter 13). The function of epinephrine has already been presented as part of the sympathetic nervous system response. In general, the hormones are involved in development of the body and in maintenance of constant conditions, homeostasis, in the adult. [Is epinephrine secreted by a duct into the bloodstream?[44]]

---

[43] All hypothalamic and pituitary hormones are peptides, and there is no protein synthesis at axon termini. Thus, ADH and oxytocin must be made in nerve cell bodies in the hypothalamus and transported down the axons to the posterior pituitary. The posterior pituitary doesn't actually make any hormones, then, it just stores ADH and oxytocin for later release.

[44] No. Endocrine hormones are not secreted through ducts.

Thyroid hormone and **cortisol** have broad effects on metabolism and energy usage. Thyroid hormone is produced from the amino acid tyrosine in the thyroid gland and comes in two forms, with three or four iodine atoms per molecule. The production of thyroid hormone is increased by thyroid stimulating hormone (TSH) from the anterior pituitary, which is regulated by the hypothalamus and the central nervous system in turn. The mechanism of action of thyroid hormone is to bind to a receptor in the cytoplasm of cells that then regulates transcription in the nucleus. The effect of this regulation is to increase the overall metabolic rate and body temperature, and, in children, to stimulate growth. Exposure to cold can increase the production of thyroid hormone. Cortisol is secreted by the adrenal cortex in response to ACTH from the pituitary. In general, the effects of cortisol tend to help the body deal with stress. Cortisol helps to mobilize glycogen and fat stores to provide energy during stress and also increases the consumption of proteins for energy. These effects are essential, since removal of the adrenal cortex can result in the death of animals exposed to even a small stress. Long-term high levels of cortisol tend to have negative effects, however, including suppression of the immune system.

- Would an inhibitor of protein synthesis block the action of thyroid hormone?[45]
- Would the production of ATP by mitochondria be stimulated or repressed by thyroid hormone?[46]
- Would thyroid hormone affect isolated mitochondria directly?[47]

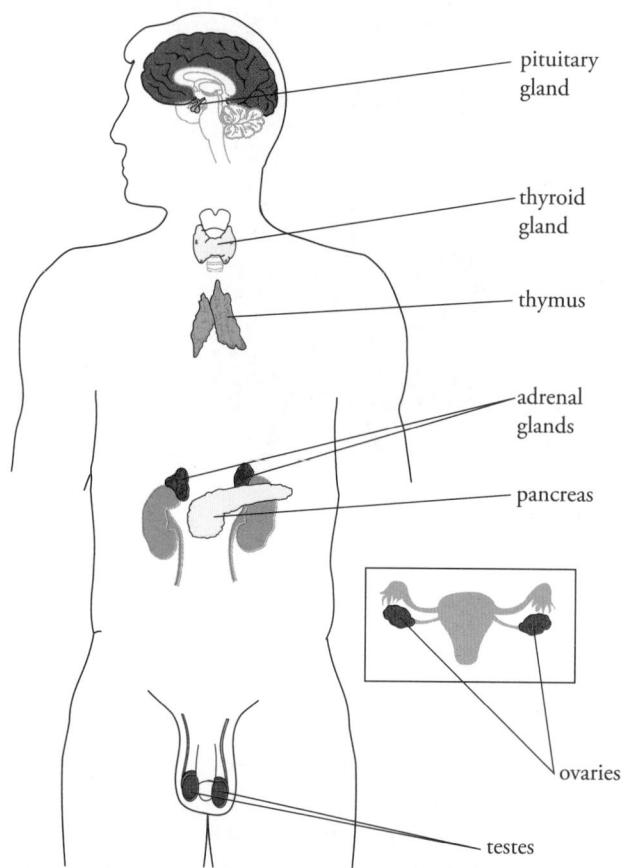

Figure 23   The Major Endocrine Glands

---

[45] Yes. Thyroid hormone binds to a receptor that regulates transcription. The mRNA stimulated by thyroid hormone receptor in the nucleus must be processed and translated before the effects of thyroid hormone can become evident.

[46] Thyroid hormone stimulates the basal metabolic rate throughout the body. More ATP will be consumed, so the mitochondria are stimulated to make more ATP.

[47] No. Thyroid hormone affects mitochondria *indirectly*, through the regulation of nuclear genes.

Table 7 Summary of the Hormones of the Endocrine System

Gland	Hormone [class]	Target/effect
Hypothalamus	releasing and inhibiting factors (peptides), posterior pituitary hormones	anterior pituitary/modify activity
Anterior pituitary	growth hormone (GH) (peptide)	↑ bone and muscle growth, ↑ cell turnover rate
	prolactin (peptide)	mammary gland/milk production
tropic	thyroid stimulating hormone (TSH) (peptide)	thyroid/↑ synthesis and release of TH
	adrenocorticotropic hormone (ACTH) (peptide)	↑ growth and secretory activity of adrenal cortex
gonadotropic	luteinizing hormone (LH) (peptide)	ovary/ovulation, testes/testosterone synth.
	follicle stimulating hormone (FSH) (peptide)	ovary/follicle development, testes/ spermatogenesis
Posterior pituitary	antidiuretic hormone (ADH, vasopressin) (peptide)	kidney/water retention
	oxytocin (peptide)	breast/milk letdown, uterus/contraction
Thyroid	thyroid hormone (TH, thyroxine) (modified amino acid)	child: necessary for physical and mental development; adult: ↑ metabolic rate and temp.
thyroid C cells	calcitonin (peptide)	bone, kidney; lowers serum $[Ca^{2+}]$
Parathyroids	parathyroid hormone (PTH) (peptide)	bone, kidney, small intestine/raises serum $[Ca^{2+}]$
Thymus	thymosin (children only) (peptide)	T cell development during childhood
Adrenal medulla	epinephrine (modified amino acid)	sympathetic stress response (rapid)
Adrenal cortex	cortisol ("glucocorticoid") (steroid)	longer-term stress response; ↑ blood [glucose]; ↑ protein catabolism; ↓ inflammation and immunity; many other
	aldosterone ("mineralocorticoid") (steroid)	kidney/↑ Na^+ reabsorption to ↑ b.p.
	sex steroids	not normally important, but an adrenal tumor can overproduce these, causing masculinization or feminization
Endocrine pancreas (islets of Langerhans)	insulin (β cells secrete) (peptide) —absent or ineffective in diabetes mellitus	↓ blood [glucose]/↑ glycogen and fat storage
	glucagon (α cells secrete) (peptide)	↑ blood [glucose]/↓ glycogen and fat storage
	somatostatin (SS—δ cells secrete) (peptide)	inhibits many digestive processes
Testes	testosterone (steroid)	male characteristics, spermatogenesis
Ovaries/placenta	estrogen (steroid)	female characteristics, endometrial growth
	progesterone (steroid)	endometrial secretion, pregnancy
Heart	atrial natriuretic factor (ANF) (peptide)	kidney/↑ urination to ↓ blood pressure
Kidney	erythropoietin (peptide)	bone marrow/↑ RBC synthesis

8.6

Chapter 8 Summary

- The neuron is the basic structural and functional unit of the nervous system. It has several specialized structures that allow it to transmit action potentials.

- Neurons receive incoming information via dendrites. Signals are summed by the axon hillock, and if the signal is greater than the threshold, an action potential is initiated.

- The action potential is an all-or-none signal that includes depolarization (via voltage-gated sodium channels) and repolarization (via voltage-gated potassium channels); it begins and ends at the cell's resting potential of −70 mV.

- Since action potentials are all-or-none events, intensity is coded by the frequency of the action potential.

- Neurons communicate with other neurons, organs, and glands at synapses. Most synapses are chemical in nature; an action potential causes the release of neurotransmitter into the synaptic cleft, and binding of the neurotransmitter to receptors on the postsynaptic cell triggers a change, either stimulatory or inhibitory, in that cell.

- The central nervous system includes the spinal cord and the brain; specialized areas control specific aspects of human behavior, movement, intelligence, emotion, and reflexes.

- The peripheral nervous system includes the somatic (voluntary) and autonomic (involuntary) subdivisions.

- The sympathetic branch of the autonomic system controls our fight-or-flight response; norepinephrine is the primary neurotransmitter of this system, and it is augmented by epinephrine from the adrenal medulla.

- The parasympathetic branch of the autonomic system controls our resting and digesting state; acetylcholine is the primary neurotransmitter of this system.

- Humans have several types of receptors (mechanoreceptors, chemoreceptors, nociceptors, thermoreceptors, electromagnetic receptors, and proprioceptors) that allow us to detect a variety of stimuli.

- The endocrine system controls our overall physiology and homeostasis by hormones that travel through the bloodstream. Hormones are released from endocrine glands, travel to distant target tissues via the blood, bind to receptors on target tissues, and exert effects on target cells.

- Peptide hormones are made from amino acids, bind to receptors on the cell surface, and typically affect target cells via second messenger pathways. Effects tend to be rapid and temporary.

- Steroid hormones are derived from cholesterol, bind to receptors in the cytoplasm or nucleus, and bind to DNA to alter transcription. Effects tend to occur more slowly and are more permanent.

CHAPTER 8 FREESTANDING PRACTICE QUESTIONS

1. Macular degeneration refers to the deterioration of the center portion of the retina, the macula, leading to vision loss. What type of receptor would you expect to see loss of in macular degeneration?

A) Deterioration of cone cells only
B) Deterioration of electromagnetic receptors found at the back of the eye
C) Deterioration of mechanoreceptors at the back of the eye
D) Deterioration of bipolar cells and ganglion cells, leading to loss of nociceptors

2. Which of the following is the correct order of events during synaptic transmission?

A) Depolarization of presynaptic membrane → Voltage-gated calcium channels open → Neurotransmitter binds to ligand-gated ion channels → Membrane depolarization of postsynaptic cell → Neurotransmitters cross the synaptic cleft
B) An action potential reaches the end of an axon at the synaptic knob → Depolarization of presynaptic membrane → Voltage-gated sodium channels open → Neurotransmitter binds to ligand-gated ion channels → Membrane depolarization of postsynaptic cell
C) Depolarization of presynaptic membrane → Neurotransmitter binds to ligand-gated ion channels → Neurotransmitter in the synaptic cleft is degraded and/or removed → An action potential reaches the end of an axon
D) An action potential reaches the end of an axon → Voltage-gated calcium channels open → Neurotransmitter binds to ligand-gated ion channels → Neurotransmitter in the synaptic cleft is degraded and/or removed

3. People who suffer from severe epilepsy are sometimes treated with a "split brain" procedure that prevents most communication between the left and right hemispheres of the brain. The structure that is most likely cut in this operation is the:

A) corpus callosum.
B) medulla.
C) thalamus.
D) pons.

4. Myasthenia gravis, an autoimmune disorder, results from the production of antibodies against acetylcholine receptors in the body. Which of the following statements is FALSE?

A) A patient may have difficulty opening his/her eyes.
B) Repeated injection of human acetylcholine receptor into an animal model will produce clinical symptoms in that animal.
C) The disease does not directly affect the release of neurotransmitter.
D) This disease only impacts the neuromuscular junction.

5. Which of the following is true about cortisol?

A) It is synthesized in the smooth ER and transported freely in the bloodstream.
B) It is synthesized in the rough ER and transported by a protein carrier in the bloodstream.
C) It is synthesized in the smooth ER and synthesized only when needed.
D) It is synthesized in the rough ER and stored in vesicles until signal for secretion is received.

6. Parathyroid adenomas are tumors that can lead to hyperparathyroidism. Which of the following can occur in a patient with a parathyroid adenoma?

    I.   Increased frequency of bone fractures
    II.   Decreased reabsorption of calcium by the kidneys
    III.   Increased serum calcium levels

A) I only
B) II only
C) I and II
D) I and III

7. All of the following hormones would activate second messenger systems to exert their effect on target cells, EXCEPT:

A) insulin.
B) glucagon.
C) epinephrine.
D) progesterone.

8. Blood levels of creatinine and urea nitrogen can be used to assess kidney function, with elevated values indicating possible kidney disease. Additionally, dehydration is known to reduce blood flow to the kidneys and elevate creatinine and urea nitrogen levels in the blood. A patient exhibits high levels of blood creatinine and blood urea nitrogen, but kidney disease is not suspected. The patient's blood pressure is also very low. Which of the following would you expect?

    I.   Increased release of ADH
    II.   Decreased release of renin
    III.   Decreased release of aldosterone

A) I only
B) II only
C) II and III only
D) I, II, and III

CHAPTER 8 PRACTICE PASSAGE

Mammalian nerve cells have on their outer surface a subtype of glutamate receptors called the *N*-methyl-D-aspartate (NMDA) receptor. The NMDA receptor binds glutamate, an amino acid neurotransmitter, which ultimately results in the inward flow of calcium ions.

The NMDA receptor has been studied by exposing nerve cells to ischemic conditions (a diminished flow of blood) which result in localized brain damage. The affected neurons demonstrate depleted energy reserves with decreased internal stores of ATP. Energy-driven Na^+/K^+ ATPase enzymes located in the cell membrane begin to fail. If the ischemic conditions continue, the neuronal cell membrane depolarizes, providing an excitatory stimulus for the release of excessive amounts of glutamate. Other nerve cells in close proximity experience sustained binding of glutamate to NMDA receptor sites, which can lead to further cell membrane depolarization.

Experiment 1:

Cultured nerve cells were exposed to normal or decreased oxygen concentrations. Differing concentrations of extracellular calcium or glutamate antagonists were also established. Intracellular calcium levels were measured after one minute. The results of this experiment are listed below:

Table 1

Extracellular environment			Intracellular calcium
Oxygen	Glutamate antagonists	Calcium	
L	−	−	N
L	−	H	I
L	+	−	N
L	+	H	N
H	−	−	N
H	−	H	N
H	+	−	N
H	+	H	N

Key: L = low concentration, H = high concentration
+ = present, − = absent
N = normal, I = increase

Experiment 2:

Several cultured neurons were bathed in a solution containing high concentrations of calcium, sodium, and chloride ions, but not oxygen. The cells experienced marked swelling and eventually an action potential was evoked. After the action potential, internal ion levels were measured every 30 seconds. Intracellular levels of both calcium and sodium were elevated.

Based on these two experiments, researchers have proposed that the initial effects of activation of the NMDA receptor can be modeled as follows:

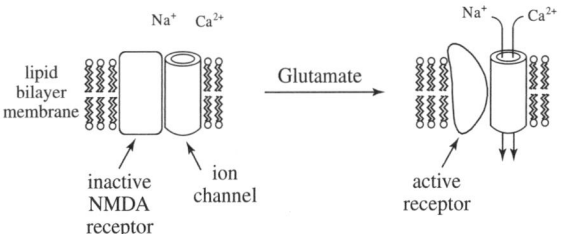

Figure 1

Further experiments suggested that the NMDA receptor also allowed K^+ to exit the cell.

1. Flow of calcium into cells is essential to which of the following processes?

A) Opening of voltage-gated sodium channels
B) Propagation of action potentials in motor neuron axons
C) Cardiac muscle contraction
D) ATP hydrolysis

2. In the increased biosynthesis of neurotransmitter receptors, activity of the rough endoplasmic reticulum increases because:

A) the cell is undergoing the process of exocytosis.
B) it is the primary site of complex lipid synthesis.
C) it is the primary site of plasma membrane protein synthesis.
D) more vesicles arrive at the rough ER from the Golgi apparatus.

3. Regarding Experiment 2, which of the following is the most likely reason that the cells experienced marked swelling?

A) Activation of the NMDA receptor due to ischemia blocked aquaporins, preventing the efflux of water from the cell.

B) The failure of the Na^+/K^+ ATPase led to osmotic influx of water.

C) The high intracellular concentrations of sodium and calcium led to the osmotic influx of water.

D) The influx of sodium due to the action potential led to the osmotic influx of water.

4. Which of the following amino acids would most likely be found in the transmembrane portion of the NMDA receptor?

A) Leu

B) Pro

C) Arg

D) Asn

5. Regarding Experiment 1, if glutamate is the only neurotransmitter that can bind to the NMDA receptor to increase the inward flow of calcium, which of the following would account for the lack of calcium flow in the presence of oxygen, extracellular calcium, and no glutamate antagonists?

A) No glutamate was supplied to the cells in the extracellular medium.

B) Other glutamate receptor subtypes inhibit the flow of calcium into the cell.

C) In the presence of oxygen, the cell does not depolarize.

D) Ischemic conditions prevent the normal functioning of the Na^+/K^+ ATPases.

SOLUTIONS TO CHAPTER 8 FREESTANDING PRACTICE QUESTIONS

1. **B** The macula contains both rods and cones; the fovea centralis is a region of the macula that contains only cones. In macular degeneration, both rods and cones would be affected (choice A is wrong). Rods and cones are electromagnetic receptors, not mechanoreceptors, at the back of the eye (choice C is wrong, and choice B is correct). Bipolar cells and ganglion cells would be affected, but they are not nociceptors (choice D is wrong).

2. **D** The correct order of events is: 1) an action potential reaches the end of an axon at the synaptic knob, 2) depolarization of presynaptic membrane, 3) voltage-gated calcium channels open, 4) neurotransmitter is released from the presynaptic cell, 5) neurotransmitter crosses the synaptic cleft, 6) neurotransmitter binds to ligand-gated ion channels on the postsynaptic membrane, 7) membrane depolarization of postsynaptic cell, 8) voltage-gated sodium channels open, 9) an action potential is initiated, and 10) neurotransmitter in the synaptic cleft is degraded and/or removed (choices A, B, and C are wrong).

3. **A** The corpus callosum is a bundle of axons that connects the left and right hemispheres of the brain and is responsible for the vast majority of the communication between the two hemispheres. Cutting this structure in half prevents the rapid cross-hemispheric communication that is observed during seizures in patients with severe epilepsy. The medulla and pons are part of the hindbrain and play roles in basic autonomic processes (choices B and D are wrong), and the thalamus is a relay station for somatic sensory stimuli located in the diencephalon (choice C is wrong).

4. **D** Acetylcholine is a neurotransmitter in several areas in the body including the neuromuscular junction, pre- and postganglionic parasympathetic neurons, and preganglionic sympathetic neurons (choice D is the false statement and the correct answer choice). As acetylcholine receptors become nonfunctional with the binding of antibody, patients have difficulty with muscle contraction, and opening of the eyes may be one possible symptom of this (choice A is a true statement and can be eliminated). Repeated injection of an acetylcholine receptor into an animal model will result in an immune response and subsequent attack of the endogenous acetylcholine receptors, producing myasthenia gravis symptoms (choice B is a true statement and can be eliminated). The antibodies attack the postsynaptic neuron receptors and do not result in a direct change in neurotransmitter release (choice C is a true statement and can be eliminated).

5. **C**   Cortisol is a steroid hormone. Steroids are synthesized in the smooth ER (choices B and D can be eliminated). It is hydrophobic, so it needs to be bound to a carrier protein (usually albumin) to travel in the bloodstream (choice A can be eliminated). Steroid hormones are synthesized only when needed, and released immediately (choice C is correct).

6. **D**   Hyperparathyroidism means having an abnormally high level of parathyroid hormone. The functions of parathyroid hormone include 1) enhancing the breakdown of bone by osteoclasts and the release of calcium into the bloodstream, 2) enhancing the reabsorption of calcium in the nephrons of the kidneys, and 3) enhancing the absorption of calcium in the small intestine. Item I is true: high PTH levels cause calcium to leave the bone and enter the bloodstream, resulting in weak bones that can fracture easily (choice B can be eliminated). Item II is false: PTH leads to increased reabsorption of calcium to increase serum calcium levels (choice C can be eliminated). Item III is true: high PTH levels cause serum calcium levels to rise since it is being removed from the bone, reabsorbed by the kidneys, and absorbed by the small intestines (choice A can be eliminated). The correct answer is choice D.

7. **D**   Make sure to highlight the word "EXCEPT" and write "A B C D" on your noteboard. Evaluate each answer choice, writing "Y" if it would activate a second messenger system or "N" if it would not. Insulin is a peptide hormone. Peptide hormones are generally unable to cross the cell membrane, so they bind to receptors on the cell surface and trigger second messenger systems (write "Y" next to "A" on the noteboard). Glucagon and epinephrine are also peptide hormones and activate second messenger systems (write "Y" next to "B" and "C" on the noteboard). Progesterone, however, is a steroid hormone, and exerts its effects on the target cell by binding to intracellular receptors that ultimately regulate DNA transcription (write "N" next to "D" on the noteboard). Since choice D stands out with an "N" instead of a "Y," it is the correct answer choice.

8. **A**   Since this is a Roman numeral question, start by analyzing the Roman numeral item that appears in exactly two of the answer choices, in this case, Item I or III. Whether it is true or false, you can eliminate half the answer choices. Item I is true: the patient is probably dehydrated if they are experiencing elevated levels of blood creatinine and urea nitrogen in the absence of kidney disease. In response to dehydration, the posterior pituitary will secrete ADH, leading to increased water retention to help counteract the dehydration (choices B and C can be eliminated). You can evaluate either Item II or III to get to the correct answer. Item II is false: the patient has low blood pressure, which stimulates the release of renin from the kidney (choice D can be eliminated, and choice A is correct). Note that Item III is also false: a downstream effect of renin release is increased release of aldosterone.

SOLUTIONS TO CHAPTER 8 PRACTICE PASSAGE

1. **C** The action potential in cardiac muscle includes the opening of slow voltage-gated calcium channels. The opening of these channels allows calcium into cardiac muscle cells, which plays a role in the release of the troponin/tropomyosin complex from actin filaments, allowing myosin heads to bind and initiate contraction. Voltage-gated sodium channels open in response to changes in membrane potential, not calcium influx, and the changes in potential are typically due to sodium influx through ligand-gated channels (choice A is wrong). Propagation of action potentials in motor neurons relies on sodium and potassium flux, not calcium (choice B is wrong), and ATP hydrolysis is not calcium-dependent (choice D is wrong).

2. **C** Neurotransmitter receptors are integral plasma membrane proteins, all of which are translated on the rough ER. Increased plasma membrane protein translation requires more activity in the rough ER. The receptors are not released via exocytosis, they are embedded in the plasma membrane (choice A is wrong), lipid synthesis occurs in the smooth ER, not the rough ER (choice B is wrong), and vesicles travel from the ER to the Golgi apparatus, not the other way around (choice D is wrong).

3. **B** The cells were kept in ischemic (low oxygen) conditions. Oxygen is required for ATP synthesis, and ATP is required to operate the Na$^+$/K$^+$ ATPase. In the absence of oxygen, the lack of ATP would cause the Na$^+$/K$^+$ ATPases to fail. One of the functions of the ATPases is to maintain osmotic equilibrium for the cell; as it pumps ions out, water doesn't want to come in. The failure of the pump would lead to osmotic influx of water (choice B is correct). There is nothing in the passage to support the idea that NMDA receptors block aquaporins, and even if they did, the movement of water through the aquaporins is not restricted to just efflux (choice A is wrong). While the increase in intracellular concentrations of sodium and calcium could lead to osmotic influx of water, this would happen after the action potential was induced, and the swelling occurred prior to the induction of the action potential (choices C and D are wrong).

4. **A** Proteins that span the plasma membrane must contain hydrophobic (nonpolar) amino acid residues in the transmembrane region. Of the amino acids listed, only leucine and proline are nonpolar; arginine and asparagine are both polar (choices C and D can be eliminated). Proline, while nonpolar, does not fit well into the alpha helical shape of most transmembrane regions, making leucine the more likely of the two to be found there (choice B can be eliminated, and choice A is correct).

5. **C** In the presence of oxygen, the Na$^+$/K$^+$ ATPases would not fail, and the cell would not depolarize. If the cell doesn't depolarize, then glutamate would not be released to stimulate the NMDA receptor and open the calcium channels (choice C is correct). It is true that no glutamate was supplied to the cells, but this was by design; the experiment was designed to test what happens with glutamate release and NMDA receptor stimulation in the absence of oxygen. Supplying glutamate in the extracellular medium would prevent any effect of ischemia from being seen since the cell would automatically be stimulated (choice A is wrong). It is also true that ischemic conditions prevent the normal activity of the ATPases, but these cells are not exposed to ischemic conditions (choice D is wrong). There is no reason to assume any other glutamate receptor subtypes (choice B can be eliminated).

Chapter 9
The Circulatory, Lymphatic, and Immune Systems

9.1 OVERVIEW OF THE CIRCULATORY SYSTEM

The cells of a multicellular organism have the same basic requirements as unicellular organisms. Living so close to billions of other cells has many advantages, but there are drawbacks too. Each cell must compete with its neighbors for nutrients and oxygen and must also cope with the waste products that are inevitable in so dense a civilization. Other requirements of community living are efficient communication and homeostasis. The circulatory system addresses these problems by accomplishing the following goals:

1) Distribute nutrients from the digestive tract, liver, and adipose (fat) tissue.
2) Transport oxygen from the lungs to the entire body and carbon dioxide from the tissues to the lungs.
3) Transport metabolic waste products from tissues to the excretory system (i.e., the kidneys).
4) Transport hormones from endocrine glands to targets and provide feedback.
5) Maintain homeostasis of body temperature.
6) *Hemostasis* (blood clotting). This does not address a need of a multicellular organism *per se*, but rather is necessitated by the presence of the circulatory system itself.

The flow of blood through a tissue is known as **perfusion**. Inadequate blood flow, known as **ischemia**, results in tissue damage due to shortages of O_2 and nutrients, and buildup of metabolic wastes. When adequate circulation is present but the supply of oxygen is reduced, a tissue is said to suffer from **hypoxia**. [What's the difference between ischemia and hypoxia?[1]]

In the following sections we will study the components of the circulatory system. We will not delve into its thermoregulatory role, which will be covered in Chapter 12 (The Respiratory System and the Skin).

Components of the Circulatory System

The functions of the circulatory system involve transport of blood throughout the body and exchange of material between the blood and tissues. The **heart** is a muscular pump that forces blood through a branching series of vessels to the lungs and the rest of the body. Vessels that carry blood away from the heart at high pressure are **arteries**, and vessels that carry blood back toward the heart at low pressure are **veins**. As arteries pass farther from the heart, the pressure of blood decreases, and they branch into increasingly smaller arteries called **arterioles**. The arterioles then pass into the **capillaries**, very small vessels, often just wide enough for a single blood cell to pass. Arterioles have smooth muscle in their walls that can act as a control valve to restrict or increase the flow of blood into the capillaries of tissues. The capillaries have thin walls made of a single layer of cells and are designed to allow the exchange of material between the blood and tissues. After passing through capillaries, blood collects in small veins called **venules**, and then into the veins leading back to the heart. Except for the largest vessels near the heart, veins lack a muscular wall. From the heart, the blood can be pumped out once again through the arteries to the capillaries in the tissues.

- If the arterioles constrict in a tissue, will material diffuse through the wall of the arterioles into the tissue?[2]

---

[1] In hypoxia, wastes are adequately removed, but in ischemia they build up. Ischemia is worse.

[2] No. All exchange of material between the blood and tissues must occur in capillaries. The walls of arterioles are too thick and muscular for exchange to occur.

The inner lining of all blood vessels is formed by a thin layer of **endothelial cells**; the walls of capillaries are formed from a single layer of such cells. These cells have important roles in a number of vascular functions such as:

- Vasodilation and vasoconstriction: The secretion of substances like nitric oxide and endothelin can regulate vessel diameter. This is important in maintaining blood pressure, tissue oxygenation, and thermoregulation.
- Inflammation: The release of inflammatory chemicals from injured tissues stimulate endothelial cells to increase their expression of adhesion molecules. These molecules allow white blood cells to adhere to the endothelial cells and ultimately enter the injured tissue.
- Angiogenesis (the formation of new blood vessels): Angiogenic growth factors stimulate endothelial cells to break free from an existing vessel and proliferate in surrounding tissues, ultimately forming new vessels altogether. This property has important implications for cancer treatments, as many tumors secrete angiogenic growth factors. The resulting vascular increase supplies oxygen and nutrients to a developing tumor to help sustain its extraordinary cell division and growth. Angiogenesis inhibitors are drugs that can be used to restrict blood flow to tumors and help reduce or halt their growth.
- Thrombosis (blood clotting): Undamaged endothelial cells secrete substances that inhibit the coagulation cascade, thus preventing the formation of potentially life-threatening clots inside undamaged or unbroken vessels.

Endothelial cell dysfunction can lead to a number of pathogenic conditions, such as hypercholesterolemia, hypertension, inappropriate clot formation, and coronary artery disease and atherosclerosis; in fact, endothelial cell dysfunction is key to the development of atherosclerosis, and predates any clinical vascular signs by several years.

To achieve both efficient oxygenation of blood in the lungs and transport of oxygenated blood to the tissues, the heart has evolved in humans to have two sides separated by a thick wall to pump blood in two separate circuits. The right side of the heart pumps blood to the lungs, and the left side of the heart pumps blood to the rest of the body. The flow of blood from the heart to the lungs and back to the heart is the **pulmonary circulation**, and the flow of blood from the heart to the rest of the body and back again is the **systemic circulation** (Figure 1, next page).

- In fish, blood passes from the heart to the gills and then to the rest of the body. Why have mammals evolved a separate circulation for the lungs?[3]

By having two separate circulations, most blood passes through only one set of capillaries before returning to the heart. There are exceptions to this, however: **portal systems**. In the hepatic portal system, blood passes first through capillaries in the intestine, then collects in veins to travel to the liver, where the vessels branch and the blood passes again through capillaries. Another example is the hypothalamic-hypophysial portal system, in which blood passes through capillaries in the hypothalamus to the portal veins, then to capillaries in the pituitary (Chapter 8). The portal systems evolved as direct transport systems, to transport nutrients directly from the intestine to the liver or hormones from the hypothalamus to the pituitary, without passing through the whole body.

---

[3] Blood is pumped away from the heart at high pressure in arteries to pass through the capillaries. If the blood is to pass through one bed of capillaries, and then through another bed of capillaries, the pressure must be very high in the first set of capillaries or blood will not have enough pressure to pass through the second set of capillaries. Having two separate circulations solves this problem.

- If the hypothalamic-hypophysial portal circulation is severed, how does this affect the function of the pituitary?[4]

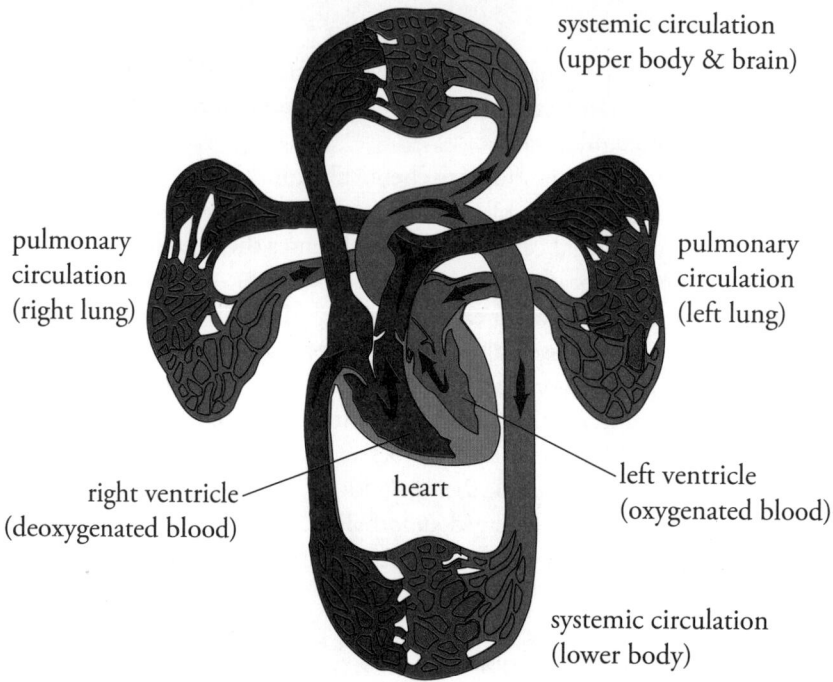

Figure 1   Pulmonary and Systemic Circuits

9.2   THE HEART

The heart has two kinds of chambers involved in pumping blood, the **atria** and the **ventricles** (Figure 2). The atria are reservoirs or "waiting rooms" where blood can collect from the veins before getting pumped into the ventricles. The muscular ventricles pump blood out of the heart at high pressures into the arteries. The systemic circulation and the pulmonary circulation are separated within the heart, so the right and left sides of the heart each have one atrium and one ventricle. The right atrium receives deoxygenated blood from the systemic circulation (from the large veins: the **inferior vena cava** and the **superior vena cava**) and pumps it into the right ventricle. From the right ventricle, blood passes through the pulmonary artery to the lungs. Oxygenated blood from the lungs returns through the pulmonary veins to the left atrium and is pumped into the left ventricle before being pumped out of the heart in a single large artery, the **aorta**, to the systemic circulation.

- Do all of the arteries of the body carry oxygenated blood?[5]

---

[4]   Normally, the pituitary receives hormones directly from the hypothalamus. If the portal system is severed, hormones must take a longer route and will be diluted and degraded before they reach the pituitary. As a result, secretion by the pituitary will not be effectively regulated by the hypothalamus.

[5]   No. The pulmonary artery carries deoxygenated blood from the heart to the lungs.

- Based on the above, you can conclude that blood flows:[6]
    A) from the lungs into the right atrium, since the right side of the heart deals with deoxygenated blood.
    B) from the right ventricle to the right atrium, since the atrium is a low-pressure chamber.
    C) from the right atrium to the left ventricle, since the right side of the heart deals with deoxygenated blood and the left side must pump blood to the body.
    D) from the lungs into the left atrium and from there to the left ventricle, since the left side of the heart deals with oxygenated blood.

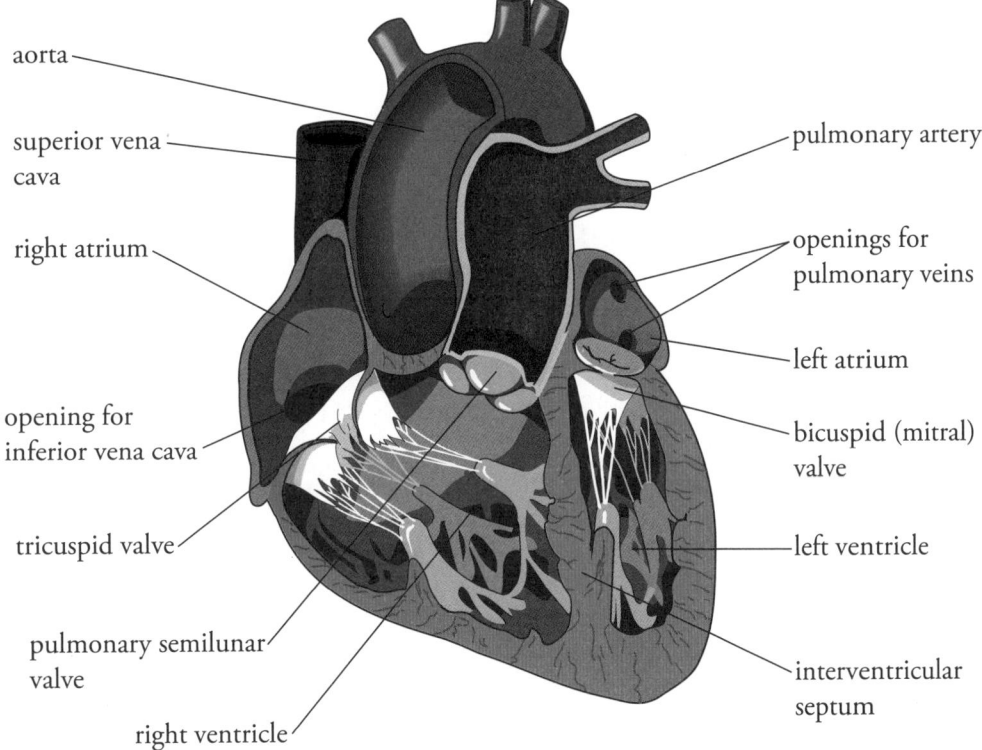

Figure 2   The Heart

The heart is a large muscular organ which requires a blood supply of its own. The very first branches from the aorta are **coronary arteries,** which branch to supply blood to the wall of the heart. They are called "coronary" because they encircle the heart, forming a crown shape. Deoxygenated blood from the heart collects in **coronary veins,** which merge to form the **coronary sinus,** located beneath a layer of fat on the outer wall of the heart. (A sinus is an open space; in the case of the cardiovascular system, it is a pool of low-pressure blood.) Blood in the coronary sinus is the only deoxygenated blood that does not end up in the inferior vena cava or superior vena cava. Instead, the coronary sinus drains directly into the right atrium.

---

[6] Oxygenated blood flows from the lungs to the left atrium (choice A is wrong), then to the left ventricle (choice **D** is right, and choice C is wrong). The atrium is a low pressure chamber, however, blood flow from the ventricles to the atria is prevented by the atrioventricular valves (choice B is wrong).

Valves

Valves are necessary to ensure one-way flow through the circulatory system. Valves in the heart are especially important, since the pressure differentials there are so extreme. In particular, ventricular pressure is very high and atrial pressure is lower. Hence, an **atrioventricular valve** (**AV valve**) between each ventricle and its atrium is necessary to prevent backflow.

The AV valve between the left atrium and the left ventricle is the **bicuspid** (or **mitral**) **valve**. [The mitral valve must withstand enormous pressures. What would happen if it ruptured?[7]] The AV valve between the right atrium and the right ventricle is the **tricuspid valve**. [What valve prevents blood flow between the left ventricle and the right ventricle?[8]]

Another set of valves is needed between the large arteries and the ventricles; these are the **pulmonary** and **aortic semilunar valves**. [Since the ventricles are ultra-high pressure chambers, why is it necessary to put valves between them and the arteries?[9]] Together these two valves are known simply as the *semilunar valves*.

There are also valves throughout the venous system. This is necessary because in passing through capillaries, blood loses its pressure. Thus, there is not much of a driving force pushing it toward the heart. Contraction of skeletal muscle becomes important, because normal body movements push and squeeze the veins, pressurizing venous blood and pushing it along. Venous valves prevent backflow; as long as the valves hold up, the blood moves toward the heart. When the valves fail, **varicose veins** result. Pregnant women often suffer from varicose veins because the growing fetus presses against the inferior vena cava, causing venous pressure in the legs to rise.

The Cardiac Cycle

The heart contracts, then relaxes, in a cycle which ends only in death. The left and right sides of the heart proceed through the same cycle at the same time. The cardiac cycle is divided into two periods, **diastole** and **systole** (pronounced dy-AS-toe-lee and SIS-toe-lee). During diastole, the ventricles are relaxed, and blood is able to flow into them from the atria. In fact, the atria contract during diastole, to propel blood into the ventricles more rapidly. [How strong is atrial compared to ventricular contraction?[10]] At the end of diastole, the ventricles contract, initiating systole. The ensuing buildup of pressure causes the AV valves to slam shut. Over the next few milliseconds, the pressure in the ventricles increases rapidly, until the semilunar valves fly open and blood rushes into the aorta and pulmonary artery. Systole is the period of time during which the ventricles are contracting, beginning at the "lub" sound and ending at the "dup." At the end of systole, the ventricles are nearly empty[11] and stop contracting. As a result, the pressure inside falls rapidly, and blood begins to flow backward, from the pulmonary artery into the right ventricle,

---

[7] The left ventricle would pump blood in both directions; out the aorta and back into the left atrium. The result will be elevated pulmonary blood pressure and pulmonary edema.

[8] None! The two ventricles are separated by a thick muscular wall. Remember: the left and right halves are separate.

[9] The ventricles are only pressurized while contracting. When they are not contracting, they must have a very low pressure so that blood can flow into them from the atria.

[10] Much weaker. The atria really only contract to ensure that most of the blood they contain passes into the ventricles. In contrast, the ventricles must propel blood through arteries, capillary beds, and veins. Therefore, the muscular walls of the atria are much thinner than those of the ventricles.

[11] Actually, only about 2/3 of the blood is normally ejected from the ventricle; this is the **ejection fraction**.

and from the aorta into the left ventricle. But very little backflow actually occurs, because the semilunar valves slam shut when the pressure in the ventricles becomes lower than the pressure in the great arteries. At this point, the heart has completed a full cardiac cycle and is back in diastole.

- Which one of the following is true during systole?[12]
    A) The bicuspid valve is open.
    B) Blood does not flow through the aortic valve.
    C) Both semilunar valves are closed.
    D) Pressure in the atria is low, and thus the atria fill with blood from the vena cava and pulmonary veins.

Heart Sounds, Heart Rate, and Cardiac Output

The "lub-dup" of the heartbeat is produced by valves slamming shut. The "lub" results from the closure of the AV valves at the beginning of systole, and the "dup" is the sound of the semilunar valves closing at the end of systole. [Based on this, which is longer: systole or diastole?[13]]

The **heart rate** (HR) or **pulse** is the number of times the "lub-dup" cardiac cycle is repeated per minute. The normal pulse rate is about one beat per second, ranging from 45 beats per minute (b.p.m.) in athletes to 80 or more beats per minute in the elderly and in children. The explanation for this variation is that a stronger heart pumps more blood each time it contracts, and thus may beat fewer times per minute and still provide adequate circulation. Athletes have strong hearts, while children and the elderly have weaker hearts. The amount of blood pumped with each systole is known as the **stroke volume** (SV). The total amount of blood pumped per minute is termed the **cardiac output** (CO), defined by the equation

$$\text{cardiac output (L/min)} = \text{stroke volume (L/beat)} \times \text{heart rate (beats/min)}$$
$$CO = SV \times HR$$

- An overweight child weighing 110 pounds, a female athlete weighing 110 pounds, and an elderly man weighing 110 pounds all require a cardiac output of about 5 L/min. But the child and the old man have a stroke volume of 1/16 L, while the athlete's stroke volume is 1/9 L. How can the child and the old man supply enough blood to their bodies?[14]
- Which is larger: the cardiac output of the right ventricle or of the left ventricle?[15]

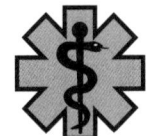

---

[12] During systole the ventricles are contracting. The bicuspid valve separates the left atrium from the left ventricle, and must be closed to prevent backflow into the left atrium (choice A is wrong). The high pressures generated during systole force blood out of the ventricles through the aortic and pulmonary semilunar valves (choices B and C are wrong). While the ventricles are contracting, the atria are resting, and blood can flow into them from the vena cava and pulmonary veins. This flow would be prevented if there were any pressure in the atria (choice **D** is correct). Note that closure of the AV valves ensures that the super-high ventricular pressure does not spread to the atria.

[13] Diastole is longer, since it occupies the space between *lub-dup* and *lub-dup*. Systole is shorter, since it occupies the space between *lub* and *dup*.

[14] The athlete's heart can provide the necessary cardiac output by pumping at a leisurely rate of 45 beats per minute. But the hearts of the child and old man will have to work hard to pump enough blood; their pulses will be 80 beats per minute.

[15] Neither; they are equal. The same amount of blood must pass through both sides of the heart or blood would back up in either the pulmonary or systemic circulatory system.

The Frank-Starling Mechanism and Venous Return

There are several ways to increase cardiac output. One is increasing heart rate, as we saw above. Also, a stronger heart has a larger stroke volume and is capable of a greater cardiac output. Another mechanism of increased stroke volume is termed the **Frank-Starling mechanism**. If the heart muscle is stretched, it will contract more forcefully. How can the heart muscle be stretched? By filling it with more blood, of course. The return of blood to the heart by the vena cava is termed **venous return**. If venous return is increased, the heart fills more. As a result, its muscle fibers are stretched, and they respond by contracting more forcefully. The result is that a larger volume of blood enters the heart *and* the heart contracts better. The stroke volume can be increased significantly in this manner. The control of cardiac output in this manner is largely automatic: the more blood the heart receives from the tissues, the more it pumps out to the tissues.

There are two principal ways to increase venous return: 1) Increase the total volume of blood in the circulatory system. The body does this by retaining water (by urinating less). 2) Contraction of large veins can propel blood toward the heart. The presence of valves throughout the venous system is essential here; without valves, contraction of the veins would cause blood to flow backward, through the venules to the capillaries. [If the arterioles in a large part of the systemic circulation dilate, how will this affect cardiac output?[16]]

Cardiac Muscle

The force of contraction in the ventricles and atria is generated by the cardiac muscle cells that form the muscular walls of the chambers of the heart. The nature of the force generation in contractile cells and the differences between skeletal muscle, cardiac muscle, and smooth muscle will be presented in Chapter 11, but it is necessary to present some aspects of cardiac muscle to understand the heart. All muscle cells, including those of cardiac muscle, share with neurons the ability to propagate an action potential across their surface. The action potential in all muscle cells, as in neurons, is a wave of depolarization of the plasma membrane. [Do ligand-gated ion channels propagate action potentials in cardiac muscle?[17]]

A difference between neurons and cardiac muscle cells is that cardiac muscle is a **functional syncytium**. A syncytium is a tissue in which the cytoplasm of different cells can communicate via gap junctions. In cardiac muscle, the gap junctions are found in the **intercalated disks**, the connections between cardiac muscle cells. The depolarization of a cardiac muscle cell can be communicated directly through the cytoplasm to neighboring cardiac muscle cells through these gap junctions. (Recall that this is an example of an electrical synapse; there are no chemical synapses between cardiac muscle cells.) As a result, once an action potential starts, it spreads in a wave of depolarization throughout the cardiac muscle tissue in the atria or the ventricles. The atria and the ventricles are separate syncytia. The action potential in the heart is transmitted from the atrial syncytium to the ventricles by the **cardiac conduction system**. Transmission of the action potential is delayed slightly as it passes through the part of the conduction system known as the A-V node (Figure 5). [Why?[18] What would happen if gap junctions in the heart were blocked, but voltage-gated ion channels remained functional?[19]]

---

[16] If the arterioles open, more blood will flow through the tissues. The more blood that flows through the tissues, the greater the venous return and the greater the cardiac output.

[17] No. Ligand-gated ion channels may help to create the threshold depolarization required to trigger an action potential but do not play a role in propagating an action potential. Propagation of action potentials requires *voltage*-gated ion channels.

[18] In order for the heart to function normally, the atria must contract first (during diastole) to completely fill the ventricles with blood before they begin contracting during systole. Thus, the action potential must be propagated through the atrial syncytium before being propagated through the ventricular syncytium.

[19] The gap junctions between cells are necessary for the propagation of action potentials in cardiac muscle. A cell with blocked gap junctions could have an action potential on its own membrane in this circumstance if it reached threshold depolarization, but it would be unable to transmit the action potential to neighboring cells.

Voltage-gated sodium channels, also called **fast sodium channels**, play an important role in cardiac muscle, as in neurons, but, in addition, another type of voltage-gated channel, the **slow calcium channel**, is involved in the cardiac muscle action potential. Like all voltage-gated channels, these channels open in response to a change in membrane potential to a specific voltage (the threshold voltage) and, when open, allow the passage of calcium down its gradient. These channels also stay open longer than the fast sodium channels do, causing the membrane depolarization to last longer in cardiac muscle than in neurons, producing a plateau phase (Figure 4, on page 339).

The nature of the action potential in cardiac muscle affects the function of this tissue. Cardiac cells, like all cells with an excitable membrane, have a period during and just after the action potential during which they are refractory to new action potentials. Another result of the long depolarization in cardiac muscle is that the contraction of muscle lasts a long time, strengthening the force with which blood is expelled. To maximize the entry of calcium in the cell, cardiac muscle has involutions of the membrane called **T tubules**. The action potentials travel down along T tubules, allow the entry of calcium from the extracellular environment, and also induce the sarcoplasmic reticulum to release calcium. The combination of intracellular and extracellular calcium causes the contraction of actin-myosin fibers. [Will the absolute refractory period, during which a cell will not fire an action potential, be longer in cardiac or neuronal cells?[20] Will the strength of contraction by cardiac muscle be affected by the extracellular concentration of calcium ions?[21]]

Rhythmic Excitation of the Heart

Once an action potential is initiated, it will spread throughout the cardiac muscle of the heart. Interestingly, the heart is *not* stimulated to contract by neuronal or hormonal influences, although these can change the rate and strength of contraction (the **contractility** of the heart). Isolated cardiac muscle cells will in some circumstances continue contracting on their own, free of any external influences. So, what initiates the action potential in heart tissue? The initiation of each action potential that starts each cardiac cycle occurs automatically from within the heart itself, in a special region of the right atrium called the **sinoatrial (SA) node**. Under normal circumstances, the cells of the SA node act as the **pacemaker of the heart**. The SA node exhibits automaticity and its action potential is commonly divided into 3 separate phases; Phase 0, Phase 3, and Phase 4. (*Note*: Other cardiac myocytes (muscle cells) additionally have Phases 1 and 2, but the SA node does *not*; see Figure 3 on the next page).

The SA node is unique in that it has an *unstable resting potential* (not really resting, huh?). This is **Phase 4** (automatic slow depolarization) and is caused by special **sodium leak channels** that are responsible for its rhythmic, automatic excitation. This inward sodium leak brings the cell potential to the threshold for voltage-gated calcium channels; when they open they cause **Phase 0**, the upstroke of the pacemaker potential. It is caused mainly by an inward flow of Ca^{2+}. (*Note*: Skeletal muscle cells and other myocytes depolarize because of a *Na*$^+$ influx, not *Ca*$^{2+}$ like the SA node.) This Ca^{2+} drives the membrane potential of the SA nodal cells toward the positive Ca^{2+} equilibrium potential. Note also that the Ca^{2+} channels operate more slowly than the Na^+ channels, leading to a more gradual upsweep in the action potential.

---

[20] The absolute refractory period is the period during the action potential in which a new action potential cannot be induced. If the membrane is still depolarized as part of an action potential, it will be refractory to new action potentials. Cardiac muscle action potentials last much longer than neuronal (or skeletal muscle) action potentials, and will therefore have a longer absolute refractory period.

[21] Yes. A significant portion of the calcium that stimulates contraction comes from the extracellular pool, entering the cell as part of the action potential.

Phase 3 is repolarization. It is caused by closure of the Ca^{2+} channels and opening of the K^+ channels, leading to an outward flow of K^+ from the cell. This loss of positively charged K^+ ions drives the membrane potential back down toward the negative K^+ equilibrium potential.

The SA node cells transmit their action potential through intercalated discs to the rest of the conduction cells in the heart (as well as to the atrial myocytes), repolarize, then start the process over again, repeated once per heartbeat for the life of the individual (Figure 3).

- Why don't potassium leak channels cause spontaneous action potentials in neurons or muscle cells?[22]

Note that while several regions of the heart can spontaneously depolarize (e.g., the AV node, Purkinje fibers), the SA node has the most Na^+ leak channels of all of the conduction system. Thus, it reaches threshold before any other region of the heart does, and sets the rate of heart contraction (that's why it's called the "**pacemaker**" of the heart). When the SA nodal cells are injured or the pathway of atrial depolarization is blocked, these other regions of the heart will take over the pacemaking responsibility, but pace the heart at a slower rate.

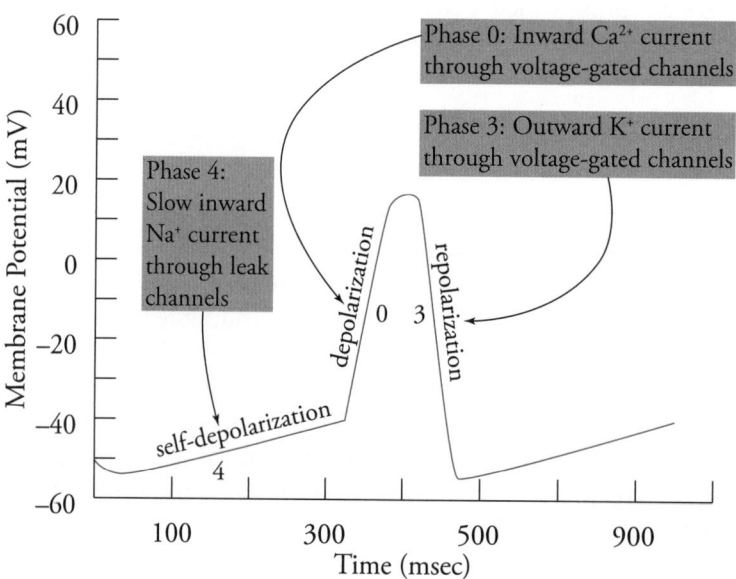

Figure 3 The Pacemaker Potential of the SA Node

The cardiac muscle cells of the heart have an action potential that differs from the SA node and the other conduction system cells. These muscle cells have a resting membrane potential of about –90 mV (very close to the K^+ equilibrium potential). The action potentials here have a long duration, up to 300 milliseconds normally. The phases of the action potential in these cells are Phases 0–4 (see Figure 4).

---

[22] Potassium leak channels allow potassium to leave the cell, down a gradient, polarizing the membrane; the *opposite* effect of sodium leak channels. Sodium is at a higher concentration outside of the cell, so sodium leak channels allow sodium to enter the cell and depolarize the membrane.

Phase 0 (depolarization) is again the upstroke of the action potential and is caused by the transient increase in Na⁺ conductance (just like in neurons). Action potentials propagating through the intercalated discs stimulate myocytes to reach threshold for voltage-gated Na⁺ channels. Once threshold is reached, the Na⁺ channels open and Na⁺ rushes into the cell.

In **Phase 1** (initial repolarization) the Na⁺ channels inactivate and K⁺ channels open. This leads to an efflux of K⁺ and a slight drop in cell potential. Furthermore, the increased potential due to the initial Na⁺ influx causes the opening of voltage-gated Ca²⁺ channels; this leads to **Phase 2**, the **plateau** phase. During the plateau, the influx of Ca²⁺ ions balance the K⁺ efflux from phase one, leading to a transient equilibrium in cell potential.

Phase 3 (repolarization) occurs when the Ca²⁺ channels close and the K⁺ channels continue to allow K⁺ to leave the cell (again, this is just like in neurons). **Phase 4** (the resting membrane potential) is the period during which inward and outward current are equal. Remember, this is dictated by action of the Na⁺/K⁺ ATPase and slow K⁺ leak channels.

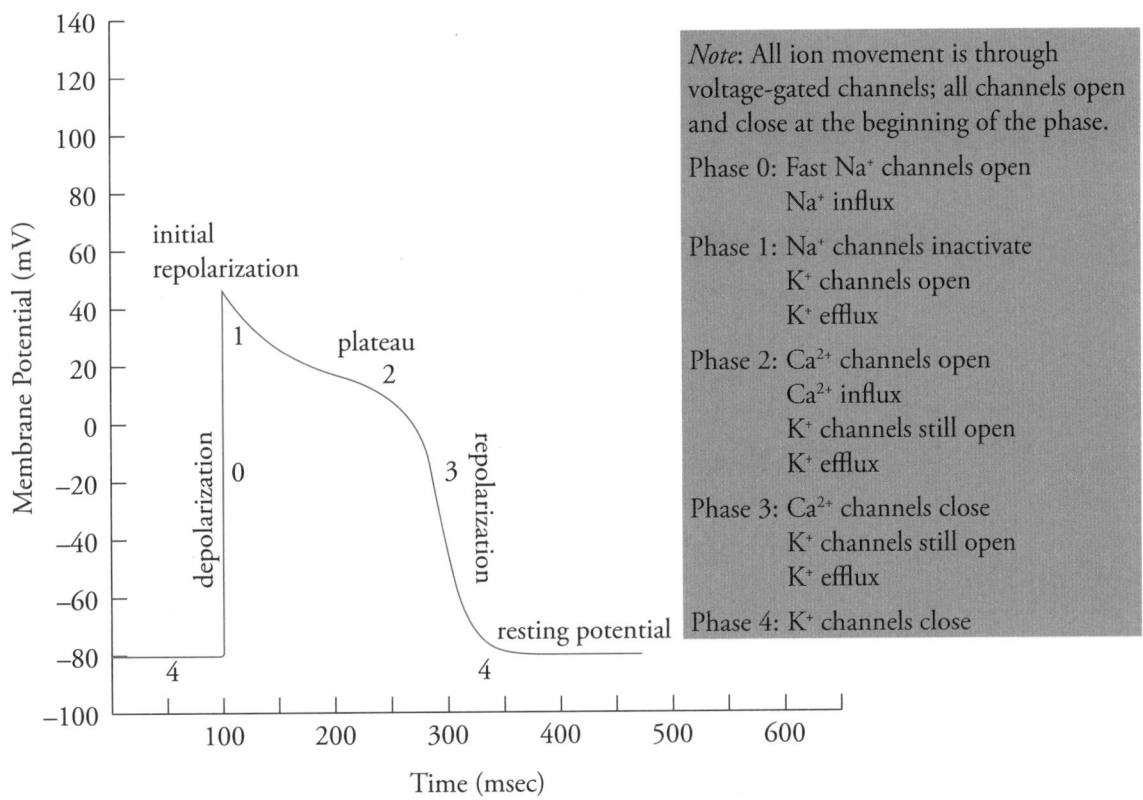

Figure 4 Phases of the Membrane Potential in a Cardiac Muscle Cell

Thus, each heartbeat begins as an action potential in the **sinoatrial (SA) node** then spreads throughout the atria, causing them to contract and fill the ventricles with blood. The action potential also spreads down the special conduction pathway which transmits action potentials very rapidly without contracting. The pathway connects the SA node to the **atrioventricular (AV) node.** Since this pathway connects the two nodes, it is referred to as the **internodal tract**. Note that while the impulse travels to the AV node almost instantaneously, it spreads through the atria more slowly, because contracting heart muscle cells pass the impulse more slowly than specialized conduction fibers. At the AV node, the impulse is delayed slightly, then passes from the node to the ventricles via the conduction pathway again. This part of the conduction pathway is known as the **AV bundle** (**bundle of His**). The AV bundle divides into the **right** and **left bundle branches**, and then into the **Purkinje fibers**, which allow the impulse to spread rapidly and evenly over both ventricles. Note that the Purkinje fibers spread over the inferior portion of the ventricles (paradoxically called the "apex" of the heart). The result is that this region of the ventricles contracts first, and blood is pushed toward the superior region of the heart (paradoxically called the "base"), where the valves and arteries are (Figure 5).

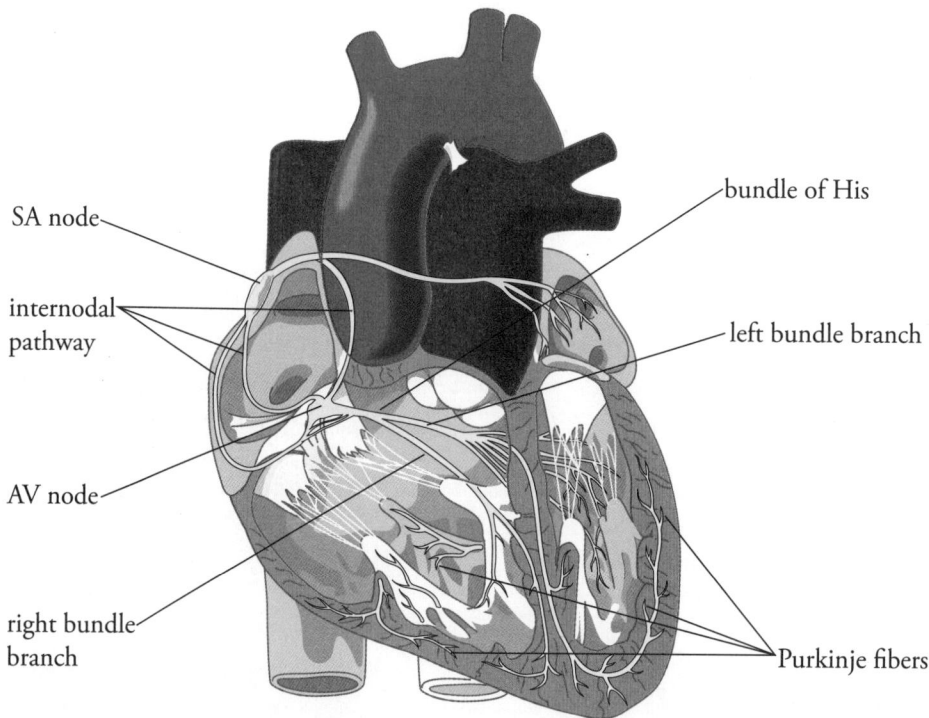

SA node

internodal
pathway

AV node

right bundle
branch

bundle of His

left bundle branch

Purkinje fibers

Figure 5 The Cardiac Conduction System

Regulation of the Heart by the Autonomic Nervous System

The autonomic nervous system does not initiate action potentials in the heart, but it does regulate the rate of contraction. The intrinsic firing rate of the SA node is about 120 beats per minute. The reason the normal heart rate is only about 60–80 beats/minute is that the parasympathetic nervous system continually inhibits depolarization of the SA node. In particular, the **vagus nerve** (a cranial nerve) contains preganglionic axons which synapse in ganglia near the SA node. The postganglionic neurons innervate the SA node, releasing acetylcholine (ACh). The ACh inhibits depolarization by binding to receptors on the cells of the SA node. The constant level of inhibition provided by the vagus nerve is known as **vagal tone**. [Does ACh always inhibit postsynaptic cells? If not, how can different responses be elicited by the same neurotransmitter?[23]] In summary, the role of the *parasympathetic* system in controlling the heart is to modulate the rate by *inhibiting rapid automaticity*.

---

[23] ACh is the neurotransmitter released by all autonomic preganglionic neurons, all parasympathetic postganglionic neurons, and all somatic motor neurons. In most cases it is stimulatory, i.e., causes an action potential to occur, causes an effect in an organ. Whether a neurotransmitter is stimulatory or inhibitory depends only on the nature of its receptor on the postsynaptic cell.

The sympathetic system can also influence the heart. At rest, however, most nervous input is from the vagus. The sympathetic system kicks in when increased cardiac output is needed during a "fight or flight" response. The sympathetic system affects the heart in two ways: first, sympathetic postganglionic neurons directly innervate the heart, releasing norepinephrine. Second, epinephrine secreted by the adrenal medulla binds to receptors on cardiac muscle cells. The effect of sympathetic activation is stimulatory. The heart rate increases, and so does the force of contraction.

The heart rate and blood pressure are tightly regulated. In any regulatory system, three components are required: input (afferent information), integration (the function of the central nervous system), and output (efferent information, discussed in the above two paragraphs). The input in this regulatory system is complex, but we can highlight one key element: in the aortic arch and in the carotid arteries there are special receptors known as **baroreceptors**, which monitor pressure (like a *baro*meter). When they notify the central nervous system that the pressure is too high, the CNS sends out information to correct the problem: increased vagal tone and decreased sympathetic input. When the pressure is too low, the opposite happens. People with high blood pressure have a poorly functioning regulatory system and must take medications designed to keep things under control.

9.3   HEMODYNAMICS

Resistance

Hemodynamics is the study of blood flow. The driving force for blood flow is a difference in pressure from arteries to veins. The force opposing flow is friction, which results when blood squeezes through many tiny branching vessels. The technical term for this opposing force is **resistance**. Ohm's law summarizes the relationship between these variables: $\Delta P = Q \times R$. Here, ΔP is the pressure gradient (in mm Hg) from the arterial system to the venous system, Q stands for blood flow (or cardiac output in L/min), and R denotes resistance. The usefulness of this simple equation is twofold: first, it shows us that blood pressure is directly proportional to both cardiac output and peripheral resistance. If either of these change, blood pressure changes similarly. [How would an increase in stroke volume change blood pressure?[24]] Second, it shows us that if we want to change blood flow, we can only change it by changing either the pressure or the resistance; those are the only independent variables in the equation.

We know that pressure can be varied by increasing the *force* (thus changing the stroke volume) or *rate* (beats per minute) of cardiac contraction. What about resistance? The principal determinant of resistance is the degree of constriction of arteriolar smooth muscle, also known as **precapillary sphincters**. If arteriolar smooth muscles contract, it becomes more difficult for blood to flow from arteries into capillaries; that is, the resistance goes up. The resistance of the entire systemic circuit is easily calculated using the above equation in the form $R = \Delta P/Q$. We can measure ΔP and Q, then solve for R. This quantity is known as the **peripheral resistance**.

---

[24] Recall that CO = SV × HR, therefore, an increase in stroke volume would increase cardiac output. Since blood pressure and cardiac output are directly proportional, an increase in cardiac output would increase blood pressure as well.

9.3

The sympathetic nervous system controls the peripheral resistance. A certain amount of pressure in the arterial system is always desirable; otherwise not all tissues would be perfused. This basal level of pressure is provided by a constant level of norepinephrine released by millions of sympathetic postganglionic axons innervating precapillary sphincters. This constant nervous input is known as **adrenergic tone**. (Adrenergic means sympathetic; the word comes from adrenaline, which is another name for epinephrine.) [Why might tense, stressed out people tend to have high blood pressure?[25]]

The sympathetic system can increase the overall peripheral resistance, thus increasing blood pressure. It can also specifically divert blood away from one tissue so that another is preferentially perfused. In particular, sympathetic activation causes precapillary sphincters in the gut to contract, while arterioles supplying skeletal muscle are allowed to relax. The result is that blood flow is diverted from the gut to skeletal muscle, which facilitates the fight or flight response.

Blood Pressure

When physicians measure blood pressure, what they are actually measuring is **systemic arterial pressure**. This is the force per unit area exerted by blood upon the walls of arteries. You may recall that a typical blood pressure reading looks like this: 120/80, pronounced "120 over 80." What do the two numbers mean? 120 mm Hg is the **systolic pressure**, and 80 mm Hg is the **diastolic pressure**. In other words, 120 mm Hg is the highest pressure that ever occurs in the circulatory system of this particular patient during the time the blood pressure is being measured. This level is attained as the ventricles contract (that is, during systole). 80 mm Hg is as low as the pressure gets between heartbeats (that is, during diastole) during the measurement. The **pulse pressure** is the difference between systolic and diastolic pressures.

The measurement is taken using a **sphygmomanometer**, or "blood pressure cuff." This is an inflatable bag attached to a manometer (pressure-measuring device). The physician wraps the cuff around the upper arm and places a stethoscope at a point below the cuff where the pulse can be heard. Then she inflates the cuff until no blood flows into the arm (silence is heard in the stethoscope). Then she gradually reduces the cuff pressure, until a pulse first becomes audible. The significance of this point is that systolic arterial pressure is just greater than the pressure of the cuff. Thus, this pressure level is written down as the systolic pressure (120 in our example above). The pulse is very loud; this sound comes from blood slamming into arteries (which are constricted by the cuff) each time the heart beats. Then the physician continues to release pressure from the cuff. At a certain level, the pulse becomes much more quiet (usually inaudible). The significance of this is that now the cuff is loose enough so that blood flows smoothly through arteries and does not create the pounding noise described above. The point at which the pulse becomes inaudible is written down as the diastolic pressure. This is the lowest arterial pressure occurring at any time during the cardiac cycle.

It is important to emphasize the last sentence: this is the lowest *arterial* pressure occurring at any time during the cardiac cycle. You must realize that throughout the cardiac cycle, the pressure in the vena cava is about *zero* mm Hg. The highest pressures in the circulatory system are achieved in the left ventricle, aorta, and other large arteries. (That's what we measured with the cuff.) But every large artery branches, giving rise to many arterioles, and every arteriole gives rise to many capillaries. The result of all this branching is that the pressure generated by the heart is dissipated (Figure 6). By the time blood reaches the vena cava, it depends on valves to prevent backflow because the driving pressure is negligible.

---

[25] Tension and stress are similar to fear. Both involve activation of the sympathetic nervous system.

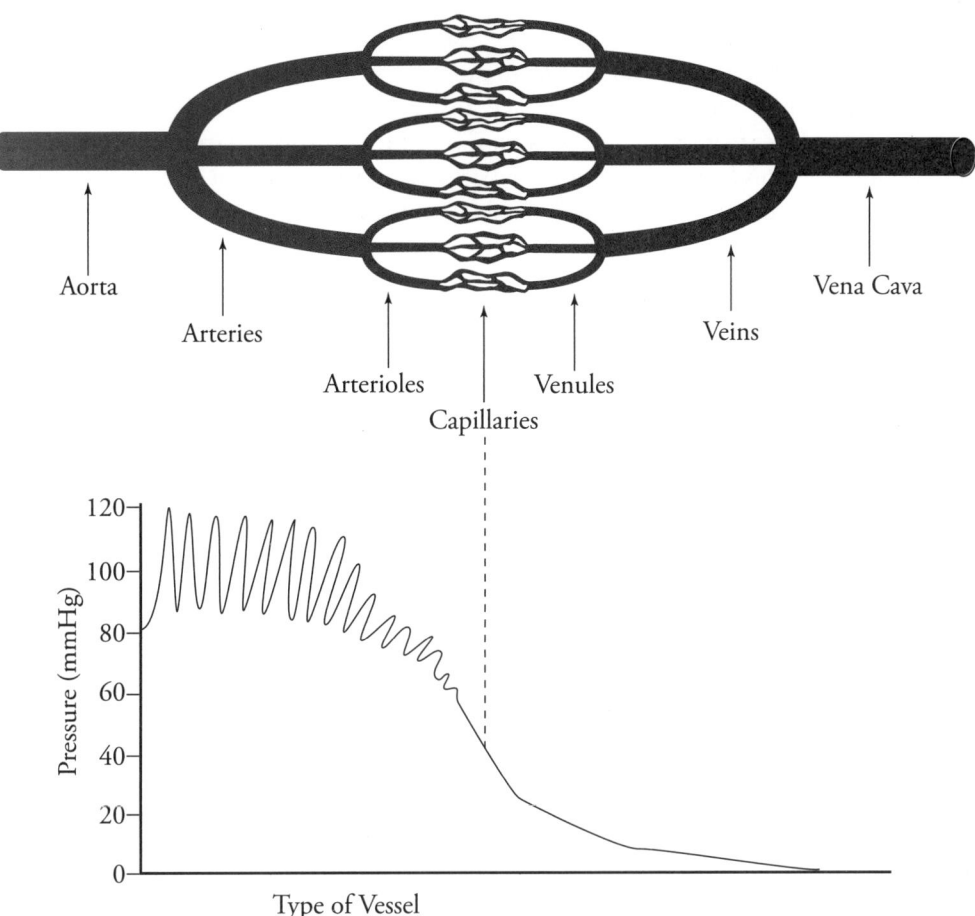

Aorta

Arteries

Arterioles

Venules

Capillaries

Veins

Vena Cava

Figure 6 Pressures Throughout the Circulatory System

Why is the diastolic arterial pressure as high as it is? In other words, between heartbeats, why does the arterial pressure remain elevated? Without the heart contracting, wouldn't you expect the pressure to fall rapidly? This is the reason arteries are highly elastic and muscular. When the heart contracts, the arteries distend like balloons. During diastole, the arteries exert pressure on the blood, just as an inflated balloon exerts pressure on the air it contains. This maintains diastolic pressure, which is important because it provides a continued driving force for blood.

- Which one of the following will increase cardiac output?[26]
  - A) Blocking sodium leak channels in the sinoatrial node
  - B) Stimulation of the heart by the parasympathetic nervous system
  - C) Significant dehydration due to prolonged exercise in the heat
  - D) Contraction of smooth muscle in the walls of the large veins

---

[26] Blocking the sodium leak channels will slow the spontaneous firing of action potentials by the sinoatrial node and slow the heart rate. Slowing the heart rate will decrease, not increase the cardiac output (choice A is wrong). The parasympathetic nervous system slows the heart rate and therefore decreases the cardiac output (choice B is wrong). Dehydration will reduce venous return and reduce the stroke volume of the heart, leading to a reduction in cardiac output (choice C is wrong). However, the large veins do have smooth muscle, although less than arteries, and can constrict in response to sympathetic stimulation. This would increase the filling pressure (the pressure gradient), driving blood into the right atrium, thus increasing venous return, stroke volume, and cardiac output (choice **D** is correct). Note that this is a difficult and complex question because we do not normally think of the veins as having smooth muscle, and furthermore, we tend to think of blood flow *reduction* when a vessel constricts. The MCAT also has difficult and complex questions. The key to answering this question correctly is to have confidence in the elimination of choices A, B, and C. Thus, choice D, however improbable it may seem, must be the correct answer.

Local Autoregulation

The nervous system does not control blood flow to every single region of the body. The amount of feedback information this would require would be huge. Instead, tissues in need of extra blood flow are able to requisition it themselves. This phenomenon is known as **local autoregulation**. The mechanism is simple: certain metabolic wastes have a direct effect on arteriolar smooth muscle, causing it to relax. Hence, when a tissue is underperfused, wastes build up, and vasodilation occurs automatically. Autoregulation is the principal determinant of coronary blood flow (blood supply to the heart); it generally overrides nervous input.

9.4 COMPONENTS OF BLOOD

Blood has a liquid portion called **plasma**, and a portion which is composed of cells. The cellular elements of blood are known as **formed elements**. Plasma accounts for 55 percent of the volume of blood, and consists of the following items dissolved in water: electrolytes, buffers, sugars, blood proteins, lipoproteins, CO_2, O_2, and metabolic waste products. **Electrolytes** refer to Na^+, K^+, Cl^-, Ca^{2+}, and Mg^{2+} ions. **Buffers** in the blood maintain a constant pH of 7.4; the principal blood buffer is bicarbonate (HCO_3^-).

- During exercise, a significant amount of lactic acid is produced by fermentation in muscles that are not receiving adequate oxygen. Despite this increase in lactic acid, the pH of the blood does not change dramatically. Why not?[27]

The principal sugar in the blood is glucose. A constant concentration must be maintained so that all the cells of the body receive adequate nutrition. The blood proteins, most of which are made by the liver, include albumin, immunoglobulins (antibodies), fibrinogen, and lipoproteins. **Albumin** is essential for maintenance of **oncotic pressure** (osmotic pressure in the capillaries due only to plasma proteins). The **immunoglobulins** are a key part of the immune system (Section 9.7). **Fibrinogen** is essential for blood clotting (hemostasis). **Lipoproteins** are large particles consisting of fats, cholesterol, and carrier proteins. Their role is to transport lipids in the bloodstream. CO_2 and O_2 are involved in respiration, of course. However, CO_2 is also important for its role in buffering the blood (see the reaction in footnote 27). The principal *metabolic waste product* is **urea**, a breakdown product of amino acids. Urea is basically a carrier of excess nitrogen. There are other important waste products too, such as **bilirubin**, a breakdown product of heme (the oxygen-binding moiety of hemoglobin, discussed below).

By centrifuging whole blood, one can separate the plasma from the formed elements, as shown below. The volume of blood occupied by the red blood cells (**erythrocytes**) is known as the **hematocrit** (Figure 7). The normal hematocrit in adult males is 40–45 percent; in females it is lower, approximately 35–40 percent. White blood cells (**leukocytes**) and platelets account for a small volume (about 1 percent). All the formed elements of the blood develop from special cells in the bone marrow, known as **bone marrow stem cells**.

If whole blood is allowed to clot, one is left with a solid clot plus a clear fluid known as **serum**. Thus, serum is similar to plasma except that it lacks all the proteins involved in clotting.

---

[27] The HCO_3^- buffer system prevents pH changes via the reaction $CO_2 + H_2O \rightleftharpoons H_2CO_3 \rightleftharpoons HCO_3^- + H^+$.

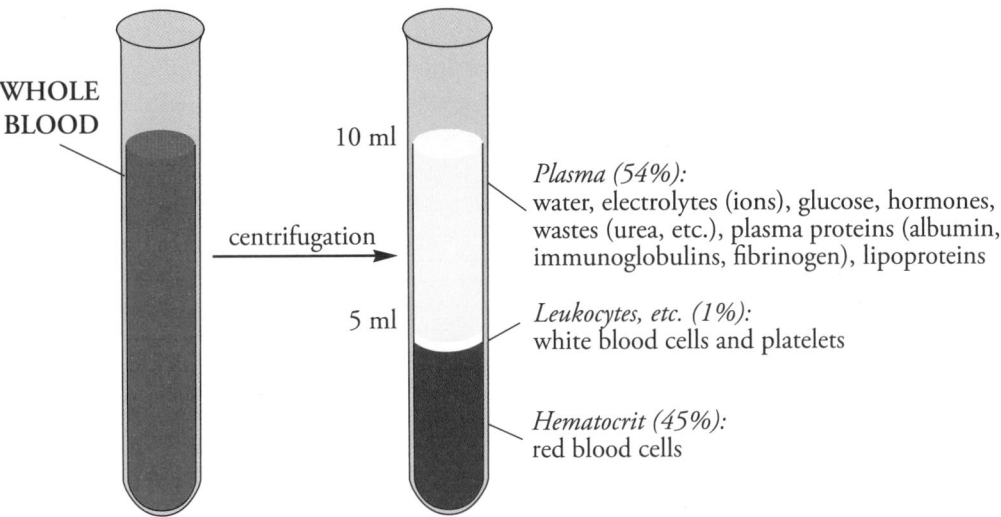

Figure 7   The Hematocrit and the Components of Blood

Erythrocytes (Red Blood Cells—RBCs)

The hormone **erythropoietin** (made in the kidney) stimulates RBC production in the bone marrow. Aged RBCs are eaten by phagocytes in the spleen and liver.

The erythrocyte is a cell, but it has no nucleus or other organelles such as mitochondria. However, it does require the energy of ATP for processes such as ion pumping and basic maintenance of cell structure during its 120-day lifetime in the bloodstream. Lacking mitochondria, the RBC relies on glycolysis for ATP synthesis. The purpose of the RBC is to transport O_2 to the tissues from the lungs and CO_2 from the tissues to the lungs. Thus, it requires a large surface area for gas exchange. A high surface-to-volume ratio is achieved by the RBC's flat, biconcave shape (like a deflated basketball or a throat lozenge, see Figure 8). The RBC is able to carry oxygen because it contains millions of molecules of **hemoglobin** (more on hemoglobin below).

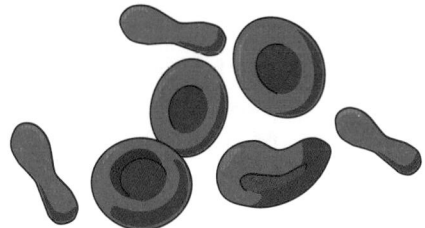

Figure 8   Red Blood Cells (Erythrocytes)

Blood Typing

Blood typing is the classification of a person's blood based on the presence or absence of certain surface antigens on their red blood cells. The two most important blood group antigens are the **ABO blood group** and the **Rh blood group**. The ABO blood group consists of glycoproteins that are coded for by three different alleles: I^A, I^B, and i. These alleles and their genotypes and phenotypes were discussed in more detail in Chapter 7 (Genetics and Evolution).

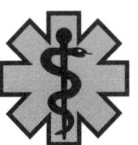

9.4

The other main antigen used in blood typing is the Rh (rhesus) factor. The expression of this antigen follows a classically dominant pattern: *RR* and *Rr* genotypes lead to the expression of the protein on the surface of the red blood cell (Rh positive), and the *rr* genotype leads to the absence of the protein (Rh negative). The combinations of the ABO alleles and the Rh alleles (and the respective antigens they code for) determine the overall blood type of an individual. Table 1 summarizes these blood types.

Table 1   Blood Group Genotypes and Phenotypes

	$I^A I^A$ or $I^A i$	$I^B I^B$ or $I^B i$	$I^A I^B$	ii
RR or *Rr*	type A+	type B+	type AB+	type O+
rr	type A-	type B-	type AB-	type O-

Determining blood type is critical when performing blood transfusions. Antibodies to the A and B antigens are produced early in infancy and can cause clumping and destruction of red blood cells bearing the incorrect antigen (called a **transfusion reaction**). For example, a person with A+ blood produces anti-B antibodies; if transfused with type B blood, these antibodies will clump and destroy the donated type B cells, possibly leading to the death of the recipient. Note that this early production of antibodies without prior exposure to the antigen is unusual; typically the immune system must be exposed to a foreign protein before it produces antibodies against it.

Antibodies to the Rh antigen do not develop unless a person with Rh– blood is exposed to Rh+ blood, an event called "sensitization"; note that this is the typical response of the immune system to a foreign protein (antigen). Subsequent exposure to Rh+ blood can then result in a transfusion reaction. This is particularly dangerous in the case of an Rh– mother carrying an Rh+ baby. Typically, if it is the first baby there are no complications (unless the mother had been previously sensitized); the mother's blood and the baby's blood do not mix during pregnancy. However, on delivery, some Rh+ cells from the child can mix with the mother's Rh– blood and lead to her sensitization. Future Rh+ babies are then at risk, since the anti-Rh antibodies can cross the placental barrier to clump and/or destroy the Rh+ baby's red blood cells. This is known as **hemolytic disease of the newborn** or *erythroblastosis fetalis*, and can be fatal. Injection of the mother at the time of birth with anti-Rh antibodies can clump and lead to the destruction of any stray Rh+ cells from the baby; this can prevent sensitization of the mother and protect any future unborn Rh+ children.

Two special blood types are AB+ and O–. Type AB+ individuals do not make antibodies to any of the blood group antigens, since their red blood cells possess all three of the antigens. Thus, type AB+ individuals are known as "**universal recipients**" because they can receive any of the other blood types without complication. Type O– individuals do not possess any of the surface antigens that could trigger a reaction in an individual with a different blood type. Thus, O– individuals are known as "universal donors" because they can donate blood to any of the other blood types, typically without complication. (Note that type O– individuals do make anti-A and anti-B antibodies, and these can sometimes cause issues in recipients. It is always best to match blood types between donors and recipients when possible.)

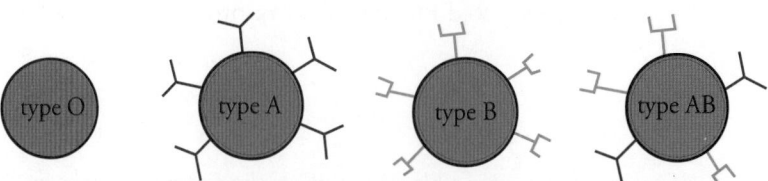

Figure 9   RBC Surface Antigens

Leukocytes

The white blood cell's role is to fight infection and dispose of debris. All white blood cells are large complex cells with all the normal eukaryotic cell structures (nucleus, mitochondria, etc.). Some white blood cells (**macrophages** and **neutrophils**) move by amoeboid motility (crawling). This is important because they are able to squeeze out of capillary intercellular junctions (spaces between capillary endothelial cells) and can therefore roam free in the tissues, hunting for foreign particles and pathogens. Some white blood cells exhibit **chemotaxis**, which means movement directed by chemical stimuli. The chemical stimuli can be toxins and waste products released by pathogens, or can be chemical signals released from other white blood cells. There are six types of white blood cells (Table 2).

Table 2   Roles of the Six Types of Leukocytes

Cell	Role
monocytes:	
macrophage	phagocytose debris and microorganisms; amoeboid motility; chemotaxis
lymphocytes:	
B cell	mature into *plasma cell* and produce antibodies
T cell	kill virus-infected cells, tumor cells, and reject tissue grafts; also control immune response
granulocytes:	
neutrophil	phagocytose bacteria resulting in pus; amoeboid motility; chemotaxis
eosinophil	destroy parasites; allergic reactions
basophil	store and release histamine; allergic reactions

Platelets and Hemostasis

Like red blood cells, platelets have no nuclei and a limited lifespan. They are derived from the fragmentation of large bone marrow cells called **megakaryocytes**, which are derived from the same stem cells that give rise to red blood cells and white blood cells. The function of platelets is to aggregate at the site of damage to a blood vessel wall, forming a **platelet plug**. This immediately helps stop bleeding. **Hemostasis** is a term for the body's mechanism of preventing bleeding.

The other component of the hemostatic response is **fibrin**. This is a threadlike protein which forms a mesh that holds the platelet plug together. When the fibrin mesh dries, it becomes a scab, which seals and protects the wound. The plasma protein **fibrinogen** is converted into fibrin by a protein called **thrombin** when bleeding occurs. A blood clot, or **thrombus**, is a scab circulating in the bloodstream. Calcium as well as many accessory proteins are necessary for the activation of thrombin and fibrinogen. Several of the proteins depend on vitamin K for their function. Defects in these proteins result in **hemophilia** ("loving to bleed"), an X-linked recessive group of diseases involving excessive bleeding.

9.5 TRANSPORT OF GASES

Oxygen

Oxygen is too hydrophobic to dissolve in the plasma in significant quantities. Therefore, RBCs are used to bind and carry O_2. RBCs are able to carry oxygen because they contain millions of molecules of **hemoglobin** (Hb). This is a complex protein composed of four polypeptide subunits. Each subunit contains one molecule of **heme**, which is a large multi-ring structure that has a single iron atom bound at its center. The role of heme with its iron atom is to bind O_2. Since each hemoglobin has four subunits and each subunit has one heme, each molecule of hemoglobin can carry four molecules of oxygen. Hemoglobin has some important properties which make it an excellent oxygen carrier.

The four subunits of hemoglobin do not bind oxygen independently of one another. When none of the subunits have oxygen bound, all four subunits assume a **tense** conformation that has a relatively low affinity for oxygen. (A *conformation* is a specific three-dimensional structure of a protein.) When one of the subunits binds oxygen, its conformation changes from a tense to a **relaxed** state that has a higher affinity for oxygen. The change in the three-dimensional structure of the subunit with oxygen bound is then communicated to the other subunits through contacts between the polypeptides to alter their conformation and increase their affinity for oxygen as well. Thus, hemoglobin is said to bind oxygen **cooperatively**.

- Myoglobin is a molecule with a structure very similar to hemoglobin, but with a single subunit that has one binding site. Does myoglobin display cooperativity in oxygen binding?[28]
- If binding of oxygen is cooperative, is it saturable?[29]
- Does hemoglobin have higher affinity for oxygen in the tissues or in the lungs?[30]

This has monumental significance for the ability of the blood to transport oxygen efficiently. The level of O_2 in active tissues is very low, because they use it in oxidative phosphorylation. Thus, in the tissues, hemoglobin has low affinity for oxygen and tends to release any oxygen which it carries. The level of O_2 in the lungs is of course very high. Hence, when a red blood cell is passing through a capillary in the lungs, the hemoglobin it contains will have higher affinity due to cooperative binding and will tend to bind oxygen very strongly. The result is that a lot of oxygen is picked up by RBCs in the lungs, and most of it is released as they pass through active tissues that need oxygen. This is an amazing example of how structural biochemistry determines physiology (or vice versa).

There is even more complexity to the hemoglobin story. It turns out that certain factors stabilize the tense configuration (which has a low O_2 affinity). These factors are:

1) decreased pH,
2) increased P_{CO_2} (level of CO_2 in the blood), and
3) increased temperature.

---

[28] Cooperativity requires more than one binding site in a protein so that one binding site can alter the affinity of another. Myoglobin cannot be cooperative in oxygen binding since it has only one binding site.

[29] There are a limited number of binding sites, even if they are cooperative, so binding will be saturated at a high concentration (partial pressure) of oxygen. There is a limit to the oxygen carrying capacity of the blood.

[30] At higher partial pressure of oxygen, more of the hemoglobin protein will have at least one of the subunits occupied with oxygen. Since binding is cooperative, the more oxygen that is bound, the higher the affinity for oxygen. The partial pressure of oxygen is higher in the lungs than in the tissues, so hemoglobin will have higher affinity for oxygen in the lungs.

The fact that these factors stabilize tense hemoglobin and thus reduce its oxygen affinity is known as the **Bohr effect**. This system is truly incredible when you realize that these three factors perfectly characterize the environment within active tissues. [What is the significance of this?[31]]

The affinity of hemoglobin for oxygen can be quantified by measurement of the fraction of O_2-binding sites which have bound O_2. If hemoglobin is in the relaxed configuration, then as more oxygen becomes available, much more of it will be bound up. But if it is in the tense configuration, the tendency to bind oxygen is reduced, and less will be bound. This can be described mathematically using the notion of **percent saturation (% sat.)**:

$$\% \text{ sat.} = (\# \text{ of } O_2 \text{ molecules bound}) \div (\# \text{ of } O_2 \text{ binding sites}) \times 100\%$$

- At a given P_{O_2}, which has a higher % sat.: tense or relaxed hemoglobin?[32]

This information can be depicted graphically, using an **O_2-Hemoglobin Dissociation Curve**, which plots % sat. vs. P_{O_2} (Figure 10). The sigmoidal shape of the curve resembles the behavior of cooperative enzymes.

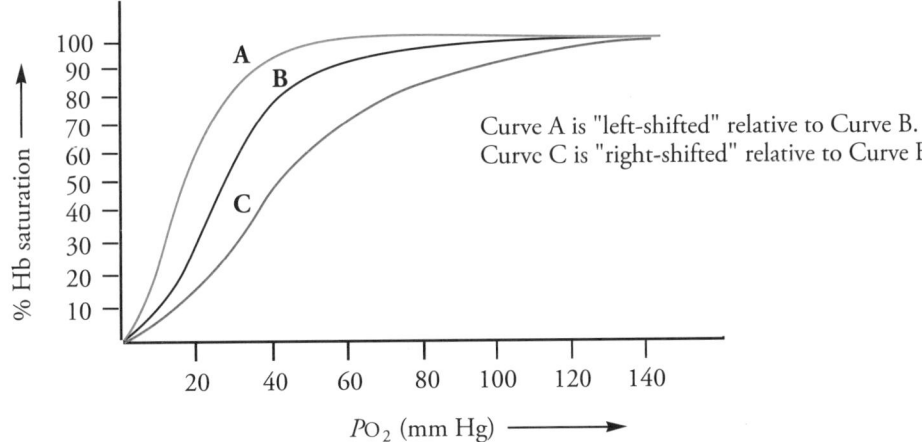

Figure 10 O_2-Hemoglobin Dissociation Curves

---

[31] When a tissue is active, its cells metabolize a lot of glucose and this results in an elevated P_{CO_2}. Soon the cells run low on oxygen and begin to perform lactic acid fermentation. The result is a drop in pH. Finally, whenever there is a lot of metabolic activity, the temperature increases. So, due to the Bohr effect, hemoglobin is most ready to release its load of oxygen in regions of the body where oxygen is most needed!

[32] Relaxed, since it has a higher affinity. This just means that at any O_2 level, relaxed hemoglobin will bind more O_2 than tense hemoglobin will.

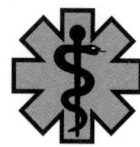

Answer all of the following questions about Figure 10 before looking at the footnote.[33]

- Curve _____ represents Hb with the highest affinity of all.
- Curve C could be the result of _____.
- Curve A would most likely be seen in what region of the body?
- Why do all the curves level off?
- It is interesting to note that fetal hemoglobin is a bit different from adult hemoglobin. The fetus must be able to "steal" oxygen away from the mother's blood. Hence, the O_2 dissociation curve for fetal hemoglobin is _____-shifted relative to the curve for adult hemoglobin.

Carbon Dioxide

Carbon dioxide is transported in the blood in three ways:

1) 73% of CO_2 transport is accomplished by the conversion of CO_2 to **carbonic acid**, which can dissociate into **bicarbonate** and a **proton** according to this reaction: $CO_2 + H_2O \rightleftharpoons H_2CO_3 \rightleftharpoons HCO_3^- + H^+$. These compounds are extremely water-soluble and are thus easily carried in the blood. The conversion of CO_2 into carbonic acid is catalyzed by an RBC enzyme called **carbonic anhydrase**. Remember that this reaction is also important as the principal plasma pH buffer.

2) Some CO_2 (~ 20%) is transported by simply being stuck onto hemoglobin. It does *not* bind to the oxygen-binding sites, but rather to other sites on the protein. Binding of CO_2 to hemoglobin is important in the Bohr effect because it stabilizes tense Hb.

3) CO_2 is somewhat more water-soluble than O_2, so a fair amount (~ 7%) can be dissolved in the blood and carried from the tissues to the lungs. Virtually no oxygen can be dissolved in the blood.

Exchange of Substances Across the Capillary Wall

The capillaries are the site of exchange between the blood and tissues. To facilitate exchange, capillaries have walls of only a single layer of flattened endothelial cells, and there are spaces (**intercellular clefts**) between the endothelial cells that make up the capillary wall. Three types of substances must be able to pass through the clefts: nutrients, wastes, and white blood cells. We will discuss each of these in turn. [Is it necessary for O_2 and CO_2 to pass through the clefts?[34]]

There are three main types of nutrients: amino acids, glucose, and lipids. Amino acids and glucose are absorbed from the digestive tract and carried by a special vein called the **hepatic portal vein** to the liver. It is called a *portal vein* because it connects two capillary beds: the one in the intestinal wall and the one inside the liver. The liver stores amino acids and glucose and releases them into the bloodstream as needed. From the bloodstream they can pass through capillary clefts into the tissues. The journey of lipids through the bloodstream is different. Fats are absorbed from the intestine and packaged into **chylomicrons**, which are a type of lipoprotein. The chylomicrons enter tiny lymphatic vessels in the intestinal wall called **lacteals**. The lacteals empty into larger lymphatics, which eventually drain into a large vein near the neck. Hence, dietary fats bypass the hepatic vein. The result is that after eating a fatty meal, a person's

---

[33] Curve A is farthest to the left and thus represents the highest affinity. Curve C could be the result of the Bohr effect. At a given O_2 level, the hemoglobin studied in Curve C has less of a tendency to bind oxygen (a lower affinity). Curve A would most likely be seen in the lungs, where there is plenty of oxygen and relaxed hemoglobin predominates. All the curves level off because 100% is the maximum degree of saturation; all the hemoglobin molecules become completely saturated. Fetal Hb has a left-shifted curve (higher affinity).

[34] No, they can pass straight through any cell by simple diffusion.

blood will appear milky. (The term for this is **lipemia**, which means "lipids flowing in the blood.") The chylomicrons are taken up by the liver and converted into another type of lipoprotein, which is released into the bloodstream. This lipoprotein carries fats to **adipocytes** (fat cells) for storage. When fats are to be used for energy, adipocyte triglycerides are hydrolyzed, and free fatty acids are released into the bloodstream. They pass easily through capillary pores and thus can be picked up by cells of various tissues.

Many wastes are produced during cellular metabolism. They diffuse through the capillary walls into the bloodstream. The liver removes many wastes and converts them into forms which can be excreted in the feces. Such compounds are passed into the gut as **bile**. Other wastes are excreted directly by the kidneys.

White blood cells must be able to pass out of capillaries in order to patrol the tissues for invading microorganisms. Two of the six types of white blood cell can squeeze through the clefts: the _____ and the _____. These are large cells which depend on _____ in order to fit through the clefts, which are too small to allow RBCs to pass.[35]

It is also important to realize that water has a great tendency to flow out of capillaries through the clefts. There are two reasons: 1) The hydrostatic pressure (fluid pressure) created by the heart simply tends to squeeze water out of the capillaries, and 2) the high osmolarity of the tissues tends to draw water out of the bloodstream. The circulatory system deals with this problem by giving the plasma a high osmolarity. [Would dissolving NaCl in the plasma accomplish this?[36]] Plasma osmolarity is provided by high concentrations of large plasma proteins, mainly albumin. Albumin is too large and rigid to pass through the clefts, so it remains in the capillaries and keeps water there too. The osmotic pressure provided by plasma proteins is given a special name: **oncotic pressure**. However, some water does leak out, resulting in an interesting cycle.

1) At the beginning of the capillary, the hydrostatic pressure is high. The result is that water squeezes out into the tissues.
2) As water continues to leave the capillary, the relative concentration of plasma proteins increases.
3) At the end of the capillary the hydrostatic pressure is quite low, but since the blood is now very concentrated, the oncotic pressure is very high. As a result, water flows back into the capillary from the tissues.

Thus, some water is lost into the tissues, but due to the oncotic pressure of the plasma proteins, the net loss is normally low. Occasionally the system breaks down and a significant amount of water is lost into the tissues. For example, during **inflammation**, capillaries dilate, increasing the size of the intercellular clefts. This allows more space for white blood cells to migrate into the tissues. The unfortunate side-effect is that plasma proteins and a lot of water are lost into the tissues. The result is water in the tissues, or swelling, termed **edema**. Small amounts of fluid loss into the tissues are normal; even some protein is normally lost. Fluid, proteins, and white blood cells in the tissues are returned to the bloodstream via the lymphatic system.

- What would occur if capillaries throughout the circulatory system were made more permeable?[37]
- Albumin is made in the liver. Alcoholics with diseased livers make insufficient amounts of albumin, and thus have insufficient plasma oncotic pressure. What result would you predict?[38]

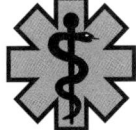

---

[35] Macrophages and neutrophils can squeeze through the clefts, even though they are larger than RBCs, because they are capable of *amoeboid motility*, as noted in Table 2. RBCs are not capable of independent motility.

[36] No, because salts can freely pass out of the capillaries.

[37] A significant volume of fluid will be lost from the plasma into tissues, decreasing the blood volume and cardiac output. Circulatory shock can result.

[38] The result is edema of the entire body, including the limbs, abdomen, and lungs.

9.6 THE LYMPHATIC SYSTEM

The lymphatic system (Figure 11) is a one-way flow system which begins with tiny lymphatic capillaries in all the tissues of the body that merge to form larger lymphatic vessels. These merge to form large lymphatic ducts. Lymphatic vessels have valves, and the larger lymphatic ducts have smooth muscles in their walls. As a result, the lymphatic system acts like a suction pump to retrieve water, proteins, and white blood cells from the tissues. The fluid in lymphatic vessels is called **lymph**. The lymph is filtered by numerous **lymph nodes**. The lymph nodes are an important part of the immune system because they contain millions of white blood cells that can initiate an immune response against anything foreign that may have been picked up in the lymph. The large lymphatic ducts merge to form the **thoracic duct**, which is the largest lymphatic vessel, located in the chest. The thoracic duct empties into a large vein near the neck. Also, lymphatic vessels from the intestines dump dietary fats in the form of chylomicrons into the thoracic duct.

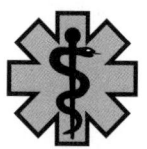

9.7 THE IMMUNE SYSTEM

The interior of the body provides a warm, protective, nourishing environment where microorganisms can flourish. We could not survive without a versatile and efficient immune system to destroy invaders without destroying the body itself. There are three types of immunity: innate, humoral, and cell-mediated.

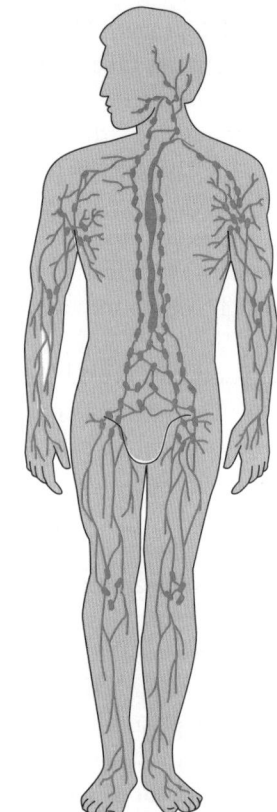

Figure 11   The Lymphatic System: Vessels and Lymph Nodes

Innate Immunity

Innate immunity refers to the general, nonspecific protection the body provides against various invaders. The simplest example of innate immunity is the barrier to the outside world known as **skin**. The skin prevents many types of pathogens from infecting us. Here is a list of the principal components of innate immunity:

1) The skin is an excellent barrier against the entry of microorganisms.
2) Tears, saliva, and blood contain **lysozyme**, an enzyme that kills some bacteria by destroying their cell walls.
3) The extreme acidity of the stomach destroys many pathogens which are ingested with food or swallowed after being passed out of the respiratory tract.
4) Macrophages and neutrophils indiscriminately phagocytize microorganisms.[39]
5) The **complement system** is a group of about 20 blood proteins that can nonspecifically bind to the surface of foreign cells, leading to their destruction.

---

[39] Do not confuse this portion of innate immunity with cell-mediated immunity. You are correct to notice that cells are involved, but this activity is placed in the "innate" category because we are referring to nonspecific phagocytosis. Humoral and cell-mediated immunity are highly specific. There is one other subtlety: when a macrophage eats an antigen which has been coated with specific antibodies, we are dealing with humoral immunity; this is different from the indiscriminate, nonspecific pathogen phagocytosis discussed above.

Humoral Immunity, Antibodies, and B Cells

Humoral immunity refers to specific protection by proteins in the plasma called **antibodies (Ab)** or **immunoglobulins (Ig)**. Antibodies specifically recognize and bind to microorganisms (or other foreign particles), leading to their destruction and removal from the body. Each antibody molecule is composed of two copies of two different polypeptides, the **light chains** and the **heavy chains**, joined by disulfide bonds (Figure 12). In addition, each antibody molecule has two regions, the **constant region** and the **variable (antigen binding) region**. There are several different classes of immunoglobulins, differentiated by their constant regions: IgG, IgA, IgM, IgD, and IgE. The classes of immunoglobulins have slightly different functions (see Table 3), with most of the antibody circulating in plasma in the IgG class. The variable regions are responsible for the specificity of antibodies in recognizing foreign particles.

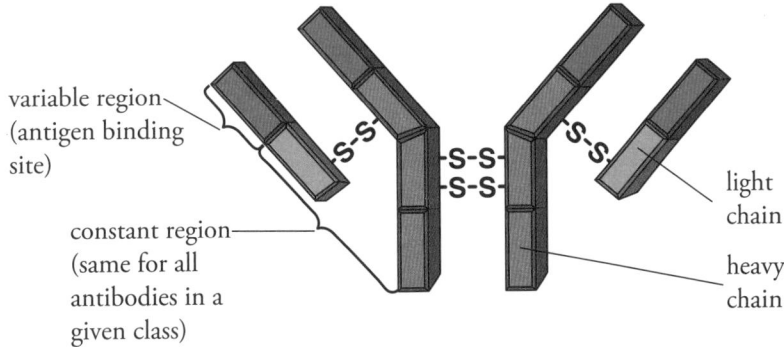

Figure 12   Antibody Structure

Constant Region Class	Location in Body	Function
IgM	blood and B cell surface	Involved in initial immune response; pentameric structure in blood, monomeric structure on B cell as antigen receptor
IgG	blood	Involved in ongoing immune response; the majority of antibody in the blood is IgG; can also cross the placental barrier
IgD	B cell surface	Serves with IgM as antigen receptor on B cells
IgA	secretions (saliva, mucus, tears, breast milk, etc.)	Secreted in breast milk; helps protect newborns, dimeric structure
IgE	blood	Involved in allergic reactions

Table 3   Classes of Antibodies

Each antibody forms a unique variable region that has a different binding specificity. The molecule that an antibody binds to is known as the **antigen (Ag)**. Examples of antigens are viral capsid proteins, bacterial surface proteins, and toxins in the bloodstream (such as tetanus toxin). [Would an antibody against a cytoplasmic bacterial protein help the immune system to remove the bacteria?[40]] The specificity of antigen binding is determined by the fit of antigen in a small three-dimensional cleft formed by the variable region of the antibody molecule (Figure 12). [If the antigen binding site is small, can antibodies recognize

---

[40]   No. Antibodies are soluble in the plasma, so they can only recognize antigens on surfaces that are accessible to them. A protein in the cytoplasm of a bacteria would never be accessible to antibodies in the plasma and therefore could not be recognized.

large proteins as antigens?[41] Why might an antibody that binds tightly to a small region of a protein, five amino acids out of 200, have very low affinity for the same five amino acids of the protein when presented as an isolated peptide?[42]] Antigens are often large molecules which have many different recognition sites for different antibodies. The small site that an antibody recognizes within a larger molecule is called an **epitope**. Very small molecules often do not elicit the production of antibodies on their own but will when bound to an antigenic large molecule like a protein. The protein in this case is called a **carrier**, and the small molecule that becomes antigenic is known as a **hapten**. When antibody binds to an antigen, the following can contribute to removal of the antigen from the body:

1) Binding of antibody may directly inactivate the antigen. For example, binding of antibody to a viral coat protein may prevent the virus from binding to cells.
2) Binding of antibody can induce phagocytosis of a particle by macrophages and neutrophils.
3) The presence of antibodies on the surface of a cell can activate the complement system to form holes in the cell membrane and lyse the cell.

Antibodies are produced by a type of lymphocyte called **B cells**. Antibodies produced by an individual B cell can recognize only one specific antigen, but B cells in general produce antibodies that recognize an immense array of antigens. How do B cells produce such a broad array of antibodies? Does the genome encode a gene for every possible antibody molecule, a million genes for a million different potential antibodies? No. Immature B cells are derived from precursor stem cells in the bone marrow. The genes that encode antibody proteins are assembled by recombination from many small segments during B cell development. Thus, there are many different B cell clones, each with a different variable region. The immature B cells express antibody molecules on their surface. When antigen binds to the antibody on the surface of a specific immature B cell, that cell is stimulated to proliferate and differentiate into two kinds of cells: **plasma cells** and **memory cells**. Plasma cells actively produce and secrete antibody protein into the plasma. Memory cells are produced from the same clone and have the same variable regions, but do not secrete antibody; they are like pre-activated, dormant B cells. The memory cells remain dormant, sometimes for years, waiting for the same antigen to reappear. If it does, the memory cells *then* become activated, and start producing antibody very quickly; so quickly that no symptoms of illness appear. This method of selecting B cells with specific antigen binding is called **clonal selection**. [In general, every cell of the body is said to possess the same copy of the genome. Is this true in the immune system?[43]]

---

[41] Yes. Antibodies often recognize proteins as antigens, but they do not recognize the whole protein. Usually antibodies recognize a small part of a protein as an antigen.

[42] In the intact protein the five amino acids assume a specific three-dimensional conformation that is recognized well by the antibody. The five amino acids as a small peptide, however, will not fold the same way and probably would not be as well recognized by the antibody.

[43] No. Recombination during development of B cells and T cells makes these an exception to the generalization that every cell contains the whole genome.

- Which one of the following best describes the mechanism by which production of specific antibody is achieved in response to antigen exposure?[44]
  - A) Immature B cell clones expressing several different antibody genes select for one gene and turn off expression of the others.
  - B) Antigen stimulates proliferation of a specific B cell clone expressing a single antibody protein that recognizes that antigen.
  - C) The variable regions of antibody proteins on an immature B cell clone form a pocket around the antigen, and the antibody genes are recombined to fit the bound antigen.
  - D) Antibody light and heavy chains are mixed on each B cell's surface in different combinations to produce different antigen recognition.

The first time a person encounters an antigen during an infection, it can take a week or more for B cells to proliferate and secrete significant levels of antibody. This is known as the **primary immune response** and is too slow to prevent symptoms of the infection from occurring. The immune response to the same antigen the second time a person is exposed, the **secondary immune response**, is much swifter and stronger, so much so that symptoms never develop, and the person is said to "be immune." This immunity can last for years and is due to the presence of the memory cells produced during the first infection. **Vaccination** is used to improve the response to infection by exposing the immune system to an antigen associated with a virus or bacterium, thus building up the secondary immune response if the live pathogen is encountered in the future. [Vaccination against some viruses is ineffective in preventing future infection, while it is highly effective against other viruses. Does the failure of vaccination to protect against some viruses indicate a failure in the ability to produce memory cells?[45]]

Cell-Mediated Immunity and the T Cell

There are two types of **T cells**: **T helpers** ("CD4 cells") and **T killers** (cytotoxic T cells, "CD8 cells").[46] The role of the T helper is to activate B cells, T killer cells, and other cells of the immune system. Hence, the T helper is the central controller of the whole immune response. It communicates with other cells by releasing special hormones called **lymphokines** and **interleukins**.[47] The T helper cell is the host of HIV, the virus that causes AIDS.

The role of the T killer cell is to *destroy abnormal host cells*, namely:

1) Virus-infected host cells
2) Cancer cells
3) Foreign cells such as the cells of a skin graft given by an incompatible donor

---

[44] Choice **B** is correct. The two key features of clonal selection in B cells are 1) recombination during development to produce many clones, each with a single antigen recognition specificity, and 2) selection of a clone out of the many clones based on specific recognition of antigen by preexisting antibody genes.

[45] No. It is probably the result of mutation by the virus. Vaccination against one form of virus and production of memory cells will not protect against a virus if the viral antigen mutates so that it is no longer recognized by the immune system.

[46] "CD" stands for "Cell Differentiation marker."

[47] *Lympho-* is short for lymphocytes, and *-kine* means move or activate. *Inter-* means between, and *-leukin* is for leukocytes or white blood cells.

9.7

The "T" in "T cell" stands for **thymus**. T cells are named after this gland because this is where they develop during childhood. Trillions of different T cells are produced in the bone marrow during childhood. Each of these is specific for a particular antigen, just as with B cells. [If a T cell is specific for an antigen, does that mean it releases antibodies that bind to the antigen?[48]] The protein on the T cell surface that can bind antigen is the **T cell receptor**.

The function of T cells is exceedingly complex. As a brief introduction, the way a T cell recognizes a bad cell is by "examining" (binding to) proteins on its surface. One important group of cell-surface proteins is known as the **major histocompatibility complex** (**MHC**). Our cells are all programmed to have MHC proteins on their surfaces so that the immune system can keep an eye on what is going on inside every cell. There are two kinds of MHCs, known as MHC class I and MHC class II, or simply **MHC I** and **MHC II**. MHC I proteins are found on the surface of every nucleated cell in the body. Their role is to randomly pick up peptides from the inside of the cell and display them on the cell surface. This allows T cells to monitor cellular contents. For example, if a cell is infected with a virus, one of its class I MHC complexes will display a piece of a virus-specific protein. When a T killer cell detects the viral protein (by binding to it) displayed on the cell's MHC I, it becomes activated and will proliferate.

The role of MHC II is more complex. Only certain special cells have MHC II. These cells are known as **antigen-presenting cells** (**APCs**). The antigen-presenting cells include macrophages and B cells. Their role is to phagocytize particles or cells, chop them up, and display fragments using the MHC II display system, which T helpers then recognize (bind to). After a T helper is activated by antigen displayed in MHC II, it will activate B cells (and stimulate proliferation of T killer cells) that are specific for that antigen. The activated B cells mature into plasma cells and secrete antibodies specific for the antigen. The complexity of this process helps explain why the primary immune response takes a week or more.

- Can a T helper cell become activated after encountering a foreign particle floating in the blood? If so, how? If not, why not, and what else is required?[49]

Note that full activation of T cells only occurs when the T cell binds to both antigen (displayed on MHC I or II) and the MHC molecule itself.

Other Tissues Involved in the Immune Response

The **bone marrow** is the site of synthesis of all the cells of the blood from a common progenitor. The cell that gives rise to all the various blood cells is called the bone marrow stem cell. **Lymph nodes** were discussed earlier in this chapter. The **spleen** filters the blood and is a site of immune cell interactions, just like lymph nodes. The spleen also destroys aged RBCs. The **thymus** is the site of T cell maturation. The thymus shrinks in size in adults since the maturation of the immune system and T cells is most active in children. The **tonsils** are masses of lymphatic tissue in the back of the throat that help "catch" pathogens which enter the body through respiration or ingestion. The **appendix** is very similar to the tonsils, both in structure and function, and is found near the beginning of the large intestine. Neither the appendix nor the tonsils are required for survival and are often removed if they become infected.

---

[48] No, only B cells make antibodies. If a T helper is specific for an antigen, it will activate B cells or T killers to destroy it.

[49] No, T helpers are only activated by antigen presented on MHC II. For a foreign particle to activate a helper T cell, the particle must first be displayed by an antigen-presenting cell (macrophage or B cell). The antigen-presenting cell must phagocytize the particle, hydrolyze it into fragments in a lysosome, and allow it to bind to an MHC II which will be displayed on the cell surface.

9.8 AUTOIMMUNITY

Ideally, the immune system will only recognize and destroy foreign antigen; it should ignore (not become activated against) all normal proteins and cell structures; this is called **tolerance**. However, the production of these trillions of different B cells and T cells with different receptors is random, and as a result, many of them will be specific for normal molecules found in the human body, or *self* antigens. Thus, B cells and T cells must go through a selection process in order to eliminate any self-reactive cells.

For B cells, this generally occurs in the bone marrow, but can also occur in lymph nodes. An immature B cell whose surface receptor binds to normal cell surface proteins (for example, MHCs or other proteins on a macrophage or other bone marrow cell) is induced to die through apoptosis. Those whose surface receptors bind to normal soluble proteins (for example, hemoglobin or lipoproteins) do not go through apoptosis, but become unresponsive or **anergic**. Only those B cells whose surface receptors bind to no normal proteins during maturation are released into the circulation. For T cells, the process is similar, but occurs in the thymus or in the lymph nodes. Immature T cells whose antigen receptors bind normal proteins in the thymus undergo apoptosis, and (because not all proteins are expressed in the thymus), some T cells are released that may bind surface proteins in the periphery; these cells become anergic. The result of this is that billions of B and T cells survive, but billions of others do not. The ones that survive go on to proliferate if stimulated by antigen in the proper context, each producing a group of identical B or T cells, all specific for a particular antigen. Such a group is known as a **B cell or T cell clone**. Clonal selection in response to antigen recognition is similar in B and T cells.

It is very important to get rid of all cells specific for self-antigen, because such cells can cause an **autoimmune reaction**, in which the immune system attacks normal body cells or proteins. Obviously, this would cause problems as normal body structures become inflamed or destroyed. Some autoimmune diseases include type I diabetes mellitus, rheumatoid arthritis, Graves' disease, myasthenia gravis, and celiac disease. Autoimmune diseases are often treated with immunosuppressant drugs or with steroids to reduce the inflammatory response.

9.8

Chapter 9 Summary

- The circulatory and lymphatic systems transport materials (O_2, CO_2, nutrients, wastes, hormones, etc.) around the body. The lymphatic system helps to filter and return tissue fluid (lymph) to the circulatory system.

- Deoxygenated blood returning from the body enters the heart at the right atrium, and is pumped to the lungs by the right ventricle. The oxygenated blood returns to the heart at the left atrium, and is pumped to the body by the left ventricle.

- AV valves (tricuspid on the right and bicuspid, or mitral, on the left) separate the atria and ventricles. Semilunar valves (pulmonary on the right and aortic on the left) separate the ventricles and the arteries.

- Veins always return blood to the heart. Most veins carry deoxygenated blood; an exception are the pulmonary veins, which return blood from the lungs to the heart.

- Arteries always carry blood away from the heart. Most arteries carry oxygenated blood; an exception are the pulmonary arteries, which carry blood from the heart to the lungs.

- Endothelial cells line the insides of blood vessels and form the walls of capillaries. They are important mediators of vasoconstriction, vasodilation, the inflammatory response, blood clotting, and angiogenesis.

- The cardiac muscle cell action potential is prolonged by the opening of voltage-gated calcium channels. The influx of calcium causes a long plateau in the action potential.

- Cardiac muscle is a functional syncytium; cells are connected by intercalated disks, which contain gap junctions. The gap junctions are electrical synapses that easily allow the transmission of the action potential, and thus contraction, to spread from cell to cell.

- The SA node is the "pacemaker" of the heart. It has an unstable resting potential that rises until threshold is reached and an action potential is fired. This action potential (and subsequent contraction) is then transmitted throughout the heart.

- Systemic blood pressure is directly proportional to cardiac output (the volume of blood pumped per minute) and to peripheral resistance (the force opposing blood flow through the vessels).

- Cardiac output is directly proportional to stroke volume and heart rate, while peripheral resistance is inversely related to vessel diameter.

- Blood is approximately 55 percent plasma, 40 to 45 percent erythrocytes (red blood cells), and 1 percent leukocytes (white blood cells) and platelets.

- ABO and Rh antigens on the surface of erythrocytes determine blood type; type AB+ is the universal recipient and type O− is the universal donor.

- Oxygen is transported in the blood bound to hemoglobin, a protein in red blood cells. Carbon dioxide is transported in the blood primarily as bicarbonate ion; some also binds to hemoglobin.

- Innate immunity is nonspecific and includes things like the skin, lysozyme, stomach acid, phagocytes, and the complement system.

- Humoral immunity is the production of antibodies by B cells that are highly specific for particular antigens (foreign molecules).

- There are five classes of antibodies: IgM (pentameric, primary immune response), IgG (secondary immune response and main blood antibody), IgA (dimeric, found in secretions like saliva and breast milk), IgD (B cell antigen receptor), and IgE (allergic reactions).

- Cell-mediated immunity is handled by T cells. Killer (cytotoxic) T cells destroy "self" cells that are displaying abnormal antigen on MHC I. Helper T cells are activated by antigen displayed on MHC II, and secrete chemicals to help activate and stimulate the proliferation of killer T cells and B cells.

- Autoimmunity occurs when the immune system targets normal body cells or tissues and destroys them. It is the result of a failure to eliminate self-reactive B cells and T cells during their development and maturation. Elimination of self-reactive lymphocytes is referred to as "developing tolerance."

CHAPTER 9 FREESTANDING PRACTICE QUESTIONS

1. The cardiac cycle is divided into systole and diastole, during which the ventricles contract and relax, respectively. During systole, blood is ejected from the ventricles and is pumped into either the aorta or pulmonary artery. The pressure in the ventricles rapidly increases; however, the volume of blood in the ventricles initially remains unchanged. This is referred to as *isovolumetric contraction*. Which of the following is the most likely reason for isovolumetric contraction?

A) Decreased ventricular contractility due to over-stretching of cardiac sarcomeres.
B) The pressure in the aorta is initially greater that of the left ventricle.
C) The pressure within the pulmonary vein is initially lower than that of the right ventricle.
D) The action potential that propagates through the bundle of His and Purkinje fibers has not yet depolarized all of the ventricles.

2. The ductus arteriosus is a shunt in the fetal circulation that diverts a portion of the blood from the pulmonary circulation into the aorta. Failure of the ductus arteriosus to close shortly after birth results in a condition referred to as a *patent ductus arteriosus* and, in severe cases, the generation of a left-to-right shunt. A left-to-right shunt would result in all of the following EXCEPT:

A) increased mixing of oxygenated blood with deoxygenated blood.
B) decreased blood flow into the systemic circulation.
C) increased blood flow into the pulmonary circulation.
D) decreased vascular pressure in the pulmonary circulation.

3. Blood pressure is directly proportional to cardiac output and peripheral resistance. Which of the following will raise blood pressure?

A) Consumption of a large meal, because it increases the heart rate
B) Exercise, because it increases cardiac output
C) Sizable blood loss, because it increases epinephrine levels due to the fear response
D) A localized allergic reaction, because it causes fluid loss to the tissue at the site

4. What are the names of the two portal systems in the body?

A) The pancreatic and the hypothalamic-hypophyseal
B) The pancreatic and the renal-urinary
C) The hepatic and the hypothalamic-hypophyseal
D) The hepatic and the renal-urinary

5. T cell antigen receptors are different from antibodies because:

A) T cell receptors must interact with antigen uniquely presented by other cells but not with free antigen.
B) T cell receptors bind various cytokines.
C) T cell receptors bind complement proteins to lyse cells.
D) T cell receptors are mediators of allergic reactions.

6. Hepatitis B is an inflammatory disease of the liver. While the virus itself is relatively benign, the body's attempt to eradicate it causes unwanted liver inflammation. Which of the following blood test results could be from an individual who has been vaccinated against Hepatitis B and does not have an active infection?

A) Negative for anti-Hepatitis B antibodies and negative for Hepatitis B antigen

B) Negative for anti-Hepatitis B antibodies and positive for Hepatitis B antigen

C) Positive for anti-Hepatitis B antibodies and positive for Hepatitis B antigen

D) Positive for anti-Hepatitis B antibodies and negative for Hepatitis B antigen

7. Individuals affected with DiGeorge syndrome have a T cell deficiency due to congenital lack, or incomplete development, of the thymus. Based on this statement, individuals affected with this syndrome will:

A) have normal humoral immunity.

B) have normal cell-mediated immunity.

C) be susceptible to infection.

D) be resistant to infection.

8. Which of the following statements about antibodies is true?

   I. Antibodies are produced by B cells.

   II. Antibodies only recognize peptide antigens.

   III. Antibodies can mark an antigen for destruction by killer T cells.

A) I only

B) II only

C) I and II

D) I and III

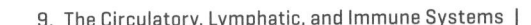

CHAPTER 9 PRACTICE PASSAGE

Endurance training, also known as aerobic exercise, causes adaptations in the cardiovascular system. The principal parameters involved in this adaptation are *maximum oxygen consumption*, *blood pressure*, and *blood flow*.

Maximum oxygen consumption is the product of cardiac output (CO) and the maximum difference in oxygen concentration between the arteries and the veins, known as the arterio-venous oxygen difference (ΔA–V_{O_2}). Figure 1 shows the ΔA–V_{O_2} before and after endurance training in a 40-year-old man.

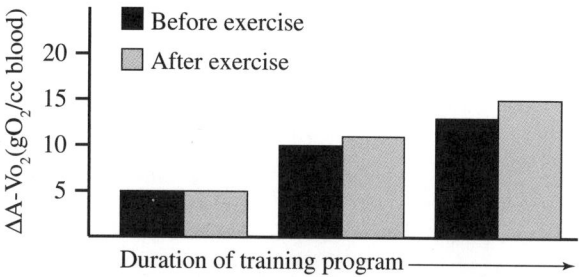

Figure 1

Blood pressure is a measure of the force per unit area with which blood pushes against the walls of the blood vessels. The pressure is determined by the pumping of the heart and by vascular *tone*. Tone refers to the level of muscular tension and is determined by sympathetic nervous input and by *autoregulation*. Autoregulation refers to changes in vascular tone determined by local factors, i.e., the buildup of metabolic end-products. It causes vessels to dilate when end products build up, indicating a need for more blood flow. The blood pressure readings of a 40-year-old man before and after an endurance training program are shown in Figure 2.

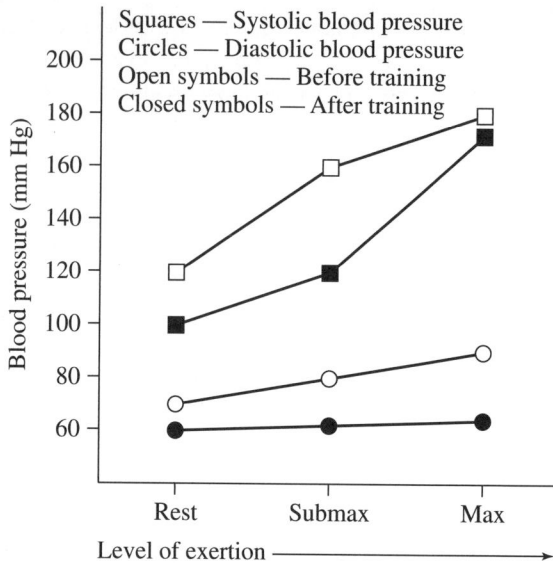

Figure 2

Blood flow is directly proportional to blood pressure, except when autoregulation is present, in which case dilation of vessels allows increased flow without increased pressure. Figure 3 shows the coronary and brain blood flow values of a 40-year-old man before and after endurance training.

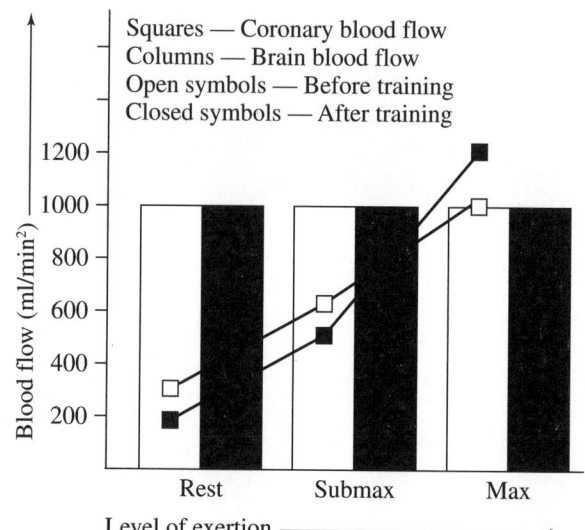

Figure 3

Adapted from *Exercise Physiology*, by George Brooks and Thomas Fahey, © 1985 by Macmillan Publishing Co.

1. Each of the following could account for the changes induced by endurance training in $\Delta A–Vo_2$ seen in Figure 1 EXCEPT increased:

A) numbers of mitochondria in muscle.
B) O_2 affinity of hemoglobin.
C) lactate buildup due to increased muscle mass.
D) muscle capillary density.

2. In Figure 2, the after-training blood pressure of the 40-year-old man at submaximal work rate is approximately:

A) 120/60.
B) 120/80.
C) 160/80.
D) 160/60.

3. Figure 3 supports which of the following conclusions?

A) The brain's oxygen requirements increase with increase in work rate.
B) The heart is more active at submax work rate after training.
C) After training, coronary metabolic requirements are greatest at maximal exercise.
D) Vasoconstriction increases in the heart during exercise.

4. Cardiac output is influenced by which of the following?

   I. Nervous input
   II. Hormones
   III. Blood pressure

A) I only
B) II only
C) I and II only
D) I, II, and III

5. It can be inferred from Figures 2 and 3 that:

A) increasing blood pressure increases brain blood flow.
B) blood pressure and blood flow are inversely proportional.
C) the brain vasculature responds to exercise differently than does cardiac muscle.
D) autoregulation leads to vasoconstriction in the heart during exercise.

6. It can be inferred from the passage that:

A) during exertion and during rest, blood pressure between heartbeats changes less than the pressure during heartbeats.
B) the maximum blood pressure measured in an individual during exercise changes more with training than the level measured during rest.
C) blood flow to the brain decreases during sleep.
D) athletes use oxygen less efficiently than people who are in poor physical shape.

SOLUTIONS TO CHAPTER 9 FREESTANDING PRACTICE QUESTIONS

1. **B**   At the start of systole the semilunar valves are closed, and although the ventricles are contracting, no blood is ejected. The semilunar valves will remain closed until the pressure within the ventricle exceeds that of the aorta or pulmonary artery (choice B is correct), at which point the semilunar valves open and blood is ejected from the ventricles. While overstretching of the cardiac sarcomeres could lead to decreased contractility (because of less overlap between actin and myosin filaments), this would not explain why the contraction is isovolumetric (choice A is wrong). It is true that the pulmonary vein has very low pressure and would be at a lower pressure than the right ventricle, but this does not explain why contraction (which pumps blood into the pulmonary artery rather than into the pulmonary *vein*) would be isovolumetric (choice C is wrong). Ventricular depolarization, initiated by the atrioventricular node, propagates through the bundle of His and Purkinje fibers and depolarizes all of the ventricles in about 120 to 200 ms. The approximate duration of ventricular contraction is 300 to 450 ms; in other words, depolarization of the ventricles is very rapid, and all of the myocytes of the ventricles have been depolarized well before the pressure within the ventricles begins to change (choice D is wrong).

2. **D**   Since the left side of the heart deals with oxygenated blood and the right side of the heart deals with deoxygenated blood, a left-to-right shunt would cause increased mixing of oxygenated and deoxygenated blood (choice A would occur and can be eliminated). A left-to-right shunt, particularly one connecting the aorta and pulmonary artery, would result in blood flow from the high-pressure aorta into the lower-pressure pulmonary artery (both choices B and C would occur and can be eliminated). This additional flow into the pulmonary artery would result in an increased blood volume in the pulmonary circulation and a subsequent increase (not decrease) in pulmonary vascular pressure (choice D would not occur and is the correct answer choice).

3. **B**   Exercise will cause muscle contraction, which pushes blood along the veins, increasing venous return to the heart. According to the Frank-Starling mechanism, the increase in venous return will increase stroke volume, increasing cardiac output and therefore blood pressure. Further, the increased heart rate due to exercise will also increase cardiac output and blood pressure. Consumption of a large meal will activate the parasympathetic nervous system (rest and digest), so the vagus nerve will be stimulated and the heart rate will decrease. This will decrease the cardiac output and decrease blood pressure (choice A is wrong). Blood loss will decrease blood volume and thus blood pressure. If the blood loss is sizable, the decrease in pressure will be larger than the increase in heart rate from the epinephrine produced by the fear response (choice C is wrong). The loss of fluid to the tissues will decrease blood volume, and thus also blood pressure (choice D is wrong).

4. **C**   A portal system consists of two capillary beds connected by a vein. The hepatic portal system connects the small intestine's nutrient absorption to the detoxification systems of the liver, and the hypothalamic-hypophyseal portal system provides a short connection for the hormones of the hypothalamus to control the hormones of the anterior pituitary. The renal system (kidney) and the urinary system (bladder) are connected by the ureter (which carries urine, not blood). Also, do not get confused by the connection of the glomerular capillaries

to the peritubular capillaries (the vasa recta); these are connected by an artery (the efferent arteriole), not a vein (choices B and D can be eliminated). The pancreas has an exocrine duct system and a single capillary bed (choice A can be eliminated).

5. **A** T cell receptors must bind antigen that is presented by MHC proteins on the surface of other cells. They are unable to bind free antigen. Cytokines have their own family of receptors and are not bound by T cell receptors or antibodies (choice B is wrong). T cell receptors do not bind complement proteins; the complement system is a set of proteins that can be activated, sometimes by antibodies, to cause nonspecific cell lysis (choice C is wrong). IgE and some other antibodies are involved with allergic reactions, but T cell receptors are not (choice D is wrong).

6. **D** Vaccination involves the introduction of non-pathogenic antigen into the body in order to trigger the production of antibodies and memory lymphocytes. Individuals who have been vaccinated against Hepatitis B would test positive for anti-Hepatitis B antibodies (choices A and B can be eliminated). Individuals who do not have an active Hepatitis B infection would test negative for Hepatitis B antigens (choice C can be eliminated, and choice D is correct).

7. **C** DiGeorge syndrome is also known as *thymic aplasia*. The T cells (or cell-mediated arm) of the immune system are affected and there is an increased susceptibility to infection (choice D is wrong), both from the lack of killer T cells (choice B is wrong), and from the lack of helper T cells and the subsequent effect on the humoral branch of the immune system (choice A is wrong).

8. **A** Item I is true: antibodies are produced by the B cells of the immune system (choice B can be eliminated). Item II is false: antibodies can recognize a great diversity of antigens which include, but are not limited to, peptides (choice C can be eliminated). Item III is false: antibodies can mark an antigen for destruction by macrophages and other phagocytes. Killer T cells do not directly destroy antigens; rather, they kill cells that are producing antigens (such as cells infected by a virus). Further, the mechanism of cell destruction by killer T cells does not involve antibodies (choice D can be eliminated, and choice A is correct).

SOLUTIONS TO CHAPTER 9 PRACTICE PASSAGE

1. **B** Figure 1 shows that as the training program progresses, the arterio-venous oxygen difference increases; in other words, after undergoing training, oxygen is extracted more efficiently from the blood. Increased numbers of mitochondria would lead to more efficient oxygen extraction (choice A could account for the changes and can be eliminated). Lactate buildup would reduce blood pH, reducing hemoglobin's affinity for oxygen and allowing oxygen to be taken from the blood more easily (choice C could account for the changes and can be eliminated). Muscle capillary density does increase during training; this would bring more blood to the muscle and make it easier for oxygen to diffuse out of the blood (choice D could account for the changes and can be eliminated). However, if hemoglobin had an increased affinity for oxygen, it would hold on to the oxygen and not release it to the muscle. This would decrease the arterio-venous oxygen difference (choice B cannot account for the changes and is the correct answer choice).

2. **A** Blood pressure is defined as systolic pressure over diastolic pressure, and the after-training values are indicated by closed symbols. The systolic value after training at submax work rate is 120 (choices C and D are wrong), and the diastolic value is 60 (choice B is wrong, and choice A is correct).

3. **C** Figure 3 shows that as the level of exertion increases, the blood flow to the brain remains constant while the blood flow to the heart increases (note that this is due to vasodilation, not vasoconstriction; choice D is wrong). This is true both before and after training. Since the brain blood flow is constant regardless of the level of exertion, its oxygen requirements must not be increasing (choice A is wrong). Coronary blood flow is higher at submax work rate before training, indicating that the heart is working harder than it is after training (choice B is wrong). Coronary blood flow is highest at maximal exercise, indicating that the metabolic requirements of the heart must be very high (need for oxygen, need to eliminate carbon dioxide, etc.; choice C is correct).

4. **D** Item I: True. Parasympathetic nerves to the SA node keep the heart rate slow when one is resting, and sympathetic stimulation increases the heart rate (choice B can be eliminated). Item II: True. Circulating hormones affect cardiac performance. The key example is epinephrine from the adrenal gland, which increases cardiac output (choice A can be eliminated). Item III: True. Increased blood pressure makes it more difficult for the heart to eject its load of blood, and decreased blood pressure impairs cardiac function when not enough blood is returned to the pumping heart (choice C can be eliminated, and choice D is correct).

5. **C** Combining Figures 2 and 3, you can see that both blood pressure and cardiac blood flow increase as exertion increases, but brain blood flow stays the same (choice C is correct, and choice A is wrong). Since both pressure and flow are increasing, they must be directly proportional, not inversely proportional (choice B is wrong). Since cardiac flow is increasing, it must be due to vasodilation, not vasoconstriction (choice D is wrong).

6. **A** Figure 2 shows that the diastolic pressure (the pressure between heartbeats) changes much less during exertion and rest than the systolic pressure (the pressure during heartbeats; choice A is correct). It also shows that the highest blood pressure reached during exercise does not change as much after training as does the resting systolic pressure (in other words, the "Max" squares are closer together than the "Rest" squares; choice B is wrong). There is no information given on brain blood flow during sleep, and if anything, you might assume it stays constant based on Figure 3 (choice C is wrong). Based on Figure 1, you can assume that athletes use oxygen more efficiently, since the arterio-venous difference is greater after training (choice D is wrong).

Chapter 10
The Excretory and Digestive Systems

10.1 OVERVIEW OF THE EXCRETORY SYSTEM

Excretion is the disposal of waste products. "The excretory system" generally refers to the kidneys, even though the liver, large intestine, and skin are involved in excretion too. Let's begin by summarizing the excretory roles of these organs to see where the kidneys fit into the picture.

Liver

The **liver** is responsible for excreting many wastes by chemically modifying them and releasing them into bile (discussed later in this chapter). In particular, the liver deals with hydrophobic or large waste products, which cannot be filtered out by the kidney. (The kidney can only eliminate small hydrophiles dissolved in plasma.) For example: in the liver, old heme units are broken down into bilirubin, which is then tagged with a molecule called glucuronate; the resulting bilirubin glucuronate is excreted with bile.

The liver is also very important in excretion because it synthesizes **urea** (Figure 1) and releases it into the bloodstream. Urea is a carrier of excess nitrogen resulting from protein breakdown. Excess nitrogen must be converted to urea because free ammonia is toxic. Urea derives its name from the fact that it is excreted in urine.

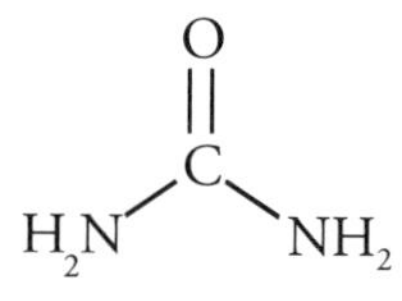

Figure 1 Urea

Colon

The **large intestine** reabsorbs water and ions (sodium, calcium, etc.) from feces. In this sense it doesn't really excrete anything, but merely processes wastes already destined for excretion. However, the colon is also capable of excreting excess ions (e.g., sodium, chloride, calcium) into the feces using active transport.

Skin

The skin produces sweat, which contains water, ions, and urea. In other words, sweat is similar to urine. In this sense, the skin is an excretory organ. However, sweating is not primarily controlled by the amount of waste that needs to be excreted, but rather by temperature and level of sympathetic nervous system activity. Therefore, the excretory role of the skin is secondary.

Kidneys

The final responsibility for excretion of hydrophilic wastes lies with the kidneys. Substances which must be excreted in the urine include urea, sodium, bicarbonate, and water. "But wait," you say, "sodium, bicarbonate, and water aren't waste products!" Actually, they sometimes are wastes, when they are present at abnormally high concentrations. You begin to see that the kidney is not like the colon, a passive container for wastes waiting to be excreted. It is a sensitive regulator that must keep concentrations at *optimum levels*, as opposed to simply dumping things.

This is the homeostatic role of the kidneys. **Homeostasis** refers to the constancy of physiological variables. For example, the normal serum Na^+ concentration is 142 mEq/L. Variations in this level greater than 15 percent are fatal due to dysfunction of neurons, cardiac muscle cells, and other cell types. There are other components to homeostasis which the kidney does not control (e.g., temperature maintenance).

Excretory and Homeostatic Roles of the Kidney

1) Excretion of hydrophilic wastes
2) Maintenance of constant solute concentration and constant pH
3) Maintenance of constant fluid volume (important for blood pressure and cardiac output)

As a simplification, we can say that these goals are accomplished via three processes:

- The first process is **filtration**. This entails the passage of pressurized blood over a filter (like a coffee filter). Cells and proteins remain in the blood (like coffee grinds), while water and small molecules are squeezed out into the **renal tubule** (like java). During filtration, water, waste products, and useful small molecules such as glucose are filtered into the renal tubule. The fluid in the tubule is called **filtrate**, and it will eventually be made into urine.
- The second process is **selective reabsorption**. Here we take back useful items (glucose, water, amino acids), while leaving wastes and some water in the tubule.
- The third process is **secretion**. This involves the addition of substances to the filtrate. Secretion can increase the rate at which substances are eliminated from the blood; because not only are the substance filtered out, more of them are added to the filtrate *after* filtration.

The last step in urine formation is **concentration and dilution**. This involves the selective reabsorption of water, and is where we decide whether to make concentrated urine or dilute urine. After this step, whatever remains in the renal tubule gets excreted as urine.

10.2   ANATOMY AND FUNCTION OF THE URINARY SYSTEM

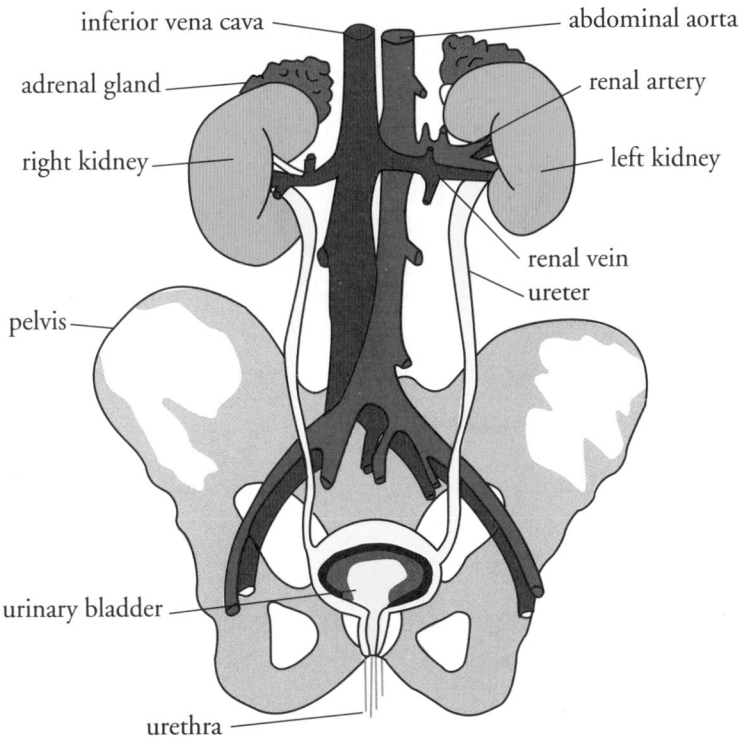

Figure 2   Gross Anatomy of the Urinary System

Each kidney is a filtration system that removes unwanted materials from the blood and passes them to the bladder for storage and eventual elimination. Blood enters the kidney from a large **renal artery**, which is a direct branch of the lower portion of the aorta (the abdominal aorta). Purified blood is returned to the circulatory system by the large **renal vein**, which empties into the inferior vena cava. Urine leaves each kidney in a **ureter**, which empties into the **urinary bladder**. The bladder is a muscular organ that stretches as it fills with urine. When it becomes full, signals of urgency are sent to the brain. There are two sphincters controlling release of urine from the bladder: an **internal sphincter** made of smooth (involuntary) muscle and an **external sphincter** made of skeletal (voluntary) muscle. The internal sphincter relaxes reflexively (and the bladder contracts) when the bladder wall is stretched. If a person decides the time is appropriate, they can relax the external sphincter, allowing urine to flow from the bladder into the urethra and out of the body.

A frontal section (separating front from back) through the kidney demonstrates its internal anatomy (Figure 3). The outer region is known as the **cortex**, and the inner region is the **medulla**. The **medullary pyramids** are pyramid-shaped striations within the medulla. This appearance is due to the presence of many **collecting ducts**. Urine empties from the collecting ducts and leaves the medulla at the tip of a pyramid, known as a **papilla** (plural: **papillae**). Each papilla empties into a space called a **calyx** (plural: **calyces**). The calyces converge to form the **renal pelvis**, which is a large space where urine collects. The renal pelvis empties into the ureter.

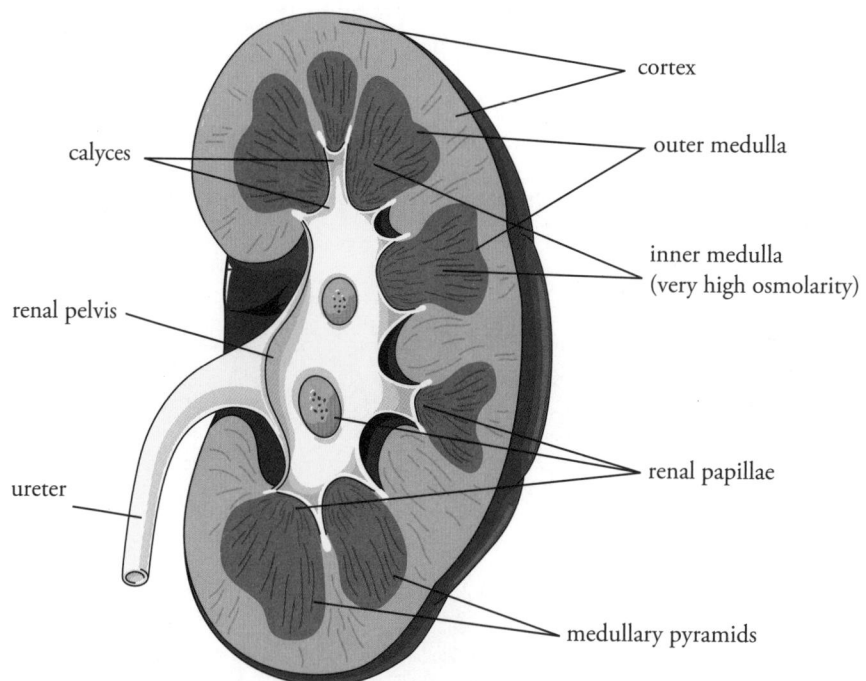

Figure 3   Internal Anatomy of the Kidney

Simplified Microscopic Anatomy and Function

The functional unit of the kidney is the **nephron**. It consists of two components:

1) a rounded region surrounding the capillaries where filtration takes place, known as the **capsule**, and

2) a coiled tube known as the **renal tubule** (Figure 4). The tubule receives filtrate from the capillaries in the capsule at one end and empties into a **collecting duct** at the other end. The collecting duct dumps urine into the renal pelvis.

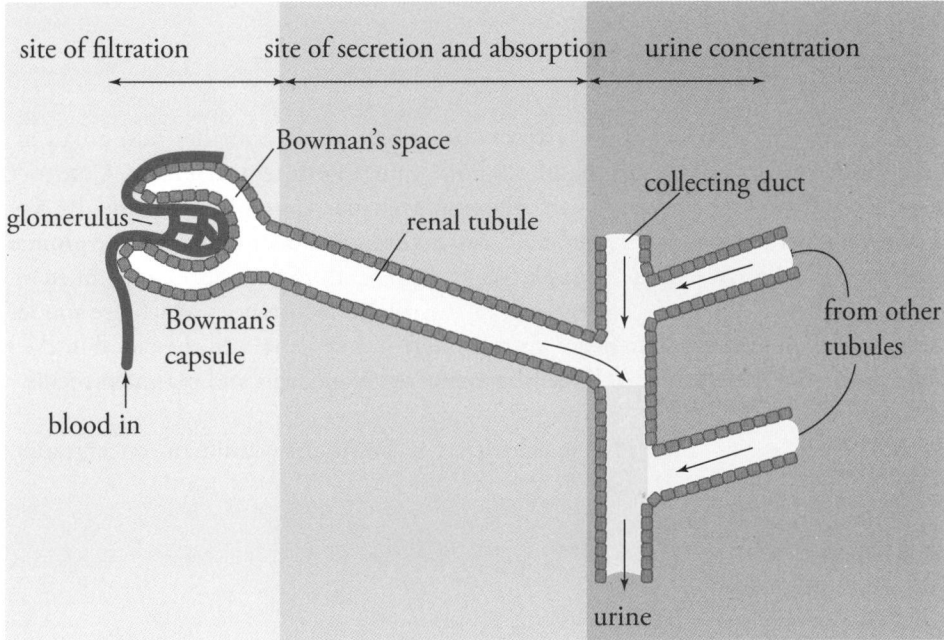

Figure 4 Simplified View of the Renal Tubule

Many blood vessels surround the nephron. They carry arterial blood toward the capillaries of the capsule for filtration, then surround the tubule to carry filtered blood and reabsorbed substances away from the tubule (Figure 5).

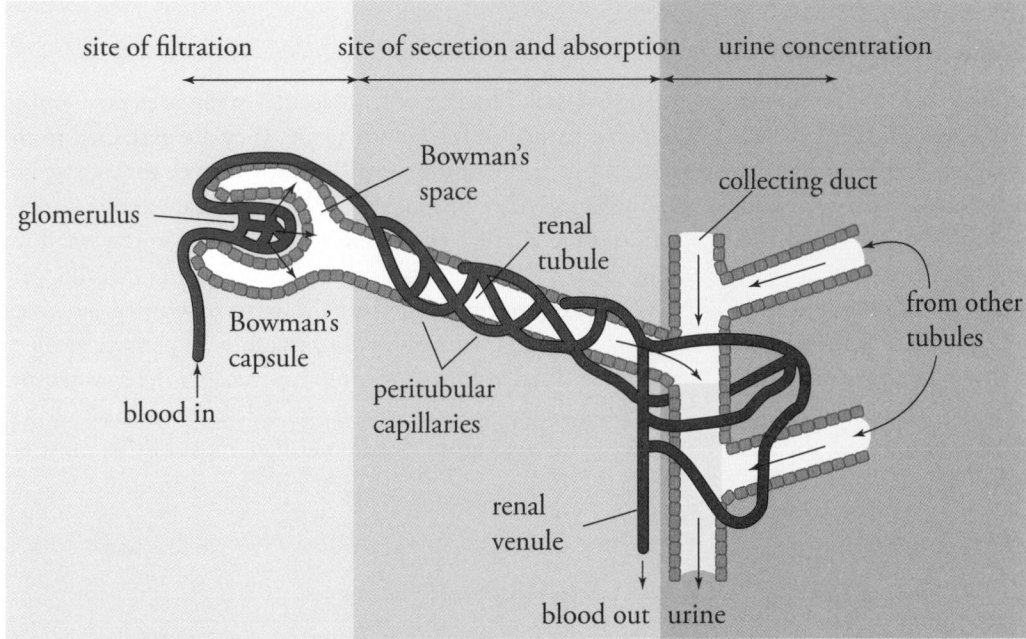

Figure 5 Simplified View of the Renal Tubule Plus Blood Vessels

Figures 4 and 5 depict most of the structures responsible for the three processes involved in urine formation. Let's go through the steps again, but this time in more detail.

Filtration

Blood from the renal artery flows into an **afferent arteriole**, which branches into a ball of capillaries known as the **glomerulus**. From there the blood flows into an **efferent arteriole**. Constriction of the efferent arteriole results in high pressure in the glomerulus, which causes fluid (essentially blood plasma) to leak out of the glomerular capillaries. The fluid passes through a filter known as the **glomerular basement membrane** and enters **Bowman's capsule**. As you can see from the figures, the lumen of Bowman's capsule is continuous with the lumen of the rest of the tubule. Substances which are too large to pass through the glomerular basement membrane are not filtered; they remain in the blood in the glomerular capillaries and drain into the efferent arteriole.[1] Examples are blood cells and plasma proteins.

- Which of the following are present in the filtrate in Bowman's capsule in concentrations similar to those seen in blood?[2]
    - I. Albumin (a plasma protein)
    - II. Glucose
    - III. Sodium

    - A) I and II only
    - B) II only
    - C) I and III only
    - D) II and III only

Selective Reabsorption

The filtrate in the tubule consists of water and small hydrophilic molecules such as sugars, amino acids, and urea. Some of these substances must be returned to the bloodstream. They are extracted from the tubule, often via active transport, and picked up by **peritubular capillaries**, which drain into venules that lead to the renal vein. For example, glucose is actively transported out of the filtrate and returned to the bloodstream by a cotransporter identical to the one involved in glucose absorption in the small intestine. A lot (most) of the reabsorption occurs in the part of the tubule nearest to Bowman's capsule, called the **proximal convoluted tubule** (**PCT**). All solute movement in the PCT is accompanied by water movement. As a result, a lot of water reabsorption occurs in this region also; roughly 70 percent of the volume of the filtrate is reabsorbed here. The amount (final volume) of urine we make is determined by much smaller fluxes taking place in the distal nephron. This makes sense if you think about it: about 5 percent of our circulating blood is continuously being filtered out of the glomerulus; most of this must be taken

---

[1] The glomerular basement membrane is actually a layer lining *each capillary* of the glomerulus.

[2] Item I: False. Plasma proteins are too large to pass through the filter. **Item II: True.** Glucose passes through into the filtrate and must be reclaimed during selective reabsorption. **Item III: True.** Sodium also passes into the filtrate. It will be reclaimed or left in the filtrate to be urinated out, depending on physiological needs. The answer is choice **D**.

back. Note that reabsorption in the PCT is selective in that it chooses what to reabsorb, but it is not overly regulated, since it reabsorbs "as much as possible," not a certain amount.

Selective reabsorption takes place further along the nephron as well, in the **distal convoluted tubule** (**DCT**). Reabsorption in this location is more regulated than in the PCT, usually via hormones (see Concentration and Dilution).

- Which one of the following best describes selective reabsorption?[3]
  - A) In normal individuals, only a small portion of the serum glucose is filtered into the tubule. Of this amount, about 50% is reabsorbed by the epithelial cells of the tubule.
  - B) In normal individuals, the concentration of glucose which is filtered into the tubule is identical to the serum [glucose]. Of the filtered glucose, 100% is reabsorbed by the epithelial cells of the tubule.
  - C) Epithelial cells of the renal tubule actively transport glucose into the filtrate.
  - D) Glucose is kept in the bloodstream by the filtering action of the glomerular basement membrane.

Secretion

Secretion is the movement of substances into the filtrate (usually via active transport) thus increasing the rate at which they are removed from the plasma. Not everything that needs to be removed from the blood gets filtered out at the glomerulus; secretion is a "back-up" method that ensures what needs to be eliminated, gets eliminated. As with reabsorption, secretion occurs all along the tubule; however unlike reabsorption, most secretion takes place in the DCT and the collecting duct. Note also that this is the primary way that many drugs and toxins are deposited in the urine.

Concentration and Dilution

Before filtrate is discarded into the ureter as urine, adjustments are made so that the urine volume and osmolarity are appropriate. This occurs in the last part of the tubule, known as the **distal nephron** (meaning the most distant part of the tubule), which includes the **DCT** and the **collecting duct**. It is controlled by two hormones: **ADH** and **aldosterone**.

1) *ADH:* When you are dehydrated, the *volume of fluid* in the bloodstream is low and the *solute concentration* in the blood is high. Therefore, you need to make small amounts of highly concentrated urine. Under these conditions (low blood volume and high blood osmolarity) **antidiuretic hormone** (**ADH** or **vasopressin**) is released by the posterior pituitary. This prevents **diuresis** (water loss in the urine) by increasing water reabsorption in the distal nephron.

---

[3] As stated in the section on filtration, glucose is small enough that all of it freely passes through the glomerular basement membrane (choice D is wrong), as are ions, amino acids, and water. However, even though glucose is filtered into the tubule, it must be reclaimed into the bloodstream or we would constantly lose glucose into the urine. 100 percent of filtered glucose is normally reclaimed (choice B is correct, and choice A is wrong), and in no instance is glucose ever transported *into* the filtrate (choice C is wrong). Note that in diabetes, the blood glucose level is so high that the cotransporters responsible for glucose reabsorption become saturated, and large amounts of glucose are left in the urine.

This is accomplished by making the distal nephron (primarily the collecting duct) permeable to water. (Without ADH, this region is impermeable to water. Note that this is the first time we have encountered a layer in the body which is impermeable to water.) As a result, water flows out of the filtrate into the tissue of the kidney, where it is picked up by the peritubular capillaries, and thus returned to the blood. [Why would water tend to flow out of the tubule into the tissue of the kidney?[4]] A drop in blood pressure can also trigger ADH release (renal regulation of blood pressure will be discussed later).

After drinking a lot of water, the plasma volume is too high, and a large volume of dilute urine is necessary. In this case, no ADH is secreted. The result is that the collecting duct is not permeable to water. This means that any water in the filtrate remains in the tubule and is lost in the urine, or *diuresed*. The reason alcohol causes people to diurese is that it inhibits ADH secretion by the posterior pituitary.

2) *Aldosterone:* When the blood *pressure* is low, **aldosterone** is released by the adrenal cortex. It causes increased reabsorption of Na^+ by the distal nephron (distal convoluted tubule and the cortical region of the collecting duct). The result is increased plasma osmolarity, which leads to increased thirst and water retention, which raises the blood pressure. (The fact that increased serum $[Na^+]$ increases blood pressure is the reason people with high blood pressure have to avoid salty foods.) When the blood pressure is high, aldosterone is not released. As a result, sodium is lost in the urine. Plasma osmolarity (and eventually blood pressure) falls. Other triggers for the release of aldosterone are low blood osmolarity, low blood volume, and **angiotensin II** (discussed below).

ADH and aldosterone work together to increase blood pressure. First, aldosterone causes sodium reabsorption, which results in increased plasma osmolarity. This causes ADH to be secreted, which results in increased water reabsorption and thus increased plasma volume.

Actual Microscopic Anatomy and Function

Up to this point we have presented a conceptual outline of kidney function, and we have referred to a simplified nephron, depicted as a straight tube. But the nephron is more complex than that (Figure 6). Bowman's capsule empties into the first part of the tubule, known as the proximal convoluted tubule (PCT). Again, *proximal* means "near" (near the glomerulus), and *convoluted* just means "twisting and turning." Both Bowman's capsule and the PCT are located in the **renal cortex**, the outer layer of the kidney. The PCT empties into the next region of the nephron, known as the **loop of Henle**. This is a long loop that dips down into the **renal medulla**, the inner part of the kidney. The part that heads into the medulla is called the **descending limb of the loop of Henle**, and the part that heads back out toward the cortex is the **ascending limb**. The descending limb is thin walled, but part of the ascending limb is thin and the other part is thick. These are referred to simply as the *thin ascending limb* and the *thick ascending limb* of the loop of Henle. [What might be the structural difference between a thick portion of the tubule and a thin portion?[5]] As we continue down the tubule, the loop of Henle becomes the distal

---

[4] Because the renal medulla has a very high osmolarity, which causes water to exit the tubule by osmosis. This will be discussed later in more detail.

[5] The two portions are composed of different types of epithelial cells. Thin portions of the tubule are composed of *squamous* (flat) epithelial cells, which are not very metabolically active. Thick portions are composed of *cuboidal* epithelial cells, which are large thick cells busily performing active transport.

convoluted tubule (DCT). The DCT dumps into a **collecting duct**. Many collecting ducts merge to form larger tributaries which empty into renal calyces. Figure 6 shows the actual anatomy and function of the nephron. You should familiarize yourself with the information in the figure, but this level of detail is too advanced to warrant extensive discussion. The conceptual material presented above is more typical of MCAT questions.

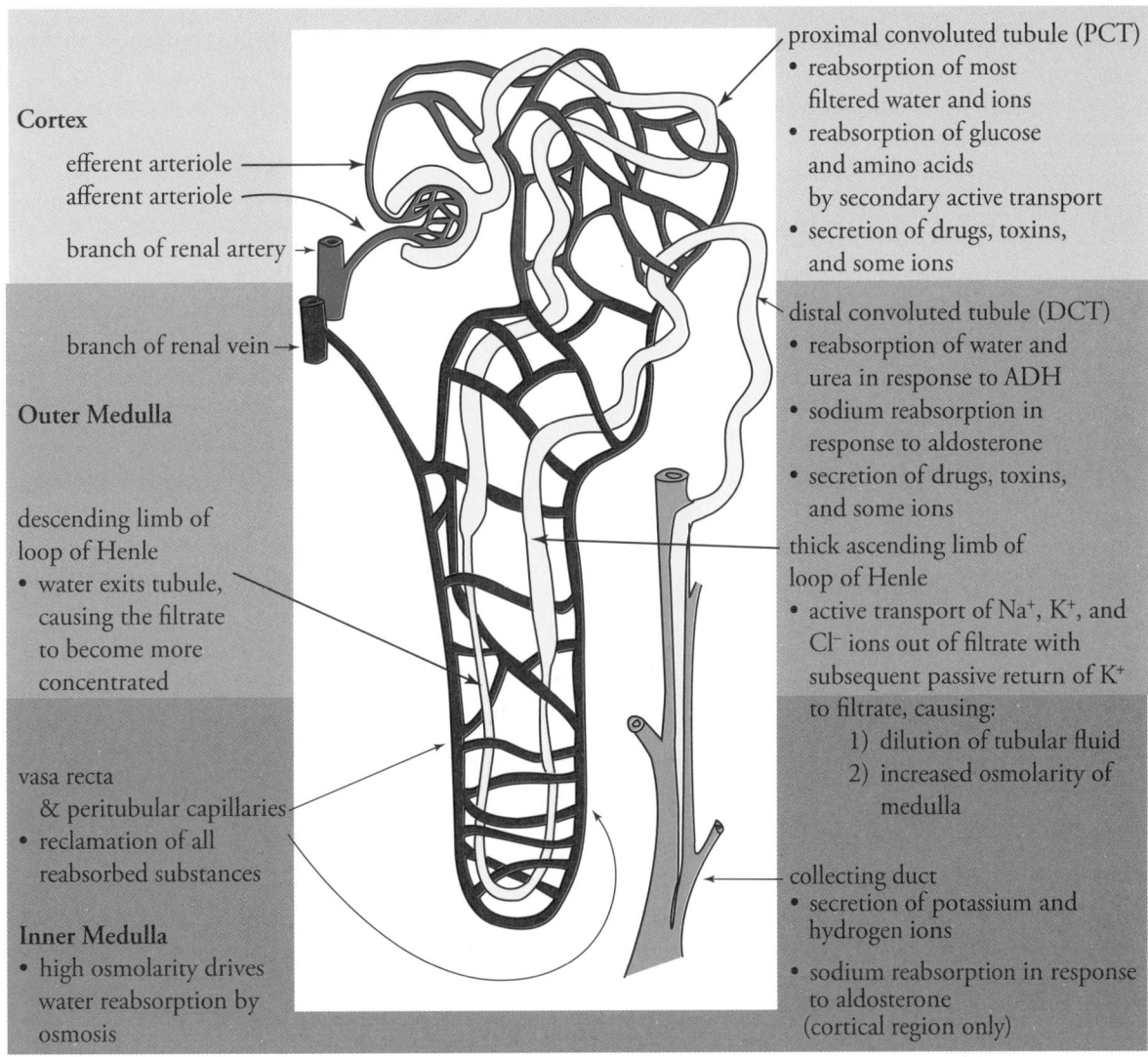

Figure 6 Regions and Functions of the Nephron

The Loop of Henle Is a Countercurrent Multiplier

Although we do not intend to go into too much detail on renal physiology, one concept is important to mention: the notion of a **countercurrent multiplier**. The significance of the loop of Henle is that the ascending and descending limbs go in opposite directions and have different permeabilities. The descending limb is permeable to water, but not to ions. Hence, water exits the descending limb, flowing into the high-osmolarity medullary interstitium.[6] Thus, the filtrate becomes concentrated. The thin ascending

---

[6]   *Interstitium* is a generic word for "tissue." It literally means "an in-between region"; in this case it means tissue in-between renal tubules.

limb is *not* permeable to water, but passively loses ions from the high-osmolarity filtrate into the renal medullary interstitium. Additionally, the thick ascending limb actively transports salt out of the filtrate into the medullary interstitium, and the medullary interstitium becomes *very* salty. This is important because the medulla will suck water out of the collecting duct by osmosis whenever the collecting duct is permeable to water (e.g., in the presence of ADH).

Don't spend too much time pondering over this now (you will in medical school). Just remember that *the loop of Henle is a countercurrent multiplier that makes the medulla very salty, and that this facilitates water reabsorption from the collecting duct. This is how the kidney is capable of making urine with a much higher osmolarity than plasma.*

The Vasa Recta Are Countercurrent Exchangers

Like the loop of Henle, the **vasa recta** form a loop that helps to maintain the high concentration of salt in the medulla. In short, the ascending portions of the vasa recta are near the descending limb of the loop of Henle and thus carry off the water that leaves the descending limb. Also, the vasa recta are branches of efferent arterioles. The vasa recta are "eager" to reabsorb water because the blood they contain is like coffee grinds which have been drained. The important thing to remember is that the vasa recta return to the bloodstream any water that is reabsorbed from the filtrate. Because the blood in the vasa recta moves in the opposite direction of the filtrate in the nephron, the vasa recta perform countercurrent exchange. Other biological systems use countercurrent exchange because it is very efficient. For example, oxygen and blood flow in opposite directions in fish gills. This mechanism increases the efficiency of the respiration process by maintaining the concentration gradient and preventing the oxygen levels from reaching an equilibrium.

10.3 RENAL REGULATION OF BLOOD PRESSURE AND pH

Since the **glomerular filtration rate** (**GFR**) depends directly on pressure, the kidney has built-in mechanisms to help regulate systemic and local (glomerular) blood pressure. The **juxtaglomerular apparatus** (**JGA**) is a specialized contact point between the afferent arteriole and the distal tubule. At this contact point, the cells in the afferent arteriole are called **juxtaglomerular** (**JG**) **cells**, and those in the distal tubule are known as the **macula densa**. The JG cells are baroreceptors that monitor systemic blood pressure. When there is a decrease in blood pressure, the JG cells secrete an enzyme called **renin** into the bloodstream. Renin catalyzes the conversion of **angiotensinogen** (a plasma protein made by the liver) into **angiotensin I,** which is further converted to **angiotensin II** by **angiotensin-converting enzyme** (**ACE**) in the lungs. Angiotensin II is a powerful vasoconstrictor that immediately raises the blood pressure. It also stimulates the release of aldosterone, which (as discussed previously) helps raise the blood pressure by increasing sodium (and, indirectly, water) retention.

The cells of the macula densa are chemoreceptors, and monitor filtrate osmolarity in the distal tubule. When filtrate osmolarity decreases (indicating a reduced filtration rate), the cells of the macula densa stimulate the JG cells to release renin. The macula densa also causes a direct dilation of the afferent arteriole, increasing blood flow to (and thus blood pressure and filtration rate in) the glomerulus.

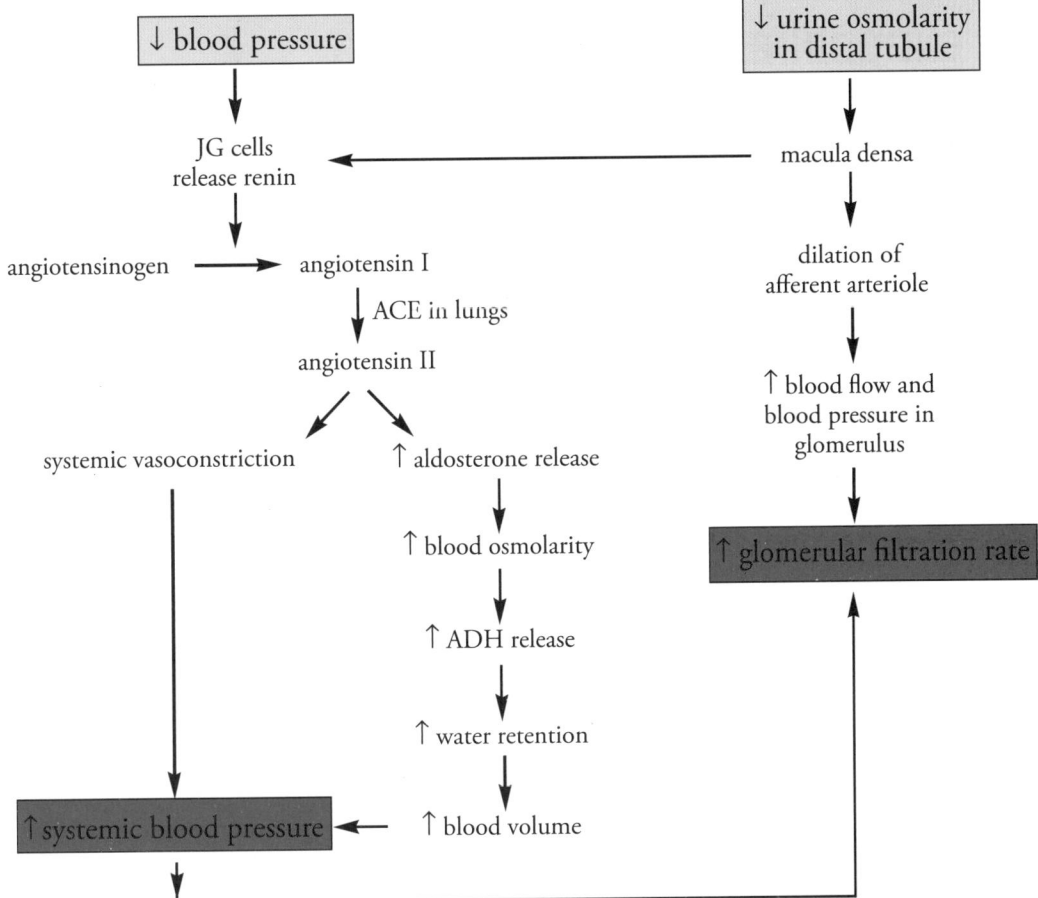

Figure 7 Regulation of Blood Pressure and GFR by the Kidney

Renal Regulation of pH

The kidney is essential for maintenance of constant blood pH. It accomplishes this by a very simple and direct mechanism: when the plasma pH is too high, HCO_3^- is excreted in the urine; when the plasma pH is too low, H^+ is excreted. We will not go into the details. Just be aware that the enzyme **carbonic anhydrase** is involved. It is found in epithelial cells throughout the nephron, except the flat (squamous) cells of the thin parts of the loop of Henle. Carbonic anhydrase catalyzes the conversion of CO_2 into carbonic acid (H_2CO_3), which dissociates into bicarbonate plus a proton. Once this reaction has taken place, the kidney can reabsorb or secrete bicarbonate or protons as needed. (Recall that carbonic anhydrase was discussed in Chapter 9, as it is found in RBCs.) Generally speaking, protons are secreted and bicarbonate is reabsorbed; the amounts are adjusted to adjust pH.

Renal pH adjustments are slow, requiring several days to return plasma pH to normal after a disturbance. The other organ important for pH regulation is the lung. By exhaling excess CO_2, the lung removes an acid (H_2CO_3) from the blood, thus raising the pH. Thus, *hyperventilation* (deep, rapid breathing) raises plasma pH. Respiratory adjustments to the plasma pH are rapid, taking effect in just minutes.

10.4 ENDOCRINE ROLE OF THE KIDNEY

Several hormones affect the kidney, and the kidney makes one as well. All are peptides except aldosterone, which is a steroid. The one made by the kidney is **erythropoietin** (**EPO**). You should know the basic role and source of each of the following hormones. You're unlikely to see very detailed memory-oriented questions on the MCAT, but as a doctor you will know this stuff like the back of your hand.

Table 1   Hormones Affecting or Secreted by Kidney

Hormone	Source	Target and effect
aldosterone	adrenal cortex	Causes sodium reabsorption and potassium secretion by increasing the synthesis of basolateral Na^+/K^+ ATPases in the distal nephron. End result: increased serum $[Na^+]$, increased blood volume (through the action of ADH), and thus increased blood pressure.
ADH	posterior pituitary	ADH is secreted when plasma volume is too low, blood pressure is too low, or plasma osmolarity is too high. It causes water reabsorption by causing epithelial cells of the distal nephron to become permeable to water, which allows water to flow out of the filtrate into the medullary interstitium. Vasa recta return this water to the bloodstream. The result is more concentrated urine, and more diluted blood. ADH and aldosterone work together to increase blood pressure: first, aldosterone causes sodium reabsorption, which results in increased plasma osmolarity; this causes ADH to be secreted, which results in increased water reabsorption and thus increased plasma volume.
calcitonin	C cells	C cells are located in the thyroid gland but do not secrete thyroid hormone. They secrete calcitonin when the serum $[Ca^{2+}]$ is too high. Calcitonin causes $[Ca^{2+}]$ to be removed from the blood by 1) deposition in bone, 2) reduced absorption by the gut, and 3) excretion in urine.
parathyroid hormone	parathyroid	There are four parathyroid glands, found embedded in the thyroid gland. The function of parathormone (PTH) is opposite that of calcitonin.
EPO	kidney	Erythropoietin (EPO) causes increased synthesis of red blood cells in the bone marrow. It is released when blood oxygen content falls.

10.5 OVERVIEW OF THE DIGESTIVE SYSTEM

Food contains molecules that are substrates in **catabolic reactions** (reactions that break down molecules to supply energy) and **anabolic reactions** (synthesis of macromolecules). Digestion is the breakdown of polymers (polypeptides, fats, starch) into their building blocks. This breakdown is accomplished by **enzymatic hydrolysis** (Figure 8). Food also contains vitamins, which are not substrates, but rather serve a catalytic role as enzyme cofactors or prosthetic groups. Digestion and absorption of foodstuffs is the primary function of the digestive system. A secondary function, which we will touch on only briefly, is protection from disease.

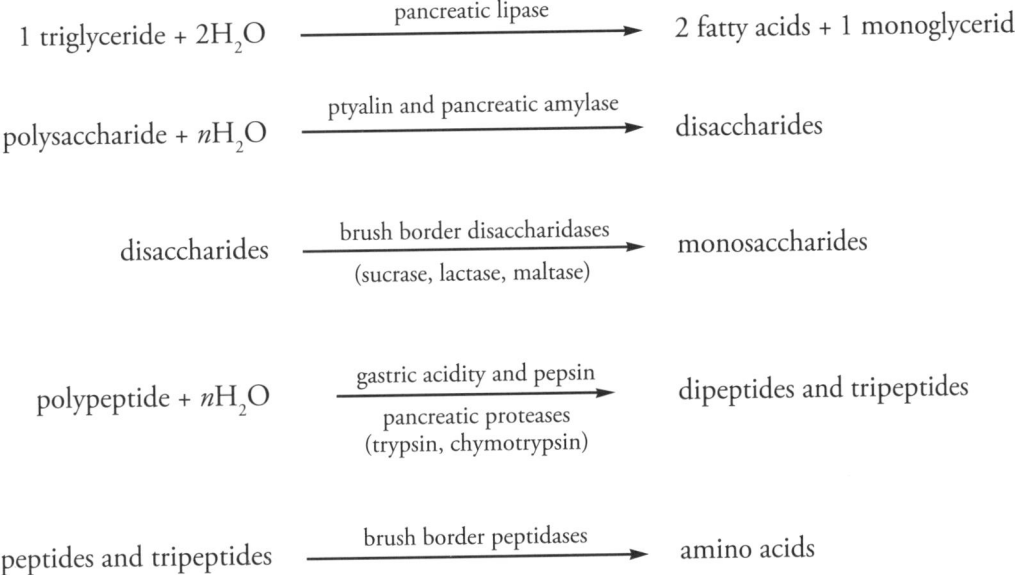

Figure 8   Enzymatic Hydrolysis of Biological Macromolecules

Digestion is accomplished along the **gastrointestinal (GI) tract**, also known as the **digestive tract**, the **alimentary canal**, or simply the **gut**. The GI tract is a long, muscular tube extending from the mouth to the anus. This tube is derived from the cavity produced by **gastrulation** during embryogenesis; the anus is derived from the **blastopore** (discussed in Chapter 13). The inside of the gut is the **GI lumen**. The lumen is continuous with the space outside the body. (Food could go from the plate into the lumen and from there into the toilet bowl without ever contacting the bloodstream, the muscles, the bones, etc.) The GI lumen is a compartment where the usable components of foodstuffs are extracted, while wastes are left to be excreted as feces. The entire GI tract is composed of specific tissue layers which surround the lumen (Figure 9).

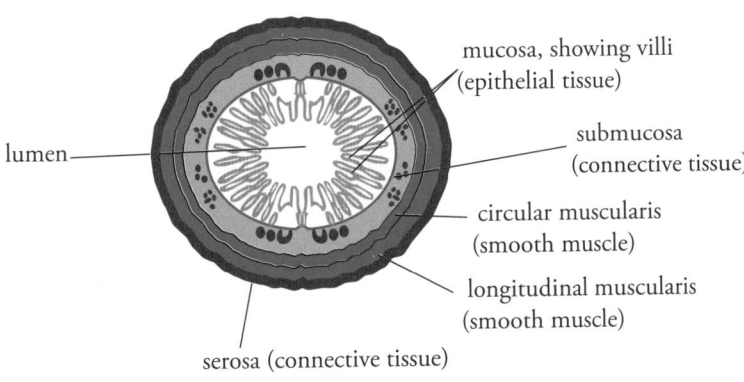

Figure 9   Layers of the GI Tract

GI Epithelium

Because it is exposed to substances from the outside world, the innermost lining of the lumen is composed of the same type of cells that line the outer surface of the body and the inner surface of the respiratory tract: epithelial cells. By definition, epithelial cells are attached to a **basement membrane**.[7] The surface of the epithelial cell which faces into the lumen is the **apical surface** (*apex* means "top"; *apical* is the adjective). In the small intestine, the apical surfaces of these cells have outward folds of their plasma membrane called **microvilli** to increase their surface area. The apical surface is separated from the remainder of the cell surface by **tight junctions**, which are bands running all the way around the sides of epithelial cells, creating a barrier that separates body fluids from the extracellular environment (see Chapter 6). The sides and bottom of an epithelial cell form the surface opposite the lumen, known as the **basolateral** surface (Figure 10). As discussed below, specialized epithelial cells are responsible for most of the secretory activity of the GI tract.

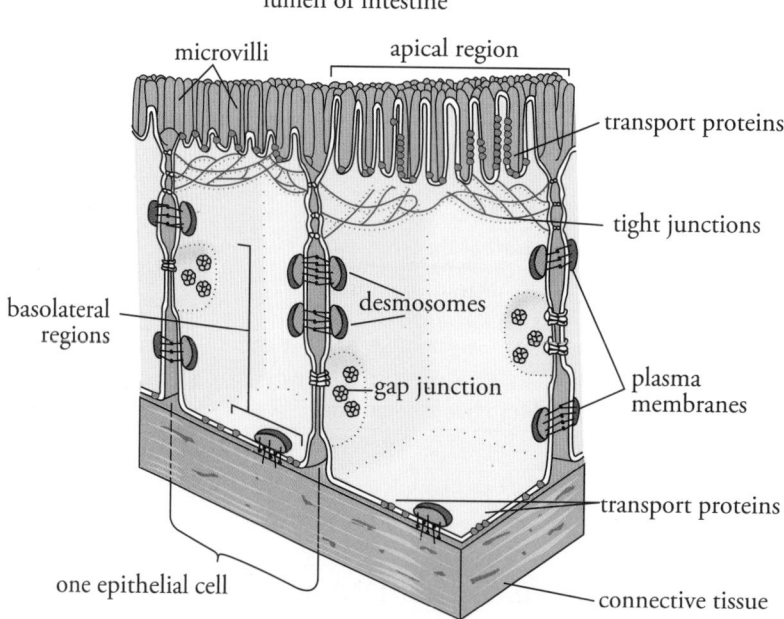

Figure 10   Epithelial Cells

GI Smooth Muscle

GI muscle is known as **smooth muscle** because of its smooth microscopic appearance. This contrasts with **striated muscle**, which appears striped under magnification. Skeletal (voluntary) muscle and cardiac (heart) muscle are striated. (The differences between smooth, skeletal, and cardiac muscle cells will be covered in Chapter 11.) Note in Figure 9 that there are two layers of smooth muscle lining the gut. The **longitudinal layer** runs along the gut lengthwise, while the **circular layer** encircles it.

GI motility refers to the rhythmic contraction of GI smooth muscle. It is determined by a complex interplay between five factors:

1)   Like cardiac muscle, GI smooth muscle exhibits *automaticity*. In other words, it contracts periodically without external stimulation, due to spontaneous depolarization.

---

[7]   *Epi-* means "upon," and *-thelial* refers to the bumpy microscopic appearance of the basement membrane (it means "nippley").

2) Like cardiac muscle, GI smooth muscle is a **functional syncytium**, meaning that when one cell has an action potential and contracts, the impulse spreads to neighboring cells.

3) The GI tract contains its own massive nervous system, known as the **enteric nervous system**. The enteric nervous system plays a major role in controlling GI motility.

4) GI motility may be increased or decreased by hormonal input.

5) The parasympathetic nervous system stimulates motility and causes sphincters to relax (allowing the passage of food through the gut), while sympathetic stimulation does the opposite.

GI motility serves two purposes: mixing of food and movement of food down the gut. Mixing is accomplished by disordered contractions of GI smooth muscle, which result in churning motions. Movement of food down the GI tract is accomplished by an orderly form of contraction known as **peristalsis** (Figure 11). During peristalsis, contraction of circular smooth muscle at point A prevents food located at point B from moving backward. Then longitudinal muscles at point B contract, with the result being shortening of the gut so that it is pulled up over the food like a sock. As a result, the food moves toward point C. Then circular smooth muscles at point B contract to prevent the food from moving backward, and longitudinal muscles at point C contract, with the result being movement of food past point C, and so on. A ball of food moving through the GI tract is called a **bolus**.

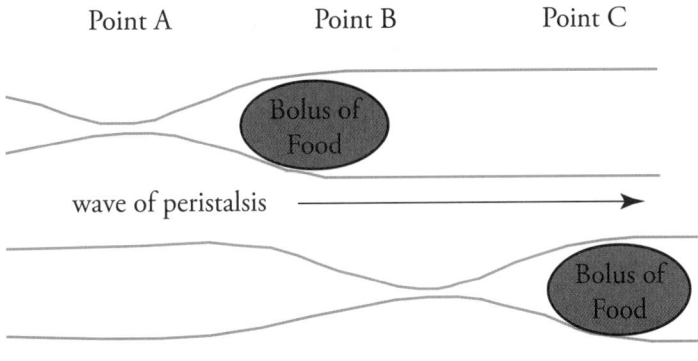

Figure 11   Peristalsis

Enteric Nervous System

The enteric nervous system is the branch of the **autonomic nervous system** that helps to control digestion via innervation of the gastrointestinal tract, pancreas, and gall bladder. Specifically, it helps to regulate local blood flow, gut movements, and the exchange of fluid from the gut to and from its lumen. This branch can operate independently of the other two branches of the autonomic nervous system, but both of those branches can modulate the activity of the enteric nervous system. [What are the two main branches of the autonomic nervous system? What effects would they have on the enteric branch?[8]]

The enteric nervous system is made up of two networks of neurons: the **myenteric plexus** and the **submucosal plexus**. The myenteric plexus is found between the circular and longitudinal muscle layers and helps primarily to regulate gut motility. The submucosal plexus is found in the submucosa and helps to regulate enzyme secretion, gut blood flow, and ion/water balance in the lumen. In areas where these functions are minimal (e.g., the esophagus or anus), the submucosal plexus is sparse.

---

[8]   The two main branches of the autonomic nervous system are the sympathetic nervous system (fight or flight) and parasympathetic nervous system (rest and digest). The sympathetic nervous system generally inhibits digestive processes and so would inhibit the enteric branch, whereas the parasympathetic nervous system stimulates the enteric branch and thus stimulates digestion.

GI Secretions

Generally speaking, GI secretion (release of enzymes, acid, bile, etc.) is stimulated by food in the gut and by the parasympathetic nervous system and is inhibited by sympathetic stimulation. There are two types of secretion: **endocrine** and **exocrine**. [What's the difference?[9]] Exocrine glands are composed of specialized epithelial cells, organized into sacs called **acini** (singular: **acinus**). Acinar cells secrete products which pass into ducts. It is important to keep the contrast between endocrine and exocrine in mind. Figure 12 shows the microscopic structure of an exocrine gland.

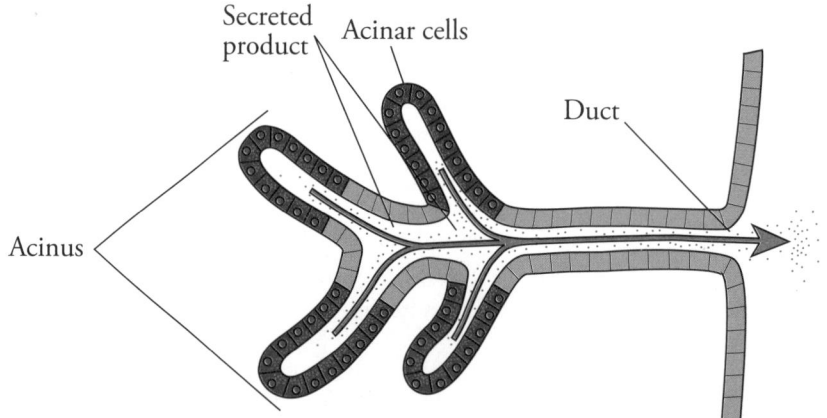

Figure 12   Exocrine Gland Structure

Most exocrine secretion in the GI tract is performed by exocrine glands within special digestive organs. These glands release enzymes into ducts (see Figure 12) that ultimately empty into the GI lumen. The digestive organs primarily involved in exocrine secretion include the liver, gallbladder, and pancreas. However, some exocrine secretion is performed by specialized individual epithelial cells in the wall of the gut itself. These cells are miniature exocrine glands, releasing secretions directly into the gut lumen. Important examples are the cells of the **gastric glands** in the stomach and specialized mucus-secreting cells called **goblet cells**. The gastric glands secrete acid and pepsinogen (a protease zymogen discussed below). Goblet cells are found along the entire GI tract. Mucus is a slimy liquid which protects and lubricates the gut; any body surface covered with mucus is known as a **mucus membrane**. One last secretion must be mentioned: water. Whenever a meal is to be digested it must be dissolved in water. Hence, each day, gallons of water are secreted into the GI lumen. Most of it is reabsorbed in the small intestine, and the colon is responsible for reclaiming whatever water is left.

Endocrine secretion is also accomplished by both specialized organs (the pancreas) and by cells in the wall of the gut. Remember that endocrine secretions (hormones) do not empty into ducts but instead are picked up by nearby capillaries. In other words, you should realize that when the same organ has both endocrine and exocrine activities, these functions are accomplished by separate cells, which are usually grouped in such a way as to be microscopically distinguishable. For example, the two principal cell types in the pancreas are: 1) exocrine cells, referred to simply as **pancreatic acinar cells**, which are organized into acini that drain into ducts, and 2) endocrine cells clumped together in groups known as **islets of Langerhans**, which are supplied with capillaries.

---

[9]   *Exocrine* glands secrete their products (digestive enzymes, etc.) into *ducts* that drain into the GI lumen. *Endocrine* glands are ductless glands; their secretions (hormones) are picked up by capillaries and thus enter the bloodstream.

10.6   THE GASTROINTESTINAL TRACT

Although the GI tract is a continuous tube, each portion is seen as a separate organ: mouth, pharynx, esophagus, etc. Here we will summarize the major structures and functions of each GI organ. The liver, gallbladder, and pancreas, known as **accessory organs**, are covered in Section 10.7. Section 10.8 details the absorptive process.

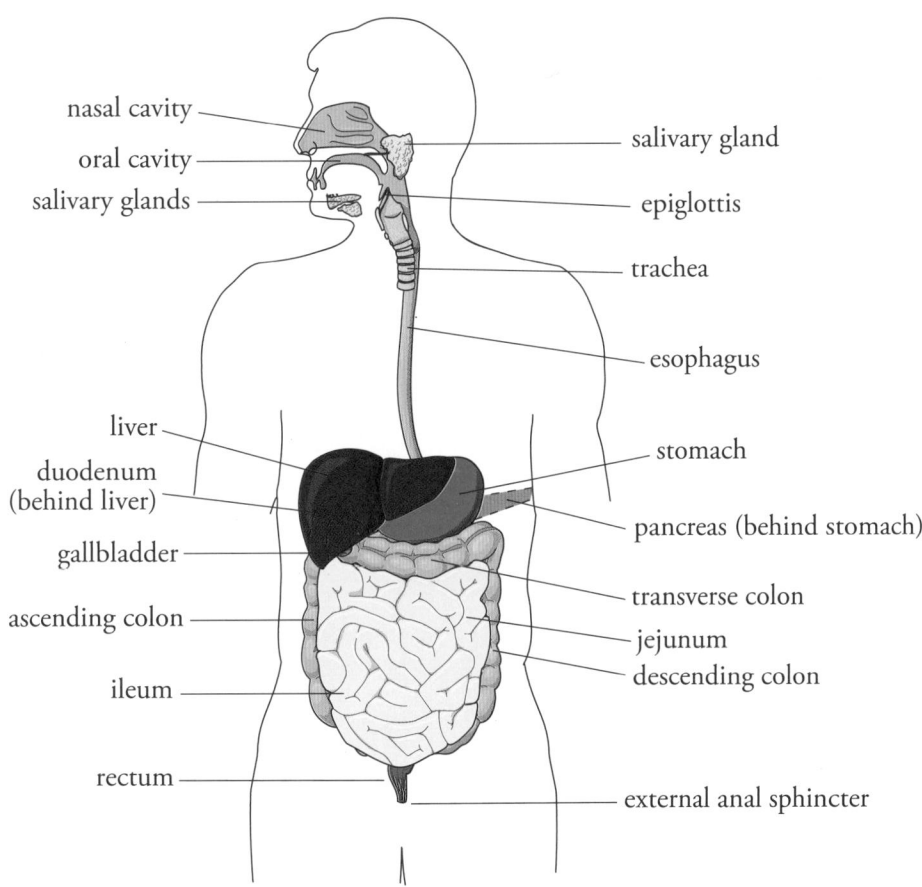

Figure 13   Organs of the Digestive System

Mouth

The mouth has three roles in the digestion of foodstuffs:

1) Fragmentation
2) Lubrication
3) Some enzymatic digestion

Fragmentation is accomplished by **mastication** (**chewing**). The **incisors** (front teeth) are for cutting, the **cuspids** (canine teeth) are for tearing, and the **molars** are for grinding.

Lubrication and some digestion are accomplished by **saliva**, a viscous fluid secreted by salivary glands. Saliva contains **salivary amylase (ptyalin)**, which hydrolyzes starch, breaking it into fragments. The smallest fragment yielded by salivary amylase is the disaccharide; digestion to monosaccharides occurs only at the intestinal brush border (discussed below). Saliva also contains a small amount of **lingual lipase** for fat digestion. No digestion of proteins occurs in the mouth. Lastly, saliva also contains **lysozyme**, which attacks _____.[10] Therefore, the mouth also participates in innate immunity.

The muscles of the mouth and the muscular tongue are important for compacting chewed food into a smooth lump which can be swallowed, a **bolus**.

10.6

- When carbohydrates are broken down by ptyalin, can they be absorbed in the mouth?[11]

Pharynx and Esophagus

The **pharynx** is what we commonly call the throat. [Key trivia: The floppy thing that hangs down at the back of the throat is called the _____.[12]] The pharynx contains the openings to two tubes: the **trachea** and the **esophagus**. The trachea is a cartilage-lined tube at the front of the neck which conveys air to and from the lungs. The esophagus is a muscular tube behind the trachea which conveys food and drink from the pharynx to the stomach. During swallowing, solids and liquids are excluded from the trachea by a flat cartilaginous flap, the **epiglottis**. A bolus of food passes through the pharynx, over the epiglottis, and into the esophagus, where it is conveyed to the stomach by peristalsis. Two muscular rings regulate movement of food through the esophagus. The **upper esophageal sphincter** is near the top of the esophagus, and the **lower esophageal sphincter** (also known as the **cardiac sphincter** since it is found near the heart) is at the end of the esophagus, at the entrance to the stomach. [Does the lower esophageal sphincter regulate movement of substances into or out of the esophagus?[13]]

Stomach

The stomach is a large hollow muscular organ which serves three purposes: partial digestion of food, regulated release of food into the small intestine, and destruction of microorganisms. The following list highlights some of the attributes and secretions that allow the stomach to accomplish these goals. **Gastric** is an adjective meaning "related to the stomach."

---

[10] bacterial cell walls. Remember, lytic phages make lysozyme too.

[11] No. Sugars are not broken down into monosaccharides until they reach the intestinal brush border. Only monosaccharides can be absorbed into the body. Absorption requires special transmembrane transporters located on the intestinal brush border; each transporter is specific for a particular monosaccharide.

[12] uvula

[13] It is there to prevent reflux from the stomach into the esophagus. There is no reason to regulate movement of substances out of the esophagus into the stomach, since nothing is stored in the esophagus; it's just a conduit.

Acidity

Gastric pH is about 2, due to the secretion of HCl by parietal cells, located in the gastric mucosa. Effects of low gastric pH include: 1) destruction of microorganisms, 2) acid-catalyzed hydrolysis of many dietary proteins, and 3) conversion of pepsinogen to pepsin.

Pepsin

This is an enzyme secreted by **chief cells** in the stomach wall. It catalyzes proteolysis (protein breakdown). Pepsin is secreted as **pepsinogen**, which is an inactive precursor that must be converted to the active form (pepsin). As noted above, this conversion is catalyzed by gastric acidity. The secretion of an inactive precursor is a common theme in the GI tract; the inactive form is known as a **zymogen**. Most zymogens are activated by proteolysis (cleavage of the protein at a specific site that activates it). Pepsinogen is unique because it is activated by _____ instead of _____.[14]

Motility

The stomach constantly churns food. Like chewing, this breaks up food particles so that they are exposed to gastric acidity and enzymes. Food mixed with gastric secretions is known as **chyme**.

Sphincters

The lower esophageal sphincter prevents reflux of chyme into the esophagus. The **pyloric sphincter** prevents the passage of food from the stomach into the duodenum. Opening of the pyloric sphincter (stomach emptying) is inhibited when the small intestine already has a large load of chyme. More specifically, stretching or excess acidity in the duodenum inhibits further stomach emptying, by causing the pyloric sphincter to contract. This effect is mediated both by nerves connecting the duodenum and stomach, and by hormones. The main hormone responsible is **cholecystokinin**, secreted by epithelial cells in the wall of the duodenum. [Is this hormone secreted into the lumen of the duodenum or into the lumen of the stomach?[15]]

Gastrin

This is a hormone secreted by cells in the stomach wall known as **G cells**. It stimulates acid and pepsin secretion and gastric motility. Gastrin secretion is stimulated by food in the stomach and by parasympathetic stimulation. The small molecule **histamine** (which is secreted in response both to stomach stretching and to gastrin) binds to parietal cells to stimulate acid release. The ulcer-healing drugs cimetidine (Tagamet) and ranitidine (Zantac) function by blocking the binding of histamine to its receptor (the "H_2 receptor") on parietal cells. This results in less gastric acidity, which allows ulcers to heal.

Small Intestine

Food leaving the stomach enters the small intestine, a tube which is about an inch wide and 10 feet long. (After death, it measures about 25 feet due to relaxation of longitudinal muscles.) The small intestine is divided into three segments: the **duodenum**, **jejunum**, and **ileum**. Digestion begins in the mouth

---

[14] Pepsinogen is unusual in that it is activated to pepsin by acidic proteolysis (autocleavage) instead of proteolytic cleavage by another enzyme.

[15] Neither! It's a hormone; by definition, it is secreted into the bloodstream.

(ptyalin), continues in the stomach, and is completed in the duodenum and jejunum. Absorption begins in the duodenum and continues throughout the small intestine. The anatomy and function of the small intestine are described below. In Section 10.8 we will detail the specific mechanisms of digestion and absorption of carbohydrates, proteins, and fats.

Surface Area

The key feature that allows the small intestine to accomplish absorption is its large surface area; this results from 1) length, 2) villi, and 3) microvilli. **Villi** (singular: **villus**) are macroscopic (multicellular) projections in the wall of the small intestine. **Microvilli** are microscopic foldings of the cell membranes of individual intestinal epithelial cells. The lumenal surface of the small intestine is known as the **brush border** due to the brush-like appearance of microvilli.

The Intestinal Villus

The villus is a finger-like projection of the wall of the gut into the lumen. It has three very important structures:

1)   The villus contains capillaries, which absorb dietary monosaccharides and amino acids. The capillaries merge to form veins, which merge to form the large **hepatic portal vein**, which transports blood containing amino acid and carbohydrate nutrients from the gut to the liver.

2)   The villus also contains small lymphatic vessels called **lacteals**, which absorb dietary fats. The lacteals merge to form large lymphatic vessels, which transport dietary fats to the thoracic duct, which empties into the bloodstream.

3)   **Peyer's patches** are part of the immune system. They are collections of lymphocytes dotting the villi that monitor GI contents and thus confer immunity to gut pathogens and toxins.

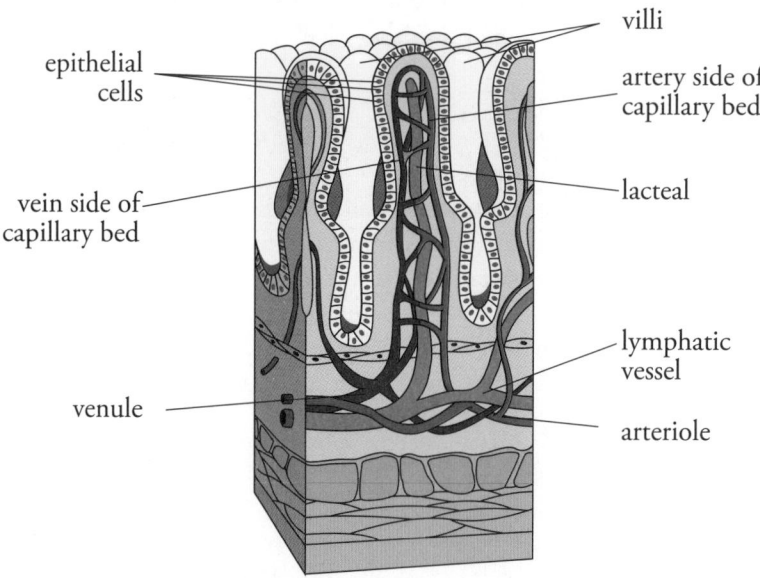

Figure 14   An Intestinal Villus

Bile and Pancreatic Secretions in the Duodenum

A key anatomical feature of the duodenum is that two ducts empty into it (Figure 15). One is the **pancreatic duct**, which delivers the exocrine secretions of the pancreas (digestive enzymes and bicarbonate). The other is the **common bile duct**, which delivers **bile**. This is a green fluid containing **bile acids**, which are made from cholesterol in the liver and are normally absorbed and recycled. Bile is stored in the **gallbladder** until it is needed. Bile has two functions: it is a vehicle for the disposal (excretion) of waste products by the liver, and it is essential for the digestion of fats, as discussed below. The bile duct and the pancreatic duct empty into the duodenum via the same orifice, known as the **sphincter of Oddi** (Figure 15).

- If a gallstone became lodged in the sphincter of Oddi, what would happen?[16]
- Bile acids secreted into the duodenum are normally reabsorbed in the ileum. Bile acid sequestrants are drugs which bind bile acids in the small intestine, causing them to remain in the GI lumen and eventually be excreted as feces. Each of the following is most likely true about such drugs EXCEPT that:[17]
  - A) they are stable at low pH levels.
  - B) they result in a decrease in the level of cholesterol in the bloodstream.
  - C) it would be reasonable to be concerned that they might disrupt fat absorption.
  - D) they would be administered intravenously (injected into a vein).

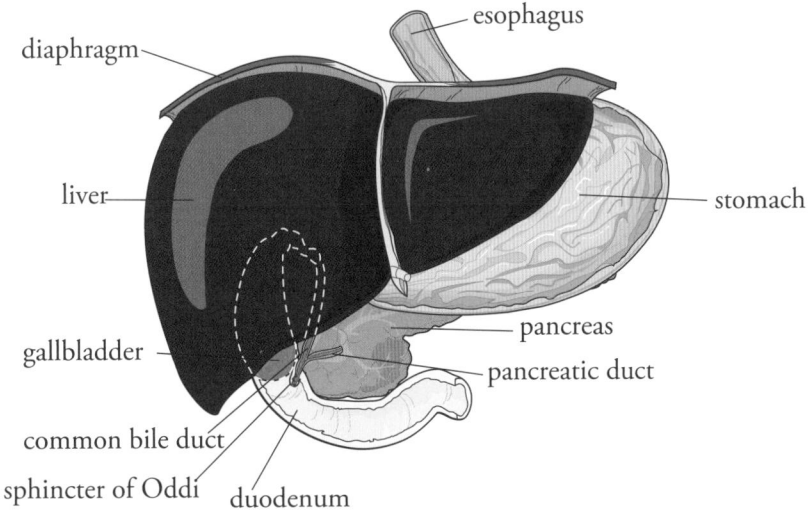

Figure 15   Anatomy around the Duodenum

---

[16]   Both the bile and the pancreatic ducts would be blocked, and digestion would be severely impaired (especially fat digestion, but also protein and carbohydrate digestion due to failure of pancreatic zymogens and amylase to reach the intestinal lumen).

[17]   Since the drugs must pass through the stomach, they should be stable at low pH levels (choice A is true and can be eliminated). The text states that bile acids are made from cholesterol and normally recycled. It is reasonable to assume that blocking this recycling would require the conversion of more cholesterol into bile acids, which would lower the serum cholesterol level. This is, in fact, what bile acid sequestrants are used for (choice B is true and can be eliminated). It would be reasonable to be concerned about fat absorption, based on the fact that bile acids are necessary for this absorption, as stated in the text (choice C is true and can be eliminated). However, the drugs would have to be *swallowed* to end up within the GI lumen, not injected (choice **D** is false and is the correct answer choice).

Duodenal Enzymes

Some duodenal epithelial cells secrete enzymes. Duodenal **enterokinase** (also known as **enteropeptidase**) activates the pancreatic zymogen **trypsinogen** to trypsin (Section 10.7). Other duodenal enzymes are peculiar in that they are not truly secreted, but rather do their work inside or on the surface of the brush border epithelial cell. These duodenal enzymes are called **brush border enzymes**. Their role is to hydrolyze the smallest carbohydrates and proteins (like disaccharides and dipeptides) into monosaccharides and amino acids (Section 10.8).

Duodenal Hormones

10.6

Other duodenal epithelial cells secrete hormones. The three main duodenal hormones are **cholecystokinin (CCK)**, **secretin**, and **enterogastrone**. CCK is secreted in response to fats in the duodenum. It causes the pancreas to secrete digestive enzymes, stimulates gallbladder contraction (bile release), and decreases gastric motility. Note that all these processes cooperate to deal with fats in the duodenum, by digesting them and preventing further stomach emptying. Secretin is released in response to acid in the duodenum. It causes the pancreas to release large amounts of a high-pH aqueous buffer, namely HCO_3^- in water. This neutralizes HCl released by the stomach. Duodenal pH must be kept neutral or even slightly basic for pancreatic digestive enzymes to function. Enterogastrone decreases stomach emptying.

Jejunum and Ileum

Substances not absorbed in the duodenum must be absorbed in these lower segments of the small intestine. The lower small intestine performs special absorptive processes. For example, absorption of vitamin B_{12} occurs only in the ileum (and only when vitamin B_{12} is complexed with **intrinsic factor**, a glycoprotein secreted by the parietal cells of the stomach). A valve called the **ileocecal valve** separates the ileum from the cecum, which is the first part of the large intestine.

- True or false? When a pancreatic exocrine cell secretes an alkaline fluid into the duodenum, a corresponding decrease in pH must occur in that cell's cytoplasm.[18]

Colon (Large Intestine)

Like the rest of the intestine, the colon is a muscular tube. It is 3 or 4 feet long and several inches wide. Its role is to absorb water and minerals, and to form and store feces until the time of defecation. Abnormalities of colon function result in poor fluid absorption and diarrhea, which can cause dehydration and death. The first part of the colon is the **cecum**. Entrance of chyme into the cecum is controlled by the ileocecal valve. The **appendix** is a finger-like appendage of the cecum. It is composed primarily of lymphatic tissue and was mentioned in the preceding chapter. The last portion of the colon is called the **rectum**. Exit of feces (**defecation**) from the rectum occurs through the **anus**. Defecation is controlled by the **anal sphincter**, which has an internal portion and an external portion. The internal anal sphincter consists of smooth muscle, which is under autonomic control. The external anal sphincter consists of skeletal muscle and is under voluntary control. (Note that this is the same arrangement as seen in the

---

[18] True. In the pancreas, CO_2 is converted to carbonic acid by carbonic anhydrase. Carbonic acid dissociates into bicarbonate (HCO_3^-) plus a proton. If the bicarbonate is secreted into the gut, the proton is left behind, thus the pH falls. Severe diarrhea may involve the loss of large amounts of bicarbonate from the gut, and this may cause a significant decrease in the plasma pH level.

urinary sphincters.) Most of the wastes from a meal are defecated about a day after it is eaten. However, the wastes from a meal are first present in stool after just a few hours and some residue of a meal is typically still present in the colon after several days.

The colon contains billions of bacteria of various species. Many are facultative or obligate anaerobes. Undigested materials are metabolized by colonic bacteria. This often results in gas, which is given off as a waste product of bacterial metabolism. **Colonic bacteria** are important for two reasons: 1) the presence of large numbers of normal bacteria helps keep dangerous bacteria from proliferating, due to competition for space and nutrients, and 2) colonic bacteria supply us with **vitamin K,** which is essential for blood clotting.

10.7   THE GI ACCESSORY ORGANS

The GI accessory organs are those that play a role in digestion, but are not actually part of the alimentary canal. They include the **pancreas, liver, gallbladder**, and the large **salivary glands** found outside the mouth. We have already discussed saliva, so the salivary glands will not be discussed further here. The pancreas and liver are essential for GI function. The gallbladder is not essential, but can become infected, obstructed, or cancerous, and is thus medically important.

Exocrine Pancreas

Pancreatic enzymes released into the duodenum are essential for digestion. **Pancreatic amylase** hydrolyzes polysaccharides to disaccharides. **Pancreatic lipase** hydrolyzes triglycerides at the surface of a micelle (see Liver and Gallbladder). **Nucleases** hydrolyze dietary DNA and RNA. Several different **pancreatic proteases** are responsible for hydrolyzing polypeptides to di- and tripeptides. Pancreatic proteases are secreted in their inactive **zymogen** forms. [Why do you suppose digestive enzymes are stored and released in an inactive form?[19]] Zymogens must be activated by removal of a portion of the polypeptide chain. **Trypsinogen** is a zymogen which is converted to the active form, **trypsin**, by **enterokinase**, an intestinal enzyme. Other pancreatic enzymes are then activated by trypsin. These include **chymotrypsinogen** (active form: **chymotrypsin**), **procarboxypeptidase** (active form: **carboxypeptidase**), and **procollagenase** (active form: **collagenase**).

Control of the Exocrine Pancreas

Two hormones discussed previously help to control pancreatic secretion. **Cholecystokinin** (CCK) secreted into the bloodstream by the duodenum causes the pancreas to secrete enzymes. **Secretin**, also released by the duodenum, causes the pancreas to secrete water and bicarbonate (high pH). Parasympathetic nervous system activation increases pancreatic secretion; sympathetic activation reduces it.

---

[19]   It is a safety mechanism. Active digestive enzymes could be dangerous to the pancreatic cells themselves.

Endocrine Pancreas

The endocrine pancreas consists of small regions within the pancreas known as **islets of Langerhans**. There are three types of cells in the islets, and each secretes a particular hormone into the bloodstream.

1) α cells secrete **glucagon** in response to low blood sugar. Glucagon functions to mobilize stored fuels by stimulating the liver to hydrolyze glycogen and release glucose into the bloodstream, and by stimulating adipocytes (fat cells) to release fats into the bloodstream.

2) β cells secrete **insulin** in response to elevated blood sugar (e.g., after a meal). Its effects are opposite those of glucagon: insulin stimulates the removal of glucose from the blood for storage as glycogen and fat.

3) δ cells secrete **somatostatin**. It inhibits many digestive processes.

Focus on Blood Glucose

1) **Lowering blood glucose:** Insulin is essential for life because it causes sugar to be removed from the bloodstream and stored. Diabetics lack insulin or have dysfunctional insulin receptors. Their blood sugar levels are extraordinarily high. The excess glucose directly destroys many physiological systems at the cellular level, including neurons, blood vessels, and the kidneys.

2) **Raising blood glucose:** Three hormones can raise the blood glucose level: glucagon (a polypeptide hormone from the pancreas), epinephrine (an amino acid derivative from the adrenal medulla), and cortisol (a steroid or glucocorticoid from the adrenal cortex). Note that of these three hormones, one is a steroid, one is a polypeptide, and one is an amino acid derivative. Also note that there is only one hormone that can lower blood glucose, while three different hormones can raise blood glucose. It makes sense to have many ways to raise blood glucose, and for it to be less easy to lower blood glucose, since low blood glucose levels are immediately fatal, while elevated blood glucose is harmless in the short term. (Over several years, however, it is harmful.)

- Which one of the following statements is true?[20]
    A) Insulin stimulates the release of glucose into the blood and also stimulates peristalsis in the small intestine.
    B) Gastrin stimulates stomach emptying and inhibits secretion of gastric acid.
    C) Cholecystokinin stimulates peristalsis in the intestine and inhibits stomach emptying.
    D) Glucagon stimulates the storage of glucose and stimulates small intestinal peristalsis.

Liver and Gallbladder

The exocrine secretory activity of the liver is simple: it secretes bile. The liver actually produces about 1 liter of bile a day. The principal ingredients of bile include bile acids (known as **bile salts** in the deprotonated—anionic—form), cholesterol, and bilirubin (from RBC breakdown). Bile emulsifies large fat particles in the duodenum, creating smaller clusters of fat particles called **micelles**. The smaller particles have a greater collective surface area than the large particles, and thus are more easily digested by hydrophilic lipases (from the pancreas). Also, bile helps fatty particles to diffuse across the intestinal mucosal membrane.

---

[20] Insulin stimulates the *removal* of glucose from the blood (choice A is false), gastrin *causes* acid secretion (choice B is false), and glucagon functions to *raise* blood glucose (choice D is false). Choice **C** is a true statement.

Bile made in the liver can go to one of two places: it is either directly secreted into the duodenum or it is stored for later use in the **gallbladder**. Bile stored in the gallbladder is concentrated, and released when a fatty meal is eaten. A **gallstone** is a large crystal formed from bile made with ingredients in incorrect proportions.

The gallbladder itself has no secretory activity. Bile release from this organ is dictated by both the endocrine system and the nervous system. Both CCK (released by the duodenal cells) and the parasympathetic nervous system stimulate contraction of the gallbladder wall.

The liver plays a more complicated role in the *processing* of absorbed nutrients than it does in digestion (breakdown). In order to understand this process, it helps to consider the **hepatic portal system**. The liver receives blood from two places. First, it receives oxygenated blood from the hepatic arteries. Second, it receives venous blood draining the stomach and intestines through the **hepatic portal vein**. (*Hepatic* means "relating to the liver.") As this blood percolates through the liver, nutrients are extracted by hepatocytes (liver cells). The hepatocytes monitor the blood and make changes to the body's physiology based on what is and is not present (much as the hypothalamus does in the hypothalamic-pituitary portal system). For example, if blood glucose is low, the liver will initiate a cascade that leads to glycogen breakdown as well as new glucose production (gluconeogenesis). The free glucose can be released to raise blood glucose levels.

Both the liver and the skeletal muscles are capable of storing glucose as glycogen and subsequently breaking glycogen down when glucose is needed. However only the liver is able to release free glucose to the bloodstream. The product of glycogen breakdown is glucose-6-phosphate; in order to move into the bloodstream, this product must be dephosphorylated, and only the liver contains the enzyme needed to accomplish this (glucose-6-phosphatase).

The waste products from protein catabolism (breakdown) are also regulated through the liver. When proteins are broken down into amino acids, and amino acids are broken down even further (e.g., to enter the Krebs cycle to generate ATP during starvation), nitrogenous by-products are released in the form of NH_3 (ammonia). Ammonia in high levels is toxic to the body, so it is transported to the liver where it is converted into urea. Urea is then absorbed into the bloodstream and excreted by the kidney in urine.

Lipid metabolism is assisted by the liver as well. Lipids exit the intestine and enter the lymphatic system in molecules called **chylomicrons**. Chylomicrons are degraded by lipases into triglycerides, glycerol, and cholesterol-rich **chylomicron remnants**. These remnants are taken up by hepatocytes and combined with proteins to make lipoproteins (HDL, LDL, VLDL, etc.). These lipoproteins then re-enter the blood and are the source of cholesterol and triglycerides for the other tissues of the body.

Many important plasma proteins (such as albumin, globulins, fibrinogens, and other clotting factors necessary to stop bleeding) are made in the liver and secreted into the plasma. People with liver disease often have problems with sealing wounds due to a lack of clotting factors. They also have a tendency to swell up; the lack of albumin allows fluid to leave the bloodstream and enter the tissues.

Finally, the liver is the major center for drug and toxin detoxification in the body. The smooth ER in hepatocytes contains enzyme pathways that break down drugs and toxins into forms that are less toxic and more readily excreted by the renal and gastrointestinal systems. Interestingly, sometimes these same enzyme pathways in hepatocytes are used to convert some drugs into their active forms. Therefore, people with liver disease must have drug levels in their blood monitored closely when they are on medications that are affected by the detoxification system of the liver.

Hormonal Control of Appetite

The desire to eat between meals is subject to hormonal control. When the stomach is empty, gastric cells produce the hormone **ghrelin** to stimulate appetite. When the colon is full, the jejunum (lower intestine) produces **peptide YY** to reduce appetite. The hormone **leptin**, produced by white adipose tissue (fat), is an appetite suppressant that acts as an "adipostat"—maintaining stable lipid content in adipose tissue. Leptin is secreted in response to increased triglyceride levels, and it works to suppress appetite until appropriate levels are restored. All three of these hormones can affect multiple target tissues, but their effects on appetite are primarily mediated by the arcuate nucleus of the hypothalamus.

Leptin has been a focus of obesity research, particularly because disruption of leptin signaling in animal models causes the animals to become obese. Disruptions include the inability to synthesize leptin or a malfunction of the leptin receptor. In humans, obesity is often associated with high levels of leptin but a lack of appetite suppression. This suggests that the hypothalamus may become resistant to leptin, possibly due to down-regulation of the receptors.

10.8

10.8   A DAY IN THE LIFE OF FOOD

In order to draw the above information together, let's trace the path of each of the three main types of dietary nutrients: carbohydrates, proteins, and fats.

Carbohydrates

You purchase a sourdough baguette and tear off a hunk. Chewing increases the bread's surface area, allowing it to soak up more saliva. Ptyalin hydrolyzes starch into fragments, while the tongue and cheeks form a bolus. As you swallow, the upper esophageal sphincter relaxes. Peristalsis carries the bolus to the stomach; the lower esophageal sphincter relaxes to let it pass. In the stomach, strong acid destroys most of the microorganisms which were present in the bread, while further hydrolyzing some polysaccharides. The stomach thoroughly churns the bread, forming acidic chyme, which is gradually released into the duodenum. In the duodenum, pancreatic amylase chops the polysaccharides into disaccharides, which diffuse to the intestinal brush border. Here the disaccharides are hydrolyzed to monosaccharides. Digestion is complete. Up to this point, none of the sugar composing the bread has entered your body; it remains on the lumenal side of GI epithelial tight junctions.

Since they are bulky and hydrophilic, monosaccharides must be taken up into the intestinal epithelial cell by active transport. An apical symport transports one sugar into the cell while allowing sodium to flow in, down its large concentration gradient (Figure 16). [Is this primary or secondary active transport?[21]] The large sodium concentration gradient is created by constant activity of Na^+/K^+ ATPases on the basolateral surface of the cell, pumping Na^+ out. As secondary active transport continues to pack the epithelial cell with monosaccharides, their concentration gets quite high. Thus, there is now a concentration gradient driving them out of the cell into nearby capillaries. This movement occurs by facilitated diffusion (uniports) at the basolateral surface of the cell. In the bloodstream, sugars dissolve into the plasma as it flows into the hepatic portal vein toward the liver.

---

[21] Secondary, since transport is powered by a pre-existing gradient, not directly by ATP hydrolysis.

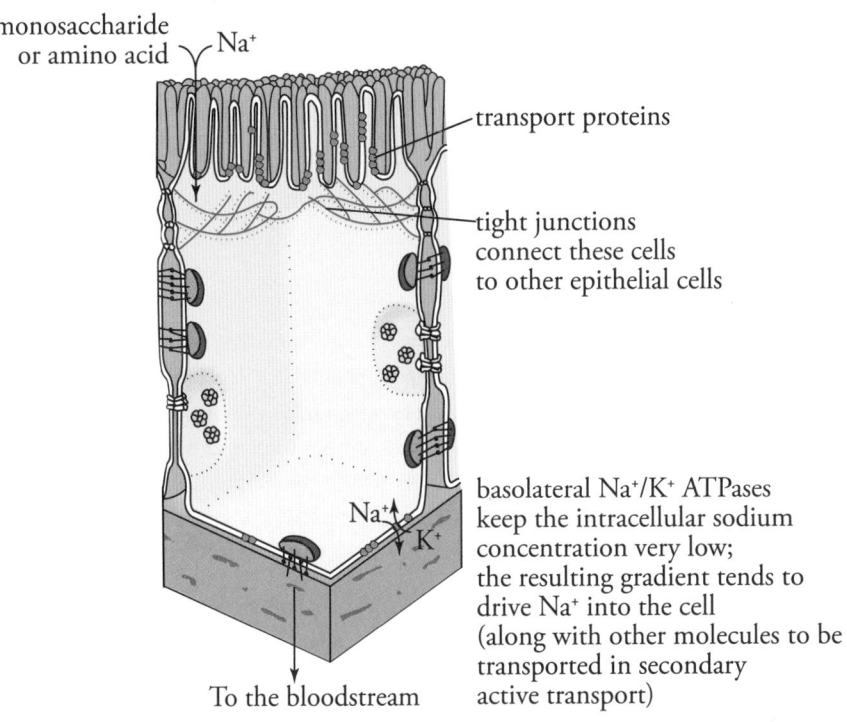

monosaccharide
or amino acid — Na⁺

transport proteins

tight junctions
connect these cells
to other epithelial cells

basolateral Na⁺/K⁺ ATPases
keep the intracellular sodium
concentration very low;
the resulting gradient tends to
drive Na⁺ into the cell
(along with other molecules to be
transported in secondary
active transport)

Na⁺

K⁺

To the bloodstream

Figure 16   Absorption of Hydrophilic Food Monomers

The liver takes up some of the sugars and begins to store them or use their energy. Nonetheless, the blood sugar level increases rather suddenly. When the pancreas is exposed to elevated blood glucose levels, the β cells of the islets of Langerhans secrete insulin. The insulin causes many different cells (liver, muscle, nerve, and fat cells) to take up, utilize, and store glucose. Soon the blood sugar level returns to normal, and you're ready for dessert.

Proteins

The next day, you're well rested from an iron-pumping session and are ready for a nice can of albacore in spring water. You buy generic because it's the same quality but cheaper (and check to make sure it's dolphin-safe).

In your mouth, the tuna is ground and mixed with saliva. No digestion of protein occurs in the mouth. A bolus is formed, and you swallow. Churning of the stomach mixes the tuna with acid, mucus, and enzymes. The low pH kills microorganisms and causes many peptide bonds to hydrolyze. Activated pepsin attacks polypeptides, breaking them into fragments. Chyme is gradually released into the duodenum.

Chyme in the duodenum causes duodenal epithelial cells to secrete CCK and secretin. As a result, the gallbladder releases concentrated bile and the pancreas secretes a basic (high pH) solution of bicarbonate plus digestive zymogens. In the gut, trypsinogen is activated to trypsin by enterokinase. Trypsin then activates other zymogens. The activated proteases go to work on polypeptides from the tuna until all that's left are dipeptides and tripeptides. These are hydrolyzed by brush border peptidases.

Amino acid absorption is similar to monosaccharide absorption: a secondary active transporter (symport) specific to each amino acid couples the uptake of an amino acid to the entrance of sodium into the cell, and a uniporter facilitates movement out of the intestinal epithelial cell into the interstitium. Just as with carbohydrates, the amino acid ends up in the liver, where it is catabolized for energy or used in synthesis (anabolism).

Fats

"Enough of sourdough and tuna fish!" you declare, as you enter an ice cream shop. The almost-pure triglycerides melt in your mouth and are swallowed. The stomach's churning mixes the triglycerides with acid and mucus to some extent, but because they are extremely hydrophobic, they end up just floating in a layer above the aqueous contents of the stomach. Eventually they are emptied into the duodenum where they stimulate CCK release into the bloodstream. Then the pancreas sends enzymes into the gut, via the sphincter of Oddi. But there is a problem: pancreatic lipase cannot digest the fats if they are organized into huge hydrophobic droplets.

Fortunately, CCK in the bloodstream also stimulates gallbladder contraction. This sends bile down the bile duct into the duodenum. Bile acids emulsify the lipids from the ice cream, forming tiny micelles. Then pancreatic lipase can go to work. It hydrolyzes triglycerides to monoglycerides plus free fatty acids, as shown below. These move into intestinal epithelial cells by simple diffusion, which they are able to do thanks to their greasy hydrophobicity and small size. Once inside, they are converted back to triglycerides, which are packaged into **chylomicrons**. These are large particles composed of fats and proteins which are designed to transport fats in the bloodstream (Figure 17).

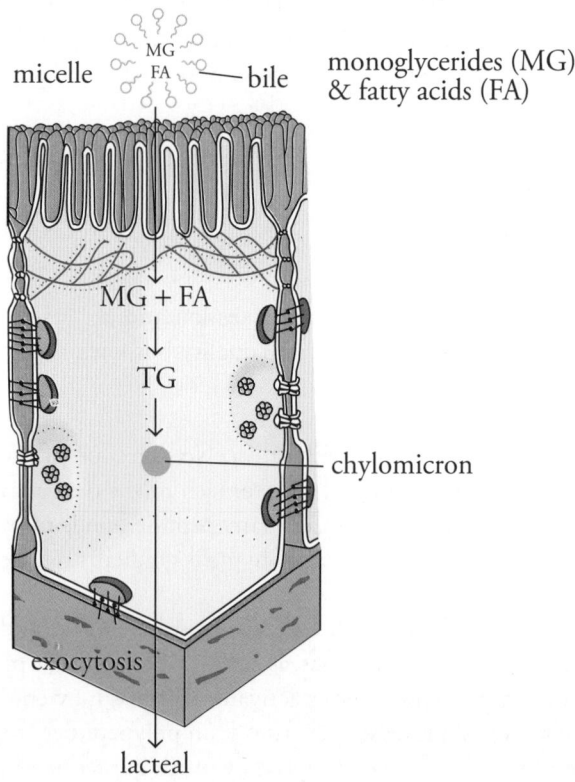

Figure 17 Fat Absorption

10.8

The chylomicrons do not enter intestinal blood capillaries. Instead, they enter tiny lymphatic capillaries known as **lacteals**. These merge to form larger lymphatic vessels, which eventually empty into the thoracic duct. This empties into a large vein near the heart. A few minutes after your sundae, huge amounts of fat are released from the thoracic duct directly into the bloodstream. Your plasma attains a milky yellow color which is easily noticeable when a blood sample is taken. The term for milky plasma is **lipemia**, meaning "fat in the blood."

The chylomicrons circulate throughout the body and are gradually whittled away by removal of fat. In particular, adipose and liver tissues contain the enzyme **lipoprotein lipase**, which hydrolyzes chylomicron triglycerides into monoglycerides and free fatty acids. These diffuse into adipocytes and liver cells, are remade into triglycerides, and then stored.

10.9 VITAMINS

Vitamins are nutrients which must be included in the diet because they cannot be synthesized in the body. They are divided into **fat-soluble** and **water-soluble** categories. Fat-soluble vitamins require bile acids for solubilization and absorption. Excess fat-soluble vitamins are stored in adipose tissue. Excess water-soluble vitamins are excreted in urine by the kidneys.

10.9

Table 2 Vitamins

Vitamin	Function
fat-soluble	
A (retinol)	A visual pigment that changes conformation in response to light
D	Stimulates Ca^{2+} absorption from the gut; helps control Ca^{2+} deposition in bones
E	Prevents oxidation of unsaturated fats
K	Necessary for formation of blood coagulation factors
water-soluble	
B_1 (thiamine)	Needed for enzymatic decarboxylations
B_2 (riboflavin)	Made into FAD, an electron transporter
B_3 (niacin)	Made into NAD^+, an electron transporter
B_6 (pyridoxine)	A coenzyme involved in protein and amino acid metabolism
B_{12} (cobalamin)	A coenzyme involved in the reduction of nucleotides to deoxynucleotides
C (ascorbic acid)	Necessary for collagen formation; deficiency results in scurvy
Biotin	Prosthetic group essential for transport of CO_2 groups
Folate	Enzyme cofactor used in the transport of methylene groups; synthesis of purines and thymine; required for normal fetal nervous system development

Chapter 10 Summary

- The kidneys filter the blood to remove hydrophilic wastes. They also play a major role in homeostasis by regulating blood pressure, pH, ion balance, and water balance.

- Urine is produced by first filtering the blood, and then by modifying the filtrate via reabsorption (moving substances from the filtrate to the blood) and secretion (moving substances from the blood to the filtrate), and finally by concentrating the filtrate to conserve body water.

- Filtration occurs at the glomerulus, most reabsorption and secretion occurs in the PCT, selective reabsorption and secretion occur in the DCT, and concentration occurs in the collecting duct.

- The loop of Henle establishes a concentration gradient in the medulla; this gradient is critical to the reabsorption of water and the creation of a concentrated urine.

- ADH increases the water permeability of the collecting duct to allow reabsorption of water, and aldosterone increases Na^+ reabsorption at the distal tubule. Both hormones work together to help regulate blood pressure.

- When systemic blood pressure falls, the kidneys release renin. Renin is an enzyme that converts the blood protein angiotensinogen into angiotensin I, which is further converted to angiotensin II. Angiotensin II is a potent vasoconstrictor, and it increases the release of aldosterone; the ultimate goal is to increase blood pressure.

- The digestive system organs are divided into two categories: the alimentary canal and the accessory organs. The alimentary canal is the long muscular tube consisting of the mouth, esophagus, stomach, small intestine, and large intestine. The accessory organs have a digestive role, but are not part of the tube. They include the salivary glands, the liver, the gallbladder, and the pancreas.

- The mouth breaks down food mechanically by chewing, and it begins starch digestion via salivary amylase.

- The stomach is primarily a storage tank for food. Mechanical digestion occurs through churning of the food, acid hydrolysis begins chemical digestion, and protein digestion is begun via pepsin.

- Almost all chemical digestion and nutrient absorption takes place in the small intestine. The large intestine primarily reabsorbs water and stores feces; no digestion takes place in the large intestine.

- The liver produces bile (secreted into the small intestine), which emulsifies fat to increase the efficiency of fat digestion. The gallbladder stores and concentrates bile.

- The pancreas secretes the majority of the digestive enzymes used in the small intestine, along with bicarbonate to help neutralize the acid entering the small intestine from the stomach. The pancreas is also a major endocrine organ, secreting insulin and glucagon to regulate blood glucose.

- The enteric nervous system consists of the myenteric plexus and the submucosal plexus. It helps to regulate gut movement, local blood flow, and ion/water exchange.

- Ghrelin is a hormone produced by gastric cells when the stomach is empty to stimulate appetite, while peptide YY is a hormone released by the jejunum when the colon is full to reduce appetite.

- Leptin is produced by fat cells and suppresses appetite when lipid levels in the blood are high.

CHAPTER 10 FREESTANDING PRACTICE QUESTIONS

1. The loop of Henle uses a countercurrent multiplier system to create an area of high ion concentration in the renal medulla. Which of the following statements about the loop of Henle is true?

A) The descending limb is permeable to ions and water.
B) The descending limb is permeable to water but not to ions.
C) The ascending limb is permeable to ions and water.
D) The ascending limb is permeable to water but not to ions.

2. All of the following would increase glomerular filtration rate EXCEPT:

A) constriction of efferent arterioles in the kidney.
B) increased circulatory volume.
C) dilation of afferent arterioles in the kidney.
D) increased filtrate osmolarity.

3. The kidneys play a role in all of the following processes EXCEPT:

A) erythropoiesis.
B) increased absorption of calcium in the intestine.
C) vasoconstriction.
D) stimulation of the sympathetic nervous system.

4. Which of the following statements about angiotensin II is true?

   I.   Angiotensin II is a vasodilator.
   II. Angiotensin II is a substrate for ACE.
   III. Angiotensin II stimulates aldosterone release from the adrenal cortex.

A) I only
B) II only
C) III only
D) II and III

5. Which of the following is *not* an effect of gastrin?

A) Promote parietal cell atrophy
B) Decrease stomach pH
C) Activate chief cells
D) Indirectly stimulate protein degradation

6. A defect in pancreatic amylase would prevent digestion of which of the following nutrients?

A) Starch
B) Maltose
C) Fructose
D) Proteins

7. Hydrochloric acid is present in the stomach, resulting in an approximate pH of 2. Which of the following is NOT a correct statement about HCl?

A) It destroys microorganisms in the stomach.
B) It is secreted by G cells.
C) It converts pepsinogen to pepsin.
D) It participates in the acid hydrolysis of proteins.

8. The hepatic portal vein carries deoxygenated blood from the alimentary canal into the liver, where it is filtered before continuing to the heart via the hepatic vein and inferior vena cava. Blood from which of the following organs does NOT drain into the hepatic portal vein?

A) Stomach
B) Small intestine
C) Colon
D) Kidneys

CHAPTER 10 PRACTICE PASSAGE

The kidneys are critical in regulating and maintaining fluid balance and blood pressure. The functional unit of the kidney is the nephron, a tubule that starts at the glomerulus, enters the cortex, descends into the medulla, loops around, and returns to the cortex. These tubules empty into collecting ducts, which empty into the renal calyces and then into the ureter. Aldosterone and vasopressin are two main hormones that affect renal function.

Aldosterone is the primary effector hormone in the *renin-angiotensin-aldosterone system* (RAAS). It is secreted in response to low blood pressure, low plasma sodium levels, and high plasma potassium levels. Renin is an enzyme secreted by the JG cells of the kidney; it converts angiotensinogen into angiotensin I, which is then converted into angiotensin II by angiotensin converting enzyme (ACE). Angiotensin II is a powerful vasoconstrictor and stimulator of aldosterone release. Aldosterone acts to increase sodium reabsorption, thereby increasing water retention.

Vasopressin is a peptide hormone and is secreted by the posterior pituitary. The main effect of vasopressin is to increase permeability of the collecting ducts to water by stimulating the insertion of *aquaporins* into the epithelial cells of these ducts. Vasopressin can also stimulate increased reabsorption of sodium in the thick ascending loop of Henle. Vasopressin release is stimulated by a decreased plasma volume (via pressure receptors), and by an increased plasma osmotic pressure (via osmoreceptors) in the hypothalamus.

Other hormones acting on or produced by the kidneys include atrial natriuretic peptide (ANP) and erythropoietin (EPO). Although EPO does not act on the kidneys, it is released by the kidneys and stimulates red blood cell production. ANP, on the other hand, is released by atrial myocytes in response to excess atrial stretch. ANP acts as a vasodilator, and increases glomerular filtration rate; this hormone also inhibits renin secretion and reduces aldosterone secretion.

Kidney function can be assessed by analyzing glomerular filtration rate (GFR). GFR is defined as the sum of the filtration rates of all functioning nephrons. An approximate value for normal GFR can be obtained by using the equation: GFR = 140 – [patient age]. Various conditions can affect GFR, as evidenced by Figure 1, which shows the prevalence of various GFR rates by function of age for patients with hyperphosphatemia and patients with hypertension.

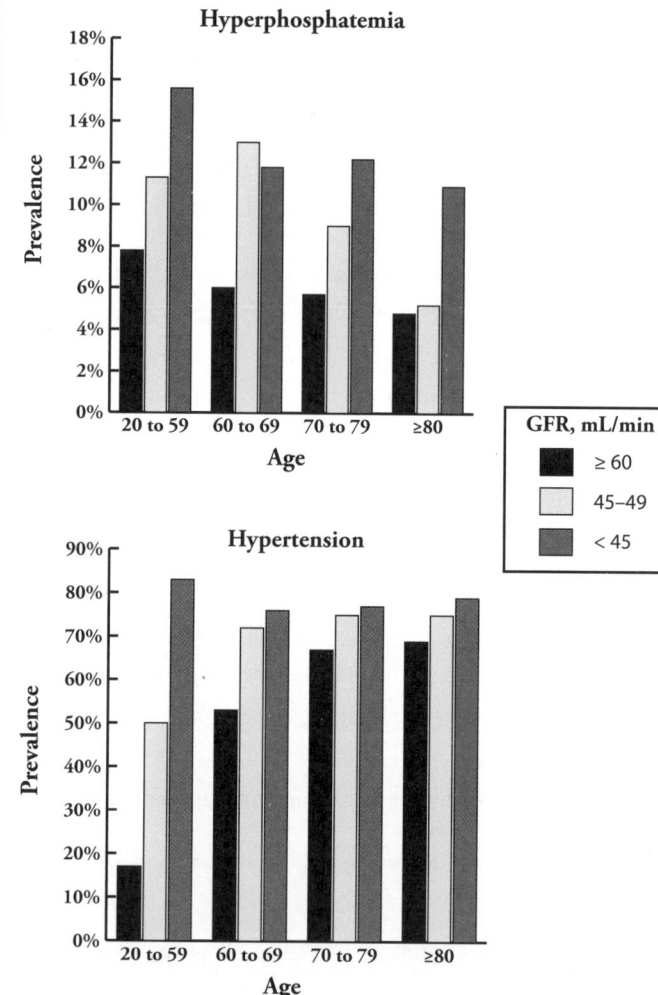

Figure 1 Prevalence of GFR rates as a function of age

Figure adapted from Bowling, Inker, Gutiérrez, Allman, Warnock, McClellan, et. al. (2011). Age-Specific Associations of Reduced Estimated Glomerular Filtration Rate with Concurrent Chronic Kidney Disease Complications. *Clinical Journal of the American Society of Nephrology, 6* (12) 2822-2828

1. Which of the following could be the result of a hormone-secreting tumor of the kidneys?

A) Increased sodium retention
B) Elevated hemoglobin
C) Concentrated urine
D) Increased thirst

2. According to Figure 1, which of the following is true?

A) In those with hypertension, it is more common for people to have a GFR of more than 60 mL/min versus less than 45 mL/min across all ages groups.

B) The prevalence of a GFR of 50 mL/min in hypertensive 50-year-old adults is approximately 85%.

C) In those with hypertension, GFR directly increases with age.

D) In those with hyperphosphatemia, the prevalence of a GFR of 60 mL/min and above is roughly similar for ages 60–69 and 70–79.

3. Which of the following statements is correct?

A) Glomeruli are circular in shape, and contain a capillary system, which separates two arterioles.

B) Vasa recta can be found accompanying the loop of Henle in the adrenal cortex.

C) The distal tubules empty into the minor calyx via the renal papilla.

D) Aldosterone acts to increase potassium reabsorption.

4. Alcohol acts as a diuretic; consumption of alcohol produces large quantities of dilute urine. Which of the following statements is NOT a possible explanation for this observation?

A) Alcohol decreases the action of ACE, thereby inhibiting the release of aldosterone from the adrenal gland and decreasing water reabsorption by the collecting duct.

B) Alcohol acts to stimulate renin release.

C) Alcohol inhibits the secretion of vasopressin, therefore diminishing the kidneys' ability to concentrate urine.

D) Alcohol stimulates the release of ANP from the atria.

5. Hyperphosphatemia refers to an elevated amount of phosphate in the blood. A 45-year-old patient with hyper-phosphatemia is tested for kidney function. His GFR value is 55 mL/min. Which of the following is/are true?

   I.   The patient would have high levels of aldosterone in his blood.

   II.   The patient's GFR would be considered normal.

   III.   The prevalence of a GFR of 55 mL/min for his age range and condition is 13%.

A) I only

B) II only

C) I and III only

D) I, II, and III

6. Which of the following statements comparing ANP and angiotensin is correct?

A) ANP increases blood pressure and urine volume, whereas angiotensin II decreases blood pressure and urine volume.

B) ANP decreases blood pressure and increases urine volume, whereas angiotensin II increases blood pressure and decreases urine volume.

C) ANP decreases blood pressure and urine volume, whereas angiotensin II increases blood pressure and urine volume.

D) ANP increases blood pressure and decreases urine volume, whereas angiotensin II decreases blood pressure and increases urine volume.

SOLUTIONS TO CHAPTER 10 FREESTANDING PRACTICE QUESTIONS

1. **B** The descending limb of the loop of Henle is permeable to water but not to ions (choice B is correct, and choice A is wrong); water leaves the filtrate, thereby concentrating it. The ascending limb is permeable to ions but not to water (choices C and D can be eliminated). Na^+, K^+, and Cl^- are actively transported out of the filtrate, and K^+ is passively transported, concentrating the renal medulla.

2. **D** Constricting efferent arterioles would restrict flow out of the glomerulus, and dilating afferent arterioles would increase flow into the glomerulus; in either case, pressure at the glomerulus would rise and filtration rate would increase (choices A and C can be eliminated). An increase in circulatory volume will increase blood pressure and further enhance this effect on a systemic level (choice B can be eliminated). However, if the filtrate osmolarity is high, the macula densa will not send signals to stimulate the juxtaglomerular cells and the GFR will not be increased (choice D would not increase GFR and is the correct answer choice).

3. **D** Erythropoietin is released by the kidneys and stimulates red blood cell production in bone marrow (the kidneys play a role in choice A, so it can be eliminated). Calcitriol (vitamin D) is activated in the kidneys and promotes the uptake of calcium in the intestines (the kidneys play a role in choice B, so it can be eliminated). Renin is released by the kidneys and triggers the production of angiotensin II, which causes vasoconstriction (the kidneys play a role in choice C, so it can be eliminated). However, sympathetic nervous system stimulation comes from the products of the adrenal glands, not the kidneys (the kidneys do not play a role in choice D, so it is the best answer choice).

4. **C** Item I is false: angiotensin II acts as a vasoconstrictor to increase blood pressure (choice A can be eliminated). Item II is false: angiotensin I is the substrate for ACE, which converts angiotensin I into angiotensin II (choices B and D can be eliminated, and choice C is correct). Item III is true: angiotensin II stimulates the release of ADH from the posterior pituitary gland and aldosterone from the adrenal cortex, thereby increasing blood pressure.

5. **A** Gastrin acts on parietal cells in a stimulatory manner, causing them to release HCl (choice B is an effect and can be eliminated). Parietal cell atrophy occurs in the *absence* of gastrin (choice A is not an effect of gastrin and is the correct answer choice). Additionally, gastrin activates chief cells to release pepsinogen (choice C is an effect and can be eliminated). The combination of pepsinogen from the chief cells and acid from the parietal cells stimulates the cleavage and activation of pepsinogen to pepsin, with subsequent degradation of proteins (choice D is an effect and can be eliminated).

6. **A** Amylase hydrolyzes starch into maltose, which is further broken down into individual glucose molecules by brush border enzymes in the small intestine (choice A is correct, and choice B is wrong). Fructose is already a monosaccharide and can be absorbed without further digestion (choice C is wrong), and proteins are digested by proteases like trypsin or pepsin (choice D is wrong).

7. **B**   Choices A, C, and D are all consistent with the function of HCl in the stomach. The statement in choice B is incorrect (and, therefore, the correct answer) because HCl is secreted by parietal cells, not G cells. G cells secrete gastrin, a hormone.

8. **D**   The stomach, small intestine, and colon (large intestine) are part of the alimentary canal, and their blood supplies drain into the hepatic portal vein to be filtered by the liver (choices A, B, and C can be eliminated). Blood that passes through the kidneys drains directly into the inferior vena cava via the renal veins (choice D is correct).

SOLUTIONS TO CHAPTER 10 PRACTICE PASSAGE

1. **B**   EPO is the only hormone secreted by the kidneys. It will act to increase red blood cell production, thus increasing hemoglobin. Don't confuse renin with a hormone! Renin is an enzyme that acts on an existing blood protein (angiotensinogen) to convert it to an active form (angiotensin). It does not bind to receptors anywhere and does not have a direct role on cellular function (as do hormones). Certainly, if the secretion of renin were increased, then all other answer choices would also occur. There would be an increase in aldosterone and a subsequent increase in sodium reabsorption. The increased sodium reabsorption would increase vasopressin release and the urine would be concentrated. Both the increased sodium and vasopressin would act to increase thirst, but since renin is not a hormone and this question specifically asks about a "hormone-secreting tumor of the kidney," choices A, C, and D are wrong.

2. **D**   In people ages 20–59 with hypertension, there is approximately an 85% prevalence of a GFR of less than 45 mL/min versus approximately 15% prevalence of a GFR of more than 60 mL/min. Since the answer choice says "across all age groups," the finding of even one age group for which this is not the case makes the answer false (choice A can be eliminated). The prevalence values are calculated for age ranges, so you cannot infer from the graph what the prevalence of the GFR for a 50-year-old specifically would be (choice B can be eliminated). The graph shows the prevalence of certain GFR values as a function of age, not the exact correlation between age and GFR (choice C can be eliminated). As shown on the graph, the prevalence of a GFR of 60 mL/min or higher in those with hyperphosphatemia is approximately 6% for both ages 60–69 and 70–79 (choice D is correct).

3. **A**   The glomeruli are small knots of capillaries, supplied with blood by the afferent arterioles and drained of blood by the efferent arterioles. Although the vasa recta do surround the loop of Henle, they are found in the medulla, not the cortex (choice B is wrong). The distal tubules empty into the collecting ducts (which then empty into the minor calyces; choice C is wrong). Aldosterone acts to increase sodium reabsorption (not potassium), and in any case, the passage states that the release of aldosterone can be triggered by high plasma potassium. If its release is triggered by high plasma potassium, aldosterone is unlikely to stimulate the reabsorption of potassium, driving the levels up even higher (choice D is wrong).

4. **B** Decreased water reabsorption means increased water elimination; in other words, the production of large quantities of dilute urine (choice A could explain the observation and can be eliminated). Similarly, since the passage describes the action of vasopressin in reclaiming water from the nephron, an inhibition of vasopressin secretion would lead to decreased water reclamation (reabsorption) and the production of dilute urine (choice C could explain the observation and can be eliminated). The passage states that ANP acts to increase glomerular filtration rate (increase urine production) and to decrease renin and aldosterone secretion; both of these would decrease water reabsorption and lead to the production of dilute urine (choice D could explain the observation and can be eliminated). However, if alcohol were to stimulate renin release, more aldosterone would be secreted, leading to the reabsorption of more water and the production of a concentrated urine (choice B does not explain the observation and is the correct answer choice). Note that the actual action of alcohol is to inhibit vasopressin, but the question only asks which of the answer choices was a *possible* explanation.

5. **C** Since this is a Roman numeral question, start by analyzing the Roman numeral item that appears in exactly two of the answer choices, in this case Item II or III. Item II is shorter, so start with that one; whether it is true or false, you can eliminate half the answers. Item II is false: the passage states that normal GFR can be approximated by subtracting a patient's age from 140; this would give an approximate GFR of 95 ml/min, which is much higher than the patient's actual GFR (choices B and D can be eliminated). Since both remaining choices include Item I, it must be true and you can evaluate Item III. Item III is true: in Figure 1, the prevalence of a GFR of 45–59 ml/min for the age range of 20–59 for those with hyperphosphatemia is approximately 13% (choice A can be eliminated, and choice C is correct). Note that Item I is in fact true: the passage states that aldosterone is secreted in response to high blood potassium levels.

6. **B** Both ANP and angiotensin II act on arteries but in opposite ways. The passage states that ANP acts as a vasodilator and thus would decrease blood pressure, but angiotensin II is a vasoconstrictor and would increase blood pressure (choices A and D can be eliminated). Angiotensin II would decrease urine volume by stimulating aldosterone (and indirectly vasopressin); the passage states that ANP reduces aldosterone secretion, and thus it would increase urine volume (choice C can be eliminated, and choice B is correct).

SEQUENTIAL NEPHRON BLOCKADE WITH COMBINED DIURETICS IMPROVES DIASTOLIC FUNCTION IN PATIENTS WITH RESISTANT HYPERTENSION

David Fouassier, Anne Blanchard, Antoine Fayol, Guillaume Bobrie, Pierre Boutouyrie, Michel Azizi, Jean-Sébastien Hulot

ESC Heart Failure 2020; 7:2561–2571 Published online 29 June 2020 in Wiley Online Library

INTRODUCTION

Heart failure with preserved ejection fraction (HFpEF) has been reported to account for almost half of all heart failure (HF) patients. HFpEF typically occurs in association with advanced age, cardiovascular, metabolic, and proinflammatory comorbidities. One of the most common comorbidities associated with HFpEF is arterial hypertension, which is thought to favour the development of left ventricular (LV) stiffening, hypertrophy, and consequent diastolic dysfunction. Patients with resistant hypertension (RHTN), defined as a failure to reach seated office systolic blood pressure < 140 mmHg or diastolic blood pressure < 90 mmHg while treated with an appropriate three drug regimen that includes a diuretic have a higher risk to develop HF, notably HFpEF.

Consequently, current European and U.S. guidelines recommend treating hypertension in HFpEF patients with diuretics, angiotensin-converting enzyme inhibitors (ACEIs)/angiotensin-II-receptor blockers (ARBs), mineralocorticoid receptor antagonists (MRAs), or beta-blockers. These anti-hypertensive drugs have different pharmacological targets with potential impact on myocardial remodelling or on the further development of cardiac dysfunction. For instance, one of the major contributors to RHTN is fluid retention, which also contributes to increase LV filling pressures. Aldosterone blockade with mineralocorticoid receptor antagonist has been shown to reduce myocardial fibrosis, an important component observed in HFpEF. Reciprocally, the use of beta-blockers in HFpEF patients is debated as potentially associated with increased risk of cardiovascular outcomes. The optimal antihypertensive strategy in patients with RHTN to both treat hypertension and improve cardiac diastolic dysfunction is thus currently undetermined.

The 'Management of Resistant Hypertension: Comparison of Two Treatment Strategies: Increase Sodium Depletion or Combined Blockage of Renin-angiotensin System (RAS)'

('PHARES trial,' NCT00224549) compared the efficacy of two different anti-hypertensive pharmacological strategies in RHTN patients. The primary results showed that sequential nephron blockade (NBD) with different diuretics (i.e., furosemide, spironolactone, and amiloride) acting on three segments of renal tubule of the nephron induced a large and well-tolerated reduction in BP compared with a strategy with combined renin-angiotensin system blockade (RASB) with irbesartan, ramipril, and bisoprolol.

In this pre-specified substudy of the PHARES trial, we aimed to evaluate and compare the changes in cardiac biomarkers (BNP) [B-type natriuretic peptide] and echocardiographic parameters of diastolic dysfunction according to the two anti-hypertensive strategies in RHTN patients.

METHODS

Study design

The design of this 12-week, single-centre, prospective, randomized, open, blinded endpoint trial with optional drug titration has been described elsewhere and will be summarized briefly here.

Briefly, eligible men or women were aged 18 to 75 years, with essential hypertension resistant to three or more antihypertensive drugs including a diuretic (supine office blood pressure BP at least 140 and or 90 mmHg). The main exclusion criteria were secondary hypertension, history of severe cardiovascular disease (cardiac surgery or percutaneous coronary angioplasty), or stroke in the past 3 months, atrial fibrillation, uncontrolled diabetes (HbA1c > 8%), and estimated glomerular filtration rates less than 40 mL/min (modification of diet in renal disease formula). The patients entered a 4-week standardized triple-therapy regimen comprising hydrochlorothiazide (12.5 mg/day), irbesartan (300 mg/day), and amlodipine (5 mg/day) (Figure 1A). After 4 weeks of the standardized triple-therapy regimen, patients with a mean daytime ambulatory systolic blood pressure ≥ 135 mmHg and/or mean daytime ambulatory diastolic blood pressure ≥ 85 mmHg were randomized 1:1 to the NBD regimen or to the RASB regimen at week 0 (W0, baseline). Treatment intensity was increased at week 4, 8, or 10 if home BP was ≥135/85 mmHg, by sequentially adding 25 mg spironolactone, 20–40 mg furosemide, and 5 mg amiloride (NBD group) or 5–10 mg ramipril and 5–10 mg bisoprolol (RASB group). No other antihypertensive drug was allowed during the study.

At W4, W8, W10, and W12, patients reported to the centre at approximately 0830 h, without having taken their morning dose, to undergo safety, office BP, and laboratory assessments.

Evaluation of cardiac biomarkers and diastolic function

BNP levels were measured at baseline and at the 12-week follow-up visit. The cut-offs BNP levels were defined in line with current guidelines in non-acute settings: BNP levels above 100 pg/mL were considered as likely indicating the presence of HF while BNP levels below 35 pg/mL were considered as invalidating the presence of HF. The grey zone was comprised between these two limits.

Trans-thoracic echocardiography was also performed at baseline (W0) and at the last follow-up visit (W12) by the same experienced operator blind to the randomization group. Cardiac dimensions including wall thickness, ventricular diameters, and left atrial area were measured. Pulse wave Doppler recordings of the LV inflow were obtained.

Haemodynamic and vascular measurements

Supine office BP was measured. Twenty four-hour ambulatory, daytime and nighttime BP and heart rate (HR) monitoring was performed.

Systemic vascular resistance (SVR) was calculated using the formula: SVR = (daytime mean arterial BP blood pressure – central venous pressure) × 79.92/cardiac output.

Mean arterial blood pressure was calculated with the formula: (daytime mean arterial systolic blood pressure + 2 × daytime mean arterial diastolic blood pressure). Cardiac output was estimated with the formula: $[\pi/2 \times$ (LV outflow tract diameter)$^2 \times$ LV outflow tract sub-valvular velocity time integral$] \times$ heart rate.

Laboratory parameters

Blood was sampled at baseline and at the last follow-up visit in fasting conditions to measure plasma renin, aldosterone, BNP, creatinine, sodium, potassium, and protein concentrations.

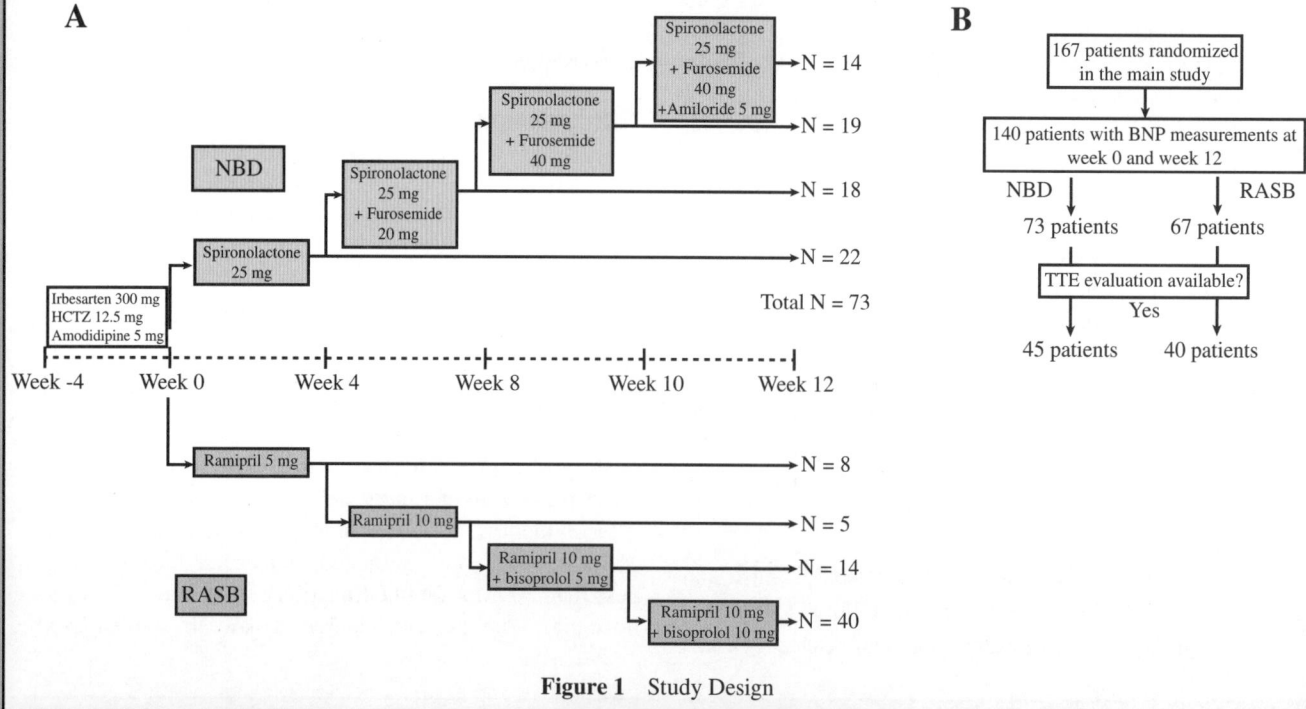

Figure 1 Study Design

Statistical analysis

Continuous variables are expressed as means ± standard deviations. Categorical variables are expressed as numbers and percentages. A Student's t-test was used for continuous variable and a χ^2 square test or Fisher's exact test for categorical variable was performed for comparison between groups and between baseline and week 12. Statistical results are presented as mean differences, with two-tailed 95% confidence intervals. To adjust for multiple testing, a P value < 0.01 was considered statistically significant.

RESULTS

Patients characteristics at randomization

Among the 167 patients randomized for the main study, the baseline characteristics, laboratory parameters, and plasma hormones (BNP, renin, and aldosterone) did not significantly differ between the NBD and the RASB groups (Tables 1 and 2). None of these patients had previous history of HF or current symptoms of congestive HF.

The proportion of patients with baseline plasma BNP concentrations < 35 pg/mL, between 35 and 100 pg/mL, and >100 pg/mL did not significantly differ between the two groups (Figure 2A and 2B). Only three (4.1%) patients of the NBD group and one (1.5%) of the RASB group had baseline plasma BNP concentrations > 100 pg/mL.

Table 1   Baseline characteristics of patients with resistant hypertension randomized to nephron blockade or renin-angiotensin system blockade group and complete BNP evaluation

n = 140	NBD group n = 73	RASB group n = 67	P
Age (years)	55.8 ± 10	53.7 ± 10.3	0.233
Men, n (%)	54 (74)	53(79)	0.475
BMI (kg/m²)	30.0 ± 4.9	28.3 ± 3.8	0.031
Obesity (BMI > 30 kg/m²), n (%)	32 (44)	24 (36)	0.334
Diabetes mellitus, n (%)	12 (15)	15 (22)	0.609
Dyslipidemia, n (%)	46 (63)	40 (60)	0.326
Duration of hypertension (years)	14.3 ± 10.3	12.7 ± 10.6	0.352
Daytime ambulatory SBP (mmHg)	148.7 ± 12.4	149.9 ± 12.1	0.569
Daytime ambulatory DBP (mmHg)	91.4 ± 10.1	93.3 ± 9.3	0.245
Daytime ambulatory HR (bpm)	79.6 ± 9.9	81.7 ± 10.2	0.375
Night-time ambulatory SBP (mmHg)	137.2 ± 13.1	135.4 ± 13.5	0.419
Night-time ambulatory DBP (mmHg)	81.0 ± 9.9	80.9 ± 9.5	0.941
Night-time ambulatory HR (bpm)	70.3 ± 8.8	69 ± 9.9	0.446

BMI, body mass index; DBP, diastolic blood pressure; PP, pulse pressure; SBP, systolic blood pressure.
Results are mean ± SD or mediane (IQR)

Table 2   Comparison between the two arms of treatment of haemodynamic and biological parameters at weeks 0 and 12

	Week 0			Week 12		
	NBD (n = 73)	RASB (n = 67)	P value	NBD (n = 73)	RASB (n = 67)	P value
Plasma BNP (pg/mL)	21 (11–33)	17 (10–27)	0.216	12 (8–22)	40 (17–64)	<0.0001
Daytime ambulatory SBP (mmHg)	148.7 ± 12.4	149.9 ± 12.1	0.569	128.0 ± 11.7	142.1 ± 17.7	<0.0001
Daytime ambulatory DBP (mmHg)	91.4 ± 10.1	93.3 ± 9.3	0.245	79.5 ± 9.9	86.1 ± 9.9	<0.0001
Systemic vascular resistance (Wood)	3064.9 ± 856.3	3131.5 ± 786.8	0.687	1396.5 ± 382.6	16423 ± 383.4	0.0024
Daytime ambulatory HR (bpm)	79.6 ± 9.9	81.7 ± 10.2	0.375	80.9 ± 9.8	68.4 ± 11.8	<0.0001
Plasma potassium (mmol/L)	3.8 ± 0.4	3.9 ± 0.4	0.199	4.3 ± 0.5	4.0 ± 0.4	<0.0001
Plasma sodium (mmol/L)	140.6 ± 2.2	140.8 ± 2.4	0.682	138 ± 3	140 ± 2	<0.0001
eGFR (ml/min per 1.73m²)	83.5 ± 18.6	89.7 ± 18.9	0.055	73 ± 20	86 ± 18	<0.0001
Plasma proteins (g/L)	69.5 ± 4.9	68.2 ± 4.2	0.122	70 ± 5	68 ± 4	0.0018
Plasma renin (mUI/M)	19 (10–39)	20.5 (9–37.8)	0.922	122 (52–327)	8 (5–29)	<0.0001
Plasma aldosterone (pmol/L)	104 (69–152)	95 (63.3–132)	0.362	270 (177–344)	91 (58–137)	<0.0001

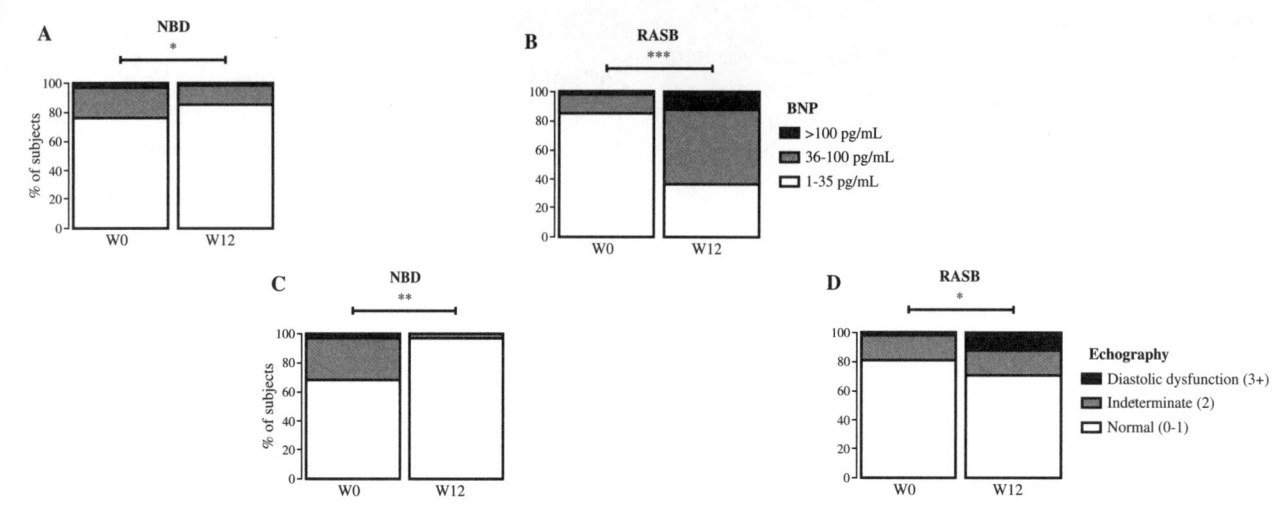

Figure 2 Evolution from randomization (W0) to week 12 (W12) of BNP and echocardiographic parameters of diastolic dysfunction in nephron blockade and renin-angiotensin system blockade arms of treatment.

Among the 140 patients with BNP measurements, 45 patients in NBD group and 40 in RASB group had TTE recordings available for analysis (Figure 1B). At baseline, there was no significant difference in echocardiographic parameters between the two groups (Table 3). A total of 21 patients (11 women and 10 men) had LV hypertrophy. The echocardiographic parameters required to score diastolic dysfunction were available in 32 patients of the NBD and 31 patients of the RASB arm. Nine patients in NBD group and five patients in RASB group had undetermined level of diastolic function, and one patient in each group had echocardiographic diastolic dysfunction (p = 0.676, Table 3, Figure 2C and 2D).

After 12 weeks, nephron blockade and renin-angiotensin system blockade had different effects on BNP levels

At 12 weeks, plasma BNP concentrations decreased significantly from baseline in the NBD group but increased in the RASB group (Figure 3 and Table 2). Consequently, the number of patients with plasma BNP concentrations between 35 and 100 pg/mL and >100 pg/ml decreased from baseline to W0 to nine (12%) and one (1.4%) patients in the NBD group, respectively, whereas it increased to 37 (55%) and 7 (10.4%) patients in the RASB group, respectively (p < 0.001; Figure 2A and 2B).

Table 3 Echocardiographic parameters at randomization (week 0) and after 12 weeks of nephron blockade or renin-angiotensin system blockade treatment

	Week 0			Week 12		
	NBD N = 45	RAS N = 40	p value	NBD n = 45	RAS n = 40	p value
LVED diameter (mm)	48.3 ± 5.2	50.7 ± 4.2	0.0244	48.4 ± 4.6	51.6 ± 5.8	0.0059
LVEF (%)	68.0 ± 8.2	66.1 ± 8.5	0.299	66.9 ± 8.1	67.0 ± 7.5	0.968
Cardiac output (l/min)	6.1 ± 1.7	5.8 ± 1.4	0.529	5.8 ± 1.5	5.3 ± 1.2	0.083
LVED volume (mL/m²)	65.9 ± 18.7	63.6 ± 11.9	0.532	66.6 ± 17.2	66.7 ± 16.6	0.977
LVES volume (mL/m²)	20.9 ± 8.3	21.9 ± 7.8	0.589	22.4 ± 9.6	22.2 ± 8.6	0.922
Left atrial area (cm²)	17.7 ± 4.2	18.5 ± 4.0	0.401	16.5 ± 3.6	19.2 ± 3.9	0.0021
	Assessment of diastolic function					
	NBD n = 32	RAS n = 31	p value	NBD n = 32	RAS n = 31	p value
Normal, n (%)	22	25	0.676	31	21	0.0048
Undetermined, n (%)	9	5		1	6	
Diastolic dysfunction, n (%)	1	1		0	4	

Full data of echographic parameters for assessment of diastolic function were available in 43% and 46% of subjects in NBD arm and RASB arm, respectively.

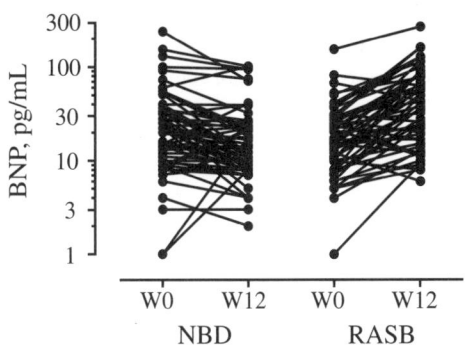

Figure 3 Evolution of BNP levels at baseline and after 12 weeks according to the nephron blockade or renin-angiotensin system blockade.

In the univariate analysis, NBD treatment was significantly associated with decrease in BNP levels over the 12 weeks of the study (Table 4). The influence of NBD treatment was also significant after adjustment on classical factors influencing BNP levels including age, sex, renal function, and BMI.

Table 4 Factors influencing difference in BNP levels between week 12 and week 0 in univariable linear regression

	B	p value
Age (years)	0.17 ± 0.36	0.636
Women	−1.02 ± 8.76	0.907
NBD versus RASB treatment	−42.51 ± 6.50	<0.0001
Difference in daytime SBP (mmHg)	1.12 ± 0.24	<0.0001
Difference in daytime PP (mmHg)	2.67 ± 0.44	<0.0001
Difference in aortic SBP (mmHg)	0.73 ± 0.22	0.0013
Difference in aortic PP (mmHg)	0.86 ± 0.34	0.0122
Difference in pulse Wave velocity (m/s)	4.55 ± 2.55	0.077
Difference in HR (bpm)	−1.68 ± 0.28	<0.0001
Difference in systemic vascular resistance (Wood)	−0.01 ± 0.01	0.924
eGFR (mL/min per 1.73m^2)	0.28 ± 0.18	0.134
BMI (kg/m^2)	0.63 ± 0.84	0.455

Nephron blockade has an independent effect on changes in BNP levels

We further looked at haemodynamics differences between the two groups that could explain the observed difference in BNP changes (Table 2). At the end of the study (week 12), the mean decrease from baseline in daytime systolic BP, diastolic BP, aortic systolic BP, and pulse pressure (PP) was significantly higher in the NBD group as compared with the RASB group (Table 2), in line with previous results in the main study. PWV tended to decrease in both groups, a trend that however did not reach significance. SVR were significantly lower after 12 weeks in the NBD

arm compared with the RASB arm (Table 2). HR was significantly lower in the RASB group than the NBD group due to bisoprolol's effect.

At week 12, patients in the NBD group had lower plasma sodium, higher potassium, and higher plasma creatinine resulting in lower estimated glomerular filtration rate than RASB group (Table 2). Similarly, renin and aldosterone plasma concentrations increased more in NBD than in RASB (Table 2). However, none of these factors has significant influence on changes in BNP levels.

Nephron blockade improved diastolic function assessed by echocardiography

After 12 weeks, we observed that LV diastolic diameter, LV mass index, and left atrial area decreased in NBD group, while these parameters slightly increased in the RASB group (Table 3). In both NBD and RASB, cardiac index did not change significantly between W0 and W12.

In line with our results on changes in BNP levels, we observed an improvement of diastolic parameters in NBD group: at week 12, 97% of patients had a normal diastolic function compared with 69% at baseline ($p = 0.001$). Only one patient in NBD group remained with undetermined diastolic function, none with diastolic dysfunction (Table 3, Figure 2C). Reciprocally, echography indicated worsening of diastolic function at week 12 in patients of the RASB group (Figure 2D). At week 12, only 68% of patients in RASB group presented normal diastolic function (Table 3, Figure 2).

DISCUSSION

We report that in patients without symptomatic HF but with RHTN as a major risk factor for HF, a 12-week treatment based on sequential NBD with combined diuretics significantly and rapidly improves biological and echocardiographic markers of diastolic function while a strategy of triple RASB (with ARB, ACEI, and beta-blocker) did not improve these markers. This study was a pre-specified substudy of the PHARES trial, a prospective, randomized, open-blinded endpoint study, where 167 patients with mean baseline daytime ambulatory blood pressure of 135 mmHg or more and/or 85 mmHg or more despite 4-week treatment with irbesartan 300 mg/day, were randomized to NBD vs. RASB. The PHARES study showed a significantly higher reduction in blood pressure and in LV mass in patients receiving NBD. In this sub-study focusing on the biological and echographic markers of cardiac function, we further show a positive and significant impact of the NBD strategy on the changes in BNP levels and cardiac parameters of diastolic dysfunction after 12 weeks of treatment. Importantly, in the multivariable analysis, the effect of NBD remained significant after adjustment for multiple factors, notably BP reduction and changes in renal function. In addition, while the RASB therapeutic strategy was also associated with BP reduction, we observed opposite effects on changes in BNP levels and echocardiographic parameters of diastolic function. This result suggests that an aggressive strategy to reduce sodium balance in patients with RHTN is preferable to rapidly reduce cardiac wall stress and improve cardiac relaxation.

RHTN combines several pathophysiological mechanisms including increased peripheral resistance, fluid retention, and salt sensitivity. RHTN is considered as major risk factor for diastolic dysfunction, a setting in which impaired relaxation is associated with an increase in telediastolic pressure, indirectly reflected by higher levels of BNP. As compared with RASB, NDB was associated with a greater reduction in blood volume as indicated by larger reduction in systemic vascular resistance and in GFR and higher increase in renin levels as compared with RASB. However, our results indicate that the improvement in cardiac function with NBD is likely explained by additional effects beyond the plasma volume reduction. A link between salt overload and increased arterial thickness has been well established experimentally and is independent of BP. Arteries play an important role in adapting to an acute sodium load by endothelium-dependent and endothelium-independent mechanisms. In a mouse model of chronic sodium loading, it was shown that the consequent increase in arterial stiffness could be partially prevented by spironolactone or amiloride. In our study, it is possible that modamide and spironolactone have induced a decrease in arterial stiffness (thus increasing compliance) leading to a greater decrease in the PP in the NBD group.

On the other hand, the achievement of a complete RASB with ARB, ACEI, and beta-blocker resulted in a significant increase of BNP levels and echographic markers of diastolic function. In the multivariable analysis, the changes in HR were significantly associated with the changes in BNP levels with lower HRs being associated with higher BNP levels. This suggests that an important part of our observation could be explained by a direct detrimental effect of beta-blockers. Beta-blockers and bisoprolol have, however, been reported to exert a positive lusitropic effect in different animal models, an observation that potentially does not translate into humans. In line with our results, it was shown in a substudy of the ASCOT clinical trial that hypertensive patients treated with atenolol displayed higher LV filling pressure and BNP levels as compared with patients receiving amlodipine while the on-treatment

BP was similar in both groups. In another study, bisoprolol improved echographic parameters of diastolic function after 3 months of treatment, but these patients did not have RHTN as in our study.

As RHTN is a major risk factor for HF, notably with HFpEF, our results can also be interpreted in the context of the different clinical studies that evaluated therapeutic strategies in patients with HFpEF. Indeed, there is currently no evidence to support a therapeutic benefit for the use of beta-blockers, ACEi, and ARB in patients with HFpEF. Furthermore, these results are in line with the ONTARGET study, which did not show any benefit of a double RAS blockade in terms of cardiovascular events or hospitalization for HF but on the contrary an increased risk of hypotension and renal failure. Reciprocally, the use of spironolactone is likely associated with a reduction in HF rehospitalization in HFpEF patients, but the effects on mortality and quality of life remain unclear. Our results further suggest that spironolactone, in combination with other diuretics, might be beneficial to prevent further development of HF, notably with preserved ejection fraction. This observation would however deserve further long-term studies.

Study limitations

The studied population has a major risk factor of HF, but none had a history of HF, so the results cannot be extrapolated to HFpEF patients. BNP and echocardiography were only available at week 0 and week 12 and in a fraction of the patients, so we could not analyse the effect of each titration of the treatment on these parameters. Moreover, some more recent echocardiographic parameters such as left atrial volume and LV longitudinal strain were not measured in our study. The scores to estimate cardiac diastolic dysfunction were derived using left atrial areas rather than volumes as lastly recommended. However, similar trends with improvement in the NBD group were also observed after deriving the scores without considering LA areas (data not shown), thus suggesting that using LA areas instead of LA volumes was not changing our overall results.

In conclusion, our data suggest that combined diuretic treatment (NBD strategy) that targets fluid retention improves diastolic dysfunction and decreases arterial stiffness. Reciprocally, our results suggest that a more complete inhibition of the renin-angiotensin system does not improve diastolic function. These differences involve mechanisms associated with BP reduction and improved ventriculararterial coupling. An intensive strategy with a combination of diuretics should be preferably considered in patients presenting RHTN.

JOURNAL ARTICLE EXERCISE 2

Remember that the science sections on the MCAT include a significant number of passages with experiments. You'll need to be able to extract information efficiently and analyze data effectively in order to do well on these passages.

This is the second of three "Journal Article Exercises" in this book. In the first exercise, we showed you the type of information you should be able to extract from the article and the sorts of things to pay attention to in the data. In this exercise, you'll do more of that on your own, and in the final exercise we'll show you how that article might get turned into an MCAT-style passage.

As a reminder, when analyzing an experiment, you should be able to:

- identify the control group(s)
- extract information from graphs and data tables
- determine how the experimental group(s) change relative to the control
- determine if the results are statistically significant
- come to a reasonable conclusion about WHY the results were observed
- consider potential weaknesses in the study
- determine how to increase the power of the study
- decide what the next most logical experiment or study should be

Again, the goal of these exercises is NOT to learn content from the articles, just to get a little more comfortable reading and extracting information from them.

For the (abridged) article on pages 403–408, try to summarize the purpose of the experiment and the methods in 4–5 sentences. Consider the following mnemonic: Oh ouR Car Won't Start (ORCWS).

- O = Organism and Organization: is the research being conducted on humans or on animals or on bacteria in a petri dish, or something else? What is being done to these organisms? Are there any unique qualities to these organisms? Are there multiple groups? Is the study conducted over a long period of time with multiple data points, or is it a short-term study? Does it have a large or small n?
- R = Results: where and how are the results presented? Is it a graph? A data table? Figures and images? What is/are the independent variable(s)? What is/are the dependent variable(s)? What are the results? Do the results show correlation or cause and effect, or both? Describe.
- C = Control and Comparison: is there a control group? How does it differ from the experimental group? Is it given a placebo or nothing at all? Is it held under different conditions? If there are multiple experimental groups, how do they differ from one another? Is it a blinded study? If so, double blind or single blind?
- W = Weirdness: does anything or do any of the results stand out as unexpected?
- S = Statistics: was any sort of statistical analysis done? How is it presented? Are there error bars on a graph? Standard errors around a mean? Are there p-values? Is there an asterisk indicating statistical significance? Is there any data that is not statistically significant?

Try interpreting the data on your own before reading the results/discussion section. When you do read the discussion, consider:

- What are the conclusions of the study?
- How are the conclusions supported by the data?
- What potential weaknesses or flaws do you see in the experimental design? Are these addressed in the discussion section?
- How might this study be potentially biased?
- How might this study be improved?
- What would be the next most logical experiment?

Let's answer the above questions for the article on pages 403–408.

1. **O = Organism and Organization:**
   - Is the research being conducted on humans or on animals or on bacteria in a petri dish, or something else?

     _____

     _____

   - What is being done to these organisms?

     _____

     _____

   - Are there any unique qualities to these organisms?

     _____

     _____

   - Are there multiple groups?

     _____

     _____

   - Is the study conducted over a long period of time with multiple data points, or is it a short-term study?

     _____

     _____

   - Does it have a large or small n?

     _____

     _____

2. **R = Results:**
   - Where and how are the results presented? Is it a graph? A data table? Figures and images?

     _____

     _____

- What is/are the independent variable(s)?

  _____

  _____

- What is/are the dependent variable(s)?

  _____

  _____

- What are the results of the study?

  _____

  _____

- Do the results show correlation or cause and effect, or both? Describe.

  _____

  _____

3. **C = Control and Comparison:**
   - Is there a control group?

     _____

     _____

   - How does it differ from the experimental group? Is it given a placebo or nothing at all? Is it held under different conditions?

     _____

     _____

   - If there are multiple experimental groups, how do they differ from one another?

     _____

     _____

   - Is it a blinded study? If so, double blind or single blind?

     _____

     _____

4. **W = Weirdness:**
   - Does anything or do any of the results stand out as unexpected?

     _____

     _____

5. **S = Statistics:**
   - Was any sort of statistical analysis done?

     _____

     _____

- How is it presented? Are there error bars on a graph? Standard errors around a mean? Are there *p*-values? Is there an asterisk indicating statistical significance?

_____

_____

- Is there any data that is not statistically significant?

_____

_____

6. **Interpreting the data:**
   - What are the conclusions of the study?

_____

_____

   - How are the conclusions supported by the data?

_____

_____

   - What potential weaknesses or flaws do you see in the experimental design? Are these addressed in the discussion section?

_____

_____

   - How might this study be potentially biased?

_____

_____

   - How might this study be improved?

_____

_____

   - What would be the next most logical experiment?

_____

_____

7. **Final Summary of Experiment and Results:**

_____

_____

_____

_____

_____

_____

SOLUTIONS TO JOURNAL ARTICLE EXERCISE 2

1. **O = Organism and Organization:**
   - Is the research being conducted on humans or on animals or on bacteria in a petri dish, or something else? *Humans (33 women, 107 men).*
   - What is being done to these organisms? *A baseline drug treatment for hypertension was given to 167 people. Of those, 140 demonstrated hypertension resistant to the treatment so they were randomized to two additional drug treatment profiles with additional medication being added depending on how their blood pressure did or did not change during the trial.*
   - Are there any unique qualities to these organisms? *No unique qualities, though the study population included those with obesity, elevated levels of lipids, and/or diabetes so comorbid conditions were not excluded.*
   - Are there multiple groups? *Yes, the treatment is split into those receiving spironolactone (plus possibly furosemide and amiloride) and those receiving ramipril (plus possibly bisoprolol).*
   - Is the study conducted over a long period of time with multiple data points, or is it a short-term study? *The initial treatment ran for four weeks and the two split treatment groups ran for 12 weeks with multiple measurements taken through the duration.*
   - Does it have a large or small *n*? *The n for the study is relatively small, but it is still reasonable given the challenges in recruiting human subjects.*

2. **R = Results:**
   - Where and how are the results presented? Is it a graph? A data table? Figures and images? *The results are presented in tables and graphs as well as a figure that combines study design with part of the results.*
   - What is/are the independent variable(s)? *Time, particular drug protocol.*
   - What is/are the dependent variable(s)? *Measurement of blood pressure, B-type natriuretic peptide (BNP), diastolic dysfunction.*
   - What are the results of the study? *The treatment with sequential nephron blockage (NBD) improved resistant hypertension, while treatment with sequential renin-angiotensin system blockade (RASB) did not.*
   - Do the results show correlation or cause and effect, or both? Describe. *The results appear to be causative as both groups were subject to the same drug treatment prior to starting either of the protocols in the study and had similar demographics and conditions. Other anti-hypertension drugs were not permitted so the cause of the improvement would have been the particular drug protocol.*

3. **C = Control and Comparison:**
   - Is there a control group? *No.*
   - How does it differ from the experimental group? Is it given a placebo or nothing at all? Is it held under different conditions? *Both groups received a drug protocol. There was not a group that was not receiving treatment or simply stayed on their current treatment.*
   - If there are multiple experimental groups, how do they differ from one another? *The difference between the two groups is the administration of the NSD protocol versus the RASB protocol.*

- Is it a blinded study? If so, double blind or single blind? *Yes, double-blinded.*

4. **W = Weirdness:**
    - Does anything or do any of the results stand out as unexpected? *The lack of effectiveness of the RASB protocol was unexpected, but it does explain why more people in that group received escalating levels of treatment.*

5. **S = Statistics:**
    - Was any sort of statistical analysis done? *Yes.*
    - How is it presented? Are there error bars on a graph? Standard errors around a mean? Are there *p*-values? Is there an asterisk indicating statistical significance? *P-values, asterisk, standard errors reported on means, error bars on graphs.*
    - Is there any data that is not statistically significant? *The RASB results were not found to make a statistically significant improvement in resistant hypertension.*

6. **Interpreting the data:**
    - What are the conclusions of the study? *For those with resistant hypertension, an NBD treatment protocol would be more effective in treatment than a RASB protocol.*
    - How are the conclusions supported by the data? *The conclusions are supported based on the improvement in diastolic function, BNP, and blood pressure measurements as seen in the NBD group in comparison to the RASB group.*
    - What potential weaknesses or flaws do you see in the experimental design? Are these addressed in the discussion section? *The protocol worked to recruit across a broad range of ages (18 to 75 years), but the study population was mostly male and the paper does not report on race, ethnicity, or descriptors of the diversity of the population. The number of subjects would need to be larger and would need to be reported to match the overall impacted patient population to make further treatment recommendations.*
    - How might this study be potentially biased? *This study may be biased based on the composition of its patient population.*
    - How might this study be improved? *A larger n with reporting done on other patient demographics.*
    - What would be the next most logical experiment? *An additional trial with a larger pool of subjects run at multiple centers.*

7. **Final Summary of Experiment and Results:**
    - *In this journal article, the effect of an NBD treatment protocol for resistant hypertension was measured in comparison to a RASB treatment protocol. The study was blinded and included male and female subjects across a range of ages and conditions. Treatments were run over the course of 12 weeks with measurements including B-type natriuretic peptide, diastolic function, and blood pressure being taken. The NBD protocol was found to make a statistically significant improvement, while the RASB protocol did not.*

Chapter 11
The Muscular and
Skeletal Systems

11.1 OVERVIEW OF MUSCLE TISSUE

There are three types of muscle which differ in cellular physiology, anatomy, and function. The type we are all familiar with is **skeletal muscle** (Section 11.2), which is also known as *voluntary* muscle, because its role is to contract in response to conscious intent. The next muscle type is called **cardiac muscle** because it is found only in the wall of the heart. Skeletal and cardiac muscle are said to be **striated** because of their microscopic appearance. The third type of muscle is **smooth muscle**, which is found in the walls of all hollow organs such as the GI tract, the urinary system, the uterus, etc. It is responsible for GI motility, constriction of blood vessels, uterine contractions, and so on. We have no conscious control over cardiac or smooth muscle because they are innervated only by the autonomic nervous system. The three types of muscle share some characteristics and differ in others. In Sections 11.3 and 11.4, we characterize cardiac and smooth muscle by comparison with skeletal muscle.

11.2 SKELETAL MUSCLE

Movement of Joints

Skeletal muscle provides voluntary movement of the body in response to stimulation by somatic motor neurons, but skeletal muscle alone cannot move the body. Skeletal muscle requires the framework of the bones of the skeleton for movement to occur. Skeletal muscles are attached at each end to two different bones. Muscles are often attached to bones by **tendons**, strong connective tissue formed primarily of collagen. By contracting, skeletal muscle can draw the points of attachment on the two bones closer together. [What effect does expansion of skeletal muscle have on the two bones the muscle is connected to?[1]] Skeletal muscles can move a joint by **flexing** (reducing the angle of the joint), **extending** (increasing the angle of the joint), by **abducting** (moving away from the body's midline) or **adducting** (moving toward the body's midline), as well as many other types of movement. [Which of these movements involve contraction of skeletal muscle?[2] Does flexing the elbow bring the hand closer to or farther from the shoulder?[3]] One of the two bones joined by a skeletal muscle is generally closer to the center of the body and tends to stay in place when the muscle contracts. The point on this bone where the muscle attaches is called the **origin** of that skeletal muscle, and the point where the muscle attaches on the bone more distant from the center of the body is referred to as the muscle's **insertion**. When a muscle contracts, its insertion point is brought closer to its origin.

An example of a skeletal muscle and its action is the flexion of the elbow joint by the biceps brachii (Figure 1). The origin of this muscle lies in the shoulder joint, and the insertion lies in the bones of the forearm. Contraction of the biceps brachii brings its insertion (the forearm) closer to its origin (the shoulder). Since muscles can only *contract* to move a joint, different muscles are necessary for flexion and extension (opposite movements) of a joint. For the elbow, the *triceps* brachii (the muscle on the back of the upper

---

[1]   None. Muscle cannot expand with force. Muscle can only contract (get shorter) to cause force on bones and movement.

[2]   All of them. It is the only way to move bones and joints: by contracting skeletal muscles.

[3]   Flexing decreases the angle of a joint. If the elbow is flexed, the hand will be closer to the shoulder.

arm) is responsible for extension. [Where is the origin of the triceps brachii?[4]] The origin and the insertion for the triceps brachii are on the opposite side of the arm as for the biceps brachii, so that contraction of the triceps has the opposite effect on the lower arm as contraction of the biceps. [Do both the biceps brachii and the triceps brachii contract vigorously simultaneously to cause movement?[5]] Muscles that are responsible for movement in opposite directions are termed **antagonistic**, while muscles that move a joint in the same direction are **synergistic**. Usually, the contraction of antagonistic muscles is coordinated by the nervous system so that one muscle relaxes while the other contracts. [Do antagonistic muscles receive stimulation by neurons that release different neurotransmitters?[6]]

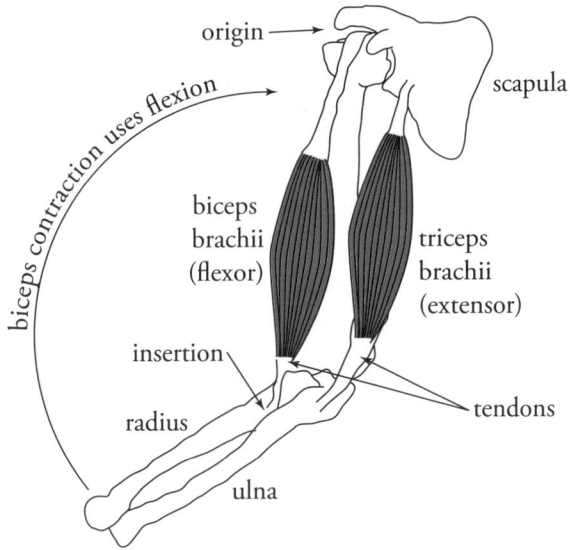

origin

scapula

biceps contraction uses flexion

biceps brachii (flexor)

triceps brachii (extensor)

insertion

radius

tendons

ulna

Figure 1   Skeletal Muscle

Structure of Skeletal Muscle

Each skeletal muscle is composed not only of muscle tissue, but also of connective tissue that holds the contractile tissue together in bundles called **fascicles** to allow flexibility within the muscle (Figure 2). Looking within each bundle, it is possible to see many fine **muscle fibers** (also called **myofibers**). Each muscle fiber is a single skeletal muscle cell. Skeletal muscle cells are **multinucleate syncytia** formed by the fusion of individual cells during development. They are innervated by a single nerve ending, and stretch the entire length of the muscle. The myofiber has a cell membrane, called the **sarcolemma**, that is made of the plasma membrane and an additional layer of polysaccharide and collagen. This additional layer helps the cell to fuse with tendon fibers. Within each skeletal muscle cell (myofiber) there are many smaller units called **myofibrils**. The myofibril in the muscle cell is like a specialized organelle; it is responsible for the striated appearance of skeletal muscle and generates the contractile force of skeletal muscle.

---

[4]   The origin of the triceps is the point of attachment nearer the center of the body, or the shoulder, on the opposite side of the biceps attachment.

[5]   Usually, no. Muscles that oppose each other's action are usually regulated by the nervous system in the opposite manner, so that one relaxes while the other contracts.

[6]   No. All skeletal muscle is innervated by somatic motor neurons which release acetylcholine at the neuromuscular junction. The difference in regulation is not the *form* of the signal (i.e., the *type* of neurotransmitter) that is sent to the muscle, but the *timing* of the signal (i.e., the *frequency* of stimulation, and thus the *amount* of neurotransmitter released).

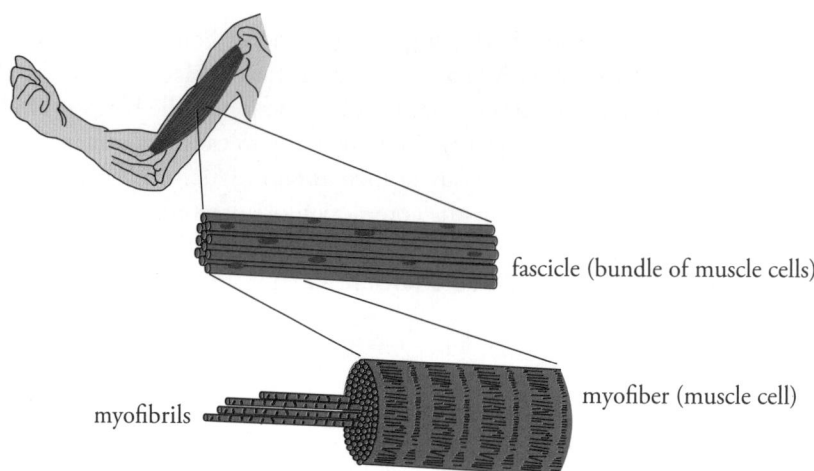

Figure 2   Levels of Skeletal Muscle Organization

The proteins in the myofibril that generate contraction are polymerized **actin** and **myosin**. Actin polymerizes to form **thin filaments** visible under the microscope, and myosin forms **thick filaments** (Figure 3). The striated appearance of skeletal muscle is due to the overlapping arrangement of bands of thick and thin filaments in **sarcomeres**. A myofibril is composed of many sarcomeres aligned end-to-end. Each sarcomere is bound by two **Z lines**. Thin filaments (actin) attach to each Z line and overlap with thick filaments (myosin) in the middle of each sarcomere; the thick filaments are not attached to the Z lines. The regions of the sarcomere composed only of thin filaments are referred to as the **I bands**. The full length of the thick filament represents the **A band** within each sarcomere; this includes both the overlapping regions of thick and thin filaments (where contraction is generated), as well as the region composed of only thick filaments (this is seen in resting sarcomeres only and is referred to as the **H zone**). See Figure 3.

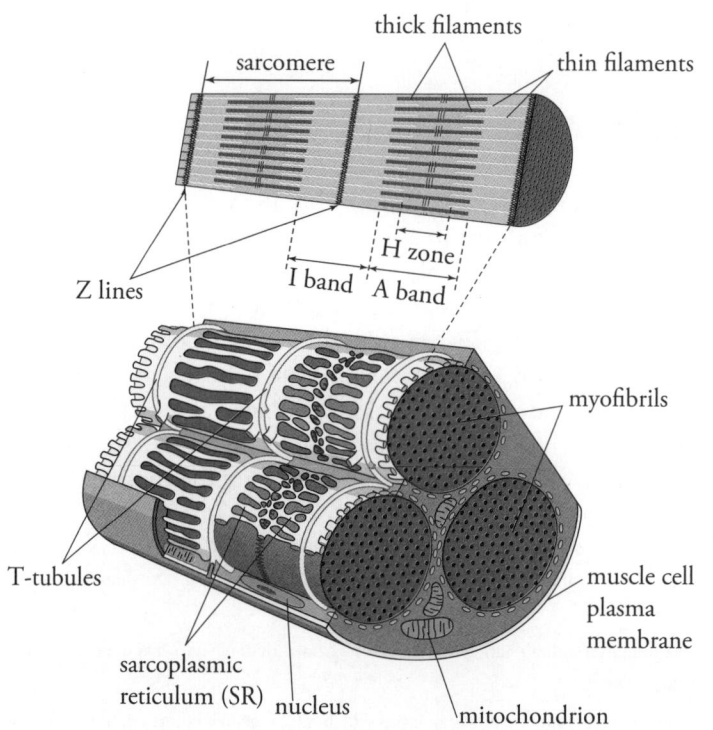

Figure 3   The Sarcomere and a Cross-Section of a Myofiber

The Sliding Filament Model of Muscle Contraction

Within each sarcomere, actin and myosin filaments overlap with each other (Figures 3 and 4). Contraction occurs when the thin and thick filaments slide across each other, drawing the Z lines of each sarcomere closer together and shortening the length of the muscle cell. [During muscle contraction, do the thin and thick filaments shorten?[7]] Filament sliding is powered by ATP hydrolysis. Myosin is an enzyme that uses the energy of ATP to create movement. (You will hear the term "myosin ATPase.") Each myosin monomer contains a **head** and a **tail**. The head attaches to a specific site on an actin molecule (the **myosin binding site**). When it is attached, myosin and actin are said to be connected by a **cross bridge**. Contraction occurs when the angle between the head and tail decreases. Filament sliding occurs in four steps. It is important to remember which step requires a new ATP molecule.

Steps of the contractile cycle:
1) Binding of the myosin head to a myosin binding site on actin, also known as **cross bridge formation**. At this stage, myosin has ADP and P_i bound.
2) The **power stroke**, in which the myosin head moves to a low-energy conformation, and pulls the actin chain toward the center of the sarcomere. ADP is released.
3) Binding of a new ATP molecule is necessary for *release* of actin by the myosin head (key!).
4) ATP hydrolysis occurs immediately and the myosin head is *cocked* (set in a high-energy conformation, like the hammer of a gun). Another cycle begins when the myosin head binds to a new binding site on the thin filament.

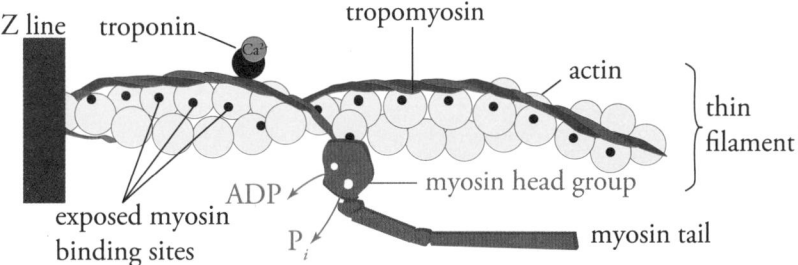

a) original position of filaments and Z line
prior to cocking of myosin head group

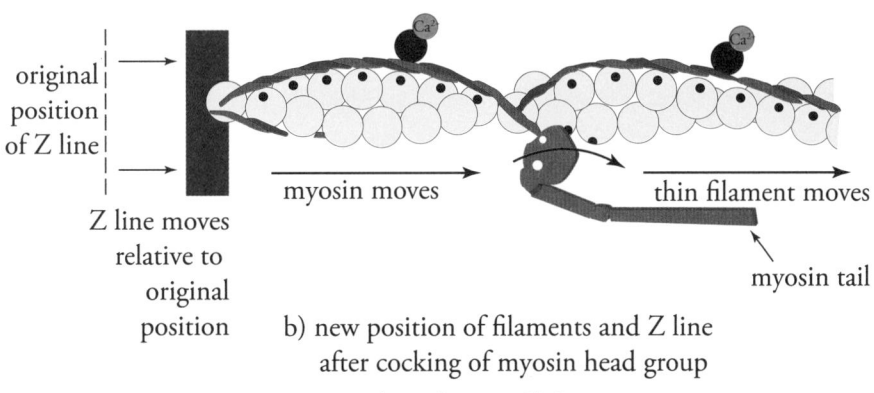

b) new position of filaments and Z line
after cocking of myosin head group

Figure 4   Filament Sliding

---

[7]   No. The thin and thick filaments slide across each other to shorten the sarcomere without themselves changing in length.

Excitation-Contraction Coupling in Skeletal Muscle

The above four steps in the contractile cycle occur spontaneously. In other words, if you put actin and myosin into a beaker and add ATP and Mg^{2+} (necessary for all reactions involving ATP), ATP will be hydrolyzed and the filaments will slide past one another. But in the myofiber, contraction occurs only when the cytoplasmic $[Ca^{2+}]$ increases. This is because in addition to polymerized actin, the thin filament contains the **troponin-tropomyosin complex** (Figure 5) that prevents contraction when Ca^{2+} is not present. **Tropomyosin** is a long fibrous protein that winds around the actin polymer, blocking all the myosin-binding sites. **Troponin** is a globular protein bound to the tropomyosin that can bind Ca^{2+}. When troponin binds Ca^{2+}, troponin undergoes a conformational change that moves tropomyosin out of the way, so that myosin heads can attach to actin and filament sliding can occur.

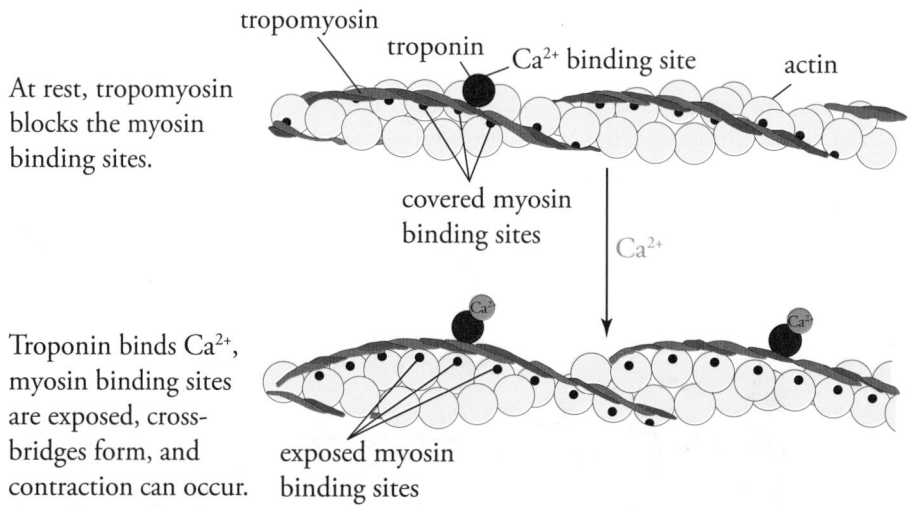

At rest, tropomyosin blocks the myosin binding sites.

Troponin binds Ca^{2+}, myosin binding sites are exposed, cross-bridges form, and contraction can occur.

Figure 5   The Troponin/Tropomyosin Complex

- What protein is responsible for ATP hydrolysis during muscle contraction?[8]
- In the absence of actin, which step in ATP hydrolysis by myosin is prevented, the hydrolysis of ATP or the release of ADP?[9]
- If troponin-tropomyosin is added to myosin and actin filaments in a test tube along with ATP, which one of the following will be true?[10]
  - A) The hydrolysis of ATP will become insensitive to the concentration of calcium.
  - B) The hydrolysis of ATP will become sensitive to the concentration of calcium.
  - C) ATP will be hydrolyzed when actin binds myosin.
  - D) ATP will be hydrolyzed during the power stroke.

---

[8]   Myosin is the protein with the ATPase activity.

[9]   In the absence of actin, myosin can still hydrolyze ATP, but it cannot release ADP after hydrolysis.

[10]   Choice **B** is correct. Without troponin-tropomyosin, ATP hydrolysis will begin as soon as ATP, actin, and myosin are mixed. In the presence of troponin-tropomyosin, myosin cannot bind actin, but if calcium is added, the troponin-tropomyosin complex allows binding and ATP hydrolysis can occur once again.

The Neuromuscular Junction and Impulse Transmission

The **neuromuscular junction** (**NMJ**) is the synapse between an axon terminus (synaptic knob) and a myofiber. The NMJ is not a single point, but rather a long trough or invagination (infolding) of the cell membrane; the axon terminus is elongated to fill the long synaptic cleft. The purpose of this arrangement is to allow the neuron to depolarize a large region of the postsynaptic membrane at once. The postsynaptic membrane (the myofiber cell membrane) is known as the **motor end plate**. ACh is the neurotransmitter at the NMJ.

Impulse transmission at the NMJ is typical of chemical synaptic transmission: an action potential arrives at the axon terminus, triggering the opening of _____ channels; the resulting increase in _____ triggers the _____ of acetylcholine.[11] The postsynaptic membrane contains ACh receptors, which are ligand-gated Na^+ channels. The ACh must reach its receptor by diffusing across the synaptic cleft. Binding of ACh to its receptor results in a postsynaptic sodium influx, which depolarizes the postsynaptic membrane. This depolarization is known as an **end plate potential** (**EPP**). The smallest measurable EPP, caused by exocytosis of a single ACh vesicle, is known as a **miniature EPP** (**MEPP**).

ACh will continue to stimulate postsynaptic receptors until it is destroyed. This is accomplished by the enzyme **acetylcholinesterase**, which hydrolyzes ACh to choline plus an acetyl unit.

As in neurons, summation is required to initiate an AP in the postsynaptic cell. In other words, a single MEPP is insufficient to cause the myofiber to contract. When a sufficient EPP occurs, threshold is reached, and _____ channels open in the postsynaptic membrane.[12] This initiates an AP in the myofiber. The AP is propagated as in neurons, by a continuing wave of voltage-gated sodium channel opening. The shape of this AP on a graph is similar to the shape of the neuronal AP (see Chapter 8).

This AP must depolarize the entire myofiber if contraction is to occur. But there is a problem: action potentials occur only at the cell surface, because they are by nature a depolarization of the cell membrane. The myofiber is so thick that an AP on its surface will not depolarize its interior. The solution is to have deep invaginations of the cell membrane, which allow the AP to travel into the thick cell. These deep infoldings are called **transverse tubules** (**T-tubules**; see Figure 3).

Another specialized membrane in the myofiber is the **sarcoplasmic reticulum** (**SR**). This is a huge, specialized smooth endoplasmic reticulum, which enfolds each myofibril in the cell (Figure 3). The SR is specialized to sequester and release Ca^{2+}. Active transporters in the SR rapidly remove calcium from the _sarcoplasm_ (myofiber cytoplasm). Then, when an AP travels down the T-tubular network, it depolarizes the cell, and with it, the SR. The SR contains voltage-gated Ca^{2+} channels, which allow Ca^{2+} to rush out of the SR into the sarcoplasm upon depolarization. The increase in sarcoplasmic $[Ca^{2+}]$ causes troponin-tropomyosin to change conformation, allowing myosin to bind actin. Actin and myosin fibers slide across each other, and the muscle fiber contracts. When the cell repolarizes, calcium is actively sequestered by the SR, and contraction is ended.

---

[11] An action potential arrives at the axon terminus, triggering the opening of **voltage-gated Ca^{2+}** channels; the resulting increase in **intracellular Ca^{2+}** triggers the **release of vesicles** of acetylcholine.

[12] voltage-gated sodium channels

Mechanics of Contraction

The smallest measurable muscle contraction is known as a muscle **twitch**. The nervous system can increase the force of contraction in two ways.

1) **Motor unit recruitment**. A motor unit is a group of myofibers innervated by the branches of a single motor neuron's axon. A muscle twitch results from the activation of one motor neuron, and a larger twitch can be obtained by activating ("recruiting") more motor neurons (and thus more myofibers).

2) **Frequency summation**. Each contraction ends when the SR returns the [Ca^{2+}] to low resting levels. If a second contraction occurs rapidly enough, however, there is insufficient time for the Ca^{2+} to be sequestered by the SR, and the second contraction builds on the first. The force of contraction increases. A rapidly repeating series of stimulations results in the strongest possible contraction, known as tetanus. This is a normal occurrence which the nervous system uses to obtain strong contractions.[13]

A note of clarification: the skeletal muscle action potential has a refractory period as does the neural AP. For frequency summation to occur, the amount of time between successive stimulations must be greater than the duration of the refractory period, but brief enough so that the cytoplasmic [Ca^{2+}] has not been returned to its low resting level.

One topic of muscle physiology which is less likely to appear on the MCAT, but worth mentioning, is the **length-tension relationship**. A muscle contracts most forcefully at an optimum length. This corresponds to a sarcomere length of 2.2 microns. The explanation is that at this length, a maximum degree of overlap between thick and thin filaments occurs. A greater sarcomere length makes the overlap smaller with fewer myosin heads able to bind to actin. A shorter length causes filaments to obstruct each other's movement by bumping together.

- The central nervous system can increase the strength of skeletal muscle contraction by:[14]
  A) increasing the size of action potentials in somatic motor neurons that innervate the muscle.
  B) increasing the number of neurons that innervate each skeletal muscle cell.
  C) increasing the number of motor neurons leading to a muscle that are firing action potentials.
  D) decreasing firing by inhibitory neurons that innervate the skeletal muscle.

Energy Storage in the Myofiber

ATP provides the energy for contraction, and supplies must be regenerated by glucose catabolism. However, glycolysis and the TCA cycle are not fast enough to keep pace with the rapid ATP utilization during

---

[13] Do not confuse this with the disease tetanus, caused by *tetanospasmin*, a bacterial toxin. The disease is an exaggerated, uncontrolled example of the normal process.

[14] Each muscle cell is innervated by a single neuron (choice B is wrong), and the more neurons that fire, the more muscle cells that will contract; the more muscle cells that contract, the greater the total force of contraction (choice **C** is correct). Action potentials are all-or-none events; the depolarization is the same size in a given neuron (choice A is wrong), and there are no inhibitory neurons that innervate the neuromuscular junction. Only acetylcholine, which is excitatory to muscle cells, is released at these synapses (choice D is wrong). (All motor neurons release a constant, small, baseline amount of ACh onto the muscle cell; this provides a baseline level of contraction that we commonly call "muscle tone." To inhibit a muscle, the amount of baseline ACh is reduced.)

extended contraction. There is a need for an *intermediate-term* energy storage molecule. **Creatine phosphate** is that molecule. During contraction, its hydrolysis drives the regeneration of ATP from ADP + P_i.

Muscle is highly aerobic tissue, with abundant mitochondria. **Myoglobin** is a globular protein and is similar to one of the four subunits of hemoglobin. The role of myoglobin is to provide an oxygen reserve by taking O_2 from hemoglobin and then releasing it as needed.

Nonetheless, during prolonged contraction, the supply of oxygen runs low, and metabolism becomes anaerobic. Lactic acid is produced and moves into the bloodstream, causing a drop in pH. The liver picks up this lactate and converts it into pyruvate, which can be used in various pathways.

Cramps may result from exhaustion of energy supplies (temporary lack of ATP) in muscle cells. **Rigor mortis** is rigidity of skeletal muscles which occurs soon after death. It results from complete ATP exhaustion; without ATP, myosin heads cannot release actin, and the muscle can neither contract nor relax.

Muscle Fiber Types

Skeletal muscle fibers generally fall into one of two categories, slow twitch fibers and fast twitch fibers. "Slow" and "fast" refer to their contractile speeds; slow twitch fibers take around three times as long as fast twitch fibers to reach their maximum tension after stimulation.

Type I Slow Twitch Fibers

These fibers are also known as **red slow twitch** or **red oxidative** fibers because of their high myoglobin content. They also have a much better blood supply than fast twitch fibers due to an extensive surrounding capillary network. The combination of good oxygen delivery from the blood stream and the ability to store oxygen on their myoglobin allows these fibers to maintain contraction for extended periods of time without fatigue. These are the fibers that allow marathoners and long distance cyclists to run or bike for hours at a time.

Type II Fast Twitch Fibers

These fibers actually fall into two subcategories according to their ability to resist fatigue. Both fiber types contract quickly, but Type IIA fast twitch fibers have more mitochondria than Type IIB fast twitch and are thus more fatigue resistant.

- *Type IIA:* also known as fast twitch oxidative fibers, these are somewhat resistant to fatigue. They cannot maintain activity for as long as slow twitch fibers can (only around 30 minutes or so), but far exceed the duration of use of the Type IIB fibers.
- *Type IIB:* also known as white fast twitch fibers due to their lack of mitochondria, these fibers contract very quickly with great force. However, they fatigue just as quickly, maxing out at around one minute of use. These are the fibers that provide the explosive force needed for jump shots and pole vaults.

Table 1 compares the three fiber types.

Table 1   Comparison of Muscle Fiber Types

Fiber type	Slow Twitch	Type IIA	Type IIB
Other names	Red slow twitch, red oxidative	Intermediate, fast twitch oxidative	White fast twitch
Speed of contraction	Slow	Intermediate	Very fast
Force generated	Low	Medium	High
Mitochondria	Many	Some	Very few
Capillaries	Very dense	Medium	Very few
Fatigue resistance	High Hours of use	Medium 30 minutes of use	Low 1 minute of use

11.3   CARDIAC MUSCLE COMPARED TO SKELETAL MUSCLE

Cardiac muscle is similar to skeletal muscle in the following ways:

1) Thick and thin filaments are organized into sarcomeres. Therefore, both cardiac and skeletal muscle are microscopically striated (striped).
2) T-tubules are present and serve the same function (transmission of APs into the interior of the large, thick cell).
3) Troponin-tropomyosin regulates contraction in the same way.
4) The length-tension relationship works the same way and is more significant in cardiac muscle. Skeletal muscle is fixed at a certain maximum length due to its attachments to bones, but cardiac muscle has no such limitations. Increasing the amount of blood that returns to the heart (e.g., through vigorous skeletal muscle contraction during exercise) can stretch cardiac muscle to optimize the length-tension relationship and maximize cardiac output, however *excess* stretch on cardiac muscle (e.g., dilation and enlargement of the heart, which can occur in heart failure) can lead to a *decrease* in contraction strength and a *decrease* in the ejection fraction (the fraction of blood the left ventricle ejects with each contraction). If the ejection fraction drops too low, death results.

Cardiac muscle is *different* from skeletal muscle in some important ways:

1) Cardiac muscle cells are not structurally syncytial (they each have only one nucleus), while skeletal muscle cells are syncytial. But all the muscle cells of the heart are interconnected by gap junctions known as **intercalated disks**, which allow action potentials to propagate throughout the entire heart without allowing nuclei and cytoplasmic contents to be shared; only small items like ions can pass. Heart muscle is thus called a ***functional* syncytium** because it acts like a syncytium (but isn't really).
2) Cardiac muscle cells are each connected to several neighbors by intercalated disks.

3) Some of the calcium required for cardiac muscle-cell contraction comes from the extracellular environment, through the voltage-gated calcium channels. In skeletal muscle, all the calcium for contraction comes from the sarcoplasmic reticulum, an intracellular structure.

4) Cardiac muscle contraction does *not* depend on stimulation by motor neurons. In fact, the most important nerve releasing ACh at chemical synapses with the heart is inhibitory! This is the vagus nerve, a parasympathetic nerve. It synapses with the sinoatrial node, where it releases ACh to inhibit spontaneous depolarization (discussed below), with the result being a slower heart rate. Contrast this with skeletal muscle innervation, in which neurons release ACh to stimulate contraction. [If neurons don't trigger cardiac contraction, what does?[15]]

5) The AP in cardiac muscle depends not only on voltage-gated sodium channels (**fast sodium channels**, as in skeletal muscle), but also on voltage-gated calcium channels. These are called **slow channels** because they respond more slowly to threshold depolarization, opening later than the fast channels and taking longer to close. The voltage-gated calcium channels cause the cardiac AP to have the distinctive plateau shown in Figure 6.

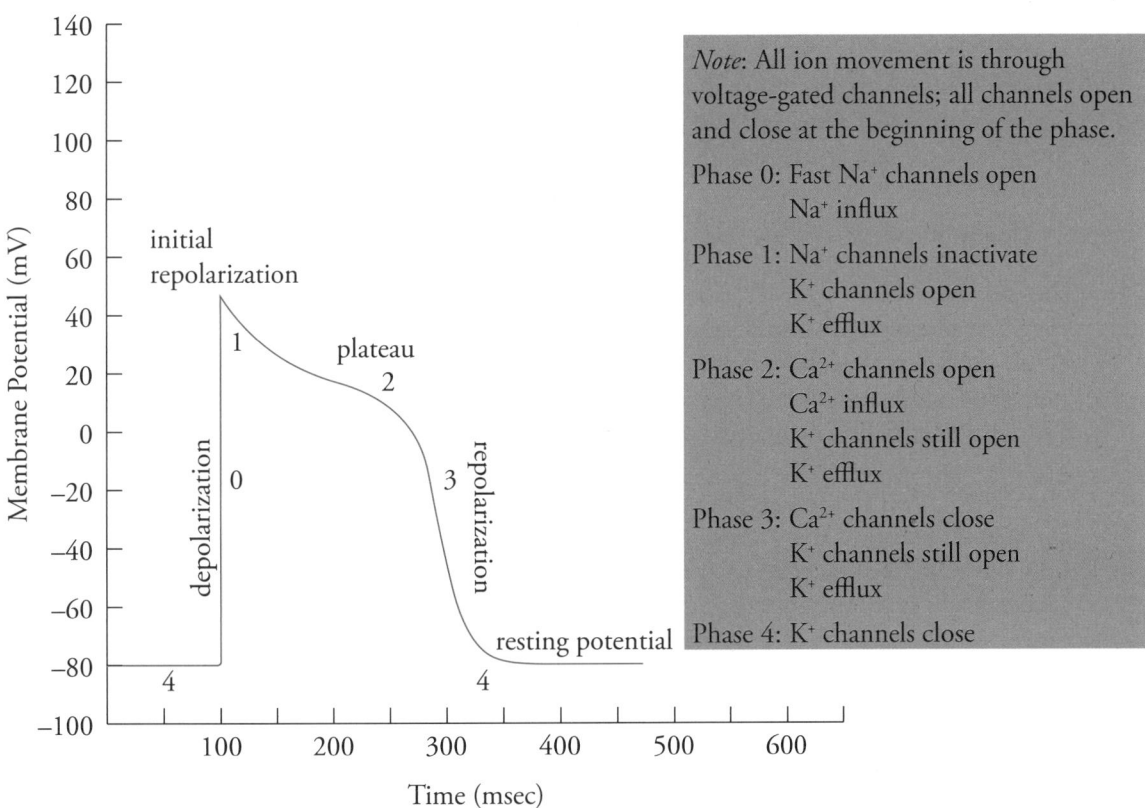

Figure 6   The Cardiac Muscle Cell Action Potential

The significance of the plateau phase is twofold: 1) a longer duration of contraction facilitates ventricular emptying (better ejection fraction), and 2) a longer refractory period helps prevent disorganized transmission of impulses throughout the heart, and makes summation and tetanus impossible. This is

---

[15]   Pacing by the sinoatrial node, as discussed in Chapter 9.

advantageous because the heart must relax after each contraction. So remember: skeletal muscle cells and neurons have the same steeply spiking AP, while cardiac muscle cells have a spike and a plateau. Figure 6 shows the phases of the cardiac action potential. This was discussed in more detail in Chapter 9.

11.4   SMOOTH MUSCLE COMPARED TO SKELETAL MUSCLE

Smooth muscle is like skeletal muscle in that contraction is accomplished by sliding of actin and myosin filaments; the four-step contractile cycle is the same. Another similarity is that contraction is triggered by an increase in cytoplasmic $[Ca^{2+}]$. Like skeletal muscle cells, smooth muscle cells do not branch. However, smooth muscle is different from skeletal muscle in many ways:

1) Smooth muscle cells are much narrower and shorter than skeletal muscle cells.
2) T-tubules are *not* present. The smooth muscle cell is so small that they are unnecessary; a depolarization on the surface can depolarize the entire cell.
3) Each smooth muscle cell has only one nucleus and is connected to its neighbors by gap junctions (like cardiac muscle cells) which allow impulses to spread from cell to cell. Thus, both smooth and cardiac muscle are functional syncytia.
4) Thick and thin filaments are not organized into sarcomeres in smooth muscle. Instead they are dispersed in the cytoplasm. This is why the cell appears smooth instead of striated (no regular A band, H zone, etc.).
5) The troponin–tropomyosin complex is not present. Instead, contraction is regulated by **calmodulin** and **myosin light-chain kinase** (**MLCK**). In brief, calmodulin binds Ca^{2+} and then activates MLCK. MLCK phosphorylates a portion of the myosin molecule, thus activating its enzymatic/mechanical activity.
6) While skeletal muscles rely heavily on Ca^{2+} from sarcoplasmic reticulum, the SR in smooth muscles is poorly developed. It stores some Ca^{2+} that can be released upon depolarization, but the cell also relies heavily on extracellular stores of Ca^{2+} for contraction.
7) The smooth muscle cell action potential varies depending on the location of the smooth muscle cell. Most smooth muscle cells can elicit action potentials (also called **spike potentials**) similar to skeletal muscle action potentials, but since smooth muscle cells have almost no sodium fast channels and their action potential is determined by slow channels only, it takes ten to twenty times as long as a skeletal muscle action potential (Figure 7).
8) Some smooth muscle that must sustain prolonged contractions (such as the uterus or vascular smooth muscle) has action potentials similar to those of cardiac muscle, although with a less-sharp spike.
9) Smooth muscles have a constantly fluctuating resting potential. Ions pass through the gap junctions between neighboring cells, causing the changes in resting potential to propagate like waves through the connected smooth muscle cells. These fluctuations in resting potential are called "slow waves." Slow waves are NOT spike potentials and do NOT elicit muscle contractions, but they are necessary to help *coordinate* the action potentials. In response to local stimuli (e.g., stretching of smooth muscle in the gut wall due to a food bolus), neurotransmitter from parasympathetic neurons is released. The neurotransmitter binds to receptors on smooth muscle cells and primes them for an action potential by pushing their electrical potential closer to threshold. Slow waves then pass through these "primed" smooth muscle cells, they reach threshold and undergo an action (spike) potential (Figure 7). The amplitude of these slow waves is increased by ACh and decreased by NE (e.g., stimulating the gut during a parasympathetic response, and slowing it down during a sympathetic one).

10) Like skeletal muscle, smooth muscles are innervated by motor neurons, but in the case of smooth muscle, they are *autonomic* motor neurons instead of somatic motor neurons. Individual neurons do activate smooth muscle cells (as in skeletal muscle), but, as mentioned previously, the action potential then spreads from cell to cell. (Recall that in skeletal muscle, each action potential is limited to one large myofiber, while the heart is one large functional syncytium in which each action potential spreads to every cell. Therefore, regarding innervation and the spread of impulses, smooth muscle shares features of both skeletal and cardiac muscle.)

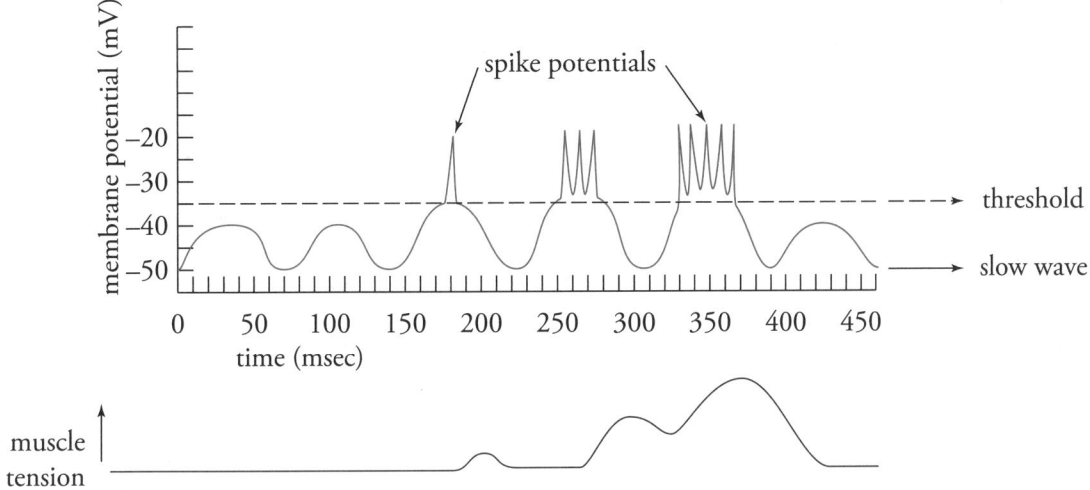

Acetylcholine increases amplitude of slow wave.
Norepinephrine decreases amplitude of slow wave.

Figure 7   The Smooth Muscle Cell Spike Potential and Slow Waves

Table 2 Comparison of Skeletal, Cardiac, and Smooth Muscle

11.4

Feature	Skeletal Muscle	Cardiac Muscle	Smooth Muscle
Appearance	Striated	Striated	No striations
Upstroke of action potential	Inward Na^+ current	Inward Ca^{2+} (SA node) Inward Na^+ (atria, ventricles, Purkinje)	Inward Na^+
Plateau	No	Yes (except for SA node)	No
Duration of AP	2–3 msec	150 msec (SA node) 300 msec (other cells)	20 msec
Calcium from	AP opens voltage-gated Ca^{2+} channels in SR, Ca^{2+} released from SR	AP opens voltage-gated Ca^{2+} channels, inward Ca^{2+} current during plateau Ca^{2+}-induced-Ca^{2+} release from SR	AP opens Ca^{2+} channels in cell membrane, inward Ca^{2+} current
Molecular basis for contraction	Ca^{2+} troponin binding	Ca^{2+} troponin binding	Ca^{2+} calmodulin binding, myosin light-chain kinase activation
Functional syncytium	No	Yes	Yes
Contraction dependent on extracellular Ca^{2+}	No	Partially	Yes

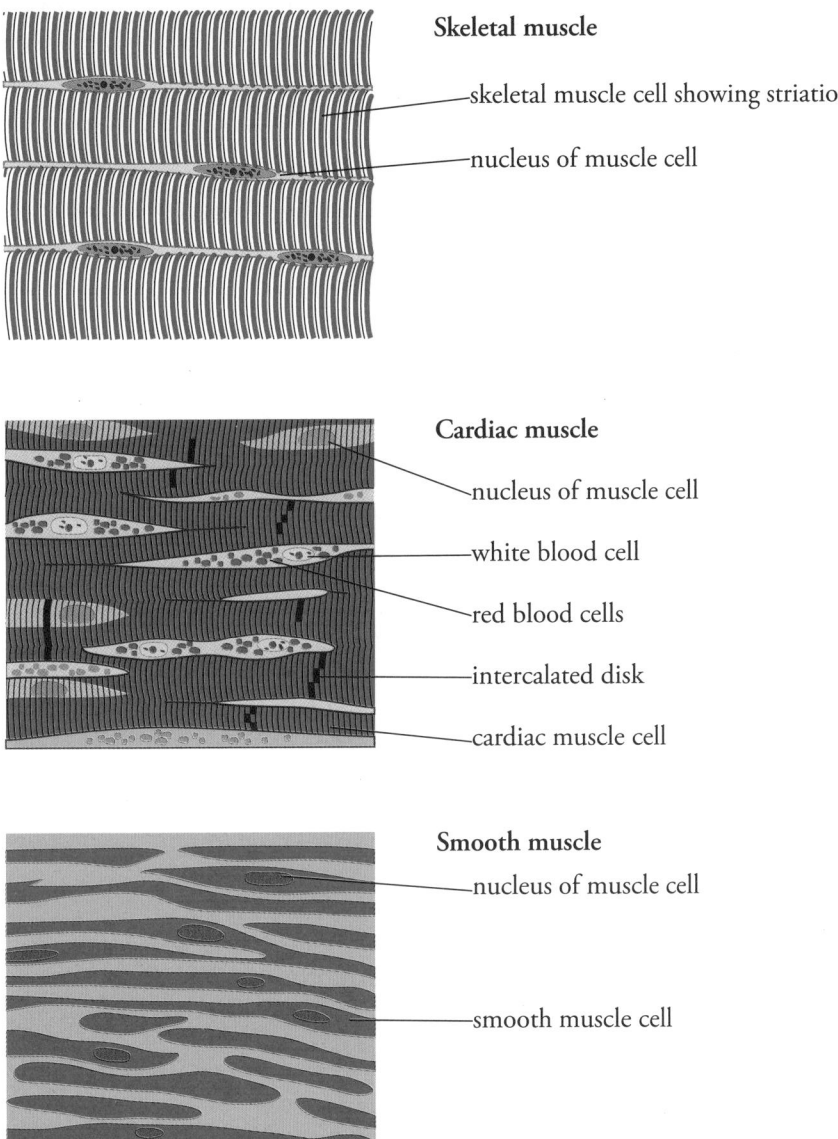

Figure 8 Three Types of Muscle Tissue

11.5 OVERVIEW OF THE SKELETAL SYSTEM

As vertebrates, we have an **endoskeleton** made of bone. This contrasts with the chitinous exoskeleton of arthropods. The vertebrate skeletal system serves five roles:

1) support the body
2) provide the framework for movement
3) protect vital organs (brain, heart, etc.)
4) store calcium
5) synthesize the formed elements of the blood (red blood cells, white blood cells, platelets). This occurs in the marrow of flat bones and is called **hematopoiesis**.

The vertebrate endoskeleton is divided into **axial** and **appendicular** components. The axial skeleton consists of the skull, the vertebral column, and the rib cage. All other bones are part of the appendicular skeleton (see Figure 9).

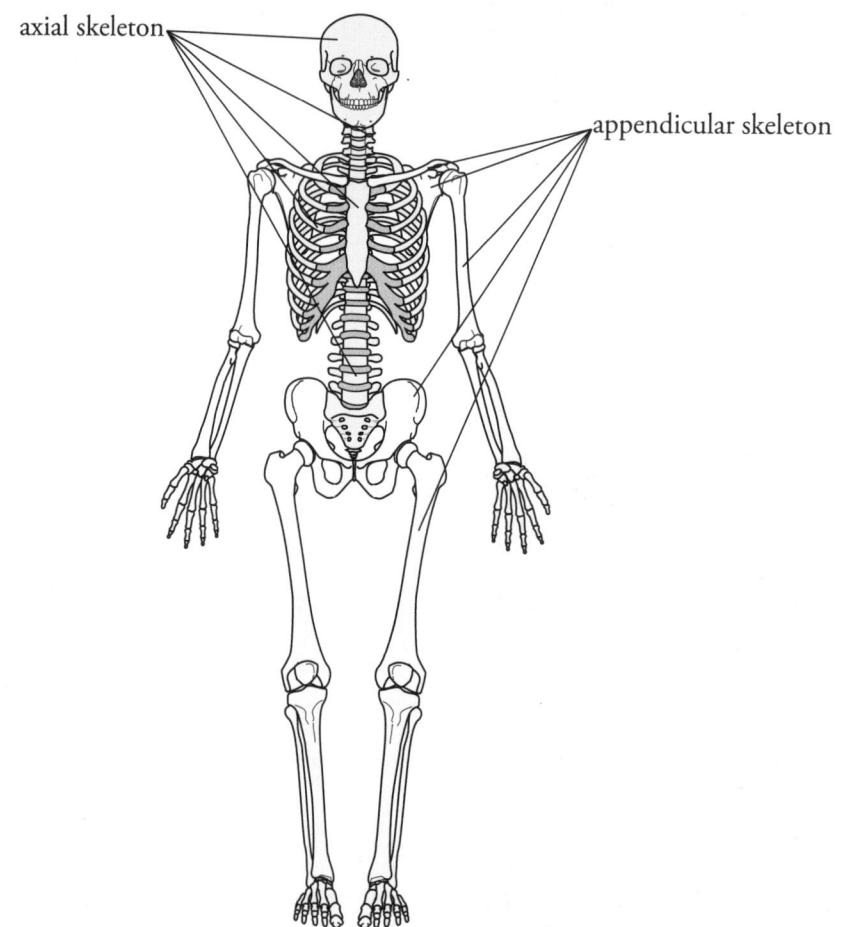

axial skeleton

appendicular skeleton

Figure 9 Axial and Appendicular Skeletons

11.6   CONNECTIVE TISSUE

Bone is an example of **connective tissue**. Connective tissue consists of cells and the materials they secrete. All connective tissue cells are derived from a single progenitor, the **fibroblast**. This name derives from its ability to secrete fibrous material such as **collagen**, a strong fibrous protein. Another important fibrous extracellular protein is **elastin**, which gives tissue the ability to stretch and regain its shape. Fibroblast-derived cells include **adipocytes** (fat cells), **chondrocytes** (cartilage cells), and **osteocytes** (bone cells).

Connective tissue differs from the other tissue types in the body (epithelial, muscle, and nervous tissue) because it is primarily extracellular material with a few cells scattered in it (the other three tissue types are the opposite; mostly cellular, with little extracellular material). The extracellular material is known as the **matrix** and consists of the fibers described above and **ground substance**, a thick, viscous material. The main ingredients of the ground substance are proteoglycans; these are large macropolymers consisting of a protein core with many attached carbohydrate chains. The carbohydrate chains are called glycosaminoglycans (GAGs) and like all carbohydrates, they are very hydrophilic. Hence, in the body, they are always surrounded by a large amount of water ("water of solvation"). This gives tissues their characteristic thickness and firmness. For example, dehydration results in saggy skin because of decreased hydration of the ground substance in the extracellular matrix.

There are two types of connective tissue: loose and dense. **Loose connective tissues** are basically packing tissues, and include areolar tissue (the soft material located between most cells throughout the body) and adipose tissue (fat). **Dense connective tissue** refers to tissues that contain large amounts of fibers (especially collagen), such as tendons, ligaments, cartilage, and bone. Cartilage and bone are sometime classified as supportive connective tissues, because of the role they play in physical support of body structures.

11.7   BONE STRUCTURE

Macroscopic

There are two primary bone shapes: **flat** and **long**. Flat bones, such as the scapula, the ribs, and the bones of the skull, are the location of hematopoiesis and are important for protection of organs. The bones of the limbs are long bones, important for support and movement. The main shaft of a long bone is called the **diaphysis**. The flared end is called the **epiphysis**.

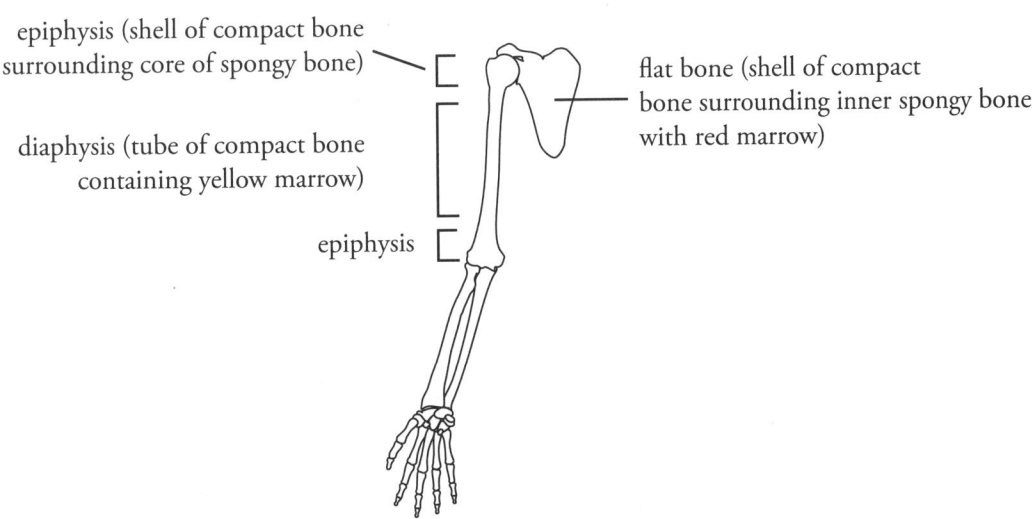

epiphysis (shell of compact bone surrounding core of spongy bone)

flat bone (shell of compact bone surrounding inner spongy bone with red marrow)

diaphysis (tube of compact bone containing yellow marrow)

epiphysis

Figure 10   Gross Anatomy of Bone

The general structure of bone may be either **compact** or **spongy**. As the names imply, compact bone is hard and dense while spongy bone is porous. Spongy bone is always surrounded by a layer of compact bone. The diaphysis of long bones is a tube composed only of compact bone.

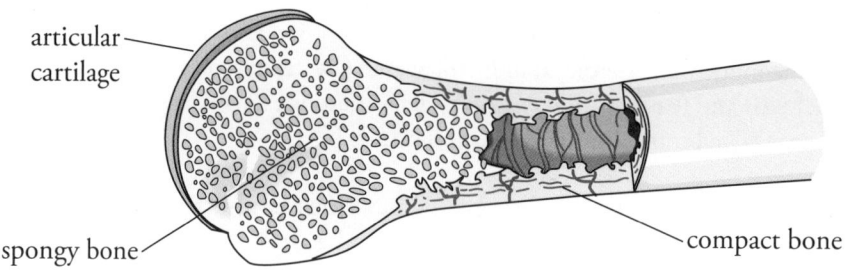

Figure 11 Compact and Spongy Bone

Bone marrow is non-bony material found in the shafts of long bones and in the pores of spongy bones. **Red marrow**, found in spongy bone within flat bones, is the site of hematopoiesis. Its activity increases in response to erythropoietin, a hormone made by the kidney. **Yellow marrow**, found in the shafts of long bones, is filled with fat and is inactive.

Microscopic

Bone is composed of two principal ingredients: collagen and **hydroxyapatite**, which is a solid material consisting of calcium phosphate crystals. During bone synthesis, collagen is laid down in a highly ordered structure. Then, hydroxyapatite crystals form around the collagen framework, giving bone its characteristic strength and inflexibility.

Spongy bone under the microscope looks like a sponge. It has a disorganized structure in which many spikes of bone surround marrow-containing cavities. The spikes of bone in spongy bone are called **spicules** or **trabeculae**.

Compact bone has a specific organization (Figure 12). The basic unit of compact bone structure is the **osteon** (sometimes referred to as a **Haversian system**). In the center of the osteon is a hole called the **central** (or **Haversian**) **canal**, which contains blood, lymph vessels, and nerves. Surrounding the canal are concentric rings of bone termed **lamellae** (which just means "sheets" or "layers"). Tiny channels, or **canaliculi**, branch out from the central canal to spaces called **lacunae** ("lakes"). In each lacuna is an **osteocyte**, or mature bone cell. Osteocytes have long processes which extend down the canaliculi to contact other osteocytes through gap junctions. This allows the cells to exchange nutrients and waste through an otherwise impermeable membrane. **Perforating** (or **Volkmann's**) **canals** are channels that run perpendicular to central canals to connect osteons.

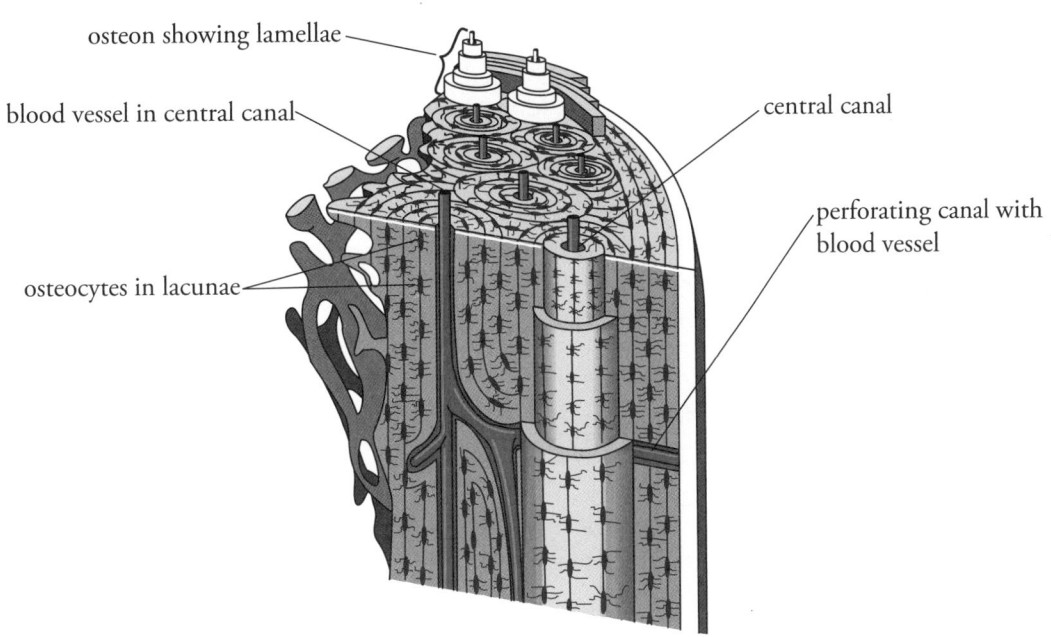

osteon showing lamellae

blood vessel in central canal

central canal

perforating canal with blood vessel

osteocytes in lacunae

Figure 12 Microscopic Structure of Compact Bone

11.8 TISSUES FOUND AT JOINTS

Cartilage

Cartilage is a strong but very flexible extracellular tissue secreted by cells called **chondrocytes**. There are three types of cartilage: hyaline, elastic, and fibrous. **Hyaline cartilage** is strong and somewhat flexible. The larynx and trachea are reinforced by hyaline cartilage, and joints are lined by hyaline cartilage known as **articular cartilage**, as shown in Figure 11. **Elastic cartilage** is found in structures (such as the outer ear and the epiglottis) that require support and more flexibility than hyaline cartilage can provide; it contains elastin. **Fibrous cartilage** is very rigid and is found in places where very strong support is needed, such as the pubic symphysis (the anterior connection of the pelvis) and the intervertebral disks of the spinal column. Cartilage is not innervated and does not contain blood vessels (it is **avascular**). It receives nutrition and immune protection from the surrounding fluid. [Why do cartilage injuries take a long time to heal?[16]]

Ligaments, Tendons, and Joints

Ligaments and tendons are strong tissues composed of dense connective tissue. **Ligaments** connect bones to other bones, and **tendons** connect bones to muscles. The point where one bone meets another is called a **joint**. Immovable joints, called **synarthroses**, are basically points where two bones are fused together. For example, the skull is formed from many fused bones. Slightly movable joints, called **amphiarthroses**, provide both movability and a great deal of support (*amphi-* means "both"). The vertebral joints are

---

[16] Cells in cartilage are not directly supplied by blood and have a low rate of metabolism. Thus, they are slow to repair damage. Often the damaged cartilage is simply removed or repaired surgically.

an example. Freely movable joints (i.e., most of the joints in the body) are called **diarthroses**. There are several types, for example, ball and socket (hip, shoulder) and hinge (elbow). All movable joints are supported by ligaments.

Movable joints are lubricated by **synovial fluid**, which is kept within the joint by the **synovial capsule**. The surfaces of the two bones that contact each other are perfectly smooth because they are lined by special **articular cartilage** (composed of hyaline cartilage). Like all cartilage, articular cartilage lacks blood vessels. Hence, it is easily damaged by overuse or infection. Inflammation of joints (**arthritis**) leads to destruction of the articular cartilage, which causes pain and stiffness.

11.9 BONE GROWTH AND REMODELING; THE CELLS OF BONE

Growth of long bones proceeds as follows: during childhood, a structure called the **epiphyseal plate** is seen between the diaphysis and the epiphysis. The epiphyseal plate is a disk of hyaline cartilage that is actively being produced by chondrocytes. As the chondrocytes divide, the epiphysis and diaphysis are forced apart. Then the cartilage is replaced by bone (ossified). This process is stimulated by growth hormone, and the rate of ossification is slightly faster than the rate of chondrocyte cell division (cartilage growth). Thus, at about the age of 18, the diaphysis and epiphyses meet and fuse together, and lengthening can no longer occur. This "fusion of the epiphyses" is easily observed in X-rays and can be used to notify adolescents when they have stopped growing taller. In adults, the fusion point is referred to as the **epiphyseal line**.

During adulthood, bones do not elongate. However, bone is continually degraded and remade in a process termed **remodeling**. The cells which make bone by laying down collagen and hydroxyapatite are called **osteoblasts**. The osteoblast synthesizes bone until it is surrounded by bone. The space it is left in is now called a lacuna, and the osteoblast is now called an **osteocyte**. Cells called **osteoclasts** continually destroy bone by dissolving the hydroxyapatite crystals. The osteoclast is a large phagocytic cousin of the macrophage. Bone destroyed by osteoclasts must be replaced by osteoblasts.

An increased ratio of osteoclast to osteoblast activity results in the liberation of calcium and phosphate into the bloodstream (and a decreased ratio has the opposite effect). Thus, activity of these cells is important not only for bone structure, but also for maintenance of proper blood levels of calcium and phosphate. The hormones **PTH (parathyroid hormone)**, **calcitonin**, and **calcitriol** (derived by the kidney from vitamin D) regulate their activity and thus blood calcium levels. PTH and calcitriol increase blood calcium, and calcitonin reduces it. The specific effects of these hormones are listed in Table 3.

Table 3 Hormonal Control of Calcium Homeostasis

Hormone	Effect on bones	Effect on kidneys	Effect on intestines
PTH	stimulates osteoclast activity	increases reabsorption of calcium, stimulates conversion of vitamin D into calcitriol	indirectly (via calcitriol) increases intestinal calcium absorption
calcitriol	may stimulate osteoclast activity, but minor effect	increases reabsorption of phosphorus	increases intestinal absorption of calcium
calcitonin	inhibits osteoclast activity	decreases reabsorption of calcium	n/a

Chapter 11 Summary

- There are three types of muscle tissue: skeletal, cardiac, and smooth.

- Skeletal muscles are voluntary, striated, multinucleate, and attached to the bones. They are individually innervated.

- The group of skeletal muscle cells controlled by a single neuron is called a motor unit, and each muscle is made of several motor units. All the cells in a motor unit contract together; to increase the strength of a contraction, additional motor units are recruited.

- Skeletal muscles are bundled into fascicles of many myofibers (cells), which are composed of myofibrils (strings of sarcomeres).

- Actin and myosin are organized into sarcomeres, which are the contractile units of the skeletal muscle cell. The arrangement of actin and myosin produces a characteristic banding pattern (striations): A band, I band, A band, I band, etc. Overlap of actin and myosin during the sliding filament theory produces sarcomere shortening.

- The four steps of the sliding filament theory involve the binding of myosin to actin (crossbridge formation), the pulling of actin toward the center of the sarcomere (power stroke), the release of actin (ATP binding), and resetting myosin to a high-energy conformation (ATP hydrolysis).

- Depolarization of the muscle cell triggers the release of calcium into the cytosol from the sarcoplasmic reticulum. Calcium binds to troponin, changing its shape, and subsequently changing the position of the tropomyosin to which the troponin is bound. This exposes the myosin binding sites on actin and allows contraction to occur. This is known as excitation-contraction coupling.

- Slow twitch fibers contract slowly, but have many mitochondria and a good blood supply, so are fatigue resistant.

- Fast twitch fibers contract quickly. Type IIA fibers have some mitochondria and are somewhat fatigue resistant, while Type IIB fibers lack mitochondria and fatigue quickly.

- Cardiac muscle is also striated, meaning that it, too, is organized into sarcomeres. Sliding filaments and excitation-contraction occur as in skeletal muscle. However, cardiac muscle is involuntary and autorhythmic. The cells are uninuclear and connected by gap junctions to form a functional syncytium.

- Cardiac muscle cells have an action potential that includes a long plateau phase. The plateau is the result of the opening of voltage-gated Ca^{2+} channels.

- Smooth muscle lacks striations and sarcomeres; however, calcium is still needed for smooth muscle cells to contract. They are involuntary.

- Bone is a dense connective tissue that functions primarily in body support and protection. Bones also play a role in mineral storage; resorption and deposition of bone is regulated by parathyroid hormone and calcitonin, respectively, to regulate blood calcium levels.

- Compact bone is organized into osteons, long cylinders of hard, dense bone. Compact bone forms the outer shell of all bones and the shaft (diaphysis) of long bones.

- Spongy bone contains much more space than compact bone and is filled with red bone marrow; this is where blood cell formation takes place. Spongy bone forms the core of flat bones and is found at the ends (epiphyses) of long bones.

CHAPTER 11 FREESTANDING PRACTICE QUESTIONS

1. Which of the following is NOT true regarding smooth muscle cells?

A) They are uninucleate and relatively small in size compared to skeletal muscle.
B) Gap junctions may exist between adjacent smooth muscle cells.
C) Ca^{2+} influx and binding to troponin results in actin and myosin binding and contraction.
D) They lack striations due to nonlinear alignment of the sarcomeres.

2. Rigor mortis, the stiffening of body limbs after death, is due to:

A) the inability of the myosin head to detach from actin due to loss of ATP.
B) the inability of the myosin head to attach to actin due to the loss of ATP.
C) the inability of the myosin head to detach from actin due to loss of ADP.
D) the inability of the myosin head to attach to actin due to the loss of ADP.

3. The neurotransmitter released at somatic axon synapses is:

A) dopamine.
B) norepinephrine.
C) acetylcholine.
D) epinephrine.

4. Lambert-Eaton syndrome is characterized by the formation of antibodies to voltage-gated calcium channels, rendering them inactive. Which of the following processes involved in generating a muscle contraction would be directly affected?

A) Saltatory conduction
B) Release of neurotransmitter at the synaptic cleft
C) Binding of neurotransmitter at the muscle end plate
D) Release of calcium from the sarcoplasmic reticulum

5. Which of the following is a possible way to distinguish between muscle types?

A) Skeletal muscle can contract via peristalsis, while smooth muscle cannot.
B) Skeletal muscle contraction depends on motor neuron stimulation, while cardiac muscle does not.
C) Cardiac muscle cells are syncytial, while smooth muscle cells are not.
D) Cardiac muscle contractions are regulated by influxes of calcium, while smooth muscle is not.

6. A young patient is found to have signs and symptoms of osteoporosis, or decreased bone density. The patient undergoes a variety of studies and is found to have a tumor secreting excessive levels of a particular hormone. What hormone could this tumor be secreting?

A) Parathyroid hormone
B) Calcitonin
C) Vitamin D
D) Thyroxine

7. Bisphosphonates are drugs that prevent the loss of bone mass and are used to treat osteoporosis and similar diseases. Which of the following is the most likely mechanism of action for this drug class?

A) Osteoblast inhibition
B) Osteoclast inhibition
C) Stimulation of PTH
D) Calcitonin inhibition

8. Synovial fluid is an essential lubricant for highly movable joints. Which of the following joints does not have synovial fluid?

A) Shoulder
B) Hip
C) Finger
D) Cranium (frontal-parietal)

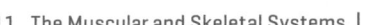

CHAPTER 11 PRACTICE PASSAGE

Peristaltic smooth muscle contractions of the small intestine are essential to digestion and are under the control of two competing neural pathways, noradrenergic and cholinergic. Stimulation of noradrenergic fibers causes the release of norepinephrine and epinephrine, which inhibit smooth muscle contractions. Stimulation of cholinergic fibers causes the release of acetylcholine (ACh), which stimulates smooth muscle contractions. These two systems work together to regulate smooth muscle contraction and digestion.

The regulatory effects of these two competing nervous pathways have been demonstrated in the laboratory. To study the effects of cholinergic and noradrenergic neural stimulation on smooth muscle contraction in the rabbit, various concentrations of ACh, norepinephrine, and epinephrine were applied to the ileum of a rabbit.

Experiment:

Step 1: A 2- to 3-cm strip of mature rabbit ileum was removed from an animal and was attached to a kymograph, a device designed especially for the study of muscle contractions. Preparation temperature was maintained between 35°C and 36°C, and the sample was kept well-aerated. Acetylcholine was applied to stimulate contractions and then epinephrine was added to the preparation in concentrations ranging from 0.4 to 0.8 μg per l00 mL of bath solution. This was done in order to determine the minimum dose required to inhibit contractions.

Step 2: The same procedure was repeated using norepinephrine in similar concentrations.

Step 3: ACh was added to restimulate muscle contractions. After a one-minute waiting period, epinephrine was added in order to determine its depressive effect. One minute later, ACh was reapplied to the preparation in order to determine its excitatory effect.

Results: When norepinephrine and epinephrine concentrations were increased relative to constant ACh levels, muscle contractions were predictably and significantly inhibited. The degree of inhibition was directly proportional to the relative amounts of noradrenergic and cholinergic neurotransmitters present.

1. Which of the following activities will NOT cause the release of epinephrine in large quantities?

A) Digesting food one hour after a large meal
B) Watching a frightening movie
C) Running in the second half of a marathon
D) Performing a difficult task under pressure

2. After a meal, when will the greatest amount of acetylcholine be released?

A) Within the first two hours
B) After 6 hours
C) After 10 hours
D) After an all-night fast

3. In the experiment, muscle contractions were significantly decreased because epinephrine causes:

A) an immediate increase in levels of ACh.
B) an increase in smooth muscle fiber nervous stimulation.
C) a decrease in the number of cholinergic fibers.
D) a decrease in the effect of acetylcholine on smooth muscle activity.

4. To conclude that both epinephrine and acetylcholine are supplied to stomach smooth muscle by nerve fibers, what information would be necessary?

A) Denervation of rabbit stomach muscle decreases food absorption.
B) Denervation of rabbit stomach muscle decreases both contractions and inhibition of contractions.
C) Epinephrine has an antagonistic effect to acetylcholine.
D) Acetylcholine and epinephrine have similar functional groups.

5. In stimulating peristaltic activity, acetylcholine is an organic molecule that has the effect of causing:

A) a decrease in actin–myosin contractions due to increased intracellular Ca^{2+} concentration.

B) a decrease in actin–myosin contractions due to decreased ATP concentration.

C) an increase in actin–myosin contractions due to increased intracellular Ca^{2+} concentration.

D) an increase in actin–myosin contractions due to decreased ATP concentration.

6. Why was the degree of inhibition in the experiment directly proportional to the relative amounts of neurotransmitters?

A) Acetylcholine and epinephrine bind to each other in the synapse in a one-to-one ratio.

B) Inhibition and excitation cause opposing ion fluxes.

C) After a certain point, acetylcholine's effects dominate over epinephrine's.

D) After a certain point, only excitatory effects are registered by the cell.

SOLUTIONS TO CHAPTER 11 FREESTANDING PRACTICE QUESTIONS

1. **C** It is important to remember that smooth muscle is activated very differently from cardiac or skeletal muscle. Smooth muscle lacks troponin and tropomyosin and utilizes other regulatory enzymes including MLCK, or myosin light-chain kinase. All the other statements are true regarding smooth muscle (choices A, B, and D can be eliminated).

2. **A** During muscle contraction, the binding of ATP to the myosin head group is required to detach myosin from the actin filament. If there is no detachment (myosin and actin remain connected), the muscles remain stiff and immovable (choices B and D are wrong). Because ATP formation is an active process that requires living cells, levels of ATP decline rapidly after death, and ADP levels rise correspondingly. Thus, it is the lack of ATP after death that leads to rigor mortis (choice A is correct, and choice C is wrong). Note that this is a two-by-two question: a single piece of information can be used to eliminate two answer choices.

3. **C** Somatic axons stimulate skeletal muscle, so the synapse under discussion is the motor end plate, and acetylcholine is always released at the motor end plate. Dopamine is a neurotransmitter used in the brain (choice A is wrong), norepinephrine is the neurotransmitter secreted by sympathetic neurons (choice B is wrong), and epinephrine is a hormone (choice D is wrong).

4. **B** Release of neurotransmitter from the axon terminal is dependent upon calcium influx from voltage-gated channels, and is greatly impaired in Lambert-Eaton syndrome (choice B is correct). Saltatory conduction is primarily dependent on sodium channels, not calcium (choice A is wrong), binding of neurotransmitter at the motor end plate does not depend on calcium (choice C is wrong), and although the calcium channels of the sarcoplasmic reticulum are voltage-gated, they are intracellular and are not likely to encounter antibodies (choice D is wrong).

5. **B** It is true that skeletal muscle contraction depends on motor neuron stimulation; remember that skeletal muscles are voluntary. However, cardiac muscle is not voluntary; contraction is controlled by the sinoatrial node. This is a possible way to distinguish between these muscle types (choice B is correct). Smooth muscle, not skeletal muscle, contracts using peristalsis, such as in the digestive tract (choice A is wrong). Cardiac muscle cells form a functional syncytium; the cells are connected by gap junctions and function as unit. Smooth muscle also functions in this manner (choice C is wrong). All muscle contractions are regulated by influxes of calcium (choice D is wrong).

6. **A** The patient is described as having signs and symptoms of decreased bone density. This could be the result of either excessive bone resorption or poor bone formation. Of the hormones listed, parathyroid is known to cause bone resorption by stimulating osteoclasts. Calcitonin functions to inhibit osteoclasts, preventing bone resorption (choice B is wrong). Excessive levels of vitamin D would result in increased calcium absorption in the small intestine and, more likely, subsequent bone formation (choice C is wrong). Thyroxine is not involved in calcium regulation (choice D is wrong).

7. **B**   Osteoporosis is a disease where bone mineral density is reduced due to increased bone resorption. The cells that are responsible for resorbing bone matrix are osteoclasts; these are stimulated by PTH and inhibited by calcitonin. In contrast, osteoblasts build bone and are stimulated by calcitonin. If bisphosphonates help prevent bone loss, they must either inhibit bone resorption or stimulate bone building. Inhibiting osteoclasts would reduce bone resorption and could be a mechanism of action of bisphosphonates (choice B is correct). Inhibiting osteoblasts is the opposite effect and would not help build bone (choice A is wrong); an increase of PTH stimulates osteoclasts and would increase bone resorption (choice C is wrong). Calcitonin reduces osteoclast activity and stimulates osteoblasts, so inhibiting calcitonin would not help bone loss (choice D is wrong).

8. **D**   Synovial fluid lubricates movable joints. Of the joints listed, the only stationary one is the frontal-parietal joint or the frontal-parietal suture (choices A, B, and C are wrong).

SOLUTIONS TO CHAPTER 11 PRACTICE PASSAGE

1. **A**   In general, the sympathetic nervous system, which releases epinephrine at postganglionic synapses, is stimulated by the "fight or flight" response. Choices B, C, and D will all stimulate the sympathetic nervous system and cause the release of epinephrine. However, digestion (choice A) stimulates the parasympathetic nervous system, which releases acetylcholine at the post-ganglionic synapse; choice A is correct.

2. **A**   Digestion quickly causes stimulation of the parasympathetic nervous system, which in turn stimulates secretion and motility in the GI tract. The response should be strongest while digestion is occurring (choice A is the best response).

3. **D**   Acetylcholine and epinephrine bind to cell-surface receptors with ligand-gated ion channels which either hyperpolarize or depolarize the membrane. Acetylcholine depolarizes the membrane, while epinephrine hyperpolarizes the membrane, causing the neurotransmitters to oppose each other (choice D is correct). Increased ACh would cause increased, not decreased contraction (choice A is wrong), and since the strip of ileum was removed from the animal, it had no neural stimulation (choices B and C are wrong).

4. **B**   If both are supplied by nerves, then it should be possible to eliminate the effect of both by denervation.

5. **C**   Acetylcholine increases peristalsis, not decreases (choices A and B are wrong). Calcium release plays a role in smooth muscle contraction (as it does in cardiac and skeletal muscle as well; choice C is correct). A decrease in ATP would lead to a decrease in contraction (choice D is wrong).

6. **B**   Neurotransmitters exert their effects on cells through opening ion channels which either depolarize or hyperpolarize the membrane. Acetylcholine and epinephrine bind to their receptors, not to each other (choice A is wrong). Neither choice C nor choice D answers the question.

Chapter 12
The Respiratory System and the Skin

12.1 FUNCTIONS OF THE RESPIRATORY SYSTEM

Single-cell eukaryotes that require oxygen to perform oxidative phosphorylation can acquire it by simple diffusion of oxygen from the surrounding medium. Even simple multicellular organisms such as coelenterates (jellyfish and hydra) can still receive sufficient oxygen by diffusion between cells and the environment. Larger organisms, such as the vertebrates, evolved a respiratory system to exchange O_2 and CO_2 between the atmosphere and the blood and a circulatory system to transport those gases between the respiratory system and the rest of the tissues of the body. Note that at the cellular level, all organisms exchange respiratory gases via simple diffusion across the plasma membrane. However, the respiratory system ensures the efficient delivery of O_2 and removal of CO_2 for all cells in a complex, multicellular animal. [What parts of glucose metabolism produce CO_2, and what point in glucose metabolism utilizes oxygen?[1]]

The simple movement of air into and out of the lungs is properly called **ventilation**, whereas the actual exchange of gases (between either the lungs and the blood or the blood and the other tissues of the body) is called **respiration**.[2] The parts of the respiratory system that participate *only* in ventilation are referred to as the **conduction zone**, and the parts that participate in actual gas exchange are referred to as the **respiratory zone**. Additional tasks performed by the respiratory system include the following:

1) *pH regulation*. In the blood, CO_2 is converted to carbonic acid by the RBC enzyme carbonic anhydrase (Chapter 9). When CO_2 is exhaled by the lungs, the amount of carbonic acid in the blood is decreased, and as a result the pH of the blood increases (becomes more alkaline). Hence, minute-to-minute variations in respiration affect blood pH. *Hyper*ventilation (too much breathing) causes alkalinization of the blood, known as **respiratory alkalosis**. *Hypo*ventilation (too little breathing) causes acidification of the blood, or **respiratory acidosis**. [Which organ regulates pH over a period of hours to days?[3]]

2) *Thermoregulation*. Breathing can result in significant heat loss. Heat loss from the respiratory system occurs through **evaporative water loss**, which functions under the same principles as sweating. The respiratory structures are necessarily moist. Liquid water absorbs heat as it changes into water vapor, and this heat is removed from the body during the process. Dogs, for example, depend on panting for the dissipation of excess heat, because they cannot sweat. Some animals manage to conserve both water and heat by utilizing **countercurrent exchange** within the nasal passages. The nasal passages warm and humidify the air entering the respiratory system, and the exiting air is cooled and de-humidified. Breathing through the mouth (as with panting, or during exercise) will bypass this mechanism and increase rates of heat loss.

3) *Protection from disease and particulate matter*. The lungs provide a large moist surface where chemicals and pathogens can do harm. The **mucociliary escalator** and alveolar macrophages, discussed below, protect us from harmful inhaled particles.

---

[1] Pyruvate dehydrogenase and the Krebs cycle produce CO_2 during oxidative respiration, and oxygen is reduced to water by the last electron carrier in electron transport, cytochrome *c* oxidase.

[2] Sometimes these terms are used interchangeably. For example, we refer to "respiratory rate" when we really mean "ventilation rate."

[3] The kidney

12.2 ANATOMY OF THE RESPIRATORY SYSTEM

The Conduction Zone

As mentioned earlier, the part of the respiratory system designed only to allow gases to enter and exit the system is called the conduction zone (Figure 1). Inhaled air follows this pathway: **nose → nasal cavity → pharynx → larynx → trachea → bronchi → terminal bronchioles → respiratory bronchioles → alveolar ducts → alveoli** (the respiratory bronchioles, alveolar ducts, and alveoli are parts of the respiratory zone and will be discussed later). The nose is important for warming, humidifying, and filtering inhaled air; nasal hairs and sticky mucus act as filters. The nasal cavity is an open space within the nose. The pharynx is the throat (a common pathway for air and food) at the bottom of which is the larynx. The larynx has three functions: 1) it is made entirely of cartilage and thus keeps the airway open, 2) it contains the **epiglottis**, which seals the trachea during swallowing to prevent the entry of food, and 3) it contains the **vocal cords**, which are folds of tissue positioned to partially block the flow of air and vibrate, thereby producing sound. The **trachea** is a passageway which must remain open to permit air flow. Rings of cartilage prevent its collapse. The trachea branches into two **primary bronchi**, each of which supplies one lung. Each bronchus branches repeatedly to supply the entire lung. Collapse of bronchi is prevented by small plates of cartilage. Very small bronchi are called **bronchioles**. They are about 1 mm wide and contain no cartilage. Their walls are made of smooth muscle, which allows their diameters to be regulated to adjust airflow into the system. The smallest (and final) branches of the conduction zone are aptly called the **terminal bronchioles**.

The smooth muscle of the walls of the terminal bronchioles is too thick to allow adequate diffusion of gases; this is why no gas exchange occurs in this region. The conduction zone is strictly for ventilation.

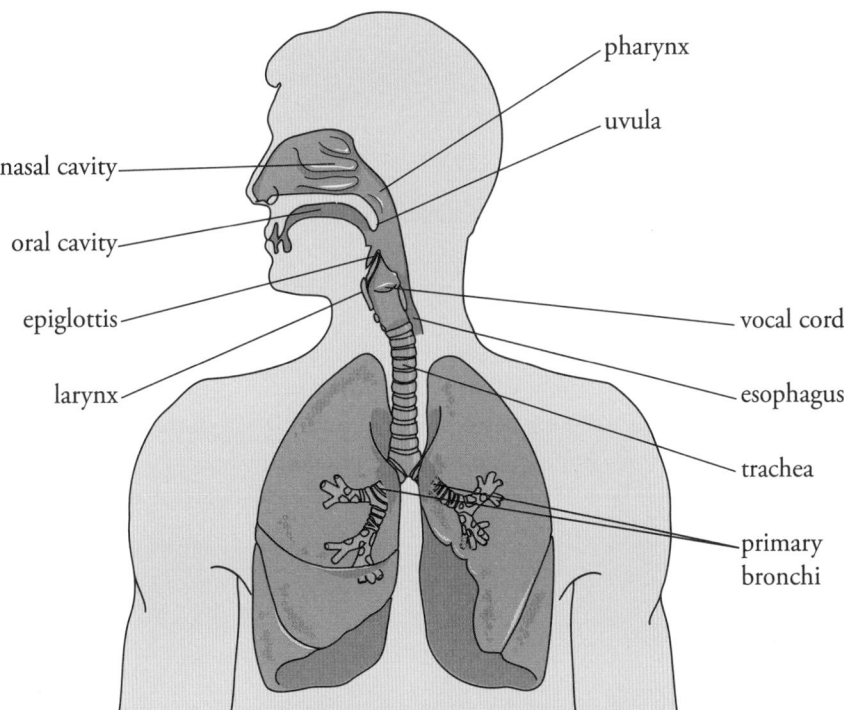

Figure 1   The Conduction Zone

The Respiratory Zone

The region of the system where gas exchange occurs is the respiratory zone (Figure 2). The actual structure across which gases diffuse is called the **alveolus** (plural: **alveoli**). Alveoli are tiny sacs with very thin walls (they're so thin that they're transparent!). The wall of the alveolus is only one cell thick, except where capillaries pass across its outer surface. The duct leading to the alveoli is called an **alveolar duct**, and its walls are entirely made of alveoli. The alveolar duct branches off a **respiratory bronchiole**. This is a tube made of smooth muscle, just like the terminal bronchioles, but with one important difference: the respiratory bronchiole has a few alveoli scattered in its walls. This allows it to perform gas exchange, so it is part of the respiratory zone.

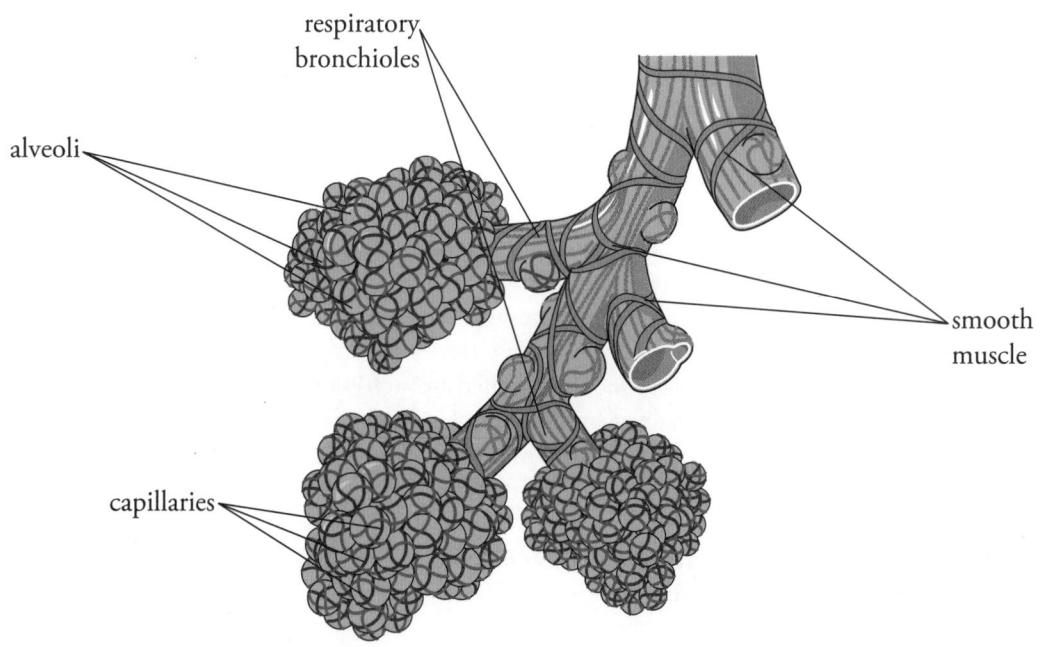

Figure 2   The Respiratory Zone

The Respiratory Epithelium: Protection from Disease and Particulate Matter

The entire respiratory tract is lined by epithelial cells. From the nose all the way down to the bronchioles, the epithelial cells are tall **columnar** (column-shaped) cells. They are too thick to assist in gas exchange; they merely provide a conduit for air. Some of these cells are specialized to secrete a layer of sticky mucus and are called **goblet cells** (just like in the gastrointestinal tract). The columnar epithelial cells of the upper respiratory tract have cilia on their apical surfaces which constantly sweep the layer of mucus toward the pharynx, where mucus containing pathogens and inhaled particles can be swallowed or coughed out. This system is known as the **mucociliary escalator**. [What would be the advantage of swallowing pathogens and particles?[4]]

---

[4]   Gastric acidity destroys many pathogens. Also, particles which would likely harm the delicate alveoli are unlikely to harm the tough lining of the GI tract.

The alveoli, alveolar ducts, and the smallest bronchioles (respiratory bronchioles) are involved in gas exchange. Oxygen and CO_2 must be able to diffuse across the layer of epithelial cells in order to pass freely between the bloodstream and the air in the lungs. Tall columnar cells with cilia would be too large to permit rapid diffusion. Thus, gas-exchanging surfaces are lined with a single layer of thin, delicate squamous epithelial cells. (Squamous means flat.) A single layer of squamous epithelial cells is called *simple squamous epithelium*. It would also be unacceptable to have a layer of mucus covering the gas exchange surface, so another method of protection from disease and inhaled particles is necessary. Alveolar macrophages fill this role by patrolling the alveoli, engulfing foreign particles.

Surfactant

Imagine a beehive made of tissue paper. If you put it in a steamy bathroom, what would happen? Would all the small air spaces remain filled with air? No, the hive would collapse into a wet ball, because the mutual attraction of water molecules would overcome the flimsy support structure provided by the fine paper fibers. The tendency of water molecules to clump together creates **surface tension**, which is the force that causes wet hydrophilic surfaces (e.g., the tissue paper) to stick together in the presence of air. Think of it this way: air is hydrophobic, so hydrophilic substances in the presence of air tend to clump together. Now imagine a beehive made of thin wax paper. If you put it into a steamy room, does it collapse? No, because the wax on the surface of the paper prevents adjacent pieces of paper from being strongly attracted. In other words, the wax destroys the surface tension.

The alveoli are as fine and delicate as tissue paper, and they too tend to collapse due to surface tension (Figure 3). This problem is solved by a soapy substance called **surfactant** (*surf*ace *acti*ve substance), which coats the alveoli. Just like the wax in our example above, surfactant reduces surface tension. Surfactant is a complex mixture of phospholipids, proteins, and ions secreted by cells in the alveolar wall. [Is it likely that these are the principal lining cells of the alveolar wall?[5]]

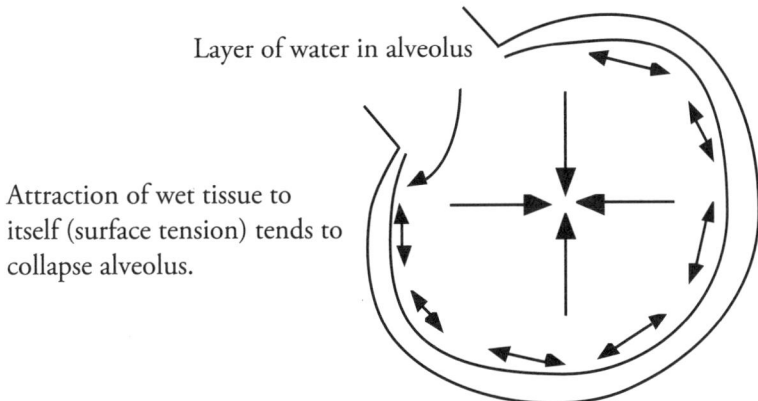

Layer of water in alveolus

Attraction of wet tissue to itself (surface tension) tends to collapse alveolus.

Figure 3   Surface Tension in an Alveolus

---

[5] No, the principal cells of the alveolar wall are thin squamous cells designed to allow diffusion of gases. Cells which actively secrete substances (i.e., surfactant) are large, metabolically active cells with many mitochondria. The basic alveolar lining cells (simple squamous epithelium) are called Type 1 alveolar cells. The fat (cuboidal) epithelial cells that secrete surfactant are called Type 2 alveolar cells.

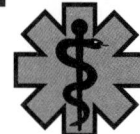

- There is not sufficient surfactant within a fetus's lungs until about the eighth month of gestation, so some premature infants lack the protective effects of surfactant when they are born. Which of the following statements best describes resulting effects upon respiration in "preemies" (babies born prematurely)?[6]
    - A) Surface tension would be abnormally low.
    - B) The alveoli would collapse.
    - C) Oxygen would be unable to diffuse through water.
    - D) Respiration is unnecessary, since the infant is dependent on the mother.

12.3 PULMONARY VENTILATION

Pulmonary ventilation is the circulation of air into and out of the lungs to continually replace the gases in the alveoli with those in the atmosphere. The drawing of air into the lungs is termed **inspiration**, and the movement of air out of the lungs is termed **expiration**. Inspiration is an active process driven by the contraction of the diaphragm, which enlarges the chest cavity (and the lungs along with the chest cavity) drawing air in. Passive expiration is driven by the elastic recoil of the lungs and does not require active muscle contraction. These processes will be described in more detail below.

The Pleural Space and Lung Elasticity

The lungs are large elastic bags that tend to collapse in upon themselves if removed from the chest cavity. However, the structures of the chest prevent this collapse and allow the lungs to remain inflated during inspiration and expiration. The lungs are not directly connected to the chest wall, however. Each lung is surrounded by two membranes, or **pleura**: the **parietal pleura**, which lines the inside of the chest cavity, and the **visceral pleura**, which lines the surface of the lungs (Figure 4). Between the two pleura is a very narrow space called the **pleural space**. The pressure in the pleural space (the **pleural pressure**) is negative, meaning that the two pleural membranes are drawn tightly together by a vacuum. This negative pressure keeps the outer surface of the lungs drawn up against the inside of the chest wall. Additionally, a thin layer of fluid between the two pleura helps hold them together through surface tension.

---

[6] In the absence of surfactant, surface tension would be high (choice **A** is wrong), and the alveoli would collapse on every exhalation like tissue-paper beehives (choice **B** is correct). It would take an enormous exertion to reopen the collapsed alveoli to get any air (oxygen) into them; the result is poor oxygen delivery to the alveoli and thus to the blood (for this reason, preemies are typically kept on ventilators until their surfactant levels are higher and they are stronger in general). Note that oxygen has some ability to diffuse through water, but choice C is wrong mostly due to irrelevance. It's not as though in the absence of surfactant the lungs suddenly fill with water. Respiration is always necessary once a baby is born; this question specifically refers to infants born prematurely (choice D is wrong).

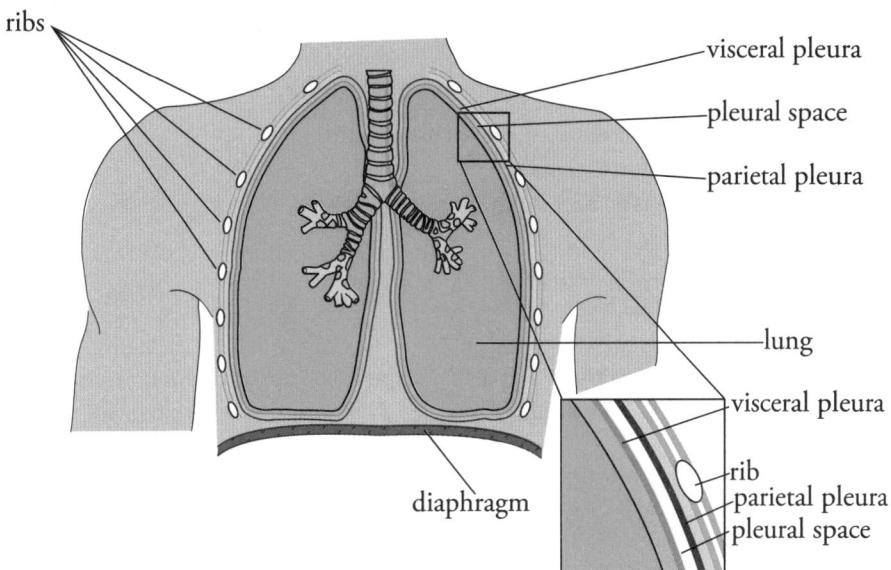

Figure 4 The Lungs and Pleura

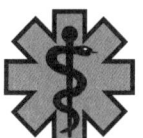

- If the pleural space is punctured, opening it to the external atmosphere, which one of the following will occur?[7]
  A) Fluid will leak out of the pleural space.
  B) Air will leak out of the pleural space.
  C) Air will leak into the pleural space.
  D) Since the pressure within the pleural space is equal to atmospheric pressure during expiration, nothing will happen.

Inspiration is caused by muscular expansion of the chest wall, which draws the lungs outward (expands them), and causes air to enter the system. The lungs expand along with the chest due to the negative pressure in the pleural space. The expansion of the chest during inspiration is driven primarily by contraction of the **diaphragm**, a large skeletal muscle that is stretched below the ribs between the abdomen and the chest cavity. When resting, the diaphragm is shaped like a dome, bulging upward into the chest cavity. When it contracts, the diaphragm flattens and draws the chest cavity downward, forcing it and the lungs (which are stuck to the inside wall of the chest cavity) to expand. The external **intercostal muscles** between the ribs also contract during inspiration, pulling the ribs upward and further expanding the chest cavity. Inspiration is an *active* process, requiring contraction of muscles to occur.

Resting expiration, by contrast, is a *passive* process (no muscle contraction required). When the diaphragm and rib muscles relax, the elastic recoil of the lungs draws the chest cavity inward, reducing the volume of the lungs and pushing air out of the system into the atmosphere. During exertion (or at other times when a more forcible exhalation is required), contraction of abdominal muscles helps the expiration process by pressing upward on the diaphragm, further shrinking the size of the lungs and forcing more air out. This is called a **forced expiration** and is an active process.

---

[7] The pleural space is always at negative pressure, or the lung would collapse. If the pleural pressure is negative, and an opening to the atmosphere is made, then air will rush into the pleural space and the lungs will collapse. The correct answer is choice **C**. (Note that choice A will probably also occur, but the amount of fluid is so minimal as to be insignificant. Choice C is the better answer.)

12.3

The pressure of air in the alveoli and the pleural pressure vary during inspiration and expiration. During inspiration, the following steps occur:

1) The diaphragm contracts and flattens (moves downward).
2) The volume of the chest cavity expands.
3) The pleural pressure decreases, becoming more negative.
4) The lungs expand outward.
5) The pressure in the alveoli becomes negative.
6) Air enters the lungs and the alveoli.

The opposite steps occur during expiration. Typically inspiration and expiration are not consciously controlled although they are mediated by voluntary muscle (which means we *can* control the processes if we want to!).

- At the beginning of inspiration, does the pleural pressure increase, decrease, or remain the same?[8]
- When is the alveolar pressure exactly zero (equal to atmospheric)?[9]
- What would be the result of a hole in the lung that allowed inhaled air to flow into the pleural cavity?[10]

Pulmonary Ventilation: Volumes and Capacities

Spirometry is the measurement of the volume of air entering or exiting the lungs at the various stages of ventilation.[11] A **spirometer** is a device used for these measurements. Data can be plotted on a **spirometric graph** (Figure 5). The volumes and capacities defined below should be familiar to you but do *not* need to be memorized.

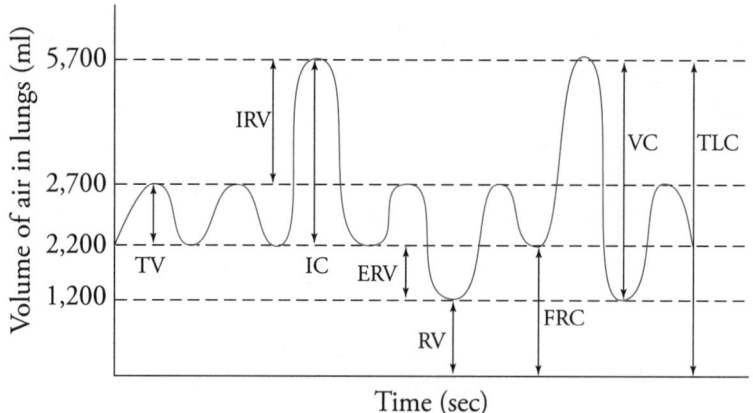

Figure 5   Lung Volumes and Capacities

---

[8] At the beginning of inspiration, pleural pressure decreases (becomes more negative), sucking the lungs open.

[9] At the end of a resting expiration, air tends to neither enter nor leave the lungs, until another inspiration begins. This is when alveolar pressure is zero. Also, just after inspiration, before expiration begins, there is an instant of zero pressure.

[10] A hole in the lung would allow air to flow into the pleural cavity, just like a hole from the pleural space to the exterior. This would cause the lung to collapse, because negative pleural pressure is the only significant force opposing lung collapse. Inspiration would be impossible.

[11] *Spir-* is from re*spir*ation.

The **tidal volume** (**TV**) is the amount of air that moves in and out of the lungs with normal light breathing and is equal to about 10 percent of the total volume of the lungs (0.5 liters out of 5–6 liters). The **expiratory reserve volume** (**ERV**) is the volume of air that can be expired after a passive resting expiration. The **inspiratory reserve volume** (**IRV**) is the volume of air that can be inspired after a relaxed inspiration. The **functional residual capacity** (**FRC**) is the volume of air left in the lungs after a resting expiration. The **inspiratory capacity** (**IC**) is the maximal volume of air which can be inhaled after a resting expiration. The **residual volume** (**RV**) is the amount of air that remains in the lungs after the strongest possible expiration. The **vital capacity** (**VC**) is the maximum amount of air that can be forced out of the lungs after first taking the deepest possible breath. The **total lung capacity** (**TLC**) is the vital capacity plus the residual volume (TLC = VC + RV).

12.4

- Is the total volume of the lungs exchanged with each breath?[12]

- In emphysema, lung elasticity is greatly reduced. Each of the following occurs EXCEPT:[13]
    A) residual volume increases.
    B) total lung capacity increases.
    C) resting expiration becomes active instead of passive.
    D) pleural pressure becomes more negative.

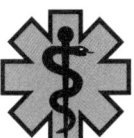

12.4 GAS EXCHANGE

The Pulmonary Circulation

Deoxygenated blood is carried toward the lungs by the pulmonary artery, which has left and right branches. These large arteries branch many times, eventually giving rise to a huge network of **pulmonary capillaries**, also called **alveolar capillaries**. Each alveolus is surrounded by a few tiny capillaries, which are just wide enough to permit the passage of RBCs, and have extremely thin walls to permit diffusion of gases between blood and alveolus. The capillaries drain into venules, which drain into the pulmonary veins. The lungs are supplied with lymphatic vessels as well.

Small increases in left atrial pressure have very little effect on the pulmonary circulation because pulmonary veins can dilate, accommodating excess blood. However, if the pressure in the left atrium increases above a certain level, the pressure will increase in pulmonary capillaries, and fluid (essentially blood plasma) will be forced out of the capillaries and into the surrounding lung tissue. Fluid in the lungs resulting from increased blood pressure is known as **pulmonary edema**. Normally, the lymphatic system prevents pulmonary edema from developing by carrying interstitial fluid out of the lungs.

---

[12]   No, some air always remains in the lungs; the FRC during relaxed breathing or the RV during deep breathing.

[13]   Typically, when the lungs are stretched on inspiration, elastic recoil draws them inward and leads to expiration. The loss of elasticity means that the lungs do not want to recoil as strongly (or at all) and remain in their stretched position (choice B would occur and can be eliminated). Thus, expiration is not as efficient and more air remains in the lungs after expiration than normal (choice A would occur and can be eliminated). In order to make expiration more efficient, contraction of internal intercostal and abdominal muscles must be used to compress the chest cavity and push air out (choice C would occur and can be eliminated). Even at rest, alveoli are typically stretched somewhat and elastic recoil tends to draw them inward; this helps create the negative pleural pressure. However, if lung elasticity is reduced, there is less of a force drawing them inward, and the pleural pressure would be less negative, not more (choice **D** would not occur and is the correct answer choice).

- Which of the following may result from increased pulmonary capillary hydrostatic pressure?[14]
    - I. Accumulation of interstitial fluid in the lungs
    - II. Fluid accumulation in the alveoli
    - III. Decreased oxygenation of the blood due to excess fluid slowing O_2 diffusion

    A) I and II only
    B) I and III only
    C) II and III only
    D) I, II, and III

The lungs are "designed" to expose a large amount of blood to a large amount of air. Thus the primary property of the lung is its enormous surface area, close to that of a tennis court. The goal is to allow O_2 from the atmosphere to diffuse into pulmonary capillaries, where it is bound by hemoglobin in RBCs. Simultaneously, CO_2 diffuses from the blood to the alveolar gas. [To review, how is CO_2 carried in the blood?[15]]

Air is a complex mixture of many gases, with nitrogen and oxygen as its primary components and other gases such as water vapor and carbon dioxide forming small percentages of the total (Table 1). In cities, poisons such as carbon monoxide may attain significant concentrations (partial pressures).

Table 1 Approximate Atmospheric Gas Compositions

Gas	% of atmosphere
N_2	80%
O_2	20%
H_2O	0.5%
CO_2	0.04%

Each gas that is part of a mixture contributes to the total pressure of the mixture in proportion to its abundance. The contribution of each individual gas to the total pressure is termed the **partial pressure**. The partial pressure of Gas X is abbreviated P_X. For example, P_{O_2} designates the partial pressure of oxygen. [If the total atmospheric pressure is 760 torr, what is the partial pressure of oxygen (P_{O_2}) in the atmosphere?[16]] The total pressure is the sum of all partial pressures.

Henry's Law

Gases in the air equilibrate with gases in liquids. If you place a beaker of water in a room, after a time the gases in the room will diffuse into the water. Therefore, partial pressures are also used to describe the amount of gases carried in the bloodstream.

---

[14] If the hydrostatic pressure is high enough, all of these will result (choice **D**).

[15] Most is transported as $HCO_3^- + H^+$ (carbonic anhydrase is the key enzyme); some is bound nonspecifically to Hb; a little can dissolve in plasma.

[16] Oxygen forms 20% of the atmosphere (Table 1). The partial pressure of oxygen in the atmosphere is 20% of 760 torr, or about 150 torr.

In order to diffuse into a cell, gas molecules from the air must dissolve into a liquid (e.g., extracellular fluid). According to **Henry's Law**, the amount of gas that will dissolve into liquid is dependent on the partial pressure of that gas as well as the solubility of that gas in the liquid. If we use oxygen as an example, Henry's Law states:

$$[O_2] = P_{O_2} \times S_{O_2}$$

where $[O_2]$ is the concentration of dissolved oxygen, P_{O_2} is the partial pressure of oxygen in the air above the fluid, and S_{O_2} is the solubility of oxygen in that liquid. Thus, an increase in pressure increases the amount of gas dissolved in a liquid.

Note that gases become less soluble in liquids as temperatures increase; this is why a soda goes flat faster on a hot day, and it is why a goldfish will gulp for air when the water is too warm. [Scuba divers breathe pressurized air. Why do they have to worry about nitrogen bubbles forming in the extracellular fluid if they ascend too quickly?[17]]

In the lungs, oxygen and carbon dioxide diffuse between the alveolar air and blood in the alveolar capillaries (Figure 6). The driving force for the exchange of gases in the lungs is the difference in partial pressures between the alveolar air and the blood. For diffusion to occur (from the air to the blood) gases must first pass across the alveolar epithelium, and then through the interstitial liquid, and finally across the capillary endothelium. These three barriers to diffusion together form the **respiratory membrane** (the pathway is obviously reversed for diffusion from the blood to the air). [Do the lipid membranes of the alveolar and capillary cells act as barriers to the diffusion of oxygen and carbon dioxide?[18]]

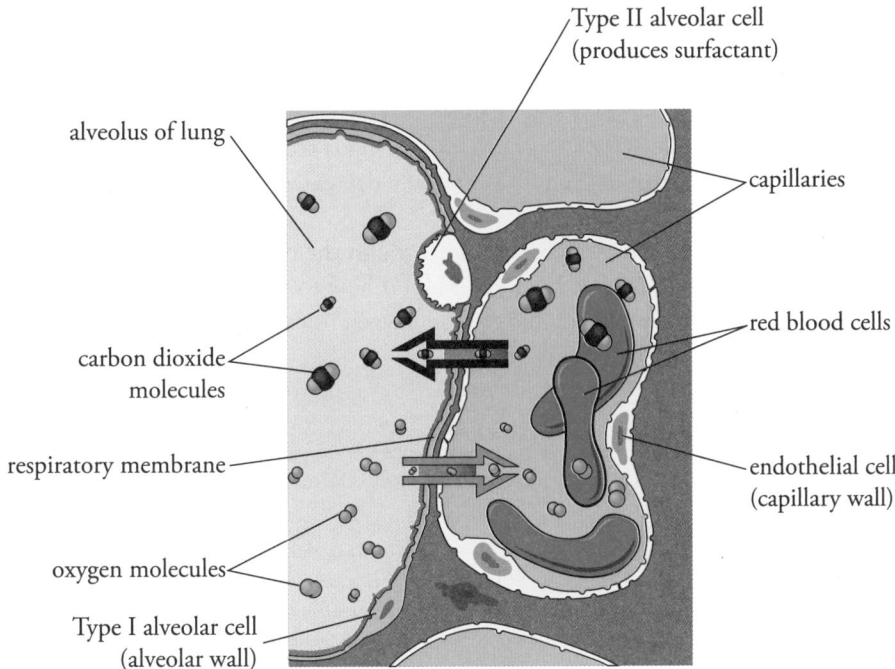

Type II alveolar cell (produces surfactant)

alveolus of lung

capillaries

carbon dioxide molecules

red blood cells

respiratory membrane

endothelial cell (capillary wall)

oxygen molecules

Type I alveolar cell (alveolar wall)

Figure 6   Diffusion of Gases Between an Alveolus and a Capillary

---

[17] Gases are more soluble in liquids at high pressures. At depth, gases dissolve into the blood and extracellular fluids more readily because of the high pressure of the surrounding water. If a diver ascends too quickly, the gases come out of solution before they can be transported to the respiratory system. This results in air bubbles that primarily contain nitrogen, the most abundant gas in the air we breathe. These bubbles tend to form most abundantly at the joints, and cause decompression sickness, a painful condition commonly known as "the bends." To treat decompression sickness, afflicted divers are put into a hyperbaric (high pressure) chamber to redissolve the gases before slowly restoring the tissues to atmospheric pressure.

[18] No, lipid bilayers do not act as barriers to the diffusion of such small hydrophobic molecules.

As blood passes through the alveolar capillaries, the oxygen pressure gradient between the alveolar air and the blood drives the net diffusion of oxygen into the blood. The arterial P_{O_2} is denoted P_aO_2.

- Is the P_{O_2} at the arterial end of pulmonary capillaries greater than, less than, or equal to the P_{O_2} in the venous end?[19]

- Although the partial pressures of oxygen and nitrogen in the atmosphere are relatively constant, the partial pressure of water vapor can vary considerably. If water vapor in the atmosphere increases, which one of the following will occur?[20]
  A) The total atmospheric pressure will increase.
  B) The partial pressures of oxygen and nitrogen will decrease.
  C) The partial pressure of oxygen will decrease, and the partial pressure of nitrogen will increase.
  D) The partial pressure of oxygen will increase, and the partial pressure of nitrogen will decrease.

- Atmospheric P_{O_2} is 150 torr, while the arterial P_{O_2} is 100 torr. Which one of the following is the best explanation for this discrepancy?[21]
  A) Due to the short amount of time blood spends in the lungs, atmospheric gases do not fully equilibrate with arterial gases.
  B) The barrier to diffusion formed by the alveolar epithelium plus the capillary endothelium prevents full equilibration of atmospheric and arterial gases.
  C) The P_{H_2O} and P_{CO_2} in the alveolus are much higher than in the atmosphere; as a result, the P_{O_2} is lower.
  D) The hydrophobic nature of oxygen prevents large amounts from dissolving in blood.

- During vigorous muscle activity, each of the following is true EXCEPT:[22]
  A) the partial pressure of oxygen in the muscle decreases; as a result, oxygen diffuses from the blood into the muscle.
  B) the flow of blood in the venous system through the muscle is reduced.
  C) arteriolar dilation increases the rate of blood flow to the muscle.
  D) myoglobin in muscle cells is able to take oxygen from RBC hemoglobin because myoglobin has a higher oxygen affinity.

---

[19] Less than. Deoxygenated blood (P_{O_2} = 40 torr) enters the pulmonary system in the pulmonary artery. As the deoxygenated blood passes through the capillaries, it becomes increasingly oxygenated until it emerges at the venous end equilibrated with the alveolar oxygen pressure (P_{O_2} = 100 torr).

[20] Total atmospheric pressure is defined as the force exerted against a surface due to the weight of the air above that surface; thus, it is determined primarily by gravitational forces and changes very little (choice A is wrong). Partial pressure, however, is defined as the portion of total pressure due to a particular gas; thus, if the partial pressure of water increases (and since the total pressure remains the same), the relative partial pressures of oxygen and nitrogen would have to decrease (choice **B** is correct, and choices C and D are wrong).

[21] The alveolar P_{O_2} is only 100 torr because water and CO_2 take up a greater proportion of gases in the alveolus than in the atmosphere. The gases in the alveolus do not have the same composition as the atmosphere since they are not fully exchanged with each breath (choice **C** is correct). While it is true that blood spends only a short amount of time in the lungs, the barrier (respiratory membrane) is extremely thin, allowing for rapid and complete equilibration of gases under normal circumstances (choices A and B are wrong). Choice D is true but irrelevant; most oxygen in the blood is carried on hemoglobin.

[22] During vigorous exertion, blood flow to the muscle through arterioles is increased (choice C is true and can be eliminated); thus, flow from the muscles through veins and venules must also increase; blood does not pool in the muscles during activity (choice **B** is false and the correct answer choice). As O_2 is used to make ATP, P_{O_2} in the muscle decreases and the resulting increased O_2 gradient from blood to muscle tissue allows oxygen to diffuse into the muscle cells (choice A is true and can be eliminated). This effect is enhanced by the fact that myoglobin has a higher affinity for oxygen than hemoglobin (choice D is true and can be eliminated).

12.5 REGULATION OF VENTILATION RATE

Proper regulation of the rate and depth of breathing is essential. Although breathing can be voluntarily controlled for short periods of time, it is normally an involuntary process directed by the **respiratory control center** in the medulla of the brain stem. The stimuli that affect ventilation rate are both mechanical and chemical (Table 2, next page).

The principal chemical stimuli that affect ventilation rate are increased P_{CO_2}, decreased pH, and decreased P_{O_2} (with CO_2 and pH being the primary regulators and O_2 secondary). These variables are monitored by special autonomic sensory receptors. **Peripheral chemoreceptors** are located in the aorta and the carotid arteries and monitor the P_{CO_2}, pH, and P_{O_2} of the blood, while **central chemoreceptors** are found in the medullary respiratory control center and monitor P_{CO_2} and pH of the cerebrospinal fluid (CSF). Recall that pH and P_{CO_2} are connected through the carbonic acid buffer system of the blood (discussed briefly in Chapters 9 and 10).

$$CO_2 + H_2O \rightleftharpoons H_2CO_3 \rightleftharpoons H^+ + HCO_3^-$$

Respiration eliminates CO_2 from the body. Thus, changes in ventilation rate can have rapid effects on pH due to the decrease or increase in P_{CO_2} and the resulting shift to maintain the above equilibrium. For example, a person hyperventilating during an anxiety attack can have an elevated pH. [Why do we give these folks a paper bag to breathe into?[23]] A person whose ventilation rate has been reduced due to extreme alcohol intoxication can become acidotic. Similarly, changes in pH can be compensated for by increasing or decreasing ventilation rate. For example, diabetics who are acidotic due to the metabolism of proteins and fats instead of glucose will have an increased ventilation rate to remove CO_2 and increase pH.

Mechanical stimuli that affect ventilation rate include physical stretching of the lungs and irritants. The mechanical stretching of lung tissue stimulates stretch receptors that inhibit further excitatory signals from the respiratory center to the muscles involved in inspiration. The walls of bronchi and larger bronchioles contain smooth muscle. Contraction of this smooth muscle is known as **bronchoconstriction**. Irritation of the inner lining of the lung stimulates irritant receptors, and reflexive contraction of bronchial smooth muscle prevents irritants from continuing to enter the passageways. This contractile response is determined by parasympathetic nerves that release ACh. During an allergy attack, mast cells release histamine, which also causes bronchoconstriction. Epinephrine opposes this; it increases ventilation by causing airway smooth muscles to relax (this is **bronchodilation**). [Asthma is caused by spasm of airway smooth muscles. Patients with asthma carry "inhalers," which are small aerosol cans whose contents they spray into their lungs during an asthma attack. Based on this discussion, what might inhalers contain?[24]]

There are also **irritant receptors** in the lung that trigger coughing and/or bronchoconstriction when an irritating chemical (such as smoke) is detected.

---

[23] Breathing into a paper bag forces them to rebreathe their exhaled CO_2. This pushes the equilibrium of the equation to the right and brings pH back down to normal.

[24] They contain epinephrine, antihistamines (drugs that block histamine receptors on smooth muscle cells), and anticholinergics (drugs that block acetylcholine receptors on smooth muscle cells).

Table 2 Factors that Regulate Ventilation Rate

Stimulus	Receptor	Effect
stretch of lung	stretch receptor in lung	inhibits inspiration
$\uparrow P_{CO_2}$	peripheral chemoreceptors and medullary respiratory center	increased P_{CO_2} causes $\downarrow$pH via carbonic anhydrase; the $\downarrow$pH is what is actually sensed (see below)
$\downarrow$pH	as above	increases respiratory rate
$\downarrow P_{O_2}$	peripheral chemoreceptors	increases respiratory rate
chemical irritation	irritant receptor in lung	coughing and/or bronchoconstriction

12.6   STRUCTURE AND LAYERS OF THE SKIN

The skin is the largest organ in the body, by size and by weight (Figure 7). Its role is to protect us from pathogens, to prevent excessive evaporation of water, and to regulate body temperature (Section 12.7). The outermost layer of the skin is called the **epidermis**; it lies upon the deeper **dermis**, which rests on **subcutaneous tissue** or **hypodermis**. The hypodermis is a protective, insulating layer of fat (adipose tissue).

The epidermis is composed of stratified (many layers of) squamous epithelial cells. These cells are constantly sloughed off and then replenished by mitosis of cells at the deepest part of the epidermis, the **stratum basale**. A cell in this layer divides, and one of the resulting daughter cells moves outward. Soon this cell will die and be pushed farther and farther outward by continued mitosis below, until it flakes away from the surface of the body. The significance of many layers of epithelial cells is that they provide a strong protective structure.

Another important facet of the stratified squamous cells of the epidermis is that they are **keratinized**. This means that as they die, they become filled with a thick coating of the tough, hydrophobic protein **keratin**. Keratin helps make the skin waterproof.

Epidermal epithelial cells also contain **melanin**. This is a brown pigment, produced by specialized cells in the epidermis termed *melanocytes*, that helps absorb the ultraviolet light of the Sun to prevent damage to underlying tissues.

Beneath the epidermis lies the **dermis**. The dermis consists of various cell-types embedded in a connective tissue matrix. It contains blood vessels that nourish both the dermis and the epidermis (the epidermis has no blood vessels of its own). The dermis also contains **sensory receptors**, which convey information about touch, pressure, pain, and temperature to the central nervous system. Also found in the dermis are **sudoriferous** (sweat) glands, **sebaceous** (oil) glands, and **hair follicles**. Hairs consist of dead epithelial cells bound tightly together. Some specialized regions of skin contain **ceruminous** (wax) glands (e.g., the external ear canal).

The sudoriferous gland is composed of a tube-like structure that originates in the dermis and leads through the epidermis to a pore on the surface of the skin. The purpose of sweat is to allow loss of excess heat by evaporation. Sweat contains water, electrolytes, and urea. Sweat glands are responsive to aldosterone. People living in hot climates must sweat a lot. In order to conserve sodium, they have a high level of aldosterone, and thus their sweat does not waste salt.

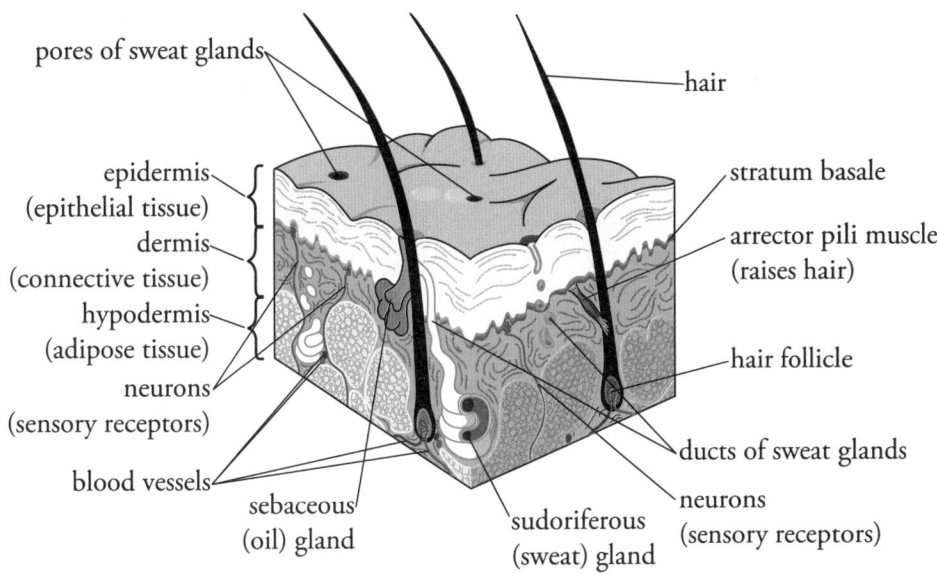

pores of sweat glands

hair

epidermis
(epithelial tissue)

stratum basale

dermis
(connective tissue)

arrector pili muscle
(raises hair)

hypodermis
(adipose tissue)

neurons
(sensory receptors)

hair follicle

blood vessels

ducts of sweat glands

sebaceous
(oil) gland

sudoriferous
(sweat) gland

neurons
(sensory receptors)

Figure 7   Skin Layers

12.7

12.7   TEMPERATURE REGULATION BY THE SKIN

Humans are **homeotherms**, meaning their body temperature is relatively constant. Heat is generated by metabolic processes and muscle contraction. Some homeotherms (e.g., bears) can maintain their temperature by burning special fat called **brown adipose tissue**; this process is called **chemical thermogenesis** or **nonshivering thermogenesis**. But this is *not* an important mechanism of temperature regulation in adult humans. Also, while it is true that an increased level of thyroid hormone can increase the metabolic rate and thus increase body temperature, this mechanism takes several weeks to kick in and is not thought to be important in day-to-day temperature regulation. So, practically, only four strategies are available to cope with cold weather:

1) Contraction of skeletal muscles produces heat, whether it is involuntary (shivering) or voluntary (jumping up and down).
2) The skin insulates us so that we conserve heat generated by metabolism. Subcutaneous (beneath the skin) tissue contains a layer of insulating fat, which helps.
3) Heat loss by conduction is minimized by constriction of blood vessels in the dermis (**cutaneous vasoconstriction**). Cutaneous vasoconstriction occurs in response to cold weather or upon activation of the sympathetic nervous system. This is why the skin becomes cold and pale when one is frightened.
4) Obviously, contrivances such as clothing and blankets help us conserve heat.

A mechanism for dissipation of excess heat is also necessary. This is accomplished by two mechanisms in the skin:

1) Sweating, which allows heat loss by evaporation
2) Dilation of blood vessels in the dermis (**cutaneous vasodilation**), which results in heat loss by conduction or convection, when air blows past the skin (as with a fan or a breeze)

Chapter 12 Summary

- The primary functions of the respiratory system are gas exchange and pH regulation. pH regulation by the respiratory system is very fast.

- The organs of the respiratory system are divided into the conduction zone and the respiratory zone.

- The conduction zone is for ventilation only and includes the nose and nasal cavity, the pharynx, the larynx, the trachea, and the respiratory tree from the primary bronchi to the terminal bronchioles.

- The larynx is made entirely of cartilage and includes the epiglottis (which separates food and air) and the vocal cords (for sound production).

- The respiratory zone is for gas exchange and includes the respiratory bronchioles, the alveolar ducts, and the alveoli.

- Surfactant reduces surface tension inside alveoli, making them easier to inflate.

- Inspiration is an active process and requires the contraction of the diaphragm to expand the chest cavity. An increase in the size of the chest cavity (and lungs) reduces their pressure, and air flows in.

- Expiration is primarily a passive process; the diaphragm relaxes and lung elastic recoil helps return them to their resting state. Forced expiration requires the contraction of the abdominal muscles to forcibly reduce the size of the chest cavity. In either case, the reduction in the size of the chest cavity increases their pressure and pushes the air out.

- Ventilation rate is determined primarily by P_{CO_2} and the need to regulate pH, according to the following equilibrium: $CO_2 + H_2O \rightleftharpoons H_2CO_3 \rightleftharpoons H^+ \rightleftharpoons + HCO^-_3$. As CO_2 levels increase, pH falls, and ventilation rate increases (the reverse is also true).

- The skin is made of three main layers: the epidermis (epithelial tissue), the dermis (connective tissue), and the hypodermis (adipose tissue).

- The epidermis provides a barrier to infection and water loss, the dermis is where sweat glands, nerves, blood vessels, and sensory receptors are found, and the hypodermis is a layer of fat for insulation and protection.

- Thermoregulation is primarily a function of the dermis. When temperatures rise, blood vessels in the dermis dilate to release heat, and sweat glands are activated. When temperature falls, blood vessels constrict to retain heat. Also, involuntary skeletal muscle contractions occur (shivering) to produce heat.

CHAPTER 12 FREESTANDING PRACTICE QUESTIONS

1. Patients injected with agents that paralyze muscles during surgeries must be artificially ventilated until they recover. These drugs interfere with which neurotransmitter?

A) Acetylcholine
B) Norepinephrine
C) Dopamine
D) GABA

2. A patient presents to the emergency room in diabetic ketoacidosis (DKA), a life-threatening complication of diabetes, which results in metabolic acidosis, as well as very high serum glucose levels. Which of the following vital signs would be expected in this patient, as compared to baseline?

A) Increased blood pressure
B) Increased respiratory rate
C) Decreased heart rate
D) Decreased respiratory rate

3. Patients can often alleviate symptoms of an asthma attack by using drugs called sympathomimetics that mimic the effects of norepinephrine. Based on this information, which is the most likely explanation for why patients with asthma have difficulty breathing?

A) Constriction of bronchial smooth muscle leads to diminished air flow.
B) Dilation of bronchial smooth muscle leads to diminished air flow.
C) Constriction of smooth muscle surrounding blood vessels leads to decreased blood flow to the lungs.
D) Interference with skeletal muscle neurons leads to decreased force of contraction of the diaphragm.

4. A middle-aged man is in a coma after a motor vehicle accident. His respiratory rate has significantly decreased due to trauma to the medulla. All of the following are true EXCEPT:

A) there will be a decrease in the [H+] of his blood.
B) normal regulation of ventilation rate has been disrupted.
C) there will be an increase in P_{CO_2} of his blood.
D) there will be a decrease in P_{O_2} of his blood.

5. All of the following are functions of the respiratory system EXCEPT:

A) regulation of pH.
B) protection from particulate matter.
C) removal of nitrogenous waste.
D) regulation of body temperature.

6. Which of the following homeostatic responses maximizes the dissipation of excess heat through the skin?

A) Increased release and evaporation of sudoriferous gland secretions and constriction of dermal blood vessels
B) Increased release and evaporation of sudoriferous gland secretions and dilation of dermal blood vessels
C) Decreased release and evaporation of sudoriferous gland secretions and constriction of dermal blood vessels
D) Decreased release and evaporation of sudoriferous gland secretions and dilation of dermal blood vessels

7. A cancer of the skin is more likely to involve which population of cells?

A) Cells in the outer (most superficial) layer of the epidermis that have uncontrolled mitosis
B) Cells in the outer (most superficial) layer of the epidermis that have uncontrolled meiosis
C) Cells in the deepest layer of the epidermis that have uncontrolled mitosis
D) Cells in the deepest layer of the epidermis that have uncontrolled meiosis

CHAPTER 12 PRACTICE PASSAGE

Occupational and environmental lung diseases are estimated to affect more than 20 million individuals in the United States alone. These diseases are generally caused by inhalation of toxic dusts and fumes and include silicosis, asbestosis, coal worker's pneumoconiosis (black lung disease), and berryliosis, as well as several diseases caused by the inhalation of dust and spores associated with agricultural businesses. Exposure to mineral dusts often leads to restrictive lung diseases (where the total lung capacity is reduced), whereas exposure to chemical agents leads to occupational asthma and other obstructive diseases (where air flow through the bronchial tubes is restricted).

Coal worker's pneumoconiosis (CWP) is a restrictive lung disease caused by long-term exposure to and inhalation of coal dust. Once inhaled, coal dust cannot be destroyed or removed, and consequently is simply engulfed by resident alveolar macrophages. These macrophages tend to aggregate and can be visualized microscopically as granular black areas that give the disease its common name. The aggregations lead to inflammation, damage to the lung tissue, fibrosis, and the formation of nodules throughout the lungs.

CWP is generally divided into simple and complicated classes. Simple CWP can develop early on from chronic exposure to coal dust; chest X-ray reveals nodules between 5 mm and 1 cm in diameter. Symptoms are similar to those experienced with cigarette smoking (cough, excess mucus, etc.). Upon continued, long-term exposure to coal dust (>10-15 years), simple CWP can progress to complicated CWP, which is characterized by lung nodules anywhere from 1 cm in diameter to the size of an entire lung lobe, significant reduction in lung volume and gas diffusion capacity, and premature mortality. Alveolar hypoxia can lead to pulmonary vasoconstriction; thus, complicated CWP can also be associated with right-side heart failure (*cor pulmonare*).

Lung function can be assessed by measurement of flow volumes during inspiration and expiration. Obstructive diseases tend to have increased total lung capacity and residual volume along with reduced flow. Restrictive diseases caused by damage to lung tissue tend to have reduced lung capacity and residual volumes, but normal flow. Restrictive diseases caused by damage to the inspiratory muscles or chest wall have reduced lung capacity, increased residual volume, and reduced flow. Figure 1 shows the expiratory flow-volume curves for four different patients.

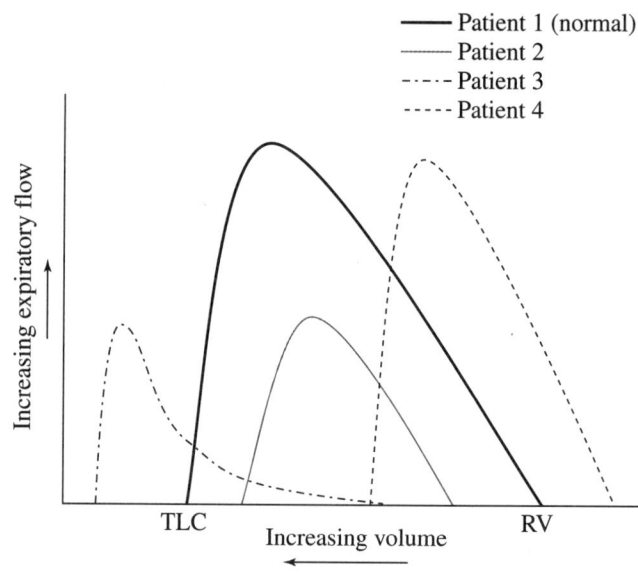

Figure 1 Expiratory flow-volume curves. Total lung capacity (TLC) and residual volume (RV) are indicated on the normal curve.

1. Agonistic drugs increase a particular response, while antagonistic drugs reduce a response. Which of the following drugs would be the best choice to treat occupational asthma?

A) Parasympathetic agonist
B) Parasympathetic antagonist
C) Sympathetic agonist
D) Sympathetic antagonist

2. The FEV_1 is a measurement of the total amount of air that can be forcibly expired in 1 second after a complete inhalation. In which of the following conditions would a reduced FEV_1 be expected?

   I.   CWP
   II. Occupational asthma
   III. Chronic obstructive pulmonary disease (COPD)

A) I only
B) II only
C) II and III only
D) I, II, and III

3. Which of the following would NOT be associated with complicated CWP?

A) Lung nodules 2–3 cm in diameter
B) Decreased pressure in the pulmonary vasculature
C) Right ventricular hypertrophy
D) Granular blackened areas in the lungs

4. Botulism is a type of food poisoning in which a toxin released by the bacteria *Clostridium botulinum* inhibits the release of acetylcholine from motor neurons. In severe cases, this can lead to paralysis of the diaphragm. Which of the following would be expected in an individual suffering from severe botulism?

A) Decreased total lung capacity, decreased residual volume, and normal flow
B) Decreased total lung capacity, increased residual volume, and decreased flow
C) Increased total lung capacity, decreased residual volume, and normal flow
D) Increased total lung capacity, increased residual volume, and decreased flow

5. Which of the following statements about the respiratory system is true?

A) The ratio of cartilage to smooth muscle decreases as the bronchial tubes branch smaller and smaller.
B) The respiratory zone participates in gas exchange only, while the conduction zone participates in both ventilation and gas exchange.
C) Contraction of the diaphragm is mediated entirely by the autonomic nervous system.
D) An increase in carbon dioxide leads to an accumulation of carbonic acid, a decrease in blood pH, and a decrease in ventilation rate.

6. Which of the patients in Figure 1 is most likely suffering from CWP?

A) Patient 1
B) Patient 2
C) Patient 3
D) Patient 4

SOLUTIONS TO CHAPTER 12 FREESTANDING PRACTICE QUESTIONS

1. **A**   The diaphragm is the primary ventilatory muscle; it is a skeletal muscle, and acetylcholine is the neurotransmitter that mediates nerve transmission to skeletal muscle (choice A is correct). Norepinephrine is the neurotransmitter used at postsynaptic synapses in the sympathetic nervous system; although interference with this neurotransmitter could affect the smooth muscle surrounding the bronchi, it would not affect the diaphragm and ventilation (choice B is incorrect). Dopamine and GABA are neurotransmitters that are found only in the central nervous system; paralysis in these patients is produced at the level of the muscle itself, not the central nervous system (choices C and D are incorrect).

2. **B**   The metabolic acidosis (decreased blood pH) would lead to hyperventilation (increased respiratory rate) in an attempt to compensate for the low pH by reducing the amount of CO_2 (thus raising the pH; choice B is correct, and choice D is wrong). It is important to remember the equation: $CO_2 + H_2O \rightleftharpoons H_2CO_3 \rightleftharpoons H^+ + HCO_3^-$. This is enough to answer the question; however, it is also true that patients in DKA have very high levels of serum glucose, which overwhelm the glucose reabsorption mechanisms of the kidney, leading to glucose in the urine. This glucose has an osmotic pressure effect and leads to severe water loss in the urine (diuresis). This in turn leads to potentially severe dehydration, which would ultimately result in lower blood pressure (choice A is incorrect), and elevated heart rates (choice C is incorrect).

3. **A**   In asthma, constriction of bronchial smooth muscle decreases the diameter of the bronchi, leading to diminished air flow. Sympathomimetics stimulate the adrenergic receptors on smooth muscle, causing the muscle to dilate and improving air flow through the bronchi (choice A is correct). Dilation of bronchial smooth muscle would improve air flow, rather than diminish it, as flow is proportional to diameter (choice B is incorrect). Norepinephrine causes constriction of smooth muscle around blood vessels, not dilation, which would lead to less blood flow to the lungs. In any case, asthma is primarily a problem of ventilation (moving air in and out), not perfusion (the flow of blood to the lungs; choice C is incorrect). Acetylcholine, not norepinephrine, is the neurotransmitter that mediates contraction of skeletal muscle (choice D is incorrect).

4. **A**   The centers that regulate respiratory rate are found in the medulla. Since the question text states his respiratory rate has significantly decreased due to trauma in this region, the normal feedback mechanisms (such as pH and P) will not be effective in restoring normal ventilatory patterns (choice B is true and can be eliminated). The reduced rate of respiration will lead to an accumulation of CO_2 and a drop in O_2 in his blood (choices C and D are true and can be eliminated). The excess CO_2 will shift the equilibrium of $CO_2 + H_2O \rightleftharpoons H_2CO_3 \rightleftharpoons H^+ + HCO_3^-$ to the right, leading to an increase in $[H^+]$ and a drop in pH (choice A is false and is the correct answer choice).

5. **C** The respiratory system participates in pH regulation via changes in the ventilation rate. An increase in ventilation (hyperventilation) will lead to rapid removal of CO_2 and, due to the carbonic anhydrase buffer system, an increase in the pH ($CO_2 + H_2O \rightleftharpoons H_2CO_3 \rightleftharpoons H^+ + HCO_3^-$). A decrease in ventilation (hypoventilation) will lead to a decrease in pH (choice A is a function of the respiratory system and can be eliminated). The mucociliary escalator protects the body from particulate matter by either swallowing or coughing out the mucus-coated particle (choice B is a function of the respiratory system and can be eliminated). Hyperventilation also leads to heat loss; in order to dissipate excess heat, dogs depend on panting (choice D is a function of the respiratory system and can be eliminated). However, the respiratory system is not involved in the removal of nitrogenous waste; that is a function of the renal excretory system (choice C is not a function of the respiratory system and is the correct answer choice).

6. **B** Sudoriferous (sweat) glands are exocrine glands found within the skin that secrete water and electrolytes. As water evaporates from the skin surface, heat is dissipated. Thus, the hotter you are, the more you sweat (choices C and D are wrong). Dilating dermal blood vessels will increase blood flow to the skin and increase conductive heat loss (choice B is correct, and choice A is wrong).

7. **C** Meiosis only occurs in sperm and ova (choices B and D are wrong). Stem cells (basal cells) located in the deepest layer of the epidermis undergo mitosis throughout an individual's life. With each mitotic event, daughter cells arise, move outward (superficially), and differentiate as they do so; eventually, they die and are sloughed off. The daughter cells that differentiate lose their ability to divide; thus, it is more likely that the stem cells (which retain their ability to divide) could develop into a cancer (choice C is a better answer than choice A).

SOLUTIONS TO CHAPTER 12 PRACTICE PASSAGE

1. **C** The passage states that occupational asthma is characterized by restricted air flow through bronchial tubes. Activation of the sympathetic nervous system leads to dilation of these tubes; thus, a sympathetic agonist would be the best choice in this case (choice C is correct, and choice D is wrong). Activation of the parasympathetic system would worsen the air flow, since it leads to bronchial constriction (choice A is wrong). While a parasympathetic antagonist might help, a sympathetic agonist would have a faster and stronger response (choice C is better than choice B).

2. **C** Reduced FEV_1 measurements are typically seen in conditions where air flow is reduced. Item I is false: coal worker's pneumoconiosis is described in the passage as a restrictive disease caused by lung-tissue damage; thus, total lung capacity would be reduced but flow would be normal (choices A and D can be eliminated). Since both remaining answer choices include Item II, Item II must be true and you can focus on Item III. Item III is true: the passage states that obstructive diseases are characterized by reduced air flow (choice B can be eliminated, and choice C is correct). Note that Item II is in fact true: occupational asthma is classified in the passage as an obstructive disease. Note: In Figure 1, the curve for Patient 3 is what would be expected for an obstructive disease; the drop to residual volume is gradual, indicating a reduced flow rate.

3. **B**   The passage states that "alveolar hypoxia can lead to pulmonary vasoconstriction," which would increase pulmonary pressures, not decrease them (choice B would not be associated with complicated CWP and is the correct answer choice). The increased pulmonary pressure could lead to a hypertrophy (increase in size) of the right ventricle in order to generate a stronger force with which to move the blood against the higher pressure (choice C could be associated and can be eliminated). Complicated CWP is associated with lung nodules greater than 1 cm in diameter (choice A can be eliminated) and both simple and complicated CWP would have granular blackened areas in the lungs (choice D can be eliminated).

4. **B**   This is a two-by-two question, in which two decisions determine the correct answer choice. The passage states that damage to the inspiratory muscles (of which the diaphragm is the primary muscle) can lead to restrictive lung disease characterized by reduced total lung capacity (choices C and D can be eliminated), increased residual volume (choice A can be eliminated), and decreased flow.

5. **A**   Most of the cartilage is found near the top of the bronchial tree. After the tertiary bronchial tubes, the cartilage disappears altogether and the tubes are formed out of smooth muscle (choice A is true and the correct answer choice). The conduction zone only participates in ventilation, not gas exchange (choice B is false and can be eliminated). The diaphragm is skeletal muscle and its contraction is predominantly mediated by somatic neurons (and is under voluntary control; choice C is false and can be eliminated). It is true that increased CO_2 would lead to an accumulation of carbonic acid and a decrease in blood pH, but that would cause an increase in ventilation rate in order to remove the excess CO_2 (choice D is false and can be eliminated).

6. **D**   Patient 1 is listed on the figure legend as "normal," so choice A can be eliminated first. CWP is a restrictive lung disease caused by damage to the lung tissue, due to chronic inhalation of coal dust. As described in the final paragraph, a patient suffering from this disease would have a reduced total lung capacity (choice C, Patient 3, has an increased total lung capacity and can be eliminated), and a reduced residual volume (choice B, Patient 2, has an increased residual volume and can be eliminated). Note that the x-axis (volume) increases to the left in this figure.

Chapter 13
The Reproductive Systems

13.1 THE MALE REPRODUCTIVE SYSTEM

Anatomy

The principal male reproductive structures that are visible on the outside of the body are the scrotum and the penis. The scrotum is essentially a bag of skin containing the male gonads, which are known as **testes** (testicles). [Does the scrotum have any active role, or is it merely a container?[1]] The testes have two roles: 1) synthesis of sperm (**spermatogenesis**), and 2) secretion of male sex hormones (**androgens**, e.g., testosterone) into the bloodstream. More detail on these topics is given later. Here we will trace the path of a sperm from its origination to its final destination.

The sites of spermatogenesis within the testes are the **seminiferous tubules**. The walls of the seminiferous tubules are formed by cells called **sustentacular cells** (also known as *Sertoli cells*). Sustentacular cells protect and nurture the developing sperm, both physically and chemically; their role will be discussed in more detail below. The tissue between the seminiferous tubules is simply referred to as testicular interstitium.[2] Important cells found in the testicular interstitium are the **interstitial cells** (also known as Leydig cells). They are responsible for androgen (testosterone) synthesis.

The seminiferous tubules empty into the **epididymis**, a long coiled tube located on the posterior (back) of each testicle (Figure 1). The epididymis from each testicle empties into a **ductus deferens** (also called the *vas deferens*), which in turn leads to the **urethra** (the tube inside the penis). To get to the urethra, the ductus deferens leaves the scrotum and follows a peculiar path: it enters the **inguinal canal**, a tunnel that travels along the body wall toward the crest of the hip bone. (There are two inguinal canals, left and right.) From the inguinal canal, the ductus deferens enters the pelvic cavity. Near the back of the urinary bladder, it joins the duct of the seminal vesicle (discussed below) to form the **ejaculatory duct**. The ejaculatory ducts from both sides of the body then join the urethra.

A pair of glands known as **seminal vesicles** is located on the posterior surface of the bladder. They secrete about 60 percent of the total volume of the **semen** into the ejaculatory duct. Semen is a highly nourishing fluid for sperm and is produced by three separate glands: the seminal vesicles, the **prostate**, and the **bulbourethral glands**. These are collectively referred to as the **accessory glands** (see Table 1). The ejaculatory duct empties into the **urethra** as it passes through the prostate gland. One final set of glands, the bulbourethral glands, contributes to the semen near the beginning of the urethra.

Table 1   The Accessory Glands

Gland and secretions	Function of secretions	% of total ejaculate volume
Seminal vesicles—mostly fructose	Nourishment of sperm	60%
Prostate gland—fructose and a coagulant	Nourishment, allows semen to coagulate after ejaculation	35%
Bulbourethral glands—thick, alkaline mucus	Lubricate urethra, neutralize acids in male urethra and in female vagina	3%
Testes—sperm	Male gamete	2%

---

[1] The scrotum is important for temperature regulation. Sperm synthesis in the testes must occur at a few degrees below normal body temperature. This is why the testes are located outside the body. Relaxation of the scrotum facilitates cooling of the testes. When the environment is cold, the scrotum contracts, pulling the testes up against the body, warming them.

[2] *Interstitium* is a term used to describe a thing or a region which is "between" other structures.

The urethra exits the body via the penis. Penile erection facilitates deposition of semen near the opening of the uterus during intercourse. Specialized **erectile tissue** in the penis allows erection. It is composed of modified veins and capillaries surrounded by a connective tissue sheath. Erection occurs when blood accumulates at high pressure in the erectile tissue. Three compartments contain erectile tissue: the **corpora cavernosa** (there are two of these) and the **corpus spongiosum** (only one).

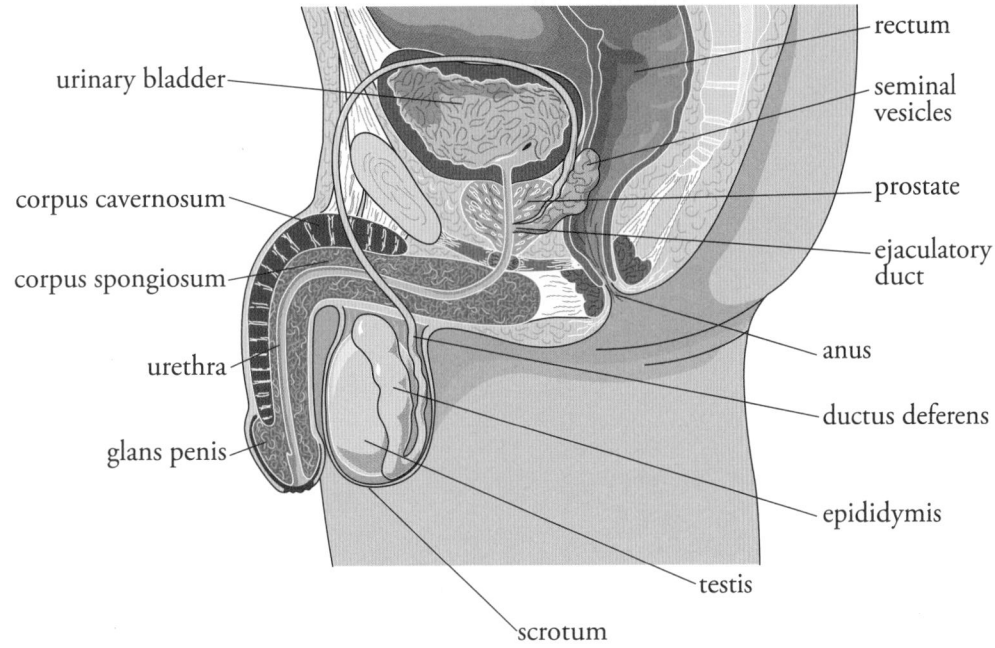

Figure 1   The Male Reproductive System

The Male Sexual Act

The three stages of the male sexual act are arousal, orgasm, and resolution. These events are controlled by an integrating center in the spinal cord, which responds to physical stimulation and input from the brain. The cerebral cortex can activate this integrating center (as in sexual arousal during sleep) or inhibit it (anxiety interferes with sexual function).

Arousal is dependent upon parasympathetic nervous input and can be subdivided into two stages: erection and lubrication. **Erection** involves dilation of arteries supplying the erectile tissue. This causes swelling, which in turn obstructs venous outflow. This causes the erectile tissue to become pressurized with blood. **Lubrication** is also a function of the parasympathetic system. The bulbourethral glands secrete a viscous mucous which serves as a lubricant.

Stimulation by the sympathetic nervous system is required for **orgasm**, which can also be divided into two stages: emission and ejaculation. **Emission** refers to the propulsion of sperm (from the ductus deferens) and semen (from the accessory glands) into the urethra by contractions of the smooth muscle surrounding these organs. Emission is followed by **ejaculation**, in which semen is propelled out of the urethra by rhythmic contractions of muscles surrounding the base of the penis. Ejaculation is actually a reflex reaction caused by the presence of semen in the urethra. Emission and ejaculation together constitute the male orgasm.

Resolution, or a return to a normal, unstimulated state, is also controlled by the sympathetic nervous system. It is caused primarily by a constriction of the erectile arteries. This results in decreased blood flow to the erectile tissue and allows the veins to carry away the trapped blood, returning the penis to a flaccid state. This typically takes 2–3 minutes.

- Name four glands that contribute to semen.[3]
- Which components of the male sexual act can occur if all sympathetic activity is blocked?[4]
- What is the difference between emission and ejaculation?[5]

13.2 SPERMATOGENESIS

What processes in a human being involve meiosis? Only one: **gametogenesis**. This is the process whereby **diploid germ cells** undergo **meiotic division** to produce **haploid gametes**. As discussed in Chapter 7, meiotic cell division fosters genetic diversity in the population (by independent assortment of genes and by recombination). The gametes produced by the male are known as **spermatozoa**, or *sperm*; females produce **ova**, or *eggs*. The role of the sperm is to swim through the female genital tract to reach the egg and fuse with it. This fusion is known as **syngamy**, and it results in a **zygote**. The gametes produced by males and females differ dramatically in structure but contribute equally to the genome of the zygote (except in the special case of the two different sex chromosomes, X and Y, given to male offspring). Although both gametes contribute equally to the genome, the egg provides *every other part of the zygote*, since the only part of the sperm which enters the egg is a haploid genome. The term for this is **maternal inheritance**. For instance, mitochondria are inherited maternally.

Sperm synthesis is called **spermatogenesis** (Figure 2). It begins at puberty and occurs in the testes throughout adult life. [Do females also make gametes throughout adult life?[6]] The seminiferous tubule is the site of spermatogenesis. The entire process of spermatogenesis occurs with the aid of the specialized sustentacular cells found in the wall of the seminiferous tubule. Immature sperm precursors are found in the outer wall of the tubule, and nearly mature spermatozoa are deposited into the lumen; from there they are transported to the epididymis. The cells that give rise to spermatogonia (and to their female counterparts, oogonia) are known as **germ cells**; under the right conditions, they *germ*inate, and give rise to a complete organism.

---

[3] Seminal vesicles, prostate, testes, and bulbourethral glands

[4] Erection and lubrication (arousal only)

[5] Emission is the movement of sperm and semen components into the urethra; ejaculation is the movement of semen from the urethra out of the body.

[6] No. This is discussed later.

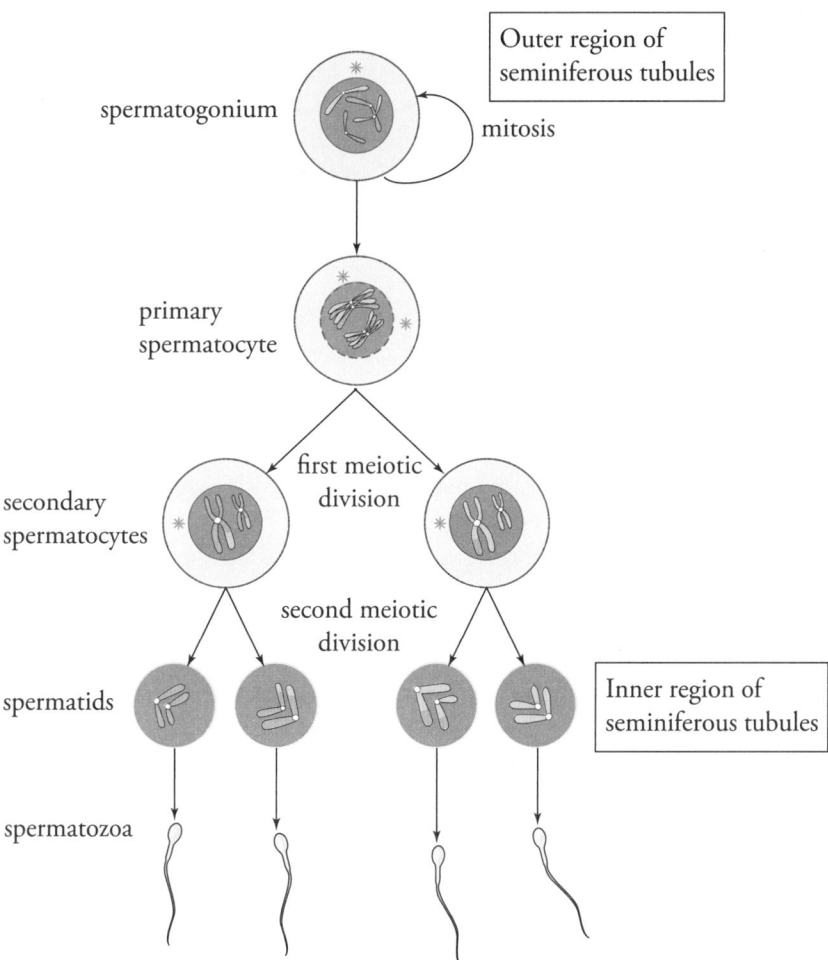

Figure 2 Spermatogenesis

Table 2 below gives the names of the sperm precursors, along with the meiotic role of each stage, and some mnemonic comments. Fill in the female version when you read that section.

Table 2 Gametogenesis

Stage	Jobs	Mnemonic	Female version
spermatogonium	1. Mitotically reproduce prior to meiosis 2. Replicate DNA in S phase of meiosis	The spermatoGONium is GONNA become a sperm.	
primary spermatocyte	Meiosis I	Any gamete precursor (male or female) with "cyte" undergoes a meiotic division.	
secondary spermatocyte	Meiosis II	The *secondary* spermatoCYTE undergoes the *second* meiotic division.	
spermatid	Turn into a spermatozoan	The spermatid's a kid, almost mature	
spermatozoan	Finish maturing: 1. in seminiferous tubule 2. in epididymis	Just remember that a mature sperm is called a spermatozoan.	

As noted in Table 2, the final stages of sperm maturation occur in the epididymis. When they first enter the epididymis, spermatozoa are incapable of motility. Many days later, when they reach the ductus deferens, they are fully capable of motility. But they remain inactive due to the presence of inhibitory substances secreted by the ductus deferens. This inactivity causes sperm to have a very low metabolic rate, which allows them to conserve energy and thus remain fertile during storage in the ductus deferens for as long as a month.

- Do spermatogonia divide by mitosis or by meiosis?[7]
- How many mature sperm result from a single spermatogonium after it becomes committed to meiosis?[8]
- Which of the following statements is/are true?[9]
  - I. During gametogenesis, sister chromatids remain paired with each other until anaphase of the second meiotic cell division.
  - II. A difference between mitosis and meiosis is that mitosis requires DNA replication prior to cell division but meiosis does not.
  - III. Recombination between sister chromatids during gametogenesis increases the genetic diversity of offspring.

Spermatids develop into spermatozoa in the seminiferous tubules with the aid of sustentacular cells. The DNA condenses, the cytoplasm shrinks, and the cell shape changes so that there is a **head**, containing the haploid nucleus and the acrosome, and a flagellum which forms the **tail**. There is also a **neck** region at the base of the tail, which contains many mitochondria. [Where do these mitochondria get their energy?[10]] The **acrosome** is a compartment on the head of the sperm that contains hydrolytic enzymes required for penetration of the ovum's protective layers. **Bindin** is a protein on the sperm's surface that attaches to receptors on the zona pellucida surrounding the ovum (discussed below).

- Concerning spermatogenesis, which of the following is/are true?[11]
  - I. Spermatocytes possess a flagellum.
  - II. Flagellar movement of sperm involves rotation of a basal structure embedded in the sperm membrane.
  - III. Spermatids possess a haploid genome.

Hormonal Control of Spermatogenesis

Testosterone plays the essential role of stimulating division of spermatogonia. **Luteinizing hormone (LH)** stimulates the interstitial cells to secrete testosterone. **Follicle stimulating hormone (FSH)** stimulates the sustentacular cells. The hormone **inhibin** is secreted by sustentacular cells; its role is to inhibit

---

[7] Mitosis. Spermatogonia undergo the meiotic S phase (replicate the genome), but the stages which undergo the actual meiotic *divisions* are called spermatocytes. *All* gamete precursors with "cyte" in their name undergo a meiotic division.

[8] Four haploid cells result from the reductive division (meiosis) of one diploid spermatogonium. Compare this to oogenesis.

[9] **Item I: True.** Meiosis I involves the pairing, recombination, and separation of homologous chromosomes. Meiosis II is like mitosis, where sister chromatids separate. Item II: False. Both require DNA replication in a preceding S phase. Item III: False. Sister chromatids don't recombine, homologous chromosomes do. (Even if sister chromatids did recombine, it would make no difference since they are identical.)

[10] From the fructose which the seminal vesicles contribute to the semen and from vaginal secretions.

[11] Item I: False. The flagellum does not begin to form until the spermatid stage. Item II: False. This describes prokaryotic flagella. **Item III: True.** Meiosis is complete by the spermatid stage. Remember, the spermatid's kid. It's just like a sperm, only immature.

FSH release. [From where, and why?[12]]

- Which of the following is/are true?[13]
  - I. Luteinizing hormone reaches its target tissue through the hypothalamic-hypophysial portal system.
  - II. The absence of luteinizing hormone does not affect spermatogenesis.
  - III. Increased testosterone levels in the blood decrease the production of follicle stimulating hormone.

13.3 DEVELOPMENT OF THE MALE REPRODUCTIVE SYSTEM

The gender of a developing embryo is determined by its sex chromosomes, either XX in females or XY in males. During the early weeks of development, however, male and female embryos are indistinguishable. Early embryos, whether male or female, have undifferentiated gonads, and possess both **Wolffian ducts** that can develop into male internal genitalia (epididymis, seminal vesicles, and ductus deferens) and **Müllerian ducts** that can develop into female internal genitalia (uterine tubes, uterus, and vagina). In the absence of a Y chromosome, Müllerian duct development occurs by default, and female internal genitalia result. Female *external* genitalia (labia, clitoris) are also the default; note that the external genitalia are not derived from the Müllerian ducts. Genetic information on the Y chromosome of XY embryos leads to the development of testes, which cause male internal and external genitalia to develop by producing testosterone and **Müllerian inhibiting factor** (**MIF**).

MIF is produced by the testes and causes regression of the Müllerian ducts; this prevents the development of female internal genitalia. Testosterone secretion by cells which will later give rise to the testes begins around week 7 of gestation. By week 9, testes are formed, and their interstitial cells supply testosterone. The testosterone that is responsible for the development of male external genitalia enters the systemic circulation and must be converted to **dihydrotestosterone** in target tissues in order to exert its effect (Figure 3 on the next page).

- If an XY genotype embryo fails to secrete testosterone, will it have testes or ovaries?[14]

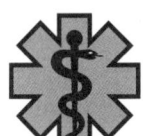

---

[12] FSH and LH are gonadotropins secreted by the anterior pituitary. The reason this occurs is to provide negative feedback.

[13] Item I: False. LH is secreted by the anterior pituitary and reaches its targets via the systemic circulation. GnRH reaches its target via the portal system. Item II: False. LH is necessary because it stimulates the interstitial cells to secrete testosterone, which is necessary for germ cell stimulation. **Item III: True.** Testosterone, estrogen, progesterone, and inhibin are all hormones that exert feedback inhibition upon the anterior pituitary and hypothalamus.

[14] Testosterone is *produced by* the embryonic testes. Their development does not depend on testosterone. Therefore, an XY embryo which didn't secrete testosterone would most likely have testes nonetheless.

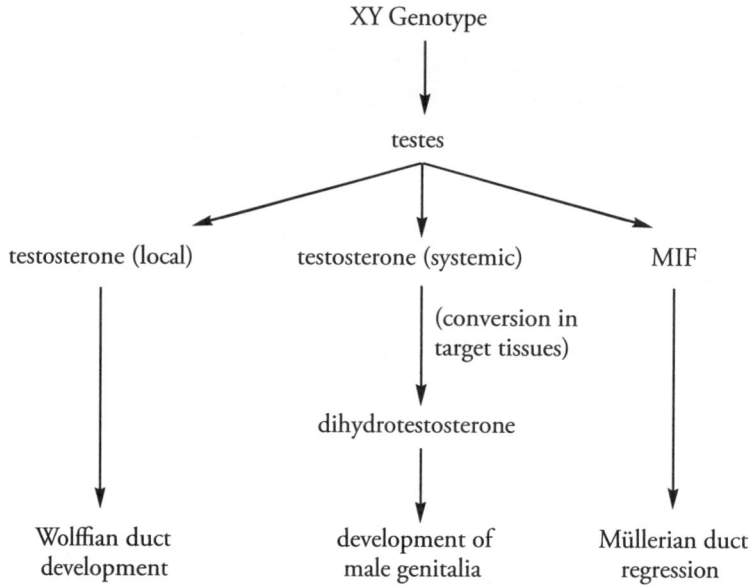

Figure 3   Control of Development of the Male Reproductive System

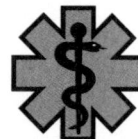

- Which one of the following would best characterize an embryo with an XY genotype that lacks the receptor for testosterone?[15]
    A) Testes, ductus deferens, and seminal vesicles are present; external genitalia are female.
    B) Ovaries, uterine tubes, and uterus are present; external genitalia are female.
    C) Testes are present; external genitalia are female; neither Müllerian nor Wolffian ducts develop.
    D) Testes and male external genitalia are present.

The development of the male and female reproductive systems is closely related. As described above, the three main fetal precursors of the reproductive organs are the Wolffian ducts, the Müllerian ducts, and the gonads. While the Wolffian ducts are the precursors of internal male genitalia, they essentially disappear in the female reproductive system. For the Müllerian ducts, this process is reversed; they essentially disappear in the male reproductive system and form the internal genitalia of the female reproductive system. Structures arising from these ducts tend to have the same function (e.g., ductus deferens in males and the uterine tubes in females both carry gametes), but because they arise from different precursors, they are considered to be **analogous structures**.

In both sexes, the gonads go on to form either the testes or the ovaries; because they are derived from the same undeveloped structure, testes and ovaries are considered homologous organs. There are a number of other homologous structures in males and females due to their common origins within the fetus (see Table 3).

---

[15] The XY genotype would lead to the development of testes (choice B is wrong), and the testes would produce MIF and testosterone. MIF would cause the degeneration of the Müllerian ducts, and no female internal genitalia would develop. However, the inability to respond to testosterone (because of the missing receptor) would prevent the development of the Wolffian ducts (choice A is wrong) as well as the male external genitalia (choice D is wrong). The external genitalia would default to female (choice **C** is correct).

Table 3 Homologous Reproductive Structures

Male Organ	Female Organ	Function
Testis	Ovary	Gamete and hormone reproduction
Penis	Clitoris	Erectile tissue, sensation
Bulbourethral glands	Greater vestibular glands	Lubrication
Scrotum	Labia majora	External skin folds

13.4 ANDROGENS AND ESTROGENS

All hormones involved in the development and maintenance of male characteristics are termed **androgens**, while those involved in development and maintenance of female characteristics are termed **estrogens**. The primary androgen produced in the testes is testosterone. It is converted into dihydrotestosterone within the cells of target tissues. The primary estrogen produced in the ovaries is estradiol.

Testosterone is required in the testes for spermatogenesis (Section 13.2). The role of testosterone in the embryonic development of the male internal and external genitalia has already been discussed. After birth the level of testosterone falls to negligible levels until puberty, at which time it increases and remains high for the remainder of adult life. Elevated levels of testosterone are responsible for the development and maintenance of male **secondary sexual characteristics** (maturation of the genitalia, male distribution of facial and body hair, deepening of the voice, and increased muscle mass). The pubertal growth spurt and fusion of the epiphyses (see Chapter 11) also result.

The role of estrogen in the female is analogous to the role of testosterone in the male. Beginning at puberty, estrogen is required to regulate the uterine cycle and for the development and maintenance of female secondary sexual characteristics (maturation of the genitalia, breast development, wider hips, and pubic hair). Estrogen causes the fusion of the epiphyses in females.

- Why are tumors derived from interstitial cells more easily diagnosed in boys than in grown men?[16]
- If testosterone levels are abnormally elevated during childhood, how will the height of the individual be affected?[17]
- How do androgens reach the cytoplasm to bind to cytoplasmic receptors?[18]
- How would an RNA polymerase II inhibitor alter the effects of dihydrotestosterone in target cells?[19]
- Which is the more abundant androgen in the blood: testosterone or dihydrotestosterone?[20]

---

[16] Interstitial cells secrete testosterone. Levels of testosterone are normally very low in boys. An abnormal increase will lead to puberty at an abnormally young age ("precocious puberty"). The results would be less obvious in an adult male.

[17] The child will undergo precocious puberty, involving an early growth spurt, so the child will be unusually tall. But then early fusion of the epiphyses will result in a shorter adult height than expected.

[18] These highly hydrophobic molecules can diffuse through the cell membrane and bind to cytoplasmic receptors.

[19] Once its ligand is bound, the steroid receptor activates transcription of specific mRNA. Messenger RNA is transcribed by RNA pol II. Therefore, we would expect inhibition of pol II to prevent the effects of all steroid hormones.

[20] The concentration of testosterone is higher. Dihydrotestosterone is produced from testosterone inside target cells. It is present in the blood in much lower concentrations than testosterone.

13.5

During puberty and adult life, sex steroid production is controlled by the hypothalamus and the anterior pituitary. **Gonadotropin releasing hormone (GnRH)** from the hypothalamus stimulates the pituitary to release the gonadotropins: follicle-stimulating hormone (FSH) and luteinizing hormone (LH). In men, LH acts on interstitial cells to stimulate testosterone production, and FSH stimulates the sustentacular cells. In women FSH stimulates the granulosa cells to secrete estrogen, and LH simulates the formation of the corpus luteum and progesterone secretion. Feedback inhibition by the steroids inhibits the production of GnRH and LH and FSH. Inhibin, produced by sustentacular cells and the granulosa cells, provides further feedback regulation of FSH production (Figure 4).

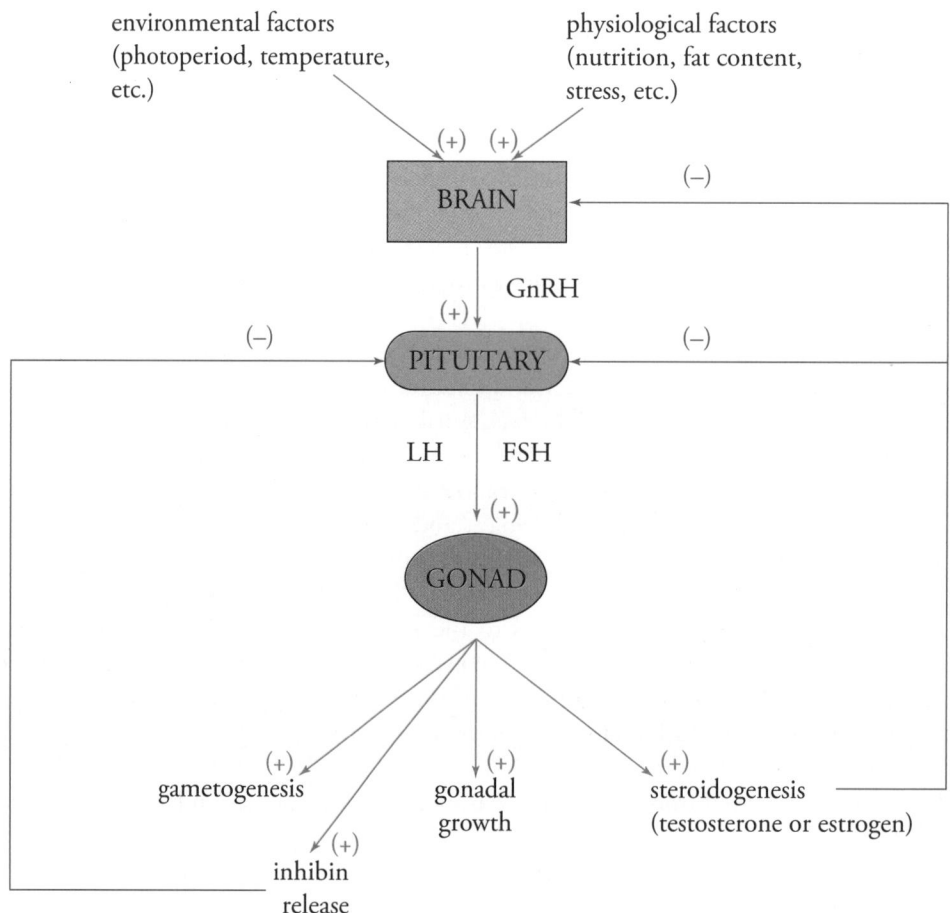

Figure 4 Regulation of Sex Steroid Production

13.5 THE FEMALE REPRODUCTIVE SYSTEM

Anatomy and Development

We mentioned in Section 13.3 that male and female genitalia are derived from a common undifferentiated precursor. Because of this, the structures of the female external genitalia are homologous to those of the male. In the female, the XX genotype leads to the formation of ovaries capable of secreting the female sex hormones (estrogens) instead of testes that secrete androgens. In the male, testosterone causes a pair of skin folds known as **labioscrotal swellings** to grow and fuse, forming the scrotum. In the female, without the influence of testosterone, the labioscrotal swellings form the **labia majora** of the vagina (labia = lips, majora = larger). The structure that gave rise to the penis in the male embryo becomes the **clitoris** in the female, located within the labia majora in the uppermost part of the vulva. Just beneath the clitoris is the **urethral opening**, where urine exits the body. Surrounding the urethral opening is another pair of skin folds called the **labia minora**.

The opening of the **vagina** is also found between the labia minora. The female internal genitalia (vagina, uterine tubes, uterus) are derived from the Müllerian ducts, so there are no homologous structures in the male. The vagina is a tube which would end in the pelvic cavity, except that another hollow organ, the **uterus**, opens into its upper portion. The part of the uterus which opens into the vagina is called the **cervix** ("neck," as in "cervical"). The innermost lining of the uterus (closest to the lumen) is the **endometrium**. It is responsible for nourishing a developing embryo, and in the absence of pregnancy, it is shed each month, producing menstrual bleeding. Surrounding the endometrium is the **myometrium**, which is a thick layer of smooth muscle comprising the wall of the uterus. The uterus ends in two **uterine tubes** (also called *fallopian tubes*), which extend into the pelvis on either side. Each uterine tube ends in a bunch of finger-like structures called **fimbriae**. The fimbriae brush up against the **ovary**, which is the female gonad. [At the time of ovulation, where does the oocyte come from and where does it go?[21]]

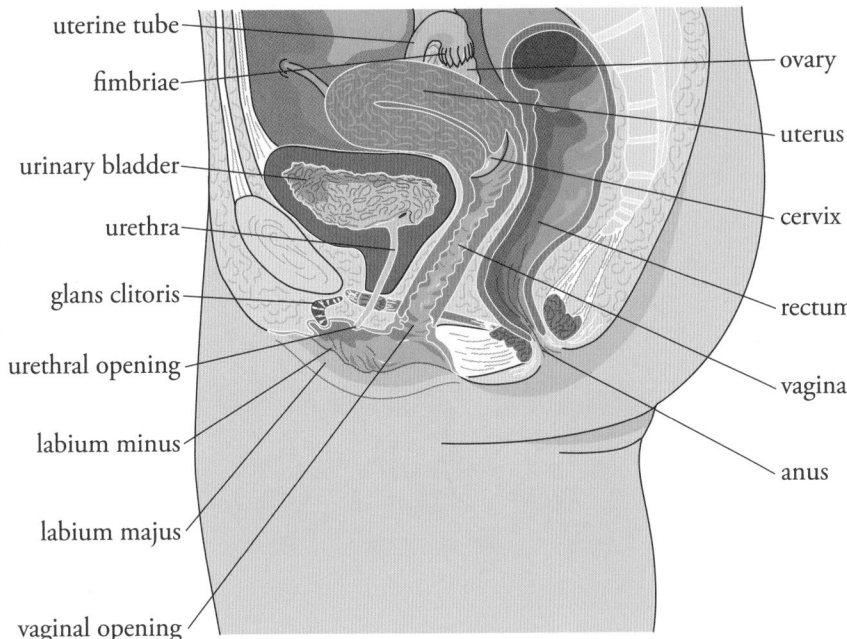

Figure 5 The Female Reproductive System

- What is the fate of the Wolffian ducts and their derivatives in the female?[22]
- Is estrogen production by the ovaries required for the development of the uterine tubes and uterus?[23]

---

[21] It emerges from the ovary (sometimes causing pain in the middle of the menstrual cycle) and must be swept into the uterine tube by a constant flow of fluid into the uterine tube caused by cilia.

[22] In the absence of testosterone, they atrophy.

[23] No, the Müllerian ducts develop into vagina, uterus, and uterine tubes by default as long as MIF is absent.

The Female Sexual Act

The stages are the same as in the male: **arousal**, **orgasm**, and **resolution**. The arousal stage, as in the male, is subdivided into erection and lubrication and is controlled by the parasympathetic nervous system. The clitoris and labia minora contain erectile tissue and become engorged with blood, just as in the male. Lubrication is provided by mucus secreted by **greater vestibular glands** and by the vaginal epithelium. Orgasm in the female is controlled by the sympathetic nervous system and involves muscle contractions, just as in the male, in addition to a widening of the cervix. (These events are thought to facilitate the movement of sperm into the uterus.) The female does not experience ejaculation. Resolution is also the same as in the male, controlled by the sympathetic system, but can take up to 20–30 minutes (compared to 2–3 minutes in the male).

13.6 OOGENESIS AND OVULATION

Oogenesis begins prenatally. In the ovary of a female fetus, germ cells divide mitotically to produce large numbers of **oogonia**. [How is this different from the male scenario?[24]] Oogonia not only undergo mitosis *in utero*, but they also enter the first phase of meiosis and are arrested in prophase I (as primary oocytes). The number of oogonia peaks at about 7 million at mid-gestation (20 weeks into fetal development). At this time mitosis ceases, conversion to primary oocytes begins, and there is a progressive loss of cells so that at birth there are only about 2 million primary oocytes. By puberty this number is further reduced to only about 400,000. Only about 400 oocytes are ever actually **ovulated** (released) in the average woman, and the remaining 99.9 percent will simply degenerate.

The primary oocytes formed in a female fetus can be frozen in prophase I of meiosis for decades, until they re-enter the meiotic cycle. Beginning at puberty and continuing on a monthly basis, hormonal changes in the woman's body stimulate completion of the first meiotic division and ovulation. This meiotic division yields a large secondary oocyte (containing all of the cytoplasm and organelles) and a small **polar body** (containing half the DNA, but no cytoplasm or organelles). The polar body (called the *first* polar body) remains in close proximity to the oocyte. The second meiotic division (i.e., completion of oogenesis) occurs *only if* the secondary oocyte is fertilized by a sperm; this division is also unequal, producing a large ovum and the second polar body. Note that if fertilization does occur, the nuclei from the sperm and egg do not fuse immediately. They must wait for the secondary oocyte to release the second polar body and finish maturing to an ootid and then an ovum. Finally, the two nuclei fuse, and a diploid ($2n$) zygote is formed.

- Is the secondary oocyte haploid?[25]
- When an oogonium undergoes meiosis, three cells result. How many of these are eggs, and why do only three cells result? (Meiosis results in four cells in the male.)[26]

Before we move on to a discussion of the menstrual cycle, you will need more background information on oogenesis. The primary oocyte is not an isolated cell. It is found in a clump of supporting cells called **granulosa cells**, and the entire structure (oocyte plus granulosa cells) is known as a **follicle**. The granulosa cells assist in maturation. [What is the male counterpart of the granulosa cell?[27]] An immature primary oocyte is surrounded by a single layer of granulosa cells, forming a **primordial follicle**.

---

[24] It only happens in *adult* males. Here, we're talking about events in the ovaries of a female while she's still in her mother's womb.

[25] Yes. After the first meiotic division, the cell is haploid; the homologous chromosomes have been separated. (They are, however, still replicated, hence the reason for meiosis II.)

[26] Only one egg results. The three cells which result are two polar bodies plus one ovum. There are only three because the first polar body does not divide. (In meiosis in the male, both cells derived from the first meiotic division go on to divide.)

[27] The cells that support and nurture developing spermatocytes are the sustentacular cells.

As the primordial follicle matures, the granulosa cells proliferate to form several layers around the oocyte, and the oocyte itself forms a protective layer of mucopolysaccharides termed the **zona pellucida**. There may be several follicles in the ovary; they are surrounded and separated by cells termed **thecal cells**. [What is the male counterpart of the thecal cells, and to which hormone do they respond?[28]] Of the several maturing follicles, only one progresses to the point of ovulation each month; all others degenerate. The mature follicle is known as a **Graafian follicle**. During ovulation, the Graafian follicle bursts, releasing the secondary oocyte with its zona pellucida and protective granulosa cells into the fallopian tube. At this point the layer of granulosa cells surrounding the ovum is known as the **corona radiata**. The follicular cells remaining in the ovary after ovulation form a new structure called the **corpus luteum** (Figure 6).

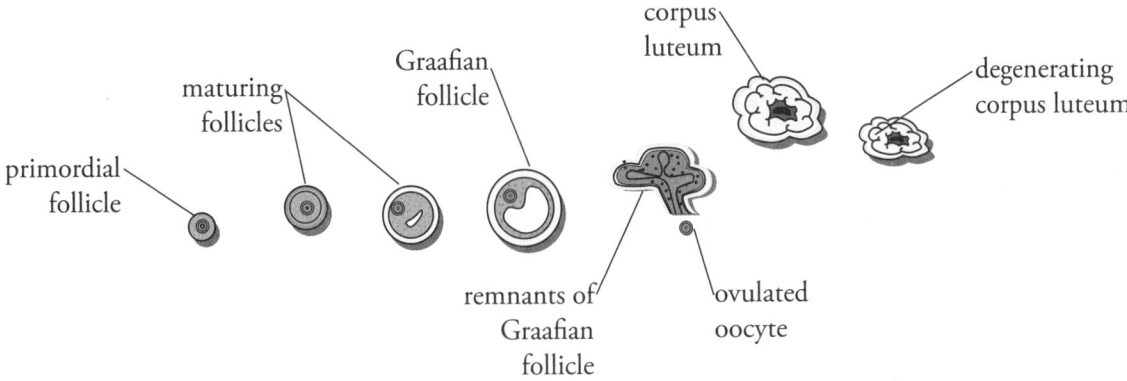

Figure 6 The Fate of a Follicle

Estrogen is made and secreted by the granulosa cells (with help from the thecal cells) during the first half of the menstrual cycle. Both estrogen and progesterone are secreted by the corpus luteum during the second half of the cycle. Estrogen is a steroid hormone that plays an important role in the development of female secondary sexual characteristics, in the menstrual cycle, and during pregnancy. [How does estrogen exert its effect on a cell?[29]] Progesterone is also a steroid hormone involved in the hormonal regulation of the menstrual cycle and pregnancy, but with different effects than estrogen.

13.7 THE MENSTRUAL CYCLE

The menstrual cycle is (on average) a 28-day cycle that includes events occurring in the ovary (discussed above and referred to as the **ovarian cycle**), as well as events occurring in the uterus (the shedding of the old endometrium and preparation of a new endometrium for potential pregnancy), referred to as the **uterine cycle**.

---

[28] They are analogous to the testicular interstitial cells. Both interstitial and thecal cells are stimulated by LH.

[29] A cytoplasmic receptor binds estrogen and binds to specific DNA elements in promoters and enhancers to regulate transcription.

The Ovarian Cycle

The ovarian cycle can be subdivided into three phases (Figure 7):

1) During the **follicular phase**, a primary follicle matures and secretes estrogen. Maturation of the follicle is under the control of follicle stimulating hormone (FSH) from the anterior pituitary. The follicular phase lasts about 13 days.

2) In the **ovulatory phase**, a secondary oocyte is released from the ovary. This is triggered by a surge of luteinizing hormone (LH) from the anterior pituitary. The surge also causes the remnants of the follicle to become the corpus luteum. Ovulation typically occurs on day 14 of the cycle.

3) The **luteal phase** begins with full formation of the corpus luteum in the ovary. This structure secretes both estrogen and progesterone and has a life span of about two weeks. The average length of the luteal phase is about 14 days.

13.7

The hormones secreted from the ovary during the ovarian cycle direct the uterine cycle.

The Uterine Cycle

The uterine cycle covers the same 28 days that were discussed above, but the focus is on the preparation of the endometrium for potential implantation of a fertilized egg. The uterine cycle can also be subdivided into three phases (Figure 7):

1) The first phase is **menstruation**, triggered by the degeneration of the corpus luteum and subsequent drop in estrogen and progesterone levels. The sharp decrease in these hormones causes the previous cycle's endometrial lining to slough out of the uterus, producing the bleeding associated with this time period. Menstruation typically lasts about 5 days.

2) During the **proliferative phase** of the menstrual cycle, estrogen produced by the follicle induces the proliferation of a new endometrium. This phase lasts about 9 days.

3) After ovulation the **secretory phase** occurs, in which estrogen and progesterone produced by the corpus luteum further increase development of the endometrium, including secretion of glycogen, lipids, and other material. If pregnancy does not occur, the death of the corpus luteum and decline in the secretion of estrogen and progesterone trigger menstruation once again. The secretory phase typically lasts about 14 days.

The menstrual cycle repeats every 28 days from puberty until menopause (at about age 50–60).

- At what stage of development is the endometrium when ovulation occurs?[30]
- Where is the secondary oocyte during the secretory phase?[31]
- If estrogen and progesterone were given to a woman without cyclic variation, how would this affect menstruation?[32]

---

[30] The endometrium is at the proliferative phase, under the influence of ovarian estrogen.

[31] The secondary oocyte is traveling down the uterine tube toward the uterus. If it fails to implant in the uterus, the secretory phase ends and menstruation begins.

[32] Menstruation occurs because the estrogen and progesterone secreted by the corpus luteum decrease suddenly when the corpus luteum degenerates. If estrogen and progesterone are kept at high levels, such as with a pill (or pregnancy), then menstruation will not occur.

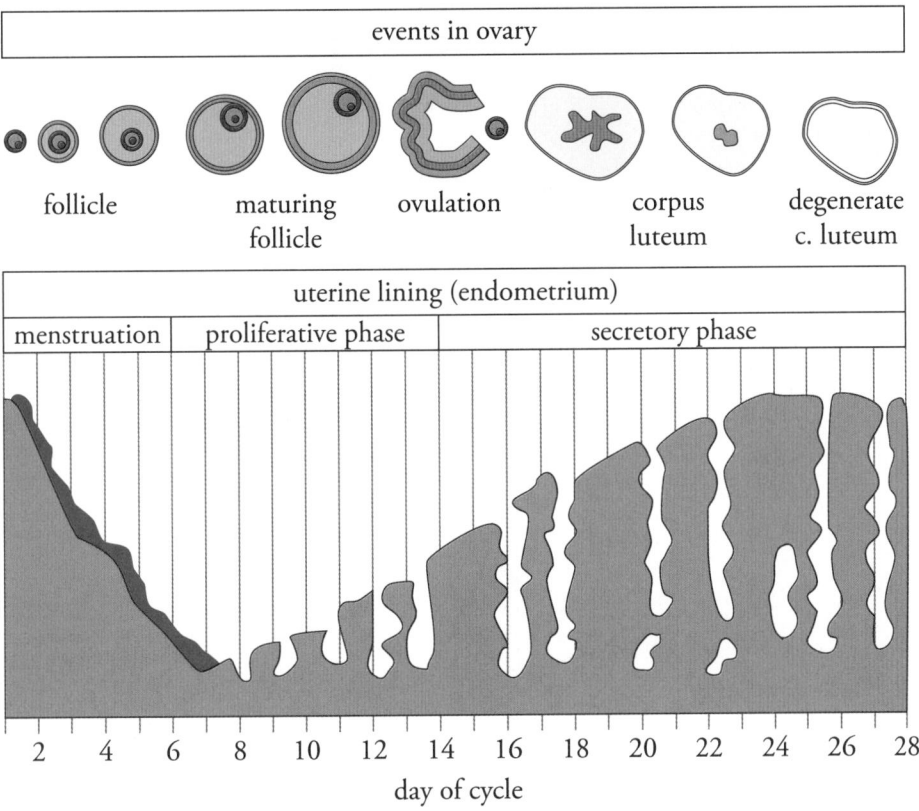

Figure 7   The Ovarian and Uterine Cycles

Focus on the Hormones

The anterior pituitary and the hypothalamus play a role in the menstrual cycle by regulating the secretion of estrogen and progesterone from the ovary (Figure 8, next page). Estrogen and progesterone then regulate the events in the uterus. The following is a summary:

1) GnRH from the hypothalamus stimulates the release of FSH and LH from the anterior pituitary.

2) Under the influence of FSH, the granulosa and thecal cells develop during the follicular phase and secrete estrogen. Secretion of GnRH, FSH, and LH is initially inhibited by estrogen; however, estrogen, which increases throughout the follicular stage, reaches a threshold near the end of this phase and has a positive effect on LH secretion.

3) This sudden surge in LH causes ovulation. After ovulation, LH induces the follicle to become the corpus luteum and to secrete estrogen and progesterone (this marks the beginning of the secretory phase). If pregnancy does not occur, the combined high levels of estrogen and progesterone feedback to strongly inhibit secretion of GnRH, FSH, and LH. When LH secretion drops, the corpus luteum regresses, no longer secretes estrogen or progesterone, and menstruation occurs.

- If LH levels remained high, how would this affect the secretion of estrogen and progesterone?[33]
- What would happen if the estrogen and progesterone levels in a woman's blood were kept artificially high for the entire month?[34]
- What would happen if the artificial hormones were suddenly taken away?[35]

13.7

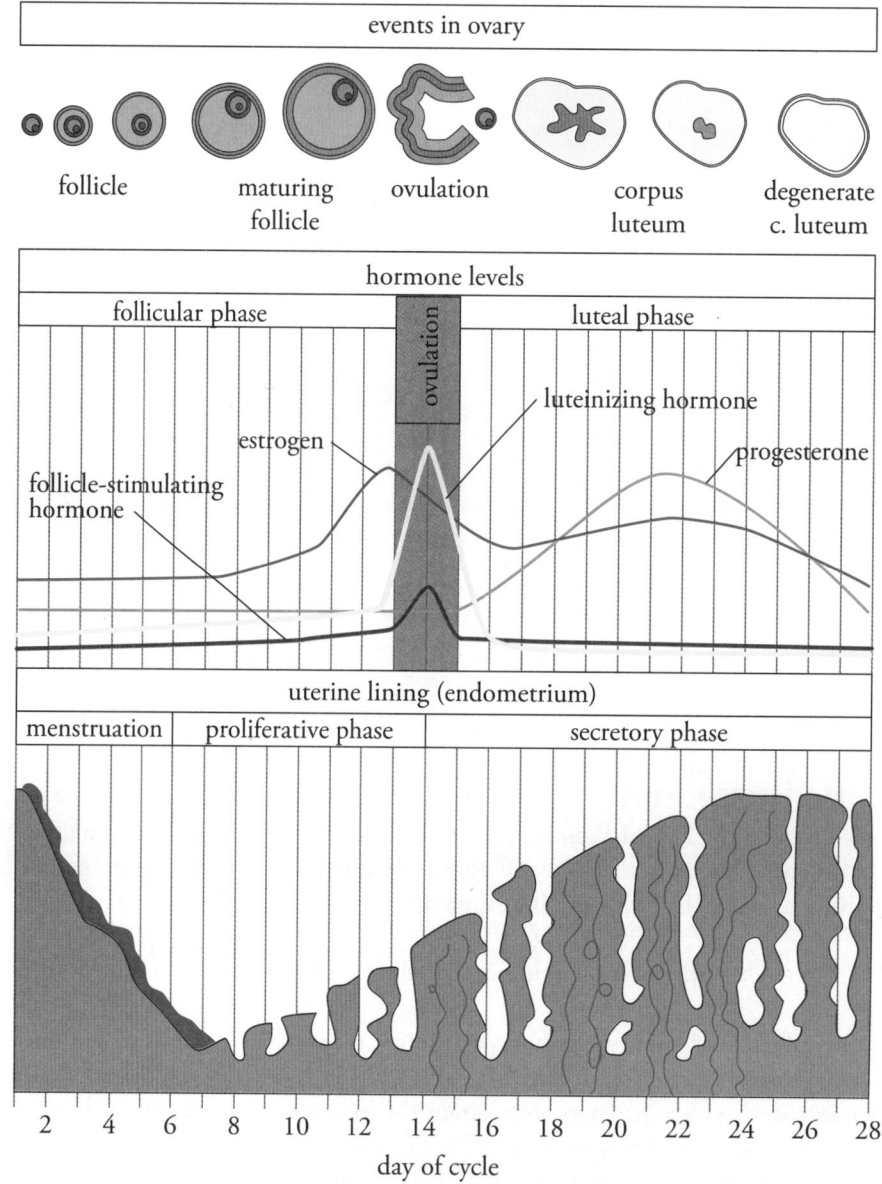

Figure 8   Pituitary and Ovarian Hormones of the Menstrual Cycle

---

[33] If LH levels remained high, the corpus luteum would not regress, and estrogen and progesterone would also remain high, thus maintaining the endometrium so that menstruation would not occur. This is, in effect, what happens if an embryo is fertilized and implants, except the hormone in this case is not LH but hCG, human chorionic gonadotropin, an LH-like hormone (see the next section).

[34] The woman would not ovulate. That's what (most) birth control pills are: estrogen and progesterone.

[35] The endometrium would slough off, and the woman would menstruate. (This is why there are 21 pills of one color and 7 pills of another color. The 7 pills contain no hormones; they are either placebos or sometimes iron supplements. If a woman took the hormone pill every day and never took the 7 placebos, she would never menstruate. Also, the placebos are actually unnecessary; these 7 pills are only present in order to help establish the habit of taking a pill every day.)

13.8 HORMONAL CHANGES DURING PREGNANCY

There are still a couple of points we have not made completely clear: how can pregnancy occur if the uterine lining is lost each month, and why does the body discard the endometrium?

Recall that the physiological reason for endometrial shedding is a decrease in estrogen and progesterone levels, which occurs as the corpus luteum degenerates. Why does the corpus luteum degenerate? Due to a decrease in luteinizing hormone. Why does LH decrease? Due to feedback inhibition from the high levels of estrogen and progesterone secreted by the corpus luteum.

Let's begin with why LH levels decrease. During pregnancy, ovulation should be prevented. The way ovulation is prevented is for the constant high levels of estrogen and progesterone seen during pregnancy to inhibit secretion of LH by the pituitary; no LH surge, no ovulation. Constant high levels of estrogen inhibit LH release. The result is pregnancy without continued ovulation. The *secondary* result is the one we were trying to explain: when the corpus luteum secretes a lot of estrogen and progesterone during the menstrual cycle, LH levels drop, causing the corpus luteum to degenerate. The point is that the corpus luteum degenerates unless fertilization has occurred.

So how can pregnancy occur? If pregnancy is to occur, the endometrium must be maintained, because it is the site of gestation (i.e., where the embryo lives and is nourished). If fertilization takes place, within a few days a developing embryo becomes **implanted** in the endometrium, and a **placenta** begins to develop. The **chorion** is the portion of the placenta that is derived from the zygote. It secretes **human chorionic gonadotropin**, or **hCG,** which can take the place of LH in maintaining the corpus luteum. In the presence of hCG, the corpus luteum does not degenerate, the estrogen and progesterone levels stay elevated, and menstruation does not occur. This answers the question of *how* pregnancy can occur. hCG is the hormone tested for in pregnancy tests because its presence absolutely confirms the presence of an embryo.

- Which of the following occur(s) during the menstrual cycle immediately prior to ovulation?[36]
    - I. A surge in luteinizing hormone release from the anterior pituitary
    - II. Completion of the second meiotic cell division by the oocyte
    - III. Shedding of the endometrium

- As a woman ages, the number of follicles remaining in the ovaries decreases until ovulation ceases. At this point, termed **menopause**, the menstrual cycle no longer occurs. Which of the following occur(s) during menopause?[37]
    - I. FSH levels drop dramatically and stay low.
    - II. Estrogen levels are abnormally high.
    - III. LH levels are very high and stay high.

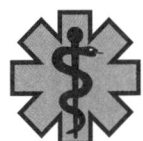

---

[36] **Item I: True.** The LH surge *causes* ovulation. Item II: False. Meiosis I is completed prior to ovulation. Meiosis II isn't completed until after fertilization. Item III: False. Ovulation occurs around day 14 of the cycle. Menstruation begins at day 1.

[37] In the absence of estrogen and progesterone secretion by follicles, there is no feedback inhibition of LH and FSH, so their levels are very high in postmenopausal women. Thus, only **item III** is true.

- Which of the following statements concerning the menstrual cycle is/are true?[38]
  - I. The proliferative phase of the endometrium coincides with the maturation of ovarian follicles.
  - II. The secretory phase of the endometrial cycle is dependent on the secretion of estrogen from cells surrounding secondary oocytes.
  - III. Luteinizing hormone levels are highest during the menstrual phase of the endometrial cycle.

13.9 FERTILIZATION AND CLEAVAGE

A secondary oocyte is ovulated and enters the uterine tube. It is surrounded by the **corona radiata** (a protective layer of granulosa cells) and the **zona pellucida** (located just outside the egg cell membrane). The oocyte will remain fertile for about a day. If intercourse occurs, sperm are deposited near the cervix, and are activated, or **capacitated**. Sperm capacitation involves the dilution of inhibitory substances present in semen. The activated sperm will survive for two or three days. They swim through the uterus toward the secondary oocyte.

Fertilization is the fusion of a spermatozoan with the secondary oocyte (Figure 9). It normally occurs in the uterine tube. In order for fertilization to occur, a sperm must penetrate the corona radiata and bind to and penetrate the zona pellucida. It accomplishes this using the **acrosome reaction**. The **acrosome** is a large vesicle in the sperm head containing hydrolytic enzymes which are released by exocytosis. After the corona radiata has been penetrated, an **acrosomal process** containing actin elongates toward the zona pellucida. The acrosomal process has **bindin**, a species-specific protein which binds to receptors in the zona pellucida. Finally, the sperm and egg plasma membranes fuse, and the sperm nucleus enters the secondary oocyte. In about twenty minutes, the secondary oocyte completes meiosis II, giving rise to an ootid and the second polar body. The ootid matures rapidly, becoming an **ovum**. Then the sperm and egg nuclei fuse, and the new diploid cell is known as a **zygote**.

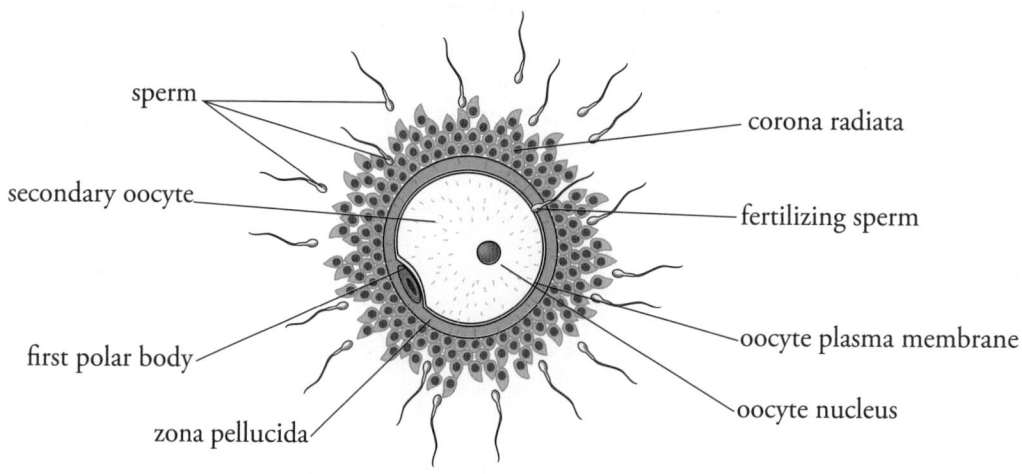

Figure 9   Fertilization

---

[38] **Item I: True.** This is explained in the text. Item II: False. It is secretion of estrogen and progesterone *by the corpus luteum* that drives the secretory phase. The corpus luteum is in the ovary, while the secondary oocyte is out in the uterine tube. Item III: False. The luteinizing hormone level peaks during the proliferative phase, since this is when ovulation occurs.

482 | For more free content, visit PrincetonReview.com

Penetration of an ovum by more than one sperm is known as **polyspermy**. It is normally prevented by the **fast block to polyspermy** and the **slow block to polyspermy**, which occur upon penetration of the egg by a spermatozoan. The fast block consists of a depolarization of the egg plasma membrane. This depolarization prevents other spermatozoa from fusing with the egg cell membrane. The slow block results from a Ca^{2+} influx caused by the initial depolarization. The slow block is also known as the **cortical reaction**. It has two components: swelling of the space between the zona pellucida and the plasma membrane, and hardening of the zona pellucida. The Ca^{2+} influx has one other noteworthy effect. It causes increased metabolism and protein synthesis, referred to as **egg activation**.

- Because of a particular disease, a man produces sperm without acrosomes. His spermatozoa are abnormal in that they:[39]
    - A) are immotile.
    - B) cannot undergo capacitation.
    - C) are incapable of fertilizing the egg.
    - D) can fertilize the eggs of many species.

- Which one of the following would NOT cause or indicate infertility?[40]
    - A) A lack of progesterone secretion during the latter half of the menstrual cycle
    - B) Failure of mitosis to occur after the male pronucleus fuses with the nucleus of the ovum
    - C) Excessively acidic pH of the vaginal secretions
    - D) A decrease in the concentration of LH after ovulation

13.9

Cleavage

The process of **embryogenesis** begins within hours of fertilization, but proceeds slowly in humans. The first stage is **cleavage**, in which the zygote undergoes many cell divisions to produce a ball of cells known as the **morula**. The first cell division occurs about 36 hours after fertilization. [The morula is the same size as the zygote, which indicates that the dividing cells spend most of their time in what phases of the cell cycle?[41] During cleavage of the zygote, do homologous chromosomes physically interact with each other?[42]]

---

[39] Acrosomal enzymes are necessary for penetration of the corona radiata, and the acrosomal process is necessary for binding to a penetration of the zona pellucida. Sperm that lack an acrosome would be unable to complete these processes, which are necessary for fertilization (choice **C** is correct, and choice D is wrong). The acrosome has nothing to do with motility (motility is the flagella's job; choice A is wrong), and capacitation is the activation of sperm in the female reproductive tract. It has nothing to do with the acrosome (choice B is wrong).

[40] Progesterone is secreted from the corpus luteum, which is formed from the remnants of the Graafian follicle after ovulation. A lack of progesterone might indicate that the corpus luteum did not form, and thus ovulation did not occur (choice A could indicate infertility and can be eliminated). The male pronucleus is just the haploid sperm nucleus. After this fuses with the ovum nucleus, the now diploid zygote must undergo cleavage (rapid mitosis) to form an embryo. If mitosis fails to occur, no embryo would develop (choice B would cause infertility and can be eliminated). Excessively acidic pH in the vagina could be harmful to sperm, which prefer a more alkaline environment. Sperm damaged by acids may not be motile, or may not be able to successfully fertilize an egg (choice C could lead to infertility and can be eliminated). However, LH normally decreases after ovulation. This is expected and not an indicator of infertility (choice **D** is the correct answer choice).

[41] They must spend most of their time during the S (synthesis) and M (mitotic) phases, skipping the G_1 and G_2 (gap or growth) phases.

[42] No. Pairing of homologous chromosomes takes place only during meiosis, which occurs only during gametogenesis.

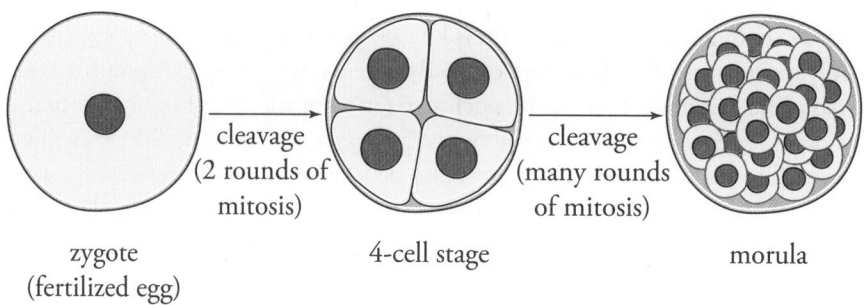

Figure 10 Cleavage

As cell divisions continue, the morula is transformed into a **blastocyst** (Figure 11). This process is known as **blastulation**. The blastocyst consists of a ring of cells called the **trophoblast** surrounding a cavity, and an **inner cell mass** adhering to the inside of the trophoblast at one end of the cavity. The **trophoblast** will give rise to the **chorion** (the zygote's contribution to the placenta). The inner cell mass will become the **embryo**.

- If two inner cell masses form in the blastula, what will the result be?[43]

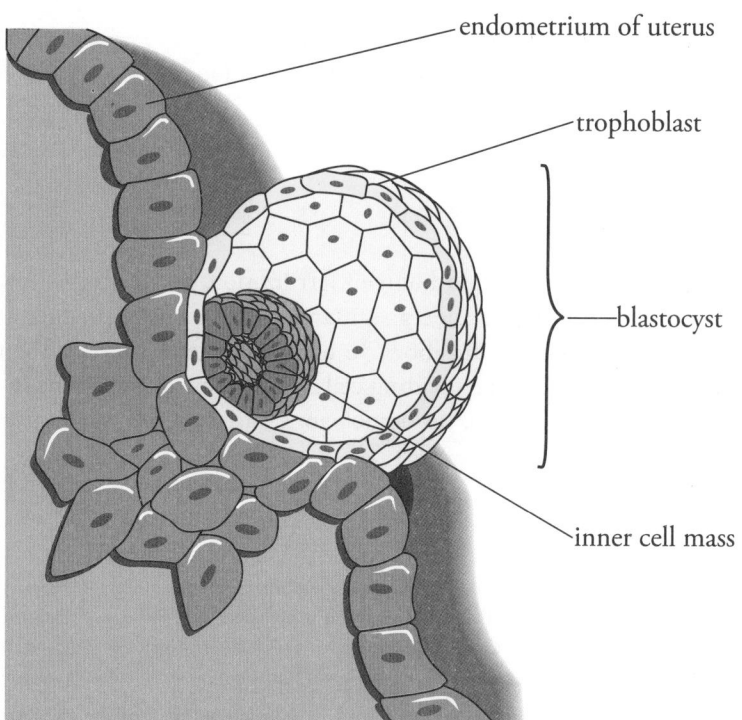

Figure 11 The Blastocyst at the Beginning of Implantation

---

[43] The inner cell mass becomes the embryo. Two inner cell masses derived from a single zygote and enclosed by the same trophoblast will result in a pair of identical twins sharing the same placenta.

13.10   IMPLANTATION AND THE PLACENTA

The developing blastocyst reaches the uterus and burrows into the endometrium, or **implants**, about a week after fertilization (Figure 11). The trophoblast secretes proteases that lyse endometrial cells. The blastocyst then sinks into the endometrium and is surrounded by it, absorbing nutrients through the trophoblast into the inner cell mass. The embryo receives a large part of its nutrition in this manner for the first few weeks of pregnancy. This is why the secretory phase of the endometrial cycle occurs: endometrial cells store glycogen, lipids, and other nutrients so that the early embryo may derive nourishment directly from the endometrium. Later, an organ develops which is specialized to facilitate exchange of nutrients, gases, and even antibodies between the maternal and embryonic bloodstreams: the **placenta**. Because it takes about three months for the placenta to develop, it is during the first trimester (three months) of pregnancy that hCG is essential for maintenance of the endometrium (Section 13.8).

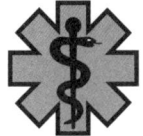

- What happens if the corpus luteum is removed during the first trimester?[44]

During the last six months of pregnancy, the corpus luteum is no longer needed because the placenta itself secretes sufficient estrogen and progesterone for maintenance of the endometrium.

The development of the placenta involves the formation of **placental villi**. These are chorionic projections extending into the endometrium, into which fetal capillaries will grow. Surrounding the villi are sinuses (open spaces) filled with maternal blood. [Does oxygen-containing blood pass from the mother into the developing fetus?[45]]

The embryo is not the only important structure derived from the inner cell mass. There are three others: amnion, yolk sac, and allantois. The **amnion** surrounds a fluid-filled cavity which contains the developing embryo. Amniotic fluid is the "water" which "breaks" (is expelled) before birth. The **yolk sac** is important in reptiles and birds because it contains the nourishing yolk. Mammals do not store yolk. Our yolk sac is important because it is the first site of red blood cell synthesis in the embryo. Finally, the **allantois** develops from the embryonic gut and forms the blood vessels of the umbilical cord, which transport blood between embryo and placenta.

- Each of the following has the same genome EXCEPT:[46]
  - A) chorion.
  - B) amnion.
  - C) yolk sac.
  - D) endometrium.

---

[44] The woman menstruates, and the embryo is lost. Remember, the role of hCG is to substitute for LH in stimulating the corpus luteum. The role of the corpus luteum is to make estrogen and progesterone, which maintain the endometrium.

[45] No. The placenta is like a lung in that it facilitates exchange of substances between the two bloodstreams without allowing actual mixing.

[46] The chorion, amnion, and yolk sac are all derived from the inner cell mass of the blastula, and therefore must have the same genome (choices A, B, and C can be eliminated). However, the endometrium is derived from the mother (it is the inner lining of the uterus), and would have a different genome than the embryo (choice **D** is correct).

13.11 POST-IMPLANTATION DEVELOPMENT

We have examined embryogenesis from fertilization through blastulation. The next phase is **gastrulation**. Gastrulation is when the three **primary germ layers** (the **ectoderm**, the **mesoderm**, and the **endoderm**) become distinct.

In primitive organisms, the **blastula** (equivalent to blastocyst) is a hollow ball of cells, and gastrulation involves the **invagination** (involution) of these cells to form layers. Imagine pushing your fist into a big soft round balloon to create an inner layer (contacting your fist) and an outer layer (contacting the air). The inner layer is the endoderm, and the outer layer is the ectoderm. The mesoderm (middle layer) develops from the endoderm. The cavity (where your fist is) is primitive gut, or **archenteron**. The opening (where your wrist is) is the **blastopore**, and will give rise to the anus. The whole structure is the **gastrula**. (Don't be confused: the *gastr*ula has a *blast*opore; the *blast*ula has no opening.)

In humans, things are a little different. The gastrula develops from a double layer of cells called the **embryonic disk**, instead of from a spherical blastula. But the end result is the same: three layers. You need to know what parts of the human body are derived from each layer.

Table 4   Fates of the Primary Germ Layers

Ectoderm	Mesoderm	Endoderm
• Entire nervous system • Pituitary gland (both lobes), adrenal medulla • Cornea and lens • Epidermis of skin and derivatives (hair, nails, sweat glands, sensory receptors) • Nasal, oral, anal epithelium	• All muscle, bone, and connective tissue • Entire cardiovascular and lymphatic system, including blood • Urogenital organs (kidneys, ureters, gonads, reproductive ducts) • Dermis of skin	• GI tract epithelium (except mouth and anus) • GI glands (liver, pancreas, etc.) • Respiratory epithelium • Epithelial lining of urogenital organs and ducts • Urinary bladder

Pay attention to what *types* of thing are derived from each layer, and you'll see that it's relatively easy to memorize. One key thing to note is that **ectoderm** and *epithelium* are not synonymous. Epithelium outside the body (epidermis) is derived from ectoderm, but epithelium inside the body (gut lining) comes from endoderm.

- Which of the following statements is/are true?[47]
  - I. Oxygen must diffuse across the chorionic membrane to reach the fetus from the mother.
  - II. Transplantation of cells from the trophoblast of one embryo to the trophoblast of another embryo will result in an infant with a mixed genetic composition.
  - III. All of the cells of the blastocyst are functionally equivalent.

The next step after gastrulation is **neurulation**, the formation of the nervous system. It begins when a portion of the ectoderm differentiates into the **neural plate**. At the edges of the plate are the **neural crest cells**; these edges thicken and fold upward (the **neural folds**), leaving the bottom of the plate to form the

---

[47] **Item I: True.** The chorion is part of the placenta. Item II: False. The trophoblast is derived from the outer cell mass and gives rise only to the chorion. The embryo is derived entirely from the inner cell mass. Item III: False. The trophoblast and the inner cell mass are both components of the blastocyst, and they have very different roles.

neural tube. The neural tube ultimately develops into the central nervous system (brain and spinal cord). During that process, the neural crest cells separate from the neural tube and the overlying ectoderm (which ultimately becomes the epidermis), then migrate to different parts of the embryo to differentiate into a variety of cell types, including melanocytes, glial cells, the adrenal medulla, some peripheral neurons, and some facial connective tissue (Figure 12). The formation of the neural tube is induced by instructions from the underlying notochord, which is mesodermal in origin. It gives rise to the vertebral column.

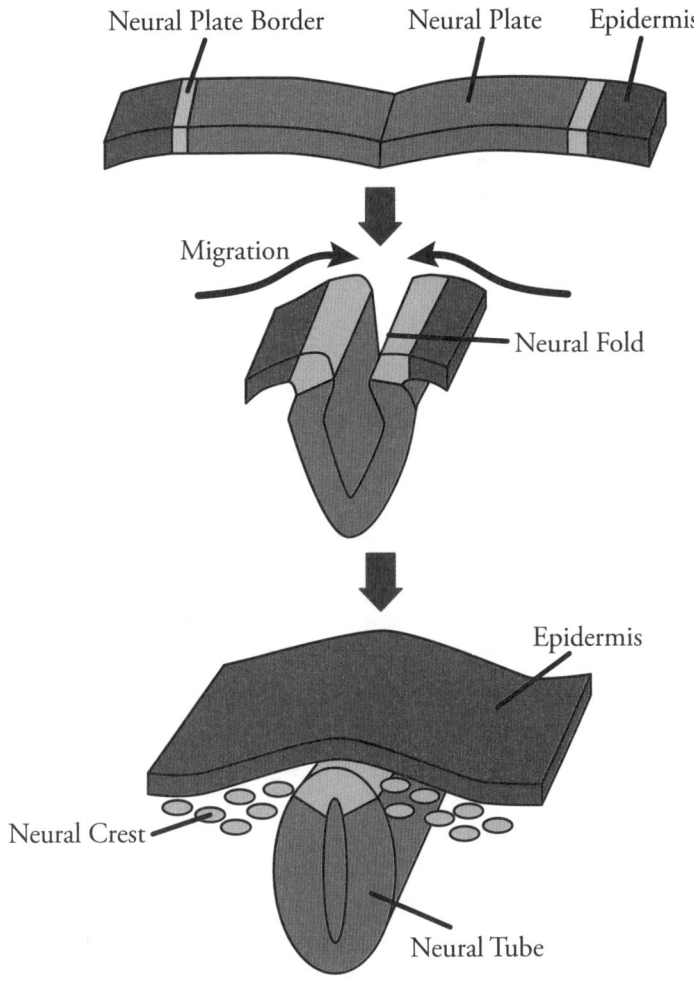

Figure 12   Neural Crest

Neurulation is one component of **organogenesis**, the development of organ systems. By the eighth week of gestation, all major organ systems are present, and the **embryo** is now called a **fetus**. Even though the developmental process has attained staggering complexity, by the end of the first trimester the fetus is still only 5 cm long. [During which trimester is the developing human most sensitive to toxins such as drugs and radiation?[48]]

---

[48]   During the first trimester, when the organs are being formed.

- A radioactive dye is detected only in the cells of placental villi. Weeks earlier, it must have been injected into the:[49]
    - A) inner cell mass.
    - B) trophoblast.
    - C) endometrium.
    - D) zygote.

- During gastrulation, do tissues derived from the trophoblast move inward to form the lining of the primitive gut?[50]

Environment-Gene Interaction

During this early time period in development, the prenatal environment can play a significant role in gene expression. For example, a lack of folic acid in the mother's diet at this time can lead to significant defects in the formation of the neural tube and central nervous system. Certain illnesses in the mother can lead to issues in the fetus; influenza has been linked to schizophrenia and German measles to deafness, eye abnormalities, and heart defects. Hypoxia in utero, such as might be caused by maternal cigarette smoking (and the resultant vasoconstriction of uterine blood vessels) can lead to a reduction in grey matter development. Fetal alcohol syndrome due to excess maternal alcohol consumption can lead to stunted fetal growth, brain damage, and other behavioral and physical problems.

13.12   DIFFERENTIATION

The specialization of cell types during development is termed **differentiation** because as cells specialize they become different from their parent cells and from each other. By specializing, a cell becomes better able to perform a particular task, while becoming less adept at other tasks. For example, a sensory neuron is the best vehicle for the transmission of a nerve impulse over great distances, but is quite incapable of obtaining nourishment on its own, or even of reproducing itself.

Primitive cells in the zygote and the morula have the potential to become any cell type in the blastocyst, including the trophoblast and the inner cell mass. They are therefore known as **totipotent** cells. Cells of the inner cell mass are more specialized and are referred to as **pluripotent**. They can differentiate into any of the three primary germ layers (ectoderm, mesoderm, or endoderm) and therefore have the capability to become any of the 220 cell types that make up an adult human. However, they cannot contribute to the trophoblast of the blastocyst (i.e., will not become the placenta).

---

[49] The placenta is derived from the chorion, which is derived from the cells of the trophoblast; thus, injecting a dye into the trophoblast would lead to its detection in the placental villi (choice **B** is correct). The inner cell mass ultimately becomes the embryo; thus, dye injected into the inner cells mass would be detected in the embryo, not the placenta (choice A is wrong). The endometrium is derived from the mother and is only the site of implantation and placental development. It does not actually contribute to the placenta; thus, dye injected into the endometrium would not be detected in the placenta (choice C is wrong). The zygote is the precursor to all embryonic and extraembryonic structures. Injecting a dye into the zygote would lead to its detection not only in the placenta, but also in the amnion, chorion, and embryo itself (choice D is wrong).

[50] No. Gastrulation involves only cells derived from the inner cell mass.

As development continues, cells continue to specialize. After gastrulation, cells from the early embryonic germ layers are each considered **multipotent**. This means they can become many, but not all, cell types. For example, cells of the mesoderm can differentiate into muscle and bone cells, but not into neurons or digestive epithelium.

In other words, totipotent cells differentiate into pluripotent cells, which specialize to become multipotent cells. Most cells in the adult have lost all potency and have become completely specialized mature cells, incapable of changing into other cell types. Adult stem cells are an exception to this, and these cells are discussed in Section A.13 of Appendix I.

Stem cells, because of their ability to become nearly any cell type in the body, are of great interest in research; they remain a potential source for regenerative medicine and tissue replacement after injury or disease. In humans, embryonic stem cells are the only pluripotent cells that have been found. These cells are isolated from the inner cell mass of the blastocyst.

There is a certain point in the development of a cell at which the cell fate becomes fixed; at this point the cell is said to be **determined**. Determination precedes differentiation. This means a cell is determined before it is visibly differentiated. Determination can be **induced** by a cell's environment, such as exposure to diffusible factors or neighboring cells, or it can be preprogrammed.

- During early embryonic development, cells near the developing notochord undergo an irreversible developmental choice to become skeletal muscle later in development, although they do not immediately change their appearance. This is an example of which of the following?[51]
  - A) Determination
  - B) Differentiation
  - C) Totipotency
  - D) Induction

13.12

There is such a thing as **dedifferentiation**. This is the process whereby a specialized cell *un*specializes and may become totipotent. If a dedifferentiated cell proliferates in an uncontrolled manner, the result can be cancer. The most important lesson you can learn from the notion of dedifferentiation is that every cell has the same genome. The specialization of cell types is a function of things in the cytoplasm and maybe proteins and RNA in the nucleus, but no genetic changes normally take place during development and differentiation.

- Can you think of two exceptions to this rule, where a particular cell type normally has a unique genome?[52]

---

[51] A cell whose fate is fixed is said to be determined, however, if it has not yet undergone a change in appearance, it has not yet been differentiated (choice **A** is correct, and choice B is wrong). Since the cell is destined to become muscle, it is no longer totipotent (choice C is wrong). Although the cells are found near the notochord, there is no reason to assume the location is the reason for their determination. They could be cytoplasmically determined (choice D is wrong).

[52] One exception is B cells and T cells of the immune system. They undergo gene (DNA!) rearrangements in the process of attaining antigen specificity. The other exception is gametes. They have unique genomes because of 1) reductive division with independent assortment, and 2) recombination.

Table 5 Stem Cells

Term	Definition	Examples
Totipotent	• Can generate trophoblast and inner cell mass	zygote; morula
Pluripotent	• Can differentiate into any of the three primary germ layers • Can generate all adult cell types (over 220 different cells)	inner cell mass of blastocyst (embryonic stem cells); IPS (induced pluripotent stem) cells
Multipotent	• Can produce many (but not all) cell types • More differentiated than pluripotent • Often tissue-specific	three primary germ layers; adult stem cells
Dedifferentiation	• Some cells can go backward and become less specialized • Example: Mature → Multipotent → Pluripotent → Totipotent	iPS cells; cancer cells

13.13   PREGNANCY

The early stages of development already discussed (gastrulation and neurulation) comprise the embryonic stage of development. These eight weeks comprise the majority of the first trimester; during this time all major organ systems appear. The stage of development from eight weeks until birth is known as the fetal stage. This stage covers the second and third trimesters of the pregnancy.

Second Trimester

During this time the organs and organ systems of the fetus continue to develop structurally and functionally. The fetus grows, typically reaching a weight of approximately 0.6 kg, and looks distinctly human.

Third Trimester

This is a stage of rapid fetal growth, including significant deposition of adipose tissue. Most of the organ systems become fully functional. A baby born 1–2 months early has a reasonably good chance of survival.

Mom

The demands placed on the mother's body increase significantly over the course of the pregnancy. Maternal respiratory rate increases to bring in additional oxygen and eliminate additional carbon dioxide. Blood volume in the mother increases by about 50% due to a drop in oxygen levels (because of the metabolic demands of the fetus) and a subsequent release of erythropoietin and renin. This is accompanied by an increase in glomerular filtration rate of a corresponding 50%. The demand for nutrients and vitamins increases by about 30%, the uterus undergoes a very significant increase in size, and the mammary glands increase in size. Additionally, secretory activity begins in the mammary glands, although this is not technically lactation.

13.14   BIRTH AND LACTATION

The technical term for birth is **parturition**. It is dependent on contraction of muscles in the uterine wall. The very high levels of progesterone secreted throughout pregnancy help to repress contractions in uterine muscle, but near the end of pregnancy uterine excitability increases. This increased excitability is likely to be a result of several factors, including a change in the ratio of estrogen to progesterone, the presence of the hormone **oxytocin** secreted by the posterior pituitary, and mechanical stretching of the uterus and cervix.

Weak contractions of the uterus occur throughout pregnancy. As pregnancy reaches full term, however, rhythmic **labor contractions** begin. It is thought that the onset of labor contractions is the result of a positive feedback reflex: the increased pressure on the cervix crosses a threshold that causes the posterior pituitary to increase the secretion of oxytocin. Oxytocin causes the uterine contractions to increase in intensity, creating greater pressure on the cervix that stimulates still more oxytocin release and even stronger contractions.

The first stage of labor is dilation of the cervix. The second stage is the actual birth, involving movement of the baby through the cervix and birth canal, pushed by contraction of uterine (smooth) and abdominal (skeletal) muscle. The third stage is the expulsion of the placenta, after it separates from the wall of the uterus. Contractions of the uterus after birth help to minimize blood loss.

During pregnancy, milk production and secretion would be a waste of energy, but after parturition it is necessary. During puberty, estrogen stimulates the development of breasts in women. The increased levels of estrogen and progesterone secreted by the placenta during pregnancy cause the further development of glandular and adipose breast tissue. But while these hormones stimulate breast development, they inhibit the release of **prolactin** and thus the production of milk. After parturition, the levels of estrogen and progesterone fall and milk production begins. Every time suckling occurs, the pituitary gland is stimulated by the hypothalamus to release a large surge of prolactin, prolonging the ability of the breasts to secrete milk. If the mother stops breast-feeding the infant, prolactin levels fall and milk secretion ceases. The converse is also true: milk secretion can continue for years, as long as nursing continues. The breasts do not leak large amounts of milk when the infant is not nursing. This is because the posterior pituitary hormone **oxytocin** is necessary for **milk let-down** (release). Oxytocin is also released when suckling occurs.

13.14

Chapter 13 Summary

- The primary sex organs produce gametes and hormones. The testes are the male primary sex organ and the ovaries are the female primary sex organ.

- Male internal genitalia are formed from Wolffian ducts and female internal genitalia are formed from Müllerian ducts.

- Spermatogenesis takes place in the seminiferous tubules and results in four haploid sperm from a single spermatogonium. It begins at puberty and continues on a daily basis for the life of the male. FSH stimulates spermatogenesis and LH stimulates testosterone production.

- Sperm travel from the seminiferous tubules to the epididymis, then to the ductus deferens, then to the urethra. Semen is a supportive fluid for sperm, produced by the seminal vesicles, the prostate, and the bulbourethral glands.

- Oogenesis begins prenatally, producing primary oocytes. It occurs again on a monthly basis, beginning at puberty and ending at menopause; this produces one secondary oocyte (which is ovulated) and the first polar body. Oogenesis is only completed if the secondary oocyte is fertilized, in which case an ovum and the second polar body will be produced.

- FSH stimulates follicle development and estrogen secretion during the first half of the menstrual cycle. LH stimulates ovulation and the formation of the corpus luteum, as well as progesterone and estrogen secretion, during the second half of the menstrual cycle.

- Estrogen stimulates growth of the endometrium during the first half of the menstrual cycle; progesterone and estrogen maintain and enhance the endometrium during the second half of the menstrual cycle. If no fertilization takes place, estrogen and progesterone levels fall, and the endometrium is sloughed off.

- Arousal is mediated by the parasympathetic nervous system, while orgasm and resolution are mediated by the sympathetic nervous system.

- Fertilization takes place in the uterine tubes, and cleavage begins 24–36 hours later. The zygote becomes a morula, the morula becomes a blatstula, and the blastula implants in the endometrium.

- The trophoblast becomes the placenta and the inner cell mass becomes the embryo.

- The first eight weeks of development are the embryonic stage, during which gastrulation (formation of the three primary germ layers), neurulation (formation of the nervous system), and organogenesis occur.

- The fetal stage begins at the eighth week of development and ends at the birth of the baby.

- Labor is a positive feedback cycle triggered by mild (initially) uterine contractions that push the baby's head on the cervix. This stimulates the release of oxytocin, which causes a stronger uterine contraction, and a bigger stretch of the cervix. This positive feedback loop will continue until the birth of the baby.

- Prolactin stimulates milk production and oxytocin stimulates milk ejection in a baby-driven cycle.

CHAPTER 13 FREESTANDING PRACTICE QUESTIONS

1. Which of the following structures undergoes mitosis?

A) Spermatid
B) Spermatogonium
C) Primary spermatocyte
D) Secondary spermatocyte

2. Which of the following statements regarding childbirth is true?

A) Release of oxytocin from the anterior pituitary, combined with increased mechanical pressure of the fetal head on the cervix, creates a positive feedback loop that increases uterine contractions.
B) Release of progesterone from the placenta, combined with increased mechanical pressure of the fetal head on the cervix, creates a positive feedback loop that increases uterine contractions.
C) Release of progesterone from the posterior pituitary, combined with increased mechanical pressure of the fetal head on the cervix, creates a negative feedback loop that increases uterine contractions.
D) Release of oxytocin from the posterior pituitary, combined with mechanical pressure of the fetal head on the cervix, creates a positive feedback loop that increases uterine contractions.

3. Which of the following is NOT a difference between spermatogenesis and oogenesis?

A) Spermatogenesis in a male begins at puberty, whereas oogenesis in a female begins when the female is an embryo.
B) Spermatogenesis produces four sperm, whereas oogenesis produces one ovum.
C) Spermatogenesis produces primary spermatocytes for a male's entire life, whereas oogenesis ceases to produce primary oocytes when a female reaches menopause.
D) Spermatogenesis occurs in the testes, whereas oogenesis occurs in the ovaries.

4. Which of the following hormones is NOT elevated during the first trimester of pregnancy?

A) Estrogen
B) Progesterone
C) GnRH
D) hCG

5. Ovulation usually occurs on the 14th day of the ovarian cycle. All of the following occur during ovulation and the days immediately following ovulation EXCEPT:

A) the ovary releases a secondary oocyte.
B) a surge of FSH from the anterior pituitary causes the follicle to become the corpus luteum.
C) the follicle secretes progesterone once it becomes the corpus luteum.
D) a surge of LH can be detected.

6. Ectopic pregnancy, where implantation of the embryo occurs in the fallopian tube rather than the uterus, is possible because:

A) though fertilization takes place in the uterus, implantation does not occur immediately and thus the embryo could migrate back up into the fallopian tubes.
B) fertilization occurs in the fallopian tubes and the embryo may fail to migrate to the uterus.
C) the fimbriae may hold the embryo in the fallopian tube rather than pushing it toward the uterus.
D) fertilization may have occurred in the ovary with subsequent implantation in the fallopian tube.

7. Postpartum women often experience mild to moderate uterine contractions when nursing. These contractions are triggered by the release of:

A) estrogen.
B) oxytocin.
C) progesterone.
D) prolactin.

8. The greater vestibular glands in the female (Bartholin's glands) have a similar function as which of the following male reproductive glands?

A) Bulbourethral glands (Cowper's glands)
B) Seminal vesicles
C) Prostate
D) Testes

CHAPTER 13 PRACTICE PASSAGE

For families struggling with infertility, IVF (in vitro fertilization) can be performed to help couples conceive. In IVF, an egg is harvested from the female partner, sperm are harvested from the male partner, and then egg and sperm are combined in a lab. The embryos are grown and observed in the lab, and then viable embryos are transferred into the uterine cavity. It is estimated that 1–2% of US births annually are via IVF.

Multiple births can develop two ways during IVF. If more than one embryo is transferred into the uterus, both could successfully implant and develop. Alternatively, a single embryo could divide into two. These two mechanisms lead to different types of twins.

Dizygotic or fraternal twins are non-identical and are formed when two genetically different eggs are fertilized by two different sperm. When fraternal twins are delivered, there are typically two placentas. Monozygotic or identical twins are formed when a zygote, morula, or blastocyst splits into two separate embryos. If the cell mass splits before day five, two embryos will develop with separate placentas and separate amniotic sacs; this occurs about 66% of the time. After day five, splitting usually leads to two amniotic sacs but one placenta; this occurs about 33% of the time. The other 1% of identical twins split even later in development.

Five sets of twins are undergoing testing to determine if they are fraternal or identical. Each set share significant physical characteristics. Each set of twins answers a questionnaire (Table 1) and undergoes RFLP genetic testing (Figure 1).

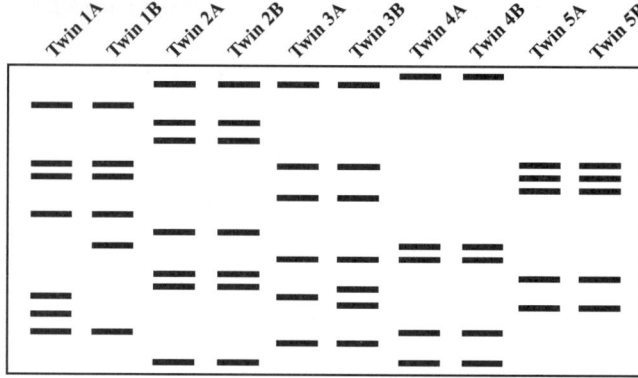

Figure 1 Twin RFLP results

	Gender	Age (years)	Placenta(s)	Amniotic Sac
Twins 1	F/M	2.2	2	2
Twins 2	M/M	14	2	2
Twins 3	F/F	0.5	2	2
Twins 4	F/F	8	1	1
Twins 5	M/M	4	1	2

Table 1 Twin questionnaire results

1. Which statement below is NOT supported by the passage?

A) It is common for identical twins to share both a placenta and an amniotic sac.
B) Monozygotic twins have identical genomic sequences and fraternal twins have different genetic information.
C) Most identical twins split before development of the three primary germ layers.
D) Twins with two placentas can be fraternal or identical.

2. A sixth set of twins was supposed to be included in the twin study described in the passage. While their questionnaire responses were appropriate, their RFLP analysis did not work. Which of the following could explain why the RFLP analysis failed?

A) High levels of RNase were detected on the sample collection tools.
B) The tubes that stored the samples were accidentally stored at 32°C for two days.
C) The tubes that stored the samples were contaminated by a DNase.
D) The twins were very young, so their samples were contaminated by proteases.

3. Which of the twins in the passage are monozygotic?

A) Twins 4 and 5
B) Twins 2, 4, 5
C) Twins 2, 3, 4, 5
D) All of the twins

4. How would carrying twins affect maternal hormone levels, compared to a single pregnancy?

A) Human chorionic gonadotropin levels stay high past 6 week of gestation.
B) Significantly more prolactin and oxytocin are made and released from the anterior pituitary.
C) Strong negative feedback inhibits estrogen synthesis and release from the posterior pituitary.
D) Twice as much progesterone is made and released from the corpus luteum and placenta.

5. Which of the following correctly ranks the order from earliest to latest the identical twins from the passage split?

A) 2 – 5 – 4
B) 2/3 – 5 – 4
C) 4 – 5 – 1/2/3
D) 4 – 5 – 2

6. Why do some identical twins have two amniotic sacs but share a placenta?

A) The placenta develops from the inner cell mass, which splits in these twins; the amnion develops from the trophoblast, which is shared in identical twins.
B) All identical twins share a trophoblast, which develops into the amnion, and an inner cell mass, which develops into the placenta.
C) The amnion develops from the inner cell mass, which splits in these twins; the placenta develops from the trophoblast, which is shared in these twins.
D) All identical twins share a trophoblast, which develops into the placenta, and an inner cell mass, which develops into the amnion.

SOLUTIONS TO CHAPTER 13 FREESTANDING PRACTICE QUESTIONS

1. **B**   The spermatogonia in the testes periodically undergo mitosis to produce both more spermatogonia and primary spermatocytes, ensuring a continual supply of primary spermatocytes for gametogenesis throughout the male reproductive lifespan. Primary spermatocytes, which are diploid, undergo meiosis I to become haploid secondary spermatocytes, which then undergo meiosis II to become (haploid) spermatids (choices C and D are wrong). Spermatids do not undergo mitosis or meiosis, but develop into mature spermatozoa (choice A is wrong).

2. **D**   Labor and delivery is one example of a positive feedback loop, in which the release of oxytocin from the posterior pituitary combined with mechanical pressure of the fetal head work together to increase uterine contractility in an effort to expel the baby from the uterus (choice D is correct, and choice A is wrong). Progesterone, released early in pregnancy from the corpus luteum and later in pregnancy from the placenta itself, decreases uterine contractility (choices B and C are wrong). Levels of progesterone are high early in pregnancy in order to keep the developing fetus inside the uterus, but levels diminish later in pregnancy in anticipation of the upcoming delivery of the baby. Note that this question is a two-by-two elimination; the role of oxytocin in delivery allows the elimination of two answer choices and determining its regulatory mechanism differentiates between the remaining two.

3. **C**   Spermatogenesis only begins once a male reaches puberty, and then continues for the rest of his life (choice C is not a difference and is the correct answer choice). Oogenesis begins when a female is an embryo, and the cells are arrested at the primary oocyte phase when she is a fetus (choice A is a difference and can be eliminated). Spermatogenesis produces four sperm from each spermatogonia, whereas oogenesis produces one ovum and two polar bodies per oogonia (choice B is a difference and can be eliminated). The testes are the male gonads and the site of spermatogenesis; the ovaries are the female gonads and the site of oogenesis (choice D is a difference and can be eliminated).

4. **C**   The corpus luteum secretes estrogen and progesterone, which help maintain pregnancy (these hormones are elevated in the first trimester; choices A and B can be eliminated). Estrogen and progesterone feedback and inhibit the secretion of GnRH from the hypothalamus (choice C would not be elevated and is the correct answer choice). hCG is a hormone secreted by the embryo that helps to maintain the corpus luteum during the first trimester until the placenta is formed (choice D would be elevated and can be eliminated).

5. **B**   During ovulation, the ovary releases a secondary oocyte (choice A is true and can be eliminated). A surge of LH, not FSH from the anterior pituitary, causes the follicle to become the corpus luteum (choice D is true and can be eliminated, and choice B is false and the correct answer choice). Once the follicle becomes the corpus luteum, it produces and secretes progesterone that stabilizes and enhances the endometrium (choice C is true and can be eliminated).

6. **B**   Fertilization occurs in the fallopian tube after an egg has been released from the ovary (choices A and D are wrong). The fimbriae sweep the egg from the ovary into the fallopian tube (not the uterus) once it has been ovulated (choice C is wrong). Choice B describes the process accurately, including the correct location of fertilization and the failure to migrate prior to implantation.

7. **B**   When suckling occurs, oxytocin is released from the posterior pituitary to trigger milk ejection from the glands toward the nipple. As this hormone is also responsible for stimulating uterine contractions during delivery, it can have a similar but less intense effect when nursing. Prolactin is involved in nursing, but is responsible for stimulating the production of milk and does not have an effect on the uterus (choice D is wrong). Estrogen and progesterone do not play a role in this situation (choices A and C are wrong).

8. **A**   The greater vestibular glands are located at the posterior of the vaginal opening, are stimulated on arousal, and secrete an alkaline mucus. This helps neutralize the acidity of the vagina to make it a more hospitable environment for sperm, which can be damaged by acids. The bulbourethral glands in the male are stimulated on arousal and secrete an alkaline mucus into the urethra. This helps neutralize any traces of acid that might remain from earlier passage of urine through that duct, and makes the urethra a more hospitable environment for sperm. The seminal vesicles and the prostate produce semen (a supportive fluid for sperm), and are stimulated at orgasm (choices B and C are wrong), and the testes are the male primary sex organs; they produce sperm and testosterone (choice D is wrong).

SOLUTIONS TO CHAPTER 13 PRACTICE PASSAGE

1. **A**   In most pregnancies, the blastocyst has formed by day 5. The passage describes four types of twins:

Twin	Definition	Genome	Extraembryonic Structures
Dizygotic or fraternal twins (non-identical)	Two genetically different eggs are fertilized by two different sperm	Different	Two amnions Two placentas
66% of monozygotic or identical twins	Single fertilization Zygote or morula splits before day 5	Same	Two amnions Two placentas
33% of monozygotic or identical twins	Single fertilization Inner cell mass of blastocyst splits after day 5	Same	Two amnions One placenta
1% of monozygotic or identical twins	Single fertilization Split later in development	Same	One amnion One placenta

Make sure to highlight the word "NOT" and write "A B C D" on the noteboard. Then evaluate each choice, writing a "Y" if it is supported and "N" if it is not. Most identical twins split early and have separate amnions and placentas (write "N" next to "A" on the noteboard). Monozygotic twins have identical genomic sequences and fraternal twins have different genetic information (write "Y" next to "B" on the noteboard). The three primary germ layers develop in gastrulation and most identical twins split before this (write "Y" next to "C" on the noteboard). All fraternal (non-identical) twins and monozygotic or identical twins that split before day 5 develop two placentas and two amnions (write "Y" next to "D" on the noteboard). Since choice A stands out with an "N" instead of a "Y," it is the correct answer choice.

2. **C**   Restriction fragment length polymorphism (RFLP) analysis uses restriction endonucleases to cut stretches of polymorphic DNA into small fragments. The resulting DNA fragments vary in size and are unique to an individual; they are separated via gel electrophoresis and analyzed. RNase enzymes degrade RNA, which is not relevant to RFLP (eliminate choice A). DNA is pretty stable and would likely survive a few days at a high temperature (eliminate choice B). DNase enzymes degrade DNA. This would destroy the samples collected from the twins and would mean no RFLP analysis is possible (choice C is correct). The age of the twins is not relevant to the quality of their DNA sample. In addition, proteases degrade proteins, and this is not relevant to RFLP (eliminate choice D).

3. **B**   Monozygotic twins are identical and have the same genetic information. Twins 1 and 3 have different RFLP patterns, so they do not have the same genome. They must be fraternal (eliminate choices C and D). Also note that twin set 1 has a male and female; these cannot be identical twins. Twin sets 2, 4, and 5 have the same RFLP patterns as each other, so these pairs must have the same genome. They are identical or monozygotic twins (eliminate choice A; choice B is correct).

4. **D**   Human chorionic gonadotropin hormones levels stay high past 6 weeks of gestation in all pregnancies (eliminate choice A). Prolactin is made and released from the anterior pituitary, but oxytocin is made in the hypothalamus and released from the posterior pituitary (eliminate choice B). Estrogen is not made in the brain (eliminate choice C). By process of elimination, the correct answer is choice D. Progesterone is made and released from the corpus luteum and placenta, and it is reasonable progesterone levels would be higher in a woman carrying multiples.

5. **A**   Twin sets 1 and 3 have different RFLP patterns, so they do not have the same genome. They must be fraternal (eliminate choices B and C). Twin sets 2, 4, and 5 have the same RFLP patterns as each other, so these pairs must have the same genome. They are identical or monozygotic twins. Based on the passage, identical twins that split early will develop separate amnions and placenta. Twins that split after day 5 usually have separate amnions and a shared placenta. This means that the small percent of twins that split even later than this (only 1% of identical twins) must share both an amnion and a placenta. Here are the results of the twin study in the passage:

	Gender	Placenta(s)	Amniotic Sac	Results	Split
Twins 1	F/M	2	2	Fraternal	n/a
Twins 2	M/M	2	2	Identical	Before day 5
Twins 3	F/F	2	2	Fraternal	n/a
Twins 4	F/F	1	1	Identical	Long after day 5
Twins 5	M/M	1	2	Identical	Shortly after day 5

This means that twins 2 must have split earliest, then twins 5, and finally twins 4 (eliminate choice D; choice A is correct).

6. **C**   The passage states that if identical twins split after day 5, there will be two amniotic sacs but one placenta. The amnion develops from the inner cell mass (eliminate choices A and B). All twins with two inner cell masses in a blastocyst will develop two separate amnions (eliminate choice D; choice C is correct). The placenta develops from the trophoblast. If a zygote or morula splits, two separate blastocysts will develop, and they will each have their own inner cells mass and trophoblast. This will lead to identical twins with separate amnions and placentas. If the inner cell mass of a blastocyst splits, identical twins will develop their own amnions but will share a placenta because they share a trophoblast.

EFFECTS OF A COMMERCIALLY AVAILABLE BRANCHED-CHAIN AMINO ACID-ALANINE-CARBOHYDRATE-BASED SPORTS SUPPLEMENT ON PERCEIVED EXERTION AND PERFORMANCE IN HIGH INTENSITY ENDURANCE CYCLING TESTS

Marco Gervasi, Davide Sisti, Stefano Amatori, Sabrina Donati Zeppa, Giosuè Annibalini, Giovanni Piccoli, Luciana Vallorani, Piero Benelli, Marco B. L. Rocchi, Elena Barbieri, Anna R. Calavalle, Deborah Agostini, Carmela Fimognari, Vilberto Stocchi & Piero Sestili

Journal of the International Society of Sports Nutrition, volume 17, Article number: 6 (2020)

BACKGROUND

Amino acids are thought to enhance athletic performance in several ways, for example modifying fuel utilization during exercise and preventing mental fatigue and overtraining. A recent (2017) position stand of the International Society of Sports Nutrition states that the three branched-chain amino acids (BCAA), leucine, isoleucine, and valine are unique among the essential amino acids for their roles in protein metabolism, neural function, blood glucose and insulin regulation. It has been suggested that the Recommended Dietary Allowance (RDA) for sedentary individuals (considering that BCAAs occur in nature in a 2:1:1 ratio, leucine: isoleucine: valine) should be 45 mg/kg/day for leucine and 22.5 mg/kg/day for both isoleucine and valine; this RDA is even higher for active individuals. Supplementation with BCAA has been proposed as a possible strategy to limit the development of central fatigue, in particular, in endurance events. Central fatigue, which pertains to the central nervous system (CNS), is a complex phenomenon arising under conditions of low energy availability, ammonia accumulation in blood and tissues, and changes in neurotransmitter synthesis—in particular, an increase in serotonin and a decrease in dopamine—which causes a state of increasing tiredness during exhaustive exercise. The presence of elevated cerebral serotonin levels observed in rats under fatigue, is the basis of a well-accepted theory to account for the onset/increase of central fatigue in humans as well. Indeed, during prolonged sustained exercise, an increased brain uptake of the serotonin precursor Tryptophan (Trp) has been observed in humans. This theory has recently been bolstered by Kavanagh et al., whose study based on paroxetine administration in humans demonstrated the influence of serotonin availability in increasing central fatigue under prolonged maximal contractions. The ability of BCAA to compete with Trp in crossing the blood brain barrier led us to hypothesize that BCAA supplementation could reduce cerebral serotonin synthesis, thus preventing/delaying the onset of central fatigue during prolonged exercise.

Carbohydrates (CHO) also play an important role in supplementation in the course of endurance events, increasing and/or maintaining energetic substrate availability, preventing and/or delaying hypoglycemia and its deleterious effects on brain functions and cognitive performance, and promoting direct anti-fatigue brain responses through the activation of sweet taste oral receptors.

In light of these findings, researchers have turned their attention to the study and development of supplements containing BCAA alone or combined with specific substances (such as CHO), assessing the efficacy of their association. Several recent investigations have shown BCAA supplementation to positively affect prolonged exercise under specific conditions. In particular, BCAA were shown to positively impact the rating of perceived exertion (RPE) and performance. However, due to the great heterogeneity of the experimental protocols and formulations used, the results of these studies are not always unequivocal; hence, the actual efficacy of BCAA – used alone or combined with other components—remains a much debated issue.

This uncertainty may generate confusion and/or false expectations regarding the efficacy of these sport supplements. To shed light on this issue, it is important to perform highly controlled and randomized studies as well as to develop and validate specific and reliable test procedures capable of determining the actual efficacy of supplements intended for use in sports after both short and long term intakes. To this end, a recent study validated a variable high intensity protocol followed by a time to exhaustion (TTE) endurance capacity test (namely high intensity endurance cycling test, HIEC) as a reliable and sensitive method to assess both performance and fatigue, providing a stable platform for the comparative analysis of the effects of different nutritional interventions. HIEC can be performed either at the beginning or at the end of training periods and protocols. In the present study, we applied HIEC to a 9-week program based on High Intensity Interval Training (HIIT), a widely used protocol to improve specific variables of endurance performance. It is worth noting that, to date, to the best of our knowledge, no study has tested the effects of the consumption of a commercially available and established BCAA-alanine-CHO based supplement on HIEC over a medium-long endurance training period.

The first aim of this randomized double-blind placebo-controlled study was to determine whether, the single or prolonged intake of a commercial BCAA, Ala and CHO formula (Friliver® Performance, FP, Dompè Farmaceutici Spa), taken according to the manufacturer's recommendations, affects RPE, performance indexes and relevant serum blood markers in young adults, at the beginning (1d) and at the end (9w) of a 9-week indoor cycling HIIT. The second aim was to verify whether a prolonged supplementation may help participants to comply with the required training load during a 9w HIIT program with progressively increasing volume.

METHODS

Participants

Thirty-two healthy university students (20 males: age 22 ± 1.7 years, height 175.5 ± 6.5 cm, weight 68.2 ± 10.9 kg, BMI 22 ± 2.7 kg/m^2; 12 females: age 21 ± 0.9 years, height 159.5 ± 4.8 cm, weight 52.5 ± 5.3 kg, BMI 21 ± 1.2 kg/m^2) were recruited. The exclusion criteria were: major cardiovascular disease risks, musculoskeletal injuries, upper respiratory infection, smoking and consumption of any medicine or protein/amino acid supplement in the past 3 months. All participants, assessed with a specific questionnaire, performed no more than one 60 min leisure walking or jogging session per week in the 3 months preceding the start of the study; their VO_{2max} values at baseline were in line with—and thus confirmed—their low level of training (see Table 2). The participants were advised to maintain their dietary routine, and to abstain from using additional

dietary supplements during the study period. They were also instructed to refrain from all training activities except for the sessions included in the experimental design. Subjects were asked to refrain from the consumption of alcohol, hypnosedative drugs and beverages containing caffeine on the 2 days prior to the trial.

Study design

This was a randomized double-blind placebo-controlled trial. In order to ensure balance, randomization for permuted blocks ($n=4$) was used. Stratification was used to ensure equal allocation by gender to each experimental condition. Study design was structured as follows: metabolic/performance (VO_{2max}, W_{peak}, W_{LT1}, W_{LT2} and TTE), biochemical (BCAA, Ala, Trp, CK serum and glucose blood levels) and RPE data were acquired before (1d) and after (9w) the incremental training period.

Supplement and supplementation regimen

FP (Dompè Farmaceutici Spa, Milan, Italy, see Table 1 for the formulation) was taken 1 h before HIEC and each training session according to the manufacturer's recommendations. BCAA and Ala content per single dose is within the range recommended by European Food Safety Authority and comparable to the dosage used in other studies. The PL group ingested a non-caloric placebo that was identical in packaging, appearance and taste to the actual supplement. FP and PL were dissolved in 500 ml of still water and ingested before each training session; neither FP nor PL was taken on rest days. Over the entire study period, the SU group received an average daily dose (total amount of each amino acid in FP/duration in days of the study) of 0.91 g leucine, 0.46 g valine, 0.46 g isoleucine and 0.91 g alanine. Importantly, as verified by the qualified medical specialist (P.B.), none of the participants experienced any side effects or adverse events as a result of the FP or placebo ingestion.

Table 1   Composition of Friliver Performance®

	Per dose	Per 100 g
Energy	71 kcal (304 kJ)	355 kcal (1520 kJ)
Total Carbohydrate	13.2 g	66 g
Sucrose	11.6 g	58 g
Polyalcohol	1.6 g	8 g
L-Leucine	1.6 g	8 g
L-Alanine	1.6 g	8 g
L-Valine	0.8 g	4 g
L-Isoleucine	0.8 g	4 g
Citric Acid	1.06 g	5 g
Orange flavor	0.8 g	4 g

Incremental test

Prior (3 days before) to the pre- and post- training experimental sessions, each subject performed an incremental test to assess individual VO_{2max}, W_{peak}, W_{LT1} and W_{LT2}. Male subjects started cycling on an electronically-braked ergometer at 75 W, and power output was increased by 25 W every 3 min, whereas female subjects started at 50 W, and power output was increased by 20 W every 3 min. All subjects continued increasing power output until volitional exhaustion or cadence dropped below 60 rpm. In the absence of specific literature, intervals were set at 3 min, which represents an appropriate compromise with previous data on incremental exercise test design. Oxygen consumption was monitored breath-by-breath and values of heart rate (HR) were recorded continuously.

Rating of perceived exertion

RPE was determined with the 0–10 OMNI-cycle scale, which combines mode-specific pictorial illustrations with a numerical rating format, using a procedure described in the literature. A standard definition of perceived exertion ("the subjective intensity of effort, strain, discomfort, and fatigue that was felt during exercise") and instructional sets for the OMNI scale were read to the subjects immediately before the exercise test. The initial exercise anchoring procedure was illustrated and performed during the incremental test (see "Incremental Test" section). Participants were asked to point to their RPE on the OMNI-cycle scale, which was in full view at all times during testing.

HIEC test

The HIEC test was performed on a power meter-provided bike. Following a warm up stage (four 5 min continuous progressive increments at a workload corresponding to 50, 60, 65 and 70% W_{peak}), participants performed ten 90 s sprints (SPR) at 90% W_{peak}, separated by 180 s recovery (REC) at 55% W_{peak}. The subjects capable of completing all the 10 SPR recovered for an additional 3 min at 55% W_{peak}, and then performed a final TTE step at 90% W_{peak}. Exhaustion was defined as the inability to maintain power output within 5 W of the target output for 15 s despite verbal encouragement; no feedback on elapsed time was provided. TTE was taken as a performance marker. Subjects were asked to maintain the same predefined cadence throughout the HIEC regardless of the power output variations (from 90 to 55% W_{peak}) introduced by the operator at each REC/SPR change. Subjects were asked to provide their RPE 10 s before the end of each of the warm up, SPR and REC steps.

Design of the 1d and 9w experimental training sessions

The 32 subjects were divided in 4 groups of 8, and they performed the HIEC test on two consecutive days (2 groups per day). On the experimental day, subjects in the first group arrived at the laboratory at 06.00 AM, 2 h before the test, in a fasted state. The second group of the day arrived 2 h later in a fasted state. All subjects had a standardized breakfast consisting of 400 ml of fruit juice and servings of jam tart adjusted according to gender caloric needs (90 g for females and 135 g for males; total breakfast calories: 612–794 kcal, 119.6–150.6 g CHO, 6–8.4 g Protein, 11.4–16.9 g Fat). The design of the experimental session is shown in Fig. 1.

Design of the experimental sessions at 1d and 9w. The experimental sessions were performed in the morning. 1 h after breakfast, participants had their first blood

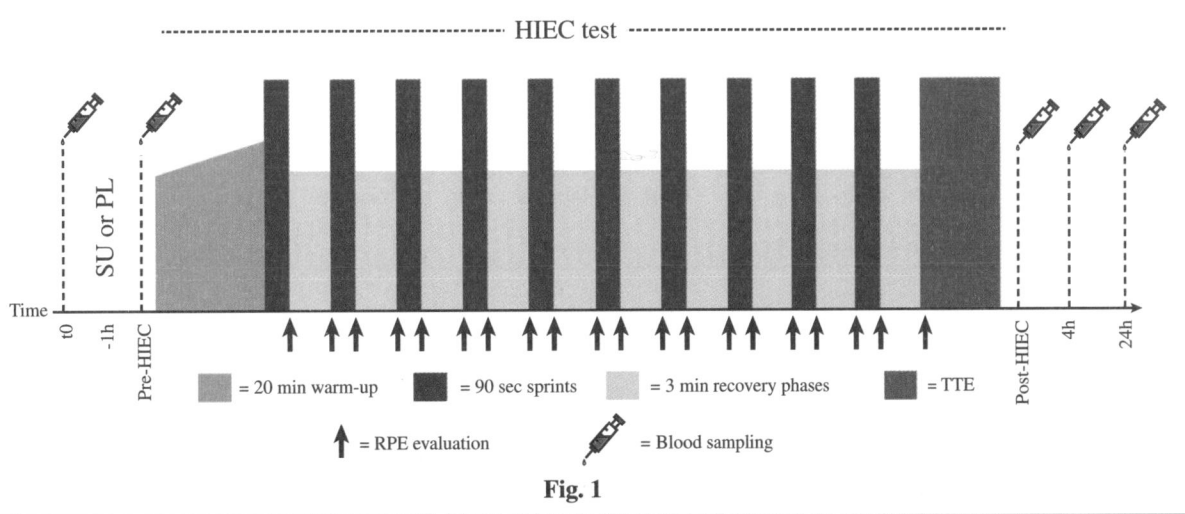

Fig. 1

draw immediately before the consumption of SU or PL; after another 1-h interval, a second blood sampling was performed immediately before the beginning of the HIEC (Pre-HIEC). In the course of the HIEC, RPE was repeatedly evaluated as indicated by the arrows. Further blood samples were collected immediately, at 4 and 24 h after the completion of the HIEC

Blood sampling and analysis

Venous blood samples (5 ml) were obtained from the antecubital vein 1 h after breakfast (immediately before FP or PL ingestion) (T0), 1 h after ingestion (immediately before exercise) (pre-HIEC), immediately post exercise (post-HIEC), after 4 h and 24 h.

Glycemia assessment

Blood glucose was measured by a portable glucometer at the following times: T0 in the fasted state; immediately and 30 min after breakfast; before the intake of FP or PL (1 h after the standardized breakfast); 30 min after intake of SU or PL; and immediately before and after the HIEC test.

Training protocol

Thirty-six indoor cycling training sessions were performed over a 9w period (see Fig. 2). The training sessions were divided into three mesocycles (see Fig. 2).

The 32 subjects were divided in two groups of 16 and trained by two expert instructors with the aim of following the same training program. Each session was choreographed based on conventional principles (warm-up, systematic high intensity interval exercise, and cool-down) widely used in the indoor cycling community. The training program of each session was designed following the same intensity distribution, based on a polarized model, with around 70% of the session time spent in zone 1, 10% spent in zone 2 and 20% spent in zone 3 (see "Incremental Test" section for zone determination). During the training sessions, the HR of each subject (instructor included) was monitored and recorded. HR values were projected onto the wall, as percentage of maximal HR (% HR_{max}), and the subjects were asked to maintain the same intensity as the instructor.

One hour before each training session, the subjects of the SU group ingested a single dose of FP, while the subjects of the PL group ingested the placebo.

Training load analysis

Lucia's TRIMP was used to calculate the Training Load for each session. The concept of Lucia's TRIMP integrates total volume, on the one hand, and total intensity relative to the intensity zones, on the other. Briefly, the score for each zone is calculated by multiplying the accumulated duration in the zone by a multiplier for that particular zone (e.g. 1 min in zone 1 is given a score of 1 TRIMP (1 X 1), 1 min in Zone 2 is given a score of 2 TRIMP (1 X 2), and 1 min in Zone 3 is given a score of 3 TRIMP (1 X 3); the total TRIMP score is then obtained by summing the results of the three zones. Finally, the mean TRIMP scores of each mesocycle performed by the SU and PL groups were compared.

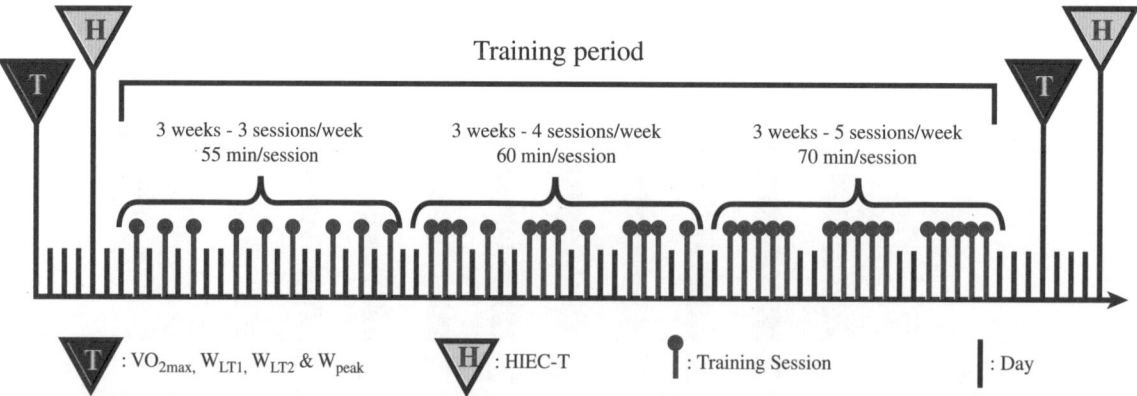

Fig. 2 Structure of training period: nine weeks divided into three mesocycles (three weeks each). The frequency and the duration of the sessions are also indicated. Key: VO_{2max}, maximal oxygen consumption; W_{LT1} and W_{LT2}, power at lactate thresholds; W_{peak}, peak power; HIEC-T, high intensity endurance cycling test.

Diet & Diet Tracking

During the entire training period, subjects' nutrition was monitored daily (by call interviews, always carried out after dinner) and data were collected and processed; macronutrients and total energy intake for experimental and control groups were finally compared in order to exclude differences in nutritional habits.

Statistical analysis

Descriptive statistics were performed using means and standard deviations. Homogeneity between groups was tested using the unpaired t-test. Daily protein, fat, carbohydrate and total caloric intake were compared between groups; the t-test and Cohen's effect size (ES) were used to quantify differences.

RESULTS

Baseline anthropometric, metabolic and biomechanical variables

Anthropometric, metabolic and biomechanical variables of participants were assessed before the beginning of the experimental session as reported in Table 2. No differences were found between the two groups in the tested parameters.

Diet monitoring

Daily caloric intake over the study period was virtually identical for both groups: 1944 ± 876 kcal in the SU group vs. 2043 ± 947 in the PL group, with no significant difference (t-test; $p > 0.05$).

Daily CHO, fat and protein intakes, supplemented vs placebo group were 49.1% vs. 51.1%; 33.4% vs 32.4%; 17.4% vs. 16.9%, respectively. No differences in specific macronutrient intake were found between groups (t-test; $p > 0.05$).

VO_{2max}, W_{peak} and power at lactate thresholds at 1d and 9w

All these variables, namely VO_{2max}, W_{peak}, W_{LT1} and W_{LT2}, were significantly different in pre vs. post 9w training as shown in Table 3. For all variables, p values were < 0.001. Results indicate that all post training values were significantly greater than pre-training ones. The effect of SU intake was not significant ($p > 0.05$) for all dependent variables.

Table 2   Anthropometric, metabolic and biomechanical variables of the participants at baseline; Mean, standard deviations and p-values for group are reported

	Supplemented Group ($n = 16$)		Placebo Group ($n = 16$)		Group (p)
Participants	Males = 10	Females = 6	Males = 10	Females = 6	
Age (yr)	22.1 ± 2.2	20.6 ± 1.0	21.0 ± 1.0	20.5 ± 0.7	0.322
Height (cm)	173.9 ± 6.0	157.2 ± 4.4	177.1 ± 6.8	161.8 ± 4.3	0.072
Weight (kg)	69.2 ± 12.7	50.3 ± 4.8	67.2 ± 6.9	54.6 ± 5.2	0.726
BMI (kg/m^2)	22.8 ± 3.4	20.3 ± 1.2	21.4 ± 1.6	20.8 ± 1.4	0.584
HR_{max} (bpm)	197.3 ± 8.2	197.5 ± 5.0	199.0 ± 7.8	199.7 ± 4.7	0.458
VO_{2max} (ml/kg/min)	42.6 ± 10.4	35.0 ± 8.5	43.9 ± 4.5	28.1 ± 3.1	0.315
W_{peak} (watt)	212.5 ± 33.9	146.7 ± 23.4	230.0 ± 28.4	133.3 ± 23.4	0.844
W_{LT1} (watt)	76.1 ± 11.3	57.7 ± 23.8	73.9 ± 22.3	40.8 ± 14.0	0.312
W_{LT2} (watt)	127.1 ± 23.4	88.2 ± 23.5	138.8 ± 27.6	74.9 ± 16.6	0.928

Table 3 VO_{2max}, W_{peak}, W_{LT1} and W_{LT2}*, in SU and PL groups at 1d and 9w

	Supplemented Group			Placebo Group		
	1d	9w	$\Delta\%$	1d	9w	$\Delta\%$
VO_{2max}	39.73 ± 10.18	44.58 ± 6.67	+12%	37.95 ± 8.82	42.93 ± 5.54	+13%
W_{peak}	187.81 ± 44.20	231.56 ± 48.91	+23%	193.75 ± 54.79	239.06 ± 56.01	+23%
W_{LT1}	69.21 ± 18.69	103.64 ± 32.95	+50%	64.83 ± 27.12	91.03 ± 26.56	+40%
W_{LT2}	112.50 ± 29.85	155.56 ± 35.34	+38%	114.83 ± 39.59	156.51 ± 40.66	+36%

Perceived exertion during HIEC test

RPE values, measured during the 20 min warm up of the HIEC tests increased progressively, showing a very similar trend in the PL and SU groups in both 1d and 9w periods (Fig. 3a and b, respectively). During the 10 SPR, each of them followed by a REC step, RPE showed an upward trend characterized by a sawtooth pattern in all the conditions tested. As expected, the RPE values reached the maximum at the end of the TTE step (11 points on OMNI cycle scale). Hence, only RPE values starting from 20 min (the end of warm up) to 65 min (prior to TTE phase) were considered for further analyses (data highlighted in grey box).

Perceived exertion at 1d (pre training HIEC test)

The linear regression equation of the curve built on SPR steps showed that intercepts ($p = 0.163$) and slopes ($p = 0.086$) were not significantly different. The linear regression equation of REC steps showed that intercepts were not significantly different ($p = 0.742$), whereas, interestingly, slopes were ($p = 0.001$). This would imply that in REC steps, the SU group showed a lower RPE (Fig. 3c e 3E).

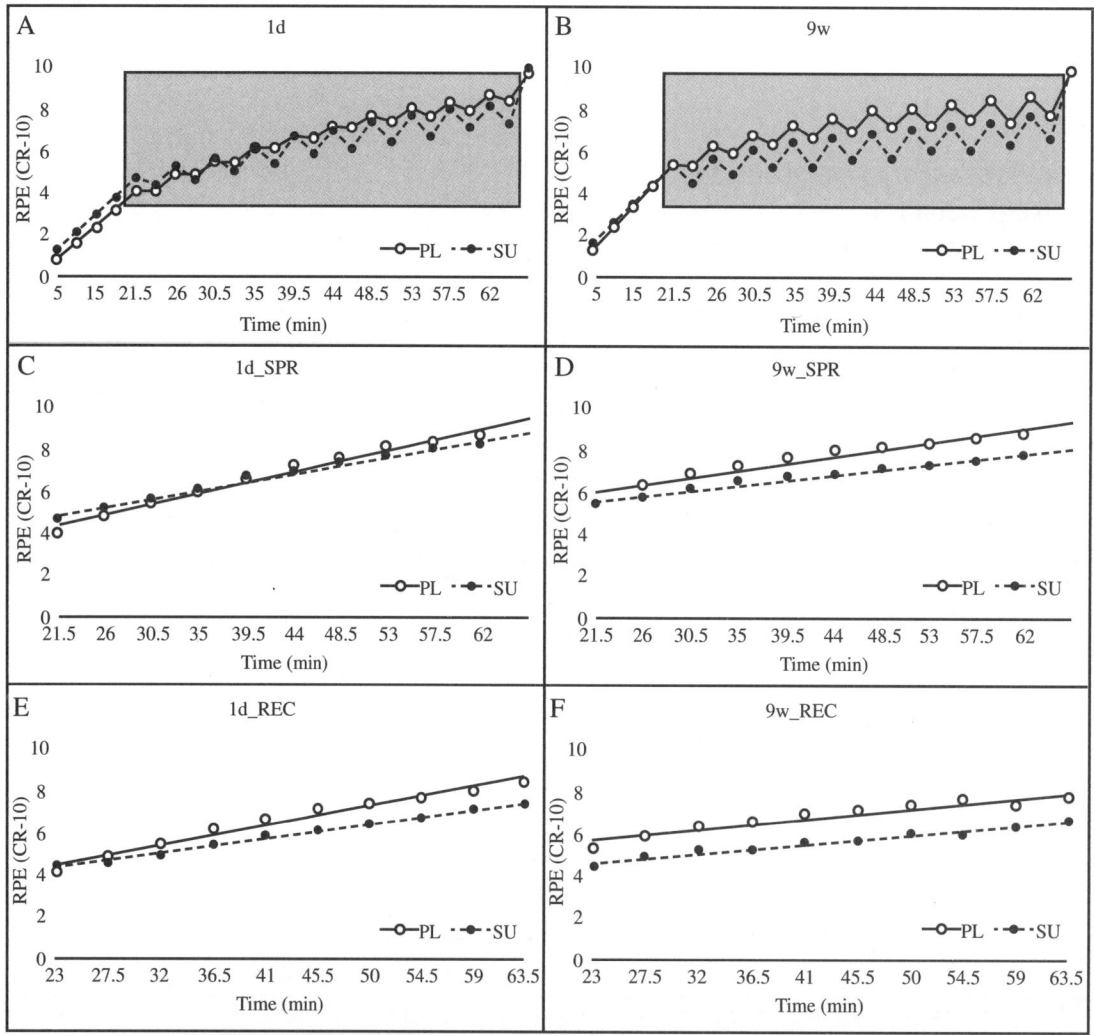

Fig. 3 Perceived exertion rate (RPE) values versus session time; a-b whole RPE time series; c-d RPE values in sprint (SPR) steps at pre-training (1d) and post training (9w) stages, respectively; e-f RPE values in REC steps at 1d and 9w, respectively. Closed circles refer to SU and open circles to the PL group.

Perceived exertion at 9w (post training HIEC test)

The linear regression equation of SPR steps showed that slopes, unlike intercepts ($p = 0.079$), were significantly different ($p = 0.017$), suggesting that in the SPR phase, the SU group showed a lower RPE. The linear regression equation of REC steps showed that slopes were not significantly different ($p = 0.371$), while an extremely significant difference was found between intercepts ($p < 0.001$). This implies that in the REC steps, the SU group showed a systematically lower RPE (Fig. 3d and f).

On the whole, RPE values increased linearly over the execution time of HIEC in both the SU and PL groups (Fig. 3a and b). Notably, the extent of the increment was significantly lower in the SU group than it was in the PL group in all the conditions tested (Fig. 3d, e and f), with the only exception of the 1d pre-training SPR phase (Fig. c); the lowest increment was observed in the 9w post-training REC phase.

Performance during HIEC test: time to exhaustion

TTE values were determined and taken as reliable performance parameters. Analysis of the 1d data failed to reveal significant differences between groups (371 ± 147 s for SU; 359 ± 177 s for PL; $p > 0.05$). On the contrary, with regard to 9w, data showed that the mean TTE was significantly longer for the SU group (517 ± 210 s) than for the PL group (321 ± 214 s) ($p = 0.025$).

Training load analysis

TRIMP represents a recognized parameter to express the extent of training load. TRIMP values were compared between groups in the course of the training period, which was divided into three different three-week mesocycles characterized by progressively increasing training loads. During the first mesocycle subjects averaged 98.4 ± 4.9 TRIMP (SU) and 97.9 ± 4.1 (PL) per session; during the second mesocycle, subjects averaged 97.9 ± 5.4 TRIMP (SU) and 96.5 ± 7.1 (PL) per session; no differences in these

mesocycles were found between groups ($p > 0.05$). Notably, during the last mesocycle TRIMP values were significantly higher ($p = 0.014$) in the SU group than they were in the PL group, with averages of 109.4 ± 5.7 vs 104.1 ± 6.4 per session, respectively. Data are shown in Fig. 4.

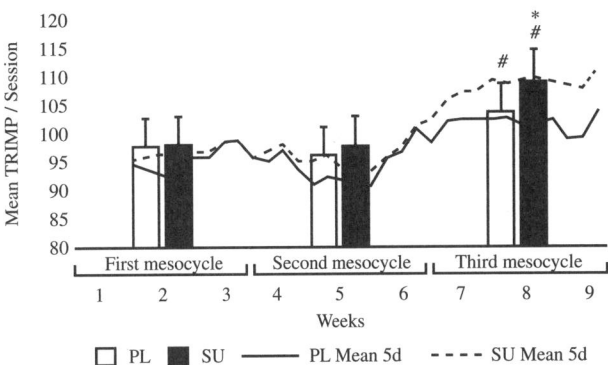

Fig. 4 Training loads in the PL and SU groups as a function of mesocycles and training progression. Bars represent the mean training impulse (TRIMP) associated with the corresponding mesocycle in the PL (white columns) and SU (black columns) groups (standard deviations are reported). Dashed lines (SU) and solid lines (PL) were obtained using a 5-day moving average. * $p < 0.05$ as compared to PL; # $p < 0.05$ as compared to an earlier time point.

Serum blood levels of BCAA and ratios of free Trp:BCAA

Blood samples were collected immediately before (T0), 1h after the ingestion (pre-HIEC) of FP or PL, and at the end of the HIEC test (post-HIEC). HPLC analysis of serum blood samples (Fig. 5) showed that total BCAA concentrations ([BCAA] is the total amount of Leu, Isoleu, and Val concentrations) before the ingestion of FP or PL powder at both 1d and 9w were similar, and that at pre-HIEC they increased significantly only in the SU group ($p < 0.05$). [BCAA] measured at post-HIEC decreased significantly in the SU group at 1d and 9w, though to a lesser extent in the latter case.

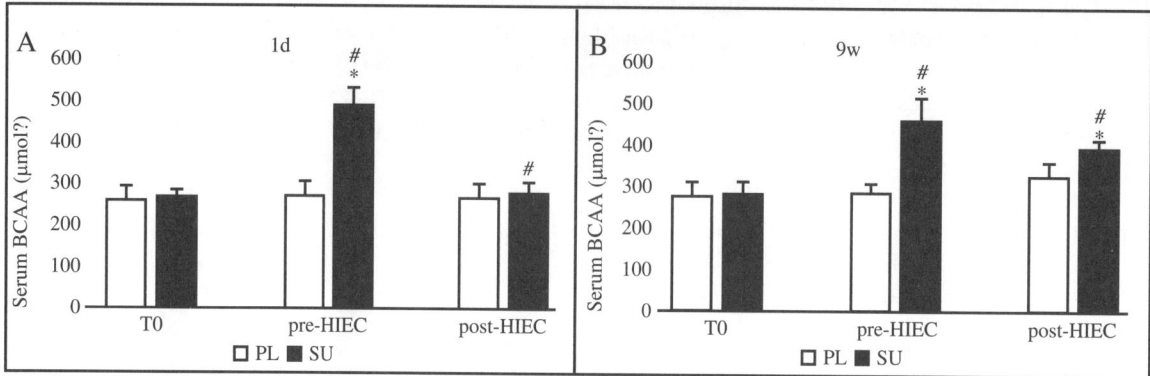

Fig. 5 Branched chain amino acids [BCAA] serum blood levels. Panels **a** and **b** show analyses performed at 1d and 9w respectively. Values for the SU (black bars) and PL (white bars) groups are reported, with mean and standard deviations. * $p < 0.05$ per group; # $p < 0.05$ per time.

Regarding Trp:BCAA ratios, at pre-HIEC they were consistently higher in the PL group than they were in the SU group (Fig. 6). At 1d, notwithstanding the time-related increase in both groups (pre- vs post-HIEC), the PL group was characterized by a higher ratio than the SU group; interestingly, at 9w a statistically significant increase could be found only in the PL group.

Glycemia

Glycemia was determined prior to breakfast (4.8 ± 0.1 and 5.3 ± 0.2 mM in SU vs PL respectively, $p > 0.05$) and at different time points up to the end of HIEC test. As expected, 30 min after breakfast, glucose levels increased (9.4 ± 1.5 and 8.5 ± 1.8 mM in the SU and PL groups respectively) and decreased thereafter, approaching basal

levels (5.7 ± 0.5 in SU vs 5.6 ± 0.6 mM in PL; $p > 0.05$). No further significant difference between groups was observed post-HIEC (6.1 ± 0.2 vs 5.8 ± 0.6 mM in SU and PL respectively; $p > 0.05$).

DISCUSSION

The effects of FP—an established, commercially available sports nutritional supplement containing BCAA, Ala and CHO—on RPE, performance and the capacity to sustain physical training were investigated in a group of 32 healthy young subjects enrolled in a randomized double-blind placebo-controlled trial. Along with RPE and performance values, a number of relevant nutritional and biological

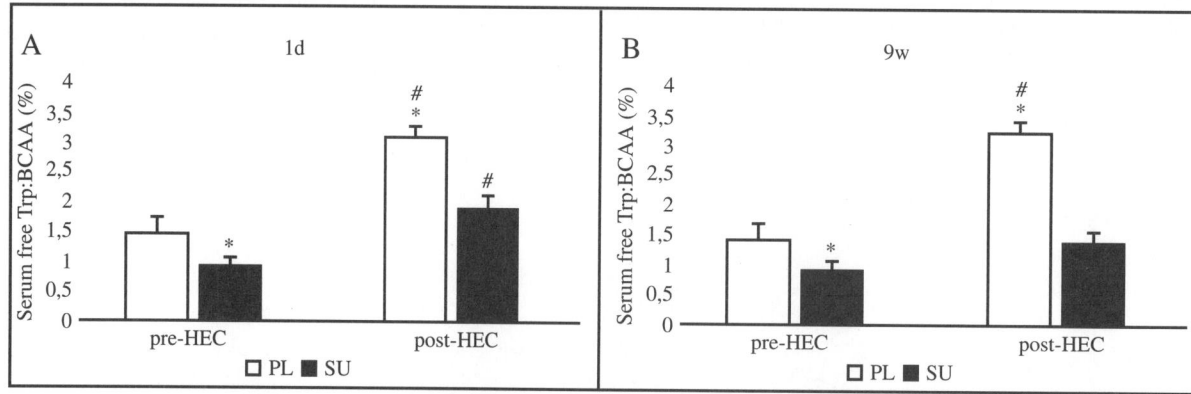

Fig. 6 Free Trp to BCAA ratios. Trp:BCAA ratios before (pre-HIEC) and after HIEC test (post-HIEC) are shown. Panel **a** shows analyses performed at 1d and panel **b** those performed at 9w. Values for the SU (black bars) and PL (white bars) groups are reported as means with standard deviations. * $p < 0.05$ between groups; # $p < 0.05$ between time points.

parameters were also determined. Notably, to the best of our knowledge, this is the first study adopting a validated and reliable HIEC protocol for these purposes.

The major finding of this study is that a single intake of FP is capable of attenuating RPE, and that its prolonged 9w consumption according to manufacturer's recommendations not only augments RPE-attenuating capacity, but also improves TTE and TRIMP, which both reflect the capacity to sustain training loads. HPLC analysis of blood sampled 1 h after FP ingestion, unlike the sample taken 1 h after PL administration, showed a significant increase in BCAA levels. This finding indicates that BCAA are rapidly absorbed after oral ingestion of FP, and that their increased serum blood concentration is likely related to the above-mentioned effects on RPE, TTE and TRIMP.

Following the first intake, the SU group showed lower RPE values only in the HIEC REC phases, while a significant RPE reduction was found following a chronic (9w) intake also in the high intensity SPR phases. Furthermore, both acute and chronic intake caused a significantly more rapid decrease in RPE observed between the SPR and corresponding REC phases compared to PL. It is worth noting that, unlike previous studies on BCAA and RPE, by virtue of the particular design of the HIEC test, this is the first investigation in which RPE associated with SPR or with REC phases was separately quantitated. This allowed us to determine that FP significantly accelerated the reduction of RPE during the recovery phases compared to PL.

Our results indicate that serum blood circulating Trp:BCAA ratios increase after HIEC in PL, and that FP consumption invariably prevented this effect. Under the conditions we observed in the PL group, namely an increased Trp:BCAA ratio, Trp is supposed to be more available for brain uptake, thus promoting an augmented synthesis of serotonin; on the contrary, a significantly lower Trp:BCAA ratio, which we did observe in the SU group, is thought to antagonize brain Trp uptake, thus limiting serotonin synthesis and availability. According to the widely held belief linking brain serotonin increases with central fatigue development, this sequence of events might have contributed to the lower RPE values we observed upon acute and/or prolonged FP supplementation.

Regarding glycemia, we did not find any variation between the two groups in the glycemic values of pre- and post-HIEC tests, suggesting that the extra CHO of FP do not significantly modify blood glucose prior to or after testing compared to PL. In this regard, it should also be considered that in our setting both groups had ingested a breakfast containing 120–150 g of CHO 1 h before HIEC, that is approximately tenfold the amount of CHO contained in FP. In light of these considerations, the CHO contribution to the functional and metabolic outcomes described thus far is probably limited. Indeed, a recent study by O'Hara et al., using the same experimental setting we adopted in the present investigation, showed that the intake of 40 g of CHO (galactose or glucose) in one liter of water, taken 30 min before HIEC, did not modify the RPE or the TTE compared to the placebo.

Finally, with respect to the possible direct effects of CHO on RPE, only in studies in which CHO were given during —and not prior to (as in our case)—endurance exercise have such effects been observed. On the whole, it can be inferred that in our conditions CHO hardly affect RPE through direct central interactions.

With regard to performance, most of the studies on BCAA-containing supplements have failed to find any significant improvements nor did we find any differences in terms of relevant metabolic parameters (VO_{2max} and Power at Lactate Thresholds) between SU and PL, either upon single (1d) or prolonged (9w) supplementation. However, even though TTE did not improve after the first, acute intake of FP, it did increase significantly following the 9w supplementation. This observation is in line with those of Kephart et al., showing that, although in a different experimental settings, 10-week BCAA supplementation results in increased peak/mean power in well-trained cyclists. Interestingly, the same study also reported a significant increase in serum blood [BCAA] and a consequent improvement in the circulating Trp:BCAA ratio, hence suggesting that performance enhancement could be related to a central fatigue-mediated mechanism. Considering that our SU group did not show any improvement in metabolic parameters or free-fat mass (not shown), we also suggest that the TTE increase might be related to the stable attenuation of RPE rather than to ergogenic or anabolic effects.

With regard to the ability to sustain training loads, our results showed that TRIMP were the same in both groups with work volumes per week <240 min. Interestingly, at higher work volumes (ca. 350 min in the third mesocycle) TRIMP values were significantly higher in the SU than in the PL group. In this regard, it is worth considering that higher TRIMP expresses an increased ability to sustain exercise at high HR values, while lower TRIMP reflects the relative inability to exercise under the same conditions.

On the whole, our data suggest that the higher TRIMP values found in SU subjects at 9w reflect their enhanced capacity to sustain training, whose volume may consequently increase over time leading to better performance than that achieved by PL subjects. Reduction in RPE, which was observed from the very beginning of the test period, is likely to play a pivotal role in the progressively enhanced capacity to sustain higher training volumes. The main limitation of the present study, as well as of similar ones, lies in the use of a multi-ingredient supplement, which makes it difficult to determine the relative impact of each component on the tested markers: as a consequence, ascertaining which of the ingredients had what effect or if there was a synergistic interaction among the ingredients remains an open question. On the other hand, the strength of this study resides in the fact that it details a multi-technique experimental approach that could be applied, in the future, to directly compare the efficacy of formulations containing different constituents (such as caffeine, electrolytes, β-alanine etc.) in attenuating RPE. This would be important because, at present, it is very hard to compare the effects of different sport supplements with different formulations on RPE because they have been studied using non-homogeneous experimental designs and approaches.

CONCLUSIONS

The main findings of this study are that the consumption of FP (a commercially available nutritional supplement containing BCAA, Ala and CHO) according to the producer's suggestions reduces RPE at all the time points tested and that, over a 9w-intake, also improves TTE and TRIMP. Although it was not possible to specifically address mechanistic issues, the effects we observed are in keeping with the theory of RPE sensitivity to serum blood Trp:BCAA ratio, while the contribution of metabolic effects seems negligible. The prolonged intake of FP, which promotes a reduction in RPE and recovery times, can enhance the capacity to sustain higher training loads and ultimately improve endurance performance. Importantly, these effects occur without affecting dietary habits and caloric intake.

Abbreviations

1d : 1 day
9w : 9 weeks
Ala: Alanine
BCAA: Branched-Chain Amino Acids
CHO: Carbohydrate
CK: Creatine Kinase
CNS: Central Nervous System
FP: Friliver Performance
HIEC: High Intensity Endurance Cycling
HIIT: High Intensity Interval Training
HR: Heart Rate
LT: Lactate threshold
PL: Placebo group
RDA: Recommended Dietary Allowance
REC: Recovery phase
RPE: Rating of Perceived Exertion
SPR: Sprint phase
SU: Supplemented group
TRIMP: Training Impulse
Trp: Tryptophan
TTE: Time To Exhaustion
VO_{2max} *:* Maximal oxygen consumption
W: Watt
W_{LT} *:* Power at lactate threshold
W_{peak} *:* Peak power

JOURNAL ARTICLE EXERCISE 3

The science sections on the MCAT include a significant number of passages with experiments. Questions for these passages often ask you to analyze data, read charts and graphs, and come to some reasonable conclusion based on the information they give you. If you don't know how to extract information efficiently and analyze data effectively, you will be at a distinct disadvantage.

There are three "Journal Article Exercises" in this book. In this final exercise, you'll read and extract information from the article, then complete an MCAT passage based on this article. After that, we'll show you the "correct" information to pull out and the answers to the passage.

As before, when analyzing an experiment, you should be able to:

- identify the control group(s)
- extract information from graphs and data tables
- determine how the experimental group(s) change relative to the control
- determine if the results are statistically significant
- come to a reasonable conclusion about WHY the results were observed
- consider potential weaknesses in the study
- determine how to increase the power of the study
- decide what the next most logical experiment or study should be

And, as before, the goal of these exercises is NOT to learn content from the articles, just to get a little more comfortable reading and extracting information from them.

For the (abridged) article on pages 499–508, summarize the purpose of the experiment and the methods in a few sentences. Remember the mnemonic: Oh ouR Car Won't Start (ORCWS).

- O = Organism and Organization
- R = Results
- C = Control and Comparison
- W = Weirdness
- S = Statistics

Try interpreting the data on your own before reading the results/discussion section. When you do read the discussion, consider:

- What are the conclusions of the study?
- How are the conclusions supported by the data?
- What potential weaknesses or flaws do you see in the experimental design? Are these addressed in the discussion section?
- How might this study be potentially biased?
- How might this study be improved?
- What would be the next most logical experiment?

Answer the above questions for the article on pages 499–508.

1. **O = Organism and Organization:**
   - Is the research being conducted on humans or on animals or on bacteria in a petri dish, or something else?

   _____

   _____

   - What is being done to these organisms?

   _____

   _____

   - Are there any unique qualities to these organisms?

   _____

   _____

   - Are there multiple groups?

   _____

   _____

   - Is the study conducted over a long period of time with multiple data points, or is it a short-term study?

   _____

   _____

   - Does it have a large or small n?

   _____

   _____

2. **R = Results:**
   - Where and how are the results presented? Is it a graph? A data table? Figures and images?

   _____

   _____

- What is/are the independent variable(s)?

  _____

  _____

- What is/are the dependent variable(s)?

  _____

  _____

- What are the results of the study?

  _____

  _____

- Do the results show correlation or cause and effect, or both? Describe.

  _____

  _____

3. **C = Control and Comparison:**
   - Is there a control group?

     _____

     _____

   - How does it differ from the experimental group? Is it given a placebo or nothing at all? Is it held under different conditions?

     _____

     _____

   - If there are multiple experimental groups, how do they differ from one another?

     _____

     _____

   - Is it a blinded study? If so, double blind or single blind?

     _____

     _____

4. **W = Weirdness:**
   - Does anything or do any of the results stand out as unexpected?

     _____

     _____

5. **S = Statistics:**
   - Was any sort of statistical analysis done?

     _____

     _____

- How is it presented? Are there error bars on a graph? Standard errors around a mean? Are there *p*-values? Is there an asterisk indicating statistical significance?

  _____

  _____

- Is there any data that is not statistically significant?

  _____

  _____

6. **Interpreting the data:**
   - What are the conclusions of the study?

     _____

     _____

   - How are the conclusions supported by the data?

     _____

     _____

   - What potential weaknesses or flaws do you see in the experimental design? Are these addressed in the discussion section?

     _____

     _____

   - How might this study be potentially biased?

     _____

     _____

   - How might this study be improved?

     _____

     _____

   - What would be the next most logical experiment?

     _____

     _____

7. **Final Summary of Experiment and Results:**

   _____

   _____

   _____

   _____

   _____

   _____

JOURNAL ARTICLE EXERCISE 3 PASSAGE

Thirty young adults who did not participate in regular exercise were recruited for a nine-week study to assess the effect of a sport nutritional supplement containing branched-chain amino acids (BCAA) on the ability to perform sustained cardiovascular activity. The protocol consisted of three, 3-week periods during which 36 indoor cycling training sessions were performed. Training sessions increased in frequency, duration, and intensity over the nine weeks. Half the participants (SU group) ingested a supplement 1 hour before each training session and the other half (PL group) ingested a non-caloric placebo. The 70 kcal supplement consisted of carbohydrates, BCAA (L, V, and I), and alanine. Participants were of similar ages and habitus. Diet was monitored carefully to ensure that calorie intake and macromolecules distribution (daily carbohydrate, protein, and fat intake) were consistent between groups.

At one day and at nine weeks, the groups performed a high-intensity endurance cycling (HIEC) test after consuming a standardized breakfast (between 600–800 kcal) and either the supplement or the placebo. The test consisted of a 20-minute warm-up, followed by ten 90-second sprints at 90% peak power, interspersed with ten 3-minute recovery periods (55% peak power). After the final recovery period, subjects cycled at 90% peak power to exhaustion, defined as the inability to maintain power output within 5 W of the target for 15 seconds. Subjects provided their rate of perceived exertion (RPE) at the end of the warm-up, and after each of the sprint and recovery steps. Results for the sprint steps are shown in Figure 1.

Prolonged exercise can lead to increased brain uptake of tryptophan. Tryptophan is a serotonin precursor, and BCAA can compete with Trp in crossing the blood-brain barrier. Increases in serotonin, as well as decreases in dopamine, lead to *central fatigue*, a complex combination of events that arise under conditions of low energy availability, in which the central nervous system is not able to supply sufficient signal to skeletal muscle. Free Trp:BCAA ratios before and after HIEC are shown in Figure 2.

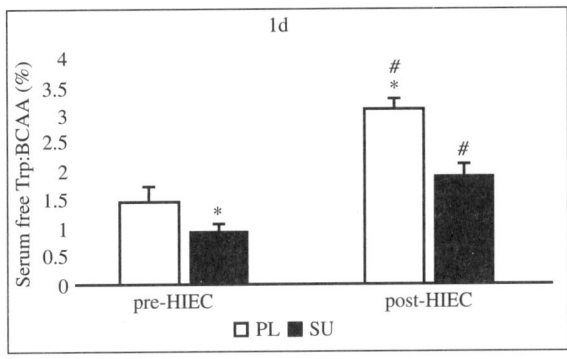

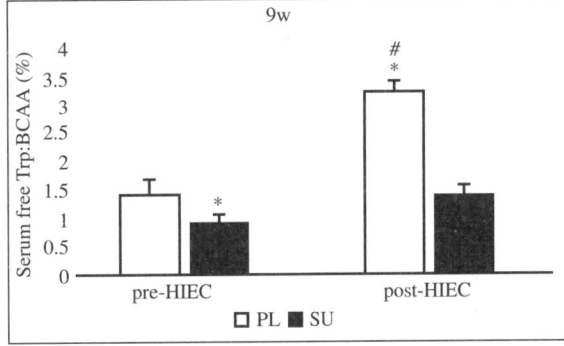

Figure 2 Free Trp to BCAA ratios before (pre-HIEC) and after HIEC test (post-HIEC) at 1d and at 9w. $*p < 0.05$ between groups; $\#p < 0.05$ between time points.

Adapted from Gervasi, M., Sisti, D., Amatori, S. *et al.* Effects of a commercially available branched-chain amino acid-alanine-carbohydrate-based sports supplement on perceived exertion and performance in high intensity endurance cycling tests. *J Int Soc Sports Nutr* 17, 6 (2020).

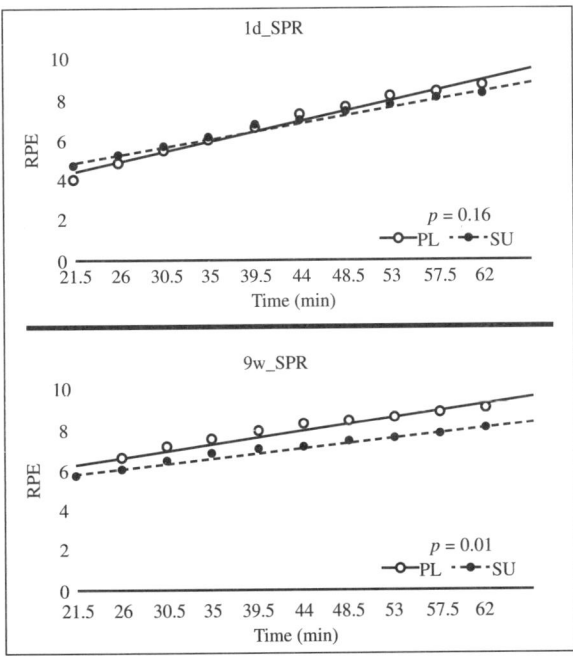

Figure 1 Sprint RPE vs. time, pre-training (1d) and post training (9w)

1. Which of the following statements is true with regard to the RPE data?

A) The placebo group had a higher RPE at 1d beginning at 39.5 minutes and for all subsequent time points.
B) The supplement group had a lower RPE for all time points measured.
C) The placebo group had a higher RPE for all time points measured at 9w.
D) The supplement group at 9w would have a longer time to exhaustion after the final recovery period.

2. Does the data in Figure 2 support the differences reported in RPE between the two groups?

A) Yes, the placebo group has a significantly higher Trp:BCAA ratio, which is correlated with the reduced RPE reported by this group.
B) Yes, the supplement group has a significantly lower Trp:BCAA ratio, which is correlated with the reduced RPE reported by this group.
C) No, the supplement group has a significantly higher Trp:BCAA ratio post-HIEC, indicating an increase in central fatigue.
D) No, lower Trp:BCAA ratios would lead to increases in serotonin, which is correlated with increases in central fatigue.

3. Which of the following is true of alanine?

A) Its side chain is reactive, so it is often found at the active sites of enzymes.
B) It was included in the experiment because it is a branched chain amino acid.
C) It would travel further up a silica gel plate in TLC than would tyrosine.
D) It can be used in gluconeogenesis because it is a ketogenic amino acid.

4. Researchers concluded that BCAAs reduce RPE and central fatigue. Which of the following casts the most doubt on their conclusion?

A) The supplement contained both carbohydrates and BCAAs.
B) RPEs were not significantly lower for the supplement group in all conditions.
C) Tryptophan was not included in the supplement to help reduce central fatigue.
D) Both groups show higher Trp:BCAA ratios post-HIEC.

SOLUTIONS TO JOURNAL ARTICLE EXERCISE 3

1. **O = Organism and Organization:**
   - Is the research being conducted on humans or on animals or on bacteria in a petri dish, or something else? *Humans.*
   - What is being done to these organisms? *They are subjected to 9 weeks of exercise, half ingest a placebo and half ingest a supplement with carbohydrates and BCAAs (branched chain amino acids).*
   - Are there any unique qualities to these organisms? *All volunteers were young adults that did not regularly participate in exercise prior to the study.*
   - Are there multiple groups? *Not initially, but they were ultimately divided into two groups.*
   - Is the study conducted over a long period of time with multiple data points, or is it a short-term study? *Medium-long time (9 weeks) with data points collected at the beginning and end of the 9 weeks.*
   - Does it have a large or small *n*? *Small n: 32 total subjects.*

2. **R = Results:**
   - Where and how are the results presented? Is it a graph? A data table? Figures and images? *Graphs and data tables.*
   - What is/are the independent variable(s)? *Time and exercise regimen, amount of supplement or placebo ingested.*
   - What is/are the dependent variable(s)? *VO_{2max}, max power, lactate threshold, RPE (rate of perceived exertion), blood BCAA, tryptophan, sugar levels.*
   - What are the results of the study? *Both the placebo and supplement groups showed a similar increase in VO_{2max}, max power, and lactate threshold, however the supplement group showed a significant reduction in RPE during recovery phases (even after a single ingestion) and a reduction in RPE during both recovery and sprint phases, as well as an increase in TTE (time to exhaustion) when consuming the supplement over the 9-week period.*
   - Do the results show correlation or cause and effect, or both? Describe. *Cause and effect. The supplement group showed reduction in RPE and the placebo group did not.*

3. **C = Control and Comparison:**
   - Is there a control group? *Yes.*
   - How does it differ from the experimental group? Is it given a placebo or nothing at all? Is it held under different conditions? *The control group consumed a non-caloric, non-supplemented drink designed to mimic the supplement in the way it looked.*
   - If there are multiple experimental groups, how do they differ from one another? *Only one experimental group.*
   - Is it a blinded study? If so, double blind or single blind? *Double blind; neither the researchers nor the participants knew whether they were ingesting the supplement or the placebo.*

4. **W = Weirdness:**
   - Does anything or do any of the results stand out as unexpected? *The fact that there was no difference in VO_{2max}, max power, and lactate thresholds between the supplement and placebo groups was unexpected. It seems like the supplement only works to reduce perceived effort.*

5. **S = Statistics:**
    - Was any sort of statistical analysis done? *Yes.*
    - How is it presented? Are there error bars on a graph? Standard errors around a mean? Are there *p*-values? Is there an asterisk indicating statistical significance? *P-values, error bars, asterisks.*
    - Is there any data that is not statistically significant? *Yes, initial characteristics of the supplement and placebo groups (age, body weight, etc.), VO_{2max}, max power, and lactate thresholds, dietary intake.*

6. **Interpreting the data:**
    - What are the conclusions of the study? *Ingestion of a BCAA supplement can lower the RPE of high-intensity cycling, allowing participants to work harder for longer with less perceived effort.*
    - How are the conclusions supported by the data? *Data on RPE show significant differences (a reduction of RPE in the supplement group) after both 1 day and 9 weeks. Also, data on Trp:BCAA ratio shows lower levels in the supplement group both after a single ingestion and after 9 weeks of supplementation; since an increased Trp:BCAA ratio is related to increased serotonin levels, and increased serotonin is related to fatigue, a lower Trp:BCAA ratio could account for less perceived exertion.*
    - What potential weaknesses or flaws do you see in the experimental design? Are these addressed in the discussion section? *The possible weakness is that the BCAAs they were testing were consumed in a supplement containing other things as well (carbohydrates, alanine). It may be that these other things could account for the observed effect, or could be acting synergistically with the BCAAs. This was addressed in the discussion section.*
    - How might this study be potentially biased? *It was a small group, and only tested on young adults.*
    - How might this study be improved? *Bigger sample size, more diversity in subjects with regard to age.*
    - What would be the next most logical experiment? *Repeat the experiment with subjects in varying age groups, repeat the experiment with single supplementation (just BCAAs, just carbohydrates, etc.), consider other supplements to test (e.g., caffeine, electrolytes, etc.).*

7. **Final Summary of Experiment and Results:**
    - *In this study a group of approximately 32 young adults were divided into two main groups, one that received a supplement prior to every exercise session over a 9-week period, and one that received a placebo. Both groups were subjected to high intensity interval training sessions that increased in intensity over the 9 weeks. At the beginning and end of the 9 weeks, subjects were asked to rate their perceived exertion during the sprint and recovery sessions of the exercise, and their time to exhaustion was measured. RPE was reduced and TTE was increased in the group receiving supplementation, even though both groups showed similar increases in $VO_{2\,max}$, max power, and lactate thresholds. The conclusion is that supplementation results in a lower RPE, which allows the subjects to work longer and harder, theoretically allowing them to sustain a harder/greater volume training load than the non-supplemented group, and this might ultimately lead to better performance.*

SOLUTIONS TO JOURNAL ARTICLE EXERCISE 3 PASSAGE

1. **C**   In Figure 1, only the data for RPE at 9w is significant, with a *p*-value of 0.01; this data shows that the placebo group had a higher RPE at all 9w time points (choice C is correct). The data for RPE at 1d has a *p*-value of 0.16, indicating that the differences between the placebo and supplement groups are not significant (even if some of the individual data points for the placebo group at 1d appear to be higher; choice A can be eliminated). Similarly, the supplement group does not have a lower RPE for the time points at 1d since the data is not significant (choice B can be eliminated). While it might seem safe to assume that the supplement group would have a longer time to exhaustion than the placebo group, given that their RPE is lower, there is no data shown to support this (choice D can be eliminated).

2. **B**   Figure 2 shows that the supplement group has a significantly lower Trp:BCAA ratio than the placebo group at all time points measured. The passage states that tryptophan is a serotonin precursor, and that increases in serotonin can lead to central fatigue. The reduced Trp:BCAA ratio means that free Trp levels are lower or BCAA levels are higher, and the passage further states that BCAA can compete with Trp in crossing the blood brain barrier. If BCAA levels are higher, less Trp will cross the blood brain barrier, and less Trp means less serotonin (choice D is wrong), which means less central fatigue and a reduced RPE (choice B is correct). Higher Trp:BCAA ratios would mean more Trp, more serotonin, more central fatigue, and a higher RPE, not a reduced RPE; furthermore the placebo group reported higher RPE than the supplement group (choice A is wrong). While choice C is technically correct (the supplement group does have a higher Trp:BCAA ratio post-HIEC at both 1 day and 9 weeks, and likely has an increase in central fatigue because of it), this answer choice does not address the differences in RPE between the groups, which is what this question is asking about (choice C is wrong).

3. **C**   Alanine is a hydrophobic amino acid that would interact more with an organic solvent in TLC than it would with the silica gel plate. Tyrosine is polar and would interact more with the plate than the solvent. Thus, alanine would travel further during TLC than tyrosine (choice C is correct). The side chain of alanine is a methyl group (choice B is wrong) and is unreactive (choice A is wrong). Ketogenic amino acids are not used in gluconeogenesis; they are converted to acetyl-CoA and contribute to ketogenesis (choice D is wrong). Note also that alanine is not ketogenic, but you did not have to know that to eliminate this answer choice.

4. **A**   The fact that the supplement contained both carbohydrates and BCAA means that the reduction in RPE might have been due to the carbohydrates and not the amino acids (choice A is correct). While it is true that the supplement group RPE were not lower than the placebo group RPE for all conditions (day 1, sprint RPE are not statistically different between supplement and placebo groups), they were lower for all other conditions, and most importantly, were lower for both sprint and recovery phases at the end of the nine-week training period. This casts less doubt on the researchers' conclusions than the carbohydrates in the supplement (choice B is wrong). The passage states that tryptophan is a serotonin precursor and that increases in serotonin contribute to central fatigue. Thus, to reduce central fatigue, tryptophan should not have been added to the supplement in order to reduce serotonin levels; in any case, tryptophan is not a branched-chain amino acid, which is what this study examined (choice C is wrong). It is true that both supplement and placebo groups show higher Trp:BCAA ratios post-HIEC, however, the conclusions of the researchers were based on the differences between supplement and placebo groups post-HIEC, not the differences between pre- and post-HIEC. The supplement group had a smaller increase in Trp:BCAA than the placebo group (choice D is wrong).

Appendix I
Some Molecular
Biology Techniques

The material in this section is not *strictly* MCAT material, thus it is presented in this appendix as a reference source; in other words, you don't need to memorize it, but you should read it for familiarity. The MCAT is a test of your ability to deal with new material like this, presented on the exam in passage form. Note also that this is a very general overview. More detail on these processes can be found in *MCAT Biochemistry Review*.

A.1 ENZYME-LINKED IMMUNO-SORBENT ASSAY (ELISA)

As the name suggests, an ELISA is a biochemical technique that utilizes antigen-antibody interactions ("immuno-sorbency") to determine the presence of either

- antigens (like proteins or cytokines), or
- specific immunoglobulins (antibodies)

in a sample (such as cells recovered from a tumor biopsy or a patient's serum). When testing for the presence of a specific antigen, the wells are coated with an antibody specific for that antigen. Then the sample is added, and if the antigen is present, it will bind to the antibodies. The wells are washed and a secondary antibody (specific for the antigen) is added; the secondary antibody is linked to a detection enzyme.

When testing for the presence of a specific antibody in a sample, the *antigen* (for which the antibody is specific) is first allowed to adhere directly to the wells. The sample is added and then mixed with enzyme-linked antibodies.

ELISA can be used to screen patients for viral infections. For example, serum from a patient suspected to be infected with HIV is loaded into wells that are coated with HIV coat proteins. If the serum contains anti-HIV antibodies (indicating infection), the antibodies will adhere to the proteins on the wells, bind enzyme-linked antibodies, and effect a color change.

A.2 RADIOIMMUNOASSAY (RIA)

RIAs are similar to ELISAs but use radiolabeled antigen and antibodies rather than enzyme-linked antibodies. Thus, the presence of target proteins or antibodies is assayed by measuring the amount of radioactivity instead of a color change. RIAs are more extensively used in the medical field to measure the relative amounts of hormones or drugs in patients' sera. A known amount of radiolabeled antigen is mixed with a known amount of antibody and the total amount of radioactivity is measured. Then unlabeled antigen is added in increasing amounts; the unlabeled antigen displaces the radiolabeled antigen so that less radioactivity is measured. This data is used to formulate a standard curve, and the steps are repeated using the patient's serum instead of the unlabeled antigen. The radioactivity is measured and compared to the standard curve to determine the amount of antigen.

A.3 ELECTROPHORESIS

Electrophoresis is a means of separating things by size (for example, nucleic acids or proteins) or by charge (for example, proteins or individual amino acids). A "gel" is made out of either acrylamide or agarose, by solubilizing the acrylamide or agarose, pouring it into a rectangular mold, and then allowing it to cool and solidify. Acrylamide and agarose form "nets" as they solidify; the more acrylamide or agarose used in the initial solution, the smaller the pores in the nets.

The mold used to pour the gel creates wells in the gel into which samples can be loaded. An electrical current is applied such that the end of the gel with the wells is negatively charged and the opposite end is positively charged. This causes the samples to migrate toward the positive pole, according to size; smaller things migrate faster (because they fit more easily through the pores of the gel) and larger things migrate more slowly.

In addition to determining their sizes, fragments of DNA (or RNA) in an electrophoresed gel can be transferred to a more solid and stable membrane in a process called "blotting." There are several types of blots used in biology laboratories.

A.4 BLOTTING

Simply put, blotting is the transfer of DNA or proteins from an electrophoresis gel to a nitrocellulose of PVDF membrane. Once transferred, further experiments can be run to isolate or detect a particular nucleic acid fragment or protein (called "probing"). Blotting is classified by the type of molecule being probed.

Southern blotting allows you detect the presence of specific sequences within a heterogeneous sample of DNA. This process also allows you to isolate and purify target sequences of DNA for further study.

Northern blotting is almost identical to Southern blotting, except that RNA is separated via gel electrophoresis instead of DNA. The rest of the process is the same; once the RNA has been separated on a gel, it is transferred to a nitrocellulose membrane and detected via radiolabeled nucleic acid probe. This technique allows you to determine whether specific gene products (normal or pathologic) are being expressed (if their mRNA is present in a cell, they are probably being translated to protein).

Western blotting allows you to detect the presence of certain proteins within a sample and also serves as a diagnostic tool. You are able to determine, for example, whether cancer cells express certain tumor-promoting growth receptors on their surface.

Several variations of Eastern blotting have been reported, but these tests are not commonly used in molecular biology labs. Eastern blots are used to analyze post-translational modification of peptides, such as the addition of lipids or carbohydrates. The details of this protocol depend on the specifics of the experiment.

A.5 RECOMBINANT DNA

In the past twenty years, a major change has occurred in biology that has allowed it to not only describe the mechanisms of life, but also to manipulate living organisms. The cloning and sequencing of genes, production of recombinant DNA, and the subsequent production of recombinant proteins for use as therapeutic agents in medicine have now become commonplace procedures. A **recombinant protein** is one which has been obtained by transcribing and translating a novel combination of DNA (**recombinant DNA**) from different organisms. For example, the gene for human insulin can be placed in a bacterial

plasmid. Bacteria with the plasmid will then produce insulin that can be used to treat diabetes. To a large extent, these advances are due to the development of new technologies for the handling of DNA, such as the discovery of restriction endonucleases that cleave particular DNA sequences.

Restriction endonucleases are bacterial enzymes that recognize specific sequences of DNA and cut the double-stranded molecule in two pieces. A **nuclease** is an enzyme that cuts nucleic acids. An ***endonuclease*** cuts in the middle of a DNA chain (contrast with ***exonucleases***, which nibble nucleotides from the ends of DNA chains). Restriction enzymes have found great use in molecular biology, where they have permitted manipulation of genes to create recombinant DNA.

A.5

Plasmids

Plasmids are small circular ds-DNA molecules found in bacteria that are capable of autonomous replication (replication that is independent of chromosome replication).

Plasmids have been manipulated by recombinant techniques to propagate and express foreign genes in bacteria. They also contain a multiple cloning site, which has restriction sites for dozens of restriction enzymes. This means the plasmid can be digested and any desired sequence with complementary ends can be ligated into the plasmid. Also, plasmids have a drug resistance gene, which helps select and isolate bacteria possessing the plasmid from other bacteria.

Bacterial expression plasmids need extra components. A prokaryotic promoter and start site allow expression of an inserted gene in the bacterial host. The promoter can be either constitutively active or inducible upon addition of a chemical.

Bacterial Transformation

Plasmids can be introduced into bacterial cells via transformation. The bacteria (or other cell types) must usually be coaxed to take up the plasmid. There are several ways to do this; the cells may be cooled in calcium chloride and then heat shocked to facilitate plasmid uptake. In another (called electroporation), an electric field is applied and this pokes holes in the membrane, which allows the plasmid to diffuse into the cell.

Once inside the bacteria, the plasmid will be exposed to the host's replication machinery, which replicates the plasmid. If you are working with an expression plasmid, the DNA is also exposed to bacterial transcription machinery. Newly synthesized mRNA can then access host ribosomes, which translate the encoded protein; on completion of translation, the cells are lysed to release the protein.

If the plasmid remains within the cytosol of the bacterium, the transformation is referred to as transient. In contrast, some plasmids are constructed to integrate within the host's genome. These stable transformations allow the plasmid to be replicated each time the bacterium replicates its own genome.

Complementary DNA

Many applications of DNA technology involve expressing eukaryotic genes in prokaryotic cells such as *E. coli*. This is conceptually simple: all you have to do is get eukaryotic DNA into a plasmid and get the plasmid into a bacterium, and the bacterium should express the gene. However, there are two main problems that need to be overcome. First, prokaryotes lack the equipment necessary for splicing out introns. Second, many eukaryotic genes are extremely long, making them hard to work with. One way to overcome these obstacles is to work with eukaryotic complementary DNA.

Complementary DNA (or cDNA) is produced from fully spliced eukaryotic mRNA. This is accomplished by a special enzyme you have encountered before: reverse transcriptase, obtained from retroviruses. This enzyme reads an RNA template and builds complementary DNA. Therefore, RNA can be isolated from a eukaryotic cell, and converted into cDNA by the addition of reverse transcriptase, some generic primers and dNTP building blocks in buffer. cDNAs carry the complete coding sequences for genes, but lack introns (and thus are smaller than the genomic sequence of the gene). Once a cDNA is ligated into a bacterial plasmid and bacteria are transformed with this plasmid, they can produce the protein encoded by the cDNA.

Artificial Chromosomes

Plasmids can only carry inserts up to a certain size. If large inserts are required, artificial chromosomes can be used. Bacterial artificial chromosomes (BACs) typically carry inserts of 100 to 350 kilobase pairs (kb), while yeast artificial chromosomes (YACs) can carry inserts between 100 and 3000 kb. In other words, BACs can easily carry up to 350,000 base pairs of DNA, and YACs can contain up to 3 million base pair inserts!

Eukaryotic Plasmids

Eukaryotic plasmids also exist. They require many of the same components as bacterial plasmids. Eukaryotes use different selection agents, usually either puromycin or neomycin. They also require different promoters in expression plasmids, as well as a poly-adenylation signal downstream of the inserted gene, to terminate transcription.

Eukaryotic plasmids can be introduced into mammalian host cells via transfection. Similar to transformation, there are several experimental options for transfection. Cells can be chemically transfected, usually using calcium phosphate precipitates, or plasmid packaging in liposomes. These lipid vesicles mask the plasmid, but deliver it to the interior of the cell by fusing with the plasma membrane. Non-chemical options for transfection include electroporation, optical transfection with lasers, or shooting the DNA coupled to a gold nanoparticle into a cell nucleus using a gene gun.

Viruses can also deliver DNA into eukaryotic cells, a process called viral transduction. Transduced cells can express genes carried by the viral vector.

A.6   POLYMERASE CHAIN REACTION

Polymerase chain reaction (PCR) is a very quick and inexpensive method for detecting and amplifying specific DNA sequences, screening hereditary and infectious diseases, cloning genes, and fingerprinting DNA. Designed to generate myriad copies of a single template sequence, PCR allows the amplification and subsequent analysis of very small samples of DNA.

Reverse Transcriptase-Polymerase Chain Reaction (RT-PCR)

This is an extension of classic PCR and is used to detect the relative expression of specific gene products. While RT-PCR does not measure the actual expression or abundance of proteins, the technique provides a gauge of gene transcription by measuring the relative amount of target mRNAs. To conduct an RT-PCR experiment, all of the mRNAs from within a cell population are first isolated, then converted into complementary DNA (cDNA) using the enzyme reverse transcriptase. This "library" of cDNAs is then subjected to PCR, using primers specific for a certain gene of interest. If the gene was actively transcribed at the time of harvest, its mRNA will have yielded a cDNA, which will be amplified by the PCR reaction and visualized on a gel.

Quantitative Polymerase Chain Reaction (qPCR)

In quantitative PCR (qPCR, also called real-time PCR), the PCR product is both detected and quantified, as either an absolute number of copies or as a relative amount normalized to a control. The amplified DNA is detected in "real time," as the reaction progresses. The detection process can either use a dye that is fluorescent and binds DNA, or a fluorescent oligonucleotide probe that hybridizes to the sequence of interest. qPCR can be performed on either DNA or cDNA templates, meaning it can give information on the presence and abundance of a particular DNA sequence in samples (if DNA is the template), or on gene expression (if the template is cDNA).

A.7   DNA SEQUENCING AND GENOMICS

DNA sequencing is a method by which scientists can determine gene sequences. This provides the basis for investigating the genetics of health and disease. Knowing gene sequences is also a critical component of other experimental techniques, for example, when constructing primers for PCR reactions.

The most widely used DNA sequencing method (the Sanger technique) hinges on a simple yet important structural characteristic of DNA molecules. The ringed ribose of a dNTP has various substituents attached to its carbons: a nitrogenous base at the 1' carbon, a hydrogen at the 2' carbon (recall that a hydroxyl group occupies this site in RNA), a hydroxyl group at the 3' carbon, and a string of three phosphates at the 5' carbon. The 3' carbon hydroxyl group serves as the binding site for another dNTP. Without a free 3' carbon hydroxyl group, dNTPs could not be linked together, and DNA synthesis would not be possible. The Sanger technique utilizes a modified dNTP, which lacks the 3' carbon hydroxyl group. These dideoxynucleotide triphosphates (ddNTPs) maintain their 5' carbon triphosphate moiety and can be incorporated normally into a growing DNA molecule, however, because they are lacking the 3' carbon hydroxyl group no further bases can be added to them. Thus, these ddNTPs terminate strand elongation at the point of their insertion. The basic protocol is as follows: a sample of DNA is obtained and denatured into single strands. All of the components necessary for replication, including radiolabeled primers, along with the DNA, are mixed in four separate test tubes. A different dideoxybase is added to each tube. Replication is allowed to proceed, and many fragments of different sizes will be produced in each tube. The fragments are separated via electrophoresis, with each dideoxybase in a separate lane, then transferred to a membrane and visualized with radiosensitive film.

Reading the film from bottom (farthest from the wells) to top (closest to the wells) indicates the sequence (in the 5' to 3' direction) of the strand.

A.7

Genomics

The genome of the bacterium *Haemophilus influenzae* was the first to be sequenced and published in 1995. Since then, the genomes of hundreds of organisms have been sequenced and published, including humans and model organisms commonly used in biology laboratories (e.g., *E. coli*, *D. melanogaster*, etc.). Researchers and clinicians have recently started sequencing the genome of many cancers, which allows comparative studies between different types and subtypes of cancer, as well as a better understanding of how the cancer genome is different from a normal one.

Genomic sequencing is generally done in two ways, which can be complementary. The first strategy is to generate a genetic linkage map, with several hundred markers per chromosome. This map is then refined to a physical map by preparing YAC or BAC libraries containing large chromosomal fragments. The library is put in order, then gradually cloned into libraries containing smaller and smaller fragments. Each of these small fragments are eventually sequenced, and assembled into an overall sequence.

The second strategy is a whole-genome shotgun approach, where chromosomes are cut into small fragments, which are cloned and sequenced. This strategy skips generating maps, and because of this, requires much more extensive analysis of sequencing data by computers in order to align fragments.

Genomic data can lead to predictions on how many genes there are in a certain organism, where they are located, how expression is controlled, and how the genome is organized. It also supports larger questions, like how evolution and speciation occur. Finally, genomic data can be used to study genetic variation within and across species. Tools for analysis of genomic data have been developed and are always being refined. Researchers can now submit several different gene or protein sequences and receive a report that predicts how related the sequences are from an evolutionary point of view. There are also tools to multiply align several sequences so we can study how similar and different they are.

A.8 DNA FINGERPRINTING

Much like visualizing subtle differences in the whorl pattern of a thumbprint, DNA fingerprinting allows scientists (and police departments!) to detect sequence variations that make each individual's DNA unique. The ability to appreciate subtle differences within different individuals' DNA comes in handy when matching a DNA sample from a murder suspect to the DNA in a drop of blood found at a crime scene, or when screening for disease-causing genes, or when doing paternity testing. Since the DNA of any two people is more than 99 percent identical, DNA fingerprinting exploits stretches of repetitive and highly variable DNA called **polymorphisms**. These intervening 2–100 base-pair sequences of DNA are structurally variable with respect to their sequence, length, multiplicity, and location within the genome. Two of the several methods of fingerprinting are described below, **restriction fragment length polymorphism** (RFLP) analysis and **short tandem repeat** (STR) analysis.

This method uses restriction endonucleases to cut 10–100 base-pair stretches of polymorphic DNA (called minisatellites) into small fragments. Because of the size variations inherent in this DNA, the resulting DNA fragments (now referred to as RFLPs) also vary in size, and are unique to an individual.

The RFLPs are separated via gel electrophoresis and transferred to a membrane. Southern blotting techniques are used to analyze the sample. The membrane is probed with radiolabeled DNA oligonucleotides that base-pair with specific RFLP sequences, and the membrane is visualized with special film. Polymorphic DNA, even though recovered from the same chromosomal region, will yield unique band distributions for each person. When RFLPs are recovered from DNA sequences within genes, mutations can be detected. For example, sickle cell disease is caused by a single base substitution in the beta chain of hemoglobin. The substituted valine at the sixth position (normally, glutamic acid is present) will introduce a novel restriction site within the gene. When cut with restriction endonucleases, the point mutation generates a different sized RFLP (when compared to the normal gene cut with the same enzymes) and will yield an anomalous banding pattern.

Short Tandem Repeat (STR) Analysis

Step 1: This method uses PCR to amplify 5–10 base-pair stretches of highly polymorphic and repetitive DNA located within noncoding (introns) regions of the genome. These STRs vary with respect to the sequence and number of repeats found at each locus. To profile an individual, a sample of DNA is obtained and the polymorphic DNA is amplified with PCR.

Step 2: The amplified STRs are separated via electrophoresis and analyzed with Southern blotting.

A.9   ADDITIONAL METHODS TO STUDY THE GENOME

Genomic sequencing is the ultimate study of the genome. However, it is very costly and takes a long time. Depending on the experiment, one of the following methods may be better suited to answering a biological question.

Exome and Targeted Sequencing

Instead of sequencing the entire genome, scientists can target only certain regions of interest. Exome sequencing involves sequencing only the exons of the genome. On a smaller scale, individual genes can be sequenced. These selective techniques involve enriching the DNA of interest (by amplification for example), followed by standard sequencing.

Karyotyping

When generating a karyotype, scientists order all the chromosomes from 1 to 22 plus the sex chromosomes, for a genome-wide view of genetic information. Chromosomes are stained to highlight structural features. Major genetic changes (involving millions of base pairs), aneuploidy (when a cell contains an abnormal number of chromosomes), and some insertions, deletions, or translocations can be revealed.

Fluorescence *in situ* Hybridization

Fluorescence *in situ* hybridization (FISH) uses fluorescently labeled probes to locate the positions of specific DNA sequences on chromosomes. This detects and localizes the presence or absence of specific DNA sequences on chromosomes. Fluorescence microscopy is used to find out where the fluorescent probe is bound to the chromosomes. For example, large chromosomal translocations have been found in several types of cancer. A translocation between chromosomes 2 and 3 is often found in follicular thyroid carcinoma. This translocation produces a fusion gene that contains the promoter from one gene and the coding sequence of another. FISH analysis using chromosome 2 and 3 probes can detect and diagnose this translocation.

A.10 ANALYZING GENE EXPRESSION

Many of the techniques discussed above give information about gene expression. For example, RT-PCR and qPCR give information on which genes are being transcribed in a given cell population. Western blot analysis can directly test protein expression, and is limited only by the amount of starting lysate and the availability of antibodies specific for the protein being studied. Additional methods have been developed to study gene expression. Each of these techniques can be used to study a certain gene and gather information about its expression and function, or to study certain cells and gain information on which genes they are expressing and how they grow and survive.

Microarrays

Microarrays can be used to study relative RNA amounts between two samples, or to compare RNA levels in one sample to a normal reference. RNA is used as a starting material. The two samples of RNA (either two different experimental samples being compared to each other, or one sample and a control) are reverse-transcribed into cDNA and labeled with fluorescent dyes of different colors, then mixed and applied to an array chip. This chip contains binding sites for every known gene, which act as probes to determine transcript levels in the samples. Microarray data is quantitative, and actual fold-changes can be calculated based on color and intensity.

In situ Hybridization

In situ hybridization (ISH) can be used to determine expression of a gene of interest in a tissue, or in an embryo. A very thin slice (or "section") of a tissue sample is mounted onto a microscope slide. The tissue is fixed to keep transcripts in place, and then permeabilized to open the cell membrane. A labeled probe, which is specific for the transcript of interest, is added to the section and binds to the transcript being studied. An enzyme-linked antibody is added and binds to the probe. When a substrate for the enzyme is added, the target transcript-probe-antibody complex is detected. In this way, it can be determined when and where transcripts are expressed on a multicellular level.

Immunohistochemistry

This technique is similar to ISH, but is specific for proteins instead of nucleic acids. As such, it gives a direct report on protein expression in a tissue. Immunohistochemistry (IHC) requires an antibody against a known protein. This antibody is recognized by a secondary antibody, which is either linked to an enzyme or a fluorescent molecule. IHC is commonly used in the clinic. For example, breast cancer biopsies from women are stained for the estrogen receptor (ER), the progesterone receptor (PR), and a plasma membrane receptor called HER2. Breast tumors are then classified as ER$^+$ or ER$^-$, PR$^+$ or PR$^-$, and HER2$^+$ or HER2$^-$. These classifications affect which therapy the patient is given.

Flow Cytometry

Flow cytometry again uses many of the same principles already discussed. Here, single cells (either from lab cultures or tissue samples) are stained for certain protein markers using specific antibodies. The antibodies are then linked to a fluorescent tag. Next, the labeled cells are suspended in a fluid stream and passed through a beam of light. Light detectors are found on the other side of, and perpendicular to, the laser. As the labeled cells pass through the light, the beam scatters and the fluorescent tag(s) on the cells can emit light. This combination of scattered and emitted light is measured to give information on cell size, and how many cells in the sample express each of the markers that were labeled. Flow cytometers can have over a dozen different light channels, so many labeled antibodies can be added to one experimental sample. In addition to being analyzed, cells can also be sorted as they go through the machine (a technique called fluorescence-activated cell sorting, or FACS). In this way, a heterogeneous mixture of cells can be sorted based on expression of markers.

A.11

A.11   DETERMINING GENE FUNCTION

Genomic sequencing has revealed thousands of genes with unknown function. There are many ways to discover the function of these genes.

Evolutionary Comparisons

Gene sequences can be compared to all other organisms sequenced. If a human gene of unknown function has much of its sequence in common with a fission yeast protein phosphatase, researchers will test if the unknown human gene may code for a phosphatase.

Protein Domains

Protein domains are conserved patterns in protein sequence and structure. These domains are typically between 25 and 500 amino acids in length and contribute to protein function. Many proteins have several structural domains and one domain can appear in a variety of different peptides from different organisms. Many domains are found in Archaea, Bacteria, and Eukarya. Some domains repeat in tandem and others are found in single copies. For example, zinc fingers are small protein domains which are DNA-binding and commonly found in transcription factors. Pleckstrin homology (PH) domains are approximately 120 amino acids long and function in lipid binding, which targets proteins to appropriate cellular compartments. As such, PH domains occur in a wide range of proteins involved in signaling pathways. Thousands of protein domains have been experimentally determined, and the presence of certain domains can shed light on protein function.

Protein Interactions

Knowing which proteins bind to a protein of interest can shed light on protein function, especially since many proteins function in complexes and pathways. Immunoprecipitations are commonly used to find protein binding partners. In this experiment, cell lysates are collected (as described above) and incubated with an antibody specific for the protein of interest (such as a green protein in Figure 1). A complex forms, including the protein of interest, its binding partners, and an antibody. An antibody binding protein covalently linked to a microscopic bead is added next. The bead can be pulled out of solution (or precipitated) by simple centrifugation (spinning the tube at high speeds). This collects bead complexes at the bottom of the tube. These complexes are then washed and purified from the lysate solution. Proteins that don't bind to the protein of interest are lost. Precipitated proteins can then be identified by Western blot analysis (if you have an idea of what proteins you're looking for), or mass spectrometry (if you have no idea what will be there). Data from these experiments can generate network maps, where protein interactions are used to elucidate functional maps of how proteins are working together in a cell.

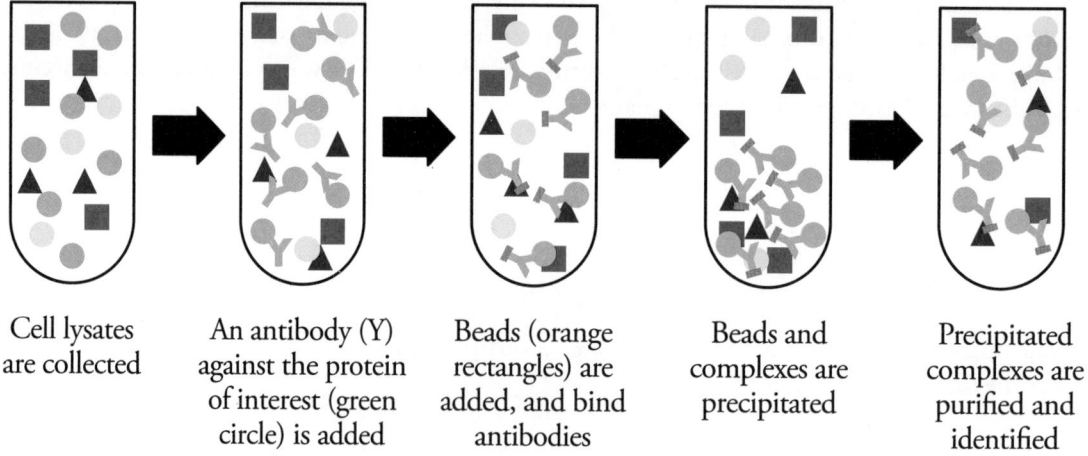

| Cell lysates are collected | An antibody (Y) against the protein of interest (green circle) is added | Beads (orange rectangles) are added, and bind antibodies | Beads and complexes are precipitated | Precipitated complexes are purified and identified |

Figure 1   Immunoprecipitation

A.11

Cellular Expression

Subcellular location can give information on protein function. To determine the subcellular location of a protein of interest, the gene for this protein can be attached to a reporter system to see where it is expressed. For example, the gene of interest can be cloned into an expression vector, and linked to a fluorescent tag such as GFP (green fluorescent protein). This effectively tags the protein with a fluorescent molecule, meaning cellular location can be determined using a fluorescent microscope. In Figure 2, the first cell (A) is expressing the GFP-tagged protein of interest on the plasma membrane, the second cell (B) expresses it in the cytoplasm, while the last cell (C) expresses it in the nucleus. In this experiment, the nucleus is also stained with a fluorescent dye called DAPI (which shows up blue under the fluorescent microscope). Since the nucleus of cell C has both blue DAPI and green protein, it shows up as a teal circle.

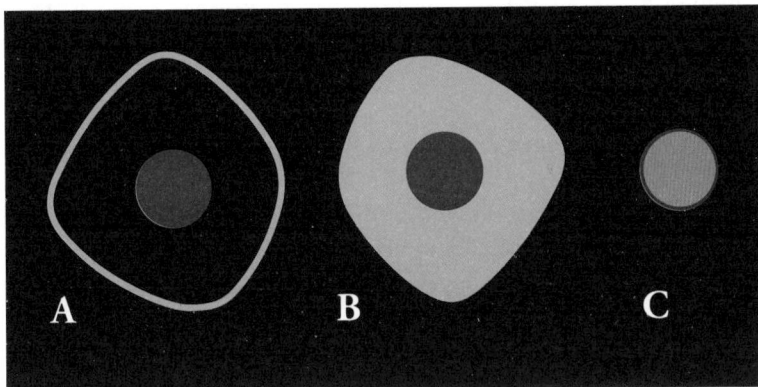

Figure 2   Using GFP-Tagged Proteins to Determine Subcellular Protein Expression

A.11

Altering Expression

Altering gene expression can also be used to help determine gene function. Gene expression can be inhibited or increased, and the subsequent phenotype can shed light on protein function.

Gene expression can be knocked down via RNA interference (or RNAi), which uses microRNA (miRNA) or small interfering RNA (siRNA). These short RNA molecules can bind to mRNAs and decrease their activity, often by promoting degradation of the mRNA transcript. Synthetic RNA has been used in both cell culture and in living organisms as a way to decrease protein expression.

The opposite experiment can also be done, where a protein of interest is over-expressed in a biological system. This can be achieved by attaching the gene of interest to a strong promoter, which will induce high levels of transcription, and therefore gene expression. This genetic construct can be on an expression plasmid or it can be recombined into the genome, either at the endogenous locus (where the gene is normally found), or at another location in the genome. These "knock-in" systems can also be made by increasing gene copy number, or increasing transcript stability (usually by decreasing transcript degradation). No matter how it is done, the cellular and biochemical effects of over-expressing a gene of interest can be investigated.

In vitro mutagenesis is when a gene is cloned, specifically mutated, then returned to a cell. Mutations can alter, destroy, or enhance gene function. These mutated genes can even be put into early multicellular embryos, to study the role of a protein in development and whole-organism function.

A.12 PROTEIN QUANTIFICATION

A good understanding of genomics has led to the field of **proteomics**, the systematic and large-scale study of protein structure and function. This is usually done in a particular context, such as in a certain biochemical pathway, organelle, cell, tissue, or organism. Often, this involves quantitative analysis of proteins. This means measuring amounts of different proteins from a functional standpoint, looking at how the amount, state, or location of a protein changes.

Many different techniques can help with studying proteins quantitatively. Some of these look at proteins in a cell, either alive (FACS, labeling a protein and looking and subcellular location) or not (immunohistochemistry, flow cytometry). Others measure proteins harvested from a cell (ELISA, Western blotting, immunoprecipitation). All these techniques are discussed earlier in this Appendix.

It's common for proteins to be grown in a biological system, then extracted and studied. Often, protein levels in lysates or purified samples must be quantified before an experiment can be started.

The most commonly used quantification method is Bradford Quantification, using UV-Vis spectrophotometers designed for biochemical analysis. This method uses a Bradford reagent containing a blue pigment called Coomassie blue. When proteins bind the pigment, it shifts the absorption peak of the sample. Absorption is measured at 600 nm. This technique is very simple and has good sensitivity.

To perform quantification, first, the negative control sample is put in the spectrophotometer, to set the zero value. Next, the samples with known concentration are applied, and the spectrophotometer generates a concentration curve. This relates absorbance of the sample with protein concentration. A new curve should be made every time proteins are being quantified. Next, the samples are put in the machine one by one. The spectrophotometer applies light in the visible and adjacent (near-UV and near-infrared) ranges. Absorbance is determined and compared to the calibration curve, and the machine usually reports both the absorbance and the subsequent protein concentration.

Affinity Chromatography

Affinity chromatography is used to separate biochemical mixtures, and it is based on highly specific interactions between macromolecules. While affinity chromatography is most commonly used to purify proteins, it can also be used on other macromolecules (such as nucleic acids). It uses many of the same principles described above: you start with a heterogeneous mixture of molecules (such as cell lysate, growth media, or blood). To isolate a protein of interest, you can either use an antibody or tag the protein with an affinity tag (for example, His-tagged proteins can be purified with nickel-based resins and slightly basic conditions; the bound proteins are eluted by adding imidazole or by lowering the pH). The target molecule is trapped on a stationary phase due to specific binding, and the stationary phase is washed to increase purity. The target protein is then released (or eluted) off the solid phase, in a highly purified state.

A.13 STEM CELLS

Stem cells are undifferentiated cells which can differentiate to become other cell types. Stem cells self-replicate by mitosis.

Embryonic Stem Cells

Embryonic stem cells (ESCs) are found in the inner cell mass of the blastocyst and are the only stem cells in humans which are pluripotent. Pluripotent cells are able to differentiate into any of the three germ layers (endoderm, mesoderm, or ectoderm), and can generate all of the over 220 cells types in the human body. ESCs can replicate indefinitely. While ESCs are the only known pluripotent cells, it's possible that other pluripotent stem cells exist in adults and have not yet been found. In addition, it's possible that multipotent stem cells could dedifferentiate into a pluripotent state, but this has not yet been demonstrated in the lab.

Adult Stem Cells

Adult stem cells are found in various tissues, and function in tissue repair and regeneration. They are multipotent, meaning they can produce many cell types. There are three sources of readily available adult stem cells: bone marrow (to regenerate blood cells), adipose tissue (to regenerate fat tissue), and blood (hematopoietic stem cells that give rise to all other blood cells). Adult stem cells are usually tissue-specific, and differentiate into slightly more differentiated progenitor cells, before completely differentiating. An understanding of this process has led to the discovery of cell hierarchies, where the pattern of maturation is characterized and traced as cells differentiate in a given tissue. It is predicted that both stem cells and progenitor cells can transform into a cancer cell, which may have major implications on the treatment and prevention of cancer.

A.13

Applications of Stem Cells

Stem cells have many important uses in biology. First, therapy using ESCs could revolutionize regenerative medicine and alleviate human suffering. Many diseases could be treated using pluripotent cells, such as blood and immune system genetic disorders, many cancers, spinal cord injuries, Parkinson's disease, juvenile diabetes, and blindness. The basic idea behind these stem cell therapies is to manipulate ESCs to become other cells for use in treatment. For example, ESCs induced to become oligodendrocytes have been used to treat patients with spinal cord injuries.

Many ESCs used in the lab come from embryos that were created for *in vitro* fertilization, but then not required. Because generating human ESC lines requires destroying the blastocyst, work on human ESCs is controversial. In addition to ethical concerns, there are additional risks of host-graft rejection, and formation of tumors from therapeutic ESCs.

Second, ESCs from model organisms (such as mice and rats) can be isolated and manipulated in the lab. These targeted ESCs can then be aggregated with a normal morula or injected into a normal blastocyst. The morula or blastocyst is then injected into the uterus of a pseudopregnant female animal, which carries the embryos to term. Pseudopregnant mice are produced by mating fertile females with vasectomized males.

A few weeks later, chimeric pups are born, which are a mix of targeted stem cells and normal stem cells. Usually animals with different coat colors are used in these experiments. For example, the ESCs used for targeting in the lab could be from a brown mouse, while the normal donor morula or blastocyst could come from an albino strain. Chimeric pups typically have a mix of white and brown fur and are screened to find "founder" animals where the germ line was derived from the targeted ESCs (see Figure 3). In this way, new transgenic lines can be generated and used for study. For example, a knock-in mouse could be made which over-expresses a gene of interest. Models are often made using tissue-specific promoters, so studies can be done on certain tissues without affecting all cells in the animal.

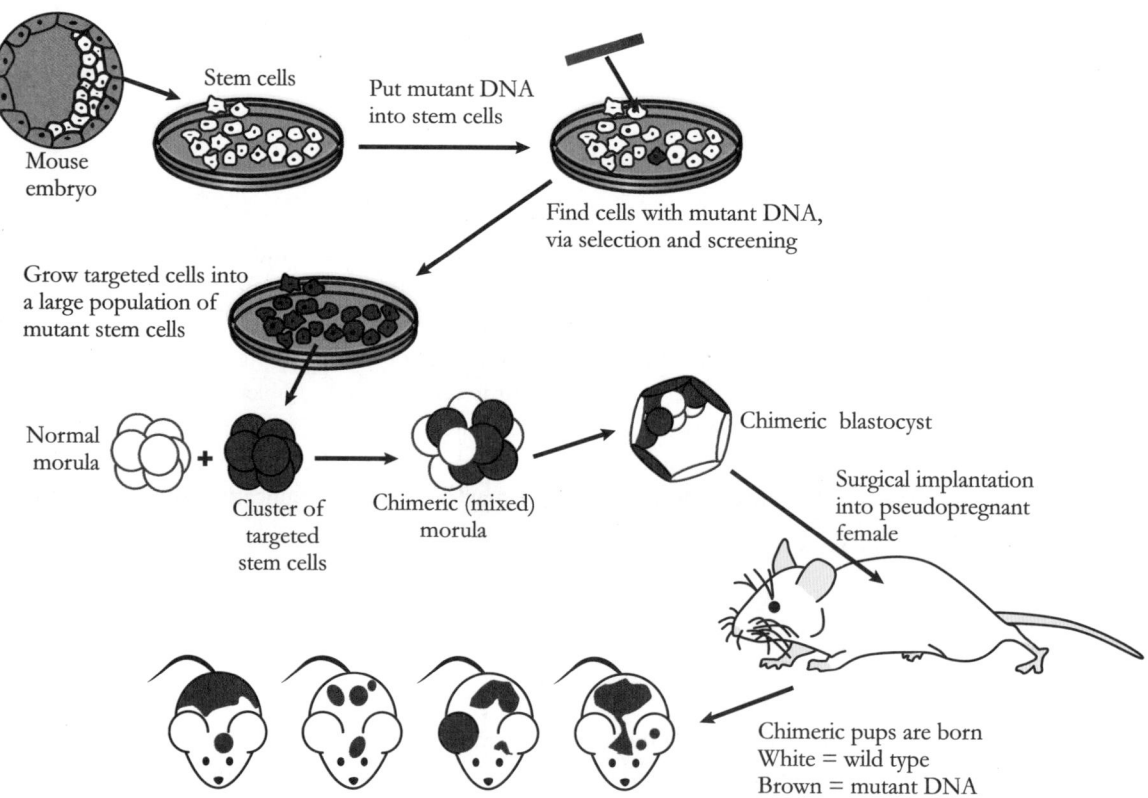

Figure 3   Gene Targeting to Generate Transgenic Mice

A.13

Because of the ethical implications of working with human ESCs, there has been a lot of excitement over induced pluripotent stem cells (iPS cells). These cells are made from adult somatic cells by inducing expression of certain genes, usually transcription factors. Induced expression of these proteins causes the somatic cells to regain pluripotency, a characteristic which only ESCs have. iPS cells have many other characteristics in common with ESCs, including morphology and replicative ability. Despite the initial excitement, however, iPS cells have not yet replaced ESCs because they are potentially tumorigenic and have low replication rates.

A.14 PRACTICAL APPLICATIONS OF DNA TECHNOLOGY

There are dozens of practical uses of DNA technology, some of which (such as forensics and paternity testing) have been already discussed. Many involve transgenic organisms. A transgenic organism is one that carries a foreign gene that has been deliberately inserted into its genome. Many useful transgenic organisms have been developed, but it is important to be aware of the ethical considerations that come with both biotechnology and genetically engineered organisms. This section discusses applications of biotechnology, while the next section discusses some ethical issues to be considered.

Pharmaceuticals

Recombinant bacteria are commonly used by pharmaceutical companies in drug production. An expression plasmid is made that contains a promoter and the gene of interest. The plasmid is transformed into competent bacteria and large cultures of the bacteria are grown in selective media. To harvest the drug of interest, the bacteria are either lysed (if the drug is produced intracellularly), or the growth media is collected and the drug is purified from solution (if the bacteria have been modified so that the drug is secreted from the cell).

Genetic engineering and biotechnology have also been important in the development of vaccines. Here, the gene for a surface protein from a harmful pathogen can be cloned into a harmless virus, which is then used as a vaccine against the pathogenic microbe. This vaccine can be safely administered, since the body will recognize the surface protein as foreign (and will therefore mount an immune response), but will not be infected by the actual pathogen. Without the ability to cut and paste segments of DNA from one source to another (using restriction enzymes, PCR, and plasmids), development of these vaccines would not be possible.

Novel vaccine delivery systems are also being developed. For example, one group has developed transgenic potato plants that express proteins from the cholera bacterium. Ingestion of these potatoes causes production of anti-cholera antibodies, meaning the potato is effectively acting like a cholera vaccine. Although not yet widely available, this could offer a major benefit to impoverished areas, where people must travel long distances to medical clinics to receive vaccination shots.

A.14

Industry

Genetically modified bacteria are also used to produce enzymes required for food processing. For example, the gene for chymosin has been cloned into both prokaryotic and eukaryotic expression plasmids, and bacteria or yeast containing these plasmids produce large amounts of the enzyme chymosin. This enzyme is then purified and used to clot milk in cheese production.

Transgenic cows are being generated to produce milk that has the same characteristics as human breast milk. Additional transgenic animals are being made to produce useful substances (such as goats that excrete silk proteins in their milk, or pigs that produce omega-3 fatty acids).

Both bacteria and plants (such as algae, corn, and poplars) have been genetically modified for use in biofuel production. Biofuel is derived from living organisms and contains energy from geologically recent carbon fixation. Bioethanol (made from carbohydrates via fermentation) and biodiesel (made from animal and plant fats) are common examples of biofuel.

Agriculture

DNA technology has had a great impact on the science of agriculture. Scientists have been able to transfer genes to plants in order to optimize crop yield. For example, some plants express a transgenic enzyme that is harmful to pests, which decreases the need for pesticide use. Others express enzymes making them resistant to diseases or herbicides.

Transgenic plants that are capable of nitrogen fixation are also in production. Most plants need large amounts of nitrate, which is produced from atmospheric nitrogen (a process call nitrogen fixation) by bacteria. Some plants, such as legumes, can fix their own nitrogen. Scientists have identified genes involved in this process and are working to develop transgenic corn and rice strains also capable of nitrogen fixation. Success in this project would mean a decrease in global fertilizer use, which could have a beneficial impact on the environment.

Food has also been modified to increase shelf life and nutritional value. For example, tomatoes have been altered to stay firm during ripening. This means green tomatoes can be picked and transported to grocery shelves without going soft. Golden rice, which contains beta-carotene, has been developed to combat vitamin A deficiency. New rice strains with higher iron content are also being developed.

While genetically modified crops are common, no genetically modified animals have yet been approved for human consumption. However, transgenic fish are in production. One project focuses on transgenic salmon that grow and mature at a faster rate than normal fish.

DNA technology has also been applied to agriculture biotechnology in the form of animal husbandry. DNA fingerprinting has been applied to certain endangered animals (such as the Puerto Rican parrot, orangutans, and some species of African livestock). This allows scientists to identify individual animals, verify their pedigree and ancestors, and track both desirable and undesirable traits. Animals can be registered, and mating pairs can be tracked to make sure the population maintains enough variation to be viable, and that deleterious traits are not passed on to offspring. This is especially important for species that have a small population. These biotechnology-based breeding programs have also been applied to common agriculture livestock species such as cattle and horses.

A.14

Environmental Applications

Bacteria are being engineered to express genes that will help cope with some environmental problems. For example, genetically engineered bacteria have been made to help with sewage treatment, and to degrade harmful compounds. Some bacteria have been made to extract heavy metals from the environment. These metals are then incorporated into different compounds that can be isolated and used to extract the metal. This means bacteria could play a role in the future of both the clean-up of toxic mining waste and the actual mining process.

Phosphorus water pollution promotes algae growth. Genetically modified pigs, which produce the enzyme phytase in their saliva, are able to break down indigestible phosphorus. These pigs may help reduce water pollution, as their manure contains about half the amount of phosphorus as normal pigs.

Genetically modified zebrafish are also being used in environmental biotechnology. For example, transgenic fish have been developed to detect aquatic pollution.

Gene Therapy

Gene therapy is when a genetic disorder is treated by introducing a gene into a cell. This is often to correct or supplement a defective gene. Gene therapy uses genetically modified viruses (such as retroviruses, adenoviruses, or lentiviruses) to deliver genes to somatic human cells. Ideally, the targeted gene will be incorporated into the genome of the cell, but this doesn't always occur. This means treatment efficacy can gradually decreases over time, and repeated treatments may be necessary. Because the targeted cells are somatic, the treatment will only affect the individual patient and will not be passed to later generations. Recent trials in gene therapy have tried to target adult stem cells as a way to increase treatment efficacy and duration.

Gene therapy-based treatments for sickle cell anemia, Parkinson's disease, cystic fibrosis, cancer, HIV, diabetes, muscular dystrophy, and heart disease are currently being developed. While the theory behind this technology is not new, it has been difficult to optimize gene therapy in practice. Because of this, gene therapy is not in widespread practice, but shows promise as a future treatment. Gene therapy of the germ line is also possible in theory, but because of ethical controversy, has not been well developed.

There are some problems associated with gene therapy. Because a foreign particle is being introduced, there is a chance the immune system will respond, and this can reduce treatment efficacy. Current gene therapies are limited to one or two genes, while many disorders are caused by many genes. Finally, there is a small chance of tumor development if the therapy DNA integrates into the genome incorrectly.

Genetic Testing

Biotechnology has also been crucial in developing DNA-based tests. You already learned how RFLP and STR analysis can be used in forensics (to compare crime scene samples to suspects for example), to establish relationships between people, or to study the evolutionary relationship between two species. Genetic testing is another application of these tests. Genetic testing can be done before birth (to look for diseases like hemophilia, cystic fibrosis, and Duchene muscular dystrophy) or after birth (to test for mutations that may lead to increased disease risk).

A.15   SAFETY AND ETHICS OF DNA TECHNOLOGY

Regulatory agencies and governments have started implementing regulations on how biotechnology can be used in industry, medicine, and agriculture. These agencies focus on assessing risk, public education, and mandating policies to protect both scientists and the public. However, with a hot topic like biotechnology, there will always be opponents. Serious considerations of risk and implications are important to mitigate any potential downsides to new technology.

Criticisms of genetically modified crops have received widespread news coverage. Opponents argue introduction of transgenic crops into ecosystems could cause unpredictable results. For example, if pesticide resistance is somehow transferred to the pest, this could cause widespread ecological problems. Biotechnology could therefore inadvertently generate new and hazardous pathogens. Opponents also point out that eating transgenic crops may not be safe, and some critics argue that they're not necessary to solve food availability issues. While there is little data supporting the hypothesis that transgenic foodstuffs are dangerous, it is important to consider that this may be the case.

Concerns over gene therapy are also common. Some are worried about the long-term implications of introducing a foreign gene into a human being. Germ line gene therapy is highly controversial, as development of this technology could lead to eugenics: a deliberate effort to control the genetic makeup of human populations. Some see germ line gene therapy as interfering with evolution. Since genetic variation is important for species survival, some argue that gene therapy is a way of decreasing alleles in a population. While this might seem like a good idea, it is possible that alleles that have a disadvantage in one situation might prove to be advantageous in another situation. If gene targeting or eugenics causes this allele to be lost, the species could suffer. A common example of an allele with multiple effects is the sickle cell allele. In the homozygous form, this allele causes sickle cell disease. However, in the heterozygous form, this allele provides some protection against malaria. What looks like a "bad allele" from one perspective, can actually be a good thing in other situations.

Working with any animal in a laboratory setting raises ethical issues. Agencies have been appointed to ensure lab animals have a good quality of life, are treated humanely, and are used in justified and important experiments. A rigorous peer-reviewed process (usually overseen by veterinarians) ensures researchers justify the use for each and every experimental animal. Despite these attempts, additional concerns exist. For example, in generating experimental animals, many labs also generate normal animals, which are sacrificed simply because they don't have the correct genotype. Also, transgenic animals typically suffer from decreased fertility and may be susceptible to conditions and diseases besides those they are bred to develop and model. Again, close monitoring of animal facilities, usually in conjunction with both local and federal regulations, ensures researchers are acting in a responsible and ethical manner when working with transgenic animals.

A.15

Appendix II
Pedigree Analysis

The AAMC has formally removed pedigree analysis from the list of MCAT topics, but they do still expect you to understand patterns of inheritance (see Section 7.6). One way to learn about and understand patterns of inheritance is by looking at and analyzing data from pedigrees. Thus, although pedigree analysis is no longer required material, we present it here to enhance your understanding of how traits are passed on from generation to generation.

PEDIGREE ANALYSIS

Often it is not possible to perform controlled genetic crosses to ascertain the nature of inheritance of a trait, particularly when people are involved. In these cases, families can be studied to determine the pattern of inheritance. Researchers organize the information learned from families into **pedigrees**, which are charts depicting inheritance of a trait (Figure 1). By studying the pedigree of families, researchers can determine the pattern of inheritance of a gene, whether it is linked to other genes, and whether an individual is likely to pass on a trait to their offspring. Pedigrees follow certain conventions in how they are drawn:

1) Males are represented by squares and females by circles.
2) A cross (mating) between a male and female is represented by a horizontal line connecting them.
3) Offspring from a cross are connected to their parents by a vertical line, and to each other by a horizontal line with vertical branches for each sibling.
4) Offspring of unknown gender (unborn children) are represented by a diamond shape.
5) Individuals afflicted with a trait being studied are shaded in; unaffected or normal individuals are not shaded in.

Many pedigrees make a common assumption: individuals mating into the family (i.e., individuals for which you have no information on their parents or grandparents) are assumed to be homozygous normal unless their phenotype tells you differently. The basis of this assumption is that the traits being studied are usually relatively rare in the human population, and therefore, it is most likely that a non-family member is homozygous for the wild-type allele.

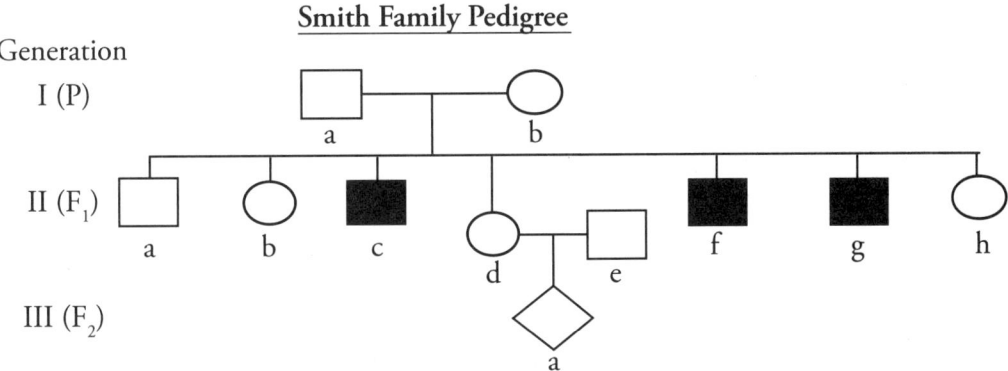

Figure 1   A Pedigree

Once drawn, a pedigree can be analyzed as follows:

Step 1: Is the allele that causes the trait dominant or is it recessive? Recessive traits commonly skip generations (affected individuals can have unaffected parents), but dominant traits do not (affected individuals must have at least one affected parent).

Step 2: Is the gene involved carried on a sex chromosome (sex-linked)? If so, there tends to be an unequal distribution of affected males (more) versus affected females (fewer). If the numbers of affected males and females are approximately equal, the gene is most likely autosomal.

Step 3: If the disease is sex-linked, is it on the X or the Y chromosome? Diseases linked to the Y chromosome will show father-to-son transmission, while diseases linked to the X chromosome will not.

Step 4: Check for mitochondrial inheritance. Affected females will have all affected children, but affected males cannot pass the trait on.

Step 5: Figure out the genotypes and calculate the probabilities of inheritance where necessary. When writing genotypes for sex-linked traits, make sure to include the chromosomes (e.g., X^AY, or X^AX^a, etc.). When writing genotypes for autosomal traits, make sure NOT to include the chromosomes (e.g., *DD* or *Dd*, etc.).

Step 6: If more than one trait is involved, go through Steps 1–5 for each.

- In the pedigree in Figure 1, the darkened squares represent individuals afflicted with a certain genetic disease. This disease is most likely caused by:[1]
    A) a dominant allele.
    B) an autosomal recessive allele.
    C) an X-linked recessive allele.
    D) a Y-linked allele.

- In the pedigree in Figure 1, what is the probability that IIIa will have the disease?[2]
    A) If male, IIIa will have the disease.
    B) Overall, there is a 1/8 chance that IIIa will have the disease.
    C) Overall, there is a 1/4 chance that IIIa will have the disease.
    D) IIIa will not have the disease.

---

[1] Since the affected individuals have unaffected parents, the disease is most likely recessive (choice A is wrong), and since the affected individuals are all male, it is most likely sex-linked (choice B is wrong). There is no father-to-son transmission (all affected males have an unaffected father), so the disease is X-linked (choice C is correct, and choice D is wrong).

[2] The disease is X-linked recessive, and IIe (IIIa's father) is not affected, so IIe cannot pass the allele on. Thus, the probability of IIIa getting the disease depends on the genotype of IId (she would have to be a carrier) and what she passes on to IIIa. It also depends on the gender of IIIa; females would not be affected because they would have to receive the allele from both IId and IIe, and IIe does not carry the disease allele. Bottom line, in order for IIIa to get the disease, IId would have to be a carrier, would have to pass the disease allele on, and IIIa would have to be male. The probability of IId being a carrier is 1/2; we know she received a good X chromosome from her father Ia (all he has is a good X chromosome), and the probability she received the affected X chromosome from her mother (Ib) is 1/2. The probability she passes the bad X chromosome on to IIIa is 1/2; she has one good X and one bad X. The probability that IIIa is male is 1/2. Finally, we can use the rule of multiplication to determine the overall probability: $1/2 \times 1/2 \times 1/2 = 1/8$ overall probability (choice **B** is correct, and choices C and D are wrong). Note that choice A is wrong because being male does not guarantee the disease; IIIa could be male (get the Y chromosome from IIe) and still be unaffected (get the good X chromosome from IId).

Below are example pedigrees for six modes of inheritance (X-linked recessive, X-linked dominant, autosomal recessive, autosomal dominant, mitochondrial, and Y-linked). For each pedigree, determine which mode of inheritance is displayed.

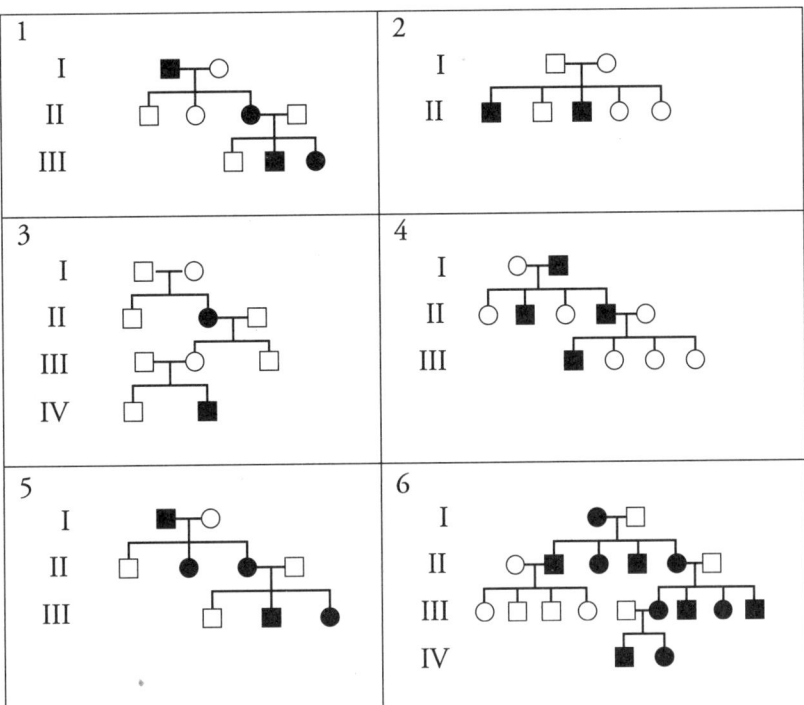

Answers

1) autosomal dominant
2) X-linked recessive
3) autosomal recessive
4) Y-linked
5) X-linked dominant
6) mitochondrial inheritance

Explanations

The easiest inheritance patterns to spot are mitochondrial (passed from mothers to all offspring) and Y-linked (passed from fathers to sons, and females are never affected). Let's start by finding these two. Since Pedigree 6 shows a trait with maternal inheritance, this must be mitochondrial inheritance. The affected father in generation II does not pass the trait to any of his children, but the affected mothers in generations I, II, and III pass the trait onto all their offspring. Pedigree 4 shows a trait with Y-linked inheritance. The trait is passed from father to all sons and does not affect females.

Next, Pedigrees 2 and 3 both show traits that skips generations. That is, there are individuals on the pedigree that are affected by the trait but who have unaffected parents. Therefore, these two pedigrees must be for recessive traits. One is autosomal and the other is X-linked.

Since the trait on Pedigree 2 affects males more than females, it is likely X-linked, and since the trait on Pedigree 3 affects males and females equally, it is probably autosomal. Let's verify this by looking more closely at Pedigree 3. If this trait is X-linked recessive, then the affected female in generation II must have the genotype X^aX^a, and would have had to receive the allele for the trait from both her parents. However, for an X-linked recessive, the unaffected male in generation I would have the genotype X^AY, and would only have X^A to donate to his daughter. Therefore, this pedigree cannot represent an X-linked recessive trait; it must represent an autosomal recessive trait. The male in generation I must have the genotype *Aa*, the female in generation I must have the genotype *Aa*, and the affected female in generation II must have the genotype *aa*. The remaining pedigree, Pedigree 2, must be X-linked recessive.

Finally, Pedigrees 1 and 5 show traits that do not skip generations. That is, affected individuals have affected parents. These are pedigrees for dominant traits; one is X-linked and one is autosomal. The only difference between these two pedigrees is the middle daughter in the second generation; in Pedigree 1 she is unaffected and in Pedigree 5 she is affected. Let's focus on her father (the male in generation I) since this is where she gets the allele for the trait. If the trait is X-linked dominant, the male in generation I would be X^AY; thus all females in generation II would inherit X^A from their father, and all of them would be affected. Since the middle daughter in Pedigree I is not affected, Pedigree 1 must show autosomal dominance and the pedigree for the X-linked dominant trait must be Pedigree 5.

Biology Glossary

After each definition, the section number in the *MCAT Biology* text where the term is discussed is given.

5' cap
A methylated guanine nucleotide added to the 5' end of eukaryotic mRNA. The cap is necessary to initiate translation of the mRNA. [**Sections 4.7 and 4.8**]

A band
The band of the sarcomere that extends the full length of the thick filament. The A band includes regions of thick and thin filament overlap, as well as a region of thick filament only. A bands alternate with I bands to give skeletal and cardiac muscle tissue a striated appearance. The A band does not shorten during muscle contraction. [**Section 11.2**]

A site
Aminoacyl-tRNA site; the site on a ribosome where a new amino acid is added to a growing peptide. [**Section 4.8**]

absolute refractory period
A period of time following an action potential during which no additional action potential can be evoked regardless of the level of stimulation. [**Section 8.1**]

absolute threshold
The minimum stimulus intensity required to activate a sensory receptor 50% of the time. [**Section 8.5**]

accessory glands
The three glands in the male reproductive system that produce semen: the seminal vesicles, the prostate, and the bulbourethral glands. [**Section 13.1**]

accessory organs
1. In the GI tract, organs that play a role in digestion, but are not directly part of the alimentary canal. These include the liver, the gallbladder, the pancreas, and the salivary glands.
2. In the reproductive systems, any organ involved in reproduction that is not a gonad (testis or ovary). [**Section 10.7**]

acetylcholine (ACh)
The neurotransmitter used throughout the parasympathetic nervous system as well as at the neuromuscular junction. [**Section 8.2**]

acetylcholinesterase (AChE)
The enzyme that breaks down acetylcholine in the synaptic cleft. [**Section 8.2**]

acid hydrolases
Enzymes that degrade various macromolecules and that require an acidic pH to function properly. Acid hydrolases are found within the lysosomes of cells. [**Section 6.2**]

acinar cells
Cells that make up exocrine glands, and that secrete their products into ducts. For example, in the pancreas, acinar cells secrete digestive enzymes; in the salivary glands, acinar cells secrete saliva. [**Section 10.5**]

acrosome
A region at the head of a sperm cell that contains digestive enzymes which, when released during the acrosome reaction, can facilitate penetration of the corona radiata of the oocyte and fertilization. [**Sections 13.2 and 13.9**]

actin
A contractile protein. In skeletal and cardiac muscle, actin polymerizes (along with other proteins) to form the thin filaments. Actin is involved in many contractile activities, such as cytokinesis, pseudopod formation, and muscle contraction. [**Sections 6.5 and 11.2**]

action potential
A localized change in a neuron's or muscle cell's membrane potential that can propagate itself away from its point of origin. Action potentials are an all-or-none process mediated by the opening of voltage-gated Na^+ and K^+ channels when the membrane is brought to the threshold potential; opening of the Na^+ channels causes a characteristic depolarization, while opening of the K^+ channels repolarizes the membrane. [**Section 8.1**]

activator proteins
Proteins that bind to enhancer sequences in eukaryotes to increase transcription. [**Section 4.9**]

active transport
The movement of molecules through the plasma membrane against their concentration gradients. Active transport requires input of cellular energy, often in the form of ATP. An example is the Na^+/K^+-ATPase in the plasma membranes of all cells. [**Section 6.4**]

adenine
One of the four aromatic bases found in DNA and RNA; also a component of ATP, NADH, and $FADH_2$. Adenine is a purine; it pairs with thymine (in DNA) and with uracil (in RNA). [**Section 4.1**]

adenohypophysis
See "anterior pituitary gland." [**Section 8.6**]

adipocyte
Fat cell. [Section 9.5]

adrenal medulla
The inner region of the adrenal gland. The adrenal medulla is part of the sympathetic nervous system, and it releases epinephrine (adrenaline) and norepinephrine into the blood when stimulated. These hormones augment and prolong the effects of sympathetic stimulation in the body. [Section 8.4]

adrenergic tone
A constant nervous input to the arteries that keeps them somewhat constricted to maintain a basal level of blood pressure. [Section 9.3]

adrenocorticotropic hormone (ACTH)
A tropic hormone produced by the anterior pituitary gland that targets the adrenal cortex, stimulating it to release cortisol and aldosterone. [Section 8.6]

afferent arteriole
The small artery that carries blood toward the capillaries of the glomerulus. [Section 10.2]

afferent neuron
A neuron that carries information (action potentials) to the central nervous system; a sensory neuron. [Section 8.3]

albumin
A blood protein produced by the liver. Albumin helps to maintain blood osmotic pressure (oncotic pressure). [Section 9.4]

aldosterone
The principal mineralocorticoid secreted by the adrenal cortex. This steroid hormone targets the kidney tubules and increases renal reabsorption of sodium. [Section 10.2]

alimentary canal
Also known as the *gastrointestinal* (GI) *tract* or the *digestive tract*, the alimentary canal is the long muscular "tube" that includes the mouth, esophagus, stomach, small intestine, and large intestine. [Section 10.5]

allele
A version of a gene. For example, the gene may be for eye color, and the alleles include those for brown eyes, those for blue eyes, those for green eyes, etc. At most, diploid organisms can possess only two alleles for a given gene, one on each of the two homologous chromosomes. [Section 7.1]

alveoli
(Singular: *alveolus*) Tiny sacs, with walls only a single cell thick, found at the end of the respiratory bronchiole tree. Alveoli are the sites of gas exchange in the respiratory system. [Section 12.2]

amino acids
The building blocks (monomers) of proteins. There are 20 different amino acids. [Section 3.1]

amino acid acceptor site
The 3' end of a tRNA molecule that binds an amino acid. The nucleotide sequence at this end is CCA. [Section 4.8]

amino acid activation
See "tRNA loading." [Section 4.8]

aminoacyl tRNA
A tRNA with an amino acid attached. This is made by an aminoacyl-tRNA synthetase, an enzyme that is specific to the amino acid being attached. [Section 4.8]

amnion
A sac filled with fluid (amniotic fluid) that surrounds and protects a developing embryo. [Section 13.10]

amylase
An enzyme that digests starch into disaccharides. Amylase is secreted by salivary glands and by the pancreas. [Section 10.6]

anabolism
The process of building complex structures out of simpler precursors (e.g., synthesizing proteins from amino acids). [Section 4.9]

analogous structures
Physical structures in two different organisms that have functional similarity due to their evolution in a common environment, but that have different underlying structure. Analogous structures arise from convergent evolution. [Section 7.10]

anal sphincter
The valve that controls the release of feces from the rectum. It has an internal part made of smooth muscle (thus involuntary) and an external part made of skeletal muscle (thus voluntary). [Section 10.6]

anaphase
The third phase of mitosis. During anaphase, replicated chromosomes are split apart at their centromeres (the sister chromatids are separated from one another) and moved to opposite sides of the cell. [Section 6.6]

anaphase I

The third phase of meiosis I. During anaphase I the replicated homologous chromosomes are separated (the tetrad is split apart) and pulled to opposite sides of the cell. [Section 7.2]

anaphase II

The third phase of meiosis II. During anaphase II, the sister chromatids are finally separated at their centromeres and pulled to opposite sides of the cell. Note that anaphase II is identical to mitotic anaphase, except that the number of chromosomes was reduced by half during meiosis I. [Section 7.2]

androgens

Male sex hormones. Testosterone is the primary androgen. [Section 13.4]

anergic

A term used to describe immune system cells that become unresponsive, but do not go through apoptosis, e.g., B cells and T cells that recognize self-antigens. [Section 9.8]

angiotensinogen

A normal blood protein produced by the liver, angiotensinogen is converted to angiotensin I by renin (secreted by the kidney when blood pressure falls). Angiotensin I is further converted to angiotensin II by ACE (angiotensin converting enzyme). Angiotensin II is a powerful systemic vasoconstrictor and stimulator of aldosterone release, both of which result in an increase in blood pressure. [Section 10.3]

antagonist

Something that acts to oppose the action of something else. For example, muscles that move a joint in opposite directions are said to be *antagonists*. [Section 11.2]

anterior pituitary gland

Also known as the *adenohypophysis*, the anterior pituitary is made of glandular tissue. It makes and secretes six different hormones: FSH, LH, ACTH, TSH, prolactin, and growth hormone. The anterior pituitary is controlled by releasing and inhibiting factors from the hypothalamus. [Section 8.6]

antibody (Ab)

Also called *immunoglobulins*, antibodies are proteins secreted by activated B cells (plasma cells) that bind in a highly specific manner to foreign proteins (such as those found on the surface of pathogens or transplanted tissues). The foreign proteins are called *antigens*. Antibodies generally do not destroy antigens directly, rather, they mark them for destruction through other methods, and can inactivate antigens by clumping them together or by covering necessary active sites. [Section 9.7]

anticodon

A sequence of three nucleotides (found in the anticodon loop of tRNA) that is complementary to a specific codon in mRNA. The codon to which the anticodon is complementary specifies the amino acid that is carried by that tRNA. [Section 4.8]

antidiuretic hormone (ADH)

Also called *vasopressin*, this hormone is produced in the hypothalamus and secreted by the posterior pituitary gland. It targets the kidney tubules, increasing their permeability to water, and thus increasing water retention by the body. [Section 8.6]

antigen (Ag)

A molecule (usually a protein) capable of initiating an immune response (antibody production). [Section 9.7]

antigen-presenting cell

Cells that possess MHC II (B cells and macrophages), and are able to display bits of ingested antigen on their surface in order to activate T cells. (See also "MHC.") [Section 9.7]

antiport

A carrier protein that transports two molecules across the plasma membrane in opposite directions. [Section 6.4]

aorta

The largest artery in the body; the aorta carries oxygenated blood away from the left ventricle of the heart. [Section 9.2]

apoptosis

Programmed cell death due to external stressors such as toxins or internal signals, such as an increase in the product of a tumor suppressor gene. Apoptosis is mediated by a family of proteins called caspases. [Section 6.7]

appendix

A mass of lymphatic tissue at the beginning of the large intestine that helps trap ingested pathogens. [Section 9.7]

aqueous humor

A thin, watery fluid found in the anterior segment of the eye (between the lens and the cornea). The aqueous humor is constantly produced and drained, and helps to bring nutrients to the lens and cornea, as well as to remove metabolic wastes. [Section 8.5]

arousal

A function in the reproductive system, controlled by the parasympathetic nervous system, that includes erection (via dilation of erectile arteries) and lubrication. [Section 13.2]

artery
A blood vessel that carries blood away from the heart chambers. Arteries have muscular walls to regulate blood flow and are typically high-pressure vessels. [**Section 9.2**]

atrioventricular (AV) bundle
Also known as the *bundle of His*, this is the first portion of the cardiac conduction system after the AV node. [**Section 9.2**]

atrioventricular (AV) node
The second major node of the cardiac conduction system (after the SA node). The cardiac impulse is delayed slightly at the AV node, allowing the ventricles to contract just after the atria contract. [**Section 9.2**]

atrioventricular valves
The valves in the heart that separate the atria from the ventricles. The *tricuspid* valve separates the right atrium from the right ventricle, and the *bicuspid* (or *mitral*) valve separates the left atrium from the left ventricle. These valves close at the beginning of systole, preventing the backflow of blood from ventricles to atria, and producing the first heart sound. [**Section 9.2**]

atrium
One of two small chambers in the heart that receive blood and pass it on to the ventricles. The right atrium receives deoxygenated blood from the body through the superior and inferior vena cavae, and the left atrium receives oxygenated blood from the lungs through the pulmonary veins. [**Section 9.2**]

attachment
The first step in viral infection. Attachment of a virus to its host is very specific and is also known as *adsorption*. [**Section 5.1**]

auditory tube
The tube that connects the middle ear cavity with the pharynx; also known as the *Eustachian tube*. Its function is to equalize middle ear pressure with atmospheric pressure so that pressure is equal on both sides of the tympanic membrane. [**Section 8.5**]

autoimmune reaction
An immune reaction directed against normal (necessary) cells. For example, type I diabetes mellitus is an autoimmune reaction directed against the β cells of the pancreas (destroying them and preventing insulin secretion), and against insulin itself. [**Section 9.8**]

autonomic nervous system (ANS)
The division of the peripheral nervous system that innervates and controls the visceral organs (everything but the skeletal muscles). It is also known as the *involuntary nervous system* and can be subdivided into the sympathetic and parasympathetic divisions. [**Section 8.4**]

autotroph
An organism that can makes its own food, typically using CO_2 as a carbon source. [**Section 5.3**]

auxotroph
A bacterium that cannot survive on minimal medium (glucose alone) because it lacks the ability to synthesize a molecule it needs to live (typically an amino acid). Auxotrophs must have the needed substance (the *aux*iliary *troph*ic substance) added to their medium in order to survive. They are typically denoted by the substance they require followed by a "−" sign in superscript. For example, a bacterium that cannot synthesize leucine would be a leucine auxotroph, and would be indicated as Leu⁻. [**Section 5.3**]

avascular
Lacking a blood supply, e.g., cartilage. [**Section 11.8**]

axon
A long projection off the cell body of a neuron down which an action potential can be propagated. [**Section 8.1**]

B cell
A type of lymphocyte that can recognize (bind to) an antigen and secrete an antibody specific for that antigen. When activated by binding an antigen, B cells mature into *plasma cells* (that secrete antibody) and *memory cells* (that patrol the body for future encounters with that antigen). [**Section 9.7**]

bacillus
A bacterium having a rod-like shape (plural = bacilli). [**Section 5.3**]

bacteriophage
A virus that infects a bacterium. [**Section 5.1**]

baroreceptor
A sensory receptor that responds to changes in pressure; for example, there are baroreceptors in the carotid arteries and the aortic arch that monitor blood pressure. [**Section 9.2**]

Bartholin's glands
See "vestibular glands." [**Section 13.5**]

basement membrane
A layer of collagen fibers that separates epithelial tissue from connective tissue. [**Section 10.2**]

basilar membrane
The flexible membrane in the cochlea that supports the organ of Corti (the structure that contains the hearing receptors). The fibers of the basilar membrane are short and stiff near the oval window and long and flexible near the apex of the cochlea. This difference in structure allows the basilar membrane to help transduce pitch. [Section 8.5]

bicarbonate
HCO_3^-. This ion results from the dissociation of carbonic acid and, together with carbonic acid, forms the major blood buffer system. Bicarbonate is also secreted by the pancreas to neutralize stomach acid in the intestines. [Section 9.5]

bicuspid valve
See "atrioventricular valve." [Section 9.2]

bile
A green fluid made from cholesterol and secreted by the liver. It is stored and concentrated in the gallbladder. Bile is an amphipathic molecule that is secreted into the small intestine when fats are present, and it serves to emulsify the fats for better digestion by lipases. [Section 9.5]

binary fission
An asexual method of bacterial reproduction that serves only to increase the size of the population; there is no introduction of genetic diversity. The bacterium simply grows in size until it has doubled its cellular components, then it replicates its genome and splits into two. [Section 5.3]

bipolar cell
A cell in the retina of the eye that receives input from photoreceptors and subsequently synapses on ganglion cells. Bipolar cells belong to a class of neurons called "bipolar neurons" that have a single dendrite and single axon extending from opposite sides of the cell body. [Section 8.5]

blastocyst
A fluid-filled sphere formed about five days after fertilization of an ovum that is made up of an outer ring of cells and an inner cell mass. This is the structure that implants in the endometrium of the uterus. [Section 13.9]

Bohr effect
The tendency of certain factors to stabilize hemoglobin in the tense conformation, thus reducing its affinity for oxygen and enhancing the release of oxygen to the tissues. The factors include increased P_{CO_2}, increased temperature, increased bisphosphoglycerate (BPG), and decreased pH. Note that the Bohr effect shifts the oxy-hemoglobin saturation curve to the right. [Section 9.5]

boiling point elevation
The increase in the boiling point of a solution due to the addition of solute. [Section 6.4]

bone marrow
A non-bony material that fills the hollow spaces inside bones. Red bone marrow is found in regions of spongy bone and is the site of blood cell production. Yellow bone marrow is found in the diaphysis (shaft) of long bones, is mostly fat, and is inactive. [Section 11.7]

bottom-up processing
A tenet of Gestalt psychology wherein the processing of sensory input begins with the sensory receptors and works up to the complex integration of information occurring in the brain. [Section 8.5]

Bowman's capsule
The region of the nephron that surrounds the glomerulus. The capsule collects the plasma that is filtered from the capillaries in the glomerulus. [Section 10.2]

bronchioles
Very small air tubes in the respiratory system (diameter 0.5–1.0 mm). The walls of the bronchioles are made of smooth muscle to help regulate air flow. [Section 12.2]

brush border enzymes
Enzymes secreted by the mucosal cells lining the intestine. The brush border enzymes are disaccharidases and dipeptidases that digest the smallest carbohydrates and peptides into their respective monomers. [Section 10.6]

bulbourethral glands
Small, paired glands found inferior to the prostate in males and at the posterior end of the penile urethra. They secrete an alkaline mucus on sexual arousal that lubricates the urethra and helps to neutralize any traces of acidic urine in the urethra that might be harmful to sperm. [Section 13.1]

Bundle of His
See "atrioventricular (AV) bundle." [Section 9.2]

calcitonin
A hormone produced by the C-cells of the thyroid gland that decreases serum calcium levels. It targets the bones (stimulates osteoblasts) and the kidneys (reduces calcium reabsorption. [Sections 8.6 and 11.9]

calcitriol
A hormone produced from vitamin D that acts to increase serum calcium levels. [Section 11.9]

calmodulin
A cytoplasmic Ca^{2+}-binding protein. Calmodulin is particularly important in smooth muscle cells, where binding of Ca^{2+} allows calmodulin to activate myosin light-chain kinase, the first step in smooth muscle cell contraction. [**Section 11.4**]

cAMP
See "cyclic AMP." [**Section 6.5**]

capacitation
An increase in the fragility of the membranes of sperm cells when exposed to the female reproductive tract. Capacitation is required so that the acrosomal enzymes can be released to facilitate fertilization. [**Section 13.9**]

capillary
The smallest of all blood vessels, typically having a diameter just large enough for blood cells to pass through in single file. Capillaries have extremely thin walls to facilitate the exchange of material between the blood and the tissues. [**Section 9.5**]

capsid
The outer protein coat of a virus. [**Section 5.1**]

carbonic anhydrase
An enzyme present in erythrocytes (as well as in other places) that catalyzes the conversion of CO_2 and H_2O into carbonic acid. [**Section 9.5**]

cardiac conduction system
The specialized cells of the heart that spontaneously initiate action potentials and transmit them to the cardiac muscle cells. The cells of the conduction system are essentially cardiac muscle cells, but lack the contractile fibers of the muscle cells, thus they are able to transmit impulses (action potentials) more quickly and efficiently than cardiac muscle tissue. The cardiac conduction system includes the SA node, the internodal tract, the AV node, the AV bundle, the right and left bundle branches, and the Purkinje fibers. [**Section 9.2**]

cardiac muscle
The muscle tissue of the heart. Cardiac muscle is striated, uninucleate, and under involuntary control (controlled by the autonomic nervous system). Note also that cardiac muscle is self-stimulatory, and autonomic control serves only to modify the intrinsic rate of contraction. [**Section 9.2**]

cardiac output
The volume of blood pumped out of the heart in one minute (vol/min); the product of the stroke volume (vol/beat) and the heart rate (beat/min). Cardiac output is directly proportional to blood pressure. [**Section 9.2**]

cardiac sphincter
See "lower esophageal sphincter." [**Section 10.6**]

carrier protein
An integral membrane protein that undergoes a conformational change to move a molecule from one side of the membrane to another. See also "uniporter," "antiporter," and "symporter." [**Section 6.4**]

cartilage
A strong connective tissue with varying degrees of flexibility. Elastic cartilage is the most flexible, forming structures that require support but also need to bend, such as the epiglottis and outer ear. Hyaline cartilage is more rigid than elastic cartilage, and forms the cartilages of the ribs, the respiratory tract, and all joints. Fibrocartilage is the least flexible of them all, and forms very strong connections, such as the pubic symphysis and the intervertebral disks. [**Section 11.8**]

caspases
A family of proteases that carry out the events of apoptosis. [**Section 6.7**]

catalase
The primary enzyme in peroxisomes; catalase catalyzes the hydrolysis of hydrogen peroxide (H_2O_2) into water and oxygen. [**Section 6.2**]

cDNA
Complementary DNA. DNA produced synthetically by reverse transcribing mRNA. Because of eukaryotic mRNA splicing, cDNA contains no introns. [**Section A.5**]

cecum
The first part of the large intestine. [**Section 10.6**]

cell surface receptor
An integral membrane protein that binds extracellular signaling molecules, such as hormones and peptides. [**Section 6.3**]

cell theory
Established by Robert Hooke in 1655, the cell theory asserts that all living organisms are composed of one or more cells and that new cells arise from preexisting, living cells. [**Section 5.3**]

central canal
The hollow center of an osteon, also known as a *Haversian canal*. The central canal contains blood vessels, lymphatic vessels, and nerves. Bone is laid down around the central canal in concentric rings called *lamellae*. [**Section 11.8**]

central chemoreceptors
Receptors in the central nervous system that monitor the pH of cerebrospinal fluid to help regulate ventilation rate. [Section 12.5]

central nervous system
The subdivision of the nervous system consisting of the brain and spinal cord. [Section 8.4]

centriole
A structure composed of a ring of nine microtubule triplets, found in pairs at the MTOC (microtubule organizing center) of a cell. The centrioles duplicate during cell division, and serve as the organizing center for the mitotic spindle. [Section 6.5]

centromere
A structure near the middle of eukaryotic chromosomes to which the fibers of the mitotic spindle attach during cell division. [Section 4.1]

cerebellum
The region of the brain that coordinates and smooths skeletal muscle activity. [Section 8.4]

cerebral cortex
A thin (4 mm) layer of gray matter on the surface of the cerebral hemispheres. The cerebral cortex is the conscious mind, and is functionally divided into four pairs of lobes: the frontal lobes, the parietal lobes, the temporal lobes, and the occipital lobes. [Section 8.4]

cerebrospinal fluid (CSF)
A clear fluid that circulates around and through the brain and spinal cord. CSF helps to physically support the brain and acts as a shock absorber. It also exchanges nutrients and wastes with the brain and spinal cord. [Section 8.4]

cervix
The opening to the uterus. The cervix is typically plugged with a sticky acidic mucus during non-fertile times (to form a barrier against the entry of pathogens), however, during ovulation, the mucus becomes more watery and alkaline to facilitate sperm entry. [Section 13.5]

channel protein
An integral membrane protein that selectively allows molecules across the plasma membrane. See also entries under "ion channel," "voltage-gated channel," and "ligand-gated channel." [Section 6.3]

chaperones
A family of proteins that assists in the folding of other proteins. [Section 4.9]

chemical synapse
A type of synapse at which a chemical (a neurotransmitter) is released from the axon of a neuron into the synaptic cleft where it binds to receptors on the next structure in sequence, either another neuron or an organ. [Section 8.2]

chemoreceptor
A sensory receptor that responds to specific chemicals. Some examples are gustatory (taste) receptors, olfactory (smell) receptors, and central chemoreceptors (respond to pH changes in the cerebrospinal fluid). [Sections 5.3 and 8.5]

chemotaxis
Movement that is directed by chemical gradients, such as nutrients or toxins. [Sections 5.3 and 9.4]

chemotroph
An organism that relies on a chemical source of energy (such as ATP) instead of using light to make ATP (like phototrophs do). [Section 5.3]

chief cells
Pepsinogen-secreting cells found at the bottom of the gastric glands of the stomach. [Section 10.6]

cholecystokinin (CCK)
A hormone secreted by the small intestine (duodenum) in response to the presences of fats. It promotes release of bile from the gallbladder and pancreatic juice from the pancreas, and reduces stomach motility. [Section 10.6]

cholesterol
A large, ring-shaped lipid found in cell membranes. Cholesterol is the precursor for steroid hormones and is used to manufacture bile salts. [Sections 3.4 and 6.3]

chondrocyte
A mature cartilage cell. [Section 11.6]

chorion
The portion of the placenta derived from the zygote. The chorionic villi secrete hCG to help maintain the endometrium during the first trimester of a pregnancy. [Section 13.8]

choroid
The darkly pigmented middle layer of the eyeball, found between the sclera (outer layer) and the retina (inner layer). [Section 8.5]

chromosome
A single piece of double-stranded DNA; part of the genome of an organism. Prokaryotes have circular chromosomes and eukaryotes have linear chromosomes. [Section 4.1]

chylomicrons
A type of lipoprotein; the form in which absorbed fats from the intestines are transported to the circulatory system. [**Sections 9.5 and 10.7**]

chyme
Partially digested, semiliquid food mixed with digestive enzymes and acids in the stomach. [**Section 10.6**]

chymotrypsin
One of the main pancreatic proteases; it is activated (from chymotrypsinogen) by trypsin. [**Section 10.7**]

cilia
A hair-like structure on the cell surface composed of microtubules in a "9 + 2" arrangement (nine pairs of microtubules surrounding 2 single microtubules in the center). The microtubules are connected with a contractile protein called *dynein*. Cilia beat in a repetitive sweeping motion, which helps to move substances along the surface of the cell. They are particularly important in the respiratory system, where they sweep mucus out of the trachea and up to the mouth and nose. [**Section 6.5**]

circular smooth muscle
The inner layer of smooth muscle in the wall of the digestive tract. When the circular muscle contracts, the tube diameter is reduced. Certain areas of the circular muscle are thickened to act as valves (sphincters). [**Section 10.5**]

clathrin
A fibrous protein found on the intracellular side of the plasma membrane (also found associated with the Golgi complex) that helps to invaginate the membrane. Typically cell surface receptors are associated with clathrin-coated pits at the plasma membrane, and binding of the ligand to the receptor triggers invagination. [**Section 6.4**]

cleavage
The rapid mitotic divisions of a zygote that begin within 24–36 hours after fertilization. [**Section 13.9**]

coccus
A bacterium having a round shape (plural = cocci). [**Section 5.3**]

cochlea
The curled structure in the inner ear that contains the membranes and hair cells used to transduce sound waves into action potentials. [**Section 8.5**]

codominance
A situation in which a heterozygote displays the phenotype associated with each of the alleles, e.g., human blood type AB. [**Section 7.4**]

codon
A group of three nucleotides that is specific for a particular amino acid, or that specifies "stop translating." [**Section 4.3**]

collagen
A protein fiber with a unique triple-helix structure that gives it great strength. Tissues with a lot of collagen fibers are typically very strong, e.g., bone, tendons, ligaments, etc. [**Section 11.6**]

collecting duct
The portion of the nephron where water reabsorption is regulated via antidiuretic hormone (ADH). Several nephrons empty into each collecting duct, and this is the final region through which urine must pass on its way to the ureter. [**Section 10.2**]

colligative properties
Properties that depend on the number of solute particles in a solution rather than on the type of particle. Colligative properties include boiling point elevation, freezing point depression, and vapor pressure depression. [**Section 6.4**]

colon
See "large intestine." [**Sections 10.1 and 10.6**]

common bile duct
The duct that carries bile from the gallbladder and liver to the small intestine (duodenum). [**Section 10.6**]

compact bone
A dense, hard type of bone constructed from osteons (at the microscopic level). Compact bone forms the diaphysis of the long bones, and the outer shell of the epiphyses and all other bones. [**Section 11.7**]

complement system
A group of blood proteins that bind non-specifically to the surface proteins of foreign cells (such as bacteria), ultimately leading to the destruction of the foreign cell. [**Section 9.7**]

cones
Photoreceptors in the retina of the eye that respond to bright light and provide color vision. [**Section 8.5**]

conjugation
A form of genetic recombination in bacteria in which plasmid and/or genomic DNA is transferred from one bacterium to the other through a conjugation bridge. [**Section 5.3**]

connective tissue
One of the four basic tissue types in the body (epithelial, connective, muscle, and nervous). Connective tissue is a supportive tissue consisting of relatively few cells scattered among a great deal of extracellular material (matrix), and includes adipose tissue (fat), bone, cartilage, the dermis of the skin, tendons, ligaments, and blood. [Section 11.6]

convergent evolution
A form of evolution in which different organisms are placed into the same environment and exposed to the same selection pressures. This causes the organisms to evolve along similar lines. As a result, they may share functional, but not structural similarity (because they possessed different starting materials). Convergent evolution produces *analogous structures.* [Section 7.9]

cooperativity
A type of substrate binding to a multi-active site enzyme, in which the binding of one substrate molecule facilitates the binding of subsequent substrate molecules. A graph of reaction rate vs. substrate concentration appears sigmoidal. Note that cooperativity can be found in other situations as well, for example, hemoglobin binds oxygen cooperatively. [Section 9.5]

copy-number variation
Structural variations in the genome that lead to different copies of certain sections of the DNA, due to duplication of those sections or deletions of those sections. [Section 4.2]

cornea
The clear portion of the tough outer layer of the eyeball, found over the iris and pupil. [Section 8.5]

corona radiata
The layer of granulosa cells that surround an oocyte after it has been ovulated. [Section 13.6]

coronary vessels
The blood vessels that carry blood to and from cardiac muscle. The coronary arteries branch off the aorta and carry oxygenated blood to the cardiac tissue. The coronary veins collect deoxygenated blood from the cardiac tissue, merge to form the coronary sinus, and drain into the right atrium. [Section 9.2]

corpus callosum
The largest bundle of white matter (axons) connecting the two cerebral hemispheres. [Section 8.4]

corpus luteum
"Yellow body." The remnants of an ovarian follicle after ovulation has occurred. The cells enlarge and begin secreting progesterone, the dominant female hormone during the second half of the menstrual cycle. Some estrogen is also secreted. [Section 13.6]

cortex
The outer layer of an organ, e.g., the renal cortex, the ovarian cortex, the adrenal cortex, etc. [Sections 8.4, 8.5, 8.6, and 10.2]

cortical reaction
See "slow block to polyspermy." [Section 13.9]

corticosteroids
Steroid hormones secreted from the adrenal cortex. The two major classes are the *mineralocorticoids* and *glucocorticoids.* Aldosterone is the principal mineralocorticoid, and cortisol is the principal glucocorticoid. [Section 8.6]

cortisol
The principal glucocorticoid secreted from the adrenal cortex. This steroid hormone is released during stress, causing increased blood glucose levels and reducing inflammation. The latter effect has led to a clinical use of cortisol as an anti-inflammatory agent. [Section 8.6]

creatine phosphate
An energy storage molecule used by muscle tissue. The phosphate from creatine phosphate can be removed and attached to an ADP to generate ATP quickly. [Section 11.2]

cross bridge
The connection of a myosin head group to an actin filament during muscle contraction (the sliding filament theory). [Section 11.2]

crossing over
The exchange of DNA between paired homologous chromosomes (tetrads) during prophase I of meiosis. [Section 7.2]

cyclic AMP (cAMP)
A cyclic version of adenosine monophosphate, where the phosphate is esterified to both the 5' and the 3' carbons, forming a ring. Cyclic AMP is an important intracellular signaling molecule, often called the "second messenger." It serves to activate cAMP-dependent kinases, which regulate the activity of other enzymes in the cell. Levels of cAMP are in part regulated by adenylyl cyclase, the enzyme that makes cAMP, and the activity of adenylyl cyclase is ultimately controlled by the binding of various ligands to cell surface receptors. [Section 6.5]

cytokinesis
The phase of mitosis during which the cell physically splits into two daughter cells. Cytokinesis begins near the end of anaphase, and is completed during telophase. [Section 6.6]

cytosine
One of the four aromatic bases found in DNA and RNA. Cytosine is a pyrimidine; it pairs with guanine. [Section 4.1]

dendrite
A projection off the cell body of a neuron that receives a nerve impulse from a different neuron and sends the impulse to the cell body. Neurons can have one or several dendrites. [Section 8.1]

dense connective tissue
Connective tissue with large amounts of either collagen fibers or elastic fibers, or both. Dense tissues are typically strong (e.g., bone, cartilage, tendons, etc.). [Section 11.6]

depolarization
The movement of the membrane potential of a cell away from rest potential in a more positive direction. [Section 8.1]

dermis
A layer of connective tissue underneath the epidermis of the skin. The dermis contains blood vessels, lymphatic vessels, nerves, sensory receptors, and glands. [Section 12.6]

desmosome
A general cell junction, used primarily for adhesion. [Section 6.5]

determination
The point during cellular development at which a cell becomes committed to a particular fate. Note that the cell is not differentiated at this point; determination comes before differentiation. Determination can be due to cytoplasmic effects or to induction by neighboring cells. [Section 13.12]

diaphragm
The primary muscle of inspiration. The diaphragm is stimulated to contract at regular intervals by the respiratory center in the medulla oblongata (via the phrenic nerve). Although it is made of skeletal muscle (and can therefore be voluntarily controlled), these stimulations occur autonomously. [Section 12.3]

diaphysis
The shaft of a long bone. The diaphysis is hollow and is made entirely from compact bone. [Section 11.7]

diastole
The period of time during which the ventricles of the heart are relaxed. [Section 9.2]

diastolic pressure
The pressure measured in the arteries while the ventricles are relaxed (during diastole). [Section 9.3]

diencephalon
The portion of the forebrain that includes the thalamus and hypothalamus. [Section 8.4]

difference threshold
The minimum noticeable difference between any two sensory stimuli, 50% of the time. [Section 8.5]

differentiation
The specialization of cell types, especially during embryonic and fetal development. [Section 13.12]

diffusion
The movement of a particle (the solute) from its region of high concentration to its region of low concentration (or *down its concentration gradient*). [Section 6.4]

diploid organism
An organism that has two copies of its genome in each cell. The paired genomes are said to be homologous. [Section 7.1]

distal convoluted tubule
The portion of the nephron tubule after the loop of Henle, but before the collecting duct. Selective reabsorption and secretion occur here; most notably regulated reabsorption of water and sodium. [Section 10.2]

divergent evolution
A form of evolution in which the same organism is placed into different environments with different selection pressures. This causes the organisms to evolve differently; to diverge from their common ancestor. The resulting (new) species may share structural (but not necessarily functional) similarity; divergent evolution produces *homologous structures*. [Section 7.9]

DNA ligase
See "ligase." [Section 4.4]

DNA polymerase
Also called DNA pol, this is the enzyme that replicates DNA. Eukaryotes and prokaryotes have different versions of this enzyme. [Section 4.4]

domain Archaea/extremophiles
One of the three main taxonomic domains, Archaea live in the world's most extreme environments (hot springs, hypersaline environments, etc.). They possess characteristics of both prokaryotes and eukaryotes. [Section 5.3]

dominant

1. The allele in a heterozygous genotype that is expressed.

2. The phenotype resulting from either a heterozygous genotype or a homozygous dominant genotype. [Section 7.1]

dorsal root ganglion

A group of sensory neuron cell bodies found just posterior to the spinal cord on either side. A pair of root ganglia exists for each spinal nerve that extends from the spinal cord. The ganglia are part of the peripheral nervous system (PNS). [Section 8.4]

downstream

Toward the 3′ end of an RNA transcript (the 3′ end of the DNA coding strand). Stop codons and (in eukaryotes) the poly-A tail are found "downstream." [Section 4.7]

ductus deferens

A thick, muscular tube that connects the epididymis of the testes to the urethra. Muscular contractions of the vas deferens during ejaculation help propel the sperm outward. Severing of the vas deferens (vasectomy) results in sterility of the male. [Section 13.1]

duodenum

The first part (approximately 5 percent) of the small intestine. [Section 10.6]

dynein

A contractile protein connecting microtubules in the "9 + 2" arrangement of cilia and eukaryotic flagella. The contraction of dynein produces the characteristic movements of these structures. [Section 6.5]

ectoderm

One of the three primary (embryonic) germ layers formed during gastrulation. Ectoderm ultimately forms external structures such as the skin, hair, nails, and inner linings of the mouth and anus, as well as the entire nervous system. [Section 13.11]

edema

Swelling. [Section 9.5]

efferent arteriole

The small artery that carries blood away from the capillaries of the glomerulus. [Section 10.2]

efferent neuron

A neuron that carries information (action potentials) away from the central nervous system; a motor neuron. [Section 8.3]

ejaculation

A subphase of male orgasm, a reflex reaction triggered by the presence of semen in the urethra. Ejaculation is a series of rhythmic contractions of muscles near the base of the penis that increase pressure in the urethra, forcing the semen out. [Section 13.1]

ejection fraction

The fraction of the end-diastolic volume ejected from the ventricles in a single contraction of the heart. The ejection fraction is normally around 60 percent of the end-diastolic volume. [Section 11.3]

elastin

A fibrous, connective-tissue protein that has the ability to recoil to its original shape after being stretched. Elastin is found in great amounts in lung tissue, arterial tissue, skin, and the epiglottis. [Section 11.6]

electrical synapse

A type of synapse in which the cells are connected by gap junctions, allowing ions (and therefore an action potential) to spread easily from cell to cell. [Section 8.2]

electron transport chain

A series of enzyme complexes found along the inner mitochondrial membrane. NADH and $FADH_2$ are oxidized by these enzymes; the electrons are shuttled down the chain and are ultimately passed to oxygen to produce water. The electron energy is used to pump H^+ out of the mitochondrial matrix; the resulting H^+ gradient is subsequently used to drive the production of ATP. [Sections 2.5, 5.1, and 6.2]

elongation factors

Proteins that assist with peptide bond formation during eukaryotic translation. [Section 4.8]

embryonic stage

The period of human development from implantation through eight weeks of gestation. Gastrulation, neurulation, and organogenesis occur during this time period. The developing baby is known as an *embryo* during this time period. [Section 13.13]

emission

A subphase of male orgasm. Emission is the movement of sperm (via the ductus deferens) and semen (via the accessory glands) into the urethra in preparation for ejaculation. [Section 13.1]

endocrine gland

A ductless gland that secretes a hormone into the blood. [Section 8.6]

endocrine system
A system of ductless glands that secrete chemical messengers (hormones) into the blood. [**Section 8.6**]

endocytosis
The uptake of material into a cell, usually by invagination. See also "phagocytosis," "pinocytosis," and "receptor-mediated endocytosis." [**Sections 5.1 and 6.4**]

endoderm
One of the three primary (embryonic) germ layers formed during gastrulation. Endoderm ultimately forms internal structures, such as the inner lining of the GI tract and some glandular organs. [**Section 13.11**]

endometrial cycle
The 28 days of the menstrual cycle as they apply to the events in the uterus. The endometrial cycle is also known as the *uterine cycle*, and has three subphases: menstruation, the proliferative phase, and the secretory phase. [**Section 13.8**]

endometrium
The inner epithelial lining of the uterus that thickens and develops during the menstrual cycle, into which a fertilized ovum can implant, and which sloughs off during menstruation if a pregnancy does not occur. [**Section 13.5**]

endospore
A bacterial structure formed in unfavorable growth conditions. Endospores have very tough outer shells made of peptidoglycan and can survive harsh conditions. The bacterium inside the endospore is essentially dormant and can become active (called germination) when conditions again become favorable. [**Section 5.3**]

endosymbiotic theory
The theory that mitochondria and chloroplasts originated as independent unicellular organisms living in symbiosis with larger cells. [**Section 6.2**]

endothelial cells
Cells that form the inner linings of arteries and veins and the walls of capillaries. Endothelial cells are involved in a number of important vascular functions. [**Section 9.1**]

endotoxin
A normal component of the outer membrane of Gram-negative bacteria. Endotoxins produce extreme immune reactions (septic shock), particularly when many of them enter the circulation at once. [**Section 5.3**]

end plate potential
The depolarization of the motor end plate on a muscle cell. [**Section 11.2**]

enteric nervous system
The nervous system of the gastrointestinal tract. It controls secretion and motility within the GI tract, and is linked to the central nervous system. [**Section 10.5**]

enterogastrone
A hormone secreted by the small intestine (duodenum) in response to the presence of food. It decreases the rate at which chyme leaves the stomach and enters the small intestine. [**Section 10.6**]

enterokinase
A duodenal enzyme that activates trypsinogen (from the pancreas) to trypsin. [**Section 10.6**]

envelope
A lipid bilayer that surrounds the capsid of an animal virus. The envelope is acquired as the virus buds out through the plasma membrane of its host cell. Not all animal viruses possess an envelope. [**Section 5.1**]

epidermis
The outermost layer of the skin. The epidermis is made of epithelial tissue that is constantly dividing at the bottom; the cells migrate to the surface (dying along the way) to be sloughed off at the surface. [**Section 12.6**]

epididymis
A long, coiled duct on the outside of the testis in which sperm mature. [**Section 13.1**]

epigenetics
Changes in gene expression that are not due to mutations, but are long-term and heritable (e.g., DNA methylation, chromatin remodeling, and RNA interference). [**Section 4.9**]

epiglottis
A flexible piece of cartilage in the larynx that flips downward to seal the trachea during swallowing. [**Sections 10.6 and 12.2**]

epinephrine
A hormone produced and secreted by the adrenal medulla that prolongs and increases the effects of the sympathetic nervous system. [**Section 8.4**]

epiphyseal plate
A band of cartilage (hyaline) found between the diaphysis and the epiphyses of long bones that allows bone growth during childhood. [**Section 11.9**]

epiphysis

One of the two ends of a long bone (pl: epiphyses). The epiphyses have an outer shell made of compact bone and an inner core of spongy bone. The spongy bone is filled with red bone marrow, the site of blood cell formation. [Section 11.7]

epistasis

A situation in which the expression of one gene prevents expression of all allelic forms of another gene, e.g., the gene for male pattern baldness is epistatic to the hair color gene. [Section 7.4]

epithelial tissue

One of the four basic tissue types in the body (epithelial, connective, muscle, and nervous). Epithelial tissue is a lining and covering tissue (e.g., skin, the lining of the stomach and intestines, the lining of the urinary tract, etc.) or a glandular tissue (e.g., the liver, the pancreas, the ovaries, etc.). [Section 12.7]

epitope

The specific site on an antigenic molecule that binds to a T cell receptor or to an antibody. [Section 9.7]

EPSP

Excitatory postsynaptic potential; a slight depolarization of a postsynaptic cell, bringing the membrane potential of that cell closer to the threshold for an action potential. [Section 8.2]

equilibrium potential

The membrane potential at which there is no driving force on an ion, and there is no net movement of ions across the membrane. [Section 8.1]

erectile tissue

Specialized tissue with a lot of space that can fill with blood upon proper stimulation, causing the tissue to become firm. Erectile tissue is found in the penis, the clitoris, the labia, and the nipples. [Section 13.1]

erythrocyte

A red blood cell; they are filled with hemoglobin, and the function of the erythrocytes is to carry oxygen in the blood. [Section 9.4]

erythropoietin

A hormone produced and released by the kidney that stimulates the production of red blood cells by the bone marrow. [Section 10.4]

estrogen

The primary female sex hormone. Estrogen stimulates the development of female secondary sex characteristics during puberty, maintains those characteristics during adulthood, stimulates the development of a new uterine lining after menstruation, and stimulates mammary gland development during pregnancy. [Section 13.4]

eukaryotic

A cell characterized by the presence of a nucleus and other membrane-bound organelles. Eukaryotes can be unicellular (protists) or multicellular (fungi, plants, and animals). [Section 6.1]

excision

The removal (and usually the activation) of a viral genome from its host's genome. [Section 5.1]

excitation-contraction coupling

The mechanism that ensures that skeletal muscle contraction does not occur without neural stimulation (excitation). At rest, cytosolic $[Ca^{2+}]$ is low, and the troponin-tropomyosin complex covers the myosin-binding sites on actin. When the muscle is stimulated by a neuron, Ca^{2+} is released from the sarcoplasmic reticulum into the cytosol of the muscle cell. Ca^{2+} binds to troponin, causing a conformation change in the troponin-tropomyosin complex that shifts it away from the myosin-binding sites. This allows myosin and actin to interact according to the sliding filament theory. [Section 11.2]

excretion

The elimination of waste products from the body. [Section 10.1]

exocrine gland

A gland that secretes its product into a duct, which ultimately carries the product to the surface of the body or into a body cavity. Some examples of exocrine glands and their products are sweat glands (sweat), gastric glands (acid, mucus, protease), the liver (bile), sebaceous glands (oil), and lacrimal glands (tears). [Section 8.6]

exocytosis

The secretion of a cellular product to the extracellular medium through a secretory vesicle. [Section 6.4]

exon

A nucleotide sequence in RNA that contains protein-coding information. Exons are typically separated by introns (intervening sequences) that are spliced out prior to translation. [Section 4.7]

exotoxin
A toxin secreted by a bacterium into its surrounding medium that help the bacterium compete with other species. Some exotoxins cause serious diseases in humans (botulism, tetanus, diphtheria, toxic shock syndrome). [**Section 5.3**]

expiration
The movement of air out of the respiratory tract. Expiration can be passive (caused by relaxation of the diaphragm and elastic recoil of the lungs) or active (caused by contraction of the abdominal muscles, which increases intraabdominal pressure and forces the diaphragm up past its normal relaxed position). [**Section 12.3**]

facilitated diffusion
Movement of a hydrophilic molecule across the plasma membrane of a cell, down its concentration gradient, through a channel, pore, or carrier molecule in the membrane. Because of the hydrophilic nature of the molecule, it requires a special path through the lipid bilayer. [**Section 6.4**]

facultative anaerobe
An organism that will use oxygen to produce energy (aerobic metabolism) if it is available, and that can ferment (anaerobic metabolism) if it is not. [**Section 5.3**]

fallopian tubes
See "uterine tubes." [**Section 13.5**]

fascicle
A bundle of skeletal muscle cells. Fascicles group together to form skeletal muscles. [**Section 11.2**]

fast block to polyspermy
The depolarization of the egg plasma membrane upon fertilization, designed to prevent the entry of more than one sperm into the egg. [**Section 13.9**]

fertilization
The fusion of a sperm with an ovum during sexual reproduction. In humans, fertilization typically occurs in the uterine tubes and requires capacitation of the sperm and release of the acrosomal enzymes. Fertilization is a species-specific process, requiring binding of a sperm protein to an egg receptor. [**Section 13.9**]

F (fertility) factor
A bacterial plasmid that allows the bacterium to initiate conjugation. Bacteria that possess the F factor are known as F⁺ "males." [**Section 5.3**]

fetal stage
The period of human development beginning at eight weeks of gestation and lasting until birth (38–42 weeks of gestation). During this stage the organs formed in the embryonic stage grow and mature. The developing baby is known as a *fetus* during this time period. [**Section 13.13**]

fibrinogen
A blood protein essential to blood clotting. The conversion of fibrinogen to its active form (fibrin) is among the final steps in clot formation, and is triggered by thrombin. [**Section 9.4**]

fibroblast
A generic connective tissue cell that produces fibers; the progenitor of all other connective tissue cell types. [**Section 11.6**]

filtration
The movement of a substance across a membrane via pressure. In the kidney, filtration refers specifically to the movement of plasma across the capillary walls of the glomerulus, into the capsule and tubule of the nephron. Filtration at the glomerulus is driven by blood pressure. [**Section 10.1**]

fimbriae
Fingerlike projections of the uterine (fallopian) tubes that drape over the ovary. [**Section 13.5**]

flagella
A long, whip-like filament that helps in cell motility. Many bacteria are flagellated, and sperm are flagellated. [**Section 5.3**]

fluid mosaic model
The current understanding of membrane structure, in which the membrane is composed of a mix of lipids and proteins (a mosaic) that are free to move fluidly among themselves. [**Section 6.3**]

follicle
A developing oocyte and all of its surrounding (supporting) cells. [**Section 13.6**]

follicle stimulating hormone (FSH)
A tropic hormone produced by the anterior pituitary gland that targets the gonads. In females, FSH stimulates the ovaries to develop follicles (oogenesis) and secrete estrogen; in males, FSH stimulates spermatogenesis. [**Section 13.2**]

follicular phase
The first phase of the ovarian cycle, during which a follicle (an oocyte and its surrounding cells) enlarges and matures. This phase is under the control of FSH from the anterior pituitary, and typically lasts from day 1 to day 14 of the menstrual cycle. The follicle secretes estrogen during this time period. [**Section 13.7**]

F_1 generation
The first generation of offspring from a given genetic cross. [Section 7.3]

formylmethionine (fMet)
A modified methionine used as the first amino acid in all prokaryotic proteins. [Section 4.8]

frameshift mutation
A mutation caused by an insertion or deletion of base pairs in a gene sequence in DNA such that the reading frame of the gene (and thus the amino acid sequence of the protein) is altered. [Section 4.5]

Frank-Starling mechanism
A mechanism by which the stroke volume of the heart is increased by increasing the venous return to the heart (thus stretching the ventricular muscle). [Section 9.2]

freezing-point depression
The decrease in the freezing point of a solution due to the addition of solute. [Section 6.4]

functional syncytium
A tissue in which the cytoplasms of the cells are connected by gap junctions, allowing the cells to function as a unit. Cardiac and smooth muscle tissues are examples of functional syncytiums. [Section 9.2]

gallbladder
A digestive accessory organ near the liver. The gallbladder stores and concentrates bile produced by the liver, and is stimulated to contract by cholecystokinin (CCK). [Section 10.6]

ganglion
A clump of gray matter (unmyelinated neuron cell bodies) found in the peripheral nervous system. [Section 8.4]

gap junction
A junction formed between cells, consisting of a protein channel called a *connexon* on each of the two cells, that connect to form a single channel between the cytoplasms of both cells. Gap junctions allow small molecules to flow between the cells, and are important in cell-to-cell communication, for example, in relaying the action potential between cardiac muscle cells, and relaying nutrients between osteocytes. [Sections 6.5 and 9.2]

gap phase
A phase in the cycle between mitosis and S phase (G_1) or between S phase and mitosis (G_2). During gap phases the cell undergoes normal activity and growth; G_1 may include preparation for DNA replication and G_2 includes preparation for mitosis. Note that non-dividing cells remain permanently in G_1, known as G_0 for these cells. [Section 6.6]

gastrin
A hormone released by the G cells of the stomach in the presence of food. Gastrin promotes muscular activity of the stomach as well as secretion of hydrochloric acid, pepsinogen, and mucus. [Section 10.6]

gastrulation
The division of the inner cell mass of a blastocyst (developing embryo) into the three primary germ layers. Gastrulation occurs during weeks 2–4 of gestation. [Section 13.11]

gene
A portion of DNA that codes for some product, usually a protein, including all regulatory sequences. Some genes code for rRNA and tRNA, which are not translated. [Sections 4.3 and 7.1]

gene pool
The sum of all genetic information in a population. [Section 7.7]

genetic code
The "language" of molecular biology that specifies which amino acid corresponds to which three-nucleotide group (a codon). [Section 4.3]

genome
All the genetic information in an organism; all of an organism's chromosomes. [Section 4.1]

genotype
The combination of alleles an organism carries. In a homozygous genotype, both alleles are the same, whereas in a heterozygous genotype the alleles are different. [Section 7.1]

glial cells
Specialized non-neuronal cells that provide structural and metabolic support to neurons; for example, the Schwann cell. [Section 8.1]

glomerulus
The ball of capillaries at the beginning of the nephron where blood filtration takes place. [Section 10.2]

glucagon
A peptide hormone produced and secreted by the α cells of the pancreas. It targets primarily the liver, stimulating the breakdown of glycogen, thus increasing blood glucose levels. [Section 10.7]

glycolipid
A membrane lipid consisting of a glycerol molecule esterified to two fatty acid chains and a sugar molecule. [Section 6.3]

goblet cells
Unicellular exocrine glands found along the respiratory and digestive tracts that secrete mucus. [Section 10.5]

Golgi apparatus
A stack of membranes found near the rough ER in eukaryotic cells that is involved in the secretory pathway. The Golgi apparatus is involved in protein glycosylation (and other protein modification) as well as sorting and packaging proteins. [Section 6.2]

gonadotropin releasing hormone (GnRH)
A hormone released from the hypothalamus that triggers the anterior pituitary to secrete FSH and LH. [Section 13.4]

gonadotropins
Anterior pituitary tropic hormones FSH (follicle stimulating hormone) and LH (luteinizing hormone) that stimulate the gonads (testes and ovaries) to produce gametes and to secrete sex steroids. [Section 13.4]

G-protein-linked receptor
A cell surface receptor associated with an intracellular protein that binds and hydrolyzes GTP. When GTP is bound, the protein is active, and can regulate the activity of adenylyl cyclase; this modifies the intracellular levels of the second messenger cAMP. When the GTP is hydrolyzed to GDP, the protein becomes inactive again. [Section 6.5]

Graafian follicle
A large, mature, ovarian follicle with a well-developed antrum and a secondary oocyte. Ovulation of the oocyte occurs from this type of follicle. [Section 13.6]

Gram-negative bacteria
Bacteria that have a thin peptidoglycan cell wall covered by an outer plasma membrane. They stain very lightly (pink) in Gram stain. Gram-negative bacteria are typically more resistant to antibiotics than Gram-positive bacteria. [Section 5.3]

Gram-positive bacteria
Bacteria that have a thick peptidoglycan cell wall, and no outer membrane. They stain very darkly (purple) in Gram stain. [Section 5.3]

granulosa cells
The majority of the cells surrounding an oocyte in a follicle. Granulosa cells secrete estrogen during the follicular phase of the ovarian cycle. [Section 13.6]

gray matter
Unmyelinated neuron cell bodies and short unmyelinated axons. [Section 8.4]

growth hormone
A hormone released by the anterior pituitary that targets all cells in the body. Growth hormone stimulates whole body growth in children and adolescents, and increases cell turnover rate in adults. [Section 8.6]

guanine
One of the four aromatic bases found in DNA and RNA. Guanine is a purine; it pairs with cytosine. [Section 4.1]

gustatory receptors
Chemoreceptors on the tongue that respond to chemicals in food. [Section 8.5]

gyrase (DNA gyrase)
A prokaryotic enzyme used to twist the single circular chromosome of prokaryotes upon itself to form supercoils. Supercoiling helps to compact prokaryotic DNA and make it sturdier. [Section 4.1]

H zone
The region at the center of an A band of a sarcomere that is made up of myosin only. The H zone gets shorter (and may disappear) during muscle contraction. [Section 11.2]

hair cells
Sensory receptors found in the inner ear. Cochlear hair cells respond to vibrations in the cochlea caused by sound waves and vestibular hair cells respond to changes in position and acceleration (used for balance). [Section 8.5]

haploid organism
An organism that has only a single copy of its genome in each of its cells. Haploid organisms possess no homologous chromosomes. [Section 7.1]

Hardy-Weinberg law

A law of population genetics that states that the frequencies of alleles in a given gene pool do not change over time. There are five assumptions required for this law to hold true: there must be no mutation, there must be no natural selection, there must be no migration, there must be random mating between individuals in the population, and the population must be large. A population meeting all of these conditions, in which the allele frequency is not changing, is said to be in *Hardy-Weinberg equilibrium*. [Section 7.7]

hCG

Human chorionic gonadotropin; a hormone secreted by the trophoblast cells of a blastocyst (i.e., a developing embryo) that prolongs the life of the corpus luteum, and thus increases the duration and amount of secreted progesterone. This helps to maintain the uterine lining so that menstruation does not occur. The presence of hCG in the blood or urine of a woman is used as a positive indicator of pregnancy. [Section 13.8]

helicase

An enzyme that unwinds the double helix of DNA and separates the DNA strands in preparation for DNA replication. [Section 4.4]

hematocrit

The percentage of whole blood made up of erythrocytes. The typical hematocrit value is between 40–45 percent. [Section 9.4]

hematopoiesis

The synthesis of blood cells (occurs in the red bone marrow). [Section 11.5]

hemizygous gene

A gene appearing in a single copy in diploid organisms, e.g., X-linked genes in human males. [Section 4.5]

hemoglobin

A four-subunit protein found in red blood cells that binds oxygen. Each subunit contains a heme group, a large multi-ring molecule with an iron atom at its center. One hemoglobin molecule can bind four oxygen molecules in a cooperative manner. [Section 9.4]

hemophilia

A group of X-linked recessive disorders in which blood fails to clot properly, leading to excessive bleeding if injured. [Section 9.4]

hemostasis

The stoppage of bleeding; blood clotting. [Section 9.4]

Henry's Law

Henry's Law states that the amount of gas that will dissolve into liquid is dependent on the partial pressure of that gas as well as the solubility of that gas in the liquid. [Section 12.4]

hepatic portal vein

A vein connecting the capillary bed of the intestines with the capillary bed of the liver. This allows amino acids and glucose absorbed from the intestines to be delivered first to the liver for processing before being transported throughout the circulatory system. [Section 9.5]

Hershey-Chase experiments

Experiments with phage and bacteria that definitively determined DNA to be the genetic information of the cell. [Section 7.1]

heterochromatin

Densely packed, tightly coiled DNA, generally inactive (i.e., not being transcribed). [Section 4.1]

heterotroph

An organism that cannot make its own food, and thus must ingest other organisms. [Section 5.3]

heterozygous

A genotype in which two different alleles are possessed for a given gene. [Section 7.3]

Hfr bacterium

High frequency of recombination bacterium. An F+ bacterium that has the fertility factor integrated into its chromosome. When conjugation takes place, it is able to transfer not only the F factor, but also its genomic DNA. [Section 5.3]

hnRNA

Heterogeneous nuclear RNA; the primary transcript made in eukaryotes before splicing. [Section 4.7]

homeostasis

The maintenance of relatively constant internal conditions (such as temperature, pressure, ion balance, pH, etc.) regardless of external conditions. [Sections 8.6 and 10.1]

homologous chromosomes

A pair of similar chromosomes that have the same genes in the same order, but may have different versions (alleles) of those genes. One of the pair of chromosomes came from Mom in an ovum, and the other came from Dad in a sperm. Humans have 23 pairs of homologous chromosomes. [Section 7.1]

homologous structures
Physical structures in two different organisms that have structural similarity due to a common ancestor, but may have different functions. Homologous structures arise from divergent evolution. [Section 7.9]

homozygous
A genotype in which two identical alleles are possessed for a given gene. The alleles can both be dominant (homozygous dominant) or both be recessive (homozygous recessive). [Section 7.3]

humoral immunity
Specific defense of the body by antibodies, secreted into the blood by B cells. [Section 9.7]

hydroxyapatite
Hard crystals consisting of calcium and phosphate that form the bone matrix. [Section 11.7]

hyperpolarization
The movement of the membrane potential of a cell away from rest potential in a more negative direction. [Section 8.2]

hypodermis
Also called subcutaneous layer, this is a layer of fat located under the dermis of the skin. The hypodermis helps to insulate the body and protects underlying muscles and other structures. [Section 12.6]

hypophysis
The pituitary gland. [Section 8.6]

hypothalamic-pituitary portal system
A set of veins that connect a capillary bed in the hypothalamus (the primary capillary plexus) with a capillary bed in the anterior pituitary gland (the secondary capillary plexus). Releasing and inhibiting factors from the hypothalamus travel along the veins to directly affect cells in the anterior pituitary. [Section 8.6]

hypothalamus
The portion of the diencephalon involved in maintaining body homeostasis. The hypothalamus also controls the release of hormones from the pituitary gland. [Section 8.6]

I band
The region of a sarcomere made up only of thin filaments. The I band is bisected by a Z line. I bands alternate with A bands to give skeletal and cardiac muscle a striated appearance. I bands get shorter (and may disappear completely) during muscle contraction. [Section 11.2]

ileocecal valve
The sphincter that separates the final part of the small intestine (the ileum) from the first part of the large intestine (the cecum). It is typically kept contracted (closed) so that chyme can remain in the small intestine as long as possible. The ileocecal valve is stimulated to relax by the presence of food in the stomach. [Section 10.6]

ileum
The 55 percent (approximately) of the small intestine. [Section 10.6]

immunoglobulins
See "antibody." [Section 9.4]

implantation
The burrowing of a blastocyst (a developing embryo) into the endometrium of the uterus, typically occurring about a week after fertilization. [Section 13.10]

imprinting
Physical change to a gene on DNA, such as methylation or histone binding, that renders it inactive, so that only one allele of the gene is expressed. [Section 4.9]

incomplete dominance
A situation in which a heterozygote displays a blended version of the phenotypes associated with each allele, e.g., pure-breeding white-flowered plants crossed with pure-breeding red-flowered plants produces heterozygous offspring plants with pink flowers. [Section 7.4]

inducible system
A system (set of genes) where the expression of those genes is stimulated by an abundance of substrate (e.g., the lac operon). [Section 4.9]

inflammation
An irritation of a tissue caused by infection or injury. Inflammation is characterized by four cardinal symptoms: redness (rubor), swelling (tumor), heat (calor), and pain (dolor). [Section 9.5]

inhibin
A protein hormone secreted by the sustentacular cells of the testes or the granulosa cells of the ovaries that acts to inhibit the release of FSH from the anterior pituitary. [Section 13.2]

initiation factors
Eukaryotic proteins that assemble in a complex to begin translation. [Section 4.8]

innate immunity
General, nonspecific protection to the body, including the skin (barrier), gastric acid, phagocytes, lysozyme, and complement. [Section 9.7]

inner cell mass
The mass of cells in the blastocyst that ultimately give rise to the embryo and other embryonic structures (the amnion, the umbilical vessels, etc.). [Section 13.9]

inspiration
The movement of air into the respiratory tract. Inspiration is an active process, requiring contraction of the diaphragm. [Section 12.3]

insulin
A peptide hormone produced and secreted by the β cells of the pancreas. Insulin targets all cells in the body, especially the liver and muscle, and allows them to take glucose out of the blood (thus lowering blood glucose levels). [Section 10.7]

integral membrane protein
A protein embedded in the lipid bilayer of a cell. These are typically cell surface receptors, channels, or pumps. [Section 6.2]

intercalated discs
The divisions between neighboring cardiac muscle cells. Intercalated disks include gap junctions, which allow the cells to function as a unit. [Section 9.2]

interleukin
A chemical secreted by a T cell (usually the helper Ts) that stimulates activation and proliferation of other immune system cells. [Section 9.7]

intermediate filaments
Cytoskeletal filaments with a diameter in between that of the microtubule and the microfilament. Intermediate filaments are composed of many different proteins and tend to play structural roles in cells. [Section 6.5]

interneuron
A neuron found completely within the central nervous system. Interneurons typically connect sensory and motor neurons, especially in reflex arcs. [Section 8.3]

internodal tract
The portion of the cardiac conduction system between the SA node and the AV node. [Section 9.2]

interphase
All of the cell cycle except for mitosis. Interphase includes G_1, S phase, and G_2. [Section 6.6]

interstitial cell
Also called *Leydig cells*, these are cells within the testes that produce and secrete testosterone. They are stimulated by luteinizing hormone (LH). [Section 13.1]

intron
A nucleotide sequence that intervenes between protein-coding sequences. In DNA, these intervening sequences typically contain regulatory sequences, however, in RNA, they are simple spliced out to form the mature (translated) transcript. [Section 4.7]

ion channel
A protein channel in a cell plasma membrane that is specific for a particular ion, such as Na^+ or K^+. Ion channels may be constitutively open (leak channels), or regulated (voltage-gated or ligand-gated). [Section 6.4]

IPSP
Inhibitory postsynaptic potential; a slight hyperpolarization of a postsynaptic cell, moving the membrane potential of that cell further from threshold. [Section 8.2]

iris
A pigmented membrane found just in front of the lens of the eye. In the center of the iris is the *pupil*, a hole through which light enters the eyeball. The iris regulates the diameter of the pupil in response to the brightness of the light. [Section 8.5]

islets of Langerhans
Also called simply "islet cells," these are the endocrine cells in the pancreas. Different cell types within the islets secrete insulin, glucagon, and somatostatin. [Section 10.5]

juxtaglomerular apparatus (JGA)
A contact point between the afferent arteriole of the glomerulus and the distal convoluted tubule of the nephron. It is involved in regulating blood pressure. [Section 10.3]

juxtaglomerular cells
The cells of the afferent arteriole at the juxtaglomerular apparatus. They are baroreceptors that secrete renin upon sensing a decrease in blood pressure. [Section 10.3]

keratin
A protein-based substance secreted by cells of the epidermis as they migrate outward. The keratin makes the cells tougher (better able to withstand abrasion) and helps make the skin waterproof. [Sections 6.5 and 12.6]

kinetochores
Multiprotein complexes that attach the spindle fibers to the centromere of a chromosome. [Section 4.1]

labia
The folds of skin that enclose the vaginal and urethral openings in females. [**Section 13.5**]

labor contractions
Strong contractions of the uterus (stimulated by oxytocin) that force a baby out of the mother's body during childbirth. Labor contractions are part of a positive feedback cycle, during which the baby's head stretches the cervix, that stimulates stretch receptors that activate the hypothalamus, that stimulates the posterior pituitary to release oxytocin, that stimulates strong uterine contractions (labor contractions) that cause the baby's head to stretch the cervix. The cycle is broken once the baby is delivered. [**Section 13.14**]

lac operon
A set of genes for the enzymes necessary to import and digest lactose, under the control of a single promoter, whose expression is stimulated by the presence of lactose (this is an inducible system). [**Section 4.9**]

lacteals
Specialized lymphatic capillaries in the intestines that take up lipids as well as lymph. [**Sections 9.5 and 10.6**]

lacunae
Small cavities in bone or cartilage that hold individual bone or cartilage cells. [**Section 11.7**]

lagging strand
The newly forming daughter strand of DNA that is replicated in a discontinuous fashion, via Okazaki fragments that will ultimately be ligated together; the daughter strand that is replicated in the opposite direction that the parental DNA is unwinding. [**Section 4.4**]

lag phase
A short period of time prior to exponential growth of a bacterial population during which no, or very limited, cell division occurs. [**Section 5.3**]

large intestine
The final part of the digestive tract, also called the colon. The primary function of the large intestine is to reabsorb water and to store feces. [**Section 10.6**]

larynx
A rigid structure at the top of the trachea made completely out of cartilage. The larynx has three main functions: (1) its rigidness ensures that the trachea is held open (provides an open airway), (2) the epiglottis folds down to seal the trachea during swallowing, thus directing food to the esophagus, and (3) this is where the vocal cords are found (voice production). [**Section 12.2**]

lawn
A dense growth of bacteria that covers the surface of a Petri dish. [**Section 5.3**]

Law of Independent Assortment
Mendel's second law, which states that genes found on different chromosomes, or genes found very far apart on the same chromosome (i.e., unlinked genes) sort independently of one another during gamete formation (meiosis). [**Section 7.3**]

Law of Segregation
Mendel's first law, also called the *Principle of Segregation*, states that the two alleles of a given gene will be separated from one another during gamete formation (meiosis). [**Section 7.3**]

leading strand
The newly forming daughter strand of DNA that is replicated in a continuous fashion; the daughter strand that is replicated in the same direction that the parental DNA is unwinding. [**Section 4.4**]

leak channel
An ion channel that is constitutively open, allowing the movement of the ion across the plasma membrane according to its concentration gradient. [**Section 6.4**]

length-tension relationship
The relationship of muscle length to its ability to generate strong contractions. Maximum tension (contraction strength) is achieved at sarcomere lengths between 2.0 and 2.2 microns. Tension decreases outside of this range. [**Section 11.2**]

leukocyte
A white blood cell; leukocytes are involved in disease defense. [**Section 9.4**]

Leydig cell
See "interstitial cell." [**Section 13.1**]

ligament
A strong band of connective tissue that connects bones to one another. [**Section 11.8**]

ligand
The specific molecule that binds to a receptor. [**Section 6.5**]

ligand-gated ion channel
An ion channel that is opened or closed based on the binding of a specific ligand to the channel. Once opened, the channel allows the ion to cross the plasma membrane according to its concentration gradient. [**Section 6.4**]

ligase
An enzyme that connects two fragments of DNA to make a single fragment; also called *DNA ligase*. This enzyme is used during DNA replication and is also used in recombinant DNA research. [**Section 4.4**]

linkage
The failure of two separate genes to obey the Law of Independent Assortment, as might occur if the genes were found close together on the same chromosome. [**Section 7.5**]

lipoproteins
Large conglomerations of protein, fats, and cholesterol that transport lipids in the bloodstream. [**Sections 3.4 and 9.4**]

liver
The largest organ in the abdominal cavity. The liver has many roles, including processing of carbohydrates and fats, synthesis of urea, production of blood proteins, production of bile, recycling of heme, and storage of vitamins. [**Section 9.5**]

local autoregulation
The ability of tissues to regulate their own blood flow in the absence of neural stimulation. This is generally accomplished via metabolic wastes (such as CO_2) that act as vasodilators. [**Section 9.3**]

log phase
The period of exponential growth of a bacterial population. [**Section 5.3**]

long bone
The most common class of bone in the body, long bones have a well-defined shaft (the diaphysis) and two well-defined ends (the epiphyses). [**Section 11.7**]

longitudinal muscle
The outer layer of smooth muscle in the wall of the digestive tract. When the longitudinal muscle contracts, the tube shortens. [**Section 10.5**]

loop of Henle
The loop of the nephron tubule that dips downward into the renal medulla. The loop of Henle sets up a concentration gradient in the kidney, so that from the cortex to the renal pelvis osmolarity increases. This gradient is ultimately used to concentrate urine at the collecting duct. [**Section 10.2**]

loose connective tissue
Connective tissue that lacks great amount of collagen or elastic fibers, e.g., adipose tissue and areolar (general connective) tissue. [**Section 11.6**]

lower esophageal sphincter
Formerly called the *cardiac sphincter*, this sphincter marks the entrance to the stomach. Its function is to prevent reflux of acidic stomach contents into the esophagus; note that it does not regulate entry into the stomach. [**Section 10.6**]

lumen
The inside of a hollow organ (e.g., the stomach, intestines, bladder, etc.) or a tube (e.g., blood vessels, ureters, etc.). [**Sections 6.2 and 10.5**]

luteal phase
The third phase of the ovarian cycle, during which a corpus luteum is formed from the remnants of the follicle that has ovulated its oocyte. The corpus luteum secretes progesterone and estrogen during this time period, which typically lasts from day 15 to day 28 of the menstrual cycle. Formation of the corpus luteum is triggered by the same LH surge that triggers ovulation. [**Section 13.7**]

luteinizing hormone (LH)
A tropic hormone produced by the anterior pituitary gland that targets the gonads. In females LH triggers ovulation and the development of a corpus luteum during the menstrual cycle; in males, LH stimulates the production and release of testosterone. [**Section 13.2**]

lymphatic system
A set of vessels in the body that runs alongside the vessels of the circulatory system. It is a one-way system, with lymphatic capillaries beginning at the tissues and ultimately emptying into the large veins near the heart. It serves to return excess tissue fluid (lymph) to the circulatory system, and filters that fluid through millions of white blood cells on its way back to the heart. [**Section 9.6**]

lymph node
A concentrated region of white blood cells found along the vessels of the lymphatic system. [**Section 9.6**]

lymphocyte
The second most common of the five classes of leukocytes. Lymphocytes are involved in specific immunity and include two cell types, B cells and T cells. B cells produce and secrete antibodies and T cells are involved in cellular immunity. [Section 9.4]

lymphokine
A chemical secreted by a T cell (usually the helper Ts) that stimulates activation and proliferation of other immune system cells. [Section 9.7]

lysogenic cycle
A viral life cycle in which the viral genome is incorporated into the host genome where it can remain dormant for an unspecified period of time. Upon activation, the viral genome is excised from the host genome and typically enters the lytic cycle. [Section 5.1]

lysosome
A eukaryotic organelle filled with digestive enzymes (acid hydrolases) that is involved in digestion of macromolecules such as worn organelles or material ingested by phagocytosis. [Section 6.2]

lysozyme
An enzyme that lyses bacteria by creating holes in their cell walls. Lysozyme is produced in the end stages of the lytic cycle so that new viral particles can escape their host; it is also found in human tears and human saliva. [Section 5.1]

lytic cycle
A viral life cycle in which the host is turned into a "virus factory" and ultimately lysed to release the new viral particles. [Section 5.1]

macrophage
A large, nonspecific, phagocytic cell of the immune system. Macrophages frequently leave the bloodstream to crawl around in the tissues and perform "clean up" duties, such as ingesting dead cells or cellular debris at an injury site, or pathogens. [Sections 6.2 and 9.4]

macula densa
The cells of the distal tubule at the juxtaglomerular apparatus. They are receptors that monitor filtrate osmolarity as a means of regulating filtration rate. If a drop is osmolarity is sensed, the macula densa dilates the afferent arteriole (to increase blood pressure in the glomerulus and thus increase filtration) and stimulates the juxtaglomerular cells to secrete renin (to raise systemic blood pressure). [Section 10.3]

maternal inheritance
Genes that are inherited only from the mother, such as mitochondrial genes (all of a zygote's organelles come only from the ovum). [Section 6.2]

mechanoreceptor
A sensory receptor that responds to mechanical disturbances, such as shape changes (being squashed, bent, pulled, etc.). Mechanoreceptors include touch receptors in the skin, hair cells in the ear, muscle spindles, and others. [Section 8.5]

medium
The environment in which or upon which bacteria grow. It typically contains a sugar source and any other nutrients that bacteria may require. "Minimal medium" contains nothing but glucose. [Section 5.3]

medulla
The inner region of an organ, e.g., the renal medulla, the ovarian medulla, the adrenal medulla, etc. [Sections 8.4 and 10.2]

medulla oblongata
The portion of the hindbrain that controls respiratory rate and blood pressure, and specialized digestive and respiratory functions such as vomiting, sneezing, and coughing. [Section 8.4]

meiosis
A type of cell division (in diploid cells) that reduces the number of chromosomes by half. Meiosis usually produces haploid gametes in organisms that undergo sexual reproduction. It consists of a single interphase (G_1, S, and G_2) followed by two sets of chromosomal divisions, meiosis I and meiosis II. Meiosis I and II can both be subdivided into four phases similar to those in mitosis. [Section 7.2]

melanin
A pigment produced by melanocytes in the bottom cell layer of the epidermis. Melanin production is increased on exposure to UV radiation (commonly called "tanning" and helps prevent cellular damage due to UV radiation. [Section 12.6]

memory cell
A cell produced when a B cell is activated by antigen. Memory cells do not actively fight the current infection, but patrol the body in case of future infection with the same antigen. If the antigen should appear again in the future, memory cells are like "preactivated" B cells, and can initiate a much faster immune response (the secondary immune response). [Section 9.7]

meninges
The protective, connective tissue wrappings of the central nervous system (the dura mater, arachnoid mater, and pia mater). [Section 8.4]

menopause
The period of time in a woman's life when ovulation and menstruation cease. Menopause typically begins in the late 40s. [Section 13.8]

menstruation
The first phase of the uterine (endometrial) cycle, during which the unused endometrium from the previous cycle is shed off. Estrogen and progesterone levels are low during this time period. Menstruation typically lasts from day 1 to day 5 of the cycle. [**Section 13.7**]

mesoderm
One of the three primary (embryonic) germ layers formed during gastrulation. Mesoderm ultimately forms "middle" structures such as the bones, muscles, blood vessels, heart, kidneys, etc. [**Section 13.11**]

metaphase
The second phase of mitosis. During metaphase, replicated chromosomes align at the center of the cell (the metaphase plate). [**Section 6.6**]

metaphase I
The second phase of meiosis I. During metaphase I the paired homologous chromosomes (tetrads) align at the center of the cell (the metaphase plate). [**Section 7.2**]

metaphase II
The second phase of meiosis II. Metaphase II is identical to mitotic metaphase, except that the number of chromosomes was reduced by half during meiosis I. [**Section 7.2**]

MHC
Major histocompatibility complex, a set of proteins found on the plasma membranes of cells that help display antigen to T cells. MHC I is found on all cells and displays bits of proteins from within the cell; this allows T cells to monitor cell contents and if abnormal peptides are displayed on the surface, the cell is destroyed by killer T cells. MHC II is found only on macrophages and B cells. This class of MHC allows these cells (known as antigen presenting cells) to display bits of "eaten" (phagocytosed or internalized) proteins on their surface, allowing the activation of helper Ts. [**Section 9.7**]

microfilament
The cytoskeleton filaments with the smallest diameter. Microfilaments are composed of the contractile protein actin. They are dynamic filaments, constantly being made and broken down as needed, and are responsible for events such as pseudopod formation and cytokinesis during mitosis. [**Section 6.5**]

microtubule
The largest of the cytoplasmic filaments. Microtubules are composed of two types of protein, α tubulin and β tubulin. They are dynamic fibers, constantly being built up and broken down, according to cellular needs. Microtubules form the mitotic spindle during cell division, form the base of cilia and flagella, and are used for intracellular structure and transport. [**Section 6.5**]

microvilli
Microscopic outward folds of the cells lining the small intestine; microvilli serve to increase the surface area of the small intestine for absorption. [**Section 10.5**]

midbrain
The portion of the brain responsible for visual and auditory startle reflexes. [**Section 8.4**]

milk let-down
The release of milk from the mammary glands via contraction of ducts within the glands. Contraction is stimulated by oxytocin, which is released from the posterior pituitary when the baby begins nursing. [**Section 13.14**]

missense mutation
A point mutation in which a codon that specifies an amino acid is mutated into a codon that specifies a different amino acid. [**Section 4.5**]

mitochondrion
An organelle surrounded by a double-membrane (two lipid bilayers) where ATP production takes place. The interior (matrix) is where PDC and the Krebs cycle occur, and the inner membrane contains the enzymes of the electron transport chain and ATP synthase. [**Section 6.2**]

mitosis
The phase of the cell cycle during which the replicated genome is divided. Mitosis has four phases (prophase, metaphase, anaphase, telophase) and includes cytokinesis (the physical splitting of the cell into two new cells). [**Section 6.6**]

mitral valve
See "atrioventricular valve." [**Section 9.2**]

monocistronic mRNA
mRNA that codes for a single type of protein, such as is found in eukaryotic cells. [**Section 4.7**]

morula
A solid clump of cells resulting from cleavage in the early embryo. Because there is very little growth of these cells during cleavage, the morula is only about as large as the original zygote. [**Section 13.9**]

motor end plate
The portion of the muscle cell membrane at the neuromuscular junction; essentially the postsynaptic membrane at this synapse. [**Section 11.2**]

motor unit
A motor neuron and all the skeletal muscle cells it innervates. Large motor units are typically found in large muscles (e.g., the thighs and buttocks) and produce gross movements. Small motor units are found in smaller muscles (e.g., the rectus muscles that control movements of the eyeball, the fingers) and produce more precise movements. [**Section 11.2**]

motor unit recruitment
A mechanism for increasing tension (contractile strength) in a muscle by activating more motor units. [**Section 11.2**]

mRNA
Messenger RNA; the type of RNA that is read by a ribosome to synthesize protein. [**Section 4.3**]

mRNA surveillance
The monitoring of mRNA transcripts to eliminate those that are defective (e.g., have no stop codon, have premature stop codons, or that have somehow stalled in translation). [**Section 4.9**]

mucociliary escalator
The layer of ciliated, mucus-covered cells in the respiratory tract. The cilia continually beat, sweeping contaminated mucus upward toward the pharynx. [**Sections 6.5 and 12.1**]

mucosa
The layer of epithelial tissue that lines body cavities in contact with the outside environment (respiratory, digestive, urinary, and reproductive tracts). [**Section 10.6**]

Müllerian ducts
Early embryonic ducts that can develop into female internal genitalia in the absence of testosterone. [**Section 13.3**]

Müllerian inhibiting factor (MIF)
A substance secreted by embryonic testes that causes the regression of the Müllerian ducts. [**Section 13.3**]

multipolar neuron
A neuron with a single axon and multiple dendrites; the most common type of neuron in the nervous system. [**Section 8.1**]

myelin
An insulating layer of membranes wrapped around the axons of almost all neurons in the body. Myelin is essentially the plasma membranes of specialized cells; *Schwann cells* in the peripheral nervous system, and *oligodendrocytes* in the central nervous system. [**Section 8.1**]

myofiber
A skeletal muscle cell, also known as a muscle fiber. Skeletal muscle cells are formed from the fusion of many smaller cells (during development), consequently they are very long and are multinucleate. [**Section 11.2**]

myofibril
A string of sarcomeres within a skeletal muscle cell. Each muscle cell contains hundreds of myofibrils. [**Section 11.2**]

myoglobin
A globular protein found in muscle tissue that has the ability to bind oxygen. Myoglobin helps to store oxygen in the muscle for use in aerobic respiration. Muscles that participate in endurance activities (including cardiac muscle) have abundant supplies of myoglobin. [**Section 11.2**]

myometrium
The muscular layer of the uterus. The myometrium is made of smooth muscle that retains its ability to divide in order to accommodate the massive size increases that occur during pregnancy. The myometrium is stimulated to contract during labor by the hormone oxytocin. [**Section 13.5**]

myosin
One of the contractile proteins in muscle tissue. In skeletal and cardiac muscle, myosin forms the thick filaments. Myosin has intrinsic ATPase activity and can exist in two conformations, either high energy or low energy. [**Section 11.2**]

myosin light-chain kinase (MLCK)
A kinase in smooth muscle cells activated by calmodulin in the presence of Ca^{2+}. As its name implies, this kinase phosphorylates myosin, activating it so that muscle contraction can occur. [**Section 11.4**]

Na^+/K^+ ATPase
A protein found in the plasma membranes of all cells in the body that uses the energy of an ATP (hydrolyzes ATP) to move three Na^+ ions out of the cell and two K^+ ions into the cell, thus establishing concentration gradients for these ions across the cell membrane. [**Section 6.4**]

natural selection
The mechanism described by Charles Darwin that drives evolution. Through mutation, some organisms possess genes that make them better adapted to their environment. These organisms survive and reproduce more than those that do not possess the beneficial genes, thus these genes are passed on to offspring, making the offspring better adapted. Over time, these genes (and the organisms that possess them) become more abundant, and the less beneficial genes (and the organisms that possess them) become less abundant. [**Section 7.7**]

ncRNA (non-coding RNA)
RNA that is not translated into protein, including tRNA, rRNA, snRNA, miRNA, etc. [Section 4.7]

negative feedback
A form of regulation in which the end result of a series of events inhibits the trigger for that series. Hormones are generally regulated via negative feedback. For example, insulin is released when blood glucose levels rise. It causes the cells of the body to take glucose out of the blood, leading to a drop in glucose levels. The fall in glucose levels stops insulin release. [Section 8.6]

nephron
The functional unit of the kidney. Each kidney has about a million nephrons; this is where blood filtration and subsequent modification of the filtrate occurs. The nephron empties into collecting ducts, which empty into the ureter. [Section 10.2]

Nernst equation
The equation that can predict the equilibrium potential for any ion based on the electrochemical gradients for that ion across the membrane. [Section 8.1]

neurohypophysis
See "posterior pituitary gland." [Section 8.6]

neuromuscular junction (NMJ)
The synapse between a motor neuron and a muscle cell. At the NMJ, the muscle cell membrane is invaginated and the axon terminus is elongated so that a greater area of membrane can be depolarized at one time. [Sections 8.2 and 11.2]

neuron
The basic functional and structural unit of the nervous system. The neuron is a highly specialized cell, designed to transmit action potentials. [Section 8.1]

neurotransmitter
A chemical released by the axon of a neuron in response to an action potential that binds to receptors on a postsynaptic cell and causes that cell to either depolarize slightly (EPSP) or hyperpolarize slightly (IPSP). Examples are acetylcholine, norepinephrine, GABA, dopamine, and others. [Section 8.2]

neurulation
The formation of the nervous system during weeks 5–8 of gestation. Neurulation begins when a section of the ectoderm invaginates and pinches off to form the neural groove, which ultimately forms the neural tube, from which the brain and spinal cord develop. [Section 13.11]

nociceptors
Pain receptors. Nociceptors are found everywhere in the body except for the brain. [Section 8.5]

nodes of Ranvier
Gaps in the myelin sheath of the axons of peripheral neurons. Action potentials can "jump" from node to node, thus increasing the speed of conduction (saltatory conduction). [Section 8.1]

nondisjunction
The failure of homologous chromosomes or sister chromatids to separate properly during cell division. This could occur during anaphase I of meiosis (homologous chromosomes), or during anaphase II of meiosis or anaphase of mitosis (sister chromatids). [Section 7.2]

nonsense mutation
A point mutation in which a codon that specifies an amino acid is mutated into a stop (nonsense) codon. [Section 4.5]

norepinephrine (NE)
The neurotransmitter used by the sympathetic division of the ANS at the postganglionic (organ-level) synapse. [Section 8.2]

nuclear envelope
The double lipid bilayer that surrounds the DNA in eukaryotic cells. [Section 6.2]

nuclear localization sequence
A sequence of amino acids that directs a protein to the nuclear envelope, where it is imported by a specific transport mechanism. [Section 6.2]

nuclear pore
A protein channel in the nuclear envelope that allows the free passage of molecules smaller than 60 kD. [Section 6.2]

nucleolus
A region within the nucleus where rRNA is transcribed and ribosomes are partially assembled. [Section 6.2]

nucleoside
A structure composed of a ribose molecule linked to one of the aromatic bases. In a deoxynucleoside, the ribose is replaced with deoxyribose. [Section 4.1]

nucleosome
A structure composed of two coils of DNA wrapped around an octet of histone proteins. The nucleosome is the primary form of packaging of eukaryotic DNA. [Section 4.1]

nucleotide
A nucleoside with one or more phosphate groups attached. Nucleoside triphosphates (NTPs) are the building blocks of RNA and are also used as energy molecules, especially ATP. Deoxynucleoside triphosphates (dNTPs) are the building blocks of DNA; in these molecules, the ribose is replaced with deoxyribose. [Section 4.1]

nucleus
An organelle bounded by a double membrane (double lipid bilayer) called the nuclear envelope. The nucleus contains the genome and is the site of replication and transcription. [Section 6.2]

obligate aerobe
An organism that requires oxygen to survive (aerobic metabolism only). [Section 5.3]

obligate anaerobe
An organism that can only survive in the absence of oxygen (anaerobic metabolism); oxygen is toxic to obligate anaerobes. [Section 5.3]

Okazaki fragments
Small fragments of DNA produced on the lagging strand during DNA replication, joined later by DNA ligase to form a complete strand. [Section 4.4]

olfactory receptors
Chemoreceptors in the upper nasal cavity that respond to odor chemicals. [Section 8.5]

oncogenes/protooncogenes
Mutated genes that cause cancer. Protooncogenes are the normal version of these genes before their mutations. [Section 6.7]

oncotic pressure
The osmotic pressure in the blood vessels due only to plasma proteins (primarily albumin). [Section 9.4]

oogonium
A precursor cell that undergoes mitosis during fetal development to produce more oogonium. These cells are then activated to produce primary oocytes, which remain dormant until stimulated to undergo meiosis I during some future menstrual cycle. [Section 13.6]

operator
A specific DNA nucleotide sequence where transcriptional regulatory proteins can bind. [Section 4.9]

operon
A nucleotide sequence on DNA that contains three elements: a coding sequence for one or more enzymes, a coding sequence for a regulatory protein, and upstream regulatory sequences where the regulatory protein can bind. An example is the lac operon found in prokaryotes. [Section 4.9]

optic disk
The "blind spot" of the eye, this is where the axons of the ganglion cells exit the retina to form the optic nerve. There are no photoreceptors in the optic disk. [Section 8.5]

optic nerve
The nerve extending from the back of the eyeball to the brain that carries visual information. The optic nerve is made up of the axons of the ganglion cells of the retina. [Section 8.5]

organ of Corti
The structure in the cochlea of the inner ear made up of the basilar membrane, the auditory hair cells, and the tectorial membrane. The organ of Corti is the site where auditory sensation is detected and transduced to action potentials. [Section 8.5]

organogenesis
The stage of human development during which the organs are formed. Organogenesis begins after gastrulation and is completed by the 8th week of gestation. [Section 13.11]

orgasm
A function of the reproductive system controlled by the sympathetic nervous system. In males, orgasm includes emission and ejaculation; in females it is mainly a series of rhythmic contractions of the pelvic floor muscles and the uterus. [Section 13.1]

origin of replication
The specific location on a DNA strand where replication begins. Prokaryotes typically have a single origin of replication, while eukaryotes have several per chromosome. [Section 4.4]

osmosis
The movement of water (the solvent) from its region of high concentration to its region of low concentration. Note that the water concentration gradient is opposite to the solute concentration gradient, since where solutes are concentrated, water is scarce. [Section 6.4]

osmotic pressure

The force required to resist the movement of water by osmosis. Osmotic pressure is essentially a measure of the concentration of a solution. A solution that is highly concentrated has a strong tendency to draw water into itself, so the pressure required to resist that movement would be high. Thus, highly concentrated solutions are said to have high osmotic pressures. [Section 6.4]

ossicles

The three small bones found in the middle ear (the *malleus*, the *incus*, and the *stapes*) that help to amplify the vibrations from sound waves. The malleus is attached to the tympanic membrane and the stapes is attached to the oval window of the cochlea. [Section 8.5]

osteoblast

A cell that produces bone. [Section 11.9]

osteoclast

A phagocytic-like bone cell that breaks down bone matrix to release calcium and phosphate into the bloodstream. [Section 11.9]

osteocyte

A mature, dormant osteoblast. [Section 11.6]

osteon

The unit of compact bone, formerly called a *Haversian system*. Osteons are essentially long cylinders of bone; the hollow center is called the *central canal*, and is where blood vessels, nerves, and lymphatic vessels are found. Compact bone is laid down around the central canal in rings (lamellae). [Section 11.7]

outer ear

The portion of the ear consisting of the pinna and the external auditory canal. The outer ear is separated from the middle ear by the tympanic membrane (the eardrum). [Section 8.5]

oval window

The membrane that separates the middle ear from the inner ear. [Section 8.5]

ovarian cycle

The 28 days of the menstrual cycle as they apply to events in the ovary. The ovarian cycle has three subphases: the follicular phase, ovulation, and the luteal phase. [Section 13.7]

ovary

The female primary sex organ. The ovary produces female gametes (ova) and secretes estrogen and progesterone. [Section 13.5]

ovulation

The release of a secondary oocyte (along with some granulosa cells) from the ovary at the approximate midpoint of the menstrual cycle (typically around day 14). Ovulation is triggered by a surge in LH. [Section 13.6]

oxytocin

A hormone released by the posterior pituitary that stimulates uterine contractions during childbirth and milk ejection during breastfeeding. [Sections 8.6 and 13.14]

P site

Peptidyl-tRNA site; the site on a ribosome where the growing peptide (attached to a tRNA) is found during translation. [Section 4.8]

pacemaker potential

A self-initiating action potential that occurs in the conduction system of the heart and triggers action potentials (and thus contraction) in the cardiac muscle cells. The pacemaker potential is triggered by the regular, spontaneous depolarization of the cells of the conduction system, due to a slow inward leak of positive ions (Na^+ and Ca^{2+}). [Section 9.2]

pancreas

An organ in the abdominal cavity with two roles. The first is an exocrine role: to produce digestive enzymes and bicarbonate, which are delivered to the small intestine via the pancreatic duct. The second is an endocrine role: to secrete insulin and glucagon into the bloodstream to help regulate blood glucose levels. [Section 10.7]

pancreatic duct

The main duct of the pancreas. The pancreatic duct carries the exocrine secretions of the pancreas (enzymes and bicarbonate) to the small intestine (duodenum). [Section 10.6]

parasite

An organism that requires the aid of a host organism to survive, and that harms the host in the process. [Section 5.1]

parasympathetic nervous system

The division of the autonomic nervous system known as the "resting and digesting" system. It causes a general decrease in body activities such as heart rate, respiratory rate, and blood pressure, an increase in blood flow to the GI tract, and an increase in digestive function. Because the preganglionic neurons all originate from either the brain or the sacrum, it is also known as the *craniosacral* system. [Section 9.3]

parathyroid hormone (PTH)
A hormone produced and secreted by the parathyroid glands that increases serum calcium levels. It targets the bones (stimulates osteoclasts), the kidneys (increases calcium reabsorption), and the small intestine (increases calcium absorption). [Section 11.9]

parietal cells
Cells found in gastric glands that secrete hydrochloric acid (for hydrolysis of ingested food) and gastric intrinsic factor (for absorption of vitamin B_{12}). [Section 10.6]

partial pressure
The contribution of an individual gas to the total pressure of a mixture of gases. Partial pressures are used to describe the amounts of the various gases carried in the bloodstream. [Section 12.4]

passive transport
Movement across the membrane of a cell that does not require energy input from the cell. Passive transport relies on concentration gradients to provide the driving force for movement, and includes both simple and facilitated diffusion. [Section 6.4]

penetrance
The percentage of individuals with a particular genotype that actually display the phenotype associated with that genotype. [Section 7.4]

penetration
The second step in viral infection, the injection of the viral genome into the host cell. [Section 5.1]

pepsin
A protein-digesting enzyme secreted by the chief cells of the gastric glands. Pepsin is secreted in its inactive form (pepsinogen) and is activated by gastric acid. It is unusual in that its pH optimum is around 1–2; most of the enzymes in the body function best at neutral pHs. [Section 10.6]

peptide hormone
A hormone made of amino acids (in some cases just a single, modified amino acid). Peptide hormones are generally hydrophilic and cannot cross the plasma membranes of cells, thus receptors for peptide hormones must be found on the cell surface. Binding of a peptide hormone to its receptor usually triggers a second messenger system within the cell. [Section 8.6]

peptidoglycan
A complex polymer of sugars and amino acids; the substance from which bacterial cell walls are made. [Section 5.3]

peptidyl transferase
The enzymatic activity of the ribosome that catalyzes the formation of a peptide bond between amino acids. It is thought that the rRNA of the ribosome possesses the peptidyl transferase activity. [Section 4.8]

perfusion
The flow of blood through a tissue. [Section 9.1]

peripheral chemoreceptors
Receptors in the carotid arteries and the aorta that monitor blood pH to help regulate ventilation rate. [Section 12.5]

peripheral membrane protein
A protein that is associated with the plasma membrane of a cell, but that is not embedded in the lipid bilayer. Peripheral proteins typically associate with embedded proteins through hydrogen bonding or electrostatic interactions. [Section 6.3]

peripheral nervous system
All parts of the nervous system except for the brain and spinal cord. [Section 8.4]

peripheral resistance
The resistance to blood flow in the systemic circulation. Peripheral resistance increases if arteries constrict (diameter decreases), and an increase in peripheral resistance leads to an increase in blood pressure. [Section 9.3]

periplasmic space
The space between the inner and outer cell membranes in Gram-negative bacteria. The peptidoglycan cell wall is found in the periplasmic space, and this space sometimes contains enzymes to degrade antibiotics. [Section 5.3]

peristalsis
A wave of contraction that sweeps along a muscular tube, pushing substances along the tube (e.g., food through the digestive tract, urine through the ureters, etc.). [Section 10.5]

peroxisome
Small organelles that contain hydrogen peroxide produced as a byproduct of lipid metabolism. Peroxisomes convert hydrogen peroxide to water and oxygen by way of the enzyme catalase. [Section 6.2]

phagocytosis
The nonspecific uptake of solid material by a cell accomplished by engulfing the particle with plasma membrane and drawing it into the cell. [Section 6.2]

pharynx
A passageway leading from behind the nasal cavity to the trachea. The pharynx is divided into three regions, named for their location. The *nasopharynx* is behind the nasal cavity, the *oropharynx* is behind the oral cavity, and the *laryngopharynx* is behind the larynx. [**Sections 10.6 and 12.2**]

phenotype
The physical characteristics resulting from the genotype. Phenotypes are usually described as dominant or recessive. [**Section 7.1**]

pheromones
Chemical signals released from one organism that result in a social response in members of the same species. [**Section 8.5**]

phospholipid
The primary membrane lipid. Phospholipids consist of a glycerol molecule esterified to two fatty acid chains and a phosphate molecule. Additional, highly hydrophilic groups are attached to the phosphate, making this molecule extremely amphipathic. [**Sections 3.4 and 6.3**]

photoreceptor
A receptor that responds to light. [**Section 8.5**]

phototroph
An organism that utilizes light as its primary energy source. [**Section 5.3**]

pilus
A long projection on a bacterial surface involved in attachment, e.g., the sex pilus attaches F+ and F- bacteria during conjugation. [**Section 5.3**]

pinocytosis
The nonspecific uptake of liquid particles into a cell by invagination of the plasma membrane and subsequent "pinching off" of a small bit of the extracellular fluid. [**Section 6.4**]

placenta
An organ that develops during pregnancy, derived in part from the mother and in part from the zygote. The placenta is the site of exchange of nutrients and gases between the mother's blood and the fetus's blood. The placenta is formed during the first three months of pregnancy. [**Section 13.10**]

placental villi
Zygote-derived projections that extend into the endometrium of the uterus during pregnancy. Fetal capillaries grow into the placental villi, which are surrounded by a pool of maternal blood. This facilitates nutrient and gas exchange between the mother and the fetus, without actually allowing the bloods to mix. [**Section 13.10**]

plaque
A clear area in a lawn of bacteria. Plaques represent an area where bacteria are lysing (dying) and a usually caused by lytic viruses. [**Section 5.3**]

plasma
The liquid portion of blood; plasma contains water, ions, buffers, sugars, proteins, etc. Anything that dissolves in blood dissolves in the plasma portion. [**Section 9.4**]

plasma cell
An activated B cell that is secreting antibody. [**Section 9.7**]

plasmid
A small, extrachromosomal (outside the genome), circular DNA molecule found in prokaryotes. [**Sections 5.3 and A.5**]

platelets
Extremely small pseudo-cells in the blood, important for clotting. They are not true cells, but are broken-off bits of a larger cell (a megakaryocyte). [**Section 9.4**]

pleura
The membranes that line the surface of the lungs (visceral pleura) and the inside wall of the chest cavity (parietal pleura). [**Section 12.3**]

pleural pressure
The pressure in the (theoretical) space between the lung surface and the inner wall of the chest cavity. Pleural pressure is negative with respect to atmospheric pressure; this keeps the lungs stuck to the chest cavity wall. [**Section 12.3**]

point mutation
A type of mutation in DNA where a single base is substituted for another. [**Section 4.5**]

polar body
A small cell with extremely little cytoplasm that results from the unequal cytoplasmic division of the primary (produces the first polar body) and secondary (produces the second polar body) oocytes during meiosis (oogenesis). The polar bodies degenerate. [**Section 13.6**]

poly-A tail
A string of several hundred adenine nucleotides added to the 3' end of eukaryotic mRNA. [**Section 4.7**]

polycistronic mRNA
mRNA that codes for several different proteins by utilizing different reading frames, nested genes, etc. Polycistronic mRNA is a characteristic of prokaryotes. [**Section 4.7**]

polymerase chain reaction (PCR)
A very quick and inexpensive method for detecting and amplifying specific DNA sequences. [**Section A.6**]

polyspermy
The fertilization of an oocyte by more than one sperm. This occurs in some animals, but in humans, blocks to polyspermy exist (the fast block and the slow block) so that only a single sperm can penetrate the oocyte. [**Section 13.9**]

population
A subset of a species consisting of members that mate and reproduce with one another. [**Section 7.7**]

pore
A pathway through a plasma membrane that restricts passage based only on the size of the molecule. Pores are made from porin proteins. [**Section 6.4**]

portal system
A system of blood vessels where the blood passes from arteries to capillaries to veins, then through a second set of capillaries, and then through a final set of veins. There are two portal systems in the body, the hepatic portal system and the hypothalamic portal system. [**Section 10.7**]

posterior pituitary gland
Also known as the *neurohypophysis*, the posterior pituitary is made of nervous tissue (i.e., neurons) and stores and secretes two hormones made by the hypothalamus: oxytocin and ADH. The posterior pituitary is controlled by action potentials from the hypothalamus. [**Section 8.6**]

postganglionic neuron
In the autonomic division of the PNS, a neuron that has its cell body located in an autonomic ganglion (where a preganglionic neuron synapses with it), and whose axon synapses with the target organ. [**Section 8.4**]

potassium leak channel
An ion channel specific for potassium found in the plasma membrane of all cells in the body. Leak channels are constitutively open and allow their specific ion to move across the membrane according to its gradient. Potassium leak channels allow potassium to leave the cell. [**Section 6.4**]

power stroke
The step in the sliding filament theory during which myosin undergoes a conformational change to its low energy state, in the process dragging the thin filaments (and the attached Z lines) toward the center of the sarcomere. Note that the power stroke requires ATP only indirectly: to set the myosin molecule in its high-energy conformation during a different step of the sliding filament theory. [**Section 11.2**]

preganglionic neuron
In the autonomic division of the PNS, a neuron that has its cell body located in the CNS, and whose axon extends into the PNS to synapse with a second neuron at an autonomic ganglion. (The second neuron's axon synapses with the target organ.) [**Section 8.4**]

primary active transport
Active transport that relies directly on the hydrolysis of ATP. [**Section 6.4**]

primary bronchi
The first branches off the trachea. There are two primary bronchi, one for each lung. [**Section 12.2**]

primary immune response
The first encounter with an antigen, resulting in activated B cells (for antibody secretion) and T cells (for cellular lysis and lymphocyte proliferation). The primary immune response takes approximately ten days, which is long enough for symptoms of the infection to appear. [**Section 9.7**]

primary oocytes
Diploid cells resulting from the activation of an oogonium; primary oocytes are ready to enter meiosis I. [**Section 13.6**]

primary spermatocytes
Diploid cells resulting from the activation of a spermatogonium; primary spermatocytes are ready to enter meiosis I. [**Section 13.2**]

primase
An RNA polymerase that creates a primer (made of RNA) to initiate DNA replication. DNA pol binds to the primer and elongates it. [**Section 4.4**]

prions
Misfolded, self-replicating proteins responsible for a class of diseases known as transmissible spongiform encephalopathies (TSEs) that cause degeneration of CNS tissues. [**Section 5.2**]

productive cycle
A life cycle of animal viruses in which the mature viral particles bud from the host cell, acquiring an envelope (a coating of lipid bilayer) in the process. [**Section 5.1**]

progesterone
A steroid hormone produced by the corpus luteum in the ovary during the second half of the menstrual cycle. Progesterone maintains and enhances the uterine lining for the possible implantation of a fertilized ovum. It is the primary hormone secreted during pregnancy. [**Section 13.6**]

prokaryote
An organism that lacks a nucleus or any other membrane-bound organelles. All prokaryotes belong to either Domain Bacteria or Domain Archaea (formerly Kingdom Monera). [Section 5.3]

prolactin
A hormone secreted by the anterior pituitary that targets the mammary glands, stimulating them to produce breast milk. [Section 13.14]

proliferative phase
The second phase of the uterine (endometrial) cycle, during which the endometrium (shed off during menstruation) is rebuilt. This phase of the cycle is under the control of estrogen, secreted from the follicle developing in the ovary during this time period. The proliferative phase typically lasts from day 6 to day 14 of the menstrual cycle. [Section 13.7]

promoter
The sequence of nucleotides on a chromosome that activates RNA polymerase so that transcription can take place. The promoter is found upstream of the *start site*, the location where transcription actually begins. [Section 4.7]

prophase
The first phase of mitosis. During prophase the replicated chromosomes condense, the spindle is formed, and the nuclear envelope breaks apart into vesicles. [Section 6.6]

prophase I
The first phase of meiosis I. During prophase I the replicated chromosomes condense, homologous chromosomes pair up, crossing over occurs between homologous chromosomes, the spindle is formed, and the nuclear envelope breaks apart into vesicles. Prophase I is the longest phase of meiosis. [Section 7.2]

prophase II
The first phase of meiosis II. Prophase II is identical to mitotic prophase, except that the number of chromosomes was reduced by half during meiosis I. [Section 7.2]

proprioceptor
A receptor that responds to changes in body position, such as stretch on a tendon, or contraction of a muscle. These receptors allow us to be consciously aware of the position of our body parts. [Section 8.5]

prostate
A small gland encircling the male urethra just inferior to the bladder. Its secretions contain nutrients and enzymes and account for approximately 35 percent of the ejaculate volume. [Section 13.1]

prosthetic group
A non-protein, but organic, molecule (such as a vitamin) that is covalently bound to an enzyme as part of the active site. [Sections 10.5 and 10.9]

proximal convoluted tubule
The first portion of the nephron tubule after the glomerulus. The PCT is the site of most reabsorption; all filtered nutrients are reabsorbed here as well as most of the filtered water. [Section 10.2]

ptyalin
Salivary amylase (see "amylase"). [Section 10.6]

pulmonary artery
The blood vessel that carries deoxygenated blood from the right ventricle of the heart to the lungs. [Section 9.2]

pulmonary circulation
The flow of blood from the heart, through the lungs, and back to the heart. [Section 9.1]

pulmonary edema
A collection of fluid in the alveoli of the lungs, particularly dangerous because it impedes gas exchange. Common causes of pulmonary edema are increased pulmonary blood pressure or infection in the respiratory system. [Section 12.4]

pulmonary vein
One of several vessels that carry oxygenated blood from the lungs to the left atrium of the heart. [Section 9.2]

pupil
A hole in the center of the iris of the eye that allows light to enter the eyeball. The diameter of the pupil is controlled by the iris in response to the brightness of the light. [Section 8.5]

purine bases
Aromatic bases found in DNA and RNA that are derived from purine. They have a double-ring structure and include adenine and guanine. [Section 4.1]

Purkinje fibers
The smallest (and final) fibers in the cardiac conduction system. The Purkinje fibers transmit the cardiac impulse to the ventricular muscle. [Section 9.2]

pyloric sphincter
The valve that regulates the passage of chyme from the stomach into the small intestine. [Section 10.6]

pyrimidine bases
Aromatic bases found in DNA and RNA that have a single-ring structure. They include cytosine, thymine, and uracil. [**Section 4.1**]

receptor-mediated endocytosis
A highly specific cellular uptake mechanism. The molecule to be taken up must bind to a cell surface receptor found in a clathrin-coated pit. [**Section 6.4**]

recessive
The allele in a heterozygous genotype that is not expressed; the phenotype resulting from possession of two recessive alleles (homozygous recessive). [**Section 7.1**]

recombination frequency (RF)
The RF value; the percentage of recombinant offspring resulting from a given genetic cross. The recombination frequency is proportional to the physical distance between two genes on the same chromosome. If the recombination frequency is low, the genes under consideration may be linked. [**Section 7.5**]

rectum
The final portion of the large intestine. [**Section 10.6**]

reflex arc
A relatively direct connection between a sensory neuron and a motor neuron that allows an extremely rapid response to a stimulus, often without conscious brain involvement. [**Section 8.3**]

relative refractory period
The period of time following an action potential when it is possible, but difficult, for the neuron to fire a second action potential, due to the fact that the membrane is further from threshold potential (hyperpolarized). [**Section 8.1**]

release factor
A cytoplasmic protein that binds to a stop codon when it appears in the A site of the ribosome. Release factors modify the peptidyl transferase activity of the ribosome, such that a water molecule is added to the end of the completed protein. This releases the finished protein from the final tRNA, and allows the ribosome subunits and mRNA to dissociate. [**Section 4.8**]

renal reabsorption
The movement of a substance from the filtrate (in the renal tubule) back into the bloodstream. Reabsorption reduces the amount of a substance in the urine. [**Section 10.1**]

renal tubule
The portion of the nephron after the glomerulus and capsule; the region of the nephron where the filtrate is modified along its path to becoming urine. [**Section 10.1**]

renin
An enzyme secreted by the juxtaglomerular cells when blood pressure decreases. Renin converts angiotensinogen to angiotensin I. [**Section 10.3**]

replication
The duplication of DNA. [**Section 4.4**]

replication bubbles
Multiple sites of replication found on large, linear eukaryotic chromosomes. [**Section 4.4**]

replication fork(s)
The site(s) where the parental DNA double helix unwinds during replication. [**Section 4.4**]

repolarization
The return of membrane potential to normal resting values after a depolarization or hyperpolarization. [**Section 8.1**]

repressible system
A system (set of genes) where the expression of those genes is inhibited by the gene product (e.g., the trp operon). [**Section 4.9**]

repressor
A regulatory protein that binds DNA at a specific nucleotide sequence (sometimes known as the operator) to prevent transcription of downstream genes. [**Section 4.9**]

residual volume
The volume of air remaining in the lungs after a maximal forced exhalation, typically about 1200 mL. [**Section 12.3**]

resolution
A function of the reproductive system (controlled by the sympathetic nervous system) that returns the body to its normal resting state after sexual arousal and orgasm. [**Section 13.1**]

respiratory acidosis
A drop in blood pH due to hypoventilation (too little breathing) and a resulting accumulation of CO_2. [**Section 12.1**]

respiratory alkalosis
A rise in blood pH due to hyperventilation (excessive breathing) and a resulting decrease in CO_2. [**Section 12.1**]

resting membrane potential

An electrical potential established across the plasma membrane of all cells by the Na^+/K^+-ATPase and the K^+ leak channels. In most cells, the resting membrane potential is approximately –70 mV with respect to the outside of the cell. [Section 6.4]

restriction endonuclease

A bacterial enzyme that recognizes a specific DNA nucleotide sequence and that cuts the double helix at a specific site within that sequence. [Section A.5]

retina

The innermost layer of the eyeball. The retina is made up of a layer of photoreceptors, a layer of bipolar cells, and a layer of ganglion cells. [Section 8.5]

retinal

A chemical derived from vitamin A found in the pigment proteins of the rod photoreceptors of the retina. Retinal changes conformation when it absorbs light, triggering a series of reactions that ultimately result in an action potential being sent to the brain. [Section 8.5]

retrovirus

A virus with an RNA genome (e.g., HIV) that undergoes a lysogenic life cycle in a host with a double-stranded DNA genome. In order to integrate its genome with the host cell genome, the virus must first reverse-transcribe its RNA genome to DNA. [Section 5.1]

reverse transcriptase

An enzyme that polymerizes a strand of DNA by reading an RNA template (an RNA dependent DNA polymerase); used by retroviruses in order to integrate their genome with the host cell genome. [Section 5.1]

ribosome

A structure made of two protein subunits and rRNA; this is the site of protein synthesis (translation) in a cell. Prokaryotic ribosomes (also known as 70S ribosomes) are smaller than eukaryotic ribosomes (80S ribosomes). The S value refers to the sedimentation rate during centrifugation. [Section 4.3]

RNA-dependent RNA polymerase

A viral enzyme that makes a strand of RNA by reading a strand of RNA. All prokaryotic and eukaryotic RNA polymerases are DNA dependent; they make a strand of RNA by reading a strand of DNA. [Section 5.1]

RNA interference (RNAi)

Small non-coding RNAs that bind to mRNAs, these double-stranded RNAs are then degraded and gene expression is reduced. [Section 4.7]

RNA polymerase

An enzyme that transcribes RNA. Prokaryotes have a single RNA pol, while eukaryotes have three; in eukaryotes, RNA pol I transcribes rRNA, RNA pol II transcribes mRNA, and RNA pol III transcribes tRNA. [Section 4.7]

RNA translocation

The movement of new mRNA transcripts to particular locations within the cell prior to their translation. [Section 4.9]

rods

Photoreceptors in the retina of the eye that respond to dim light and provide us with black and white vision. [Section 8.5]

rough endoplasmic reticulum

A large system of folded membranes within a eukaryotic cell that has ribosomes bound to it, giving it a rough appearance. These ribosomes synthesize proteins that will ultimately be secreted from the cell, incorporated into the plasma membrane, or transported to the Golgi apparatus or lysosomes. [Section 6.2]

rRNA

Ribosomal RNA; the type of RNA that associates with ribosomal proteins to make a functional ribosome. It is thought that the rRNA has the peptidyl transferase activity. [Section 4.7]

rule of addition

A statistical rule stating that the probability of either of two independent (and mutually exclusive) events occurring is the *sum* of their individual probabilities. [Section 7.3]

rule of multiplication

A statistical rule stating that the probability of two independent events occurring together is the *product* of their individual probabilities. [Section 7.3]

saltatory conduction

A rapid form of action potential conduction along the axon of a neuron in which the action potential appears to jump from node of Ranvier to node of Ranvier. [Section 8.1]

sarcolemma

The plasma membrane of a muscle cell. [Section 11.2]

sarcomere

The unit of muscle contraction. Sarcomeres are bounded by Z lines, to which thin filaments attach. Thick filaments are found in the center of the sarcomere, overlapped by thin filaments. Sliding of the filaments over one another during contraction reduces the distance between Z lines, shortening the sarcomere. [Section 11.2]

sarcoplasmic reticulum (SR)
The smooth ER of a muscle cell, enlarged and specialized to act as a Ca^{2+} reservoir. The SR winds around each myofibril in the muscle cell. [**Section 11.2**]

Schwann cell
One of the two peripheral nervous system supporting (glial) cells. Schwann cells form the myelin sheath on axons of peripheral neurons. [**Section 8.1**]

sclera
The white portion of the tough outer layer of the eyeball. [**Section 8.5**]

sebaceous glands
Oil-forming glands found all over the body, especially on the face and neck. The product (sebum) is released to the skin surface through hair follicles. [**Section 12.6**]

secondary active transport
Active transport that relies on an established concentration gradient, typically set up by a primary active transporter. Secondary active transport relies on ATP indirectly. [**Section 6.4**]

secondary immune response
A subsequent immune response to previously encountered antigen that results in antibody production and T cell activation. The secondary immune response is mediated by memory cells (produced during the primary immune response) and is much faster and stronger than the primary response, typically taking only a day or less. This is not long enough for the infection to become established; symptoms do not appear, thus the person is said to be "immune" to that particular antigen. [**Section 9.7**]

secondary oocyte
A haploid cell resulting from the first meiotic division of oogenesis. Note that the cytoplasmic division in this case is unequal, producing one large cell with almost all of the cytoplasm (the secondary oocyte) and one smaller cell with virtually no cytoplasm (the first polar body). The secondary oocyte, along with some follicular cells, is released from the ovary during ovulation. [**Section 13.6**]

secondary sexual characteristics
The set of adult characteristics that develop during puberty under the control of the sex steroids. In males, the secondary sex characteristics include enlargement and maturation of the genitalia, growth of facial, body, and pubic hair, increased muscle mass, and lowering of the voice. In females, the characteristics include the onset of menstruation and the menstrual cycle, enlargement of the breasts, widening of the pelvis, and growth of pubic hair. [**Section 13.4**]

secondary spermatocytes
Haploid cells resulting from the first meiotic division of spermatogenesis. Secondary spermatocytes are ready to enter meiosis II. [**Section 13.2**]

second messenger
An intracellular chemical signal (such as cAMP) that relays instructions from the cell surface to enzymes in the cytosol. [**Section 6.5**]

secretin
A hormone secreted by the small intestine (duodenum) in response to low pH (e.g., from stomach acid). It promotes the release of bicarbonate from the pancreas to act as a buffer. [**Section 10.6**]

secretion
1. The secretion of useful substances from a cell, either into the blood (endocrine secretion) or into a cavity or onto the body surface (exocrine secretion).
2. In the nephron, the movement of substances from the blood to the filtrate along the tubule. Secretion increases the rate at which substances can be removed from the body. [**Sections 10.2 and 10.5**]

secretory phase
The third phase of the uterine (endometrial) cycle, during which the rebuilt endometrium is enhanced with glycogen and lipid stores. The secretory phase is primarily under the control of progesterone and estrogen (secreted from the corpus luteum during this time period), and typically lasts from day 15 to day 28 of the menstrual cycle. [**Section 13.7**]

semen
An alkaline, fructose-rich fluid produced by three different glands in the male reproductive tract and released during ejaculation. Semen is very nourishing for sperm. [**Section 13.1**]

semicircular canals
Three loop-like structures in the inner ear that contain sensory receptors to monitor balance. [**Section 8.5**]

semiconservative replication
DNA replication. Each of the parental strands is read to make a complementary daughter strand, thus each new DNA molecule is composed of half the parental molecule paired with a newly synthesized strand. [**Section 4.4**]

semilunar valves
The valves in the heart that separate the ventricles from the arteries. The pulmonary semilunar valve separates the right ventricle from the pulmonary artery, and the aortic semilunar valve separates the left ventricle from the aorta. These valves close at the end of systole, preventing the backflow of blood from arteries to ventricles, and producing the second heart sound. [**Section 9.2**]

seminal vesicles
Paired glands found on the posterior external wall of the bladder in males. Their secretions contain an alkaline mucus and fructose, among other things, and make up approximately 60 percent of the ejaculate volume. [**Section 13.1**]

seminiferous tubules
Small convoluted tubules in the testes where spermatogenesis takes place. [**Section 13.1**]

senescence
The process of biological aging at the cellular (and organismal) level. [**Section 6.7**]

Sertoli cells
See "sustentacular cells." [**Section 13.1**]

serum
Plasma with the clotting factors removed. Serum is often used in diagnostic tests since it does not clot. [**Section 9.4**]

sex-linked trait
A trait determined by a gene on either the X or the Y chromosomes (the sex chromosomes). [**Section 7.4**]

Shine-Dalgarno sequence
The prokaryotic ribosome-binding site on mRNA, found 10 nucleotides 5' to the start codon. [**Section 4.8**]

signal recognition particle (SRP)
A cytoplasmic protein that recognizes the signal sequences of proteins destined to be translated at the rough ER. It binds first to the ribosome translating the protein with the signal sequence, then to an SRP receptor on the rough ER. [**Section 6.2**]

signal sequence
A short sequence of amino acids, usually found at the N-terminus of a protein being translated, that directs the ribosome and its associated mRNA to the membranes of the rough ER where translation will be completed. Signal sequences are found on membrane-bound proteins, secreted proteins, and proteins destined for other organelles. [**Section 6.2**]

signal transduction
The intracellular process triggered by the binding of a ligand to its receptor on the cell surface. Typically this activates second messenger pathways. [**Section 6.5**]

silent mutation
A point mutation in which a codon that specifies an amino acid is mutated into a new codon that specifies the same amino acid. [**Section 4.5**]

simple diffusion
The movement of a hydrophobic molecule across the plasma membrane of cell, down its concentration gradient. Since the molecule can easily interact with the lipid bilayer, no additional help (such as a channel or pore) is required. [**Section 6.4**]

single nucleotide polymorphisms (SNPs)
Variations in a single nucleotide from one person's DNA gene sequence to another's. These minor mutations can produce changes in phenotype. [**Section 4.2**]

single strand binding proteins
Proteins that bind to and stabilize the single strands of DNA exposed when helicase unwinds the double helix in preparation for replication. [**Section 4.4**]

sinoatrial (SA) node
A region of specialized cardiac muscle cells in the right atrium of the heart that initiate the impulse for heart contraction; for this reason the SA node is known as the "pacemaker" of the heart. [**Section 9.2**]

sister chromatid
Identical copies of a chromosome, produced during DNA replication and held together at the centromere. Sister chromatids are separated during anaphase of mitosis. [**Section 6.6**]

skeletal muscle
Muscle tissue that is attached to the bones. Skeletal muscle is striated, multinucleate, and under voluntary control. [**Section 11.2**]

sliding filament model
The mechanism of contraction in skeletal and cardiac muscle cells. It is a series of four repeated steps: (1) myosin binds actin, (2) myosin pulls actin toward the center of the sarcomere, (3) myosin releases actin, and (4) myosin resets to its high-energy conformation. [**Section 11.2**]

slow block to polyspermy
Also known as the *cortical reaction*, the slow block occurs after a sperm penetrates an oocyte (fertilization). It involves an increase in intracellular [Ca^{2+}] in the egg, which causes the release of cortical granules near the egg plasma membrane. This results in the hardening of the zona pellucida and its separation from the surface of the egg, preventing the further entry of more sperm into the egg. [**Section 13.9**]

slow twitch fibers
Skeletal muscle cells that contract slowly but are fatigue resistant due to a high concentration of myoglobin and a good blood supply. [**Section 11.2**]

small intestine
The region of the digestive tract where virtually all digestion and absorption occur. It is subdivided into three regions: the duodenum, the jejunum, and the ileum. [**Section 10.6**]

smooth endoplasmic reticulum
A network of membranes inside eukaryotic cells involved in lipid synthesis (steroids in gonads), detoxification (in liver cells), and/or Ca^{2+} storage (muscle cells). [**Section 6.2**]

smooth muscle
Muscle tissue found in the walls of hollow organs, e.g., blood vessels, the digestive tract, the uterus, etc. Smooth muscle is nonstriated, uninucleate, and under involuntary control (controlled by the autonomic nervous system). [**Section 11.4**]

soma
The cell body of a neuron. [**Section 8.1**]

somatic nervous system
The division of the peripheral nervous system that innervates and controls the skeletal muscles; also known as the *voluntary nervous system*. [**Section 8.3**]

spatial summation
Integration by a postsynaptic neuron of inputs (EPSPs and IPSPs) from multiple sources. [**Section 8.2**]

spermatid
A haploid but immature cell resulting from the second meiotic division of spermatogenesis. Spermatids undergo significant physical changes to become mature sperm (spermatozoa). [**Section 13.2**]

spermatogenesis
Sperm production; occurs in human males on a daily basis from puberty until death. Spermatogenesis results in the production of four mature gametes (sperm) from a single precursor cell (spermatogonium). For maximum sperm viability, spermatogenesis requires cooler temperatures and adequate testosterone. [**Section 13.2**]

spermatogonium
A diploid cell that can undergo mitosis to form more spermatogonium, and can also be triggered to undergo meiosis to form sperm. [**Section 13.2**]

S (synthesis) phase
The phase of the cell cycle during which the genome is replicated. [**Sections 4.4 and 6.6**]

sphincter of Oddi
The valve controlling release of bile and pancreatic juice into the duodenum. [**Section 10.6**]

sphygmomanometer
A blood pressure cuff. [**Section 9.3**]

spirochete
A bacterium having a spiral shape (plural = spirochetes). [**Section 5.3**]

spleen
An abdominal organ that is considered part of the immune system. The spleen has four functions: (1) it filters antigen from the blood, (2) it is the site of B cell maturation, (3) it stores blood, and (4) it destroys old red blood cells. [**Section 9.7**]

spliceosome
A complex made of many proteins and several small nuclear RNAs (snRNAs) that assembles around an intron to be spliced out of the primary transcript. [**Section 4.7**]

splicing
One type of eukaryotic mRNA processing in which introns are removed from the primary transcript and exons are ligated together. Splicing of transcripts can be different in different tissues. [**Section 4.7**]

spongy bone
A looser, more porous type of bone tissue found at the inner core of the epiphyses in long bones and all other bone types. Spongy bone is filled with red bone marrow, important in blood cell formation. [**Section 11.7**]

start site
The location on a chromosome where transcription begins. [**Section 4.7**]

steroid hormone
A hormone derived from cholesterol. Steroids are generally hydrophobic and can easily cross the plasma membranes of cells, thus receptors for steroids are found intracellularly. Once the steroid binds to its receptor, the receptor-steroid complex acts to regulate transcription in the nucleus. [**Section 8.6**]

stomach
The portion of the digestive tract that stores and grinds food. Limited digestion occurs in the stomach, and it has the lowest pH in the body (pH 1–2). [**Section 10.6**]

stop codon
A group of three nucleotides that does not specify a particular amino acid, but instead serves to notify the ribosome that the protein being translated is complete. The stop codons are UAA, UGA, and UAG. They are also known as *nonsense codons*. [**Section 4.3**]

striated muscle
See "skeletal muscle." [**Section 11.2**]

stroke volume
The volume of blood pumped out of the heart in a single beat (contraction). [**Section 9.2**]

submucosa
The layer of connective tissue directly under the mucosa of an open body cavity. [**Section 10.5**]

submucosal plexus
A network of neurons found in the submucosa of the gut; it helps to regulate enzyme secretion, gut blood flow, and ion and water flow in the lumen. Part of the enteric nervous system. [**Section 10.5**]

sudoriferous gland
A sweat gland located in the dermis of the skin. Sweat consists of water and ions (including Na⁺ and urea) and is secreted when temperatures rise. [**Section 12.6**]

summation
1. The integration of input (EPSPs and IPSPs) from many presynaptic neurons by a single postsynaptic neuron, either temporally or spatially. Summation of all input can either stimulate the postsynaptic neuron and possibly lead to an action potential, or it can inhibit the neuron, reducing the likelihood of an action potential.
2. The integration of single muscle twitches into a sustained contraction (tetany). [**Sections 8.2 and 11.2**]

surfactant
An amphipathic molecule secreted by cells in the alveoli (type 2 alveolar cells) that reduces surface tension on the inside of the alveolar walls. This prevents the alveoli from collapsing upon exhale and sticking together, thus reducing the effort required for inspiration. [**Section 12.2**]

sustentacular cells
Cells that form the walls of the seminiferous tubules and help in spermatogenesis. Sustentacular cells are also called *Sertoli cells*, and respond to FSH. [**Section 13.1**]

symbiotic bacteria
Bacteria that coexist with a host, where both the bacteria and the host derive a benefit. [**Section 5.3**]

sympathetic nervous system
The division of the autonomic nervous system known as the "fight or flight" system. It causes a general increase in body activities such as heart rate, respiratory rate, and blood pressure, and an increase in blood flow to skeletal muscle. It causes a general decrease in digestive activity. Because all of its preganglionic neurons originate from the thoracic or lumbar regions of the spinal cord, it is also known as the *thoracolumbar* system. [**Section 8.4**]

symport
A carrier protein that transports two molecules across the plasma membrane in the same direction. For example, the Na⁺-glucose cotransporter in intestinal cells is a symporter. [**Section 6.4**]

synapse
A neuron-to-neuron, neuron-to-organ, or muscle cell-to-muscle cell junction. [**Section 8.2**]

synapsis
Pairing of homologous chromosomes in a diploid cell, as occurs during prophase I of meiosis. [**Section 7.2**]

synaptic cleft
A microscopic space between the axon of one neuron and the cell body or dendrites of a second neuron, or between the axon of a neuron and an organ. [**Section 8.1**]

synaptonemal complex
A structure that forms in early prophase I that mediates synapsis (pairing of homologous chromosomes). [**Section 7.2**]

syncytium
A large multinucleate cell, typically formed by the fusion of many smaller cells during development (e.g., a skeletal muscle cell), or formed by nuclear division in the absence of cellular division. [**Sections 10.5 and 11.3**]

synergist
Something that works together with another thing to augment the second thing's activity. For example, a muscle that assists another muscle is said to be a synergist. An enzyme that helps another enzyme is a synergist. [**Section 11.2**]

synovial fluid
A lubricating, nourishing fluid found in joint capsules. [**Section 11.8**]

systemic circulation
The flow of blood from the heart, through the body (not including the lungs), and back to the heart. [**Section 9.1**]

systole
The period of time during which the ventricles of the heart are contracted. [**Section 9.2**]

systolic pressure
The pressure measured in the arteries during contraction of the ventricles (during systole). [**Section 9.3**]

T cell
A type of lymphocyte. The major subtypes of T cells are the helper T cells (CD4) and the killer T cells (CD8, or cytotoxic T cells). Helper T cells secrete chemicals that help killer Ts and B cells proliferate. Killer T cells destroy abnormal self-cells (e.g., cancer cells) or infected cells. [**Sections 9.4 and 9.7**]

tandem repeats
Regions of the genome where short sequences of nucleotides are repeated one after the other, anywhere from three to 100 times. [**Section 4.2**]

telencephalon
The cerebral hemispheres. [**Section 8.4**]

telomere
A specialized region at the ends of eukaryotic chromosomes that contains several repeats of a particular DNA sequence. These ends are maintained (in some cells) with the help of a special DNA polymerase called *telomerase*. In cells that lack telomerase, the telomeres slowly degrade with each round of DNA replication; this is thought to contribute to the eventual death of the cell. [**Sections 4.1, 4.4, and 6.7**]

telophase
The fourth (and final) phase of mitosis. During telophase the nuclear envelope reforms, chromosomes decondense, and the mitotic spindle is disassembled. [**Section 6.6**]

telophase I
The fourth phase of meiosis I. Telophase I is identical to mitotic telophase, except that the number of chromosomes is now reduced by half. After this phase the cell is considered to be haploid. Note, however, that the chromosomes are still replicated, and the sister chromatids must still be separated during meiosis II. [**Section 7.2**]

telophase II
The fourth and final phase of meiosis II. Telophase II is identical to mitotic telophase, except that the number of chromosomes was reduced by half during meiosis I. [**Section 7.2**]

temporal summation
Summation by a postsynaptic cell of input (EPSPs or IPSPs) from a single source over time. [**Section 8.2**]

tendon
Strong bands of connective tissue that connect skeletal muscle to bone. [**Section 11.2**]

testcross
A genetic cross between an organism displaying a recessive phenotype (homozygous recessive) and an organism displaying a dominant phenotype (for which the genotype is unknown), done to determine the unknown genotype. [**Section 7.3**]

testes
The primary male sex organ. The testes are suspended outside the body cavity in the scrotum and have two functions: (1) produce sperm, and (2) secrete testosterone. [**Section 13.1**]

testosterone
The primary androgen (male sex steroid). Testosterone is a steroid hormone produced and secreted by the interstitial cells of the testes. It triggers the development of secondary male sex characteristics during puberty (including spermatogenesis) and maintains those characteristics during adulthood. [**Section 13.2**]

tetanus
A smooth sustained muscle contraction, such as occurs in skeletal muscle when stimulation frequency is high enough (this is the normal type of contraction exhibited by skeletal muscle). [**Section 11.2**]

tetrad
A pair of replicated homologous chromosomes. Tetrads form during prophase I of meiosis so that homologous chromosomes can exchange DNA in a process known as "crossing over." [**Section 7.2**]

thalamus
The central structure of the diencephalon of the brain. The thalamus acts as a relay station and major integrating area for sensory impulses. [**Section 8.4**]

thecal cells
A layer of cells surrounding the granulosa cells of the follicles in an ovary. Thecal cells help produce the estrogen secreted from the follicle during the first phase of the ovarian cycle. [**Section 13.6**]

thermoreceptor
A receptor that responds to changes in temperature. [**Section 8.5**]

theta replication
DNA replication in prokaryotes, so named because as replication proceeds around the single, circular chromosome, it takes on the appearance of the Greek letter theta. [**Section 4.4**]

thick filament
In skeletal and cardiac muscle tissue, a filament composed of bundles of myosin molecules. The myosin head groups attach to the thin filaments during muscle contraction and pull them toward the center of the sarcomere. [**Section 11.2**]

thin filament
In skeletal and cardiac muscle tissue, a filament composed of actin, tropomyosin, and troponin. Thin filaments are attached to the Z lines of the sarcomeres and slide over thick filaments during muscle contraction. [**Section 11.2**]

thrombus
A blood clot that forms in an unbroken blood vessel. Thrombi are dangerous because they can break free and begin traveling in the bloodstream (become an *embolus*). Emboli ultimately become stuck in a small vessel and prevent adequate blood delivery to tissues beyond the sticking point, leading to tissue death. A brain embolism can lead to stroke, a heart embolism to a heart attack, and a pulmonary embolism to respiratory failure. [**Section 9.4**]

thymine
One of the four aromatic bases found in DNA. Thymine is a pyrimidine; it pairs with adenine. [**Section 4.1**]

thymus
An immune organ located near the heart. The thymus is the site of T cell maturation and is larger in children and adolescents. [**Section 9.7**]

thyroid stimulating hormone (TSH)
A tropic hormone produced by the anterior pituitary gland that targets the thyroid gland, stimulating it to produce and release thyroid hormone. [**Section 8.6**]

thyroxine
Also called *thyroid hormone*, thyroxine is produced and secreted by follicle cells in the thyroid gland. It targets all cells in the body and increases overall body metabolism. [**Section 8.6**]

tidal volume
The volume of air inhaled and exhaled in a normal, resting breath, typically about 500 mL. [**Section 12.3**]

tight junction
Also called *occluding junctions*, tight junctions form a seal between cells that prevents the movement of substances across the cell layer, except by diffusion through the cell membranes themselves. Tight junctions are found between the epithelial cells lining the intestines and between the cells forming the capillaries in the brain (the blood-brain barrier). [**Section 6.5**]

tolerance
The unresponsiveness of the immune system to normal proteins. [**Section 9.8**]

tolerant anaerobe
An organism that can survive in the presence of oxygen (oxygen is not toxic), but that does not use oxygen during metabolism (anaerobic metabolism only). [**Section 5.3**]

top-down processing
A tenet of Gestalt psychology where the brain applies experience and expectations to interpret sensory information. [**Section 8.5**]

topoisomerase
An enzyme that cuts one or both strands of DNA to relieve the excess tension caused by the unwinding of the helix by helicase during replication. [**Section 4.4**]

total lung capacity
The maximum volume of air that the lungs can contain. Total lung capacity is the sum of the vital capacity and the residual volume, and is typically about 6000 mL (6 L). [**Section 12.3**]

totipotent
Having the ability to become anything, e.g., a zygote is totipotent. [**Section 13.12**]

trachea
The main air tube leading into the respiratory system. The trachea is made of alternating rings of cartilage and connective tissue. [**Sections 10.6 and 12.2**]

transcription
The enzymatic process of reading a strand of DNA to produce a complementary strand of RNA. [**Sections 4.3 and 4.7**]

transduction
The transfer by a lysogenic virus of a portion of a host cell genome to a new host. [**Section 5.1**]

transition mutation
A point mutation in which a pyrimidine is substituted for a pyrimidine, or a purine is substituted for a purine. [**Section 4.5**]

translation
The process of reading a strand of mRNA to synthesize protein. Protein translation takes place on a ribosome. [**Sections 4.3 and 4.7**]

transmembrane domain
The portion of an integral membrane protein that passes through the lipid bilayer. [**Section 6.2**]

transposons
Segments of the genome that can "jump" from one location to another. Can lead to mutations depending on the final location of the transposon. [**Section 4.5**]

transverse tubule
See "T tubules." [**Section 11.2**]

transversion mutation
A point mutation in which a pyrimidine is substituted for a purine, or vice versa. [**Section 4.5**]

tricuspid valve
See "atrioventricular valve." [**Section 9.2**]

tRNA
Transfer RNA; the type of RNA that carries an amino acid from the cytoplasm to the ribosome for incorporation into a growing protein. [**Section 4.7**]

tRNA loading
The attachment of an amino acid to a tRNA (note that this is a specific interaction). tRNA loading requires two high-energy phosphate bonds. [**Section 4.8**]

trophoblast
The outer ring of cells of a blastocyst. The trophoblast takes part in formation of a placenta. [**Section 13.9**]

tropic hormone
A hormone that controls the release of another hormone. [**Section 8.6**]

tropomyosin
A helical protein that winds around actin helices in skeletal and cardiac muscle cells to form the thin filament of the sarcomere. In the absence of Ca^{2+}, tropomyosin covers the myosin-binding sites on actin and prevents muscle contraction. When calcium is present, a conformational change in tropomyosin occurs so that the myosin-binding sites are exposed and muscle contraction can occur. [**Section 11.2**]

troponin
A globular protein that associates with tropomyosin as part of the thin filament of the sarcomere. Troponin is the protein that binds Ca^{2+}, which causes the conformational change in tropomyosin required to expose the myosin-binding sites on actin and initiate muscle contraction. [**Section 11.2**]

trp operon
A set of genes for the enzymes necessary to synthesize tryptophan, under the control of a single promoter, the expression of which is inhibited by the presence of tryptophan (this is a repressible system). [**Section 4.9**]

trypsin
The main protease secreted by the pancreas; trypsin is activated (from trypsinogen) by enterokinase, and subsequently activates the other pancreatic enzymes. [**Section 10.7**]

T-tubules
Also called *transverse tubules*, these are deep invaginations of the plasma membrane found in skeletal and cardiac muscle cells. These invaginations allow depolarization of the membrane to quickly penetrate to the interior of the cell. [**Section 11.2**]

tumor suppressor genes
Genes that produce proteins that are the inherent defense system in cells to prevent the conversion of the cell into a cancer cell. p53 is a well-known tumor suppressor gene. [**Section 6.7**]

tympanic membrane
The membrane that separates the outer ear from the middle ear. The tympanic membrane is also known as the *eardrum*. [**Section 8.5**]

type I fibers
Also known as red slow twitch or red oxidative fibers, these are skeletal muscle cells that contract slowly and are extremely resistant to fatigue. [**Section 11.2**]

type IIA fibers
Also known as fast twitch oxidative fibers, these are skeletal muscle cells that contract quickly and are somewhat resistant to fatigue. [**Section 11.2**]

type IIB fibers
Also known as white fast twitch fibers, these are skeletal muscle cells that contract quickly and fatigue quickly. [**Section 11.2**]

umbilical cord

The cord that connects the embryo of a developing mammal to the placenta in the uterus of the mother. The umbilical cord contains fetal arteries (carry blood toward the placenta) and veins (carry blood away from the placenta). The umbilical vessels derive from the *allantois*, a structure that develops from the embryonic gut. [**Section 13.10**]

uniport

A carrier protein that transports a single molecule across the plasma membrane. [**Section 6.4**]

universal acceptor (recipient)

A person with blood type AB$^+$. Because this person's red blood cells possess all of the typical blood surface proteins, they will not display an immune reaction if transfused with any of the other blood types. [**Section 9.4**]

universal donor

A person with blood type O$^-$. Because this person's red blood cells possess none of the typical blood surface proteins, they cannot initiate an immune reaction in a recipient. [**Section 9.4**]

upstream

Toward the 5' end of an RNA transcript (the 5' end of the DNA coding strand). The promoter and start sites are "upstream." [**Section 4.7**]

uracil

One of four aromatic bases found in RNA. Uracil is pyrimidine; it pairs with adenine. [**Section 4.7**]

urea

A waste product of protein breakdown, produced by the liver and released into the bloodstream to be eliminated by the kidney. [**Sections 9.4 and 10.1**]

ureters

The tubes that carry urine from the kidneys to the bladder. [**Section 13.11**]

urethra

The tube that carries urine from the bladder to the outside of the body. In males it also carries semen and sperm during ejaculation. [**Section 13.1**]

urinary sphincter

The valve that controls the release of urine from the bladder. It has an internal part made of smooth muscle (thus involuntary) and an external part made of skeletal muscle (thus voluntary). [**Section 10.6**]

uterine cycle

The shedding of the old endometrium and preparation of a new endometrium for potential pregnancy. [**Section 13.7**]

uterine tubes

Also called *fallopian tubes*, these tubes extend laterally from either side of the uterus and serve as a passageway for the oocyte to travel from the ovary to the uterus. This is also the normal site of fertilization. Severing of the uterine tubes (tubal ligation) results in sterility of the female. [**Section 13.5**]

uterus

The muscular female organ in which a baby develops during pregnancy. [**Section 13.5**]

vaccination

The deliberate exposure of a person to an antigen in order to provoke the primary immune response and memory cell production. Typically the antigens are those normally associated with pathogens, thus if the live pathogen is encountered in the future, the secondary immune response can be initiated, preventing infection and symptoms. [**Section 9.7**]

vagal tone

The constant inhibition provided to the heart by the vagus nerve. Vagal tone reduces the intrinsic firing rate of the SA node from 120 beats/minute to around 80 beats/minute. [**Section 9.2**]

vagina

The birth canal; the stretchy, muscular passageway through which a baby exits the uterus during childbirth. [**Section 13.5**]

vagus nerves

Cranial nerve pair X. The vagus nerves are very large mixed nerves (they carry both sensory input and motor output) that innervate virtually every visceral organ. They are especially important in transmitting parasympathetic input to the heart and digestive smooth muscle. [**Section 8.4**]

van't Hoff factor

The van't Hoff factor (or ionizability factor, i) tells us how many ions one unit of a substance will produce in a solution. For example, glucose is non-ionic (does not dissociate) so i = 1, however NaCl dissociates into Na$^+$ and Cl$^-$, therefore i = 2. [**Section 6.4**]

vasa recta

The capillaries that surround the tubules of the nephron. The vasa recta reclaims reabsorbed substances, such as water and sodium ions. [**Section 10.2**]

vas deferens

See "ductus deferens." [**Section 13.1**]

vein
A blood vessel that carries blood toward the heart chambers. Veins do not have muscular walls, have valves to ensure that blood flows in one direction only, and are typically low-pressure vessels. [**Section 9.1**]

vena cava
One of two large vessels (superior and inferior) that return deoxygenated blood to the right atrium of the heart. [**Section 9.2**]

venous return
The amount of blood returned to the heart by the vena cavae. [**Section 9.2**]

ventricle
One of two large chambers in the heart. The ventricles receive blood from the atria and pump it out of the heart. The right ventricle has thin walls and pumps deoxygenated blood to the lungs through the pulmonary artery. The left ventricle has thick walls and pumps oxygenated blood to the body through the aorta. [**Section 9.2**]

vestibular glands
Paired glands near the posterior of the vaginal opening that secrete an alkaline mucus upon sexual arousal. The mucus helps to reduce the acidity of the vagina (which could be harmful to sperm) and lubricates the vagina to facilitate penetration. [**Section 13.5**]

villi
(Singular: *villus*.) Folds of the intestinal mucosa that project into the lumen of the intestine; villi serve to increase the surface area of the intestine for absorption. [**Section 10.6**]

viroids
Short pieces of circular single-stranded RNA that do not code for proteins but interfere with normal gene expression. Mostly they cause diseases in plants; the only human disease linked to viroids is hepatitis D. [**Section 5.2**]

virus
A nonliving, intracellular parasite. Viruses are typically just pieces of nucleic acid surrounded by a protein coat. [**Section 5.1**]

vital capacity
The maximum amount of air that can be forcibly exhaled from the lungs after filling them to their maximum level, typically about 4500 mL. [**Section 12.3**]

vitamin
One of several different nutrients that must be consumed in the diet, and generally not synthesized in the body. Vitamins can be hydrophobic (fat-soluble) or hydrophilic (water-soluble). [**Section 10.9**]

vitreous humor
A thick, gelatinous fluid found in the posterior segment of the eye (between the lens and the retina). The vitreous humor is only produced during fetal development and helps maintain intraocular pressure (the pressure inside the eyeball). [**Section 8.5**]

voltage-gated ion channel
An ion channel that is opened or closed based on the electrical potential across the plasma membrane. Once opened, the channel allows ions to cross the membrane according to their concentration gradients. [**Section 6.4**]

Weber's law
Weber's law states that two stimuli must differ by a constant proportion in order for their difference to be perceptible. [**Section 8.5**]

white matter
Myelinated axons. [**Section 8.4**]

Wolffian ducts
Early embryonic ducts that can develop into male internal genitalia under the proper stimulation (testosterone). [**Section 13.3**]

X-chromosome inactivation
The silencing of one of the two X chromosomes in female cells, so that only one is active. [**Section 4.7**]

yolk sac
An embryonic structure particularly important in egg-laying animals because it contains the yolk, the only source of nutrients for the embryo developing inside the egg. In humans, the yolk sac is very small (since mammals get their nutrients via the placenta) and is the site of synthesis of the first red blood cells. [**Section 13.10**]

Z lines
The ends of a sarcomere. [**Section 11.2**]

zona pellucida
A thick, transparent coating rich in glycoproteins that surrounds an oocyte. [**Section 13.6**]

zygote
A diploid cell formed by the fusion of two gametes during sexual reproduction. [**Section 13.9**]

zymogen
An inactive precursor of an enzyme, activated by various methods (acid hydrolysis, cleavage by another enzyme, etc.). [**Sections 4.9 and 10.6**]

NOTES

NOTES

NOTES

NOTES

NOTES

NOTES

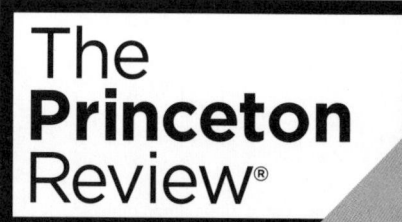
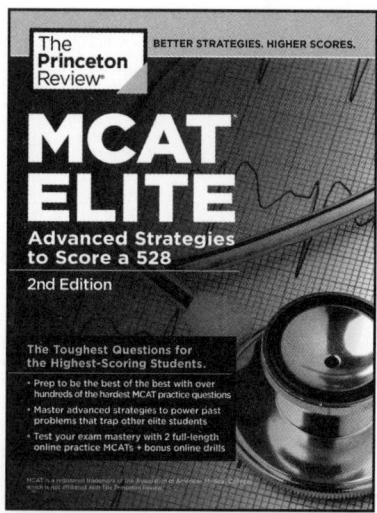
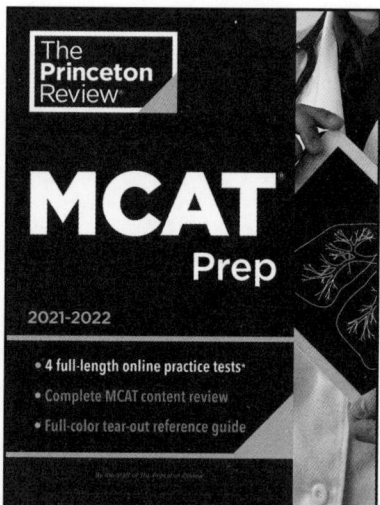
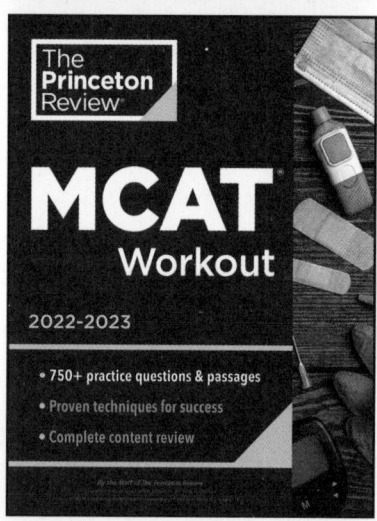
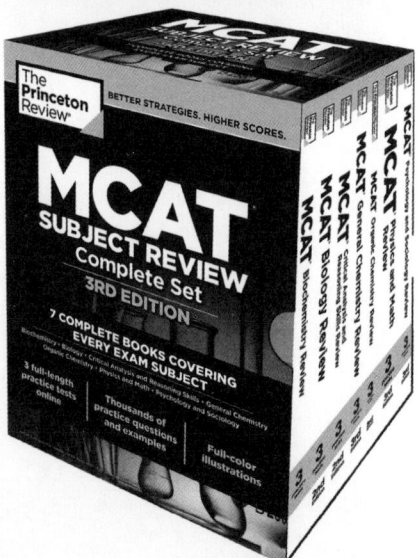

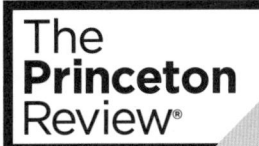
The
Princeton
Review®

MCAT®

Physics and Math Review

4th Edition

The Staff of The Princeton Review

Penguin
Random
House

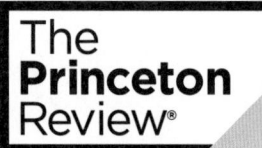

The Princeton Review
110 E. 42nd Street
New York, NY 10017

Published in the United States by Penguin Random
House LLC, New York, and in Canada by Random House
of Canada, a division of Penguin Random House Ltd.,
Toronto.

Terms of Service: The Princeton Review Online Companion Tools ("Student Tools") for retail books are available for only the two most recent editions of that book.
Student Tools may be activated only once per eligible
book purchased, for a total of 24 months of access.
Activation of Student Tools more than once per book
is in direct violation of these Terms of Service and may
result in discontinuation of access to Student Tools
Services.

The material in this book is up-to-date at the time of
publication. However, changes may have been instituted by the testing body in the test after this book was
published.

If there are any important late-breaking developments,
changes, or corrections to the materials in this book,
we will post that information online in the Student Tools.
Register your book and check your Student Tools to see
if there are any updates posted there.

Every attempt has been made to obtain permission
to reproduce material protected by copyright. Where
omissions may have occurred the editors will be happy
to acknowledge this in future printings.

ISBN: 978-0-593-51627-0
ISSN: 2150-8895

MCAT is a registered trademark of the Association of
American Medical Colleges.

The Princeton Review is not affiliated with Princeton
University.

Editor: Selena Coppock
Production Artist: Deborah Weber
Production Editors: Wendy Rosen, Emily Epstein White

Manufactured in China.

10 9 8 7 6 5 4 3 2 1

4th Edition

The Princeton Review Publishing Team
Rob Franek, Editor-in-Chief
David Soto, Senior Director, Data Operations
Stephen Koch, Senior Manager, Data Operations
Deborah Weber, Director of Production
Jason Ullmeyer, Production Design Manager
Jennifer Chapman, Senior Production Artist
Selena Coppock, Director of Editorial
Aaron Riccio, Senior Editor
Meave Shelton, Senior Editor
Chris Chimera, Editor
Orion McBean, Editor
Patricia Murphy, Editor
Laura Rose, Editor
Alexa Schmitt Bugler, Editorial Assistant

Penguin Random House Publishing Team
Tom Russell, VP, Publisher
Alison Stoltzfus, Senior Director, Publishing
Brett Wright, Senior Editor
Emily Hoffman, Assistant Managing Editor
Ellen Reed, Production Manager
Suzanne Lee, Designer
Eugenia Lo, Publishing Assistant

For customer service, please contact
editorialsupport@review.com,
and be sure to include:

- full title of the book

- ISBN

- page number

CONTRIBUTORS

Steven A. Leduc
Senior Author

TPR MCAT Physics Development Team:
Jon Fowler, M.A., Senior Editor, Lead Developer

Edited for Production by:
Judene Wright, M.S., M.A.Ed.
National Content Director, MCAT Program, The Princeton Review

The TPR MCAT Physics Team and Judene would like to thank the following people for their contributions to this book:

Khawar Chaudry, B.S., Doug Couchman, James Hudson, B.S., B.A., Ryan Katchky, Jason N. Kennedy, M.S.,
Brendan Lloyd, B.Sc., M.Sc., Travis Mackoy, B.S., Ashley Manzoor, Ph.D., Al Mercado, Gina Passante, Chris Pentzell, M.S.,
Mark Shew, H.BSc, Gillian Shiau, M.D., Teri Stewart, B.S.E., Dylan Sweeney, Carolyn J. Shiau, M.D., Felicia Tam, Ph.D.,
Tom Watts, B.A., Barry Weliver, Hesham Zakaria.

JOURNAL ARTICLE PERMISSIONS

PERIODIC TABLE OF THE ELEMENTS

1																		18
1 **H** 1.0	2												13	14	15	16	17	**2** **He** 4.0
3 **Li** 6.9	**4** **Be** 9.0												**5** **B** 10.8	**6** **C** 12.0	**7** **N** 14.0	**8** **O** 16.0	**9** **F** 19.0	**10** **Ne** 20.2
11 **Na** 23.0	**12** **Mg** 24.3	3	4	5	6	7	8	9	10	11	12		**13** **Al** 27.0	**14** **Si** 28.1	**15** **P** 31.0	**16** **S** 32.1	**17** **Cl** 35.5	**18** **Ar** 39.9
19 **K** 39.1	**20** **Ca** 40.1	**21** **Sc** 45.0	**22** **Ti** 47.9	**23** **V** 50.9	**24** **Cr** 52.0	**25** **Mn** 54.9	**26** **Fe** 55.8	**27** **Co** 58.9	**28** **Ni** 58.7	**29** **Cu** 63.5	**30** **Zn** 65.4		**31** **Ga** 69.7	**32** **Ge** 72.6	**33** **As** 74.9	**34** **Se** 79.0	**35** **Br** 79.9	**36** **Kr** 83.8
37 **Rb** 85.5	**38** **Sr** 87.6	**39** **Y** 88.9	**40** **Zr** 91.2	**41** **Nb** 92.9	**42** **Mo** 95.9	**43** **Tc** (98)	**44** **Ru** 101.1	**45** **Rh** 102.9	**46** **Pd** 106.4	**47** **Ag** 107.9	**48** **Cd** 112.4		**49** **In** 114.8	**50** **Sn** 118.7	**51** **Sb** 121.8	**52** **Te** 127.6	**53** **I** 126.9	**54** **Xe** 131.3
55 **Cs** 132.9	**56** **Ba** 137.3	**57** ***La** 138.9	**72** **Hf** 178.5	**73** **Ta** 180.9	**74** **W** 183.9	**75** **Re** 186.2	**76** **Os** 190.2	**77** **Ir** 192.2	**78** **Pt** 195.1	**79** **Au** 197.0	**80** **Hg** 200.6		**81** **Tl** 204.4	**82** **Pb** 207.2	**83** **Bi** 209.0	**84** **Po** (209)	**85** **At** (210)	**86** **Rn** (222)
87 **Fr** (223)	**88** **Ra** (226)	**89** **†Ac** (227)	**104** **Rf** (267)	**105** **Db** (268)	**106** **Sg** (271)	**107** **Bh** (270)	**108** **Hs** (269)	**109** **Mt** (278)	**110** **Ds** (281)	**111** **Rg** (282)	**112** **Cn** (285)		**113** **Nh** (286)	**114** **Fl** (289)	**115** **Mc** (289)	**116** **Lv** (293)	**117** **Ts** (294)	**118** **Og** (294)

*Lanthanoids	**58** **Ce** 140.1	**59** **Pr** 140.9	**60** **Nd** 144.2	**61** **Pm** (145)	**62** **Sm** 150.4	**63** **Eu** 152.0	**64** **Gd** 157.3	**65** **Tb** 158.9	**66** **Dy** 162.5	**67** **Ho** 164.9	**68** **Er** 167.3	**69** **Tm** 168.9	**70** **Yb** 173.0	**71** **Lu** 175.0
†Actinoids	**90** **Th** 232.0	**91** **Pa** (231)	**92** **U** 238.0	**93** **Np** (237)	**94** **Pu** (244)	**95** **Am** (243)	**96** **Cm** (247)	**97** **Bk** (247)	**98** **Cf** (251)	**99** **Es** (252)	**100** **Fm** (257)	**101** **Md** (258)	**102** **No** (259)	**103** **Lr** (266)

MCAT PHYSICS CONTENTS

MCAT MATH CONTENTS

Get More (Free) Content
at **PrincetonReview.com/prep**

As easy as **1・2・3**

1 Go to PrincetonReview.com/prep or scan the **QR code** and enter the following ISBN for your book: **9780593516270**

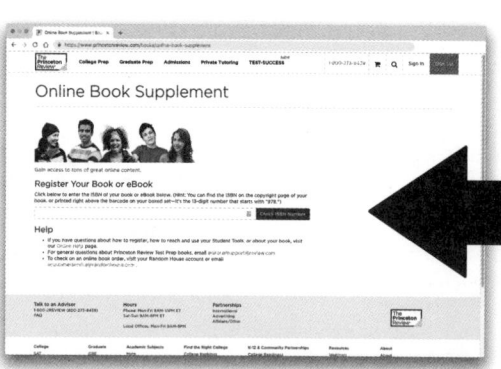

2 Answer a few simple questions to set up an exclusive Princeton Review account. *(If you already have one, you can just log in.)*

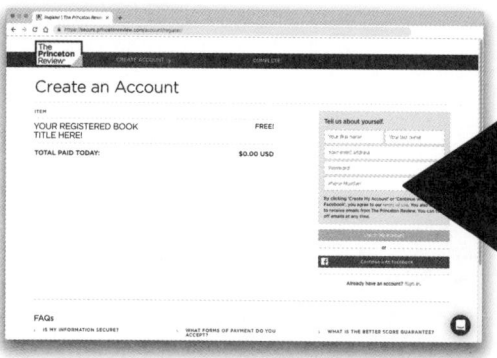

3 Enjoy access to your **FREE** content!

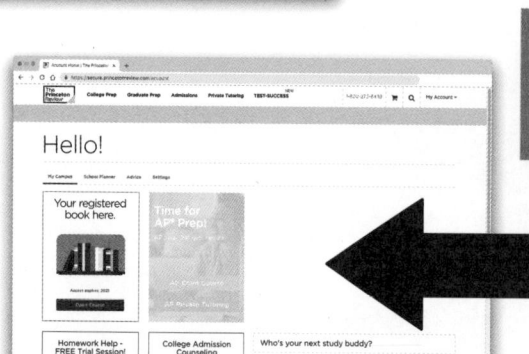

Once you've registered, you can...

- Take **3** full-length practice MCAT exams

- Find useful information about taking the MCAT and applying to medical school

- Check to see if there have been any corrections or updates to this edition

- Get our take on any recent or pending updates to the MCAT

Need to report a potential content issue?

Contact **EditorialSupport@review.com** and include:

- full title of the book
- ISBN
- page number

Need to report a technical issue?

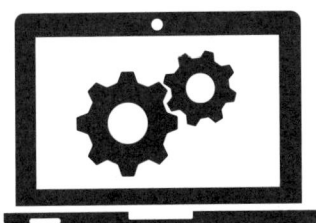

Contact **TPRStudentTech@review.com** and provide:

- your full name
- email address used to register the book
- full book title and ISBN
- Operating system (Mac/PC) and browser (Chrome, Firefox, Safari, etc.)

Chapter 1
MCAT Basics

SO YOU WANT TO BE A DOCTOR

So...you want to be a doctor. If you're like most premeds, you've wanted to be a doctor since you were pretty young. When people asked you what you wanted to be when you grew up, you always answered "a doctor." You had toy medical kits, bandaged up your dog or cat, and played "hospital." You probably read your parents' home medical guides for fun.

When you got to high school you took the honors and AP classes. You studied hard, got straight As (or at least really good grades!), and participated in extracurricular activities so you could get into a good college. And you succeeded!

At college you knew exactly what to do. You took your classes seriously, studied hard, and got a great GPA. You talked to your professors and hung out at office hours to get good letters of recommendation. You were a member of the premed society on campus, volunteered at hospitals, and shadowed doctors. All that's left to do now is get a good MCAT score.

Just the MCAT.

Just the most confidence-shattering, most demoralizing, longest, most brutal entrance exam for any graduate program. At about 7.5 hours (including breaks), the MCAT tops the list. Even the closest runners up, the LSAT and GMAT, are only about 4 hours long. The MCAT tests significant science content knowledge along with the ability to think quickly, reason logically, and read comprehensively, all under the pressure of a timed exam.

The path to a good MCAT score is not as easy to see as the path to a good GPA or the path to a good letter of recommendation. The MCAT is less about what you know, and more about how to apply what you know...and how to apply it quickly to new situations. Because the path might not be so clear, you might be worried. That's why you picked up this book.

We promise to demystify the MCAT for you, with clear descriptions of the different sections, how the test is scored, and what the test experience is like. We will help you understand general test-taking techniques as well as provide you with specific techniques for each section. We will review the science content you need to know as well as give you strategies for the Critical Analysis and Reasoning Skills (CARS) section. We'll show you the path to a good MCAT score and help you walk the path.

After all, you want to be a doctor. And we want you to succeed.

WHAT IS THE MCAT...REALLY?

Most test-takers approach the MCAT as though it were a typical college science test, one in which facts and knowledge simply need to be regurgitated in order to do well. They study for the MCAT the same way they did for their college tests, by memorizing facts and details, formulas and equations. And when they get to the MCAT they are surprised...and disappointed.

It's a myth that the MCAT is purely a content-knowledge test. If medical-school admission committees want to see what you know, all they have to do is look at your transcripts. What they really want to see is how you *think*, especially under pressure. *That's* what your MCAT score will tell them.

The MCAT is really a test of your ability to apply basic knowledge to different, possibly new, situations. It's a test of your ability to reason out and evaluate arguments. Do you still need to know your science content? Absolutely. But not at the level that most test-takers think they need to know it. Furthermore, your science knowledge won't help you on the Critical Analysis and Reasoning Skills (CARS) section. So how do you study for a test like this?

You study for the science sections by reviewing the basics and then applying them to MCAT practice questions. You study for the CARS section by learning how to adapt your existing reading and analytical skills to the nature of the test (more information about the CARS section can be found in the *MCAT Critical Analysis and Reasoning Skills Review*).

The book you are holding will review all the relevant MCAT Physics and Math content you will need for the test, and a little bit more. It includes hundreds of questions designed to make you think about the material in a deeper way, along with full explanations to clarify the logical thought process needed to get to the answer. It also comes with access to three full-length online practice exams to further hone your skills.

MCAT NUTS AND BOLTS

Overview

The MCAT is a computer-based test (CBT) that is *not* adaptive. Adaptive tests base your next question on whether or not you've answered the current question correctly. The MCAT is *linear*, or *fixed-form*, meaning that the questions are in a predetermined order and do not change based on your answers. However, there are many versions of the test, so that on a given test day, different people will see different versions. The following table highlights the features of the MCAT exam.

Registration	Online via www.aamc.org. Begins as early as six months prior to test date; available up until week of test (subject to seat availability).
Testing Centers	Administered at small, secure, climate-controlled computer testing rooms.
Security	Photo ID with signature, electronic fingerprint, electronic signature verification, assigned seat.
Proctoring	None. Test administrator checks examinee in and assigns seat at computer. All testing instructions are given on the computer.
Frequency of Test	Many times per year distributed over January, April, May, June, July, August, and September.
Format	Exclusively computer-based. NOT an adaptive test.
Length of Test Day	7.5 hours
Breaks	Optional 10-minute breaks between sections, with a 30-minute break for lunch.
Section Names	1. Chemical and Physical Foundations of Biological Systems (Chem/Phys) 2. Critical Analysis and Reasoning Skills (CARS) 3. Biological and Biochemical Foundations of Living Systems (Bio/Biochem) 4. Psychological, Social, and Biological Foundations of Behavior (Psych/Soc)
Number of Questions and Timing	59 Chem/Phys questions, 95 minutes 53 CARS questions, 90 minutes 59 Bio/Biochem questions, 95 minutes 59 Psych/Soc questions, 95 minutes
Scoring	Test is scaled. Several forms per administration.
Allowed/ Not allowed	No timers/watches. Noise reduction headphones available. Laminated noteboard and wet-erase marker given at start of test and taken at end of test. Locker or secure area provided for personal items.
Results: Timing and Delivery	Approximately 30 days. Electronic scores only, available online through AAMC login. Examinees can print official score reports.
Maximum Number of Retakes	The test can be taken a maximum of three times in one year, four times over two years, and seven times over the lifetime of the examinee. An examinee can be registered for only one date at a time.

Registration

Registration for the exam is completed online at www.aamc.org/students/applying/mcat/reserving. The AAMC opens registration for a given test date at least two months in advance of the date, often earlier. It's a good idea to register well in advance of your desired test date to make sure that you get a seat.

Sections

There are four sections on the MCAT, all of which consist of multiple-choice questions:

Section	Concepts Tested	Number of Questions and Timing
Chemical and Physical Foundations of Biological Systems	Basic concepts in chemistry and physics, including biochemistry; scientific inquiry; reasoning; research methods; and statistics.	59 questions in 95 minutes
Critical Analysis and Reasoning Skills	Critical analysis of information drawn from a wide range of social science and humanities disciplines.	53 questions in 90 minutes
Biological and Biochemical Foundations of Living Systems	Basic concepts in biology and biochemistry, scientific inquiry, reasoning, research methods, and statistics.	59 questions in 95 minutes
Psychological, Social, and Biological Foundations of Behavior	Basic concepts in psychology, sociology, and biology, research methods, and statistics.	59 questions in 95 minutes

Most questions on the MCAT (44 in the science sections, all 53 in the CARS section) are passage-based; the science sections have 10 passages each and the CARS section has 9. A passage consists of a few paragraphs of information on which several following questions are based. In the science sections, passages often include graphs, figures, and experiments to analyze. CARS passages come from literature in the social sciences, humanities, ethics, philosophy, cultural studies, and population health, and do not test content knowledge in any way.

Some questions in the science sections are freestanding questions (FSQs). These questions are independent of any passage information and appear in four groups of about three to four questions, interspersed throughout the passages. About 15 of the questions in the science sections are freestanding, and the remainder are passage-based.

Each section on the MCAT is separated by either a 10-minute break or a 30-minute lunch break. We recommend that you take these breaks.

Section	Time
Test Center Check-In	Variable, can take up to 40 minutes if center is busy.
Tutorial	10 minutes
Chemical and Physical Foundations of Biological Systems	95 minutes
Break (optional)	10 minutes
Critical Analysis and Reasoning Skills	90 minutes
Lunch Break (optional)	30 minutes
Biological and Biochemical Foundations of Living Systems	95 minutes
Break (optional)	10 minutes
Psychological, Social, and Biological Foundations of Behavior	95 minutes
Void Option	5 minutes
Survey (optional)	5 minutes

The survey includes questions about your satisfaction with the overall MCAT experience, including registration, check-in, etc., as well as questions about how you prepared for the test.

Scoring

The MCAT is a scaled exam, meaning that your raw score will be converted into a scaled score that takes into account the difficulty of the questions. There is no guessing penalty. All sections are scored from 118–132, with a total scaled score range of 472–528. Because different versions of the test have varying levels of difficulty, the scale will be different from one exam to the next. Thus, there is no "magic number" of questions to get right in order to get a particular score. Plus, some of the questions on the test are considered "experimental" and do not count toward your score; they are just there to be evaluated for possible future inclusion in a test.

At the end of the test (after you complete the Psychological, Social, and Biological Foundations of Behavior section), you will be asked to choose one of the following two options: "I wish to have my MCAT exam scored" or "I wish to VOID my MCAT exam." You have five minutes to make a decision, and if you do not select one of the options in that time, the test will automatically be scored. If you choose the VOID option, your test will not be scored (you will not now, or ever, get a numerical score for this test), medical schools will not know you took the test, and no refunds will be granted. You cannot "unvoid" your scores at a later time.

So, what's a good score? The AAMC is centering the scale at 500 (i.e., 500 will be the 50th percentile), and recommends that application committees consider applicants near the center of the range. To be on the safe side, aim for a total score of around 510. Remember that if your GPA is on the low side, you'll need higher MCAT scores to compensate, and if you have a strong GPA, you can get away with lower MCAT scores. But the reality is that your chances of acceptance depend on a lot more than just your MCAT scores. It's a combination of your GPA, your MCAT scores, your undergraduate coursework, letters of recommendation, experience related to the medical field (such as volunteer work or research), extracurricular activities, your personal statement, etc. Medical schools are looking for a complete package, not just good scores and a good GPA.

GENERAL LAYOUT AND TEST-TAKING STRATEGIES

Layout of the Test

In each section of the test, the computer screen is divided vertically, with the passage on the left and the range of questions for that passage indicated above (e.g. "Passage 1, Questions 1–5"). The scroll bar for the passage text appears in the middle of the screen. Each question appears on the right, and you need to click "Next" to move to each subsequent question.

In the science sections, the freestanding questions are found in groups of 3–4, interspersed with the passages. The screen is still divided vertically; on the left is the statement "Questions [X–XX] do not refer to a passage and are independent of each other," and each question appears on the right as described above.

CBT Tools

There are a number of tools available on the test, including highlighting, strike-outs, the Flag for Review button, the Navigation and Review Screen buttons, the Periodic Table button, and of course, the noteboard booklet. All tools are available with both mouse control (buttons to click) or keyboard commands (Alt+ a letter). As everyone has different preferences, you should practice with both types of tools (mouse and keyboard) to see which is more comfortable for you personally. The following is a brief description of each tool.

1) **Highlighting:** This is done in the passage text (including table entries and some equations, but excluding figures and molecular structures), in the question stems, and in the answer choices (including Roman numerals). Select the words you wish to highlight (left-click and drag the cursor across the words), and in the upper left corner click the "Highlight" button to highlight the selected text yellow. Alternatively, press "Alt+H" to highlight the words. Highlighting can be removed by selecting the words again and in the upper left corner clicking the down arrow next to "Highlight." This will expand to show the "Remove Highlight" option; clicking this will remove the highlighting. Removing highlighting via the keyboard is cumbersome and is not recommended.

2) **Strike-outs:** This can be done on the answer choices, including Roman numeral statements, by selecting the text you want to strike out (left-click and drag the cursor across the text), then clicking the "Strikethrough" button in the upper left corner. Alternatively, press "Alt+S" to strikeout the words. The strike-out can be removed by repeating these actions. Figures or molecular structures cannot be struck out, however, the letter answer choice of those structures can.

3) **Flag for Review button:** This is available for each question and is found in the upper right corner. This allows you to flag the question as one you would like to review later if time permits. When clicked, the flag icon turns yellow. Click again to remove the flag. Alternatively, press "Alt+F."

4) **Navigation button:** This is found near the bottom of the screen and is only available on your first pass through the section. Clicking this button brings up a navigation table listing all questions and their statuses (unseen, incomplete, complete, flagged for review). You can also press "Alt+N" to bring up the screen. The questions can be sorted by their statuses, and clicking a question number takes you immediately to that question. Once you have reached the end of the section and viewed the Review screen (described below), the Navigation screen is no longer available.

5) **Review Screen button:** This button is found near the bottom of the screen after your first pass through the section, and when clicked, brings up a new screen showing all questions and their statuses (either incomplete, unseen, or flagged for review). Questions that are complete are assigned no additional status. You can then choose one of three options by clicking with the mouse or with keyboard shortcuts: Review All (Alt+A), Review Incomplete (Alt+I), or Review Flagged (Alt+R); alternatively, you can click a question number to go directly back to that question. You can also end the section from this screen.

6) **Periodic Table button:** Clicking this button will open a periodic table (or press "Alt+T"). Note that the periodic table is large, covering most of the screen. However, this window can be resized to see the questions and a portion of the periodic table at the same time. The table text will not decrease, but scroll bars will appear on the window so you can center the section of the table of interest in the window.

7) **Noteboard Booklet (Scratch Paper):** At the start of the test, you will be given a spiral-bound set of four laminated 8.5″ × 14″ sheets of paper and a wet-erase marker to use as scratch paper. You can request a clean noteboard booklet at any time during the test; your original booklet will be collected. The noteboard is only useful if it is kept organized; do not give in to the tendency to write on the first available open space! Good organization will be very helpful when/if you wish to review a question. Indicate the passage number, the range of questions for that passage, and a topic in a box near the top of your scratch work, and indicate the question you are working on in a circle to the left of the notes for that question. Draw a line under your scratch work when you change passages to keep the work separate. Do not erase or scribble over any previous work. If you do not think it is correct, draw one line through the work and start again. You may have already done some useful work without realizing it.

General Strategy for the Science Sections

Passages vs. FSQs in the Science Sections: What to Start With

Since the questions are displayed on separate screens, it is awkward and time-consuming to click through all of the questions up front to find the FSQs. Therefore, go through the section on a first pass and decide whether to do the passage now or to save it for later, basing your decision on the passage text and the first question. Tackle the FSQs as you come upon them. More details are below.

Here is an outline of the procedure:

1) For each passage, write a heading on your noteboard with the passage number, the general topic, and its range of questions (e.g. "Passage 1, thermodynamics, Q 1–5" or "Passage 2, enzymes, Q 6–9). The passage numbers do not currently appear in the Navigation or Review screens, thus having the question numbers on your noteboard will allow you to move through the section more efficiently.

2) Skim the text and rank the passage. If a passage is a "Now," complete it before moving on to the next passage (also see "Attacking the Questions" below). If it is a "Later" passage, first write "SKIPPED" in block letters under the passage heading on your noteboard and leave room for your work when you come back to complete that passage. (Note that the specific passages you skip will be unique to you; in the Bio/Biochem section, you might choose to do all Biology passages first, then come back for Biochemistry. Or in Chem/Phys you might choose to skip Experiment Presentation passages. Know ahead of time what type of passage you are going to skip and follow your plan.)

3) Next, click on the "Navigation" button at the bottom to get to the Navigation screen. Click on the first question of the next passage; you'll be able to identify it because you know the range of questions from the passage you just skipped. This will take you to the next passage, where you will repeat steps 1–3.

4) Once you have completed the "Now" passages, go to the Review screen and click the first question for the first passage you skipped. Answer the questions, and continue going back to the Review screen and repeating this procedure for other passages you have skipped.

Attacking the Questions

As you work through the questions, if you encounter a particularly lengthy question, or a question that requires a lot of analysis, you may choose to skip it. This is a wise strategy because it ensures you will tackle all the easier questions first, the ones you are more likely to get right. If you choose to skip the question (or if you attempt it but get stuck), write down the question number on your noteboard, click the Flag for Review button to flag the question in the Review screen, and move on to the next question. At the end of the passage, click back through the set of questions to complete any that you skipped over the first time through, and make sure that you have filled in an answer for every question.

General Strategy for the CARS Section

Ranking and Ordering the Passages: What to Start With

Ranking: Since the questions are displayed on separate screens, it is awkward and time consuming to click through all of the questions before ranking each passage as "Now" (an easier passage), "Later" (a harder passage), or "Killer" (a passage that you will randomly guess on). Therefore, rank the passage and decide whether or not to do it on the first pass through the section based on the passage text, skimming the first 2–3 sentences.

Ordering: Because of the additional clicking through screens (or use of the Review screen) that is required to navigate through the section, the "Two-Pass" system (completing the "Now" passages as you find them) is likely to be your most efficient approach. However, if you find that you are continuously making a lot of bad ranking decisions, it is still valid to experiment with the "Three-Pass" approach (ranking all nine passages up front before attempting your first "Now" passage).

Here is an outline of the basic Ranking and Ordering procedure to follow.

1) For each passage, write a heading on your noteboard with the passage number and its range of questions (e.g. Passage 1, Q 1–5). The passage numbers do not currently appear in the Navigation or Review screen, thus having the question numbers on your noteboard will allow you to move through the section more efficiently.

2) Skim the first 2–3 sentences and rank the passage. If the passage is a "Now," complete it before moving on to the next. If it is a "Later" or "Killer," first write either "Later" or "Killer" and "SKIPPED" in block letters under the passage heading on your noteboard and leave room for your work if you decide to come back and complete that passage. Then click through each question, flagging each one and filling in random guesses, until you get to the next passage.

3) Once you have completed the "Now" passages, come back for your second pass and complete the "Later" passages, leaving your random guesses in place for any "Killer" passages that you choose not to complete. You can go to the Review screen and use your noteboard notes on the question numbers. Click on the number of the first question for that passage to go back to that question, and proceed from there. Alternatively, if you have consistently flagged all the questions for passages you skipped in your first pass you can use "Review Flagged" from the Review screen to find and complete your "Later" passages.

4) Regardless of how you choose to find your second pass passages, unflag each question after you complete it, so that you can continue to rely on the Review screen (and the "Review Flagged" function) to identify questions that you have not yet attempted.

Previewing the Questions

The formatting and functioning of the tools makes previewing the questions effective! Having each question on a separate screen will encourage you to really focus on that question. Even more importantly, you can highlight in the question stem and in the answer choices.

Here is the basic procedure for previewing the questions:

1) Start with the first question, and if it has lead words referencing passage content, highlight them. You may also choose to jot them down on your noteboard. Once you reach and preview the last question for the set on that passage, THEN stay on that screen and work the passage (your highlighting appears and stays on every passage screen, and persists through the whole 90 minutes).

2) Once you have worked the passage and defined the Bottom Line—the main idea and tone of the entire passage—work **backward** from the last question to the first. If you skip over any questions as you go (see "Attacking the Questions" below), write down the question number on your noteboard. Then click **forward** through the set of questions, completing any that you skipped over the first time through. Once you reach and complete the last question for that passage, clicking "Next" will send you to the first question of the next passage. Working the questions from last to first the first time through the set will eliminate the need to click back through multiple screens to get to the first question immediately after previewing, and will also make it easier and more efficient to do the hardest questions last (see "Attacking the Questions" below).

3) Remember that previewing questions is a CARS-only technique. It is not efficient to preview questions in the science sections.

Attacking the Questions

The question types and the procedure for actually attacking each type will be discussed later. However, it is still important **not** to attempt the hardest questions first (potentially getting stuck, wasting time, and discouraging yourself).

So, as you work the questions from last to first (see "Previewing the Questions" above), if you encounter a particularly difficult and/or lengthy question (or if you attempt a question but get stuck) write down the question number on your noteboard (you may also choose to Flag it) and move on backward to the next question you will attempt. Then click **forward** through the set and complete any that you skipped over the first time through the set, unflagging any questions that you flagged that first time through and making sure that you have filled in an answer for every question.

Pacing Strategy for the MCAT

Since the MCAT is a timed test, you must keep an eye on the timer and adjust your pacing as necessary. It would be terrible to run out of time at the end only to discover that the last few questions could have been easily answered in just a few seconds each.

In the science sections you will have about one minute and thirty-five seconds (1:35) per question, and in the CARS section you will have about one minute and forty seconds (1:40) per question, not taking into account the time spent reading the passage before answering the questions.

Section	# of Questions in passage	Approximate time (including reading the passage)
Chem/Phys, Bio/Biochem, and Psych/Soc	4	6.5 minutes
	5	8 minutes
	6	9.5 minutes
CARS	5	8.5 minutes
	6	10 minutes
	7	11.5 minutes

When starting a passage in the science sections, make note of how much time you will allot for it, and the starting time on the timer. Jot down on your noteboard what the timer should say at the end of the passage. Then just keep an eye on it as you work through the questions. If you are near the end of the time for that passage, guess on any remaining questions, make some notes on your noteboard, Flag the questions, and move on. Come back to those questions if you have time.

For the CARS section, keep in mind that many people will maximize their score by *not* trying to complete every question or every passage in the section. A good strategy for test takers who cannot achieve a high level of accuracy on all nine passages is to randomly guess on at least one passage in the section, and spend your time getting a high percentage of the other questions right. To complete all nine CARS passages, you have about ten minutes per passage. To complete eight of the nine, you have about 11 minutes per passage.

To help maximize your number of correct answer choices in any section, do the questions and passages within that section in the order *you* want to do them in. See "General Strategy" above.

Process of Elimination

Process of elimination (POE) is probably the most useful technique you have to tackle MCAT questions. Since there is no guessing penalty, POE allows you to increase your probability of choosing the correct answer by eliminating those you are sure are wrong.

1) Strike out any choices that you are sure are incorrect or that do not address the issue raised in the question.
2) Jot down some notes to help clarify your thoughts if you return to the question.
3) Use the "Flag for Review" button to flag the question for review. (Note, however, that in the CARS section, you generally should not be returning to rethink questions once you have moved on to a new passage.)

4)   Do not leave it blank! For the sciences, if you are not sure and you have already spent more than 60 seconds on that question, just pick one of the remaining choices. If you have time to review it at the end, you can always debate the remaining choices based on your previous notes. For CARS, if you have been through the choices two or three times, have re-read the question stem and gone back to the passage, and you are still stuck, move on. Do the remaining questions for that passage, take one more look at the question you were stuck on, then pick an answer and move on for good.

5)   Special Note: if three of the four answer choices have been eliminated, the remaining choice must be the correct answer. Don't waste time pondering *why* it is correct, just click it and move on. The MCAT doesn't care if you truly understand why it's the right answer, only that you have the right answer selected.

6)   More subject-specific information on techniques will be presented in the next chapter.

Guessing

Remember, there is NO guessing penalty on the MCAT. NEVER leave a question blank!

QUESTION TYPES

In the science sections of the MCAT, the questions fall into one of three main categories.

1)   Memory questions: These questions can be answered directly from prior knowledge and represent about 25 percent of the total number of questions.

2)   Explicit questions: These questions are those for which the answer is explicitly stated in the passage. To answer them correctly, for example, may just require finding a definition, or reading a graph, or making a simple connection. Explicit questions represent about 35 percent of the total number of questions.

3)   Implicit questions: These questions require you to apply knowledge to a new situation; the answer is typically implied by the information in the passage. These questions often start "if.... then...." (for example, "if we modify the experiment in the passage like this, then what result would we expect?"). Implicit style questions make up about 40 percent of the total number of questions.

In the CARS section, the questions fall into four main categories:

1)   Specific questions: These either ask you for facts from the passage (Retrieval questions) or require you to deduce what is most likely to be true based on the passage (Inference questions).

2)   General questions: These ask you to summarize themes (Main Idea and Primary Purpose questions) or evaluate an author's opinion (Tone/Attitude questions).

3)   Reasoning questions: These ask you to describe the purpose of, or the support provided for, a statement made in the passage (Structure questions) or to judge how well the author supports his or her argument (Evaluate questions).

4)   Application questions: These ask you to apply new information from either the question stem itself (New Information questions) or from the answer choices (Strengthen, Weaken, and Analogy questions) to the passage.

More detail on question types and strategies can be found in Chapter 2.

TESTING TIPS

Before Test Day

- Take a trip to the test center at least a day or two before your actual test date so that you can easily find the building and room on test day. This will also allow you to gauge traffic and see if you need money for parking or anything like that. Knowing this type of information ahead of time will greatly reduce your stress on the day of your test.
- During the week before the test, adjust your sleeping schedule so that you are going to bed and getting up in the morning at the same times as on the day before and morning of the MCAT. Prioritize getting a reasonable amount of sleep during the last few nights before the test.
- Don't do any heavy studying the day before the test. This is not a test you can cram for! Your goal at this point is to rest and relax so that you can go into test day in a good physical and mental condition.
- Eat well. Try to avoid excessive caffeine and sugar. Ideally, in the weeks leading up to the actual test you should experiment a little bit with foods and practice tests to see which foods give you the most endurance. Aim for steady blood sugar levels during the test: sports drinks, peanut-butter crackers, trail mix, etc. make good snacks for your breaks and lunch.

General Test Day Info and Tips

- On the day of the test, arrive at the test center at least a half hour prior to the start time of your test.
- Examinees will be checked in to the center in the order in which they arrive.
- You will be assigned a locker or secure area in which to put your personal items. Textbooks and study notes are not allowed, so there is no need to bring them with you to the test center.
- Your ID will be checked, a scan of your palm will be taken, and you will be asked to sign in.
- You will be given a noteboard booklet and a wet-erase marker, and the test center administrator will take you to the computer on which you will complete the test. You may not choose a computer; you must use the computer assigned to you.
- Nothing is allowed at the computer station except your photo ID, your locker key (if provided), and a factory sealed packet of ear plugs; not even your watch.
- If you choose to leave the testing room at the breaks, you will have your palm scanned again, and you will have to sign in and out.
- You are allowed to access the items in your locker, except for notes and cell phones. (Check your test center's policy on cell phones ahead of time; some centers do not even allow them to be kept in your locker.)
- Don't forget to bring the snack foods and lunch you experimented with in your practice tests.
- At the end of the test, the test administrator will collect your noteboard and clean off your notes.
- Definitely take the breaks! Get up and walk around. It's a good way to clear your head between sections and get the blood (and oxygen!) flowing to your brain.
- Ask for a clean noteboard at the breaks if you want a fresh one.

A NOTE ABOUT FLASHCARDS

For most of the exams you've taken previously, flashcards were likely very helpful. This was because those exams mostly required you to regurgitate information, and flashcards are pretty good at helping you memorize facts. However, the most challenging aspect of the MCAT is not that it requires you to memorize the fine details of content knowledge, but that it requires you to apply your basic scientific knowledge to unfamiliar situations: flashcards alone may not help you there.

Flashcards can be beneficial if your basic content knowledge is deficient in some area. For example, if you don't know Big 5 kinematics equations, flashcards can certainly help you memorize these facts. Or, maybe you are unsure of the rules for waves. You might find that flashcards can help you memorize these. But unless you are trying to memorize basic facts in your personal weak areas, you are better off doing and analyzing practice passages than carrying around a stack of flashcards.

Chapter 2
Physics Strategy
for the MCAT

2.1 SCIENCE SECTIONS OVERVIEW

There are three science sections on the MCAT:

- Chemical and Physical Foundations of Biological Systems
- Biological and Biochemical Foundations of Living Systems
- Psychological, Social, and Biological Foundations of Behavior

The Chemical and Physical Foundations of Biological Systems section (Chem/Phys) is the first section on the test. It includes questions from General Chemistry (about 30%), Physics (about 25%), Organic Chemistry (about 15%), Biochemistry (about 25%), and Biology (about 5%). Further, the questions often test chemical and physical concepts within a biological setting; for example, pressure and fluid flow in blood vessels. A solid grasp of math fundamentals is required (arithmetic, algebra, graphs, trigonometry, vectors, proportions, and logarithms); however, there are no calculus-based questions.

The Biological and Biochemical Foundations of Living Systems section (Bio/Biochem) is the third section on the test. Approximately 65% of the questions in this section come from biology, approximately 25% come from biochemistry, and approximately 10% come from Organic and General Chemistry. Math calculations are generally not required on this section of the test; however, a basic understanding of statistics as used in biological research is helpful.

The Psychological, Social, and Biological Foundations of Behavior section (Psych/Soc) is the fourth and final section on the test. About 65% of the questions will be drawn from Psychology (and about 5% of these will be Biological Psychology), about 30% from Sociology, and about 5% from Biology. As with the Bio/Biochem section, calculations are generally not required; however, a basic understanding of statistics as used in research is helpful.

Most of the questions in the science sections (44 of the 59) are passage-based, and each section has ten passages. Passages consist of a few paragraphs of information and include equations, reactions, graphs, figures, tables, experiments, and data. Four to six questions will be associated with each passage.

The remaining 25% of the questions (15 of 59) in each science section are freestanding questions (FSQs). These questions appear in approximately four groups interspersed between the passages. Each group contains three to four questions.

95 minutes are allotted to each of the science sections. This breaks down to approximately one minute and 35 seconds per question.

2.2 SCIENCE PASSAGE TYPES

The passages in the science sections fall into one of three main categories: Information and/or Situation Presentation, Experiment/Research Presentation, or Persuasive Reasoning.

Information and/or Situation Presentation

These passages either present straightforward scientific information or describe a particular event or occurrence. Generally, questions associated with these passages test basic science facts or ask you to predict outcomes given new variables or new information. Here is an example of an Information/Situation Presentation passage:

Figure 1 shows a portion of the inner mechanism of a typical home smoke detector. It consists of a pair of capacitor plates which are charged by a 9-volt battery (not shown). The capacitor plates (electrodes) are connected to a sensor device, D; the resistor R denotes the internal resistance of the sensor. Normally, air acts as an insulator and no current would flow in the circuit shown. However, inside the smoke detector is a small sample of an artificially produced radioactive element, americium-241, which decays primarily by emitting alpha particles, with a half-life of approximately 430 years. The daughter nucleus of the decay has a half-life in excess of two million years and therefore poses virtually no biohazard.

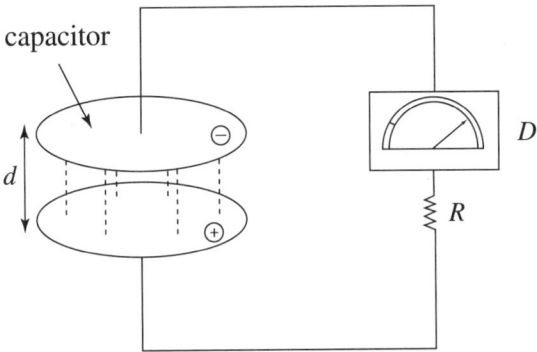

Figure 1   Smoke detector mechanism

The decay products (alpha particles and gamma rays) from the ^{241}Am sample ionize air molecules between the plates and thus provide a conducting pathway which allows current to flow in the circuit shown in Figure 1. A steady-state current is quickly established and remains as long as the battery continues to maintain a 9-volt potential difference between its terminals. However, if smoke particles enter the space between the capacitor plates and thereby interrupt the flow, the current is reduced, and the sensor responds to this change by triggering

the alarm. (Furthermore, as the battery starts to "die out," the resulting drop in current is also detected to alert the homeowner to replace the battery.)

$$C = \varepsilon_0 \frac{A}{d}$$

Equation 1

where ε_0 is the universal permittivity constant, equal to 8.85×10^{-12} C^2/(N·m^2). Since the area A of each capacitor plate in the smoke detector is 20 cm^2 and the plates are separated by a distance d of 5 mm, the capacitance is 3.5×10^{-12} F = 3.5 pF.

Experiment/Research (or Data) Presentation

These passages present the details of experiments and research procedures. They often include data tables and graphs. Generally, questions associated with these passages ask you to interpret data, draw conclusions, and make inferences. Here is an example of an Experiment/Research Presentation passage:

The development of sexual characteristics depends upon various factors, the most important of which are hormonal control, environmental stimuli, and the genetic makeup of the individual. The hormones that contribute to the development include the steroid hormones estrogen, progesterone, and testosterone, as well as the pituitary hormones FSH (follicle-stimulating hormone) and LH (luteinizing hormone).

To study the mechanism by which estrogen exerts its effects, a researcher performed the following experiments using cell culture assays.

Experiment 1:

Human embryonic placental mesenchyme (HEPM) cells were grown for 48 hours in Dulbecco's Modified Eagle Medium (DMEM), with media change every 12 hours. Upon confluent growth, cells were exposed to a 10 mg per mL solution of green fluorescent-labeled estrogen for 1 hour. Cells were rinsed with DMEM and observed under confocal fluorescent microscopy.

Experiment 2:

HEPM cells were grown to confluence as in Experiment 1. Cells were exposed to Pesticide A for 1 hour, followed by the 10 mg/mL solution of labeled estrogen, rinsed as in Experiment 1, and observed under confocal fluorescent microscopy.

Experiment 3:

Experiment 1 was repeated with Chinese Hamster Ovary (CHO) cells instead of HEPM cells.

Experiment 4:

CHO cells injected with cytoplasmic extracts of HEPM cells were grown to confluence, exposed to the 10 mg/mL solution of labeled estrogen for 1 hour, and observed under confocal fluorescent microscopy.

The results of these experiments are given in Table 1.

Table 1 Detection of Estrogen (+ indicates presence of Estrogen)

Experiment	Media	Cytoplasm	Nucleus
1	+	+	+
2	+	+	+
3	+	+	+
4	+	+	+

After observing the cells in each experiment, the researcher bathed the cells in a solution containing 10 mg per mL of a red fluorescent probe that binds specifically to the estrogen receptor only when its active site is occupied. After 1 hour, the cells were rinsed with DMEM and observed under confocal fluorescent microscopy. The results are presented in Table 2.

The researcher also repeated Experiment 2 using Pesticide B, an estrogen analog, instead of Pesticide A. Results from other researchers had shown that Pesticide B binds to the active site of the cytosolic estrogen receptor (with an affinity 10,000 times greater than that of estrogen) and causes increased transcription of mRNA.

Table 2 Observed Fluorescence and Estrogen Effects (G = green, R = red)

Experiment	Media	Cytoplasm	Nucleus	Estrogen effects observed?
1	G only	G and R	G and R	Yes
2	G only	G only	G only	No
3	G only	G only	G only	No
4	G only	G and R	G and R	Yes

Based on these results, the researcher determined that estrogen had no effect when not bound to a cytosolic, estrogen-specific receptor.

Persuasive (Scientific) Reasoning

These passages typically present a scientific phenomenon along with a hypothesis that explains the phenomenon, and may include counter-arguments as well. Questions associated with these passages ask you to evaluate the hypothesis or arguments. Persuasive Reasoning passages in the science sections of the MCAT tend to be less common than Information Presentation or Experiment-based passages. Here is an example of a Persuasive Reasoning passage:

Two theoretical chemists attempted to explain the observed trends of acidity by applying two interpretations of molecular orbital theory. Consider the pK_a values of some common acids listed along the conjugate base:

acid	pK_a	conjugate base
H_2SO_4	< 0	HSO_4^-
H_2CrO_4	5.0	$HCrO_4^-$
H_2PO_4	2.1	$H_2PO_4^-$
HF	3.9	F^-
HOCl	7.8	ClO^-
HCN	9.5	CN^-
HIO_3	1.2	IO_3^-

Recall that acids with a $pK_a < 0$ are called strong acids, and those with a $pK_a > 0$ are called weak acids. The arguments of the chemists are given below.

Chemist #1:

"The acidity of a compound is proportional to the polarization of the H—X bond, where X is some nonmetal element. Complex acids, such as H_2SO_4, $HClO_4$, and HNO_3 are strong acids because the H—O bonding electrons are strongly drawn towards the oxygen. It is generally true that a covalent bond weakens as its polarization increases. Therefore, one can conclude that the strength of an acid is proportional to the number of electronegative atoms in that acid."

Chemist #2:

"The acidity of a compound is proportional to the number of stable resonance structures of that acid's conjugate base. H_2SO_4, $HClO_4$, and HNO_3 are all strong acids because their respective conjugate bases exhibit a high degree of resonance stabilization."

MAPPING A PASSAGE

"Mapping a passage" refers to the combination of on-screen highlighting and noteboard notes that you take while working through a passage. Typically, good things to highlight include the overall topic of a passage, unfamiliar terms and their definitions, familiar terms in unfamiliar contexts, repeated phrases in a paragraph (highlight the first instance), extreme or exclusive terms (most/least, maximum/minimum, always/never, except, etc.), italicized terms and their definitions, numerical values floating in text, hypotheses or causal terms, and results or effects terms. Noteboard notes can be used to copy given equations and equations from memory (when none are given), to copy and label simplified figures or to draw diagrams of something described in words but not pictured, to summarize the paragraphs, and to jot down important facts and connections that are made when reading the passage. More details on passage mapping will be presented in Section 2.5.

2.3 SCIENCE QUESTION TYPES

Each question in the science sections is generally one of three main types: Memory, Explicit, or Implicit.

Memory Questions

These questions can be answered directly from prior knowledge, with little need to reference the passage or question text. Memory questions represent approximately 25 percent of the science questions on the MCAT. Usually, Memory questions are found as FSQs, but they can also be tucked into a passage. Here's an example of a Memory question:

Which of the following acetylating conditions will convert diethylamine into an amide at the fastest rate?

A) Acetic acid / HCl
B) Acetic anhydride
C) Acetyl chloride
D) Ethyl acetate

2.3

Explicit Questions

Explicit questions can be answered primarily with information from the passage, along with basic prior knowledge. They may require data retrieval, graph analysis, or making a simple connection. Explicit questions make up approximately 35–40 percent of the science questions on the MCAT; here's an example (taken from the Information/Situation Presentation passage on page 17):

> The sensor device D shown in Figure 1 performs its function by acting as:
>
> A) an ohmmeter.
> B) a voltmeter.
> C) a potentiometer.
> D) an ammeter.

Implicit Questions

These questions require you to take information from the passage, combine it with your prior knowledge, apply it to a new situation, and come to some logical conclusion. They typically require more complex connections than do Explicit questions, and may also require data retrieval, graph analysis, etc. Implicit questions usually require a solid understanding of the passage information. They make up approximately 35–40 percent of the science questions on the MCAT; here's an example (taken from the Experiment/Research Presentation passage on page 18):

> If Experiment 2 were repeated, but this time exposing the cells first to Pesticide A and then to Pesticide B before exposing them to the green fluorescent-labeled estrogen and the red fluorescent probe, which of the following statements will most likely be true?
>
> A) Pesticide A and Pesticide B bind to the same site on the estrogen receptor.
> B) Estrogen effects would be observed.
> C) Only green fluorescence would be observed.
> D) Both green and red fluorescence would be observed.

The Rod of Asclepius

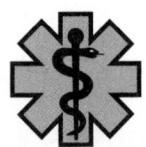

You may notice this Rod of Asclepius icon as you read through the book. In Greek mythology, the Rod of Asclepius is associated with healing and medicine; the symbol continues to be used today to represent medicine and healthcare. You won't see this on the actual MCAT, but we've used it here to call attention to medically related examples and questions.

2.4 PHYSICS ON THE MCAT

Of all the sciences on the MCAT, Physics relies the least on information recall and the most on problem-solving and reading comprehension skills. This is in part because the subject matter lends itself to these kinds of problems. Perhaps more importantly, though, the subject content in Physics pertains less to the material you will ultimately study in medical school, whereas the critical thinking that Physics demands fits with what you will encounter (particularly during your clinical years). In many ways, your ability to formulate an "approach" to a tough problem is one of the most useful skills you can develop along the path to medicine.

The science sections of the MCAT have 10 passages and 15 freestanding questions (FSQs). Physics makes up about 25% of the questions in the Chemical and Physical Foundations of Biological Systems section (Chem/Phys). The remaining 75% of the questions are divided up as General Chemistry (30%), Organic Chemistry (15%), Biochemistry (25%), and Biology (5%) questions.

2.5 TACKLING A PASSAGE

Passage Types as They Apply to Physics

Information/Situation Presentation

These passages tend to fall into two types for Physics. The first type consists of straightforward descriptions of phenomena you should already understand well, such as a passage comparing the function of a nerve cell to a DC circuit with a battery, a capacitor, a couple of switches, and a few resistors in parallel combinations. Common question types include solving for unknown quantities using given values and memorized formulas, definition questions about physical laws, and comparisons of the "real" to the "ideal."

The second type of passage consists of elaborations of phenomena you know something about, such as a passage about an electrocardiogram circuit with resistors, a capacitor, and a number of operational amplifiers (circuit elements that multiply input voltage) that provides equations for the time-dependent voltage input from the body and output by the device. These more complex passages are often marked by several new equations and possibly graphs, followed by paragraphs defining the variables and constants, or perhaps a few new conceptual definitions. Common question types for these passages include algebraic manipulation or proportion questions using the new equations, graph generation or interpretation questions, and implicit conceptual questions.

Experiment or Data Presentation

These passages often include data tables or numerically labeled graphs; if there is data, the passage usually covers an experiment or multiple experiments. The subject matter in experimental passages is typically familiar, though the concepts might be extended somewhat beyond basic knowledge, for example, measuring the viscosity in a fluid or the resistance of a conducting wire as a function of temperature. These passages tend *not* to push your understanding of content as much as the technical passages or heavily conceptual passages. Rather, the implicit questions found in experiment presentation passages are usually of the form, "If another trial were conducted changing [some set of parameters], then the resulting value of [another parameter] would be…." Such questions require you to interpret a given equation or to read numbers from the tables and extrapolate their functional dependence on the altered parameters.

Persuasive (Scientific) Reasoning

Persuasive reasoning passages on the Physics portion of the MCAT are largely conceptual: They describe some particular phenomenon about which you most likely have no prior knowledge, offering one or more theories as to its causes and effects, and they do so mostly with words (as opposed to using figures, equations, and numbers). These are generally the hardest passages for most people, as they rely heavily on reading comprehension as well as the ability to recall and synthesize physics concepts and equations from different topics (e.g., atomic structure, magnetism, and standing waves). You can expect questions in which both the question text and the answer choices are themselves entirely in words. This means you must be comfortable translating sentences into proportions, ratios, or equations, and then translating them back into sentences. Moreover, it may not be enough to be a careful reader with a good memory for formulas: Conceptual passages will test whether you know the conditions under which equations apply (such as the conditions for an ideal fluid or when to hold Q or V constant in $Q = CV$).

Reading a Physics Passage

Don't let our heading here deceive you; "reading" in the sense we commonly use the word is seldom the best way to use physics passages effectively. A kind of "informed skimming" is usually the best strategy. A quick holistic scan of the passage, including reading its first sentence, should be enough to tell you its topic and type; this will help you decide whether to do it now or postpone it until you've tackled easier passages (for example, if you dislike circuits, or if a lot of reading comprehension slows you down, by all means leave those passages until later!). Once you decide to do a passage, use the following techniques to find what you need to know quickly.

1. Read the first sentence again carefully. It will probably define the main idea of the passage and might inform your answer to one of the questions directly. Similarly, if the passage describes a set of experimental procedures, read the first sentences in each subsection so you understand precisely what is being done and why.
2. Look for the familiar Physics terms within the passage and highlight the ones used in new contexts (not every instance of a physics term should be highlighted or you will over-highlight the passage). Remember that the questions on the MCAT can come directly from anything mentioned by the AAMC topics list, or they can come from a reading-comprehension topic in a passage. And in fact, many Physics passages may not seem to be about a particular Physics topic at first glance. For example, a passage about ultrasound scans may be about waves, or sound, or fluid dynamics, or all of those topics at the same time! If you can identify the relevant physics within the passage text, you can focus in on that text and topic rather than getting stuck on the paragraph about, say, the historical perspective of how we measure heart rate.
3. Look for any new terms. These are often italicized but not always, so scan for long unfamiliar phrases (phrases like "aeroelastic flutter" stick out in a paragraph even in plain type). Highlight them along with their definitions.

4.   Look for cause-effect language such as "causes," "because," "due to," "results in," etc., as well as extreme or exclusive language like "always," "never," "most," "least," "greatest," "only," "except," etc. Highlight the phrase and the text that it modifies.

5.   Find the equations and figures. You might start with these to figure out the topic quickly. The text immediately before or after them tends to define terms or provide numerical values (measurements in a diagram or values of constants in an equation). If the diagrams are basically complete or the equations make sense to you, *skip this text*: There's no good reason to read a paragraph describing the circuit diagram for a defibrillator if the picture already tells the whole story.

6.   Look for numbers. These are sometimes worth highlighting or jotting down on your noteboard and they are easy to find (however, if a passage gives you a whole pile of values, just highlight them so you can find those you need for the questions). There are a couple of key things to remember about numbers:

   a.   Numbers on the MCAT are always accompanied by their units, either immediately following the number, or in the heading of the table where the numbers appear. If there are no units, the number must be unitless.

   b.   Highlighting can be done with a left-click and drag, then clicking the highlighting icon, but keep in mind that numbers in figures may not be in a format that allows for highlighting. In these cases, use your noteboard to note numbers.

7.   Finally, for lengthy Persuasive (Scientific) Reasoning passages, you may need to spend time fruitfully highlighting the text and dealing with complicated figures by redrawing a simplified version or carefully studying it on the screen. The fact that this will take longer is a legitimate reason to leave conceptual passages for last, but don't make the common error of thinking you have to understand everything you read! This is a multiple choice test, not an essay exam: you often don't need to understand this sort of question to be able to eliminate all but one answer choice.

Mapping a Physics Passage

Physics work should be done on paper; there are very few answers on the test that can be found without writing something down. Thus, your noteboard is your primary tool, whether solving FSQs or mapping a passage. "Mapping" involves the highlighting described above and preparing your noteboard to help you to answer the questions efficiently without having to fish for information. Here are some mapping strategies:

1.   Label your noteboard with the passage number and question numbers. Staying organized saves time and avoids errors.

2.   Write down any given equations with space below to work on them. The chances that you will *not* end up using some equation given to you in a passage are low, so it's worth the time to prepare for the algebra and estimation the questions will require. Moreover, merely copying the equations helps you to understand them better than you would just looking at them.

3.   If there are any simple diagrams, copy them down and label any values (some will be given in the text around the diagram and not labeled directly in the version on your screen). Again, you might resist this as a potential waste of time, but it is important to be able to manipulate the figures to answer the questions. For example, in a passage where forces are important (e.g., for most of mechanics, buoyancy in fluids, charges interacting with electric or magnetic fields, or simple harmonic oscillators), you should put the forces on your diagram *before* you do the questions. By doing so, you will probably anticipate the answers to one or more questions even before they are asked. Overall, this should both save you time and increase your percentage of right answers.

2.5

4. If the passage is conceptual or has conceptual parts to it, translate any mathematical statements written as sentences into symbols and treat those as you would equations given in a more technical passage. For example, if you were reading a passage on Poiseuille's law applied to blood flow and came across the sentence, "Poiseuille's law shows that the flow rate of a viscous fluid through a pipe with circular cross section is inversely proportional to the fourth power of its radius," you would jot down $f \propto 1/r^4$.

5. Especially for passages that don't include many diagrams or equations, write down the equations and basic ideas you recall about the passage topic. This will give you something tangible with which to tackle the questions. For example, a passage might describe a centrifuge spinning several test tubes at a constant rate for some period of time, and you might write down $a = v^2/r$ and "constant rpm $\rightarrow$ v/r = constant."

Practice all of these strategies with the passages in this book to see which work best for you; then make those strategies a part of your standard repertoire. Give yourself about two minutes to map a passage before you look at the questions. Many passage maps will take less time than this, a few might take longer. Don't worry that you're spending time not answering questions; practice will make you more efficient.

Another, more advanced study technique you might use once you feel more comfortable about your passage mapping is to map a couple of passages, put those maps aside for an hour or so while you do something else (practice FSQs), then go back to the passages, cover up their text, and try to do the questions with just your map. You shouldn't necessarily be able to answer all the questions without referring to the passage, but if you find that you're unable to answer any but those that rely on memory of basic concepts, then you need to improve your mapping technique. Below is an example of these strategies applied to a passage.

Blood flow through the vascular system of the human body is controlled by several factors. The rate of flow, Q, is directly proportional to the pressure differential, ΔP, between any two points in the system and inversely proportional to the resistance, R, of the system:

$$Q = \Delta P/R$$

Equation 1

The resistance, R, is dependent on the length of the vessel, L, the viscosity of blood, η, and the vessel's radius, r according to the equation

$$R = \frac{8\eta L}{\pi r^4}$$

Equation 2

Under normal conditions, vessel length and blood viscosity do not vary significantly. However, certain conditions can cause changes in blood content, thereby altering viscosity. Veins are generally more compliant than arteries due to their less muscular nature. The flow of blood through the major arteries can be approximated by the equations of ideal flow.

The dynamics of fluid movement from capillaries to body tissue and back to capillaries is also driven by pressure differentials. The net filtration pressure is the difference between the hydrostatic pressure of the blood in the capillaries, P_c, and the hydrostatic pressure of tissue fluid outside the capillaries, P_i. The oncotic pressure is the difference between the osmotic pressure of the capillaries, Π_c (approximately 25 torr), and the osmotic pressure of the tissue fluids, Π_i (negligible). Whether fluid moves into or out of the capillary network depends on the magnitudes of the net filtration and oncotic pressures. The direction of fluid movement can be determined by calculating the following pressure differential:

$$\Delta P = (P_c + \Pi_i) - (P_i + \Pi_c)$$

Equation 3

The sum in the first set of parentheses gives the pressure acting to move fluid out of the capillaries, while the sum in the second set of parentheses gives the pressure acting to move fluid into the capillaries.

Capillaries are porous, and the blood pressure on the arterial end of a capillary bed is enough to push fluid out of the capillaries and into the surrounding tissues. However, blood proteins and cells are too big to fit through the pores. Consequently, as the blood travels across the capillary bed, it becomes relatively more concentrated in proteins and cells; this leads to an osmotic influx of fluid on the venous side of the capillary bed. Note, however, that the volume of fluid lost to the tissues due to pressure is greater than the volume of fluid returned to the blood due to osmosis, so there is a net outward flow of fluid to the tissues. This excess fluid is recaptured and returned to the cardiovascular system via the lymphatic vessels.

Sample Passage Analysis and Mapping

Highlight the key phrase, "blood flow." Note that this passage is heavily laden with equations (three), has several potentially unfamiliar terms, and has no tabular data. This is best characterized as a technical Information Presentation passage, not as obscure as some if you understand the underlying biology and physics, but still challenging.

The overall lack of numbers is obvious, so just highlight the 25 torr for the osmotic pressure of the capillaries and be done with it. Some people might be more comfortable drawing a simple figure of blood moving from capillaries to tissues to capillaries and including pressures there, but that's up to you: this isn't a case in which a force diagram or simplified circuit will shed tremendous light on the phenomenon.

A few possibly unfamiliar terms like "net filtration pressure" and "oncotic pressure" appear and should be highlighted with their definitions. The definitions of some given variables are worth highlighting both because the symbols can be confusing (Q for flow rate, R for flow resistance) and in case you encounter a question that uses the words without the algebraic symbols. You should copy the three given equations on your noteboard, noting mentally the difference between this flow rate equation and the one you know from memory ($f = Av$). Remember, a new equation in a passage is always more important than a memorized equation for any questions that deal explicitly with the phenomenon described in the passage. At this point it may also be worthwhile to write down the continuity equation ($A_1v_1 = A_2v_2$). You should have committed to memory the rules for ideal fluid flow (including negligible viscosity) and know therefore that Bernoulli's equation would not apply except to the case of "major arteries."

The third paragraph presents perhaps the greatest mapping challenge for this passage. You might be tempted to highlight the entire paragraph because it describes an unfamiliar phenomenon. However, highlighting is not the same as comprehension; further, none of the terminology here is specialized. Thus, it's better to skip highlighting the paragraph entirely or to follow the rule to highlight causal phrases (as shown). It's worth noting that the passage doesn't actually mention what "certain conditions" are, so this paragraph lacks the information necessary to answer Explicit questions.

Your noteboard map should thus look something like this:

P3, Q11–16, Fluids

$$Q = \Delta P/R \qquad\qquad R = \frac{8\eta L}{\pi r^4} \qquad\qquad \Delta P = (P_c + \Pi_i) - (P_i + \Pi_c)$$

$$\Pi_c = 25 \text{ torr}, \ \Pi_i = 0$$

2.6 PHYSICS QUESTION TYPES

As stated previously, the questions in this section of the MCAT fall into one of three main categories:

1. **Memory questions**: Answered from concepts and equations you know walking into the test with just brute facts from the questions or passage, such as numbers or vector directions.
2. **Explicit questions**: Answered from information stated explicitly in the passage. To answer them correctly may require finding a definition, reading a graph, or manipulating a given equation.
3. **Implicit questions**: Answered by applying knowledge to a new situation or making more complex connections. Often the answer is implied by the information in the passage but requires logical reasoning on your part.

Note that the way you categorize questions on the MCAT will depend on how much knowledge you bring to the test in the first place. The more confident you are about the basic material outlined in the list of Physics topics, the less you will have to rely on the passage and question text to answer questions. This will ultimately save you those few precious seconds that can be better used for answering the tougher questions. For example, a passage may explicitly state the formula for the relationship of potential difference to the electric field and physical parameters of a parallel plate capacitor (i.e., $V = Ed$), but if you already know this formula, you will not need your map of the passage to find it when you need it to answer a question. That changes the type of question for you from Explicit to Memory.

Physics Memory Questions

These questions are often the easiest to answer. They follow a format that is more familiar for most students; typical Physics course work requires the memorization of formulas and facts, as well as their applications. Since Memory questions rely minimally if at all on information from the passage, they are similar to the freestanding questions on the MCAT.

Consider a question about the flow speed of blood in the major arteries taken from the previous blood flow passage. The following is an example of a Memory question.

The cross sectional area of the aorta is approximately 4 cm^2 and the total cross sectional area of the major arteries is 20 cm^2. If the speed of the blood in the aorta is 30 cm/sec, what is the average blood speed in the major arteries?

A)   5 cm/sec
B)   6 cm/sec
C)   120 cm/sec
D)   150 cm/sec

The equation to solve this question ($A_1v_1 = A_2v_2$) is not included in the passage.

Physics Explicit Questions

You need information directly from the passage in order to answer Explicit questions. It is critical to have a solid passage map so that information from the passage is easy to find and use. Even when you have inherent knowledge about the topic, it is important to read for information more specific to the precise situation in question.

Here's an example of an Explicit question from the blood flow passage:

Blood flow to the various systems in the body is regulated by the dilation and constriction of the blood vessels. After a person has eaten a large meal, the blood vessels supplying the digestive system dilate, increasing their radii by 50%. As a result of this blood vessel dilation, the flow of blood to the digestive system will:

A)   increase to 500% of the original flow.
B)   increase to 225% of the original flow.
C)   increase to 150% of the original flow.
D)   decrease to 50% of the original flow.

The equation needed to answer this question is given in the passage (Equation 2) and should be one that you recorded in your map. Note that you will always have to include information from the passage for an Explicit question.

Sometimes Explicit questions require more basic facts or principles from memory. In order to get the correct answer, you need to merge information from the passage with information you already know. For example, the passage gives an equation for a familiar variable in a new situation, and that must be blended with an understanding of the significance of that variable generally, or of other equations featuring that variable. These questions can appear straightforward but may be deceptively difficult, and it would certainly be justifiable to think of them as Implicit questions in some cases (the lines between the types are sometimes blurry).

The following is an example of an Explicit question using the blend of passage information and a bit of knowledge from memory:

> At the venular end of skeletal muscle capillaries, the hydrostatic pressure of the capillary is 17 torr and the hydrostatic pressure of the surrounding tissue is 1 torr. Fluid movement is from:
>
> A) the capillary to the tissue, at a rate proportional to 7 torr.
> B) the tissue to the capillary, at a rate proportional to 7 torr.
> C) the capillary to the tissue, at a rate proportional to 9 torr.
> D) the tissue to the capillary, at a rate proportional to 9 torr.

This asks about the pressure differential and the direction of fluid flow. This requires remembering that fluids move from high to low pressure (or correctly interpreting the final paragraph), but also requires using Equation 3 from the passage and the given values of osmotic pressures to solve for the numerical rate.

Physics Implicit Questions

This is the most difficult question type. Implicit questions often require information from memory, combined with information from the passage, and all applied to a new situation. They rely most heavily on critical reasoning skills, but also require a solid map, since information from the passage is usually needed. Most often, the answer choices for these questions contain a lot of words, but they can also sometimes be algebraic expressions or graphs. Note also that for many of these questions, you might be able to devise sound explanations that are not among the answer choices. However, there is always only *one* answer choice that *best* answers the question of all the options.

On Information and/or Situation passages, Implicit questions are often of the form "Which of the following best describes how [a parameter not mentioned in the passage] would change the [real world parameter described in the passage] from its present value?" The answers are verbal descriptions of increasing and decreasing values. Consider this example from the blood flow passage:

> Adaptation to life at high altitudes is characterized by polycythemia (high red blood cell count). Excluding other physiological compensations, what is the effect of this change on the flow of blood?
>
> A) Flow is decreased because viscosity is decreased.
> B) Flow is increased because viscosity is decreased.
> C) Flow is decreased because viscosity is increased.
> D) Flow is increased because viscosity is increased.

The correct answer would be selected by using background knowledge about viscosity and applying it to Equation 2, which describes the flow rate.

On Experiment/Research passages, Implicit questions are often of the form "Which of the following changes to the experiment would result in a change to [an experimental parameter]?" and are followed by verbal descriptions of changes to the apparatus, process, or mechanism of the experiment described in the passage. Suppose the following paragraph were added to the end of the Experiment/Research Presentation Passage example in Section 2.2.

> Confocal fluorescent microscopy relies on a light source of frequency tuned to the absorption frequencies of fluorescing compounds in the sample, focused through a pinhole using a converging mirror. This light illuminates the sample at specific focal planes, which are determined by a lens that focuses light both at the sample and eyepiece. Filters remove wavelengths other than those emitted by the fluorophores, and a semi-reflective mirror diverts the light to a pinhole, which is used in order to eliminate out-of-focus light from the image detector.

The following then is an example of an Implicit question in which the change to the apparatus is described in the answer choices:

> Which of the following changes if made without any additional changes would be LEAST LIKELY to affect the observed results of the experiments described in the passage?
>
> A) Using a fluorescing compound with a different wavelength dependence.
> B) Changing the index of refraction of the lens without changing its curvature or position.
> C) Decreasing the frequency of the light source from blue to yellow.
> D) Rotating the sample 180°.

This question requires recall of the principles of optics and properties of fluorescence, as well as some understanding of the apparatus described in the passage addendum.

On Persuasive or Scientific Reasoning passages, Implicit questions are often of the form "Which of the following phenomena best exemplifies or analogizes to the [physics concept]?" and are followed by verbal descriptions of physics phenomena. Often selecting the right answer requires a combination of eliminating wrong answers by logical reasoning (or common sense) and revisiting the passage for the precise definition of the principle in question. Consider the blood flow passage: it's really more of a technical Information Presentation passage than a Persuasive or Scientific Reasoning passage, but this example suits either.

An example of an Implicit question is

According to the following schematic diagram of
systemic circulation, which of the following is true?

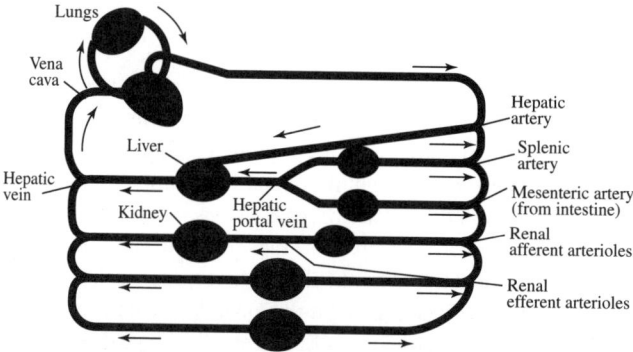

A) Vascular architecture of organs is in series so total
     peripheral resistance is greater than the resistance of
     individual organs.
B) Vascular architecture of organs is in parallel so total
     peripheral resistance is greater than the resistance of
     individual organs.
C) Vascular architecture of organs is in series so total
     peripheral resistance is less than the resistance of
     individual organs.
D) Vascular architecture of organs is in parallel so total
     peripheral resistance is less than the resistance of
     individual organs.

This question requires both understanding the analogy between resistance in blood flow and resistance in
circuits and remembering the rules for adding resistors.

The physics question types discussed so far categorize questions based on where to find the information
for the answer. There is another way to categorize questions based on *how* you achieve the answer once
you have the information.

Question Types by Technique

Algebraic Manipulation questions: These require use of one or several equation(s) to solve algebraically for a variable. Typically they have either numeric answer choices (e.g., "5 newtons") or algebraic
equations for answer choices (i.e. "$F_c = F_G + F_N$"). Another twist on algebraic manipulation questions
would be a question that asks for the units of an unfamiliar term (e.g., "What are the units for viscosity?")
followed by answer choices with a variety of units of measure.

Estimation/Computation questions: Are there numerical answer choices? It's likely you need to do some computation/approximation with a given or memorized equation (though *not necessarily:* be on the lookout for numbers directly implied by the scenario, such as the work done by a magnetic field always being zero). Just remember when you start plugging in numbers to check for shortcuts. Do all the answer choices have the same coefficient multiplied by different powers of ten? Then focus on the powers of ten and assume the coefficient comes out as given! Is your calculation coming out at 100 – (something hard to estimate)? Then the answer is <100 and all other choices can be eliminated. You can find more on approximation in chapter 15.

Functional Dependence/Proportionality questions: These require the use of one or more equations, graphs, or data tables to calculate proportions and changes in variables or values. These can have numeric answer choices, algebraic answer choices (e.g., "$a_{car} = -2a_{truck}$"), or verbal answer choices (e.g., "The radius doubles," or "The range increases from launch angle of 0° to launch angle of 45°, then decreases from launch angle of 45° to launch angle of 90°.").

Graph Generation or Interpretation questions: These require use of one or more equations, graphs, or data tables to create a graph of two variables; or they require you to locate points on a curve, the slope of a curve, or the area under a curve.

Conceptual questions: Is the question a paragraph and are all of the answer choices sentences? Such questions often require you to narrow down your choices by eliminating choices that express non-physical scenarios, like gravity having a horizontal component or a resistor dissipating more energy than was output by the only battery in its circuit. They can also require you to eliminate choices that aren't supported by the passage, such as choices that contradict a definition given for an italicized term.

2.7 SUMMARY OF THE APPROACH TO PHYSICS

As with all the science sections, when tackling the Chemical and Physical Foundations of Biological Systems section of the MCAT, it is best to do the easy questions first; typically, the freestanding questions are easier Memory questions, so when you get to them as you progress through the test, do them all. As mentioned previously, the best strategy for tackling passages is to decide quickly whether each passage in sequence is a "Do Now" or a "Do Later." Skip the "Do Later" ones, write "skip" on your noteboard next to the passage header you wrote for that passage so you can be sure to come back to it, then return to the skipped passages once you've gotten to the end of the test. Within each passage, again, save especially difficult questions until last, and make sure to fill in answers for ALL the questions before moving to the next passage. If you find a question or two especially difficult, make your best guess and be sure to click the "Flag for Review" button so that you can review the question later.

Since you will be skipping some questions within the test, it is important to keep your noteboard organized. Clearly indicate the passage and question number beside the work that you do for that question. If you think you've made an error in calculation, draw a line through your work and start again.

Notes

After reading the text of the question, you may need to draw a quick sketch or diagram. This step is particularly useful for freestanding questions. Don't waste time or space on ornate drawings; just sketch enough to record the basic vectors and the positive direction, and make sure that your drawing is big enough for you to add vectors or numbers to it.

Try to predict the physics formula you'll need to answer the question before looking at the answer choices. This will either be an equation from memory or from the passage. Write this formula (or formulas) on your noteboard by the label for the question. This will help when you want to review a previously flagged question. Instead of having to search for the information all over again, you have an indicator on your noteboard of where to start.

2.7

Avoid Confusion

When analyzing a question, remember that the situation will be ideal only when stated. Most of the concepts and equations you have memorized are for the ideal world. If the question asks for an approximation, the ideal world formulas are valid. If the question asks you to take the real world into consideration, look for a new formula or description in the passage that addresses the issue.

Remember to use the correct units! All calculations should be done with the "m.k.s." unit system (meters, kilograms, and seconds) unless otherwise specified. If you can't remember the formula, a unit analysis can help you regenerate or confirm the correct formula (for example, if you are solving a uniform circular motion question and you can't remember if velocity or radius is squared in the centripetal force equation, a quick unit analysis will show that velocity must be squared and the radius must *not* be squared in order to get an answer in newtons). Also, evaluating units may help you to quickly eliminate choices that have the wrong units. Finally, don't forget the "powers of 10": you may calculate the correct answer in meters, but if the answer choices are in millimeters, you will need to convert your results.

It can be helpful to form your own idea of the answer before looking at the choices. The MCAT tries to offer you similar-sounding answer choices that can muddle your thinking. Knowing what you are looking for before you read the answer choices keeps your POE focused.

Process of Elimination

Process of Elimination (POE) is paramount! Use the strikeout tool to indicate answer choices you have eliminated. Aggressively use process of elimination to improve your chances of guessing a correct answer even if you are not able to narrow it down to one choice. Remember each of the following POE strategies:

1. Eliminate answer choices that are clearly false or that do not answer the question.
2. If you think an answer choice is correct, double-check the remaining choices to confirm that they are incorrect. There may be two true statements in the answer choices, but only one best answer to the question; make sure the answer you choose addresses the issue in the question.
3. Remember that if two answer choices are essentially the same, neither can be correct, and both can be eliminated immediately.

4. Roman numeral questions: Whenever possible, start by evaluating the Roman numeral item that shows up in exactly two answer choices. This allows you to quickly eliminate two wrong answer choices regardless of whether the item is true or false. Typically then, you will only have to assess one of the other Roman numeral items to determine the correct answer. Always work between the I-II-III items and the answer choices. Once an item is found to be true (or false) strike out answer choices which do not contain (or do contain) that item number. Make sure to strike out the actual Roman numeral item as well, and highlight those items that are true.
5. LEAST/EXCEPT/NOT questions: Don't get tricked by these questions that ask you to pick that answer that doesn't fit (the incorrect or false statement). Make sure to highlight the words "LEAST," "EXCEPT," or "NOT" in the question stem. It's often good to use your noteboard and write "A B C D" with a T or F next to each answer choice. The one that stands out as different is the correct answer!
6. Work backwards, trying each answer choice to see if it correctly answers the question. This is particularly useful for questions such as "An increase in which of the following results in an increase in [some parameter] except...." Track these on your noteboard so you can see the work done for each answer choice tried.
7. If you have eliminated three answer choices, the fourth choice must be the correct choice. Don't waste time pondering why it is correct.

2.8 EXAMPLES OF STRATEGY IN USE

Below is an example of these strategies applied to the blood flow passage we mapped earlier.

1. The cross sectional area of the aorta is approximately 4 cm^2 and the total cross sectional area of the major arteries is 20 cm^2. If the speed of the blood in the aorta is 30 cm/sec, what is the average blood speed in the major arteries?

    A) 5 cm/sec
    B) 6 cm/sec
    C) 120 cm/sec
    D) 150 cm/sec

This is a memory computation question. Your initial reaction to the question might well be to check the given equations in the passage for a possible route, but you should quickly notice that none of them has a flow-speed term. The equation for flow speed in terms of area is the Continuity equation: $A_1 v_1 = A_2 v_2$. Solving for v_2 yields $\dfrac{A_1 v_1}{A_2} = \dfrac{\left(4 \text{ cm}^2\right)\left(30 \text{ cm/s}\right)}{\left(20 \text{ cm}^2\right)} = 6 \text{ cm/s}$. Nothing to it but plugging and chugging once you've identified that this might as well be a freestanding question. The correct answer is choice B.

2. Blood flow to the various systems in the body is regulated by the dilation and constriction of the blood vessels. After a person has eaten a large meal, the blood vessels supplying the digestive system dilate, increasing their radii by 50%. As a result of this blood vessel dilation, the flow of blood to the digestive system will:

A) increase to 500% of the original flow.
B) increase to 225% of the original flow.
C) increase to 150% of the original flow.
D) decrease to 50% of the original flow.

This is an explicit proportionality question. The question mentions a fractional change to the radius of the blood vessels and asks for a fractional change in blood flow rate (both expressed as percentages), which should immediately suggest to you that you want a proportion. Equations 1 and 2 combine to express just such a proportion, so directly under them on your mapping you can write $Q \propto 1/R$ and $R \propto 1/r^4$, thus $Q \propto r^4$. If r goes to 1.5 times its original value (immediately eliminating choice D), then Q goes to $(1.5)^4$ times its original value (eliminating choice C). Since $1.5^2 = 2.25$, choice B is eliminated, so the answer must be choice A.

3. Adaptation to life at high altitudes is characterized by polycythemia (high red blood cell count). Excluding other physiological compensations, what is the effect of this change on the flow of blood?

A) Flow is decreased because viscosity is decreased.
B) Flow is increased because viscosity is decreased.
C) Flow is decreased because viscosity is increased.
D) Flow is increased because viscosity is increased.

This is an implicit functional-dependence question with a 2x2 answer choice pattern, that is, two variables vary between two possible values or trends (flow and viscosity are increasing or decreasing). With such questions, it is best to focus on one variable at a time. In this case, the question implies by stating that red blood cell count increases that viscosity will increase (eliminating choices A and B): this relies on commonsense reasoning (more stuff floating around in the fluid will make it more viscous) more than explicit knowledge of the passage or memory of a specific equation. On an implicit question like this, you're being asked to rely on your intuition and logic when you have no specific equations or definitions to apply. If viscosity η increases, then according to Equations 1 and 2 combined (as with the previous question), Q will decrease (there's an inverse proportionality between flow rate and viscosity, $Q \propto 1/\eta$). Thus choice C is correct.

4. At the venular end of skeletal muscle capillaries, the hydrostatic pressure of the capillary is 17 torr and the hydrostatic pressure of the surrounding tissue is 1 torr. Fluid movement is from:

A)   the capillary to the tissue, at a rate proportional to 7 torr.
B)   the tissue to the capillary, at a rate proportional to 7 torr.
C)   the capillary to the tissue, at a rate proportional to 9 torr.
D)   the tissue to the capillary, at a rate proportional to 9 torr.

This is an explicit computation question, with some dependence on basic outside knowledge. Like question 3, it has a 2x2 pattern of answer choices. Applying Equation 3 (we recommend you do your work directly below where you wrote the equation on your mapping) with the numbers given in the question stem and the passage, we get $\Delta P = (17 + 0) - (1 + 25) = -9$ torr (eliminating choices A and B). If the pressure differential is negative, then there is greater pressure acting to move fluid into the capillaries (this is stated explicitly in the final paragraph, but you should also have basic knowledge that fluid naturally flows from high to low pressure). The correct answer is choice D.

2.8

5. According to the following schematic diagram of systemic circulation, which of the following is true?

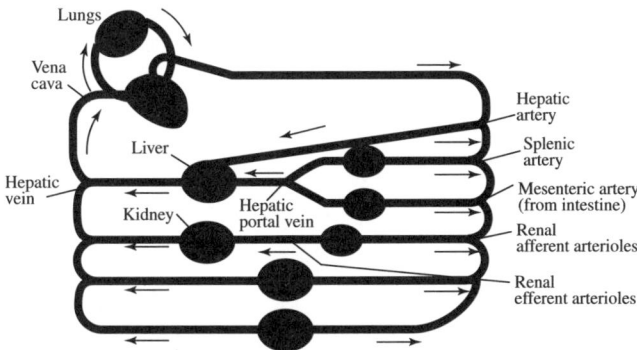

A)   Vascular architecture of organs is in series so total peripheral resistance is greater than the resistance of individual organs.
B)   Vascular architecture of organs is in parallel so total peripheral resistance is greater than the resistance of individual organs.
C)   Vascular architecture of organs is in series so total peripheral resistance is less than the resistance of individual organs.
D)   Vascular architecture of organs is in parallel so total peripheral resistance is less than the resistance of individual organs.

This is an implicit conceptual question. It requires you to make an analogy between fluid flow rate and current flow, an analogy justified by the similarity between Equation 1 and by Ohm's Law, $I = V/R$. The answer choices are once again in a 2x2 pattern, with the two variables being configuration (series or parallel) and total resistance (greater or less than the resistance of a single element, in this case an organ). Visual inspection of the provided diagram shows that the configuration (or "vascular architecture") is in parallel, because there are multiple paths the flow can take from and back to the heart. This eliminates choices A and C. At this point you must remember that resistors in parallel add reciprocally, so that the total resistance is always less than any given resistive element. Choice D is correct.

2.8

Chapter 3
Kinematics

3.1 UNITS AND DIMENSIONS

Before we begin our study of physics, we'll briefly go over metric units. Scientists —and the MCAT—use the Système International d'Unités (the International System of Units), abbreviated **SI**, to express the measurements of physical quantities. The **base units** of the SI that we'll be interested in (at least for most of our study of MCAT Physics) are listed below:

SI base unit	abbreviation	measures	dimension
meter	m	length	L
kilogram	kg	mass	M
second	s	time	T

This system of units is also referred to as the **mks system** (m̲ for meters, k̲ for kilograms, and s̲ for seconds). Each **dimension** is simply an abbreviation for the quantity that is being measured; it does not depend on the particular unit that's used. For example, we could measure a distance in miles, meters, or furlongs—to name a few—but in all cases, we're measuring a *length*. We say that distance has the dimensions of length, L. As another example, we could measure an object's speed in miles per hour, meters per second, or furlongs per fortnight; but regardless what units we use, we're always dividing a length by a time. Therefore, speed has dimensions of length per time (L/T).

Any physical quantity can be written in terms of the SI base units. Here are some examples:

quantity	symbol	units	dimensions
speed	v	m/s	L/T
density	ρ	kg/m^3	M/L^3
work	W	$kg \cdot m^2/s^2$	ML^2/T^2

Multiples of the base units that are powers of ten are often abbreviated and precede the symbol for the unit. For example, "n" is the symbol for nano-, which means 10^{-9} (one billionth). Thus, one billionth of a second, 1 nanosecond, would be written as 1 ns. The letter "M" is the symbol for mega-, which means 10^6 (one million), so a distance of one million meters, 1 megameter, would be abbreviated as 1 Mm.

Some of the most common power-of-ten prefixes are given in the following list:

prefix	symbol	multiple
pico-	p	10^{-12}
nano-	n	10^{-9}
micro-	μ	10^{-6}
milli-	m	10^{-3}
centi-	c	10^{-2}
kilo-	k	10^{3}
mega-	M	10^{6}
giga-	G	10^{9}

You should memorize this list.

On the MCAT, you won't need to convert between the American system of units (which uses things like inches, feet, yards, and pounds) and the metric system, so don't bother memorizing conversions like 2.54 cm = 1 inch or 39.37 inches = 1 meter, etc. You will need to be able to convert within the metric system using the powers-of-ten prefixes.

Example 3-1: Express a density of 5500 kg/m³ in g/cm³.

Solution: All we want to do with this physical measurement is to change the units in which it's expressed. For that, we need conversion factors. A **conversion factor** is simply a fraction whose value is 1, that multiplies a measurement in one set of units to give the equivalent measurement in a different set of units. In this case, we'd write

$$\rho = 5.5 \times 10^3 \, \frac{\text{kg}}{\text{m}^3} \times \left(\frac{10^3 \, \text{g}}{1 \, \text{kg}}\right) \times \left(\frac{1 \, \text{m}}{10^2 \, \text{cm}}\right)^3 = 5.5 \frac{\text{g}}{\text{cm}^3}$$

Notice that each of these conversion factors is written so that the unit we want to change (that is, the unit we want to eliminate) cancels out. The fraction

$$\frac{1 \, \text{kg}}{10^3 \, \text{g}}$$

is also a conversion factor for mass, but writing it like this would not have been helpful in this particular problem because then the "kg" would not have canceled.

Example 3-2: If a ball is dropped from a great height, then the force of air resistance it feels at any point during its descent is given by the equation $F = KD^2v^2$, where D is the diameter of the ball and v is its speed. If the units of F are kg·m/s², what are the units of K?

Solution: If the equation $F = KD^2v^2$ is to be valid, then the units of the left-hand side must be the same as the units of the right-hand side. To specify the unit of a quantity, we put brackets around it; for example, $[F]$ denotes the units of F; that is, $[F] = \text{kg·m/s}^2$. So we need to make sure that $[F] = [KD^2v^2]$, which means

$$[F] = [K][D]^2[v]^2$$
$$\frac{\text{kg} \cdot \text{m}}{\text{s}^2} = [K] \cdot \text{m}^2 \cdot \left(\frac{\text{m}}{\text{s}}\right)^2$$
$$= [K] \cdot \frac{\text{m}^4}{\text{s}^2}$$
$$\text{kg} \cdot \text{m} = [K] \cdot \text{m}^4$$
$$\therefore [K] = \frac{\text{kg}}{\text{m}^3}$$

3.2 KINEMATICS

Kinematics is the description of motion in terms of an object's position, velocity, and acceleration. The MCAT will expect not only that you can answer mathematical questions about these quantities but also that you know the definitions of these quantities.

Displacement

The **displacement** of an object is its change in position. For example, let's say we were measuring an object moving along a straight line by laying a meter stick along the object's line of motion. If the object starts at, say, the *10 cm* mark on the meter stick and moves to the *70 cm* mark, then its position changed by 70 cm − 10 cm = 60 cm, so we'd say its displacement is 60 cm.

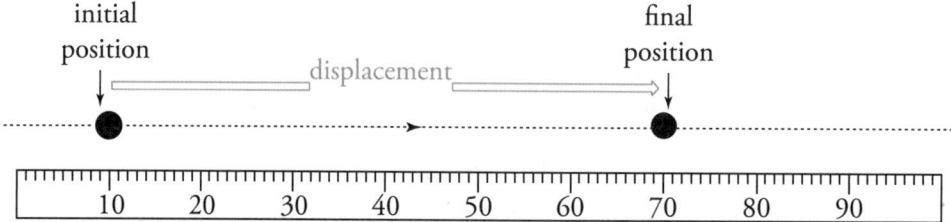

We find the displacement by subtracting the object's initial position from its final position:

$$\text{displacement} = \Delta(\text{position}) = \text{position}_{\text{final}} - \text{position}_{\text{initial}}$$

Now, what if the object moved from the *70 cm* mark on the meter stick to the *10 cm* mark? Then its displacement would be 10 cm − 70 cm = −60 cm.

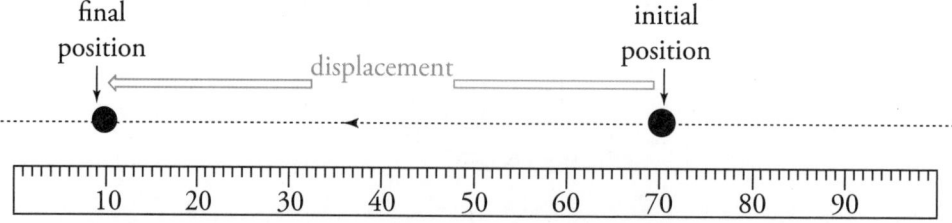

In both cases, the object moved a distance of 60 cm, but in the first case it moved to the right, and in the second case, it moved to the left. Displacement is a vector, so it takes direction into account. If we call *to the right* the positive direction (hence *to the left* automatically becomes the negative direction) then in the first case, we'd say the displacement is +60 cm, and in the second case, it's −60 cm.

The motion of the object can be more complicated. For example, what if the object started at the *10 cm* mark, moved to the *50 cm* mark, back to the *40 cm* mark, and then over to the *70 cm* mark?

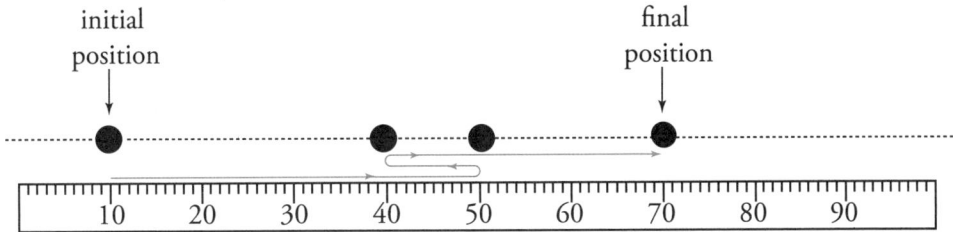

This example brings up a crucial point about displacement. The *total* distance that the object travels is (40 cm) + (10 cm) + (30 cm) = 80 cm, but the object's displacement is still

displacement $\quad= \Delta(\text{position}) = \text{position}_{\text{final}} - \text{position}_{\text{initial}}$

$\qquad\qquad = (70 \text{ cm}) - (10 \text{ cm})$

$\qquad\qquad = +60 \text{ cm}$

Displacement gives us the *net* distance traveled by the object, which may very well be less than the total distance. So, the displacement is a vector that always points from the object's initial position to its final position, *regardless of the path the object took*, and whose magnitude is the *net* distance traveled by the object. There are multiple different symbols that are used to represent the displacement vector, such as $\Delta\mathbf{s}$, but the most common one is the single letter $\mathbf{d}$. Sometimes, we use $\Delta\mathbf{x}$ if we know the displacement is horizontal or $\Delta\mathbf{y}$ if we know the displacement is vertical. Be aware that the MCAT also uses the word *displacement* to mean just the magnitude of the displacement vector (that is, just the net distance traveled by the object without regard for direction); the question will make it clear which meaning is intended.

Displacement

$$\mathbf{d} = \text{position}_{\text{final}} - \text{position}_{\text{initial}} = \text{net distance plus direction}$$

For example, if a sprinter runs 400 meters around a circular track and returns to her starting point, she has covered a *total* distance of 400 meters, but her *displacement* is zero. If a sprinter runs 300 meters north, then 400 meters east, he's covered a total distance of 700 m, but his displacement is only 500 meters.

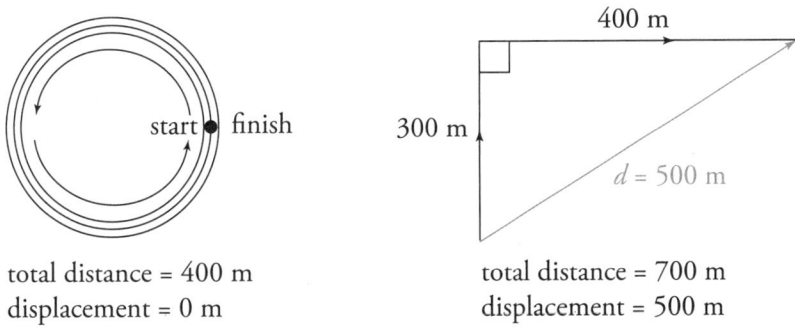

total distance = 400 m
displacement = 0 m

total distance = 700 m
displacement = 500 m

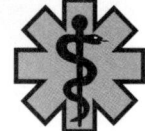

Example 3-3: Though the total length of all pathways of the human circulatory system is on the order of 10^8 m, a typical red blood cell may complete a circuit of about 3 meters in one minute.

    a)   What is the total distance traveled by a red blood cell in an hour?

    b)   What is its total displacement in that time?

Solution:

    a)   If 3 m are traveled in a minute, then 3 m/min × 60 min/hour = 180 m will be traveled in an hour.

    b)   Displacement is the net change in position. If a circuit is completed, regardless of the number of times, the displacement is 0 m.

Velocity

Displacement tells us how much an object's position changes. **Velocity** tells us how *fast* an object's position changes. If you're in a car traveling at 60 miles per hour along a long, straight highway, then this means your position changes by 60 miles every hour. To calculate velocity, simply divide how much the position has changed by how much time it took for it to change; in other words, divide displacement by time.

Average Velocity

$$\text{average velocity} = \frac{\text{displacement}}{\text{time}}$$

$$\bar{\mathbf{v}} = \frac{\Delta x}{\Delta t} = \frac{\mathbf{d}}{\Delta t}$$

This is actually the definition of **average velocity**, and we place a bar above the $\mathbf{v}$ to signify that it's an *average*. So, $\mathbf{v}$ is velocity and $\bar{\mathbf{v}}$ is average velocity. (If the velocity happens to be constant, then there's no distinction between *velocity* and *average velocity*, and we don't need the bar.) Notice right away that velocity is a vector; after all, we're dividing a vector (the displacement, $\mathbf{d}$) by a number, so we're left with a vector. In fact, because Δt is always positive, $\bar{\mathbf{v}}$ always points in the same direction as $\mathbf{d}$.

The magnitude of the velocity vector is called the **speed**. Speed is a scalar; it has no direction and can never be negative. (Notice that the speedometer in your car is well-named; it only tells you how fast the car is moving, not the direction of motion. It's not a "velocity-o-meter.") Velocity is a vector that specifies both speed and direction.

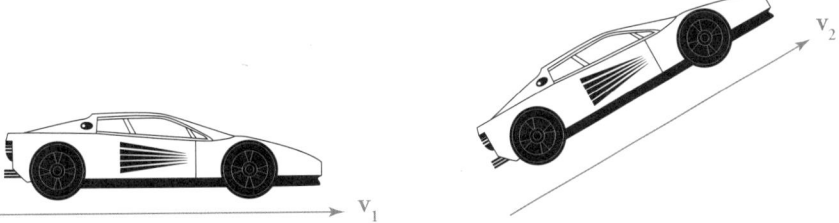

Velocity

$$\mathbf{v} = \text{speed \& direction}$$

In the figure below, each vector represents the car's velocity. Both cars have the same speed (let's say 20 m/s), so the magnitudes of their velocity vectors are the same. Nevertheless, they have different velocities, because the directions are different. (By the way, if the car on the right looks bigger than the car on the left, it's an optical illusion. Grab a ruler and check it for yourself. They're the same size!)

These two cars have the same speed but different velocities. Is it possible for two cars to have the same velocity but different speeds? No. Velocity is speed plus direction, so if the velocities are the same, then the speeds (and the directions) are the same.

Example 3-4: Though the total length of all pathways of the human circulatory system is on the order of 10^8 m, a typical red blood cell may complete a circuit of about 3 meters in one minute.

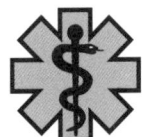

a) What is the average velocity of this red blood cell?
b) What is its average speed?

Solution:

a) In example 3-3(b) we determined that the displacement of the red blood cell was 0 m. Thus by definition the average velocity must be 0 m/s.
b) Average speed is not the magnitude of average velocity. (Confusing, though this example should make clear why this must be the case.) Rather, it is by definition the total distance traveled divided by time. In this case, $v = (3 \text{ m/min})(1 \text{ min}/60 \text{ sec}) = 1/20$ m/s or 0.05 m/s.

Example 3-5: A sprinter runs 300 meters north, then 400 meters east, which takes 100 seconds.

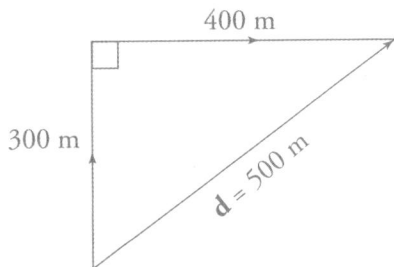

What was his average speed? What was the magnitude of his average velocity?

Solution: The sprinter's average speed was (700 m)/(100 s) = 7 m/s. However, because his displacement is 500 m, his average velocity has a magnitude of (500 m)/(100 s) = 5 m/s.

Example 3-6: An object moves from Point A to Point B in 4 seconds.

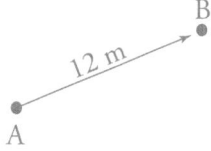

What was the object's velocity?

   A.   3 m/s
   B.   8 m/s
   C.   6 m/s
   D.   48 m/s

Solution: Notice that the question is asking for velocity (which is a vector) but all the choices are scalars. Strictly speaking, the answer should include the correct direction as well as the magnitude. However, the MCAT (as well as textbook authors and teachers) will often use the word *velocity* when they mean *speed*; usually, it won't cause confusion. From the choices given, we know it's the magnitude of the velocity that is the desired quantity, and this is

$$v = \frac{\Delta x}{\Delta t} = \frac{12 \text{ m}}{4 \text{ s}} = 3 \text{ m/s}$$

Choice A is the answer we'd choose.

Acceleration

Velocity tells us how fast an object's position changes. **Acceleration** tells us how fast an object's *velocity* changes.

> **Average Acceleration**
>
> $$\text{average acceleration} = \frac{\text{change in velocity}}{\text{time}}$$
>
> $$\overline{\mathbf{a}} = \frac{\Delta \mathbf{v}}{\Delta t}$$

Acceleration is a little trickier than velocity. Even though both involve how fast something changes, acceleration is how fast velocity changes, and an object's velocity changes if the speed *or* the direction changes. So, for example, an object can be accelerating even if its speed is constant. This is a very important point and a potential MCAT trap.

In everyday language, we use the word *acceleration* to describe what happens when we step on the gas pedal and go faster. Well, that's certainly an example of acceleration even from the "proper" physics perspective, but it isn't the only example of acceleration.

What happens when you step on the brake? You slow down. Is that acceleration? Yes, although we might also call it a *deceleration*, because our speed changes.

Now, imagine that you set the car on cruise control at, say, 60 miles per hour. Up ahead you see a curve in the road, so as you approach it, you slowly turn the wheel to stay on the road. Even though your speed remains constant, your direction of motion changes, which means your velocity vector changes. Thus, you experience an acceleration.

Let's try this one. Throw a baseball straight up into the air. It rises, gets to the top of its path, then falls back down. At the moment it's at the top of its path, its velocity is zero. What is the ball's acceleration at this point?

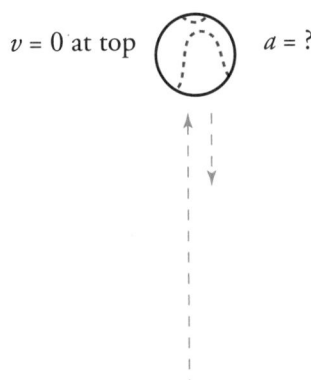

$v = 0$ at top　　$a = ?$

A common answer is, "If the velocity is 0, then the acceleration is 0 too." Let's see why this isn't the case here. What's happening to the baseball's velocity at the top of the path? Its direction is changing from up to *down*. The fact that the velocity is changing means there's an acceleration, so the acceleration can't be zero at the top of the path. Here's another way of looking at it: What if the acceleration *were* zero at the top? Zero acceleration means no change in velocity, so if $a = 0$ at a certain point, then whatever velocity there is at that point will stay constant. Does the velocity of the baseball remain zero? No, because the ball immediately starts to fall toward the ground.

Example 3-7: The velocity of an object moving along a straight line changes from $v_i = 4$ m/s at time $t_i = 0$ to $v_f = 10$ m/s at time $t_f = 2$ sec.

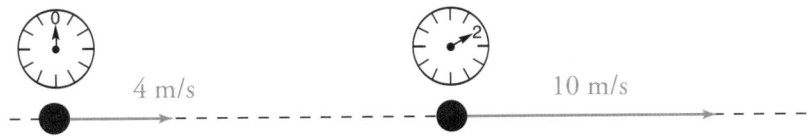

4 m/s　　10 m/s

What was the object's average acceleration during this time interval?

Solution: By definition of average acceleration, we have

$$\bar{\mathbf{a}} = \frac{\Delta \mathbf{v}}{\Delta t} = \frac{\mathbf{v}_f - \mathbf{v}_i}{t_f - t_i} = \frac{10 \text{ m/s} - 4 \text{ m/s}}{(2 \text{ s}) - 0 \text{ s}} = 3 \text{ m/s}^2$$

Notice that $\bar{\mathbf{a}}$ is positive, which means that it points to the right, just like $\mathbf{v}_i$. If the acceleration points in the *same* direction as the initial velocity, then the object's speed is *increasing*.

Example 3-8: The velocity of an object moving along a straight line changes from $\mathbf{v}_i$ = 7 m/s at time t_i = 0 to $\mathbf{v}_f$ = 1 m/s at time t_f = 3 sec.

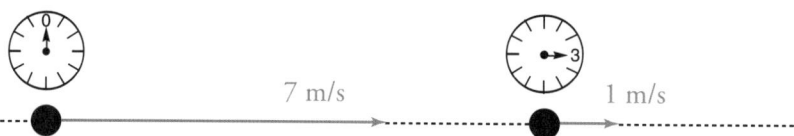

What was the object's average acceleration during this time interval?

Solution: By definition of average acceleration, we have

$$\bar{\mathbf{a}} = \frac{\Delta \mathbf{v}}{\Delta t} = \frac{\mathbf{v}_f - \mathbf{v}_i}{t_f - t_i} = \frac{1 \text{ m/s} - 7 \text{ m/s}}{(3 \text{ s}) - 0 \text{ s}} = -2 \text{ m/s}^2$$

Notice that $\bar{\mathbf{a}}$ is negative, which means that it points to the left, in the direction opposite to $\mathbf{v}_i$. If the acceleration points in the direction *opposite* to the initial velocity, then the object's speed is *decreasing*.

Example 3-9: The velocity of an object moving along a straight line changes from $\mathbf{v}_i$ = −2 m/s at time t_i = 0 to $\mathbf{v}_f$ = −5 m/s at time t_f = 2 sec.

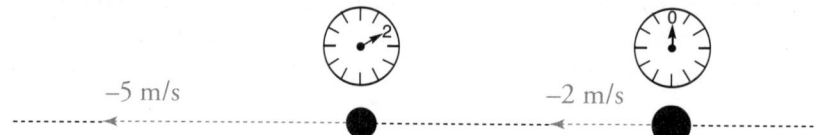

What was the object's average acceleration during this time interval?

Solution: By definition of average acceleration, we have

$$\bar{\mathbf{a}} = \frac{\Delta \mathbf{v}}{\Delta t} = \frac{\mathbf{v}_f - \mathbf{v}_i}{t_f - t_i} = \frac{-5 \text{ m/s} - (-2 \text{ m/s})}{(2 \text{ s}) - 0 \text{ s}} = -1.5 \text{ m/s}^2$$

Notice that $\bar{\mathbf{a}}$ is negative, which means that it points to the left, just like $\mathbf{v}_i$. If the acceleration points in the *same* direction as the initial velocity, then the object's speed is *increasing*.

Example 3-10: The velocity of an object changes from $\mathbf{v}_1$ at time $t_i = 0$ to $\mathbf{v}_2$ at time $t_f = 2$ sec.

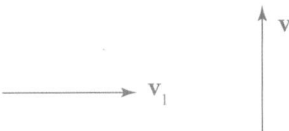

Which of the following best illustrates the object's average acceleration during this time interval?

A. ↑

B. ↘

C. ↗

D. ↘

Solution: By definition of average acceleration, we have

$$\overline{\mathbf{a}} = \frac{\Delta \mathbf{v}}{\Delta t} = \frac{\mathbf{v}_2 - \mathbf{v}_1}{t_f - t_i} = \frac{\mathbf{v}_2 - \mathbf{v}_1}{2\,\text{s}}$$

The direction of $\overline{\mathbf{a}}$ is (always) the same as the direction of $\Delta \mathbf{v} = \mathbf{v}_2 - \mathbf{v}_1 = \mathbf{v}_2 + (-\mathbf{v}_1)$. The following diagram shows how we find $\mathbf{v}_2 + (-\mathbf{v}_1)$:

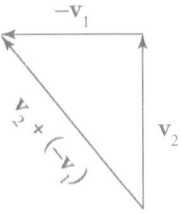

Therefore, choice B is the best answer.

The direction of **a** tells **v** how to change; the following diagrams summarize the possibilities:

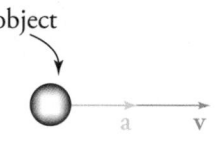

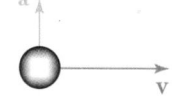

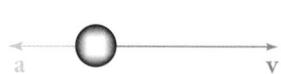

a in the same direction as **v** means object's speed is increasing.

a perpendicular to **v** means object's speed is constant.

a in the opposite direction from **v** means object's speed is decreasing.

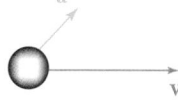

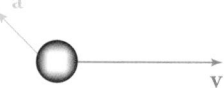

a at an angle between 0° and 90° to **v** means object's speed is increasing and direction of **v** is changing.

a at an angle between 90° and 180° to **v** means object's speed is decreasing and direction of **v** is changing.

Example 3-11: The velocity and acceleration of an object at a certain point are shown in the diagram below.

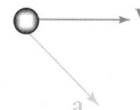

Describe the object's velocity a short time later.

Solution: We split the acceleration vector into components, one along the direction of **v** and one perpendicular to the direction of **v**:

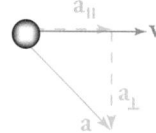

The component $\mathbf{a}_{\parallel}$ points along the line of the object's motion, so the *speed* of the object will change; in particular, the speed will *increase*, since $\mathbf{a}_{\parallel}$ points in the *same* direction as **v**. The component of **a** that's perpendicular to **v**, $\mathbf{a}_{\perp}$, will make the *direction* of **v** change; in particular, it will turn downward (since $\mathbf{a}_{\perp}$ points downward). Therefore, we'd expect the object to increase in speed as it turns downward.

3.3 [A]CCELERATED MOTION

In the las[t] [...] [p]rincipal quantities of kinematics: displacement, velocity, and acceleration. In t[...] [characte]rize the mathematical relationships between them in the special but
important [...] [acc]elerated motion. This is motion in which the object's acceleration, **a**, is
constant.

The defini[tion] [...] $\mathbf{v} = \Delta\mathbf{s}/\Delta t$. We can rewrite this equation without a fraction like this:
$\Delta\mathbf{s} = \overline{\mathbf{v}}\Delta t$. [...] [notatio]n, let's agree to (1) use **d** for displacement, (2) use t, rather than Δt, for
the time interval, and (3) abandon the bolding for vectors (although we'll still specify the direction of a
vector by either a plus or a minus sign). With this change in notation, the equation reads simply $d = \overline{v}t$.
In the case of uniformly accelerated motion (which means a is constant), the average velocity, $\overline{v}$ is just the
average of the initial and final velocities: $\frac{1}{2}(v_i + v_f)$. Using t instead of Δt for the time interval means that
we're setting the initial time, t_i, equal to 0 and that we're letting t stand for the final time, t_f (notice that
$\Delta t = t_f - t_i = t - 0 = t$). The initial velocity is then the velocity at time 0, which we write as v_0 (pronounced
"v zero" or "v naught") and the final velocity is v (dropping the subscript "f" on v_f just like we're dropping
the subscript "f" on t_f). Therefore, the average velocity can be written as $\overline{v} = \frac{1}{2}(v_0 + v)$, and the equation
for d becomes $d = \frac{1}{2}(v_0 + v)t$.

The definition of average acceleration is $\overline{a} = \Delta v/\Delta t$. We can rewrite this equation without a fraction like
this: $\Delta v = \overline{a}\Delta t$. Now, since we are specifically looking at uniformly accelerated motion (motion in which
the acceleration is constant), then there's no need for the bar on the **a**. After all, if **acceleration** is a constant, there's no distinction between **a** and $\overline{a}$. So, removing the bar and using the simplified notation
described in the last paragraph, the equation becomes $\Delta v = at$, or $v = v_0 + at$.

The two equations $d = \frac{1}{2}(v_0 + v)t$ and $v = v_0 + at$ follow directly from the definitions of average velocity
and acceleration. There are three other equations that relate these quantities, but they would require more
algebra to derive them. Instead of boring you with the details, we'll just state them. Since there are five
equations, we call them **The Big Five**:

The Big Five

1. $d = \frac{1}{2}(v_0 + v)t$ missing a

2. $v = v_0 + at$ missing d

3. $d = v_0 t + \frac{1}{2}at^2$ missing v

4. $d = vt - \frac{1}{2}at^2$ missing v_0

5. $v^2 = v_0^2 + 2ad$ missing t

3.3

Notice that these equations involve *five* quantities—d, v_0, v, a, and t—and there are *five* equations. Each equation has exactly one of those quantities missing, and this is how you decide which equation to use in a particular problem. A quantity is *missing* from the problem if it's *not given and not asked for*. For example, if a question does not give or ask for v, then use Big Five #3; if a question does not give or ask for t, then use Big Five #5. On the MCAT, the Big Five equations that are used most frequently are #2, #3, and #5.

Example 3-12: An object has an initial velocity of 3 m/s and a constant acceleration of 2 m/s² in the same direction. What will the object's velocity be at $t = 6$ s?

Solution: We're given v_0, a, and t, and asked for v. Since the displacement, d, is neither given nor asked for, we use Big Five #2:

$$v = v_0 + at = 3 \text{ m/s} + (2 \text{ m/s}^2)(6 \text{ s}) = 15 \text{ m/s}$$

Example 3-13: A particle has an initial velocity of 10 m/s and a constant acceleration of 3 m/s² in the same direction. How far will the particle travel in 4 seconds?

Solution: We're given v_0, a, and t, and asked for d. Since the final velocity, v, is missing, we use Big Five #3:

$$d = v_0 t + \tfrac{1}{2} at^2 = (10 \text{ m/s})(4 \text{ s}) + \tfrac{1}{2}(3 \text{ m/s}^2)(4 \text{ s})^2 = 64 \text{ m}$$

Example 3-14: An object starts from rest and travels in a straight line with a constant acceleration of 4 m/s² in the same direction until its final velocity is 20 m/s. How far does it travel during this time?

Solution: We're given v_0, a, and v, and asked for d. Since the time, t, is neither given nor asked for, we use Big Five #5. Because the object starts from rest, we know that $v_0 = 0$, so we get

$$v^2 = v_0^2 + 2ad \;\rightarrow\; v^2 = 2ad \;\rightarrow\; d = \frac{v^2}{2a} = \frac{(20 \text{ m/s})^2}{2(4 \text{ m/s}^2)} = 50 \text{ m}$$

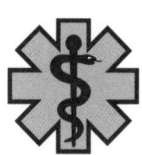

Example 3-15: A particular red blood cell traveling through the aorta has a peak speed of 92 cm/s after accelerating for 98 ms at a rate of 470 cm/s². What was its speed before undergoing this acceleration?

Solution: We're given a, v, and t, and asked for v_0. Since the displacement, d, is neither given nor asked for, we use Big Five #2:

$$v = v_0 + at \rightarrow v_0 = v - at = (92 \text{ cm/s}) - (470 \text{ cm/s}^2)(0.098 \text{ s}) \approx 45 \text{ cm/s}$$

3.4 KINEMATICS WITH GRAPHS

The MCAT expects you to be able to interpret graphs as well as to be able to apply equations. In general, you will need to be able to extract three forms of information from graphs: individual points, slopes, and areas. Below we consider these in two types of graphs: the **position vs. time** graph and the **velocity vs. time** graph.

Consider the following graph, which gives an object's position, x, as a function of time, t:

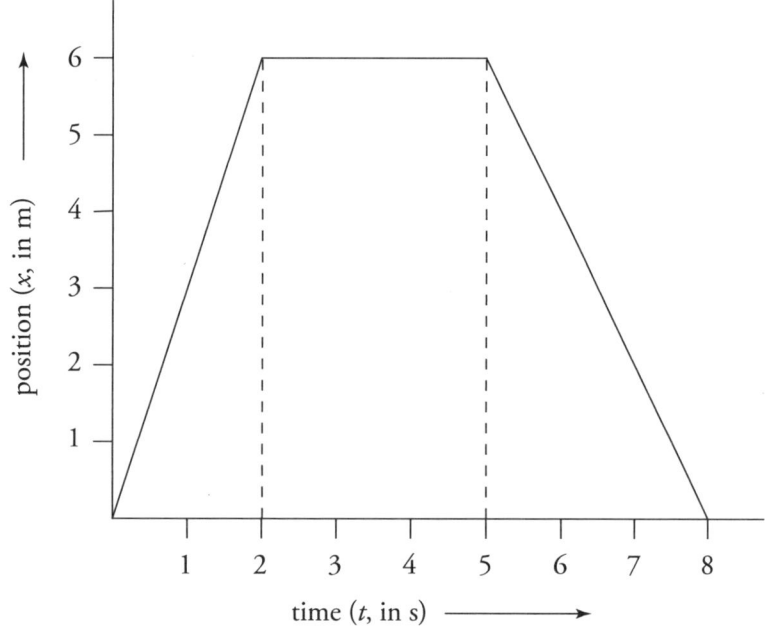

The object starts at $x = 0$, then moves to $x = 6$ m at $t = 2$ s. From $t = 2$ s to $t = 5$ s, it remains at position $x = 6$ m. Then, from $t = 5$ s to $t = 8$ s, the object moves from $x = 6$ m back to $x = 0$.

Let's figure out its velocity during these time intervals. From $t = 0$ to $t = 2$ s, its velocity is

$$v = \frac{\Delta x}{\Delta t} = \frac{x - x_0}{t_f - t_i} = \frac{(6 \text{ m}) - (0 \text{ m})}{2 \text{ s}} = 3 \text{ m/s}$$

Note that Δx is the vertical change in this graph and Δt is the horizontal change, from $t = 0$ to $t = 2$ s. Dividing a vertical change by the corresponding horizontal change gives the *slope* of a graph. So, we have this rule:

The slope of a position vs. time graph gives the velocity.

From $t = 2$ s to $t = 5$ s, the object remained at position $x = 6$ m. Since the object didn't move, we expect its velocity during this time interval to be zero. Also, notice that the graph is flat here, and the slope of a flat line is 0.

Finally, from $t = 5$ s to $t = 8$ s, the velocity is

$$v = \frac{\Delta x}{\Delta t} = \frac{x - x_0}{t_f - t_i} = \frac{(0 \text{ m}) - (6 \text{ m})}{(8 \text{ s}) - (5 \text{ s})} = -2 \text{ m/s}$$

This is the slope of the graph from $t = 5$ s to $t = 8$ s.

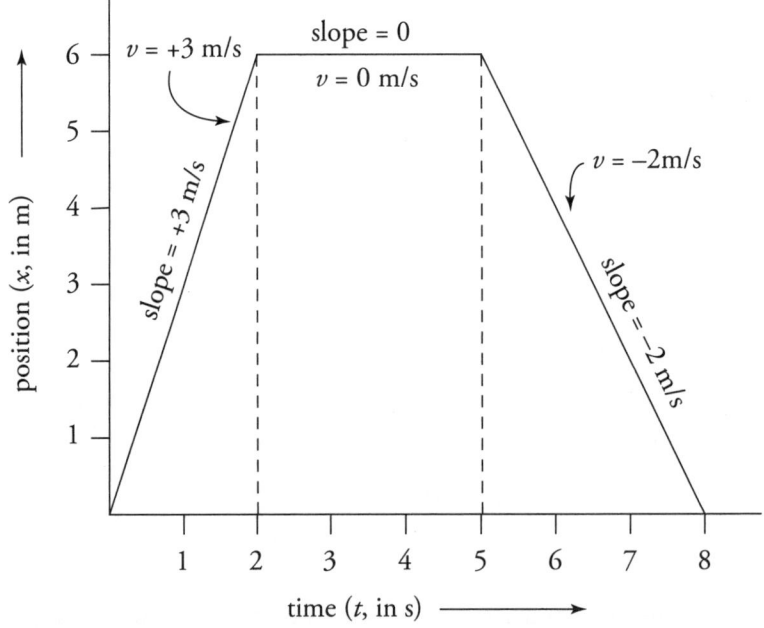

Now consider the following graph, which gives an object's velocity, v, as a function of time, t:

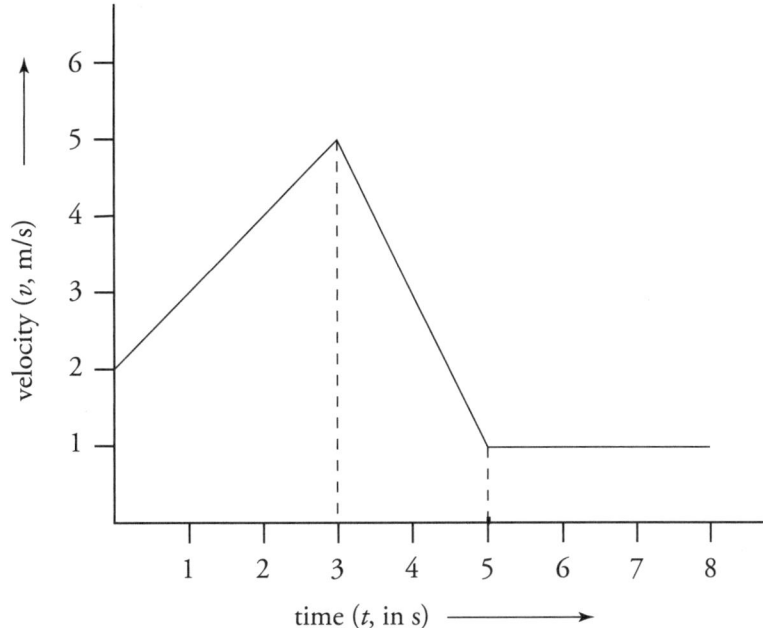

The object's velocity at $t = 0$ is $v = 2$ m/s, and steadily increases to $v = 5$ m/s at time $t = 3$ s. From $t = 3$ s to $t = 5$ s, the velocity decreases to $v = 1$ m/s. Then, from $t = 5$ s to $t = 8$ s, the object's velocity remains constant at $v = 1$ m/s.

Let's figure out the object's acceleration during these time intervals. From $t = 0$ to $t = 3$ s, its acceleration is

$$a = \frac{\Delta v}{\Delta t} = \frac{v - v_0}{t} = \frac{\left(5 \text{ m/s}\right) - \left(2 \text{ m/s}\right)}{3 \text{ s}} = 1 \text{ m/s}^2$$

Note that $\Delta \mathbf{v}$ is the vertical change in this graph and Δt is the horizontal change, from $t = 0$ to $t = 3$ s. Once again, dividing a vertical change by the corresponding horizontal change gives the slope of a graph. So, we have this rule:

> The slope of a velocity vs. time graph gives the acceleration.

From $t = 3$ s to $t = 5$ s, the acceleration is

$$a = \frac{\Delta v}{\Delta t} = \frac{v - v_0}{t - t_0} = \frac{\left(1 \text{ m/s}\right) - \left(5 \text{ m/s}\right)}{5 \text{ s} - 3 \text{ s}} = -2 \text{ m/s}^2$$

This is the slope of the graph from $t = 3$ s to $t = 5$ s.

Finally, from $t = 5$ s to $t = 8$ s, the object's velocity remained constant at $v = 1$ m/s. Since the object's velocity didn't change, we expect its acceleration during this time interval to be zero. The graph is flat here, and the slope of a flat line is 0.

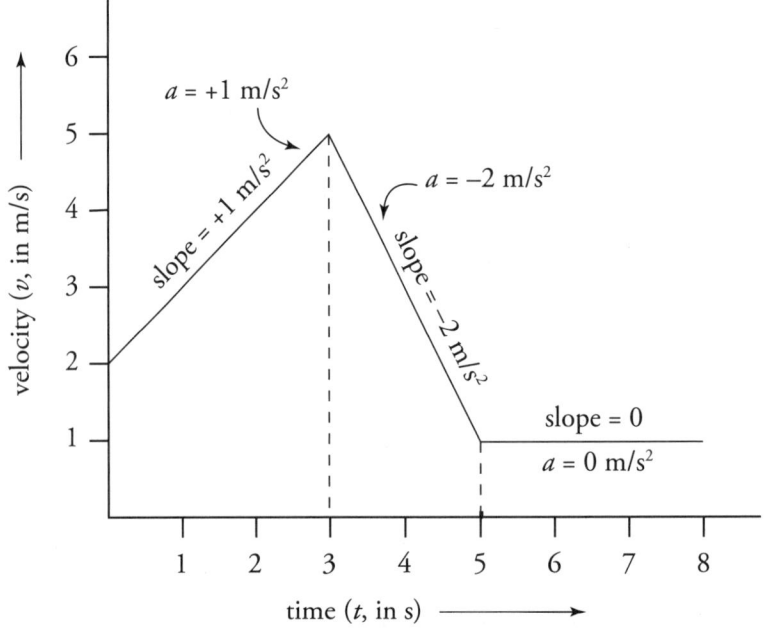

Besides asking about the object's acceleration, there's an additional type of question we could be asked given an object's velocity vs. time graph. For example, what was the object's *displacement* from $t = 5$ s to $t = 7$ s? Since the object's velocity was a constant $v = 1$ m/s, we just use the basic equation *distance = rate × time* (which is really just Big Five #1 in the case where v is constant) to find that $d = (1$ m/s$)(2$ s$) = 2$ m. But if we look at the graph, we realize that what we've just found is the *area* under the graph from $t = 5$ s to $t = 7$ s. After all, the area under the graph is just a rectangle for which the height is a velocity and the base is a time. The area of a rectangle is *base × height* (*bh*), so we're multiplying velocity × time, and that gives us displacement. The same rule applies even if the graph isn't flat:

> The area under a velocity vs. time graph gives the displacement.

What is the object's displacement from $t = 0$ to $t = 3$ s? It will be the area under the velocity vs. time graph from $t = 0$ to $t = 3$ s. The figure below shows that we can split this area into two pieces: a triangle whose area is $\frac{1}{2}bh = \frac{1}{2}(3\,\text{s})(3\,\text{m/s}) = \frac{9}{2}$ m, and a rectangle whose area is $bh = (3\,\text{s})(2\,\text{m/s}) = 6$ m. Therefore, the object's displacement from $t = 0$ to $t = 3$ s, which is the *total* area under the graph between $t = 0$ and $t = 3$ s, is $\left(\frac{9}{2}\,\text{m}\right) + (6\,\text{m}) = 10.5\,\text{m}$.

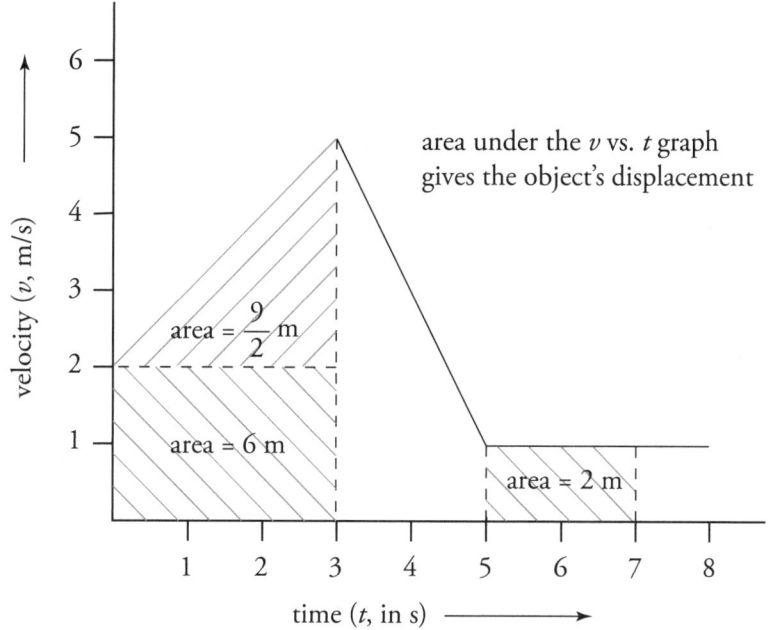

We can check this result using Big Five #1:

$$d = \frac{1}{2}(v_0 + v)t = \frac{1}{2}(2 \text{ m/s} + 5 \text{ m/s})(3 \text{ s}) = 10.5 \text{ m}$$

Example 3-16: For the object whose velocity vs. time graph is shown below, what is its displacement from $t = 2$ s to $t = 5$ s?

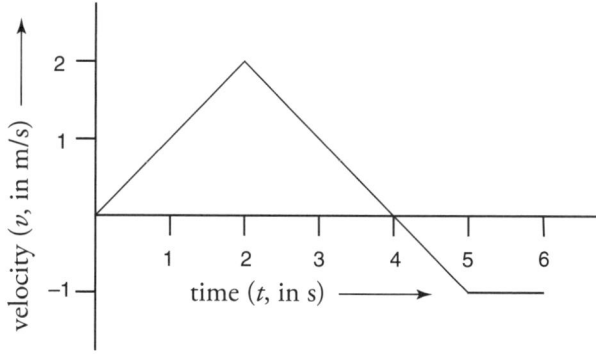

Solution: The area under the graph (or, more precisely, the area between the graph and the t-axis) gives the object's displacement. The area under the graph from $t = 2$ s to $t = 4$ s is $\frac{1}{2}bh = \frac{1}{2}(2 \text{ s})(2 \text{ m/s}) = 2$ m. After $t = 4$ s, the graph is *below* the t-axis, so any area here counts *negatively*. From $t = 4$ s to $t = 5$ s, the area is $\frac{1}{2}bh = \frac{1}{2}(1 \text{ s})(-1 \text{ m/s}) = -0.5$ m. Therefore, the total area between the graph and the t-axis, from $t = 2$ s to $t = 5$ s, is $(2 \text{ m}) + (-0.5 \text{ m}) = 1.5$ m.

3.5 FREE FALL

The Big Five are used only in situations where the acceleration is constant. The most important "real life" situation in which motion takes place under constant acceleration is **free fall**, which describes an object moving only under the influence of gravity (ignoring any effects due to the air, such as air resistance and buoyancy).

Near the surface of the earth, the magnitude of **g**, the **gravitational acceleration**, is approximately equal to 9.8 m/s². *For the MCAT, we can use the simpler approximation of 10 m/s².* The term "free fall" might make you think that The Big Five apply only to objects that are actually falling, but if we throw a baseball up into the air (and ignore effects due to the air), then the ball is still experiencing the downward acceleration due to gravity, so it, too, would be considered in free fall. So, think of free fall not as a description of a downward velocity but as a description of a downward *acceleration*.

The way we decide which Big Five equation to use is to figure out which one of the five kinematics quantities (d, v_0, v, a, or t) is missing from the question, and then use the equation that does not involve this missing quantity. Often, in questions asking about objects in free fall, the acceleration will not be given because it's known implicitly. As soon as you realize the question involves an object moving under the influence of gravity, then you know that a is automatically known; on Earth, the magnitude of this a is about 10 m/s².

However, there is one thing you will have to decide on once you've selected which Big Five equation to use. Gravitational acceleration, like any acceleration, is a vector, so it has magnitude and direction. We know the magnitude is 10 m/s² and the direction is downward, but is *down* the positive direction or the negative direction? The answer is: it's up to you. We suggest letting the direction of the object's displacement be the positive direction in every problem (this is almost always the simplest, most intuitive, decision). If the object's displacement is *down*, then call *down* the positive direction, and use $a = +g = +10$ m/s² in whichever Big Five equation you've selected. If the object's displacement is *up*, call *up* the positive direction (and thus *down* is automatically the negative direction) and use $a = -g = -10$ m/s².

It's important to remember that once you make your decision about which direction, up or down, is the positive direction, your decision applies to all other vectors in that problem: namely, v_0, v, and d. Therefore, if *down* is positive, for example, then in addition to the downward acceleration being positive, a downward initial velocity is positive, a downward final velocity is positive, and a downward displacement is positive. (This would mean that an upward initial velocity is negative, an upward final velocity is negative, and an upward displacement is negative.) Of course, if you follow the suggestion of always calling the direction of the displacement positive, then d will always be positive.

Example 3-17: An object is dropped from a height of 80 m. How long will it take to strike the ground?

Solution: We're given v_0, a, and d, and asked for t. Since the final velocity, v, is neither given nor asked for, we use Big Five #3. Because the object is falling, its displacement is downward, so let's call *down* the positive direction; this means that $a = +g = +10$ m/s². Since the term *dropped* means that the object's initial velocity is 0 m/s, we find that

$$d = v_0 t + \tfrac{1}{2}at^2 \rightarrow d = \tfrac{1}{2}at^2 \rightarrow t = \sqrt{\frac{2d}{a}} = \sqrt{\frac{2d}{+g}} = \sqrt{\frac{2(80 \text{ m})}{+10 \text{ m/s}^2}} = 4 \text{ s}$$

Example 3-18: An object is dropped from a height of 80 m. What is its velocity as it strikes the ground?

Solution: (Don't make the common mistake of thinking that the answer is 0 because once the object hits the ground, it stops. The question is really asking for the velocity of the object *as* it slams into the ground, and this won't be zero.) We're given v_0, a, and d, and asked for v. Since the time, t, is neither given nor asked for, we use Big Five #5. Because the object is falling, its displacement is downward, so let's call *down* the positive direction. This means that $a = +g = +10$ m/s^2. Since the term *dropped* means that the object's initial velocity is 0, we find that

$$v^2 = v_0^2 + 2ad \rightarrow v^2 = 2ad \rightarrow v = \sqrt{2ad} = \sqrt{2(+g)d} = \sqrt{2(+10 \text{ m/s}^2)(80 \text{ m})} = 40 \text{ m/s}$$

Example 3-19: A ball is thrown straight upward with an initial speed of 30 m/s. How high will it go?

Solution: We're given v_0, a, and v, and asked for d. (We know v because the question is asking how high the ball will go; at the top of the ball's path, its velocity at this point is 0.) Since the time, t, is missing, we use Big Five #5. Since we're interested only in the object's upward motion, let's call *up* the positive direction. This means that $v_0 = +30$ m/s and $a = -g = -10$ m/s^2. Because the velocity of the ball is 0 at its highest point, we find that

$$v^2 = v_0^2 + 2ad \rightarrow 0 = v_0^2 + 2ad \rightarrow d = -\frac{v_0^2}{2a} = -\frac{v_0^2}{2(-g)} = -\frac{(+30 \text{ m/s})^2}{2(-10 \text{ m/s})} = 45 \text{ m}$$

Notice that the displacement d turned out to be positive; that's because we chose *up* to be our positive direction, and the ball moves *up* to its highest position.

Example 3-20: A ball of mass 10 kg and a ball of mass 1 kg are dropped simultaneously from a tower of height 45 m. If air resistance could be ignored, which ball will hit the ground first and how long does it take?

Solution: We're given v_0, a, and d, and asked for t. Since the final velocity, v, is missing, we use Big Five #3. Because each object is falling, their displacement is downward, so let's call *down* the positive direction. This means that $a = +g = +10$ m/s^2. Remembering that the term *dropped* means that $v_0 = 0$, Big Five #3 becomes $d = \frac{1}{2}at^2$, so

$$t = \sqrt{\frac{2d}{a}} = \sqrt{\frac{2d}{+g}} = \sqrt{\frac{2(45 \text{ m})}{+10 \text{ m/s}^2}} = 3 \text{ s}$$

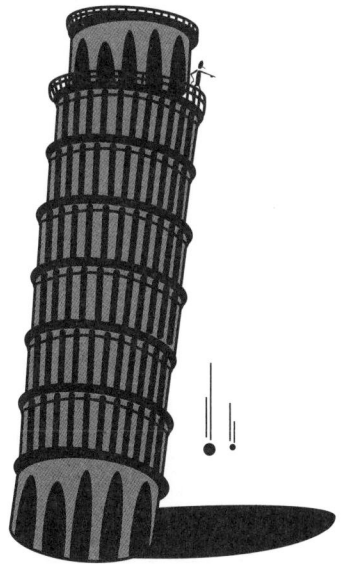

Because none of the Big Five equations involves the *mass* of the object, this is how long it takes *each* ball to strike the ground. The free-fall acceleration of an object does not depend on its mass (or size or shape), so in the absence of effects due to the air, both objects will hit the ground *at the same time.*

3.6 PROJECTILE MOTION

The examples we've worked through so far have involved objects that move along a straight line, either horizontal or vertical. However, if we were to throw a baseball up at an angle to the ground, the path the ball would follow (its **trajectory)** would not be a straight line. If we neglect effects due to the air, the path will be a *parabola*.

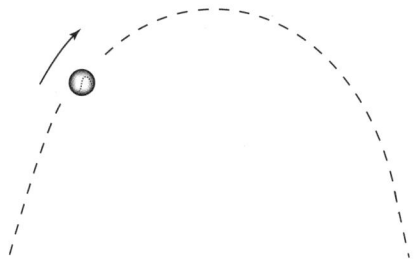

In this case, the motion of an object, experiencing only the constant, downward acceleration due to gravity (free fall), is called **projectile motion**. This is also a case of uniformly accelerated motion.

Because the projectile is experiencing both horizontal and vertical motion, we'll need to analyze both. But the trick is to analyze them *separately*. We'll use The Big Five to look at the horizontal motion, simply specializing the variables to horizontal motion; for example, we'll use x instead of d, we'll use v_{0x} and v_x instead of v_0 and v, and we'll use a_x instead of a. The same will be true for the vertical motion. We'll use The Big Five to look at the vertical motion, too, and simply specialize the variables to vertical motion; we'll use y instead of d, v_{0y} and v_y instead of v_0 and v, and a_y instead of a. In this case, a_y will be equal to the gravitational acceleration.

In order to make an object follow a parabolic path, we'll need to launch the object at an angle to the horizontal. Therefore, the initial velocity vector $\mathbf{v}_0$ will have a nonzero horizontal component (v_{0x}) *and* a nonzero vertical component (v_{0y}). In terms of the **launch angle**, θ_0, which is the angle the initial velocity vector makes with the horizontal, we have $v_{0x} = v_0 \cos \theta_0$ and $v_{0y} = v_0 \sin \theta_0$.

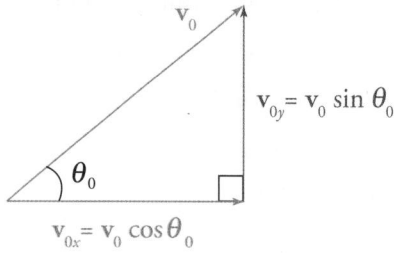

Let's first take care of the horizontal motion. This is the easier of the two for one important reason: once the projectile is launched, it no longer experiences a horizontal acceleration. That is, a_x will be zero throughout the projectile's flight. If the horizontal acceleration is zero throughout the projectile's flight, then *the horizontal velocity will be constant throughout the flight.* If the horizontal velocity does not change, then whatever it was initially is all it'll ever be; that is, the horizontal velocity of the projectile at any point during its flight will be equal to the initial horizontal velocity, v_{0x}. Finally, if a_x is always equal to 0, then by using Big Five #3, we have $x = v_{0x}t$ (this is just *distance = rate × time* in the case where the rate is constant).

For the vertical motion, we realize that there *is* an acceleration; after all, the gravitational acceleration is vertical. In order to write down the equations for the vertical motion, we need to make a decision about which direction is positive. Let's call *up* the positive direction, so that *down* is the negative direction; this will mean that $a_y = -g$. Big Five #2 now tells us that the vertical component of the velocity, v_y, will be $v_{0y} + a_y t = v_{0y} + (-g)t$ at time t. Big Five #3 tells us that the vertical displacement of the projectile, y, will be $v_{0y}t + \frac{1}{2}a_y t^2 = v_{0y}t + \frac{1}{2}(-g)t^2$.

Projectile Motion

	Horizontal Motion	Vertical Motion
displacement:	$x = v_{0x}t$	$y = v_{0y}t + \frac{1}{2}(-g)t^2$
velocity:	$v_x = v_{0x}$ (constant!)	$v_y = v_{0y} + (-g)t$
acceleration:	$a_x = 0$	$a_y = -g$
	$(v_{0x} = v_0 \cos\theta_0)$	$(v_{0y} = v_0 \sin\theta_0)$

In addition to these formulas (which are really nothing new, since they're just a few of the Big Five equations), there are a couple of other facts worth knowing. The first involves the projectile's velocity at the top of its trajectory. Since the top of the parabola is the parabola's turning point, and an object's velocity is always tangent to its path (whatever the shape of the trajectory), the projectile's velocity will be horizontal at the top of the parabola. This means that the vertical velocity is zero. (*Be careful* not to say that the velocity is zero at the top. For a projectile moving in a parabolic path, it's only the *vertical* velocity that's zero at the top; the horizontal velocity is still there!)

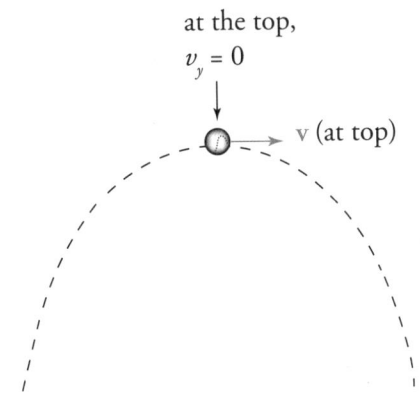

at the top,
$v_y = 0$
v (at top)

The second fact reflects the symmetry of the parabolic shape of the path. If we were to draw a vertical line up from the ground through the top point on the parabola, we'd notice that the left and right sides are just mirror images of each other. One of the consequences of this observation is that the time the projectile takes to reach the top will be the same as the time it takes to drop back down (to the same height from which it was launched). Therefore, *the projectile's total flight time will be twice the time required to reach the top.* So, for example, if the time it takes the projectile to reach the top of the parabola is 3 seconds, then the total flight time will be 6 seconds, because it'll take another 3 seconds to come back down.

Example 3-21: A cannonball is shot from ground level with an initial velocity of 100 m/s at an angle of 30° to the ground.

3.6

a) How high will the cannonball go?
b) What is the cannonball's velocity at the top of its path?
c) What will be the cannonball's total flight time?
d) How far will the cannonball travel horizontally?

Solution:

a) The maximum height reached by the projectile is the displacement y at the moment the cannonball is at the top of the parabola. What does it mean for the projectile to be at the top of the parabola? It means the vertical velocity is zero. So, we'll set the vertical velocity equal to zero. (Note that since we don't care about flight time for this particular question, we could ignore it and simply use Big Five #5.)

$$v_y = v_{0y} + (-g)t \text{ with } v_y = 0 \rightarrow v_{0y} + (-g)t = 0 \rightarrow t = \frac{v_{0y}}{g} = \frac{v_0 \sin\theta_2}{g}$$

This is how long it'll take the projectile to reach the top. If we plug in $v_0 = 100$ m/s, $\theta_0 = 30°$, and $g = 10$ m/s², we find that

$$t = \frac{v_0 \sin\theta_0}{g} = \frac{(100 \text{ m/s})\sin 30°}{10 \text{ m/s}^2} = 5 \text{ s}$$

So now the question is, "What is y when $t = 5$ s?" All we need to do is take the equation for the vertical displacement of the projectile and plug in $t = 5$ s:

$$y = v_{0y}t + \tfrac{1}{2}(-g)t^2$$
$$= (v_0 \sin\theta_0)t + \tfrac{1}{2}(-g)t^2$$

$$\therefore y \text{ (at } t = 5 \text{ s)} = (100 \text{ m/s} \cdot \sin 30°)(5 \text{ s}) + \tfrac{1}{2}(-10 \text{ m/s}^2)(5 \text{ s})^2 = 125 \text{ m}$$

b) At the top of its path, the cannonball's velocity is horizontal, and the horizontal velocity is the same throughout the flight, equal to the initial horizontal velocity:

$$v_x = v_{0x} = v_0 \cos\theta_0 = (100 \text{ m/s})\cos 30° \approx (100 \text{ m/s})(0.85) = 85 \text{ m/s}$$

c) The projectile's total flight time is just equal to twice the time required for it to reach the top. Since we found in part (a) that it takes 5 seconds for the cannonball to reach the top, its total flight time will be $2 \times (5 \text{ s}) = 10 \text{ s}$.

d) The question is asking for the horizontal displacement at the time when the cannonball strikes the ground. We found in part (b) that the cannonball's horizontal velocity is a constant 85 m/s, and we found in part (c) that the cannonball's total flight time is 10 seconds. Therefore, the total horizontal displacement is

$$x = v_{0x}t = (85 \text{ m/s})(10 \text{ s}) = 850 \text{ m}$$

(The total horizontal displacement is called the **range** of the projectile.)

Example 3-22: The archerfish is able to use a spit stream of water to knock insects off of branches overhanging the swamps and rivers they inhabit. Suppose the archerfish shoots at an insect with a spit speed of 8 m/s at a launch angle of 60°. What is the maximum height of the insect at which it could be knocked into the water?

Solution: The maximum height of a projectile occurs at the apex of the trajectory, at which point $v_y = 0$ m/s, and of course gravitational acceleration $a_y = -g = -10 \text{ m/s}^2$. The question implies the initial vertical velocity,

$v_{0y} = v_0 \sin 60° = (8 \text{ m/s})\left(\dfrac{\sqrt{3}}{2}\right) = 4\sqrt{3} \text{ m/s}$. The question asks for vertical displacement y, and the missing

variable is time t, so we use Big Five #5 adjusted for the vertical direction:

$$v_y^2 = v_{0y}^2 + 2a_y y \rightarrow y = \frac{v_y^2 - v_{0y}^2}{2a_y} = \frac{0 - \left(4\sqrt{3} \text{ m/s}\right)^2}{-20 \text{ m/s}} = \frac{48}{20} \approx 2.5 \text{ m}$$

Example 3-23: A rock is thrown horizontally, with an initial speed of 10 m/s, from the edge of a vertical cliff. It strikes the ground 5 s later.

a) How high is the cliff?

b) How far from the foot of the cliff does the rock land?

Solution:

a) The height of the cliff will be the vertical distance the rock falls. Because the rock is thrown horizontally, it has no initial vertical velocity: $v_{0y} = 0$. Therefore, the equation for the projectile's vertical displacement becomes $y = \frac{1}{2}(-g)t^2$. Considering the time it takes the rock to fall is $t = 5$ s, we have $y = \frac{1}{2}(-10 \text{ m/s}^2)(5 \text{ s})^2 = -125 \text{ m}$. This tells us that the rock falls 125 m in 5 s, so the height of the cliff is 125 m.

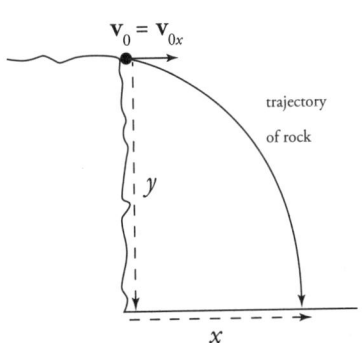

b) The horizontal displacement of the rock is given by the equation $x = v_{0x}t$. Since $v_{0x} = 10$ m/s and $t = 5$ s, we get
$$x = \left(10 \text{ m/s}\right)\left(5 \text{ s}\right) = 50 \text{ m}$$

Summary of Formulas

displacement: $d - \Delta x - [\text{final position}] - [\text{initial position}] = net \text{ distance [plus direction]}$

average velocity: $\bar{v} = \dfrac{\Delta x}{\Delta t} = \dfrac{d}{\Delta t}$

average acceleration: $\bar{a} = \dfrac{\Delta v}{\Delta t}$

The **BIG FIVE** [for Uniformly Accelerated Motion: $a = \text{constant}$]:

$$d = \frac{1}{2}\left(v_0 + v\right)t$$

$$v = v_0 + at$$

$$d = v_0 t + \frac{1}{2}at^2$$

$$d = vt - \frac{1}{2}at^2$$

$$v^2 = v_0^2 + 2ad$$

Position [x] vs. time [t] graph: slope = velocity [v]

Velocity [v] vs. time [t] graph: slope = acceleration [a]

area under graph = displacement [d]

Projectile Motion :

[Downward = Negative Direction]

	Horizontal Motion	**Vertical Motion**
displacement:	$x = v_{0x}t$	$y = v_{0y}t + \frac{1}{2}[-g]t^2$
velocity:	$v_{0x} = v_x$ [constant!]	$v_y = v_{0y} + [-g]t$
acceleration:	$a_x = 0$	$a_y = -g$
	$[v_{0x} = v_0 \cos\theta_0]$	$[v_{0y} = v_0 \sin\theta_0]$

$v_y = 0$ at the top of the trajectory

$v_x \neq 0$ at the top of the trajectory

Total flight time = [time from launch to top] + [time from top to landing]

CHAPTER 3 FREESTANDING PRACTICE QUESTIONS

1. In a crash simulation, a car traveling at x m/s can stop at a distance d m with a maximum deceleration. If the car is traveling at $2x$ m/s, which of the following statements is/are true, assuming a maximum deceleration?

   I. The stopping time is doubled.
   II. The stopping distance is doubled.
   III. The stopping distance is quadrupled.

A) I and II only
B) I and III only
C) II only
D) III only

2. A ball is thrown in a projectile motion trajectory with an initial velocity v at an angle θ above the ground. If the acceleration due to gravity is $-g$, which of the following is the correct expression of the time it takes for the ball to reach its highest point, y, from the ground?

A) $v^2 \sin\theta / g$

B) $-v\cos\theta / g$

C) $v\sin\theta / g$

D) $v^2 \cos\theta / g$

3. A surfer searching for the perfect wave paddles out to sea on her surfboard. She heads west from her beach spot and paddles at a rate of 8 meters per minute. There is a constant current in the water that day, pulling the surfer south at 6 meters per minute. After 5 minutes of paddling, how far is the surfer from her original beach spot?

A) 40 m west
B) 40 m southwest
C) 50 m southwest
D) 70 m southwest

4. A bubble in a glass of carbonated water rises from the bottom of the glass to the surface (a depth of 12 cm) in 4 seconds. What constant acceleration did it experience during this time?

A) 0 cm/s^2
B) 1.5 cm/s^2
C) 3 cm/s^2
D) 6 cm/s^2

5. A cart is moving along a frictionless track in a straight line. Which of the following graphs represents a completed round trip, returning to the starting point?

A)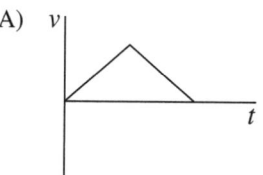

B)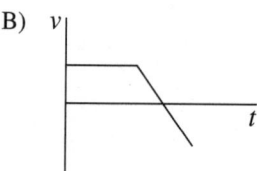

C)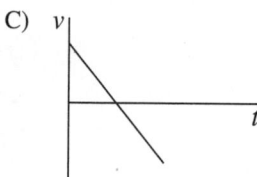

D)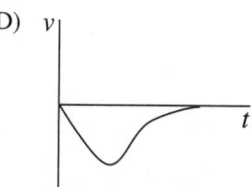

6. Two friends run toward one another in a straight line across a field. If they start 100 m apart and one friend runs at a constant speed of 9 m/s while the other friend runs at a constant speed of 6 m/s, how far will the faster friend run before they meet?

A) 50 m
B) 60 m
C) 67 m
D) It is impossible to determine with the information given.

7. The position x of an object is plotted as a function of time t. What is the acceleration of the object from $t = 2$ s to $t = 4$ s?

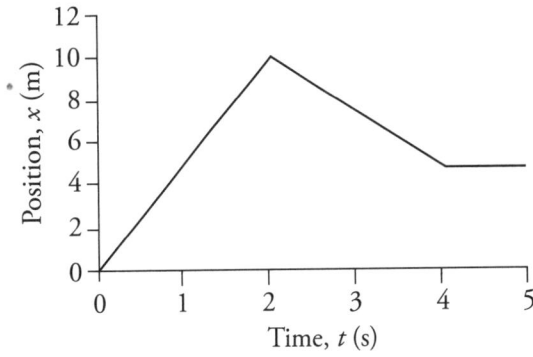

A) -2.5 m/s^2
B) 0 m/s^2
C) 2.5 m/s^2
D) 5 m/s^2

CHAPTER 3 PRACTICE PASSAGE

An airplane is susceptible to substantial deflection off course due to wind. A pilot calls the engines' contribution the *airspeed*. This motion relative to the air, combined with the wind velocity, results in the *ground speed*, or velocity relative to fixed terrestrial objects.

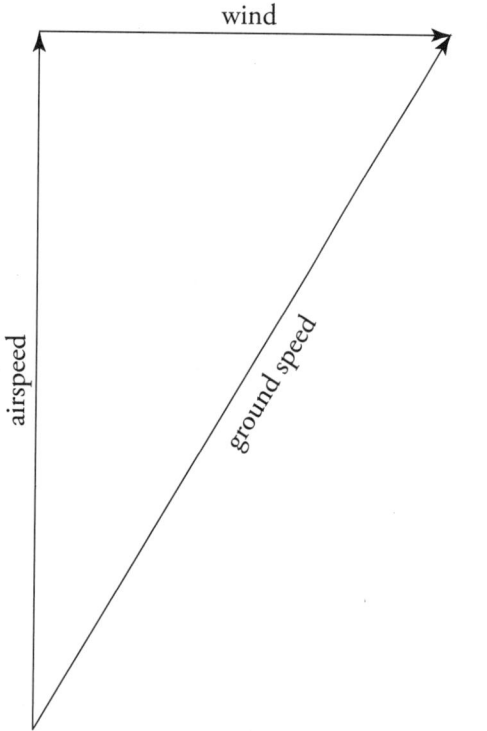

Figure 1

When a parachutist typically leaves an airplane, it is not so much a jump as a drop. He steps out of a door or lets go of a strut under the wing, not giving him any significant velocity relative to the airplane. He becomes subject to gravity without the lift of the wings. Air resistance allows the plane to get ahead of him. If we neglect this drag effect, then the parachutist's constant horizontal velocity and constant vertical acceleration gives him a trajectory resembling half of an inverted parabola. This is a reasonable assumption for the free fall before the parachute is engaged.

1. A pilot wanting to travel northeast in a wind blowing from the west at a speed similar to her airspeed should direct her airplane in which direction?

   A) north
   B) south
   C) east
   D) west

2. If an airplane has an airspeed of 100 km/hr southwest but is traveling 140 km/hr south relative to the ground, what is the wind velocity?

   A) 40 km/hr to the east
   B) 100 km/hr to the southeast
   C) 100 km/hr to the east
   D) 170 km/hr to the southeast

3. An airplane capable of an airspeed of 100 km/hr is 60 km off the coast above the sea. If the wind is blowing from the coast out to sea at 40 km/hr, what is the least amount of time it will take for the plane to get to shore?

   A) 26 minutes
   B) 36 minutes
   C) 60 minutes
   D) 100 minutes

4. Neglecting air resistance, what is the total velocity of a parachutist just before engaging her parachute, 8 s after dropping from an airplane flying horizontally at 60 m/s?

   A) 60 m/s
   B) 80 m/s
   C) 100 m/s
   D) 140 m/s

5. Which graph correctly represents the vertical speed of a dropped object with respect to time?

A)

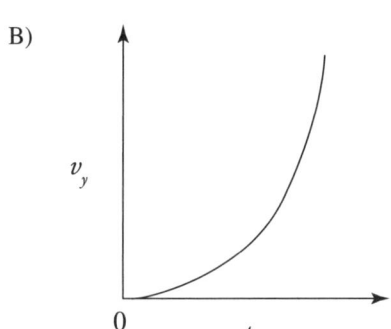

B)

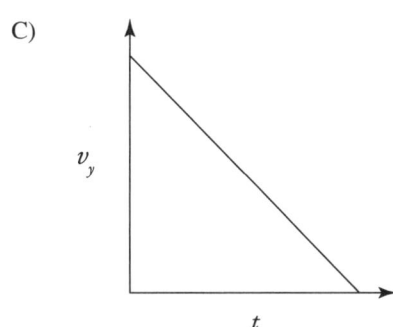

C)

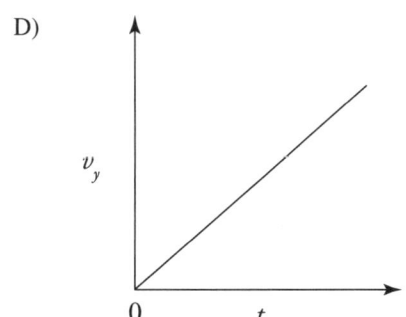

D)

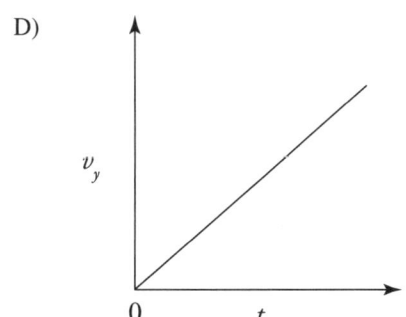

6. Relative to the typical dropping parachutist, one who thrusts himself downward on exiting the airplane (ignoring air resistance and assuming both parachutists open their parachutes after the same amount of time) will have:

A) lower acceleration but the same velocity just before engaging his parachute.
B) the same acceleration and the same velocity just before engaging his parachute.
C) the same acceleration but greater velocity just before engaging his parachute.
D) greater acceleration and greater velocity just before engaging his parachute.

SOLUTIONS TO CHAPTER 3 FREESTANDING PRACTICE QUESTIONS

1. **B** According to the formula $v^2 = v_0^2 + 2ad$, the initial velocity, v_0, can be related to the stopping distance, d. If v is zero, and the equation is rearranged for d, it becomes $d = v_0^2/2a$. Since the car is decelerating, a is negative. Therefore, if v_0 is doubled, the stopping distance, d, is quadrupled. To determine the relationship between v_0 and t, the formula $v = v_0 + at$ is used. Since v is zero, and the equation is rearranged for t, it becomes $t = -v_0/a$. Similar to the above scenario, a is negative. Therefore, if v_0 is doubled, the stopping time, t, is doubled. Only Items I and III are correct, and the correct answer is choice B.

2. **C** At the highest point from the ground, the ball has a velocity of zero. Therefore, applying the formula $v_y = v_{0y} + a_y t$ and rearranging for t, it becomes $t = -v_{0y}/-g$. Substituting $v_{0y} = v \sin \theta$ into the equation, $t = v \sin \theta / g$. Therefore the correct answer is C.

3. **C** The surfer is paddling west. That component of displacement can be calculated using the formula distance = (rate)(time) = (8 m/min)(5 min) = 40 m. So the surfer has traveled 40 m west on her own. The water current is constantly moving her south. That component of displacement can be calculated using the same formula, so distance = (6 m/min)(5 min) = 30 m. Each of these displacements are vectors and can be added together tip-to-tail. The result is a right triangle as shown below.

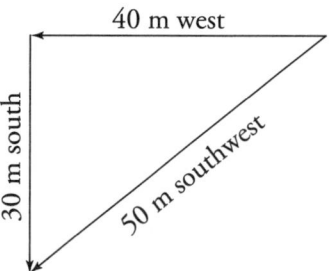

The triangle is a 3-4-5 triangle, so the total displacement is 50 m southwest (the total distance can also be found using the Pythagorean theorem, where $c^2 = a^2 + b^2$). The correct answer is choice C.

4. **B** The bubble starting from the bottom of the glass can be presumed to have started from rest. Thus the three given kinematics values are $v_0 = 0$ cm/s, $d = 12$ cm, and $t = 4$ s. We want acceleration a, so final velocity is missing and we use Big Five equation 3:

$$d = v_0 t + \tfrac{1}{2}at^2 \xrightarrow{v_0=0} a = \frac{2d}{t^2} = \frac{2(12 \text{ cm})}{(4 \text{ s})^2} = \frac{24 \text{ cm}}{16 \text{ s}^2} = 1.5 \frac{\text{cm}}{\text{s}^2} .$$

5. **C** For an object to return to its starting point, it must have a displacement of zero. Displacement is the total area between the velocity and time curve and the horizontal axis (because displacement is the product of average velocity and time), so we want the curve where that total area is zero. Only choice C, with its equivalent positive and negative areas (above and below the horizontal axis), can fulfill that condition.

6. **B** There are two approaches to this question. The more direct approach is to recognize that the two friends must run a total of 100 m combined in order to meet, and that each runs for the same amount of time as the other. Thus since $d = vt$ for motion at constant speed, $9t + 6t = 15t = 100$ m, so $t = (100/15)$ s. The faster friend running 9 m/s during that time will cover a distance $d = (9 \text{ m/s})(100/15 \text{ s}) = (3 \times 100/5)$ m = 60 m. Alternatively, you could reason that, because the faster friend is running at 1.5 times the speed of the slower friend, they must cover 1.5 times the distance. Call the distance the slower friend runs d, and the total distance is thus $d + 1.5d = 100$ m $\rightarrow 2.5d = 100$ m, so $d = 40$ m and the faster friend must have run $1.5(40 \text{ m}) = 60$ m.

7. **B** From $t = 2$ s to $t = 4$ s, the object is moving at a constant velocity, since the slope of the position vs. time graph does not change over this interval. Since the velocity of the object is constant, it is therefore not experiencing any acceleration.

SOLUTIONS TO CHAPTER 3 PRACTICE PASSAGE

1. **A**   We are given the resultant airspeed and asked for a different component. You must subtract the wind velocity (or add its negative) to the desired ground speed. Alternatively, just draw out the vectors and reason which way would be required to get the addition resultant northeast. Beware that "from the west" means "pointing to the east."

2. **B**   When you draw a vector diagram, remember that you are given the resultant and one of the components and asked for the other component. You must subtract the airspeed (or add its negative) to the resulting ground speed. This makes for a 1-1-$\sqrt{2}$ triangle, so the wind must also be 100 km/hr. It is southeast to counteract the westerly element of the airspeed and contribute more to the southerly component. There is more than just counteracting (like choices A or C). Mixing up the hypotenuse and sides might lead to choice D.

3. **C**   The airspeed and opposing wind superimpose to result in a ground speed of 60 km/hr toward the coast, so the 60 km will take 1 hour (60 minutes) to traverse. If you add the velocity vectors to a total of 140 km/hr then you would calculate choice A. If you surmised that 100 km/hr was the relevant velocity, you would calculate choice B. If you thought the resultant velocity was 40 km/hr, you might select choice D.

4. **C**   This first requires the calculation of the vertical component of velocity starting from rest and accelerating at 10 m/s^2 for 8 s. According to Big Five #2, the parachutist will be falling at 80 m/s (choice B). Her horizontal velocity will be constant at 60 m/s (choice A). Adding these two components is easy if you recognize that it is a 3-4-5 triangle multiplied by 20, so the hypotenuse is 100 m/s. Both of the individual components are listed as distractions. Linear (rather than vector) addition would result in choice D.

5. **D**   Though the passage does say that the trajectory will be half of a parabola, this question is asking about velocity, not displacement. Do not be fooled by the quadratic forms of choices A and B. The question asks for the speed, or magnitude of velocity. This magnitude will increase linearly as the object falls. Choice C would be an object slowing down at a constant negative acceleration.

6. **C**   This parachutist gives himself higher initial vertical velocity, whereas the typical one starts from rest in the vertical. They will both be subject to the same acceleration due to gravity, so choices A and D can immediately be eliminated. Starting at a higher velocity will, however, result in a greater final velocity.

Chapter 4
Mechanics I

4.1 MASS, FORCE, AND NEWTON'S LAWS

In the preceding chapter, we studied kinematics, which is the description of motion in terms of an object's position, velocity, and acceleration. In this chapter, we'll begin our study of **dynamics**, which is the *explanation* of motion in terms of the forces that act on an object.

Simply put, a **force** is a push or pull exerted by one object on another. If you pull on a rope attached to a crate, you create a *tension* in the rope that pulls the crate. When a sky diver is falling through the air, the Earth exerts a downward pull called the *gravitational force*, and the air exerts an upward force called *air resistance*. When you stand on the floor, the floor provides an upward, supporting force called the *normal force*. If you slide a book across a table, the table exerts a *frictional force* against the book, so the book slows down and eventually stops. Static cling provides a simple example of the *electrostatic force*. (In fact, all of the forces mentioned above, with the exception of gravity, are due ultimately to the electromagnetic force.)

> ### Newton's First Law
> An object's state of motion—its *velocity*—will not change unless a net force acts on the object.
>
> That is, if no net force acts on an object, then:
>
> > **if the object is at rest, it will remain at rest**
> >
> > *and*
> >
> **if the object is moving, then it will continue to move with constant velocity**
> >
> > (constant speed in a straight line).
>
> Or, more simply: **no net force** = **no acceleration**.

How forces affect motion is described by three physical laws, known as **Newton's laws**. They form the foundation of mechanics, and you should memorize them.

The first law says that objects naturally resist changing their velocity. In other words, objects at rest don't just suddenly start moving all on their own. Some external source must exert a force to make them move. Also, an object that's already moving doesn't change its velocity. It doesn't go faster, or slower, or change direction all by itself; something must exert some force on it to make any of these changes happen. This property of objects, their natural resistance to change in their state of motion, is called **inertia**. In fact, the first law is often referred to as the *law of inertia*.

It's important to note that the first law applies when there is no *net* force on an object. This could mean there are no forces at all, though that couldn't happen in our universe; more commonly, it means the forces on an object balance out, in other words, the total of all the forces, in each dimension, is zero. We'll work examples of computing net force when we get to Newton's second law.

The **mass** of an object is the quantitative measure of its inertia; intuitively, mass measures how much matter is contained in an object. Mass is measured in *kilograms*, abbreviated kg. (Note: An object whose mass is 1 kg weighs a little more than 2 pounds on Earth, but be careful not to confuse mass with weight; they're different things.) Compared to an object whose mass is just 1 kg, an object whose mass is 100 kg has 100 times the inertia. Intuitively, we'd find it 100 times more difficult to cause the same change in its motion than we would with the 1 kg object. This point will be clearer after we state the second of Newton's laws.

Newton's Second Law

If $\mathbf{F}_{net}$ is the net—or total—force acting on an object of mass m, then the resulting acceleration of the object, $\mathbf{a}$, satisfies this simple equation:

$$\mathbf{F}_{net} = m\mathbf{a}$$

Notice that the first law is really just a special case of the second law: the case in which $\mathbf{F}_{net} = 0$.

Forces are represented by vectors, because a force has a magnitude and a direction. If two different forces (let's call them $\mathbf{F}_1$ and $\mathbf{F}_2$) act on an object, then the total—or *net*—force on the object is the sum of these individual forces: $\mathbf{F}_{net} = \mathbf{F}_1 + \mathbf{F}_2$. Since forces are vectors, they must be added as vectors; that is, their directions must be taken into account. The following figures show some examples of obtaining $\mathbf{F}_{net}$ from the individual forces that act on an object:

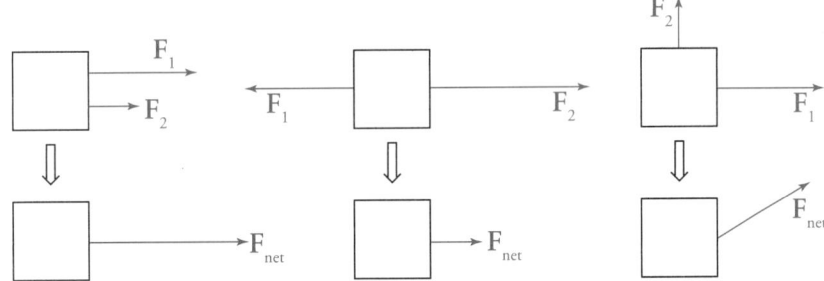

Note the following facts about the equation $\mathbf{F}_{net} = m\mathbf{a}$:

1. $\mathbf{F}_{net}$ is the sum of all the forces that act *on* the object; namely, the object whose mass, m, is on the other side of the equation. Any force exerted *by* the object is *not* included in $\mathbf{F}_{net}$.

2. Because m is a *positive* number, the direction of $\mathbf{a}$ is always the same as the direction of $\mathbf{F}_{net}$. Therefore, an object will accelerate in the direction of the net force it feels. This does not mean that an object will always *move* in the direction of $\mathbf{F}_{net}$. Be sure that this distinction makes sense, because it can be a source of confusion, and therefore a potential MCAT trap. Newton's second law tells us about the direction of an object's *acceleration* but does not define the direction of an object's velocity.

3. What if $\mathbf{F}_{net} = 0$? Then $\mathbf{a} = 0$. What does $\mathbf{a} = 0$ mean? It means that the object's velocity does not change, which is also what Newton's *first* law says. But how about this question: Does $\mathbf{F}_{net} = 0$ mean that $\mathbf{v} = 0$? Not necessarily! $\mathbf{F}_{net} = 0$ means that an object won't *accelerate*, not that it won't move. This is a key point and another potential MCAT trap. If the object is already moving at, say, 100 m/s toward the north, then it will continue to move at 100 m/s toward the north as long as the net force on the object remains zero.

4. Because $\mathbf{F}_{net} = m\mathbf{a}$ is a vector equation, it automatically means that the components of both sides must be the same. In other words, $\mathbf{F}_{net}$ could be written as the sum of a force in the horizontal direction, $(\mathbf{F}_{net, x})$ plus a force in the vertical direction $(\mathbf{F}_{net, y})$; these would be the horizontal and vertical components of $\mathbf{F}_{net}$. The equation $\mathbf{F}_{net} = m\mathbf{a}$ would then tell us that $\mathbf{F}_{net, x} = m\mathbf{a}_x$ and $\mathbf{F}_{net, y} = m\mathbf{a}_y$. So, dividing the horizontal component of the net force by m gives us the horizontal component of the object's acceleration, and dividing the vertical component of the net force by m gives us the vertical component of the object's acceleration.

5. The unit of force is equal to the unit of mass times the unit of acceleration:

$$[F] = [m][a] = \text{kg} \cdot \text{m/s}^2$$

A force of 1 kg·m/s² is called 1 **newton** (abbreviated N). A force of 1 N is about equal to a quarter of a pound, or about the weight of a medium-sized apple (on Earth).

Newton's Third Law

If Object 1 exerts a force, $\mathbf{F}_{1\text{-on-}2}$, on Object 2, then Object 2 exerts a force, $\mathbf{F}_{2\text{-on-}1}$, on Object 1. These forces, $\mathbf{F}_{1\text{-on-}2}$ and $\mathbf{F}_{2\text{-on-}1}$, have the same magnitude but act in opposite directions, so

$$\mathbf{F}_{1\text{-on-}2} = -\mathbf{F}_{2\text{-on-}1}$$

and they act on different objects. These two forces are said to form an **action–reaction pair**.

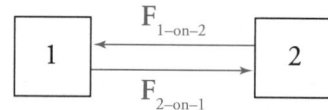

This is the law commonly stated as, "For every action, there is an equal but opposite reaction." Unfortunately, this popular version of Newton's third law can lead to confusion. Essentially, Newton's third law says that the *forces* in an action–reaction pair have the same magnitude and act in opposite directions (and on "opposite" objects). It does *not* say that the *effects* of these forces will be the same. For example, suppose that two skaters are next to and facing each other on a skating rink. Let's say that Skater 1 has a mass of 50 kg and Skater 2 has a mass of 100 kg. Now, what if Skater 1 pushes on Skater 2 with a force of 50 N? Then $\mathbf{F}_{1\text{-on-}2} = 50$ N and $\mathbf{F}_{2\text{-on-}1} = -50$ N, by Newton's third law.

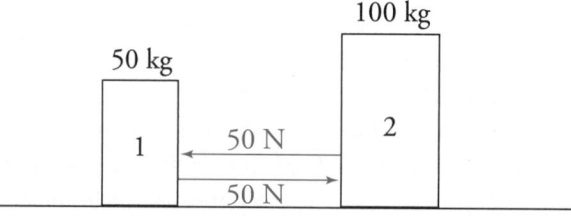

But will the *effects* of these equal-strength forces be the same? No, because the masses of the objects are different. The accelerations of the skaters will be

$$a_1 = \frac{F_{2\text{-on-}1}}{m_1} = \frac{-50 \text{ N}}{50 \text{ kg}} = -1 \text{ m/s}^2 \quad \text{and} \quad a_2 = \frac{F_{1\text{-on-}2}}{m_2} = \frac{+50 \text{ N}}{100 \text{ kg}} = +0.5 \text{ m/s}^2$$

So, Skater 2 will move away with an acceleration of 0.5 m/s², while Skater 1 moves away, in the opposite direction, with an acceleration of twice that magnitude, 1 m/s².

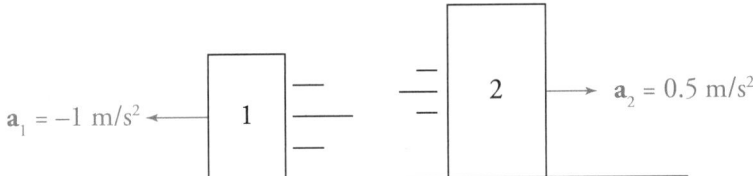

Therefore, while the forces are the same (in magnitude), the effects of these forces—that is, the resulting accelerations (and velocities)—are not the same, because the masses of the objects are different. Newton's third law says nothing about mass; it only tells us that the action and reaction forces will have the same magnitude. So, the point is not to interpret "equal but opposite reaction" as meaning "equal but opposite effect," because if the masses of the interacting objects are not the same, then the resulting accelerations (and velocities) of the objects will not be the same.

The key to distinguishing Newton's second law from Newton's third law is to focus on the description of the forces. In Newton's second law, all of the forces must be acting on a *single* object; thus, the net force on a single object is calculated by adding those vectors. However, in Newton's third law, each force must be acting on a *different* object in an action-reaction pair.

There are two aspects of Newton's third law that frequently give students trouble. First, just because two forces are equal and opposite does *not* mean they form an action-reaction pair; the forces also have to be from two objects acting on each other, not two objects acting on a third object. Second, the third law applies even when the objects are accelerating; even if one object is accelerating, the second object pushes or pulls just as hard on the first as the first pushes or pulls on the second.

Example 4-1: An object of mass 50 kg moves with a constant velocity of magnitude 1000 m/s. What is the net force on this object?

Solution: If the object moves with constant velocity, then the net force it feels must be zero, regardless of the object's mass or speed.

Example 4-2: The net force on an object of mass 10 kg is zero. What can you say about the speed of this object?

Solution: If the net force on an object is zero, all we can say is that it will not accelerate; its velocity may be zero, or it may not. Without more information, we cannot determine the object's speed; all we know is that whatever the speed is, it will remain constant.

Example 4-3: For 6 seconds, you push a 120 kg crate along a frictionless horizontal surface with a constant force of 60 N parallel to the surface. If the crate was initially at rest, what will its velocity be at the end of this 6-second time interval?

Solution: Using Newton's second law, we find that the acceleration of the crate is $a = F/m = (60 \text{ N})/(120 \text{ kg}) = 0.5 \text{ m/s}^2$. Using Big Five #2, we now find that $v = v_0 + at = 0 + (0.5 \text{ m/s}^2)(6 \text{ s}) = 3 \text{ m/s}$.

Example 4-4: For 6 seconds, you pull a 120 kg crate along a frictionless horizontal surface with a constant force of 60 N directed at an angle of 60° to the surface. If the crate was initially at rest, what will its horizontal velocity be at the end of this 6-second time interval?

Solution: To find the horizontal velocity, we need the horizontal acceleration.

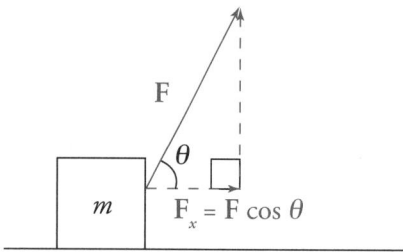

Using Newton's second law, we find that the horizontal acceleration of the crate is $a_x = F_x/m = (F\cos\theta)/m = (60\ N)(\cos 60°)/(120\ kg) = (30\ N)/(120\ kg) = 0.25\ m/s^2$. Using Big Five #2, we now find that $v_x = v_{0x} + a_x t = 0 + (0.25\ m/s^2)(6\ s) = 1.5\ m/s$.

Example 4-5: Two crates are moving along a frictionless horizontal surface. The first crate, of mass $M = 100$ kg, is being pushed by a force of 300 N. The first crate is in contact with a second crate, of mass $m = 50$ kg.

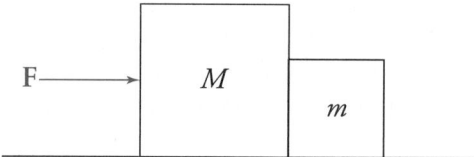

a)   What's the acceleration of the crates?
b)   What's the force exerted by the larger crate on the smaller one?
c)   What's the force exerted by the smaller crate on the larger one?

Solution:

a)   The force **F** is pushing on a combined mass of 100 kg + 50 kg = 150 kg, so by Newton's second law, the acceleration of both crates will be $a = (300\ N)/(150\ kg) = 2\ m/s^2$.

b)   Because M and m are in direct contact, each is pushing on the other with a certain force. Let $\mathbf{F_2}$ be the force that M exerts on m. Then we must have $F_2 = ma$, so $F_2 = (50\ kg)(2\ m/s^2) = 100\ N$.

c)   By Newton's third law, if the force that M exerts on m is $\mathbf{F_2}$, then the force that m exerts on M must be $-\mathbf{F_2}$. So, if we call "to the right" our positive direction, then the force that m exerts on M is -100 N. We can check that this is correct by looking at all the forces acting on M. We have $\mathbf{F}$ pushing to the right and $-\mathbf{F_2}$ pushing to the left. The net force on M is therefore $\mathbf{F_{net\ on\ M}} = \mathbf{F} + (-\mathbf{F_2}) = (300\ N) + (-100\ N) = 200\ N$. If this is correct, then $F_{net\ on\ M}$ should equal Ma. Since $M = 100$ kg and $a = 2\ m/s^2$, we get $Ma = 200$ N, which does match what we found for $F_{net\ on\ M}$. (In effect, what's happening here is that M is using 200 N of the 300 N force from **F** for its own motion and passing the remaining 100 N along to m, so that both move together with the same acceleration.)

Example 4-6: Two forces act on an object of mass $m = 5$ kg. One of the forces has a magnitude of 6 N, and the other force, perpendicular to the first, has a magnitude of 8 N. What's the acceleration of the object?

Solution: Forces are vectors, and when we find the net force on this object, we see that it's the hypotenuse of a 6-8-10 right triangle.

$$F_{net} = 10\ N \qquad F_2 = 8\ N$$
$$m \qquad F_1 = 6\ N$$

Since $F_{net} = 10$ N, the acceleration of the object will be $a = F_{net}/m = (10\ \text{N})/(5\ \text{kg}) = 2\ \text{m/s}^2$.

Example 4-7: When a doctor injects someone with a hypodermic needle, she exerts about 15 N of force to pierce adult skin. Once the skin has been pierced, considerably less force is required to push the needle deeper. If a force of 5 N on the plunger is required to initiate the injection, how hard should one pull back on the barrel to minimize risk of hematoma to the patient once the needle is inserted into the vein?

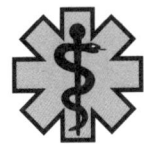

Solution:

According to Newton's second law, $\mathbf{F}_{net} = m\mathbf{a}$. Minimizing risk of hematoma implies that the acceleration of the stationary needle should be zero (so it won't move deeper in or out of the vein during the injection). Thus $\mathbf{F}_{net} = 0$, and $F_{plunger} = F_{barrel}$, or $F_{barrel} = 5$ N.

Example 4-8: According to Newton's third law, every force is "accompanied by" an equal but opposite force. If this is true, shouldn't these forces cancel out to zero? How could we ever accelerate an object?

Solution: The answer does not involve the masses of the objects; Newton's third law says nothing about mass. The key is to remember what $\mathbf{F}_{net}$ means; it's the sum of all the forces that act *on* an object, not *by* the object. Let's say we have a pair of objects, 1 and 2, and an action–reaction pair of forces between them, and we wanted to find the acceleration of Object 2. We'd find all the forces that act on Object 2. One of these forces is $\mathbf{F}_{1\text{-on-}2}$. The reaction force, $\mathbf{F}_{2\text{-on-}1}$, is *not* included in $\mathbf{F}_{net\text{-on-}2}$ because it doesn't act on Object 2; it's a force *by* Object 2. So, the reason why the two forces in an action–reaction pair don't cancel each other is that we'd never add them in the first place because they don't act on the same object.

4.2 THE FORCE OF GRAVITY

The mass of an object is a measure of its inertia, its resistance to acceleration. We'll now look at the related concept of an object's weight.

Although in everyday language the terms *mass* and *weight* are sometimes used interchangeably, in physics they have very different technical meanings. The **weight** of an object is the gravitational force exerted on it by the earth (or by whatever planet it happens to be on or near). **Mass** is an intrinsic property of an object and does not change with location. Put a baseball in a rocket and send it to the moon. The baseball's *weight* on the moon is less than its weight here on Earth, but you'd have as much "baseball stuff" there as you would here; that is, the baseball's *mass* would *not* change.

Since weight is a force, we can use $\mathbf{F} = m\mathbf{a}$ to compute it. What acceleration would the gravitational force (which is what *weight* means) impose on an object? The gravitational acceleration, of course! Therefore, setting $\mathbf{a} = \mathbf{g}$, the equation $\mathbf{F} = m\mathbf{a}$ becomes

$$\mathbf{w} = m\mathbf{g}$$

This is the equation for the weight, $\mathbf{w}$, of an object of mass m. (Weight is often symbolized by $\mathbf{F}_{grav}$, rather than $\mathbf{w}$; we'll use both notations.) Note that mass and weight are proportional but not identical. Furthermore, mass is measured in kilograms, while weight is measured in newtons.

Example 4-9:

  a) Find the weight of an object whose mass is 50 kg.
  b) Find the mass of an object whose weight is 50 N.

Solution:

  a) To find an object's weight, we multiply its mass by g. Using $g = 10$ m/s^2 (or, equivalently, $g = 10$ N/kg), we find that $w = mg = (50 \text{ kg})(10 \text{ N/kg}) = 500$ N.
  b) To find an object's mass, we divide its weight by g. With $g = 10$ N/kg, we find that $m = w/g = (50 \text{ N})/(10 \text{ N/kg}) = 5$ kg.

Most of the time, we'll use the formula $w = mg$ to find the weight of an object whose mass is m. However, the value of g can change, and if we're not near the surface of Earth (where we know that g is approximately 10 m/s^2), we may not know the value of g. In that case, we'll invoke another law discovered by Newton: Newton's Law of Gravitation.

Newton's Law of Gravitation

Every object in the universe exerts a gravitational pull on every other object. The magnitude of this gravitational force is proportional to the product of the objects' masses and inversely proportional to the square of the distance between them. The constant of proportionality is denoted by G and known as Newton's universal gravitational constant.

$$F_{grav} = G\,\frac{Mm}{r^2}$$

distance between centers

The value of G is roughly 6.7×10^{-11} N·m²/kg², but don't bother memorizing this constant. *The AAMC has removed gravitation from the list of topics subject to memory questions, so the main point of this section is to make connections between basic physics principles and to anticipate certain problem-solving techniques.*

One of the most important features of Newton's law of gravitation is that it's an **inverse-square law**. This means that the magnitude of the gravitational force is *inversely* proportional to the *square* of the distance between the centers of the objects. Another important physical law, Coulomb's law (for the electrostatic force between two charges), which we'll see later, is also an inverse-square law.

Also notice that the forces illustrated in the box above form an action–reaction pair. Even if M and m are different, the gravitational force that M exerts on m has the same magnitude as the gravitational force that m exerts on M. (If the directions of the force vectors in the box above seem backward, remember that gravity is always a *pulling* force; therefore, in the figure above, $\mathbf{F}_{M\text{-on-}m}$ pulls to the left, toward M, while $\mathbf{F}_{m\text{-on-}M}$ pulls to the right, toward m.) Of course, the accelerations of the objects will have different magnitudes if the masses are different, as we discussed earlier when we studied Newton's third law.

Example 4-10: What will happen to the gravitational force between two objects if the distance between them is doubled? What if the distance is cut in half?

Solution: Since the gravitational force obeys an inverse-square law, if r increases by a factor of 2, then F_{grav} will *decrease* by a factor of $2^2 = 4$. On the other hand, if r decreases by a factor of 2, then F_{grav} will *increase* by a factor of $2^2 = 4$.

Notice that the two formulas given in this section, $w = mg$ and $F_{grav} = GMm/r^2$, are really formulas for the same thing. After all, weight *is* gravitational force. Therefore, we could set these expressions equal to each other:

$$mg = G\,\frac{Mm}{r^2}$$

Then, dividing both sides by m, we get

$$g = G\frac{M}{r^2}$$

This formula tells us how to find the value of the gravitational acceleration, g. On Earth, we know that $g \approx 10$ m/s². If we were to go to the top of a mountain, then the distance r to the center of the earth would increase, but compared to the radius of the earth, the increase would be very small. As a result, while the value of g *is* less at the top of a mountain than at the earth's surface, the difference is small enough that it can usually be neglected. However, at the position of a satellite orbiting the earth, for example, the distance to the center of the earth has now increased dramatically (for example, many satellites have an orbit radius that's over 6.5 times the radius of the earth), and the resulting decrease in g would definitely need to be taken into account.

This formula for g also shows us why g changes from planet (or moon) to planet. For example, on Earth's moon, the value of g is only about 1.6 m/s² (about a sixth of what it is on Earth) because the mass of the moon is so much smaller than the mass of the earth. It's true that the radius of the moon is smaller than the radius of the earth, which would, by itself, make g bigger, but M is *much* smaller, and this is why the value of g on the surface of the moon is smaller than its value on the surface of the earth. So, while big G is a universal gravitational constant, the value of little g depends on where you are.

Example 4-11: The radius of Earth is approximately 6.4×10^6 m. What's the mass of Earth?

Solution: We can use the formula $g = GM/r^2$ to solve for M:

$$M = \frac{gr^2}{G} = \frac{(10 \text{ m/s}^2)(6.4 \times 10^6 \text{ m})^2}{6.7 \times 10^{-11} \frac{\text{N} \cdot \text{m}^2}{\text{kg}^2}} \approx 6 \times 10^{24} \text{ kg}$$

Example 4-12: The mass of Mars is about 1/10 the mass of Earth, and the radius of Mars is about half that of Earth. Is the value of g on the surface of Mars less than, greater than, or equal to the value of g on Earth?

Solution: We'll use the formula $g = GM/r^2$ to compare the two values of g:

$$\frac{g_{\text{Mars}}}{g_{\text{Earth}}} = \frac{G\dfrac{M_{\text{Mars}}}{r_{\text{Mars}}^2}}{G\dfrac{M_{\text{Earth}}}{r_{\text{Earth}}^2}} = \frac{M_{\text{Mars}}}{M_{\text{Earth}}} \cdot \left(\frac{r_{\text{Earth}}}{r_{\text{Mars}}}\right)^2 = \frac{1}{10} \cdot 2^2 = 0.4$$

Therefore, the value of g on Mars is only about 40% of its value here.

Example 4-13: A long, flat, frictionless table is set up on the surface of the moon (where $g = 1.6$ m/s^2). An object whose mass on Earth is 4 kg is also transported there.

a) What is the object's mass on the moon?
b) What is the object's weight on the moon?
c) If we drop this object from a height of $h = 20$ m, with what speed will it strike the lunar surface?
d) If we wish to push this object across the table to give it an acceleration of 3 m/s^2, how much force must we exert? Would this force be different if the table and object were back on Earth?

Solution:

a) The mass is the same, 4 kg.
b) The weight of the object on the moon is $w = m \cdot g_{moon} = (4 \text{ kg})(1.6 \text{ m/s}^2) = 6.4$ N. Notice that the object's weight on the moon is different from its weight on Earth.
c) Calling *down* the positive direction and using Big Five #5 with $v_0 = 0$ and $a = g_{moon} = 1.6$ m/s^2, we find that

$$v^2 = v_0^2 + 2ad \rightarrow v^2 = 2gh \rightarrow v = \sqrt{2gh} = \sqrt{2(1.6 \text{ m/s}^2)(20 \text{ m})} = 8 \text{ m/s}$$

d) Using $F = ma$, we get $F = (4 \text{ kg})(3 \text{ m/s}^2) = 12$ N. Since Newton's second law depends only on mass (not on weight, because there's no g in Newton's second law), we'd need this same force even if the object and table were back on Earth.

Example 4-14: The human body can only withstand a vertical *g-force* of about 5g before the body has difficulty pumping blood out of the feet and into the brain. Approximately how much upward force could be applied to a 60 kg person at sea level before that person risked fainting? (The phrase "g-force" is a misnomer, because it actually refers to acceleration: the real *force* involved is the normal force from the surface of contact. A person in free fall experiences "zero gees.")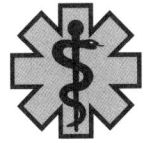

Solution: A person standing motionless on flat ground experiences a normal force equal to his weight, *mg*. That corresponds to 1g. Thus the additional upward force from the surface should provide an additional 4g of acceleration. According to Newton's second law $\mathbf{F}_{net} = m\mathbf{a} = 60 \text{ kg} \times 40 \text{ m/s}^2 = 2400$ N.

4.3 FRICTION

Some of the examples in the preceding sections described a frictionless surface. Of course, there's no such thing as a truly frictionless surface, but when a problem uses a term like *frictionless*, it simply means that friction is so weak that it can be neglected. Having frictionless surfaces also made those examples easier, so we could become comfortable with Newton's laws while first learning to apply them. However, there are cases in which friction cannot be ignored, so we need to learn how to handle such situations.

When two materials are in contact, there's an electrical attraction between the atoms of one surface with those of the other; this attraction will make it difficult to slide one object relative to the other. In addition, if the surfaces aren't perfectly smooth, the roughness will also increase the force required to slide the objects against each other. **Friction** is the term we use for the combination of these effects. Fortunately, the forces due to all those intermolecular forces and to the interactions of surface irregularities can be expressed by a single equation.

The MCAT will expect you to know about two big categories of friction; they're called **static friction** and **kinetic** (or **sliding**) **friction**.[1] When there's no relative motion between the surfaces that are in contact (that is, when there's no sliding) we have static friction; when there *is* relative motion between the surfaces (that is, when there *is* sliding) we have kinetic friction.

Now, in order to state the equations we'll use to figure out these frictional forces, we first need to discuss another contact force, the one known as the normal force.

Place a book on a flat table. Assuming that the book isn't too heavy and the tabletop isn't made of, say, tissue paper, the book will remain supported by the table. One force acting on the book is the downward gravitational force. If this were the only force acting on the book, then the book would fall through the table. Hence, there must be an upward force acting on the book that cancels out the book's weight. This supporting force, which acts perpendicular to the tabletop, is called the **normal force**. It's called the *normal* force because it is, by definition, perpendicular to the surface that exerts it. The word *normal* means *perpendicular*. We'll denote the normal force by $\mathbf{N}$ or by $\mathbf{F_N}$. [Don't confuse $\mathbf{N}$ (or its magnitude, N) with the abbreviation for the newton, N.] In the case of an object simply lying on a flat surface, the magnitude of the normal force is just equal to the object's weight. As a result, the book feels a downward force of magnitude $w = mg$ and an upward force of magnitude $N = mg$, so the net force on the book is 0.

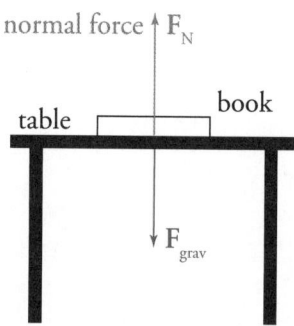

Example 4-15: Do the normal force and the gravitational force described in the preceding paragraph form an action–reaction pair?

Solution: No. While these forces *are* equal but opposite, they do not form an action–reaction pair, because they act on the same object (namely, the book). The forces in an action–reaction pair always act on different objects. So, while it's true that the forces in an action–reaction pair are always equal but opposite, it is not true that any pair of equal but opposite forces must always form an action–reaction pair. The reaction force to $\mathbf{F}_\text{table-on-book}$, which is the normal force, is $\mathbf{F}_\text{book-on-table}$. The reaction force to $\mathbf{F}_\text{Earth-on-book}$, which is the weight of the book, is $\mathbf{F}_\text{book-on-Earth}$. The force $\mathbf{F}_\text{table-on-book}$ is not the reaction to $\mathbf{F}_\text{Earth-on-book}$.

For an object on a horizontal surface that feels no other vertical forces, the normal force will be equal to the weight of the object. However, there are many cases in which the normal force isn't equal to the weight of the object. For example, suppose we place a book against a vertical wall and push on the book with a horizontal force $\mathbf{F}$. Then the magnitude of the normal force exerted by the wall will be equal to F, which may certainly be different from the weight of the book. Here's another example (which we'll look at in more detail in the next section): If we place a book on an inclined plane (e.g., a ramp), then the normal force exerted by the ramp on the book will not be equal to the weight of the book. What we can say is the general definition of the normal force: *The normal force is the perpendicular component of the contact force exerted by a surface on an object.*

We had to discuss the normal force here, because the force of friction exerted by a surface on an object in contact with is related to the normal force. In the case of sliding (kinetic) friction, the magnitude of the force of friction is directly proportional to the magnitude of the normal force. The constant of proportionality depends on what the surface is made of and what the object is made of; this constant is called the **coefficient of kinetic friction**, denoted by μ_k (the Greek letter *mu*, with subscript k), where the k denotes kinetic friction. For every pair of surfaces, the coefficient μ_k is an experimentally determined positive number with no units, and the greater its value, the greater the force of kinetic friction. For example, the value of μ_k for rubber-soled shoes on ice is only about 0.1, while for rubber-soled shoes on wood, the value of μ_k is much higher; it's about 0.7 for your sneakers, but could be greater than 1 if you walk around in rock-climbing shoes.

Notice carefully that this is *not* a vector equation. It is only an equation giving the *magnitude* of $\mathbf{F}_\text{f}$ in terms of the *magnitude* of $\mathbf{F}_\text{N}$.

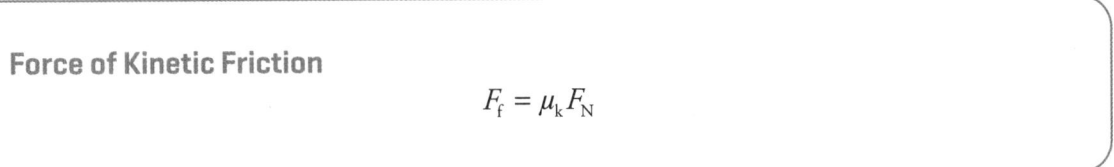

Force of Kinetic Friction

$$F_\text{f} = \mu_\text{k} F_\text{N}$$

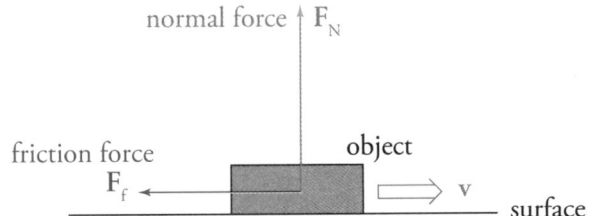

The magnitude of the force of kinetic friction is given by the equation $F_f = \mu_k F_N$. The direction of the force of kinetic friction is always parallel to the surface and in the opposite direction to the object's velocity (relative to the surface).

Example 4-16: A book of mass $m = 2$ kg slides across a flat tabletop. If the coefficient of kinetic friction between the book and table is 0.4, what's the magnitude of the force of kinetic friction on the book?

Solution: Because the magnitude of the normal force is $F_N = mg = (2 \text{ kg})(10 \text{ m/s}^2) = 20$ N, the magnitude of the force of kinetic friction is $F_f = \mu_k F_N = (0.4)(20 \text{ N}) = 8$ N.

The formula for static friction is similar to the one for kinetic friction, but there are two important differences. First, given a pair of surfaces, there's a **coefficient of static friction** between them, μ_s (the subscript s now denotes static friction), and on the MCAT, it's always greater than the coefficient of kinetic friction. This is equivalent to saying that, in general, static friction is capable of being stronger than kinetic friction. To illustrate this, imagine there's a heavy crate sitting on the floor and you want to push the crate across the room. You walk up to the crate and push on it, harder and harder until, finally, it "gives" and starts sliding. Once the crate is sliding, it's easier to keep it sliding than it was to get it started in the first place. The friction that resisted your initial push to get the crate moving was static friction. Because it was easier to keep it sliding than it was to get it started sliding, kinetic friction must be weaker than the maximum static friction force.

The second difference between the formula for kinetic friction and the one for static friction is that there's actually no general formula for the force of static friction. All we have is a formula for the *maximum* force of static friction. It's important that you understand this distinction. Let's go back to that heavy crate sitting on the floor. Let's say you know by previous experience that it'll take 400 N of force on your part to get that crate sliding. So, what if you push with a force of 100 N? Well, obviously, the crate won't move. Therefore, there must be another 100 N acting on the crate, opposite to your push, to make the net force on the crate zero. Okay, what if you now push on the crate with a force of 200 N? The crate still won't move, so there must now be another 200 N acting on the crate, opposite to your push, to make the net force on the crate zero. Whatever force you exert on the crate, as long as it's less than 400 N, will cause the force of static friction to cancel you out. Static friction is capable of supplying any necessary force, but only up to a certain maximum. That's why we can't write down a general formula for the force of static friction, only a formula for the maximum force of static friction. The formula looks just like the one above, except we replace μ_k by μ_s, and add the word "max" to denote that all this formula gives is the maximum force of static friction.

Maximum Force of Static Friction

$$F_{f,\,max} = \mu_s F_N$$

The maximum magnitude of the force of static friction is given by the equation $F_{f,\,max} = \mu_s F_N$. The direction of the force of static friction (maximum or not) is always parallel to the surface and in the opposite direction to the object's intended velocity. The magnitude of the force of static friction is whatever value, up to the maximum given by the equation, it takes exactly to cancel out the force(s) that are trying to make the object slide.

Example 4-17: A crate that weighs 1000 N rests on a horizontal floor. The coefficient of static friction between the crate and the floor is 0.4. If you push on the crate with a force of 250 N, what is the magnitude of the force of static friction?

Solution: The answer is not 400 N. The *maximum* force of static friction that the floor could exert on the crate is $F_{f,\,max} = \mu_s F_N = (0.4)(1000\ N) = 400\ N$. However, if you exert a force of only 250 N on the crate, then static friction will only be 250 N. (Just imagine what would happen to the crate if you pushed on it with a force of 250 N and the floor pushed it back toward you with a force of 400 N!)

Example 4-18: You push a 50 kg block of wood across a flat concrete driveway, exerting a constant force of 300 N. If the coefficient of kinetic friction between the wood and concrete is 0.5, what will be the acceleration of the block?

Solution: The normal force acting on the block has a magnitude of $F_N = mg = (50\ kg)(10\ m/s^2) = 500\ N$. Therefore, the force of kinetic friction acting on the sliding block has a magnitude of $F_f = \mu_k F_N = (0.5)(500\ N) = 250\ N$. This means that the net force acting on the block (and parallel to the driveway) is equal to $F - F_f = (300\ N) - (250\ N) = 50\ N$. If $F_{net} = 50\ N$ and $m = 50$ kg, then $a = F_{net}/m = (50\ N)/(50\ kg) = 1\ m/s^2$.

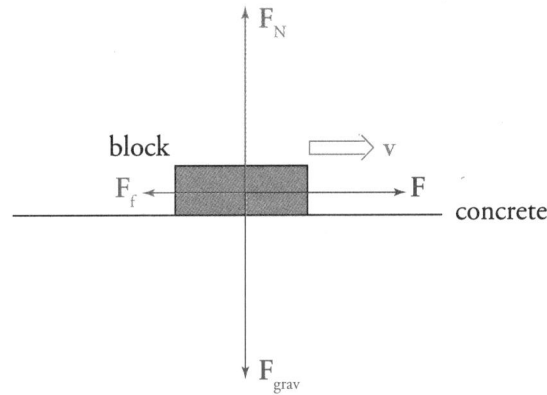

Example 4-19: Instead of pushing the block by a force that's parallel to the driveway, you wrap a rope around the block, sling the rope over your shoulder, and walk it across the driveway. If the rope makes an angle of 30° to the horizontal, and the tension in the rope is 300 N (the same force you exerted on the block in the last example), what will the block's acceleration be now?

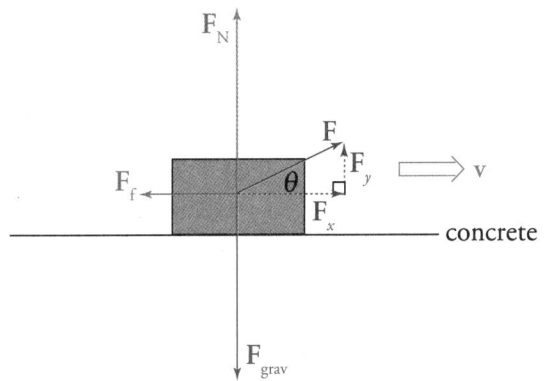

Solution: This is a tough question, but it uses a lot of the material we've covered so far. First, we'll need the normal force to find the friction force. The net vertical force on the block is 0 (because we're not lifting the block off the ground or watching it fall through the concrete). Therefore, $F_N + F_y = F_{grav}$, so $F_N = F_{grav} - F_y$. (Here's another example of the normal force not equaling the weight of the object.) Since $F_y = F \sin \theta = F \sin 30° = (300 \text{ N})(0.5) = 150$ N, we have $F_N = (500 \text{ N}) - (150 \text{ N}) = 350$ N. (Intuitively, the normal force is less than the weight of the block because the vertical component of the tension in the rope is "taking some of the pressure" off the surface.) Therefore, $F_f = \mu_k F_N = (0.5)(350 \text{ N}) = 175$ N. Now, the horizontal force that you provide is $F_x = F \cos \theta = F \cos 30° \approx (300 \text{ N})(0.85) = 255$ N. Therefore, the net force acting on the block, parallel to the driveway, is equal to $F_x - F_f = (255 \text{ N}) - (175 \text{ N}) = 80$ N. If $F_{net} = 80$ N and $m = 50$ kg, then $a = F_{net}/m = (80 \text{ N})/(50 \text{ kg}) = 1.6 \text{ m/s}^2$. (Notice that you get the block moving faster—even exerting the same force—by doing it this way!)

4.4 INCLINED PLANES

So far, we've had practice problems where the object is moving along a flat, horizontal surface. However, the MCAT will also expect you to handle questions in which the object is on a ramp, or, in fancier language, an **inclined plane**.

The figure below shows an object of mass m on an inclined plane; the angle the plane makes with the horizontal (the **incline angle**) is labeled θ. If we draw the vector representing the weight of the object, we notice that it can be written in terms of two components: one parallel to the ramp and one perpendicular to it. The diagram on the left shows that the magnitudes of the components of the object's weight, **w** = m**g**, are $mg \sin \theta$ (parallel to the ramp) and $mg \cos \theta$ (perpendicular to the ramp).

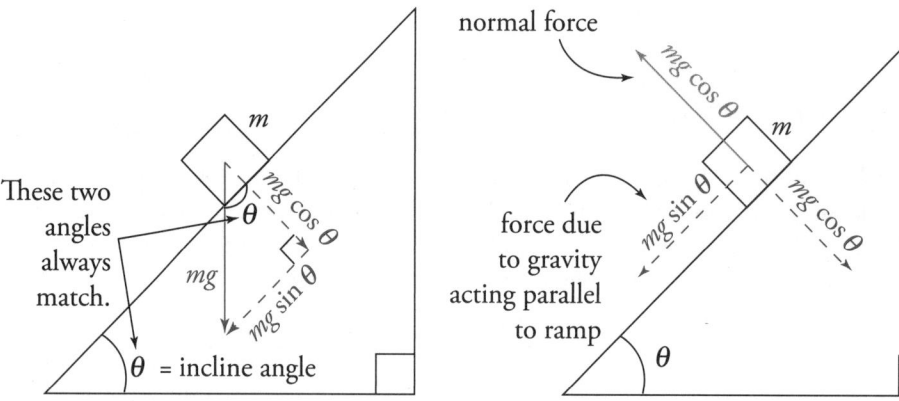

Therefore, as illustrated in the diagram on the right,

the force due to gravity acting parallel to the inclined plane = $mg \sin \theta$

the force due to gravity acting perpendicular to the inclined plane = $mg \cos \theta$

where θ is measured between the incline and horizontal. **You should memorize both of these facts.**

Incidentally, any time we see an angle in an MCAT problem we'll probably be breaking a vector (say a force, a velocity, or an acceleration) into components. When we looked at projectile motion we broke the projectile's initial velocity into horizontal and vertical components; here, we're breaking the force of gravity into a component parallel to and one perpendicular to the surface of the incline. Why the difference? In general, the components you'll use will be vertical and horizontal, *unless* the object can only move along one possible line; in that case, the components to use will be the direction of (possible) travel (in this case, parallel to the incline) and, the direction perpendicular to that.

Example 4-20: A block of mass $m = 4$ kg is placed at the top of a frictionless ramp of incline angle 30° and length 10 m.

a) What is the block's acceleration down the ramp?
b) How long will it take for the block to slide to the bottom?

Solution:

a) Because the force due to gravity acting parallel to the ramp is $F = mg \sin \theta$, the acceleration of the block down the ramp will be

$$a = \frac{F}{m} = \frac{mg \sin \theta}{m} = g \sin \theta = \left(10 \text{ m/s}^2\right) \sin 30° = 5 \text{ m/s}^2$$

b) Using Big Five #3 with $d = 10$ m, $v_0 = 0$, and $a = 5$ m/s², we find that

$$d = v_0 t + \frac{1}{2} a t^2 = \frac{1}{2} a t^2 \rightarrow t = \sqrt{\frac{2d}{a}} = \sqrt{\frac{2(10 \text{ m})}{5 \text{ m/s}^2}} = 2 \text{ s}$$

Notice that the block's mass was irrelevant to both of these questions. That's because all of the forces were directly proportional to mass, but so was the object's inertia; in effect, mass canceled out of both sides of $F = ma$. This is common in problems in which the forces on an object are all functions of gravity.

Example 4-21: A block of mass m slides down a ramp of incline angle 60°. If the coefficient of kinetic friction between the block and the surface of the ramp is 0.2, what's the block's acceleration down the ramp?

Solution: There are now two forces acting parallel to the ramp: $mg \sin \theta$ (directed downward along the ramp) and F_f, the force of kinetic friction (directed upward along the ramp). Therefore, the net force down the ramp is $F_{net} = mg \sin \theta - F_f$. To find F_f, we multiply F_N by μ_k. Since $F_N = mg \cos \theta$, we have

$$F_{net} = mg \sin \theta - \mu_k mg \cos \theta$$

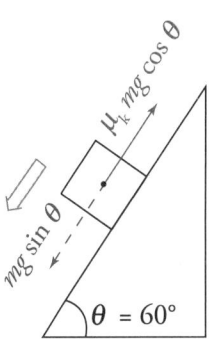

Dividing F_{net} by m gives us a:

$$a = \frac{F_{net}}{m} = \frac{mg\sin\theta - \mu_k mg\cos\theta}{m} = g(\sin\theta - \mu_k\cos\theta)$$

Putting in the numbers, we get

$$a = (10 \text{ m/s}^2)(\sin 60° - 0.2\cos 60°) \approx (10 \text{ m/s}^2)(0.85 - 0.2 \cdot \tfrac{1}{2}) = 7.5 \text{ m/s}^2$$

Example 4-22: A block of mass m is placed on a ramp of incline angle θ. If the block doesn't slide down, find the relationship between μ_s (the coefficient of static friction) and θ.

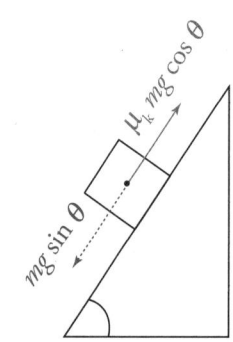

Solution: If the block doesn't slide, then static friction is strong enough to withstand the pull of gravity acting downward parallel to the ramp. This means that the *maximum* force of static friction must be greater than or equal to $mg\sin\theta$. Since $F_{f(static), max} = \mu_s F_N$, and $F_N = mg\cos\theta$, we have $F_{f(static), max} = \mu_s mg\cos\theta$. Therefore,

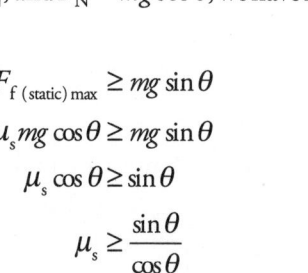

$$F_{f(static)max} \geq mg\sin\theta$$

$$\mu_s mg\cos\theta \geq mg\sin\theta$$

$$\mu_s \cos\theta \geq \sin\theta$$

$$\mu_s \geq \frac{\sin\theta}{\cos\theta}$$

$$\therefore \mu_s \geq \tan\theta$$

4.5 PULLEYS

A **pulley** is a device that changes the direction of the **tension** (the force exerted by a stretched string, cord, or rope) that pulls on the object that the string is attached to. (We'll use $\mathbf{F_T}$ or $\mathbf{T}$ to denote a tension force.) For example, in the picture below, if we pull *down* on the string on the right with a force of magnitude F_T, then the tension force on the left side of the pulley will pull *up* on the block with the same magnitude of force, F_T.

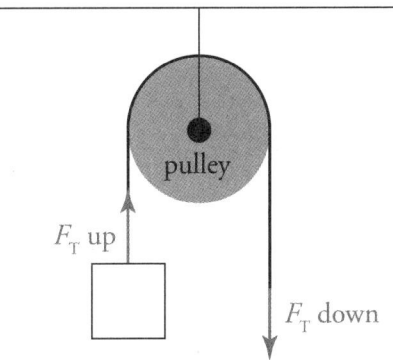

Pulleys can also be used to decrease the force necessary to lift an object. For example, consider the pulley system illustrated on the left below. If we pull down on the string on the right with a force of magnitude F_T, then we'll create a tension force of magnitude F_T throughout the entire string. As a result, there will be *two* tension forces, each of magnitude F_T, pulling up to lift the block (and the bottom pulley, too, but we assume that the pulleys are massless; that is, the mass of any pulley is small enough that it can be ignored). Therefore, we only need to exert half as much force to lift the block! This simple observation, that a pulley system (with massless, frictionless pulleys) causes a constant tension to exist through the entire string, which can lead to multiple tension forces pulling on an object, is the key to many MCAT problems on pulleys.

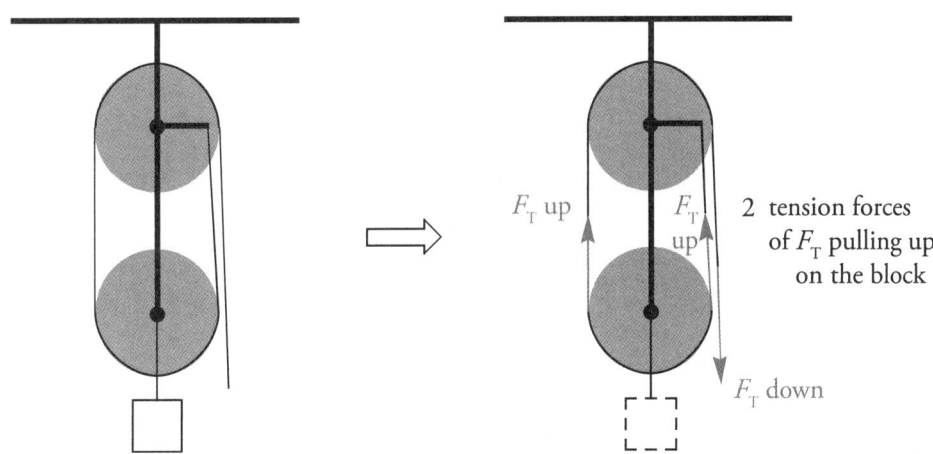

Pulley systems like this multiply our force by however many strings are pulling on the object.

Notice carefully that the tension force is applied wherever a string (or rope, or cable, or whatever) comes in contact with a pulley, which means that there will often be *two* tension forces on a single pulley, one on each side. You can see this in the right-hand diagram above.

Example 4-23: In the figure below, how much force would we need to exert on the free end of the cord in order to lift the plank (mass M = 300 kg) with constant velocity? (Ignore the masses of the pulleys.)

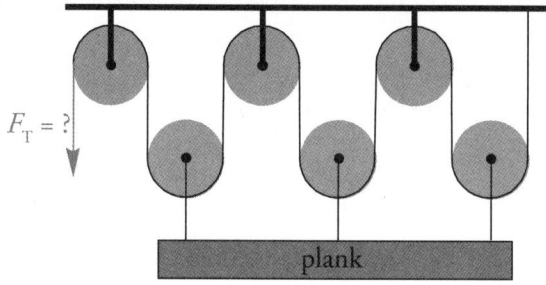

Solution: As a result of our pulling downward, there will be 6 tension forces pulling up on the plank:

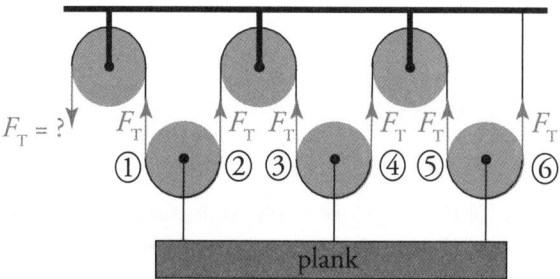

In order to lift with constant velocity (acceleration = zero), we require the net force on the plank to be zero. Therefore, the total of all the tension forces pulling up, $6F_T$, must balance the weight of the plank downward, Mg. This gives us

$$6F_T = Mg \rightarrow F_T = \frac{Mg}{6} = \frac{(300 \text{ kg})(10\frac{\text{N}}{\text{kg}})}{6} = 500 \text{ N}$$

Example 4-24: Two blocks are connected by a cord that hangs over a pulley. One block has a mass, M, of 10 kg, and the other block has a mass, m, of 5 kg. What will be the magnitude of the acceleration of the system of blocks once they are released from rest?

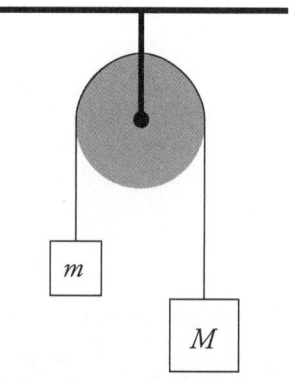

Solution: We'll solve this by a step-by-step approach using a **force diagram**. To apply Newton's second law, $\mathbf{F}_{net} = m\mathbf{a}$, to any problem, we follow these steps:

Step 1   Draw all the forces that act *on* the object. (That is, draw the force diagram.)

Step 2:   Choose a direction to call *positive* (simply take the direction of the object's motion to be positive; it's almost always the easiest, most natural decision).

Step 3:   Find $\mathbf{F}_{net}$ and set it equal to $m\mathbf{a}$.

We have effectively done these steps in the solutions to the examples we have seen already, but now that we have a situation involving two accelerating objects, it is even more important to make sure that we have a systematic plan of attack. When you have more than one object to worry about, just make sure that the Step-2 decision you make for one object is compatible with the Step-2 decision you make for the other one(s). On the left below are the force diagrams for the blocks on the pulley. Notice that we call *up* the positive direction for m (because that's where it's going), and we call *down* the positive direction for M (because that's where *it's* going); these decisions are compatible, because when m moves in its positive direction, so does M.

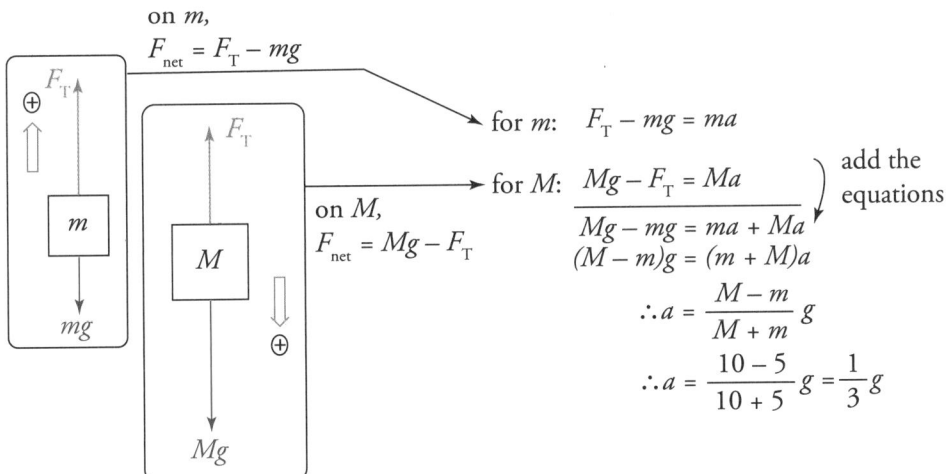

Because *up* is the positive direction for little m, the force F_T on m is positive and the force mg is negative; therefore, for little m, we have $F_{net} = F_T + (-mg) = F_T - mg$. Since *down* is the positive direction for big M, the force Mg on M is positive and the force F_T is negative; therefore, for big M, we have $F_{net} = Mg + (-F_T) = Mg - F_T$. On the right above, we've written down F_{net} = mass × acceleration for each block. There are two equations, but we have two unknowns (F_T and a), so we *need* two equations. To solve the equations, the trick is simply to *add the equations*. Notice that this makes the F_T's drop out, so all we're left with is one unknown, a, which we can solve for immediately. The calculation shown above gives $a = g/3$, so we get $a = 3.3 \text{ m/s}^2$.

If the question had asked for the tension in the cord, we could now use the value we found for a and plug it back into either of our two equations (we'd get the same answer no matter which one we used). Using $F_T - mg = ma$, we'd find that

$$F_T = ma + mg = m(a + g) = m(\tfrac{1}{3}g + g) = \tfrac{4}{3}mg = \tfrac{4}{3}(5 \text{ kg})(10 \tfrac{\text{N}}{\text{kg}}) = 67 \text{ N}$$

Example 4-25: In the figure below, the block of mass m slides up a frictionless inclined plane, pulled by another block of mass M that is falling. If $\theta = 30°$, $m = 20$ kg, and $M = 40$ kg, what's the acceleration of the block on the ramp?

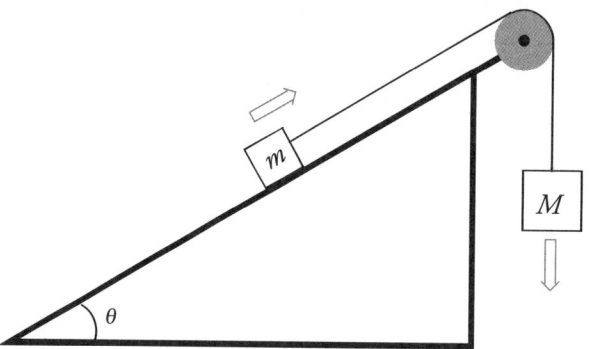

Solution: On the left below are the force diagrams for the blocks. Notice that we call *up the ramp* the positive direction for m (because that's where it's going), and we call *down* the positive direction for M (because that's where *it's* going); these decisions are compatible, because when m moves in its positive direction, so does M.

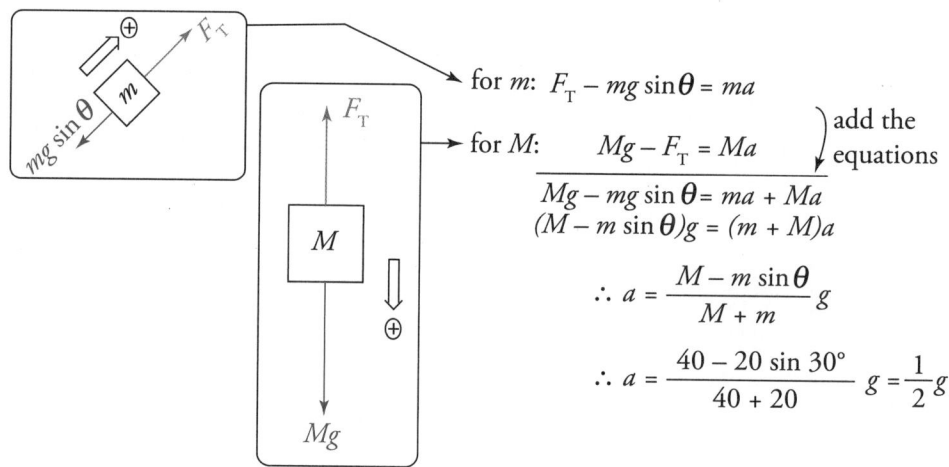

for m: $F_T - mg \sin\theta = ma$

for M: $Mg - F_T = Ma$

$\left.\right\}$ add the equations

$$Mg - mg \sin\theta = ma + Ma$$
$$(M - m \sin\theta)g = (m + M)a$$

$$\therefore a = \frac{M - m \sin\theta}{M + m}g$$

$$\therefore a = \frac{40 - 20 \sin 30°}{40 + 20}g = \frac{1}{2}g$$

Because *up the ramp* is the positive direction for little m, the force F_T on m is positive and the force due to gravity along the ramp, $mg \sin\theta$, is negative; therefore, for little m, we have $F_{net} = F_T + (-mg \sin\theta) = F_T - mg \sin\theta$. Since *down* is the positive direction for big M, the force Mg on M is positive and the force F_T is negative; therefore, for big M, we have $F_{net} = Mg + (-F_T) = Mg - F_T$. On the right above, we've written down $F_{net} =$ mass × acceleration for each block. As in the preceding example, there are two equations, (and two unknowns, F_T and a). Again using the trick of adding the equations, the F_T's drop out, and all we're left with is one unknown, a, to solve for. The calculation shown above gives $a = g/2$, so we get $a = 5$ m/s^2.

Summary of Formulas

NEWTON'S LAWS:

First law: $\mathbf{F}_{net} = 0 \Leftrightarrow \mathbf{v} = $ constant

Second law: $\mathbf{F}_{net} = m\mathbf{a}$

Third law: $\mathbf{F}_{1\text{-on-}2} = -\mathbf{F}_{2\text{-on-}1}$

Weight: $\mathbf{w} = m\mathbf{g}$

Gravitational force: $F_{grav} = G\,\dfrac{Mm}{r^2}$ given that $w = F_{grav}$, we get $g = G\,\dfrac{M}{r^2}$.

Kinetic friction: $F_f = \mu_k F_N$

Static friction: $F_{f,max} = \mu_s F_N$

$$\mu_s > \mu_k$$

Direction of friction is opposite to the direction of motion (or intended direction of motion).

Force due to gravity acting parallel to inclined plane: $mg \sin \theta$

Force due to gravity acting perpendicular to inclined plane: $mg \cos \theta$, where θ is measured between the incline and horizontal.

CHAPTER 4 FREESTANDING PRACTICE QUESTIONS

1. The gravitational force the Sun exerts on Earth is *F*. Mars is 1.5 times further from the Sun than Earth and its mass is $\frac{1}{6}$ of Earth's mass. Given that Newton's Law of Universal Gravitation states that the gravitational force is directly proportional to the masses and inversely proportional to the square of the distance separating the masses, what is the gravitational force that the Sun exerts on Mars?

   A) $\frac{2}{27} F$

   B) $\frac{1}{9} F$

   C) $9 F$

   D) $\frac{27}{2} F$

2. You have four frictionless, massless pulleys, arranged as shown below. If you have enough force to lift a 40 kg object without any pulleys, what is the maximum mass of the couch that can be raised with the pulley system?

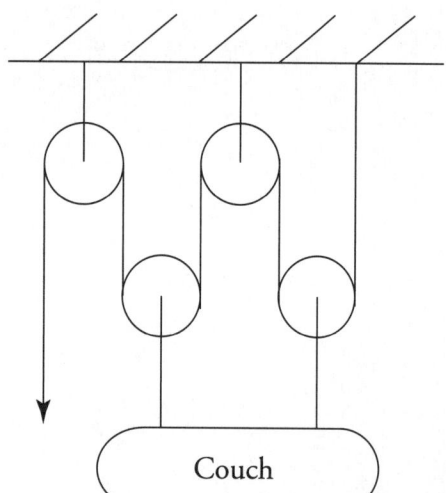

Couch

   A) 80 kg
   B) 120 kg
   C) 160 kg
   D) 240 kg

3. When an object falls from a very large height, it accelerates towards Earth because of the force of gravity. Air resistance also acts on the object as it falls, and the air resistance increases as the speed of the object increases. Eventually, the force due to air resistance equals that of gravity and the object reaches terminal velocity. What best describes this situation?

   A) The acceleration of the object at terminal velocity is the largest it will ever be.
   B) The speed of the object increases until it hits the ground.
   C) The speed of the object at terminal velocity is zero.
   D) The acceleration of the object at terminal velocity is zero.

4. A person starting from rest begins walking to the north. During their first step, the best description of the frictional force acting on the foot in contact with the ground is a:

   A) static frictional force to the north.
   B) static frictional force to the south.
   C) kinetic frictional force to the north.
   D) kinetic frictional force to the south.

5. A 100 g block is sitting at rest on a horizontal table. According to Newton's third law, which of the following indicates the correct action-reaction pair of the two forces?

   A) The gravitational force exerted by the table on the block and the normal force exerted by the block on the table
   B) The gravitational force exerted by the block on Earth and the normal force exerted by the table on the block
   C) The weight of the block and the normal force exerted by the table on the block
   D) The weight of the block and the gravitational force exerted by the block on Earth

6. A person is pulling a block of mass m with a force equal to its weight directed 30° above the horizontal plane across a rough surface, generating a friction f on the block. If the person is now pushing downward on the block with the same force 30° below the horizontal plane across the same rough surface, what is the friction on the block? (μ_k is the coefficient of kinetic friction across the surface.)

A) f
B) $1.5f$
C) $2f$
D) $3f$

7. Attempting to move a heavy couch ($m = 100$ kg) resting on sliders (assume negligible friction), two people apply pushing forces on perpendicular sides. One pushes to the north with a force of 150 N, and the other pushes to the east with a force of 200 N. If the couch starts from rest, how far does it move in the first two seconds while both forces are applied?

A) 3 m
B) 4 m
C) 5 m
D) 7 m

CHAPTER 4 PRACTICE PASSAGE

When an object is falling through air, it experiences a drag force due to the frictional effects of the air. The drag force is always directed opposite the direction of motion of the object. For a spherical object, the drag force can be calculated using Stokes' law:

$$F_D = 6\pi\eta r v$$

Equation 1

where F_D is the drag force, η is the coefficient of viscosity of the air, r is the radius of the sphere, and v is the velocity of the sphere.

Since the drag force is related to the velocity of the sphere, as the sphere's velocity increases, so does the drag force. After a certain time, the drag force will be large enough that the net force acting on the sphere is zero. At this point, the sphere falls with a constant velocity, known as the terminal velocity, v_T.

A student experiments with different spherical objects falling on Earth in order to test Stokes' law. The experiment involves dropping a variety of spheres from the balcony of a building. The relative mass and radius for each sphere are listed in Table 1.

Object	Mass	Radius
Beach ball	m	$20r$
Bowling ball	$20m$	$10r$
Golf ball	m	r
Ping pong ball	$0.25m$	r

Table 1 Mass and radius of spheres

1. Ignoring air resistance, which ball will hit the ground first?

A) The beach ball, since it has the largest radius.
B) The bowling ball, since it has the largest mass.
C) The golf ball, since it has the smallest radius and more mass than the ping pong ball.
D) All the balls will hit at the same time.

2. Considering air resistance, which ball will take the longest time to reach the ground when dropped, assuming none of the balls reaches its terminal velocity?

A) Beach ball
B) Bowling ball
C) Golf ball
D) Ping pong ball

3. For the experiment conducted, let v_1 be the velocity of the golf ball after 10 seconds when dropped from height, h. Let v_2 be the velocity of the ping pong ball after 10 seconds when dropped from the same height, h. How do v_1 and v_2 compare?

A) $v_1 < v_2$
B) $v_1 = v_2$
C) $v_1 > v_2$
D) It cannot be determined without information on the drag force.

4. How does the drag force on the beach ball compare to the drag force on the bowling ball when the velocities of the two balls are the same?

A) The drag force on the beach ball is 20 times the drag force on the bowling ball.
B) The drag force on the beach ball is 2 times the drag force on the bowling ball.
C) The drag force on the beach ball is $\frac{2}{3}$ the drag force on the bowling ball.
D) The drag force on the beach ball is $\frac{1}{2}$ the drag force on the bowling ball.

5. Which of the following gives an equation for the terminal velocity for the balls?

A) $v_T = mg - 6\pi\eta r$

B) $v_T = mg + 6\pi\eta r$

C) $v_T = \dfrac{mg}{6\pi\eta r}$

D) $v_T = \dfrac{6\pi\eta r}{mg}$

6. Which ball has the greatest terminal velocity?

A) Beach ball
B) Bowling ball
C) Golf ball
D) Ping pong ball

SOLUTIONS TO CHAPTER 4 FREESTANDING PRACTICE QUESTIONS

1. **A** The gravitational force in this case can be written as $F \propto m/r^2$. Using the given factor changes between the Earth and Mars yields $F \propto \dfrac{m}{r^2} \rightarrow \dfrac{1/6}{\left(3/2\right)^2} = \dfrac{1/6}{9/4} = \dfrac{4}{54} = \dfrac{2}{27} F.$

2. **C** With four pulleys you have four times the tension force acting upwards, allowing you to lift four times the weight. Since the maximum tension force is (40 kg)(10 m/s²) = 400 N, the maximum force that can be applied to the couch is 4 × 400 N = 1600 N. This corresponds to a mass of 160 kg.

3. **D** The net force on the object is the difference between the force due to gravity and the force due to air resistance. Therefore, as the force due to air resistance grows larger, the net force decreases, as does the acceleration, eliminating choice A. When the force due to air resistance equals that of gravity, the net force is zero, as is the acceleration (according to Newton's second law), which makes choice D correct. When there is zero acceleration, velocity is constant, eliminating choice B and the object does not stop moving once it reaches terminal velocity, eliminating choice C.

4. **A** Note the 2x2 pattern among the answer choices and use process of elimination. First, consider that in normal walking motion, a person's feet (or shoes) *grip* the ground without slipping. This means that the force is static friction, not kinetic; just because the person is moving *does not mean* that the contact surfaces are slipping relative to one another: this is a critical point about static versus kinetic friction (choices C and D can be eliminated). Next, consider that the person is accelerating to the north if they're starting from rest and moving north. By Newton's second law, this means that the net force points to the north. Since friction is the source of the horizontal force, friction points north (choice B can be eliminated and choice A is correct). Don't assume that static friction resists all motion: it only resists slipping motion at the point of contact between the surfaces. The best way to get the direction of the static frictional force is to apply Newton's laws.

5. **D** Since the answers could be confusing, a good strategy would be to identify all the correct action–reaction pairs, and match them to the answer choices. Here are the correct action–reaction pairs in question:

   a. The weight of the block and the gravitational force exerted by the block on Earth
   b. The normal force exerted by the block on the table and the normal force exerted by the table on the block
   c. The gravitational force exerted by the table on the block and the gravitational force exerted by the block on the table

   Of all the answer choices, only choice D matches the pairs described above.

6. **D** The friction f on the block is represented by the formula $f = \mu_k N$, where N is the normal force acting on the block. When the force is applied 30° above the horizontal, $N = mg - mg \sin 30°$. Since $\sin 30°$ is 0.5, $N = mg - 0.5mg = 0.5mg$. Substituting N into the formula for friction, it becomes $f_1 = 0.5\mu_k mg$. When the force is applied 30° below the horizontal, $N = mg + mg \sin 30° = mg + 0.5mg = 1.5mg$. Substituting N into the formula for friction, it becomes $f_2 = 1.5\mu_k mg = 3f$.

Therefore, the correct answer is choice D.

7. **C** To find the displacement of the couch, first determine its acceleration via Newton's second law. For two perpendicular forces, the net force must be the vector sum, and the net force therefore is the hypotenuse of the right triangle formed by the north and east forces. The Pythagorean theorem gives the length of the hypotenuse, but you should recognize the 3-4-5 ratio in this case: 150 N to 200 N to 250 N! Thus we have $F_{net} = ma \rightarrow a = \dfrac{250 \text{ N}}{100 \text{ kg}} = 2.5 \dfrac{\text{m}}{\text{s}^2}$. Add to that the initial velocity $v_0 = 0$ and $t = 2$ s, and we're missing the final velocity, so we use kinematics Big Five equation 3 to solve for d: $d = v_0 t + \frac{1}{2}at^2 = \frac{1}{2}\left(2.5\dfrac{\text{m}}{\text{s}^2}\right)(2 \text{ s})^2 = 5 \text{ m}$.

SOLUTIONS TO CHAPTER 4 PRACTICE PASSAGE

1. **D** For ideal conditions with no friction, the drag force will not exist (it is a frictional force). The acceleration of each ball can be calculated from $F_{net} = ma$. The only force acting on the ball is its weight, so $mg = ma$ and $a = g$ so the acceleration on each ball will be the acceleration from gravity, g. Since all balls are dropped from the same height and have the same acceleration, they will hit the ground at the same time.

2. **A** The acceleration of each ball can be calculated from $F_{net} = ma$. Since the net displacement of the balls is down, F_G is in the positive direction and $F_G - F_D = ma$ so $mg - 6\pi\eta rv = ma$ and $a = g - 6\pi\eta rv/m$. The only values in the equation that change for the different balls are the mass and radius. The larger the ratio of r/m, the larger amount that is subtracted from g, and the slower the ball's acceleration. The question asks for the longest time, which is the slowest acceleration. The beach ball has the largest radius/mass ratio ($20r/m$) and so the slowest acceleration and the longest time.

3. **C** The acceleration of each ball can be calculated from $F_{net} = ma$. Since the net displacement of the balls is down, F_G is in the positive direction and $F_G - F_D = ma$ so $mg - 6\pi\eta rv = ma$ and $a = g - 6\pi\eta rv/m$. The only value in the equation that changes for the different balls is the mass. The larger the mass, the smaller the amount that is subtracted from g, and the larger the ball's acceleration, so the larger the ball's velocity. Since the golf ball has the larger mass, it will have the larger velocity, v_1.

4. **B** Using Equation 1, the drag force on the beach ball is F_D, beach ball $= 6\pi\eta(20r)v$. The drag force on the bowling ball is F_D, bowling ball $= 6\pi\eta(10r)v$. Thus, the drag force on the beach ball is twice the drag force on the bowling ball.

5. **C** The passage states that terminal velocity is reached when the net force on the sphere is zero, so $F_{net} = 0$. The only two forces acting on the sphere are the force of gravity and the drag force, so these forces must be equal when the terminal velocity is reached. Starting with the equation $F_G = F_D$ and plugging in Equation 1 yields $mg = 6\pi\eta rv$. Solving this equation for the velocity, which in this case is the terminal velocity, yields $v = (mg)/(6\pi\eta r)$. Notice the equations in choices A and B include the sum and difference with the weight of the ball, which is not a velocity, so these two choices can be eliminated, leaving choice C as the correct answer.

6. **B** The passage states that terminal velocity is reached when the net force on the sphere is zero, so $F_{net} = 0$. The only two forces acting on the sphere are the force of gravity and the drag force, so these forces must be equal when the terminal velocity is reached. Starting with the equation $F_G = F_D$ and plugging in Equation 1 yields $mg = 6\pi\eta rv$. Solving this equation for the velocity, which in this case is the terminal velocity, yields $v = (mg)/(6\pi\eta r)$. The sphere with the largest terminal velocity will have the largest ratio of mass/radius. The bowling ball has the largest mass/radius ratio ($2m/r$) and so will have the largest terminal velocity.

AN ANALYSIS OF THE FORCES REQUIRED TO DRAG SHEEP OVER VARIOUS SURFACES

J.T. Harvey, J.Culvenor, W.Payne, S.Cowley, M.Lawrance, D.Stuart, R.Williams

Abstract

Some occupational health and safety hazards associated with sheep shearing are related to shearing shed design. One aspect is the floor of the catching pen, from which sheep are caught and dragged to the shearing workstation. Floors can be constructed from various materials, and may be level or gently sloping. An experiment was conducted using eight experienced shearers as participants to measure the force exerted by a shearer when dragging a sheep. Results showed that significant changes in mean dragging force occurred with changes in both surface texture and slope. The mean dragging forces for different floor textures and slopes ranged from 359N (36.6 kg) to 423N (43.2 kg), and were close to the maximum acceptable limits for pulling forces for the most capable of males. The best floor tested was a floor sloped at 1:10 constructed of timber battens oriented parallel to the path of the drag, which resulted in a mean dragging force 63.6N (15%) lower than the worst combination. © 2002 Elsevier Science Ltd. All rights reserved.

INTRODUCTION

Sheep shearing is an arduous occupation involving a range of physically demanding tasks: catching and tipping the sheep, dragging the sheep into position, fleece removal, and guiding the shorn sheep away. Shearing has proved difficult to mechanise, and still has significant occupational hazards involving manual handling (Australian Workers' Union (Vic.), 1993; Health and Safety Organisation, Victoria, 1995; National Occupational Health and Safety Commission, 1990). Cole and Foley (1995) reported that injuries to shearers included fractures and sprains (66.4%), musculoskeletal injuries (15.0%), and contusions/burns (8.5%). The most common bodily location for these injuries was the hand, finger and thumb (22%) and back (19.0%). Back injuries were reported at a frequency of 100.6 cases per 1,000,000 h worked. According to Culvenor et al. (1997), Australian shearers suffer injuries at six times the all-industry average (per worker or per hour) and injuries are on average between 70% and 140% more costly than in other industries. Other studies have confirmed that shearing is intensive in terms of its energy demand (Stuart, 1991; Webster and Lush, 1991).

In the study of which the work reported in this paper formed part (Payne et al., 1998), industry focus groups identified the effort required to drag sheep as an issue, indicating that many shearers suffered back injuries during sheep dragging. Alternative sheep delivery systems such as elevated races (Freeman, 1991) eliminate dragging, but require substantial financial investment. This study focussed on identifying simple and inexpensive ways to reduce risks, and to quantify the impact of these methods in order to encourage their adoption.

Shearing involves repeated loading of the tissues of the low back to apparently submaximal levels. McGill (1997) reported that cumulative trauma from sub-failure magnitude loads causes a slow degradation of the failure tolerance due to the prolonged stoop posture loading the posterior ligaments of the spine and posterior fibres of the intervertebral disc, causing creep deformation, possibly to the point of micro-failure. It is possible that failure tolerance is reduced by repeated stooping during shearing, rendering the shearer more susceptible to back injury when dragging.

The aim of the current study was to examine the range of floor surfaces and angles identified by industry focus groups, and to determine the combination of floor surface and angle which minimised the forces required during sheep dragging. A second aim was to assess the forces measured in comparison to those considered acceptable from a health and safety perspective.

METHODOLOGY

Subjects

The study involved eight male shearers, as described in Table 1, and five sheep. The data were collected on 2 days, with four shearers attending on each day. The sheep weighed 50–55 kg and had approximately 8 months' wool. Shearers gave their informed consent to participate and the study was approved by the ethics committee of the University of Ballarat.

Table 1 Subject Details			
Shearer	Height (cm)	Mass (kg)	Full-time/ Part-time
1	194	87	PT
2	178	72	FT
3	185	97	PT
4	178	76	FT
5	178	85	FT
6	182	101	PT
7	182	110	FT
8	172	82	PT
Mean	181	89	
SD	6.5	13	

Experimental factors: floor surfaces and slopes

Five types of flooring material were investigated:

1. Wood battens oriented parallel to the drag.
2. Wood battens oriented at right angles to the drag.
3. Plastic battens oriented parallel to the drag.
4. Plastic battens oriented at right angles to the drag.
5. Steel mesh.

The wood battens were 45 mm wide with a 15 mm gap, chamfered to mimic the profile of a worn batten. The plastic "battens" were tiles 800 × 400 mm, with slots that gave a directional character. The steel mesh was woven of 5 mm wire with square holes at 25 mm centres. The floor slopes tested were horizontal (0°) and 1:10 (5.6°).

Interchangeable sections of flooring were constructed from each of the five materials, and with both slopes. The sections could be attached to a force plate, together with matching panels in front of and behind the force plate (see Fig. 1.)

Experimental design

The combination of the two factors (five surfaces, two slopes) with each of the five sheep resulted in a repeated measures design with 50 trials for each of the eight shearers, or 400 trials in all. The order of the experiment was randomised within some practical constraints. Time-consuming slope changes were minimised, with no slope in the morning of day one and with the slope in the afternoon. This order was reversed on day two. Within each session, a random order of textures was used, then a random order of sheep, and lastly a random order of shearer. This schedule minimised the chance of any shearer undertaking two trials in succession. On the few occasions that this occurred, a rest period of a least 3 min separated the trials to minimise the potential confounding effect of fatigue.

Experimental procedure

The shearers wore 'shearing moccasins' and were instructed to drag the sheep at constant speed across the force plate. Force was measured with a 900 × 600 mm Kistler 9287 3D force plate, fitted beneath the centre panel of flooring (see Fig. 1). Data collection software was AP30 (Pearce, 1996). All data were represented in a global co-ordinate system relative to the ground (see Fig. 1). Force in the horizontal longitudinal (x), horizontal lateral (y) and vertical (z) directions was sampled for two seconds at 1000 Hz (2000 samples per trial). Data analysis was carried out using Microsoft ExcelV6 and MinitabV9. Each trial was videotaped.

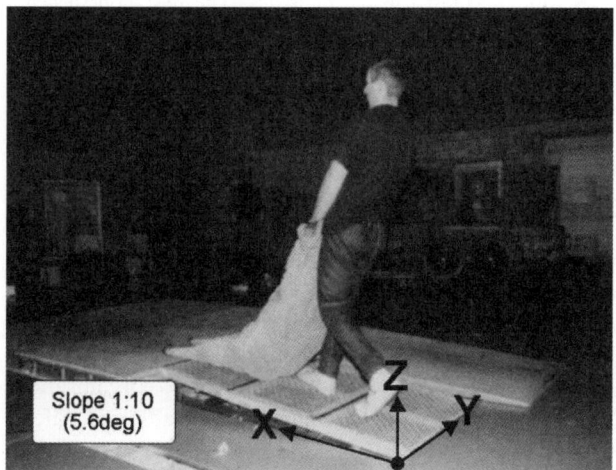

Figure 1. Shearer on force plate and XYZ co-ordinates.

Response variables

Three key response variables were derived and analysed:

1. Dragging force.
2. Maximum vertical ground reaction on the shearer.
3. Maximum rate of increase of the vertical ground reaction on the shearer.

Variable 1 was derived from data collected with the sheep on the force plate and variables 2 and 3 from data collected while the shearer was on the force plate.

Dragging force: The primary variable was the dragging force F being exerted by the shearer on the sheep (see Fig. 2). It was not feasible to measure this force directly. Rather, it was derived indirectly from force plate measurements of the ground reaction forces R and weights W. Because the sheep was being passively dragged, data collected while the sheep was on the force plate were less subject to impulse effects than data collected while the shearer was on the force plate. For this reason, sheep-based data were used to estimate a steady-state average dragging force.

The dragging force F was calculated as follows:

$$F = \sqrt{R_x^2 + R_y^2 + (W - R_z)^2} \tag{1}$$

where R is the ground reaction force and W the weight of the sheep.

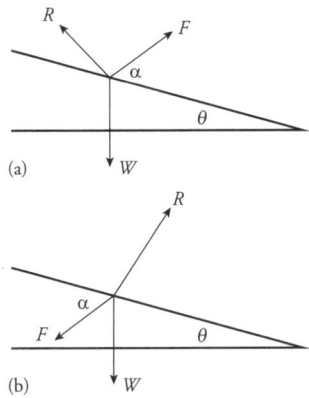

Figure 2. Force diagrams. (a) Forces on Sheep. (b). Forces on Shearer. F = dragging force; R = ground reaction; W = weight; y = angle of inclination of floor; a = angle of inclination of drag to floor.

This best available estimate of the force being applied by the hands of the shearer is predicated on the assumptions that the sheep were inelastic and moving at constant velocity. Both assumptions are regarded as reasonable approximations. A trace of this variable, plotted over the 2000 ms of data collection, was visually inspected to identify a section of 100 ms duration in which the process was in a steady state, and a mean value was calculated.

Maximum vertical ground reaction on shearer and Maximum rate of increase of vertical ground reaction on shearer: The data measured while the shearer was on the plate had a more dynamic characteristic. The maximum value of the vertical ground reaction R_z and the maximum rate of increase of R_z were chosen as indicators of the impulsive forces exerted on the shearer's body. The maximum vertical ground reaction was estimated directly from the trace of R_z; after first smoothing it with a moving window of 40 ms duration to remove any spurious high frequency transients induced within the measurement

equipment. The smoothed trace R_z of was then differenced and the maximum rate of increase determined from the difference trace.

Ancillary variables

Four further variables were calculated for the purpose of biomechanical modelling and to enable further exploration of the behaviour of the three key variables. These were:

4. Coefficient of kinetic friction.
5. Vertical angle of application of dragging force.
6. Normal component of ground reaction force on sheep.
7. Speed of shearer.

Coefficient of kinetic friction: The coefficient of kinetic friction μ_k is determined by the characteristics of the floor material and the wool of the sheep in sliding contact. It is the ratio of the parallel and normal components of the ground reaction force. It was calculated using the following formula.

$$\mu_k = \frac{\sqrt{(R_x \cos\theta + R_z \sin\theta)^2 + R_y^2}}{R_z \cos\theta - R_x \sin\theta} \tag{2}$$

where R is the ground reaction force, and θ the angle of inclination of the surface ($0°$ or $5.6°$).

Angle of application of dragging force: This is the angle between the dragging force vector and its projection onto the floor surface (see Fig. 3), calculated by

$$\alpha = \tan^{-1}\left(\frac{R_x \sin\theta - (R_z - W)\cos\theta}{\sqrt{(R_x \cos\theta + (R_z - W)\sin\theta)^2 + R_y^2}}\right) \tag{3}$$

where R is the ground reaction force, W the weight of the sheep, and θ the angle of inclination of the surface ($0°$ or $5.6°$).

Normal component of ground reaction force on sheep: This variable is the denominator of the formula for μ_k:

$$R_n = R_z \cos\theta - R_x \sin\theta \tag{4}$$

where R is the ground reaction force, and θ the angle of inclination of the surface ($0°$ or $5.6°$).

Speed of shearer: Videotapes of each trial were examined and the shearer's average speed was calculated by measuring the time (the number of video frames) taken by an identifiable point on the body of the sheep to traverse the test surface.

RESULTS

Not unexpectedly, there were statistically significant differences between shearers and between sheep for all dependent variables. When the heights and weights of shearers were incorporated as covariates, they accounted for much of the differences between shearers.

Dragging force

Table 2 shows results for the dragging force by texture and slope. There were significant differences between textures ($F(4,379) = 31.70$, $p < 0:0005$). Using the Tukey HSD criterion, any two means that differ by more than 8.8 N were significantly different at the 0.05 level. Thus the mean for wooden battens at right angles did not differ significantly from either of the two means for plastic battens. All other pairwise differences were statistically significant.

The texture with the lowest mean dragging force was wooden battens parallel to the drag (horizontal: 388 N; slope: 359 N). The texture with the highest mean dragging force was steel mesh (horizontal: 423 N; slope: 394 N).

Coefficient of kinetic friction

Table 3 shows results for the coefficient of friction by texture and slope. There are significant differences between textures ($F(4,379) = 907.36$, $p < 0:0005$). Using Tukey HSD, any two means which differed by more than 0.019 were significantly different at the 0.05 level.

Table 2 Dragging force on sheep (N): by texture and slope[a]

Texture	Slope = 0°		Slope = 5.6°		Both slopes
	Mean	**SD**	**Mean**	**SD**	**Mean**
Wood: parallel	388.2	28.0	359.2	31.8	373.7
Wood: at right angles	400.4	22.4	376.4	29.2	388.4
Plastic: parallel	395.6	26.4	370.1	30.9	382.9
Plastic: at right angles	405.4	24.7	378.9	31.4	392.2
Steel mesh	422.8	21.2	394.1	26.3	408.4
All textures	402.5		375.7		

[a]Sample size $n = 40$ for each of the 10 texture-slope combinations.

Table 3 Coefficient of friction: by texture and slope[a]

Texture	Slope = 0°		Slope = 5.6°		Both slopes
	Mean	**SD**	**Mean**	**SD**	**Mean**
Wood: parallel	0.507	0.045	0.484	0.047	0.496
Wood: at right angles	0.606	0.035	0.585	0.040	0.595
Plastic: parallel	0.620	0.034	0.596	0.025	0.608
Plastic: at right angles	0.688	0.049	0.645	0.043	0.666
Steel mesh	0.928	0.066	0.858	0.081	0.893
All textures	0.670		0.633		

[a]Sample size $n = 40$ for each of the 10 texture-slope combinations.

DISCUSSION

The discussion has been formulated with reference to the conceptual model of Hoozemans et al. (1998). This model integrates exposure to external factors (work situation, actual working method, posture, movement and external forces), resultant internal (mechanical) exposure, acute responses, long-term effects and work capacity. The discussion will also acknowledge the frameworks outlined by Winkel and Mathiassen (1994) and Hoozemans et al. (1998). Winkel and Mathiassen (1994) proposed that exposure to work related factors can be explored through examining work intensity (amplitude and direction), frequency and duration. The review by Hoozemans et al. (1998) outlined the perspectives of epidemiology, psychophysics, physiology and biomechanics.

In terms of these frameworks, it can be seen that the current study was motivated by epidemiological evidence, and sought to understand work intensity during shearing through modifying aspects of external exposure and examining aspects of both external and internal exposure. Specifically, the study sought to determine the impact of factors that alter the actual work situation (floor slope and texture) on the forces exerted, as aspects of external exposure, and the resultant internal exposure. The exerted forces were explored via an examination of psychophysical factors. That is, the forces exerted when performing the work task under the various floor slope and texture conditions, were related to the maximum acceptable forces. Internal exposure was examined via the biomechanical estimation of L5/S1 compression. Specific physiological measures were not made during the study.

Psychophysical perspectives

Dragging force

The minimum mean dragging force was achieved using a sloping surface constructed of wooden battens arranged parallel to the direction of the drag. But whilst the central aim of the study was to compare the different floor surfaces, the actual magnitude of the forces also warrants examination. Since the number of sheep shorn per day by a professional shearer can be in excess of 200, injuries are more likely to be the result of the sustained nature of the work-task rather than the impact of a single instantaneous act.

Thus dragging sheep repetitively is a difficult task, within the capability of only the most able men, and too physically demanding for almost all women. Clearly, the forces involved are at the extreme of what is acceptable for an occupational activity. The findings here, which substantiate a difference in the order of 15% between the best floor tested and the worst floor tested, are thus of great practical importance.

Some caution must be exercised in drawing these conclusions. The results obtained were based on an indirect estimate of the force exerted by the shearer, which is predicated on the assumption of an inelastic sheep being dragged at constant velocity. Whilst every effort was made to ensure that the latter condition was achieved, no quantitative assessment has been made of the effect of any departures from either of these assumptions.

Another issue is that the initial force required to begin motion exceeds the steady–state dragging force. Calculation of this initial force from force plate measurements was infeasible because estimates of acceleration and elasticity of the sheep would be required. From this perspective, our conclusions are clearly conservative, since our results underestimate the peak stresses.

Relationship between coefficient of kinetic friction and dragging force

The effect of floor surface and slope on the coefficient of friction was examined in order to understand the factors affecting the dragging force. On both sloping and horizontal floors, the coefficient of friction increased by some 80 percent from its minimum value for parallel wooden battens to its maximum value for steel mesh, compared to an increase of only 10 percent in the dragging force. We now explore the reason for this difference.

On a horizontal surface, the relationship between the dragging force F; coefficient of friction μ_k; sheep weight W; and drag angle α is given by

$$F = \frac{\mu_k W}{\cos \alpha + \mu_k \sin \alpha} \tag{5}$$

when $\alpha = 90°$ (i.e. lifting the sheep), F reaches a maximum value equal to W; and is independent of the coefficient of friction. At the opposite extreme, when $\alpha = 0°$ (i.e. a horizontal force), then $F = \mu_k W$: This is a lower force (providing $\mu_k < 1$) but requires a posture not conducive to dragging. If shearers did drag sheep in this manner, the force required on different surfaces would change in direct proportion to the coefficient of friction.

In fact, the dragging force in all cases was applied only some 10–15° away from the vertical (Table 4), that is, with a substantial component of lift. Because the body angle adopted by the shearers, consistent with comfort and efficiency, was close to the vertical, the dragging force is not greatly dependent on the coefficient of friction, hence the relatively smaller differences between dragging forces on different surfaces.

Dependence of the coefficient of kinetic friction on slope

For each floor texture, the coefficient of friction was found to be some 5–10 percent lower on the 5.6° slope than on the horizontal (Table 2). This is thought to be due to greater compaction of the wool on the sloping floor. Because shearers maintained the same drag angle relative to the vertical under both conditions (Table 4), the drag angle relative to the normal to the floor surface was less when the floor was sloping, resulting in an increase in the component of the ground reaction force normal to the floor surface in this case (Table 5), and hence, it is conjectured, increased compaction of the wool.

Table 4 Vertical angle of dragging force (degrees from vertical): by texture and slope[a]

Texture	Slope = 0°		Slope = 5.6°[b]		Both slopes
	Mean	SD	Mean	SD	Mean
Wood: parallel	11.0	2.9	12.2	2.4	11.6
Wood: at right angles	11.8	2.4	11.6	2.6	11.7
Plastic: parallel	12.9	3.3	13.1	2.7	13.0
Plastic: at right angles	13.1	3.2	12.8	2.7	13.0
Steel mesh	14.8	3.1	16.2	3.3	15.5
All textures	12.7		13.2		

[a]Sample size n = 40 for each of the 10 texture-slope combinations.
[b]For the sloped floor, the angles to the normal to the floor plane are approximately 5.6° less than these figures.

Table 5 Normal component of ground reaction force on sheep (N): by texture and slope[a]

Texture	Slope = 0°		Slope = 5.6°		Both slopes
	Mean	SD	Mean	SD	Mean
Wood: parallel	145.2	32.3	166.8	31.2	156.0
Wood: at right angles	134.4	23.8	150.8	28.9	142.4
Plastic: parallel	140.7	29.5	156.2	25.4	148.4
Plastic: at right angles	131.5	24.2	148.0	29.7	139.9
Steel mesh	117.8	23.2	137.2	26.5	127.4
All textures	133.9		151.9		

[a]Sample size n = 40 for each of the 10 texture-slope combinations.

CONCLUSION

In conclusion, of the range of floor surfaces and angles examined, the optimum floor is a sloping surface (1:10 as tested) constructed of wooden battens arranged parallel to the direction of the drag. These relatively inexpensive modifications have the potential to substantially improve the safety of shearing as it is likely that the risk of injury will be reduced through a reduction of dragging force by up to 15%.

It is recommended that such a floor be installed where practicable. Both a slope and a change to the orientation of battens require some alteration to the sub-floor structure, but this should not be very difficult or expensive. However, the ramifications of a slope, insofar as it affects the way sheep enter the pen and the way gates operate may be more problematic. These issues relate to individual shearing sheds and would have to be addressed on an individual basis.

JOURNAL ARTICLE EXERCISE 1

The science sections on the MCAT include a significant number of passages with experiments or quantitative data. In the Chem/Phys section, questions for these passages often ask you to analyze numerical data from tables and graphs, interpret an apparatus, and come to some reasonable conclusion based on the information they give you. If you don't know how to extract information efficiently and analyze data effectively, you will be at a distinct disadvantage.

There are three "Journal Article Exercises" in this book. In this first exercise, we'll show you the type of information you should be able to extract from the article and the sorts of things to pay attention to in the data. In subsequent exercises, you'll do more of that on your own, and in the final exercise we'll show you how that article might get turned into an MCAT-style passage.

When analyzing a physics article, you should be able to:

- find the research question(s),
- identify the independent and dependent variables,
- determine the significance of any equations and recognize any familiar terms therein,
- interpret the experiment design in terms of basic physical principles,
- analyze any experiment apparatus,
- extract information from graphs and data tables,
- observe trends in the data,
- interpret the hypotheses in terms of the research questions and data, and
- assess the strengths and limitations of the study.

The goal of these exercises is NOT to learn content from the articles, just to get a little more comfortable reading and extracting information from them.

For the (abridged) article on pages 103–108, try to summarize the purpose, methods, results, and assumptions of the study. Consider the following questions:

- **Topic(s) of the research**: where does this research fit within the subject matter covered within Chem/Phys? Is more than one discipline or topic pertinent to this research?
- **Research question(s)**: what are the researchers trying to determine? How are their methods informed by the question(s)?
- **Data collection**: how do the authors get their information? What is the experimental procedure, the apparatus, the measurement device?
- **Data analysis**: how do the authors make sense of the numbers? If there are stated equations, what are the inputs and outputs, the independent and dependent variables? What descriptive statistics are used?
- **Data presentation**: how do the authors show their work? Are there figures showing the apparatus? How do these relate to the data? Are there tables or graphs? If so, what quantities/units are shown? What trends are evident? What do these reveal about the significance of the findings?
- **Conclusions/hypotheses**: what does the research mean? How does it answer the research questions? What does it *not* answer, and how do the authors acknowledge its limitations? Are there any unacknowledged limitations you can see?
- **Assumptions**: what do the authors implicitly or explicitly take as given in the ways they design their research, interpret their data, or argue for the significance of their findings? Do these assumptions seem justified, given your knowledge of the underlying science?

SOLUTIONS TO JOURNAL ARTICLE EXERCISE 1

Let's answer the above questions for the article on pages 103–108.

1. **Topic:**
   - Where does this research fit within the subject matter covered within Chem/Phys? *Physics, specifically dynamics related to the friction force*
   - Is more than one discipline or topic pertinent to this research? *No*

2. **Research questions:**
   - Where what are the researchers trying to determine? *What "combination of floor surface and angle minimized the forces required during sheep dragging, [and how do the] forces measured [compare] to those considered acceptable from a health and safety perspective?"*
   - How are their methods informed by the question(s)? *The selection of surfaces and slopes was informed by those used in the sheep shearing industry.*

3. **Data collection:**
   - What is the experimental procedure? *Eight male shearers dragged five sheep across ten different combinations of slopes and surfaces over two days.*
   - What is the experiment apparatus and the measurement device? *Five different flooring types were each placed at two different angles (0° and 5.6°), and a force plate was mounted in the midst of the flooring. The force plate data were sampled over a period of two seconds at a rate of 1000 Hz.*

4. **Data analysis:**
   - What are the independent and dependent variables in the stated equations? *Forces on the sheep and the shearers moving at constant speeds were measured in three dimensions using the force plate, and these independent variables were used to determine the net dragging forces exerted by the shearers as well and the maximum vertical forces and maximum rates of change of vertical forces from the ground on the shearers. The coefficients of kinetic friction for each surface at each angle were also computed, as were the vertical angle of application of dragging force, the normal component of ground reaction force on sheep, and the speeds of each shearer.*
   - What descriptive statistics are used? *Means and standard deviations of dragging forces and coefficients of kinetic friction were calculated.*

5. **Data presentation:**
   - Are there figures showing the apparatus? How do these relate to the data? *Yes, the figure showing the forces acting on the sheep and the shearer explains the equations for the dragging force and kinetic friction coefficient.*
   - Are there tables or graphs? If so, what quantities/units are shown? What trends are evident? *Tables show calculated dragging forces in newtons, coefficients of kinetic friction, vertical angle of dragging forces, and normal forces in newtons. The dragging forces and coefficients of friction trend slightly upward from wood to plastic to steel mesh.*
   - What do these reveal about the significance of the findings? *There is a statistically significant difference between the optimal dragging force condition and the worst condition.*

6. Conclusions/hypotheses:

- How does the research answer the research questions? *The data show that the some surfaces do indeed minimize the forces exerted by the shearers in dragging the sheep.*
- What does it *not* answer, and how do the authors acknowledge its limitations? *Given that none of the calculated dragging forces exceeds recommended limits, it's plausible but not definitive that the recommended change in dragging surfaces would be worth the investment (the authors say only that "it is likely that the risk of injury will be reduced" by the recommended changes, but do not quantify that likelihood).*
- Are there any unacknowledged limitations you can see? *The sample size is relatively small—eight people dragging five sheep—and it is not stated whether they were sampled from a wide region or were more likely a local convenience sample, so it could be that other shearers-sheep combinations would have different dragging techniques that would yield significantly different data.*

7. Assumptions:

- What do the authors implicitly or explicitly take as given in the ways they design their research, interpret their data, or argue for the significance of their findings? *The authors base all of their biomechanical and physiological conclusions (some results not shown in abridged article) on indirect evidence and previous work by other researchers: no direct measurements of loads on the body were taken, for example. Also, the authors assume the coefficient of kinetic friction to be independent of the dragging speed: they measure the speed but do not use it in their calculations. "The results obtained were based on an indirect estimate of the force exerted by the shearer, which is predicated on the assumption of an inelastic sheep being dragged at constant velocity. Whilst every effort was made to ensure that the latter condition was achieved, no quantitative assessment has been made of the effect of any departures from either of these assumptions."*
- Do these assumptions seem justified, given your knowledge of the underlying science? *The friction assumption certainly fits the standard equation for the coefficient of kinetic friction, but given that the authors acknowledge that the friction coefficient changes with the slight change in slope of the floor and guess that this has to do with the compaction of the wool, it seems possible that the velocity was also relevant, and this would require further investigation.*

Chapter 5
Mechanics II

5.1 CENTER OF MASS AND GRAVITY

In the examples we looked at in the preceding chapter, objects were treated as though they were each a single particle. In fact, in the step-by-step solution to one of the pulley problems, we drew a force diagram showing all the forces acting on the objects in the system. To make that step go faster, we sometimes just represent each object by a dot and draw the force arrows on the dot. For example, the force diagram in the solution to Example 4-24 could have been drawn like this:

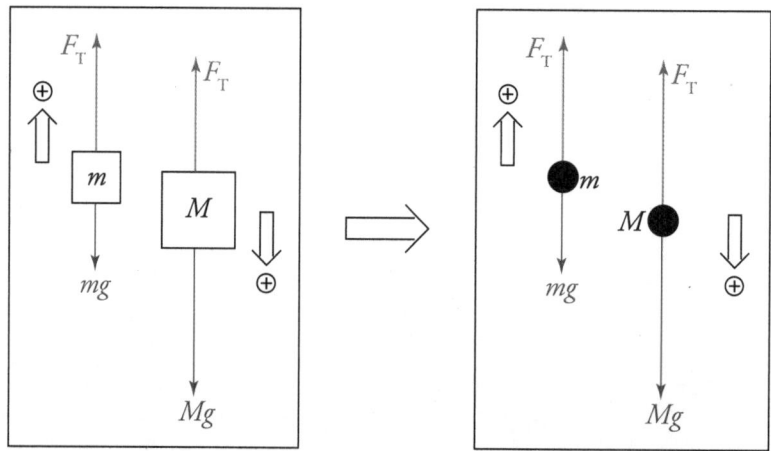

Each dot really denotes the *center of mass* of the object (or "center of gravity": the terms are interchangeable on the MCAT), which we'll now describe and define.

Imagine the following series of experiments. You walk into a large room with a friend, a hammer, and a glow-in-the dark (phosphorescent) sticker. After shining light on the sticker (so that it will glow), stick it on the metal head of the hammer. Hand the hammer to your friend, stand back, and turn off the light. Ask your friend to flip and toss the hammer across the room so that you can watch its trajectory. You'll see only the glow-in-the-dark sticker, and it will, in general, trace out some complicated loopy path as the hammer tumbles and flies through the air.

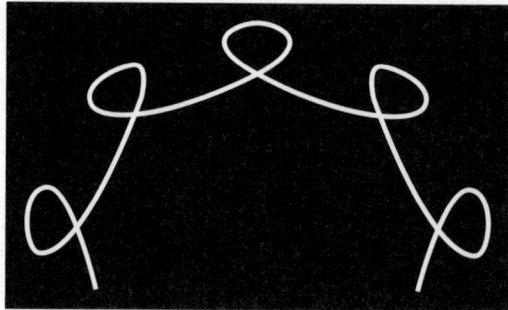

Repeat the experiment with the sticker attached to the end of the handle of the hammer. Once again, when your friend flips and tosses the hammer across the room so that you can watch it face on, you'll see only the glow-in-the-dark sticker, and it'll trace out another complicated loopy path.

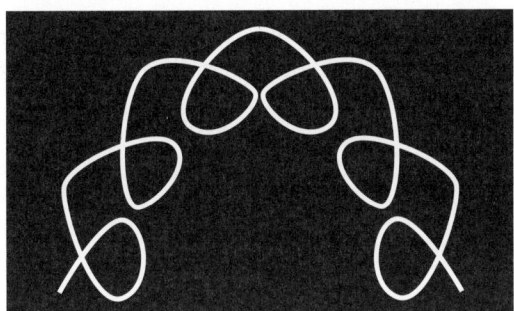

Now let's try this one more time, but rather than attaching the sticker at some random spot on the hammer, first find the point where the hammer just balances on the tip of your finger. Put the sticker on that spot and hand the hammer to your friend. Turn off the light, and watch as the hammer is tossed across the room. This time you'll see the sticker trace out a nice parabola, no loops.

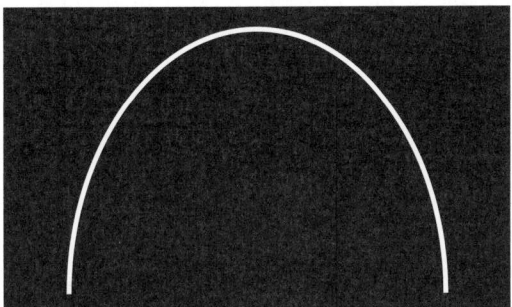

Apparently there was something special about the final location of the sticker. Most points on the hammer traced out complicated loopy trajectories, but this final point traced out a simple parabolic path, just as a single particle would. It is this one point that behaves as if the object (whether it's a block or a hammer or whatever) was a single particle. This special point is the **center of mass**. Another way of looking at it is to say that the center of mass is the point at which we could consider all the mass of the object to be concentrated. It's the dot in our simplified force diagrams.

For a simple object such as a sphere, block, or cylinder, whose density is constant (that is, for an object that's *homogeneous*), the center of mass is where you'd expect it to be—at its geometric center.

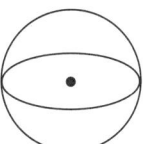 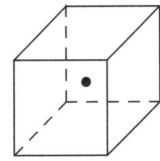 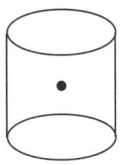

Note that in some cases, the center of mass isn't even located within the body of the object:

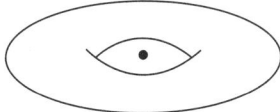 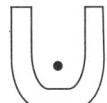

For a nonhomogeneous object, such as a hammer, whose density *does* vary from point to point, there's no single-step way mathematically to calculate the location of the center of mass.

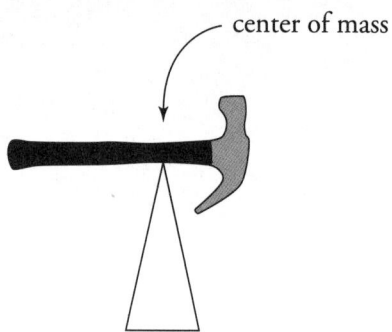

center of mass

However, there is a simpler type of problem on which the MCAT *will* expect you to locate the center of mass. The situation involves a series of masses arranged in a line. For example, imagine that you had a stick with several blocks hanging from it. Where should you attach a string to the stick so that this mobile would balance?

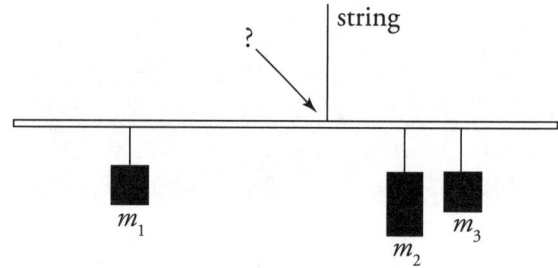

For a problem like this, in which each individual mass can be considered to be at a single point in space, here's the formula for the location of the center of mass:

Center of Mass for Point Masses

$$x_{CM} = \frac{m_1 x_1 + m_2 x_2 + m_3 x_3 \ldots}{m_1 + m_2 + m_3 \ldots}$$

(The location of the center of mass is often denoted by $\bar{x}$ as well. We'll use both notations.) To use this formula, follow these steps:

Step 1: Choose an origin (a reference point to call $x = 0$). The locations of the objects will be measured relative to this point. Often the easiest point to use will be at the location of the left-hand mass, but any point is fine; if a coordinate system is given in the problem, use it.

Step 2: Determine the locations (x_1, x_2, x_3, etc.) of the objects.

Step 3: Multiply each mass by its location ($m_1 x_1$, $m_2 x_2$, $m_3 x_3$, etc.) then add.

Step 4: Divide by the total mass ($m_1 + m_2 + m_3 + \ldots$).

Example 5-1: In the figure below, three blocks hang below a massless meter stick. Block m_1 hangs from the *20 cm* mark, block m_2 hangs from the *70 cm* mark, and block m_3 hangs from the *80 cm* mark. If m_1 = 2 kg, m_2 = 5 kg, and m_3 = 3 kg, at what mark on the meter stick should a string be attached so that this system would hang horizontally?

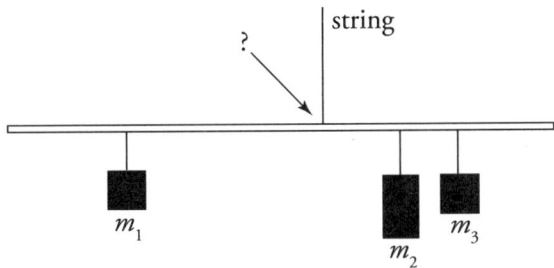

Solution: The first step is to choose an origin, a reference point to call x = 0. We are free to choose our zero mark anywhere we want, but the simplest choice here is the one implicitly mentioned in the question itself. The question wants to know at what mark on the meter stick we should attach the string; in other words, how far from the left end of the meter stick should we attach the string? Since the question asks essentially, "How far from the *left end*...?" the best place to choose our zero mark is at the *left end*. We now can write x_1 = 20 cm, x_2 = 70 cm, and x_3 = 80 cm. Using the formula above, we find that

$$x_{CM} = \frac{m_1 x_1 + m_2 x_2 + m_3 x_3}{m_1 + m_2 + m_3}$$

$$= \frac{(2 \text{ kg})(20 \text{ cm}) + (5 \text{ kg})(70 \text{ cm}) + (3 \text{ kg})(80 \text{ cm})}{(2 \text{ kg}) + (5 \text{ kg}) + (3 \text{ kg})}$$

$$= \frac{630 \text{ kg} \cdot \text{cm}}{10 \text{ kg}}$$

$$\therefore x_{CM} = 63 \text{ cm}$$

What if we had instead chosen the center of the meter stick (the *50 cm* mark) to be our origin? In that case, we would have found x_1 = –30 cm (because m_1 hangs from the *20 cm* mark, and *20 cm* is 30 cm to the *left*—hence the minus sign—of *50 cm*), x_2 = 20 cm, and x_3 = 30 cm. The formula would have told us that

$$x_{CM} = \frac{m_1 x_1 + m_2 x_2 + m_3 x_3}{m_1 + m_2 + m_3}$$

$$= \frac{(2 \text{ kg})(-30 \text{ cm}) + (5 \text{ kg})(20 \text{ cm}) + (3 \text{ kg})(30 \text{ cm})}{(2 \text{ kg}) + (5 \text{ kg}) + (3 \text{ kg})}$$

$$= \frac{130 \text{ kg} \cdot \text{cm}}{10 \text{ kg}}$$

$$\therefore x_{CM} = 13 \text{ cm}$$

Well, 13 cm to the *right* (because x_{CM} is *positive*) of the *50 cm* mark is the *63 cm* mark, the same answer we found before.

Example 5-2: Falls are one of the most serious medical issues among the elderly. Falls result when the center of mass of a person's body is not located over a base of support (determined largely by one's foot placement) and the person is unable to correct for the imbalance with sufficient speed and coordination. Center of mass when standing still is determined by body shape and weight distribution. It's important to keep in mind that when people move, they redistribute their body mass and thus change the location of their centers of mass. What are some likely physical (as opposed to physiological, neurological, or environmental) risk factors for falling, and some possible avoidance strategies?

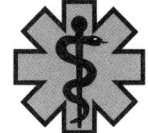

Solution: One risk factor for falling is obesity: not only does this shift the center of mass while standing still, but because it can affect walking motion, the obese individual may be more likely to experience a shift of the center of mass outside the base of support while moving and be less able to prevent the fall once it begins. Another is posture. For example, people often develop a head protrusion and thoracic kyphosis (a hump in the upper back) as they age, shifting the center of mass forward.

Many ways of shifting the body's center of mass closer to the feet and thus making it more likely that the center of mass will remain above the base of support (at least while both feet are planted) are impractical: heavy shoes and pants, for example. However, apart from exercises and physical therapies to avoid or alleviate the risk factors mentioned above, one common risk avoidance strategy is to increase the size of the support base with a cane or a walker. Both of these have the effect of providing a larger total area that the center of mass can occupy without causing imbalance.

Example 5-3: An ammonia molecule (NH_3) contains 3 hydrogen atoms that are positioned at the vertices of an equilateral triangle. The nitrogen atom lies 38 pm (1 pm = 1 picometer = 10^{-12} m) directly above the center of this triangle. If the N:H mass ratio is 14:1, how far below the N atom is the center of mass of the molecule?

Solution: The objects in this system (the four atoms) are not arranged in a line, so how can we hope to determine the center of mass? The key to the answer is to realize that we don't need to include all four of these objects in a single calculation; we can divide the problem into stages. Since the three H atoms have equal masses and are symmetrically arranged at the corners of an equilateral triangle, the center of mass of just these 3 H's is at their geometric center: namely, the center of the triangle. Therefore, by definition of center of mass, the 3 H atoms behave as if all their mass were concentrated at the center of the triangle. This now turns the problem into computing the center of mass of 2 objects (which obviously lie on a line): the 3 H atoms at the center of the triangle and the N atom:

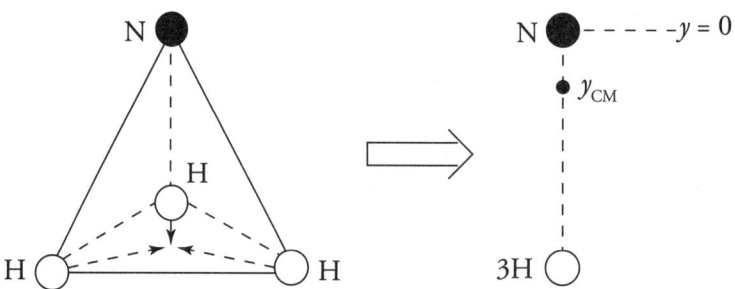

Because the question asks for the center of mass of the molecule relative to the N atom, we'll let the position of the N atom be our zero mark. (It's labeled y in the diagram on the right simply because the way the system is drawn, the objects are arranged along a *vertical* line.) The formula now gives us

$$
\begin{aligned}
y_{CM} &= \frac{m_N x_N + m_{3H} x_{3H}}{m_N + m_{3H}} \\[2mm]
&= \frac{(14)(0 \text{ cm}) + (3 \cdot 1)(38 \text{ pm})}{(14) + (3 \cdot 1)} \\[2mm]
&= \frac{114 \text{ pm}}{17} \\[2mm]
\therefore y_{CM} &= 7 \text{ pm}
\end{aligned}
$$

Therefore, the center of mass of the NH_3 molecule is 7/38, or about 1/6 of the way down from the nitrogen atom toward the plane of the hydrogens. Because the nitrogen atom is more massive than the hydrogens, we expect the center of mass to not be at the geometric center but, rather, much closer to the nitrogen atom. (This is just like the balancing point of the hammer: Since the metal head is much heavier [because it's denser] than the rest of the hammer, we expect the hammer's center of mass to be not at the geometric center, but, instead, closer to the heavier end.)

You may have noticed in Example 5-1 that we applied the point mass formula to a system that didn't include only point masses: The stick's mass was spread along its entire length. What we did in that problem is what we can *always* do with a collection of homogenous (i.e., constant density) masses: First, find the center of mass of each piece; second, apply the point mass formula, assuming that each piece's mass is concentrated at its own center of mass.

It's possible (though unlikely) that on the MCAT you'll have to find the center of mass of a two-dimensional collection of masses. In Example 5-3 on the previous page, we were able to simplify the problem to reduce it to a single dimension, but that might not always be the case. If you can't simplify the problem in this way, do what we always do with multidimensional problems: break it into components, and consider the components separately. In other words, first find the center of mass in, say, the x-direction, using only the x-components of position; then do the same in the y-direction.

5.2 UNIFORM CIRCULAR MOTION

So far, we've analyzed motion that takes place along a straight line (horizontal, vertical, or slanted) or along a parabola. The MCAT will also require that you know how to analyze an object that moves in a circular path.

The title of this section is Uniform Circular Motion (often abbreviated UCM). What does *uniform* mean here? When we talk about uniform acceleration, we mean constant acceleration; uniform density means constant density; *uniform* is a term used in physics to denote something that remains constant. What property of an object undergoing uniform circular motion is constant? The radius of its path is constant, but that's already in the definition of *circular*, so it must be something else.

> An object moving in a circular path is said to execute
>
> **uniform circular motion**
>
> if its *speed* is constant.

Notice right away that this does *not* mean the object's *velocity* is constant. Velocity is a vector: It has both speed and direction. If an object is moving in a circular path, then it's constantly turning, so its direction is constantly changing. A changing direction, even at constant speed, automatically means a changing velocity. An object's velocity vector is always tangent to its path, regardless of the shape of the path (parabola, circle, figure-8, or whatever) so in the figure below, you can see that the object will have a different velocity vector at every point on the circle, even though the magnitudes of these vectors are all the same.

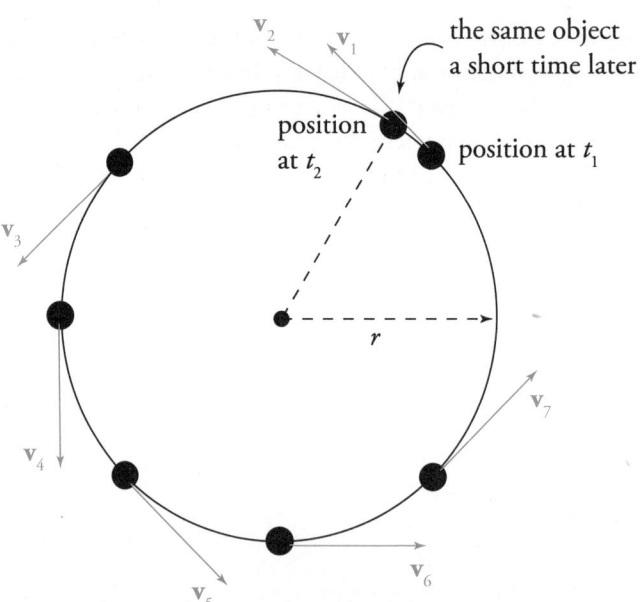

The first thing that should come to mind when you see an object's velocity changing is that the object is experiencing acceleration. The acceleration of an object undergoing uniform circular motion is not affecting the *speed* of the object; this acceleration is only changing the direction of the velocity in order to keep the object moving in a circle.

In the figure below, the velocity vectors of the object are drawn at two close points in its path; they're labeled $\mathbf{v}_1$ and $\mathbf{v}_2$. By definition, the direction of the acceleration is the same as the direction of the velocity change (remember the definition: $\mathbf{a} = \Delta\mathbf{v}/\Delta t$). So, the acceleration of the object has the same direction as $\Delta\mathbf{v} = \mathbf{v}_2 - \mathbf{v}_1$. Notice that $\mathbf{v}_2 - \mathbf{v}_1$, which is $\mathbf{v}_2 + (-\mathbf{v}_1)$, points toward the center of the circle. Therefore, the acceleration of the object always points toward the center of the circle. (This will be true no matter where on the circle we look.)

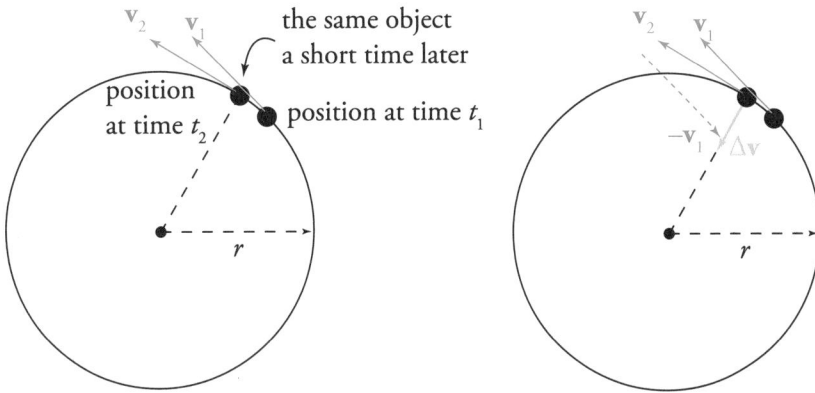

The acceleration of an object undergoing uniform circular motion always points toward the center of the circle. The term **centripetal** (from the Latin, meaning *to seek the center*) is therefore used to describe the acceleration of an object undergoing UCM. We'll denote centripetal acceleration by $\mathbf{a}_c$.

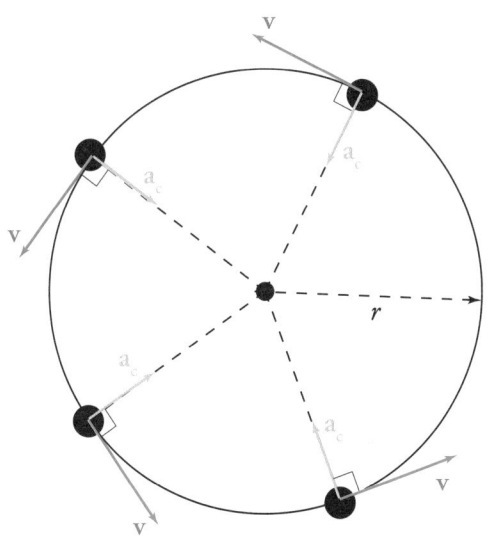

Since $\mathbf{v}$ is always tangent to the circle, and $\mathbf{a}_c$ always points to the center of the circle, $\mathbf{v}$ and $\mathbf{a}_c$ are always perpendicular to each other at any position of the object.

(*Note*: In the figure above, all the velocity vectors are different—because they point in different directions—so they really shouldn't all be labeled by the same **v**. The same is true for the centripetal acceleration vectors. However, adding subscripts to distinguish all the **v** vectors and all the $\mathbf{a}_c$ vectors would have made the picture look too confusing.)

We now know the *direction* of the centripetal acceleration at any point on the circle; what is its *magnitude*? If v is the speed of the object and r is the radius of the circular path, then the magnitude of the centripetal acceleration, a_c, is v^2/r.

Magnitude of Centripetal Acceleration

$$a_c = \frac{v^2}{r}$$

If an object is accelerating, then it must be feeling a force (after all, $\mathbf{F}_{net} = m\mathbf{a}$, so you can't have an acceleration without a force). Since $\mathbf{F}_{net}$ and $\mathbf{a}$ always point in the same direction, no matter what the path of the object, the net force on an object undergoing UCM must, like $\mathbf{a}$, point toward the center. So, guess what we call it? **Centripetal force** (denoted $\mathbf{F}_c$). This is the *net* force directed toward the center that acts on an object to make it execute uniform circular motion. And since $F_{net} = ma$, we'll have $\mathbf{F}_c = m\mathbf{a}_c$ and $F_c = ma_c$, so the magnitude of the centripetal force is mv^2/r, where m is the mass of the object that's moving around the circle.

Magnitude of Centripetal Force

$$F_c = ma_c = \frac{mv^2}{r}$$

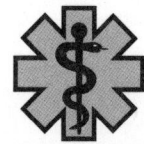

Example 5-4: Separating blood plasma from the solid bodies in blood (blood cells and platelets) by rapid sedimentation requires use of a *centrifuge* to produce the necessary accelerations on the order of 5000g. In one approach, the blood is placed in a bag inside a rigid container and mounted to the end of a horizontal rotor (so that it extends out beyond the rotor), which then spins up to several thousands of revolutions per minute. Suppose the rotor has a radius of 30 cm and rotates at a maximum rate of 5000 rpm, and that the bag is 10 cm long. Note that translational velocity $v = r\omega$, where ω is in radians/second.

a) What will be the centripetal acceleration at the middle of the bag?

b) Will the centripetal acceleration increase or decrease for the blood further from the axis of rotation?

Solution:

a) First we convert rpm to rad/s: 5000 rev/min $\times$ 2π rad/rev $\times$ 1/60 min/s $\approx$ 500 rad/s. Now $v = r\omega = (0.30 \text{ m} + 0.05 \text{ m})(500 \text{ rad/s}) = 175$ m/s. Thus for the centripetal acceleration we have

$$a_c = \frac{v^2}{r} = \frac{(175 \text{ m/s})^2}{0.35 \text{ m}} \approx \frac{(200 \text{ m/s})^2}{0.5 \text{ m}} = 8 \times 10^4 \text{ m/s}^2$$

This is 8000g, so more than enough acceleration to achieve separation of blood.

b)   Your first instinct upon reading this question might be to say, "I know that centripetal acceleration is inversely proportional to the radius, so increasing the distance from the central axis should decrease the acceleration." That would be wrong: such reasoning implicitly (and falsely) assumes that speed is constant as radius increases, but for a *rigid rotator* like a centrifuge or a merry-go-round, translational speed is proportional to the radius according to the equation $v = r\omega$, (the constant is the angular speed ω). If you're having trouble picturing this, imagine what happens when you're on a merry-go-round: standing at the center, you are spinning in place and thus have a translational speed of zero (your position isn't changing with time). The further you get from the center, the faster you are moving. Thus because of the v^2 term in the numerator, $a_c \propto r$, and centripetal acceleration increases for blood further from the axis of rotation.

Example 5-5: If an object undergoing uniform circular motion is being acted upon by a constant force toward the center, why doesn't the object fall into the center?

Solution: Actually, it *is* falling toward the center, but because of its speed, the object remains in a circular orbit around the center. Remember: the direction of **v** is not necessarily the same as the direction of $\mathbf{F}_{net}$. So, just because $\mathbf{F}_{net}$ points toward the center does not mean that **v** must point toward the center. It's the direction of the *acceleration*, not the velocity that always matches the direction of $\mathbf{F}_{net}$. Let's look at the motion of the object at a certain point in its circular path:

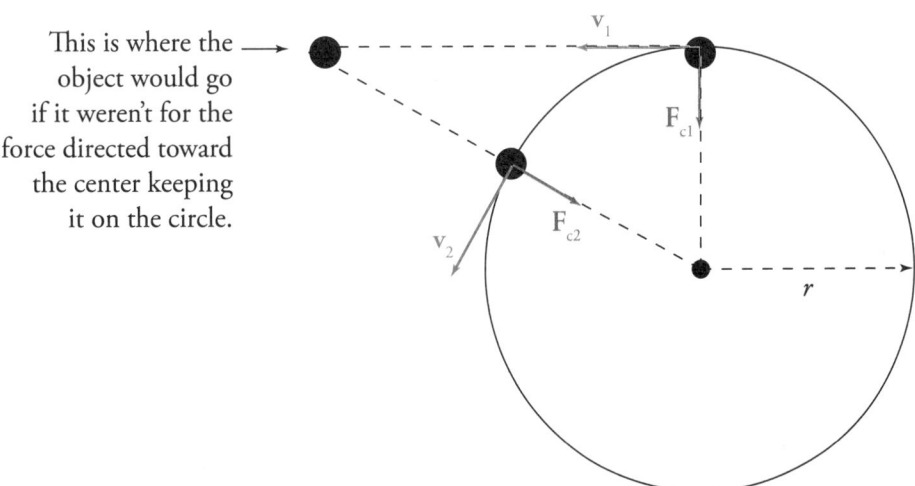

In this figure, the net force on the object at Position 1 points downward (toward the center of the circle). Therefore, it's telling $\mathbf{v}_1$ to move downward a little, so that at the next moment, at Position 2, the velocity will point downward slightly. Notice that this is just what we want in order to keep the object traveling in a circle! If it weren't for this force pointing toward the center (that is, if the centripetal force were suddenly removed), then the object's velocity wouldn't change. It would not continue to move in a circle but would instead fly off in a straight line, tangent to the circle at the point where the force was removed.

Example 5-6: How would the net force on an object undergoing uniform circular motion have to change if the object's speed doubled?

Solution: Centripetal force, mv^2/r, is proportional to the *square* of the speed. So, if the object's speed increased by a factor of 2, then the magnitude of $\mathbf{F}_c$ would have to increase by a factor of $2^2 = 4$.

Solving circular motion problems often involves something more than simply using the formulas $a_c = v^2/r$ or $F_c = mv^2/r$. The key to solving such problems is to answer this question:

What provides the centripetal force?

In other words, what force(s) act in the dimension toward the center of the circle?

Centripetal force is not some new kind of force like gravity or tension. It's simply the name for the net force directed toward the center of the circular path. The vector sum of forces such as gravity and tension is what gets *called* centripetal force, when those forces, or components of them, are directed toward the center of the circle. When drawing a force diagram for an object undergoing UCM, here are a couple of tips:

1. Do not add a force called $\mathbf{F}_c$ in your picture; forces such as gravity, tension, normal force, etc. *do* go in your picture, but $\mathbf{F}_c$ doesn't. Remember, $\mathbf{F}_c$ is what the forces toward the center have to add up to.
2. Always call *toward the center* the positive direction. Any forces toward the center are then positive forces, and any forces directed away from the center are negative. You'll need this to find F_{net} and then set the result equal to F_c.

Example 5-7: The moon orbits the earth in a (nearly) circular path at (nearly) constant speed. If M is the mass of the earth, m is the mass of the moon, and r is the radius of the moon's orbit, find an expression for the speed of the moon's orbit. Recall that the force of gravity between two masses is given by $F_{grav} = GMm/r^2$, where G is the universal gravitational constant.

Solution: We begin by answering the question, *What provides the centripetal force?* The answer is the gravitational pull by the earth. We now simply translate our answer into an equation, like this:

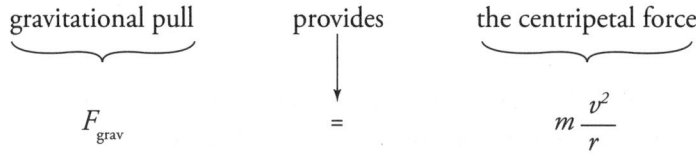

Since we know $F_{grav} = GMm/r^2$, we get

$$F_{grav} = F_c \;\rightarrow\; G\frac{Mm}{r^2} = m\frac{v^2}{r} \;\rightarrow\; G\frac{M}{r} = v^2 \;\rightarrow\; \therefore v = \sqrt{G\frac{M}{r}}$$

Notice that the mass of the moon, m, cancels out. So, any object orbiting at the same distance from the earth as the moon must move at the same speed as the moon.

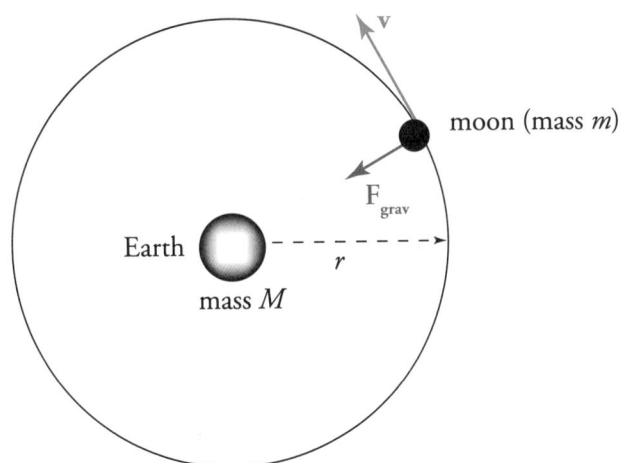

Example 5-8: A string is tied around a rock of mass 0.2 kg, and the rock is then whirled at a constant speed v in a horizontal circle of radius 0.4 m, as shown in the figure below. If $\sin \theta = 0.4$ and $\cos \theta = 0.9$, what's v?

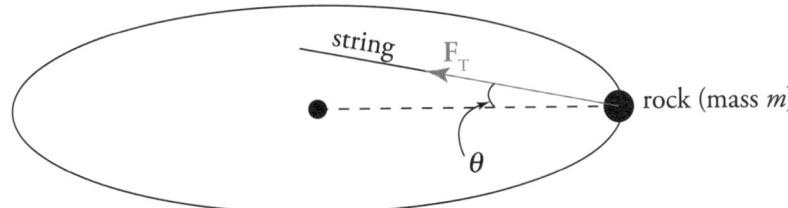

Solution: First, let's draw a bigger force diagram:

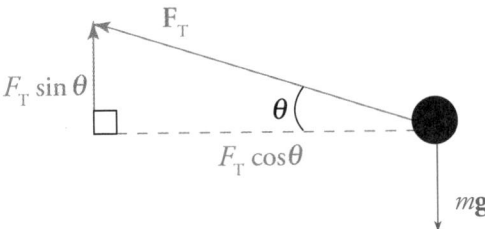

(This figure also shows why the end of the string is slightly above the center of the circle. The string has to point upward a little in order for there to be an upward component of the tension to cancel out the weight of the rock and allow the rock to revolve in a *horizontal* circle.) Because the rock is moving in a horizontal circle and not accelerating vertically, we know that the net vertical force must be zero. Therefore, the vertical component of the string's tension, $F_y = F_T \sin \theta$, must balance out the weight of the rock, mg:

$$F_T \sin \theta = mg$$

From this, we can figure out that

$$F_T = \frac{mg}{\sin\theta} = \frac{(0.2 \text{ kg})(10\frac{\text{N}}{\text{kg}})}{0.4} = 5 \text{ N}$$

Now, let's look at the circular motion: *What provides the centripetal force?* As the diagram shows, there's only one force directed toward the center of the circle (namely, the horizontal component of the tension, $F_x = F_T \cos\theta$) so this must be it:

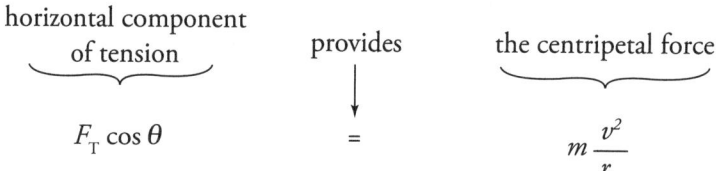

We now just plug in the value we found for F_T to get v:

$$F_T \cos\theta = m\frac{v^2}{r} \rightarrow v = \sqrt{\frac{rF_T \cos\theta}{m}} = \sqrt{\frac{(0.4 \text{ m})(5 \text{ N})(0.9)}{0.2 \text{ kg}}} = 3 \text{ m/s}$$

Example 5-9: A rope of length 60 cm is tied to the handle of a bucket (whose mass is 3 kg), and the bucket is then whirled in a vertical circle. At the bottom of its path, the tension in the rope is 50 N. What is the speed of the bucket at this point?

Solution: First, let's draw a diagram.

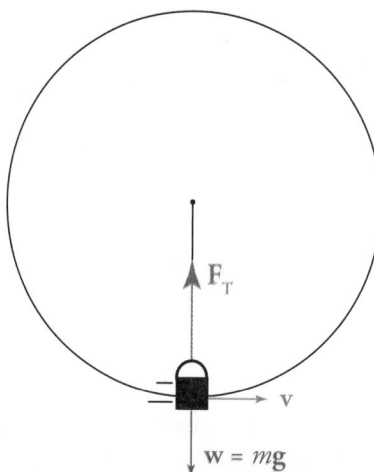

Because we call *toward the center* the positive direction when doing circular motion problems, we see that the tension, $\mathbf{F}_T$, is a positive force, and the bucket's weight, $\mathbf{w}$, is a negative force. (Because $\mathbf{w}$ points *away* from the center, we count it as negative.) Therefore, the net force on the bucket at this point is $F_T - w$. Because the net force directed toward the center is called the centripetal force, we'd write

$$F_T - w = F_c$$

Because $w = mg$ and $F_c = mv^2/r$, this equation becomes

$$F_T - mg = m\frac{v^2}{r}$$

We now just use this equation and the numbers we were given to figure out v, realizing that the radius of the circle is equal to the length of the rope (so $r = 0.6$ m):

$$v = \sqrt{\frac{r(F_T - mg)}{m}} = \sqrt{\frac{(0.6 \text{ m})[50 \text{ N} - (3 \text{ kg})(10\frac{\text{N}}{\text{kg}})]}{3 \text{ kg}}} = 2 \text{ m/s}$$

Example 5-10: For the situation described in the preceding example, what is the tension force on the bucket when the bucket is at the position shown below?

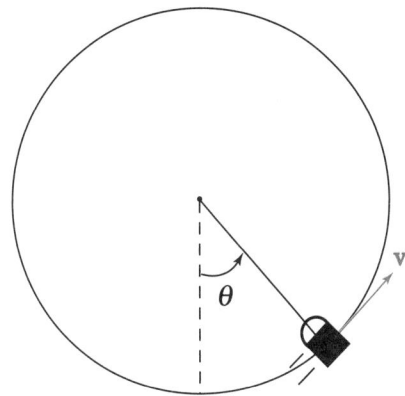

Solution: Here's the force diagram:

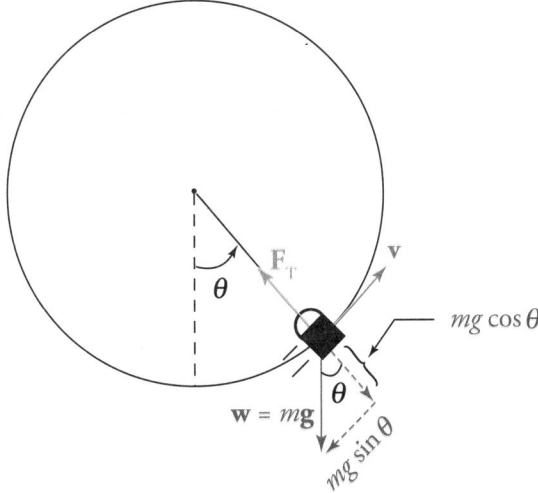

Because there's a force of F_T pointing toward the center and a force of $mg \cos \theta$ pointing *away* from the center, the net force toward the center of the circle (which is the centripetal force) is

$$F_{net\ toward\ center} = F_c = F_T - mg \cos\theta$$

Let's examine this situation a little more closely. Notice that at the position of the bucket shown, we also have a force component *tangent* to the circle (*mg* sin θ), which *opposes* the direction of the bucket's velocity. As a result, the bucket's speed will be reduced. Centripetal acceleration only makes an object turn so that it moves in a circular path; it does not change the speed. **Tangential** acceleration, on the other hand, *does* change the speed. Therefore, the bucket's speed will decrease as it rises to the top of the circle, and we wouldn't call the entire motion of the bucket "uniform." However, even if the speed of an object moving in a circle changes, there will always be a component of the net force that points toward the center of the circle; this is the centripetal force. The mathematical translation of the statement "the net force toward the center provides the centripetal force" becomes

$$F_\text{T} - mg\cos\theta = m\frac{v^2}{r} \rightarrow F_\text{T} = m\frac{v^2}{r} + mg\cos\theta$$

Because *v* decreases as the bucket rises (because of the downward tangential force, *mg* sin θ) and since cos θ decreases as the bucket rises (because the angle θ increases from 0° to 180°), this final equation for F_T shows us that the tension in the rope will decrease as the bucket rises.

It's not often that we need to worry about both centripetal and tangential acceleration in an MCAT problem, but the example above shows how to deal with it when we do encounter such a situation: Ignore the tangential components of force and acceleration when calculating the centripetal force and acceleration. This is really just another example of the general principle: In MCAT-level Physics, you can always consider the components of motion separately.

5.3 TORQUE

We can tie a rope to a bucket and make it move in a circular path, but how would we make the bucket itself spin? One way would be to grab the handle and then rotate our hand, or we could place our hands on opposite sides of the bucket and then, by moving our hands in opposite directions, rotate the bucket. In order to make an object's center of mass accelerate, we need to exert a force. In order to make an object *spin*, we need to exert a *torque*.

Torque is the measure of a force's effectiveness at making an object spin or rotate. (More precisely, it's the measure of a force's effectiveness at making an object *accelerate* rotationally.) If an object is initially at rest, and then it starts to spin, something must have exerted a torque. And if an object is already spinning, something would have to exert a torque to get it to stop spinning. In this section, we'll begin by looking at two different (but entirely equivalent) ways of figuring out torque.

All systems that can spin or rotate have a "center" of turning. This is the point that does not move while the remainder of the object is rotating, effectively becoming the center of the circle. There are many terms used to describe this point, including **pivot point** and **fulcrum**.

Let's say we want to tighten a bolt with a wrench. The figure below illustrates the situation.

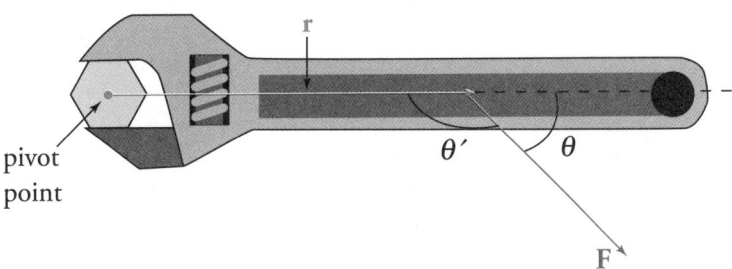

If we applied the force **F** to the wrench, would we make the wrench and the bolt rotate? Yes, because this force **F** has *torque*. (Notice: Torque is not a force; it's a property of a force.) To say how *much* torque **F** provides, we need a couple of preliminary definitions. First, the vector from the center of rotation (the **pivot point**) to the point of application of the force is called the **radius vector, r**. The angle between the vectors **r** and **F** is called θ. Now notice in the figure above that the angle between the vectors **r** and **F** at the point where they actually meet is denoted by θ'. This is because the angle between two vectors is actually the angle they make *when they start at the same point*. But in the figure, the vector **r** starts at the pivot point (which is where **r** always starts), and **F** starts at the *end* of **r** (which is where **F** always starts). One way to find the correct angle between these vectors is to imagine sliding **r** over so that it does start where **F** starts; the dashed line in the figure shows the line along which such a translated **r** vector would lie and the resulting correct angle θ. However, all this fuss about which angle is the correct one doesn't really matter, as you'll soon see.

The amount of torque a force **F** provides depends on three things: the magnitude of **F**, the length of **r**, and the angle θ.

Torque

$$\tau = rF \sin\theta$$

(The letter we use for torque is τ, the Greek letter *tau*.) From this equation, we can immediately figure out the unit of torque:

$$[\tau] = [r][F] = \text{m·N} = \text{N·m}$$

There's no special name for this unit; it's just a newton-meter.[1]

For example, let's say that $F = 20$ N, $r = 10$ cm, and $\theta = 30°$. Then the torque provided by this force would be $\tau = rF \sin\theta = (0.1 \text{ m})(20 \text{ N}) \sin 30° = 1$ N·m. Notice that if we had instead used θ', we would have gotten the same answer, since $\theta' = 150°$ and $\sin 150° = \sin 30°$. This is why we don't have to worry about which angle, θ or θ', is the true angle between **r** and **F** when we calculate torque, because θ and θ' will

---

[1] In Chapter 6 we'll encounter another newton-meter and rename it the joule. What's the difference? Torque has a direction, like a vector (though technically it's what's called a pseudovector), while the joule, a unit of energy, is a scalar. For the MCAT, there's no need to worry about this; just calculate torque in newton-meters, and then label it clockwise or counterclockwise.

always be *supplements* (they'll add up to 180°) and the sine of an angle is always equal to the sine of its supplement. Therefore, $\tau = rF \sin \theta = rF \sin \theta'$.

Look at this force on the wrench:

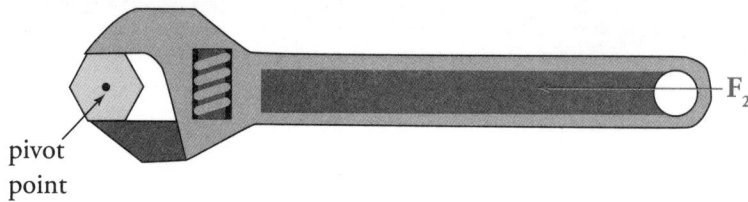

Our intuition tells us that this force would not make the wrench (or bolt) rotate. Therefore, we expect that this force has zero torque. Using the definition, we can see that this is true. If we were to draw the **r** vector from the pivot to the point where F_2 is applied, we'd see that the value of $\sin \theta$ is 0, so $\tau_2 = 0$. Forces with no torque (like this one) cannot increase (or decrease) the rotational speed of an object.

How about this force on the wrench?

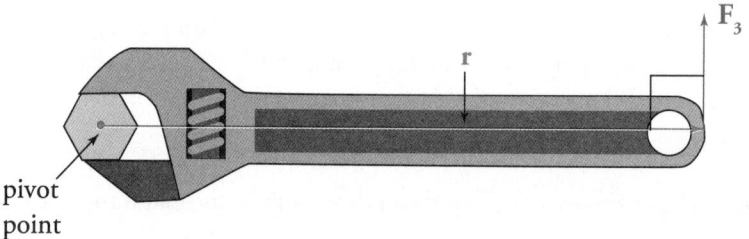

The force F_3 is perpendicular to its **r** vector, so $\theta = 90°$ and $\sin \theta = 1$, its maximum value. Therefore, when $\mathbf{r} \perp \mathbf{F}$, we get the maximum torque for a given r and F, and the equation for torque gives us simply $\tau_3 = rF_3$. (This situation is very common, by the way.)

$$\text{If } \mathbf{r} \perp \mathbf{F}, \text{ then } \tau = rF.$$

The force F_3 above would produce counterclockwise rotation, so we say that it produces a **counterclockwise (CCW)** torque. The force F_4 below would produce clockwise rotation, so we say it produces a **clockwise (CW)** torque.

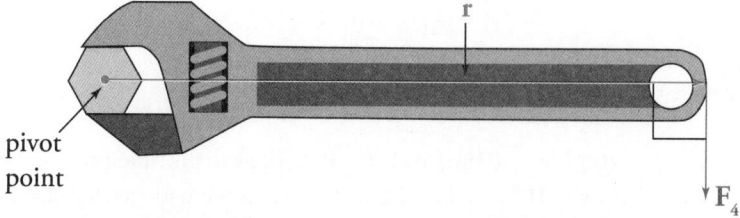

If $F_3 = F_4$, then these forces produce the same amount of torque, but one is clockwise and the other is counterclockwise. If we want to distinguish between them mathematically, we can say that $\tau_3 = +rF_3$ and $\tau_4 = -rF_4$, since it's customary to specify CCW rotation as positive and CW as negative.

The other method for calculating torque, which gives the same answer as the method we've just described, is based on the *lever arm* of a force. Let's look again at the first picture of our wrench:

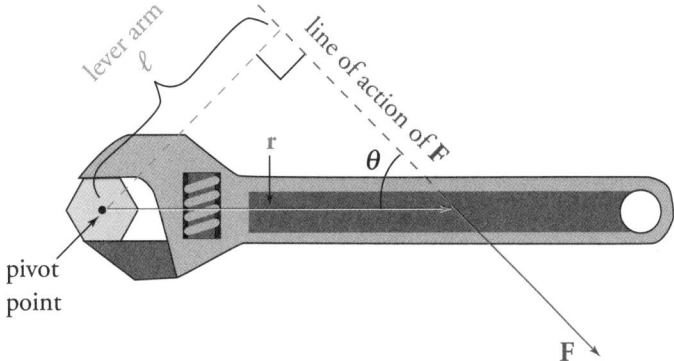

This time, however, rather than measuring the distance from the pivot to the *point* where the force is applied (the length *r*), we'll measure the shortest distance from the pivot to the *line* along which **F** is applied. This distance, which is always perpendicular to the line of action of F, is called the **lever arm** of **F**, written as ℓ or *l*.

Once we know the lever arm, ℓ, the definition of the torque of **F** is then simply $\tau = \ell F$.

Torque

$$\tau = \ell F$$

To see that this gives the same value for the torque as the formula $\tau = rF \sin\theta$, just notice that in the picture above, the lever arm, ℓ, is the side opposite the angle θ in a right triangle whose hypotenuse is *r*; therefore, $\ell = r \sin\theta$. So, $\tau = \ell F$ is the same as $\tau = (r \sin\theta)F$. Because you can use either formula for calculating the torque, use whichever one is more convenient in a particular problem. In general, it's convenient to use the lever arm method if the length of the lever arm is obvious from the situation; otherwise, use $\tau = rF \sin\theta$.

For the force $\mathbf{F}_5$ shown below, our intuition tells us that this force would not make the wrench (or bolt) rotate. Therefore, we expect that this force has zero torque. Using the definition of lever arm, we can see that this is true. The line of action of $\mathbf{F}_5$ passes right through the pivot point, so the level arm of the force is zero, and $\tau_5 = \ell_5 F_5 = (0)F_5 = 0$.

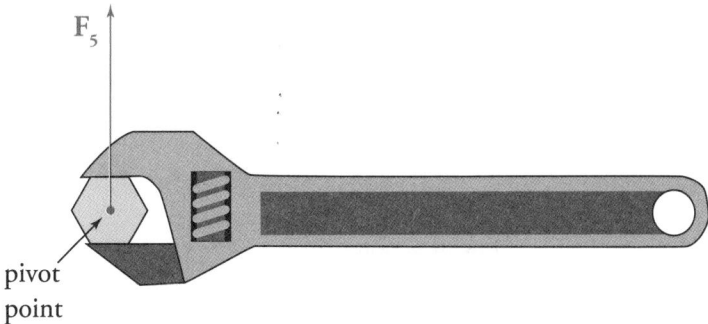

In general, if a force acts at the pivot or along a line through the pivot, then its torque is zero.

Example 5-11: A square metal plate (of side length s) rests on a flat table, and we exert a force **F** at one corner, parallel to one of the sides, as shown below. What is the torque of this force? (Use the center of the plate as the pivot point.)

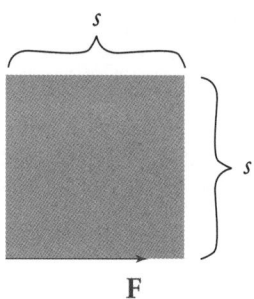

Solution: We'll calculate the torque of **F** by two different methods: first using the formula $\tau = rF \sin \theta$, and then using the formula $\tau = \ell F$.

Method 1. We draw in the **r** vector, which points from the pivot to the point where the force is applied. The angle between **r** and **F** can be taken to be $\theta = 45°$. If s is the length of each side of the square, then the length of **r** is $\frac{1}{2}s\sqrt{2}$ (because r is the hypotenuse of a 45°-45° right triangle, it's $\sqrt{2}$ times the length of each leg).

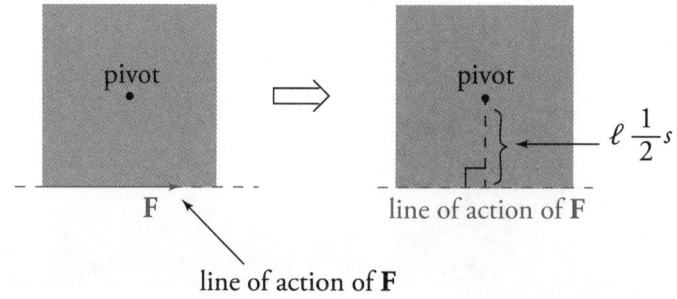

This gives $\tau = rF \sin \theta = \left(\frac{1}{2}s\sqrt{2}\right)(F)\sin 45° = \left(\frac{1}{2}s\sqrt{2}\right)(F)\left(\frac{\sqrt{2}}{2}\right) = \frac{1}{2}sF$.

Method 2. The line of action of the force **F** is simply the bottom side of the square. The perpendicular distance from the pivot to the side of the square is half the length of the square, $\frac{1}{2}s$, so this is the lever arm, ℓ.

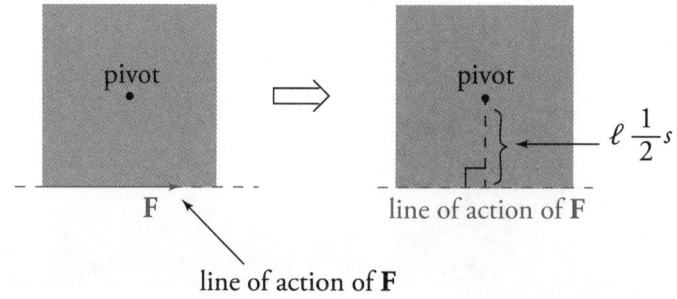

Therefore, $\tau = \ell F = \frac{1}{2}sF$.

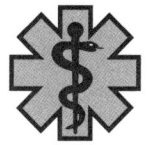

In this situation, the formula using the lever arm is the easier way to calculate the torque. That's because you can look at the diagram and see the length of the lever arm right away. If you find yourself having to *calculate* the length of the lever arm, you probably should just be using $\tau = rF \sin \theta$.

Example 5-12: Which of the following best explains why people with biceps attachment points farther from their elbows tend to have greater elbow flexion strength, and thus an improved ability to perform a dumbbell curling exercise?

   A.   An attachment point that is farther from the elbow increases the force provided by muscle contraction.

   B.   An attachment point that is farther from the elbow decreases the force provided by muscle contraction.

   C.   An attachment point that is farther from the elbow results in a greater torque produced by the biceps as it contracts.

   D.   An attachment point that is closer to the hand results in a lesser torque produced by the biceps as it contracts.

Solution: The first two answer choices discuss a difference in the muscle's contraction force. This force is a function of the muscle fibers, not its point of attachment to the forearm, which eliminates choices A and B. An attachment point farther from the elbow increases r, the distance from the pivot point (elbow) to where the force is applied (at the attachment), so according to the equation for torque, $\tau = rF \sin\theta$, this would increase the torque created by the biceps contraction, which makes choice C correct. The distance to the hand is a trap answer: there are two torques acting on someone curling a dumbbell or other mass, one provided by the contraction of the biceps muscle and an opposing one from the weight of the dumbbell acting downward at the hand. Both torques depend on the radial distance from the pivot point, which is the elbow.

Example 5-13: In the figure below, three blocks hang below a massless meter stick. Block m_1 hangs from the 20 cm mark, block m_2 hangs from the 70 cm mark, and block m_3 hangs from the 80 cm mark. If $m_1 = 2$ kg, $m_2 = 5$ kg, and $m_3 = 3$ kg, at what mark on the meter stick should a string be attached so that this system would hang horizontally?

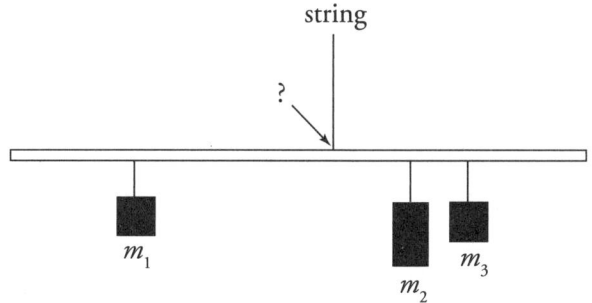

Solution: Look familiar? This is the same example we solved in the Center of Mass section. Let's see how we can answer this same question by balancing the torques. Let the pivot be the point where the string is attached to the stick. (Consider that the string is attached at the x cm mark, so that it's x cm from the left end of the stick.) Then the weight of mass m_1 produces a counterclockwise torque (τ_1), and the weights of m_2 and of m_3 each produce a clockwise torque (τ_2 and τ_3). If the counterclockwise torque (τ_1) balances the total clockwise torque ($\tau_2 + \tau_3$), the stick will remain level.

5.3

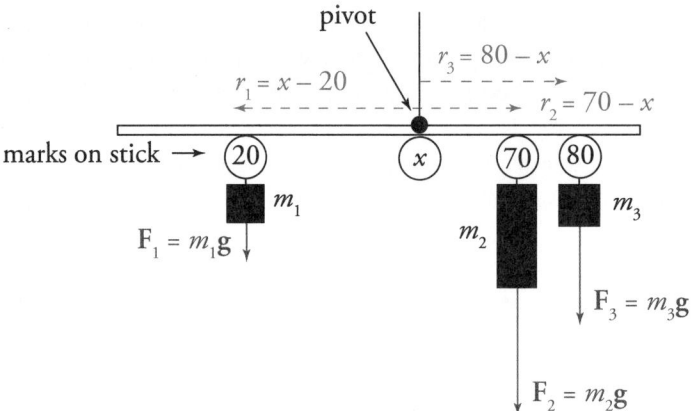

For each force, we need to find its corresponding r. For F_1, we have $r_1 = (x - 20)$ cm; for F_2, we have $r_2 = (70 - x)$ cm; and for F_3, we have $r_3 = (80 - x)$ cm. The equation that balances the torques is

$$\tau(CCW) = \tau(CW)$$

$$r_1 \cdot m_1 g = r_2 \cdot m_2 g + r_3 \cdot m_3 g$$

$$r_1 m_1 = r_2 m_2 + r_3 m_3$$

$$(x - 20)(2 \text{ kg}) = (70 - x)(5 \text{ kg}) + (80 - x)(3 \text{ kg})$$

$$\therefore x = 63 \text{ cm}$$

This is the same answer we found before. (By the way, the torque exerted by the tension in the string is equal to zero [which is why we ignored it] because the tension acts *at* the pivot.)

Example 5-14: A homogeneous rectangular sheet of metal lies on a flat table and is able to rotate around an axis through its center, perpendicular to the table. Four forces, all of the same magnitude, are exerted on the sheet as shown below:

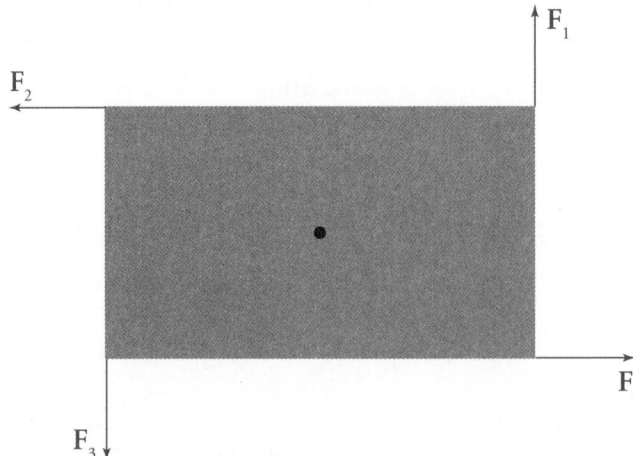

Which one of the following statements is true?

A. The net force is zero, but the net torque is not.
B. The net torque is zero, but the net force is not.
C. Neither the net force nor the net torque is zero.
D. Both the net force and the net torque equal zero.

Solution: There are two vertical forces that point in opposite directions (so they cancel), and two horizontal forces that point in opposite directions (so *they* cancel). Therefore, the net force, $\mathbf{F}_{net} = \mathbf{F}_1 + \mathbf{F}_2 + \mathbf{F}_3 + \mathbf{F}_4$, is zero. Eliminate choices B and C.

Now for the torques. In the figure below, each force has its corresponding lever arm. Notice that each force produces a counterclockwise (CCW) torque. As a result, the total, or net, torque cannot be zero. (The net torque is zero only when the total counterclockwise torque balances the total clockwise torque.) Therefore, the answer is A.

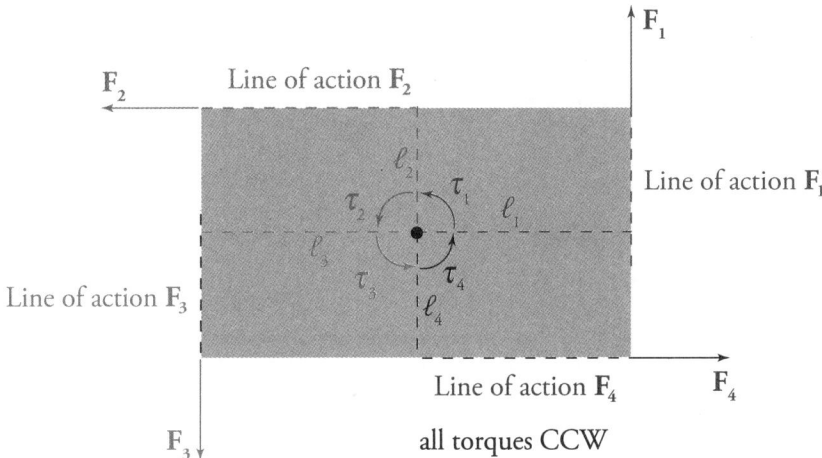

5.4 EQUILIBRIUM

As it's used in physics, the term **equilibrium** means *zero acceleration*. Notice that this does not mean zero velocity. As long as the velocity of the system remains constant (no change in speed or direction), then we can say that the system is in equilibrium. If the velocity happens to be zero, then we say the system is in **static** equilibrium.

There are actually two kinds of equilibrium, because there are two kinds of acceleration. There's *translational* equilibrium and *rotational* equilibrium. A system is said to be in **translational equilibrium** if the forces cancel; if $F_{net} = 0$, then the translational acceleration (*a*) is zero. A system is in **rotational equilibrium** if the torques cancel; if $\tau_{net} = 0$, then the rotational acceleration (denoted by α, the Greek letter *alpha*) is zero. If the term *equilibrium* is used without specifying which type, then it's assumed that the system is in *both* translational and rotational equilibrium.

Example 5-13 (the blocks balancing on the stick) involved a system in equilibrium. We balanced the torques to ensure rotational equilibrium. We didn't explicitly analyze the translational equilibrium, but in the example of the blocks hanging from the stick, the upward tension in the supporting string balanced the total weight of the blocks.

We'll now look at a couple of other examples of systems in equilibrium.

Example 5-15: A barber pole of mass 10 kg hangs from the end of a homogeneous rod of mass 40 kg that sticks out horizontally from the side of a vertical wall. The end of the rod, where the barber pole is attached, is connected to the upper part of the wall by a taut cable. For the angle θ, it is known that $\sin \theta = 0.6$ and $\cos \theta = 0.8$.

a) What's the tension in the cable?

b) What force is exerted by the wall on the rod?

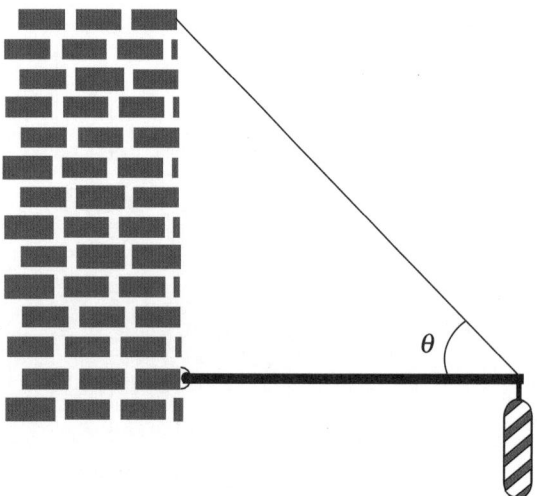

Solution:

a) First, let's draw a diagram of all the forces acting on the rod.

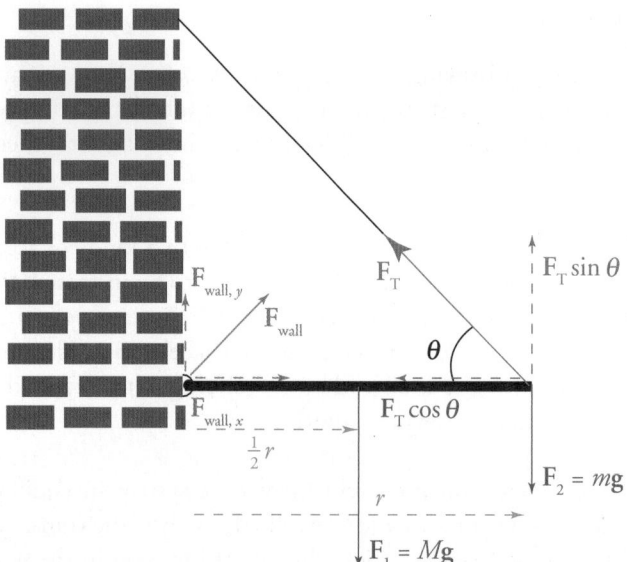

Notice that because the rod is in contact with the wall, the wall is exerting a force on the rod. However, at the start of the problem, we have no way of knowing what this force looks like (in other words, what either its magnitude or its direction are), so we break the force F_{wall} into a horizontal component and a vertical component. We do the same with the tension force, F_T, (which must act along the direction of the cable), and we can write these components as $F_{T,x} = F_T \cos\theta$ and $F_{T,y} = F_T \sin\theta$.

The system is in static equilibrium, so there must be no net torque and no net force. If we try to balance out all the forces, we find that we have too many unknowns. To balance the vertical forces, we'd write $F_{wall,y} + F_T \sin\theta = Mg + mg$, and to balance the horizontal forces, we'd write $F_{wall,x} = F_T \cos\theta$. We have three unknown ($F_{wall,x}$, $F_{wall,y}$, and F_T) but only two equations.

The trick is to balance the *torques* first and to choose our pivot to be the point of contact between the rod and wall. Notice that the torques of the components of the force exerted by the wall will both be zero (because they're applied *at* the pivot), so they won't even appear in the equation. As a result, our "balance-the-torques" equation will have just one unknown, F_T. That's why we chose to put the pivot point at the wall end of the rod: There are two unknown force components there, and only one at the other end.

So, with our pivot so chosen, we have three forces exerting torque: $\mathbf{F}_{T,y}$ produces a counter-clockwise torque, and each of the weight vectors, $M\mathbf{g}$ and $m\mathbf{g}$, produces a clockwise torque. These torques balance to keep the rod level.

$$\tau_{CW} = \tau_{CCW}$$

$$r \cdot F_T \sin\theta = \tfrac{1}{2} r \cdot Mg + r \cdot mg$$

$$F_T \sin\theta = \tfrac{1}{2} Mg + mg$$

$$F_T = \frac{(\tfrac{1}{2}M + m)g}{\sin\theta}$$

$$= \frac{(\tfrac{1}{2} \cdot 40 \text{ kg} + 10 \text{ kg})(10 \tfrac{N}{kg})}{0.6}$$

$$\therefore F_T = 500 \text{ N}$$

b) Now that we've answered part (a) and found F_T, the tension in the cable, we can now find $F_{wall,x}$ and $F_{wall,y}$. We use the "balance-the-horizontal-forces" equation, $F_{wall,x} = F_T \cos\theta$, to get

$$F_{wall,x} = F_T \cos\theta = (500 \text{ N})(0.8) = 400 \text{ N}$$

Then we use the "balance-the-vertical-forces" equation to find $F_{wall,y}$:

$$F_{wall,y} + F_T \sin\theta = Mg + mg$$

$$F_{wall,y} = Mg + mg - F_T \sin\theta$$

$$= (40 \text{ kg})(10 \tfrac{N}{kg}) + (10 \text{ kg})(10 \tfrac{N}{kg}) - (500 \text{ N})(0.6)$$

$$\therefore F_{wall,y} = 200 \text{ N}$$

Finally, the magnitude of the force exerted by the wall on the rod can be found using the Pythagorean theorem:

$$\left(F_{wall}\right)^2 = \left(F_{wall,\,x}\right)^2 + \left(F_{wall,\,y}\right)^2 \rightarrow F_{wall} = \sqrt{\left(F_{wall,\,x}\right)^2 + \left(F_{wall,\,y}\right)^2} \rightarrow F_{wall} = \sqrt{(400\text{ N})^2 + (200\text{ N})^2} \approx 447\text{ N}$$

Whew! Let's now look at a problem that's more MCAT-like in terms of the amount of calculation:

Example 5-16: In the figure below, a block of mass 40 kg is held in place by two ropes exerting equal tension forces. If $\cos\theta = 2/3$, what's the tension in each rope?

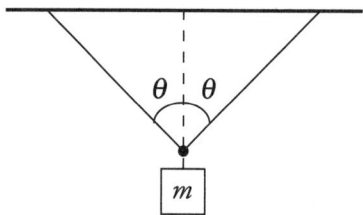

Solution: At the point where the mass is attached to the two ropes, we balance the forces. The horizontal forces automatically balance (we have $F_T \sin\theta$ pointing to the left and $F_T \sin\theta$ pointing to the right). For the vertical forces, we notice that there's the vertical component of the tension in the left-hand rope plus the vertical component of the tension in the right-hand rope ($F_T \cos\theta + F_T \cos\theta = 2F_T \cos\theta$), to balance out the weight of the block, mg. This gives us:

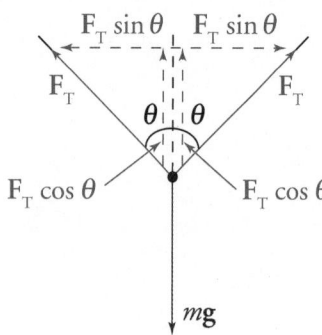

$$2F_T \cos\theta = mg$$

$$F_T = \frac{mg}{2\cos\theta}$$

$$= \frac{(40\text{ kg})(10\,\frac{\text{N}}{\text{kg}})}{2\left(\frac{2}{3}\right)}$$

$$\therefore F_T = 300\text{ N}$$

Summary of Formulas

Center of mass: $x_{CM} = \dfrac{m_1 x_1 + m_2 x_2 + m_3 x_3 \ldots}{m_1 + m_2 + m_3 \ldots}$

Center of gravity: $x_{CG} = \dfrac{w_1 x_1 + w_2 x_2 + w_3 x_3 \ldots}{w_1 + w_2 + w_3 \ldots}$

in uniform gravitational field (g constant), $x_{CM} = x_{CG}$

Centripetal acceleration: $a_c = \dfrac{v^2}{r}$ (directed toward center of circle)

Centripetal force: $F_c = ma_c = \dfrac{mv^2}{r}$

$F_c = F_{\text{net towards center}}$

Torque: $\tau = rF \sin\theta$ (θ = angle between **r** and **F**)

$\tau = \ell F$ (ℓ = lever arm of force)

Equilibrium: $F_{\text{net}} = 0$ (translational equilibrium)

$\tau_{\text{net}} = 0$ (rotational equilibrium)

static equilibrium means:

$F_{\text{net}} = 0$

$\tau_{\text{net}} = 0$

v = 0

CHAPTER 5 FREESTANDING PRACTICE QUESTIONS

1. A 100 kg skier's knee can withstand a lateral torque of 500 N·m before dislocating. As the skier loses control going around a corner, one ski comes up off the snow and the other boot and lower leg remain vertical, such that the knee starts to bend laterally. If the distance from the skier's knee to his center of mass is 1 m, at what angle θ from vertical will the knee dislocate due to the torque of gravity alone?

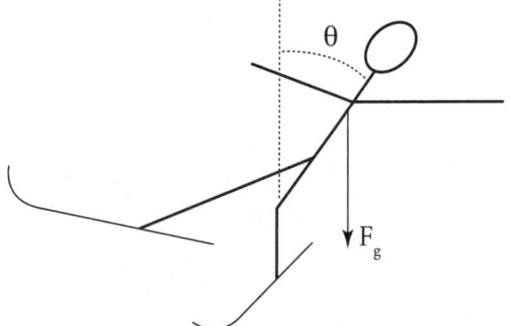

A) 30°
B) 45°
C) 60°
D) 90°

2. When rapidly turning a corner on a flat road, a cyclist leans into the center of the turn. The frame of the bike is nearly parallel to which vector?

A) The force of gravity on the bicycle and rider
B) The normal force on the pair
C) The centripetal force
D) The sum of the normal and friction forces

3. A 1000 kg gondola is operated on a cable between two towers 340 m apart. When the gondola is exactly between the towers, it is 100 m below their height. What is the tension in the cable at this midpoint?

A) 5 kN
B) 8 kN
C) 10 kN
D) 20 kN

4. Which of the following concerning uniform circular motion is true?

A) The centrifugal force is the action-reaction pair of the centripetal force.
B) Unlike the centrifugal force, the centripetal force is a type of force akin to that of friction, gravity, and tension forces.
C) The velocity of the object in motion changes, whereas the acceleration of the object is constant.
D) A satellite undergoing uniform circular motion is falling towards the center in a circular path.

5. When spinning a coin on a flat surface, two equal forces with opposite directions are applied to the opposite sides of a coin. Which of the following is true about the coin after it leaves the hand? (Assume ideal frictionless motion.)

A) The coin does not rotate because equal but opposite forces cancel each other out.
B) The coin does not rotate because equal but opposite torques cancel each other out.
C) The coin rotates and the rotational acceleration is zero.
D) The coin rotates and the rotational acceleration is equal to the nonzero net torque divided by the moment of inertia.

6. In human legs, 20% of the body's mass is in the upper legs (acting at 20 cm from the hip), 10% is in the lower legs (acting at 90 cm), and 3% is in the feet (acting at 120 cm). Find the center of mass of an outstretched leg for a person who is 70 kg.

A) 30 cm from the hip
B) 40 cm from the hip
C) 50 cm from the hip
D) 60 cm from the hip

7. Maria and Ali want to play on a teeter totter (a plank balanced atop a fulcrum, where each child sits on opposite ends of the plank and moves up and down by pushing off the ground in turns). They have a 4 m long, 10 kg plank and a round boulder to serve as a fulcrum. If Maria weighs 650 N and Ali weighs 350 N, how far from Maria's seat should they balance the plank in order to make the game as fair as possible?

A) 1.5 m
B) 167 cm
C) 1.8 m
D) 233 cm

CHAPTER 5 PRACTICE PASSAGE

As part of a school project, a group of physics students goes on a trip to an amusement park. The students who went on the trip were told to enjoy all the rides, but to be prepared to explain the physics behind two particular rides.

The first ride is a rotating cylinder that spins the riders uniformly in a circle. The passengers initially stand along the outer rim of the cylinder, at a radius $r = 4$ m. When the ride is started up, the cylinder begins to rotate, with its axis of rotation at its center. When a certain speed (v) is achieved, the floor of the ride drops away entirely, leaving the riders suspended against the wall.

In order for the passengers to be suspended, the coefficient of static friction (μ_s) of the wall needs to be large. The larger the coefficient of static friction, the slower the ride needs to spin in order to keep the riders suspended. Normally, $\mu_s = 0.50$. Because of its unique mechanism of action, the riders do not need to be restrained to the wall during the ride (see Figure 1).

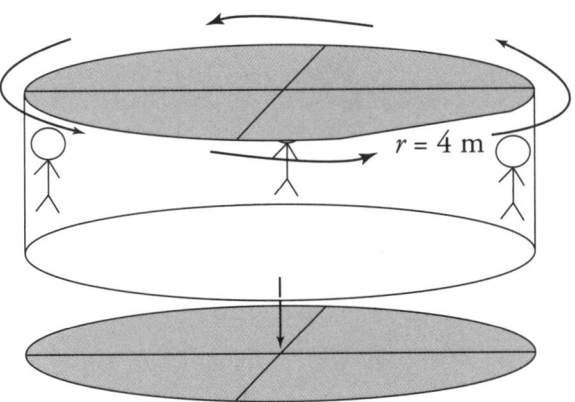

Figure 1 The first ride

The second ride consists of a carriage with mass 300 kg and with maximum occupancy of 300 kg. The carriage is attached to a mechanical arm of length $L = 5$ m that is capable of rotation. The arm is able to provide the torque necessary to swing the riders back and forth on a circular path. Initially, the trips back and forth are very small, but with each trip the swings become larger. Eventually, the riders have enough kinetic energy to swing 360° around, performing a complete circle. In order to partake in this ride, the passengers must be restrained to their seats (see Figure 2).

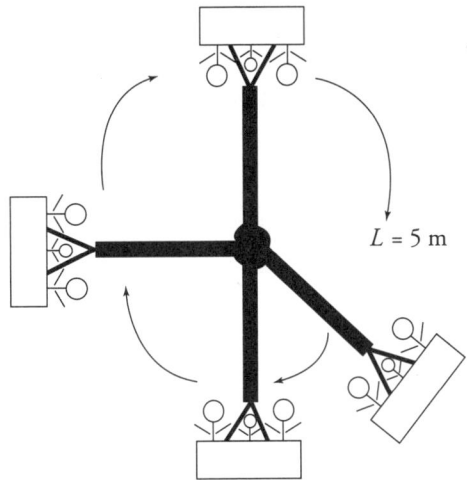

Figure 2 The second ride

1. In the first ride, what is the minimum tangential speed required to suspend a 50 kg man?

A) 7 m/s
B) 8 m/s
C) 9 m/s
D) 10 m/s

2. In the first ride, when spinning at a speed v, a person with mass m is successfully suspended. If a person with mass $3m$ rides, the ride would have to spin at a speed of:

A) v
B) $3v$
C) $6v$
D) $9v$

3. With a full carriage, the second ride suffers a power outage with the mechanical arm parallel to the ground. How much torque must the mechanical arm provide in order to prevent the passengers from swinging down? (Assume the mechanical arm itself does not require any torque support.)

A) 0 N·m
B) 3×10^4 N·m
C) 18×10^4 N·m
D) 24×10^4 N·m

4. Assume the riders in the second ride are undergoing uniform circular motion. Which of the following is true?

A) The normal force and the centripetal force are at their maximum values at the bottom of the swing.
B) The normal force and the centripetal force are at their maximum values at the top of the swing.
C) The normal force is at maximum value at the bottom of the swing, while the centripetal force value does not change.
D) The normal force is at maximum value at the top of the swing, while the centripetal force is constantly changing.

5. With its carriage full, the second ride goes through the top of its swing. What is the value of the normal force if its speed is 20 m/s?

A) 42 kN
B) 48 kN
C) 54 kN
D) 60 kN

6. In the second ride, a mass of 200 kg is placed on the mechanical arm 3 meters from the center of rotation. In this setup, where is the center of mass relative to the center of rotation? (Assume that the mechanical arm itself has no mass and that the carriage is full.)

A) 3.5 m
B) 4.0 m
C) 4.25 m
D) 4.5 m

SOLUTIONS TO CHAPTER 5 FREESTANDING QUESTIONS

1. **A** Rearranging the formula for torque, we find that $\sin \theta = \tau/rF$. The force of gravity is acting at the center of mass, 1 m from the knee, which is the fulcrum. Substituting the values, being careful to use 1000 N of gravitational force rather than 100 kg, we find that $\sin \theta = 0.5$. Therefore, $\theta = 30°$.

2. **D** A free body diagram is a very important first step here. Gravity always acts downward meaning choice A cannot be correct. The normal force is always perpendicular to the surface, so up in this case, eliminating choice B. The centripetal force will be toward the center of the turn, which will be horizontal on a flat road, so choice C is wrong. The answer is choice D because the friction is the source of that horizontal centripetal force and the normal force is up. If you add them, the resultant will be similar to the angle at which the bike leans.

3. **C** A diagram is vital here. Looking at the symmetrical triangles formed by the cable, one finds that the top side is 170 m on each, while the vertical displacement of the gondola is 100 m. This is a 1-2-$\sqrt{3}$ triangle, so the hypotenuse must be 200 m, though the actual distance does not matter, just the proportion. We find that the gravitational force is 10,000 N, which is divided evenly between the vertical components of the two tensions, giving each a T_y of 5000 N. Do not stop here; that would give you choice A, which is wrong. Because of the nature of the triangle, we know that the total tension is twice the value of this vertical component. So each tension must be 10,000 N. Note that if you add up the tension of the two spans acting on the gondola, which is not what the question is asking, then you get choice D.

4. **D** This requires an understanding of the basic concepts of uniform circular motion and the forces at work. The centripetal force is a name given to the net force of an object undergoing uniform circular motion. Therefore, it is not a separate force and does not have an action-reaction pair. This eliminates choices A and B. The speed of the object in uniform circular motion is constant, but its direction changes, therefore the velocity changes with time. However, the acceleration also changes because the direction of the centripetal acceleration always points to the center of the circle. This eliminates choice C. A satellite undergoing uniform circular motion is in fact falling towards the center, but never accomplishes its goal due to its tangential velocity. Its velocity changes as a result, but it would always form a tangent to its circular path.

5. **C** This is a two-by-two question. Although two equal forces with opposite directions are applied, giving a zero translational acceleration, the net torque is the sum of the two torques, resulting in a rotation of the coin. This eliminates choices A and B. However, after the coin leaves the hand, it undergoes rotational equilibrium, as no net torque is applied. In this case, the rotational acceleration is zero, with the coin undergoing a constant angular rotation.

6. **C** Using the hip as the reference point, center of mass can be calculated using the formula: $x_{CM} = (m_1x_1 + m_2x_2 + \ldots + m_nx_n) / (m_1 + m_2 + \ldots + m_n)$.

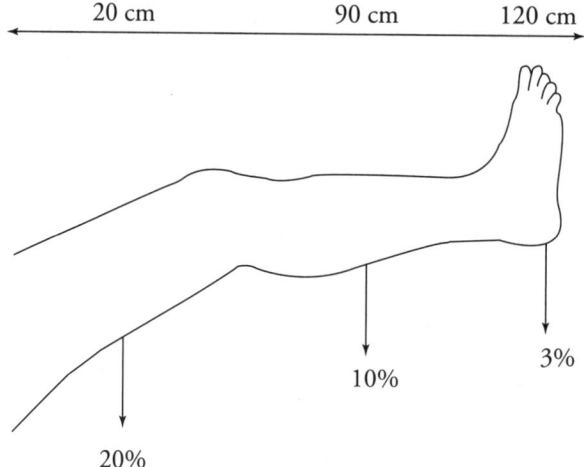

The points where the mass is centered for each body part can be used as the distances. Note that the mass of 70 kg does not affect the solution since it is in every term so it factors out of both the numerator and denominator.

$$x_{CM} = \frac{(0.03)(70)(120) + (0.1)(70)(90) + (0.2)(70)(20)}{(0.03)(70) + (0.1)(70) + (0.2)(70)} \approx 50 \text{ cm}.$$

7. **B** The fulcrum should be at the center of mass to balance the teeter totter. Calculate the center of mass the standard way or pick an arbitrary point x and balance the torques about that point. For the sake of this calculation, Maria's location will be called $x_1 = 0$ m and Ali's $x_2 = 4$ m; note that their respective masses are just the given weights divided by $g = 10$ m/s^2. That makes the location of the plank's center of mass $x_3 = 2$ m. The center-of-mass equation then yields

$$x_{CM} = \frac{m_1x_1 + m_2x_2 + m_3x_3}{m_1 + m_2 + m_3} = \frac{(65 \text{ kg})(0) + (45 \text{ kg})(4 \text{ m}) + (10 \text{ kg})(2 \text{ m})}{(65 + 45 + 10) \text{ kg}}$$

$$= \frac{(180 + 20) \text{ kg} \cdot \text{m}}{120 \text{ kg}} = \frac{200}{120} \text{ m} = \frac{5}{3} \text{ m} \approx 167 \text{ cm}$$

SOLUTIONS TO CHAPTER 5 PRACTICE PASSAGE

1. **C** In the first ride, the riders are undergoing uniform circular motion, therefore $F_c = mv^2/r$. The cause of the centripetal force is actually the normal force F_N of the wall on the rider: $F_N = F_c = mv^2/r$. To suspend the man, the force of gravity (F_{grav}) must be counteracted by the force of static friction (F_f). Therefore, to find the minimum tangential speed (and thus the minimum normal force), we presume the maximum static frictional force corresponding to that normal force:

$$F_f = F_{grav} \rightarrow \mu_s F_N = mg \rightarrow \mu_s \frac{mv^2}{r} = mg$$

$$v = \sqrt{\frac{gr}{\mu_s}} = \sqrt{\frac{10 \cdot 4}{0.5}} = \sqrt{80} \approx 9 \text{ m/s}$$

2. **A** As in the previous problem, any rider will be suspended only if friction counteracts their weight: $F_f = F_{grav}$. The normal force from the wall provides the centripetal force keeping them moving in a circular path, so $F_N = F_c = mv^2/r$.

$$F_f = F_{grav} \rightarrow \mu_s F_N = mg \rightarrow \mu_s \frac{mv^2}{r} = mg \rightarrow v = \sqrt{\frac{gr}{\mu_s}}$$

Because mass does not appear in this expression, the necessary tangential speed of the ride to suspend a rider doesn't change.

3. **B** If the arm is stuck parallel to the ground, then the mechanical arm must provide enough torque to cancel out the torque produced by the gravitational force.

$$\tau = rF \sin\theta = mgr = (m_{carriage} + m_{passengers})gr = (300 + 300) \times 10 \times 5 = 3 \times 10^4 \, \text{N} \cdot \text{m}$$

4. **C** If the riders are undergoing uniform circular motion, then $F_c = mv^2/r$ with constant speed v. Since mass m and radius r are also constant, then F_c must also be constant, eliminating all options except choice C. Even though F_c may be constant during rotation, the normal force is not. The centripetal force is the sum of the forces radially, which include the tension force of the mechanical arm as well as the force of gravity. At the bottom of the swing, the normal force is opposite to the force of gravity, as opposed to at the top of the swing where the normal force and gravity are facing the same direction. Therefore, at the bottom of the swing, the normal force must be at a maximum, in order to cancel out the force of gravity, while at the top of the swing the normal force is at a minimum, because gravity is working with the normal force.

5. **A** At the top of the swing, $F_c = F_G + F_N$, since both are pointing radially and in the same direction. Therefore:

$$F_c = F_G + F_N = \frac{mv^2}{r}$$

$$6000 + F_N = \frac{600 \times 20^2}{5}$$

$$F_N = 48,000 - 6000 = 42 \text{ kN}$$

6. **D** For a two mass system, $x_{CM} = (m_1 x_1 + m_2 x_2)/(m_1 + m_2)$. For this question, we shall measure the position from the center of rotation (although other centers are usable as well). For the carriage (m_1), $x_1 = 5$ m. For the second mass (m_2), $x_2 = 3$. Thus,

$$x_{CM} = \frac{m_1 x_1 + m_2 x_2}{m_1 + m_2}$$

$$= \frac{600 \times 5 + 200 \times 3}{800}$$

$$= 4.5 \text{ m}$$

Chapter 6
Mechanics III

6.1 WORK

Imagine a constant force **F** pushing a crate through a displacement **d**, as shown below:

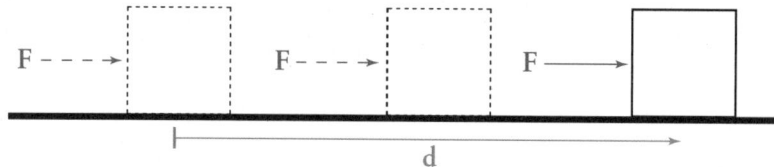

(Notice that the force **F** here doesn't just act momentarily at the initial position of the crate, with the crate then sliding across the floor with **F** removed; the force **F** is assumed to act constantly over the entire displacement.) We say that the **work** done by **F** is the product of F and d: Work $W = Fd$.

For example, if the magnitude of **F** is 20 N and the magnitude of **d** is 5 m, then the work done by the force **F** in the situation pictured above is (20 N)(5 m) = 100 N·m. When it's used to measure work, the newton-meter (N·m) is renamed the **joule**, abbreviated J. Therefore, we have $W = 100$ J.

The situation pictured above is quite special, however, because the vectors **F** and **d** point in the same direction. What if **F** and **d** do not point in the same direction? For example, what if we tie one end of a rope around the crate, sling the other end over our shoulder and pull the crate across the floor? Then our force **F** (which is actually the tension in the rope) will be at an angle to the displacement:

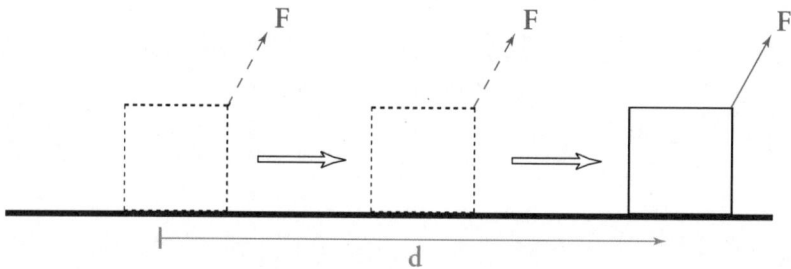

In this case, the work done by **F** is not the product of F and d. It's only the component of the force in the direction of **d** that does work. If θ is the angle between **F** and **d**, then the component of **F** that's parallel to **d** has magnitude $F\cos\theta$. Therefore, the work done by **F** is $(F\cos\theta)(d)$.

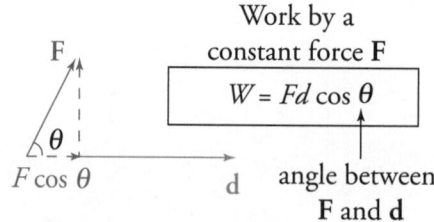

Work by a
constant force **F**

$$W = Fd\cos\theta$$

angle between
F and **d**

Work by a Constant Force, F

$$W = Fd\cos\theta$$

where θ = angle between **F** and **d**

Notice that the formula $W = Fd \cos \theta$ includes the formula $W = Fd$ as a special case. After all, if **F** and **d** do point in the same direction, then $\theta = 0°$, and $\cos \theta = \cos 0° = 1$, so $Fd \cos \theta$ becomes Fd. Therefore, the formula $W = Fd \cos \theta$ covers all cases of a constant force **F** acting through a displacement **d**.

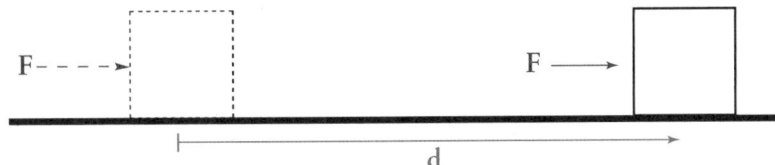

Example 6-1: In the situation pictured above, assume the mass of the crate, m, is 20 kg and the coefficient of kinetic friction between the crate and the floor is 0.4. If $F = 100$ N and $d = 6$ m,

a) How much work is done by **F**?
b) How much work is done by the normal force?
c) How much work is done by gravity?
d) How much work is done by the force of friction?
e) What is the total work done on the crate?

Solution:

a) Because **F** is parallel to **d**, the work done by **F** is simply $Fd = (100 \text{ N})(6 \text{ m}) = 600$ J.
b) The normal force is perpendicular to the floor, and to **d**. Since the angle between $\mathbf{F}_N$ and **d** is $\theta = 90°$, and $\cos 90° = 0$, the work done by $\mathbf{F}_N$ is zero.
c) The gravitational force is also perpendicular to the floor, and to **d**. Because the angle between $\mathbf{F}_{grav}$ and **d** is $\theta = 90°$, and $\cos 90° = 0$, the work done by $\mathbf{F}_{grav}$ is zero, too.
d) First, since $F_N = mg = (20 \text{ kg})(10 \text{ N/kg}) = 200$ N, we have $F_f = \mu_k F_N = (0.4)(200 \text{ N}) = 80$ N. However, the direction of the vector $\mathbf{F}_f$ is opposite to the direction of **d**, so the angle between $\mathbf{F}_f$ and **d** is $\theta = 180°$. Because $\cos 180° = -1$, the work done by the friction force is $(80 \text{ N})(6 \text{ m})(-1) = -480$ J.
e) To find the total work done on the crate, we just add up the work done by each of the forces that acts on the crate. In this case, then, we'd have

$$W_{total} = W_{by\ F} + W_{by\ F_N} + W_{by\ F_{grav}} + W_{by\ F_f} = (600 \text{ J}) + (0 \text{ J}) + (0 \text{ J}) + (-480 \text{ J}) = 120 \text{ J}$$

Here are a couple of things to notice about Example 6-1:

1) Although work depends on two vectors for its definition (namely, **F** and **d**), work itself is *not* a vector. *Work is a scalar.* W may be positive, negative, or zero, but work has no direction.
2) In this example, there were four forces acting on the crate: the pushing force **F**, gravity, the normal force, and friction. Each force does its own amount of work, which is why each part had to specify for which force we wanted the work. Only in the last part, where the total work is desired, can we omit the specific force we're looking at (because we're considering them all).

Example 6-2: In the situation described in Example 6-1, what is the net force on the crate? How much work is done by $\mathbf{F}_{net}$?

Solution: The normal force cancels out the gravitational force, so the net force on the crate is just $\mathbf{F} + \mathbf{F}_f =$ (100 N) + (−80 N) = +20 N, where the + indicates that $\mathbf{F}_{net}$ points to the right. Now, since $\mathbf{F}_{net}$ is parallel to $\mathbf{d}$, the work done by $\mathbf{F}_{net}$ is just the product, $F_{net}d$ = (20 N)(6 m) = 120 J. Notice that this is the same as the total amount of work done on the crate, as we figured out in part (e) of Example 6-1. This wasn't a coincidence. The total work done (found by adding up the values of the work done by each force separately) is always equal to the work done by the net force.

Remember that work is a scalar and it can be positive, zero, or negative. Now here's how to know *when* W will be positive, zero, or negative. Because $W = Fd \cos \theta$, and F and d are magnitudes (which means they're positive), the sign of W depends entirely on the sign of $\cos \theta$.

The diagrams below show the three cases.

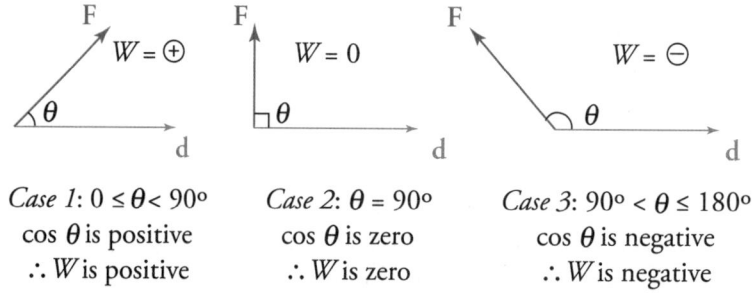

Case 1: $0 \leq \theta < 90°$
cos θ is positive
∴ W is positive

Case 2: $\theta = 90°$
cos θ is zero
∴ W is zero

Case 3: $90° < \theta \leq 180°$
cos θ is negative
∴ W is negative

In Case 1, the angle between $\mathbf{F}$ and $\mathbf{d}$ is less than 90° (an acute angle); since the cosine of such an angle is positive, the work done by this force will be positive.

In Case 2, the angle between $\mathbf{F}$ and $\mathbf{d}$ is 90°; since the cosine of 90° is zero, the work done by this force will be zero.

In Case 3, the angle between $\mathbf{F}$ and $\mathbf{d}$ is greater than 90° (an obtuse angle); since the cosine of such an angle is negative, the work done by this force will be negative.

Example 6-1 illustrated all three cases. The force that pushed the crate across the floor did positive work, gravity and the normal force did zero work, and sliding friction did negative work.

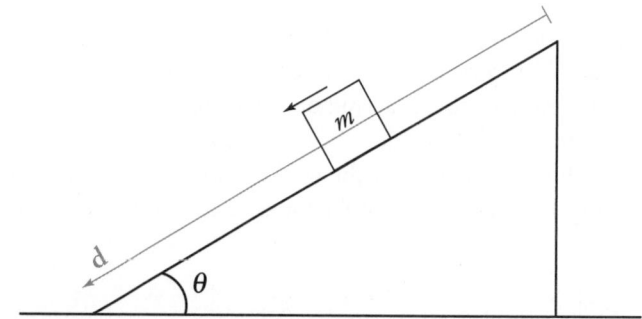

Example 6-3: In the situation pictured on the previous page, assume the mass of the block, *m*, is 20 kg and the coefficient of kinetic friction between the block and the ramp is 0.4. If *d* = 10 m and *θ* = 30°,

a) How much work is done by the normal force?
b) How much work is done by the force of friction?
c) How much work is done by gravity?
d) What is the total work done on the block?

Solution:

a) The normal force is perpendicular to the ramp, and to **d**. Since the angle between $\mathbf{F_N}$ and **d** is *θ* = 90°, and cos 90° = 0, the work done by $\mathbf{F_N}$ is zero. Forces acting perpendicular to the direction of travel always do zero work.

b) First, we know that since the block is on a ramp, we'll have $F_N = mg \cos \theta$, where *θ* is the incline angle of the ramp. The magnitude of $\mathbf{F_f}$, the force of kinetic friction, is $\mu_k F_N$, so we get $F_f = (0.4)(20 \text{ kg})(10 \text{ N/kg}) \cos 30°$, which is approximately $(0.4)(200 \text{ N})(0.85) = 68$ N. Now, since the vectors $\mathbf{F_f}$ and **d** point in opposite directions (because **d** points down the ramp and $\mathbf{F_f}$ points up the ramp), the work done by $\mathbf{F_f}$ will be $-F_f d = -(68 \text{ N})(10 \text{ m}) = -680$ J.

c) There are two ways we can answer this part. One way is to remember that the force due to gravity acting parallel to the ramp is $mg \sin \theta$, where *θ* is the incline angle. Since this component of the gravitational force is parallel to **d**, we can simply multiply $mg \sin \theta$ by *d* to find the work done by gravity: $W = (mg \sin \theta)(d) = (20 \text{ kg})(10 \text{ N/kg})(\sin 30°)(10 \text{ m}) = 1000$ J. Here's another way: The force $\mathbf{F_{grav}} = m\mathbf{g}$ points straight down, and the angle between $\mathbf{F_{grav}}$ and **d** is *β*, where *β* is the angle shown below. It's the complement of the incline angle *θ*; that is, $\beta = 90° - \theta$.

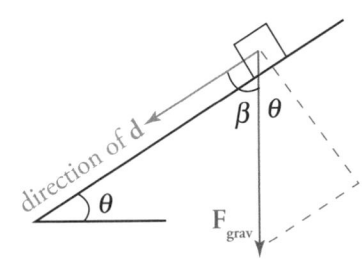

Since *θ* = 30°, we have *β* = 60°. Therefore, the work done by $\mathbf{F_{grav}}$ is $F_{grav} d \cos \beta = mgd \cos \beta = (20 \text{ kg})(10 \text{ N/kg})(10 \text{ m})(\cos 60°) = 1000$ J. You need to be very careful here; the formula for work reads, "$W = Fd \cos \theta$," but the *θ* in this formula is *not* the same as the *θ* labeled in the figure. The angle in the formula for *W* is the angle between **F** and **d**, and this is not the same as the incline angle.

d) To find the total work done on the block, we just add up the work done by each of the forces that acts on the block. In this case, then, we'd have

$$W_{\text{total}} = W_{\text{by } F_N} + W_{\text{by } F_f} + W_{\text{by } F_{grav}} = (0 \text{ J}) + (-680 \text{ J}) + (1000 \text{ J}) = 320 \text{ J}$$

The formula $W = Fd \cos\theta$ can only be used if the force is constant during the motion. What if the force changes? In general, calculus is required, which is not needed for the MCAT. However, if a graph of force vs. position is given (assuming $\theta = 0$), then the work done by that force is equal to the area *under the curve.*

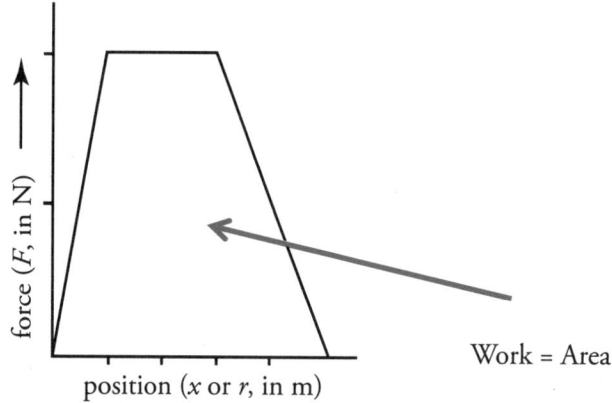

In Chapter 11, we will apply this to find the work required to compress or stretch a spring.

6.2 POWER

Power measures how fast work gets done. For example, if a force does 100 J of work in 20 seconds, then work is being done at a *rate* of

$$\frac{100 \text{ J}}{20 \text{ s}} = 5 \text{ J/s}$$

This is the power.

We use the letter P to denote power, and from the sample calculation above, we can see that the unit of power is the joule-per-second. This unit has its own name: the **watt**, abbreviated W. Therefore, power is measured in watts: $[P] = \text{J/s} = \text{W}$. (Don't confuse the abbreviation for the watt, W, with the usual variable used for work, W.)

The term *watt* makes most of us think of light bulbs, but the watt is used to measure the power of anything, not just light bulbs. After all, should the unit *horsepower* make us think that only horses can provide power? By the way, 1 hp (1 horsepower) is equal to about 750 W.

The sample calculation on the previous page also shows us how we should define P in general:

> **Power**
>
> $$P = \frac{\text{work}}{\text{time}} = \frac{W}{t}$$

What if 100 J of work is done over a time interval of just 2 seconds? Then the power would be 50 W; it's easy to see that the faster work gets done, the greater the power.

A handy formula that you can also use to calculate P uses the fact that $v = d/t$:

$$P = \frac{W}{t} = \frac{Fd}{t} = F\frac{d}{t} = Fv \rightarrow P = Fv$$

(We're assuming here that **F** is parallel to **d**, so that $W = Fd$, and that the object's speed, v, is constant.) To see how this formula would be used, let's answer this question: How much power must be provided to a model rocket of mass 50 kg to keep it moving upward at a constant speed of 40 m/s? Ignoring air resistance, the engine thrust must provide an upward force that's equal to the weight of the rocket: $F = mg = (50 \text{ kg})(10 \text{ N/kg}) = 500 \text{ N}$. Therefore, $P = Fv = (500 \text{ N})(40 \text{ m/s}) = 20{,}000 \text{ W} = 20 \text{ kW}$.

From the definition of power, we can see that

> $$W = Pt$$

This equation is used as often on the MCAT as the definition $P = W/t$. For example, if a machine has a power output of 200 W, how much work can it do in 1 hour? Multiplying power by time (and remembering to change 1 hour into $(60)(60) = 3600$ seconds) gives the work:

$$W = Pt = (200 \text{ W})(3600 \text{ s}) = 720{,}000 \text{ J} = 720 \text{ kJ}$$

Example 6-4: A force of magnitude 40 N pushes on an object of mass 8 kg through a displacement of 5 m for 10 seconds. What's the power provided by this force?

Solution: Power is equal to work divided by time, so

$$P = \frac{W}{t} = \frac{Fd}{t} = \frac{(40 \text{ N})(5 \text{ m})}{10 \text{ s}} = 20 \text{ W}$$

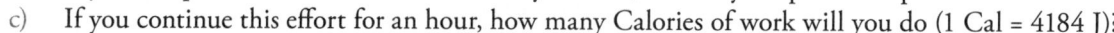

6.2

Example 6-5: You're lifting bricks, each with a mass of 2 kg, from the floor up to a shelf that is 1.5 m high.

   a)   How much work do you perform lifting each brick?
   b)   If you can place 20 bricks on the shelf every minute, what is your power output?
   c)   If you continue this effort for an hour, how many Calories of work will you do (1 Cal = 4184 J)?

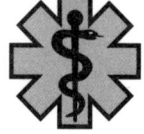

Solution:

   a)   The force you must provide to lift a brick is equal to the weight of the brick, which is mg = (2 kg)(10 N/kg) = 20 N. Since this force must act over a distance of 1.5 m to lift it up to the shelf, the work required is $W = Fd$ = (20 N)(1.5 m) = 30 J.

   b)   If you can place 20 bricks on the shelf every 60 seconds, then on average you're lifting one brick every 3 seconds. If the work performed in 3 seconds is 30 J—as we found in part (a)—then your power output is

$$P = \frac{W}{t} = \frac{30 \text{ J}}{3 \text{ s}} = 10 \text{ W}$$

   c)   In an hour a power of 10 W amounts to $W = Pt$ = 10 J/s × 3600 s/hr = 36,000 J. Unfortunately, that's only 36,000 J × 1/4184 Cal/J ≈ 9 Cal. However, our bodies are far from perfectly efficient, so we have to burn many more Calories than that to achieve that much work output. Moreover, there's a lot more to making a human body move than ideal work done against gravity in a frictionless process. After all, if you run for an hour on a horizontal treadmill, you have accomplished zero physical work, but obviously you will burn a lot of Calories!

Example 6-6: A car of mass 2000 kg accelerates from rest to a speed of 30 m/s in 9 seconds. Given that the engine does a total of 900,000 J of work, what is the average power output of the car's engine?

Solution: Since we're given the amount of work done and the time interval, we can find the average power output of the engine simply by dividing work by time:

$$P = \frac{W}{t} = \frac{900,000 \text{ J}}{9 \text{ s}} = 100,000 \text{ W} = 100 \text{ kW}$$

Notice that neither the mass of the car, nor its final speed, were needed to answer the question because the required information (work and time) was given.

Example 6-7: One month, your electric bill states that you used 500 kWh of electricity, at a cost of 8¢ per kWh. What is a kWh, and how much is your electric bill that month?

Solution: A kilowatt (kW) is a thousand watts; it's a unit of power. An hour (h) is a time interval. Therefore, a kilowatt-hour, kWh, obtained by multiplying power times time, Pt, has units of work. (1 kWh = (1000 W)(3600 s) = 3.6×10^6 J = 3.6 MJ.) The electric company performed 500 kWh of work pushing and pulling the electrons within the wires in your home to make electrical devices function, at a cost to you of (500 kWh)(8¢/kWh) = $40.

6.3 KINETIC ENERGY

An intuitive way to describe **energy** is that it's the ability to do work. Objects that move have this ability, since they can crash into something and thus exert a force over a distance. Therefore, objects that move have energy; specifically, we say they have **kinetic energy**, the energy due to motion.

To figure out how much kinetic energy a moving object has, imagine that an object of mass m is initially at rest (and thus has no kinetic energy). To get it moving, we have to exert a force **F** on it, over some distance d. (Let's assume, to keep things simple, that **F** points in the same direction as **d**.) How fast will the object be moving as a result? The acceleration is a constant $a = F/m$, so, using Big Five #5, we get

$$v^2 = v_0^2 + 2ad \rightarrow v^2 = 2ad \rightarrow v^2 = 2\frac{F}{m}d$$

Therefore, the final speed, v, will be $\sqrt{2Fd/m}$

Now let's do a little algebra and rewrite the last equation above like this:

$$Fd = \tfrac{1}{2}mv^2$$

We recognize the product Fd as the work done by the force. So, we did work on the object to get it moving, and now because it's moving, it has kinetic energy. How much kinetic energy? This last equation tells us that we should consider the amount of kinetic energy to be $\tfrac{1}{2}mv^2$.

Kinetic Energy

$$KE = \frac{1}{2}mv^2$$

In words, this definition says that the kinetic energy of an object whose mass is m and whose speed is v is equal to one-half m times the square of the speed. Since $\frac{1}{2}mv^2$ is equal to the work Fd, we see right away that the unit of KE should also be the joule. In addition, like work, kinetic energy is a scalar.

Example 6-8: An object of mass 10 kg moves with a velocity of 4 m/s to the north. What is its kinetic energy? What would happen to the kinetic energy if the speed of the object doubled?

Solution: Kinetic energy is a scalar that cares only about the speed of an object; the direction of the object's velocity is irrelevant. So we find that

$$KE = \tfrac{1}{2}mv^2 = \tfrac{1}{2}(10 \text{ kg})(4 \text{ m/s})^2 = 80 \text{ J}$$

Because KE is proportional to v^2, if v were to increase by a factor of 2 then KE would increase by a factor of $2^2 = 4$.

The Work-Energy Theorem

The use of Big Five #5 on the previous page (to motivate the definition $KE = \frac{1}{2}mv^2$) assumed that the initial speed of the object was zero. But what if the initial speed wasn't zero? Then we'd have

$$v^2 - v_0^2 = 2\frac{F}{m}d$$

$$v^2 = v_0^2 + 2ad \rightarrow v^2 - v_0^2 = 2ad \rightarrow \frac{1}{2}m(v^2 - v_0^2) = Fd$$

$$Fd = \frac{1}{2}mv^2 - \frac{1}{2}mv_0^2$$

$$W = KE_{final} - KE_{initial}$$

In other words, the total work done on the object is equal to the change in its kinetic energy. This fact is important enough that it's given a name:

Work-Energy Theorem

$$W_{total} = \Delta KE$$

This formula gives you another way to calculate work. You don't even need to know the force or the displacement! If you know the change in an object's kinetic energy, then you automatically know the total amount of work that was done on it.

Look back on page 150 at the set of three diagrams showing when the work done by a force is positive, zero, or negative. In Case 1, the force is pulling in roughly the same direction as the object's displacement (more formally, the force **F** has a component that's in the same direction as **d**). We can think of such a force as "helping" the object move, and therefore causing its speed to increase. More technically, the work done on an object *transfers* energy from the environment into the object. In the case of positive work being done, and according to the work-energy theorem, positive work would automatically imply a positive change in kinetic energy. If the kinetic energy increases, then the speed increases.

In Case 3, the force is pulling in roughly the opposite direction from the object's displacement (more formally, the force **F** has a component that's in the opposite direction from **d**). We can think of such a force as "hindering" the object's motion, and therefore causing its speed to decrease. This is also consistent with the work-energy theorem because Case 3 was the case of negative work being done on the object, transferring energy out of the object into the environment. According to the work-energy theorem, negative work automatically implies a negative change in kinetic energy. If the kinetic energy decreases, then the speed decreases.

Example 6-9: An object of mass 10 kg whose initial speed is 4 m/s is accelerated until it achieves a final speed of 9 m/s.

a) How much work was done on this object?
b) If the acceleration took place over a displacement **d** of magnitude 13 m, and the force **F** exerted on it was constant and parallel to **d**, what was F?

Solution:

a) Although neither **F** nor **d** is given, we can still figure out the work done by using the work-energy theorem:

$$
\begin{aligned}
W_{total} &= \Delta KE \\
&= KE_f - KE_i \\
&= \tfrac{1}{2}mv^2 - \tfrac{1}{2}mv_0^2 \\
&= \tfrac{1}{2}m(v^2 - v_0^2) \\
&= \tfrac{1}{2}(10 \text{ kg})\left[\left(9 \text{ m/s}\right)^2 - \left(4 \text{ m/s}\right)^2\right]
\end{aligned}
$$

$$\therefore W = 325 \text{ J}$$

b) Because **F** is parallel to **d**, we know that $W = Fd$. We just found W in part (a), and since we now know d, we can find F:

$$W = Fd \rightarrow \quad F = \frac{W}{d} = \frac{325 \text{ J}}{13 \text{ m}} = 25 \text{ N}$$

Example 6-10: An object of mass 10 kg is moving at a speed of 9 m/s. How much work must be done on this object in order to stop it?

Solution: Once again, we're asked to find W without being given **F** and **d**, so we use the work-energy theorem. If we want to stop the object, we want to bring its final kinetic energy to zero. Therefore,

$$
\begin{aligned}
W &= \Delta KE \\
&= \tfrac{1}{2}mv^2 - \tfrac{1}{2}mv_0^2 \\
&= 0 - \tfrac{1}{2}mv_0^2 \\
&= -\tfrac{1}{2}(10 \text{ kg})(9 \text{ m/s})^2
\end{aligned}
$$

$$\therefore W = -405 \text{ J}$$

The work that must be done on the object has to be negative, because only negative work causes a decrease in speed.

Example 6-11: Recall the centrifuge Example 5-4 from the preceding chapter. Suppose the mass of blood in one bag is 0.5 kg.

    a)   What's the magnitude of the net force on the blood?

    b)   How much work is done by the net force during each revolution of the centrifuge?

Solution:

    a)   The net force on an object undergoing uniform circular motion (UCM) is the centripetal force:

$$F_c = m\frac{v^2}{r} = (0.5 \text{ kg})\frac{(175 \text{ m/s})^2}{0.35 \text{ m}} \approx 4 \times 10^4 \text{ N}$$

    b)   We can answer this part in two ways. The centripetal force points toward the center of the circular path, so it's always perpendicular to the blood's velocity:

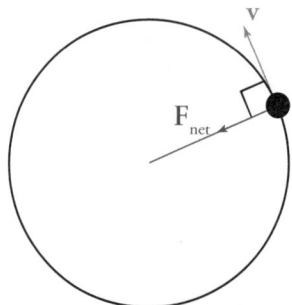

    The work done by a force that's perpendicular to the blood's motion is *zero* (remember Case 2 depicted in Section 6.1: $\mathbf{F} \perp \mathbf{d}$ means $W = 0$.)

    Another way is to use the work-energy theorem. Since the blood's speed is constant, its kinetic energy is constant, too. No change in kinetic energy means no work is being done.

Example 6-12: A box of mass 4 kg is initially at rest on a frictionless horizontal surface. A horizontal force **F** of magnitude 32 N is exerted on the object and then removed. If the speed of the object is then 2 m/s, over what distance did **F** act?

Solution: By the work-energy theorem, the work done by **F** was

$$W = \Delta KE = KE_f - KE_i = KE_f = \tfrac{1}{2}mv^2 = \tfrac{1}{2}(4 \text{ kg})(2 \text{ m/s})^2 = 8 \text{ J}$$

The question now is, "Given that **F** is parallel to **d** (so $W = Fd$), what's d?"

$$W = Fd \rightarrow d = \frac{W}{F} = \frac{8 \text{ J}}{32 \text{ N}} = 0.25 \text{ m}$$

Example 6-13: Consider the block described in Example 6-3. If the initial speed of the block was zero, what is the block's speed when it reaches the bottom of the ramp?

Solution: We figured out in part (d) of that example that the total work done on the block was 320 J. By the work-energy theorem, we find that

$$W = \Delta KE = KE_f - KE_i = KE_f = \tfrac{1}{2}mv^2 \rightarrow v = \sqrt{\frac{2W_{total}}{m}} = \sqrt{\frac{2(320\,\text{J})}{20\,\text{kg}}} = \sqrt{32\,\text{m}^2/\text{s}^2} \approx 5.6\,\text{m/s}$$

Example 6-14: Consider the crate described in Example 6-1.

a)   If the initial speed of the crate was zero, what was the speed once the force **F** was removed after acting through the given displacement **d**?

b)   How far would the crate slide before coming to rest?

Solution:

a)   We figured out in part (e) of that example that the total work done on the crate was 120 J. The work-energy theorem then tells us that

$$W = \Delta KE = KE_f - KE_i = KE_f = \tfrac{1}{2}mv^2 \rightarrow v = \sqrt{\frac{2W_{total}}{m}} = \sqrt{\frac{2(120\,\text{J})}{20\,\text{kg}}} = \sqrt{12\,\text{m}^2/\text{s}^2} \approx 3.5\,\text{m/s}$$

b)   Once the force **F** is removed, the only force acting on the crate that doesn't do zero work is friction. The work done by friction will be $-F_f d'$, where d' is the distance the crate will slide before coming to rest. By the work-energy theorem, we have

$$W = \Delta KE = KE_f - KE_i = 0 - KE_i$$
$$-KE_i = -F_f d'$$
$$F_f d' = KE_i$$
$$d' = \frac{KE_i}{F_f}$$

Since the crate had 120 J of kinetic energy right when the force **F** was removed, using the equation $F_f = \mu_k F_N = \mu_k mg$ gives us

$$d' = \frac{KE_i}{F_f} = \frac{KE_i}{\mu_k mg} = \frac{120\,\text{J}}{(0.4)(20\,\text{kg})(10\,\tfrac{\text{N}}{\text{kg}})} = 1.5\,\text{m}$$

6.4 POTENTIAL ENERGY

In the preceding section, we defined kinetic energy as the energy an object has due to its motion. **Potential energy** is the energy an object has by virtue of its *position*. There are different "kinds" of potential energy because there are different kinds of forces. For example, in our study of MCAT physics, we'll look at three types of potential energy: gravitational, electrical, and elastic. In this chapter, we'll study the first of these: *gravitational* potential energy.

Imagine a brick lying on the ground. Now, pick it up and place it on a shelf. You've just changed the position of the brick, and, since potential energy is the energy an object has by virtue of its position, you might expect that you've changed the brick's potential energy as well. You did. The brick's gravitational potential energy has been changed, because its position in a gravitational field has changed.

Now, let's be more specific. By *how much* did the brick's gravitational potential energy change? To find the answer, we need to look at the work done by the gravitational force (this is gravitational potential energy, after all). While the brick was being lifted, gravity did work on the brick. Let m be the mass of the brick, and let h be the height from the ground up to the shelf. The gravitational force on the brick is $\mathbf{F}_{\text{grav}} = m\mathbf{g}$, pointing downward; the displacement of the brick is h, upward.

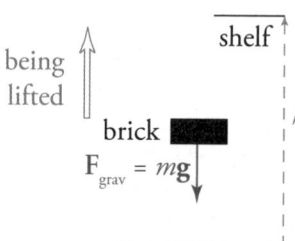

Because the force $\mathbf{F}_{\text{grav}}$ and the displacement $\mathbf{h}$ point in opposite directions, we know that the work done by $\mathbf{F}_{\text{grav}}$ will be the negative of F_{grav} times h: $W_{\text{by } \mathbf{F}_{\text{grav}}} = -F_{\text{grav}}h = -mgh$. The change in gravitational potential energy is defined to be the opposite of the work done by the gravitational force:

$$\Delta PE_{\text{grav}} = -W_{\text{by } \mathbf{F}_{\text{grav}}}$$

In this case, then, we have $\Delta PE_{\text{grav}} = -(-mgh) = mgh$. If the brick had *fallen* from the shelf to the floor, so that its height *decreased* by h, then we would have had $W_{\text{by } \mathbf{F}_{\text{grav}}} = -F_{\text{grav}}h = mgh$ and $\Delta PE_{\text{grav}} = -mgh$. In summary, then, we have

Change in Gravitational Potential Energy

$$\Delta PE_{\text{grav}} = \begin{array}{l} +mgh, \text{ if the height of } m \text{ is increased by } h \\ -mgh, \text{ if the height of } m \text{ is decreased by } h \end{array}$$

where it's assumed that we're close enough to the surface of the earth that g can be considered a constant.

The formulas on the previous page give the *change* in the gravitational potential energy of an object of mass *m*. If we designate the ground as our "PE_{grav} = 0" level, then we can say that the gravitational potential energy of an object at height *h* is equal to *mgh*.

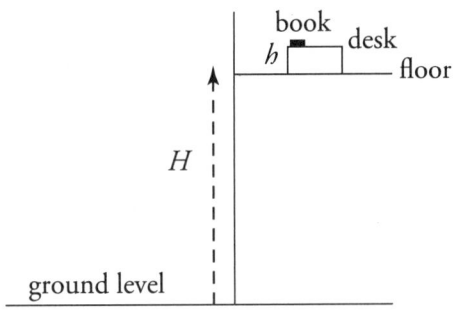

Potential energy is relative. Consider a book sitting on the desk in a second-floor office. Relative to the floor, the height of the book might be, say, half a meter. So, if the book has a mass of 1 kg, its gravitational potential energy is *mgh* = (1 kg)(10 N/kg)(0.5 m) = 5 J. But what if we were to measure the height of the book above the *ground*? Relative to the ground, the floor of the office might be at height *H* = 5 m, so the height of the book above the ground would be *H* + *h* = 5.5 m, and the book's gravitational potential energy is *mg*(*H* + *h*) = (1 kg)(10 N/kg)(5.5 m) = 55 J. Whenever we talk about "the" potential energy of an object, we must specify where we're choosing our "*PE* = 0" level.

The fact that potential energy is relative typically doesn't matter because only *changes* in potential energy are important and physically meaningful. Let's go back to our book on the office desk example. If the book falls off the desk to the floor, what is the change in its potential energy? To the person who calls the floor of the office their "*PE* = 0" level, the change in the book's potential energy will be

$$\Delta PE_{grav} = PE_f - PE_i = 0 - mgh = -mgh = -(1 \text{ kg})(10 \tfrac{N}{kg})(0.5 \text{ m}) = -5 \text{ J}$$

Now, to the person who calls the ground their "*PE* = 0" level, the change in the book's potential energy will be the same:

$$\Delta PE_{grav} = PE_f - PE_i = mgH - mg(H + h) = -mgh = -(1 \text{ kg})(10 \tfrac{N}{kg})(0.5 \text{ m}) = -5 \text{ J}$$

Both people will always agree on the *change* in an object's potential energy, even if they disagree about what the potential energy *is* at a certain height (because they choose different "*PE* = 0" levels).

Example 6-15: A brick that weighs 25 N is lifted from the ground to a shelf that's 2 m high. What is its change in gravitational potential energy?

Solution: Because *mg* = 25 N, we have ΔPE_{grav} = *mgh* = (25 N)(2 m) = 50 J. Notice that since the brick was lifted *up*, its change in gravitational potential energy is *positive*.

Example 6-16: A 1 N apple in a tree is at a height 4 m above the ground. The apple falls off its branch and lands on a branch that's only 1 m above the ground. What is the change in the apple's potential energy?

Solution: Because the apple *falls* a distance of $h = 4 - 1 = 3$ m, the change in its gravitational potential energy is $-mgh = -(1 \text{ N})(3 \text{ m}) = -3$ J. We could also have answered the question like this: First, we choose, say, the ground to be our "$PE = 0$" level. Then the initial potential energy of the apple is $PE_i = mgh_i = (1 \text{ N})$ $(4 \text{ m}) = 4$ J, and the final potential energy of the apple is $PE_f = mgh_f = (1 \text{ N})(1 \text{ m}) = 1$ J. The change in the potential energy is, therefore, $\Delta PE = PE_f - PE_i = (1 \text{ J}) - (4 \text{ J}) = -3$ J. Note that because the apple *falls*, the change in its gravitational potential energy must be *negative*.

Example 6-17: Which has more gravitational potential energy: an object of mass 2 kg at a height of 50 m, or an object of mass 50 kg at a height of 2 m? (Set $PE_{grav} = 0$ at the ground for both objects.)

Solution: Since the ground is the $PE_{grav} = 0$ level, then at height h an object's gravitational potential energy is $PE_{grav} = mgh$. The potential energy of the 2 kg object is

$$PE_1 = m_1 g h_1 = (2 \text{ kg})(10 \tfrac{\text{N}}{\text{kg}})(50 \text{ m}) = 1000 \text{ J}$$

and the potential energy of the 50 kg object is

$$PE_2 = m_2 g h_2 = (50 \text{ kg})(10 \tfrac{\text{N}}{\text{kg}})(2 \text{ m}) = 1000 \text{ J}$$

Therefore, these two objects have the *same* gravitational potential energy relative to the ground.

Gravity Is a Conservative Force

Suppose we want to move a brick from the floor up to a shelf. One way we could do it would be to simply lift the brick straight up. Another way would be to set up a ramp and then push the brick up the ramp to the shelf. Let's figure out how much work gravity does in each of these cases. We'll assume that the brick has a mass of 3 kg and that the shelf is 2 m high.

The first case is easy. The gravitational force on the brick is $mg = (3 \text{ kg})(10 \text{ N/kg}) = 30$ N, directed straight downward. Since the displacement **h** of the brick is straight upward (that is, in the opposite direction from F_{grav}), we know that the work done by gravity is negative F_{grav} times h:

$$W_{\text{by } F_{grav}} = -F_{grav} h = -(30 \text{ N})(2 \text{ m}) = -60 \text{ J}$$

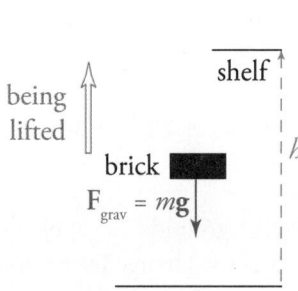

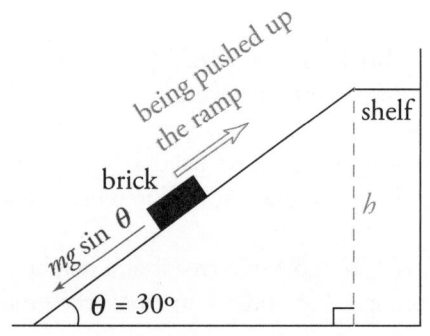

Now, let's look at the second case. Let's use a ramp whose incline angle θ is 30°. The gravitational force acting parallel to the ramp has magnitude $mg \sin \theta$, directed downward along the ramp. Because the displacement **d** is upward along the ramp (that is, in the opposite direction), we know the work done by gravity is negative, and equal to $-(mg \sin \theta)(d)$. Since the height of the shelf is $h = 2$ m, the length of the ramp (i.e., the hypotenuse of the right triangle) must be $d = h/(\sin \theta) = (2 \text{ m})/(\sin 30°) = 4$ m. Therefore, the work done by the gravitational force as the block is pushed up the ramp is

$$W_{\text{by } F_{\text{grav}}} = -(mg \sin \theta)(d) = -(30 \text{ N})(\sin 30°)(4 \text{ m}) = -(15 \text{ N})(4 \text{ m}) = -60 \text{ J}$$

This is the same answer as we found before! Since the change in the gravitational potential energy is defined to be the opposite of the work done by the gravitational force, $\Delta PE_{\text{grav}} = -W_{\text{by } F_{\text{grav}}}$, we can say that $\Delta PE_{\text{grav}} = -(-60 \text{ J}) = 60 \text{ J}$ in either case.

In the first case (lifting the brick straight upward), we exert a greater force over a smaller distance, while in the second case (moving the brick up a ramp), we exert a smaller force over a greater distance. However, the work done is the same in both cases.

These examples illustrate the following:

> *The work done by gravity*
>
> *depends only on the initial and final heights of the object,*
>
> *not on the path the object follows.*

Another way of saying this is to state that gravity is a **conservative** force. (In fact, it is the conservative nature of the gravitational force that allows us to define gravitational potential energy.)

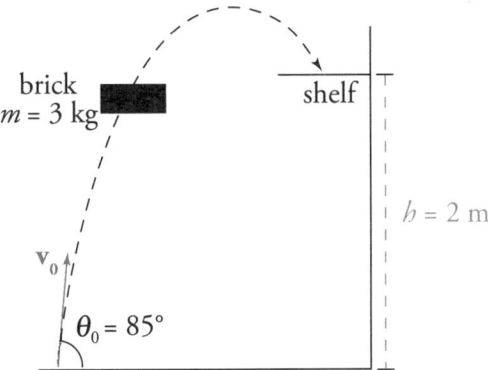

Example 6-18: In the situation pictured above, a brick is projected upward with an initial velocity $\mathbf{v}_0$ that makes an angle of 85° with the horizontal. The brick follows the path indicated and lands on the shelf. How much work did the gravitational force do on the brick?

Solution: The work done by gravity depends only on the initial and final positions of the object, not on the particular path the object takes. Since the initial height was $h_i = 0$ and the final height was $h_f = 2$ m, the change in the brick's gravitational potential energy is $\Delta PE_{grav} = mgh_f - mgh_i = mgh_f - 0 = mgh_f = (3$ kg$)$ $(10$ N/kg$)(2$ m$) = 60$ J. Therefore, the work done by the gravitational force is

$$W_{by\ \mathbf{F}_{grav}} = -\Delta PE_{grav} = -60\ J$$

just as we found before.

Friction Is NOT a Conservative Force

Gravity is a conservative force because the work done by gravity depends only on the initial and final positions of the object, not on the path taken. We'll now show that friction is *not* a conservative force; the work done by kinetic friction *does* depend on the path taken.

Consider a flat tabletop and mark two points on it, A and B. We're going to slide a block from Point A to Point B along two different paths; the work done will be different for the two paths, which will show that friction is not a conservative force. The figure below shows the two points, A and B, separated by a distance of 5 m. Another way to get from A to B is to move from A to C and then from C to B; I've chosen a point C that's 3 m from A and 4 m from B.

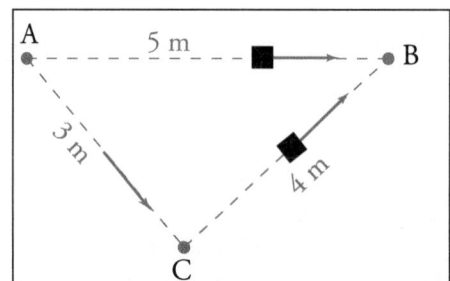

Assume the block has a mass of 1 kg; then its weight is $w = mg = (1$ kg$)(10$ N/kg$) = 10$ N, so the normal force on the block has magnitude 10 N also. If the coefficient of kinetic friction between the block and tabletop is 0.4, then, as the block slides, the magnitude of the force of kinetic friction is $F_f = \mu_k F_N = (0.4)$ $(10$ N$) = 4$ N, always directed opposite to the direction in which the block is sliding.

Let's first figure out how much work friction does as we slide the block directly from A to B:

$$W_{\substack{by\ F_f \\ A \to B}} = -F_f \cdot d_{A \to B} = -(4\ N)(5\ m) = -20\ J$$

Now let's figure out how much work friction does as we slide the block from A to B by way of C:

$$W_{\substack{by\ F_f \\ A \to C \to B}} = W_{\substack{by\ F_f \\ A \to C}} + W_{\substack{by\ F_f \\ C \to B}} = (-F_f \cdot d_{A \to C}) + (-F_f \cdot d_{C \to B}) = (-4\ N)(3\ m)\ + (-4\ N)(4\ m) = -28\ J$$

Even though we started at A and ended at B in both cases, we got a different amount of work done by friction for two different paths from A to B. Therefore, friction is *not* a conservative force. This means that there's no such thing as "frictional potential energy," because potential energy can be defined only for conservative forces.

6.5 TOTAL MECHANICAL ENERGY

Now that we've defined kinetic energy and potential energy, we can define an object's **total mechanical energy**, E. It's just the sum of the object's kinetic energy and potential energy:

Total Mechanical Energy
$$E = KE + PE$$

For example, consider an object of mass m sitting on a shelf that's at height h above the floor. Then, relative to the floor (where we'll set PE_{grav} equal to 0), the object's total mechanical energy is

$$E = KE + PE = 0 + mgh = mgh$$

Now, what if this same object falls off the shelf? What is its total mechanical energy when its height is, say, $h/2$? If v is the object's speed at this point, then the object's total mechanical energy is

$$E = KE + PE = \tfrac{1}{2}mv^2 + mg\tfrac{h}{2}$$

Example 6-19: An object of mass m is projected straight upward with an initial speed of v_0 at time $t = 0$.

a) What is the object's total mechanical energy at time $t = 0$?
b) At what time t will the object reach its maximum height?
c) What is the maximum height?
d) What is the object's total mechanical energy at this point?

Solution:

a) If we take the object's height at $t = 0$ to be $h = 0$, then its initial total mechanical energy is

$$E = KE + PE = \tfrac{1}{2}mv_0^2 + mg(0) = \tfrac{1}{2}mv_0^2$$

b) When the object reaches the highest point in its vertical path, its velocity is 0. Using Big Five #2 with $a = -g$, we find that

$$v = v_0 + at \rightarrow 0 = v_0 + \left(-g\right)t \rightarrow t = \frac{v_0}{g}$$

c) Using Big Five #5, we can find the object's maximum height:

$$v^2 = v_0^2 + 2ad \rightarrow (0)^2 = v_0^2 + 2(-g)d \rightarrow d = -\frac{v_0^2}{2(-g)} = \frac{v_0^2}{2g}$$

6.5

d) The object's total mechanical energy at this point is

$$E = KE + PE = \tfrac{1}{2}mv^2 + mgh = \tfrac{1}{2}m(0)^2 + mg\left(\tfrac{v_0^2}{2g}\right) = 0 + m\tfrac{v_0^2}{2} = \tfrac{1}{2}mv_0^2$$

Notice in this example that the answer to part (d) is the same as the answer to part (a): the object's total mechanical energy at its highest point is the same as it was at the object's initial point. This illustrates a very important concept: the **Conservation of Total Mechanical Energy**. If the only forces acting on an object during its motion are conservative (that means, for example, *no friction*), then the object's total mechanical energy will remain the same throughout the motion. Pick any two positions (or times) during the object's motion; for example, we could pick the initial position (initial time) and the final position (final time). Then

$$E_i = E_f$$

Writing E as $KE + PE$, we have

Conservation of Total Mechanical Energy
(no nonconservative forces)

$$KE_i + PE_i = KE_f + PE_f$$

Example 6-20: An object of mass m is projected straight upward with an initial speed of v_0 at time $t = 0$. Use Conservation of Total Mechanical Energy to find its maximum height.

Solution: If we take the object's height at $t = 0$ to be $h = 0$, then its initial total mechanical energy is

$$E = KE_i + PE_i = \tfrac{1}{2}mv_0^2 + mgh = \tfrac{1}{2}mv_0^2 + mg(0) = \tfrac{1}{2}mv_0^2$$

When the object reaches the highest point in its vertical path, its velocity is 0. Calling this height h, the object's total mechanical energy at this point is

$$E = KE_f + PE_f = \frac{1}{2}mv_0^2 + mgh = \frac{1}{2}m(0)^2 + mgh = mgh$$

Therefore, by Conservation of Total Mechanical Energy, we have

$$E_i = E_f$$
$$\tfrac{1}{2}mv_0^2 = mgh$$

$$\therefore h = \frac{v_0^2}{2g}$$

This is the same answer we found in Example 6-19(c) using the Big Five equations.

Another way to think about this problem is in terms of an energy *transformation*. At the moment the object was shot upward, it had only *KE*; at the top of its path, however, it has only *PE*. In other words, kinetic energy was transformed into gravitational potential energy:

$$KE \rightarrow PE \rightarrow \quad \frac{1}{2}mv_0^2 = mgh \quad \rightarrow \quad \therefore h = \frac{v_0^2}{2g}$$

It can be very helpful to think of Conservation of Total Mechanical Energy in terms of energy transformation between *KE* and *PE*. (The MCAT likes to ask questions about such energy transformations.)

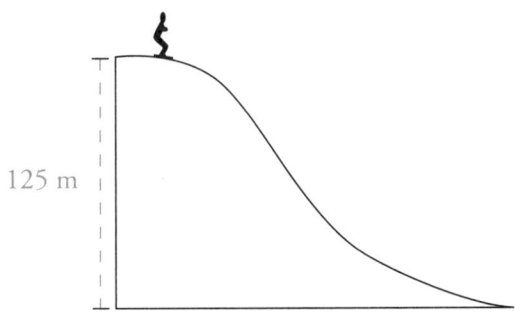

Example 6-21: A skier begins at rest at the top of a hill of height 125 m. If friction between her skis and the snow is negligible, what will be her speed at the bottom of the hill?

Solution: Let the bottom of the hill be $h = 0$, and call the top of the hill the skier's initial position and the bottom of the hill her final position. Then we have

$$KE_i + PE_i = KE_f + PE_f$$
$$0 + mgh = \tfrac{1}{2}mv^2 + 0$$
$$v = \sqrt{2gh}$$
$$= \sqrt{2(10 \text{ m/s}^2)(125 \text{ m})}$$
$$\therefore v = 50 \text{ m/s}$$

We could also think about this problem in terms of an energy transformation. At the top of the hill, the skier had only *PE*; at the bottom of the hill, she has only *KE*. In other words, gravitational potential energy was transformed into kinetic energy:

$$PE \rightarrow KE \rightarrow \quad mgh = \frac{1}{2}mv_0^2 \quad \rightarrow \quad \therefore v = \sqrt{2gh}$$

Example 6-22: A roller-coaster car drops from rest down the track and enters a loop. If the radius of the loop is *R*, and the initial height of the car is *5R* above the bottom of the loop, how fast is the car going at the top of the loop? Assume that *R* = 15 m and ignore friction.

Solution: Let's call the bottom of the loop our *h* = 0 level. At the car's initial position, we have $h_i = 5R$ and $v_i = 0$ (so $KE_i = 0$). At the top of the loop (the "final" position, for purposes of this question), we have $h_f = 2R$. The question is to find the car's speed, *v*, at this point. Using Conservation of Total Mechanical Energy, we get

$$KE_i + PE_i = KE_f + PE_f$$

$$0 + mgh_i = \tfrac{1}{2}mv^2 + mgh_f$$

$$gh_i = \tfrac{1}{2}v^2 + gh_f$$

$$v = \sqrt{2g(h_i - h_f)}$$

$$= \sqrt{2g(5R - 2R)}$$

$$= \sqrt{2g \cdot 3R}$$

$$= \sqrt{2(10 \text{ m/s}^2) \cdot 3(15 \text{ m})}$$

$$\therefore v = 30 \text{ m/s}$$

For extra practice, show that the car's speed when it's at the "9 o'clock" position within the loop is $\sqrt{1200}$ m/s ≈ 35 m/s, and that the car's speed when it's at the bottom of the loop is $\sqrt{1500}$ m/s ≈ 39 m/s.[1]

---

[1] For even more practice, compute the centripetal acceleration at these points, and show that the amusement park operator is in danger of being sued. (As a benchmark, consider that fighter pilots with the benefit of pressurized suits risk blacking out at accelerations greater than about $9g \approx 88$ m/s^2.)

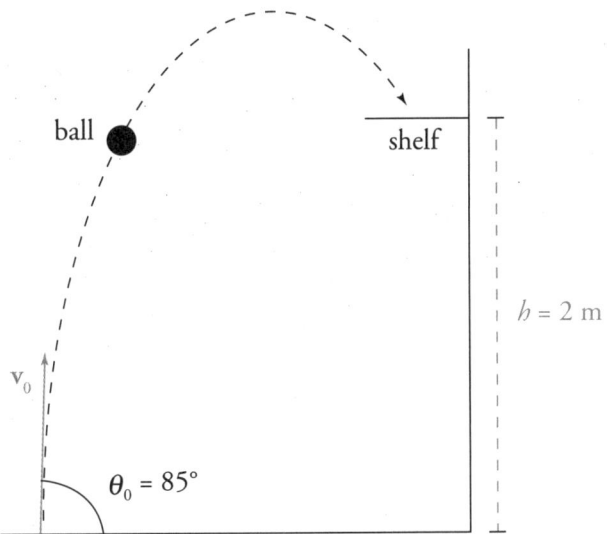

Example 6-23: In the situation pictured above, a ball is projected upward from the floor with an initial velocity $\mathbf{v}_0$ of magnitude 12 m/s that makes an angle of 85° with the horizontal. The ball follows the path indicated and lands on the shelf. How fast is the ball traveling as it hits the shelf? (Ignore air resistance.)

Solution: Let's call the floor our $h = 0$ level. At the object's initial position, we have $h_i = 0$ (so $PE_i = 0$). At the shelf (the final position), we have $h_f = 2$ m. The question is to find the speed of the ball, v, at this point. Using Conservation of Total Mechanical Energy, we get

$$KE_i + PE_i = KE_f + PE_f$$

$$\tfrac{1}{2}mv_0^2 + 0 = \tfrac{1}{2}mv^2 + mgh_f$$

$$\tfrac{1}{2}v_0^2 = \tfrac{1}{2}v^2 + gh_f$$

$$v = \sqrt{v_0^2 - 2gh_f}$$

$$= \sqrt{(12 \text{ m/s}^2)^2 - 2(10 \text{ m/s}^2)(2 \text{ m})}$$

$$\therefore v \approx 10 \text{ m/s}$$

Notice that the direction of the initial velocity vector (given to be "at an angle of 85° with the horizontal") was irrelevant here. One of the most useful attributes of solving problems by Conservation of Total Mechanical Energy is that KE, PE, and E are all *scalars*. This makes it easier to solve questions because we don't have to worry about direction.

Using the Energy Method when There Is Friction

If friction acts during an object's motion, then total mechanical energy is no longer conserved. Consider this example: We give a block of mass 2 kg an initial speed of 6 m/s across a flat surface, where the coefficient of kinetic friction between the block and the surface is $\mu_k = 0.2$.

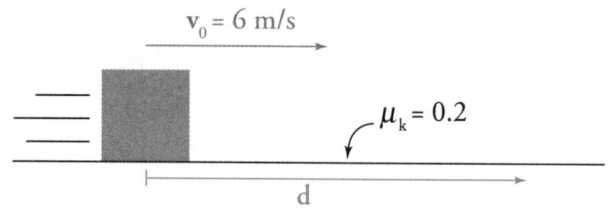

Kinetic friction will do work as the block slides. If d is the distance the block slides, then the work done by friction will be

$$W_{\text{by } F_f} = -F_f \cdot d = -\mu_k F_N d = -\mu_k mgd = -(0.4)(2 \text{ kg})(10\tfrac{\text{N}}{\text{kg}})d = -(4 \text{ N})d$$

In particular, when d = 9 m, the work done by friction will be

$$W_{\text{by } F_f} = -(4 \text{ N})d = -(4 \text{ N})(9 \text{ m}) = -36 \text{ J}$$

Since the initial kinetic energy of the block was

$$KE_i = \tfrac{1}{2}mv_0^2 = \tfrac{1}{2}(2 \text{ kg})(6 \text{ m/s})^2 = 36 \text{ J}$$

then the work-energy theorem tells us that the final kinetic energy of the block will be 0:

$$W = \Delta KE = KE_f - KE_i \rightarrow \quad KE_f = KE_i + W = \left(36 \text{ J}\right) + \left(-36 \text{ J}\right) = 0 \text{ J}$$

The block lost KE (and, therefore, E) as it moved because of friction. So, when friction acts, total mechanical energy is not a constant; in other words, it's not conserved.

Despite the fact that total mechanical energy is no longer conserved if friction acts, we can use a *modified* version of the Conservation of Total Mechanical Energy equation to handle questions with friction (or any force besides gravity). We can write this modified equation either in the form

$$E_i + W_{\text{by } \mathbf{F}} = E_f$$

or as:

**Conservation of Total Mechanical Energy
(with outside forces)**

$$KE_i + PE_i + W_{\text{by } \mathbf{F}} = KE_f + PE_f$$

Since $W_{\text{by } F_f}$ is negative, E_f will be less than E_i, just as we expect, since friction takes away mechanical energy.

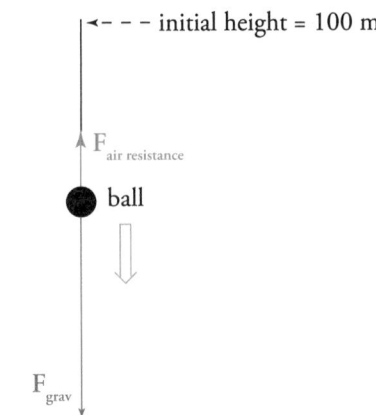

initial height = 100 m

$F_{air\ resistance}$

ball

F_{grav}

Example 6-24: A ball of mass 2 kg is dropped from a height of 100 m. As it falls, the ball feels an average force of air resistance of magnitude 4 N. What is the ball's speed as it strikes the ground?

Solution: Let's call the ground our $h = 0$ level. At the object's initial position, we have $h_i = 100$ m and $v_0 = 0$ (so $KE_i = 0$). As it hits the ground (the final position), we have $h_f = 0$ m (so $PE_f = 0$). The question is to find the speed of the ball, v, as it strikes the ground. Because the air resistance is given, and air resistance is friction exerted by the air on the moving object, we need to use the modified version of the energy equation, the one that includes the work done by friction.

Let's figure out the work done by the force of air resistance. Since the displacement of the ball is downward, the force of air resistance is upward; the opposite direction. This tells us that the work done by air resistance is negative, as we expect:

$$W_{by\ F_f} = -F_f \cdot h = -(4\ \text{N})(100\ \text{m}) = -400\ \text{J}$$

Therefore, using the modified equation for Conservation of Total Mechanical Energy, we find that

$$KE_i + PE_i + W_{by\ F_f} = KE_f + PE_f$$

$$0 + mgh + (-400\ \text{J}) = \tfrac{1}{2}mv^2 + 0$$

$$v = \sqrt{2gh - \frac{800\ \text{J}}{m}}$$

$$= \sqrt{2(10\ \text{m/s}^2)(100\ \text{m}) - \frac{800\ \text{J}}{2\ \text{kg}}}$$

$$= \sqrt{1600\ \text{m}^2/\text{s}^2}$$

Without air resistance, you can check that the ball's speed at impact would have been greater:

$$\sqrt{2000}\ \text{m/s} \approx 45\ \text{m/s}$$

6.5

6.6 SIMPLE MACHINES AND MECHANICAL ADVANTAGE

Simple machines are tools that allow us to accomplish a variety of tasks with less applied force. Some examples of common simple machines are inclined planes, pulleys, levers, screws, and wheel and axle systems. These machines generally have few or no moving parts. If the simple machine is used in the "ideal world" where there are only conservative forces (i.e., no loss of energy to friction, heat, etc.), the work done to complete the task using the machine is equal to the work that would be required to complete the task without the machine. The difference is that with less applied or effort force, a larger distance must be covered to satisfy the work requirements.[2]

Let's consider the task of lifting a 3 kg brick up to a shelf that is 2 m above the ground.

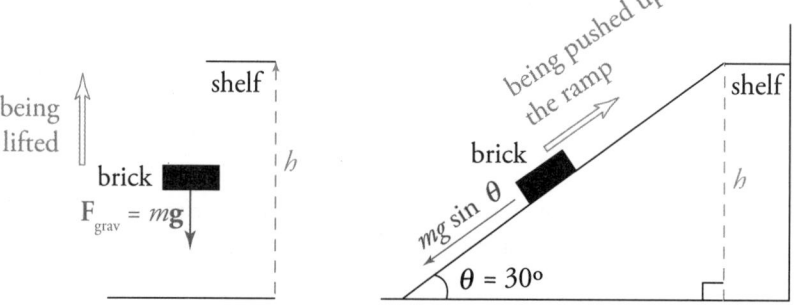

To move a mass straight upward, the applied force, $F_{\text{app}_{\text{lift}}}$, would need to be at least equal to the force of gravity acting on the mass. Thus, $F_{\text{app}_{\text{lift}}} \geq F_{\text{grav}} = mg = (3 \text{ kg})\left(10 \ \frac{\text{N}}{\text{kg}}\right) = 30 \text{ N}$. The minimum amount of work to lift the brick upward is

$$W_{\text{lift}} = F_{\text{app}_{\text{lift}}} \cdot d = mgh = 60 \text{ J}$$

Now, let's consider the inclined plane shown above. The plane allows us to push the brick up the ramp. If this is a frictionless ramp, the applied force on the ramp, $F_{\text{app}_{\text{ramp}}}$ would need to overcome the component of F_{grav} parallel to the plane. Thus,

$$F_{\text{app}_{\text{ramp}}} \geq mg \sin\theta = (3 \text{ kg})(10 \ \tfrac{\text{N}}{\text{kg}})(\sin 30°) = 15 \text{ N}$$

which will be less than $F_{\text{app}_{\text{lift}}} = mg$ (because the maximum value for sin θ is 1). However, compared to lifting the box straight up through a distance h, the ramp requires you to push the brick over a longer distance, $d = \dfrac{h}{\sin\theta}$. Therefore, the work done to push the brick up the ramp is

$$W_{\text{ramp}} = F_{\text{app}_{\text{ramp}}} \cdot d = (mg \sin\theta) \cdot \left(\frac{h}{\sin\theta}\right) = mgh = 60 \text{ J}$$

---

[2] Simple machines are also used to *increase* distance (and therefore speed) while *decreasing* force; this does not change the way we analyze the situation.

The work required to move a brick to a height of h is the same, regardless of whether you lift it straight upward or push it up a ramp.

The fact that the inclined plane allows your effort force or applied force to be decreased in comparison to the straight lift is called **mechanical advantage**. Mechanical advantage can be quantified into a factor that describes precisely how much less force is required when using that particular simple machine. In other words, mechanical advantage tells us the factor by which the mechanism multiplies the input or effort force.

> **Mechanical Advantage**
>
> $$\text{mechanical advantage } (MA) = \frac{\text{resistance force}}{\text{effort force}} = \frac{F_{\text{resistance}}}{F_{\text{effort}}}$$

Resistance force is the force that would be applied if no machine were being used, and *effort force* is the force applied with the machine. Mechanical advantage is also sometimes expressed as $F_{\text{out}} / F_{\text{in}}$.

For the previous example of the inclined plane, the mechanical advantage of the ramp would be

$$MA = \frac{F_{\text{resistance}}}{F_{\text{effort}}} = \frac{mg}{mg \sin \theta} = \frac{1}{\sin 30°} = \frac{1}{\frac{1}{2}} = 2$$

Therefore, this specific inclined plane with an angle of $\theta = 30°$ has a mechanical advantage of 2, allowing it to "multiply" the input force $F_{\text{app}_{\text{ramp}}} = 15 \text{ N}$ by a factor of 2 to give the force that would have been required without the machine, $F_{\text{app}_{\text{lift}}} = 30 \text{ N}$.

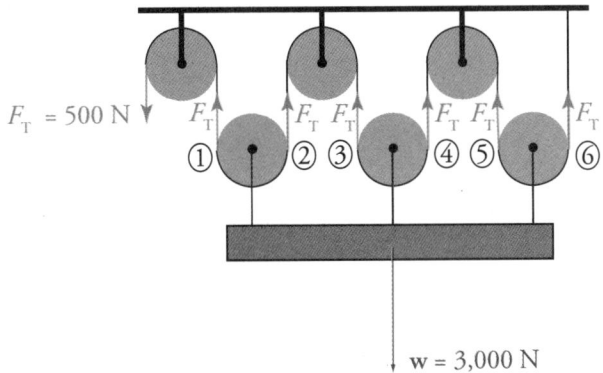

As another example, look back at Example 4-23 which shows a system consisting of 6 pulleys used to lift a plank. The plank weighs 3000 N, but we only have to exert a force of 500 N to lift it. The mechanical advantage is therefore equal to 3000 N/500 N = 6.

Efficiency

So far, we have described simple machines that are used in the ideal world. However, if the machine is used in the real world, we have to take into consideration the possibility of energy losses to the surroundings. In general, the actual mechanical advantage of a machine is less than its ideal mechanical advantage. The fact that the machine does not work as well in the real world leads us to the concept of **efficiency**. The efficiency of any machine measures the degree to which friction and other factors reduce the actual work output of the machine from its theoretical maximum. This can be calculated by examining the ratio of the useful energy output versus the supplied or input energy.

Efficiency

$$\text{Efficiency (\%)} = \frac{W_{output}}{Energy_{input}}$$

A machine that operates in the ideal world has an efficiency of 100% because it has no loss of energy to its surroundings. However, a machine with an efficiency of 50% has an output only one-half of its theoretical output. By calculating a machine's efficiency, we can determine what percentage of energy is being lost to heat, sound, light, etc.

How does an efficiency of less than 100% affect mechanical advantage? For the inclined plane example, the presence of friction would reduce the efficiency, since some of the work done to push the block up would be lost as heat. In terms of force, the minimum applied force (the effort force) would now have to be enough to balance the component of gravity down the inclined plane plus the force of kinetic friction.

$$F_{effort} = mg\sin\theta + F_f = mg\sin\theta + \mu_k mg\cos\theta$$

Since $MA = F_{resistance} / F_{effort}$, and the resistance force remains the same, the mechanical advantage will decrease. This makes sense conceptually, since the purpose of using the inclined plane is to reduce force. There will be less of an advantage to using a plane with friction.

Summary of Formulas

Work: $W = Fd\cos\theta$ [$\theta =$ angle between **F** and **d**]

Power: $P = \dfrac{W}{t}$

    $P = Fv$ if **F** is parallel to **v** and constant

Kinetic Energy: $KE = \dfrac{1}{2}mv^2$

Work-energy theorem: $W_{total} = \Delta KE$

Gravitational Potential Energy: $\Delta PE_{grav} = -W_{by\, F_{grav}} = +mg\Delta h$ [if g is constant]

    Gravity is a conservative force [path independent]

    Friction is NOT a conservative force [path dependent]

Total Mechanical Energy: $E = KE + PE$

Conservation of Total Mechanical Energy: $KE_i + PE_i = KE_f + PE_f$

    If non-conservative forces [i.e., friction] act: $KE_i + PE_i + W_{other} = KE_f + PE_f$

Simple Machines:

    Mechanical Advantage $= \dfrac{F_{resistance}}{F_{effort}}$

    Efficiency [%] $= \dfrac{W_{output}}{Energy_{input}}$

CHAPTER 6 FREESTANDING PRACTICE QUESTIONS

1. How much work is needed to lift a box of mass 2 kg up a height of 3 m using a pulley system with 75% efficiency?

   A) 4 J
   B) 8 J
   C) 45 J
   D) 80 J

2. An automobile with a certain shape experiences a drag force due to air resistance that is, in Newtons, equal to one-third the square of the car's speed, in meters per second. How much power would the engine have to supply to the wheels to balance this drag force when the car is moving at a constant speed of 30 m/s?

   A) 10 W
   B) 300 W
   C) 9 kW
   D) 27 kW

3. A young child is sliding down a hill at an incline of 30° on a sled with total combined mass of 10 kg. If the coefficient of friction between the hill and the sled is 0.3 and the length of the hill is 50 m, how much work has been done by gravity when the child reaches the bottom of the hill?

   A) 1000 J
   B) 2500 J
   C) 3535 J
   D) 4330 J

4. A physically fit person has a mechanical efficiency of 25%, meaning that 25% of the chemical potential energy converted in the body during a given physical task is output as useful work (the remaining energy is predominantly wasted as heat). Suppose that she has a mass of 50 kg and climbs stairs at a constant speed, moving upward at a rate of 25 cm/s. At what rate is she consuming energy?

   A) 500 W
   B) 125 W
   C) 6.25 W
   D) 1.56 W

5. A 200 kg roller coaster starts from rest 50 m above the ground. It falls toward the ground without any friction, then once it reaches ground level, the brakes are applied over 30 m in order to bring the coaster to a complete stop. How much work is done by the brakes?

   A) 10×10^4 J
   B) 10×10^5 J
   C) -10×10^4 J
   D) -10×10^5 J

6. A 7 kg ball is dropped from 20 m. If the speed just before it hits the ground is 18 m/s, what is the work done by air resistance?

   A) 266 J
   B) 13 J
   C) −13 J
   D) −266 J

CHAPTER 6 PRACTICE PASSAGE

Alice is playing with her little brother Jeff at an ice-skating rink that is entirely flat except for a ramp at one end that is at an upward incline of 30 degrees. Alice is pushing Jeff on a little toboggan that has blades on the bottom, so it glides along the surface of the ice without the effects of friction. Alice has a mass of 60 kg, Jeff has a mass of 28 kg and the mass of the toboggan is 2 kg.

Alice is pushing Jeff around the rink and decides that she wants to push him right up until the incline, then let go and see how far up the incline he goes. They start from rest 10 meters from the incline and she pushes him with a force that varies with the distance (Figure 1). Jeff goes speeding up the incline with a velocity of 2 m/s, travels a certain distance and then comes speeding down. At the bottom of the incline, Jeff's toboggan collides with Alice and the two of them travel across the ice.

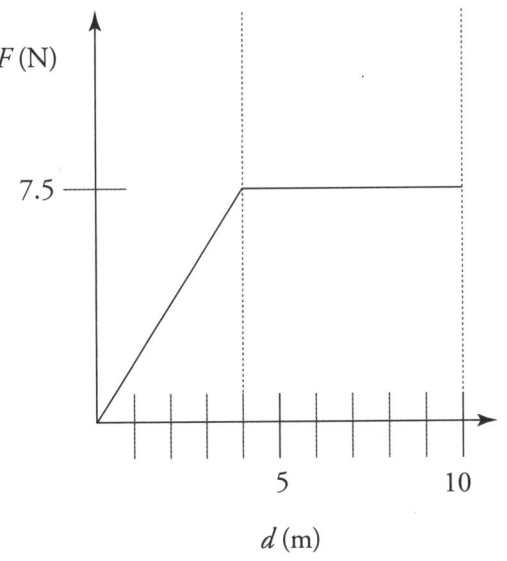

Figure 1 Graph of force vs. distance

Alice and Jeff keep sliding on the ice until the toboggan crashes into the end of the rink. One of the blades on the bottom of the toboggan has come loose in the crash and it no longer glides effortlessly on the ice. Alice once again pushes Jeff with a force given by Figure 1 and lets go just as they reach the incline. This time Jeff travels 10 centimeters less up the incline than he did before the toboggan broke.

1. How much work does Alice do from the moment she begins to push Jeff 10 m from the incline until she lets go just before the incline?

A) 60 J
B) 75 J
C) 0 J
D) There is not enough information to answer the question.

2. The first time Jeff goes up the incline, what distance along the incline does the toboggan travel before it comes to rest?

A) 0.2 m
B) 0.3 m
C) 0.4 m
D) 0.5 m

3. Once the toboggan has broken, if Jeff goes up the incline with the same initial velocity v as he did the first time, how much energy has been lost?

A) 1.0 J
B) 1.5 J
C) 10 J
D) 15 J

4. If Alice did 10 J of work while pushing Jeff in 5 seconds, and the force of friction due to the broken toboggan did −2 J of work, how much power did Alice exert?

A) 50 W
B) 2 W
C) 1.6 W
D) 1.5 W

5. If Jeff brought his friend Jeremy out to play with him and Alice pushes both of them from rest on the toboggan with the same force as given in Figure 1, how would the distance they travel up the incline and their initial velocity change from when just Jeff was being pushed (ignoring friction)?

A) The velocity would be greater and they would go farther.
B) The velocity would be greater and they would go less far.
C) The velocity would be less and they would go farther.
D) The velocity would be less and they would go less far.

SOLUTIONS TO CHAPTER 6 FREESTANDING QUESTIONS

1. **D**   Without the pulley system, lifting this box would require doing the work to increase the potential energy by *mgh*, which is (2)(10)(3) = 60 J. With a pulley system that has less than 100% efficiency, it will require more work, so the answer has to be greater than 60 J. Choice D is the only answer large enough. As a quick check, a 75% efficiency means that 75% of the work done would need to be put in to complete the task regardless, and 25% of the work goes to overcoming friction and other inefficiencies in the system. In this case, 75% of 80 J is 60 J, and this matches that the task would require 60 J without the pulleys. Be careful not to multiply the work required by 75% and choose C! That would be the right answer if the question told us that the pulley system required 60 J of work and asked how much work would be needed without the pulley system.

2. **C**   The word-equation given in the first sentence of the question stem can be expressed as

    $F_{drag} = \dfrac{1}{3} v^2$. (Neglect the dimensional incorrectness of the equation; the stem indicates that

    speed units of m/s will give force units of N here.) The question asks for power, and the rela-

    tionship between force and power is $P = Fv$, so $P = (\dfrac{1}{3} v^2)(v) = \dfrac{1}{3} v^3$. Plug in the number given:

    $P = \dfrac{1}{3} (30)^3 = 9000$. Thus, the answer is 9 kW.

3. **B**   There are a couple of ways to approach this problem:

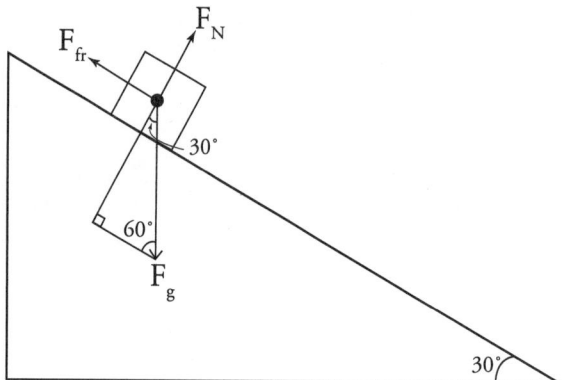

    Number 1:

    The formula for work is $W = Fd \cos \theta$, where W is the work, F is the force, d is the displacement and θ is the angle between the force and displacement vectors. To determine the work done by gravity, we use gravitational force and the length of the hill to get: $W = (mg)(d) \cos 60°$, where $60°$ is from the direction of gravitational force vertically down and d is along the ramp. Thus, $W = (10)(10)(50)(0.5) = 2500$ J.

Number 2:

We can resolve the F and d to be in the same direction, that is, take the component of the force acting in the same direction as the child's movement down the hill, eliminating the $\cos \theta$ (since $\cos 0° = 1$) from the equation. Then, we have, $F = mg \sin \theta$, where $\theta = 30°$. Thus, $W = Fd = (mg \sin \theta)d = (10)(10)(0.5)(50) = 2500$ J.

4. **A** The output work in running up stairs at a constant speed ($\Delta KE = 0$) is due to the increase in gravitational potential energy: $W_{\text{against gravity}} = \Delta PE_{\text{gravity}} = mg\Delta h = (50 \text{ kg})$ $(10 \text{ m/s}^2)(0.25 \text{ m}) = 125$ J every second. Thus power output $P_{\text{output}} = W_{\text{out}} / t = 125$ J/s $= 125$ W. With an efficiency of 25%, the rate at which energy is being consumed (energy input as converted chemical potential, e.g., ATP in muscle tissues) is given by

$$\eta = \frac{W_{\text{output}}}{E_{\text{input}}} \rightarrow E_{\text{input}} = \frac{W_{\text{output}}}{\eta} = \frac{125 \text{ W}}{0.25} = 500 \text{ W} \,.$$

5. **C** This question requires you to use the work-kinetic energy theorem, which states that $W = \Delta KE$. The kinetic energy at the bottom is equal to the potential energy at the top, by conservation of energy, which is $mgh = (200)(10)(50) = 10^5$ J. The change in kinetic energy is the final kinetic energy minus the initial. Therefore, the work done by friction to bring the roller coaster to a stop is equal to $\Delta KE = -10^5$ J $= -10 \times 10^4$ J.

6. **D** The initial energy is $mgh = (7)(10)(20) = 1400$ J. The final energy is completely kinetic, $1/2(mv^2) = 1134$ J. The equation for conservation of energy with friction is $E_i + W_{\text{by friction}} = E_f$. Thus, the work done by friction is negative and equal to $1134 - 1400 = -266$ J.

SOLUTIONS TO CHAPTER 6 PRACTICE PASSAGE

1. **A** There are two methods of solving this problem. First, the work done by Alice is equal to the area under the graph given in Figure 1. This can be calculated in two steps. From $d = 0$ m to $d = 4$ m the work done is the area of the triangle: $\dfrac{(7.5 \text{ N})(4 \text{ m})}{2} = 15$ J. From $d = 4$ m to $d = 10$ m the work done is the area of the rectangle: $(7.5 \text{ N})(6 \text{ m}) = 45$ J. Therefore the total work is 60 J. The second method involves understanding that the work done by Alice is equal to the kinetic energy gained by the sled. This is equal to $(1/2)mv^2 = (1/2)(30 \text{ kg})(2 \text{ m/s})^2 = 60$ J.

2. **C** Jeff's initial kinetic energy can be computed by using the mass and velocity given and it is equal to $\dfrac{1}{2}(30 \text{ kg})(2 \text{ m/s})^2 = 60$ J. All of this energy is converted to potential energy at the top of the incline, therefore $60 \text{ J} = mgh$. This tells us that the height above the ground is 0.2 m. However, the question asks for the ground the toboggan covers, which is along the incline. So the correct answer is $\dfrac{(0.2 \text{ m})}{\sin(30°)} = 0.4$ m.

3. **D** The initial kinetic energy remains the same in both cases, therefore the potential energy at the top of the hill is the initial kinetic energy minus the energy lost. The change in potential energy, $mg\Delta h$, is equal to the energy lost. The difference in height is sin 30° multiplied by the change in distance traveled, which is $(\sin 30°)(0.1 \text{ m}) = 0.05$ m. The energy lost is then $(30 \text{ kg})(10 \text{ m/s}^2)(0.05) = 15$ J.

4. **B** The amount of work done by friction does not matter in this question. The power exerted by Alice is the work she does divided by the time it takes her. $\dfrac{(10 \text{ J})}{5 \text{ s}} = 2 \text{ J/s} = 2$ W.

5. **D** This is a two-by-two question, meaning that two pieces of information are required in order to reach the correct answer. The work done is the same in both cases, so by the work-energy theorem, the kinetic energy is the same in both cases, and since the mass is larger in the second case, the velocity must be smaller. This eliminates choices A and B. All the kinetic energy is being converted to potential energy at the top of the hill, so the potential energy at the top of the hill is also the same in both cases. Again, since the mass is greater in the second case, the resulting height is less and that eliminates choice C.

Chapter 7
Thermodynamics

7.1 SYSTEMS, THERMAL PHYSICS, AND THERMODYNAMICS

As we've seen so far, work can be done on or by a physical system—a box on a ramp, a car's engine block hooked to several loops of rope attached to two pulleys, or a satellite launched into orbit are just a few examples—thereby increasing or decreasing the energy in that system. Broadly speaking, work is a *transfer of mechanical energy into or out of a system, from or to the environment.*

We ought to be careful here with our terms. In physics, as in chemistry and biology, you will hear a lot about *systems*. For our purposes, it is enough to define a system as the object or objects under examination, e.g., the things you want to answer questions about to do well on the MCAT. The *environment* is just the other objects and external forces outside the system. The environment may or may not be able to interact with the system. If the system is *closed*, then the environment cannot contribute matter to it; if the system is *isolated*, then the environment cannot contribute either matter or energy to it. If the system is *open*, then it is free to interact with the environment. This leads to a crucial point: systems obey conservation laws. Within the system, different forms of energy can *transform from one type to another but cannot spontaneously appear or cease to exist.* In other words, the only way the total energy in a system can change is if energy is *transferred* into or out of the system.

Consider a tennis ball in your hand. If you want to focus exclusively on the ball itself, you might call the ball "the system" and everything else "the environment." This is an open system; if you drop the ball, an external force in the environment (gravity) will do work on the ball, contributing to its increase in kinetic energy as it falls. Alternatively, you might want to look at the ball + the earth + gravity (the interaction between those two objects) as the system. In that case, when you drop the ball, one form of energy (gravitational potential energy) is transformed into another (kinetic energy).

But what about some other factors? For one thing, you could choose to throw the ball up in the air instead of just letting it idly drop to the ground. If we counted you as part of the environment, then we would say that the work you did on the ball in throwing it upward increased its kinetic energy: you transferred energy into the system. If we counted you as part of the system, we would have to explain the energy transformation in terms of the ATP turning to ADP and then AMP as your muscles contracted to allow you to throw the ball, and thus chemical potential energy was transformed into kinetic energy (for more on that, consult the *MCAT Biology Review*!). What about the air resistance the ball experiences as it falls through the air? As a frictional force, air resistance does what we have previously called "nonconservative" work on the ball, as it causes the ball to move more slowly (i.e., to have less kinetic energy) than it would if there were no air. Is this a violation of what we have said so far about energy conservation or transferring to and from the environment?

It is not. The problem is that so far we have considered only a limited number of kinds of energy, and we have neglected an important mode of energy transfer. Consider the tennis ball a bit more closely. Even as it sits apparently still in your hand, on the molecular level there is a tremendous amount of random motion. This is another form of energy internal to the system, which we'll call *thermal energy* (or sometimes just *internal energy*, though as you know from chemistry, there are other forms of internal energy such as chemical or nuclear energies). **Temperature (*T*)** is the macroscopic measure of this thermal energy per molecule. As the tennis ball falls, the frictional effects of air resistance do negative work on the ball, slowing it down, but they also cause the temperature of the ball to increase, because all of those tiny collisions between the air molecules and the molecules in the ball increase the thermal energy of the ball's molecules (as well as that of the air molecules that interact with the ball directly). That is to say, the individual molecules of the surface of the ball are moving faster than before, but in random directions (in addition to all moving toward the ground while the ball is falling). If you were to catch and hold the now slightly warmer ball in your hand, over time it would cool back to the temperature of the surrounding air. Its thermal energy would decrease, but it would be sitting perfectly still, so clearly it wasn't doing any work. It transferred energy to the environment by means of heat. **Heat** (Q) is the transfer of thermal energy between a system and its environment: $Q > 0$ when heat transfers *into* the system, $Q < 0$ when heat transfers *out* of the system. Please note this important distinction between *temperature* and *heat*, words that we use everyday in ways that can make them seem interchangeable. When we say *"it's hot* outside today," we're referring to the temperature, an indicator of the relatively high thermal energy per molecule of the local atmospheric system. When we then say "this weather *is making me hot* and sweaty," we're talking about heat, the transfer of the thermal energy from the atmosphere into our bodies. Note the difference in units as well: heat, as with energy, is measured in joules, whereas absolute temperature is measured in kelvins. Another important difference between temperature and thermal energy contained within a system (and transferable as heat) is that temperature is an *intensive* property whereas thermal energy is an *extensive* one. That is to say, temperature (like density, for example) does not depend on the amount of a material present, but thermal energy (like mass) does. Imagine a block of stone at a temperature of 300 kelvins and containing 20,000 joules of thermal energy. If you split it in half, each half would still be 300 kelvins (not 150), but each would contain only 10,000 joules of thermal energy.

Thermodynamics concerns how macroscopic systems transfer and transform energy. As such, it is perhaps the broadest subject you'll study in preparation for physics on the MCAT, taking into account not only everything we've looked at so far in this text, but also extending into all the other science topics on the exam.

7.2 THE ZEROTH LAW OF THERMODYNAMICS

Thermal physics depends upon the quantity *temperature* being well defined in such a way that, if we stick thermometers on two different objects and get the same reading, we know there is something fundamentally similar about those two objects. This is unlike, say, length: a 2 m long metal rod does not have anything fundamentally in common with a 2 m long wooden plank. The **zeroth law of thermodynamics** provides this definition. It states that if one object is in thermal equilibrium with a second object, and that second object is in thermal equilibrium with a third object, then the first and third objects are in thermal equilibrium with each other. By *thermal equilibrium* we mean that, though the two bodies are in contact in such a way that heat is free to pass between them, no heat actually does so (or, more precisely, the same amount of heat passes each way). Practically, what this means is that Objects 1 and 3 are the same temperature. Technically, this *defines* temperature as a fundamental property, or *state variable,* of a system. It tells us that if we measured the temperatures of two objects (like our metal rod and wooden plank) to be the same, we would know that when we put the two in contact with each other, no net heat would be transferred between them.

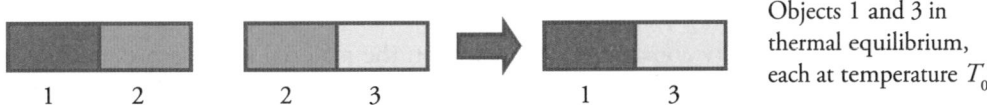

Objects 1 and 3 in thermal equilibrium, each at temperature T_0

The other *state variables* include pressure, volume, moles, and entropy. On the MCAT as in your college coursework, discussion of these variables crosses over between physics and chemistry (and possibly other disciplines), and the connections among those discussions can be confusing. One unifying idea you should keep in mind in all applications is that these variables define a *state function* for a system, which means they are macroscopic properties that reflect the microscopic conditions of that system and predict the future behavior of the system. The specific relation between the microscopic average kinetic energy per atom of a monatomic ideal gas (wherein kinetic energy is the only form of energy) is given by the following equation, sometimes called the equipartition of energy equation for ideal gases (k_B is the Boltzmann constant and is equal to 1.38×10^{-23} J/K).

$$\frac{1}{2}mv_{avg}^2 = \frac{3}{2}k_B T$$

Heat Transfer

In stating the zeroth law of thermodynamics, we relied upon the idea that bodies can achieve thermal equilibrium by heat transfer, the movement of thermal energy from one point to another. There are three mechanisms by which this is achieved.

Conduction

An iron skillet is sitting on a hot stove, and you accidentally touch the handle. You notice right away that there's been a transfer of thermal energy to your hand. The process by which this happens is known as **conduction**. The highly agitated atoms in the handle of the hot skillet bump into the atoms of your hand, making them vibrate more rapidly, thus heating up your hand.

Example 7-1: The rate at which materials conduct heat varies widely. Metals conduct heat well, meaning that heat moves through them rapidly. Materials like fiberglass, which is often used to provide thermal insulation in buildings, conduct heat very poorly. The *conduction rate* is described by the equation

$$P_{cond} = \frac{\Delta Q}{\Delta t} = -kA\frac{\Delta T}{\Delta x} = kA\frac{T_i - T_f}{L}$$

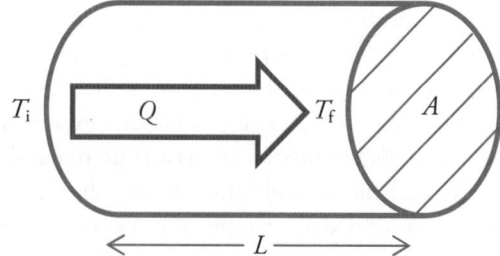

where k is a thermal conductivity constant dependent upon the material and the power P indicates the rate of thermal energy transfer. This energy is measured in joules as usual. (This is not an equation the

MCAT would expect you to have memorized.) Window glass typically has a thermal conductivity of $k = 1$ watt per meter per kelvin (recall that kelvins are a measure of absolute temperature with a scale equal to that of degrees Celsius). How many joules per second of heat are transferred out of a room at 25°C to an outside environment of at 0°C if there are two 2 × 1 meter single-paned windows in the room with a thickness of half a centimeter? Assume the walls are perfectly insulated.

Solution: Find the total area A by multiplying the dimensions of the windows and their total number: $A = 2 \times 2 \times 1 = 4 \text{ m}^2$. Applying the given equation then yields

$$\frac{\Delta Q}{\Delta t} = kA\frac{T_i - T_f}{L} = (1)(4)\frac{25-0}{0.5\times10^{-2}} = 200\times10^2 = 2\times10^4 \text{ J/s}$$

This is quite a bit of power, which is why it is a good idea to use double-paned or otherwise insulated windows in climates where it gets cold outside!

Convection

As the air around a candle flame warms, it expands, becomes less dense than the surrounding cooler air, and thus rises due to buoyancy. (We'll study buoyancy in the next chapter.) As a result, heat is transferred away from the flame by the large-scale (from the atoms' point of view anyway) motion of a fluid (in this case, air). This is (natural) **convection**.

Example 7-2: During circulation, the relatively warm blood moves from the heart to the extremities, where it cools slightly before returning to the heart. What best describes this process?

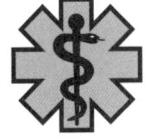

A. This is a natural convection process, as warm blood rises to the head while relatively cold blood sinks to the feet.
B. This is a natural convection process, as the expansion of the warm blood in the heart pushes blood out to the extremities via the arteries, whereas cooler blood at the extremities condenses and sinks toward the heart via the veins.
C. This is a forced convection process where the pumping action of the heart forces blood heated by the body's metabolic processes out to the extremities, which in turn forces the cooler blood back toward the heart (during which time it is heated).
D. This is a forced convection process where the pumping action of the heart compresses and thereby heats the blood. Its motion to the extremities is a result of this pressurization.

Solution: The heart is a pump: you should know that blood's motion through the body is caused by the heart, not by some passive physical process. Choices A and B are eliminated for not making sense: don't ignore your biology knowledge when answering physics questions if it's pertinent! Along that line of thought, the heart is not a pressure cooker: the heat of our bodies is produced by metabolic processes, the conversion of chemical energy to other forms (such as kinetic energy in the contraction of muscles throughout the body, which is why you feel hotter when exercising vigorously). Choice D doesn't adequately explain this and is therefore eliminated. Choice C is correct: the movement of the warm fluid and displacement of the cooler fluid is convection, but it is *forced convection* due to the pumping action. The process by which a convection oven works is analogous: the forced movement of the fluid (air) in the oven due to a fan results in faster heat transfer than in a normal oven that relies on natural convection and conduction.

7.3

Radiation

Sunlight on your face warms your skin. Radiant energy from the sun's fusion reactions is transferred across millions of kilometers of essentially empty space via electromagnetic waves. Absorption of the energy carried by these light waves defines heat transfer by **radiation**.

Thermal Expansion

Another response of materials to temperature difference is to change their physical dimensions, i.e., length and volume. Most materials expand as their temperature increases: this is why, for example, bridges have expansion slots, the metal grates you drive over every 10 meters or so. If the bridge got longer in response to an increase in temperature but had no room to expand, it would buckle and crack. The formula for linear thermal expansion is $\Delta L = \alpha L_0 \Delta T$, where ΔL is the change in length of the object, L_0 is its original length, and α is the coefficient of linear expansion of the material the object is made of. This is not typically an equation the MCAT expects you to have memorized.

7.3 THE FIRST LAW OF THERMODYNAMICS

Having defined two ways in which energy can transfer between the environment and a system (heat and work), as well as a way to measure the energy internal to the system (temperature), we are now ready to make a broader statement about conservation of energy than the ones we made in the preceding chapter. The first law of thermodynamics is just this statement: it says that *the total energy of the universe is constant.* Energy may be transformed from one form to another, but it cannot be created or destroyed.

The first law of thermodynamics can be expressed both tangibly and mathematically. To do this, consider the physical aspects of transferring energy to an object. Since energy cannot be created or destroyed, it must be transferred into some other form such as heat (Q) or work (W). Thus, we have the following mathematical statement of the first law:

First Law of Thermodynamics

$$\Delta E = Q - W$$

Pay close attention to the sign conventions we're using. Q is considered positive when heat is moving into the system, negative when it is coming out of the system. W is considered positive when the work is *being done by the system on the environment.* W is considered negative when the work is *being done by the environment on the system.* Unfortunately, this convention for work is opposite what is typically used in chemistry books, so you may remember the formula as $\Delta E = Q + W$, or with U in place of E, or with lower case letters. As long as you remember how the variables are being defined, when they are positive and negative, you shouldn't have any problems.

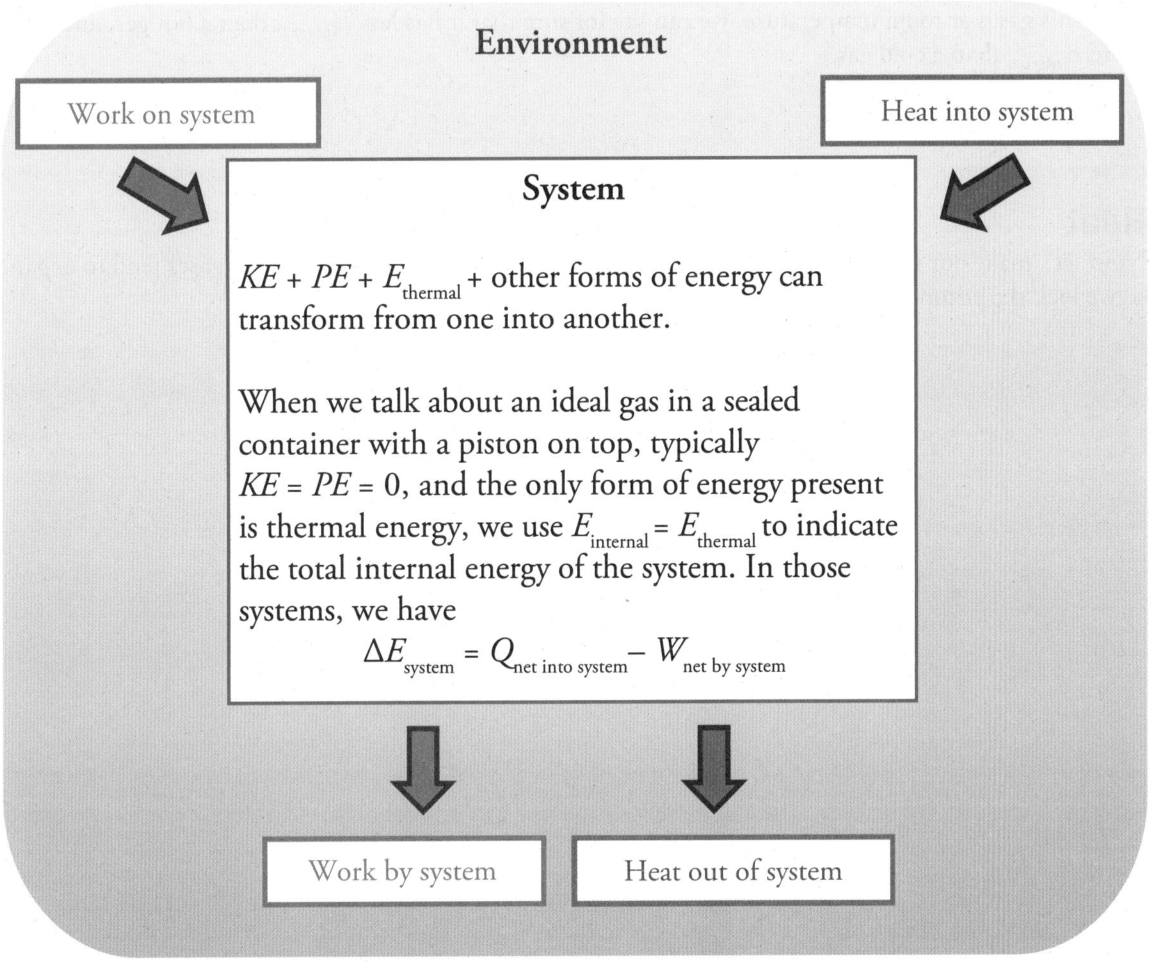

Environment

| Work on system | | Heat into system |

System

$KE + PE + E_{thermal}$ + other forms of energy can transform from one into another.

When we talk about an ideal gas in a sealed container with a piston on top, typically $KE = PE = 0$, and the only form of energy present is thermal energy, we use $E_{internal} = E_{thermal}$ to indicate the total internal energy of the system. In those systems, we have

$$\Delta E_{system} = Q_{net\ into\ system} - W_{net\ by\ system}$$

| Work by system | Heat out of system |

To analyze the First Law equation, let's take a sample of ideal gas at room temperature and put it into a container to make a closed (but not isolated) system. Let's use a metal cylinder that's welded shut at one end and sealed on the other end with a piston.

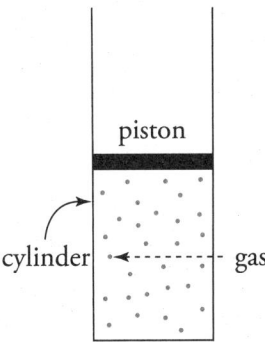

Starting with the energy component of the equation, we can consider the internal energy of the system. Again recall that for an ideal gas, the only form of internal energy is the kinetic energy of the atoms or molecules. The internal energy, $E_{internal}$, is proportional to the object's absolute temperature, T:

$$E_{internal} \propto T$$

Since this gas is at room temperature, we can say for sure that it has less $E_{internal}$ than a hot gas, and it has more $E_{internal}$ than a cold gas.

Heat

Now, let's make our gas hot. But before we do that, we learned somewhere that hot gases tend to expand, so we lock the piston in a fixed position to prevent it from moving:

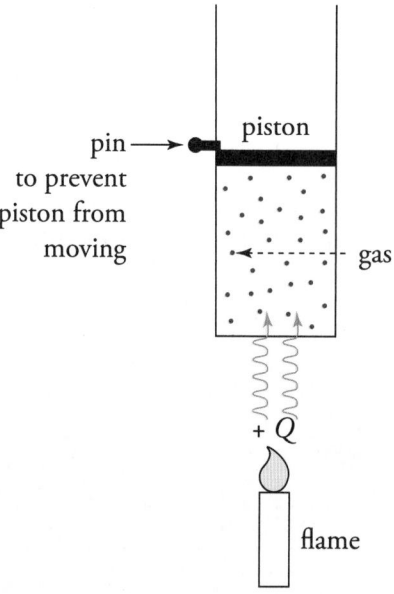

We gently apply the flame, and heat the cylinder and the gas inside. Since the piston does not move, no work is done, but energy is transferred as heat. We can sum up what's happening as

$$\Delta E_{internal} = Q, \; Q > 0$$

where we know that $E_{internal}$ has to increase because we feel that the gas and cylinder are getting hotter, and the additional energy is added to our system in the form of heat, Q.

If we let the hot gas and hot cylinder just sit on a table, what's going to happen over time? The hot cylinder and gas will cool down as they lose heat to the room, until they're at room temperature again. So, for this cooling down process, we'll have

$$\Delta E_{internal} = Q, \; Q < 0$$

where we know that $E_{internal}$ has to decrease because we feel that the gas and cylinder are cooling down, and energy is lost from our system in the form of heat, Q.

Work

Let's make the gas hot again. This time, let's remove the lock on the piston and allow it to move.

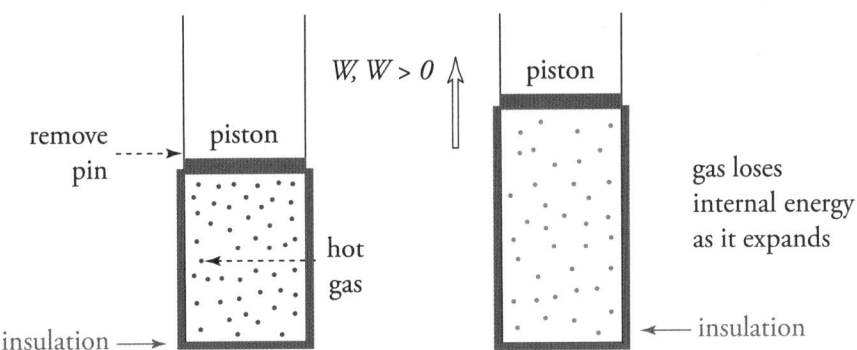

The hot gas pushes the piston up. Our gas is doing work, W, because it's applying a *force* and moving the piston a certain *distance*. As the piston moves, the volume of the gas increases since gases expand to fill their containers. Therefore, the ΔV in this example is positive. To quantify the work in a system, we not only need to know how much the volume of the system changes, but we also need to know how much pressure the gas exerts upward on the piston. Therefore, work can be defined as

$$W = P\Delta V$$

Due to an increase in volume, the work described in the case above has a positive value. A positive W is defined as work done *by* the system. When the weight on our piston moves up, it gains potential energy (the h in mgh is getting larger). Conservation of energy states that energy cannot be created or destroyed, but is simply moved around. Therefore, the energy gained by the weight must come from something else (the hot gas!). As long as the piston is well insulated, such that no heat (Q) can go in or out, we have

$$\Delta E_{internal} = -W, \ W > 0$$

where $E_{internal}$ of our gas has to decrease because energy is lost from our system in the form of doing work, W. Because the gas is losing energy as it expands and raises the piston, and we learned earlier that $\Delta E_{internal}$ is proportional to temperature, the *gas cools as it expands.*

Now, if after our gas has expanded and cooled as far as it's going to, we add more weight on the piston so that the piston and weights move down and compress the gas,

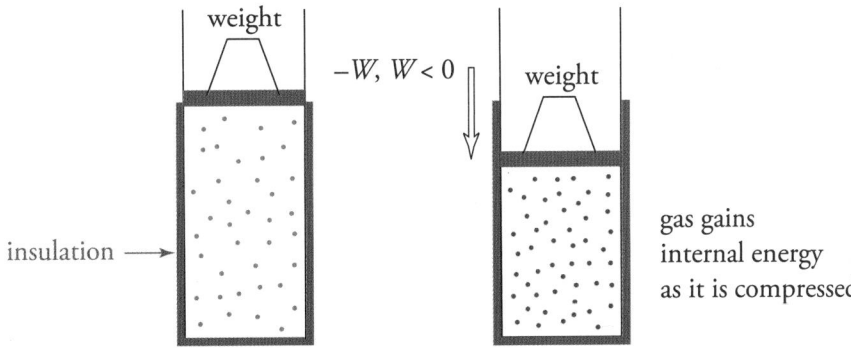

we have the situation for which

$$\Delta E_{internal} = W,\ W < 0$$

Now, because ΔV is a negative value (because our gas has been compressed), this will lead to negative work being done *by the gas* (which is the same as *positive* work being done *on the gas*). In this situation, $E_{internal}$ has to increase because energy is gained by our system. Here, we'd see that our *gas warms as it is compressed*.

Thus, for processes in which no heat is exchanged between the gas and the environment, in general expanding gases cool and compressed gases warm. This is the principle behind how a steam engine, refrigerator, and air conditioner work.

Case 1: An Isobaric Process

An **isobaric** process is one that occurs at constant pressure. Consider heating our cylinder such that the volume of gas expands, pushing the piston upward, but the pressure remains constant because the weight on the piston is held constant, and that force divided by the area of the piston remains constant. If we plot pressure vs. volume for this process, the graph would look like this:

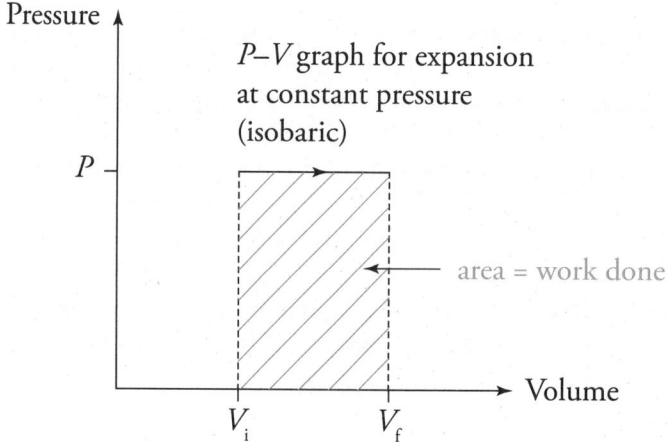

and the area under the curve would be equal to the work done by the gas on the piston. This means we can easily calculate W, without the use of calculus, since $W = P\Delta V$. Note that this is positive because ΔV is positive; when the arrow goes backward in the graph indicating $\Delta V < 0$, the area should be considered negative.

Case 2: An Isochoric Process

An **isochoric** process maintains a constant volume. Heating the gas with a locked piston would result in increasing pressure but no change in volume:

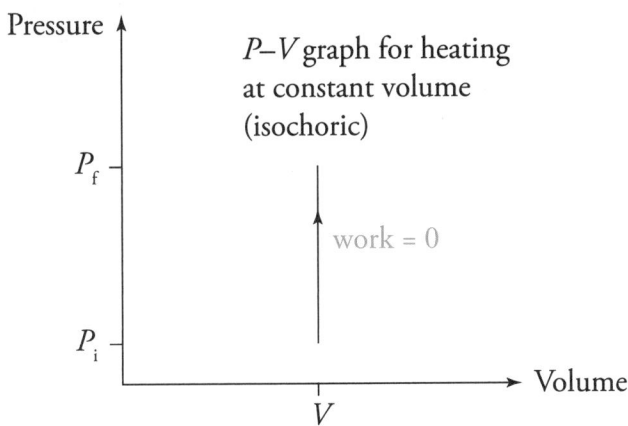

Therefore, no work is done. You can see this either by noticing that the area under the P-V graph is zero (since the graph is just a vertical line), or by realizing that if the volume didn't change, then the piston didn't move, and if there's no displacement of the piston, then there was no work done on the piston. Because $W = 0$, we know that $\Delta E = Q$.

Case 3: An Isothermal Process

When heat is allowed to pass freely between a system and its environment, an **isothermal** process can occur, where the temperature of the system remains constant. For example, for our gas to expand at constant temperature, the pressure must decrease (as governed by Boyle's law).

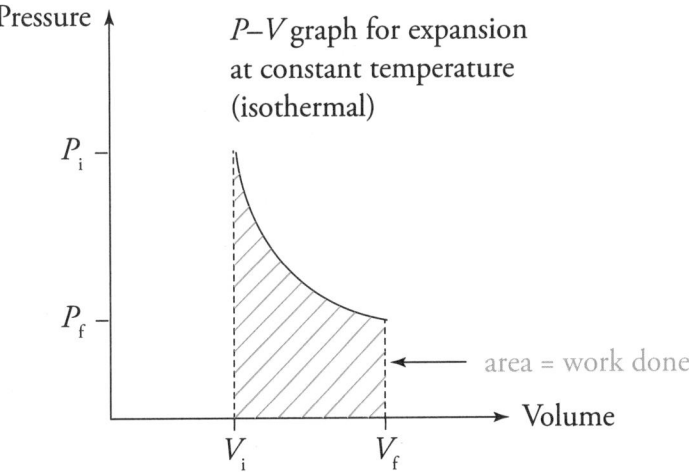

Again, the work done by the gas on the piston will be equal to the area under the curve. Since we know that E is directly proportional to T, we can say that in an isothermal process, $\Delta E = 0$ and $Q = W$.

Case 4: An Adiabatic Process

An **adiabatic** process occurs when no heat is transferred between the system and the environment, and all energy is transferred as work: the previous example with the insulated container is one instance. Another imperfect but real-world example is a rapidly expanding gas, which drops its pressure precipitously and simultaneously cools. This is the principle behind the release of compressed water vapor in a snow-making machine. The process happens so quickly that theoretically no heat is transferred; since $Q = 0$, we get $\Delta E_{internal} = -W$ (here the positive work done by the expanding gas is simply the pushing of the surrounding atmosphere out of the way).

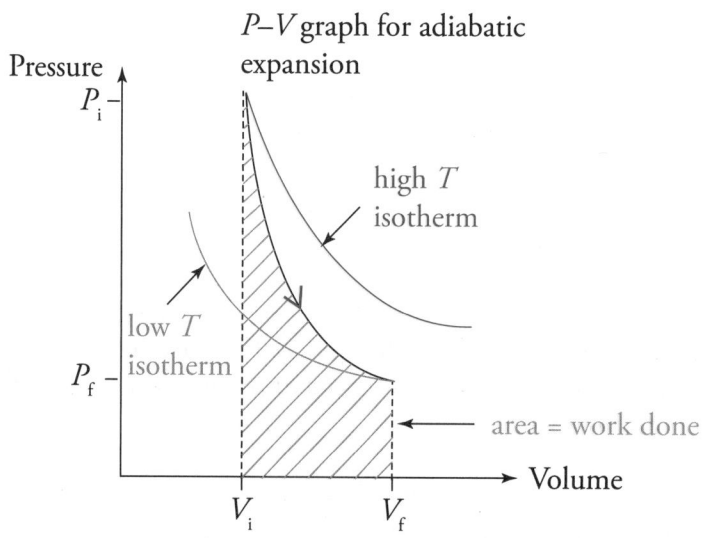

P–V graph for adiabatic expansion

Example 7-3: For a perfectly insulated system, what are the values of $\Delta E_{internal}$ and Q if $W = +100$ J?

A. $\Delta E_{internal} = -100$ J and $Q = 0$
B. $\Delta E_{internal} = 0$ and $Q = -100$ J
C. $\Delta E_{internal} = +100$ J and $Q = 0$
D. $\Delta E_{internal} = 0$ and $Q = +100$ J

Solution: A perfectly insulated system allows no heat transfer (adiabatic), so $Q = 0$; this eliminates choices B and D. Now, by the first law of thermodynamics, $\Delta E_{internal} = Q - W = 0 - (+100 \text{ J}) = -100$ J, so the answer is A.

Example 7-4: Suppose you want to raise the temperature of an ideal gas while adding the lowest possible amount of heat and doing no work on the gas. Which process should you use?

A. Isobaric
B. Isochoric
C. Isothermal
D. Adiabatic

Solution: An isothermal process will not raise the temperature of the gas at all by definition, so choice C is eliminated. An adiabatic process will not allow the transfer of heat into the gas, so choice D is eliminated. If you add heat during an isochoric process, the change in internal energy of the gas (which is directly proportional to the change in temperature) will be $\Delta E = Q$, whereas during an isobaric process it will be $\Delta E = Q - P\Delta V$, because the gas will expand as it increases in temperature; rearranging gives

$Q = \Delta E + P\Delta V$. Thus the isochoric process will require less heat to increase E and therefore T by some arbitrary amount. The correct choice is B.

This example illustrates the difference between two ideal gas heating processes. This distinction is quantified by the difference between *molar specific heats*. An ideal gas at constant volume will increase in temperature according to $Q = nC_V\Delta T$, where n is the number of moles and C_V is called the constant volume molar specific heat. An ideal gas at constant pressure, on the other hand, will increase in temperature according to $Q = nC_P\Delta T$, where C_P is called the constant pressure molar specific heat. The units of molar specific heat are $[C] = [Q] / [n][T] = $ J/mol-K. The exact values of the molar specific heats depend upon the type of gas (monatomic, diatomic, polyatomic), and you are unlikely to need to know them. However, as you already know from the preceding example that a constant pressure process requires more heat for an equal change in temperature than a constant volume process, it is worth noting that, in general, $C_P = C_V + R$, where R is the gas constant.

Example 7-5: The PV curve below represents a thermodynamic *cycle*, a series of reversible processes through which an ideal gas passes that return it to its initial state function. What area represents the net work done by the gas from steps 1 to 2 to 3 to 4 back to 1?

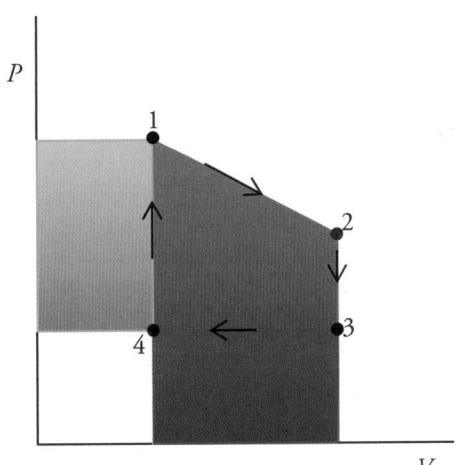

A. The blue trapezoid
B. The red rectangle
C. The blue trapezoid and the red rectangle
D. The blue trapezoid and both the red and green rectangles

Solution: The isochores 2→3 and 4→1 do no work, so we can ignore them. The process 1→2 does positive work $W_{1\to2} = P\Delta V$, which is the sum of the blue and red areas. The process 3→4 does negative work, because the volume decreases (this would correspond to the piston moving down, compressing the gas), $W_{3\to4} = P\Delta V$, which is the negative of the red area. Thus the sum of the four processes yields (blue + red) + 0 + (−red) + 0 = blue. The correct choice is A.

This example illustrates a couple of important facts about *thermodynamic cycles,* sequences of processes that lead a gas back to its original state function. This means that $\Delta E = 0$ for the overall cycle, and thus $Q = W$. During a cycle, the system either converts heat to work (for a clockwise cycle, like the one shown) or work to heat (for a counterclockwise cycle). Thermodynamic cycles are important as models of ideal heat engines. Indeed, many of the breakthroughs in the science of thermodynamics were made by engineers attempting to understand how to make more efficient engines.

Example 7-6: An ideal gas is held under pressure in an isolated container behind a thin membrane opposite which is vacuum, like an inflated balloon in a large evacuated room. The membrane is suddenly ruptured, like popping the balloon. What happens next?

 A. Nothing: the membrane ruptures but the gas is unaffected.
 B. The pressure and temperature both decrease rapidly.
 C. The temperature decreases rapidly but the pressure stays constant.
 D. The pressure decreases rapidly, but the temperature remains constant, since no heat is exchanged and no work is done.

Solution: If a gas is held under pressure and the source of the pressure is released, like suddenly removing the piston from the canister in the examples discussed previously, the pressure will spontaneously decrease to match that of the surroundings (this will be discussed in more detail in the next chapter on fluids). This eliminates choice A. The phenomenon described in this question is a special type of adiabatic process called a *free expansion:* it is nearly instantaneous, so there is no time for heat transfer, but because the membrane ruptures and there is nothing to push against, no work is done either. Applying the First Law equation thus yields

$$\Delta E = Q - W = 0 - 0 = 0.$$

Therefore there is no change in temperature either, and the correct choice is D. It might seem to you counterintuitive that something like popping a balloon could have such small apparent effect on the thermodynamic state of the system. You'd be right: something *does* increase, namely the *entropy* of the system.

7.4   THE SECOND LAW OF THERMODYNAMICS

As we have seen, the first law of thermodynamics is an expanded statement of conservation of energy, a principle we're familiar with from the realm of balls rolling down hills and blocks sliding across tables, as well as (now) gases being heated and expanding, doing work in the process. However, now that we have expanded our view of what counts as energy, it becomes apparent that many situations we would never expect to see do not in fact violate the principle of energy conservation. Imagine, for example, that you are looking at a wooden block resting on a normal horizontal table. All of the sudden, it begins sliding to the right. You'd be pretty surprised, and you'd probably start looking for the string (or the camera), because you would think that would violate the conservation of energy. However, suppose the block had a thermometer attached to it, and you noticed that as the block began to slide, its temperature began to lower. In that case, conservation of energy might not be violated: thermal energy was just transforming into kinetic energy. You would likely continue to object; it's one thing for a sliding block to slow down and stop due to friction, heating up in the process, but this doesn't typically work in reverse. Why *don't* things go backward? What directs the *arrow of time*? One answer is **entropy** and the **second law of thermodynamics.**

Entropy is a measure of the *disorder* of a system. What does this mean? Imagine the Great Pyramid of Giza, built so carefully of stacked stones that it has stood for over 4500 years. Now imagine those same six billion kilograms of stone scattered around hundreds of square kilometers of desert. The pyramid is ordered, the scattered stone is disordered. A microscopic analogy would be a diamond crystal, with its extremely regular and predictable organization of carbon atoms, versus the carbon atoms in pencil shavings scattered on a desk. The carbon atoms in the pencil shavings have much greater entropy than those in the crystal.

Without stating any equations you won't need to know, we can say qualitatively that *predictability* is one measure of order. If I tell you the first five cards in a deck are the ace, 2, 3, 4, and 5 of spades, you will probably feel pretty comfortable guessing the next card will be the 6 of spades, a lot more comfortable than if I shuffled the deck and asked you to predict the sixth card (technically, this is a function of information entropy and not physical entropy, but the details aren't important). By analogy, the entropy will be lower whenever there's a higher likelihood that, given you know the locations and velocities of some particles, you can deduce the same of other particles. Under this criterion, solids, with their regular arrays of atoms, have greater order and therefore less entropy than liquids, which have in turn less entropy than gases. Entropy is another *state variable*, one whose value corresponds to the microscopic order of the particles making up the system, just as temperature corresponds to the microscopic kinetic energy of those particles. The MCAT doesn't care about the mathematical details of this correspondence, and you are really likely to see quantitative entropy problems only in chemistry or biochemistry, not in physics.

The second law of thermodynamics states that the *entropy of an isolated system either stays the same or increases during any thermodynamic process*. If the system is closed, its entropy can decrease, but not without a corresponding greater increase in the entropy of the surrounding environment. Over a thermodynamic cycle, the rules are slightly different. If the entropy stays the same over a thermodynamic cycle, the cycle is said to be reversible, meaning that you could return from each state to the previous state by the same path in reverse (think of these paths as the curves on a *PV* graph), and that on returning there would be no indication of any change.

This means also that it is impossible for a system to convert all of the input heat (disordered energy) into work (ordered energy) during a thermodynamic cycle: it must always output some heat as well. Similarly, it is impossible to move heat from a colder system to a hotter one without inputting some work (work which, we've just discovered, must itself involve some output of heat). If the entropy increases over a series of processes (thereby making it not a true cycle), this indicates the process is *irreversible*. In the real world, all macroscopic processes are irreversible due to friction and other "loss" effects. A wooden block sliding on a horizontal table comes to a stop due to friction. Energy is conserved, converted from kinetic to thermal, but entropy increases, which is why you will never see the block spontaneously accelerate backward from whence it came. Things really can't go back to just the way they were.

Summary of Formulas

Energy flow into a system has a positive sign. Energy flow out of a system has a negative sign.

Temperature is defined by $\frac{1}{2}mv_{avg}^2 = \frac{3}{2}k_bT$ for a monatomic ideal gas.

The first law of thermodynamics states that energy cannot be created or destroyed. Based on this, $\Delta E = Q - W$.

The internal energy of an object is proportional to its temperature: $\Delta E \propto T$.

Work done by a gas: $W = P\Delta V$.

For an adiabatic process, $Q = 0$.

An isobaric process occurs at constant P, isothermal at constant T, and isochoric at constant V.

The change in absolute temperature of an ideal gas when heated is given by $Q = nC_V \cdot T$ or $Q = nC_P \cdot T$, depending upon whether the gas is heated at constant volume or constant pressure. $C_P = C_V + R$.

The second law of thermodynamics states that all processes tend toward maximum disorder, or entropy (S). It further states that heat cannot flow from a colder to a warmer object unless some work is done on the system to make it do so. Equivalently, the law says that heat cannot be converted totally to work by any cycle.

CHAPTER 7 FREESTANDING PRACTICE QUESTIONS

1. The linear thermal expansion of a metal rod is given by $\Delta L = \alpha L_0 \Delta T$. By how many degrees Celsius would the temperature of a rod have to increase for the rod's length to increase by 20%?

A) $\alpha L_0 / 5$
B) $1/5\alpha$
C) It depends on the original length of the rod.
D) Cannot be determined because kelvins must be used for ΔT.

2. An amount of heat Q is added to a system. Which of the following can result?

   I. Its temperature increases.
   II. Its phase changes.
   III. It undergoes isothermal expansion.

A) I only
B) I or II only
C) I or III only
D) I, II, or III

3. An expanding spring pushes a rigid cylinder of gas across a horizontal frictionless table. Consider the system to be the gas inside the cylinder. Which of the following sets of relations best describes what happens?

A) $W_{\text{on system}} > 0, Q > 0, \Delta KE > 0$
B) $W_{\text{on system}} = 0, Q = 0, \Delta KE = 0$
C) $W_{\text{on system}} > 0, Q = 0, \Delta KE > 0$
D) $W_{\text{on system}} > 0, Q < 0, \Delta KE > 0$

4. During adiabatic compression of a gas the temperature:

A) increases because no heat is transferred.
B) remains constant because heat is transferred.
C) remains constant because no heat is transferred.
D) decreases because heat is transferred.

5. A closed system consisting of a balloon expands by 5×10^{-2} L at constant temperature in an environment with a pressure of 1.0×10^5 Pa. What is the value of heat transfer in this process?

A) -5.0 J
B) -5.0 kJ
C) 5.0 J
D) 5.0 kJ

6. In the thermodynamic cycle shown below, the processes connecting points 2 and 3 and points 1 and 4 are adiabatic. What statement below is true?

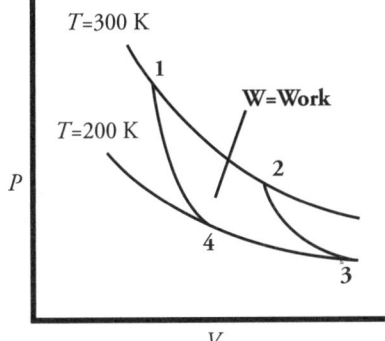

A) Work is done on or by the gas at every step.
B) Heat is exchanged only on processes 1-2 and 3-4.
C) The internal energy of the system returns to the same value after completing a cycle.
D) All of the above

CHAPTER 7 PRACTICE PASSAGE

Figure 1 shows a thin-walled, cylindrical metal container fitted with a tight-fitting but freely movable lightweight plastic piston and containing 0.25 mol of helium at 0°C and a pressure of 1 atm.

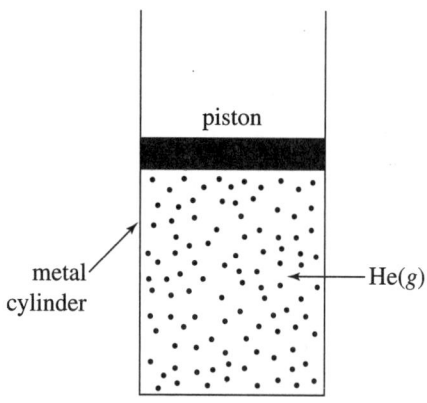

Figure 1

The volume, pressure, and temperature of the gas can be changed by various processes, such as by adding weights to the top of the piston or by heating the cylinder with a flame. The heat exchanged between the confined helium gas and the surroundings will be denoted by Q, where a positive value of Q indicates that the heat has been transferred *into* the gas; if Q is negative, heat has been transferred *out* of the gas. The work done on the gas will be denoted by W, where a positive value of W indicates that the gas does work on its surroundings; if W is negative, this means that the surroundings do work on the gas. The change in the internal energy of the gas is given by the equation.

$$\Delta E = Q - W$$

Equation 1

A student conducts the following series of experiments in a chemistry lab.

Experiment 1

The student measures the volume of the gas in the cylinder, places a known mass m on top of the piston, and then increases the temperature of the gas at constant pressure to 273°C.

Experiment 2

After the gas is allowed to cool back to 0°C at 1 atm pressure, the student locks the piston in place, and then increases the temperature of the gas to 273°C.

Experiment 3

After Experiment 2 is completed, the student unlocks the piston and a computer-controlled heat source maintains the temperature at a constant 273°C.

Experiment 4

After Experiment 2 is completed, the cylinder is completely wrapped in insulation before the piston is unlocked.

1. Experiment 4 is an example of an adiabatic process. Which of the following will always be true of an adiabatic process?

   A) The temperature will remain constant.
   B) $Q = W$
   C) $Q = -W$
   D) $Q = 0$

2. How do the pressure and volume of the gas change as a result of the procedures in Experiment 2?

   A) The pressure doubles, but the volume remains the same.
   B) The pressure stays the same, but the volume doubles.
   C) The pressure and volume both double.
   D) The pressure and volume both remain the same.

3. Which of the following best describes how the pressure and volume of the gas change as a result of Experiment 3?

   A) The pressure decreases, but the volume increases.
   B) The pressure increases, but the volume decreases.
   C) The pressure and volume both decrease.
   D) The pressure and volume both increase.

4. The student repeats Experiment 1 with a different cylinder and piston and finds that the volume increases from 0.025 m³ to 0.1 m³ at a constant pressure of 40 kPa. What is the value of W?

   A) −3000 J
   B) −300 J
   C) +300 J
   D) +3000 J

5. Let Q_3 and Q_4 denote the value of the heat transferred in Experiments 3 and 4, respectively, and let ΔE_3 and ΔE_4 represent the change in the internal energy of the gas in Experiments 3 and 4, respectively. Which one of the following statements is true?

    A) $Q_3 < Q_4$ and $\Delta E_3 < \Delta E_4$
    B) $Q_3 < Q_4$ and $\Delta E_3 > \Delta E_4$
    C) $Q_3 > Q_4$ and $\Delta E_3 < \Delta E_4$
    D) $Q_3 > Q_4$ and $\Delta E_3 > \Delta E_4$

6. After Experiment 4 is completed, the student places a 200-gram block on top of the piston, which pushes it down by 5 cm. As a result, the student should find that the internal energy of the gas:

    A) decreases by 1 J.
    B) decreases by 0.1 J.
    C) increases by 0.1 J.
    D) increases by 1 J.

SOLUTIONS TO CHAPTER 7 FREESTANDING QUESTIONS

1. **B** An increase of 20% in length is the same as saying $\Delta L/L_0 = 0.20$. This eliminates choice C. Substituting into the given equation yields

   $$\alpha\Delta T = \Delta L/L_0 = 0.2 \rightarrow \Delta T = 0.2/\alpha = 1/5\alpha.$$

   Choice D is eliminated because the scale of degrees Celsius and kelvins is the same, they just have different zeros ($-273°C = 0$ K).

2. **D** Obviously heat can raise the temperature of a system, and Item I is true (which doesn't eliminate anything). Heat can also melt a solid or boil a liquid without raising its temperature, so Item II is true, eliminating choices A and C. Heat additionally can expand a gas while it maintains constant temperature, so Item III is true, eliminating choice B. The point of the question is to reinforce that heat is a form of energy, not just something that makes other things "hot."

3. **C** An expanding spring exerts a force that causes a mass (the gas and its container, but even the gas has mass on its own) to displace, so it does positive work on the system, eliminating B. This work done on the system is mechanical, and because the gas is neither expanded nor compressed, simply translated, its kinetic energy increases. There is no friction and no mention of a temperature differential that would move heat into or out of the system, so $Q = 0$, eliminating choices A and D.

4. **A** During an adiabatic process, no heat is exchanged between the system and its surroundings ($Q = 0$). This eliminates choices B and D. For adiabatic processes, the change in internal energy of the system is equivalent to the negative work done by or positive work done on the system. When a gas is compressed, work is done on the gas. The temperature of the gas increases as a result.

5. **C** For a closed system at constant pressure, the magnitude of work can be calculated as $W = P\Delta V$. In this problem liters must be converted to m^3 as shown here:

   $$W = (1.0 \times 10^5 \text{ Pa})(5 \times 10^{-2} \text{ L})$$

   $$W = (1.0 \times 10^5 \text{ J/m}^3)(5 \times 10^{-2} \text{ L} \times 10^{-3} \text{ m}^3 /\text{L})$$

   $$W = (1.0 \times 10^5 \text{ J/m}^3)(5 \times 10^{-5} \text{ m}^3) = 5.0 \text{ J}$$

   The balloon is expanding at constant temperature so work is being done by the balloon on the surroundings, so $W > 0$. Since the question asks for the heat transferred when $\Delta T = 0$, in an isothermal system $Q = W$. Therefore, $Q = +5.0$ J.

6. **D** Because every curve has a nonzero area beneath it, the statement in choice A is true; only vertical isochores describe processes in which $W = 0$. By definition, no heat is exchanged during adiabatic processes, but heat is exchanged in all other processes, so the statement in choice B is true. That's enough to make choice D correct, but it's also worth noting that the statement in choice C is true: a cycle that returns a gas to the same point on the PV diagram must return all state variables to the same value.

SOLUTIONS TO CHAPTER 7 PRACTICE PASSAGE

1. **D** If no heat is exchanged between the system and the surroundings, then $Q = 0$. Choice A is a trap: A process in which the temperature remains constant is called *isothermal*; do not confuse adiabatic with isothermal. The internal energy of the gas can be increased either by an exchange of heat or by work being performed on or by the gas. If Q is 0 but W is not, then ΔE will not be zero; as a result, the temperature of the gas will change.

2. **A** Since the piston is locked in place, the volume of the gas cannot change; this eliminates choices B and C. From the Ideal-Gas law, $PV = nRT$, we see that P is proportional to T. Since the absolute temperature doubles (from 0°C = 273 K to 273°C = 546 K), so does the pressure.

3. **A** Once the piston is unlocked, the hot gas can expand. Since a constant temperature is maintained, the gas expands isothermally. In an isothermal expansion of a gas, the pressure decreases while the volume increases.

4. **D** Because the volume of the gas increases, the gas does positive work against the piston, pushing it upwards. Because the gas does work on its surroundings, the value of W must be positive; this eliminates choices A and B. Since the pressure is constant, the force exerted by the gas is constant, so the expression $P\Delta V$ gives the magnitude of the work (it's just the area of a rectangle of base ΔV and height P). In this case, we have $W = P\Delta V = (40 \times 10^3 \text{ Pa})(0.075 \text{ m}^3) = 3000$ J.

5. **D** In Experiment 3, T is constant, so E is constant (because the internal energy of a gas is directly proportional to its absolute temperature); thus, $\Delta E_3 = 0$. Since the gas does work pushing the piston upwards, W_3 is positive; as a result, $Q_3 = \Delta E_3 + W_3$ is positive. Experiment 4 describes an adiabatic process, so $Q_4 = 0$. Since the gas does work pushing the piston upwards, W_4 is positive, so $\Delta E_4 = Q_4 - W_4$ is negative. Therefore, $Q_3 > Q_4$ and $\Delta E_3 > \Delta E_4$.

6. **C** The weight on the piston pushes it down, and thus does work on the gas. The force is equal to the weight, $F = mg = (0.2 \text{ kg}) \times (10 \text{ N/kg}) = 2$ N. Multiplying this by the distance, $d = 0.05$ m, we find that the work done on the gas is $W = Fd = 0.1$ J. Remember that $-W_{\text{on gas}} = W_{\text{by gas}} = -0.1$ J. Because no heat is exchanged in Experiment 4, we have $\Delta E = Q - W = 0 - (-0.1 \text{ J}) = +0.1$ J, so the internal energy of the gas increases by 0.1 J.

JOURNAL ARTICLE 2

QUANTIFYING THE COOLING EFFICIENCY OF AIR VELOCITY BY HEAT LOSS FROM SKIN SURFACE IN WARM AND HOT ENVIRONMENTS

Chenqiu Du, Baizhan Li, Hong Liu, Yifan Wei, Meilan Tan

Abstract

In warm and hot environments, the possibility of increasing air velocity reduces energy consumption without compromising occupants' thermal comfort; whereas the cooling efficiency pertains to the temperature limits. To address the coupling effect of air velocity and temperature on thermal comfort and evaluate the cooling efficiency objectively, 9 experimental conditions with side air supply (piston flow) were conducted in a well-controlled climate chamber, covering temperatures from warm (28 °C) to hot (34 °C). Both skin temperatures and questionnaires were measured on 20 subjects. The results showed the cooling efficiency by airflow was significantly affected by temperatures. Subjects' mean skin temperatures (MST) and thermal sensations (TSV) were improved by increasing air velocities when temperature was lower than or equal to 32 °C, but no significant differences were found between different air velocities at each temperature level (except for MST at 28 °C). The air velocity failed to modify subjects' thermal responses but caused negative thermal and pressure due to higher air temperature and airflow at 34 °C. Thanks to the uniform air movement, subjects' total heat loss from skin surface(Q_{skin}) was quantified that significantly reduced from 46.98 W/m² at 28 °C/0 m/s, to 31.45 W/m² at 34 °C/1.4 m/s, indicating the poor cooling efficiency of air velocity in hot environments. The relation between air velocity and temperature with a prerequisite of neutral thermal sensation was obtained based on Q_{skin}, which can reserve as a reference for air velocity design in warm and hot environments considering thermal comfort, cooling efficiency and energy savings.

INTRODUCTION

An incentive for utilizing air movement to achieve indoor thermal comfort is that using air movement to raise room temperature set-points enables substantial HVAC energy savings. Buildings employing fan cooling could promise substantial savings in HVAC energy more than 30% below that of conventionally conditioned buildings. Using simulation for fifty-four cases covering six cities, Schiavon concluded that a cooling energy between 17% and 48% was saved by fan through increasing air velocity.

However, in hot environments, the air velocity cannot alleviate the discomfort caused by higher temperatures, and thus the considerations of energy efficiency are not any longer necessary. Therefore, it is primary to determine the temperature ranges in which the cooling efficiency of air velocity is applicable and the energy savings can be considered. The majority of research on the cooling performance of increasing air velocity are based on the lab experiments and the results show that in the warm sides, the boundaries of acceptable temperatures fluctuate in the range of 26 °C–32 °C, and the preferred air velocity varies from 0.4 m/s to 2.0 m/s. However, human perceptions of air movement depend on many factors, including the levels and directions of air velocity, air temperature and humidity, the personal factors of clothes, activity levels, thermal experiences and so on. The cooling efficiency of air velocity was thus less examined and no consistent findings were obtained reporting the thresholds above which a satisfactory thermal comfort cannot be achieved by elevated air velocity.

Therefore, the aims of this study are twofold. Firstly, to what extent the air velocity can be elevated to offset the increasing temperature in hot environments is explored based on subjects' thermal responses via a climate chamber experiment. Secondly, how to evaluate the cooling efficiency of air movement objectively through theoretical indices from the views of body heat exchange and how to bridge the relations between human thermal comfort and thermal environment parameters using such indices are investigated. The outcomes are expected to guide the air velocity designs reasonably in warm and hot environments, instead of stubbornly increasing air velocity with lower cooling efficiency.

METHOD

Climate chamber

All the experiments were conducted in a well-controlled climate chamber, with the size of 4 m × 3 m × 3 m (L × W × H), as shown in Fig. 1(a). The envelope of the climate chamber used 100 mm thick double color steel plate with polyurethane filling in the middle, to ensure the internal environment was unaffected by the external environments. The temperature ranges in the chamber can be controlled from 10 °C to 40 °C within an accuracy of ± 0.3 °C and from –5 °C to 10 °C within an accuracy of ± 0.5 °C. The relative humidity is designed with different levels from 10% to 90%, with an accuracy of ± 5%. In addition, a variety forms of air distribution could be created via different air supply terminals. In this study, to ensure the subjects were exposed to uniform air movement, the air was designed to be supplied from side perforated plate, and returned on the other side with perforated plate, forming a piston flow in the whole room. Fig. 1(b) shows the sketch of air distribution in experiments from front view and the supply-air outlet used in experiments (Fig. 1(c)). Besides, an adjacent room with dimensions of 5.15 m × 4.2 m × 3 m (L × W × H) was maintained at neutral thermal environment (26 °C) for the preparation work before the experiments.

Experimental conditions

Given the purpose of this study was to examine the cooling efficiency of air velocity and the upper temperature limits, all experimental conditions were designed with four temperature levels in warm and hot environments, as listed in Table 1. In Table 1, the relative humidity was designed at normal level of 60%. Referring to previous studies, most subjects were accepted when the temperature was at 28 °C, and thus the air velocity of 0 m/s was designed as a comparative condition at 28 °C. According to ASHRAE 55, the upper limits of air velocities of 0.8 m/s without personal control and 1.2 m/s with personal control are suggested when the temperature is higher than 30 °C, which were adopted as the low and high air velocity at 32 °C. However, to make the consistent increment of air velocity at each temperature level, an added middle air velocity of 1.0 m/s was considered at 32 °C. Besides, in Table 1 the temperature of 34 °C is considered as the critical upper boundary, considering that it is defined as extreme hot environments when the temperature is above 35 °C, and that increasing air movement is not be beneficial when the air temperature is above skin temperatures, due to the suppressed convective heat loss and sweating evaporations. At 34 °C, as the form of air supply in this study was different from the previous personal ventilation researches, where the local body parts were exposed to air movement, a pilot test was conducted and the upper limit of air velocity of 1.4 m/s was finally determined.

Subjects

Based on the experimental design, a total of 20 college students, between 20 and 30 years of age were recruited for participation in all the designed experiments (Table 1), with a healthy condition, no colds, fever and other symptoms. Meanwhile, in order to reduce the error caused by the differences in gender, 10 males and 10 females were included in this investigation. The experiments were performed in accordance with the ethical standards of the 1964 Declaration of Helsinki. They were paid to participate in all the experiments, and before the experiments, written informed consent was obtained from these participants. Table 2 shows the physical characteristics of all subjects. To note, since the clothes would have significant effect on the heat exchange between subjects and surroundings, the uniform summer clothes (cotton short-sleeved T-shirt, shorts and slippers, with clothing insulation of 0.32clo) were provided for subjects during the tests.

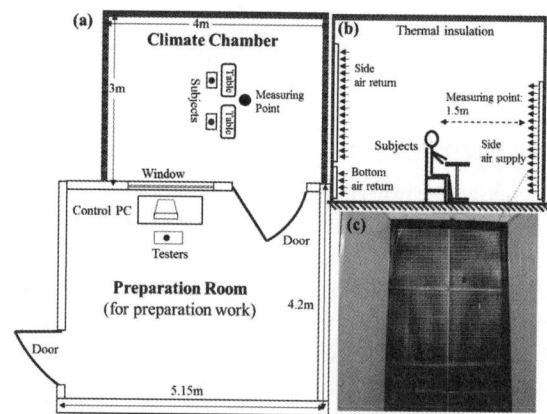

Figure 1. The schematic diagram in chamber.

Table 1 The designed environment conditions

Conditions	Air Temperature (°C)	Relative Humidity (%)	Air Velocity (m/s)		
			Case 1	Case 2	Case 3
1	28°C	60%	0	0.4	
2	30°C		0.6	0.8	
3	32°C		0.8	1.0	1.2
4	34°C		1.2	1.4	

Table 2 Physical characteristics of 20 subjects (mean ± SD)

Gender	Number	Age (year)	Height (cm)	Weight (kg)	$A_D (m^2)$
male	10	23.3 ± 0.9	173.6 ± 5.5	63.6 ± 4.9	1.76 ± 0.09
female	10	24.5 ± 0.6	162.1 ± 6.9	49.9 ± 6.3	1.51 ± 0.12
total	20	23.9 ± 1.0	167.9 ± 8.5	56.8 ± 8.9	1.64 ± 0.16

Questionnaires

The questionnaire was designed to cover thermal sensation, air movement sensation, environmental expectation and so on. The thermal sensation was quantified using ASHRAE 55 7-point scale (i.e. –3 cold, –2 cool, –1 slightly cool, 0 neutral, +1 slightly warm, +2 warm, +3 hot). In a similar vein, subjects evaluated their air movement sensation based on 7-point scale (–3 too still, –2 still, –1 slight still, 0 just right, +1 slight windy, +2 windy, +3 too windy). Here to note, in some situations when the subjects had some difficulties in expressing judgements, he was allowed to use middle votes (e.g., +1.5 between +1 and + 2). Besides, environmental expectations for temperatures and air velocity were designed by 3-point scale (–1, temperature/ air velocity down, 0 unchanged, +1 up), to evaluate the satisfaction of subjects for temperature and air movement.

Experimental process

Before each experiment, testers were asked to arrive at the chamber 1 h in advance. During this period, they would preset the thermal environments (i.e., air temperature, air velocity) in the climate chamber to the designed conditions and prepare for the instruments for measurements. Subjects were asked to arrive at the preparation room 30 min (see Fig. 1(a)) in advance to eliminate the effect of outdoor environments and previous thermal experiences. Then subjects were asked to change the clothes and attach the thermocouples on the local skin surfaces from eight left parts of body, including forehead, left chest, left back, left upper arm, left lower arm, left hand, right anterior thigh and anterior calf, using surgical, water permeable, adhesive tapes. The logging interval was set at 0.5/s and recorded by the multi-channel physiological acquisition system. The mean skin temperatures (MST) were calculated using an eight-point formula, based on the area-weighted averages of local skin temperatures, as expressed in Equation (1).

$$MST = 0.07*T_{forehead} + 0.175*T_{chest} + 0.175*T_{back}$$
$$+ 0.07*T_{upperarm} + 0.07*T_{lowerarm} + 0.05*T_{hand}$$
$$+ 0.19*T_{thigh} + 0.2*T_{calf} \tag{1}$$

The formal test lasted 60 min after subjects left the preparation room and entered the climate chamber and sat down. To note, before they entered the chamber, the environmental temperature and air velocity had been kept at the designed level. During the test, the physical parameters including air temperature, relative humidity, black-bulb temperature around the subjects were measured by Thermal Comfort Monitoring Station instrument, MI6401, Germany, Accuracy: air temperature: ± 0.2 °C, relative humidity: ± 2%, globe bulb temperature: ± 0.15 °C). The instrument was placed 1.5 m far from the supply-air outlet (Fig. 1(b)) and the probe was at a height of 0.6 m above the floor and 0.5 m away from subjects. Data were recorded every 10 min and exported after experiments. To measure the air velocity accurately, the Air Distribution Measuring System (AirDistSys 5000, Sensor Electronic, Poland, range: 0.05 m/s – 5m/s, accuracy: ± 0.02 m/s ± 1% reading data) was used with a sampling interval of 0.1/s.

To make sure the whole body of subjects were exposed to uniform air movement, subjects were sedentary in front of outlet 1.5 m away during the whole 60 min. For each test, two subjects were involved. Over the period of test, subjects' local skin temperatures were measured continuously. Besides, their subjective thermal perceptions were investigated by identical questionnaires every 10 min. Only light activities like reading, listening and talking softly were allowed, to keep a steady state condition (the metabolic rate was appropriately 1 met).

RESULTS

Thermal environments in experiments

Table 3 shows the measured thermal environments during tests. From Table 3, the measured air temperature and air velocity near subjects were close to that of designed condition. As denoted in Fig. 1(a), the chamber had the insulated inner enclosure structure and there was only an inner window for investigation. And the heat from subjects and lamps was strictly controlled by the air-conditioning system. Therefore, in Table 3, the measured black-globe temperature was much close to the air temperature, the difference of which was less than 0.3 °C. Therefore, in the following analysis, it mainly focused on the air temperature and the radiant temperature was assumed being equal to the air temperature.

Subjects' thermal responses to air temperatures and air velocities

Mean skin temperatures (MST)

Fig. 2 shows the differences of subjects' MST under different air velocity conditions, averaged by all 20 subjects at steady state. Significant differences were found for different temperature levels: with the temperature increasing, subjects' MST increased, regardless of the different air velocity levels. When the temperature was 28 °C, the MST of subjects were higher without airflow and significantly decreased when the air velocity was available at 0.4 m/s ($p < 0.05$). However, when the temperatures were at 30 °C and 32 °C, there were some decreases of MST to different extent with increasing air velocity, but no significant differences were found ($p > 0.05$). Besides, when the temperature was higher, the decrement of MST caused by the same increment of air velocity was small. For example, at 32 °C, the MST decreased by 0.11 °C when air velocity was from 0.8 m/s to 1.0 m/s, while the value was just 0.02 °C from 1.0 m/s to 1.2 m/s. When the temperature increased to 34 °C, the subjects' MST increased significantly, and the higher air velocity of 1.2 m/s and 1.4 m/s failed to decrease the MST. It manifests that when the environmental temperatures were lower, increasing air velocity was effective to enhance heat loss and reduce skin temperatures. However, when the temperatures were higher, the air temperature, instead of air velocity, had dominant effect on body physiological responses, and thus the elevated air velocity was unable to offset the increases of MST.

Thermal sensation votes (TSV)

Fig. 3 shows the changes of subjects' mean thermal sensation (TSV). Being similar to subjects' MST in Fig. 2, subjects' TSV significantly increased with increasing temperatures. Subjects felt neutral (nearly 0 for TSV) at 28 °C and there was no significant difference with and without air movement. This might, on the one hand, attributed to subjects' long-term thermal adaptations and improved thermal tolerance, considering the experiment was conducted at the height of summer. On the other hand, it attributed to the light clothes (0.32 clo) in experiments, which was lower than the recommended standard clothes (0.5 clo) in summer in standard. The TSV increased at 30 °C but were still under 0.5 with the available air movement. The higher air velocity of 0.8 m/s reduced the TSV by 0.11, regardless of the not significant difference. However, when the temperature increased to 32 °C, the TSV were higher than 0.5, and the increased air velocity from 0.8 m/s to 1.2 m/s led to slight decrease of TSV from 0.85 to 0.57 ($p > 0.05$). This indicates that under higher air temperatures the cooling efficiency of air movement was limited and the higher air velocity failed to alleviate subjects' thermal discomfort. It was further verified at 34 °C where the subjects' TSV were around 2.0, even though they were exposed to higher air velocity of 1.2 m/s and 1.4 m/s. It may because the convective and evaporative heat dissipation were weakened due to the smaller temperature differences between skin and surroundings. However, it is interestingly found that when the temperature was 34 °C, the change trends of TSV with increased air velocity were opposite from that under other temperature levels. The air velocity of 1.4 m/s conversely increased subjects' TSV, as marked in red rectangle in Fig. 3. Since the environmental temperature was close to subjects' skin temperatures at 34 °C, the isothermal air supply and higher air velocity caused the additional thermal effect on subjects' sensation. As a result, when the air velocity was 1.2 m/s, the additional effect was lightened so that subjects' TSV decreased.

Overall, subjects' TSV are not only affected by air velocity itself, but also couple with air temperatures. That is, the cooling performance of increasing air velocity is significant when the air temperature is equal to or under 32 °C. However, the thermal discomfort takes the first place under higher temperatures that the isothermal airflow is less efficient to improve subjects' TSV.

Table 3   The measured environmental parameters at each condition (mean ± SD)

Designed conditions		Experimental conditions			
Temp. (°C)	Air Velocity (m/s)	T_{air}/°C	RH/%	V/m/s	T_{glob}/°C
28	0	28.0 ± 0.2	60.2 ± 0.9	0.05 ± 0.02	28.3 ± 0.2
28	0.4	28.0 ± 0.2	59.6 ± 1.0	0.40 ± 0.02	28.2 ± 0.1
30	0.6	30.0 ± 0.0	60.5 ± 0.2	0.60 ± 0.02	30.2 ± 0.0
30	0.8	30.0 ± 0.0	60.4 ± 0.2	0.80 ± 0.02	30.2 ± 0.0
32	0.8	32.0 ± 0.0	60.9 ± 0.5	0.80 ± 0.01	32.1 ± 0.0
32	1.0	32.2 ± 0.2	59.5 ± 0.9	1.00 ± 0.06	32.1 ± 0.2
32	1.2	32.0 ± 0.0	60.9 ± 0.4	1.19 ± 0.02	32.1 ± 0.0
34	1.2	34.0 ± 0.0	60.8 ± 0.2	1.19 ± 0.03	34.1 ± 0.0
34	1.4	34.0 ± 0.0	60.8 ± 0.2	1.43 ± 0.04	34.1 ± 0.0

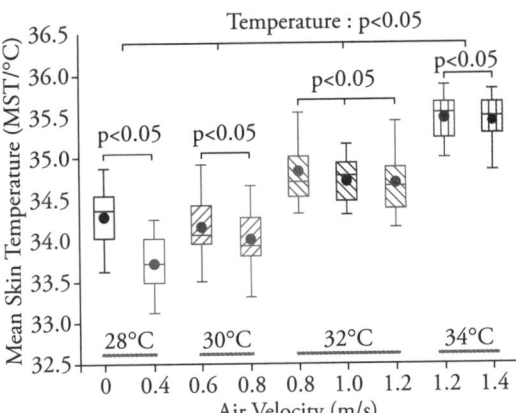

Figure 2. Subjects' MST at steady-state under different conditions.

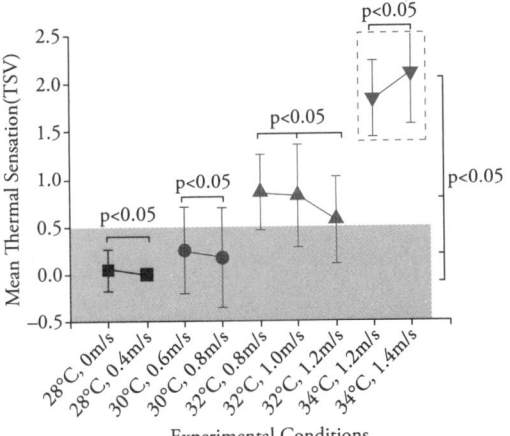

Figure 3. Subjects' TSV at steady-state under each condition.

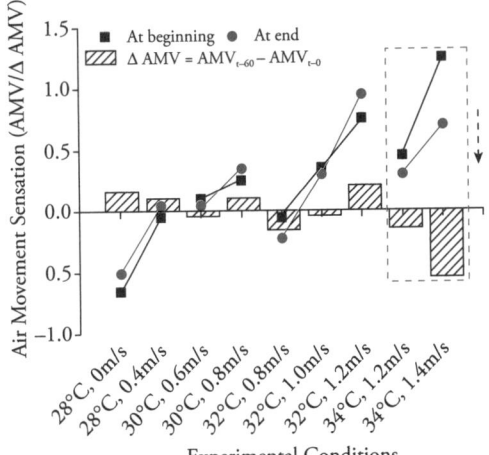

Figure 4. Changes of subjects' AMV at beginning and end of the test under each condition.

Air movement sensation votes (AMV)

Air movement sensation (AMV) is a useful index for evaluating the perceived air movement and reflecting the sensitivity to airflow. Fig. 4 demonstrates the changes of subjects' AMV with time and air velocity, where the black ones represent the subjects' AMV at $t = 0$ min and the red ones at $t = 60$ min. It is clearly seen that unlike TSV, the AMV significantly increased with increasing air velocity at each temperature level. The higher the air velocity was, the higher the AMV was, suggesting subjects' sensations to air movement were mainly related to air velocity rather than temperatures. However, the AMV were slightly different comparing subjects' AMV at initial stage of exposure to the end of exposure, as shown in bar in Fig. 4. When the temperatures were under 32 °C, at the end of tests, subjects' AMV increased slightly compared to that at beginning. It deduces that after a long term exposure to air movements, the heat balance of subjects in warm environments was rebuilt and thus subjects who were in neutral thermal status became fatigued to and more sensitive to airflow, feeling the air velocity higher. On the contrary, when the temperature was 34 °C, subjects' AMV decreased at end under both two air velocity levels and the differences were enlarged under higher air velocity of 1.4 m/s, as marked in arrow in Fig. 4. By contrast, in hot environments, the cooling efficiency of air movement was weaker and thus the body heat storage of subjects increased with prolong exposure time. In that case, subjects psychologically judged the air movement far from enough, leading to a decreased AMV on air velocity.

Subjects' heat loss from skin and its relation to thermal environments

Total heat loss from skin surface (Q_{skin})

Since the heat exchange were difficult to be evaluated objectively in the previous personal ventilation studies, the uniform air movement and thin clothes (0.32clo) of subjects in this study took advantages to calculate the whole heat loss between skin surface and surroundings. In this line of approach, the total heat loss from skin surface was projected as an objective index evaluating the cooling efficiency. Because the ASHRAE's method (shown in Equation (2)) is not very complicated and the items can be obtained expediently, which is useful for application, here it is also adopted to calculate the sensible and latent heat loss from subjects' skin surface.

$$Q_{skin} = Q_{con} + Q_{rad} + E_{sk}$$

$$= (t_{sk} - t_o)/[R_{cl} + 1/(f_{cl} h)] + w(p_{sk,s} - p_a)/[R_{e,cl} + 1/(f_{cl} h_e)] \quad (2)$$

Where Q_{skin} = the total heat loss, W/m²; Q_{con} = the convective heat loss, W/m²; Q_{rad} = the radiant heat loss, W/m²; E_{sk} = the evaporative heat loss, W/m²; t_{sk} = the skin temperature, °C; t_o = the operative temperature, °C, here is equal to air temperature; R_{cl} = the thermal resistance of clothing in m²K/W, here is 0.0496 m² °C/W; f_{cl} = the clothing area factor, here is 1.096; h = heat transfer coefficient, W/m² °C, here is calculated by the sum of convective and radiative heat transfer coefficient; w is skin wettedness, here is 1; $p_{sk,s}$ = the water vapor pressure at skin, here is assumed to be that of saturated water vapor at t_{sk}, kPa; $R_{e,cl}$ = the evaporative heat transfer resistance of clothing, m²Pa/W, here is equal to R_{cl}; h_e = the evaporative heat transfer coefficient, W/m²kPa, here is equal to h_c.

In Equation (2), the radiative heat transfer coefficient of 4.7 W/m² °C was used. The convective heat transfer coefficient was calculated for seated people based on Equation (3).

$$h_c = \begin{cases} 3.1 & 0 < v < 0.2 \\ 8.3 \times v^{0.6} & 0.2 < v < 4.0 \end{cases} \tag{3}$$

Taken together, based on the physical parameters and subjects' measured skin temperatures from experiments, the total heat loss from skin (Q_{skin}) was calculated by Equations (2) and (3) under different experimental conditions. There were slight fluctuations of Q_{skin} during the whole process for each condition. However, the total Q_{skin} decreased significantly with increasing air temperatures, from 46.98 W/m² at t = 60 min at 28 °C/0 m/s, to 31.45 W/m² at 34 °C/1.4 m/s, indicating that the heat dissipation caused by air velocity was restrained significantly with increasing temperatures.

To examine the cooling efficiency of air velocity, note that when the temperature was equal to or under 32 °C, the variation of heat loss was significant owing to the enhanced heat transfer between skin surface and the surrounding environments, which was similar to those reported in previous research. For example, the Q_{skin} increased by nearly 1.7 W/m² when the air velocity increased from 0 m/s to 0.4 m/s at 28 °C. It was more significant at 30 °C: when the air velocity increased from 0.6 m/s to 0.8 m/s, the total Q_{skin} increased by nearly 3.3 W/m², demonstrating the stronger cooling efficiency of air movement at 30 °C. The similar trend was found at 32 °C but the decrement of Q_{skin} caused by the increment of air velocity (0.2 m/s) reduced. When the temperature was 34 °C, though the air velocity was high (1.2 m/s and 1.4 m/s

respectively), the total Q_{skin} was much smaller (30 W/m²), indicating that depending on air velocity to maintain body heat balance was not enough anymore.

Relations between total Q_{skin} and air velocity and temperature

In theory, the air velocity enhances the convective and evaporative heat exchange between human body and surroundings, thus improving thermal comfort. From Equation (4), the Q_{skin} is determined by both air velocity and air temperature. Compared to air temperature, the Q_{skin} is more sensitive to air velocity: when the temperature changes by 1 °C, the Q_{skin} would change 4.25 W/m²; while it would change 13.26 W/m², for example, when the air temperature is 30 °C and air velocity increases by 1 m/s. Besides, the interactive influence between temperature and air velocity exists but it is slight (slope: 0.99). To note, since the model was regressed from experimental data, the ranges of air temperature and air velocity should be limited to experiments. In particular, the average heat loss from skin surface should be much less than the body heat generation at stable state (58.15 W/m²), accounting for appropriately 97% without air movement. Under such cases, the lower limits of air temperature in Equation (4) should be higher than 25.16 °C.

$$Q_{skin} = 162.93 - 4.25*T + 42.96*V - 0.99*T*V \tag{4}$$

where Q_{skin} is the total heat loss from skin surface, W/m², T is the air temperature, °C; V is the air velocity around human body, m/s.

Relation between TSV and temperature and air velocity based on Q_{skin}

Since the body heat balance is the main driving force affecting human thermal perceptions, the Q_{skin} can be a robustly theoretical index to evaluate thermal sensation. Fig. 5 demonstrates the relationship between subjects' Q_{skin} and their thermal sensations. Here to note, Fig. 5 presents the Q_{skin} and the correlated TSV during the whole process (t = 0 min, 10 min, ..., 60 min) under different conditions. It is clearly seen that the subjects' TSV changed linearly with Q_{skin}: the TSV deceased significantly when the heat loss from skin surface increased.

The relation between TSV and Q_{skin} is obtained in Equation (5). It indicates that the TSV would decrease by 0.11 unit when the Q_{skin} increase by 1 W/m². When the TSV fluctuate under 0.5, the heat of nearly 43 W/m² should be removed from skin surface to maintain comfort. Here considering subjects' thermal sensations in this study are mostly above

0, the relation between TSV and Q_{skin} is reserved when the TSV is below 0, which should be studied further.

$$TSV = 5.24 - 0.11*Q_{skin} \qquad (R^2 = 0.94) \qquad (5)$$

In practice, people all prefer much the direct index to the indirect index to evaluate thermal environments. Fig. 5 shows a close relation between human thermal sensation and the theoretical heat loss from skin surface, which bridges the correlation between human thermal sensation and environmental parameters. Through introducing the intermediate variable Q_{skin} (Equation (4)), the Equation (5) can be redefined as follows (Equation (6)).

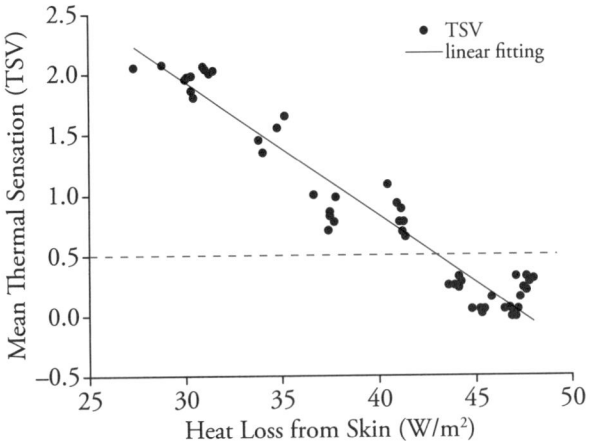

Figure 5. The relationship between Q_{skin} and TSV.

$$TSV = 0.47*T - 4.73*V + 0.11*T*V - 12.68 \qquad (6)$$

Based on Equation (6), the thermal sensation can be predicted under certain temperature and air velocity levels. When the required thermal sensation is given, the relation between temperature and the corresponding air velocity can be obtained from Equation (6). However, to note here, due to the limited experimental data regressing the Equations (4) and (5), coupled with the deviations caused by the transformation and integration, Equation (6) provides a referring method for guiding thermal environment design, but it should be further improved on prediction performance.

DISCUSSION

Overall, the Equation (6) provides a method for application in practice conveniently when designing thermal environments. However, some limitations should be considered. The limited experimental conditions and sample capacity may cause some deviations of prediction performance on Equations (4)–(6). However, thanks to a simplified thermoregulation model of human body based on a variety of lab experiments on Chinese in our recent research, it enable us to predict human skin temperature and calculate the heat loss more accurately using the physiological model. In this line of thoughts, for in-depth research, our following study would relate the TSV to the human body thermoregulation model through a variety of experimental, and thus improve the obtained model between TSV and Q_{skin}, with a wide range of air temperatures and air velocities in Equation (6) (e.g., isothermal and non-isothermal air movement, local heat loss and local thermal comfort, etc.), in order for better application in future and achieving energy efficiency guidance.

Cooling efficiency of air movement in warm and hot environments

In warm and hot environments, the air velocity acts as a useful way to improve human thermal comfort, but the cooling efficiency is dependent. In our study, the total Q_{skin} reduces gradually when the air temperature is above 30 °C and the increasing air velocity plays a negative effect on subjects' TSV at 34 °C (Fig. 3). Our study [shows] that the cooling efficiency of air velocity would be weakened significantly at higher temperatures, leading to the preferred air velocity of occupants being conservative at that case. In fact, there were slight differences of Q_{skin} between two air velocity levels at 34 °C, and subjects' thermal sensations were diversely lower under lower air velocity of 1.2 m/s. This suggests that in hot environments the thermal discomfort caused by temperature plays the dominant role and that the isothermal air movement may increase pressure on skin surface, block breathing, cause dizziness symptom, etc., deteriorating human thermal sensation. In such cases, increasing air velocity would make no sense but increase energy consumption, meantime increase the risk of uncomfortable "thermal draught". Therefore, when the temperature is beyond 30 °C, the non-isothermal air supply should be considered to enhance cooling efficiency, and the air conditioning is suggested to put into application if the temperature exceeds 32 °C.

To point out, even for the appropriate air velocity, occupants' perceptions would vary with some non-environmental and individual factors, like gender, ages, the transient or stationary, length of exposure or stay time. Studies show the thermal sensation would be stabilized within 10 min after the thermal environment changes (e.g., local and whole body cooling). Gong studied the human thermal responses to facial airflow under short-term (15 min) and long-term (90 min) exposures. The results showed the subjects were almost settled in their steady state of thermal sensation after an hour of adaptation that the final values were similar to that of short-term exposures. The "alliesthesia" model, which was first proposed by Cabanac and then revisited by de Dear, emphasizes such phenomenon that the hedonic, or pleasurable sensations are generated by perceiving a given external stimulus and restoring a bodily stress toward a neutral interior condition. Taking into account a number of cold and warm receptors on the skin, the airflow on the subjects' skin surface can create cool sensations through stimulating the cold receptors and increasing heat loss from body, and temporarily change the local skin temperatures. However, when subjects are exposed to the constant air velocity after a certain period of time (60 min), the skin thermoreceptors would adapt to the airflow and send other information to the central system than the temperature sent initially. As a result, subjects' skin temperatures have slight changes over time, so is the total heat loss from skin surface. Meanwhile, the discomforts and fatigues of subjects occur over time that they would like to reduce the air velocity. In such cases, if people are potentially exposed to airflow for long time, the dynamic and periodic airflow is recommended to create and sustain an awareness of cooling sensation of body meanwhile prevent thermoreceptors adaptation to enhance the heat loss on the skin surface.

CONCLUSION

The present study examines the human thermal responses to isothermal air movement under warm and hot environments based on a series of experiments in chamber, and presents an objective index evaluating the cooling efficiency of air movement. Some conclusions are thus drawn as follows:

1) The MST and TSV are improved by increasing air velocities at temperatures under or equal to 32 °C. The higher air velocity at 34 °C fails to reduce subjects' MST and TSV but leads to additional effect of thermal and pressure, deteriorating the thermal comfort;

2) The cooling efficiency of air velocity is quantified by total heat loss from skin surface (Q_{skin}) that the Q_{skin} reduces significantly with increased temperature from 46.98 W/m^2 at 28 °C/0 m/s, to 31.45 W/m^2 at 34 °C/1.4 m/s. The relation between Q_{skin} and temperature and air velocity is obtained, quantifying the coupled effect of air velocity and air temperature on body heat dissipation;

3) The negative linear relation is built between subjects' TSV and Q_{skin}, which bridges the relation between subjective thermal sensation and the temperature and air velocity. The appropriate air velocity in response to air temperature is presented with the given neutral thermal sensation (0), which can be instructive for thermal environment design considering cooling efficiency and energy saving of air movement.

JOURNAL ARTICLE EXERCISE 2

The science sections on the MCAT include a significant number of passages with experiments or quantitative data. On the Chem/Phys section, questions for these passages often ask you to analyze numerical data from tables and graphs, interpret an apparatus, and come to some reasonable conclusion based on the information they give you. If you don't know how to extract information efficiently and analyze data effectively, you will be at a distinct disadvantage.

There are three "Journal Article Exercises" in this book. In the first exercise, we showed you how to extract important information from an abridged article about forces, specifically frictional forces. In this second exercise, you get the opportunity to practice extracting the vital information from an abridged peer-reviewed journal article related to thermodynamics on your own. In the final exercise, we'll show you how a scientific journal article can be translated into an MCAT passage.

As a reminder, when analyzing a physics article, you should be able to:

- find the research question(s),
- identify the independent and dependent variables,
- determine the significance of any equations and recognize any familiar terms therein,
- interpret the experiment design in terms of basic physical principles,
- analyze any experiment apparatus,
- extract information from graphs and data tables,
- observe trends in the data,
- interpret the hypotheses in terms of the research questions and data, and
- assess the strengths and limitations of the study.

The goal of these exercises is NOT to learn content from the articles, just to get a little more comfortable reading and extracting information from them.

For the (abridged) article on pages 203–210, try to summarize the purpose, methods, results, and assumptions of the study. Note that this article, being written by nonnative speakers of English, contains some awkward phrasing and grammatically incorrect sentences. This is not uncommon in scientific publications and should not be taken to reflect poorly on the science. Answer the following questions:

1. **Topic:**
   - Where does this research fit within the subject matter covered within Chem/Phys?

   _____

   _____

   - Is more than one discipline or topic pertinent to this research?

   _____

   _____

2. **Research questions:**
   - What are the researchers trying to determine?

   _____

   _____

   - How are their methods informed by the question(s)?

   _____

   _____

3. **Data collection:**
   - What is the experimental procedure?

   _____

   _____

   - What is the experiment apparatus and the measurement device?

   _____

   _____

4. **Data analysis:**
   - What are the independent and dependent variables in the stated equations?

   _____

   _____

   - What descriptive statistics are used?

   _____

   _____

5. **Data presentation:**
   - Are there figures showing the apparatus? How do these relate to the data?

   _____

   _____

- Are there tables or graphs? If so, what quantities/units are shown? What trends are evident?

  _____

  _____

- What do these reveal about the significance of the findings?

  _____

  _____

6. **Conclusions/hypotheses:**
   - How does the research answer the research questions?

     _____

     _____

   - What does it not answer, and how do the authors acknowledge its limitations?

     _____

     _____

   - Are there any unacknowledged limitations you can see?

     _____

     _____

7. **Assumptions:**
   - What do the authors implicitly or explicitly take as given in the ways they design their research, interpret their data, or argue for the significance of their findings?

     _____

     _____

   - Do these assumptions seem justified, given your knowledge of the underlying science?

     _____

     _____

SOLUTIONS TO JOURNAL ARTICLE EXERCISE 2

Let's answer the above questions for the article on pages 203–210.

1. **Topic:**
   - Where does this research fit within the subject matter covered within Chem/Phys? *Physics, specifically thermodynamics of heat transfer*
   - Is more than one discipline or topic pertinent to this research? *Not in this case, though in thermodynamics generally that is true*

2. **Research questions:**
   - What are the researchers trying to determine? *How do variations in ventilation air speeds at various room temperatures affect office workers' skin temperatures and perceived comfort?*
   - How are their methods informed by the question(s)? *Because comfort is subjective, participants in the study were surveyed about their perceptions of temperature and air movement, and these data were coupled with measured skin temperatures and calculated heat loss.*

3. **Data collection:**
   - What is the experimental procedure? *Ten male and ten female healthy college students were placed in pairs in the climate chamber with experimentally controlled temperatures, relative humidity levels, and air speeds over a period of one hour, during which time skin temperatures at eight different points on the body were measured. Participants also filled out identical questionnaires about thermal and air movement sensations as well as environmental expectations every ten minutes.*
   - What is the experiment apparatus and the measurement device? *Participants sat in the thermally insulated Climate Chamber at a table wearing light clothing 1.5 m from the air vents with thermocouples attached to the skin, which sampled temperatures at a rate of 2 Hz. "During the test, the physical parameters including air temperature, relative humidity, black-bulb temperature around the subjects were measured by Thermal Comfort Monitoring Station instrument (Accuracy: air temperature: ±0.2 °C, relative humidity: ±2%, globe bulb temperature: ±0.15 °C). The instrument was placed 1.5m far from the supply-air outlet and the probe was at a height of 0.6m above the floor and 0.5m away from subjects. Data were recorded every 10 min and exported after experiments. To measure the air velocity accurately, the Air Distribution Measuring System (accuracy: ±0.02 m/s ± 1% reading data) was used with a sampling interval of 0.1/s."*

4. **Data analysis:**
   - What are the independent and dependent variables in the stated equations? *Independent variables include room temperature, relative humidity, air speed, and clothing thermal factors. Dependent variables include the 8-point skin temperatures used to calculate the Mean Skin Temperature, that and other variables to calculate total heat loss from the skin, as well as the questionnaire responses to gauge Thermal Sensation, Air Movement Sensation, and Environmental Expectation (the latter meaning basically "are you comfortable, too cold, or too hot?").*
   - What descriptive statistics are used? *Means and standard deviations of the independent variables as well as skin temperatures were calculated.*

5. **Data presentation:**
   - Are there figures showing the apparatus? How do these relate to the data? *Yes, the figure showing the Climate Chamber explains the control and verifying measurements of the independent variables.*
   - Are there tables or graphs? If so, what quantities/units are shown? What trends are evident? *Tables show the experimental conditions and participants' characteristics. Graphs show the objectively measured mean skin temperature as a function of environment temperature (in °C) and air speed (in m/s), the subjective questionnaire values of mean thermal sensation and air movement sensation as functions of temperature and air speed, and a linear fit between mean thermal sensation and calculated heat loss from the skin (in W/m^2). Some trends are subtle, but the most obvious and interesting include that participants felt cooler with greater air speed, except at 34 °C, where faster air speed created a warmer sensation, and that heat loss from skin is negatively correlated with sensation of warmth. The latter is not surprising (a person should feel cooler if they are losing more heat), but does at least confirm that thermal sensation is not arbitrary.*
   - What do these reveal about the significance of the findings? *Though the differences are not statistically significant (see $p > 0.05$ in Figure 4), it does seem that faster air speed is not always correlated with a sensation of cooling.*

6. **Conclusions/hypotheses:**
   - How does the research answer the research questions? *The data show that there are limits to the usefulness of air movement to create comfort in warm and hot office environments for sedentary workers. The authors derive an empirical relation between heat loss from the skin—which correlates to thermal sensation—and temperature and air speed, which provides the possibility of optimizing the work environment for certain initial conditions.*
   - What does it not answer, and how do the authors acknowledge its limitations? *The experimental conditions (size of the space, lack of interior temperature variation) could limit the validity of the empirically derived equations relating skin heat loss and thermal sensation to environment temperature and air speed. Skin heat loss was not directly measured but based upon an extant equation that relies on a number of assumptions about human anatomy and physiology, as well as the clothing characteristics.*
   - Are there any unacknowledged limitations you can see? *The sample size is both small and fairly uniform: it may well be, for example, that an older cohort would report quite different thermal sensations.*

7. **Assumptions:**
   - What do the authors implicitly or explicitly take as given in the ways they design their research, interpret their data, or argue for the significance of their findings? *Apart from the direct measurements of mean skin temperature, the authors do not measure any of the characteristics related to skin heat loss, thus presuming that the hypothetical human model underlying the borrowed equation is accurate for their participants. The authors also use a fairly crude instrument to measure people's perceptions of thermal sensation and air movement. The fact that they use these questionnaire data in the same way they use objectively measured or calculated data requires significant assumptions that, for example, participants understood the questions and rating scale in the same way as the authors and each other, and that their answers were not influenced by the artificial conditions. When they derive empirical formulas relating skin heat loss and thermal sensation, these assumptions compound.*

- Do these assumptions seem justified, given your knowledge of the underlying science? *The heat loss equation begins from sound principles in counting loss by two modes of heat transfer and one of heat and mass transfer (evaporation), but it's difficult to accept completely without more explanation the multi-term expansion of equation 2. The assumption of a "mean human" in terms of thermal sensations and preferences seems a stretch without knowing more about the range of human responses to heat and wind.*

Chapter 8
Fluids and Elasticity
of Solids

8.1 HYDROSTATICS: FLUIDS AT REST

In this section and the next, we'll discuss some of the fundamental concepts dealing with substances that can flow, which are known as **fluids**. *Both liquids and gases are fluids*, but there are distinctions between them. At the molecular level, a substance in the liquid phase is similar to one in the solid phase in that the molecules are close to, and interact with, one another. The molecules in a liquid are able to move around a little more freely than those in a solid, in which the molecules typically only vibrate around relatively fixed positions. By contrast, the molecules of a gas are not constrained and fly around in a chaotic swarm, with hardly any interaction. On a macroscopic level, there is another distinction between liquids and gases. If you pour a certain volume of a liquid into a container of a greater volume, the liquid will occupy its original volume, whatever the shape and size of the container. However, if you introduce a sample of gas into a container, the molecules will fly around and fill the *entire* container.

Density and Specific Gravity

The **density** of a substance is the amount of mass contained in a unit of volume. In SI units, density is usually expressed in kg/m^3 or g/cm^3.

$$\text{density} = \frac{\text{mass}}{\text{volume}}$$

$$\rho = \frac{m}{V}$$

There is one substance whose density you should memorize: The density of liquid water is taken to be $1000 \ kg/m^3$ or $1 \ g/cm^3$. (Another useful version of the same value: $1 \ kg/L$, where L stands for a liter; a liter is $1000 \ cm^3$.)

Sometimes the MCAT mentions **specific gravity**. This (poorly named) unitless number tells us how dense something is compared to water:

$$\text{specific gravity} = \frac{\text{density of substance}}{\text{density of water}}$$

$$\text{sp. gr.} = \frac{\rho}{\rho_{H_2O}}$$

For solids, density doesn't change much with surrounding pressure or temperature. For example, the density of marble is pretty close to 2700 kg/m³ under most conditions. Liquids behave the same way: the density of water is pretty close to 1000 kg/m³ under all conditions at which it's a liquid. However, the density of a gas changes markedly with pressure and temperature. (The ideal gas law tells us that $PV = nRT$, so the density of a sample of an ideal gas is given by the equation $\rho_{gas} = m/V = mP/nRT$, which depends on P and T.)

Example 8-1: Turpentine has a specific gravity of 0.9. What is the density of this liquid?

Solution: By definition, we have

$$\rho_{turpentine} = (sp.\ gr._{turpentine})(\rho_{H_2O}) = (0.9)(1000\tfrac{kg}{m^3}) = 900\tfrac{kg}{m^3}$$

Example 8-2: A 2 cm³ sample of osmium, one of the densest substances on Earth, has a mass of 45 g. What's the specific gravity of this metal?

Solution: The density of osmium is

$$\rho = \frac{m}{V} = \frac{45\ g}{2\ cm^3} = 22.5\tfrac{g}{cm^3}$$

Since this is 22.5 times the density of water (which is 1 g/cm³), the specific gravity of osmium is 22.5.

Example 8-3: A cork has volume of 4 cm³ and weighs 0.01 N. What is its density? What is its specific gravity?

Solution: Because the cork weighs 10^{-2} N, its mass is

$$m = \frac{w}{g} = \frac{10^{-2}\ N}{10\ \tfrac{N}{kg}} = 10^{-3}\ kg$$

Therefore, its density is

$$\rho_{cork} = \frac{m}{V} = \frac{10^{-3}\ kg}{4\ cm^3} \times \left(\frac{10^2\ cm}{1\ m}\right)^3 = \tfrac{1}{4} \times 10^3\ \tfrac{kg}{m^3} = 2.5 \times 10^2\ \tfrac{kg}{m^3}$$

and its specific gravity is

$$sp.\ gr._{cork} = \frac{\rho_{cork}}{\rho_{H_2O}} = \frac{\tfrac{1}{4} \times 10^3\ \tfrac{kg}{m^3}}{10^3\ \tfrac{kg}{m^3}} = \tfrac{1}{4} = 0.25$$

Force of Gravity for Fluids

When solving questions involving fluids, it is often handy to know how to find the force of gravity acting on the fluid itself or objects that are immersed in the fluid. In previous chapters, we have used $F_{grav} = mg$ without too much difficulty. However, with fluids, it is more difficult to remove a portion of fluid from a tank, place it on a scale, and find its mass. Using the relationship between mass, volume, and density, we can redefine the magnitude of F_{grav} for fluids questions:

$$\rho = \frac{m}{V} \rightarrow m = \rho V \rightarrow \therefore F_{grav} = mg = \rho V g$$

With this new formula $F_{grav} = \rho V g$, it is important to make sure that the density (ρ) and the volume (V) describe the properties of the correct object or fluid.

Pressure

If we place an object in a fluid, the fluid exerts a contact force on the object. If we look at how that force is *distributed* over any small area of the object's surface, we have the concept of **pressure**:

Pressure

$$P = \frac{\text{force}_\perp}{\text{area}} = \frac{F_\perp}{A}$$

The subscript $\perp$ (which means "perpendicular") indicates that pressure is defined as the magnitude of the force acting *perpendicular* to the surface, divided by the area. We don't need to worry very much about this, because (for MCAT purposes) at any given point in a fluid the pressure is the same in all directions, which means that the force does not depend on the orientation of the force.

Although the formula for pressure involves "force," pressure is actually a *scalar* quantity, because the perpendicular force is the same for all orientations of surface. The unit of pressure is the N/m^2, which is called a **pascal** (abbreviated **Pa**). Because 1 N is a pretty small force and 1 m^2 is a pretty big area, 1 Pa is very small. Often, you'll see pressure expressed in kPa (or even in MPa). For example, at sea level, normal atmospheric pressure is about 100 kPa.

Let's imagine we have a tank of water with a lid on top. Suspended from the lid is a string attached to a thin metal sheet. The figures on the following page show you two views of this.

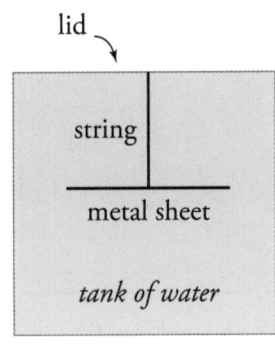

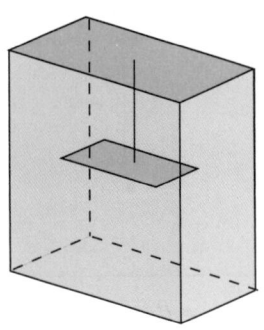

front view   side corner view

The weight of the water above the metal sheet produces a force that pushes down on the sheet. If we divide this force by the area of the sheet, w/A, we get the pressure, due to the water, on the sheet. The formula for calculating this pressure depends on the density of the fluid in the tank (ρ_{fluid}), the depth of the sheet (D), and the acceleration due to gravity (g).

$$P = \frac{w_{\text{fluid}}}{A} = \frac{m_{\text{fluid}}g}{A} = \frac{\rho_{\text{fluid}}V_{\text{fluid}}g}{A} = \frac{\rho_{\text{fluid}}ADg}{A} = \rho_{\text{fluid}}Dg$$

Hydrostatic Gauge Pressure

$$P_{\text{gauge}} = \rho_{\text{fluid}}gD$$

This formula gives the pressure due only to the fluid (in this case, the water) in the tank. This is called **hydrostatic gauge pressure**. It's called hydro*static*, because the fluid is at rest, and *gauge* pressure means that we don't take the pressure due to the atmosphere into account. If there were no lid on the water tank, then the water would be exposed to the atmosphere, and the *total* pressure at any point in the water would be equal to the atmospheric pressure pushing down on the surface *plus* the pressure due to the water (that is, the gauge pressure). So, below the surface, we'd have

$$P_{\text{total}} = P_{\text{atm}} + P_{\text{gauge}}$$

If the tank were closed to the atmosphere, but there were a layer of gas above the surface of the water, then the total pressure at a point below the surface would be the pressure of the gas pushing down at the surface plus the gauge pressure: $P_{\text{total}} = P_{\text{gas}} + P_{\text{gauge}}$. In general, we'll have

$$P_{\text{total}} = P_{\text{at surface}} + P_{\text{gauge}}$$

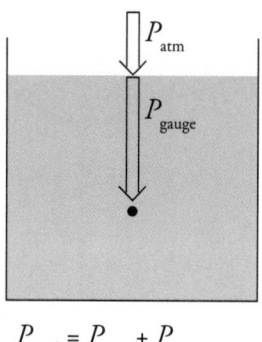

$$P_{\text{total}} = P_{\text{atm}} + P_{\text{gauge}}$$

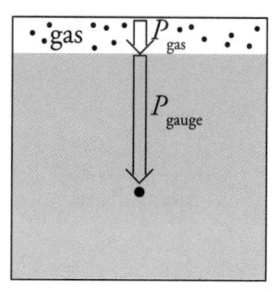

$$P_{\text{total}} = P_{\text{gas}} + P_{\text{gauge}}$$

in either case:

$$P_{\text{total}} = P_{\text{at surface}} + P_{\text{gauge}}$$

Notice that hydrostatic gauge pressure, $P_{\text{gauge}} = \rho_{\text{fluid}} g D$, is proportional to both the depth and the density of the fluid. *Total* pressure, however, is *not* proportional to either of these quantities if $P_{\text{on surface}}$ isn't zero.

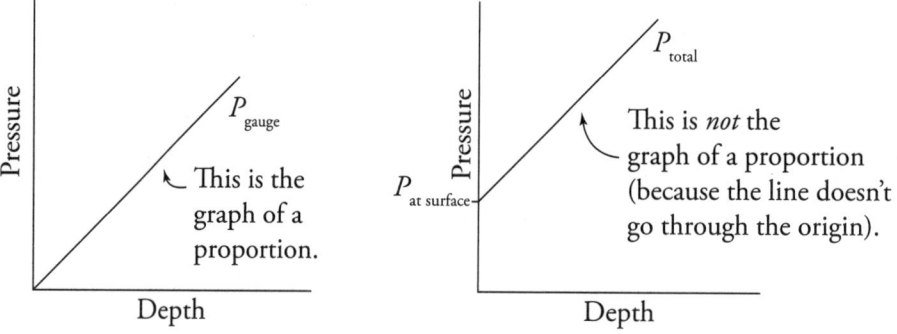

The lines in these graphs will be straight as long as the density of the liquid remains constant as the depth increases. Actually, ρ increases as the depth increases, but the effect is small enough that we generally consider liquids to be **incompressible**; that is, that the density of a liquid remains constant (so, in particular, the density doesn't increase with depth).

Example 8-4: The density of seawater is 1025 kg/m³. Consider a point X that's 10 m below the surface of the ocean.

    a)   What's the gauge pressure at X?

    b)   If the atmospheric pressure is 1.015×10^5 Pa, what is the total pressure at X?

    c)   Consider a point Y that's 50 m below the surface. How does the gauge pressure at Y compare to the gauge pressure at X? How does the total pressure at Y compare to the total pressure at X?

Solution:

    a)   The gauge pressure at X is

$$P_{gauge} = \rho_{fluid} gD = (1025\tfrac{kg}{m^3})(10\tfrac{N}{kg})(10 \text{ m}) = 1.025 \times 10^5 \text{ Pa}$$

    b)   The total pressure at X is the atmospheric pressure plus the gauge pressure:

$$P_{total\ at\ X} = P_{atm} + P_{gauge} = (1.015 \times 10^5 \text{ Pa}) + (1.025 \times 10^5 \text{ Pa}) = 2.04 \times 10^5 \text{ Pa}$$

    c)   Since P_{gauge} is proportional to D, an increase in D by a factor of 5 will mean the gauge pressure will also increase by a factor of 5. Therefore, the gauge pressure at Y will be $5(P_{gauge\ at\ X}) = 5.125 \times 10^5$ Pa. The total pressure at Y is equal to the atmospheric pressure plus the gauge pressure at Y, so

$$P_{total\ at\ Y} = P_{atm} + P_{gauge} = (1.015 \times 10^5 \text{ Pa}) + (5.125 \times 10^5 \text{ Pa}) = 6.14 \times 10^5 \text{ Pa}$$

Notice that $P_{total\ at\ Y}$ is not 5 times $P_{total\ at\ X}$. *Total* pressure is *not* proportional to depth.

Example 8-5: A large storage tank fitted with a tight lid holds a liquid. The space between the surface of the liquid and the lid of the tank is filled with molecules of the stored liquid in the gaseous phase. At a depth of 40 m, the total pressure is 520 kPa, while at a depth of 50 m, the total pressure is 600 kPa. What's the pressure of the gas above the surface of the liquid?

Solution: Let P_{gas} be the pressure that the gas exerts on the surface of the liquid. Then we have

$$P_{total\ at\ D_1 = 40\ m} = P_{gas} + \rho_{fluid} gD_1 = P_{gas} + \rho_{fluid} g(40 \text{ m}) = 520 \text{ kPa}$$
$$P_{total\ at\ D_1 = 50\ m} = P_{gas} + \rho_{fluid} gD_2 = P_{gas} + \rho_{fluid} g(50 \text{ m}) = 600 \text{ kPa}$$

We have two equations and two unknowns (P_{gas} and ρ_{fluid}). If we subtract the first equation from the second, we get $\rho_{fluid} g(10 \text{ m}) = 80 \text{ kPa}$, which tells us that $\rho_{fluid} g = 8\dfrac{\text{kPa}}{\text{m}}$. Plugging this back into either one of the equations will give us P_{gas}. Choosing, say, the first one, we find that

$$P_{gas} + \left(8\,\frac{\text{kPa}}{\text{m}}\right)(40 \text{ m}) = 520 \text{ kPa} \rightarrow P_{gas} = 200 \text{ kPa}$$

Example 8-6: The containers shown below are all filled with the same liquid. At which point (A, B, C, D, E, or F) is the gauge pressure the lowest?

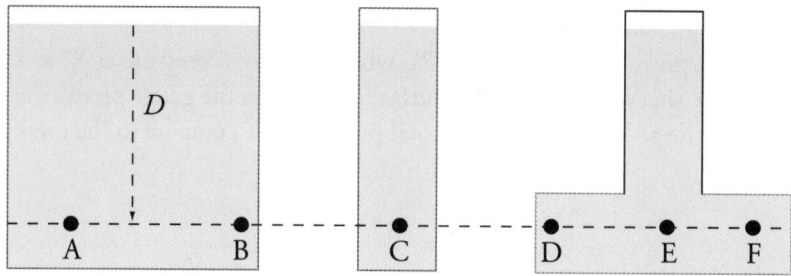

Solution: It's important to remember that the formula $P_{gauge} = \rho_{fluid}gD$ applies regardless of the shape of the container in which the fluid is held. If all the containers are filled with the same fluid, then the pressure is the *same* everywhere along the horizontal dashed line. This is because every point on this line (and within one of the containers) is at the same depth, D, below the surface of the fluid. The fact that the first container is wide, the second container is narrow, and the third container is wide at the base but has a narrow neck makes no difference. Even the fact that Points D and F (in the third container) aren't *directly* underneath a column of fluid of height D makes no difference.

Pressure is the magnitude of the force per area, so pressure is a *scalar*. Pressure has no direction. The force *due to the pressure* is a vector, however, and the direction of this force on any small surface is always perpendicular to that surface. For example, in the figure below, the pressure at Point A is the same as the pressure at Point B, because they're at the same depth. But, as you can see, the direction of the force due to the pressure varies depending on the orientation of the surface (and even which side of the surface) the force is pushing on.

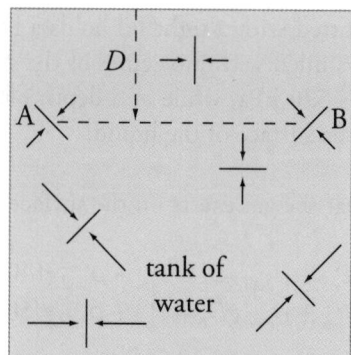

Buoyancy and Archimedes' Principle

Let's place a wooden block in our tank of water. Since the pressure on each side of the block depends on its average depth, we see that there's more pressure on the bottom of the block than there is on the top of it. Therefore, there's a greater force pushing up on the bottom of the block than there is pushing down on the top. The forces due to the pressure on the other four sides (left and right, front and back) cancel out, so the net fluid force on the block is upward. This net upward fluid force is called the **buoyant** force (or just **buoyancy** for short), which we'll denote by F_{Buoy} (or F_B).

We can calculate the magnitude of the buoyant force using Archimedes' principle:

> **Archimedes' Principle**
>
> *The magnitude of the buoyant force
> is equal to
> the weight of the fluid displaced by the object.*

When an object is partially or completely submerged in a fluid, the volume of the object that's submerged, which we call V_{sub}, is the volume of the fluid displaced.

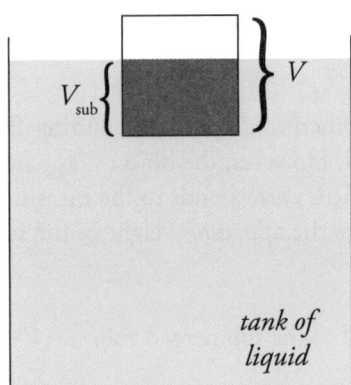

tank of liquid

By multiplying V_{sub} by the density of the fluid, we get the *mass* of the fluid displaced; then, multiplying this mass by g gives us the weight of the fluid displaced. So, here's Archimedes' principle as a mathematical equation:

> **Archimedes' Principle**
>
> $$F_{Buoy} = \rho_{fluid} V_{sub} g$$

When an object floats, its submerged volume is just enough to make the buoyant force it feels balance its weight. That is, for a floating object, we always have $w_{object} = F_{Buoy}$. If an object's density is ρ_{object} and its volume is V, its weight will be $\rho_{object} V_{object} g$. The buoyant force it feels is $\rho_{fluid} V_{sub} g$.

Setting these equal to each other, we find that

Floating Object in Equilibrium on Surface

$$w_{object} = F_{Buoy}$$

$$\frac{V_{sub}}{V} = \frac{\rho_{object}}{\rho_{fluid}}$$

So, if $\rho_{object} < \rho_{fluid}$, then the object will float; and the fraction of its volume that's submerged is the same as the ratio of its density to the fluid's density. *This is a very helpful fact to know for the MCAT.* For example, if the object's density is 3/4 the density of the fluid, then 3/4 of the object will be submerged (and vice versa).

If an object is denser than the fluid, then the object will sink. In this case, even if the entire object is submerged (in an attempt to maximize the buoyant force), the object's weight is still greater than the buoyant force. This leaves a net force in the downwards direction, causing the object to sink by accelerating downwards. If an object just happens to have the same density as the fluid, it will be happy hovering (in static equilibrium) underneath the fluid.

For an object that is completely submerged in the surrounding fluid, the actual weight of the object ($w_{object} = \rho_{object}Vg$) remains unchanged. However, the object's "apparent" weight is less due to the buoyant force "buoying" the object upwards. This corresponds to the measurement of a scale placed at the bottom of a tank of liquid in order to measure the apparent weight of the submerged object, or the normal force acting on the object.

Since the volume of the object is equal to the submerged volume ($V = V_{sub}$), the buoyant force F_{Buoy} on the object is equal to $\rho_{fluid}Vg$. Therefore,

$$\frac{w_{object}}{F_{Buoy}} = \frac{\rho_{object}Vg}{\rho_{fluid}Vg} = \frac{\rho_{object}}{\rho_{fluid}}$$

If the fluid in which the object is submerged is water, the ratio of the object weight to the buoyant force is equal to the specific gravity of the object.

Example 8-7: Ethyl alcohol has a specific gravity of 0.8. If a cork of specific gravity 0.25 floats in a beaker of ethyl alcohol, what fraction of the cork's volume is submerged?

    A. 4/25
    B. 1/5
    C. 1/4
    D. 5/16

Solution: Because the cork has a lower density than the ethyl alcohol, we know that the cork will float. Furthermore, the fraction of the cork's volume that will be submerged is

$$\frac{V_{sub}}{V} = \frac{\rho_{object}}{\rho_{fluid}} = \frac{(0.25)\rho_{H_2O}}{(0.8)\rho_{H_2O}} = \frac{0.25}{0.8} = \frac{\frac{1}{4}}{\frac{4}{5}} = \frac{5}{16}$$

Therefore, the answer is D.

Example 8-8: The density of ice is 920 kg/m^3, and the density of seawater is 1,025 kg/m^3. Approximately what percent of an iceberg floats above the surface of the ocean (in other words, how much is "the tip of the iceberg")?

A. 5%
B. 10%
C. 90%
D. 95%

Solution: Because the ice has a lower density than the seawater, we know that the iceberg will float. Furthermore, the fraction of the iceberg's volume that will be submerged is

$$\frac{V_{sub}}{V} = \frac{\rho_{object}}{\rho_{fluid}} = \frac{920 \frac{kg}{m^3}}{1025 \frac{kg}{m^3}} \approx \frac{900}{1000} = 90\%$$

However, the answer is not C. The question asked what percent of the iceberg floats *above* the surface. So, if 90% is submerged, then 10% is above the surface, and the answer is B. Watch for this kind of tricky wording; it is a common MCAT tactic.

Example 8-9: A glass sphere of specific gravity 2.5 and volume 10^{-3} m^3 is completely submerged in a large container of water. What is the apparent weight of the sphere while immersed?

Solution: Because the buoyant force pushes up on the object, the object's *apparent weight*, $w_{apparent} = w - F_{Buoy}$, is less than its true weight, w. Because the sphere is completely submerged, we have $V_{sub} = V$, so the buoyant force on the sphere is

$$
\begin{aligned}
F_{Buoy} &= \rho_{fluid} V_{sub} g \\
&= \rho_{H_2O} V g \\
&= (1000 \tfrac{kg}{m^3})(10^{-3} \text{ m}^3)(10 \tfrac{N}{kg}) \\
&= 10 \text{ N}
\end{aligned}
$$

The true weight of the glass sphere is

$$w = \rho_{glass}Vg$$

$$= (\text{sp. gr.}_{glass} \times \rho_{H_2O})Vg$$

$$= (2.5 \times 1000 \ \tfrac{kg}{m^3})(10^{-3} \ m^3)(10 \ \tfrac{N}{kg})$$

$$= 25 \ N$$

Therefore, the apparent weight of the sphere while immersed is

$$w_{apparent} = w - F_{Buoy} = 25 \ N - 10 \ N = 15 \ N$$

Example 8-10: One way of measuring a person's body fat percentage is by comparing his weight in air to his weight while completely submerged in water. The principle is that fat is less dense than water (sp. gr. = 0.94) whereas bone and other tissues (average sp. gr. = 1.1) are more dense than water. If someone weighs 1050 N when weighed in air and 50 N when weighed fully submerged (with as little air in the lungs as possible), approximately what is his body fat percentage?

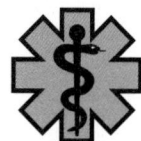

If the person has an apparent weight of 50 N when submerged, the buoyant force acting on him must be $w_{apparent} = w - F_B \rightarrow F_B = w - w_{apparent} = 1{,}050 \ N - 50 \ N = 1{,}000 \ N$. According to Archimedes' principle, the ratio of the man's weight to the buoyant force while completely submerged yields the ratio of his density to that of the fluid (in this case, water).

$$\frac{w}{F_B} = \frac{\rho_{man}}{1{,}000 \ kg/m^3} \rightarrow \frac{1{,}050 \ N}{1{,}000 \ N} = 1.05 = \frac{\rho_{man}}{1{,}000 \ kg/m^3} \rightarrow \rho_{man} = 1{,}050 \ kg/m^3$$

To achieve this density, the man must be some fraction of lean mass and the rest fat (note that we convert the given specific gravities of lean mass and fat to densities by multiplying by 1,000). Calling X the fraction of lean mass and omitting units for clarity:

$$1{,}100X + 940(1 - X) = 1{,}050 \rightarrow 1{,}100X - 940X = 160X = 110 \rightarrow X = \frac{110}{160} \approx \frac{2}{3}$$

Thus the man is about 70% lean mass and is 30% body fat mass.

Example 8-11: A balloon that weighs 0.18 N is then filled with helium so that its volume becomes 0.03 m³. (Note: The density of helium is 0.2 kg/m³.)

a) What is the net force on the balloon if it's surrounded by air? (Note: The density of air is 1.2 kg/m³.)

b) What will be the initial upward acceleration of the balloon if it's released from rest?

Solution:

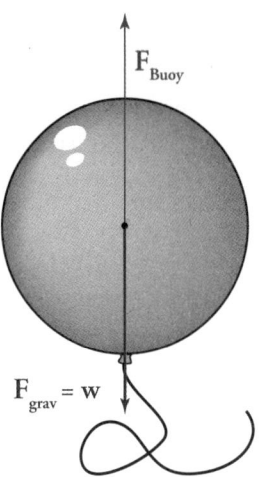

a) Remember that gases are fluids, so they also exert buoyant forces. If an object is immersed in a gas, the object experiences a buoyant force equal to the weight of the gas it displaces. In this case, the balloon is completely immersed in a "sea" of air (so $V_{sub} = V$), and Archimedes' principle tells us that the buoyant force on the balloon due to the surrounding air is

$$F_{Buoy} = \rho_{fluid} V_{sub} g$$
$$= \rho_{air} V g$$
$$= (1.2 \tfrac{kg}{m^3})(0.03 \text{ m}^3)(10 \tfrac{N}{kg})$$
$$= 0.36 \text{ N}$$

The weight of the inflated balloon is equal to the weight of the balloon material (0.18 N) plus the weight of the helium:

$$w_{total} = w_{material} + w_{helium}$$
$$= w_{material} + \rho_{helium} V g$$
$$= 0.18 \text{ N} + (0.2 \tfrac{kg}{m^3})(0.03 \text{ m}^3)(10 \tfrac{N}{kg})$$
$$= 0.18 \text{ N} + 0.06 \text{ N}$$
$$= 0.24 \text{ N}$$

Because $F_{Buoy} > w_{total}$, the net force on the balloon is upward and has magnitude
$$F_{net} = F_{Buoy} - w_{total} = (0.36 \text{ N}) - (0.24 \text{ N}) = 0.12 \text{ N}$$

b) Using Newton's second law, $a = F_{net} / m$ we find that

$$a = \frac{F_{net}}{m} = \frac{F_{net}}{\frac{w}{g}} = \frac{0.12 \text{ N}}{\left(\frac{0.24 \text{ N}}{10 \text{ m/s}^2}\right)} = \frac{(0.12 \text{ N}) \cdot (10 \text{ m/s}^2)}{0.24 \text{ N}} = \frac{10 \text{ m/s}^2}{2} = 5 \text{ m/s}^2$$

Pascal's Law

Pascal's law is a statement about fluid pressure. It says that a confined fluid will transmit an externally applied pressure change to all parts of the fluid and the walls of the container without loss of magnitude. In less formal language, if you squeeze a container of fluid, the fluid will transmit your squeeze perfectly throughout the container. The most important application of Pascal's law is to hydraulics.

Consider a simple hydraulic jack consisting of two pistons resting above two cylindrical vessels of fluid that are connected by a pipe. If you push down on one piston, the other one will rise. Let's make this more precise. Let F_1 be the magnitude of the force you exert down on one piston (whose cross-sectional area is A_1) and let F_2 be the magnitude of the force that the other piston (cross-sectional area A_2) exerts upward as a result.

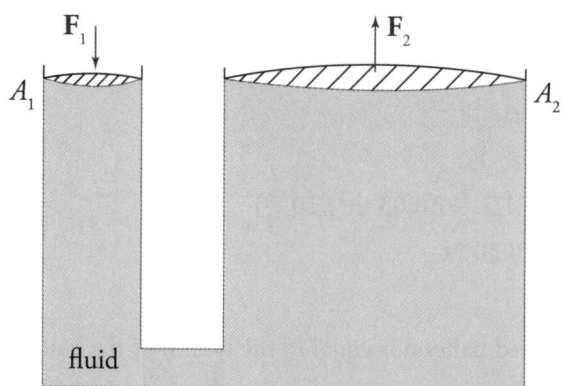

Pushing down on the left-hand piston with a force F_1 introduces a pressure increase of F_1 / A_1. Pascal's law tells us that this pressure change is transmitted, without loss of magnitude, by the fluid to the other end. Since the pressure change at the other piston is F_1 / A_1, we have, by Pascal's law,

$$\frac{F_1}{A_1} = \frac{F_2}{A_2}$$

Solving this equation for F_2, we get

$$F_2 = \frac{A_2}{A_1} F_1$$

So, if A_2 is greater than A_1 (as it is in the figure), then the ratio of the areas, A_2 / A_1, will be greater than 1, so F_2 will be greater than F_1; that is, *the output force, F_2, is greater than your input force, F_1*. This is why hydraulic jacks are useful; we end up lifting something very heavy (a car, for example) by exerting a much smaller force (one that would be insufficient to lift the car if it were just applied directly to the car).

This seems too good to be true; doesn't this violate some conservation law? No, since there's no such thing as a "Conservation of Force" law. However, there *is* a price to be paid for the magnification of the force. Let's say you push the left-hand piston down by a distance d_1, and that the distance the right-hand piston moves upward is d_2. Assuming the fluid is incompressible, whatever fluid you push out of the left-hand cylinder must appear in the right-hand cylinder. Since volume is equal to cross-sectional area times distance, the volume of the fluid you push out of the left-hand cylinder is $A_1 d_1$, and the extra volume of fluid that appears in the right-hand cylinder is $A_2 d_2$.

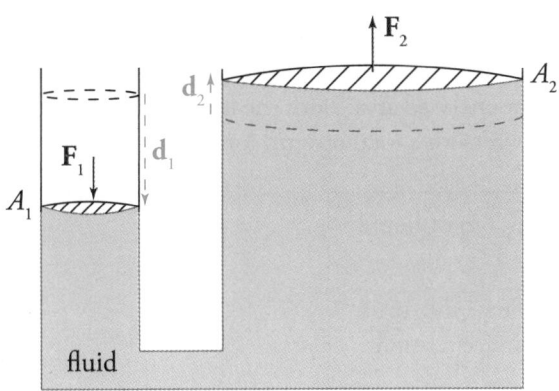

But these volumes have to be the same, so $A_1 d_1 = A_2 d_2$. Solving this equation for d_2, we get

$$d_2 = \frac{A_1}{A_2} d_1$$

If the area of the right-hand piston (A_2) is greater than the area of the left-hand piston (A_1), the ratio A_1 / A_2 will be *less* than 1, so d_2 will be less than d_1. In fact, the decrease in d is the same as the increase in F. For example, if A_2 is five times larger than A_1, then F_2 will be five times greater than F_1, but d_2 will only be *one-fifth* of d_1. We can now see that the product of F and d will be the same for both pistons:

$$F_2 d_2 = \left(\frac{A_2}{A_1} F_1 \right) \cdot \left(\frac{A_1}{A_2} d_1 \right) = F_1 d_1$$

Recall that the product of F and d is the amount of work done. What we have shown is that the work you do pushing the left-hand piston down is equal to the work done by the right-hand piston as it pushes upward. Just as when we discussed simple machines and mechanical advantage in Chapter 6, we can't cheat when it comes to work. True, we can do the same job with less force, but we will always pay for that by having to exert that smaller force through a greater distance. This is the whole idea behind all simple machines, not just a hydraulic jack.

Surface Tension

To complete our section on fluids at rest, we introduce the phenomenon of **surface tension**. We have all seen long-legged bugs that can walk on the surface of a pond or have watched a slowly-leaking faucet form a drop of water that grows until it finally drops into the sink. Both of these are illustrations of surface tension. The surface of a fluid can behave like an elastic membrane or thin sheet of rubber. A liquid will form a drop because the surface tends to contract into a sphere (to minimize surface area); however, when you see a drop hanging precariously from a faucet, its spherical shape is distorted by the pull of gravity. In fact, the reason it eventually falls into the sink is that the force due to surface tension causing the drop to cling to the head of the faucet is overwhelmed by the increasing weight of the drop. It can't hang on, and away it goes.

A standard way to define the surface tension is as follows. Imagine a rectangular loop of thin wire with one side able to slide up and down freely, thereby changing the enclosed area. If this apparatus is dipped into a fluid, a thin film will form in the enclosed area. Both the front face and the back face of the film are pulling upward on the free horizontal wire with a total upward force **F** against the wire's weight.

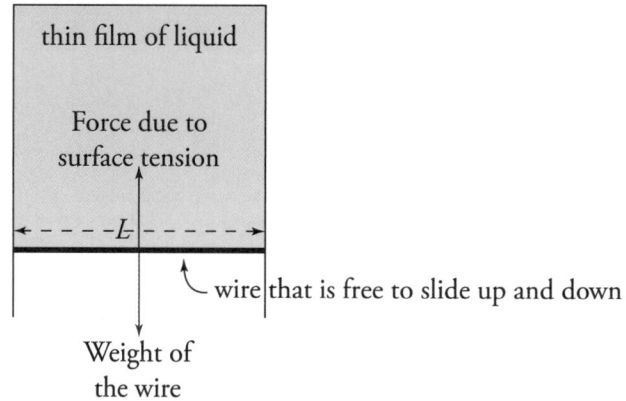

The strength of the surface tension force depends on the particular liquid and is determined by the *coefficient of surface tension*, γ, which is the force per unit length. Since there are *two* surfaces here (the front and the back), each of which acts along a length L, the force F due to surface tension acts along a total length of $2L$. The coefficient of surface tension is defined to be $\gamma = F/2L$, so $F_{\text{surf tension}} = 2\gamma L$. To give you an idea of the values of γ, the surface tension coefficient of water is 0.07 N/m at room temperature (and decreases as the temperature increases). A fluid with one of the highest surface tension coefficients is mercury. Its surface tension coefficient is nearly seven times greater than that of water: $\gamma_{\text{Hg}} = 0.46$ N/m at room temperature. Note that these values are really quite small. The surface of a pond of water can support the weight of a bug, but a frog isn't about to walk across the pond supported by surface tension.

8.2 HYDRODYNAMICS: FLUIDS IN MOTION

Flow Rate and the Continuity Equation

Consider a pipe through which fluid is flowing. The **flow rate**, f, is the volume of fluid that passes a particular point per unit time, like how many liters of water per minute are coming out of a faucet. In SI units, flow rate is expressed in m³/s. To find the flow rate, all we need to do is multiply the cross-sectional area of the pipe at any point, A, by the average speed of the flow, v, at that point:

Flow Rate

$$f = Av$$

Be careful not to confuse flow rate with flow speed; flow rate tells us how *much* fluid flows per unit time; flow speed tells us how *fast* the fluid moves. There's a difference between saying that a hose ejects 4 liters of water every second (that's flow rate) and saying that the water leaves the hose at a speed of 4 m/s (that's flow speed).

If a pipe is carrying a liquid, which we assume is **incompressible** (that is, its density remains constant), then the flow rate must be the same everywhere along the pipe. Choose any two points in a flow tube carrying a liquid, Point 1 and Point 2. If there aren't any sources or sinks between these points (i.e., no leaks and no additional liquid), then the liquid that flows by Point 1 must also flow by Point 2, and vice versa. In other words, $f_1 = f_2$, or, since $f = Av$, we get $A_1 v_1 = A_2 v_2$; this is called the

---

Continuity Equation

$$A_1 v_1 = A_2 v_2$$

This tells us that when the tube narrows, the flow speed will increase; and if the tube widens, the flow speed will decrease. In fact, we can say that the flow speed is inversely proportional to the cross-sectional area (or to the square of the radius) of the pipe.

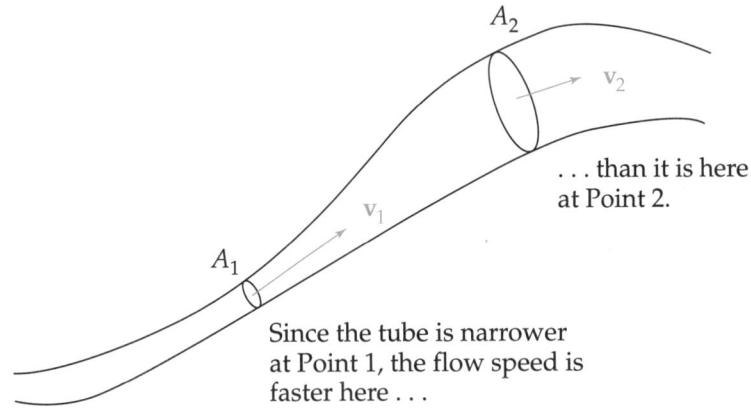

A_2

v_2

. . . than it is here
at Point 2.

A_1

v_1

Since the tube is narrower
at Point 1, the flow speed is
faster here . . .

Example 8-12: In the pipe shown above, if $A_2 = 9A_1$, then which of the following will be true?

A. $v_1 = 9v_2$
B. $v_1 = 3v_2$
C. $v_2 = 9v_1$
D. $v_2 = 3v_1$

Solution: If the cross-sectional area at Point 2 is 9 times the cross-sectional area at Point 1, then the flow speed at Point 2 will be 1/9 the flow speed at Point 1. That is, $v_2 = v_1 / 9$, or, solving for v_1, we get $v_1 = 9v_2$ (choice A).

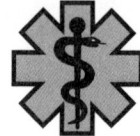

Example 8-13: Before using a hypodermic needle to inject medication into a patient, a nurse tests the needle by shooting a small amount of the liquid into the air. The barrel of the needle is 1 cm in diameter, and the tip is 1 mm in diameter. If the nurse pushes the piston with a speed of 2 cm/s, how fast does the liquid come out the tip?

    A.   4 cm/s
    B.   20 cm/s
    C.   40 cm/s
    D.   200 cm/s

Solution: Cross-sectional area is proportional to the square of the diameter of the flow tube. In this case, the diameter decreases by a factor of 10 (from 1 cm to 1 mm), so the cross-sectional area decreases by a factor of $10^2 = 100$. Now, according to the continuity equation, if A decreases by a factor of 100, then v increases by a factor of 100. Therefore, the speed of the liquid coming out of the tip is $100 \times (2 \text{ cm/s}) = 200$ cm/s, choice D.

Example 8-14: A pipe of nonuniform diameter carries water. At one point in the pipe, the radius is 2 cm and the flow speed is 6 m/s.

    a)   What's the flow rate?
    b)   What's the flow speed at a point where the pipe constricts to a radius of 1 cm?

Solution:

    a)   At any point, the flow rate, f, is equal to the cross-sectional area of the pipe multiplied by the flow speed; therefore,

$$f = Av = \pi r^2 v = \pi (2 \times 10^{-2} \text{ m})^2 (6 \text{ m/s}) \approx 75 \times 10^{-4} \text{ m}^3/\text{s} = 7.5 \times 10^{-3} \text{ m}^3/\text{s}$$

    b)   By the continuity equation, we know that v, the flow speed, is inversely proportional to A, the cross-sectional area of the pipe. If the pipe's radius decreases by a factor of 2 (from 2 cm to 1 cm), A decreases by a factor of 4 because A is proportional to r^2. If A decreases by a factor of 4, then v will increase by a factor of 4. So, the flow speed at a point where the pipe's radius is 1 cm will be $4 \times (6 \text{ m/s}) = 24$ m/s.

Bernoulli's Equation

The most important equation in fluid dynamics is Bernoulli's equation, but before we state it, it's important to know under what conditions it applies. Bernoulli's equation applies to **ideal fluid** flow. A fluid must satisfy the following four requirements in order to be considered an ideal fluid:

- *The fluid is incompressible.*
  This works very well for liquids; gases are quite compressible, but it turns out that we can use the Bernoulli equation for gases provided the pressure changes are small.

- *There is negligible viscosity.*
  Viscosity is the force of cohesion between molecules in a fluid; think of it as internal friction for fluids. For example, maple syrup is more viscous than water, and there's more resistance to a flow of maple syrup than to a flow of water. (While Bernoulli's equation gives good results when applied to a flow of water, it would not give good results if it were applied to a flow of maple syrup.)

- *The flow is laminar.*
  In a tube carrying a flowing fluid, a *streamline* is just what it sounds like: a "line" in the stream. If we were to inject a drop of dye into a clear glass pipe carrying, say, water, we'd see a streak of dye in the pipe, indicating a streamline. The entire flow is called streamline (as an adjective) or laminar if the individual streamlines don't cross. When the flow is laminar, the fluid flows *smoothly* through the tube.

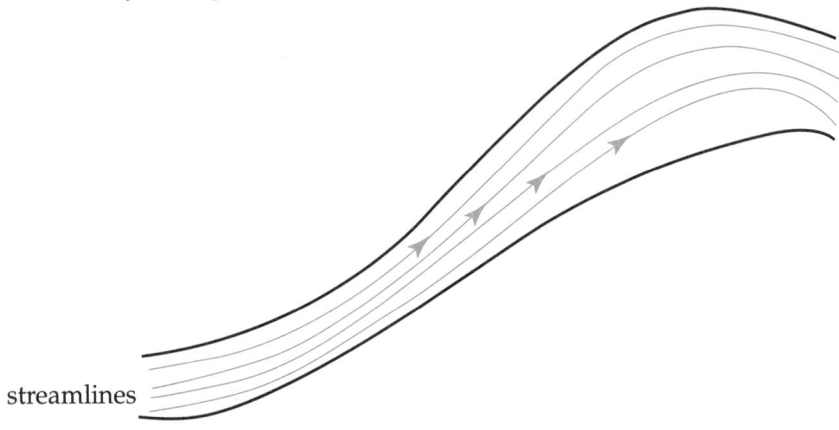

streamlines

The opposite of streamline flow is called **turbulent flow**. In this case, the flow is not smooth; it is chaotic (unpredictable). Turbulence is characterized by whirlpools and swirls (vortexes). At high enough speeds, all real fluids experience turbulent flow, and no simple equation can be applied to such a flow.

- *The flow rate is steady.*
  That is, the value of f is constant. If we're analyzing the water flowing through a garden hose connected to a faucet sticking out of the side of the house, turn the faucet handle to a particular setting and then leave it there. The flow rate through the hose must be steady while we're taking our measurements.

If these conditions hold—(1) the fluid is incompressible, (2) the flow is smooth (laminar), (3) there's no friction (viscosity), and (4) the flow rate is steady—then total mechanical energy will be conserved. *Bernoulli's equation is the statement of conservation of total mechanical energy for ideal fluid flow.* On the MCAT, you will often be told to consider a fluid to be ideal, allowing you to use Bernoulli's equation.

Bernoulli's Equation

$$P_1 + \tfrac{1}{2}\rho v_1^2 + \rho g y_1 = P_2 + \tfrac{1}{2}\rho v_2^2 + \rho g y_2$$

In this equation, ρ is the density of the flowing fluid, P_1 and P_2 give the pressures at any two points along a streamline within the flow, v_1 and v_2 give the flow speeds at these points, and y_1 and y_2 give the heights of these points above some chosen horizontal reference level.

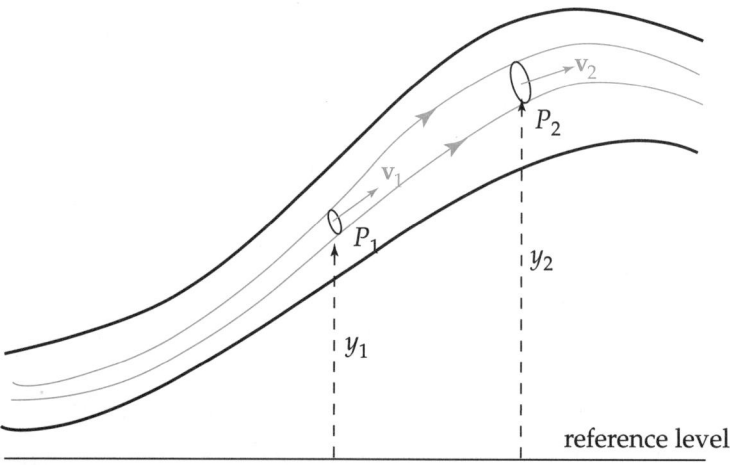

Although the equation may look complicated, notice that the two sides are the same, except all the subscripts on the left-hand side are 1's while all the subscripts on the right-hand side are 2's. Also, each $\dfrac{1}{2}\rho v_1^2$ term looks very much like the kinetic energy (sometimes it's referred to as kinetic energy density), and each term $\rho g y$ looks very much like gravitational potential energy. So, just take the equation you already know for conservation of total mechanical energy, $KE_1 + PE_1 = KE_2 + PE_2$, change the m's to ρ's, add P to both sides, and you've got Bernoulli's equation.

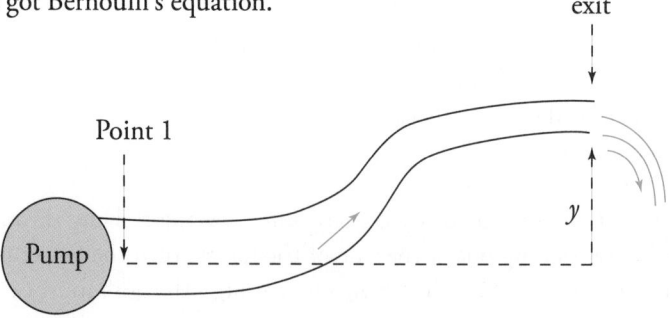

Example 8-15: In the figure above, a pump forces water at a constant flow rate through a pipe whose cross-sectional area, A, gradually decreases. At the exit point, A has decreased to 1/3 its value at the beginning of the pipe. If $y = 60$ cm and the flow speed of the water just after it leaves the pump (Point 1 in the figure) is 1 m/s, what is the gauge pressure at Point 1?

Solution: We'll apply Bernoulli's equation to Point 1 and the exit point, which we'll call Point 2. We'll choose the level of Point 1 as our horizontal reference level; this makes $y_1 = 0$. Now, because the cross-sectional area of the pipe decreases by a factor of 3 between Points 1 and 2, the flow speed must increase by a factor of 3; that is, $v_2 = 3v_1$. Since the pressure at Point 2 is P_{atm}, Bernoulli's equation becomes

$$P_1 + \tfrac{1}{2}\rho v_1^2 = P_{atm} + \tfrac{1}{2}\rho v_2^2 + \rho g y_2$$

This tells us that

$$
\begin{aligned}
P_1 - P_{atm} &= \rho g y_2 + \tfrac{1}{2}\rho v_2^2 - \tfrac{1}{2}\rho v_1^2 \\
&= \rho g y_2 + \tfrac{1}{2}\rho (3v_1)^2 - \tfrac{1}{2}\rho v_1^2 \\
&= \rho(g y_2 + 4v_1^2) \\
&= (1000\ \tfrac{kg}{m^3})[(10\ m/s^2)(0.6\ m) + 4(1\ m/s)^2]
\end{aligned}
$$

$$\therefore P_{gauge\ at\ 1} = 10^4\ Pa$$

Imagine that we punch a small hole in the side of a tank of liquid. We can use Bernoulli's equation to figure out the *efflux speed,* that is, how fast the liquid will flow out of the hole.

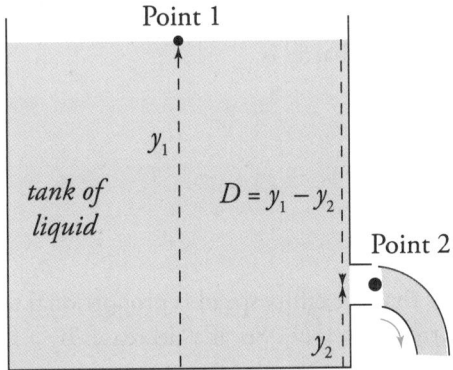

Let the bottom of the tank be our horizontal reference level, and choose Point 1 to be at the surface of the liquid and Point 2 to be at the hole where the water shoots out. First, the pressure at Point 1 is at atmospheric pressure; and the emerging stream at Point 2 is open to the air, so it's at atmospheric pressure, too. Therefore, $P_1 = P_2$, and these terms cancel out of Bernoulli's equation. Next, since the area at Point 1 is so much greater than at Point 2, we can assume that v_1, the speed at which the water level in the tank drops, is much lower than v_2, the speed at which the water shoots out of the hole. (Remember that by the continuity equation, $A_1 v_1 = A_2 v_2$; since $A_1 \gg A_2$, we'll have $v_1 \ll v_2$.) Because $v_1 \ll v_2$, we can say that $v_1 \approx 0$ and ignore v_1 in this case. So, Bernoulli's equation becomes

$$\rho g y_1 = \tfrac{1}{2}\rho v_2^2 + \rho g y_2$$

Crossing out the ρ's, and rearranging, we get

$$\frac{1}{2}v_2^2 = g(y_1 - y_2)$$
$$= gD$$
$$v_2 = \sqrt{2gD}$$

That is, $v_{\text{efflux}} = \sqrt{2gD}$, where D is the distance from the surface of the liquid down to the hole. This is called **Torricelli's result**. This equation should look familiar; it's basically the same formula that tells us how fast an object is going after it has fallen a distance h from rest.

Example 8-16: The side of an above-ground pool is punctured, and water gushes out through the hole. If the total depth of the pool is 2.5 m, and the puncture is 1 m above ground level, what is the efflux speed of the water?

Solution: We apply Torricelli's result, $v = \sqrt{2gD}$, where D is the distance from the surface of the pool down to the hole. If the puncture is 1 m above ground level, then it's $2.5 - 1 = 1.5$ m below the surface of the water (because the pool is 2.5 m deep). Therefore, the efflux speed will be

$$v = \sqrt{2gD} = \sqrt{2(10 \text{ m/s}^2)(1.5 \text{ m})} = \sqrt{30 \text{ m/s}^2} \approx 5.5 \text{ m/s}$$

Example 8-17: A hole is opened at the bottom of a full barrel of liquid. When the efflux speed has decreased to 1/2 the initial efflux speed, the barrel is:

A. 1/4 full
B. $1/\sqrt{2}$ full
C. 1/2 full
D. 3/4 full

Solution: Torricelli's result tells us that the efflux speed is proportional to the square root of the height to the surface of the liquid in the barrel: $v \propto \sqrt{D}$. So, if v decreases by a factor of 2, then D has decreased by a factor of 4, and the answer is A.

Example 8-18: What does Bernoulli's equation tell us about a fluid at rest in a container open to the atmosphere?

Solution: Consider the figure below:

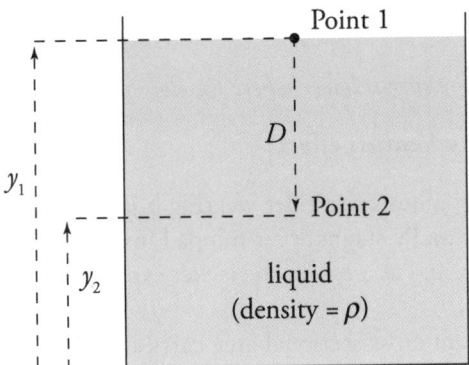

Because the fluid in the tank is at rest, both v_1 and v_2 are zero, and Bernoulli's equation becomes

$$P_1 + \rho g y_1 = P_2 + \rho g y_2$$

Since $P_1 = P_{atm}$, if we solve this equation for P_2, we get

$$P_2 = P_{atm} + \rho g(y_1 - y_2) = P_{atm} + \rho g D$$

which is the same formula we found earlier for hydrostatic pressure.

The Bernoulli or Venturi Effect

Consider the two points labeled in the pipe shown below:

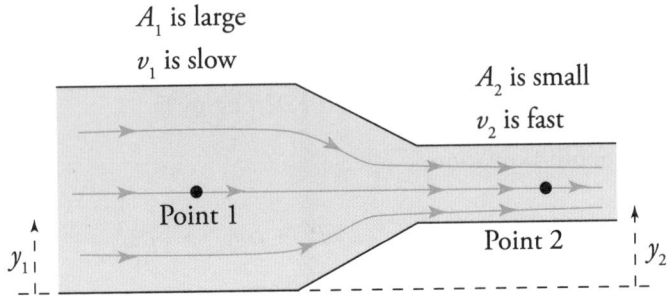

Since the heights y_1 and y_2 are equal in this case, the terms in Bernoulli's equation that involve the heights will cancel, leaving us with

$$P_1 + \tfrac{1}{2}\rho v_1^2 = P_2 + \tfrac{1}{2}\rho v_2^2$$

8.2

We already know from the continuity equation ($f = Av$) that the speed increases as the cross-sectional area of the pipe decreases. Since $A_2 < A_1$, we know that $v_2 > v_1$, and the equation above then tells us that $P_2 < P_1$. That is,

The pressure is lower where the flow speed is greater.[1]

This is known as the **Bernoulli** or **Venturi effect**.

You may have seen a skydiver or motorcycle rider wearing a jacket that seems to puff out as they move rapidly through the air. The essentially stagnant air trapped inside the jacket is at a much higher pressure than the air whizzing by outside, and as a result, the jacket expands outward.

Example 8-19: A pipe of constant cross-sectional area carries water at a constant flow rate from the hot-water tank in the basement of a house up to the second floor. Which of the following will be true?

A.   The speed at which the water arrives at the second floor must be lower than the speed at which it left the water tank.
B.   The speed at which the water arrives at the second floor must be greater than the speed at which it left the water tank.
C.   The water pressure at the second floor must be lower than the water pressure at the tank.
D.   The water pressure at the second floor must be greater than the water pressure at the tank.

Solution: Because the flow rate is constant and the cross-sectional area of the pipe is constant, the flow speed will be constant (this follows from the continuity equation, $f = Av = $ constant). This eliminates choices A and B. Now, if the flow speeds v_1 and v_2 are the same, Bernoulli's equation becomes

$$P_1 + \rho g y_1 = P_2 + \rho g y_2$$

Because $y_2 > y_1$, it must be true that $P_2 < P_1$ (choice C).

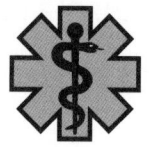

Example 8-20: In a healthy adult standing upright, blood pressure in the arms and legs should be roughly equal. Suppose the height difference between elbow and ankle is 1 m. If one assumes that blood is an ideal fluid flowing through smooth rigid pipes of equal diameter, what would be the pressure difference between the arm and leg (the density of blood is about 1,025 kg/m³)?

Solution: According to Bernoulli's equation,

$$P_{arm} + \rho g y_{arm} + \tfrac{1}{2}\rho v_{arm}^2 = P_{leg} + \rho g y_{leg} + \tfrac{1}{2}\rho v_{leg}^2$$

The question stem states that the diameter of the pipes (the arteries and veins) should be assumed constant, so according to the continuity equation, $v_{arm} = v_{leg}$. Thus we have

$$\Delta P = P_{leg} - P_{arm} = \rho g y_{arm} - \rho g y_{leg} = \rho g(y_{arm} - y_{leg})(1{,}025\ \text{kg/m}^3)(10\ \text{m/s}^2)(1\ \text{m}) = 10{,}250\ \text{Pa}$$

---

[1]   Note that this is not a *causal* statement: faster flow speed does not cause lower pressure. Indeed, as you should know from gases, a pressure gradient causes a force on a parcel of a fluid that accelerates the fluid toward the lower pressure, so if anything, that suggests that lower pressure along a streamline causes faster flow speed. Neither explanation captures the reality of fluid flow, which is complex beyond the scope of the exam. On the MCAT, it will suffice for you to associate faster fluid flow with lower pressure within a continuous ideal fluid. If other examples seem to violate this application of Bernoulli's law, keep in mind that this is a simplification only!

For reference, this is about 80 torr, a huge pressure difference compared to typical healthy values of 120/80 torr. Clearly this result is suspicious. There are several reasons why one cannot validly apply Bernoulli's equation to blood flow, including the fact that the heart is a pump (the flow is not under a constant pressure), the flexibility of the venous system, and the presence of valves in the circulatory system. However, one extremely important reason having to do with blood is its viscosity: blood is about 4 times more viscous than water (though the viscosity of blood varies depending upon several factors). This viscosity contributes to a resistance to flow, which leads to a pressure drop effect as blood gets further from the heart. One statement of *Poiseuille's law* for viscous fluid flow gives this pressure drop per unit length as

$$\frac{\Delta P}{L} = \frac{8\eta f}{\pi r^4}$$

where η is the viscosity coefficient of the fluid, f is flow rate, and r is the radius of the pipe.

8.3 THE ELASTICITY OF SOLIDS

Support beams for a building are compressed slightly under the heavy load they support; thick steel cables may be stretched in the construction of a bridge; and the ends of a connecting rod in a structure can be pushed or pulled in opposite directions, causing the rod to bend. These are some examples of the type of problem we'll look at in this section: the relationship between the forces applied to a solid object and the resulting change in the object's shape.

Stress

We'll look at three ways forces can be applied to an object: **tension** (stretching) forces, **compression** (squeezing) forces, and **shear** (bending) forces:

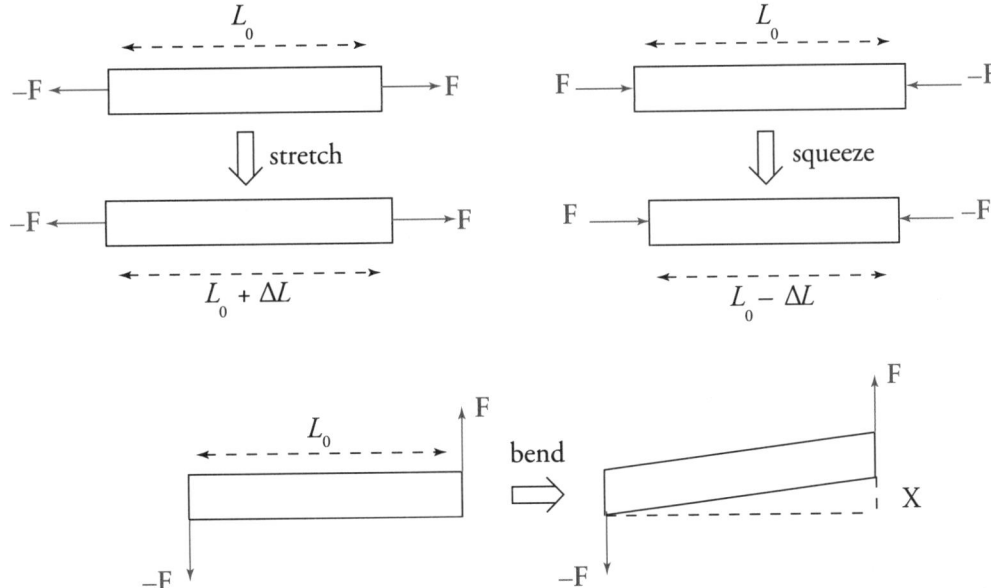

The magnitude of the force at either end, F, divided by the area over which it acts is called the **stress**:

Stress

$$\text{stress} = \frac{\text{force}}{\text{area}} = \frac{F}{A}$$

Stress is much like pressure, but they're not the same, because the force in the stress equation doesn't have to be perpendicular to the area over which it acts. For example, a shear force acts *parallel*, not perpendicular, to the areas at the ends. Nevertheless, we're still dividing a force by an area, so the unit of stress is the N/m^2, or pascal (Pa). It's *very important* to notice that stress is inversely proportional to the cross-sectional area, or, for an object with circular cross sections, inversely proportional to the *square* of the cross-sectional radius or diameter.

Strain

As a result of these forces, the object's shape will change. The ratio of the appropriate change in the length to the object's original length (see the figure above) is called the **strain**:

Strain

Tensile or Compressive

$$\text{strain} = \frac{\text{change in length}}{\text{original length}} = \frac{\Delta L}{L_0}$$

Shear Strain

$$\text{strain} = \frac{\text{distance of shear}}{\text{original length}} = \frac{X}{L_0}$$

The following mnemonic (though imprecise) may be helpful:

*St**ress** is p**ress**ure. Str**ain** is ch**ange**.*

Hooke's Law

The idea is simple: *Stress causes strain*. As long as the stress isn't too large—so that we don't permanently deform the object once the stress is removed (that is, allowing the object to display some *elasticity*)—then *stress and strain are proportional*. This is known as **Hooke's law**. For a tensile or compressive stress, the constant of proportionality is called **Young's modulus**; for a shear stress, it's called (what else?) the **shear**

modulus. The modulus depends on the type of material the object is made of; generally, the stronger the intermolecular bonds, the greater the modulus. A material's modulus can also depend on the type of stress the material is subjected to. For example, for the kind of steel used in building construction, the shear modulus is less than half its Young's modulus; this tells us that structural steel is weaker when subjected to shear forces than to tension or compression forces (that is, it's easier to bend steel than it is to stretch or compress it). It's even possible to have a Young's modulus for tension and a different one for compression. For example, human bone has two Young's moduli: The value of the modulus for compact bone under a tensile stress is about twice the value of the modulus for a compressive stress. Bone is more resistant to tension than to compression.

Hooke's Law

$$\text{stress} = \text{modulus} \times \text{strain}$$

Young's modulus is denoted by the letter Y or by E, while shear modulus is denoted by S or by G. Using E for Young's modulus (for tension and compression) and G for shear modulus, Hooke's law yields the following easy-to-remember formulas for tension/compression and for shear:

Tension/Compression

$$\frac{F}{A} = E\frac{\Delta L}{L_0}$$

$$\therefore \Delta L = \frac{FL_0}{EA}$$

Shear

$$\frac{F}{A} = G\frac{X}{L_0}$$

$$\therefore X = \frac{FL_0}{AG}$$

We call these the *Flea* and *Flag* formulas.

8.3

Example 8-21: A piece of rubber, originally 18 cm long, is stretched to a length of 20 cm. What strain has it undergone?

Solution: The change in length is $\Delta L = 20 \text{ cm} - 18 \text{ cm} = 2 \text{ cm}$. Therefore, the strain is

$$\frac{\Delta L}{L_0} = \frac{2 \text{ cm}}{18 \text{ cm}} = \frac{1}{9}$$

Example 8-22: What are the units of Young's modulus and the shear modulus?

Solution: Hooke's law says that stress = modulus × strain. Because strain has no units (we're dividing a length by a length), the units of the modulus must be the same as the units of stress: pascals.

Example 8-23: Two cylindrical rods with circular cross sections are identical except for the fact that Rod 2 has four times the diameter of Rod 1. If these two rods are subjected to identical compressive forces, how will the compression of Rod 2 compare to that of Rod 1?

Solution: First, the fact that Rod 2 has 4 times the diameter of Rod 1 means that Rod 2 has $4^2 = 16$ times the cross-sectional area. Therefore, if both rods experience identical compressive forces, the stress on Rod 2 will be 1/16 the stress on Rod 1 (because stress = force/area). Since the rods are made of the same material, their Young's moduli are the same, so, by Hooke's law, the strain on Rod 2 will be 1/16 the strain on Rod 1. Finally, because the rods had the same original length, the change in length of Rod 2 will be 1/16 of the change in length of Rod 1.

Example 8-24: Two objects are subjected to identical tensile stresses. The object with the greater value of Young's modulus will undergo:

    A. a smaller change in length.
    B. a greater change in length.
    C. less strain.
    D. greater strain.

Solution: Hooke's law says that stress = modulus × strain. If stress is a constant, then the strain is inversely proportional to the modulus. Therefore, the object with the greater value of Young's modulus will experience less strain (choice C). Notice that we can't say that choice A is correct, since we don't know the original lengths of the objects.

Example 8-25: Which material has the greater Young's modulus: rubber or glass?

Solution: Hooke's law says that stress = modulus × strain. Or, using the *Flea* formula, $\Delta L = FL_0 / EA$, and solving for E, we get $E = FL_0 / A\Delta L$. Now let's say we had a piece of glass and an identical piece of rubber: same original length, width, and height. If we apply the same force to both the glass and the rubber, which one will experience the greater change in length? The rubber, of course. Since E is *inversely* proportional to ΔL, we'd expect that E for rubber will be lower than E for glass. Or, equivalently, the value of E is greater for glass than for rubber. (In fact, the value of E for glass is nearly ten thousand times the value of E for rubber.) In general, the greater the value of E, the more difficult it is to stretch or compress the material; similarly, the greater the value of G (the shear modulus), the more difficult it is to bend the material.

Example 8-26: Two metal beams have the same length and cross-sectional area, but Beam X has twice the shear modulus of Beam Y. If each beam is subjected to the same shear forces, which beam will bend more and by what factor?

A. Beam X, by a factor of 2
B. Beam X, by a factor of 4
C. Beam Y, by a factor of 2
D. Beam Y, by a factor of 4

Solution: If the beams have the same cross-sectional area and are subjected to the same shear forces, the shear stress on the beams will be the same (since stress = force/area). By Hooke's law, then, the strain is inversely proportional to the modulus. If Beam X has twice the shear modulus, it will undergo 1/2 the strain. Since the beams had the same original length, Beam Y will bend more, by a factor of 2 (choice C).

Example 8-27: Hooke's law for a spring says that the magnitude of the force required to stretch or compress the spring from its natural length is given by the simple formula $F = kx$, where k is a constant (which depends on the spring) and x is the amount by which the spring is stretched or compressed. Is this formula for Hooke's law the same as the one given in this section?

Solution: Yes. Some of the letters may be different, but the idea is exactly the same: The force of tension or compression is proportional to the amount of stretch or compression. Let's take Hooke's law as given in this section, express it in the form of the *Flea* formula, $\Delta L = FL_0 / EA$, and rewrite it like this: $F = \left(EA / L_0 \right) \cdot \Delta L$. Now, notice that this equation has exactly the same form as the equation $F = kx$:

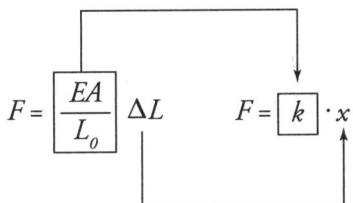

Summary of Formulas

HYDROSTATICS

Assume liquids are incompressible unless otherwise stated

Standard atmospheric pressure = 1 atm = 760 mmHg = 760 torr ≈ 100 kPa

Density: $\rho = \dfrac{m}{V}$

Specific gravity: $sp.gr. = \dfrac{\rho}{\rho_{H_2O}}$

$$\left(\rho_{H_2O} = 1000\,\tfrac{kg}{m^3} \text{ or } 1\,\tfrac{g}{cm^3} \text{ or } 1\,\tfrac{kg}{L} \right)$$

Force of gravity: $mg = \rho Vg$

Pressure: $P = \dfrac{F_\perp}{A}$

Hydrostatic gauge pressure: $P_{gauge} = \rho_{fluid}gD$

Hydrostatic gauge pressure is proportional to depth. Total hydrostatic pressure increases with increasing depth but is NOT proportional to depth.

Total hydrostatic pressure: $P_{total} = P_{at\,surface} + P_{gauge}$

Archimedes' principle: $F_{Buoy} = \rho_{fluid}V_{sub}g$

Buoyant force is equal to the weight of the displaced fluid.

Floating object: $\rho_{object} < \rho_{fluid} \rightarrow w_{object} = F_{Buoy}$

$$\dfrac{V_{sub}}{V} = \dfrac{\rho_{object}}{\rho_{fluid}}$$

Apparent weight of submerged object: $w_{apparent} = w_{object} - F_{Buoy}$

Pascal's law: $\dfrac{F_1}{A_1} = \dfrac{F_2}{A_2}$

HYDRODYNAMICS

Conditions for ideal fluid:

- incompressible

- negligible viscosity

- laminar (non-turbulent)

- steady flow (satisfies continuity equation)

Flow rate: $f = Av$

Continuity equation: $A_1 v_1 = A_2 v_2$

Bernoulli's equation (ideal fluid):

- total energy (density) within all parts of an ideal fluid is the same

$$P_1 + \tfrac{1}{2}\rho v_1^2 + \rho g y_1 = P_2 + \tfrac{1}{2}\rho v_2^2 + \rho g y_2$$

Venturi or Bernoulli effect ($y_1 = y_2$)

$$P_1 + \tfrac{1}{2}\rho v_1^2 = P_2 + \tfrac{1}{2}\rho v_2^2$$

- Fast flowing fluids have low pressure.

- Slow flowing fluids have high pressure.

Toricelli's result: $v_{efflux} = \sqrt{2gD}$

Poiseuille's law for flow rate of a viscous fluid: $\dfrac{\Delta P}{L} = \dfrac{8\eta f}{\pi r^4}$.

ELASTICITY OF SOLIDS

Stress: stress $= \dfrac{F}{A}$

Strain: strain $= \dfrac{\Delta L}{L_0}$

Hooke's law: stress = modulus × strain

Tension or compression: $\Delta L = \dfrac{FL_0}{EA}$

Shear: $X = \dfrac{FL_0}{AG}$

CHAPTER 8 FREESTANDING PRACTICE QUESTIONS

1. Which of the following is true?

A) Compression in length increases with an increased area of applied force.
B) Compression in length increases with a decreased area of applied force.
C) Compression in length is larger with a smaller original length.
D) Compression in length is larger with a smaller Young's modulus.

2. A person is leaning on his elbow on a table. If the amount of force the table must exert to keep the person upright is F, the area of contact between the person and the table is A, and the angle that the person's arm makes with the table's surface is θ, how much pressure is exerted by the person on the table?

A) $\dfrac{F}{A}$

B) $\dfrac{F\sin\theta}{A}$

C) $\dfrac{F\cos\theta}{A}$

D) Since the force exerted by the person on the table is not given, the pressure exerted by the person on the table cannot be determined.

3. What is the maximum weight of an object that a 50 kg person could lift by standing on one piston of a hydraulic jack, if the jack's pistons are circular and have radii of 5 m and 10 m?

A) 500 N
B) 1000 N
C) 2000 N
D) 4000 N

4. If the blood in the body is taken to be an ideal fluid, which of the following is true of blood flow in arteries?

A) The flow speed of blood is the same through the complete peripheral vascular system at any given moment, but it varies over time.
B) The flow speed of blood is the same through the complete peripheral vascular system and does not vary over time.
C) The flow rate of blood is the same through the complete peripheral vascular system at any given moment, but it varies over time.
D) The flow rate of blood is the same through the complete peripheral vascular system and does not vary over time.

5. If the density of a person is approximately the density of water and the density of air is approximately 1 kg/m^3, how many times greater is the weight of the person than the buoyant force from the air on the person?

A) 10
B) 100
C) 1000
D) 10000

6. Will an object with more mass but the same volume as another object sink faster in a non-viscous fluid?

A) No, because acceleration due to gravity is independent of the mass of the object being accelerated.
B) No, because the buoyant force is greater on an object with more mass.
C) Yes, because it weighs more, and the weight itself induces greater acceleration for the heavier object than for the lighter one.
D) Yes, because the buoyant force impedes the downward acceleration of a greater mass less than it does a lesser mass.

7. A particular eucalyptus tree has a density of 667 kg/m^3 and a mass of 6000 kg. What volume of the tree would float above the surface of water?

A) 3 m^3
B) 5 m^3
C) 6 m^3
D) 9 m^3

CHAPTER 8 PRACTICE PASSAGE

Students are performing experiments in the laboratory using their knowledge of hydrostatics and hydrodynamics.

Experiment 1

Students are given five liquid substances and they are asked to find their densities. They also have a test block that they measure to have a mass of 50 g and a volume of 100 cm³. They place the test block into each liquid and measure how much of the test block is submerged in the water. Table 1 summarizes their results.

Liquid	Volume submerged	Float?
1	80 cm³	Yes
2	75 cm³	Yes
3	100 cm³	No
4	50 cm³	Yes
5	100 cm³	Yes

Table 1   Test block placed in different liquids

Experiment 2

The students are given four different complex objects that all have the same density. They place each object in a test liquid that has a specific gravity of 2. They record the submerged volume of the object by measuring the displacement of the liquid. Their results are summarized in Table 2.

Object	Volume of displaced liquid
A	150 cm³
B	90 cm³
C	75 cm³
D	110 cm³

Table 2   Complex objects in a test liquid

Experiment 3

Students must create an irrigation system that takes water from a reservoir 80 cm deep to a wave pool across the room. A perfectly leveled, horizontal tube with constant circumference takes water from the bottom of the reservoir to the wave pool.

1. From Experiment 1, which liquid has the lowest density?

A) Liquid 4
B) Liquid 3
C) Liquid 5
D) Liquids 3 and 5

2. What is the specific gravity of Liquid 1?

A) 7/2
B) 5/8
C) 8/5
D) 2/7

3. What is the buoyant force acting on the test block in Liquid 5?

A) 2500 N
B) 500 N
C) 5 N
D) 0.5 N

4. Which object from Experiment 2 has the greatest mass?

A) Object A
B) Object B
C) Object C
D) Object D

5. During Experiment 3, one student lowers the wave pool to the floor, 1.5 meters below the aperture in the reservoir. The water then flows through the tubing to the wave pool. As it flows, how does the flow speed at the reservoir aperture compare to the flow speed leaving the tubing into the wave pool?

A) $v_{\text{wave pool}} = \sqrt{v_{\text{reservoir}}^2 + 3g}$

B) $v_{\text{wave pool}} = \sqrt{v_{\text{reservoir}}^2 - 3g}$

C) $v_{\text{wave pool}} = v_{\text{reservoir}}$

D) Cannot be determined without knowing the instantaneous depth of the water in the reservoir and the wave pool.

6. Two objects made from the same material with the same mass are placed in a liquid, base first. The base of Object 2 is three times that of Object 1. What best describes the buoyant force on the objects?

A) Object 1 has a greater buoyant force acting on it because it has a larger volume submerged.

B) Object 2 has a greater buoyant force acting on it because it has a larger volume submerged.

C) Object 2 has a greater buoyant force acting on it because it has a larger area at its base.

D) The buoyant force acting on both objects is the same.

SOLUTIONS TO CHAPTER 8 FREESTANDING QUESTIONS

1. **D** The formula for change in length is $\Delta L = FL_0 / EA$, where ΔL is the change in length, F is the applied force, L_0 is the original length, E is the Young's modulus and A is the area of applied force. Choice B could be eliminated first because from our everyday knowledge, the more force is applied, the more compressed an object is. Of the remaining choices, only choice D fits the relationship described by the above formula.

2. **B** First, eliminate D because the force exerted by the table on the person, given as F, is equal in magnitude to the force exerted by the person on the table, according to Newton's third law. Next, the way that pressure, force, and area are related is $P = \dfrac{F_\perp}{A}$. Since the given angle is between the arm and the table, the vertical component of the force will be related to the sine of that angle. Thus, $P = \dfrac{F \sin \theta}{A}$. Choice A is wrong because it would be the pressure if the force were not at an angle, and choice C is wrong because it would be the pressure if the angle given were between the arm and a line perpendicular to the table's surface.

3. **C** Pascal's law states that $\dfrac{F_1}{A_1} = \dfrac{F_2}{A_2}$. Thus, $F_2 = \dfrac{F_1 A_2}{A_1}$. For the greatest force, A_1 should be small and A_2 should be large (that is, the person should stand on the smaller piston and put the object on the larger). If the person is standing on the piston, then the force applied is the person's weight, and the area of the circular pistons is πr^2, so $F_2 = \dfrac{(mg)(\pi r_2^{\,2})}{\pi r_1^{\,2}}$. Cancel π and plug in: $F_2 = \dfrac{(50 \times 10)(10^2)}{5^2}$. This comes out to 2000 N. Choice A is wrong because it is just the person's weight, and choice B is wrong because the force is proportional to the area, not to the radius. Choice D is wrong because volume (which would involve cubing the radius and gives this result) is not relevant here.

4. **C** This is a two-by-two question: determining whether the flow speed or flow rate is the relevant quantity will eliminate two answers, and determining whether the flow varies over time or not will eliminate the final wrong answer. The continuity equation states that flow rate is the same in a pipe, and arteries are enough like pipes that the same applies to them. The only assumption in the continuity equation is that the fluid is incompressible, and the question stem states that this fluid is an ideal liquid. Thus, eliminate choices A and B, because it is flow rate, not flow speed, that is the same through the complete peripheral vascular system. The difference between choices C and D is time variation, and the heart's pumping definitely is not steady. Between heartbeats, blood experiences much less pumping than it does during heartbeats. Therefore, the flow rate should vary over time, which eliminates choice D.

5. **C** The weight of a person, in terms of density, is $w_p = \rho_p Vg$, where V is the volume of the person. The buoyant force from air on the person is $F_B = \rho_{air} Vg$, where V is again the volume of the person because the whole person is submerged in air. This means that the only difference is the density of the person as compared to the density of air, and since we are told that the density of the person is approximately the density of water (1000 kg/m³) and air has a density of approximately 1 kg/m³, the relevant factor is 1000.

6. **D** Begin by setting up the forces and finding the acceleration. $F_{net} = ma$, as always, so (defining the sinking direction as positive) $w - F_B = ma$. Next, specify weight and the buoyant force: $mg - \rho_f V_{sub} g = ma$. Divide by m, which yields $a = g - \frac{\rho_f V_{sub} g}{m}$. For a larger mass, the subtracted buoyant force will be less, and subtracting less means ending up with a greater number, so yes, the acceleration is greater for an object with greater mass, provided that the compared objects are sinking in the same fluid on the same planet (that is, ρ_f and g are the same for the two objects) and they have the same volume (as the stem indicates they do). Notice that it is the buoyant force term that makes the difference here: mass canceled in the weight term. Objects fall at the same rate in a vacuum, so it can't be the weight itself that is causing this effect, which is the reason that choice C is wrong. It is the buoyant force that is responsible for the difference in accelerations. Choices A and B are wrong for their "No" answers; choice A gives a true justification (acceleration due to gravity is independent of the mass of the object being accelerated), but it neglects the effect of the buoyant force, and choice B gives an incorrect reason, since equal volumes mean that the magnitude of the buoyant force on each object is the same.

7. **A** Recall that for floating objects $\frac{\rho_o}{\rho_f} = \frac{V_{sub}}{V}$. Since the density of the object is 667 kg/m³ and the density of water is 1000 kg/m³, two-thirds of the object will be submerged and one-third will be above the surface of the water. Since $\rho = \frac{m}{V}$, then $V = \frac{m}{\rho} = \frac{6000}{667} = 9 \text{ m}^3$. The total volume of the object is 9 m³, and one-third of that is 3 m³.

SOLUTIONS TO CHAPTER 8 PRACTICE PASSAGE

1. **B** An object will only sink if its density is greater than the density of the liquid. Since the test object is the same for all liquids, and only sank in Liquid 3, then Liquid 3 has the lowest density.

2. **B** The specific gravity is equal to ρ_{fl}/ρ_{water}, and the density of water is 1 g/cm^3. The density of the fluid is $\rho_{obj}V/V_{sub} = m_{obj}/V_{sub}$, therefore, the density of Liquid 1 is (50 g)/(80 cm^3), and the specific gravity is 5/8.

3. **D** The buoyant force is equal to $\rho_{fl}'V_{sub}'g$. The density of Liquid 5 is given by $m_{obj}/V_{sub} = 0.5$ g/cm^3. Thus the buoyant force is equal to (50 g)(10 m/s^2) = (0.05 kg)(10 m/s^2) = 0.5 N.

4. **A** Using the equation for objects floating on the surface $V_{sub}/V_{obj} = \rho_{obj}/\rho_{fluid}$, we know that V_{sub} is proportional to $V_{obj}'\rho_{obj} = m_{obj}$. Since V_{sub} is the only variable, we know that the object with the largest submerged volume has the greatest mass, which is Object A.

5. **C** Don't make the mistake of applying the Bernoulli equation in cases when it would contradict the continuity principle! The passage states that the tubing has a constant circumference, from which you can deduce that it has a constant cross-sectional area (if the tubing were to become pinched, that would change the area, but the MCAT would never ask you to deduce that behavior). Because the flow rate remains constant and the area remains constant, so must the flow speed, by $f = Av$.

6. **D** The buoyant force is given by $\rho_{fl}V_{sub}g$. Since the blocks have the same density, they will have the same volume submerged, and thus, they will have the same buoyant force acting on them.

Chapter 9
Electrostatics

9.1 ELECTRIC CHARGE

An atom is composed of a central nucleus (which is itself composed of protons and neutrons) surrounded by a cloud of one or more electrons. The fact that an atom is held together as a single unit is due to the fact that protons and electrons have a special property: They carry **electric charge**, which gives rise to an attractive force between them.

Electric charge exists in two varieties, which are called **positive** and **negative**. By convention, we say that protons carry positive charge and electrons carry negative charge. (Neutrons are well-named: They're neutral, because they have no electric charge.) The charge of a proton is +e, where e is called the **elementary charge**, and the charge of an electron is –e. Notice that the proton and the electron carry exactly the same amount of charge; the only difference in their charges is that one is positive and the other is negative.

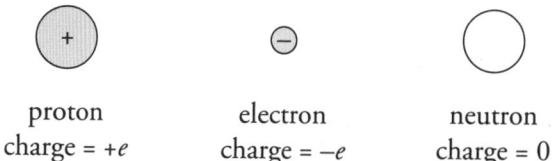

proton
charge = +e

electron
charge = –e

neutron
charge = 0

In SI units, electric charge is measured in **coulombs** (abbreviated **C**), and the value of the elementary charge, e, is 1.6×10^{-19} C.

Elementary Charge

$$e = 1.6 \times 10^{-19} \text{ C}$$

When an atom (or any other object) contains the same number of electrons as protons, its total charge is zero because the individual positive and negative charges add up and cancel. So, when the number of electrons (#e) equals the number of protons (#p), the object is *electrically neutral*. We say that an object is **charged** when there's an imbalance between the number of electrons and the number of protons. When an object has one or more extra electrons (#e > #p), the object is *negatively charged*, and when an object has a deficit of electrons (#e < #p), the object is *positively charged*. If a neutral atom has electrons removed or added, we say that it has been **ionized**, and the resulting electrically charged atom is called an **ion**. A positively charged ion is called a **cation**, and a negatively charged ion is called an **anion**. (An object can also become charged by gaining or losing protons, but these are usually locked up tight within the nuclei of the atoms. In virtually all cases, objects become charged by the transfer of *electrons*.)

Because an object can become charged only by losing or gaining electrons or protons, which can't be "sliced" into smaller pieces with fractional amounts of charge, the charge on an object can only be a whole number of ±e's; that is, charge is **quantized**. So, for any object, its charge is always equal to n(±e), where n is a whole number. To remind us that charge is *quantized*, electric charge is usually denoted by the letter q (or Q).

Charge is Quantized

$$q = n(\pm e)$$

where $n = 0, 1, 2...$

It is interesting to note that this quantization of charge applies to all fundamental particles either found in nature or created in the laboratory (e.g., muons, pions, etc.).

In chemistry, it's common to talk about the charge of an atom in terms of whole numbers like +1 or −2, etc. For example, we say that the charge of the fluoride ion, F^-, is −1, and the charge of the calcium ion, Ca^{+2}, is +2. This is just a convenient way of saying that the charge of the fluoride ion is −1 elementary unit (in other words, $-1e$), and the charge of the calcium ion is +2 elementary units, $+2e$. When we want to find the electric force between ions, we will express their charges in the proper unit (coulombs), and say, for example, that the charge of the fluoride ion is $-1e = -1.6 \times 10^{-19}$ C and the charge of the calcium ion is $+2e = +3.2 \times 10^{-19}$ C.

Finally, total electric charge is always conserved; that is, the total amount of charge before any process must always be equal to the total amount of charge afterward.[1]

Example 9-1: When you pet a cat, you rub electrons off the cat's fur, which are transferred to your hand. Assuming that you transfer 5×10^{10} electrons to your hand, what is the electric charge on your hand? What's the charge on the cat?

Solution: Because each electron carries a charge of $-e = -1.6 \times 10^{-19}$ C, and you've gained 5×10^{10} of them, the charge on your hand will be

$$(5 \times 10^{10})(-e) = (5 \times 10^{10})(-1.6 \times 10^{-19} \text{ C}) = -8 \times 10^{-9} \text{ C}$$

Since the cat has lost 5×10^{10} electrons, the charge on the cat will be

$$(-5 \times 10^{10})(+e) = (-5 \times 10^{10})(-1.6 \times 10^{-19} \text{ C}) = +8 \times 10^{-9} \text{ C}$$

Notice that the *net* charge before and after petting the cat was zero; all you've done is transfer charge.

---

[1] This does not mean that electric charge cannot be created or destroyed, which happens all the time. For example, in the reaction $e^- + e^+ \rightarrow \gamma + \gamma$ an electron (e^-) and its antiparticle (the positron, e^+, which is, in effect, a positively charged electron) meet and annihilate each other, producing energy in the form of two gamma-ray photons (γ), which carry no charge. Charge has been destroyed, but the total charge (zero, in this case) has been conserved. Conversely, charge can be created in the opposite process, when energy is converted to mass and charge (but always with zero total charge).

Example 9-2: How much positive charge is contained in 1 mole of carbon atoms? How much negative charge? What is the total charge?

Solution: Every atom of carbon contains 6 protons, so the amount of positive charge in one carbon atom is $q_+ = +6e$. Therefore, if N_A denotes Avogadro's number, the total amount of positive charge in 1 mole of carbon atoms is

$$Q_+ = N_A \times q_+ = N_A \times (+6e) = (6.02 \times 10^{23}) \times (6)(+1.6 \times 10^{-19} \text{ C}) = +6 \times 10^5 \text{ C}$$

Because every neutral carbon atom also contains 6 electrons, the amount of negative charge in a carbon atom is $q_- = 6(-e) = -6e = -q_+$ so the total amount of negative charge in 1 mole of carbon atoms is $Q_- = N_A \times q_- = -Q_+ \approx -6 \times 10^5 \text{ C}$. The total charge on the carbon atoms, $Q_+ + Q_-$, is zero.

9.2 ELECTRIC FORCE AND COULOMB'S LAW

If two charged particles are a distance r apart,

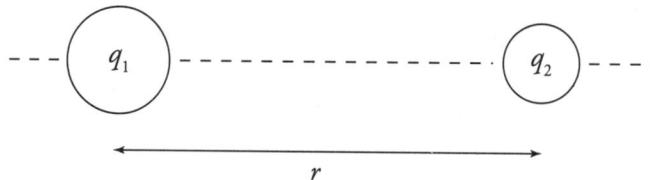

then the electric force between them, $\mathbf{F}_E$, is directed along the line joining them. The magnitude of this force is proportional to the charges (q_1 and q_2) and inversely proportional to r^2, as given by

> **Coulomb's Law**
>
> $$F_E = k\frac{|q_1 q_2|}{r^2}$$

The proportionality constant is k, and in general, its value depends on the material between the particles. However, in the usual case where the particles are separated by empty space (or by air, for all practical purposes), the proportionality constant is denoted by k_0 and called **Coulomb's constant**. This is a fundamental constant of nature (equal in magnitude, by definition, to 10^{-7} times the speed of light squared), and its value is $k_0 = 9 \times 10^9$ N·m²/C²:

> ### Coulomb's Constant
>
> $$k_0 = 9 \times 10^9 \; \tfrac{\text{N·m}^2}{\text{C}^2}$$

This is the value of k you should use unless you're specifically given another value (which would happen only if the charges were embedded in some insulating material that weakens the electric force).

The absolute value sign in the formula gives the magnitude of the force, whether repulsive or attractive. If direction (e.g., + or −) needs to be assigned, it should be done based on the fact that like charges (two positives or two negatives) repel each other, and opposite charges (one positive and one negative) attract. Note that the two electric forces in each of the following diagrams form an action–reaction pair.

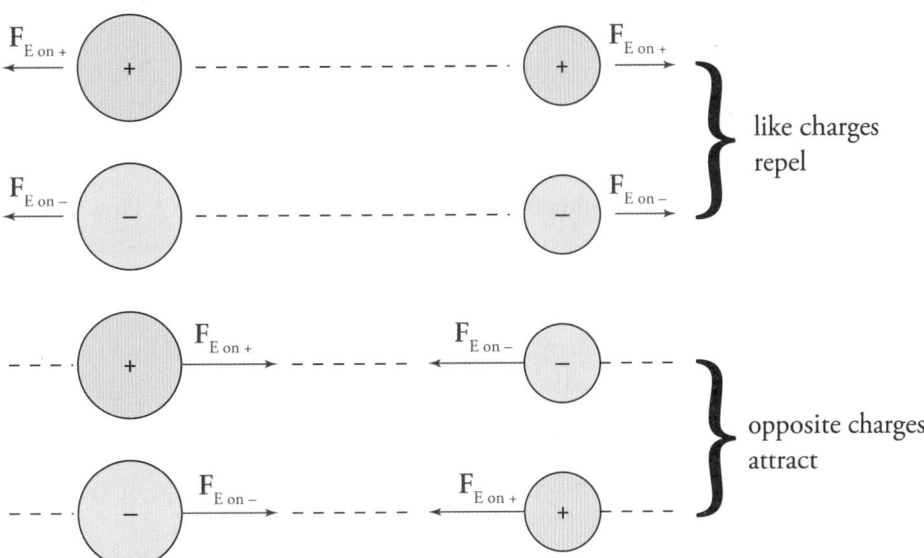

Example 9-3: Two charges, $q_1 = -2 \times 10^{-6}\,\text{C}$ and $q_2 = +5 \times 10^{-6}\,\text{C}$, are separated by a distance of 10 cm. Describe the electric force between these particles.

Solution: Using Coulomb's law, we find that

$$F_E = k_0 \frac{|q_1 q_2|}{r^2} = (9 \times 10^9 \; \tfrac{\text{N·m}^2}{\text{C}^2}) \frac{(2 \times 10^{-6}\,\text{C})(+5 \times 10^{-6}\,\text{C})}{(10^{-1}\text{m})^2} = 9\,\text{N}$$

Since one charge is positive and one is negative, the force is attractive, and each charge feels a 9 N force toward the other.

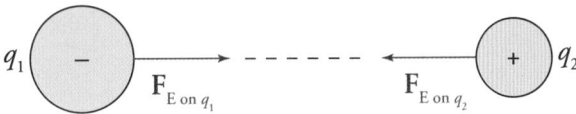

Example 9-4: A coulomb is a *lot* of charge. To get some idea just how much, imagine that we had two objects, each with a charge of 1 C, separated by a distance of 1 m. What would be the electric force between them?

Solution: Using Coulomb's law, we'd find that

$$F_E = k_0 \frac{|q_1 q_2|}{r^2} = (9 \times 10^9 \text{ } \frac{\text{N} \cdot \text{m}^2}{\text{C}^2}) \frac{(1 \text{ C})(1 \text{C})}{(1 \text{ m})^2} = 9 \times 10^9 \text{ N}$$

To write this answer in terms of a more familiar unit, let's use the fact that 1 pound (1 lb) is about 4.5 N, and 1 ton is 2000 lb:

$$F_E = (9 \times 10^9 \text{ } \frac{\text{N} \cdot \text{m}^2}{\text{C}^2}) \cdot \frac{1 \text{ lb}}{4.5 \text{ N}} \cdot \frac{1 \text{ ton}}{2000 \text{ lb}} = \text{one million tons}$$

That's roughly equivalent to the weight of the Golden Gate Bridge! It's now easy to understand why most real-life situations deal with charges that are very tiny fractions of a coulomb; the *microcoulomb* (1 μC = 10^{-6} C) and the *nanocoulomb* (1 nC = 10^{-9} C) are more common "practical" units of charge.

Example 9-5: Consider a charge, $+q$, initially at rest near another charge, $-Q$. How would the magnitude of the electric force on $+q$ change if $-Q$ were moved away, doubling its distance from $+q$?

Solution: Coulomb's law is an inverse-square law, $F_E \propto 1/r^2$, so if r increases by a factor of 2, then F_E will *decrease* by a factor of 4 (because $2^2 = 4$).

Example 9-6: Consider two plastic spheres, 1 meter apart: a little sphere with a mass of 1 kg and an electric charge of +1 nC, and a big sphere with a mass of 11 kg and an electric charge of +11 μC.

a) Find the electric force and the gravitational force between these spheres. Which force is stronger?
b) If the big sphere is fixed in position, and the little sphere is free to move, describe the resulting motion of the little sphere if it's released from rest.

Solution:

a) Using Coulomb's law, we find that the electric force between the spheres is

$$F_E = k_0 \frac{Qq}{r^2} = (9 \times 10^9 \text{ } \frac{\text{N} \cdot \text{m}^2}{\text{C}^2}) \frac{(11 \times 10^{-6} \text{ C})(1 \times 10^{-9} \text{ C})}{(1 \text{ m})^2} = 9.9 \times 10^{-5} \text{ N} \approx 10^{-4} \text{ N}$$

Using Newton's law of gravitation, the gravitational force between them is

$$F_G = G \frac{Mm}{r^2} = (6.7 \times 10^{-11} \text{ } \frac{\text{N} \cdot \text{m}^2}{\text{kg}^2}) \frac{(1 \text{ kg})(11 \text{ kg})}{1 \text{ m}^2} \approx 7.4 \times 10^{-10} \text{ N}$$

Which force is stronger? It's no contest: The electric force is *much* stronger than the gravitational force. So, even though the spheres experience an attraction due to gravity, it is many orders of magnitude weaker than their electrical repulsion and can therefore be ignored.

b)   The net force on the little sphere is essentially equal to the electrical repulsion it feels from the big sphere (since the gravitational force is *so* much smaller, it can be ignored). Therefore, the initial acceleration of the little sphere is

$$a = \frac{F_E}{m} = \frac{10^{-4} \text{ N}}{1 \text{ kg}} = 10^{-4} \text{ m/s}^2$$

directed away from the big sphere. Notice that as the little sphere moves away, its acceleration does not remain constant. Because the electric force is inversely proportional to the square of the distance between the charges, as the little sphere moves away, the repulsive force it feels weakens, so its acceleration decreases. Therefore, the little sphere moves directly away from the big sphere with decreasing acceleration.

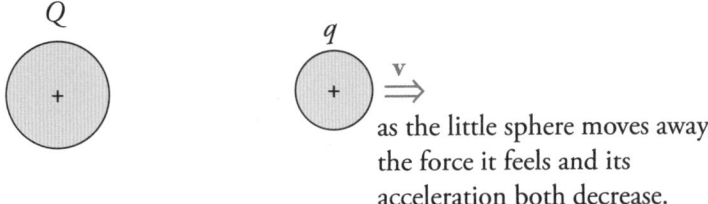

as the little sphere moves away, the force it feels and its acceleration both decrease.

Nevertheless, because the acceleration of the little sphere always points in the same direction (namely, away from the big sphere), the speed of the little sphere is always increasing, although the rate of increase of speed gets smaller as the little sphere gets farther away.

The Principle of Superposition for Electric Forces

Coulomb's law tells us how to calculate the force that one charge exerts on another one. What if two (or more) charges affect a third one? For example, what is the electric force on q_3 in the following figure?

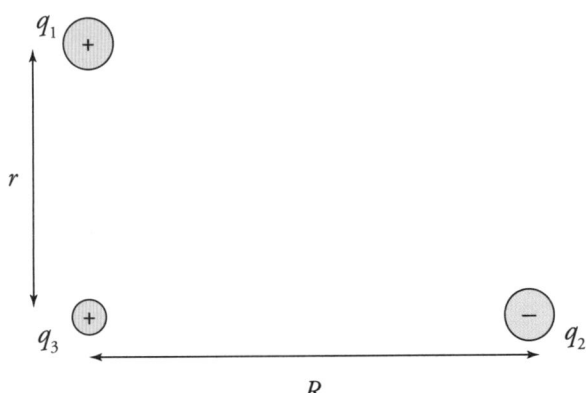

Here's the answer: If $\mathbf{F}_{1\text{-on-}3}$ is the force that q_1 *alone* exerts on q_3 (ignoring the presence of q_2) and if $\mathbf{F}_{2\text{-on-}3}$ is the force that q_2 *alone* exerts on q_3 (ignoring the presence of q_1), then the total force that q_3 feels is simply the vector sum $\mathbf{F}_{1\text{-on-}3} + \mathbf{F}_{2\text{-on-}3}$. The fact that we can calculate the effect of several charges by considering them individually and then just adding the resulting forces is known as the **principle of superposition**. (This important property will also be used when we study electric field vectors, electric potential, magnetic fields, and magnetic forces.)

The Principle of Superposition

The net electric force on a charge (q) due to a collection of other charges (Q's)

is equal to

the sum of the individual forces that each of the Q's alone exerts on q.

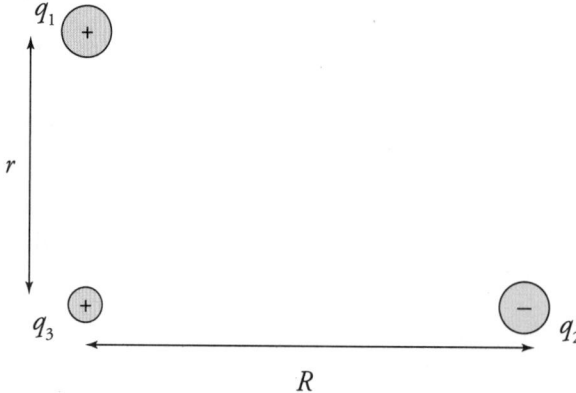

Example 9-7: In the figure above, assume that $q_1 = 2$ C, $q_2 = -8$ C, and $q_3 = 1$ nC. If $r = 1$ m and $R = 2$ m, which one of the following vectors best illustrates the direction of the net electric force on q_3?

A. ↖   C. ↘

B. ↗   D. ↙

Solution: The individual forces $\mathbf{F}_{1\text{-on-}3}$ and $\mathbf{F}_{2\text{-on-}3}$ are shown in the figure on the following page. Adding these vectors gives $\mathbf{F}_{\text{on }3}$, which points down to the right, so the answer is C.

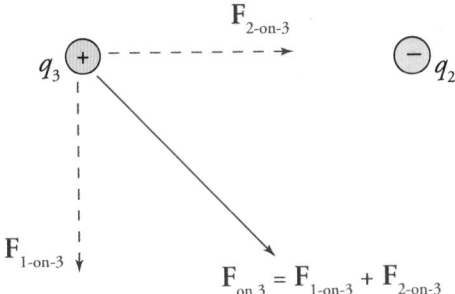

$$F_{1-on-3} = k_0 \frac{q_1 q_3}{r^2} = \left(9 \times 10^9 \ \frac{N \cdot m^2}{C^2}\right) \frac{(2 \ C)(1 \times 10^{-9} \ C)}{(1 \ m)^2} = 18 \ N$$

(repulsive; away from q_1)

$$F_{2-on-3} = k_0 \frac{|q_2| q_3}{R^2} = \left(9 \times 10^9 \ \frac{N \cdot m^2}{C^2}\right) \frac{(8 \ C)(1 \times 10^{-9} \ C)}{(2 \ m)^2} = 18 \ N$$

(attractive; toward q_2)

If the question had asked for the magnitude of the net electric force on q_3, then we'd use the Pythagorean theorem to find the length of the vector $\mathbf{F}_{on\,3}$. The vector $\mathbf{F}_{on\,3}$ is the hypotenuse of the right triangle whose legs are $\mathbf{F}_{1-on-3}$ and $\mathbf{F}_{2-on-3}$, so the magnitude of $\mathbf{F}_{on\,3}$ is found like this:

$$
\begin{aligned}
(\mathbf{F}_{on\,3})^2 &= (\mathbf{F}_{1-on-3})^2 + (\mathbf{F}_{2-on-3})^2 \\
&= 18^2 + 18^2 \\
&= (18^2)(2) \\
\therefore \mathbf{F}_{on\,3} &= 18\sqrt{2} \approx 25 \ N
\end{aligned}
$$

Example 9-8: In the figure below, assume that $q_1 = 1 \ C$, $q_2 = -1 \ nC$, and $q_3 = 8 \ C$. If q_4 is a negative charge, what must its value be in order for the net electric force on q_2 to be zero?

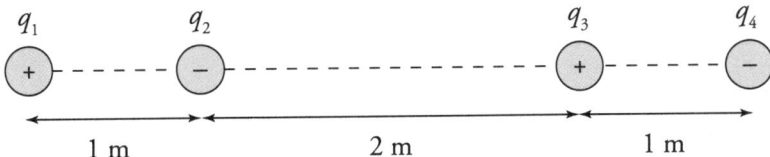

Solution: The individual forces $F_{1\text{-on-}2}$, $F_{3\text{-on-}2}$, and $F_{4\text{-on-}2}$ are shown in the figure below. Notice that $F_{1\text{-on-}2}$ and $F_{4\text{-on-}2}$ point to the left, while $F_{3\text{-on-}2}$ points to the right.

If we let $q_4 = -x$ C, then the magnitudes of the individual forces on q_2 are

$$F_{1\text{-on-}2} = k_0 \frac{q_1 |q_2|}{(r_{1-2})^2} = (9 \times 10^9 \, \tfrac{\text{N·m}^2}{\text{C}^2}) \frac{(1 \, \text{C})(1 \, \text{nC})}{(1 \, \text{m})^2} = 9 \, \text{N}$$

$$F_{3\text{-on-}2} = k_0 \frac{|q_2||q_3|}{(r_{2-3})^2} = (9 \times 10^9 \, \tfrac{\text{N·m}^2}{\text{C}^2}) \frac{(1 \, \text{nC})(8 \, \text{C})}{(2 \, \text{m})^2} = 18 \, \text{N}$$

$$F_{4\text{-on-}2} = k_0 \frac{|q_2||q_4|}{(r_{2-4})^2} = (9 \times 10^9 \, \tfrac{\text{N·m}^2}{\text{C}^2}) \frac{(1 \, \text{nC})(x \, \text{C})}{(3 \, \text{m})^2} = x \, \text{N}$$

In order for the net electric force on q_2 to be zero, the sum of the magnitudes of $F_{1\text{-on-}2}$ and $F_{4\text{-on-}2}$ must

be equal to the magnitude of $F_{3\text{-on-}2}$. That is, $9 \, \text{N} + x \, \text{N} = 18 \, \text{N}$ so $x = 9$. Therefore, $q_4 = -x$ C $= -9$ C.

9.3 ELECTRIC FIELDS

There are several advantages to regarding electrical interactions in a slightly different way from the simple "charge Q exerts a force on charge q" mode of thinking. In this more sophisticated interpretation, the very existence of a charge (or a more general distribution of charge) alters the space around it, creating what we call an **electric field** in its vicinity. If a second charge happens to be there or to roam by, it will feel the effect of the field created by the original charge. That is, we think of the electric force on a second charge q as exerted *by the field*, rather than directly by the original charge(s). Qualitatively, we can represent electrical interactions as follows:

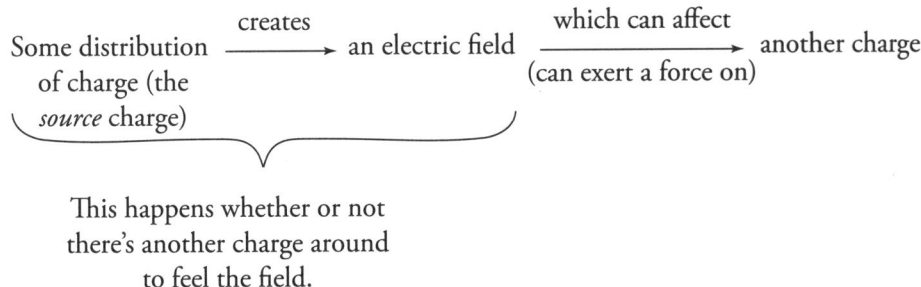

The charge(s) creating the electric field is/are called the **source charge(s)**; they're the source of the electric field. You may like to think of a source charge as a spider and its electric field as the spider's web. After a spider creates a web, when a small insect roams by, it is the web that ensnares the unfortunate bug, not the spider directly.

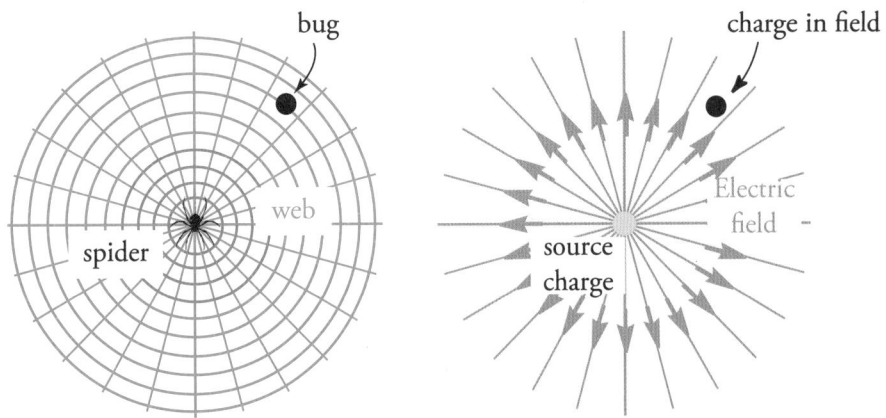

The figure on the right above illustrates one way to picture an electric field, but a few words of explanation are needed. First: An electric field is a **vector field**, which means that at each point in space surrounding the source charge, we associate a specific vector. The length of this vector will tell us the magnitude, or strength, of the field at that point, and the direction of the vector will tell us the direction of the resulting electric force that a *positive* test charge would feel if it were placed at that point. That's the convention: Although the charge that finds itself in an electric field can of course be positive or negative, for purposes of *illustrating* the field, we always think of a *positive* test charge. Because of this convention, *electric field vectors always point away from positive source charges and toward negative ones*. Also, the closer we are to the source charge, the stronger the resulting electric force a test charge would feel (because Coulomb's law is an *inverse*-square law). So, we expect the electric field vectors to be long at points close to the source charge and shorter at points farther away. The following figures illustrate the electric field due to a positive source charge and the electric field due to a negative source charge.

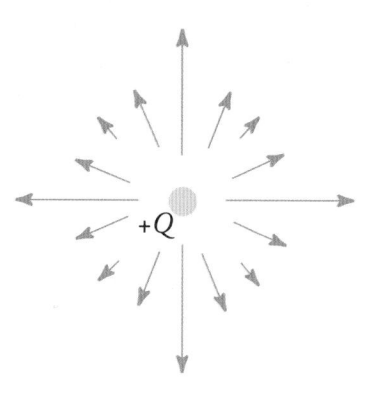

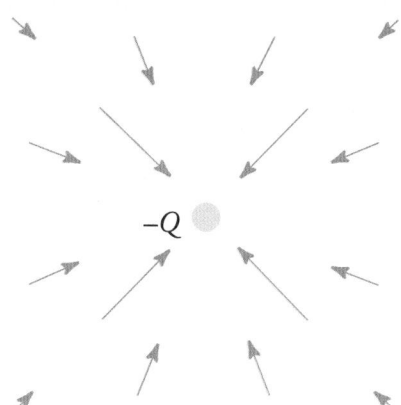

Electric field vectors
point away from
a positive source charge.

Electric field vectors
point toward
a negative source charge.

We can use Coulomb's law to find a formula for the strength of the electric field due to a point charge. Remember that a source charge creates an electric field whether or not there's another charge in the field to feel it. It takes *two* charges to create an electric *force*, but it takes only *one* (the source charge) to create an electric *field*. So, let's imagine we have a single source charge, Q, and another charge, q, at a distance r from Q.

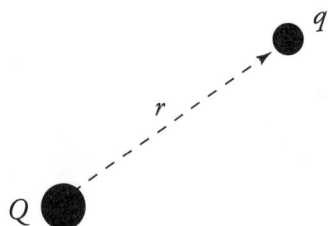

The force by Q, on the charge q, is, by Coulomb's law,

$$F_{\text{by } Q} = k\frac{|Q||q|}{r^2}$$

Now we ask, "What if q weren't there? Do we still have something?" The answer is *yes*, we have the electric field created by the source charge, Q. "So, if q weren't there, what if we removed q from the formula for the force exerted on it by Q? Would we still have something?" The answer is *yes*, we'd have the formula for the electric field, **E**, created by the single source charge Q.

Electric Field

$$E_{\text{by } Q} = k\frac{|Q|}{r^2}$$

In the formula for the force by Q on q, the variable r represents the distance from Q to q. However, if q is not there, what does r mean now? Answer: It's simply the distance from Q to the point in space where we want to know the electric field vector.

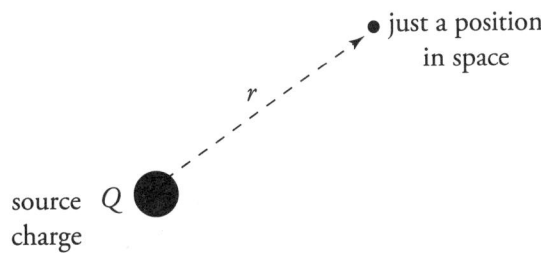

Example 9-9: Let Q = +4 nC be a charge that is fixed in position at the origin of an x-y coordinate system. What is the magnitude and direction of the electric field at the point (10 cm, 0)? At the point (–20 cm, 0)?

Solution: In the figure below, the point A is (10 cm, 0), which is 10 cm directly to the right of Q, and B is the point (–20 cm, 0), which is 20 cm directly to the left of Q.

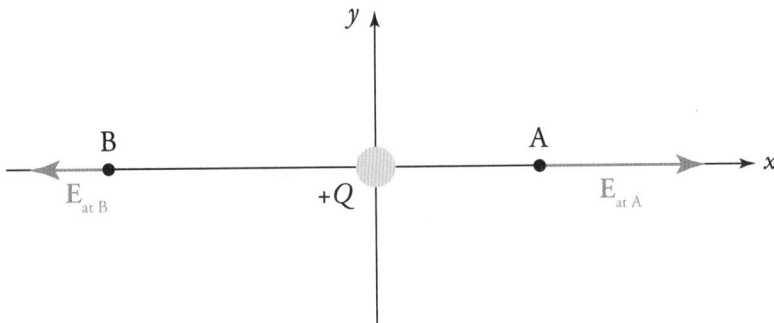

The electric field at point A is

$$E_{\text{at A}} = k_0\frac{Q}{(r_{\text{to A}})^2} = (9\times10^9 \ \tfrac{\text{N·m}^2}{\text{C}^2})\frac{(4\times10^{-9} \ \text{C})}{(10^{-1} \ \text{m})^2} = 3600\tfrac{\text{N}}{\text{C}}$$

Since Q is positive, this means the electric field vector, $\mathbf{E}_{\text{at A}}$, points away from the source charge. Therefore, $\mathbf{E}_{\text{at A}}$ points in the positive x direction, which is usually written as the direction $\mathbf{i}$. So, if we wanted to write the complete electric field vector at point A, we'd write $\mathbf{E}_{\text{at A}}$ = (3600 N/C)$\mathbf{i}$.

9.3

The electric field at point B is

$$E_{\text{at B}} = k_0 \frac{Q}{(r_{\text{to B}})^2} = (9 \times 10^9 \tfrac{\text{N·m}^2}{\text{C}^2}) \frac{(4 \times 10^{-9} \text{ C})}{(2 \times 10^{-1} \text{ m})^2} = 900 \tfrac{\text{N}}{\text{C}}$$

Once again, $\mathbf{E}_{\text{at B}}$ points away from the source charge. Therefore, $\mathbf{E}_{\text{at B}}$ points in the negative x direction, which is usually written as the direction $-\mathbf{i}$. So, if we wanted to write the complete electric field vector at point B, we'd write $\mathbf{E}_{\text{at B}} = (900 \text{ N/C})(-\mathbf{i})$ or $-(900 \text{ N/C})\mathbf{i}$.

Notice from the formula $E = k|Q|/r^2$ that the electric field obeys an inverse-square law, like the electric force. So the strength of an electric field from a single source charge decreases as we get farther from the source; in particular, $E \propto 1/r^2$. Also, for a given source charge Q, the electric field strength depends only on r, the distance from Q. So at every point on a circle (or more generally a sphere) of radius r centered on the source charge, the electric field strength is the same. In the electric field vector diagram below on the left, all the field vectors at the points on the smaller dashed circle have the same length, indicating that the electric field magnitude is the same at all points on this circle. Similarly, all the field vectors at the points on the larger dashed circle have the same length, indicating that the electric field magnitude is the same at all points on *this* circle. (Note that the field vectors at the points on the larger circle are shorter than those at the points on the smaller circle.) However, notice that the magnitude may be the same at every point on each circle (because they're all the same distance r from the source charge) but the directions of the electric field vectors are all different on each circle. Therefore, we're forced to say that the electric field isn't the same at every point a distance r from Q because the directions are all different.

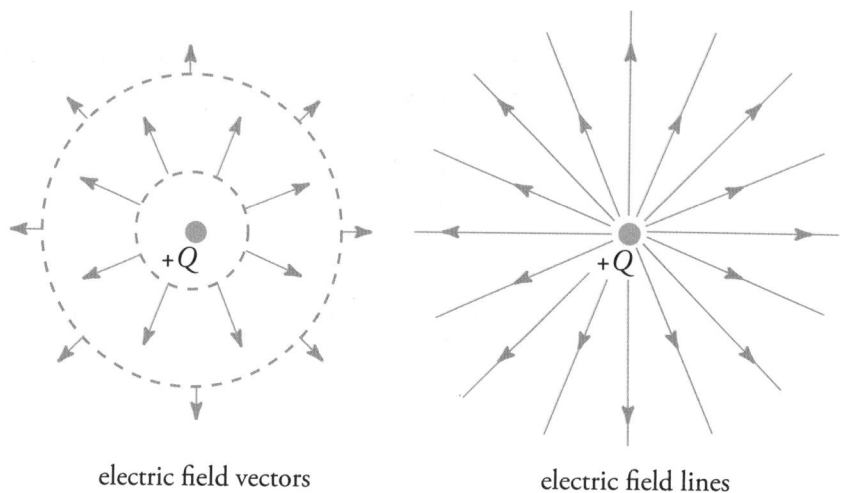

electric field vectors   electric field lines

The diagram on the left above and the two given earlier for the electric field produced by a positive source charge and by a negative source charge show the field represented by individual vectors. However, this is not the easiest way to draw an electric field.

Instead of drawing a bunch of separate vectors, we instead draw *lines* through them, like in the diagram on the right above. This drawing depicts the electric field using **field lines**. The direction of the field is indicated as usual; remember that, by convention, the electric field points away from positive source charges and toward negative ones and indicates the direction of the electric force that a positive test charge would feel if it were placed in the field.

Now that we've eliminated the separate vectors, it seems as though we've lost some information, namely, where the field is strong and where it's weak because we got this information from the lengths of the individual vectors. (Where the vectors were long, the field was strong, and where the vectors were shorter, the field was weaker.) However, we can still get a general idea of where the field is strong and where it's weak by looking at the *density* of the field lines: Where the field lines are cramped close together, the field is stronger; where the field lines are more spread out, the field is weaker.

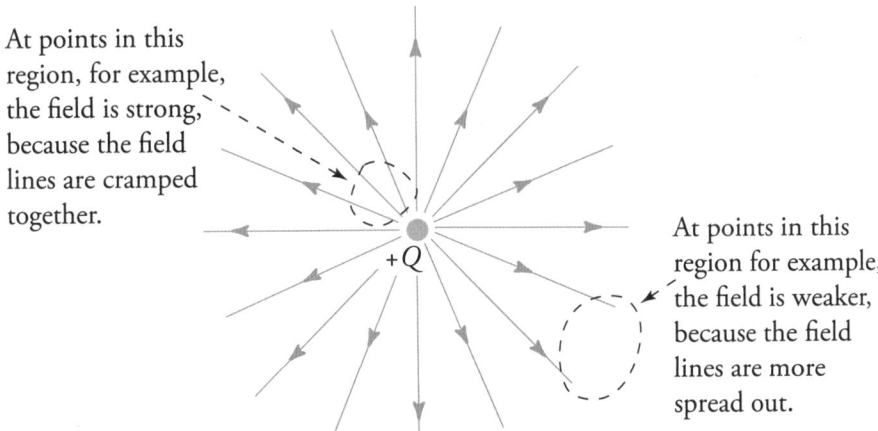

At points in this region, for example, the field is strong, because the field lines are cramped together.

$+Q$

At points in this region for example, the field is weaker, because the field lines are more spread out.

Now, let's imagine that we have a source charge Q creating an electric field, and another charge, q, roams in to the field. What force will q feel? We want to find an equation for the force on q due to the electric field. Recall the formulas above: $F_{on\,q} = k|Qq|/r^2$ and $E_{by\,Q} = k|Q|/r^2$. What would we need to do to E to get F? Just multiply it by q! That is, $F_{on\,q} = |q|E_{by\,q}$. It turns out that this very important formula works not just for the electric field created by a single source charge; it works for *any* electric field:

Electric Force and Field

$$\mathbf{F}_{on\,q} = q\mathbf{E}$$

Note that the absolute value symbol is useful when solving for the magnitude of force and electric field. The vector equation, $\mathbf{F}_E = q\mathbf{E}$, contains directional information and therefore does not need absolute values. Notice also from this formula that $E = F/|q|$, so the units of E are N/C, which you saw in Example 7-9. The equation $\mathbf{E} = \mathbf{F}/q$ also gives us the definition of the electric field: It's the force per unit charge.

Finally, before we get to some more examples, realize that we've had two important (boxed) formulas in this section on the electric field: $E = k|Q|/r^2$ and $\mathbf{F} = q\mathbf{E}$. In the first formula, Q is the charge that *makes* the field, while in the second formula, q is the charge that *feels* the field.

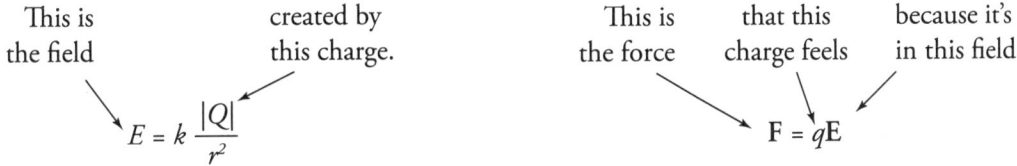

This is the field   created by this charge.   This is the force   that this charge feels   because it's in this field.

$$E = k\frac{|Q|}{r^2}$$

$$F = q\mathbf{E}$$

9.3

Example 9-10: The magnitude of the electric field at a distance r from a source charge $+Q$ is equal to E. What will be the magnitude of the electric field at a distance $4r$ from a source charge $+2Q$?

Solution: The first sentence tells us that $kQ/r^2 = E$. Now, if we change Q to $2Q$ and r to $4r$, we find that E decreases by a factor of 8, because

$$E' = k\frac{Q'}{(r')^2} = k\frac{2Q}{(4r)^2} = \frac{2}{16}\cdot k\frac{Q}{r^2} = \frac{1}{8}E$$

Example 9-11: A particle with charge $q = 2\ \mu C$ is placed at a point where the electric field has magnitude 4×10^4 N/C. What will be the strength of the electric force on the particle?

Solution: From the equation $F_{on\ q} = qE$, we find that

$$F = (2\times10^{-6}\ C)(4\times10^4\ \tfrac{N}{C}) = 8\times10^{-2}\ N$$

Notice that we didn't need to know what created the field. If E is given, and the question asks for the force that some charge q feels in this field, all we have to do is multiply, $F = qE$, and we're done.

Example 9-12: In the diagram on the left below, the electric field at Point A points in the positive y direction and has magnitude 5×10^6 N/C. (The source charge is not shown.) If a particle with charge $q = -3\ nC$ is placed at point A, what will be the electric force on the particle?

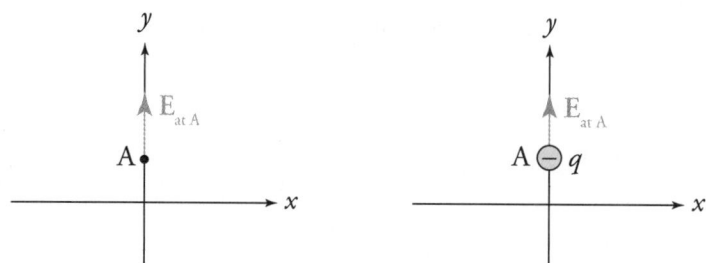

Solution: $\mathbf{E}_{at\ A}$ points in the positive y direction, which is usually written as the direction $\mathbf{j}$, so $\mathbf{E}_{at\ A} = (5\times10^6\ N/C)\mathbf{j}$. The equation $\mathbf{F}_{on\ q} = q\mathbf{E}$ then gives us

$$\mathbf{F} = (-3\times10^{-9})(5\times10^6\ \tfrac{N}{C})\mathbf{j} = (1.5\times10^{-2}\ N)(-\mathbf{j})$$

That is, the force will have magnitude 1.5×10^{-2} N and point in the negative y direction ($-\mathbf{j}$). Notice that whenever q is negative, the force $F_{\text{on } q}$ will always point in the direction *opposite* to the electric field.

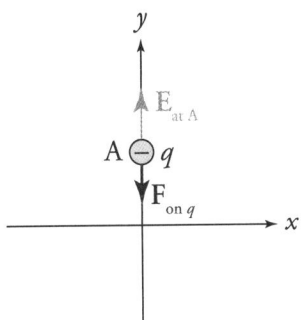

Example 9-13: A particle of mass m and charge q is placed at a point where the electric field is **E**. If the particle is released from rest, find its initial acceleration, **a**.

Solution: The acceleration of the particle is the force it feels divided by its mass: $\mathbf{a} = \mathbf{F}/m$. Because $\mathbf{F} = q\mathbf{E}$, we get

$$\mathbf{a} = \frac{\mathbf{F}}{m} = \frac{q\mathbf{E}}{m}$$

Notice that if q is negative, then **F** (and, consequently, **a**) will be directed *opposite* to the electric field **E**. Also, the question asked only for the *initial* acceleration, because once the particle starts moving, it will most likely move through locations where the electric field is different (in magnitude or direction or both), so the force on the particle will change; and if the force on the particle changes, so will the acceleration.

If a region contains a *uniform* electric field (i.e., same magnitude and direction at all points within the region), then the electrostatic force and the particle's acceleration will likewise be uniform. The Big 5 kinematics equations can therefore be used to solve for final velocity, time, etc. In addition, the formula $W = Fd \cos\theta$ can also be used to calculate the work done by or against the electrostatic force to move a charge from one position to another. A large conducting plate that is charged (or a parallel plate capacitor, as detailed in the next chapter) creates an electric field that is approximately uniform.

Example 9-14: A uniform electric field of strength 4×10^6 N/C points to the left as shown in the figure on the next page. A particle with charge $q = -20$ nC and mass $m = 10$ g is initially placed at point B.

a)   If the particle is released from rest, toward which point will it move and how fast will it be traveling when it arrives?

9.3

b) If the particle is again placed at point B and is now moved to point D, how much work is done "by the field"? (Note: In reality, forces do work, not fields; work done "by the field" is a commonly used expression.)

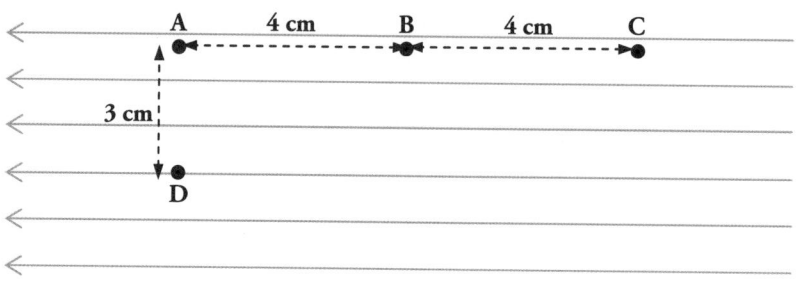

Solution:

a) Negatively charged particles feel a force opposite the direction of the electric field, therefore the particle will move to point C. To find the final speed, the acceleration must first be calculated using Newton's Second Law:

$$|q|E = ma$$

$$a = |q|E\,/\,m = (20 \times 10^{-9}\ \text{C})(4 \times 10^{6}\ \text{N/C})\,/\,(10 \times 10^{-3}\ \text{kg}) = 8\ \text{m/s}^2$$

Using Big 5 #5,

$$v^2 = v_0{}^2 + 2ad = 0 + 2(8\ \text{m/s}^2)(0.04\ \text{m}) = 0.64\ \text{m}^2/\text{s}^2$$

v is therefore 0.8 m/s.

b) $W = Fd\cos\theta = |q|Ed\cos\theta$. Since $\theta > 90°$ the work done by the field is negative. ΔBAD is a 3-4-5 triangle, so $d = 5$ cm. More importantly, $\cos\theta = -4/5$. Therefore,

$$W = (20 \times 10^{-9}\ \text{C})(4 \times 10^{6}\ \text{N/C})(0.05\ \text{m})(-4/5) = -3.2 \times 10^{-3}\ \text{J}$$

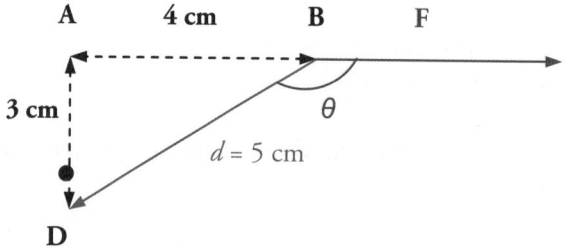

Notice that the work done by the field from point B to point D is the same as if the particle were moved from point B to point A. The field will only do work (whether positive or negative) if there is displacement in the direction of the electric field or opposite the field. This is similar to gravity, which only does work if there is displacement up or down. And as with gravity, the work done by the field is also path independent. This will be discussed in more depth later in the chapter.

The Principle of Superposition for Electric Fields

The pictures we've drawn so far have been of electric fields created by a single source charge. However, we can also have two or more charges whose electric fields overlap, creating one combined field. For example, let's consider an **electric dipole**, which, by definition, is a pair of equal but opposite charges:

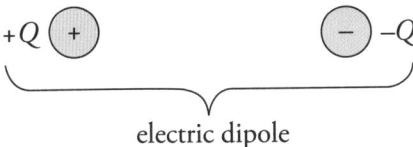

electric dipole

What if we regarded *both* of them as source charges; how would we find the electric field that they create together? By using the principle of superposition. If we wanted to find the electric field vector at, say, the point P in the diagram below,

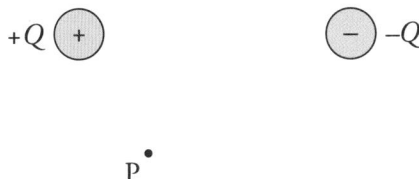

we'd first find the electric field vector, $\mathbf{E}_+$, at P due to the $+Q$ charge alone (ignoring the presence of the $-Q$ charge) and then we'd find the electric field vector, $\mathbf{E}_-$, at P due to the $-Q$ charge alone (ignoring the presence of the $+Q$ charge). The net electric field vector at P will then be the vector sum, $\mathbf{E}_+ + \mathbf{E}_-$.

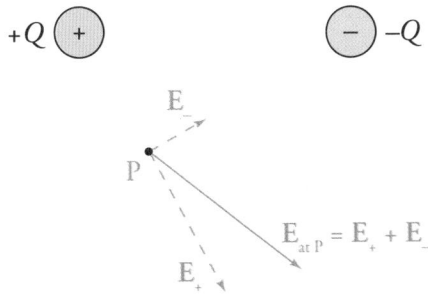

We can do this for as many points as we like and obtain a diagram of the electric field as a collection of vectors. The diagram in terms of electric field lines would look like this:

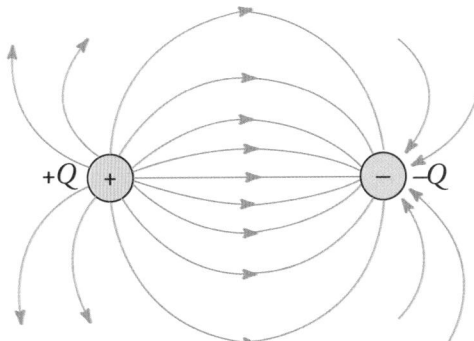

Notice that between the charges, where the field lines are dense, the field is strong; and as we move away from the charges, the field lines get more spread out, indicating that the field gets weaker.

Example 9-15: An electric dipole consists of two charges, $+Q$ and $-Q$, where $Q = 4\ \mu C$, separated by a distance of $d = 20$ cm. Find the electric field at the point midway between the charges.

Solution: The electric field at P due to the positive charge is $E_+ = k_0 Q / \left(\frac{1}{2}d\right)^2$, pointing away from $+Q$, and the electric field at P due to the negative charge is $E_- = k_0 Q / \left(\frac{1}{2}d\right)^2$, pointing toward $-Q$ (which is in the same direction as $\mathbf{E}_+$).

$$+Q \ \bigoplus \qquad\qquad \mathrm{P}\underset{E_-}{\overset{E_+}{\cdot\longrightarrow}} \qquad\qquad \bigominus -Q$$

$$\underset{\frac{1}{2}d}{\longleftrightarrow} \quad \underset{\frac{1}{2}d}{\longleftrightarrow}$$

By the principle of superposition, the net electric field at P is the sum: $\mathbf{E} = \mathbf{E}_+ + \mathbf{E}_-$. The magnitude of $E_{\text{at P}}$ is $E_+ + E_- = k_0 Q / \left(\frac{1}{2}d\right)^2 + k_0 Q / \left(\frac{1}{2}d\right)^2 = 2k_0 Q / \left(\frac{1}{2}d\right)^2$:

$$E = 2k_0 \frac{Q}{(\frac{1}{2}d)^2}$$
$$= 2(9 \times 10^9\ \tfrac{\mathrm{N \cdot m^2}}{\mathrm{C^2}}) \frac{4 \times 10^{-6}\ \mathrm{C}}{(1 \times 10^{-1}\ \mathrm{m})^2}$$
$$= 7.2 \times 10^6\ \tfrac{\mathrm{N}}{\mathrm{C}}$$

The direction of $\mathbf{E}_{\text{at P}}$ is away from $+Q$ and toward $-Q$:

$$+Q \ \bigoplus \qquad\qquad \underset{\mathrm{P}}{\cdot}\overset{E}{\longrightarrow} \qquad\qquad \bigominus -Q$$

Example 9-16: A positive charge, $+q$, is placed at the point labeled P in the field of the dipole shown below. Describe the direction of the resulting electric force on the charge. Do the same for a negative charge, $-q$, placed at the point labeled N.

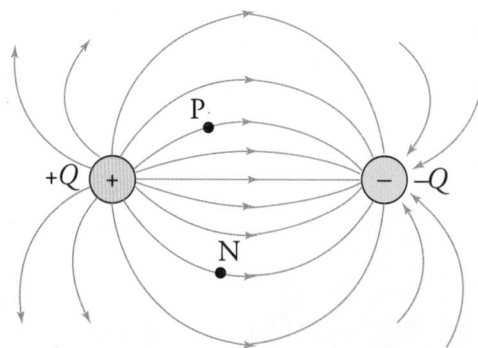

Solution: The electric field vector at any point is always *tangent* to the field line passing through that point and its direction is the same as that of the field line. Since $\mathbf{F} = q\mathbf{E}$, the force on a positive charge is in the same direction as $\mathbf{E}$ and the force on a negative charge is in the opposite direction from $\mathbf{E}$. The directions of $\mathbf{F}_{\text{on } q}$ and $\mathbf{F}_{\text{on } -q}$ are shown in the figure below.

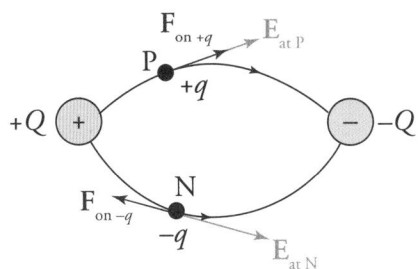

Conductors, Insulators, and Polarization

Most everyday materials can be classified into one of two major categories: *conductors* or *insulators* (also known as *dielectrics*). A material is a **conductor** if it contains charges that are free to roam throughout the material. Metals are the classic and most important conductors. In a metal, one or more valence electrons per atom are not strongly bound to any particular atom and are thus free to roam. If a metal is placed in an electric field, these free charges (called **conduction electrons**) will move in response to the field. Another example of a conductor would be a solution that contains lots of dissolved ions (such as saltwater).

Here's an interesting property of conductors: Imagine that we place a whole bunch of electrons on a piece of metal. It's now negatively charged. Since electrons repel each other, they'll want to get as far away from each other as possible. As a result, all this excess charge moves (rapidly) to the surface. Any net charge on a conductor resides on its surface. Since there's no excess charge within the body of the conductor, there cannot be an electrostatic field inside a conductor. You can block out external electric fields simply by surrounding yourself with metal; the free charges in the metal will move to the surface to shield the interior and keep $\mathbf{E} = 0$ inside.

By contrast, an **insulator** (**dielectric**) is a material that doesn't have free charges. Electrons are tightly bound to their atoms and thus are not free to roam throughout the material. Common insulators include rubber, glass, wood, paper, and plastic.

Now, let's study this situation: Start with a neutral metal sphere and bring a charge (a positive charge) Q nearby without touching the original metal sphere. What will happen? The positive charge will attract free electrons in the metal, leaving the far side of the sphere positively charged. Since the negative charge is closer to Q than the positive charge, there'll be a net attraction between Q and the sphere. So, even though the sphere as a whole is electrically neutral, the separation of charge induced by the presence of Q will create a force of electrical attraction between them.

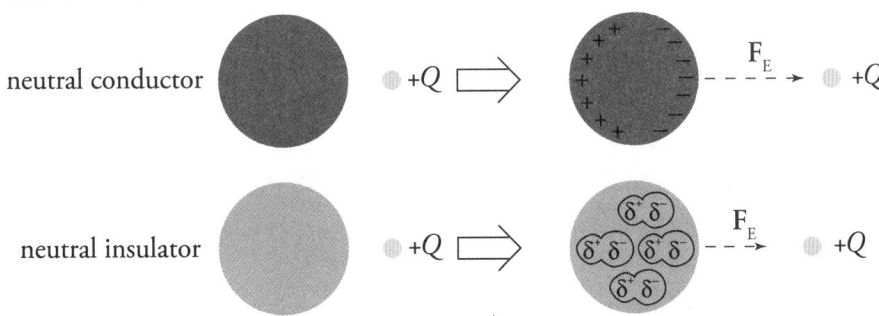

Now what if the sphere was made of glass (an insulator)? Although there aren't free electrons that can move to the near side of the sphere, the atoms that make up the sphere will become **polarized**. That is, their electrons will feel a tug toward Q, causing the atoms to develop a partial negative charge pointing toward Q (and a partial positive charge pointing away from Q). The effect isn't as dramatic as the mass movement of free electrons in the case of a metal sphere, but the polarization is still enough to cause an electrical attraction between the sphere and Q. For example, if you comb your hair, the comb will pick up extra electrons, making it negatively charged. If you place this electric field source near little bits of paper, the paper will become polarized and will then be attracted to the comb.[2]

9.4 ELECTRIC POTENTIAL AND POTENTIAL ENERGY

So far, we have viewed the electric field due to a source charge (or a more general charge distribution, such as a pair of charges or a plate) as a collection of vectors. This point of view allowed us to answer questions about other *vector* quantities, like force and acceleration. The basic equations for finding these quantities were $\mathbf{F} = q\mathbf{E}$ and $\mathbf{a} = \mathbf{F}/m = q\mathbf{E}/m$.

What if we wanted to answer questions about *scalar* quantities, like energy, work, or speed? It turns out that the easiest way to answer these questions is to view the electric field in a different way, in terms of a scalar field. First, it is useful to review a few facts about gravitational potential energy. As you'll recall, if an object of mass m is dropped from rest from a height h and hits the ground, $W_{\text{by grav}} = +mgh$ while $\Delta PE_{\text{grav}} = -mgh$. Similarly, if the object is lifted from the ground to a height h, $W_{\text{by grav}} = -mgh$, $W_{\text{against grav}} = +mgh$ and $\Delta PE_{\text{grav}} = +mgh$.

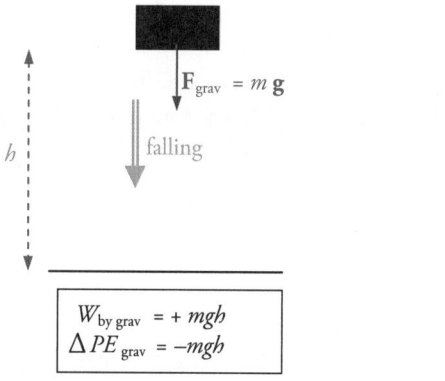
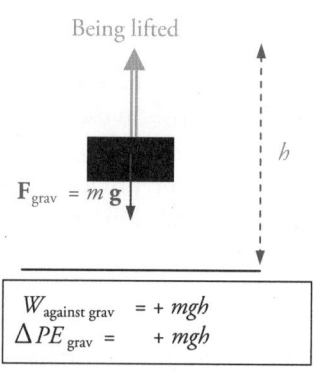

If an object moves "with nature" (i.e., in the direction that gravity points), then potential energy decreases. If an object moves "against nature," then potential energy increases. This is an important fact to remember going forward, as it will be applied to electric potential energy as well.

---

[2] The same phenomenon, in which the presence of a charge tends to cause polarization in a nearby collection of charges, is responsible for a kind of intermolecular force: Dipole-induced dipole forces are caused by a shifting of the electron cloud of a neutral molecule toward positively charged ions or away from a negatively charged ion; in each case, the resulting force between the ion and the atom is attractive.

The **London dispersion force**, in which electrically neutral molecules temporarily induce polarization in each other, is a much weaker version of the same phenomenon—again, electron clouds shift a little bit to create dipoles.

In the example below, a positively charged particle is fixed in place and a negatively charged particle is moved from point A to point B.

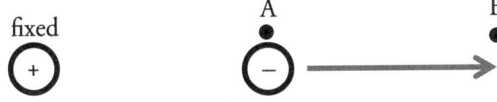

Without knowing the formula for electric potential energy, we can say that $\Delta PE_{elec} > 0$, since the particle is being moved "against nature."

Mathematically, we see that $W_{by\ grav} = -\Delta PE_{grav}$ and that $W_{against\ grav} = +\Delta PE_{grav}$. Similarly, we will be able to make an analogous statement about the relationship between the work done by or against the electric field and the change in electric potential energy. We will also be able to answer questions involving speed by using Conservation of Mechanical Energy.

To find the equation for electric potential energy, it is useful to first consider that charged particles not only create a vector field (i.e., the electric field), they also create a scalar field.

This scalar field has a name: it's called **electric potential** (or just **potential** for short).

Let Q be a point source charge. At any point P that's a distance r from Q, we say that the electric potential at P is the scalar given by this formula:

Electric Potential

$$\phi = k\frac{Q}{r}$$

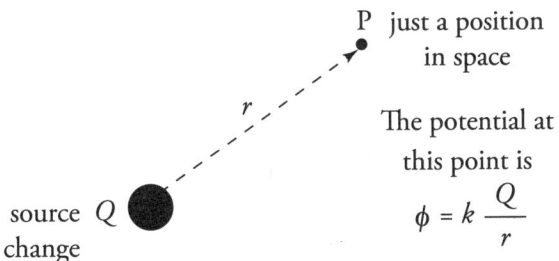

P just a position in space

The potential at this point is

$\phi = k\dfrac{Q}{r}$

source Q change

Notice the differences between this formula and the one for the electric field. First, the potential is kQ divided by r, while the electric field is kQ divided by r^2. Second, the electric field has a specific direction at each point (because it's a vector quantity); the potential, on the other hand, is not a vector, so it has no direction. For this reason, no absolute value symbol is needed. The sign of the potential is important in determining the behavior of nearby charges if they are placed in the field. While the electric field has the same magnitude at every point a distance r from Q, the field has a different direction at every point on the circle (or, more generally, the sphere) of radius r centered on Q. Therefore, we're forced to say that the electric field isn't the same at every point a distance r from Q because the directions are all different. The potential, however, is easier because it has no direction: The potential *is* the same at every point that's a distance r from Q.

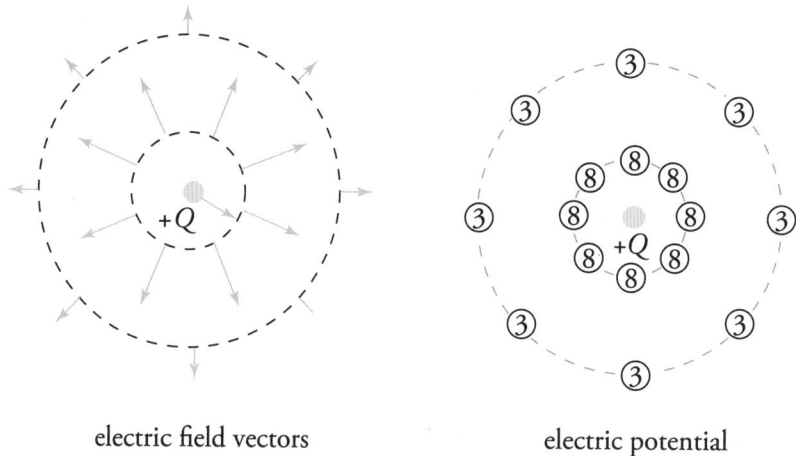

electric field vectors   electric potential

The dashed circles shown in the figure on the right above are called **equipotentials** ("equal potentials"), because the potential is the same at every point on them. For example, the potential is equal to 8 units everywhere on the inner dashed circle, and equal to 3 units everywhere on the outer dashed circle. As we move around on either dashed circle, the electric field changes (because the direction of **E** changes), but the potential doesn't change. This example of the electric field vectors and the electric equipotentials for a point charge also illustrates a general rule for the relation between the two fields: *electric field vectors point from higher to lower potentials*. You should memorize this rule: it is consistent with what you've already learned about electric fields created by source charges and what we will discuss below about the tendencies of free charges within potential gradients, but it is also something true on its own that you can use to answer MCAT questions where you do not know the charge configuration in a region of space.

The formula given on the previous page for the potential, $\phi = kQ/r$, assumes that the potential decreases to 0 as we move far away from the source charges (that is, as $r \to \infty$); this is the standard, conventional assumption. With this formula, you can see that if Q is a positive charge, then the values of the potential due to this source charge are also positive (if Q is positive, then kQ/r is positive); on the other hand, the values of the potential due to a negative source charge are negative (if Q is negative, then kQ/r is negative). The sign of the potential (that is, whether it's positive or negative) is not an indication of a direction; remember, potential is a scalar, so it has no direction.

Before we get to some examples, it's important to mention that while there's no special name for the unit of electric field, there *is* a special name for the unit of electric potential:

$$[\phi] = [k]\frac{[Q]}{[r]} = \left(\tfrac{\text{N} \cdot \text{m}^2}{\text{C}^2}\right)\frac{\text{C}}{\text{m}} = \frac{\text{N} \cdot \text{m}}{\text{C}} = \frac{\text{J}}{\text{C}}$$

A joule per coulomb (J/C) is called a **volt**, abbreviated V.

Example 9-17: What is the electric potential at a distance of $r = 30$ cm from a source charge $Q = -20$ nC?

Solution: Using the formula $\phi = k_0 Q / r$, we find that

$$\phi = k_0 \frac{Q}{r} = (9 \times 10^9 \ \tfrac{N \cdot m^2}{C^2}) \frac{-20 \times 10^{-9} \ C}{30 \times 10^{-2} \ m} = -600 \ V$$

9.4

Example 9-18: In the figure below, the potential at Point A is 1,000 V. What's the potential at Point B?

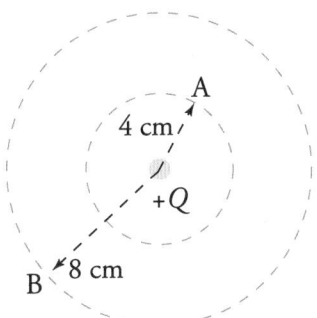

Solution: From the formula $\phi = k_0 Q / r$, we see that the potential is inversely proportional to r: Thus, $\phi \propto 1 / r$. Because the distance from Q to B is twice the distance from Q to A, the potential at B should be half the potential at A. Therefore, $\phi_{at\,B} = 500\,V$. (Notice that because the potential at A is 1,000 V, the potential at *every* point on the inner circle is 1,000 V; and since the potential at B is 500 V, the potential at *every* point on the outer circle is 500 V.)

Now that we know how to calculate electric potential, how do we use it to answer questions about the scalar quantities energy, work, and speed? The applications of electric potential all follow from this one fundamental equation:

Change in Electrical Potential Energy
$$\Delta PE = q\Delta\phi = qV$$

That is, the change in potential energy of a charge q that moves between two points whose potential difference is $\Delta\phi$ is just given by the product, $q\Delta\phi$; it also can be expressed as qV, where V is defined as the change in potential and is known as the *voltage*. For example, let's say a charge $q = +0.03$ C moves from a point on the inner circle to a point on the outer circle in the figure accompanying the preceding example:

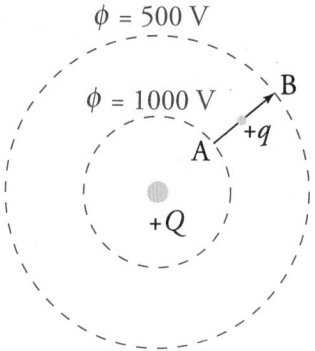

Then the change in the electrical potential energy of the charge q is

$$\Delta PE_{A \to B} = q\Delta\phi_{A \to B} = q(\phi_B - \phi_A) = (+0.03\,\text{C})(500\,\text{V} - 1000\,\text{V}) = -15\,\text{J}$$

We expected that the change in potential energy would be negative (that is, the potential energy would decrease), because the positive charge is moving farther from the positive source charge (i.e., "with nature"). Because q moves in a way it naturally "wants" to move (since the positive charge q is naturally repelled by the positive charge Q), its potential energy should decrease.

If the charge q were instead pushed (by some outside force) from Point B to Point A (i.e., "against nature"), then its potential energy would increase:

$$\Delta PE_{B \to A} = q\Delta\phi_{B \to A} = q(\phi_A - \phi_B) = (+0.03\,\text{C})(1000\,\text{V} - 500\,\text{V}) = +15\,\text{J}$$

What if the charge q were moved from one point on the outer circle (Point B, say) to another point on the outer circle, B′?

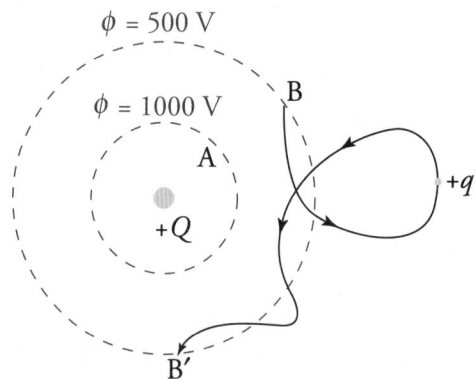

Its potential energy would not change. Because the potential is the same everywhere on the outer circle, the potential at B is the same as the potential at B′, so the potential *difference* between Points B and B′ is zero; and if $\Delta\phi = 0$, then $\Delta PE = 0$ as well. *A charge experiences no change in potential energy when its initial and final positions are at the same potential.*

The figure above also illustrates that the path taken by the charge is irrelevant. Like the gravitational force, the electric force is conservative; all that matters is where the charge began and where it ended; the specific path it takes doesn't matter.

Example 9-19: A charge $q = -8$ nC is moved from a position that's 10 cm from a charge $Q = +2$ µC to a position that's 20 cm away. What is the change in its electrical potential energy?

Solution: Let A be the initial point and B the final point; then the change in potential from Point A to Point B is

$$\Delta\phi = \phi_B - \phi_A = \frac{k_0 Q}{r_B} - \frac{k_0 Q}{r_A} = k_0 Q \left(\frac{1}{r_B} - \frac{1}{r_A}\right)$$

$$= (9 \times 10^9 \tfrac{\text{N·m}^2}{\text{C}^2})(2 \times 10^{-6} \text{ C})\left(\tfrac{1}{0.2 \text{ m}} - \tfrac{1}{0.1 \text{ m}}\right)$$

$$= -9 \times 10^4 \text{ V}$$

Therefore, the change in potential energy of the charge q is

$$\Delta PE = q\Delta\phi = (-8 \times 10^{-9} \text{ C})(-9 \times 10^4 \text{ V}) = 7.2 \times 10^{-4} \text{ J}$$

We've seen that all charged particles naturally move to positions of lower potential energy. To accomplish this, notice in the preceding examples that *positively charged particles naturally tend toward lower potential and negatively charged particles tend toward higher potential.* To verify this mathematically, we have learned that $\Delta PE = q\Delta\phi$ or $\Delta\phi = \Delta PE / q$. Moving "with nature" or spontaneously **always** means that ΔPE is negative. So if q is positive, then $\Delta\phi$ is (–)/(+) = (–), which means that potential decreases. If q is negative, then $\Delta\phi$ is (–)/(–) = (+), which means that potential increases. *This shows how charges are different from masses.* The gravitational field here on Earth always points down, and since there are no negative masses, anything dropped will spontaneously fall downward, *with the field.* However, unlike mass, charge can be negative, and negative charge will "fall upward," that is, move spontaneously *against the field.* Remember, though, that this is still a case of moving spontaneously toward lower potential energy: that tendency will always be true.

Now that we've seen examples of how to calculate changes in potential energy in an electric field by using the concept of electric potential, how do we answer questions about work or kinetic energy? By using equations we already know from mechanics.

What if we want to find the work done by the electric field as a charge moves? If we move objects around in a *gravitational* field, we remember that the change in gravitational potential energy is equal to the opposite of the work done by the gravitational field. That is, $\Delta PE_{grav} = -W_{by\,gravity}$, which is the same as $W_{by\,gravity} = -\Delta PE_{grav}$. Applying this same idea to an electric field, we can say that the work done by the electric field is equal to $-\Delta PE_{elec}$:

Work Done by Electric Field

$$W_{by\,electric\,field} = -\Delta PE_{elec}$$

Now what about kinetic energy? Well, if there's no friction (which will be the case for charges moving around in empty space) or other forces doing work as a charge moves, then mechanical energy is conserved; that is $KE + PE$ will remain constant. And if $KE + PE$ is constant, then $\Delta(KE + PE)$ will be zero. That is, ΔKE will be equal to $-\Delta PE$. Since we know how to calculate ΔPE, we can calculate ΔKE by just changing the sign of ΔPE:

$$\Delta KE = -\Delta PE$$

So, as long as you remember the fundamental formula for potential energy changes in an electric field, $\Delta PE = q\Delta\phi$, you can answer questions about work or kinetic energy in an electric field by just using the formulas above.

Example 9-20: In the figure below, a particle whose charge q is +4 nC moves in the electric field created by a negative source charge, $-Q$.

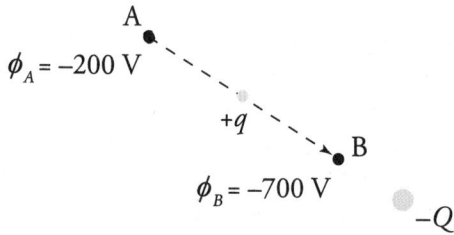

Find:

a) the change in potential energy,
b) the work done by the electric field, and
c) the change in kinetic energy of the particle as it moves from position A to position B.
d) If the mass of the particle is 10^{-8} kg and it started from rest at Point A, what will be its speed as it passes through Point B?

Solution:

a) $\Delta PE = q\Delta\phi = q\left(\phi_B - \phi_A\right) = \left(4 \times 10^{-9}\,\text{C}\right)\left[\left(-700\,\text{V}\right) - \left(-200\,\text{V}\right)\right] = -2 \times 10^{-6}\,\text{J}$

b) $W_{\text{by electric field}} = -\Delta PE_{\text{elec}} = -\left(-2 \times 10^{-6}\,\text{J}\right) = 2 \times 10^{-6}\,\text{J}$

c) $\Delta KE = \Delta PE_{elec} = -\left(-2 \times 10^{-6} \text{ J}\right) = +2 \times 10^{-6} \text{ J}$

d) If the particle started from rest at Point A, then $PE_{atB} = \Delta KE = +2 \times 10^{-6} \text{ J}$, so

$$\frac{1}{2}mv_B^2 = 2 \times 10^{-6} \text{ J} \rightarrow v_B^2 = \frac{2(2 \times 10^{-6} \text{ J})}{m} \rightarrow v_B = \sqrt{\frac{4 \times 10^{-6} \text{ J}}{10^{-8} \text{ kg}}} = \sqrt{400 \text{ m}^2/\text{s}^2} = 20 \text{ m/s}$$

Example 9-21: An electric field pulls an electron from one position to another such that the change in potential is +1 V. By how much does the electron's kinetic energy change?

Solution: The change in potential energy is

$$\Delta PE = q\Delta\phi = (-1.6 \times 10^{-19} \text{ C})(+1 \text{ V}) = -1.6 \times 10^{-19} \text{ J}$$

so the change in kinetic energy is the opposite of this, $+1.6 \times 10^{-19}$ C. This amount of energy is known as 1 **electron volt (eV)**. In fact, the abbreviation for this unit makes the definition easy to remember: An electron (e^-) moving through a potential difference of 1 V experiences a kinetic energy change of $-q\Delta\phi = (e)(1 \text{ V}) = 1.6 \times 10^{-19} \text{ J} = 1 \text{ eV}$. While the joule is the SI unit for energy, it's too big to be convenient when discussing atomic-sized systems. The electron volt is commonly used instead.

Example 9-22: An electric field pushes a proton from one position to another such that the change in potential is –500 V. By how much does the kinetic energy of the proton increase, in electron volts?

Solution: The change in potential energy is

$$\Delta PE = q\Delta\phi = (+e)(-500 \text{ V}) = -500 \text{ eV}$$

so the change in kinetic energy, ΔKE, is $-\Delta PE = -(-500 \text{ eV}) = +500$ eV.

The Principle of Superposition for Electric Potential

The formula $\phi = kQ/r$ tells us how to find the potential due to a single point source charge, Q. To find the potential in an electric field that's created by more than one charge, we use the principle of superposition. In fact, applying this principle is even easier here than for electric forces and fields because potential is a scalar. When we add up individual potentials, we're simply adding numbers; we're not adding vectors.

9.4

Let's illustrate with an example. In the figure below, the source charges Q_1 = +10 nC and Q_2 = –5 nC are fixed in the positions shown; the charges and the two points, A and B, form the vertices of a rectangle. What is the potential at Point A? at Point B?

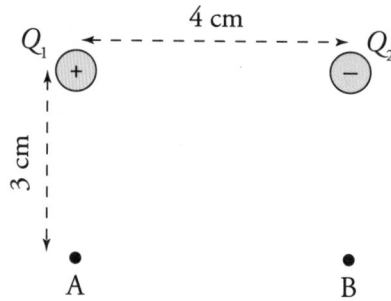

The potential at Point A due to Q_1 alone (ignoring the presence of Q_2) is

$$\phi_{A1} = k_0 \frac{Q_1}{r_{A1}} = (9 \times 10^9 \tfrac{\text{N} \cdot \text{m}^2}{\text{C}^2}) \frac{+10 \times 10^{-9} \text{ C}}{3 \times 10^{-2} \text{ m}} = 3000 \text{ V}$$

Since Point A is 5 cm from Q_2 (it's the hypotenuse of a 3-4-5 right triangle), the potential at Point A due to Q_2 alone (ignoring the presence of Q_1) is

$$\phi_{A2} = k_0 \frac{Q_2}{r_{A2}} = (9 \times 10^9 \tfrac{\text{N} \cdot \text{m}^2}{\text{C}^2}) \frac{-5 \times 10^{-9} \text{ C}}{5 \times 10^{-2} \text{ m}} = -900 \text{ V}$$

Therefore, the total electric potential at Point A, due to both source charges, is

$$\phi_A = \phi_{A1} + \phi_{A2} = (3000 \text{ V}) + (-900 \text{ V}) = 2100 \text{ V}$$

Similarly, the total electric potential at Point B is

$$\phi_B = \phi_{B1} + \phi_{B2} = k_0 \frac{Q_1}{r_{B1}} + k_0 \frac{Q_2}{r_{B2}}$$
$$= (9 \times 10^9 \tfrac{\text{N} \cdot \text{m}^2}{\text{C}^2}) \frac{+10 \times 10^{-9} \text{ C}}{5 \times 10^{-2} \text{ m}} + (9 \times 10^9 \tfrac{\text{N} \cdot \text{m}^2}{\text{C}^2}) \frac{-5 \times 10^{-9} \text{ C}}{3 \times 10^{-2} \text{ m}}$$
$$= (1800 \text{ V}) + (-1500 \text{ V})$$
$$= 300 \text{ V}$$

Example 9-23: A charge $q = 1$ nC is moved from position A to position B, along the path labeled a in the figure below. Find the work done by the electric field. How would your answer change if q had been moved from position A to position B, along the path labeled b?

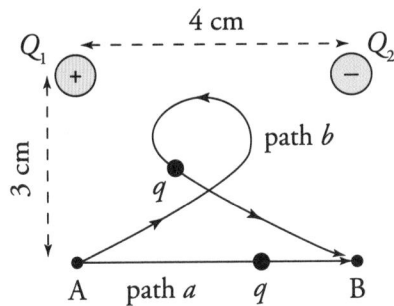

Solution: Path a begins at Point A, where $\phi_A = 2100\,\text{V}$, and ends at Point B, where $\phi_B = 300\,\text{V}$, so $\Delta\phi_{A\to B} = \phi_B - \phi_A = 300\,\text{V} - 2100\,\text{V} = -1800\,\text{V}$. Therefore, the change in potential energy of the charge q is

$$\Delta PE = q\Delta\phi = (1\times10^{-9}\ \text{C})(-1800\ \text{V}) = -1.8\times10^{-6}\ \text{J}$$

This means that the work done by the electric field, $W_{\text{by E}}$, is equal to $-\Delta PE = 1.8\times10^{-6}$ J. If q had followed path b, the change in potential energy and the work done by the electric field would have been the same as for path a. The shape or length of the path is irrelevant; all that matters is the initial point and the ending point, and both paths begin at Point A and end at Point B.

We can't use the formula "work = force × distance" here, because the force is not constant during the object's displacement. To calculate work in an electric field, we use electric potential and the formula $W_{\text{by E}} = -\Delta PE_{\text{elec}}$.

Example 9-24: The figure below shows two source charges, $+2Q$ and $-Q$. What is the minimum amount of work that must be done by some outside force against the electric field to move a negative charge, $-q$, from position A to position B along the semicircular path shown?

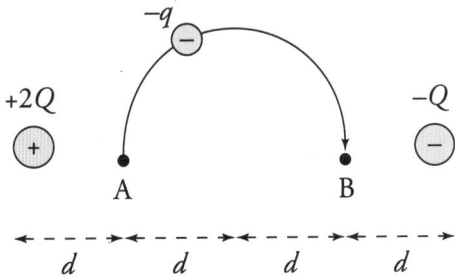

Solution: First, remember that neither the shape nor the length of the path matters; the fact that the path is a semicircle is irrelevant. All that matters is the initial point and the ending point of the path. Using the principle of superposition, the potentials at Points A and B are

$$\phi_A = \frac{k(+2Q)}{d} + \frac{k(-Q)}{3d} = \frac{5kQ}{3d} \quad \text{and} \quad \phi_B = \frac{k(+2Q)}{3d} + \frac{k(-Q)}{d} = -\frac{kQ}{3d}$$

Therefore, the change in potential energy of the charge $-q$ as it's moved from A to B is

$$\Delta PE = (-q)(\phi_B - \phi_A) = (-q)\left(\frac{-kQ}{3d} - \frac{5kQ}{3d}\right) = \frac{2kQq}{d}$$

Since the change in PE is positive, we know that the charge $-q$ is not moving as it would naturally on its own (after all, we can see from the figure that it's being moved from a point near a positive source charge, to which it's attracted, to a point near a negative charge, from which it's repelled). Therefore, some outside force is pushing this charge, doing work against the electric field. Since the work done *by* the electric field is $-\Delta PE = -2kQq/d$, the work done *against* the electric field by some outside force must be the opposite of this: $2kQq/d$.

Example 9-25: An electric dipole consists of a pair of equal but opposite charges, $+Q$ and $-Q$, separated by a distance d. What is the electric potential at the point (call it P) that's midway between these source charges?

Solution: The potential at P due to the positive charge alone is $k(+Q)/\left(\frac{1}{2}d\right)$, and the potential at P due to the negative charge alone is $k(-Q)/\left(\frac{1}{2}d\right)$. Adding these, we get zero, which is the potential at P due to both charges. (Notice that although the potential at P is zero, the electric field at P is *not* zero. We can have the "opposite" situation as well; that is, it's possible to have a point where the electric field is zero, but the potential is not. For example, if we had two equal source charges of the *same* sign, say $+Q$ and $+Q$, separated by a distance d, then the potential at the point that's midway between them would not be zero [it would be $2k(+Q)/\left(\frac{1}{2}d\right)$] but the electric field there *would* be zero.)

Example 9-26: An electric dipole consists of a pair of equal but opposite charges, $+Q$ and $-Q$, separated by a distance d. The dashed curves in the figure below are equipotentials. (Notice that the equipotentials are always perpendicular to the electric field lines, wherever they intersect. This is true for *any* electrostatic field, not just for the field created by a dipole.)

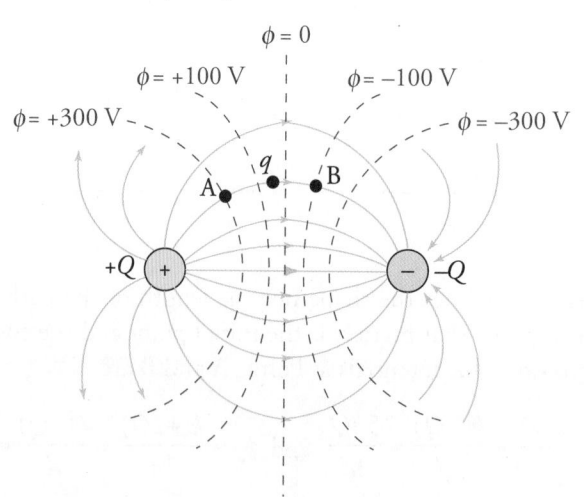

If a particle of mass $m = 1 \times 10^{-6}$ kg and charge $q = 5$ nC starts from rest at Point A and moves to Point B,

a)   How much work is done by the electric field?

b)   What is the speed of the particle when it reaches Point B?

Solution:

a)   The work done by the electric field is equal to the opposite of the change in the particle's elec-

trical potential energy $W_{by\ E} = -\Delta PE_{elec}$. Since the potential at Point A is $\phi_A = +300\,V$

(because A lies on the $\phi = +300\,V$ equipotential) and the potential at Point B is $\phi_B = -100\,V$

(because B lies on the $\phi = -100\,V$ equipotential), the change in potential from A to B is

$\phi_B - \phi_A = \left(-100\ V\right) - \left(300\ V\right) = -400\ V$. Therefore,

$$W_{by\ E} = -\Delta PE_{elec} = -q\Delta\phi = -(5\times 10^{-9}\ C)(-400\ V) = 2\times 10^{-6}\ J$$

b)   Since the total work done on the particle is equal to its change in kinetic energy (the work-

energy theorem), we have $\Delta KE = 2 \times 10^{-6}\ J$. Because the particle started from rest at Point A,

we have $KE_{at\ B} = \Delta KE_{A\rightarrow B} = 2\times 10^{-6}\ J$, so

$$\frac{1}{2}mv_B^2 = 2\times 10^{-6}\ J \rightarrow v_B = \sqrt{\frac{2\left(2\times 10^{-6}\ J\right)}{1\times 10^{-6}\ kg}} = 2\tfrac{m}{s}$$

Example 9-27: The figure below shows several point source charges, $+Q_1$, $+Q_2$, $-Q_3$, and $-Q_4$, and the electric potential at various points (A, B, C, Z, Y, and Z) in the electric field they produce:

The difference in electric potential between two points is called the **voltage**, V. That is, $V = \Delta\phi$. For example, the voltage from Point A to Point B is $\phi_B - \phi_A = (+200\,V) - (+100\,V) = +100\,V$, and the voltage from X to Y is $V = (-300\,V) - (-100\,V) = -200\,V$.

a) How much work does the electric field do on a charge $q = +2\,\mu C$ as q is moved from Point X to Point C?

b) True or false? If the charge q is placed at Point Z, it will remain at this point because the electric potential is 0 V.

Solution:

a) The work done by the electric field is equal to the opposite of the change in the electrical potential energy $W_{by\,E} = -\Delta PE_{elec}$. Since $\Delta\phi = V$, the fundamental equation $\Delta PE = q\Delta\phi$ becomes simply

$$\Delta PE = qV$$

Since $V_{X\to C} = \phi_C - \phi_X = (+400\,V) - (-100\,V) = +500\,V$, we have

$$\Delta PE = qV = (2 \times 10^{-6}\,C)(5 \times 10^2\,V) = 1 \times 10^{-3}\,J$$

Therefore, $W_{by\,E} = -1 \times 10^{-3}\,J$. (Does it make sense that ΔPE is positive and $W_{by\,E}$ is negative? *Yes*, because a positive charge q would have to be pushed by some outside force from Point X (which is near a negative charge) to Point C (which is near a positive charge). When an external force has to do positive work against the electric field, the electrical potential energy increases and the work done by the electric field is negative.)

b) False. If q were placed at a point where the *electric field* was zero, *then* it would feel no force and remain there. However, if q is placed at a point where the electric potential is zero, it will be accelerated toward a point where the potential is lower (because q is positive; recall Example 7-21). In this case, q would be accelerated by the electric field toward the negative source charge $-Q_3$.

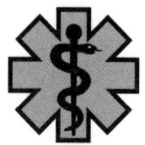

Example 9-28: During the active phase of the sodium-potassium pump, Na$^+$ ions are moved out of the cell against a potential difference of about 70 mV. How much work per sodium ion is done against the electric field during this process?

Solution: The work done against a field (or on a system, to use a more familiar phrasing for the same concept) is given by $W_{against\,E} = \Delta PE_{elec} = q\Delta\phi$. In this instance that yields $q\Delta\phi = (1.6 \times 10^{-19}\,C)(7 \times 10^{-2}\,V) \approx 11 \times 10^{-21}\,J = 1.1 \times 10^{-20}\,J$.

Summary of Formulas

Elementary charge: $e = 1.6 \times 10^{-19}$ C

   charge of proton = $+e$; charge of electron = $-e$

Charge is quantized: $e = 1.6 \times 10^{-19}$ C

Coulomb's law: $F_{elec} = k \dfrac{|Q||q|}{r^2}$

   Opposite charges attract, like charges repel.

Coulomb's constant: $k_0 = 9 \times 10^9 \ \frac{N \cdot m^2}{C^2}$

Principle of Superposition:

The net force, electric field, or electric potential on a charge q (for force) or point P (for electric field or electric potential) due to a collection of other charges (Qs) is equal to the sum of individual effects of each Q.

Electric field due to point charge Q: $E = k \dfrac{|Q|}{r^2}$

Direction of electric field:

   Positive charges want to move in the direction of the electric field (**E**).

   Negative charges want to move opposite the direction of the electric field (**E**).

Electric force and field: $\mathbf{F} = q\mathbf{E}$

Electric potential: $\phi = k\dfrac{Q}{r}$

(a scalar, not a vector)

Positive charges want to move to regions of lower potential

Negative charges want to move to regions of higher potential

Change in electrical PE: $\Delta PE_{elec} = q\Delta\phi = qV$

Work done by electric field: $W_{by\,E} = -\Delta PE_{elec}$

Change in KE: $\Delta KE = -\Delta PE$

For conductors, charge rests on the outer surface and the electric field inside is zero.

CHAPTER 9 FREESTANDING PRACTICE QUESTIONS

1. How far apart are two charges ($A = 10\ \mu C$ and $B = 12\ \mu C$) if the electric potential measured at point C midway between them is 10 V?

A) 2×10^{-5} m
B) 2×10^{5} m
C) 4×10^{-4} m
D) 4×10^{4} m

2. In a certain region of space, one equipotential of –100 V lies above another equipotential of –20 V. Between these two regions, what best describes the direction of the electric field?

A) Pointing upward
B) Pointing downward
C) Pointing horizontally
D) There is no field because the two potential regions are both negative.

3. Two equally positive charges are r distance apart. If the amount of charge on A is doubled and the distance between the charges is doubled, what is the ratio of new electric force to old electric force?

A) 1/4
B) 1/2
C) 2
D) 4

4. The amount of work required to move a charge in an electric field depends:

A) only on the change in potential and not the path traveled.
B) on both the change in potential and the path traveled.
C) only on the path traveled and not the change in potential.
D) on neither the path traveled nor the change in potential.

5. Which of the following pairs of electric forces form an action-reaction pair?

   I. Two positive charges, of different masses, placed at a distance d apart.
   II. Two negative charges, of equal masses, placed at a distance d apart.
   III. One positive charge and one negative charge, of equal masses, placed at a distance d apart.

A) I and II only
B) II and III only
C) III only
D) I, II and III

6. A hollow metal sphere of radius 0.5 m has a net charge of 2.0×10^{-6} C. A solid metal sphere of radius 0.5 m has a net charge of 4.0×10^{-6} C. The centers of the spheres are placed a distance 2 m apart and equilibrium is established. Compared to the electric field at the center of the hollow sphere, the electric field at the center of the solid sphere is:

A) twice the magnitude.
B) four times the magnitude.
C) half the magnitude.
D) equal in magnitude.

7. Starting from rest, a sphere of mass 2 kg and charge –0.1 C slides across a frictionless horizontal plane through a potential difference of 220 V. Determine the instantaneous velocity of the sphere the moment it has rolled through this potential.

A) 4.7 m/s
B) 5.1 m/s
C) 5.5 m/s
D) 6.1 m/s

CHAPTER 9 PRACTICE PASSAGE

Electroreception refers to the capacity of an organism to sense changes in the local electric field, typically for purposes of prey locating or predator avoidance, as the muscle contractions of nearby organisms disrupt the ambient electric field. The phenomenon is particularly well studied in several types of fishes, though it has also been explored more recently in marine and aquatic mammals. As long ago as 1678, Italian physician Stefano Lorenzini described pores with long tubes ending in bulbs, or *ampullae*, around the heads of sharks that were later confirmed to be electroreceptors.

Recent studies have shown that multiple species have independently evolved electroreception, the anatomy usually involving tubes of various orientations in the epidermal and dermal layers filled with an electrolytic gel or mucus. Though the precise mechanism of electroreception varies and the details are not well understood in all cases, the general requirement is a potential difference between the opening of the tube and its base. In the case of ampullae of Lorenzini in sharks, the signal mechanism involves low-threshold voltage-gated calcium channels triggered by a potential difference across receptor cell epithelium, where an influx of calcium ions depolarizes the membrane. Voltage-gated potassium channels allow K^+ efflux rates that vary with voltage, allowing for repetitive stimulation.

Many experiments have been conducted to determine voltage sensitivity thresholds among various aquatic electroreceptive organisms. One study with dolphins, which are highly trainable due to their intelligence, involved placing the dolphin's head inside a hoop while it rested its snout on a small platform so that its closest electroreceptive organs were 10 cm below a dipole electrode. The dolphin was trained to leave the hoop when an electrical signal was present and to remain when there was no such signal. The following data were obtained, where the voltage per centimeter was calculated at the location of the sense organs and the hit rate and false alarm rate correspond to the number of times that dolphin left the hoop when there was or was not an electric field present, respectively.

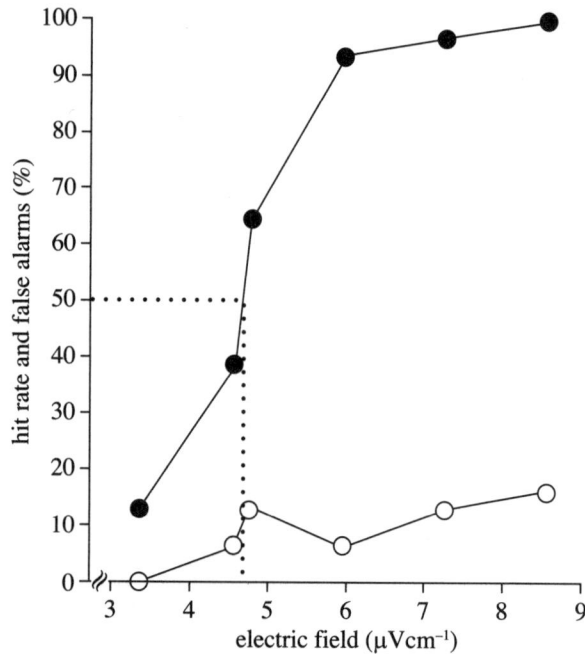

Figure 1 Successful (black circles) and false-positive (white circles) detection rates for a dolphin exposed to electric fields of different strengths

Figure adapted from: Czech-Damal NU, Liebschner A, Miersch L, Klauer G, Hanke FD, Marshall C, Dehnhardt G, Hanke W. *Electroreception in the Guiana dolphin (Sotalia guianensis).* Proc Biol Sci. 2012 Feb 22;279(1729):663-8.

1. Suppose that the net charge inside a receptor cell is to remain constant. Neglecting any other ion channels, which of the following must be the case?

A) The influx rate of calcium ions must be twice the efflux rate of potassium ions.
B) The influx rate of calcium ions must be the same as the efflux rate of potassium ions.
C) The influx rate of calcium ions must be half the efflux rate of potassium ions.
D) It is not possible for the charge to remain constant during the flow of calcium and potassium ions.

2. In examining the anatomy of saltwater and freshwater electroreceptive fishes, scientists discover that the electroreceptor tubes in saltwater fishes are generally much longer—the distance between the pores and base of the ampullae is greater—than those of freshwater fishes. What most likely explains this?

A) The conductivity of salt water is greater than that of fresh water, so the potential difference between two points in a given electric field is generally less than it would be in fresh water.

B) The conductivity of salt water is less than that of fresh water, so the potential difference between two points in a given electric field is generally less than it would be in fresh water.

C) The conductivity of salt water is greater than that of fresh water, so the potential difference between two points in a given electric field is generally greater than it would be in fresh water.

D) The conductivity of salt water is less than that of fresh water, so the potential difference between two points in a given electric field is generally greater than it would be in fresh water.

3. The data from the dolphin electroreception experiment support which of the following conclusions?

   I. Dolphins' sensory threshold for electric fields occurs at 4.7 µV/cm.
   II. Dolphins' sensitivity to electric fields increases monotonically with field strength within the given domain, once the sensory threshold is reached.
   III. The dolphin never left the hoop at a signal voltage of 3.3 µV/cm.

A) I only
B) I and II only
C) I and III only
D) II and III only

4. The electric field generated by a dipole electrode decreases roughly as the cube of the distance from the dipole axis. Suppose the experiment was repeated with a distance of 20 cm between the dipole electrode and the dolphin's electroreceptors. By what factor would the experimenters need to change the magnitude of the electrode charge to achieve the same electric field strengths as shown in Figure 1?

A) 10^{-3}
B) 1/8
C) 8
D) 10^3

5. Suppose a shark was swimming north into a uniform electric field pointing south. Which of the following best characterizes the sensory effects in its ampullae of Lorenzini?

A) In a northward-facing tube, the electric potential is higher at the pore than at the ampulla base.
B) In a southward-facing tube, the electric potential is higher at the pore than at the ampulla base.
C) In an eastward-facing tube, the electric potential is higher at the pore than at the ampulla base.
D) In an upward-facing tube, the electric potential is higher at the pore than at the ampulla base.

SOLUTIONS TO CHAPTER 9 FREESTANDING PRACTICE QUESTIONS

1. **D** This question requires us to remember the electric potential formula. The question stem tells us that C is the midway point between A and B, so if we can determine the distance between A and C (or B and C), we can double that distance to determine the distance between A and B. Since $\phi_{elec} = kQ / r$ is a scalar quantity, when we use the Principle of Superposition for Electric Potential, it is straight addition. Let C be the distance between A and C (note that it is also the distance between B and C since C is midway between A and B). Thus,

$$\phi_{elec} = \frac{kQ_A}{C} + \frac{kQ_B}{C}$$
$$C = (kQ_A + kQ_B) / \phi_{elec}$$
$$= [(9 \times 10^9)(10 \times 10^{-6}) + (9 \times 10^9)(12 \times 10^{-6})] / 10$$
$$= [(90 \times 10^3) + (108 \times 10^3)] / 10$$
$$= 1.98 \times 10^4 \text{ m} \approx 2 \times 10^4 \text{ m}$$

Now that we know how far apart A and C are (and also therefore how far apart B and C are), we double this distance to calculate how far apart A and B are (i.e., $2 \times (2 \times 10^4 \text{ m}) = 4 \times 10^4 \text{ m}$).

2. **A** Differences in electric potential induce electric fields in the direction from higher to lower potential: you can remember this rule by recalling that positive charges tend to move toward regions of lower potential (going "downhill" in potential), and positive charges also experience electrostatic forces in the direction of the electric field. Remember that electric potential is a scalar and the sign matters: since –20 V is greater than –100 V, the electric field points from –20 V to –100 V, which is upward.

3. **B** The MCAT loves proportion questions, as they require us to remember the formula for specific quantities. In this question, we need to recall the formula for electric force and how it varies with respect to the variable of distance. Given that $F_E = \frac{kq_1q_2}{r^2}$, the (original F_E) = $\frac{kq^2}{r^2}$ and the (new F_E) = $\frac{k(2q)(q)}{(2r)^2} = \frac{2kq^2}{4r^2} = \frac{kq^2}{2r^2} = \frac{1}{2}\left(\frac{kq^2}{r^2}\right) = \frac{1}{2}$ (original F_E). Therefore, the ratio of (new F_E)/(original F_E) = $(\frac{1}{2}$ original F_E)/(original F_E) = $\frac{1}{2}$.

4. **A**   The amount of work required to move a charge in an electric field depends only on the change in potential and is independent of the path traveled. Remember, like the gravitational field, the electric field is conservative.

5. **D**   The electric force is a force in the same sense as gravity and friction are forces. In each of these three cases the pairs of forces are acting on the two separate objects, thereby satisfying Newton's third law. As such, each forms an action-reaction pair. Note that the mass in each case is irrelevant as the electric force is independent of the mass.

6. **D**   The electric field inside of an electrostatic conductor is always zero. Therefore, the electric fields at the centers of the solid and hollow sphere are both equal in magnitude.

7. **A**   Since $\mathbf{v}_0 = 0$ (the sphere starts at rest), we need to calculate the kinetic energy gained by the sphere and use this to determine v_F. $\Delta PE = q\Delta\phi = -0.1\ \text{C}\ (220\ \textbf{V}) = -22\ \text{J}$. Using $\Delta PE = -\Delta KE$, $\Delta KE = 22\ \text{J}$. Finally, $\Delta KE = mv^2/2$, so $v = \sqrt{22}$. The MCAT does not expect you to have this square root memorized, but notice that it is less than $\sqrt{25}$, which is 5. We know that $\sqrt{22}$ is less than $\sqrt{25}$ so we can eliminate choices B, C and D.

SOLUTIONS TO CHAPTER 9 PRACTICE PASSAGE

1. **C** Calcium ions are Ca^{2+}, meaning that each has a charge of +2e. Potassium ions, K^+, have a charge of +1e. Thus half as many calcium ions must flow into the cell to account for the charge of the potassium ions flowing out of the cell.

2. **A** Notice the 2x2 pattern of these answer choices and approach with process of elimination. Though there are equations that apply to the situation, qualitative reasoning should suffice. First note that the passage indicates that electroreception depends upon the potential difference between the opening of the tube and its base, so a greater potential difference is logically going to meet the threshold of sensation more easily. Thus a longer tube is necessary if the potential difference between any two points is less than it would be in freshwater, eliminating choices C and D. From chemistry, we know that electrolytes in solution make a liquid conductive, and that eliminates choice B. We also know from physics that a perfect conductor contains zero electric field because the charges redistribute until the field is canceled out, and that also logically eliminates choice B.

3. **B** It helps for this question to have reviewed sensory processing in psychology. This is a Roman numeral question, so start by assessing the item that appears precisely twice among the answer choices. In this case, that is Item II or Item III, and Item III is shorter, so start there. Item III is false: the passage states that both hit rate and false alarms correspond to the dolphin leaving the hoop during the experiment, and hit rate is not zero anywhere on the graph (choices C and D can be eliminated). Since both remaining answer choices include Item I, it must be true and you can focus on Item II. Item II is true: "sensitivity" and "hit rate" are synonyms, and the graph clearly shows an increase, or positive slope, in hit rate throughout the domain of increasing electric field strength (choice A can be eliminated and choice B is correct). Note that Item I is in fact true: the standard experimental definition of sensory threshold is a signal can be detected at least 50% of the time, and the hit rate of 50% is indicated on the graph at about 4.7 μV/cm.

4. **C** The passage states that the original distance from the electrode to the dolphin's electroreceptors was 10 cm, so increasing that to 20 cm means doubling the distance. Since the electric field decreases as the cube of the distance, this would mean with the same original charge as generated the fields shown in the graph for 10 cm, the field strength would decrease by a factor of $2^3 = 8$. To cancel out this effect, the charge on the dipole must be increased by a factor of 8. Note that this presumes that the dipole field is directly proportional to the charge, which it in fact is, and that's a reasonable assumption given that the electric field from a point charge is proportional to the charge.

5. **A** Electric field lines point from higher to lower electric potential, so if the electric field is pointing south, locations to the north will have higher potentials than those to the south. If the tube is facing north, the pore (the front of the tube) will therefore have a higher potential than the ampulla base at the back (choice A is correct).

Chapter 10
Electricity and Magnetism

10.1 ELECTRIC CIRCUITS

An electric circuit is a pathway for the movement of electric charge, consisting of a voltage source, connecting wires, and other components.

Current

Current can be defined as the movement of charge, but for the purposes of analyzing an electric circuit, we need a more precise definition. For example, imagine picking up a metal paper clip and untwisting it to make it relatively straight. If we could look inside this piece of metal wire at the individual atoms, we would see a lattice with about one electron per atom free to roam freely, unbound to any particular atom. These free electrons are known as **conduction electrons**. (Recall the discussion of metallic bonding in *MCAT General Chemistry*.) The conduction electrons in a metal are zooming around throughout the lattice at very high speeds. However, we only have a current when there is a *net* movement of charge. Let's look at this a little more closely.

The figure below shows an imagined magnified view inside a metal wire. The conduction electrons move at an average speed on the order of a million meters per second ($v \sim 10^6$ m/s). If we chose any cross-sectional slice of the wire, we would see that these conduction electrons cross from left to right as often as they cross from right to left. So, while there is movement of charge, there's no *net* movement of charge; that is, there's no current.

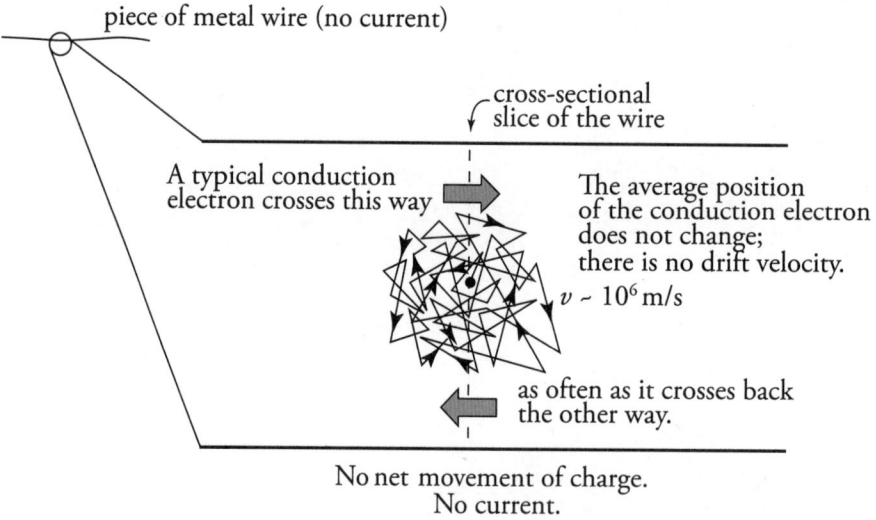

So how would this same piece of wire look if there *were* current in it? Superimposed on the conduction electrons' going-nowhere-fast zooming, we would see that there's a slight drift in one particular direction. This is known as the electrons' **drift velocity** (v_d). If we chose any cross-sectional slice of the wire, we'd see that these conduction electrons move across it from, say, left to right more often than they cross back. Thus, the average positions of the conduction electrons do change and there is a *net* movement of charge (in the case pictured below, negative charge to the right). This is **current**.

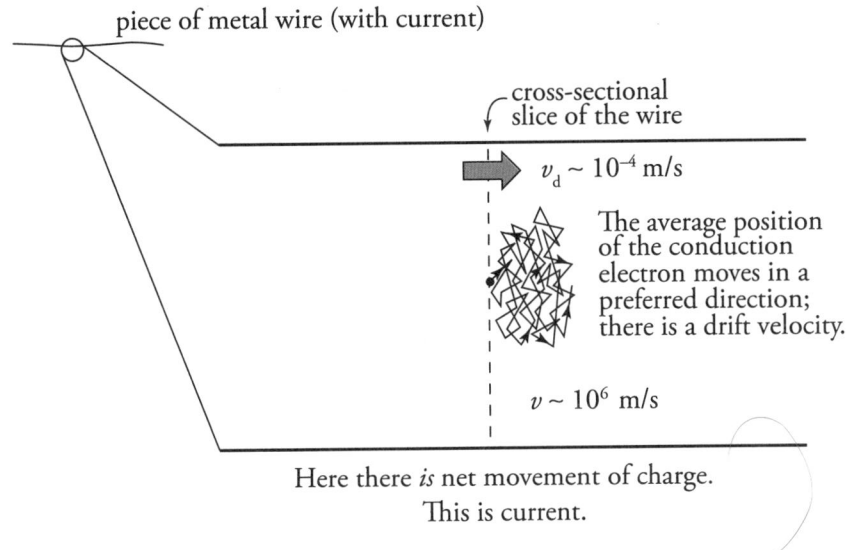

piece of metal wire (with current)

cross-sectional slice of the wire

$v_d \sim 10^{-4}$ m/s

The average position of the conduction electron moves in a preferred direction; there is a drift velocity.

$v \sim 10^6$ m/s

Here there *is* net movement of charge.
This is current.

In the first figure, there was no drift velocity and, therefore, no preferred direction for the movement of charge and no current. In the figure above, however, there is a drift velocity, so there is a flow of charge: a current.

Now, how do we measure current? Since current is the flow of charge, it makes sense to measure current as the amount of charge that moves past a certain point per unit time. Current is denoted by the letter I, and is equal to charge (Q) divided by time (t):

Current

$$I = \frac{Q}{t}$$

The unit of current is the coulomb per second (C/s), which has its own special name: the **ampère** (or just **amp**, for short), abbreviated **A**. Thus, 1 A = 1 C/s.[1] Since we know that one coulomb is a lot of charge (recall Example 9-4 in the preceding chapter), we would expect that one amp is a lot of current. The following table shows that even a small fraction of a coulomb is enough to kill you.

Current	Physiological Effect
~ 0.01 A	slight tingling
~ 0.02 A	painful; muscles may contract around source (can't let go)
~ 0.05 A	painful; can't let go; breathing difficult
~ 0.1 to 0.2 A	ventricular fibrillation (potentially fatal arrhythmia)
> 0.2 A	severe burning; breathing stops; heart stops (may be restarted)

---

[1] Notice that current is defined in about the same way that we defined *flow rate* in Chapter 8: amount of stuff per unit time. You can think of current as the flow rate of charge.

Example 10-1: Within a metal wire, 5×10^{17} conduction electrons drift past a certain point in 4 seconds. What is the magnitude of the current?

Solution: The magnitude of charge that passes the point in $t = 4$ seconds is

$$Q = ne = (5 \times 10^{17})(1.6 \times 10^{-19} \text{ C}) = 8 \times 10^{-2} \text{ C}$$

Therefore, the value of the current is

$$I = \frac{Q}{t} = \frac{8 \times 10^{-2} \text{ C}}{4 \text{ s}} = 0.02 \text{ A}$$

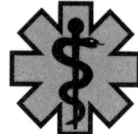

Example 10-2: A typical ion channel in a cellular membrane might allow the passage of 10^7 sodium ions to flow through in one second. What is the magnitude and direction of this ionic current?

Solution:

$$I = \frac{Q}{t} = \frac{(10^7)1.6 \times 10^{-19} \text{ C}}{1 \text{ s}} = 1.6 \times 10^{-12} \text{ A}$$

Because sodium ions are positive, the direction of current flow is the same as the one in which the charges are moving. (It is interesting to note that this current of ions into and out of the cell does not obey Ohm's Law generally, so predicting the current based upon voltage difference across the membrane is impossible.)

Voltage

Now that we know how to measure current, the next question is, *What causes it?* Look back at the picture of the wire in which there was a current. What would make an electron drift to the right? One answer is to say that there's an electric field inside the wire, and since negative charges move in the direction opposite to the electric field lines, electrons would be induced to drift to the right if the electric field pointed to the left:

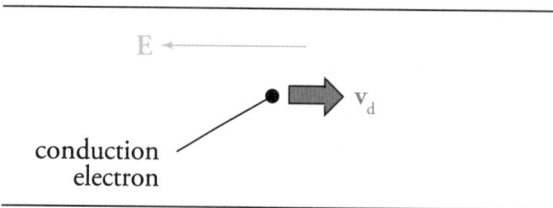

Another (equivalent) answer to the question, "What would make an electron drift to the right?" is that there's a potential difference (a voltage) between the ends of the wire. Because we know that negative charges naturally move toward regions of higher electric potential, electrons would be induced to drift to the right if the right end of the wire were maintained at a higher potential than the left end.

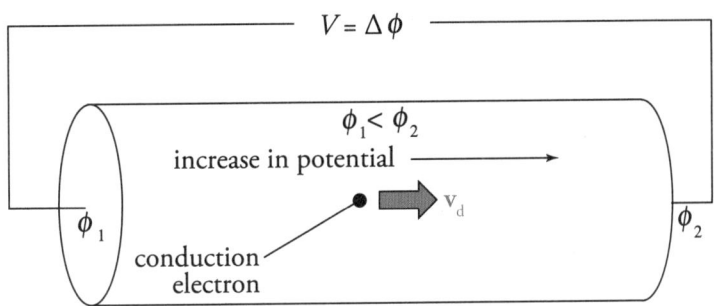

For our purposes in analyzing circuits, this second interpretation of the answer will be the one we use: that is, *it is a voltage that creates a current*. If there's no voltage (no potential difference), then the conduction electrons will just zoom around their original positions, going essentially nowhere; without a potential difference, they'd have no reason to do anything differently.

It is not uncommon to see the voltage that creates a current referred to as **electromotive force** (**emf**), since it is the cause that sets the charges into motion in a preferred direction. Notice, however, that calling it a "force" really isn't correct; it's a potential difference. Along similar lines, you will often encounter phrasing referring to "voltage drop" or "voltage increase" in descriptions of circuits. Some sources use V to refer to electric potential and then ΔV to refer to a change in electric potential, that is, what we're calling "voltage." Don't let this confuse you: the word "voltage" as used here *means* a "change in electric potential," so a phrase like "voltage drop" is redundant.

Resistance

Now that we know what current is, how to measure it, and what causes it, the next question is, *How much do we get?* The answer is, *It depends*. If we took a paper-clip wire and touched its two ends to the terminals of a battery, we'd get a measurable current. Now imagine picking up a rubber band and cutting it, so that it becomes essentially a straightened out "wire" of rubber. If we took this rubber wire and touched its two ends to the terminals of the same battery, we'd get essentially zero current. What's the difference? The metal wire and the rubber wire have very different **resistances**. Metals are conductors and rubber is an insulator. That is, metals have a very low intrinsic resistance, while insulators (like rubber) have a very high intrinsic resistance to the flow of charge. Since insulators have very few free electrons, there's going to be virtually no current, even with an applied voltage, which is why we got essentially zero current with our rubber wire.

Let V be the voltage applied to the ends of an object, and let I be the resulting current. By definition, the resistance of the object, R, is given by this equation:

Resistance

$$R = \frac{V}{I}$$

The unit of resistance is the volt per amp (V/A), which has its own special name: the **ohm**, abbreviated Ω (the Greek letter capital *omega*—get it? "ohmega"). Thus, $1\,\Omega = 1$ V/A. Notice from the definition that for a given voltage, a large I means a small R, and a small I means a big R; that is, for a fixed voltage, resistance and current are inversely proportional.

Example 10-3: When the potential difference between the ends of a wire is 12 V, the current is measured to be 0.06 A. What's the resistance of the wire?

Solution: Using the definition of resistance, we find that

$$R = \frac{V}{I} = \frac{12\text{ V}}{0.06\text{ A}} = 200\,\Omega$$

There's another way to calculate the resistance, using a formula that does not depend on V or I. Instead, it expresses the resistance in terms of the material's *intrinsic* resistance, which is known as its **resistivity** (and denoted by ρ, not to be confused with the material's density):

Resistance and Resistivity

$$R = \rho\frac{L}{A}$$

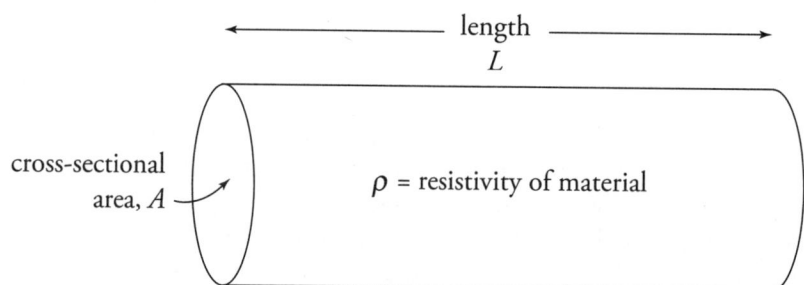

length
L

cross-sectional
area, A

ρ = resistivity of material

Notice that resistance and resistivity are not the same thing. Each material has its own resistivity; its *intrinsic* resistance. However, the resistance R depends on how we shape the material. For example, if we had two aluminum wires, one that was long and thin and another that was short and thick, both would have the same resistivity (because they're both made of the same material, aluminum), but the wires would have different resistances. The long, thin wire would have the greater resistance because R is proportional to L and inversely proportional to A.

Example 10-4: Consider two copper wires. Wire #1 has three times the length and twice the diameter of Wire #2. If R_1 is the resistance of Wire #1 and R_2 is the resistance of Wire #2, then which of the following is true?

    A. $R_2 = (2/3)R_1$
    B. $R_2 = (4/3)R_1$
    C. $R_2 = 6R_1$
    D. $R_2 = 12R_1$

Solution: We're told that $L_1 = 3L_2$, and since $d_1 = 2d_2$, we know that $A_1 = 4A_2$ (because area is proportional to the *square* of the diameter). Since both wires have the same resistivity (because they're both made of the same material), we find that

$$\frac{R^2}{R^1} = \frac{\rho L_2 / A_2}{\rho L_1 / A_1} = \frac{L_2}{L_1} \cdot \frac{A_1}{A_2} = \frac{1}{3} \cdot 4 = \frac{4}{3} \rightarrow R_2 = \frac{4}{3} R_1$$

Thus, the answer is B.

Example 10-5: The wire used for lighting systems is usually No. 12 wire, in the American Wire Gauge (AWG) system. The diameter of No. 12 wire is just over 2 mm (which means a cross-sectional area of 3.3×10^{-6} m²). What would be the resistance of half a mile (800 m) of No. 12 copper wire, given that the resistivity of copper is 1.7×10^{-8} Ω·m?

Solution: Using the equation $R = \rho L / A$, we get

$$R = \rho \frac{L}{A} = (1.7 \times 10^{-8} \ \Omega \cdot m) \frac{8 \times 10^2 \ m}{3.3 \times 10^{-6} \ m^2} \approx 4 \ \Omega$$

If we wanted to give a more precise formula for the resistance in terms of resistivity, we would have to include the temperature dependence. The resistivity of conductors generally increases slightly with temperature. However, unless specifically mentioned otherwise, assume that the MCAT will treat resistivity as a constant.

Ohm's Law

The definition of resistance, $R = V/I$, is usually written more simply as $V = IR$, and known as **Ohm's law**.

> **Ohm's Law**
>
> $$V = IR$$

However, the actual statement of Ohm's law isn't $V = IR$; rather, it's a statement about the behavior of certain conductors, and it isn't true for all materials. A material is said to obey Ohm's law if its resistance, R, remains constant as the voltage is varied; another requirement is that the current must reverse direction if the polarity of the voltage is reversed.[2] On the MCAT, you can assume that materials are "ohmic" unless you are specifically told otherwise.

---

[2] Some materials don't behave this way, and the relationship between voltage and current is more complex; on the MCAT, however, it's safe to assume that $V = IR$ applies unless you're told otherwise.

Resistors

A resistor is a component in an electric circuit that has a specific (and usually known) resistance. When we analyze a circuit, we generally ignore the resistance of the connecting metal wires and think of the resistance as being concentrated solely in the resistors placed in the circuit. We can do this because metal wires are such good conductors, i.e., their resistance is very low. Recall that in Example 8-4, we calculated that even half a mile of household wire has a resistance of only 4 Ω.

In the real world, a resistor is typically a little cylinder filled with an alloy (of carbon or of nickel and copper) and often encircled by colored bands to indicate the numerical value of its resistance, like this:

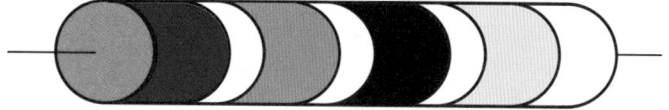

In circuit diagrams, however, a resistor is denoted by the following symbol:

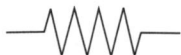

Electric circuits on the MCAT may contain just one resistor, but it's more likely that they'll have two or more. There are two ways the MCAT will combine resistors: in series or in parallel. Two or more resistors are said to be in **series** if each follows the others along a single connection in a circuit. For example, these two resistors are in series, because R_2 directly follows R_1 along a single path.

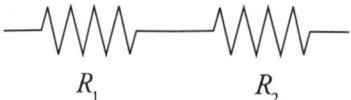

Resistors in Series

On the other hand, two or more resistors are said to be in **parallel** if they provide alternative routes from one point in a circuit to another. For example, the following two resistors are in parallel, because we get from Point P to Point Q in the circuit *either* by traveling through R_1 *or* by traveling through R_2; we don't go through both resistors like we would if they were in series.

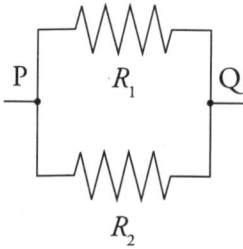

Resistors in Parallel

Typically, we analyze a circuit by first transforming it into a simpler one, one that contains just a single resistor. Therefore, we need a way to turn combinations of resistors (series combinations and parallel combinations) into a single, equivalent resistor; that is, one resistor that provides the same overall resistance as the combination.

Here are the formulas:

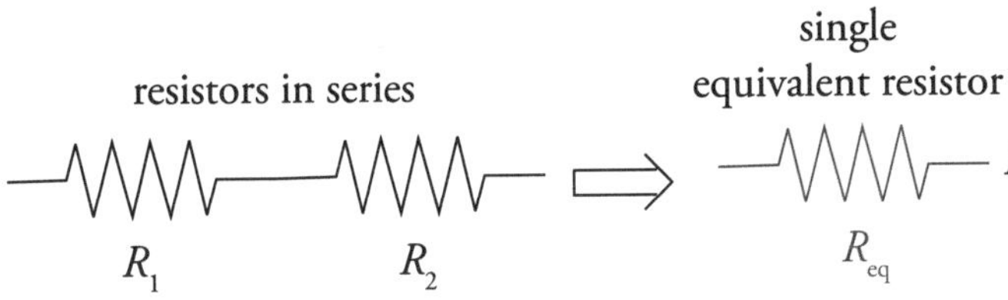

single
equivalent resistor

resistors in series

$$R_{eq} = R_1 + R_2 (+ R_3 + \cdots)$$

resistors in parallel

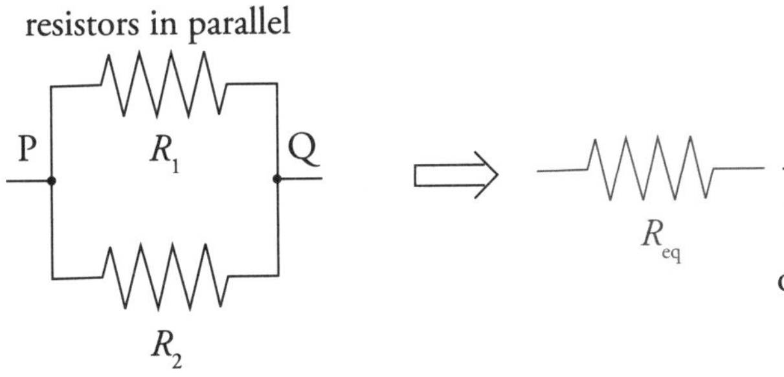

$$\frac{1}{R_{eq}} = \frac{1}{R_1} + \frac{1}{R_2}\left(+\frac{1}{R_3} + \cdots\right),$$

or only for 2 resistors, $R_{eq} = \dfrac{R_1 R_2}{R_1 + R_2}$

So, for resistors in series, we simply add the resistances. For example, if a 20 Ω resistor is in series with a 30 Ω resistor, this combination is equivalent to a single 50 Ω resistor, because 20 + 30 = 50. Notice that for a series combination, the equivalent resistance is always greater than the largest resistance in the combination; that's why the "R" is bigger in the figure above for the series combination.

For resistors in parallel, the formula is a little more complicated. If we have two resistors in parallel, we get the equivalent resistance by taking the product of the resistances ($R_1 R_2$) and dividing this by their sum ($R_1 + R_2$). For example, if a 3 Ω resistor is in parallel with a 6 Ω resistor, this combination is equivalent to a single 2 Ω resistor, because (3 × 6) divided by (3 + 6) is equal to 2. Alternatively, you can add the fractions and then take the reciprocal of the sum: $1/R_{eq}$ = 1/3 + 1/6 = 2/6 + 1/6 = 3/6 = 1/2, so R_{eq} = 2 Ω. For a parallel combination, the equivalent resistance is always less than the smallest resistance in the combination; that's why the "R_{eq}" is smaller in the figure above for the parallel combination.

The "product over sum" formula for parallel resistors only works for *two* resistors. If you have three or more resistors in parallel, use the reciprocal equation. Here's an example:

$$\frac{1}{R_{eq}} = \frac{1}{12\ \Omega} + \frac{1}{6\ \Omega} + \frac{1}{12\ \Omega} = \frac{1+2+1}{12\ \Omega} = \frac{4}{12\ \Omega} = \frac{1}{3\ \Omega} \to R_{eq} = 3\ \Omega$$

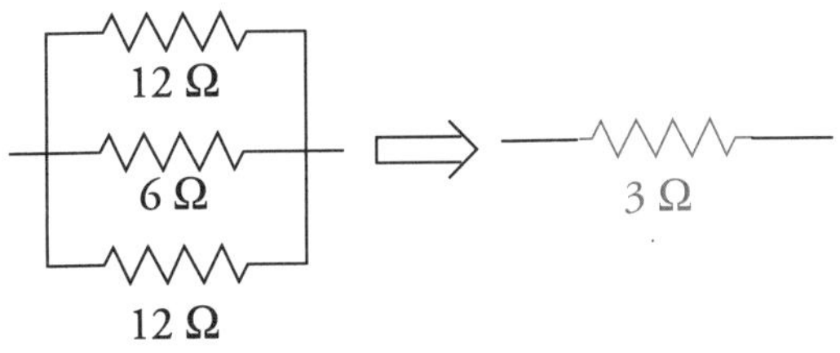

Example 10-6: Show that the equivalent resistance of two identical resistors in series is twice the resistance of either resistor, but the equivalent resistance of two identical resistors in parallel is half the resistance of either resistor.

Solution: Let the resistance of each resistor be R. Then, if two such resistors are in series, the equivalent resistance is $R_{eq} = R + R = 2R$. However, if two such resistors are in parallel, then their equivalent resistance is

$$R_{eq} = \frac{R \cdot R}{R + R} = \frac{R^2}{2R} = \frac{R}{2}$$

Example 10-7: What is the equivalent or total resistance of the following combination of resistors?

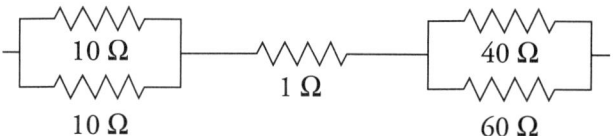

Solution: Here we have a mixture of parallel *and* series combinations. There's a parallel combination (the pair of 10 Ω resistors) that's in series with both a 1 Ω resistor and another parallel combination (the 40 Ω and 60 Ω resistors). To simplify this, we work in steps:

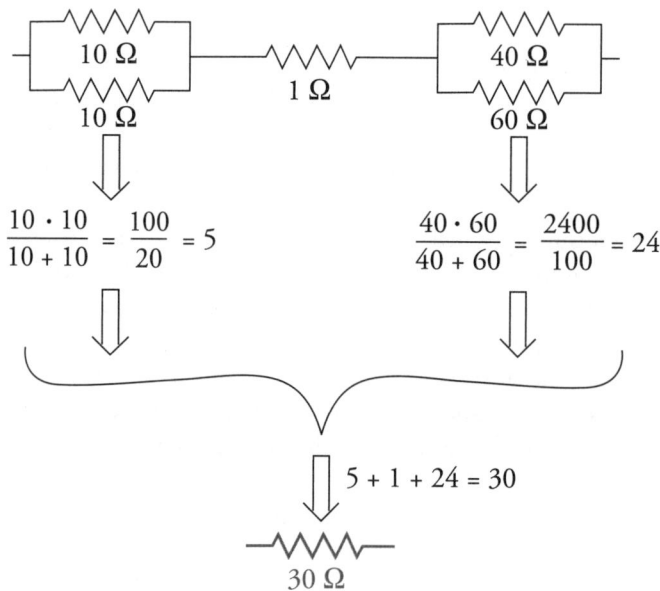

Therefore, the given combination of resistors is equivalent to a single 30 Ω resistor.

DC Circuits

Now that we know how to simplify series and parallel combinations of resistors, we're ready to analyze circuits. The simplest circuit consists of a voltage source (most commonly, it's a battery), a connecting wire between the terminals of the voltage source, and a resistor. As an example, imagine hooking up a light bulb to a typical flashlight battery; one wire connects the positive terminal of the battery to one of the "leads" on the light bulb, and another wire connects the other lead on the bulb to the negative terminal of the battery. This completes the circuit. The diagram on the right below shows the way this real-life circuit would be drawn schematically.

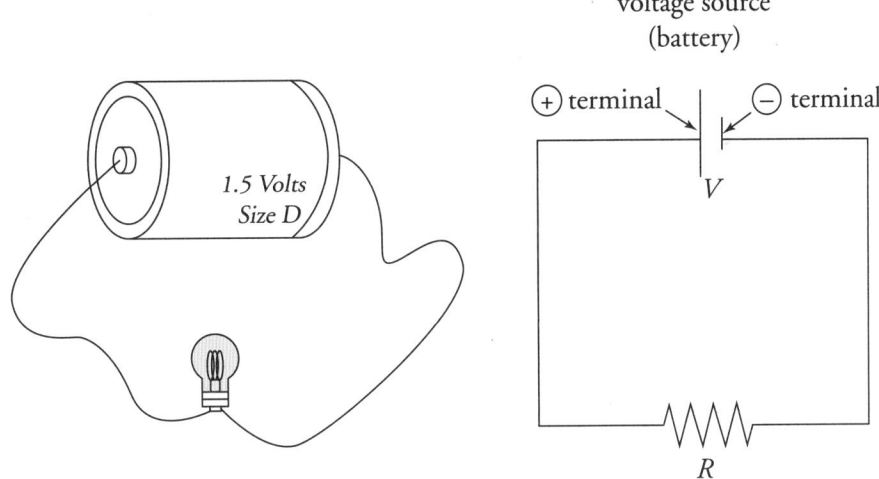

The pair of adjacent parallel lines denotes the voltage source. The job of the voltage source is to maintain a potential difference (a voltage) between its terminals; the value of this voltage is denoted by V or sometimes by ε, for emf (electromotive force). Remember that a voltage is needed to create a current. The terminal that's at the higher potential is denoted by the longer line and called the **positive terminal**; the terminal that's at the lower potential is denoted by the shorter line and called the **negative terminal**.

Once the circuit is set up, we know what will happen inside the metal wires: conduction electrons will drift toward the higher potential terminal; that is, they'll drift away from the negative terminal, toward the positive terminal. The direction of the flow of conduction electrons would be clockwise in the diagram as drawn. However, there is a convention that is followed when discussing the direction of the current. *The direction of the current is taken to be the direction that <u>positive</u> charge carriers would flow, even though the actual charge carriers that do flow might be negatively charged.* (Sounds like the convention for defining the direction of the electric field, doesn't it? "The direction of the electric field is taken to be the direction of the force that a positive charge would feel, even if the actual charge that gets placed in the field isn't positive." In fact, that's the reason for the convention about the direction of the current; to keep things consistent.) Even though we know electrons are drifting clockwise in this circuit, we'd say that the current, I, flows counterclockwise from the positive terminal around to the negative terminal.

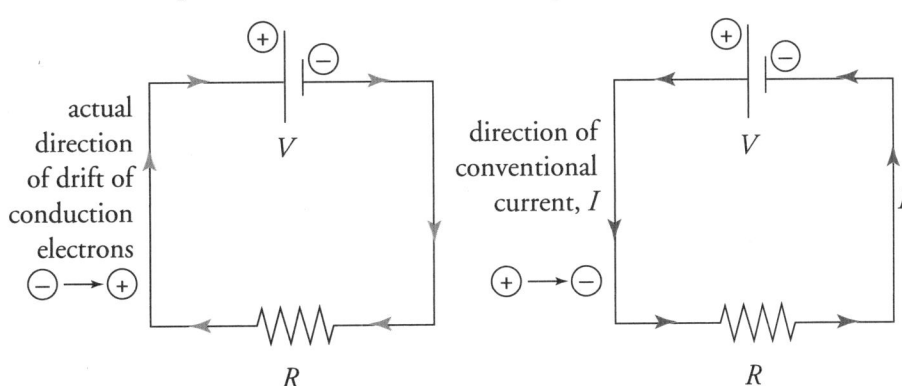

If we were asked for the value of the current in this circuit, this question would be easy to answer. We know V and R, and we want I. Using the equation $V = IR$, we'd say that

$$I = \frac{V}{R}$$

For example, if $V = 1.5$ V and $R = 150\ \Omega$, then $I = 0.01$ A. So, what made this problem so easy? The answer: There was only one resistor. This will usually be our goal: to simplify a circuit with multiple resistors into a circuit with just a single equivalent resistor. (We say "usually" because there are some question types that can be answered without changing the circuit into one with just a single resistor; we'll show you some examples of those, too.)

In order to simplify a circuit with multiple resistors, we first need a way to turn resistors in series and resistors in parallel into a single equivalent resistor; this we already know how to do. However, there are two other important quantities in circuits besides R; namely, I and V. We also need to know what happens to these other quantities when we convert a series or parallel combination of resistors into a single resistor. The following figure contains this needed information:

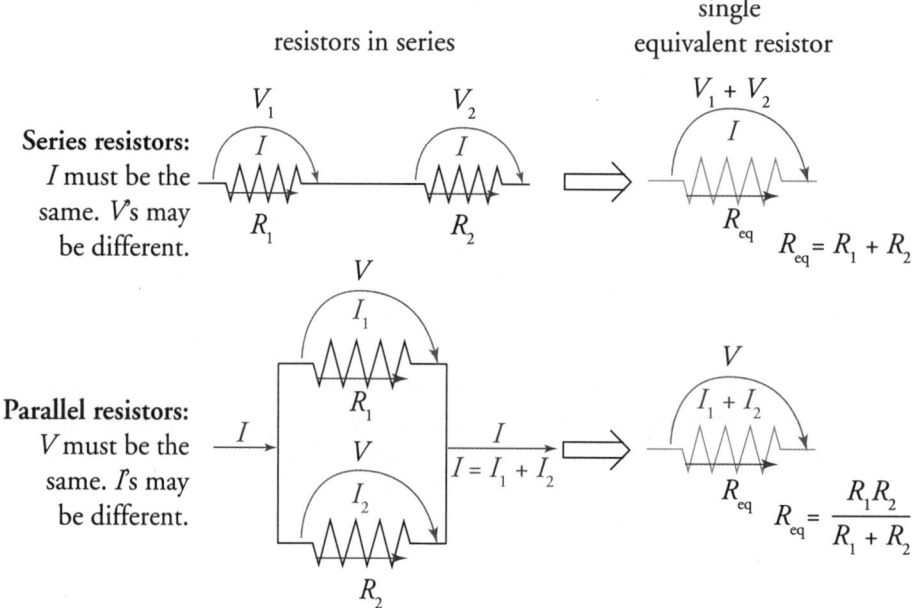

Resistors in series always share the same current, and resistors in parallel always share the same voltage drop. However, the voltage drops across series resistors will be different (and the currents through parallel resistors will be different) if the resistances are different.

With all this information at hand, we're ready to tackle an example.

Consider the following circuit:

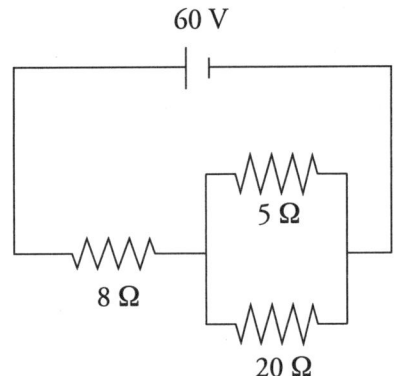

We'll find the current in the circuit, the current through each resistor, and the voltage across each resistor. The first stage of the solution involves simplifying this multiple-resistor circuit into a circuit with just a single equivalent resistor, like this:

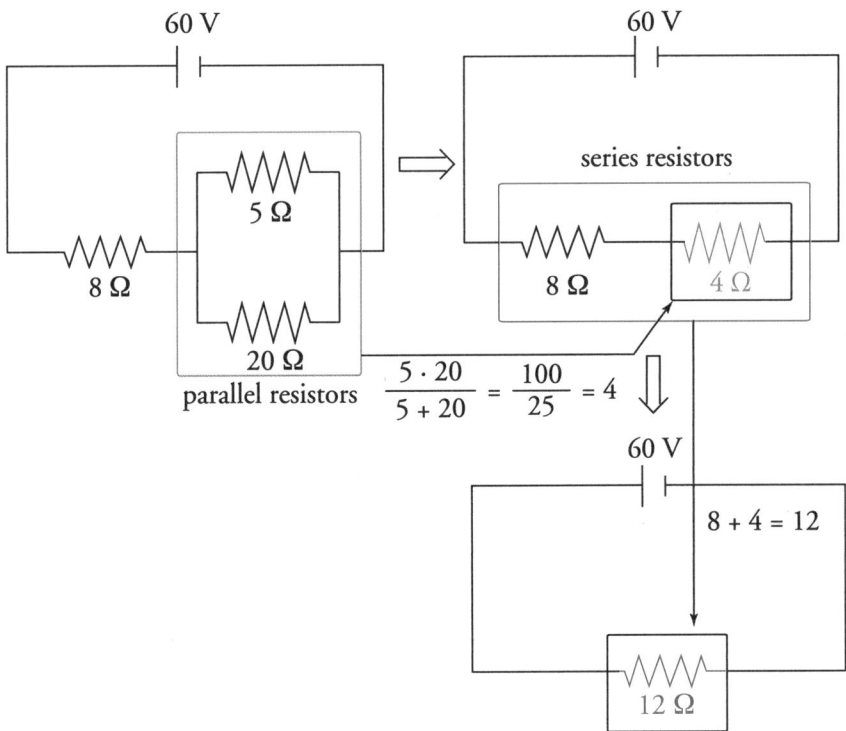

Now that we have an equivalent circuit with just one resistor, we can find the current:

$$I = \frac{V}{R} = \frac{60 \text{ V}}{12 \text{ } \Omega} = 5 \text{ A}$$

If we want to find the currents through (and the voltages across) the individual resistors in the original circuit, we have to work backward. The key to "working backward" is to ask at each stage: "What am I going back to?" If the answer is, "a *series* combination," then the value you bring back is the *current*, because series resistors share the same current. If the answer is, "a *parallel* combination," then the value you bring back is the *voltage*, because parallel resistors share the same voltage.

going back to series combination → bring *I*

going back to parallel combination → bring *V*

Let me illustrate this "working backward" technique with our circuit above. You should read this figure starting at the bottom, then up, then to the left... in other words, in the *reverse* order from what we did before because now we're working backward:

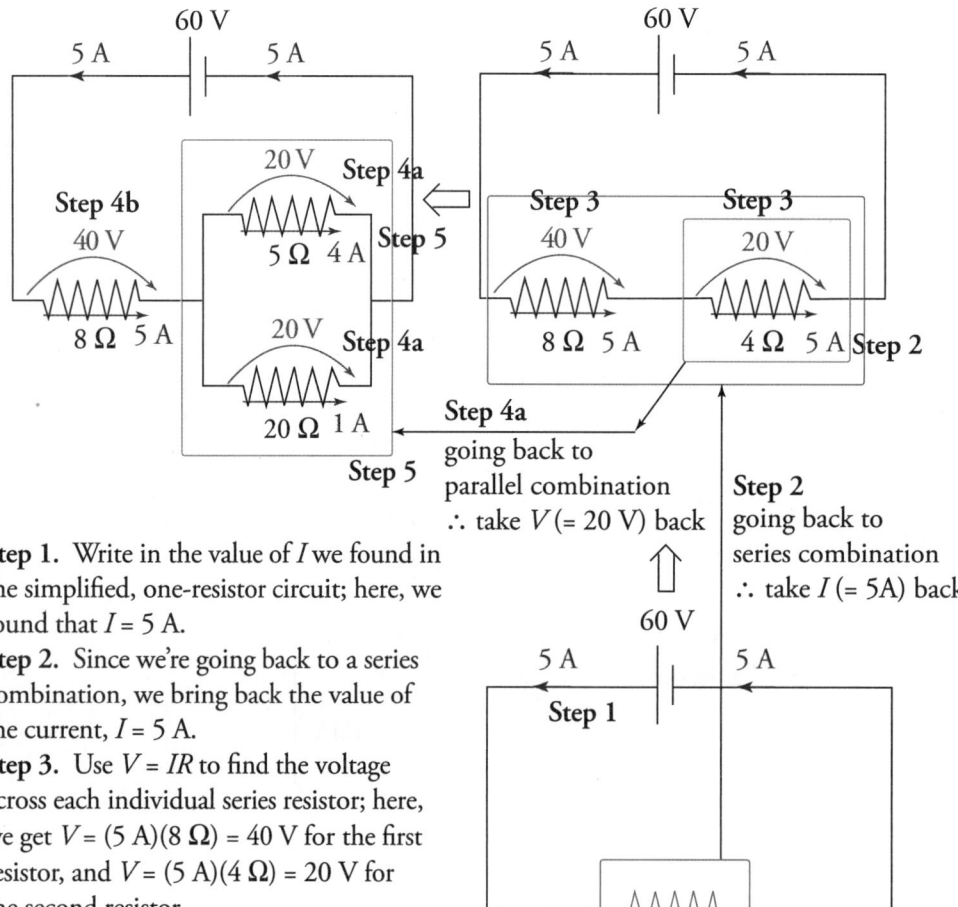

Step 1. Write in the value of *I* we found in the simplified, one-resistor circuit; here, we found that *I* = 5 A.

Step 2. Since we're going back to a series combination, we bring back the value of the current, *I* = 5 A.

Step 3. Use *V* = *IR* to find the voltage across each individual series resistor; here, we get *V* = (5 A)(8 Ω) = 40 V for the first resistor, and *V* = (5 A)(4 Ω) = 20 V for the second resistor.

Step 4a. Since we're going back to a parallel combination, we bring back the value of the voltage, *V* = 20 V.

Step 4b. Simply copy the information for the 8 Ω resistor, since that resistor doesn't change when we go back.

Step 5. Use *I* = *V/R* to find the current across each individual parallel resistor; here, we get *I* = (20 V)/(5 Ω) = 4 A for the top resistor, and *I* = (20 V)/(20 Ω) = 1 A for the bottom resistor.

Now that we have found all the information for the original circuit,

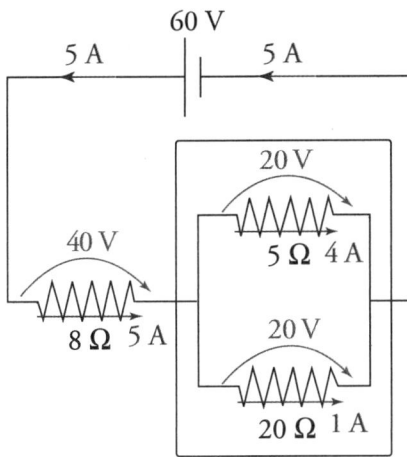

there are a couple of important things to notice, things that will hold true in any circuit. They are consequences of **Kirchhoff's laws** (pronounced "Keer-koff").

- *For a circuit containing one battery as the voltage source, the sum of the voltage drops across the resistors in any complete path starting at the (+) terminal and ending at the (–) terminal matches the voltage of the battery.*

For our circuit above, we have 40 V + 20 V = 60 V. (We don't add the 20 V twice, because these resistors are in parallel; each charge carrier moving through the circuit would go *either* across the 20 V voltage as it drifts through the top resistor in the parallel combination *or* across the 20 V voltage as it drifts through the bottom resistor; it doesn't go through both resistors.)

- *The amount of current entering the parallel combination is equal to the sum of the currents that pass through all the individual resistors in the combination.*

For our circuit above, we have 5 A = 4 A + 1 A.

Besides asking about resistance, current, and voltage, the MCAT can also ask about power. When current passes through a resistor, the resistor gets hot: it dissipates heat. The rate at which it dissipates heat energy is the **power dissipated by the resistor**. The formula used to calculate this power, *P*, is known as the **Joule heating law**.

Power Dissipated by a Resistor: Joule Heating Law

$$P = I^2 R$$

So, for our circuit above, we find that:

the power dissipated by the 8 Ω resistor is I^2R = (5 A)^2(8 Ω)   = 200 W
the power dissipated by the 5 Ω resistor is I^2R = (4 A)^2(5 Ω)   = 80 W
the power dissipated by the 20 Ω resistor is I^2R = (1 A)^2(20 Ω)   = 20 W
the total power dissipated by all resistors is the sum: 300 W

The power *supplied* to the circuit by the voltage source (like a battery) is given by this formula: $P = IV$. So, for our circuit above, we find that

power supplied by the 60 V battery is $P = IV$ = (5 A)(60 V) = 300 W

Notice that these answers match:

power dissipated by all resistors = 300 W = power supplied by the battery

This is simply a consequence of Conservation of Energy, so it will be true in general:

* *The total power dissipated by the resistors is equal to the power supplied by the battery.*

Sometimes, a circuit may contain more than one battery, and in some of these cases, the battery with the lower voltage will be *absorbing* power from the battery with the higher voltage (that is, from the "boss battery" that supplies the power to the circuit). The power *absorbed* by a battery is also given by the formula $P = IV$, and the italicized statement above should then read:

* *The total power dissipated by the resistors and absorbed by other voltage sources (i.e., the total power used by the circuit) is equal to the power supplied to the circuit by the highest-voltage power source.*

One more note: The Joule heating law, $P = I^2R$, can be written as $P = I(IR) = IV$, so, in fact, we need just one formula for the power dissipated or supplied by *any* component in a circuit:

Power

$$P = IV$$

However, if you use the formula $P = IV$ to find the power dissipated by a resistor, *be careful* that you only use the *V for that resistor*, and not the *V* for the entire circuit. So, for our circuit above, we'd find that:

the power dissipated by the 8 Ω resistor is IV = (5 A)(40 V) = 200 W
the power dissipated by the 5 Ω resistor is IV = (4 A)(20 V) = 80 W
the power dissipated by the 20 Ω resistor is IV = (1 A)(20 V) = 20 W

giving us the same answers we found before when we used the formula $P = I^2R$.

Along with questions about power, there could also be questions about energy. Simply remember the definition: power = energy/time, so

$$\text{energy} = \text{power} \times \text{time}$$

For example, how much energy is dissipated in 5 seconds by the 5-ohm resistor in the circuit above? We calculated that the power dissipated by this resistor is $P = 80\ \text{W} = 80\ \text{J/s}$; so the energy dissipated in $t = 5$ seconds is $Pt = (80\ \text{J/s})(5\ \text{s}) = 400\ \text{J}$.

In some circuits (in practice, most of them), one or more of the resistors are actually doing something useful besides just heating up. However, the circuit diagrams and the calculations we do will be the same. For example, a motor will be shown as a resistor in an MCAT circuit; so will a light bulb (which is really just a resistor that happens to get so hot that some of the energy dissipated is emitted as light rather than heat). In either case, the calculations for these components are the same as treating each as a regular resistor. Notice that if you want to calculate the work that can be done by a motor, you'll wind up multiplying power by time.

Finally, a common and useful model/analogy for an electric circuit is a stream of water traveling down a series of waterfalls, with a pump in the collecting pool at the bottom to take the water back up to the top again. The battery (voltage source) is like the pump, and the voltage of the battery is the height it lifts the water. The current is the water, and each resistor is a waterfall. Resistors in series share the same current, because however much water drops down one waterfall must drop down the next one in the line (it has nowhere else to go); the heights of these waterfalls can of course be different, which is why the voltage drops for series resistors may be different. Parallel resistors are parallel waterfalls: They provide different paths for the water to drop from one point in the stream to a lower point. Because such waterfalls connect the same higher point to the same lower point, their heights must be the same; this is why parallel resistors always share the same voltage drop. One waterfall in parallel might be very narrow and only allow a small amount of water to flow down, while another waterfall in the same parallel (side-by-side) combination might be wide and thus allow more water to flow down; this is why resistors in parallel may have different currents. However, the total amount of water entering the top of the parallel waterfall combination must go down all the waterfalls in that combination (again, the water has nowhere else to go); this illustrates why the amount of current entering the parallel combination is equal to the total amount of current that passes through all the resistors in the combination. Finally, the total height of the waterfalls must be the same as the height through which the pump lifts the water from the collecting pool at the bottom; this illustrates why the total voltage drop across the resistors matches the voltage of the battery.

circuit	stream of water flowing down waterfalls with pump at the bottom
current	the flow rate of the water
resistor	waterfall
series	one waterfall after another
parallel	side-by-side waterfalls
voltage	for resistor: height of waterfall (distance water falls)
	for battery: total height the pump lifts the water to start a new cycle
resistance	relative width of channel in the water circuit (narrower width = higher resistance; wider = lower resistance)

Here's a diagram of the water stream and waterfalls that would be analogous to the circuit we analyzed above.

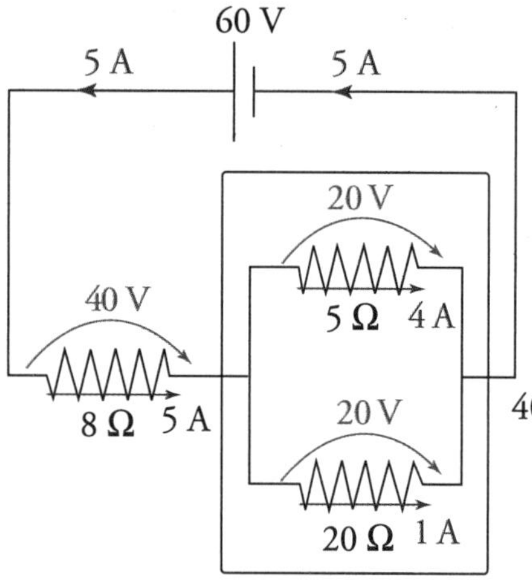

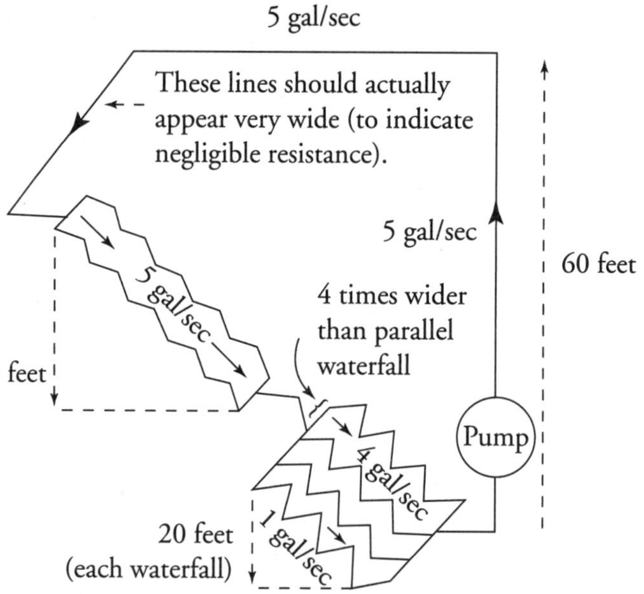

Example 10-8: Verify that the formulas $P = IV$ and $P = I^2R$ are dimensionally correct by showing that the product of current and voltage (IV) and the product of current squared and resistance (I^2R), both have the same units of power.

Solution: First, because $[I] = C/s$ and $[V] = J/C$, we have

$$[IV] = [I][V] = \frac{C}{s} \cdot \frac{J}{C} = \frac{J}{s} = W = \text{watt} = [P]$$

Next, because $[I] = C/s$ and $[R] = \Omega = V/A$, we have

$$[I^2R] = [I]^2[R] = \left(\frac{C}{s}\right)^2 \cdot \frac{V}{A} = \frac{C^2}{s^2} \cdot \frac{\frac{J}{C}}{\frac{C}{s}} = \frac{C^2}{s^2} \cdot \frac{J \cdot s}{C^2} = \frac{J}{s} = W = \text{watt} = [P]$$

Example 10-9: A portion of a circuit is shown below:

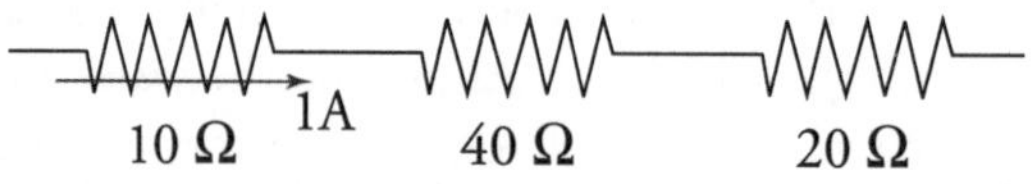

If the current through the 10-ohm resistor is 1 A, what is the current through the 20-ohm resistor?

A. 0.25 A
B. 0.5 A
C. 1 A
D. 2 A

Solution: Because these resistors are in series, they all share the same current. If the current in the first resistor is 1 A, then the current through each of the other resistors is also 1 A. The answer is C.

Example 10-10: A portion of a circuit is shown below:

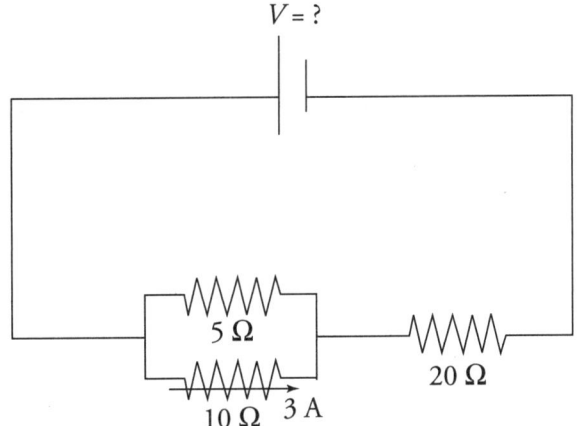

If the current through the 12-ohm resistor is 1 A, what is the value of the current I?

Solution: The voltage drop across the top resistor is $V = IR = (1 \text{ A})(12 \text{ }\Omega) = 12$ V. Because the resistors are in parallel, the voltage drop across the bottom resistor must also be 12 V. Using $I = V/R$, we find that the current through the bottom resistor is $(12 \text{ V})/(4 \text{ }\Omega) = 3$ A. Therefore, the total amount of current passing through the parallel combination is $1 \text{ A} + 3 \text{ A} = 4 \text{ A}$.

Example 10-11: With the information given in the circuit diagram below, what is the voltage of the battery?

A.   150 V
B.   210 V
C.   240 V
D.   300 V

Solution: The voltage drop across the bottom resistor in the parallel combination is $V = IR = (3 \text{ A})(10 \text{ }\Omega)$ = 30 V. Because the top and bottom resistors in this combination are in parallel, the voltage drop across the top resistor must also be 30 V. Using $I = V/R$, we find that the current through the top resistor is $(30 \text{ V})/(5 \text{ }\Omega) = 6$ A. Therefore, the total amount of current passing through the parallel combination is 6 A + 3 A = 9 A. Since this much current flows through the 20-ohm resistor, the voltage drop across the 20-ohm resistor is $V = IR = (9 \text{ A})(20 \text{ }\Omega) = 180$ V. Because the total voltage drop across the resistors must match the voltage of the battery, we have $V = 30 \text{ V} + 180 \text{ V} = 210 \text{ V}$, so the answer is B. (Remember: We don't add the 30 V voltage drop twice here; choice C is a trap.)

Example 10-12: A portion of a circuit is shown below:

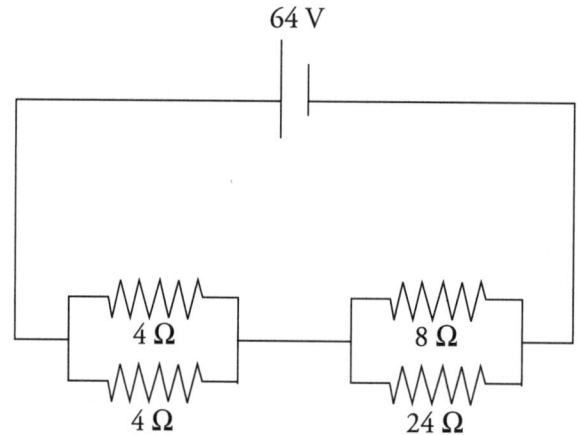

If the current entering the parallel combination is 12 A, how much current flows through the 120-ohm resistor?

Solution: Because the 60-ohm bottom resistor has half the resistance of the 120-ohm top resistor, twice as much current will flow through the bottom resistor as through the top one. So, if we let X stand for the current in the top resistor, then the current in the bottom resistor is $2X$. Because 12 A enters the parallel combination, we must have $X + 2X = 12$ A, so $X = 4$ A. Therefore, the current in the top resistor is 4 A (and the current in the bottom resistor is 8 A). Notice that the voltage drop across the top resistor is $V = IR = (4 \text{ A})(120 \ \Omega) = 480$ V, and the voltage drop across the bottom resistor is $V = IR = (8 \text{ A})(60 \ \Omega) = 480$ V. The fact that these voltages match (as they must for parallel resistors) verifies that our answer is correct.

Example 10-13: How much energy is dissipated in 10 seconds by the 24-ohm resistor in the following circuit?

A. 480 J
B. 640 J
C. 720 J
D. 960 J

Solution: The pair of parallel 4-ohm resistors is equivalent to a single 2-ohm resistor [because $(4 \times 4)/(4 + 4) = 2$], and the parallel 8-ohm and 24-ohm resistors are equivalent to a single 6-ohm resistor [because $(8 \times 24)/(8 + 24) = 192/32 = 6$]. These equivalent resistors are in series, so the overall equivalent resistance for the circuit is $2 \ \Omega + 6 \ \Omega = 8 \ \Omega$. This means the current in the circuit is $I = V/R_{eq} = 64/8 = 8$ A. When these 8 amps enter the second parallel combination (the one with the 8-ohm and 24-ohm resistors), it must split up in such a way that the current through the 8-ohm resistor is 3 times the current through the 24-ohm resistor. (Because the 8-ohm resistor has 1/3 the resistance of the 24-ohm resistor, it will get 3 times the current.) So, if we let X stand for the current in the 24-ohm resistor, then the current through the 8-ohm resistor is $3X$; this gives $X + 3X = 8$ A, so $X = 2$ A. Thus, the current in the 24-ohm resistor is 2 A. [The current in the 8-ohm resistor is $3X = 6$ A. The voltage drop across the 8-ohm resistor is (6 A)(8 Ω) = 48 V, and the voltage drop across the 24-ohm resistor is (2 A)(24 Ω) = 48 V; the fact that these match verifies that our calculation is correct.] Since the current in the 24-ohm resistor is 2 A, the power dissipated by this resistor is $P = I^2R = (2^2)(24) = 96$ W. Therefore, the energy dissipated by this resistor in 10 seconds is (96 W)(10 s) = 960 J, and the answer is D.

Example 10-14: What is the current in the 100-ohm resistor shown below?

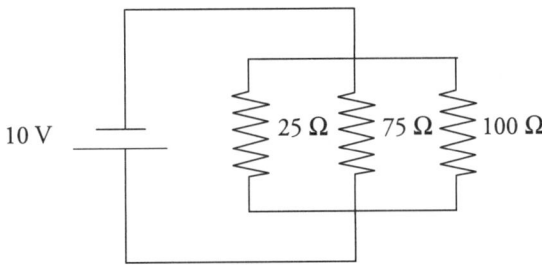

Solution: For this question, we don't need to begin by finding the single equivalent resistance of the given parallel combination, because we already know the voltage across the 100-ohm resistor. The parallel combination is attached directly to the terminals of the battery, so the voltage across each of the resistors must be 10 V. Because we know both V and R, we can find I in one step: $I = V/R = (10 \text{ V})/(100 \text{ Ω}) = 0.1$ A.

Example 10-15: What is the current in the circuit below?

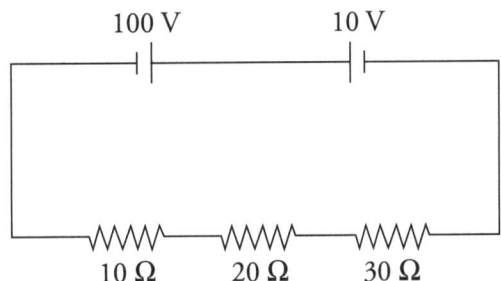

Solution: This circuit contains two batteries. The 100-volt battery wants to send current clockwise. (Remember: We consider current as the directed motion of positive charge, and positive charge carriers would move away from the positive terminal, around the circuit to the negative terminal.) However, the 10-volt battery would want to send current the opposite way: counterclockwise. Since the 100-volt battery has the higher voltage (or, equivalently, the greater emf), it's the "boss" battery. Therefore, current will flow clockwise, but the effective emf will be reduced to $100 - 10 = 90$ V, because the 10-volt battery is opposing the 100-volt boss battery. The equivalent resistance is $10 + 20 + 30 = 60$ Ω (the resistors are in series), so the current in the circuit will be $I = V/R_{eq} = (90 \text{ V})/(60 \text{ Ω}) = 1.5$ A. (Note: The 10-volt battery is being charged by the 100-volt boss battery.)

Example 10-16: A toaster oven is rated at 720 W. If it draws 6 A of current, what is its resistance?

Solution: Here, we're given P and I, and asked for R. Since $P = I^2R$, we find that

$$R = \frac{P}{I^2} = \frac{720 \text{ W}}{(6 \text{ A})^2} = 20 \ \Omega$$

Example 10-17: Current passes through an insulated resistor of resistance R, mass m, and specific heat c. The voltage across this resistor is V. If the resistor absorbs all the heat it generates, find an expression for the increase in temperature of the resistor after a time t. (All values are expressed in SI units.)

Solution: The amount of heat energy generated (and absorbed) by the resistor is $Q = Pt$, where $P = IV = (V/R)V = V^2/R$. (Here, Q stands for heat not charge.) Now, using the fundamental equation $Q = mc\Delta T$ (from general chemistry), we have

$$\Delta T = \frac{Q}{mc} = \frac{Pt}{mc} = \frac{\frac{V^2}{R}t}{mc} = \frac{V^2t}{Rmc}$$

All real batteries have **internal resistance**, which we denote by r. Let ε denote the emf of the battery; this is its "ideal" voltage (i.e., the voltage between its terminals when there's no current). Once a current is established, the internal resistance causes the voltage between the terminals to be different from ε. If the battery is supplying current I to the circuit, then the **terminal voltage**, V, is less than ε and given by $V = \varepsilon - Ir$. (On the other hand, if the circuit is *supplying* current to the battery [charging it up] then the terminal voltage is greater than ε and given by the equation $V = \varepsilon + Ir$.) The internal resistance is actually *between* the terminals in a real battery, but in circuit diagrams, the internal resistance is drawn next to the battery, like this:

terminal voltage
V

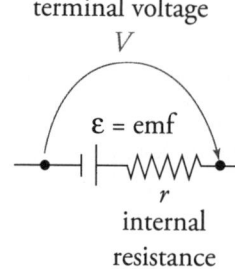

$\varepsilon = $ emf

r
internal
resistance

However, unless you are told otherwise, you may assume that all batteries are ideal and have no internal resistance.

Example 10-18: The battery shown in the circuit below has an emf of 100 V and an internal resistance of 5 Ω. What is its terminal voltage in this circuit? (*Note:* It's not uncommon to see a dashed box drawn around the battery and its internal resistance; this emphasizes that r is actually inside the battery.)

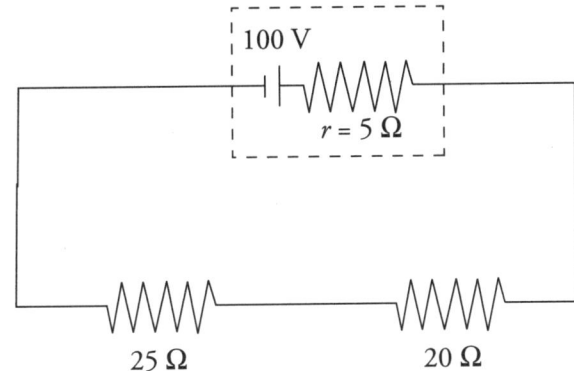

A. 80 V
B. 90 V
C. 100 V
D. 110 V

Solution: The three resistors in this circuit are in series, so the equivalent resistance for the circuit is 5 + 25 + 20 = 50 Ω. Because the emf is 100 V, the current in the circuit is

$$I = \varepsilon / R = (100 \text{ V})(50 \text{ Ω}) = 2 \text{ A}$$

The terminal voltage is therefore

$$V = \varepsilon - Ir = (100 \text{ V}) - (2 \text{ A})(5 \text{ Ω}) = 90 \text{ V}$$

The answer is B. (*Note:* You could eliminate choices C and D immediately; the terminal voltage must be *less* than the emf because the battery is supplying current to the circuit.)

Example 10-19: The diagram below shows a point X held at a potential of $\phi = 60$ V connected by a combination of resistors to a point (denoted by G) that is **grounded**. *The **ground** is considered to be at potential zero.* What is the current through the 100-ohm resistor?

Solution: The parallel resistors are equivalent to a single 20 Ω resistor, which is then in series with the 100 Ω resistor, giving an overall equivalent resistance of 20 + 100 = 120 Ω. Since the potential difference between points X and G is $V = \phi_X - \phi_G = 60 - 0 = 60$ V, the current in the circuit (and through the 100-ohm resistor) is

$$I = V/R = (60 \text{ V})/(120 \text{ Ω}) = 0.5 \text{ A}$$

Example 10-20: The diagram below shows a battery with an emf of 100 V connected to a circuit equipped with a switch, S.

a) What is the current in the circuit when the switch is open?
b) What is the current in the circuit when the switch is closed?

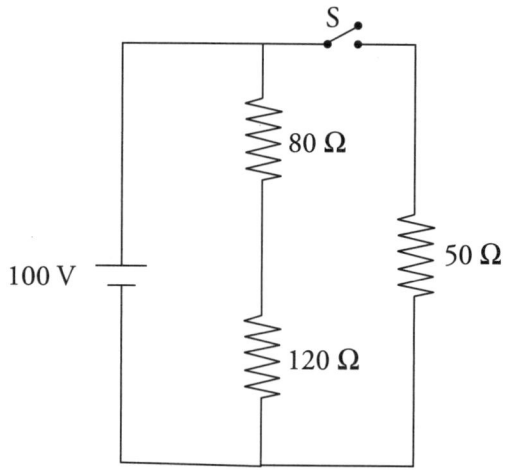

Solution:

a) With the switch open (as pictured above) the 50 Ω resistor is effectively taken out of the circuit; no current will flow in that branch. Current will flow only in the part of the circuit shown below:

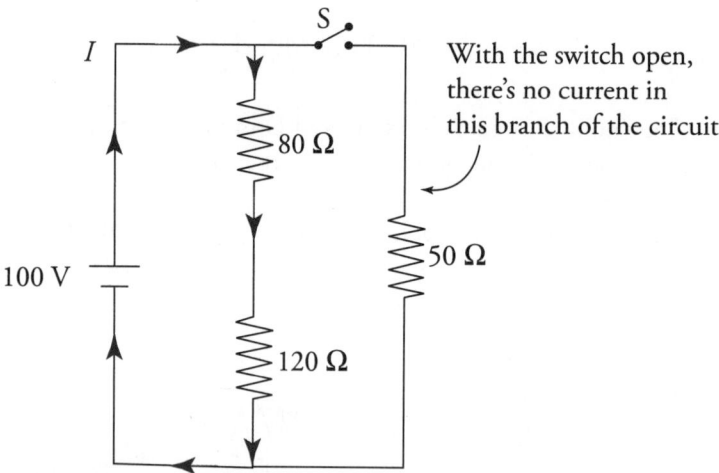

With the switch open, there's no current in this branch of the circuit.

The two resistors that *are* in the circuit when the switch is open are in series, so the total equivalent resistance is 80 + 120 = 200 Ω; thus, the current is

$$I = V / R = (100 \text{ V})/(200 \text{ Ω}) = 0.5 \text{ A}$$

b) With the switch closed, all the resistors are part of the circuit, and there will be current in all the branches. Let's find the equivalent resistance. The 80 Ω and 120 Ω resistors are in series, so they're equivalent to a single 80 + 120 = 200 Ω resistor, which is then in parallel with the 50 Ω resistor. This gives an overall equivalent resistance of 40 Ω because $(200 \times 50)/(200 + 50)$ is equal to 40. Therefore, the current supplied to the circuit in this case is $I = V/R_{eq} = (100 \text{ V})/(40 \text{ Ω}) = 2.5$ A.

Example 10-21: Three identical light bulbs are connected to a battery, as shown:

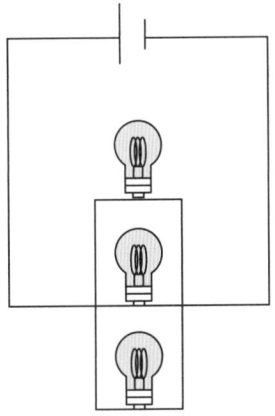

What will happen if the middle bulb burns out?

A. The other two bulbs will go out.
B. The light intensity of the other two bulbs will decrease, but they won't go out.
C. The light intensity of the other two bulbs will increase.
D. The light intensity of the other two bulbs will remain the same.

Solution: Let V be the voltage of the battery, and let R be the resistance of each light bulb. The current through each light bulb (that is, through each resistor) is $I = V/R$. If the middle bulb burns out, then the middle branch of the parallel combination is severed; but current can still flow through the top and bottom bulbs, and the current through each will still be $I = V/R$. Because the intensity of the light is directly related to the power each one dissipates, the fact that the current doesn't change means that $P = I^2R$ won't change, so the light intensity of the other two bulbs will remain the same. The answer is D. [What *will* change if the middle bulb burns out? Before the middle bulb burns out, the current through each of the three bulbs is $I = V/R$, so the battery must be providing a total current of $3I = 3V/R$. After the middle bulb burns out, the current through each of the other two bulbs is still $I = V/R$, so the battery need only provide a total current of $2I = 2V/R$. That is, the total current through the circuit will decrease (since, after all, there are only two bulbs to light, not three). In addition, the power supplied by the battery will also decrease, from $P = (3I)(V) = 3V^2/R$ to $P = (2I)(V) = 2V^2/R$, and the battery will last longer. Finally, notice that if the three bulbs were wired in *series* rather than in parallel, then if any one of the bulbs burned out, they'd all go out because the circuit would be broken.]

Measuring Circuit Values

To verify that a circuit is operating properly, or to troubleshoot one that is malfunctioning, we need to be able to measure the voltage and current in different parts of the circuit. **Voltmeters** are used to measure the potential difference between two points in a circuit, and **ammeters** are used to measure the current through a particular point in the circuit. At the core of each of these devices is a **galvanometer**.

A galvanometer on its own is an apparatus that sensitively measures current using the interaction between currents and magnetic fields (discussion of the particulars of this interaction is left to the final section of this chapter). Current enters the galvanometer and travels through a coil that is wound around the base of a needle. The coil is situated in an external magnetic field in such a way that whenever current runs through the coil, magnetic forces deflect the galvanometer needle. The degree of deflection indicates the amount of current running through the device.

To construct an ammeter, we need to have a small, known fraction of the current we are trying to measure running through the galvanometer (because the galvanometer is very sensitive, a large current will overload it). For instance, let's take a look at the circuit we discussed earlier in this section. Say that we want to measure the current flowing through each of the resistors. To do so, all we need to do is connect the ammeter in series with the resistor of interest.

To measure the current through the 8 Ω resistor:

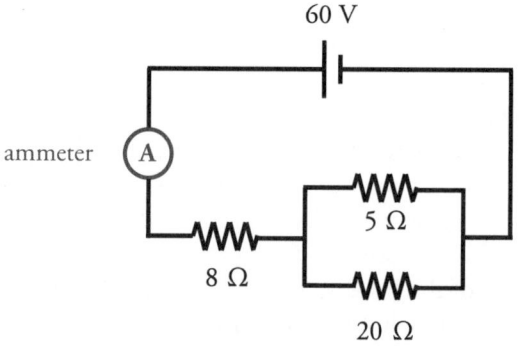

To measure the current through the 5 Ω resistor:

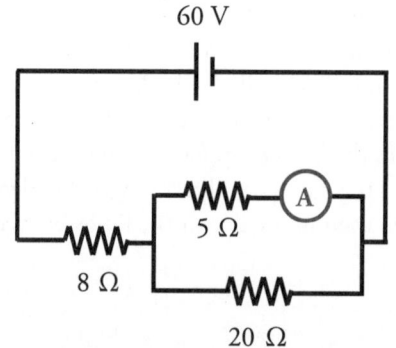

When we connect the ammeter to the circuit, we are adding an additional resistance to the circuit, known as the *internal resistance, r,* of the meter. In reality, this internal resistance is roughly equal to a small *shunt resistance, R_s,* connected in parallel with the ideal galvanometer (G) and its own much larger series resistance, R_g, used to ensure that only a small current actually passes through the galvanometer (the internal resistance of the galvanometer itself is approximated to be zero, a sound assumption given the large value of the R_g).

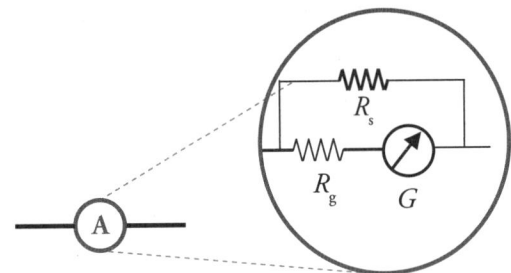

Since we don't want the ammeter to interfere with the circuit in the process of measuring it, we want our ammeter to have as low of an internal resistance as possible so that there is as little voltage dropped over this resistor as possible. The way to achieve this is for the shunt resistance to be very small, because the shunt resistance is very close to the total internal resistance of the ammeter:

$$r = \frac{R_s R_g}{R_s + R_g} = R_s \times \frac{R_g}{R_s + R_g} \xrightarrow{R_g \gg R_s} R_s \times 1 = R_s$$

Another way to think about this is that we want the equivalent resistance of the combination of the ammeter's internal resistance and the resistor of interest to be as close to the original resistance of the resistor as possible.

Example 10-22: A typical ammeter might have an internal resistance of $r = 0.1$ mΩ. If we are measuring the current through the 5 Ω resistor in the circuit above, what would be the equivalent resistance of the ammeter and resistor connected in series?

Solution: Just add the resistances: $R_{eq} = 5\ \Omega + 1 \times 10^{-4}\ \Omega \approx 5\ \Omega$.

Although a galvanometer is intrinsically a current-measuring device, it can also be used to measure voltage, since we know that current and voltage are proportional. To do this, we'll want to connect the voltmeter across the resistor of interest, so that it can measure the potential difference from one side of the resistor to the other.

To measure the voltage across the 8 Ω resistor:

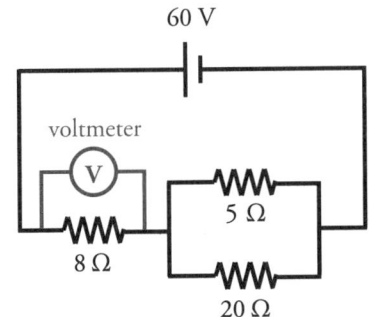

To measure the voltage across the 5 Ω resistor:

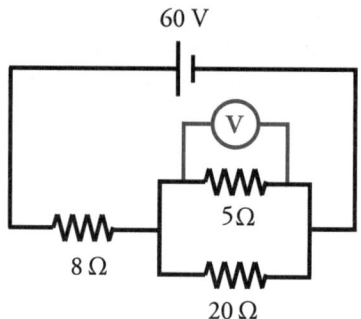

Just like an ammeter, a voltmeter also has an internal resistance. In this case, however, the internal resistance is connected in parallel to the resistor of interest. Again, we want to minimize any impact to the original circuit, so for the voltmeter we'll want the internal resistance to be as large as possible to minimize any current going through the voltmeter. A typical voltmeter might have an internal resistance of 10 MΩ. This is achieved by using a large resistance R_g in series with the galvanometer, as shown below. If we again assume the resistance of G is negligible, then $r = R_g$.

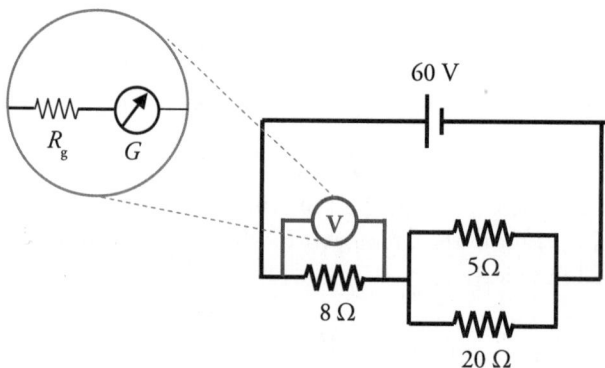

Example 10-23: When connecting a voltmeter to a circuit, we want the equivalent resistance of the combination to be as close to the original resistance as possible. In the circuit above, if $r = R_g = 10$ MΩ when measuring the voltage across the 8 Ω resistor, find

a)   the equivalent resistance of the voltmeter and resistor, and
b)   the measured voltage.

Solution:

a)   The equivalent resistance is given by the product over sum rule for resistors in parallel:
$R_{eq} = (10 \times 10^6 \ \Omega)(8 \ \Omega)/(10 \times 10^6 \ \Omega + 8 \ \Omega) \approx (10 \times 10^6 \ \Omega)(8 \ \Omega)/(10 \times 10^6 \ \Omega) = 8 \ \Omega.$

b) This is the same circuit we solved previously in the beginning of the subsection on DC circuits, when we found that the voltage across the 8 Ω resistor was 40V. (This would be a good time to confirm you remember how to solve for currents and resistances across circuit elements by solving for this result again.) Because we have just confirmed that the voltmeter does not appreciably affect the resistance across this circuit element, the measured value will be the same as the calculated value.

10.2   CAPACITORS

A pair of conductors that can hold equal but opposite charges is known as a **capacitor**. The conductors can be of any shape, but the most common capacitor consists of a pair of parallel metal plates; it's known as a **parallel-plate capacitor**:

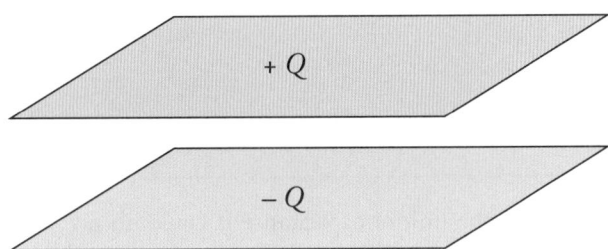

Notice that one plate carries a positive charge and the other plate carries an equal amount of negative charge. Therefore, the *net* charge on a capacitor is zero. However, whenever we talk about the "charge on a capacitor," we always mean the magnitude of charge on either plate, which is $+Q$.

In circuit diagrams, a capacitor is denoted by either of these two symbols:

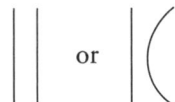

The first question we'll answer is, "How do we create a charged capacitor?" Take an uncharged parallel-plate capacitor, and hook the plates to the terminals of a battery. Conduction electrons in the connecting wires will be repelled from the negative terminal and flow to one plate, while electrons from the other plate will be attracted toward the positive terminal of the battery. The current rises quickly at first, but it gradually dies out as the plates acquire charge. The plate that's connected to the positive terminal becomes positively charged, and the plate that's connected to the negative terminal becomes negatively charged. Since the positive plate has a higher potential than the negative plate, the potential difference between the plates opposes the potential difference of the battery. Charge will stop flowing when the potential difference between the plates matches the voltage of the battery because at that point the circuit will look like one that has two opposing voltage sources.

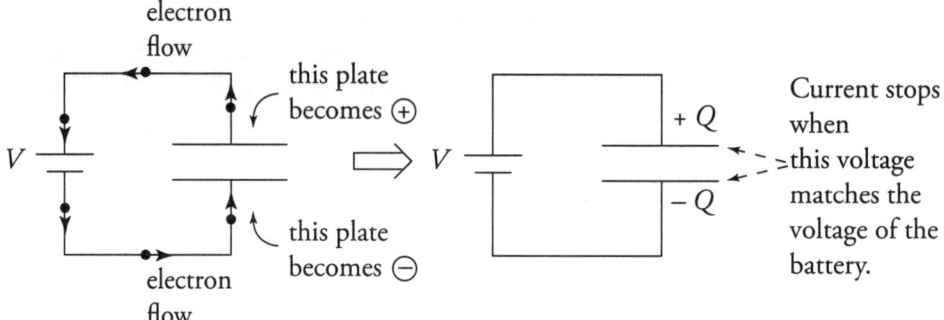

If V is the potential difference between the plates of a charged capacitor, and Q is the charge on the capacitor, then Q and V are proportional. The proportionality constant, C, is called the **capacitance**:

Charge on a Capacitor

$$Q = CV$$

From this equation we can see that the unit of capacitance is coulomb per volt (C/V), which has its own name: the **farad**, abbreviated F. Therefore, 1 C/V = 1 F. Because a coulomb is a lot of charge, we'd expect a farad to be a lot of capacitance. Most real-life capacitors have capacitances that are on the order of a few microfarads.

The capacitance is determined only by the sizes of the plates and how far apart they are (and, as we'll see a little later, whether there's anything between the plates). For a parallel-plate capacitor with empty space between the plates, C is given by the following equation:

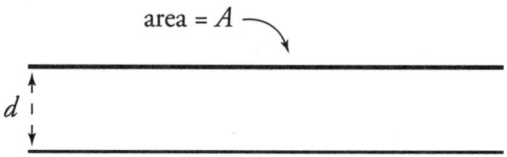

Capacitance of a Parallel Plate Capacitor

$$C = \varepsilon_0 \frac{A}{d}$$

---

where A is the area of each plate, d is their separation, and ε_0 is a fundamental constant of nature. (The constant ε_0 is known as the **permittivity of free space**; it's equal to $1/(4\pi k_0)$, where k_0 is Coulomb's constant, so the approximate numerical value of ε_0 is 8.85×10^{-12} F/m.)

The capacitance C depends only on A and d. Although $Q = CV$, the capacitance C does not depend on either Q or V; it only tells us how Q and V will be related. If you were given an uncharged capacitor, you could determine C without charging it up, by using the formula $C = \varepsilon_0 A/d$.

Intuitively, capacitance measures the plates' "capacity" for holding charge at a certain voltage. Let's say we had two capacitors with different capacitances, and we wanted to store as much charge as we could while keeping V low. We'd choose the capacitor with the greater capacitance because it would be able to hold more charge per volt.

Example 10-24: A capacitor has a capacitance of 2 nF. How much charge can it hold at a voltage of 150 V?

Solution: We're given C and V, and asked for Q. Using the equation $Q = CV$, we find that

$$Q = CV = (2 \times 10^{-9} \text{ F})(150 \text{ V}) = 3 \times 10^{-7} \text{ C}$$

(This means that the positive plate will have a charge of $+Q = 3 \times 10^{-7}$ C, and the negative plate will have a charge of $-Q = -3 \times 10^{-7}$ C.)

Example 10-25: A charged capacitor has charge Q, and the voltage between the plates is V. What will happen to C if Q is doubled?

Solution: Nothing. For a given capacitor, C is a constant. Because $Q = CV$, we see that Q is proportional to V. Doubling Q will not affect C; what *will* happen is that V will double.

Example 10-26: What will happen to the capacitance of a parallel-plate capacitor if the plates were moved closer together, halving the distance between them?

Solution: From the equation $C = \varepsilon_0 A/d$, we see that C is inversely proportional to d. Thus, if d is decreased by a factor of 2, then C will increase by a factor of 2.

Example 10-27: How big would the plates of a parallel-plate capacitor need to be in order to make the capacitance equal to 1 F, if d = 8.85 mm?

Solution: We'll start with the equation $C = \varepsilon_0 A/d$ and solve for A:

$$A = \frac{Cd}{\varepsilon_0} = \frac{(1 \text{ F})(8.85 \times 10^{-3} \text{ m})}{8.85 \times 10^{-12} \frac{\text{F}}{\text{m}}} = 10^9 \text{ m}^2$$

(If the plates were squares, they'd have to be nearly 20 miles on each side to make $A = 10^9$ square meters! Now you can see that 1 F is a *lot* of capacitance.)

Now that we know the basic equation for capacitance ($Q = CV$) and how to calculate it ($C = \varepsilon_0 A/d$), the next question is, "What's a capacitor used for?" For MCAT purposes, a parallel-plate capacitor should be associated with the rapid storing and releasing of charge (batteries also store and release charge over a much longer period, but for physics purposes, their main property is maintaining a constant *voltage*). This accumulation of charge has two important consequences:

1. It creates a uniform electric field, and
2. It stores electrical potential energy.

Let's go over each one.

When we studied electric fields in the preceding chapter, we noticed that the electric field created by one or more point source charges varied, depending on the location. For example, as we move farther from the source charges, the field gets weaker. Even if we stay at the same distance from, say, a single source charge, the direction of the field changes as we move around. Therefore, we could never obtain an electric field that was constant in both magnitude and direction throughout some region of space from point-source charges. However, the electric field that's created between the plates of a charged parallel-plate capacitor *is* constant in both magnitude and direction throughout the region between the plates; in other words, a charged parallel-plate capacitor can create a *uniform* electric field. The electric field, **E**, always points from the positive plate toward the negative plate, and it's the same magnitude at every point between the plates, whether we choose a point closer to the positive plate, closer to the negative plate, or right in the middle between them.

Because **E** is so straightforward (it's the same everywhere between the plates), the equation for calculating it is equally straightforward. The strength of **E** depends on the voltage between the plates, V, and their separation distance, d. We call the equation "Ed's formula":

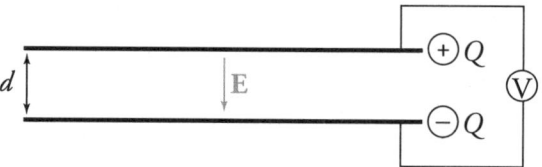

Ed's Formula

$$V = Ed$$

The equation $F = qE$ showed us that the units of E are N/C (because $E = F/q$). Ed's formula now tells us that the units of E are V/m (because $E = V/d$). You'll see both newtons-per-coulomb and volts-per-meter used as units for the electric field; it turns out that these units are exactly the same.

Example 10-28: The charge on a parallel-plate capacitor is 4×10^{-6} C. If the distance between the plates is 2 mm and the capacitance is 1 µF, what's the strength of the electric field between the plates?

Solution: Since $Q = CV$, we have $V = Q/C = (4 \times 10^{-6}$ C$)/(10^{-6}$ F$) = 4$ V. Now, using the equation $V = Ed$, we find that

$$E = \frac{V}{d} = \frac{4\ \text{V}}{2 \times 10^{-3}\ \text{m}} = 2000\ \tfrac{\text{V}}{\text{m}}$$

Example 10-29: The plates of a parallel plate capacitor are separated by a distance of 2 mm. The device's capacitance is 1 µF. How much charge needs to be transferred from one plate to the other in order to create a uniform electric field whose strength is 10^4 V/m?

Solution: Because $Q = CV$ and $V = Ed$, we find that

$$Q = CEd = (1 \times 10^{-6}\ \text{F})(10^4\ \tfrac{\text{V}}{\text{m}})(2 \times 10^{-3}\ \text{m}) = 2 \times 10^{-5}\ \text{C}$$

Example 10-30: A proton (whose mass is m) is placed on top of the positively charged plate of a parallel-plate capacitor, as shown below.

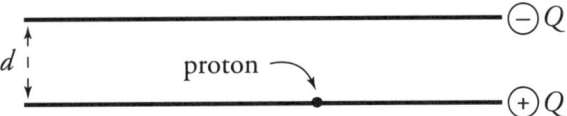

The charge on the capacitor is Q, and the capacitance is C. If the electric field in the region between the plates has magnitude E, which of the following expressions gives the time required for the proton to move up to the other plate?

A. $d\sqrt{\dfrac{eQ}{mC}}$

B. $d\sqrt{\dfrac{m}{eQC}}$

C. $d\sqrt{\dfrac{2eQ}{mC}}$

D. $d\sqrt{\dfrac{2mC}{eQ}}$

Solution: Once we find the acceleration of the proton, we can use Big Five #3, with $v_0 = 0$ (namely, $y = \frac{1}{2}at^2$) to find the time it will take for the proton to move the distance $y = d$. The acceleration of the proton is F/m, where $F = qE = eE$ is the force the proton feels; this gives $a = eE/m$. (We're ignoring the gravitational force on the proton because it is so much weaker than the electric force.) Now, since $E = V/d$ and $V = Q/C$, the expression for a becomes $a = eQ/mdC$. Substituting eQ/mdC for a, and d for y, Big Five #3 gives us

$$y = \frac{1}{2}at^2 \;\rightarrow\; d = \frac{1}{2}\cdot\frac{eQ}{mdC}t^2 \;\rightarrow\; t = d\sqrt{\frac{2mC}{eQ}}$$

The answer is D. Another way we could have attacked this question is to look at the answer choices and see if they make sense. If choice A were correct, then it would imply that a greater charge Q would *increase* the time required for the proton to move to the top plate. This doesn't make sense because a greater Q would create a greater force on the proton, giving it a greater acceleration, thus making it move faster, and causing t to decrease. We can also see that choice C can't be correct, for the same reason. Choice B could be eliminated because the units don't work out to be seconds, as shown below; therefore, the answer *had* to be D.

$$[d]\sqrt{\frac{[m]}{[e][Q][C]}} = m\sqrt{\frac{kg}{C\cdot C\cdot \frac{C}{V}}} = m\sqrt{\frac{kg}{C\cdot C\cdot \frac{C}{J/C}}} = \frac{m}{C^2}\sqrt{kg\cdot J} = \frac{m}{C^2}\sqrt{kg\cdot \frac{kg\cdot m^2}{s^2}} = \frac{kg\cdot m^2}{C^2\cdot s} \neq s$$

Example 10-31: An electron is projected horizontally into the space between the plates of a parallel-plate capacitor, as shown below, where the electric field has a magnitude of 56 V/m. The initial velocity of the electron is horizontal and has a magnitude of $v_0 = 5 \times 10^6$ m/s.

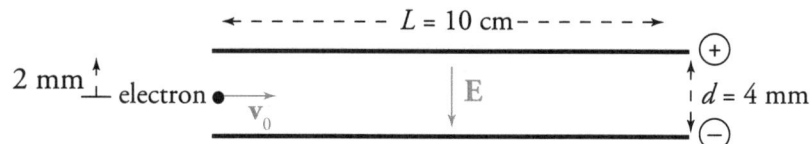

a) What is the force on the electron while it's in the region between the plates? (Neglect gravity.) What's the acceleration of the electron in this region? (Note: electron mass $\approx 9 \times 10^{-31}$ kg.)

b) How long would it take the electron to cover the horizontal distance L through the capacitor?

c) Describe the electron's trajectory through this region.

Solution:

a) Because the electric field **E** is constant between the plates, the force on the electron is also constant and given by $\mathbf{F} = q\mathbf{E} = -e\mathbf{E}$; this force points upward, in the direction opposite to the electric field (because q is negative), toward the positively charged top plate. Substituting in the numerical values gives $F = eE = (1.6 \times 10^{-19}$ C$) \times (56$ N/C$) = 9 \times 10^{-18}$ N. If the mass of the electron is m, then its acceleration, **a**, is $\mathbf{F}/m$. Like **F**, the acceleration is uniform and vertical, pointing upward, toward the top plate. The magnitude of **a** is $a = F/m = (9 \times 10^{-18}$ N$)/(9 \times 10^{-31}$ kg$) = 10^{13}$ m/s^2.

b) Because the acceleration of the electron is vertical, the electron's horizontal velocity will not change. Because v_{0x} is always equal to v_{0x}, the time required to traverse the 10 cm horizontal distance through the region between the plates is

$$x = v_x t \;\rightarrow\; t = \frac{x}{v_x} = \frac{x}{v_{0x}} = \frac{L}{v_{0x}} = \frac{10 \times 10^{-2} \text{ m}}{5 \times 10^6 \text{ m/s}} = 2 \times 10^{-8} \text{ s}$$

c) Because the acceleration is constant, we can use The Big Five to describe the motion of the electron. In fact, the motion of the electron between the plates is just like the motion of a projectile whose initial velocity is horizontal. The only difference is that while a projectile would curve downward in a half-parabola, the electron in the figure above will curve upward. Adapting Big Five #3 to vertical motion (in the y direction), we have $y = v_{0y}t + \frac{1}{2}a_y t^2$. Because $v_{0y} = 0$, this equation simplifies to $y = \frac{1}{2}a_y t^2$. Now, in the time t that the electron moves through the region between the plates (which we found in part b) its vertical displacement will be $y = \frac{1}{2}(10^{13}\,\text{m/s}^2)(2 \times 10^{-8}\,\text{s})^2 = 2 \times 10^{-3}\,\text{m} = 2\,\text{mm}$. Therefore, the electron will just hit the right edge of the top plate.

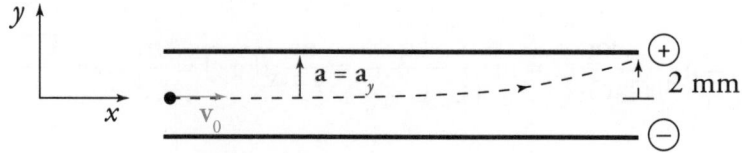

Now let's look at the second important use of a capacitor: as a storage device for electrical potential energy. We can think of the process of charging a capacitor as a transferal of electrons from one plate to the other. The plate that the electrons are taken from is left positively charged, and the plate the electrons are transferred to becomes negatively charged. Also, because we're simply transferring charge from one plate to the other, we are always assured at each moment that the plates carry equal but opposite charges.

During this charging process, an outside agent (the voltage source) must do work against the electric field that's created between the plates of the capacitor. Once we begin the process of transferring electrons from one plate to the other, it becomes increasingly difficult to transfer more. After all, it takes effort to remove more electrons from the plate that is left positively charged, *and* it takes effort to place them on the plate that is negatively charged. The fact that we have to "fight" against the system means we're storing potential energy.

This transferal is fighting against the electric field.

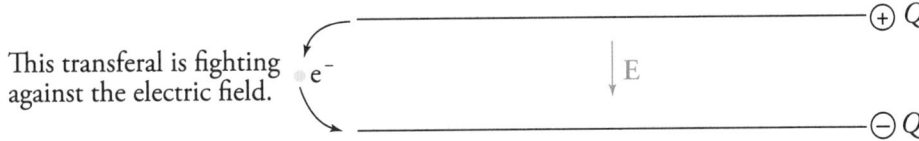

To increase the charge on the capacitor, work is required to remove extra electrons from the positive plate and move them to the negative plate. This work against the electric field is stored as electrical potential energy.

Because it requires more work to transfer more charge, we'd expect that the amount of potential energy stored should depend on Q, the final charge on the capacitor; that is, as Q increases, so should the *PE*. We'd also expect that the amount of stored *PE* should depend on the voltage between the plates. After all, we defined potential difference, V, by the equation $\Delta PE = qV$, where q was the charge that moved between the points whose potential difference was V. Hence, the higher voltage V leads to an increase in stored potential energy. If the final charge on the capacitor is Q and the final resulting voltage is V, then *PE* is proportional to both Q and V. Here's how we can intuitively find the formula for *PE* in this case: We transferred a total amount of charge equal to Q, fighting against the voltage that prevailed at each stage. If the final voltage is V, then the average voltage during the charging process is $\frac{1}{2}V$. Since ΔPE is equal to charge times voltage, we get $\Delta PE = Q \cdot \left(\frac{1}{2}V\right) = \frac{1}{2}QV$. At the beginning of the charging process, when there was no charge on the capacitor, we had $PE_i = 0$, so $\Delta PE = PE_f - PE_i = PE_f - 0 = PE_f$. Therefore, we have $PE_f = \frac{1}{2}QV$:

Electrical PE Stored in a Capacitor

$$PE = \tfrac{1}{2}QV$$

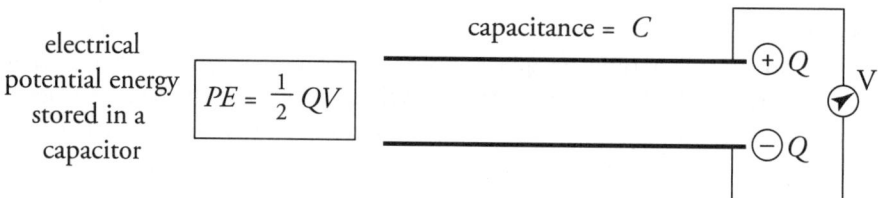

electrical potential energy stored in a capacitor

$$PE = \frac{1}{2} QV$$

capacitance = C

Using the fundamental equation $Q = CV$, we can rewrite this equation in terms of C and V, or in terms of Q and C:

$$PE = \frac{1}{2}QV = \frac{1}{2}CV^2 = \frac{Q^2}{2C}$$

If you lift a rock off the ground, you do work against the gravitational field of the earth, and, as a result, you store gravitational potential energy. To recapture this stored energy, you let the rock fall back to the ground, transferring the gravitational potential energy into mechanical kinetic energy. Similarly, if you transfer electrons from one plate of a capacitor to the other, you do work against the electric field of the capacitor, and, as a result, you store electrical potential energy. To recapture this stored electrical energy, you let the electrons go back to their original plate, effectively **discharging** the capacitor. The movement of electrons can be used in a productive manner by providing a path for them and placing some electrical devices along the way. As a result, the electrons that return to the plate end up passing through, say, a light bulb, and the current causes the bulb to light. We've been able to tap into the energy stored in the capacitor to do useful work. When we connect the charged capacitor plates by a wire with some resistor(s) along it, the charge drains off rapidly at first, but the rate at which the charge leaves gradually decreases as time goes on. The same is true of the resulting current; it too starts off high and then gradually drops to zero as the capacitor discharges.

Discharging a Capacitor

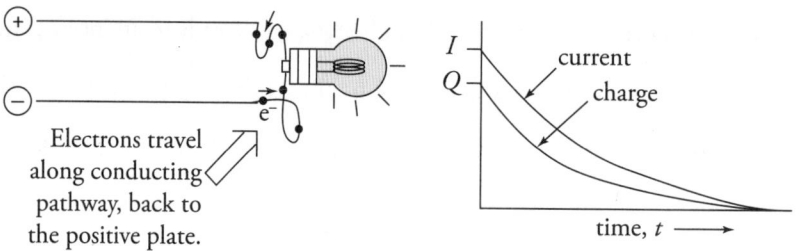

Electrons travel along conducting pathway, back to the positive plate.

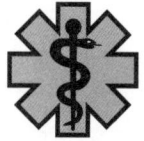

Example 10-32: A defibrillator contains a circuit whose primary components are a battery, a capacitor, and a switch. When the heart is undergoing ventricular fibrillation, the normally ordered electrical signals that organize the heart's pumping behavior are out of sync. The strong current delivered by the conducting paddles of the defibrillator can depolarize the entirety of the heart and potentially reset its orderly pumping triggered by the SA node. The defibrillator circuit first charges the capacitor with the battery. During the application and discharging of the circuit, a switch is closed to allow the capacitor to discharge through the paddles and the patient's tissue. Which of the following graphs best illustrates the voltage between the capacitor plates during this latter process?

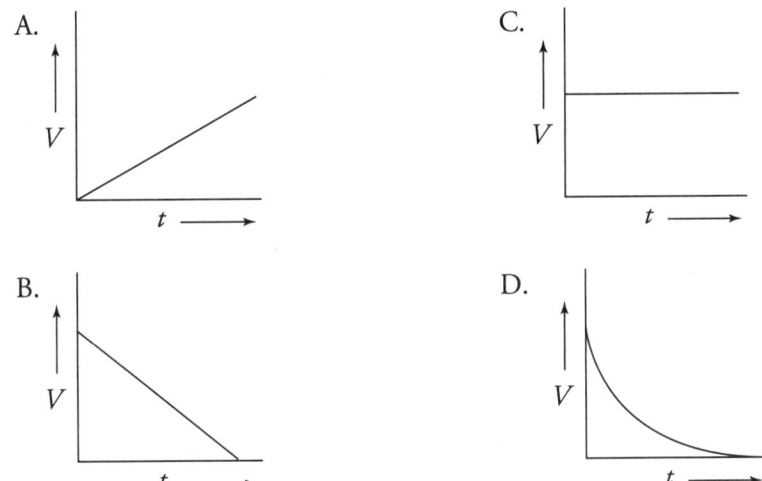

Solution: As the capacitor loses charge, Q decreases. Since $V = Q/C$, we know that V must decrease, too. This eliminates choices A and C. The charge drains off rapidly at first, but the rate at which the charge leaves gradually decreases as time goes on; therefore, the decrease in Q (and therefore in V also) is not linear. Thus, the best graph is the one in choice D. (The defibrillator circuit will also feature an *inductor* or *solenoid*, described later in this chapter. This has the effect of slowing the discharge of the capacitor and prolonging the application of current sufficiently to completely depolarize the heart.)

Dielectrics

If the plates of a capacitor were touching at the start of the charging process, then we'd effectively have a single conductor, not a pair, and no transferal of electrons from one plate to the other could begin; it wouldn't work as a capacitor. And if the plates were ever allowed to touch during the charging process, the capacitor would discharge almost immediately, since the transferred electrons would have a direct route back to the positive plate. All the electrical potential energy that had been stored would be lost in an instant, without any useful work being done by the stored energy. So for a capacitor to be useful, we need to keep the plates from touching.

Let's consider ways to do that. One way would be to mount them on separate insulating handles, like this:

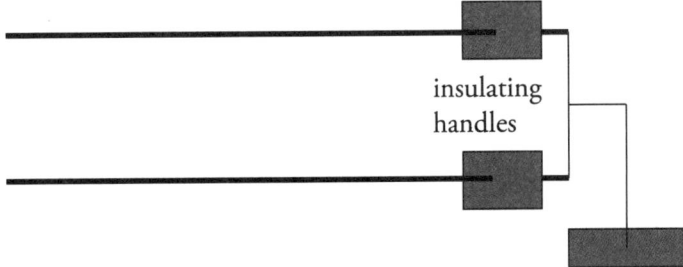

insulating
handles

That could work, but the way it's typically done is to sandwich a slab of insulating material between the plates. Such an insulator is known as a **dielectric**:

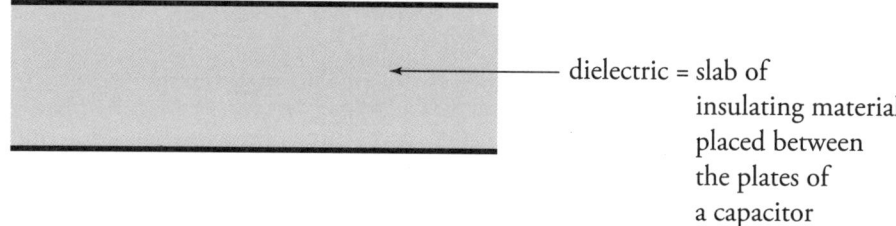

dielectric = slab of insulating material placed between the plates of a capacitor

Not only does a dielectric keep the plates from touching, but there's also a bonus: *The presence of a dielectric always increases the capacitance.* For the capacitor whose plates are mounted on insulating handles, with vacuum (or, for all practical purposes, air) between the plates, the capacitance is given by the equation we gave earlier: $C = \varepsilon_0 A/d$. However, if the capacitor is fitted with a dielectric, the capacitance is multiplied by a unitless factor of K, where K is known as the **dielectric constant** of the insulating material.[3] For example, wax paper is a dielectric, with a dielectric constant of about 3.5. If a parallel-plate capacitor were fitted with wax paper as a dielectric, the capacitance would be multiplied by 3.5. Other common dielectrics are teflon and certain plastics and ceramics.

Here's the formula for the capacitance of a parallel-plate capacitor with a dielectric:

Capacitance of a Parallel-Plate Capacitor with a Dielectric

$$C_{\substack{\text{with} \\ \text{dielectric}}} = K \cdot C_{\substack{\text{without} \\ \text{dielectric}}} = K\varepsilon_0 \frac{A}{d}$$

The value of K for vacuum is exactly 1, which makes sense since having empty space between the plates means there's *no* dielectric. The MCAT will assume that $K = 1$ for air as well because the actual value of K for air (~1.0005) is so close to 1. A capacitor with just air between its plates is known simply as an *air capacitor*. K is never less than 1, which is the reason dielectrics always increase capacitance.

Example 10-33: The area, A, of each plate of a parallel-plate capacitor satisfies the equation $\varepsilon_0 A = 10^{-10}$ F·m. If the plates are separated by a distance of 2 mm and this space is filled by a sheet of mica with a dielectric constant of 6, what is the capacitance of this capacitor?

Solution: The presence of the mica increases the capacitance by a factor of 6, so:

$$C_{\substack{\text{with} \\ \text{dielectric}}} = K \cdot C_{\substack{\text{without} \\ \text{dielectric}}} = K\varepsilon_0 \frac{A}{d} = 6 \cdot \frac{10^{-10} \text{ F} \cdot \text{m}}{2 \times 10^{-3} \text{ m}} = 3 \times 10^{-7} \text{ F}$$

---

[3] A note about notation: We're using a capital K for the dielectric constant, where some sources use the Greek letter κ and others use a lowercase k (which can be especially confusing given that Coulomb's constant is also k or k_0). You often also see a lowercase Greek ε to represent the permittivity of a material, that is what we're calling the product $K\varepsilon_0$. The lesson is that you should be prepared to encounter unfamiliar notation on the MCAT and not let that confuse you as to the underlying physics an equation represents, which will reliably be the same as you're learning now!

Example 10-34: The capacitance of a certain air capacitor whose plates are separated by a distance of 1 mm is 4 pF. If the plates are moved apart to a distance of 2.2 mm to accommodate a slab of porcelain of thickness 2.2 mm that is then inserted between them, the capacitance becomes 12 pF. What is the dielectric constant of porcelain?

Solution: The capacitance without the porcelain is $C_{without\ dielectric} = \varepsilon_0 A / d_1$, and the capacitance with the porcelain is $C_{with\ dielectric} = K\varepsilon_0 A / d_2$. The ratio of these values is

$$\frac{C_{with\ dielectric}}{C_{without\ dielectric}} = \frac{K\varepsilon_0 A / d_2}{\varepsilon_0 A / d_1} = K\frac{d_1}{d_2} = K\frac{1\ mm}{2.2\ mm} = \frac{K}{2.2}$$

Now, because the capacitance increased by a factor of 3, we have

$$\frac{K}{2.2} = 3 \rightarrow \quad \therefore K = 6.6$$

The presence of a dielectric can affect other properties of a capacitor besides capacitance. However, the ways a dielectric affects the charge, voltage, and electric field depend on whether the capacitor is connected or disconnected from the battery that charged it.

Let's begin by looking at the case in which a capacitor without a dielectric is charged by a battery and then disconnected from it. What happens if we then insert a dielectric between the plates? First, since the capacitor is disconnected from the battery, the charge that exists on the plates is trapped and cannot change. Therefore, Q remains constant. Because the capacitance C increases, the equation $Q = CV$ tells us that the voltage will decrease; in fact, because Q stays constant and C increases by a factor of K, we see that V will decrease by a factor of K. Next, using the equation $V = Ed$, we see that because V decreases by a factor of K, so does E. Finally, using the equation $PE = \frac{1}{2}QV$, we conclude that since Q stays constant and V decreases by a factor of K, the stored electrical potential energy decreases by a factor of K.

We can look at this a little more closely: First, why does the electric field strength, E, decrease in this case? The dielectric is an insulator, so although the field between the plates won't move any free electrons through the material, it will polarize the molecules. That is, the electric field will create tiny dipole moments in the molecules of the insulator, with the negative (δ^-) ends closer to the positive plate and the positive (δ^+) ends closer to the negative plate. As a result, we'll have a layer of negative charge at the surface of the dielectric that's near the positive plate and a layer of positive charge at the surface of the dielectric that's near the negative plate. These layers of induced charge on the opposite surfaces of the dielectric are the source of a new electric field through the dielectric, $\mathbf{E}_{induced}$, a field that points in the opposite direction from the electric field created by the charged capacitor plates themselves (because electric fields always point from positive and toward negative source charges).

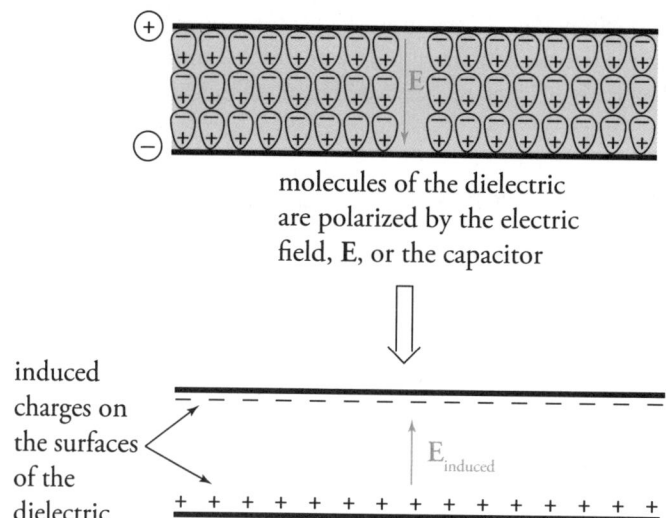

molecules of the dielectric
are polarized by the electric
field, **E**, or the capacitor

induced
charges on
the surfaces
of the
dielectric

The total electric field between the plates is then the sum of the field created by the plates, **E**, and the field created by the layers of induced charge on the surfaces of the dielectric, $\mathbf{E}_{induced}$. Because $\mathbf{E}_{induced}$ points in the direction *opposite* to **E**, the *net* field strength is reduced to $E - E_{induced}$. This is the physical reason why the electric field magnitude is reduced in this case.

We also found that the potential energy would be reduced if we inserted a dielectric after disconnecting the capacitor from the charging battery. Where did this energy go? Most of it is stored as electrical potential energy inside those induced dipoles in the dielectric. (Unfortunately, that stored energy is hard to recapture in a useful way.) You would notice that as you began to place the dielectric between the plates, the electric field would actually pull it in; thus, some of the stored potential energy turns into kinetic energy of the dielectric as it is pulled into the space between the capacitor plates. Finally, there would be some heat production (the usual MCAT answer to "Where did the energy go?").

Now let's examine the case in which a capacitor without a dielectric is first charged up and then while it's still connected to its voltage source, we insert a dielectric between its plates. First, since the capacitor is still connected to the battery, the voltage between the plates must match the voltage of the battery. Therefore, V will not change.[4] Because the capacitance C increases, the equation $Q = CV$ tells us that the charge Q must increase; in fact, because V doesn't change and C increases by a factor of K, we see that Q will increase by a factor of K. Next, using the equation $V = Ed$, we see that because V doesn't change, neither will E. Finally, using the equation $PE = \frac{1}{2}QV$, we conclude that since V doesn't change and Q increases by a factor of K, the stored electrical potential energy increases by a factor of K. An important point to notice is that V doesn't change because the battery will transfer additional charge to the capacitor plates. This increase in Q offsets any momentary decrease in the electric field strength when the dielectric is inserted (because the molecules of the dielectric are polarized, as above) and brings the electric field strength back to its original value. Furthermore, as more charge is transferred to the plates, more electrical potential energy is stored.

---

[4] This analysis assumes that the circuit has no resistance, so the newly increased capacitance can be "filled up" instantaneously. In practice, voltage in the capacitor would drop at first but then rise quickly until it was again equal to the battery's voltage.

The following figure summarizes the effects on the properties of a capacitor with the insertion of a dielectric in the two cases:

charge capacitor
to voltage V

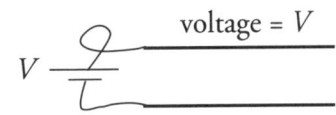

charge capacitor
to voltage V

then disconnect battery
and insert dielectric

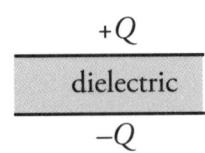

keep battery connected
and insert dielectric

- C increases by factor of K
- Q stays the same
- V decreases by a factor of K
- E decreases by a factor of K

- C increases by factor of K
- Q increases by factor of K
- V stays the same
- E stays the same

Example 10-35: An air capacitor is charged and disconnected from the battery. The electric field between the plates is **E**. Now, a dielectric with dielectric constant $K = 4$ is inserted between the plates. What is the electric field created by the layers of induced charges on the surfaces of the dielectric?

A. $3E/4$ opposite the direction of **E**
B. $E/4$ opposite the direction of **E**
C. $E/4$ in the same direction of **E**
D. $3E/4$ in the same direction of **E**

Solution: The question is asking for $\mathbf{E}_{induced}$. First, $\mathbf{E}_{induced}$ points in the *opposite* direction from **E**, so the answer must be either A or B. To find the magnitude of $\mathbf{E}_{induced}$, we use the fact that $E - E_{induced} = E/K$; since $K = 4$, we see that $E_{induced} = 3E/4$. Thus, the answer is A.

Example 10-36: A parallel-plate capacitor, with air between the plates, is charged to a voltage of $V = 1000$ V by a battery. The values of Q, E, and PE are also measured. The battery is then disconnected from the capacitor and a dielectric with dielectric constant $K = 4$ is inserted between the plates. The values of V, Q, E, and PE are measured again. Which of these values did *not* change?

A. V
B. Q
C. E
D. PE

Solution: Since the battery was disconnected from the capacitor after charging, the value of Q does not change: there's nowhere for charges to go and no source of new charges. The values of V, E, and PE will all decrease by a factor of K. The answer is B.

Example 10-37: A particular cell membrane has a dielectric number of about 9. If the internal potential of the cell is about 70 mV lower than the external potential, how much charge could accumulate on a square micrometer of phospholipid layer with a thickness of 8 nanometers ($\varepsilon_0 \approx 9 \times 10^{-12}$ F/m)?

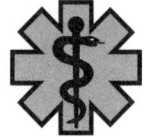

Solution:

$$C = \frac{K\varepsilon_0 A}{d} = \frac{9\left(9\times10^{-12}\right)\left(1\ \mu m^2 \times \left(\dfrac{10^{-6}\ m}{\mu m}\right)^2\right)}{8\times10^{-9}\ m} \approx 10^{-14}\ F$$

Now the charge this cell membrane capacitor can hold at the given voltage is $Q = CV = (10^{-14}$ F$)$ $(70 \times 10^{-3}$ V$) = 7 \times 10^{-16}$ C. This may not seem like much, but considering that the charge of one sodium or potassium ion is 1.6×10^{-19} C, this amounts to about 4 thousand ions. This is NOT what actually happens to a living cell, mind you, because a living cell is not a passive participant in its local environment (and there are chemical considerations in addition to electrical ones).

Dielectric Breakdown

Dielectrics have another purpose besides keeping the plates apart and increasing the capacitance. The illustration earlier for a discharging capacitor showed the plates connected by a conducting wire; the electrons on the negative plate used this pathway to travel back to the positive plate. This type of controlled discharge is necessary if we are to tap into the motion of these electrons to do useful work (like lighting a light bulb). But why don't the extra electrons on the negative plate just jump across the gap to the positive plate, without traveling through a conducting wire pathway? They can, but only under extreme circumstances.

For an air capacitor, the maximum electric field strength is about 3 million volts per meter. If the value of E were to exceed this maximum value, the air would no longer act as an insulator. Electrons would be pulled out of the molecules, ionizing the air, and the electrons on the negative plate would then have a conducting pathway through the air; we'd see a spark as the capacitor discharged very rapidly. When the electric field strength between the plates becomes so strong that the dielectric (which is supposed to act as an insulator) is ionized, providing a route for the electrons on the negative plate to return to the positive plate, we say that the dielectric has suffered **dielectric breakdown**. This is essentially what causes lightning. The bottom region of a thundercloud is negatively charged and the surface of the earth below the cloud is positively charged; these surfaces act as the oppositely charged plates in a huge parallel-plate capacitor. When the voltage V becomes so great that $E = V/d$ exceeds 3 million volts per meter, the air is ionized, and charge is transferred in a spectacular bolt of lightning.

The presence of a dielectric increases this maximum electric field strength. As a result, capacitors with dielectrics can hold more charge (and thus store more potential energy) without the threat of dielectric breakdown. For example, wax paper has a **dielectric strength** that's about 5 times greater than that of air; in other words, the maximum electric field that a piece of wax paper can withstand is about 15 million volts per meter, 5 times what air could withstand. If the maximum E is increased by a factor of 5, the maximum V that the plates can support is increased by a factor of 5 (since V is proportional to E). Because $PE = \frac{1}{2}CV^2$, a capacitor with wax paper as a dielectric not only has a capacitance 3.5 times greater than an air capacitor (because $K = 3.5$ for wax paper), but its maximum V is increased by 5. Therefore, a capacitor with a wax paper dielectric can store $(3.5) \times 5^2 = 87.5$ times more potential energy than the same capacitor with just air between the plates.

Except for enjoying a great lightning display or causing a spark to jump across the gap in your car's spark plugs, dielectric breakdown is something that you typically want to avoid. In electrical devices that contain capacitors, if any of the capacitors suffer dielectric breakdown this generally means that a hole is burned through the dielectric, and the capacitor must then be replaced.

Example 10-38: An air capacitor has a capacitance of 1 µF. If its plates are separated by a distance $d = 1$ mm, what is the maximum amount of charge the capacitor could hold before dielectric breakdown occurs? (Dielectric strength of air = 3 million volts per meter)

Solution: Because $V = Ed$, we can find the maximum voltage that the capacitor can withstand:

$$V_{max} = E_{max}d = \left(3 \times 10^6 \, \tfrac{v}{m}\right)\left(10^{-3}\, m\right) = 3000\, V. \text{ Now, because } Q = CV, \text{ we find that}$$

$$Q_{max} = CV_{max} = (1 \times 10^{-6} \text{ F})(3000 \text{ V}) = 3 \times 10^{-3} \text{ C}$$

Combinations of Capacitors

Like resistors, capacitors can also be placed in series and in parallel within a circuit. In this section, we'll see how to find the equivalent capacitance for each of these cases.

Capacitors in **parallel** all have the same voltage (like *resistors* in parallel), but the equivalent capacitance is the sum of the individual capacitances (like resistors in *series*):

equivalent capacitance
for capacitors in parallel
$$\boxed{C_{eq} = C_1 + C_2 + C_3 + \ldots}$$

For example, in the figure below, the equivalent capacitance, C_{eq}, is 2 µF + 3 µF + 4 µF = 9 µF:

capacitors in parallel

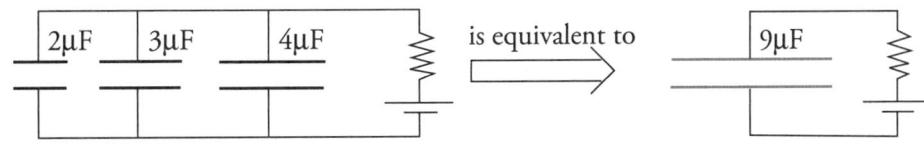

Capacitors in **series** all have the same charge (similar to *resistors* in series all having the same current), but the equivalent capacitance is found from the same formula that we used for resistors in *parallel*:

$$\begin{array}{l} \text{equivalent capacitance} \\ \text{for capacitors in series} \end{array} \quad \boxed{\frac{1}{C_{eq}} = \frac{1}{C_1} + \frac{1}{C_2} + \frac{1}{C_3} + \cdots}$$

Equivalently, we could simplify the capacitors two at a time using the expression *product/sum*. For example, in the figure below, the equivalent capacitance, C_{eq}, is 2 μF, because 1/12 + 1/6 + 1/4 = 1/2. (We could also calculate it as (12 × 6)/(12 + 6) = 4 and (4 × 4)/(4 + 4) = 2.)

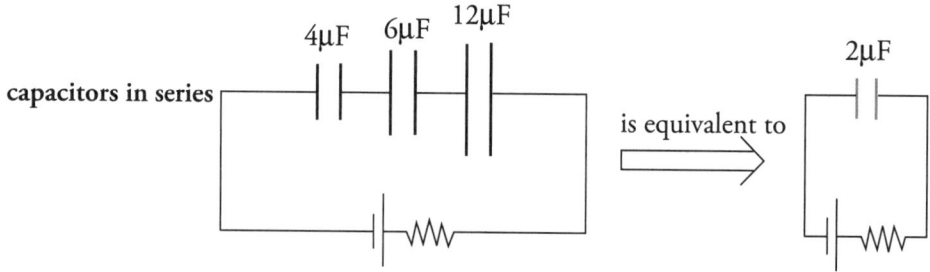

Example 10-39: Three uncharged capacitors are arranged in a circuit as shown.

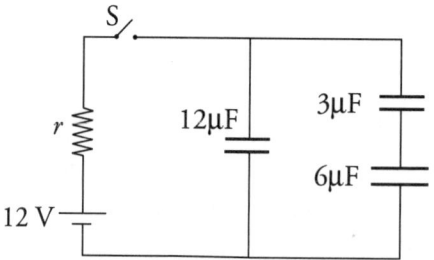

After the switch S has been closed for a long time and electrostatic equilibrium is reached, how much charge is on the 6 μF capacitor?

Solution: The 3 μF and 6 μF capacitors are in series, so they're equivalent to a single 2 μF capacitor, because (3 × 6)/(3 + 6) = 2. Therefore, the circuit shown above is equivalent to

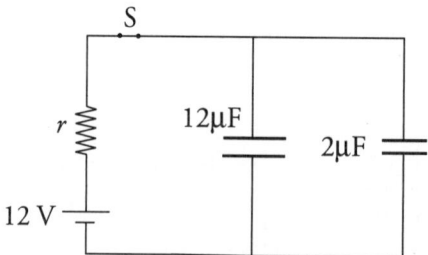

These two capacitors are in parallel, so both will have the same voltage: 12 V, since the plates of each are connected to the terminals of a 12 V battery. Now, using the equation $Q = CV$, we see that the charge on the 2 μF capacitor will be

$$Q = (2 \text{ μF})(12 \text{ V}) = 24 \text{ μC}$$

Since the 2 μF capacitor is equivalent to the series combination consisting of the 3 μF and 6 μF capacitors, the charge on each of these capacitors must be the same, 24 μC—this is equivalent to saying that two resistors in parallel must have the same current (Kirchhoff's current rule). (For extra practice, you may wish to verify the final voltages and charges on each of the three capacitors in the original circuit; the answers are shown below.)

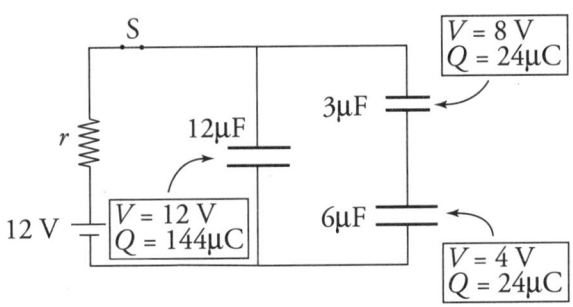

10.3 ALTERNATING CURRENT

In Section 8.1, we discussed circuits in which the current flowed in one direction only; such current is called **direct current** (DC). However, the electrical current that we use in our homes and offices every day is **alternating current** (AC), because the direction of the current changes: first one way, then the opposite way, then back again, and so on. The electrons that drift in the wires (and whose flow constitutes the current) are constantly forced to shuttle back and forth. While this may seem a little silly, producing an alternating voltage (and thus an alternating current) on a scale that supplies electricity to entire cities is far easier than producing a steady, direct voltage.

An AC generator creates a sinusoidally varying voltage. The voltage starts at, say, zero, and climbs to a peak value (called the amplitude), then falls back to zero; at this point, the polarity reverses, and the voltage again rises to its peak value then falls back to zero, and the cycle starts again. When we graph this time-varying voltage, we show the first half of the cycle as positive and the second half as negative; the negative voltage simply means that it "points" in the opposite direction from the voltage in the first half of the cycle. Thus, when the voltage is positive, the current flows in one direction. When the voltage is negative, the current flows in the opposite direction. In cases where the circuit contains only a source of alternating voltage and resistors, the current is in phase with the voltage, and we also consider Ohm's law to hold: That is, the voltage and current are related by $v = iR_{eq}$, where R_{eq} is the equivalent resistance of the circuit.

Note: It's customary when discussing time-varying voltages and currents to use lower-case letters; *v* and *i*, rather than *V* and *I*. The capital letters then denote the *maximum* values of *v* and *i*.

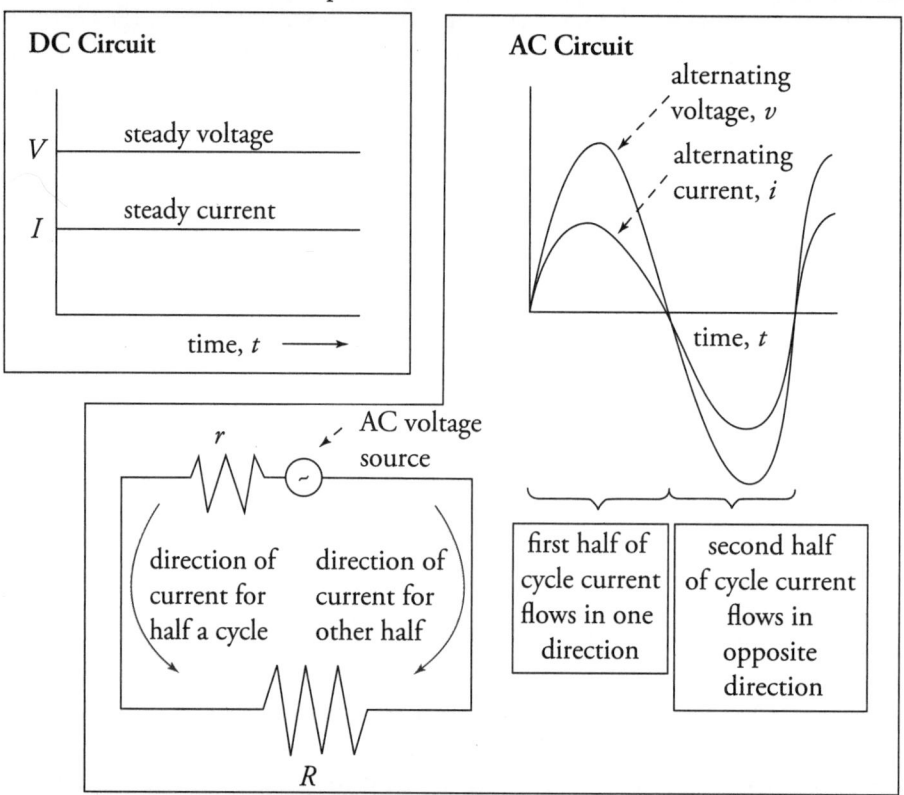

Notice that since *v* and *i* are constantly changing in an AC circuit, we can't talk about *the* voltage or *the* current. Instead, we talk about a kind of average voltage and average current. The particular average that is most useful is known as the **root-mean-square**, abbreviated **rms**. To form the rms of a quantity, we square it, average it over a cycle (that is, find the mean), then take the square root; it's the *root* of the *mean* of the *square* (hence root-mean-square). Fortunately, what all this boils down to is that the rms of a quantity is equal to its maximum divided by $\sqrt{2}$.

RMS Voltage and RMS Current

$$V_{rms} = \frac{v_{max}}{\sqrt{2}} = \frac{V}{\sqrt{2}} \quad \text{and} \quad I_{rms} = \frac{i_{max}}{\sqrt{2}} = \frac{I}{\sqrt{2}}$$

Recall that the power dissipated by a resistor in a DC circuit is given by the equation $P = I^2R$ and the power supplied by a voltage source is given by $P = IV$. For an AC circuit, we say that the average power dissipated by a resistor is $\bar{P} = I_{rms}^2 R$ and the average power supplied by the voltage source is $\bar{P} = I_{rms}V_{rms}$. This is why the rms average is one we use; it keeps the formulas the same as they were for DC circuits.

Example 10-40: Homes are typically supplied with 110 V rms.

a) What's the maximum voltage?
b) How much energy (in kWh) is used in 2 hours by a device whose resistance is 110 ohms?
c) How much would this cost if the electric company charges you 8¢ per kWh?

Solution:

a) Since 110 V is the rms voltage, we find the maximum voltage by multiplying V_{rms} by $\sqrt{2}$:

$$v_{max} = \sqrt{2} \cdot V_{rms} \approx (1.4)(110 \text{ V}) = 154 \text{ V}$$

b) Energy is power × time, so we can find the energy consumed by this device by multiplying the average power it consumes by the time. Since

$$\bar{P} = I_{rms}^2 R = \left(\frac{V_{rms}}{R}\right)^2 R = \frac{V_{rms}^2}{R} = \frac{(110 \text{ V})^2}{110 \text{ }\Omega} = 110 \text{ W}$$

we have

$$\text{energy} = \bar{P} \times t = (110 \text{ W})(2 \text{ h}) = 220 \text{ Wh} = 0.220 \text{ kWh}$$

c) To calculate how much this would cost, we multiply this by 8¢/kWh:

$$\text{cost} = 0.220 \text{ kWh} \times \frac{\$0.08}{\text{kWh}} = \$0.0175 = 1\tfrac{3}{4} \text{ cents}$$

10.4   MAGNETIC FIELDS AND FORCES

Electric fields are created by electric charges; **magnetic fields** are created by *moving* electric charges. If a charge is at rest, it produces an electric field in the surrounding space. If this charge were to move, it would create an additional force field, a magnetic field, in the surrounding space. Since charge in motion constitutes a current, we can also say that magnetic fields are produced by electric currents. A permanent bar magnet is a source of a magnetic field because of the multitude of microscopic currents due to motions of the orbiting electrons within the metal; therefore, even a bar magnet's magnetic field is ultimately due to charges in motion.

If we place a charge q in a given electric field, **E**, the force that the field will exert on this charge is given by the equation $\mathbf{F}_E = q\mathbf{E}$. We now need a similar formula to tell us the force that a magnetic field would exert on a charge q. First, a magnetic field can only exert a force on a charge that is *moving* through the field. A magnetic field is produced by moving charges and it exerts a force only on other moving charges. A magnetic field will exert no force on a charge that's at rest. The letter **B** is used to denote a magnetic field.

The formula for the force that a magnetic field exerts on a charge q is as follows:

10.4

Magnetic Force

$$\mathbf{F}_B = q(\mathbf{v} \times \mathbf{B})$$

where $\mathbf{v}$ is the velocity of the charge q. Notice that if $\mathbf{v} = 0$ (that is, if the charge is at rest), then $\mathbf{F}_B$ will also be 0.

The formula $\mathbf{F}_B = q(\mathbf{v} \times \mathbf{B})$ involves the *cross product* of $\mathbf{v}$ and $\mathbf{B}$. You don't need to worry about calculating the vector components of the cross product; there is a much simpler way of finding $\mathbf{F}_B$ that is more than adequate for the MCAT. First, the magnitude of $\mathbf{F}_B$ is given by this equation:

Magnitude of Magnetic Force

$$F_B = |q|vB \sin\theta$$

where θ is the angle between $\mathbf{v}$ and $\mathbf{B}$. Notice that if $\mathbf{v}$ is parallel to $\mathbf{B}$, then $\theta = 0°$, and, since $\sin 0° = 0$, we get $\mathbf{F}_B = 0$. So, a charge could be moving through a magnetic field and yet feel no force if its direction of motion is parallel to the magnetic field lines. The same will be true if $\mathbf{v}$ is anti-parallel to $\mathbf{B}$ (that is, if the direction of $\mathbf{v}$ is exactly opposite to the direction of $\mathbf{B}$), since in this case, we have $\theta = 180°$ and $\sin 180° = 0$, so again we get $\mathbf{F}_B = 0$. If $\mathbf{v} \perp \mathbf{B}$, then $\theta = 90°$, and since $\sin 90° = 1$, the magnitude of $\mathbf{F}_B$ becomes simply $F_B = |q|vB$. From this equation, we can find the SI unit for magnetic field strength:

$$[B] = \frac{[F_B]}{[q][v]} = \frac{N}{C \cdot m/s} = \frac{N}{\frac{C}{s} \cdot m} = \frac{N}{A \cdot m}$$

One newton per amp-meter (1 N/A·m) is renamed one **tesla**, abbreviated **T**. That is, B is measured in teslas.

Now that we know how to find the magnitude of $\mathbf{F}_B$, all we need is a way to find the direction. The direction of $\mathbf{F}_B$ will depend on whether the charge q that moves through the field is positive or negative. Just like the force due to an electric field, the force due to a magnetic field also depends on the sign of the charge: If $\mathbf{B}$ exerts a force in a particular direction on a charge $+q$ moving with velocity $\mathbf{v}$, then it would exert a force in the opposite direction on $-q$ moving with velocity $\mathbf{v}$. In addition, magnetic forces have the following strange property: *The direction of $\mathbf{F}_B$ is always perpendicular to both $\mathbf{v}$ and $\mathbf{B}$.* For example, if we had a magnetic field whose field lines pointed across this page (say, from left to right), and a positive charge q travels down the page, then the direction of the force $\mathbf{F}_B$ that q feels would be out of the plane of the page. The direction of $\mathbf{F}_B$ will always be perpendicular to the plane containing the vectors $\mathbf{v}$ and $\mathbf{B}$. Since we're now dealing with a situation in which we'll have vectors in *three* dimensions, we need a notation to indicate when a vector points into, or out of, the plane of the page.

Here are the symbols:

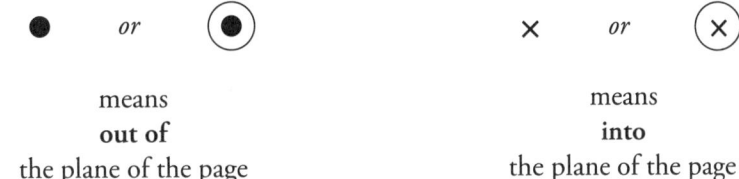

means
out of
the plane of the page

means
into
the plane of the page

Now let's learn how to find the direction of the magnetic force, $\mathbf{F_B}$, acting on a particle of charge q moving with velocity **v** through a magnetic field **B**. It involves the **right-hand rule** and the **left-hand rule**. You use the right-hand rule if the charge q moving through the field is positive, and the left-hand rule if q is negative.[5] Here's how the rules work.

First, determine whether the charge moving through the magnetic field is positive or negative.

If q is *positive*, use your *right* hand and the *right*-hand rule.

If q is *negative*, use your *left* hand and the *left*-hand rule.

Whether you use the right-hand rule or the left-hand rule, you will always follow these steps:

1. Orient your hand so that your thumb points in the direction of the velocity **v.**
2. Point your fingers in the direction of **B**.
3. The direction of $\mathbf{F_B}$ will then be perpendicular to your palm.

Think of your palm pushing with the force $\mathbf{F_B}$; the direction it pushes is the direction of $\mathbf{F_B}$.

Right-Hand Rule:

For determining the direction of the magnetic force, $\mathbf{F_B}$, on a *positive* charge

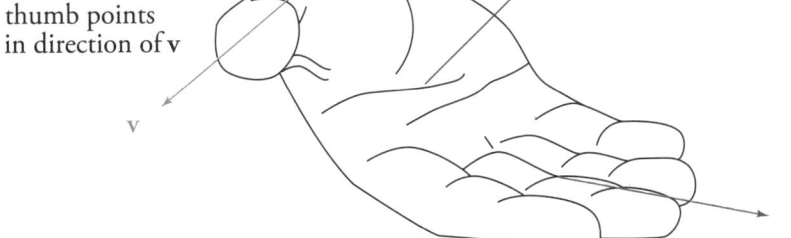

direction of $\mathbf{F_B}$ is perpendicular to your palm

thumb points in direction of **v**

fingers point in direction of **B**

---

[5] Another method which many people prefer is always to use the right-hand rule, and then reverse the result (in other words, solve for the direction of the force on a positive charge, and then realize that the force on a negative charge is in exactly the opposite direction).

Left-Hand Rule:

For determining the direction of
the magnetic force, $\mathbf{F}_B$,
on a *negative* charge

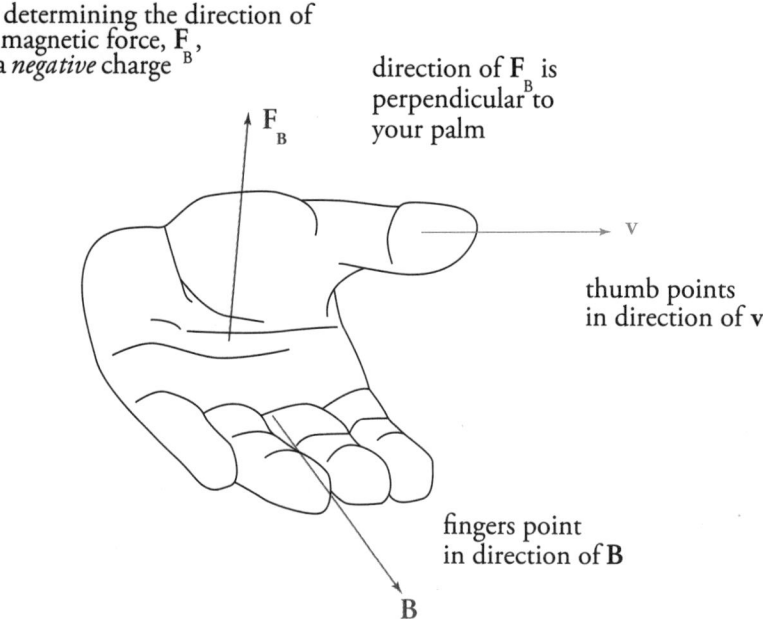

For example, let's say we have a positive charge q moving with velocity $\mathbf{v}$ to the right across the plane of this page through a magnetic field $\mathbf{B}$ directed toward the top of the page. How would you find the direction of the resulting magnetic force on this moving charge? Since q is positive, use your right hand, and lay it flat on this page with your palm facing up; notice that in this orientation, your thumb points to the right (as it should since your thumb always points in the direction of the particle's velocity, $\mathbf{v}$) and your fingers point up toward the top of the page (as they should since your fingers always point in the direction of the magnetic field, $\mathbf{B}$). The direction of $\mathbf{F}_B$ is perpendicular to your palm, pointing out of the plane of the page, and so we symbolize the direction of $\mathbf{F}_B$ by ⊙. In this case, the charged particle would start curling out of the plane of the page as a result of the magnetic force it feels.

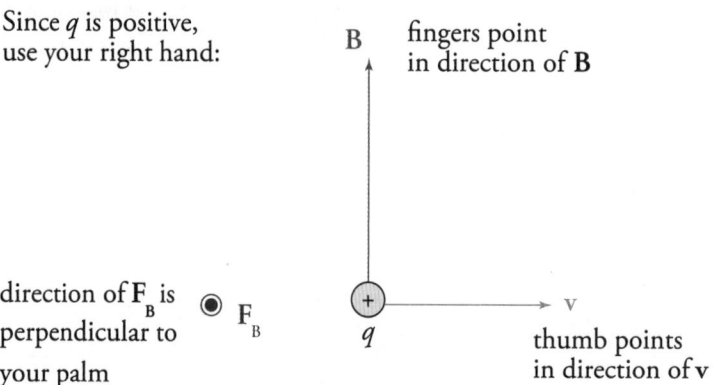

Now let's examine what would happen in the previous example if the charged particle had been *negative*. That is, we have a *negative* charge q moving with velocity $\mathbf{v}$ to the right across the plane of this page through a magnetic field $\mathbf{B}$ directed toward the top of the page. How would you find the direction of the resulting magnetic force on this moving charge? Since q is negative, use your *left* hand, and lay it flat on this page with your palm facing *down*; notice that in this orientation, your thumb points to the right (as it should since your thumb always points in the direction of the particle's velocity, **v**) and your fingers point up toward the top of the page (as they should since your fingers always point in the direction of the magnetic field, **B**). The direction of F_B is perpendicular to your palm, pointing *into* the plane of the page, and so we symbolize the direction of F_B by $\otimes$. In this case, the charged particle would start curling into the plane of the page as a result of the magnetic force it feels.

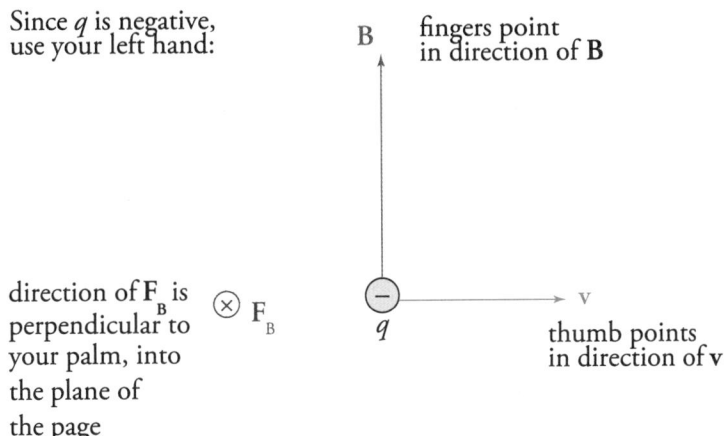

Practice the right- and left-hand rules and verify each of the following:

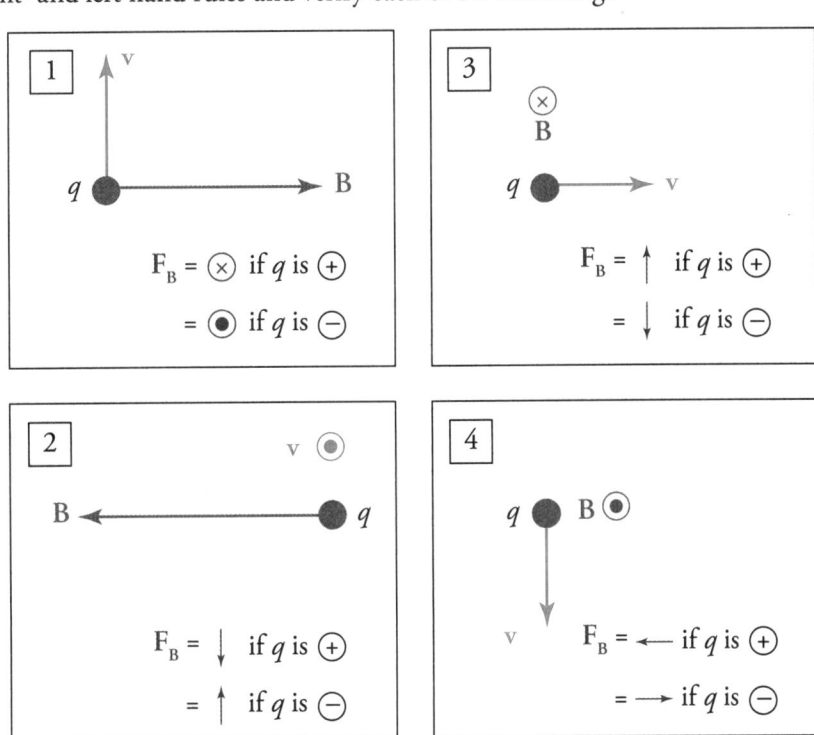

Because the magnetic force a charge feels is always perpendicular to the velocity of the charge, *magnetic forces do no work*. Recall that if a force **F** is perpendicular to the displacement **d** of an object, then this force **F** does zero work, because $W = Fd \cos \theta$ and $\theta = 90°$; since $\cos 90° = 0$, we get $W = 0$. Since magnetic forces never do work, they can never change the kinetic energy of a particle, meaning that KE is constant. (This follows from the work-energy theorem, $W = \Delta KE$.) Since magnetic forces cannot change the kinetic energy of a particle, they can't change the speed of a particle. All magnetic forces can do is make charged particles change their direction; they can't make them speed up or slow down.

The formula given earlier for the magnitude of the magnetic force is $|q|vB\sin\theta$, where θ is the angle between $\mathbf{v}$ and $\mathbf{B}$. On the MCAT, it's most common to have a constant magnetic field and $\mathbf{v} \perp \mathbf{B}$; in this case, $\theta = 90°$, and because $\sin 90° = 1$, the magnitude of $\mathbf{F}_B$ becomes $F_B = |q|vB$. Further, if $\mathbf{v} \perp \mathbf{B}$, the subsequent motion of the charged particle will be uniform circular motion, with the magnetic force providing the centripetal force. Recall that in uniform circular motion, the centripetal force is always perpendicular to the particle's velocity and the particle's speed is constant; all the particle does is continuously change direction as it moves in a circular path. This is consistent with what we said in the previous paragraph about magnetic forces: they don't change the speed of a particle, only its direction. The case of a charged particle executing uniform circular motion in a constant magnetic field is so important for the MCAT, that we'll do the following example in detail.

Example 10-41: A proton is injected with velocity $\mathbf{v}$ into a region of constant magnetic field $\mathbf{B}$ that points out of the plane of the page. The direction of $\mathbf{v}$ is to the right, in the plane of the page, as shown in the diagram below:

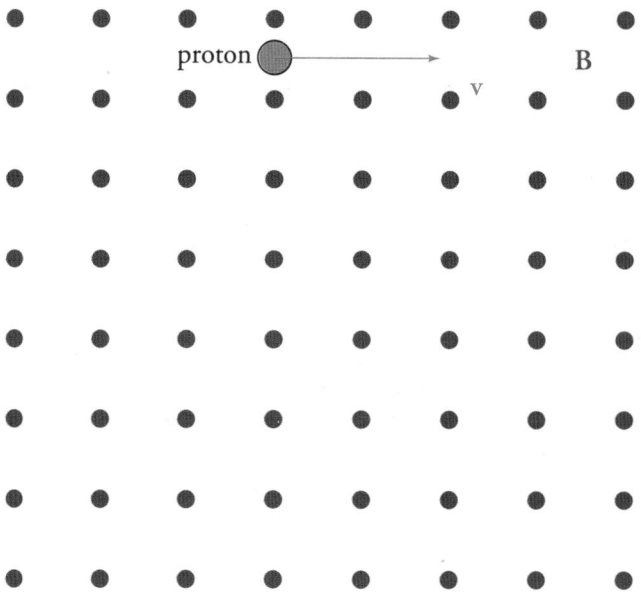

a)   Describe the subsequent motion of the proton.
b)   Find the radius of the circular trajectory it follows.

Solution:

a)   Because the proton is a positive charge, we use the *right*-hand rule to find the direction of the magnetic force it feels. With $\mathbf{v}$ to the right and $\mathbf{B}$ out of the page, we find that $\mathbf{F}_B$ points downward in the plane of the page:

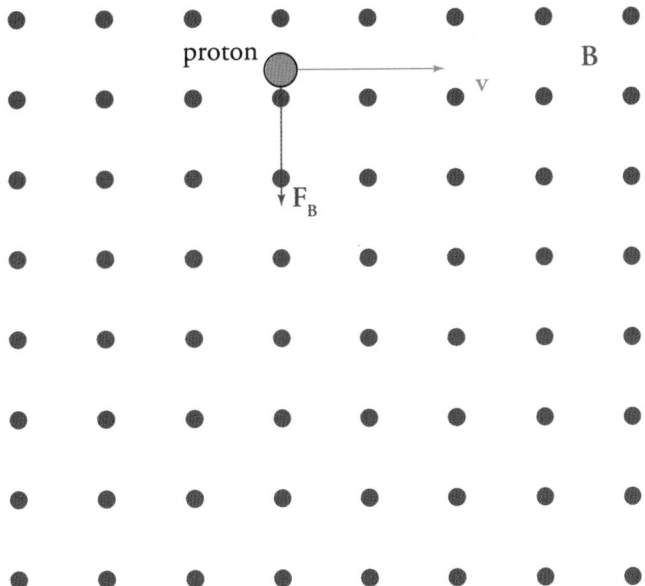

As a result, the proton will curve downward, and as it does, it is still continuously acted on by the magnetic force, but because the direction of **v** changes, so will the direction of $\mathbf{F_B}$. For example, when the proton is at the position shown in the following figure, the direction of $\mathbf{F_B}$ will be to the left:

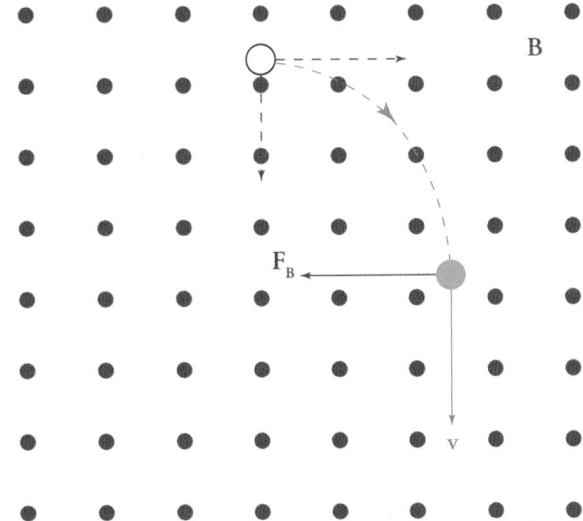

10.4

We can now see that the proton will continue to curve in a circular path, traveling clockwise:

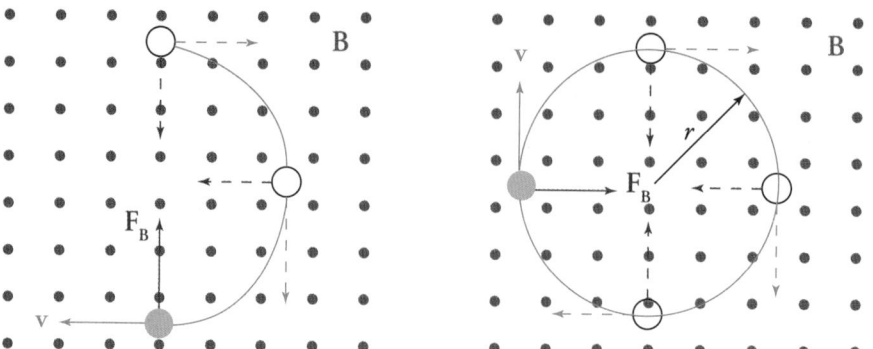

b) To find the radius of the circular path, we use the fact that the magnetic force provides the centripetal force to write

$$qvB = \frac{mv^2}{r}$$

where m is the mass of the proton. (We can drop the absolute value signs on the charge q because q is positive here.) Substituting $q = e$ (remember, it's a proton), then canceling one v from the right-hand side and solving for r, we get

$$r = \frac{mv}{eB}$$

Example 10-42: A particle with positive charge q and mass m moving with speed v undergoes uniform circular motion in a constant magnetic field **B**. If the radius of the particle's path is r, which of the following expressions gives the particle's orbit period (in other words, the time required for the particle to complete one revolution)?

A. $2\pi/qvB$
B. $2\pi m/qB$
C. $qvB/2\pi m$
D. $qB/2\pi m$

Solution: Since the magnetic force provides the centripetal force, we have

$$qvB = \frac{mv^2}{r}$$

Canceling one v from the right-hand side and solving for r, we get $r = mv/qB$. The time required for the particle to complete one revolution is equal to the total distance traveled by the particle in one revolution (the circumference, $2\pi r$) divided by the particle's speed, v. This gives

$$T = \frac{2\pi r}{v} = \frac{2\pi \cdot \dfrac{mv}{qB}}{v} = \frac{2\pi m}{qB}$$

Therefore, the answer is B. (*Note:* T is called the *cyclotron period*. Notice that it does *not* depend on r or v. Whether the particle moves rapidly in a large circle or more slowly in a smaller circle, it doesn't matter: the orbit period is determined solely by the mass and charge of the particle, and the magnitude of the magnetic field.)

Example 10-43: A particle with negative charge $-q$ moving with speed v_0 enters a region containing a uniform magnetic field **B**. If the vector $\mathbf{v}_0$ makes an angle of 30° with **B**, what is the particle's speed 8 seconds after entering the field?

    A. $v_0/4$
    B. v_0
    C. $2v_0$
    D. $4v_0$

Solution: Since magnetic forces do no work, the kinetic energy (and thus the speed) of the particle will be unchanged. The answer is B.

Example 10-44: The figure below shows a charged parallel-plate capacitor with a uniform electric field, **E**, in the space between its plates. A uniform magnetic field, **B**, is also produced in the space between the capacitor plates by another device.

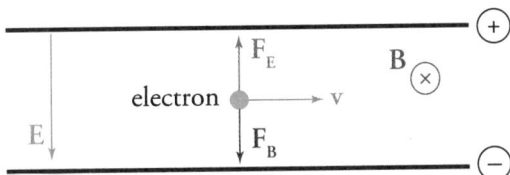

At what speed would an electron need to travel between the plates in order to pass through undeflected? (Ignore gravity.)

    A. E/B
    B. B/E
    C. EB
    D. EB^2

Solution: In between the plates, the direction of the electric force, $\mathbf{F}_E$, on the electron is upward. Using the left-hand rule (because the particle carries a negative charge), we find that the direction of the magnetic force, $\mathbf{F}_B$, is downward.

Therefore, these two forces point in opposite directions. They'll cancel (giving $\mathbf{F}_{net} = 0$) and allow the particle to pass through undeflected if these forces have the same magnitude. The magnitude of the electric force is $F_E = |q|E = |-e|E = eE$, and the magnitude of the magnetic force is $F_B = |q|vB = |-e|vB = evB$. Therefore, we'll have $F_B = F_E$ when $evB = eE$. Solving this equation for v, we find that $v = E/B$, choice A.

Example 10-45: A uniform magnetic field **B** exerts a force $\mathbf{F}_B$ on a particle with charge q moving with velocity **v** through the field. Which of the following gives the magnetic force that the same field would exert on a particle of charge $2q$ moving with velocity $-2\mathbf{v}$?

A. $-8\mathbf{F}_B$
B. $-4\mathbf{F}_B$
C. $4\mathbf{F}_B$
D. $8\mathbf{F}_B$

Solution: If **B** exerts a force of $\mathbf{F}_B$ on a charge q moving with velocity **v**, then it would exert a force of $-\mathbf{F}_B$ on a charge q moving with velocity $-\mathbf{v}$. Now, because F_B is proportional to q and to v, if q and v both double, then F_B will be multiplied by a factor of $2 \cdot 2 = 4$. Therefore, the force that **B** would exert on a particle of charge $2q$ moving with velocity $-2\mathbf{v}$ is $-4\mathbf{F}_B$, choice B.

Example 10-46: The figure below shows a simple mass spectrometer. It consists of a source of ions that are accelerated from rest through a potential difference V and then enter a region containing a uniform magnetic field **B** that points out of the plane of the page and is perpendicular to the initial velocity, **v**, of the ion as it enters. Once an ion enters the magnetic field, it travels in a semicircular path until it strikes the detector, which records its arrival and the distance, d, from the opening.

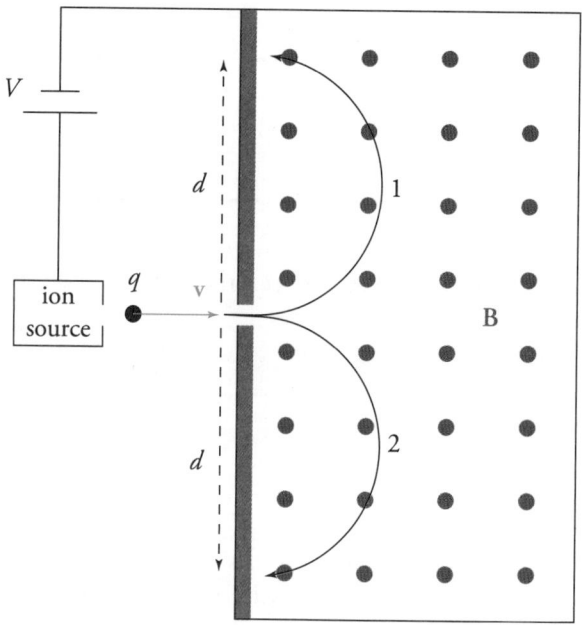

a)   An ion of charge $+q$ and mass m will enter the magnetic field with what speed? Write v in terms of q, m, and V.

b)   Which semicircular path would a cation follow: 1 or 2?

c)   If you were using this device in a lab to analyze a sample containing various isotopes of an element, how would you find the mass of a cation striking the detector if all you knew were q, V, B, and d?

Solution:

a) The ion loses electrical potential energy in the amount qV, and as a result, gains kinetic energy, $\frac{1}{2}mv^2$. Therefore, $\frac{1}{2}mv^2 = qV$, so $v = \sqrt{2qV/m}$.

b) The right-hand rule (for a positive charge) tells us that if **v** points to the right and **B** points out of the plane of the page, then $\mathbf{F_B}$ points downward:

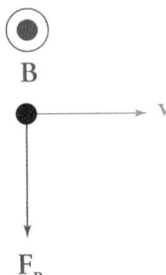

Since $\mathbf{F_B}$ points downward when the particle is at the opening, a cation would follow path 2, because $\mathbf{F_B}$ provides the centripetal force and thus points toward the center of the path. The following diagram illustrates this:

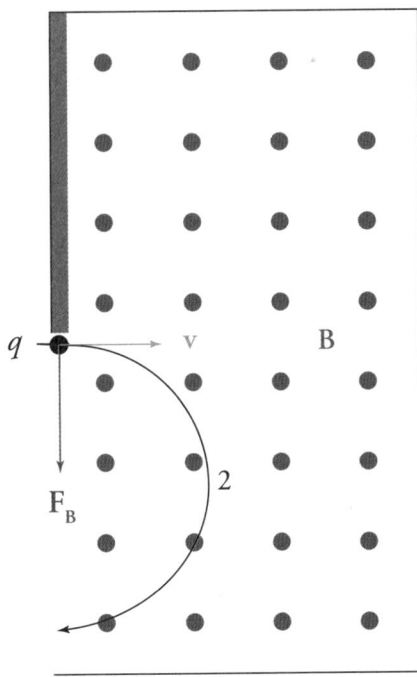

c) Since the magnetic force provides the centripetal force, we have

$$qvB = \frac{mv^2}{r}$$

Canceling one v from the right-hand side and solving for m (the mass of the cation) gives

$$m = \frac{qBr}{v}$$

10.4

From the diagram, we see that $r = \frac{1}{2}d$, and from part (a), $v = \sqrt{2qV/m}$, so we get

$$m = \frac{qB \cdot \frac{1}{2}d}{\sqrt{2qV/m}}$$

Squaring both sides and solving for m, we find that the mass of the cation is

$$m = \frac{qB^2 d^2}{8V}$$

Sources of Magnetic Fields

Now that we know how a given magnetic field affects a charged particle, we'll now look at how the magnetic field was created in the first place. Recall that charges *in motion* produce a magnetic field. A current is charge in motion, so electric currents produce magnetic fields. Let's take the simplest possible case: An electric current moving in a straight line. The magnetic field lines created by the current wrap around the current, forming closed loops. To find the direction of these magnetic field loops, we use the right-hand rule because by convention we consider a current I to be the direction that positive charges would move.[6] Imagine grabbing the wire in your right hand in such a way that your thumb points in the direction of the velocity of the charges (that is, in the direction of I). The way that your fingers wrap around the wire gives the direction of the magnetic field. Verify the directions of the **B**-field loops for the wires shown below; remember, magnetic field "lines" are actually circles that wrap around the wire. (That's the end of the right-hand rule in this situation. We are not trying to figure out the direction of the magnetic force that a given magnetic field exerts on a charged particle; we're now finding the magnetic field. Your thumb and fingers mean the same thing now as they did before: Your thumb points in the direction of the motion of the relevant charge (the charge making the field) and your fingers point in the direction of the magnetic field, **B**.)

current-carrying wire perpendicular to page with current coming *out* of the plane of the page

current-carrying wire perpendicular to page with current going *into* the plane of the page

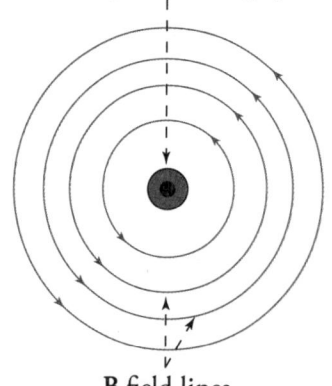

B field lines

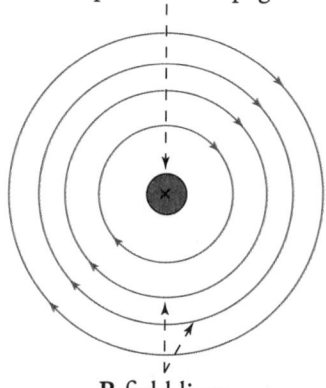

B field lines

---

[6] Though it's uncommon on the MCAT, it's possible you'll be asked about the field produced by a single moving charge, not a current. If the charge is positive you simply use the method given here; if the charge is negative you could use the left-hand rule, or use the right-hand rule and then reverse the direction of the answer; in other words, the field lines created by a negative charge circle in the opposite direction from those created by a positive charge.

In these next two diagrams, the **B**-field circles look like ellipses because of perspective; here the current-carrying wires lie in the plane of the page, and the **B**-field circles are perpendicular to the page, going into (or out of) the page above the wire and out of (or into) the page below the wire.

With the current pointing to the left, the **B** field lines go into the page above the wire . . .

With the current pointing to the right, the **B** field lines come out of the page above the wire . . .

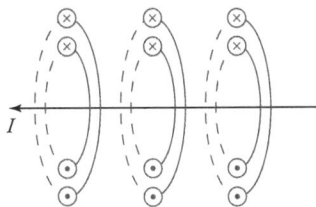

and come out of the page below the wire.

and go into the page below the wire.

The magnitude of the magnetic field created by a straight wire carrying a current I is proportional to I and inversely proportional to the distance r from the wire:

$$B \propto \frac{I}{r}$$

Hence, the magnetic field will be stronger if the current is increased or if we are positioned closer to the wire.

Circular wire loops that carry current also create magnetic fields. In the figure below, notice that the field lines are nearly vertical near the center of the circular wire loop that lies along the central axis. At the center of the loop, the magnitude of **B** is proportional to the current, I, and inversely proportional to the radius of the wire loop ($B \propto I/r_{loop}$). If the current in the wire loop had been traveling in the opposite direction (that is, clockwise), then each of the arrows on the **B**-field lines would point in the opposite direction.

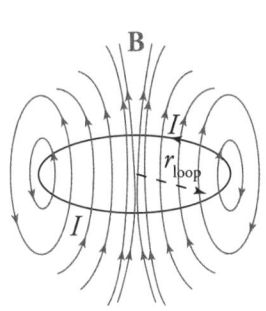

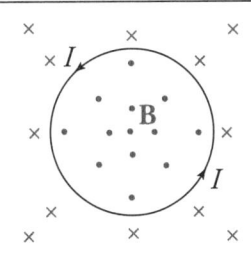

counterclockwise current: **B** field points out of page inside the loop and points into the page outside the loop

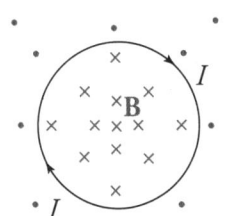

clockwise current: **B** field points into page inside the loop and points out of the page outside the loop

Imagine taking a long wire and wrapping it tightly around a cylinder, like a paper-towel tube. The result will look like a spring; we can also consider it to be like a lot of circular loops close together. Such a helical coil of wire is called a **solenoid**. The magnetic field it produces inside the cylinder is parallel to the central axis and achieves its maximum magnitude *on* the central axis, getting weaker as we move away from the center, closer to the coils:

10.4

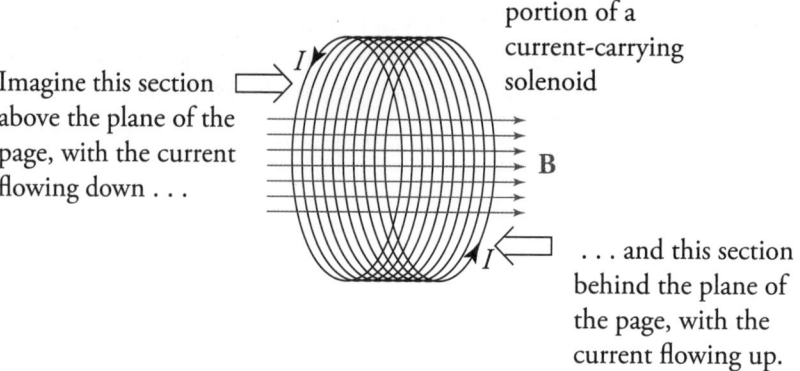

Imagine this section above the plane of the page, with the current flowing down . . .

portion of a current-carrying solenoid

. . . and this section behind the plane of the page, with the current flowing up.

If the solenoid has many windings and if the length is much greater than its diameter, then the magnetic field in the interior is nearly uniform and is proportional to the current (I) and to the number of turns per unit length (N/L): $B \propto I(N/L)$. Hence, the magnetic field will be stronger if the current is increased or if the solenoid wire loops are tightly packed.

Example 10-47: The figure below shows a long straight wire carrying a current, I. An electron is projected above the wire and initially parallel to it.

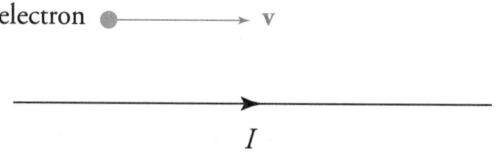

Which of the following best illustrates the direction of the magnetic force on the electron at the position shown?

Solution: Since the current in the wire points to the right, the direction of the magnetic field **B** above the wire is out of the plane of the page. Using the left-hand rule (since the electron is a negative charge),

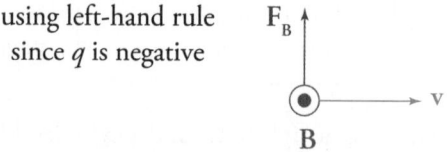

using left-hand rule since q is negative

we find that the direction of the magnetic force $\mathbf{F_B}$ is upward, away from the wire, so choice D is correct.

Example 10-48: The figure below shows two long, straight wires carrying current. The top wire carries a current $I_1 = I$ to the left, while the bottom wire carries a current $I_2 = 2I$ to the right.

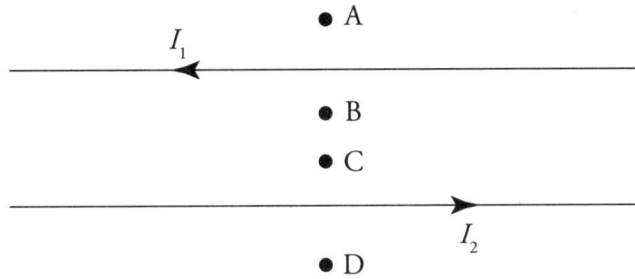

Points A and B are equidistant from the top wire, and Points C and D are equidistant from the bottom wire. Furthermore, the distance between Points B and C is the same as the distance between B and the top wire, which is also the same as the distance between C and the bottom wire. Of these four points, where is the total magnetic field the weakest?

Solution: First, we notice that the magnetic field created by the top wire, $\mathbf{B_1}$, encircles the wire, with the magnetic field circles centered on the top wire and pointing into the plane of the page above the wire and out of the page below it. Similarly, the magnetic field created by the bottom wire, $\mathbf{B_2}$, also encircles the wire, with the magnetic field circles centered on the bottom wire and pointing out of the plane of the page above the wire and into the page below it:

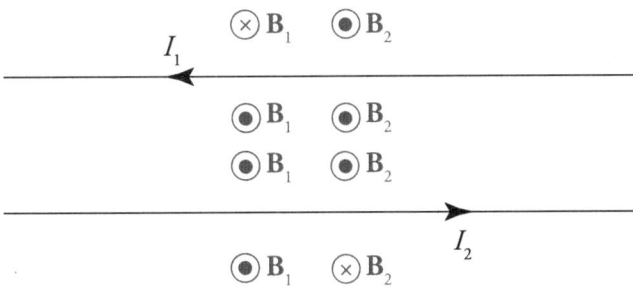

So, we can immediately rule out choices B and C; between the wires, the individual magnetic fields point in the same direction, so their magnitudes add, giving a strong field in this region. However, above the top wire and below the bottom wire, the individual magnetic fields point in opposite directions, so their magnitudes subtract; therefore, of the choices given, the field is weakest at either Point A or Point D. Because $I_2 = 2I$, Point D is closer to the higher-current wire, so to calculate the net **B** field at Point D, we'd subtract a small quantity (the contribution from the weaker-current, which is also farther away) from a large quantity (the contribution from the close higher-current). By contrast, to calculate the net **B** field at Point A, the quantity we'd subtract is larger than the one we subtracted to find the field at Point D and the positive term here is smaller than the positive term in the calculation of the field at Point D. Therefore, we expect the field at Point A to be weaker than at Point D.

If this "intuitive" argument is unconvincing, let's do some math to back it up:

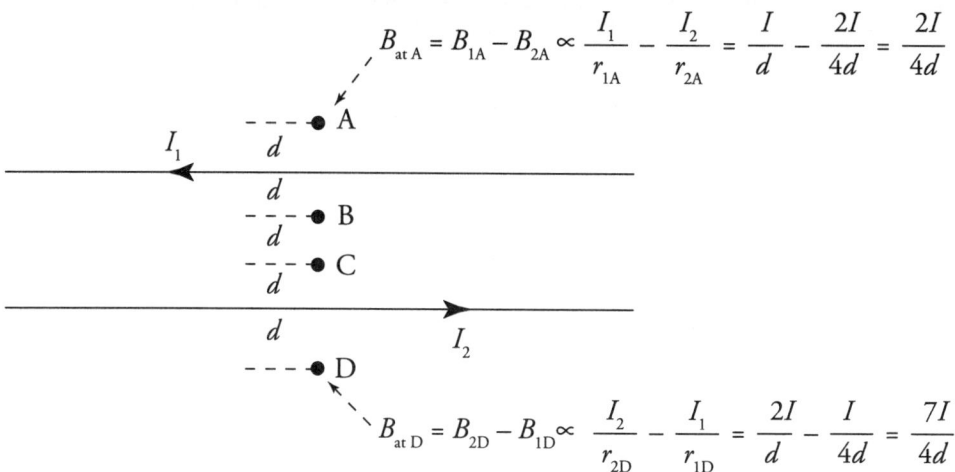

$$B_{at\ A} = B_{1A} - B_{2A} \propto \frac{I_1}{r_{1A}} - \frac{I_2}{r_{2A}} = \frac{I}{d} - \frac{2I}{4d} = \frac{2I}{4d}$$

$$B_{at\ D} = B_{2D} - B_{1D} \propto \frac{I_2}{r_{2D}} - \frac{I_1}{r_{1D}} = \frac{2I}{d} - \frac{I}{4d} = \frac{7I}{4d}$$

Example 10-49: The figure below shows a circular loop of wire in the plane of the page, carrying a current I. A proton is projected with velocity **v**, such that **v** lies in a plane slightly above and parallel to the plane of the loop, as shown:

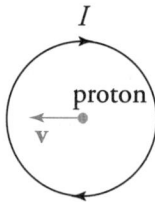

Which of the following best illustrates the direction of the magnetic force on the proton at the position shown?

A. ↑   C. ⊗

B. ⊙   D. ↓

Solution: Since the current in the loop travels clockwise, the direction of the magnetic field **B** above the center of the loop points *into* the plane of the page. Using the right-hand rule (since the proton is a positive charge),

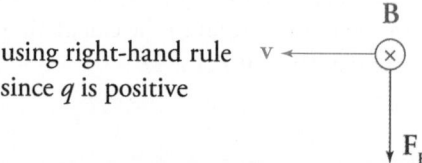

using right-hand rule
since q is positive

we find that the magnetic force $\mathbf{F}_B$ is in the plane above and parallel to the plane of the loop and with a direction as illustrated by choice D.

Example 10-50: The figure below shows a portion of a long narrow solenoid carrying a current, *I*. An alpha particle (α) is projected with velocity **v** down the central axis of the solenoid, as shown:

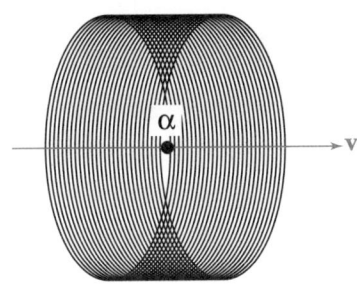

Which of the following best illustrates the direction of the magnetic force on the alpha particle?

A. ↓   C. ↑

B. ⊙   D. None of the above

Solution: At the position of the alpha particle, the magnetic field **B** created by the current-carrying solenoid is directed along the central axis; that is, either in the same direction as **v** or in the opposite direction from **v**, depending on the direction of the current in the wire loops. In either case, though, the magnetic force will be zero. (Remember that if **v** is parallel or anti-parallel to **B**, then $\mathbf{F_B} = 0$.) The answer is D.

Magnets

A permanent bar magnet creates a magnetic field that closely resembles the magnetic field produced by a circular loop of current-carrying wire:

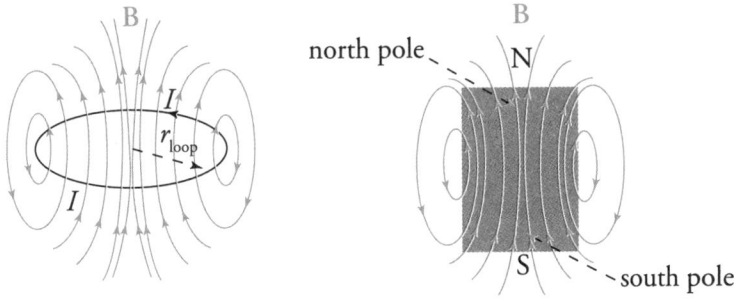

By convention, the magnetic field lines emanate from the end of the magnet designated the **north pole** (**N**) and then curl around and re-enter the magnet at the end designated the **south pole** (**S**). The magnetic field created by a permanent bar magnet is due to the electrons; they have an intrinsic spin (remember the spin quantum number, m_s, from general chemistry) and they orbit their nuclei; therefore, they are charges in motion, the ultimate source of all magnetic fields. If a piece of iron is placed in an external magnetic field (for example, the one created by a current-carrying solenoid) the individual magnetic dipole moments of the electrons will be forced to more or less line up. Because iron is *ferromagnetic*, these now-aligned magnetic dipole moments tend to retain this configuration, thus permanently magnetizing the bar and causing it to produce its own magnetic field.

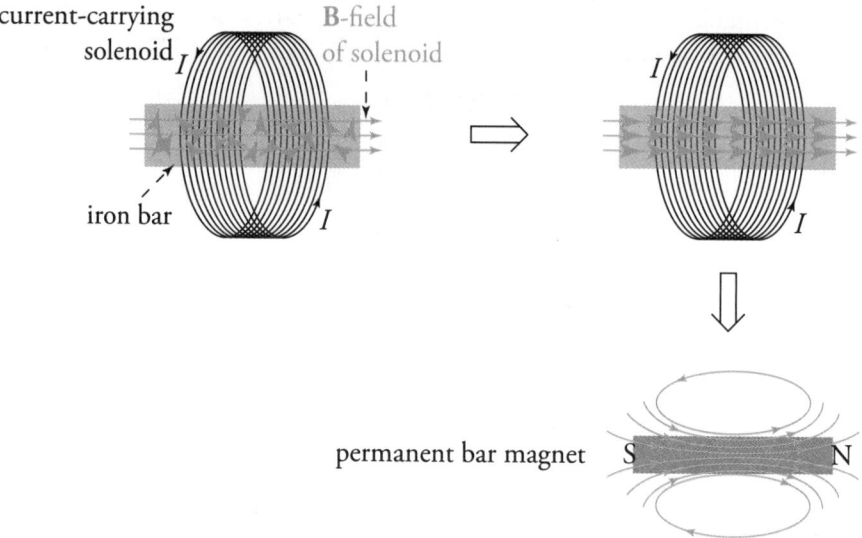

As with electric charges, like magnetic poles repel each other, while opposite magnetic poles attract each other:

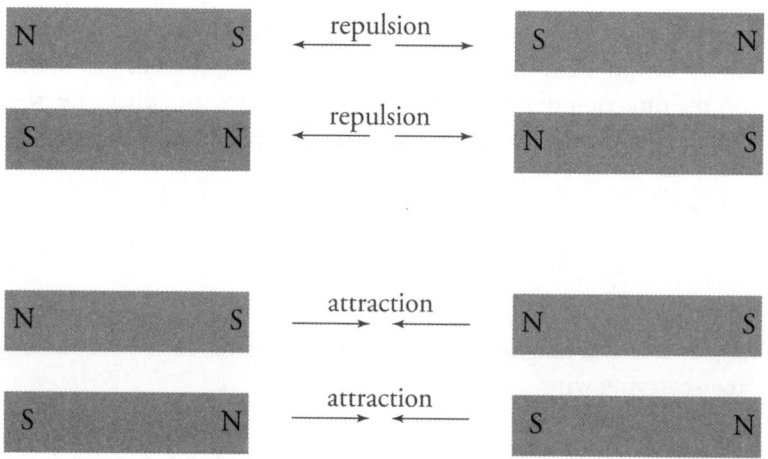

However, while you can have a positive electric charge all by itself, you can't have a single magnetic pole all by itself: the existence of a lone magnetic pole has never been confirmed. That is, there are no magnetic *monopoles*; magnetic poles always exist *in pairs*. If you cut a bar magnet into two pieces, you wouldn't get a piece with just an N and another piece with just an S; you'd get two separate and complete magnets, each with a N–S pair:

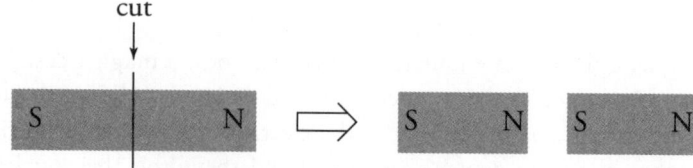

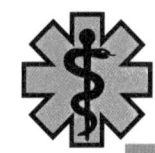

Example 10-51: An MRI scanner functions according to some subtle quantum mechanical principles, but at its most basic, it takes advantage of the fact that spinning protons (namely the two hydrogen nuclei in every water molecule in your body) function as tiny magnets. An extremely powerful, constant external magnetic field $\mathbf{B}_0$ is applied to the body, causing these proton magnets to align. Why? When a magnet is placed in a magnetic field, it tends to align with the field (or, slightly less likely, exactly opposite it), so that the vector from the S pole to the N pole of the magnet is parallel to the field lines.

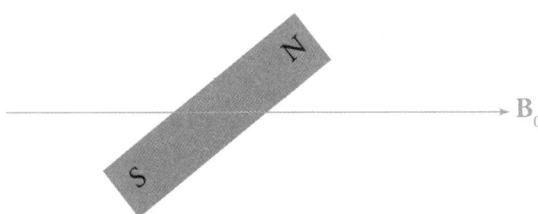

Given that the uniform magnetic field $\mathbf{B}_0$ in the figure above exerts the same magnitude of force on the N pole as it does on the S pole and the magnetic force on a pole is along the field line, what can you say about the net force and net torque on the magnet?

Solution: Because the $\mathbf{B}_0$ field will exert a force $\mathbf{F}_B$ on the N pole and a force of $-\mathbf{F}_B$ on the S pole, the net force on the magnet will be zero ($\mathbf{F}_B + -\mathbf{F}_B = 0$). However, the net torque will not be zero, since the magnetic force produces a clockwise torque on each pole, tending to align the magnet parallel to the field line.

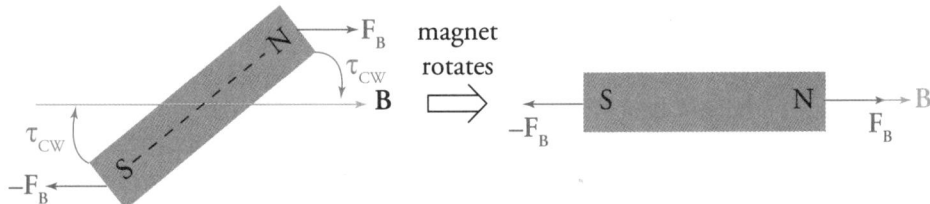

The tiny proton magnets don't actually align statically with the external field, but rather precess around that alignment, the way a teetering spinning top does before it falls over. It is the frequency of this precession that is ultimately utilized to make the protons emit radio waves, which are then detected and translated into images by the MRI machine.

The rotating Earth itself is the source of a (nonuniform) magnetic field, which surrounds the planet and traps electrons and protons emitted by the Sun, making them spiral throughout curved regions called the Van Allen belts. (Protons tend to be confined in Van Allen belts close to Earth's surface, while electrons spiral around in belts farther from the surface. These energetic trapped protons can ionize nitrogen and oxygen in the upper atmosphere, creating cations and electrons. When these cations and electrons recombine, energy is emitted. This is the source of the light that produces the aurora borealis [and, in the southern hemisphere, the aurora australis].) The magnetic poles are *near*, but not *at*, the geographic poles; also notice that it's the magnetic *south* pole that's near the geographic North Pole, and the magnetic *north* pole that's near the geographic South Pole. After all, the magnetic north pole of a compass needle points (roughly) toward geographic north, but we know that it's *opposite* magnetic poles that attract, so the compass needle must be attracted to the magnetic south pole.

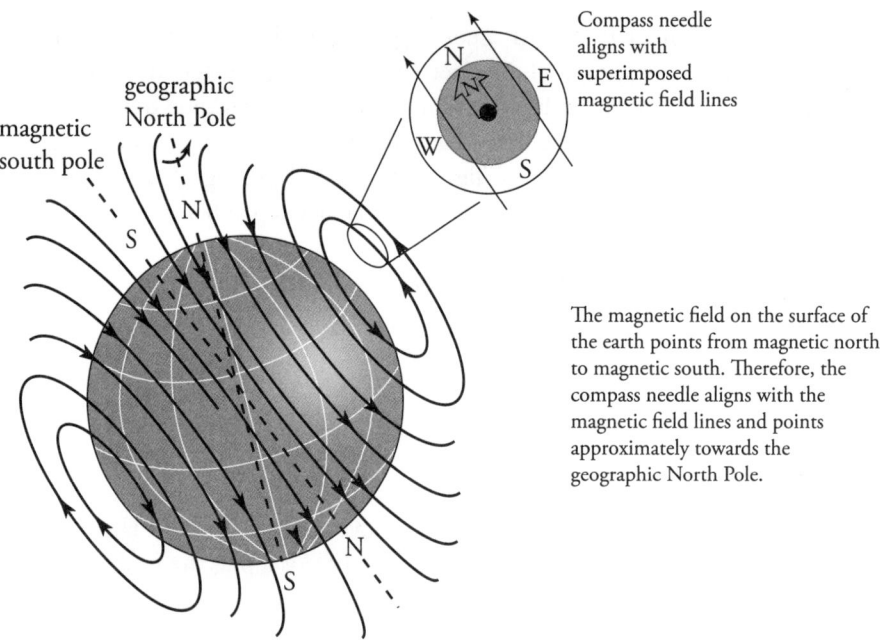

The magnetic field on the surface of the earth points from magnetic north to magnetic south. Therefore, the compass needle aligns with the magnetic field lines and points approximately towards the geographic North Pole.

Example 10-52: The magnitude of Earth's magnetic field is roughly 1 gauss (1 G) at the surface; the **gauss** is a very common (non-SI) unit of magnetic field strength, with 1 G equal to 10^{-4} T. If a proton moving with speed $v = 5 \times 10^6$ m/s in the atmosphere experiences a magnetic field strength of 0.5 G, what force (magnetic or gravitational) has the greater effect? (*Note*: mass of proton ≈ 1.7×10^{-27} kg.)

Solution: The gravitational force on the proton is

$$F_{grav} = mg = (1.7 \times 10^{-27} \text{ kg})(10 \tfrac{\text{N}}{\text{kg}}) = 1.7 \times 10^{-26} \text{ N}$$

The maximum magnetic force on the proton is

$$F_B = qvB = evB = (1.6 \times 10^{-19} \text{ C})(5 \times 10^6 \tfrac{\text{m}}{\text{s}})(0.5 \times 10^{-4} \text{ T}) = 4 \times 10^{-17} \text{ N}$$

Since $F_B \gg F_{grav}$, we see that it's the magnetic force that is chiefly responsible for the proton's motion through Earth's atmosphere.

Example 10-53: Two bar magnets are fixed in position, and a proton is projected with velocity **v** into the region between adjacent opposite poles, as shown below:

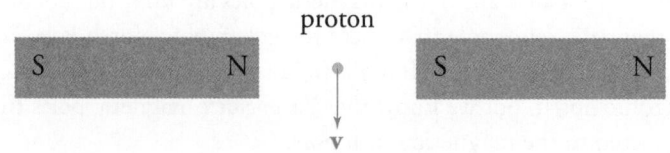

Which of the following best illustrates the direction of the magnetic force on the proton at the position shown?

A. ⟵   C. ⊗

B. ⊙   D. ⟶

Solution: On the outside of the magnet(s), **B** points from the N pole to the S pole.

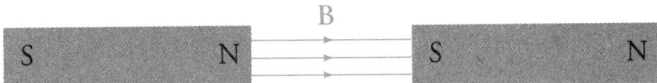

Using the right-hand rule (for a positive charge) where **B** points to the right and **v** is downward, then F_B points out of the plane of the page:

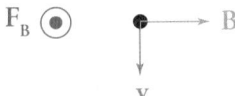

Therefore, the answer is B.

Example 10-54: The following figure shows an electromagnet with an iron core. Since iron is ferromagnetic, the magnetic field created by the current-carrying coil aligns the magnetic dipole moments of electrons in the iron, creating a magnetic field throughout the iron.

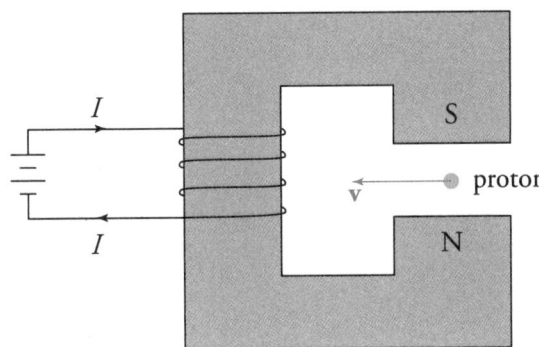

If a proton is projected with velocity **v** between the poles as shown, which of the following best illustrates the direction of the magnetic force on the proton at the position shown?

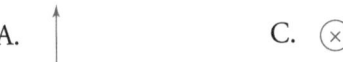

A. ↑   C. ⊗

B. ⊙   D. ↓

Solution: Because outside the magnet the B field always points from the N pole to the S pole, the direction of the **B** field at the position of the proton is upward:

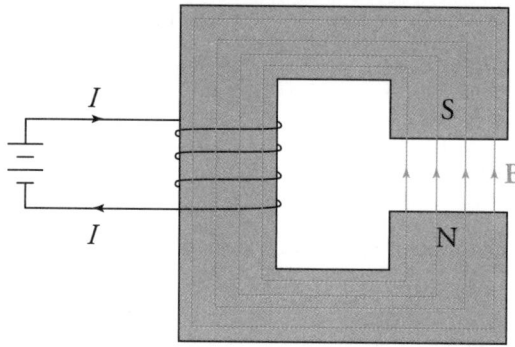

The right-hand rule (for a positive charge) tells us that if **B** points upward and **v** is directed to the left, then **F**$_B$ points into the plane of the page:

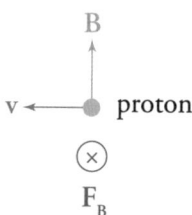

Therefore, the answer is C.

Summary Of Formulas

CIRCUITS

Current: $I = \dfrac{Q}{t}$

- in the direction of "flow of positive charge"

- actual flow of electrons is in the opposite direction

Resistance: $R = \rho \dfrac{L}{A}$ [ρ = resistivity, not density]

Ohm's law: $V = IR$ [where R is constant as V varies]

Resistors in series: $R_{eq} = R_1 + R_2 + \ldots$

Resistors in parallel: $\dfrac{1}{R_{eq}} = \dfrac{1}{R_1} + \dfrac{1}{R_2} + \ldots$ or $R_{eq} = \dfrac{R_1 R_2}{R_1 + R_2}$ [two at a time]

Current is the same for resistors in series; voltage is the same for resistors in parallel.

Kirchhoff's Rules:

- The sum of the voltage-drops across the resistors in any complete path is equal to the voltage of the battery.

- The amount of current entering a parallel combination of resistors is equal to the sum of the currents that pass through the individual resistors.

Power of circuit element: $P = IV = I^2 R = \dfrac{V^2}{R}$

Total power supplied by a battery equals the total power dissipated by the resistors.

The ground is at potential zero [potential = 0].

Root-mean-square quantities for AC circuit:

$$V_{rms} = \frac{V_{max}}{\sqrt{2}}, \quad I_{rms} = \frac{I_{max}}{\sqrt{2}}$$

Average power of circuit element in AC circuit:

$$\overline{P} = \left(I_{rms}\right)^2 R = I_{rms}V_{rms}$$

PARALLEL PLATE CAPACITORS

Charge on a capacitor: $Q = CV$

- The capacitance does not depend on voltage or charge. It is determined by the formula below.

Capacitance:

no dielectric: $C = \varepsilon_0 \dfrac{A}{d}$

with dielectric: $C_{with\ dielectric} = KC_{without\ dielectric} = K\varepsilon_0 \dfrac{A}{d}$ [K = dielectric constant]

- Inserting a dielectric always increases the capacitance. If the battery remains attached, V is constant; if the battery is taken away Q is constant.

Electric field in parallel-plate capacitor:

$$V = Ed$$

Stored potential energy in capacitor:

$$PE = \frac{1}{2}QV = \frac{1}{2}CV^2 = \frac{Q^2}{2C}$$

- The work done by the battery to charge the capacitor = PE.

Capacitors in series: $\dfrac{1}{C_{eq}} = \dfrac{1}{C_1} + \dfrac{1}{C_2} + \ldots$ or $C_{eq} = \dfrac{C_1 C_2}{C_1 + C_2}$ [two at a time]

Capacitors in parallel: $C_{eq} = C_1 + C_2 + \ldots$

MAGNETIC FORCE AND FIELD

Magnetic force on moving charge q:

$$\mathbf{F}_B - q(\mathbf{v} \times \mathbf{B})$$

$$F_B = |q| vB \sin\theta \quad (\theta = \text{angle between } \mathbf{v} \text{ and } \mathbf{B})$$

Direction of $\mathbf{F}_B$: use right-hand rule if q is positive; use left-hand rule if q is negative (or use right-hand rule and reverse the answer)

 $\mathbf{F}_B$ is always perpendicular to both $\mathbf{v}$ and $\mathbf{B}$

 $\mathbf{B}$ created by long, straight current-carrying wire: $B \propto I / r$

 $\mathbf{B}$ created by a solenoid: $B \propto I \dfrac{N}{L}$ (L = length of solenoid, N = number of coils)

The magnetic force never changes the speed of a particle, and does NO work on the particle.

 Magnetic field lines created by a magnet will point north to south.

The north pole of a magnet wants to line up with the direction of an external magnetic field; the south pole wants to line up opposite the field.

CHAPTER 10 FREESTANDING PRACTICE QUESTIONS

1. A helium nucleus traveling at speed v feels a magnetic force of magnitude F_B due to a solenoid that produces a magnetic field. If the number of turns per unit length in the solenoid is doubled while the current is kept constant, what is the magnitude of the force that the helium nucleus feels if it is traveling with the same speed in the same direction?

A) $0.5F_B$
B) $1F_B$
C) $2F_B$
D) $4F_B$

2. Capacitor C_1 has a capacitance of 5 F and holds an initial charge $Q_{1,i} = 40$ C. Capacitor C_2 has a capacitance of 15 F and holds an initial charge $Q_{2,i} = 60$ C. The two capacitors are in a circuit with an open switch S between them, as shown in the figure below. When the switch closes, the charges on the capacitors will redistribute. What is the quantity of charge, $Q_{1,f}$ and $Q_{2,f}$, on each capacitor a long time after the switch closes?

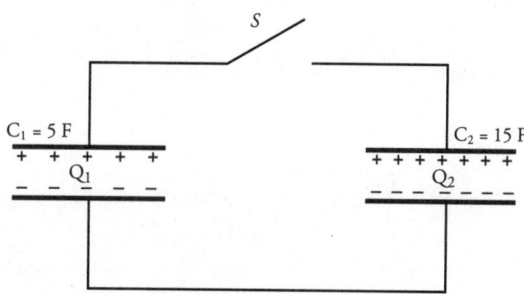

A) $Q_{1,f} = 25$ C, $Q_{2,f} = 75$ C
B) $Q_{1,f} = 75$ C, $Q_{2,f} = 25$ C
C) $Q_{1,f} = 50$ C, $Q_{2,f} = 50$ C
D) $Q_{1,f} = 40$ C, $Q_{2,f} = 60$ C

3. An air capacitor stores potential energy. If you wanted the potential energy to double by adding a dielectric between the plates while keeping the voltage constant, what would have to be the value of the dielectric constant?

A) 0.5
B) 2
C) 4
D) 8

4. Determine the total power dissipated through the circuit shown below in terms of V, R_1, R_2, and R_3.

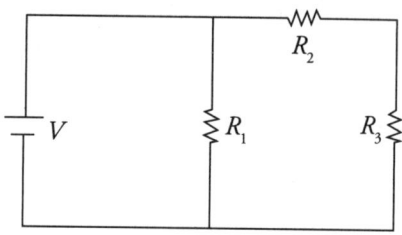

A) $\dfrac{V^2}{R_1 + R_2 + R_3}$

B) $\dfrac{R_1 + R_2 + R_3}{V^2}$

C) $\dfrac{R_1(R_2 + R_3)}{V^2(R_1 + R_2 + R_3)}$

D) $\dfrac{V^2(R_1 + R_2 + R_3)}{R_1(R_2 + R_3)}$

5. Lightning is an atmospheric discharge of electricity that can propagate at speeds of up to 60,000 m/s and can reach temperatures of up to 30,000°C. A single lightning strike lasts for approximately 250 ms and can transfer up to 500 MJ of energy across a potential difference of 2×10^7 volts. Estimate the total amount of charge transferred and average current of a single lightning strike.

A) 6.25×10^{-4} coulombs, 8×10^7 amps
B) 6.25×10^{-4} coulombs, 2.5×10^{-3} amps
C) 25 coulombs, 100 amps
D) 25 coulombs, 8×10^7 amps

6. Which of the following changes will increase the resistance of a closed circuit system?

    I. Replacing the wire with one made of the same metal that has a smaller cross sectional area

    II. Placing a voltmeter in series with the rest of the circuit

    III. Doubling the wire length in the closed circuit

A) III only
B) I and III only
C) II and III only
D) I, II and III

7. If the resistance of a wire in a household appliance becomes 4 times its original value, which of the following statements is/are correct?

    I. The voltage of the wire becomes quadrupled.
    II. The current through the wire becomes 1/4th the original value.
    III. The power consumed by the appliance becomes quadrupled.

A) I only
B) II only
C) I and III only
D) II and III only

CHAPTER 10 PRACTICE PASSAGE

A current-carrying wire will generate a magnetic field around the wire that varies with current in the wire, i, and the distance from the wire, r. The strength of the magnetic field generated can be calculated using the equation

$$B = \mu_0 i / 2\pi r$$

Equation 1

where B is the magnitude of the magnetic field generated and μ_0 is a constant known as the permeability of free space. The direction of the magnetic field generated will always be circular around the wire.

A physics student is conducting an experiment to test the effects on charged particles of the magnetic field created by wires. Two long wires are stretched parallel to each other a distance 20 cm apart. Each wire is connected to a voltage source and a grounded point so that a current will flow through the wire. Three separate test paths are established and marked in Figure 1. The wires are fixed in place, so any forces experienced by the wires will not cause them to move.

The charged particle used in the experiment is a lightweight (mass, m) negatively charged (charge, $-q$) metal marble. For each experiment, the marble is injected along the test path with a constant initial velocity, v, which is parallel to the wires. The magnetic field created by the wires exerts a magnetic force on the marble, causing the velocity to change direction from the initial velocity direction. Because the marble rolls without slipping, frictional effects are assumed to be negligible.

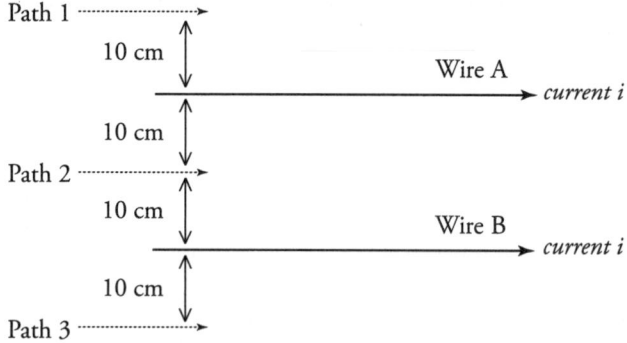

Figure 1 Complete setup for Trial 1 with the three test paths marked

In the first trial of the experiment, the student has the same voltage drop across both wires and the current, i, in both wires is going from left to right, as shown in Figure 1. The metal marble was injected along each test path, and its initial change in direction recorded in Table 1. In the second trial of the experiment, the current in Wire A remained the same, but the current in Wire B was doubled. Again, the metal marble was injected along each test path, and its initial change in direction recorded in Table 1.

Table 1

Trial	Test Path	Initial Change in Direction of Marble
1	1	Up, away from Wire A ($\uparrow$)
1	2	No change in direction, marble passes straight along path 2 ($\rightarrow$)
1	3	Down, away from Wire B ($\downarrow$)
2	1	Up, away from Wire A ($\uparrow$)
2	2	Up, toward Wire A and away from Wire B ($\uparrow$)
2	3	Down, away from Wire B ($\downarrow$)

1. Which of the following best explains why the marble on Path 2 did not change direction in Trial 1 of the experiment?

A) The net magnetic force acting on the marble was zero because the net magnetic field was zero along Path 2 since the magnetic field created from Wire A was equal in magnitude and opposite in direction from the magnetic field created from Wire B.

B) The net magnetic force acting on the marble was zero because the magnetic fields created by the two wires along Path 2 resulted in forces that were an action-reaction pair.

C) The net magnetic force acting on the marble was not zero, but the magnetic fields created by the two wires resulted in forces on the marble that were parallel to the wires and kept the marble on Path 2.

D) The net magnetic force acting on the marble was not zero because the marble increased velocity as it traveled on Path 2.

2. What is the magnitude and direction of the magnetic field on Path 2 in Trial 2 if $i = 6$ A?

A) magnitude is 30 μ_0/π direction is into the page
B) magnitude is 30 μ_0/π direction is out of the page
C) magnitude is 60 μ_0/π direction is into the page
D) magnitude is 60 μ_0/π direction is out of the page

3. How much work is done by the magnetic force on the marble on Path 3 in Trial 2 in terms of the variables given in the passage?

A) $qv\mu_0 i/2\pi$
B) $qv\mu_0 i/2\pi r$
C) $qv\mu_0 ir/2\pi$
D) 0

4. Assuming the same voltage drop is used for both trials of the experiment, how might the student double the current in Wire B in Trial 2?

A) Increase the resistance by a factor of 2
B) Decrease the resistance by a factor of 2
C) Increase the resistance by a factor of 4
D) Decrease the resistance by a factor of 4

5. Which of the following best describes the negative charge on the metal marble?

A) The negative charge means the electric field inside the marble points in, toward the center of the marble.
B) The negative charge means the electric field inside the marble points out, away from the center of the marble.
C) There is no electric field inside the marble since the negative charge is spread evenly on the surface of the marble.
D) There is no electric field inside the marble since conductors absorb charge and neutralize it.

6. The student wanted to conduct a Trial 3 of the experiment where the current in Wire A is the same as in Trial 1, and the current in Wire B is the same magnitude as Wire A but in the opposite direction. Predict the results of Trial 3 of the experiment.

   I. The initial change in direction of the marble on Path 1 is up, away from Wire A (↑)
   II. The initial change in direction of the marble on Path 2 is no change in direction (→)
   III. The initial change in direction of the marble on Path 3 is up, toward Wire B (↑)

A) I only
B) I and II only
C) I and III only
D) I, II, and III

SOLUTIONS TO CHAPTER 10 FREESTANDING QUESTIONS

1. **C** The magnetic field generated by a solenoid is proportional to IN/L, so doubling the number of turns per unit length will double the magnetic field. The magnitude of the force in a magnetic field is proportional to the magnetic field strength, therefore it will double if the magnetic field strength doubles.

2. **A** The sum of the charges, Q_{tot}, on the two capacitors is 100 C. After Switch S is closed, capacitors C_1 and C_2 are connected together and must have the same terminal voltage V. Q_{tot} remains 100 C. After a long time, the charge has become redistributed between the two capacitors. If the final charge on C_1 is $Q_{1,f}$, then the final charge on C_2 is $Q_{2,f} = Q_{tot} - Q_{1,f}$. Therefore $V = Q_{1,f}/C_1 = Q_{2,f}/C_2 = (Q_{tot} - Q_{1,f})/C_2$. Solving for $Q_{1,f}$ gives $Q_{1,f} = Q_{tot}/4 = 25$ C and $Q_{2,f} = 75$ C.

3. **B** The potential energy is equal to $1/2\ QV = 1/2\ (CV)V$. When you add a dielectric, the capacitance gets multiplied by the dielectric constant K, giving $1/2\ KCV^2$. Therefore, in order to increase the potential energy by a factor of 2, K must be 2 if V is to stay constant.

4. **D** Power can be expressed as $P = V^2/R$. Therefore, begin by determining total resistance of the circuit, R_{TOT}. In this circuit, R_2 and R_3 are connected in series, and are connected in parallel to R_1. R_2 and R_3 can be reduced to $R_{EQ} = R_2 + R_3$. This equivalent resistor connects in parallel to R_1, and can be further reduced to $R_{TOT} = R_1\ (R_2 + R_3)/(R_1 + R_2 + R_3)$. Use this equation for total resistance in the equation for power to yield $P = V^2/R_{TOT}$, or choice D.

5. **C** Change in electrical potential energy is given by the equation $\Delta PE = qV$. The problem states that there is an energy transfer of 500 megajoules across a potential difference of 20 megavolts. Solving for q yields a charge transfer of 500 MJ / 20 MV, or 25 coulombs. The problem states that the time over which the charge is transferred is 250 msec, or 0.25 seconds. Using the equation $I = Q/t$, the average current can be calculated as 25 coulombs / 0.25 seconds, or 100 amps.

6. **D** Item I is correct because the electrical resistance of a metal wire is inversely proportional to its cross sectional area (choices A and C can be eliminated). Note that since both remaining choices include Item III, Item III must be correct and we only need to evaluate Item II. Item II is also correct. The internal resistance of a voltmeter is very high, and thus adding a voltmeter will increase the resistance of the whole system (choice B can be eliminated and choice D is correct). Item III is in fact correct. According to the formula $R = \rho L/A$, the resistance of the wire is directly proportional to its length L. Therefore, as the length of the wire increases, so does the overall resistance of the system.

7. **B** Item I is false. The voltage is the electromotive force that drives the current through the wire. Therefore, it remains constant and unaffected by the increase in resistance (choices A and C can be eliminated). Note that the remaining choices both include Item II so Item II must be true: according to the equation $V = IR$, when V is constant, the current I is inversely proportional to the resistance R. Item III is false. The power P is expressed by the equation $P = IV$, where I is the current through the wire and V is the voltage that drives the current. Since V stays constant, and I becomes 1/4 of the original value, the power P would be $1/4\ I \times V = 1/4\ IV$, which is 1/4 the original power output (choice D is wrong and choice B is correct).

SOLUTIONS TO CHAPTER 10 PRACTICE PASSAGE

1. **A** In Trial 1 along Path 2, the magnitude of each magnetic field can be calculated using Equation 1. Since the current is the same in each wire, and along Path 2 the distance from each wire is the same, the magnitude of the magnetic field created by each wire is the same. The direction of the magnetic field created by the wires can be found by using the right hand rule. Pointing the thumb of the right hand in the direction of the current (to the right) and curling the fingers around the wire shows the direction of the magnetic field created. Along Path 2, Wire A creates a magnetic field that is into the page. The magnetic field created by Wire B along Path 2 is out of the page. So the magnetic field created by Wire A is equal in magnitude and opposite in direction from the magnetic field created by Wire B, and the net magnetic field along Path 2 is zero. The magnetic force, F, exerted by a magnetic field, B, on a particle moving with velocity, v, and charge q, is calculated as $F = |q|vB \sin \theta$ where θ is the angle between v and B. Since $B = 0$ along Path 2, then $F = 0$. By Newton's second law, $F = ma$ where a is the acceleration. Since $F = 0$ then $a = 0$ and the velocity is constant in both magnitude and direction. Choices C and D are incorrect, since the net force on the marble is zero. Choice B is incorrect because there is no action-reaction pair since all forces are acting on the same object. The correct answer is choice A.

2. **B** In Trial 2 along Path 2, the magnitude of each magnetic field can be calculated using Equation 1. The magnetic field created by Wire A is $\mu_0 i/2\pi r = \mu_0 6/2\pi (0.1) = 30 \mu_0/\pi$ and the magnetic field created by Wire B is $\mu_0 i/2\pi r = \mu_0 6(2)/2\pi (0.1) = 60 \mu_0/\pi$. The direction of the magnetic field created by the wires can be found by using the right hand rule. Pointing the thumb of the right hand in the direction of the current (to the right) and curling the fingers around the wire shows the direction of the magnetic field created. Along Path 2, Wire A creates a magnetic field that is into the page. The magnetic field created by Wire B along Path 2 is out of the page. Since the magnetic fields created by each wire are in opposite directions, the net field is in the direction of the field with the larger magnitude. The field created by Wire B has the larger magnitude, so the net field is out of the page. This eliminates choices A and C. The magnitude of the net field is the difference in the two magnitudes. So $60 \mu_0/\pi - 30 \mu_0/\pi = 30 \mu_0/\pi$. The correct answer is choice B.

3. **D** The work done by magnetic forces is always zero. The magnetic force on an object is always perpendicular to the velocity of the object. The work done is always calculated by multiplying the force times the distance traveled times the cosine of the angle between them. Since the angle between the force and the distance will always be 90°, then $\cos 90° = 0$, and the work will always be zero. The correct answer is choice D.

4. **B** The current in a wire can be calculated using $V = IR$ where V is the voltage, I is the current, and R is the resistance. Since the voltage is constant in this case, then the resistance needs to be decreased in order to increase the current. This eliminates choices A and C. In order to increase current by a factor of 2, then the resistance needs to be decreased by a factor of 2. The correct answer is choice B.

5.　**C**　The metal marble is a spherical conductor, and the excess charge will be distributed evenly around the surface of the marble. (Since the metal is a conductor, the charges are free to move. Since the individual negative charges oppose each other, they move to be as far from each other as possible.) With the charges distributed evenly on the surface of the sphere, there is no electric field inside the sphere, eliminating choices A and B. Choice D is false. The correct answer is choice C.

6.　**C**　The direction of the magnetic field created from Wire A is found using the right hand rule: the direction of the magnetic field created by Wire A is out of the page on Path 1, and into the page on Path 2 and Path 3. The direction of the magnetic field created from Wire B is also found using the right hand rule: the direction of the magnetic field created by Wire B is into the page on Path 1 and Path 2, and out of the page on Path 3. On both Path 1 and Path 3, the magnetic fields generated by each wire are in opposite directions from each other, so the net magnetic field direction is determined by the magnetic field with the largest magnitude. Since current is the same in both wires, then, using Equation 1, the magnetic field magnitude is largest where the distance from the wire is least. For Path 1, the magnetic field created from Wire A will have the least distance and so the largest magnitude, therefore the net magnetic field will be out of the page. For Path 3, the magnetic field created from Wire B will have the least distance and so the largest magnitude, therefore the net magnetic field will be out of the page. This information is summarized below.

Path	Direction of Magnetic Field Created by Wire A	Direction of Magnetic Field Created by Wire B	Direction of Net Magnetic Field
1	Out of Page	Into Page	Out of Page
2	Into Page	Into Page	Into Page
3	Into Page	Out of Page	Out of Page

The direction of the magnetic force from the magnetic field on the moving negatively charged marble can be found using the left hand rule (remember e"left"ron so negative charges use the left hand). For Path 1 and Path 3, the magnetic field is out of the page, so the force is up (↑). So Items I and III are correct. This eliminates choices A and B. For Path 2, the magnetic field is into the page, so the force is down (↓), and Item II is not correct. This eliminates choice D. The correct answer is choice C.

BIOMECHANICAL ENERGY HARVESTING: GENERATING ELECTRICITY DURING WALKING WITH MINIMAL USER EFFORT

J. M. Donelan, Q. Li, V. Naing, J. A. Hoffer, D. J. Weber, A. D. Kuo

Abstract

We have developed a biomechanical energy harvester that generates electricity during human walking with little extra effort. Unlike conventional human-powered generators that use positive muscle work, our technology assists muscles in performing negative work, analogous to regenerative braking in hybrid cars, where energy normally dissipated during braking drives a generator instead. The energy harvester mounts at the knee and selectively engages power generation at the end of the swing phase, thus assisting deceleration of the joint. Test subjects walking with one device on each leg produced an average of 5 watts of electricity, which is about 10 times that of shoe-mounted devices. The cost of harvesting—the additional metabolic power required to produce 1 watt of electricity—is less than one-eighth of that for conventional human power generation. Producing substantial electricity with little extra effort makes this method well-suited for charging powered prosthetic limbs and other portable medical devices.

Humans are a rich source of energy. An average-sized person stores as much energy in fat as a 1000-kg battery. People use muscle to convert this stored chemical energy into positive mechanical work with peak efficiencies of about 25%. This work can be performed at a high rate, with 100 W easily sustainable. Many devices take advantage of human power capacity to produce electricity, including hand-crank generators as well as wind-up flashlights, radios, and mobile phone chargers. A limitation of these conventional methods is that users must focus their attention on power generation at the expense of other activities, typically resulting in short bouts of generation. For electrical power generation over longer durations, it would be desirable to harvest energy from everyday activities such as walking.

It is a challenge, however, to produce substantial electricity from walking. Most energy harvesting research has focused on generating electricity from the compression of the shoe sole, with the best devices generating 0.8 W. A noteworthy departure is a spring-loaded backpack that harnesses the vertical oscillations of a 38-kg load to generate as much as 7.4 W of electricity during fast walking. This device has a markedly low "cost of harvesting" (COH), a dimensionless quantity defined as the additional metabolic power in watts required to generate 1 W of electrical power

$$COH = \frac{\Delta \text{ metabolic power}}{\Delta \text{ electric power}} \qquad (1)$$

where Δ refers to the difference between walking while harvesting energy and walking while carrying the device but without harvesting energy. The COH for conventional power generation is simply related to the efficiency with which (i) the device converts mechanical work to electricity and (ii) muscles convert chemical energy into positive work

$$\text{COH for conventional generation} = \frac{\Delta \text{ metabolic power}}{\Delta \text{ electric power}}$$

$$= \frac{1}{\text{device eff} \times \text{muscle eff}} \qquad (2)$$

The backpack's device efficiency is about 31%, and muscle's peak efficiency is about 25%, yielding an expected COH of 12.9. But the backpack's actual COH of 4.8 ± 3.0 (mean $\pm$ SD) is less than 40% of the expected amount. Its economy appears to arise from reducing the energy expenditure of walking with loads. No device has yet approached the power generation of the backpack without the need to carry a heavy load.

We propose that a key feature of how humans walk may provide another means of economical energy harvesting. Muscles cyclically perform positive and negative mechanical work within each stride (Fig. 1A). Mechanical work is required to redirect the body's center of mass between steps and simply to move the legs back and forth. Even though the average mechanical work performed on the body over an entire stride is zero, walking exacts a metabolic cost because both positive and negative muscle work require metabolic energy. Coupling a generator to leg motion would generate electricity throughout each cycle, increasing the load on the muscles during acceleration but assisting them during deceleration (Fig. 1B). Although generating electricity during the acceleration phase would exact substantial metabolic cost, doing so during the deceleration phase would not, resulting in a lower COH than for conventional generation. An even lower COH could be achieved by selectively engaging the generator only during deceleration (Fig. 1C), similar to how regenerative braking generates power while decelerating a hybrid car. Here, "generative braking" produces electricity without requiring additional positive muscle power. If implemented effectively, metabolic cost could be about the same as that for normal walking, so energy would be harvested with no extra user effort.

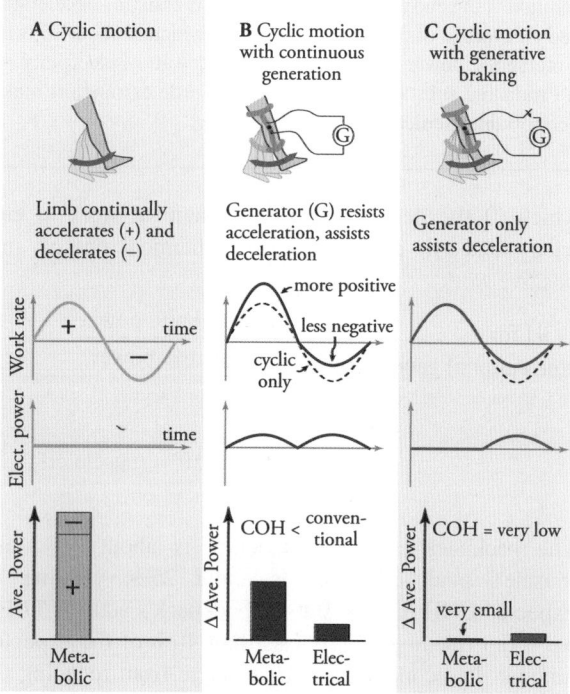

Figure 1. Theoretical advantages of generative braking during cyclic motion, comparing the back-and-forth motion of the knee joint without power generation (A) against a generator operating continuously (B) and against a generator operating only during braking (C). Each column of plots shows the rate of work performed by muscles (work rate) and the electricity (elect. power) generated over time, as well as the average metabolic power expended by the human and the resulting average electrical power (ave. power bar graphs). In (B) and (C), work rate is compared against that for (A), denoted by dashed lines, and average power is shown as the difference (Δ ave. power) with respect to (A). COH is defined as the ratio of the electrical to metabolic Δ ave. powers.

We developed a wearable, knee-mounted prototype energy harvester to test the generative-braking concept (Fig. 2). Although other joints might suffice, we focused on the knee because it performs mostly negative work during walking. The harvester comprises an orthopedic knee brace configured so that knee motion drives a gear train through a one-way clutch, transmitting only knee extension motion at speeds suitable for a debrushless motor that serves as the generator. For convenient testing, generated electrical power is then dissipated with a load resistor rather than being used to charge a battery. The device efficiency, defined as the ratio of the electrical power output to the mechanical power input, was empirically estimated to be no greater than 63%, yielding an estimated COH for conventional generation of 6.4 (Eq. 2). A potentiometer senses knee angle, which is fed back to a computer controlling a relay switch in series with the load resistor, allowing the electrical load to be selectively disconnected in real time. For generative braking, we programmed the harvester to engage only during the end of the swing phase (Fig. 3), producing electrical power while simultaneously assisting the knee flexor muscles in decelerating the knee. We compared this mode against a continuous-generation mode that harvests energy whenever the knee is extending. We could also manually disengage the clutch and completely decouple the gear train and generator from knee motion. This disengaged mode served as a control condition to estimate the metabolic cost of carrying the harvester mass, independent of the cost of generating electricity.

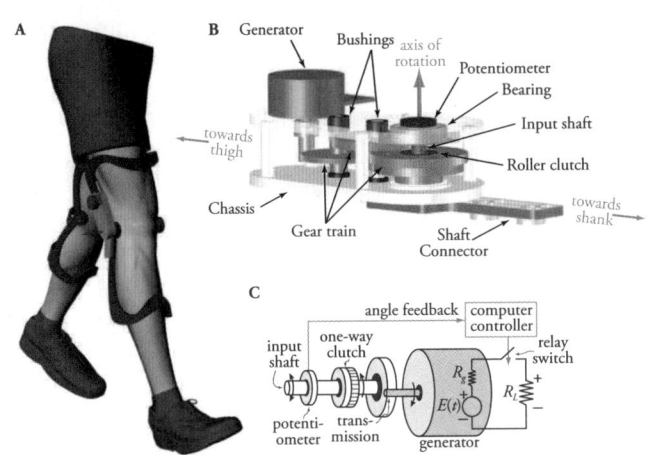

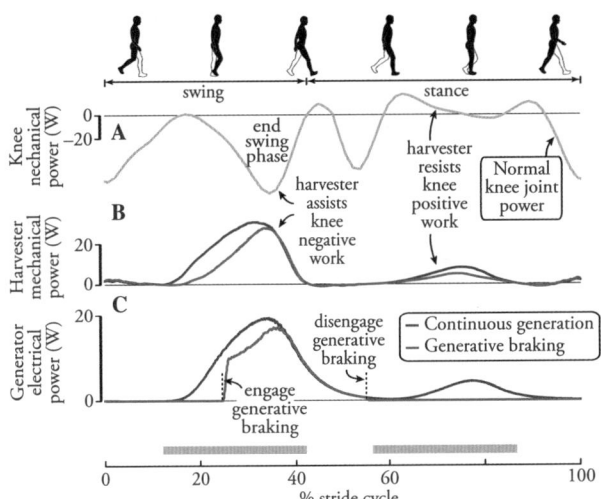

Figure 2. Biomechanical energy harvester. (A) The device has an aluminum chassis (green) and generator (blue) mounted on a customized orthopedic knee brace (red), totaling 1.6-kg mass, with one worn on each leg. (B) The chassis contains a gear train that converts low velocity and high torque at the knee into high velocity and low torque for the generator, with a one-way roller clutch that allows for selective engagement of the gear train during knee extension only and no engagement during knee flexion. (C) The schematic diagram shows how a computer-controlled feedback system determines when to generate power using knee-angle feedback, measured with a potentiometer mounted on the input shaft. Generated power is dissipated in resistors. R_g, generator internal resistance; R_L, output load resistance; $E(t)$, generated voltage.

Figure 3. Timing of power generation during walking. Time within a stride cycle, beginning with the swing phase, is shown at the bottom. The shaded bars indicate when the knee is extending and the energy harvester's clutch is engaged. (A) The pattern of knee mechanical power during normal walking illustrates that the knee typically generates a large amount of negative power at the end of the swing phase. (B) Mechanical power performed on the harvester over time, shown for continuous generation (red line) and generative braking (blue line). (C) Generated electrical power over time, also for both types of generation.

Energy-harvesting performance was tested on six male subjects who wore a device on each leg while walking on a treadmill at 1.5 m s⁻¹. We estimated metabolic cost using a standard respirometry system and measured the electrical power output of the generator (Fig. 3C). In the continuous-generation mode (Fig. 4A), subjects generated 7.0 ± 0.7 W of electricity with an insignificant 18 ± 24 W ($P = 0.07$) increase in metabolic cost over that of the control condition. In the generative-braking mode (Fig. 4B), subjects generated 4.8 ± 0.8 W of electricity with an insignificant 5 ± 21 W increase in metabolic cost as compared with that of the control condition ($P = 0.6$). For context, this electricity is sufficient to power 10 typical cell phones simultaneously. The results demonstrate that substantial electricity could be generated with minimal increase in user effort.

The corresponding COH values highlight the advantage of generative braking (Fig. 4). Average COH in generative braking was only 0.7 ± 4.4; less than 1 W of metabolic power was required to generate 1 W of electricity. This is significantly less than the COH of 6.4 expected for conventional generation ($P = 0.01$). The COH in continuous generation, 2.3 ± 3.0, was also significantly lower than that for conventional generation ($P = 0.01$), indicating that the former mode also generated some of its electricity from the deceleration of the knee. The difference between the two modes, 2.2 ± 0.7 W of electricity, came at a difference in metabolic cost of 13 ± 12 W ($P = 0.05$). A COH taken from the average ratio of these differences yields 5.7 ± 6.2, which is nearly the same as that expected of conventional generation ($P = 0.4$). This indicates that continuous generation of power at the knee during walking produces electricity partially by conventional generation with a high COH and partially by generative braking with a very low COH. But generative braking, with less than one-eighth the COH of conventional generation, benefits almost entirely from the deceleration of the knee.

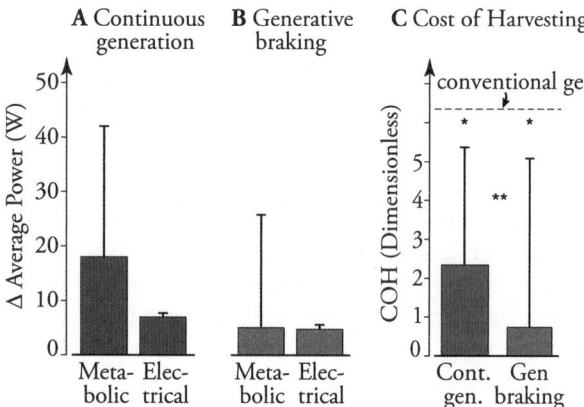

Figure 4. Average metabolic cost and generated electricity for continuous generation (A) and generative braking (B), with change in metabolic cost (Δ average power) shown relative to the control condition. (C) COH (see Fig. 1) for continuous generation and generative braking as compared against that for conventional generation (dashed line). In both modes, a fraction of the harvested energy is generated from the deceleration of the knee rather than directly from muscle action. Error bars in (A) to (C) indicate SD. Asterisks indicate significant differences with conventional generation (*) and between continuous generation and generative braking (**) ($P < 0.05$ for all comparisons).

This preliminary demonstration could be improved substantially. We constructed the prototype for convenient experimentation, leading to a control condition about 20% more metabolically costly than normal walking: The disengaged-clutch mode required an average metabolic power of 366 ± 63 W as compared with 307 ± 64 W for walking without wearing the devices. The increase in cost is due mainly to the additional mass and its location, because the lower a given mass is placed, the more expensive it is to carry. Although the current increase in metabolic cost is unacceptably high for most practical implementations, revisions to improve the fit, weight, and efficiency of the device can not only reduce the cost but also increase the generated electricity. A generator designed specifically for this application could have lower internal losses and require a smaller, lighter gear train. Commercially available gear trains can have much lower friction and higher efficiency, in more compact and lightweight forms. Relocating the device components higher would decrease the metabolic cost of carrying that mass. A more refined device would also benefit from a more form-fitting knee brace made out of a more lightweight material such as carbon fiber.

Several potential applications are especially suited for generative braking. These include lighting and communications needs for the quarter of the world's population who currently live without electricity supply. Innovative prosthetic knees and ankles use motors to assist walking, but battery technology limits their power and working time. Energy harvesters worn on human joints may prove useful for powering the robotic artificial joints. In implantable devices, such as neurostimulators and drug pumps, battery power limits device sophistication, and battery replacement requires surgery. A future energy harvester might be implanted alongside such a device, perhaps in parallel with a muscle, and use generative braking to provide substantial power indefinitely. Generative braking might then find practical applications in forms very different from that demonstrated here.

JOURNAL ARTICLE EXERCISE 3

The science sections on the MCAT include a significant number of passages with experiments or quantitative data. On the Chem/Phys section, questions for these passages often ask you to analyze numerical data from tables and graphs, interpret an apparatus, and come to some reasonable conclusion based on the information they give you. If you don't know how to extract information efficiently and analyze data effectively, you will be at a distinct disadvantage.

There are three "Journal Article Exercises" in this book. In this final exercise, you'll read and extract information from the article, then complete a passage related to the article. Following that, we'll show you the information we would pull from the article as well as the solutions to the passage.

As a reminder, when analyzing a physics article, you should be able to:

- find the research question(s),
- identify the independent and dependent variables,
- determine the significance of any equations and recognize any familiar terms therein,
- interpret the experiment design in terms of basic physical principles,
- analyze any experiment apparatus,
- extract information from graphs and data tables,
- observe trends in the data,
- interpret the hypotheses in terms of the research questions and data, and
- assess the strengths and limitations of the study.

The goal of these exercises is NOT to learn content from the articles, just to get a little more comfortable reading and extracting information from them.

For the (abridged) article on pages 375–378, try to summarize the purpose, methods, results, and assumptions of the study. Answer the following questions:

1. **Topic:**
   - Where does this research fit within the subject matter covered within Chem/Phys?

   _____

   _____

   - Is more than one discipline or topic pertinent to this research?

   _____

   _____

2. **Research questions:**
   - What are the researchers trying to determine?

   _____

   _____

   - How are their methods informed by the question(s)?

   _____

   _____

3. **Data collection:**
   - What is the experimental procedure?

   _____

   _____

   - What is the experiment apparatus and the measurement device?

   _____

   _____

4. **Data analysis:**
   - What are the independent and dependent variables in the stated equations?

   _____

   _____

   - What descriptive statistics are used?

   _____

   _____

5. **Data presentation:**
   - Are there figures showing the apparatus? How do these relate to the data?

   _____

   _____

- Are there tables or graphs? If so, what quantities/units are shown? What trends are evident?

_____

_____

- What do these reveal about the significance of the findings?

_____

_____

6. **Conclusions/hypotheses:**
   - How does the research answer the research questions?

   _____

   _____

   - What does it *not* answer, and how do the authors acknowledge its limitations?

   _____

   _____

   - Are there any unacknowledged limitations you can see?

   _____

   _____

7. **Assumptions:**
   - What do the authors implicitly or explicitly take as given in the ways they design their research, interpret their data, or argue for the significance of their findings?

   _____

   _____

   - Do these assumptions seem justified, given your knowledge of the underlying science?

   _____

   _____

JOURNAL ARTICLE EXERCISE 3 PASSAGE

Biomechanical energy harvesting, the transformation of the energy of the body's movement into electrical energy for immediate use or storage, has become more feasible with the development of strong, lightweight materials and rechargeable batteries with greater storage capacities. Whether tiny devices implanted in the body to harvest the continuous motion of the heart to power a pacemaker or large removable devices used to charge external devices like personal electronics when electricity is unavailable, biomechanical energy harvesters use *generators* of various types to transform kinetic energy into electric energy. The efficacy of such devices can be measured by their *Cost of Harvesting* (*COH*), the metabolic power cost to a user per watt of electric power produced:

$$COH = \frac{\Delta p_{\text{metabolic}}}{\Delta p_{\text{electrical}}}$$

Equation 1

where the Δ refers to the difference between the power produced when the harvesting device is activated and the power produced when the device is installed but deactivated.

One such biomechanical energy harvester involves a knee brace fitted with a gear train that drives a generator when the wearer walks. A one-way clutch prevents power from being generated during knee flexion, so electrical power is only produced during the extension portion of the knee motion (see figure 1). The mechanism is fitted with a *potentiometer*—a rotational position-sensitive variable resistor—that sends a signal to a computer, which in turn can disengage the generator except when the forces at the knee are doing negative work to decelerate the leg. In contrast with a continuous power generation setting, in which the generator is constantly engaged and takes mechanical power from the extending knee whether it is doing positive or negative work, this *generative braking* setting assists the knee to slow the leg when the generator is active, but does not hinder the knee in accelerating the leg forward during that portion of the swing (beyond the passive burden of bearing the weight and internal friction of the brace).

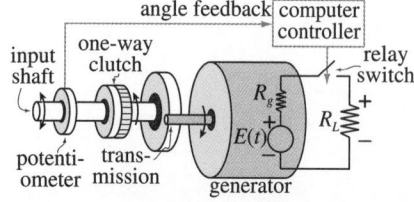

Figure 1   The generative-braking biomechanical energy harvester gearing and circuitry

In an experiment to test the generative-braking device, six adults wearing the orthopedic knee brace energy harvesters walked on treadmills at a steady pace of 1.5 m/s while their metabolic power consumption and the electrical power output by the energy harvester were measured. Measurements were taken with the generator disengaged, with the generator continuously engaged, and with the generative-braking circuit engaged. Results showed that the generative braking mode has significantly lower *COH* than does a continuously-engaged energy harvester, averaging a *COH* of 0.7 versus 2.3, respectively. During the experiment, the electrical power output by the generator (voltage $E(t)$) was dissipated across a load resistor, R_L, and the generator's smaller internal resistance, R_g.

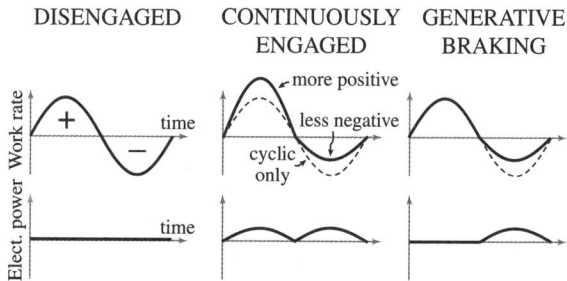

Figure 2   Biomechanical work and generated electrical power with the generator disengaged, continuously engaged, and in the generative-braking mode (dashed lines represent the comparative work rate in the disengaged case)

1. The following data were obtained from the experiment: the average metabolic power when using the brace was 366 W when the generator was disengaged, compared with 307 W without wearing the brace. When the generator was continuously engaged, the average metabolic power was 384 W. Approximately how much electrical power was being generated with the generator continuously engaged?

A) 7.8 W
B) 18 W
C) 21.7 W
D) 33.5 W

2. The efficiency of mechanical-to-electrical power conversion for the device is given by the product of the efficiency of the generator, η_g, and the efficiency of the gear train, η_t. The generator efficiency is the ratio of the usable electrical power provided to the load to the total electrical power dissipated by the generator circuit resistance. Which of the following expressions is equivalent to the total efficiency of the biomechanical energy harvester when the generator is engaged?

A) $\eta_t \dfrac{R_g}{R_L}$

B) $\eta_t \dfrac{R_g R_L}{R_g + R_L}$

C) $\eta_t \dfrac{R_g}{R_g + R_L}$

D) $\eta_t \dfrac{R_L}{R_g + R_L}$

3. During the experiment, a 75 kg person walks in place on the treadmill at a speed of 1.5 m/s in the "generator disengaged" condition. Supposing that each leg has a mass of 15 kg and neglecting non-conservative forces like kinetic friction, how much net work is done by the leg muscles in moving the leg over a complete stride if the total stride length is 1 m? Assume that a complete stride begins with the leg aligned vertically with the hips and includes moving the leg forward, backward, and then forward again into alignment with the hips.

A) 0 J
B) 75 J
C) 150 J
D) 750 J

4. Which of the following changes to the experiment would be most likely to increase the value of $E(t)$, the output voltage of the generator?

A) Decreasing the load resistance, R_L
B) Increasing the weight of the participants
C) Increasing the treadmill speed
D) Disconnecting the potentiometer from the computer control

SOLUTIONS TO JOURNAL ARTICLE EXERCISE 3

Let's answer the above questions for the article on pages 375–378.

1. **Topic:**
   - Where does this research fit within the subject matter covered within Chem/Phys? *Physics, covering circuits as well as work-energy mechanics*
   - Is more than one discipline or topic pertinent to this research? *Definite intersection with biology in the discussion of muscles and joints as well as metabolic energy*

2. **Research questions:**
   - What are the researchers trying to determine? *How can we design a biomechanical energy harvester that generates continuous power during normal activities without burdening the user?*
   - How are their methods informed by the question(s)? *Because the question is more one of engineering than of physical hypothesis confirmation, the methods are basically a proof of concept with the actual design and implementation of the generative braking knee brace, and the data are taken to show just how much power the device generates and at what cost to the user.*

3. **Data collection:**
   - What is the experimental procedure? *Six male participants wore the generative power devices on both legs while walking on a treadmill. The knee brace was set alternately on continuously engaged and generative-braking (engaged in power harvesting only during the negative-work deceleration of the lower leg) modes, or with the generator fully disengaged for a control. Metabolic cost, mechanical power on the device, and electrical power were measured.*
   - What is the experiment apparatus and the measurement device? *The knee brace itself was equipped with a potentiometer circuit that enabled it to engage and disengage the generator according to the portion of the knee swing, so that in the generative braking power harvesting mode it was only engaged during deceleration. The generator itself was connected to a load resistor in order to dissipate the generated power for convenience. Metabolic cost was measured "using a standard respiratory system" and electrical power generated was measured via the circuitry (the exact device is not mentioned: presumably a voltmeter across the load resistor would suffice).*

4. **Data analysis:**
   - What are the independent and dependent variables in the stated equations? *The study is not an experiment in the traditional sense of manipulating independent variables to see the effects on dependent variables (for example, the subjects are not asked to walk or run at different speeds on the treadmill). The condition manipulated by the researchers is the setting of the knee brace energy harvester to fully disengaged, engaged continuously, or engaged selectively during deceleration of the leg (generative braking). The measured/calculated variables are metabolic, mechanical, and electrical power.*
   - What descriptive statistics are used? *Means and standard deviations of the power values are provided.*

5. **Data presentation:**
   - Are there figures showing the apparatus? How do these relate to the data? *Yes, there are several figures picturing and representing the apparatus in action, as well as its gearing and electrical generation circuitry.*
   - Are there tables or graphs? If so, what quantities/units are shown? What trends are evident? *Bar graphs show the metabolic and electrical power averages comparing the different conditions, and line graphs show mechanical and electrical powers as a function of position in the stride cycle.*
   - What do these reveal about the significance of the findings? *P values are given for each average and standard deviation value in the text (most are less than 0.05, and the text notes where values are insignificant), and Figure 4 comparing the continuous versus generative braking conditions regarding calculated Cost of Harvesting values shows the significance of the comparisons to be P < 0.05.*

6. **Conclusions/hypotheses:**
   - How does the research answer the research questions? *The study shows that the knee brace energy harvester set to generative braking mode (engaging during deceleration and assisting the knee in that process) has a lower Cost of Harvesting energy than a traditional full-cycle energy harvester while providing consistent and significant energy during normal walking motion. Both settings have a significantly lower Cost of Harvesting than a conventional biomechanical energy harvester like a hand-crank charger, which generates power only during the positive work portion of motion (during which time the user is actively pushing the crank arm to turn it).*
   - What does it *not* answer, and how do the authors acknowledge its limitations? *The prototype device conditions, namely the mass and location on the leg of the brace, add enough to the metabolic cost of wearing the energy harvester to make it impractical for actual use as currently configured. Though they project possible upgrades, they cannot offer a completely practical means of harvesting and utilizing or storing biomechanical energy.*
   - Are there any unacknowledged limitations you can see? *The problem is viewed almost entirely from an engineering perspective, so that the authors cannot speak to whether actual people would be willing to implement such energy harvesters in their day-to-day lives. There might be concerns apart from design practicality or metabolic cost that they have not considered.*

7. **Assumptions:**
   - What do the authors implicitly or explicitly take as given in the ways they design their research, interpret their data, or argue for the significance of their findings? *Given that they do not elaborate upon them, the authors must assume that their means of measuring metabolic costs and electrical power output are accurate without testing against some other measure. This may have something to do with a uniform and small set of participants.*
   - Do these assumptions seem justified, given your knowledge of the underlying science? *Probably: standardized measures for quantities like these are typical in scientific research. It may be that field tests would vary more widely in terms of input and output power measurements versus reality.*

SOLUTIONS TO JOURNAL ARTICLE EXERCISE 3 PASSAGE

1. **A** Using to Equation 1 from the passage, we find $\Delta p_{\text{electrical}} = \dfrac{\Delta p_{\text{metabolic}}}{COH}$. The passage defines the delta as the difference between the device being activated and the device being worn but deactivated. The $\Delta p_{\text{metabolic}}$ is therefore 384 W – 366 W = 18 W. The passage gives a value of COH = 2.3 for the continuously engaged energy harvester, yielding $\Delta p_{\text{electrical}} = \dfrac{18 \text{ W}}{2.3} \approx 7.8 \text{ W}$.

2. **D** The question stem states that the efficiency of the generator is the ratio of electrical power provided to the load to the total electrical power dissipated by the circuit. This means that $\eta_g = \dfrac{P_{\text{load}}}{P_{\text{total}}} = \dfrac{I^2 R_L}{I^2 R_{\text{total}}} = \dfrac{R_L}{R_g + R_L}$; note that the currents are equivalent and the resistances sum for the total resistance because Figure 1 shows a series circuit. The question stem also states that that total efficiency of the device is the product of the generator and gear train efficiencies, $\eta_g \times \eta_t$, yielding choice D.

3. **A** Looking at the graph in Figure 2 of the disengaged condition, you should observe that the positive and negative work curves are symmetric, showing that in total, no work is done for a complete cycle. Alternatively, recall that work is the product of force and displacement. Walking on a treadmill at the set speed does not result in any displacement of a person's center of mass. Moreover, since a complete stride returns the leg to its original position, whatever forces acted upon it during the process must do zero net work.

4. **C** This question is best to approach with process of elimination. The output voltage of a generator, like that of a battery, determines the current in a circuit as a function of its equivalent resistance, not the other way around (eliminate choice A). Similarly, a generator, like a battery, will generate a voltage whether it is connected to a closed circuit or not. This means we can eliminate choice D, which would have the effect of leaving the relay switch closed throughout the process (the continuous generation condition); don't be fooled by the Figure 2 graphs into thinking that more total electrical energy over an entire cycle entails a greater generator voltage! There's no reason to think that the weight of the participants affects the functioning of the generator; it would likely affect their metabolic power cost, but that doesn't causally determine the electrical power or voltage (eliminate choice B). Choice C is correct: increasing the treadmill speed would increase the speed at which the knee was extending per stride, which would in turn cause the gearing to turn faster. The voltage output by a generator is a function of this spin rate; though this is not something you'd be expected to recall, you should associate more work per unit time with greater power, and greater power for a circuit would mean a greater voltage to resistance ratio by $P = \dfrac{V^2}{R}$. Since the resistance hasn't changed, the voltage must increase.

Chapter 11
Oscillations and Waves

11.1 OSCILLATIONS

Any motion that regularly repeats is referred to as **periodic** or **harmonic motion**. Common examples include an object undergoing uniform circular motion, a mass oscillating on a spring and a pendulum. This type of motion can be characterized by its **period** or **frequency**.

Period

The time it takes an object to move through one full cycle of motion is called the period. For an object undergoing uniform circular motion, the period is the time it takes to make one revolution. For a mass on a spring or a pendulum, it is the time it takes to make a round trip (i.e., the final position and velocity must be the same as the initial values). The period is denoted by T and is measured in seconds.

Example 11-1: The bob on a pendulum moves from point A to point B in 0.5 seconds. What is the period of oscillation?

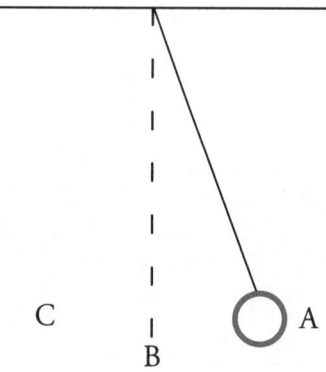

Solution: A to B represents one-quarter of a period. A full period is the time it takes for the bob to move from A to B to C to B and back to A. So $T = 4(0.5\ \text{s}) = 2\ \text{s}$.

Frequency

Rather than timing one cycle to find the period, we can instead count the number of cycles that occur in one second. This is known as the frequency, denoted by f. The units of f are cycles per second, or **hertz** (Hz).

Now the first thing we notice is that period and frequency are reciprocals. After all, the period is "the number of seconds per cycle," and the frequency is "the number of cycles per second." So, we have these fundamental relationships:

Period and Frequency

$$f = \frac{1}{T} \quad \text{and} \quad T = \frac{1}{f}$$

Every type of oscillation has a period and a frequency, but there is a special class of oscillations in which these quantities have a unique property. This "ideal" type of oscillatory motion is referred to as **simple harmonic motion** (often abbreviated SHM). A mass oscillating on a spring exhibits SHM.

The spring in the series of diagrams below is fixed at its left end and has a block attached to its right end. When the spring is neither stretched nor compressed (i.e., when it's at its natural length, as shown in Diagram 1 below) we say the spring is at its **equilibrium position**. In general, the point at which the net force on the block is zero, which in this case is when the spring is at its natural length, is called the equilibrium position, and we label it $x = 0$.

Now, imagine that we stretch the spring (Diagram 1 to Diagram 2), and let go. Once released, the spring pulls back to the left, going through its equilibrium position and then to the point of maximum compression. From here, the spring pushes back to the right, passing again through its equilibrium position, and returning to the point of maximum extension. If friction is negligible, this back-and-forth motion will continue indefinitely, and the time it takes for the block to go through one period, for example, from Diagram 2 to Diagram 6, is a constant.

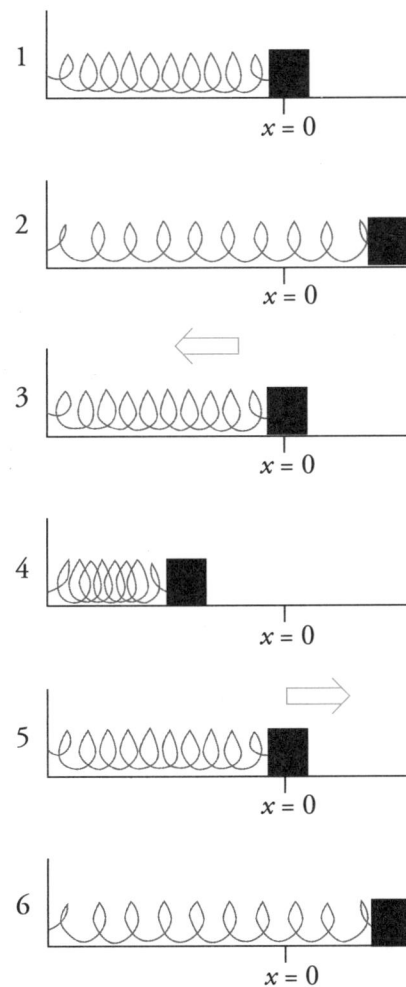

The Dynamics of SHM

Force

Let's first describe the motion of the block attached to the spring from the point of view of the force it feels. The spring exerts a force on the block that's proportional to its displacement. If we call the equilibrium position $x = 0$, then the force exerted by the spring is given by

---

Hooke's Law

$$\mathbf{F} = -k\mathbf{x}$$

The proportionality constant, k, called the **spring constant**, tells us how strong the spring is; the greater the value of k, the stiffer (and stronger) the spring.

As we can see from Hooke's Law, the units of k are newton/meter. Since a meter is a large distance to stretch or compress a spring, the values for k are often large.

What is the role of the minus sign in Hooke's law? Look back at the diagrams on the previous page. Since we're calling the equilibrium position $x = 0$, when the block is to the right of equilibrium, its position, x, is positive. At this point, the stretched spring wants to pull back to the left; because the direction of the force of the spring is to the left, we indicate this direction by calling it negative. Similarly, when the block is to the left of equilibrium, its position, x, is negative. At this point, the compressed spring wants to push back to the right; because the direction of the force of the spring is to the right, we indicate this direction by calling it positive. We see that the direction of the spring force is always directed opposite to its displacement from equilibrium, and for this reason, the minus sign is needed in Hooke's law. Furthermore, because the spring is always trying to restore the block to equilibrium, we say that the spring provides the **restoring force**; it's this force that maintains the oscillations. The fact that the restoring force exerted by the spring obeys Hooke's Law (i.e., the force is directly proportional to the distance from equilibrium) is the reason why the block undergoes simple harmonic motion.

Energy

Unfortunately, knowing an equation for the force doesn't allow us to solve directly for other things, such as the speed of the block at some later time or the work done by or against the spring: The force changes as the block moves, so acceleration is not uniform. However, there is a way to figure out these quantities by using energy. When we pull on the spring to get the oscillations started, we're exerting a force over a distance; that is, we're doing work. Because we're doing work against the spring, the spring stores potential energy, called **elastic potential energy**. If we once again call the equilibrium position of the spring $x = 0$, then the potential energy of a stretched or compressed spring is given by this equation:

Elastic Potential Energy

$$PE_{\text{elastic}} = \tfrac{1}{2}kx^2$$

It follows that $W_{\text{by spring}} = -\Delta PE_{\text{elastic}}$ and $W_{\text{against spring}} = \Delta PE_{\text{elastic}}$. To justify this, imagine an external force is stretching a spring from $x = 0$ to $x = X$. The minimum force required to do this is opposite the spring force: $+kx$. From mechanics, we learned that the work done by a variable force is equal to the area under the force vs. position graph.

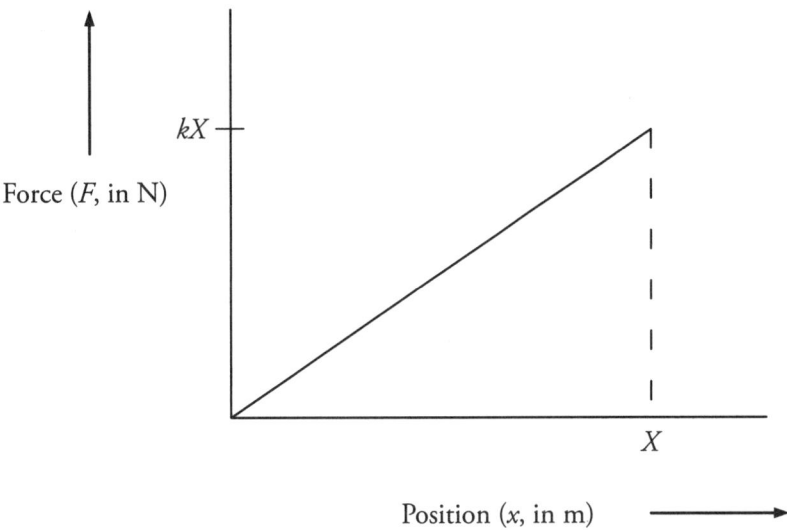

The area under the curve is the area of a triangle with base equal to X and height equal to kX. So $PE = W_{\text{against spring}} = (1/2)bh = (1/2)(X)(kX) = (1/2)kX^2$.

We can also use conservation of energy to find the speed of a oscillating mass on a spring at any given position.

When we release the block from rest in Diagram 2 from page 389, the spring is stretched and the block isn't moving, so all the energy is in the form of elastic potential energy. This potential energy turns into kinetic energy, until at $x = 0$ (equilibrium), all the energy has been converted to kinetic energy. As the block rushes past equilibrium, this kinetic energy gradually turns back into elastic potential energy until the point where the spring is at maximum compression and it's all transformed back to potential energy. The compressed spring then pushes outward, converting its potential energy back to kinetic; the block rushes through equilibrium again, and kinetic energy is transformed back to potential energy, until it reaches its starting point (Diagram 6 from page 389) at maximum extension. At this instant, we're back to our full reserve of elastic potential energy (and no kinetic energy), and the process is ready to repeat.

As a result, we can look at the motion of the block from the point of view of the back-and-forth transfer between elastic potential energy and kinetic energy.

The maximum displacement of the block from equilibrium is called the **amplitude**, denoted by A. This positive number tells us how far to the left and right of equilibrium the block will travel. So, in the series of diagrams above, the block's position at maximum extension is $x = +A$, and its position at maximum compression is $x = -A$.

We can summarize the dynamics of the oscillations in this table:

	at $x = -A$	at $x = 0$	at $x = +A$
magnitude of restoring force	max	0	max
magnitude of acceleration	max	0	max
$PE_{elastic}$ of spring	max	0	max
KE of block	0	max	0
speed (v) of block	0	max	0

Because we're ignoring any frictional forces during the oscillations of the block, total mechanical energy will be conserved. That is, the sum of the block's kinetic energy, $\frac{1}{2}mv^2$, and the spring's potential energy, $\frac{1}{2}kx^2$, will be a constant. We can use this fact to figure out the maximum speed of the block. At the instant the block is passing through equilibrium, all the potential energy of the spring has been transformed into kinetic energy of the block. If the amplitude of the oscillations is A, then the maximum elastic potential energy, $\frac{1}{2}kA^2$ (the value of $\frac{1}{2}kx^2$ when $x = \pm A$), is completely converted to maximum kinetic energy at $x = 0$. This gives us:

$$PE_{elastic,\ max} \rightarrow KE_{max}$$

$$\tfrac{1}{2}kA^2 = \tfrac{1}{2}mv^2$$

$$\therefore v_{max} = A\sqrt{\frac{k}{m}}$$

Example 11-2: A block of mass m attached to a spring with constant k oscillates horizontally on a frictionless surface with amplitude A. In which case does the spring do more work, moving the mass from $x = A$ to $x = A/2$ or from $x = A/2$ to $x = 0$?

Solution: In both cases the spring does positive work, since the restoring force is in the same direction as the motion of the block. Since the force is not constant, we cannot use the formula $W = Fd\cos\theta$. Instead, the work done by the spring is given by $W = -\Delta PE_{elastic} = -(PE_{final} - PE_{initial})$.

From $x = A$ to x to $A/2$:

$$W = -(\frac{1}{2}k[A/2]^2 - \frac{1}{2}kA^2) = -(\frac{1}{8}kA^2 - \frac{1}{2}kA^2) = \frac{3}{8}kA^2$$

From $x = A/2$ to $x = 0$:

$$W = -(\frac{1}{2}k[0]^2 - \frac{1}{2}k[A/2]^2) = -(0 - \frac{1}{8}kA^2) = \frac{1}{8}kA^2$$

Notice that even though the distance traveled is the same in each case, the average force exerted by the spring is greater from $x = A$ to $x = A/2$ than it is from $x = A/2$ to $x = 0$, and therefore the work done by the spring is also greater.

Example 11-3: A block of mass 200 g is oscillating on the end of a horizontal spring of spring constant 100 N/m and natural length 12 cm. When the spring is stretched to a length of 14 cm, what is the acceleration of the block?

Solution: When the spring is stretched by 2 cm, Hooke's law tells us that the force exerted by the spring has a magnitude of $F = kx = (100 \text{ N/m})(0.02 \text{ m}) = 2 \text{ N}$. Therefore, by Newton's second law, the acceleration of the block will have a magnitude of $a = F/m = (2 \text{ N})/(0.2 \text{ kg}) = 10 \text{ m/s}^2$.

Example 11-4: If the block in Example 11-3 above were replaced with a block of mass 800 g, how would its maximum speed change?

Solution: The equation derived above, $v_{max} = A\sqrt{k/m}$, tells us that v_{max} is inversely proportional to the square root of the mass of the oscillator. Therefore, if m increases by a factor of 4, v_{max} will decrease by a factor of 2.

The Kinematics of SHM

Earlier it was mentioned that a mass oscillating on a spring exhibits "ideal" oscillatory motion, which is called simple harmonic motion, and that this motion is the result of Hooke's Law (i.e., the restoring force is directly proportional to the distance from equilibrium). But what makes this motion different than non-ideal oscillations? It turns out (using calculus) that the frequency and period only depend on the spring constant, k, and the mass of the block, m.

$$f = \frac{1}{2\pi}\sqrt{\frac{k}{m}} \quad \text{and} \quad T = 2\pi\sqrt{\frac{m}{k}}$$

Notice that neither f nor T depends on A, the amplitude. This is why we call the motion of the block on the spring *simple* harmonic motion. This is not an obvious statement. If a mass on a spring is pulled back 1 cm or pulled back 10 cm (assuming the spring is still within its elastic limit), the time it takes to complete one cycle is exactly the same. As an example of an oscillating system that does not exhibit simple harmonic motion, imagine a ball bouncing. Removing air resistance and assuming that the bounces are completely elastic, the ball will continue to bounce to the same height from which it was released. However, dropping the ball from 1 cm will take less time to fall and rise than dropping it from 10 cm (which can be proven with the Big 5 equations).

It's possible for a system to oscillate because of a restoring force that is not directly proportional to the displacement. If this were the case, the frequency and period would depend on the amplitude; we'd still call the motion *harmonic*, which just means back-and-forth, but we wouldn't call it *simple* harmonic.

Example 11-5: Suppose that the block shown in the series of diagrams on the first page of this chapter requires 0.25 sec to move from Diagram 4 to Diagram 6. What is the frequency of the oscillations?

Solution: The interval from Diagram 4 to Diagram 6 represents *half* a cycle, which requires *half* a period to complete. If half a period is 0.25 sec, then the period is 0.5 sec. Therefore, the frequency, *f*, is $1/T = 1/(0.5 \text{ s}) = 2$ Hz.

So far we have examined the simple harmonic motion of a mass on a horizontal spring, where the system is in equilibrium when the spring is at its rest length. If the spring is now rotated so that it is suspended vertically and a mass is attached, will the oscillations still be simple harmonic? The answer is yes. The formulas for period and frequency are exactly the same. The force of gravity, however, does affect the situation. The weight of the block will naturally stretch the spring so that equilibrium ($F_{net} = 0$) no longer occurs when the spring is at its rest length. The new equilibrium position is when the upward force of the spring exactly balances the weight: $kx = mg$. When the spring is stretched beyond this point and released, the mass will oscillate around the new equilibrium position. It is often convenient to rename the new equilibrium position $x = 0$. This enables us to "ignore gravity". In other words, measuring *x* from equilibrium instead of measuring from the rest length of the spring, it becomes exactly like a horizontal spring, but with a longer rest length. We can therefore still use the equations

$$-kx = ma \text{ and } v_{max} = A\sqrt{\frac{k}{m}}$$

Pendulums

Besides the spring-block simple harmonic oscillator, there's another oscillator that the MCAT will expect you to know about: the simple pendulum. If the connecting rod or string between the suspension point and the object at the end of a pendulum has negligible mass (so that all the mass is in the object at the end of the rod or string), and if there is no friction at the suspension point during oscillation, we say the pendulum is a **simple pendulum**.

The displacement of the mass is not taken as a distance from equilibrium (as in the spring-block case), but rather as the angle it makes with the vertical. The vertical (shown as a dashed line in the figure below) is the equilibrium position, $\theta = 0$. The restoring force here is gravity; specifically, it's equal to $mg \sin \theta$, which is the component of the object's weight in the direction toward equilibrium.

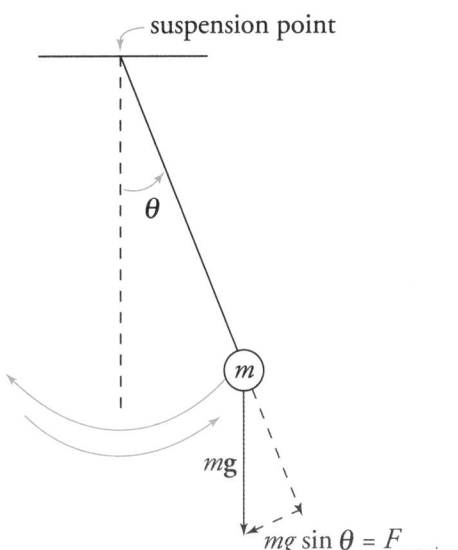

Strictly speaking, a pendulum does not undergo simple harmonic motion because the restoring force is not proportional to the displacement ($mg \sin \theta$ is not exactly proportional to θ). However, if the angle is small, then $\sin \theta \approx \theta$ (in radians), so the restoring force can be approximated as $mg\theta$, which is proportional to θ.[1] In this case, we can treat the motion as simple harmonic, and the frequency and period are given by the following equations:

$$f = \frac{1}{2\pi}\sqrt{\frac{g}{l}} \text{ and } T = 2\pi\sqrt{\frac{l}{g}}$$

where l is the length of the pendulum and g is the acceleration due to gravity. Observe that in the case of simple harmonic motion of a simple pendulum, the mass of the swinging object does not affect the frequency or period of oscillation.

Example 11-6: The bob (mass = m) of a simple pendulum is raised to a height h above its lowest point and released. Find an expression for the maximum speed of the pendulum.

Solution: When the bob is at height h above its lowest point, it has gravitational potential energy equal to mgh (relative to its lowest point). As it passes through the equilibrium position, all this potential energy is converted to kinetic energy. Therefore, $mgh = \frac{1}{2}mv_{max}^2$, and we get $v_{max} = \sqrt{2gh}$. This is the speed of the bob as it passes through equilibrium, which is where it attains its maximum speed.

---

[1] The conversion between degrees and radians is as follows: 180 degrees = π radians. If the angle is given in degrees, the restoring force is approximately $mg\,\theta(\pi/180°)$, which is still proportional to θ.

11.2 WAVES

A **mechanical wave** is a series of disturbances (i.e., oscillations) within a medium that transfers energy from one place to another. The medium itself is not transported, just the energy. Examples included a vibrating string or sound. Mechanical waves cannot exist without a medium. In a later chapter we will discuss **electromagnetic waves**, which do not need a medium. This is because the electric and magnetic fields oscillate rather than physical matter.

Transverse Waves

Perhaps the simplest example of wave is one we can create by wiggling one end of a long rope:

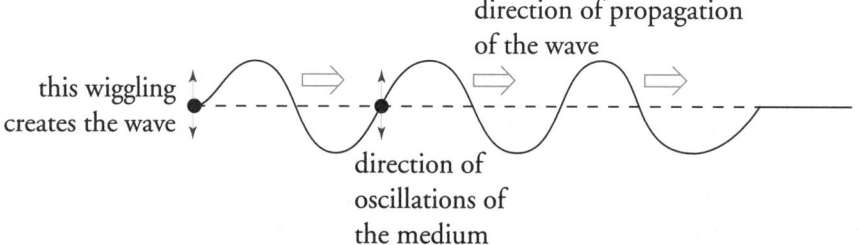

This wave uses the rope as the medium, traveling from one end to the other. Notice that the wave is moving horizontally, but the rope itself is moving up and down. That's why this is called a **transverse** wave: The wave travels (propagates) in a direction that's *perpendicular* to the direction in which the medium is vibrating.

Frequency and Period

The most fundamental characteristic of a wave is its frequency. If we pick a spot on the rope and count how many times it moves up and down (the number of round trips it makes) in one second, we've just measured the **frequency**, f, which we express in hertz (cycles per second).

The **period** of a wave, T, is the reciprocal of the frequency, and is the amount of time it takes any spot on the rope to complete one cycle (in this case, one up-and-down round trip).

These definitions for frequency and period are same as for a mass on a spring or a pendulum. Each particle of rope oscillates up and down with simple harmonic motion. However, we can also think of the frequency and period of a wave in a different way. Instead of focusing on the oscillations, we can observe "pulses" moving the right. Frequency can be thought as the number of pulses that pass a given point per unit time and period is the time it takes between pulses.

Wavelength and Amplitude

The figure below identifies the **crests** (**peaks**) and **troughs** of the wave. The distance from one crest to the next (i.e., the length of one cycle of the wave) is called the **wavelength**, denoted by λ, the Greek letter lambda. We can also measure the wavelength by measuring the distance from one trough to the next, or, in fact, between any two consecutive corresponding points along the wave.

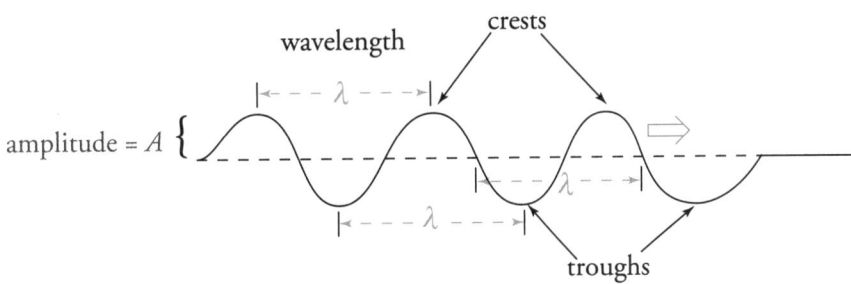

The **amplitude** of a wave, A, is the maximum displacement from equilibrium that any point in the medium makes as the wave goes by. In the case of a wave on a rope, the amplitude is the distance from the original horizontal position of the rope up to a crest; it's also the distance from the horizontal position down to a trough.

Wave Speed

To figure out how fast the wave travels, we just notice that the wave travels a distance of λ in time T; that is, λ is the length of one wave cycle, and T, the period, is the time required for one wave cycle to go by. Since distance = rate × time, we get $\lambda = vT$. Solving this for v gives us $\lambda(1/T) = v$ and since $f = 1/T$, the equation becomes $v = \lambda f$. *This is the most important equation for waves and one of the most important equations for the MCAT.*

Wave Equation

$$v = \lambda f$$

Two Big Rules for Waves

Notice that the second equation for the wave speed shows that v does not depend on f (or λ). While this may seem to contradict the first equation, $v = \lambda f$, it really doesn't. The speed of the wave depends on the characteristics of the rope: how tense it is, and what it's made of. We can wiggle the end at any frequency we want, and the speed of the wave we create will be a constant. However, because $\lambda f = v$ must always be true, a higher f will mean a shorter λ (and a lower f will mean a longer λ). Thus, changing f doesn't change v: It changes λ. This brings up our first big rule for waves:

> **Big Rule 1:** The speed of a wave is determined by the type of wave and the characteristics of the medium, *not* by the frequency.

For example, the speed of a transverse wave on a rope is given by:

$$v = \sqrt{\frac{\text{tension}}{\text{linear density}}}$$

The linear density of a rope is its mass per unit length. Notice that the tension and linear density are properties of the medium, and that this equation is independent of wave properties of frequency, wavelength, and amplitude.

Note that two different types of waves can move with different speeds through the same medium; for example, sound and light move through air with very different speeds. There are exceptions to Big Rule 1, but the only one the MCAT will expect you to know about is *dispersion*, which is discussed in Chapter 13, on Optics. Any other exception would be discussed in the passage; otherwise, you can assume the rule applies.

Our second big rule for waves concerns what happens when a wave passes from one medium into another. Because wave speed is determined by the characteristics of the medium, a change in the medium implies a change in wave speed, but the frequency won't change.

> **Big Rule 2:** When a wave passes into another medium, its speed changes, but its frequency does *not*.

The reasoning behind this makes sense if you focus on a wave as a series of pulses. Frequency is the number of pulses that pass by per unit time. It stands to reason that, if a certain number of pulses per second arrives at the boundary between two different media, then the same number of pulses per second must leave, passing into the new medium. In other words, rate in = rate out. This is similar to the Equation of Continuity in fluids and the rule for electric current passing through resistors in series.

Because f is constant, Rule 2 tells us that the wavelength is proportional to wave speed.

Notice that Rule 1 applies to different waves in one medium, while Rule 2 applies to a single wave in different media. Memorize these rules. The MCAT loves waves.

Example 11-7: A transverse wave of frequency 4 Hz travels at a speed of 6 m/s along a rope. What would be the speed of a 12 Hz wave along this same rope?

Solution: Big Rule 1 for waves says that the speed of a wave is determined by the type of wave and the characteristics of the medium, not by the frequency. If all we do is change the frequency, the wave speed will not change: The wave speed will still be 6 m/s. (What *will* change? The wavelength. Because $\lambda = v/f$, a change in f with no change in v will change λ.)

Example 11-8: Which one of the following statements is true concerning the amplitude of a wave?

   A. Amplitude increases with increasing frequency.
   B. Amplitude increases with increasing wavelength.
   C. Amplitude increases with increasing wave speed.
   D. None of the above.

Solution: The amplitude is determined by how much energy we put into the wave to get it started. If we wiggle the rope up and down through a large distance (a large amplitude), this takes more energy on our part, and as a result, the wave carries more energy. However, the amplitude doesn't depend on f, λ, or v. The answer is D.

Example 11-9: A wave of frequency 12 Hz has a wavelength of 3 m. What is the speed of this wave?

Solution: Using the equation $v = \lambda f$, we find that $v = (3 \text{ m})(12 \text{ Hz}) = 36$ m/s.

Example 11-10: An electrocardiogram responds to changes in the electric potential of the heart from a number of different angles and distances, and represents a different pair combinations of these signals (voltages) as deflections of several needles under which runs graph paper moving horizontally at a constant speed. Suppose a patient has a resting heart rate of 60 beats per minute and the tape runs through the machine at 4 cm/s. What is the wavelength over which the pattern should repeat?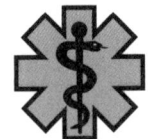

Solution: 60 beats/min = 1 beat/s, or a period of 1s and frequency of 1 Hz. The wave speed, v, is simply the speed at which the tape runs under the needle: $v = 4$ cm/s. Thus $\lambda = v / f = 4$ cm/s / 1 Hz = 4 cm.

Example 11-11: What happens when the wave shown below passes from the thick, heavy rope into the thinner, lighter rope?

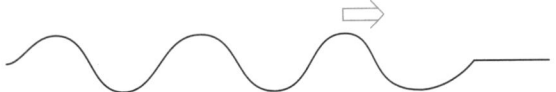

Solution: According to Big Rule 2 for waves, when a wave passes into another medium, its speed changes, but its frequency does not. How does the speed change? Because the rope is lighter (i.e., it has a lower linear density), the equation for wave speed on a string (given above) tells us that v will *increase*. So, if v increases but f doesn't change, then λ will also increase because $\lambda = v/f$.

Example 11-12: A certain rope transmits a 2 Hz transverse wave of amplitude 10 cm with a speed of 1 m/s. What would be the wavelength of a 5 Hz transverse wave of amplitude 8 cm on this same rope?

Solution: First, ignore the amplitudes; they're included in the question only to make things seem more complicated than they are. The amplitude of a wave indicates how much energy the wave transports, but it has nothing to do with wavelength, period, frequency, or wave speed (recall Example 11-8 above). Now, if a

2 Hz transverse wave has a speed of 1 m/s on this rope, then a transverse wave of *any* frequency will have a speed of 1 m/s on this rope; that's what Big Rule 1 for waves tells us. Thus, if $f = 5$ Hz and $v = 1$ m/s, then

$$\lambda = \frac{v}{f} = \frac{1 \text{ m/s}}{5 \text{ Hz}} = 0.2 \text{ m}$$

Example 11-13: How long will it take a wave of wavelength λ and period T to travel a distance d?

A. $\lambda T d$

B. $\dfrac{\lambda d}{T}$

C. $\dfrac{T d}{\lambda}$

D. $\dfrac{\lambda T}{d}$

Solution: First, let's see if we can eliminate any choices because the units don't work out correctly. We're being asked for an amount of time, so the answer must have the dimension (and units) of time. Choice A can't be correct, since it has units of $[\lambda][T][d] = \text{m·sec·m} = \text{m}^2\text{·sec}$. Notice that both λ and d have units of meters, which we don't want in the answer, so these units must cancel. Therefore, B can't be correct either since λ and d are multiplied by each other, rather than being divided as they should to make their units cancel.

One difference between the two remaining choices is that in C, the distance d is in the numerator, while in D, the distance d is in the denominator. Now, let's think about this: More time will be required for the wave to travel a greater distance. In other words, the bigger d is, the greater the travel time should be. Therefore, we can eliminate D; after all, since d is in the denominator in choice D, a larger d will result in a smaller amount of time, which doesn't make sense. Thus, the answer must be C.

Here's an alternate solution using equations. Because *distance = speed × time* ($d = vt$), we know that $t = d/v$. We can find v using the wave equation $v = \lambda f$, and since $f = 1/T$, we find that

$$t = \frac{d}{v} = \frac{d}{\lambda f} = \frac{d}{\lambda} \cdot \frac{1}{f} = \frac{d}{\lambda} \cdot T = \frac{T d}{\lambda}$$

The answer is indeed C, just as we figured out by checking units and using logic.

11.3 INTERFERENCE OF WAVES

When two or more waves are superimposed on each other, they will combine to form a single resultant wave. This is called **interference**. The amplitude of the resultant wave will depend on the amplitudes of the combining waves *and* on how these waves travel relative to each other.

If crest meets crest, and trough meets trough, we say that the waves are **in phase** with each other. Their amplitudes will *add*, and we say the waves interfere **constructively**. However, if the crest of one wave coincides with the *trough* of the other (and vice versa), we say that the waves are exactly **out of phase** with each other. In this case, their amplitudes *subtract*, and we say that the waves interfere **destructively**.

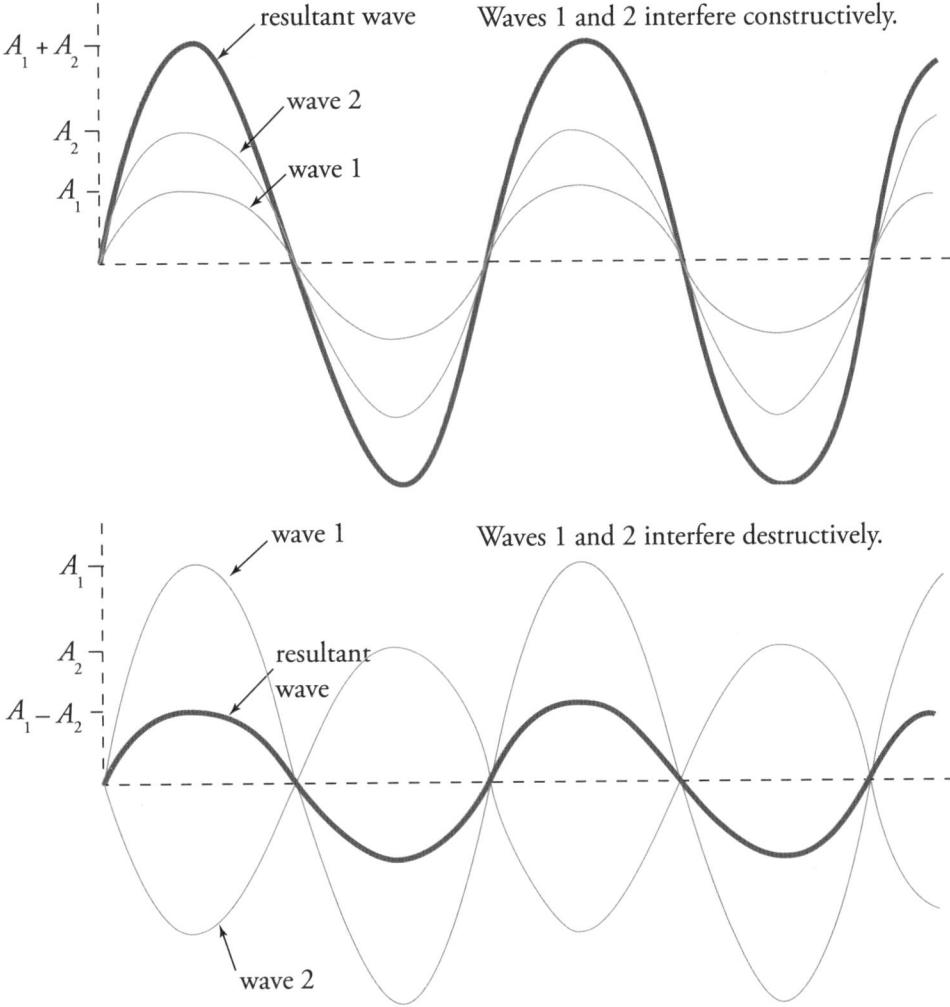

A passage might also say that waves that are directly opposite each other in amplitude are *180 degrees out of phase*, or *π radians out of phase*; it is common to refer to a whole cycle or wave as being 360 degrees or 2π radians, as if it were a circle. If the waves aren't exactly in phase ($0°$, $360°$, or 2π radians) or exactly out of phase ($180°$ or π radians), the amplitude of the resultant wave will be somewhere between the difference and the sum of the amplitudes of the interfering waves.

The interfering waves may also have different wavelengths. These waves will produce a more complicated-looking resultant wave, but we'd still say the waves interfere constructively where they reinforce each other, and destructively where they tend to cancel each other out.

11.3

The preceding pictures of waves that are in phase and out of phase can also be thought of as graphs representing the displacement at a fixed location as a function of time. As an example, imagine a cork floating in calm water. Source 1 creates a wave, which travels through the water, causing the cork to bob up and down. A graph of the cork's motion as a function of time would be sinusoidal (i.e., it looks like Wave 1 in the picture except that the distance from maximum to maximum is the period rather than the wavelength).

Similarly, if Source 2 were acting alone, Wave 2 would cause the cork to bob up and down. The graph of this motion as a function of time would look similar to the picture of Wave 2. If Wave 1 and Wave 2 both arrive at the cork, they will interfere. If the waves are in phase when they arrive at the cork (i.e., crests arrive at the same time, troughs arrive at the same time, etc.) or if they are 180° out of phase when they arrive at the cork (i.e., the crest of one wave arrives simultaneously with the trough of the other), the graph of the cork's motion as a function of time would look like the resultant waves in the picture. Note that if the waves have different frequencies (and wavelengths), then the graph of the cork's motion will not look like a sine or cosine, but will be more complicated. An example of this is **beats**, which are discussed in the next chapter.

Be careful on the MCAT. If you see a picture of a sine or cosine, make sure you can determine whether it is an actual wave (pictured at a fixed time), or a graph of one particle's motion as a function of time.

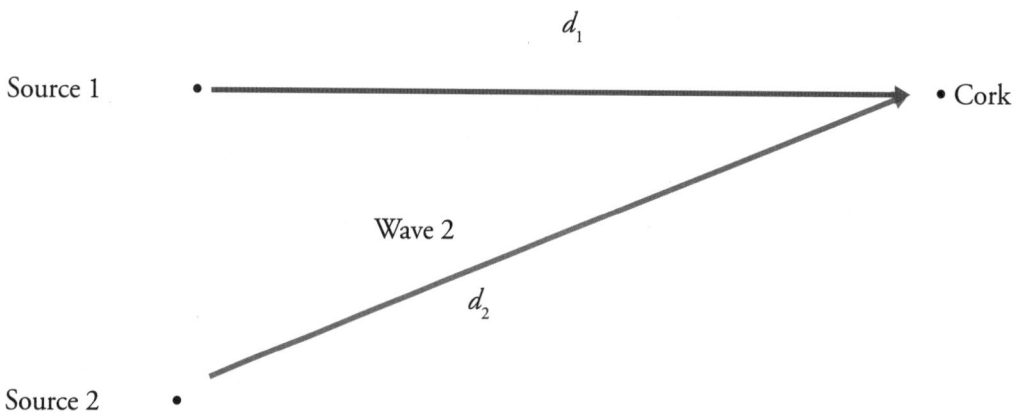

How can you determine whether two waves are in phase, 180° out of phase or something in between? One way is to look at *path difference*. In the above picture, imagine Source 1 and Source 2 emit identical waves that are exactly in phase. Just because they are initially in phase does not mean they will be in phase when they arrive at the cork. The reason is because Wave 2 had to travel a larger distance than Wave 1. The path difference = $d_2 - d_1$. The general rule is:

- If the path difference = $n\lambda$ and, ($n = 0, 1, 2, \ldots$), the waves will be in phase and will therefore constructively interfere.
- If the path difference = $(n + \frac{1}{2})\lambda$, the waves will be 180° out of phase and will therefore destructively interfere.

If Wave 2 travels an integer number of wavelengths farther than Wave 1, the crests from each will still arrive at the same time. If Wave 2 travels $\lambda/2$, $3\lambda/2$, $5\lambda/2$, etc. farther than Wave 1, the crest from one wave will arrive simultaneously with a trough from the other wave. Note that if the cork in the picture experiences constructive interference, it does not mean than neighboring corks will. The distance from the sources to the other corks would be different. An example of this is Young's Double-Slit experiment, where the two sources are small holes in a screen emitting light that is in phase. On the opposite wall is a screen that features alternating bright and dark fringes. Bright fringes are the result of constructive interference and dark fringes are the result of destructive interference. They alternate, since the path difference changes as you move up or down the screen.

11.4 STANDING WAVES

Let's say that we have a long rope with one end in our fingers and the other end attached to a wall. We wiggle the rope up and down at a certain frequency, f, and create waves of frequency f that travel down the length of the rope. When they hit the wall, they'll be reflected. We now have two waves on the same rope (the wave we continue to generate plus the reflected wave) with the same frequency and amplitude but traveling in opposite directions. These waves will interfere. If the frequency is just right, the resulting wave seems to stand still; the rope continues to vibrate up and down, but the resultant wave no longer travels. The combination of these traveling waves produces a **standing wave**, with the horizontal positions of the crests and troughs remaining fixed.

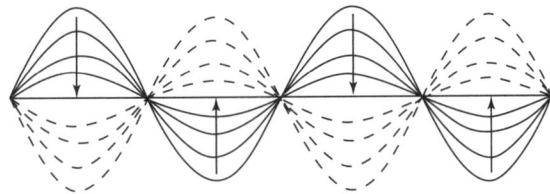

Notice that each point along the rope has its own amplitude. Some points don't vibrate up and down at all; these points are called **nodes** (points of <u>no</u> displacement). Halfway between any two consecutive nodes are points where the amplitude is maximized; these positions are called **antinodes**. Every other point has an amplitude that's smaller than the amplitude at the antinode positions.

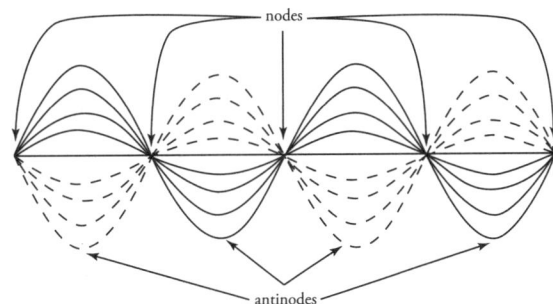

To figure out the conditions under which a standing wave will be formed, we'll look at the three simplest standing waves. In the figure at the top of the next page, we have a rope of length L. The first picture shows the simplest standing wave that can form if we have nodes at the two ends; the second and third pictures show the next simplest standing waves that the rope could support.

The distance between any two consecutive nodes is always one-half of the wavelength. The first picture shows us that one of these half-wavelengths is equal to L; in the second picture, two half-wavelengths are equal to L; and in the third picture, three half-wavelengths are equal to L.

Notice the pattern that emerges relating the length of the rope and the wavelength of the standing wave.

First
Harmonic
(Fundamental)

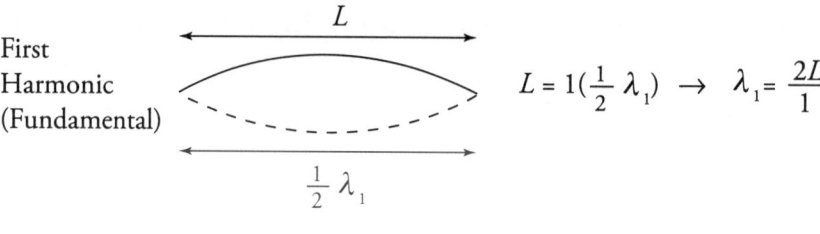

$$L = 1\left(\tfrac{1}{2}\lambda_1\right) \;\rightarrow\; \lambda_1 = \frac{2L}{1}$$

Second
Harmonic

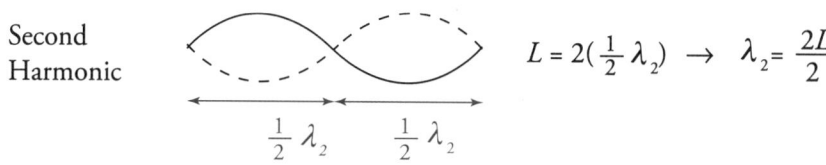

$$L = 2\left(\tfrac{1}{2}\lambda_2\right) \;\rightarrow\; \lambda_2 = \frac{2L}{2}$$

Third
Harmonic

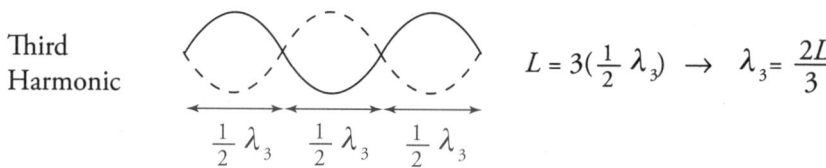

$$L = 3\left(\tfrac{1}{2}\lambda_3\right) \;\rightarrow\; \lambda_3 = \frac{2L}{3}$$

The only standing waves that can be supported are those for which the length of the rope is equal to a whole number of half-wavelengths, so the wavelength must be twice the length of the rope divided by a whole number:

> **Standing-Wave Wavelengths for Two Fixed Ends**
>
> $$\lambda_n = \frac{2L}{n} \quad \text{where} \quad n = 1, 2, 3\ldots$$

The number n is called the **harmonic number**. The first harmonic is usually called the **fundamental** because once we know the **fundamental wavelength**, λ_1, we automatically know all the other harmonic wavelengths, because we can write λ_n in terms of λ_1, like this: $\lambda_n = \lambda_1/n$.

Because the equation $v = \lambda f$ must always be true, and only certain wavelengths are allowed for a standing wave, then only certain frequencies will give standing waves. To find the harmonic frequencies, we just write $\lambda_n f_n = v$, and solve for f_n:

> **Standing-Wave Frequencies for Two Fixed Ends**
>
> $$f_n = \frac{n}{2L}v \quad \text{where} \quad n = 1, 2, 3\ldots$$

In the same way that the fundamental wavelength can be used to figure out all the other harmonic wavelengths, the fundamental frequency can be used to figure out all the other harmonic frequencies: $f_n = nf_1$. Memorizing this equation is helpful for the MCAT.

It is possible to create standing waves with only one fixed end (node) and one non-fixed end (antinode), but the appropriate formulas to find frequency and wavelength for this situation are discussed in Chapter 12. Regardless of the type of standing wave, the formula to find the appropriate harmonic from the fundamental frequency still holds ($f_n = nf_1$).

Example 11-14: If a rope of length 6 m supports a standing wave with exactly four nodes (which includes the ends of the rope), what is the wavelength of the standing wave?

Solution: Draw the standing wave. It should look just like the third harmonic drawn on the previous page. Therefore, the wavelength is $\lambda_3 = 2L/3 = 2(6 \text{ m})/3 = 4$ m.

Example 11-15: The speed of a transverse traveling wave along a certain 4-meter-long rope is 24 m/s. Which of the following frequencies could cause a standing wave to form on this rope, assuming both ends of the rope are fixed?

    A.   32 Hz
    B.   33 Hz
    C.   34 Hz
    D.   35 Hz

Solution: The fundamental frequency for this rope is $f_1 = (1/2L)v = 3$ Hz. All harmonic frequencies are whole-number multiples of the fundamental, so any frequency that could cause a standing wave to form on the rope must be a multiple of 3 Hz. Of the choices given, only choice B, 33 Hz, is a multiple of 3 Hz.

Example 11-16: For a particular rope, it's found that the fundamental frequency is 6 Hz. What's the third-harmonic frequency?

Solution: From the equation $f_n = nf_1$, we get $f_3 = 3f_1 = 3(6 \text{ Hz}) = 18$ Hz.

Example 11-17: For a particular rope, it's found that the second-harmonic frequency is 8 Hz. What's the fifth-harmonic frequency?

Solution: The equation $f_n = nf_1$ gives us $f_2 = 2f_1$. This means that $f_1 = f_2/2 = (8 \text{ Hz})/2 = 4$ Hz. Therefore, $f_5 = 5f_1 = 5(4 \text{ Hz}) = 20$ Hz.

Example 11-18: The second-harmonic wavelength for a rope fixed at both ends is 0.5 m. How fast do transverse waves travel along this rope if the fundamental frequency is 4 Hz?

Solution: Using the equation $\lambda_n = \lambda_1/n$, we get $\lambda_2 = \lambda_1/2$. This means that $\lambda_1 = 2\lambda_2 = 2(0.5 \text{ m}) = 1$ m. Now, multiplying any harmonic wavelength by its corresponding harmonic frequency will give us the wave speed. In particular, we have $v = \lambda_1 f_1$, so $v = (1 \text{ m})(4 \text{ Hz}) = 4$ m/s.

Summary of Formulas

Simple Harmonic Motion [SHM] requires:

- dynamics condition: restoring force is directly proportional to displacement from equilibrium ($x = 0$) and points towards that equilibrium point

- kinematics condition: frequency and period are independent of the amplitude of oscillations

Hooke's law [spring]: $F = -kx$

Elastic potential energy [spring]: $PE_{elastic} = \frac{1}{2}kx^2$

Spring-block oscillator frequency: $f = \dfrac{1}{2\pi}\sqrt{\dfrac{k}{m}}$

Simple pendulum frequency [small oscillations]: $f = \dfrac{1}{2\pi}\sqrt{\dfrac{g}{l}}$

Period/frequency
[all harmonic motion and waves]: $T = 1/f$

Wave equation: $v = \lambda f$

Two Big Rules for Waves to be used with wave equation:

1] Wave speed v depends on wave type and the medium, not on frequency

2] A single wave passing between media maintains a constant frequency

Standing wave on a rope [both ends fixed nodes]

Standing-wave wavelengths: $\lambda_n = \dfrac{2L}{n}$ $(n = 1, 2, 3, \ldots)$

$\lambda_n = \dfrac{\lambda_1}{n}$

Standing-wave frequencies: $f_n = \dfrac{n}{2L}v$ $(n = 1, 2, 3, \ldots)$

$f_n = nf_1$

CHAPTER 11 FREESTANDING PRACTICE QUESTIONS

1. A 2 kg mass is attached to a massless, 0.5 m string and is used as a simple pendulum by extending it to an angle $\theta = 5°$ and allowing it to oscillate. Which of the following changes will increase the period of the pendulum?

A) Replacing the mass with a 1 kg mass
B) Changing the initial extension of the pendulum to a 10° angle
C) Replacing the string with a 0.25 m string
D) Moving the pendulum to the surface of the moon

2. A 100 kg bungee jumper attached to a bungee cord jumps off a bridge. The bungee cord stretches and the man reaches the lowest spot in his descent before beginning to rise. The force of the stretched bungee cord can be approximated using Hooke's law, where the value of the spring constant is replaced by an elasticity constant, in this case, 100 kg/s². If the cord is stretched by 30 m beyond its vertical equilibrium length at the lowest spot of the man's descent, then what his acceleration at the lowest spot?

A) 0 m/s²
B) 10 m/s²
C) 20 m/s²
D) 30 m/s²

3. A physics student is doing a wave experiment with a 1 m long cord stretched across the lab table. In the middle of the cord, a 1 cm section is painted red. A specially designed machine creates vibrations so that a sine wave will travel on the cord from the east side of the table to the west side of the table. The vibrations of the sine wave are parallel to the table and peak at the north side of the table and the south side of the table. Which of the following best describes the motion of the red spot?

A) The spot moves from east to west along the sine wave.
B) The spot moves from west to east along the sine wave.
C) The spot remains in a fixed location on the table.
D) The spot vibrates between the north side and south side of the table.

4. A parent is pushing a young child on a swing at the playground. When the parent stops pushing, the child's swinging motion continues without assistance. Assume the chain on the swing has negligible mass and any friction is negligible. Which of the following would need to be true in order for the child's motion on the swing to be considered simple harmonic motion?

   I. The mass of the child is not too large
  II. The child is not swinging too high, so the angle between the swing and the vertical is not too big
 III. The tension in the chain of the swing is negligible

A) I only
B) II only
C) I and III
D) I, II, and III

5. Immediately before a performance, a musician breaks a guitar string. The only string available to repair the guitar is twice the linear density of the string normally used. How can the musician adjust the new string so that it will still have the correct frequency? (Note: $v = (\text{Tension}/\mu)^{0.5}$, where μ = linear mass density.)

A) The tension of the new string should be twice the tension of the old string.
B) The tension of the new string should be half the tension of the old string.
C) The amplitude of the new string should be twice the amplitude of the old string.
D) The amplitude of the new string should be half the amplitude of the old string.

6. The speed of a 2 kg mass on a spring is 4 m/s as it passes through its equilibrium position. What is its frequency if the amplitude is 2 m?

A) 1/5 Hz
B) 1/3 Hz
C) 3 Hz
D) 5 Hz

7. The distance from a trough to a crest is 20 cm on a 3 m rope of 1 kg. If the tension in the rope is 3 N, what is the period? (Note: $v = $ [tension/linear density]$^{0.5}$)

A) 1/15 s
B) 2/15 s
C) 15/2 s
D) 15 s

CHAPTER 11 PRACTICE PASSAGE

A physics student conducts an experiment to study pendulums. Using an apparatus known as *Newton's cradle*, the student conducts two different trials. The Newton's cradle apparatus consists of five identical steel balls of equal size and mass. Each ball is suspended from two wires that connect it to a frame, so that the ball is in the air and can move side to side in a single plane. The balls are suspended so that they are touching each other and are free to move individually or as a group. Each ball can be considered a simple pendulum since the hanging wires have negligible mass. Assume there is no friction in the pendulum mechanism.

For the first trial, Ball A is raised at an angle, θ, from the vertical and let go. The ball swings down and hits Ball B. Kinetic energy is transferred through Balls B, C, and D to Ball E, causing Ball E to swing up to a maximum angle, θ, from the vertical on the right while Balls A, B, C, and D are stationary. Then Ball E swings down and hits Ball D, transferring kinetic energy through Balls D, C, and B to Ball A, causing Ball A to swing up again to the same maximum angle, θ, from the vertical while Balls E, D, C, and B are stationary. The period for this motion is measured to be 1.5 seconds.

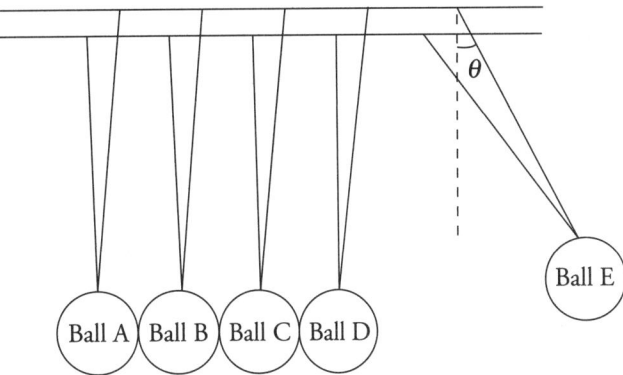

Figure 2 Newton's Cradle Apparatus after transfer of kinetic energy to Ball E during Trial 1

For the second trial, both Ball A and Ball B are lifted together to the same angle, θ, as in the first trial. The result of the swing is that both Ball D and Ball E swing up on the right with the same displacement angle, θ.

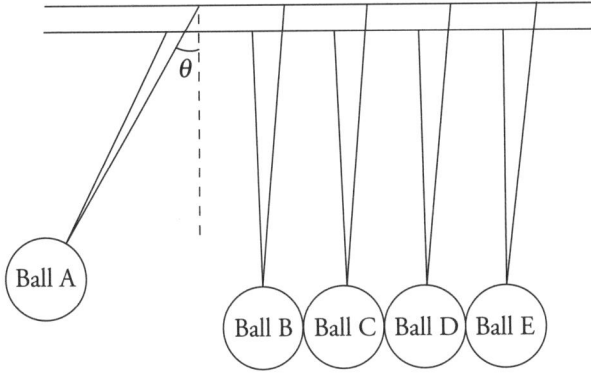

Figure 1 Newton's Cradle Apparatus with Ball A raised at the start of Trial 1

1. Which of the following is true when Ball E is at half of its maximum height as measured from its lowest point?

   I. The kinetic energy is half of the total mechanical energy.
  II. The velocity is half of the maximum velocity of the ball.
 III. The time elapsed from the time Ball E started in motion to the time it reached half of its maximum height is half of the period.

A) I only
B) I and III
C) II and III
D) I, II, and III

2. What should be the measured period in Trial 2?

A) 1.0 seconds
B) 1.5 seconds
C) 2.0 seconds
D) 3.0 seconds

3. For Ball E, how does the maximum velocity in Trial 2, v_2, compare to the maximum velocity in Trial 1, v_1?

A) $v_2 = (1/2)v_1$
B) $v_2 = \left(1\sqrt{2}\right)v_1$
C) $v_2 = v_1$
D) $v_2 = 2v_1$

4. To help record results, the student attached pens of negligible mass to balls A and E and scrolled paper perpendicular to the axis of motion of the Newton's cradle. The paper scrolls at a rate of 20 cm/s underneath the pens during the trials. What is the wavelength of the resulting wave graphed in Trial 1 (assume the pens are rigged to align parallel to the paper when the cradle isn't in motion)?

A) 13 cm
B) 20 cm
C) 30 cm
D) 33 cm

5. If L is the length of each string, what is the maximum height of Ball E in Trial 1 above its lowest position?

A) $L - \cos\theta$
B) $L - L\cos\theta$
C) $L + L\cos\theta$
D) $L\cos\theta$

SOLUTIONS TO CHAPTER 11 FREESTANDING QUESTIONS

1. **D** Based on the equation $T = 2\pi\sqrt{\frac{L}{g}}$, we know that the period does not depend on either the mass or the initial angle of extension, eliminating choices A and B. Furthermore, we know that decreasing the length of the string will decrease the period, eliminating choice C. Moving the pendulum to the surface of the moon will lower the gravitational acceleration, which would increase the period. Therefore, choice D is correct.

2. **C** A force diagram of the jumper at the lowest spot is shown below.

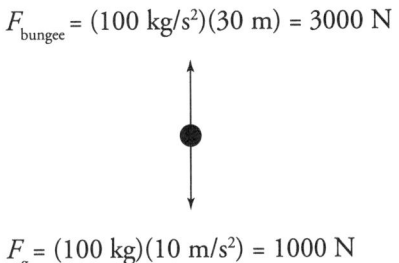

$$F_{\text{bungee}} = (100 \text{ kg/s}^2)(30 \text{ m}) = 3000 \text{ N}$$

$$F_g = (100 \text{ kg})(10 \text{ m/s}^2) = 1000 \text{ N}$$

Since the force up is greater than the force down, there is a net upward force of 2000 N on the jumper and an upward acceleration. Acceleration = F/m = (2000 N)/(100 kg) = 20 m/s^2.

3. **D** A sine wave is a transverse wave, so the vibration direction is perpendicular to the direction of propagation. The question states that the wave vibrates between the north and south and propagates from east to west. The red spot is simply a part of the cord and will vibrate in the same direction the cord is vibrating (choice C is wrong), namely between the north and south. Since a wave only transports energy, not material, it would be impossible for the spot to propagate along the wave, eliminating choices A and B and leaving choice D as the correct answer.

4. **B** Simple harmonic motion is by definition when the restoring force is proportional to the displacement of the object. In this case, the swing is similar to a simple pendulum (a simple pendulum has no mass in the material connecting the end of the pendulum to the rotation point, and the question states the chain has negligible mass). For a simple pendulum to experience simple harmonic motion, the restoring force must be proportional to the displacement. In this case, the displacement is the angle, θ, between the swing and the vertical. The restoring force is the component of the weight directed toward the vertical. For a child of mass, m, the restoring force is $mg \sin \theta$. If the angle is small, then $\sin \theta$ approximates θ, so the motion is considered simple harmonic motion. Thus, Item II is true, eliminating choices A and C. Item I is false: The mass of the child will impact the magnitude of the restoring force, but will not indicate whether the motion is simple harmonic motion (choice D can be eliminated and choice B is correct). Item III is also false: The tension in the chain will have a variable value that depends upon the component of the weight directed along the chain, but it will have no impact on whether the motion is simple harmonic motion.

5. **A**   The amplitude of the wave on the string will not impact the frequency of the wave or the wave speed, eliminating choices C and D. Since the frequency = wave speed / wavelength, in order to keep the frequency constant, the wave speed should be kept constant. Wave speed is proportional to the square root of tension / linear density ($v = (\text{Tension}/\mu)^{0.5}$) and since linear density is doubled, then tension should also be doubled in order to keep wave speed constant. The correct answer is choice A.

6. **B**   The kinetic energy is at a maximum at the equilibrium position, and is equal to the potential energy at the amplitude: $\frac{1}{2}kA^2 = \frac{1}{2}mv_{max}^2$. This equation can be solved for the spring constant, $k = 8$ N/m. The spring constant and the mass are all you need to determine the frequency from $f = \frac{1}{2\pi}\sqrt{k/m}$, giving a frequency of approximately 0.33 Hz.

7. **B**   The speed of the wave is $\sqrt{3/(\frac{1}{3})} = 3$ m/s. From $v = f\lambda$, and knowing that the wavelength is 40 cm $= \frac{2}{5}$ m, the frequency is 15/2 Hz, making the period $\frac{2}{15}$ s.

SOLUTIONS TO CHAPTER 11 PRACTICE PASSAGE

1. **A**   When Ball E is at its maximum height, all of its energy is potential energy and

   $E_{total} = PE_{max} = mgh_{max}$. When Ball E is at half of its maximum height, its potential energy is

   $mg(\frac{1}{2})h_{max} = (\frac{1}{2})PE_{max} = (\frac{1}{2})E_{total}$. Since the total mechanical energy is the sum of the po-

   tential energy and the kinetic energy, then the other half of the total energy must be kinetic

   energy. Item I is true (choice C can be eliminated). When the ball is at its lowest point, all

   of its mechanical energy will be kinetic energy and $E_{total} = KE_{max} = \frac{1}{2}mv^2_{max}$. As discussed

   above, at half the maximum height, half the total mechanical energy is kinetic energy. So

   $\frac{1}{2}E_{total} = \frac{1}{2}KE_{max} = \frac{1}{4}mv^2_{max} = KE_{half}$. The kinetic energy can also be calculated using the

   velocity at the half height, v_{half}. So $KE_{half} = \frac{1}{2}mv^2_{half} = \frac{1}{4}mv^2_{max}$ and $v_{half} = \frac{1}{\sqrt{2}}v_{max}$. Item

   II is false (choice D can be eliminated). The period is the time for one full cycle. This is

   the time from Ball A dropping, through Ball E rising, Ball E dropping, and Ball A rising

   again. The entire time Ball E is moving is half of the period. The time for it to rise half way

   is approximately 1/8 of the entire period. Item III is false (choice B can be eliminated). The

   correct answer is choice A.

2. **B**   Period depends on the length of the wire and the acceleration due to gravity $T = 2\pi\sqrt{\frac{L}{g}}$.
   Neither of these changed between Trial 1 and Trial 2, so the period should be the same in
   Trial 2 as in Trial 1. The correct answer is choice B.

3. **C**   For a pendulum, the maximum velocity is at the lowest point (when $\theta = 0$). For Ball E, this
   occurs after the collision of Ball A, and again after falling from its maximum height. For
   both trials, since the angle of displacement is the same for Ball E, then the height of the ball
   is the same, the maximum potential energy is the same, the maximum kinetic energy is the
   same, and the maximum velocity is the same. The correct answer is choice C. (Note: The
   total mechanical energy for the system will be doubled in Trial 2 compared to Trial 1, but
   the question is asking specifically about Ball E, not the whole system.)

4. **C**   The rate of the paper is the rate of propagation of the wave. Since $v = f\lambda$, and $f = 1/T$, we
   have that $\lambda = vT$. Then, $\lambda = (20 \text{ cm/s})(1.5 \text{ s}) = 30$ cm. The correct answer is choice C.

5.   **B**   The easiest way to solve this is to remember that at $\theta = 0°$ the height = 0. Plugging in 0° for the angle in each of the answer choices, only choice B gives the correct value of height = 0, eliminating choices A, C, and D. Another (longer) way solve the question is using a sketch like the one below.

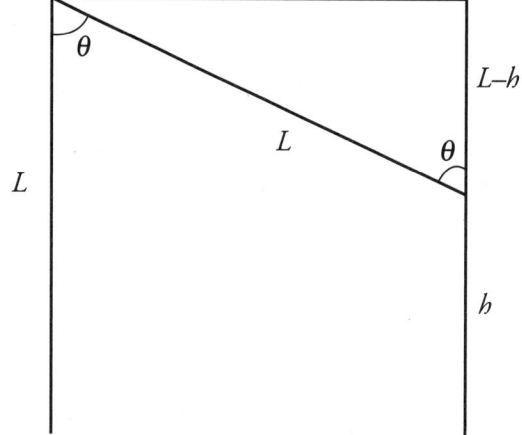

Using the sketch and basic trigonometry the equation is $\cos \theta = (L - h)/L$ and $h = L - L \cos \theta$. The correct answer is choice B.

Chapter 12
Sound

12.1 SOUND WAVES

Sound waves don't travel in the same way that waves on a rope do. The waves we've looked at so far are transverse waves: The direction in which the particles of the conducting medium oscillate is perpendicular to the direction in which the wave travels. If, however, the direction in which the particles of the conducting medium oscillate is *parallel* to the direction in which the wave travels, we call the wave **longitudinal**. Sound waves (also known as compression waves) are longitudinal waves in gas, liquid, or solid; when a compression wave's frequency is between 20 Hz and 20 kHz, humans can perceive it as what we commonly call sound.

Let's take a closer look at sound waves. As a stereo speaker, vocal fold, or tuning fork vibrates, it creates regions of high pressure (**compressions**) that alternate with regions of low pressure (**rarefactions**). These pressure waves are transmitted through the air (or some other medium) and can eventually reach our ears and brain, which translate the vibrations into sound.

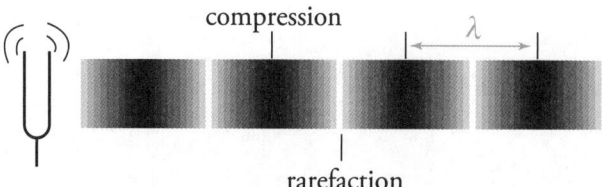

Like other waves, a longitudinal compression wave has a wavelength, a speed, a frequency, a period, and an amplitude. The equation $v = \lambda f$ holds, as do the two Big Rules for waves.

Sound can travel in any medium: gas, liquid, or solid. Its speed depends on two things: the medium's resistance to compression (quantified by its *bulk modulus B*) and its density, according to the equation $v_{sound} = \sqrt{\dfrac{B}{\rho}}$.

On the MCAT, knowing the relationship is good enough—you won't have to calculate the speed of sound in a given medium. However, you should know that in general, *sound travels slowest through gases, faster through liquids, and fastest through solids.* The speed of sound in air is about 340 m/s (that's about 760 miles per hour), but it varies slightly with temperature, pressure, and humidity.

Example 12-1: A sound wave of frequency 440 Hz (this note is *concert A*, or the A above middle C) travels at a speed of 344 m/s through the air in a concert hall. How fast would a note one octave higher, 880 Hz, travel through the same concert hall?

- A. 172 m/s
- B. 344 m/s
- C. 516 m/s
- D. 688 m/s

Solution: Altering the frequency will not affect the wave speed. Remember Big Rule 1 for waves. Therefore, the answer is B.

Example 12-2: A siren produces sound waves in the air. If the frequency of the waves is gradually decreasing, which of the following changes to the waves is most likely also occurring?

    A. The wavelength is increasing.
    B. The wave speed is decreasing.
    C. The amplitude is decreasing.
    D. The period is decreasing.

Solution: Because the wave speed is set by the medium (the air, in this case), the wave speed is a constant. Since $v = \lambda f$, this means that λ and f are inversely proportional. So, if f is decreasing, then λ must be increasing, choice A.

Example 12-3: What is the wavelength of a sound wave of frequency 170 Hz if the wave speed is 340 m/s?

Solution: Using $v = \lambda f$ we find that $\lambda = v/f = (340 \text{ m/s})/(170 \text{ Hz}) = 2$ m.

Example 12-4: A typical medical ultrasound scan uses frequencies in the MHz range. What would happen to an ultrasound signal as it passed from air into body tissues?

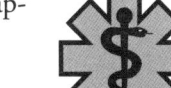

    A. Its wavelength and speed would both decrease.
    B. Its wavelength and speed would both increase.
    C. Its wavelength would decrease and its speed would increase.
    D. Its wavelength would increase and its speed would decrease.

Solution: When a wave passes into a new medium, its frequency does not change (the specific frequency range is irrelevant). Therefore, when traveling through the body, the frequency of the sound wave will be the same as it was in the air. However, we know that sound waves generally travel faster through liquids and solids than they do through gases, so we'd expect the wave speed through the body to be faster. Because the equation $v = \lambda f$ is always true, the same f at a faster v means a greater wavelength. Therefore, the answer is B. (Note that almost all of the ultrasound wave would reflect off the skin if it were incident on it from air: this is why a gel is first applied to the skin before the emitter/detector is placed on the skin, so that no air interrupts the signal.)

Example 12-5: When a longitudinal compression wave of frequency 700 Hz travels through a brass rod, its wavelength is 5 m. How fast does sound travel through brass?

Solution: Using $v = \lambda f$, we find that $v = (5 \text{ m})(700 \text{ Hz}) = 3500$ m/s.

12.2 STANDING SOUND WAVES IN PIPES

Just as we can have standing waves on a rope caused by the interference of two oppositely directed transverse waves with equal amplitudes, standing sound waves in a pipe can be caused by the interference of two oppositely directed longitudinal waves of equal amplitude.

The analysis of these standing waves is similar to that of a string attached at each end. In that case, the ends correspond to nodes (because there is no motion). Since the distance between nodes is some whole number of half-wavelengths, this gave us formulas for the different frequencies and wavelengths that the standing waves can have. In the case of pipes, we also need to know what corresponds to each end. The ends of a pipe can either be open to the atmosphere or closed.

It turns out that the open end of a pipe (technically, just beyond it) corresponds to an antinode. To be more specific, these are often referred to as displacement antinodes (maximum displacement). They are also called pressure nodes (constant pressure). The closed end of a pipe corresponds to a displacement node (no motion) or a pressure antinode (maximum pressure fluctuations). The pressure varies most where there is no motion and the motion varies most where there is constant pressure.

Pipes are often classified as *open pipes* (open on each end) or *closed pipes* (open on one end and closed on the other).

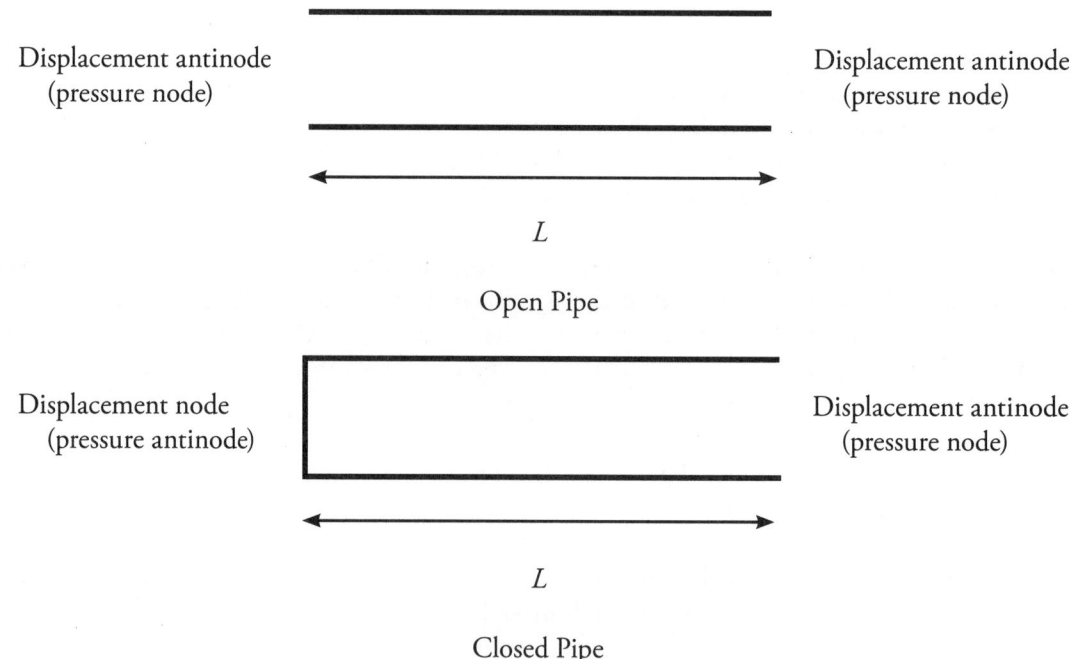

Displacement antinode (pressure node) — Displacement antinode (pressure node)

L

Open Pipe

Displacement node (pressure antinode) — Displacement antinode (pressure node)

L

Closed Pipe

In the case of the open pipe, the distance between displacement antinodes (or pressure nodes) is equal to a whole number of half-wavelengths. The formulas for wavelength and frequency are therefore the same as for the string attached at each end: $\lambda_n = 2L / n$ and $f_n = nv / 2L$, where the harmonic number, n, is any positive whole number, and v now refers to the speed of sound in air.

To visualize the harmonic modes, it is convenient to represent the standing waves as transverse.

L

First Harmonic (Fundamental)

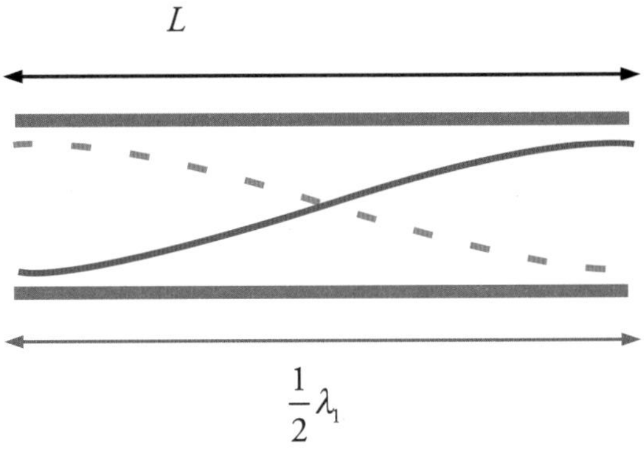

$$L = 1\left(\frac{1}{2}\lambda_1\right) \rightarrow \lambda_1 = \frac{2L}{1}$$

$\frac{1}{2}\lambda_1$

Second Harmonic

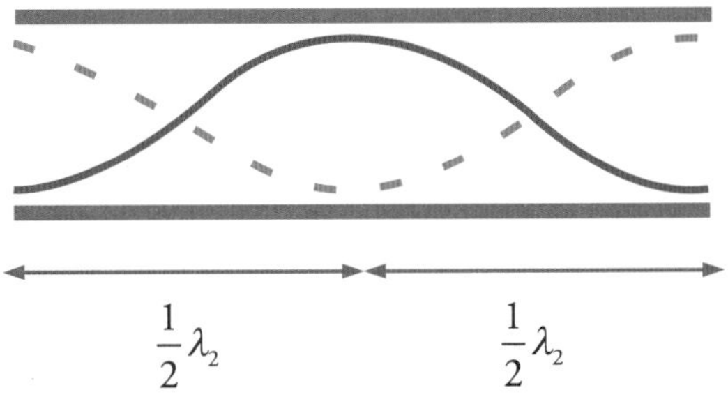

$$L = 2\left(\frac{1}{2}\lambda_2\right) \rightarrow \lambda_2 = \frac{2L}{2}$$

$\frac{1}{2}\lambda_2$ $\frac{1}{2}\lambda_2$

Third Harmonic

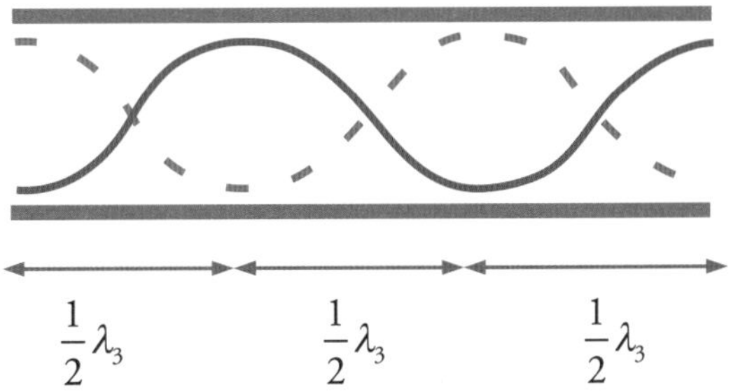

$$L = 3\left(\frac{1}{2}\lambda_3\right) \rightarrow \lambda_3 = \frac{2L}{3}$$

$\frac{1}{2}\lambda_3$ $\frac{1}{2}\lambda_3$ $\frac{1}{2}\lambda_3$

In the case of the closed pipe, the distance between a displacement antinode (or pressure node) and a displacement node (or pressure antinode) is equal to an *odd* number of *quarter*-wavelengths. As a result, $\lambda_n = 4L / n$ and $f_n = nv / 4L$, where n (which is still called the harmonic) is an *odd* number.

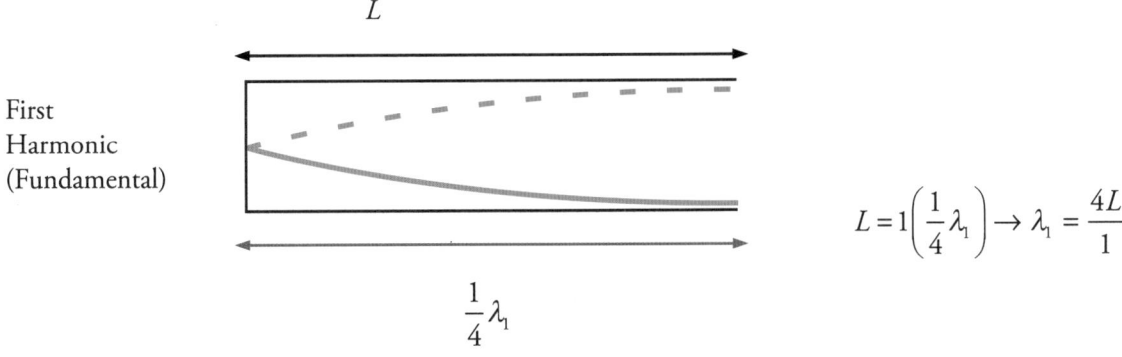

L

First Harmonic (Fundamental)

$$L = 1\left(\frac{1}{4}\lambda_1\right) \rightarrow \lambda_1 = \frac{4L}{1}$$

$\frac{1}{4}\lambda_1$

12.3

Third
Harmonic

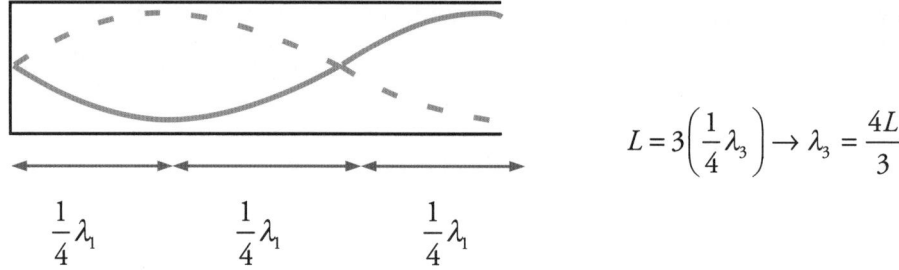

$$L = 3\left(\frac{1}{4}\lambda_3\right) \rightarrow \lambda_3 = \frac{4L}{3}$$

$\frac{1}{4}\lambda_1$ $\frac{1}{4}\lambda_1$ $\frac{1}{4}\lambda_1$

Note that for all types of resonance, $f_n = nf_1$ and $\lambda_n = \lambda_1 / n$.

Example 12-6: An organ pipe that is closed at one end has a length of 3 m. What is the second-longest harmonic wavelength for sound waves in this pipe?

   A.   3 m
   B.   4 m
   C.   6 m
   D.   9 m

Solution: Because one end of the pipe is closed, the length of the pipe, L, must be an *odd* number of *quarter*-wavelengths: $L = 1(\lambda/4), 3(\lambda/4), 5(\lambda/4)\ldots$, in order to support standing waves. Therefore, the possible harmonic wavelengths are $\lambda = 4L/1, 4L/3, 4L/5$, and so on. The second longest is $\lambda = 4L/3 = 4(3\text{ m})/3 = 4$ m, choice B.

Example 12-7: An organ pipe that is open at both ends has a length of 3 m. What is the second-longest harmonic wavelength for sound waves in this pipe?

   A.   3 m
   B.   4 m
   C.   6 m
   D.   9 m

Solution: Because both ends of the pipe are open, the length of the pipe, L, must be a whole number of half-wavelengths: $L = 1(\lambda/2), 2(\lambda/2), 3(\lambda/2)\ldots$, in order to support standing waves. Therefore, the possible harmonic wavelengths are $\lambda = 2L/1, 2L/2, 2L/3$, and so on. The second longest is $\lambda = 2L/2 = L = 3$ m, choice A.

12.3 BEATS

In the previous chapter, it was mentioned that if two waves with different frequency interfere, the resultant wave will be complicated. If the two waves are sound waves with slightly different frequencies (the difference is less than about 10 Hz), the product is a pulsating, "wobbling" resultant wave. This produces the phenomenon known as **beats**. Because the frequencies don't match, sometimes the waves are in phase and sometimes they're out of phase. When they're in phase, their amplitudes add; when they're out of phase, their amplitudes subtract. The combined waveform reaches its maximum amplitude when the waves interfere constructively and its minimum amplitude when they interfere destructively, and these points alternate. Maximum amplitude sounds loud and minimum amplitude sounds soft, so we hear loud, soft, loud, soft, etc. The resulting equally spaced moments of constructive interference (the loud moments) are the beats.

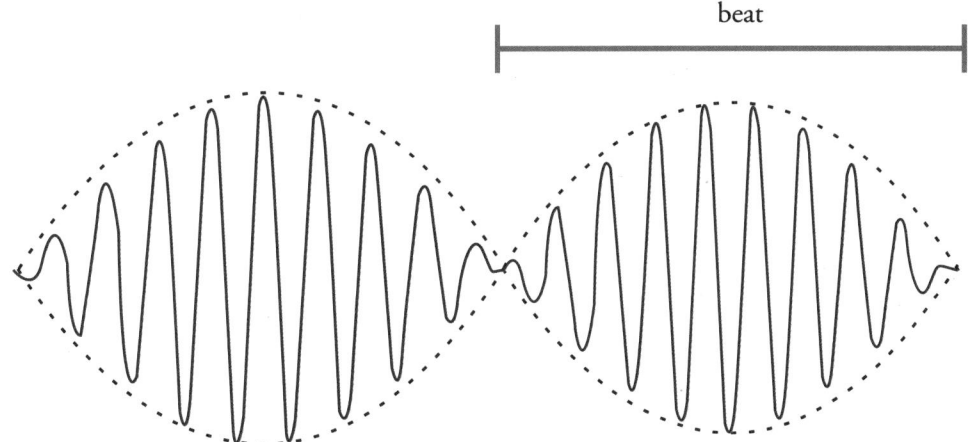

The frequency at which the beats are heard (the **beat frequency**) is equal to the difference between the frequencies of the two original sound waves. Therefore, if one of these waves has frequency f_1 and the other has frequency f_2, then $f_{beat} = |f_1 - f_2|$.

Beat Frequency

$$f_{beat} = |f_1 - f_2|$$

Example 12-8: A piano tuner strikes a tuning fork at the same time he strikes a piano key with a note of similar pitch. If he hears 3 beats per second, and the tuning fork produces a standard 440 Hz tone, then what must be the frequency produced by the struck piano string?

    A.   437 Hz
    B.   443 Hz
    C.   437 Hz or 443 Hz
    D.   434 Hz or 446 Hz

Solution: If f_{beat} = 3 Hz, then the frequencies of the tuning fork and piano string are "off" by 3 Hz. The frequency produced by the piano string might be 3 Hz lower or 3 Hz higher than the tuning fork; without more information, we don't know which one. If the tuning fork produces a tone of frequency 440 Hz, the piano string produces a frequency of either 440 − 3 = 437 Hz or 440 + 3 = 443 Hz. Choice C is the answer.

12.4 INTENSITY AND INTENSITY LEVEL

Intensity and intensity level are closely related quantities. The **intensity** of a sound wave (or, indeed, any wave) is the energy it transmits per second (the power) per unit area. It is measured in W/m^2. For a point source (i.e., one that creates waves that travel uniformly in all directions), the area in the equation is the surface area of a sphere, which equals $4\pi r^2$. Each wavefront in the figure below can be thought of as a bundle of energy that is expanding in size, much like a balloon being blown up. The farther a detector is from the source, the larger the bundle of energy will be, and therefore the detector will receive a smaller fraction of it.

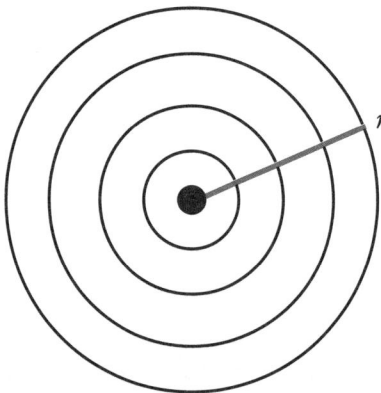

Mathematically, the important fact to remember is that, for a point source, intensity varies inversely as the square of the distance r from that source: $I \propto 1/r^2$. If the detector of a wave doubles his distance from the source, the power produced by the wave will spread out over an area that is $2^2 = 4$ times larger, causing the detector to receive ¼ as much. Intensity is also proportional to the square of the amplitude of a wave.

Since the intensity that we can hear spans an impressively large range (about twelve orders of magnitude!), we use logarithms to make the numbers easier to handle. The **threshold of hearing**, which is roughly the lowest intensity the human ear can perceive as sound at the common middle frequencies, is equal to 10^{-12} W/m^2; this intensity is denoted by I_0. The **intensity level** (or **sound level**) of a sound wave whose intensity is I is equal to the base-10 logarithm of the ratio I/I_0. The unit of intensity level is the **bel**, abbreviated **B**. Usually, we multiply this by 10 to get the intensity level, β, in **decibels** (dB):

Intensity Level in Decibels

$$\beta = 10 \log_{10} \frac{I}{I_0}$$

The most important relationship to get from this equation can be summarized as follows:

Every time we *multiply* I by 10, we *add* 10 to β.

Every time we *divide* I by 10, we *subtract* 10 from β.

For example, if the intensity is multiplied by 10,000, which is $10 \times 10 \times 10 \times 10$, the intensity level in decibels is increased by adding $10 + 10 + 10 + 10 = 40$. If we divide by the intensity by, say, $100,000 = 10^5$, then the decibel level decreases by 50.

Example 12-9: At a distance of 1 m, the intensity level of a soft whisper is about 30 dB, while a normal speaking voice is about 60 dB. How many times greater is the power delivered per unit area by a normal-speaking voice than by a whisper?[1]

 A. 2.5
 B. 30
 C. 1000
 D. 3000

Solution: The normal speaking voice has an intensity level that's 30 dB greater than the whisper. Therefore, the intensity must be $10 \times 10 \times 10 = 10^3 = 1000$ times greater. Since "power delivered per unit area" *is* intensity, the answer is C.

Example 12-10: A person listening to music on a stereo system experiences a sound level of 70 dB. If the volume dial is turned up to increase the intensity by a factor of 500, what sound level would this person hear now?

 A. 97 dB
 B. 105 dB
 C. 115 dB
 D. 120 dB

Solution: If the intensity had increased by a factor of 100, which is 10×10, the sound level would have increased by $10 + 10 = 20$ dB. If the intensity had increased by a factor of 1000, which is $10 \times 10 \times 10$, the sound level would have increased by $10 + 10 + 10 = 30$ dB. The fact that the intensity increased by a factor of 500, which is between 100 and 1000, means that the sound level increased by between 20 dB and 30 dB. If the original sound level was 70 dB, then the new sound level must be between $70 + 20 = 90$ dB and $70 + 30 = 100$ dB. Only choice A falls in this range.

Example 12-11: Suppose one moves 10 times further away from a loud siren of constant power. What is the resultant decrease in sound level?

 A. 10 dB
 B. 20 dB
 C. 40 dB
 D. 100 dB

Solution: Increasing distance by a factor of 10 decreases intensity by a factor of 100, which is 10×10. Therefore, sound level will be reduced by $10 + 10 = 20$ dB, choice B.

---

[1] Our perception of loudness is completely different from both intensity and intensity level. Roughly speaking, a difference in intensity level of 10 dB (and therefore a factor of 10 in intensity) corresponds to a perceived loudness difference of a factor of 2.

12.5 THE DOPPLER EFFECT

Suppose a train that is loudly sounding its horn is approaching a passenger waiting on a platform. As the train is approaching, the person hears the pitch at a higher frequency than does the engineer on the train. As the train is moving away, the person on the platform hears a lower frequency than does the engineer. These differences in frequency are the result of the **Doppler effect**, which arises whenever a source of waves is moving relative to the detector. The result is that the *detected* frequency will be different from the frequency of the sound that was emitted from the *source*.

Normally when a sound is emitted from a source, the rate of the compressions (or frequency, f) emitted from the source is the same as the rate received at the detector. The most important fact to remember is that if the source and detector are moving *closer* together (no matter which is moving), the detected frequency with be *higher* than the emitted frequency. Similarly, if the source and detector are moving *farther apart*, the detected frequency will be *lower* than the emitted frequency.

Doppler Effect

approaching ↔ higher detected frequency

receding ↔ lower detected frequency

For sound, if the detector moves toward the source or if the source moves toward the detector, the detected frequency will be higher than the emitted frequency. But the reasons are different.

If a detector moves toward (or away from) a stationary source, the *relative* speed of sound changes. As an example, if a sound wave is moving toward the detector at 340 m/s and the detector moves toward the source at 20 m/s, the wave will be moving at 360 m/s in the detector's frame of reference. Similarly, if the detector is moving away from the source at 20 m/s, the wave will move at 320 m/s. The wavelength (i.e., the spacing between wavefronts) will not change. According to the wave equation, $v = \lambda f$, an increase (or decrease) in measured wave speed with a constant wavelength will cause an increase (or decrease) in detected frequency.

If the source moves, the waves themselves become distorted. Say a source emits a pulse that spreads out in all directions. The wavefront is a sphere, though in two dimensions it looks like a circle. If the source moves to the right the next pulse it emits would again look like a circle, but whose center is to the right of the previous pulse's center. The wavefronts bunch up on the right and spread out on the left. The wavelength has therefore changed. If the detector is at rest, then the speed of the wave hasn't changed. According to the wave equation, $v = \lambda f$, an increase (or decrease) in wavelength with a constant wave speed will result in a decrease (or increase) in frequency.

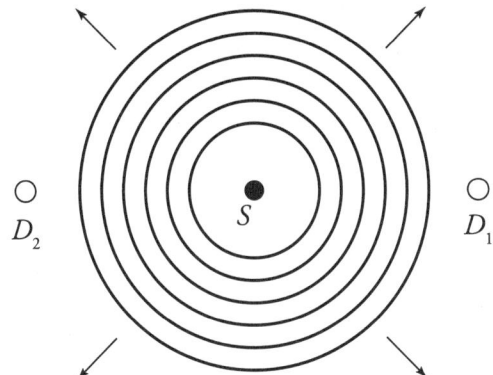

No relative motion between the source (S) and detectors (D_1 and D_2)

Each wave compression emitted by S arrives at the same speed when perceived by D_1 and D_2. The frequency is the same.

No Doppler shifts.

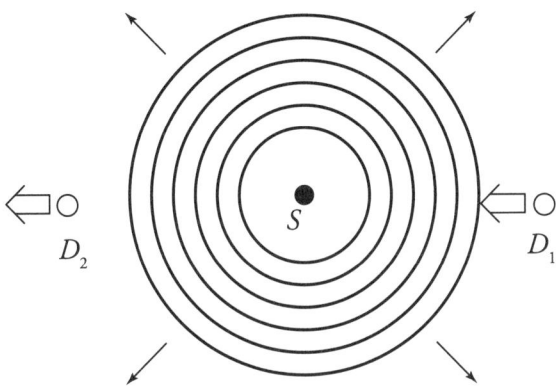

Here, there *is* relative motion between the source (S) and detectors (D_1 and D_2).

D_1 is approaching S, so each compression of the wave emitted from S requires less time to reach D_1. The measured wave speed at D_1 is faster, and thus the frequency at D_1 is higher.

D_2 is receding from S, so each compression of the wave requires more time to reach D_2. The measured wave speed at D_2 is slower, and thus the frequency is lower.

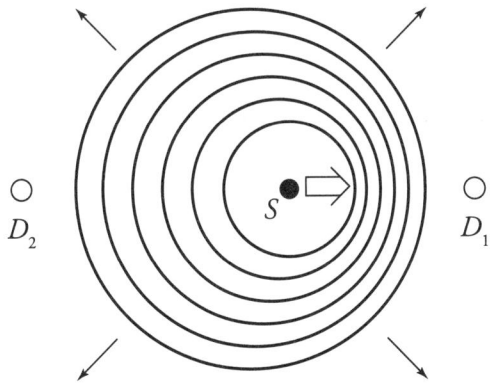

Here, there *is* relative motion between the source (S) and detectors (D_1 and D_2).

S is approaching D_1, so the compressions of the wave emitted from S are closer together. The wavelength at D_1 is shorter, and thus the frequency at D_1 is higher.

S is receding from D_2, so the compressions of the wave emitted from S are farther apart. The wavelength at D_2 is longer, and thus the frequency at D_2 is lower.

To predict exactly what the detected frequency will be, we need an equation. Despite the fact that there are lots of individual cases to consider (whether the source and/or the detector are stationary or in motion), we can summarize everything in a single equation:

Doppler Effect

$$f_D = f_S \frac{v \pm v_D}{v \mp v_S}$$

In this equation:

f_D = the frequency heard by the detector
f_S = the frequency emitted by the source
v_D = the speed at which the detector is moving
v_S = the speed at which the source is moving
v = the speed of the wave

What we need to do to make this one equation fit all the possible cases is use the conceptual relationships given in the box on the previous page to decide whether to use the + or − in the numerator and whether to use + or − in the denominator.

Notice that we have written ± in the numerator and ∓ in the denominator; one way to memorize the sign conventions for this equation is by the mnemonic "top sign is toward." When the motion of the detector is toward the source, you use the top of ±, or the "+" sign, in the numerator. When the motion of the source is toward the detector, you use the top of ∓, or the "−" sign, in the denominator.

For example, suppose the source is stationary and the detector is moving toward it. Because $v_S = 0$, there's no decision to make in the denominator. Now, we know that f_D will be higher than f_S in this case. Therefore, we choose the + in the numerator, to make the fraction multiplying f_S bigger, to give the higher f_D we expect:

$$f_D = f_S \frac{v + v_D}{v} \text{ (adding } v_D \text{ makes the numerator bigger)}$$

If the detector is moving away from the stationary source, we know that f_D will be lower than f_S in this case. Therefore, we choose the − in the numerator to make the fraction multiplying f_S smaller, to give the lower f_D we expect:

$$f_D = f_S \frac{v - v_D}{v} \text{ (subtracting } v_D \text{ makes the numerator smaller)}$$

Now, suppose the detector is stationary and the source is moving toward it. Since $v_D = 0$, there's no decision to make in the numerator. We know that f_D will be higher than f_S in this case. Therefore, we choose the—in the denominator, to make the denominator smaller, and thus make the fraction multiplying f_S bigger, to give the higher f_D we expect:

$$f_D = f_S \frac{v}{v - v_S} \text{ (subtracting } v_S \text{ makes the denominator smaller)}$$

If the source is moving away from the stationary detector, we know that f_D will be lower than f_S in this case. Therefore, we choose the + in the denominator, to make the denominator bigger, and thus make the fraction multiplying f_S smaller, to give the lower f_D we expect:

$$f_D = f_S \frac{v}{v + v_S} \text{ (adding } v_S \text{ makes the denominator bigger)}$$

If both the source and the detector are moving, we have two decisions to make (one in the numerator and one in the denominator). The key is to make the two decisions separately. For example, let's say you're the detector, driving in your car following a police car whose siren is wailing. In this case, both the source (the police car) and the detector (you) are moving. To decide what to do in the numerator, ask yourself: *what's the detector doing?* It's approaching the source, so its "contribution" to the Doppler effect should be an increase in frequency. Therefore, we'd choose the + in the numerator. Now, *what's the source doing?* It's receding from the detector, so its "contribution" to the Doppler effect should be a *decrease* in frequency. Therefore, we'd choose the + in the denominator.

$$f_D = f_S \frac{v + v_D}{v + v_S}$$

If your speed is greater than that of the police car, you're gaining on it, so the relative motion is motion *toward*. We'd expect f_D to be greater than f_S. If $v_D > v_S$, then the fraction multiplying f_S is bigger than 1, so f_D will indeed be greater than f_S. On the other hand, if your speed is less than that of the police car, it's pulling away from you, so the relative motion is motion *away*. In this case, we'd expect f_D to be lower than f_S. Further, if $v_D < v_S$, then the fraction multiplying f_S is less than 1, so f_D will indeed be lower than f_S. Finally, it's important to notice what happens if your speed is the same as the police car's speed. If $v_D = v_S$, then the fraction multiplying f_S is equal to 1, so $f_D = f_S$. Therefore, even though you're both moving, there's no Doppler shift because there's no *relative* motion between you.

The Doppler effect also applies to electromagnetic waves, such as visible light. The same qualitative relationships continue to hold: motion *toward* results in a frequency shift upward, while motion *away* results in a frequency shift downward. An astronomer observing a star moving away from the earth observes the light emitted as being shifted downward in frequency, toward the red end of the visible spectrum (in fact, this is known as the **redshift**). Furthermore, by measuring the shift, the astronomer can calculate how fast the star is moving away from us.[2]

Example 12-12: A speaker emitting a sound with a constant frequency approaches a detector. Which of the following wave characteristics will have a greater value at the detector than at the source?

   I.   Frequency
  II.   Wavelength
 III.   Speed

---

[2] For light waves, the equation that is used to calculate the magnitude of the Doppler effect is different. This is because of a postulate of special relativity: the speed of light is the same in all frames of reference. The detector, therefore, cannot perceive the speed of light to be faster or slower than 3×10^8 m/s. Another way of saying this is that we can always treat the detector as being at rest while the source may move.

Solution: Since the source is approaching the detector, the detected frequency will be higher than the emitted frequency. The wavelength will be shorter, and the wave speed will be the same. Therefore, only characteristic I will have a greater value at the detector than at the source.

Example 12-13: When you push the "star" key on your cell phone, a tone whose frequency is about 1080 Hz is emitted. However, the button gets stuck and the tone is continuous. Exasperated, you drop the broken phone off a bridge. What is the frequency of the tone you hear at the instant the phone's speed is 20 m/s (speed of sound in air = 340 m/s)?

Solution: Since you (the detector) are stationary, $v_D = 0$. Now, because the source of the sound (the broken phone) is moving away from you, we use the plus sign on v_S in the denominator of the Doppler effect equation to find that

$$f_D = f_S \frac{v}{v + v_S} = (1080 \text{ Hz}) \cdot \frac{340 \text{ m/s}}{340 \text{ m/s} + 20 \text{ m/s}} = (1080 \text{ Hz}) \cdot \frac{340}{360} = (3 \text{ Hz}) \cdot 340 = 1020 \text{ Hz}$$

Note that, because the phone is *accelerating* away from you, the magnitude of v_S is increasing as the phone falls, and thus the frequency you detect is *decreasing* as a function of time.

Example 12-14: As a high-speed chase begins, a police car travels at a speed of 40 m/s directly toward the suspect's getaway car, which is traveling at a speed of 70 m/s, trying to outrun the pursuing police. The frequency that the suspect hears will be what percentage of the frequency of the police car's siren? (speed of sound = 340 m/s)

Solution: Use the Doppler effect equation, choosing the signs carefully. The suspect in the getaway car is the detector (so v_D = 70 m/s), moving *away* from the source. The source is the police car (v_S = 40 m/s), moving *toward* the detector. Therefore,

$$f_D = f_S \frac{v \pm v_D}{v \mp v_S} = f_S \frac{340 \text{ m/s} - 70 \text{ m/s}}{340 \text{ m/s} - 40 \text{ m/s}} = f_S \frac{270}{300} = f_S \frac{90}{100} = (90\%) f_S$$

In order to find the correct value of f_D, it was necessary to plug in the values for v_D and v_S, and to change the top and the bottom of the equation separately; we couldn't just use the relative velocity of 30 m/s. However, if all the problem had asked for was the qualitative effect (i.e., whether the detected frequency was higher or lower than that of the source), then we could have worked out that the frequency was lower simply by noticing that the detector was getting farther away from the source.

Example 12-15: A technician is using his ultrasound scanner to detect a fetal heartbeat. The scanner emits short pulses of frequency 5 MHz, which then bounce off the beating heart and return to the scanner (functioning as a detector). The detector compares the final received frequency, f_2, with the original emitted frequency, f_1, and converts the difference in frequency into the speed and direction of the heart's motion. The difference in frequency, $\Delta f = f_2 - f_1$, is equal to $\pm 2vf_1/v_{sound}$, where v is the speed of the heart and $v_{sound} = 1500$ m/s is the speed of the ultrasound pulses. If $\Delta f = -100$ Hz, then the observed heart is:

A. expanding at 1.5 cm/s.
B. contracting at 1.5 cm/s.
C. expanding at 7.5 cm/s.
D. contracting at 7.5 cm/s.

Solution: First, the fact that Δf is negative means that f_2 is lower than f_1, and if the final detected frequency is *lower* than the frequency emitted by the source, then the heart surface must be moving *away from* the source (i.e., contracting). This eliminates choices A and C. Now, to figure out the value of the heart's speed, v, we just use the given formula:

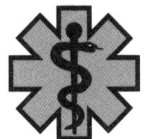

$$\Delta f = -\frac{2vf_1}{v_{sound}} \rightarrow v = -\frac{v_{sound}\Delta f}{2f_1} = -\frac{(1{,}500 \text{ m/s})(-100 \text{ Hz})}{1 \times 10^7 \text{ Hz}} = 1.5 \times 10^{-2} \text{ m/s}$$

This is equal to 1.5 cm/s, and choice B is correct.

Summary of Formulas

Standing Waves in a Tube:

Both ends open: $\lambda_n = \dfrac{2L}{n}$

$$f_n = \dfrac{n}{2L} v \; (n = 1, 2, 3, ...)$$

One end closed: $\lambda_n = \dfrac{4L}{n}$

$$f_n = \dfrac{n}{4L} v \; (n = 1, 3, 5, ...; \textit{odd } n \text{ only})$$

Beats, Intensity, Doppler Effect:

Beat frequency: $f_{beat} = \left| f_1 - f_2 \right|$

Intensity: $I = \dfrac{\text{power}}{\text{area}}$

I is inversely proportional to r^2 (where r = distance from source), and directly as the square of the wave amplitude.

Sound intensity level (in decibels, dB): $\beta = 10 \log_{10} \dfrac{I}{I_0}$

(where $I_0 = 10^{-12} \, \text{W/m}^2 = 0$ threshold of hearing)

multiply I by 10 $\leftrightarrow$ *add* 10 to β.

divide I by 10 $\leftrightarrow$ *subtract* 10 from β.

Doppler effect: describes the change in frequency between a source and a detector due to relative motion of both

relative motion toward $\leftrightarrow$ frequency increase ($f_D > f_S$)

relative motion away $\leftrightarrow$ frequency decrease ($f_S > f_D$)

For constant velocities, this shift is constant. The frequency is not increasing or decreasing with time, but is simply a higher or lower constant at the detector than at the source. Relative acceleration creates an increasing or decreasing frequency.

Doppler effect (for waves other than light): $f_D = f_S \dfrac{v \pm v_D}{v \mp v_S}$

CHAPTER 12 FREESTANDING PRACTICE QUESTIONS

1. When all the finger holes on a clarinet are closed, it can be approximated as a hollow tube with one closed end (mouthpiece) and one open end. When all the finger holes on a clarinet are closed, the lowest pitch that can be produced corresponds to the G-flat below middle C (185 Hz). How long is the clarinet? (assume the speed of sound in air is 340 m/s).

A) 90 cm
B) 70 cm
C) 46 cm
D) 30 cm

2. A 37.5 cm glass pipe that is open at both ends is placed next to a student a cappella group. It was observed that the pipe first resonates when the choir produces a note at 450 Hz. At which subsequent frequencies will resonance again be observed? (The speed of sound through the pipe is 340 m/s.)

A) 675 Hz and 900 Hz
B) 675 Hz and 1350 Hz
C) 900 Hz and 1350 Hz
D) 900 Hz and 1800 Hz

3. Two pianos play the same key, but while one is in perfect tune, the other is sharp (out of tune to the higher frequency end). If the in-tune note has a wavelength in air of 3.091 m and a beat frequency of 2 Hz is heard, what is the frequency of the sharp note? Use a speed of sound of 340 m/s.

A) 0.009 Hz
B) 100 Hz
C) 112 Hz
D) 442 Hz

4. An airplane is traveling 157 m/s north on a runway and is producing a sound of frequency f. A woman is seated in a car moving 43 m/s to the south, away from the airplane. What frequency will she observe? (assume the speed of sound in air is 343 m/s)

A) $1/2 f$
B) $3/5 f$
C) f
D) $2f$

5. A man standing 1 m away from an omnidirectional speaker is exposed to a sound of 140 dB. How far would he have to travel in order to no longer be in pain (the threshold of pain is about 120 dB), given $I = P/A$ and $\beta = 10\log(I / I_0)$, where $I_0 = 10^{-12}$ W/m^2.

A) 9 m
B) 10 m
C) 20 m
D) 100 m

6. A stationary cat is purring. Which of the following correctly explains why its owner hears a frequency that is higher than that which is produced by the cat?

A) The owner is moving towards the cat.
B) The owner is moving away from the cat.
C) Both are on an accelerating train.
D) Both are on a decelerating boat.

7. A herpetologist studying alligators at the Kennedy Space Center is 1000 m from the launch pad, when a siren sounds, signaling 30 minutes to launch. After running away for 4000 m, the herpetologist turns to watch the launch. How does the intensity of sound produced by the siren at his new location compare to the original intensity, I_1, given $I = P/A$?

A) $5 I_1$
B) $1/5 I_1$
C) $1/25 I_1$
D) $1/50 I_1$

CHAPTER 12 PRACTICE PASSAGE

Sound waves propagate away from a source in spherical wavefronts, lines that connect the points on a sound wave that were emitted at the same time. When the source is stationary, these wave fronts are concentric spheres centered about the source. However, when the source begins to move with a velocity v_0, the wavefronts get closer together in the direction of v_0 and are spread farther apart in the opposite direction.

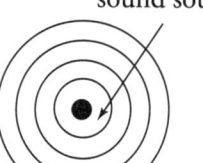
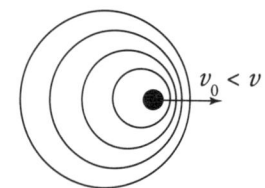

Figure 1 Wavefronts generated by sound sources that are stationary and moving with a speed less than the speed of sound.

As a result of the change in the distance between wavefronts, a listener standing ahead of or behind the object will hear a frequency different from the original emitted frequency, a phenomenon known as the Doppler effect, according to the equation:

$$f_D = f_S \frac{v \pm v_D}{v \mp v_S}$$

Equation 1

where f_D and f_S are the detected and emitted frequencies, respectively, v is the speed of sound, and v_D and v_S are the velocities of the detector and the source, respectively.

Some jets have been designed to fly at speeds greater than the speed of sound. There speeds are usually given as a Mach number, $M = v_0/v$, which indicates the jet's speed relative to the speed of sound in the surrounding air. Because the speed of sound in air increases as the temperature increases, the jets flying with the same Mach number can be traveling at different speeds. When a jet flies at exactly Mach 1, the wavefronts build up just in front of the object, creating an intense shock wave. Flight at this speed is incredibly turbulent. Interestingly, in this case an observer ahead of the jet would not hear it until the jet itself arrived, since the first wavefront and the jet arrive at the same time. Jets can also fly faster than the speed of sound, at supersonic speeds. When this happens, the jet actually advances ahead of the shock wave it creates. The intense sound heard when a shockwave passes by an observer is known as a sonic boom.

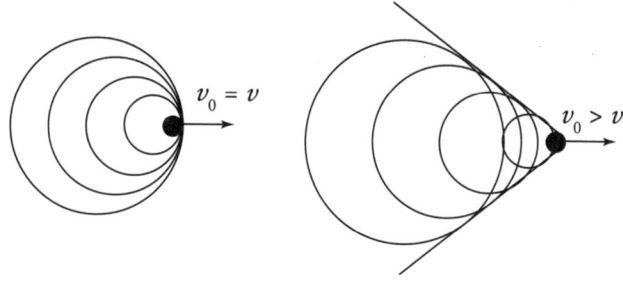

Figure 2 Wavefronts created by a jet flying at the speed of sound and at a supersonic speed.

1. Two jets are flying at Mach 3, one close to sea level, the other at 50,000 ft where the air temperature is cooler. Compared to the jet at sea level, the one flying at 50,000 ft is traveling:

A) at the same speed.
B) at a lower speed because the speed of sound decreases at altitude due to the lower air temperature.
C) at a greater speed because the speed of sound decreases at altitude due to the lower air temperature.
D) at a greater speed because the speed of sound increases at altitude due to the greater air temperature.

2. While driving down the road at 10 m/s, a driver hears a 330 Hz siren from police car approaching from behind. If the frequency emitted by the siren is 300 Hz, how fast is the police car going?

A) 9 m/s
B) 10 m/s
C) 20 m/s
D) 40 m/s

3. A stationary observer is standing on a sidewalk when a police car emitting a 300 Hz siren passes by on the road at 20 m/s. Just as the police car passes her, what is the frequency she hears?

A) 283 Hz
B) 300 Hz
C) 318 Hz
D) 340 Hz

4. If the sonic boom that the jet produces when it goes supersonic is 60 dB louder than acceptable limits for the people on the base below, at minimum how many times farther away should it be from the base when it goes supersonic?

A) 10^3
B) 10^4
C) 10^5
D) 10^6

5. As a siren approaches an observer at a constant velocity, the observer hears a sound that is:

A) increasing in frequency.
B) at a constant frequency that is higher than the emitted frequency.
C) at a constant frequency that is lower than the emitted frequency.
D) decreasing in frequency.

6. What is a possible explanation for why flying at Mach 1 results in incredibly turbulent flight?

A) The transverse motion of the air molecules of the sound wave jostle the vessel up and down.
B) The transverse motion of the air molecules of the sound wave make it difficult for the pilot to steer.
C) The build-up of sound waves in front of the jet creates an extreme pressure front.
D) Jets are increasingly structurally unstable the faster they travel.

SOLUTIONS TO CHAPTER 12 FREESTANDING QUESTIONS

1. **C**   The clarinet with all its finger holes closed approximates a hollow tube with one closed end and one open end, and can be diagrammed as below:

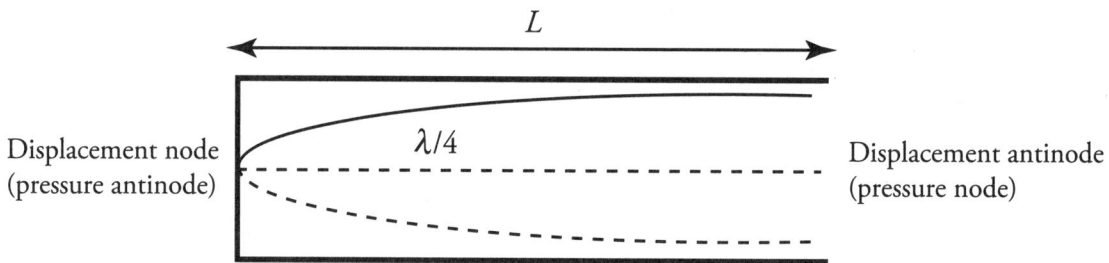

L

Displacement node
(pressure antinode)

$\lambda/4$

Displacement antinode
(pressure node)

There is only one quarter (not one half) of a wavelength, and so the length of the pipe must be one-quarter the wavelength of the sound wave. The first (or fundamental) harmonic of a pipe with one closed end is $f_1 = v/4L$, where L is the length of the pipe. Rearranging this formula: $L = v/4 f_1 = 340$ m/s / $[(4)(185)]) = 0.46$ m.

2. **C**   If the pipe first resonated at 450 Hz, then the fundamental frequency (f_1) of the standing wave in the pipe is 450 Hz. The subsequent frequencies that will produce resonance are $f_2, f_3, f_4, \ldots f_n$. These can be calculated using the equation $f_n = nf_1$. Since f_1 is given to us, the next resonance will be at $f_2 = (2)(450) = 900$ Hz, and the resonance after that will be $f_3 = (3)(450) = 1350$ Hz.

3. **C**   First convert the given wavelength for the in-tune note using the wave speed equation: $v = \lambda f \rightarrow f = \dfrac{340 \text{ m/s}}{3.091 \text{ m}} \approx 110 \text{ Hz}$. Note that you do not need to get this exact answer: it is enough to recognize that the answer must be larger than 100 but not by very much, because 300/3 = 100. Since the in-tune note has a frequency of about 110 Hz, the sharp note must have a higher frequency given by the beat frequency equation:

$$f_{\text{beat}} = |f_1 - f_2| = 2 \text{ Hz} \rightarrow f_{\text{sharp}} = f_{\text{correct}} + 2 \text{ Hz} = (110 + 2) \text{ Hz} = 112 \text{ Hz}.$$

4. **B**   This is a Doppler shift question, and thus begins with using the Doppler equation:

$$f_D = f_s \frac{v \pm v_D}{v \mp v_S}$$

The speed of the detector (v_D) is subtracted in the numerator because the car is moving away from the source, and thus the frequency observed will be lower than that produced. Addition is used in the denominator because the source, the airplane, is moving away from the detector and thus the frequency needs to be decreased. Subsequently plugging into the equation yields

$$f_D = f_s \frac{343 \text{ m/s} - 43 \text{ m/s}}{343 \text{ m/s} + 157 \text{ m/s}} \approx f_s \frac{300 \text{ m/s}}{500 \text{ m/s}} \approx \frac{3}{5} f$$

which gives choice B as correct. Both choices C and D can be eliminated because when two objects are moving apart, the frequency needs to decrease. (Note that if addition were used in the numerator and subtraction in the denominator, thus reversing the relationship and causing the frequency to increase, the answer would approximate 390/190 or approximately $2f$, which is choice D.)

5. **A**   A difference of 20 dB means a decrease in intensity of 10^2. This can either be gathered from the given logarithmic equation [$20 = 10 \log(I/I_0) \rightarrow 2 = \log(I/I_0)$ and therefore $I = 10^2$)] or by remembering that for every time 10 is added or subtracted from β, 10 is multiplied or divided from I, respectively. Knowing that I decreased by a factor of 100 means that the area would have had to increase by a factor of 100, since the power stays constant (from $I = P/A$). Since $A \propto r^2$, the radius must increase by a a factor of 10. Since the man was already 1 m from the source, he will have to travel 9 m. Choice B is a trap answer which ignores the original 1 m. Choice C is simply the number of dB dropped. Choice D is a trap which is equal to the factor that intensity is reduced.

6. **A**   Choices C and D are both incorrect; they will have no effect on the frequency heard since the action is occurring to both the observer and the source. Choice B is backwards, because approaching objects will experience an increase in frequency (choice A is correct).

7. **C**   Since the new radius is 5 times the original radius, the area will increase by 25 times (remembering that A is proportional to r^2). Since the area will increase by a factor of 25, the intensity will decrease by that factor (they are inversely proportional), giving choice C. Choice A can be eliminated because it assumes a direct, rather than inverse, relationship between the intensity and the area. Choice B is a trap; it is the correct answer if one forgets to square the multiple of the radius.

SOLUTIONS TO CHAPTER 12 PRACTICE PASSAGE

1. **B** Since $M = v_0/v$, for a given Mach number, v_0 and v are directly related. The passage indicates that the speed of sound increases with increasing air temperature. Thus, at 50,000 ft where the air is cooler, the speed of sound is lower than at sea level. As a result the jet flying at 50,000 ft must be flying more slowly than the jet flying at sea level, even though they are traveling at the same Mach number.

2. **D** Since the detected frequency is greater than the emitted frequency, choices A and B would be eliminated since these velocities would not result in the siren approaching the observer. Using the fact that the detector is moving away from the source and that the source is approaching the detector, we obtain the equation $f_D = f_S (v - v_D)/(v - v_S)$. Plugging the given values into the equation yields 330 Hz = 300 Hz (340 m/s – 10 m/s)/(340 m/s – v_S) → 330 = 300 (330)/(340 – v_S) → 340 – v_S = 300 → v_S = 40 m/s.

3. **B** As the siren is passing the observer, the siren is neither moving towards nor away from the listener. As a result, there is no difference between the detected and the emitted frequencies.

4. **A** In order to decrease the sound by 60 dB, the intensity of the sonic boom must be decreased by a factor 10^6. Although this result makes choice D a tempting answer choice, it must be remembered that intensity is proportional to $1/r^2$. As a result, in order to decrease the intensity by a factor of 10^6, the radius only has to increase by a factor of 10^3.

5. **B** If a sound source is approaching the observer, the frequency should increase, which eliminates choices C and D. If the siren is moving at a constant velocity, then as it approaches, the fraction $(v - v_D)/(v - v_S)$, which indicates the frequency shift, is constant, not continually increasing, which eliminates choice A.

6. **C** Since sound is a pressure wave, a buildup of many sound waves does create an extreme pressure front. Choices A and B cannot be correct since sound is not a transverse wave. Although there may be some regime in which jets do become more structurally unstable the faster they fly, it does not answer the question since the passage mentions that the extreme turbulence is felt at exactly Mach 1, not at all speeds greater than Mach 1, indicating that choice D cannot explain this particular phenomenon.

Chapter 13
Light and Geometrical Optics

13.1 ELECTROMAGNETIC WAVES

We've seen that if we oscillate one end of a long rope, we generate a wave that travels down the rope and whose frequency is the frequency with which we oscillate.

You can think of an electromagnetic wave in a similar way: An oscillating electric charge generates an **electromagnetic (EM)** wave, which is composed of oscillating electric and magnetic fields. These fields oscillate with the same frequency at which the electric charge that created the wave oscillated. The fields oscillate in phase with each other, perpendicular to each other and to the direction of propagation. For this reason, electromagnetic waves are transverse waves. The direction in which the wave's electric field oscillates is called the direction of **polarization** of the wave.

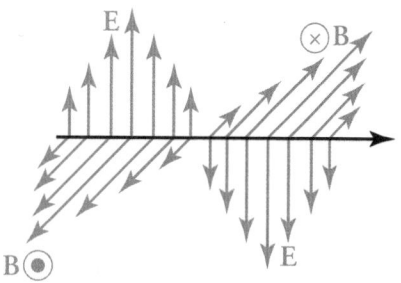

Most EM waves have electric fields oscillating in all perpendicular directions to propagation equally and are thus *unpolarized*.

Unlike waves on a rope or sound waves, electromagnetic waves do not require a material medium to propagate; they can travel through empty space (vacuum). When an EM wave travels through vacuum, its speed is a constant. It is one of the fundamental constants of nature and a value you should memorize for the MCAT:

Speed of Light in Vacuum

$$c = 3 \times 10^8 \, \tfrac{m}{s}$$

All electromagnetic waves, regardless of frequency, travel through vacuum at this speed. The most important equation for waves, $v = \lambda f$, is also true for electromagnetic waves. For EM waves traveling through vacuum, $v = c$, so the equation becomes $c = \lambda f$.

The frequencies for electromagnetic waves span a huge range, and different ranges have been given specific names. This assignment of names to specific regions based on frequency (or wavelength) is known as the **electromagnetic spectrum** and is shown here.

Notice that visible light occupies only a small part of the electromagnetic spectrum. When waves from all over the visible spectrum are mixed together, the resulting light is perceived as white. You should memorize the order of the colors of the visible spectrum from lowest frequency (longest wavelength) to highest frequency (shortest wavelength): ROYGBV ("Roy-Gee-Biv"), which stands for r̲ed, o̲range, y̲ellow, g̲reen, b̲lue, and v̲iolet. In terms of wavelengths, violet light has a wavelength (in vacuum) of about 400 nm and red light has a wavelength of about 700 nm; the other colors are in between.

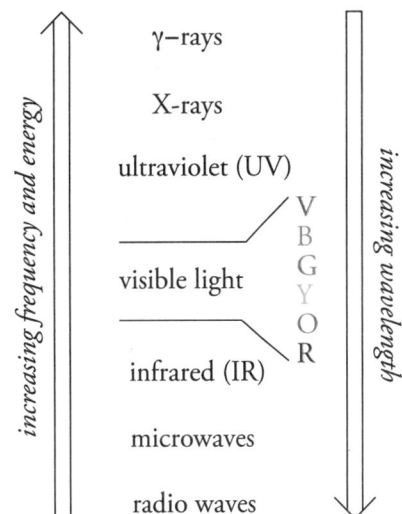

Photons

When electromagnetic radiation interacts with matter (absorption and emission), we find that it carries energy, and that the energy is quantized. That is, the energy associated with EM radiation is absorbed or emitted by matter in "packets"; individual bundles. Each such bundle of energy is called a **photon**, and the energy of a photon is directly proportional to the frequency:

Photon Energy

$$E = hf = h\frac{c}{\lambda}$$

The constant of proportionality, h, is called **Planck's constant**. (In SI units, its value is about 6.6×10^{-34} J·s.)

The fact that electromagnetic radiation carries energy in packets (photons), which we can think of as "particles of light," gives rise to the idea of **wave-particle duality** for electromagnetic radiation: EM radiation travels like a wave but interacts with matter like a particle. One peculiarity of this duality is that, for waves, energy is proportional to the square of amplitude (recall the intensity relation from the previous chapter), whereas for particles (photons), energy is proportional to frequency. In Chapter 11, we noted that these two properties were independent of one another. Thus, the wave and particle models for light differ significantly in their predictions, and yet each is sometimes true.

Example 13-1: Which one of the following statements is true regarding red photons and blue photons traveling through vacuum?

    A. Red light travels faster than blue light and carries more energy.
    B. Blue light travels faster than red light and carries more energy.
    C. Red light travels at the same speed as blue light and carries more energy.
    D. Blue light travels at the same speed as red light and carries more energy.

Solution: All electromagnetic waves, regardless of frequency, travel through vacuum at the same speed, *c*. This eliminates choices A and B. Now, because blue light has a higher frequency than red light (remember ROYGBV, which lists the colors in order of increasing frequency), photons of blue light have higher energy than photons of red light. Therefore, the answer is D.

13.2 REFLECTION AND REFRACTION

When a beam of light strikes the boundary between two transparent media, some of the light will be reflected from the surface. In the figure below, some of the sunlight will be reflected off the water in the tank.

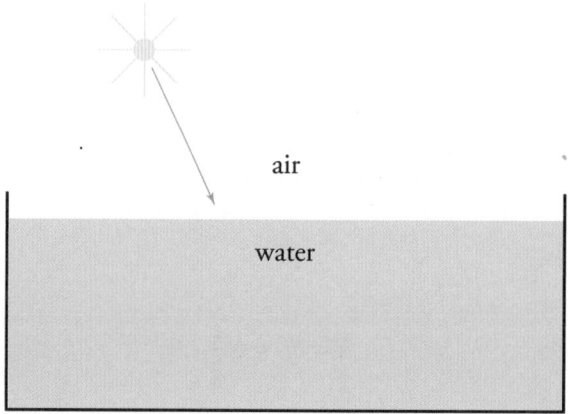

When a ray of light passing through one medium is reflected from the surface of another, the angle at which it bounces off the new medium is equal to the angle at which it strikes. In other words, *the angle of reflection is equal to the angle of incidence*. This fact is known as the **law of reflection**. Notice that, by definition, the angles of incidence and reflection are measured with reference to a line that's perpendicular to the plane of interface between the two media; that is, the angle of incidence and the angle of reflection are the angles that the incident and reflected rays make with *the normal*, not with the surface.

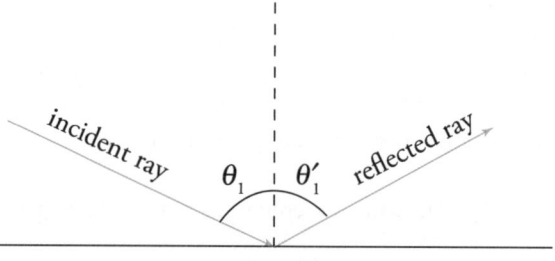

angle of incidence = angle of reflection
$$\theta_1 = \theta_1'$$

Example 13-2: In the figure above, assume that a ray of sunlight strikes the water, making an angle of 60° with the surface. What is the angle of reflection?

   A. 15°
   B. 30°
   C. 60°
   D. 90°

Solution: Be careful. If the incident ray makes an angle of 60° with the surface, then it makes an angle of 30° with the normal. Therefore, the angle of incidence is 30°. By the law of reflection, the angle of reflection is 30° also. Choice B is the answer.

In the figure below, not all of the sunlight that encounters the surface of the water is reflected; some is transmitted into the water. Unless the angle of incidence is 0°, the light will be *bent* as it enters the water. The bending is called **refraction**. The **angle of refraction** is the angle that the **transmitted** (or **refracted**) ray makes with the line that's perpendicular to the plane of interface between the two media.

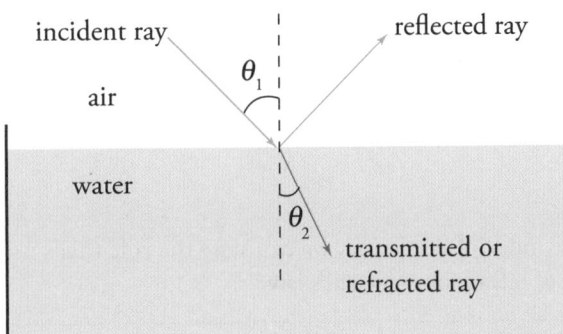

If $\theta_1 = 0°$ (that is, if the incident ray is perpendicular to the boundary), then $\theta_2 = 0°$. However, if θ_1 is any other angle, then θ_2 will be different from θ_1; that is, the ray bends as it's transmitted. In order to figure out the angle of refraction, we first need to discuss a medium's index of refraction.

Index of Refraction

Light travels at speed $c = 3 \times 10^8$ m/s when traveling in a vacuum. However, when light travels through a material medium such as water or glass, its transmission speed is less than c. Every medium, in fact, has an **index of refraction** that tells us how much more slowly light travels through that medium than through empty space.

Index of Refraction

$$\text{index of refraction} = \frac{\text{speed of light in vacuum}}{\text{speed of light in medium}}$$

$$n = \frac{c}{v}$$

The index of refraction of vacuum is, by definition, exactly equal to 1. Because the index for air is very close to 1, we simply use $n = 1$ for air as well. (The MCAT will use this approximation unless otherwise specified.) Notice that n has no units, it's never less than 1, and the greater the value of n for a medium, the slower light travels through that medium. For most materials, the value of n is between 1 and 2.5. Glass has an index of refraction of about 1.5 (but varies depending on the type of glass) while diamond has a particularly high value of n, about 2.4. Values of n above 2.5 are rare.

Example 13-3: Light travels through water at an approximate speed of 2.25×10^8 m/s. What is the refractive index of water?

    A.   0.75
    B.   1.33
    C.   1.50
    D.   2.25

Solution: First, eliminate choice A: The index of refraction is never less than 1. Now, by definition,

$$n = \frac{c}{v} = \frac{3 \times 10^8 \text{ m/s}}{2.25 \times 10^8 \text{ m/s}} = \frac{3}{2.25} = \frac{3}{2\frac{1}{4}} = \frac{3}{\frac{9}{4}} = 3 \cdot \frac{4}{9} = \frac{4}{3} \approx 1.33$$

Therefore, the answer is B.

Now that we know about the index of refraction, we can state the rule that's used to figure out the angle of refraction. It's called the law of refraction, or Snell's law:

> ## Law of Refraction (Snell's Law)
>
> $$n_1 \sin \theta_1 = n_2 \sin \theta_2$$

In this equation, n_1 is the refractive index of the medium through which the incident ray is traveling, and n_2 is the refractive index of the medium through which the transmitted (or refracted) ray is traveling.

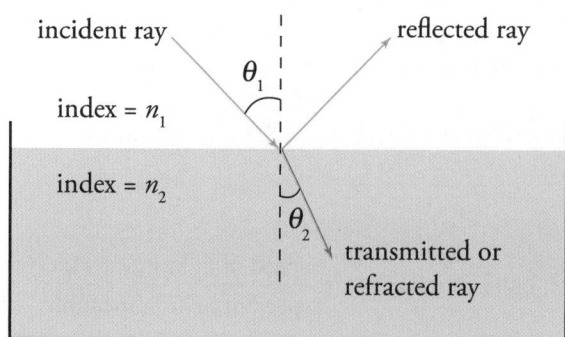

It follows from Snell's law that if $n_2 > n_1$, then $\theta_2 < \theta_1$. That is, if the transmitting medium has a higher index of refraction than the incident medium, then the ray will bend *toward* the normal. Similarly, if $n_2 < n_1$, then $\theta_2 > \theta_1$. That is, if the transmitting medium has a lower index of refraction than the incident medium, then the ray will bend *away from* the normal. You should memorize both of these facts.

Example 13-4: A ray of light traveling through air is incident on a piece of glass whose refractive index is 1.5. If the sine of the angle of incidence is 0.6, what's the sine of the angle of refraction?

Solution: Using the law of refraction, we find that

$$n_1 \sin\theta_1 = n_2 \sin\theta_2 \rightarrow (1)(0.6) = (1.5)(\sin\theta_2) \rightarrow \sin\theta_2 = \frac{0.6}{1.5} = \frac{6}{15} = \frac{2}{5} = 0.4$$

Notice that $\sin\theta_2$ is less than $\sin\theta_1$; this immediately tells us that $\theta_2 < \theta_1$. The light is traveling from air ($n_1 = 1$) into glass, whose refractive index is higher. If the transmitting medium (i.e., the second one) has a higher index of refraction than the incident medium (i.e., the first one), then θ_2 *will* be less than θ_1; that is, the ray will bend toward the normal.

Example 13-5: Consider the diagram below, showing an incident ray, reflected ray, and transmitted ray:

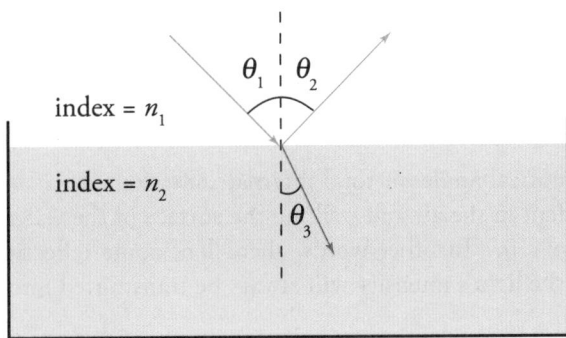

What information is needed to find θ_2?

A. n_1, n_2, and θ_1
B. n_1, n_2, and θ_3
C. n_1 only
D. θ_1 only

Solution: The angle labeled θ_2 is the angle of reflection. To find it, all we need to know is the angle of incidence, θ_1. (By the law of reflection, we find that $\theta_2 = \theta_1$.) The answer is D. (This unconventional labeling of the angles is a common MCAT tactic, by the way.)

Total Internal Reflection

When a light ray traveling in a medium of high refractive index approaches a medium of lower refractive index (for example, a light ray traveling in water towards the interface with the air), it may or may not escape into the second medium. If the ray's angle of incidence exceeds a certain **critical angle**, the light ray will undergo **total internal reflection**: All of the incident ray's energy will be reflected back into its original medium; there will be no refracted ray.

Critical Angle for Total Internal Reflection

$$\sin\theta_{crit} = \frac{n_2}{n_1}$$

In this equation, n_1 is the refractive index of the medium through which the incident ray is traveling, and n_2 is the refractive index of the medium on the other side of the boundary. The angle θ_{crit} is the critical angle. What this means is that if the angle of incidence, θ_1, is greater than θ_{crit}, then total internal reflection will occur.[1] However, if θ_1 is less than θ_{crit}, then total internal reflection will not occur. (If θ_1 just happens to equal θ_{crit}, then the refracted beam skims along the boundary with $\theta_2 = 90°$.)

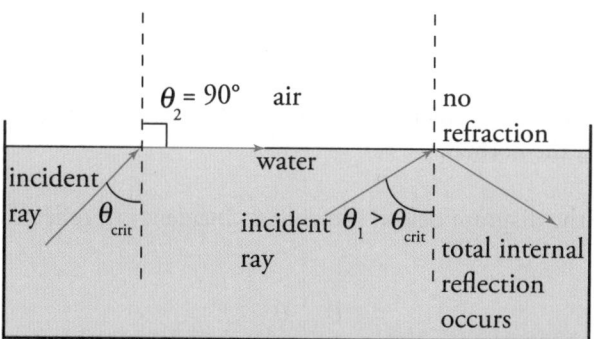

Notice that there can be a critical angle for total internal reflection *only if n_1 is greater than n_2*. For example, a beam of light incident in the air and striking the surface of the water can never experience total internal reflection because $n_1 < n_2$. In other words, there'll be some reflection and some refraction, as usual. In this case, some of the light's intensity will always be transmitted into the water.

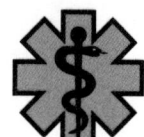

Example 13-6: A beam of light is incident on the boundary between air and a piece of glass whose index of refraction is $\sqrt{2}$. When would total internal reflection (TIR, for short) of this beam occur?

Solution: First, in order to have TIR, the beam would have to start in the glass, trying to exit into the air. (If the beam were traveling in the air and incident on the glass, then TIR could not occur.) Furthermore, the angle of incidence would have to be greater than the critical angle, which we calculate as follows:

$$\sin\theta_{crit} = \frac{n_2}{n_1} = \frac{1}{\sqrt{2}} = \frac{\sqrt{2}}{2} \;\rightarrow\; \theta_{crit} = 45°$$

Total internal reflection is a vital technology for medicine because it is the underlying principle of fiber optics, used in endoscopy for laparoscopic and arthroscopic surgeries. Without the ability to see clearly inside the body with a thin, flexible tube through which light travels both into and out of the body (after reflecting off of organs and other tissues), many surgical procedures would still require large incisions and long recovery times.

---

[1] If you forget the formula for the critical angle, there's another way to know that total internal reflection occurs: If you plug numbers into the law of refraction and find that $\sin\theta > 1$ (which is impossible), that tells you there is no angle of refraction, so there must be total internal reflection.

13.3 WAVE EFFECTS

Diffraction

Simply put, waves, whether they're water waves, sound waves, EM waves, etc., don't always travel in a single direction when they encounter an obstruction. This redistribution of the wave's intensity is known as **diffraction**. Water waves bend around a rock sticking up out of the water, for example. The "obstruction" can even be a hole. For example, water or light incident on a hole in a barrier will pass through and *spread out* beyond the barrier. These effects are observed when the size of the object or opening is comparable to the wavelength of the waves.

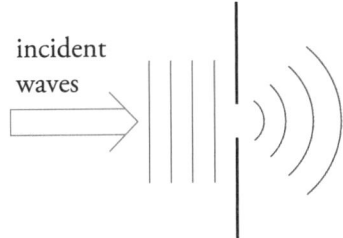

Polarization

Normally, the electric-field components of the waves in a beam of light vibrate in *all* planes. **Polarized** light is light whose direction of polarization has been restricted somehow. For example, all the waves in a beam of **plane-polarized** light have their electric-field components vibrating in a single plane.

It is possible to transform unpolarized light into polarized light by several methods. One method is the use of a *polarizing filter*. The filter has a polarization axis, so that when unpolarized light strikes the filter, only the portion of the waves vibrating in that direction pass through while the portion of the waves vibrating perpendicular to the axis is absorbed. The light that emerges is now polarized in the direction of the axis and has half the intensity of the original unpolarized light.

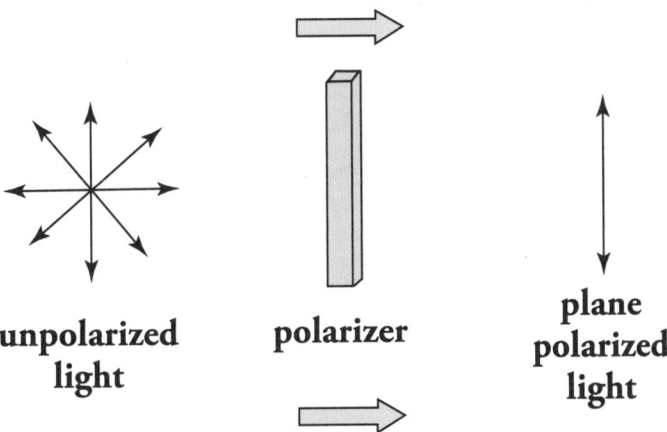

If polarized light passes through a second polarizer, the amount of light that passes through or is absorbed depends on the angle between the direction of polarization of the incident light and the axis of the polarizer. As an example, if vertically polarized light is incident upon a horizontally polarizing filter, none of the light will pass through.

If two light waves of equal amplitude vibrate perpendicular to each other and have a 90° phase difference (the "crest" of one wave interferes with the "0" of the other), the light is *circularly polarized*.

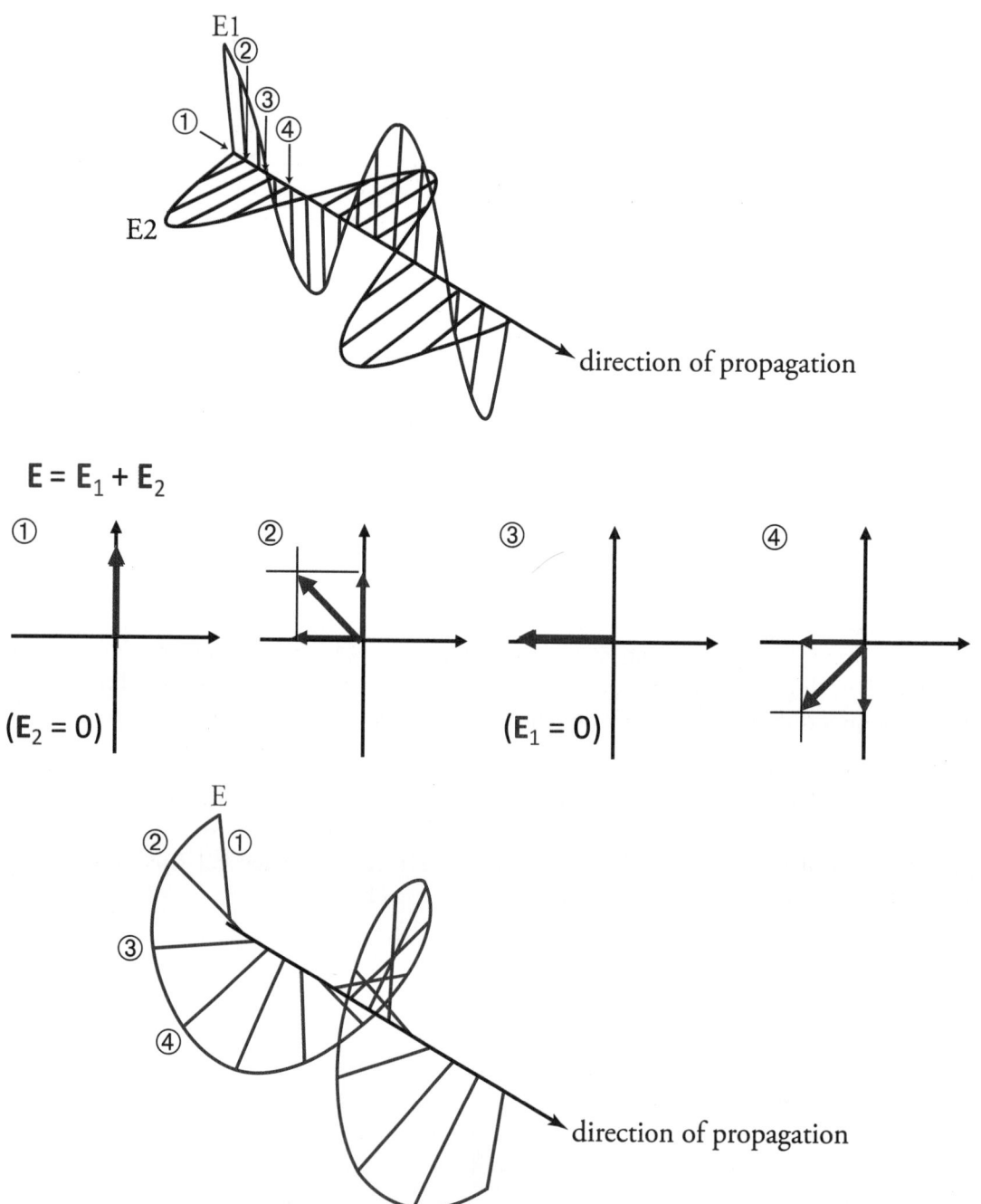

As a result, the electric field appears to be rotating.

Dispersion

When light moves from one medium to another, some wavelengths are bent more than others. The reason for this is that electromagnetic waves of different frequencies travel at slightly different speeds when traveling through a material medium like glass or water. Although Big Rule 1 for waves states that the speed of a wave is determined by the medium, not by the wave's frequency, light waves traveling through a material medium are an exception to this rule.[2] (In fact, they're the only exception that's at all likely to appear on the MCAT.) When light travels through a material (not vacuum), different frequencies will have different speeds. Thus, when we say that the index of refraction for a piece of glass is 1.5, what is really true is that the index varies slightly as the color of the light varies. For example, the index of refraction of the glass could be 1.47 for red light but 1.54 for violet light.[3] Because different colors have different refractive indexes, they will have different angles of refraction. This is why when white light passes through a prism, the beam is broken into its component colors. Each color leaves the prism at its own angle of refraction.[4] We call this variation in wave speed for different frequencies (and the effects this variation produces) **dispersion**.

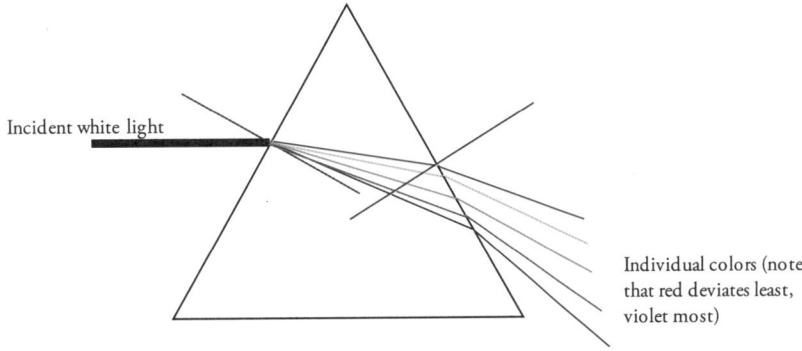

Incident white light

Individual colors (note that red deviates least, violet most)

13.4 MIRRORS

A **mirror** is a surface, usually made of glass or metal, that forms an image of an object by *reflecting* light.

Plane Mirrors

A **plane** mirror is an ordinary flat mirror. If you put an object in front of a plane mirror, the image will appear to be behind the mirror. The image will be the same size as the object and will appear to be as far behind the mirror's surface as the object is in front of it. The image will also appear upright; it won't be inverted.

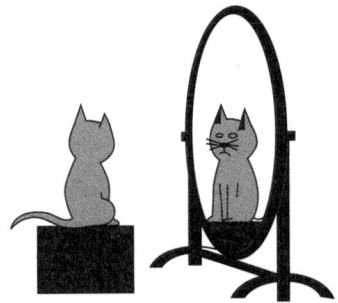

---

2 This isn't the case when electromagnetic waves travel through vacuum, where *all* frequencies travel at the same speed, *c*.

3 In general, as in this example, the higher the frequency of the light, the lower the speed. However, there are complicated exceptions to this rule of thumb, and there's no need to memorize it or learn about the exceptions for the MCAT.

4 The greater the index of refraction, the more the light will be bent on entering the medium from air or vacuum, so high-frequency violet light will generally bend more than red light.

Curved Mirrors

We all have experience with plane mirrors, but a **curved** mirror presents us with images that are less familiar. The purpose of this section is to find a systematic way to describe the images formed by curved mirrors.

There are essentially two types of curved mirrors: concave and convex. The shiny (reflecting) surface of a **concave** mirror appears like the entrance to a "cave" from the point of view of the object. The reflecting surface of a **convex** mirror bends away from the object. As a simple demonstration of the difference, imagine holding a polished spoon. If you look into the spoon, you're looking at a concave surface; if you turn it around and look at the back of the spoon, you're looking at a convex surface.

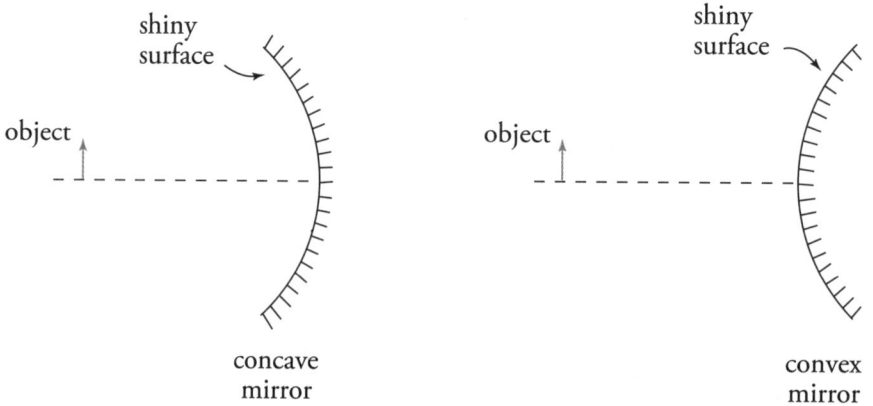

The curved mirrors we'll consider could be termed **spherical** mirrors, because near the center of the mirror, the surface is spherical (that is, part of a sphere).

When light parallel to the central **axis** of a concave mirror strikes the surface, the reflected rays *converge* at a point called the **focus** (or **focal point**), denoted by F. This point is halfway to the **center of curvature**, C, of the mirror, which is the center of the sphere that the mirror is "cut from." The distance between the center of curvature and the mirror is called the **radius of curvature**, *r*. Because the focal point is halfway between the mirror and C, the distance from the mirror to the focal point, the all-important **focal length**, *f*, is half the radius of curvature: $f = \frac{1}{2}r$.

When light parallel to the central axis of a *convex* mirror strikes the surface, the reflected rays *diverge* directly *away from* the **focal point** behind the mirror.

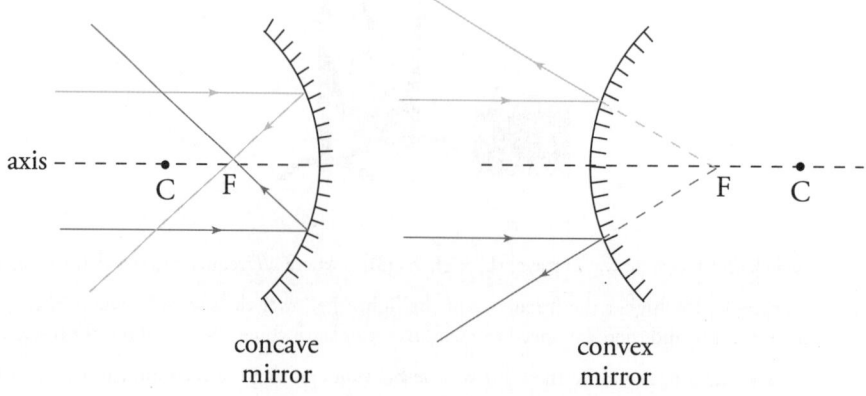

We see an image in a mirror at the point where the rays reflected off the mirror intersect in front of the mirror *or* at the point from where the reflected rays seem to intersect (and therefore emanate from) behind the mirror. When a very distant object has its light reflected from a mirror, the light rays that strike the mirror are approximately parallel, like the rays shown on the previous page. This illustrates the significance of the focal point. *The image of a distant object will appear at the focal point for all curved mirrors.* This turns out to be true for thin lenses as well. But what if the object is not distant?

The following figures illustrate the process of image formation by curved mirrors:

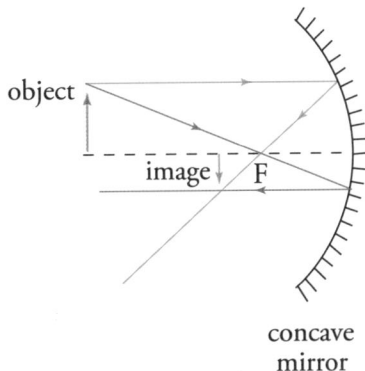

concave
mirror

The ray diagram for the concave mirror shows two incident rays reflecting off the mirror. One ray, parallel to the axis, is reflected through the focal point. Another ray, which goes through the focal point, is reflected parallel to the axis. The intersection point of these reflected rays determines the location of the image.

Note that the light rays still cross after reflecting off the mirror, but the image is located behind the focal point. If the object is moved closer to the mirror (i.e., inside the focal point), the reflected rays no longer cross and the image forms behind the mirror.

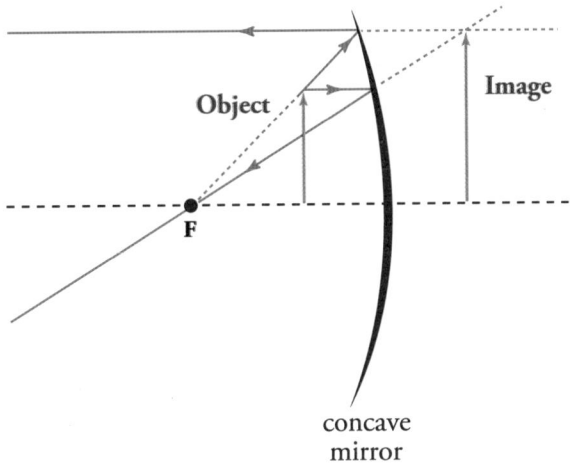

concave
mirror

One ray, parallel to the axis, is again reflected through the focal point. Another ray, which is directed as if it came from the focal point, is reflected parallel to the axis.

The ray diagram for the convex mirror also shows two incident rays reflecting off the mirror. One ray, parallel to the axis, is reflected directly away from the focal point. Another ray, which hits the center of the mirror (the point where its axis of symmetry intersects the mirror surface), is reflected at the same angle below the axis. Following these reflected rays back behind the mirror, their intersection point determines the location of the image.

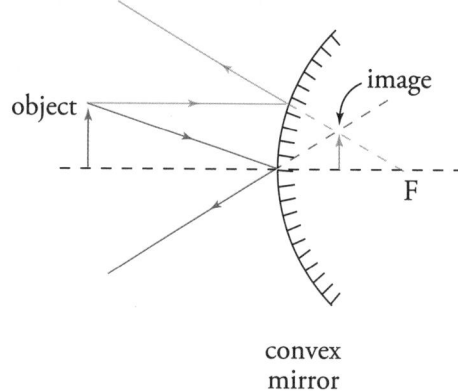

convex
mirror

Ray diagrams (like the ones drawn in the figures above) can be used to determine the approximate location of the image, but they usually can't give precise answers to all the questions we may be asked about the image formed by a mirror. Moreover, it is both impractical and unnecessary to draw ray diagrams when taking the MCAT! What we want is a systematic way to get precise answers to these four questions:

1. Where is the image?
2. Is the image real or is it virtual?
3. Is the image upright or is it inverted?
4. How large is the image compared to the object?

Before we discuss how to answer these questions, let's first define the terms *real* and *virtual*. An image is said to be **real** if light rays actually focus at the position of the image. A real image can be projected onto a surface. An image is said to be **virtual** if light rays don't actually focus at the apparent location of the image. For example, look back at the figures above, showing the formation of images by a concave mirror and by a convex mirror. The image formed by the concave mirror in the first diagram is real: light rays actually intersect at the image location. However, the images formed by the concave mirror in the second diagram and by the convex mirror are virtual: no light rays intersect at its location; they just seem to come from that location.

The Mirror Equation

To answer the first two questions given above, we use the mirror (and lens) equation:

Mirror (and Lens) Equation

$$\frac{1}{o} + \frac{1}{i} = \frac{1}{f}$$

Here, o stands for the object's distance from the mirror and is always positive. The value of f represents the focal length of the mirror. The value of i that satisfies this equation gives us the image's distance from the mirror. Both f and i are positive if they are on the same side as the human observer in relation to the mirror or lens. In the case of a mirror, the human observer is on the same side as the object. In the case of a lens, the human observer is on the opposite side of the lens from the object. Using the mirror (and lens) equation, we can find the location of the image, answering the first question.

The second question is also answered using the mirror equation. If we get a *positive* value for i, that tells us that the image is in front of the mirror and it's *real*; a *negative* value for i means the image is behind the mirror and is *virtual*. For example, let's say that $o = 2$ cm and $f = 6$ cm. Substituting these values into the mirror equation, we find that $i = -3$ cm. Therefore, the image is 3 cm behind the mirror and it's virtual. Note that you can use any unit for the measurement of distance, as long as it is the same unit for o, i, and f.

The Magnification Equation

To answer the last two questions, we then use the magnification equation:

Magnification Equation

$$m = -\frac{i}{o}$$

The value of m is the **magnification factor**; multiplying the size in any dimension (e.g., height or width) of the object by m gives us the size of the image. The sign of m tells us whether the image is upright or inverted. If m is *positive*, the image is *upright*; if m is *negative*, the image is *inverted*. To illustrate this, let's continue our example above, with $o = 2$ cm and $f = 6$ cm. We found that $i = -3$ cm. Therefore, the magnification factor is $m = -(-3 \text{ cm})/(2 \text{ cm}) = +1.5$. This tells us that the height of the image is 1.5 times the height of the object, and (because m is positive) the image is upright.

The object distance, o, is always positive. If i is positive, then m is negative; if i is negative, then m is positive. In other words,

Real images are inverted, and virtual images are upright.

Now, the only thing that's left to do is to find the way to "tell" the mirror equation whether we have a concave mirror or a convex mirror. The rule is simple: for any *converging* optic, the focal length is *positive*, and for any *diverging* optic, the focal length is *negative*. Therefore, the focal length of a *concave* mirror is a *positive* number, and the focal length of a *convex* mirror is a *negative* number. Here's a summary of mirrors:

Mirrors

Concave mirror f is positive

Convex mirror f is negative

$$\frac{1}{o} + \frac{1}{i} = \frac{1}{f}$$

i positive $\longrightarrow$ real image (in front of mirror)

i negative $\longrightarrow$ virtual image (behind mirror)

$$m = -\frac{i}{o}$$

m positive $\longrightarrow$ image upright

m negative $\longrightarrow$ image inverted

- Concave mirrors can create real and virtual images
- Convex mirrors can only create virtual images

Example 13-7: Describe the image formed in a plane mirror.

- A. Real and upright
- B. Real and inverted
- C. Virtual and upright
- D. Virtual and inverted

Solution: First, eliminate choices A and D; *real* always goes with *inverted*, and *virtual* always goes with *upright*. We know from common experience that the image formed in a flat mirror is upright, so the answer must be C.

Example 13-8: If an object is placed very far from a concave mirror, where will the image be formed?

- A. Halfway between the focal point and the mirror
- B. At the focal point
- C. At the center of curvature
- D. At infinity

Solution: Use the mirror equation. "The object is placed very far from a mirror" means that we take $o = \infty$, so $1/o = 0$. The mirror equation then says $1/i = 1/f$, so $i = f$. That is, the image is formed at the focal point of the mirror, choice B.

Example 13-9: An object is placed 40 cm in front of a concave mirror with a radius of curvature of 60 cm. Locate and describe the image.

Solution: Because $f = \dfrac{1}{2}r$, we know that $f = 30$ cm. The mirror equation now gives

$$\frac{1}{40 \text{ cm}} + \frac{1}{i} = \frac{1}{30 \text{ cm}} \rightarrow \frac{1}{i} = \frac{1}{30} - \frac{1}{40} = \frac{4-3}{120} = \frac{1}{120} \rightarrow \therefore i = 120 \text{ cm}$$

(Be careful: The MCAT often gives the radius of curvature, r. What you want is f, the focal length, which is half of r.) Since i is positive, we know the image is real; also, it's located 120 cm in front of the mirror. (*Virtual* images are located *behind* the mirror.) Since $m = -i/o = -(120 \text{ cm})/(40 \text{ cm}) = -3$, we know that the image is 3 times the height of the object and inverted.

Example 13-10: An object is placed 40 cm in front of a convex mirror with a radius of curvature of –60 cm. Locate and describe the image.

Solution: Because $f = \dfrac{1}{2}r$, we know that $f = -30$ cm. The mirror equation now gives

$$\frac{1}{40 \text{ cm}} + \frac{1}{i} = \frac{1}{-30 \text{ cm}} \rightarrow \frac{1}{i} = \frac{1}{-30} - \frac{1}{40} = \frac{-4-3}{120} = \frac{-7}{120} \rightarrow \therefore i = -\frac{120}{7} \text{ cm}$$

Since i is negative, we know the image is virtual; also, it's located $120/7 \approx 17$ cm behind the mirror. Since $m = -i/o = -(-\frac{120}{7} \text{ cm})/(40 \text{ m}) = +3/7$, we know that the image is 3/7 times the height of the object and upright. Comparing this example to the preceding one, notice how critical the sign of f was. It changed everything about the image.

Example 13-11: A convex mirror forms an upright image 12 cm behind the mirror when an object of height 15 cm is placed 20 cm in front of it. What is the height of the image?

Solution: To find the height of the image, we need the magnification. We're given that $o = 20$ cm and $i = -12$ cm. (We know that i is negative because not only do convex mirrors only form virtual images but the question also says that the image is formed "behind the mirror." Images formed behind the mirror are virtual.) Therefore, $m = -i/o = -(-12 \text{ cm})/(20 \text{ cm}) = 3/5$. Multiplying the height of the object by the magnification gives the height of the image. Therefore, the height of the image is $(3/5)(15 \text{ cm}) = 9$ cm.

13.5 LENSES

A **lens** is a thin piece of clear glass or plastic that forms an image of an object by *refracting* light. The purpose of this section is to find a systematic way to describe the images formed by lenses.

There are essentially two types of lenses: converging and diverging. **Convex, converging** lenses are thicker in the middle than they are at the ends, and they refract light rays that are parallel to the axis *toward* the focal point on the other side of the lens. **Concave, diverging** lenses are thinner in the middle than they are at the ends, and they refract light rays that are parallel to the axis *away from* the "imaginary" focal point that's in front of the lens.

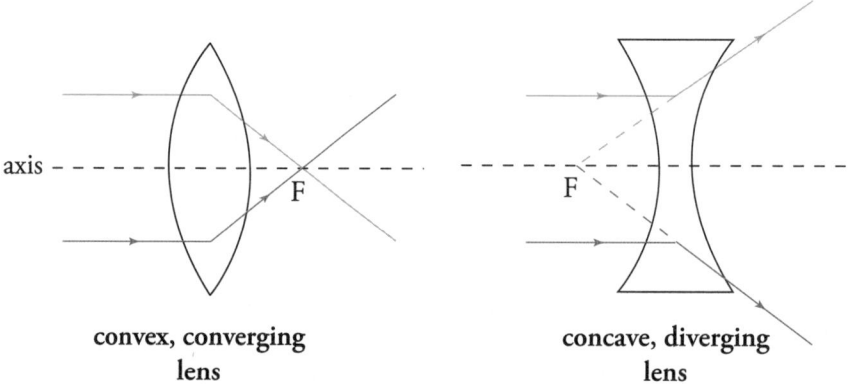

convex, converging
lens

concave, diverging
lens

We want to be able to answer the same four questions for lenses as we did for mirrors. Fortunately, *virtually everything we did for mirrors carries over unchanged to lenses.* For example, the mirror equation is also the lens equation, and the magnification equation is also the same. The conventions for positive and negative i and m are also the same for lenses as they are for mirrors.

We distinguish between the two types of lenses in the same way we distinguished between the two types of mirrors. When using the lens equation, the focal length of a *converging* lens is a *positive* number, and the focal length of a *diverging* lens is a *negative* number.

Here's an important note. The MCAT uses the terms *concave* and *convex* to refer to different mirrors and lenses. The diagrams above show us that a converging lens is convex and a diverging lens is concave. You may have noticed that this is the opposite of what we saw with mirrors. For a concave *mirror*, f is positive; and for a convex *mirror*, f is negative. When these terms are applied to lenses, things necessarily switch: For a concave *lens*, f is negative; and for a convex *lens*, f is positive. *Be careful* when you see the words *concave* or *convex*.

Besides the fact the lenses form images by refracting light (rather than by reflecting light, as is the case for mirrors), there's really only one difference: For lenses, *real* images are formed on the *opposite* side of the lens from the object while *virtual* images are formed on the *same* side of the lens as the object.

Here's a summary of lenses:

Lenses

Converging lens   Diverging lens
(convex lens)   (concave lens)
f is positive f is negative

$$\frac{1}{o} + \frac{1}{i} = \frac{1}{f}$$

i positive $\Rightarrow$ real image (other side of lens)
i negative $\Rightarrow$ virtual image (same side of lens as object)

$$m = -\frac{i}{o}$$

m positive $\Rightarrow$ image upright
m negative $\Rightarrow$ image inverted

- Converging (convex) lenses can create real and virtual images.
- Diverging (concave) lenses can create only virtual images.

Example 13-12: If an object is placed 10 cm in front of a diverging lens with a focal length of −40 cm, then the image will be located:

A. 5 cm in front of the lens
B. 5 cm behind the lens
C. 8 cm in front of the lens
D. 8 cm behind the lens

Solution: We use the lens equation to find i:

$$\frac{1}{10 \text{ cm}} + \frac{1}{i} = \frac{1}{-40 \text{ cm}} \rightarrow \frac{1}{i} = \frac{1}{40} - \frac{1}{10} = \frac{-1-4}{40} = \frac{-5}{40} = -\frac{1}{8} \rightarrow \therefore i = -8 \text{ cm}$$

This eliminates choices A and B. Because i is negative, the image is virtual, and for lenses, virtual images are formed on the same side of the lens as the object. Therefore, the answer is C.

Example 13-13: An object of height 10 cm is held 50 cm in front of a convex lens with a focal length of magnitude 40 cm. Describe the image.

Solution: The fact that the lens is convex means that it's a converging lens with a *positive* focal length; therefore, $f = +40$ cm. The lens equation now gives us i:

$$\frac{1}{50 \text{ cm}} + \frac{1}{i} = \frac{1}{40 \text{ cm}} \rightarrow \frac{1}{i} = \frac{1}{40} - \frac{1}{50} = \frac{5-4}{200} = \frac{1}{200} \rightarrow \therefore i = 200 \text{ cm}$$

13.5

Because i is positive, we know the image is real; also, it's located 200 cm from the lens on the *opposite* side of the lens from the object. Because $m = -i/o = -(200 \text{ cm})/(50 \text{ cm}) = -4$, we know that the image is 4 times the height of the object and inverted.

Lens Power

A lens with a short focal length refracts light more (i.e., through larger angles) than a lens with a longer focal length. We say that the lens of short focal length has a greater *power* than a lens with a longer focal length.

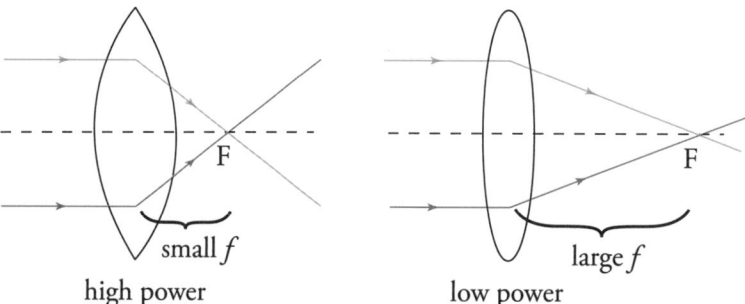

The **power** of a lens is defined to be the reciprocal of f, the focal length. When f is expressed in *meters*, the unit of lens power is called the **diopter** (abbreviated **D**).

Lens Power

$$P = \frac{1}{f} \text{ where } f \text{ is in meters}$$

For example, to find the power of a lens whose focal length is 40 cm, we first write f in meters: $f = 0.4$ m. Since $0.4 = 2/5$, the reciprocal of 0.4 is $5/2 = 2.5$. Therefore, the power of this lens is 2.5 diopters. Since the focal length of a converging lens is positive, the power of a converging lens is positive. Similarly, since the focal length of a diverging lens is negative, the power of a diverging lens is negative.

If two (or more) lenses are placed side by side, the power of the lens combination is equal to the sum of the powers of the individual lenses. In the case of two lenses, $P = P_1 + P_2$. For example, if we place a converging lens with a power of 3 D right next to a converging lens with a power of 1 D, then the power of the lens combination will be 4 D.

Example 13-14: A lens has a focal length of −20 cm. Is the lens converging or diverging? What is the power of this lens?

Solution: The fact that the lens has a negative focal length means that it's a diverging (or concave) lens. Rewriting f in meters, we have $f = -\frac{1}{5} \text{ m}$. Therefore, the power of this lens is

$$P = \frac{1}{f} = \frac{1}{-\frac{1}{5} \text{ m}} = -5 \text{ D}$$

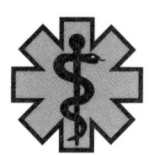

The Basics of Eyesight Correction

Let's now look at the fundamental use of auxiliary lenses to correct the two most common types of eye defects: myopia and hyperopia. **Myopia** is the technical name for *nearsightedness*; myopic individuals cannot focus clearly on distant objects. **Hyperopia** (or **hypermetropia**) is the technical name for *farsightedness*; in contrast to myopes, hyperopic individuals cannot focus clearly on objects that are near the eye. (As we age, most of us will be afflicted with *presbyopia*, in which the eyes' ability to *accommodate* is compromised by the loss of elasticity in the lens of the eye. **Accommodation** refers to the ability to focus on nearby objects through the action of the ciliary muscles, which essentially squeeze the lens of the eye, increasing its curvature and decreasing its focal length. However, the correction for presbyopia is the same as that for hyperopia.)

13.5

Correcting Myopia: Light rays from objects whose distance from the eye is greater than about 6 m are essentially parallel to the axis of the lens of the eye, so a relaxed eye will focus these rays at the focal point. Because the diameter of a myopic eye is greater than the focal length of the lens of the eye, the image of the object is focused not on the retina but in front of it. As a result, a myopic individual receives a blurred image of distant objects. To correct this defect, a lens that "delays" the focusing is required. In essence, what is needed is a lens to diverge the parallel rays before they enter the lens of the eye so that they will focus beyond the focal point of the unaided eye, specifically on the retina. Because diverging lenses have negative focal lengths, they have negative powers (this follows from the definition $P = 1/f$). The greater the distance between the focal point of the lens of the myopic eye and the retina, the more the auxiliary lens must diverge the incoming parallel rays; that is, the more powerful the corrective lens (and the more negative the lens power).

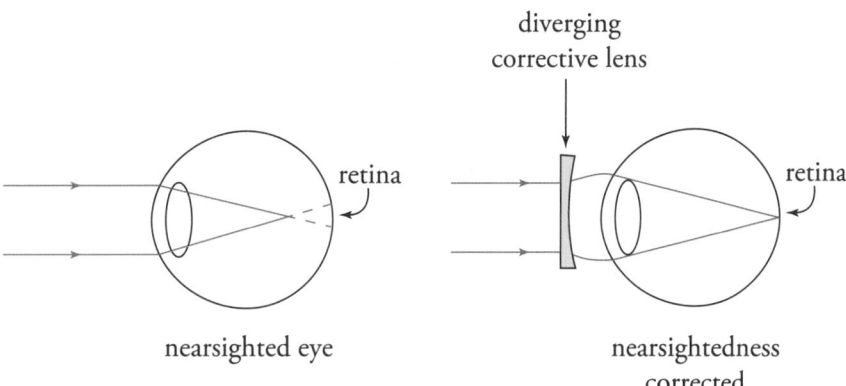

Correcting Hyperopia or Presbyopia: In these cases, light rays would be focused beyond the retina, either due to the diameter of the eye being smaller than the focal length of the lens of the eye or the inability of the ciliary muscles to decrease the focal length of the lens of the eye. To correct this defect, a lens that "accelerates" the focusing is required. In essence, what is needed is a lens to converge the rays before they enter the lens of the eye so that they will focus in front of the focal point of the unaided eye, specifically, on the retina. Because converging lenses have positive focal lengths, they have positive powers. (This follows from the definition $P = 1/f$.) The greater the distance between the focal point of the lens of the hyperopic eye and the retina, the more the auxiliary lens must converge the incoming rays; that is, the more powerful the corrective lens (and the more positive the lens power).

13.5

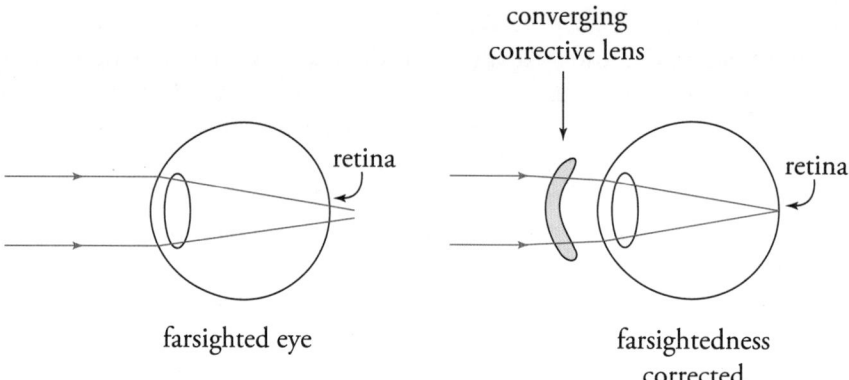

farsighted eye

converging
corrective lens

farsightedness
corrected

If you wear eyeglasses or contacts, check the prescription. If you have trouble seeing faraway objects, then you're nearsighted (myopic), and your corrective lenses are diverging and will have a negative power. On the other hand, if you have trouble seeing objects that are close-up, then you're farsighted (hyperopic), and your corrective lenses are converging and will have a positive power. Also, if the power of your left corrective lens is different from the power of your right corrective lens, the lens with the power of greater *absolute value* corresponds to the weaker eye. For example, if your left eye requires a lens of power −3.5 D while your right eye requires a lens of power −3.25 D, then your left eye is weaker because 3.5 > 3.25.

Summary of Formulas

Light acts as both a wave and a particle depending on the circumstance. In the former, energy is a function of amplitude; in the latter, energy is a function of frequency.

$$c = 3 \times 10^8 \text{ m/s for light in a vacuum}$$

- All angles for reflection and refraction formulas are measured from the normal to the surface.

Photon energy: $E = hf = h\dfrac{c}{\lambda}$

Law of reflection: $\theta_1 = \theta_1'$

Index of refraction: $n = \dfrac{c}{v}, n \geq 1$

Law of refraction (Snell's law): $n_1 \sin\theta_1 = n_2 \sin\theta_2$

Total internal reflection: If $n_1 > n_2$ and $\theta_1 > \theta_{crit}$, where $\sin\theta_{crit} = \dfrac{n_2}{n_1}$

Total internal reflection (meaning no light is transmitted from the incident medium through the boundary) can occur for incident angles greater than θ_{crit} and only when the incident medium has a larger index of refraction (n) than that of the medium beyond the boundary.

Mirror/lens equation: $\dfrac{1}{o} + \dfrac{1}{i} = \dfrac{1}{f}$

Magnification: $m = -\dfrac{i}{o}$

Converging mirror or lens (concave mirror or convex lens) $\leftrightarrow$ f positive

Diverging mirror or lens (convex mirror or concave lens) $\leftrightarrow$ f negative

Note o is always positive.

Real, inverted image $\leftrightarrow$ positive i

Virtual, upright image $\leftrightarrow$ negative i

Lens power: $P = \dfrac{1}{f}$ (P in diopters when f is expressed in meters)

CHAPTER 13 FREESTANDING PRACTICE QUESTIONS

1. In optics, spontaneous parametric down conversion is often used to create two photons from one photon. Thus, it is possible for a blue photon with a frequency of 700 THz to be split into two identical red photons when incident on a nonlinear crystal. What is the wavelength of the red photons with respect to the blue photon, λ_B, given that energy is conserved?

A) $2\lambda_B$
B) $4\lambda_B$
C) $1/2\lambda_B$
D) $1/4\lambda_B$

2. If the magnification of a mirror is 2, where are the focal point and the image?

A) The image is on the same side of the mirror as the object and the focal point is twice as far from the mirror as the object.
B) The image is on the same side of the mirror as the object and the focal point is half as far from the mirror as the object.
C) The image is on the opposite side of the mirror as the object and the focal point is twice as far from the mirror as the object.
D) The image is on the opposite side of the mirror as the object and the focal point is half as far from the mirror as the object.

3. Glasses that correct for nearsightedness have a negative power associated with them. Are these lenses diverging or converging, and do they have a focal length that is positive or negative?

A) Diverging lens with positive focal length
B) Converging lens with negative focal length
C) Diverging lens with negative focal length
D) Converging lens with positive focal length

4. An object is placed in front of a convex mirror. If the object is moved closer to the mirror, the image will move:

A) farther from the mirror and become smaller.
B) farther from the mirror and become larger.
C) closer to the mirror and become smaller.
D) closer to the mirror and become larger.

5. A physics student looking into a carnival funhouse mirror sees that his image is upright but his head appears twice as big as normal and his feet look half as big as normal. Let o represent the distance from the student to the mirror, f_{top} represent the focal length of the top of the mirror (where the student's head appears), and f_{bottom} represent the focal length of the bottom of the mirror (where the student's feet appear). What combination of curved mirrors is necessary to create the illusion?

A) The mirror top is concave with $f_{top} = 2o$ and the mirror bottom is convex with $f_{bottom} = -(1/2)o$.
B) The mirror top is concave with $f_{top} = 2o$ and the mirror bottom is convex with $f_{bottom} = -o$.
C) The mirror top is concave with $f_{top} = 3o$ and the mirror bottom is convex with $f_{bottom} = -(1/3)o$.
D) The mirror top is convex with $f_{top} = -o$ and the mirror bottom is concave with $f_{bottom} = (1/2)o$.

6. For a plane mirror, the object distance from the mirror is o, the image distance from the mirror is i, the focal point distance from the mirror is f, and the magnification of the mirror is m. Which of the following is true of the plane mirror?

I. Since f approaches infinity, then $i = -o$.
II. Since $f = 0$, then $i = -o$.
III. Since $i = -o$, then $m = 1$ and the image is the same size as the object.

A) I only
B) II only
C) I and III
D) II and III

7. A beam of light passing through crown glass ($n = 1.5$) strikes the surface between the glass and air and experiences Total Internal Reflection. Which of the following changes to the experiment would ensure that the beam of light continues to experience this phenomenon?

A) Have the light originate in air
B) Decrease the angle of incidence
C) Immerse the glass in water ($n = 1.33$)
D) Decrease the wavelength of light

CHAPTER 13 PRACTICE PASSAGE

Optical instruments, such as mirrors and lenses, are often used to converge or diverge light. When more than one optical instrument bends light in succession, it is sometimes useful to consider the image produced by the first mirror or lens to be the object from which the light comes to the second mirror or lens. In such cases, the virtual object for the second instrument is sometimes on the opposite side of the instrument as the incoming light. The convention for these objects is that their distances are negative in optics equations.

One example of the use of multiple optical instruments together can be found in vision correction. For an object to appear in focus, light from that object must converge on the retina at the back of the eye, roughly 2 cm away from the front in most humans. Normally, the cornea and crystalline lens (together effectively constituting one converging lens, with an index of refraction of about 1.4) at the front of the eyeball do this. When this does not occur, eyeglasses can often be used to fix the problem. Eyeglasses are made of converging or diverging lenses in frames, and they change the angle of the incoming light that reaches the lens at the front of the eye, which then is able to focus the differently angled light at the retina.

A lens bends light by refraction, so the refractive index of the lens material is one of the determinants of the focal length of the lens. For a lens with circular curvatures on either side, the radius of curvature of each side is another determinant. In a vacuum or air, the thin lens equation gives the focal length of a lens of minimal thickness, index of refraction n, radius of curvature of the side nearest the source of light R_1, and radius of curvature of the side opposite the source of light R_2:

$$\frac{1}{f} = (n-1)\left(\frac{1}{R_1} - \frac{1}{R_2}\right)$$

Equation 1

1. If a certain eye can only focus on objects at least 50 cm away, which of the following lenses, if placed in front of the eye, would allow it to focus on an object 25 cm away?

A) A converging lens with focal length 17 cm
B) A diverging lens with focal length 17 cm
C) A diverging lens with focal length 50 cm
D) A converging lens with focal length 50 cm

2. Which of the following is true of a nearsighted eye's native lens?

A) Its lens power is too small, causing the light rays to converge before they reach the retina.
B) Its lens power is too small, causing the light rays not to have converged even when they reach the retina.
C) Its lens power is too great, causing the light rays to converge before they reach the retina.
D) Its lens power is too great, causing the light rays not to have converged even when they reach the retina.

3. Which of the following describes the image formed in a typical human eye from light rays from an object 10 cm away?

A) The image is virtual and 0.4 cm away from the lens.
B) The image is real and 2 cm away from the lens.
C) The image is real and 2.5 cm away from the lens.
D) The image is virtual and 2.5 cm away from the lens.

4. What is the speed of light in the lens of the eye?

A) 1.5×10^8 m/s
B) 2.1×10^8 m/s
C) 3.0×10^8 m/s
D) 4.2×10^8 m/s

5. A person notices that an object at a given distance is clearly in focus when viewed in air, but when the same object at the same distance is viewed in clear water, it appears blurry. Which of the following best explains this phenomenon?

A) The water absorbs much of the light energy coming from the object.
B) The index of refraction of water is different from that of air.
C) Dispersion in the water causes only a few of the light rays from the object to reach the eyes.
D) The water acts as a polarizing filter.

6. How will the lens power of a thin lens with a greater index of refraction compare to that of a thin lens with a smaller index of refraction, if the two lenses have all the same radii of curvatures?

A) It will be greater.
B) It will be equal.
C) It will be less.
D) It cannot be determined.

SOLUTIONS TO CHAPTER 13 FREESTANDING QUESTIONS

1. **A**   The energy of a photon is $E = hf = hc/\lambda$. Since $E_B = 2E_R$ we know that $f_B = 2f_R$, and consequently, $\lambda_R = 2\lambda_B$.

2. **C**   The magnification equation is $m = -i/o$. Since $m = 2$, i is negative, which tells us the image is on the opposite side of the mirror as the object, a virtual image. This question is a two-by-two, meaning that we need two pieces of information to answer correctly. The fact that the image is virtual eliminates choices A and B. Using the mirror equation we find that $f = 2o$. Therefore, the focal point is twice as far from the mirror as the object.

3. **C**   For lenses, negative focal length is a property of a diverging lens and a positive focal length is a property of a converging lens. This eliminates choices A and B. The second piece of information comes from the fact that the power of nearsighted corrective glasses is negative, indicating a negative focal length since $P = 1/f$.

4. **D**   Ray tracing is not necessary to solve this problem. The mirror and the magnification equations can be used, but without numbers they could be time consuming. A simple method would be to choose the initial object distance to be very large ($o \approx \infty$). For any mirror (except the plane mirror) or lens, the image of a distant object forms at the focal point (Note: the mirror equation, $1/o + 1/i = 1/f$, backs this up; for large o, $1/o \approx 0$, so $i \approx f$). It also stands to reason that the image of a very distant object will be very small (by the magnification equation, $m = -i/o \approx 0$). The final object distance can be chosen as almost 0 (i.e., when the object is pressed up against the mirror. From experience, if an object is pressed up against any mirror, the image will also be pressing up against the mirror and appear to be the same size as the object. The image therefore moves from the focal point to the mirror, eliminating choices A and B, and goes from being very small to the size of the object, eliminating choice C.

5. **B**   Since the image is always upright, the magnification, m, is always positive. For the top of the mirror, $m = 2 = -i/o$ and $i = -2o$. Plugging this into the mirror equation $1/f = 1/i + 1/o = 1/(-2o) + 1/o = 1/(2o)$ and $f = 2o$. A positive focal length corresponds to a concave mirror. For the bottom of the mirror, $m = 1/2$ and $i = -(1/2)o$. Plugging this into the mirror equation $1/f = 1/i + 1/o = -2/o + 1/o = -1/o$ and $f = -o$. A negative focal length corresponds to a convex mirror. The correct answer is choice B.

6. **C**   For a plane mirror, the image size is the same as the object size, and the object is upright. So $m = -i/o = 1$ and $i = -o$. So Item III is true, eliminating choices A and B. Both Items I and II have $i = -o$, so plugging this into the mirror equation gives $1/f = 1/i + 1/o = 1/(-o) + 1/o = 0$ and f = something very large. So Item I is true, eliminating choice D. Notice that Item II cannot be true because if $f = 0$ then $1/f = 1/0$ which is not defined. The correct answer is choice C.

7. **D**   For light to experience total internal reflection, two conditions must be met. First, the light must originate in the slower medium (i.e., the one with the larger index of refraction), which eliminates choice A; second, the angle of incidence must be greater than the critical angle. While decreasing the angle of incidence may result in total internal reflection, it is not guaranteed since the angle could be smaller than or equal to the critical angle. This eliminates choice B. The formula for the *critical angle* is given by $\theta_c = \sin^{-1}(n_2 / n_1)$. Immersing the glass in water would increase n_2, which would increase the critical angle. This may cause the angle of incidence to be less than the critical angle, eliminating choice C. Due to *dispersion*, the shorter the wavelength of light, the slower it travels in glass, and therefore the more it will bend. Another way of thinking about this is that n_1 slightly increases for shorter wavelength. This would decrease the critical angle, and therefore make it impossible for refraction to occur.

SOLUTIONS TO CHAPTER 13 PRACTICE PASSAGE

1. **D**   According to the first paragraph, the lens needs to create an image where the object ought to be (50 cm away from the eye), and then the image becomes the "object" for the eye's lens, which converges the light on the retina. In other words, the object is at a distance of 25 cm and the image at a distance of 50 cm, and since the image is going to be on the same side of the lens as the object, the image will be virtual. Next, apply $\dfrac{1}{f} = \dfrac{1}{o} + \dfrac{1}{i}$ and plug in: $\dfrac{1}{f} = \dfrac{1}{25} + \dfrac{1}{(-50)} = \dfrac{1}{50}$, so the focal length is 50 cm.

2. **C**   In this question, one can eliminate two answers by deciding whether the lens power is too great or too small and eliminate the final wrong answer by determining whether the light rays converge too soon or too late. Nearsighted eyes can see near things well (the light of which is already diverging: look back at the diagram for correcting myopia), but cannot focus on faraway things (the light of which is arriving in parallel rays). This suggests that the eyes converge too strongly, which is a too-great lens power (eliminate choices A and B). Second, if the lens converges too strongly, the light rays must converge before they reach the retina (eliminate choice D). Note: This question can be answered without any information from the passage.

3. **B** According to the second paragraph, the retina is about 2 cm away from the lens in most humans. Also, the light rays actually converge on the retina. That describes the formation of a real image. Thus, the image is real (eliminate choices A and D) and is about 2 cm away from the lens (eliminate choice C). Be careful not to select choice C! This would be the correct answer if the distance between the retina and the lens were the focal length, but this does not match the passage's description; the position of the light rays actually converging (or where they would be traced back to converge, for a virtual image) is the image distance, not the focal length.

4. **B** Apply $n = \dfrac{c}{v}$. According to the second paragraph, in the lens, the index of refraction is 1.4, so $v = \dfrac{c}{n} \approx \dfrac{3 \times 10^8}{1.4} \approx 2.1 \times 10^8$ m/s. Note that light cannot travel faster than c, so choice D can be eliminated immediately.

5. **B** The lens in the eye works by refraction (like all lenses). If the eye does not change, but the medium from which the light is coming changes, then the angle of refraction will change (as in $n_1 \sin \theta_1 = n_2 \sin \theta_2$: modify n_1 while holding n_2 and θ_1 constant, and θ_2 will change). If the angle of refraction changes, then the light will not focus on the retina anymore. Note: This could be determined without reference to the passage, but if necessary, the fact that the light must converge on the retina can be found in the second paragraph, and the fact that refraction is involved is in the third paragraph.

    Alternatively, use process of elimination. Even if choice A were true, it would mean that less light energy would reach the eye, reducing the intensity of light; that dims the image but does not blur it. In choice C, dispersion refers to differences in a material's index of refraction for different frequencies of light (different colors); this can blur an image as different colors have slightly different focal lengths, but it would not significantly diminish the total amount of light reaching the eye. In choice D, polarization does not blur light, and water does not normally polarize light.

6. **A** Recall that lens power is given by $P = \dfrac{1}{f}$, and combining this with Equation 1 yields $P = (n-1)(\dfrac{1}{R_1} - \dfrac{1}{R_2})$. Thus, P is directly proportional to $(n - 1)$, and when n increases, so does P.

Chapter 14
Quantum Physics

14.1 QUANTIZATION

In the previous chapter, we learned that electromagnetic radiation can behave as a wave or as a particle called a photon. The discovery of this wave-particle duality of light was one of the first important results of the new **quantum physics** around the turn of the twentieth century. The word "quantum" refers to a specific amount of something measurable, like mass, charge, wavelength, momentum, energy, etc. Quantum physics, then, is the physics associated with discrete values and changes in the values of such quantities; that is, their **quantization**. We've already encountered an example of this phenomenon with charge: only charges that are integer multiples of the elementary charge $e = 1.6 \times 10^{-19}$ coulombs will ever be observed, because you can't have half a proton or two thirds of an electron. Thus charge is **quantized**.

Quantum physics is a complex and fascinating field that describes myriad strange phenomena and underlies many of our most important technological advances, such as computers, MRIs, and lasers. For MCAT purposes, you will need to understand the basic quantum model of the atom and the Pauli exclusion principle, the quantization of EM energy and the photoelectric effect, and the Heisenberg uncertainty principle.

14.2 THE BOHR MODEL OF THE ATOM

When a diffuse elemental gas is energized by heating or passing a current through it, the gas glows with a particular hue. If that light is passed through a prism, then dispersion will cause the light to separate into its component colors, corresponding to frequencies and wavelengths. This pattern of distinct bright lines of color is called the element's **emission spectrum**.

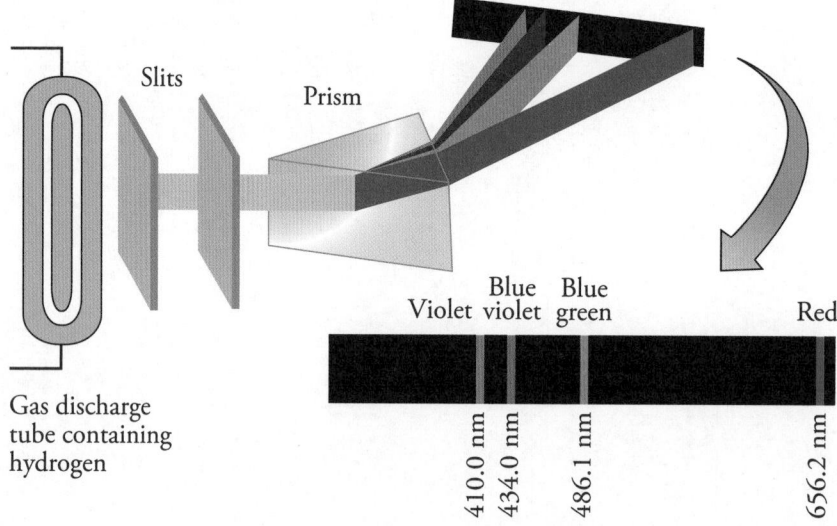

Recall that the energy of a photon is given by

$$E_{photon} = hf = hc \ / \ \lambda$$

where h is Planck's constant, 6.63×10^{-34} joule-seconds. Thus, one can use the measured wavelengths of light to determine the energies of the atomic transitions that produced the light. The assumption is that the particular frequencies of photons emitted by the atoms in the gas correspond to the energy losses of the atoms as their electrons transition from higher to lower energy states. Because only these characteristic frequencies are observed for a given element under normal conditions, this indicates that only certain electron transitions can occur.

Example 14-1: The wavelength of the red Hα spectral line characteristic of the visible hydrogen spectrum is 656 nm. How much energy does a hydrogen atom lose when it emits an Hα photon? Use $h = 6.63 \times 10^{-34}$ J·s.

Solution: Use the equation for the energy of a photon in terms of wavelength:

$$E_{photon} = \frac{hc}{\lambda} = \frac{\left(6.63 \times 10^{-34} \text{ J·s}\right)\left(3 \times 10^{8} \text{ m/s}\right)}{656 \times 10^{-9} \text{ m}} \approx 3 \times 10^{-19} \text{ J}$$

The energy of the emitted photon corresponds exactly to the energy lost by the hydrogen atom.

Danish physicist Niels Bohr explained these discrete and characteristic emission spectra by modifying the classical Rutherford atomic model, which depicted the atom as a planetary system, with a tiny but massive central positive charge orbited by distant electrons. The Rutherford model explained many experimental results, but it failed to account for the discrete emission spectra. Scientists knew that accelerating charges emitted EM waves, but because there were no restrictions on the orbital radii of the electrons in the Rutherford model, there was no reason that the emission spectra shouldn't include all wavelengths instead of the discrete few actually observed. To fix this problem, Bohr's model proposed that the angular momentum of the orbiting electrons was quantized, restricted to multiples of the Planck constant:

Quantization of Angular Momentum

$$mvr = nh \ / \ 2\pi$$

where $n = 1, 2, 3 \ldots$

Note that this angular momentum for a circular orbit is simply the familiar linear momentum $p = mv$ multiplied by the orbital radius r. Note that as of 2015, the MCAT stopped testing linear and angular momentum as memorized concepts. We present this formula and explanation here because it is required to explain how Bohr arrived at his quantum model of the atom.

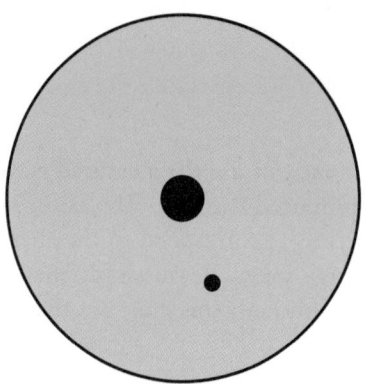 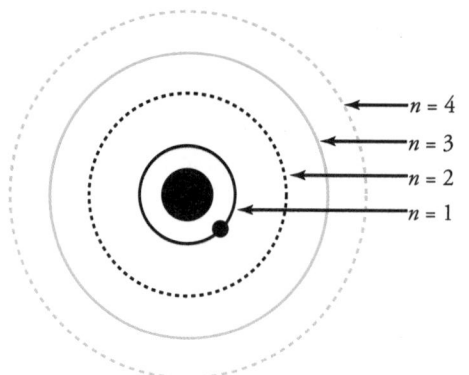

Rutherford Model
Electrons assume arbitrary orbits

Bohr Model
Electrons assume quantized orbits

The Bohr model assumes that atoms have electron orbitals with quantized energy levels and that a transition between levels requires the absorption or emission of a photon:

Energy of a Photon Emitted or Absorbed under the Bohr Model

$$E_{\text{photon}} = |\Delta E_{\text{atom}}|$$

Bohr's model retained two classical assumptions built into the Rutherford model: conservation of energy and the idea that the Coulomb force provided the centripetal acceleration for the electrons. For the sake of simplicity, the equations below apply to a hydrogen atom with a single proton and electron.

Total orbital energy: $\quad E = KE + PE = \frac{1}{2}mv^2 - k\dfrac{e^2}{r}$

Centripetal force: $\quad F_c = \dfrac{mv^2}{r} = k\dfrac{e^2}{r^2}$

Example 14-2: Find the orbital radius of an electron in the nth orbital of a hydrogen atom.

Solution: First solve for the orbital speed v using the angular momentum quantization equation

$$mvr = \frac{nh}{2\pi} \rightarrow v = \frac{nh}{2\pi mr}$$

Now substitute this value for v into the centripetal force equation and solve the resulting equation for r

$$\frac{mv^2}{r} = k\frac{e^2}{r^2} \rightarrow \frac{m\left(n^2h^2\right)}{r\left(4\pi^2 m^2 r^2\right)} = \frac{n^2h^2}{4\pi^2 mr^3} = \frac{ke^2}{r^2}$$

$$r_n = \frac{n^2h^2}{4\pi^2 km_{\text{electron}}e^2}$$

Example 14-3: What is the diameter of a hydrogen atom in the ground state according to the Bohr model? Use 9×10^{-31} kg for the mass of the electron.

Solution: The ground state of an atom corresponds to a value of $n = 1$, and the diameter is just twice the radius. Thus we can substitute values into the equation for the radius found in Example 14-2 on the previous page.

$$r_1 = \frac{h^2}{4\pi^2 k m_{electron} e^2} = \frac{\left(6.63 \times 10^{-34}\right)^2}{4\left(\pi\right)^2 \left(9 \times 10^9\right)\left(9 \times 10^{-31}\right)\left(1.6 \times 10^{-19}\right)^2} \approx$$

$$\frac{44 \times 10^{-68}}{4 \times 9 \times 9 \times 9 \times 2.5 \times 10^{-60}} \approx \frac{10^{-68}}{200 \times 10^{-60}} = 5 \times 10^{-11} \text{ m}$$

Thus the diameter of the hydrogen atom in the ground state is about 1×10^{-10} meters (also called one angstrom).

Example 14-4: What is the energy of the nth orbital of a hydrogen atom in terms of n and known constants?

Solution: Solve the centripetal force equation for mv^2 and substitute into the energy equation:

$$\frac{mv^2}{r} = \frac{ke^2}{r^2} \rightarrow mv^2 = \frac{ke^2}{r}$$

$$E = KE + PE = \tfrac{1}{2}mv^2 - k\frac{e^2}{r} = \frac{1}{2}\frac{ke^2}{r} - \frac{ke^2}{r} = -\frac{ke^2}{2r}$$

Now substitute the expression for r_n into the result:

$$E_n = -\frac{ke^2}{2r_n} = -\frac{ke^2}{2n^2 h^2} \times 4\pi^2 k m_{electron} e^2 = -\frac{2\pi^2 k^2 m_{electron} e^4}{n^2 h^2}$$

If you plug in values for the constants, you find that $E_n = -2.17 \times 10^{-18}$ J/n^2. More commonly, the energy of the atomic energy levels is expressed in terms of electron-volts (eV), that is, the product of the elementary charge e with volts V. Because the elementary charge is equal to 1.6×10^{-19} C, converting from joules to eV requires dividing by this number. This yields

Energy Level of a Hydrogen Atom

$$E_n = -13.6 \text{ eV} / n^2$$

where $n = 1, 2, 3 \ldots$

Be sure you understand why this energy is negative. Electrons orbiting a nucleus are energetically bound to it and must absorb more energy to move further from that nucleus or to escape (thereby ionizing the atom). Thus the energy of the orbital has to become increasingly positive as n increases, up to zero as n approaches infinity (which means ionization has occurred).

Bohr's model thus explains the emission spectra of hydrogen and, by extension, the other elements: any single change in n entails a discrete change in energy according to

$$\Delta E = -13.6 \text{ eV}\left(\frac{1}{n_{final}^2} - \frac{1}{n_{initial}^2}\right)$$

This change in energy between two states will correspond to the emission (if the change is negative) or absorption (if the change is positive) of a photon. The energy of that photon will therefore be given by

The Energy of a Photon Emitted or Absorbed by a Hydrogen Atom

$$hf = |\Delta E| = \left|13.6 \text{ eV}\left(\frac{1}{n_{final}^2} - \frac{1}{n_{initial}^2}\right)\right|$$

Example 14-5: What is the frequency of a photon that, when absorbed, will ionize a hydrogen atom that begins in the $n = 2$ state? Planck's constant is $h = 4.14 \times 10^{-15}$ eV·s

Solution: When an atom is ionized, its final state is $n \to \infty$, so applying the preceding equation yields

$$hf = \left|13.6 \text{ eV}\left(0 - \frac{1}{2^2}\right)\right| = 3.4 \text{ eV}$$

$$f = \frac{3.4 \text{ eV}}{4.14 \times 10^{-15} \text{ eV·s}} \approx 8 \times 10^{14} \text{ Hz}$$

Example 14-6: The red Hα line has a wavelength of 656 nm. If the final state in the atomic transition that produces this line is $n = 2$, what was the initial state?

Solution: According to the solution to Example 14-1, the energy of the Hα photon is roughly 3×10^{-19} J. First convert this value to eV by dividing by $e = 1.6 \times 10^{-19}$ C to get about 2 eV. Then apply the equation for the energy change associated with a hydrogen energy-level transition:

$$|\Delta E| = 2 \text{ eV} = \left|13.6 \text{ eV}\left(\frac{1}{2^2} - \frac{1}{n_{initial}^2}\right)\right|$$

$$\frac{2}{13.6} = \frac{1}{4} - \frac{1}{n_{initial}^2} \to \frac{1}{7} - \frac{1}{4} = -\frac{1}{n_{initial}^2}$$

$$\frac{4}{28} - \frac{7}{28} = -\frac{3}{28} \approx -\frac{1}{9} = -\frac{1}{n_{initial}^2}$$

$$n_{initial}^2 = 9 \to n_{initial} = 3$$

14.3 THE PAULI EXCLUSION PRINCIPLE

A few years after Bohr refined his model, Wolfgang Pauli devised an explanation for the fact that the elements exhibited patterns of chemical behavior related to the number of electrons. For example, atoms with even numbers of electrons are in general more chemically stable than those with odd numbers. Pauli determined that these groupings of elements and their behaviors could be explained that so long as only one electron was allowed to occupy a particular *quantum state*, defined not only by the principal quantum number n but three additional quantum numbers. For MCAT purposes, understanding the **Pauli exclusion principle** usually means recognizing that each atomic orbital can hold only two electrons of opposite *spin*, a quantum number that defines the intrinsic angular momentum of the electron. However, the Pauli exclusion principle applies to protons and neutrons as well, and asserts more broadly that there is a limit to how many such particles can be confined in a small space.

14.4 THE PHOTOELECTRIC EFFECT

In the late nineteenth century, long before Bohr's quantum atomic model, it was noticed that a spark would jump between two charged plates when a strong light was shone on the negative plate, and that the spark would diminish or disappear altogether when a filter was used to block the ultraviolet component of the light. Because the light is giving rise to an electric current, the effect is called the **photoelectric effect**. Below is a picture of the apparatus used to measure this effect.

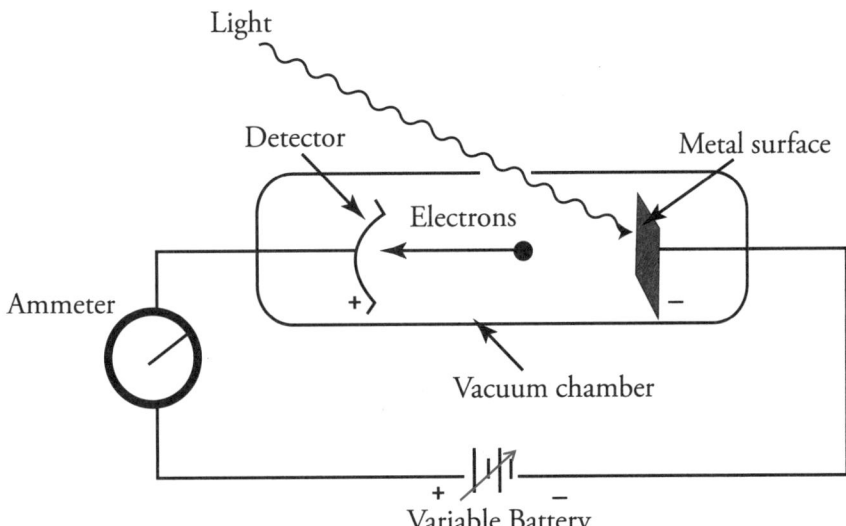

The ammeter will register a current only when *photoelectrons* (that is, electrons ejected by the incident light) pass from the metal surface to the detector. Note that the voltage of the battery can be varied and that its polarity can be reversed.

According to the classical theory of light as a wave, the energy absorbed by the metal surface depends only upon the amplitude of the light wave, i.e., the light's brightness. The energy delivered by this continuous wave increases with time; the longer a light of a given intensity shines on a surface, the more energy will be absorbed. It was also well known by the time the photoelectric effect was first observed that some of the electrons normally bound to a metal would be ejected when the metal was heated. This is analogous to a pot of water on the stove: individual water molecules are bound to the volume of liquid water, but due to thermal effects, some will occasionally evaporate off the surface. This effect increases as the water is heated to boiling. The binding energy of the metal for its surface electrons (the ones most likely to be ejected) is called the metal's **work function**, ϕ.

Based upon the wave theory and the thermal ejection of electrons, one would expect the following:

- a brighter light would yield a stronger current than a dimmer one, regardless of color/frequency;
- because the light takes some time to heat the metal, there would be a delay between the time the light first shines on the metal and when a current is detected; and
- if the polarity of the battery were reversed, so that electrons ejected from the metal surface were repelled by the detector and only the more energetic among them would reach the detector, increasing the brightness of the light would increase the maximum potential difference the ejected electrons could overcome to reach the detector. In other words, when light of a certain brightness is shone on the metal surface, there will be some negative potential at the detector at which the measured current drops to zero. This is called the **stopping voltage**, V_{stop}. According to the wave theory of light, increasing the brightness of the light should increase the magnitude of this stopping voltage.

Surprisingly, each of these expectations was contradicted by experimental results. Though increasing the brightness of the light did yield more current when there was a current to begin with, light below a certain frequency would not generate *any* current, regardless of brightness. Current was detected instantaneously when the light illuminated the metal surface. Finally, the intensity of the light had no effect on the measured stopping voltage, but the frequency of the light did affect V_{stop}. The wave theory of light was at an impasse.

In 1905, Einstein published the paper that explained these findings (the paper for which he later won the Nobel Prize). Einstein's explanation of the photoelectric effect developed the photon model of light previously mentioned. There are three important points in this model that explain the experimental results better than does the wave model of light.

- Electromagnetic radiation (i.e., light) of a certain frequency is made up of discrete bundles of energy (now called "photons"), each with energy $E = hf$.
- Photons of light are absorbed or emitted as single instantaneous interactions (as opposed to the mechanism provided by the wave model for gradually absorbing or emitting energy).
- When a photon strikes the surface of a metal, it interacts with a single electron, imparting all of its energy in the form of increased kinetic energy for the electron. If this energy is greater than the work function of the metal, the electron will be ejected from the metal with kinetic energy given by the following expression (note the subscript indicating that this is the maximum kinetic energy for an ejected electron: many electrons ejected will be "deeper" in the metal and thus will lose more energy in the process of ejection).

Kinetic Energy of a Photoelectron

$$KE_{max} = hf - \phi$$

Let's consider how the photon model resolves the three problems with the experiment previously described. First, if the individual photons interact with individual electrons, then a single photon must provide enough energy for the electron to overcome the work function of the metal, or that electron will remain bound and no photoelectric current will be measured. A brighter light means there are more photons, but the energy of *each individual photon remains the same unless the frequency/color of the light is changed.* Therefore, as was observed, making the light brighter will increase the measured current if there is some current to being with, but a frequency of light that doesn't create any current of photoelectrons will never do so, no matter how bright it is.

The photon-electron interaction also explains why the photoelectric current is measured instantaneously instead of after a delay for the metal to absorb enough light energy. Photons deliver their energy all at once instantaneously, so as soon as photons of sufficient energy hit the metal, some electrons will be ejected and will begin to strike the detector.

To understand the relevance of Einstein's explanation for the determination of the stopping voltage, it helps to consider the requirements for a photoelectron to reach the detector. When the detector is connected to the positive terminal of the battery and there is a positive voltage difference between the metal surface and the detector (as shown in the figure), it will attract all the photoelectrons ejected from the metal surface. On the other hand, when the polarity of the battery is reversed so that the detector is connected to the negative terminal of the battery, then the detector repels the photoelectrons. In that case, in order for the ammeter to measure a current, the detected photoelectrons must overcome the negative voltage difference between the metal surface and the detector. As that negative voltage is increased in magnitude, eventually it will be large enough that no photoelectrons will reach the detector. At that point, the current will drop to zero.

Stopping Voltage for the Photoelectric Effect

$$-eV_{stop} = KE_{max}$$

Remember that we've defined V_{stop} as a negative voltage, so the term on the left must have an additional negative sign to equal a necessarily positive kinetic energy.

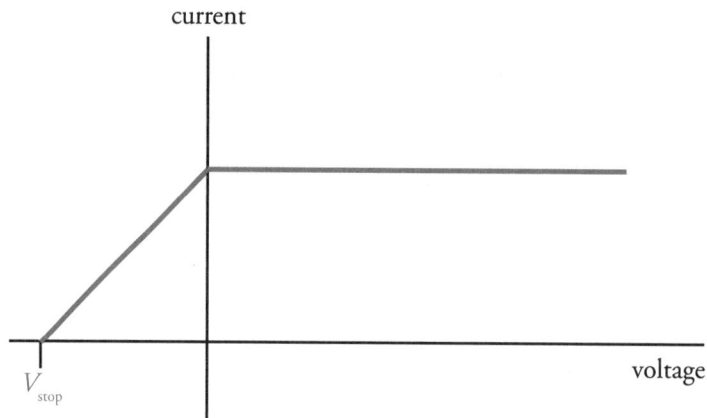

Current through the Ammeter as a Function of Applied Voltage

Example 14-7: The photon model of light is necessary to explain each of the following experimentally observed effects EXCEPT:

A. The ejection of electrons from a metal surface with light shining upon it
B. The stopping voltage as a function of light frequency
C. The instantaneous detection of a current following the application of light to the metal surface
D. The fact that an intense infrared light may result in no measured current where a dim ultraviolet light results in measured current

Solution: Refer back to the list of three expected outcomes of the photoelectric experiment given the wave theory of light. The wave theory of light predicts that the stopping voltage should be a function of intensity, not frequency, eliminating choice B. It also predicts a delay between the application of light to the metal surface and a detection of a current (providing adequate time for the plate to energize and eject electrons). This eliminates choice C. Moreover, the wave theory predicts that the ejection of electrons at all depends purely upon the intensity of the light applied to the metal surface, not on its frequency. This eliminates choice D. Choice A is correct because the ejection of electrons by the application of light is perfectly predictable according to the classical wave theory: it's just the *manner* in which they are ejected that requires the photon theory.

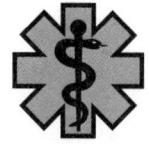

Example 14-8: Almost all modern medical imaging (that doesn't rely on actual film) relies on a simple principle: translating electromagnetic or ionizing radiation signals from the imaging device into electrical signals, which can then be translated into an image on a screen. In the operation of a positron emission tomography (*PET*) scan, for example, a radioactive tracer is injected into a patient. The tracer undergoes β^+ decay, and the positrons annihilate electrons in their vicinity in a matter-antimatter interaction that releases gamma radiation. The gamma radiation is then picked up by a so-called "gamma camera" composed of an array of scintillating crystals (which absorbs the gamma photon and reemits a photon of lower energy) and *photomultiplier tubes* (which absorb these secondary photons). The principle of operation of the photomultiplier tubes is the photoelectric effect: incident photons are converted to photoelectrons, which are absorbed and amplified as a cascading electric current measured and recorded by a computer. These flashes of current are eventually composed into an image.

Suppose the photomultiplier tubes in a gamma camera use cesium to absorb the incident photons. Cesium has a work function of 2.1 eV. What is the maximum wavelength of incident light that would eject a photoelectron from cesium?

Solution: First, recognize that the *maximum* wavelength of light will correspond to the *minimum* frequency and therefore energy. The minimum kinetic energy an electron could have when ejected would be 0, meaning the electron just barely overcame the work function of the metal. Applying the equation for the kinetic energy of the ejected photoelectron yields

$$0 = hf_{min} - \phi = \left(4.1 \times 10^{-15} \text{ eV}\right) f_{min} - 2.1 \text{ eV}$$

$$f_{min} = \frac{2.1}{4.1 \times 10^{-15}} \approx 5 \times 10^{14} \text{ Hz}$$

Now convert this minimum frequency into a maximum wavelength:

$$c = f\lambda \rightarrow \lambda_{max} = \frac{c}{f_{min}} = \frac{3 \times 10^8}{5 \times 10^{14}} = 6 \times 10^{-7} \text{ m}$$

Example 14-9: Suppose a photoelectric experiment is conducted and the applied voltage is varied over a range of values to generate a graph of current versus voltage similar to that shown above. If the intensity of the light is increased but all other aspects of the experiment are kept the same, which of the following aspects of the generated graph would change?

   I.   The slope of the line from V_{stop} to $V = 0$
   II. The location of V_{stop}
  III. The maximum value of the current

   A. I only
   B. II only
   C. I and III only
   D. I, II, and III

Solution: The stopping voltage depends upon the maximum kinetic energy of the photoelectrons, which in turn depends upon the *frequency* of the incident light and the work function of the metal target. Therefore, changing the *intensity* of the incident light will not alter the stopping voltage, so Item II is false, eliminating choices B and D. Increasing the intensity will, however, increase the number of photons striking the target, and therefore will increase the number of photoelectrons and therefore the maximum current, meaning Item III is true, eliminating choice A. Choice C is correct, and Item I is true because if the stopping voltage stays the same but the maximum current increases, the slope of the line from V_{stop} up to the now higher *y*-intercept must be greater.

Example 14-10: Now suppose the experiment were repeated and both the applied voltage and frequency of the incident light were varied by the experimenter (but not the intensity of the light). For each set frequency, the experimenter would increase the negative voltage of the variable battery until no current was measured in the ammeter (sufficiently low frequencies would produce zero current even for positive voltages). What would the experimenter's graph of stopping voltage versus incident frequency look like?

Solution: Consider that only electrons that have at least as much kinetic energy as the potential energy gap they must cross can be detected as current. This is analogous to tossing balls in the air in a room with a high ceiling: you can weakly toss up a million balls, but none of them will be detected as a "current" of thumps against the ceiling unless you toss some with enough energy to reach the height of the ceiling. Mathematically, this means:

$$KE_{max} = -\Delta PE \rightarrow hf - \phi = -eV_{stop} \rightarrow -V_{stop} = \frac{h}{e}f - \frac{\phi}{e}$$

Note that we've solved for $-V_{stop}$: that is simply because we are more accustomed to reading graphs predominantly in the first quadrant (this just means that values above the horizontal axis indicate negative voltages of the variable battery). The graph of this function looks like this (note the dashed line below the horizontal, representing a linear extrapolation of the work function: no data points could be discovered below the threshold frequency):

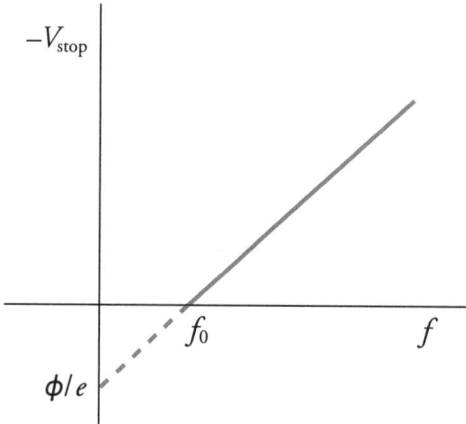

14.5   THE HEISENBERG UNCERTAINTY PRINCIPLE

In 1927, Werner Heisenberg was working with Niels Bohr in Copenhagen to further develop the new quantum physics. While Bohr was away skiing, Heisenberg recognized a surprising but critical consequence of wave-particle duality: uncertainty. To measure the position of a particle extremely accurately, one had to shine a very short wavelength light on it, because the wavelength itself is a limitation on the determination of position. A short wavelength corresponds to a high frequency and high energy, and when a high energy photon interacts with a particle like an electron, it imparts some of its energy and momentum to the particle. (The relation between energy and momentum is given by $E = p^2/2m$.) This means the momentum of the particle changes, which introduces an uncertainty into the measure of the momentum. Conversely, a longer wavelength, lower energy light beam would allow one to measure the momentum of the particle it interacted with to greater precision, but the long wavelength means a greater uncertainty in the position of the particle. Using capital deltas to represent the uncertainty in a quantity, Heisenberg's uncertainty relation can be written as

> ### The Heisenberg Uncertainty Relation
>
> $$\Delta x \Delta p \geq h/2\pi$$

where x represents the position of the particle (or object more generally) and h is Planck's constant.[1]

Example 14-11: Driving through M-k-sopolis, you are pulled over by a policeman for doing 30 m/s in a 25 m/s speed limit zone. Trying to talk your way out of the ticket, you ask the officer how he knows you were in 25 m/s zone. He replies that he used a high frequency laser detector to determine your position to within 10^{-7} m. Given this precision in position, is the minimum uncertainty in his measurement of your momentum large enough that you can argue you might have been going 25 m/s? Assume your car has a mass of 1000 kg, and use $h = 6.63 \times 10^{-34}$ J·s.

Solution: The uncertainty in the position of your car is $\Delta x = 10^{-7}$ m. Plugging this into the Heisenberg uncertainty relation yields

$$\Delta x \Delta p \geq \frac{h}{2\pi} \rightarrow \Delta p \geq \frac{6.63 \times 10^{-34}}{2\pi \times 10^{-7}} \approx 10^{-27} \text{ kg} \cdot \text{m/s}$$

Using momentum $p = mv$, the uncertainty in velocity is thus $\Delta p = m\Delta v \rightarrow \Delta v = 10^{-27}/10^3 = 10^{-30}$ m/s. Since this is much, MUCH less than 5 m/s (the difference between your measured speed and the speed limit), you'll have to bite the bullet and pay the ticket!

Heisenberg's uncertainty relation has far-reaching consequences. For one, though it is often explained using the language of measurement, you should not interpret it to mean that a particle like an electron *really* has an exact position and momentum, but we just can't find out what they are. The reality is far stranger than that: uncertainty isn't just a matter of what we can *know*, but rather a matter of *what really is the case!* In quantum physics, quantities like position and momentum, energy and time, are fundamentally probabilistic. This means that they have most likely values, but not exact values; if one attempted to determine the exact value of one of the quantities, the other would become entirely uncertain. In other words, if you were to describe *exactly* how fast an electron was moving, the uncertainty in its position would be the entire universe: it could be anywhere with equal likelihood! Practically speaking, this would be impossible, because to measure any quantity requires using a beam that has wave properties, and no wave can have a wavelength of 0 or infinity. This uncertainty affects biomedical research into very small objects, because it limits the extent to which microscopic structures can be imaged by light but also opens up possibilities for imaging them with particles like electrons. More theoretically, Heisenberg's uncertainty relation explains, for example, why the ground state of a hydrogen atom is the smallest orbital, i.e., why there can't be a smaller one. This is something that the Bohr model did not explain.

---

[1] You will also see the Heisenberg Uncertainty Relation expressed with $h/4\pi$, and possibly other ways as well depending upon the source and how the relation was derived and interpreted. The nuances will not matter for the MCAT, nor are you likely to be asked to do a precise calculation using this inequality. The basic concept should be your focus.

Example 14-12: Determine the uncertainty of the momentum of an electron in the $n = 1$ state.

Solution: We previously determined that the diameter of the hydrogen atom in the ground state was about 10^{-10} m. An electron in the $n = 1$ state therefore could be found anywhere within that diameter, meaning $\Delta x = 10^{-10}$ m. The uncertainty of its momentum is therefore given by

$$\Delta x \Delta p \geq \frac{h}{2\pi} \rightarrow \Delta p \geq \frac{6.63 \times 10^{-34}}{2\pi \times 10^{-10}} \approx 10^{-24} \text{ kg} \cdot \text{m/s}$$

Though the math is slightly beyond the level of the MCAT, it is straightforward to show using the relation $E = p^2/2m$ that, given this uncertainty in momentum, were the electron to be confined to a smaller radius, the uncertainty in its energy would necessarily be greater than 13.6 eV, the energy of the hydrogen ground state. In other words, a "lower" state than the ground state would, according to the Heisenberg uncertainty principle, have to have a *higher* energy. This is a contradiction, proving that the ground state in the Bohr model of hydrogen indeed must be the lowest energy state.

Summary of Formulas

Energy of a photon: $E_{photon} = hf = hc/\lambda$

Bohr model of the atom assumes:

The atom is made up of a dense, massive positive nucleus orbited by negative electrons (like the Rutherford model)

The energy levels of an atom are quantized. They are determined by the discrete orbital states of the electrons, numbered n = 1, 2, 3.... The higher numbered states correspond to higher energies. The lowest state, n = 1, is the *ground* state, and is stable over time.

Atoms can change quantized energy states by absorbing or emitting a photon. The energy of the photon must correspond exactly to the energy difference between the two states: $E_{photon} = |\Delta E_{atom}|$

Atoms can also change energy states thermally by interacting with other particles. As with the case of photon absorption, though, the changes in atomic energy are quantized, and excited atoms will tend to return to the ground state by emitting photons (this is why a heated metal glows, for example).

Bohr model of the hydrogen atom: $E_n = -13.6 \text{ eV} / n^2$, where n = 1, 2, 3...

Photons absorbed or emitted by a hydrogen atom: $hf = \left| 13.6 \text{ eV} \left(\dfrac{1}{n_{final}^2} - \dfrac{1}{n_{initial}^2} \right) \right|$

The Pauli exclusion principle states that no two electrons, protons, or neutrons can occupy the same quantum state (have the same quantum numbers) within a small space.

The photoelectric effect occurs when light incident upon a metal surface causes electrons to be ejected by that surface. Individual photons provide energy hf to individual electrons, and if that energy is enough to overcome the binding energy of the metal, the electrons are ejected.

The maximum kinetic energy of the ejected electrons is $KE_{max} = hf - \phi$.

The stopping voltage necessary to prevent the most energetic electrons from reaching a negatively-charged plate is given by $-eV_{stop} = KE_{max}$

The Heisenberg uncertainty principle sets a limit on the precision with which position and momentum are determined: $\Delta x \Delta p \geq h/2\pi$

CHAPTER 14 FREESTANDING QUESTIONS

1. A red photon and a blue photon both strike a piece of unknown material at the same acute angle of incidence. Any of the following could happen EXCEPT:

A) The blue photon ejects an electron but the red photon does not.
B) The blue photon passes through the material at a faster speed than does the red photon.
C) The blue photon is reflected while the red photon is transmitted.
D) Both photons eject electrons from the material.

2. An electromagnetic beam with wavelength λ_0 is incident upon an unknown metal. If electrons are ejected with maximum kinetic energy K, what is the work function of the metal?

A) hc/λ_0
B) $h\lambda_0/c$
C) $hc/\lambda_0 - K$
D) $h\lambda_0/c - K$

3. According to the *de Broglie hypothesis*, wave-particle duality extends to all particles, not just photons. The wavelength of any particle is a function of the particle's momentum p according to the equation $\lambda = h/p$. An electron orbiting a proton can thus be considered a standing wave that forms a closed loop around the nucleus: only modes producing integer wavelengths are permitted. What is the wavelength of the ground state, fundamental mode of the electron in this simple Bohr atom (let m_e represent the mass of the electron)?

A) $\dfrac{h^2}{4\pi^2 m_e k e^2}$

B) $\dfrac{h^2}{2\pi m_e k e^2}$

C) $\dfrac{h^2}{\pi m_e k e^2}$

D) $\dfrac{2\pi m_e k e^2}{h^2}$

4. A series of trials are conducted using the standard photoelectric experiment set up, with the variable voltage at the detector set to a high positive difference from the target metal surface. In each trial, a filter is used to allow only light of a certain frequency to shine on the metal target's surface. Over the course of five trials, five different frequencies of increasing value are allowed to strike the target. If we assume that the intensity of the light striking the target remains constant over all the trials, which of the following graphs represents the most likely outcome of measured current as a function of frequency?

A)

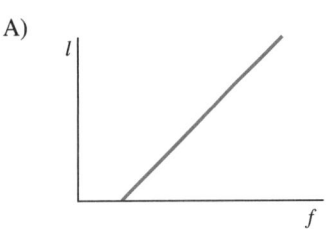

B)

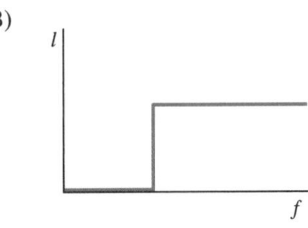

C)

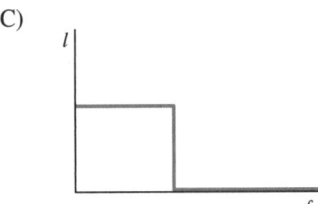

D)

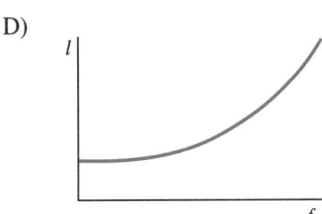

5. Which of the following changes to the photoelectric experiment could change the value of the stopping voltage?

   I.   Increasing the duration of the experiment
   II. Changing the wavelength of the incident light
   III. Changing the material used for the metal target

A) I only
B) II only
C) I and III only
D) II and III only

6. A singly ionized helium atom behaves the same way as a hydrogen atom, the important difference being that there are two protons in the nucleus instead of one. What would be the energy of the photon released by an He$^+$ ion as it transitioned from the $n = 2$ state to the $n = 1$ state?

A) 10.2 eV
B) 13.6 eV
C) 20.4 eV
D) 40.8 eV

7. When you breathe in, oxygen molecules from the atmosphere enter small sacs in your lungs called alveoli. These sacs have an average diameter of 250 μm when inflated. If an oxygen molecule has a mass of about 5.3×10^{-26} kg, what is the minimum uncertainty in the speed of an O_2 molecule confined in an alveolus?

A) 8×10^{-9} m/s
B) 8×10^{-6} m/s
C) 8×10^{-3} m/s
D) 8 m/s

CHAPTER 14 PRACTICE PASSAGE

Cells of malignant tumors may be destroyed by various types of radiation or particles, including X-rays, protons and positrons (the positively-charged antiparticle of the electron). Ultimately, the mechanism of cell destruction is the photon or particle transferring energy to a molecule, breaking a bond in the molecule. As this occurs, the photon or particle loses energy.

For high-energy charged particles (such as protons and positrons, but *not* X-rays) moving through matter, the rate at which they lose energy to atoms in the matter was worked out by Hans Bethe and Felix Bloch in the 1930s, soon after the discovery of quantum mechanics. For protons the rate is given in Figure 1 as a function of proton momentum. (This is actually $\Delta E/\rho\Delta x$, the energy loss per centimeter divided by the density of the matter through which the particle passes.) As the proton loses energy, its momentum decreases and it moves along the curve to the left.

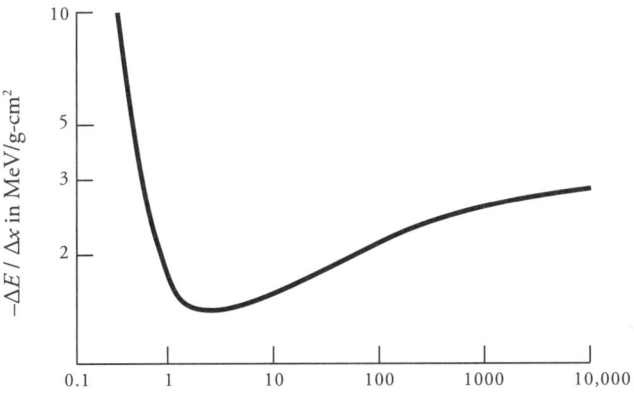

Figure 1

X-rays are created by accelerating electrons to high energy and then slamming them into a high-density metal. As the electrons decelerate rapidly, about 1% of their energy is radiated as X-ray photons, and the remainder heats the metal.

In the following, h represents Planck's Constant, with a value of 6.6×10^{-34} J-s.

1. Compared to a lower-energy X-ray photon, a higher-energy X-ray photon will have:

A) higher frequency and higher wavelength.
B) higher frequency and lower wavelength.
C) lower frequency and higher wavelength.
D) lower frequency and lower wavelength.

2. Using the Bethe-Bloch formula, a radiation technician can calculate the energy of a proton that would *range out* (its momentum would reach zero) after traversing enough body tissue to reach an interior tumor. An advantage of using protons of this energy is:

A) the proton will disintegrate in the tumor, causing more damage to the tumor.
B) the proton will deposit more energy (thus causing more damage) in the tumor than in the material in front of the tumor.
C) the proton will deposit less energy (thus causing more damage) in the tumor than in the material in front of the tumor.
D) the proton has the minimum possible energy when it enters the body, causing less damage to healthy tissue.

3. Suppose 400 kJ/mole is required to break a bond, disintegrating a particular molecule. What is the lowest possible frequency of a single photon that could possibly break the bond?

A) 10^9 Hz
B) 10^{12} Hz
C) 10^{15} Hz
D) 6×10^{39} Hz

4. An electron knocked out of a molecule by passing radiation may bind to a neutral hydrogen atom making H^-, with one proton and two electrons. In the ground state, will both electrons have the same energy?

A) No, because the Pauli exclusion principle forbids two electrons having the same energy.
B) Yes, because the Pauli exclusion principle allows a maximum of two electrons with the same energy.
C) Yes, but the two electrons must have opposite spin to satisfy the Pauli exclusion principle.
D) No, the Pauli exclusion principle makes both energies uncertain, so they cannot be equal.

5. A proton has a certain momentum as it passes through a certain cell. For which momentum will the proton cause the least damage to molecules in the cell?

A) 0.8 GeV/c
B) 3.0 GeV/c
C) 52 GeV/c
D) 1000 GeV/c

6. A photon is most effective at breaking molecules if it is not much bigger than the molecules; that is to say, if its positional uncertainty is on the same scale as the molecule. If a 1.7×10^{-22} kg protein has a linear dimension of about 6 nm, what is the minimum *transverse momentum* (i.e., momentum in a direction perpendicular to the main direction of propagation) of a photon that could be small enough to break the protein?

A) 2.2×10^{-20} cm/s
B) 1.6×10^{8} GeV/c
C) 3×10^{-15} kg-m/s
D) 3.3×10^{-25} kg-m/s

SOLUTIONS TO CHAPTER 14 FREESTANDING QUESTIONS

1. **B** According to the explanation of the photoelectric effect, an electron can be ejected from a material by a photon whenever the photon energy hf is greater than the work function of the material. In this case, where the work function is unknown, all we can assume is that a more energetic, higher frequency photon is more likely to eject an electron than is a less energetic, lower frequency photon. Because blue light is higher frequency than red light, the blue photon is more likely to eject an electron. This is consistent with choices A and D, eliminating them. The phenomenon of dispersion entails that blue light experiences a higher index of refraction than does red light when it moves through a material. This means that blue light is more likely to undergo total internal reflection when it strikes the interface between two materials than red light: $\sin \theta_{crit} = n_2 / n_1$, where n_2 is the index of refraction of the unknown material and n_1 would be the index for the medium of incidence (which would have to have a higher index than the unknown material for any TIR to occur). This eliminates choice C. Choice B is correct because a higher index of refraction for blue light means that the blue photon will travel more slowly than the red one.

2. **C** The principle of conservation of energy tells us that the initial energy of the photon, $hf = hc/\lambda$, must equal the final energy of the system, which is the sum of the potential energy represented by the work function ϕ and the kinetic energy of the electron, K.

$$\frac{hc}{\lambda_0} = \phi + K \rightarrow \phi = \frac{hc}{\lambda_0} - K$$

3. **B** The key to answering this question is to realize that, if integer multiples of wavelengths are required for the de Broglie electron standing waves, then the ground state, the fundamental mode, must have a wavelength equal to the circumference of that circular orbit: $\lambda_1 = 2\pi r_1$. The value for r_n was found in example 14-2: we follow the same procedure here. Beginning with the equation for quantized angular momentum yields

$$mvr = \frac{nh}{2\pi} \rightarrow v_1 = \frac{(1)h}{2\pi m r_1}$$

Now substitute this value for v into the centripetal force equation and solve the resulting equation for r_1

$$\frac{mv^2}{r} = k\frac{e^2}{r^2} \rightarrow \frac{m_{electron}\left(h^2\right)}{r_1\left(4\pi^2 m_{electron}^2 r_1^2\right)} = \frac{h^2}{4\pi^2 m_{electron} r_1^3} = \frac{ke^2}{r_1^2}$$

$$r_1 = \frac{h^2}{4\pi^2 k m_{electron} e^2}$$

Finally, substitute this equation into the formula for λ_1:

$$\lambda_1 = 2\pi\left(\frac{h^2}{4\pi^2 k m_{electron} e^2}\right) = \frac{h^2}{2\pi k m_{electron} e^2}$$

4. **B**   In the photoelectric experiment, when the frequency of the incident light is too low, no pho-toelectrons will be ejected. In this case, no current will be measured: this eliminates choice C. As the frequency increases, the energy of the incident photons increases, until at some point it is sufficient to begin ejecting photoelectrons. At that point, because the detector is positively polarized, all the ejected electrons will be collected, which will be represented in the current measured. The question also states that the intensity of the light is kept constant, so the number of photons remains basically the same, as therefore does the number of pho-toelectrons. This means the current will remain constant for all frequencies so long as the frequency is sufficiently high to eject any photoelectrons, which is shown by graph B.

5. **D**   The photoelectric effect is essentially instantaneous, so increasing the duration of the experi-ment should not affect the determination of the stopping voltage, which depends upon the maximum kinetic energy of the ejected photoelectrons. $eV_{stop} = KE_{max}$. Thus I is false, elimi-nating choices A and C. The remaining choices are distinguished entirely by whether III is true, so you should focus on that. Changing the material used for the target will change the work function, ϕ. Because the maximum kinetic energy of ejected photoelectrons depends upon this value according to $KE_{max} = hf - \phi$, this would indeed affect the value of the stop-ping voltage, meaning III is true and the correct choice is D.

6. **D**   The important difference between a hydrogen atom and a singly ionized helium ion is the charge of the nucleus: it is twice as great for the He$^+$. Without repeating the calculations shown in examples 14-2 and 14-4, it should be evident that the expression for the energy levels in hydrogen

$$E_n = -\frac{ke^2}{2r_n} = -\frac{ke^2}{2n^2h^2} \times 4\pi^2 km_{electron}e^2$$

will introduce two additional factors of 2 when accounting for the two protons in the He$^+$ ion. The e^2 in the numerator of the first energy expression will be $2e^2$, and the second e^2 from the radius term will also be $2e^2$. Thus the energy levels for He$^+$ will be equal to four times the equivalent levels for hydrogen:

$$E_n = 4(-13.6 \text{ eV}/n^2) = -54.4 \text{ eV}/n^2$$

And therefore the equation for photon energies emitted by He$^+$ as it transitions between energy levels is

$$\Delta E = hf = \left|54.4 \text{ eV}\left(\frac{1}{n_{final}^2} - \frac{1}{n_{initial}^2}\right)\right| \rightarrow \Delta E_{2-1} = \left|54.4 \text{ eV}\left(\frac{1}{1^2} - \frac{1}{2^2}\right)\right| = 54.4 \times \frac{3}{4} = 40.8 \text{ eV}$$

Note that there is a short cut: if you remember that 10.2 eV is the energy difference for the hydrogen atom transitioning between $n = 2$ and $n = 1$, multiplying that by four for the rea-sons explained above yields the answer.

7. **B** Apply the Heisenberg uncertainty principle:

$$\Delta x \Delta p = \frac{h}{2\pi} \rightarrow \Delta p = \frac{h}{2\pi \Delta x} \rightarrow \Delta v = \frac{h}{2\pi \Delta x \times m} = \frac{6.63 \times 10^{-34}}{2\pi \left(250 \times 10^{-6}\right)\left(5.3 \times 10^{-26}\right)} \approx$$

$$\frac{1}{1300} \times 10^{-2} \approx 8 \times 10^{-6} \text{ m/s}$$

Note that the answer choices all have the same coefficient, so you're really just trying to figure out the order of magnitude. In such cases, don't stress over the numbers, make quick estimations!

SOLUTIONS TO CHAPTER 14 PRACTICE PASSAGE

1. **B** We know immediately that frequency energy corresponds to higher energy, according to the relation $E = hf$. So the answer must be either choice A or choice B. Because the speed of the wave is fixed at c, the frequency and wavelength are inversely proportional, according to the relation $f\lambda = c$. So as the frequency increases, the wavelength must decrease.

2. **B** According to Figure 1, as a proton approaches the end of its passage through tissue (toward the left side of the curve), the less momentum a proton has, the more energy it loses per unit length. This means that, per centimeter, the amount of energy the proton gives to the matter (and hence the amount of molecular damage it can cause, eliminating choice C) increases as the proton nears stopping. Choice A cannot be right because protons are stable; they do not disintegrate. Choice D is not right because, depending on the exact numbers, a lower-energy proton (which would necessarily have less momentum as well) may do more damage than a higher-energy proton.

3. **C** If it takes a certain amount of energy to break a mole of bonds, we must divide by Avogadro's number to get the energy needed to break a single bond. The lowest-energy photon that could break the bond would be one that gives up all of its energy to the molecule, giving just enough energy to break the bond. From the relation $E = hf$, the frequency corresponding to this minimum-energy photon is

$$f_{\min} = \frac{E_{\text{binding}}}{N_A \times h} = \frac{4 \times 10^5 \, \dfrac{\text{J}}{\text{mol}}}{\left(6 \times 10^{23} \, \dfrac{1}{\text{mol}}\right)\left(6.63 \times 10^{-34} \text{ J} \cdot \text{s}\right)} \approx \frac{4}{40} \times 10^{16} = 10^{15} \text{ Hz}$$

4. **C** The Pauli exclusion principle allows states with two electrons in which at least one quantum number is different, which is consistent with choice C. This is the case for a filled $n = 1$ shell; the principle doesn't expressly forbid any two electrons from having the same energy, so choice A is wrong. Choice B is incorrect for basically the same reason; recall from chemistry that for a given $n > 1$, there are more than two states at the same energy because there are more than two electrons per shell. Choice D is incorrect because the Pauli exclusion principle does not deal with uncertainty.

5. **B** Damage to cells happens when molecular bonds are broken by energy transferred from the proton. Figure 1 shows a minimum in energy loss, i.e., energy transferred to molecules in the cell, of around 3 to 4 GeV/c.

6. **D** When a question mentions a linear dimension, then asks about a momentum, this should make you think of the uncertainty principle. If the momentum were known to precision Δp, the location of the photon would be smeared out over a length $\Delta x = h/2\pi\Delta p$. So we actually want more momentum uncertainty to get enough position certainty to match the size of the molecule. The momentum must be at least as large as its uncertainty, so the momentum must be at least

$$\Delta p = \frac{h}{2\pi\Delta x} = \frac{6.63 \times 10^{-34}}{2\pi \times 3 \times 10^{-9}} \approx 3.3 \times 10^{-25} \text{ kg} \cdot \text{m/s}$$

Although A and B have different units than C and D, only choice A can be eliminated due to having the wrong dimension. The units in choices B, C and D all have dimensions of momentum, that is, the product of mass and velocity.

Glossary

After each definition, the section of the *MCAT Physics* text where the term is discussed is given.

acceleration
The rate of change of velocity: $\overline{\mathbf{a}} = \Delta\mathbf{v}/\Delta t$. **[Section 3.2]**

action-reaction pair
The two forces described by Newton's third law: If Object 1 exerts a force, $\mathbf{F}_{\text{1-on-2}}$, on Object 2, then Object 2 exerts a force, $\mathbf{F}_{\text{2-on-1}}$, on Object 1. These forces—known as an action-reaction pair—have the same magnitude but point in opposite directions, so $\mathbf{F}_{\text{2-on-1}} = -\mathbf{F}_{\text{1-on-2}}$, and act on different objects. **[Section 4.1]**

adiabatic
Describes a thermodynamic process in which there is no heat exchange. **[Section 7.3]**

alternating current (AC)
Current whose direction reverses (usually many times per second) during the operation of the circuit. **[Section 10.3]**

ammeter
A device for measuring current in a circuit. **[Section 10.1]**

ampere (or amp)
The SI unit of current: 1 ampere (amp) = 1 A = 1 coulomb per second = 1 C/s. **[Section 10.1]**

amplitude
The maximum displacement of an oscillator from its equilibrium position, or the maximum displacement of a wave from equilibrium. **[Section 11.1, 11.2]**

angles of incidence, reflection, and refraction
In optics, the angles that the incident beam, reflected beam, and transmitted beam make with the normal to the boundary between the two media. **[Section 13.2]**

antinode
A point where a standing wave has its maximum amplitude. **[Section 11.4]**

Archimedes' principle
The magnitude of the buoyant force on an object is equal to the weight of the fluid displaced. So, if the density of the fluid is ρ_{fluid} and the volume of the object that is submerged is V_{sub}, then the magnitude of the buoyant force is given by $F_{\text{Buoy}} = \rho_{\text{fluid}} V_{\text{sub}} g$. **[Section 8.1]**

beats
The variation in amplitude of the resultant wave created by the interference of two waves with different frequencies. If f_1 and f_2 are the frequencies of the two waves, then the beat frequency is given by $f_{\text{beat}} = |f_1 - f_2|$. **[Section 12.3]**

Bernoulli effect
The lowering of fluid pressure as the flow speed increases; also known as the *Venturi effect*. **[Section 8.2]**

Bernoulli's equation
The statement that follows from the Conservation of Mechanical Energy applied to ideal fluid flow. **[Section 8.2]**

Bohr model of the atom
The description of the atom as having quantized orbitals associated with discrete energies and energy level transitions. **[Section 14.2]**

buoyant force
The upward force exerted by a fluid on an object partly or completely submerged in it. If the density of the fluid is ρ_{fluid} and the volume of the object that is submerged is V_{sub}, then the magnitude of the buoyant force is given by $F_{\text{Buoy}} = \rho_{\text{fluid}} V_{\text{sub}} g$. **[Section 8.1]**

capacitance
The ratio of charge to voltage for a capacitor:
$C = Q/V$. **[Section 10.2]**

center of gravity
For an extended object or system, the point where the gravitational force acts. In a uniform gravitational field, the center of gravity is the same as the center of mass. **[Section 5.1]**

center of mass
The point that behaves as if all of an object's mass were concentrated there. **[Section 5.1]**

centripetal acceleration
The acceleration of an object that undergoes uniform circular motion; if the speed of the object is v and the radius of its circular path is r, then its centripetal acceleration points toward the center of the circle and has magnitude $a_c = v^2 / r$. **[Section 5.2]**

centripetal force
The net force on an object that undergoes uniform circular motion: $\mathbf{F}_c = m\mathbf{a}_c$, where $\mathbf{a}_c$ is the object's centripetal acceleration. Its magnitude is $F_c = mv^2 / r$ if the speed of the object is v and the radius of the circular path is r. **[Section 5.2]**

coefficient of friction
A positive unitless number that describes the strength of the friction force between two surfaces in contact. The coefficient of kinetic friction is usually denoted μ_k, and the coefficient of static friction by μ_s; in virtually all cases, $\mu_s > \mu_k$ for a given pair of surfaces. **[Section 4.3]**

compression
1. A type of stress applied to an object that decreases its length. **[Section 8.3]**

2. A compression is also a region where the local density and pressure is momentarily increased from standard due to the passage of a sound wave. **[Section 12.1]**

concave
1. A concave mirror is a mirror whose reflecting surface is curved toward the object so that its center is furthest away from the object; it has a positive focal length. **[Section 13.4]**

2. A concave lens is a diverging lens; it has a negative focal length. **[Section 13.5]**

conduction
A mode of heat transfer in which the medium does not move during the transfer of thermal energy. **[Section 7.2]**

conductor
A material with a very low resistivity, which therefore allows charge to flow through it easily. Metals are conductors. **[Section 9.3]**

conservative force
If the work done by a force depends only on the initial and final positions of the object that the force is acting on, and not on the particular path between the positions, the force is said to be conservative. The gravitational and electric forces are examples of conservative forces; friction is non-conservative. **[Section 6.4]**

continuity equation
For ideal fluid flow, the amount of fluid per unit time (the flow rate) passing one point in a flow tube must be the same as the amount passing through another point: $f_1 = f_2$ (or $A_1 v_1 = A_2 v_2$). **[Section 8.2]**

convection
A mode of heat transfer in which the medium moves during the transfer of thermal energy. **[Section 7.3]**

converging lens
A lens that is thicker in the middle than at its edges. A converging lens causes incident parallel rays of light to converge to the focal point after passing through the lens. **[Section 13.5]**

convex
1. A convex mirror is a mirror whose reflecting surface is curved away from the object; it has a negative focal length. **[Section 13.4]**

2. A convex lens is a converging lens; it has a positive focal length. **[Section 13.5]**

coulomb
The SI unit of electric charge, abbreviated C; the fundamental electric charge (the charge on a proton or the magnitude of the charge on an electron) is defined to be $e = 1.6 \times 10^{-19}$ C. Therefore, one coulomb is equal to the total charge on 6.25×10^{18} protons. **[Section 9.1]**

Coulomb's law
The law that gives the magnitude of the electric force between two charged objects: $F_E = k|q_1 q_2|/r^2$. **[Section 9.2]**

critical angle
The angle at which an incident beam of light refracts at an angle of 90°. If n_1 is the refractive index of the incident medium and n_2 is the index of the refracting medium (and $n_1 > n_2$), then the critical angle, θ_{crit}, is defined by the equation sin $\theta_{crit} = n_2 / n_1$. **[Section 13.2]**

current
A net flow of electric charge; more precisely, it's the net amount of charge that passes a given point per unit time: $I = Q/t$. **[Section 10.1]**

decibel
A unit of sound level. If I is the intensity of a sound wave, then the sound level (in decibels, dB) is defined as $\beta = 10 \log (I/I_0)$, where I_0 is the threshold of hearing (a reference intensity, 10^{-12} W/m²). **[Section 12.4]**

density
The ratio of an object's mass to its volume: density $= \rho = m/V$. **[Section 8.1]**

dielectric
An insulating material sandwiched between the plates of a capacitor; a capacitor always has a higher capacitance when a dielectric is present. **[Section 9.3, 10.2]**

diffraction
The redistribution of a wave's energy as it encounters and moves beyond an obstruction (or hole). **[Section 13.3]**

diopter
The unit of lens power: 1 diopter = 1 D = 1 m⁻¹. **[Section 13.5]**

direct current
Current whose direction remains steady during the operation of an electric circuit. **[Section 10.1, 10.3]**

dispersion
The variation of the speed of a wave as the frequency changes. For the MCAT, the only example of dispersion you should know is the variation of the speed of light through a material medium, such as glass. The colorful spectrum that is seen exiting a glass prism is an example of this dispersion. **[Section 13.3]**

displacement
The change in position of an object. The magnitude of an object's displacement gives the net distance traveled by the object. **[Section 3.2]**

diverging lens
A lens that is thinner in the middle than at its edges. A diverging lens causes incident parallel rays of light to diverge away from the focal point after passing through the lens. **[Section 13.5]**

Doppler effect
The perceived change in frequency of a wave due to relative motion between the source of a wave and the detector. When the source and detector are in relative motion toward each other, the detected frequency is higher than the emitted frequency; when the source and detector are in relative motion away from each other, the detected frequency is lower than the emitted frequency. **[Section 12.5]**

efficiency
The percentage of the useful work that a machine does in comparison to its theoretical maximum, or $W_{output}/Energy_{input}$. **[Section 6.6]**

elastic potential energy
The energy stored in a stretched or compressed spring: $PE_{elastic} = \frac{1}{2}kx^2$, where k is the spring constant. **[Section 11.1]**

electric field
A force field created by one or more electric charges. **[Section 9.3]**

electric force
The force exerted by an electric field; if a charge q is in an electric field **E**, then the electric force on q is given by the equation $\mathbf{F}_E = q\mathbf{E}$. **[Section 9.2, 9.3]**

electric potential
The electric potential at a point P is equal to the work required to bring a unit charge from infinity to P, divided by that charge. If P is a distance r away from a point charge Q, then the electric potential at P is a scalar quantity given by $\phi = kq/r$ where k is Coulomb's constant. **[Section 9.4]**

electric potential energy
The energy stored in the field surrounding a configuration of charged objects. A charge q experience and electric potential ϕ has an electric potential energy given by $PE = q\phi$. **[Section 9.4]**

electromagnetic (EM) spectrum
The full range of electromagnetic radiation, where different ranges of frequencies (and wavelengths) are categorized. Such categories include (in order of increasing frequency): radio waves, microwaves, infrared (IR) light, visible light, ultraviolet light, x-rays, and gamma rays. **[Section 13.1]**

electron
A fundamental subatomic particle with a negative electric charge (equal to $-e$, the negative of the elementary electric charge) that orbits the nucleus of an atom. **[Section 9.1]**

entropy
The measure of disorder of a thermodynamic system. **[Section 7.4]**

equilibrium
An object or system is said to be in translational equilibrium if the net force on it is zero. An object or system is said to be in rotational equilibrium if the net torque on it is zero. An object or system is said to be in equilibrium if it is in both translational and rotational equilibrium. **[Section 5.4]**

For an oscillator, the equilibrium position is the point at which the restoring force is zero. **[Section 11.1]**

equipotential
A curve or surface on which the electric potential remains constant. **[Section 9.4]**

equivalent resistance
The single resistance that provides the same overall resistance as a combination of resistors. **[Section 10.1]**

farad
The SI unit of capacitance: 1 farad = 1 coulomb per volt = 1 C/V. **[Section 10.2]**

flow rate
The amount of fluid that flows per unit time; it is equal to the cross-sectional area of the flow tube multiplied by the flow speed: $f = Av$. **[Section 8.2]**

fluid
A substance that can flow, or more precisely, a substance that cannot withstand a shear stress. Both liquids and gases are fluids. **[Section 8.1]**

focal length
The distance from a mirror or lens to its focal point along the axis of curvature. Concave mirrors and converging lenses have positive focal lengths; convex mirrors and diverging lenses have negative focal lengths. **[Section 13.4, 13.5]**

focal point (or focus)
The point where any curved mirror or lens focuses the image of a distant object. For a concave mirror or a converging lens, the focal point (or focus) is the point *to* which rays of light that are initially parallel to the optical axis are focused after contact with the mirror or lens. For a convex mirror or a diverging lens, the focal point is the point *from* which rays of light that are initially parallel to the optical axis are diverged after contact with the mirror or lens. **[Section 13.4, 13.5]**

force
Intuitively, a push or pull exerted by one object on another. This may result in an acceleration if the forces on the object are not balanced. **[Section 4.1]**

frequency
The number of oscillations (or cycles) per second. **[Section 11.1, 11.2, 12.1, 13.1]**

friction
The friction force is the parallel component of the contact force exerted by a surface on an object. **[Section 4.3]**

fundamental frequency
The lowest permissible frequency, or longest permissible wavelength, of a standing wave; also referred to as the *first harmonic*. **[Section 11.4]**

gravitational acceleration
The acceleration produced by the gravitational pull of a body, directed toward the center of the body. The magnitude of the gravitational acceleration, g, produced by the earth is approximately 10 m/s^2 near the surface. **[Section 3.5]**

gravitational force
In Newton's theory of gravitation, every object exerts a force, a gravitational pull, on every other object. If the masses of the two objects are m_1 and m_2, and if their centers of mass are separated by a distance r, then the magnitude of the gravitational force between them is given by $F_{grav} = Gm_1m_2 / r^2$. **[Section 4.1, 4.2]**

heat
The transfer of thermal energy between a system and its environment. **[Section 7.1]**

Heisenberg uncertainty principle
The quantum physics principle that restricts the precision with which position and momentum of a particle can be defined: $\Delta x \Delta p \geq h / 2\pi$ **[Section 14.5]**

hertz
The SI unit of frequency; 1 hertz = 1 Hz = 1 cycle (or oscillation) per second. **[Section 11.1]**

Hooke's law
The magnitude of the force exerted by a stretched or compressed object or spring is proportional to the distance by which it is stretched or compressed from equilibrium: $F_{rest} = -kx$. **[Section 8.3, 11.1]**

hydrostatic gauge pressure
The pressure at a point below the surface of a fluid at rest, due to the weight of the fluid above it: $P_{gauge} = \rho_{fluid} gD$, where D is the depth. **[Section 8.1]**

index of refraction
The index of refraction for a medium is equal to the ratio of the speed of light in vacuum to the speed of light through the medium: $n = c/v$. **[Section 13.2]**

inertia
Resistance to acceleration; an object's inertia is measured by its mass and is the ratio of the net force on an object to its acceleration: inertia $= m = F_{net} / a$. **[Section 4.1]**

insulator
A material with a very high resistivity that does not permit charge to flow through it easily. Glass and wood are examples of insulators. **[Section 9.3]**

intensity
The intensity of a wave is the power it transmits per unit area; the units of I are therefore W/m^2. Intensity is related directly to the wave's amplitude and diminishes with the square of the distance from the source. **[Section 12.4]**

interference
The combination of two or more waves. When the waves are in phase (crest meets crest, trough meets trough), this is *constructive* interference, and the amplitude of the resultant wave is equal to the sum of the individual amplitudes; when the waves are *out of phase* (crest meets trough, trough meets crest), this is *destructive* interference, and the amplitude of the resultant wave is equal to the difference between the individual amplitudes. **[Section 11.3]**

isobaric
Describes a thermodynamic process in which pressure is held constant. **[Section 7.3]**

isochoric
Describes a thermodynamic process in which volume is held constant. **[Section 7.3]**

isothermal
Describes a thermodynamic process in which temperature is held constant. **[Section 7.3]**

joule
The SI unit of work and energy; 1 joule = 1 J = 1 N·m = 1 kg·m^2/s^2. **[Section 6.1]**

kinetic energy
The energy due to motion; for an object of mass m and speed v, the kinetic energy is $KE = \frac{1}{2}mv^2$. **[Section 6.3]**

kinetic friction
Also known as sliding friction, it is the friction that results when there is relative motion between the two surfaces; that is, when one surface slides across the other. If F_N is the magnitude of the normal force and μ_k is the coefficient of kinetic friction between the two surfaces, then the force of kinetic friction is directed opposite to the direction of the sliding and its magnitude is $F_f = \mu_k F_N$. **[Section 4.3]**

Kirchhoff's laws
1. The total amount of current entering a junction in a circuit must be equal to the total amount of current leaving the junction.

2. The sum of the voltages around a closed loop in a circuit must be zero. **[Section 10.1]**

lens
A thin piece of glass or plastic that forms an image by refracting light. **[Section 13.5]**

lever arm
Denoted by ℓ, it is the perpendicular distance from the pivot (reference) point to the line of action of a force. **[Section 5.3]**

longitudinal wave
A wave in which the oscillations of the medium are parallel to the direction of propagation of the wave. Sound waves are longitudinal. **[Section 12.1]**

magnetic field
The force field created by a *moving* electric charge. **[Section 10.4]**

magnetic force
The force exerted by a magnetic field on a moving charge. If a charge q moves with velocity **v** through a magnetic field **B**, then the magnetic force on q is given by $\mathbf{F} = q(\mathbf{v} \times \mathbf{B})$. The magnitude of **F** is $|q|vB\sin\theta$ (where θ is the angle between **v** and **B**), and the direction of **F** is given by the right-hand rule if q is positive and by the left-hand rule if q is negative. **[Section 10.4]**

magnification
The ratio of the height of the image to the height of the object; a negative value for the magnification means that the image is inverted relative to the object. For a mirror or lens, the magnification is given by the equation $m = -i/o$, where i and o are the distances from the mirror or lens to the image and the object, respectively. **[Section 13.4, 13.5]**

mass
The quantitative measure of an object's inertia; intuitively, we think of mass as measuring the amount of matter in an object. In SI units, mass is expressed in kilograms (kg) and is the ratio of the net force on an object to its acceleration: mass $= m = F_{net}/a$. **[Section 4.1]**

mechanical advantage
The factor by which a machine or mechanism multiplies the input or effort force. This term is applied to simple machines such as inclined planes, pulley systems, and levers. **[Section 6.6]**

mirror
A surface that forms an image by reflecting light. **[Section 13.4]**

net force
The sum of all the forces that act on an object. **[Section 4.1]**

neutron
A subatomic particle with zero electric charge that is a constituent of atomic nuclei. **[Section 9.1]**

newton

The SI unit of force: 1 newton = 1 N = 1 kg·m/s^2. **[Section 4.1]**

Newton's laws of motion

1. If $\mathbf{F}_{net}$ = 0, then the object's velocity will not change.

2. $\mathbf{F}_{net}$ = $m\mathbf{a}$

3. If Object 1 exerts a force, $\mathbf{F}_{1\text{-on-}2}$, on Object 2, then Object 2 exerts a force, $\mathbf{F}_{2\text{-on-}1}$, on Object 1. These forces (known as an action-reaction pair) have the same magnitude but point in opposite directions, so $\mathbf{F}_{2\text{-on-}1} = -\mathbf{F}_{1\text{-on-}2}$, and act on different objects. **[Section 4.1]**

node

A point where a standing wave has zero amplitude. **[Section 11.4]**

normal

As an adjective, it means *perpendicular*. As a noun, a normal is a line that's perpendicular to a surface. **[Section 4.3, 13.2]**

normal force

For an object in contact with a surface, the normal force is the component of the force exerted by the surface that is perpendicular to the surface. **[Section 4.3]**

north pole of magnet

The pole from which the magnetic field lines emerge from a magnet. **[Section 10.4]**

ohm

The unit of resistance: 1 ohm = 1 Ω = 1 volt per amp = 1 V/A. **[Section 10.1]**

Ohm's law

A material is said to obey Ohm's law if its resistance remains constant as the voltage across it varies; thus, for such a material, $V = IR$, where R is a constant. **[Section 10.1]**

parallel resistors

Resistors in a circuit are said to be in parallel if they provide alternate routes for current to flow from one point in the circuit to another; parallel resistors always share the same voltage drop. **[Section 10.1]**

pascal

The unit of pressure: 1 pascal = 1 Pa = 1 newton per square meter = 1 N/m^2. **[Section 8.1]**

Pascal's law

A confined fluid transmits an externally applied change in pressure to all parts of the fluid equally. **[Section 8.1]**

Pauli exclusion principle

The quantum physics rule that restricts the number of particles that can occupy the same quantum state within a small proximity; the principle that explains how electron orbitals fill in the elements. **[Section 14.3]**

period

The time required for one complete oscillation (or cycle). **[Section 11.1, 11.2]**

periodic (or harmonic) motion

Any motion that regularly repeats, such as uniform circular motion or oscillatory motion. **[Section 11.1]**

photoelectric effect

The effect wherein photons eject individual electrons from a metal. **[Section 14.4]**

photon

Light travels as a wave, but interacts with matter as a stream of particles; these "particles," each an indivisible quantum of energy, are photons. Photons have no mass and move at the speed of light. The energy carried by each photon is proportional to the frequency of the light: E_{photon} = hf, where h is a constant of nature known as Planck's constant. **[Section 13.1, 14.2]**

polarized

1. A transverse wave is polarized if the direction of its oscillations is constant (or is confined to vary in a particular way). For a plane-polarized electromagnetic wave, the direction of polarization is the direction of oscillation of the electric field.

2. Circular polarization is the result of two perpendicular waves with a 90° phase difference interfering, and resulting in the apparent rotation of the electric field. **[Section 13.1, 13.3]**

potential energy

The energy of an object (or system) due to its position or configuration. There are different forms of potential energy, depending on the force involved; for the MCAT, the three most important forms are gravitational *PE*, electrical *PE*, and elastic *PE*. **[Section 6.4, 9.4, 11.1]**

power

1. In mechanics, power is the rate at which work is done or energy is used. Power is thus equal to work (or energy) divided by time, and its SI unit is the watt, where 1 watt = 1 W = 1 J/s. **[Section 6.2]**

2. In optics, lens power is a measure of the focusing strength of a lens. By definition, lens power is equal to the reciprocal of the focal length of the lens: $P = 1/f$. If f is expressed in meters, then lens power has units of diopters, where 1 diopter = $1\ D = 1\ m^{-1}$. **[Section 13.5]**

pressure

A scalar quantity equal to the magnitude of the perpendicular force per unit area. **[Section 7.2, 7.3, 8.1]**

projectile motion

The motion of a particle moving under the influence of uniform (constant) acceleration; if the object's initial velocity is not purely vertical, the path of the object will be a parabola. **[Section 3.6]**

proton

A subatomic particle with a positive electric charge (equal to the elementary electric charge, $+e$) that is a constituent of atomic nuclei. **[Section 9.1]**

quantized

A quantity is said to be quantized if it exists only in discrete amounts. Examples: (1) Electric charge on an object can only be an integer multiple of the basic unit of electric charge, e. (2) Electromagnetic radiation of frequency f can be absorbed only in whole number multiples of the photon energy, hf. **[Sections 9.1, 14.1]**

quantum physics

The physics associated with discrete values and changes in the values of such quantities; associated strongly with wave-particle duality. **[Section 14.1]**

radiation

1. Energy emitted or absorbed due to propagation of waves (electromagnetic waves, unless a different kind of wave is specially mentioned). **[Section 13.1]**

2. A mode of heat transfer via electromagnetic waves. **[Section 7.2]**

rarefaction

A region where the local density and pressure is momentarily decreased from standard due to the passage of a sound wave. **[Section 12.1]**

real image

An image formed by a mirror or lens where light rays actually do intersect. Unlike a virtual image, a real image can be projected onto a screen. **[Section 13.4]**

reflection

When waves or particles "bounce off" a surface on which they are incident, the return of these waves or particles is called reflection. **[Section 13.2]**

refraction

The change in direction of a wave when it passes from one medium into another. **[Section 13.2]**

resistance
The ratio of the voltage to current: $R = V/I$. [**Section 10.1**]

resistivity
The intrinsic resistance of a material. [**Section 10.1**]

resistor
A component of an electrical circuit that provides resistance to the flow of current. [**Section 10.1**]

restoring force
For an object undergoing oscillation, the force on the object that is directed toward equilibrium. [**Section 11.1**]

series resistors
Resistors in a circuit are said to be in series if current must flow through each of them, one after the other; series resistors always share the same current. [**Section 10.1**]

shear stress
The magnitude of the shearing force exerted on an object divided by the area parallel to which it acts. [**Section 8.3**]

simple harmonic motion
Periodic (oscillatory) movement where the period and frequency of the oscillations do not depend on the amplitude, caused by a restoring force that is proportional to the displacement from equilibrium. [**Section 11.1**]

Snell's law
The law of refraction in optics, $n_1 \sin \theta_1 = n_2 \sin \theta_2$, where n_1 and n_2 are the refractive indexes of the incident and refracting media (respectively), and θ_1 is the angle of incidence and θ_2 the angle of refraction. [**Section 13.1, 13.2**]

sound level
A measurement, in decibels, of the intensity of a sound wave. The sound-level for a wave of intensity I is given by the equation $\beta = 10 \log_{10} (I/I_0)$, where I_0 is the threshold of hearing. [**Section 12.4**]

south pole of magnet
The pole into which the magnetic field lines enter a magnet. [**Section 10.4**]

specific gravity
The unitless ratio of the density of a substance to the density of water: sp. gr. = $\rho_{substance}/\rho_{water}$. [**Section 8.1**]

speed
The magnitude of an object's velocity. [**Section 3.2**]

standing wave
A wave caused by the superposition of two oppositely directed traveling waves, for which the resulting crests and troughs do not travel. [**Section 11.4**]

state function or state variable
The measure of an intrinsic, macroscopic property of a thermodynamic system that defines the present attributes of the system, independent of past processes. [**Section 7.2**]

static friction
The friction that results when there is no relative motion between the two surfaces; that is, when neither slides across the other. If F_N is the magnitude of the normal force and μ_s is the coefficient of static friction between the two surfaces, then the force of static friction is directed opposite to the direction of the intended motion and its *maximum* magnitude is $F_{f,\,max} = \mu_{s,\,max} F_N$. [**Section 4.3**]

stopping voltage
In the photoelectric experiment, the negative voltage necessary to prevent the most energetic photoelectrons ejected from the metal surface from reaching the detector. [**Section 14.4**]

strain
The ratio of the change in one of an object's dimensions to the original, caused by an applied stress. For a compressive or tensile stress, the strain is equal to (the magnitude of) the change in the object's length divided by the original length. For a shear stress, the strain is equal to the distance the object is deformed perpendicular to the shear stress divided by the length perpendicular to the direction of the bend. **[Section 8.3]**

stress
The magnitude of the force acting on an object, divided by the area over which it acts. **[Section 8.3]**

superposition
The addition principle that applies to several different physical phenomena, such as electric forces, fields, potentials, and waves, where the result is simply equal to the sum of the individual vector or scalar values. **[Section 9.2, 9.3, 9.4]**

system
The object or substance—or objects or substances and the interactions among them—that are the focus of study. Contrasted with the environment, which is everything else. **[Section 7.1]**

temperature
A thermodynamic state function that corresponds to the internal, random kinetic energy of the constituent particles of a system. **[Section 7.1, 7.2]**

tension
A type of force applied to a solid object that tends to increase its length. Tension is also used to describe the pulling force exerted by a stretched string, rope, chain, or spring. **[Section 4.1, 4.5, 8.3]**

tesla
The SI unit of magnetic field strength:
1 tesla = 1 T = 1 newton per amp-meter = 1 N/A·m. **[Section 10.4]**

thermodynamics
The study of how macroscopic systems transfer or transform energy. **[Section 7.1]**

Thermodynamic laws
0th law: Two objects in thermal equilibrium with the same third object are in thermal equilibrium with each other. Defines temperature as a state function. **[Section 7.2]**

1st law: The total quantity of energy in the universe is conserved. More specifically, the energy into and out of a system equals its change in internal energy; $\Delta E = Q - W$ **[Section 7.3]**

2nd law: The entropy of a closed system will either stay the same or increase. **[Section 7.4]**

threshold of hearing
The lowest intensity the human ear can detect; denoted I_0, it is defined as 10^{-12} W/m^2. **[Section 12.4]**

torque
A quantity associated with a force that measures how effective the force is at producing rotational acceleration. If **r** is the vector from the pivot point to the point of application of a force **F**, and the angle between **r** and **F** is θ, then the torque of the force is defined to be $\tau = rF \sin\theta$. **[Section 5.3]**

Torricelli's result
The equation giving the speed of efflux for a static fluid from a small hole in a large open container: $v = \sqrt{2gD}$, where D is the depth of the hole below the surface of the fluid. **[Section 8.2]**

total internal reflection
When an incident beam of light strikes the surface of a medium with a lower index of refraction, the beam will experience total internal reflection (TIR) if the angle of incidence is greater than the critical angle. In this case, none of the beam's energy is transmitted to the other medium; it is only reflected. **[Section 13.2]**

total mechanical energy
The sum of an object's kinetic energy and potential energy: $E = KE + PE$. **[Section 6.5]**

transverse wave
A wave in which the oscillations that make up the wave are perpendicular to the direction of the wave's propagation. Waves on a rope and electromagnetic waves are transverse. **[Section 11.2]**

velocity
The rate of change of an object's position: $\bar{\mathbf{v}} = \Delta\mathbf{s}/\Delta t = \mathbf{d}/\Delta t$. An object's velocity gives both the speed and the direction of motion of the object. **[Section 3.2]**

virtual image
An image formed by a mirror or lens where light rays don't actually intersect. Unlike a real image, a virtual image cannot be displayed on a screen. Convex mirrors and diverging (concave) lenses form only virtual images. **[Section 13.4]**

viscosity
The internal friction of a fluid; an ideal fluid is one whose viscosity is negligible. **[Section 8.2]**

volt
The SI unit of electric potential and voltage; 1 volt = 1 V = 1 joule per coulomb = 1 J / C. **[Section 9.4]**

voltage
The difference in electric potential between two points. **[Section 9.4, 10.1]**

voltmeter
A device for measuring the voltage across a circuit element. **[Section 10.1]**

watt
The SI unit of power; 1 watt = 1 W = 1 joule per second = 1 J / s. **[Section 6.2]**

wave
A propagating oscillation that carries energy from one position to another. **[Section 11.2]**

wavelength
The distance (denoted by λ) between consecutive crests (or between consecutive troughs) of a wave. **[Section 11.2]**

weight
The gravitational force exerted on an object: $\mathbf{w} = m\mathbf{g}$. **[Section 4.2]**

work
The work done by a constant force $\mathbf{F}$ as it acts through a displacement $\mathbf{d}$ is given by the equation $W = Fd\cos\theta$, where θ is the angle between $\mathbf{F}$ and $\mathbf{d}$. For an ideal gas in a container, work can be expressed as the product of its change in volume and its pressure, $W = P\Delta V$. Work is a scalar quantity, and its SI unit is the joule, where 1 joule = 1 J = 1 kg-m^2/s^2. **[Section 6.1, 7.3]**

work-energy theorem
The total amount of work done on an object is equal to the change in the object's kinetic energy: $W = \Delta KE$. **[Section 6.3]**

work function
The binding energy of a metal for its free electrons, overcome during the photoelectric effect. **[Section 14.4]**

MCAT Physics
Formula Sheet

KINEMATICS

The Big Five

if a is constant:

1. $d = vt = \dfrac{1}{2}(v_0 + v)t$

2. $v = v_0 + at$

3. $d = v_0 t + \dfrac{1}{2} at^2$

4. $d = vt - \dfrac{1}{2} at^2$

5. $v^2 = v_0^2 + 2ad$

Projectile Motion

<u>Horizontal</u>	<u>Vertical</u>
$x = v_{0x} t$	$y = v_{0y} t - \dfrac{1}{2} gt^2$
$v_x = v_{0x}$	$v_y = v_{0y} - gt$
$a_x = 0$	$a_y = -g$

$$v_{0x} = v_0 \cos\theta_0$$
$$v_{0y} = v_0 \sin\theta_0$$

θ	$\cos\theta$	$\sin\theta$
0°	$\sqrt{4}/2$	$\sqrt{0}/2$
30°	$\sqrt{3}/2$	$\sqrt{1}/2$
45°	$\sqrt{2}/2$	$\sqrt{2}/2$
60°	$\sqrt{1}/2$	$\sqrt{3}/2$
90°	$\sqrt{0}/2$	$\sqrt{4}/2$
120°	$-\sqrt{1}/2$	$\sqrt{3}/2$
135°	$-\sqrt{2}/2$	$\sqrt{2}/2$
150°	$-\sqrt{3}/2$	$\sqrt{1}/2$
180°	$-\sqrt{4}/2$	$\sqrt{0}/2$

$$\sqrt{2} \approx 1.4 \qquad \sqrt{3} \approx 1.7$$

INCLINED PLANE

θ = incline angle to horizontal

Force due to gravity parallel to ramp = $mg\sin\theta$

Force due to gravity perpendicular to ramp = $mg\cos\theta (= F_N)$

CENTER OF MASS (= CENTER OF GRAVITY)

$$x_{CM} = \frac{m_1 x_1 + \dots + m_n x_n}{m_1 + \dots + m_n} = \frac{w_1 x_1 + \dots + w_n x_n}{w_1 + \dots + w_n} = x_{CG}$$

WORK, ENERGY, POWER

Work: $W = Fd\cos\theta$

Kinetic energy: $KE = \dfrac{1}{2}mv^2$

Work-Energy theorem: $W_{total} = \Delta KE$

Power: $P = \dfrac{W}{t}$, $P = Fv$ if $\mathbf{F} \parallel \mathbf{v}$, and $\mathbf{v}$ is constant.

Potential energy: $PE_{grav} = mgh$ (if $h \ll r_{Earth}$)

Mechanical energy: $E = KE + PE$

Conservation of Mechanical Energy:
$E_i = E_f$ or $KE_i + PE_i = KE_f + PE_f$
If non-conservative (nc) forces—like friction—act during the motion: $E_i + W_{\text{by nc forces}} = E_f$

THERMODYNAMICS

First law: $\Delta E = Q - W$

Work: $W = P\Delta V$

Temp. of monatomic ideal gas: $\dfrac{1}{2}mv_{avg}^2 = \dfrac{3}{2}k_B T$

Heat and Temp for an ideal gas: $Q = nC_V \Delta T$ (constant volume) or $Q = nC_P \Delta T$ (constant pressure)

DYNAMICS

Newton's Laws

1. $\mathbf{F}_{net} = \mathbf{0} \rightarrow \mathbf{v} = $ constant
2. $\mathbf{F}_{net} = m\mathbf{a}$
3. $\mathbf{F}_{2\text{-on-}1} = -\mathbf{F}_{1\text{-on-}2}$

GRAVITY

$F_{grav} = w = mg$ $\qquad$ $F_{grav} = G\dfrac{Mm}{r^2}$

$g = G\dfrac{M}{r^2}$ $\qquad$ $g_{Earth} \approx 10\dfrac{\text{m}}{\text{s}^2}$

FRICTION

F_N = magnitude of normal force

$F_{f,static,max} = \mu_s F_N$

$F_{f,kinetic} = \mu_k F_N$

UNIFORM CIRCULAR MOTION

Centripetal acceleration: $a_c = \dfrac{v^2}{r}$

Centripetal force: $F_c = ma_c = m\dfrac{v^2}{r}$

TORQUE

$\tau = rF\sin\theta = lF$

STRESS AND STRAIN

Stress = $\dfrac{F}{A}$

Strain = $\dfrac{\Delta L}{L}$

Hooke's law: $\Delta L = \dfrac{FL}{EA}$

FLUIDS

Density: $\rho = \dfrac{m}{V}$, $\rho_{H_2O} = 1000\dfrac{\text{kg}}{\text{m}^3}$

Specific gravity: sp. gr. = $\dfrac{\rho}{\rho_{H_2O}}$

Pressure: $P = \dfrac{F_\perp}{A}$

Total Hydrostatic pressure: $P = P_0 + \rho gD = P_{\text{atm}} + \rho gD$
(if $P_0 = P_{\text{atm}}$)

Gauge pressure: $P_{\text{gauge}} = \rho_{fluid}gD$

Archimedes' principle: $F_{\text{Buoyant}} = \rho_{\text{fluid}}V_{\text{sub}}g$

Pascal's law: $\dfrac{F_1}{A_1} = \dfrac{F_2}{A_2}$

Volume flow rate: $f = Av$

Continuity equation: $A_1v_1 = A_2v_2$

Bernoulli's equation:

$P_1 + \rho gy_1 + \dfrac{1}{2}\rho v_1^2 = P_2 + \rho gy_2 + \dfrac{1}{2}\rho v_2^2$

OSCILLATIONS AND WAVES

Hooke's law: $\mathbf{F}_S = -k\mathbf{x}$

$PE_S = \dfrac{1}{2}kx^2$

frequency and period: $f = \dfrac{1}{T}, T = \dfrac{1}{f}$

$f = \dfrac{1}{2\pi}\sqrt{\dfrac{k}{m}}, T = 2\pi\sqrt{\dfrac{m}{k}}$

$f_{\text{simple pendulum}} = \dfrac{1}{2\pi}\sqrt{\dfrac{g}{L}}$

$\lambda f = v$

$v = \sqrt{\dfrac{F_T}{\mu}} = \sqrt{\dfrac{F_T}{m/L}}$

Harmonic frequencies: $f_n = n\dfrac{v}{2L}, f_n = nf_1$

Harmonic wavelengths: $\lambda_n = \dfrac{2L}{n}, \lambda_n = \dfrac{1}{n}\lambda_1$

CAPACITORS

Capacitance: $C = \dfrac{Q}{V}$

$C_{\text{parallel-plate}} = \varepsilon_0\dfrac{A}{d}$

$C_{\text{with dielectric}} = K \cdot C_{\text{without}}$

electric field between plates: $E = \dfrac{V}{d}$

$PE_E = \dfrac{1}{2}QV = \dfrac{1}{2}CV^2 = \dfrac{Q^2}{2C}$

Capacitors in series: $\dfrac{1}{C_S} = \dfrac{1}{C_1} + \dfrac{1}{C_2} + ...$

Capacitors in parallel: $C_P = C_1 + C_2 + ...$

ELECTRIC CIRCUITS

Current: $I = \dfrac{Q}{t}$

Resistance: $R = \dfrac{V}{I}$ ("Ohm's law": $V = IR$)

Resistance: $R = \rho\dfrac{L}{A}$

Resistors in series: $R_S = R_1 + R_2 + ...$

Resistors in parallel: $\dfrac{1}{R_P} = \dfrac{1}{R_1} + \dfrac{1}{R_2} + ...$

Power in circuit: $P = IV = I^2R = \dfrac{V^2}{R}$

Power in AC circuit: $\bar{P} = I_{\text{rms}}V_{\text{rms}} = \dfrac{I_{\text{max}}}{\sqrt{2}} \cdot \dfrac{V_{\text{max}}}{\sqrt{2}}$

SOUND

$$v = \sqrt{\frac{B}{\rho}}$$

Intensity: $I = \dfrac{\text{Power}}{\text{Area}}$

Intensity-level (in dB): $\beta = 10 \log \dfrac{I}{I_0}$

Harmonic f's and λ's:

Open ends: $f_n = \dfrac{nv}{2L}$, $\lambda_n = \dfrac{2L}{n}$

Closed ends: $f_n = \dfrac{nv}{4L}$, $\lambda_n = \dfrac{4L}{n}$ (odd n)

$f_{\text{beat}} = |f_1 - f_2|$

Doppler effect: $f_D = \dfrac{v \pm v_D}{v \mp v_S} f_S$

Approaching $\longleftrightarrow$ higher f

Receding $\longleftrightarrow$ lower f

ELECTROSTATICS AND MAGNETISM

Coulomb's law: $F_E = k \dfrac{|Q||q|}{r^2}$

Electric field due to Q: $E = k \dfrac{|Q|}{r^2}$

Electric force by field: $\mathbf{F}_E = q\mathbf{E}$

Electric potential due to Q: $\phi = k \dfrac{Q}{r}$

$\Delta PE_E = q\Delta\phi = qV$

magnetic force: $\mathbf{F}_M = q(\mathbf{v} \times \mathbf{B})$

$F_M = qvB \sin\theta$

LIGHT AND OPTICS

$c = 3.0 \times 10^8$ m/s

index of refraction: $n = \dfrac{c}{v}$

Law of reflection: $\theta_1 = \theta_1'$

Law of refraction (Snell's law): $n_1 \sin\theta_1 = n_2 \sin\theta_2$

TIR: if $\theta_1 > \theta_{\text{crit}}$, where $\sin\theta_{\text{crit}} = \dfrac{n_2}{n_1}$

Mirror-Lens equation: $\dfrac{1}{o} + \dfrac{1}{i} = \dfrac{1}{f}$

Focal length: $f = \dfrac{r}{2}$

Magnification: $m = -\dfrac{i}{o}$

Lens power: $P = \dfrac{1}{f}$; $P_{\text{combination}} = P_1 + P_2$

QUANTUM PHYSICS

$E_{\text{photon}} = hf = \dfrac{hc}{\lambda}$

Photoelectron Energy: $KE_{\text{max}} = hf - \phi$

Stopping Voltage: $-eV_{\text{stop}} = KE_{\text{max}}$

Heisenberg Uncertainty Principle:

$\Delta x \Delta p \geq h/2\pi$

CONSTANTS AND UNITS

Constants

magnitude of gravitational acceleration near the surface of Earth: $g = 9.8 \text{ m/s}^2 \approx 10 \text{ m/s}^2$

density of water: $\rho_{water} = 1000 \text{ kg/m}^3 = 1 \text{ g/cm}^3$

elementary electric charge: $e = 1.6 \times 10^{-19} \text{ C}$

Coulomb's constant: $k_0 = 9 \times 10^9 \text{ N·m}^2 / \text{C}^2$

threshold of hearing: $I_0 = 10^{-12} \text{ W/m}^2$

speed of light in vacuum: $c = 3 \times 10^8 \text{ m/s}$

atmospheric pressure: $P_{atm} = 10^5 \text{ Pa}$

speed of sound in air: $v_{sound} = 340 \text{ m/s}$

visible light wavelengths: 400 nm to 700 nm

SI Units

distance: $[d]$ = meters = m

mass: $[m]$ = kilograms = kg

time: $[t]$ = seconds = s

velocity, speed: $[v]$ = meters per second = m/s

acceleration: $[a]$ = meters per second squared = m/s^2

force: $[F]$ = newtons = kg·m/s^2

torque: $[\tau]$ = newton-meters = N·m

work: $[W]$ = joules = J = kg·m^2/s^2

energy: $[KE] = [PE] = [E]$ = joules = J = kg·m^2/s^2

power: $[P]$ = watts = W = J/s

pressure: $[P]$ = pascals = Pa = N/m^2

density: $[\rho]$ = kilograms per cubic meter = kg/m^3

flow rate: $[f]$ = m^3/s

electric charge: $[q]$ = coulombs = C

electric field: $[E]$ = newtons per coulomb = N/C (or volts per meter = V/m)

electric potential: $[\phi]$ = volts = V = J/C

voltage: $[V]$ = volts = V = J/C

current: $[I]$ = amps = A = C/s

resistance: $[R]$ = ohms = Ω = V/A

resistivity: $[\rho]$ = ohm-meters = Ω·m

capacitance: $[C]$ = farads = F = C/V

magnetic field: $[B]$ = teslas = T = N/A·m

frequency: $[f]$ = hertz = Hz = s^{-1}

period: $[T]$ = seconds = s

sound level: $[\beta]$ = decibels = dB

lens power: $[P]$ = diopters = D = m^{-1}

MCAT Math for Physics

PREFACE

The MCAT is primarily a conceptual exam, but you should expect some mathematical computation and reasoning. Any math that is on the MCAT is fundamental: just arithmetic, algebra, and trigonometry. There is absolutely no calculus. The purpose of this section of the book is to go over some math topics with which you may feel a little rusty.

This text is intended for reference and self-study. Therefore, there are lots of examples, all completely solved. Practice working through these examples and master the fundamentals!

Chapter 15
Arithmetic, Algebra, and Graphs

15.1 THE IMPORTANCE OF APPROXIMATION

Since you aren't allowed to use a calculator on the MCAT, you need to practice doing arithmetic calculations by hand again. Fortunately, the amount of calculation you'll have to do is small, and you'll also be able to approximate. For example, let's say you were faced with simplifying this expression:

$$\frac{\sqrt{5 \times 10^{-7}}}{(3.1 \times 10^{-2})^2}$$

Our first inclination would be to reach for our calculator, but we don't have one available. Now what? Realize that on the Chemical and Physical Foundations of Biological Systems section of the MCAT, there are 95 minutes for 67 questions, or approximately 1.4 minutes per question, so there simply cannot be questions requiring lengthy, complicated computation. Instead, we'll figure out a reasonably accurate (and fast) approximation of the value of the expression above:

$$\frac{\sqrt{5 \times 10^{-7}}}{(3.1 \times 10^{-2})^2} = \frac{\sqrt{50 \times 10^{-8}}}{(3.1)^2 \times (10^{-2})^2} \approx \frac{\sqrt{50} \times \sqrt{10^{-8}}}{10 \times 10^{-4}} \approx \frac{7 \times 10^{-4}}{10 \times 10^{-4}} = \frac{7}{10} = 0.7$$

So, if the answer to an MCAT question was the value of the expression above, and the four answer choices were, say, 0.124, 0.405, 0.736, and 1.289, we'd know right away that the answer is 0.736. The choices are far enough apart that even with our approximations, we were still able to tell which choice was the correct one. Just as importantly, we didn't waste time trying to be more precise; it was unnecessary, and it would have decreased the amount of time we had to spend on other questions.

If you find yourself writing out lengthy calculations on your scratch paper when you're working through MCAT questions that contain some mathematical calculation, it's important that you recognize that you're not using your time efficiently. Say to yourself, "I'm wasting valuable time trying to get a precise answer, when I don't need to be precise." Which of the following calculations for figuring out the value of 23.6×72.5 is faster?

$$
\begin{array}{r}
23.6 \\
\times\ 72.5 \\
\hline
1180 \\
472 \\
1652 \\
\hline
1711.00
\end{array}
\qquad \text{or} \qquad
\begin{array}{r}
25 \\
\times\ 70 \\
\hline
1750
\end{array}
$$

In the one-step calculation on the right, we approximated: $23.6 \approx 25$ and $72.5 \approx 70$, and the answer we got in just a few seconds differs from the precise answer by only 2%. For the MCAT, you should always strive to make such approximations so that you can do the math quickly.

Try this one: What's 1583 divided by 32.1? (You have five seconds. Go.)

For the previous practice exercise, you should have written (or done in your head):

$$\frac{1500}{30} = 50$$

15.2 SCIENTIFIC NOTATION, EXPONENTS, AND RADICALS

It's well known that very large or very small numbers can be handled more easily when they're written in **scientific notation**, that is, in the form $\pm\, m \times 10^n$, where $1 \le m < 10$ and n is an integer. For example:

$$602,000,000,000,000,000,000,000 = 6.02 \times 10^{23}$$

$$-35,000,000,000 = -3.5 \times 10^{10}$$

$$0.000000004 = 4 \times 10^{-9}$$

Quantities like these come up all the time in physical problems, so you must be able to work with them confidently. Since a power of ten (the term 10^n) is part of every number written in scientific notation, the most important rules for dealing with such expressions are the Laws of Exponents:

Laws of Exponents

Illustration (with b = 10 or a power of 10)

Law 1	$b^p \times b^q = b^{p+q}$	$10^5 \times 10^{-9} = 10^{5+(-9)} = 10^{-4}$
Law 2	$b^p/b^q = b^{p-q}$	$10^5/10^{-9} = 10^{5-(-9)} = 10^{14}$
Law 3	$(b^p)^q = b^{pq}$	$(10^{-3})^2 = 10^{(-3)(2)} = 10^{-6}$
Law 4	$b^0 = 1$ (if $b \ne 0$)	$10^0 = 1$
Law 5	$b^{-p} = 1/b^p$	$10^{-7} = 1/10^7$
Law 6	$(ab)^p = a^p b^p$	$(2 \times 10^4)^3 = 2^3 \times (10^4)^3 = 8 \times 10^{12}$
Law 7	$(a/b)^p = a^p/b^p$	$[(3 \times 10^{-6})/10^2]^2 = (3 \times 10^{-6})^2/(10^2)^2 = 9 \times 10^{-16}$

Example 15-1: Simplify each of the following expressions, writing your answer in scientific notation:
a) $(4 \times 10^{-3})(5 \times 10^9)$
b) $(4 \times 10^{-3})/(5 \times 10^9)$
c) $(3 \times 10^{-4})^3$
d) $[(1 \times 10^{-2})/(5 \times 10^{-7})]^2$

Solution:
a) $(4 \times 10^{-3})(5 \times 10^9) = (4)(5) \times 10^{-3+9} = 20 \times 10^6 = 2 \times 10^7$
b) $(4 \times 10^{-3})/(5 \times 10^9) = (4/5) \times 10^{-3-9} = 0.8 \times 10^{-12} = 8 \times 10^{-13}$
c) $(3 \times 10^{-4})^3 = 3^3 \times (10^{-4})^3 = 27 \times 10^{-12} = 2.7 \times 10^{-11}$
d) $[(1 \times 10^{-2})/(5 \times 10^{-7})]^2 = (1 \times 10^{-2})^2/(5 \times 10^{-7})^2 = (1 \times 10^{-4})/(25 \times 10^{-14}) = (1/25) \times 10^{-4-(-14)}$
       $= (4/100) \times 10^{10} = 4 \times 10^8$

Another important skill involving numbers written in scientific notation involves changing the power of 10 (and compensating for this change so as not to affect the original number). The approximation carried out in the very first example in this chapter is a good example of this. To find the square root of 5×10^{-7}, it is much easier to first rewrite this number as 50×10^{-8}, because then the square root is easy:

$$\sqrt{50 \times 10^{-8}} = \sqrt{50} \times \sqrt{10^{-8}} \approx 7 \times 10^{-4}$$

Other examples of this procedure are found in Example 15-1 above; for instance,

$$20 \times 10^{6} = 2 \times 10^{7}$$
$$0.8 \times 10^{-12} = 8 \times 10^{-13}$$
$$27 \times 10^{-12} = 2.7 \times 10^{-11}$$

In writing $\sqrt{50 \times 10^{-8}} = \sqrt{50} \times \sqrt{10^{-8}} \approx 7 \times 10^{-4}$, I used a familiar law of square roots, that the square root of a product is equal to the product of the square roots. Here's a short list of rules for dealing with radicals:

Laws of Radicals

Illustration

Law 1 $\sqrt{ab} = \sqrt{a} \cdot \sqrt{b}$ $\sqrt{9 \times 10^{12}} = \sqrt{9} \times \sqrt{10^{12}} = 3 \times 10^{6}$

Law 2 $\sqrt{a/b} = \sqrt{a}/\sqrt{b}$ $\sqrt{(4 \times 10^{-6})/10^{-18}} = \sqrt{(4 \times 10^{-6})}/\sqrt{10^{-18}} = (2 \times 10^{-3})/10^{-9} = 2 \times 10^{6}$

Law 3 $\sqrt[q]{a^{p}} = a^{p/q}$ $\sqrt[3]{(8 \times 10^{6})^{2}} = (8 \times 10^{6})^{2/3} = 8^{2/3} \times 10^{(6)(2/3)} = 4 \times 10^{4}$

A couple of remarks about this list: First, Laws 1 and 2 illustrate how to handle square roots, which are the most common. However, the same laws are true even if the index of the root is not 2. (The **index** of a root [or radical] is the number that indicates the root that's to be taken; it's indicated by the little q in front of the radical sign in Law 3. Cube roots are index 3 and written $\sqrt[3]{\ }$; fourth roots are index 4 and written $\sqrt[4]{\ }$; and square roots are index 2 and written $\sqrt[2]{\ }$, although we hardly ever write the little 2.) Second, Law 3 provides the link between exponents and radicals.

Example 15-2: Approximate each of the following expressions, writing your answer in scientific notation:

a) $\sqrt{3.5 \times 10^{9}}$

b) $\sqrt{8 \times 10^{-11}}$

c) $\sqrt{\dfrac{1.5 \times 10^{-5}}{2.5 \times 10^{-17}}}$

Solution:

a) $\sqrt{3.5\times10^9} = \sqrt{35\times10^8} = \sqrt{35}\times\sqrt{10^8} \approx \sqrt{36}\times\sqrt{10^8} = 6\times10^4$

b) $\sqrt{8\times10^{-11}} = \sqrt{80\times10^{-12}} = \sqrt{80}\times\sqrt{10^{-12}} \approx \sqrt{81}\times\sqrt{10^{-12}} = 9\times10^{-6}$

c) $\sqrt{\dfrac{1.5\times10^{-5}}{2.5\times10^{-17}}} = \dfrac{\sqrt{1.5\times10^{-5}}}{\sqrt{2.5\times10^{-17}}} = \dfrac{\sqrt{15\times10^{-6}}}{\sqrt{25\times10^{-18}}} \approx \dfrac{\sqrt{16}\times\sqrt{10^{-6}}}{\sqrt{25}\times\sqrt{10^{-18}}} = \dfrac{4\times10^{-3}}{5\times10^{-9}} = 0.8\times10^6 = 8\times10^5$

Example 15-3: Approximate each of the following expressions, writing your answer in scientific notation:

a) The mass (in grams) of 4.7×10^{24} molecules of CCl_4: $\dfrac{(4.7\times10^{24})(153.8)}{6.02\times10^{23}}$

b) The electrostatic force (in newtons) between the proton and electron in the ground state of hydrogen:

$$\frac{(8.99\times10^9)(1.6\times10^{-19})^2}{(5.3\times10^{-11})^2}$$

c) The diameter (in cm) of a 1 kg sphere of gold: $200\sqrt[3]{\dfrac{3}{4\pi}\dfrac{1}{19,300}}$

Solution:

a) $\dfrac{(4.7\times10^{24})(153.8)}{6.02\times10^{23}} \approx \dfrac{5(150)}{6}\times10^{24-23} = 5(25)\times10 = 1.25\times10^3$

b) $\dfrac{(8.99\times10^9)(1.6\times10^{-19})^2}{(5.3\times10^{-11})^2} \approx \dfrac{9(1.6)^2\times10^{9+(-19)(2)}}{(5.3)^2\times10^{(-11)(2)}} \approx \dfrac{(9)3\times10^{-29}}{27\times10^{-22}} = 1\times10^{-7}$

c) $200\sqrt[3]{\dfrac{3}{4\pi}\dfrac{1}{19,300}} \approx 200\sqrt[3]{\dfrac{1}{4}\dfrac{1}{20,000}} = \dfrac{200}{\sqrt[3]{80\times10^3}} = \dfrac{200}{\sqrt[3]{80}\times10} \approx \dfrac{200}{4\times10} = 5$

Two notes about the approximation in part (c). First, we canceled the 3 and the π in the first fraction; this is fine since $\pi \approx 3.14$. Second, we had to approximate $\sqrt[3]{80}$. Since 80 is between $64 = 4^3$ and $125 = 5^3$, the cube root of 80 is between 4 and 5. And, since 80 is closer to 64 than it is to 125, the cube root of 80 is closer to 4. In general, to approximate the nth root of a number that isn't an nth power, simply locate the given number between successive n^{th} powers and approximate from there. For example, $\sqrt{42}$ is not an integer since 42 is not a perfect square. However, 42 is between $36 = 6^2$ and $49 = 7^2$, so $\sqrt{42}$ is between 6 and 7. And since 42 is about halfway between 36 and 49, the square root of 42 is about halfway between 6 and 7: $\sqrt{42} \approx 6.5$.

15.3 FRACTIONS, RATIOS, AND PERCENTS

A **fraction** indicates a division; for example, 3/4 means 3 divided by 4. The number above (or to the left of) the fraction bar is the numerator, and the number below (or to the right) of the fraction bar is called the denominator.

$$\frac{3}{4} \xleftarrow{\text{numerator}} \xrightarrow{} 3/4$$

Our quick review of the basic arithmetic operations on fractions begins with the simplest rule: the one for multiplication:

$$\frac{a}{b} \times \frac{c}{d} = \frac{ac}{bd}$$

In words, just multiply the numerators and then, separately, multiply the denominators.

Example 15-4: What is 4/9 times 2/5?

Solution: $\dfrac{4}{9} \times \dfrac{2}{5} = \dfrac{4 \times 2}{9 \times 5} = \dfrac{8}{45}$

The rule for dividing fractions is based on the reciprocal. If $a \ne 0$, then the **reciprocal** of a/b is simply b/a; that is, to form the reciprocal of a fraction, just flip it over. For example, the reciprocal of 3/4 is 4/3; the reciprocal of $-2/5$ is $-5/2$; the reciprocal of 3 is 1/3; and the reciprocal of $-1/4$ is -4. (The number 0 has no reciprocal.) As a result of this definition, we have the following basic fact: The product of any number and its reciprocal is 1.

Example 15-5: Find the reciprocal of each of these numbers:
  a)   2.25
  b) 5×10^{-4}
  c) 4×10^5

Solution:
  a)   2.25 is equal to 2 + (1/4), which is 9/4. The reciprocal of 9/4 is 4/9.

  b) $\dfrac{1}{5 \times 10^{-4}} = \dfrac{1}{5} \times \dfrac{1}{10^{-4}} = 0.2 \times 10^4 = 2 \times 10^3$

  c) $\dfrac{1}{4 \times 10^5} = \dfrac{1}{4} \times \dfrac{1}{10^5} = 0.25 \times 10^{-5} = 2.5 \times 10^{-6}$

Now, in words, the rule for dividing fractions reads: *multiply by the reciprocal of the divisor*. That is, flip over whatever you're dividing by, and then multiply:

$$\frac{a}{b} \div \frac{c}{d} = \frac{a}{b} \times \frac{d}{c}$$

Example 15-6: What is 4/9 divided by 2/5?

Solution: $\dfrac{4}{9} \div \dfrac{2}{5} = \dfrac{4}{9} \times \dfrac{5}{2} = \dfrac{4 \times 5}{9 \times 2} = \dfrac{20}{18} = \dfrac{10}{9}$

Finally, we turn to addition and subtraction. In elementary and junior-high school, you were probably taught to find a common denominator (preferably, the *least* common denominator, known as the LCD), rewrite each fraction in terms of this common denominator, then add or subtract the numerators. If a common denominator is easy to spot, this may well be the fastest way to add or subtract fractions:

$$\frac{1}{2} + \frac{3}{4} = \frac{2}{4} + \frac{3}{4} = \frac{2+3}{4} = \frac{5}{4}$$

However, there is an efficient method for adding and subtracting fractions by making use of the following rules:

Here's what the arrows in the top line represent: "Multiply *up* (*d* times *a* gives *ad*), multiply *up* again (*b* times *c* gives *bc*), do the adding or subtracting of these products, and place the result over the product of the denominators (*bd*)." The length of this last sentence hides the simplicity of the rule, but it describes the recipe to follow. For example,

$$\frac{4}{9} + \frac{2}{5} = \frac{20+18}{45} = \frac{38}{45} \qquad\qquad \frac{4}{9} - \frac{2}{5} = \frac{20-18}{45} = \frac{2}{45}$$

Example 15-7:

a) Approximate the sum $\dfrac{1}{2.4 \times 10^5} + \dfrac{1}{6 \times 10^4}$

b) What is the reciprocal of this sum?

c) Simplify: $\dfrac{1}{2 \times 10^{-8}} - \dfrac{2}{5 \times 10^{-7}}$

15.3

Solution:

a) Using the rule illustrated above, we find that

$$\frac{1}{2.4 \times 10^5} + \frac{1}{6 \times 10^4} = \frac{(6 \times 10^4) + (2.4 \times 10^5)}{(2.4 \times 10^5)(6 \times 10^4)} = \frac{(6 \times 10^4) + (24 \times 10^4)}{(2.4 \times 10^5)(6 \times 10^4)} = \frac{(6 + 24) \times 10^4}{(2.4)(6) \times 10^{5+4}} \approx \frac{30 \times 10^4}{15 \times 10^9} = 2 \times 10^{-5}$$

b) The reciprocal of this result is $\dfrac{1}{2 \times 10^{-5}} = \dfrac{1}{2} \times \dfrac{1}{10^{-5}} = 0.5 \times 10^5 = 5 \times 10^4$.

c) $\dfrac{1}{2 \times 10^{-8}} - \dfrac{2}{5 \times 10^{-7}} = \dfrac{(5 \times 10^{-7}) - (2 \times 10^{-8})(2)}{(2 \times 10^{-8})(5 \times 10^{-7})} = \dfrac{(50 \times 10^{-8}) - (4 \times 10^{-8})}{(2)(5) \times 10^{-8+(-7)}} = \dfrac{(50 - 4) \times 10^{-8}}{10 \times 10^{-15}} = 46 \times 10^6$

$$= 4.6 \times 10^7$$

Let's now move on to ratios. A **ratio** is another way of saying *fraction*. For example, the ratio of 3 to 4, written 3:4, is equal to the fraction 3/4. Here's an illustration using isotopes of chlorine: The statement *the ratio of ^{35}Cl to ^{37}Cl is 3:1* means that there are 3/1 = 3 times as many ^{35}Cl atoms as there are ^{37}Cl atoms.

A particularly useful way to interpret a ratio is in terms of parts of a total. A ratio of *a*:*b* means that there are *a* + *b* total parts, with *a* of them being of the first type and *b* of the second type. Therefore, *the ratio of ^{35}Cl to ^{37}Cl is 3:1* means that if we could take all ^{35}Cl and ^{37}Cl atoms, we could partition all them into 3 + 1 = 4 equal parts such that 3 of these parts will all be ^{35}Cl atoms, and the remaining 1 part will all be ^{37}Cl atoms. We can now restate the original ratio as a ratio of these parts to the total. Since ^{35}Cl atoms account for 3 parts out of the 4 total, the ratio of ^{35}Cl atoms to all Cl atoms is 3:4; that is, 3/4 of all Cl atoms are ^{35}Cl atoms. Similarly, the ratio of ^{37}Cl atoms to all Cl atoms is 1:4, which means that 1/4 of all Cl atoms are ^{37}Cl atoms.

Example 15-8: The formula for the compound TNT (trinitrotoluene) is $C_7H_5N_3O_6$.
  a) What fraction of the atoms in this compound are nitrogen atoms?
  b) If the molar masses of C, H, N, and O are 12 g, 1 g, 14 g, and 16 g, respectively, what is the ratio of the mass of all the nitrogens to the total mass?

Solution:
  a) There are a total of 7 + 5 + 3 + 6 = 21 atoms per molecule. The ratio of N atoms to the total is 3:21, or, more simply, 1:7. Therefore, 1/7 of the atoms in this compound are nitrogen atoms.
  b) The desired ratio of masses is calculated like this:

$$\frac{\text{mass of all N atoms}}{\text{total mass of molecule}} = \frac{3(14)}{7(12) + 5(1) + 3(14) + 6(16)} = \frac{42}{227} \approx \frac{40}{220} = \frac{2}{11}$$

Example 15-9: In a simple hydrocarbon (molecular formula C_xH_y), the ratio of C atoms to H atoms is 5:4, and the total number of atoms in the molecule is 18. Find *x* and *y*.

Solution: Since the ratio of C atoms to H atoms is 5:4, there are 5 parts C atoms and 4 parts H atoms, for a total of 9 equal parts. These 9 equal parts account for 18 total atoms, so each part must contain 2 atoms. Thus, C (which has 5 parts) has 5 × 2 = 10 atoms, and H (which has 4 parts) has 4 × 2 = 8 atoms. Therefore, *x* = 10 and *y* = 8.

Example 15-10: The ratio of O atoms to C atoms in each molecule of triethylene glycol is 2:3, and the ratio of O atoms to the total number of C atoms and H atoms is 1:5. If there are 24 atoms (C, H, and O only) per molecule, find the formula for this compound.

Solution: The ratio of O to C atoms is 2:3, which tells us there are 2 parts O atoms and 3 parts C atoms, for a total of 5 parts C and O. Since the ratio of O to (C *and* H) atoms is 1:5, there are 5 times as many C and H atoms as there are O atoms. But, we have found that there are 2 parts O atoms, so C and H must account for 5 times as many: 10 parts. And, because there are 3 parts C atoms, there must be $10 - 3 = 7$ parts H atoms. We therefore have $2 + 3 + 7 = 12$ parts total, accounting for 24 atoms, which means 2 atoms per part. So, there must be $2 \times 2 = 4$ O atoms, $3 \times 2 = 6$ C atoms, and $7 \times 2 = 14$ H atoms. The formula is $C_6H_{14}O_4$.

The word **percent**, symbolized by %, is simply an abbreviation for the phrase "out of 100." Therefore, a percentage is represented by a fraction whose denominator is 100. For example, 60% means 60/100, or 60 out of 100. The three main question types involving percents are as follows:

1. What is y% of z?
2. x is what percent of z?
3. x is y% of what?

Fortunately, all three question types fit into a single form and can all be answered by one equation. Translating the statement *x is y% of z* into an algebraic equation, we get

$$x \text{ is } y\% \text{ of } z$$
$$\Downarrow$$
$$x = \underbrace{\frac{y}{100}}_{\substack{\text{is} \quad y\% \quad \text{of}}} \cdot z$$

So, if you know any two of the three quantities x, y, and z, you can use the equation above to figure out the third.

Example 15-11:
a) What is 25% of 200?
b) 30 is what percent of 150?
c) 400 is 80% of what?

Solution:
a) Solving the equation $x = (25/100) \times 200$, we get $x = 25 \times 2 = 50$.
b) Solving the equation $30 = (y/100) \times 150$, we get $y = (30/150) \times 100 = (1/5) \times 100 = 20$.
c) Solving the equation $400 = (80/100) \times z$, we get $z = (100/80) \times 400 = 100 \times 5 = 500$.

It's also helpful to think of a simple fraction that equals a given percent, which can be used in place of $y/100$ in the equation above. For example, 25% = 1/4, 50% = 1/2, and 75% = 3/4. Other common fractional equivalents are: 20% = 1/5, 40% = 2/5, 60% = 3/5, and 80% = 4/5; 33.3% = 1/3 and 66.7% = 2/3; and $10n\% = n/10$ (for example, 10% = 1/10, 30% = 3/10, 70% = 7/10, and 90% = 9/10).

Example 15-12:
  a)   What is 60% of 35?
  b)   12 is 75% of what?
  c)   What is 70% of 400?

Solution:
  a)   Since 60% = 3/5, we find that $x = (3/5) \times 35 = 3 \times 7 = 21$.
  b)   Because 75% = 3/4, we solve the equation $12 = (3/4) \times z$, and find $z = 12 \times (4/3) = 16$.
  c)   Since 70% = 7/10, we find that $x = (7/10) \times 400 = 7 \times 40 = 280$.

Example 15-13:
  a)   What is the result when 50 is increased by 50%?
  b)   What is the result when 80 is decreased by 40%?

Solution:
  a)   "Increasing 50 by 50%" means adding (50% of 50) to 50. Since 50% of 50 is 25, increasing 50 by 50% gives us 50 + 25 = 75.
  b)   "Decreasing 80 by 40%" means subtracting (40% of 80) from 80. Since 40% of 80 is 32, decreasing 80 by 40% gives us 80 − 32 = 48.

Example 15-14:
  a)   What is 250% of 60?
  b)   2400 is what percent of 500?

Solution:
  a)   Solving the equation $x = (250/100) \times 60$, we get $x = 25 \times 6 = 150$.
  b)   Solving the equation $2400 = (y/100) \times 500$, we get $2400 = 5y$, so $y = 2400/5 = 480$.

Example 15-15: There are three stable isotopes of magnesium: ^{24}Mg, ^{25}Mg, and ^{26}Mg. The relative abundance of ^{24}Mg is 79%. Consider a sample of natural magnesium containing a total of 8×10^{24} atoms.
  a)   About how many atoms in the sample are ^{24}Mg atoms?
  b)   If the number of ^{25}Mg atoms in the sample is 8×10^{23}, what is the relative abundance (as a percentage) of ^{25}Mg?
  c)   What's the relative abundance of ^{26}Mg?

Solution:
  a)   Since the question is asking, *What is 79% of 8×10^{24}?*, we have

$$x = \frac{79}{100} \times (8 \times 10^{24}) \approx \frac{80}{100} \times (8 \times 10^{24}) = 6.4 \times 10^{24}$$

  b)   The question is asking, *8×10^{23} is what percent of 8×10^{24}?*, so we write

$$8 \times 10^{23} = \frac{y}{100} \times (8 \times 10^{24}) \Rightarrow \frac{y}{100} = \frac{8 \times 10^{23}}{8 \times 10^{24}} = \frac{1}{10} \Rightarrow y = 10 \Rightarrow \text{relative abundance} = 10\%$$

  c)   Assuming that these three isotopes account for all naturally occurring magnesium, the sum of the relative abundance percentages should be 100%. Therefore, we need only solve the equation 79% + 10% + *Y*% = 100%, from which we find that *Y* = 11.

Example 15-16: What is the percentage by mass of carbon in $C_7H_5N_3O_6$? (Given: Molar mass of compound = 227 g.)

A. 26%
B. 37%
C. 49%
D. 62%

Solution: Once the fraction of the total molar mass of the compound that's contributed by carbon is calculated, we obtain a percentage by multiplying this fraction by 100%. Since the molar mass of carbon is 12 g, and the molecule contains 7 C atoms, we have

$$\%C, \text{ by mass } = \frac{7(12)}{227} = \frac{84}{227} \approx \frac{100}{250} = \frac{2}{5} = \frac{2}{5} \times 100\% = 40\%$$

Therefore, choice B is best.

15.4 EQUATIONS AND INEQUALITIES

You may have several questions on the MCAT that require you to solve—or manipulate—an algebraic equation or inequality. Fortunately, these equations and inequalities won't be very complicated.

When manipulating an algebraic equation, there's basically only one rule to remember: *Whatever you do to one side of the equation, you must do to the other side.* (Otherwise, it won't be a valid equation anymore.) For example, if you add 5 to the *left*-hand side, then add 5 to the *right*-hand side; if you multiply the *left*-hand side by 2, then multiply the *right*-hand side by 2, and so forth.

Inequalities are a little more involved. While it's still true that whatever you do to one side of an inequality you must also do the other side, there are a couple of additional rules, both of which involve flipping the inequality sign—that is, changing > to < (or vice versa) or changing ≥ to ≤ (or vice versa).

1. *If you multiply both sides of an inequality by a negative number, then you must flip the inequality sign.*
   For example, let's say you're given the inequality $-2x > 6$. To solve for x, you'd multiply both sides by $-1/2$. Since this is a negative number, the inequality sign must be flipped: $x < -3$.

2. *If both sides of an inequality are positive quantities, and you take the reciprocal of both sides, then you must flip the inequality sign.*
   For example, let's say you're given the inequality $2/x \leq 6$, where it's known that x must be positive. To solve for x, you can take the reciprocal of both sides. Upon doing so, the inequality sign must be flipped: $x/2 \geq 1/6$, so $x \geq 1/3$.

Example 15-17:

a) Solve for T: $PV = nRT$

b) Solve for t (given that t is positive): $y = (1/2)gt^2$

c) Solve for x (given that x is positive): $4x^2 = 2.4 \times 10^{-11}$

d) Solve for B: $h = k + \log(B/A)$

e) If $mg = GMm/r^2$ and r is positive, solve for r in terms of g, G, and M.

f) If $f = \pi r^2 v$, solve for r in terms of f and v.

g) If $\lambda f = c$ and $n\lambda = 2L$, solve for n in terms of L, f, and c.

h) If $1/f = (1/o) + (1/i)$, solve for i in terms of o and f.

i) Assume that $p = p_0 + 10\rho D$, where p_0 and ρ are constants. If $p = 300$ when $D = 10$ and $p = 400$ when $D = 15$, find the value of p when $D = 30$.

j) Solve for x: $3(2 - x) < 18$

k) Find all positive values of λ that satisfy $\dfrac{2 \times 10^{-25}}{\lambda} \geq 4 \times 10^{-19}$

Solution:

a) Dividing both sides by nR, we get $T = PV/(nR)$.

b) Multiply both sides $2/g$, then take the square root: $t = \sqrt{\dfrac{2y}{g}}$.

c) $4x^2 = 2.4 \times 10^{-11} \Rightarrow x^2 = 6 \times 10^{-12} \Rightarrow x = \sqrt{6} \times 10^{-6} \approx 2.5 \times 10^{-6}$

d) $h = k + \log\dfrac{B}{A} \Rightarrow \log\dfrac{B}{A} = h - k \Rightarrow 10^{h-k} = \dfrac{B}{A} \Rightarrow B = 10^{h-k}A$ [see Section 19]

e) $mg = G\dfrac{Mm}{r^2} \Rightarrow g = G\dfrac{M}{r^2} \Rightarrow r^2 = G\dfrac{M}{g} \Rightarrow r = \sqrt{G\dfrac{M}{g}}$

f) $f = \pi r^2 v \Rightarrow r^2 = \dfrac{f}{\pi v} \Rightarrow r = \sqrt{\dfrac{f}{\pi v}}$

g) Since $\lambda = c/f$, we get $n\dfrac{c}{f} = 2L \Rightarrow n = \dfrac{2Lf}{c}$.

h) $\dfrac{1}{f} = \dfrac{1}{o} + \dfrac{1}{i} \Rightarrow \dfrac{1}{i} = \dfrac{1}{f} - \dfrac{1}{o} = \dfrac{o-f}{fo} \Rightarrow i = \dfrac{fo}{o-f}$

i) Let's plug in the given information: $300 = p_0 + 100\rho$ and $400 = p_0 + 150\rho$. If we subtract the first equation from the second one, the p_0's cancel and we get $100 = 50\rho$, so $\rho = 2$. Plugging $\rho = 2$ back into either one of the equations, we find that $p_0 = 100$. Therefore, $p = 100 + 20D$. So, when $D = 30$, we get $p = 100 + (20)(30) = 700$.

j) $3(2 - x) < 18 \Rightarrow 2 - x < 6 \Rightarrow -x < 4 \Rightarrow x > -4$

k) $\dfrac{2 \times 10^{-25}}{\lambda} \geq 4 \times 10^{-19} \Rightarrow \dfrac{\lambda}{2 \times 10^{-25}} \leq \dfrac{1}{4 \times 10^{-19}} \Rightarrow \lambda \leq \dfrac{2 \times 10^{-25}}{4 \times 10^{-19}} = 0.5 \times 10^{-6} \Rightarrow \lambda \leq 5 \times 10^{-7}$

15.5 THE X-Y PLANE, LINES, AND OTHER GRAPHS

The figure below shows the familiar *x-y* **plane**, which we use to plot data and draw lines and curves showing how one quantity is related to another one:

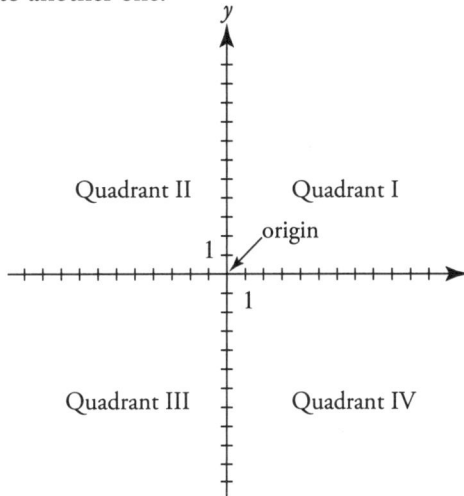

The *x-y* plane is formed by intersecting two number lines perpendicularly at the origins. The horizontal axis is generically referred to as the *x*-**axis** (although the quantity measured along this axis might be named by some other letter, such as time, *t*), and the vertical axis is generically known as the *y*-**axis**. The axes split the plane into four **quadrants**, which are numbered consecutively in a counterclockwise fashion. Quadrant I is in the upper right and represents all points (x, y) where x and y are both positive; in Quadrant II, x is negative and y is positive; in Quadrant III, x and y are both negative; and in Quadrant IV, x is positive and y is negative.

Suppose that two quantities, x and y, were related by the equation $y = 2x^2$. We would consider x as the **independent variable**, and y as the **dependent variable**, since for each value of x we get a unique value of y (that is, y *depends* uniquely on x). The independent variable is plotted along the horizontal axis, while the dependent variable is plotted along the vertical axis. Constructing a graph of an equation usually consists of plotting specific points (x, y) that satisfy the equation—in this case, examples include $(0, 0)$, $(1, 2)$, $(2, 8)$, $(-1, 2)$, $(-2, 8)$, etc.—and then connecting these points with a line or other smooth curve. The first coordinate of each point—the x coordinate—is known as the **abscissa**, and the second coordinate of each point—the y coordinate—is known as the **ordinate**.

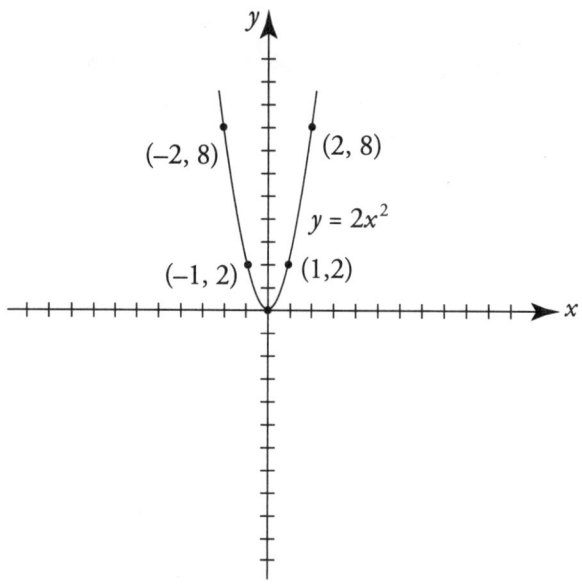

Lines

One of the simplest and most important graphs is the (straight) **line**. A line is determined by its slope—its steepness—and one specific point on the line, such as its intersection with either the x- or y-axis. The **slope** of a line is defined to be a change in y divided by the corresponding change in x ("rise over run"). Lines with positive slope rise to the right; those with negative slope fall to the right. And the greater the magnitude (absolute value) of the slope, the steeper the line.

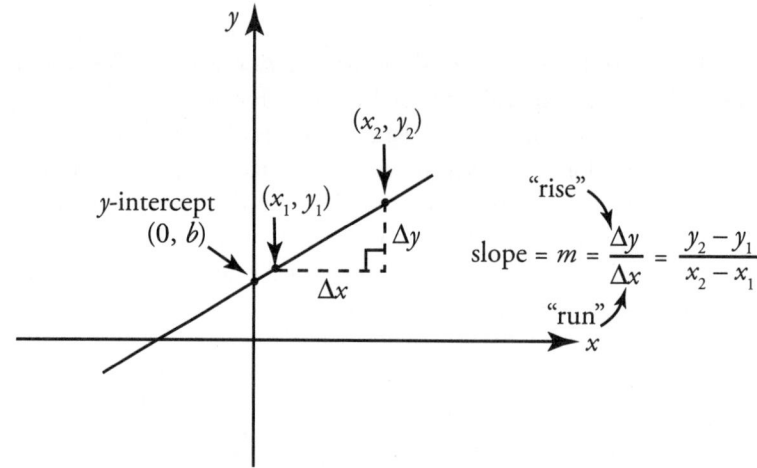

Perhaps the simplest way to write the equation of a line is in terms of its slope and the y-coordinate of the point where it crosses the y-axis. If the slope is m and the y-intercept is b, the equation of the line can be written in the form

$$y = mx + b$$

The only time this form doesn't work is when the line is vertical, since vertical lines have an undefined slope and such a line either never crosses the y-axis (no b) or else coincides with the y-axis. The equation of every vertical line is simply $x = a$, where a is the x-intercept.

Example 15-18:

a) Where does the line $y = 3x - 4$ cross the y-axis? the x-axis? What is its slope?

b) Find the equation of the line that has slope -2 and crosses the y-axis at the point $(0, 3)$.

c) Find the equation of the line that has slope 4 and crosses the y-axis at the origin.

d) A *linear* function is a function whose graph is a line. Let's say it's known that some quantity p is a linear function of x. If $p = 50$ when $x = 0$ and $p = 250$ when $x = 20$, find an equation for p in terms of x. Then use the equation to find the value of p when $x = 40$.

Solution:

a) The equation $y = 3x - 4$ matches the form $y = mx + b$ with $m = 3$ and $b = -4$. Therefore, this line has slope 3 and crosses the y-axis at the point $(0, -4)$. To find the x-intercept, we set y equal to 0 and solve for x: $0 = 3x - 4$ implies that $x = 4/3$. Therefore, this line crosses the x-axis at the point $(4/3, 0)$.

b) We're given $m = -2$ and $b = 3$, so the equation of the line is $y = -2x + 3$.

c) We're given $m = 4$ and $b = 0$, so the equation of the line is $y = 4x$.

d) Since p is a linear function of x, it must have the form $p = mx + b$ for some values of m and b. Because $p = 50$ when $x = 0$, we know that $b = 50$, so $p = mx + 50$. Now, since $p = 250$ when $x = 20$, we have $250 = 20m + 50$, so $m = 10$. Thus, $p = 10x + 50$. Finally, plugging in $x = 40$ into this formula, we find that the value of p when $x = 40$ is $(10)(40) + 50 = 450$.

Example 15-19: An insulated 50 cm^3 sample of water has an initial temperature of $T_i = 10°C$. If Q calories of heat are added to the sample, the temperature of the water will rise to T, where $T = kQ + T_i$. When the graph of T vs. Q is sketched (with Q measured along the horizontal axis), it's found that the point $(Q, T) = (200, 14)$ lies on the graph.

a) What is the value of k?

b) How much heat is required to bring the water to 20°C?

c) If $Q = 2200$ cal, what will be the value of T?

Solution:

a) The equation $T = kQ + T_i$ matches the form $y = mx + b$, so k is the slope of the line. To find the slope, we evaluate the *rise-over-run* expression—which in this case is $\Delta T / \Delta Q$—for two points on the line. Using $(Q_1, T_1) = (0, 10)$ and $(Q_2, T_2) = (200, 14)$, we find that

$$k = \text{slope} = \frac{\Delta T}{\Delta Q} = \frac{T_2 - T_1}{Q_2 - Q_1} = \frac{14 - 10}{200 - 0} = \frac{1}{50}$$

b) We set T equal to 20 and solve for Q:

$$T = kQ + T_i \Rightarrow T = \frac{1}{50}Q + 10 \Rightarrow 20 = \frac{1}{50}Q + 10 \Rightarrow Q = 500 \text{ (cal)}$$

c) Here we set $Q = 2200$ and evaluate T:

$$T = kQ + T_i \Rightarrow T = \frac{1}{50}Q + 10 \Rightarrow T = \frac{1}{50}(2200) + 10 = 44 + 10 = 54 \text{ (°C)}$$

(Technical note: The equation for the temperature of the water, $T = kQ + T_i$, is valid as long as no phase change occurs.)

Besides lines, there are a few other graphs and features you should be familiar with.

The equation $y = kx^2$, where $k \neq 0$, describes the basic **parabola**, one whose turning point (**vertex**) is at the origin. It has a U shape, and opens upward if k is positive and downward if k is negative. The graph of the related equation $y = k(x - a)^2$ is obtained from the basic parabola by shifting it horizontally so that its vertex is at the point $(a, 0)$. The graph of the equation $y = kx^2 + b$ is obtained from the basic parabola by shifting it vertically so that its vertex is at the point $(0, b)$. Finally, the graph of the equation $y = k(x - a)^2 + b$ is obtained from the basic parabola in two shifting steps: First, shift the basic parabola horizontally so that its vertex is at the point $(a, 0)$; next, shift this parabola vertically so that the vertex is at the point (a, b). These parabolas are illustrated below for positive a, b, k, and x:

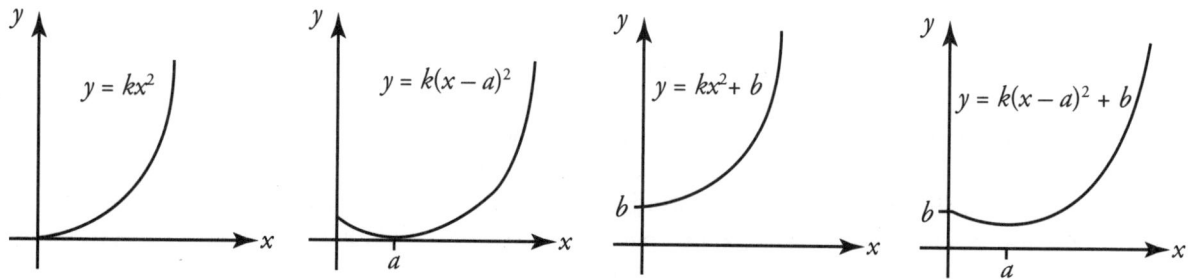

The equation $y = k/x$, where $k \neq 0$, describes a **hyperbola**. It is the graph of an inverse proportion (see Section 18.2). For small values of x, the values of y are large; and for large values of x, the values of y are small. Notice that the graph of a hyperbola approaches—but never touches—both the x- and y-axes. These lines are therefore called **asymptotes**.

The equation $y = k/x^2$, where $k \neq 0$, has a graph whose shape is similar to a hyperbola but it approaches its horizontal asymptote faster and vertical asymptote slower than a hyperbola does (because of the square in the denominator).

The graph of the equation $y = Ae^{-kx}$ (where k is positive) is an **exponential decay curve**. It intersects the y-axis at the point $(0, A)$, and, as x increases, the value of y decreases. Here, the x-axis is an asymptote.

The graph of the equation $y = A(1 - e^{-kx})$, where k is positive, contains the origin, and as x increases, the graph rises to approach the horizontal line $y = A$. This line is an asymptote.

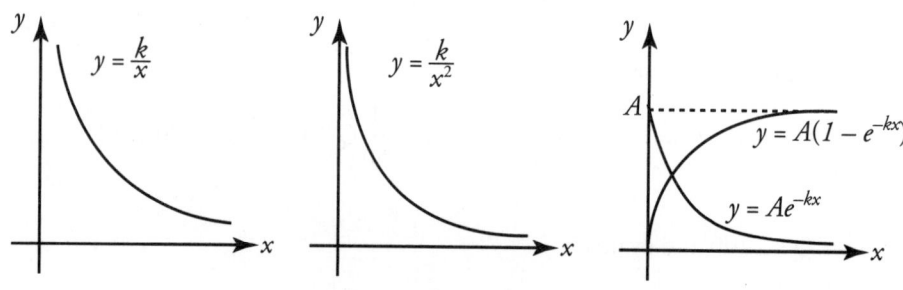

Chapter 16
Trigonometry

16.1 INTRODUCTION

Let me begin by saying that you will *not* need to know the countless identities that pervade this subject, equations you may have studied in high school like $\sin^2 \theta = (1 - \cos 2\theta)/2$. The MCAT requires only that you know the important basics. The term **trigonometry** literally means *triangle measurement*, and this is where the basics start.

Consider a *right* triangle; that is, a triangle with a 90° (right) angle. Let's call the triangle ABC and let C be the vertex of the right angle. Then sides AC and BC are called the **legs**, and side AB is called the **hypotenuse**. If the lengths of sides BC, AC, and AB are a, b, and c, respectively, then the *Pythagorean theorem* tells us that $a^2 + b^2$ must be equal to c^2.

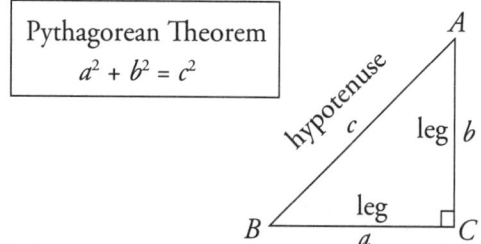

Three positive numbers a, b, and c that satisfy the Pythagorean theorem and can therefore be the lengths of the sides of a right triangle, are known as a **Pythagorean triple**. The most familiar of these is the triple 3, 4, 5. (It's easy to check that $3^2 + 4^2 = 5^2$.) The legs have lengths 3 and 4, and the hypotenuse (which is always the longest side of any right triangle) has length 5. Other examples of Pythagorean triples are 5, 12, 13 and 7, 24, 25, but the list is endless. An important and useful fact about Pythagorean triples is this: Any multiple of a Pythagorean triple is another Pythagorean triple. For example, since 3, 4, 5 is such a triple, so are 6, 8, 10 (obtained from 3, 4, 5 by multiplying the lengths by 2) and 9, 12, 15 (by multiplying by 3) and 1.5, 2, 2.5 (by multiplying by one-half).

Example 16-1:
   a)   Is 5, 6, 8 a Pythagorean triple?
   b)   If a, 16, 20 is a Pythagorean triple and $a < 20$, what is a?

Solution:
   a)   Since $5^2 + 6^2 = 25 + 36 = 61$ but $8^2 = 64$, the sum $5^2 + 6^2$ does *not* equal 8^2. Therefore, 5, 6, 8 is not a Pythagorean triple. No right triangle could have sides whose lengths are 5, 6, and 8.
   b)   Because $a < 20$, we know that a is not the length of the longest side of the triangle, so it's not the hypotenuse. The hypotenuse must be 20. Therefore, we want to solve the equation $a^2 + 16^2 = 20^2$. Since $16^2 = 256$ and $20^2 = 400$, we find that $a^2 = 400 - 256 = 144$, so $a = 12$. Notice that the Pythagorean triple 12, 16, 20 is just four times the triple 3, 4, 5.

We can also use a right triangle to make a crucial observation. Consider a magnified version of right triangle ABC. Each angle of the larger triangle (let's call it DBE) is equal to the corresponding angle in the smaller one. These triangles are said to be **similar**, and each side of the larger triangle is the *same* multiple of the corresponding side in the smaller triangle. For example, if leg BE is twice the length of leg BC, then leg DE is twice the length of leg AC, and hypotenuse DB is twice the length of hypotenuse AB. One of the consequences of this is that certain ratios of the lengths of the sides of the triangle are the same, regardless of the size of the triangle. For example, let's say that each side of triangle DBE is k times the corresponding side of triangle ABC, so BE = $k \cdot$ BC, DE = $k \cdot$ AC, and DB = $k \cdot$ AB. Now consider, for example, AC/AB, the ratio of leg AC to the hypotenuse AB. It will be equal to the ratio DE/DB, because

$$\frac{DE}{DB} = \frac{k \cdot AC}{k \cdot AB} = \frac{AC}{AB}$$

Similarly, we'll have

$$\frac{BE}{DB} = \frac{BC}{AB} \quad \text{and} \quad \frac{DE}{BE} = \frac{AC}{BC}$$

These three ratios are therefore uniquely determined by the *angles* of the triangle, regardless of the size of the triangle, and they're given special names: **sine**, **cosine**, and **tangent** (respectively).

Triangle DBE is a magnified version of triangle ABC, which means:

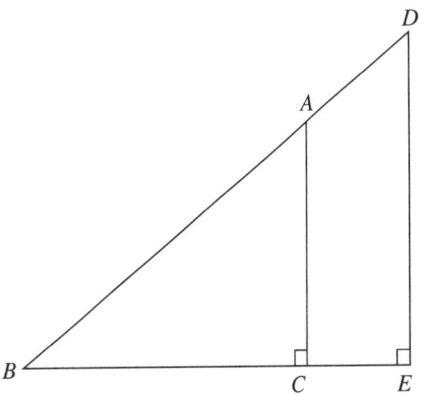

$$\frac{DE}{AC} = \frac{BE}{BC} = \frac{DB}{AB}$$

Therefore,

$$\frac{AC}{AB} = \frac{DE}{DB} \qquad \leftarrow \text{this ratio is the sine of angle B}$$

$$\frac{BC}{AB} = \frac{BE}{DB} \qquad \leftarrow \text{this ratio is the cosine of angle B}$$

$$\frac{AC}{BC} = \frac{DE}{BE} \qquad \leftarrow \text{this ratio is the tangent of angle B}$$

So, for an arbitrary acute angle θ in a right triangle, we have the following definitions:

sine of θ: $\qquad \sin\theta = \dfrac{\text{opp}}{\text{hyp}} = \dfrac{b}{c}$

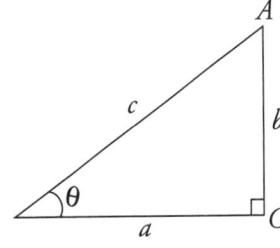

cosine of θ: $\qquad \cos\theta = \dfrac{\text{adj}}{\text{hyp}} = \dfrac{a}{c}$

tangent of θ: $\qquad \tan\theta = \dfrac{\text{opp}}{\text{adj}} = \dfrac{b}{a}$

The abbreviation *opp* stands for *opposite*, *adj* stands for *adjacent*, and *hyp* stands for *hypotenuse*. So, for example, the sine of an acute angle in a right triangle, opp/hyp, is equal to the length of the side opposite the angle divided by the length of the hypotenuse. Some people remember the definitions of the sine, co-sine, and tangent of an acute angle in a right triangle by this mnemonic:

SOH CAH TOA

where the letters stand for the following: $\underline{S}$ine = $\underline{O}$pp/$\underline{H}$yp, $\underline{C}$osine = $\underline{A}$dj/$\underline{H}$yp, $\underline{T}$angent = $\underline{O}$pp/$\underline{A}$dj.

Example 16-2: In a 3-4-5 right triangle ABC, let A be the smaller acute angle and let B be the larger acute angle.
  a) What are $\sin A$, $\cos A$, and $\tan A$?
  b) What are $\sin B$, $\cos B$, and $\tan B$?

Solution: Because A is the smaller acute angle, the side opposite A is the shorter leg (of length 3); there-fore, the side opposite the larger acute angle, B, has length 4.

  a) By definition, $\sin A = 3/5$, $\cos A = 4/5$, and $\tan A = 3/4$
  b) By definition, $\sin B = 4/5$, $\cos B = 3/5$, and $\tan B = 4/3$

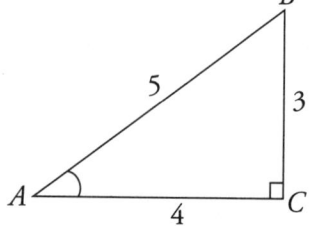

Example 16-3: In right triangle ABC, the right angle is at C. If $\sin A = 1/3$ and $AB = 6$, what are the lengths of the legs of the triangle?

Solution: The triangle is sketched to the right. By defini-tion, $\sin A = BC/AB$; from this equation, we immediately get $BC = AB \cdot \sin A = 6 \cdot (1/3) = 2$. Now, by the Pythagorean the-orem, $AC^2 + BC^2 = AB^2$, so $AC^2 = 6^2 - 2^2 = 32$, which gives $AC = \sqrt{32} = 4\sqrt{2}$.

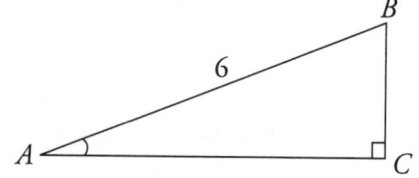

Example 16-4: In right triangle DEF, the right angle is at F. If $\tan E = 2$ and $EF = 2$, what's the length of the hypotenuse?

Solution: The triangle is sketched to the right. By definition, $\tan E = DF/EF$; from this equation, we get $DF = EF \cdot \tan E = 2 \cdot 2 = 4$. Now, by the Pythagorean theorem, $DF^2 + EF^2 = DE^2$, so $DE^2 = 4^2 + 2^2 = 20$, which gives $DE = \sqrt{20} = 2\sqrt{5}$.

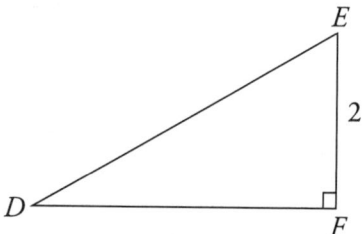

How would you find the sine of an angle whose measure is, say, 20°? Here's a way that only requires the definitions we've gone over so far, plus a protractor and a ruler:

Step 1: Draw a horizontal line segment, AC.
Step 2: Place a protractor so that its center is at the left end-
point (A) of the line segment drawn in Step 1.
Step 3: Draw a line from A through the 20° mark on the
protractor.
Step 4: Draw a line segment up from C that's perpendicular
to AC. Let B be the point where it intersects the line
drawn in Step 3.
Step 5: Use a ruler to measure the lengths of BC and AB.
Step 6: sin 20° = sin A = BC/AB

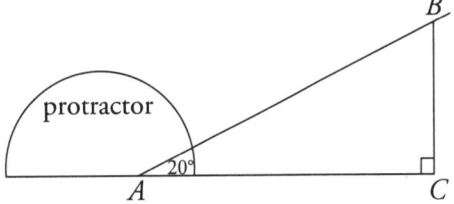

If you try this with a horizontal line segment AC whose length is 3 inches, you'll find that BC ≈ 1 1/16" and AB ≈ 3 3/16" , so

$$\sin A = \sin 20° \approx \frac{1\frac{1}{16}}{3\frac{3}{16}} = \frac{1}{3}$$

But what if you don't have a protractor and ruler? Then without some fancy (and time-consuming) math, it's going to be pretty tough. But the MCAT won't require you to know the sine of 20°. The MCAT will expect that you'll know the values of the sine, cosine, and tangent of angles that are multiples of 30° and 45° only.

If we take a square of side length 1 and cut it in half down a diagonal, we end up with a pair of isosceles right triangles.

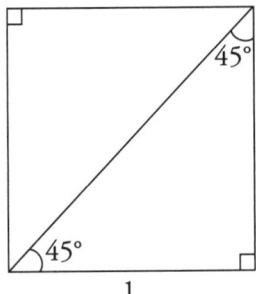 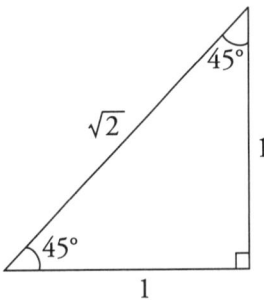

In each triangle, both acute angles are 45°. By the Pythagorean theorem, the hypotenuse has length

$$\sqrt{1^2 + 1^2} = \sqrt{2}$$

It's now easy to apply the definitions to find that

Memorize

$$\sin 45° = \frac{1}{\sqrt{2}} = \frac{\sqrt{2}}{2} \qquad \cos 45° = \frac{1}{\sqrt{2}} = \frac{\sqrt{2}}{2} \qquad \tan 45° = \frac{1}{1} = 1$$

If we take an equilateral triangle of side length 2 and cut it from a corner into two equal pieces, we end up with a pair of 30°-60° right triangles.

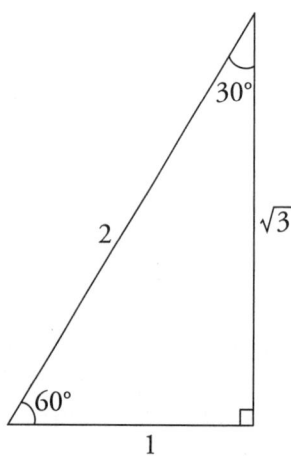

The shorter leg in each right triangle has length 1 (half the length of the hypotenuse), so by the Pythagorean theorem, the length of the longer leg is

$$\sqrt{2^2 - 1^2} = \sqrt{3}$$

It's now easy to apply the definitions to find that

Memorize

$$\sin 30° = \frac{1}{2} \qquad\qquad\qquad \sin 60° = \frac{\sqrt{3}}{2}$$

$$\cos 30° = \frac{\sqrt{3}}{2} \qquad\qquad\qquad \cos 60° = \frac{1}{2}$$

$$\tan 30° = \frac{1}{\sqrt{3}} = \frac{\sqrt{3}}{3} \qquad\qquad \tan 60° = \frac{\sqrt{3}}{1} = \sqrt{3}$$

Example 16-5: In right triangle *ABC*, the right angle is at *C* and angle *A* = 60°. If BC = 2, what are AB and AC?

Solution: The triangle is sketched to the right. By definition, sin *A* = BC/AB; from this equation, we immediately get

$$AB = \frac{BC}{\sin A} = \frac{2}{\sin 60°} = \frac{2}{\frac{1}{2}\sqrt{3}} = \frac{4\sqrt{3}}{3}$$

To find the other leg, AC, we now have several options. Here's one: Since cos *A* = AC/AB, we get

$$AC = AB \cdot \cos A = \frac{4\sqrt{3}}{3} \cdot \cos 60° = \frac{4\sqrt{3}}{3} \cdot \frac{1}{2} = \frac{2\sqrt{3}}{3}$$

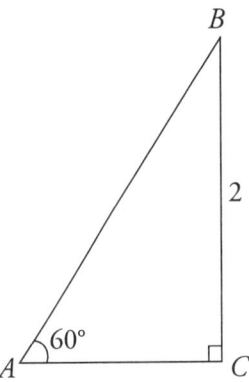

16.2 EXTENDING THE DEFINITIONS

In the preceding section, we gave the definitions of the trig functions sine, cosine, and tangent only for an *acute* angle (that is, an angle whose measure is between 0° and 90°) in a right triangle. However, for many important uses of trig, we won't want such a restriction. The purpose of this section is to extend the definitions of these trig functions to an angle of *any* measure.

Consider the usual *x-y* coordinate system and imagine a ray starting at the origin and lying along the positive *x*-axis. We can generate an angle, *θ*, of any size we want by rotating this ray about the origin. If we rotate it counterclockwise, we'll call the generated angle positive; if we rotate clockwise, we'll call it negative. To figure out the values of the trig functions of this angle, we choose any point P (other than the origin) on the terminal side of the angle—that is, on the final position of the rotated ray—and then drop a perpendicular from P to the *x*-axis. Let (*x*, *y*) denote the coordinates of the point P, and let *r* be the distance from the origin to P. The trig functions of *θ* are then defined in terms of *x*, *y*, and *r* as follows:

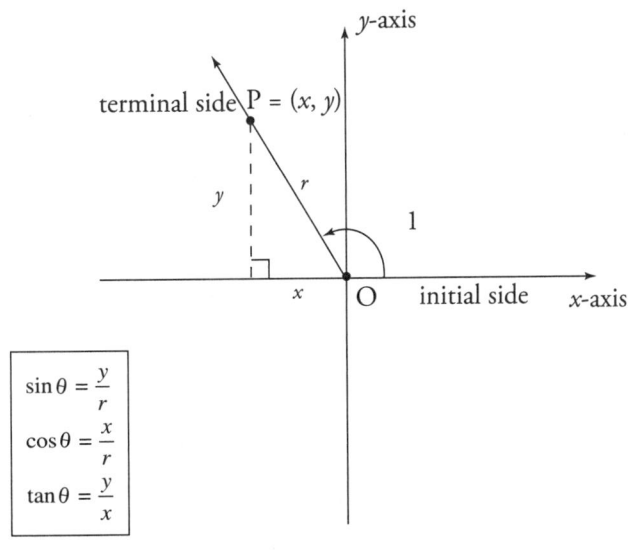

Notice that if θ is a positive, acute angle, then these definitions in terms of x, y, and r give the same values as those involving the lengths designated adjacent, opposite, and hypotenuse in a right triangle. The advantage of the definitions above is that they apply to *any* angle, not just to acute angles in right triangles.

The terminal side of the angle θ pictured above lies in Quadrant II, so we say the angle itself is in Quadrant II. So, for the point P, the x coordinate is negative and the y coordinate is positive. (The value of r is *always* positive.) Therefore, the value of $\sin \theta$ is positive, but the values of $\cos \theta$ and $\tan \theta$ are negative.

Similarly, if θ lies in Quadrant III, then both x and y will be negative, so $\tan \theta$ will be positive, but both $\sin \theta$ and $\cos \theta$ will be negative. If θ lies in Quadrant IV, then x is positive and y is negative, so $\cos \theta$ is positive, but $\sin \theta$ and $\tan \theta$ will be negative. If θ lies in Quadrant I, then $\sin \theta$, $\cos \theta$, and $\tan \theta$ will all be positive.

If θ lies on either the x- or y-axis, then either y or x will be zero. For example, if $\theta = 90°$, then θ lies on the positive y axis, so $x = 0$. In this case, we can see right away that $\cos \theta = \cos 90° = x/r = 0/r = 0$, $\sin 90° = y/r = y/y = 1$, and $\tan 90°$ is undefined (because we can't divide by 0). Any angle—like 90°, 180°, etc.—whose terminal side lies along either the x- or the y-axis is called a **quadrantal** angle.

Example 16-6: Find $\sin \theta$, $\cos \theta$, and $\tan \theta$ for each of the following angles:
- a) $\theta = 120°$
- b) $\theta = 180°$
- c) $\theta = 225°$
- d) $\theta = 330°$

Solution:

a) The figure below shows an angle of 120°. Since the right triangle that's formed by dropping a perpendicular to the x-axis is a 30°-60° right triangle, we know that we can take $x = -1$, $y = \sqrt{3}$, and $r = 2$. Therefore,

$$\sin 120° = \frac{y}{r} = \frac{\sqrt{3}}{2} ; \quad \cos 120° = \frac{x}{r} = \frac{-1}{2} = -\frac{1}{2} ;$$

$$\tan 120° = \frac{y}{x} = \frac{\sqrt{3}}{-1} = -\sqrt{3}$$

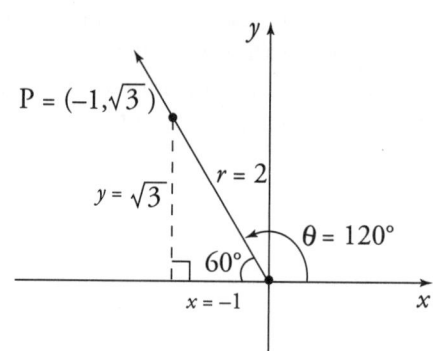

b) The figure below shows an angle of 180°. Here, no triangle is formed, but that doesn't matter. We simply choose a point P on the terminal side of the angle, say, P = (−1, 0). Since $x = -1$, $y = 0$, and $r = 1$, we have

$$\sin 180° = \frac{y}{r} = \frac{0}{1} = 0 ; \quad \cos 180° = \frac{x}{r} = \frac{-1}{1} = -1 ;$$

$$\tan 180° = \frac{y}{x} = \frac{0}{-1} = 0$$

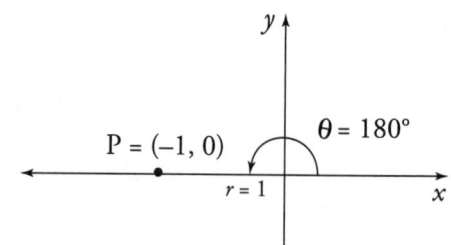

c)   The figure at the right shows an angle of 225°. Since the right triangle that's formed by dropping a perpendicular to the x-axis is a 45°-45° right triangle, we know that we can take $x = -1$, $y = -1$, and $r = \sqrt{2}$. Therefore,

$$\sin 225° = \frac{y}{r} = \frac{-1}{\sqrt{2}} = -\frac{\sqrt{2}}{2}; \quad \cos 225° = \frac{x}{r} = \frac{-1}{\sqrt{2}} = -\frac{\sqrt{2}}{2};$$

$$\tan 225° = \frac{y}{x} = \frac{-1}{-1} = 1$$

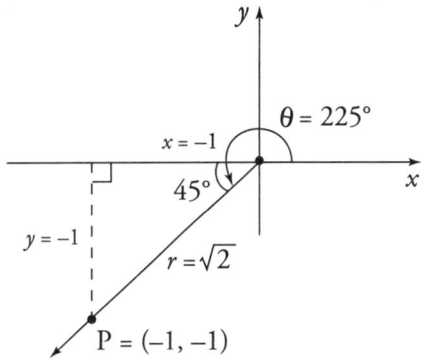

d)   The figure at the right shows an angle of 330°. Since the right triangle that's formed by dropping a perpendicular to the x-axis is a 30°-60° right triangle, we know that we can take $x = \sqrt{3}$, $y = -1$, and $r = 2$. Therefore,

$$\sin 330° = \frac{y}{r} = \frac{-1}{2} = -\frac{1}{2}; \quad \cos 330° = \frac{x}{r} = \frac{\sqrt{3}}{2};$$

$$\tan 330° = \frac{y}{x} = \frac{-1}{\sqrt{3}} = -\frac{\sqrt{3}}{3}$$

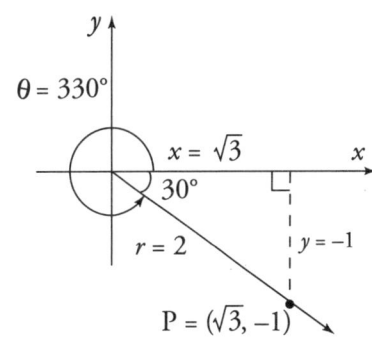

Example 16-7: Find $\sin \theta$, $\cos \theta$, and $\tan \theta$ for each of the following angles:

a) $\theta = 270°$
b) $\theta = 420°$
c) $\theta = -150°$

Solution:

a)   The figure below shows an angle of 270°. Here, no triangle is formed, but that doesn't matter. We simply choose a point P on the terminal side of the angle, say, P = (0, –1). Since $x = 0$, $y = -1$, and $r = 1$, we have

$$\sin 270° = \frac{y}{r} = \frac{-1}{1} = -1; \quad \cos 270° = \frac{x}{r} = \frac{0}{1} = 0;$$

$$\tan 270° = \frac{y}{x} = \frac{-1}{0} \text{ is undefined}$$

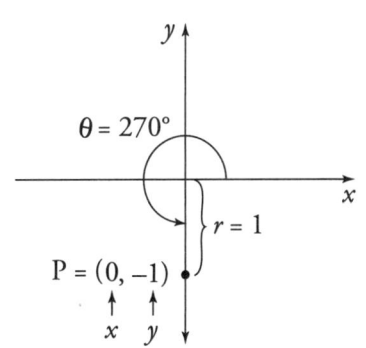

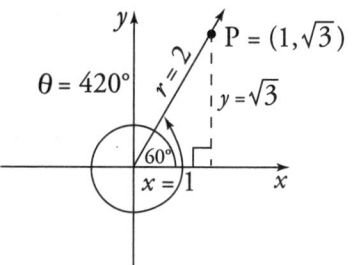

b) The figure at the right shows an angle of 420°. Notice that the angle is formed by making one complete revolution (360°) plus an additional 60°. Since the right triangle that's formed by dropping a perpendicular to the x-axis is a 30°-60° right triangle, we know that we can take $x = 1$, $y = \sqrt{3}$, and $r = 2$. Therefore,

$$\sin 420° = \frac{y}{r} = \frac{\sqrt{3}}{2}; \quad \cos 420° = \frac{x}{r} = \frac{1}{2};$$

$$\tan 420° = \frac{y}{x} = \frac{\sqrt{3}}{1} = \sqrt{3}$$

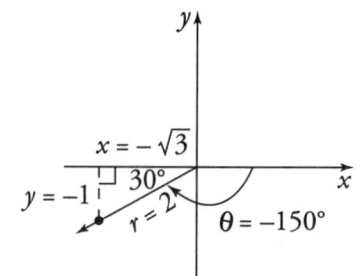

c) The figure at the right shows an angle of –150°. Because the angle is *negative*, we must perform a *clockwise* rotation (rather than a counterclockwise one) to generate it. Since the right triangle that's formed by dropping a perpendicular to the x-axis is a 30°-60° right triangle, we know that we can take $x = -\sqrt{3}$, $y = 1$, and $r = 2$. Therefore,

$$\sin (-150°) = \frac{y}{r} = \frac{-1}{2} = -\frac{1}{2}; \quad \cos (150°) = \frac{x}{r} = \frac{-\sqrt{3}}{2} = -\frac{\sqrt{3}}{2};$$

$$\tan (150°) = \frac{y}{x} = \frac{-1}{-\sqrt{3}} = \frac{\sqrt{3}}{3}$$

Example 16-8: If $\sin \theta = -\sqrt{3}/2$ and $\cos \theta = 1/2$, what is the value of $\tan \theta$?

Solution: One way to answer this question is to try to find θ. Since $\sin \theta$ is negative and $\cos \theta$ is positive, the terminal side of θ must lie in Quadrant IV. A quick sketch will show that $\theta = 300°$, where we take the point P = $(1, -\sqrt{3})$ on the terminal side. Therefore, $\tan \theta = \tan 300° = y/x = -\sqrt{3}$). Another solution is to notice the simple and important identity $\tan \theta = (\sin \theta)/(\cos \theta)$ [which is true because $y/x = \frac{y}{r} / \frac{x}{r}$], so $\tan \theta = -\frac{\sqrt{3}}{2} / \frac{1}{2} = -\sqrt{3}$.

16.2

16.3 RADIAN MEASURE

So far we've been measuring angles in degrees. By definition, a complete rotation (revolution) is equal to 360°, or, equivalently, a right angle has a measure of 90°. But why should a complete rotation be equal to 360 units? Why not, say, 100?

Actually, the ancient Babylonians started this system (called the sexagesimal system) basing angle measurement on the number 60. A degree can be split into 60 equal parts, each called a *minute*, and each minute can be further divided into 60 equal parts called *seconds*. (For example, an angle whose measure is 20° 30′ is 20.5° [the prime denotes minutes]; an angle whose measure is 20° 30′ 15″ is equal to 20° 30 1/4′ [the double prime denotes seconds].) One theory is that a complete revolution was called 360° because a year (one revolution around the Sun, although the Babylonians didn't know about the earth orbiting the sun) is approximately 360 days. So, each day of the year corresponded to 1 degree. Whatever the reason, it's clear that 360 was an arbitrary choice with no real mathematical basis. But what of an ancient civilization on another planet, whose year has 500 days? They might have started measuring angles in some other unit, *reegeds*, where a complete revolution is equal to 500 reegeds (500^∂), and a right angle would have a measure of 125^∂. If we were to communicate with this civilization, our angle measurements would be incompatible. What we'd want is a truly universal unit for measuring angles, one which is natural in the sense that an intelligent civilization on another planet will devise the same system (without regard to, say, how many days their year is). This universal unit for measuring angles is called the **radian**.

Draw a circle and construct an angle whose vertex is at the center such that when the sides of the angle hit the circle, the length of the subtended arc is equal to the radius of the circle. The measure of such an angle is, by definition, one radian.

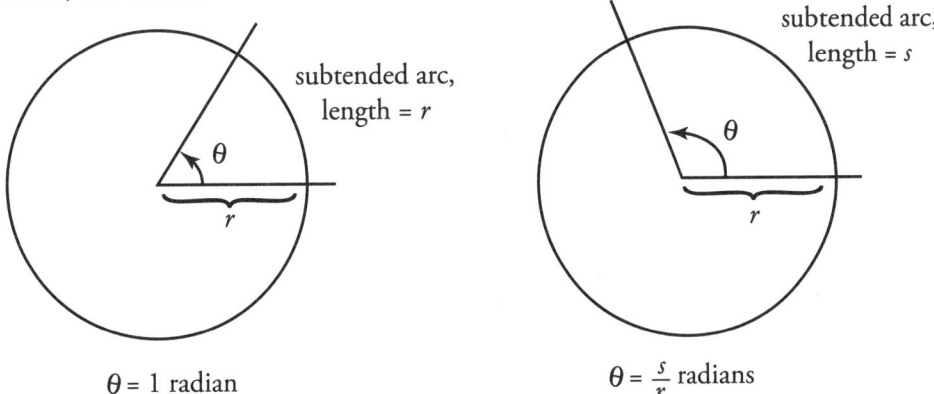

$$\theta = 1 \text{ radian} \qquad\qquad \theta = \frac{s}{r} \text{ radians}$$

For a general angle, if s is the length of the subtended arc and the radius of the circle is r, then the radian measure of the angle is the ratio s/r. The size of a radian is not arbitrary and it doesn't even depend on the size of the circle you draw. It's a natural unit for measuring angles.

So, what is the connection between degrees and radians? A complete rotation is 360°. What is a complete rotation in radians? The length of the arc subtended by a complete rotation is equal to the entire circumference of the circle, which is $s = 2\pi r$. Dividing this by r to get the radian measure, we see that a complete rotation is equal to 2π (or about 6.3) radians. (By the way, this means that 1 radian is equal to $360°/2\pi \approx 57.3°$.) So, the conversion between radians and degrees is this: 2π radians = 360°, or, if you prefer, divide both sides of this equation by 2 to get

$$\pi \text{ radians} = 180°$$

16.3

This way, every time you see an angle written in radians and there's a π there, just mentally substitute 180° for the π and you're back in degree mode. For example, an angle whose radian measure is $\pi/3$ is equal to 180°/3 = 60°. Since angles that are multiples of 30° and 45° are so common, it's useful to memorize the following conversions between degrees and radians:

$$30° \leftrightarrow \frac{\pi}{6} \qquad 45° \leftrightarrow \frac{\pi}{4} \qquad 60° \leftrightarrow \frac{\pi}{3} \qquad 90° \leftrightarrow \frac{\pi}{2} \qquad 180° \leftrightarrow \pi$$

When faced with an angle in radian measure like $2\pi/3$, just think of it as $2(\pi/3)$, which is $2(60°) = 120°$. Similarly, if you needed to convert an angle like 150° to radians, think of it this way: $150° = 5(30°) = 5(\pi/6)$. In general, here are the formulas for converting between degrees and radians:

$$(\theta \text{ in radians}) \times \frac{180°}{\pi} = (\theta \text{ in degrees}) \qquad (\theta \text{ in degrees}) \times \frac{\pi}{180°} = (\theta \text{ in radians})$$

Finally, notice that in the definition of radian measure, $\theta = s/r$, we're dividing a length by a length. Therefore, the ratio θ has no units. Radian measure is actually unitless. So, if you see an equation like $\theta = 2$ (no units), you'll know that the "2" means 2 radians. If you want to express the measure of an angle in degrees, you *must* put in the degree sign; $\theta = 2°$ means an angle of measure 2 degrees. But if you want to express the measure of an angle in radians, no unit is required; writing the word *radians* after the number is optional. In fact, because radian measure is unitless, we can interpret an expression like sin $\pi/6$ either as the sine of an angle whose measure is $\pi/6$ radians, or simply as the sine of the *number $\pi/6$*.

Example 16-9:
a)   Convert from radians to degrees: $3\pi/4$; $3\pi/2$; $4\pi/3$; 2
b)   Convert from degrees to radians: 180°; 210°; 225°; 300°
c)   Evaluate: sin $(\pi/6)$; cos π; tan $(7\pi/4)$
d)   Evaluate: sin $(-5\pi/6)$; cos $(2\pi/3)$; tan 3π

Solution:
a) $3\pi/4 = 3(\pi/4) = 3(45°) = 135°$; $3\pi/2 = 3(\pi/2) = 3(90°) = 270°$;
     $4\pi/3 = 4(\pi/3) = 4(60°) = 240°$; $2 \cdot (180°/\pi) = (360/\pi)° \approx 115°$
b) $180° = \pi$ radians; $210° = 7(30°) = 7(\pi/6) = 7\pi/6$ radians;
     $225° = 5(45°) = 5(\pi/4) = 5\pi/4$ radians; $300° = 5(60°) = 5(\pi/3) = 5\pi/3$ radians
c)   sin $(\pi/6)$ = sin 30° = 1/2; cos π = cos 180° = –1 (look back at Example 16-6b)
     tan $(7\pi/4)$ = tan $[7(45°)]$ = tan 315° = –1
d)   sin $(-5\pi/6)$ = sin $[-5(30°)]$ = sin $(-150°)$ = –1/2 (look back at Example 16-7c)
     cos $(2\pi/3)$ = cos $[2(60°)]$ = cos 120° = –1/2 (look back at Example 16-6a)
     tan 3π = tan $[3(180°)]$ = tan 540° = 0 (look back at Example 16-6b)

Chapter 17
Vectors

17.1 SCALARS AND VECTORS

Some quantities are completely described simply by a number (possibly with units). Examples include constants (like –2, 9.8, 0, and π) and physical quantities such as mass, length, time, speed, energy, power, density, volume, pressure, temperature, charge, potential, resistance, capacitance, frequency, sound level, and refractive index. All of these quantities are known as **scalars**, which you can think of as just a fancy word for *numbers*.

On the other hand, there are other quantities which are completely specified only when they're described by a number *and a direction*. Examples include displacement, velocity, acceleration, force, and electric and magnetic fields. All of these quantities are known as **vectors**. A vector is a quantity that involves *both* a number (its magnitude, which is a scalar) *and* a direction.

Here's an example: If I say the wind is blowing at 5 m/s, I'm giving the wind's *speed*, which is a *scalar*. However, if I say the wind is blowing at 5 m/s to the east, I'm giving the wind's *velocity*, which is a *vector*. (By the way, the distinction between speed and velocity is easy to remember: **s**peed is a **s**calar, while **v**elocity is a **v**ector.)

Since a vector is determined by a number and a direction, we represent a vector by an arrow. The length of the arrow we draw represents the number, and the direction of the arrow represents the direction of the vector. For example, the wind velocity *5 m/s to the east* might be drawn as an arrow like this:

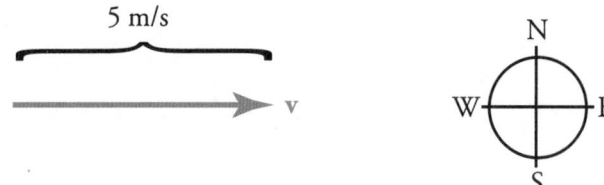

The symbol **v** is the name of this vector. In books, vector names are written as boldface letters; in handwritten work, we'd put a small arrow over the letter—like this: $\vec{v}$ or $\vec{v}$ —to signify that the quantity is a vector.

The number (or scalar) associated with a vector is its **magnitude**; it's the length of the arrow. For instance, for the vector **v** = 5 m/s to the east, the magnitude would be the scalar 5 m/s. Here's another example: If we push on something with a force of 10 N to the left,

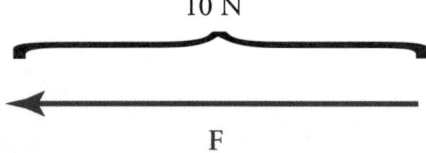

then the magnitude of the vector **F** = *10 N to the left* would be 10 N. Magnitudes are never negative.

There are two common ways to denote the magnitude of a vector. The first is to change the bold letter for the vector to an italic letter. Using this notation, the magnitude of the vector **v** would be written as *v*. As another example, the magnitude of the vector **F** would be written as *F*. The second way to denote the magnitude of a vector is to put absolute-value signs around the letter name of the vector. In this notation, the magnitude of the vector **v** would be written as $|\mathbf{v}|$ (or, in handwritten work, as $|\vec{v}|$) and the magnitude of the vector **F** would be $|\mathbf{F}|$.

17.2 OPERATIONS WITH VECTORS

For the MCAT, the three most important operations we perform with vectors are (1) addition of vectors, (2) subtraction of vectors, and (3) multiplication of a vector by a scalar.

Vector Addition

To add one vector to another vector, we use the **tip-to-tail method**. The **tail** of a vector is the starting point of the arrow, and the **tip** of a vector is the ending point (the sharp point of the arrow head):

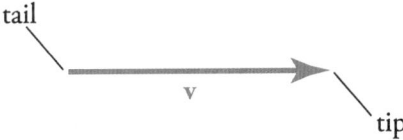

To add two vectors, we first put the tip of one of the vectors at the tail of the other one (tip-to-tail). Then we connect the exposed tail to the exposed tip; that vector is the sum of the vectors. The following figure shows this process for adding the vectors **A** and **B** to get their sum, **A + B**:

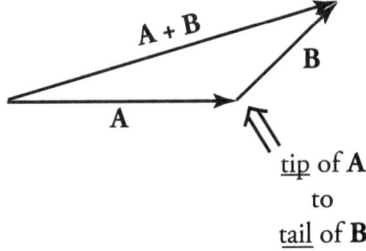

We could have put the tip of **B** at the tail of **A**, and the answer would have been the same:

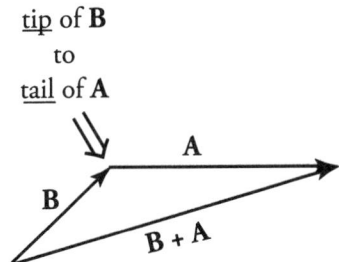

We can see from these two figures that the vector **A + B** has the same length *and* the same direction as the vector **B + A**. Therefore, the vectors are the same: **A + B = B + A**. We say that vectors obey the *commutative law for addition*; this means we can add them in either order, and the result is the same. (Actually, vectors *automatically* obey the commutative law for addition, by definition; that is, if **A** and **B** are vectors, then **A + B** will always be the same as **B + A**. There actually are quantities that are specified by a number and a direction but which do not obey the law **A + B = B + A**. Because of this failure, these quantities are not called vectors. However, you won't have to worry about such peculiar quantities for the MCAT.)

Vector Subtraction

To subtract one vector from another vector, we use the familiar *scalar* equation $a - b = a + (-b)$ as motivation. That is, for any two vectors **A** and **B**, we say that **A** − **B** is equal to **A** + (−**B**). So, we first have to answer the question: Given a vector **B**, how do we form the vector −**B**? By definition, the vector −**B** has the same magnitude as **B** but the opposite direction:

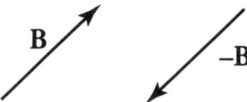

Therefore, to form the vector difference **A** − **B**, we just add −**B** to **A**:

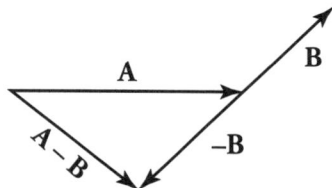

The following figure shows how to form the vector difference **B** − **A**, which is **B** + (−**A**):

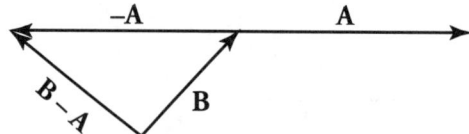

Notice that **B** − **A** is *not* the same as **A** − **B**, because their directions are not the same. That is, in general, **B** − **A** ≠ **A** − **B**; vector *subtraction* is generally *not* commutative. In fact, **B** − **A** will always be the *opposite* of **A** − **B** (same magnitude, opposite direction): **B** − **A** = −(**A** − **B**).

Another procedure you can use to subtract the vectors **A** and **B** is to put the tail of **A** at the tail of **B**, then connect the tips. (Vector *addition* uses the *tip*-to-tail method; vector *subtraction* (by this alternate procedure) uses the *tail*-to-tail method.) If you draw the resulting vector from the tip of **B** to the tip of **A**, you've constructed the vector **A** − **B**. On the other hand, if you draw the resulting vector from the tip of **A** to the tip of **B**, you've drawn the vector **B** − **A**.

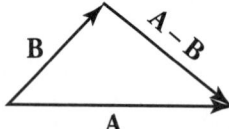 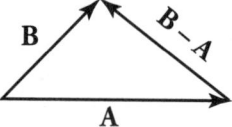

Notice that the figure on the left also illustrates the tip-to-tail vector addition **B** + (**A** − **B**) = **A**, while the figure on the right illustrates the tip-to-tail vector addition **A** + (**B** − **A**) = **B**.

Scalar Multiplication

To multiply a vector by a scalar, we consider three cases: that is, whether the scalar is positive, negative, or zero.

If k is a positive scalar, then $k\mathbf{A}$, the product of k and some vector $\mathbf{A}$, is a vector whose magnitude is k times the magnitude of $\mathbf{A}$ and whose direction is the same as that of $\mathbf{A}$. In short, multiplying a vector by a positive scalar k just changes the magnitude by a factor of k (but leaves the direction of the vector unchanged). If k is less than 1, the scalar multiple $k\mathbf{A}$ is shorter than $\mathbf{A}$; if k is greater than 1, then $k\mathbf{A}$ is longer than $\mathbf{A}$.

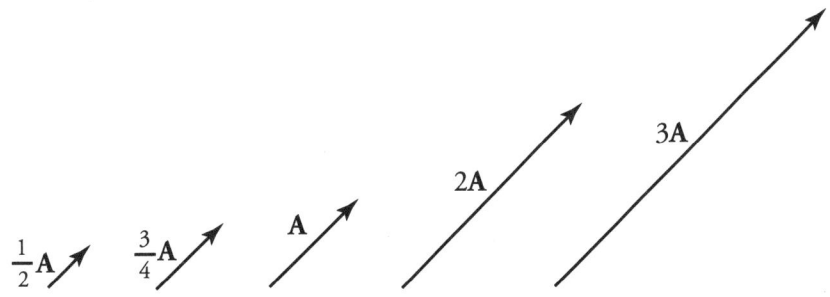

If k is a negative scalar, then $k\mathbf{A}$, the product of k and some vector $\mathbf{A}$, is a vector whose magnitude is the *absolute value* of k times the magnitude of $\mathbf{A}$ and whose direction is *opposite* the direction of $\mathbf{A}$. In short, multiplying a vector by a negative scalar k changes the magnitude by a factor of $|k|$ and reverses the direction of the vector.

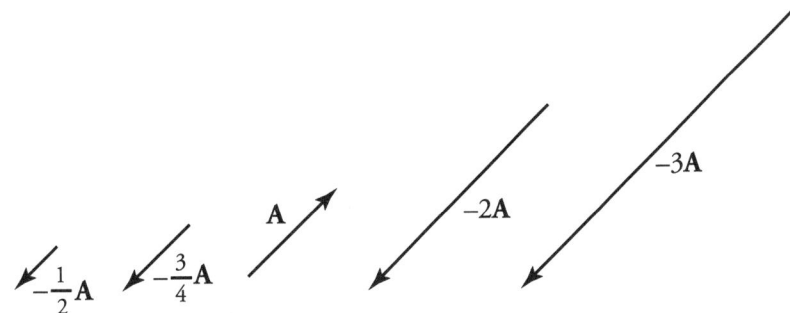

If k is zero, then the product $k\mathbf{A}$ gives **0**, the **zero vector**. This unique vector has magnitude 0 and has no direction. Rather than being pictured as an arrow, the zero vector is simply pictured as a dot.

$$\mathbf{A}\nearrow \quad \bullet\, 0\mathbf{A} = 0$$

Example 17-1: Consider the vectors **A**, **B**, and **C** shown below:

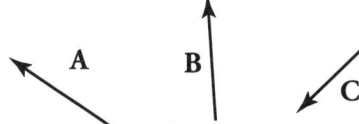

Construct each of the following vectors:

a)   **A + B**

b)   **A − 2C**

c) $\frac{1}{2}$**A − B + 3C**

Solution:

a)   Using the tip-to-tail method for vector addition gives

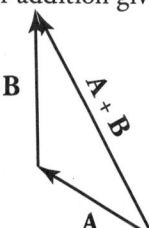

b)   Since **A − 2C = A + (−2C)**, we first multiply **C** by −2, then add the result to **A**:

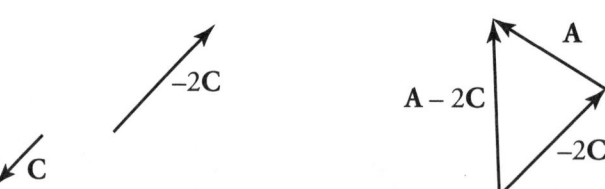

c)   We multiply **A** by 1/2, then **B** by −1, then **C** by 3, and add the three results:

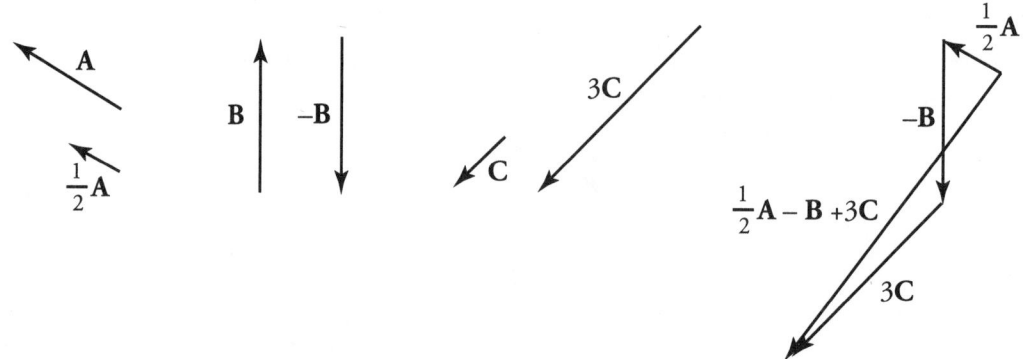

Example 17-2: Consider the vectors **A**, **B**, and **C** shown below:

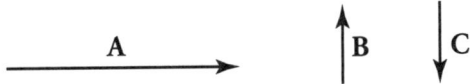

Construct each of the following vectors:

a) −**A** + **B**;
b) **B** + **C**;
c) **A** + 2**B**

Solution:

a) Multiplying **A** by −1 then using the tip-to-tail method to add the result to **B**, we get

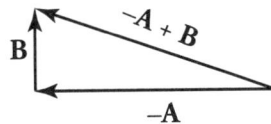

b) Since **C** has the same length as **B** but the opposite direction, **C** is equal to −**B**. So, adding **B** + **C** gives us **B** + (−**B**), which is **0**, the zero vector. You can also see that the sum of **B** and **C** will be **0** using the tip-to-tail method for vector addition: If we put the tip of **B** at the tail of **C**, then the tail of **B** *coincides* with the tip of **C**, so the vector sum is **0**.

c) Multiplying **B** by 2 then using the tip-to-tail method to add the result to **A**, we get

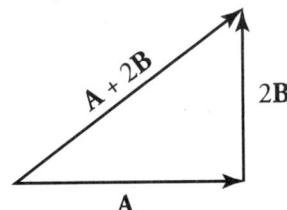

Example 17-3: Add these four vectors:

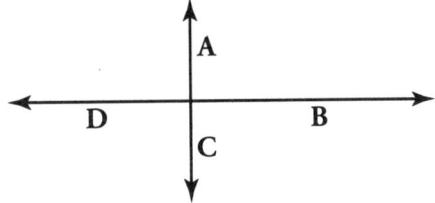

Solution: The vectors **A** and **C** have equal magnitudes but opposite directions, so **A** + **C** is **0**; that is, **A** and **C** cancel each other out. Now, since **D** points in the direction opposite to **B**, if we place the tail of **D** at the tip of **B**, then connect the tail of **B** to the tip of **D**, we get **B** + **D**, which is a vector in the same direction as **B**, but much shorter. This vector is **B** + **D**, which is also the sum **A** + **B** + **C** + **D** (since **A** + **C** = **0**):

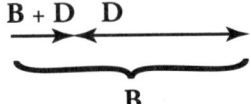

17.3 VECTOR PROJECTIONS AND COMPONENTS

In the preceding section, we performed the basic vector operations geometrically. In this section, we'll see how we can perform these operations with algebra and trig.

Let's imagine a vector **A** in a standard *x-y* coordinate system, with the tail of **A** at the origin. We construct perpendicular segments from the tip of **A** to the *x*-axis and to the *y*-axis. The resulting **vector projections** of **A** are denoted by A_x and A_y; the vector A_x is the horizontal projection of **A**, and A_y is the vertical projection. Notice that $A = A_x + A_y$. Therefore, *any vector **A** in the x-y plane can be written as the sum of a horizontal vector and a vertical vector (namely, its horizontal and vertical projections).*

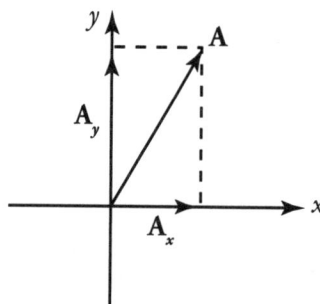

We now want to find a way to write A_x and A_y algebraically. Since any vector is specified by giving its magnitude and its direction, we need an algebraic way of describing the directions of these vectors. We do this by constructing two special vectors, one of which points in the horizontal direction, the other in the vertical direction. These two vectors are called **i** and **j**, and each has length 1:[1]

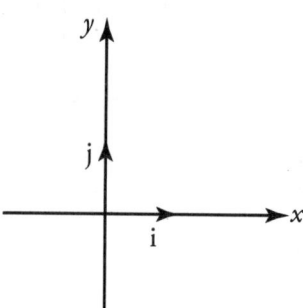

Any horizontal vector is some multiple of **i** ($A_x = A_x\mathbf{i}$), and any vertical vector is some multiple of **j** ($A_y = A_y\mathbf{j}$). Therefore, *any vector **A** in the x-y plane can be written as the sum of a multiple of **i** plus a multiple of **j**:*

$$A = A_x\mathbf{i} + A_y\mathbf{j}$$

These multiples, A_x and A_y, are called the **components** of **A**. Notice that projections are vectors, while components are scalars.

---

[1] While you are extremely unlikely to encounter this **i, j** notation on the MCAT, we include it here to simplify the discussion of algebraic decomposition of vectors. It's a useful tool.

For example, the horizontal vector of magnitude 3 that points to the right is 3**i**, and the horizontal vector of magnitude 3 that points to the left is 3(−**i**) or −3**i**. The vertical vector of magnitude 4 that points upward is 4**j**, and the vertical vector of magnitude 4 that points downward is 4(−**j**) or −4**j**. For the vector **A** = −3**i** + 4**j**, we would say that its horizontal projection is −3**i** and its horizontal component is −3; similarly, its vertical projection is 4**j** and its vertical component is 4.

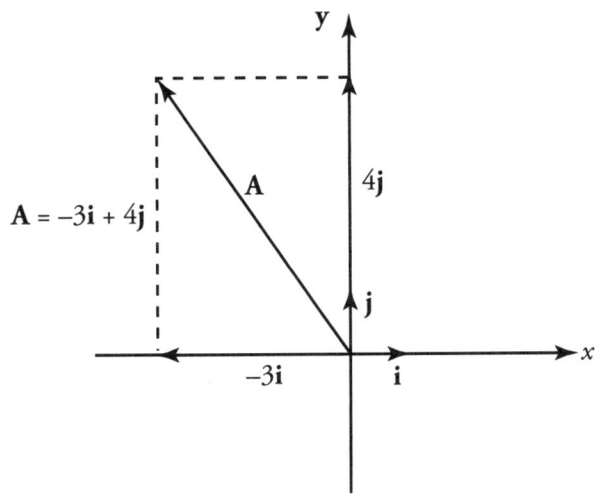

The great advantage of writing vectors algebraically is that it gives us the ability to perform vector operations quickly and precisely without having to draw the vectors (and using such procedures as the tip-to-tail method).

Magnitude

The magnitude of a vector can be found from its horizontal and vertical components using the Pythagorean theorem:

$$A = \sqrt{(A_x)^2 + (A_y)^2}$$

For example, the magnitude of the vector **A** = −3**i** + 4**j** is $A = \sqrt{(-3)^2 + 4^2} = 5$.

Direction

The direction of a vector can be described by giving the angle, θ, which the vector makes with the positive *x*-axis. Since the components of a vector **A** are given by the formulas

$$A_x = A\cos\theta$$

$$A_y = A\sin\theta$$

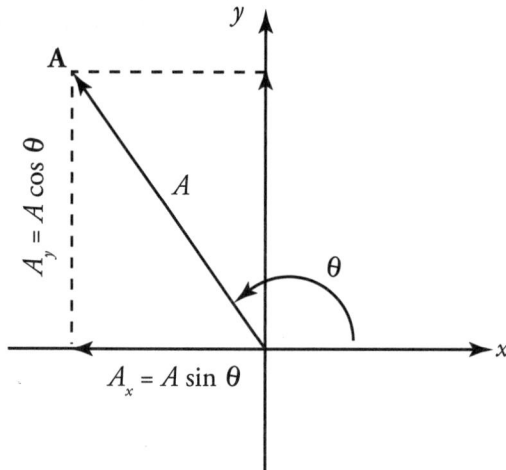

we see that

$$\frac{A_y}{A_x} = \frac{A\sin\theta}{A\cos\theta} = \tan\theta \;\rightarrow\; \theta = \tan^{-1}\frac{A_y}{A_x}$$

Vector Addition and Subtraction

The operations of addition and subtraction of vectors is made especially easy by the use of components. To add the vector $\mathbf{A} = A_x\mathbf{i} + A_y\mathbf{j}$ to the vector $\mathbf{B} = B_x\mathbf{i} + B_y\mathbf{j}$, we simply add the horizontal components and add the vertical components; and to subtract the vectors, we just subtract their components:

$$\mathbf{A} + \mathbf{B} = (A_x + B_x)\mathbf{i} + (A_y + B_y)\mathbf{j}$$
$$\mathbf{A} - \mathbf{B} = (A_x - B_x)\mathbf{i} + (A_y - B_y)\mathbf{j}$$

Scalar Multiplication

To multiply a vector by a scalar, just multiply each component by the scalar:

$$k\mathbf{A} = (kA_x)\mathbf{i} + (kA_y)\mathbf{j}$$

Example 17-4: Let **A** = –22**i** + 16**j**, **B** = 30**j**, and **C** = –10**i** – 10**j**. Find each of the following vectors:

a) **A** + **B**

b) **A** – 2**C**

c) $\dfrac{1}{2}$**A** – **B** + 3**C**

Solution:
a) **A** + **B** = (–22 + 0)**i** + (16 + 30)**j** = –22**i** + 46**j**

b) Since 2**C** = 2(–10**i** – 10**j**) = –20**i** – 20**j**, we get:

   A – 2**C** = [–22 – (–20)]**i** + [16 – (–20)]**j** = –2**i** + 36**j**

c) Since $\dfrac{1}{2}$**A** = $\dfrac{1}{2}$(–22)**i** + $\dfrac{1}{2}$(16)**j** = –11**i** + 8**j** and 3**C** = 3(–10**i** – 10**j**) = –30**i** – 30**j**, we find that

   $\dfrac{1}{2}$**A** – **B** + 3**C** = (–11 – 0 – 30)**i** + (8 – 30 – 30)**j** = –41**i** – 52**j**

Compare this example (and its results) with Example 17-1.

Example 17-5: What's the magnitude and direction of the vector **A** = 3**i** – 3**j**?

Solution: If we draw the vector starting at the origin, then

the vector points down into Quadrant IV. Its magnitude is

$A = \sqrt{3^2 + (-3)^2} = 3\sqrt{2}$, and its direction is given by

$\theta = \tan^{-1}\dfrac{A_y}{A_x} = \tan^{-1}(\dfrac{-3}{3}) = \tan^{-1}(-1) = 315°$ or $-45°$

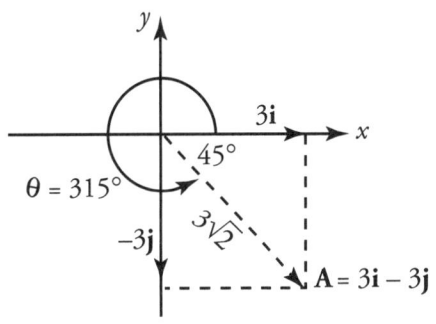

Example 17-6: Let **A** be the vector of magnitude 6 that makes an angle of 150° with the positive *x*-axis. Sketch this vector, determine its components, and write **A** in terms of **i** and **j**.

Solution: The figure at the right is a sketch of this vector.

Its components are

$$A_x = A\cos\theta = 6\cos 150° = 6(-\dfrac{\sqrt{3}}{2}) = -3\sqrt{3}$$

$$A_y = A\sin\theta = 6\sin 150° = 6(\dfrac{1}{2}) = 3$$

Therefore, since for any vector **A** we have **A** = A_x**i** + A_y**j**, we can write

$$\mathbf{A} = -3\sqrt{3}\mathbf{i} + 3\mathbf{j}$$

Example 17-7: The figure below shows a vector **W** of magnitude 100 and its projections, **W**$_1$ and **W**$_2$, onto two mutually perpendicular directions, such that **W** = **W**$_1$ + **W**$_2$. Find the magnitudes of **W**$_1$ and **W**$_2$.

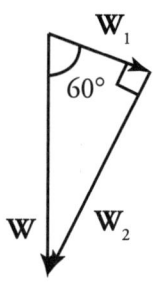

Solution: By definition of the sine and cosine, we have

$$W_1 = W\cos\theta = 100\cos 60° = 100(\frac{1}{2}) = 50$$

$$W_2 = W\sin\theta = 100\sin 60° = 100(\frac{\sqrt{3}}{2}) = 50\sqrt{3}$$

Chapter 18
Proportions

The concept of proportionality is fundamental to analyzing the behavior of many physical phenomena and is a common topic for MCAT questions.

18.1 DIRECT PROPORTIONS

If one quantity is always equal to a constant times another quantity, we say that the two quantities are **proportional** (or **directly** and **linearly proportional**, if emphasis is desired). For example, if k is some nonzero constant and the equation $A = kB$ is always true, then A and B are proportional, and k is called the **proportionality constant**. We express this fact mathematically by using this symbol: $\propto$, which means *is proportional to*. So, if $A = kB$, we'd write $A \propto B$. Of course, if $A = kB$, then $B = (1/k)A$, so we could also say that $B \propto A$.

Here are a few examples:

Example 18-1: The circumference of a circle is equal to π times the diameter: $C = \pi d$. Therefore, $C \propto d$.

Example 18-2: The gravitational potential energy of an object of weight w can be written as $PE = wh$, where h is the altitude of the object (if it's much smaller than the radius of the earth). Therefore, $PE \propto h$.

Example 18-3: The force exerted on a particle of charge q moving with speed v through a magnetic field of magnitude B is $F = qvB$, if the velocity **v** is perpendicular to **B**. Therefore, $F \propto v$.

The most important fact about direct proportions is this:

> *If $A \propto B$, and B is multiplied by a factor of b, then A will also be multiplied by a factor of b.*

After all, if $A = kB$, then $bA = k(bB)$.

Example 18-4: Since the circumference of a circle is proportional to its diameter, $C \propto d$, then, if the diameter is doubled, so is the circumference. If the diameter is cut in half, so is the circumference. If the diameter is tripled, so is the circumference.

Example 18-5: Since the gravitational potential energy of an object of weight w is proportional to its altitude, $PE \propto h$, then if the altitude is doubled, so is the potential energy. If the altitude is quadrupled, so is the potential energy. If the altitude is divided by 3 (which is the same as saying it's multiplied by 1/3), then the potential energy will also decrease by a factor of 3.

Example 18-6: Since the force exerted on a particle of charge q moving with speed v perpendicular to a magnetic field of magnitude B is $F = qvB$, we know that $F \propto v$. If the particle's speed is decreased by a factor of 2, the force F it feels will also be decreased by a factor of 2. If the speed is increased by a factor of 5, the force F will also increase by a factor of 5.

It's important to notice that the actual numerical value of the proportionality constant was irrelevant in the statements made above. For example, the fact that π is the proportionality constant in the equation $C = \pi d$ did not affect the conclusions made above. If C and d were some other quantities and C happened to always be equal to $(17,000)d$, we'd still say $C \propto d$, and all the conclusions made in Example 18-4 above would still be correct.

Graphically, linear proportions are easy to spot. If the horizontal and vertical axes are labeled linearly (as they usually are), then *the graph of a linear proportion is a straight line through the origin.* Be careful not to make the common mistake of thinking that any straight line is the graph of a proportion. If the line doesn't go through the origin, then it's *not* the graph of a proportion.

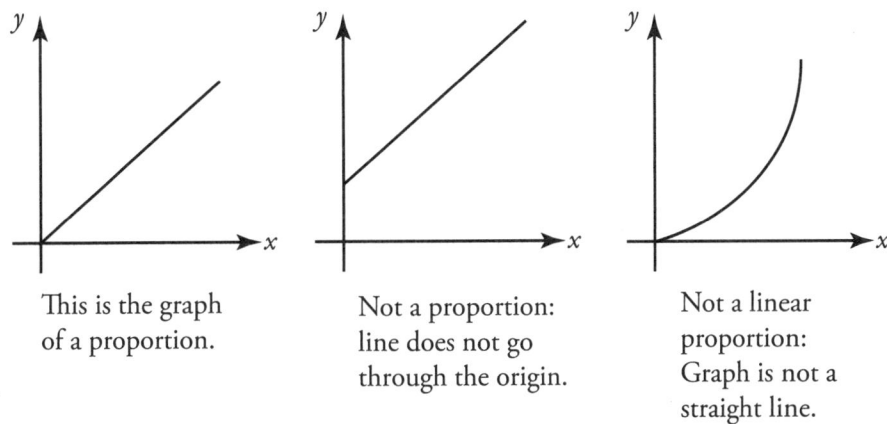

This is the graph of a proportion.

Not a proportion: line does not go through the origin.

Not a linear proportion: Graph is not a straight line.

The examples we've seen so far have been the equations $C = \pi d$, $PE = wh$, and $F = qvB$. Notice that in all of these equations, all the variables are present to the first power. But what about an equation like this: $KE = \frac{1}{2}mv^2$? This equation gives the kinetic energy of an object of mass m moving with speed v. So, if m is constant, KE is proportional to v^2. Now, what if v were multiplied by, say, a factor of 3, what would happen to KE? Because $KE \propto v^2$, if v increases by a factor of 3, then KE will increase by a factor of 3^2, which is 9. (By the way, this does not mean that if we graph KE versus v, we'll get a straight line through the origin. KE is not proportional to v; it's proportional to v^2. If we were to graph KE vs. v^2, *then* we'd get a straight line through the origin.) Here's another example using the same proportion, $KE \propto v^2$: If v were decreased by a factor of 2, then KE would decrease by a factor of $2^2 = 4$.

Here are a few more examples:

Example 18-7: The volume of a sphere of radius r is given by the equation $V = \frac{4}{3}\pi r^3$. Therefore, the volume is proportional to the radius cubed: $V \propto r^3$. So, for example, if r were doubled, then V would increase by a factor of $2^3 = 8$. If r were decreased by a factor of 3, then V would decrease by a factor of $3^3 = 27$.

Example 18-8: Consider an object starting from rest and accelerating at a constant rate of a in a straight line. Let the distance it travels be x and its final velocity be v. Then it's known that $x = v^2/2a$, which means x is proportional to v squared: $x \propto v^2$. If v were quadrupled, then x would increase by a factor of $4^2 = 16$. If v were reduced by a factor of 5, then x would be reduced by a factor of $5^2 = 25$. Now, how about this: What if x were increased by a factor of 9, what would happen to v? Since x is proportional to v^2, if x increases by a factor of 9, then v^2 also increases by a factor of 9; this means that v increases by a factor of 3.

Example 18-9: The intensity of energy radiated by an object of absolute temperature T is given by the formula $I = \sigma T^4$, where σ is a constant. Therefore, $I \propto T^4$. If T were increased by a factor of 3, then I would increase by a factor of $3^4 = 81$. In order to reduce I to 1/16 its original value, the temperature T would have to be reduced by a factor of 2, since $\dfrac{1}{16} = (\dfrac{1}{2})^4$.

18.2 INVERSE PROPORTIONS

If one quantity is always equal to a nonzero constant *divided* by another quantity (that is, if $A = k/B$, where k is some constant), we say that the two quantities are **inversely proportional**. Here are two equivalent ways of saying this:

(i)   If the product of two quantities is a constant ($AB = k$), then the quantities are inversely proportional.

(ii) If A is proportional to $1/B$ [that is, if $A = k(1/B)$], then A and B are inversely proportional.

In fact, we'll use this final description to symbolize an inverse proportion. That is, if A is inversely proportional to B, then we'll write $A \propto 1/B$. (There's no commonly accepted single symbol for *inversely proportional to*.) Of course, if $A = k/B$, then $B = k/A$, so we could also say that $B \propto 1/A$.

Here are a few examples:

Example 18-10: The electric potential, ϕ, at a distance r from a point charge q is given by the equation $\phi = kq/r$, where k is a constant. Therefore, ϕ is inversely proportional to r. $\phi \propto 1/r$.

Example 18-11: The pressure P and volume V of a sample containing n moles of an ideal gas at a fixed temperature T is given by the equation $PV = nRT$, where R is a constant. Therefore, the pressure is inversely proportional to the volume: $P \propto 1/V$.

Example 18-12: For electromagnetic waves traveling through space, the wavelength λ and frequency f are related by the equation $\lambda f = c$, where c is the speed of light (a universal constant). Therefore, wavelength is inversely proportional to frequency: $\lambda \propto 1/f$.

The most important fact about inverse proportions is this:

If $A \propto 1/B$, and B is multiplied by a factor of b, then A will be multiplied by a factor of $1/b$.

After all, if $A = k/B$, then $(1/b)A = k/(bB)$. Intuitively, if one quantity is *increased* by a factor of b, the other quantity will *decrease* by the same factor, and vice versa.

Example 18-13: Since the electric potential is inversely proportional to the distance from the source charge, $\phi \propto 1/r$, then, if the distance is doubled, the potential is cut in half. If the distance is cut in half, the potential is doubled. If the distance is tripled, the potential is multiplied by 1/3.

Example 18-14: Since the pressure of an ideal gas at constant temperature is inversely proportional to the volume, $P \propto 1/V$, then if the volume is doubled, the pressure is reduced by a factor of 2. If the volume is quadrupled, the pressure is reduced by a factor of 4. If the volume is divided by 3 (which is the same as saying it's multiplied by 1/3), then the pressure will increase by a factor of 3.

Example 18-15: Because for electromagnetic waves traveling through space, the wavelength is inversely proportional to frequency, $\lambda \propto 1/f$, if f is increased by a factor of 10, λ will decrease by a factor of 10. If the frequency is decreased by a factor of 2, the wavelength will increase by a factor of 2.

The graph of an inverse proportion is a *hyperbola*. In the graph below, $xy = k$, so x and y are inversely proportional to each other.

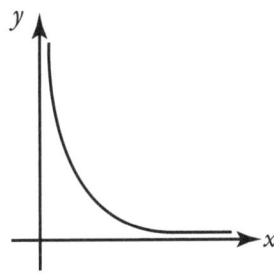

This is the graph of
an inverse proportion.

The examples we've seen so far have been where one quantity is inversely proportional to the first power of another quantity. But what about an equation like this:

$$F = G\frac{Mm}{r^2}$$

This equation gives the gravitational force between two objects of masses M and m separated by a distance r. (G is the universal gravitational constant.) So, if M and m are constant, F is inversely proportional to r^2. Now, what if r were increased by, say, a factor of 3, what would happen to F? Because $F \propto 1/r^2$, if r increases by a factor of 3, then F will decrease by a factor of 3^2, which is 9. Here's another example using the same proportion, $F \propto 1/r^2$: If r were decreased by a factor of 2, then F would increase by a factor of $2^2 = 4$.

Example 18-16: The electrostatic force between two charges Q and q separated by a distance r is given by the equation $F = kQq/r^2$, where k is a constant. Therefore, the electrostatic force is inversely proportional to the distance squared: $F \propto 1/r^2$. So, for example, if r were doubled, then F would decrease by a factor of $2^2 = 4$. If r were decreased by a factor of 3, then F would increase by a factor of $3^2 = 9$.

Example 18-17: The frequency of a simple harmonic oscillator consisting of a block of mass m attached to a spring of force constant k is given by the formula $f = 1/2\pi\sqrt{k/m}$. Therefore, the frequency is inversely proportional to the square root of the block's mass: $f \propto 1/\sqrt{m}$. So, if m were multiplied by 4, f would be multiplied by 1/2, since $1/\sqrt{4} = 1/2$. If m were increased by a factor of 36, then f would decrease by a factor of 6. If we wanted f to increase by a factor of 3, we'd have to decrease m by a factor of 9.

Example 18-18: An object starting from rest travels a distance given by $d = at^2/2$ in a time t if it undergoes a constant acceleration a.
   a)   If t is doubled, then what happens to d?
   b)   If t is tripled, what happens to d?

Solution:
   a)   Since $d \propto t^2$, if t increases by a factor of 2, then d increases by a factor of $2^2 = 4$.
   b)   Since $d \propto t^2$, if t increases by a factor of 3, then d increases by a factor of 9.

Example 18-19: The kinetic energy of an object of mass m traveling with speed v is given by the formula $KE = mv^2/2$.
   a)   If v is increased by a factor of 6, what happens to KE?
   b)   In order to increase KE by a factor of 6, what must happen to v?

Solution:
   a)   Since $KE \propto v^2$, if v increases by a factor of 6, then KE increases by a factor of $6^2 = 36$.
   b)   Since $KE \propto v^2$, it follows that $\sqrt{KE} \propto v$. So, if KE is to increase by a factor of 6, then v must be increased by a factor of $\sqrt{6}$.

Example 18-20: The area of a circle of radius r is given by $A = \pi r^2$.
   a)   If r is halved, then what happens to A?
   b)   If r increases by 50%, by what percentage will A increase?
   c)   If the *diameter* of the circle is halved, what happens to A?

Solution:
   a)   Since $A \propto r^2$, if r decreases by a factor of 2, then A will decrease by a factor of $2^2 = 4$.
   b)   If r increases by $r/2$ (which is 50% of r) to $3r/2$, then r increases by a factor of 3/2. Therefore, A increases to $(3/2)^2 = 9/4 = 225\%$ times its original value. This represents an increase of $225\% - 100\% = 125\%$.
   c)   Since $d = 2r$, we know that $d \propto r$. Therefore, if d is halved, then so is r, and A decreases by a factor of 4 [just as in part (a)]. Alternatively, we could first write the formula for the area of a circle in terms of d, its diameter, as follows:

$$A = \pi r^2 = \pi\left(\frac{1}{2}d\right)^2 = \frac{1}{4}\pi d^2$$

Therefore, $A \propto d^2$, so if d is decreased by a factor of 2, then A will be decreased by a factor of $2^2 = 4$.

Example 18-21: A metal rod of length L will be stretched by a distance $\Delta L = mgL/EA$ when a weight $w = mg$ is suspended from it.

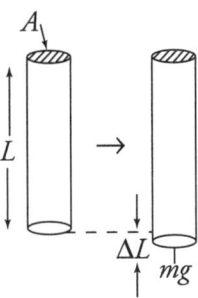

In this formula, E is a constant (depending on the material of which the rod is made) and $A = \pi r^2$ is the rod's cross-sectional area.

a) How will ΔL change if the mass m is doubled?

b) If identical weights are suspended from two metal rods of the same initial length and made of the same material, but with the radius of Rod #1 being twice that of Rod #2, which rod will be stretched more, and by what factor?

Solution:

a) Since $\Delta L \propto m$, if m increases by a factor of 2, then so does ΔL.

b) Because $A \propto r^2$, it follows that $\Delta L \propto 1/r^2$. Since the radius of Rod #2 is half the radius of Rod #1, the stretch of Rod #2 will be $\dfrac{1}{\left(\frac{1}{2}\right)^2} = 4$ times that of Rod #1.

Example 18-22: Newton's law of gravitation states that the force between two objects is given by $F = GMm/r^2$, where M and m are the masses of the objects, r is the distance between them, and G is the universal gravitational constant.

a) If both masses are doubled, and the distance between them is also doubled, what happens to F?

b) If r is decreased by 50%, what happens to F?

Solution:

a) If both masses are doubled, then the product Mm increases by a factor of $(2)(2) = 4$. If the distance r is doubled, then r^2 increases by a factor of 4. Since $F \propto Mm/r^2$ and both Mm and r^2 increase by the same factor (in this case, 4), F will remain unchanged:

$$F' = G\frac{(2M)(2m)}{(2r)^2} = G\frac{4Mm}{4r^2} = G\frac{Mm}{r^2} = F$$

b) If r decreases by 50%, then r changes to $r - (r/2) = r/2$; that is, r decreases by a factor of 2. Since $F \propto 1/r^2$, if r decreases by a factor of 2, F will increase by a factor of $2^2 = 4$.

Example 18-23: Consider the equation $xy = z$.

a) If z is a constant, how are x and y related?

b) If x is constant, how are y and z related?

c) If x is a positive constant, and we increase y by adding 2, by what factor does z increase?

Solution:

a) If z is a constant, then x and y are inversely proportional: $x \propto 1/y$.

b) If x is constant, then y and z are (directly) proportional: $z \propto y$.

c) If x is constant, then $z \propto y$. If we add 2 to y, we can say that z will increase by some amount, but we cannot say by what factor. If we *multiplied* y by 2, *then* we could say that z will increase by a factor of 2. But *adding* 2 to y does not allow us to say by what *factor* z will increase. Predictions can be made with proportions only when we're told the factor by which some quantity changes (that is, what the quantity is *multiplied* by).

Chapter 19
Logarithms

19.1 THE DEFINITION OF A LOGARITHM

A **logarithm** (or just **log**, for short) is an exponent.

For example, in the equation $2^3 = 8$, 3 is the exponent, so 3 is the logarithm. More precisely, since 3 is the exponent that gives 8 when the base is 2,

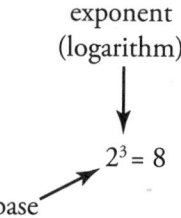

we say that the base-2 log of 8 is 3, symbolized by the equation $\log_2 8 = 3$.

Here's another example: Since $10^2 = 100$, the base-10 log of 100 is 2; that is, $\log_{10} 100 = 2$. The logarithm of a number to a given base is the exponent the base needs to be raised to give the number. What's the log, base 3, of 81? It's the exponent we'd have to raise 3 to in order to give 81. Since $3^4 = 81$, the base-3 log of 81 is 4, which we write as $\log_3 81 = 4$.

The exponent equation $2^3 = 8$ is equivalent to the log equation $\log_2 8 = 3$; the exponent equation $10^2 = 100$ is equivalent to the log equation $\log_{10} 100 = 2$; and the exponent equation $3^4 = 81$ is equivalent to the log equation $\log_3 81 = 4$. For every exponent equation, $b^x = y$, there's a corresponding log equation: $\log_b y = x$, and vice versa. To help make the conversion, use the following mnemonic, which I call the *two arrows method*:

$$\log_2 8 = 3 \iff 2^3 = 8$$

$$\log_b y = x \iff b^x = y$$

You should read the log equations with the two arrows like this:

$$\log_2 8 = 3 \iff 2 \xrightarrow{\text{to the}} 3 \xrightarrow{\text{equals}} 8 \iff 2^3 = 8$$

$$\log_b y = x \iff b \xrightarrow{\text{to the}} x \xrightarrow{\text{equals}} y \iff b^x = y$$

Always remember: The log is the exponent.

19.2 LAWS OF LOGARITHMS

There are only a few rules for dealing with logs that you'll need to know, and they follow directly from the rules for exponents (given earlier, in Chapter 15). After all, logs *are* exponents.

In stating these rules, we will assume that in an equation like $\log_b y = x$, the base b is a positive number that's different from 1, and that y is positive. (Why these restrictions? Well, if b is negative, then not every number has a log. For example, $\log_{-3} 9$ is 2, but what is $\log_{-3} 27$? If b were 0, then only 0 would have a log; and if b were 1, then every number x could equal $\log_1 y$ if $y = 1$, and *no* number x could equal $\log_1 y$ if $y \neq 1$. And why must y be positive? Because if b is a positive number, then b^x [which is y] is always positive, no matter what real value we use for x. Therefore, only positive numbers have logs.)

Laws of Logarithms

Law 1   The log of a product is the sum of the logs:
$$\log_b (yz) = \log_b y + \log_b z$$

Law 2   The log of a quotient is the difference of the logs:
$$\log_b (y/z) = \log_b y - \log_b z$$

Law 3   The log of (a number to a power) is that power times the log of the number:
$$\log_b (y^z) = z \log_b y$$

We could also add to this list that *the log of 1 is 0*, but this fact just follows from the definition of a log: Since $b^0 = 1$ for any allowed base b, we'll always have $\log_b 1 = 0$.

For the MCAT, the two most important bases are $b = 10$ and $b = e$. Base-10 logs are called **common** logs, and the "10" is often not written at all:

$$\log y \quad \text{means} \quad \log_{10} y$$

The base-10 log is useful because we use a *decimal* number system, which is based on the number 10. For example, the number 273.15 means $(2 \cdot 10^2) + (7 \cdot 10^1) + (3 \cdot 10^0) + (1 \cdot 10^{-1}) + (5 \cdot 10^{-2})$. In physics, the formula for the decibel level of a sound uses the base-10 log. In chemistry, the base-10 log has many uses, such as finding values of the pH, pOH, pK_a, and pK_b.

Base-e logs are known as **natural** logs. Here, e is a particular constant, approximately equal to 2.7. This may seem like a strange number to choose as a base, but it makes calculus run smoothly—which is why it's called the *natural* logarithm—because (and you don't need to know this for the MCAT) the only numerical value of b for which the function $f(x) = b^x$ is its own derivative is $b = e = 2.71828....$ Base-e logs are often used in the mathematical description of physical processes in which the rate of change of some quantity is proportional to the quantity itself; radioactive decay is a typical example. The notation "ln" (the abbreviation, in reverse, for **n**atural **l**ogarithm) is often used to mean $\log_e$:

$$\ln y \quad \text{means} \quad \log_e y$$

The relationship between the base-10 log and the base-e log of a given number can be expressed as $\ln y \approx 2.3 \log y$. For example, if $y = 1000 = 10^3$, then $\ln 1000 \approx 2.3 \log 1000 = 2.3 \cdot 3 = 6.9$. You may also find it useful to know the following approximate values:

$\log 2 \approx 0.3$	$\ln 2 \approx 0.7$
$\log 3 \approx 0.5$	$\ln 3 \approx 1.1$
$\log 5 \approx 0.7$	$\ln 5 \approx 1.6$

Example 19-1:

a) What is $\log_3 9$?

b) Find $\log_5 (1/25)$.

c) Find $\log_4 8$.

d) What is the value of $\log_{16} 4$?

e) Given that $\log 5 \approx 0.7$, what is the value for $\log 500$?

f) Given that $\log 2 \approx 0.3$, find $\log (2 \times 10^{-6})$.

g) Given that $\log 2 \approx 0.3$ and $\log 3 \approx 0.5$, find $\log (6 \times 10^{23})$.

Solution:

a) $\log_3 9 = x$ is the same as $3^x = 9$, from which we see that $x = 2$. So, $\log_3 9 = 2$.

b) $\log_5 (1/25) = x$ is the same as $5^x = 1/25 = 1/5^2 = 5^{-2}$, so $x = -2$. Therefore, $\log_5 (1/25) = -2$.

c) $\log_4 8 = x$ is the same as $4^x = 8$. Since $4^x = (2^2)^x = 2^{2x}$ and $8 = 2^3$, the equation $4^x = 8$ is the same as $2^{2x} = 2^3$, so $2x = 3$, which gives $x = 3/2$. Therefore, $\log_4 8 = 3/2$.

d) $\log_{16} 4 = x$ is the same as $16^x = 4$. To find x, you might notice that the square root of 16 is 4, so $16^{1/2} = 4$, which means $\log_{16} 4 = 1/2$. Alternatively, we can write 16^x as $(4^2)^x = 4^{2x}$ and 4 as 4^1. Therefore, the equation $16^x = 4$ is the same as $4^{2x} = 4^1$, so $2x = 1$, which gives $x = 1/2$.

e) $\log 500 = \log (5 \cdot 100) = \log 5 + \log 100$, where we used Law 1 in the last step. Since $\log 100 = \log 10^2 = 2$, we find that $\log 500 \approx 0.7 + 2 = 2.7$.

f) $\log (2 \times 10^{-6}) = \log 2 + \log 10^{-6}$, by Law 1. Since $\log 10^{-6} = -6$, we find that $\log (2 \times 10^{-6}) \approx 0.3 + (-6) = -5.7$.

g) $\log (6 \times 10^{23}) = \log 2 + \log 3 + \log 10^{23}$, by Law 1. Since $\log 10^{23} = 23$, we find that $\log (6 \times 10^{23}) \approx 0.3 + 0.5 + 23 = 23.8$.

Example 19-2: In each case, find y.

a) $\log_2 y = 5$

b) $\log_2 y = -3$

c) $\log y = 4$

d) $\log y = 7.5$

e) $\log y = -2.5$

f) $\ln y = 3$

Solution:

a) $\log_2 y = 5$ is the same as $2^5 = y$, so $y = 32$.

b) $\log_2 y = -3$ is the same as $2^{-3} = y$, which gives $y = 1/2^3 = 1/8$.

c) $\log y = 4$ is the same as $10^4 = y$, so $y = 10,000$.

d) $\log y = 7.5$ is the same as $10^{7.5} = y$. We'll rewrite 7.5 as $7 + 0.5$, so $y = 10^{7+(0.5)} = 10^7 \times 10^{0.5}$. Because $10^{0.5} = 10^{1/2} = \sqrt{10}$, which is approximately 3, we find that $y \approx 10^7 \times 3 = 3 \times 10^7$.

e) $\log y = -2.5$ is the same as $10^{-2.5} = y$. We'll rewrite -2.5 as $-3 + 0.5$, so $y = 10^{-3+(0.5)} = 10^{-3} \times 10^{0.5}$. Because $10^{0.5} = 10^{1/2} = \sqrt{10}$, which is approximately 3, we find that $y \approx 10^{-3} \times 3 = 0.003$.

f) $\ln y = 3$ means $\log_e y = 3$; this is the same as $y = e^3$ (which is about 20).

Example 19-3: If a sound wave has intensity I (measured in W/m^2), then its loudness level, β (measured in decibels), is found from the formula

$$\beta = 10\log\frac{I}{I_0}$$

where I_0 is a constant equal to 10^{-12} W/m^2. What is the loudness level of a sound wave whose intensity is 10^{-5} W/m^2?

Solution: Using the given formula, we find that

$$\beta = 10\log\frac{10^{-5}}{10^{-12}} = 10\log(10^7) = 10 \cdot 7 = 70 \text{ decibels}$$

Example 19-4: The definition of the pH of an aqueous solution is

$$pH = -\log [H_3O^+] \text{ (or } -\log [H^+])$$

where $[H_3O^+]$ is the hydronium ion concentration (in M).

Part I: Find the pH of each of the following solutions:
a)   coffee, with $[H_3O^+] = 8 \times 10^{-6}\ M$
b)   seawater, with $[H_3O^+] = 3 \times 10^{-9}\ M$
c)   vinegar, with $[H_3O^+] = 1.3 \times 10^{-3}\ M$

Part II: Find $[H_3O^+]$ for each of the following pH values:
d)   pH = 7
e)   pH = 11.5
f)   pH = 4.7

Solution:
a)   pH = $-\log (8 \times 10^{-6}) = -[\log 8 + \log (10^{-6})] = -\log 8 + 6$. We can now make a quick approximation by simply noticing that log 8 is a little less than log 10; that is, log 8 is a little less than 1. Let's say it's 0.9. Then pH $\approx -0.9 + 6 = 5.1$.
b)   pH = $-\log (3 \times 10^{-9}) = -[\log 3 + \log (10^{-9})] = -\log 3 + 9$. We now make a quick approximation by simply noticing that log 3 is about 0.5 (after all, $9^{0.5}$ *is* 3, so $10^{0.5}$ is close to 3). This gives pH $\approx -0.5 + 9 = 8.5$.
c)   pH = $-\log (1.3 \times 10^{-3}) = -[\log 1.3 + \log (10^{-3})] = -\log 1.3 + 3$. We can now make a quick approximation by simply noticing that log 1.3 is just a little more than log 1; that is, log 1.3 is a little more than 0. Let's say it's 0.1. This gives pH $\approx -0.1 + 3 = 2.9$.

*Note 1:** We can generalize these three calculations as follows: If $[H_3O^+] = m \times 10^{-n}\ M$, where $1 \le m < 10$ and n is an integer, then the pH is between $(n - 1)$ and n; it's closer to $(n - 1)$ if $m > 3$ and it's closer to n if $m < 3$. (We use 3 as the cutoff since log 3 $\approx$ 0.5.)

d)   If pH = 7, then $-\log [H_3O^+]$ = 7, so $\log [H_3O^+]$ = -7, which means $[H_3O^+]$ = 10^{-7} M.

e)   If pH = 11.5, then $-\log [H_3O^+]$ = 11.5, so $\log [H_3O^+]$ = -11.5, which means $[H_3O^+]$ = $10^{-11.5}$ = $10^{(0.5)-12}$ = $10^{0.5} \times 10^{-12} \approx 3 \times 10^{-12}$ M.

f)   If pH = 4.7, then $-\log [H_3O^+]$ = 4.7, so $\log [H_3O^+]$ = -4.7, which means $[H_3O^+]$ = $10^{-4.7}$ = $10^{(0.3)-5}$ = $10^{0.3} \times 10^{-5} \approx 2 \times 10^{-5}$ M. ($10^{-0.3} \approx 2$ follows from the fact that $\log 2 \approx 0.3$.)

---

*Note 2: We can generalize these last two calculations as follows: If pH = $n.m$, where n is an integer and m is a digit from 1 to 9, then $[H_3O^+] = y \times 10^{-(n+1)}$ M, where y is closer to 1 if $m > 3$ and closer to 10 if $m < 3$. (We take $y = 5$ if $m = 3$.)

Example 19-5: The definition of the pK_a of a weak acid is

$$pK_a = -\log K_a$$

where K_a is the acid's ionization constant.

Part I: Approximate the pK_a of each of the following acids:
   a)   HBrO, with $K_a = 2 \times 10^{-9}$
   b) HNO_2, with $K_a = 7 \times 10^{-4}$
   c)   HCN, with $K_a = 6 \times 10^{-10}$

Part II: Approximate K_a for each of the following pK_a values:
   d) $pK_a = 12.5$
   e) $pK_a = 2.7$
   f) $pK_a = 9.2$

Solution:
   a) $pK_a = -\log (2 \times 10^{-9}) = -[\log 2 + \log (10^{-9})] = -\log 2 + 9$. We can now make a quick approximation by remembering that log 2 is about 0.3. Then $pK_a = -0.3 + 9 = 8.7$. Because the formula to find pK_a from K_a is exactly the same as the formula for finding pH from $[H^+]$, we could also make use of Note 1 in the solution to Example 19-4. If $K_a = m \times 10^{-n}$ M, where $1 \le m < 10$ and n is an integer, then the pK_a is between $(n - 1)$ and n; it's closer to $(n - 1)$ if $m > 3$ and it's closer to n if $m < 3$. In this case, $m = 2$ and $n = 9$, so the pK_a is between $(n - 1) = 8$ and $n = 9$. And, since $2 < 3$, the pK_a will be closer to 9 (which is just what we found, since we got the value 8.7). Given a list of possible choices for the pK_a of this acid, just recognizing that it's a little less than 9 will be sufficient.
   b)   With $K_a = 7 \times 10^{-4}$, we have $m = 7$ and $n = 4$. Therefore, the pK_a will be between $(n - 1) = 3$ and $n = 4$. Since $m = 7$ is greater than 3, the value of pK_a will be closer to 3 (around, say, 3.2).
   c)   With $K_a = 6 \times 10^{-10}$, we have $m = 6$ and $n = 10$. Therefore, the pK_a will be between $(n - 1) = 9$ and $n = 10$. Since $m = 6$ is greater than 3, the value of pK_a will be closer to 9 (around, say, 9.2).

d) If $pK_a = 12.5$, then $-\log K_a = 12.5$, so $\log K_a = -12.5$, which means $K_a = 10^{-12.5} = 10^{(0.5)-13}$ $= 10^{0.5} \times 10^{-13} \approx 3 \times 10^{-13}$. We could also make use of Note 2 in the solution to Example 19-4. If $pK_a = n.m$, where n is an integer and m is a digit from 1 to 9, then $K_a = y \times 10^{-(n+1)}$ M, where y is closer to 1 if $m > 3$ and y is closer to 10 if $m < 3$. In this case, with $pK_a = 12.5$, we have $n = 12$ and $m = 5$, so the K_a value is $y \times 10^{-(12+1)} = y \times 10^{-13}$, with y closer to 1 (than to 10) since $m = 5$ is greater than 3 (this agrees with what we found, since we calculated that $K_a \approx 3 \times 10^{-13}$).

e) With $pK_a = 2.7$, we have $n = 2$ and $m = 7$. Therefore, the K_a value is $y \times 10^{-(2+1)} = y \times 10^{-3}$, with y close to 1 since $m = 7$ is greater than 3. We can check this as follows: If $pK_a = 2.7$, then $-\log K_a = 2.7$, so $\log K_a = -2.7$, which means $K_a = 10^{-2.7} = 10^{(0.3)-3} = 10^{0.3} \times 10^{-3} \approx 2 \times 10^{-3}$.

f) With $pK_a = 9.2$, we have $n = 9$ and $m = 2$. Therefore, the K_a value is $y \times 10^{-(9+1)} = y \times 10^{-10}$, with y closer to 10 (than to 1) since $m = 2$ is less than 3. We can say that $K_a \approx 6 \times 10^{-10}$.

Example 19-6:
a) If y increases by a factor of 100, what happens to $\log y$?
b) If y decreases by a factor of 1000, what happens to $\log y$?
c) If y increases by a factor of 30,000, what happens to $\log y$?
d) If y is reduced by 99%, what happens to $\log y$?

Solution:
a) If y changes to $y' = 100y$, then the log increases by 2, since
$$\log y' = \log(100y) = \log 100 + \log y = \log 10^2 + \log y = 2 + \log y$$

b) If y changes to $y' = y/1000$, then the log decreases by 3, since
$$\log y' = \log\left(\frac{y}{1000}\right) = \log y - \log 1000 = \log y - \log 10^3 = \log y - 3$$

c) If y changes to $y' = 30{,}000y$, then the log increases by about 4.5, since
$$\log y' = \log(30000y) = \log 3 + \log 10000 + \log y \approx 0.5 + 4 + \log y = 4.5 + \log y$$

d) If y is reduced by 99%, that means we're subtracting $0.99y$ from y, which leaves $0.01y = y/100$. Therefore, y has decreased by a factor of 100. And if y changes to $y' = y/100$, then the log decreases by 2, since
$$\log y' = \log\left(\frac{y}{100}\right) = \log y - \log 100 = \log y - \log 10^2 = \log y - 2$$

Example 19-7: A radioactive substance has a half-life of 70 hours. For each of the fractions below, figure out how many hours will elapse until the amount of substance remaining is equal to the given fraction of the original amount.
a) 1/4
b) 1/8
c) 1/3

Solution:
a) After one half-life has elapsed, the amount remaining is 1/2 the original (by definition). After another half-life elapses, the amount remaining is now 1/2 of 1/2 the original amount, which is 1/4 the original amount. Therefore, a decrease to 1/4 the original amount requires 2 half-lives, which in this case is 2(70 hr) = 140 hr.

b) The fraction 1/8 is equal to 1/2 of 1/2 of 1/2; that is, $1/8 = (1/2)^3$. In terms of half-lives, a decrease to 1/8 the original amount requires 3 half-lives, which in this case is equal to 3(70 hr) = 210 hr. *In general, a decrease to $(1/2)^n$ the original amount requires n half-lives.*

c) The fraction 1/3 is not a whole-number power of 1/2, so we can't directly apply the fact given in the italicized sentence in the solution to part (b). However, 1/3 is between 1/2 and 1/4, so the time to get to 1/3 the original amount is between 1 and 2 half-lives. Since one half-life is 70 hr, the amount of time is between 70 and 140 hours; the middle of this range (since 1/3 is roughly in the middle between 1/2 and 1/4) is about 110 hours. The most general formula for calculating the elapsed time involves a logarithm: If $x < 1$ is the fraction of a radioactive substance remaining after a time t has elapsed, then

$$t = \frac{\log \frac{1}{x}}{\log 2} \times t_{1/2}$$

where $t_{1/2}$ is the half-life. (If you want to use this formula, remember that $\log 2 \approx 0.3$.)

Appendix: Statistics and Research Methods

The MCAT tests your knowledge of basic research methods and statistical concepts within the context of passages and questions about the social and behavioral sciences. The MCAT will not test your knowledge about statistics, *per se*, but will test whether you are able to *apply* statistical concepts and an understanding of research methodology within the context of answering content-related questions, especially in the Psychological, Social, and Biological Foundations of Behavior section. Application questions might include

- Graphical analysis and interpretation

- Determining whether results are supported by data presented in figures

- Demonstrating an understanding of basic statistics and research methods

- Interpreting data presented in graphs, figures, and tables

- Drawing conclusions about data and methodology

What is statistics?

Statistics is a tool to organize data. On the MCAT, statistics is often employed to organize data sets and present data in a logical manner such that the data can be analyzed and conclusions can be drawn. Data often include numerical information collected through research. The different types of statistical data that you might encounter on the MCAT are described in this Appendix.

DESCRIPTIVE STATISTICS

Descriptive statistics quantitatively describe a population or set of data; in behavioral fields, descriptive statistics will often provide information about the data involved in the study, such as: number of subjects (or sample size), proportion of subjects of each sex, average age (or weight, or height, or IQ...whatever is relevant to the study) of the sample. Descriptive statistics include **measures of central tendency** (such as mean, median, mode) and **measures of variability** (such as range and standard deviation).

A.1 MEASURES OF CENTRAL TENDENCY

Measures of central tendency summarize or describe the entire set of data in some meaningful way.

Mean

The mean is the average of the sample. The average is derived from adding all of the individual components and dividing by the number of components. The mean is not necessarily a number provided in the sample. You should be able to recognize what the mean of a given data set is, and be able to calculate the mean.

Example Mean Question:

Subject	Starting Weight (in pounds)	Final Weight (in pounds)
Subject 1	184	176
Subject 2	200	190
Subject 3	221	225
Subject 4	235	208
Subject 5	244	225

Table 1   Starting and Final Weights for Study Subjects

What is the average amount of weight lost in pounds for all five subjects whose data is represented in Table 1, rounded to the nearest pound?

Solution:

In order to answer this question, you must first calculate how much weight each subject lost, and then divide by the number of subjects (in this case, five).

Subject	Starting Weight (in pounds)	Final Weight (in pounds)	Weight Lost (in pounds)
Subject 1	184	176	8
Subject 2	200	190	10
Subject 3	221	225	-4*
Subject 4	235	208	27
Subject 5	244	225	19

* Subject 3 gained 4 pounds

Total weight lost is 60 pounds (remember to subtract 4 pounds for subject 3, not add), divided by 5 subjects is 12 pounds. The average weight lost is **12 pounds**.

Note: the mean can be both useful and deceptive. Using the example above, what sort of conclusions could be drawn from the fact that the subjects lost an average of 12 pounds? One might conclude that the subjects were successful at losing weight. However, the mean does not reflect the fact that one of the participants, Subject 3, actually gained weight. Nor does it reflect that one the participants, Subject 4, was very successful, losing over twice the mean. Consider another example: if ten people are in a room together and all of them earn salaries at or below minimum wage, but one of them is a billionaire, the mean salary for the ten people might make it seem like they were all quite wealthy. Therefore, use caution when making assumptions about a data set when given just the mean.

Median

The median is the middle number in a data set. The median is determined by putting the numbers in consecutive order and finding the middle number. If there is an odd number of numbers, there will be a single number that is the median. If there is an even number of numbers, the median is determined by averaging the two middle numbers. Therefore, the median is not necessarily one of the numbers in the data set. You should be able to recognize what the median of a given data set is, and be able to calculate the median.

Example Median Question:

Subject	Height (in inches)
Subject 1	67
Subject 2	61
Subject 3	72
Subject 4	70
Subject 5	66
Subject 6	68

Table 2   Height of Study Subjects

Is Subject 6 taller than the median for all subjects whose height is displayed in Table 2?

Solution:

In order to determine the median height for all six subjects, their heights must first be organized in ascending order: 61, 66, 67, 68, 70, 72. The middle two numbers are 67 and 68; when averaged, this produces a median of **67.5 inches**. Subject 6 is taller than the median.

Note: the median can be useful in gauging the midpoint of the data, but will not necessarily tell you much about the **outliers** (a numerical observation that is far removed from the rest of the observations). Using the example where nine people earn salaries at or below minimum wage and the tenth is a billionaire, the median will give you a pretty good idea about the income for most of the people in the room, but will not indicate that one person makes much more than the rest. Therefore, also use caution when making assumptions about a data set when given just the median.

Mode

The mode is the most frequently recurring number in the data set. If there are no numbers that occur more than once, there is no mode. If there are multiple numbers that occurs most frequently, each of those numbers is a mode. The mode must be one of the numbers in the sample, and modes are never averaged. You should be able to recognize what the mode of a given data set is, and be able to calculate the mode.

Example Mode Question:

In the following set of test scores, what is the mode?

Test Scores: 32, 65, 66, 67, 68, 68, 69, 70, 71, 72, 73, 75, 75, 75, 75, 78, 82

Solution:

The most frequently recurring number in the set above is **75**.

Note: like the mean and median, the mode is only useful is describing some types of data sets. Mode is particularly useful for scores (such as test scores). For example, looking at the test scores above, the mean is 69.5 and the median is 71. Using all three measures you could conclude that while the mean was low, most of the students in the class scored above the mean, and the most common score was 75. There was one very low score that brought down the mean, but there were no very high scores.

A.2 MEASURES OF VARIABILITY

Knowing information about the central tendency of a data set can be useful, but it is also useful to know something about the variation in the data set. In other words, how similar or diverse are the data?

Range

The range is the difference between the smallest and largest number in a sample. You should be able to recognize what the range of a given data set is, and be able to calculate the range.

Example Range Question:

In the following set of values, what is the range? Values: –5, 8, 11, –1, 0, 4, 14

Solution:

The smallest value in the set above is –5, and the largest is 14. The difference between these two is the range, which is **19**.

Note: the range only provides limited information about a data set, however. Returning to the example of the ten people in a room, the range of incomes might be 3 billion dollars, but that provides relatively little information about the individual salaries of the people in the room. Knowing just the range does not tell us that the majority of the people in the room all have salaries around minimum wage.

Standard Deviation

The standard deviation is more useful than the range for calculating how much the data vary. It can determine if numbers are packed together or dispersed because it is a measure of how much each individual number differs from the mean. The best way to understand standard deviation is to consider a normal distribution (also called a bell-shaped curve). You will not need to calculate standard deviation, but you should understand what it is and should be able to make assumptions and draw conclusions from standard deviation data.

Normal Distributions

A normal distribution is a very important class of statistical distributions for the study of human behavior, because many psychological, social, and biological variables are normally distributed. Large sets of data (such as heights, weights, test scores, IQ) often form a symmetrical, bell-shaped distribution when graphed by frequency (number of instances). For example, if you took the weight of all 25-year-old males in America and plotted the weight on the *x*-axis and the frequency on the *y*-axis, the results will be normally distributed.

Standard Deviation

Standard deviation describes the degree of variation from the mean. A low standard deviation reflects that data points are all similar and close to the mean, while a high standard deviation reflects that the data are more spread out. For the purposes of the MCAT, you should be familiar with a normal distribution (or bell-shaped curve) and should be able to determine what a standard deviation means for a set of data. You will not be expected to calculate the standard deviation. Figure 1 demonstrates the relationship between a normal distribution and standard deviation.

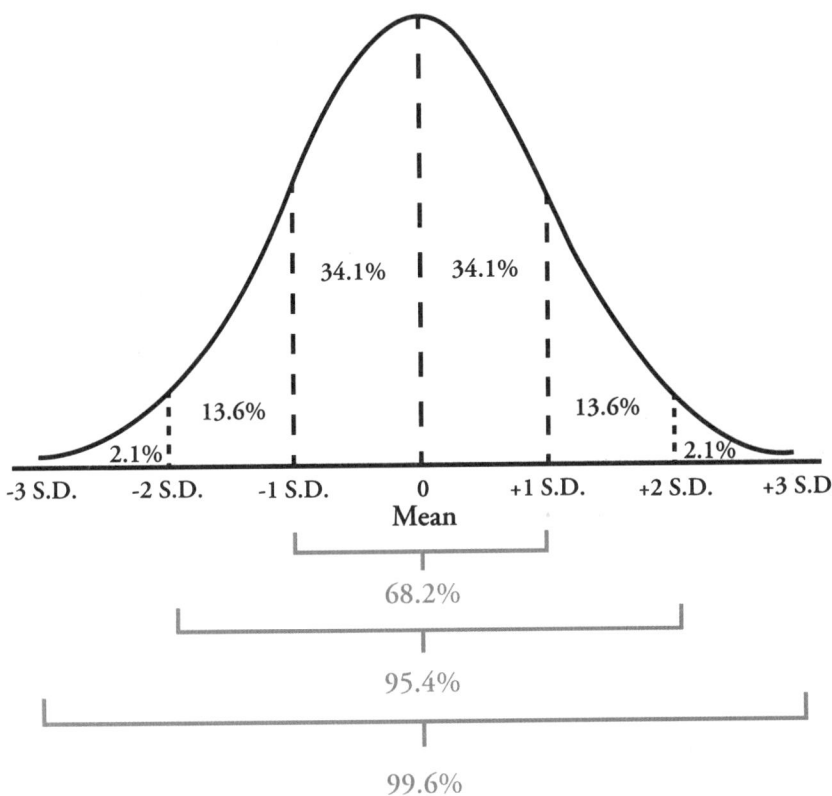

Figure 1 Normal Distribution and Standard Deviation Rules

All normal distributions have the following properties:

- 34.1% of the data will fall within one standard deviation above or below the mean, thus 68.2% of the data will fall within one standard deviation of the mean,
- 13.6% of the data will fall between one and two standard deviations above or below the mean, thus 95.4% of the data will fall within two standard deviations of the mean,
- 2.1% of the data will fall between two and three standard deviations above or below the mean, thus 99.6% of the data will fall within three standard deviations of the mean,
- 0.2% of the data will fall beyond three standard deviations above or below the mean, thus 0.4% of the data will fall beyond three standard deviations of the mean.

So for a normal distribution, almost all of the data lie within **3 standard deviations** of the mean.

Example Standard Deviation Question:

Suppose that 1,000 subjects participate in a study on reaction time. The reaction times of the subjects are normally distributed with a mean of 1.3 seconds and a standard deviation of 0.2 seconds. How many subjects had a reaction time between 1.1 and 1.5 seconds? How many participants had reaction times faster than 1.9 seconds? A reaction time of 0.9 seconds is within how many standard deviations of the mean?

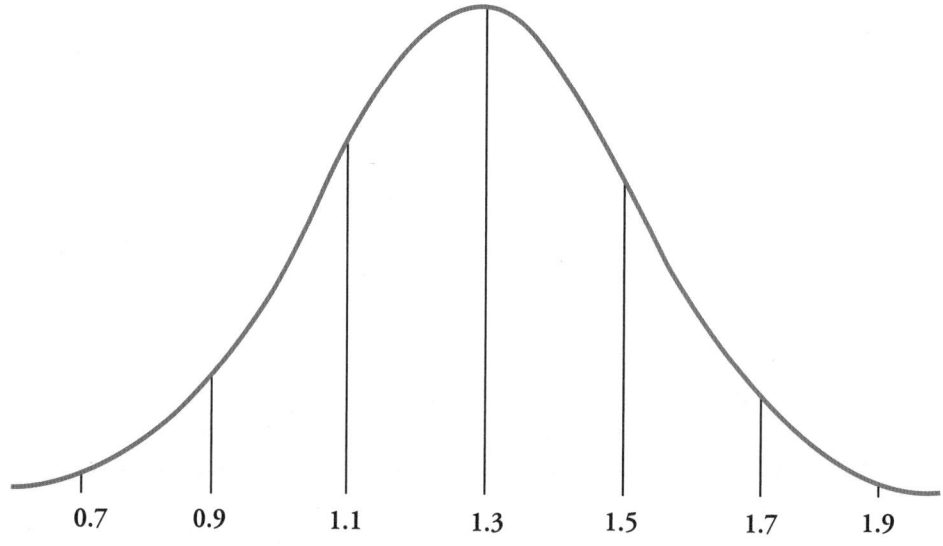

Figure 2 Subjects' Reaction Time

Solution:

Subjects' reaction times would produce a normal distribution like the one above. Reaction times within 1.1 and 1.5 seconds would include all of the data within one standard deviation of the mean (or, in other words, one standard deviation above and below the mean). 68.2% of the data fall within one standard deviation of the mean (34.1% above and 34.1% below), so **682** subjects have a reaction time between 1.1 and 1.5 seconds.

0.2% of the data will fall above 3 standard deviations of the mean, so only **2** subjects will have a reaction time faster than 1.9 seconds.

A reaction time of 0.9 seconds is **two standard deviations below the mean**.

Percentile

Percentiles are often used when reporting data from normal distributions. Percentiles represent the area under the normal curve, increasing from left to right. A percentile indicates the value or score below which the rest of the data falls. For example, a score in the 75th percentile is higher than 75% of the rest of the scores. Each standard deviation represents a fixed percentile as follows:

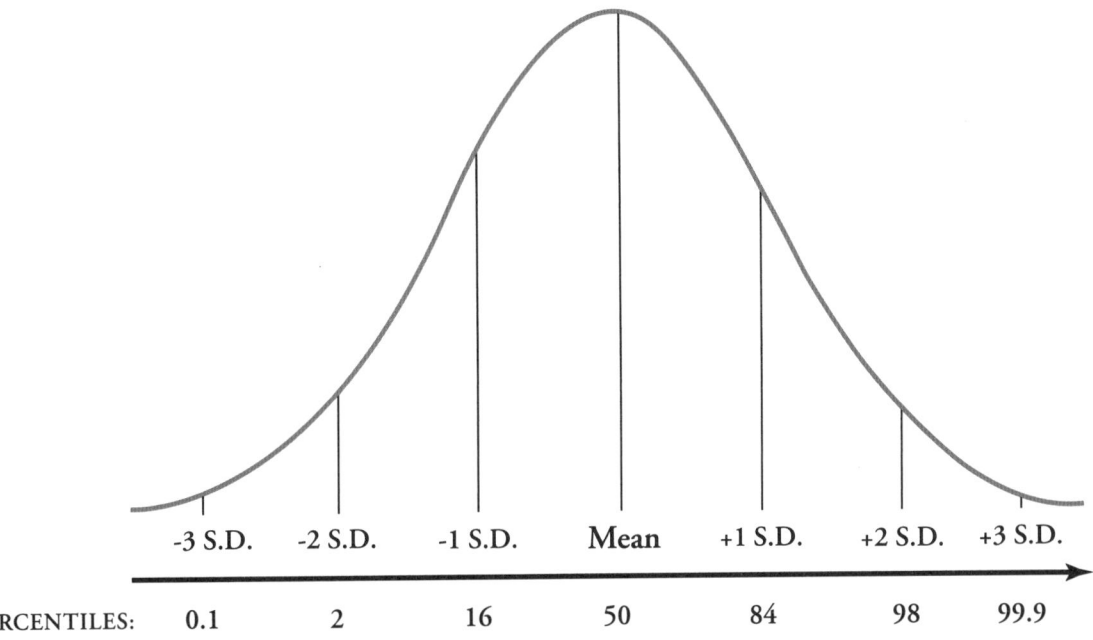

Figure 3   Normal Distribution and Percentiles

- 0.1th percentile corresponds to three standard deviations below the mean
- 2nd percentile corresponds to two standard deviations below the mean
- 16th percentile corresponds to one standard deviation below the mean
- 50th percentile correspond to the mean
- 84th percentile corresponds to one standard deviation above the mean
- 98th percentile corresponds to two standard deviations above the mean
- 99.9th percentile corresponds to three standard deviations above the mean

Example Percentile Question:

If the scores for an exam are normally distributed, the mean is 20 and the standard deviation is 6, a score of 14 would be what percentile? What score would correspond to the 99.9th percentile?

Solution:

A score of 14 would be one standard deviation below the mean, which corresponds to the **16th percentile**. The 99.9th percentile is three standard deviations above the mean, which would correspond to a score of **38**.

A.3 INFERENTIAL STATISTICS

Beyond merely describing the data, inferential statistics also allows inferences or assumptions to be made about data. Using inferential statistics, such as a regression coefficient or a *t*-test, you can draw conclusions about the population you are studying. Inferential statistics starts with a hypothesis and checks to see if the data prove or disprove that hypothesis. You will not be expected to calculate any of the following statistical measures on the MCAT, but you will be expected to recognize these statistical analyses and apply information about these various measures.

Variables

Variables are the things that statistics is designed to test; more specifically, statistics measures whether or not a change in the independent variable has an effect on the dependent variable. An **independent variable** is the variable that is manipulated to determine what effect it will have on the dependent variable. A **dependent variable** is a function of the independent variable, as the independent variable changes, so does the dependent variable. Typically, the independent variable is the one altered by the scientist in a behavioral experiment and the dependent variable is the one measured by the scientist. Common independent variables in behavioral sciences include: age, sex, race, socioeconomic status, and other group characteristics. Standardized measures and scores are also common independent variables. Dependent variables could be any number of things, such as test scores, behaviors, symptoms, and the like.

Example Variable Question:

> Two scientists want to measure the impact of caffeine consumption on fine motor performance. Therefore, they devise an experiment where a treatment group receives 50 mg of caffeine (in the form of a sugar-free beverage) 20 minutes before performing a standardized motor skills test, and the control group receives an non-caffeinated sugar-free beverage 20 minutes before performing a standardized motor skills test. What is the independent variable in this example? What is the dependent variable?

Solution:

> The independent variable is caffeine because the researchers are attempting to determine the impact of this variable on another, the dependent variable (which in this example is performance on the standardized motor skills test).

Sample Size

Sample size refers to the number of observations or individuals measured. Simply enough, if an experiment involves 100 people, the sample size is 100. Sample size is typically denoted with: N (the total number of subjects in the sample being studied) or n (the total number of subjects in a subgroup of the sample being studied). While larger sample sizes always confer increased accuracy, in practicality, particularly for behavioral research where it is likely impossible to test *all* of the people in the country who are clinically depressed, the sample size used in a study is typically determined based on convenience, expense, and the need to have sufficient **statistical power** (which is essentially the likelihood that you have enough subjects to accurately prove the hypothesis is true within an acceptable margin of error). Bigger sample sizes are always better; the larger the sample size, the more likely that you can draw accurate inferences about the population that the sample was drawn from.

Random Samples

In statistics, especially in the behavioral sciences, where (as previously mentioned), it is often not possible to test everyone in the population, it is crucial to select a random sample from the larger population in order to conduct research. A **random sample** is a subset of individuals from within a statistical population that can be used to estimate characteristics of the whole population. A population can be defined as including all of the people with a given condition or characteristic that you wish to study. Except under the rarest of circumstances, it will not be possible to study everyone with a given characteristic or condition, so a subset of the population is selected. If the subset is not selected randomly, then this non-randomness might unintentionally skew the results (which is called **sampling bias**). A classic example of this occurred during the 1948 Presidential Election in the U.S.: a survey was conducted by randomly calling households and asking people who they were planning to vote for, Harry Truman or Thomas Dewey. Based on this phone survey, Dewey was projected to win, but Truman actually did. What could have possibly gone wrong? Well it turns out that in 1948 having a phone was not such a common thing; in fact, only wealthier households were likely to have a telephone. So the "random" selection of telephone numbers was in fact not a representative random sample of the U.S. population, because many people (of whom a large proportion were clearly voting for Truman) did not have telephone numbers. For the purposes of the MCAT, you should be able to identify the following types of sampling biases:

1) The bias of selection from a **specific real area** occurs when people are selected in a physical space. For example, if you wanted to survey college students on whether or not they like their football team, you could stand on the quad and survey the first 100 people that walk by. However, this is not a completely random sample, because people who don't have class that day at that time are unlikely to be represented in the sample.

2) **Self-selection bias** occurs when the people being studied have some control over whether or not to participate. A participant's decision to participate may affect the results. For example, an Internet survey might only elicit responses from people who are highly opinionated and motivated to complete the survey.

3) **Pre-screening** or **advertising** bias occurs often in medical research; how volunteers are screened or where advertising is placed might skew the sample. For example, if a researcher wanted to prove that a certain treatment helps with smoking cessation, the mere act of advertising for people who "want to quit smoking" could provide only a sample of people who are highly motivated to quit and would be likely to quit without the treatment.

4) **Healthy user bias** occurs when the study population is likely healthier than the general population. For example, recruiting subjects from the gym might not be the most representative group.

t-test and p-values

The *t*-test is probably one of the most common tests in the social sciences, because it can be used to calculate whether the means of two groups are significantly different from each other statistically. For example, if you have a control group and a treatment group both take a standardized test, the means of the two groups can be compared statistically. Furthermore, *t*-tests are also often used to calculate the difference between a pre-treatment measure and a post-treatment measure for the same group. For example, you could have a group of subjects take a survey before and after some sort of treatment, and statistically compare the means of the two tests.

The *t*-test is most often applied to data sets that are normally distributed. You will not be required to know how to perform a t-test, but you will need to understand what **significance** is. For the purposes of most experiments, two samples are considered to be significantly different if the *p*-value is below ± 0.05 (the *p*-value can be found using a table of values from the *t*-test). If two data sets are determined to be statistically significantly different (the *p*-value is below ± 0.05), then it can be concluded with 95% confidence that the two sets of data are actually different, instead of containing data that could be from the same data set.

Correlation

Expressing a relationship between two sets of data using a single number, the correlation coefficient (if represented at all, the correlation coefficients will usually be represented as R or r). This value measures the direction and magnitude of linear association between these two variables. A correlation coefficient can have a maximum value of 1 and a minimum value of –1. A **positive correlation** (meaning a coefficient greater than 0) indicates a *positive* association between the two variables; that is, when one variable increases the other also tends to increase as well (similarly, as one variable decreases, the other tends to decrease). A **negative correlation** (meaning a coefficient that is less than 0) indicates a negative association between the two variables; that is, when one increases, the other tends to decrease (or vice versa). A correlation coefficient of exactly 0 indicates that there is no linear relation between the two variables.

Example Correlation Question:

Psychologists studied 500 male infants from birth to age 16. Infants were measured on "agreeableness" at age one using a standardized questionnaire given to the parents (with scores ranging from 0 to 5). As the infants aged, the psychologists would collect standard measures of behavior problems (including cheating, fighting, getting put in detention, and later delinquency, smoking, and drug use) every two years. Overall behavior problems were summed. The psychologists found a correlation between agreeableness and later behavior problems of – 0.6 (Figure 4). What does a higher "agreeableness" score correlate to? An "agreeableness" score of 4.0 corresponds to roughly how many accumulated behavior problems by age 16? What conclusions can we draw about the causes of behavior problems?

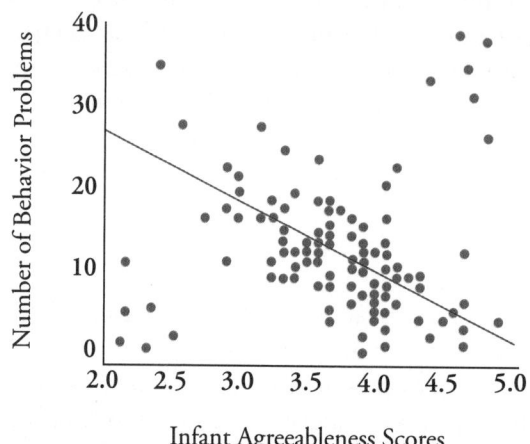

Figure 4 Correlation Between Infant Agreeableness and Later Behavior Problems (R = −0.6)

Solution:

Because the two variables are inversely correlated, as scores for "agreeableness" increase, behavioral problems decrease (this is also demonstrated by Figure 4).

An "agreeableness" score of 4.0 corresponds to approximately 10 accumulated behavior problems by age 16; note that correlations are not best used to make assumptions about people's behavior like this in behavioral psychology and medicine, though they may be used for generalizations.

Note: We can draw no conclusions about behavioral problems based on a correlation! A very important concept in statistics is that **correlation does not imply causation**. A famous example is this one: In New York City, the murder rate is directly correlated to the sale of ice cream (as ice cream sales increase, so do murders). Does this mean that buying ice cream somehow causes murders? Of course not! When two variables are correlated (especially two variables that are as complex as measures of human behavior), there are always a number of other factors that could be influencing either one. In the ice cream/murder example, a logical third factor might be temperature; as the temperature rises, more crimes are committed, but people also tend to eat more cold food, like ice cream.

Reliability

Reliability is the degree to which a specific assessment tool produces stable, consistent, and replicable results. The two types of reliability you should be able to recognize on the exam are test-retest reliability and inter-rater reliability.

- **Test-retest reliability** is a measure of the reliability of an assessment tool in obtaining similar scores over time. In other words, if the same person takes the assessment five times, their scores should be roughly equal, not wildly different.
- **Inter-rater reliability** is a measure of the degree to which two different researchers or raters agree in their assessment. For example, if two different researchers are collecting observational data, their judgments of the same person should be similar, not wildly different.

Validity

Generally, **validity** refers to how well an experiment measures what it is trying to measure. There are three important type of validity: internal, external, and construct. For the purposes of the MCAT, you should know what each type of validity is, and should be able to recognize threats to internal and external validity.

1) **Internal validity** refers to whether the results of the study properly demonstrate a causal relationship between the two variables tested. Highly controlled experiments (with random selection, random assignment to either the control or experimental groups, reliable instruments, reliable processes, and safeguards against confounding factors) may be the only way to truly establish internal validity. **Confounding factors** are hidden variables (those not directly tested for) that correlate in some way with the independent or dependent variable and have some sort of impact on the results.

2) **External validity** refers to whether the results of the study can be generalized to other situations and other people. Generalizability is limited to the independent variable, so the following must be controlled for in order to protect the external validity:
   - sample must be completely random (any of the sampling errors discussed above will threaten external validity)
   - all situational variables (treatment conditions, timing, location, administration, investigator) must be tightly controlled
   - cause and effect relationships may not be generalizable to other settings, situations, groups, or people.

3) **Construct validity** is used to determine whether a tool is measuring what it is intended to measure; for example, does a survey ask questions clearly? Are the questions getting at the intended construct? Are the correct multiple choices present? And so on.

A.4 CONDUCTING EXPERIMENTS ON HUMANS

It is complicated to conduct studies on humans because it is infinitely harder to manipulate all of the variables; it is much, much harder to make causal conclusions. Therefore, one of your best tools for questions of this nature (which are likely to show up in the Psychological, Social, and Biological section) will be healthy skepticism; if an answer choice seems too obvious, too general, or too strong, it probably is! Furthermore, the only real type of research conducted on humans that can produce information about the effectiveness of treatment or therapy on a particular disease or condition is a **double-blinded randomized controlled trial**.

In a **randomized controlled trial**, there are two groups: a treatment group and a control group. The treatment group receives the treatment under investigation and the control group either receives no treatment, a placebo, or (in the case of most medical studies) the current standard of care. Randomized controlled trials can answer questions about the effectiveness of different therapies or interventions. Randomization helps avoid selecting a sample that is biased, and having a control group allows for a comparison. However, in human research there are many instances where a randomized controlled trial cannot be utilized; for example, you cannot randomly assign people to different socioeconomic classes, and it would not be ethical to inject healthy subjects with some sort of disease.

Double-blindedness is an especially stringent way of conducting an experiment which attempts to eliminate subjective, unrecognized biases held by the subjects *and* the researchers. In a **double-blind experiment**, neither the participants nor the researchers know which participants belong to the control group, as opposed to the test group. Only after all data have been recorded (and in some cases, analyzed) do the researchers learn which participants were which. Performing an experiment in double-blind fashion can greatly lessen the power of preconceived notions or physical cues (for example, the placebo effect, observer bias, experimenter's bias) to distort the results (by making researchers/participants behave differently than they would in everyday life). Random assignment of test subjects to the experimental and control groups is a critical part of any double-blind research design. The key that identifies the subjects and which group they belonged to is kept by a third party, and is not revealed to the researchers until the study is over. Double-blind methods can be applied to any experimental situation in which there is a possibility that the results will be affected by conscious/unconscious bias on the part of researchers, participants, or both.

NOTES

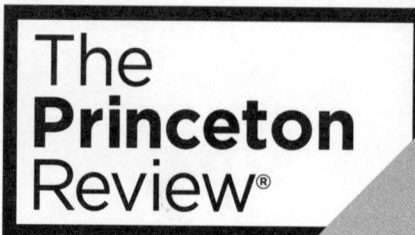
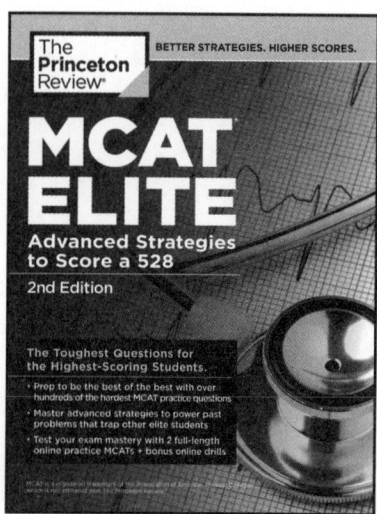
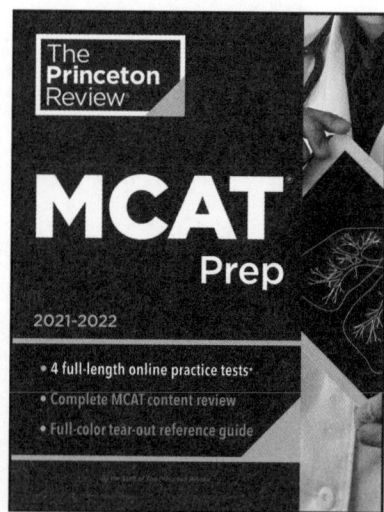
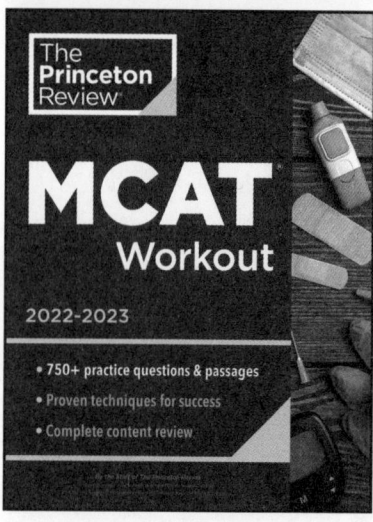
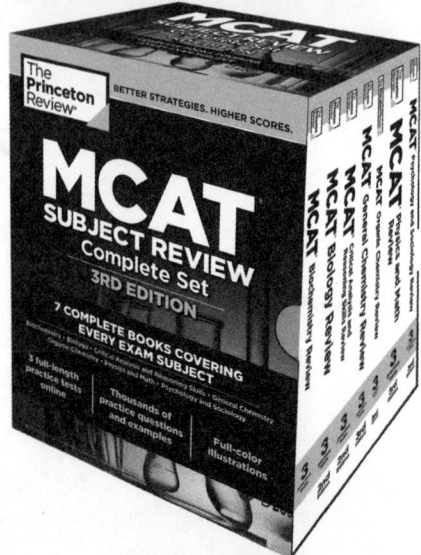